Textbook of
Postgraduate Psychiatry

Textbook of Postgraduate Psychiatry

Third Edition

Volume 1

Editors

JN Vyas
MBBS DPM MNAMS MAPA (USA) DIPLO WPA

Professor and Head
Department of Psychiatry
National Medical College and Teaching Hospital
Birgunj, Nepal

Former Superintendent
PBM Group of Hospitals, Bikaner and
Psychiatric Center, Jaipur

Former Principal and Controller
SP Medical College and Associated Group of Hospitals, Bikaner
Former Head
Department of Psychiatry, SMS Medical College, Jaipur
Dr SN Medical College, Jodhpur and SP Medical College, Bikaner

Former Head, Department of Psychiatry
Mahatama Gandhi National Institute of Medical Sciences, Jaipur, Rajasthan, India

Former Head, Department of Psychiatry
Universal College of Medical Sciences, Bhairahwa, and
Nepalgunj Medical College, Nepalgunj, Nepal

Shree Ram Ghimire
MBBS (TU) MD (TU) MPH/MHID (Flinders University, Australia)

Consultant Psychiatrist
Transcultural Psychosocial Organization Nepal
Baluwatar, Kathmandu, Nepal

Former Lecturer, Department of Psychiatry
National Medical College and Teaching Hospital, Birgunj, Nepal

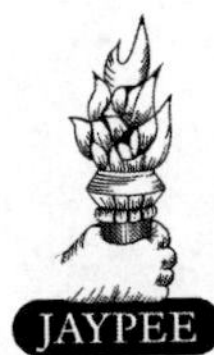

JAYPEE BROTHERS MEDICAL PUBLISHERS
The Health Sciences Publisher
New Delhi | London

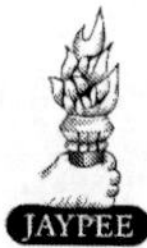

Jaypee Brothers Medical Publishers (P) Ltd

Headquarters
EMCA House
23/23-B, Ansari Road, Daryaganj
New Delhi 110 002, India
Landline: +91-11-23272143, +91-11-23272703
+91-11-23282021, +91-11-23245672
E-mail: jaypee@jaypeebrothers.com

Corporate Office
4838/24, Ansari Road, Daryaganj
New Delhi 110 002, India
Phone: +91-11-43574357
Fax: +91-11-43574314
E-mail: jaypee@jaypeebrothers.com

Overseas Office
J.P. Medical Ltd
83 Victoria Street, London
SW1H 0HW (UK)
Phone: +44 20 3170 8910
E-mail: info@jpmedpub.com

EU GPSR Authorised Representative
Logos Europe, 9 rue Nicolas Poussin
17000, La Rochelle, France
Phone: +33 (0) 6 67 93 73 78
E-mail: contact@logoseurope.eu

Website: www.jaypeebrothers.com
Website: www.jaypeedigital.com

Inquiries for bulk sales may be solicited at: jaypee@jaypeebrothers.com

Inquiries for bulk sales may be solicited at: jaypee@jaypeebrothers.com

Textbook of Postgraduate Psychiatry (2 Volumes)

First Edition : 1992
Second Edition : 1999
Third Edition : **2016**
Reprint: **2026**

ISBN 978-93-5152-910-1

Printed at: Samrat Offset Pvt. Ltd.

Dedicated to

My beloved mother Smt Lal Kaur Devi and father, (Late) Shri KN Vyas and to my grandchildren—Abhishek, Eshita, Om Narain and Hari Narain

– JN Vyas

My beloved parents, brother, sister, wife, children (Smriti, Ritu, Pratik and Aarush), all mentally ill patients and their family members

– Shree Ram Ghimire

Contributors

Abhinav Tandon
Consultant Psychiatrist
Neuropsychiatric Centre
Allahabad, Uttar Pradesh, India

Abhishek Pathak
Senior Resident
Department of Psychiatry
Institute of Medical Sciences
Banaras Hindu University
Varanasi, Uttar Pradesh, India

Adarsh Tripathi
Assistant Professor
Department of Psychiatry
King George's Medical University
Lucknow, Uttar Pradesh, India

A Das
Resident
Department of Psychiatry
Jawaharlal Nehru Medical College
Wardha, Maharashtra, India

Ajit Avasthi
Professor
Department of Psychiatry
Postgraduate Institute of Medical
Education and Research (PGIMER)
Chandigarh, India

AK Agarwal
Former Professor and Head
Department of Psychiatry
King George's Medical University
Lucknow, Uttar Pradesh, India

Alakananda Dutt
Senior Resident
Department of Psychiatry
Postgraduate Institute of Medical
Education and Research (PGIMER)
Chandigarh, India

Allen De Souza
Research Assistant
Desousa Foundation
Mumbai, Maharashtra, India

A Mulmule
Resident
Department of Psychiatry
Jawaharlal Nehru Medical College
Wardha, Maharashtra, India

AN Basu
Consultant Psychoanalyst
Girindra Sekar Clinic
Kolkata, West Bengal, India

Andrea-Sylvia Winkler
Registrar
King's Healthcare NHS Trust
Mapother House
King's College Hospital
Denmark Hill, London, UK

Anjali Chabbria
Lecturer
Department of Psychological Medicine
Dr RN Cooper Hospital and KEM
Group of Hospitals
Mumbai, Maharashtra, India

Anjanik Kumar Ranjan
Senior Resident
Central Institute of Psychiatry
Ranchi, Jharkhand, India

Anushul Khichy
Senior Resident
Central Institute of Psychiatry
Ranchi, Jharkhand, India

Aparna Garg
Assistant Professor
Department of Physiology
Mahatma Gandhi Medical College
and Hospital
Jaipur, Rajasthan, India

AP Behere
Consultant (Attending) Child and
Adolescent Psychiatrist
Mid Coast Mental Health Centre and
Pen Bay Psychiatry
Rockland, Belfast, USA

AP Dadhich
Professor and Head
Department of Pharmacology
Christian Medical College
Ludhiana, Punjab, India

A Prasad
Assistant Professor
Department of Neurology
Institute of Human Behaviour and
Allied Sciences, New Delhi, India

A Puri
Formerly Clinical Psychologist
Department of Pediatrics
Postgraduate Institute of Medical
Education and Research (PGIMER)
Chandigarh, India

AR Garg
Former Professor and Head
Department of Psychiatry
Jawaharlal Nehru Medical College
Ajmer, Rajasthan, India

Asha Krishnan
Senior Resident
Central Institute of Psychiatry
Ranchi, Jharkhand, India

Ashok Singhal
Assistant Professor
Department of Psychiatry
SP Medical College
Bikaner, Rajasthan, India

Avinash De Souza
Research Associate
Department of Psychiatry
Lokmanya Tilak Municipal
Medical College
Mumbai, Maharashtra, India

AW Jagdeesh
Resident
Department of Psychiatry
National Institute of Mental Health and
Neurosciences
Bengaluru, Karnataka, India

Baljit Singh Saluja
Department of Psychiatry
Postgraduate Institute of Medical Education and Research
Chandigarh, India

Bhoomika Sachacher
Research Officer
Project HIFAZAT
Regional Technical Training Centre
Ranchi, Jharkhand, India

Bikramaditya Jaiswal
Senior Resident
Central Institute of Psychiatry
Ranchi, Jharkhand, India

BK Singh
Professor and Head
Department of Psychiatry
Patna Medical College and Hospital
Patna, Bihar, India

BN Gangadhar
Professor
Department of Psychiatry
National Institute of Mental Health and Neurosciences
Bengaluru, Karnataka, India

B Reddy
Senior Resident
Department of Psychiatry
Jawaharlal Institute of Postgraduate Medical Education and Research
Puducherry, India

BS Bhogle
Professor and Head
Department of Psychiatry
Medical College
Belgaum, Karnataka, India

BS Chavan
Professor and Head
Department of Psychiatry
Government Medical College
Chandigarh, India

Chittaranjan Andrade
Professor
Department of Psychiatry
National Institute of Mental Health and Neurosciences
Bengaluru, Karnataka, India

Christoday RJ Khess
Director
Professor and Head
Central Institute of Psychiatry
Ranchi, Jharkhand, India

CR Chandrashekar
Additional Professor
Department of Psychiatry
National Institute of Mental Health and Neurosciences
Bengaluru, Karnataka, India

CR Mukundan
Professor and Head
Department of Psychiatry
Neuropsychology Laboratory
National Institute of Mental Health and Neurosciences
Bengaluru, Karnataka, India

Deyashini Lahiri Tikka
Assistant Professor
Department of Clinical Psychology
Central Institute of Psychiatry
Ranchi, Jharkhand, India

Dhanesh K Gupta
Assistant Professor
Department of Psychiatry
All India Institute of Medical Sciences
New Delhi, India

Dilip R Patel
Professor
Department of Pediatrics
Michigan State University
Kalamazoo Center for Medical Studies
Oakland, USA

Dinesh Mohan Das
Senior Resident
Department of Psychiatry
Dr RN Cooper Hospital and
Seth GS Medical College
Mumbai, Maharasthra, India

Dinesh Tyagi
Consultant Psychiatrist
Senior Resident
Department of Psychiatry
Institute of Human Behaviour and Allied Sciences
New Delhi, India

DK Kochar
Professor
Department of Medicine
Neurology Section
SP Medical College
Bikaner, Rajasthan, India

DN Nandi
Consultant Psychiatry
Garindra Sekar Clinic
Kolkata, West Bengal, India

Eesha Sharma
Lecturer
Department of Psychiatry
King George's Medical University
Lucknow, Uttar Pradesh, India

Gayatri Saraf
Post Doctoral Fellow in Consultation Liaison Psychiatry and Senior Resident
Department of Psychiatry
National Institute of Mental Health and Neurosciences
Bengaluru, Karnataka, India

GC Munjal
Formerly Professor and Head
Department of Psychiatry
GB Pant Hospital and
Maulana Azad Medical College
New Delhi, India

Geeta Mehta
Professor and Head
Department of Microbiology
Lady Hardinge Medical College
New Delhi, India

GN Saxena
Principal
Professor of Medicine
Mahtama Gandhi Institute of Medical Sciences
Jaipur, Rajasthan, India

G Prasad Rao
Professor and Head
Department of Psychiatry
Bhaskar Medical College
Director
Schizophrenia and Psychopharmacological Division
Asha Hospital
Hyderabad, Telangana, India

Hemant Vyas
Former Senior Demonstrator
Department of Community Medicine
Mahatma Gandhi Institute of Medical Sciences
Jaipur, Rajasthan, India

Hitesh Khurana
Senior Resident
Department of Psychiatry
Postgraduate Institute of Medical Education and Research
Chandigarh, India

Indira Sharma
President
Indian Psychiatric Society
President
SAARC Psychiatric Foundation
Vice President
Asian Federation of Psychiatric Associations
Professor and Head
Department of Child and Adolescent Psychiatry Unit
Institute of Medical Sciences
Banaras Hindu University
Varanasi, Uttar Pradesh, India

Issy Pilowsky
Professor
Department of Psychiatry
The University of Adelaide
Royal Adelaide Hospital Adelaide
South Australia

Jagadisha Thirthalli
Additional Professor
Department of Psychiatry
National Institute of Mental Health and Neurosciences
Bengaluru, Karnataka, India

Jayati Simlai
Additional Professor and Head
Department of Psychiatry
Ranchi Institute of Neuro-Psychiatry and Allied Sciences
Ranchi, Jharkhand, India

Jayesh Ranjan
Consultant Neuropsychiatrist
Ranchi Mental Hospital
Ranchi, Jharkhand, India

JN Vyas
Professor and Head
Department of Psychiatry
National Medical College and Teaching Hospital
Birgunj, Nepal
Former Superintendent
PBM Group of Hospitals, Bikaner and Psychiatric Center
Jaipur
Former Principal and Controller
SP Medical College and Associated Group of Hospitals
Bikaner
Former Head
Department of Psychiatry
SMS Medical College, Jaipur
Dr SN Medical College, Jodhpur and
SP Medical College
Bikaner
Former Head
Department of Psychiatry
Mahatama Gandhi National Institute of Medical Sciences
Jaipur, Rajasthan, India
Former Head
Department of Psychiatry
Universal College of Medical Sciences
Bhairahwa and
Nepalgunj Medical College
Nepalgunj, Nepal

Johnson Pradeep R
Assistant Professor
Department of Psychiatry
St. John's Medical College Hospital
St. John's National Institute of Health Sciences
Bengaluru, Karnataka, India

Joyita Sinha
Senior Resident
Central Institute of Psychiatry
Ranchi, Jharkhand, India

Jyoti Ahuja
Clinical Psychologist
National Institute of Mental Health and Neurosciences
Bengaluru, Karnataka, India

KA Khurshid
Senior Resident
Department of Psychiatry
All India Institute of Medical Sciences (AIIMS)
New Delhi, India

KE Sadanandan Unni
Assistant Professor
Department of Psychiatry
Jawarhar Lal Institute of Medical Education
Puducherry, India

KK Verma
Assistant Professor
Department of Psychiatry
SP Medical College
Bikaner, Rajasthan, India

K Ray Chaudhuri
Consultant Neurologist and Senior Lecturer
Department of Neurology
King's Healthcare NHS Trust
Mapother House
King's College Hospital
Denmark Hill, London, UK

KS Anand
Associate Professor
Department of Neurology
Institute of Human Behaviour and Allied Sciences
New Delhi, India

Late JK Trivedi
Formerly Professor
Department of Psychiatry
King George's Medical College
Lucknow, Uttar Pradesh, India

Late V Ramachandran
Formerly Professor
Department of Psychiatry
Madras Medical College, Chennai
Formerly Neuropsychiatrist
Institute of Mental Health
Chennai, Tamil Nadu, India

Laura Murray
Clinical Psychologist
Michigan State University
Kalamazoo Center for Medical Studies
Oakland, USA

LN Gupta
Professor
Department of Psychiatry
SMS Medical College
Jaipur, Rajasthan, India

Malavika Kapur
Professor
Department of Psychiatry
National Institute of Mental Health and Neurosciences
Bengaluru, Karnataka, India

Manju Mehta
Additional Professor
Department of Clinical Psychology
All India Institute of Medical Sciences (AIIMS)
New Delhi, India

Manoj Dhungana
Senior Psychiatrist
Former Assistant Professor
Universal Medical College
Bhairahawa, Nepal

Mridula Vyas
Professor and Head
Department of Mathematics
Vivekananda Institute of Technology
Jaipur, Rajasthan, India

M Behere
Psychiatric Social Worker
Department of Psychiatry
Jawaharlal Nehru Medical College
Wardha, Maharashtra, India

Munish Aggarwal
Senior Resident
Department of Psychiatry
Postgraduate Institute of Medical
Education and Research (PGIMER)
Chandigarh, India

Naveen Kumar C
Assistant Professor
Department of Psychiatry
National Institute of Mental Health and
Neurosciences
Bengaluru, Karnataka, India

Neena Bohra
Former Senior Psychiatrist
Professor
Department of Psychiatry
Lady Hardinge Medical College
New Delhi, India

Neha Singh
Senior Resident
Central Institute of Psychiatry
Ranchi, Jharkhand, India

Nikhil Jain
Senior Resident
Department of Psychiatry
Dr SN Medical College
Jodhpur, Rajasthan, India

Nilesh Shah
Professor and Head
Department of Psychiatry
Lokmanya Tilak Municipal Medical
College, Mumbai, Maharashtra, India

Nimesh G Desai
Professor and Head
Department of Psychiatry
Institute of Human Behaviour and
Allied Sciences, New Delhi, India

Niraj Ahuja
Assistant Professor
Department of Psychiatry
Jawaharlal Institute of Postgraduate
Medical Education and Research
Puducherry, India

NK Bohra
Director
Neuropsychiatric Center
New Delhi, India
Director
Delhi Academy of Practicing
Psychaitrists
Former President, Association of
Private Psychiatrists of India
Former President of Indian Association
of Biological Psychiatry

NK Singh
Professor and Head
Department of Psychiatry
Patna Medical College and Hospital
Patna, Bihar, India

N Parvez
Senior Resident
Central Institute of Psychiatry
Ranchi, Jharkhand, India

N Sanjay Kumar Rao
Royal Edinburgh Hospital
Edinburgh, UK

PB Behere
Director
Research and Development (R&D)
Professor and Head
Department of Psychiatry
Jawaharlal Nehru Medical College
Datta Meghe Institute of Medical
Sciences, Wardha, Maharashtra, India
Visiting Professor
University of Chester, UK
Adjunct Faculty, Georgia Southern
University, USA

Prabha S Chandra
Professor
Department of Psychiatry
National Institute of Mental Health and
Neurosciences
Bengaluru, Karnataka, India

Pramodh Bhardhwaj
Former Professor and Head
Department of Psychiatry
Rabindra Nath Tagore Medical College
Udaipur, Rajasthan, India

Priti Arun
Senior Lecturer
Department of Psychiatry
Government Medical College
Chandigarh, India

PSDV Prasadarao
Assistant Professor
Department of Clinical Psychology
National Institute of Mental Health and
Neurosciences
Bengaluru, Karnataka, India

RA Bumb
Professor and Head
Department of Dermatology,
Venereology and Leprosy
SP Medical College
Bikaner, Rajasthan, India

Radha Prabhu
Clinical Psychologist
National Institute of Mental Health and
Neurosciences
Bengaluru, Karnataka, India

Rajesh Sagar
Assistant Professor
Department of Psychiatry
All India Institute of Medical Sciences
New Delhi, India

Raju Sedhain
Pediatrics Consultant
Mechi Hospital, Jhapa, Nepal

Rakesh Lal
Additional Professor
Department of Psychiatry
All India Institute of Medical
Sciences (AIIMS)
New Delhi, India

Raminder Kalra
Tutor
Rajkumari Amrit Kaur
College of Nursing, New Delhi, India

R Chandrasekaran
Professor and Head
Department of Psychiatry
Jawaharlal Institute of Postgraduate
Medical Education and Research
Puducherry, India

RC Chowdhary
Professor and Head
Department of Community Medicine
Mahatma Gandhi National Institute
of Medical Sciences
Jaipur, Rajasthan, India

RC Jiloha
Professor and Head
Department of Psychiatry
GB Pant Hospital and
Maulana Azad Medical College
New Delhi, India

RD Mehta
Assistant Professor
Department of Dermatology,
Venereology and Leprosy
SP Medical College
Bikaner, Rajasthan, India

RK Chadda
Professor
Department of Psychiatry
All India Institute of Medical Sciences
New Delhi, India

RK Solanki
Senior Professor and Head
Department of Psychiatry
Dr SN Medical College
Jodhpur, Rajasthan, India

Roshan V Khanande
Senior Resident
Central Institute of Psychiatry
Ranchi, Jharkhand, India

RP Agarwal
Assistant Professor
Department of Medicine
SP Medical College
Bikaner, Rajasthan, India

Sachchidanand Singh
Senior Resident
Central Institute of Psychiatry
Ranchi, Jharkhand, India

Sai Krishna Tikka
Senior Resident
Central Institute of Psychiatry
Ranchi, Jharkhand, India

Sandeep Grover
Associate Professor
Department of Psychiatry
Postgraduate Institute of Medical
Education and Research
Chandigarh, India

Sandeep M
Senior Resident
Central Institute of Psychiatry
Ranchi, Jharkhand, India

Santosh K Chaturvedi
Professor
Department of Psychiatry
National Institute of Mental Health and
Neurosciences
Bengaluru, Karnataka, India

Sarita Parajuli
Chakrabarti Habi Nursing College
Bhaktapur, Nepal

SC Bhargav
Professor
Department of Psychiatry
Medical College
Rohtak, Haryana, India

SC Gupta
Reader
Department of Psychiatry
King George's Medical College
Lucknow, Uttar Pradesh, India

SC Malik
Formerly Professor and Head
Department of Psychiatry
Lady Hardinge Medical College
New Delhi, India

SC Pradhan
Senior Resident
Institute of Human Behaviour and
Allied Sciences
New Delhi, India

Shashi Kiran
Formerly Assistant Professor
Department of Psychiatry
National Institute of Mental Health and
Neurosciences
Bengaluru, Karnataka, India
Currently Child and Adolescent
Psychiatry Consultant
County Durham and Darlington
Priority Services NHS Trust
Durham, UK

Shaswat Saxena
Senior Resident
Department of Psychiatry
King George's Medical University
Lucknow, Uttar Pradesh, India

Sheela Jain
Associate Professor
Department of Anatomy
SP Medical College
Bikaner, Rajasthan, India

Shivananda Jena
Assistant Professor
Department of Psychiatry
GB Pant Hospital and
Maulana Azad Medical College
New Delhi, India

Shivanshu Shrivastava
Research Assistant and Observer
Department of Psychiatry
Lokmanya Tilak Municipal
Medical College
Mumbai, Maharashtra, India

Shree Ram Ghimire
Consultant Psychiatrist
Transcultural Psychosocial
Organization Nepal
Baluwatar, Kathmandu, Nepal
Former Lecturer
Department of Psychiatry
National Medical College and Teaching
Hospital
Birgunj, Nepal

Shubhakaran
Senior Registrar
SP Medical College
Bikaner, Rajasthan, India

S Kalyanasundaram
Principal and Professor
Department of Psychaitry
The Richmond Fellowship Post
Graduate College for Psychosocial
Rehabilitation
Bengaluru, Karnataka, India

SK Pandey
Senior Psychiatrist
Carewell Family Clinic
Jaipur, Rajasthan, India

SK Verma
Additional Professor
Department of Clinical Psychology
Postgraduate Institute of Medical
Education and Research
Chandigarh, India

SN Ali
Central Institute of Psychiatry
Ranchi, Jharkhand, India

Somnath Sen Gupta
Associate Professor
Department of Psychiatry
Kasturba Medical College and Hospital
Manipal, Karnataka, India

Sourav Khanra
Senior Resident
Central Institute of Psychiatry
Ranchi, Jharkhand, India

SS Nathawat
Former Professor and Head
Department of Psychology
University of Rajasthan
Jaipur, Rajasthan, India

Sudhir Hebbar
Senior Resident
Department of Psychiatry
Jawaharlal Institute of Postgraduate
Medical Education and Research
Puducherry, India

Sudhir Kumar CT
Senior Resident
Department of Psychiatry
National Institute of
Mental Health and Neurosciences
Bengaluru, Karnataka, India

Sujata Malik
Senior Occupational Therapist
Safdarjung Hospital
New Delhi, India

Sumant Khanna
Former Professor
Department of Psychiatry
National Institute of Mental Health and
Neurosciences
Bengaluru, Karnataka, India

Sunila Chadda
Professor and Head
Department of Pathology
Dr SN Medical College, Jodhpur
SP Medical College
Bikaner, Rajasthan, India

Suresh Bada Math
Additional Professor
Department of Psychiatry
National Institute of Mental Health and
Neurosciences
Bengaluru, Karnataka, India

Swarnali Bose
Clinical Psychologist and Training
Co-ordinator
Project HIFAZAT
Regional Technical Training Centre
Ranchi, Jharkhand, India

TS Sathyanarayana Rao
Editor
Indian Journal of Psychiatry
Chief Advisor
Indian Journal of Psychological
Medicine, Indian Journal of Geriatric
Psychiatry, Indian Journal of Social
Psychiatry, Indian Journal of Private
Psychiatry, Andhra Pradesh Journal of
Psychological Medicine
President Elect
Indian Association for Geriatric
Mental Health
Professor
Department of Psychiatry
JSS Medical College and Hospital
Mysuru, Karnataka, India

Uma Joshi
Professor
Department of Physiology
Mahatma Gandhi Institute of Medical
Sciences
Jaipur, Rajasthan, India

Umesh S
Senior Resident
Central Institute of Psychiatry
Ranchi, Jharkhand, India

Urvakhsh Mehta
Assistant Professor
Department of Psychiatry
National Institute of Mental Health and
Neurosciences
Bengaluru, Karnataka, India

V Balasubramaniam
Department of Neurosurgery
Institute of Medical Sciences
Banaras Hindu University
Varanasi, Uttar Pradesh, India

Varun S Mehta
Senior Resident
Central Institute of Psychiatry
Ranchi, Jharkhand, India

Veena Vyas
Social Scientist
Jaipur, Rajasthan, India

Vijaya S Nathawat
Department of Psychology
University of Rajasthan
Jaipur, Rajasthan, India

V Kumaraiah
Professor and Head
Department of Clinical Psychology
National Institute of Mental Health and
Neurosciences
Bengaluru, Karnataka, India

VK Verma
Formerly Professor and Head
Department of Psychiatry
Postgraduate Institute of Medical
Education and Research (PGIMER)
Chandigarh, India

VN Vahiya
Professor and Head
Department of Psychiatry
Dr RN Cooper Municipal Medical
College and General Hospital
Mumbai, Maharashtra, India

VS Chadda
Former Professor an Head
Department of Medicine
SP Medical College
Bikaner, Rajasthan, India

VS Randhawa
Assistant Professor
Department of Microbiology
Lady Hardinge Medical College
New Delhi, India

W Balati
Department of Psychiatry
National Institute of Mental Health and
Neurosciences
Bengaluru, Karnataka, India

Preface to the Third Edition

Textbook of Postgraduate Psychiatry (3rd edition, 2 vols) is assimilated with all modern developments in psychiatry and their effects on clinical practice. It incorporates over 10,000 references with some of the original data on which modern evidence-based medicine depends. There are a few new chapters on clinical epidemiology, genetics in psychiatry, neuropsychiatry, special areas of interest and others. This is a highly readable and comprehensive package of modern psychiatry. It places emphasis on detailed clinical descriptions of both common and rare psychiatric disorders and their places within 10th revision of the International Statistical Classification of Diseases and Related Health Problems (ICD-10), Diagnostic and Statistical Manual of Mental Disorders, 4th Edition (DSM-IV) and Diagnostic and Statistical Manual of Mental Disorders, 5th Edition (DSM-5). Clinical management is given due prominence, with extensive accounts of modern drug management, cognitive therapy, psychosocial approaches and current guidelines such as those published in American Psychiatric Association (APA) and National Institute for Health and Clinical Excellence (NICE). Easy to read with over 400 tables and boxes summarizing information, this is an essential text for trainees studying for their MD (Psychiatry), DNB, DMP and MRC Psychiatry examinations. It is also a best reference book for established practitioners across the world. We hope that readers will welcome this edition with the same spirit with which they liked the previous two editions. We welcome any suggestions for further improvements to be incorporated in future.

JN Vyas
Shree Ram Ghimire

Preface to the First Edition

It has been a long-felt need of the postgraduate resident in psychiatry in India for a textbook that covers this subject matter comprehensively, with up-to-date references, and is in a simple language and easily comprehensible. The 'Western' textbooks are either too lengthy or make difficult reading, or are not comprehensive and integrated, or are not adequately referenced, or lack internal citations in the text. Moreover, they are exorbitantly priced, and do not take note of the psychiatric research done in the Indian subcontinent.

The time was, therefore, ripe for *Textbook of Postgraduate Psychiatry*. It attempts to cover clinical psychiatry and allied subjects comprehensively in a lucid style, making it easily understandable and interesting. It is replete with references and each chapter provides a 'further reading' list. Though comprehensive, it is yet concise, avoiding circumstantial explanations. Indian research work in psychiatry is adequately covered, and it is not merely compiled but cited in the context of world literature on the subject.

Textbook of Postgraduate Psychiatry is addressed primarily to the postgraduate student in psychiatry and allied mental health fields, but it should equally serve as a good source of revision and reference to psychiatrists, who have already completed their training, and to practitioners and clinicians, and other mental health professionals.

Such an exhaustive textbook cannot be justifiably written by one or two authors. The contributors include renowned authorities in the various subspecialties of psychiatry with original work to their credit as well as young, zealous psychiatrists, who are actively involved in academic life. We wish to express our deep appreciation to the contributors who worked with enthusiasm and cooperated fully in the preparation of the textbook.

The preparation of the book was a major endeavor that involved the efforts of several persons, too numerous to be mentioned individually. In particular, we wish to thank *Padma Shree* Dr SR Mehta, Ex-Principal, SMS Medical College, Jaipur, Rajasthan; Dr Rajeshwar Sharma, Ex-Principal, SMS Medical College, Jaipur; Dr GC Munjal, Director-Professor and Head, Department of Psychiatry, GB Pant Hospital and Maulana Azad Medical College, New Delhi; Dr SC Malik, Professor and Head, Department of Psychiatry, SK Hospital and Lady Hardinge Medical College, New Delhi; Dr Neena Bohra, Head, Department of Psychiatry, RML Hospital, New Delhi; and Dr SK Khandelwal, Associate Professor, and Dr K Chandiramani, Assistant Professor, Department of Psychiatry, All India Institute of Medical Sciences (AIIMS), New Delhi, India; for their constructive advice and comments. Dr Pradeep Sharma, Assistant Professor, Department of Psychiatry, SMS Medical College, Jaipur, helped in the initial stages of this project.

We are grateful to the publishers, BI Churchill Livingstone, for their useful suggestions and editorial assistance. We are also thankful to Remson Press for their efficient typesetting and to Ram Printograph, India, for their neat and speedy printing.

Textbook of Postgraduate Psychiatry would not have seen the light of the day without constant encouragement and support from our respective families.

The book must finally be assessed by the reader, for whom it is meant. We intend to revise and update it at regular intervals in the light of newer developments.

We welcome suggestions and critical comments from the reader.

JN Vyas
Niraj Ahuja

Acknowledgments

Textbook of Postgraduate Psychiatry is not the effort of a single hand but of multiple contributors. I am especially thankful to them for their laudable efforts, and I am particularly indebted to Drs Shree Ram Ghimire and Jayati Simlai, whose team stood by me at every step and put in hard labor. I would like to thank all contributors and advisors for their coordination and hard work. I would like to thank Dr Jainuruddin Ansari, Chairman, National Medical College and Teaching Hospital, Birgunj, Nepal; Dr Basuruddin Ansari, Managing Director, National Medical College; Drs SN Hissaria, KN Singh, Mohamad Aslam and Abid Hussain Ansari, for their kind blessing and support. I thank all wellwishers, advisors, and contributors. The outstanding coordination, cooperation and patience of the publisher, M/s Jaypee Brothers Medical Publishers (P) Ltd, New Delhi, India, is always gratefully acknowledged. I would also like to thank my family members including my wife Manju, sons Hemant and Kapil, and daughters-in-law Mridula and Veena for their consistent moral support. Last but not least, I am very much thankful to Drs Sarita Parajuli, Jyoti Dahal, Kiran Dahal and Niranjan Chaudhary for their help in editing the book, without whose contribution, the publication of the book would not have been possible. Readers are the best critics of any book. All creative minds are most welcome to critically analyze the book, and provide their feedback through email us at: *drsrghimire@gmail.com* or *jnvyas2012@gmail.com*. Critical feedback is always appreciated to improve standard of the book.

JN Vyas

Contents

VOLUME 1

SECTION 1
Clinical Examination in Psychiatry and Epidemiology of Mental Disorder

SECTION 2
Organic Mental Disorder and Substance Related Disorders

SECTION 3
Schizophrenia, Other Psychotic Disorders and Mood Disorder

SECTION 4
Anxiety Disorders

SECTION 5
Stress Related Disorders

SECTION 6
Psychosomatic Medicine, Somatoform Disorder, Dissociative Disorder and Other Related Disorders

SECTION 7
Personality Disorder, Sexual Disorder, Sleep Disorder and Eating Disorders

SECTION 8
Pregnancy and Menstruation Related Disorders

SECTION 9
Liaison Psychiatry, Neuropsychiatry, Psychiatric Aspect of Medical Disorders and Other Related Conditions

Section 10
Emergency in Mental Health

VOLUME 2

SECTION 11
Child and Adolescent Psychiatry

SECTION 12
Basic Sciences and Imaging in Psychiatry

SECTION 13
Neuropsychology, Research Methods, Statistics and Genetics in Psychiatry

SECTION 14
Biological Therapies

SECTION 16
Geriatric Psychiatry: Life Stress, Sociology, and Psychiatry

SECTION 17
Mental Health Issues in Women and Indian Minorities

SECTION 18
Culture, Spirituality, Anthropology and Psychiatry

SECTION 19
Community Psychiatry and Psychiatric Nursing

SECTION 20
Special Area of Interest

SECTION 21
Forensic Psychiatry and Mental Health Legislation

SECTION 22
Ethics and History of Psychiatry

CHAPTER 1 Clinical Examination in Psychiatry

Somnath Sen Gupta

Every mentally-ill person is a special problem in diagnosis and treatment. Every mental patient is a unity, a unique example, suffering from some particular combination of events that has broken or is breaking his adaptations to life. The first task of the physician in determining the cause or the nature of the illness is the collection of pertinent data. Securing the record of the subjective complaints and the physical examination of the patient are arts, the systematic method of sorting and classifying the data and the making of a diagnosis from the facts secured is a science, and treatment is a combination of science and art. Errors in judgment, errors in analysis, errors in data, and above all errors in technique are among the reasons or sources of a mistaken diagnosis.

PSYCHIATRIC INTERVIEWING

Types

Interviewing remains the most basic skill of clinical examination in psychiatry. This is inspite of the major advances in understanding of the biological basis of mental illness.

Most psychiatrists, like other clinicians, are less proficient in their essential clinical skills than they realize. Interviewing, is a practical skill that the trainee can acquire by carrying out interviews under supervision and watching experienced interviewers at work. A sound knowledge of normal and abnormal mental phenomena is also essential.

Psychiatric interviews could be diagnostic or therapeutic. The former focuses on obtaining historical information and eliciting psychopathology that help the clinician to attempt diagnostic formulations. Therapeutic interviews, on the other hand, intend to bring about desirable change in mental and behavioral problems and are beyond the scope of this chapter.

The diagnostic interviews are essentially of two types. A *freeform interview* is directed by the clinician, allows the patient narrate his/her own story and fosters therapeutic relationship. However, with inexperienced interviewers, this may deteriorate into a social conversation and important themes may be forgotten. In *standardized interviews*, the wording of the questions is fixed. In semi-structured interviews, e.g. Schedules for Clinical Assessment in Neuropsychiatry (SCAN),[1] there is an opportunity for interviewers to further explore the symptoms in order to determine their positive rating. No such explorations are allowed in structured interviews, e.g. Composite International Diagnostic Interview (CIDI)[2] where the content, order and wording of the questions are fixed and as a result the patient may sometimes feel being interrogated. The standardized interviews are useful in research.

The constraint of time always provides a structuring framework for every interview. The interviewer should have a framework of questionnaire in mind while allowing the patient to tell his/her own story initially. As the story unfolds, it is fitted into the framework so that the gaps are filled up with further questioning.

Goals

Psychological experiences are private and personal. A patient would not normally share them with a clinician unless an atmosphere of trust and openness builds up between them, and the patient becomes aware of the confidentiality of the relationship. This relationship manifests in rapport (spontaneous emotional resonance between the client and interviewer) and lays the foundation for the subsequent interviewing tasks (collection of information, giving feedback, etc.). The relationship is established through an interpersonal interaction between the doctor and the patient. A desire to be helped enables the patient to expose his intimate thoughts and feelings. However, the following characteristics in the interviewer's approach to the patient contribute to the building of the relationship: respect for others, calm manner, genuine caring, nonjudgmental attitude, dependability, openness, warmth, honesty and consistency.

The interviewer must fully respect the patient regardless of his/her values, beliefs and social class. He cannot be the judge of the patient's life. Concern and interest should be expressed with a nonjudgmental attitude. The clinician should be open to all kinds of queries from the patient and at the same time should be spontaneous in his own enquiry. He should be honest, and consistent throughout the interaction.

These elements are useful even when the patient denies suffering and need for help as a result of lack of insight into the illness. Further aims of psychiatric interview are shown in Table 1.

Techniques

Patients may be afraid that everyone else will hear about their problems. The interview should be conducted in a quiet room, relatively free from distractions. The chair of the patient should be ideally on the left side of a right handed individual and at the same level with that of the interviewer. This kind of *setting puts* the patient at ease and helps the interviewer take notes during the interview.

Patients should be given an opportunity to talk and be listened to attentively, particularly while describing the presenting problems. *Attentive listening* would encourage the patient to express thoughts and feelings. In order to listen effectively the examiner should face the patient, make eye contact, give full attention, nod head, say something like "I see", so that the patient knows he is listened to. The interviewer should not let himself be distracted as far as possible.

The clinician must *ask questions* calmly and slowly. He should be thoughtful about what he asks and think about how the patient may feel in answering him. It is often useful to let the patient talk at his own pace.

The types of questions frequently asked in diagnostic interviews are shown in Table 2. Recent works[3] favor the use of open ended questions in eliciting accurate information. The open ended question with checks and probes are to be used most liberally, e.g. to open the interview the examiner may ask " tell me what brings you to the hospital". Closed ended question need to be asked to review systems and to guide those patient who tends to talk profusely.

The interviewer may lead the conversation to get information but should continue to follow the patient's train of thought. If the patient talks about restlessness, he should be encouraged to describe the behavior further. He then should be asked what thought occurred to him, followed by how did he feel at that time.

Information about feelings are more difficult to obtain because many cultures discourage expression of feelings openly. When a safe environment is provided and the examiner appears caring and listens closely, most people would open up about their feelings. The examiner may recognize and respond to the patient's emotions in several ways that may seem appropriate during the course of the interview. The nonverbal cues may be recognized as "you appear tearful, your hands are trembling when you talked about your marriage". Patients may be directly asked, "how do you feel". Finally, the interviewer may enquire about any emotionally charged events in the family (e.g. quarrel, violence, drunken behavior, cruelty and neglect). The clinician must never assume that he knows how the person feels, rather he should listen to what the person has to say.

The interviewer should *empathize* with the patient by trying to imagine himself in the patient's position and understand how that person sees the world. The interviewer may ask himself—how does this person feel about his life, how does he view the world, what is best for this person to do?

It is possible to *facilitate expression* of the patient by telling him "please continue," " tell me more about it", "I see". Nonverbally, the examiner may sit slightly leaning forward, maintain eye contact, nod and smile appropriately.

Table 1: Goals of psychiatric interview

1.	To build relationship of trust and openness
2.	To collect historical information in details relevant to the presenting problems
3.	To assess personality of the patient
4.	To conduct a mental status examination and assess psychopathology
5.	To write a diagnostic formulation and list the differential diagnoses
6.	To explain to the patient what the clinician thinks is wrong with him and discuss the action he intends to take

Table 2: Type of questions used in psychiatric interview

Type	*Example*	*Likely responses*	*Remarks*
Open ended	How are you feeling?	Narrative unfocused	To be used at the beginning and while opening a new area in the history
Checks (Conjunction to open question)	Tell me more about it	Narrative	Used for clarification
Closed ended	Do you feel sad?	Focussed, Yes/No	To be used at the beginning to check the extent of symptoms; toward the end as screening questions
Probes (Conjunction to open and closed questions)	Has it been mild, moderate or severe? How much of the time were you low?	Specific details or examples	Clarifying and screening questions
Leading	How sad do you feel?	Confusion	To be used rarely with over talkative patients
Double	How are your sleep and appetite?	Confusion	To be avoided
Multiple choice	Do you feel happy, sad or angry?	Confusion	To be avoided

Sometimes, the interview may not progress as smoothly as expected since the patient may not come out spontaneously with his problems or may like to raise unnecessary topics. The interviewer should try to control the interview in order to maintain the focus on the relevant issues. For example, calm manner and reassurance are particularly needed for an over anxious patient, whereas techniques of verbal and nonverbal facilitation should be used more with a taciturn patient. An over talkative patient may be initially told about the time limit, may need to be interrupted at the natural breaks and asked more direct questions. When the patient is hostile and resentful, the interviewer should talk about the circumstances of referral and try to persuade the patient that the interview is intended to be in his own interest. Some people may like to dominate the interview when the interviewer should interrupt gently and firmly, and ensure what is being said is relevant to the present problems.

Interviewing Relatives

The psychiatrist should see the patient first and obtain his permission before speaking with a family member. If any information provided by the patient needs to be discussed with the family member, the psychiatrist should also obtain the patient's permission first. Wherever possible, the patient should be present during discussion with the family. Patients with psychosis and delirium are the exceptions to these rules. Moreover, if the psychiatrist cannot obtain the patient's permission to reveal a plan for suicide or homicide and if the patient refuses hospitalization, the psychiatrist has an obligation to advice and to recommend commitment to an inpatient unit.

PSYCHIATRIC HISTORY

Table 3 shows the organization of psychiatric history.

Sociodemographic Data

This includes the patient's name, age, sex, marital status, occupation, income (of patient and family), language, religion, nationality, and a brief statement about the patient's place of residence and the circumstances of living. Omission of one or more of these items in written records could be a result of lack of thoroughness or countertransference problem of the interviewer. These data are useful in ascertaining the social class to which patient belongs.[4,5] The relationship between mental illness and social class are reviewed elsewhere.[6]

Source and Reasons of Referral

This is to be mentioned clearly whenever applicable since such information provides useful background of the patient's illness and treatment.

Table 3: Organization of psychiatric history
Sociodemographic data Source and reasons of referral Chief complaints
History of present illness
Patient's version Informant's version
Past history
Physical illness Psychiatric illness Forensic history
Family history
Education, occupation and personality of the parents and siblings. Quality of relationship with the patient, family history of mental illness, social support system
Personal history
Prenatal period Early childhood Middle childhood Late childhood (adolescence)
Psychosexual history Occupational history Menstrual history Marital history Premorbid personality

Chief (Presenting) Complaints

Chief complaints are those for which the patient seeks professional help. These should be recorded in the patient's own words in chronological order.

History of Present Illness

Patient's version: The history begins with the examiner's impression of the reliability of the information provided. This is judged on the basis of consistency and coherence of the history, and its concordance with that of the informant. The interviewer should make an attempt to establish the nature of the problems volunteered by the patient. The problems revealed by questioning should, however, be separately mentioned. Once this is over, the following details have to be elicited.

Onset: The patient should be asked when he was entirely well or when he first sought medical or other help. Sometimes, use of anchor dates like birth days and marriage anniversary can improve the accuracy of recall. However, there will be no clear dating of onset of the problems emerging from personality disorders.

Precipitating factors: These are the events that occur shortly before the onset of the illness or appear to have induced it.

The interviewer should find out whether the patient considers that any physical (seizure, trauma, substance misuse, prescribed drugs) or psychosocial (stressful life events) factor was related to the onset of the illness. While doing this the interviewer must remember that the patient's recall of life events may be poor or he may causally link his problems to an event which could very well be a result of his illness, e.g. losing a job during a depressive episode. In order to minimize these effects the clinician should set limits to the period (one, three or six months), accurately determine the onset of the illness, concentrate on the events 'independent' of the illness, (e.g. birth or death) and use semi-structured interview schedules like Presumptive Stressful Life Events Scale (PSLES).[7]

Recognizing precipitating factors, when present, helps in reaching a diagnosis, formulating treatment and in preventing the illness in future.

Mode of onset: This may be abrupt, acute, sub-acute or insidious. Mode of onset often gives clue to the cause and has implications in prognosis.

Development of symptoms (and their change in frequency and intensity over time, and whether they co-vary or take an independent course).

This may indicate whether there is a single or multiple disorders.

Effects of the symptoms on the following:

- *Self*: Giving rise to euphoria or distress.
- *Other mental functions*: Leading to impairments like lack of concentration, inefficient thinking, poor recall, indecisiveness, anxiety or depression.
- *Biological functions*: Sleep, appetite, bowel and bladder habits, sexual function.
- *Social functioning*: Leading to disabilities like decreased ability to work, managing day to day chores, enjoying hobbies, or making use of leisure.
- *Interpersonal relations*: Any change in the quality of relationships with family members.
- *Law*: Any legal problems, arrests, ongoing cases in the court.

The extent of these problems would determine the severity of the illness.

Any *perpetuating factor* of the illness, which may be again physical (concomitant illness), or psychosocial (chronic stressors or conflicts) or consequences of the illness (secondary gain, relief drinking in alcoholism).

A *negative history* has then to be taken by enquiring about the physical or mental symptoms not elicited so far. This is necessary while making comorbid diagnoses or arranging the symptoms in a hierarchical order.

Treatment history: Nature and duration of treatment, any hospitalization and any response to treatment given so far have to be recorded. This could be obtained from the referral letter and other papers of previous consultations. At this stage, the examiner should be able to make certain diagnostic impressions in his mind so as to keep the rest of the interview most relevant and meaningful.

Informant's version: A remark should be made on the reliability of the information. Informant's observation on the patient's behavior, functioning, lifestyle and habits should be recorded here. A careful amalgamation of patient's and informant's versions is to be done while writing the diagnostic formulation. Information by an independent observer is of crucial importance in Psychiatry than in other branches of Medicine, since patients may deny illness due to lack of insight, or provide information distorted by psychopathology, or have poor appraisal of personality in cases of personality disorders.

Past History

Physical illness: Date, duration of illness, operation, accidents, etc. nature of treatment and any sequele.

Psychiatric illness: Symptoms, date, duration, nature of treatment, any hospitalization and response to treatment. All the prescriptions and the reports of investigations available should be utilized in this regard. Past history may greatly contribute to diagnosis, which depends on both longitudinal and cross-sectional profile of the illness.

Forensic history: Any history of delinquency, criminal offenses, illicit drug use, including punishments received. This may throw light on the personality and, on occasion, such behavior may be a manifestation of mental disorder.

Family History

Here onwards, begins the biography of the patient. This throws light on the hereditary and environmental forces influencing the development of the individual. This indicates predisposing factors toward the illness.

The interviewer should draw the family tree (*family of origin*) preferably covering at least three generations (this will indicate the nature of heredity). The interviewer should record the following details about the first degree relatives (parents and siblings).

If alive, present age. If dead, age at death and the cause of death. This may be relevant to the diagnosis, e.g. loss of mother below the age of eleven, in case of female patients, seems to contribute to later development of depressive illness. The cause of death, e.g. suicide, alcohol related accident or liver disease could suggest a familial illness. Similarly, family history of death of a brother from heart failure due to rheumatic heart disease may explain the patient's concern about chest pain. Reaction of the patient at the time of parent's death needs to be enquired into.

Separation, divorce or remarriage of the parents needs to be enquired about. Was there any prolonged absence of the parents through illness, service or marital discord? What was the nature of marital discord? In case of separation or divorce, how did the patient respond to this event? Did it cause any particular problems? If brought up by others, how did he react?

Educational background and occupational history of the first degree relatives should be asked. This will indicate the intellectual and social adjustment with which patient's own attainments could be contrasted. If there is a discrepancy, this will need to be explained.

Personality and quality of relationship to the patient may be elicited through the following enquiries, e.g. tell me about your father? What sort of person was he? What kind of person was your mother? How well did they get long? Was there any major disagreement between them? How did you get on with each one of them? Were they warm and supportive toward you? Could you confide anything in them? How would they respond? Were you encouraged to become independent?

Some personality characteristics may have definitive impact on the personality development and contribute to later development of deviant behavior or neurotic disorder, e.g. parental violence, misuse of alcohol, criminal behavior, unduly punitive, restrictive or inconsistent attitudes, or undue leniency.

The interviewer should next enquire about the family history of any illness, viz. mental illness, mental retardation, suicide, abnormal personality, alcoholism and drug abuse, epilepsy, movement disorder, dementia, and early death. Nature of the symptoms, duration of the illness, any hospitalization, impact on social and occupational functioning, treatment received and the outcome must be detailed from the patient or a key informant.

It is necessary to go into the various components of the support system, viz. sources (family, friends and organizations), types (instrumental, i.e. material or tangible, and emotional or esteem enhancing), actual behavior (who did or said what when support was last needed) versus perceived support (who you feel you can call on when need arises), and negative versus positive aspects of support. Some kinds of emotional support may hinder recovery and render relapse more likely. Taking over the roles of the patient that is more than justified by the illness, fussing over the patient, getting too involved in his problems, non-acceptance of the illness of the patient, and showing negative emotions may be harmful to the patient. Assessment of the support system is relevant to the management and rehabilitation of the patient.

Personal History

The interviewer must collect some information on all the areas and expand on other pertinent areas as it is impossible to obtain the complete history of a person's life. Personal history needs to be recorded in the following way.

Prenatal history: The psychiatrist should find out whether the patient was a planned/wanted child, any problems during mother's pregnancy or delivery, any evidence of defect or injury at birth, and the parents' reaction to the gender of the patient.

Early childhood (0–5 years): It is customary to ask about the developmental milestones[8] from the mother. The details are particularly required in cases of developmental disorders. The quality of mother and child interaction during feeding is more useful than finding out whether the patient was breastfed or bottle-fed.

Could the baby single out the mother? What was the activity level? Was there any early disturbance in the sleep pattern? Was there any problem in the resolution of stranger anxiety? What was the age of gaining control over bladder and bowel? Was there any problem in toilet training? How was the early play with body parts and toys? Who were living in the patient's home? What were their roles in upbringing of the patient? Was there any serious illness during this time, especially affecting the central nervous system (CNS), e.g. febrile seizures, exanthematous fever or any head trauma that might have interfered with normal development.

Middle childhood (5–11 years): The quality of relationship of the patient with his siblings. If any, may influence the social adaptation of the patient. It is necessary to ask about any sibling rivalry as well as positive or supporting relation with the siblings. The latter may be occurring when the patient was rejected by the parents. Death of a sib before the birth of the patient or during the formative years, may lead to emotional disorder of the mother who may be unable to offer emotional nourishment to other children.

Play is a useful area to explore in studying the growing capacity for social adaptation and developing ego structures, which will indicate the future personality. The ability to concentrate, tolerate frustration, cooperate with peers, understand and comply with the rules, and any intellectual play should be enquired.

Unmet emotional needs as well as exaggerated power struggles give rise to the various problems in childhood, including thumb sucking, temper tantrums, tics, nightmares, fears, eating disorders, excessive masturbation, bed wetting and nail biting. The predictive validity of these early neurotic traits to later mental disorders is, however, not known.

Schooling provides important clues regarding intellectual, social and moral development of the patient. How did he take the first separation from mother? Did he make friends easily? Was he popular? Did he belong to gangs or groups? How did he perceive his teachers? How did he compare himself with other children? Was there any problem with discipline? Was there any failure or discontinuation or change in school. If so, what were the reasons? Was there any prolonged absence? What were the reasons? How was the ability to read, write and learn, and ability to concentrate on the task at hand? How was the activity level? Early patterns of assertion, impulsiveness, aggression, passivity, anxiety or antisocial behavior often emerge in the context of school relationships.

Later childhood (adolescence): The unfolding and consolidation of adult personality occurs during later childhood. During this time, through relations with peers and group activity, a person begins to develop independence from his parents. The psychiatrist should attempt to define the values of his social group and whom he idealized. To what extent did he become independent from the parents?

The progress in secondary education should be explored. Was there problem with teacher, peers or rules? Any discrepancy between potential and achievement should be noted with reasons. Results in public examinations and subsequent higher education, achievements, and any disruption should be noted.

Adolescence is also the time of experiencing various problems, like emotional problems (anxiety, inferiority feelings), physical problems (weight loss or gain) and behavioral problems (experimentation with drugs, antisocial behavior, running away from home).

Psychosexual history: The interviewer should use discretion regarding how much to ask in this area. The questions should be asked in a matter-of-fact manner, e.g. "do you mind if I ask you regarding physical aspects of relationship?" Enquiries should be made about any infantile sexuality, sexual curiosity or sexual games during early childhood, or any history of sexual transgression on the patient during childhood? How did he react? How did he learn about sex? Was he instructed adequately? Did he have any misconceptions? What was the attitude of the parents to sex and its development? How does he recall his reaction to achieving a true sense of sexual identity and maturity; any problems did it give rise to? How did he feel about the onset of puberty and secondary sexual changes? Was there any precocity or any embarrassment? Did he masturbate? What did he use to think at that time? Any dating, heterosexual experiences, any inclination toward his own sex, or any homosexual relations? Whenever necessary, interviewer should ask about any promiscuity, incestuous behavior and asexual deviant practices, and any history of contracting sexually transmitted disease?

Occupational record: Type of jobs the patient has had, duration, reasons for changes, any period of unemployment, income at different stages (provide guide to his progress), ways of coping with his work, e.g. overconscientious, difficulty in delegating to others, tendency of double checking, reluctant to take holidays, level of job satisfaction. For retired people, the way time is spent and satisfaction with work, if any, should be asked. Occupational record may indicate the level of stress at work, as well as personality traits. Was there any service or war experience, promotion, awards received or any disciplinary problems?

Menstrual history: Age of menarche, attitude to periods, regularity and amount, any dysmenorrhea, premenstrual tensions, age of menopause, any symptoms, and date of last menstruation. How did she learn about menstruation?

Marital history: The time the couple had known each other, previous relationships and marriage engagements, ages and occupation at marriage (indicate their compatibility), parental consent, health, present age, occupation and personality of the spouse. The quality of marital relationship is indicated by (a) adequacy of sexual relationship, (b) methods of contraception/family planning, (c) the way in which roles are allocated between the partners-sharing of decisions and responsibilities, (d) extent to which each partner is involved in outside interests and relationships, (e) possibility of extramarital relationship to be considered with discretion, and (f) present couple living as nuclear/extended/joint family-relationship with others. Date of birth of the children and their age, health, education, occupation, any problem in their development and in relationship, and any illness during pregnancies in case of women.

Premorbid Personality

The patient's personality consists of his life-long persistent and enduring characteristics and attitudes, including ways of thinking (cognition), feeling (affectivity) and behaving (impulse control, and ways of relating to others and handling interpersonal relation). Personality traits may contribute to or influence the manifestations of a mental disorder in several ways. Personality may change following severe emotional trauma, brain damage, or mental disorder, when it becomes imperative to know about premorbid personality.

Premorbid personality may be assessed from the patient (recall may be distorted due to illness particularly when the illness is recurrent and thus certain allowance should be given to this), close relatives and colleagues who know him well, and observing his behavior at interview.

Premorbid personality should be described under the following headings:

Self: How does he describe himself? What kind of person is he? What are his strengths and abilities? What are his shortcomings? Does he see himself as worthwhile? Can he plan ahead ? How resilient is he in the face of adversity? How assertive is he? What are his hopes and ambitions?

Relations: Does he prefer company or solitude? Is he shy or makes friends easily? Are the relationships close or lasting? How is his relation with people of his own or opposite sex? How does he handle others' mistakes or inconsistencies? Does he always want to be the center of attraction? How does he tolerate others' criticisms?

Work and leisure: How is his relations with workmates or superiors (vide occupational record)? What are his hobbies and interests? Is he affiliated to any society, club or organization?

Mood: What is his mood like? How changeable is it? How quickly the mood changes appear, how long they last, do they follow life events? Can he express feelings of love, anger, frustration or sadness? Does he ever lose control over his feelings? Has he ever been violent? Is he usually anxious, cheerful, despondent, optimistic, pessimistic or self-depreciating?

Character: While taking the personal history, the interviewer will already have gathered some impression of character. Further information should he sought by asking whether he was reserved, timid, self-conscious, sensitive or suspicious, resentful or jealous, irritable, selfish, or self-centered.

Attitudes and standards: Attitudes to the body, health and illness, as well as religious and moral standards should be asked for. Personal history would have indicated about some of these.

Habits: Use of tobacco, alcohol, drugs, and food habit should be asked for.

It is not a must that the personality of the patient has to resemble any of those described in the present classificatory systems. In fact, a person is likely to have a mixture of various traits. However, the examiner should always try to make a balanced assessment of the positive and negative attributes of the personality of the patient. If there is any doubt of abnormal personality further assessment may be done with International Personality Disorder Examination (IPDE).[9]

Mental Status Examination

Mental status examination (MSE) is defined as a standardized format (Table 4) in which the clinician records the psychiatric signs and symptoms present at the time of the interview. This appears to correspond to the physical examination in medical cases. MSE reveals conscious mental experiences (*phenomenological data*) and several of them rely on the subjective information provided by the patient. Physical examination, on the other hand, is done in a much more objective way. MSE conducted efficiently generates reliable data of high diagnostic utility. However, the fact that a small sample of behavior of the patient is observed in a rather artificial situation tends to limit the scope of MSE.

The techniques involved in doing MSE are shown in Table 5. It is evident that the interviewer will have gathered information on most of the areas of the mental state whilst taking the history. The clinician should offer a lucid account of his observations to substantiate his conclusions. This makes the MSE a reliable document for potential use by other clinicians in future. The observations made in the MSE should be evaluated against the background information from the family members who have observed the patient in real life situation.

The nursing and occupational staffs may observe an in-patient over a greater length of time. Their reports include the behavior in the ward, interpersonal behavior, any variability from time to time over day, and any difficulties over a given task. The psychiatrist should pay a great deal of attention to these reports while interpreting his own observation.

Mental status examination should describe all the areas of mental functioning. However, some areas may deserve differential emphasis according to the clinical impressions that may arise from the history, e.g. it is necessary to expand

Table 4: Mental status examination

Consciousness	
	Alertness Awareness
General appearance and behavior	
	Appearance Grooming Facial expression and posture Social behavior and attitude Rapport Motor behavior
Speech	
Mood and affect	
Thought	
	Stream Form Possession Content
Perception	
	Sense distortions Sense deceptions Other psychotic phenomena: Somatic passivity phenomena Other experiences: Derealization and depersonalization Body image disturbances
Cognitive functions	
	Attention and concentration Language functions Orientation Memory Intelligence Fund of general knowledge Abstract thinking Judgment
Insight	

Table 5: Differential contribution of various components of clinical examination to assessment of psychopathology

Mental function	*Historical information*	*Observation of nonverbal behavior*	*Active enquiry*	*Formal tests*
Consciousness	++	+	++	++
Appearance and behavior	+	++	–	–
Language	++	–	++	++
Orientation	++	+	++	++
Memory	++	–	++	++
Abstraction	–	–	++	++
Judgment	++	++	+	–
Thought	++	+	++	+
Mood and affect	++	++	+	–
Perception	++	+	++	–

on mood and thought in depression, while cognitive functions and mood need more emphasis in dementia.

Mental status examination is a hierarchical examination and cannot be approached haphazardly. If inattention is missed early in MSE, memory and higher cognitive functions may be improperly judged. Similarly, if aphasia is missed, the thought content may be misinterpreted as psychosis. The outline of MSE followed here is shown in Table 5.

Consciousness

Consciousness is best conceptualized as having two components viz. alertness and awareness. The former refers to the readiness to respond to a stimulus and is maintained by the state of activation (arousal) of the cortex by the reticular activating system. Awareness (content of consciousness) refers to the higher cognitive and emotional functioning, and is sub served by the faculty of attention. Alertness and awareness can vary independently and the final level of consciousness represents a dynamic balance between cortical and ascending reticular activating system. In neurological sense, only alertness is assessed whereas a true appreciation of the level of consciousness must include assessment of both the components.

There are three aspects in the *assessment of the level of alertness*. First, the intensity of stimulation needed to arouse the patient should be indicated: calling the patient's name in a normal conversational tone, calling in a loud voice, light touch on the arm, vigorous shaking of the shoulder, painful stimulation. Second, the highest level of responses should be described. This is best done with the Glasgow Coma scale[10] in which a numeric value is given to the best response in each of the three categories (eye opening, verbal, motor). Third, it is helpful to make a chart in the progress notes so that a rapid assessment of changing levels of consciousness can be made. This can be done objectively with the Glasgow Coma scale at regular intervals and plotted as a graph.

Most clinicians distinguish five principal levels of alertness representing different points on a continuum: normal alertness, somnolence, obtundation, stupor and coma.

Early or subtle changes in consciousness may only involve awareness of the environment with little or no change in alertness. This predominantly manifests in impairment of attention and other cognitive functions. Thus, the assessment includes behavioral observations (viz. neglect of appearance and needs, slowed responses, losing thread of conversation, episodes of incontinence and altered sleep wakeful cycle), formal tests of attention as well as comprehension, orientation, memory, other changes in mental status such as illusions, hallucinations (visual and tactile mainly), fleeting delusions, perplexity and euphoria, and any change in the mental state over the day.

In psychiatry, global assessment of consciousness is important with an emphasis on altered awareness. Following disorders of consciousness are relevant in psychiatry: delirium, clouding of consciousness, twilight state and stupor. The interested reader is referred to references.[11,12]

General Appearance and Behavior

Although MSE is based on mainly what the patient says, observation of nonverbal behavior can offer a great deal of diagnostic clues.[13] In doing this, however, the examiner must not forget to take into account the nuances of personality and sociocultural background of the patient, as these to a great extent shape the customs of grooming and social behavior.

Appearance

The examiner should note the appearance of the patient for chronological age and his body build. Height and weight need to be recorded in certain cases. A lean and thin appearance with clothes that appear too loose might suggest recent weight loss and may occur in physical illness (e.g. malignancy), anorexia nervosa and depression.

Personal cleanliness (indicated by the state of skin, hair, nails, teeth and beard), the dress and grooming, and their appropriateness to the situation should be described next. Self-neglect suggested by untidy dress and dirty look may be associated with several conditions such as dementia, schizophrenia, depression and substance use disorders. Patients with mania may prefer colorful dress and make excessive use of cosmetics (women). Dress inappropriate for sex, e.g. men wearing women's clothes and make-up may suggest transvestism or trans-sexualism. Any asymmetry in cleanliness or dress, e.g. unshaven left side of the face, undone hair of the left side, may indicate sensory inattention due to nondominant parietal lobe lesion.

Facial expression, eye contact and posture are the most obvious nonverbal indices of the patient's mood. The examiner should describe the facial expression as well as its mobility during the conversation. In depression, the patient's eyes are often downcast with medial ends of the brows raised obliquely, vertical furrows in the forehead and down turning of the corners of the mouth. In severe depression, this look of misery may be unchanging. The patient sits with the shoulders hunched up, head bent forward, with arms kept close to the body. A still, expressionless face may be seen in chronic schizophrenia as well as in parkinsonism (idiopathic or drug induced). Anxiety in general may be associated with raised eye brows, widening of the palpebral fissures, mydriasis and the presence of horizontal furrows on the forehead. The patient sits upright on the edge on the chair with head erect, with fine tremor of the hands and perspiration over the face.

Social Behavior and Attitude

The examiner should note how the patient relates to him. For example, an anxious patient may relate in a tense manner. A depressed patient may be withdrawn, may not exhibit the usual social smile, and make few social contacts with the examiner. Increased social contact, with over familiarity and disinhibition, may characterize the manner of relating in a manic patient. A schizophrenic patient may be guarded or aggressive during the interview. Inappropriate, odd responses may be seen in mental retardation, dementia or delirium. The attitude of the patient may be assessed in the areas of cooperativeness, friendliness, trust, purposefulness, seductiveness, ingratiation, hostility, evasiveness and guardedness.

Rapport

An instantaneous emotional resonance between the patient and the interviewer usually develops early in the interview (vide supra). It is necessary to indicate whether rapport is established or not. It is difficult to establish rapport with patients with psychosis (e.g. schizophrenia) and certain personality disorders (e.g. antisocial personality). A positive rapport is necessary for a constructive therapeutic alliance.

Motor Behavior (Conation)

This can be assessed by observing the patient enter the interview room as well as his movements during the interview.

Usually, the gait is examined in a neurological sense. However, observation of gait is worthwhile in several psychiatric conditions. This is done as the patient enters the interviewer's room. Unusually, slow gait may occur in depression. Slow rigid gait with short shuffling steps, with loss of automatic associated movements, is associated with parkinsonism. Manic patients may walk relatively fast. In schizophrenia, gait may be abnormal due to mannerism, ambitendency or blocking of the movements. Broad-based staggering gait, with tendency to collapse at intervals and to cling to the nearest person for support, is seen in dissociative paraplegia (*astasia-abasia*).

A normal individual may change the posture to get more comfortable, use gestures appropriate to his needs and context of conversation. An exaggeration of normal movements is seen in anxiety disorder (fidgeting with an object and frequent change in posture). The examiner should make following observations of the patient's motor behavior: How fast does the patient initiate and carry out the movements? Is the speed uniform throughout the movement? Are the movements goal-directed? Does the patient show appropriate gestures? Do the movements occur spontaneously or in response to any stimulus?

Underactivity may be due to psychomotor retardation (as in retarded depression) or obstruction (as in catatonia). The former uniformly slows down the movements. Whereas, the movements are rather irregularly interrupted in catatonia. Increased goal directed activities occur in mania as well as in obsessive compulsive disorder (compulsive acts). Aimless increased activity is seen in severe agitation (wringing of the hands, pacing up and down, etc.), in depression and in akathisia (constant movements of the legs) due to neuroleptic drugs.

Certain catatonic features become obvious on inspection during the interview, e.g. stereotypy, echolalia, echopraxia, while other catatonic features such as automatic obedience, waxy flexibility, cooperation, and negativism may have to be elicited. Presence of catatonia indicates organic as well as functional psychoses.

Hallucinatory behavior in the form of muttering to self, making gestures at imaginary figures, keeping the head tilted at an angle while listening to the voices should also be described here.

Tardive dyskinesia (central or peripheral), tremor, dystonia, chorea, athetosis, tics and other involuntary movements should be described according to the following points: parts of the body affected, present only at rest, on movement or both, does voluntary movements increase or suppress it, is it affected by emotion, is it altered by eye closure, does it persist in sleep, if the patient is aware of it, can he describe its onset, and is it present when the patient does not know he is being observed.

Speech

Speech can be described in terms of its quantity, rate of production, and quality. The patient may be described as talkative, garrulous, voluble, taciturn, unspontaneous, or normally responsive to cues from the interviewer. Speech can be rapid or slow, pressured, hesitant, emotional, dramatic, monotonous, loud, whispered, slurred, staccato or mumbled. Speech impairment such as stuttering, are included in this section. Any unusual rhythms or accent should be noted. The patient's speech may be spontaneous.

Mood and Affect

DSM IV[25] defines mood as 'a pervasive and sustained emotion that colors the perception of the world.' Common examples include depression, elation, anger and anxiety.

The assessment of mood includes:
Quality: This is assessed in two ways: (a) subjectively—by asking the patient 'how do you feel in yourself' or 'how do you feel in your spirits,' (b) objectively—this is to be based on history, general appearance, behavior, posture and speech. Types of quality include euthymia, euphoria, elation, dysphoria and irritability among others.

Stability: To what extent mood is consistent over the day.

Reactivity: Change of mood with external events.

Persistence: How long does the mood last, i.e. days, weeks, months.

According to DSM IV, affect is a pattern of observable behavior that is the expression of a subjectively experienced feeling state (emotion). Affect is a variable over time in response to changing emotional states, whereas mood refers to a pervasive and sustained emotion.

The following aspects of affect need evaluation:
Quality: (vide supra)

Range: The spectrum of emotional changes displayed over a period of time in reference to various themes or topics during the interview. It is interpreted as full, increased (in mania), or constricted (in depression or schizophrenia).

Appropriateness: Congruity of emotion to the prevailing thought or speech. A normal person usually shows various emotions in relation to the various topics. For example, when the subject giggles on the matters of recent death of mother, it is an inappropriate affect which is hardly communicated to the interviewer. This is seen in schizophrenia (e.g. hebephrenic type).

Mobility: The ease with which affect changes from one mode to the other. This is decreased in depression (monotonic affect) and increased in mania. Rapid changes of affect from one mode to the other is called lability. This may occur in organic brain syndrome (e.g. dementia, pseudobulbar palsy), drug intoxications, early in schizophrenia, and some types of neurotic or personality disorders.

Relatedness (communicability): Capacity to connect with the interviewer, usually present in mania with infectious jocularity but absent in schizophrenia.

Intensity of expression (depth of affect): Increased in mania, and certain personality disorders, and decreased (blunted) or absent (flat) in schizophrenia.

What is considered the normal range of the expression of affect varies considerably both within and among different cultures. It is thus essential to describe affect under several parameters so as to minimize the examiner's bias or error in assessment.

Thought

Speech (verbal behavior) is the vehicle of thought. Thus speech, language and communication become essential parts of the examination of thought. There are four aspects of thought: stream, form, possession and content. The interviewer must document verbatim samples of speech and, if required, written samples in order to substantiate the inferences.

Stream: The examiner should comment on rate, reaction in, quality, volume and tone of speech.

Rate of speech refers to the number of words spoken in a given time. Decreased rate with increased pauses in between the sentences is associated with retarded depression and dementia. In the process, the reaction time (interval between question asked and responses from the patient) may be prolonged. Rate may be increased with shortened reaction time (acceleration) in mania.

Quantity of speech may be reduced in depression and in schizophrenia with negative symptoms. In extreme form, speech may be reduced to monosyllabic answers. Decreased quantity is also seen in shy and less intelligent people. Quantity is increased in mania either in the form of volubility (copious amount of goal directed speech) (logorrhea) or pressure of speech (uninterruptible). Increased quantity without acceleration may be seen in anxiety disorders, anankastic personality and hypochondriasis.

Volume is low in depression, often punctuated by sighing with a drop in volume, giving an impression of mournful cadence. Manics speak in volume louder than necessary. Restricted normal variation of tone with low pitched voice is seen in depression. A monotonous voice without low pitch occurs in negative schizophrenia and parkinsonism.

Form: Normal form indicates that thought is logical, coherent and sequential, makes use of symbols and is goal directed. Disorder of form of thought may mean abnormalities in language, communication or thought *per se*. The diagnostic specificity of thought disorders is rather low. This is in contrast to the previous views.

Doubts about abnormal form is raised when the patient's speech is poorly understandable. This could be either reported by the informant or recognized by the interviewer. It is also tested by asking the patient to describe verbally or in writing a neutral topic that is unrelated to the delusional system of thinking, e.g. patient's profession, religion, climate etc. at length. While analyzing the sample, the examiner should look for the following characteristics.

Are there logical and meaningful (semantic) connections between the successive ideas? If not, there is likely to be shift between two sentences or in the middle of a sentence. Then the examiner should check whether these shifts are based on some understandable and superficial (e.g. phonetic) connections like clang association (words rhyming), punning (words with more than one meaning), assonance (words sounding similar), word association or any external cues. If so, that will indicate flight of ideas which, when associated with pressured speech, is often seen in mania. When no such connections (semantic or phonetic) are found but the grammatical structure (syntax) is preserved, the shifts between the ideas make the speech difficult to understand and indicate *loosening of association* (*derailment*), which is seen in some cases of chronic schizophrenia. When the grammatical structure is also lost, the speech is reduced to a string of unrelated words called *verbigeration* (*word salad, incoherence*).

Are the responses relevant to the question? If there is a shift between the question and the answer, the reply is made in an oblique, irrelevant manner (*tangentiality*).

Is the amount of speech more than the information it conveys so that the content becomes vague and lacks in focus (*poverty of content of speech*)?

How goal directed is the speech? Does it reveal tedious, boring details and is long winded in reaching the goal (*circumstantially*)?

Is the patient able to shift focus whenever required? If not, there will be persistent repetition of words, ideas, or subjects beyond the point of relevance (*preservation*).

Is there any coinage of a new word or a known word used in a personal way (*neologism*)?

A written sample of speech could be further subjected to certain linguistic tests: (i) *type/token ratio*: ratio of different words to the total number of words.[14] A low score means limited language repertoire. (ii) *cloze score*: every fifth word in the paragraph is obliterated and normal people are asked to guess the deleted word.[15] The cloze score is the ratio of number of correct guesses to the number of words deleted and measures the readability of language, (iii) *contextual constraint* refers to the extent the language is grammatically correct.[16] The practical utility of such tests is limited at present, although they were originally used to explain thought disorder in schizophrenia.

There are further tests for thought disorder. Inability to maintain conceptual boundaries (over inclusive thinking) is tested by asking the patient to make conceptually similar sortings from several dissimilar objects. Impaired abstraction (vide supra) is tested by proverb test. Idiosyncratic personal constructs based on Kelly's personal construct theory is tested by Bannister and Fransella grid test.[17]

For detailed reading on the various types of thoughts disorder, the reader is referred to further references.[18-21]

Possession: Normally, the subject experiences his thinking as having two qualities: sense of personal possession and sense of control over his thinking. Disorder of the former is alienation experiences and of the latter indicate obsessions and compulsions. However, these are currently subsumed under content of thought.

Content of thought: This includes:

- *Preoccupation*: It is repetitive reference to one major idea. This could be normal or morbid. The latter has the quality of worries, i.e. unpleasantness, not being controlled with diversion of mind, and excessive to the topic worried about. The content of the preoccupation could be ideas of reference, persecution, grandeur, worthlessness, hopelessness, sin, guilt, nihilism, wishes, suicidal ideas, impoverishment, hypochondriasis, or dysmorphophobia.
- *Phobia*: Patient should be asked, when people get anxious and panicky they often feel their heart beating fast, or they start shaking or sweating, or cannot get their breath. Have you had feeling like that? Does it occur only in certain situations? If the patient says yes, their exact nature has to be clarified. While describing phobia, the examiner should mention, the extent of avoidance, anticipatory anxiety, any generalization to other innocuous situations and other commonly associated anxiety symptoms, viz. panic attacks and free floating anxiety.
- *Obsession*: Do you have any thoughts which keep coming to your mind. Are they unpleasant or unwanted thoughts? Do you try to resist them? Do you ever find you have to do anything repeatedly like washing things repeatedly that are already clean? How do you feel about it? How much does it interfere with your daily life? The examiner should describe the obsession with its content (ideas, thoughts, doubts impulses, imagery, rumination, phobia, symmetry and the orderliness), associated compulsions (motor or mental, yielding or neutralizing), along with slowness (primary or secondary). The most important quality of obsession is the ego dystonic quality (that they are intrusive and inappropriate and they are not normally expected to occur in mind, not merely a part of worries about day-to-day events, and cause distress). Ego syntonic obsession-like ideas occur in anankastic personality, schizotypal disorder and in psychosis as a symptom.
- *Somatization*: Although this must have been indicated from history, it is important to ask about all the somatoform symptoms.
- *Abnormal beliefs*: (including overvalued ideas and delusions). These have to be viewed in relation to the beliefs prevalent in the social, cultural, political and religious group the patient belongs to.

An *overvalued idea* is an unreasonable belief maintained with less than delusional intensity (i.e. the person is able to acknowledge the possibility that the belief is not true) and held idiosyncratically (i.e. not shared by the members of his sociocultural group). However, it is understandable in terms of the circumstances and the development of a particular personality. Such ideas, sometimes, may be normal.

A *delusion* is a false, incorrigible (briefly or not at all susceptible to change by experience or evidence to the contrary) conviction or judgment based on incorrect inference about external reality, and out of keeping with socially shared beliefs. Primary delusions are incomprehensible in terms of life history and personality of the patient (delusional mood, sudden delusional idea and delusional perception) and are usually characteristic of acute schizophrenia. Secondary delusions arise from either a morbid mood state (when they may be mood-congruent or mood-incongruent) or personality trait like suspicion. There could be delusional elaboration of a primary phenomenon like hallucination or thought alienation experience. Induced delusions mean that the delusion of a psychotic patient is shared with a previously normal person(s) when they are emotionally dependent on each other over a long period of time. This may involve two (*folie a deux*), three (*folie a trois*) or four (*folie a quatre*) people. Once a half-a-dozen or more people share a belief, it is likely to be subcultural and within the range of normal behavior.

Delusions would have been indicated from the history. When not, certain screening questions should be asked to the patient.

Primary delusions: Have you had the feeling that something odd is going that you cannot explain? Do you feel puzzled by strange happenings that are difficult to account for (delusional mood)? Did the idea occur to you fully formed (sudden delusional idea)? When you saw... the event (an example of misinterpretation) how did you know what it meant? Is there any explanation (delusional perception)?

Other questions: Can you think clearly or does there seem to be some kind of interference with your thoughts? Are you fully in control of your thoughts and actions? Have you felt that people are unduly interested in you? Have you felt that things were arranged so as to have a special meaning, or even that harm may come to you?

Once the content (reference, persecution, grandiosity, erotomania, jealousy, guilt, control, thought broadcast, thought insertion, etc.) is clear, it is important to go on assessing the following aspects of delusions.

a. *Degree of conviction*: By confronting the patient with evidence to the contrary. The level of certainty may vary or may be concealed. At times it is inferred from the behavioral responses
b. *Systematization*: A delusion often has an organizing nucleus and a system of other ideas to support it. Systematization refers to what extent the system is logical and internally consistent, thus, when the basic idea is accepted, the rest should get automatically explained
c. *Bizarreness*: This indicates to what extent the patient's culture would regard the phenomenon of his delusion as implausible
d. *Involvement* of other areas of life and relationships
e. *Affective responses*
f. *Acting upon* the delusions
g. A delusion without d, e, f, is described as *encapsulated*.

When multiple delusions are present it is important to find out the interconnectedness of these delusions or whether they are multiple. This could be of diagnostic importance.

Perception

Perception refers to the process of being aware of a sensory experience and being able to recognize it by comparing it with the previous experiences. Disorders of perception include the following:

Sense distortions: (a) changes in intensity, e.g. hyper- or hypoesthesia, (b) change in quality, e.g. colored perception of the visual stimuli, (c) change in spatial form (dysmegalopsia), e.g. micropsia or macropsia.

The interviewer should ask the following questions in relation to this area. Do things seem to change in size or shape or color in a puzzling way? Have things looked gray or flat lacking their usual color and detail? Do surroundings seem unnaturally clear, objects look vividly colored, or pattern seem particularly vivid and interesting?

Experiences of sense distortion may occur in depression (decreased intensity), mania (increased intensity), prodromal phase of schizophrenia, drug induced states and in delirium.

Sense deceptions: This includes illusion and hallucination. Behavior suggestive of experiencing hallucinations would have been indicated in the history or from the nurses' report in case of inpatients. In other cases, the interviewer should open the area tactfully. The patient may be asked, 'do you ever seem to hear noises or voices when there is nobody about or see or feel things that others cannot'? Once the modality is clear, it is essential to ask about other modalities, if relevant. The interviewer should look for the following features: (a) continuous or discontinuous (frequency), (b) three dimensionality—voices can be located to a point, at a distance, visual images have the three dimensional qualities, (c) clarity and veridicality, i.e. life like qualities, (d) control—when the experience can be started or stopped by the subject on his will, (e) objective or subjective space: whether the experience occurs within the inner space of the mind or from external space, (f) content and emotional reaction, (g) elementary, partially formed or formed, (h) insight: whether the experience is true or a product of imagination.

Based on above characteristics, distinction has to be made among true hallucination (which has true-to-life quality, occurs in the objective space, cannot be controlled and the person lacks insight), pseudohallucination (lacks clarity and vividness, occurs in the subjective space, cannot be controlled and the person retains insight) and imagery (has the qualities of pseudohallucination and is in the person's control). In case of auditory hallucination, further enquiries have to be made on the lines of Schneiderian hallucinations. Do your hear voices commenting on thoughts, repeat what you are reading or doing? Do you hear single or multiple voices? Does the voice refer to you in second (as you) or third (he or she) person? Do the voices talk among each other about you? Second person auditory hallucination should be distinguished from delusion of reference. In case of visual hallucination, it is necessary to distinguish it from illusion. Dissociative experiences (talking to, seeing other well-known persons in the context of religion) should be distinguished from true hallucination.

Enquiries about special types of hallucination also have to be made (autoscopy, synesthesia, cenesthopathic, fantastic, functional, reflex hallucination).

Other Psychotic Phenomena (Somatic Passivity)

This may be elicited by asking the patient "do you feel that your will has been replaced by that of some force or power outside yourself, e.g. voice, action, thought, impulse, affect? Do you feel some sensations are caused by external agencies?"

Other experiences: (derealization, depersonalization and body image disturbances).

Have you felt that the world is unreal only like a stage set, cardboard cutout? Did other people seem to be acting a part like actors in a play or have you felt you yourself were not a real person. Do you experience time seems to have changed? Does it go fast or slow? Interviewer should try to clarify with examples from the patient. When the patient appears to have a conviction of such experience, this should be recorded as delusion under content of thought.

Body image: Have you worried too much about putting on weight or getting too fat? Do others think you are too fat? Do they think you are too thin?

Cognitive Functions

Attention and Concentration

The capacity to attend to a stimulus is an integral part of consciousness (vide supra). Attention has four qualities: to focus and discriminate, to mobilize, to sustain and to shift. Concentration (vigilance) is the ability to sustain the focus over an extended period.

Valid information regarding the patient's attentiveness may be obtained by observing his ability to continue coherent sequence of conversation and noting any evidence of distractibility, and any fluctuation in the level of attention over the day. Attention is tested in the following ways:

Digit span test: Present one digit per second in a normal tone, the patient should listen carefully and repeat them after the examiner. An example with a two number sequence should be given and continued until the patient fails. Numbers should be presented randomly without any natural sequence. A normal person can repeat five to seven digits without any difficulty. Inability to repeat three digits or more suggests poor attention. Digit span may be asked to be repeated in a backward fashion with increasing span till the patient fails.

Vigilance can be tested by uttering (one letter per second) a long series of letters. The patient should tap the desk the moment he hears the letter 'A'. Three types of errors may occur in organic brain syndromes viz. omission (failure to tap), commission (tapping with letters other than 'A') and preservation (failure to stop tapping on subsequent presentation of letters). The two tests mentioned above cannot be done in patients with aphasia.

Serial subtraction test, e.g. counting backward from 100–7 until the remainder is <7. The time taken together with the number of errors are noted. This test is not useful when the patient has poor arithmetic skills. Alternative tests exist, e.g. serial subtraction by threes from 40, counting 1 to 20, months of the year, days of the week forward and backward.

Language Functions

Language is the building block of the cognitive functions. Its integrity needs to be established in order to assess cognitive functions. Several aspects of language are required to be assessed, viz. articulation, fluency, comprehension, repetition, naming, word finding, reading, writing and prosody. Invaluable information is obtained from the spontaneous speech of the patient. Some additional tests may be necessary in certain cases.

Handedness: This is allied to cerebral dominance for language function. Besides, this may have to be determined in two other situations, (a) for interpretation of neuropsychological test findings, (b) while assessing the patient for unilateral electroconvulsive therapy. The examiner should try to assess handedness of the patient by asking him (a) whether he is right or left handed, (b) to demonstrate which hand he uses to hold a knife, throw a ball, and flip a coin, (c) any tendency to use the opposite hand for any skilled movement, and (d) any family history of left handedness or ambidexterity. An accurate picture is obtained by asking questions from Annett handedness questionnaire.[22]

Articulation may be tested by asking the patient to pronounce tonguie twisters like "West Register Street", "The Leith Police dismisseth us" or from the local language.

Fluency: Patient is asked open questions about his work, hobby or weather, and to write spontaneously on a topic or on dictation. The examiner should look for grammatical errors, word finding difficulties, uses of nouns and verbs, and any word substitution (paraphasia).

Comprehension is tested by asking the patient: (a) to point to the objects in room or articles from the pocket of the examiner in increasing sequences. Brain damaged persons fail to point to more than four objects in a sequence, (b) questions that can be answered with "Yes" or "No" at random, e.g. is it your right eye? do you take lunch before dinner? is this a school?, (c) to corn carry out two steps or three step commands (*Marie's 3 paper test*—three pieces of papers of different sizes are put before the patient, he is told to take the biggest one and hand it to the examiner; take the smallest one, throw it to the ground; and take the middle sized one, put it in his pocket), (d) to read a written material and explain.

Repetition: To begin with monosyllables, going to sentences.

Naming and word finding: Patient should have different categories of objects in the room. Asking to describe objects and actions in a picture could test his word finding ability. The reader is referred to further reference[11] for formal test of language.

Orientation

Important information is obtained from nurses' report on the behavior of the patient in the ward as well as that during the interview. Orientation to time (time, day, date, month, year, season), place (ward, building, floor), person (self and others) should be described. The sense of passage of time may be assessed by asking a question "how long do you think has passed since we have started talking?"

Memory

Any difficulty in remembering day-to-day events would have been asked while taking the history. In MSE, each of the aspects of memory should be assessed in some detail. This will allow the examiner to distinguish the type of memory deficit (if any), the degree of memory loss, and the impact of the memory deficit on the patient's ability to function in a vocational or social role.

Immediate memory is tested by digit span test (vide supra).

Recent memory (new learning ability) is assessed by:

- Recall of the events of last 24–48 hours and by corroborating it from a reliable informant. Particular attention needs to be paid to the temporal sequencing of the events, any confabulation or false memories in the retrieval, any selective loss of memory about any special incident or theme, any anterograde or retrograde amnesia in case of patients with head injury, epilepsy or those on treatment with electroconvulsive therapy, and the attitude of the patient to the loss of memory like indifference, concern or distress.
- Recent verbal memory is tested by the interviewer introducing himself carefully and then asking the patient to repeat his name once to ensure that he has registered it. Then continuing the interview for 3–5 minutes, he asks the patient to repeat his name. An amnesic patient may not recall or may deny having been told the name at all.

  The examiner may present an address with five facts, the patient is asked to repeat it and then after 3–5 minutes of continued interview. Failure to recall less than three facts indicate impairment in recent memory. Once the digit span is determined, then the ability to extend the list by one or two items is assessed by repeated presentation. Amnesic subjects can perform adequately on the straight forward digit span test, but show a breakdown in performance as soon as this is exceeded. This is called as *supradigit span test.*
- Recent visual memory is tested by presenting 3 or 5 unrelated objects. Interviewer should ask the patient to name all of these to exclude nominal aphasia and visual agnosia. Then, he should hide the objects in different places while allowing the patient to watch. After a gap of 3–5 minutes of conversation on other topics, he should ask the patient to tell and take out the objects from the respective places. Less than 3 recall is abnormal.

  Patient may be asked to reproduce a simple geometric figure after an interval of 5 minutes (Fig. 1).

Remote memory is tested by asking the patient about:

- Personal events, e.g. to describe the day he married, his first child was born, he joined the job or resigned from the job and so on. It is important to ask "can you describe the day of your marriage rather than the date of your marriage?" The first question requires mobilization of actual memories.
- Impersonal events, e.g. well known, political, public events in country, state or locality.

Important information may be also obtained from the observation made by the nurses and occupational therapists, how he learns daily routine, names of staff and other patients, forgetting where he has put things, where to find his bed and so on.

Topographic memory: The ability to trace the path back home and the layout of the wards are to be tested historically as well as on observation.

Memory of skills: Playing cards or chess, cooking, tailoring, computer skills, mainly to be obtained from the history.

Fig. 1: Simple geometric figure

Intelligence

Intelligence is the ability to think and act logically and rationally. This is to be interpreted from education, occupational history (these will throw light on adaptive functioning-ability to adjust in novel situation and to cope with the challenges), clinical behavior and test performance on comprehension, abstraction, judgment, general information and calculation.

General information: To be assessed with reference to the subject's background. For illiterate people may be asked about local rivers, well known religious places, local or state politics, panchayats, important festivals, seasons, and agricultural market prices.

Calculation: Verbal and written—one or two step problem.

Whenever necessary, patients should be referred for standardized psychological assessment. The above battery of tests can often be abbreviated when responses are accurate from the start. It is important, however, to gain a clear understanding of the patient's capacities under each of these headings whatever form the presenting illness may take. The headings presented above are not, of course, mutually exclusive. Orientation and memory, e.g. are interrelated. Moreover, some of these factors are impaired in organic as well as in functional disorders (e.g. attention and concentration). However, memory and orientation have been shown to discriminate, relatively better, organic from functional states.[23]

Abstract Thinking

An ability to think in the abstract depends on education, level of intelligence and an abstract attitude. This is tested by:

- *Proverb interpretation*: The patient is first enquired whether he has heard of proverbs. If yes, a proverb may be presented with the instruction that it has a literal and inner meaning. He is required to give the inner meaning. About 5 proverbs need to be asked. In case he is not familiar with those presented by the examiner, he may be asked to recall a proverb on his own and offer the interpretation. The interpretation may be concrete, semiabstract or abstract.[24]
- *Test of similarity and dissimilarity* between two overtly dissimilar situations, which requires analysis of relationships, formation of verbal concepts and logical thinking, e.g. car-airplane, poem-novel.

Poor abstraction is difficult to interpret as there is wide variation in normal interpretation. However, poor abstraction may occur in dementia, mental retardation and schizophrenia—in the former two it could be purely concrete, in the latter personalized or delusional meaning may be given.

Judgment

This refers to the ability to differentiate between internal and external reality, plan ahead and show responses appropriate to the situations. Three types of judgment are to be described.

- *Social*: This is inferred from historical information and observation of behavior in the ward (vide social manners)
- *Personal*: Personal logic about present and future. How do you explain the present state, what is your plan about future?
- *Test*: Responses in test situations; a letter on the road or house on fire; this component, has poor validity.

Insight

Insight is a patient's degree of awareness and understanding about being ill. It usually becomes clear by this time about the patient's awareness of the morbid phenomena or illness. There are three components of insight that require to be assessed.

Does the patient feel that his thoughts, and emotions are excessive, experiences are morbid, out of the ordinary?

Does he recognize he is ill, if so, what is the nature of illness (physical or mental)? Does he feel he needs help?

Insight need to be described and recorded as present, partial or absent.

FURTHER EVALUATION

Physical Examination and Higher Cortical Function Tests

The associations between physical and mental illness could be causal, coincidental and consequential, and so carrying out a complete physical examination is mandatory at the time of first assessment of the patient. A detailed neurological examination including the higher cortical functions[11] is essential, especially when any kind of brain insult is suspected. Some of these functions (consciousness, attention, language, orientation and memory) have been already described. The rest is briefly mentioned here:

Apraxia is an inability to perform purposive volitional acts which does not result from paresis, incoordination, sensory loss or involuntary movements. Constructional apraxia and visuospatial agnosia are tested in a similar way. Patient is asked to construct geometric designs (star, pentagon) with

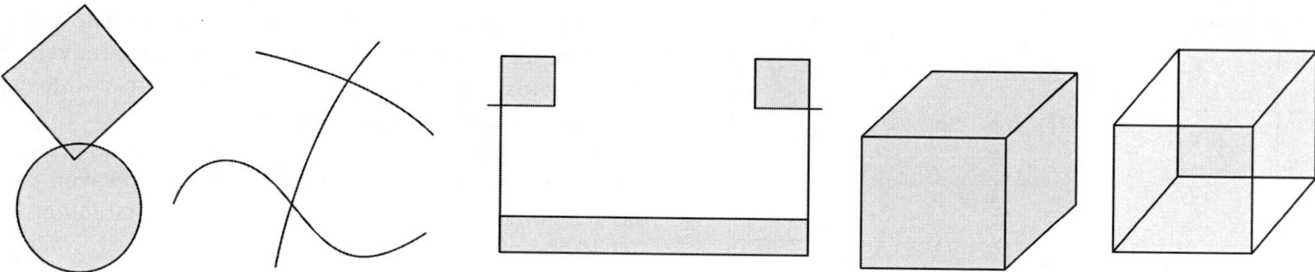

Fig. 2: Geometric designs including two- or three-dimensional figures

match sticks or copy certain two or three dimensional figures of increasing complexity (Fig. 2). Inability to put on items of clothing indicates dressing apraxia. Ideomotor apraxia refers to inability to perform single step motor acts, viz. "blow out a match" , "flip a coin", "kick a ball". Failure to perform motor acts of multiple steps suggest ideational apraxia and is tested by, for example, asking the patient to fold a letter, place it in an envelope, seal it, addressing it and place a stamp on the envelope.

Agnosia is an inability to interpret and recognize the significance of sensory information which does not result from impairment of sensory pathways, mental deterioration, disorder of consciousness and attention. Agnosia can occur in any sensory modality. In astereognosis objects cannot be recognized by palpation. A graphesthesia is present if the patient is unable to identify with closed eyes, numbers or letters traced on his palm. In finger agnosia, patient is unable to recognize individual fingers, either his or another person's, with eyes closed. Agnosia for colors indicate inability to name colors perfectly although color sense is still present.

Right-left orientation is the ability to point to the objects around him on the right or on the left, or touching right ear with left hand and so on.

Body image disturbances: Hemiasomatognosia is present when the patient feels that a limb (which is present) is missing. Phantom limb indicates continued awareness of a missing limb.

Tests of dynamic organization of the motor act: The subject is required to perform a series of movements whose components follow in a connected alternating sequence, e.g. alternately changing the position of the hands on the table, one with fist and the other with fingers extended; tapping the table twice with the right hand and once with the left hand in an ongoing alternating sequence; making fist and ring alternately with the same hand.

Physical Tests

In clinical situation, there are three aims for carrying out the laboratory tests: (i) to look for organic etiology, e.g. endocrine disorders, CNS infections, psychoactive substance use, etc; (ii) to check for physical complications of psychiatric disorders, e.g. nutritional deficiency, organ damage in substance use disorders; (iii) to detect metabolic disorders which may influence pharmacotherapy, e.g. renal function tests must precede lithium therapy.

A range of tests may be relevant to the investigations in psychiatric illnesses, e.g. tests of blood, urine and cerebrospinal fluid; imaging techniques like electro-encephalography, event related potentials, computerized tomography and magnetic resonance imaging; finally, karyotyping in case of developmental disorders. However, in a given case, the nature of symptoms and differential diagnoses would indicate such investigations.

Psychological Assessment

Neuropsychological Tests

These are standardized measurement of cognition and behavior. The primary aim is to measure the deficits and impairments, as well as the preserved strengths and abilities in patients with brain damage. The second aim is to differentiate organic (e.g. dementia) from psychiatric conditions (e.g. depressive pseudodementia). A third aim is to monitor the neuropsychological status of the patients who have undergone treatment (medical or surgical). The fourth aim is to identify developmental disorders including learning difficulties.

Tests of Clinical Psychology

Various types of tests are available to assess intelligence, personality traits, thought disorder, ego functions, and intrapsychic and interpersonal conflicts.

Several rating scales (self-rated, observer-rated, or interview-based) are now available to quantity psychopathology. These are useful to monitor change in response to interventions.

Clinical Assessment of Ego Functions

This is relevant while attempting a psychodynamic formulation and planning dynamically-oriented psychotherapy. The following clinical parameters are useful:

- Ability to resolve intrapsychic conflicts and cope with stressors, and bring down anxiety. This is mediated by automatic psychological processes called defence mechanisms.[25,26] Preponderance of mature over primitive defenses, patient's resilience under stress and his ability not to regress to more immature levels of defence organization is a sign of healthy ego

- Ability to postpone gratification of drivers, control impulses and tolerate the resulting sense of frustration and tension
- Capacity for deep relationship with others as manifested by mutual love, sharing and empathy coupled with an ability to tolerate normal frustration and anger evoked within the relationship
- A sense of self-worth and self-confidence enough to obtain gratification of needs, reasonable control over life and to ensure survival. Fluctuating sense of self-worth is a sign of ego weakness
- Capacity to organize mental functions in a disorganizing environment, e.g. to read and concentrate in noisy surroundings
- Ability to release the perceptual and cognitive attention in order to allow for new experiences in pleasurable areas, e.g. sex, music, art, food, literature, sleep, creative imagery, falling in love
- Ability to discriminate between internal and external reality, i.e. whether a given stimulus originates from inside or outside, to be aware that one is the thinker of one's thought, perception of self and how one is viewed by others
- Intact functioning of primary autonomy of ego that includes language, motor function, conceptualization, memory, concentration, attention, judgment, and capacity to integrate new experiences with reconciliation of inconsistencies.

In summary, ego strength means good capacities that are well developed and unimpaired by conflict.

SPECIAL INTERVIEWS

Emergency Evaluation

General Guidelines

Psychiatric symptoms could be manifestations of medical, neurological and psychiatric disorders. The clinician should be broad and open-minded in his approach to a patient. The examiner should have a direct, calm, nonthreatening and nonjudgmental attitude and one of showing concern. The examiner may have to rely more on supplementary information from the accompanying persons or police mainly, in case of uncooperative patients. A skill of rapid clinical assessment is essential. The examiner should be able to decide what to enquire and what to defer in history and mental status examination. An efficient, physical examination with discrete use of laboratory tests is needed since the evaluation in emergency is more time limited than in other settings.

Homicidal and Aggressive Patient

The interview should not be conducted in a cramped room situated in an isolated place. The patient and the examiner should be positioned in such a way that both have access to the door. The examiner should be preferably towards the door. The examiner should be vigilant about the signs of impending violence: loud and threatening speech, increased muscle tension—sitting on the edge of the chair or gripping the arms, pacing up and down, slamming the doors or knocking over furniture, carrying weapons, and alcohol or drug intoxication.

The examiner must take certain steps to minimize harm, e.g. patient must surrender the weapons, if any, before interview proceeds; four or five persons should be around, sometimes the presence itself is enough to make the patient calm down; and keep the available means of restraint (physical or sedatives) ready.

The examiner should show concern and should not be humiliate the patient. His requests should be treated in a forthright manner, e.g. where he should take a seat and asking for a glass of water. The examiner should develop some rapport with the patient before asking specific question about violence. Questions about violence should be direct and honest. The patient should be assured of all kinds of help for him to stay in control of violent impulses. If necessary, limits may be set by talk, sedation or physical restraint.

Potentially Suicidal Patient

All suicidal threats should be taken seriously. If a patient refuses to discuss suicidality at all, it is helpful to ask the friends and family about the patient's behavior.

Suicide is a personal matter. The patient must be approached in an empathic and circumspect manner. Rapport needs to be established before direct questions are asked about suicide. It is better to talk to the patient alone and whenever in doubt to enquire from the relatives. It is an error to avoid the subject of suicidality for fear of doing so. In fact, patient feels relieved when he is allowed to talk about it. Patient should not be given premature reassurance as this may be perceived by the patient as a sign of lack of empathy. The clinician should listen, evaluate and then make a decision.

Patient with Altered Sensorium

A more medical approach is useful, e.g. examining his pulse and blood pleasure, taking the temperature. It is wise to assess the cognitive functions directly. If the patient is hyperkinetic, it is right to defer the interview and to interview another informant.

Unresponsive Patient

History should be obtained from a reliable informant. A detailed physical examination is to be conducted and level of consciousness has to ascertained. Psychiatric examination should be done following the format of Kirby (1921).[27]

In case of mutism, it is necessary to find out whether it is elective, situational or in relation to some persons only.[28] Does the patient attempt to communicate by signs? Is there any distress in the patient? Does he write when offered a pen ? Is partial vocalization preserved? Are there any lip movements or coughing? Does he speak very occasionally or chiefly on restricted themes, or after a long delay?

Primary Care Interview

Patients usually present with physical symptoms in the primary care setting and the psychological basis of these complaints is likely to be missed by the primary care physicians.[29] The physician should have a positive attitude to mental illness. He should be aware that bodily symptoms could occur out of psychosocial problems and may be the presenting features of anxiety and depression, and underlie misuse of alcohol and drugs. Moreover, he should be oriented to the basic interviewing skills (vide supra) in order to be able to correctly establish the nature of presenting symptoms.

REFERENCES

1. World Health Organization. Schedules for Clinical Assessment in Neuropsychiatry. Geneva: WHO; 1992.
2. Robins LN, Wing JK, Wittch HU, et al. The Composite International Diagnostic Interview. Arch Gen Psychiatry. 1988; 45:1069-77.
3. Hersen M, Turner SM (Eds). Diagnostic Interviewing. New York: Plenum; 1985.
4. Kuppuswamy B. Socioeconomic Status Scale (Urban). Delhi: Manasayan; 1984.
5. Trivedl G, Pareek U. Socioeconomic Status Scale (Rural). Delhi: Manasayan; 1964.
6. Gallagher III BJ. Sociology of Mental illness. 3rd edition, New Jersey: Prentice-Hall, Englewood Cliffs, 1993. pp. 260-80.
7. Singh G, Kaur D, Kaur H. Presumptive stressful life events scale (PSLES). Indian J Clin Psychol. 1981;8:173.
8. Hurlock EB. Child Development. Delhi: McGraw-Hill Book Company; 1978. pp. 107-90.
9. Loranger AW, Sartorius N, Andreoli A, et al. The International Personality Disorder Examination: The World Health Organization/Alcohol, Drug Abuse and Mental Health Administration International Pilot Study of Personality Disorders. Arch Gen Psychiatry. 1994;51:215.
10. Teasdale G, Jennett B. Assessment of coma and impaired consciousness. Lancet. 1974;2:81.
11. Strub RL. Mental disorders in brain disease. In: Frederiks JAM (Ed). Handbook of Clinical Neurology. Neurobehavioural disorders, Amsterdam: Elsevier Science Publishers. 1985; 2(46): 413-41.
12. Plum F, Posner J. Diagnosis of Stupor and Coma. 3rd edition. Philadelphia: FA Davis; 1982.
13. Left JP, Isaacs AD. Psychiatric Examination in Clinical Practice. 3rd edition. Oxford: Blackwell Scientific; 1990.
14. Fairbanks H. The quantitiative differentiation of samples of spoken language. Psychol Monographs. 1944;56:19-38.
15. Taylor WL. Cloze procedure: A new-tool tor measuring readability. Journalism Quart. 1953;30:415-33.
16. Miller GA, Selfridge JA. Verbal context and recall of meaningful material. Am J Psychol. 1950;63:176-85.
17. Bannister D, Fransella F. A grid test schizophrenic thought disorder. Br J Soc Clin Psychol. 1966;5:95-102.
18. Fish FJ. Schizophrenia. Bristol: Wright; 1962.
19. Chapman LJ, Chapman JP. Disordered Thought in Schizophrenia. New York: Appleton-Century-Crofts; 1973.
20. Andreasen NC. Thought, language and communication disorders. Arch Gen Psychiatry. 1979;36:1315-30.
21. Cutting J. The Psychology of Schizophrenia. Edinburgh: Churchill Livingstone; 1985. pp. 243-265 and pp. 309-48.
22. Annett M. Classification of hand preference by association analysis. Br J Psychol. 1970;61:303-21.
23. Lishman WA. Organic Psychiatry. 2nd edition. Delhi: Oxford University Press; 1987. pp. 78-125.
24. Strub RL, Black FW. The Mental Status Examination in Neurology. 3rd edition. Delhi: Jaypee Brothers Medical Publisher; 1995. pp. 121-49.
25. American Psychiatric Association. Diagnostic and Statiscal Manual of Mental Disorders. 4th edition. Washington DC: Americal Psychiatric Association; 1994.
26. Vaillant G. Adaptive ego mechanisms. Arch Gen Psychiatry. 1971;24:107-18.
27. Slater E, Roth M. Clinical Psychiatry. 3rd edition. Delhi: Jaypee Brothers Medical Publisher; 1986. pp. 46-47.
28. Oyebode F. Sims' symptoms in mind: an introduction to descriptive psychopathology. Elsevier Saunders, London; 2008.
29. Carr S. Interview technique in psychiatry. Macmillan, London; 2013. pp. 11-67.

CHAPTER 2

Neurological Examination in Psychiatry

KS Anand, A Prasad, SC Pradhan

Like in any other branch of medicine, neurological examination forms a cornerstone of total management of the patient in psychiatry. Very often a neurological disorder has to be excluded while making a final psychiatric diagnosis.

'Neuropsychiatry' deals with the study of psychiatric problems in neurological disorders and the neurological problems in the classical psychiatric disorders. Ideally, a detailed neurological examination should be performed in every case in psychiatry, but because of the peculiar nature of psychiatric disorders (i.e. the lack of insight into their problems and non-cooperativeness), the detailed examinations is often deferred until the patient becomes more amenable for it.

In the absence of a definitive guideline for the neurological examination in psychiatric patients, here we mention a tentative format for the basic neurological testing, especially appropriate in an emergency psychiatric setting.[1]

In the discussion, we have limited ourselves to the higher mental functions briefly, examination of the functions of different lobes of brain, language assessment, and some of the psychiatric states that may mimic neurological disorders, along with certain tests to differentiate malingering from true neuropsychiatric conditions.

HIGHER MENTAL FUNCTIONS

Higher mental functions (HMF) should be tested in all cases; there are specific observations and bedside tests to be conducted.[1] The details of the HMF test can be found in any textbook for psychiatric examinations. However, for the bedside assessment a scale that has been frequently used is mini-mental state examination (MMSE).[2] The maximum score of the scale is 30. This scale is a screening examination for a wide range of cognitive functions. Although abnormal results in MMSE do not provide information about organicity or cause, they do provide a reliable screening of cognitive functions that can be followed over time. Psychotic patients may have abnormal MMSE results because of poor cooperation or cognitive deficits.

LOBE FUNCTION TESTS

The results of the examinations of different lobes of the brain often provide useful information for diagnosis of subtle neurological deficits. These are enumerated under the following headings (Table 1).

Frontal Lobe Disorders

These can be discussed under the following subheadings:
- Orbitofrontal syndrome.
- Medial frontal lobe syndrome.
- Frontal convexity syndrome.

Orbitofrontal Syndrome (Synonym: Pseudopsychopathic State)

It consists of impulsiveness, loss of tact, lack of empathy and lack of concern for the feelings of others. The mood is typically irritable and labile, with insensitive humor (*Witzelsucht*).

Medial Frontal Lobe Syndrome (MFLS) (Synonym: Pseudoapathetic State)

It is characterized predominantly by apathy. The severity may extend from akinetic mutism at one end to a mild lack of motivation at the other end. In akinetic mutism, patients are typically alert, have their eyes open and exhibit ocular movement following environmental events. This syndrome has been reported following bilateral anterior cerebral artery occlusion, trauma, hydrocephalus, bilateral thalamic infarction, etc. With left-sided lesions, the patients manifest transcortical motor aphasia, having little speech initiation, nonfluent output, intact comprehension and preserved repetition.

Table 1: Lobar tests

A. Frontal lobe tests
• Attention and concentration (Digit forward and digit backward test, 100-7, 40-3, random letter test, letter cancellation test, word generation list) • Alternate sequences (rhythm tapping, visual pattern completion, fist-palm-side test, fist-ring test, reciprocal test). • Perseveration • Soft signs and release reflexes • Apathy • Aprosody • Abstract reasoning • Judgment • Proverb interpretation • Similarity and differences • Gait apraxia • Conceptual series completion • General intelligence and information • Frontal lobe syndrome
B. Parietal lobe tests
• Alexia • Agraphia • Anomia • Acalculia • Anosognosia • Autopagnosia • Asomatognosia • Amorphosynthesis • Right/Left disorientation • Hemineglect/unilateral inattention • Astereognosis • Finger agnosia • Two point discrimination • Extinction • Agraphesthesia • Impaired spatial ability • Gerstmann syndrome • Apraxia (constructional, ideomotor, ideational, kinesthetic, dressing) • Tactile agnosia
C. Temporal lobe tests
• Memory (immediate, recent, remote, orientation) • New learning ability • Language (handedness, comprehension, reading, writing, spelling, naming, spontaneous speech, dysarthria, dysphasia) • Auditory illusion/hallucination • Auditory agnosia • Auditory verbal agnosia • Amusia • Adversive seizures • Aggressive outburst • Kluver-Bucy syndrome • Temporal lobe personality (hypergraphia, hyposexuality, viscosity, circumstantially, hypermorality, hyper-religiosity, philosophical ideation)
D. Occipital lobe tests
• Color anomia • Color agnosia • Prosopagnosia • Metamorphopsia • Allesthesia • Asthenopia (visual fatigue) • Visual illusion/hallucination • Anton's syndrome • Balint's syndrome (simultanognosia, ocular apraxia, optic ataxia) • Visual agnosia.

Frontal Convexity Syndrome

It is characterized predominantly by executive deficits, i.e. perseveration, impersistence, impaired serial order behavior. Some of the later deficits are impairment in shifting from the set, disturbances of programming sequential motor acts, like alternating programs, reciprocal programs, multiple loops and serial hand sequences. Schizophrenia is often considered to be a frontal convexity syndrome (FCS). Another feature of this FCS is the appearance of release reflexes (frontal release reflexes) and various soft neurological signs.

Parietal Lobe Disorders

These can be divided into:
- Left parietal lobe syndrome
- Right parietal lobe syndromes.

Left Parietal Lobe Syndrome

It consists of:
- Alexia and agraphia
- Alexia, agraphia, and anomia
- Gerstmann syndrome (agraphia, acalculia, right left disorientation and finger agnosia)
- The various combinations of the above are also seen in left parietal lobe syndrome.

Right Parietal Lobe Syndrome

It consists of:
- Constructional impairment (apraxia)
- Dressing apraxia
- Geographic disorientation
- Astereognosis on the left side
- Calculation and writing problems as a result of grossly distorted placement or production of the actual letters and numbers
- Denial and neglect of the left side, both of the body and of the environment.

Temporal Lobe Disorders

Temporal lobe not only serves as the cortical area for auditory input, but it also functions as the auditory processor for language reception. The various aphasic disturbances are directly related to the damage of the left temporal lobe. The right temporal lobe is intimately associated with high-level visual processing and the damage produces defects in visual perceptions and visio-motor integration. Temporal lobes are also implicated in the behavioral changes that are seen in patient with temporal lobe epilepsy. A characteristic temporal lobe personality has also been described.

Occipital Lobe Disorders

The occipital lobe syndromes are predominantly manifested by visual symptoms.

Anton's Syndrome

It is a combination of cortical blindness, usually secondary to bilateral posterior cerebral artery occlusion and denial of any loss of vision by the patients.

Balint's Syndrome

Bilateral temporoparietal lesions cause ataxia of optically guided movements, inability to refix the eyes after fixation without first closing the eyes, and inability to see more than one object at a time.

LANGUAGE ASSESSMENT

The assessment of the language is crucial to both the patients' general functioning and cognitive functioning. Accordingly, the integrity of the language function must be evaluated early during the course of mental status examination.

Below we present a tentative format for quick assessment of the language functions (Mnemonics: CNS-RRW).

Handedness

Handedness and cerebral dominance for language are closely related and should be assessed before language testing. The patient can be asked whether he is left or right handed, or he has been forced to change the hands because of family or school pressure. Family history of left handedness or ambidexterity is also important. A final observation can be made by asking patients to write by using paper and pencil.

Spontaneous Speech

Ask an open-ended question like "tell me something about your work" or "how is life", and observe for the following:
- Is the speech output present?
- Is the speech dysarthric?
- Is there evidence of aphasia?

Comprehension

Comprehension is assessed by asking the patient, either to point a single named object in the room (single word comprehension) or to a task of increased complexity (general comprehension). The questions can be graded from simple to complex matters. Several questions should be used and the correct answers should alternate randomly from yes to no (to check for perseveration).

Repetition

As repetition of the words is affected by a variety of language disorders, the impaired repetition performance is clinically significant but not pathognomonic of a specific language disturbance. Testing should be carried out with verbal material of increasing difficulty. Record the level of complexity, at which the patient failed to repeat accurately.

Object Naming

Several categories of objects should be used, as some aphasics display a differential impairment for color and shapes. Paraphasias are errors in word usage that are common in aphasia.

Reading and Writing

After evaluation of the verbal language, a brief clinical assessment should be made of the patient's ability to read and write. The initial reading should be of single simple words, progressing to phrases and then sentences. Similarly, the writing can be tested.

An interesting clinical problem is to distinguish between a schizophrenic with thought and language disorders (e.g. neologism, word salad) from true aphasics. But in practice, it is rarely a difficult problem as schizophrenia is usually associated with other cardinal symptoms of the disease (e.g. first rank symptoms, personality deterioration, etc.).

PSYCHIATRIC DISORDERS MASQUERADING AS NEUROLOGICAL STATES

Dementia versus Pseudodementia

Often the dementia syndrome, characterized by forgetfulness and affective dysregulation, is seen in depression. However, a careful look at the following features would differentiate the conditions. In depressive pseudodementia, the onset is fairly well demarcated, with rapid progression, and a history of previous psychiatric disorders or life events. Whereas in dementia, the onset is often insidious, with slow progression of the disorder. In the former, the complaints are often elaborate and associated with affective changes whereas in the later, patient himself does not complain of cognitive loss and the affect is typically apathetic and shallow. On examination, the pseudodemented patient often answers "I do not know" before even trying. Whereas patients with true dementia will be struggling with the cognitive task given to them. Memory loss for the recent events is worse than the remote, in demented patients.

Conversion and Dissociation Reactions versus Neurologic Disorders

Patients with conversion reaction classically demonstrate special sensory or voluntary motor problems, such as blindness, hemiparesis, paraparesis or anesthesia, but can have behavioral problems as well.

An uncommon conversion reaction is seen in hospitalized patient is 'simulated coma', also known as *'psychiatric unresponsiveness'*. A complete physical, neurologic and laboratory screening can distinguish between two conditions. The 'psychiatric coma' patient very often has completely normal results on examination and often looks 'too healthy' for his depressed level of consciousness.

Another condition that mimics an organic state is amnesia. The *'psychogenic amnesia'* is most often seen in people under severe stress and is associated with anxiety. It affects mostly the memory of events that took place prior to the onset of the stress (retrograde amnesia). Often the personal details are lost. Whereas the organic amnesia is of anterograde type and hardly involves the past personal details.

Another important condition that requires meticulous examination is *'seizures versus pseudoseizures'* ('nonepileptic attack disorders' or NEAD). Table 2 distinguishes between the two.

NEUROLOGICAL ASPECTS OF CLASSICAL PSYCHIATRIC DISORDERS

There is a growing body of evidence to suggest that the classical psychiatric syndromes have subtle but definite neurological and neuropsychological abnormalities. Many clinicians tend to view schizophrenia as a neurological disorder, as the neurological abnormalities are found in more than 50% of schizophrenics.

Table 2: Differential diagnosis of true seizure vs pseudoseizure

Features	*True seizure*	*Pseudoseizure*
Aura	Common stereotyped	Rare
Timing	Nocturnal common	Only when awake
Incontinence	Common	Rare
Cyanosis	Common	Rare
Postictal confusion	Yes	No
Body movement	Tonic-clonic	Nonstereotyped and asynchronous
Self-injury	Common	Rare
EEG	May be abnormal	Normal
Affected by suggestion	No	Yes
Secondary gain	No	Yes

Although the localization of these abnormalities is often inconclusive, the frontal lobe abnormality as the substrate for negative schizophrenic symptoms is receiving much attention from the treatment and prognosis point of view. The important soft neurological signs that are often evaluated include the following:

- Dominance
- R-L discrimination
- Hopping
- Standing balance
- Abnormal Romberg's sign
- Abnormal tandem gait
- Abnormal finger-thumb opposition
- Extinction
- Graphesthesia
- Astereognosis
- Face-hand test
- Fist-ring test
- Fist-edge-palm test
- Fist stretch, among several others.

Neurological History

The following items should be asked:

- *Perinatal events:* Prematurity, complicated labor, infections, seizures, APGAR score (if available).
- Developmental milestones.
- Head injury or infection in childhood.
- Family history of epilepsy, dementia, or other neurological disorders, etc.

Motor System Examination

The following abnormalities are common:

- Loss of natural graceful body movements (early feature).
- Choreoathetoid movements of extremities.
- Apraxia (i.e. difficulty in carrying out a purposive task, in the absence of any sensory or motor abnormalities).

Abnormal Eye Signs

Two major abnormalities seen, both in the patients and their first-degree relatives, are:

- Frequent blinking (reflects dopaminergic overactivity)
- *Abnormality in smooth pursuit eye movement (SPEM)*: Abnormal rapid eye movements (saccades) are seen in 50 to 80% of the patients and approximately 40% of their first-degree relatives (compared to 8% of the normal population).

Nonlocalizing Neurological Signs

Sometimes, these are called as *'soft neurological signs'* and are present more frequently than normal. A partial list was mentioned earlier. Soft neurological sign is subtle abnormalities in sensory perceptual motor or other CNS function. They may not cause functional impairment e.g. clumsiness, motor incoordination, motor overflow, poor balance or coordination, etc.

Speech Disorders

As described earlier, the right left disorientation, apraxias, and the loss of the prosody of the speech are the common speech problems of the schizophrenics that are due to parietal lobe damage.

Autonomic Abnormalities

Autonomic overactivity, i.e. dilated pupils, moist palms, tachycardia, and systolic hypertension may be present in the absence of emotional excitation, and these can be considered as intrinsic to psychoses.

Neuropsychological Testing

Certain neuropsychological tests sensitive to subtle brain damage are enumerated below:

- *Attentional deficits*: Selective impairment is often found in nonparanoid patients. These impairments can be related to frontal lobe dysfunctions and are unrelated to chronicity.
- *Memory impairment*: Dysfunctional working memory, unrelated to attentional deficits, motivations or cooperativeness is often found in schizophrenics.
- *Impaired executive function*: Planning, sequencing, concept formation or cognitive set shifting (frontal lobe dysfunction) are often impaired in chronic schizophrenics.
- *Abnormal motor functioning*: Delayed reaction time, impaired finger tapping, etc. are suggestive of brain damage.
- *IQ assessment*: Increased scatter between verbal and performance IQ is often considered to be due to brain damage. The verbal IQ is normally more than performance IQ, and the difference is not more than 15.

TESTS TO DIFFERENTIATE MALINGERING AND PSYCHOGENIC SYMPTOMS FROM TRUE NEUROLOGIC DISORDERS

The golden rule is to suspect a psychogenic origin of the deficit, if the observation defies the laws of neuroanatomy. For example, preserved temperature sensation but lost pain perceptions, or a changing pattern of the deficits (e.g. patient with paraplegia walks when not observed).

Below are given certain tests commonly employed to differentiate among psychogenic symptoms and malingering versus true neurological deficits (Table 3).

Table 3: Specific procedures for distinguishing among neurological illness, dissociative/conversion disorder (Hysteria), and malingering

Nature of disturbance	*Neurological illness*	*Dissociative/conversion disorder (hysteria)*	*Malingering*
I. Special Senses			
A. Sight			
i. Total blindness	Atrophy of optic disc; absent/feeble pupillary response to light, optokinetic nystagmus, absent visual evoked response	Normal fundus and pupillary responses; no optokinetic nystagmus; positive visual evoked response	Same as hysteria; may draw up forehead to inhibit pupillary reflex to sudden light
ii. Monocular blindness	Same as above for affected eye; consensual pupillary light reflex; no diplopia to pressure on unaffected eye	Same as above; pressure on unaffected eye may produce diplopia or polyopia	Same as above
	Shows appropriate response to 'Harmon's Diaphragm test', based on two facts: (a) If both eyes open, patient is unable to tell with which eye objects are seen; (b) objects on right side are seen by left eye, and conversely-therefore, patient with monocular blindness can see contralateral half of letters with "Drane's test"	No clinical data	Sees all letters or those on ipsilateral side
	Prism placed before defective eye does not impair reading	Impaired reading when prism placed before defective eye	Same as hysteria
iii. Reduced vision	Determine how many large letters patient can read at distance of 20 feet from Snellen chart placed in front of large mirror—then move patient 10 feet closer to mirror with chart on his chest with letters naturally reversed—according to laws of reflection, he should only be able to read same number of letters	No clinical data	May be induced to read twice number of letters on Snellen chart
	Perimetry or gross examination of field defects reveals consistent responses and wider field of vision, in conformance with visual angle, as object is moved farther away	Tubular or gun-barrel vision with expanding field as object recedes; hemianopia rare; usually smaller field on anesthetic or hemiparetic side; with continued testing occasionally get concentrically contracted field	Inconsistent response to perimetry on gross field examination
iv. Ptosis	Eyebrow generally higher than on unaffected side with secondary contraction of frontalis	Eyebrow generally lower than on unaffected side without secondary compensatory contraction of frontalis	Same as hysteria
B. Hearing			
i. Bilateral deafness	Auditory averaged evoked responses should be absent	Evoked responses should be present	Evoked responses should be present
	No impairment or subjective disturbance in reading out loud with delayed auditory feedback into affected ear(s)	Impaired reading out loud with delayed auditory feedback into affected ear(s) but probably without subjective disturbance	Probably same as hysteria but with subjective disturbance
ii. Unilateral deafness	Sound from vibrating turning fork placed on frontal bone near unaffected ear will be carried by bone conduction to affected ear when unaffected ear is plugged	No clinical data	Will deny hearing sound transmitted by bone conduction

Contd...

Contd...

Nature of disturbance	*Neurological illness*	*Dissociative/conversion disorder (hysteria)*	*Malingering*
C. Smell			
	Can identify stringent stimuli (e.g. ammonia) which excite cranial nerves I and V, but cannot name	Denies smell	No clinical data
II. Motor power			
i. All muscle groups	"Erben test" is based on physiological principle that during fine movements agonists and contracting antagonists act in synergy so that movements can be executed with precision during gross movements; agonists alone contract and antagonists become relaxed, thereby making action of agonist more effective; muscle groups are evaluated by requesting patient to move part against resistance; slow course tremor may appear	Antagonist muscles contract when patient told to move part; no tremor	Same as hysteria
ii. Paresis/paralysis	Characteristic physiological and compensation responses, such as circumduction of affected leg, wide gait, consistent weakness pattern	Astasia-abasia with flailing legs and no falling; may be able to run but not walk; can move legs while in recumbent position; no circumduction of paretic leg from hip; can maintain spasms or contractures	Indicates cannot stand or walk or move legs in recumbent position with when requested to walk on or not simulated lame gait may forget to limp support self on good leg when getting up from kneeling position
	Reduced or exaggerated deep tendon reflexes	Normal reflexes	Normal reflexes
	"Hoover test" for unilateral leg paralysis principle that when supine patients try to lift on a leg against resistance, there is compensatory downward thrust of other leg which can be detected by examiner's hand under heel-downward heel pressure can be measured objectively with bathroom scale	No downward thrust of patient attempts to move affected leg; also, shows downward thrust of affected leg when attempts to move affected leg; also, shows downward thrust of affected leg when attempts to move unaffected leg	No clinical data
iii. Aphonia	Paralysis of vocal cords with inability to perform normal speech movements	Can whisper with formal movement of lips, tongue, pharynx, and vocal cords during respiration, can cough on request, indicating intact vocal nerves; may have absent or reduced pharyngeal reflex and hypesthesia of larynx	No clinical data
III. Analgesia deficits			
	Conforms to anatomical principles (heminanesthesias and hemianalgesias uncommon)	Nonanatomical distribution with midline or sharp demarcation; often associated with other complaints, such as paralysis; usually annular or total; impossible claim of deficits in all sensations	Rare complaints
	Japanese illusion test—cross both hands palm-to-palm, interlock fingers, and invert-consistent responses to testing of anesthetic hand	Responses may be consistent or inconsistent	Inconsistent responses more probable inconsistent

Contd...

Contd...

Nature of disturbance	*Neurological illness*	*Dissociative/conversion disorder (hysteria)*	*Malingering*
	Stocking-glove anesthesia rare	Stocking-glove anesthesia—may move up limb with repeated testing and suggestibility	Rare complaint
	Vibratory sense loss at mid-ulna or mid-tibia is a physiological impossibility since solid structures vibrate as a whole. Vibratory sense will be transmitted by solid structures to abnormal side whichever side of sternum or frontal bone tested	Will deny perception of vibration on anesthetic side when affected bone tested but will acknowledge perception when this is done over normal side. Cornea not insensitive on hemianesthetic side	No clinical data
	Distal deficits more severe than proximal	Proximal deficits may be more severe than distal	
	No pain in response to intradermal histamine	Pain in response to intradermal histamine over anesthetic area	
i. Pain	Pressure over or movement of painful part may lead to temporary increase of pulse rate from 10–30 beats per minute (Mannkopf's sign), and also pupil dilation, sudden flushing and sweating	No clinical data	No increase in pulse rate or dilation of pupils
IV. Coordination			
i. Ataxia	Worse with eyes closed; when patient lying on back, ataxic limb will not be lifted straight and steadily in vertical plane—it is abducted or adducted, rotated inwards or outwards, oscillates, and does not come down vertically	Different pattern from true ataxia	As severe with eyes closed; different pattern from true ataxia
ii. Romberg test	Makes every effort to maintain equilibrium and keep from falling, tendency of plantar surfaces of feet to grip floor	Pattern probably between organic and malingering responses	Starts to fall before eyes closed and makes little effort to maintain equilibrium or grasp floor
	When sitting in bed, will show less sway with upper torso because of broader base for balance		May fall backward when sitting; no change in sway from standing

SUGGESTED READING

1. Bhatia MS, Jagawat T, Pradhan SC. A Comprehensive and Practical Guide to Psychiatric Interview and Examination. New Delhi: CBS Publishers, 1997.
2. Bickerstaff ER, Spillane JA. Neurological Examinations in Clinical Practice. V Ed. Delhi: Oxford University Press, 1989.
3. Cummings JL. Neuropsychiatry and behavioural neurology. In: Kaplan HI, Sadock BJ (Eds). Comprehensive Textbook of Psychiatry, 6th edition. Baltimore: Williams and Wilkins, 1995.
4. Dejong RN. The Neurologic Examination, 5th edition. Hagerstown: Harper and Row, 1992.
5. Folstein MF, Folstein S, McHugh PR. Mini-mental state: A practical method for grading the cognitive state of patients for the clinician. J Psychiatr Res. 1975;12:189.
6. Kaplan HI, Sadock BJ. Pocket Handbook of Emergency Psychiatric Medicine. New Delhi: BI Publications, 1993.
7. Kauffman DM. Clinical Neurology for Psychiatrists. Philadelphia: WB Saunders, 1995.
8. Snell SR. Clinical Neuroanatomy, 7th edition. Lippincott William & Wilkins. 2010.
9. Spillane J. Bickerstaff's Neurological Examination Clinical Practice. Blackwell Science. 2012.
10. Standring S. Grays's Anatomy, 39th edition. London. Elsevier Churchil Livingstone. 2005.
11. Strub RL, Black FW. Mental Status Examination in Neurology. Philadelphia: FA Davis, 1977.
12. Strub RL, Black FW. Neurobehavioural Disorders: A Clinical Approach. New Delhi: Jaypee Brothers, 1990.
13. Walsh K. Neuropsychology: A Clinical Approach. New Delhi: BI Churchill Livingstone, 1994.

CHAPTER

3 Epidemiology of Mental Disorders

R Chandrasekaran, Sudhir Kumar CT

DEFINITION

The term *epidemiology* is derived from the Greek words, *epi* (upon) and *deme* (the people). It is the quantitative study of the distribution and determinants of mental disorders in the human population. Instead of individuals, population subgroups are studied in epidemiology. The differences in the frequency of mental disorders in the population subgroups are assessed by quantitative methods. Epidemiology also throws light on the causative or risk factors associated with a particular morbidity. If the characteristic risk factors are identified, interrupting them may reduce the occurrence of the illness.

PROBLEMS IN PSYCHIATRIC EPIDEMIOLOGY

Several problems have been identified in psychiatric epidemiology; the foremost among them being nosology. The psychiatric diagnosis is essentially based on the signs and symptoms, and the course and treatment response. The causal factors are not clearly identified in most of the psychiatric disorders. This invariably results in heterogeneity among the diagnostic groups. If varied conditions are included, then this leads to the dilution of diagnostic groups and the risk factors like biological and psychosocial variables associated with the particular diagnosis cannot be identified with certainty. The lack of a valid and reliable method for making a standard psychiatric diagnosis was clearly highlighted by the US-UK diagnostic project.[1]

In the absence of a well-defined nosology, case detection becomes difficult. Further, while developing case detection instruments, the minimum that is expected of an instrument is to have face validity and diagnostic specificity. In the past, questionnaires of unproven reliability and validity have been used to assess the psychological problems in the community. However, standardized clinical interview methods have replaced the older methods to improve the case detection techniques. Difficulties have also arisen while studying chronic conditions in psychiatric epidemiology. These include time-disease relationship, uncertainty about the role of causal factors and uncertain prodromal period.[2] Research towards identifying modifiable risk factors in psychiatric disorders is lacking and this affects the prospects of reducing the occurrence of new cases.

USES OF EPIDEMIOLOGY

Morris[3] has defined the various uses of epidemiology and they are as follows:

- *Study of historical trends:* The study of the decrease or increase of a disorder over time or a changing rate of incidence can give clues about the role of environmental factors or recent social change as etiological factors
- *Community diagnosis:* A minority of patients seeks treatment in the hospital. The study, which includes the untreated ill persons in a community, can give a better estimate of the disorder
- *Individual risks:* The risk of an individual suffering a disorder is important in planning care and prevention
- *Operational research:* This is to study in detail to get information on the health services in operation and the population utilizing or not utilizing such services. The information, thus obtained, will provide clues on the effectiveness of economics of health care
- *Completing the clinical picture:* This improves the understanding of the full clinical picture of a disorder. In particular, this helps one to understand the early signs of a disorder and the mixed and atypical varieties of a particular disorder. This information can be used for early intervention and control or prevention of a full-blown disorder
- *Identification of syndromes:* This provides an opportunity to identify syndromes, which have not been previously recognized. To cite an example, agoraphobia without history of panic disorder occurs more in the general population than in a clinical sample

- *Clues to cause:* Study of populations with high and low rates of mental disorders can provide clues to the causative or protective factors related to the disorders.

EPIDEMIOLOGICAL METHODS

The basic approach to studying the epidemiology of psychiatric disorders is similar to that of a chronic disease. It may be useful to define certain epidemiological terms before proceeding to understanding the method. Point prevalence is defined as that proportion of the population that has the disorder being studied at a given point of time. This is calculated regardless when the disorder started. Incidence is the rate at which new cases of a disorder occur in a population at risk over a specified time interval. The annual incidence rate is the usual one reported. Incidence density refers to an average incidence over the time period of interest. This rate is more precise as it takes into account the number of dropouts from the population sample at risk during the study. The period prevalence is the proportion of the population that either has a disorder at the beginning of specified time interval or has developed it over the interval. This does not distinguish between incidence and prevalence. Lifetime prevalence is defined as that proportion of the population considered at a point in time who have ever had the disorder under the study. This measure has its own limitations. It is based on subjective recall and may include population who had not completed the risk period or reached the risk period. The true differences in incidence rates in different age groups are also obscured. One way of overcoming this problem is to work out age specific incidence of psychiatric disorders. Treated prevalence refers to point prevalence rate of the treatment receiving population.

Descriptive Methods

Sampling is to be done from 'population' which is to be explicitly stated and this sample should be representative of the population. The community population is more commonly studied. When sampling is done from a clinical population like a hospital, the selection bias always occurs. Different clinical populations when studied can cause a discrepancy in the results. Hence, the investigator has to decide what population is available for the study that matches the desired objective so that a sample can be derived.

Simple random sample uses random numbers to draw subjects from a list of the entire study population. For example, if one wants to select cases from a series of consecutive admissions from a hospital, all patients are rostered and a sample is selected randomly. If the population to be studied is not homogenous, different sections of the population which are homogenous within them are to be sampled. A useful procedure in such a situation will be stratified random sampling. Here the population is divided into a number of sections called strata. A random sample is to be selected from each stratum so that the whole population is adequately represented and the variability in each stratum is taken care of.

Systematic sampling offers a convenient technique while dealing with a large sampling scheme. In this sampling method, every nth case is chosen from a list of cases. This can be done even when the list is not available. Investigators can use cluster sampling when the whole population consists of many natural groups called clusters. Cluster sampling is often possible when a large population in a community is surveyed. Selection of clusters can be done at village level, block level and household level. But in cluster sampling, confidence intervals are larger and hence the estimates are less precise.

A discrepancy found between the characteristics of the sample actually obtained and that of the base population is referred to as sampling error. With the help of standard error, investigators will be able to arrive at the range of point estimates at 95% confidence interval. In epidemiological studies, larger samples are preferred as they provide more stable point estimates.

Assessment Instruments

The assessment instruments are developed only after the diagnostic criteria can be unambiguously stated. In the field of psychiatry, nosology has been one of the main topics of interest. Wing et al.[4] have dealt on the issue of 'what is a case' and its significance in epidemiological approach. In spite of this, any diagnostic procedure should be carefully scrutinized for any source of error. Safety, feasibility, reliability and validity are the important characteristics of diagnostic instruments. The safety of the instrument for establishing psychiatric diagnosis need not be emphasized as so far no problems have been reported with regard to the safety of the instrument. Feasibility includes issues like sample size, subject availability and adequate financial support.

Reliability assumes importance because several sources of variance are likely to contribute to the unreliability of diagnosis. Consistency in diagnostic assessment between examiners, is known as inter-rater reliability and between examinations, test-retest reliability. The measure of agreement expressed in percentage is no more valid as agreements can occur by chance. The most widely used measure of agreement for reliability is kappa, a measure that corrects for the proportion of chance agreement. Values above 0.75 are regarded as excellent. Values between 0.40 and 0.75 are good and values below 0.40 are poor. If the condition being assessed is rare, the use of kappa is not advocated. In split half reliability, items in a test are divided into two halves. If all the items are measuring the same characteristic, a high correlation is observed between the two halves. This is a measure of internal reliability. This can be further improved by estimating the correlation between all the items.

Validity of the instrument is assessed by whether it is able to measure accurately. Several types of validity have been described. Face validity is based on the judgment by an expert that a particular instrument can be employed in a given situation. But this type of validity lacks accuracy. Similarly, content validity refers to a judgment by an expert that the item of the test covers the appropriate domains of knowledge relevant for the purposes of the test. In criterion validity, the result of the test instrument is compared with the result of another well-known accurate instrument. In psychiatry, this is largely practised to assess the accuracy of the instrument. There are several measures of criterion validity. Sensitivity is a measure of the instrument's ability to detect true cases and specificity is a measure of the instrument's ability to detect noncases as identified by the criterion instrument. The false positive rate is the proportion of true noncases mistakenly identified by the new instrument. The false negative rate is the proportion of true cases missed by the instrument. The most difficult form of validity to establish is the construct validity of the instrument. The procedure is to make sure that the thing being measured exists in the same way that the instrument designed to measure it assumes it does. Predictive validity assesses the ability of the instruments to accurately identify subjects who will at some future points be shown to have the disorder. Procedural validity combines both reliability and validity measure. This is relevant in situations where a nonclinician can use a particular instrument as effectively as a psychiatrist. Many epidemiological studies have used the services of nonspecialists in the initial screening of the population.

Analytic Methods

Analytical studies are employed to identify risk factors associated with morbidity. A cross-sectional evaluation-like point prevalence, though easy to carry out, has its own limitations. No information is available regarding the duration of the illness. There can be an over-representation of chronic cases. And further, all the sick patients might not have had access to effective treatment so that they remain more disabled than an individual who had access to treatment. To overcome some of these problems, incidence studies are helpful. The risk factors can be studied for new cases emerging in the population over a period of time. Ideally the incidence rates are studied in the following manner: A sample from the population who are younger than the typical age of onset of a particular disorder is selected. People who have already developed the disorder are excluded. Potential risk factors are studied at the beginning and the subjects are re-examined after a considerable period of time to identify those who have developed the illness. By considering the incidence rates in different groups, like socioeconomic characteristics, the relative risks can be obtained. If an elevated relative risk is identified, further investigations can be done to identify high-risk group with factors contributing to the same. Prospective longitudinal studies are usually expensive and time consuming.

Case control study, another design, is employed for rare disorders and also as a substitute for prospective longitudinal studies. In this method, known cases are identified from hospitals or medical records. A group not having the illness is matched for age, sex, socioeconomic status or other characteristics and used for comparison. The relative risk is estimated by calculating odds ratio. Danish adoption study[5] is an example of case control study. The results of this study done on 5483 adoptees indicated a genetic contribution to schizophrenia. Analytical studies are likely to be flawed by various biases. Poor sample selection-sampling (sampling bias), invalid instrument (observation bias), noninclusion of certain causal factors related to risk factors (confounding bias) are some of the biases which can affect the findings of the study. Further the association between a risk factor and an illness does not support the causal nature and interaction can occur in both directions. The epidemiologist has to further look for temporal relationship and the findings require replication.

PSYCHIATRIC EPIDEMIOLOGY

Considerable advances have been made in the area of diagnostic assessment to attempt to approximate clinical diagnosis in large-scale community studies. In spite of this, reliability in diagnostic assessments suffers because of certain potential sources of error. Information variance is one such error, if examiners collect different information from subjects for assessing psychiatric morbidity. Observer variance refers to the different interpretations made by different examiners on the same data, e.g. depressed mood and blunted affect. If different examiners use different sets of criteria to arrive at a diagnosis with the same data, the problem is one of criterion variance.

Two approaches are used to minimize these problems. One is to apply standardized protocols guiding the interview of the subjects. The protocol specifies the information to be obtained by the examiner and provides a glossary defining the terms. Examiners are also trained so that information elicited remains constant.[6] The other approach is to develop a set of specified criteria to be used in assigning diagnosis to research subjects.[7]

Instruments for Assessing Psychiatric Symptoms

Present State Examination (PSE-9)[6]

This is designed for experienced clinicians who have been trained in its use. There are 140 items and each symptom is rated on three or four points scale. The patient symptomatology is covered during the previous four weeks. A manual gives the definition of the symptoms to be rated and indicates the levels of symptomatology for each point in the scale. The CATEGO program is a computer program available for using information derived from PSE to make a diagnosis. Reliability for most section is satisfactory, though reliability for items covering behavior during interview is low. A past history schedule is also described which can be used prior to the administration of PSE. Based on PSE data, an index of definition (ID)[8] has been developed. Using a computer program, a patient can be allocated to an ID from 1 to 8. An ID of 5 or above indicates that the patient has a psychiatric illness. This is helpful in identifying "cases" in the community surveys. Many drawbacks have been identified in this system. Historical information is not covered. Organic psychoses, subcultural or psychosomatic conditions, mental retardation, personality disorders, substance abuse and chronic disability are not dealt in detail. The system does not provide diagnosis according to established classificatory systems. This has been recently overcome by updating PSE to reflect criteria according to DSM-III-R[9] and ICD-10.[10] A short 40-item version for non-patient population and a ten-item version for community studies are also available.

General Health Questionnaire[11]

This is a self-rated questionnaire. 60, 30, 28, and 20 item versions are available. In the full version of 60 items questionnaire, a score of 11 discriminates 'cases' from 'non-cases'. The questionnaire can be used in community settings, primary care or general medical patients. The questionnaire is not suitable for detecting psychosis. A 28-item scaled version[12] is also available. The four sub-scales include somatic symptoms, anxiety and insomnia, social dysfunction and severe depression. Each question has four possible responses; less than usual, no more than usual; rather more than usual or much more than usual.

Schedule for Affective Disorders and Schizophrenia[13]

Endicott and Spitzer developed a structured interview to differentiate schizophrenia from affective disorders. The symptoms are assessed on a seven-point scale. A score of 3 or more is regarded as clinically significant. Schedule for affective disorders and schizophrenia (SADS) has two parts. Part 1 rates symptoms during two periods: the week before the interview and one week period during the past year when symptoms were at their worst. Part II covers past history and treatment history. The interview schedule describes each symptom and the criteria for rating. There are three versions of the instrument SADS, SADS-L (lifetime version) and SADS-C (change version). The diagnosis is based on Research Diagnostic Criteria.[14] Though it is recommended for hospital-based population, few epidemiological studies have been conducted using this instrument.

Diagnostic Interview Schedule[15]

The diagnostic interview schedule (DIS), developed by Robins et al. (1981), is a highly structured interview that was designed for use by lay interviewers in epidemiological studies. Computer diagnoses are possible according to DSM-III,[16] Feighner's criteria[7] and Research Diagnostic Criteria.[14] The schedule elicits the symptoms, the severity, the frequency, the distribution over time and whether or not the symptom can be explained by physical illness, drug or alcohol abuse. There is precoding for the interview and answers can be directly entered into the computer. It takes 45 minutes to 1 hour to administer the schedule. Diagnosis can be generated both currently (last two weeks, 1 month, 6 months, 1 year and lifetime). It has certain advantages like that it neither requires a psychiatrist to administer the schedule nor a lengthy training program for the investigator.

Composite International Diagnostic Interview[17]

It has the same structural characteristics of DIS. The version 1.1 of composite international diagnostic interview (CIDI) is a comprehensive interview schedule, designed for the assessment of major diagnostic categories according to ICD-10[9] and DSM-III-R.[10] It is a highly structured instrument, which can be used by trained lay interviewers. There is a probing system for positive answers to determine the psychiatric significance of the responses. The symptom is considered to be of psychiatric relevance if a doctor ever attributed a psychological etiology to it, found no physical basis for it, or if the respondent reports that there was at least one occasion when its occurrence was not explained by physical illness, use of alcohol and drugs, injury and other medical conditions. The instrument consists of 288 symptom questions and skip rules are available. The CIDI core version 1.1 consists of: (a) interview schedule covering demographics and various psychiatric disorders, (b) researcher's manual, (c) interviewer's manual, (d) computer manual, and (e) data entry and computer diagnosis programs for ICD-10 and DSM-III-R diagnosis. A computerized version of CIDI core version 1.1, CIDI-auto[18] enables self-administration and thereby shortens administration time. The probing of positive answers to symptom questions is also simplified in this. Another version, Quick CIDI,[19] is based on the Quick Diagnostic Interview Schedule IIIR. This is a computerized version, with a skipping facility. The CIDI–PHC[20] version is a modification of the CIDI core version 1.1, and has been developed keeping in mind the type of psychological problems one is likely to come across in patients of general health care settings. The University of Michigan version of CIDI (UM-CIDI[21]) covers most of the diagnoses included in CIDI core version 1.1, with the exception of somatization disorder. This version has been used in a collaborative epidemiological investigation of the prevalence, course and consequence of mental morbidity and comorbidity in the United States. A version of CIDI, that has incorporated DSM-IV,[22] is also available. One of the major drawbacks of the schedule is its over-reliance on the subject's self-report at the cost of examiner's observation and judgment.

Schedules for Clinical Assessment in Neuropsychiatry[23]

Schedules for clinical assessment in neuropsychiatry (SCAN) is primarily designed for use by the trained psychiatrists and clinical psychologists, and meant for patients in clinical settings. Professionals in field studies have, however, used it. The instrument consists of: (1) an interview schedule,[24] 10th edition of PSE, (2) glossary of definitions, (3) item group checklist, and (4) clinical history schedule. The SCAN interview schedule has two main parts. Part I covers non-psychotic phenomena and includes many sections. Part II contains sections covering psychotic, cognitive disorders, and abnormalities of behavior, speech and affect. The glossary provides definitions of symptoms and signs to be assessed by the interviewer. Item group checklist is available to rate the psychopathology item from sources, like medical records or an informant. There is a provision to enter data relevant to the broader clinical and social history, and rate the presence or absence of disorders in Clinical History Schedule. It also consists of sections on childhood education to age 16, intellectual level, social roles and performance, disability, disorders of adult personality and behavior, physical illnesses, and disabilities not coded elsewhere. The rater has an option to rate the patient's present state, present episode, or the 'lifetime ever'. CATEGO-5, a computer program, can categorize patients according to the diagnoses on ICD-10 or DSM-III-R. The SCAN also has provision for axial formulation. The CAPSE[25] has a computer program that allows the interviewer to directly enter the data.

Indian Psychiatric Survey Schedule[26] *(IPSS)*

Indian researchers have frequently used this schedule. A modified version of the Indian psychiatric interview schedule (IPIS)[27] is designed to enquire about the presence or absence of 124 psychiatric symptoms and items of historical information. A symptom is defined as an item of behavior, mood, speech, thinking or sensorium that represents a change from the usual pattern for the individual and is distressful to the subject or those around him or both. The interview focuses on symptoms at the time of interview and the symptoms during the preceding one-week. Nonmedical investigators, following a short training, can conduct a large part of the enquiry. Section 1 consists of a preliminary enquiry, which has ten sub-sections. The enquiry can be conducted by nonmedical investigators. Sections 2 and 3 cover detailed enquiry from the subjects and the relatives respectively. Section 4 allows the psychiatrists to observe and record the presence of signs. The sections 2 to 4 are to be conducted by psychiatrists. Section 5 deals with detailed enquiry about sociopathic items.

Surveys of Clinical Populations

Social Class and Mental Illness

Hollingshead and Redlich,[28] in the 1950s, conducted a study in New Haven, Connecticut to determine the number of patients seen in the various health treatment settings, including private clinics. The patients in treatment, within a six-month period for any mental disorder, were estimated to be 8/1000 residents in the community. The researchers, based on income, education and occupation divided the class structure into 5 groups. Class I represented the highest class and class V represented the lowest class. A definite relation between social class and mental disorders was identified. Neuroses were found to be more prevalent in high socioeconomic groups and psychoses in the lower socioeconomic groups. Overall, the morbidity rate in the highest social classes was found to be 5–7/1000, and 17/1000 in the lower social classes. But, this study failed to establish any true association between social class and mental disorder.

Chicago Study[29]

This study involved examination of 35,000 admissions to mental hospitals in Chicago between 1922 and 1934. Based on this study, a 'drift hypothesis' was postulated, which meant that impaired individuals suffering from chronic illness slide down the socioeconomic state. The other hypothesis called 'segregation hypothesis' tries to explain how schizophrenics try to insulate themselves from the demands of the society by living in isolation. Although, it is accepted that there is a relationship between schizophrenia and social class indices, the nature of the relationship in cause and effect terms still remains a subject of debate. This is often referred to as 'social causation and social selection theories'.[30] Evidence till date favors the view that low status is a social consequence of schizophrenia than a social cause.

Surveys of Community Population

Sterling County Study[31]

This study surveyed 1010 adult residents in a rural Canadian county of 20,000 people. One of the highlights of the study was that DSM-I[32] was applied following a structured interview to arrive at a diagnosis. 57% had evidence of symptom patterns on a lifetime prevalence basis, which could be diagnosed according to DSM-I. 20% of the population were in need of psychiatric attention for a diagnosable mental disorder. High rates of illness were found in areas of social and economic deterioration. This study gave a lot of impetus to develop instruments like DSM-III[16] and DIS,[15] using explicit criteria for mental disorders.

Midtown Manhattan Study

Srole et al.[33] studied the impact of urban life on mental health by interviewing more than 1000 adult residents, selected by probability sampling in mid-town Manhattan, New York. Psychologists and social workers used a structured interview to obtain information from the residents. 81.5% of the population had at least mild impairment from psychological symptoms and 23.4% had significant impairment. The importance of using more rigorous criteria became apparent, as this study identified less than 20% of the population as healthy.

Recent Epidemiological Studies

The NIMH-Epidemiological Catchment Area Program[34-38]

The objective of this program was to determine the prevalence of mental disorders as defined in DSM-III, DSM-IIIR or DSM-IV, and to establish the longitudinal data on the course of various mental disorders. The epidemiological catchment area (ECA) program was conducted at five sites: New Haven, Connecticut; Baltimore, Maryland; St. Louis, Missouri; Durham, North Carolina; and Los Angeles, California. In all the five sites put together, a community population of 200,000 was appropriately sampled and a total of 18,571 were included for the interview. In addition, 500 respondents from institutional settings like prisons, nursing homes, etc. were included. A minimum of 3000 adults aged 18 or older from each area were interviewed during initial examination. The diagnostic interview schedule (DIS) was the major instrument used by a trained lay interviewer to interview each subject. In addition to this, information was collected on use of health and mental health services in 6 to 12 months preceding the interview. A telephone interview was conducted 6 months after the initial interview enquiring about the use of mental health services during the intervening period. A follow-up personal interview was conducted 12 months after the initial visit to repeat the procedure followed during the initial interview.

The estimates of one month, six-month and lifetime prevalence rates for any DIS/DSM-III disorder were 15.14%, 19.1% and 32.2% respectively. The ECA survey brought out the following facts. Almost 1 in 5 was found to have one or more DIS/DSM-III disorders. There were significant differences in socioeconomic status groups, with the lowest two groups having significantly higher overall rates of disorders than the high socioeconomic groups. Schizophrenia, panic disorders and cognitive impairment were found more frequently (8 to 11 times) in the low socioeconomic groups. In terms of marital status, the separated/divorced groups had the highest rate for most of the disorders. Affective, anxiety and somatization disorders were significantly higher in females, while substance use disorders and antisocial personality disorders were significantly more in males. The depressive disorders were lowest in the elderly age group. Mental disorders occurred together, which could not be explained just by their prevalence rates.

National Comorbidity Survey[21]

Based on findings of the ECA study, 8,089 respondents, aged between 18 and 55 years, were interviewed with CIDI. The study revealed a lifetime rate of mental disorders of 48% and one year rate of 29.5%. The lifetime rates of major depressive episodes were 17.1% for all respondents and 21.3% for women. The higher rates found in this study compared to the ECA study again raise issues like sampling and case identification methods. Further, it is also possible that a genuine change might have occurred in the population. The survey also concurred with the view that major depression occurs with earlier age at onset with younger generation.

The Taiwan Psychiatric Epidemiological Project[39]

The project was conducted from 1982 to 1986, using the multi-site random sampling method with 5005, 3004 and 2995 subjects selected respectively from metropolitan area, small town area and rural village area. Chinese modified DIS was used for case identification. The lifetime prevalence of any disorders defined by a DIS (CM) was 16.3%, 28% and 21.5% in metropolitan, town and rural samples, respectively. The differences in lifetime prevalence between the three sampling areas were significant for 8 disorders. Generalized anxiety disorders, alcohol abuse, tobacco dependence and cognitive impairment had higher prevalence rates in small towns and rural samples. The authors explained the differences based on socioeconomic and cultural factors, living conditions in metropolitan and nonmetropolitan areas, as well as biological and personality factors.

National Psychiatric Morbidity Surveys of Great Britain[40, 41]

Four separate surveys were carried out in this study, which included private household samples, a sample of institution caring for the mentally ill, a sample of homeless people, and a supplementary sample of patients with psychosis living in private households. A two-stage assessment procedure was used, in which lay interviewers administered the Revised

Clinical Interview Schedule (CIS-R) with a cutoff score of 12, to assess neurotic symptoms and disorders. A psychosis screen, including psychosis-screening questionnaire, was also used. Psychiatrists, using SCAN,[23] interviewed those who were positive on psychosis screen.

In the household survey, 10,108 adults aged 16-65 were interviewed. This survey provided information regarding the prevalence of neurotic disorders on a nation-wide sample of Great Britain. The one-week prevalence rate of neurotic disorder was found to be 12.3% in males and 19.5% in females. Unmarried, single parents, people living on their own and unemployed had high rates of neurotic disorders. Social class 1 had lower rates of disorder. The higher rates in blacks could be explained by other factors like age, family type and social class. The one-year prevalence rates of functional psychosis were 4 per 1000. Alcohol and drug dependence was found to be more prevalent in males.

PSYCHIATRIC EPIDEMIOLOGY IN INDIA

Field survey studies for psychiatric morbidity in India have come a long way since they were started nearly four decades ago. Surya,[42] in Pondicherry, conducted one of the early field survey studies of mental morbidity. Following this, many epidemiological studies have been conducted in various parts of the country. The Table 1 shows the prevalence rates of psychiatric disorders reported in the various studies. A majority of these studies covered a population size ranging from 1000 to 5000. The prevalence rates show a wide variation of 9.5/1000[42] to 370/1000[47]. Few studies have been carried out in the recent past to study the epidemiological aspects of priority psychiatric disorders, as the concept is closely linked to primary mental health care. These disorders include schizophrenia, organic psychosis, manic depressive psychosis, epilepsy and mental retardation.

Epidemiological research on psychiatric morbidity in special population subgroups has also been carried out. Studies have been conducted to identify the mental morbidity in a slum area,[61] industrial area with predo-minantly low-income group[62] and beggar's colony.[63] The neuropsychiatric morbidity in these studies ranged between 22.6/1000 and 131.09/1000. The highest morbidity found in the beggar's colony[63] (131.09/1000) points to the role of poverty, overcrowding and social disorganization in mental illnesses.

Table 1: Prevalence of psychiatric morbidity in some general population studies

S.No.	*Investigator*	*Year*	*Center*	*Location*	*Population*	*Prevalence/1000*
1.	Surya[42]	1964	Pondicherry	U	2731	9.5
2.	Sethi et al.[43]	1967	Lucknow	U	1733	72.7
3.	Gopinath[44]	1970	Bangalore	R	423	16.54
4.	Dube[45]	1970	Agra	M	29,468	18
5.	Elnagar et al.[46]	1971	Hoogly	R	1393	27
6.	Sethi, et al.[47]	1972	Lucknow	R	2691	39.4
7.	Kapur[48]	1973	Kota	R	1233	370
8.	Vergheese et al.[49]	1973	Vellore	U	1887	66.5
9.	Thacore[50]	1973	Lucknow	U	1977	81.6
10.	Sethi et al.[51]	1974	Lucknow	U	4481	67.0
11.	Nandi et al.[52]	1975	West Bengal	R	1060	109
12.	Shah et al.[53]	1980	Ahmedabad	U	—	47.3
13.	Bhide[54]	1982	Ootacamund	R	1658	184
14.	Mehta et al.[55] (PPD)	1985	Vellore	R	5941	14.5
15.	Sachdeva et al.[56] (PPD)	1986	Faridkot	R	1989	22.12 (PPD)
16.	Trivedi et al.[57]	1988	Pondicherry	R	4467	203.7
17.	Premarajan et al.[58]	1993	Pondicherry	U	1115	99.4
18.	Verghese et al.[59]	1993	Ernakulam	R	1699	12.95
19.	Shaji et al.[60] (PPD)	1995	Ernakulam	R	5284	14.57
20.	Sharma and Singh[61]	2001	Goa	M	4022	60.2

R = Rural
U = Urban
M = Mixed
PPD = Priority Psychiatric Disorders

Attempts have been made to study mental morbidity among students. A prevalence rate of 9.8/1000 among medical students[64] and 19.6% among high school students[65] have been reported. Another study[66] used Goldberg's 60-item questionnaire as a screening tool to assess mental morbidity among 1160 postgraduate and research students. According to the survey, 16.68% were found to have mental morbidity. The authors have suggested that dissatisfaction arising from living arrangements, financial problems, poor extracurricular activities, poor social relationships and poor staff student contact could have contributed to mental morbidity. Incidence studies are few in numbers. Nandi et al.[67] carried out an incidence study in West Bengal and reported a rate of 17.66/1000 which covered all cases. The other studies have focused mainly on the incidence rates of schizophrenia.[68-70]

A Selective Review of Indian Field Studies

The first field survey of mental morbidity was conducted by Surya[42] in Pondicherry. He personally surveyed a population of 2731 from 510 households in an urban slum of Pondicherry town. He used a simple screening questionnaire. No depressive disorder was identified in the study. Further, a very low prevalence rate of alcoholism was reported. Dube[45] carried out a prevalence study of mental illness in a population of 29,468, comprising of rural and semirural population. He defined an 'active case' as one suffering from mental illness during 1½ years preceding the date of first psychiatric interview, and an 'inactive case' as one who suffered from mental disorders at any time prior to 18 months but since then had no active symptoms. Elnagar et al.[46] conducted a three stage procedure while studying the morbidity pattern. During the first stage, a house to house survey was conducted. During the second stage, detailed case histories of suspected cases were done. During the third stage, a psychiatrist confirmed the diagnosis. Sethi et al.[43,47] have carried out surveys, both in urban and rural populations. The rates of subnormality and epilepsy were higher in the rural population while schizophrenia, psychoneuroses and depression were significantly more in urban population. Verghese et al.[49] in a major epidemiological study, used a stratified sampling technique. He also used a validated mental item health sheet comprising of 60 common psychiatric symptoms. Mental retardation scale of Cornell Medical Index for adults and Seguin Form Board for children were used to identify mental retardation.

Nandi et al.[52] defined a 'case' as a manifest disturbance of mental functioning, specific enough in clinical character to be consistently recognizable as conforming to a clearly defined standard pattern and severe enough to cause at least partial loss of working or social capacity or both, of a degree which can be specified in terms of degrees in quality or quantity of work, or of taking legal or other social action.

Kapur and Carstairs[26] developed Indian Psychiatric Survey Schedule for field surveys in Indian studies. Carstairs and Kapur used this schedule for a cross-cultural field survey of mental disorder among three caste groups, viz. *brahmins*, *bants* and *mogers* (fishermen) in the South-West coastal village of Kota in Karnataka. Another highlight of the study was that the groups studied had different patterns of inheritance. The *brahmins* followed patrilineal inheritance whereas *bants* and *mogers* followed matrilineal inheritance. When the matrilineal system was declared illegal by the Government of India, this proved to be stressful to the community, especially women, who followed matrilineal inheritance. The study also developed the 'need scale', that is the need for help, by combining the criteria of consultation sought by the individual, inability to cope and number of symptoms. Using this scale, 6% of the population was identified as highest need category. *Bants* and *moger* women were found to fall in a higher need category.

Schizophrenia

The various prevalence studies in schizophrenia are given in Table 2. The prevalence rate on an average is 2 to 3 per 1000. Urban, rural and mixed populations have been studied. Indian epidemiological studies, so far, have largely focused on the prevalence and incidence aspects of schizophrenia. Studies conducted later have used standardized instruments and computer analysis of data. The varying rates found in Indian studies could be due to variation in sample size, different methodologies and different sets of criteria for the diagnosis of schizophrenia. A study, done at Madras,[72] covered a large urban population of more than 100,000. A two-stage procedure was adopted to detect the cases. Using IPSS,[26] a complete enumeration door to door survey was conducted to screen the cases by trained field staff. The probable cases were further subjected to clinical examination by psychiatrists and confirmed by present state examination. The age corrected prevalence rate was found to be 3.87/1000, which was comparable to other studies.[43,73]

Incidence studies are few in numbers. In an earlier study,[67] an incidence rate of 0.93/1000 of schizophrenia was reported in a rural population. Other major studies[68-70] reported an incidence rate of 3–4.2/10,000. The incidence rate fell to 1/10,000 when more rigorous criteria were applied for diagnosing schizophrenia.[69] 'Leakage study' nearly doubled the incidence rate of schizophrenia in another study.[70] Precise estimates of lifetime prevalence rate for schizophrenia are not available at present. Higher prevalence rates have been found to be associated with lower socioeconomic status, age range of 15 to 45 years, those living alone, the unemployed and illiterate.[71] The onset of illness and number of cases occurring in relation to gender require further investigation. It is not possible to propose any causality with available data, as these studies have relied heavily on association rather than making a concerted effort to identify the high-risk groups. Multicentric epidemiological studies, covering large

Table 2: Prevalence rates of neuropsychiatric disorders in some general population studies*

Authors	Schizophrenia	Affective disorders	Organic disorders	Mental retardation	Neuroses
Surya[42]	1.5	—	2.2	0.7	5.0
Sethi et al.[43,51]	2.3/2.5	6.9/7.8	—	22.5/10.5	42.5/37.1
Gopinath[44]	2.36	7.0	23.6	4.72	2.36
Dube[45]	1.49	0.51	2.88	3.7	12.7
Elnagar et al.[46]	4.31	2.9	4.35	1.45	14.4
Sethi et al.[47]	1.1	1.5	—	25.3	10.4
Verghese[49]	2.6	0.5	2.6	3.2	47.6
Thacore[50]	1.9	1.5	2.7	3.7	71.4
Nandi et al.[52]	2.83	37.74	10.38	2.83	35.8
Shah et al.[53]	1.5	14.8	—	1.8	29.2
Mehta et al.[55]	1.9	0.5	7.9	3.2	—
Sachdeva et al.[56]	2.01	13.07	4.52	2.5	—
Trivedi et al.[57]	2.87	20.78	—	15.5	103
Premarajan[58]	2.5	20.2	—	18.3	53
Verghese et al.[59]	2.94	1.77	1.77	2.35	1.18
Shaji et al.[60]	3.6	3.02	—	2.84	—

* Prevalence rates are expressed per 1000 population.

populations, are required to study the role of various risk factors in schizophrenia, giving due importance to cultural factors.

Affective Disorders

The prevalence rates for depression range from 1.5/1000[47] to 37.74/1000.[52] Surya[42] did not report any affective disorder in his study. The rates for manic depressive psychosis, as included under ICD-9, range from 0.51/1000[45] to 20.78/1000[57] (Table 2). There is a marked variability in the rate of depression across the studies. This is partly because of the heterogeneity of the disorder as well as nonuse of reliable diagnostic instruments and standardized criteria A variety of nomenclatures have been used while describing the prevalence of affective disorders. The terms include affective disorders, affective psychoses, involutional melancholia, and depression. Higher rates of depression have been reported in North India than in South India. According to Sethi and Sharma,[74] this could be due to diagnostic practice, researchers' bias, tolerance of symptoms, and genuine differences arising from biological and sociocultural differences. Similarly, higher rates of depression are reported in rural compared to urban population.[52,75] Preponderance of females in depressive disorders is a consistent finding. The rates show marked variation when analyzed according to different age groups, because the studies have included all types of depression.

Substance Abuse Disorders

In India, drug abuse has been studied in the general population and specific populations from an epidemiological point of view. The prevalence of drug abuse, in three different rural settings conducted in Punjab and in an urban setting from Madhya Pradesh, were found in the range of 30 to 78%.[76-79] From the state of Uttar Pradesh, the prevalence figures were found to show less variation. The figures range between 18 and 22%.[80-82] Lower rates have been reported from West Bengal.[46,52]

Among students, medical students, high school students and college students have been studied. In one study,[83] 7 out of 10 students had used some drug in the past. A majority of students were polydrug users. The prevalence of daily use was found to be low, the highest being for tobacco and alcohol. In another study[84] that compared drug use among physicians and medical students, undergraduate students had higher rate of multiple drug use. In both these studies, the lifetime prevalence was found to be in the range of 70 to 80%. Chakraborty et al.[85] identified 3.2% of medical students using drugs on a regular basis. Sethi et al.[86] adopting a criteria of indulgence in a drug with a frequency of at least once a month, found that 25% of the medical students surveyed used a drug at least once a month. In this particular study, it should be noted that the minor tranquilizers were more abused than alcohol. Another study[87] applied similar criteria and identified 22.67% of internees as alcohol abusers. A recent study[88] used a standardized drug survey instrument[89] for detecting drug abuse among medical students. The most common substance ever used was betel nut. Daily use was reported for tobacco smoking only. A study by Mohan et al.[90] estimated the overall prevalence rate of drug abuse as 32.2% among Delhi University students. Alcohol and tobacco were the more frequently abused drugs, followed by cannabis in males and painkillers in females. A similar trend was observed among high school students, wherein 12.7% students were current abusers of alcohol.[91] Verma et al.[92] in his evaluation of college students, detected 1.47% of the study population dependent mostly on drugs, like amphetamine and methaquolone.

Studies have also been conducted in the underprivileged sections of the society. A high prevalence of alcohol and tobacco abuse was identified among rickshaw pullers.[93] In an urban slum in Delhi, Mohan et al.[94] interviewed the head of the household (key informant method), with an instrument containing questions based on DSM-III criteria of dependence, and estimated 26% of the respondents as drug abusers. Another study has high-lighted the problems of substance abuse among child laborers.[95] The child laborers, according to the study, used tobacco (chewing and smoking) more regularly than other drugs. It is also encouraging to note that, with sustained efforts, it was possible to bring down the prevalence of drug abuse.[96]

The various epidemiological studies conducted in India on drug abuse reveal that a minority of the population abused drugs regularly and, probably, they suffer from signs and symptoms of dependence. A significant proportion of the population experiment on drugs but gives up the habit later. At any point of time, nonabusers are found to be a majority. Though the studies have identified alcohol, tobacco and cannabis as the common drugs abused in the population, the preference for a particular drug may depend on various factors.

Alcohol Use Disorders

Alcohol deserves a special mention as it has been identified as one of the most common substances abused. The public health problem caused by alcohol can be measured by per capita consumption, lifetime prevalence, current users, and morbidity and mortality rates. Studies of the prevalence of alcohol are hard to evaluate because of lack of uniformity in the diagnosis of alcoholism and heterogeneous sub-populations. There is a wide variation in the reported prevalence of alcoholism/alcohol abuse in community studies (Tables 3 and 4). Two recent studies from Pondicherry, in both urban and rural populations,[57,58] have reported a higher prevalence rate than what was reported in an earlier study[42] three decades ago. These studies have primarily focused on various psychiatric disorders, like psychosis and neurosis, and it is likely that the problems related to alcoholism might have been overlooked. Singh,[104] in a review, has identified various methodological problems in epidemiological studies of alcohol abuse. These include different methods of data collection and lack of uniformity in the definition of terms and categorization of alcohol users. Terms like 'current users', 'ever used', 'normal drinkers', and 'daily/weekly/monthly users' come in the way of comparing the results of various studies. Very few studies have employed a screening instrument or used the definition of alcohol dependence syndrome according to an established classification system.[100,103] The most consistent finding, in the general population surveys of alcohol use in India, is that the proportion of female users is very low. The studies carried out in the student populations have found prevalence rates for alcohol ranging between 10 and 32%.[105-107] Sethi and Manchanda[86] reported a much higher prevalence of alcohol use among medical students. In spite of growing evidence that alcoholism/alcohol abuse is a major problem in India, information regarding its

Table 3: Surveys of alcohol use (psychiatric morbidity surveys)

Authors	*Prevalence rates/1000*	*Categorization*	*Location*
Surya[42]	3.6	Alcoholism	Pondicherry
Gopinath[44]	2.36	Alcoholism	Bangalore
Verghese et al.[49]	4.8	Alcoholism	Vellore
Dube and Handa[97]	1.38	Habitual use	Agra
Elanagar et al.[46]	13	Addiction	West Bengal
Nandi et al.[52]	0.94	Addiction	West Bengal
Premarajan et al.[58]	34.5	Alcoholism	Pondicherry
Trivedi et al.[57]	61.7	Alcoholism	Pondicherry

Table 4: Surveys of alcohol use (general population surveys)

Authors	*% of current users of alcohol*	*Center*
Varma et al.[98]	23.7	Punjab
Sethi and Trivedi[81]	21.4	Uttar Pradesh
Lal and Singh[99]	49.6	Punjab
Ponnudurai et al.[100]	16.7	Tamil Nadu
Chakravarty[101]	26 to 50	Rural Tamil Nadu
Mathrubhootam[102]	33	Rural Tamil Nadu
Mohan et al.[94]	26	Delhi
ICMR-CAR-CMH[103]	1.15	Bangalore
Mohan et al.[76]	32.9	Punjab
Ghulam et al.[79]	26.5	Madhya Pradesh

prevalence is fragmented and imprecise. Differing concepts and methodologies have contributed to the existing problems. One has to define what constitutes an alcohol use problem in the Indian context before further studies are attempted.

Neuroses

The prevalence rates of neurosis are given in Table 3. The term neurosis has been deleted from the official nomenclature. Depressive reaction, anxiety states and dissociative disorders identified in the various epidemiological studies have been included under the term neurosis. Like in other areas, there is a wide variation in the prevalence rates. The common neurotic disorders identified include neurotic depression, anxiety and hysteria. Though none of the general morbidity surveys have identified obsessive compulsive disorders, specific studies have shown prevalence rates of 0.4% in a rural population and 3.38% in an urban population.[108]

Child Psychiatry

Epidemiological measures, like prevalence rates of mental morbidity, in children have been carried out in general population surveys. The findings show that the prevalence rate is 25.9 to 127.7/1000 (Table 5). Higher prevalence rates have been shown in studies done exclusively in children (20.3 to 33.7%).[110-113] The multicentric WHO sponsored study on children in four developing countries, including India, has reported a prevalence rate of 12 to 29%.[114] In addition to this, hospital-based studies also provide information on the mental morbidity of children.[115,116] The common child psychiatric disorders identified in these studies include nocturnal enuresis, mental retardation and hyperkinetic syndrome.[117] Emotional problems and conduct disorders have also been identified. Large-scale epidemiological studies, adopting currently used classificatory systems and standardized instruments, are necessary to arrive at a valid conclusion regarding the extent of psychiatric problems in children in India.

Table 5: Prevalence studies of mental disorders in children

Authors	*Prevalence rates/1000*
Nandi, et al[52]	25.9
Sethi, et al (Rural)[43]	80.9
Sethi, et al (Urban)[47]	94.4
Verghese, et al[49]	82.0
Lal and Sethi[109]	172.7
Trivedi, et al[57]	41.82
Premarajan, et al[58]	58.6

Geriatric Psychiatry

Early reports on prevalence of mental illness in the aged are based on hospital studies and general epidemiological studies. Ramachandran et al.[118] carried out an epidemiological study in a geriatric population and found a prevalence rate of 276.2/1000. 6% of the subjects above 60 years of age suffered from organic disorders. The prevalence rates for functional psychosis and neurotic disorders were 1.7 and 1.6 respectively. Widowhood was found to have significant association with mental morbidity. In addition to this, the study also identified that many elderly had physical ailments like hypertension, diabetes, cataracts and otosclerosis. Venkoba Rao and Madhavan[118] chose a semiurban area with a population of 15668 and conducted a door to door survey to assess the psychiatric and physical morbidity in those aged 60 and above. The prevalence of psychiatric morbidity was estimated at 89/1000. A significant number (48.84%) suffered from physical morbidity. Depressive illness accounted for 67% of total psychiatric morbidity and a prevalence rate of 60/1000. This figure was much higher than the figure derived from clinic-based studies. The authors explained that there is a large segment of invisible depression in the community. A more recent study[119] involved door to door survey of two villages. A case detection schedule was used to identify the cases. The total sample of elderly population above 60 years of age was 183. A high prevalence rate of mental morbidity was reported (612/1000), depression being the most common with a rate of 522/1000 population. Women had higher morbidity rates than men. The rate of dementia (16/1000) reported in this study is quite low compared to other studies where higher rates have been reported.[118,120]

Meta-analysis

Policy-makers are haunted by major discrepancies in the prevalence of mental disorders. Unfortunately, there is no sharp boundary between mental disorders and normalcy. Weak agreement at the level of diagnosis continues to threaten the credibility of estimates of prevalence.[121] However, efforts to overcome these discrepancies through meta-analysis and adding prevalence of individual disorders helped give meaning to the data, thereby enabling policy-makers to plan service delivery.

A meta-analysis of 13 epidemiological studies consisting of 33,572 persons, who met the following criteria: Door to door survey, all age groups included and prevalence rate for urban and rural being available,[122] reported a total morbidity of 58.2 per 1000. Though meta-analysis has its own limitations, this was the first attempt to analyze the epidemiological studies. Another meta-analysis of epidemiological studies reported a total morbidity of 73 per 1000.[123] The difference noted in the two available meta-analyses is due to the methodology of selecting the papers for the review.

PREVALENCE OF PSYCHIATRIC DISORDERS: COMPARISON WITH INTERNATIONAL STUDIES

NIMH-Epidemiological Catchment Area study[124,125] of the US reported psychiatric morbidity as follows; one year incidence of 60/1000 population, one month prevalence of 151/1000 population and lifetime prevalence of 322/1000 population. National Comorbidity Study of the US[126] reported 12 months prevalence of 277/1000 population and lifetime prevalence of 487/1000 population. On comparing the Indian epidemiological studies to any international epidemiological studies, it is found that prevalence rates reported in India are very low.

Low prevalence of psychiatric disorders in india can be attributed to the following reasons: Available evidence supports the first possibility of the under-reporting by Indian epidemiological studies. However, the remote possibility of genuine low prevalence of psychiatric disorders in the Indian population cannot be disregarded because of low rates of substance use in the general population compared to Western countries and good outcome of psychiatric disorders due to various factors like better coping skills, religious, cultural, social and family support. Is the prevalence rate of psychiatric disorders stable or changing? Does globalization and recession play a role in the mental health of individuals? Does changing family structure (joint family to nuclear) influence psychiatric morbidity? Unfortunately, we do not have any long-term epidemiological studies to answer these questions.

Disasters and Mental Health

India has been traditionally vulnerable to natural disasters on account of its unique geoclimatic conditions. Both natural and manmade disasters occur quite regularly in India like many in the developing world.[126-131] About 60% of the Indian landmass is prone to earthquakes of various intensities; over 40 million hectares are prone to floods; about 8% of the total area is prone to cyclones and 68% of the areas are susceptible to drought.[127]

The first well-documented research study in this area in India was on the survivors of a fire disaster and this revealed not only the symptoms of mental disturbances but also the reduced coping behavior of the families of the deceased.

The Bhopal gas tragedy (1984) was the most important disaster to draw national attention due to its severe impact and the sensitivity of the politicoeconomic issues involved therein. The psychosocial impact was studied systematically although intervention programs were more psychiatric in nature. The Marathawada earthquake (1993) and the Andhra Pradesh supercyclone (1996) were disasters in which mental health professionals took an active part in terms of providing mental health services and undertaking research to study the psychosocial impact of these disasters.

Natural Disasters

A study conducted a month after the Latur earthquake found psychiatric morbidity in 59%; post-traumatic stress disorder (PTSD) in 23% and major depression in 21% being the common diagnoses.[133] Another study following Latur earthquake in Marathawada revealed that survivors had PTSD (74%), major depression (89%), generalized anxiety disorder (GAD) (42%) and panic disorder (28%).[126] An Indian Council of Medical Research (ICMR) study in Latur found that 21.5% of adult males in the affected group received a psychiatric diagnosis compared to 13.1% in the controls; corresponding figures for adult females were 14.9% and 5.1% respectively.[134]

The psychiatric sequelae of the Orissa super-cyclone in 1999 suggested that 80.4% of the subjects had probable psychiatric disorder. PTSD was found in 44.3%; anxiety disorder in 57.5% and depression in 52.7%. A considerable proportion (63.4%) of victims with psychiatric disorder had comorbidity. Children and adolescents, elderly persons, lower socioeconomic status (SES), lower educational levels, unemployment, physical injury, degree of exposure, need for evacuation, death in the family, fear of imminent death during the event, hopelessness, increased stress before disaster and past psychiatric history were associated with adverse psychological sequelae. Increase in suicidality was observed.[132]

Around one year after the super-cyclone in Odisha, a study on adolescents found that the prevalence of PTSD was 26.9%, depression 17.6%, and GAD 12.0%. Proportion of adolescents with any diagnosis was 37.9%. Comorbidity was found in 39.0% of adolescents with a psychiatric diagnosis. Adolescents from middle SES were more affected. Prolonged periods of helplessness and lack of adequate postdisaster psychological support were perceived as probable influencing factors other than the severity of the disaster.[135] Another study on children following the super-cyclone, found that PTSD presentations were similar to that in other cultures. It was felt that, though highly prevalent, PTSD might be missed without clinical screening. PTSD was present in 30.6%, and an additional 13.6% had subsyndromal PTSD. Parents or teachers reported mental health concerns in 7.2% subjects, who were only a minor proportion (12.8%) of subjects with any syndromal diagnosis. Significantly more (43.7%) children in high-exposure areas had PTSD than those (11.2%) in low-exposure areas. Depression was significantly associated with PTSD. High exposure, lower educational level and middle SES significantly predicted PTSD. Extreme fear and perceived threat to life during disaster, death in family, damage to home, stay in shelters were not significantly associated with PTSD in children.[136]

The prevalence rates for psychiatric disorders (27.2%) and psychological symptoms (79.7%) around six to nine months following the Tsunami in coastal Tamil Nadu have been considerable. The most common psychiatric disorder was depression, followed by alcohol use disorders in males and anxiety disorders in females. The rate of PTSD, 12.5/1000, was found to be lower than expected. It was perceived that the psychological symptoms get taken care of by the informal social mechanism and counselors working with non-governmental organizations (NGOs) and that the specialist psychiatric services are required for a smaller proportion of populations.[137]

In a study of Tsunami-affected males in Kanyakumari, 43% had clinically significant psychological distress, and 31% had very high levels of psychological distress. Individuals with higher frequency of personal prayer, better quality of marital life, job satisfaction were relatively protected; whereas substance abuse and severe disaster experience such as losing a family member were risk factors for severe psychological distress.[138]

Initial assessment in the Andaman and Nicobar Islands during the early phase of the 2004 Tsunami disaster revealed 5 to 8% of the population was suffering from significant mental health problems. The authors expected that the psychiatric morbidity would be around 25 to 30% in the disillusionment phase. High resilience was seen in the joint family system of the tribal Nicobarese.[139] Psychiatric morbidity in these islands during the first three months following the earthquake and Tsunami was significantly more (5.2%) in the displaced population than (2.8%) the nondisplaced. The overall psychiatric morbidity was 3.7%. The disorders included panic disorder, unspecified anxiety disorder, and somatic complaints. The existence of an adjustment disorder was significantly higher in the nondisplaced survivors. Depression and PTSD were distributed equally in both groups.[140]

The most common psychiatric morbidities in children and adolescents as primary (exposed directly to Tsunami and earthquake) and secondary (those with close family and personal ties with primary survivors) survivors in the Andaman and Nicobar were adjustment disorder (13.5%), depression (13.5%), panic disorder (10.8%), PTSD (10.8%), schizophrenia (2.7%), and other disorders (43.2%). Sub-clinical syndrome was present in the majority of the primary and secondary survivors. A majority of survivors required community-based group interventions.[141]

Fire disasters are common in India. A study in a Delhi slum following a fire disaster reported that the prevalence of psychiatric disorders was significantly higher (7.8%) compared to that (2.2%) in the control group; prevalence of psychological ill health was also higher (23.2% vs 5.0% respectively). The common psychiatric disorders were depression, substance use disorders, GAD and somatoform disorder. Age and participation in relief work were found to be strong predictors and physical injuries were found to be a weak predictor of mental health morbidity.[134]

Following a fire disaster in Bangalore in 1981, 35.8% of the bereaved relatives had psychiatric symptoms requiring treatment.[134,142] In another study, following Mandi Dabwali fire disaster 56% of children had PTSD after two months.[143]

Industrial Disasters

A study conducted within three months of the Bhopal gas tragedy yielded a 22.6% prevalence of mental disorders. Most of the patients were females (81.1%), and under 45 years of age (74%). The main diagnoses were anxiety neurosis (25%), depression (20%) and adjustment reaction with predominant disturbance of emotions (16%). Cases of psychosis were rare.[124,144]

In a community-based study of a representative sample of the gas-exposed population, the prevalence of psychiatric morbidity in the exposed population after one and a half years of disaster was found to be significantly higher in comparison to control group (9.4% vs 2.5%).[134,145]

Man-made Disasters

Following the Mumbai riots in 1992-93, a study on hospitalized victims found them in a state of shock, fear and helplessness; 33% expressed anger; 2% of these (all female who saw the mangled bodies of their husbands) had attempted suicide; 21% of those interviewed had severe anxiety, 41% had paranoid thinking and obsessional symptoms and majority had loss of libido. PTSD features scored very high; and a few were emotionally dumb; and 36% had suicidal thoughts.[124,146]

Within days of a bomb blast (1996) in a bus in a terrorist activity in Dausa, Rajasthan, 35.5% had psychiatric morbidity, 19.4% had acute stress reaction, 9.7% had depression and 6.5% dissociative amnesia. The most commonly reported symptoms were depersonalization, derealization, sleep disturbances, especially generalized sleep loss, loss of appetite, nightmares, situational anxiety, depression, mental irritability, dullness of feelings, self-blame, guilt, loss of interest, suicidal ideas, and worry about money, spouse, work and children.[147]

Four years after exposure to communal violence in Ahmedabad PTSD was found in 4.7% of children and adolescents; and 9.4% had major depression. PTSD was associated with age older than 12 and residence in Ahmedabad, the worst affected city; it was not associated with gender, religion, change of residence, income or education.[148,149]

CONCLUSION

Large-scale community surveys so far have identified the distribution of mental disorders in the population. Research has to focus on the role of the etiological factors in these disorders. In the past, knowledge of risk factors associated with pellagra psychosis and general paresis had led to preventive efforts of the underlying disorders. One has to remember that most psychiatric disorders have multiple etiological factors. Emphasis should be laid on factors that can be modified (e.g. stress), so that a fall in incidence of psychiatric disorders can be achieved. Disciplines-like genetic epidemiology, may throw more light on the inherited causes of mental disorders. Psychiatric epidemiology is expected to make substantial contributions towards better understanding of mental disorders.

REFERENCES

1. Cooper JE, Kendell RE, Gurland BJ, et al. A Comparative Study of Mental Hospital Admissions. Maudsley Monographs No. 20. London: Oxford University Press; 1972.
2. Regier DA, Burke JD. Epidemiology. In: Kaplan HI, Sadock BJ (Eds). Comprehensive Textbook of Psychiatry, 6th edition. Vol. 1. Baltimore: Williams and Wilkins; 1995. pp. 378.
3. Morris JN. Uses of Epidemiology, 3rd edition. Edinburgh: Churchill Livingstone; 1975.
4. Wing JK, Mann SA, Leff JA, Nixon JM. The concept of a 'case' in psychiatric population surveys. Psychol Med. 1978;8:203-17.
5. Kety SS. Mental illness in the biological and adoptive relatives of schizophrenic adoptees: Findings relevant to genetic and environmental factors in aetiology. Am J Psychiatry. 1983;140: 720-7.
6. Wing JK, Cooper JE, Sartorius N. The Measurement and Classification of Psychiatric Symptoms. New York: Cambridge University Press; 1974.
7. Feighner JP, Robins E, Guze SB, et al. Diagnostic criteria for use in psychiatric research. Arch Gen Psychiatry. 1972;26:57-63.
8. Peck DF. Measurement in psychiatry. In: Kendell RE, Zealley AK (Eds). Companion to Psychiatric Studies, 5th edition. Edinburgh: Churchill Livingstone; 1993. pp. 171.
9. World Health Organization. The ICD-10 Classification of Mental and Behavioural Disorders. Clinical Description and Diagnostic Guidelines. Geneva: WHO; 1992.
10. American Psychiatric Association. Diagnostic and Statistical Manual of Mental Disorders, 3rd edition. Rev Washington DC: APA; 1987.
11. Goldberg DP. The Detection of Psychiatric Illness by Questionnaire. Maudsley Monograph 21. London: Oxford University Press; 1972.
12. Goldberg DP, Hilier VP. A scaled version of the General Health Questionnaire. Psychol Med. 1979;9:139-45.
13. Endicott J, Spitzer RL. A diagnostic interview: The schedule of affective disorders and schizophrenia. Arch Gen Psychiatry. 1978;35:783-7.
14. Spitzer RL, Endicott J, Robins E. Research Dianostic Criteria, 3rd edition. New York: New York State Psychiatric Institute, Biometrics Research Division; 1978.
15. Robins LN, Helzer JE, Croughan, et al. National Institute of Mental Health Diagnostic Interview Schedule: Its history, characteristics and validity. Arch Gen Psychiatry. 1981;38: 381-9.
16. American Psychiatric Association. Diagnostic and Statistical Manual of Mental Disorders, 3rd edition. Washington DC: APA; 1980.
17. World Health Organisation. The Composite International Diagnostic Interview, Core version 1.1. Geneva: World Health Organisation; 1993.
18. World Health Organisation. Computerised CIDI (CIDI-Auto). Geneva: World Health Organisation; 1993.
19. Marcus S, Robins LN, Bucholz KK. Quick Diagnostic Interview Schedule III-R version 1.0. St. Louis: Washington University, School of Medicine. Department of Psychiatry; 1991.
20. Sartorius N, Ustun TB, Costa E Silva JA, et al. An international study of psychological problems in primary care. Arch Gen Psychiatry. 1993;50:819-24.
21. Kessler RC, McGonsgle KA, Zhao S, et al. Lifetime and twelve months prevalence of DSM III R psychiatric disorders in the United States. Arch Gen Psychiatry. 1994;51:8-19.
22. American Psychiatric Association. Diagnostic and Statistical Manual of Mental Disorders, 4th edition. Washington DC: APA; 1994.
23. World Health Organisation. Schedules for Clinical Assessment in Neuropsychiatry (SCAN). Geneva: World Health Organization; 1992.
24. Wing JK, Cooper JE, Sartorius N. Measurement and Classification of Psychiatric Symptoms: Instruction Manual for the PHC and CATEGO programme. London: Cambridge University Press; 1974.
25. World Health Organisation. Schedules for Clinical Assessment in Neuropsychiatry: Computer manual (draft version). Geneva: Wold Health Organisation; 1992.
26. Kapur RL, Carstairs GM. Indian Psychiatric Survey Schedule. Social Psychiatry. 1974;9:71-6.
27. Kapur RL, Kapur M, Carstairs GM. Indian Psychiatric Interview Schedule (IPIS). Social Psychiatry. 1974;9:61-9.
28. Hollingshead AB, Redlich FD. Social Class and Mental Illness. New York: John Wiley; 1958.
29. Faris REL, Dunham HW. Mental Disorders in Urban Areas: An Ecological Study of Schizophrenia and Other Psychosis. Chicago: University of Chicago Press; 1939.
30. Dohrenwend BP, Dohrenwend BS. Social Status and Psychological Disorder. New York: John Wiley; 1969.
31. Leighton DC, Harding JS, Macklin DB, et al. The Character of Danger, Stirling County Study No. 3. New York: Basic Books; 1963.
32. American Psychiatric Association. Diagnostic and Statistical Manual of Mental Disorders. (DSM-I) Washington DC: American Psychiatric Association; 1952.

33. Srole L, Langner TS, Michael ST, et al. Mental Health in the Metropolis: The Midtown Manhattan Study. Vol. 1. New York: McGraw Hill; 1962.
34. Regier DA, Myers JK, Kramer M, et al. The NIMH Epidemiologic Catchment Area Program. Arch Gen Psychiatry. 1984;41: 934-41.
35. Eaton WW, Holzer CE, Von Korff M, et al. The design of the Epidemiologic Catchment Area surveys. Arch Gen Psychiartry. 1984;41:942-8.
36. Robins LN, Helzer JE, Weissman MM, et al. Lifetime prevalence of specific psychiatric disorders in three sites. Arch Gen Psychiatry. 1984;41:949-58.
37. Myers JK, Weissman MM, Tischler, et al. Six-month prevalence of psychiatric disorders in three communities. Arch Gen Psychiatry. 1984;41:959-67.
38. Eaton WW, Kessler LG (Eds). Epidemiological Field Methods in Psychiatry: The NIMH Epidemiologic Catchment Area Program. New York: Academic Press; 1985.
39. Hwy HG, Yeh EK, Chang LY. Prevalence of psychiatric disorders in Taiwan defined by the Chinese Diagnostic Interview Schedule. Acta Psychiatr Scand. 1989;79:136-47.
40. Genkins R, Bebbington T, Brugha M, et al. The national psychiatric morbidity surveys of Great Britain-strategies and methods. Psychol Med. 1997;27:765-74.
41. Genkins R, Bebbington T, Brugha M, et al. The national psychiatric morbidity surveys of Great Britain: Initial findings from the household survey. Psychol Med. 1997;27:775-89.
42. Surya NC. Mental Morbidity in Pondicherry. Transaction 4. Bangalore: All India Institute of Mental Health; 1964.
43. Sethi BB, Gupta SC, Rajkumar S. Three hundred urban families: A psychiatric study. Indian J Psychiatry. 1967;9:290-302.
44. Gopinath PS. Epidemiology of mental illness in an Indian village: Prevalence survey for mental illness and mental deficiency in Sakalwara. MD thesis submitted to Bangalore University; 1968.
45. Dube KC. A study of prevalence and bio-social variables in mental illness in a rural and urban community in Uttar Pradesh, India. Acta Psychiatr Scand. 1970;46:327-59.
46. Elnagar MM, Maitra P, Rao M. Mental health in an Indian Community. Br J Psychiatry. 1971;118:499.
47. Sethi BB, Gupta SC, Rajkumar S, et al. A psychiatric survey of 500 rural families. Indian J Psychiatry. 1972;14:183.
48. Kapur RL. An illustrative presentation of population survey of mental disorders: A cross-cultural study in an Indian settings. WHO seminar on the organisation of mental health services. Addis Ababa; 1973.
49. Verghese A, Beig A, Sensman JA, et al. A social and psychiatric study of representative group of families in Vellore town. Indian J Med Res. 1973;61:608-20.
50. Thacore VR. Mental Illness in an Urban Community. Allahabad: United Publishers; 1973.
51. Sethi BB, Gupta SC, Mahendru RK, et al. Mental health and urban life: A study of 850 families. Br J Psychiatry. 1974;124: 243-6.
52. Nandi DN, Ajmany S, Ganguly H, et al. Psychiatric disorders in a rural community in West Bengal: An epidemiological study. Indian J Psychiatry. 1975;17:87-92.
53. Shah AV, Goswami UA, Maniar RG, et al. Prevalence of psychiatric disorders in Ahmedabad: An epidemiological study. Indian J Psychiatry. 1980;22:384-8.
54. Bhide A. Prevalence of psychiatric morbidity in a closed community in South India. MD thesis submitted to Bangalore University; 1982.
55. Mehta P, Joseph A, Verghese A. An epidemiological study of psychiatric disorder in rural area in Tamil Nadu. Indian J Psychiatry. 1985;27:153-8.
56. Sachdeva JS, Singh S, Sidhu BS, et al. An epidemiological study of psychiatric disorders in rural Faridkot (Punjab). Indian J Psychiatry. 1986;28:317-23.
57. Trivedi S, Chandrasekaran R, Venugopal M, et al. An epidemiological study of psychiatric morbidity in a rural area of Pondicherry. Abstracts, 41st Annual Conference of Indian Psychiatric Society; 1988.
58. Premarajan KC, Danabalan M, Chandrasekaran R, et al. Prevalence of psychiatric morbidity in urban community of Pondicherry. Indian J Psychiatry. 1993;35:99-102.
59. Verghese J, Thomas V, Jacob KS. Psychiatric Morbidity in a rural community in Kerala. Indian J Psychol Med. 1993;16:5-7.
60. Shaji S, Verghese A, Promodu K, et al. Prevalence of priority psychiatric disorders in a rural area in Kerala. Indian J Psychiatry. 1995;37:91-6.
61. Gehlot PS, Purohit DR, Jain TP, et al. Mental morbidity survey of a slum area of Udaipur. J Rajasthan Psychiatr Soc. 1979;2: 27-34.
62. Katagade VL. A study of mental morbidity in low income group families of a residential industrial area. MD thesis submitted to Banaras Hindu University, Varanasi.
63. Sharma PSVN, Muralidhar D, Gopinath PS. Neuropsychiatric morbidity in a beggars' colony. Indian J Psychiatry. 1985;27: 303-10.
64. Thacore VR, Gupta SC. Psychiatric morbidity among medical students. Indian J Psychiatry. 1972;14:339.
65. Rao PN. Psychiatric morbidity in adolescence. MD thesis submitted to Bangalore University, Bangalore.
66. Chandrasekar CR, Shamasundar C, Kapur RL, et al. Mental morbidity among graduates and research students: An epidemiological study. Indian J Psychiatry. 1980;22:89-93.
67. Nandi DN, Ajmany S, Ganguly H, et al. The incidence of mental disorders in one year in a rural community in West Bengal. Indian J Psychiatry. 1976;18:79-87.
68. Rajkumar S, Padmavathy R, Thara R, Sarada Menon M. Incidence of schizophrenia in an urban community. Indian J Psychiatry. 1993;35:18-21.
69. Wig NN, Varma VK, Mattoo SK, et al. An incidence study of schizophrenia in India. Indian J Psychiatry. 1993;35:11-7.
70. Sartorius N, Jablensky A, Korten A, et al. Early manifestation and first contact incidence of schizophrenia in different cultures. Psychol Med. 1986;16:909-28.

71. Carstairs GM, Kapur RL. The Great Universe of Kota: Stress: Change and Mental Disorder in an Indian Village. London: The Hogarth Press; 1976.
72. Padmavathy R, Rajkumar S, Kumar N, et al. Prevalence of schizophrenia in an urban community in Madras. Indian J Psychiatry. 1987;31:233-9.
73. Dube KC, Kumar N. Epidemiological study of schizophrenia. J Biosocial Science. 1971;4:187-95.
74. Sethi BB, Sharma N. Depressive disorders in the developing world. Social Psychiatry. 1985;31:217-22.
75. Kapoor R, Singh G. An epidemiological study of prevalence of depressive illness in rural Punjab. Indian J Psychiatry. 1983;25: 110-14.
76. Mohan D, Sundaram KR, Sharma RK, et al. Prevalence of drug abuse in young rural males in Punjab. Indian J Med Res. 1978; 68:689-94.
77. Deb PC, Jindal RB. Drinking in rural areas: A study in selected villages of Punjab. Monograph by Punjab Agricultural University, Ludhiana; 1974.
78. Lal B, Singh G. Drug abuse in Punjab. Br J Addiction. 1979;74: 427-41.
79. Ghulam R, Rahman I, Naqir S, et al. An epidemiological study of drug abuse in an urban population of Madhya Pradesh. Indian J Psychiatry. 1996;38:160-5.
80. Thacore VR. Drug abuse in India with special reference to Lucknow. Indian J Psychiatry. 1972;14:257-61.
81. Sethi BB, Trivedi JK. Drug abuse in rural population. Indian J Psychiatry. 1979;21:211-6.
82. Deb KC. Drug abuse in Northern India: Observation concerning Delhi and Agra. Bulletin Narcotics. 1972;24:49-53.
83. Singh G. Drug use among medical students. Prevalence and pattern of use. Indian J Psychiatry. 1979;21:332-8.
84. Singh G, Singh R, Jindal KC. Drug use among physician and medical students. Indian J Med Res. 1981;73:594-602.
85. Chakraborthy AK, Ray M, Ganguly SS. Drug abuse in medical students in Calcutta, a preliminary study. Indian J Med Res. 1990;71:455-61.
86. Sethi BB, Manchanda R. Drug abuse among medical students. Indian J Psychiatry. 1977;19:31-5.
87. Ponnudurai R, Somasundaram O, Indira TP, et al. Alcohol and drug abuse among internees. Indian J Psychiatry. 1984;26: 128-32.
88. Zulfikar Ali RV, Vancar GK. Psychoactive substance among medial students. Indian J Psychiatry. 1994;36:138-40.
89. Johnston LD, Bachman JG, O'Molley PM. Student Drug Use, Attitudes and Beliefs. Rockwille, MD: National Institute of Drug Abuse; 1982.
90. Mohan D, Prabhakar AK, Sharma PN. Prevalence and patterns of drug abuse among Delhi University students. Indian J Med Res. 1977;66:627-34.
91. Mohan D, Thomas MG, Prabhu GG. Prevalence of drug abuse among high school population. Indian J Psychiatry. 1978;20: 20-4.
92. Verma VK, Gosh A. Drug abuse amongst college students. Indian J Psychiatry. 1977;19:1-10.
93. Gupta R, Narang RL, Singh S, et al. Drug abuse among rickshaw pullers in the industrial town of Ludhiana. Indian J Psychiatry. 1986;28:145-9.
94. Mohan D, Desai NG, Chopra A, et al. A rapid survey on substance abuse disorders in the urban slum of New Delhi. Indian J Med Res. 1992;96:122-7.
95. Bansal RK, Banerjee S. Substance use by child labourers. Indian J Psychiatry. 1993;35:159-62.
96. Mahanta J, Chaturvedi H K, Phukan RK. Opium addiction in Assam: A trend analysis. Indian J Psychitry. 1997;39:143-6.
97. Dube KC, Handa SK. Drug use in health and mental illness in an Indian population. Br. J Psychiatry. 1971;118:345-9.
98. Verma VK, Singh A, Singh S, et al. Extent and pattern of alcohol use and alcohol related problems in North India. Indian J Psychiatry. 1980;22:331-7.
99. Lal B, Singh G. Alcohol consumption in Punjab. Indian J Psychiatry. 1978;20:212-6.
100. Ponnudurai R, Jayakar J, Raju B, et al. An epidemiological study of alcoholism. Indian J Psychiatry. 1991;33:176-9.
101. Chakravarthy C. Community workers estimate of drinking and alcohol related problems in rural areas. Indian J Psychol Med. 1990;13:49-56.
102. Mathrubootham N. Epidemiological study of drinking behaviour in a rural population. PhD thesis submitted to University of Madras.
103. ICMR-CAR-CMH. Longitudinal study of mental health problems in a PHC area. Indian Council of Medical Research Centre for advanced research on community mental health. NIMHANS, Bangalore, Unpublished report.
104. Singh G. Epidemiology of alcohol abuse in India. In: Ray R, Pickens RW (Eds). Proceedings of the Indo-US Symposium on Alcohol and Drug Abuse. NIMHANS Publication No 20, Bangalore; 1989. pp. 3-11.
105. Mohan D. In: Mohan D, Sethi SH, Tongue E (Eds). Current research in drug abuse in India. New Delhi: Japyee Brothers; 1981.
106. Dube KC, Kumar A, Kumar N, et al. Prevalence and patterns of drug use among college students. Acta Psychatr Scand. 1978;57:336-56.
107. Verma VK, Dang R. Non-medical use of drugs amongst school and college students. Indian J Psychiatry. 1979;21:228-34.
108. Guruswamy R, Khanna S. Prevalence of obsessive compulsive disorders in rural population in Karnataka. Abstracts of scientific papers. 48th Annual National Conference of the Indian Psychiatric Society, Bangalore; 1996.
109. Lal N, Sethi BB. Estimate of mental ill health in children in an urban community. Indian J Pediatr; 4. pp. 55-64.
110. Jiloha RC, Murthy RS. An epidemiological study of psychiatric problems in school children. Child Psychiatr Quart. 1981;3:28.
111. Deivasigamani TR. Psychiatric morbidity in school children: An epidemiological study. Indian J Psychiatry. 1990;32:235-40.

112. Banerjee T. Psychiatric morbidity among rural primary school children in West Bengal. Indian J Psychiatry. 1997;39:130-35.
113. Misra G, Tandon SK, Tripathi KN, et al. Psychiatric morbidity in children: An epidemiological study. Indian J Behav Sci. 1994;4: 109-13.
114. Giel R, DeArango MV, Climent GE, et al. Childhood mental disorders in primary health care: Results of observation in 4 developing countries. Paediatrics. 1981;68:677-83.
115. Srinivasamurthy R, Ghose A, Verma VK. Behaviour disorders in childhood and adolescence. Indian J Psychiatry. 1974;16: 229-37.
116. Chandra R, Srinivasan S, Chandrasekaran R, et al. The prevalence of mental disorders in school age children attending a general paediatric department in Southern India. Acta Psychiatr Scand. 1993;87:192-6.
117. Ramachandran V, SaradaMenon M, Ramamurty B. Psychiatric disorders in subjects aged over 50. Indian J Psychiatry. 1979;22: 193-8.
118. VenkobaRao A, Madhavan T. Geropsychiatric morbidity survey in a semi-urban area near Madurai. Indian J Psychiatry. 1982; 24:258-67.
119. Nandi PS, Banerjee G, Mukherjee SP, et al. A study of psychiatric morbidity of elderly population of a rural community in West Bengal. Indian J Psychiatry. 1997;39:122-9.
120. Shaji S, Promodu K, Abraham T, et al. An epidemiological study of dementia in a rural community in Kerala, India. Br J Psychiatry. 1996;168:745-9.
121. Norris F, Friedman M, Watson P. 60,000 disaster victims speak, Part I: An empirical review of the empirical literature, 1981-2001. Psychiatry. 2002;65:207-39.
122. Reddy MV, Chandrasekar CR. Prevalence of mental and behavioural disorders in India: A metaanalysis. Indian J Psychiatry. 1998;40:149-57.
123. Ganguli HC. Epidemiological finding on prevalence of mental disorders in India. Indian J Psychiatry. 2000;42:14-20.
124. Gururaj G, Girish N, Isaac MK. Mental, neurological and substance abuse disorders: Strategies towards a systems approach, NCMH Background Papers-Burden of Disease in India. Ministry of Health and Family Welfare, New Delhi; 2005.
125. World Health organization. India. Viewed 6 October 2013, <http://whoindia.org/en/section102/section201_888.htm>
126. Kar GC. Disaster and mental health. Indian J Psychiatry. 2000;42:3-13.
127. Mohandas E. Roadmap to Indian Psychiatry. Indian J Psychiatry. 2009;51:173-9.
128. Shastri PC. Promotion and prevention in child mental health. Indian J Psychiatry. 2009;51:88-95.
129. Reddy IR. Making psychiatry a household word. Indian J Psychiatry. 2007;49:10-8.
130. Rao TSS. Managing impact of natural disasters: some mental health issues. Indian J Psychiatry. 2004;46:289-92.
131. Desai NG. Public mental health: An evolving imperative. Indian J Psychiatry. 2006;48:135-7.
132. Khandelwal SK. The joy of mental health: Some popular writings of Dr. NN Wig Book Review. Indian J Psychiatry. 2006;48:207-8.
133. Kar N, Jagadisha T, Sharma PS, Murali N, Mehrotra S. Mental health consequences of the trauma of supercyclone 1999 in Orissa. Indian J Psychiatry. 2004;46:228-37.
134. Sharan P, Chaudhary G, Kavathekar SA, Saxena S. Preliminary report of psychiatric disorders in survivors of a severe earthquake. Am J Psychiatry. 1996;153:556-8.
135. Desai NG, Gupta DK, Srivastava RK. Prevalence, pattern and predictors of mental health morbidity following an intermediate disaster in an urban slum in Delhi: A modified cohort study. Indian J Psychiatry. 2004;46:39-51.
136. Kar N, Bastia BK. Post-traumatic stress disorder, depression and generalised anxiety disorder in adolescents after a natural disaster: A study of comorbidity. Clin Pract Epidemiol Mental Health. 2006;2:17.
137. Kar N, Mohapatra PK, Nayak KC, Pattnaik P, Swain SP, Kar HC. Post-traumatic stress disorder in children and adolescents one year after a super-cyclone in Orissa, India: Exploring cross-cultural validity and vulnerability factors. BMC Psychiatry. 2007;7:8.
138. Nambi S, Desai NG, Shah S. Mental health morbidity and service needs in Tsunami affected population in coastal Tamil Nadu. Indian J Psychiatry. 2007;49:S2-3.
139. George C, Sunny G, John J. Disaster experience, substance abuse, social factors and severe psychological distress in male survivors of the 2004 Tsunami in South India. Indian J Psychiatry. 2007;49S:47.
140. Math SB, Girimaji SC, Benegal V, Uday Kumar GS, Hamza A, Nagaraja D. Tsunami: Psychosocial aspects of Andaman and Nicobar islands. Assessments and intervention in the early phase. Int Rev Psychiatry. 2006;18:233-9. [PubMed]
141. Math SB, John JP, Girimaji SC, Benegal V, Sunny B, Krishnakanth K, et al. Comparative study of psychiatric morbidity among the displaced and non-displaced populations in the Andaman and Nicobar Islands following the Tsunami. Prehosp Disaster Med. 2008;23:29-34. [PubMed]
142. Math SB, Tandon S, Girimaji SC, Benegal V, Kumar U, Hamza A, et al. Psychological impact of the Tsunami on children and adolescents from the andaman and nicobar islands: Prim Care Companion. J Clin Psychiatry. 2008;10:31-7.
143. Narayanan HS, Sathyabati K, Nardev G, Thakar S. Grief reaction among bereaved relatives following a fire disaster in a circus. NIMHANS J. 1987;5:13-21.
144. Sharma A, Rao S, Srinivas S. Mandi Dabwali fire disaster. Psychological impact on school children after two months-preliminary findings. Indian J Psychiatry. 1998;40S:51-2.
145. Murthy RS. In: Proceedings of National workshop on psychosocial consequences of disasters. Bangalore: NIMHANS; 1997. Psychological consequences of Bhopal disaster.
146. Bhiman A. Mental health consequences of Bhopal gas tragedy. Paper presented in the 17th World Congress of Social Psychiatry, Agra; 2001.

147. Shetty H, Chhabria A. In Proceedings of National workshop on Psychosocial consequences of disasters. Bangalore: NIMHANS; 1997. Bombay riots.
148. Gautam S, Gupta ID, Batra L, Sharma H, Khandelwal R, Pant A. Psychiatric morbidity among victims of bomb blast. Indian J Psychiatry. 1998;40:41-5.
149. Vankar GK, Banwari G, Parikh V, Shah H. PTSD in children and adolescents: Four years after the communal violence. Indian J Psychiatry. 2007;49S:4.

SUGGESTED READING

1. D'Netto TB. Psychiatric first aid in community disasters, with special reference to Nuclear warfare. Indian J Psychiatry. 1963;3:176-80.
2. Falconer DS. Introduction of Quantitative Genetics. New York: John Wiley; 1989.
3. Feinstein A. Clinical Epidemiology. Philadelphia: WB Saunders; 1985.
4. Freedman DX. Psychiatry epidemiology counts. Arch Gen Psychiatry. 1984;41:931-3.
5. Kar N, Misra BN. Mental health care following disasters. Bhubaneswar: Quality of Life Research and Development Foundation; 2008.
6. Kar N. Psychosocial issues following a natural disaster in a developing country: A qualitative longitudinal observational study. Int J Disaster Med. 2006;4:169-76.
7. Murali N, Kar N. Jagadisha Recognition and clinical assessment of childhood PTSD. Indian J Psychiatry 2002;44:82-3. [PMC free article] [PubMed]
8. Murthy RS, Isaac MK. Mental health needs of Bhopal disaster victims and training of medical officers in mental health aspects. Indian J Med Res. 1987;86:51-8. [PubMed]
9. Murthy RS, Kar N, Sekar K, Swain S, Mishra V, Daniel U. Evaluation report on psychosocial care of survivors of supercyclone in Orissa. Bhubaneswar: Sneha Aviyan, Action Aid; Bangalore: NIMHANS; 2003.
10. Murthy RS. Introduction to psychiatry: Book Review. Indian J Psychiatry. 2009;51:72.
11. Park K. Preventive and Social Medicine. Pub: M/S Banarsidas Bhanot, Jabalpur, India; 2012.
12. Rajkumar AP, Premkumar TS, Tharyan P. Coping with the Asian Tsunami: Perspectives from Tamil Nadu, India on the determinants of resilience in the face of adversity. Soc Sci Med. 2008;67:844-53.
13. Rao K. Lessons learnt in mental health and psychosocial care in India after disasters. Int Rev Psychiatry. 2006;18:547-52.
14. Sahu RN, Naik GP, Dusad A, Agrawal VK. Neurocognitive function in women affected by the Bhopal gas disaster. Indian J Psychiatry. 2005;47:51-3.
15. Sham P. Genetic epidemiology. Br Med Bulletin. 1996;52: 408-33.
16. Shethi BB, Sharma M, Trivedi JK, Singh H. Psychiatric morbidity in patients attending clinics in gas affected areas in Bhopal. Indian J Med Res. 1987;86S:45-50.
17. Shetty H. Awakening the kundalini of humour. Indian J Psychiatry. 2006;48:267-71.
18. Shetty H. In: Proceedings of National workshop on Psychosocial consequences of disasters. Bangalore: NIMHANS; 1997. Marathawada earthquake.
19. Vijayakumar L, Kannan GK, Ganesh Kumar B, Devarajan P. Do all children need intervention after exposure to Tsunami? Int Rev Psychiatry. 2006;18:515-22. [PubMed]
20. Vijaykumar L, Thara R, John S, Chellappa S. Psychosocial interventions after Tsunami in Tamil Nadu, India. Int Rev Psychiatry 2006;18:225-31. [PubMed]

CHAPTER 4

Organic Mental Disorders

S Kalyanasundaram, Johnson Pradeep R

INTRODUCTION

Organic mental disorders are group of conditions caused directly by abnormalities of the brain structures or by alterations of brain neurochemistry or neurophysiology. They are traditionally called as organic mental disorders or organic brain disorders to distinguish them from the functional disorders such as schizophrenia or depression. This terminology "functional" and "organic" has been removed from most of the classificatory systems since neurodiagnostics and neurobiological evidences have found that every psychiatric condition had a biological component. With the advent of newer technologies and new evidences; newer etiologies are discovered and newer medications are manufactured. In a country like India, where the population is increasing and there are significant improvements in economic and health care, the quantum of dementia and other cognitive disorders are increasing. Global prevalence of dementia in 2010 was estimated to be 35.6 million and in India it is 3.7 million. It is projected to double every 20 years, to 65.7 million in 2030 and 115.4 million in 2050 and has been attributed to increase in the numbers of people with dementia in LIMC. Hence, it is important to identify these disorders and consider early management to prevent further complications and disability.

HISTORY

In the 5th century BC, the father of medicine Hippocrates described for the first time the conditions of "phrenitis" and "paraphrenitis" which in the present day is related to delirium. He referred to a term called as lethargus to describe inertia and a dulling of the senses and suggested that lethargus can turn into phrenitis and back again into lethargus. The term "delirium" was coined by Aulus Cornelius Celsus (greatest Roman medical writers) to describe mental disorders. "Delirare" translated from Latin means "to be off the track" or "to go wrong" and was used to define general mental illness. Organic mental disorders were divided into acute and chronic type by Aretaeus of Cappadocia. Later Galen introduced the concept of primary and secondary brain diseases. Also the concept of hyper- and hypoactive forms of delirium have been described by Galen. Karl Bonhoeffer (1909) made a significant contribution to the concept of organic mental disorders. He stated that the brain reacts to exogenic irritants in a nonspecific manner and that the number of such reactions is limited and depends on the constitution of a person. Based on this, authors have suggested that completely different etiological phenomena may evoke similar psychotic symptoms. Bonhoeffer had suggested five acute brain reactions which include delirium, amentia, a twilight state (or epileptic type), excitement and acute hallucinosis. In 1913, a German, psychiatrist and philosopher Karl Jaspers gave more clarity to mental illness and was the first who described consciousness disorder symptoms. Eugen Bleuler gave a detailed definition of organic brain syndrome and Manfred Bleuler described symptoms of organic brain disorder. The modern concept of delirium was provided by an American psychiatrist Zbigniew J Lipowski in 1980. He sub-classified delirium into increased, reduced, or mixed motor activity during delirium. Philippe Pinel was credited to give detailed description of dementia. There has been a varied course in the evolution of the concept of organic mental disorders. With the enormous development of neuroimaging, genetic studies, biomarkers and understanding of these disorders, the conceptualization of organic mental disorders may change.

DEFINITIONS

Confusion

It refers to clinical signs and symptoms where patient is unable to think with clarity and coherence. It can manifest in both psychiatric and organic conditions. Cognitive impairment is preferred than confusion and is one of the earliest symptom of insult to the brain. In acute conditions the confusion is due to impairment of consciousness, however in chronic condition it is due to disruption of thought processes due to structural brain damage. Sometimes confusion can present without any structural damage in psychiatric conditions such as heightened emotional reactions and early stages of psychotic conditions.

Clouding of Consciousness

Clouding of consciousness is also known as brain fog or mental fog. There is mild global impairment of cognitive functions in addition to decreased awareness of environment. It is described as an abnormality in the "regulation" of the "overall level of consciousness that is mild and less severe than a delirium. It is the mildest form of impairment of consciousness. The sufferer experiences a subjective sensation of mental clouding described as feeling "foggy". This may affect performance on virtually any cognitive task. According to Jasper, they may have additional phenomenon such as vivid affects, hallucinations and fantasies.

Minimally Conscious State

The criterion for minimally conscious state (MCS) was proposed by Aspen group to categorize patients who are not in a vegetative state but are unable to communicate consistently. It is a condition where the patients show limited but clear evidence of awareness of themself or their environment, on a reproducible or sustained basis, by at least one of the following behaviors: following simple commands, gestural or verbal yes/no response (regardless of accuracy), intelligible speech, purposeful behavior (including movements or affective behavior that take place in relation to stimuli in the environment and are not due to reflexive activity). According to[1] emergence from the minimally conscious state is defined by the ability to communicate or use objects functionally and they further improvement occurs better than in vegetative states.[2,3]

Locked-in Syndrome

Locked-in syndrome is defined by sustained eye opening, awareness of the environment, aphonia or hypophonia, quadriplegia or quadriparesis, and vertical or lateral eye movement or blinking of the upper eyelid to signal yes/no responses. The main method of communication is by eyes or eyelid movements. The term was introduced by Plum and Posner to describe the quadriplegia and anarthria resulting from the disruption of corticospinal and corticobulbar pathways, respectively.[4,5]

Vegetative State

The patients in this state are awake but are unaware of themselves or their environment. The term vegetative is defined as "an organic body capable of growth and development but devoid of sensation and thought". There are two terms related to vegetative states. "Persistent vegetative state" which is a reversible state and defined as a vegetative state remaining 1 month after acute traumatic or non-traumatic brain damage and "permanent vegetative state" which is irreversible and present if the vegetative state is prolonged for 3 months after nontraumatic brain damage or 12 months after traumatic injury.[6-9]

Twilight States

It is one of the forms of exogenous reaction to pathogenic factors according to Bonhoeffer's. It is a condition where there is an interruption in the continuity of consciousness and it has an abrupt onset and termination. There is clouding and narrowing of consciousness, but patients may be able to perform certain activities like driving, walking, etc. and they have amnesia for the event. It usually occurs in patients with epilepsy, head injury, alcoholism, dissociative disorders, etc. It may lead to violent behaviors and such patients who are vulnerable to this phenomenon may have pre-existing organic brain pathology. The duration may last from few hours to weeks. Oneiroid state is a similar clinical phenomenon where there is narrowing of consciousness with multiple scenic hallucinations but in this condition they remember the events compared to twilight states. This condition is perceived as strange and dream-like and has been found in patients who are very dependent on others and schizophrenic patients. It is used to describe hysterical manifestations in addition to acute organic reactions.

Coma

It is a state of unresponsiveness characterized by the absence of arousal and consciousness. In this condition the patient lies with the eyes closed, cannot be aroused, and has no awareness of self and surroundings. They will not produce spontaneous periods of wakefulness or eye-opening with significant stimulation. In order to distinguish it from syncope, concussion, or other states of transient unconsciousness, coma must persist for at least one hour. Patient who survive the coma gradually improve within 2 to 4 weeks but the recovery may progress to vegetative or minimally conscious state before a complete consciousness state is achieved.[4]

Delirium

It is a neuropsychiatric syndrome characterized by disturbances in the baseline cognitions such as consciousness, orientation, memory, perception, thought and behavior; not explained by pre-existing or evolving neurocognitive disorder. It is a reversible condition and has an acute onset, fluctuating course within the day and worsening in the evening or night due to decreased stimuli. The etiology could be substance withdrawal, medication use, exposure to toxins or abnormalities of metabolic parameters. It is associated with high morbidity and mortality. They manifest with features of irritability, anger, euphoria, aggression, sleep wake disturbances, screaming, moaning and sometimes they may be apathetic and silent.

Dementia

Dementia is a syndrome due to disease of the brain—usually of a chronic or progressive nature—in which there is disturbance of multiple higher cortical functions, including memory, thinking, orientation, comprehension, calculation, learning capacity, language, and judgement. Consciousness is not clouded. The impairments of cognitive function are commonly accompanied, and occasionally preceded, by deterioration in emotional control, social behavior, or motivation. This syndrome occurs in a large number of conditions primarily or secondarily affecting the brain. The four most common subtypes in order of frequency are Alzheimer's disease, vascular dementia (VaD), dementia with Lewy bodies (DLB), and frontotemporal dementia (FTD).[10,11]

CLASSIFICATION

In DSM-4, the term "organic mental disorder" was removed for the first time. The disorders were divided into three groups: (1) delirium, dementia, amnestic disorders, and other cognitive disorder (2) mental disorders due to general medical conditions and (3) substance-related disorders. Previous classifications such as organic mood or organic anxiety disorders were subsumed under second category as mentioned above.[12]

In the DSM-5,[13] dementia and amnestic disorders are subsumed under neurocognitive disorders and delirium is retained. The delirium has further specifiers such as acute or persistent course and type of delirium (hyperactive, hypoactive and mixed). The neurocognitive disorders (NCD) include group of disorders in which the primary clinical deficit is in cognitive functions, which are acquired rather than developmental. Even though the psychiatric disorders also have cognitive dysfunctions, only those disorders whose core features are cognitive are included in this category. The NCD is further divided into major and minor. The criteria for the major NCD is given below and has specifiers of the etiological factors and further specifiers such as severity and association of behavioral disturbances. The difference between major and minor NCD are the time course, severity of cognitive impairment, characteristic domains affected and associated symptoms. In DSM-5, new separate criterias are presented for frontotemporal, Lewy body, traumatic brain injury, substance/medication, HIV infection, prion disease, Parkinson's disease, Huntington's disease and other medical conditions.

- Evidence of significant cognitive decline from a previous level of performance in one or more area of cognitive domains (complex attention, executive function, learning and memory, language, perceptual-motor or social cognition) based on:
  - Concern of the individual, a knowledgeable informant or the clinician that there has been a significant decline in cognitive function
  - Substantial impairment in cognitive performance, preferably documented by standardized neuro-psychological testing or, in its absence, another quantified clinical assessment.
- The cognitive deficits interfere with independence in everyday activities.
- The cognitive deficits do not occur exclusively in the context of a delirium.
- The cognitive deficits are not better explained by another mental disorder (e.g. major depressive disorder, schizophrenia).

In India, the International Classification of Diseases (ICD)[14] system of classification is used commonly. It has similar flaws such as the preliminary editions of DSM and retains the psychotic and nonpsychotic dichotomy. In the ICD-10 version, the term "organic mental disorder" continues to find its place and has introduced a new term called "mild cognitive disorder" which has been associated with acquired immunodeficiency syndrome (AIDS).

With the advent of newer evidences, newer classificatory systems would evolve and lead to better understanding of the psychiatric conditions. However, we should not forget the value of classical teaching of phenomenology because even with advanced neuroimaging diagnostic abilities of these newer methods are only complimentary and not confirmatory.

DELIRIUM

Delirium is one of the most common and serious medical illness. Many terminologies have been used to describe it such as "acute confusional state", acute brain syndrome or toxic metabolic syndrome; however, the "acute confusional state" is accepted as the synonym for delirium. Delirium has been derived from the word *delirare* which means to become "crazy or to rave". This term was first used by Celsus in 1st AD. It has been documented and described in the literature for more than 2000 years. Hippocrates described the subtypes of delirium hyperactive as phrenitis and hypoactive as lethargus. The outcome of delirium is usually adverse due to poor diagnosis and fluctuating nature of the syndrome.[15]

Epidemiology

The prevalence of delirium in the community is lower and is estimated to be 1 to 2%. However, the rates are higher in hospitalized patients, it has varied from 10 to 31% during the time of admission and an incidence of 3 to 29% during the hospitalization. There have been significantly increased prevalence rates in different settings in the hospitals. In the intensive care units a prevalence of 80%, in palliative care units the rates are 85% and in surgical settings an incidence of 10 to 70% after surgery.[16]Also, there has been higher rates are noticed in especially in patients undergoing cardiothoracic surgery, emergency orthopedic procedures (repair of a hip fracture), vascular surgery, or cataract removal.[17] In India, the prevalence of delirium has varied from 3 to 27% in hospitalized patients (>65 years) and an incidence of 4.3% in postcataractomy patients in a year. Grover et al. found a prevalence of 30 to 38% for all ages and 48 % in patients more than 60 years.[18,19]

Clinical Types

Three clinical forms of delirium have been described, they include hyperactive, hypoactive, and mixed, based on psychomotor behavior. Even though ICD-10 or DSM-IV do not recognize this classification, several studies have confirmed the existence. The *hyperactive subtype* is most easily identified and manifests as increased psychomotor activity, hypervigilance, restlessness, agitation, aggression, mood lability, disruptive behavior hallucinations and delusions.[20] However, the *hypoactive form* is the most common type in the elderly and manifests as withdrawn behavior, drowsiness, lethargy, apathy, confusion and decreased psychomotor. They have reduced spontaneity and answer slowly to questions and without. In a study by Khurana et al, they found a high prevalence of 65% of hypoactive delirium elderly delirious patients who were hospitalized. This subtype is usually difficult to recognize and can be easily missed.[18] *Mixed subtype* is the most common subtype and consists of features of both the types mentioned above. *Persistent delirium* defined as delirium present on admission and at the time of discharge or beyond.[15] *Excited delirium syndrome* is a syndrome with uncertain, likely multiple, etiologies. It is characterized by delirium, agitation, acidosis, and hyperadrenergic autonomic dysfunction, typically in the setting of acute-on-chronic drug abuse or serious mental illness.[21]

Subsyndromal Delirium

Recently a new concept of subsyndromal deliruim has emerged. It is defined as the presence of one or more core diagnostic symptoms (inattention, altered level of consciousness, disorientation and perceptual disturbances) that do not meet the full criteria for delirium and may not progress to full blown delirium.[22] In intensive care units, the prevalence rates of 30–50% have been reported and the incidence rate was 5.2 per 100 person-weeks of follow-up.[23] The risk factors for this type are also similar to the delirium. This variety needs detailed attention and early identification and treatment. Subsyndromal delirium occurs in 21 to 76% of hospitalized elderly people in long-term care elderly residents, with dementia, the occurrence was 48.4 or 50.3%, depending on the criteria used. A recent cohort study has found that 68 of the 104 residents had incident subsyndromal delirium during 6 months of observation. The risk factors for subsyndromal delirium are similar to those for classical overt *delirium.*[24]

Clinical Features

Delirium has been defined as "the rapid onset of symptoms that tend to fluctuate even during the same day with an altered level of consciousness, global disturbance of cognition or perceptual abnormalities and evidence of physical cause, substance intoxication or withdrawal, or multiple etiologies" according to APA.[25] The diagnosis is based on detailed history, physical examination, mental state examination and laboratory investigations. The central features of delirium are sudden or acute onset, fluctuating course and inattention. The symptom fluctuations are unpredictable, intermittent, and often worse at night.

Disturbance in consciousness: It is one of the earliest symptoms and fluctuates frequently. The disturbances may be from mild drowsiness to coma in advanced cases. However, in hyperactive delirium as such in alcohol or sedative withdrawal, hypervigilance and hyperactivity may be noticed. The disturbance is seen mainly in the evening when environmental stimulation is at its lowest. Patients also present with disorientation to time first and then to place. In terms of memory, they have deficits in short-term memory and retrieval of information.

Disturbance in psychomotor activity: It is also another important clinical feature of delirium it may be increased or decreased.

Disturbances in thought also present with disorganized thinking, which can present as incoherent speech, irrelevant conversation or illogical flow of ideas. They have difficult in taking appropriate decisions or do simple tasks. The patients can have poor judgment and insight. They can also present with delusions in 30% of patients and they are predominantly paranoid or persecutory in nature.

Disturbances in perception also present with perceptual disturbances. They may include illusions, misinterpretations and hallucinations (visual). The content of the hallucinations may range from simple colors, lines, or shapes to dangerous animals or bizarre images. They also present with emotional disturbances, such as anxiety, fear, irritability, anger, depression, and euphoria.

Other symptoms found delirium include sleep-wake cycle disturbance, characterized by an excessive daytime sleepiness with insomnia at night, sleep fragmentation, reduction of sleep or complete sleep-cycle reversal and disturbance of circadian rhythm. Sundowning syndrome seen in delirium and is characterized by worsening of disruptive behavior in the late afternoon or evening. This aspect has been attributed to sleep fragmentation, disturbance of circadian rhythm, fatigue and reduced sensory input toward the evening.

In children and adolescents, the most common symptoms included sleep-wake cycle disturbance and impaired orientation. The other symptoms which they presented were impaired attention (89.5%), impaired short-term memory (84.2%), agitation (68.4%), and lability of affect (60.5%). However, delusions and hallucinations were only in few. The pathology detected in them includes infection of various types, followed by neoplasms.[18]

Pathophysiology

The exact pathophysiology of delirium is not clear. However various theories have been proposed. Based on the current understanding and evidence neurotransmission disruption has been proposed. In the neurotransmitter hypothesis, cholinergic deficits and dopaminergic excess has been implicated in the development of delirium.[26] There has been a strong evidence for the role of cholinergic system in the pathophysiology of delirium based on the evidence that the cholinergic system has an important role in cognition and attention and anticholinergic properties may precipitate delirium in vulnerable individuals based on this hypothesis a surrogate marker called "serum anticholinergic activity" (SAA) has been developed to detect anticholinergic activity and there is a relationship between SAA levels and development of delirium.[27]

Excessive dopamine has also been implicated in the pathophysiology of delirium. It has been found that the dopamine plays a significant role in the motor activity and cognitive functions and based on the evidence that dopaminergic drugs cause delirium in Parkinson's disease. Also, excess dopamine has been associated with emergence of psychotic symptoms. All these evidences reinforce the fact that excessive dopamine could have a role in delirium.[28]

Researchers have found evidence for increased production of cytokines after trauma, infection or postoperative which may induce delirium in vulnerable patients. A recent review of older adults suggested that increase in cytokines lead to development of cognitive dysfunction which is observed in delirium.[29] These evidences suggest an inflammatory hypothesis for the pathophysiology of delirium. Other hypothesis proposed are hypercortisolemia, medication induced (valproate) and lower plasma cholinesterases.[30,31]

Risk Factors

The identification of risk factors are important for the prevention and early management of delirium. The etiology of delirium could be a single factor (as in alcohol withdrawal) or multifactorial. Researchers have categorized the risk factors into predisposing (vulnerability to develop delirium) and precipitating (acute factors triggering delirium). The predisposing factors have been found to contribute more to the development of delirium than precipitating factors. The predisposing factors are advanced age, pre-existing dementia (second most common), male gender, pre-existing depression, visual and hearing impairment, functional dependence, dehydration and malnutrition, poly pharmacy (mainly psychoactive drugs), alcohol abuse and coexistence of multiple, and severe medical conditions. The most common precipitating factors are intercurrent illnesses (e.g. infections), iatrogenic complications, metabolic derangements, primary neurological conditions (e.g. acute stroke), surgery, drugs (benzodiazepines, narcotic analgesics, drugs with anticholinergic effects and uncontrolled pain have also been associated with the development of delirium.[17]

Prognosis

Delirium is usually reversible within 10 to 12 days but can vary in some cases and persist for more than 2 months. In a study, they found that one-third of patients continued to remain in delirium for almost 6 months. Delirium has been associated with increased hospital stay, cognitive decline, functional decline, institutionalization and mortality.[32] The incident delirium was found to accelerates the trajectory of cognitive decline in hospitalized elderly patients with Alzheimer's disease.

Diagnosis

The diagnosis of delirium is purely clinical and there are no specific diagnostic tests. It is made based on clinical history, observation and comprehensive physical and a detailed mental state examination. History obtained from family members, nursing staff and care givers may be very valuable. Even thogh there are around 11 scales to identify delirium the confusion assessment method (CAM) has the most evidence for its use as a bedside tool. However, the minimental status examination (MMSE) was found to have the least useful test for identifying delirium.[33] An attempt should be made by the physician to identify the underlying cause for the delirium. Some of the important investigations to be considered include complete blood count, blood urea, creatinine levels, electrolytes, blood sugar, C-reactive protein, liver function, thyroid function and plasma ammonia. EEG and imaging may be warranted in cases where the physicians are suspecting a intracranial pathology.

DSM-5 Diagnostic Criteria for Delirium

a. A disturbance in attention (i.e. reduced ability to direct, focus, sustain, and shift attention) and awareness (reduced orientation to the environment).
b. The disturbance develops over a short period of time (usually hours to a few days), represents a change from baseline attention and awareness, and tends to fluctuate in severity during the course of a day.
c. An additional disturbance in cognition (e.g. memory deficit, disorientation, language, visuospatial ability, or perception).
d. The disturbances in criteria a and c are not better explained by another pre-existing, established, or evolving neurocognitive disorder and do not occur in the context of a severely reduced level of arousal, such as coma.
e. There is evidence from the history, physical examination, or laboratory findings that the disturbance is a direct physiological consequence of another medical condition, substance intoxication or withdrawal (i.e. due to a drug of abuse or to a medication), or exposure to a toxin, or is due to multiple etiologies.

Specify whether

Substance intoxication delirium: This diagnosis should be made instead of substance intoxication when the symptoms in criteria a and c predominate in the clinical picture and when they are sufficiently severe to warrant clinical attention.

PREVENTION

Studies report that one-third of delirium episodes could be prevented and prevention as a cost-effective strategy.[34,35] In the Yale Delirium Prevention Trial, the intervention was focussed towards minimizing 6 risk factors in elderly patients (≥70 years of age) who were at risk for developing delirium. Some of the interventions used included orientation activities for the cognitively impaired, early mobilization, preventing sleep deprivation, minimizing the use of psychoactive drugs, use of eyeglasses and hearing aids, and treating volume depletion. In the intervention group, the delirium incidence had reduced to 9.9% compared with 15% in the usual care. In another study, patients with post hip fractures who were randomized to either standard care versus the addition of a geriatrics consultation preoperatively or immediately after hip repair, providing recommendations based on a structured protocol. They found that the incidence of delirium reduced to 32% in the geriatrics consultation group versus 50% in the standard care group.[36,37]

Regarding the role of medication in the prevention of delirium, a Cochrane review found 6 RCT in hospitalized surgical patients and found that low-dose haloperidol prophylaxis was effective in reducing the severity, duration of delirium and reduced the length of hospital stay in hip surgery patients, but it did not prevent delirium occurrence. Another review by Campbell et al. evaluated 9 studies and found that use of a single-dose risperidone after cardiac surgery decreased delirium incidence compared to placebo.[38-40]

Treatment

Delirium is a medical emergency and an attempt should be made to identify the underlying cause. The first line of treatment is nonpharmacological intervention and this involves providing supportive care, preventing complications and treating behavioral problems. Supportive care involves close monitoring and care by nursing staff. They need to take care of the patient's airway, adequate nutrition, correction and prevention of dehydration vital sign monitoring, attention to oral intake, prevention of aspiration, encourage of mobility, and ensuring a good sleep pattern. It is also important to involve the family and caregivers. They can assist the health professionals in facilitating effective communication, reorientating the patient, calm, protect, and support older people.[34,35] Physical restraint has to use mainly to control violent behavior or to prevent the removal of important devices, such as endotracheal tubes.[34]

Environmental manipulation such as ensuring that there is a big clock and a calendar in the room; verbal reminders of the time, day, and place frequently; avoiding change in paramedical/nursing staff changes; transferring the patient to an isolated room, if possible; obtaining familiar possessions from home (e.g. family picture); avoiding sensory deprivation (e.g. windowless room) or sensory overload (e.g. too much noise); reducing sensory impairment (including vision and hearing loss) by the use of corrective devices.

The pharmacological interventions should be considered mainly in the management of behavioral disturbances. Haloperidol or olanzapine, lower doses and for a short period are recommended, however, it is better avoided in Parkinson's disease or DLB patients.[35] In alcohol and benzodiazepine withdrawal, or neuroleptic malignant syndrome, benzodiazepines have been recommended. Regarding the use of cholinesterase inhibitors no specific evidence from controlled trials that donepezil or rivastigmine are effective in the treatment of this medical condition.[41]

DEGENERATIVE DEMENTIAS

DEMENTIA

Aging is a worldwide phenomenon. Health facilities in the past few years have increased the life expectancy and are providing better health care. However, it has increased the burden of noncommunicable disorders such as dementia and psychiatric illnesses. The word dementia is derived from the Latin word "dementatus" meaning out of one's mind. Dementia is not part of normal aging but a syndrome due to disease of the brain, usually of a chronic or progressive nature, in which there is an intact consciousness but there is disturbance of multiple higher cortical functions, including memory, thinking, orientation, comprehension, calculation, learning capacity, language, and judgment.[42]

Epidemiology

There have been improvements in the data related to dementia and Alzheimer's Disease International (ADI) in 2005, commissioned a panel of experts to review all available epidemiological data and reach a consensus estimate of prevalence in each of 14 world regions.[43] They estimated that the prevalence of dementia in people aged 60 years and above was 24.3 million in 2001, 60% were living in low middle income countries (LMIC). The global prevalence of dementia in 2010 was estimated to be 35.6 million people worldwide were living. It is projected to double every 20 years, to 65.7 million in 2030 and 115.4 million in 2050 and has been attributed to increase in the numbers of people with dementia in LIMC.[44]

Late Onset Dementia

Among the global burden of disease (GBD) study 2010, Western Europe had highest prevalence of dementia (7.0 million), followed by East Asia (5.5 million), South Asia (4.5 million) and North America (4.4 million). In terms of countries with a prevalence of one million or more, China had 5.4 million, USA (3.9 million), India (3.7 million), Japan (2.5 million), Germany (1.5 million), Russia (1.2 million), France (1.1 million), Italy (1.1 million) and Brazil (1.0 million).

Indian Scenario

In Indian, the reporting of prevalence rates of dementia has improved significantly. Based on the quality of data and the methodology, using survey diagnosis or clinical diagnosis of DSM 4 or ICD 10 the estimated prevalence of dementia in people above 60 years ranged from 0.6% to 3.5% in rural areas and 0.9–4.8% in urban areas. It was estimated that 3.7 million Indian people aged over 60 have dementia (2.1 million women and 1.5 million men) in 2010. However, these rates are higher than previously reported estimates by Delphi consensus.[43] In the Indian states, Trivandrum (Kerala) and Thirupur (Tamil Nadu) had highest rates, where as Ballabgarh and Vellore have the lowest based on an study involving 42,000 older people studied in eight centres (5 urban and 4 rural areas).[45-49]

Young Onset Dementia

It is defined as typically as onset of dementia before the age of 65 years. So far only four major studies have attempted to estimate the prevalence in young onset dementia (YoD), they include European Collaboration on Dementia group (EUROCODE), two registry-based studies from the United Kingdom and The Rotterdam study (1995); but the expert did not attempt a meta-analysis in view of scarcity of data and variability of the estimates. Using the Delphi consensus, estimates were attempted with the data of two United Kingdom studies, one carried out in Cambridgeshire and four London boroughs. They found prevalence of persons aged 45–64 of about 120/100 000 (London) and 101/100 000 (Cambridgeshire) for males and 77/100 000 (London) and 61/100 000 (Cambridgeshire) for females. Also the expert's consensus was that the prevalence increased exponentially with increasing age, roughly doubling every five years from 9/100 000 at age 30 to 156/100 000 at age 60–64 years. They also reported that 68% of all YoD were aged 55 and above and males predominated over females (gender ratio of 1.7 to 1) in India, prevalence of YOD were as low as those seen in high-income population-based surveys: 328/100 000 (60–64 years) in Kerala *(24)*, 249/100 000 in Ballabgarh (55–64 years), and 63/100 000 (50–59 years) and 280/100 000 (60–64 years) in Mumbai.[50-52]

Clinical Features

Cognitive Impairment

The memory is significantly affected in persons with dementia (PwD). In early stages of dementia the short-term memory is impaired. It is manifested by forgetting recent interactions, events and conversations, repetitive questions related to recent events (even they forget that they have eaten their meals and demand to be given food), they forget important dates and appointments, they misplace commonly used objects and, lose money or costly items. They have difficulty learning new information or new skills. In later aspect of the disease long-term memory starts becoming impaired and they will have difficulty recall their past memories and will forget previously highly learned material. However, they are able to preserve the procedural memory for longer time.

Apraxia

Apraxia is the inability to carry out motor activities, even if the motor functions are normal. The apraxia presents as difficulty in using familiar objects (i.e. cooking, washing) or skills which have been previously acquired (i.e. using machinery, cycling). As the disease progresses they have difficulties in dressing, bathing, or feeding which affect their activities of daily living.

Agnosia

Agnosia is defined as the failure to recognize or identify objects in spite of having normal perception and sensory functions. It presents as difficulty in recognize familiar objects, familiar people and in end stages one's face may not be recognized. Visuospatial dysfunction manifests as difficulty navigating around their familiar surroundings, they may be confused and lose their way and sometimes wander away. There is also significant executive dysfunction manifested by problems in planning, organizing, sequencing, and abstracting. They have difficulty performing complex tasks or activities such as managing money, medications and hence lead to poor judgment.

Behavioral Disturbance

In most of the dementias, behavioral disturbance is common and manifests as disinhibition, agitation, aggressive behavior, uncooperative behavior, and wandering. There is significant agitation which is worse in the evenings or night as the sensory stimuli reduces.

Personality Changes

There have been different types of personality changes manifestations in dementia. It is very common in Frontotemporal dementia. They often presents with disinhibition and impulsivity. The PwD present as inappropriate jokes, overfamiliarity with strangers, social norms are violated, sexual disinhibition or behaviors and impulsive buying. Also, depending on the dementia and involvement of brain structures apathy syndrome with a motivation and withdrawal Alzheimer's disease and vascular dementia. Exaggerated of pre-existing personality traits may occur in some cases. Also, personality change was particularly associated with severity of cognitive impairment, longer duration of illness, and neurological signs. The findings emphasize the biological basis of personality changes in dementia. Also associated with it, PwD have disturbances of self-awareness.[53]

Psychiatric Manifestations

About 10% of the PwD may have mood symptoms and depression is the common presentation (10–25%) especially early phase.[54] Depressive symptoms are associated with greater temporal lobe and cingulate gyrus hypometabolism. Suicidal attempts may also occur in them, especially in those with milder cognitive impairment and those who have insight about the disease. Anxiety disorders are also very common and reported to be more than 50%. It manifests as fear of being alone, have "catastrophic reactions" when cognitively challenged and they would expect the family members to be with them always. Manic is less common and the estimated prevalence is less than 5%.[55] Psychotic symptoms are also common and occur in the middle phase of dementia. They have delusions that their belongings have been stolen and accuse neighbors or relatives. These paranoia may be associated with their primary cognitive dysfunctions. In the latter aspects, hallucinations become were prominent and are associated with delusions. In fact, visual type are the most common compared to auditory or olfactory or tactile. They see small animals or people and they are complex in nature. They also have misidentification syndromes, commonly associated with their family members.

Normal Aging vs Dementia

There are no clear cut criteria to distinguish the both. Some authors suggest that it is a continuum. Normal aging (NA) occurs due to physiological processes over a person's lifetime. Some persons can have successful aging without cognitive dysfunction while others may develop mild dysfunction which may not be pathological. The "threshold hypothesis" of normal aging, suggests that the cognitive reserve slowly diminishes and a critical level may be reached and vice versa someone may start with a low reserve and more easily reach the threshold for the clinical manifestation of dementia as they age. In normal aging, they complain of memory loss often and provide considerable details on how they forgot but PwD may complain of memory problems only if specifically asked for and not able recall instances. In normal aging, they are more concerned about alleged forgetfulness than are close family members but in PwD the close family members much more concerned. The recent memory for important events, affairs, conversations not impaired in NA whereas in PwD have significant cognitive decline on testing. NA have occasional word-finding difficulties, but PwD have frequent word-finding pauses and substitutions. NA are able to operate common appliances even if not willing to learn how to operate new devices but PwD are unable to operate common appliances; unable to learn to operate even simple new appliances. PwD may get lost easily due to cognitive dysfunction but NA may not. PwD may exhibits loss of interest in social activities and inappropriate behaviors but NA may not.[56]

In view of the above, many terms were used such as "benign senescent forgetfulness" "age associated mental impairment" (AAMI) and "mild cognitive impairment (MCI)". The criteria for AAMI, which includes 50 years of age, complaints of memory loss in everyday life, memory performance on standardized tests at least one standard deviation below the average for young adults, and the absence of dementia. But this is not used widely. The MCI is widely used on early cognitive deficits indicating an illness that leads to dementia and have been adopted to indicate alternative interpretations of cognitive decline with increasing age. They performance in memory tasks is 1.5 standard deviations below age-matched controls that cover the spectrum between normal aging and dementia. 4–12% of MCI patients are expected to develop AD each year.[57,58]

Etiology

There are multiple etiological factors involved in dementia. They can be classified into neurodegenerative, vascular, intracranial space occupying lesions, metabolic, endocrine, traumatic brain injury, epilepsy, infections, toxic, hypoxia, vitamin deficiency and rare causes. The dementias can also be classified into primary and secondary based on the etiological. The types are listed in Table 1. Neurodegenerative causes are the most common globally and in that Alzheimer's disease is the most common and prototypical of all dementias. Other common dementias include vascular dementia (VaD), dementia with Lewy bodies (DLB), and frontotemporal dementia (FTD).[59] The presentations and clinical features are different in most for the dementia. Based on the current diagnostic guideline, we can make a probable diagnosis and only postmortem studies are confirmative.

Protective Factors in Dementia

The psychosocial protective factors in dementia include higher education, rich social network, mentally stimulating activity, active social engagement and regular physical exercise and vascular factors in late life include use of antihypertensive, use of NASID's and light to moderate alcohol use. Higher education was associated with reduced incidence of dementia. This was supported by two meta-analysis which found 60% increased risk of dementia with lowest education. This evidence supports the "cognitive reserve" hypothesis which proposes that higher education improves the cognitive reserve and which provides compensatory mechanisms to cope with the degenerative pathology and therefore delay

Table 1: Primary and secondary dementias

Primary dementias

Definition: Primary degenerative disease are defined as those dementias in which there is selective and progressive loss of specific populations of neurons for reasons that in most cases remain unknown.

- Cortical
  - Alzheimer's disease
  - Vascular dementias
  - Prion disorders (including Creutzfeldt–Jakob disease (CJD)
  - Dementia with Lewy bodies (DLB)
  - Frontotemporal dementias (including Pick's disease)
  - Behavioral variant of FTD (bvFTD)
  - Semantic dementia (SD)
  - Progressive nonfluent aphasia (PNFA)
- Subcortical
  - Parkinson's disease
  - Huntington's disease
  - Progressive supranuclear palsy
  - Idiopathic basal ganglia calcification (Fahr's disease)
  - Spinocerebellar degeneration
  - Thalamic degeneration
  - Progressive subcortical gliosis

Secondary dementias

Dementias in which there is no degenerative process and for which there are causative agents or related to medical illness.

Endocrine and metabolic disorders

- Thyroid disease
- Parathyroid disease
- Adrenal disease
- Panhypopituitarism
- Prolonged hypoglycemia
- Pancreatitis
- Chronic obstructive pulmonary disease
- Congestive heart failure
- Hypoxia
- Hepatic encephalopathy

Contd...

Contd...

- Hyponatremia
- Hypernatremia
- Uremia
- Dialysis

Nutritional disorder

- Folate, niacin, thiamine and vitamin B_{12} deficiency

Toxin and drug induced disorders

- Alcohol related syndromes
- Drugs and toxins

Infection related disorders

- Chronic meningtidis (fungal, tuberculosis, viral, bacterial)
- Neurosyphilis
- Neurobrucellosis
- Lyme neuroborreliosis
- Brain abscess
- Human immunodeficiency virus
- Arbovirus encephalitis
- Progressive rubella panencephalitis
- Progressive multifocal leukoencephalopathy
- Subacute sclerosing panencephalitis
- Creutzfeldt-Jakob disease
- Gerstmann-Straussler disease
- Postviral encephalitic syndromes
- Kuru
- Alpers' disease
- Whipple's disease
- Behçet's syndrome

Collagen vascular disorders

- Systemic lupus erythematosus
- Temporal arteritis
- Rheumatoid vasculitis
- Sarcoidosis
- Thrombotic thrombocytopenic purpura
- Granulomatous angiitis
- Idiopathic hypereosinophilic syndrome

Miscellaneous disorders and conditions

- Multiple sclerosis
- Brain tumor
- Radiation-induced
- Limbic encephalitis
- Subdural hematoma
- Hydrocephalus
- Sequelae of open and closed head injury
- Atrial myxoma

the dementia.[60,61] Systematic reviews have shown that poor social network or engagement in late life is associated with increased risk of dementia.[62] Rich social network or high level of social engagement has been hypothesized to improve social networks and resources which provides intellectual stimulations that affect cognitive and other health outcomes. Mentally stimulating activities, especially complex work with data or people have been associated with reduced risk of dementia. Again this supports the cognitive reserve hypothesis. A neuroimaging study also found that higher levels of complex activity was correlated with reduced rate of hippocampal atrophy.[63]

A higher level of physical activity was found to reduce the risk of dementia by 30–45%.[64] Regular physical exercise may promote vascular and circulatory health by reducing the blood pressure, serum lipids, obesity and blood glucose levels. Using antihypertensives especially angiotensin receptor blockers for a long-term has been found have beneficial effect in preventing dementia. Also, fewer neuritic plaques and neurofibrillary tangles in medicated hypertensive than in nonhypertensives.[65] Initial studies on dietary factors showed promising effects of antioxidants, vitamin B_{12} and folic acid in reducing the risk of dementia, later studies were did not support. Independent of vascular risk factor and physical activity, the Mediterranean diet (higher intake of fish, fruits and vegetables rich in antioxidants) has been found to reduce the risk of dementia.[66,67] Heavy alcohol use has been associated with three fold increase in AD and dementia especially in those with APOE epsilon 4 allele. However, two meta-analysis found that light to moderate alcohol use (1–3 drinks per day) was protective against dementia and cognitive decline (30–40% reduced in risk).[68]

Diet

Diets high in fish, fruit and vegetables are high in antioxidants and polyunsaturated fatty acids (PUFAs). In some observational population-based studies, people who had a high intake of vitamins E and C (both antioxidants) were less likely to show cognitive decline and had a lower AD risk than individuals with a low intake of these vitamins. By contrast, other large prospective studies of the effects of vitamins on AD risk found no such associations, and investigations examining the effect of dietary PUFAs on the risk of cognitive dysfunction proved inconclusive. Indeed, while several studies showed that the consumption of PUFAs led to reductions in the risks of dementia and AD, MCI and age-related cognitive decline, other studies found no association between dietary PUFAs and cognitive impairment. Scarmeas et al. reported that consumption of a Mediterranean-type diet (MeDi)—a diet characterized by a high intake of plant foods and fish (with olive oil as the primary source of monounsaturated fat), a moderate intake of wine and a low intake of red meat and poultry—reduced the incidence of AD and showed a trend towards reducing the risk of MCI. These effects were independent of levels of physical activity and vascular comorbidity. In a subsequent cohort study in France, MeDi was found not to alter performance on the Isaacs Set Test, the Benton Visual Retention Test or the Free and Cued Selective Reminding Test, but was associated with high MMSE scores, providing some support for the findings from the initial studies of this diet. In a meta-analysis of 15 prospective studies exploring the effect of alcohol on dementia risk, light to moderate alcohol consumption was associated with a reduction in the risk of AD and dementia.

Most RCTs examining the effects of antioxidant supplementation have found no association with cognitive performance. To date, prospective clinical trial data for dietary supplementation with omega-3 PUFAs have shown no overall effect on cognition in patients with MCI or AD, but have suggested that docosahexaenoic acid supplementation has a beneficial effect on cognitive function in people harboring the APOE ε4 allele and in the earliest stages of AD.

Reactive oxygen species are clearly associated with neuronal damage in AD; however, whether the presence of these molecules reflects a primary or secondary event in the neurotoxic process remains unclear. Deposition of Aβ, which is an early event in AD, leads to a decrease in cerebral iron and copper concentrations, resulting in oxidative stress and neuronal damage. Evidence from *in vitro* studies indicates that vitamin E reduces the extent of Aβ-induced lipid peroxidation and cell death. In addition, carotenes and vitamin C protect against lipid peroxidation. Furthermore, vitamin C reduces the formation of nitrosamines and may affect catecholamine synthesis. Evidence also exists that antioxidant intake reduces AD risk through a reduction in the risk of cerebrovascular disease. Besides reducing oxidative stress, PUFAs have favorable effects on neuronal and vascular functions and inflammatory processes.

Physical Activity

Epidemiological and experimental data suggest that physical exercise may promote brain health. Conflicting results have, however, emerged from cross-sectional and longitudinal observational studies that examined the relationship between exercise levels and cognitive decline or dementia: while some studies indicated that physical activity has a beneficial effect on brain health, others showed no association between these variables.

Physical activity could affect cognition via multiple mechanisms. An improvement in aerobic fitness increases cerebral blood flow, oxygen extraction and glucose utilization, and activates growth factors that promote structural brain changes, such as an increase in capillary density. In addition, rodent studies suggest that physical activity decreases the rate of amyloid plaque formation. RCTs exploring the effects of exercise on cognitive function in healthy elderly individuals have yielded conflicting results. A recent meta-analysis that included 11 RCTs involving cognitively healthy people aged >55 years suggested that undertaking of aerobic physical activities improves selective cognitive functions, including cognitive speed, as well as auditory and visual attention.

Intellectual Activity

Following initial reports that elderly people with higher levels of education had a lower incidence of dementia than individuals with no education, cognitive activity was suggested to decrease the risk of cognitive decline by increasing cognitive reserve. Several prospective studies subsequently found that both young and old people who engage in cognitively stimulating activities, such as learning, reading or playing games, were less likely to develop dementia than individuals who did not engage in these activities.

RCTs have shown a beneficial effect of intellectual interventions on cognitive function in elderly, dementia-free individuals. The benefits of cognitive training seem to be domain specific, however. Several trials found that while cognitive training can improve memory, reasoning and mental processing speed in older adults, cognitive training did not have an effect on all cognitive domains, and did not affect day-to-day functioning. In addition, one study found that among elderly individuals, those with memory impairment showed less improvement in cognition through memory training than those without such impairment. Consequently, in elderly people, the effect of cognitive training on the risk of dementia is unclear, but several trials are underway.[69]

Diagnosis

Dementia is a syndrome like delirium. Hence careful attention has to be given and a detailed history from the patient and an informant, in addition to mental state examination and cognitive testing is recommended. In the history, look for the type of onset of cognitive impairment (insidious or sudden), course (gradual or stepwise, progressive or episodic, or fluctuating), duration of impairment, any accompanying symptoms (like mood, psychotic symptoms or personality changes). Efforts should be made to look for evidence of treatable causes in the history, so the focus of physical examinations and investigations can be planned. Past and family history will give leads into the genetic etiology. Also, past history of psychiatric or neurological disorders may be helpful in further management. Also, an attempt should be made to look for any abuse during the physical examination.

The mental state examination is a very valuable and very important to diagnose and categorize the type of dementia. It may be painstaking and time consuming to do a MSE with elderly patients but the amount of time invested will give fruitful evidence for further management. In the general appearance, patient's attire, cleanliness and rapport will help in suggesting the severity of dementia. Cognitive tests are the key to diagnosis but PwD may not co-operate for the full assessment and hence the interview sessions have to be split and time should be given for them to complete tasks. It is important to remember the age of the patient, disabilities due to aging (such as vision and hearing deficits) intellectual capacity, socioeconomic background, educational background, rural or urban settings and premorbid personality. The tests as general fund of information, similarities and differences and tests of abstraction also have to be accommodative of all these factors to appropriately diagnose the deficits. Extended cognitive tests may be required if there are any confusion or it is historically evident but not picked up by bedside cognitive tests. There are lots of scales to evaluate and have their own limitations. The DSM-IV diagnosis of dementia and amnestic disorder are subsumed under newely named entity major neurocognitive disorder (NCD) in DSM-5.

DSM-5 Criteria for Major Neurocognitive Disorder

a. Evidence of significant cognitive decline from a previous level of performance in one or more cognitive domains (complex attention, executive function, learning and memory, language, perceptual-motor, or social cognition) based on:
   1. Concern of the individual, a knowledgeable informant, or the clinician that there has been a significant decline in cognitive function; and
   2. A substantial impairment in cognitive performance, preferably documented by standardized neuropsychological testing or, in its absence, another quantified clinical assessment.
b. The cognitive deficits do not interfere with independence in everyday activities (i.e., at a minimum, requiring assistance with complex instrumental activities of daily living such as paying bills or managing medications).
c. The cognitive deficits do not occur exclusively in the context of a delirium.
d. The cognitive deficits are not better explained by another mental disorder (e.g. major depressive disorder, schizophrenia).

Specify whether due to:

• Alzheimer's disease	Frontotemporal lobar degeneration
• Lewy-body disease	Vascular disease
• Traumatic brain injury	
• Substance/medication use	HIV infection
• Prion disease	Parkinson's disease
• Huntington's disease	Another medical condition
• Multiple etiologies	Unspecified

Coding note: Code based on medical or substance etiology. In some cases, there is need for an additional code for the etiological medical condition, which must immediately precede the diagnostic code for major neurocognitive disorder, as shown in Table on pp. 302-304.

Contd...

Contd...

Specify:

Without behavioral disturbance: If the cognitive disturbance is not accompanied by any clinically significant behavioral disturbance

With behavioral disturbance (specify disturbance): If the cognitive disturbance is accompanied by a clinically significant behavioral disturbance (e.g. psychotic symptoms, mood disturbance, agitation, apathy, or other behavioral symptoms).

Specify current severity:

Mild: Difficulties with instrumental activities of daily living (e.g. housework, managing money).

Moderate: Difficulties with basic activities of daily living (e.g. feeding, dressing).

Severe: Fully dependent.

DSM-5 Criteria for Mild Neurocognitive Disorder

a. Evidence of modest cognitive decline from a previous level of performance in one or more cognitive domains (complex attention, executive function, learning and memory, language, perceptual-motor, or social cognition) based on:
   1. Concern of the individual, a knowledgeable informant, or the clinician that there has been a mild decline in cognitive function.
   2. A modest impairment in cognitive performance, preferably documented by standardized neuropsychological testing or, in its absence, another quantified clinical assessment.

b. The cognitive deficits do not interfere with capacity for independence in everyday activities (i.e. complex instrumental activities of daily living such as paying bills or managing medications are preserved, but greater effort, compensatory strategies, or accommodation may be required).

c. The cognitive deficits do not occur exclusively in the context of a delirium.

d. The cognitive deficits are not better explained by another mental disorder (e.g. major depressive disorder, schizophrenia).

Specify whether due to:

- Alzheimer's disease
- Frontotemporal lobar degeneration
- Lewy body disease
- Vascular disease
- Traumatic brain injury
- Substance/medication use
- HIV infection
- Prion disease
- Parkinson's disease
- Huntington's disease
- Another medical condition
- Multiple etiologies
- Unspecified

Coding note: For mild neurocognitive disorder due to any of the medical etiologies listed above, code 331.83 (G31.84). Do not use additional codes for the presumed etiological medical conditions. For substance/medication-induced mild neurocognitive disorder, code based on type of substance; see "Substance/Medication-Induced Major or Mild Neurocognitive Disorder." For unspecified mild neurocognitive disorder, code 799.59 (R41.9).

Contd...

Contd...

Specify: Without behavioral disturbance: If the cognitive disturbance is not accompanied by any clinically significant behavioral disturbance.

With behavioral disturbance (specify disturbance): If the cognitive disturbance is accompanied by a clinically significant behavioral disturbance (e.g. psychotic symptoms, mood disturbance, agitation, apathy, or other behavioral symptoms).

Laboratory and Investigations

Once a detailed history is collected and physical examination has been completed. Laboratory investigations need to be considered to corroborate the history and to identify the etiology of some treatable dementias and to look into comorbid physical disorders. In this aspect the investigations can be classified into three aspects:

To Corroborate the Diagnosis

Neuroimaging is very importance to rule out infarcts, mass lesions, tumors, and hydrocephalus. It is also very vital to identify the pattern of neuronal damage and also may provide clues to the diagnosis. Computed tomography without contrast or magnetic resonance imaging may be useful in the essential work-up of PwD.

Rule Out Treatable or Contributory Causes of Dementia

Complete blood count, serum electrolytes, renal and hepatic function, blood glucose, albumin and protein, vitamin B_{12} and folate, rapid plasma reagin or VDRL (syphilis), thyroid-stimulating hormone, urinalysis are important investigations to be considered to rule out treatable causes of dementia.The dementias can be classified into reversible and irreversible types based on the reversible causes such as infections, vitamin deficiencies, etc. The list of types of reversible and irreversible dementias are given in Table 2.

However, sensitive tests such as VDRL, HIV and HBsAG may be required in suspected cases of exposure to STD and patients with personality changes associated with dementia due to high-risk behavior.

The CSF analysis also may be important when suspecting neurosyphilis, cysticercosis, viral, fungal infections and CSF pressure analysis in normal pressure hydrocephalus.

Specialized tests such as drug screen, toxins level, electrolytes are very important especially when the history is not clear or there is delirium superimposed on dementia. It should be based on clinical suspicion and need to consider the cost effectiveness of the tests especially in a country like India.

Table 2: Reversible and irreversible causes of dementia

Irreversible	*Reversible*
• Alzheimer disease • Frontotemporal dementia • Vascular dementia • Parkinson diseases • Lewy-body disease • Huntington's dementia • Wilson's disease • Multiple system atrophy • Progressive supranuclear palsy	*Neuroinfections and inflammations* • Meningitis (tubercular, fungal, malignant) • Encephalitis (limbic, HIV, herpes) • Sarcoidosis • Cerebral vasculitis • Cerebral cysticercosis • Neurosyphilis • Lyme's disease • Whipple's disease *Metabolic conditions* • Hypo- and hyperthyroidism, • Hashimoto's encephalitis • Hypo- and hyperparathyroidism • Pituitary insufficiency • Hypercalcemia • Cushing's disease • Addison's disease • Hypoglycemia • Vitamin deficiencies (B_1, B_6, B_{12}, and folate) • Hepatic disorders (Chronic liver failure) • Chronic respiratory failure • Chronic renal failure *Neurosurgical conditions* • Subdural hematoma • Normal pressure hydrocephalous • Intracranial empyema or abscess • Benign brain tumors (meningioms) *Others* • Depression (Pseudodementia) • Epilepsy • Drugs (antipsychotics, anticholinergic, antihypertensive agents, anticonvulsants, antineoplastic therapies and steroids) • Heavy metal intoxication • Alcohol abuse • Limbic encephalitis (neoplastic/autoimmune) • Porphyria

Only with neuropathological investigation of the brain through either brain biopsy or autopsy a definitive diagnosis of dementia type but there is no clinical indication for the same.

General Medical Conditions of PwD

It is also important to do certain laboratories tests such as ECG, EEG, chest X-ray and ESR for the evaluation of normal health status.

Neuropsychological Assessment

There are several scales to screen and assess the severity of dementia. The commonly used are given below:

The **mini-mental state examination (MMSE)**[70] is best known and most widely used measure of cognition globally. This scale assesses cognitive function in the areas of orientation, memory, attention and calculation, language and visual construction. Patients score between 0 and 30 points, and cut-offs of 23/24 have typically been used to show significant cognitive impairment. It is widely translated and used.

Abbreviated Mental Test Score

The abbreviated mental test score (AMTS)[71] is a 10-item scale derived from a longer scale introduced previously.[72] It has been found to assesses orientation, registration, recall and concentration, and scores of 6 or below (from maximum of 10) have been shown to screen effectively for dementia,

Montreal Cognitive Assessment

The Montreal Cognitive Assessment[73] assesses attention/concentration, executive functions, conceptual thinking, memory, language, calculation and orientation. A score of

25 or lower (from maximum of 30) is considered significant cognitive impairment. It performs at least as well as MMSE, including in screening for dementia. It is particularly useful for patients with vascular impairment, including vascular dementia since it also assesses executive function.

Addenbrookes Cognitive Assessment

The addenbrookes cognitive assessment (ACE)[74] and its commonly used revision the ACE-R[75] was originally developed as a screening test for dementia which, unlike the MMSE, would rely less on verbal than on executive abilities. It has been shown to have very high reliability and excellent diagnostic accuracy, and it is a practical option for clinical services intent on precision in diagnoses.

Longer Cognitive Assessments

Alzheimer's Disease Assessment Scale: Cognitive Section

The Alzheimer's Disease Assessment Scale: Cognitive section (ADAS-Cog)[76] is a detailed cognitive assessment for dementia covers all cognitive areas in dementia.

Cambridge Assessment of Memory and Cognition

The Cambridge Assessment of Memory and Cognition[77] is the cognitive section of the comprehensive CAMDEX assessment. It covers a range of cognitive functions, including orientation, language, memory, attention, praxis, calculation, abstract thinking and perception. It takes around 25 to 40 minutes for a clinician to administer and requires a modest degree of training. It performs well against MMSE with no ceiling effects and conventional cutoffs of 79/80 have demonstrated excellent sensitivity and specificity for dementia.[78] Its combination of breadth and relative brevity make it suitable for clinical use, particularly new assessments of patients in memory clinics. It has the added advantage of including questions to generate an MMSE score.

Overall Dementia Severity

Clinical Dementia Rating

The Clinical Dementia Rating scale[79] helps in more reliable staging of dementia than MMSE, and is based on caregiver accounts of problems in daily functional and cognitive tasks. It classifies people with dementia into questionable, mild, moderate and severe.

Global Deterioration Scale

The Global Deterioration Scale[80] is essentially for staging dementia and takes only 2 minutes once relevant clinical information has been collated. It has been well validated and classifies cases into seven stages from no complaints through to very severe.

Clinicians Global Impression of Change

The Clinicians Global Impression of Change (CIBIC-Plus)[81] is a global measure of detectable change in cognition, function and behavior, usually requiring separate interviews with patients and carers. It is therefore conceptually attractive for assessing progression, but requires a trained clinician and 10–40 minutes of interview time so may be unsuited to routine clinical practice.

Differential Diagnosis

There are many clinical conditions which can mimic dementia. It is difficult to collect a detailed history and if needed substitute with neuroimaging and other laboratory investigations to rule out other conditions. Some of the common disorders which needs to be ruled out before dementia is diagnosed include 4 "D"s Delirium, Depression, mild cognitive Decline and Drugs. Delirium can be differentiated by an acute onset, altered levels of consciousness, fluctuating levels of alertness, sundowning effect, sleep wake cycle disturbances, significant impairment of cognition and perceptual abnormalities whereas in dementia they usually have a gradual onset, progressive loss of cognitive functions. Delirium can be superimposed on dementia. Infact the risk factor for delirium is dementia. However, if cognitive dysfunctions persist beyond one month with adequate treatment, than dementia needs to be considered. The differences between demetia and delirium are given in Table 3.

The next important condition is depression. Again, depressive disorders have usually gradual onset and improve within few weeks to months compared to dementia which has a progressive course. Cognitive impairment is common in depression and is present in 50% of the patients. This concept was called as "pseudodementia" and was coined by Leslie Kiloh in 1961. Depressed patients complain of memory problems themselves but in PwD the caregivers notice the memory problems. Even though both the groups can have low mood, reduced concentration and psychomotor slowing, depressive or negative cognitions such as ideas of worthlessness, ideas of hopelessness, helplessness, guilt feelings and death wishes differentiate them from PwD. On testing the depressed patients do not co-operate easily, they produce incomplete answers; give "I don't know" answers. A long-term study of depressive pseudodementia in the elderly in UK found that 71.4% in the moderate-to-severe depression group converted to dementia compared to only 18.2% in the cognitively intact elderly, suggesting that moderate to severe depression are strong predictors of dementia.[82]

Table 3: Comparison of the features of Delirium and Dementia

Features	*Delirium*	*Dementia*
Onset	Acute (hours to days)	Insidious (months to years)
Course	Fluctuates hourly, lucid periods in a day confusion usually worsens at night, stable throughout the day	Chronic; progresses slowly
Duration	Days to months; often reversible	Months to years; Progressive and irreversible; progresses to death
Consciousness	Altered (hyperalert, alert or hypoalert)	Clear until late in the course of the illness (can have intermittent fluctuation if delirium is superimposed)
Hallucinations	Gross distortions, frequent hallucinations, usually visual or visual and auditory	Often absent in early stages; in later stages may have hallucinations, especially visual (some types of dementia it can present early, e.g. Lewy-body dementia)
Paranoid ideas	Fleeting, poorly systematized	Present sometimes
Attention/concentration	Impaired normal	Except in late stages
Orientation	Usually impaired	Impaired as disease progresses
Memory	Immediate and short-term memory impaired	Memory impaired, gradually worsening as disease progresses
Psychomotor activity	Increased, reduced or shifting unpredictably	Agitation may be present
Speech	Often incoherent; slow or rapid	Usually coherent until late stage
Thinking	Disorganized or incoherent	Limited and vague
Sleep/wake cycle	Disturbed; may change hourly	Disturbed; day/night reversal

Mild cognitive impairment is a new concept and is impairment of cognitive functions in one or more domains without functional impairment but not adequate enough to make a diagnosis of dementia. They have objective memory impairment but able to function at the same level as they always did. However, they are at higher risk of developing dementia.

Drugs or medications can also mimic dementia. Medications such as anticholinergics, antiparkinsonian, antiepileptics can impair cognitive functions and resemble dementia. Identification and removal or substitution of these medications can reverse the cognitive impairments. Also substances such as alcohol, cannabis, inhalants, opioids, Hallucinogens can cause cognitive impairments.

Caregivers Burden

Family members are very important aspect of caring the PwD at home. They also experience psychological problems and burnout associated while taking care of PwD. It is called caregiver's burden when they experience "enduring stress and frustration".[83] Due to above reasons they have poor outcomes such as depression, illness and reduced quality of life.[84] Caregiver's burden is defined as "a multidimensional response to physical, psychological, emotional, social and financial stressors associated with the caregiving experiences.[85] Just caregiving is different from caregivers burden, where they just provide assistance and do not have the psychological distress.

As the disease progresses they PwD become more dependent on the caregivers. They may need to manage difficult behaviors and sometimes physical or verbal abuses. It can be very traumatizing if they have insomnia or delirium. Caregiver's burden can lead to inadequate care and can increase the risk factor for abuse and neglect of the demented patient. Hence, treatment approaches to PwD should also include strategies to reduce caregiver's burden. Family interventions programs have been found to reduce the depression and stress among CG. It included education, stress management and coping skills. A meta-analysis by[86] concluded studies with multicomponent interventions reduce CG burden.

Nonpharmacological Approaches

Education

In the very beginning of the any interventions in PwD, it is important to spend valuable time with the family members of PwD in explaining about the diagnosis, prognosis, treatment possibilities, and course of dementia. This should be done in a staged manner and gradually. Initially it may be a shock and many families will not accept the diagnosis and would be in denial. It would take some time for them to understand the nuances of dementia and its therapeutic process. Currently online educational materials and NGOs like ARDSI and other support groups' agencies provide support and care for the PwD and their caregivers.

Behavioral Therapy

There are significant behavioral disturbance in PwD especially when the later stages of disease and associated with other psychiatric conditions. Behavioral therapy becomes a very important nonpharmacological intervention for the same. Classically this therapy is based on principles of conditioning and learning theory. However, currently non-aversive and positive programming methodologies have been developed to cater to the PwD for improving functional behaviors.[87] In behavioral therapy (BT), antecedents, behaviors and their consequences are identified and a relationship with it is made clear to PwD. Then the therapist formulates a intervention program to tackle the maladaptive behaviors. Three important features are to be considered while formulating an intervention are taking account of the individual's preferences; changing the context in which the behavior takes place; and using reinforcement strategies and schedules that reduce the behavior.[88] The efficacy of BT in PwD have been shown only in few studies and found evidence for successful reductions in wandering, incontinence and other forms of stereotypical behaviors.[89]

Reality Orientation

It is a widely used therapy for people with memory loss and disorientation by reminding them of facts about themselves and their environment in a group or individual format.[90] In this therapy they are oriented to their environment using a range of materials and activities. They use orientation devices such as photographs, notices and signposts. By doing this it is thought that it would provide the person with a greater understanding of their surroundings, possibly resulting in an improved sense of control and self-esteem. However, this therapy has been criticized that it has been applied in a mechanical fashion, is insensitive to the needs of the individual and constant relearning of material can actually contribute to mood and self-esteem problems. A systematic review by Cochrane database concluded that this therapy is effective for cognition and behavior for dementia sufferers but needs to be continued to sustain the potential benefits.[91]

Validation Therapy

This therapy was developed by Naomi Feil, as an antidote to perceived lack of efficacy of reality orientation. The therapy attempts at communicate with PwD by empathising with the feelings and meanings hidden behind their confused speech and behavior. It is the emotional content which is more important than the person's orientation to the present. Naomi Feil classified individuals with cognitive impairment as having one of four stages in a continuum of dementia which include malorientation, time confusion, repetitive motion and vegetation. It is based on the general principle of validation, the acceptance of the reality and personal truth of another's experience, and incorporates a range of specific techniques. Studies have found that this therapy promotes contentment, results in less negative affect and behavioral disturbance, produces positive effects and provides the individual with insight into external reality,[92,93] evaluated validation therapy in a systematic review and found only three studies which were included in the final analysis but did not find any statistical significane between validation and social contact or usual therapy.

Reminiscence Therapy

This therapy aims at helping a PwD to relive past experiences, especially those that might be positive and personally significant. It allows discussion of past activities, events and experiences with another person or group of people. They use photographs, household items, music and archived sound recordings. Participants are encouraged to talk about past events at least once a week; guided in sequence through life experiences and encouraged to evaluate them and lead to produce a life story book. Here, the role of caregivers is important and are actively involved. It is highly appreciated by staff and family members and there are evidence that it increases the levels of well-being and provides pleasure and cognitive stimulation. A systematic review by Woods et al.[94] found that there was a statistically significant improvement in for cognition (at follow-up), mood (at follow-up) and on a measure of general behavioral function (at the end of the intervention period). The improvement on cognition was evident in comparison with both no treatment and social contact control conditions. Not only PwD benefitted from this therapy but also the care-giver strain showed a significant decrease.

Cognitive Stimulation

It provides a general stimulation for thinking, concentration and memory usually in a social setting, such as a small group using a range of enjoyable activities the basic idea behind this therapy is that lack of cognitive activity hastens cognitive decline. Even though it has its roots in reality orientation, this therapy is implemented in a sensitive, respectful and person-centered manner. A recent Cochrane review by Woods et al.,[95] they concluded that there was consistent evidence from multiple trials that cognitive stimulation programs benefit cognition in people with mild-to-moderate dementia over and above any medication effects.

Creative Art Therapies

Creative arts therapy includes music, art, dance/movement, drama, and bibliotherapy (literature and poetry). These are a group of therapies which involves the increasing or improving the activity levels of PwD through various methods such as exercise, dance, sport and drama. It has been found that physical exercise or simple repetitive exercises can have health benefits such as improve blood circulation, prevent falls and fractures; mental health and sleep[96-98].Perrin[99] described an interesting approach to dance therapy known as 'jabadeo', which allows the participants to engage with each other in an interactive movement. This also improves non-sexual physical contact which many people with dementia find soothing Art therapy has been found to improve meaningful stimulation, social interaction and levels of self-esteem.[100] Painting, drawing, collage or other activities provide them opportunity to express themselves and gives a chance to them to exercise some choice in terms of the colors and themes of their creations. A recent case report has found it to be useful in reducing the stress in PwD.[101]

The music therapy allows PwD to engagement in a musical activity (e.g. singing or playing an instrument), or merely listening to songs or music and has many studies have found to be of benefitted to PwD.[100] It has been found to reduce agitation, increases in levels of well-being, better social interaction and improvements in autobiographical memory.[102,103]

Activities of Daily Living

In PwD the activities of daily living are compromised due to the disease and their dependence on caregivers. The Basic daily activities such as brushing, bathing, dressing, grooming and toileting all get affected as the disease progresses. Hence, it is important to consider it early to schedule the activities as part of the daily routine so the dependence on staff and caregivers can be reduced and also their self-esteem improves when they are able to cater to these activities themselves. Kalyansundaram[104] has suggested few simple tips to improve them. They include reminding and supervising the PwD, use positive reinforcement for completing the tasks, to use simple charts with labels or symbols placed in a prominent position for the patient to see; to show their achievements even though they are in small steps.

Pet and Therapeutic Touch Therapy

This is a very old therapy but has been currently revalidated for its use in PwD. This therapy has been found to improve agitation and mood of the residents.[105] Therapeutic touch has been found to provide clients with benefits.[106]

Services for the Care of Dementia in India

In developed countries, the services are in place to screen for dementia earlier and intervene earlier. They are usually covered with health insurance and these take care of the cost of medicine and care of the patients for long-term. However, in India it is different situation. The estimated prevalence of people with dementia in India is 3.7 million and will increase significantly. Also, they are major impact of this disorder on family and caregivers in terms of finance, time, psychological issues and burnout in them. The service gap for dementia in India is estimated to be much over 90%.[107]

Currently Available Services in India

Alzheimer's and Related Disorders Society of India (ARDSI) along with other organizations like Helpage India, Dignity Foundation, Nightingales Trust, the Dementia Society of Goa, Sangath, Silver Innings Foundation, Christian Medical College Vellore, St. John's Medical College Bengaluru and Voluntary Health Services Chennai are involved in the care and support of people with Dementia. However, ARDSI has taken up the responsibility of having dedicated services for the care, support and research of dementia. ARDSI has around 14 chapters around India and has made efforts to map the dementia services available in India.

Residential care: In India, currently five full time residential care facilities for persons with dementia (PwD) they include four homes in Kerala [Harmony Home (Kottapadi), Malabar Harmony Home (Calicut), Snehasadanam (Trivandrum) and Cochin Harmony Home (Cochin)]; one in Karnataka [Nightingales Dementia Care, Bengaluru, Karnataka) and one in Maharashtra (Dignity Lifestyle Home (Neral)). Various health professionals monitor the health of the patients in these homes. The staffs are trained to provide therapies like reminiscence, music, art, pet, yoga, light exercises, cognitive stimulation exercises and reality orientation. Several are also practiced.

Day care center: There are around 10 day care centers in India. It is designed for those persons with dementia who do not require institutionalization and need medical attention and supervision. They are looked after during the day, after which they return home. They are also give similar therapies as mentioned above. Apart from ARDSI, Dignity Foundation (Mumbai) and the Nightingales Trust (Bengaluru) are also running day care services for PwD.

Domiciliary care services: There are around 6 domiciliary care services, which basically provide care at their residence. It is usually provided by geriatric home nurses, part time staff, social workers or volunteers who visit families of PwD and provide assistance in the form of counseling, guidance and sometimes physical help (like bathing, grooming, and simple exercises), education, providing tips on caregiving to actual formal care.

Support groups: These are a collection of people (Caregivers) who have someone in the family or relatives with dementia and have gone through the difficult experiences, not only help themselves but also help others and they provide solace and support to other caregiver and family members.

Memory clinics: They are specialized clinics which provide evaluation, support, information and advice to those with memory problems and their caregivers. There are around 100 such clinics in India.

Help lines: These are freely accessible phone numbers which are handled by trained personnel to address the queries on dementia. They are around 10 such helplines and mainly run by ARDSI. There are available in Cochin, Kolkata, Mumbai, Bengaluru, New Delhi and Hyderabad. Considering a lack of facilities and opportunities for the PwD and caregivers, there is a great demand for improving the services, training and research in dementia in India. Alzheimer's and Related Disorders Society of India (ARDSI) looked into this matter and prepared a comprehensive report in this regard called The Dementia India Report, 2010.[108] This report has compiled the available services and addresses, the need for improving the current scenario in India. It has come up with few recommendations, they include:

- Make dementia a national priority
- Increase funding for dementia research
- Increase awareness about dementia
- Improve dementia identification and care skills
- Develop community support
- Guarantee carer support packages
- Develop comprehensive dementia care models
- Develop new National Policies and Legislation for PwD.

ALZHEIMER'S DEMENTIA

It is a neurodegenerative type of dementia and one of the most common dementia seen globally. It is characterized by significant deterioration in memory, cognitive functions; progressive impairment of activities of daily living and associated with neuropsychiatric symptoms. It is named after Alois Alzheimer in 1906.

Definitions

The below definitions are adapted from the position statement of the American Association for Geriatric Psychiatry.

Dementia resulting from Alzheimer's disease or DAT is characterized by decline primarily in cortical aspects of cognition (i.e. memory, language, praxis) and follows a characteristic time course of gradual onset and progression.

Alzheimer's disease is a specific degenerative brain disease characterized by senile plaques, neuritic tangles, and progressive loss of neurons, the presumptive cause of Alzheimer's disease.[109]

Current Diagnostic Revisions

National Institute on Aging and the Alzheimer's Association workgroup has proposed the classification of individuals with dementia caused by AD: (1) Probable AD dementia, (2) Possible AD dementia, and (3) Probable or possible AD dementia with evidence of the AD pathophysiological process. They have given detailed criteria with inclusion of biomarkers in the diagnostic workup. The AD biomarkers can be divided into two classes based on the biology which they measure. They include biomarkers of brain amyloid-beta (Ab) protein deposition which are low CSF Ab42 and positive PET amyloid imaging. Next group belongs to biomarkers of downstream neuronal degeneration or injury which include elevated CSF tau (total tau and phosphorylated tau (p-tau), decreased 18-fluorodeoxyglucose (FDG) uptake on PET in temporo-parietal cortex; and disproportionate atrophy on structural MRI imaging in medial, basal, and lateral temporal lobe, and medial parietal cortex. Those who meet the core clinical criteria for probable AD dementia biomarker evidence may increase the certainty the etiology of clinical dementia syndrome is the AD pathophysiological process. However they do not recommend the use of AD biomarker tests for routine diagnostic purposes.[110-113]

DSM-5: Criteria for major or mild neurocognitive disorder due to Alzheimer's disease

a. The criteria are met for major or mild neurocognitive disorder.
b. There is insidious onset and gradual progression of impairment in one or more cognitive domains (for major neurocognitive disorder, at least two domains must be impaired).
c. Criteria are met for either probable or possible Alzheimer's disease as follows:

For major neurocognitive disorder:

Probable Alzheimer's disease is diagnosed if either of the following is present; otherwise, possible Alzheimer's disease should be diagnosed.

1. Evidence of a causative Alzheimer's disease genetic mutation from family history or genetic testing.
2. All three of the following are present:
   a. Clear evidence of decline in memory and learning and at least one other cognitive domain (based on detailed history or serial neuropsychological testing).
   b. Steadily progressive, gradual decline in cognition, without extended plateaus.
   c. No evidence of mixed etiology (i.e., absence of other neurodegenerative or cerebrovascular disease, or another neurological, mental, or systemic disease or condition likely contributing to cognitive decline).

For mild neurocognitive disorder:

Probable Alzheimer's disease is diagnosed if there is evidence of a causative Alzheimer's disease genetic mutation from either genetic testing or family history.

Contd...

Contd...

Possible Alzheimer's disease is diagnosed if there is no evidence of a causative Alzheimer's disease genetic mutation from either genetic testing or family history, and all three of the following are present:

1. Clear evidence of decline in memory and learning.
2. Steadily progressive, gradual decline in cognition, without extended plateaus.
3. No evidence of mixed etiology (i.e. absence of other neurodegenerative or cerebrovascular disease, or another neurological or systemic disease or condition likely contributing to cognitive decline).

d. The disturbance is not better explained by cerebrovascular disease, another neurodegenerative disease, the effects of a substance, or another mental, neurological, or systemic disorder.

Coding note: For probable major neurocognitive disorder due to Alzheimer's disease, with behavioral disturbance, code first 331.0 (G30.9) Alzheimer's disease, followed by 294.11 (F02.81) major neurocognitive disorder due to Alzheimer's disease. For probable neurocognitive disorder due to Alzheimer's disease, without behavioral disturbance, code first 331.0 (G30.9) Alzheimer's disease, followed by 294.10 (F02.80) major neurocognitive disorder due to Alzheimer's disease, without behavioral disturbance.

For possible major neurocognitive disorder due to Alzheimer's disease, code 331.9 (G31.9) possible major neurocognitive disorder due to Alzheimer's disease. (Note: Do not use the additional code for Alzheimer's disease. Behavioral disturbance cannot be coded but should still be indicated in writing.)

For mild neurocognitive disorder due to Alzheimer's disease, code 331.83 (G31.84). (Note: Do not use the additional code for Alzheimer's disease. Behavioral disturbance cannot be coded but should still be indicated in writing.)

Types of Alzheimer's Disease

There are two types of AD, they are (1) Early-onset Familial and (2) Late-onset sporadic. In early onset type patients with AD develop symptoms before the age of 65 years. Around 10% of them have familial etiology and it is transmitted as an autosomal dominant trait. In as late-onset Alzheimer disease, symptoms develop after the age of 65 years. It is present in 5% of the population aged over 65 years and more than 20% of the population over 85 years.

Epidemiology

Global

The current prevalence of dementia is around 15 million around the world and estimated to rise to 25 million by 2050. The prevalence of DAT in Europe was 4.4% (age-standardized), it increased with age by 0.6% for those aged 65–69 years and 22.2% for those aged 90 years or older.[114] The prevalence of DAT in 2000 in United States was around 4.5 million people and the incidence rates one per 1,000 person-years among individuals aged 60–64 years and 25 per 1,000 person-years among those older than age 85 years.[115,116]

India

In India, the prevalence is around 3.7 million people (2.1 million are women 1.5 million men) aged over 60 have dementia.[117] In the Indian states, the prevalence rate for Trivandrum (4.8%) (Kerala) and Thiropour (3.5%) (Tamil Nadu) have the highest while the Ballabgarh (Haryana) (1.1%) (Delhi) and Vellore (0.6%)(Tamil Nadu) have the lowest prevalence rates whilst.[118,119] Based on the Delphi Consensus study the global incidence is 4.6 million new cases of dementia every year however the data in India is limited and one study reported 3.24 per 100000 for people aged over 65 years in rural Ballabgarh (Haryana).[117,120]

Symptoms

Cognitive symptoms: They include Amnesia, dysphasia, apraxia and agnosia. Amnesia is an early symptom seen in AD. Amnesia is typically for recent events but there is sparing of remote memory and relative sparing of working memory. In AD, the forgetting of new memories is greater in AD than in other groups and the most probable reason for this is due to deficits in encoding and storing memories rather than failure to retrieve or to primary loss of memories. As the disease progresses there is deficits in the episodic memory and visuospatial deficits. Semantic memory is initially preserved but as the disease progresses it worsens. Visuospatial deficits manifest as becoming disoriented in strange places and getting lost in familiar places. Aphasias: Patients may present with word finding difficulty, incomplete sentences, grammatical errors and poor use of tenses. Later, they present with receptive difficulties, perseverations, echolalia and decreased fluency. Apraxia—They manifest difficulties in complex motor tasks withouta primary motor difficulties. Patients present with difficulty in enacting a command in a detailed and goal directed acts. This can manifest as poor self-care, poor ADL and can harm themselves. Agnosia—Difficulty in correctly interpreting sensory input is common in AD patients. They have auto prosopagnosia, which is inability to recognize one's own face. Executive dysfunction is also found to occur early in AD. It was related to frontal lobe dysfunction. AD patients also have significant disturbances in their ADL. Initially they may have difficulties in finding personal belongings, later it progresses to difficulties only in demanding circumstances such as at work, in terminal stages they may bedbound.

Behavioral and Psychological Symptoms of Dementia

Behavioral and psychological symptoms of dementia (BPSD) are common in AD and are the core features of AD. Alzheimer highlighted the importance of these symptoms in AD. They can be categorized into psychotic, mood and activity related.

Psychotic Symptoms

Delusions are more common in AD; a particularly delusion of theft is the most common. These are associated with the Amnesia which is a primary symptom. Visual hallucinations are more common followed by auditory, olfactory and then tactile. They typically have hallucination of small animals or people. AD patients are less reactive to the hallucination because they do have an insight that these are abnormal experience and not normal perceptions. Misidentification syndromes are also found in AD, especially related to the family members. Candidate association studies have found that variations in serotonin receptors are associated with risk of hallucinations and variation in dopamine receptors with risk of delusions.[121-123]

Affective Symptoms

Depression is a common diagnosis in AD. It can be easily confused for pseudodementia. The prevalence of major depression in AD has been estimated to be 10% but minor depression is around 30%. One of the scales used for identifying depression in AD patient is Cornell Scale for Depression in Dementia,[124] because it may be difficult to segregate depressive symptoms from dementia in different stages of the disease. There has been evidence of loss of neurons in the locus coeruleus and dorsal raphe suggesting noradrenergic or serotonergic dysfunction in AD patients with depression anxiety disorders are more common in AD patients and a prevalence of more than 50% have been reported in studies. The prevalence of mania has been found to be less than 5%.

Activity

The most common activity symptoms include Circadian rhythm disturbance (30–80%), agitation (30–70%) and the least common was aggression (20–40%), apathy (15–40%) and wandering (15–40%).[125]

Assessment of Cognitive Functions in Alzheimer's Dementia

Mini mental state examination (MMSE) is commonly used for the assessment of cognitive functions in many countries. Specifically in AD patients Alzheimer disease assessment scale (ADAS) has been used and it measures cognitive functioning, memory, concentration, mood, behavioral disturbances. Severe impairment battery (SIB) is used to asses cognitive functioning in patients with severe AD, multidimensional observation scale for elderly subjects (MOSES) is used to assess cognitive and psychosocial functioning and Cohen-Mansfield Agitation Inventory (CMAI) is used for assessment of manifestation and frequency of agitation in patients with dementia. Neuropsychiatric inventory (NPI) is a scale used for assessment of psychopathology in patients with dementia.[126-129]

Pathophysiology

The gross pathology of the brain reveals gross cerebral atrophy. The key lesions are found only histopathologically and include extracellular neuritic plaques and intracellular neurofibrillary tangles. Both are found in frontal and temporal lobes (including Hippocampus); however in advanced cases it is found in most of the cortex which includes parietal and occipital lobes. The plaques are insoluble extracellular deposits composed of amino acid peptide called beta-amyloid and they are derived from a larger protein, beat-amyloid precursor protein (APP). There are two types of plaques; they are diffuse type and classical type. The classical type contains densely aggregated beta-amyloid and are associated with degeneration and neuronal cell loss. However, diffuse plaques are amorphous aggregates of beta-amyloid and not associated with neuronal cell loss. Tangles are intracellular deposits of microtubules associated protein tau found inside the dystrophic neurons and binds to tubulin monomers and affect the presumed cellular transport and axonal growth. In AD cases, it is found in hyperphosphorylated state and leads to less effective binding to microtubules. However, it is not clear whether plaques and tangles are biomarkers of AD or is a consequence of the disease. Apart from this they may have significant synaptic loss due to the accumulation of plaques and tangles. Synaptic loss and neuronal loss are attributed to the clinical features of AD. The other lesions noticed in AD cases but the significance of it is not known still includes granulovacuolar body (an intraneuronal change, found often in pyramidal neurones) and extensive nonamyloid atherosclerotic change.

Neurochemistry

AD has been currently thought as a disorder of cholinergic system. This hypothesis is based on the evidence that there is a predominant loss of cholinergic neurons and the first ones to be lost in AD and the fact that cholinergic system is required for memory. However, it is only part of the story. A review by Lyness, et al.[130] found that there is extensive loss of noradrenergic and serotonergic neurones and with the loss of noradrenergic neurons being as extensive as loss of cholinergic tracts. Even though decreased glutamate *in vivo* from MRS studies have been found, however, the evidence is not convincing.

Etiology/Risk Factors

Age is one of the important risk factors associated with DAT. Other possible risk factors include gender, marital status, lower education, Down syndrome (trisomy 21), hypertension, midlife high cholesterol level, head injury, head trauma, traumatic brain injury (TBI) and living in an urban area have been associated. Higher educational status had lower risk and was associated with older age at onset probably attributed to brain and cognitive reserve.

Genetic risk factors include presenilin I, presenilin II, and APP. They are associated with early-onset variant and account for 5% of AD cases. They probably work through increased production of Ab peptides and are associated with familial cases of AD. APOe4 allele (APOe4) is the only proven genetic risk factor for the late form of the disease. In the general population the risk for AD is around 20%, however, for those who are 85 years and homozygous for the APOe4 allele have 50–90% chance and those heterozygous have 45% chance. The late onset AD cases (onset after the age of 65) occur in the absence of one of the causative genes and without family history. Some of the protective factors associated with AD are lifestyle changes such as intellectual, physical, recreational and social activities and social network size which play a role in preserving cognitive functioning.[131]

Modification of the Amyloid Cascade Hypothesis

One of the most important theories so far was "Amyloid Cascade Hypothesis" to explain the pathogenesis of Alzheimer's disease (AD). It proposed that the deposition of β-amyloid (Aβ) is the initial pathological event in AD leading to the formation of senile plaques (SPs) and then to neurofibrillary tangles (NFTs) death of neurons, and ultimately dementia. However, there were many questions related to the cause and effect NFT and SP. Based on the current evidence a modification of the original amyloid cascade hypothesis (ACH) has been proposed by Armstrong.[132] He suggested that the essential trigger to the development of AD is aging of the brain and associated risk factors called as "allostatic load" (head trauma, vascular disease, and systemic disease)[133] exacerbate processes leading to cell death. As neurons degenerate, various proteins are upregulated leading to the formation of extracellular A β deposits and intracellular tau, the latter resulting in the development of neurofibrillary tangles. They may be toxic and initiate a secondary degeneration phase that accelerates the neuronal loss leading to dementia. In this modified hypothesis, genetic factors, rather than initiating disease, indirectly influence the formation and composition of peptides formed when neurons degenerate. Hence, the modified ACH incorporates information suggesting a more complex relationship between SPs and NFTs and proposes that the lesions are essentially reactive rather than causal.

Head Injury

Repeated head injury with and without loss of consciousness is associated with cases of AD. Post mortem studies of people dying of head injury showed increased amounts of amyloid peptide deposition. The impact of the injury in vulnerable groups such as boxers leads to significant damage and leads to tau aggregations similar to those of AD and also deposition of amyloid peptide.[134] The deposition of amyloid has been found to be increased in people having at least one APOEε4 allele and that clinical response to brain injury is APOE dependent.[135]

Inflammation

The amyloid-β peptide (Aβ) seen in neuritic plaques has been found to promote an inflammatory response mediated by microglia and astrocytes, thus activating signaling pathways and induction of proinflammatory molecules thus leading to synaptic damage, neuronal loss, and the activation of other inflammatory participants. The accumulation of amyloid activates caspases and transcription factors such as NF-κB and AP-1, which produce numerous inflammation amplifiers (IL-1β, TNF-α, and IL-6). These proinflammatory cytokines, could act directly on the neuron and induce apoptosis. The TNF-α and IL-1β can activate astrocytes and which in turn release factors that have the capacity to activate microglia.APP, BACE1, and PSEN expression is up regulated by the presence of proinflammatory cytokines. Increased amyloid production and microglia-mediated activation of inflammation is contributed by inflammatory mediators acting on neurons and the microglia-neuron communication amplifies the production of factors that contribute to AD-type pathology. The IL-1β may cause neuronal death, which activates microglia and later increases the release of IL-1β, thus generating a self-sustaining mechanism that is amplified by itself. This gradual but steady inflammation state, generated for long periods in the brain eventually can destroy neurons and contribute to the clinical symptoms observed in the disease.[136]

Diabetes

Type 2 diabetes mellitus has been found to have an increased risk and has been found to have a strong interaction of other factors such as hypertension, dyslipidemia and ApoE genotype. Various pathophysiological mechanisms have been proposed with diabetes which includes glycemia, insulin resistance, oxidative stress, advanced glycation endproducts, inflammatory cytokines, and microvascular and macrovascular disease.

Oxidative Stress

There has been evidence of an increased oxidation of macromolecules—lipids, carbohydrates, proteins, and DNA and oxidative stress products has been found in senile plaques and neurofibrillary tangles. The biomarkers of oxidation have been found even in peripheral tissues (e.g. blood cells) and biological fluids (e.g. urine) of individuals affected by AD. It is not clear whether Aβ peptide deposition is the cause or the result of the oxidative stress. However, researchers propose that initially Aβ peptide deposition and the formation of neurofibrillary tangles are consequences of oxidative stress and may protect neurons against oxidative damage but as the disease progresses they form into prooxidants driving a self-sustained "autodestructive" process and the progression of the disease.

Air Pollution

Studies have found that olfactory dysfunction occurred in 90% of patients in the early stages of AD and it results from the extensive cell loss and neurofibrillary tangles formation associated with AD which precede Aβ peptide deposition. Entry of infective agents and pollutants through the nose to the brain through the olfactory epithelium has been suggested in the pathology of AD. Animal and cellular studies found that individuals exposed to high levels of air pollution show damage in the olfactory mucosa, olfactory bulb, and frontal cortex region tissues which are all similar to brain pathology in AD. A few studies in human have shown that exposure to air pollution impaired cognitive function and caused cerebrovascular damage. The evidence of neocortical hyperphosphorylated tau with pretangle material and amyloid-β diffuse plaques in the frontal cortex of subjects exposed to urban air pollution suggests a link between oxidative stress, neuroinflammation, neurodegeneration, and chronic exposure to high concentrations of air pollution. Also, air pollution was found to accelerate amyloid beta-42 (Aβ-42) accumulations, which is associated with the neuronal dysfunction that precedes the formation of Aβ peptide plaques and neurofibrillary tangles. Based on all the evidence researcher suggest a hypothesis that interaction of age, genetic vulnerability and exposure to air pollution may lead to development AD.[137]

Metal Toxins

There is evidence of unusual distribution of iron, copper, zinc and aluminum in AD brains which show degeneration. Aluminum and iron have been implicated in the pathogenesis of not only in AD but also in other neurodegenerative disorders. There is evidence that metal ion exposure to aluminum or iron triggers changes in gene expression, preceded by reactive oxygen species (ROS) as seen in AD. Aluminum has been found to impair mitochondrial bioenergetics leading to the progressive accumulation of oxidative modified cellular proteins, affects cell functions, rapidly promotes compaction of biological molecules, affects metabolism of calcium and magnesium and it binds to A-T rich regions of DNA and has been postulated to play a role in gene silencing. Aluminum sulfate alone appeared to induce ROS-mediated up-regulation of an NF-kB-sensitive miRNA-146a that down-regulates the expression of complement factor H (CFH), an important repressor of inflammation and the NF-kB-miRNA-146a-CFH signaling circuit is affected by Aβ42 peptides in the same way as aluminum sulfate, and the circuit also is abnormal in the AD brain. These findings suggest the role of ROS induction by metal-catalyzed reactions in the regulation of genetic mechanisms of AD pathogenesis.[138,139]

Neuroimaging

CT and MRI may reveal cerebral atrophy present but it may not help in confirming the diagnosis of AD. A special focus on the medial temporal lobe has found to be diagnostic and of prognostic value and in particular the hippocampal volume which has been found to be reduced in early in AD and can be easily distinguished from normal controls. Using this Scheltens, et al.[140] after reviewing the a series of studies reported that the sensitivity and specificity for detection of mild to moderate AD compared with controls was 85% and 88%. It has been found that the both cerebral blood flow and oxygen utilization was reduced in gray and white matter, significantly in the parietal and temporal regions was demonstrated using PET. As the AD worsens there is frontal hypometabolism however the visual cortex and the primary sensorimotor cortex were relatively spared. Hypometabolism of brain has been confirmed using FDG-PET in AD and it correlates with amyloid burden. The sensitivity and specificity of FDG-PET's role in the diagnosis of AD was found to be 86% and 86%, respectively.[141] Also, reduced *N*-acetylaspartate (NAA) (marker of neuronal integrity) and increased myoinositol (marker of glial cells) using proton magnetic resonance spectroscopy (1H-MRS) have been well established in AD cases. The levels of NAA correlated with plaque density and neuro fibrillary tangles and reductions in NAA/creatine and phosphocreatine correlated with disease severity.[142]

Primary Prevention

The prevention of subsequent dementia in cognitively normal subjects and is the ultimate goal for AD management. As we know that some risk factors such as age, gender and gentic aspect cannot be modified and hence the epidemiological approach has been focussed towards modifiable risk factors such as hypertension, smoking, diabetes, atrial fibrillation and obesity and head injury. Even though initial efforts were promising, such as "Women's'Health Initiative Memory Study" which is a large, prospective, placebo-controlled trial which used estrogen plus progestin in post-menopausal women and treatment of hypertension trial did not show any significant clinical benefit.[143-145]

Secondary Prevention

The prevention of development of AD in non-demented subjects with some evidence of cognitive impairment is the main aim in secondary prevention. Many RCTs of cholinesterase inhibitors (ChEIs) have been undertaken in mild cognitive impairment (MCI), where the primary outcome was conversion of MCI to dementia. Even though multiple drugs have been tried so far; such as ChEIs, aspirin, vitamin E, *Gingko Biloba* and anti-inflammatories, none of them have been found to be demonstrated efficacy for preventing or delaying development of AD in MCI subjects.[146,147]

Treatment of Established Alzheimer's Dementia

Cholinesterase Inhibitors

They were the first drugs to be approved by the FDA for the treatment of AD. Even though Tacrine was the first to be approved due to its adverse effects and significant hepatotoxicity, it is not used commonly. The three drugs which have shown efficacy on cognitive function, global outcome and ADL in patients with mild-to-moderate AD include donepezil, rivastigmine and galantamine. Most of the studies have been for short-term. However, Donepezil has shown evidence for long-term efficacy (1–3 years). Even though there are only few head on comparisons, currently, there is no evidence of better efficacy of one cholinesterase inhibitors over another.[148] They are usually well tolerated, however, they have minor adverse symptoms such as nausea, diarrhea, and vomiting.

Rivastigmine is the only drug in which cytochrome P450 isoenzymes is not involved in its metabolism and hence few drug-drug interactions. Also, it is transdermal patch preparation has been found to have lower side effects but with equal efficacy to oral preparation.[149]

Galantamine, is a selective acetylcholinesterase inhibitor and extracted from the flowers and bulbs of lilies and daffodils. It is found to improve cognitive dysfunction and affords neuronal protection, preventing the cytotoxicity caused by aggregation of Aβ. It is also believed to enhance central neurotransmission.[150,151]

Huperzine A is an alkaloid from a plant named *Huperzia serrate and* an effective AChE Inhibitor which can cross the blood-brain barrier (BBB). It provides neuroprotection against neuronal damage.[152]

Memantine is an uncompetitive antagonist of NMDA receptor and it was approved for the treatment of moderate severity AD. It shows both shows neuroprotective effects and cognition-enhanced properties. It has a moderating effect with other medication and protects the brain from the toxic levels of calcium, allows normal signaling among brain neurons.[153] Even though it has a positive effect in cognitive functions in all severities of AD, but its effect on activities of daily living and behavior was only moderate. Agitation/aggression and irritability were the most responsive symptoms with this medication. Addition to cholinesterase inhibitors did not show any evidence of benefit.

M1 Receptor Agonists

There are two M_1 receptor agonists, xanomeline and milameline. The M_1 muscarinic receptors are intact in the AD brain and hence, a potential target for AD treatment. They usually reduce the symptoms of AD and also delay the disease's progression. Xanomeline is a selective muscarinic M_1 and M_4-preferring receptor agonist which can cross blood-brain barrier. Preliminary studies have shown significant improvement in the cognitive function of patients but they had some important side effects such as gastrointestinal response and cardiovascular adverse reactions.[154]

Other Drugs

Many drugs have been suggested to be helpful in AD. They include non-steroidal anti-inflammatory drugs (NSAIDs), estrogens, statins and *Ginkgo biloba* extract. Even though vitamin E (1000 IU, twice a day over 2 years) has been found to delay the time to primary outcome measures in moderate AD, but there has been negative results with mild cognitive impairment. Also a Cochrane review is that, there is insufficient evidence for the efficacy of vitamin E in the treatment of AD or MCI.[155] NSAIDs and cyclo-oxygenase-2 inhibitors had negative results with serious adverse effects in AD and MCI. They have been a trial of some novel compound in AD such as piracetam, nicergoline, selegiline, vinpocetine, pentoxifylline and Cerebrolysin. However, currently Cochrane review of the efficacy of most of the compounds has been negative.[148,156,157]

Vaccines

Dale Schenk and his colleagues invented the vaccination therapy for AD in 1999. Immunotherapy was one of the approaches to prevent aggregation of Aβ. Preliminary studies have shown that anti-Aβ antibodies are effective in clearing Aβ deposits. Even though, it was very promising and a breakthrough, the studies very halted because few of the subjects developed subacute meningoencephalitis. Currently, there are passive immunization clinical trials using anti-Aβ antibodies in AD.[158]

Management of Behavioral Symptoms

It is important to identify the cause for the behavioral or psychological symptoms. Efforts should be taken to use non-pharmacological treatments before considering pharmacological treatments. Cholinesterase inhibitors have been used for mild behavioral problems, but it has not been consistent. Typical and atypical antipsychotics have been used in aggression/psychotic symptoms and has demonstrated significant efficacy, especially risperidone. However, the side effects associated with antipsychotics have to be considered. Typical antipsychotics have the advantage of lesser metabolic syndrome; can be used in parenteral forms in emergency management compared to atypicals. Some of the major concerns with typicals are cognitive symptoms, extrapyramidal symptoms and falls associated with it. However, there is no evidence that typical antipsychotics are safer with regard to risk of stroke or mortality than atypicals. It is preferable to use low dose and monitor for side effects. Carbamazepine has also been found to useful in aggression. Antidepressants may be useful in patients with depressive symptoms.[159-162]

Non-Pharmacological Treatments

Non-pharmacological treatments have been found to be useful, versatile and potentially cost-effective approach to improve outcomes and quality of life in AD for both the patients and the care givers. Various techniques have been used. They include cognitive training, behavioral interventions, cognitive stimulation, transcutaneous electrical stimulation, physical exercise, use of music, reminiscence, ADL training, massage and touch, recreation therapy, use of light, multisensory stimulation, support and psychotherapy, validation, acupuncture, transcranial magnetic stimulation, muscle relaxation and multicomponent and have been tried in AD patients.[163]

To improve cognition: It has been found that training of specific cognitive abilities in small groups were helpful in improve specific cognitive abilities. Also, teaching of memory strategies conducted daily or twice weekly improved the verbal and visual learning. Significant improvement in measures of attention, memory, orientation, language and general cognition was found when the cognitive stimulation group sessions were combined with multicomponent interventions (e.g. relaxation). Cognitive stimulation with medications (Donepezil) was more effective than even medications alone when it was delivered by the caregivers.[164]

To improve the ADL: ADL training was found to be effective. Some of the interventions included such as scheduling and prompting used to reduce urinary incontinence; graded assistance to improve individual autonomy; prompting and reinforcement during meals to improve eating independence and a specific way-finding intervention to assist residents in locating a dining room.[165-168]

To improve the quality of life: A RCT using community occupational therapy, where adapting home environment to AD patients capabilities and providing continuous counseling and support to the caregivers improved quality of life as rated by the AD patients.[169]

VASCULAR DEMENTIA

Currently, all forms of cognitive impairment related to vascular disease in the brain are termed as *vascular cognitive impairment* (VCI). This term was introduced by O'Brien, et al.[170] and includes: VCI no dementia, vascular dementia, and AD with a vascular component. VCI no dementia constitutes the most prevalent VCI subgroup in persons younger than 85 years of age. Vascular dementia (VaD) is the loss of cognitive functions to a degree that interferes with ADLs, resulting from ischemic or hemorrhagic cerebrovascular disease (CVD) or from cardiovascular or circulatory disturbances that injure brain regions that are important for memory, cognition, and behavior.[171]

Epidemiology

Globally, vascular dementia (VD) is the second most common dementia affecting the elderly. The prevalence of VD is 15–20%, however, higher rates of 40–50% have been reported in few studies.[172,173] It is more common in men, especially before the age 75 years.

In India, most of the studies have found the VD to be the second most common dementia.[174] In an epidemiological survey (3-year) for dementia in an urban community-resident population in Mumbai (Bombay) found that the prevalence of vascular dementia was 22% (n = 23). In a memory clinic based follow-up, VD was found to be the second most common subtype of dementia and the prevalence was 25.4%. The subcortical type was the most common subtype of VD and found in nearly 50% of the patients. They were found to be younger than the Alzheimer's group and were predominantly male.[175] However, a study by Shaji, et al. (2005) found a higher prevalence of 39% of VD in his subjects in Kerala. In a sample of 42 patients with VD, they found that the subcortical dementia was the most common type (52.4%), followed by cortical-subcortical (26.2%), strategic infarcts in (14.3%), and cortical dementia (7.1%).[176]

Risk Factors

The risk factors for vascular dementia include advanced age, long-term, untreated arterial hypertension, isolated systolic hypertension in the elderly, diabetes mellitus, cigarette smoking, hyperlipidemia, hyperhomocysteinemia, hyperfibrinogenemia, congestive heart failure, atrial fibrillation, other cardiac arrhythmias, complicated stroke, recurrent stroke, orthostatic hypotension, obstructive sleep apnea, major surgery in the elderly, and coronary artery bypass graft surgery. In an epidemiological survey from Kolkata, they found a strong correlation with vascular risk factors and MCI.[177] A study by Ray, et al.[178] found that alterations in homocysteine and Lipoprotein (a) in serum are indicators of vascular pathology in AD or VD (increased). A study by Alladi[176] in a hospital dementia registry, in a series of 42 patients with VD; found that stroke (81%), hypertension (71.4%), and diabetes (35.7%) were some of the important risk factors. Also, they found that the small artery disease was the underlying vascular mechanism in 42.9%; intracranial large artery disease, in 16.7%; extracranial disease, in 2.3%; cardioembolism, in 2.3%; multiple mechanisms, in 19%; and unknown, in 16.7%.

Clinical Forms and Pathology of Vascular Dementia

The current classification of VD can be classified into acute and sub-acute according to Roman.[179]

Acute Vascular Dementia (Poststroke, Postictal, or Postapoplectic VD)

This categories involve patients with new onset of dementia after an acute cerebrovascular event, usually resulting from a single strategic stroke resulting from occlusion (or rupture) of a large-size vessel or a symptomatic subcortical lacunar stroke caused by occlusive small-vessel disease. Approximately, 20% of ischemic stroke (> 65 year) develop in poststroke VD. The large-vessel forms of poststroke VD may resemble the cortical dementias and have stroke-related cortical cognitive deficits, such as agnosia, apraxia, alexia, aphasia, often without motor deficit.[180] The patients with this type do not have significant amnesia and some of the patients recover their independence in ADLs and do not fulfil the criteria for dementia. Main features of acute-onset VD syndromes associated with large-vessel stroke follows.

Posterior Cerebral Artery

Patient presents with amnesia (25%) due to damage to the hippocampus, isthmus, endorhinal and perirhinal cortex, and parahippocampal gyrus. Bilateral damage gives rise to global amnesia whereas unilateral lesions cause material-specific memory loss (verbal amnesia with left-sided lesions and loss of visuospatial memory and right side lesions with memory deficits for locations). Patients with mesial temporal lobe lesions sometimes present with episodic anterograde amnesia.[181] They are unable to encode and consolidate new verbal material, facts; events, short stories, names, and concepts their but working memory and procedural memory are intact; confabulations are uncommon.[182] Patients with PCA strokes present with visual signs (80%) which usually accompany the memory deficits.

Basal Forebrain Infarction

Patients with ischemic injury to basal forebrain present with severe anterograde amnesia for verbal or visuospatial material, along with severe apathy, lack of initiative and spontaneity, and executive dysfunction.[183] Most subjects with VD perform better on story recall and wordlist learning (California and the Rey verbal learning tests). They are usually able to respond to cues and have superior free recall and relatively minor deficits of verbal long-term memory.[184] Patients with VD retain speech and calculation longer than those with AD.

Thalamic Vascular Dementia (VaD)

This rare condition was described by Castaigne et al.[185] It has been noticed after ischemic strokes occurred to paramedian thalamic structures. The patients usually presented with impairments in attention, motivation, initiative, executive functions, memory and reduced levels of consciousness that gradually improves within days to weeks. They also showed dramatic verbal and motor slowness and apathy.[186] Visual abnormalities include vertical gaze paresis, medial rectus paresis, and absent convergence. They may present with Dysarthria and mild hemiparesis when the lesions extend to the subthalamic and midbrain tegmentum. Left thalamic lesions are associated with memory deficits and visual memory loss. Right-sided lesions are associated with visual amnesia. Bilateral lesions or in those with simultaneous damage to the mamillothalamic tract and the inferior thalamic peduncle are associated with global amnesia. They also have anterograde episodic amnesia plus retrograde amnesia.[180]

Inferior Genu Stroke

This syndrome was associated with lacunar infarcts of inferior genu of the internal capsule and was described by Tatemichi and colleagues.[187] The patients present with sudden onset of cognitive function, fluctuating attention, confusion, abulia, striking psychomotor retardation, inattention, executive dysfunction, memory loss and with mild focal findings, such as hemiparesis or dysarthria. Right-sided infarcts caused visuospatial memory loss and left-sided infarcts have severe verbal memory loss.[188,189]

Caudate Strokes

They present with memory loss consisting of recall difficulties even with cues but with normal recognition.[53] The interruption of frontal connections may be associated with typical abulia.[190]

Subacute Vascular Dementia

Lacunar State

This syndrome is associated with multiple brain lacunes. Small areas of ischemic necrosis and liquefaction of less than 15 mm diameter is called as lacunes. They are located in basal ganglia, internal capsule, thalamus, pons, corona radiata, and centrum semiovale, and commonly seen in chronic cavitated stage.[191] Lacunar strokes are caused by occlusion of the arterial lumen of small arterioles (also including deep thalamoperforating and long medullary arterioles). The number of lacunes does not correlate better with cognitive deficits, however, the extent of white matter lesions in patients with subcortical lacunes. In a series of elderly US population; in around 89%, even though the lacunes were clinically silent, the participants had gait problems and subtle cognitive impairments, which was not recognized as stroke.[192]

Binswanger's Disease

The Binswanger's disease was first described by Binswanger in 1894 with the title 'encephalitis subcorticalis chronica progressiva'. The clinical presentation is manifested by subacute progression of dementia associated with focal neurological deficits in hypertensive patients in their 50s or 60s, associated with prominent motor signs and usually by pseudobulbar palsy. The deficits progress over weeks or months, then stabilizing with long plateau periods lasting for months or occasionally years. The cognitive symptoms include executive dysfunction, loss of verbal fluency, slowing of motor function with perseveration, impersistence, inattention, difficulties with set shifting, and abnormal Luria's kinetic melody tests. The memory deficitsis characterized by poor retrieval and intact recognition. The motor symptoms include mild residual hemiparesis, a peculiar short-stepped gait *(marche à petits pas),* dysarthria, pseudobulbar palsy, extrapyramidal features such as inexpressive facies, slowness of movement, axial rigidity, loss of postural reflexes, frequent falls, increased urinary frequency, and nocturia.[193] Apathy, depression, and behavioral problems are common. The main pathology noted were in the long perforating vessels to the deep white matter and subcortical nuclear masses, resulting in multiple small areas of infarction (lacunes) together with the cardinal feature of diffuse demyelination of the white matter due to subacute hypertensive encephalopathy. There is typically sparing of the arcuate subcortical U fibers, which is a hallmark of this condition. The other mechanism proposed is chronic hypoperfusion in the watershed area between the territories of the cortical medullary arteries and the long-perforating branches to the white matter.[194] The cortical areas are relatively spared.

Cerebral Autosomal Dominant Arteriopathy with Subcortical Infarcts and Leukoencephalopathy

Cerebral autosomal dominant arteriopathy with subcortical infarcts and leukoencephalopathy (CADASIL) is an autosomal dominant disorder of cerebral small vessels associated with chromosome 19q12. It was originally called familial Binswanger's disease. The clinical symptoms are TIAs and strokes (80%), cognitive deficits and VD (50%), migraine with focal deficits (40%), mood disorders (30%), and epilepsy (10%). The age of onset is early adulthood (mean age 46 year and it leads to dementia and death by 20 years after the onset of the symptoms. The dementia is slow, subcortical and frontal in nature, associated with gait and urinary disturbances, and pseudobulbar palsy. The main pathology involves nonamyloid nonatherosclerotic microangiopathy involving arterioles (100–400 μ in diameter) and capillaries, primarily in the brain. Skin biopsy is used for the diagnostic workup and confirmed by immunostaining with a *Notch3* monoclonal antibody.[195-197] Yadav, et al. reported the first family of Indian origin known to be affected by (CADASIL). Five of the 17 members were genetically confirmed carriers of the *Notch3* gene *R141C* mutation in exon 4 (421(C→T) and 141(Cys→Arg)) of the family spanning 3 generations who had neurologic syndromes compatible with CADASIL.[198]

Cerebral Amyloid Angiopathy

This disorder presents with recurrent or multiple lobar hemorrhages, cognitive deterioration, and ischemic strokes. The pathological lesions include deposition of amyloid in the walls of leptomeningeal and cerebral cortical blood vessels.

Diagnosis of Vascular Dementia

Various clinical criteria have been considered in the diagnosis of Vascualr dementia, they include NINDS-AIREN, ICD 10, ADDTC, DSM IV, DSM-5 and Mayo clinic. A Hachinski ischemic score is a screening tool used to differentiate vascular dementia from degenerative forms of the disorder. A score of 7 or higher are more likely to have a vascular dementia, while low score is less likely to indicate vascular dementia. This is because ischemic lesions severe enough to produce a dementia would be expected to be severe enough to cause the accompanying neurologic changes and elevate the index.[199]

Treatment and Prevention of Vascular Dementia

Risk factor modifications is one the important measures in primary prevention. There has been good results with calcium channel blocker nitrendipine, ACE inhibitors, and diuretics.[200,201] Of all antihypertensives, angiotensin II receptor blockers have been particularly effective because of their direct effects on the brain (Mogi, 2009). However, the Syst-Eur study found that calcium channel blockers used as antihypertensives have reduced the incidence of dementia by 50% in elderly patients. But, it is important to keep in mind that lowering blood pressure in the elderly can have adverse effect on the brain by causing ischemic damage to these brains, affected by impaired cerebral autoregulation.[202] In the event of cognitive decline following a stroke, important protective measures against further strokes should be initiated. Patients treated with aspirin (325 mg/day) in a RCT in multi-infarct dementia were having significantly higher cognitive symptoms than those without aspirin. However, currently there are no drug has been approved for the treatment of VaD. Despite, trying approved anti-AD drugs in VD, including the cholinesterase inhibitors (ChEIs), and memantine, all had only small effect sizes. Physical activity has been found to prevent VCI.[203]

DEMENTIA IN PARKINSON'S DISEASE

Parkinson's disease (PD) is a neurodegenerative disorder. The diagnosis is made based on the characteristic motor disturbance such as bradykinesia, resting tremor, rigidity, and postural instability; asymmetrical symptom onset, and good response to levodopa.[204] One out 100 people aged more than 60 years are affected in the industrialized countries with PD.[205] They do present with cognitive impairment consisting of deficits in executive functions, memory and visuospatial and dementia, these features can be independent of motor deficits.[206] Clinical dementia in this disorder affects the functional outcome and reduces the life expectancy in patients.[206] The prevalence estimated in the general population is 2–3%. There is a risk of 3–5 times in Parkinson's disease patients to develop dementia. The cumulative prevalence of Parkinson's disease population range from 75% to 90%, since it is associated with mortality.[207,208]

Diagnosis

There is a no consistent evidence for a clear entity of Dementia in Parkinson's disease. Also, there is no evidence whether development of cognitive deficits early in the Parkinson's disease will develop dementia. The Queen Square Brain Bank criteria describes Parkinson's dementia as a syndrome that manifests in two or more cognitive domains with a decline in levels of functioning and that causes social and occupational impairment; deficits such as fluctuating attention, executive dysfunction, free recall, and visuospatial function.

Clinical Features

They usually present with mild forgetfulness, memory difficulties, bradyphrenia, impaired planning, lack of organization of goal-directed activity, problems with set shifting, visuospatial deficits, fluctuation in attention and cognition, personality instability and learning and memory difficulties.[209] Following the worsening of motor symptoms of PD, the cognitive symptoms of DPD worsens, however, the language and praxis remain stable till the last stage. This suggests the role in subcortical regions in the pathophysiology of dementia.[210]

Pathology

The cognitive symptoms seen in dementia in Parkinson's disease are related to dementia with Lewy bodies, even though they both are different from Alzheimer's disease. The pathological changes such as Lewy bodies, plaques, and vascular changes are present in both dementia in Parkinson's disease and dementia with Lewy bodies. There is significant atrophy of the brain, especially, it is more particularly in the frontal, temporal, and occipital cortices and in subcortical regions in established cases of DPD.[211,212] Reduced grey matter in the bilateral occipital region was able to differentiate Parkinson's disease dementia from Parkinson's disease and in another study, reduced blood flow in the precuneus (parieto-occipital regions) found in DPD patient and not in Alzheimer's disease.[213,214] A new hypothesis which is supported by clinicopathological finding suggest that increased amyloid and α-synuclein concentrations have been found in patients with dementia in Parkinson's disease of shorter disease duration than longer duration. Lewy body accumulation and degeneration of the Basal forebrain (frontal, parietal, and temporal cortices and the amygdala) and ascending ascending cholinergic pathways have been found more in the DPD than in Alzheimer'sDisease or PD. Also, significant degeneration of basal forebrain cholinergic system was associated with onset of dementia.[215] These suggest a cholinergic hypothesis in the pathophysiology of DPD and experience with cholinesterase inhibitors have a moderate benefits on Patients with DPD. Patients with Parkinson's disease with visual hallucinations have been found to develop rapid cognitive deterioration and dementia onset. Visual hallucinations are associated with cortical Lewy bodies (temporal regions) and Hippocampal atrophy. Patients with visual hallucinations also have frontal hypermetabolism and orbitofrontal atrophy which correlates with visual memory deficits.[216-220]

Risk Factors

The risk factors for developing Parkinson's disease dementia include old age, comorbid depression, and nicotine misuse, hallucinations early on in the disease course and the akinetic-rigid type of Parkinson's disease.

Genetic Risk

Although, there is a family history of Parkinson's disease and lots of genetic studies have been done, genetic risk studies have not found a single gene or a cluster. The apolipoprotein E (*e4*) which predicts cholinergic deficits has been associated with DPD, (Williams-Gray, 2009). The glucocerebrosidase mutations which has been implicated in Lewy body formation may increase the risk for DPD.[221] It has been found that the patient DPD carrying both the *APOE* (*e4*) allele and the butyrylcholinesterase gene (*BCHE*) K allele might worsen their cognitive symptoms rapidly than those without.[222]

Treatment

Various molecules have been tried for DPD. Only few medications have been helpful. Rivastigmine has been found to improve activities of daily living in Parkinson's disease dementia relative to baseline. Donepezil, also improve cognition, as measured by mini-mental state examination scores and clinicians' interview-based impression of change with caregiver input, without exacerbating Parkinsonism. Memantine has been found to ameliorated cognitive impairment in Parkinson's disease dementia in recent trials. A novel initiative of using atomoxetine, a norepinephrine-reuptake inhibitor improved the executive function, attention, and verbal memory in patients with Parkinson's disease in an 8-week, dose-flexible pilot study. It is very important to be aware of the adverse effects of some medication on the cognition such as pramipexole and anticholinergic drugs, which have typically been used to target tremor in Parkinson's disease.[222-225]

Nonpharmacological Interventions

Apart from medications, they would also require non-pharmacological interventions such as psychosocial support and cognitive rehabilitation. A study which was conducted in PD patients without dementia found that cognitive training which focused on attention, abstract reasoning, and visuospatial abilities improved aspects of cognition (especially frontal function). Also, this study showed lasting improvements verbal fluency and recall.[226]

HUNTINGTON'S DISEASE

Huntington's disease is an autosomal dominant inherited and neurodegenerative disease. The age of onset is between 30 to 50 years, however, juvenile onset (< 20 years) and older onset (>70 years) are also common. It was initially described by George Huntington in 1872 and one of the most remarkable in the history of medicine for its brevity, clarity and comprehensiveness. The worldwide prevalence of HD is 5 to 8 per 100,000 populations. The prevalence is highest in European countries and lowest in Africa, China, Japan and Finland. The prevalence rate in the US is 4.1 to 8.4 per 100,000 population.[227] The prevalence in India has also been found to be high and closer to Western Europe due to the admixture of Caucasians in the native population.[227] A recent meta-analysis has estimated an incidence of 0.38 per 100,000 population per year worldwide and they found lower incidence in Asia compared to Europe, North America and Australia.[228] The outcome in HD is fatal and the death is due to significant immobility. They develop significant disability and communication problems requiring full time care. They have a longer course of 15–20 years compared to other primary dementing illnesses.

HD is caused by a mutation encoding an abnormal expansion of CAG-encoded polyglutamine repeats in a protein (htt). The Gene for HD is present on chromosome 4p16.3 and comprises 67 exons and 3144 amino acids. Normally, the repeat length in the *htt* gene is 36 or less however more than 40 codons causes HD. A study by Uday Murgod found an. Mean (SD) of 48.4 (8.7) CAG repeats in the abnormal allele.[229] *Htt* protein is expressed more intensely in neurons than in glial cells; it is accumulation which is proteolytic; triggers a cascade that leads to increasing neuronal dysfunction through oxidative injury, transcriptional dysregulation, glutamate excitotoxicity, apoptotic signals, mitochondrial dysfunction and energy depletion.[230-232] The neuroanatomical sites involved are caudate and putamen while the interneurons and afferent terminals are largely spared. The striatal projection neurons are affected and it leads to large decreases in striatal GABA concentrations while somatization and dopamine concentrations are relatively preserved.[233]

The clinical manifestations include motor, cognitive and psychiatric symptoms. The predominant motor symptom is chorea which is a rapid, jerky, dyskinetic, irregular, purposeless, arrhythmic and asymmetric movement that occur both at rest and during voluntary movements. It leads to difficulty walking, speaking and swallowing. The other motor symptoms include tics, loss of coordination and balance, slurred speech, jaw clenching or teeth grinding, difficulty swallowing or eating, continual muscular contractions and stumbling or falling.

Cognitive symptoms develop within the first year of overt motor signs. Initially, they have difficulties in sustained attention, problem solving, verbal fluency and memory retrieval later.[234] Language functions, comprehension and general knowledge are spared in the disease. This suggests that the Huntington dementia is more of subcortical pathology than cortical.

The psychiatric manifestations occur after the onset of motor disorders and the most common include affective disorders. The major depression is very high (50%)[235] and mania or hypomania (12%).[236] The symptoms associated with putative subcortical dementias, such as apathy, irritability and impulse control problems, have also been observed in HD patients.[237] There may also be a relatively high rate of violent behavior and criminality and explosive disorder. The schizophrenia-like psychosis has been termed as'delusional–hallucinatory states' because of origin of psychotic symptoms from a pervasive delusional mood.

The personality change consisted of aggression, violence, suspiciousness and outbursts of temper against the relatives or spouse. The prevalence was around 42% of 65 patients in the Oxfordshire region.[238] Another behavioral alteration of HD is decreased sex drive.

The risk of suicide associated with HD is around 7% [239] and they are three times more likely to commit suicide than general population. The gene carriers who are nearing the point of diagnosis and those who are beginning to lose their functional ability and independence have highest suicidal ideation.[240]

Juvenile or childhood type of HD has its onset during childhood or adolescent and is usually associated with paternal transmission. They present with muscular rigidity and tremors than choreiform movements. They may demonstrate clumsiness, ataxia and dysarthria. They perform badly in the school and shows difficulties with concentration. 50% of them have epileptic seizures. The mortality rate is higher in the first decade.

The treatment in HD is multidisciplinary in nature. There are currently no FDA approved medications for HD. Dopamine antagonist or depleters (Tetrabenazine) are effective in reducing involuntary movements such as chorea.[241] Antidepressants and mood stabilizers have been used in depressed patients. Antipsychotics have been effective in controlling psychotic symptoms and aggressive behavior. Botulinum antitoxin has been helpful in reducing dystonia in HD. Other novel treatments such as vitamin E, stem cell therapy are in research phase and may be helpful in the future for the HD cases.[242] Psychological support for the patient and caregivers are also important aspects of treatment.

CREUTZFELDT-JAKOB DISEASE

Introduction

Creutzfeldt-Jakob disease (CJD) is a rare, fatal neurological disorder, rapidly developing form of dementia. This disorder was first described by a German neurologist named Hans Gerhard Creutzfeldt in 1920 and afterwards by Alfons Maria Jakob and thus the name Creutzfeldt-Jakob. Also, familial CJD was described by an German psychiatrist and neurologist Friedrich Meggendorfer (1880–1953). It is caused by infectious proteinaceous particles called prions. Prions which are normally present in the brain cause disease when they take on a mis-shapen form accumulate in the brain and kill the brain cells.

CJD belongs to a group of disease's which affect man and animals called transmissible spongiform encephalopathies which is a fatal progressive neurological illness, and presents with a characteristic neuropathological changes, and a causal agent which does not require a nucleic acid template. Apart from CJD which is common in Humans, other forms include Kuru, Gerstmann-Sträussler-Scheinker disease and fatal familial insomnia. One of the unusual features of this group of disease is that they are very resistant to routine sterilization procedures.

Four different varieties have been reported and include Sporadic (sCJD), familial (fCJD), iatrogenic (iCJD), and variant forms of CJD (vCJD). The most common is of CJD cases are sporadic (85–95%) and 5–15% of CJD cases are due to fCJD and only 1% are due to iCJD. CJD occurs at the rate of about 1 case per million population per year globally. It occurs more commonly in the age group of 55–65 years but can also occur above 90 years or below 55 years. Few case reports case series have been reported in India.[243,244]

Modes of Transmission

The mode of transmission for sporadic CJD is not known and one of the hypothesis suggested is *de novo* spontaneous generation of self-replicating protein has been hypothesized. Familial CJD (fCJD) is transmitted through inheritance. The variant (vCJD) even though the exact mode is not known, it is probably linked to consumption of contaminated foods of bovine origin and secondary transmission by blood transfusion. The iatrogenic CJD infection is usually transmitted from an infected case with sCJD in the course of medical/surgical treatment, e.g. human pituitary hormone therapy, human duramater grafts, corneal grafts or neurological instruments.

Sporadic Creutzfeldt-Jakob Disease

This form of CJD is the most common of all CJD. Even though it is rare, although it is rare, the incidence is around 1.2 per million per annum and most of them develop the disease around 60–75 years old. Both genders are equally vulnerable. It is characterized by a rapidly-progressive dementing illness, leading to akinetic mutism. Initially, they present with depressive symptoms, memory disturbances, lack of interest and significant social withdrawal. Later, they present with neurological features which include myoclonus, cerebellar ataxia, pyramidal and extrapyramidal signs and cortical blindness. In the end, they become mute and unable to move. The duration of the illness is 4–5 months and 70% of them die within 6 months after the onset of symptoms. The clinical diagnosis of sCJD depends on clinical features, characteristic periodic triphasic sharp wave complexes (EEG) seen in two-thirds of patients) and CSF protein electrophoresis findings of raised 14-3-3 protein. The CT, PET or SPECT do not reveal valuable information in these patients. MRI reveals characteristic marked hyperintensity of the caudate head and putamen is seen in 70–80% of cases and it is has 90% specificity.[245,246]

Variant Creutzfeldt-Jakob Disease

In 1996, the UK National CJD Surveillance Unit in Edinburgh reported new variety CJD known as variant CJD (vCJD). This particular variety is more common in UK. It is characterized by a younger age of onset (median 29 years), longer duration of disease (median 14 months), with florid plaques in the brain, widespread accumulation of abnormal prion protein (PrP) and thalamic gliosis. The clinical symptoms consist of sensation of cold or paraesthesia, depressive symptoms, withdrawn behavior, fleeting delusions. They also present with neurological symptoms such as cerebellar signs, abnormal eye movements, and involuntary movements (myoclonus, chorea, dystonia). They have astrocytosis and neuronal loss prominent in the pulvinar of the thalamus and with characteristic "florid plaques" seen in the cerebral cortex in histopathology samples. In vCJD, a characteristic hyperintensity in the pulvinar of the thalamus is found. The hyperintensity is greater than that seen in the putamen or cortical gray matter called 'pulvinar sign' and it is best visualized on axial scans. In they have hyperintensities in the dorsomedial nuclei of the thalamus giving a 'hockey-stick' appearance.[247]

Familial Creutzfeldt-Jakob Disease

This variety of CJD is an inherited form and results from several types of mutations on prion gene. The other forms of genetic prion disease include Gerstmann-Sträussler-Scheinker syndrome, and fatal familial insomnia and all of these are inherited as autosomal dominant disorders with a high degree of penetrance. The onset is usually at the age of 52, the incidence of this type is less than in 5 cases each year in UK. The symptoms and course of familial CJD will vary depending on the type of PrP mutation involved. The symptoms are consisting of dementia and neurological problems such as unsteadiness; sometimes they have similar symptoms of sporadic type. The course of the disease is often longer and the patient may survive for several years after the onset of symptoms. FCJD have a range of mutations within the open reading frame of the prion protein gene (*PRNP*) on chromosome 20. Now, the mutations in the PrP gene can be easily identified with a blood test.[248]

Iatrogenic Creutzfeldt-Jakob Disease

Till around 2010, around 420 cases were reported. Most of the cases occurred in france and Japan and were transmitted by human duramatter grafts and human growth hormone treatment. The mean incubation period was is generally long and usually more than 12 months. The clinical features of iCJD are similar to spasmodic type except in those cases treated with of human growth hormone treatment where it is characterized by progressive cerebellar ataxia with or without dementia. If dementia develops, then it occurs late. The macroscopic changes reported are similar to sporadic type with spongiform changes, neuronal loss and gliosis and amyloid plaque formation (with accumulation of abnormal forms of prion protein. However, in human growth hormone recipients cerebellar atrophy is prominent.[249] Microscopic features are similar to spaordic type except in Japan, where a subset of cases had florid plaques in the cerebral cortex and basal ganglia. In UK, kuru-type plaques occurred in patients who are heterozygous at codon 129 of the *PRNP* gene.[249]

Treatment

Currently, there is no medication approved for the treatment of CJD. However, many medications have been tried on experiment basis. Pentosan polysulphate (PPS), which is used to treat interstitial cystitis was infused into the patient's lateral ventricle within the brain. Even though, PPS was able to slow the progression, it did not help the subjects overall. Amphotericin B and doxorubicin have been investigated but they are currently no strong evidence for its efficacy against CJD. A preliminary study showed that an anti-malarial medications Quinacrine, permanently cleared abnormal prion proteins from cell cultures, but results are not promising. Astemizole which has an anti-prion activity has been proposed to help in Creutzfeldt-Jakob disease. However, more clinical studies looking into the efficacy are required. Apart from medication, researchers have looked at other measures of curbing CJD, Shalu, et al. suggested that religious standards and government Policies in India are helpful in curbing the CJD.[250]

FRONTOTEMPORAL DEMENTIAS

It is a neurodegenerative type of dementia, which involves the degeneration of the anterior parts (frontal and temporal) of the brain and with preservation of the posterior cerebral region; hence the name frontotemporal dementias (FTD). The clinicopathological spectrum of the above is termed as frontotemporal lobar degeneration (FTLD). It is the second most common cause of young onset dementia. It is very important in psychiatry because of the behavioral and personality changes which can mimic psychiatric disorders. The term Pick's disease is used for patients of FTLD with intraneuronal argyrophilic inclusions, the so called Pick bodies, which consist of abnormal three-repeat tau protein (FTLD-tau).

Epidemiology

The exact prevalence of FTD is not clear. It has varied from 3 to 22 per 100,000 population in the age range of 45–64 years.[251-253] In India, a study by Alladi et al. in a Hospital based memory clinic with 347 dementia patients found a prevalence of frontotemporal dementia syndromes in around 18.7%.[254] In another study by Shankar et al. in West Bengal in young onset dementia patients, they found that the prevalence was 27% and it was the second most common dementia and 20% had a positive family history.[255] The incidence of FTD was found to be between 3.5–4.1 cases per 100,000 person-years in the age group of 45–65 years. There were no gender differences.[256,257] The age of onset varies between 45–64 years, around 10% of them had it after 70 years.[258]

Clinical Features

There are three distinct clinical syndromes with a distinct topographical cerebral involvement and characteristic histopathology. They include the behavioral variant of FTD (bvFTD) and the language variants, semantic dementia (SD) and progressive non-fluent aphasia (PNFA). There is also overlap of FTD with motor neuron disease (FTD-MND or FTD-ALS), as well as the parkinsonian syndromes, progressive supranuclear palsy (PSP) and corticobasal syndrome (CBS).[259] All the types have insidious onset, progressive course but a variable decline.

Behavioral-variant Frontotemporal Dementia

They present with marked changes in personality and behavior. They can be further divided into three varieties apathy, disinhibition and stereotyped-compulsive syndrome.[260,261] Apathy is characterized by social withdrawal, loss of interest in personal affairs and responsibilities. As the disease advances, there is loss of awareness of personal hygiene and sphincter control. Atrophy and dysfunction of right anterior cingulate cortex and superior frontal gyrus has been associated with apathy.[262] Disinhibition is characterized by socially inappropriate behaviors, including confrontation seeking, making hurtful or insensitive remarks to others, engaging in frankly sociopathic behaviors (e.g. shop-lifting, traffic violations) or rarely physical assault.[263,264] They are not empathetic and appear cold, showing little concern for the effect of their behavior on loved ones.[265] They also show no insight and a very shallow recognition of a cognitive problem (often described as mild memory problems or word-finding difficulties). Dramatic changes in religious beliefs, political convictions, or dress and social style, personality changes that are so profound they have been described as a "change in self".[266]

Right subgenual cingulate and orbitofrontal cortex have been implicated in with disinhibition.[262,267,268] Hyperorality, overeating, loss of table manners, idiosyncratic hoarding, collecting and repetitive motor behaviors (e.g. rubbing, picking, throat clearing, pacing and wandering) have been reported.[269,270] Orbitofrontal-striatal circuit has been associated with overeating.[271] Behavioral disturbance are more prominent than cognitive disturbance in these group of patients. The common cognitive symptoms include inattentiveness, distractibility, loss of planning, poor judgment, loss of planning ability and disorganization.[272]

Semantic Dementia

It is also referred to as temporal-variant of FTLD. Fluent speech progressive impairment of single-word comprehension, preserved articulatory abilities and behavioral changes in the setting of marked, often asymmetric degeneration of the anterior temporal lobes. Patients with primarily left-sided atrophy present initially with progressive loss of 'semantic' knowledge about words, objects and concepts. This is manifest as a fluent aphasia with impoverished speech content and semantic paraphasic errors, but intact syntax, prosody and motor speech. Loss of meaning follows a hierarchical pattern; for example, patients may first lose their ability to differentiate between types of dogs, and later become unable to distinguish dogs from other animals. Eventually, all animals may be referred to as 'things'. With time, loss of knowledge extends beyond language, and patients develop features of a multimodal agnosia. On cognitive testing, patients perform poorly on tests of confrontation naming, word-to-picture matching and category fluency, while episodic memory (particularly visual memory), spatial abilities and executive functions are spared.Left-sided SD patients outnumber right-sided patients 3:1 in most series. Patients with predominant right anterior temporal atrophy present with a behavioral syndrome that overlaps with bvFTD. Rigidity is common and manifests with strict schedules and routines, clock watching and restrictive dieting or food fads. Patients with right-sided SD typically develop the semantic-loss characteristic of the left temporal variant after a mean of 3 years, as the disease spreads to the contralateral temporal pole, while patients with left temporal SD develop the behavioral changes associated with right temporal disease within a similar timeframe.

Progressive Non-fluent Aphasia (PNA)

Patients present with slow, effortful and decreased production of speech, agrammatism and motor speech deficits. They have a characteristic apraxia of speech, consisting of difficulty initiating speech, a slow rate of speech or incorrect sequencing or omission of phonemes. They may also have phonemic paraphasic errors and mild anomia. Comprehension is spared for single words and for all but the most complex syntactic structures. Reading is nonfluent and effortful, while writing is agrammatic and features phonemic paraphasias. The main pathology is atrophy, hypometabolism and hypoperfusion of the left frontal operculum, premotor and supplementary motor areas and anterior insula. The psychological test may show aphasia, mild deficits in working memory and executive function, with sparing of episodic memory and visuospatial function.[273]

Histopathology

The major pathological hallmark of FTLD is selective atrophy of the frontal and temporal cortex, with neuronal loss, gliosis and spongiosis of the superficial layers, especially of layer II. On microscopic examination, there is loss of pyramidal neurons and microvacuolar degeneration in layers II and III of the frontal and temporal cortex, with a variable degree of cortical gliosis.[272] The FTLD can be further classified into: (i)

FTLD with tau inclusions (FTLD-Tau) and (ii) FTLD with tau-negative, ubiquitin and TDP-43-positive inclusions (FTLD-TDP) based on presence or absence of specific inclusion bodies. Pick's disease, the prototypical of FTLD with tau inclusions (FTLD-TAU) is characterized by Pick bodies, which are solitary, round or oval, argyrophilic inclusions found in the cytoplasm of neurons. Pick bodies are most commonly found in the dentate gyrus of hippocampus, amygdala, and frontal and temporal neocortex.[274] They are stained by Bielschowsky but not Gallyas stains, and are most readily detected by tau immune-histochemistry.

Genetics

BvFTD type of FTD have 30–50% of positive family history compared to SD and PNFA. Around 10–27% of FTD patients have been found to have an autosomal dominant mode of inheritance. Microtubule-associated Protein Tau Gene Mutations *(MAPT)* was identified as the causal gene in FTDP-17 families with tau-positive histopathology and mutations in the Progranulin Gene Mutations (*PGRN)* gene were found to account for FTDP-17 families with tau-negative histopathology.[275,276] In an international genome-wide association study (GWAS) with pathologically proven FTLD-TDP patients has demonstrated a significant association with three SNPs within the *TMEM106B* gene on chromosome *7p21.203 TMEM106B* variants also contribute to genetic risk for FTLD-TDP in individuals with *GRN* gene mutations.[277]

Treatment

Pharmacological

There is a strong evidence for the deficiency of serotonergic neurotransmitters in FTLD. There has been an evidence decrease in 5-HT1A and 5-HT2A receptors in the frontal cortex both in pathological specimens and *in vivo* using PET studies. Also studies have found a significant response with SSRI and SNRIs to behavioral disturbances and stereotypical movements.[278] However, in patients with severe behavioral disturbances and patients refractory to SSRIs; uses of atypical antipsychotics have been preferred. The patients need to be monitored for extrapyramidal side effects because they are very vulnerable to these side effects. Acetyl cholinesterase inhibitors use in FTD patients had mixed results. Memantine, a noncompetitive NMDA antagonist has been found to be promising but more studies are required to confirm its usefulness.[279]

Nonpharmacological

A structured program for these patients is more valuable than pharmacological interventions because they have only modest effect and significant adverse effects. These programs should include environmental, behavioral and physical interventions designed to minimize the occurrence and consequences of undesired behaviors. The interventions should also include physical, occupational and speech therapy, home safety evaluations and the implementation of augmentative communication devices. Interventions for family and caregivers would be very valuable.[280]

DEMENTIA WITH LEWY BODIES

The term "Dementia with Lewy Bodies (DLB)" was proposed in the first International Workshop of the Consortium on DLB in 1996. Previously the term Lewy body was named after the the person who first described the abnormal intracytoplasm inclusions in 1912 Frederick Lewy. Later, Kosaka, Yoshimura, Ikeda and Budka in 1984 reviewed the literature and proposed a new disease entity called 'diffuse Lewy body disease'. Currently, DLB is part of a spectrum of Lewy body diseases, i.e. PD, PD with dementia (PDD) and DLB since Lewy body is found in other disorders also. The prevalence of DLB compared to other dementias is 3.6–6.6% in people older than 65 and 1.7–30.5% in dementia patients older than 65.[281-282]

Diagnostic Criteria

The core feature of progressive cognitive decline which interferes with daily functioning is essential for diagnosis for DLB. The time duration suggested for the onset of dementia is one year within 12 months of the motor features for DLB. Some of the additional core features required for diagnosis include fluctuating cognition with pronounced variations in attention and alertness, recurrent visual hallucinations that are well-formed and detailed, and/or spontaneous features of parkinsonism. A diagnosis of possible DLB is made if one of these features is present, while probable DLB is identified if two of these features are present. However, three suggestive features were included in 2005 to assist with a diagnosis of DLB; they include rapid eye movement (REM) sleep behavior disorder, severe narcoleptic sensitivity and low dopamine transporter uptake in basal ganglia demonstrated by SPECT or PET. These criteria were revised in 2005 following the 3rd DLB International Workshop.[283]

Clinical Features

The symptoms starts with cognitive and/or psychiatric symptoms and they present within the first year (or from the beginning compared to cognitive deficits and/or dementia develop only if the full motor symptoms of Parkinson's have been present for a minimum of one year.[284] They have fluctuations in cognition, which may reflect periods of unresponsiveness while awake (e.g. blanking out), episodes of excessive sleep in the day time somnolence, or periods of daytime behavioral confusion with limited awareness of surroundings alternating with normal or below normal function. They have visual hallucinations, which are well-formed and recurrent; consisting of people, children or animals in three dimensions. They also have illusions very commonly.[285] Sometimes, few of subjects with visual hallucinations may have auditory hallucinations and delusions. Auditory hallucinations are usually elementary in nature (banging, knocking, sizzling, a doorbell or footsteps). Delusional themes include strangers or intruders in the home or the belief that deceased friends or family members are visiting.[286] These complex visual image generations have been associated with the Lewy body counts in the anterior and inferior temporal lobe, claustrum and the amygdala.[287-289] In DLB, the extrapyramidal signs usually occur spontaneously or occur subsequent to dementia and they also present with postural instability, gait difficulty and facial immobility. However, the resting tremors of the limbs and levodopa responsiveness are less common.[290-292] Patients with DLB with probable REM sleep behavior disorder have an earlier onset of other symptoms (parkinsonism and visual hallucinations), a more rapid disease course and less AD but similar Lewy-related pathologies compared with DLB patients who do not have REM sleep behavior disorder. Also, REM sleep behavior disorder has been taken as an important component supportive of the diagnosis of DLB. These evidences suggest that REM sleep behavior disorder in patients with DLB may indicate a particular subtype of DLB. DLB patients (30–50%) are very sensitive to neuroleptics and have been attributed to dysfunction of dopamine D2 receptors. It manifests as a sudden onset of drowsiness, increased confusion, immobility, and muscle rigidity.[293,294] It has been useful to show low dopamine transporter uptake in the basal ganglia, using SPECT imaging or PET, is clinically useful in distinguishing DLB from AD and it has been reported that DaTSCAN findings were concordant with the outcome clinical DLB diagnosis in 95% cases in a retrospective study.[283,295-297]

Pathology

Lewy bodies are concentric, intracytoplasmic neuronal inclusions bodies. In the subcortical region the Lewy bodies are distributed in the dorsal motor nucleus of the vagus, medullary magnocellular reticular nuclei, locus coeruleus, raphe nucleus, midbrain tegmentum, hypothalamus and basal forebrain.[298-301] In the neocortical areas they are found to be less eosinophilic, less circumscribed, and are better detected by α-synuclein immunohistochemistry (gold standard)[298] The "cortical" Lewy bodies are more common in limbic and temporal regions than frontal and posterior cortical regions.[300-303] Compared to AD, DLB has very little cortical involvement and shows a discrete cluster of gray matter loss in the cholinergic-rich regions of the nucleus basalis of Meynert in the basal forebrain and dorsal midbrain. The α-synuclein positive inclusions called Lewy neurites (LN) are found widespread in the neural processes, and preferentially affect limbic and temporal lobe structures.[299,304] Some DLB cases have AD-type pathology that include neurofibrillary tangles (NFTs) and neuritic plaques.[305,306] However, the plaques in Lewy body disease are typically diffuse (though some may contain a core), and are primarily composed of Ab42 with a paucity or absence of tau-positive neuritis.[307-311]

Genetics

Based on the evidence from autopsy confirmed studies, the researchers have found that DLB has a significant family history and runs in family in an autosomal dominant inheritance pattern.[312,313] Also they suggest a genetic contribution in this disease and analysis of genetic material have found that there are variants in all three members of the synuclein gene family, α-, β-, and γ-synuclein which have a risk of developing DLB.[314] The nonamyloidogenic homolog of α-synuclein called β-Synuclein has been found to be associated with DLB and not PD and the V70M and P123H mutations in the same gene predisposes to DLB.[315] Even though mutations in α-synuclein gene are most commonly associated with PD, with or without dementia, an E46K mutation in it has been found in one Spanish family with DLB[316] and triplication of the α-synuclein gene occurs in a Swedish American family with early-onset parkinsonism and dementia,[317] consistent with current DLB diagnostic criteria.[318,319] Researchers have found a common genetic factors for the susceptibility of these LRP disorders in the glucocerebrosidase (GBA) gene.[320]

Pharmacologic Treatment

Quetiapine has been found to be very helpful in DLB patients with episodic confusion, hallucinations, delusions and agitation compared to AD.[321] This molecule is especially help since the patients with DLB are very sensitive traditional and to some atypical neuroleptics and it does not reverse on stopping the medications.[322] Olanzapine also has been found to helpful by not worsening the parkins parkinsonism,[323] however its anticholinergic properties may worsen cognitive impairment.[324]

Cholinesterase inhibitors are recommended as a first-line treatment for DLB in view improved in cognition and it causes reduced extrapyramidal effects and there is a significantly low brain acetylcholine in the early stages of DLB. Care should be taken to avoid anticholinergic drugs in patients with DLB to avoid worsening of cognition and delirium.[325]

Sleep disturbances in RBD and other sleep disturbances are best treated with clonazepam and melatonin.[188,189] Daytime somnolence due to RBD can be managed with agents such as modafinil and methylphenidate[190] even though it can worsen the hallucinations or delusions.[326,327]

Nonpharmacologic Treatment

It is important to understand the behavior of the patient; they may be actually communicating to us some vital information. It is important understand and then use non-pharmacological methods before trying chemical or physical restraints. Some of the techniques proposed are modifying the environment (e.g. adjusting the illumination, reducing noise), clear communication and response to behavior (e.g. apologizing, reassuring the patient, avoid correcting or quizzing the patient, model calm, avoid trying to "reality orient"), examining task demands (e.g. providing structure and routine, providing repetitive tasks, providing exercise, breaking down tasks into more manageable parts, focus on successes and not failures, refrain from giving tasks that are too hard).

It is also very important to educate the family and caregivers about the diagnosis, expected behaviors and how to handle the behaviors. It is also important help them to overcome their burnout. It is also important to utilize the resources and help available locally. Respite care is also important to reduce the burnout in families.

NEUROSYPHILIS

Syphilis is a sexually transmitted disease and is caused by the bacterium *Treponema pallidum*. The prevalence of syphilis in developed countries is very less however the prevalence in Africa is very high. It is estimated to be 350 cases per 100,000 populations and more common in males than females. However, it is re-emerging especially after the spread of the AIDS pandemic. Around 4–9% of the untreated cases of syphilis go on to develop neurosyphilis (NS).[328,329] NS can occur in any stage of infection of the syphilis. In India, a study in Chandigarh reported 25 cases of neurosyphilis over a period of 13 years from 630 positive patients[330] and in another study by Ashok, et al.[331] who followed up patients, found 14 definite cases of NS in a span of 2 years.

Neurosyphilis can be divided into two stages early and late. Early stages are usually seen in the first week of infection to a year and characterized by the involvement of mesodermal structures (meninges and vessels) and the late stage occurs many years after the infection and involves brain and spinal cord parenchyma.[329] The clinical syndromes of neurosyphilis include asymptomatic CNS infection, acute syphilitic meningitis, meningovascular syphilis, Tabes Dorsalis, general paresis of the insane (GPI) and optic atrophy.

Meningovascular Syphilis

It clinically manifests as stroke involving middle cerebral artery or basilar artery territory in young adults and subacute encephalitic syndrome where they present with headache, vertigo, insomnia, seizures, change in personality and intellectual deterioration followed by a gradually progressive vascular syndrome. The main pathology consists of endarteritis and perivascular inflammation of the medium-sized and small intracranial vessels. They usually manifest within few months to years after infection (7 years). There is fibroblastic proliferation of the intima, thinning of the media, and fibrous and inflammatory changes with lymphocytic and plasma cell infiltration in the adventitia. Also they have gummas which are leptomeningeal granulomas which are formed due to response to cell-mediated immune *Treponema pallidum*. In view of narrowing of the lumina, it predisposes to cerebrovascular events such as ischemia and infarction. They usually have good prognosis only with adequate treatment and if there are no significant cerebral infarction. In few cases, they have reported seizures, hydrocephalus or permanent intellectual impairment.[328,329]

Syphilitic Encephalitis (General Paresis Dementia Paralytica, General Paralysis of the Insane)

The older term general paresis of the insane (GPI) is outdated and a new term has been suggested called "syphilitic encephalitis." There is no core or particular symptomatology in GPI, but it has features of chronic progressive fronto-temporal meningoencephalitis. They present with initially features of episodic forgetfulness and later they have disturbances in concentration and cognitive slowing. They gradually progress dementia with severe impairment of memory, judgment and other cognitive functions. They frequently present with agitated delirium, psychosis and prominent paranoid ideation and hallucinations, both auditory and verbal, and with extreme motor restlessness. They do present with personality change, depressive symptoms, memory impairment and hostility.[332] On neurological evaluation they reveal prominent primitive reflexes with hyper-reflexia, Argyll Robertson pupils (even though not pathognomonic). However, the grandiose form is the prototype of the GPI. The typical symptoms include euphoric mood, increased jocularity, disinhibited behavior, excessive boasting of the past, expansive ideas, delusions of power, wealth or social position. The simple dementing type has now taken over the grandiose type and is now becoming more common. It has been represented in various studies and the percentage has varied from 20% to 60% series. They present with global impairment of cognitive dysfunction such as impairment of memory, slowed thinking and early loss of insight. They also present with episodes of impairment of consciousness. They usually have mild euphoria but they are also found with dull and apathetic behavior. They also develop fleeting and ill systematized delusions of persecutory nature.[333-335] In the depressive type, they may present with symptoms of depression, however if the dementia has already set in then the mood may be shallow. However, their mood readily lifts than what is seen in the nonorganic affective disorders. This variety was the most common the[334] series with a prevalence of 27%. They also present with nihilistic delusions and hypochondriacal delusions. The juvenile general paresis is very rare and associated with infection transmitted via the placenta. It is usually recognized in the childhood or adolescent and the age of onset is between 6 and 21 years. They present with learning difficulties, which leads to mental impairment later. The adolescence onset leads to simple dementing type. Seizure fits are common in this group.

The course of untreated GPI is associated with significant physical and psychological worsening. They may have periods of remission for a short period and later worsening. They become childish, apathetic and rarely aggressive. There is significant clearing of delusions as the disease progresses. They also have episodes of 'congestive attacks' consisting of sudden episodes of loss of consciousness, hemiplegia, monoplegia, aphasia or hemianopia, which increase the process of the disease. In the end, they have ataxia and spastic paralysis and are usually confined to bed. Mortality occurs 4–5 years of symptoms presentation.

This is only syphilitic disorder where *Treponema pallidum* can be directly be demonstrated in the brain tissue. It is typically associated with cerebral atrophy and ventricular dilatation in proportion to the degree of atrophy. The sometimes demonstrate pachymeningitis hemorrhagica which is the thickening of the dura mater and chronic subdural hemorrhage which forms a thick membrane over the brain. Histopathology may reveal cortical thinning in the frontal and parietal regions and may show frosted granular appearance due to the neuroglial proliferation. They also show inflammatory features all over the cortex due to irritation by the spirochetes. They also present with "Rod cells" (enlarged microglial cells) arranged in rows and they stained with Prussian blue to show iron-containing pigments in their cytoplasm, this reaction is found pathognomonic for general paresis.

Treatment in Neurosyphilis

It has shown that the therapy may stop the progression of the disease and improve cognitive and psychiatric disturbances.[336] Aqueous crystalline penicillin G is currently recommended therapy for neurosyphilis. The dosage is 12–24 mU daily for 10–14 days, or procaine penicillin, 2.4 mU daily plus probenecid, 500 mg p.o. four times a day, both for 10-days.[337] These treatment regimens improves the penicillin levels in CSF above the minimal treponemicidal concentration of 0.018 µg/mL during treatment.[338] However, benzathine penicillin does not achieve detectable levels in the CSF, hence it is not recommended.[339] However, due to concerns regarding the persistence of slowly dividing organisms after therapy, some experts do recommend benzathine penicillin G (2.4 mUi.m.) weekly for 3 weeks following the completion of intravenous (i.v.) or i.m. therapy.[337]

HIV-ASSOCIATED NEUROLOGICAL DISEASE (HAND)

HIV infection is associated with disturbances in cognitive functions and is currently termed as HIV-associated neurological disease (HAND). The diagnostic nosology was revised based on the recommendations from the US National Institutes of Health working group. It is classified as (1) asymptomatic neurocognitive impairment (ANI), (2) mild neurocognitive disorder (MND), and HIV-associated dementia (HAD).[340] The current prevalence of neurocognitive abnormalities without comorbidities vary between 18% and 52% compared to 83% with comorbities in different settings.[341] HIV, subtype clade C is responsible for more than 50% of all HIV-1 infections causing rapidly growing epidemics in India, China, Brazil, and southern and eastern parts of Africa. HIV clade C therefore infects the largest populations in the world. The subtype distribution in India was confirmed to be predominantly clade C in a study that employed a subtype-specific PCR1. In India, AIDS dementia complex has been reported in 4 (13%) of AIDS participants and in another study, they found higher prevalence of HAD in HIV clade C infected population.[342,343]

Asymptomatic Neurocognitive Impairment (ANI)

It is most common neurocognitive disorders and has been found in over 50% diagnosed cases. Patients present with symptoms of mild slowing of mental acuity and loss of concentration; with acquired impairment in at least two cognitive domains, quantified as less than 1 standard deviation (SD) below the mean of demographically adjusted normative scores in the presence of intact everyday functioning. It is best assessed with the use of neuropsychological tools. Early detection could lead to identify patients early and to intervene to prevent further progression of the neurocognitive dysfunction.

Mild Neurocognitive Disorder (MND)

This refers at least 1 SD below the mean of demographically adjusted normative scores. To satisfy the diagnostic criteria, such impairment should occur in at least 2 cognitive domains with perceived interference with daily function to at least a mild degree (work inefficiency, reduced mental acuity). The requirement of mild functional impairment is satisfied when at least 2 of the following criteria are met: (i) patient or informant report of decline in at least 2 instrumental activities of daily living (bathing, dressing or financial management); (ii) unemployment or a significant reduction in job responsibilities secondary to reduced cognitive abilities; (iii) decline in vocational functioning (e.g. increased errors, decreased productivity, or greater effort required to achieve prior levels of productivity); (iv) patient or informant report of increased problems in at least 2 cognitive ability areas in day-to-day life (this criterion cannot be used if based only on the self report of an individual with current depression, since depression may bias self-report); and (v) scores of 1 SD below the mean on a performance-based laboratory measure of everyday functioning (e.g. medication management).

HIV-associated Dementia

It is the most severe form of HAND. It continues to be a significant cause of morbidity with a prevalence of 15–50%, despite the HAART treatment.[344] It is a subcortical type of dementia and characterized by memory impairment, the inability to manipulate acquired knowledge, apathetic personality changes, and generalized slowing of thought processes.[345] The diagnostic criteria includes moderate to severe cognitive impairment that represents less than 2 SD below demographically adjusted normative means in at least 2 cognitive domains, in addition to a marked decline in the ability to complete activities of daily living. The functional impairment due to HIV-associated dementia (HAD) is particularly impairing. Two of the following functional deficits are required to fulfill the diagnostic criteria: (i) unemployment due to cognitive impairment; (ii) patient or informant report of dependence in at least 2 activities of daily living related to cognitive problems; (iii) patient or informant report of declines in at least 4 cognitive ability areas in day-to-day life; and (iv) performance at least 2 SD below the mean on a performance-based laboratory measure of everyday functioning (or 1 SD below the mean on 2 functional tests).[346]

Cognitive Deficits in HIV Patients

Receptive and expressive language functions are minimally affected and there may be worsening of the expressive language deficits in the later aspect of the disease.[347] The verbal fluency is the most frequently identified language deficit (40%) in HIV. The patients also present with difficulties in communication, poor lexical selection and turn taking during communication.[348,349] Initially there is a mild deficit in the basic attentional processes but as the disease progresses it becomes worse. In the working memory, the visual and verbal working memory difficulties have been found. Also, studies have concluded that the attention/working memory deficits are the strongest predictors of medication adherence, predictive of cognitive complaints in HIV-positive patients and significantly associated with driving abilities and dependence on activities of daily living.[350] Episodic memory deficits are very highly prevalence and most studies ranging from 40% to 60%. The verbal and visual memory deficits in episodic memory are sensitive indicators of HAND. Mild to moderate impairment with many omission and perseverative errors have been found in HIV-positive individuals during the performance based testing of prospective memory. The difficulties in prospective memory can affect activities of daily living, employment, household activities, social functioning and health care in terms of medication compliance.[351] In HAD, there is a mild deficit in the semantic memory (famous people faces and public events.[16] Also in HAD, there is significant movement abnormalities in the form of bradykinesia, hypomania, tremors, bradyphrenia and hand agility.[346] There a lot of neuropsychological screening instruments which are effective in detecting the cognitive disorders early and for effective treatment. The International HIV Dementia Scale (IHDS) has been recommended for screening in HAND, it is a brief tool, can be completed in 2-3 minutes, specialized instruments are not required, can be performed by non-neurologist and patient need not know English to conduct the test. This instrument has been used in India and it is recommended for it specifically for resource-limited settings, however validation studies are needed to confirm it.[343] MMSE may not be useful for HAND, since subcortical functions are affected and milder forms of HAND cannot be detected.

Neuropathogenesis of HAND

The HIV invades and replicates in the parenchyma of the brain. The infection is predominantly in the brain perivascular macrophages, endogenous microglia and very less in astrocytes. This leads to inflammation and immune activation of glia and finally leads to reversible and irreversible neuronal injury. The persistence of high-risk for HAND despite better treatment options cannot be clearly explained and some authors have suggested factors such as effects of aging on brain vulnerability, persistence of HIV replication in brain macrophages, evolution of highly neurovirulent CNS HIV strains, and even long-term CNS toxicity of ART.

Treatment

The mainstay of the treatment for HAND is HAART therapy. It has dramatically helped in reducing the incidence of HAND. Most studies have found the benefits of HAART regimens for the full range of HIV-associated neurocognitive symptoms.[352,353] Of all the symptoms, most consistent improvement has been noticed in psychomotor processing speed. There are certain concerns in the use of HAART; which include crossing the blood brain barrier to achieve adequate HIV-1 inhibitory concentrations in the CNS. Only some medications can penetrate the blood brain barrier effectively they include nucleoside/nucleotide reverse-transcriptase inhibitors (NRTIs) zidovudine, stavudine, lamivudine, and abacavir, the non-nucleoside reverse transcriptase inhibitor (NNRTI) nevirapine and indinavir (protein inhibitors (PIs). Various other neuroprotective agents which have been tried include pentoxifylline, a tumor necrosis factor-alpha inhibitor; nimodipine, a calcium channel blocker; memantine, an N-methyl-D-aspartate receptor antagonist; selegiline, a monoamine oxidase type B inhibitor, antioxidant, and antiapoptotic and platelet-activating factor antagonists, methylphenidate and dextroamphetamine (psychostimulants) and modafinil and lithium.[354,355]

NORMAL PRESSURE HYDROCEPHALUS

Normal-pressure hydrocephalus (NPH) is characterized with a clinical triad of symptoms: cognitive impairment, gait difficulty and urinary incontinence. It is one of the few causes of dementia that is potentially reversible. It was the first treatable cause ever described and described by S. Hakim in 1963.[356,357] However, in 1965, Hakim and Adams, first described the classical clinical triad.[358] Currently for the diagnosis of NPH, even two cardinal symptoms or just one is also suggested in view of early interventions to prevent further complications.

Epidemiology

The prevalence of NPH ranged from 3.3 per 100,000 for people 50–59 years of age, to 49.3 per 100,000 for people 60–69 years of age, to 181.7 per 100,000 for people 70–79 years of age. The incidence was found to be 5.5 per 100,000 in a study by Brean and Eidein 2008.[359]

Clinical Features

Gait Disturbance

Most commonly patients present with "shuffling," "magnetic," or "wide-based" gait. They also have disequilibrium, slowness of gait (due to short steps and gait apraxia) and slowness of both upper and lower extremities. As the disease approaches middle stages they gait becomes broad-based, slow, short-stepped, and glue-footed (a gait disturbance of the abasia-astasia type). In later stages, with cognitive deficits patients have difficulty in walking and become bed ridden. The latter two improve with shunting. In 40% of patients with NPH appendicular tremor is noticed.[360-363]

Urinary Incontinence

The urinary symptoms usually presents as urinary frequency, urgency and incontinence. It has been attributed to detrusor overactivity and has proven with urodynamic evidence of detrusor over activity in 95% of NPH.

Dementia

The initial signs of in NPH include frontal and subcortical deficits (psychomotor slowing and impaired attention, executive, and visuospatial dysfunction).[11] Global tests of cognition may reveal marked deficits even though screening tests may not detect higher levels of deficits. However, there is marked improvement in memory symptoms with shunting.[364,365]

Neuroimaging

The typical findings seen in NPH are disproportionate widening of the ventricles in comparison to the cerebral sulci (inner vs. outer CSF spaces). A narrow subarachnoid space surrounding the outer surface of the brain (a "tight convexity") and narrow medial cisterns are seen in the coronal section at the level of the posterior commissure. The third ventricle is usually enlarged but the fourth ventricle may or may not be enlarged.[366]

Invasive Diagnostic Testing

To improve the prognostic accuracy above 80% with the clinical and radiological findings, it is suggested to consider invasive diagnostic testing such as (i) Spinal tap test: where lumbar puncture is done with the removal of 30–70 mL of CSF. This can be repeated on two or three consecutive days. (ii) Continuous spinal drainage of 150–200 mL of CSF per day for 2 to 7 days. These tests are positive if the number of steps taken in a 10 m gait test, and the time needed to walk 10 m, are reduced by at least 20%, and/or psychometric tests show an improvement of at least 10%. CSF dynamics (R_{out}, compliance) can be measured with infusion tests also have been helpful.[367,368]

Pathophysiology

One of the important hypothesis to explain idiopathic NPH is poor venous compliance which impairs CSF absorption and pulsation through arachnoid granulations. However, a frequent accompany of NPH is cerebrovascular disease and Alzheimer's disease, which has been found to make a new model in which these three conditions are causally interrelated. All these conditions cause a loss of the Windkessel effect in the skull base arteries. This loss of elasticity which is a consequence of low craniospinal compliance leads to prevention of expansion of the arteries at the skull base. This results in higher compressive stress and greater shearing forces, which develop in the brain parenchyma, leads to tissue damage and loss physical and physiological differences between superficial and deep (periventricular) brain tissue. This manifests as ventriculomegaly. Also another consequence of loss of the

Windkessel effect is a lowering of cerebral blood flow (which explains the common simultaneous occurrence of iNPH and cerebral hypoperfusion) lowers CSF turnover. It has been hypothesized that low CSF turnover impairs the clearance of toxic metabolites and thereby contributes to the pathogenesis of Alzheimer's disease.[366,369]

Treatment

In NPH, various CSF shunting procedures, including ventriculoperitoneal, ventriculopleural, or ventriculoatrial shunting have been tried. This leads to significant clinical improvement in NPH symptoms in approximately 70–90% of NPH patients. The guidelines recommend use of adjustable shunt valves in the treatment of NPH because this enables fine tuning of the ventricular drainage and prevents the need for reoperation.[370,371]

WERNICKE'S ENCEPHALOPATHY

Wernicke's encephalopathy is a medical emergency and an acute, reversible neuropsychiatric condition characterized by global confusion, ataxia, nystagmus and ophthalmoplegia and caused by overwhelming metabolic demands on braincells that have depleted intracellular thiamine (vitamin B1).[372,373] It was first described by Wernicke in 1881 under the title 'polio-encephalitis hemorrhagica superior'. It causes Korsakoff's syndrome in 85% and mortality in 20% of cases. Most of the cases are missed and identified only after the postmortem. The prevalence is 1 and 2.8% in the general population and 12 and 14% in the alcohol misusing population. The WE remains one of the most important encephalopathy due to a single vitamin deficiency (thiamine).

Etiology

Majority of cases of WE are reported for alcoholism. Other etiologies include malignant disease, gastrointestinal disease and surgery, fasting, starvation, malnutrition, use of unbalanced diets and postbariatric surgery.[374] Cases of hyperemesis gravidarum presenting with WE and a case of hemorrhagic Wernicke's encephalopathy following gastric surgery due to acute deficiency of thiamine have reported in India.[375-377]

Diagnosis

Thomson and Marshall had added important recommendation to the guidelines created by The Royal College of Physicians for the diagnosis of WE and suggested that patients with presumptive diagnosis should be treated with thiamine. A presumptive diagnosis of WE is made if the patients have a history or signs of chronic alcohol misuse and any of the following unexplained symptoms: acute confusion (not due to intoxication) or delirium tremens, decreased conscious level, memory disturbance, ophthalmoplegia, nystagmus, ataxia (not due to intoxication) and hypothermia with hypotension.[373,378]

Caine et al. proposed an operational criteria for the diagnosis of WE and KS (Wernicke-Korsakoff syndrome) among alcoholics to improve the precision of clinical diagnosis. According to them two out of the four following have to be present for diagnosis: (1) dietary deficiency, (2) oculomotor abnormalities (eye signs), (3) cerebellar dysfunction (cerebellar signs) or (4) altered mental state or mild memory impairment.

Clinical Features

The triad of confusion, ataxia and ophthalmoplegia confers high diagnostic value to this syndrome. However, all the features of the classical triad may not be present in all the patients, it was present only in 16%. Around, 28% had two signs, 37% had only one sign and 19% had no features of the triad. Men are affected twice compared to women.

The onset of symptoms can be abrupt and sometimes in few cases it takes few days for the manifestations of all the symptoms. *Ocular signs:* The common symptoms are nystagmus, sixth nerve palsies producing lateral rectus weakness (usually bilateral), or some form of conjugate gaze paralysis. The nystagmus is typically evoked by horizontal gaze to both sides. The pupils showed little more than sluggishness of reactions. It was found in 96% of the cases. It is the first symptom to improve following treatment with thiamine.

Ataxia

It has varied from difficulty in standing to mild difficulties on heel-toe walking. It may be due to combination of polyneuropathy, cerebellar involvement and vestibular dysfunction. Patients in whom it is not severe walk with a wide based gait. It is found in 82% of the cases and responds to treatment within the first week but may take about 1–2 months to resolve.

Mental Abnormalities

They presented with global confusion, disorientation, indifference, inattentiveness, apathy and derangement of memory and found in 90% of the patients. Untreated patients may progress to coma and later death.[379] Even though most of them were drowsy there were easily arousable. They were found to be having reduced speech output, irrational, reduced responsivity and fatigued. Some of them had delirium consisting of perceptual disturbances, sleep disturbances, deluded and hyperactivity. Some of them had confabulation early in the disorder which improved as the confusion cleared. With treatment, the global confusion mprove after 2–3 weeks but usually takes 1–3 months to clear.

Other signs or symptoms: Patients presented with peripheral neuropathy with subjective complaints of weakness, pain and paresthesia. Some of the patients had signs of malnutrition such as papillary atrophy of the tongue, cheilosis, angular stomatitis, telangiectases, and dryness and discoloration of the skin. Other symptoms include vestibular dysfunction without hearing loss and hypothermia.

Pathology

The gross pathology includes symmetrical lesions near the walls of the third ventricle, the periaqueductal region, the floor of the fourth ventricle, certain thalamic nuclei (including especially the paraventricular parts of the medial dorsal nuclei, the anteromedial nuclei and the pulvinar), the mammillary bodies, the terminal portions of the fornices, the brainstem, and the anterior lobe and superior vermis of the cerebellum. Convolutional atrophy was a significant finding in 27% of their cases who came to postmortem.[372] An atypical case of WE was reported in a case of nonalcoholic starvation showing symmetrical lesions in substantia nigra in addition to the classical neuro radiological findings.[380]

The microscopical lesions involved all neural elements–neurones, axis cylinders, blood vessels and glia. The myelinated fibers tend to be affected more severely than the neurones themselves. There is significant proliferation of astrocytes, tissue destruction and gliosis and in the areas of parenchymal loss, the astrocytic and histiocytic proliferation was found. In the chronic histopathological changes of WE, are often confined to the mamillary bodies and the dorsomedial nuclei of the thalami, the major difference in the acute presentation of Wernicke's encephalopathy and chronic Korsakoff's syndrome is the chronicity of the glial and vascular reactions.

Investigations

It is important to do thiamine levels in suspected cases of WE before thiamine is administered to know the severity of thiamine deficiency and the sample should not be exposed to sunlight. The thiamine pyrophosphate analysis has been replaced by direct measurement of thiamine and its phosphate esters in human blood by high-performance liquid chromatography (HPLC) and is commercially available in most countries. This normal range in adults is 60–220 nM.[381] Instead of CT, MRI would be recommended to locate the lesions and follow-up in WE cases.[374]

Treatment

Most of the reviews and RCT's suggest using higher doses of thiamine (200 mg three times a day) in the form of intravenous injections instead of intramuscular. Also, the normal diet should be initiated after thiamine therapy. Thiamine is safe and rarely anaphylactic reactions have been reported but the exact cause is not linked to thiamine. Also prophylactic thiamine is recommended especially before carbohydrate infusions. Supplementing thiamine with alcoholic beverages may not benefic in prophylaxis in prevention of WE in alcohol dependent subjects.[374]

The current recommendation for the dosage of thiamine therapy as recommended by the British National Formulary and the Royal College of Physicians, London (2001) is Thiamine 500 mg IV three times daily for 2–3 days and 250 mg IV daily for the next 3–5 days given as an infusion over 30 min, diluted in 50–100 mL of normal saline. Later thiamine 100 mg orally three times daily for the rest of the hospital stay and during outpatient treatment and multivitamins IV are suggested. Also it is important to monitor for electrolytes, blood pressure, magnesium and renal function and replace fluid and electrolyte losses.

KORSAKOFF'S SYNDROME

Introduction

Korsakoff's syndrome (KS) is defined as "an abnormal mental state in which memory and learning are affected out of all proportion to other cognitive functions in an otherwise alert and responsive patient".[382] It is usually preceded by Wernicke's encephalopathy (WE) but can be missed easily and progresses to KS. This condition is irreversible and can only be prevented if detected early at the stage of Wernicke's encephalopathy. The incidence of the Korsakoff syndrome has been found to be increased in Netherlands and in Scotland and probably due to poor diet, increased per capita consumption of alcohol, reduced prescription of prophylactic parenteral vitamins in alcohol-dependent individuals.[383-385]

Clinical Features

They present with profound anterograde (inability to acquire new episodic memories) and retrograde amnesia, disorientation to time and place and a significant lack of insight. They also present with peripheral neuropathy, nystagmus and ataxia which are associated with Wernicke's encephalopathy. Sometimes the patient invent 'fictions' in their discourse (confabulations), and these false recollections often represented as real memories jumbled up and out of sequence with time. In KS, they usually have 'momentary' or 'provoked' confabulation, in which fleeting intrusion errors or distortions are seen in response to a challenge to memory, such as a memory test.[386,387]

Neuropathology

The postmortem brain analysis have found petechial hemorrhages, endothelial proliferation, focal areas of parenchymal necrosis, demyelination, gliosis and variable degrees of neuronal loss in the paraventricular and peri-aqueductal gray matter, cerebellum, and the walls of the third and fourth ventricle. The mammillary bodies and the thalamus are among the sites commonly affected. They found shrinkage and brownish discoloration of the mammillary bodies and dilatation of the ventricular system. However, the most striking feature is gliosis that results due to increase in packing density of cells due to atrophy of these regions surrounding the third and fourth ventricles. The exact location of the lesions for memory deficits is not clear. Some authors suggest a disruption of the circuit which consists of the hippocampus, entorhinal and perirhinal cortex, mammillary bodies, mammillothalamic tract and the anterior nucleus of the thalamus. A study attempted to look into this aspect and found that neuronal loss in the anterior thalamic nuclei was found consistently only in the Korsakoff's group and not in Wernicke's group without amnesia.[388] This suggested that damage in the anterior thalamic is critical for the development of amnesia.[389]

Genetics

It has been hypothesized that there is a genetic vulnerability to thiamine deficiency in Wernicke Korsakoff syndrome. However, a single gene could not be associated. As we know that thiamine is not synthesized in humans, hence it needs to be ingested from an outside source. Many authors have hypothesized that there could be deficits in the thiamine transporter system in humans. Thiamine is carried to cells by specific carriers called the thiamine transporter-1 and transporter-2, respectively which are the products of the SLC19A2 and SLC19A3 genes. The gene SLC19A2 has been implicated with thiamine-responsive megaloblastic anemia syndrome (TRMA), an autosomal recessive disorder[390] and SLC19A3 was associated with familial Wernicke's encephalopathy caused by two different mutations in the SLC19A3 (K44E and E320Q) responsible for a reduction of intracellular trafficking and thiamine transporter activity. However, more studies in this regard are still required.

Neuroimaging

A series of neuroimaging studies in KS patients have confirmed the involvement of third ventricles, thalamus and mammillary bodies. In one study, they found that the level of third ventricular enlargement (may reflect thalamic and hypothalamic pathology) correlated significantly with the severity of memory impairment. In another study, they found significant correlations between thalamic volume (MRI based) and anterograde memory performance. Later, they found significantly reduced thalamic volumes on MRI in Korsakoff patients with evidence of mammillary body atrophy, whereas the temporal lobes, hippocampi and parahippocampal gyri did not differ significantly from healthy controls. Fluoro-deoxyglucose PET studies in KS patient have revealed white matter hypermetabolism and hypometabolism in the diencephalic and medial frontal gray matter.

Neuropsychology

Korsakoff patients have an extensive retrograde memory loss. It manifests as memory difficulties for public or semantic information, facts about their own life, and autobiographical memory for incidents or events from the patient's past and severe deficit in explicit memories (acquiring consciously aware memories for events or episodes) and preserved implicit memory and semantic memory (relative). They also have executive dysfunction.[391-394]

Outcome

Outcome studies in Korsakoff's patients are very rare and difficult. In a follow-up study of KS patients (of alcoholic etiology) they found that 25% of them recovered, 50% showed improvement through time and 25% remained unchanged.[382] According to some authors the improvement takes a long time to occur and occurs in 75% if they are completely abstinent from alcohol. However, impairments in memory and learning improve very slowly than the acute clinical features of Wernicke's encephalopathy.[395] Cognitive and social functioning improved if patients are in placed in a specialist rehabilitation center than in nursing homes or long stay homes. Also, 50% of the 104 KS patients who underwent rehabilitation program were placed in the community after 1-2 years after their discharge from the hospital.[396]

Improving the Brain Functions in KS Patients

The IQ in KS patients is usually intact, since there working memory, procedural memory and semantic memory are usually preserved.[391] New learning is possible in KS patients especially if the information is cued. Also they are able to recall new information over a long period of time if they are not allowed to guess and it is possible if they are in calm, well structured environment and a supportive psychologist.[397] They perform poorly in the tests of frontal lobe function especially tests of executive functioning and impairments in spatiotemporal processing have been reported.[398] Also some authors suggest good nutrition especially with thiamine and magnesium will help in the process of recovery.

Conclusion

The Korsakoff syndrome is a preventable amnestic disorder. It causes significant disability for the patients. Early recognition and treatment of Wernicke's encephalopathy can prevent KS.

TRANSIENT GLOBAL AMNESIA

Transient global amnesia (TGA) is a very intriguing clinical phenomenon and it is defined by a sudden onset of an anterograde and retrograde amnesia that lasts up to 24 hours. Initial case reports of TGA was described by Bender (1956) and Guyotat and Courjon (1956) even before Fisher and Adams could introduce the terminology in 1965. The incidence of TGA has been estimated to be between 3 and 8 per 100,000 people per year based on various epidemiological studies.[399-401] Most of the attacks (75%) occur in people aged 50–75 years and it rare below the age of 40 years. There is male or female preponderance. The recurrence rate of second episode and third episode was found to be between 6–10% according to a recent meta-analysis.[402]

TGA is primarily diagnosed by clinical features. It classically presents with an abrupt onset of severe anterograde amnesia, accompanied by repetitive questioning and without any focal neurological symptoms. Even though the patients usually remain alert, attentive, and cognition is not impaired, they are disoriented to time and place. The TGA attacks usually last for 1–8 hours. 50–90% of people with TGA have experienced precipitating events before an attack. The precipitating events frequently described include sudden immersion in cold or hot water, physical exertion, emotional or psychological stress, pain, medical procedures, sexual intercourse, and valsalva-associated maneuvers.[403] Also they found that patients who had psychological or emotional instability had increased risk of TGA. Also, patients with personal or family history of psychiatric disorders or phobic traits had increased occurrence of TGA. There is significant anterograde amnesia and patients are unable to register new memories and they also have retrograde amnesia of variable period. Patients are usually alert and carryout complex tasks. Sometimes the TGA is accompanied by headache, dizziness, nausea and vomiting. After the attack has stopped, there is complete return of anterograde memory and minor difficulties may persist for sometime. However, retrograde memory returns slowly.[404]

However, with the help of diagnostic criteria of Caplan[405] and Hodges[406] it would be more specific. The criteria includes (i) presence of an anterograde amnesia that is witnessed by an observer, (ii) no clouding of consciousness or loss of personal identity, (iii) cognitive impairment limited to amnesia, (iv) no focal neurological or epileptic signs, (v) no recent history of head trauma or seizures, and (vi) resolution of symptoms within 24 hours.

In TGA various pathophysiological mechanisms have been suggested; they include migraine-related mechanisms, hypoxic–ischemic events, venous flow abnormalities, psychological mechanisms, and epilepsy-related activity.[407] One of the important structures implicated is mesial temporal structures or specifically the hippocampus. Based on the evidence with stress responses in animals; it has been shown that acute emotional or behavioral stress impairs long-term potentiation and enhances long-term depression in CA1 neurons, leading to a disruption of hippocampus-dependent memory. Also it has been shown that CA1 synaptic mechanisms involved in learning and memory are modulated by acute stress. The acute stress leads to enhanced glutamatergic transmission and increased calcium influx in CA1 neurons which is mediated by increased levels of corticotropin-releasing hormone, neurosteroids, β-adrenoceptor agonists, and corticosterone acting via CA1 mineralocorticoid and glucocorticoid receptors. This response increases the risk for CA1 neurons with regard to an increased metabolic vulnerability and thus potentially impairing their structural integrity. These mechanisms are involved in the pathophysiology and could selectively affect hippocampal CA1 neurons with a subsequent perturbation of memory pathways, which might result in acute TGA.[408-411]

The neuroimaging studies from the PET and SPECT have been difficult to compare and interpret; however, MRI has been promising. The evidence from recent neuroimaging studies report that transient perturbation of hippocampal function is the correlate of TGA, as focal lesions can be reliably detected in the CA1 field of the cornu ammonis by use of DWI. The maximum period of detection after the onset of the lesions is 24–72 hours. Hence, neuroimaging may be used as a supplement tot the clinical diagnosis of TGA.[412-414]

Investigating a patient with TGA is important even though TGA is a self-remitting phenomenon it is important to rule out other conditions with similar acute phenomenon. The differential diagnosis which should be considered include ischemia in the posterior cerebral circulation, intoxication, adverse drug side-effects, complex focal seizures, transient epileptic amnesia, postictal conditions, psychogenic fugue, dissociative disorders, post-traumatic amnesia and hypoglycemia. MRI, magnetic resonance angiography, EEG, ECG, ECHO (with bubble study), holter and toxicology screen may be required to rule out other causes or atypical presentations.[415]

Current there are no specific treatment indicated for a typical episode of TGA. However, other possibilities of such as TIA, epilepsy or migraine should be considered and treated appropriately.

NONCOGNITIVE PSYCHOPATHOLOGICAL MANIFESTATIONS OF BRAIN DYSFUNCTION

Organic Mental Disorders

It is a group of disorders where there is decreased mental function due to a medical disease, other than a psychiatric illness. In ICD-10 they need to have the below features to qualify for the diagnosis. If only conditions (a) and (b) are present, then a provisional diagnosis is made but if all the four conditions are present, the certainty of diagnostic classification is significantly increased.

- Evidence of cerebral disease, damage or dysfunction or of systemic physical disease, known to be associated with one of the listed syndromes
- A temporal relationship (weeks or a few months) between the development of the underlying disease and the onset of the mental syndrome
- Recovery from the mental disorder following removal or improvement of the underlying presumed cause
- Absence of evidence to suggest an alternative cause of the mental syndrome (such as a strong family history or precipitating stress).

Organic Hallucinosis

It is a disorder of perception where there is a persistent or recurrent hallucination, usually visual or auditory, that occurs in clear consciousness and may or may not be recognized by the subject as such. There may be delusional elaboration of the hallucinations but insight is not infrequently preserved. Also, there should be no clouding of consciousness; no significant intellectual decline; no predominant disturbance of mood; and no predominance of delusions (ICD-10). Auditory hallucinations which are common in psychiatric conditions can also occur in organic conditions, especially in patients with pontine lesions.[416] Gustatory hallucinations are usually unpleasant and are often associated with temporal lobe lesions and uncinate gyrus fits.[417] Olfactory hallucinations are reported in temporal lobe epilepsy, tumors of the brain and migraine. It has also been sometimes associated with olfactory referential syndrome. Airborne toxins like herbicides or pesticides can also affect the way smell is perceived. Kinesthetic hallucinations, perceptions that unmoving body parts are moving, may involve amputated body parts (collectively called as somatosensory hallucinations) are common in seizure disorders.[417]

Visual hallucinations can be associated with organic conditions such as cerebral lesions, sensory deprivation, the administration of psychedelics (e.g. LSD and mescaline) and migraine. In occipital lobe epilepsy, elementary visual hallucinations and negative hallucinations of visual loss are common. Well-formed visual hallucinations have been reported in Parkinson's disease (PD), lewy body dementia,[418] "Charles Bonnet syndrome" which is described as complex visual hallucinations with preserved insight regardless of whether the experiences are the result of cerebral lesions, metabolic disturbance or eye disease.[419] Lesions of the upper brainstem or thalamus can sometimes present as vivid, elaborate, and well-formed visual hallucinations called as peduncular hallucinosis. Palinopsia, the persistence or recurrence of visual stimulus after the disappearance of the stimulus, have been associated with drugs (cannabis, trazodone, nefazodone, etc.), seizures (temporal and occipital), focal cerebral lesions, and Creutzfeldt-Jakob disease.

Some of the psychoactive substances which can cause Hallucinosis include alcohol abuse (alcoholic hallucinosis), amphetamine and related sympathomimetics, cocaine, Hallucinogens, e.g. LSD and flashback phenomena (associated with use of hallucinogens). Medications which can cause the above include amantadine, bromocriptine, ephedrine, levodopa and lisuride. Intracranial causes include brain tumors, Huntington's disease, head injury, migraine, infections, e.g. neurosyphilis, epilepsy – particularly temporal lobe epilepsy. Endocrine causes include hypothyroidism (myxedematous madness). It has also been seen in patients who have sensory deprivation such as deafness, poor vision, e.g. cataracts and in people who have been tortured, e.g. in prisoners of war.

Organic Anxiety Disorder

It is an anxiety disorder characterized by the features of a generalized anxiety disorder or panic disorder or a combination of both, but arising as a consequence of an organic disorder capable of causing cerebral dysfunction (e.g. temporal lobe epilepsy, thyrotoxicosis, or pheochromocytoma). They usually present with symptoms of tremors, paresthesia, choking, palpitations, chest pain, dry mouth, nausea, abdominal pain ('butterflies'), loose motions and increased frequency of micturition.

The causes of organic anxiety disorders include many factors. Psychoactive substance use such as alcohol and drug withdrawal, amphetamine and related sympathomimetics, cannabis and caffeine withdrawal causes the above. Medications such as penicillin, aspirin, levodopa, tricyclic antidepressants, bupropion, fluoxetine, isoniazid thyroid hormones and sulphonamides can cause the anxiety symptoms. Toxic substances such as arsenic, mercury, organophosphates, phosphorus and benzene can cause anxiety disorders. Intracranial causes include brain tumors, head injury, migraine, cerebrovascular disease, subarachnoid hemorrhage, multiple sclerosis, hepatolenticular degeneration (Wilson's disease), Huntington's disease, epilepsy. Infections causes include encephalitis, neurosyphilis, mononucleosis, tuberculosis and cerebral malaria. Endocrine causes include pituitary dysfunction, thyroid dysfunction, parathyroid dysfunction, adrenal dysfunction, pheochromocytoma, hypoglycemia and virilization disorders of females. Inflammatory disorders include systemic lupus erythematosus, rheumatoid arthritis. Polyarteritis nodosa and temporal arteritis. Vitamin deficiency related causes include Vitamin B12 deficiency and pellagra (nicotinic acid deficiency). Other systemic disorders causes include hypoxia, cardiovascular disease (mitral valve prolapse, atrial fibrillation), pulmonary insufficiency, anemia, carcinoid syndrome, systemic neoplasia, febrile illnesses and chronic infections, porphyria, infectious mononucleosis (glandular fever), posthepatic syndrome,

Uremia and premenstrual syndrome. Left anterior cortical lesions are associated with poststroke anxiety. There is a significant relationship has been found between anxiety or panic and (right sided) temporal lobe lesions.[420]

Organic Mood Disorder

These are mood (affective) disorders characterized by a change in mood or affect, usually accompanied by a change in the overall level of activity. The etiology of these disorders is their presumed direct causation by a cerebral or other physical disorder whose presence must either be demonstrated independently (e.g. by means of appropriate physical and laboratory investigations) or assumed on the basis of adequate history information. It must meet the criteria for the requirements for a diagnosis of one of the mood or affective disorders. It is not just be judged to represent an emotional response to the patient's knowledge of having, or having the symptoms of a concurrent brain disorder (ICD-10). The prevalence of depression is highly prevalent in both gender (slightly higher in men). In patient with medical disorders and patients with secondary mania have negative family and personal histories of mood disorder.

The causes of organic depressive disorders include psychoactive substance use such as amphetamine and related sympathomimetics, hallucinogens (e.g. LSD), medication such as corticosteroids, levodopa, centrally acting antihypertensives—clonidine, methyldopa, reserpine, and Rauwolfia alkaloids, cycloserine, estrogens - hormone replacement therapy, oral contraceptives, clomifene; endocrine disorders include hypothyroidism, hyperthyroidism, Addison's disease, cushing's syndrome, hypoglycemia, diabetes mellitus, hyperparathyroidism and hypopituitarism. Other systemic disorders include pernicious anemia, hepatic failure, renal failure, rheumatoid arthritis and systemic lupus erythematosus; neoplastic conditions which include carcinoma of the pancreas and carcinoid syndrome; viral infections—e.g. influenza, pneumonia, infectious mononucleosis (glandular fever), hepatitis; intracranial causes such as Alzheimer's disease and frontotemporal dementias, extrapyramidal disorders like Parkinson's disease and Huntington's disease, cerebrovascular diseases, cerebral neoplasms, cerebral trauma, CNS infections like viral encephalitis, epilepsy.[421]

The prevalence of secondary mania is more common in multiple sclerosis, Huntington's disease and HIV infection and after closed head injury. Following closed head injury they present with symptoms of irritability, aggression and hypersexuality. One of the important brain structures associated with mania after traumatic brain injury is anterior temporal lesions.

The treatment in organic mood disorders should aim at identifying the underlying organic factor and making attempts to treat the primary conditions. However, it may be difficulty to treat the primary causes such as head injury, stroke or degenerative causes. In conditions where it may be difficulty to treat the primary causes, attempt should be made to manage the behavioral problems. In poststroke depression. Nortriptyline and trazodone have been found effective.[422] Also, in traumatic brain injury, sertraline and desipramine have been found very helpful in treating depression.[423,424] In secondary mania, lithium, clonidine, valproate, carbamazepine and antipsychotics have been found to be effective. Medications should be started at lower dosages and increased gradually to avoid potential side effects.

Organic Personality Disorder

This disorder has been described from the beginning of the XXth century under the heading of "frontal lobe syndrome", later with the development of psychiatric nosology did the term "organic personality disorder" emerge in the middle of the XXth century. The classical case of Phineas Gage's case confirmed findings that damage to the prefrontal cortex could result in personality changes while leaving other neurological functions intact. This disorder is characterized by a significant alteration of the habitual patterns of premorbid behavior. The expression of the individual's emotions, needs, and impulses are affected. The individual's cognitive functions may be defective mainly or even exclusively in the areas of planning and anticipating the likely personal and social consequences, as in the so called frontal lobe syndrome. However, it is now known that this syndrome occurs not only with frontal lobe lesions but also with lesions to other circumscribed areas of the brain.[425] In the DSM-5, it is classified on the basis of the predominant symptom presentation into labile, disinhibited, aggressive, apathetic, paranoid, other, combined and unspecified subtypes.[426]

The clinical manifestations of OPD depends on the age, premorbid personality, intelligence, location of the lesion, severity of brain damage and any past psychiatric history. Three distinct prefrontal syndromes have been described, they include—dysexecutive type, disinhibited type, and apathetic type. The dysexecutive type present with diminished judgment, planning, insight and temporal organization; cognitive impersistence, motor programming deficits, and diminished self-care and involves the dorsal convexity system. The disinhibited type manifest with stimulus driven behavior, diminished social insight, distractibility and emotional lability and involve orbitofrontal system; and the apathetic type manifest as diminished spontaneity, verbal output and motor behavior; urinary incontinence, lower extremity weakness and sensory loss; and increased response latency and due to lesions in the mesial frontal system.

One of the important causes of OPD is head injury. However, there are other conditions which include brain tumors, brain abscesses, subarachnoid hemorrhage, neurosyphilis and epilepsy, Huntington's disease, hepatolenticular degeneration (Wilson's disease) and medication such as corticosteroids, psychoactive substance use; endocrine conditions (e.g. hypothyroidism, hypo- and hyperadrenocorticism), and autoimmune conditions (e.g. systemic lupus erythematosus), may cause personality changes. Strokes of the right hemisphere present with unilateral spatial neglect, anosognosia, motor impersistence, and other neurological deficits with personality changes where as left sided present with paranoid symptoms. However, patients with right hemispheric lesions early in the life develop a typical personality characterized by shyness, depression, isolation and schizoid behavior.

Pharmacological treatment includes psychostimulants for attentional deficits; antipsychotics, benzodiazepines, buspirone, carbamazepine, trazodone, propranolol, valproate, and lithium for disinhibited behavior;[427] and psychostimulants and dopaminergic agents for apathy. It should be combined with psychoeducation to the family, family therapy, individual therapy, occupational therapy and cognitive remediation (if cognitive dysfunction is present) as appropriate for the underlying condition.

TRAUMATIC BRAIN INJURY

Traumatic brain injury (TBI) is the leading cause of morbidity and mortality worldwide. The incidence of TBI in Europe is 235 hospitalized cases per 100000 populations and in US it is estimated to be around 150. In India, about 1.5–2 million persons are injured and 1 million expire every year. The leading cause of TBI includes road traffic accidents, followed by falls (20–25%) and violence (10%).[428-431] About 30–80% of TBI patients have neurobehavioral sequelae (NBS). Most of the studies suggest that the cognitive symptoms improve within 3–12 months. Around 15% of the mild TBI patients can have NBS persisting beyond three months and cause significant socio-occupational dysfunction. WHO collaborating Center Task Force has given guidelines on the diagnosis of TBI related NBS, they suggest a presence of at least 3 or more of the following eight symptoms; they include headache, dizziness, fatigue, irritability, insomnia, concentration, memory difficulties and intolerance to stress, emotions or alcohol.

Neuropsychiatric Sequelae

Cognitive disorders: Severity of the injury determines the persistence of cognitive symptoms. Studies have reported significant impairment of attention, concentration, efficiency and speed of information processing, memory and executive functions. Patients with frontal lobe injuries have reported difficulties in sustained attention, divided attention deficits planning, switching parameters, organizing or sequencing.[432] Attention is very important in the assessment of further cognitive functioning; impaired attention could affect retention of memory. Impairment of alertness has been found in severe cases of head injury. Patients were found to have deficient short-term storage and were slower to learn. The long-term storage and retrieval were adequate. Depth of encoding and automaticity of encoding were poorer in quality though present in patients. Patients remembered better when the encoding was semantic and the retrieval cue was congruent. Storage and encoding deficits were not related.

Overall cognitive deficits can be be divided into four groups according to when they occur in relation to the phases of the TBI.[20,21] The first is the period immediately after the injury and presents as loss of consciousness or coma (lasts from few days to one month), followed by a second stage characterized by a mixture of cognitive and behavioral abnormalities (agitation, confusion, disorientation, and alteration in psychomotor activity). During this period it is characterized by inability to recall events, sequence time, and learn new information and there is a rapid recovery of cognitive function, followed by plateauing of recovery over 12–24 months subsequent to the injury. In the last phase, which is termed as "dementia due to head trauma" is characterized by patients having permanent cognitive sequelae such as problems in speed of information-processing, attention and vigilance, short- and long-term memory deficits, verbal and nonverbal deficits, and problems with executive functions and mental inflexibility.[433-435]

Mood Disorders

Around 25% of patients with TBI can present with major depression. Initially they present with feelings of loss, discouragement, guilt and demoralization and later present with persistent low mood, easy fatigue, irritability, suicidal ideation, anhedonia, disinterest, and insomnia are seen in most patients for duration of 6–24 months. Some important risk factors for depression include poor premorbid level of functioning and past history of psychiatric illness. One of the mechanisms purported in the formation of depression in TBI is the disruption of biogenic amine-containing neurons as they pass through the basal ganglia or frontal-subcortical white matter and also injuries to the left dorsolateral frontal and left basal ganglia lesions. The treatment proposed for the depression secondary to TBI is similar to the treatment of major depressive disorder and includes antidepressants, psychostimulants, and electroconvulsive therapy (ECT).[436-439]

However, Mania is less common (9%) in TBI compared to depression, but more than in the general population. They usually present with irritability, euphoria, insomnia, agitation, aggression, impulsivity and aggression. Some of the risk factors include positive family history of affective disorder and subcortical atrophy prior to TBI is added risk factors. Also mania is commonly seen in patients with right-hemispheric limbic structure lesions. Treatment includes anticonvulsants such as carbamazepine or valproate, which are may be more effective than lithium.[440,441]

Anxiety Disorders

All varieties of anxiety disorders are seen, they include generalized anxiety disorder, panic disorder, phobic disorders, post-traumatic stress disorder, and obsessive-compulsive disorder. The prevalence of anxiety disorder has varied from 11% to 70%. Some of the proposed mechanism for this condition includes increased activity of the aminergic system and decreased activity of the GABA inhibitory network. More than left sided, right-hemispheric lesions are more often associated with anxiety disorder. Medications such as SSRIs, buspirone and naltrexone are promising in the treatment of anxiety disorders. However, caution is required with benzodiazepines and antipsychotics since they may cause memory impairment, disinhibition, and delayed neuronal recovery.[442-445]

Psychosis

The prevalence of schizophrenia-like psychosis in patients with TBI was estimated to be 0.7% to 9.8%. They may manifest as acute or chronic, transient or persistent, and may or may not be associated with mood disturbances. They psychotic symptoms include delusions, hallucinations, illogical thinking, agitation, ideas of reference, grimacing, silly giggling, expression of odd ideas, regression, and aggressiveness. Both hemispheres have been implicated in the development of psychotic symptoms. A rational approach to treatment of psychotic disorders anticonvulsant for left-temporal involvement, for delusional can benefit from dopaminergics.[446-448]

Personality Change

Personality change can be classified into three type and they can present with a mixer of these symptoms depending on the location of the injury. The orbitofrontal syndrome or pseudopsychopathic manifests with disinhibition, antisocial behavior, affective lability, hyperactivity, sexual preoccupation without overt sexual aggression, impulsivity, distractibility and poor insight. Frontal convexity syndrome or pseudodepressed manifests as with apathy, indifference, decreased initiative, psychomotor retardation, inflexibility, impersistence and perseveration. Medial frontal syndrome is characterized by akinesia, sparse verbal output and incontinence. Behavioral management is advised before any pharmacological interventions. Antipsychotics of lower doses could be considered for orbitofrontal syndrome.[449-451]

Apathy

Apathy is a syndrome of disinterest, disengagement, inertia, lack of motivation, and absence of emotional responsivity and may be secondary to mesial frontal lobe lesions. Around 60% have some degree of apathy and depression following TBI and 10% of patients tend to have apathy without depression. The treatment suggested includes psychostimulants, dextroamphetamine, amantadine, or bromocriptine.[452-454]

REFERENCES

1. Giacino JT. Untitled. J Head Trauma Rehab. 2000;15(1):9-10.
2. Giacino JT. Disorders of consciousness: Differential diagnosis and neuropathologic features. Semin Neurol. 1997;17(2): 105-111.
3. Giacino JT, Ashwal S, Childs N, et al. The minimally conscious state:Definition and diagnostic criteria. Neurology. 2002;58(3):349-53.
4. Plum F, Posner JB. The diagnosis of stupor and coma, 3rd ed. Philadelphia: FA avis; 1983.
5. American Congress of Rehabilitation Medicine. Recommendations for use of uniform nomenclature pertinent to patients with severe alterations of consciousness. Arch Phys Med Rehabil. 1995;76(2):205-9.
6. Jennett B. The vegetative state:Medical facts, ethical and legal dilemmas. Cambridge:Cambridge University Press; 2002.
7. The Multi-Society Task Force on Persistent Vegetative State. Medical aspects of the Persistent Vegetative State (1). The Multi-Society Task Force on PVS. N Engl J Med. 1994;330(21):1499-508.
8. Menon DK, Owen AM, Williams EJ, et al. Cortical processing in persistent vegetative state: Wolfs on Brain Imaging Centre Team. Lancet. 1998;352(9123):200.
9. Wilson BA, Gracey F, Bainbridge K. Cognitive recovery from "persistent vegetative state": psychological and personal perspectives. Brain Inj. 2001;15(12):1083-92.
10. Van Drimmelen-Krabbe JJ, Bradley WG, Orgogozo JM, et al. The application of the International Statistical Classification of Diseases to neurology:ICD-10 NA. J Neurol Sci. 1998;161(1):2-9.
11. World Health Organization and Alzheimer's disease International. Dementia:A Public Health Priority. Geneva, WHO Press; 2012.
12. American Psychiatric Association (APA). Diagnostic and Statistical Manual of Mental Disorders, 4th edn. text revision (DSM IV-TR). Washington, DC:American Psychiatric Association; 2000.
13. American Psychiatric Association (APA). Diagnostic and Statistical Manual of Mental Disorders, 5th edn. text revision (DSM-5). Washington, DC:American Psychiatric Association; 2012.
14. World Health Organization. ICD-10 Classifications of Mental and Behavioural Disorder:Clinical Descriptions and Diagnostic Guidelines. Geneva: World Health Organization; 1992.

15. Cole MG, Ciampi A, Belzile E, et al. Persistent delirium in older hospital patients: A systematic review of frequency and prognosis. Age Ageing. 2009;38(1):19-26.
16. Martins S, Fernandes L. Delirium in elderly people:A review. Frontiers in Neurology. 2012;3:1-12.
17. Saxena S, Lawley D. Delirium in the elderly: A clinical review. Postgrad Med J. 2009;85:405-13.
18. Grover S, Subodh BN, Avasthi A, et al. Prevalence and clinical profile of Delirium: A Study from a tertiary care hospital in Nor the India. Gen Hosp Psychiatry. 2009;31:25-9.
19. Khurana P, Sharma PSVN, Avasthi A. Prevalence of delirium in geriatric hospitalized general medical population. Indian J Psychiatry. 2002;44:41-6.
20. Lipowski ZJ. Delirium updated. Compr Psychiatry. 1980;21: 190-6.
21. Vilke GM, DeBard ML, Chan TC, et al. Excited delirium syndrome (ExDS): Defining based on a review of the literature. J Emerg Med. 2012;43(5):897-905.
22. Voyer P, Richard S, Doucet L, et al. Detecting Delirium and sub syndromal delirium using different diagnostic criteria among demented long-term care residents. J Am Med Dir Assoc. 2009;10:181-8.
23. Cole MG, McCusker J, Voyer P, et al. Sub syndromal delirium in older long-term care residents:Incidence, risk factors, and outcomes. J Am Geriatr Soc. 2011;59:1829-36.
24. Cole M, McCusker J, Dendukuri N, et al. The prognostic significance of subsyndromal delirium in elderly medical inpatients. J Am Geriatr Soc. 2003;51:754-60.
25. American Psychiatric Association (APA). Diagnostic and statistical manual of mental disorders DSM- IV-TR. 4th edn. text revision. Arlington: American Psychiatric Publishing; 2000.
26. Trzepacz P. Is there a final common neural pathway in delirium? Focus on acetyl choline and dopamine. Semin Clin Neuropsychiatry. 2000;5(2):132-48.
27. Mussi C, Ferrari R, Ascari S, et al. Importance of serum anticholinergic activity in the assessment of elderly patients with delirium. J Geriatr Psychiatry Neurol 1999;12(2):82-6.
28. Ramirez-Bermudez J, Ruiz-Chow A, Perez-Neri I, et al. Cerebrospinal fluid homovanillic acid is correlated to psychotic features in neurological patients with delirium. Gen Hosp Psychiatry. 2008;30(4):337-43.
29. Simone MJ, Tan ZS. The role of inflammation in the pathogenesis of delirium and dementia in older adults:A review. CNS Neurosci Ther. 2011;17(5):506-13.
30. Cerejeira J, Batista P, Nogueira V, et al. Low preoperative plasma cholinesterase activity as a risk marker of postoperative delirium in elderly patients. Age Ageing. 2011;40:621-6.
31. Pradeep RJ. Valproate monotherapy induced-delirium due to hyperammonemia:A report of three adult cases with different types of presentation. Indian J Psychiatry. 2008;50(2):121-3.
32. Shi Q, Presutti R, Selchen D, et al. Delirium in acute stroke:A systematic review and meta-analysis. Stroke. 2012;43(3):645-9.
33. Wong CL, Holroyd-Leduc J, Simel DL, et al. Does this patient have delirium? Value of bedside instruments. JAMA. 2010;304(7):779-86.
34. Marcantonio ER. In the clinic. Delirium. Ann Intern Med 2011;154(11): ITC6-1, ITC6-2, ITC6-3, ITC6-4, ITC6-5, ITC6-6, ITC6-7, ITC6-8, ITC6-9, ITC6-10, ITC6-11, ITC6- 12, ITC6-13, ITC6-14, ITC6-15;quizITC6-16.
35. National Institute for Health and Care Excellence. Delirium: Diagnosis, Prevention and Management. (Clinical Guideline103). London; National Institute for Health and Care Excellence: 2010. Available from:www.nice.org.uk/CG103.
36. Inouye SK, Bogardus ST Jr, Charpentier PA, et al. A multi component intervention to prevent delirium in hospitalized older patients. N Engl J Med. 1999;340(9):669-76.
37. Marcantonio ER, Flacker JM, Wright RJ, et al. Reducing delirium after hip fracture:A randomized trial. J Am Geriatr Soc. 2001;49(5):516-22.
38. Kalisvaart KJ, de Jonghe JF, Bogaards MJ, et al. Haloperidol prophylaxis for elderly hip-surgery patients at risk for delirium:A randomized placebo-controlled study. J Am Geriatr Soc. 2005;53(10):1658-66.
39. Prakanrattana U, Prapaitrakool S. Efficacy of risperidone for prevention of postoperative delirium in cardiac surgery. Anaesth Intensive Care. 2007;35(5):714-9.
40. Campbell N, Boudtani MA, Avub A, et al. Pharmacological management of delirium in hospitalized adults:A systematic evidence review. J Gen Intern Med. 2009;24(7): 848-53.
41. Gamberini M, Bolliger D, Lurati-Buse GA, et al. Rivastigmine for the prevention of postoperative delirium in elderly patients undergoing elective cardiac surgery-a randomized controlled trial. Crit Care Med. 2009;37(5):1762-8.
42. World Health Organization. ICD-10 Classifications of Mental and Behavioural Disorder: Clinical Descriptions and Diagnostic Guidelines. Geneva: World Health Organization; 1992.
43. Ferri CP, Prince M, Brayne C, et al. Global prevalence of dementia: A Delphi consensus study. Lancet. 2005;366(9503): 2112-7.
44. World Alzheimer's Report 2009. London:Alzheimer's disease International; 2009.
45. Prince M. Methodological issues for population-based research into dementia in developing countries: A position paper from the 10/66 Dementia Research Group. Int J Geriatr Psychiatry. 2000;15(1):21-30.
46. Prince M, Ferri CP, Acosta D, et al. The protocols for the 10/66 dementia research group population-based research programme. BMC Public Health. 2007;7:165.
47. Mathers C, Matilde Leonardi. Global burden of dementia in the year 2000. Summary of methods and data sources. World Health Organization. Ref Type: Generic; 2004.
48. Asia Pacific Members of Alzheimer's Disease International. Dementia in the Asia Pacific Region: The Epidemic is Here; 2006.
49. Dewey ME, Saz P. Dementia, cognitive impairment and mortality in persons aged 65 and over living in the community:A systematic review of the literature. Int J Geriatr Psychiatry. 2001;16(8):751-61.

50. Shaji S, Promodu K, Abraham T, et al. An epidemiological study of dementia in a rural community in Kerala, India. Br J Psychiatry. 1996;168(6):745-9.
51. Chandra V, Ganguli M, Pandav R, et al. Prevalence of Alzheimer's disease and other dementias in rural India:The Indo-US study. Neurology. 1998;51(4):1000-8.
52. Vas CJ, Pinto C, Panikker D, et al. Prevalence of dementia in an urban Indian population. International Psychogeriatrics. 2001;13(4):439-50.
53. Aitken L, Simpson S, Burns A. Personality Change in Dementia. International Psychogeriatrics. 1999;11(3):263-71.
54. Li Y, Meyer JS, Thornby J. Depressive symptoms among cognitively normal versus cognitively impaired elderly subjects. Int J Geriatr Psychiatry. 2001;16(5):455-61.
55. Lyketsos CG, Corazzini K, Steele C. Mania in Alzheimer's disease. J Neuropsychiatry Clin Neurosci. 1995;7(3):350-2.
56. AHCPR Clinical Practice Guidelines. No. 19. Publication #97-0702, Washington, DC, US Department of Health and Human Services, November; 1996.
57. Paykel ES, Brayne C, Huppert FA, et al. Incidence of dementia in a population older than 75 years in the United Kingdom. Arch Gen Psychiatry. 1994;51:325-32.
58. Brayne C, Gill C, Huppert FA, et al. Incidence of clinically diagnosed subtypes of dementia in an elderly population. Cambridge Project for Later Life. Br J Psychiatry. 1995;167: 255-62.
59. Kalyanasundaram S, Srinivasan K. Organic Mental Disorders. In:Vyas JN, Ahuja N, eds. Post graduate psychiatry. New Delhi:B.I. Churchill Livingstone;1992. p.10.
60. Stern Y. Cognitive reserve and Alzheimer disease. Alzheimer Dis Assoc Disord. 2006;20(3 Suppl 2):S69-74.
61. Fratiglioni L, Wang HX. Brain reserve hypothesis in dementia. J Alzheimer's Dis. 2007;12(1):11-22.
62. Fratiglioni L, Paillard-Borg S, Winblad B. An active and socially integrated lifestyle in late life might protect against dementia. Lancet Neurol. 2004;3(6):343-53.
63. Valenzuela MJ, Sachdev P, Wen W, et al. Lifespan mental activity predicts diminished rate of hippocampal atrophy. PloS one. 2008;3(7):e2598.
64. Hamer M, Chida Y. Physical activity and risk of neuro-degenerative disease:A systematic review of prospective evidence. Psychol Med. 2009;39(1):3.
65. Hoffman LB, Schmeidler J, Lesser GT, et al. Less Alzheimer disease neuropathology in medicated hypertensive than nonhypertensive persons. Neurology. 2009;72(20):1720-6.
66. Scarmeas N, Stern Y, Tang MX, et al. Mediterranean diet and risk for Alzheimer's disease. Annals of neurology. 2006;59(6):912-21.
67. Scarmeas N, Luchsinger JA, Schupf N, et al. Physical activity, diet, and risk of Alzheimer disease. JAMA. 2009;302(6):627-37.
68. Anstey KJ, Mack HA, Cherbuin N. Alcohol consumption as a risk factor for dementia and cognitive decline: Meta-analysis of prospective studies. Am J Geriatr Psychiatry. 2009;17(7):542-55.
69. Reitz C, Brayne C, Mayeux, R. Epidemiology of Alzheimer Disease:Risk and protective factors. Nat Rev Neurol. 2011; 7(3):1-32.
70. Folstein MF, Folstein SE, McHugh Pr. 'Mini-Mental State':A practical method for grading the cognitive state of patients for the clinician. J Psychiatr Res. 1975;12:189-98.
71. Qureshi KN, Hodkinson HM. Evaluation of a 10 question mental test of the institutionalized elderly. Age Ageing. 1974;3(3):152-7.
72. Hodkinson M. Evaluation of a mental test scores for assessment of mental impairment in the elderly. Age Ageing. 1972;1(4):233-8.
73. Nasreddine ZS, Phillips NA, Bédirian V, et al. The Montreal Cognitive Assessment MoCA: A brief screening tool for mild cognitive impairment. J Am Geriatr Soc. 2005;53(4):695-9.
74. Mathuranth PS, Nestor PJ, Berrios GE, et al. A brief cognitive test battery to differentiate Alzheimer's disease and frontotemporal dementia. Neurology. 2000;55:1613-20.
75. Mioshi E, Dawson K, Mitchell J, et al. The Addenbrooke's Cognitive Examination Revised (ACE-R): A brief cognitive test battery for dementia screening. Int J Geriatr Psychiatry. 2006;21:1078-85.
76. Rosen WG, Mohs RC, Davis KL. A new rating scale for Alzheimer's disease. Am J Psychiatry. 1984;141:1356-64.
77. Roth M, Tym E, Mountjoy CQ, et al. CAMDEX. A standardized instrument for the diagnosis of mental disorder in the elderly with special reference to the early detection of dementia. Br J Psychiatry. 1986;149:698-709.
78. Huppert FA, Brayne C, Gill C, et al. CAMCOG - a concise neuropsychological test to assist dementia diagnosis: Socio-demographic determinants in an elderly population sample. Br J Clin Psychol. 1995;34(Pt4):529-41.
79. Morriss J. The CDR:Current version and scoring rules. Neurology. 1993;43(11):2412-3.
80. Reisberg B, Ferris SH, de Leon MJ, et al. Global Deterioration Scale (GDS) for assessment of primary degenerative dementia. Am J Psychiatry. 1982;139(9):1136-9.
81. Schneider LS, Olin JT, Doody RS, et al. Validity and reliability of the Alzheimer's Disease cooperative study-clinical global impression of change. Alzheimer Dis Assoc Disord. 1997;11:S1-S12.
82. Sáez-Fonseca JA, Lee L, Walker Z. Long-term outcome of depressive pseudodementia in the elderly. J Affect Disord. 2007;101(1-3):123-9.
83. Butcher HK, Holkup PA, Buckwalter KC. The experience of caring for a family member with Alzheimer's disease. West J Nurs Res. 2001;23(1):33-55.
84. Schulz R, Boerner K, Shear K, et al. Predictors of complicated grief among dementia caregivers: A prospective study of bereavement. Am J Geriatr Psychiatry. 2006;14(8):650-8.
85. Kasuya RT, Polgar-Bailey P, Takeuchi R. Caregiver burden and burnout: A guide for primary care physicians. Postgrad Med. 2000;108(7):119-23.

86. Acton GJ, Kang J. Interventions to reduce the burden of caregiving for an adult with dementia: meta-analysis. Res Nurs Health. 2001;24(5):349-60.
87. LaVigna GW, Donnellan AM. Alternatives to punishment: Solving behavior problems with non-aversive strategies. New York: Irvington;1986.
88. Emerson E. Working with people with challenging behaviour. In: Emerson EC, Hatton J, Bromley, et al, eds. Clinical Psychology and People with Intellectual Disabilities.Chichester: John Wiley; 1998.pp.127-53.
89. Woods RT. Psychological Problems of Ageing. Chichester: John Wiley; 1999.
90. Holden UP, Woods RT. Positive Approaches to Dementia Care. III Ed. Edinburgh: Churchill Livingstone; 1995.
91. Spector A, Orrell M, Davies S, et al. Reality orientation for dementia. Cochrane Database Syst Rev. 2000;(4):CD001119.
92. Hitch S. Cognitive therapy as a tool for caring for the elderly confused person. J Clin Nurs. 1994;3(1):49-55.
93. Neal M, Briggs M. Validation therapy for dementia. Cochrane Database Syst Rev. 2003;(3):CD001394.
94. Woods B, Spector A, Jones C, et al. Reminiscence therapy for dementia. Cochrane Database Syst Rev. 2005;(2):CD001120.
95. Woods B, Aguirre E, Spector AE, et al. Cognitive stimulation to improve cognitive functioning in people with dementia. Cochrane Database Syst Rev. 2012;2:CD005562.
96. King A, Oman R, Brassington G, et al. Moderate intensity exercise and self-rated quality of sleep in older adults:A randomised controlled trial. JAMA. 1997;277:32-7.
97. Buchner DM, Larson EB. Falls and fractures in patients with Alzheimer-type dementia. JAMA. 1987;257:1492-5.
98. Myers AH, Robbinson EG, Van Natta ML, et al. Hip fractures among the elderly:factors associated with in hospital mortality. Am J Epidemiol. 1991;134:1128-37.
99. Perrin, T. Lifted into a world of rhythm and melody. J Dementia Care. 1998;6:22-4.
100. Killick J, Allan K. The arts in dementia care: Tapping a rich resource. J Dementia Care. 1999;7:35-8.
101. Mimica N, Kalinić D. Art therapy may be beneficial for reducing stress-related behaviours in people with dementia case report. Psychiatr Danub. 2011;23(1):125-8.
102. Lord T, Garner E. Effects of music on Alzheimer patients. Perceptual and Motor Skills. 1993;76:451-5.
103. Gerdner LA. Effects of individualized versus classical "relaxation" music on the frequency of agitation in elderly persons with Alzheimer's disease and related disorders. International Psychogeriatrics. 2000;12(1):49-65.
104. Kalyanasundaram S. Non-Pharmacological approaches: Patient centered approaches. In: Krishnamoorthy ES, Cummings J and Prince M, eds. Dementia:A global approach. Cambridge: Cambridge University Press; 2010. p.117-21.
105. Zisselman MH, Rovner BW, Shmuely Y, et al. A pet therapy intervention with geriatric psychiatry inpatients. Am J Occup Ther. 1996;50:47-51.
106. Whall AL, Gillis GL, Yankou D, et al. Disruptive behavior in elderly nursing home staff. J Gerontol Nurs. 1992;18:13-7.
107. Dias A, Patel V. Closing the treatment gap for dementia in India. Indian J Psychiatry. 2009;51(5):93-7.
108. Shaji KS, Jotheeswaran AT, Girish N, et al. The Dementia India Report: Prevalence, impact, costs and services for Dementia. New Delhi: Alzheimer's & Related Disorders Society of India; 2010.
109. Lyketsos CG, Colenda CC, Beck C, et al. Position statement of the American Association for Geriatric Psychiatry regarding principles of care for patients with dementia resulting from Alzheimer disease. Am J Geriatr Psychiatry. 2006;14(7):561-72.
110. Jack CR Jr, Lowe VJ, Senjem ML, et al. 11C PiB and structural MRI provide complementary information in imaging of Alzheimer's disease and amnestic mild cognitive impairment. Brain. 2008;131:665-80.
111. Chetelat G, Villemagne VL, Bourgeat P, et al. Relationship between atrophy and beta-amyloid deposition in Alzheimer disease. Ann Neurol. 2010;67:317-24.
112. Hyman BT, Trojanowski JQ. Consensus recommendations for the post-mortem diagnosis of Alzheimer disease from the National Institute on aging and the Reagan Institute Working Group on diagnostic criteria for the neuropathological assessment of Alzheimer disease. J Neuropatho Exp Neurol. 1997;56:1095-7.
113. McKhann GM, Knopman DS, Chertkow H, et al. The diagnosis of dementia due to Alzheimer's disease: Recommendations from the National Institute on Aging-Alzheimer's Association workgroups on diagnostic guidelines for Alzheimer's disease. Alzheimer's Dement. 2011;7(3):263-9.
114. Lobo A, Launer LJ, Fratiglioni L, et al. Prevalence of dementia and major subtypes in Europe: A collaborative study of population-based cohorts. Neurologic diseases in the elderly research group. Neurology. 2000;54(Suppl 5):S4-9.
115. Hebert LE, Scherr PA, Bienias JL, et al. Alzheimer disease in the US population: Prevalence estimates using the 2000 census. Arch Neurol. 2003;60(8):1119-22.
116. Van Duijn CM. Epidemiology of the dementias:Recent developments and new approaches. J Neurol Neurosurg Psychiatry. 1996;60:478-88.
117. Ferri CP, Prince M, Brayne C, et al. Global prevalence of dementia: A delphi consensus study. Lancet. 2005;366(9503): 2112-7.
118. Prince M. Methodological issues for population-based research into dementia in developing countries:A position paper from the 10/66 dementia research group. Int J Geriatr Psychiatry. 2000;15(1):21-30.
119. Mathuranath PS, Cherian PJ, Mathew R, et al. Dementia in Kerala, South India: Prevalence and influence of age, education and gender. Inter J Geriatr Psychiatry. 2010;25(3):290-7.
120. Chandra V, Pandav R, Dodge HH, et al. Incidence of Alzheimer's disease in a rural community in India: The Indo-US study. Neurology. 2001;57(6):985-9.

121. Rocchi A, Micheli D, Ceravolo R, et al. Serotoninergic polymorphisms (5-HTTLPR and 5-HT2A): Association studies with psychosis in Alzheimer disease. Genet Test. 2003;7(4):309-14.
122. Holmes C, Smith H, Ganderton R, et al. Psychosis and aggression in Alzheimer's disease: The effect of dopamine receptor gene variation. J Neurol Neurosur Psychiatry. 2001;71(6):777-9.
123. David A, Fleminger S, Kopelman M, et al. eds. Lishman's organic psychiatry, A textbook of neuropsychiatry. John Wiley and Sons; 2009.
124. Alexopoulos GS, Abrams RC, Young RC, et al. Cornell scale for depression in dementia. Biological psychiatry. 1988;23(3): 271-84.
125. McCurry SM, Gibbons LE, Logsdon RG, et al. Anxiety and nighttime behavioral disturbance: Awakenings in patients with Alzheimer's disease. Journal of Gerontological Nursing. 2004;30(1):12-20.
126. Chow TW, Hynan LS, Lipton AM. MMSE scores decline at a greater rate in front temporal degeneration than in Alzheimer's Disease. Dement Geriatr Cogn Disord. 2006;22:194-9.
127. Thavichachart N, Phanthumchinda K, Chankrachang S, et al. Efficacy study of galantamine in possible Alzheimer's disease with or without cerebrovascular disease and vascular dementia in Thai patients:A slow-titration regimen. Int J Clin Pract. 2006;60(5):533-40.
128. Tariot PN, Farlow MR, Grossberg GT, et al. Memantine treatment in patients with moderate to severe Alzheimer disease already receiving donepezil: A randomized controlled trial. JAMA. 2004;291(3):317-24.
129. Fuh JL, Wang SJ, Cummings JL. Neuropsychiatric profiles in patients with Alzheimer's disease and vascular dementia. J Neurol Neurosurg Psychiatry. 2005;76(10):1337-41.
130. Lyness SA, Zarow C, Chui HC. Neuron loss in key cholinergic and aminergic nuclei in Alzheimer disease: A meta-analysis. Neurobiol Aging. 2003;24(1):1-23.
131. Lye TC, Shores EA. Traumatic brain injury as a risk factor for Alzheimer's disease:A review. Neuropsychol Review. 2000;10(2):115-29.
132. Armstrong RA. The Pathogenesis of Alzheimer's Disease:A Re-evaluation of the "Amyloid Cascade Hypothesis". Int J Alzheimers Dis. 2011;2011:630865.
133. Carroll BJ. Ageing, stress and the brain. Novartis Found Symp. 2002;242:26-36.
134. Roberts GW, Gentleman SM, Lynch A, et al. βA4 amyloid protein deposition in brain after head trauma. Lancet. 1991;338(8780):1422-3.
135. Horsburgh K, McCarron MO, White F, et al. The role of apolipoprotein E in Alzheimer's disease, acute brain injury and cerebrovascular disease:Evidence of common mechanisms and utility of animal models. Neurobiol Aging. 2000;21(2):245-55.
136. Meraz-Ríos MA, Toral-Rios D, Franco-Bocanegra D, et al. Inflammatory process in Alzheimer's disease. Front Integr Neurosci. 2013;7:59.
137. Moulton PV, Yang W. Air pollution, oxidative stress, and Alzheimer's disease. J Environ Public Health. 2012;2012:472751.
138. Lukiw WJ. Evidence supporting a biological role for aluminum in chromatin compaction and epigenetics. J Inorg Biochem. 2010;104(9):1010-2.
139. Bonda DJ, Lee HG, Blair JA, et al. Role of metal dyshomeostas is in Alzheimer's disease. Metallomics. 2011;3(3):267-70.
140. Scheltens P, Fox N, Barkhof F, et al. Structural magnetic resonance imaging in the practical assessment of dementia: Beyond exclusion. Lancet Neurology. 2002;1(1):13-21.
141. Patwardhan MB, McCrory DC, Matchar DB, et al. Alzheimer Disease:Operating Characteristics of PET—A Meta-Analysis 1. Radiology. 2004;231(1):73-80.
142. Jessen F, Block W, Träber F, et al. Proton MR Spectros copy detects a relative decrease of N-acetylaspartate in the medial temporal lobe of patients with AD. Neurology. 2000;55(5): 684-8.
143. McGuinness B, Craig D, Bullock R, et al. Statins for the prevention of dementia. Cochrane Database Syst Rev. 2009;2:CD003160.
144. Shumaker SA, Legault C, Kuller L, et al. Conjugated equine estrogens and incidence of probable dementia and mild cognitive impairment in postmenopausal women:Women's Health Initiative Memory Study. JAMA. 2004;291:2947-58.
145. Peters R, Beckett N, Forette F, et al. Incident dementia and blood pressure lowering in the Hypertension in the Very Elderly Trial cognitive function assessment (HYVET-COG): A double-blind, placebo controlled trial. Lancet Neurol. 2008;7:683-9.
146. DeKosky ST, Williamson JD, Fitzpatrick AL, et al. Ginkgo biloba for prevention of dementia: A randomized controlled trial. JAMA. 2008;3009(19):2253-62.
147. Hort J, O'Brien JT, Gainotti G, et al. EFNS guidelines for the diagnosis and management of Alzheimer's disease. Eur J Neurol. 2010;17:1236-48.
148. Birks J, Flicker L. Selegiline for Alzheimer's disease. Cochrane Database Syst Rev. 2003;1:CD000442.
149. Grossberg GT, Schmitt FA, Meng X, et al. Reviews:Effects of transdermal rivastigmine on ADAS-cog items in mild-to-moderate Alzheimer's disease. Am J Alzheimer's Dis Other Demen. 2010;25:627-33.
150. Ago Y, Koda K, Takuma K, et al. Pharmacological aspects of the acetylcholinesterase inhibitor galantamine. J Pharmacol Sci. 2011;116:6-17.
151. Seltzer B. Galantamine-ER for the treatment of mild-to moderate Alzheimer's disease. Clin Interv Aging. 2010;5:1-6.
152. Zheng R, Su YF. Research progress of clinical use of Huperzine A. Pract Pharm Clin Remedies. 2008;11:107-8.
153. Tanovic A, Alfaro V. Glutamate-related excitotoxicity-neuroprotection with memantine, an uncompetitive antagonist of NMDA-glutamate receptor, in Alzheimer's disease and vascular dementia. Rev Neurol. 2006;42:607-16.
154. Jakubik J, Michal P, Machova E, et al. Importance and prospects for design of selective muscarinic agonists. Physiol Res. 2008;57(Suppl 3):S39-47.
155. Isaac MG, Quinn R, Tabet N. Vitamin E for Alzheimer's disease and mild cognitive impairment. Cochrane Database Syst Rev. 2008;3:CD002854.

156. Flicker L, Grimley Evans G. Piracetam for dementia or cognitive impairment. Cochrane Database Syst Rev. 2001;2:CD001011.
157. Wei ZH, He QB, Wang H, et al. Meta analysis:The efficacy of nootropic agent Cerebrolysin in the treatment of Alzheimer's disease. J Neural Transm. 2007;114:629-34.
158. Xing XN, Zhang WG, Sha S, et al. Amyloid β 3-10 DNA vaccination suggests a potential new treatment for Alzheimer's disease in BALB/c mice. Chin Med J (Engl). 2011;124:2636-41.
159. De Deyn PP, Katz IR, Brodaty H, et al. Management of agitation, aggression, and psychosis associated with dementia: A pooled analysis including three randomized, placebo-controlled double blind trials in nursing home residents treated with risperidone. Clin Neurol Neurosurg. 2005;107:497-508.
160. Katz I, de Deyn PP, Mintzer J, et al. The efficacy and safety of risperidone in the treatment of psychosis of Alzheimer's disease and mixed dementia: A meta-analysis of 4 placebo controlled clinical trials. Int J Geriatr Psychiatry. 2007;22:475-84.
161. Schneider LS, Dagerman KS, Insel P. Risk of death with atypical antipsychotic drug treatment for dementia: Meta-analysis of randomized placebo-controlled trials. JAMA. 2005;294:1934-43.
162. Gill SS, Bronskill SE, Normand SL, et al. Antipsychotic drug use and mortality in older adults with dementia. Ann Intern Med. 2007;146:775-86.
163. Olazarán J, Reisberg B, Clare L. Nonpharmacological therapies in Alzheimer's Disease: A systematic review of efficacy. Dement Geriatr Cogn Disord. 2010;30:161-78.
164. Spector A, Thorgrimsen L, Woods B, et al. Efficacy of an evidence-based cognitive stimulation therapy programme for people with dementia: A randomised trial. Br J Psychiatry. 2003;183:248-54.
165. Schnelle JF. Treatment of urinary incontinence in nursing home patients by prompted voiding. J Am Geriatr Soc. 1990;38:356-60.
166. Tappen RM. The effect of skill training on functional abilities of nursing home residents with dementia. Res Nurs Health. 1994;17:159-65.
167. Coyne ML, Hoskins L. Improving eating behaviours in dementia using behavioral strategies. Clin Nurs Res. 1997;6:275-90.
168. McGilton KS, Rivera TM, Dawson P. Can we help persons with dementia find their way in a new environment? Aging Ment Health. 2003;7:363-71.
169. Graff MJ, Vernooij-Dassen MJ, Thijssen M, et al. Effects of community occupational therapy on quality of life, mood, and health status in dementia patients and their caregivers:A randomized controlled trial. J Gerontol A Biol Sci Med Sci. 2007;62:1002-9.
170. O'Brien JT, Erkinjuntti T, Reisberg B, et al. Vascular cognitive impairment. Lancet Neurology. 2003;2(2):89-98.
171. Román GC. Vascular dementia revisited:Diagnosis, pathogenesis, treatment, and prevention. Med Clin N Am. 2002;86(3):477-99.
172. Kuller LH, Lopez OL, Jagust WJ, et al. Determinants of vascular dementia in the cardiovascular health cognition study. Neurology. 2005;64(9):1548-52.
173. Román GC. Vascular dementia may be the most common form of dementia in the elderly. J Neurologic Scie. 2002;203–204:7-10.
174. Chicot JV, Charles P, Dilip P, et al. Prevalence of Dementia in an Urban Indian Population. Int Psychogeriatr. 2001;13(4):439-50.
175. Alladi S, MekalaS, Chadalawada KS, et al. Subtypes of dementia: A study from a memory clinic in India. Dement Geriatr Cogn Disord. 2011;32(1):32-8.
176. Alladi S, Kaul S, Meena AK, et al. Pattern of vascular dementia in India: Study of clinical features, imaging, and vascular mechanisms from a hospital dementia registry. J Stroke Cerebrovasc Dis. 2006;15(2):49-56.
177. Das SK, Bose P, Biswas A, et al. An epidemiologic study of mild cognitive impairment in Kolkata, India. Neurology. 2007;68(23):2019-26.
178. Ray L, Khemka VK, Behera P, et al. Serum homocysteine, dehydroepiandrosterone sulphate and lipoprotein (a) in Alzheimer's disease and vascular dementia. Aging Dis. 2013;4(2):57-64.
179. Roman GC. Vascular dementia today. Rev Neurol (Paris). 1999;155(Suppl):S64-S72.
180. Ferro JM. Hyperacute cognitive stroke syndromes. J Neurol. 2001;248(10):841-9.
181. Brandt T, Steinke W, Thie A, et al. Posterior cerebral artery territory infarcts:Clinical features, infarct topography, causes and outcome. Multi centre results and a review of the literature. Cerebrovasc Dis. 2000;10(3):170-82.
182. Kopelman MD. Disorders of memory. Brain. 2002;125(10): 2152-90.
183. Phillips S, Sangalang V, Sterns G. Basal forebrain infarction: A clinicopathologic correlation. Arch Neurol. 1987;44(11):1134-8.
184. Looi JC, Sachdev PS. Differentiation of vascular dementia from AD on Neuropsychological tests. Neurology. 1999;53(4):670-8.
185. Castaigne P, Lhermitte F, Buge A, et al. Paramedian thalamic and midbrain infarcts: Clinical and neuropathological study. Ann Neurol. 1981;10(2):127-48.
186. Ghika-Schimid F, Bogousslavsky J. The acute behavioral syndrome of anterior thalamic infarction: A prospective study of 12 cases. Ann Neurol. 2000;48(2):220-7.
187. Tatemichi TK, Desmont DW, ProhovnikI, et al. Confusion and memory loss from capsular genu infarction: A thalamocortical disconnection syndrome? Neurology. 1992;42(10):1966-79.
188. Madureira S, Guerreiro M, Ferro JM. A follow-up study of cognitive impairment due to inferior capsular genu infarction. J Neurol. 1999;246(9):764-9.
189. Pantoni L, Basile AM, Romanelli M, et al. Abulia and cognitive impairment in two patients with capsular genu infarct. Acta Neurol Scand. 2001;104(3):185-90.
190. Kumral E, Evyapan D, Balkir K. Acute caudate vascular lesions. Stroke. 1999;30(1):100-8.
191. Fisher CM. Lacunes: Small deep cerebral infarcts. Neurology. 1965;15:774-84.
192. Longstreth WT Jr, Bernick C, Manolio TA, et al. Lacunar infarcts defined by magnetic resonance imaging of 3660 elderly people: The cardiovascular health study. Arch Neurol. 1998;55(9):1217-25.

193. Román GC. Senile dementia of the Binswanger type: A vascular form of dementia in the elderly. JAMA. 1987;258(13):1782-8.
194. Loizou LA, Kendall BE, Marshall J. Subcortical arteriosclerotic encephalopathy: A clinical and radiological investigation. J Neurol Neurosurg Psychiatry. 1981:44(4):294-304.
195. Tournier-Lasserve E, Joutel A, Melki J, et al. Cerebral autosomal dominant arteriopathy with subcortical infarcts and leukoencephalopathy maps to chromosome 19q12. Nat Genet. 1993;3(3):256-9.
196. Joutel A, Vahedi K, Corpechor C, et al. Strong clustering and stereotyped nature of mutations in CADASIL patients. Lancet. 1997;350(9090):1511-5.
197. Dichgans M, Herzog J, Gasser T. NOTCH3 mutation involving three cysteine residues in a family with typical CADASIL. Neurology. 2001;57(9):1714-7.
198. Yadav S, Bentley P, Srivastava P, et al. The first Indian-origin family with genetically proven cerebral autosomal dominant arteriopathy with subcortical infarcts and leukoencephalopathy (CADASIL). J Stroke Cerebrovasc Dis. 2013;22(1):28-31.
199. Moroney JT. Meta-analysis of the Hachinski Ischaemic Score in pathologically verified dementias. Neurology. 1997;49:1096-105.
200. Shah K, Qureshi SU, Johnson M, et al. Does use of anti hypertensive drugs affect the incidence or progression of dementia? A systematic review. Am J Geriatr Pharmacother. 2009;7(5):250-61.
201. Forette F, SeuxML, Staessen JA, et al. The prevention of dementia with antihypertensive treatment: New evidence from the systolic hypertension in Europe (Syst-Eur) study. Arch Intern Med. 2002;162(18):2046-52.
202. McGuinness B, Todd S, Passmore P, et al. Blood pressure lowering inpatients without prior cerebrovascular disease for prevention of cognitive impairment and dementia. Cochrane Database Syst Rev. 2009;(4):CD004034.
203. Middleton L, Kirkland S, Rockwood K. Prevention of CIND by physical activity: Different impact on VCI-ND compared with MCI. J Neurol Sci. 2008;269(1):80-4.
204. Litvan I, Bhatia KP, Burn DJ, et al. Movement Disorders Society Scientific Issues Committee report: SIC Task Force appraisal of clinical diagnostic criteria for Parkinsoni an disorders. Mov Disord. 2003;18(5):467-86.
205. de Lau LM, Breteler MM. Epidemiology of Parkinson's disease. Lancet Neurol. 2006;5(6):525-35.
206. Levy G, Tang MX, Louis ED, et al. The association of incident dementia with mortality in PD. Neurology. 2002;59:1708-13.
207. Hely MA, Reid WG, Adena MA, et al. The Sydney multicenter study of Parkinson's disease:The inevitability of dementia at 20 years. Mov Disord. 2008;23(6):837-44.
208. Yip AG, Brayne C, Matthews FE. Risk factors for incident dementia in England and Wales: The Medical Research Council Cognitive Function and Ageing Study. A population-based nested case-control study. Age Ageing. 2006;35(2):154-60.
209. Rana AQ, Yousuf MS, Naz S, et al. Prevalence and relation of dementia to various factors in Parkinson`s disease. Psychiatry Clin Neurosci. 2012;66(1):64-8.
210. Marttila RJ, Rinne UK. Dementia in Parkinson's disease. Acta Neurol Scand. 1976;54(5):431-41.
211. Burton EJ, McKeith IG, Burn DJ, et al. Brain atrophy rates in Parkinson's disease with and without dementia using serial magnetic resonance imaging. Mov Disord. 2005;20(12):1571-6.
212. Junque C, Ramirez-Ruiz B, Tolosa E, et al. A mygdalar and hippocampal MRI volumetric reductions in Parkinson's disease with dementia. Mov Disord. 2005;20(5):540-4.
213. Burton EJ, McKeith IG, Burn DJ, et al. Cerebral atrophy in Parkinson's disease with and without dementia:A comparison with Alzheimer's disease, dementia with Lewy bodies and controls. Brain. 2004;127(4):791-800.
214. Firbank MJ, Colloby SJ, Burn DJ, et al. Regional cerebral blood flow in Parkinson's disease with and without dementia. Neuroimage. 2003;20(2):1309-19.
215. Ruberg M, Villageois A, Bonnet AM, et al. Acetyl cholinesterase and butyryl scholinesterase in frontal cortex and cerebrospinal fluid of demented and non-demented patients with Parkinson's disease. Brain Res. 1986;362(1):83-91.
216. Burn D, Emre M, McKeith I, et al. Effects of rivastigmine in patients with and without visual hallucinations in dementia associated with Parkinson's disease. Mov Disord. 2006;21(11):1899-907.
217. Moretti R, Torre P, Vilotti C, et al. Rivastigmine and Parkinson dementia complex. Expert Opin Pharmacother. 2007;8(6):817-29.
218. Ibarretxe-Bilbao N, Ramirez-Ruiz B, Tolosa E, et al. Hippocampal head atrophy predominance in Parkinson's disease with hallucinations and with dementia. J Neurol. 2008;255(9):1324-31.
219. Nagano-Saito A, Washimi Y, Arahata Y, et al. Visual hallucination in Parkinson's disease with FDG PET. Mov Disord. 2004;19(7):801-6.
220. Sanchez-Castaneda C, Rene R, Ramirez-Ruiz B, et al. Frontal and associative visual areas related to visual hallucinations in dementia with Lewy bodies and Parkinson's disease with dementia. Mov Disord. 2010;25(5):615-22.
221. Neumann J, Bras J, Deas E, et al. Glucocerebrosidase mutations in clinical and pathologically proven Parkinson's disease. Brain. 2009;132(7):1783-94.
222. Ballard C, Morris C, Kalaria R, et al. The k variant of the butyrylcholinesterase gene is associated with reduced phosphorylation of tau in dementia patients. Dement Geriatr Cogn Disord. 2005;19(5-6):357-60.
223. Aarsland D, Laake K, Larsen JP, et al. Donepezil for cognitive impairment in Parkinson's disease: A randomised controlled study. J Neurol Neurosurg Psychiatry. 2002;72(6):708-12.
224. Emre M, Cummings JL, Lane RM. Rivastigmine in dementia associated with Parkinson's disease and Alzheimer's disease: Similarities and differences. J Alzheimers Dis. 2007;11(4): 509-19.
225. Litvinenko IV, Odinak MM, Mogil'naya VI, et al. Use of memantine (Akatinol) for the correction of cognitive impairments in Parkinson's disease complicated by dementia. Neurosci Behav Physiol. 2010;40(2):149-55.

226. Sinforiani E, BanchieriL, Zucchella C, et al. Cognitive rehabilitation in Parkinson's disease. Arch Gerontol Geriatr 2004;(Suppl 9):387-91.
227. Harper PS. The epidemiology of Huntington's disease. Hum Genet. 1992;89:365-76.
228. Pringsheim T, Wiltshire K, Day L, et al. The incidence and prevalence of Huntington's disease: A systematic review and meta-analysis. Movement Disorders. 2012;27(9):1083-91.
229. Murgod UA, Saleem Q, Anand A, et al. A clinical study of patients with genetically confirmed Huntington's disease from India. J NeurolSci. 2001;190(1):73-8.
230. Jarabek BR, Yasuda RP, Wolfe BB. Regulation of proteins affecting NMDA receptor-induced excitotoxicity in a Huntington's mouse model. Brain. 2004;127:505-16.
231. Li JY, Plomann M, Brundin P. Huntington's diseases a synaptopathy? Trends Mol Med. 2003;9(10):414-20.
232. Reiner A, Albin RL, Anderson KD. Differential loss of striatal projection neurons in Huntington's disease. Proc Natl Acad Sci USA. 1988;85(15):5733-7.
233. Vonsattel JP, Meyers RH, Stevens TJ, et al. Neuropathological classification of Huntington's disease. J Neuropathol Exp Neurol. 1985;44(6):559-77.
234. Caine ED, Hunt RD, Weingartner H, et al. Huntington's dementia. Clinical and neuropsychological features. Arch Gen Psychiatry. 1978;35(3):377-84.
235. Hebb C. CNS at the cellular level: Identity of transmitter agents. Annu Rev Physiol. 1970;32:165-92.
236. Folstein SE, Jensen B, Leigh RJ, et al. The measurement of abnormal movement: Methods developed for Huntington's disease. Neurobehav Toxicol Teratol. 1983;5(6):605-9.
237. Burns A, Folstein S, Brandt J, et al. Clinical assessment of irritability, aggression, and apathy in Huntington and Alzheimer disease. J Nerv Ment Dis. 1990;178(1):20-6.
238. Watt DC, Seller A. A clinico-genetic study of psychiatric disorder in Huntington's chorea. Psychol Med. 1993;23(Suppl):1-46.
239. Reddy HP, Willams M, Tagle DA. Recent advances in understanding the pathogenesis of Huntington's disease. Trends Neurosci. 1999;22(6):248-54.
240. Paulsen JS, Hoth KF, Nehl C, et al. Critical periods of suicide risk in Huntington's disease. Am J Psychiatry. 2005;162(4):725-31.
241. Dalby MA. Effect of tetrabenazine in extrapyramidal movement disorders. Br Med J. 1969;2(5654):422-3.
242. ShoulsonI, Odoroff C, Oakes D, et al. A controlled trial of baclofen as protective therapy in early Huntington's disease. Ann Neurol. 1989;25(3):252-9.
243. Gadgil NM, Chaudhari CS, Gohil SD, et al. Creutzfeldt-Jacob disease:An autopsy case report in tertiary care hospital. Indian J Pathol Microbiol. 2012;55(1):97-9.
244. Mehndiratta MM, Bajaj BK, Gupta M, et al. Creutzfeldt-Jakob disease: Report of 10 cases from North India. Neurol India. 2001;49(4):338-41.
245. Finkenstaedt M, Szudra A, Zerr I, et al. MR imaging of Creutzfeldt-Jakob disease. Radiology. 1996;199:793-8.
246. Schroter A, Zerr I, Henkel K, et al. Magnetic resonance imaging in the clinical diagnosis of Creutzfeldt-Jakob disease. Arch Neurology. 2000;57(12):1751-7.
247. Will RG, Ironside JW, Zeidler M, et al. A new variant of Creutzfeldt-Jakob disease in the UK. Lancet. 1996;347(9006): 921-5.
248. Delacourte A, Evers C. Familial CJD.Available from:http:// *www.alzheimer-europe.org/Dementia/Other-forms-of-dementia/Infectious-Diseases/Human-Prion-Diseases/Familial-CJD?#fragment-1.*
249. Satoh K, Muramoto T, Tanaka T, et al. Association of an 11-12 kDa protease-resistant prion protein fragment with subtypes of dura graft-associated Creutzfeldt-Jakob disease and other prion diseases. J Gen Virol. 2003;84(Pt 10):2885-93.
250. Darshan S, Krewski D, Karyakina N, et al. Preventive risk management strategies for bovine spongiform encephalopathy and variant Creutzfeldt-Jakob disease in India. Int J Risk Assessment and Management. 2010;14(3-4):239-53.
251. Bird T, Knopman D, Vanswieten J, et al. Epidemiology and genetics of frontotemporal dementia/Pick's disease. Annals of Neurology. 2003;54(Suppl 5):S29-S31.
252. Ratnavalli E, Brayne C, Dawson K, et al. The prevalence of Frontotemporal dementia. Neurology. 2002;58(11):1615-21.
253. Harvey RJ, Skelton-Robinson M, Rossor MN. The prevalence and causes of dementia in people under the age of 65 years. J Neurol Neurosurg Psychiatry. 2003;74(9):1206-9.
254. Alladi S, Mekala S, Chadalawada SK, et al. Subtypes of Dementia: A study from a memory clinic in India. Dement Geriatr Cogn Disord. 2011;32(1):32-8.
255. Shankar NP, Atanu B, Sandip P, et al. Clinical profile of young-onset dementia: A study from Eastern India. Neurology Asia. 2007;13(2):103-8.
256. Knopman DS, Petersen RC, Edland SD, et al. The incidence of frontotemporal lobar degeneration in Rochester, Minnesota, 1990 through 1994. Neurology. 2004;62(3):506-8.
257. Mercy L, Hodges JR, Dawson K, et al. Incidence of early-onset dementias in Cambridgeshire, United Kingdom. Neurology. 2008;71(19):1496-9.
258. Seelaar H, Kamphorst W, Rosso SM, et al. Distinct genetic forms of frontotemporal dementia. Neurology. 2008;71(16):1220-6.
259. Kertesz A, McMonagle P, Blair M, et al. The evolution and pathology of frontotemporal dementia. Brain. 2005;128: 1996-2005.
260. Snowden JS, Neary D, Mann DMA. Fronto-temporal lobar degeneration: Frontotemporal dementia, progressive aphasia, semantic dementia. New York:Churchill Livingstone; 1996.
261. Neary D, Snowden JS, Gustafson L, et al. Frontotemporal lobar degeneration: A consensus on clinical diagnostic criteria. Neurology. 1998;51(6):1546-54.
262. Zamboni G, Huey ED, Krueger F, et al. Apathy and disinhibition in frontotemporal dementia: Insights into their neural correlates. Neurology. 2008;71(10):736-42.

263. Miller BL, Darby A, Benson DF, et al. Aggressive, socially disruptive and antisocial behaviour associated with frontotemporal dementia. Br J Psychiatry. 1997;170:150-4.
264. Mendez MF, Chen AK, Shapira JS, et al. Acquired sociopathy and frontotemporal dementia. Dement Geriatr Cogn Disord. 2005;20(2-3):99-104.
265. Rankin KP, Baldwin E, Pace-Savitsky C, et al. Self-awareness and personality change in dementia. J Neurol Neurosurg Psychiatry. 2005;76(5):632-9.
266. Miller BL, Seeley WW, Mychack P, et al. Neuroanatomy of the self: Evidence from patients with frontotemporal dementia. Neurology. 2001;57(5):817-21.
267. McMurtray AM, Chen AK, Shapira JS, et al. Variations in regional SPECT Hypoperfusion and clinical features in frontotemporal dementia. Neurology. 2006;66(4):517-22.
268. Peters F, Perani D, Herholz K, et al. Orbitofrontal dysfunction related to both apathy and disinhibition in frontotemporal dementia. Dementia Geriatric Cogn Disord. 2006;21:373-9.
269. Mendez MF, Shapira JS, Miller BL. Stereotypical movements and frontotemporal dementia. Mov Disord. 2005;20(6):742-5.
270. Ikeda M, Brown J, Holland AJ, et al. Changes in appetite, food preference, and eating habits in frontotemporal dementia and Alzheimer's disease. J Neurol Neurosurg Psychiatry. 2002;73(4):371-6.
271. Woolley JD, Gorno-Tempini ML, Seelev WW, et al. Binge eating is associated with right orbitofrontal-insular-striatal atrophy in frontotemporal dementia. Neurology. 2007;69(14):1424-33.
272. Gregory CA, Serra-Mestres J, Hodges JR. Early diagnosis of the frontal variant of frontotemporal dementia: How sensitive are standard neuroimaging and neuropsychologic tests? Neuropsychiatry Neuropsychol Behav Neurol. 1999;12(2):128-35.
273. Gorno-Tempini ML, Dornkers NF, Rankin KP, et al. Cognition and anatomy in three variants of primary progressive aphasia. Ann Neurol. 2004;55(3):335-46.
274. Dickson DW. Neuropathology of Pick's disease. Neurology. 2001;56:S16-20.
275. Goldman JS, Farmer JM, Wood EM, et al. Comparison of family histories in FTLD subtypes and related tauopathies. Neurology. 2005;65(11):1817-9.
276. Seelaar H, Kamphorst W, Rosso SM, et al. Distinct genetic forms of frontotemporal dementia. Neurology. 2008;71(16):1220-6.
277. Van Deerlin VM, Sleiman PM, Martinez-Lage M, et al. Common variants at 7p21 are associated with frontotemporal lobar degeneration with TDP-43 inclusions. Nat Genet. 2010;42(3):234-9.
278. Bowen DM, Procter AW, Mann DM, et al. Imbalance of a serotonergic system in frontotemporal dementia: Implication for pharmacotherapy. Psychopharmacology (Berl). 2008;196(4):603-10.
279. Swanberg MM. Memantine for behavioral disturbances in frontotemporal dementia: A case series. Alzheimer Dis Assoc Disord. 2007;21(2):164-6.
280. Merrilees J. A model for management of behavioral symptoms in frontotemporal lobar degeneration. Alzheimer Dis Assoc Disord. 2007;21(4):S64-9.
281. Mollenhauer B, Förstl H, Deuschl G, et al. Lewy body and parkinsonian dementia: common, but often misdiagnosed conditions. Dtsch Ärztebl Int. 2010;107(39):684.
282. Zaccai J, McCracken C, Brayne C. A systematic review of prevalence and incidence studies of dementia with Lewy bodies. Age Ageing. 2005;34(6):561-6.
283. McKeith I, O'Brien J, Walker Z, et al. Sensitivity and specificity of dopamine transporter imaging with 123I-FP-CIT SPECT in dementia with Lewy bodies: A phase III, multi centre study. Lancet Neurol. 2007;6(4):305-13.
284. Huang Y, Halliday G. Can we clinically diagnose dementia with Lewy bodies yet? Translational Neurodegeneration. 2013;2(4):1-9.
285. Uchiyama M, Nishio Y, Yokoi K, et al. Pareidolias: Complex visual illusions in dementia with Lewy bodies. Brain. 2012; 135(8):2458-69.
286. Bonanni L, Thomas A, Tiraboschi P, et al. EEG comparisons in early Alzheimer's disease, dementia with Lewy bodies and Parkinson's disease with dementia patients with a 2-year follow-up. Brain. 2008;131(pt 3):690-705.
287. Harding AJ, Stimson E, Henderson JM, et al. Clinical correlates of selective pathology in the amygdala of patients with Parkinson's disease. Brain. 2002;125(Pt 11):2431-45.
288. Harding AJ, Lakay B, Halliday GM. Selective hippocampal neuron loss in dementia with Lewy bodies. Ann Neurol. 2002;51(1):125-8.
289. Yamamoto R, Iseki E, Murayama N, et al. Correlation in Lewy pathology between the claustrum and visual areas in brains of dementia with Lewy bodies. Neurosci Lett. 2007;415(3):219-24.
290. Molloy S, McKeith IG, O'Brien JT, et al. The role of levodopa in the management of dementia with Lewy bodies. J Neurol Neurosurg Psychiatry. 2005;76(9):1200-3.
291. Lucetti C, Logi C, Del Dotto P, et al. Levodopa response in dementia with Lewy bodies: A 1-year follow-up study. Parkinsonism Relat Disord. 2010;16(8):522-6.
292. McKeith I. Dementia with Lewy bodies and Parkinson's disease with dementia: Where two worlds collide. Pract Neurol. 2007;7(6):374-82.
293. Hassan I. Consultation-liaison psychiatry and prevention of severe neuroleptic sensitivity reactions in dementia with Lewy bodies. Australas Psychiatr. 2011;19(6):536-7.
294. Aarsland D, Perry R, Larsen JP, et al. Neuroleptic sensitivity in Parkinson's disease and Parkinsonian dementias. J Clin Psychiatry. 2005;66(5):633-7.
295. Tiraboschi P, Salmon DP, Hansen LA, et al. What best differentiates Lewy body from Alzheimer's disease in early stage dementia? Brain. 2006;129(pt 3):729-35.
296. Klein JC, Eggers C, Kalbe E, et al. Neurotransmitter changes in dementia with Lewy bodies and Parkinson disease dementia in vivo. Neurology. 2010;74(11):885-92.

297. Kemp PM, Clyde K, Holmes C. Impact of 123I-FP-CIT (DaTSCAN) SPECT on the diagnosis and management of patients with dementia with Lewy bodies: A retrospective study. Nucl Med Commun. 2011;32(4):298-302.
298. Dickson DW, Davies P, Mayeux R, et al. Diffuse Lewy body disease. Neuropathological and biochemical studies of six patients. Acta Neuropathol. 1987;75(1):8-15.
299. Dickson DW, Feany MB, Yen SH, et al. Cytoskeletal pathology in non-Alzheimer degenerative dementia: New lesions in diffuse Lewy body disease, Pick's disease, and corticobasal degeneration. J Neural Transm Suppl. 1996;47:31-46.
300. Kosaka K, Yoshimura M, Ikeda K, et al. Diffuse type of Lewy body disease: Progressive dementia with abundant cortical Lewy bodies and senile changes of varying degree—a new disease? Clin Neuropathol. 1984;3(5):185-92.
301. Braak H, Braak E. Pathoanatomy of Parkinson's disease. J Neurol. 2000;247(Suppl 2):II3-I10.
302. Kosaka K. Diffuse Lewy body disease in Japan. J Neurol. 1990;237:197-204.
303. Braak H, Del Tredici K, Rub U, et al. Staging of brain pathology related to sporadic Parkinson's disease. Neurobiol Aging. 2003;24(2):197-211.
304. Dickson DW, Schmidt ML, Lee VM, et al. Immunoreactivity profile of hippocampal CA2/3 neurites in diffuse Lewy body disease. Acta Neuropathol. 1994;87(3):269-76.
305. Hansen L, Salmon D, Galasko D, et al. The Lewy body variant of Alzheimer's disease: A clinical and pathologic entity. Neurology. 1990;40(1):1-8.
306. Lippa CF, Smith TW, Swearer JM. Alzheimer's disease and Lewy body disease: A comparative clinicopathological study. Ann Neurol. 1994;35:81-8.
307. Lippa CF, Smith TW, Perry E. Dementia with Lewy bodies: Choline acetyltransferase parallels nucleus basalis pathology. J Neural Transm. 1999;106(5-6):525-35.
308. Dickson DW, Crystal H, Mattiace LA, et al. Diffuse Lewy body disease: Light and electron microscopic immunocytochemistry of senile plaques. Acta Neuropathol. 1989;78:572-84.
309. Dickson DW. The pathogenesis of senile plaques. J Neuropathol Exp Neurol. 1997;56:321-39.
310. Armstrong RA, Cairns NJ, Lantos PL. Beta-amyloid deposition in the temporal lobe of patients with dementia with Lewy bodies: Comparison with non-demented cases and Alzheimer's disease. Dement Geriatr Cogn Disord. 2000;11(4):187-92.
311. Jellinger KA. Morphological substrates of mental dysfunction in Lewy body disease: An update. J Neural Transm Suppl. 2000;59:185-212.
312. Woodruff BK, Graff-Radford NR, Ferman TJ, et al. Family history of dementia is a risk factor for Lewy body disease. Neurology. 2006;66(12):1949-50.
313. Harding AJ, Das A, Kril JJ, et al. Identification of families with cortical Lewy body disease. Am J Med Genet B Neuropsychiatr Genet. 2004;128B(1):118-22.
314. Nishioka K, Wider C, Vilarino-Guell C, et al. Association of alpha-, beta-, and gamma-Synuclein with diffuse Lewy body disease. Arch Neurol. 2010;67(8):970-5.
315. Ohtake H, Limprasert P, Fan Y, et al. Beta-synuclein gene alterations in dementia with Lewy bodies. Neurology. 2004;63(5):805-11.
316. Zarranz JJ, Alegre J, Gomez-Esteban JC, et al. The new mutation, E46K, of alphasynucle in causes Parkinson and Lewy body dementia. Ann Neurol. 2004;55(2):164-73.
317. Singleton AB, Farrer M, Johnson J, et al. Alpha-Synucleinlocus-triplication causes Parkinson's disease. Science. 2003; 302(5646):841.
318. Higuchi S, Arai H, Matsushita S, et al. Mutation in the alpha-synuclein gene and sporadic Parkinson's disease, Alzheimer's disease, and dementia with Lewy bodies. Exp Neurol. 1998;153(1):164-6.
319. El-Agnaf OM, Curran MD, Wallace A, et al. Mutation screening in exons 3 and 4 of alpha-synucleinin sporadic Parkinson's and sporadic and familial dementia with Lewy bodies cases. Neuroreport. 1998;9(17):3925-7.
320. Meeus B, Verstraeten A, Crosiers D, et al. DLB and PDD:A role for mutations in dementia and Parkinson disease genes? Neurobiol Aging. 2012;33(3):629 e5-629 e18.
321. Juncos JL, Roberts VJ, Evatt ML, et al. Quetiapine improves psychotic symptoms and cognition in Parkinson's disease. Mov Disorders. 2004;19(1):29-35.
322. McKeith I, Fairbairn A, Perry R, et al. Neuroleptic sensitivity in patients with senile dementia of Lewy body type. BMJ. 1992;305(6855):673-8.
323. Cummings JL, Street J, Masterman D, et al. Efficacy of olanzapine in the treatment of psychosis in dementia with Lewy bodies. Dement Geriatr Cogn Disord. 2002;13(2):67-3.
324. Mulsant BH, Gharabawi GM, Bossie CA, et al. Correlates of anticholinergic activity in patients with dementia and psychosis treated with risperidone or olanzepine. J Clinical Psychiatry. 2004;65(12):1708-14.
325. Samuel W, Caligiuri M, Galasko D, et al. Better cognitive and psychopathologic response to donepezil in patients prospectively diagnosed as dementia with Lewy bodies: A preliminary study. Int J Geriatr Psychiatry. 2000;15(9):794-802.
326. Boeve B, Silber MH, Ferman TJ. Melatonin for treatment of REM sleep behavior disorder in neurologic disorders:Results in 14 patients. Sleep Med. 2003;4(4):281-4.
327. Boeve B, Silber MH, Ferman TJ. Rem sleep behavior disorder in Parkinson's disease and dementia with lewy bodies. J Geriatr Psychiatry Neurol. 2004;17(3):146-57.
328. Estanislao LB, Pachner AR. Spirochetal infections of the nervous system. Neurol Clin. 1999;17(4):783-800.
329. Knudsen PR, Menezes MS de. Neurosyphilis.eMedicine>Neurology>Neurological infections. Eds: Pruitt AA, Talavera F, Thomas FP, Benbadis SR, Lorenzo N. Last updated. 2005; 1-10.

330. Sethi S, Das A, Kakkar N, et al. Neurosyphilis in a tertiary care hospital in north India. Indian J Med Res. 2005;122(3):249-53.
331. Kayal AK, Goswami M, Das M, et al. Clinical spectrum of neurosyphilis in North East India. Neurology India. 2011;59(3):344.
332. Roberts MC, Emsley RA. Psychiatric manifestations of neurosyphilis. S Afr Med J. 1992;82(5):335-7.
333. David A, (Ed). Lishman's organic psychiatry:A textbook of neuropsychiatry. John Wiley; 2009.
334. Dewhurst K. The neurosyphilitic psychoses today: A survey of 91 cases. Br J Psychiatry. 1969;115:31-8.
335. Fröshaug H, Ytrehus A. A study of general paresis with special reference to the reasons for the admission of these patients to hospital. Acta Psychiatr Neurol Scand. 1956;31(1):35-60.
336. Solbrig MV, Healy JF, Jay CA. Infections of the nervous System. In:Bradley WG, Daroff RB, Gerald MF, Marsden CD, eds. The Neurological Disorders, 3rd edn. Boston: Butterworth-Heinemann. 2000. pp.1317-51.
337. Centers for Disease Control and Prevention. 1998 guidelines for treatment of sexually transmitted diseases. Morbid Mortal Weekly Rep. 1998;47:28-49.
338. Schoch PE, Wolters EC. Penicillin concentrations in serum and CSF during high-dose intravenous treatment for neurosyphilis. Neurology. 1987;37(7):1214-6.
339. Polnikorn N, Witoonpanich R, Vorachit M, et al. Penicillin concentrations in cerebrospinal fluid after different treatment regimens for syphilis. Br J Vener Dis. 1980;56(6):363-7.
340. Antinori A, Arendt G, Becker JT, et al. Updated research nosology for HIV-associated neurocognitive disorders. Neurology. 2007;69(18):1789-99.
341. Cysique LA, Brew BJ. Prevalence of non-confounded HIV-associated neurocognitive impairment in the context of plasma HIV RNA suppression. J Neurovirol. 2011;17(2):176-83.
342. Kothari K, Goyal S. Clinical profile of AIDS. J Assoc Physicians India. 2001;49:435-8.
343. Riedel D, Ghate M, Nene M, et al. Screening for human immunodeficiency virus (HIV) dementia in an HIV clade C–infected population in India J Neuro Virology. 2006;12(1):34-8.
344. Nath A, Schiess N, Venkatesan A, et al. Evolution of HIV dementia with HIV infection. Int Rev Psychiatry. 2008;20(1): 25-31.
345. McArthur JC, Brew BJ, Nath A. Neurological complications of HIV infection. Lancet Neurol. 2005;4(9):543-55.
346. Woods SP, Moore DJ, Weber E, et al. Cognitive neuropsychology of HIV-associated neurocognitive disorders. Neuropsychol Rev. 2009;19(2):152-68.
347. Iudicello JE, Woods SP, Weber E, et al. Cognitive mechanisms of switching in HIV-associated category fluency deficits. J Clin Exp Neuropsychol. 2008;30(7):797-804.
348. Troyer AK. Normative data for clustering and switching on verbal fluency tasks. J Clin Exp Neuropsychol. 2000;22(3):370-8.
349. McCabe P, Sheard C, Code C. Pragmatic skills in people with HIV/AIDS. Disabil Rehabil. 2007;29(16):1251-60.
350. Reger M, Welsh R, Razani J, et al. A meta-analysis of the neuropsychological sequelae of HIV infection. J Int Neuropsychol Soc. 2002;8(3):410-24.
351. Martin EM, Nixon H, Pitrak DL, et al. Characteristics of prospective memory deficits in HIV-seropositive substance-dependent individuals:Preliminary observations. J Clin Exp Neuropsychol. 2007;29(5):496-504.
352. Ferrando S, van Gorp W, McElhiney M, et al. Highly active antiretroviral treatment in HIV infection:Benefits for neuropsychological function. AIDS. 1998;12(8):F65-F70.
353. Ferrando SJ, Rabkin JG, van Gorp W, et al. Longitudinal improvement in psychomotor processing speed is associated with potent combination antiretroviral therapy in HIV-1 infection. J Neuropsychiatry Clin Neurosci. 2003;15(2):208-14.
354. Dana Consortium on Therapy for HIV Dementia and Related Cognitive Disorders. Clinical confirmationof the American Academy of Neurology algorithm for HIV-1 associated cognitive/motor disorder. Neurology. 1996;47(5):1247-53.
355. Cohen MA, Gorman JM, eds. Comprehensive textbook of AIDS psychiatry. Oxford:Oxford University Press; 2008.
356. Relkin N, Marmarou A, Klinge P, et al. Diagnosing idiopathic normal-pressure hydrocephalus. Neurosurgery. 2005; 57(Suppl 3):S4-16.
357. Deutsche Gesellschaft für Neurologie:Leitlinie Normal druckhydrocephalus. Available from: *http://www.dgn.org/images/stories/dgn/leitlinien/LL2008/ll08kap_017.pdf.*
358. Hakim S, Adams RD. The special clinical problem of symptomatic hydrocephalus with normal cerebrospinal fluid pressure; Observations on cerebrospinal fluid hydrodynamics. J Neurol Sci. 1965;2(4):307-27.
359. Brean A, Eide PK. Prevalence of probable idiopathic normal pressure hydrocephalus in a Norwegian population. Acta Neurol Scand. 2008;18(1):48-53.
360. Marmarou A, Young HF, Aygok GA, et al. Diagnosis and management of idiopathic normal-pressure hydrocephalus:A prospective study in 151 patients. J Neurosurg. 2005;102(6): 987-97.
361. Bugalho P, Guimaraes J. Gait disturbance in normal pressure hydrocephalus: A clinical study.Parkinsonism Relat Disord. 2007;13(7):434-7.
362. Nowak DA, Topka HR. Broadening a classic clinical triad:The hypo kinetic motor disorder of normal pressure hydrocephalus also affects the hand. Exp Neurol. 2006;198(1):81-7.
363. Krauss JK, Regel JP, Droste DW, et al. Movement disorders in adult hydrocephalus. Mov Disord. 1997;12(1):53-60.
364. Iddon JL, Pickard JD, Cross JJ, et al. Specific patterns of cognitive impairment in patients with idiopathic normal pressure hydrocephalus and Alzheimer's disease: A pilot study. J Neurol Neurosurg Psychiatry. 1999;67(6):723-32.
365. Mataro M, Matarin M, Poca MA, et al. Functional and magnetic resonance imaging correlates of corpus callosum in normal pressure hydrocephalus before and after shunting. J Neurol Neurosurg Psychiatry. 2007;78(4):395-8.

366. Greitz D. Radiological assessment of hydrocephalus:New theories and implications for therapy. Neurosurg Rev. 2004; 27(3):145-65.
367. Weerakkody RA, Czosnyka M, Schuhmann MU, et al. Clinical assessment of cerebrospinal fluid dynamics in hydrocephalus:Guide to interpretation based on observational study. Acta Neurol Scand. 2011;124(2):85-98.
368. Ishikawa M, Hashimoto M, Kuwana N, et al. Guidelines for management of idiopathic normal pressure hydrocephalus. Neurol Med Chir (Tokyo). 2008;48(Suppl):S1-23.
369. Bateman GA:Vascular compliance in normal pressure hydrocephalus. AJNR Am J Neuroradiol. 2000;21(9):1574-85.
370. Hebb AO, Cusimano MD. Idiopathic normal pressure hydrocephalus: a systematic review of diagnosis and outcome. Neurosurgery. 2001;49(5):1166-84.
371. Lavinio A, Harding S, Van Der Boogaard F, et al. Magnetic field interactions in adjustable hydrocephalus shunts. J Neurosurg Pediatr. 2008;2(3):222-8.
372. Victor M, Adams RD, Collins GH. The Wernicke-Korsakoff syndrome: A clinical and pathological study of 245 patients, 82 with post-mortem examinations. Contemporary Neurology Series. 1971;7:1-206.
373. Thomson AD, Cook CC, Touquet R, et al. The royal college of physicians report on alcohol: Guidelines for managing Wernicke's encephalopathy in the accident and emergency department. Alcohol Alcohol. 2002;37(6):513-21.
374. Galvin R, Bråthen G, Ivashynka A, et al. EFNS guidelines for diagnosis, therapy and prevention of Wernicke encephalopathy. European Journal of Neurology. 2010;17(12):1408-18.
375. Kotha VK, De Souza A. Wernicke's encephalopathy following Hyperemesis gravidarum. A report of three cases. Neuroradiol J. 2013;26(1):35-40.
376. Chitra S, Lath KV. Wernicke's encephalopathy with visual loss in a patient with Hyperemesis gravidarum. J Assoc Physicians India. 2012;60:53-6.
377. Renna R, Plantone F, Plantone D. A case of hemorrhagic Wernicke's encephalopathy following gastric surgery. Neurol India. 2012;60(4):453-4.
378. Thomson AD, Marshall EJ. The treatment of patients at risk of developing Wernicke's encephalopathy in the community. Alcohol Alcohol. 2006;41(2):159-67.
379. Victor M, Adams RD, Collins GH. The Wernicke-korsakoff syndrome and related neurologic disorders due to alcoholism and malnutrition. Philadelphia: FA Davis;1989.
380. Kalidass B, Sunnathkal R, Rangashamanna V, et al. Atypical Wernicke's encephalopathy showing involvement of substantianigra. J Neuroimaging. 2012;22(2):204-7.
381. Lu J, Frank EL. Rapid HPLC measurement of thiamine and its phosphate esters in whole blood. Clin Chem. 2008;54(5):901-6.
382. Victor M, Adams RD, Collins GH. The Wernicke-Korsakoff syndrome: A clinical and pathological study of 245 patients, 82 with post-mortem examinations. Contemporary Neurology Series. 1971;7:1-206.
383. Smith I, Hillman A. Management of alcohol Korsakoff syndrome. Adv Psychiatr Treat. 1999;5:271-8.
384. Kok AF. Developments in the care of Korsakoff patients. Tijdschriftvoor Alcohol, Drugs en Andere Psychotropic Stoffen. 1991;17:3-9.
385. Ramayya A, Jauhar P. Increasing incidence of Korsakoff's psychosis in the east end of Glasgow. Alcohol Alcohol. 1997;32: 281-5.
386. Berlyne N. Confabulation. Br J Psychiatry. 1972;120(554):31-9.
387. Kopelman MD. Two types of confabulation. J Neurol Neurosurg Psychiatry. 1987;50:1482-7.
388. Harding A, Halliday G, Caine D, et al. Degeneration of anterior thalamic nuclei differentiates alcoholics with amnesia. Brain. 2000;123(1):141-54.
389. Von Cramon DY, Hebel N, Schuri U. A contribution to the anatomical basis of thalamic amnesia. Brain. 1985;108(4): 993-1008.
390. Guerrini I, Thomson AD, Gurling HM. Molecular genetics of alcohol-related brain damage. Alcohol Alcohol. 2009;44(2): 166-70.
391. Jacobson RR, Lishman W. Selective memory loss and global intellectual deficits in alcoholic Korsakoff 's syndrome. Psychol Med. 1987;17(3):649-55.
392. Kopelman MD, Lasserson D, Kingsley D, et al. Structural MRI volumetric analysis in patients with organic amnesia, 2: Correlations with anterograde memory and executive tests in 40 patients. J Neuro Neurosur Psychiatr. 2001;71: 23-8.
393. Colchester A, Kingsley D, Lasserson D, et al. Structural MRI volumetric analysis in patients with organic amnesia, 1: Methods and findings, comparative findings across diagnostic groups. J Neuro Neurosurge Psychiatr. 2001;71:13-22.
394. Reed LJ, Lasserson D, Marsden P, et al. FDG-PET findings in the Wernicke-Korsakoff syndrome. Cortex. 2003;39(4-5): 1027-45.
395. Day E, Bentham P, Callaghan R, et al. Thiamine for Wernicke-Korsakoff syndrome in People at risk from alcohol abuse. Cochrane Database Syst Rev. 2004;(1):CD004033.
396. Lennane KJ. Management of moderate to severe alcohol related brain damage (Korsakoff's syndrome). Med J Aust. 1986;145(3-4):136,141-3.
397. Wilson BA, Baddeley A, Evans J, et al. Errorless learning in the rehabilitation of memory impaired people. Neuropsychol Rehabil. 1994;4(3):307-26.
398. Kopelman MD. Remote and autobiographical memory, temporal context memory and frontal atrophy in Korsakoff and Alzheimer patients. Neuropsychologia. 1989;27(4):437-60.
399. Miller JW, Petersen RC, Metter EJ, et al. Transient global amnesia: Clinical characteristics and prognosis.Neurology. 1987;37:5733-7.
400. Hodges JR, Warlow CP. The aetiology of transient global amnesia: A case-control study of 114 cases with prospective follow-up. Brain. 1990;113(3):639-57.

401. Berli R, Hutter A, Waespe W, et al. Transient global amnesia -not so rare after all. Swiss Med Wkly. 2009;139(19-20): 288-92.
402. Quinette P, Guillery-Girard B, Dayan J, et al. What does transient global amnesia really mean? Review of the literature and thorough study of 142 cases. Brain. 2006;129(7):1640-58.
403. Rosler A, Mras GJ, Frese A, et al. Precipitating factors of transient global amnesia. J Neurol. 1999;246(1):53-4.
404. Owen D, Paranandi B, Sivakumar R, et al. Classical diseases revisited: Transient global amnesia. Postgrad Med J. 2007;83: 236-9.
405. Caplan L. Transient global amnesia. In:Vinken PJ, Bruyn GW, Klawans HL, Eds. Handbook of Clinical Neurology. Amsterdam: Elsevier. 1985;45:205-18.
406. Hodges JR, Warlow CP. Syndromes of transient amnesia: Towards a classification. A study of 153 cases. J Neurol Neurosurg Psychiatry. 1990;53(10):834-43.
407. Sander K, Sander D. New insights into transient global amnesia: Recent imaging and clinical findings. Lancet Neurol. 2005;4(7):437-44.
408. Howland JG, Wang YT. Synaptic plasticity in learning and memory: Stress effects in the hippocampus. Prog Brain Res. 2008;169:145-58.
409. Kim JJ, Foy MR, Thompson RF. Behavioral stress modifies hippocampal plasticity through N-methyl-D-aspartate receptor activation. Proc Natl Acad Sci USA. 1996;93(10):4750-3.
410. Yang CH, Huang CC, Hsu KS. Behavioral stress enhances hippocampal CA1 long-term depression through the blockade of the glutamate uptake. J Neurosci. 2005;25(17): 4288-93.
411. Joels M. Stress, the hippocampus, and epilepsy. Epilepsia. 2009;50(4):586-97.
412. Bartsch T, Deuschl G. Transient global amnesia: Functional anatomy and clinical implications. Lancet Neurol. 2010;9(2): 205-14.
413. Cianfoni A, Tartaglione T, Gaudino S, et al. Hippocampal magnetic resonance imaging abnormalities in transient global amnesia. Arch Neurol. 2005;62(9):1468-9.
414. Nakada T, Kwee IL, Fujii Y, et al. High-field, T2 reversed MRI of the hippocampus in transient global amnesia. Neurology. 2005;64(7):1170-4.
415. Sandson TA, Price BH. Transient global amnesia. Semin Neurol. 1995;15:183-7.
416. Douen AG, Bourque PR. Musical auditory hallucinosis from *Listeria* rhombencephalitis. Can J Neurol Sci. 1997;24(1):70-2.
417. Kolb LC, Brodie HKH. Modern clinical psychiatry. Philadelphia: WB Saunders; 1982.
418. Fénelon G, Mahieux F, Huon R, et al. Hallucinations in Parkinson's disease Prevalence, phenomenology and risk factors. Brain. 2000;123(4):733-45.
419. Ffytche DH. Visual hallucinations and the Charles Bonnet syndrome. Curr Psychiatry Rep. 2005;7(3):168-79.
420. Capwell RR, Carter R. Organic anxiety syndrome secondary to metastatic brain tumor. Psychosomatics. 1991;32(2):231-3.
421. Cummings JL, Mega MS. Neuropsychiatry and Behavioral Neuroscience. Oxford, Oxford University Press, 2003.
422. Lipsey J, Pearlson G, Robinson R, et al. Nortriptyline treatment of post-stroke depression: A double-blind study. Lancet. 1984;323(8372):297-300.
423. Wrobleski BA, Joseph AV, Cornblatt RR. Antidepressant pharmacotherapy and the treatment of depression in patients with severe traumatic brain injury: A controlled prospective study. J Clin Psychiatry. 1996;57:582-7.
424. Fann JR, Uomoto JM, Katon WJ. Sertraline in the treatment of major depression following mild traumatic brain injury. J Neuropsychiatry Clin Neurosci. 2000;12:226-32.
425. World Health Organization. ICD-10 Classifications of Mental and Behavioural Disorder:Clinical Descriptions and Diagnostic Guidelines. Geneva:World Health Organization;1992.
426. American Psychiatric Association (APA). Diagnostic and Statistical Manual of Mental Disorders, 5 Edn. text revision (DSM-5). Washington, DC: American Psychiatric Association; 2012.
427. Silver JM, Yudofsky SC. Psychopharmacological approaches to the patient with affective and psychotic features. J Head Trauma Rehabil. 1994;9(3):61-77.
428. Tagliaferri F, Compagnone C, Korsic M, et al. A systematic review of brain injury epidemiology in Europe. Acta Neurochir. 2006;148:255-68.
429. Kraus JF, Chu LD. Epidemiology. In: Silver JS, McAllister TW, Yudofsky SC, Eds. Neuropsychiatry of traumatic brain injury. Washington: American Psychiatric Press; 2005. pp.3-26.
430. Gururaj G. Epidemiology of traumatic brain injuries:Indian scenario. Neurol Res. 2002;24(1):24-8.
431. Sudarsanan BS, Chaudhary S, Pawar AA, et al. Psychiatric effects of traumatic brain injury. MJAFI. 2006;62:259-63.
432. Mishra S, Rao SL. Divided attention in head injury. NIMHANS Journal. 1994;12:157-62.
433. Kwentus JA, Hart RP, Peck ET, et al. Psychiatric complications of closed head trauma. Psychosomatics. 1985;26:8-15.
434. Levin HS. Neurobehavioral sequelae of head injury, In: Cooper PR, Ed. Head Injury, 2nd edn. Baltimore: Williams & Wilkins; 1987.
435. Cripe LI. The neuropsychological assessment and management of closed head injury: General guidelines. Cogn Rehabil. 1987;5:18-22.
436. Fedoroff JP, Starkstein SE, Forrester AW, et al. Depression in patients with traumatic brain injury. Am J Psychiatry. 1992;149:918-23.
437. Jorge RE, Robinson RG, Arndt SV, et al. Comparison between acute and delayed-onset depression following traumatic brain injury. J Neuropsychiatry Clin Neurosci. 1993;5(1):43-9.
438. Hinkeldy NS, Corrigan JD. The structure of head-injured patients' neurobehavioral complaints: Preliminary studies. Brain Inj. 1990;4(2):115-33.
439. Van Zomeran AH, van den Burg W. Residual complaints of patients two years after severe head injury. J Neurol Neurosurg Psychiatry. 1985;48:21-8.

440. Jorge RE, Robinson RG, Starksein SE, et al. Secondary mania following traumatic brain injury. Am J Psychiatry. 1993;150(6): 916-21.
441. Stuart JT, Hemsath RH. Bipolar illness following TBI: Treatment with lithium and carbamazepine. J Clin Psychiatry. 1988;49(2):74-5.
442. Paul SM. Anxiety and depression: A common neurobiological substrate. J Clin Psychiatry. 1988;49(Suppl):13-6.
443. Jorge RE, Robinson RG, Starkstein SE, et al. Depression and anxiety following TBI. J Neuropsychiatry Clin Neurosci. 1993;5:369-74.
444. Tennant FS, Wild J. Naltrexone treatment for postconcussional syndrome. Am J Psychiatry. 1987;144(6):813-4.
445. Gualiteri CT. Buspirone: Neuropsychiatric effects. J Head Trauma Rehabil. 1988;6:90-2.
446. Davison K, Bagley CK. Schizophrenia-like psychosis associated with organic disorder of the CNS. Br J Psychiatry. 1969;4(Suppl):113-84.
447. Nasrallah HA, Fowler RC, Judd LL. Schizophrenia-like illness following head injury. Psychosomatics. 1981;22(4):359-61.
448. Feeney DM, Sutton RL. Pharmacotherapy for recovery of function after brain injury. Crit Rev Neurobiol. 1997;3: 135-97.
449. Cummings JL. Clinical Neuropsychiatry. New York: Grune and Stratton; 1985. pp.29-43.
450. Drummond LM, Gravestock S. Delayed emergence of obsessive compulsive neurosis following head injury. Br J Psychiatry. 1988;153:839-42.
451. Brooks N, Campsie L, Symington C, et al. The five year outcome of severe blunt head injury: A relative's view. J Neurol Neurosurg Psychiat. 1986;49:764-70.
452. Kant R, Duffy JD, Pivovarnik A. The prevalence of apathy following head injury. Brain Inj. 1988;12(1):87-92.
453. Duffy JD, Campbell JJ. The regional prefrontal syndromes: A theoretical and clinical overview. J Neuropsychiatry Clin Neurosci. 1994;6(4):379-87.
454. Gualtieri CT. Neuropsychiatry and Behavioral Pharmacology. New York: Springer-Verlag; 1991.

Acknowledgments

We would like to thank God for giving us an opportunity to write this chapter. We would like to whole heartedly thank Mrs Nalini Gururaj, Chief Librarian and Ms Shobha HS, Assistant. Librarian, from The Richmond Fellowship Postgraduate College for Psychosocial Rehabilitation for the help provided in editing, formatting and finalizing the manuscript. Last but not the least; we would also like to thank our family members for allowing us to take away their quality time for the preparation of this chapter.

CHAPTER 5

Substance Use Disorders

Nimesh G Desai, Dhanesh K Gupta, KA Khurshid, RK Solanki, Ashok Singhal, G Prasad Rao

5.1. CLASSIFICATION AND EPIDEMIOLOGY

Nimesh G Desai, Dhanesh K Gupta, KA Khurshid

Substance-related disorders have become matters of global concern because of impact on individual health, familial and social consequences, criminal and legal problems, and the effects on the national productivity and economy. The range of problems from occasional use of a substance through regular use to dependent use is wide and persons may slide across the spectrum of use as well as from softer substances to the more harmful substances on the spectrum of substances. All the problems along the two spectra, i.e. from use to dependence and from the most innocuous substance-like tea and coffee to the most hard substances, contribute to the cost that the human society or a particular nation has to bear.

In India, although alcohol use in ancient times and cannabis and *affim* (raw opium) in more recent times have been known and reported for sometime, substance use problems have been recognized to have a significant importance as a public health problem and in various other facets of life only very recently. In respect of the illicit drugs, especially heroin, India has changed from being a transit country to a user country and with increasing use of alcohol and tobacco, substance abuse problems have spread across strata of the society. They are of particular concern among slum dwellers, transport workers and youth. An additional concern about substance use disorders has occurred because of their relationship with the infection by human immunodeficiency virus (HIV) and acquired immunodeficiency syndrome (AIDS). The relationship between HIV spread and substance use disorder in its extreme form has been seen and recorded in the North Eastern State of Manipur, with explosive patterns of rise in rates of injection heroin users and seropositivity.

As such a comprehensive approach, to eradicate or minimize the occurrence of substance use disorders and their impact on various aspects of the society, will have to include strategies covering many fields of interest. In its most broad-based conceptualization, such an approach consists of two major streams of strategies aimed at supply curtailment and demand reduction. Supply curtailment includes strategies of total prohibition of alcohol, restricted hours of sale and other such strategies to ensure reduced supply of licit drugs-like alcohol and tobacco as well as legislation, law enforcement and legal punitive measures for offenders of the laws relating to supply and trafficking of illicit drugs.

Treatment and rehabilitation of persons with substance abuse problems, preventive education in schools and colleges, awareness campaigns in the community and involvement of youth in health promotion activities are some of important strategies for demand reduction.

The entire range of activities that occur in the field of demand reduction cover many varied fields of interest and expertise. While it will be useful for those involved in substance use related work on a regular basis to be familiar with all these activities, it is necessary for all mental health professionals, indeed all health professionals, to be well conversant with the hard core clinical issues of diagnosis, clinical features and management of various substance use disorders. This chapter is largely focused on these clinical issues which are necessary for clinical mental health professionals, but also touches upon some of the important aspects of the other issues in the field of demand reduction for generating awareness about the complex and interconnected nature of the solutions to the problems associated with the use of chemical substances.

DEFINITIONS AND CLASSIFICATION

Although the common clinical phenomena, like tolerance and withdrawal as well as their underlying mechanisms, had been found to be similar in basic science and clinical research for alcohol and some drugs of abuse, the group of clinical syndromes with various substances with abuse potential remained uncertain in their classification. The diagnostic and classificatory groupings have gone through many changes and revisions in the past few decades during which problems associated with use of chemical substances have been studied. Some of the important fallacies prevalent in the past, contributing to the divergence and chaos in this field are highlighted here:

- Definitions or diagnostic criteria for dependence were posited by different groups of researchers and clinical teams from varying perspectives. Many of these descriptions were predominantly social, psychological or medical in their orientation
- Alcohol dependence syndrome was recognized as a clinical syndrome very early and for quite sometime remained the only well-delineated description of dependence. Although the physical dependence to opioids was well-known, the clinical description of opioid dependence or for other illicit drugs of abuse remained unclear and the problems associated with illicit drug use were considered separately from the alcohol-related problems
- Categories of abuse and addiction for some illicit drugs remained uncertain, based on the distinction between psychological and physical dependence. This was more so for cannabis, stimulants and sedatives
- Substances, like nicotine (in tobacco) and caffeine (in tea, coffee or cola soft drinks), which were not only licit but also widely used and socially sanctioned were, not considered to have significant abuse potential
- *Abuse* of drugs was seen differently from the *misuse* of prescription drugs, and as such it was considered incorrect to view these two types of substance use together.

It is important to understand that while some of these concepts about different classes of chemical substances, do still have relevance in specific aspects like the degree of dependence, harmful effects, the pattern of use, etiological factors and the strategies for prevention, they are not considered valid or relevant for defining the group of disorders related to use of chemical substances and classifying them. In the current time, the term *substance* refers to the commonly known drugs of abuse like cannabis and opioids, legal substances like alcohol and tobacco, medicinal compounds with abuse liability like tranquilizers and sedatives, and other chemicals like volatile solvents. The 1992 International Classification of Diseases-10th edition (ICD-10) by the World Health Organization (WHO)[1] has identified 10 classes of *psychoactive substances* which lead to mental and behavioral disorders. These classes of substances are:

- *Alcohol*: Usually only ethyl alcohol, except in illicit beverages which sometimes contain methyl alcohol along with other congeners and adulterants
- *Opioids*: Includes morphine and the other alkaloids from the poppy plant, semisynthetic compounds like heroin, hydromorphine and oxycodeine, as well as synthetic compound, like pentazocine, pethidine and buprenorphine
- *Cannabinoids*: Plant products from the cannabis sativa and indica plants, e.g. marihuana (*ganja*), *hashish*, *charas* and *bhang*
- *Sedatives or hypnotics*: The medicinal drugs, which are generally prescribed for their sleep inducing properties and which often have anxiolytic effects also. These include barbiturates, benzodiazepines and methaquilone
- *Cocaine*
- *Stimulants including caffeine*: Includes amphetamines, methylphenidate, pemoline and caffeine
- *Hallucinogens*: Includes LSD, dimethyl tryptamine, psilocybin, psilocin, and mescaline
- *Tobacco*: Including all forms of use by smoking (cigarettes, pipes, cigars, beedies) and nonsmoking routes (*zarda*, *khaini*, *naswar*, *snuff*, etc.)
- *Volatile solvents*: Includes toluene, ethyl acetate, trichloroethane, butane, propane, nitrous oxide, ethyl chloride, acetone, isopropylnitrite, amyl nitrite
- Multiple drug use.

The 1994 American Psychiatric Association's Diagnostic and Statistical Manual, IV edition (DSM-IV) also enlists the same classes, but separates caffeine and PCP, leading to eleven classes of substances.

In both classification systems, the first step in classification is to specify the substance or the class of substance that is involved. This identification has to be, necessarily, based on the basis of self-report data, report from informants, characteristic clinical symptoms and signs, and objective analysis of specimens of biological fluids like urine and blood. This classification is to be made on the basis of the most important substance used, since many of the drug users do take more than one substance.

As a next step, the disorder which is clinically observed and inferred, is to be added to the substance abused, with sub-classification where applicable. Research in basic and clinical sciences has led to important convergence of ideas not only in considering all chemical use of substances on similar paradigm, but also in the classification of the disorders related to substance use. This convergence is also reflected in the two most commonly used classificatory systems, although the terms used are different. The ICD-10 uses the term, *disorders due to psychoactive substance use,* for a wide variety of disorders that differ in severity from uncomplicated intoxication and harmful use to obvious psychotic disorders and dementia but are all attributable to the use of one or more psychoactive substances. The DSM-IV describes this group of disorders as *substance-related disorders*. The ICD-10 considers all such disorders in one common list, but the DSM-IV divides them into two groups, i.e. *substance use disorders* (*substance dependence* and *substance abuse*) and *substance induced disorders*. The *substance abuse disorder* of DSM-IV, a relatively wide concept does not find a corresponding category in ICD-10, which has a restrictive category of *harmful use*. The substance induced disorders of DSM-IV are by and large also found in the list of disorders due to *psychoactive substance use* of ICD-10, and additionally recognizes sleep disorder and sexual dysfunction related to substance use as specific categories (Table 1).

As such, ICD-10 and DSM-IV classificatory systems are more similar than they were earlier, with certain positive landmarks. All substances are considered as one group, with classes of the substances used and the disorders due to substance use are also considered similarly across the various classes of substances. This system has the support of scientific research about the biopsychosocial approach to these disorders and the advantage of uniformity across various classes of substances, but also has an important caveat. According to such a system, any of the disorders can be linked to any of the class of substances, whereas in reality, not all the disorders occur with all the substances. Psychotic disorder or dementia are not seen to occur with tobacco or sedative-hypnotics. On the other hand, amnestic disorder has been clearly established to occur only with alcohol, and been described to occur possibly with sedative-hypnotics.

Table 1: Substance-related disorders in ICD-10 and DSM-IV

ICD-10	*DSM-IV*
Disorders due to psychoactive substance use	*Substance-related disorders*
	I. *Substance use disorder*
1. Acute intoxication	1. Dependence
2. Harmful use	2. Abuse
	II. *Substance induced disorders*
3. Dependence syndrome	3. Intoxication
4. Withdrawal state	4. Withdrawal
5. Withdrawal state with delirium	5. Withdrawal delirium
6. Psychotic disorder Schizophrenia-like • Predominantly delusional • Predominantly polymorphic • Predominantly depressive symptoms • Predominantly manic symptoms • Mixed	6. Persisting dementia
7. Amnestic syndrome	7. Persisting amnestic disorder
8. Residual and late-onset psychotic disorders • Flashbacks	8. Psychotic disorder with delusions with hallucinations
• Personality or behavior disorder	9. Mood disorder
• Residual affective disorder	10. Anxiety disorder dementia
• Other persisting cognitive impairment	11. Sexual dysfunction
• Late onset psychotic disorder	12. Sleep disorders
9. Other mental and behavioral disorders	
10. Unspecified mental and behavioral disorder	

Nonetheless, the application of common definition of some of the disorders like withdrawal state, acute intoxication, dependence and abuse/harmful use across all the classes of substances is possible and useful. The consensus in the concepts in the definition of these disorders is evident also in the similarity of the diagnostic criteria for dependence in DSM-IV and the diagnostic guidelines in ICD-10. The striking aspect of the description in both the systems is that they are well balanced in their biopsychosocial emphasis while outlining the important components of dependence. The only difference in the two descriptions is that compulsive use is one of the features of *dependence syndrome* in ICD-10, and this is not included in the diagnostic criteria in DSM-IV (Table 2).

In the fifth edition of the *Diagnostic and Statistical Manual of Mental Disorders* (DSM-5), the revised chapter of "Substance-Related and Addictive Disorders" includes substantive changes to the disorders grouped there plus changes to the criteria of certain conditions.

Substance use disorder in DSM-5 combines the DSM-IV categories of substance abuse and substance dependence into a single disorder measured on a continuum from mild to severe. Each specific substance (other than caffeine, which cannot be diagnosed as a substance use disorder) is addressed as a separate use disorder (e.g. alcohol use disorder, stimulant use disorder, etc.), but nearly all substances are diagnosed based on the same overarching criteria. In this overarching disorder, the criteria have not only been combined, but strengthened. Whereas a diagnosis of substance abuse previously required only one symptom, mild substance use disorder in DSM-5 requires two to three symptoms from a list of 11. Drug craving will be added to the list, and problems with law enforcement will be eliminated because of cultural considerations that make the criteria difficult to apply internationally.

In DSM-IV, the distinction between abuse and dependence was based on the concept of abuse as a mild or early phase and dependence as the more severe manifestations. In practice, the abuse criteria were sometimes quite severe. The revised substance use disorder, a single diagnosis, will better match the symptoms that patients experience. Additionally, the diagnosis of dependence caused much confusion. Most people link dependence with "addiction" when in fact dependence can be a normal body response to a substance.

Table 2: Description of dependence in ICD-10 and DSM-IV

ICD-10		*DSM-IV*	
Diagnostic guidelines for dependence syndrome		*Diagnostic criteria for substance dependence disorder*	
Three or more of the following criteria are met at any time during the last year:		Three or more of the following criteria are met at any time during the same 12 month period:	
1.	A strong desire or sense of compulsion to take the substance	1.	Tolerance defined by either need for markedly increased amounts of substance to achieve intoxication or desired effect or markedly diminished effect with continued use of the same amount of substance
2.	Difficulties in controlling substance taking behavior in terms of its onset, termination, or levels of use	2.	Withdrawal as evidenced by either of the following characteristic withdrawal syndrome for the substance or the same (or closely related) substance is taken to relieve or avoid withdrawal symptoms
3.	Physiological withdrawal state when substance use has ceased longer intended	3.	The substance is often taken in larger amounts over a or been reduced, as evidenced period of time than was by either of the following: the characteristic withdrawal syndrome for the substance or use of some (or closely related) substance to relieve the withdrawal symptoms
4.	Tolerance as evidenced by increased doses of substance required to achieve the same effects as originally produced by lower doses	4.	Persistent desire or repeated unsuccessful efforts to cut down or control substance use
5.	Progressive neglect of alternative pleasurable activities or interests and increasd amount of time spent to obtain or take the substance, or recover from its effects	5.	A great deal of time is spent in activities necessary to obtain the substance, use the substance or to recover from its effects
6.	Persistent substance use despite clear evidence of overtly harmful consequences (physical or mental)	6.	Important social, occupational, or recreational activities given up or reduced because of substance use
		7.	Continued substance use despite knowledge of having had a persistent or recurrent physical or psychological problem that was likely to have been caused or exacerbated by the substance

DSM-5 Diagnostic criteria for alcohol use disorder
A problematic pattern of alcohol use leading to clinically significant impairment or distress, as manifested by at least two of the following, occurring within a 12-month period:
1. Alcohol is often taken in larger amounts or over a longer period than was intended.
2. There is a persistent desire or unsuccessful efforts to cut down or control alcohol use.
3. A great deal of time is spent in activities necessary to obtain alcohol, use alcohol, or recover from its effects.
4. Craving, or a strong desire or urge to use alcohol.
5. Recurrent alcohol use resulting in a failure to fulfill major role obligations at work, school, or home.
6. Continued alcohol use despite having persistent or recurrent social or interpersonal problems caused or exacerbated by the effects of alcohol.
7. Important social, occupational, or recreational activities are given up or reduced because of alcohol use.
8. Recurrent alcohol use in situations in which it is physically hazardous.
9. Alcohol use is continued despite knowledge of having a persistent or recurrent physical or psychological problem that is likely to have been caused or exacerbated by alcohol.
10. Tolerance, as defined by either, of the following: a. A need for markedly increased amounts of alcohol to achieve intoxication or desired effect. b. A markedly diminished effect with continued use of the same amount of alcohol.
11. Withdrawal, as manifested by either of the following: a. The characteristic withdrawal syndrome for alcohol (refer to Criteria A and B of the criteria set for alcohol withdrawal, pp. 235-236). b. Alcohol (or a closely related substance, such as a benzodiazepine) is taken to relieve or avoid withdrawal symptoms.

Contd...

Contd...

Specify if: *In early remission:* After full criteria for alcohol use disorder were previously met, none of the criteria for alcohol use disorder have been met for at least 3 months but for less than 12 months (with the exception that Criterion A4, "Craving, or a strong desire or urge to use alcohol," may be met). *In sustained remission:* After full criteria for alcohol use disorder were previously met, none of the criteria for alcohol use disorder have been met at anytime during a period of 12 months or longer (with the exception that Criterion A4, "Craving, or a strong desire or urge to use alcohol," may be met).
Specify if: *In a controlled environment:* This additional specifier is used if the individual is in an environment where access to alcohol is restricted. *Code based on current severity:* Note for ICD-10-CM codes: If an alcohol intoxication, alcohol withdrawal, or another alcohol-induced mental disorder is also present, do not use the codes below for alcohol use disorder. Instead, the comorbid alcohol use disorder is indicated in the 4th character of the alcohol-induced disorder code (see the coding note for alcohol intoxication, alcohol withdrawal, or a specific alcohol-induced mental disorder). For example, if there is comorbid alcohol intoxication and alcohol use disorder, only the alcohol intoxication code is given, with the 4th character indicating whether the comorbid alcohol use disorder is mild, moderate, or severe: F10.129 for mild alcohol use disorder with alcohol intoxication or F10.229 for a moderate or severe alcohol use disorder with alcohol intoxication.
Specify current severity: *305.00 (F10.10) Mild:* Presence of 2 to 3 symptoms. *303.90 (F10.20) Moderate:* Presence of 4 to 5 symptoms. *303.90 (F10.20) Severe:* Presence of 6 or more symptoms.

DSM-5 Diagnostic criteria for alcohol intoxication
A. Recent ingestion of alcohol.
B. Clinically significant problematic behavioral or psychological changes (e.g. inappropriate sexual or aggressive behavior, mood lability, impaired judgment) that developed during, or shortly after, alcohol ingestion.
C. One (or more) of the following signs or symptoms developing during, or shortly after, alcohol use: 1. Slurred speech. 2. Incoordination. 3. Unsteady gait. 4. Nystagmus. 5. Impairment in attention or memory. 6. Stupor or coma.
D. The signs or symptoms are not attributable to another medical condition and are not better explained by another mental disorder, including intoxication with another substance.
Coding note: The ICD-9-CM code is 303.00. The ICD-10-CM code depends on whether there is a comorbid alcohol use disorder. If a mild alcohol use disorder is comorbid, the ICD-10-CM code is F10.129, and if a moderate or severe alcohol use disorder is comorbid, the ICD-10-CM code is F10.229. If there is no comorbid alcohol use disorder, then the ICD-10-CM code is F10.929.

Other Alcohol-induced Disorders

The biopsychosocial approach to the diagnosis of dependence disorder encompasses all the aspects of the clinical disorder, although the importance of neuroadaptation and physical dependence is well accepted. The phenomenon of physical dependence is central to the definition of dependence disorder, but not a prerequisite. Diagnosis of dependence disorder can be made in the absence of physical dependence to the substance (either tolerance or withdrawal). Compulsive use, use despite harm having occurred, and the other

DSM-5 Diagnostic criteria for alcohol withdrawal
A. Cessation of (or reduction in) alcohol use that has been heavy and prolonged.
B. Two (or more) of the following, developing within several hours to a few days after the cessation of (or reduction in) alcohol use described in Criterion A: 1. Autonomic hyperactivity (e.g. sweating or pulse rate greater than 100 bpm). 2. Increased hand tremor. 3. Insomnia. 4. Nausea or vomiting. 5. Transient visual, tactile, or auditory hallucinations or illusions. 6. Psychomotor agitation. 7. Anxiety. 8. Generalized tonic-clonic seizures.
C. The signs or symptoms in Criterion B cause clinically significant distress or impairment in social, occupational, or other important areas of functioning.
D. The signs or symptoms are not attributable to another medical condition and are not better explained by another mental disorder, including intoxication or withdrawal from another substance.
Specify if: *With perceptual disturbances:* This specifier applies in the rare instance when hallucinations (usually visual or tactile) occur with intact reality testing, or auditory, visual, or tactile illusions occur in the absence of a delirium.
Coding note: The ICD-9-CM code is 291.81. The ICD-10-CM code for alcohol withdrawal without perceptual disturbances is F10.239, and the ICD-10-CM code for alcohol withdrawal with perceptual disturbances is F10.232. Note that the ICD-10-CM code indicates the comorbid presence of a moderate or severe alcohol use disorder, reflecting the fact that alcohol withdrawal can only occur in the presence of a moderate or severe alcohol use disorder. It is not permissible to code a comorbid mild alcohol use disorder with alcohol withdrawal.

Table 3: Definitions of the basic concepts in dependence
Neuroadaptation: The phenomenon of altered neuronal response to persistent exposure to a substance, manifesting in physical and/or psychological dependence on the substance.
Physical dependence: It is a state characterized by the occurrence of tolerance and/or withdrawal due to persistent use of a substance.
Tolerance: Process whereby effects of initial drug doses become ineffective leading to a markedly diminished effect with continued use of the same amount of the substance or creating a need for markedly increased amount of the substance to achieve the desired effect.
Withdrawal: It is a group of time limited and substance specific signs and symptoms, that occur when a substance is reduced in amount or discontinued following persistent use.
Psychological dependence: A state characterized by compulsive use, craving and the other behavioral features of dependence on a substance, with or without the physical dependence.

diagnostic features of dependence disorder, are the specific cognitive and behavioral patterns of substance seeking nature described as manifestations of the phenomenon of psychological dependence (Table 3).

While the definition of dependence is well accepted and more or less uniform, the concept of problem use not amounting to dependence is not very well agreed upon. Such problem use or abuse has been quite extensively studied in case of alcohol use and to a lesser extent for tobacco and other substances. This lack of clarity is evident in the approach of the two classificatory systems to the category of non-dependent use disorder. ICD-10 recognizes only *harmful use* as a disorder, with a stringent requirement of actual damage to physical or mental health having been caused. The DSM-IV description of *substance abuse* is more in keeping with the biopsychosocial approach to these disorders and the current research literature (Table 4).

Table 4: Description of nondependent use disorder		
ICD-10	*DSM-IV*	
Diagnostic guidelines for harmful use	*Diagnostic criteria for substance abuse*	
A pattern of psychoactive substance use that is causing damage to health; the damage may be to physical or mental health	A.	A maladaptive pattern of substance use leading to clinically significant impairment or distress, as manifested by one (or more) of the following occurring within a 12-month period: 1. Recurrent substance use, resulting in a failure to fulfill major role obligations at work, school or home 2. Recurrent substance abuse in situations that are physically hazardous 3. Recurrent substance abuse related legal problem 4. Continued substance abuse despite having persistent or recurrent social or interpersonal problems caused or exacerbated by the effects of the substance.
	B.	Has never met the criteria for substance dependence for this class of substance.

EPIDEMIOLOGY

In view of the public health importance of substance-related disorders, it is necessary to have information on direct epidemiological indicators like the incidence and the prevalence rates for different substances. It has generally been difficult to arrive at accurate assessment of these direct indicators due to specific problems in epidemiological studies of substance-related disorders, in addition to the general problems in epidemiology. Some of these problems in studying the direct epidemiology of substance-related disorders, until recently, were:

- *Concepts and definitions*: The concepts of disorder in problems related to use of substances have been evolving and the definitions of the 'disorder' have been undergoing modification. It is only in recent time that a consensus has emerged for the definition of dependence disorder. The studies carried out till recently have employed variable definitions of dependence disorder. The issue of definition becomes more difficult about the nondependent use and the other categories of use. Many surveys on epidemiology of drug abuse in India have enquired into 'ever use' or examined abuse in ill-defined terms. At times, the rates arrived at in such surveys have been quoted for estimating the rates of drug abuse
- *Reliability of information*: The major source of information in epidemiological studies is the report provided by the concerned individuals. The reliability of the information does remain questionable because respondents tend to be cautious while reporting about use of illicit substances and the sociocultural practices also influence the accuracy of the report
- *Lack of objective diagnosis*: The fact that the diagnosis of these disorders is not supported by objective laboratory-based tests does reduce the reliability of the epidemiological studies. Such laboratory-based tests and test batteries have been utilized for diagnosis of alcoholism in community-based epidemiological studies with modest success. In the other categories of substances, such objective diagnosis is not very feasible. Screening of biological fluids for the substance or its metabolite is informative about one time cross-sectional evaluation and can, at best, be seen to be a supportive tool and not as a diagnostic test of a disorder

- *Lack of stability of diagnosis*: It is well known that persons move from one locus on the spectrum of use to another as part of natural course. Hence, the diagnosis does not remain as stable as in physical or other psychiatric disorders. The category of dependence has more stability as compared to the other substance-related disorders, which makes it more difficult to estimate rates of these disorders
- *Changing trends of use*: The choice of the substance and the use pattern are known to undergo rapid changes over relatively short periods of time, especially with the illicit drug of abuse on the street
- *Overlap with psychiatric disorders*: The substance-related disorders have significant overlap with other psychiatric disorders on Axis I as well as on Axis II. This overlap makes accurate assessment difficult because of misdiagnosis and the possible unsuitable nature of the instruments used
- *Sampling technique*: The relatively low frequency of the observation (prevalence rate) and the tendency of users of illicit drugs to form subcultures in social isolation, render the standard sampling technique of selecting a statistically representative sample with scientific random method ineffective for an accurate estimate of the rates of various disorders
- *Geographical variations*: The patterns and the rates of substance use and hence the related disorders are known to vary across geographical regions, with in a nation or state. Such variations make it difficult to generalize rates from one study to adjoining areas, even if they are based on statistically representative samples. The fact that the rates of substance-related disorders are also influenced by sociocultural factors, availability and other external factors places significant restriction on extrapolating the observations on prevalence rates from one setting to another
- *Resources*: The difficulties involved and the resultant need for total sampling as well as the trained manpower escalate the cost of studies for direct epidemiological indicators enormously
- *Time lag*: The time required for completing research studies which can provide reliable estimates is large, usually running into one or two years, and by the time the research data are analyzed and made available their relevance may be compromised. This is more true for the pattern of illicit drug use because of the rapidly changing trends.

The above-mentioned problems or difficulties in the field of direct epidemiology of substance-related disorders have restricted the possibility of arriving at reliable and accurate estimates. In the absence of reliable direct indicators and to supplement them, indirect indicators have been used to estimate the magnitude of the substance-related problems. Indirect indicators are elicited from the data already available at some source and require no specific resources except for secondary analysis. Morbidity and mortality rates of conditions linked to specific substance use like liver cirrhosis for alcohol, hepatitis B for parenteral drug use and overdose deaths for opioids, are some good examples of indirect indicators. The other indirect indicators, which have been utilized for illicit drugs, are seizures of heroin and the number of persons seeking help at treatment centers.

The Drug Abuse Warning Network (DAWN) and Drug Abuse Reporting Program (DARP) in USA, and Home Office Addicts Notification Index and Regional Drug Misuse Database in the UK are well-known examples of reporting systems based on the principle that the data about persons presenting at the treatment centers can provide useful indirect information about the magnitude of the drug abuse population in the community. Additionally, these reporting systems have also provided early indicators of changes in the drug abuse pattern, in terms of new drugs being introduced or change in the preferred route of administration. Reporting systems have been operationalized and in existence for many years in the developed countries like USA, UK, Sweden and other European countries, as well as some of the South East Asian countries.

In India, pilot testing of a reporting system was carried out in a research project funded by the Indian Council of Medical Research (ICMR) from 1989 to 1992, at Delhi, Lucknow and Jodhpur. The drug abuse monitoring system (DAMS) developed for this research project has been reported to be feasible. It does seem that such reporting systems are workable and useful in countries with large financial resources, strong administrative support for such programs, participation of the various treatment agencies or at least the advantage of small size.

The usefulness of indirect indicators in case of illicit drugs is limited because the activities related to these drugs from street sale to treatment seeking remain underground and hidden. On the other hand, the indirect indicators of the magnitude of the problems with illicit drugs like alcohol and tobacco have more utility. The sales data for alcohol or the rates of deaths due to cirrhosis reflect the magnitude of the problem more closely. Some indirect indicators are useful not only in arriving at estimates of the magnitude of the problem but are well correlated to the rates of disorder. About 10–20% of people, who drink alcohol excessively, develop cirrhosis of liver. Therefore, deaths from cirrhosis can be used as a means of estimating rates of alcohol abuse.

The relationship between total alcohol consumption in a community and the distribution of consumption amongst its members was first studied by a Frenchman, Lederman, in 1956. He produced a graph, now known as *Lederman curve*, which represents the relationship between these two variables. The curve is lognormal, i.e. natural logarithms of consumption and not the raw data are normally distributed. It is positively skewed, i.e. with increase in total consumption, the proportion of heavy drinkers will also rise. Relationships between overall alcohol consumption and alcohol-related problems have been demonstrated in the UK, Sweden and the USA.

These indirect indicators are more useful in situations in which no direct indicators are available, or if available are not reliable, or to supplement the information available from direct indicators. They were developed in situations, which existed in large parts of the world a few decades ago, wherein direct indicators were not available at all or were not reliable. In the developing countries, with the inadequacy of direct indicators persisting, these indirect indicators may be the only or one of the few sources of information on the epidemiology and must be utilized. The developed countries have, with advancements in research methodology and huge resource allocations, overcome the limitations of direct epidemiology and reliable rates for many of the important categories of substance-related disorders, from studies on direct indicators, have been available in the recent past. Many countries have been able to report on use pattern as well as the rates of clinical disorders in the recent past.

Large surveys in households with scientific random sampling as well as surveys in schools and colleges have been carried out in USA over the years, focusing on monthly, yearly and lifetime use pattern. The National Institute on Drug Abuse (NIDA) survey data suggest that while the drug use in college students and young adults was high in 1986, it has progressively declined since then (Table 5). There has been a decline in the overall illicit drug use, especially in the reported use of heroin, cocaine and sedative-hypnotics but with increase in marihuana and hallucinogens in the USA.

The National Household Survey on Drug Abuse (NHSDA) of USA has been carried out, at regular periodic intervals since 1971, with the objective of measuring the prevalence of use of illicit drugs, alcohol, tobacco products, and non-medical use of prescription drugs based on a stratified multi-stage area probability sample. The monthly, annual and lifetime prevalence rates of illicit drug use are provided in Table 6. As is evident, the prevalence rates are higher in males as compared to females.

Table 5: Prevalence rates of illicit drug use in college students and young adults in USA (NIDA Survey Data)

	1986	*1991*	*1992*
Monthly	25.89%	15.1%	14.8%
Annual	41.9%	27.0%	28.3%
Lifetime	70.5%	62.2%	60.2%

Table 6: Prevalence rates of illicit drug use in general population in USA (NHSDA Data,1996)

	Total	*Male*	*Female*
Monthly	6.1	8.1	4.2
Annual	10.8	13.9	8.0
Lifetime	34.8	40.0	29.9

In UK, there is a consistent finding that one-third of young adults have tried illegal drugs. According to Health Education Authority Survey, 25% of 16–19-year-old have tried cannabis, 6% have tried LSD and 3% have tried ecstasy, 5% have tried amphetamines, 3% have sniffed solvents and less than 1% have tried heroin, cocaine or *crack*. In both USA and UK, the 1990s have seen a substantial growth in the levels of cocaine use which have stabilized and an upsurge in use of marihuana and amphetamines. Methamphetamines, in particular, have been seen to have become popular and there has been widespread popularity of LSD (lysergic acid diethylamide) and ecstasy (methylenedioxymethampheta-mine; MDMA).

The proportion of drug users who develop drug dependence seems to vary considerably from one drug category to another and most likely determined by factors such as drug availability and the reinforcing functions served by these drugs. Currently available data suggest that the risk of developing drug dependence is just under 1% per year for adults in USA; the one year prevalence of drug dependence is between 1.4% and 2.2% in the age group of 15–54 years.

The one year prevalence of drug dependence is some two to four times the annual incidence of drug dependence. This relationship between one year prevalence and annual incidence is consistent with the concept of drug dependence as a persistent psychiatric disturbance with a duration of more than one year. For every newly developed incident case of drug dependence in the adult population at present, there are several other adults whose drug dependence started some years back and who continue to be burdened by its complications in their current lives. Recent estimates for the lifetime prevalence of drug dependence indicate a broad range from under 1% in some countries, like Korea and Puerto Rico, to above 3% in other locales, like Christchurch (New Zealand), Edmonton (Canada), and Los Angeles (USA).

Since alcohol use is a common sociocultural behavior in most American and European countries, there have been many studies from differing sociological and medical perspectives to assess the extent of drinking, problem drinking and alcoholism. It is generally believed that more than 60 to 70% of the population drinks at least once in a year and more than 5% of the population reports drinking 8 or more drinks in a day, at least once a week. The NHSDA 1996 data (Table 7) suggest that the rates of use in past one month, one year or lifetime are higher in males as compared to females, although the gender difference seems to be not as marked for use of alcohol as it is for illicit drugs (Tables 6 and 7).

In UK, the General Household Survey (GHS) conducted by the Office of Population Censuses and Surveys (OPCS) has documented data on the trends of alcohol use based on their own definitions of 'sensible' levels of drinking (i.e. 21 units/week for men and 14 Units/week for women). According to this definition, 25–26% of men and 9–10% of women drink alcohol above the 'sensible' level. The proportion of persons who drink above the sensible levels are more in the age group of 18–45 years.

Table 7: Prevalence rates of alcohol use in general population in USA (NHSDA Data,1996)

	Total	*Male*	*Female*
Monthly	51.0	58.9	43.6
Annual	64.9	70.0	60.2
Lifetime	82.6	86.6	78.8

Surveys that include information on use pattern in different time frames and the presence of abuse or dependence provide a good holistic picture of the range of substance related problems. The Epidemiological Catchment Area (ECA) Program has been the only epidemiological study that has sought to estimate prospectively the prevalence and incidence for drug dependence for general population using standardized diagnostic assessment in the context of an epidemiologic field survey. By means of a prospective study design and taking advantage of repeatedly administered assessments, ECA surveys, conducted in five American communities, have provided evidence on the occurrence of drug dependence in adulthood, measured as cumulative annual incidence estimate of 1.09% for the diagnostic category of drug dependence combined with drug abuse. Approximately 40% of the identified cases in the ECA survey have been found to qualify for a diagnosis of drug abuse without drug dependence and the remaining 60% qualified for drug dependence. Thus, assuming generalizability of these estimates from the ECA sites to the nation as a whole, for adults living in US during the early 1980s, an estimated 0.6% or 6 per thousand were found to become incident cases of drug dependence during a one year interval of observation (Table 8).

In view of the limitations of the standard epidemiological survey methods, other survey techniques have been employed for estimating the prevalence of substance use disorders in the community. The two most commonly employed techniques are the key informant technique and the snowball technique. The key informant technique elicits information on substance use and its profile in the persons under survey, from a number of key informants. Such key informants can be Head of the Household (HOH) for community-based household surveys, or teachers for surveys in schools or colleges. The major advantage of this technique is the time and the money saved, although the reliability and validity of information obtained may be suspect to an extent. Rapid and less expensive surveys of this kind have been carried out, with adequate reliability and validity.

The *snowball technique* begins with a few identified users who provide information about the other users in their contact; the newly identified users, in turn, leading to other users; ultimately broadening the net of identifying the users to cover all the users in the area. The snowball technique is particularly useful in surveys for illicit drug use, which are not very reliable due to the phenomenon of many of these users remaining hidden in their own 'subcultures' or underground due to the other illegal activities associated with such drug use. This technique has been used to complement the information obtained from standard surveys. Direct relevance for policy planning has led to attempts of arriving at the population estimates, i.e. total number of persons with use or disorder for any class of substance in a country.

Table 8: Prevalence rates of alcohol and other drug disorders in USA (ECA Data)

Disorders	*1-month (SEM)*	*6-month (SEM)*	*Lifetime (SEM)*
Any substance use disorder	3.8 (0.2)	6.1 (0.3)	16.7 (0.4)
Any alcohol disorder	2.8 (0.2)	4.8 (0.2)	13.5 (0.4)
Dependence	1.7 (0.1)	2.8 (0.2)	7.9 (0.3)
Abuse only	1.1 (0.1)	1.9 (0.2)	5.6 (0.2)
Any other drug disorder	1.3 (0.1)	2.0 (0.1)	6.1 (0.2)
Dependence	0.8 (0.1)	1.2 (0.1)	3.5 (0.2)
Abuse only	0.5 (0.1)	0.9 (0.1)	2.6 (0.2)

In arriving at these figures, the prevalence rates from standard data are used along with the other survey data available and the indirect indicators. Population estimates from the NHSDA (1996) data clearly suggest that although illicit drug users do form a large part of the overall problem of substance use, alcohol and tobacco rank higher. It also indicates clearly that not all of tobacco use in USA is in the form of smoking (Table 9).

The gross estimates of prevalence rates and the total number of abusers in the world in the 1990s for the illicit substances have been provided, by combining the information received from many sources using the above-mentioned techniques, by the United Nations International Drug Control Program (UNDCP) in 1998. The annual prevalence of heroin abuse has been cited as 0.14% of the total population, with a population estimate of 8.0 million. Cannabis has been estimated to have an annual prevalence rate of 2.45%, with total number of abusers estimated at 141.2 million. The abuse of sedative type substances has been estimated to be the highest, with an annual prevalence rate of 3.92% of the total population and population estimate of abusers of 227.4 million persons.

Alcohol-use disorders are common in all developed countries, and are more prevalent in men than women, with lower, but still substantial rates in developing countries. Although rates of these disorders are lower in Mediterranean countries (e.g. Greece, Italy and Israel), and higher in northern and eastern Europe (e.g. Russia and Scandinavia), they are responsible for a large proportion of the healthcare burden in almost all populations.

Table 9: Population estimates of alcohol, tobacco and illicit drug use in USA (in millions) (NHSDA Data, 1996)

	Alcohol	*Tobacco (Smoking)*	*Tobacco (Smokeless)*	*Illicit drugs*
Monthly	109.15	61.76	6.81	13.03
Annual	138.91	69.10	10.03	23.18
Lifetime	176.71	153.25	36.36	74.39

As many as 80% of men and 60% of women in developed countries drink at sometime during their lives. In any year, between half and two-thirds of individuals who were drank are likely to have stopped because of medical concerns. 30 to 50% of people who drank in the past year experience at least one adverse alcohol-related problem during their lifetime, such as missing work or school, driving after drinking, or interpersonal problems. The lifetime risk of alcohol-use disorders for men is more than 20%, with a risk of about 15% for alcohol abuse and 10% for alcohol dependence. The risk of developing an alcohol-use disorder in the previous year is about 10% overall.

Only about a quarter of people with alcohol-use disorders ever seek help for these conditions, with higher proportions for women than men. Most receive care from their general practitioner, where they represent about a fifth of patients seen: the proportions seen for diabetes and hypertension are similar. The challenge for the clinician is to learn enough about these disorders to identify them, since missing an alcohol-use disorder can complicate the assessment and treatment of other medical and psychiatric issue.

Epidemiology in India

The earliest information on epidemiology of substance abuse in India has been available from the surveys carried out in the 1960s and early 1970s for mental illnesses. The questionnaires of these surveys included items on alcohol or illicit drug use and problems associated with such use. In the late 1970s and the early part of the 1980s, many surveys were conducted on drug use (including alcohol use) in school and college students as well as some general population surveys.

Most of the studies of this period, in general population, have been carried out in small and nonrepresentative samples, enquiring into use or abuse that was not well-defined. There has been an extremely wide variation in the rates reported from these studies because of these methodological issues (Table 10). Notwithstanding these limitations, the conclusions from the studies in the general population are that the prevalence rates vary but the problem of drug abuse does exist in rural as well as urban areas and the most common drugs are tobacco, alcohol and cannabis. The large number of studies in student populations, including medical students, from 1963 to 1984, have varied greatly in their definition of drug use/abuse, methodology followed and

Table 10: Summary of the early studies on epidemiology of drug use/abuse in India

Drug	*Surveys on mental illness*	*Surveys in general population*	*Surveys in students*
Cannabis	0.4–1.0%	1.9–33.0%	1.7–66.0%
Opiates	0.04–0.1%	0.7–24.8%	4.5–12.7%
Alcohol	–	2.9–82.5%	5.2–58.0%
Tranquilizers	–	3.5–53.8%	3.5–61.0%
Overall	1.30–2.77%	28.77%	5.0–56.21%

Table 11: Summary of the studies on epidemiology of alcohol use in India

	General population	*Students*	*Medical professionals*
Ever use	25.6–74.2%	21.6–58.4%	8.5–66.7%
Use in last one year	19.0–82.5%	–	–
Use in last one month	–	9.3–12.7	–

the period of enquiry. The studies reveal that the prevalence rates of use in students varied from 5.0 to 56.2%, the rates being higher in medical students, and tobacco, alcohol, pain-killers, tranquilizers and cannabis being the commonly used drugs.

The studies on alcohol use epidemiology also have reported similar variations, although the differences in the methods employed are more striking in this group of studies (Table 11). It was concluded in a review of the studies till the mid 1980s that alcohol use was predominantly seen in males and the rates for female users of alcohol were very low and less than 5% of all the females. It was also concluded that the rates of alcohol use, and heavy use at that, were higher in the medical professionals as compared to general population.

A report by the Ministry of Health and Family Welfare, Government of India (1995) has stated that epidemiological studies on representative general population in the late 1970s showed a period prevalence for opium addiction between 6.3 and 18.9%. The prevalence rate of opium use has been reported to be 1.3% in Jodhpur, 0.1% in Delhi and none in Lucknow, from area survey multicentric ICMR study. One ICMR sponsored study has examined the feasibility of using the key informant technique, by assessing the agreement between the report of the individual subjects and the head of the household (HOH) about the drug dependence of the individuals. The HOH-based survey was found to be a valid and reliable method of assessing the prevalence rates of drug dependence in the community and a representative sample of general population survey in the megapolis of Delhi was undertaken.

In another ICMR study, the prevalence rate of heroin dependence was found to be 0.5% in a high prevalence slum population of Delhi. The report suggested that based on crude estimate of 0.3–0.5% prevalence rate, there would be about 2-3 lakh users in the country. As per the study on Drug Abuse Monitoring System (DAMS), it has been seen that in the early 1990s about two-thirds of the patients registered at the treatment centers in Delhi were heroin users, and 33–50% of the patients in the cities of Lucknow and Jodhpur were heroin users. These studies carried out in the late 1980s and the early 1990s had found very little evidence, if at all, for Injection Drug Use (IDU). Reports of injection use have been accumulating from different cities after the first report of increasing injection use of buprenorphine patients at a treatment clinic in Calcutta.

There has been an exponential rise in the patients, at treatment centers, who report with primary dependence on injection use or injection use as part of multidrug use pattern. Indeed, the profile of drug use pattern also has been seen to be undergoing a significant change from one drug dependence and use to multidrug use and dependence. A very large part of such injection use involves the use of buprenorphine. This increase in the number of injection users poses a grave danger for HIV transmission not only among the high-risk groups but also to the general population.

Injection Drug Use in India

The scenario of injection drug use and HIV seroprevalence in the North Eastern State of Manipur is well-known. The State of Manipur and its neighboring parts of the other States have been affected by injection use of heroin since the early part of the 1980s. Huge amounts of heroin are reportedly transported to other parts of the world from Myanmar, Thailand and Laos in South East Asia, notoriously known as the '*Golden triangle*', and as part of the well-known phenomenon of '*fall-out*' en route, the North Eastern Indian States of Manipur, Nagaland and Mizoram have had significant injection heroin use in the late 1970s and the early 1980s. The explosive rise in the rate of HIV seropositivity has led to a serious problem of a grave nature. None of the 2,322 IDUs seen from 1986 to 1989 in Manipur were seropositive, but the seroprevalence increased to more than 50% in 6 months time from September, 1989 and is now believed to have stabilized between 60 and 70%. The seroprevalence rates in the neighboring States of Nagaland and Mizoram are 50% and 6–10% respectively. In view of the increasing reports of injection drug use from different cities, the epidemic of HIV and IDU seen in Manipur may well be repeated in many parts of the country.

The Manipur experience was decidedly quite drastic and although it did receive some attention, it continues to be in need of attention. Some of the facts of the HIV epidemic in Manipur and the surrounding states have been quite commonly discussed and made available. Much of the assistance for HIV prevention with substance users has remained exclusively focused on the North Eastern region. It had become almost axiomatic that this region has a major problem of IDUs and HIV, and the other parts of the country need not focus on this issue too much, since this was a problem localized and specific to the North Eastern region.

Two research studies carried out from 1989 to 1992 as Task Force Projects of ICMR focused on epidemiological information. A collaborative project on 'Monitoring of narcotic drugs and psychotropic substances' in the cities of Delhi, Lucknow and Jodhpur developed a method for Drug Abuse Monitoring System (DAMS) for reporting on patients of drug dependence or abuse reaching the various treatment centers. The project also included a Community Area Survey Component, which collected information on the frequency and the pattern of alcohol and narcotic drug and psychotropic substances in a 'high-prevalence' community area, with a purposive sampling method, in each of these three cities. Report of these studies make no mention of injecting drug use. In another study on 'Survey on drug dependence in the community (urban megapolis Delhi)', carried out in the 72 residential colonies of Delhi, injecting drug use was not focused on or reported.

The major epidemiological studies on drug abuse in the late 1980s and the early 1990s did not report of any injection use, but it must be recognized that it was not enquired into, as it was not considered significant at all in parts of India other than the North Eastern States. In the subsequent years, reports of IDUs, especially with buprenorphine, have been accumulating from many cities in the other parts of India.

In a report from the Eastern city of Calcutta, Chowdhury and Chowdhury observed that while no cases of buprenorphine abuse was reported in 1987 at the de addiction clinic, in 1988, of the 498 outpatient opiate addicts, 24 (4.08%) were of buprenorphine addiction, twenty (4%) of these 24 patients used intramuscular route. In the year 1989, the clinic saw 18 patients (17.8%) of injection buprenorphine and 9 patients (3.2%) of tablet buprenorphine use. The preference for the intramuscular route reported in this study was also found in a report from another eastern city of Ranchi.

In a later sample of 45 IDUs from Chandigarh in the North, Malhotra, et al reported that both the routes were reported by patients who were using cocktail injections, mainly with buprenorphine. A report from Patna found significant buprenorphine use and explored the reasons for the same. Easy availability, low cost, and purity were the common reasons for such use in this study, as well as in almost all other studies.

Reporting from the Southern city of Bangalore, a study of the patients seen at the National Institute of Mental Health and Neuro Sciences (NIMHANS), from 1991 to 1994, confirmed the rising trends of buprenorphine abuse, with a noticeable shift from heroin to buprenorphine.

In a prospective study carried out at the Drug Dependence Treatment Centre of the All India Institute of Medical Sciences

(AIIMS) in Delhi, in a serial sample of 100 patients with current or past diagnosis of opioid dependence syndrome from amongst the 136 first contact outpatients seen in July and August, 1995, drug use patterns and reasons thereof were ascertained in detail for multiple substance use pattern. There was significant multidrug pattern including alcohol, tobacco, cannabis, benzodiazepines and antihistaminics. Of the 100 patients, 66 patients were dependent on only one substance, if nicotine was excluded from the analysis. Of these, 51 were using heroin through the 'chasing' route (inhaling the smoke with indirect heat to heroin powder on a silver or aluminium foil), 2 were using raw opium, and 13 were using only injection buprenorphine. Nine patients were using various injection cocktails with buprenorphine (with diazepam in seven patients, with pentazocine in one patient, and with both pentazocine and diazepam in one patient). Of the 34 other patients with more than one drug use, 10 patients had dependence on injection buprenorphine use alongside dependence on other injections or noninjection drug use. Fifteen patients had multiple drug use, with ten of these patients using the injection route occasionally or frequently. All in all, dependence on injection use was seen in 22% of the cases and injection use as part of multidrug use pattern in another 20% of the cases, leading to a figure of 42% injecting users.

This pattern of injecting users in 1995 was more striking in view of the fact that, as per the collective opinion of the staff members, there were only a few injecting drug users amongst the patients at this center in the initial years since the center was established in 1988, up until 1992 or 1993. Only to verify this opinion and provide a chronological background to the prospective data collected in 1996, outpatient records for the month of January, 1991 were scrutinized for injection drug use pattern. Of the 98 patients, 70 had opioid dependence. Of these, two patients reported dependence on injecting drug use (pentazocine) and two other patients reported injection use as part of multiple drug use pattern.

A survey, by a nongovernmental organization (NGO) in the slums of South Delhi, identified 307 intravenous drug addicts. A majority of these addicts were in the age group of 21 to 40 years, literate, and from lower income groups. Most of these addicts were drivers, motor mechanics or manual laborers by occupation. Easy availability and economic considerations were the most common reasons cited by most of these addicts.

Although direct epidemiological indicators are inadequate, there are sufficient indirect indicators of increasing trends of IDUs from many cities in parts of India, other than the North East. There is some conflicting evidence about the preferred route for injection, but most reports emphasize the predominant use of buprenorphine alone or in cocktails. The general maxim is that the number of drug addicts who reach the hospital are only a small fraction of the addicts in the general population, and the common international research finding is of injecting drug users getting marginalized and remaining underground and not coming into contact with treatment services. By these and the indirect indicators described, it is reasonable to infer that the towns and cities of India, particularly the megapolises of Delhi, Bombay, Madras and Calcutta are witnessing increasing trends of injecting drug users which form high-risk groups for HIV infection.

Recent Regional Studies

Studies between 1968 until 2006 have been primarily on alcohol use. They have varied in terms of populations surveyed (ranged from 115 to 16,725), sampling procedures (convenient, purposive and representative), focus of enquiry (alcohol use, habitual excessive use, alcohol abuse, alcoholism, chronic alcoholism, alcohol and drug abuse and alcohol dependence), location (urban, rural or both, slums), in the screening instruments used (survey questionnaires and schedules, semistructured interviews, quantity frequency index, Michigan Alcohol Screening Test (MAST), etc. Alcohol 'use/abuse' prevalence in different regions has thus varied from 167/1000 to 370/1000; 'alcohol addiction' or 'alcoholism' or 'chronic alcoholism' from 2.36/1000 to 34.5/1000; alcohol and drug use/abuse from 21.4 to 28.8/1000. A meta-analysis by Reddy and Chandrashekhar (1998) revealed an overall substance use prevalence of 6.9/1000 for India with urban and rural rates of 5.8 and 7.3/1000 population. The rates among men and women were 11.9 and 1.7% respectively. Regional studies between 2001 and 2007 continue to reflect this variability. Currently, the interest is to look at hazardous alcohol use. A study in Southern rural India showed that 14.2% of the population surveyed had hazardous alcohol use on the AUDIT. A similar study in the tertiary hospital showed that 17.6% admitted patients had hazardous alcohol use.

The only incidence study on alcohol use from Delhi found that annual incidence of nondependent alcohol use and dependent alcohol use among men was 3 and 2 per 1000 persons in a total cohort of 2,937 households.

Recent National Studies

The National Household Survey of Drug Use in the country is the first systematic effort to document the nationwide prevalence of drug use. Alcohol (21.4%) was the primary substance used (apart from tobacco) followed by cannabis (3.0%) and opioids (0.7%). Seventeen to 26% of alcohol users qualified for ICD 10 diagnosis of dependence, translating to an average prevalence of about 4%. There was a marked variation in alcohol use prevalence in different states of India (current use ranged from a low of 7% in the Western state of Gujarat (officially under prohibition) to 75% in the North-Eastern state of Arunachal Pradesh. Tobacco use prevalence was high at 55.8% among males, with maximum use in the age group 41 to 50 years. The National Family Health Survey (NFHS) provides some insights into tobacco and alcohol use. The changing trends between NFHS 2 and NFHS 3 reflect an increase in alcohol use among males since the NFHS 2, and an increase in tobacco use among women.

The Drug Abuse Monitoring System, which evaluated the primary substance of abuse in inpatient treatment centers found that the major substances were alcohol (43.9%), opioids (26%) and cannabis (11.6%).

Patterns of Substance Use

Rapid situation assessments (RSAs) are useful to study patterns of substance use. An RSA by the UNODC in 2002 of 4648 drug users showed that cannabis (40%), alcohol (33%) and opioids (15%) were the major substances used. A Rapid Situation and Response Assessment (RSRA) among 5800 male drug users revealed that 76% of the opioid users currently injected buprenorphine, 76% injected heroin, 70% chasing and 64% using propoxyphene. Most drug users concomitantly used alcohol (80%). According to the World Drug Report, of 81,802 treatment seekers in India in 2004–2005, 61.3% reported use of opioids, 15.5% cannabis, 4.1% sedatives, 1.5% cocaine, 0.2% amphetamines and 0.9% solvents.

Comorbidity

The coexistence of substance use disorder and psychiatric disorder in the same patient at a point in time, best referred to as comorbidity, has been of interest from two perspectives. In patients of psychiatric disorders, the abuse or dependence of chemical substances has been studied and found to be quite high, for alcohol as well as for the illicit drugs. These patients have been termed as *mentally ill chemical abuser* (MICA), *mentally ill substance abuser* (MISA) or *chemical abusing mentally ill* (CAMI). The professionals in the field of substance abuse have been concerned about the proportion of their patients who manifest psychiatric symptoms or disorders. These patients have often been referred to as *dual diagnosis patients* and treated as a separate group of patients since the treatment strategies are quite different from the ones used in the treatment of substance use disorder patients. It has been found that the prevalence rates of those in treatment are double the rates for those who were not in treatment. In the US settings, these dual diagnosis patients often represent about half of the patients seen in psychiatric emergency services and are considered more difficult to assess and treat.

The early studies were carried out in alcoholism and very often in hospital inpatient samples. In a review of these studies, in 1987 of the extant international literature, revealed that the prevalence rates of alcoholism among psychiatric inpatients have ranged from 19 to 32% and, with broader definition of excessive drinking, rates are found to be as high as 50%. The review also found that the prevalence rates of depression, the most common psychiatric disorder amongst hospital samples of patients of alcoholism, varied widely according to the method of assessment, i.e. case note diagnosis (rate 9.8%), rating scales (rate 78%) and structured interviews (rate 38%). It was concluded from the review of these studies that a very high percentage of alcoholism patients display depressive symptoms, but only half of that number meet the criteria for a diagnosis of depression. In studies on opiate-dependent patients, who are seeking help, depression has been found in a little more than half the patients, being the most common diagnosis. It is quite possible that being in depressive mood state increases the motivation for treatment and so higher rates of current depression are seen in treatment-seeking patients as compared to nontreatment-seeking patients.

The real comorbidity can be established with community-based studies. The first landmark community-based study on comorbidity of substance abuse and psychiatric disorders was reported in 1980. This study reported lifetime prevalence of at least one other mental disorder in 70% of the persons with any alcohol disorder, depression being the most common at 44%. Two large scale community-based studies in the US, the ECA study by NIMH and the National Comorbidity Survey (NCS), have concluded that the prevalence of comorbid psychiatric illnesses and substance use disorders is high with respect to the general population.

The ECA study has concluded that 76% of the men and 65% of the women, who met the criteria for drug abuse or dependence, received at least one additional diagnosis and also found that more than half (53%) of the persons, who abuse drugs other than alcohol, have at least one comorbid mental illness. Of the persons with a psychiatric disorder, substance use disorder was found to be 15.7% in the past month and 32.7% for the lifetime prevalence. In an analysis of the ECA data for comorbidity, it has been reported that among those with an alcohol disorder, 37% had a comorbid disorder. The ECA data reports on the base prevalence rates for individual disorders and the lifetime prevalence rates for comorbid disorder.

The odds ratios (ORs) indicate the proportion of the comorbid diagnosis rates within each major diagnostic group, with the rates of same diagnosis in the rest of the population without the major diagnosis. Thus, it is possible to examine the base rates of any disorder in the persons with another disorder and also to estimate the odds ratio of the occurrence of the comorbidity (Tables 12 and 13) While assessing the comorbidity of various mental disorders among persons with any alcohol disorder diagnosis or any other drug disorder diagnosis (Table 12) schizophrenia has a prevalence rate of only 3.8% among those with alcohol disorders; but the disorder is seen more than three times as often in this group and has an odds ratio of 3.3. Although anxiety disorders are most prevalent in those with alcohol disorders (19.4%), the high base rate of anxiety disorders in the general population results in an odds ratio of 1.5. On the other hand, the

Table 12: Lifetime prevalence (%) and odds ratios (ORs) of mental disorders with substance diagnosis, ECA

Comorbid disorder	*Any alcohol disorder*		*Any other drug disorder*	
	% (SE)	*OR*	*% (SE)*	*OR*
Any mental disorder	36.6 (1.4)	2.3	53.1 (2.0)	4.5
Schizophrenia	3.8 (0.6)	3.3	6.8 (0.9)	6.2
Any affective disorder	13.4 (0.9)	1.9	26.4 (1.8)	4.7
Any anxiety disorder	19.4 (1.0)	1.5	28.3 (1.8)	2.5
Antisocial personality disorder	14.3 (1.0)	21.0	17.8 (1.6)	13.4

Table 13: Lifetime prevalence (%) and odds ratios (ORs) of alcohol and other drug disorders with schizophrenia and affective disorders (ECA)

Comorbid disorder	*Schizophrenia*		*Any affective disorder*	
	% (SE)	*OR*	*% (SE)*	*OR*
Any substance abuse or dependence	47.0 (4.0)	4.6	32.0 (1.7)	2.6
Any alcohol diagnosis	33.7 (4.4)	3.3	21.8 (1.4)	1.9
Alcohol dependence	24.0 (3.7)	3.8	14.9 (1.1)	2.2
Alcohol abuse only	9.7 (2.7)	1.9	6.9 (0.9)	1.3
Any other drug diagnosis	27.5 (3.2)	6.2	19.4 (1.4)	4.7
Any other dependence	12.9 (2.6)	4.2	11.3 (1.0)	4.4
Any drug abuse only	14.6 (3.0)	6.9	8.1 (1.1)	4.3

prevalence of antisocial personality disorder is only slightly lower at 14.3%, this disorder is associated with the highest OR of 21. In Table 13, although the prevalence rates of any alcohol diagnosis and any other drug diagnosis are very similar for schizophrenia as well as any affective disorder, the odds ratio of any drug disorder diagnosis is double or a little more than double as compared to the odds ratio for any alcohol diagnosis. Among those with a mental disorder, the odds ratio of having some addictive disorder was 2.7 in the ECA sample. The odds of having a mental disorder, as compared to general population, is approximately two and a half times greater in patients of alcohol use disorder, and four and a half times higher in patients of any other drug disorder. Interestingly, the ECA data also provide information on lifetime prevalence of coexisting substance use disorder diagnosis and suggest that for those with either an alcohol or any other drug disorder, the odds of having other addictive disorder were seven times greater than in the general population.

The relationship of the two or more disorders in the comorbid condition is very intricate and many clinical situations difficult to analyze. The comorbid or dual diagnosis cases can be categorized into many groups based on the drug of abuse, the purpose that the drug serves, the nature of psychiatric symptomatology and the etiological significance. Broadly, without getting into the finer aspects of etiology debate, this group of patients can be seen to occur in the following four groups. These groups have support, most often from the clinical research and at times also from basic science research. It is also helpful to apply this categorization to individual cases in clinical practice, to be established by the chronological order of the appearance of the symptoms, influence of periods of remission in one of the disorders on the symptom profile and the severity of the other disorder, as well as the common clinical observations of the link between various disorders:

- *Primary substance use disorder with secondary psychiatric disorder*: The occurrence of depression in many of the cases of alcoholism has been seen as being caused by the secondary psychological and social effects. Davidson and Ritson concluded that the most common cause of depressive symptomatology in alcohol dependent subjects was adjustment disorder or alcohol induced mood disorder. In fact, many of the substance-related disorders of DSM-IV are eligible to be considered under this category, with alcohol induced hallucinosis and other psychotic disorders being good examples
- *Primary psychiatric disorder with secondary substance use disorder*: The occurrence of alcohol abuse or dependence in cases of generalized anxiety disorder or phobic disorder is demonstrative of this category. Indeed, the possibility of abuse or dependence for alcohol or nicotine should be a common clinical consideration. Mood disorder leading to a pattern of use of alcohol that may amount to abuse or dependence and schizophrenia contributing to cannabis use disorder are the other examples
- *Primary psychiatric disorder with substance use disorder as part of the clinical syndrome*: In many instances, the substance use disorder occurs as a part of the overall clinical profile of the psychiatric disorder. Nearly a third of the patients of mood disorder, in the depressive or the manic phase, are prone to escalate their alcohol use to an extent that they meet the criteria for dependence. This is also commonly seen in Axis II diagnoses of personality disorders, in which the substance use is only an epiphenomenon of the psychiatric disorder. About 70% of the patients of antisocial personality disorder are known to have alcohol abuse or dependence. Among patients of alcohol or other drug dependence, the rates for antisocial personality disorder have ranged from 18 to 60.8% and up to 91% of polydrug users have been found to have a mean of four DSM-III-R axis II disorders
- *Two primary coexisting disorders*: Although it was believed earlier that it was always possible and necessary to differentiate into primary and secondary disorders in cases of comorbidity, it is no longer considered so. It is

Table 14: Indian studies on prevalence rates of psychiatric disorders and symptoms in alcoholism

Study and sample size	*Setting and method*	*Psychiatric disorder*	*Psychosis*	*Depressive signs symptoms*	*Depressive disorder*
Desai, et al (n = 72)	NIMHANS Prospective DSM-III	46.0%	16.6%	48.6%	23.6%
Ray (n = 147)	NIMHANS Charts DSM-III	40.0%	29.2%	45.0%	8.8%
Kumar Kumar, Desai, Kapoor (n = 40)	AIIMS Prospective CPRS and DSM-III	12.5%	10.0%	27.5%	0%

well recognized, by now, that two disorders can coexist in some persons without one having led or contributed significantly towards the other. Common etiological basis had earlier been hypothesized for some of the comorbid conditions like depression and alcoholism. It has been conclusively documented that these are two distinct and separate disorders.

Indian Studies on Comorbidity

Some Indian studies are available on the issue of comorbidity with alcohol. The studies suggest that in the patient samples from psychiatric hospitals settings the prevalence rates of psychiatric disorders are higher than the rates in patient samples from specialized drug dependence treatment center settings. The higher proportion of depressive symptoms as compared to depressive disorder is also seen in the studies available (Table 14).

ETIOLOGY AND PHARMACOLOGY

ETIOLOGY

The etiology of substance related disorders is complex and multifactorial having biopsychosocial components. Over the past few decades, the disease concept of substance use disorders, particularly alcoholism, has become well accepted.

Genetics

Most of the information on genetics relates to alcoholism. The results of family, twin and adoption studies in alcoholism, when taken together, provide evidence for the importance of genetic factors in the etiology of this disorder.

Family studies have shown that rates of alcoholism are substantially higher in relatives of alcoholics than in relatives of nonalcoholics, with children of alcoholics demonstrating 3–4 times increased risk for developing the disorder, as compared to the other children. Familial aggregation of such a disorder can also result from the shared social and developmental influences of being raised in the same environment. As such, family studies do not provide conclusive evidence of genetic basis.

Twin studies provide more definitive argument for the genetic basis of the disorder. In Sweden, Kay had found that the concordance rate for alcoholism in monozygotic twins was almost double of that in dizygotic twins (58% vs 28%). Several other studies have also revealed higher concordance rates in monogygotic twins than that in dizygotic twins. Thus, twin studies do provide more definitive evidence for alcoholism being genetically influenced and yet the fact that the concordance rates in dizygotic twins are in the range of 50–60%, suggest that although heritability factors play a role, the occurrence of the disorder results from an interaction of the genetic and the environmental factors.

Adoption studies assess the interaction between the genetic and environmental influences by examining the rates of disorder in children of affected parents, who have been adopted out. Goodwin et al. found that the sons of alcoholics were about 4 times more likely to be alcoholic than sons of nonalcoholics, and that being raised by either nonalcoholic adoptive parents or by biologic parents did not affect this increased risk.

Based on the genetic factors in etiology, alcoholism has been subtyped by Cloninger et al. into familial and non-familial types. Type 1, the *nonfamilial alcoholism*, or the '*milieu-limited*' variety is characterized by onset of alcohol use or loss of control of drinking after the age of 25, pronounced environmental reactivity to drinking, minimal associated criminality, higher degree of associated psychopathology and 'passive-dependent personality traits', marked by high degree of harm avoidance, low levels of novelty seeking and is known to predominate among female alcoholics and their male relatives.

Type 2, the *familial type of alcoholism* is '*male-limited*' and has an inheritance pattern less dependent on environmental factors for phenotypic expression and has an earlier age of onset, severe levels of dependence, more associated criminal behavior, and personality traits that run opposite those of the prototypic 'milieu-limited' alcoholics.

Different study approaches have been used to identify populations at elevated risk for developing alcoholism, usually evaluating children and grown up children of alcoholic fathers. Various biochemical and electrophysiological markers have been identified for alcoholism; the feasibility of these markers, as linking the phenotype and the genotype, remains to be seen. Advances in molecular genetics might soon add important information to our understanding of the biological factors associated with the susceptibility to alcoholism.

Genetic factors have also been found operating in cigarette smoking. Carmelli, et al. reported moderate genetic influences on lifetime smoking prevalence. These genetic influences are found significant even when the rates are adjusted for covariates like alcohol consumption.

Neurobiology

The neurobiological mechanisms, which have been studied for understanding the etiology of substance use disorders, are wide-ranging and also vary according to the substance. Some of the mechanisms are applicable across different classes of substances and some remain specific to the substance for which they have been studied.

Brain-reward Mechanisms

Animal experiments have been designed to study the drug-taking behavior of animals. In self-administration paradigm in laboratory animals, alternating drug-intake and drug-abstinence periods, continuing for months, have been shown to occur. These periods markedly resemble the alternating binge and abstinence patterns of human substance abuse.

It has also been shown in animal experiments that chronic indwelling intracranial stimulating electrodes in specific brain loci have been associated with repetitive self-stimulation for reward. In such stimulation, hungry animals ignore food and thirsty animals ignore water to get the substance. It has been hypothesized that drug-reward and brain-stimulation reward activate the same brain locations.

Crow had suggested in the early 1970s that activation of mesolimbic and mesostriatal dopamine (DA) systems was rewarding. In the later years, a number of brain reward circuits have been delineated. The primary brain reward relevant portion appears to be a subset of the mesolimbic projections originating in the ventral tegmental area (DA nucleus area-10) and terminating in the nucleus accumbens. Perturbations of the dopaminergic brain reward system, leading to increased vulnerability to drug taking behavior, have been inferred. It has been hypothesized that genetically imparted DA reward perturbations leading to increased vulnerability to drug taking behavior are operative in substance abusing patients.

The substances which are commonly abused seem to have two characteristics across the different classes. These are that they are voluntarily self-administered by nonhuman mammals, and they acutely enhance brain reward mechanisms. It is generally believed that these substances act on brain circuits that evoked to subserve the normal reinforcement functions of the central nervous system, like biologically essential behavior of feeding. It has been suggested that substance abusers have a defect in their ability to capture reward and pleasure from everyday experience, so called 'reward deficiency syndrome'. A basic hypofunctionality in brain mechanisms subserving normal reward and pleasure functions has important implications for treatment strategies.

Neuroregulator Systems

Animal experiments have also suggested that the reinforcing effects of the substances of abuse, including alcohol, are mediated by increased dopamine release in the subcortical regions, mainly the nucleus accumbens. The axonal terminal projections in the nucleus accumbens have been considered the primary neuropharmacological site of action wherein the substances act to produce their intensely rewarding effects and also possibly the site where some neural aspects of the genetic vulnerability are encoded. These axonal terminal projections are heavily innervated and modulated by numerous synaptic inputs including GABAergic, glutamatergic, serotonergic, opioid peptidergic and other neural systems.

Studies, in which serotonin function was increased by means of brain or peripheral injections of serotonin or its precursors, serotonin uptake inhibitors, serotonin releasers or serotonin agonists, have found that an increase in the serotonergic function leads to decrease in alcohol consumption. Conversely, the hypothesis that a decrease in serotonin function should lead to an increase in alcohol consumption, did not find support from studies in which serotonin function was decreased by means of serotonergic neurotoxins, electrolytic lesions of serotonergic pathways. Nonetheless, some studies with serotonergic drugs on alcohol discrimination suggest that serotonin has a role in alcohol reinforcement. It has been amply demonstrated by electrophysiological and neurochemical studies that serotonin modulates the activity of dopamine neurons.

Since the time of discovery of the opioid peptides and receptors in the 1970s, exciting possibilities have been explored for explaining the mechanisms of dependence. It was observed early that tolerance and physical dependence develop to pharmacological doses of opioid peptides. It has also been observed that chronic administration of opiate agonists leads to decrease in the synthesis and/or release of endorphins. Attempts have been made to correlate these experimental situations of tolerance and dependence with specific changes in opiate receptor sites. The failure of such attempts at correlation has shifted the focus to the events in the postreceptor cascade. It has been demonstrated that chronic morphine use causes a compensatory increase in all the components of the cAMP signal transduction pathway, i.e. G proteins, adenylate cyclase, cAMP-dependent protein kinase and several protein kinase substrates in the locus ceruleus. An important role of NMDA (N-methyl-D-aspartate) receptor has been discovered in the development of opioid tolerance in recent times.

The role of opiate systems in the development of alcohol dependence has also been proposed, with the major hypothesis that these persons are deficient in the activity of their opiate systems and the intake of alcohol compensates for such deficiency.

Craving

Craving is an irresistible urge to use a substance that compels drug seeking behavior. The concept of craving is beset with numerous controversies, but it is important in drug seeking behavior and in relapse. It is not entirely clear whether it is a desire to experience a pleasurable state, avoid an anxious state or whether it is an irresistible state. Craving has been linked to the changes in the concentrations of neurotransmitters in the brain, like that of dopamine and endorphins in regions like nucleus accumbens and hippocampus. Changes in the dopamine levels have been found to be associated with craving for cocaine and stimulant use, and changes in endorphin and serotonin levels have been linked to craving for alcohol. Hippocampus is one of the anatomical sites suggested for craving, which has basis in the fact that the hippocampus is a seat for learning, memory and conditioned response. Kindling has also been proposed as a mechanism of craving.

Membrane Studies

A large part of the research on the membrane mechanisms for development of tolerance and dependence has been focusing on the alcohol-induced changes in the membrane lipids. In the recent times, it has become clear that the alcohol-induced changes in the membrane lipids or the fluidity of the membrane are too insignificant to be important in the development of tolerance and dependence. The attention has shifted from the effects on membrane lipids to the effects on membrane receptors and intracellular signalling systems. In studies on acute effects, glycine, NMDA, AMPA, and kainate receptors have emerged as the possible sites of alcohol action. Some of these sites have also been found to have changed with chronic alcohol exposure, alongside changes in the ion channels. It has been suggested that chronic alcohol exposure produces a fascinating example of 'molecular rewiring' of the brain, but the question does remain as to which of the many neurochemical and molecular changes demonstrated are really important for the development of tolerance and dependence.

Behavioral Conditioning Factors

External and internal cues, that are associated with substance use, can acquire the ability to later elicit special drug-related responses. The external cues may be a TV-advertisement or meeting a drug using friend. The internal cues may be depressed or anxious mood, or anger, which often precede substance use. These external and internal cues (CS) get conditioned to the substance related events (UCS), like the direct euphoriant action of the drug. Such conditioning contributes to the ability of these external or internal cues to lead a person to use of the substance. These cues are important secondary reinforcers or maintaining factors. The conditioning of these cues occurs not only with the pleasant effects of the substance but also with some other substance related experiences like the withdrawal syndrome. The phenomenon of *'conditioned withdrawal'* is the physiological conditioned response to a conditional stimulus, wherein an external cue like the smell of a familiar nature of substance, site of a needle or any other injection equipment in a person who had been dependent earlier, triggers a withdrawal syndrome. This phenomenon is different from the withdrawal syndrome in that it is not linked to recent cessation or reduction in the dose of a substance, and is known to occur even after a considerable period of abstinence. It has been seen to be clearly operative in opiate dependence patients, and may trigger substance use and relapse.

Behavioral cues have been found to be operative in the development of dependence to smoking. It has been extensively studied that the behavioral cues of the sight of a pack of cigarettes or a cigarette, the act of lighting a matchstick or holding a cigarette between the fingers, contribute to repetitive smoking, as much as, if not more than, the pharmacological effects of nicotine.

Psychodynamic Factors

Early Psychoanalytic Theories

Freud considered addiction as substitution for regressive infantile autoeroticism, which was first experienced as pleasurable, and then unpleasurable, the vicious cycle of most addictions. In this cycle, the wish for pleasure becomes gratified, but only with accompanying guilt and loss of self-esteem. These feelings produce unbearable anxiety, which in turn leads to repetition of the act in order to find relief. Karl Abraham stressed the role of alcohol in reducing sexual inhibitions in men. He theorized that male alcoholics have intense conflicts about homosexuality and that alcohol allows them to express these unconscious feelings in a way that is socially acceptable.

Rado had suggested that addicts take drugs to find relief from a specific type of depression. Glover had proposed addiction as a way of expressing aggressive and sadistic instincts. Balint characterized the alcoholics as having a basic character flaw, which he called the 'basic fault', and suggested that a patient resorts to alcohol as a means of correcting the fault that he feels within himself.

Recent Psychodynamic Theories

Winnicott described the object relationships of the early developmental period. The early experiences of the child with the mother have become increasingly important in understanding the etiology of the addictive core of the self. Thus, psychoanalysis of substance abuse has centered on stages of structural development, including appropriate functions of the ego and a secure sense of self. As traumatized adults, these individuals seek self-regulation outside of themselves through alcohol or other drugs or via addictive relationships.

Wieder and Kaplan emphasized that the dominant conscious motive for substance use is reduction in distress that the individual can not achieve by his own psychic efforts. Rothschild had stated that in substance abusers, the improvements of ego functions are typically defended against by denial.

Defense Mechanisms

The primary role of psychodynamic factors in the etiology of substance use disorders is not believed in as strongly now as it was some decades ago. The perpetuating role of some of the defense mechanisms, conscious or unconscious or partially both, in persons with substance use disorders is well accepted. Some of the common defense mechanisms of this kind have been identified and described by workers from many perspectives. These can be considered to have a consensual agreement in the field of substance use disorders.

Denial: It is one of the most common and the strongest defense mechanisms by which the person denies the use pattern (amount or frequency of use), the problems associated with the use, the loss of control over one's use pattern and the need for external help.

Minimization: The person may accept the use pattern or the associated pattern, but minimizes the magnitude or severity.

Rationalization: The person believes in and provides an apparently logical explanation for the substance use or its pattern, based on the circumstances and other persons around.

Projection: The person perceives and attributes the origin and/or perpetuation of substance use pattern or the related problems as emanating from some other person or source, instead of being part of one's own behavior.

Sociocultural Factors

The genetic susceptibility, the possible underlying neurobiological mechanisms and the psychological theories do not detract from the fact that the occurrence of substance use as well as use disorders is linked to the social and the cultural factors, including the political and economic factors. The availability of one or more substances, the cultural patterns of use and attitudes, the legal controls as well as the sociological stress are some of the important factors in this respect. It has been amply demonstrated that although the genetic susceptibility and the neurobiological mechanisms for the development of tolerance and dependence to alcohol are crucial, the permissiveness of a given community and the availability of alcohol determines the prevalence of alcohol use disorders. The change in the attitude to smoking, in large parts of the Western world and particularly USA, from it being considered a necessary part of the masculine behavior to one of being seen as an act of socially inappropriate behavior has made significant impact in lowering the rates of abuse and dependence to nicotine. It has also been established that the problem of illicit drug use is directly linked to the rate of social change. It has been found that the societies with a higher pace of social change undergo a more manifest problem of illicit drug use. The problem of illicit drug use has also been linked to the process of economic or other social marginalization of a groups within the society.

In the American context, it has been seen that the rates of illicit drug use as well as drug-related problems are seen more in the inner cities which have predominantly African-American populations. It has even been suggested that most of the 'gains' of declining rates of drug use, documented by the national household surveys and the other surveys, have occurred outside the inner cities where most of the severe drug problems have been concentrated. This process of 'ghettoization' is believed to have harmed the clientele and the treatment programs. A shift towards less stable forms of family, rising unemployment, rising costs of housing and shelter, changing social values towards individuation and hedonism have been identified as some of the aspects of the social change that contribute to increased problem of illicit drug use.

In India, the cultural tradition and permissiveness of alcohol use in Punjab has been seen to be associated with higher rates of alcohol use disorders in epidemiological studies. In places like Goa and Bangalore, where the availability of alcohol and the permissiveness is high, indirect indicators, like the number of patients seen at treatment centers, do suggest a higher proportion of alcohol use disorders. The need for help for individuals with abuse or dependence for raw opium or '*affim*', which is consumed by ingestion, has been documented in Rajasthan where the use of the substance is not only socially approved, but very often encouraged.

Family Dynamics

The nature versus nurture debate in the etiology of substance use disorders has been active for some time and has been accentuated by the evidence from the genetic studies for alcoholism. The family, twin and adoption studies, by implication, suggest an important role for environmental factors in the etiology of substance use disorders. Family studies document that many alcoholics do not have alcoholic near-relatives. The monozygotic concordance rates for alcoholism and other substance use disorders do not approach unity. The specific environmental variables that contribute to the etiology of substance use disorders have not been well delineated. There are certain environmental conditions that characterise alcoholic homes and families of persons with substance use disorders. The relationship between these characteristics and the substance use disorders may be causal but is more likely to be bidirectional. The primary etiological role of such family or environmental characteristics is difficult to be proven, but their contribution as perpetuating factors is more tenable and possible to be studied.

The influence of the substance use and related attitudes in the parents are known to influence the use pattern and the development of disorders in children by modeling or identification. Conversely, children of alcohol or drug use disorder parents have been known to be teetotallers and have strong negative attitudes towards substance use. The quality of marital relationship contributing towards the development of substance use disorder in the spouses of either gender has also been documented. Interestingly, interaction with growing up children with oppositional traits or disorder can perpetuate the development of substance use disorders in their parents.

Family interaction and family environment, that commonly prevails in the families of some of the persons with substance use disorders, can be related to the ongoing substance use and the problems caused by the substance use. The extent to which 'family rituals', like celebrating holidays and taking vacations, are disrupted by the drinking pattern of the alcoholic parent, has been studied by semistructured interviews. The families have been classified as 'distinctive' (little or no disruption of family rituals), 'subsumptive' (family rituals subsumed by alcoholism), and 'intermediate' (some family rituals subsumed while others were spared). It was found that subsumptive families and, to a lesser extent, intermediate families tended to produce alcoholic offsprings while distinctive families did not. It has also been shown that there is great heterogeneity in the interaction patterns among alcoholic families and alcohol serves a variety of adaptive functions in different families. These adaptive functions may be of uniting, deflection, masking, rebellion and revenge.

Studies of alcoholic families indicate that alcoholic families report lower levels of family cohesion, expressiveness, independence, intellectual cultural orientation and higher levels of conflict compared to nonalcoholic families. It has also been shown that alcoholic families show impaired problem solving and more negative and hostile communications as compared to nonalcoholic families.

As the persons with substance use disorders do, their families also develop and sustain the defence mechanisms of denial, minimization, rationalization and projection which perpetuate the disorder. The family members of the persons with substance use disorders often tend to get caught up in their own reasoning or sense of responsibility or experience of shame or guilt. These factors lead to the behavior of family members which directly helps the substance use (by providing money or other support) or indirectly contributes to it by shielding or covering up and helping out in situations of the difficulties associated with substance use without any effort at helping the person realize the responsibility for one's actions. Such direct and indirect contribution to the development or sustenance of the problematic substance use, by the family members (or any closely involved persons, like friends or colleagues) has been termed as *enabling*. It has been suggested and seems plausible that such enabling is more operative in cultures and families with higher degree of involvement.

Some of these emerging ideas over the many decades about the experiences of the family members of substance use persons have coalesced into the concept of 'co-dependence'. It has been described as any suffering and/or dysfunction that is associated with or results from focusing on the needs and behavior of others. Family members of substance using persons have been found to have become so preoccupied with these persons that they neglect the healthy needs of their ownselves. Co-dependence has been defined as "a multidimensional condition manifested by any suffering and dysfunction that is associated with or due to focusing on the needs of others." It can mimic, be associated with, and aggravate many physical, psychological and spiritual conditions. It has been said that co-dependence is addiction to looking elsewhere. There has been a large amount of research from the American centers in the recent past on various aspects of co-dependence, in respect of substance use disorders as well as other conditions. The concept of co-dependence has begun to be studied in the other cultures and its applicability and usefulness in different cultures remains to be examined.

CLINICAL PHARMACOLOGY

Alcohol

Pharmacokinetics

When taken orally, alcohol is absorbed rapidly, predominantly in small intestine. It is highly lipid soluble and diffusible. Absorption is delayed by solutions above 20% of alcohol (decreased gastric peristalsis), and food, especially milk. Alcohol is distributed uniformly throughout all tissues and tissue fluids. It passes across the placental barrier, is found in all physiological fluids (urine, blood, CSF, breast milk, saliva). Any of these fluids is suitable for determining the concentration of alcohol.

The metabolism of ethanol (ethyl alcohol, the only legal constituent of alcoholic beverages), which shows genetic polymorphism, is catalyzed primarily by alcohol dehydrogenase with zero-order kinetics.

$$\text{Ethanol} \xrightarrow{\text{Alcohol dehydrogenase}} \text{Acetaldehyde} \xrightarrow{\text{Acetaldehyde dehydrogenase}} \text{Acetic acid}$$
$$NAD^+ \longrightarrow NADH \quad NAD^+ \longrightarrow NADH$$

The rate-limiting factor in the metabolism of ethanol is the availability of NAD^+.

Ethanol is not metabolized by cytochrome P-450 enzymes. However, it is metabolized to a certain extent by the microsomal ethanol-oxidizing system (MEOS). Ethanol inhibits microsomal drug metabolizing system and increases the rate of its synthesis. Thus, acute substantial dose of alcohol (binge drinking) inhibits hepatic drug metabolism whereas repeated exposure to alcohol leads to induction of hepatic drug metabolizing enzymes. Alcohol in alveolar air is in equilibrium with that in pulmonary capillary blood and reliable, easily handled devices have been devised to measure the presence of alcohol in the breath. The devices available can also indicate the blood alcohol concentration (BAC) and have been used in enforcement of law about safe limits for driving, in the industry as well as in treatment centers.

Pharmacodynamics

The mechanism of action involves interaction with membrane lipids leads to ionic fluxes across the membranes; increase in the GABA-stimulated flux of chloride through receptorgated membrane ion channels, a receptor subtype effect that may be involved in motor impairment caused by alcohol; and increase in endorphin production.

Ethanol is a CNS depressant and obeys the law of descending depression, in that it first inhibits the cerebral cortex, then the cerebellum, spinal cord, and medullary centers. Hyperactivity or hyperarousal, when it occurs, is due to removal of cortical inhibitory effects. The usefulness of alcohol as a 'social lubricant', has its basis in this loss of inhibition, besides the euphoriant effects which do occur with lower concentrations. With increasing doses, the subject passes through all the stages of general anesthesia and may die of respiratory depression. Loss of consciousness occurs at blood concentrations around 300 mg/dL, and death at about 400 mg/dL. But the usual cause of death in acute alcohol poisoning is inhalation of vomit, and not the direct toxic effect of alcohol.

Alcohol inhibits the secretion of antidiuretic hormone by posterior pituitary gland and causes diuresis. Alcohol produces dilation of the skin vessels, flushing and a sensation of warmth. This response to acute doses of ethanol is genetically determined and has been found to be more pronounced in Asian population, especially Japanese, as compared to Caucasians. Earlier, this flushing response of some racial groups had been hypothesized as a protective factor against the development of dependence. Alcohol also interferes with the normal cutaneous vasoconstriction in response to cold. The body heat is, therefore, lost very rapidly and the internal temperature consequently falls. The widely circulated belief about the protective use of alcohol in extreme cold climates is not supported by the physiological studies on alcohol. At toxic alcohol levels, the hypothalamic temperature-regulating mechanism becomes depressed and fall in body temperature becomes pronounced.

As a gastric secretagogue, alcohol stimulates the secretion of gastric juice, which is rich in acid and pepsin. Alcohol, in small quantities, has been used as an appetite stimulant. It is debatable if it should be used for this purpose, but alcohol consumption is contraindicated in subjects with acid peptic disease.

Poisoning and Toxicity

Acute poisoning may be characterized by inebriation, muscular incoordination, blurred vision, impaired reaction time, excitement due to loss of inhibition, impaired consciousness, coma, tachycardia, and slow respiration. A blood alcohol level of 80 mg/dL can produce recognizable features of drunkenness; a level above 300 mg/dL is life-threatening. Acute poisoning is treated with gastric aspiration and lavage combined with intensive supportive therapy, including measures to prevent respiratory failure and aspiration. In cases of very severe poisoning, peritoneal dialysis or hemodialysis may be necessary.

Chronic alcoholism produces pathologic changes, such as chronic gastritis, cirrhosis of liver, alcoholic cardiomyopathy, Korsakoff's syndrome, flabby muscles, fine tremors, and impaired memory. Although, the possible role of nutritional and other lifestyle factors in human subjects cannot be discounted, the direct tissue toxicity of long-term alcohol exposure has been established to contribute in a large measure to these chronic effects.

Opioids

The opium alkaloids are grouped into *phenanthrene derivatives*: morphine (1–10%), codeine (0.7–2.5%), and thebaine (0.5–1.5%), and *isoquinoline derivatives*: papaverine (1%) and noscapine (5–10%). The term *opiates* was used to describe those compounds with opium like properties which were derived from the poppy plant. The term *opioid* is now used to include all the plant products as well as the synthetic compounds with opium like properties.

Table 15: Agonist (+) and antagonist (–) activity at different opioid receptor subtypes

Compound	*μ receptor*	*κ receptor*	*δ receptor*
Morphine	Agonist (+++)	Agonist (+)	No affinity (0)
Pentazocine	Partial agonist	Agonist (++)	No affinity (0)
Methadone	Agonist (+++)	No affinity (0)	No affinity (0)
Buprenorphine	Partial agonist	Antagonist (–)	?
Naloxone	Antagonist (–)	Antagonist (–)	Antagonist
Naltrexone	Antagonist (–)	Antagonist (–)	Antagonist

Opioid Receptors

The opioids produce a large variety of pharmacological actions by interacting with multiple opioid receptors. These receptors are distributed widely throughout CNS, but the highest density is found in the limbic structures, thalamic nuclei, and neural areas important for visceral functioning. Opioid receptor subtypes have been delineated with different functions. The mu, kappa, and sigma receptor subtypes have all been implicated in the mediation of analgesia. Mu and kappa opioids have opposite effects on motor behavior, i.e. activation or sedation, and on fluid regulation, i.e. antidiuretic or diuretic effects, respectively. The agonist and antagonist activity of some of the opioids and other related compounds is shown in Table 15.

Pharmacodynamics

The prototype agent, morphine, depresses the cerebral cortex, hypothalamus, and medullary centers. These effects are responsible for suppressing pain perception, depressing the cough center, the chemoreceptor trigger zone (CTZ) or vomiting center, and the respiratory center.

Morphine stimulates certain parts of the CNS, like the vomiting center, and emesis occurs early in cases of intoxication. Depression of the vomiting center then ensues later in intoxication. Morphine stimulates the vagus nerve, causing bradycardia, and also stimulates the nucleus of the third cranial nerve (oculomotor), causing miosis.

Analgesia brought about by morphine is selective and other sensory modalities (touch, vibration, vision, hearing, etc.) are not obtunded. It exerts its analgesic effects by altering patient's reactions to pain and by elevating the pain threshold. It induces analgesia by activating the opioid, adrenergic, and serotonergic systems. Analgesia results from activation of those systems within the dorsal horn of the spinal cord that depress the transmission of pain sensation to the brain. This is accomplished by decreasing the release of pain transmitters (such as substance P), or by hyperpolarizing the interneurons within the dorsal horn, or both. Morphine activates these mechanisms by interacting with the μ receptors located on neurons in the dorsal cord.

Morphine alters a person's reaction to pain. It has been reported that the sensation of pain often exists, but, under the influence of morphine, the person feels more at ease and comfortable. Euphoria occurs in 90–95% of persons, and dysphoria may occur in the other 5–10%.

Morphine depresses respiration by decreasing the responsiveness of respiratory center to carbon dioxide.

Morphine decreases the secretion of hydrochloric acid, delays gastric emptying, decreases peristaltic waves and decreases the defecation reflex. These actions collectively lead to constipation. Morphine causes peripheral vasodilation and orthostatic hypotension via histamine release.

Tolerance develops to the narcotic and the analgesic actions of morphine, so that increasingly larger doses are needed to render persons pain free. Tolerance develops to many of morphine's effects, such as analgesia, euphoria, narcosis, respiratory depression, hypotension and antidiuresis, but no tolerance develops to morphine-induced miosis or constipation. Tolerance is lost on discontinuation of morphine use.

Therapeutic Uses

Many opioid compounds have a range of therapeutic uses, although the possibility of abuse and dependence must always be kept in mind, especially in view of the cases of iatrogenic dependence in individual cases, and also the public health consequences of over-the-counter sale of these drugs.

Morphine, in relatively small doses of 5–10 mg, relieves the constant but dull pain originating from the viscera, such as that of coronary, pulmonary, and biliary origin. In somewhat larger doses (10–20 mg), it relieves the sharp, lancinating, and intermittent pain resulting from fractures and other physical injuries. Morphine was earlier used for the control of diarrhea and still continues to be used for this purpose in cases of infants in some rural areas of Rajasthan, Uttar Pradesh, Punjab and Harayana, in the form of raw opium.

Pentazocine, a mixed agonist and a weak antagonist, has analgesic potency about a third that of morphine. It has been used in injection form for analgesic effect.

Codeine has an analgesic and antitussive action, the analgesic activity being one-sixth that of morphine. It forms an important constituent of most of the marketed formulations of cough mixtures.

Meperidine has minimal antitussive and antidiarrheal effects and is used as an analgesic during diagnostic procedures.

Dextropropoxyphene is structurally similar to methadone, with analgesic potency two-thirds that of codeine. It is often used for analgesic effect and for detoxification.

Methadone, with longer onset and duration of action, and being effective orally, is used in detoxification and maintenance treatment, and in the management of pain.

Buprenorphine is a semisynthetic derivative from thebaine, which has antagonist and partial agonist properties and is 25–50 times more potent than morphine in analgesic effect. It has become popular for analgesic effect in sublingual as well as injection form, and is also used for detoxification as well as substitution maintenance.

Pharmacology of Opioid Receptor Antagonists

Naloxone reverses the CNS and respiratory depressant actions of narcotics. It is not effective orally but only through IM or IV route, and has a short half-life of 2–4 hours. One milligram of naloxone can counter the effects of 25 mg of heroin. It has been used for the treatment of opioid overdose and diagnosis of dependence due to its property to precipitate an abstinence syndrome when administered to persons who are dependent. It is not useful in the long-term treatment due to its pharmacokinetic profile. It is not yet available in the Indian market.

Naltrexone is a pure opioid antagonist, which is orally effective, with a plasma half-life of 3–4 hours and an even longer duration of action (72–96 hours) because of the sustained receptor binding. It has been extensively researched into for long-term antagonist treatment of opioid dependence and is now also available in Indian market.

Cannabis

Cannabis is obtained from the annual plant, Cannabis sativa and Cannabis americana. The preparations that are smoked are called *marihuana* (*grass, pot, weed*, etc.) and consist of crushed leaves and flowers. The resin scraped off the plant is called *hashish* (*charas*). The dried leaves of the Indian plant, *bhang*, are used in the various forms in different parts of India and Asia.

There are various pharmacologically active compounds in cannabis, important being the oily cannabinoids, the chief compound being 9-d-tetrahydrocannabinol (9-d-THC). The THC content of the preparations varies; most marihuana varies from 1 to 5% in its THC content (*hashish* 10%, *hashish* oil 15–30%). Smoke from a cannabis cigarette delivers 25–50% of the THC content to the respiratory tract. THC is lipid soluble and rapidly absorbed after inhalation. It is metabolized in liver to active 11-hydroxy-THC and inactive 9-hydroxy-THC. Blood levels of THC peak in 30 minutes and then decline and become undetectable in 3–4 hours. The mechanism of action of cannabinoids is by inhibition of adenylate cyclase activity, centrally.

Pharmacodynamics

The effect of cannabis begin with in minutes of starting to smoke and lasts for 2–3 hours. The effect of *bhang*, through the intestinal route, depends on many factors, but generally begins in half an hour and last for 6–12 hours.

THC produces effects on mood, memory, motor coordination, cognitive ability, sensorium, time sense and self-perception. Most commonly, there is euphoria, sleepiness or spontaneous laughter. Short-term memory is impaired, and depersonalization also occurs. Decrease in muscle strength and hand steadiness can be demonstrated. More complex processes (including perception, attention, and information processing), which are involved in driving and flying, are impaired by doses equivalent to one or two cigarettes.

Marihuana smokers frequently report increased hunger, dry mouth and throat, more vivid visual imagery, and a keener sense of hearing. Clarity of sequential dialogue is impaired, and irrelevant ideas and words intrude into the stream of communication. Altered perception of time is a consistent effect of cannabinoids. Time seems to pass more slowly; minutes may seem like hours. Marihuana decreases REM sleep.

Higher doses of THC can induce frank hallucinations, delusions and paranoid feelings. Thinking becomes confused and disorganized; depersonalization and altered time sense are accentuated. Anxiety, reaching panic proportions, may replace euphoria, often as a result of the feeling that the drug-induced state will never end. With high doses, the clinical picture is that of a toxic psychosis with hallucinations, depersonalization and loss of insight. It can occur acutely or after months of use.

Chronic marihuana users may exhibit apathy, dullness, impaired judgment, concentration and memory, and loss of interest in personal appearance and pursuit of conventional goals. This has been called *amotivational syndrome*. It may be due in part to factors other than the use of cannabis.

Hallucinogens

Hallucinogens produce mental changes that resemble those of some psychotic states. These include LSD, PCP, mescaline, and psilocybin.

An effective oral dose of 30 mg of LSD produces visual hallucinations. Its half-life is 2–3 hours. The mechanism of action is believed to be through the agonist effect at presynaptic 5-HT receptors in the CNS. Tachyphylaxis (acute tolerance) occurs to LSD. Psychological dependence can occur, though physical dependence does not occur. LSD induces analgesia and indifference. Serious psychotic reaction with suicide can occur. LSD produces interesting effects in animals experiments with higher doses producing convulsion and death.

PCP (*angeldust*) was produced in search for a better intravenous anesthetic. It is structurally related to pethidine. PCP was found to induce analgesia without unconsciousness, but with amnesia, in man. Psychiatric disturbances in the form of agitation, hallucinations, and 'abreaction' occur with PCP use, and it has been used in experimental therapy.

Stimulants

Cocaine

It is derived from cocoa leaves and causes psychological but no physical dependence. Cocaine (*snow*) is used as snuff (snorting), swallowed, smoked or injected intravenously. Cocaine-free base is smoked (*crack*). Immediately following administration of cocaine, the user may experience intense pleasure, referred to as *rush* or *flash*. Intranasal use of cocaine produces euphoria (high) but not *rush*. The *rush* is followed in a few minutes by dysphasia. This leads to repeated use called *run*. After the *run* follows the *crash* (i.e. dysphoria, irritability, hypersomnia) lasting hours to days. After the *crash*, there may be depression (*cocaine blues*) and anhedonia for days to weeks.

Intranasal use causes mucosal vasoconstriction, anosmia, and eventually necrosis and perforation of nasal septum. Inhalation with breath holding allows pulmonary absorption that is about as rapid as an injection. It induces an intense euphoric state. The mouth and pharynx become anesthetized. Cocaine may be mixed with heroin (*speedball*). Cocaine is metabolized to plasma esterases and the half-life is 30 to 50 minutes.

The psychotropic effects of cocaine are due to block-ade of the reuptake of dopamine at CNS synapses, which increases its concentration at receptors and produces the characteristic '*high*'.

Fetal growth is retarded by maternal use, but teratogenicity is uncertain.

Amphetamines

These drugs include dextroamphetamine, methamphetamine, phenmetrazine, methylphenidate, etc. These drugs act by releasing catecholamines from interneuronal stores and prevent subsequent reuptake. The effects are similar to those of cocaine but longer lasting. Acute intoxication from amphetamine-like drugs is characterized by dizziness, tremor, irritability, confusion, hallucinations, chest pain, palpitations, hypertension, sweating and cardiac arrhythmias. Death is preceded by hyperpyrexia, convulsions and shock.

After long-term use of either cocaine or amphetamines, abrupt cessation is commonly followed by depression, anxiety and craving for the drug, that is soon followed by general fatigue and a need for sleep. Mood returns to normal over a period of days although in some cases dysphasia and anhedonia may persist for weeks.

Methylene-dioxy-methamphetamine

In the past few years, one of the amphetamines, which has become highly popular in some parts of the North American region, is methylene-dioxy-methamphetamine (MDMA) or known briefly as methamphetamine with the street name of *ecstasy*. It appeared in the street traffic in the 1970s and was used by some psychotherapists who believed it to be promoter of intimacy and communication. It is becoming popular as a party drug among the rich classes in the megapolises of India.

MDMA is usually taken orally, although intranasal application is also known. It is available in capsules and the usual dose is 100–150 mg. MDMA is metabolized to MDA (methylene-dioxy-amphetamine) in the body and the effects are mediated by MDA.

MDMA damages serotonergic axons in the hypothalamus and cerebral cortex in experimental animals. It has been demonstrated that the serotonergic function is altered in persons using MDMA. The effects occur in 20–60 minutes, often with a *rush*, which has been compared by some to cocaine. The period of rush merges into a state of euphoria that may last for 2–3 hours. Many users experience insomnia and fatigue that may persist for one or two days.

Nicotine

Pharmacokinetics

Nicotine in cigarette smoke, suspended on minute particles of 'tar', is quickly absorbed from the lung, almost with the efficiency of IV administration. It reaches the brain within 0.8 seconds after inhalation. It is absorbed through mucous membranes in a highly pH dependent fashion. Nicotine in cigarette smoke is somewhat acidic and is not well absorbed from the mouth. The peak plasma concentrations of nicotine in the plasma after a cigarette is smoked are typically 25 to 50 ng/mL. Regular smokers are able to, very often without conscious knowledge or effort, calibrate the plasma concentrations by regulating the puff volume, interpuff interval and the amount of smoke inhaled. The half-life is half an hour to two hours. It is largely metabolized to inert substances, e.g. cotinine, though some is excreted unchanged in the urine. Cotinine is used as a marker for nicotine intake in smoking surveys, because it has a half-life of half an hour to 20 hours.

Pharmacodynamics

Nicotine causes release of catecholamines in the CNS, as well as of serotonin, ADH, corticotrophin and growth hormone. On the cardiovascular system, the effects are those of sympathetic autonomic stimulation. There is vasoconstriction in the skin and vasodilation in muscles, tachycardia and a rise in blood pressure of about 15 mm Hg systolic and 10 mm Hg diastolic, and increased plasma noradrenaline. Ventricular extrasystoles may occur and cardiac output, work and oxygen consumption increase. Nicotine increases platelet adhesiveness, an effect that may be clinically significant in atheroma and thrombosis. Nicotine increases metabolic rate and stopping smoking may lead to weight gain. Tolerance develops to some of the effects of nicotine, taken repeatedly over few hours.

Nicotine is an agonist to receptors at the ends of peripheral cholinergic nerves whose cell bodies lie in the CNS, i.e. it acts at autonomic ganglia and at the voluntary, neuromuscular junction. Higher doses paralyze the same points. The CNS is stimulated, including the vomiting center, and tremors and convulsions may occur. As with peripheral actions, depression follows stimulation.

Caffeine

It is 1,3,7 trimethylxanthine which is found mainly in coffee and tea, and also in soft drinks, cocoa, chocolates and a number of prescription drugs.

Caffeine is absorbed from the gastrointestinal tract rapidly and completely. Peak plasma levels tend to occur within 30–45 minutes. Following absorption, the drug readily crosses the blood brain barrier, and ingested dosages are closely correlated with brain concentrations. Clinical and animal studies indicate that CNS stimulation is what most consumers of caffeine actively seek. Paraxanthine is an active metabolite of caffeine and has many equivalent pharmacological effects.

Caffeine increases CNS norepinephrine secretions, inhibits cAMP and cGMP breakdown, and increases cortisol. Caffein's stimulant or anxiety-inducing actions appear to be secondary to adenosine antagonism. Caffeine antagonises adenosine induced vasodilation and this may account for caffeine withdrawal headaches, as well as for its efficacy in treating migraine headache.

Caffeine has been reputed to increase verbal and motor output, reduce fatigue, and induce insomnia. Caffeine can induce some deleterious actions in many physiological systems, like tachycardia, arrhythmias, peptic ulceration, and diuresis.

CLINICAL FEATURES

In one restrictive sense, substance use disorders are merely disorders of behavior or '*behavioral disorders*'. The specific behavior that causes the problem is consumption of psychoactive substances in quantity, frequency and situations that results in distress and/or disability to the individual and family members, and causes problem to the society at large. All the other features, like intoxication, drug seeking behavior or the neglect of one's obligations, can be seen as the consequences of this fundamental behavior problem. Many behavioral scientists have looked at the clinical features of substance use disorders in this behaviorist perspective.

On the other hand, in the recent past, these disorders have been seen in an extremely wide perspective as problems of lifestyle and described as '*lifestyle disorders*'. The balanced perspective of a large number of professionals, and consensual opinion in the form of diagnostic guidelines, views substance use disorders as one more set of biopsychosocial disorders. It is believed that the disorders, besides being multifactorial in their etiology, manifest themselves clinically in different aspects. So, although the central feature is consumption of psychoctive substance, the various facets of these disorders are seen in biological features, such as tolerance and withdrawal, medical hazards of long-term use; psychological features, such as the experience of craving, preoccupation with drug seeking and other drug use related activities, salience of drug consumption over other activities; and social features, such as neglect of familial, social and occupational obligations as well as the other social consequences of drug use.

It should be evident that there is a large degree of overlap between the clinical features or presentation of substance use disorders and the consequences or the complications of long-term use. In the biopsychosocial perspective, the clinical features of substance use disorders are best described and understood, alongside the complications. As such, this section describes the complications along with the clinical features, firstly for the broad-spectrum of substance disorders in general, and in the later part the clinical features and the complications specific to each of the important classes of substances.

GENERAL CLINICAL FEATURES

The general clinical features can be well-understood in the context of the emerging phase of substance use and also cannot be divested from the description of the sequential manner in which the substance use occurs. As such, the general clinical features are described here in the vein of how initial substance use leads to more regular pattern, and onward to disorders.

Initiation of drug use, in some persons, leads to a more frequent use due to the reinforcement which can be a feeling of euphoria, relief from anxiety or any other effect of the substance (*primary reinforcers*). In respect of the substances with low or moderate abuse liability, like alcohol or tobacco, many of the persons in these early stages do manage to discontinue the use of the substance or maintain it as infrequent use. Some of the other persons progress gradually, to more regular frequency and use pattern. Based on the legal and social attitudes and use pattern, they may begin to be secretive about their use, start changing their association from nonusers to users, start spending extra-money on substances, and spend less time with the family. Such behaviors certainly occur more clearly in cases of illicit drugs, like heroin or cocaine, and can be considered as early indicators of substance use which requires attention. Nonetheless, it needs to be recognized that some persons in the community do have *substance related disorders*, like intoxication, in the absence of use disorder, in these early stages of use.

With increasing duration, the tolerance begins to develop, and the person requires and argues for more of the substance. The increase in the dose is generally noticeable and the people around (e.g. friends, family members and others) express their reservation, disapproval or objection in different ways. Arguments or tiffs over this or related issues becomes more common. Further, biobehavioral changes result in the occurence of *secondary reinforcers* like appearance of withdrawal symptoms, relief from craving for the drugs leading to more regular and increasingly heavy consumption of substances. Compulsive use and loss of control over the substance use also occur, and the drug seeking behavior becomes more intense and socially evident. The drug seeking behavior also increases the time spent in all drug-related activity, alongside curtailment of the routine activities of daily life and neglect of obligations. There is progressive decline in the quality of social interactions, financial resources, and the peer group consists of other substance users. All these changes, with the salience of substance use, contributes to a gradual narrowing of the repertoire of the person's life. Moreover, often the person gets involved in unlawful activities due to the activities in obtaining illicit drugs, or fights in states of withdrawal or intoxication, or road traffic accidents. There is a general decline in the health status of the persons who have dependent use or regular heavy use.

Important changes occur in the use pattern in some cases of dependence with the progression of the disorder. Tolerance and withdrawal phenomena contribute to these changes. The decreased effect due to tolerance, in some instances, leads to the change of route from nonparenteral to parenteral, or use of combination of drugs for potentiation effects. The use of combination of drugs or substitution of substances occurs also because of the experience of withdrawal and the need for overcoming the withdrawal, as well as the compulsive use and craving. The use of tranquilizers and other prescription drugs, along with other substance use, is determined by these factors as well as their easy availability and relatively lower cost as compared to the illicit drugs.

Many of the medical and psychiatric complications of substance use disorders become part of the clinical features of these disorders and the specific complications for each class of substance have been described later. It is useful to note that in general, the occurrence of repeated infections, injuries due to road traffic, work place or other accidents, and problems with the law, are seen frequently in many of the patients of substance use disorders.

COMMON CLINICAL PRESENTATIONS

The patients of substance use disorders do present in many different settings in various ways. It is important that all professionals and paraprofessionals in different settings are aware of these presentations, so as to be able to identify these cases and manage or refer them appropriately. Psychiatrists and other mental health professionals will do well to not only be alert to these varied presentations for rendering effective prevention and treatment services but also to orient the other professionals to these presentations. In addition to the persons who visit or are brought to the specialized treatment centers for substance use disorders with various presentations, some of the other common clinical presentations are listed here. This list is illustrative and not exhaustive.

- Hospital emergency services
  - Overdose
  - Intoxication
  - Withdrawal syndrome
  - Road traffic or other accidents
  - Medical/psychiatric complications of substance use, e.g. alcoholic cirrhosis or bleeding peptic ulcer or esophageal varices, cannabis psychosis
  - Battered child (or wife) syndrome
- Medical and other speciality services
  - *Medical complications*: As listed above, and also specific to each speciality, e.g. stroke or peripheral neuropathy (neurology services), gastritis (gastroenterology services), bronchitis or lung cancer (general medical services)
  - *Repeated infections*: Especially of the lungs and the liver (with opioid, alcohol or cannabis use; more with parenteral use)
  - The HIV seropositive persons
- General psychiatry services
  - *Comorbidity*: Depression, anxiety, psychotic disorders and other comorbid conditions, associated with any substance use.
  - *Psychiatric disorder in significant others*: Psychiatric disorder in significant others, which is linked to the substance use disorder in one of the family members, even if it is not a definitive causal link. A female patient with chronic or recurrent depressive disorder with alcohol or other substance use disorders in the husband.
  - *Recurrent or treatment refractory conditions*: This kind of clinical course is at times undetected associated substance use disorder. Patients of anxiety with tobacco, caffeine, alcohol or benzodiazepine use, or of depressive disorder, or bipolar disorder with alcohol use.
- Welfare and other social service agencies
  - Persons with financial, employment or other social problems
  - Families with frequent interpersonal or other problems
  - Marital units with frequent separations
- Police and other law enforcement agencies
  - Driving under influence (DUI) and other traffic offences
  - Persons with drug trafficking or other petty crimes.

Table 16: General complications of substance use disorders

Financial	*Occupational*	*Familial*	*Social*	*Legal*
• Spending money over drugs instead of family • Financial obligations not fulfilled • Exhausting savings • Borrowing money • Selling personal articles • Selling household article and coercing money from family members • Selling immovable property • Financial bankruptcy and destitution	• Inefficiency due to decreased performance • Impunctuality • Fights, quarrels, thefts • Absenteeism • Accidents at work place • Getting warnings • Suspension from job • Loss of job • Frequent changes in job • Declining status in job • Loss of work habit • Loss of skills • Longtime unemployment • Unsuitability for being meaningfully employed	• Arguments over drug use • Neglect of family obligations • Role change and conflict • Quarrels and physical violence • Long absences from home • Frequent marital separation • Divorce • Ostracization by family	• Peer alienation • Misbehavior with others • Arguments, fights • Decreased social reputation • Loss of position • Social isolation • Involvement in drug 'subcultures' • Social ostracization	• Violation of rules • Driving under influence (DUI) • Thefts and petty crimes • Involvement in drug trafficking • Arrests and court cases • Involvement in criminal gangs, and the underworld • Conviction and imprisonment

GENERAL COMPLICATIONS

The complications of substance use disorders are, to quite an extent, specific to each substance and are described later. The very nature of the disorders, specifically dependence, causes complications which are similar, regardless of the substance. Many of the general complications arise because of the priority of the substance use over the other activities of life and the lifestyle changes that form a part of the disorder. These general complications are listed in Table 16, but it must be understood that not all of these complications occur in all the cases. The general complications have been described in the order of severity and usually in each patient, these occur in the increasing order of severity.

SPECIFIC CLINICAL FEATURES

The specific clinical features are described in this section as use pattern, intoxication, withdrawal syndrome and the complications for each class of substances (i.e. alcohol, opioids, cocaine, cannabis, nicotine, caffeine as well as multidrug use). The substance-specific complications are discussed with the clinical features, since one or more of these complications occur in most cases of abuse or dependence. As such, clinical presentation of many cases of substance use disorders are associated with one or more of this complications.

It must also be understood that some of these complications of substance use in the medical sense, have been seen as alcohol or drug use related disabilities and in the current classificatory system will qualify for *substance related disorder*.

Korsakow's psychosis or amnestic disorder is an example of many such conditions. It can be seen as a medical complication of long-term regular alcohol use, has been seen broadly as an alcohol-related disability, and will be identified in the current classificatory system as an alcohol-related disorder.

Alcohol-related Disorders

Use Pattern

The use of alcohol starts as a social phenomenon, leading to abuse or dependent use in some of the individuals. The occurrence of alcohol-related disorders is not necessarily associated with abuse or dependent use. In fact, the average person with alcohol-related problems is likely to be neatly dressed, to have no severe signs of alcohol withdrawal, to have a job and good family support, and may have physical or psychiatric complications. In alcohol abuse, there is impairment of social, legal, interpersonal, and occupational functioning. The amount of alcohol intake, frequency, pattern of alcohol intake, type of liquor and response of person show great variability. One person may take alcohol occasionally or nightly only and yet show severe alcohol-related complications, whereas another person may take alcohol daily, throughout the day and yet show no impairment.

An alcohol-dependent person has a broad array of problems, including impairment in many areas of life due to alcohol use, compulsive intake of alcohol, evidence of tolerance and physical withdrawal. In most cases, drinking occurs around the clock to the exclusion of most, if not all, of the other activities of life. The origin of the term 'alcoholism' from the words 'alcohol' and 'ism' is explanatory about the salience of alcohol and alcohol-related activities over all the other aspects of life.

It has been found that persons who are severely dependent or those who are on the road to dependence, tend to drink alone, steal drinks, hide and drink, camouflage their drinks,

Table 17: CNS effects at different blood alcohol concentrations (BAC)

Blood alcohol concentration (BAC)	*CNS effects*
20–30 mg/dL	Slowed motor performance and decreased thinking ability
30–80 mg/dL	Increase in motor and cognitive problems
80–200 mg/dL	Increased incoordination and errors in judgement, mood lability, deterioration in cognition
200–300 mg/dL	Nystagmus, marked slurring of speech and alcohol black-outs
>300 mg/dL	Impaired vital signs and possible death

drink before going to parties and are most inclined to deny or justify their pattern of use. As the person slides across the spectrum towards dependence and a more severe level of dependence, his choice and quality of beverage tends to go down from high-quality liquors to illicit liquors.

Alcohol Intoxication

Alcohol depresses the CNS and the extent of depression corresponds to blood alcohol concentration (BAC) (Table 17). Evidence of behavioral changes (inappropriate excitation, aggression, overt sexual behavior), a slowing in motor performance and inability to think clearly are seen with blood alcohol levels of 20–30 mg/dL. Blood alcohol levels of 80 mg/dL or higher have pronounced effects on driving abilities. In nontolerant person, a level above 300 mg/dL is life-threatening and level above 400 mg/dL causes respiratory failure, coma and death.

Alcohol Withdrawal

Cessation or rapid decrease in the amount of alcohol in the body of an alcohol dependent person is most likely to produce a number of symptoms which are characteristic features of the withdrawal or abstinence syndrome. These are coarse tremors of hands and body, insomnia, anxiety, increased blood pressure and heart rate, increased sweating and body temperature and increased respiratory rate. These symptoms usually start within 8–12 hours of the last dose and peak on the second or the third day, and markedly diminish by the fourth or the fifth day. Disturbances of mood, notably anxiety and dysphoria amounting to depressed mood and irritability, are common during this phase. These mood changes are also associated with similar cognitive changes.

Auditory hallucinations, which are more often ill-formed and of the second person variety, in the absence of delirium or any sensorium disturbance, are distinctive features of alcohol withdrawal syndrome. These do not occur as commonly as tremors or autonomic disturbances, but do occur in a sizeable number of patients. These hallucinations occur usually after 12–24 hours after the last drink and convulsions (*rum fits*) occur after about 24–48 hours.

The alcohol withdrawal syndrome is not a uniform entity. It varies significantly in clinical manifestations and severity. Symptoms can range from mild insomnia to delirium tremens (DTs). The first symptoms and signs occur within hours of the last drink and peak within 24–48 hours. They include restlessness, tremor, sweating, anxiety, nausea, vomiting, loss of appetite, and insomnia. Tachycardia and systolic hypertension are also evident. Generalized seizures occur rarely, usually within 24 hours of cessation. In most alcohol-dependent individuals symptoms of alcohol withdrawal are mild-to-moderate and disappear within 5–7 days after the last drink. In more severe cases (approximately 5% of cases), DTs may develop.

Delirium tremens is a toxic confusional state that occurs when alcohol withdrawal symptoms are severe, and is often associated with medical illness. It is a life-threatening condition with a mortality of approximately 5%. The classic triad of symptoms includes clouding of consciousness and confusion, vivid hallucinations affecting every sensory modality, and marked tremor. Clinical features also include paranoid delusions, agitation, sleeplessness and autonomic hyperactivity (tachycardia, hypertension, sweating, and fever). Symptoms of DTs typically peak between 72 and 96 hours after the last drink. Prodromal symptoms usually include night-time insomnia, restlessness, fear, and confusion. Treatment of DTs requires early diagnosis and prompt transfer to the general medical setting where intravenous diazepam can be given, medical disorders treated, fluids and electrolytes replaced, and thiamine and other vitamins administered.

Risk Factors for Delirium Tremens and Seizures

- Severe alcohol dependence
- Past experience of DTs
- Long history of alcohol dependence with multiple previous episodes of inpatient treatment
- Older age
- Concomitant acute medical illness
- Severe withdrawal symptoms when presenting for treatment.

Wernicke's encephalopathy is quite often associated with, and triggered by, alcohol withdrawal syndrome. It had been found in 1950s and 1960s that tremors and the autonomic disturbances occur in more than 80% of the cases, auditory hallucinations in about 50% of the cases and the convulsions in less than 10–20% of the cases. The triad of WE is ataxia, confusion and ophthalmoplegia. The phenomenological aspects and the time course of the alcohol withdrawal syndrome seem to have undergone a change over the years. The cases seen at treatment centers as well as hospital emergency rooms do not seem to be as florid in their phenomenology as they were earlier. Greater awareness among primary care physicians, shorter time lag for reaching the hospital centers and prompt initiation of the treatment regimens can be considered as some of the reasons for the change in the phenomenology and the time course.

Generally, all the physical and psychological symptoms and signs of alcohol withdrawal remit in a period of two weeks, even if untreated. In treated cases, it can be expected that the symptoms and signs will last for no longer than a week or ten days. In a small number of cases, some of the withdrawal symptoms can persist be the period of two weeks, and sometimes up to 3–6 months. The common symptoms of such *protracted withdrawal syndrome* in case of alcohol are headache and insomnia.

In some cases, the withdrawal syndrome may be complicated by disorientation or confusion, along with visual or other hallucinations. Convulsions, coma, and occasionally death, have been reported as complications. The convulsions, which occur as part of the alcohol withdrawal, are quite like the seizures that occur in the patients of grand mal epilepsy. They are more often isolated, not associated with EEG changes suggestive of epilepsy, except for postictal slowing and can be traced to have occurred during the descending phase of alcohol level.

These complications can occur in the absence of delirium or as part of one of the severe forms of alcohol withdrawal that is associated with delirium, i.e. *delirium tremens* (DT). The clinical features of DT include restlessness and agitation, marked disorientation and altered consciousness, hallucinations in auditory and visual modalities, illusions and intense fear, sleeplessness, hypotension and tachycardia, and sometimes grand mal convulsions. Clover-shaped ST changes in the ECG are evident.

DT is infrequent and when it occurs, it is often associated with medical illnesses (e.g. hepatic decompensation, pneumonia, subdural hematoma, pancreatitis and fractures) and biochemical factors (e.g. hypomagnesemia, respiratory alkalosis). It typically begins 48–72 hours after the last drink and subsides within 1–5 days. The treatment of patients during a DT episode includes administration of another CNS depressant, usually diazepam or chlordiazepoxide or oxazepam. Other supportive medications and dietary management are also essential.

Medical Complications

- *Gastrointestinal complications*
  - *Gastritis and acid peptic disease*: Although alcohol is absorbed mainly from the small intestine, the direct effect on the gastric mucosa that alcohol produces during the gastric emptying time is adequate to lead to acute gastritis in many of the patients. Repetitive bouts of acute gastritis occur in these patients, also contributed by the neglect of food and the other lifestyle patterns. Attacks of acute gastritis often lead to vomiting and does occur with isolated instances of heavy drinking, in the absence of abuse or dependent use. Precipitation of acid peptic disease by long-term alcohol use, sometimes even with short-term heavy use, has been established. The role of alcohol use in the causation of peptic ulceration has been suggested but not proven.
  - *Alcoholic liver disease (ALD)*: The effect on the liver is possibly the most common and most serious complication of long-term alcohol use. The stages of ALD have been identified as *alcoholic fatty change* (stage 1), *alcoholic hepatitis* (stage 2), *alcoholic precirrhosis* (stage 3), and *alcoholic cirrhosis* (stage 4).

    The fact that the rates of cirrhosis related deaths have been considered as one of the best indirect indicators of the magnitude of alcohol related problems is noteworthy. Most persons with alcohol dependence do manifest ALD and a decreasing proportion of these persons progress from stage 1 to stage 4. The stage of ALD can be best determined only by histopathology following biopsy, which is an invasive procedure. In clinical practice, the severity of ALD is determined by the signs and symptoms as well as the biochemical assay of liver enzymes. Gamma glutayl tansaminase (GGT) is the most sensitive indicator of liver cell damage and is considered a good marker for ALD, indeed alcoholism, in the absence of any other possible cause of liver cell damage.

    A large part of the liver dysfunction has been seen to be reversible, as indicated by the biochemical tests, in a period of 3 to 4 weeks of abstinence. The changes seen as part of the first three stages revert towards normal functional and structural status with abstinence. The fourth stage of cirrhosis is the only irreversible stage of ALD.

    The cirrhotic stage, and at times the precirrhotic stage, of ALD leads to portal hypertension which may manifest as ascites, caput meduse, hematemesis and malena due to esophageal varices and bleeding per rectum due to hemorrhoids.
  - *Malabsorption syndrome*: It occurs due to alcohol induced pancreatic dysfunction and hemorrhagic lesions of duodenum, but is often not identified in clinical practice.
  - *Pancreatitis*: Acute pancreatitis is often triggered by a heavy bout of drinking, presenting as acute abdomen with excruciating pain. Chronic pancreatitis has also been known to be associated with alcohol use.
  - *Mellory Weiss syndrome*: Chronic heavy drinking, if associated with violent vomiting, can produce a

longitudinal tear in the mucosa at gastroesophageal junction.

- *Cardiovascular complications:* Long-term alcohol use causes cardiomyopathy, with symptoms ranging from unexplained arrhythmias in the presence of left ventricular impairment to heart failure with dilatation of all the four heart chambers and hypocontractility of heart muscle.

  There is an association between cerebrovascular accidents and alcoholism, especially within 24 hours of heavy drinking.
- *Hematological complications:* Alcohol exerts multiple reversible acute and chronic effects on blood cells. There is an increase RBC size (MCV) usually without anemia. Associated folic acid deficiency, leads to hypersegmented neutrophils, reticulocytopenia, hyperplastic bone marrow, and sideroblastic changes due to coexisting malnutrition.

  Long-term alcohol use has been documented to lead to a decreased production of WBCs and impaired delayed hypersensitivity response to new antigens. Toxic granulocytosis and mild thrombocytopenia have also been described.
- *Neuromuscular complications:* Peripheral neuropathy, more commonly of the sensory type, numbness, tingling and paresthesias in distal parts of the limbs, occurs in 5 to 15% of the patients. In addition to the direct toxic effects of alcohol, thiamine deficiency, malnutrition and demyelination contribute to these changes, which are also reversible with abstinence.

  Alcoholic myopathy occurs in the larger proximal limb muscles than in the smaller distal muscles and more in the lower limbs. The clinical picture is generally characterized by acute pain in the thigh muscles, often with myositis and raised levels of creatine phosphokinase (CPK) in the blood, and rarely myoglobinemia and myoglobinuria. Myopathy occurs with peripheral neuropathy or in isolation.
- *Endocrinological abnormalities:* Long-term alcohol use induces an increase in serum cortisol levels, which remain elevated during heavy drinking. The clinical presentation is often of pseudo-Cushing's syndrome.

  It also causes inhibition of vasopressin secretion at rising blood alcohol concentrations and an opposite effect is seen at falling blood alcohol concentrations. The final result is that most patients are likely to be slightly over-hydrated. It also induces a modest and reversible decrease in serum thyroxine (T4) and a more marked decrease in serum tri-iodothyronine (T3).

  Male heavy drinkers have been noted for many years to be liable to two distinct endocrine syndromes. These syndromes are of feminization and hypogonadism. Patients often display some features of both the syndromes. The syndrome of feminization results from the acquisition of the characteristics induced by the female hormone (estrogen). Thus, apart from biochemical evidence of hyperestrogenization, the alcoholic male may develop gynecomastia, a female habitus, and increased hypogastric and pelvic fat pads. Spider angiomata is considered by some to be a sign of hyperestrogenization. The syndrome of hypogonadism is as a result of damage to both spermatogenesis as well as androgenesis (hormone production). Reduced spermatogenesis results in small testes, reduced ejaculatory volume, oligospermia, and ultimately infertility. Failure of androgen production results in reduced libido, loss of acquired postpubertal secondary sexual characteristics. Thus, prostatic and seminal vesicular size will be reduced. Facial, pubic and axillary hair growth will be reduced or absent.
- *Sexual dysfunction:* The sexual changes induced by alcohol may have profound somatic effects on the male patients and these effects are not necessarily dependent upon the presence of long-standing advanced liver disease. The sexual dysfunction as evident in the form of decreased or lost libido, erectile impotence and infertility. The lifestyle, and familial as well as social, complications of long-term alcohol use, and the comorbidity with depression further compound these sexual dysfunctions.
- *Fetal alcohol syndrome:* It consists of facial malformations, small teeth, microcephaly with mental retardation, cardiac atrial or ventricular septal defects.
- *Methanol poisoning:* It is usually accidental, due to its ingestion as a partial or total substitute during use of illicitly manufactured and marketed alcohol beverages, or as a result of consumption of denatured ethanol. Instances of methanol poisoning occur more in situations of total prohibition and during periods of very tight legal controls. The effects of methanol occur due to the two toxic metabolic products, viz. formaldehyde and formic acid. The toxicity of these two compounds is most pronounced on the cells in retina and optic nerve. The severe acidosis which develops also contributes to the symptoms of headache, dizziness, nausea and vomiting, vasomotor disturbances, central nervous system depression and respiratory failure.

  These symptoms set in after 12–24 hours of ingestion of methanol. Visual disturbances are almost universal and permanent retinal damage leading to total blindness is common.
- *Neuropsychiatric complications*
  - *Blackouts*: In addition to the acute behavioral effects, an episode of heavy drinking may be accompanied by forgetting (*anterograde amnesia*) all or part of what occurred during drinking when the patient was inebriated but awake. The blackout is temporary and involves a short period of time. Blackout occurs in 30 to 40% of men in their late teens and early 20s,

most of whom do not develop serious and pervasive alcohol related problems.

Two types of blackouts have been described (i.e. en-bloc and fragmentary). In *en-bloc type*, events covering a period of many hours of drinking are not remembered when the person becomes sober. In *fragmentary type* of blackout, sober recall for drinking events is impaired but not absent and forgotten incidents may be remembered during a subsequent drinking bout. This has been attributed to *state dependent learning*. Blackouts are more correlated with blood alcohol levels than the alcohol dependence process itself.

- *Wernicke's encephalopathy/syndrome*: It consists of a triad of confusion, ataxia and opthalmoplegia (sixth nerve palsy). It is caused by deficiency of thiamine, and perhaps niacinamide. It is easily treatable with thiamine supplement and recovers fully.
- *Korsakof's state/syndrome*: It consists of only memory loss which is characterized by profound short-term memory loss which is of the anterograde type. This state often occurs following Wernicke's syndrome. One fourth of Korsakof's patients achieve full recovery, one half experience partial recovery, and the other one-fourth show no improvement with thiamine.
- *Neurocognitive deficits and dementia:* Long-term alcohol use is known to lead to deterioration in neurocognitive functions, which can be identified by bedside screening instruments or neuropsychological tests. The deficits have been shown in abstracting ability, frontal lobe functions, and perception and memory for nonverbal material. These deficits have been found to be correlated with the evidence for cortical atrophy and gray matter loss on CT and MRI scan. These neurocognitive deficits, as well as the CT and MRI changes, have been found to be reversible with abstinence. In social drinkers too, similar reversible neurocognitive deficits have been demonstrated. More severe and manifest form of these neurocognitive deficits has been seen in the form of alcoholic dementia, which is similar to the dementia of Alzheimer's type and distinctly different from the Korsakow's state or alcoholic amnestic syndrome.
- *Cerebellar degeneration*: It occurs in about 1% of alcoholics with associated malnutrition. It is a syndrome of progressive unsteady stance and gait, often accompanied by mild nystagmus. Cerebellar atrophy is seen on CT or MRI, but CSF is normal.
- *Central pontine myelinosis*: It is characterized by impaired arousal, quadriparesis and pseudobulbar signs due to demyelination of the base of the pons. CT or MRI scan confirm the diagnosis and the response to thiamine is poor.

Psychiatric Complications

- *Alcohol-induced mood disorders:* Alcoholism patients present with a variety of depressive syndromes/symptoms both during intoxication and during withdrawal. All the cases, which have depressive symptoms, do not qualify for a syndrome or disorder diagnosis. Many of the patients who have depressive symptoms at the beginning phase of detoxification do not continue with these symptoms. In a study of 191 patients, it was found that of the 42% of the patients who had depressive symptoms at the time of intake in an inpatient treatment program, only 6% continued to have some depressive symptoms at the end of a period of four weeks.

  As a general rule, it is good to remember not to diagnose depressive disorder or start antidpressant therapy during the period of detoxification, except for a very few cases in which the evidence for a diagnosis of a disorder is convincing. The hospital-based studies have reported rates ranging from 4 to 98% of patients of alcoholism to have depressive disorder, depending on the method of assessment used. The ECA data reported a prevalence rate of 13.4% for affective disorder in those with alcohol disorders as against a prevalence of 7.5% in the general population, leading to an odds ratio of 1.9. Thus, it can be said from the community-based data that the odds of having an affective disorder in patients of alcohol use disorder are twice greater than the general population. The ECA data also confirmed the earlier impression that this comorbidity is higher in females than in males. While 44% of the male subjects with alcohol used disorder had a comorbid depressive diagnosis, 65% of the female subjects had a comorbid depressive diagnosis.

  Although a large part of the comorbidity is apparent comorbidity, some of it is real comorbidity, and is associated with the unipolar and bipolar disorder. It must also be borne in mind that not all the cases depression with alcoholism are necessarily alcohol induced mood disorders. Suicide rates among alcoholism patients are higher than among the general population.
- *Alcohol-induced psychotic disorder:* About 3% of chronic heavy drinkers develop psychotic symptoms. The psychotic symptoms are varied and may range from transient fleeting elementary hallucinations to fully organized hallucinations and delusions. Auditory hallucinations or delusions of paranoid type often form the symptom complex. Their symptoms may resemble those seen in schizophrenia. When the symptoms occur only in the context of heavy drinking, they are likely to clear spontaneously on cessation of alcohol intake, and recur if heavy drinking is resumed.
- *Alcohol-induced jealousy:* In these cases, the patients suspect their spouses of infidelity and the belief is morbid enough to influence various aspects of personal and social

life. It is less common than a nondelusional suspicious attitude to the spouse.

Opioid-related Disorders

Use Pattern

There is a variety of opioids, licit and illicit, which are used by different routes. Some drugs and routes are preferred, depending on various factors like availability, regional use pattern, drug subcultures, etc. The form of oral use of '*affim*' (raw opium) or '*doda*' (opium husk) that is prevalent in certain areas of some States in India, like Rajasthan, Punjab and Uttar Pradesh, is not only culturally acceptable and approved, but at times actively encouraged. There are instances of groups of persons belonging to one or more families using opium only during harvesting season or festivals and functioning adequately without any opium use subsequently. In these geographical regions, there are subgroups of persons who consume opium everyday and yet function adequately without any overt opioid related problems or disorder.

Heroin use, in Indian towns and cities, has followed the pattern of being smoked or '*chased*' through the nasal route. Some persons start with the smoking route and move on to chasing and some others initiate their heroin use with the chasing route. This route is generally preferred over the smoking route due to the more rapid onset of action, the possibility of calibrating the dose and the economic advantage of using small amounts over many occasions. Unlike the European and the American cities, the use of heroin through injection route has not been one of the popular routes in most parts of India, except for the North Eastern states. The increasingly popular use of buprenorphine injections among the users of illicit opioids in the towns and cities of India has also brought forth more underground drug use in groups and 'shooting galleries' have existed in the major cities, since the early and middle of 1990s.

The heroin chasers also undergo the experience of increasing amounts used, but this phenomenon is quite difficult to be ascertained due to the marked variation in the quality of street preparations of heroin (*smack*) from time to time and in different parts of the same city. Heroin dependent persons may exhibit a marked heterogeneity in their life-styles. Some are quite stable socially, avoid criminality, have good occupational functioning. At the other extreme are those persons who live exclusively with drug-related and other illicit activities, are socially isolated, have some criminal record and have their own drug subculture. They may be involved with prostitution, theft, violent crimes and other activities in order to procure the money needed for drugs. A third group is an intermediate group who identify with both cultures partially and keep moving from one to the other lifestyle.

Health professionals and other iatrogenic induced dependent users of injection users of opioids like morphine, pethidine, pentazocine, etc. do not form subgroups. Their drug use is generally carried out as individual activity and quite often remains hidden for long periods.

Opioid Intoxication

Despite a high degree of tolerance that develops to opioids, overdose toxicity is not uncommon among opioid addicts. This is known to occur due to change of the drug used, the alteration in the street preparation, and miscalculation of the dose.

The characteristic signs of acute intoxication include clouded consciousness, severe respiratory depression, and pinpoint pupils. There may be pulmonary edema associated with respiratory depression. Death from intoxication is due to respiratory failure. Blood pressure is usually well maintained, if the patient is supine, until anoxia causes circulatory failure. At this end stage, the pupils are dilated.

Opioid Withdrawal

The opioid withdrawal syndrome consists of a range of signs and symptoms across various systems. They are dysphoric mood, nausea and vomiting, muscle aches and joint pains, lacrimation and rhinorrhea, frequent yawning, pupillary dilation, piloerection and sweating, marked diarrhea, restlessness and insomnia.

The time course and severity of withdrawal syndrome vary with the opioid and the degree of dependence. Drugs such as heroin, morphine have short half lives and after sudden cessation of their use, the onset of observable withdrawal occurs within 8–12 hours, reaches its peak with in 48 hours and subsides over a period of 5–7 days. With longer acting drugs, like codeine and methadone, peak withdrawal may occur after 4– 6 days and persist for more than 14 days.

Many opioid dependent persons continue to experience some unwanted symptoms after the acute withdrawal is over. Such symptoms range from vague sense of not feeling well through continuing bodyache and irritability, to feelings of anxiety and sadness. These have been referred to as *protracted abstinence syndrome* and it may contribute to relapse.

Opioid Use-related Complications

Due to the illicit nature of substance use and the lifestyle changes, many of the complications of opioid use are in the realm of the familial, social, legal, and occupational complications, already described in the section on general complications. The psychiatric complications have also been described under the section on comorbidity. The major complications of opioid use are linked to the immunosuppression that occurs with all long-term opioid use and the complications of injection use.

Medical Complications of Injection Drug Use

These complications arise mainly due to the use of repeated injections and the related problems of sepsis, but also due to the immunosuppression and the nutritional deficiencies. Some of these complications do occur in injection use with any substance and some are also seen in nonparenteral users of opioids.

- *Infections*: Infections are the most important medical complications in these patients. Examples are cellulitis, candidiasis, septic arthritis, fasciitis, osteomyelitis, endocarditis, pneumonia, pulmonary tuberculosis, STDs (like chancroid, gonorrhea, syphilis, HIV). The rates of HIV infection (seropositivity) and AIDS are higher among injection substance users, as compared to the nonparenteral substance users as well as the general population. The injection users are high risk groups in the spread of HIV in the second and third phases of the epidemic. The spread is not only through the injection route but also through sexual contacts of these patients. The sexual route is important for the spread from the substance users to the general population, and many of the HIV seropositive women and children in the community have been linked to injection users. Some of the patients of injection use and HIV seropositive status also have a comorbid psychiatric disorder. These cases are termed as *triple diagnosis patients* and are beginning to be seen in the American, European and African settings.
- *Hepatic complications*: Acute hepatitis, hepatic failure, chronic hepatitis, cirrhosis.
- *Renal complications*: Glomerulonephritis, renal failure.
- *Cardiovascular complications*: Thrombophlebitis, arrhythmias, mycotic aneurysms.
- *Pulmonary complications*: Pulmonary edema, pneumothorax.
- *Gastrointestinal complications*: Motility disorders, constipation.
- *Neuromuscular complications*: Epidural abscess, subdural abscess, brain abscess, transverse myelitis, myositis.
- *Miscellaneous overdose toxicity*: Allergic reactions, needle embolus, necrotizing angiitis.
- *Immunologic abnormalities*: Patients with substance use disorders in general and opioid users, in particular, have various immunological abnormalities. Most of these are due to the immunosuppressant effects of the opioids or the other substances. It has been argued that these changes are contributed to by changes in the liver function and the nutritional deficits. These immunological changes have been documented even in the absence of HIV infection, as well as in nonparenteral users. Some of these include generalized lymphadenopathy, lymphocytosis, reduced Natural Killer cell activity, delayed type-IV immune response, false positive serological tests, and increased levels of serum immunoglobulins.

Cocaine-related Disorders

Use Pattern

The pattern of cocaine use varies widely. Cocaine may be used continuously for days in '*runs*' or '*binges*', or at regular intervals when a paycheck is received. Others may use once or twice in a month, while still others use daily for prolonged periods of months or years. The acute intake of cocaine leads to intense pleasure referred to as '*rush*' that is followed by dysphoria, sleepiness, etc. referred to as '*crash*' in order to avoid this unpleasant state, patients go on repetitively using cocaine referred to as a '*run*'. This is followed by dysphoria, irritability, sadness of mood called '*cocaine blues*', that is usually self-limiting.

Cocaine users come from all social strata, all races and both sexes. Cocaine addicts tend to be young (12–39 years of age), are dependent on at least three drugs including alcohol, and are predominantly male. In ECA study, 84% of those with cocaine dependence were also alcohol dependent.

Cocaine Intoxication

Acute intoxication with high doses of cocaine is characterized by rambling speech, headache, transient ideas of reference and tinnitus. Paranoid ideation, auditory hallucinations in a clear sensorium and tactile hallucinations (*cocaine bugs*), visual hallucinations (*snow lights*) also occur with acute intoxication. Tachycardia, hypertension and coronary vasospasm are the infrequent cardiovascular signs. Extreme anger with threats or acting out behavior, mood changes like depression, suicidal ideation, irritability, emotional lability or disturbances in sensorium are also common.

Cocaine Withdrawal

The symptoms include decreased energy, dysphoric and anhedonic mood changes, psychomotor retardation, fatigue, insomnia and unpleasant dreams, and increased appetite. These symptoms are mild to begin with and increase over 48–72 hours.

Complications

Medical complications: The common complications are cardiovascular (including arrhythmias and myocardial infarction), respiratory (such as chest pain and respiratory failure), neurological effects (such as headache and seizures), and gastrointestinal (like nausea and abdominal pain).

Body packers and stuffers—In order to smuggle the drug across international borders, carefully prepared packages are swallowed by the users. Rupture of these packages can cause death due to overdose and intestinal obstruction can also occur. As against these *body packers*, who swallow carefully prepared packets, the *body stuffers* tend to rapidly swallow cocaine to avoid being apprehended.

Psychiatric complications: The neuropsychiatric complications include toxic paranoid psychosis, panic attacks, suicide, as well as delirium and memory deficits.

Cannabis-related Disorders

Use Pattern

Drug preparations from the plant vary widely in quality and potency. These are smoked, eaten or drunk. Most experimental users discontinue cannabis use after a few trials, but some continue to use it once or twice a week. A still smaller fraction of initial users become regular users, consuming the drug several times per week, and a still smaller group eventially become daily or almost daily users, who may smoke up to 20 marijuana cigarettes per day, or use *bhang* or *charas* through the day.

Some tolerance develops to the cardiovascular and mood-elevating psychological effects of cannabis. It is thought that brief effects that occur after cannabis smoking are sufficient to maintain the behavior. Such effects include euphoria, an apparent slowing of time, enhancement and distortion of sensations, and perceptions and, in some circumstances, increased sexual arousal.

Cannabis Intoxication

The clinical picture is variable, but usually takes the form of acute onset of excited and violent behavior, with changes in perception, mood, cognition and psychomotor performance. The perceptual change may be in the form of depersonalization, derealization, sensory distortions and altered time perception. The mood changes are in the form of euphoria and inappropriate laughing. The cognitive impairments include disorientation, poor concentration and short-term memory dysfunction. The psychomotor impairment is manifest as inability to carry out complex mental and motor activities, e.g. driving, design, copying, calculations, etc. The judgement is often impaired. The effects may be attenuated or altered by the concurrent use of other substances, like alcohol.

Cannabis Withdrawal

A cannabis withdrawal syndrome has been documented is animal experiments. Discontinuation of cannabis use is humans may be followed by anxiety, insomnia, and other symptoms resembling sedative anxiolytic withdrawal. The relationship of this generally mild syndrome to the perpetuation of cannabis use is uncertain.

Complications of Cannabis Use

Medical complications: Chronic use of cannabis effects a number of organ systems. The lungs show chronic inflammatory changes, partly due to concurrent tobacco smoking. Cannabis is suspected to reduce fertility through alterations in LH and FSH. Cannabis has been shown to induce chromosomal anomalies in animal experiments and also to increase fetal loss. Cananabis increases the risk of cardiovascular problems in patients with hypertension, coronary artery disease and cerebrovascular disorders. Chronic cannabis use has also been associated with cerebral atrophy, on CT scan studies.

Psychiatric complications: Cannabis use can induce anxiety, paranoid states, and recurrence of schizophrenic symptoms. Many clinicians and researchers believe that chronic cannabis use is associated with *amotivational syndrome,* that is characterized by lethargy, reduced drive, mild depression and loss of interest. The occurrence of *acute cannabis psychosis* or short-term psychosis is well accepted. These psychotic states are known to occur in chronic users of cannabis, who have had no past history or family history any psychiatric disorder. The consensus is that these acute psychotic states occur following a recent increase in the dose of cannabis and the symptom complex is quite amorphous, i.e. an admixture of confusional, paranoid, schizophrenic and excitation symptoms. These psychotic states are also known to recover with discontinuation of cannabis use, even without antipsychotic treatment.

The etiological role of cannabis in chronic psychoses is more uncertain. It has been argued that chronic forms of psychosis occur in those cannabis users who were already suffering from schizophrenic or other psychotic disorders or carried the vulnerability in terms of genetic loading in the family. The course of the psychotic disorders in these patients has also not been linked to use or discontinuation of cannabis. These disorders have been termed as *cannabis triggered psychotic states*, rather than cannabis related disorders.

Nicotine-related Disorders

Use Pattern

Tobacco cigarette smoking is the most common substance use disorder. Most smokers begin their habit in their teens. The habit is acquired mainly through social contacts, and the risk is increased if the family members and friends also smoke. The prevalence rates of smoking are higher in psychiatric patients. Smokeless tobacco, in the form of snuff or chewing tobacco, forms a less frequent but sizeable portion of tobacco use.

Nicotine and tar intake can not be determined by the amount smoked, since dose is affected by the manner of smoking. Smokers can puff harder, deeper or more frequently to obtain significant amounts of nicotine from fewer cigarettes or from low nicotine cigarettes. Patterns of use may also depend upon social factors. Suppression of smoking in forbidden areas like hospitals, religious places, aircrafts, etc. forces smokers to alter their pattern of intake to accommodate periods of deprivation.

After a period of experimental smoking follows a period of initiation, during which the person smokes less than one cigarette per week. During experimental smoking, peers often provide social reinforcement. Smoking serves as a means, whereby adolescence express an image of toughness, precocity and sociability. Experimental smoking is followed by habituation in which person smokes at least one cigarette per week and acquires the skill of inhalation and regulation of the dose of nicotine. With habituation, consumption may increase to a pack of cigarettes or more per day. Habituation progresses to development of dependence.

Intoxication

In novice smokers, nicotine causes dizziness or light headedness and sometimes vertigo. With higher doses, nausea and then vomiting supervene. These effects can also occur in chronic smokers with forced rapid smoking. Nicotine also increases the physiological tremor due to release of catecholamines and sympathetic stimulation.

Acute nicotine poisoning is seen occassionally. The symptoms include nausea, salivation, pallor, weakness, abdominal pain, vomiting or diarrhea, dizziness, headache and cold sweats. There may also be inability to concentrate, confusion, various sensory disturbances, severe elevations in blood pressure, and a weak and rapid pulse. At lethal doses, death is usally caused by respiratory paralysis.

Withdrawal

After daily use of nicotine for several weeks, abrupt cessation of nicotine use, or reduction in the amount of nicotine taken, is followed by nicotine withdrawal. It occurs within 24 hours, often in 6–8 hours, of the last dose. It comprises of a number of characteristic signs which are more among persons who smoke cigarettes as compared to those who use other nicotine containing products. The characteristic signs of nicotine withdrawal include mood changes, physiological symptoms and physiological signs. The mood changes include dysphoric or depressed mood, irritability, and impatience. The physiological symptoms include restlessness, difficulty in concentration, constipation, sleep disturbance, drowsiness, fatigue, lightheadedness, headache, hunger, urge to smoke and craving. The physiological signs decrease in heart rate, increased peripheral circulation, sweating and mouth ulcers.

Complications

The complications arise as a result of acute effects of smoking tobacco and from effects of chronic smoking.

The complications due to the *acute effects* include increased airway resistance (due to nonspecific effects of submicronic particles, e.g. carbon particles of less than one micrometer diameter). Initially, ciliary activity is stimulated and then depressed, and the particles are removed from the lungs more slowly. Carbon monoxide absorption is clinically important in the presence of coronary heart disease, which is worsened.

The complications due to *chronic smoking* include cancer. The risk of death from lung cancer is related to the number of cigarettes smoked and the age of starting. Pecentage of men aged 35 who smoke 25 or more cigarettes per day are three times more likely to die before the age of 65, as compared to the percentage of men aged 35 who do not smoke. The risk of smokers developing cancer of the mouth, throat and esophagus is 5–10 times greater than that of nonsmokers. The cancer of pancreas, kidney and urinary tract is also more common in smokers.

The incidence of ischemic heart disease is markedly higher in smokers as compared to nonsmokers. Atherosclerotic narrowing of the smallest coronary arteries is enormously increased in heavy and even in moderate smokers. Smoking also causes increased platelet adhesiveness that increases the readiness with which the thrombi form. Death from the aneurysm of the aorta is five times more common in smokers as compared to nonsmokers. Disease of the arteries of legs is even more closely related to smoking, more than 95% of these patients being smokers.

Chronic mucous hypersecretion leading to chronic bronchitis is seen more often in smokers. Chronic obstructive lung disease originates chiefly in small airways and is related to smoking.

Smokers have an increased risk of spontaneous abortion, bleeding during pregnancy and development of various placental abnormalities. The babies of women, who smoke, are lighter and there is an increased prevalence of low birth weight in women who smoke regularly.

Caffeine-related Disorders

Use Pattern

Caffeine is the most widely consumed psychoactive agent. Intake starts in early childhood and steadily increases during adolescence. The majority of persons have moderate consumtion and as many as one of five adults consume doses generally considered large enough to cause clinical symptoms.

A cup of tea provides approximately 50 mg of caffeine and a cup of coffee has about 75–100 mg of caffeine. Most of the marketed cola drinks have about 50 mg of caffeine and an average sized bar of chocolate has between 25 and 50 mg of caffeine. It has been estimated that the global daily average consumption of caffeine is 50 mg/person and average American consumption is 200 mg/person/day. Intake exceeding 500 mg/day represents the best marker of high risk for caffeine-related disorders. 20–30% of North Americans meet this criterion. An estimated 10% are believed to qualify for the diagnosis of caffeine intoxication, a higher rate than for most other substances of abuse.

Caffeine Intoxication

Caffeinism is the term used to describe the clinical syndrome produced by acute or chronic overuse of caffeine. It is usually characterized by anxiety, psychomotor alterations, sleep disturbances, mood changes and other psychophysiological complications. Patient may take more caffeine with intention of relieving such distressing symptoms but that only leads to further increase in the symptoms.

Acute or chronic caffeine intoxication often simulates panic or generalized anxiety disorders. There is also evidence that panic disorder patients are more sensitive to the anxiogenic and other stimulant effects of caffeine.

Caffeine intoxication is also associated with diuresis, nausea, headache, chest pain, and delirium. Focal and generalized seizures, and deaths have also been reported after acute ingestion of massive doses of caffeine. The acute lethal dose of caffeine is 5–10 g.

Caffeine Withdrawal

The symptoms of caffeine withdrawal include headache (most common), irritability, inability to concentrate, drowsiness, yawning, fatiguability, nausea and craving. The withdrawal syndrome develops within 2–4 hours of the last dose and lasts usually for 18–24 hours.

Complications

The complications of long-term caffeine use are sleep disturbances, frequent headache and diarrhea, and mood changes of dysphoria, irritability and anxiety. The relationship between caffeine use and mood disturbances, particularly anxiety is very controversial and requires to be understood more clearly.

Multiple Drug Use

Use Pattern

Multidrug use is the use of more than one drug at the same time or in close temporal proximity. Some specific use patterns have been described for multidrug use. These patterns are not necessarily stable patterns in all the patients, and the same patients shift from one pattern to another over lifetime.

- *Sequential use*: Specific pattern of use over a 24 hour cycle, based on the specific actions of each drug. Although the sequential pattern varies across different patients, generally the pattern remains the same for each patient. One of the popular pattern is of use of stimulants in the morning, alcohol in the later part of the day, and sedative drugs at night.
- *Ancillary use*: In these patients, there is generally one primary drug of abuse which is preferred. The other drugs are used for potentiating the effects of the primary drug, for overcoming or reducing the unwanted effects of the primary drug or to substitute partially or totally for the nonavailability of the primary drug.
- *Concurrent use*: The pattern of use is not really not based on any specific reasons for the effects or on any one primary drug. The use of more than one drug is not necessarily at the same time, but occurs the same time period. Often, it is difficult to identify any of the drugs used as the primary drug and the drugs used and their pattern are not fixed.

Multiple drug use is seen more commonly with opioid use and cocaine use as compared to other drugs, and is more associated with parenteral use. Various combinations of opioids, antihistaminics, sedatives, phenothiazines as 'cocktail' injections are quite common in patients attending treatment centers in India. The use of sedative-hypnotics with alcohol or cannabis, as well as alcohol and cannabis together, has also been seen in many patients. One of the predictors of multidrug use in later life is early onset of substance use in adolescence.

Intoxication

Patients with multidrug use are more prone to instances of intoxication due to miscalculation of the dose, as well as the additive and synergistic effects of the substances used. The clinical features of the intoxication will be determined by the primary drug of abuse or the most recent use of one or more drug. Since the commonly used drugs in many of these patients are CNS depressants, the clinical features of coma and respiratory depression must be kept in mind.

Withdrawal

In multiple substance users with one primary substance of dependence, the characteristic withdrawal syndrome of that substance will be evident clinically. It is, by now, well recognized that in patients with dependence on more than one drug, the withdrawal symptoms of all the drugs on which the patient is dependent are manifestly seen.

Complications

The specific complications of each of the substances with dependence or regular use can be expected in these patients. It is also worth noting that since many of these patients use injection as one of the common routes, all the complications of injection use, listed above, should be expected.

MANAGEMENT

Management will essentially include assessment as well as treatment, and although they have been described separately, they should not be considered as compartmentalized, but as phases that merge with each other and are complementary. Often, acute treatment is necessary to be initiated alongside brief initial assessment, to be followed by a more comprehensive assessment after treatment for acute conditions like intoxication or withdrawal symptoms has been taken care of. Conversely, the process of building a therapeutic alliance begins during the phase of assessment and the foundation for many of the therapeutic interventions, like motivation enhancement, is best laid in this phase.

Barriers in Assessment

It is useful to understand some specific issues about the interaction and the relationship of the clinician with the patients and their family members.

Clinicians need to be aware of these issues since they usually act as barriers to a good therapeutic relationship but also influence the accuracy of the assessment and, consequently, the treatment. The following phenomena in patients and their family members can become barriers in assessment.

- Denial of the problem, as well as ambivalence about the need for external help
- Guilt about the substance use and the use related behavior patterns
- Feelings of shame about having been 'weak' or a 'failure'
- Stigmatization of the patient and the family
- Dilemmas about physician's role and reactions
- Apprehension of possible legal and other punitive consequences.

The clinician characteristics and phenomena also contribute significantly as barriers in assessment. Some of the important ones are:

- Lack of correct scientific knowledge about the field of substance use disorders.
- Judgmental attitude to persons with substance use and related disorders.
- False opinion of therapeutic nihilism.
- Fear of inability to manage substance use disorders.

Remedies for Barriers in Assessment

The barriers in assessment can be effectively overcome by some remedial measures in the clinician's approach to the assessment of patients with substance use and related disorders, for example:

- Ensuring privacy and confidentiality
- Remaining nonjudgmental and nonmoralistic
- Showing nonpossessive warmth and concern
- Expressing empathy and optimism
- Readiness to listen and understand before reaching conclusions
- Avoiding ambiguous messages
- Being clear and firm regarding one's own role, functions, abilities and limitations
- Introspective ability of clinician and its application to practice.

ASSESSMENT

Purpose

The purpose of assessment is not merely arriving at a diagnosis or labeling, but also to ascertain the severity and extent of the problem as well as the patient's biological, psychological and social resources. Identification of both the problems and resources will help to choose appropriate treatment alternatives. It must be noted that many times, the interview carried out for assessment does have therapeutic use, e.g. establishing therapeutic alliance, monitoring transference phenomena and motivational interviewing.

Setting

Assessment is required to be done in different clinical settings, like emergency rooms, psychiatric services, specialized treatment centers, and general medical or surgical services. The overall extent of the assessment and the relative emphasis on various components of assessment varies according to the setting in which the assessment is carried out and also according to the condition of the patient.

In some settings, like specialized treatment centers, assessment is carried out by multiple health care professionals including physicians, clinical psychologists, social workers and counselors. Patients and their families should be appraised of this well in time and the roles of multiple carers should be explained to enhance their cooperation. Proper maintenance of clinical records by multiple assessors should be ensured for assimilation of information within the team.

Sources of Information

Information required for assessment is to be obtained from multiple sources, although mainly from the patient. The information obtained from the other sources, like family members (preferably spouse), friends or peers, and from the institutional sources (like employers, school teachers, jail authorities) is useful to corroborate as well as to supplement the information provided by the patient. The information from these other sources become even more important and indispensable, for intoxicated patients, acutely ill patients and those with cognitive deficits.

Treatment and other medical records of patients are very helpful in reviewing overall long-term impact of treatment, response to specific treatment methods and understanding the comorbid medical or psychiatric condition.

Components of the Assessment

Assessment includes the components of history, examination (including general physical, systemic and mental state examination), as well as laboratory investigations, like the standard format for any medical or psychiatric assessment (Table 18). However, certain aspects require special attention and these apsects specific to the assessment of cases of substance use and related disorders are described here, along with a semistructured format for assessment.

It is useful to realize that while such a format has been found useful by most clinical teams and treatment centers, there can be and has been a valid argument for the format of assessing these cases requiring to be quite different from the standard clinical format. Clinical teams and treatment centers find this format useful, owing to their own professional background and familiarity with this type of format. Long-term rehabilitation centres, counseling centers for early problem users or families of users do follow their own method of assessment and recording.

History Taking

Chief complaints: The chief complaints (or the purpose of consultation), as reported by patient and family members, are often discrepant or contradictory. Such discrepancies about the clinical problems of patient, the manner in which the complaints are presented provides indication of motivation and attitude of the patient, perception and attitude of the family members and family dynamics, and presence of barriers like denial.

History of present illness: This should include details of substance use pattern, complications related to substance use, abstinence attempts and treatment history. The order of eliciting information on these different points will vary according to the problems presented by the patient or the family, the co-operativeness of the patient and the immediate clinical need. The semistructured format can be useful to ensure that all the important aspect of the history are covered and for the purpose of recording the history in a systematic manner.

- *Substance use pattern*: As per the standard format of a medical case history, the use pattern for the current substance use is recorded in this part and the details of life time substance use pattern are recorded in the section on past history. Some clinicians and teams have preferred to consider the lifetime use pattern, alongwith the current the pattern in continuity and record it as part of the history of present illness. This approach can be seen as a major departure from the standard format, but has the advantage of understanding the patient's substance use and related disorders in a coherent manner. It does remain to be a choice of a particular clinician or a team, to use either of these two methods but the latter approach is recommended.
- *Complications of substance use*: Adequate queries should be made to assess the complications of drug use and related behavior in different spheres, like physical and mental health, occupational, financial and social life as well as legal complications. The physical and mental health complications will vary according to the substance(s) of use, the route of administration and severity of substance use. The other complications are often similar across the patients of different substance use disorders depending upon the severity of substance use, the available resources and support systems. A detailed assessment of the complications is required for a comprehensive understanding of the life situations of the patients and their families so as to plan appropriate treatment and other intervention strategies.
- *Abstinence attempts*: Details of attempts at abstinence, self-imposed (SIA) or treatment related (TRA), are helpful in planning appropriate treatment strategies, as well as in prognosticating the likely outcome. Successful attempts at abstinence as well as unsuccessful abstinence attempts need to be recorded, along with the contributing factors.
- *Treatment history*: All the details of the treatment history, with details of the patient's compliance and adherence to the treatment and the outcome of treatment must be assessed and recorded.

Past history: Any history of long-term physical illness, chronic pain, and long term medical prescription is important to be inquired into and recorded.

Family history: The evidence in the history for any substance use disorder in the parents, siblings or genetically linked family members must be clearly elicited and recorded, with a genogram. A detailed exploration of the familial factors, which could be contributing to the onset and maintenance of substance use, will cover primary family dysfunction, attitude and responses of the family members as well as possible 'enabling' by the family members. The impact of substance use disorder on the family functioning will be helpful in understanding the attitudes and responses of the family. This understanding, along with an assessment of the strengths and

Table 18: Semistructured format for assessment at intake

1.	*Chief (or presenting) complaints* As reported by the patient, and family members or other informants, specifically about the following: *From the patient*: Experience of withdrawal symptoms and other dependence features, physical health complications, reasons for treatment contact, and goal of treatment. *From the family members (or other informants)*: Physical health complications, intoxication, withdrawal and other dependence features, family's role in treatment contact.
2.	*History of present illness (HOPI)* a. *Substance use pattern* *Onset*: First use of any substance and the following items for each substance in chronology. Age at first use, reasons for use and the situation, amount and frequency, route of administration, initial experience with the substance or the effects. *Progression*: Reasons for subsequent use of substance, change in amount and frequency and reasons thereof, route of administration, development of tolerance, first appearance of withdrawal symptoms, occurrence of compulsive use and the other features of dependent use, viz. drug use getting priority over other activities, neglect of responsibility and obligations, use despite knowledge of harm, etc. HIV risk practices of substance use, like parenteral cocktails, needle sharing, needle re-use, use in 'shooting galleries', pattern of multi-drug use, if any, attempts to cut down use or shifting to other substances of routes and reasons thereof, periods of heavy use and its psychosocial concomitants. *Recent drug use*: Most preferred substance during last one month, dose frequency, heaviest use, withdrawal symptoms, date and time of last use, specifying the substance and route.
	b. *Complications of drug use*, with details, in the areas of physical health, mental health, occupational functioning, family functioning, social functioning, financial complications, and legal complications
	c. *Abstinence attempts*: Self-imposed or treatment related period(s) of abstinence, any other substance use during the period of abstinence, reasons for relapse, shift to other substances and reasons there of, positive factors which contributed to abstinence.
	d. *Treatment history*: Number of treatment attempts, duration of treatment, compliance with and adherence to treatment, outcome of treatment, viz. dropout, failure, relapse, abstinence, duration of abstinence, use of other drugs during abstinence, level of social and occupational functioning achieved during each period of abstinence.
3.	*Past history* a. Psychiatric illness, especifically mood disorders and anxiety disorders, evidence for antisocial personality disorder or traits.
	b. Chronic physical illness or chronic pain, refractory surgical problem.
	c. Long-term medication for a valid indication or misuse after initial prescription.
4.	*Family history:* Family history of substance use, disorders, psychiatric illness, personality disorders, suicide, with a genogram.
	Current living arrangement: Family structure and composition, broad indicators of family environment, roles, communication patterns and problem solving skills.
	Social support system: Availability and future potential.
	Influence of substance use on family, perception and attitudes of the family members about patient's substance use, their willingness and suitability for participation in treatment.
5.	*Personal history* *Early childhood and development*: Problems in parenting, emotional deprivation, school performance, truancy or other antisocial traits.
	Adolescence: Crisis, nonconformist attitude, influence of peers on behavior, evidence for conduct disorder.
	Educational history: The level of education achieved, effect of substance use over education (e.g. dropout).
	Sexual history: Sexual beliefs and attitudes, any sexual problems prior to or consequent to drug use, sex with multiple partners, unprotected sex.
	Marital history: Marital factors maintaining drug use, co-dependence, quality of marital relationship, primary or secondary marital discord, separations, current attitude of the spouse to patient's substance use, and willingness to participate in treatment.
	Occupational history: All jobs/self-employment period in which patient had been engaged till date, frequent changes and reasons thereof, current skills and potential for meaningful employment, influence of peers at work for substance use.
6.	*Premorbid personality:* Specific traits of anxiety, dysphoria, dependence, avoidance or antisocial personality profile, evidence of personality disorder, locus of control, strengths and weaknesses in the profile.
7.	*Physical examination* a. Vital signs
	b. General physical examination
	c. *Systemic examination*: For routine assessment and for specific needs with different substances. *i. For patients with alcohol use*: Signs of liver dysfunction and portal hypertension, signs of neuromyopathy, signs of CNS dysfunction (Wernicke's signs), signs of gastric dysfunction (acid peptic disease). *ii. For patients with opioid use*: Signs of infections, specifically of chest and liver, signs of immunocompromised status. *iii. For patients with tobacco use*: Signs of chest infections and malignancies in smokers and signs of precancerous oral lesions and submucous fibrosis in nonsmoking tobacco users. *iv. For patients with injection use*: Phlebothrombosis, injection marks, injection abscesses or carbuncles, signs of infections, signs of immunocompromised status.
8.	*Mental state examination:* Signs elicited and their severity, temporal relationship in detoxification phase, cognitive functions, insight and motivation for treatment.
	Diagnosis: Current and past, specifying the primary drug as far as possible.

weaknesses of the families, will help in ensuring participation in treatment.

Personal history: Specific aspects of the personal history, which could be contributing to the substance use, require to be highlighted. In different patients, the emphasis will be required variably on factors in developmental, educational, occupational or aspects of the personal history. Detailed assessment of relationship with peers and peer groups, especially in the context of its influence on personal behavior, can go a long way in understanding the genesis of the substance use disorder and in planning appropriate treatment strategy.

A thorough assessment of the marital and occupational history, including the strengths and the potential for resource mobilization, will be necessary for formulating a comprehensive treatment plan. In view of importance of the sexual route of transmission of HIV, in parenteral as well as nonparenteral substance users, a detailed sexual history has to be an integral part of the assessment.

Premorbid personality: Assessment of premobid personality functioning should include an assessment of specific character traits, behavior patterns suggestive of personality traits, and their relationship with substance use. Although antisocial personality disorder is not uncommonly associated with substance use disorders, the mistake of considering report of antisocial behavior during substance use career, as evidence for antisocial personality disorder must be carefully avoided. Detailed assessment should be made to ascertain whether antisocial behavior has occurred only during the period of substance use as a consequence of compulsive use or other dependence phenomena, or it is a part of an overall pattern of antisocial traits.

Physical examination: It should be as thorough as in any medical case. However, specific signs corresponding to presenting symptoms and to the physical complications, withdrawal syndrome, intoxication of the reported or suspected substance(s) should be looked for and recorded.

Mental state examination: All patients should be specifically examined for attitude and behavior towards clinician, depressed or anxious mood, level of sensorium, deficits in cognitive functions and patient's motivation for treatment. In patients with comorbid psychiatric condition, a thorough mental state examination should be carried out.

Laboratory Investigations

Two categories of laboratory investigations are generally required in patients with substance use disorders, viz. screening for substances of use and investigations for assessment of physical health complications.

Screening for Substance of Use

By and large, substance use history as given by patients and corroborated by family members, is reliable. However, laboratory screening at intake assessment provides an objective measure of all the substances used in the recent past. Such screening is also useful when performed during various phases of treatment including the abstinence phase. A negative result of screening supports the self-report of abstinence, while a positive result must alert the clinician to the possibility of relapse. Screening for occasional lapses during the treatment or after care, when handled appropriately, can provide an opportunity for patient and the clinician to discuss issues of adherence to treatment.

Indications for screening for substances or their metabolites in clinical practice can be considered to be:

- At the time of intake for reported substances used and for the substances suspected to have been used.
- During the detoxification and treatment phases:
  - Frequent periodic routine screening.
  - Recurrence of withdrawal symptoms after being controlled adequately.
  - Suspected substance use reported by family members or other informants.
  - Any other indirect indicator of substance use.
- During the after-care phase:
  - Infrequent periodic routine screening.
  - Any evidence of lapse or relapse.

The most commonly used method for screening is *thin layer chromatography* (TLC) which is less expensive, quicker and available more readily. It can yield more false negative results due to low sensitivity but has a high specificity, leading to lower rates of false positive results.

Gas liquid chromatography (GLC) is highly sensitive but time consuming and expensive. Other techniques are *radioimmunoassay* (RIA), and *high performance liquid chromatography* (HPLC). Qualitative screening is most commonly done on urine samples and also on blood samples, when it is suspected that the patient is tampering with the urine sample. Quantitative assays are more reliably carried out on blood samples. Methods for screening saliva and hair samples are also available but have not become common in clinical practice.

Methods for qualitative assay for alcohol, as well as estimation of the blood alcohol concentration (BAC), have been standardized for blood samples as well as for exhaled air in the breath. Breath analysis, with commercially available *breath analyzers*, is the preferred method because of the readiness for use and its noninvasive nature but requires the cooperation of the patient. Breath analyzers have been used by law enforcement officials for traffic and other offences in India and some other countries for some time. Their use in treatment settings, as per the indications listed above, can be

Table 19: Biological Markers of alcoholism

1.	Aspartate aminotransferase (AST)	If raised indicates liver cell injury of any cause. In the absence of other causes, increased in up to 75% of alcoholics. Useful as an adjunct when combined with other tests.
2.	Alanine aminotransferase (ALT)	Similar to AST. AST/ALT>2 is highly correlated with alcoholic liver disease.
3.	Ratio of m-AST to total AST	Proposed parameter to distinguish alcoholic hepatitis from other liver diseases. However, recent population based studies do not favor it.
4.	Gamma glutamyl transferase (GGT)	Most commonly used test. Increased activity in 35–38% alcoholics or heavy drinkers. Non-specific for alcoholism (also increased in other diseases). Useful as a combined test; also as adjunct to monitoring treatment or in motivating patients.
5.	Mean corpuscular volume (MCV)	Less sensitive but more specific than GGT. A useful adjunctive test, used with GGT.
6.	Adenylate cyclase (Platelet)	This enzymes activity is lower in alcoholics. Long lasting change detectable in alcoholics. If combined with another test, has sensitivity and specificity of approximately 75%.
7.	Erythrocyte aldehyde dehydrogenase	Decreased activity in chronic alcoholics. Low sensitivity.
8.	Carbohydrate deficient transferrin (CDT)	Increased level in alcoholics. Can distinguish recent excessive consumption from abstinence or very light drinking.

very useful. Blood sample assays are more useful in research settings and emergency room situations, or for forensic purposes.

It must be remembered that screening for substance is a useful additional tool in assessment and treatment. Although it cannot be considered indisposable, it is necessary part of specialized treatment settings.

Laboratory investigations for assessment of physical health complications include routine investigations (hemogram, blood counts, urine examination, blood sugar, blood urea, X-ray chest), specific investigations according to the indications (like liver function tests, lipid profile, test for HBsAg and HIV—after pretest counseling, EKG, CT head, EMG studies, urine/blood culture, sputum for AFB), psychological testing (for comorbid disorders, personality traits/disorders, suitability for treatment methods), and neuropsychological tests (for cognitive deficits, amnestic disorder, dementia).

Biological Markers

Biological markers are certain biological parameters, alteration in which is associated with specific disorders. These markers can be trait markers or state markers. *Trait markers* indicate the vulnerability of developing a particular disorder begins and does remain so even after an individual recovers from disorder. *State markers* indicate the psychological, pathological and biochemical changes occurring during the presence of disorders and hence, they are present only during the period of clinically manifest illness.

In the field of substance use disorders, the biological markers of alcoholism have been studied in great details, and a number of trait markers as well as state markers in alcoholism have been identified. The study of these markers helps in better understanding of biology of alcohol use disorders as well as many of these markers, specifically the state markers have been found to be useful to identify the patients with alcohol use disorders in epidemiological studies as well as in clinical practice. A list of some useful state markers in alcoholism is provided in Table 19. Many of these markers have been found more useful with increased sensitivity and specificity when used in combination in the form of test batteries.

Table 20: Screening instruments and rating scales

i.	Screening	MAST (Michigan Alcoholism Screening Test) CAGE Questionnaire AUDIT (Alcohol Use Disorders Inventory Test) DAST (Drug Abuse Screening Test)
ii.	Withdrawal rating scale	SOWS (Short Opiate Withdrawal Scale) CIWA-A (Clinical Institute Withdrawal Assessment-Alcohol Scale)
iii.	Scales for assessment of severity	ASI (Addiction Severity Index) SODQ (Severity of Opiate Dependence Questionnaire) SADQ (Severity of Alcohol Dependence Questionnaire)

Use of Screening Instruments and Rating Scales

A number of screening instruments and rating scales are available in the field of substance use and related disorders (Table 20). The screening instruments, mostly for alcohol use disorders, are used in epidemiological studies, where large populations are to be screened for the presence of substance use disorders. They are also useful in clinical settings like medical and surgical outpatient departments, where detailed history of substance use in every patient is difficult to obtain due to time constraints. The rating scales for the severity of dependence and withdrawal symptoms can be used in day-to-day clinical practice, though some experts recommend their use in research context only (Table 21).

One should be aware that the usefulness of these instruments and scales in routine clinical practice is limited, because most of these refer to only one group of substance and are of limited use in patients using multiple substances. Another potential problem with instruments is that the interviewer may relate to the instrument rather than to the patient.

CAGE

C—Have you ever felt you should cut down on your drinking?
A—Have people annoyed you by criticizing your drinking?
G—Have you ever felt bad or guilty about your drinking?
E—*Eye opener*: Have you ever had a drink first thing in the morning to steady your nerves or to get rid of a hangover?

The CAGE can identify alcohol problems over the lifetime. Two positive responses are considered a positive test and indicate further assessment is warranted.

Table 21: Alcohol use disorders identification test (AUDIT)

Score (0-4)		
1.	How often do you have a drink containing alcohol?	Never (0) to more than four per week (4)
2.	How many drinks containing alcohol do you have on a typical day?	One or two (0) to more than ten (4)
3.	How often do you have six or more drinks on one occasion?	Never (0) to daily of almost daily (4)
4.	How often during the last year have you found that you were not able to stop drinking once you had started?	Never (0) to daily of almost daily (4)
5.	How often during the last year have you failed to do what was normally expected from you because of drinking?	Never (0) to daily of almost daily (4)
6.	How often during the last year have you needed a first drink in the morning to get yourself going after a heavy drinking session?	Never (0) to daily of almost daily (4)
7.	How often during the last year have you had a feeling of guilt or remorse after drinking?	Never (0) to daily of almost daily (4)
8.	How often during the last year have you been unable to remember what happened the night before because you had been drinking?	Never (0) to daily of almost daily (4)
9.	Have you or someone else been injured as a result of your drinking?	No (0) to yes, during the last year (4)
10.	Has a relative, friend, doctor or other health worker been concerned about your drinking or suggested that you should cut down?	No (0) to yes, during the last year (4)
The AUDIT score is the sum of the response values. A score of 8 or more identifies heavy drinkers and those with alcohol-use disorders.		

MICHIGAN ALCOHOLISM SCREENING TEST (MAST)

It contains 24 questionnaires with YES NO Points

0. Do you enjoy drinking now and then? ___ ___
1.* Do you feel you are a normal drinker? ("normal"—drink as much or less than most other people) (2)
2. Have you ever awakened the morning after some drinking the night before and found that you could not remember a part of the evening? (2)
3. Does your wife, husband, a parent, or other near relative ever worry or complain about your drinking?(1)
4.* Can you stop drinking without a struggle after one or two drinks? (2)
5. Do you ever feel guilty about your drinking? (1)
6.* Do friends or relatives think you are a normal drinker? (2)
7.* Are you able to stop drinking when you want to? (2)
8. Have you ever attended a meeting of Alcoholics Anonymous(AA)? (5)
9. Have you gotten into physical fights when drinking? (1)
10. Has you drinking ever created problems between you and your wife, husband, a parent, or other relative? (2)
11. Has your wife, husband (or other family members) ever gone to anyone for help about your drinking? (2)
12. Have you ever lost friends because of your drinking? (2)
13. Have you ever gotten into trouble at work or school because of drinking? (2)
14. Have you ever lost a job because of drinking? (2)
15. Have you ever neglected your obligations, your family, or your work for two or more days in a row because you were drinking? (2)
16. Do you drink before noon fairly often? (1)
17. Have you ever been told you have liver trouble? Cirrhosis? (2)
18.** After heavy drinking have you ever had Delirium Tremens (D.T.s) or severe shaking, or heard voices, or seen things that are really not there? (2)
19. Have you ever gone to anyone for help about your drinking? (5)
20. Have you ever been in a hospital because of drinking? (5)
21. Have you ever been a patient in a psychiatric hospital or on a psychiatric ward of a general hospital where drinking was part of the problem that resulted in hospitalization? (2)
22. Have you ever been seen at a psychiatric or mental health clinic or gone to any doctor, social worker,

* Alcoholic response is negative.
** 5 points for delirium tremens.

or clergyman for help with any emotional problem, where drinking was part of the problem? (2)

23.*** Have you ever been arrested for drunk driving, driving while intoxicated, or driving under the influence of alcoholic beverages?(If YES, How many times?) (2)

24.*** Have you ever been arrested, or taken into custody even for a few hours, because of other drunk behavior? (If YES, How many times? (2)

SCORING

Add up the points for every question you answered with YES, for Q23 and Q24 multiply the number of times by points:

- 0–3—No apparent problem
- 4—Early or middle problem drinker
- 5 or more—Problem drinker (Alcoholic)

Programs using the above scoring system find it very sensitive at the five point level an it tends to find more people alcoholic than anticipated. However, it is a screening test and should be sensitive at its lower levels.

TREATMENT

The treatment of substance use disorders has traditionally aimed at helping the person achieve and maintain abstinence and over time has also been enlarged in its scope to include the goals of treatment of complications, improving the social and psychological functioning and preventing relapse. Such a broad based purpose of treatment can be achieved well by a comprehensive treatment plan executed by multidisciplinary team with good motivation and adherence to treatment on part of the patients and support and participation of the family members.

Development of an effective treatment plan will be based on the findings of the assessment, and the availability of treatment settings and modalities. The selection of treatment setting will depend on the treatment goals in the immediate, short-term and long-term time frames. These treatment goals will be determined by severity of disorder, the patient's current condition and motivation, as well as the presence of physical and/or psychiatric comorbidity. The treatment goals and the suitability in different patients, will help in choosing from the available treatment modalities for each phase of the treatment.

Treatment Settings

The patients of substance use disorders receive treatment in a wide variety of hospital, nonhospital residential and community settings. The hospital settings range from specialized treatment centers for substance use disorders, through psychiatric hospitals or centers, and psychiatric services in a general hospital to the medical services (in many speciality disciplines) in general hospitals. These settings, in public as well as private health care sector, provide inpatient treatment and/or outpatient treatment.

The belief about inpatient setting being the preferred or the only one suitable for patients of substance use disorders had been a part of clinical opinion until recently and still continues to be held. It is certainly true that inpatient settings have the advantages of 'restrictive care', continuous monitoring of the patients adherence to treatment and a more intensive contact with the treating team, but the outpatient treatment has the merits of being closer to natural settings, increased confidence of the patients about their mastery over substance use, and more active participation of the family in treatment. Research data does not support the belief about the superiority of inpatient treatment over outpatient treatment. It is important to be able to choose inpatient or outpatient treatment as per the suitability of the patients and guidelines are provided in Table 22.

The nonhospital residential settings of halfway homes, residential rehabilitation centres and therapeutic communities provide alternative settings for treatment or as settings for after case of the patients treated in the hospital settings. Many of these settings do operate on principles which are different from the principles followed in hospital settings, but can be complementary. A wide range of community settings have been offered and utilized for treatment of substance use disorders. Some patients avail of the services in any one of these settings as the only treatment and many others as part of the multimodal treatment program.

Most patients move through many of these different settings over their career and many patients avail of the services in more than one setting during a particular treatment attempt. This phenomenon is not only permissible but also desirable, and should be encouraged as part of a multi-modal treatment plan. The need for active cooperation, if not collaboration, amongst the agencies and the professionals in these different settings has begun to be seen as a necessity for the maximal benefits of treatment to the patient.

It has been demonstrated that more intensive treatment is not necessarily more effective. Treatment in primary care settings or simple treatment in counseling centers can be as effective as treatment in tertiary care centers or specialized treatment settings, in group comparisons. The benefit of treatment in individual patient depends on many factors, one of them being the choice of appropriate treatment setting. Psychiatrists, physicians and other health professionals will do well to be sensitive to the possibility of patients benefiting from a variety of settings.

Although recent trend in most countries is to favor specialized drug dependence treatment facilities, the availability of such specialized care facilities is low in many countries including India. There is need to treat these patients in other settings, like general medical services and psychiatry

*** 2 points for each arrest.

Table 22: Guidelines for inpatient and outpatient treatment

A.	Indications for inpatient treatment 1. Heavily intoxicated patients 2. Patients having severe or complicated withdrawal syndrome, e.g. delirium tremens, withdrawal seizures 3. Patients having significant physical complications requiring inpatient management, e.g. Wernicke's encephalopathy, multiple abscesses, hematemesis 4. Patients with acute or chronic general medical condition that makes outpatient detoxification unsafe, e.g. patients with cardiac disease 5. Patient with significant psychopathology 6. Unsuccessful attempts at outpatient treatment 7. Parenteral substance use or/and multiple substance use 8. Crisis in social support system 9. Geographical distance consideration 10. Academic and research reason
B.	Indications for outpatient treatment 1. Mild or moderate level of dependence 2. Short duration of dependence 3. Minimal health damage 4. Good social support system
C.	Unsuitability for inpatient treatment 1. Antisocial personality disorder or traits 2. Significant criminal record 3. Earlier instances or disciplinary problems during inpatient treatment 4. Several aborted treatment attempts in inpatient setting

services. The description of the various treatment modalities in this chapter may give an impression that treatment of substance use disorders is too complex and specialized to be carried out in general settings by general physicians. However, if the basic principles in the management of a case of substance use disorder are applied by physicians, many of these patients can be effectively treated. In countries like India with limited resources, treatment of substance use disorders need to be integrated with general health care system.

Some of the important factors in the decision regarding the setting of treatment are:

- Patient's capacity and willingness to cooperate with treatment,
- Patient's capacity to care for himself or herself,
- Need for structure, support, and supervision in order to remain safe, and pursue treatment away from environment and activities that promote substance use,
- Need for specific treatment for comorbid medical or psychiatric conditions,
- Need for particular treatment modality that may be available only in certain settings
- Preference of the patient or the clinician for particular treatment setting(s).

Goals of Treatment

The goals of treatment vary according to the time frame and the scope envisaged. They will also differ across individual patients and can be revised from time to time. *Immediate goals* can be detoxification, treatment of acute medical sequele and crisis intervention; *short-term goals* usually target treatment of comorbid medical or psychiatric conditions, maintaining abstinence, family reintegration and vocational placement; and the *long-term goals* focus on the larger issues of relapse prevention, occupational rehabilitation, social reintegration, abstinent life-style and improvement of quality of life.

Although total abstinence is one of the most common goals of treatment, it is becoming clear that there is a need for considering alternate goals. The alternate goals are based mostly on the principle of harm reduction or minimization, which refers to 'minimizing the direct and indirect effects of substance use'. The alternate goals include controlled or responsible use and substitution maintenance. While substitution maintenance for opioid and nicotine dependence is being increasingly accepted, the goal of controlled use has been more controversial. There has been some evidence of controlled use in early problem drinkers of alcohol being a feasible goal in some patients, it requires further evidence.

Phases of Treatment

The detoxification phase being considered as treatment in itself is a common misconception, not only in the patients and their families but also in health professionals. It must be emphasized that detoxification is one of the phases of treatment. In the pretreatment phase, the preparation and acceptance on part of the patient about the problem and the need for external help occurs as a long-term process. The role of peers, family members and primary care providers is highly important in this phase, which may last from a few days to many weeks or months. The detoxification phase usually runs from 2 to 4 weeks, followed by the active treatment phase during which the short-term goals are focused upon and the plan for the long-term goals are made. This phase runs from 3 to 12 months or more, and involves the process of choosing from amongst the many pharmacological and psychosocial modalities of treatment. It has been suggested and proven in research studies, that for early problem drinkers, and possibly cases of mild degree of dependence on any substance, do not require too much of the active phase of treatment and can be treated with simple advice or minimal treatment. The post-treatment or after-care phase focuses on the long-term objectives being realized and can be seen to continue for 3–5 years or even longer. In this phase too, the role of the family and the other social agencies is more active and necessary.

Treatment Methods

Treatment of substance use disorders is essentially multi-modal, a combination of two or more treatment methods to deal with the disorder comprehensively. In the past few decades, a large number of pharmacological and non-pharmacological modalities of treatment have been described and practised, many having evolved in isolation, with strong claims of effectiveness. Most of them have been found to be useful to a certain extent but the relative superiority of one over the others has not been proven and the effectiveness of each one has been found to be satisfactory or less than satisfactory when used alone, and none of them is suitable for all the patients. Different treatment modalities have different applicability and limitations and suit different patients. Different modalities pursue different paths to bring about desirable changes in one or the other aspect of substance use behavior and its determinants. As such, various treatment modalities described should not be seen as antagonistic or even competitively different from each other but as complementary to each other. The current knowledge suggests that there is a need to develop treatment strategy which combines various treatment modalities meaningfully. These treatment modalities can be executed simultaneously as well as sequentially in phases. This chapter provides an overview of the various treatment modalities since the details of each one of these are beyond the scope of this chapter.

Detoxification

The literal meaning of detoxification is 'elimination of toxin (usually a poison) from the body' and the term has been used in the treatment of dependence, as this phase involves the treatment of intoxication or overdose and the treatment of withdrawal syndrome in the process of achieving a substance free state. This evolution of the term is misleading in that detoxification is sometimes seen as a process of flushing out the toxins which accumulate with long-term substances use and no more than that. A much more comprehensive concept of detoxification refers to an initial phase of treatment of substance dependence which includes treatment of withdrawal syndrome, assessment of health and psychosocial complications with treatment of those requiring acute treatment, and building up of a therapeutic relationship between the patient and treating team.

There are many approaches to the task of helping a dependent person, achieve abstinence from the substance. It can be done by abrupt cessation of the substance and prescription of specific agents or by means of gradually tapering off the substance by decreasing amounts. The purpose is to alleviate subjective discomfort and minimize observable or measurable withdrawal signs, so as to prevent the person continuing to use the substance, which is a frequent occurrence in the early fast of detoxification or self-imposed abstinence.

Methods of detoxification: Detoxification for nicotine has been mostly carried out by nicotine replacement through other routes and many clinicians still favor gradual reduction method in detoxification of benzodiazepines, specially of long acting benzodiazepines. Some treatment teams and centres prefer the method of abrupt cessation without any medication, i.e. the '*cold turkey*', and herbal methods are still in use for inducing vomiting. By and large, abrupt total cessation of the primary drug of dependence and control of withdrawal syndrome to a tolerable level by suitable medication is the widely accepted method. The methods of detoxification include:

- Gradual reduction of the substance in decreasing amounts
- Abrupt cessation with specific medication which:
  - Have cross tolerance to the substance of use, e.g. benzodiazepines for alcohol withdrawal, dextropropoxyphene, buprenorphine or methadone for opioid withdrawal
  - Have some specific pharmacological properties to suppress withdrawal, e.g. carbamazepine for alcohol withdrawal, clonidine for opiate withdrawal.
  - Provide general symptomatic relief, e.g. hypnotics (benzodiazepine as well as nonbenzodiazepines, antiemetics, antidiarrheals, etc).

Use of antipsychotic or antiepileptics agents is not recommended to control withdrawal, though they may be require to treat comorbid psychiatric or seizure disorders. Similarly use of IV fluids and parenteral drugs to control withdrawal is not recommended, until there are specific indications, e.g. presence of severe dehydration, delirium tremens.

Doses of medicines for detoxification: Doses of medicines should be decided according to the expected severity of withdrawal syndrome; which will vary according to the substance abused (its potency, half-life), the time elapsed since the last dose, severity of dependence (duration, consumption, route of administration, etc), the concomitant use of other drugs, the presence of general medical or psychiatric disorder and individual biological and psychological variables.

The aim is to make the experience of withdrawal state tolerable rather than to suppress all symptoms of withdrawal. The principle 'least possible amount of medicines for the shortest possible time' should be followed as majority of the drugs used for detoxification themselves have moderate to high abuse liability. Explanation of this principle to the patient at the outset, along with support and reassurance to the patient goes a long way in ensuring better compliance to treatment. However, one should be willing to modify the dosage schedule according to the withdrawal symptoms throughout the detoxification phase.

Duration of detoxification: Usually alcohol detoxification can be completed in 7–10 days and opioid detoxification requires 2–3 weeks. However, the duration will depend on severity of dependence, drug of dependence (its half-life), drugs used for detoxification (their half-life). This will be longer in elderly patients, and debilitated and medically or surgically ill patients. Management of protracted withdrawal takes longer duration of weeks or months (even up to 6 months) and various nonpharmacological methods like relaxation therapy, cognitive behavior therapy may need to be used.

Table 23 provides a summary of detoxification agents for various substances. The details of the detoxification methods for the common clinical situations are described thereafter.

Detoxification of Individual Substances

Alcohol withdrawal: The management of alcohol withdrawal has been reviewed elsewhere and is summarized in Table 23. It must be emphasized again that the benzodiazepines are the drugs of choice in management of alcohol withdrawal, complicated as well uncomplicated. Usually daily doses of 20–60 mg of diazepam or 40–120 mg of chlordiazepoxide are required. The use of antipsychotics or antiepileptics, except carbamazepine, has no role and hence not recommended. Patients with any of the clinical features of Wernicke's syndrome must be treated immediately with IV thiamine HCl, 100 mg twice in a day, for the first five days. Parenteral administration of thiamine in every patient is not necessary, but oral administration of thiamine in all the patients for prevention of Wernicke's syndrome is justified. Carbamazepine has been found to be effective in place of benzodiazepines; the phenomenon of 'kindling' has been hypothesized to be the mechanism behind this effect. Chlormethiazole is another compound found to be effective and is used widely in Europe. Use of loading dose of diazepam has been reported by some to reduce the total amount of diazepam and duration of withdrawal syndrome, but is not proven more effective and advantageous.

Delirium tremens (DT) or impending DT should be treated as an emergency (20–50% mortality in untreated cases and 5–10% mortality even with treatment). Immediate hospitalization is indicated. Treatment of choice is intravenous diazepam, which needs to be given in doses of 10 mg every 20 minutes till patient is sedated or signs and symptoms of withdrawal subside significantly. Patient may require further doses of diazepam (oral or intravenous), depending upon the withdrawal symptoms that may reappear subsequently up to two weeks. Supportive treatment comprises of parenteral thiamine in all patients, and correction of fluid depletion and electrolyte imbalances. The environment needs to be protective, safe, helpful to orient the patient and should provide low sensory stimuli, as in case of any delirious patient. With treatment, the features of DT are usually controlled

Table 23: Summary of detoxification agents

	Category of medication	Opiate withdrawal	Alcohol withdrawal	BDZ withdrawal	Nictotine withdrawal
1.	Cross tolerant medicines[a]	Tincture opium[b] Methadone[b] Dextropropoxyphene Buprenorphine	Oral benzodiazepines Dizepam Chlordiazepoxide Oxazepam[c]	Long acting benzodiazepines	Nicotine gums Nicotine transdermal patches
2.	Medicines having no cross tolerance but supresses specific withdrawal syndromes	α-2 adrenergic agonists, e.g. clonidine	Carbamazepine β-blockers[d]	—	Benzodiazepines
3.	General symptomatic medications[d]	Antidiarrheals hypnotics	—	—	—
4.	Medicines for complicated withdrawal	—	Injection benzodiazepines in DT, seizures	—	—
5.	Others	Naltrexone and clonidine	Loading dose of diazepam	—	—

[a]Also used in long-term maintenance therapy in opioid dependence and nicotine dependence
[b]Not used/available in India.
[c]Useful in cases with significant hepatic impairment.
[d]Used as an adjunct only.

within 2–3 days, though patient usually requires to continue under inpatient treatment for at least a week.

Opioid withdrawal: The various medicines recommended are summarized in Table 23. The starting dose of medication needs to be decided according to amount of opioid consumed by a patient in the 24 hours period, converted into equivalent doses of compound used for detoxification. Subsequent doses needs to be adjusted according to the fluctuation in the severity of withdrawal symptoms, e.g. peak during 3rd–7th days of heroin withdrawal. Usually the doses required are 1.2–3.0 mg buprenorphine or 60–120 mg of methadone. The medicines should be tapered off by a rate of 5–25% each day, with greater reductions at initial high dose levels. Usually, detoxification medicines in opioid withdrawal are required for 2–3 weeks, though there are detoxification programs of longer duration also, e.g. 180 days methadone detoxification program. In cases of pretreated withdrawal symptoms, like insomnia restlessness and mild bodyaches persist even after 3 weeks, and can be managed symptomatically by sedatives and non-narcotic analgesics as well as nonpharmacological treatments like relaxation therapy, etc.

In accelerated detoxification, low doses of naltrexone are given to precipitate withdrawal symptoms and clonidine in usual or higher doses is used to control symptoms. This method reduces the detoxification period remarkably to 4–5 days and can be useful in patients selected for long-term naltrexone therapy.

Sedative hypnotic withdrawal: Sedative hypnotic withdrawal is managed on the lines of gradual tapering of the substance of dependence. In cases of mild-to-moderate dependence, an outpatient detoxification by tapering of the drug, with weekly reduction in doses can be carried out in well motivated patients. In patients with severe dependence, particularly with dependence on short-acting benzodiazepines, the indoor detoxification is preferred. In indoor setting, the drugs can be tapered off at a rate of 10% a day. In patients dependent on short or intermediately acting benzodiazepines like oxazepam, alprazolam, etc. risk of withdrawal seizures should be kept in mind and to prevent the seizures, detoxification is started with equivalent doses of long-acting benzodiazepines, which then should be tapered off as usual. Usually, detoxification in indoor is over within 2 weeks; however, sometimes, protracted withdrawal requires longer detoxification medication. In cases where only insomnia persists, the nonbenzodiazepine hypnotics, like zopiclone alone or with relaxation exercises, should be tried.

Nicotine withdrawal: There is no specific medication for nicotine withdrawal syndrome, which is not very florid or distressing. It is possible to tide over this period with psychological intervention, with or without benzodiazepines for a period of week or so. Use of nicotine chewing gum as a substitute over long-term makes the detoxification easier and this is recently made available in India.

Multiple substance withdrawal: In patients, where dependence to more than one substance has been clearly identified, the specific medication for each category of the substance of dependence shall be given. Frequently, patient requires inpatient treatment and the period of detoxification is longer than in patients with single substance dependence.

Long-term Pharmacological Treatment

This is intended to help patients maintain abstinence after completion of detoxification, with the use of medically prescribed drugs. As has been mentioned earlier, the treatment of substance dependence goes beyond the phase of detoxification, and the long-term pharmacological treatment must form an important part of the overall treatment, whenever it is feasible and suitable. The possibility of modifying or reverting the underlying process of neuroadaptation, which is the basis of dependence, seems unrealistic, at the current time. As such 'cure' of dependence is improbable but successful treatment with pharmacological agents is possible.

The long-term medication helps in preventing the occurrence of relapse. The other rationale for use of 'drugs' for treatment of 'drugs' is that when the patients are able to maintain abstinence, even if it is with the help of medication, they are able to overcome the psychosocial and physical consequences and get reintegrated more easily. It is expected that the learning, that occurs in this period, will continue to help on patients even after the duration of medication. In some instances, this is not possible and the medication continues for indefinite period running into many years.

Based on the mechanism which operates for maintenance of abstinence, the pharmacological agents used in long-term treatment can be classified in four categories as illustrated in Table 24.

Table 24: Pharmacological agents for long-term treatment

A	Deterrent agents	Disulfiram, citrated calcium carbimide, metronidazole, and compounds like nitrefezole
B	Substitution agents	Methadone, LAAM, buprenorphine, nicotine replacement (nasal solution, gum, dermal patch)
C	Antagonist agents	Naltrexone
D	Anticraving agents	Fluoxetine, fluvoxamine

Deterrent Agents

Alcohol sensitizing drugs act through definite chemical mechanism(s) to deter the person from drinking and hence, they are called deterrent agents. The most prominent example in this category is disulfiram (tetraethylthiuram disulfide), which is discussed here in some detail. The other agents have been used in some geographical regions at times, but have not gained wider acceptance.

Disulfiram

Disulfiram has been used in many countries for treatment of alcoholism for over forty years and extensive clinical and pharmacological information is available.

Mechanism of action: Disulfiram and its active metabolites inhibit irreversibly the activity of aldehyde dehydrogenase (ALDH), the enzyme that metabolizes acetaldehyde, the first metabolic breakdown product of alcohol. In the presence of disulfiram pretreatment, alcohol use results in the accumulation of toxic levels of acetaldehyde in liver and systemic blood circulation, which causes a host of unpleasant, potentially dangerous and rarely lethal signs and symptoms. Many metabolites of disulfiram have been proposed to be responsible for the action, but, the most important active metabolite is diethylthiomethyl carbamate (Mc-DTC). The *acetaldehyde syndrome*, as a result of the effect of disulfiram treated individuals when they consume alcohol, has been termed as *disulfiram ethanol reaction* (DER). Although it has been suggested that the effectiveness of disulfiram is only as a placebo, there is evidence for the effectiveness being linked to the DER, due to the pharmacological action, and the operant conditioning model.

The cognitive awareness of occurrence of DER and/or any previous experience of DER with use of alcohol while on disulfiram therapy, prevents a drinking response when exposed to alcohol use related cues (like persuasion by friends, company of other users social gatherings and parties). Prevention of drinking response helps to maintain abstinence. Additionally, the patient gets on opportunity to learn and practice the coping skills to restrain himself on exposure to such cues. It should be remembered that disulfiram does not reduce the craving but prevents response to craving.

Side effects and adverse reactions: The commonly experienced side effects are of drowsiness and gastric irritation. The adverse effects which occur most commonly with use of disulfiram are hepatic, neurological, skin reactions and psychosis. Few systematic investigations exist amongst many case reports. The 124 spontaneous reports from Danish physicians between 1968 and 1991, reporting to the Danish Committee on Adverse Drug Reactions (ADRs), reported 154 ADRs, the most common adverse reactions were hepatotoxicity and peripheral neuropathy. The safety of disulfiram, estimated on the amount produced and the number of reactions reported, corresponds to an intermediate rate of adverse reaction (1 per 200–2000 treatment year). The death rate with disulfiram is estimated at per 25,000 treatment year.

Contraindications: Many of the adverse reactions of disulfiram therapy are also long-term health complications of alcohol use and must be considered as contraindications for disulfiram therapy. Hepatic dysfunction, peripheral neuropathy, and psychosis are the common relative contraindications. The other relative contraindication presence of cognitive deficits because of the inability to understand and remember the consequences of alcohol use while on disulfiram. Use in first trimester of pregnancy is perhaps the only absolute contraindication.

Clinical regimen: Disulfiram should always be given after obtaining informed consent and after baseline investigations for monitoring the side effects. The usual dose is 250 mg/day; however due to metabolic differences, some patients may require a higher dose 500–750 mg/day to experience DER. It is generally dispersed in a single daily dose in the morning but a bedtime single dose has also been used.

Supervised disulfiram therapy: Disulfiram works well when its use is supervised as it ensures better compliance. Supervision can be most effective when done by spouse, though it can be done by an other family member or a supervisor at work place. Supervision also ensures that the possibility of DER is reduced. Some training of supervisor in the detection of the techniques of evasion, which the patients use, is desirable. Disulfiram in dissolved form can help decrease evasion. Unsupervised use in-well motivated patients is also in practice widely, but several randomized controlled trials have shown that disulfiram can make statistically and clinically significant contribution to treatment outcome only if its administration is carefully supervised.

Education of the patient and the supervisor: Disulfiram therapy should be initiated only after the patient and the supervisor have been informed about the rationale for its use as well as the necessary precautions, and an informed consent of patient obtained. Patient and family members should be educated about the signs and symptoms of DER, and the actions required to be taken if they notice these symptoms and/or signs.

It should be explained that DER can occur with alcohol intake even in small doses. It is a good practice that the patients be provided small cards containing the sign and symptoms of DER and necessary first aid methods in case of occurrence of DER. DER does not occur in the first week of disulfiram use and if alcohol is consumed after 5–7 days of stopping disulfiram, but can occur even up to two weeks after stopping disulfiram.

Ethanol challenge test: A challenge test by administering a small dose of ethyl alcohol to the patient, in controlled conditions in hospital setting, has been recommended by some clinicians on the premise that actual experience of the DER is likely to be more effective than the mere cognitive awareness of DER. The clinical opinion varies considerably about the usefulness of such an ethanol challenge and definitive research information is lacking. It is recommended that the option of undergoing a challenge test should be with the patient after adequate explanation. In any case, proper explanation of the rationale to the patient should be an essential prerequisite to obtaining the consent for the challenge test. The challenge test is to be carried out after a minimum of five days of disulfiram therapy at the initial daily dose of 250 mg.

Alcohol is administered, generally in the form of spirits (like whisky or rum) which have approximately 40% volume by volume content of absolute ethyl alcohol, starting with 15 mL and further supplements of 15 mL every 15 minutes up to a maximum of 90 mL. The patient's vital data are to be closely monitored all through the test, alongside maintaining a patent intravenous line should a need arise for vasopressor administration for a precipitous fall in the blood pressure. The purpose of the test is to get the patient to experience DER significantly to leave an impression. At any point of time while supplementing alcohol, if the symptoms and signs of DER are significant or the subjective discomfort of the patient is high, subsequent alcohol administration should be withheld. If it is not possible to achieve a significant DER with 250 mg of disulfiram, the dose can be increased to 500 mg and the challenge test be repeated. The dose may be required to be increased to 750 mg in some cases to obtain a good DER. It can be argued that since it is known that some patients do require higher dose of disulfiram than other patients and there is no other way of identifying these patients, challenge test is helpful in identifying these patients.

Treatment of DER: In case of a DER induced by a challenge test, the resuscitation should be and is usually available but the occurrence of a DER in uncontrolled situations is more likely to be fatal. Prompt treatment in such situations is necessary although it is mainly supportive and for controlling the fall in blood pressure. If DER is mild, assurance and oral fluids suffice. In patients with moderate or severe DER, intravenous fluids and, in some patients, dopamine infusion is necessary to control the severe hypotension. The use of antihistamines also has been recommended. The use of 4-methylpyrazole, which blocks formation at acetaldehyde, has been found to be successful but is still not common in clinical practice.

Compliance and efficacy: Although disulfiram has been in use for over forty years, it has been underused. The reasons for this include the misgivings about combining pharmacological and psychosocial methods in the treatment of alcoholism, or any other substance use disorder, as well as the myth about the lack of evidence for the effectiveness of disulfiram. In the recent years, the effectiveness of disulfiram therapy has been extensively researched into, especially the role of supervised disulfiram therapy. Azrin et al. reported on a series of studies comparing supervised and unsupervised disulfiram therapy, with a package of essentially behavioral interventions termed as *community reinforcement therapy* (CRT). The effectiveness of disulfiram therapy was demonstrated, if it is properly supervised. Another study examined the treatment outcome in a sample of 68 patients who accepted mandatory disulfiram therapy, of the 73 patients who had been offered the therapy. In this uncontrolled study, the outcome had been predefined in different categories and 27 patients (40%) had total success, 12 patients (18%) had partial success, 20 patients (29%) were considered to have failed and the outcome remained undetermined in 9 (13%) patients. The evidence for the effectiveness of supervised disulfiram therapy from these two and the other American studies has been confirmed in a multicenter British study by Chick et al., in which supervised disulfiram therapy was compared with supervised vitamin C. The results have clearly favored the disulfiram group with significant reductions in several measures of drinking behavior, including the level of GGT in the disulfiram group, compared to no reductions in these measures in the vitamin C group. A review of controlled clinical trials with disulfiram concluded that there is 'unopposed evidence for its effectiveness'.

Substitution Agents

Substitution maintenance programs derive their philosophy from the methadone maintenance program, initiated by Dole and Nyswander in 1964, as an experiment with six heroin addicts. It was suggested that high frequency of relapse in heroin addicts is due to intense craving for narcotics and it might be appropriate to target at rehabilitation rather than abstinence in these patients. It was recommended that narcotic medication (e.g. methadone), if used in these patients to satisfy their craving, will help in controlling illicit drug use and related behavior thereby making them accessible to rehabilitation. Successful initial experiment with methadone and positive outcome of subsequent use with more and more number of patients in a number of methadone programs established it as the most commonly used pharmacological treatment for heroin addiction in the US. The British experience with heroin substitution was not as much of a success, and the methadone programs have become more popular and are widely used in England and Europe as well as in many other countries.

In India, substitution maintenance program had been practised though the opium registry, wherein registered opium addicts were disbursed a certain amount of tincture opium till it was discontinued in 1959. In the period of heroin dependence in India, there has been no officially approved substitution maintenance program and the treatment has been mainly focused on the goal of total abstinence and helping the patients achieve a life style free of any substance use.

The issue of using drugs for the treatment of drugs has become very sharp and accentuated about the treatment strategy of substitution maintenance programs. Use of medications as maintenance for the control or suppression of chronic medical illness and metabolic deficiencies is well accepted. However, in spite of the recognition of substance dependence as a chronic disease which is not amenable to 'cure', many people, including psychiatrists and physicians, do not feel comfortable with the idea of maintenance therapy with substitution agents, by the same logic. Although substitution of morphine, raw opium or heroin with another opioid, which is prescribed medically, has been practised in one or other form in various countries in this century, reservations have been expressed by many people about prescribing 'addictive' drugs to addicts. The reservations have been about the moral and ethical issues involved in such a treatment strategy and about the sociopolitical considerations of the expense involved in making the lifestyle of these addicts more comfortable by providing another addictive drug. Methadone programs and the idea of substitution maintenance programs have remained somewhat controversial among treatment providers, health professionals, policy makers and the general public. This controversial position and the argument, that the science is succumbing to the vicarious needs of the socially deviant persons, has limited the benefits of substitution maintenance programs reaching larger groups, despite the positive opinion of many of the patients and the professionals involved in such programs.

In the recent years, two developments have reinforced the debate in favor of maintenance programs in general and the methadone program in particular. These are the proposition and wider research based acceptance of the biological rationale for substitution maintenance programs and the proof of their effectiveness in terms of the change in the observable outcome indicators, also based on hard research data. Biological rationale for maintenance medication is that adequate oral doses of substitution medication (methadone) will relieve the persistent narcotic craving or hunger without creating euphoria, sedation, analgesia or impaired mental or physical performance and without modifying emotional reactions. Meanwhile, the narcotic medication (methadone) will keep the body system cross tolerant to other narcotics including those abused earlier. By developing this narcotic cross tolerance or 'blockade', it blocks the narcotic effect (e.g. euphoria) of normal street doses of short-acting narcotics such as heroin. Thus, it decreases the reinforcement of heroin and the heroin taking behavior in the patient. As tolerance to methadone remains quite static, it is possible to maintain patients on the same dose for many years or even indefinitely this biological rationale has been strengthened by the research findings of many of these patients being deficient in endorphins and the evidence that by substituting the substance this deficiency is being taken care of.

Research data for the effectiveness of methadone program on outcome indicators has been accumulating for sometime and by now there is convincing evidence for significant change in the indicators of heroin use during treatment, time spent in dealing with drugs, treatment duration, crime free periods, employment, injection drug use and HIV seroconversion rates. There is also clear evidence that the cost of treatment with methadone programs is considerably lower than the cost to the society due to the active heroin addiction.

It is important that the merits and the demerits of the substitution maintenance programs be understood for making appropriate choices in individual patients as well as for larger policy decisions in the context of each region or country.

The merits of and arguments in support of substitution maintenance treatment are as follows:

- Reduction in illicit drug consumption.
- Avoidance of medical complications of impurities in street preparations, and the complications of parenteral administration and overdose.
- Better nutritional and health status, with regular monitoring.
- Decrease in criminal behavior.
- An increase in productive social behavior and psychological well-being.
- Medical management replacing penal management resulting in better retention in treatment.
- Cost effectiveness.

The demerits and arguments against substitution maintenance treatment are as follows:

- Moral issues in giving addictive drugs to addicts.
- Problem of drug use other than narcotics, e.g. alcohol, cocaine (usually injectable).
- Societal control over person who may be only socially deviant.
- State's support of opioid use and its tacit approval
- Not affecting the psychosocial disabilities of the individual addicts.
- Illegal diversion of the licit maintenance compound.

Criteria for Patient Selection

Although some treatment programs, and even countries tend to favor substitution maintenance as the treatment strategy for all the patients of opioid dependence, and some others do not use them at all, it is reasonable to consider this strategy in some patients based on the following criteria:

- Severe dependence of long duration, with significant psychosocial disability

- Past record of unsuccessful treatment attempts (at least three)
- No possibility of achieving a drug-free style
- Not in early age, preferably not below 25 years

Patient characteristics associated with success in substitution maintenance treatment are as follows:

- Age over 25 years.
- Minimal criminal involvement.
- Emotional and psychiatric stability.
- Intact social support network.
- Positive employment history at some point in time.

Substances Used for Long-term Maintenance Therapy

Opioid agonists

a. *Methadone:* It is the most commonly used agonist for maintenance therapy. It is orally effective, has long half-life, is medically safe, and does not result in euphoria and cognitive impairment. The majority of the patients require 80–120 mg/day of methadone, in a single dose. Doses below 60 mg/day have been repeatedly proven to be ineffective.

   Utility of plasma levels of methadone to decide the adequacy of doses is still controversial and is indicated in few of the selected patients. Side effects of methadone usually occur during initial phases of therapy and are minor. They include constipation, sweating, transient skin reaction, weight gain and water retention.

b. *LAAM*: Levo-alpha-acetylmethadol, a methadone derivative, is a μ opioid agonist. LAAM and active metabolites (nor-LAAM and dinor LAAM) have long half-life of 48–96 hours and hence a three times a week schedule is required, which is more convenient. LAAM has the advantage of having a lesser potential for street diversion.

Opiate partial agonists: Buprenorphine, a partial μ receptor agonist produces submaximal effect in maximally effective doses. It also has Kappa opioid receptor antagonistic properties. Since the early studies of Jasinki and Mello and Mendelson, there have been a number of studies establishing the role of buprenorphine in the treatment of opiate dependence, including its role as substitution therapy. Although it has a short plasma half-life of three hours, its duration of action has been longer, due to its slow dissociation from opioid receptors. This prolonged action of buprenorphine makes it effective when dispensed in once daily dosage or even on alternate days. Side effects of buprenorphine are sedation, drowsiness and constipation. Tolerance to these effects can be expected to develop during continued buprenorphine therapy. No apparent health risk has been reported in studies involving long-term buprenorphine therapy. Due to partial agonist property, there is a ceiling effect on the side effects, reducing the risk of severe drug induced respiratory depression. Buprenorphine is less likely than other partial agonists, to precipitate opioid withdrawal in patients already maintained on opioid agonists, such as methadone. It also eases transfer to opioid antagonist treatment.

Due to all these properties and evidence from clinical trials, there has been a strong recommendation about the use of buprenorphine as a maintenance agent in case of opioid dependence. The dosage schedule is 2–8 mg/day. In India too, many experts working in the field of drug dependence, also hold the same view on the basis of their clinical experience. However, buprenorphine does produce physical dependence. There has been a concern about increasing sublingual and parenteral use of buprenorphine, which enhances the risk of illicit channelization of buprenorphine disposed as a maintenance agent. A combination product containing buprenorphine and naloxone for sublingual use, is in experiment stages and may be become a promising agent for opioid substitution therapy, but it also has the potential of being diverted for parenteral use.

Maintenance Therapy in Other Substance Use Disorders

- *Nicotine replacement*: Use of nicotine replacement with gums or patches, is based essentially on the principle of substitution therapy and has been found to be useful in conjunction with behavioral techniques.
- *Oral substitution in parenteral substance users*: In broader term, the substitution of a more harmful route by a less harmful route (e.g. oral) without changing the substance of abuse, can be termed as substitution therapy. It will minimize the harmful consequences of use.

Maintenance Program in India

In India, the health policies do not approve any kind of substitution treatment program using agonist agents despite the opinions of experts working in this field. The need for maintenance program of this nature has been emphasized even by the Expert Committee on Drug Dependence Services in 1986. Buprenorphine can be promising as substitution therapy. However, there is need for further research in this area.

Antagonist Agents

Opioid antagonists are substances that bind to opioid receptors but do not produce morphine like effects. If an individual stabilized on opiate antagonist, consumes an opiate agonist like heroin, he will not experience the euphoric effects as the opioid receptors are already occupied and hence not available for the opiate agonist. In this manner, over time, the operantly reinforced drug seeking behavior become extinct.

In addition, due to constant occupation of opioid receptors by antagonists, physical dependence is not re-established and the conditioned withdrawal symptoms becomes extinct. These phenomena help patients in achieving a drug-free life style and brings the ideal of finding a pharmacological agent for 'cure' one step closer.

Various antagonists (like naloxone, cyclazocine and nalorphine) had been tried but were not found suitable due to their short half-life, severe side effects or lack of effectiveness through oral administration. However, the introduction of naltrexone in the early 1980s, which is effective orally, with long duration of potent antagonist action and minimal side effects, has revolutionized this approach (also called as the medical corrective method).

Naltrexone is available as 50 mg tablets, is well absorbed from the GI tract. Although its plasma half-life is about 6–8 hours, effective receptor blockade is sustained for 48–72 hours. This pharmacodynamic property of naltrexone makes it easy to be administered in simple and convenient regimens. There are three common regimens suggested, namely *daily* (50 mg/day), *thrice a week* (100 mg on Mondays and Wednesdays, and 150 mg on Fridays), *twice a week* (150 mg on Mondays and 200 mg on Thursdays).

The daily dose regimen is generally preferred over the other regimens. Naltrexone therapy should be started, only after detoxification has been completed, which can be confirmed by naloxone challenge tests. This is necessary as there is a risk of precipitation of severe withdrawal features resulting in patient's noncompliance. The common side effects of naltrexone are mild opiate withdrawal like symptoms (nausea, abdominal pain, dyspepsia), skin rash and derangement in liver function test in obese persons. The only important contraindication of naltrexone therapy is the presence of hepatic failure, though minor abnormalities in liver function need not be a contraindication. Baseline liver function tests are mandatory before starting naltrexone therapy. The duration of naltrexone therapy has been recommended to be of 6–12 months, but longer duration of this therapy has also been suggested.

The theoretical rationale for use of naltrexone and its properties had generated a high amount of optimism in the professionals working and thus field at the time of its introduction. It has been realized over the years of its clinical use that the acceptance of this therapy by the patients is low, especially since they have been aware of the substitution agents and some of the patients have had experience with substitution agents. This is understandable in view of the fact that, unlike agonists or substitution agents, the antagonists like naltrexone do not provide any effect of a 'high'. In large multimodal programs, only 5–10% of opioid dependent patients show an interest in naltrexone at a given point of time and many patients drop out early. These patients stop taking naltrexone before they have recognized the relapse factors and before they have learned the methods to handle these factors. It has been seen that appropriate patient selection and explanation of need for adequate duration of therapy can reduce the drop-out rate. The naltrexone therapy is suitable for and recommended for patients with the following characteristics:

- Younger age
- Shorter duration of dependence
- Patients with good premorbid adjustment for whom drug free life style or total abstinence is a feasible goal
- Patients who have no major underlying emotional problems
- Patients whose substance use is mainly due to environmental or conditional factors
- Patients who are health care professionals and paraprofessionals
- Patients who have been on substitution maintenance agents and are willing to shift to antagonist agents.

Naltrexone has also been reported to have modest success in the treatment of alcohol dependence in some studies. Two alternative hypotheses have been proposed for this clinical effect, viz opioid deficiency hypothesis and opioid surfeit hypothesis. This is particularly useful and worth a trial in patients who have contraindications for disulfiram therapy and in patients who are dependent on alcohol and opioid simultaneously.

Anticraving Agents

Selective serotonin reuptake inhibitors (SSRIs) have proved valuable in treatment of alcohol dependence and possibly in treatment of opioid dependence. Several animal studies had demonstrated these drugs to the effective in reducing alcohol intake, by up to 80% in some instances. Results in human studies have been favorable but more modest. Fluoxetine has been studied more extensively in clinical population and the initial impressions are of good beneficial effects in patients with definite experience of craving.

Psychosocial Treatment Methods

Psychosocial treatments for substance use disorders include a number of diverse nonpharmacological interventions, aimed at effective and comprehensive management of these disorders. These should not be seen to be at variance with pharmacological treatment methods but as complementary treatment methods which help each other. The short-comings of even the most powerful pharmacotherapies, delivered without psychosocial methods have been convincingly demonstrated. Even in situations where the principal treatment is seen as pharmacological, the psychosocial interventions are needed to complement the pharmacotherapy by:

- Enhancing motivation to take prescribed medicine,
- Providing guidance for use of medicines and their side effects
- Providing the relationship element.

Psychosocial treatments are essential for maintaining long-term abstinence and to bring about a change in lifestyle leading to complete rehabilitation.

Though some of psychosocial interventional skills require specially trained professionals, most of these skills can be acquired by general physicians, nurses, social workers and counselors making it possible to offer these interventions in a number of settings, including primary health care facilities and nongovernmental organizations working in the community. Psychosocial treatment methods include a wide range of individual therapies, group therapies, family and marital therapies, etc. All of these approaches are not to be applied concurrently in a ritualized fashion for every patient. Nonetheless, many of these modalities can be employed in various phases of treatment in the same patient. Individualized patient and family assessments hold the key to an appropriate selection of therapies.

Individual Psychotherapies

Psychoanalytically oriented individual psychotherapies tried in patients of substance use disorders before 1960 were not successful due to problems of premature termination, reaction to anxiety arousing interpretations with resumption to drug use, erratic attendance at sessions, difficulty posed by attending sessions while intoxicated, and failure to pay fees because money was spent on drugs.

However, individual psychotherapies have again been in use since the 1980s, partly as a result of the modifications in psychodynamic therapies, brief psychodynamic models to deal above problems and development of a number of other individual therapies (like supportive expressive, interpersonal and cognitive behavior therapies), as well as due to the realization of the limitations of pharmacotherapies when used alone.

Currently the use of individual psychotherapies is recommended:

- To introduce and engage a patient in treatment to enhance motivation for treatment
- To treat patients with mild severity of dependence in primary care settings
- To impart the coping skills for tackling relapse situations
- To change reinforcement contingencies, from substance use related rewards to sobriety related rewards
- To help patient improve interpersonal functioning and enhancing social support
- To help patient solidify the gains following achievement of abstinence.

Most of the individual psychotherapeutic models currently in use, viz. brief psychotherapy, supportive expressive therapy, interpersonal therapy, behavior therapy and cognitive behavior therapy, have been found to be useful as adjunctive treatment for the above-mentioned aims, with none having significant superiority over the others. The more commonly practised brief psychotherapy and behavior and cognitive behavior therapies are described here.

Brief psychotherapies: Brief psychotherapeutic interventions comprise of 1–4 sessions and are popular as they are cost beneficial. The sessions are aimed to deglamorize drug use, correct misconceptions regarding drug use and treatment, install optimism in the patient and provide a realistic feedback of the harms already caused. It simultaneously emphasizes the potential reversibility of the conditions and talks regarding need to abstain and treatment planning.

Cognitive and cognitive behavior therapies: These therapies primarily focus on individual thoughts and behaviors. These structured, focused, collaborative approaches are based on the assumption that substance abuse is mediated by complex cognitive and behavioral processes, which can be modified to decrease the drug using and other related behaviors. These therapies can be predominantly cognitive or behavioral, or can have equal emphasis on both cognition and behavior. Some of these are summarized in Table 25.

Table 25: Models of cognitive and behavior therapies for substance use disorders

	Model	*Focus*
1.	Cognitive therapy of Beck et al	Reduction in drug used by identifying and modifying maladaptive thinking patterns
2.	Relapse prevention model of Marlatt and Gordon	Cognitive behavioral approach to help patients develop greater self control in order to avoid relapse
3.	Motivational interviewing of Miller and Rollnick	Motivating patient by cognitive approach to his problem and its solutions
4.	Operant behavior therapy by Higgins et al	Involve operant rewarding or punishing of patients for desirable (e.g. adherence to treatment) or undesirable (relapse) behaviors
5.	Contigency management by Anker and Crowley	A kind of operant behavioral therapy based on use of predetermined positive or negative consequences to reward abstinence or punish drug related behaviors
6.	Cue exposure treatment	Based on Pavlovian extinction paradigm. Exposure to craving inducing cues and prevention of drug use response leads to extinction of dependence
7.	Aversion therapy	Coupling drug or alcohol use with unpleasant experience (e.g. chemically induced vomiting) to result aversion to use of alcohol/drugs. Not much in use currently

Group Therapies

Group therapy for drug dependents can be defined as "an assembly of chemically dependent patients usually 5–10 in number, who meet regularly under guidance of a professional leader (usually a professional therapist or an addiction counselor), for the purpose of promoting abstinence from all mood altering chemicals and recovery from addiction". Group is used as a medium or strategy for whatever therapeutic interventions are to be delivered.

The groups can be homogenous according to diagnosis, age, gender and treatment modality (or the target intervention e.g. relapse prevention) or heterogeneous. A good guiding principle is to allow maximum tolerable heterogenicity. The groups can be open or closed depending upon whether membership is open to new patients or not during the group process.

The therapist or the group leader is simultaneously a participant-observer and a manager of group activities, who assumes responsibility for a variety of 'executive' or group management tasks. These tasks include the following:

- Defining and maintaining adherence to the group rules
- Screening and selecting new members and preparing them for group entry, if required through one or two individual sessions prior to group therapy
- Managing problematic members, like antagonistic, argumentation, sarcastic members or silent non-participating members or intoxicated members
- Formulating specific treatment goals
- Guiding the group through sequential stages of the treatment and recovery process including management of early resistance, peer confrontation and 'slips'

The treatment goals in group therapy for substance dependents patients are as follows:

- Enhancing motivation
- Establishing abstinence
- Psychoeducation
- Establishing stable familial, social and occupational functioning
- Preventing relapse
- Addressing specific psychosocial issues identified.

Therapeutic or curative factors operating during the process of group therapy are multiple and include mutual identification, acceptance, role modeling and confrontation, reality testing and immediate feedback; positive peer pressure, affiliation, cohesiveness and social support; structure, discipline and limit setting; experiential learning and exchange of factual learning and instillation of hope. These are very similar to the curative factors operating in interactional model described by Yalom.

Due to multiple therapeutic processes involved and better time efficiency and cost-effectiveness, group therapies are regarded as a useful part of any comprehensive treatment program for drug-dependent patients. Unfortunately in India, these therapies have not been followed as much as they can be or should be followed. Our cultural characteristics of sharing life intimately with large number of people can be utilized by adopting the available models group approaches to our needs.

Family Therapy

The role of family transcends genesis, maintenance, treatment seeking, recovery as well as relapse of substance use disorders. There is a vicious cycle in which the patient's drug use adversely affects the family's well-being and coping resources. Dysfunctional and burdened families have strongly negative responses towards patients, resulting in increased substance use by patient. To break this vicious cycle, involvement of family members is needed during all the phases of treatment for substance use disorders. This is more true in the Indian context, because of the intact family systems and support, with family members having an important say in the matters of an individual and peculiar intrafamilial characteristics of the Indian families.

The kind of family therapy and the degree of family involvement in the treatment will vary according to the issues to be addressed. Mainly, one can differentiate four levels of family involvement in the treatment of substance use disorders, based on an appropriate assessment of family functioning and its relationship with the substance use.

- If the chemical dependence seems to be mainly owing to dysfunctional patterns in the family, '*family as a unit*' need to be treated with intensive family or marital therapy.
- If chemical dependence has led to dysfunction in the family, then a less intensive but active and constant participation of family members shall be sought to treat the patient while focusing on '*family as context*'.
- In all other cases, the minimum objective should be to involve family members to help and support the patient in achieving sobriety and maintaining it. This can be approved by:
  - Educating family members about the medical model of the patient's substance use disorders
  - Encouraging family support
  - Involving family members to provide necessary information about patient's attitudes, compliance, social and vocational adjustment, and degree of abstinence. The most feasible and meaningful strategy is to involve a key family member preferably the spouse of the patient, who will act as a useful ally for the treating team and a sympathetic but watchful observer for the patient.
- Family intervention is also indicated in cases where patient's abstinence upsets a previously well established but maladaptive style of family interaction and where other family members need help in adjusting to a new set of individual and goals, attitudes and behaviors. If these

issues are not identified and handled adequately through appropriate family interventions, the efforts at abstinence will be compromised, due to high probability of relapse, as family will covertly and overtly strive and work for early (mal)adjustment level to ward off the stress caused by the new set of circumstances during abstinence phase.

Relapse Prevention

Recovery, Lapse and Relapse

Recovery from a substance use disorder is the process of initiating and maintaining abstinence from the substance or substances as well as making intrapsychic and interpersonal changes towards an improvement in the quality of life. The process of recovery is not stable and is fraught with substance use, intrapsychic and interpersonal disturbances. The occasions of substance use need to be differentiated as lapses or relapses. Isolated instances of substance use are considered as lapses and relapse is defined as return to the previous pattern of use or dependent use following a period of abstinence. It is a common error on part of the patient, family members or the treating team to consider any lapse as a relapse, leading to the reactions to a relapse. It has been argued that such reactions lead to a process whereby a lapse turns to a relapse. Realistic acceptance of occasional lapses during the recovery process is necessary.

Relapse must also be differentiated from failure of treatment, which follows soon after dropout from treatment or completion of treatment. Recognition of relapse as an important phenomenon in the course of the disorder and the recovery process, which can be tackled meaningfully, can help in avoiding the sense of dejection and helplessness that surrounds the patient family or the treating team, if it is seen as a failure of treatment. The patient, the family members and the treating team can be in a better position to help in the total process of recovery if they can accept the phenomenon of relapse, alongside working towards preventing relapse.

Need and Scope

Numerous reviews of treatment outcome literature have documented high rates of relapse up to 65–80% in the first year of treatment among substance dependance disorder patients. Efforts at ensuring total abstinence in all or a majority of the patients in treatment programs have not been successful. The emphasis in recent years, has been on strategies for preventing relapse. While it can be considered unrealistic to aim at eliminating the possibility of relapse, the scope of relapse prevention should be on:

- Decreasing the number and frequency of relapses over the period of recovery
- Delaying individual instances of relapse
- Ensuring timely and appropriate management of relapses, if and when they do occur.

Strategies

Relapse prevention (RP) generally refers to two type of treatment strategies:

1. RP gets incorporated in any treatment plan aimed at helping a patient maintain abstinence. All the long-term pharmacological treatment methods and many of the psychosocial treatment methods aim to help the patient remain substance free and prevent relapse.
2. Specific strategies for relapse prevention, which incorporate the lesson learnt about the risk for relapse and the interventions or approaches which help in reducing this risk. The focus of these specific RP models is to help the patient identify the potential precipitants of relapse and the possible coping skills.

Specific Models

Many models of relapse prevention have been described in the literature and the two models commonly followed are, Daley's psychoeducative model and Marlatt's cognitive behavioral model. The various models of relapse prevention do have commonalities in the objectives and the components of the programs and focus on relapse precipitants specifically.

Objectives

The objectives of many of the relapse prevention models are:

- To develop new coping skills for handling high risk situations and relapse warning signs
- To make lifestyle changes to decrease the need for substances
- To increase healthy activities
- To prepare for interrupting lapses, so that they do not end in a full blown relapse
- To prepare for managing relapses, so that the adverse consequences can be minimized.

Components

The components of different relapse prevention models have been identified:

- Help the patient identify their high risk relapse factors and develop strategies to deal with them
- Help the patient understand relapse as a process and as an event
- Help the patient understand and deal with alcohol or drug cues, craving and social pressures to use substances
- Help the patient develop and enhance a supportive social network
- Help the patient develop methods of coping with negative emotional states

- Assess the patient for psychiatric disorders and facilitate treatment, if needed
- Facilitate the patient to learn methods to cope with cognitive distortions
- Help the patient work towards a balanced lifestyle
- Help the patient develop a plan to manage a lapse or relapse.

Relapse Precipitants

Marlatt and Gordon have classified determinants of relapse into two broad categories, intrapersonal and interpersonal determinants.

- *Intrapersonal factors* contributing to relapse include negative emotional states (most common), negative physical states, positive emotional states, testing of personal control over urges and temptations.
- *Interpersonal factors* of relapse include relationship conflict, social pressure to use substances, and positive emotional states associated with some type of interaction with others.

According to Daley, relapse can be understood as resulting from an interaction of client, family, social and treatment related factors. These include as follows:

- *Affective variables*: Negative or positive mood states.
- *Cognitive variables*: Attitudes towards recovery, self-perception of ability to cope with high risk situations.
- *Behavioral variables*: Coping skills or social skills deficits, impulsivity.
- *Environmental variables*: Lack of social or family interpersonal stability, social pressure variables to use substances, lack of leisure time/recreational activities.
- *Physiological variables*: Craving, protracted withdrawal syndrome, chronic illness or physical pain
- *Psychiatric variables*: Presence of comorbid psychiatric illness, sexual trauma.
- *Spiritual variables*: Excessive guilt and shame, sense that life lacks meaning.
- *Treatment related variables*: Negative attitudes of caregivers, inadequate after care services, lack of integrated services of dual diagnosis patients.

The focus on relapse precipitants in the research on relapse and in clinical practice with individual patients has become highly important. The role of life events in relapse has also been studied and found to be important.

Relapse Management

Management of relapse will essentially be focused on:

- Detoxification and assessment of consequences of substance use
- Assessment of the reasons and precipitants for current relapse and the past history of relapses
- Assessment of the reactions of the patient and the family members to the relapse
- Assessment of the recovery process, specifically the periods of abstinence and the factors contributing to abstinence
- Intervention for the relapse precipitants and the reaction
- Preparation for future relapses.

Indeed, the management of relapse will have to cover all aspects of the patients life situations before, during and after be relapse. It can well be said that a 'perirelapse' assessment is a cornerstone for effective relapse management.

Other Approaches to Treatment of Substance Use Disorders

The treatment modalities discussed so far, operate within the health care approach to the treatment of substance use disorders, based on the disease concept of substance dependence disorders. There are three other major treatment approaches of substance use disorders which are commonly availed of by the persons in need of help:

1. Self-help approach.
2. Social correctional approach.
3. Moralistic-religious approach.

These approaches are based on different concepts about the substance use disorders and so use different techniques. Although these are some treatment programs which adhere to one of these approaches, by and large many treatment programs and agencies do utilize techniques from more than one of these approaches. Patients do on their own, and sometimes with consent and even active encouragement of the professionals and paraprofessionals involved, avail of the services offered by agencies and programs simultaneously.

Self-help Approach

This approach can be defined as the coming together of people with similar problems to form voluntary, small groups for mutual aid. These groups, called 'self-help groups', are self-sufficient groups providing mutual assistance to members in satisfying a common need, overcoming a common handicap or life disrupting problem and bringing about desired social and personal change.

Self-help group approach in the field of substance use disorders began with the formation of alcoholic anonymous (AA) fellowship in 1935, in Europe by two persons afflicted with alcoholism, one of them being a physician. With increasing popularity and success of AA, many other programs on similar ideology developed, viz. Narcotic anonymous (NA), cocaine anonymous (CA). Similar self-help groups for the family members, friends and children of the patients (Al Anon, Al Teen, Alafam, Nar-Alon, Al Atot) for helping them cope with the substance use problem have also been popular for many years.

During last the two decades, a few new self-help groups have developed, with ideologies different from that of AA. These are Women for Sobriety (WFS), Rational Recovery (RR), Modern Management (MM), etc. However in this chapter, the ideology and approach of AA and similar groups will be discussed, as they are the most influential the world over, including India.

The programs of AA: Self-help group approach of AA is reflected in its preamble "AA is a fellowship of men and women who share their experience, strength and hope with each other that may solve their common problem and help others to recover from alcoholism". The only requirement for membership is a desire to stop drinking. Groups may or may not allow simultaneous treatment from other treatment facilities for psychiatric comorbidity, detoxification, etc.

The AA meetings are of different types, as described here. *Closed meetings,* which are meant only for AA members, i.e. persons who admit to an alcohol problem, *open meetings,* in which nonalcoholics also can participate; *speaker meetings,* in which members speak out their stories; *discussion meetings,* where brief experiences are narrated followed by detailed discussion; and *step meetings,* in which one or other of the 'twelve steps' are discussed.

All groups have many basic similarities described below:

- *Twelve traditions*: All AA groups are careful to adhere to 'twelve traditions', which are intended to preserve the integrity of AA program. These traditions reflect about the organization and policy aspects of the AA groups, by emphasizing the importance of unity, autonomous nature of the group, nonprofessional nature of the group, noninvolvement in outside issues, and anonymity, i.e. to place principles before personality.
- *Twelve steps:* The programs of AA consist of studying and following the twelve steps of AA. These steps are seen as necessary tools to be used by each AA member in the process of recovery and hence, these steps offer the person, a satisfying way of life without alcohol. It is suggested that new members start at step one and proceed sequentially at their own pace through the remaining steps. The steps involve admission of complete defeat against alcohol use; belief of dependence on 'higher power'; intensive self-evaluation and admission; self forgiveness and correction of the shortcomings/wrongs, attitudes and behaviors towards self and others; maintaining this corrected behavior; and helping others in the same way as they have been through these steps.
- *Difference from professional treatment:* In AA groups, alcoholism provides a bond among various members, while professional relationship establishes a boundary between doctor and patient. Mutual sharing of similar experiences between AA members and equality of relationship in AA members is grossly lacking in professional treatment. Moral culpability of the patient and moral superiority of helper is quite obvious in professional treatment.

Ideology of AA: The AA views alcoholism as a disease or a spiritual illness and drinking as a symptom of that illness. The central spiritual defect in 'alcoholics' is described as an excessive preoccupation with self. Treatment of the preoccupation with self is the core of AA's approach.

The theory of AA is that addiction is not a property of the drugs (alcohol) but a characteristic of the addict 'being powerless over drugs'. Indeed an 'addict' remains an addict (termed as recovering addict) even when not using drugs. Abstinence is the primary goal but the ultimate goal is the transformation of 'alcoholic' into the 'type' of person who does not drink. 'Emotional sobriety', rather than mere physical sobriety, is the goal. In fact, the twelve steps are directed mainly towards such a spiritual transformation rather than towards alcohol abstinence directly.

The dynamics of AA: There are many dynamic processes, which are presumed to be contributing towards the effectiveness of AA. These are described below:

- AA offers a nonjudgemental setting, with unconditional acceptance of the alcoholic, without inducing any guilt in him.
- The deceptively simple twelve steps provide a concrete, tangible course of action. Working through these steps triggers cognitive processes previously unformed, unfocused or abandoned, and it may encapsulate powerful dynamics capable of having an impact on craving, conditioning and character.
- Many elements of group therapy can be found operating in the group process at AA meetings. These are hope instillation by associating with sobriety, maintaining recovering alcoholics, imitation of these fellows, universality due to mutual sharing of experiences, information through conversation and group discussions, catharsis, learning of social skills, cohesiveness
- A successful deflation of pathological narcissism through twelve steps and twelve tradition might be another factor behind effectiveness of AA.

Efficacy of AA: The widespread popularity of AA and the other self-help groups the world over, in itself is an indication of the benefit they provide. Innumerable individual accounts and collective impressions have been documented about the efficacy of these approaches. Systematic evaluation for outcome, as per the models of modern science, like controlled studies have not been feasible. The AA and other groups have become sensitive to the need for systematic evaluation and collaborative research is ongoing.

The efficacy depends on retention of members and extent of participation of AA meetings. AA involvement is associated with a more stable social adjustment, more active religious life, internal locus at control and better employment adjustment.

Implications for health professionals: The indifference, bordering on distrust and antagonism between the supporters and practitioners of self-help group approach and the health care approach, has been gradually replaced by an increased sensitivity to the usefulness of each other's approach.

Despite lack of conclusive scientific evidence to support its efficacy, clinical experience does suggests that participation in self-help groups can be an important adjunct to treatment for better outcome in many patients with substance use disorders. Patients, who have experienced 'loss of control', believe in the need to abstain, have no significant psychopathology, are socially stable and show signs of religiosity, should be referred to self-help groups, besides the treatment they are receiving.

Limitations of AA: AA does not:

- Furnish initial motivation
- Provide detoxification, hospitalization, medical and psychiatric treatment, nursing care and other services which might be required during different phases of treatment
- Follow-up patients or try to control drop-outs
- Deal with the problem of multiple substance use
- Appreciate that many problem drinkers have difficulties that precede the onset of alcohol use and persists after abstinence (e.g. anxiety, depression)

Self-help groups in India: Started since 1957, at present AA meetings are held in many cities and in some towns in India. During the past decade, NA meetings have also begun in some cities. As very often these meetings are held in Churches in India, a mistaken impression is generated that these are Christianity based. It must be understood that the underlying rationale is not religion based, but rests on 'faith'. It is necessary to encourage more active referrals to AA and the other self-help groups.

Social Correctional Approach

The social correctional approach is based on the underlying premise that problematic substance use is a form of social deviance and requires only correctional methods. Many residential programs with youth in difficult circumstances and juvenile delinquents follows this premise. The therapeutic communities (TCs) have been the most prominent and well known model based on the social correctional approach.

Therapeutic community: Therapeutic community (TC) has been founded on a social learning model that fosters behavioral and attitudinal change brought by behavioral modeling and peer pressure as a result of the client's membership in a residential community (TC).

Treatment of TC is primarily indicated for patients whose lives and social interactions have come to focus exclusively on substance use and who currently lack sufficient motivation and/or drug free social support to remain abstinent in other settings of treatment. For such patients, TC provides a safe and drug-free environment in which residents learn individual and group living skills.

In TC, the person learns social values and addresses self-destructive, antisocial behavioral patterns through an intensive peer-based interactions. The person is made to learn and use social skills and assume responsibilities (take up work tasks) to help maintain the TC. As the person progresses in the treatment, more challenging and responsible assignments are earned with a higher level of status. In addition, 'morning meetings', 'encounter groups', seminars, request groups provide the opportunity to learn. Thus, TC is a powerful concept designed to provide its clients with the tools for growth in an emotional spiritual and intellectual plane.

Duration of treatment in a TC is be dictated by the time necessary to achieve specific utilization criteria that would predict a successful transition to a less structured, less restrictive treatment setting. Various studies suggest that optimum length of stay is 6 to 12 months.

Because only 15–25% of clients complete the program, the overall effectiveness is difficult to be commented upon. However, treatment completors at TCs have lower rates of relapse and better outcome at one year follow-up than do patients entering outpatient treatment.

Currently, apart from adopting social correctional approach, most of TCs has been able to modify themselves to suit the changing needs of clients. Thus, they do provide a number of other services to address issues, like medical and psychiatric comorbidity, HIV infection, educational and vocational rehabilitation.

Reasonable candidates for treatment in TC include patients who need a highly structural setting in which to initiate treatment, and patients whose level of denial is such that interpersonal and group confrontation is deemed an important part of initial approach to treatment.

Moralistic-religious Approach

These approaches are based on the premise that problem use of a substance occurs due to a moral weakness and/or due to lack of adequate religious roots. Help for problematic use is provided through religious retention and moral reduction or strengthening. Many programs and agencies have become sensitive to incorporating the themes of moral values and religion in their activities. Unfortunately, characteristics like religious commitment, religious affiliation and religiosity has been analyzed for their 'behavior predictive' value rather than being examined as significant elements potentiating recovery, maintaining sobriety, and encouraging social reaffiliation. In the countries like India, where religious faith is widely prevalent, the religiously oriented treatment approach or assessments of the nature can be suitable in the treatment of many substance use disorder patients. The full potential of this aspect remains to be understood and exploited.

Treatment of Substance-related Disorders Other than Dependence

The treatment of dependence disorders has generally been the major focus of treatment in the conceptualization and the practice of health professionals, mainly because of the proximity of the treatment methods for dependence to the medical model and the relatively well defined category of dependence disorder. The treatment of some of the other disorders due to psychoactive substance use as outlined in the ICD-10 or the substance related disorders as described in DSM-IV, do get focused on as part of treatment of dependence disorder, but often gets overlooked. The persons with use disorders like abuse or harmful use do not form a large part of the patient population seen at treatment centers or in hospital services. These persons are often found in the client population at the social services offered by the non-governmental organizations (NGOs) in the community and to the general medical services in the hospital. The comorbidity patients and the persons with substance use related medical conditions often reach the general psychiatry or the general medical services. It is necessary that the needs of the persons with all these disorders and the treatment strategies required for them are better understood than they are at present.

Treatment of Problem Use

Although these persons do not quality for any disorder in the classification systems, the persons or their families often feel the need for professional help for individual instances of problem use, e.g. road traffic accident, or acute gastritis, or substance use that interferes with one particular area of life, e.g. occupational or marital problems. Usually, the preventive methods at various levels are sufficient to help such persons tackle their problems which, if unnoticed and unmanaged, can result in more severe and diagnosable problems along the spectrum of use. The measures consists of minimal advice or single session counseling of education and provision of alternative ways of recreation or conflict resolution, development of social skills to handle peer pressure, and to cope with. It is necessary to rule out any affective, anxiety or personality disorder and treat them, if found to be present. These persons can be effectively managed by general practitioners or family physicians and counselors. Problem use in persons, who have genetically linked family members with dependence, should be focused on more intensively.

Treatment of Substance Abuse or Harmful Use

If substance use results into maladaptive socio-occupational functioning, but still does not qualify for dependence, it needs to be treated before it progresses to dependence and before the maladaptive functioning causes significant deterioration in socio-occupational life. It is generally not easy for the patients with abuse disorder to agree to the heed for treatment. It is necessary to motivate the patients to understand the concept of abuse and the possibility of progression to dependence.

The treatment methods for these patients vary considerably across different settings, but many of these patients can be managed by psychosocial interventions. They may report lack of adequate self-control despite good motivation and the presence of environmental factors maintaining the substance drug use as impediments. As such, most of the well described treatment methods are behaviorally oriented. Although it can be generally agreed that abstinence should be the goal of treatment for these patients, the debate about the feasibility of controlled use as a treatment goal assumes more validity. There is considerable scientific evidence for the goal of controlled use being achieved in many of the patients with abuse or harmful use. The patients also often do not find the goal of total abstinence necessary in the absence of dependence disorder. The issue of whether the goal of total abstinence is to be followed only with dependence disorder patients remains open.

Long-term pharmacological treatment methods, like disulfiram or naltrexone, also traditionally seem to be seen as appropriate only in cases with dependence. There is no basis for this being an absolute rule. In patients with abuse or harmful use, who may be considered fit for and accept these treatment methods, there is no reason not to use them.

Treatment of Overdose

Overdose or intoxication can occur in any user, although it is seen more commonly in abuse and dependence. Patients with overdose are often seen in emergency services and medical services, though they do present directly at the specialized treatment centers also.

General principles: The first priority in the treatment of overdose is to provide general supportive care in a safe and monitored environment and carrying out resuscitative measures. Airway obstruction, adequacy of ventilation, vital signs, cardiac rhythm and level of consciousness should be evaluated, and attended to immediately, as per the need. A complete systematic history and examination is frequently impractical in these patients. However, the initial determination of severity of overdose should be attempted by taking note of patient's general condition and the level of consciousness, suspended substance involved, its dose and route of administration, and complicated clinical situations specific to the substance. Emergency laboratory screening for substances of abuse, if available, can be useful, but it is not mandatory as it is possible to ascertain the drug overdose and to decide the management based on the clinical features.

Apart from supportive and resuscitative measures, the management of overdose should also be directed towards hastening the removal of substances from the body either by halting absorption into the body (e.g. by gastric lavage) or by increasing the excretion of these drugs or their active metabolites. In some instances, it is possible to reverse the effects of overdose by administering specific drugs that antagonize the effects of abused substance (e.g. naloxone in opioid overdose).

Principles in treatment of overdose of specific substances are:

- *Treatment of opioid overdose*: Opioid overdose should be treated as a medical emergency, as death can occur due to respiratory and CNS depression. Naloxone (0.4 mg) should be given intravenously and repeated after every 5–10 minutes till cardiorespiratory depression is reversed. Thereafter, naloxone infusion at 0.4 mg/hour should be given for a minimum of 12 hours. Emergency rooms and specialized treatment centers must ensure availability of naloxone injections. Ipecac-induced emesis or gastric lavage, followed by administration of activated charcoal, is indicated in cases of overdoses by recent ingestion. Patients having pulmonary edema require intubation, positive pressure ventilation, and intensive care.

  Opioid overdoses should not be treated by naltrexone, because it can precipitate severe withdrawal symptoms in cases of overdose in opiate dependents.
- *Treatment of alcohol intoxication*: It is largely supportive after ruling out head injury, concomitant overdoses of other drugs like barbiturates, opioids and other benzodiazepines and other causes of similar clinical picture.
- *Treatment of benzodiazepines overdose:* It is largely supportive, aimed at preventing respiratory and cardiovascular collapse. Ruling out other causes of intoxication is necessary. A benzodiazepine antagonist (flumazenil) is useful, but is not available in India.
- *Treatment of pathological intoxication*: It is supportive and symptomatic, by parenteral sedatives and physical restraint.

Treatment of Medical Complications

Most of these are direct sequele of use of substance(s) but the entire spectrum of human disease may be encountered. Management of these medical conditions is a necessary component of overall management of drug-dependence and can be even more significant in the management of harmful substance use. The medical treatment has to be selected and delivered according to the specific medical complications/ ailments (e.g. infection, nutritional deficiency, Wernicke's encephalopathy, etc.) found in a particular patient. Some of the general principles in management of medical conditions are as follows:

- The clinician should be able to understand and assess the medical and surgical problems in the patient with substance use disorders, as linked to and as a part of substance-related disorder, and hence should include the treatment of these problems in the overall treatment strategy. This is specially true for complications of parenteral substance use which should not be overlooked during assessment and treatment.
- Treatment of serious physical conditions should take priority over other components of management of drug-dependence (viz. detoxification, motivation enhancement, etc.), which might need to be postponed till the seriousness of physical condition is managed.
- Patients with severe medical complications can be better managed in general medical or surgical wards than at specialized treatment centers. However, treatment of substance use disorder (e.g. detoxification, counseling etc.) can be carried out there together with treatment of physical condition, in the medical or surgical ward.
- At the specialized treatment centers for substance use disorders, adequate facility of referral and management of physical conditions not requiring intensive care, but due medical alteration should be ensured.
- Detoxification should usually proceed slowly in these patients as they have more severe and protracted withdrawal syndromes.
- The relationship between the substance use and physical complications should be emphasized to the patient, along with the further risk of continued drug use.
- Management of medical illnesses is required more often during the initial phases of treatment but such need can arise at any phase of treatment including the aftercare phase.
- Feedback about improved health status with abstinence, e.g. improvement in liver function tests should be provided to the patient for motivation enhancement.

Treatment of Patients with Dual Diagnosis

As described earlier, a number of patients of substance use disorders have another psychiatric disorder on axis I or axis II. Management of these patients puts a tough challenge at all phases, viz evaluation, early treatment, long-term treatment for maintenance of abstinence and rehabilitation. The treatment of psychiatric disorder also requires more planning and efforts. In these patients, clinicians need not only to assess and treat the state of substance dependence/abuse and the symptoms of comorbid psychiatric illness but also to explore and monitor the possible causal relationship between the two problems.

Problem in evaluation of patients with dual diagnosis: In all patients, careful evaluation of the premorbid personality, presenting psychopathology, the characteristics and sequele of substance use and the relationship of the substance and psychopathology must be carried out. Clinicians should be particularly sensitive to the possibility of psychosis, depression, anxiety, panic attacks, suicidality, cognitive impairment and personality problems, as these phenomena are seen to occur commonly in patients with dual diagnosis. Difficulties in evaluating these patients are:

- Ascribing a particular behavior (e.g. irritability) to drug use or psychiatric illness
- Understanding the socio-occupational deterioration in the context of substance use disorder and the other psychiatric disorder
- Differentiating dependence from abuse and problem use, protracted withdrawal from symptoms of psychiatric illnesses (like anxiety and depressive disorders)
- Need for eliciting information from multiple sources
- Correlating the fluctuations in psychotic symptoms with the changing patterns of substance use.

Problems in early treatment of patients with dual diagnosis: It is difficult to find a balance between urgency and importance of the interventions required. Following guidelines are helpful to decide:

- In most of the cases, treatment of withdrawal symptoms should be administered concurrently with the treatment of severe psychotic symptoms that might interfere with early treatment compliance. Aggressive treatment of acute severe symptoms of psychosis, severe depression, and anxiety will enhance patient's ability to participate in treatment program of substance dependence.
- In a few cases, acute florid psychotic symptoms (like agitation, violent behavior, etc.) should be treated urgently, even before medication for detoxification can be given, especially when nature and severity of withdrawal syndrome is difficult to be predicted.
- In cases, where psychiatric diagnosis is still unclear and psychiatric symptoms are tolerable, one should wait till withdrawal is completed and then assess psychopathology and reach a psychiatric diagnosis before starting treatment for psychiatric illness. The same holds true for the cases where psychotic symptoms (e.g. sadness, hallucinations) are likely to be due to drug use or withdrawal.

Problems in long-term treatment of patients with dual diagnosis

- Difficulty in patient's active participation in psychosocial interventions, like psychoeducative groups, relapse prevention programs, etc.
- Difficulties in socio-occupational rehabilitation due to residual psychiatric symptoms.
- Inadequate compliance with treatment results in worsening of one disorder which in turn leads to exacerbation of the other.

Treatment of specific comorbid conditions: There are many clinical situations of dual diagnosis in various combinations of substance use and other psychiatric disorders but some of the common and important clinical situations are discussed here.

Alcoholism Patients with Depressive Symptoms/Syndrome

- *Alcoholism patients with depressive symptoms*: In the initial few days of detoxification, many patients of alcoholism experience subjective symptoms and/or demonstrate objective signs of depressive nature. These abate at a rapid pace in a majority of the patients and the initial levels of the symptomatology is not predictive of the course of symptoms. Brown and Schuckit in a study of 191 patients, found that the proportion of patients with depressive symptoms declined from 42% at intake of 6% after four weeks of inpatient stay without any specific treatment for these symptoms. It is crucial that any decision of diagnosing these symptoms or initiating pharmacological treatment be deferred for a minimum of two weeks, preferably for four weeks. In a small group of patients, who continue to have depressive symptoms, these have the potential of being 'relapse triggers'. Appropriate psychosocial treatment methods, if possible group therapy, must be considered for the management of these symptoms as well as for relapse prevention.
- *Alcoholism patient with major depression*: Although it is necessary to observe the depressive features in patients of alcoholism for a period of two to four weeks before arriving at a diagnosis, in some clinical situations, the imperative need for diagnosis and treatment is overriding, viz. in cases of major depression (DSM-IV) or depressive disorder-moderate/severe (ICD-10). Evidence from the past history as well as the family history can be helpful in reaching the diagnosis in such patients. Antidepressants must be considered in all these patients.

  The traditionally used tricyclic antidepressants have been recognized to have limitation in such clinical situation due to their sedation, cardiac toxicity and low safety profile. The never antidepressants, specifically the ones like fluoxetine and tianeptine acting through the serotonergic system, are more appropriate and are also being researched into.

  Disulfiram is known to have significant mood altering effects. In patient with significant depressive recurrences, use of disulfiram as treatment for alcoholism should be therefore considered sparingly and under regular close supervision. On the other hand, recurrence of a depressive episode can trigger a relapse of alcoholism.

- *Alcoholism patients with dysthymic disorder*: Dysthymic disorder (DSM-IV) or depressive disorder (mild) require careful evaluation for the need for use of antidepressants. Psychosocial therapies, particularly supportive psychotherapy or cognitive behavior therapy must be considered according to the suitability and feasibility. The course in these patients is marked with frequent relapses and the prognosis of alcoholism is not too favorable.

Depression Patients with Alcohol Use/Disorder

- *Major depression with alcohol dependence*: The concept of secondary alcoholism is well documented from such situations and it is quite possible to arrive at the diagnosis through careful history and examination. In the active phase of treatment for depression, the chance of the suicidal attempt will have to be recognized and guarded against. The alcohol dependence does manifest in these patients also with withdrawal features, although these may be masked or overlooked. Specific treatment for these withdrawal features must be initiated particularly thiamine supplementation. The short-term as well as long term neuropsychiatric complications of alcoholism are very often missed or recognized late due to the neglect in the depressed by the attending clinician.

  The prophylactic management in bipolar disorder with lithium can be expected to have beneficial effect on the course of alcoholism, by attenuating the euphoria with the use of alcohol. The research evidence on the use of lithium does not support the drug in primary alcoholism, but is in good support for depression with secondary alcoholism. In such patients, the problem of drug compliance can be of danger and must be attended to specifically. In unipolar disorder, if the need for prophylaxis has been established, a combination of lithium and fluoxetine seems preferred. Adequate therapeutic and prophylactic management of the affective disorder should need no major intervention for alcoholism except for a monitoring of the alcohol use pattern. If the dual diagnosis has been explained and discussed with the patient and the family members, and the affective episodes are effectively prevented, ensuring abstinence is not too difficult.
- *Major depression with alcohol use/abuse*: All the considerations for patients of major depression with alcohol dependence, about long-term management, will be highly relevant for patients of major depression with alcohol use or abuse. The task of ensuring abstinence is more difficult in these cases, owing of the weakness of the alcohol diagnosis, lack of clear management guidelines and the possibility of inadequate attention to the alcohol use patterns by the attending clinician. Indeed, in routine clinical management of depressive disorders, these aspects are often overlooked entirely or partially. The possibility of suicidal attempts has been found to be high in such cases, if not managed effectively. The treatment guidelines and programs, which have been found useful for early problems drinkers, must be considered for this group of patients. These include brief counseling, behavior therapy packages and minimal advice. They should be implemented after successful treatment of the depressive disorder.
- *Dysthymic disorder with alcohol use/abuse*: These patients have unfavorable prognosis and are often neglected in services. In view of both the disorders being of a soft and debatable nature, the patient and the physician factors contribute to the difficulty in management. Individualized treatment programs, targeting both the disorders, must be actively considered and implemented. Clinical experience as well as research information is very necessary to be generated by this group of patients.

Treatment of Anxiety and Alcohol-related Disorders

- *Treatment of anxiety in alcoholism*: Anxiety symptoms in alcoholism vary from anxiety states related to acute and protracted withdrawal to comorbid anxiety disorders. Prevalence rates for anxiety disorders in studies performed on patients in alcohol treatment programs range from 16 to 60%.

  A proper assessment of symptomatology and its temporal relationship with alcohol use is essential. It may be good to delay any definite diagnosis of an additional anxiety disorder till the patient has abstained from alcohol for 2 weeks. The main classes of medications used in anxiety disorders, which include monoamine oxidase inhibitors, tricyclic antidepressants and benzodiazepines, are all contraindicated in patients who are abusing alcohol. Patients who take benzodiazepines along with alcohol, even in small amounts, are at risk for developing increased tolerance and dependence on both the alcohol and benzodiazepines. For patients, who had moderated or stopped drinking, guidelines similar to treatment of anxiety syndromes should be used. Anxiolytic agents should be administered to patients who experience anxiety disorders separately from any problems related to alcohol. However, it is vital to prescribe short courses where symptoms are closely monitored, and in combination with psychological treatments. Longer acting benzodiazepines are preferred because of lower abuse liability, though daytime drowsiness and cumulative toxicity is a problem.

  It has been proposed that there is no clear evidence that alcohol interacts with buspirone and this drug can be used in the treatment of anxiety syndromes in alcoholics.
- *Treatment of alcohol use in anxiety disorder*: On the other hand, alcohol-related disorders can occur in patients with anxiety disorders. It has been shown that 28% of patients with panic disorder have a history of alcohol problems. It has also been found that 17.3% of patients

with agoraphobia, panic, simple or social phobia, and generalized anxiety disorder scored in the alcoholic range on MAST.

In patients with anxiety disorders, who also abuse alcohol for its anxiolytic properties or other reasons, management should involve patient education and advice envisaging total abstinence. If abstinence cannot be achieved on outpatient basis, then patient may be treated in an inpatient setting wherein both the goals of proper management of anxiety symptoms and abstinence from alcohol can be achieved. The subsequent treatment of anxiety disorders should be carried out with pharmacological and/or relaxation and behavioral techniques, along with patient education at avoiding alcohol self-medication.

Treatment of Patients with Cannabis Use and Other Psychiatric Disorders

- *Psychosis in cannabis use*: Acute psychosis has been found to be associated with heavy cannabis use or increased cannabis use in individuals having history of chronic cannabis use in low doses. Acute psychosis in cannabis users commonly is characterized by amorphous mixed type of picture along with altered sensorium and is self-limiting with in few hours to few days. This does not require any specific treatment, except benzodiazepines. Antipsychotics should be avoided as far as possible in initial few weeks and if necessary, patient should be hospitalized in a restrictive setting. If the symptoms persist beyond initial two weeks then antipsychotics should be started and should be withdrawn after 3–6 months.
- *Cannabis use in psychosis*: Cannabis use can trigger psychosis in psychosis prone individuals, can worsen the symptoms in individuals with preexisting psychosis, and can compromise the effectiveness of treatment in patients already on treatment. At this stage, the patient is not amenable to any counseling or advice regarding control of cannabis use and hence, it is warranted that patient is put under restrictive inpatient care to achieve abstinence from cannabis. After abstinence is ensured and psychotic symptoms have been well controlled, it is possible to educate and counsel the patient about the role of cannabis use in the worsening of his psychiatric condition and the need for total abstinence.

Patients with Substance Use Disorders and Personality Disorders

Treatment of these patients is difficult in terms of the relationship problems and adherence to the treatment. These patients tend to carry their personality traits to the treatment setting and repeatedly test limits with the individual treating members and the team. It is generally difficult to treat these patients effectively in general medical or even general psychiatric settings. It is possible to plan treatment in general psychiatric setting, if treatment setting can be restrictive and structured, and it can be ensured that the entire treating team is able to maintain a consistent policy of limit setting with empathy and concern. Even with these provisions, many hospital-based treatment centers are not in a position to ensure the retention of such patients in treatment and it is prudent to accept the limitation of health care approach to treatment. These patients should be more appropriately managed in treatment programs based on social correctional approach entirely or following treatment in a hospital setting. Residential rehabilitation programs in therapeutic community model or other models are suitable for the treatment and rehabilitation of this group of patients.

Treatment Issues in Special Groups

- *Women patients*: Women with substance use disorders have been stigmatized intensely, which has lead to increased barriers to their treatment and excessive victimization of these women. Even the research has discriminated, as most of the studies have used male population exclusively. Recent focus on dependent women has revealed that there are certain differences in the course and pattern of substance use disorders in women and treatment of women patients needs to focus on certain issues specific to women.

  It has been found that women start substance use at a later age but appear for treatment at about the same age as male patients do. The quantity of substance use is less in women and they more often tend to use licit substances. Many women coming for treatment are likely to have a spouse with substance use disorder.

  They are more likely to have comorbid axis I illness, depression being the commonest one.

  Specific issues in the management of women patients include a comprehensive diagnostic assessment, evaluation and treatment of family members, education about maternal and child health issues in relation to substance use, parenting education and child care services. Treatment outcome studies have found no significant difference in the outcome of treatment in women as compared to men.
- *Physician patients*: Physicians and other health care professionals, who are dependent on substance(s), require different treatment strategies and their rehabilitation in the same profession poses difficult problems. No specialized facilities exist in India for such patients. The general attitudinal barriers in physicians and the other health professionals about their own health needs and the defences specific to the issue of substance use makes the treatment of such patients a more challenging task. All the same, the attitude of the treating team needs to be

empathic and rooted strongly in the disease model of use disorders.

- *Ex-patients on treatment team*: The phenomenon, so common in the West, of ex-patients continuing to work on treatment teams or health care professionals recovering from dependence also continuing to function on treatment teams, is still very uncommon in India. Some voluntary agencies have ex-patients on their teams. Some problems of such an arrangement can be raised, but clearly there are many advantages for the team and the individuals in particular. The phenomenon is likely to catch on and some precautions need to be planned and implemented to avoid counterproductive results.
- *Children of patients*: With the proliferation of substance abuse problem in general and the increased population of women patients in particular, there has been a recognition of a distinct population, the children of substance abusers who are known to have unique characteristics, that require special attention. It is being increasingly documented that these children are at risk for serious educational, medical and emotional problems and have the potential for abusing substances as well as an increased risk for HIV infection. Comprehensive drug treatment services must include services for parents as patients and must address the special needs of the children of patients through services, like day care facilities, parenting skill training and school facilities.

SUMMARY OF NICE GUIDANCE

Alcohol dependence affects 4% of people aged between 16 and 65 years in England (6% of men and 2% of women), and over 26% of all adults (38% of men and 16% of women) consume alcohol in a way that is potentially or actually harmful to their health or well-being. Yet currently only 6% of people who are alcohol-dependent receive treatment. Alcohol dependence is characterized by withdrawal, craving, impaired control, and tolerance of alcohol and is associated with a higher rate of mental and physical illness and a wide range of social problems. Harmful drinking is a pattern of alcohol consumption that can lead to psychological problems such as depression, accidents, injuries, and physical health problems such as pancreatitis. Alcohol misuse is also an increasing problem in children and young people, with over 24000 treated in the NHS for alcohol related problems in 2008 and 2009. Hospital admissions related to alcohol consumption increased by 81% between 2003 and 2009. Harmful drinking and alcohol dependence therefore represent a considerable burden to individuals, their families, and wider society.

This chapter summarizes the most recent recommendations from the National Institute for Health and Clinical Excellence (NICE) on the diagnosis, assessment, and management of harmful drinking and alcohol dependence.

Recommendations

The NICE recommendations are based on systematic reviews of best available evidence and explicit consideration of costeffectiveness. When minimal evidence is available, recommendations are based on the Guideline Development Group's experience and opinion of what constitutes good practice.

Identification and Initial Assessment

- Staff working in services provided and funded by the NHS should be competent to identify harmful drinking and alcohol dependence and to initially assess the need for an intervention; if they are not competent, they should refer people who misuse alcohol to a service that can provide such an assessment. Validated tools such as the alcohol use disorders identification test (AUDIT) are effective in identifying harmful drinking and alcohol dependence in nonspecialist settings such a primary care and acute hospitals.
- Consider a comprehensive assessment for all adults referred to specialist alcohol services who score more than 15 on the identification test This should assess multiple areas of need, be structured in a clinical interview, and cover:
  - Alcohol use, including consumption and patterns of drinking; severity of dependence (using the severity of alcohol dependence questionnaire (SADQ) or Leeds dependence questionnaire (LDQ)); and alcohol-related problems (using the alcohol problems questionnaire (APQ))
  - Misuse of other drugs, including over the counter-medication
  - Physical health problems
  - Psychological and social problems
  - Cognitive function (using, for example, the minimental state examination)
  - Readiness and belief in ability to change.

All Interventions for Harmful Drinking and Alcohol Dependence

- All interventions for harmful drinking and alcohol dependence should be delivered by appropriately trained and competent staff. Drug interventions should be administered by specialist and competent staff. Base psychological interventions on a relevant evidence-based treatment manual, which should guide the structure and duration of the intervention.
- Carry out a motivational intervention as part of the initial assessment to help engage the person in treatment from first contact. The intervention should include helping people to recognize problems related to drinking and resolve ambivalence; encouraging positive change;

and adopting a persuasive and supportive rather than argumentative and confrontational position.

- For all interventions, staff should:
  - Receive regular supervision from individuals competent in both the intervention and supervision
  - Routinely use outcome measurements to ensure that the person who misuses alcohol is involved in reviewing the effectiveness of their treatment
  - Monitor and evaluate the person's adherence to treatment and their own practice competence for example, by using videotapes and audiotapes and external audit.

Psychological Interventions for Harmful Drinking and Mild Alcohol Dependence

For harmful drinkers and people with mild alcohol dependence, offer a psychological intervention (such as cognitive behavioral therapies, behavioral therapies, or social network and environment based therapies) focused specifically on cognitions, behavior, problems, and social networks that are related to alcohol.

Assessment for Assisted Alcohol Withdrawal

- For those who typically drink over 15 units of alcohol a day and/or score 20 or more on the identification test, consider offering:
  - Assessment for and delivery of a community-based assisted withdrawal, or
  - Assessment and management in inpatient care if you have safety concerns about a community-based assisted withdrawal.
- Consider inpatient or residential assisted withdrawal if the person meets one or more of the following criteria:
  - Drinks over 30 units of alcohol a day
  - Has a score of more than 30 on the severity of alcohol dependence questionnaire
  - Has a history of epilepsy or of withdrawal related seizures or delirium tremens during previous assisted withdrawal programs
  - Needs concurrent withdrawal from alcohol and benzodiazepines
  - Regularly drinks 15–20 units of alcohol a day and has psychiatric or physical comorbidities (for example, chronic severe depression, psychosis, malnutrition, congestive cardiac failure, unstable angina, chronic liver disease) or a learning disability or cognitive impairment.

Interventions for Moderate and Severe Alcohol Dependence

- After a successful withdrawal for people with moderate and severe alcohol dependence, consider offering a camprosate or oral naltrexone in combination with an individual psychological intervention (cognitive behavioral therapies, behavioral therapies, or social network and environment-based therapies) that focuses specifically on alcohol misuse. At the time of publication (mid-February 2011), oral naltrexone did not have UK marketing authorization for this indication. Obtain and document informed consent before prescribing.
- Consider offering interventions to promote abstinence and prevent relapse as part of an intensive and structured community-based intervention for people with moderate and severe alcohol dependence who have:
  - Very limited social support (for example, they are living alone or have very little contact with family or friends)
  - Complex physical or psychiatric comorbidities
  - Not responded to initial community-based interventions to promote abstinence or moderate drinking.

Interventions for Children and Young People Aged 10–17 Years Who Misuse Alcohol

- For those with limited comorbidities and good social support, offer individual cognitive behavioral therapy
- For those with significant comorbidities and/or limited social support, offer multicomponent programs (such as multidimensional family therapy, brief strategic family therapy, functional family therapy or multisystemic therapy).

Interventions for Depression or Anxiety Disorders in Alcohol Misuse

Treat the alcohol misuse first as this may lead to improvement in the depression or anxiety. If depression or anxiety continues after three to four weeks of abstinence from alcohol, assess the depression or anxiety and consider referral and treatment in line with the relevant NICE guideline for the particular disorder.

Overcoming Barriers

Poor recognition of alcohol misuse is a major barrier to effective treatment and requires a service—wide approach to improve case identification. Current service delivery also fragmented, with access pathways to services unclear to both patients and professionals. To clarify care pathways and properly implement this and other NICE guidance that relates to alcohol uses NICE is currently developing an integrated care pathway for the three pieces of guidance.

Limited availability of specialist alcohol services also hinders effective guideline implementation—for example, there is a lack of skilled staff to deliver evidence-based psychological interventions and support intensive

Table 26: Some important myths and facts about treatment of substance use disorders

1.	Myth	Detoxification is equivalent to treatment
	Fact	Detoxification is only the initial phase in the long-term process of treatment
2.	Myth	Inpatient treatment is necessary and outpatient treatment does not work
	Fact	Outpatient treatment is feasible and is effective in selected patients
3.	Myth	More intensive treatment is more likely to succeed
	Fact	Shor-term, less intensive treatment or minimal treatment can be effective in some patients
4.	Myth	Total abstinence is the only treatment goal for dependance disorder
	Fact	Other treatment goals like controlled use or substitution maintenance age feasible and worth pursuing in suitable patients
5.	Myth	Relapse indicates that the treatment has failed
	Fact	Relapse is a part of the recovery process and not failure of treatment
6.	Myth	Any one treatment method is superior to other treatment method(s)
	Fact	Different treatment methods suit different patients and no one method is superior to the others for all patients
7.	Myth	Combining more than one treatment method has no advantage
	Fact	Multimodal treatment is superior to any single treatment method
8.	Myth	It is an individual's problem and the treatment has to be focussed on the individual
	Fact	Involvement of a key family member, preferably the spouse helps in the treatment
9.	Myth	Uniform structured programs for all patients are more effective
	Fact	Structured programs with flexibility for individual needs and matching of patients with treatment methods are more effective
10.	Myth	Patients who join treatment do so either entirely voluntarily or due to coercion and those who join voluntarily fare better in treatment
	Fact	There is some element, in varying degrees, of voluntariness and coercion in all patients and there are no group differences in the outcome of voluntary and coerced patients

community-based assisted withdrawal, and limited prescribing of cost effective medication, such as a camprosate and oral naltrexone to prevent relapse in moderate to severely dependent drinkers. Guideline recommendations on these interventions will need to be supported by effective commissioning.

Myths about Treatment

Although some of the issues in the field of substance use disorders are getting classified, quite a few myths continue to prevail. These myths abound not only amongst the patients and their family members but also in health professionals, including psychiatrists. Table 26 provides some of these myths and facts, as per the current scientific knowledge. These are fine points and gray areas about some of these issues, but by and large the consensus is clear enough to be record these as facts. It is important to clarify these myths for psychiatrists as well as primary care physicians and counselors.

NATURAL HISTORY AND OUTCOME

NATURAL HISTORY OF DRUG USE

Experimental drug use may be a form of normal adolescent risk-taking behavior. The nature of the initial experience and peer group influences determine whether the individual moves from experimental to more regular use.

The consumption of one drug increases the likelihood of consuming other drugs, so that those who consume tobacco are more likely to take cannabis and those who use cannabis are more likely to consume other illicit substances but this relationship is neither causative nor predictable. Heroin and cocaine are similar to nicotine in their reinforcing properties and regular use is more likely to be associated with dependence. The longitudinal study of Jessor cohort indicates that growth into adult responsibilities or jobs, marriages and children is a conveyance towards social conformity, which is associated with less drug use and less problem drug use. This is postulated as the maturing out hypothesis by Winnick. In a 20-year follow-up of 100 heroin addicts in New York by Vaillant, it was found that 23% were dead, 35% were stable and abstinent and 25% have continued using opiates. In a recently completed 22-year follow-up study of London heroin addicts, 56% were off opiates, 21% were using and 10% were dead. All long-term follow-up studies agree about the high mortality from drug use related complications as well as a higher proportion of maturing out of drug use among heroin 'addicts', who have been in treatment as well as in those who were not in treatment contact.

Similar findings have also been reported for persons with regular cocaine use. The natural history of alcohol use disorders has been studied more extensively but the findings continue to be variable. The recent research has shown that the course of alcoholism is a process of flux. It is a relapsing and remitting disorder, rather than one that is necessarily progressive. It was demonstrated in a review of 13 treatment samples that remission rates ranged from 21–80%, over a follow-up period of 8–20 years. In the longer term, improvements in drinking behavior appear to be related to improvements in psychosocial functioning. Most clinics and treatment programs demonstrate a degree of improvement in the short-term, but six months or a year of abstinence does not necessarily equate with long-term abstinence.

Need for Treatment Evaluation

There are great variations in program size, setting, organization, approach, services and funding among various treatment modalities described in previous section. There is a need to evaluate the effectiveness of treatment of substance use disorders, as well as to evaluate the comparative effectiveness of different treatment modalities and approaches to approve their use while planning substance use control strategies at macro level and to help clinician deciding their patients' treatment strategies at micro level. Treatment evaluation is also required to study various factors in terms of patient characteristics and treatment characteristics which influence the treatment outcome and hence knowledge of these factors helps in better matching of the treatment with patients, Lastly, critical evaluation of effectiveness at each of the treatment components of a particular treatment modality or approach is helpful in improving the effectiveness of individual treatment modalities.

Summary of the Outcome Findings

The findings of outcome studies in 1970s were discouraging. The Rand report on the outcome of interventions for control of alcohol drinking concluded that "relatively uniform and low rates of remission for different treatment modes tend to contradict theories that alcoholism must be treated by dealing with deeper psychological problems". Edwards et al. came to even more sceptical conclusion that adequate treatment of whatever form was no better than simple advice. Similarly, high rate of relapse after treatment for dependence another substances were reported in many outcome studies. All these findings resulted into therapeutic nihilism, which prevailed among the health professionals and others working in this area during that period and people started thinking whether there is a need of any treatment of these patients, as there was general impression that the outcome after treatment in these patients was no different from that of the natural history of substance dependence. It was believed that the outcome with intervention as well as outcome in natural history was a result of maturing out effect with the increasing age and increasing social obligations. This held specially true for heroin and cocaine dependence.

However, during last two decades, the picture is changing. Three national multiprogram studies have been developed to described the effectiveness of various treatment modalities in USA. These are the drug abuse reporting program (DARP), the treatment outcome studies (DATOS). In addition, there has been a number of studies of individual programs. Common outcome criteria used in most of these studies are decrease in use of substances, decrease in crime and increase in socio-occupationally productive activity. The overwhelming weight of the evidence from these studies and carefully designed epidemiologic outcome studies is that treatment contributes significantly to change in patients behavior during and after treatment. The major reviews of treatment outcome studies have concluded that treatment is effective. A more limited number of studies indicate that the benefits of these changes considerably out weight the cost of treatment. However comparative costeffectiveness at one treatment modality over others has not been conclusively proven.

Various Predictors of Outcome

Clinicians as well as researchers are interested to know the various factors which can predict the outcome of the treatment. Out of these factors that predict the outcome, the patient and disease variables have been studied extensively and are found to exert a crucial influence on the outcome. Some of the important factors are locus of control, intrinsic and extrinsic motivational factors, premorbid adjustment, stressful life situations, and post-treatment stress score, marital status and social support, age at onset of dependence, duration of dependence, experience of treatment related abstinence and presence of associated psychopathology.

Variables Affecting Treatment Process

Treatment of substance use disorders as currently rendered is a complex, multifaceted process delivered in a variety of contexts and environments to clients having different characteristics and undergoing behavioral and cognitive changes at different rates. A number of factors influence independently as well as interactively the process of treatment as well as its outcome. The information about these factors can be useful in choosing the suitable treatment modality by treatment matching, determining the overall management strategy and in enhancing the treatment effectiveness by modifying these factors wherever possible.

Due to inherent long standing bias in medical health care model of considering the patient to be responsible for efficacy of treatment, until recently, patient characteristics were the main focus of attention of professionals while studying the factors in treatment process and outcome.

However, healthcare settings and the professionals therein possess their own characteristics that may influence the process of treatment favorably or otherwise. Often either of them is taken into consideration individually and sometimes they are considered together. In reality, there is a complex interplay of these variables during the treatment process which can be better understood by a three dimensional model of treatment process. The relevance and the applicability of such a three-dimensional model for the treatment process and outcome have been high in the Indian context also, based on clinical experience.

This 3D model categorizes the variables on factors influencing the treatment process into patient variables, treatment variables and therapist variables (Table 27). The model proposes that the treatment process be understood as an interplay of these factors in three-dimensions occurring in the context of the society which could be conceived as fourth dimension or as a larger background.

PREVENTION

In view of the adverse socioeconomic, legal and health consequences of substance use disorders and the chronic relapsing nature of these disorders making their cure difficult, it is apparent that prevention is the most useful approach to the menace of substance abuse. Prevention of substance use has been conceptualized in terms of supply and demand reduction models and as primary, secondary and tertiary prevention. Each encompasses a different aspect of prevention and has substantially different operational implications.

Supply Curtailment and Demand Reduction

Supply curtailment strategies are based on the assumption that by controlling the availability of substances, their use can be decreased. These strategies aim to decrease the use by one of the following:

- Measures to break the cycle of drug production from source to consumer by:
  - Crop eradication/control.
  - Substitution and alternative development of the cultivation areas.
  - Detection of illicit laboratories.
  - Suppression of illicit trafficking.

Table 27: Variables affecting treatment process and outcome

Patient variables		*Treatment variables*		*Therapist variables*	
A.	*Sociodemographic variables* 1. Age 2. Gender 3. Education 4. Occupation 5. Employment 6. Marital status 7. Social support	1. 2. 3. 4. 5. 6. 7. 8.	Settings Nature of treatment viz inpatient versus outpatient Type of treatment Single versus multimodel treatment Duration of treatment Availability of aftercare services Laboratory facilities Participatory nature of treatment	A.	*Personal variables* 1. Sociocultural background 2. Familial origins 3. Moral values 4. Attitudes 5. Personality characteristics 6. Use or dependence
B.	*Disease variables* 1. Age of onset 2. Duration of dependence 3. Severity of dependence 4. Type of drugs 5. Single or multiple drug use 6. Route of administration 7. Physical health damage 8. Associated psychopathology 9. Criminality 10. Previous treatment attempts 11. Expectancy from treatment 12. Motivation for treatment	9.	Flexibility of treatment program	B.	*Professional variables* 1. Professional speciality 2. Conceptual framework 3. Length and nature of professional experience 4. Administrative support 5. Carrier prospects and benefits

- Market disruption strategies aimed at dismantling criminal organizations.
- Effective monitoring of sale/dispensing of medically used abusable drugs, e.g. injection morphine and licit substances like tobacco and alcohol.

Demand reduction strategies aim to reduce the need or demand of the substance of abuse by dissuading, discouraging and deterring the individuals from either using drugs or desiring to use drugs. The following measures are included in demand reduction strategies.

- Prevention of the onset of substance use.
- Provision of help and encouragement to those who have already taken substances to discontinue use and maintain abstinence.
- Provision of advice and treatment for problem or dependent users whereby the harm to the users themselves and to society can be limited.

The supply and demand reduction model of substance use control can also be viewed in the context of classical public health model for disease control in terms of interaction among the triad of host, agent and environment. While the supply curtailment measures can be seen as analogous to the measures for control of agent, the demand reduction measures focus mainly on the host factors, and to some extent, on the environmental factors. It is also worth highlighting that the agents, i.e. substances targeted in supply reduction strategies are predominantly the illicit substances while the health hazards are documented conclusively to be more frequent and severe with the use of illicit substances like tobacco and alcohol which are tactically kept out of supply control measures due to the major revenue returns for the governments of most of the countries. This is the '*prevention paradox*' and needs to be corrected with some measures to limit the supply of licit substances, if not their complete prohibition.

Levels of Prevention

The various demand reduction measures can operate at the levels of primary, secondary or tertiary prevention.

- *Primary prevention*: Interventions to prevent the occurrence of the substance abuse and hence these are designed to reach individuals before they have developed specific substance use disorders. The focus of primary prevention is to provide information and educate various target groups within the general population about psychoactive substances and the risks associated with their use. Educational services aim to strengthen the individual's self-esteem and resistance to peer pressure, promote healthy lifestyles and provide a supportive environment and the opportunity to develop skills. Some of the important aspects of primary prevention are discussed in later part of this section.
- *Secondary prevention*: Early detection and appropriate treatment of those already affected by substance use disorders. It includes counseling services to motivate them to cease the substance use and various treatment regimens. These aspects have been discussed at length in the section on treatment.
- *Tertiary prevention*: Preventing the progression of a well established disorder to the point of disability, and rehabilitation of the substance users and their reintegration in the society. Various strategies and measures to reduce the adverse consequences of substances abuse falls under tertiary prevention. The medical strategies and technologies for this purpose have been described to some extent in the earlier section on treatment of medical complications and follow the general principles of medical management. Details of these are beyond the scope of this chapter, but the harm reduction perspective, which is not commonly discussed or understood, merits elaboration. This perspective has been briefly described in a later part of this section.

Primary Prevention

Strategies for Primary Prevention

The strategies for primary prevention of substance use disorders, or substance use itself, have evolved over the past few decades, based on the changing needs in the context of the emerging problems from time-to-time, the experience with prevention programs which have been implemented and the theoretical understanding of the complex process of bringing about behavior change. There is no unitary or final answer to the question of which strategy is most effective for substance use prevention. The lessons from the experiences gained can provide some indication of what strategies are likely to be effective or otherwise. Some of the important strategies which have been used in this field have been described here.

Information dissemination: Based on a rational model of human behavior, this approach assumes that exposure to factual information about adverse consequences of substance use will bring changes in attitudes which, in turn, will lead to nonsubstance use behavior. Various public information campaigns through mass media, health exhibitions, seminars and school programs through guest lectures, postures, educational films are examples of this approach. Over time, the focus of the information has changed from scare techniques and moral appeals through impartial intellectual information to the positive aspects of substance free life. The empirical researches about the effectiveness of information dissemination approaches indicate that they increase the knowledge but do not reduce or prevent the substance use. Some studies have even suggested that this approach may lead to increased use, possibly due to stimulation of adolescents curiosities.

Extensive experience and research, in the international field over the past few decades, with the strategies which are only information based, has led to the conclusion that they are unlikely to yield desirable effects for behavior change if used independently. As such, mere awareness campaigns or information based prevention programs, although useful in disseminating the knowledge, cannot serve the purpose of bringing about change in substance use.

Affective education: This strategy focuses on increasing self-understanding and acceptance through activities like values clarification and responsible decision making, improving interpersonal relations by fostering effective communication, peer counseling and assertiveness, and increasing individual ability to fulfill their basic needs through existing social institutions. This strategy did generate some enthusiasm and has been utilized often, but the research evidence for the effectiveness of this strategy has been equivocal. There is some evidence for the technique of peer counseling being well accepted and effective.

Providing alternatives to substance use: This strategy aims at restructuring the environment to provide individuals the alternatives to substance use and activities associated with substance use with assumption that if they are provided with real life experiences which are as appealing as substance use, their involvement in these activities will prevent their involvement in substance use. The basic premise is the acceptance of the psychobiological need that young persons have for exciting experiences and providing the nonchemical means for meeting with this need. It is also necessary that the young persons are aware of this possibility of an 'alternate high' and are encouraged to choose the alternate means of achieving a high instead of the use of abusable substances. Music, sports, religious activities are some of the common means of achieving an alternate high and the availability and promotion of various youth centers, sports and hobby clubs, community centers is helpful in channelizing the energy of the youth in more adaptive means. It has been pointed out that alternatives which are appropriate to prevent substance use are likely to be those which would have the least interest for individuals at high risk for using substances. As such, this strategy will require to be devised carefully keeping in mind the belief systems and needs of the youth and will have to be appealing enough to be chosen over the activity of substance use. The experience with this strategy has been very positive and it has been suggested to be incorporated in all youth development activities and programs.

Resistance skills training: This strategy is based on the influence of social factors, specifically the peer influences, in the initiation and continuation of substance use. The influence of the peers or other social groups, in a real life situation of substance use, operates through persuasion, challenging the masculine image, isolation or even coercion. The basic human need to belong to a group and acceptance in a group, alongside the influence that the glamorization of substance use in the audiovisual media, makes the peer influence and the other social influences effective. The resistance skills training strategy not only includes the awareness of these influences so that individuals are able to recognize and avoid the situations in which these influences are likely to be operating, but also preparing the individuals in the skills to resist the influences. These skills include the various practical aspects of tackling such situations by communicating refusal in an effective manner and asserting one's right to choose if one uses the substance or not. The effectiveness of resistance skills training has been well documented.

Personal and social skills training: This strategy used either alone or in combination with resistance skills training aims to impart a number of generic skills for coping with life as a whole. The skills include general problem solving and decision making skills, anxiety and stress relieving skills, general assertive skills and general social skills. Individuals can be taught to apply these skills for dealing with many of the challenging situations including those which can lead to substance use. Evaluation studies of this strategy have demonstrated significant behavior change effects. To maximize the effectiveness, this strategy should be used in combination of resistance skills training.

Health promotion: This strategy focuses on the larger issue of health promotion, by encouraging the choice of healthy lifestyles and reducing the unhealthy lifestyles or behaviors like substance use. The strategy has the advantages of being integrative and not focusing on one isolated issue like substance use, but requires a very different perspective and a collaborative effort from many disciplines and agencies. The experience with this strategy has been rewarding and it has been suggested that while specific targeted prevention strategies for substance use will need to be continued, all efforts should be made to integrate the issues of substance use prevention in the larger programs on health promotion.

Implementation of the Prevention Strategies

The implementation of the prevention strategies needs to be done based on the aims, the scope and the availability of resources.

- *Institution based*: Prevention programs in institutions like the educational institutions, factories, jails and other such places, have to be carried out with the active administrative support of the institutions, but have the advantage of a preexisting infrastructure and organization. The implementation can be swift and comprehensive services can be delivered at less of a cost and evaluations are easily possible to be carried out. The needs of these groups can be met within a uniform program easily, but the reach of the program remains limited.

- *Target group based*: Organizations devoted to specific population groups like women, youth and other such groups which have their distinctive needs can be encouraged to implement programs for substance use prevention. These programs quite often in the voluntary sector or the nongovernmental organizations (NGOs), working with these population groups and can become a part of their larger framework.
- *Risk group based*: Prevention programs targeted at specific vulnerable groups like the children of substance abusers, children of broken families, children in difficult circumstances (e.g. street children), unemployed youth, drivers, commercial sex workers and other such risk groups require a broader base for implementation since these groups are widely distributed in the community. The reach of these programs is larger, but evaluation of these programs are more difficult and expensive.
- *Community based*: The target in broad based prevention programs can be entire community and the reach is aimed to be the widest. These programs are expensive, difficult to evaluate and implement, and by necessity become reductionist since the needs of all the varied groups in the community have to be met with. Campaigns through the mass media, outreach prevention programs and legislative controls (e.g. about not smoking in public places) are some of the examples of such large scale community based programs. Integrating substance use preventive measures with the existing programs in health, social services, youth development or juvenile correction also serve the same purpose of community based prevention.

Harm Reduction Perspective

The improbable nature of the goal of making human existence drug-free for individuals in treatment and for community or sometimes in larger prevention efforts, has been realized in some ways since the later part of the 19th century and the early part of the 20th century. The morphine maintenance programs in USA in early 20th century, the program in UK in the middle of this century and the opium registry in India in the first half of this century are indicative of the underlying assumption that is better for both the individual and the safety for four on reducing the risk and the farms of continued drug use than to four solely on making people drug free. The American experience of total population of alcohol in the 1920s and its failure leading to its retraction in the early 1930s is a phenomenon reflective of the improbable task of making a society free of a substance of abuse. The human propensity for chemical substance use for pleasure or relief from unpleasant mental states, the fiscal and political issues involved in eradicating alcohol due to the huge revenue involved and in eradicating drug use due to the global pattern of relief drug market as well as the spread of the HIV pandemic have accentuated the debate about the attempt to eradicates substance use as against adopting realistic strategy for reducing the harm associated with substance use. The recognition in the mode 1980s, that injecting drugs with shared needles spreads HIV was the most important event that made harm reduction official drug policy in United Kingdom, Australia, Switzerland and many parts of Europe. There was a clear affirmation of what the British Advisory Council on Misuse of Drugs stated "HIV is a great threat to public and individual health than drug misuse" and that AIDS prevention efforts should be integrated with antidrug efforts with emphasis on the former.

Substitution maintenance programs, needle and syringe exchange programs and the more controversial strategy of legalizing cannabis so as to 'decriminalize' its use are the prominent harm reduction strategies. It must be noted that strategies based on the harm reduction perspective have been advocated and practised in the field of prevention, beyond the illicit drugs. Low nicotine content cigarettes and campaigning against 'drunken driving' are programs in the genre. The larger perspective of harm reduction reflects a paradigm shift from viewing substance use disorders as phenomena caused by individual psychological factors to potential causes of extensive social problems are threats to public health. Such a paradigm shift brings about the goal of limiting the medical and social consequences of dependence disorder (e.g. substitution maintenance programs) and the goal of limiting the length and severity of substance related disorders as the goal in secondary prevention (e.g. needle exchange programs). In this perspective, the primary prevention is aimed at the absolute prevention of dependence disorder, but not of substance use per se. (e.g. decriminalization of cannabis). The tertiary prevention strategies in this perspective like the substitution maintenance program are gaining acceptance, mainly based on the impressive data generated on the outcome measures in methadone maintenance programs. The secondary prevention strategies like needle exchange programs also have a research database support, but have remained fairly controversial. It is the primary prevention strategies in this perspective like the suggestion to legalize and decriminalize cannabis which have remained much more controversial. These aspects were require to be considered whole applying the harm reduction strategies to cultures other than the European cultures in which they have originated and been practised. Even the American scientists have expressed the caution for applying these strategies in their culture without adequate adaptation. Obviously, the need for examining the adaptability and the potential efficacy of these strategies in India, before they are actively considered, is high. The other major difficulty in implementing harm reduction strategies is about the methodological limitations. In evaluating their effectiveness by reliable data collection and analysis about personal, intimate behavior in fine degrees.

It must be understood that the harm reduction perspective does not legitimize or glamorize substance use but merely acknowledges that it cannot be totally eliminated. It does not have to be seen as disavowing abstinence, but addresses the problem of substance related disorders in a pragmatic manner. Nonetheless, it does get overshadowed by the global 'war on drugs' slogans which aim at drug-free or substance free human society. It can be hoped that in the rest few years, the differential application of the totalitarian perspective and the harm reduction perspective in different situations and contexts will become possible, based on the experience and the research which is being currently generated.

HIV INFECTION AND SUBSTANCE USE

International Scenario of Injecting Drug Use and HIV Infection

The problem of HIV infections in drug users is a major route for transmission of HIV in the US, and is the principal means by which infection has spread in Italy, Spain, Thailand and North East India. IDUs have been identified as major vectors for the spread of AIDS to the general population. Since a great majority of the IDUs are heterosexual, they form a primary source for heterosexual and *in utero* transmission to the general population.

The greatest risk for IDUs is associated with injection risks such as sharing contaminated needles. Many studies have described the situational nature of needle sharing, supporting the idea that peer behavior heavily influences needle sharing behavior. Several studies have also indicated the importance of not only needle and syringe sharing practices in HIV transmission but the sharing of drug containers, cotton and other injection paraphernalia. Furthermore, use of contaminated needles may entail not only sharing, but also pooling of needles. Virological studies have indicated that HIV can survive in ordinary tap water for extended periods of time and thus shared rinse water represents a considerable potential transmission risk.

The sexual risk behavior contributing to HIV transmission in IDUs are multiple sex partnerships and unprotected sex. In most of the studies on IDUs in Europe and USA, IDUs have been reported to have higher chance of multiple sex partners and low frequency of condom use. Most studies of HIV seroprevalence among IDUs do not show any significance of sexual behavior after controlling for drug use and demographic characteristics. Some studies on the contrary, have heterosexual contact with other IDUs to be an independent risk factor for HIV infection when drug use and demographic factors were controlled statistically. It has been pointed out that the heterosexual transmission of HIV may be relatively more important for younger IDUs who are more sexually active and engage in lower levels of drug using risk behaviors. The relative roles of needle sharing and sexual transmission may differ depending on the seropositivity level of the community. As IDUs increasingly adopt safer needle using practices, sexual transmission can be expected to play an increasingly more important role in the spread of HIV among heterosexual IDUs, unless corresponding changes in high risk sexual behaviors are also made.

Treatment of Drug Abuse as an HIV Prevention Strategy and the Harm Reduction Approach

In many countries, the drug abuse problem is approached with drug-free treatment programs on the one hand, and law enforcement on the other. Generally, this results in a limited number of drug abusers in the treatment programs and marginalization and criminalization of drug users. Treatment programs often actively pursue the goal of persuading drug users to abstain from the use of drugs. Although there have been advances in the therapeutic treatment approaches, success in terms of the number of people achieving long-term abstinence is limited. Abstinence-oriented programs provide excellent services to those who are motivated to stop using the drugs. The question remains as to what should be done about the 80–90% who are not. The answer to this question might be found by adopting a harm-reduction approach. The rationale of harm reduction is "if it is not possible to cure drug users, one should at least try to minimize the harm that is being done both to them and the wider social environment". The drug taker is helped through a difficult phase in life, while it is hoped that in the longer term addiction may be overcome, either by treatment or natural recovery. The effects of problem drug use, the spread of diseases and the problems for neighborhoods caused by drug-related crimes, are targets of the harm reduction approach.

Abstinence-oriented drug abuse treatment has been traditionally considered a principal means by which disease prevention objectives might be attained. As such, drug abuse treatment addresses HIV risk behavior indirectly through abstinence from drugs of abuse. As desirable as drug abuse treatment is for those willing and able to benefit from it, relying on drug abuse treatment as a sole means of HIV prevention in IDUs has some fundamental problems. They are: (i) due to the illegal nature and nearly universal condemnation of the practice, injecting drug use is very much an underground activity. Many of the IDUs do not wish to enter treatment. (ii) drug addiction or dependence has been shown in many studies to be a chronic and relapsing condition, refractory to treatment.

HIV specific individual counseling or group counselling approaches can and do form a part of the drug abuse treatment services, but have very limited and short-lasting effects. As such, along with continuing the emphasis on drug abuse treatment, specific interventions aimed at HIV prevention in drug users in general and injecting drug users in specific require to be developed, implemented and evaluated. The recommendations of a Technical Review meeting on 'AIDS and Intravenous Drug Use' at the National Institute on Drug Abuse (NIDA) clearly state that "From the Public Health point of view, and to contain the spread of HIV, it is essential that the goal of drug abuse abstinence and the goal of HIV prevention be recognized as separate issues. Abstinence is the most effective means of HIV prevention, and it is desirable to help IV drug abusers to stop using drugs. However, it must be recognized that many IV drug abusers will be unwilling or unable to stop. Thus, interventions with IV drug abusers who are not in treatment should have a dual focus-encouraging risk reduction efforts and entry into treatment." A paper from the Global Program on AIDS, WHO, Geneva suggests that "Accepting the priority of HIV prevention over that of drug use control is essential in adopting an integrated approach to HIV risk reduction".

Strategies for HIV Prevention among IDUs

Interventions aimed at HIV prevention among IDUs have been in the form of:

- Individual or group counseling for in-treatment drug users, with short lasting and limited success.
- Needle and syringe exchange programs, argued for cities or states which have already reached a high level of HIV seroprevalence among IDUs. New York city, Amsterdam, Edinburgh have reported success with such programs. The suitability and need for such programs is for the developed societies and high seroprevalence areas. Their relevance for developing nations is still considered low.
- Preventive intervention programs aimed at modifying the high risk behavior of IDUs and thereby preventing HIV infection among the IDUs and transmision to the general population. There is a very wide range of programs and approaches of this genre, varying according to the objectives, the theoretical model, the program and the target group of IDUs.

Effectiveness of HIV Prevention in IDUs

Persuasive evidence from different settings is accumulating to the effect that HIV prevention among IDUs does lead to change in high-risk behavior, maintained over longtime.

Besides the positive evidence from individual studies, reports on pooled data from two sources support the claim of HIV prevention in IDUs being effective in reducing the risk behavior. In the USA, the National Institute on Drug Abuse (NIDA) funded street outreach prevention efforts as part of the National AIDS Demonstration Research (NADR) projects. Longitudinal data on 13,475 IDUs and 1,637 sexual partners from 28 NADR programs indicated significant changes over 6 months period in HIV-related risk behaviors among IDUs, including frequency of injecting drugs, the use of non-injecting drugs, the use of borrowed injection equipment and the number of sexual partners. In particular, changes in the risky needle-related behaviors were more dramatic than the changes in the risky sexual behaviors. Nevertheless, there were significant numbers of subjects who did not reduce their AIDS risk behavior. WHO Collaborative Study Group also reported similar findings from a large study in 13 cities.

In a critical review of 27 published studies on risk reduction interventions targeting injecting drug users, Booth and Watters arranged the studies in four groups in the order of their methodological strength, from weakest to strongest, based on their capability of controlling for threats to validity.

- Post-test only nonequivalent group design.
- One group pretest post-test design.
- Independent cross-section design.
- Pretest-Post-test control group design.

In the first generation studies, there were serious methodological problems. Interventions were credited with producing the behavior change despite a lack of information on intervention exposure or a comparison group that did not receive the intervention. Among the nine studies with pretest-post-test control group design, only two found consistent and significant differences between groups. Booth and Watters concluded that "the findings are not unequivocal" and that "in the studies with a more powerful design, the failure to detect differences between interventions may have been more a failure of the research than of the intervention." Some more recent studies continue to report significant reductions in risk behavior with no group effect between intervention group and no intervention group.

Many researchers and policy makers have identified the conclusions that can be drawn from all the available research and suggested future directions for research. Some of the important conclusions are:

- *Effectiveness:* Behavior change is possible in IDUs targeting specifically at risk behaviors, with intervention programs, as compared to HIV counseling which has limited success in behavior change.
- *Outreach:* Community based street or outreach services have been found to be necessary and effective and are strongly recommended.
- *Specific behaviors:* HIV prevention in IDUs requires to be seen as an issue of high public health importance alongside drug abuse treatment services and interventions, should focus on harm-reduction in specific high risk behaviors and entry into treatment.
- *Timing:* HIV prevention needs to be started early in the development of the epidemic, with low seroprevalence

to be effective in preventing or stabilizing the epidemic; reversing a well established epidemic with high to very high seroprevalence is a formidable task.

- *Research evaluation:* It may not be possible to evaluate with powerful research design all service programs, systematic research evaluation will have to be carried out in the initial stages. The evaluation parameters will require to be focused at the planning stage.
- *Social process:* The focus of attention needs to enlarge from assessing and modifying individual risk behavior to understanding and intervening at the level of larger social processes or the context of risk behavior. The intrinsic social and peer-influenced nature of injection practices and sexual practices require to be recognized as intrinsic to the attempt at modifying them. This may be one of the reasons for consistently limited effects with the interventions that have been evaluated.

Table 28: Awareness, risk behavior and willingness to change in injection and noninjection drug users

S. No.	*Parameters*	*Injection users (N = 28)*		*Noninjection users (N = 34)*	
		Yes	No	Yes	No
1.	*Awareness*				
	a. About HIV/AIDS	26	2	26	8
	b. About routes of transmission	10	18	22	12
2.	*Risk behavior-sexual*				
	a. Multiple sex partners	20	8	16	18
	b. Unprotected sex*	17	3	8	8
3.	*Risk behavior-injection*	22	6	—	—
4.	*Willingness to change*				
	a. Sexual practices*	7	13	6	10
	b. Injection practices*	17	5	—	—

* Note: Only where applicable, so that the total in each row does not add up to the sample size (N) of the Groups.

Awareness, HIV Seroprevalence and Prevention in IDUs in India

These issues in respect of the IDUs in the North Eastern States have been extensively reported in the literature, widely known among concerned groups of professionals and have been reviewed in this project proposal. In view of the increasing trends of injection drug use and the general low levels of awareness with highly prevalent unsafe sexual practices, there is a need to review the existing state of knowledge on these issues in other parts of India.

In a study using qualitative research method, from the Drug Dependence Treatment Centre of AIIMS, detailed in-depth interviews were carried out by the clinical consultant in regular contact with the patients of injection and non-injection use to elicit information on awareness about HIV/AIDS, needle use and sexual practices and willingness to change. The sample comprised of 34 noninjection heroin users and 28 patients with primary or multidrug dependence, including injection use, seen between 1993 and 1995. A majority of injection and noninjection users were aware about HIV/AIDS, but the awareness about the routes of HIV transmission was more among noninjection users (n = 22) and less common in the injection users (n = 10). A majority of the injection users also had unprotected sex with multiple sex partners while less than half (n = 16) of the noninjection users had multiple sex partners and half of these were regularly using condoms (Table 28). As part of the counseling, willingness to change was assessed and it was found that the willingness to change sexual practices was limited in both the groups, but the a majority of the injection users were willing to change their injection practices.

These findings reveal patterns of awareness and risk behavior similar to the trends reported to have existed in the early part of the epidemic in the North East, but different from the existing practices among the injection users in Manipur. In their study on ethnographic observations of drug injecting in Manipur and Calcutta, Chatterjee et al. have significant, differences in awareness and practices across the two settings. The patterns they report for Calcutta are similar to the observations from the hospital sample in Delhi, viz. low levels of awareness and high risk behavior being common. In the sample of 307 intravenous drug addicts in South Delhi, by a team from NGO, only 83 addicts (27% were aware about AIDS and the other 224 (73%) had no awareness about AIDS or HIV.

In a sample from a tertiary hospital clinic in Chandigarh, Malhotra et al. reported on a sample of 45 injection users (IDUs) seen between December 1989 and June 1992. Eighteen (40%) of the 45 IDUs admitted to needle sharing and a majority of the IDUs reported having multiple sex partners. It was also reported that one of these 45 IDUs was found to be seropositive, yielding a prevalence of 2.2% in the group of IDUs. Information on HIV seroprevalence among IDUs in parts of India, other than the North East are few.

Bollinger et al. concluded in their comprehensive review that "although intravenous drug use is less common in other areas of India, an HIV seroprevalence of 1.1-3.4% has been documented in intravenous drug users in Bizalae and Bombay."

Intervention targeted at IDUs in other parts of India remains at the level of hospital based services and a few initial experiments in outreach services. One of the teams actively involved in the North-Eastern Region for many years has emphasized the need for such intervention. Sarkar et al. have opined that "in spite of limited available data on HIV among the injecting population in other parts of India, there is a possibility that the prevalence would be low. However, in recent times there has been a phenomenal rise (5–13 times in last two years) of the injecting behaviors among drug addict population in cities like Calcutta where 15 to 46% of the substance users (mainly heroin smokers) have reportedly switched to injecting behaviors from less than 1% in 1986. Similar reports are also available from Madras, another metropolitan city in South India. We must mobilize urgently all political and social support towards launching socially targeted intervention efforts for all the areas with injecting population".

EPILOGUE

As should be evident from the Chapter, the clinical issues in substance use disorders are quite wide ranging and complex. The interface with biomedical on the one hand and the social sciences on the other, makes the field more difficult but also challenging. The clinical and the treatment issues of this field are not the exclusive domain of psychiatrists but will remain the major component of the discipline. The belief that the psychiatrists and the other mental health professionals can fulfil the obligation of providing leadership in these issues has held true over time. It has also been clear that the larger issues of prevention of substance use disorders will have to benefit from the inputs of not only the public health professionals, but also a variety of social scientists and the policy makers. This larger scenario of the field of substance use can be daunting, but the expertise required in the clinical and treatment issues of substance use disorders, for psychiatrists is undebatable. This Chapter has been aimed at fulfilling this need. There is an increasing realization of the usefulness of being alert and sensitive to the other larger issues of the field. This need, it is hoped, will also be met within this chapter.

As in many other fields in Psychiatry and Mental Health, there are exciting directions being charted in the field of substance use disorders from the basic sciences to the applied therapeutics. The scientific research and the cumulative clinical experience in the field till now, as well as the HIV pandemic and the other developments in public health are contributing to a significant reorientation. The developments in India, indeed in South East Asia, in this respect can be more contemporary and in keeping with the global scenario.

5.2 ALCOHOL USE DISORDER

RK Solanki

INTRODUCTION

The alcohol-use disorder consist of alcohol dependence, alcohol abuse, and dependence of harmful use. These are common and potentially lethal disorders that mimic and exacerbate a wide range of additional medical and psychiatric conditions, and therapy shorten the lifespans of affected people by more than a decade. However, most people with alcohol-use disorder are hard to identity, since they are likely to have jobs and families, and present with general complaints such as malaise, insomnia, anxiety, sadness, or a range of medical problems.

Both primary-care physicians and specialists can help to screen for these disorders, institute brief interventions, and refer patients for more intensive care if needed. This seminar presents a selective update of clinical developments regarding alcohol-use disorders that are relevant to practicing physicians, and focus on skills that they already have or can easily acquire.

EPIDEMIOLOGY

Alcohol-use disorders are common in all developed countries, and are more prevalent in men than women, with lower, but still substantial rates in developing countries. Although rates of these disorders are lower in Mediterranean countries (e.g. Greece, Italy and Israel), and higher in northern and eastern Europe (e.g. Russia and Scandinavia), they are responsible for a large proportion of the healthcare burden in almost all populations.As many as 80% of men and 60% of women in developed countries drink at some time during their lives. In any year, between half and two-thirds of individuals who were drank are likely to have stopped because of medical concerns. 30 to 50% of people who drank in the past year experience at least one adverse alcohol-related problem during their lifetime, such as missing work or school, driving after drinking, or interpersonal problems. The lifetime risk of alcohol-use disorders for men is more than 20%, with a risk of about 15% for alcohol abuse and 10% for alcohol dependence. The risk of developing an alcohol-use disorder in the previous year is about 10% overall.

Only about a quarter of people with alcohol-use disorders ever seek help for these conditions, with higher proportions for women than men. Most receive care from their general practitioner, where they represent about a fifth of patients seen: the proportions seen for diabetes and hypertension are similar. The challenge for the clinician is to learn enough about these disorders to identify them, since missing an alcohol-use disorder can complicate the assessment and treatment of other medical and psychiatric issue.

DIAGNOSIS

Criteria for Screening and Diagnosis

Clinicians should screen for unhealthy drinking (e.g. more than three or four standard drinks per day), just as they counsel their patients for other risky behaviors such as being 10% overweight. A standard drink is defined as 8 g of ethanol in the UK and about 10 g in the USA. Both the US-based 4th Diagnostic and Statistical Manual (DSM-IV) and the 10th International Classification of Disease (ICD10) describe alcohol dependence as the more severe condition, associated with major physiological consequences and life impairment. Dependence can be identified as repetitive problems, affecting three or more areas of life, and about 80% of people who are diagnosed with dependence at any point still have alcohol-related problems when assessed a year or more later. Dependence criteria are reliable across different ages, sexes, and most cultural groups. The concordance between ICD and DSM approaches to diagnosis is about 80% (Panel 1). Alcohol abuse and harmful use, however, have different definitions from dependence. The DSM-IV defines alcohol abuse as one or more problems with functioning in a 12-month period in a person without dependence; failure in obligations; alcohol use in hazardous situations; recurrent legal problems; or continued use despite social or interpersonal problems. The ICD10 defines harmful use as either a physical or mental problem associate with alcohol in a 12-month period or both. The ICD10 label of harmful use is not as reliable as that for abuse, and the two diagnostic systems have low agreement. People who abuse alcohol drink smaller quantities than those with dependence do, but the abuse label predicts a risk of about 50% for continued problems. Only 10% of those with alcohol abuse go on to dependence.

Questionnaires

Although they are not a substitute for a careful clinical interview, a range of self-administered questionnaires can be used to screen for heavy drinking and alcohol-use disorders in clinical settings. The shortest of the most widely-used instruments is the CAGE questionnaire, which is an acronym for whether a patient has ever felt the need to cut down on drinking; felt Annoyed when criticized about alcohol use; felt guilty about drinking, or ever needed an eye-opener on awakening. Results vary across different subgroups (with highest accuracy in man and white people). The cut-off score of two of a possible four positive response has a sensitivity of between 53% (in heavy drinkers) and 77% in patients who have alcohol dependence, with specificities of 80% or higher. The sensitivity measures the proportion of actual positives who are correctly identified as such; and the specificity measures the proportion of negative who are correctly identified. This short test might operate best in medical and surgical settings, especially when combined with blood test for heavy drinking. Another questionnaire is the ten-item version of the Michigan Alcohol Screening Test, in which five to six affirmative answers indicate a possible alcohol-use disorder (with sensitivity and specificity of about 80%), and seven indicates a probable alcohol-use disorder. Table 21 shows questions for the ten-item alcohol-use identification test (AUDIT), in which a score of eight or above identifies both heavy drinkers and those with alcohol-use disorders with a sensitivity of 50–90%, and a specificity of about 80% although a lower sensitivity has been reported in women and elderly people. Four of the AUDIT items are used for the shorter fast alcohol screening test (FAST), which has similar accuracy to the full AUDIT test. Another short instrument is the TWEAK questionnaire, which asks about Tolerance, Worry about drinking by friends, eye-opener drinks in the morning, Amnesia about drinking, and feeling the need to cut down.

Blood Tests

Although not as sensitive a questionnaires, blood tests for markers that are likely to change in the context of heavy drinking can also help to identify patients who consumer hazardous amounts of alcohol (Table 29). These tests can be especially useful if the veracity of the history is in doubt, and can also be used to help the patient recognize that alcohol has adversely affected their health. These markers of heavy drinking indicate relatively high amounts or mark of alcohol (e.g. five or more standard drinks per day) consumed on a regular basis (e.g. for 5 days or more). High values are likely to return to normal within several weeks of abstinence, an evanescence that can be useful in monitoring adherence to treatment. Values are likely to be highest in the heaviest drinkers, and might have the greatest sensitivities and specificities for men and for patients who are not grossly overweight, diabetic, or smokers.

DSM-5: It does not separate the diagnoses of substance abuse and dependence as in DSM-IV. Rather criteria are provided for substance use disorder, accompanied by criteria for intoxication, withdrawal, etc.

One such marker is the serum activity of γ-glutamyl transferase, and enzyme important in amino acid transport, Results of at least 35 units per L γ-glutamyl transferase indicate the probability of heavy drinking. This test is available in most chemistry laboratories, is inexpensive, and has sensitivities and specificities that approach 60% in men, although the sensitivity might be closer to 50% in women.

A second useful test is for carbohydrate-deficient transferring, which measures a change in the structure

Panel 1: Criteria for diagnosis of alcohol dependence, according to diagnostic and statistical Manual (DSM.IV) and international Classification of Diseases (ICD10)	
Diagnostic and Statistical Manual (DSM-IV)	
•	Tolerance to alcohol
•	Withdrawal syndrome
•	Greater alcohol use than intended
•	Desire to use alcohol and inability to control use
•	Devotion of large proportion of time to getting and using alcohol, and recovering from alcohol use.
•	Neglect of social work, or recreational activities
•	Continued alcohol use despite physical or psychological problems
International Classification of Diseases (ICD-10)	
•	Strong desire or compulsion to use alcohol
•	Inability to control use
•	Withdrawal syndrome
•	Tolerance to alcohol
•	Neglect to pleasures of interest
•	Continued alcohol use despite physical or psychological problems

Table 29: State markers of heavy drinking

	Suggested cut value
Gamma glutamyltransferase (GGT)	>35 u/L
Carbohydrate deficient transferin (CDT)	>20 G/L or > 2.6%
Alanine aminotransferase (ALT)	>67 u/L
Aspartate aminotransferase (AST)	>65 u/L

of a proportion of transferring that is likely to occur with heavy drinking over a long period; a result of 20 units per L or more indicates heavy drinking. The sensitivities for identification of heavy drinking and alcohol-use disorders range from 30 to 75% across studies (with higher figures for men), and specificities are as high as 90%, although results might be difficult to interpret in the context of iron deficiency. Test of liver function that measure alanine and aspartate aminotransferases can identify heavy drinking and alcohol-use disorders with sensitivities of between 25% and 45% and specificities as high as 90%. A ratio of aspartate aminotransferase to alanine aminotransferase of greater than 2, especially if concentrations for each of these enzymes do not exceed 400 units per L, raises the possibility of alcoholic hepatitis. Finally, very high blood alcohol (e.g. 35 mmol/L or higher) should raise suspicion of alcohol dependence, especially if encountered in emergency departments and trauma-room settings.

DSM-5 Criteria for alcohol use disorder	
A.	A problematic pattern of alcohol use leading to clinically significant impairment or distress, as manifested by at least two of the following, occurring within a 12-month period:
	1. Alcohol is often taken in larger amounts or over a longer period than was intended.
	2. There is a persistent desire or unsuccessful efforts to cut down or control alcohol use.
	3. A great deal of time is spent in activities necessary to obtain alcohol, use alcohol, or recover from its effects.
	4. Craving, or a strong desire or urge to use alcohol.
	5. Recurrent alcohol use resulting in a failure to fulfill major role obligations at work, school, or home.
	6. Continued alcohol use despite having persistent or recurrent social or interpersonal problems caused or exacerbated by the effects of alcohol.
	7. Important social, occupational, or recreational activities are given up or reduced because of alcohol use.
	8. Recurrent alcohol use in situations in which it is physically hazardous.
	9. Alcohol use is continued despite knowledge of having a persistent or recurrent physical or psychological problem that is likely to have been caused or exacerbated by alcohol.
	10. Tolerance, as defined by either, of the following: a. A need for markedly increased amounts of alcohol to achieve intoxication or desired effect. b. A markedly diminished effect with continued use of the same amount of alcohol.
	11. Withdrawal, as manifested by either of the following: a. The characteristic withdrawal syndrome for alcohol (refer to Criteria A and B of the criteria set for alcohol withdrawal, pp. 235-236). b. Alcohol (or a closely related substance, such as a benzodiazepine) is taken to relieve or avoid withdrawal symptoms.
Specify *if:* **In early remission:** After full criteria for alcohol use disorder were previously met, none of the criteria for alcohol use disorder have been met for at least 3 months but for less than 12 months (with the exception that Criterion A4, "Craving, or a strong desire or urge to use alcohol," may be met). **In sustained remission:** After full criteria for alcohol use disorder were previously met, none of the criteria for alcohol use disorder have been met at any time during a period of 12 months or longer (with the exception that Criterion A4, "Craving, or a strong desire or urge to use alcohol," may be met).	
Specify *if:* **In a controlled environment:** This additional specifier is used if the individual is in an environment where access to alcohol is restricted. **Code based on current severity:** Note for ICD-10-CM codes: If alcohol intoxication, alcohol withdrawal, or another	

Contd...

Contd...

alcohol-induced mental disorder is also present, do not use the codes below for alcohol use disorder. Instead, the comorbid alcohol use disorder is indicated in the 4th character of the alcohol-induced disorder code (see the coding note for alcohol intoxication, alcohol withdrawal, or a specific alcohol-induced mental disorder). For example, if there is comorbid alcohol intoxication and alcohol use disorder, only the alcohol intoxication code is given, with the 4th character indicating whether the comorbid alcohol use disorder is mild, moderate, or severe: F10.129 for mild alcohol use disorder with alcohol intoxication or F10.229 for a moderate or severe alcohol use disorder with alcohol intoxication.
Specify current severity:
305.1 (F10.10) Mild: Presence of 2–3 symptoms.
303.90 (F10.20) Moderate: **Presence of 4 to 5 symptoms.**
303.90 (F10.20) Severe: Presence of 6 or more symptoms.

Clinical Course

The course of an alcohol-use disorder is as predictable as most medical or psychiatric disorders, with differences across subgroups (e.g. men vs women) that reflect more general characteristics of each group in society. However, most studies of the clinical course and treatment of alcohol-use disorders focus on patients who do not have major comorbid psychiatric disorders. Therefore, these issues are not as well understood in people with severe anxiety, mood, or psychotic disorder. Therefore, these issues are not as well understood in people with severe anxiety, mood, or psychotic disorders. Overall, women who have alcohol-use disorders have a slightly shorter time between onset of problems and seeking help than men do, and are less likely to be violent or arrested. Similarly, compared with younger people, older people with alcohol-use disorders have more medical problems, less violence, and are less likely to be employed.

Moreover, although children who have persistent conduct disorders and adults who have antisocial personalities have similar alcohol problems to other with alcohol-use disorders, they exhibit more drug dependence and criminality, and the combination of problems is sometimes referred to as type 2 or type B alcoholism.

The usual age of first drinking, independently of the family, is about 15 years (although this varies across cultural groups), and has not changed much in decades. This age does not differ much for those who go on to develop alcohol-use disorders and those who do not, although an earlier onset of regular drinking is associated with a greater likelihood of later problems. The period of heaviest drinking is usually between 18 and 22 years of age, and also does not differ much between those with future alcohol-use disorders and the general population. More than 60% of teenagers, even those without alcohol-use disorders, have experienced drunkenness by the age of 18 years, and about 30% have either given up events such as school or work to drink, or have driven while intoxicated. Alcohol abuse and dependence often begin in the early to mid-20s, at a time when most people begin to moderate their drinking as their responsibilities increase.

Repeated heavy drinking in alcohol-use disorders is associated with a 40% risk of temporary depressive episodes, associated suicidal ideas and attempts, and severe anxiety and insomnia. However, many of these forms of psychopathology are substance-induced, and likely to improve within 2–4 weeks of abstinence. Additional comorbidities include use, abused, and dependence on illicit drugs, especially for patients who have very early-onset alcohol-use disorders and antisocial personalities (i.e. type 2 or type B subtypes of dependence). As many as 80% of alcohol-dependent people are regular smokers, a co-occurrence that could reflect either use of the second drug to deal with effects of the first of overlapping genetic predispositions. These comorbidities can make treatment more difficult.

As is true of many chronic relapsing disorders (e.g. hypertension), the course of alcohol-use disorders fluctuates over time. Abstinence often develops after a crisis, and the subsequent days to months of sobriety are often followed by temporary controlled drinking, which carries a subsequent enhanced likelihood of increasing intake and problems. This fluctuating course relates to the controversy about whether a person with an alcohol-use disorder can return to long-term controlled nonproblematic drinking. Abstinence is the usual goal for treatment of dependence in the USA, although efforts to control drinking, or reduce harm, are more often deemed appropriate goals in the UK and other parts of Europe. Some studies have reported that about 20% of those with alcohol dependence were able to drink moderately without problems in the previous year, but this is often temporary, and other studies indicate that fewer than 10% ever develop long periods of nonproblematic drinking.

Another element in the course of alcohol-use disorders is the 20–39% rate of long-term remission of alcohol-related problems in the absence of formal treatment of self-help programmes. Remission is usually associated with deteriorating health, new life-partners, parenthood, a new job, or maturation over time, and once achieved, is likely to remain stable.

Continued alcohol problems increase the rate of early death by three or four times. The most common causes are early onset of heart disease, stroke, and cancers; and a high risk of accidents, suicide, and liver cirrhosis (although about 80% of people with alcohol-use disorders do not have this disorder). Alcohol-related mortality contributes to 2–4% of all deaths in adults, with the highest rate in the first decade after treatment.

PATHOPHYSIOLOGY

Causes and Origins

About 40–60% of the risk of alcohol-use disorders is explained by genes and the rest through gene-environment associations. The environment includes the availability of alcohol, attitudes towards drinking and drunkenness, peer pressures, levels of stress and related coping strategies, models of drinking, and laws and regulatory frameworks.

Recent advances in our understanding for genes that operate through intermediate characteristics (or phenotypes) to affect the risk of alcohol-use disorders can help parents with alcohol-use disorders to identify children who might be at high risk of alcohol-use disorders. These could contribute to preventive approaches in the future through early intervention in those at highest risk, even before problems develop. First, variations (polymorphisms) in genes for enzymes that metabolize alcohol are generally associated with a lower risk of alcohol-use disorders, since they increase sensitivity to alcohol. At least one variant of aldehyde dehydrogenase (the ALDH2*2 allele), produces an aversive response to alcohol. Second, gene forms associated with impulsivity, disinhibition, and sensation-seeking contribute the vulnerability to both drug-use and alcohol-use disorders in people with type 2 and type B disorders, perhaps through impaired judgment and difficulty learning from mistakes that could reduce control of alcohol intake. Relevant polymorphisms include variations in receptors for γ-aminobutyric acid (e.g. GABRA2), acetylcholine (e.g. CHRM2), and dopamine (e.g. DRD2). Third, people who have low responsiveness (or low sensitivity) to alcohol are more likely to drink more on each occasion to get the desired effect, which increases their risk of alcohol-use disorders, but not other drug-related disorders. Relevant genes include those that encode an allele of the serotonin transporter (SLC6A4), some potassium channels (e.g. KCNMA1), variations in γ-aminobutyric acid receptors (e.g. GABRA6), second messenger systems (e.g. AC9), and genes that affect glutamate receptors (GRM3), Additional genetic mechanisms might operate via genes that regulate dopamine-reward systems.

Alcohol Metabolism

Although 2–10% of alcohol is excreted through the lungs, urine, and sweat, the remainder is metabolized to acetaldehyde, mainly by alcohol dehydrogenase (ADH). This metabolite is then quickly converted to carbon dioxide and water, primarily through the actions of aldehyde dehydrogenase (ALDH). The wild type forms of ADH decrease the concentration of alcohol blood by about 4–5 mmol/L ethanol/h (this is the equivalent of about one drink/h).

At least two variations of ADH genes (ADH1B*2) and (ADHIC*1) produce a slightly more rapid breakdown of alcohol, and therefore potentially faster production of acetaldehyde. ALDH*2, the form most relevant for acetaldehyde metabolism, then rapidly destroys this product. However, about 40% of Asian people (Japanese, Chinese, and Koreans) have an inactive ALDH*2*2, mutation that results in much more acetaldehyde after drinking than normal. About 10% of people who are homozygous for this gene form cannot drink alcohol without becoming sick, and have almost no risk of alcohol-use disorders, whereas those who are heterozygous have a relatively low rate of alcohol-use disorders.

Effects on the Brain

Even low doses of alcohol enhance activity in the inhibitory γ-aminobutyric acid systems throughout the brain. These sedating effects cause muscle relaxation, somnolence, and intoxicated feelings. Adaptations in these systems are prominent in the development of tolerance to alcohol, and diminished activity of γ-aminobutyric acid contributes to anxiety and insomnia during acute and protracted alcohol withdrawal. Having an alcoholic drink also diminishes the activity of the stimulating glutamate N-methyl-D-aspartate (NMDA) receptor system, and withdrawal is associated with enhanced activity of these pathways.

Drinking releases dopamine and increases activity at related synapses. Such brain changes, especially in the nucleus accumbens and the ventral tegmental areas, contribute to the rewarding effects of this drug, and might contribute to both craving and disinhibition drug intoxication. Drinking also enhances the release of opioid peptides (e.g. is β endorphin) that are not only rewarding but also associated with dopamine release, which potentially contributes to sensitization to alcohol and craving.

Alcohol also stimulates the serotonergic system; low concentrations of serotonin in the synapse are associated with a diminished effect of alcohol and, perhaps, a propensity towards consumption of this drug. Additional effects are seen for epinephrine, cannabinol receptors, adenosine systems, acetylcholine, and stress-relates system such as corticotrophin-releasing hormone.

Alcohol-related Organ Damage

In the nervous system, the severe anterograde amnesia of Wernicke-Korsakoff syndrome is seen in fewer than 1% of those with alcohol dependence (usually in the context of transketolase deficiency). However, mild anterograde amnesias (alcoholic blackouts) are common, as are temporary cognitive deficits, including difficulties in problem-solving, abstraction, memory, and learning. Cognitive deficits, such as problems with memory, learning, and problem-solving, usually reverse within weeks to months of abstinence, as do related brain-imaging findings such as sulcal widening and ventricular enlargement. Other common problems with heavy drinking include intensification of sleep apnea, trouble falling asleep, and frequent awakenings in the second half of the night, complaints that enhance the risk of a return to heavy drinking. Also, 15% of those with alcohol dependence develop peripheral neuropathy (alcoholic polyneuropathy) associated with numbness, paresthesias, and decreases in vibration and position sense, especially in the legs.

Heavy drinking affects the cardiovascular system. Three or more drinks per day increase both blood pressure and LDL cholesterol, and also enhance the risk of cardiomyopathy. Heavy drinking is associated with temporary arrhythmias (so-called holiday heart), which are usually atrial in origin, but sometimes ventricular and associated with increased dispersion of QT intervals.

Cancer is the second leading cause of early death in people with alcohol-use disorders, even after controlling for the effect of smoking. Almost 75% of patients who have head and neck cancers have alcohol-use disorders, and alcohol-use disorders also double the risk of cancer of the esophagus, rectum, and breast. These findings could reflect alcohol-induced impairment of the immune system.

Other disorders related to heavy drinking included acute hemorrhagic gastritis, pancreatitis, and liver changes ranging from fatty infiltration to alcoholic hepatitis and cirrhosis. Alcohol-induced immune dysfunction can exacerbate the course of hepatitis C and complicate the treatment of AIDS. Furthermore, heavy drinking is associated with a decrease in bone density, and enhanced vulnerability to hip fractures, and alterations in blood-producing system that decrease with blood cells, platelets, and granulocyte mobility.

Additional problems include heavy drinking associated with fatal accidents. Furthermore, a pregnant woman who drinks heavily can cause adverse effects on her developing fetus, including low birth weight, spontaneous abortions, premature deliveries, fetal-alcohol syndrome, and fetal alcohol spectrum disorders. Fetal-alcohol spectrum disorders include abnormalities in facial features, such as an absent philtrum, a flattened nose, and shortened palpebral fissures; ventricular septal heart deficits; syndactyly; and mental retardation.

Treatment

Despite perceptions of the contrary, efforts to help patients decrease heavy drinking commonly result in change in behaviors, and most patients with alcohol-use disorders do well after treatment. About 50 to 60% of men and women with alcohol dependence abstain or show substantial improvements in functioning the year after treatment, and such outcomes are excellent predictors of their status at 3–5 years. Although anyone in treatment might do well, better outcomes are associated with more intense treatment, less severe alcohol problems, less cognitive impairment, higher self-confidence about outcome, and fewer comorbid psychiatric disorders. The figure sets out the process of treatment, in which clinicians first identify alcohol-use disorders and share their concerns with patients, and then follow through with brief interventions, treatment, and referral to the specialist if problems are severe. For most clinicians, the goal of treatment for severe alcohol dependence is abstinence, and only a few favor teaching control of drinking. At the same time, individuals who drink unhealthy amounts (e.g. more than 35 g absolute ethanol per day) and those with alcohol abuse who refuse to abstain might benefit form approaches that emphasize moderation of drinking.

Treatment centers on clinicians' interactions with patients to help them to recognize their problems, and enhance motivation for change and implementation of change.

Intervention

The intervention step effectively starts the process of recovery and can be delivered by the general physician. The process incorporates the principles of motivational interviewing, brief interventions, or both, to help a patient recognize their problem and take steps to minimize future difficulties. Interventions can be offered both to those who seek help and to patients with excessive drinking or alcohol-use disorders who are opportunistically identified.

In motivational interviewing, clinicians explore the assets and liabilities of the drinking pattern, offer feedback no risk, encourage patients to take responsibility for change, offer advice, give a menu of options, interact in an empathetic way, and enhance self-efficacy or the ability to take responsibility for change; this combination is summarized by the acronym FRAMES. Brief interventions are broader in scope, and use a range of tools to educate the patient about the norms of consumption, and help to identify and avoid situations in which heavy drinking is most likely to occur.

Both approaches aim to increase patients motivations for change, elicit their perceptions of the situation and what needs to be done, and offer suggestion. Reluctance to change should be explored through discussions, to gauge when the patient is ready to implement the necessary steps. Motivational interviewing of brief interventions can be used in sessions of 15 to 30 min, and the time spent generates more savings than cost. One approach for the more directive brief interventions offers information about the patients' risk of problems, education about the dangers of continued heavy drinking, and a discussion of the benefit of change. Steps include the suggestion that a patient keeps a diary of behaviors, provision of reading materials, and a follow-up several weeks later by nursing or counseling staff.

Detoxification

About 50% of alcohol-dependent patients develop clinically relevant symptoms of withdrawal. These represent a rebound from the usual effects of alcohol intoxication, begin about 8 h after a pronounced decrease in blood-alcohol concentrations, peak on day 2, and are substantially reduced by day 4 or 5. A syndrome associated with protracted abstinence can persist for several months, it consists of mild anxiety, insomnia, and autonomic dysfunction, including modest elevations in blood pressure, pulse and respiratory rates; and sweating, tremor, anxiety, and insomnia. Fewer than 5% of alcohol-dependent people ever have a grand mal seizure during withdrawal (usually on day 2), or a severe agitated confusion (delirium tremens). Such seizures required care by a specialist, usually in a hospital setting, where the intensity of withdrawal can be closely monitored, including through the clinical-observer-based Clinical institute withdrawal assessment for alcoholism scale.

A physical examination is essential for patients with withdrawal symptoms (since risks of seizures and delirium rise with medical problems), followed by education and reassurance about the temporary nature of the symptoms. Doses of oral multivitamins, including oral thiamine (about 10 mg per day) can be beneficial; intramuscular or intravenous routes and higher doses are needed for the rare Wernicke-Korsakoff syndromes, which are much less likely to be seen in general-practice settings. Withdrawal symptoms are most safely and efficiently diminished by prescribing depressants (e.g. drugs that boost γ-aminobutyric acid); benzodiazepines are the most cost-effective approach. Anticonvulsants confer no additional benefit, are more expensive, and have more side-effects; β blockers or α-adrenergic agonists can mask signs of withdrawal that might highlight impending seizures of delirium.

Detoxification can begin with 25 mg chlordiazepoxide every 4–6 h for 1 day, deleting a dose if the patient is sleeping or resting comfortably, along with a supplementary 25–50 mg if a severe tremor or autonomic dysfunction is seen about 1 h after the schedule dose. Higher doses of benzodiazepines can be used if needed, depending on the level of autonomic dysfunction. Over the next 5–7 days, the dose used on day 1 should be decreased by 15–20% each day, or maintained at the same dose if symptoms worsen. If a shorter-acting benzodiazepine (e.g. lorazepam, 2–4 mg, four times a day) is used, it must be given on a strict schedule to avoid a higher risk of withdrawal seizures if concentrations of benzodiazepine in blood fluctuate. The average patient with a stable social situation, no severe medical problems, and no previous history or indicators of impending delirium of seizures can usually be treated with similar outcomes but less cost as an outpatient. Alternative approaches include higher does on day 1 and more rapid decreases, and a more fluid sliding scale with doses triggered by direct scoring of symptoms, but these are more complex and might be better reserved for specialists.

Rehabilitation

The goals of rehabilitation for alcohol-use disorders are the same as for any chronic relapsing disorder; to help to keep motivation high, change attitudes toward recovery, and diminish the risk of relapse. Cognitive-behavioral steps can help people to change how they think about alcohol and its role in their lives (the cognitive component); learn new behaviors for development and maintenance of abstinence of diminished drinking; and avoid relapses.

The alcoholics antonymous program offers support, emphasizes changes in attitudes and behavior, helps to rebuild life in the absence of alcohol, and decreases the demand for more expensive care. In fact, incorporation of the key elements of the alcoholics anonymous program through 12-step facilitation has been reported to increase the likelihood of a positive outcome.

Rehabilitation can be offered through groups in which participants are encourage to talk about their alcohol-related problems, consider how alcohol contributed to the difficulties, develop supportive peers, improve their relationships, deal with stress, make the most of work and free time, and avoid relapse. Such groups encourage patients to use their own and others experiences to identify situations that are associated with a risk of relapse, to learn how to avoid them and how to re-establish sobriety if heavy drinking resumes. Although outpatient rehabilitation is often successful, the better outcome with more intensive treatment indicates that some patients might need inpatient of residential-based care. Stages of treatment use depicted in Flow chart 1.

Flow chart 1: Stages of treatment

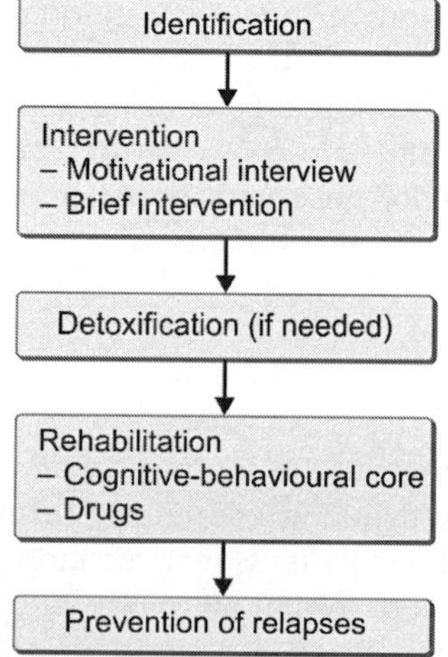

Table 30: Drugs dosage* for rehabilitation of alcohol-use disorders	
Naltrexone	
Oral	50–100 mg per day
Intramuscular injection	380 mg per month
Acamprosate	666 mg three times per day
Naltrexone-acamprosate	Same doses as above
Disulfiram	250 mg per day
*These drug are usually prescribed for 3–12 months	

Role of Drugs

Although many clinicians believe that medications are helpful, the core of treatment rests with motivational interviewing, brief interventions, and cognitive-behavioral approaches. Placebo-controlled studies are important for assessment of drugs because alcohol-use disorders have a high rate of spontaneous remission and fluctuating courses that contribute to outcomes, even with placebo. Table 30 lists drug shown on have probable effectiveness across most placebo-controlled trials.

Naltrexone is used in the USA for alcohol rehabilitation, but is not licensed in the UK. This opioid antagonist decreases drinking in animals, and might help alcohol-dependent-patients by diminishing craving and feelings of reward or pleasure when drinking. Given at 50–100 mg per day (or 150 mg three times a week), most studies report a longer time before relapse of lower alcohol intake on drinking days, with an outcome that is improved by a modest 20%. Some studies show a person's family history or μ-opioid-receptor genotype. Naltrexone can be given as an intramuscular dose of 380 mg once a month, which, although more expensive, optimizes compliance and has shown some promising results. Naltrexone's side-effects include increased liver function tests, possible interference with pain control, and a potential blunting of mood.

Acamprosate is structurally similar to γ-aminobytyric acid, but with actions that inhibit the N-methyl-D-aspartic acid-glutamate receptor hyperactivity that occurs during protracted wihtdrawal. Most trials report that this drug increases the time to relapse, decreases the number of drinks per drinking day, or helps maintain abstinence, with a rate of improved outcome similar to naltrexone. Side effects include gastrointestinal upset and diarrhea, which rarely cause patients to stop use of the drug. Combined naltrexone and acamprosate might be slightly better than either drug alone, although not all studies agree.

Disulfiram and calcium carbimide inhibit ALDH2 so that acetaldehyde increases dramatically after drinking, to produce nausea, vomiting, diarrhea, rapid heart rate, and changes in blood pressure. Several weeks are needed after discontinuation of disulfiram for ALDH to return to normal; calcium carbimide has a more rapid onset and a shorter action. More than 500 mg per day of disulfiram are needed for maximum inhibition of ALDH, but that dose would produce unacceptable side effects. This drug is best given under observation, to ensure compliance. The efficacy of ALDH inhibitors is controversial, perhaps because the anticipation of obverse effects after drinking could contribute to the outcome even with placebo. At the same time, disulfiram has both relatively benign side effects (a bad taste, sedation, a rash, and temporary impotence) and rarer but more severe sequelae (neuropathies, depression, psychotic symptoms, and increase in liver function tests, and severe hepatitis). In one study, the risk of fatal disulfiram-related hepatitis was one in every 25,000 patients per year with as many as one in 200 patients per year having adverse drug reactons. The potentially severe reaction to alcohol in individuals who take these drugs precludes their prescription to patients with diabetes, heart disease stroke, psychosis, or those who are pregnant; they should be used with caution for patients who have liver disease.

No other drugs have yet been shown to be more effective than placebo for alcohol-use disorders in sufficient large and broad-based studies. However, a 14-week placebo-controlled trail of 300 mg per day of the anticonvulsant topiramate reported up to a 16% reduction in heavy drinking days, although the rate of modest side-effects was high.

CONCLUSION

The criteria for alcohol dependence are reliable, patients face substantial morbidity and mortality, and resources are available to identify patients with unhealthy drinking or alcohol-use disorders, and to offer treatment. Treatment can include motivational interviewing to help people to evaluate their situations, brief interventions to facilitate more healthy behaviours, cognitive-behavioral therapies, and the judicious use of drugs to improve outcomes for alcohol-use disorder.

5.3 DIAGNOSIS, ASSESSMENT AND MANAGEMENT OF ALCOHOL USE DISORDER—NICE GUIDELINES

RK Solanki

Alcohol dependence affects 4% of people aged between 16 and 65 years in England (6% of men and 2% of women), and over 26% of all adults (38% of men and 16% of women) consume alcohol in a way that is potentially or actually harmful to their health or well-being. Yet currently only 6% of people who are alcohol dependent receive treatment. Alcohol dependence is characterized by withdrawal, craving, impaired control, and tolerance of alcohol and is associated with a higher rate of mental and physical illness and a wide range of social problems. Harmful drinking is a pattern of alcohol consumption that can lead to psychological problems such as depression, accidents, injuries, and physical health problems such as pancreatitis. Alcohol misuse is also an increasing problem in children and young people, with over 24000 treated in the NHS for alcohol related problems in 2008 and 2009. Hospital admissions related to alcohol consumption increased by 81% between 2003 and 2009. Harmful drinking and alcohol dependence therefore represent a considerable burden to individuals, their families, and wider society.

This chapter summarizes the most recent recommendations from the National Institute for Health and Clinical Excellence (NICE) on the diagnosis, assessment, and management of harmful drinking and alcohol dependence.

Recommendations

The NICE recommendations are based on systematic reviews of best available evidence and explicit consideration of cost-effectiveness. When minimal evidence is available, recommendations are based on the Guideline Development Group's experience and opinion of what constitutes good practice. Evidence levels for the recommendations are in the full version of this article on bmj.com.

Identification and Initial Assessment

- Staff working in services provided and funded by the NHS should be competent to identify harmful drinking and alcohol dependence and to initially assess the need for an intervention; if they are not competent, they should refer people who misuse alcohol to a service that can provide such an assessment. Validated tools such as the alcohol use disorders identification test (AUDIT) are effective in identifying harmful drinking and alcohol dependence in nonspecialist settings such a primary care and acute hospitals.
- Consider a comprehensive assessment for all adults referred to specialist alcohol services who score more than 15 on the identification test. This should assess multiple areas of need, be structured in a clinical interview, and cover:
  - Alcohol use, including consumption and patterns of drinking; severity of dependence (using the severity of alcohol dependence questionnaire (SADQ) or Leeds dependence questionnaire (LDQ)); and alcohol related problems (using the alcohol problems questionnaire (APQ))
  - Misuse of other drugs, including over the counter medication
  - Physical health problems
  - Psychological and social problems
  - Cognitive function (using, for example, the mini-mental state examination)
  - Readiness and belief in ability to change.

All Interventions for Harmful Drinking and Alcohol Dependence

- All interventions for harmful drinking and alcohol dependence should be delivered by appropriately trained and competent staff. Drug interventions should be administered by specialist and competent staff. Base psychological interventions on a relevant evidence based treatment manual, which should guide the structure and duration of the intervention.
- Carry out a motivational intervention as part of the initial assessment to help engage the person in treatment from first contact. The intervention should include helping people to recognize problems related to drinking and resolve ambivalence; encouraging positive change; and adopting a persuasive and supportive rather than argumentative and confrontational position.
- For all interventions, staff should:
  - Receive regular supervision from individuals competent in both the intervention and supervision
  - Routinely use outcome measurements to ensure that the person who misuses alcohol is involved in reviewing the effectiveness of their treatment
  - Monitor and evaluate the person's adherence to treatment and their own practice competence for

example, by using videotapes and audiotapes and external audit.

Psychological Interventions for Harmful Drinking and Mild Alcohol Dependence

- For harmful drinkers and people with mild alcohol dependence, offer a psychological intervention (such as cognitive behavioral therapies, behavioral therapies, or social network and environment based therapies) focused specifically on cognitions, behavior, problems, and social networks that are related to alcohol.

Assessment for Assisted Alcohol Withdrawal

- For those who typically drink over 15 units of alcohol a day and/or score 20 or more on the identification test, consider offering:
  - Assessment for and delivery of a community based assisted withdrawal, or
  - Assessment and management in inpatient care if you have safety concerns about a community based assisted withdrawal.
- Consider inpatient or residential assisted withdrawal if the person meets one or more of the following criteria:
  - Drinks over 30 units of alcohol a day
  - Has a score of more than 30 on the severity of alcohol dependence questionnaire
  - Has a history of epilepsy or of withdrawal related seizures or delirium tremens during previous assisted withdrawal programs
  - Needs concurrent withdrawal from alcohol and benzodiazepines
  - Regularly drinks 15–20 units of alcohol a day and has psychiatric or physical comorbidities (for example, chronic severe depression, psychosis, malnutrition, congestive cardiac failure, unstable angina, chronic liver disease) or a learning disability or cognitive impairment.

Interventions for Moderate and Severe Alcohol Dependence

- After a successful withdrawal for people with moderate and severe alcohol dependence, consider offering a camprosate or oral naltrexone in combination with an individual psychological intervention (cognitive behavioral therapies, behavioral therapies, or social network and environment based therapies) that focuses specifically on alcohol misuse. At the time of publication (mid-February 2011), oral naltrexone did not have UK marketing authorization for this indication. Obtain and document informed consent before prescribing.
- Consider offering interventions to promote abstinence and prevent relapse as part of an intensive and structured community based intervention for people with moderate and severe alcohol dependence who have:
  - Very limited social support (for example, they are living alone or have very little contact with family or friends)
  - Complex physical or psychiatric comorbidities
  - Not responded to initial community based interventions to promote abstinence or moderate drinking.

Interventions for Children and Young People Aged 10–17 years who Misuse Alcohol

- For those with limited comorbidities and good social support, offer individual cognitive behavioural therapy.
- For those with significant comorbidities and/or limited social support, offer multicomponent programs (such as multidimensional family therapy, brief strategic family therapy, functional family therapy or multisystemic therapy).

Interventions for Depression or Anxiety Disorders in Alcohol Misuse

Treat the alcohol misuse first as this may lead to improvement in the depression or anxiety. If depression or anxiety continues after three to four weeks of abstinence from alcohol, assess the depression or anxiety and consider referral and treatment in line with the relevant NICE guideline for the particular disorder.

Overcoming Barriers

Poor recognition of alcohol misuse is a major barrier to effective treatment and requires a service -wide approach to improve case identification. Current service delivery also fragmented, with access pathways to services unclear to both patients and professionals. To clarify care pathways and properly implement this and other NICE guidance that relates to alcohol uses NICE is currently developing an integrated care pathway for the three pieces of guidance.

Limited availability of specialist alcohol services also hinders effective guideline implementation-for example, there is a lack of skilled staff to deliver evidence based psychological interventions and support intensive community based assisted withdrawal, and limited prescribing of cost effective medication such as a camprosate and oral naltrexone to prevent relapse in moderate to severely dependent drinkers. Guideline recommendations on these interventions will need to be supported by effective commissioning.

5.4 DIAGNOSIS AND CLINICAL MANAGEMENT OF ALCOHOL USE DISORDER

RK Solanki

Continued hazardous and harmful drinking can result independence and tolerance, with risk of alcohol withdrawal syndrome on abrupt reduction or cessation; it may also result in damage to almost any organ or system in the body. Hazardous and harmful drinkers are commonly encountered among hospital patients, with 8,63,300 alcohol-related admissions to hospital in 2007–08, an increase of 69% since 2002–03. The cost to the NHS of treating acute and chronic drinking is estimated to be as much as £2.7 billion a year.

This article summarizes recommendations made in the recent guidance from the National Institute for Health and Clinical Excellence (NICE) for the diagnosis and clinical management of alcohol-related physical complications in adults and children (aged over 10 years). That guideline should be read in conjunction with the NICE public health guidance on the prevention and early identification of alcohol use disorders in adults and young people and the forthcoming NICE clinical guideline on the management of alcohol dependence and harmful alcohol use.

RECOMMENDATIONS

NICE recommendations are based on systematic reviews of best available evidence and explicit consideration of cost effectiveness. When minimal evidence is available, recommendations are based on the Guideline Development Group's experience and opinion of what constitutes good practice. Evidence levels for the recommendations are in the full version of this article on bmj.com,

ACUTE ALCOHOL WITHDRAWAL

Admission to Hospital

- For people in acute alcohol withdrawal with alcohol withdrawal seizures or delirium tremens, or for those at high risk (for example, those who have a history of alcohol withdrawal seizures or delirium tremens) of developing either condition, offer admission to hospital for medically-assisted alcohol withdrawal
- For young people aged under 16 years, who are in acute alcohol withdrawal, offer admission to hospital for physical and psychosocial assessment, in addition to medically-assisted alcohol withdrawal
- For people who are alcohol dependent but not admitted to hospital, offer advice to avoid a sudden reduction in alcohol intake (as this may result in severe withdrawal) and information about how to contact local alcohol support services.

Assessment and Monitoring

People in acute alcohol withdrawal should be assessed immediately on admission to hospital by a health care professional skilled in the management of alcohol withdrawal.

Treatment for Acute Alcohol Withdrawal

- Offer pharmacotherapy for the symptoms of acute alcohol withdrawal as follows:
  - Consider offering a benzodiazepine or carbamazepine
  - Consider offering clomethiazole as an alternative to a benzodiazepine or carbamazepine. However, use this with caution and in inpatient settings only.
- Follow a symptom triggered regimen (box) for drug treatment for people in acute alcohol withdrawal who are either in hospital or in other settings where 24 hours assessment and monitoring is available.

Management of Delirium Tremens

In people with delirium tremens, offer oral lorazepam as first-line treatment. If symptoms persist or oral medication is declined, give parenteral lorazepam, haloperidol, or olanzapine.

Management of Alcohol Withdrawal Seizures

In people who are having or who have had an alcohol withdrawal seizure, consider offering an immediate dose of quick acting benzodiazepine (such as lorazepam) to reduce the likelihood of further seizures.

Wernicke's Encephalopathy

- Be highly alert to the possibility of Wernicke's encephalopathy (clinical features include global confusion, eye muscle weakness, and ataxia), particularly if the person is intoxicated.

- Offer thiamine to people at risk of developing Wernicke's encephalopathy (those with harmful or hazardous drinking, malnutrition, or decompensated liver disease). Thiamine should be given in doses towards the upper end of the range recommended in the British National Formulary and given orally or parenterally as described in the full guideline.
- Offer parenteral thiamine to people with suspected Wernicke's encephalopathy for a minimum of five days, unless Wernicke's encephalopathy is excluded. Follow parenteral treatment with oral thiamine.

ALCOHOL-RELATED LIVER DISEASE

Assessment and Diagnosis

- Refer people to a specialist experienced in the management of alcohol-related liver disease to confirm a clinical diagnosis of such disease
- In people with suspected acute alcohol-related hepatitis whose suspected hepatitis is severe enough to require corticosteroid treatment, consider a liver biopsy to confirm the diagnosis.

Referral for Consideration of Liver Transplantation

Refer patients with decompensated liver disease (Jaundice, ascites, or encephalopathy) for assessment for liver transplantation if they still have decompensated liver disease after best management and three months' abstinence from alcohol and are otherwise suitable candidates for liver transplantation according to guidelines.

Corticosteroid Treatment for Alcohol-related Hepatitis

Otter corticosteroid treatment to people with severe acute alcohol-related hepatitis and a poor prognosis as determined by Maddrey's discriminant function of ≥ 32. This is calculated as 4.6 × [prothrombin time-control prothrombin time (seconds)] + either (bilirubin in mg/dL) or (bilirubin in µmol/L divided by 17).

Nutritional Support for Alcohol-related Hepatitis

Assess the nutritional requirements of people with acute alcohol-related hepatitis. Offer nutritional support if needed, and consider using nasogastric tube feeding.

Pancreatic Surgery versus Endoscopic Therapy for Chronic Alcohol-related Pancreatitis

- Refer people with pain from chronic alcohol-related pancreatitis to a specialist center for multidisciplinary assessment
- Offer surgery rather than endoscopic therapy to people with pain from large duct (obstructive) chronic alcohol-related pancreatitis.

Enzyme Supplementation for Chronic Alcohol-related Pancreatitis

- Offer pancreatic enzyme supplements to people with chronic alcohol-related pancreatitis who have symptoms of steatorrhea or poor nutritional status as a result of exocrine pancreatic insufficiency
- Do not prescribe pancreatic enzyme supplements to people with chronic alcohol-related pancreatitis if pain is their only symptom.

Overcoming Barriers

Implementing symptom triggered dosing regimens for acute alcohol withdrawal (where 21: hour assessment and monitoring is available) may require additional training and staff time. However, importantly, the clinical evidence review and economic analysis suggest that symptom triggered regimens are associated with positive outcomes such as lower doses of medication and a reduced length of hospital stay. The impact of the recommendation on referral for liver transplantation is difficult to assess, but referral rates may increase if patients are currently being asked to abstain for longer than three months before referral. There commendations to refer patients with alcohol-related liver disease and with pain associated with chronic pancreatitis may lead to a small but noticeable increase in the number of referrals.

5.5 ADVERSE HEALTH EFFECTS OF NONMEDICAL CANNABIS USE

RK Solanki, Ashok Singhal

SUMMARY

For over two decades, cannabis, commonly known as marijuana, has been the most widely used illicit drug by young people in high-income countries, and has recently become popular on a global scale. Epidemiological research during the past 10 years suggests that regular use of cannabis during adolescence and into adulthood can have adverse effects. Epidemiological, clinical, and laboratory studies have established an association between cannabis use and adverse outcomes. We focus on adverse health effects of greatest potential public health interest—that is, those that are most likely to occur and to affect a large number of cannabis users. The most probable adverse effects include a dependence syndrome, increased risk of motor vehicle crashes, impaired respiratory function, cardiovascular disease, and adverse effects of regular use on adolescent psychosocial development and mental health.

INTRODUCTION

Psychoactive preparations of *Cannabis sativa* have been used for over 4000 years for medical and religious purposes. Over the past 50 years, they have been increasingly adopted by adolescents and young adults for recreational use—in social settings to increase sociability and produce euphoric and intoxicating effects. Since cannabis use was first reported over 40 years ago by US college students, its recreational or nonmedical use has spread globally, first to high-income countries, and recently to low-income and middle-income countries.

Uncertainties exist about the number of people who use cannabis because of lack of timely, good-quality data in most countries. The UN Office on Drugs and Crime has estimated that in 2006 cannabis was used by 166 million adults (3.9% of the global population aged 15–64 years). Use was the highest in the USA, Australia, and New Zealand, followed by Europe. These countries reported higher rates of cannabis use than did the Middle East and Asia. Some African countries are also thought to have high rates of cannabis use. Because of their large populations, 31%, 25%, and 24% of the world's cannabis users are estimated to be from Asia, Africa, and the Americas, respectively, compared with 18% in Europe and 2% in Oceania.

Pattern of Cannabis Use

In the USA, rates of cannabis use in young adults peaked in 1979, which was followed by a long decline until the early 1990s, when use increased again, before levelling off towards the end of the decade. A similar rise in its use in the early 1990s, followed by decline or stabilization in recent years, has been reported in Australia and Western Europe.

Research in the USA has indicated that about 10% of those who ever use cannabis become daily users, and 20–30% become weekly users. Cannabis use in the USA typically begins in the middle to late teenage years and peaks in the early and middle 1920s. Use declines steeply after young people enter full-time employment, marry, and have children.

No reliable information exists about the concentration of Δ-9-tetrahydrocannabinol and other cannabinoids (e.g. cannabidiol) in commonly used cannabis products. In epidemiological studies, heavy or regular cannabis use is usually defined as every day or almost every day use. This pattern, when continued over years, predicts an increased risk of some adverse health effects. This review summarizes the most probable adverse health effects of cannabis use during the years since the last review in 1997 by WHO.

Cannabis

The effects of cannabis depend on the dose received, the mode of administration, the user's previous experience with this drug, and the set and setting, i.e. the user's expectations, attitudes towards the effects of cannabis, the mood state, and the social setting in which it is used. The main reason why most young people use cannabis is to experience a so-called high: mild euphoria, relaxation, and perceptual alterations, including time distortion and intensification of ordinary experiences such as eating, watching films, listening to music, and engaging in sex. When used in a social context, the so-called high could be accompanied by infectious laughter, talkativeness, and increased sociability. These effects typically occur 30 minutes after smoking and last for 1–2 hours.

The primary psychoactive constituent of cannabis preparations is Δ-9-tetrahydrocannabinol (THC). THC produces psychological and physical effects that are similar to those that users report after smoking cannabis, and drugs that block the effects of THC on brain receptors also block the effects of cannabis in animals and human beings. The effects of THC can be modulated by cannabidiol (CBD), a nonpsychoactive cannabinoid present in many cannabis products.

THC acts on at least two types of cannabinoid receptors (CB_1 and CB_2) in the brain. The CB_1 receptor is widely distributed in brain regions involved in cognition, memory, reward, pain perception, and motor coordination. It also responds to a naturally occurring (or endogenous) ligand—anandamide—which produces effects similar to THC but is less potent and shorter acting. Neuroimaging studies indicate that THC increases activity in the frontal and paralimbic regions and in the cerebellum of the human brain.

The THC content is highest in the flowering tops of the female cannabis plant. Marijuana (THC content 0·5–5%) comprises the dried flowering tops and leaves of the plant. Hashish (THC content 2–20%) consists of dried cannabis resin, and hash oil is an oil-based extract of hashish (THC content 15–50%). In the USA, THC content of cannabis increased from less than 2% in 1980 to 4·5% in 1997 and 8·5% in 2006. THC content also increased in the Netherlands and probably in other countries. No data are available on changes in CBD content.

Cannabis is usually smoked in a joint or a water pipe (sometimes with tobacco added) because this is the most efficient way to achieve the desired psychoactive effects. The amount of THC delivered to the lungs varies between 20 and 70%, and 5–24% reaches the brain. A dose of 2–3 mg of THC will produce a high in occasional users who typically share a single joint with others. Regular users might smoke up to 3–5 joints of potent cannabis a day for several reasons, including development of tolerance and to experience stronger effects.

Health Effects of Cannabis

We looked for evidence: that an association exists between cannabis use and outcomes in case—control and prospective studies; that reverse causation was an implausible explanation of the association (evidence from prospective studies that cannabis use preceded the outcome); from prospective studies that controlled for potential confounding variables (such as other drug use and characteristics on which cannabis users differed from nonusers); and that a causal association was biologically plausible. Our focus was on adverse health effects that are of greatest potential public health interest—that is, those with the greatest probability of affecting a substantial proportion of cannabis users.

Acute Effects

The dose of THC that kills rodents is very high and the estimated fatal human dose is between 15 g and 70 g, 9, 15 which is much higher than that smoked by a heavy user. The most common acute adverse effects are anxiety, panic reactions, and psychotic symptoms, all of which are most often reported by naïve users.

In the laboratory, cannabis and THC produce dose-related impairment in reaction time, information processing, perceptual—motor coordination, motor performance, attention, and tracking behavior. These effects can increase the risk of accidents if users drive while intoxicated. Studies of the effects of cannabis upon on-road driving found more modest impairments than those caused by intoxicating doses of alcohol because cannabis-affected people drive more slowly and take fewer risks. Nonetheless, some experimental studies have shown diminished driving performance in response to emergency situations. Epidemiological studies also suggest that cannabis users who drive while intoxicated are at increased risk of crashes. Gerberich and colleagues found that cannabis users had higher rates of hospital admission for injury from all causes than had former cannabis users or non-users in a group of 64,657 patients from a health maintenance organization. The risk of motor vehicle accidents (relative risk 1·96) persisted after statistical adjustment in men. Mura and colleagues showed a similar relation in a study of THC in the serum of 900 individuals admitted to a French hospital for motor vehicle injuries and 900 age-matched and sex-matched controls. Drummer and colleagues, who assessed THC in the blood in 1420 Australian drivers killed in accidents, showed that cannabis users were more likely to be culpable than were nonusers (odds ratio [OR] 2·5). Individuals with blood THC concentrations greater than 5 μg/mL had a higher accident risk (OR 6·6) than those without THC. Laumon and colleagues compared blood THC concentrations in 6766 culpable and 3006 nonculpable drivers in France between October, 2001 and September, 2003. The investigators showed increased culpability in drivers with THC concentrations of more than 1 μg/mL (OR 2·87). A dose—response relation between THC and culpability persisted after controlling for blood alcohol concentration, age, and time of accident. They estimated that 2·5% of fatal accidents in France can be attributed to cannabis and 29% to alcohol. Driving after having taken cannabis might increase the risk of motor vehicle crashes 2–3 times compared with 6 to 15 times with alcohol. The policy challenge is to specify a concentration of THC in the blood that legally defines impaired driving.

Reproductive Effects

High doses of cannabis cause growth retardation and malformations in animals, but epidemiological studies have given scarce evidence for an increased risk of birth defects in women who use cannabis during pregnancy. Interpretation of the few associations that have been reported is difficult because cannabis users are also more likely to use tobacco, alcohol, and other illicit drugs during pregnancy,and less likely to seek antenatal care and have poorer nutrition than women who do not use cannabis. Zuckerman and colleagues reported that no increased risk of birth defects could be seen in a large group of women who use cannabis. Cannabis use in pregnancy has been most consistently associated with reduced birthweight in large epidemiological studies. A meta-analysis showed that regular cannabis smoking during pregnancy decreased birth weight, although less so than tobacco smoking, probably through the effects of carbon monoxide on the developing fetus.

Mild developmental abnormalities have been reported in children born to women who used cannabis during pregnancy. These include developmental delay in the visual system shortly after birth, and increased tremor and startle; however, no effects were seen at 1 month, or on ability tests at 6 and 12 months. Behavioral effects were subsequently reported at 36 and 48 months but not at 60 and 72 months. At 12 years of age, children who were exposed to cannabis did not differ on full-scale intelligence quotient (IQ) scores from those not exposed, but there were small differences in higher cognitive processes (e.g. perceptual organisation and planning).

Other studies have given mixed results. Tennes and colleagues found no differences at 1 year between children of users and those of nonusers. Day and colleaguesfollowed up children born to 655 women in Pittsburgh between 1990 and 1995, and found poorer performances on memory and verbal skills of the Stanford-Binet intelligence scale in 3-year-old children of cannabis users. By 10 years of age, children born to cannabis users showed increased delinquency and behavioural problems.

Postnatal behavioural effects of prenatal cannabis exposure seem modest.The causal interpretation of any such effects is weakened by the inability of these studies to control for the confounding effects of other drug use during pregnancy, poor parenting, and genetic factors.

Chronic Effects

With no data for THC and other cannabinoids, chronic cannabis use has usually been defined as almost daily use over a period of years. Epidemiological studies cited below have reported associations between this pattern of cannabis use during adolescence and various adverse health outcomes. The major challenge in the interpretation of these studies is to rule out alternative explanations of the associations. Cannabis use is highly correlated with use of alcohol, tobacco, and other illicit drugs, all of which adversely affect health. Regular cannabis users also differ from nonusers before they use cannabis in ways that could affect their risk of some outcomes, especially behavioural ones. Statistical control of confounding has been used to assess these relations but some epidemiologists doubt the success of this strategy.

Cannabis dependence is characterised by impaired control over cannabis use and difficulty in ceasing use despite its harms. In Australia, Canada, and the USA, cannabis dependence is the most common type of drug dependence after that on alcohol and tobacco. It has affected 1–2% of adults in the past year, and 4–8% of adults during their lifetime. The lifetime risk of dependence in cannabis users has been estimated at about 9%, rising to one in six in those who initiate use in adolescence. The equivalent lifetime risks are 32% for nicotine, 23% for heroin, 17% for cocaine, 15% for alcohol, and 11% for stimulant users. Those at highest risk of cannabis dependence have a history of poor academic achievement, deviant behavior in childhood and adolescence, rebelliousness, poor parental relationships, or a parental history of drug and alcohol problems.

Animals and human beings develop tolerance to many of the effects of THC. The cannabinoid antagonist SR141716A causes a withdrawal syndrome in rats, mice, and dogs that is reversed by THC. Cannabis users seeking help to stop report withdrawal symptoms that include anxiety, insomnia, appetite disturbance, and depression. Over the past 20 years, increasing numbers of people have sought help in the USA, Europe, and Australia to stop using cannabis. Some of this escalation might be explained by increased treatment of users as a legal requirement; however, a rise has also occurred in the Netherlands where cannabis use has been decriminalised. Cognitive—behavioral therapy reduces cannabis use and cannabis-related issues, but only 15% of people remain abstinent 6 to 12 months after treatment.

Effects of long-term cannabis smoking on respiratory function are less clear. Regular cannabis smokers report more symptoms of chronic bronchitis (wheeze, sputum production, and chronic coughs) than do nonsmokers. The immunological competence of the respiratory system in cannabis-only smokers is also impaired, increasing their health service use for respiratory infections. A longitudinal study of 1037 young people in New Zealand followed until the age of 26 years found impaired respiratory function in cannabis-dependent users, but this finding was not replicated in longer-term follow-up of US users. Chronic cannabis smoking did not increase the risk of emphysema in follow-up studies over 8 years in cannabis-only smokers in the USA and New Zealand. Cannabis smoke contains many of the same carcinogens as does tobacco smoke, with some in higher concentrations. It is also mutagenic and carcinogenic in the mouse skin test, and chronic cannabis smokers show pathological changes in lung cells that precede the development of lung cancer in tobacco smokers.

Case-control studies of lung cancer have produced more consistent associations with cannabis use but their interpretation is uncertain because of confounding by cigarette smoking. A Tunisian case—control study of 110 cases of hospital-diagnosed lung cancer and 110 community controls indicated an association of lung cancer with cannabis use (OR 8·2) that persisted after adjustment for cigarette smoking. A pooled analysis of three Moroccan case—control studies also showed an increased risk of lung cancer in cannabis smokers, all of whom also smoked tobacco. A New Zealand case—control study of lung cancer in 79 adults under the age of 55 years and 324 community controls found a dose—response relation between frequency of cannabis use and lung cancer risk. A US case—control study showed a simple association between cannabis smoking and head and neck and lung cancers, but these associations were not significant after controlling for tobacco use. Larger cohort and better designed case—control studies are needed to clarify whether any such risks from chronic cannabis smoking exist.

Evidence exists to support the adverse cardiovascular effects of cannabis use. Cannabis and THC increase heart rate in a dose-dependent way. These drugs marginally affect healthy young adults who quickly develop tolerance, but concern exists about adults with cardiovascular disease. A case-crossover study by Mittleman and colleagues of 3882 patients who had had a myocardial infarction showed that cannabis use can increase the risk of myocardial infarction 4·8 times in the hour after use. A prospective study of 1913 of these individuals reported a dose—response relation between cannabis use and mortality over 3·8 years. Risk increased 2·5 times for those who used cannabis less than once a week to 4·2 times in those who used cannabis more than once a week. These findings are supported by laboratory studies that indicate that smoking cannabis provokes angina in patients with heart disease.

CNS Effects

Poor cognitive functioning is a risk factor for regular cannabis use; however, whether chronic cannabis use impairs cognitive performance is not clear. Studies that matched users and nonusers on estimated intellectual function before cannabis use or on cognitive performance assessed before cannabis use have found subtle cognitive impairments in frequent and long-term cannabis users.

Deficits in verbal learning, memory, and attention are most consistently reported in heavy cannabis users, but these have been variously related to duration and frequency of use, and cumulative dose of THC. Debate continues about whether these deficits are caused by acute drug effects, residual drug effects, or the effects of cumulative THC exposure. Whether cognitive function recovers after cessation of cannabis use is also unclear. Solowij showed partial recovery after 2 years of abstinence but brain event-related potential measures still showed impaired information processing that was correlated with years of use. Bolla and colleagues found indications of persistent dose-related impairment in neurocognitive performance after 28 days of abstinence in heavy young users (5 years of use) but Pope and colleagues reported recovery after 28 days' abstinence.

Acute and chronic cannabis use is associated with changes in brain function that can be detected by cerebral blood flow, positron emission tomography (PET), and electroencephalography (EEG). Block and colleagues, for example, showed that, after 26 hours of abstinence, regular users had lower resting brain blood flow than had controls in the posterior cerebellum and prefrontal cortex. Functional imaging studies have shown less activity in brain regions involved in memory and attention in chronic cannabis users than in nonusers, even after 28 days of abstinence. Changes in cannabinoid receptor activity in the hippocampus, prefrontal cortex, and cerebellum have been seen in chronic cannabis users. Yücel and colleagues reported reduced volumes of the hippocampus and the amygdala in 15 long-term users who had smoked five or more joints a day for 10 or more years. These reductions increased with the duration of use. More functional brain imaging studies on larger samples of long-term users are needed to see if cognitive impairments in long-term users are correlated with structural changes in brain areas implicated in memory and emotion.

Psychosocial Effects

Cannabis use is associated with poor educational attainment. However, whether cannabis use is a contributory cause of poor school performance, is a consequence of poor educational attainment, or poor educational attainment is the result of common factors is unclear. The first two possibilities could both be true if poor school performance increased cannabis use, which further impaired school performance.

Longitudinal studies have shown a relation between cannabis use in young individuals before the age of 15 years and early school leaving that has persisted after adjustment for confounders. The most plausible hypothesis is that impaired educational outcomes are attributable to a combination of higher pre-existing risk, effects of regular cannabis use on cognitive performance, increased affiliation with peers who reject school, and a strong desire to make an early transition into adulthood. Adolescent cannabis users who leave school early are more likely to be unemployed and depend on social welfare, and are less satisfied with their lives and their relationships than are peers in their late 1920s.

Other Illicit Drug Use

In the USA, Australia, and New Zealand, regular cannabis users were most likely to later use heroin and cocaine, and the earlier the age at which a young person uses cannabis, the more likely they are to use heroin and cocaine. Three explanations have been given for these patterns of drug involvement: cannabis users have more opportunities to use other illicit drugs because cannabis is supplied by the same black market; those who are early cannabis users are more likely to use other illicit drugs for reasons that are unrelated to their cannabis use; and pharmacological effects of cannabis increase the propensity to use other illicit drugs.Young people in the USA who have used cannabis report more opportunities to use cocaine at an early age. Socially deviant young people (who are more likely to use cocaine and heroin) start using cannabis at an earlier age than do their peers. A simulation study has shown that the second (common cause) hypothesis, if true, would reproduce all the associations between cannabis and other illicit drug use.

The common causal hypothesis has been assessed in longitudinal studies to see whether cannabis users are more likely to report heroin and cocaine use after statistically controlling for confounders. Adjustment for confounders (including unmeasured ones with fixed-effects regression) has weakened but not eliminated the associations between regular cannabis use and the use of other illicit drugs. Studies of discordant twins have tested the hypothesis that the association is explained by a shared genetic vulnerability to use cannabis and other illicit drugs. Lynskey and colleagues assessed the association between cannabis and other illicit drug use in 136 monozygotic and 175 dizygotic twin pairs in which one twin had used cannabis before the age of 17 years, and the other had not. The twin who had used cannabis was more likely to have used other illicit drugs than was their co-twin who had not, and the association persisted after controlling for nonshared environmental factors.

Animal studies suggest some ways in which the effects of cannabis could predispose cannabis users to use other illicit drugs. First, cannabis, cocaine, and heroin all act on the brain reward centre in the nucleus accumbens. Second, the cannabinoid and opioid systems in the brain interact with each other.

Cannabis and Mental Health

Cannabis use has been associated with increased risk of psychiatric disorders. A 15-year follow-up of 50,465 Swedish male conscripts reported that those who had tried cannabis by age 18 years were 2·4 times more likely to be diagnosed with schizophrenia than those who had not. Risk increased with the frequency of cannabis use and remained significant after statistical adjustment for a few confounding variables. Those who had used cannabis ten or more times by 18 years of age were 2·3 times more likely to be diagnosed with schizophrenia than those who had not. Zammit and colleagues reported a 27-year follow-up of the same cohort. These investigators also showed a dose—response relation between frequency of cannabis use in individuals aged 18 years and risk of schizophrenia during the follow-up, and this association persisted after controlling for the effects of other confounding factors. They estimated that 13% of schizophrenia cases could be averted if cannabis use was prevented. These findings have been supported by longitudinal studies in the Netherlands, Germany, and New Zealand, all of which indicated that the association persisted after adjustment for confounders.

A meta-analysis of these longitudinal studies reported a pooled OR of 1·4 (95% CI 1·20-1·65) of psychotic symptoms or psychotic disorders in those who had ever used cannabis. Risk of psychotic symptoms or disorders was higher in regular users than in nonusers (OR 2·09, 95% CI 1·54-2·84). Reverse causation was addressed in most of these studies by exclusion of cases reporting psychotic symptoms at baseline or by statistically adjusting for pre-existing psychotic symptoms. The common causal hypothesis was difficult to exclude because the association between cannabis use and psychosis was attenuated after statistical adjustment for potential confounders, and no study assessed all major confounders.

Evidence is conflicting on whether incidence of schizophrenia increases as cannabis use increases in young adults, as would be expected if the association was causal. An Australian study did not show clear evidence of increased psychosis incidence despite steep increases in cannabis use during the 1980s and 1990s. A similar study suggested that it was too early to see any increased incidence in England and Wales in the 1990s. A British and a Swiss study reported increases in the incidence of psychoses in recent birth cohorts but another British study failed to do so.

Nonconsistent and weak associations have been reported between cannabis use and depression. Fergusson and Horwood, for example, found a dose—response relation between frequency of cannabis use in individuals aged 16 years and depressive disorder, but the association was not significant after adjusting for confounders. A meta-analysis of these studies reported an association between cannabis use and depressive disorders (OR 1·49, 95% CI 1·15-1·94). The investigators argued, however, that these studies had not controlled for confounders and had not convincingly excluded the possibility that depressed young people are more likely to use cannabis.

Several case-control studies have shown a relation between cannabis use and suicide in adolescents, but whether this is causal is unclear. For example, a New Zealand case-control study of serious suicide attempts resulting in hospitalization found that 16% of the 302 people attempting suicide met criteria for cannabis dependence or abuse compared with 2% of the 1028 community controls. Controlling for social disadvantage, depression, and alcohol dependence substantially reduced, but did not eliminate, the association (Odd Ratio 2).

The evidence from prospective studies is mixed. Fergusson and Horwood, for example, found a dose-response relation between frequency of cannabis use in individuals aged 16 years and a self-reported suicide attempt, but the association did not persist after controlling for confounders. Patton and colleagues reported that cannabis was associated with self-harmful behavior in women but not in men, after controlling for depression and alcohol use. A meta-analysis reported that these studies were too heterogeneous to estimate risk, and few had excluded reverse causation or properly controlled for confounding.

Increased THC Content in Cannabis Products

Concerns have been expressed over the past 20 years about putative increases in the potency of cannabis products, which recent studies suggest may have occurred during the late 1990s. It is unclear whether increased THC content has been accompanied by any changes in CBD content. Any health effects of increased potency depend on whether users are able and willing to titrate their dose of THC, and might also vary with the experience of users. A high THC content can increase anxiety, depression, and psychotic symptoms in naive users, while increasing the risk of dependence and psychotic symptoms if regular users do not titrate their dose. Adverse effects on respiratory and cardiovascular systems could be reduced if regular users titrate the dose of THC and reduce the amount they smoke. Increased potency could also increase the risk of road traffic crashes if users drive while heavily intoxicated.

Panel 2: Acute and chronic adverse effects of cannabis use	
Acute adverse effects	
•	Anxiety and panic, especially in naive users
•	Psychotic symptoms (at high doses)
•	Road crashes if a person drives while intoxicated
Chronic adverse effects	
•	Cannabis dependence syndrome (in around one in ten users)
•	Chronic bronchitis and impaired respiratory function in regular smokers
•	Psychotic symptoms and disorders in heavy users, especially those with a history of psychotic symptoms or a family history of these disorders
•	Impaired educational attainment in adolescents who are regular users
•	Subtle cognitive impairment in those who are daily users for 10 years or more

Panel 3: Possible adverse effects of regular cannabis use with unknown causal relation
• Respiratory cancers
• Behavioral disorders in children whose mothers used cannabis while pregnant
• Depressive disorders, mania, and suicide
• Use of other illicit drugs by adolescents

CONCLUSION

Acute adverse effects of cannabis use include anxiety and panic in naive users, and a probable increased risk of accidents if users drive while intoxicated (Panel 2). Use during pregnancy could reduce birth weight, but does not seem to cause birth defects. Whether cannabis contributes to behavioural disorders in the offspring of women who smoked cannabis during pregnancy is uncertain.

Chronic cannabis use can produce a dependence syndrome in as many as one in ten users. Regular users have a higher risk of chronic bronchitis and impaired respiratory function, and psychotic symptoms and disorders, most probably if they have a history of psychotic symptoms or a family history of these disorders. The most probable adverse psychosocial effect in adolescents who become regular users is impaired educational attainment. Adolescent regular cannabis users are more likely to use other illicit drugs, although the explanation of this association remains contested. Regular cannabis use in adolescence might also adversely affect mental health in young adults, with the strongest evidence for an increased risk of psychotic symptoms and disorders.

Some other adverse effects are associated with regular cannabis use (Panel 3), but whether they are causal is not known because of the possible confounding effects of other drugs (tobacco for respiratory cancers; tobacco, alcohol, and other drugs for behavioral disorders in children whose mothers smoked cannabis during pregnancy). In the case of depressive disorders and suicide, the association with cannabis is uncertain. For cognitive performance, the size and reversibility of the impairment remain unclear. The focus of epidemiological and clinical research should be on clarifying the causative role of cannabis for these adverse health effects.

The public health burden of cannabis use is probably modest compared with that of alcohol, tobacco, and other illicit drugs. A recent Australian study estimated that cannabis use caused 0·2% of total disease burden in Australia—a country with one of the highest reported rates of cannabis use. Cannabis accounted for 10% of the burden attributable to all illicit drugs (including heroin, cocaine, and amphetamines). It also accounted for around 10% of the proportion of disease burden attributed to alcohol (2·3%), but only 2·5% of that attributable to tobacco (7·8%).

5.6 TOBACCO ADDICTION

G Prasad Rao

INTRODUCTION

Lung cancer was confirmed to be caused by cigarette smoking over 50 years ago, and since then several other diseases have been added to the list of diseases caused by smoking and involuntary exposure to cigarette smoke. However, the worldwide production and consumption of cigarettes has continued to increase unabated during this period. There are about 1.2 billion smokers in the world, half of whom will die from diseases caused by smoking. Smoking causes 5 million deaths per year and if present trends continue. 10 million smokers per year are projected to die by 2025. The prevalence varies greatly, from less than 5% to more than 55% in different countries. It also varies greatly between men and women. So prevalence in both sexes needs to be examined separately.

On the basis of analyses of the WHO and American Cancer Society database, Table 31 shows the distribution of prevalence of smoking in men and women in different countries of the world. These prevalence rate are not strictly comparable - samples might not be representative of the population of the country, the may refer to different time periods, the definitions of smoking might be different (e.g. smoking at least 100 cigarettes in a lifetime), and even age cutoffs might differ. Despite restrictions, they are the best data available.

More men smoke than do women. In men, prevalence seems to be moderate to low in industrialized countries and in sub-Saharan Africa. Prevalence seems generally high in Eastern Europe and Asia. About 45% of the world wide population lives in countries where the prevalence of smoking in men is greater than 45% and about 92% of the population lives where prevalence in men is more than 25%. By contrast, only about 10% of the female population worldwide lives in a country where the prevalence is greater than 24%. The prevalence in women is low in some of the most highly population countries of the world (China, India, Indonesia, and Nigeria) and in most countries of Asia, whereas high prevalence is reported from several industrialized countries.

The main determinant to substantially reduce the accelerated increase of morbidity related to tobacco in the short-term would be if smokers were able to quit smoking. This seminar will provide descriptions for the diagnosis of tobacco addiction, the biobehavioral basis for this addiction, and evidence-based treatments.

DIAGNOSIS

The 1988 US Surgeon General's report—The Health Consequences of Smoking, Nicotine Addiction—described three major conclusions: cigarettes and other forms of tobacco are addictive, nicotine is the drug that causes this addiction, and the pharmacological and behavioral processes that determine tobacco addiction are similar to those that determine addiction to drugs such as heroin and cocaine. The primary difference between nicotine addiction and addiction to other drugs is the absence of behavioral disruption associated with tobacco use; but the lack of this drug effect by no means signifies diminished addictive capabilities of nicotine.

Criteria for nicotine dependence have been described in the Diagnostic and Statistical Manual IV (DSM-IV) and the International Classification of Diseases, 10th revision (ICD-10). Core features include a repeated or compulsive administration of the drug, impaired control over use as manifested by continued use despite negative effects or by

Table 31: Smoking prevalence in men and women

	Number of countries (%)	*Combined population across countries (% of population)*	*Examples of large countries*
Men			
<25%	26 (18%)	467405158 (8%)	Nigeria, Iran, Sudan, Tanzania, Canada
25–35%	30 (20%)	1733797361 (30%)	India, USA, France, UK, Italy, Colombia, Morocco
35–45%	39 (27%)	988527769 (27%)	Brazil, Pakistan, Germany, Egypt, Thailand, Burma
45–55%	28 (19%)	2017020322 (35%)	China, Bangladesh, Japan, Philippines, Vietnam, Turkey
>55%	24 (16%)	590227532 (10%)	Indonesia, Russia, Ukraine, Kenya
Women			
<4%	36 (24%)	3220581420 (55%)	China, India, Indonesia, Nigeria, Vietnam, Iran, Thailand
4–14%	37 (25%)	1031593028 (18%)	Pakistan, Russia, Japan, Philippines, Turkey, Congo
14–24%	43 (29%)	1022297825 (18%)	USA, Bangladesh, Egypt, France, Italy, Burma
>24%	33 (22%)	572828144 (10%)	Brazil, Germany, UK, Spain, Kenya

repeated relapse to use after quit attempts, a high motivation to seek the drug, a higher value given to the use of the drug than to other activities, and manifestation of physical dependence, i.e. tolerance and withdrawal (Panel 4). Whether the DSM-IV and ICD-10 diagnostic criteria are sufficiently valid measures of nicotine dependence is debated. Studies have shown that these diagnostic criteria do not have adequate predictive validity. Such as their ability to predict relapse to smoking. Diagnosis made on the basis of these criteria is also restricted because of its one dimensional and categorical nature, rather than reflecting the potentially multidimensional and continuous aspects of addiction.

The most widely used dependence measure is the Fagerstrom tolerance questionnaire, or the recent modified version, the Fagerstrom test for nicotine dependence (Table 32). Although this scale tends to be one-dimensional, it often predicts relapse to smoking. The items that contribute most to the prediction of relapse are the number of cigarettes smoked and time to first cigarette after waking. These two items, which constitute the heaviness of smoking scale, can be a useful measure of dependence in a clinic-office setting and helpful in establishment of the dose of nicotine replacement treatments (e.g. nicotine lozenge or gum). Irrespective of whether or not a smoker meets DSM-IV or ICD-10 criteria for nicotine dependence or scores high on the Fagerstrom test for nicotine dependence, all smokers should be provided with treatment for smoking cessation.

Panel 4: Characteristics of nicotine dependence based on the Diagnostic and Statistical Manual Version IV (DSM-IV) and the International Classification of Diseases Revision 10 (ICD-10)

DSM-IV criteria	
Three or more of the following at any time in the same 12-month period:	
•	Tolerance—smoker needs increased amount of nicotine to achieve desired effect, or diminished effect with continued use of same amount.
•	Withdrawal symptoms
•	Nicotine often taken in larger amounts or over a longer period than intended
•	Persistent or unsuccessful efforts to cut down or control use
•	Great deal of time spent in activities necessary to obtain nicotine or recover from its effects
•	Important social, occupational, or recreational activities given up or reduced because of nicotine use
•	Nicotine use continued despite knowledge of having a persistent or recurrent physical or psychological problem that is likely to have been caused or exacerbated by it
ICD-10 criteria	
•	A cluster of behavioral cognitive and psychological occurrences that develop after repeated use
•	Increased tolerance
•	Sometimes physical withdrawal symptoms
•	A strong desire to take nicotine
•	Difficulty controlling use
•	Higher priority given to nicotine use than to other activities and obligations
•	Persisting use-despite harmful effects

Table 32: The Firestorm test for nicotine dependence

	Points
How soon after you wake up do you smoke your first cigarette?	
Within 5 min	3
6–30 min	2
31–60 min	1
After 60 min	0
Do you find it difficult–refrain from smoking in places where it is forbidden, e.g. in church, at the library, in cinema, etc.?	
Yes	1
No	0
Which cigarette would you have most–give up?	
The first one in the morning	1
All others	0
How Many cigarettes per day do you smoke?	
<10	0
11–20	1
21–30	2
>31	3
Do you smoke more frequently during the first hours after waking than you do during the rest for the day?	
Yes	1
No	0
Do you smoke if you are so ill that you are in bed most of the day?	
Yes	1
No	0
Maximum score is 10 with higher scores indicating greater dependences	

PATHOPHYSIOLOGY

Nicotine, when inhaled; enters the lungs where a large surface area of small airways and alveoli exists, undergoes dissolution in pulmonary fluid at a high pH is transported to the heart, and then immediately passes to the brain. The rapid rate of nicotine absorption and high amounts of nicotine attained in the brain from smoking is two crucial factors that promote and sustain nicotine addiction. The rate of nicotine metabolism can also greatly affect the circulating concentrations of nicotine in a smoker and the amount of nicotine which reaches the brain, and can vary between individuals. Nicotine targets various subtypes of nicotinic acetylcholine receptor, which are found in the periphery and in the CNS. Members of the so-called bungarotoxin-insensitive subtypes have been extensively implicated in the behavioral effects of nicotine, including its effects related to dependence, such as nicotine self-administration and in neurotransmitter release such as dopamine. Nicotinic acetylcholine receptors that are sensitive to bungarotoxin-such as the homomeric alpha-7 subtype seem to affect the release of the excitatory transmitter, glutamate.

Neuronal interactions and the circuitry involved in nicotine dependence are being progressively elucidated. For example, differential effects of nicotine at its receptors on neurons containing gamma-aminobutyric acid (GABA), which mediate inhibition, and on glutamate containing cells has been implicated in extending the effects of drug on synaptic function. Nicotine administration also increases the extracellular nor-adrenaline in specific parts of the brain, however, the effects of nicotine on neurotransmitters such as serotonin or other CNS neurotransmitter systems such as the endocannabinoids and neuropeptides have been less studied. The release of all these various neurotransmitters leads to the arousal, mood modulation, performance enhancement, and analgesic and weight-loss effects associated with tobacco use.

With chronic or even acute administration of nicotine, neural adaptations occur to attain homeostasis resulting from the increased activity on the nicotinic acetylcholine receptor sites and increased concentration of neurotransmitters. Although some, subtypes of nicotinic acetylcholine receptor are upregulated by chronic nicotine treatment (i.e. their numbers increase), receptors also become desensitized or inactivated, which is one potential mechanism leading to the development of tolerance. Because the body develops a homeostatic response, smokers have withdrawal symptoms on abstinence from the drug. These withdrawal symptoms include negative affect such as irritability, frustration or anger, anxiety dysphoric or depressed mood, restlessness, difficulty concentrating, insomnia, decreased heart rate, and increased appetite. Other possible symptoms can include constipation, cough, dizziness, increased dreaming, and mouth sores.

Withdrawal symptoms, with the exception of weight, peak during the first week of abstinence and then gradually drop to baseline levels by 2–4 weeks, although further studies have shown withdrawal to be persistent and elevated for several months after quitting. However, weight might increase over the course of 6 months, and then decrease or become sustained. Studies have also shown individual variations in the intensity, slope, and variability predict relapse to smoking and those of craving and negative affect were the most likely to be associated with relapse. Withdrawal symptoms can make abstaining smokers more reactive to environmental events that engender emotional reactions.

In addition to the physiological basis for addiction, behavioral or learning factors also sustain addiction. Stimuli in the environment become associated with the positive reinforcing effects of nicotine and withdrawal symptoms. With time and associative learning, these stimuli begin to control behavior, such that when a smoker is exposed to these stimuli, they evoke craving for the drug or drug-seeking behavior. These stimuli could include smoking cues such as other smokers, an ashtray, or a lighter, negative affect such as irritability, depressed mood, or anxiety; situational cues such as a bar or after finishing a meal; alcohol use: or sensory cues from smoking such as the harshness in the throat and lungs and the taste. This associative learning has been regarded by some to make an equally important contribution to nicotine addiction as do the direct effects of the drug itself. Nicotine has also been noted to enhance the reinforcing effects of stimuli or other reinforcers that are not associated with the administration of nicotine, which is an effect that also contributes to the addictive nature of nicotine.

SUSCEPTIBILITY

Apart from the effect of nicotine on the brain, the experience of nicotine withdrawal, and the associative learning processes, other factors contribute to whether tobacco use is started or sustained. These factors include the environmental culture (access and availability of tobacco products, bans on tobacco use, cost, social acceptability and modeling (e.g. parental or peer smoking) and the characteristics of the individual (e.g. genes, comorbid psychiatry disorders, and personality features). For factors related to an individual's characteristics, initiation of smoking behavior and transition to dependence (i.e. persistent smoking) have shown strong heritability. The reported heritability coefficients range from 30% to greater than 80% (with a mean of roughly 60% for initiation and 70% for progression to dependence). The potential candidate gene variants include cholinergic nicotine receptor genes such as *CHRNB3* (β3 nicotinic receptor subunit) and *CHRNA5* (α5 nicotinic receptor subunit); dopamine pathway genes such as dopamine D2 and D4 receptor *(DRD2 and DRD4)* and dopamine transport *(DAT)* genes; serotonin pathway genes such as tryptophan hydroxylase, *TPH* (associated with serotonin biosynthesis), and serotonin transporter. *5HTTLPR* (associated with serotonin reuptake) genes; monoamine oxidase (MAO-A) and dopamine beta hydroxylase genes affecting norepinephrine pathways; and genes associated with the metabolism of nicotine such as P540 *CYP2A6*.

What is inherited might be differences in response to nicotine, differences in responsiveness of the various neurotransmitter pathways, or behavioural traits such as novelty or sensation seeking, impulsivity hostility, or harm avoidance. Furthermore, comorbid psychiatric disorders can predispose a smoker to begin or persist in smoking. A population survey showed that 41% of individuals with mental illness smoked cigarettes. People with a mental illness in the previous month were estimated to smoke over 40% of total cigarettes smoked by the sample. Similarly, in a large study, nicotine-dependent individuals with comorbid psychiatric disorder accounted for 34% of all cigarettes smoked in the USA. Studies have recorded a higher prevalence of alcohol and drug dependence depression, and anxiety disorders in daily or dependent smokers than in nonsmokers or nondependent smokers, the more severe the dependence, the greater the likelihood of psychiatric disorders.

TREATMENTS

Treatments are targeted towards dealing with the physical addiction to nicotine, the psychological reliance on the effects of nicotine, and the behavioural aspects of tobacco use. Several meta-analyses and public-health guidelines have described evidence-based treatment approaches.

Physician's Role

In the USA, although more than 70% of smokers want to quit every year and 45% make an attempt to quit, less than 5% in the general population are successful. Proportions are much the same in the UK. Although most smokers will give up on their own. Physicians and other health care professionals can have a powerful effect in helping to stop the use of tobacco products and can enhance cessation rates by three fold to five-fold above 5%. Even brief advice to quit by a health care professional leads to a small (2.5%) but significant increased absolute rate of cessation compared with no advice. In the USA 70% of smokers see primary care physicians each year, and in the UK 78% of the population see a family doctor every year. Therefore, health care providers are in an extraordinary position to provide effective treatments. The US public Health Service clinical-practice guidelines recommend provision of evidence-based counselling and pharmacotherapies (if not contraindicated) for all smokers and also institutional changes that would help with the provision of these services. Institutional changes can involve a system that routinely identifies people who use tobacco and documents status of tobacco use at every clinic visit. They also include other system-wide changes in health systems such as providing education, resources, and feedback to promote provider intervention, dedicating staff to provide treatment in for tobacco dependence and assess the delivery of this treatment in staff performance evaluations, promoting hospital polices that support and provide inpatient services for tobacco dependence, including treatments for tobacco dependence (both counseling and pharmacotherapy), identified as reflective in the Public Health Service clinical practice guideline. Health care providers can also provide their patients with a brief intervention that has been described as the "five As". Assistance for cessation includes both counseling (ideally, four or more sessions) and pharmacotherapies.

Counseling

Counseling involves motivating tobacco users to quit by examination of the results from smoking. It includes educating tobacco users about the beneficial health effects from stopping smoking, which can happen even when cessation occurs at an older age. Components of effective counseling include problem solving and skills training—i.e., discussing methods and coping skills to deal with high-risk situations for tobacco use, and providing social support as part of treatment. When physician care or personnel to provide smoking cessation are unavailable, tobacco users can be referred to specialists in smoking cessation or telephone quite lines, which are most effective if they proactively provide frequent personal counseling. One major advantage of quit lines, besides their effectiveness, is that they are accessible and can reach a large population of diverse tobacco users. In the USA, a national network of quite lines for tobacco cessation has been established that can refer tobacco users to their own regional quite line. The UK and Australia also have such systems.

Pharmacotherapies

Pharmacotherapies for nicotine dependence can enhance quit rates by about two-three fold. Therefore, according to the UK and US Public Health Service guidelines, all smokers should be considered for pharmacotherapies, but with special consideration or exception given to smoker with specific medical conditions, to those who smoke less than ten cigarette per day, to pregnant or breast feeding women, and to adolescents. Table 33 describes the various medicinal treatment that are available to treat smoking addiction. The UK clinical practice guidelines recommend nicotine replacement therapies (NRTs) and bupropion as a first-line treatment although bupropion is recommended as a second-line therapy in New Zealand and Germany. In the USA first-line therapies are drug that have been approved by the US Food and Drug Administration (FDA) and include NRTs (except nicotine microtab) bupropion, and varenicline. Second-line treatments—including clonidine and nortriptyline—have shown efficacy but have not been approved by the FDA.

Nicotine Replacement Therapies

NRTs are given transdermally, orally (gum, lozenge or sublingual tablets, inhaler), or nasally. Medicinal nicotine is mainly used to replace nicotine in tobacco users to maintain some of its effects while also reducing the addiction potential (e.g. reducing the amount and speed of nicotine deliver) and toxic effects associated with tobacco use. The use of medicinal nicotine leads to a decrease in withdrawal symptoms.

Table 33: Pharmacotherapies

Dose		*Instructions for use*	*Most frequent side effects (at all doses)*	*Precautions (at all doses)*
First-line therapies				
Nicotine-replacement therapies				*Cardiac diseases, recent myocardial infarction, serious arrhythmias, unstable angina pectoris; peptic ulcers; insulin-dependent diabetes; uncontrolled hypertension, drug treatment for depression or asthma, pregnancy or lactation; hyperthyroidism, pheochromocytoma or type 1 diabetes mellitus.
Nicotine patch	21 mg,14 mg, 7 mg, 15 mg, 10 mg, 5 mg, 22 mg, 11 mg	24 application: 21 mg for 4–6 weeks, 14 mg for 2 weeks, 7 mg for 2 weeks, 16 hours application: 15 mg 6 weeks, 10 mg 2 weeks, 5 mg 2 weeks, 22 mg and 11 mg (light smokers) for 8 weeks	Local skin reaction, sleep disruption	Allergy to tape or dermatological condition
Nicotine gum	2 mg (<25 cpd): 4 mg (25 cpd)	1 piece every 1–2 hours for 6 weeks, every 2–4 hours for 3 weeks, and every 4–8 hours for 3 weeks. Maximum 24 pieces.	Jaw ache, mouth soreness, dyspepsia, hiccups	Dental conditions exacerbated by chewing gum: history of esophageal, oral or pharyngeal inflammation.
Nicotine inhaler	10 mg cartridge (4 mg delivered)	6–16 cartridges per day for 12 weeks gradual reduction for final 6–12 weeks	Local irritation of mouth and throat, coughing and rhinitis	Allergy to menthol, bronchospastic disease
Nicotine nasal spray	0.5 mg in each nostril	1–2 doses per hours, 12–26 weeks of treatment Maximum 40 doses per day	Nasal and airway irritation	Severe reactive airway disease, chronic nasal disorder
Nicotine lozenge	2 mg (>30 min to first cigarette in morning): 4 mg (<30 min to first cigarette in morning)	1 lozenge every 1–2 hours for 6 weeks, every 2–4 hours for 3 weeks, and every 4–8 hours for 3 weeks, Maximum 20 per day	Hiccups, mouth or throat irritation, heartburn or dyspepsia	Severe reactive airway disease, chronic nasal disorder
Nicotine microtab	2 mg	1 (< 20 cigarettes per day) – 2 (> 20 cigarettes per day) per hour for 12 weeks followed by gradual reduction Maximum 40 per day		
Non-nicotine products				
Bupropion	150 mg twice a day**	1–2 weeks before cutting, 150 mg every morning for 3 days then 150 mg twice a day, 7–12 weeks of treatment, may consider extending treatment to 6 months (150 mg per day)	Dry mouth, insomnia	Seizure disorder or predisposition towards seizure disorder concomitant use of wellbutrin, diagnosis of bulimia or anorexia nervosa, concomitant or recent use of monoamine oxidase inhibitors
Varenicline	1 mg twice a day	1 week before quitting, 0.5 mg once a day for days 1–3, 0.5 mg twice per day for days 4–7, 1 mg twice per day for 12 weeks, and an option of additional 12 weeks for quitters	Nausea/ vomiting, sleep disturbance, flatulence	Severe renal impairment, pregnancy, can impair ability to drive or to operate heavy machinery

Contd...

Contd...

Dose		*Instructions for use*	*Most frequent side effects (at all doses)*	*Precautions (at all doses)*
Second-line therapies				
Clonidine	Oral = 0.15–0.75 mg per day. Patch = 0.1–0.2 mg per day	Start on quit date or up to 3 days before quit date, initial dose 0.1mg twice a day orally or 0.1 mg per day transdermally, increasing by 0.1 mg per day per week, 3–10 weeks of treatment, down titrate dose over 2–4 days	Dry mouth, drowsiness, dizziness, sedation, constipation, lower blood pressure, rebound hypertension	Pregnancy
Nortriptyline	75–150 mg per day	Initial dose 25 mg per day and up titrate to 75–150 mg per day 10–28 days before quit date, 12 weeks of treatment, may consider treatment for up to 6 months	Dry mouth, sedation, blurred vision, urinary retention, light headedness, shaky hands, cardiotoxicity with overdose	Cardiovascular disease, pregnancy, monoamine oxidase inhibitors, may impair ability to drive or to operate heavy machinery.

Information from reference 68,83 and 84 cigarettes per day.
**Treatment with nicotine patches has been examined with smokers who have cardiovascular disease and the drugs have been found in to be safe.*
***No significant differences in cessation rates were recorded between the recommended 300 mg dose and the 150 mg dose (OR 1-07, 95% 937-1.32).*

Furthermore, medicinal nicotine, particularly transdermal patches, might be associated with desensitization of nicotinic receptors, resulting in reduced reinforcement from cigarette smoking. Table 33 details general and drug-specific precautions and sideeffects for NRTs.

The Cochrane meta-analysis pools studies of all types of NRT with follow-up of 6 months or longer using sustained and validated outcomes when available. It includes both earl efficacy studies and pragmatic trials in various settings and populations, with different levels of common behavioral support. Table 34 shows estimated pooled odds ratios derived from applying the quit rates of active nicotine drug to the median long-term quit rate, for the placebo groups receiving only behavioral support. Table 34 also shows estimates of the abstinence rates achievable if the estimated odds ratios are applied to a range of quit rates in the control group. The quit rates that can be expected without pharmacotherapy will depend on the motivation and level of dependence of the smokers and the amount of behavioral support provided, as well as the definition of abstinence and follow-up time. The meta-analysis includes any type of NRT product, and the odds ratios for different types are not statistically different.

Table 34: Estimates of efficacy of pharmacotherapies

	Odds ratio (95% CI)	*Median (IQR) abstinence rate* with placebo and support*	*Estimated abstinence rate of (95% CI) with pharmacotherapy*
Nicotine replacement therapy (104 studies)	1.8 (1.8–1.9)	11% (7–17)	18% (17–19)
Bupropion (31 studies)	1.9 (1.7–2.2)	10% (6–14)	17% (15–19)
Varenicline (four studies)	3.2 (2.4–4.3)	7% (5–9)	18% (15–23)
Nortriptyline (six studies)	2.3 (1.6–3.4)	10% (6–14)	21% (15–28)
Clonidine (six studies)	1.9 (1.3–2.7)	13% (11–22)	22% (17–30)

**Abstinence rates from control groups of trials with 6 months or more follow-up; strictest available criteria for abstinence with losses to follow-up treated as smokers. Estimated abstinence rates with 95% CI obtained from applying the odds ratio (95% CI) to median placebo quit rate.*

A randomized clinical trial comparing gum, patch, nasal spray, and inhaler reported no significant differences at the 3-month follow-up, with 12-week continuous abstinence rates ranging from 20 to 24.%. Studies examining the effects of 4 mg versus 2 mg nicotine gum in smokers who are highly nicotine dependent have shown that 4 mg gum is more efficacious than 2 mg gum (four studies, odds ratio

Table 35: Efficacy of nicotine lozenge

	Active (n=450–459)	*Placebo (n=450–459)*	*Odds ratio*
Low dependence (2 mg lozenge)	24.2%	14.4%	2.8 (1.4–2.8)
High dependence (4 mg lozenge)	23.6%	10.2%	2.8 (1.9–4.0)

[OR] 2.2, 95% CI 1.5–3.3). Trials comparing two patches with one patch for heavy smokers suggest only *a* small benefit (six studies, OR 1.2, 1.0–1.4). In a clinical trial investigating the nicotine lozenge, smokers with low dependence (time to first cigarette 30 min or greater) were randomly assigned to 2 mg nicotine lozenge or placebo, and highly-dependent smokers to 4 mg nicotine lozenge or placebo. Quit rates were lower in the high-dependence placebo group than in the low-dependence placebo group, and in both groups efficacy improved with the active drug (Tables 34 and 35).

Non-nicotine-based Treatments

Bupropion sustained release is a non-nicotine-based drug that is also being used as an antidepressant. Bupropion is thought to target the neurochemistry of nicotine addiction by blocking the reuptake of dopamine and noradrenalin which increases their concentrations in the synapse. It is also considered to function as a noncompetitive antagonist of the nicotinic acetylcholine receptor. The second line-treatments clonidine and nortriptyline also effect the noradrenergic system. Clonidine, which is an adrenergic autoreceptor agonist, decreases nordrenaline but also serotonin. Nortriptyline is a reuptake inhibitor, mainly or noradrenaline but also serotonin. Meta-analyses of results from clinical trials show much the same odds ratios, ranging from 1.9 to 3.2 across these non-nicotine pharmacotherapies (Tables 34 and 35).

Indirect comparisons of odds ratios from meta-analysis suggest that NRT, bupropion and nortriptyline have much the same effcacy. Clonidine is noted to be as efficacious as the other drugs in promotion of cessation, but the high frequency of sideeffects might be a deterrent for this drug being considered as a primary therapy. One report stated that clonidine should be potentially targeted to a subgroup of smokers who can benefit from the sedative side effects, such as those who report having anxiety, or agitation when they stop smoking.

The FDA and other national licensing authorities have approved varenicline—a drug- that targets a specific nicotinic receptor subtype. This drug is a potent α4 β2 partial agonist, which provides tobacco withdrawal relief by its agonist action and blocks the reinforcing effects of nicotine by its antagonist action.

Table 35 shows efficacy of nicotine lozenge:continuous abstinence rates at 6 months.

In early 2008, the FDA added serious neuropsychiatric symptoms to the warnings section of the prescribing information for varenicline. This measure was taken because symptoms such as changes in behavior, agitation, depressed mood, suicidal ideation, and attempted and completed suicide were recorded in patients taking varenicline or after taking varenicline. Although these symptoms are rare, they should be carefully monitored.

Combination Drugs

Studies have also examined combinations of drugs to improve efficacy. The combination of nicotine patches (which can provide a steady concentration of nicotine throughout the day) and the use of ad labitum nicotine (which can help to deal with high-risk situations or effects from increased craving) has led to better efficacy than have single products (seven studies, OR 1.4, 1.1–1.8). One study showed that a combination of bupropion and nicotine patches was more efficacious than were patches only, but not bupropion alone. However, three other trials comparing a combination, with patches alone have not replicated this result, primarily in populations of adolescents and schizophrenics. A combination of nortriptyline and nicotine patches resulted in higher success rate than, did nicotine patches alone (23% vs 10% at 6 months) but another study showed inconsistent effects of a combination of nicotine patch and nortriptyline compared with nicotine patch alone, with 'significant differences' in the short term but not in the long-terms. Up until now, the results suggest that there is no evidence to strongly support the combination of a nicotine and non-nicotine treatment over immunotherapy, however the combination of nicotine patches with an ad labium form of NRT could confer some benefit.

Relapse Prevention or Extended Drug Use

Pharmacotherapies could also be considered for relapse prevention, i.e. use of drugs to sustain abstinence rates. In a study examining the use of bupropion in individuals who quit smoking, use of bupropion for 1 year led to significantly higher rates of success than did placebo during treatment assignment. However, this study and another did not show that bupropion would sustain long-term abstinence after treatment with the drug (OR 1.2. 0.8–1.7). In other studies, no differences were recorded between bupropion versus placebo both during and after intervention to prevent relapse. Hall et al. reported that 1 year's continued use of nortriptyline seemed to improve continuous abstinence rates throughout the year compared with 8 weeks of nortriptyline (plus treatment with nicotine patches for 8 weeks in both conditions): however no differences were recorded in point prevalence abstinence at

1 year. What was remarkable in this study was that extended treatment, which included psychological counselling and pharmacotherapy, resulted in an abstinence rate (50%) that is substantially higher than in the published work.

Varenicline has also shown some efficacy in prevention of relapse. In a clinical trial examining sustained abstinence, smokers were assigned to 12 weeks' treatment with varenicline, and those who achieved abstinence were then randomly assigned to a double blind trial of varenicline versus placebo for 12 weeks. The continuous abstinence rates from weeks 13 to 24 and weeks 13 to 52 were significantly higher for varenicline than for placebo but the effect was fairly modest (OR at 52 weeks 1.3, 1.1–1.7) and there was some indication that the extended treatment deferred rather than prevented relapse. Up until now, there was no strong evidence to suggest that extended use of pharmacotherapy was necessary, except perhaps for people trying to maintain abstinence. However, the recent US treatment guidelines reported that the long-term (>14 weeks) use of gum might be more effective than a shorter (6–14 weeks) course and that long-term (14 weeks) patch use plus ad libitum gum or spray produced one of the largest effects on abstinence rates compared with other pharmacotherapies.

Recycling Smokers

Recycling drugs can be indicated in smokers who have relapsed, as would be the case in-treatment of many other diseases. Studies have examined repeated use of the same drug or use of different drugs for die subsequent attempts to quit. So, far repeated use of nicotine patches shortly after previous cessation failure with patches did not lead to significant cessation rates (sustained abstinence at 26 weeks 0-1-6%). However, repeated of use of bupropion in smokers who had previously failed to quit with this drug led to significantly greater continuous abstinence rates than did placebo 1(12% vs 14.2%). One study showed that smokers who reported previous use of treatments (nicotine gum, patch, inhaler, and bupropion) showed as much success with nicotine lozenge compared with placebo as did those without a previous history with drugs for smoking cessation. Similarly, in another study, smokers who reported a past history of NRT showed as much efficacy with bupropion alone, nicotine patches alone; and bupropion plus nicotine patches as did those without a past history of NRT: and in those who previously used nicotine replacements, the active drugs led to significantly better results than die placebo.

However, in one prospective study, treating smokes who have not been successful with nicotine replacement agents with bupropion did not show significant increases in efficacy compared with placebo. nor did treating smokers who were not successful with bupropion with a NRT. Perhaps the differences in these findings can be accounted for partly because of differences in participant recruitment—smokers who failed abstinence in previous clinical trial versus smokers with and without a history of prior drug use who are entering a new clinical trial. These results suggest that smokers who are highly motivated to make another attempt to quit, even with previous cessation failures with a drug, can benefit from another, course of pharmacotherapy.

Cigarette Reduction

Some smokers might not be ready or want to quit, Another method of intervention is to reduce cigarette consumption through the use of pharmacotherapies. The use of nicotine replacement agents compared with placebo has led to more smokers achieving a 50% reduction in cigarette smoking, although the extent of reduction is unlikely to confer beneficial health effects. Smokers engage in substantial compensatory smoking (e.g. deeper inhalation per cigarette) so that a reduction in cigarette consumption of 50% or more results only in a 30% decrease in biomarkers for toxicant exposure and modest reductions in biomarkers for cardiovascular risk. Epidemiological, longitudinal studies have shown that cigarette reductions of 50% or greater do not lead to a significantly reduced risk of fatal and nonfatal myocardial infarction compared with smokers who did not reduce their cigarette smoking (hazard ratio [HR] 1 .2, 95% Cl 0.9–1.4) or reduced risk of admissions for chronic obstructive pulmonary disease (0.9. 0.7–1.2). However, smokers who reduced cigarette consumption did have a reduced risk of lung cancer compared with continuous smokers, but only by 25% (0.7, 0.5–1.0).

Other studies have shown either an improved or no effect on disease risk with cigarette reduction. Therefore, reduction in smoking might be seen as a stepping stone towards cessation, and studies show that recommendation of cigarette reduction has not conferred any detrimental effects and a potential facilitation of smoking cessation. The use of nicotine gum and nicotine inhaler has been approved for cigarette reduction as a means for cessation in several European countries.

Future Directions: Novel Drugs and Pharmacokinetics

Although available pharmacotherapies can improve success rates, the absolute cessation rate remains fairly low at around 20%. Several other drugs have undergone clinical trials and many others that target specific neurotransmitters or metabolic enzymes (e.g. GABAergic drug or monoamine oxidase inhibitors) or specific nicotinic receptor subtypes (e.g. $\alpha 7$) are undergoing development or testing in phase I or II trials. Two drugs are noteworthy because of their novel mechanism of action or target site and promising results. The first is the nicotine vaccine, which stimulates the immune system to develop antinicotine antibodies. Study results have shown that the nicotine vaccine reduces the early distribution of nicotine to the brain in rats, by up to 65%, in clinically relevant acute and chronic nicotine doses. Several preliminary studies in human beings have been done. One such study showed that the vaccine was safe and well-tolerated and, although not intended as a treatment study, the highest dose of the vaccine (200 μg) led to significantly higher 4-week continuous abstinence rates than did the other vaccine doses and placebo.

Another promising drug that has undergone large clinical trials is a selective cannabinoid CB1 receptor antagonist, rimonabant. This drug reduces the increase induced by nicotine in dopamine turnover in the nucleus accumbens and nicotine self-administration in animals, and reduces nicotine-seeking behavior in response to cues related to nicotine after weeks of abstinence from it. Rimonabant is marketed in some European countries to treat metabolic syndrome and is being considered for the treatment of smoking. Three large double-blind, placebo controlled clinical trials have been undertaken in the USA and Europe. In a pooled analysis of these trials, significant effects at the end of treatment were noted after 10 weeks of treatment with 20 mg Rimonabant compared with placebo (22.0% vs 15.0%, $p = 0.0003$), and a significantly decreased weight gain in nonobese people who abstained. (0.8 kg vs 2.5 kg, $p < 0.0003$.

One area of research that is receiving considerable attention is pharmacogenetics-matching treatment on the basis of the genotypes. Up until now, the little research has shown that polymorphisms on specific genes associated with neurobiological effects of nicotine or metabolism of nicotine might affect treatment response to some drugs. Pharmacogenetics for tobacco addiction is an evolving and fairly new area and, therefore, genotyping smokers at this point is premature; however, this area of research will probably provide valuable data for a potential method for matching patients to treatment.

CONCLUSION

Nicotine or tobacco addiction should be treated as a chronic disorder. Treatment can need persistent efforts to try to assist tobacco users in their attempts at quitting. Relapse should be seen as a probable event. In smokers who quit without treatment, the proportion who can achieve abstinence for at least 1 week is 25–51% and at least 3 months is 10–20%. By 6 months, only 3–5% have achieved long lasting abstinence. Treatment can improve these outcomes. Treatment can include the use of various avenues of counseling and different types of pharmacotherapy. It might also involve the use of many drugs. Clearly effective treatments are available and promising new treatments are being developed. The most crucial component of care is the actual delivery of such treatments. Delivery of treatments can be eased by development of the infrastructure to promote the identification to smokers at every clinic visit, by training healthcare professionals on treatments for nicotine addiction, by providing medicinal products for smoking cessation on the formulary, and by providing healthcare coverage for tobacco cessation.

BIBLIOGRAPHY

Classification and Epidemiology

1. Alati R, Mamun AA, Williams GM. In utero alcohol exposure and predication of alcohol disorders in early adulthood. Arch Gen Psychiatry. 2006;63:1009-16.
2. Alati R, Mamun AA, Williams GM. In utero alcohol exposure and predication of alcohol disorders in early adulthood. Arch Gen Psychiatry. 2006;63:1009-16.
3. Alte D, Ludemann J, Piek M, et al. Distribution and dose response of laboratory markers to alcohol consumption in a general population: Results of the Study of Health in Pomerania (SHIP). J Stud Alcohol. 2003;64:75-82.
4. American Psychiatric Association. Desk Reference to the Diagnostic Criteria from DSM-5. Washington DC; 2013
5. American Psychiatric Association. Diagnostic and Statistical Manual of Mental Disorders, 4th edition. Washington DC: APA; 1994.
6. American Psychiatric Association. Practice guidelines for the treatment of patients with substance use disorders: Alcohol, cocaine, opioids. Am J Psychiatry. 1995;152(Suppl):1-59.
7. Anglin MD, Hser Y. Treatment of drug abuse. In: Torry M, Wilson JQ (Eds). Drugs and crime. Chicago: University of Chicago Press; 1990. pp. 393-460.
8. Anker A, Crowley T. Use of contingency contracts in speciality clinics for cocaine abuse. NIDA Res Monogr 41. 1982. pp. 452-9.
9. Anthony JC, Helzer JE. Epidemiology of drug dependence. In: Tsuang MT, Tohan M, Zahner GEP (Eds). Text book of Psychiatric Epidemiology. New York: John Wiley; 1995. pp. 361-406.
10. Anton RF, Youngblood M. Factors affecting % CDT status at entry into a multisite clinical treatment trial: experience from the COMBINE study. Alcohol Clin Exp Res. 2006;30:1878-83.
11. Arif A, Westermeyer J. Manual of Drug and Alcohol Abuse. Guidelines for Teaching in Medical Health Institutions. New York: Plenum Publishing Corporation, 1988.
12. Armor DJ, Polich JM, Stambul HB. Alcoholism and Treatment. Santa Monica: Rand Corporation; 1976.
13. Azrin NH, Sissons R, Myer SR, et al. Alcoholism treatment by disulfiram and community reinforcement therapy. J Behav Ther Exp Psychiatr. 1982;13:105-12.
14. Babor T, Higgins-Biddle J, Dauser D, et al. Brief interventions for at-risk drinking: patient outcomes and cost-effectiveness in managed care organizations. Alcohol. 2006;41:624-31.
15. Babor T, Higgins-Biddle J, Dauser D, et al. Brief interventions for at-risk drinking: patient outcomes and cost-effectiveness in managed care organizations. Alcohol Alcohol. 2006;41: 624-31.

16. Babor TF, Hofmann M, DelBOca FK, et al. Types of alcoholics, I: Evidence for an empirically derived typology based on indicators of vulnerability and severity. Arch Gen Psychiatry. 1992;49:599-608.
17. Babor TF. Management of alcohol use disorders in developing and developed countries. In: Ray R, Pickens RW (Eds). Proceedings of Indo-US Symposium on Alcohol and Drug Abuse. NIMHANS Publication No. 20. Bangalore: NIMHANS; 1989. pp. 131-83.
18. Ball JC, Ross A. The effectiveness of methadone maintenance treatment: Patients, programs, services and outcomes. New York: Springer Verlag, 1991.
19. Banys P. The clinical use of disulfiram (Antabuse): a review. J Psychoactive Drugs. 1988;20:243-51.
20. Barr C, Newman T, Becker M, et al. Serotonin treanspoter gene variation is associated with alcohol sensitivity in rhesus macaques exposed to early-life stress. Alcohol Clin Exp Res. 2005;27:812-17.
21. Battjes RJ, Leukefield CG, Amsel Z. Community prevention efforts to reduce the spread of AIDS associated with intravenous drug use. In: Leukefield CG, Battjes RJ, Amsel Z (Eds). AIDS and Intravenous Drug Use: Community Intervention and Prevention. NIDA Res Monogr 93. Rockville, MD: NIDA, 1990.
22. Battjes RJ, Pickens RW, Amsel Z, et al. Heterosexual transmission of human immunodeficiency virus among intravenous drug users. J Infect Dis. 1990;162:1007-11.
23. Bean MH. Alcoholics Anonymous: AA. Psychiatr Ann. 1975;5: 3-64.
24. Beck AT, Wright FD, Newman CF, et al. Cognitive Therapy of Substance Abuse. New York: Guilford Press; 1993.
25. Beeder AB, Milman RB. Patients with psychopathology: Management of medical conditions associated with substance abuse. In: Lowinson JH, Ruiz P, Millman RB, et al (Eds). Substance Abuse: A Comprehensive Textbook, 3rd edition. Baltimore: Williams and Wilkins; 1997. pp. 551-63.
26. Benegal V, Gururaj G, Murthy P. Report on a WHO Collaborative Project on Unrecorded Consumption of Alcohol in Karnataka, India. Bangalore, India: National Institute of Mental Health and Neurosciences; 2003.
27. Berner MM, Kriston L, Bentele M, Harter M. The Alcohol Use Identification Test for detecting at-risk drinking: a systematic review and meta-analysis. J Stud Alcohol Drug. 2007;68:461-73.
28. Bickel WK, Amass L. Buprenorphine treatment of opioid dependence: a review. Exp Clin Psychopharmacol. 1995;3: 477-89.
29. Bodin M, Romelsjo A. Predictors of abstinence and nonproblem drinking after 12-steps treatment in Sweden. J Stud Alcohol. 2006;67:139-46.
30. Bollinger RC, Tripathy SP, Quinn TC. The Human Immunodeficiency Virus Epidemic in India: Current Magnitude and Future Projections. Medicine (Baltimore). 1995;74:97-106.
31. Booth RE, Watters JK. How effective are risk reduction interventions targeting injecting drug users? AIDS. 1994;8:1515-24.
32. Bottlender M, Soyka M. Outpatient alcoholism treatment: predictors of outcome after 3 years. Drugs Alcohol Depend. 2005;80:83-9.
33. Bottlender M, Soyka M. Outpatient alcoholism treatment: predictors of outcome after 3 years. Drugs Alcohol Depend. 2005;80:83-9.
34. Botvin GJ, Botvin EM. School based programs: Prevention and education. In: Lowinson JH, Ruiz P, Millman RB, et al (Eds). Substance Abuse: A Comprehensive Textbook, 3rd edition. Baltimore: Williams and Wilkins; 1997. pp. 764-75.
35. Bowen RC, Cipywny KD, D' Arcy C, et al. Alcoholism, anxiety disorders and agoraphobia. Alcoholism Clin Exp Res. 1984;8: 48-50.
36. Brehm NM, Khantzian EJ. Psychodynamics: Determinants and perpetuators of substance abuse. In: Lowinson JH, Ruiz P, Millman RB, et al (Eds). Substance Abuse: A Comprehensive Textbook, 3rd edition. Baltimore: Williams and Wilkins; 1997. pp. 90-100.
37. Brewer C. Combining pharmacological antagonists and behavioral psychotherapy in treating addictions: why it is effective but unpopular. Br J Psychiatry. 1990;157:34-40.
38. Brewer C. Controlled trials of antabuse in alcoholism: the importance of supervision and adequate dosage. Acta Psychiat Scand. 1992;86(Suppl):51-8.
39. Brill L. The treatment of drug abuse: Evolution of a perspective. Am J Psychiatry. 1977;134:157-60.
40. Brown SA, Schuckit MA. Changes in depression among abstinent alcoholics. J of Stud on Alcohol. 1988;49:412-7.
41. Brown SA, Schuckit MA. Changes in depression among abstinent alcoholics. J Stud Alcohol. 1988;49:412-7.
42. Cahalan D. An Ounce of Prevention. San Francisco: Jossey-Bass; 1992.
43. Carmelli D, Swan GE, Robinette D, et al. Genetic influences on smoking: A study of male twins. N Engl J Med. 1992;327:829-33.
44. Carroll K, Ball S, Nich C, et al. Motivational interviewing to improve treatment engagement and outcome in individuals seeking treatment for substance abuse: a multisite effectiveness study. Drug Alcohol Depend. 2006;81:301-12.
45. Carroll K, Ball S, Nich C, et al. Motivational interviewing to improve treatment engagement and outcome in individuals seeking treatment for substance abuse: a multisite effectiveness study. Drug Alcohol Depend. 2006;81:301-12.
46. Castaneda R, Cushman P. Alcohol withdrawal: A review of clinical management. J Clin Psychiatry. 1989;50:278-84.
47. Catalano R, Howard M, Hawkins J, et al. Relapse in the addiction-rates, determinants and promising prevention strategies. In: 1988 Surgeon General's report on health consequences of smoking. Washington DC: Office of Smoking and Health , Govt. Printing office; 1988.
48. Chagas Silva M, Gaunekar G, Patel V, Kukalekar DS, Fernandes J. The prevalence and correlates of hazardous drinking in industrial workers: A community study from Goa, India. Alcohol. 2003;38:79-83. [PubMed]
49. Chang G, Kosten TR. Detoxification, evaluation and early treatment. In: Lowinson JH, Ruiz P, Millman RB, et al (Eds).

Substance Abuse: A Comprehensive Textbook, 3rd edition. Baltimore: Williams and Wilkins; 1997. pp. 377-85.

50. Channabasavanna SM. Epidemiology of drug abuse in India: An overview. In: Ray R, Pickens RW (Eds). Proceedings of the Indo-US Symposium on Alcohol and Drug Abuse. NIMHANS Publication No. 20. Bangalore: NIMHANS; 1989. pp. 43-56.
51. Chatterjee A, Zomi GT, Hangzo CZ. Ethnographic observations of drug injecting in Manipur and Calcutta: Implications for intervention. Abstracts of the 48th Annual National Conference of Indian Psychiatric Society, Bangalore; 1996.
52. Chaturvedi HK, Phukan RK, Mahanta J. Sociocultural diversity and substance use pattern in Arunachal Pradesh, India. Drug Alcohol Depend. 2004;74:97-104. [PubMed]
53. Chavan B, Arun P, Bhargava R, Singh GP. Prevalence of alcohol and drug dependence in rural and slum population of Chandigarh: A community survey. Indian J Psychiatry. 2007;49:44-8. [PMC free article] [PubMed]
54. Chick J, Gough K, Falbowski W, et al. Disulfiram treatment in alcoholism. Br J Psychiatry. 1992;161:84-90.
55. Childress A, Ehrman R, McLellan A, et al. Update on behavioral treatments for substance abuse. NIDA Res Monogr 90. 1988. pp. 183-92.
56. Choi K, Coates TJ. Prevention of HIV Infection. AIDS. 1994; 8:1371-89.
57. Chowdhury AN, Chowdhury S. Buprenorphine abuse: Report from India. Br J Addict. 1990;85:1349-50.
58. Clark DB. The natural history of adolescent alcohol use disorders: addiction. 2004;99:5-22.
59. Cloninger CR, Sigvardsson S, Reich T, et al. Inheritance of risk to develop alcoholism. In: Braude MC, Chao HM (Eds). Genetic and biological markers in drug abuse and alcoholism. NIDA Research Monograph 66, Rockville MD: DHHS;1986.
60. Cohen G, Fleming NF, Glatter KA, et al. Epidemiology of substance use. In: Friedman L, Fleming NF, Roberts DH, et al. (Eds). Source Book of Substance Abuse and Addiction. Baltimore: Williams and Wilkins; 1996. pp. 17-40.
61. Conigrave KM, Degenhardt LJ, Whitfield JB, et al. CDT, GGT, and AST as markers of alcohol use: The WHO/ISBRA Collaborative Project. Alcohol Clin Exp Res. 2002;26:332-9.
62. Cook TAR, Luczak SE, Shea SH, et al. Association of ALDH2 and ADH1B genotypes with response to alcohol in Asian Americans. J Stud Alcohol. 2005;66:196-204.
63. Cox WM, Roseberg H, Hazel C, et al. United Kingdom and United States healthcare providers recommendations of abstinence versus controlled drinking. Alcohol Alcohol. 2004; 39:130-34.
64. Crawford MJ, Patton R, Touquet R, et al. Screening and referral for brief intervention of alcohol-misusing patients in an emergency department; a pragmatic randomized controlled trial. Lancet. 2004;364:1334-9.
65. Crawford MJ, Patton R, Touquet R, et al. Screening and referral for brief intervention of alcohol misusing patients in an emergency department; a pragmatic randomized controlled trial. Lancet. 2004;364:1334-9.
66. Cutting J. Alcohol dependence and alcohol related disabilities. In: Granville-Grossman K (Eds). Recent Advances in Clinical Psychiatry, 3rd edition. London: Churchill Livingstone; 1979. pp. 225-50.
67. Daley D. Five perspectives on relapse in chemical dependency. J Chem Depend Treat. 1989;2:23-6.
68. Daley D. Relapse: A guide for successful recovery. Bradenton FL: Human Serivces Institute; 1987.
69. Daley DC, Marlatt GA. Relapse prevention: Treatment approaches. In: Lowinson JH, Ruiz P, Millman RB, et al (Eds). Substance Abuse: A Comprehensive Textbook, 3rd edition. Baltimore: Williams and Wilkins; 1997. pp. 458-67.
70. Darke S, Hath W, Swift W. Prevalence, symptoms and correlates of antisocial personality disorder among methadeno maintenance clients. Drugs and Alcohol Dependence. 1994; 34:253-7.
71. Davidson K, Ritson EB. The relationship between alcohol dependence and depression. Alcohol and Alcoholism. 1993;28: 147-55.
72. Dawson DA, Grant BF, Stinson FS, et al. Recovery from DSM-IV alcohol dependence: United States, 2001–2002 edition. 2005;100:281-92.
73. DeJong CAJ, Brink VD, et al. Personality disorders in alcoholics and drug addicts. Compr Psychiatry. 1993;34:87-94.
74. DeLeon GD, Wexler HK, Jainchilli N. The therapeutic community: Success and improvement rates 5 years after treatment. Int J Addict. 1982;17:703-47.
75. Department of Health and Human Services. Methadone maintenance treatment: Translating research into policy. Rockville, Washington: National Institute of Drug Abuse, 1995.
76. Department of Health and Human Services. National Household Survey on Drug Abuse: Population Estimates; 1996. Rockville, Maryland: DHHS; 1997.
77. Deren S, Davis WR, Beardsley M, et al. Outcomes of a risk-reduction intervention with high-risk populations: The Harlem AIDS Project. AIDS Education and Prevention. 1995; 75: 379-90.
78. Desai NG, Chavan BS, Jhingan HP. Drug dependence treatment: A three-dimensional model of understanding its process in health care settings. In: Paul MC (Ed). Drugs, Youth and Society. Delhi: Madhu Deep Publication; 1996. pp. 189-202.
79. Desai NG, Gupta DK, Kishore C, et al. Injection drug use among outpatient sample of drug dependence in Delhi, India. Abstracts of the NIDA Meeting on Building International Research in Drug Abuse, Nashville, USA; 1997. pp. 40.
80. Desai NG, Murthy P, Channabasavana SM. A clinical cross-sectional study of alcohol dependence and other concurrent diagnosis on DSM-III multiaxial classification. Paper presented at 40th Annual National Conference of Indian Psychiatric Society, Cuttack; 1988.
81. Desai NG. Alcohol and depression. In: Proceedings of the Annual Continuing Medical Education. Madras: Indian Psychiatric Society; 1995. pp. 19-28.
82. Desai NG. HIV Risk Behavior in a Delhi Hospital Sample of injection and noninjection drug users. Paper presented at the

Indo-US Workshop on "Social and Behavioral Research for Injectable Drug Abuse and HIV Prevention, Delhi; 1996.

83. Desai NG. Treatment of drug and alcohol dependence: Contemporary issues and future possibilities. In: Kumar KA (Ed). Facets of Substance Abuse: An Update. Proceedings of National CME Conference on Drug Abuse and Dependence. Trivandrum Medical College; 1992. pp. 310-35.
84. Des Jarlais DC, Friedman SR, Woods JS. Intravenous drug use and AIDS. In: Ostrow DG (Ed). Behavioral Aspects of AIDS. New York: Plenum Medical Book Company; 1990.
85. Des Jarlais DC, Friedman SR. AIDS and the use of injected drugs. Sci Am. 1994;270:56-62.
86. Dick DM, Bierut L, Hinrichs A, et al. The role of GABRA 2 in risk for conduct disorder and alcohol and drug dependence across developmental stages. Behave Genet. 2006;36:577-90.
87. Duncan D, et al. Chlormethiazole or chlordiazepoxide in alcohol detoxification. Psychiatr Bull. 1996;20:599-601.
88. Edwards G, Orford J, Egert S, et al. Alcoholism: A controlled trial of 'treatment' and 'advice.' J Stud Alcoholism. 1977;34:112-32.
89. Ellickson PL, Bell RM. Prospects for preventing drug abuse among young adolescents. Science. 1990;247:1299-305.
90. Emrick C. Alcoholics Anonymous: Affiliation processes and effectiveness as treatment. Alcoholism (NY). 1987;11:416-23.
91. Eugenia E, Kosten TR, Kleber HD. Clinical utility of rapid clonidine-naltrexone detoxification for opioid abusers. Br J Addict. 1988;83:567-75.
92. Feeney G, Connor J, Young R, Tucker J, McPherson A. Combined acamprosate and naltrexone, with cognitive behavioural therapy is superior to either medication alone for alcohol abstinence: a single centres experience with pharmacotherapy. Alcohol Alcohol. 2006;41:321-7.
93. Fram DH, Marmo J, Holden R. Naltrexone treatment: The problem of patient acceptance. J Subst Abuse Treat. 1989;6: 119-22.
94. Fuller FK, Gordis E. Does disulfiram have a role in alcoholism treatment today? Addition. 2004;99:21-4.
95. Gardener EL. Brain reward mechanisms: Determinants and perpetuators of substance abuse. In: Lowinson JH, Ruiz P, Millman RB, et al (Eds). Substance Abuse: A Comprehensive Textbook, 3rd edition. Baltimore: Williams and Wilkins; 1997. pp. 51-85.
96. Gelernter J, Gueorgulieva R, Kranzler HR, et al. Opioid receptor gene (OPRM1, OPRK1, and OPRD1) variants and response to naltrexone treatment for alcohol dependence: result from the VA Cooperative Study. Alcohol Clin Exp Res. 2007;31:555-63.
97. Gerstein DR, Harwood HJ (Eds). Treating Drug Problems. Washington, DC: National Academy Press; 1990.
98. Ghulam R, Rahman I, Naqi S, Gupta SR. An epidemiological study of drug abuse in urban population of Madhya Pradesh. Indian J Psychiatry. 1996;38:160–5. [PMC free article] [PubMed]
99. Goodwin DW. Alcoholism and heredity. Arch Gen Psychiatry. 1979;36:57-61.
100. Gossop M, et al. A Short Alcohol Withdrawal Scale (SAWS): development and psychometric properties. Addict Biol. 2002; 7:37-43.
101. Gossop M, Johns A, Green L. Opiate withdrawal: inpatient versus outpatient programs and preferred versus random assignment to treatment. Br Med J. 1986;293:103-4.
102. Granville-Grossman K. Psychiatric aspects of cannabis use. In: Recent Advances in Clinical Psychiatry. Vol. III. London: Chuchill Livvingstone; 1979. pp. 251-70.
103. Granville-Grossman K. Psychiatric aspects of cannabis use. In: Recent Advances in Clinical Psychiatry. Vol. III. London: Churchill Livingstone; 1979. pp. 251-70.
104. Gray RF, Ferry A, Jaular P. Emergence of buprenorphine dependence. Br J Addict. 1989;84:1373-4.
105. Greenstein RA, Amdt IC, McLellan AT, et al. Naltrexone: a clinical perspective. J Clin Psychiatry. 1984;45:25-8.
106. Greenstein RA, Fudela PJ, O'Brain CP. Alternative pharmacotherapies for opiate addition: treatment approaches. In: Lowinson JH, Ruiz P, Millman RB, et al (Eds). Substance Abuse: A Comprehensive Textbook, 3rd edition. Baltimore: Williams and Wilkins; 1997. pp. 415-25.
107. Gross PL. Toxicologic Emergencies. In: Wilkins WE (Ed). Textbook of Emergency Medicine, 2nd edition. Baltimore: Williams and Wilkins; 1989. pp. 395-422.
108. Gupta DK, Desai NG, Kishore C, et al. Pattern of multiple substance use in heroin dependent individuals. Abstracts of the 48th Annual National Conference of the Indian Psychiatric Society, Bangalore. Indian J Psychiatry. 1996;38(Suppl):82.
109. Gupta PC, Saxena S, Pednekar M. Alcohol consumption among middle-aged and elderly men: A community study from Western India. Alcohol Alcohol. 2003;38:327-31. [PubMed]
110. Gururaj G, Girish N, Benegal V, Chandra V, Pandav R. Burden and Socioeconomic impact of alcohol, The Bangalore Study, World Health Organization, South East Asia Regional Office, New Delhi; 2006.
111. Gururaj G, Isaac MK, Girish N, Subbukrishna DK. Final report of the pilot study establishing health behaviour surveillance in respect of mental health. Report submitted to Ministry of Health and Family Welfare, Government of India and WHO India Country Office, New Delhi; 2004.
112. Hammersley R, Forsyth A, Lavelle T. The criminality of new drug users. Br J Addict 1990;85:1583-94.
113. Harford T, Ye-Yi H, Hilton M. Alcohol abuse and dependence in college and noncollege samples: a ten-years prospective follow-up in a national survey. J Stud Alcohol. 2006;67:803-9.
114. Harwood HJ, Hubbard RL, Collins JJ, et al. The cost of crime and the benefits of drug abuse treatment: a cost-benefit analysis using TOPS data. In: Leukefeld CG, Time FM (Eds). Compulsory Treatment of Drug Abuse: Research and Clinical Practice. NIDA Research Monograph Series 86. Rockville MD: National Institute of Drug Abuse, 1988.
115. Hasin DS, Stinson FS, Ogburn E, et al. Prevalence, correlates, disability, and comorbidity of DSM-IV alcohol abuse and dependence in the United States. ArchGen Psychiatry. 2005; 64;830-42.
116. Hawks R, Chiang CN. Buprenorphine-naloxone combination drug for the treatment of drug addiction. NIDA Res Monograph. 153.1995. pp. 165.

117. Hayashida M, Alterman AL, McLellan AT, et al. Comparative effectiveness and costs of inpatient and outpatient detoxification of patients with mild to moderate alcohol withdrawal syndromes. N Engl J Med. 1989;320:358-65.
118. Hazarika NC, Biswas D, Phukan RK, Hazarika D, Mahanta J. Prevalence and pattern of substance abuse at bandardewa, a border area of Assam and Arunachal Pradesh. Indian J Psychiatry. 2000;42:262-6. [PMC free article] [PubMed]
119. Health Education Authority Survey. Today's Young Adults. London: Health Education Authority; 1992.
120. Heather N, Brodie J, Wale S, et al. A randomized controlled trial of moderation-oriented cue exposure. J Stud Alcohol. 2000; 61:561-70.
121. Heather N, Brodie J, Wale S, et al. A randomized controlled trial of moderation-oriented cue exposure. J Stud Alcohol. 2000;61: 561-70.
122. Hietala J, Kiovisto H, Anttila P, Niemela O. Comparison of the combined marker GGT - CDT and the conventional laboratory markers of alcohol abuse in heavy drinkers, moderate drinkers and abstainers. Alcohol Alcohol. 2006;41:528-33.
123. Higgins ST, Delaney DD, Budney AJ, et al. A behavioral approach to achieving initial cocaine abstienence. Am J Psychiatry. 1991; 148:1218-24.
124. Hilbon ME, Hjelm-Jager M. Should alcohol withdrawal be treated with antiepileptic drugs? Acta Neurol Scand. 1984;69: 39-42.
125. Hnckers AS, Laucht M, Schmidt MH, et al. Low level of response to alcohol as associated with serotonin transporter genotype and high alcohol intake in adolescents. Boil Psychiatry 2006; 60:282-7.
126. Holder H, Longabaugh R, Miller W, et al. The cost effectiveness of treatment for alcoholism: a first approximation. J Stud Alcohol. 1991;52:517-40.
127. Ho MP, Yo CH, Liu CM, Chen CL, Lee CC. Refractive hypotension in a patient with disulfiram-ethanol reaction. Am J Med Sci. 2007;333:53-5.
128. Hubbard RL. Evaluation and outcome of treatment: Treatment approaches. In: Lowinson JH, Ruiz P, Millman RB, et al (Eds). Substance Abuse: A Comprehensive Textbook, 3rd edition. Baltimore: Williams and Wilkins; 1997. pp. 449-511.
129. Hughes JR, Kalman D. Do smokers with alcohol problems have more difficulty quitting? Drug Alcohol Depend. 2006;82:91-102.
130. Humphreys K, Moos R, Encouraging posttreatment self-help group involvement to reduce demand for continuing care services: two-year clinical and utilization outcomes. Alcohol Clin Exp Res. 2007;31:64-8.
131. Humphreys K, Moos R, Encouraging posttreatment self-help group involvement to reduce demand for continuing care services: two-year clinical and utilization outcomes. Alcohol Clin Exp Res. 2007;31:64-8.
132. Hunt W, Barnett L, Branch L. Relapse rates in addiction programs. J Clin Psychol. 1971;27:455-6.
133. Hunt W, Barnett L, Branch L. Relapse rates in addiction programs. J Clin Psychol. 1971; 27: 455-6.
134. Irwin M, Baird S, Smith T, Schuskit MA. User of laboratory tests to monitor heavy drinking by alcoholic men discharged from a treatment program. Am J Psychiatry. 1988;145: 595-9.
135. Jasinski DR, Pevnick JS, Griffith JD. Human pharmacology and abuse potential of the analgesic buprenorphine. Arch Gen Psychiatry. 1978;35:501-16.
136. Jessor R, Jessor SL. Problem behavior and psychosocial development: A longitudinal study of youth. New York: Academic Press; 1977.
137. John A, Barman A, Bal D, Chandy G, Samuel J, Thokchom M, et al. Hazardous alcohol use in rural southern India: Nature, prevalence and risk factors. Natl Med J India. 2009;22:123-5. [PubMed]
138. Johnson BA, Koob GF, Schuckit MA, et al. Understanding and treating alcohol dependence. Alcohol Clin Exp Res. 2006;30: 567-84.
139. Johnson BD, Muffler J. Socio-cultural: Determinants and perpetuators of substance abuse. In: Lowinson JH, Ruiz P, Millman RB, et al (Eds). Substance Abuse: A Comprehensive Textbook, 3rd edition. Baltimore: Williams and Wilkins; 1997. pp. 107-17.
140. Johnson RE, Fudala PJ. Development of buprenorphine for the treatment of opioid dependence. NIDA Res Monograph. 1997; 121:120-41.
141. Jones KA, Porjesz B, Almasy L, et al. A cholinergic receptor gene (CHRM2) affects event-related oscillations. Behav Genet. 2006;36:627-39.
142. Jonston LD, O' Malley PM, Batchman JG, Schulenberg JE. Monitoring the future national survey results on drug use, 1975-2006: Vol 1, Secondary school students (NIH Publication No. 06-5727). Bethesda, MD, USA: National Institute on drug Abuse; 2007.
143. Kandell D, Davies M, Kraus D, et al. The consequences in young adulthood of adolescent drug involvement. Arch Gen Psychiatry 1986;43:746-54.
144. Kaukonen JP, Luthje IN, Luthje P, et al. Acute alcohol use among patients with acute hip fractuires: a descriptive incidence study in southeastern Finland. Alcohol. 2006;41:345-8.
145. Kay L. Studies on etiology and sequel of abuse of alcohol. Lund, Sweden: University of Lund Press; 1960.
146. Kendell RE. The beneficial consequences of United Kingdom's declining per capita consumption of alcohol in 1979 to 1982. Alcohol and Alcoholism. 1984;19:271-6.
147. Kendler K, Kuo PWT, Kalsi G, et al. A joint genomewide linkage analysis of symptoms of alcohol dependence and conduct disorder. Alcohol Clin Exp Res. 2006;30:1972–7.
148. Kiefer F, Jahn H, Tarnaske T, et al. Comparing and combining naltrexone and acamprosate in relapse prevention of alcoholism: a double-blind, placebo-controlled study, Arch Gen Psychiatry. 2003;60:92-9.
149. Kinder B, Pape N, Walfish S. Drug and alcohol education programs: A review of outcome studies. Int J Addict. 1980;15:1035-54.

150. Kodituwakku PW, Adams CM, Hay A, et al. Letter and category fluency in children with fetal alcohol syndrome from a community in south Africa. J Stud Alcohol Drugs. 2007;68: 502-9.
151. Kodituwakku PW, Adams CM, Hay A, et al. Letter and category fluency in children with fetal alcohol syndrome from a community in south Africa. J Stud Alcohol Drugs. 2007; 68:502-9.
152. Krampe H, Stawicki S, Wagner T, et al. Follow-up of 180 alcoholic patients for up to 7 years after outpatient treatment; impact of alcohol deterrents on outcome. Alcohol Clin Exp Res. 2006;30:86-95.
153. Kranzler H. Koob G, Gastifriend D, Swift R, Willenbring M, Advances in the pharmacotherapy of alcoholism: Challenging misconceptions. Alcohol Clin Exp Res. 2006;30:272-81.
154. Kraus ML, Gottlieb LD, Horwitz RI, et al. Randomized clinical trials of atenolol in alcohol withdrawal. N Engl J Med. 1985; 313:905-9.
155. Krishna-Sarin S. Krystal JH, Shi J, et al. Family history of alcoholism influences naltrexone induced reduction in alcohol drinking. Biol Psychiatry. 2007;62:694-7.
156. Kumar MS. Rapid Assessment Survey of Drug Abuse in India. United Nations Office on Drugs and Crime Regional Office for South Asia and Ministry of Social Justice and Empowerment, Government of India. New Delhi, India. Available from: http://www.unodc.org/india/ras.html [cited in 2012]
157. Kumar S, Desai NG, Kapoor V. Depression in alcohol dependence syndrome. Paper presented at 44th Annual National Conference of Indian Psychiatric Society, Delhi; 1992.
158. Kumar S. Associated psychopathology in alcoholism. MD thesis. AIIMS, New Delhi; 1991.
159. Kumar V, Singh BK. Reasons behind increasing buprenorphine abuse. Abstracts of the 48th Annual National Conference of the Indian Psychiatric Society, Bangalore. Indian J Psychiatry. 1996; 38(Suppl):82-3.
160. Kuperman S, Chan G, Kramer JR, et al. Relationship of age of first drink to child behavioral problems and family psychopathology. Alcohol Clin Exp Res. 2005;29:1869-76.
161. Laucht M, Becker K, Blomeyer D, Schmidt M. Novelty seeking involved in mediating the association between to dopamine D4 receptor gene exon III polymorphism and heavy drinking in male adolescents: results from a high-risk community sample. Boil Psychiatry. 2007;61:87-92.
162. Lemke S, Schutte K, Brennan P, Moos R. Sequencing the lifetime onset of alcohol-related symptoms in order adults: is there evidence for disease progression? J Stud Alcohol. 2005; 66:756-65.
163. Lieber CS. Alcohol and the liver: Update. Hepatology. 1984;4: 1243-460.
164. Liepman MR, Nirenberg TD, Porges RE, et al. Depression associated with substance abuse. In: Cameron OG (Ed). Presentations of Depression and Depressive symptoms in Medical and Psychiatric Disorders. New York: John Wiley; 1987. pp. 131-67.
165. Lindros KO, Stowell A, Pikkarainen P, et al. The disulfiram (Antabuse) alcohol reaction in male alcoholics: its efficient management by 4-methylpryazole. Alcoholism Clin Exp Res. 1981;5:528-30.
166. Lingford-Hughes AR, et al. Evidence-based guidelines for the pharmacological management of substance misuse, addiction and comorbidity: recommendations from the British Association for Psychopharmacology. J Psychopharmacol. 2004;18:293-335.
167. Lingford-Hughes AR, Welch S, Nutt DJ. Evidence-based guidelines for the pharmacological management of substance misuse, addition and comorbidity: recommendations from the British Association for Psychopharmacology. J Psychopharmacol. 2004;18:293-335.
168. Lingford-Hughes AR, Welch S, Nutt DJ. Evidence-based guidelines for the pharmacological management of substance misuse, addition and comorbidity: recommendations from the British Association for Psychopharmacology. J Psychopharmacol. 2004;18:293-335.
169. Li T - K. The biological bases of nicotine and alcohol co-addiction. Boil psychiatry. 2007;61:1-3.
170. Lowinson JH, Payte JT, Salsitz E, et al. Methadone maintenance: treatment approaches. In: Lowinson JH, Ruiz P, Millman RB, et al (Eds). Substance Abuse: A Comprehensive Textbook, 3rd edition. Baltimore: Williams and Wilkins; 1997. pp. 405-15.
171. Maddrey WC. Alcohol-induced liver disease. Clin Liver Dis. 2000;4:115-31.
172. Maisto S, Clifford P, Stout R, Davis C. Drinking in the year after treatment as a predictor of three-year drinking outcomes. J Stud Alcohol. 2006;67:823-32.
173. Malhotra A, Balaji M, Basu D, et al. HIV screening and risk behavior in psychoactive substance users. Ind J Med Res [A]. 1993;97:231-3.
174. Malhotra A, Balaji M, Basu D, et al. HIV screening and risk behavior in psychoactive substance users. Ind J Med Res [A]. 1993;97:231-3.
175. Mann K, Lehert P, Morgan MY. The efficacy of acamprosate in the maintenance of abstinence in alcohol-dependent individuals: results of a mata-analysis. Alcohol Clin Exp Res. 2004;28:51-63.
176. Mann K, Schafer DR, Langle G, Ackermann K, Croissant B. The long-term course of alcoholism, 5, 10 and 16 years after treatment. Addiction. 2005;100:797-805.
177. Marlatt GA, Gordon JR. Relapse Prevention: Maintenance strategies in the treatment of addictive behavior. New York: Guilford Press; 1995.
178. Mason B, Goodman A, Chabac S, Lehert P. Effect of oral acamprosate on abstinence in patients with alcohol dependence in a double-bline, placebo-controlled trail: the role of patient motivation. J Psychiatr Res. 2006;40: 383-93.
179. Mayfield D, Maclead G, Hall S. The CAGE Questionnaire: validation of new alcoholism screening instrument. Am J Psychiatry. 1974;131:1121-3.

180. Mayo-Smith MF. Pharmacological management of alcohol withdrawal. A meta-analysis and evidence-based practice guideline. American Society of Addiction Medicine Working Group on Pharmacological Management of Alcohol Withdrawal. JAMA. 1997;278:144-51.
181. McDermott N, Mathews S (Eds). Residential treatment guidelines—January. A collaboration of ten therapeutic communities. New York: Therapeutic Communities of New York; 1994.
182. McKellar JD, Harris AH, Moos RH. Predictors of outcomes for patients with substance-use disorders five years after treatment dropout. J Stud Alcohol. 2006;67:685-93.
183. McKellar JD, Harris AH, Moos RH. Predictors of outcomes for patients with substance - use disorders five years after treatment dropout. J Stud Alcohol. 2006;67:685-93.
184. McLellan AT, Amdt IC, Metzger DS, et al. The effects of psychosocial services in substance abuse treatment. JAMA. 1993;269:1953-9.
185. McLellan AT, Luborsky L, Erdlen FR, et al. Addiction Severity Index: A diagnostic evaluation profile of substance abuse patients. In: Goltheil E, McLellan AT, Druley KA (Eds). Substance Abuse and Psychiatric Illness. New York: Pergamon Press; 1980. pp. 151-9.
186. Meena, Khanna P, Vohra AK, Rajput R. Prevalence and pattern of alcohol and substance abuse in urban areas of Rohtak city. Indian J Psychiatry. 2002;44:348-52. [PMC free article] [PubMed]
187. MeetensJ, Weisner C, Ray G, Fireman B, Walsh K. Hazardous drinkers and drugs user in HMO primary care: prevalence, medical conditions and costs. Alcohol Clin Exp Res; 2005
188. Mello NK, Mendelson JH. Burprenorphine suppresses herois use by heroin addicts. Science. 1980;207:657-9.
189. Metzger DS, Woody GE, McLellan AT, et al. Human immunodeficiency virus seroconversion among intravenous drug users in and out of treatment: An 18 month prospective follow-up. J AIDS. 1993;6:1049-56.
190. Miller WR, Rollnick S. Motivational Interviewing: Preparing People to Change Addictive Behavior. New York: Guilford Press; 1991.
191. Ministry of Health and Family Welfare, Government of India. Drug Abuse, Consequences and Responses: India Country Report. Draft Report. New Delhi: Ministry of Health and Family Welfare, Government of India; 1995.
192. Ministry of Health and Family Welfare. Expert Committee Report on Drug Dependence Services. New Delhi: Ministry of Health and Family Welfare Govt. of India; 1986. pp. 23.
193. Mohan D, Chopra A, Sethi H. Incidence estimates of substance use disorders in a cohort from Delhi, India. Indian J Med Res. 2002;115:128-35. [PubMed]
194. Mohan D, Desai NG, Chopra A, et al. A rapid survey on substance abuse disorders in the urban slums of New Delhi. Indian J Med Res(B). 1992;96:122-7.
195. Mohan D, Ray R, Sitholey P, et al. Collaborative study on narcotic drugs and psychotropic substances: Project component-Monitoring. Report submitted to the Indian Council of Medical Research, Delhi; 1993.
196. Moos R, Finney J, Moos B. Inpatient substance abuse care and the outcome of subsequent community residential and outpatient care. Addiction. 2000;95:833-46.
197. Moos R, Finney J, Moos B. Inpatient substance abuse care and the outcome of subsequent community residential and outpatient care. Addiction. 2000;95:833-46.
198. Moos RF, Moos BS. Rates and predictors of relapse after natural and treated remission from alcohol use disorders. Addiction. 2006;39:212-22.
199. Moyer A, Finney JW, Swearingen CE, et al. Brief interventions for alcohol problems: a meta-analytic review of controlled investigations in treatment-seeking and non-treatment-seeking populations. Addiction. 2002;97:279-92.
200. Moyer A, Finney JW, Swearingen CE, et al. Brief interventions for alcohol problems: a meta-analytic review of controlled investigations in treatment-seeking and nontreatment-seeking populations. Addiction. 2002;97:279-92.
201. Mundt M, French M, Roebuck M, Manwell L, Barry K, Brief physician advice for problem drinking among older adults; an economic analysis of costs and benefits. J Stud Alconol 2005; 66:380-94.
202. Mundt M, French M, Roebuck M, Manwell L, Barry K, Brief psysician advice for problem drinking among older adults; an economic analysis of costs and benefits. J Stud Alconol. 2005; 66:380-94.
203. Nadelman E, McNeely J, Drucker E. International Perspectives: Background. In: Lowinson JH, Ruiz P, Millman RB, et al (Eds). Substance Abuse: A Comprehensive Textbook, 3rd edition. Baltimore: Williams and Wilkins; 1997. pp. 22-40.
204. Narain HP. HIV/AIDS in South-East Asia: An update. Delhi: WHO, Regional office for South-East Asia; 1995.
205. Naranjo CA, Kadlec KE, Sanhueja P, et al. Fluoxetine differentially alters alcohol intake and other consummatory behaviors in problem drinkers. Clin Pharmacol Ther. 1990;47:490-8.
206. National Family Health Survey India-3. Available from: http://www.nfhsindia.org/nfhs3.html [Accessed on 2012 20 December].
207. Niaua R, Abrams D, Demuth B, et al. Responses to smoking related stimuli and early relapse to smoking. Addict Behav. 1989;144:419-28.
208. Niemela O. Biomarkers in alcoholism. Clin Chim Acta. 2007; 377:39-49.
209. Nizamie SH, Sharma LN. Buprenorphine abuse: A case report. Indian J Psychiatry. 1990;32:198-200.
210. Norstrom T. Per capita alcohol consumption and all - cause mortality in Canada, 1950–1998. Addiction. 2004;99:1274-8.
211. Nusnberger JI Jr, Bierut LJ. Seeking the connections: alcoholism and our genes. Sci Am. 2007;296:46-53.
212. Oppenheimer E, Tobutt C, Taylor C, et al. Death and survival in a cohort of heroin addicts from London clinics: A 22 year follow up study. Addiction. 1994;89:1299-308.

213. O'Malley SS, Garbutt JC, Gastfriend Dr, Dong Q, Kranzler HR. Efficacy of extended release naltrexone in alcohol-dependent patients who are abstinent prior to treatment. J Clin Psychopharmacology. 2007;27:507-12.
214. O'Malley SS, Jaffe AJ, Chang G, et al. Naltrexone and coping skills therapy for alcohol dependence: A controlled study. Arch Gen Psychiatry. 1992;49:881-7.
215. Palmieri VO,Cicco G, Minerva F, et al. Red blood cells (RBC) deformability and aggregability: alterations in alcoholism. Adv Exp Med Biol. 2006;578:125-31.
216. Palmieri VO,Cicco G, Minerva F, et al. Red blood cells (RBC) deformability and aggregability: alterations in alcoholism. Adv Exp Med Biol. 2006;578;125-31.
217. Parker AJR, Marshall EJ, Bll DM. Diagnosis and management of alcohol use disorders. BMJ. 2008;496-501.
218. Pastor R, Aragon C. The role of opioid receptor subtypes in the development of behavioural sensitization to ethanol. Neuropsychopharmalogy. 2006;31:1489-99.
219. Peace K, Mellsop G. Alcoholism and psychiatric disorders. ANZ J Psychiatry. 1987;21:94-101.
220. Petersen EN. The pharmacology and toxicology of disulfiram and its metabolites. Acta Psychiat Scand. 1992;86(Suppl):7-13.
221. Poulsen HE, Loft S, Anderson JR, et al. Disulfiram therapy: adverse drug reactions and interactions. Acta Psychiat Scand. 1992;86(Suppl):59-66.
222. Powell BJ, Penick EC, Othermer E, et al. Prevalence of additional psychiatric syndromes among male alcoholics. J Clin Psychiatry. 1982;43:10.
223. Ray R. Alcohol diagnosis and phenomenology. In: Ray R, Pickens RW (Eds). Proceedings of the Indo-US symposium on alcohol and drug abuse. NIMHANS Publication No. 20. Bangalore: NIMHA-NS; 1989. pp. 71-82.
224. Ray R. The Extent, Pattern and Trends of Drug Abuse in India, National Survey, Ministry of Social Justice and Empowerment, Government of India and United Nations Office on Drugs and Crime, Regional Office for South Asia; 2004.
225. Reddy MV, Chandrashekhar CR. Prevalence of mental and behavioural disorders in India: A meta-analysis. Indian J Psychiatry. 1998;40:149-57. [PMC free article] [PubMed]
226. Regier DA, Boyd JH, Burke JD, et al. One month prevalence of mental disorders in the United States based on five Epidemiologic Catchment Area sites. Arch Gen Psychiatry. 1988;45:977-86.
227. Regier DA, Farmer ME, Rae DS, et al. Comorbidity of mental disorders with alcohol and other drug abuse. JAMA. 1990;264: 2511-8.
228. Reich J, Chaudry D. Personality of panic disorder alcohol abusers. J Nerv Ment Dis. 1987;175:224-8.
229. Reinert DF, Allen JP. The alcohol use disorders identification test: an update of research findings. Alcohol Clin Exp Res. 2007; 31:185-99.
230. Reoux JP, Miller K. Routine hospital detoxification practice compared to symptom triggered management with an objective withdrawal scale (CIWA - Ar). J Addiction. 2000;9:135-44.
231. Reoux JP, Miller K. Routine hospital detoxification practice compared to sympyom triggered management with an objective withdrawal scale (CIWA - Ar). J Addiction. 2000;9: 135-44.
232. Ritson B, Chick JD, Strang J. Dependence on alcohol and other drugs. In: Kendell RE, Zelley AK (Eds). Companion to Psychiatric Studies. Edinburgh: Churchill Livingstone; 1993. pp. 359-95.
233. Rivara FP, Garrison MM, Ebel B, McCarty CA, Christakis DA. Mortality attributable to harmful drinking in the United States, 2000. J Stud Alcohol. 2004;65:530-6.
234. Romelsjo A, Agren G. Has mortality related to alcohol decreased in Sweden? Br Med J. 1985;291:167-70.
235. Romero-Gemez M, Grande L, Nogales MC, et al. Chronic alcohol use enhances the hepatitis C virus load in the liver. Alcohol Research. 2002;7:66.
236. Rosenbloom Mj, Sullivan EV, Sassoon SA, et al. Alcoholism, HIV infection, and their comorbidity: factors affecting self-rated health-related quality of life. J Stud Alcohol Drugs 2007; 68:115–25.
237. Rounsaville BJ, Carroll KM. Individual psychotherapy: Treatment approaches. In: Lowinson JH, Ruiz P, Millman RB, et al (Eds). Substance Abuse: A Comprehensive Textbook, 3rd edition. Baltimore: Williams and Wilkins; 1997. pp. 430-39.
238. Rounsaville BJ, Dolinsky ZS, Babor TF, et al. Psychopathology as a predictor of treatment outcome in alcoholics. Arch Gen Psychiatry. 1987;44:505-13.
239. Rumpf HJ, Biscjof G, Hapke U, Meyer C, John U. Stability of remission from alcohol dependence without formal help. Alcohol Alcohol. 2006;41:311-4.
240. Sampath SK, Chand PK, Murthy P. Problem drinking among male inpatients in a rural general hospital. Indian J Community Med. 2007;32:93.
241. Sannibale C, Fucito L, O' Connor D, Curry K. Process evaluation of an out-patient detoxification services. Drug Alcohol Review. 2005;24:475-81.
242. Sannibale C, Fucito L, O' Connor D, Curry K. Process evaluation of an out-patient detoxification services. Drug Alcohol Review. 2005;24:475-81.
243. Sarkar S, Mookerjee P, Roy A. Descriptive epidemiology of intravenous heroin users: A new risk group for transmission of HIV in India. J Inf. 1991;23:201-7.
244. Sarkar S, Panda S, Das N, et al. Rapid spread of HIV among infecting drug users in North-Eastern states of India. CARC Calling. 1993;6:23-8.
245. Saxena S. Alcohol, Europe, and developing countries. Addiction. 1997;92(suppl 1):48
246. Schellenberg F, Schwan R, Mennetrey L, et al. Dose-effect relation between daily ethanole intake in the range 0–70 grams and % CDT value: validation of a cut-off value. Alcohol. 2005;40:532-4.
247. Schuckit MA, Smith TL, Danko GP, et al. Prospective evaluation of the four DSM–IV criteria for alcohol abuse in a large population, Am J Psychiatry. 2005;162:350-60.

248. Schuckit MA, Smith TL, Pierson J, et al. Externalizing disorders in the offspring from the San Diego Prospective Study of alcoholism. J Spychiatric Reasearch. 2008;46:644-52.
249. Schuckit MA. Alcohol and drug interactions with antianxiety medications. Am J Med. 1987;82:27-33.
250. Schuckit MA. Alcohol related disorders. In: Kaplan HI, Sadock BJ (Eds). Comprehensive Textbook of Psychiatry, 6th edition. Baltimore: Williams and Wilkins; 1995. pp. 775-91.
251. Schuckit MA. Biological vulnerability to alcoholism. J Consult Clin Psychol. 1987;55:301-9.
252. Schuckit MA. Comorbidity between substance use disorders and psychiatric conditions. Addiction. 2006;101:76-88.
253. Schuckit MA. Genetic and clinical implications of alcoholism and affective disorders.Am J Psychiatry. 1986;143:140-7.
254. Schuckit MA. Genetic and clinical implications of alcoholism and affective disorders. Am J Psychiatry. 1986;143:140-7.
255. Schuckit MA. Smith TL. An evaluation of the level of responses to alcohol, externalizing symptoms, and depressive symptoms as predictors of alcoholism. J Stud Alcohol. 2006;67:215-27.
256. Schuckit MA. Vulnerability factors for alcoholism. In: Davis K, (Ed). Neuropsychopharmacology: the fifth generation of progress. Baltimore, MD, USA: Lippincott Willians & Wilkams; 2002. pp. 1399-1411.
257. Sellers EM, Naranjo CA, Harrison M, et al. Diazepam loading: simplified treatment of alcohol withdrawal. J Stud Alcohol. 1977;39:2096-8.
258. Sellers EM. Clinical Institute Withdrawal Assesssment-Alcohol (CIWA-A) Scale. Toronto: Alcoholism and Drug Addiction Research Foundation, 1980.
259. Selzer ML. The Michigan Alcoholism Screening Test: The quest for a new diagnostic instrument. Am J Psychiatry. 1971;127: 1653-8.
260. Sereny G, Sharma V, Holt J, et al. Mandatory supervised antabuse therpay in an outpatient alcoholism program: a study. Alcoholism Clin Exp Res. 1986;10: 290-2.
261. Sharma S, Singh MM. Prevalence of mental disorders: An epidemiological study in Goa. Indian J Psychiatry. 2001;43:118-26.
262. Simon EJ. Opiates: Neurobiology. In: Lowinson JH, Ruiz P, Millman RB, et al (Eds). Substance Abuse: A Comprehensive Textbook, 3rd edition. Baltimore: Williams and Wilkins; 1997. pp. 148-58.
263. Singh G. Epidemiology of alcohol in India. In: Ray R, Pickens RW (Eds). Proceedings of the Indo-US Symposium on Alcohol and Drug Abuse. NIMHANS Publication No. 20. Bangalore: NIMHANS; 1989. pp. 3-11.
264. Singh G. Epidemiology of alcohol in India. In: Ray R, Pickens RW (Eds). Proceedings of the Indo-US Symposium on Alcohol and Drug Abuse. NIMHANS Publication No. 20. Bangalore: NIMHANS; 1989. pp. 3-11.
265. Singh RB, Ghosh S, Niaz MA, Rastogi V, Wander GS. Validation of tobacco and alcohol intake questionnaire in relation to food intakes for the five city study and proposed classification for indians. J Physicians India. 1998;46:587-91. [PubMed]
266. Sisk JE, Hatziandren EJ, Hughes R. The effectiveness of drug abuse treatment: Implication for controlling AIDS/HIV infection. Washington DC: Office of Technology Assessment; 1990.
267. Sitholey P, Mohan D, Purohit DR, et al. Collaborative study on narcotic drugs and psychotropic substances: Project component-Area Survey. Report submitted to the Indian Council of Medical Research, Delhi; 1993.
268. Skinner HA. The drug abuse screening instrument. Addict Behav. 1982;7:363-71.
269. Smith TL, Volpe FR, Hashima JN, Schuckit MA. Impact of a stimulant-focused enhanced program on the outcome of alcohol - and/or stimulant-dependent men. Alcohol Clin Exp Res. 1999;23:1772-9.
270. Smith TL, Volpe FR, Hashima JN, Schuckit MA. Impact of a stimulant-focused enhanced program on the outcome of alcohol - and/or stimulant-dependent men. Alcohol Clin Exp Res. 1999;23:1772-9.
271. Society for Promotion of Youth and Masses. Intravenous Drug Addicts: A Study in South Delhi Slums. New Delhi: SPYM; 1995.
272. Society for Promotion of Youth and Masses. Intravenous Drug Addicts: A Study in South Delhi Slums. New Delhi: SPYM; 1995.
273. Srisurapanont M, Jarusuraisin N, Naltrexone for the treatment of alcoholism: a met-analysis of randomized controlled trials. Int J Neuropsychopharmacol. 2005;8:267-80.
274. Stahlbrandt H, Jonsson KO, Berglund M. Two-year outcome of alcohol interventions in Swedish university halls of residence: a cluster randomized trial of a brief skills training program, twelve-step-influenced intervention, and controls. Alcohol Clin Exp Res. 2007;31:458-66.
275. Stahlbrandt H, Jonsson KO, Berglund M. Two-year outcome of alcohol interventions in Swedish university halls of residence: a cluster randomized trial of a brief skills training program, twelve-step-influenced intervention, and controls. Alcohol Clin Exp Res. 2007;31:458-66.
276. Stanton MD, Thomas TC. Family Therapy of Drug Abuse and Addiction. New York: Guilford Press; 1982.
277. Stecker T, Curran GM, Han X, Booth BM. Patterns of health services use associated with Veterans Affairs outpatient substances-use treatment. J Stud Alcohol Drugs. 2007;68: 510-18.
278. Stecker T, Curran GM, Han X, Booth BM. Patterns of health services use associated with Veterans Affairs outpatient substances-use treatment. J Stud Alcohol Drugs. 2007;68: 510-18.
279. Steensland P, Simms JA, Holgate J, et al. Varenicline, an alpha4beta2 nicotinic acetylcholine receptor partial agonist, selectively decreases ethanol consumption and seeking. PNAS. 2007;104:12518-23.
280. Steinglass P. The alcoholic family in the interaction laboratory. J Nerv Ment Dis. 1979;167:428-36.
281. Stephens RC, Alemagno SA. Injection and sexual risk behaviors of male heterosexual injecting drug users. In: Battjes RJ, Sloboda Z, Grace WC (Eds). The Context of HIV Risk Among

Drug Users and Their Sexual Partners. NIDA Res Monogr 143. Rockville, MD: NIDA, 1994.

282. Stockwell J, Hodgson R, Edwards G, et al. The development of a questionnaire to measure severity of alcohol dependence. Br J Addict. 1979;74:79-87.
283. Strain EC, Preston KL, Liebson IA, et al. Acute effects of buprenorphine, hydronorphine, and naloxone in methadone maintained volunteers. J Pharmacol Exp Ther. 1992;261: 985-93.
284. Stryker J, Coates TJ, De Carlo P, et al. Prevention of HIV Infection: Looking Back, Looking Ahead. JAMA. 1995;273:1143-8.
285. Suh JJ, Pettinati HM, Kampman KM, O'Brine CP. The status of disulfiram: a half of a century later. J Clin Psychopharmacol. 2006;26:290-302.
286. Sutherland G, Edwards G, Taylor C, et al. The measurement of opiate dependence. Br J Addict. 1987;81:485-94.
287. Szucs S, Sarvary A, McKee M, Adany R. Could the high level of cirrhosis in central and eastern Europe be due partly to the quality of alcohol consumed? An exploratory investigation. Addiction. 2005;100:536-42.
288. Tawil O, Vester A, O'Reilly KR. Enabling approaches for HIV/AIDS Prevention: Can we modify the environment and minimise the risk? AIDS. 1995;9:1299-306.
289. Taylor C. What happens over long-term. Br Med Bull. 1994; 50:50-67.
290. Tchuckit MA. Drug and alcohol abuse: a clinical guide to diagnosis and treatment, 6th edn. New york, U.S.A. Springer; 2006
291. Teesson M, Baillie A, Lynskey A, Manor B, Degenhardt L. Substance use, dependence and treatment seeking in the United States and Australia: a cross-national comparison. Drug alcohol Depent. 2006;81:149-55
292. Thomson AD, et al. The treatment of patients at risk of developing Wernicke's encephalopathy in the community. Alcohol Alcohol. 2006; 41:159-67.
293. Thomson AD et al. The Royal College of Physicians report on alcohol: guidelines for managing Wernicke's encephalopathy in the accident and emergency department. Alcohol Alcohol. 2002;37:513-21.
294. Thyer BA, Panish RT, Himle J, et al. Case histories and short communication alcohol abuse among clinically anxious patients. Behev Res Ther. 1986;24:357-9.
295. Timberlake DS, Hopfer CJ, Rhee SH, et al. College attendance and its effect on drinking behaviors in a longitudinal study of adolescents. Alcohol Clin Exp Res. 2007;31:1020-30.
296. Umesh Babu SB, Chaturvedi SK. Changing patterns in opiate abuse with a focus on buprenorphine. Abstracts of 47th Annual National Conference of the Indian Psychiatric Society, Patna. Indian J Psychiatry. 1995;37(Suppl):23.
297. United Nations Drug Control Program. World Drug Report. New York: Oxford University Press; 1997.
298. United Nations International Drug Control Program. Report of the United Nations General Assembly Special Session on the World Drug Problem, New York, Information Sheet No. 2.
299. Vaillant GE. A 20 year follow up of New York narcotic addicts. Arch Gen Psychiatry. 1973;29:237-41.
300. Valenzuela CF, Harris RA. Alcohol: Neurobiology: Substances of abuse. In: Lowinson JH, Ruiz P, Millman RB, et al (Eds). Substance Abuse: A Comprehensive Textbook, 3rd edition. Baltimore: Williams and Wilkins; 1997. pp. 119-42.
301. van den Wildenberg E, Wiers R, Dessers J, et al. A functional polymorphism of the u-opioid receptor gene (OPRM) influences cue-induced craving for alcohol in male heavy drinkers. Alcohol Clin Exp Res. 2007;31:1-10.
302. Vasilaki E, Hosier S, Cox M. The efficacy of motivational interviewing as a brief intervention for excessive drinking: a meta-analytic review. Alcohol Alcohol. 2006;41:328-36.
303. Vasilaki E, Hosier S, Cox M. The efficacy of motivational interviewing as a brief intervention for excessive drinking: a meta-analytic review. Alcohol Alcohol. 2006;41:328-36.
304. Vaswani M, Desai NG. Biological markers of alcoholism. Ann Natl Acad Med Sci (India). 1997;33:173-84.
305. Verge C, Lucena KI, Lopez-Torres F, et al. Adverse hepatic reactions associated with calcium carbimide and disulfiram therapy: is there still a role for these drugs? World J Gastroenterol. 2006;21:5078-78.
306. Volpicelli JR, Alterman AI, Hayashide M, et al. Naltrexone in the treatment of alcohol dependence. Arch Gen Psychiatry. 1992;49:876-80.
307. Walsh SL, Preston KL, Sitzer ML, et al. Clinical pharmacology of buprenorphine: ceiling effects at high doses. Clin Pharmacol Ther. 1994;55:569-80.
308. Washton AM. Structured outpatient group therapy: treatment approaches. In: Lowinson JH, Ruiz P, Millman RB, et al (Eds). Substance Abuse: A Comprehensive Textbook, 3rd edition. Baltimore: Williams and Wilkins; 1997. pp. 440-48.
309. Watters JK, Guydish J. HIV/AIDS Prevention for Drug Users in Natural Settings. In: Di Clemente RJ, Peterson JL (Eds). Preventing AIDS: Theories and Methods of Behavioral Interventions. New York: Plenum Press; 1994.
310. Weinshenker D, Schroeder JP. There and back again: a tale of norepinephrine and drug addition. Neuropsychopharmacology. 2007;32:1433-51.
311. Weisman MM, Myers JH, Harding PS. Prevalence and psychiatric heterogeneity of alcoholism in a United States urban community. J Stud Alcohol. 1980;41:672-81.
312. Winick C. Maturing out of narcotic addiction. Bull Narcotics 1962;142:1-7.
313. Witkiewitz K Marlatt G. Relapse prevention for alcohol and drug problems. Am Psychol. 2004;59:224-35.
314. Witkiewitz K Marlatt G. Relapse prevention for alcohol and drug problems. Am Psychol. 2004;59:224-35.
315. Wolin SJ, Bennett LA, Noonan DL. Family rituals and the recurrence of alcoholism over generations. Am J Psychiatry. 1979;136:589-93.
316. World Health Organisation. ICD-10 Classification of Mental and Behavioral Disorders: Clinical Descriptions and Diagnostic Guidelines. Geneva: WHO; 1992.

317. World Health Organisation. The Alcohol Use Disorders Inventory Test (AUDIT): Guidelines for use in primary health care. Geneva: WHO, 1989.
318. Yalom ID. The Theory and Practice of Group Psychotherapy, 2nd edition. New York: Basic Books; 1975.

Alcohol-use Disorder

319. Alati R, Mamun AA, Williams GM. In utero alcohol exposure and predication of alcohol disorders in early adulthood. Arch Gen Psychiatry. 2006;63:1009-16.
320. Alte D, Ludemann J, Piek M, et al Distribution and dose response of laboratory markers to alcohol consumption in a general population: Results of the Study of Health in Pomerania (SHIP). J Stud Alcohol. 2003;64:75-82.
321. American Psychiatric Association. Desk Reference to the Diagnostic Criteria from DSM-5. Washington DC, 2013.
322. American Psychiatry Association. Diagnostic and statistical manual of mental disorder—text revision (DSM-IV), 4th edition. Washington, DC,USA: American Psychiatry Association; 2000.
323. Anton RF, Youngblood M. Factors affecting % CDT status at entry into a multisite clinical treatment trial: experience from the COMBINE study. Alcohol Clin Exp Res. 2006;30:1878-83.
324. Babor T, Higgins-Biddle J, Dauser D, et al. Brief interventions for at-risk drinking: patient outcomes and cost-effectiveness in managed care organizations. Alcohol. 2006;41:624-31.
325. Babor TF, Hofmann M, DelBOca FK, et al. Types of alcoholics, I: Evidence for an empirically derived typology based on indicators of vulnerability and severity. Arch Gen Psychiatry. 1992;49:599-608.
326. Barr C, Newman T, Becker M, et al. Serotonin transporter gene variation is associated with alcohol sensitivity in rhesus macaques exposed to early-life stress. Alcohol Clin Exp Res. 2005;27:812-7.
327. Bartsch AJ, Homola G, BillerA. Manifestations of early brain recovery associated with abstinence from alcoholism. Brain. 2007;130:36-47.
328. Berner MM, Kriston L, Bentele M, Harter M. The Alcohol Use Identification Test for detecting at-risk drinking: a systematic review and meta - analysis. J Stud Alcohol Drug. 2007;68:461-73.
329. Blednov YA, Cravatt BF, Boehn SL II, et al. Role of endocannabinoids in alcohol consumption and intoxication: studies of mice lacking fatty acid amide hydrolase. Neuropsychopharmacology. 2007;32:1433-51.
330. Bodin M, Romelsjo A. Predictors of abstinence and nonproblem drinking after 12-steps treatment in Sweden. J Stud Alcohol. 2006;67:139-46.
331. Borgheses CM, Ali DN, Bleck V, et al. Acetylcholine and alcohol sensitivity of neuronal nicotinic acetylcholine receptors: mutations in transmembrane domains. Alcohol Clin Exp Res. 2002;26:1764-72.
332. Bottlender M, Soyka M. Outpatient alcoholism treatment: predictors of outcome after 3 years. Drugs Alcohol Depend. 2005;80:83-9.
333. Carroll K, Ball S, Nich C, et al. Motivational interviewing to improve treatment engagement and outcome in individuals seeking treatment for substance abuse: a multisite effectiveness study. Drug Alcohol Depend. 2006;81:301-12.
334. Clark DB. The natural history of adolescent alcohol use disorders: addiction. 2004;99:5-22.
335. Conigrave KM, Degenhardt LJ, Whitfield JB, et al. CDT, GGT, and AST as markers of alcohol use: The WHO/ISBRA Collaborative Project. Alcohol Clin Exp Res. 2002;26:332-39.
336. Conroy DA, Arnedt JT, Brower KJ, et al. Perception of sleep in recovering alcohol-dependent patients with insomnia: relationship with future drinking. Alcohol Clin Exp Res. 2006;30:1992-9.
337. Cook TAR, Luczak SE, Shea SH, et al. Association of ALDH2 and ADH1B genotypes with response to alcohol in Asian Americans. J Stud Alcohol. 2005;66:196-204
338. Cox WM, Roseberg H, Hazel C, et al. United Kingdom and United States healthcare providers recommendations of abstinence versus controlled drinking. Alcohol. 2004;39: 130-4.
339. Crawford MJ, Patton R, Touquet R, et al. Screening and referral for brief intervention of alcohol-misusing patients in an emergency department; a pragmatic randomized controlled trial. Lancet. 2004;364:1334-9.
340. Dawson DA, Grant BF, Stinson FS, et al, Recovery from DSM-IV alcohol dependence: United States, 2001–2002. addition. 2005;100:281-92.
341. Dick DM, Bierut L, Hinrichs A, et al. The role of GABRA 2 in risk for conduct disorder and alcohol and drug dependence across developmental stages. Behave Genet. 2006;36:577-90.
342. Dickson P, James M, Health A, et al. Effects of variation at the ALDH2 locus on alcohol metabolism, sensitivity, consumption, and dependence in Europeans. Alcohol Clin Exp Res. 2006;30:1093-100.
343. Duranceaux NCE, Schuckit MA, Eng MY, et al. Associations of variations in alcohol dehydrogenase genes with the level of response to alcohol in non-Asians. Alcohol Clin Exp Res. 2006;30:1470-8.
344. Enoch M, Schwartz L, Albaugh B, Vikkunen M, Goldman D. Dimensional anxiety mediates linkage of GABRA2 haplotypes with alcoholism. Am J Med Genet. 2006;141:599-607.
345. Fatjo F, Sancho-Bru P, Fernandez-Sopla J, et al. Up-regulation of myocardial L-type Ca2+ channel in chronic alcoholic subjects without cardiomyopathy. Alcohol Clin Exp Res. 2007;31:1099-105.
346. Feeney G, Connor J, Young R, Tucker J, McPherson A. Combined acamprosate and naltrexone, with cognitive bheavioural therapy is superior to either medication alone for alcohol abstinence: a single centres experience with pharmacotherapy. Alcohol. 2006;41:321-7.
347. Fuller FK, Gordis E. Does disulfiram have a role in alcoholism treatment today? Addition. 2004;99:21-4.
348. Gelernter J, Gueorgulieva R, Kranzler HR, et al. Opioid receptor gene (OPRM1, OPRK1, and OPRD1) wariants and response to

naltrexone treatment for alcohol dependence: result from the VA Cooperative Study. Alcohol Clin Exp Res. 2007;31:555-63.

349. Hamilton SP, Slager S, Baisre de Leon A, et al. Evidence for a genetic linkage between a polymorphism in the adenosine 2A receptor and panic disorder. Neuropsychopharmacology. 2004;29:558-65.
350. Harford T, Ye - Yi H, Hilton M. Alcohol abuse and dependence in college and noncollege samples: a ten-years prospective follow-up in a national survey. J Stud Alcohol. 2006;67:803-9.
351. Hasin D, Grant BF, Cottler L, et al. Nosological comparisons of alcohol and drug diagnoses: a multisite, multi-instrument international study. Drug Alcohol Depend. 1997;47:217-26.
352. Hasin DS, Stinson FS, Ogburn E, et al. Prevalence, correlates, disability, and comorbidity of DSM-IV alcohol abuse and dependence in the United States. ArchGen Psychiatry. 2005; 64;830-42.
353. Heather N, Brodie J, Wale S, et al. A randomized controlled trial of moderation-oriented cue exposure. J Stud Alcohol. 2000;61:561-70.
354. Hietala J, Kiovisto H, Anttila P, Niemela O. Comparison of the combined marker GGT - CDT and the conventional laboratory markers of alcohol abuse in heavy drinkers, moderate drinkers and abstainers. Alcohol Alcohol. 2006;41:528-33.
355. Hnckers AS, Laucht M, Schmidt MH, et al. Low level of response to alcohol as associated with serotonin transporter genotype and high alcohol intake in adolescents. Boil Psychiatry. 2006;60:282-7.
356. Ho MP, Yo CH, Liu CM, Chen CL, Lee CC. Refractive hypotension in a patient with disulfiram-ethanol reaction. Am J Med Sci. 2007;333:53-5.
357. Hsin D, Li Q, McCloud S, Endicott J. Agreement between DSM-III, DSM-III-R, DSM-IV and ICD-10 alcohol diagnoses in US community-sample heavy drinkers. Addition. 1996;91:1517-27.
358. Hughes JR, Kalman D. Do smokers with alcohol problems have more difficulty quitting? Drug Alcohol Depend. 2006;82:91-102.
359. Humphreys K, Moos R, Encouraging posttreatment self-help group involvement to reduce demand for continuing care services: two-year clinical and utilization outcomes. Alcohol Clin Exp Res. 2007;31:64-8.
360. Irwin M, Baird S, Smith T, Schuskit MA. User of laboratory tests to monitor heavy drinking by alcoholic men discharged from a treatment program. Am J Psychiatry. 1988;145:595-99.
361. Johnson BA, Koob GF, Schuckit MA, et al. Understanding and treating alcohol dependence. Alcohol Clin Exp Res. 2006;30:567-84.
362. Johnson BA, Rosenthal N, Capece JA, et al. Torpiramate for treating alcohol dependence: a randomized controlled trial: JAMA. 2007;298:1641-51.
363. Jones KA, Porjesz B, Almasy L, et al. A cholinergic receptor gene (CHRM2) affects event - related oscillations. Behav Genet. 2006;36:627-39.
364. Jonston LD, O' Malley PM, Batchman JG, Schulenberg JE. Monitoring the future national survey results on drug use, 1975-2006: Vol 1, Secondary school students (NIH Publication No. 06-5727). Bethesda, MD, USA: National Istitute on drug Abuse; 2007.
365. Kalivas K, Volkow N. The neuroal bais of addiction: a pathology of motivation and choice. Am J Psychiatry. 2005;162:1403-13.
366. Kaukonen JP, Luthje IN, Luthje P, et al. Acute alcohol use among patients with acute hip fractures: a descriptive incidence study in southeastern Finland. Alcohol. 2006;41:345-8.
367. Kendler K, Kuo PWT, Kalsi G, et al. A joint genomewide linkage analysis of symptoms of alcohol dependence and conduct disorder. Alcohol Clin Exp Res. 2006;30:1972-7.
368. Kiefer F, Jahn H, Tarnaske T, et al. Comparing and conbining naltrexone and acamprosate in relapse prevention of alcoholism: a double-blind, placebo-controlled study. Arch Gen Psychiatry. 2003;60:92-9.
369. Kodituwakku PW, Adams CM, Hay A, et al. Letter and category fluency in children with fetal alcohol syndrome from a community in south Africa. J Stud Alcohol Drugs. 2007;68:502-9.
370. Krampe H, Stawicki S, Wagner T, et al. Follow-up of 180 alcoholic patients for up to 7 years after outpatient treatment; impact of alcohol deterrents on outcome. Alcohol Clin Exp Res. 2006;30:86-95.
371. Kranzler H, Koob G, Gastifriend D, Swift R, Willenbring M, Advances in the pharmacotherapy of alcoholism: Challenging misconceptions. Alcohol Clin Exp Res. 2006;30:272-81.
372. Krishna-Sarin S, Krystal JH, Shi J, et al. Family history of alcoholism influences naltrexone induced reduction in alcohol drinking. Biol Psychiatry. 2007;62:694-7.
373. Krystal J, Staley J, Manson G, et al. Gamma aminobutyric acid type A receptors and alcoholism. Arch Gen Psychiatry. 2006;63:957-68.
374. Kuperman S, Chan G, Kramer JR, et al. Relationship of age of first drink to child behavioural problems and family psychopathology. Alcohol Clin Exp Res. 2005;29:1869-76.
375. Laucht M, Becker K, Blomeyer D, Schmidt M. Novelty seeking involved in mediating the association between to dopamine D4 receptor gene exon III polymorphism and heavy drinking in male adolescents: results from a high-risk community sample. Boil Psychiatry. 2007;61:87-92.
376. Lemke S, Schutte K, Brennan P, Moos R. Sequencing the lifetime onset of alcohol-related symptoms in order adults: is there evidence for disease progression? J Stud Alcohol. 2005;66:756-65.
377. Lingford-Hughes AR, Welch S, Nutt DJ. Evidence-based guidelines for the pharmacological management of substance misuse, addition and comorbidity: recommendations from the British Association for Psychopharmacology. J Psychopharmacol. 2004;18:293-335.
378. Li T-K. The biological bases of nicotine and alcohol co-addiction. Boil pychiatry. 2007;61:1-3.
379. Maddrey WC. Alcohol-induced liver disease. Clin Liver Dis. 2000;4:115-31.

380. Maisto S, Clifford P, Stout R, Davis C. Drinking in the year after treatment as a predictor of three-year drinking outcomes. J Stud Alcohol. 2006;67:823-32.
381. Mann K, Lehert P, Morgan MY. The efficacy of acamprosate in the maintenance of abstinence in alcohol-dependent individuals: results of a meta-analysis. Alcohol Clin Exp Res. 2004;28:51-63.
382. Mann K, Schafer DR, Langle G, Ackermann K, Croissant B. The long-term course of alcoholism, 5, 10 and 16 years after treatment. Addiction. 2005;100:797-805.
383. Mason B, Goodman A, Chabac S, Lehert P. Effect of oral acamprosate on abstinence in patients with alcohol dependence in a double-bline, placebo-controlled trail: the role of patient motivation. J Psychiatr Res. 2006;40:383-93.
384. McKellar JD, Harris AH, Moos RH. Predictors of outcomes for patients with substance-use disorders five years after treatment dropout. J Stud Alcohol. 2006;67:685-93.
385. MeetensJ, Weisner C, Ray G, Fireman B, Walsh K. Hazardous drinkers and drugs user in HMO primary care: prevalence, medical conditions and costs. Alcohol Clin Exp Res; 2005.
386. Moos R, Finney J, Moos B. Inpatient substance abuse care and the outcome of subsequent community residential and outpatient care. Addiction. 2000;95;833-46.
387. Moos RF, Moos BS. Rates and predictors of relapse after natural and treated remission from alcohol use disorders. Addiction. 2006;39:212-22.
388. Moyer A, Finney JW, Swearingen CE, et al. Brief interventions for alcohol problems: a meta-analytic review of controlled investigations in treatment-seeking and non-treatment-seeking populations. Addiction. 2002;97:279-92.
389. Mundt M, French M, Roebuck M, Manwell L, Barry K, Brief physician advice for problem drinking among older adults; an economic analysis of costs and benefits. J Stud Alconol. 2005;66:380-94.
390. Nelson EC, Health AC, Bucholz KK, et al. Genetic epidemiology of alcohol-induced blackouts. Arch Gen Psychiatry. 2004;61:257-63.
391. Niemela O. Biomarkers in alcoholism. Clin Chim Acta. 2007;377:39-49.
392. Norstrom T. Per capita alcohol consumption and all-cause mortality in Canada, 1950–1998. Addiction 2004; 99: 1274-8.
393. Nusnberger JI Jr, Bierut LJ. Seeking the connections: alcoholism and our genes. Sci Am. 2007;296:46-53.
394. O'Malley SS, Garbutt JC, Gastfriend Dr, Dong Q, Kranzler HR. Efficacy of extended release naltrexone in alcohol-dependent patients who are abstinent prior to treatment. J Clin Psychopharmacology. 2007;27:507-12.
395. Palmieri VO, Cicco G, Minerva F, et al. Red blood cells (RBC) deformability and aggregability: alterations in alcoholism. Adv Exp Med Biol. 2006;578;125-31.
396. Parker AJR, Marshall EJ, Bll DM. Diagnosis and management of alcohol use disorders. BMJ. 2008;496-501.
397. Pastor R, Aragon C. The role of opioid receptor subtypes in the development of behavioural sensitization to ethanol. Neuropsychopharmacology. 2006;31:1489-99.
398. Peters TJ, Kotowicz J, Nyka W, et al. Treatment of alcoholic polyneuropathy with vitamin B complex: a randomized controlled trial. Alcohol. 2006;41:636-42.
399. Pitel AL, Beaunieux H, Witkowski T, et al. Genuine episodic memory deficits and executive dysfunctions in alcoholic subjects early in abstinence. Alcohol Clin Exp Res. 2007;31:1169-1178.
400. Polednak AP. Recent trends in incidence rates for selected alcohol-related cancers in the United States. Alcohol. 2005;40:234-38.
401. Ramstedt M. Alcohol and pancreatitis mortality in the population level: experiences from 14 western countries. Addiction. 2004;99:1255-61.
402. Reinert DF, Allen JP. The alcohol use disorders identification test: an update of research findings. Alcohol Clin Exp Res. 2007;31:185-99.
403. Reoux JP, Miller K. Routine hospital detoxification practice compared to symptom triggered management with an objective withdrawal scale (CIWA – Ar). J Addiction. 2000;9:135-44.
404. Rivara FP, Garrison MM, Ebel B, McCarty CA, Christakis DA. Mortality attributable to harmful drinking in the United States, 2000. J Stud Alcohol. 2004;65:530-6.
405. Romero-Gemez M, Grande L, Nogales MC, et al. Chronic alcohol use enhances the hepatitis C virus load in the liver. Alcohol Research. 2002;7:66.
406. Rosenbloom Mj, Sullivan EV, Sassoon SA, et al. Alcoholism, HIV infection, and their comorbidity: factors affecting self-rated health-related quality of life. J Stud Alcohol Drugs. 2007; 68:115-25.
407. Rumpf HJ, Biscjof G, Hapke U, Meyer C, John U. Stability of remission from alcohol dependence without formal help. Alcohol. 2006;41:311-4.
408. Rush AJ Jr, Pincus HA, First MB, et al. Handbook of Psychiatric Measures: Task Force for the Handbook of Psychiatric Measures. Washington, DC, USA: American Psychiatric Association; 2000.
409. Sannibale C, Fucito L, O' Connor D, Curry K. Process evaluation of an out-patient detoxification services. Drug Alcohol Review. 2005;24:475-81.
410. Saremi A, hason RL, Williams DE, et al. Validity of the CAGE questionnaire in an American Indian population. J Stud Alcohol. 2001;62:294-300.
411. Saxena S. Alcohol, Europe, and developing countries. Addiction. 1997:92(suppl 1):43-8
412. Schellenberg F, Schwan R, Mennetrey L, et al. Dose-effect relation between daily ethanole intake in the range 0-70 grams and %CDT value: validation of a cut-off value. Alcohol Alcohol. 2005;40:532-34.
413. Schuckit MA, Smith TL, Danko GP, et al. Prospective evaluation of the four DSM-IV criteria for alcohol abuse in a large population, Am J Psychiatry. 2005;162:350-60.
414. Schuckit MA, Smith TL, Kalmijn J. The search for genes contributing to the low level of response to alcohol: patterns of findings across studies. Alcohol Clin Exp Res. 2004;28: 1449-58.

415. Schuckit MA, Smith TL, Pierson J, et al. Externalizing disorders in the offspring from the San Diego Prospective Study of alcoholism. J Spychiatric Reasearch. 2008;46:644-52.
416. Schuckit MA. Comorbidity between substance use disorders and psychiatric conditions. Addiction. 2006;101:76-88.
417. Schuckit MA. Smith TL. An evaluation of the level of responses to alcohol, externalizing symptoms, and depressive symptoms as predictors of alcoholism. J Stud Alcohol. 2006;67:215-27.
418. Schuckit MA. Vulnerability factors for alcoholism. In: Davis K (Ed). Neuropsychopharmacology: the fifth generation of progress. Baltimore, MD, USA: Lippincott Willians & Wilkams; 2002. pp. 1399-411.
419. Schumann G, Saam C, Heinz A Mann K, Treutlein J. The NMDA receptor for alcoholism. Nervenarzt. 2005;76:1355-62.
420. Smith TL, Volpe FR, Hashima JN, Schuckit MA. Impact of a stimulant-focused enhanced program on the outcome of alcohol-and/or stimulant-dependent men. Alcohol Clin Exp Res. 1999;23:1772-9.
421. Srisurapanont M, Jarusuraisin N, Naltrexone for the treatment of alcoholism: a met-analysis of randomized controlled trials. Int J Neuropsychopharmacol. 2005;8:267-80.
422. Stahlbrandt H, Jonsson KO, Berglund M. Two - year outcome of alcohol interventions in Swedish university halls of residence: a cluster randomized trial of a brief skills training program, twelve-step-influenced intervention, and controls. Alcohol Clin Exp Res. 2007;31:458-66.
423. Stecker T, Curran GM, Han X, Booth BM. Patterns of health services use associated with Veterans Affairs outpatient substances-use treatment. J Stud Alcohol Drugs. 2007;68:510-8.
424. Steensland P, Simms JA, Holgate J, et al. Varenicline, an alpha4beta2 nicotinic acetylcholine receptor partial agonist, selectively decreases ethanol consumption and seeking. PNAS. 2007;104:12518-23.
425. Suh JJ, Pettinati HM, Kampman KM, O'Brine CP. The status of disulfiram: a half of a century later. J Clin Psychopharmacol. 2006;26:290-302.
426. Szucs S, Sarvary A, McKee M, Adany R. Could the high level of cirrhosis in central and eastern Europe be due partly to the quality of alcohol consumed? An exploratory investigation. Addiction. 2005;100:536-42.
427. Tchuckit MA. Drug and alcohol abuse: a clinical guide to diagnosis and treatment, 6th edition. New york, U.S.A. Springer; 2006.
428. Teesson M, Baillie A, Lynskey A, Manor B, Degenhardt L. substance use, dependence and treatment seeking in the United States and Australia: a cross-national comparision. Drug alcohol Depent. 2006;81:149-55
429. Thomson AD, Marshall EJ. The natural history and pathophysiology of Wernicke's encephalopathy and Korsakoffs psychosis. Alcohol. 2006;41:151-9.
430. Timberlake DS, Hopfer CJ, Rhee SH, et al. College attendance and its effect on drinking behaviors in a longitudinal study of adolescents. Alcohol Clin Exp Res. 2007;31:1020-30.
431. Uyarel H, Ozdol C, Gencer AM, Okmen E, Cam N. Acute alcohol intake and QT dispersion in healthy subjects. J Stud Alcohol. 2005;66:555-8.
432. van den Wildenberg E, Wiers R, Dessers J, et al. A functional polymorphism of the u-opioid receptor gene (OPRM) influences cue-induced craving for alcohol in male heavy drinkers. Alcohol Clin Exp Res. 2007;31:1-10.
433. Van Reen E, Jenni OG, Carskadon MA. Effects of alcohol on sleep and the sleep electroencephalogram in healthy young women. Alcohol Clin Exp Res. 2006;30:974-81.
434. Vasilaki E, Hosier S, Cox M. The efficacy of motivational interviewing as a brief intervention for excessive drinking: a meta-analytic review. Alcohol. 2006;41:328-36.
435. Verge C, Lucena KI, Lopez-Torres F, et al. Adverse hepatic reactions associated with calcium carbimide and disulfiram therapy: is there still a role for these drugs? World J Gastroenterol. 2006;21:5078-8.
436. Volkow N, Wang G, Begleiter H, et al. High levels of dopamine D2 receptors in unaffected members of alcoholic families. Arch Gen Psychiatry. 2006;63:999-1008.
437. Weinshenker D, Schroeder JP. There and back again: a tale of norepinephrine and drug addition. Neuropsychopharmaco-logy. 2007;32:1433-51.
438. WHO. ICD - 10 classification of mental and behavioural disorders: clinical descriptions and diagnostic guidelines. Geneva, Switzerland: World Health Organization, 1992.
439. Witkewitz K, Lpses following alcohol treatment: modeling and falls from the wagon. J Alcohol Drugs. 2008;69:594-604.
440. Witkiewitz K, Marlatt G. Relapse prevention for alcohol and drug problems. Am Psychol. 2004;59:224-35.

Diagnosis, Assessment and Management of Alcohol Use Disorder—Nice Guidelines

441. Babor TF, Higgins-Biddle JC, Saunders JB, Monteiro MG. AUDIT—the alcohol use disorders identification test: guidelines for use in primary care. 2nd edition. World Health Organization, 2001. http://whqlibdoc.who.int/hq/2001/who_msd_msb_01.6a,pdf.
442. Drummond CD. The relationship between alcohol dependence and alcohol-related problems in a clinical population. Br J Addict. 1990;85:357-66.
443. Drummond DC, Oyefeso N, Phillips T, Cheeta S, Deluca R, Perryman K, et al. Alcohol needs assessment research project: the 2004 national alcohol needs assessment for England. Department of Health, 2005. www.dh.gov.uk/en/Publicationsandstatistics/Publications/PublicationsPolicyAndGuidance/DH_41222341.
444. Folstein MF, Folstein SE, McHugh PR. "Mini-mental state". A practical method for grading the cognitive state of patients for the clinician./Psychiatr Res. 1975;12:189-98.
445. Fuller E. Drug use, smoking and drinking among young people in England in 2007. National Centre for Social Research.

National Foundation for Educational Research, 2008. www.ic.nhs.uk/pubs/sdd07fullreport.

446. National Institute for Health and Clinical Excellence. Alcohol-used is orders: diagnosis and clinical management of alcohol related physical complications. (Clinical guideline CG100.)2010. http:// guidence.nice.org.uk/CG100.
447. National Institute for health and Clinical Excellence. Alcohol-use disorders: preventing the development of hazardous and harmful drinking. (Public health guideline PH24.) 2010. http:// guidance.nice.org.uk/PH24.
448. National Institute for Health and Clinical Excellence. Alcohol use disorders: diagnosis assessment and management of harmful drinking and alcohol dependence. (Clinical guideline CG115.) 2011. http://guidance.nice.org.uk/CG115.
449. National Institute for Health and Clinical Excellence. Depression: the treatment and management of depression in adults. (Clinical guideline90.) 2009, http://guidance.nice.org.uk/CG90.
450. National Institute for Health and Clinical Excellence. Generalised anxiety disorder and panic disorder (with or without a goraphobia) in adults; management in primary secondary and community care. (Clinical guideline 113.) 2011, http://guidance.nice.org,uk/CG113.
451. National Institute for Health and Clinical Excellence. Obsessive-compulsive disorder: core interventions in the treatment of obsessive compulsive disorder and body dysmorphic disorder. (Clinical guideline31.) 2005.http://guidance.nice.org.uk/CG31.
452. National Institute for Health and Clinical Excellence. Post-traumatic stress disorder (PTSD): the management of PTSD in adults and children in primary and secondary care. (Clinicalguideline 26), 2005.http://guidance.nice.org,uk/CG26.
453. North West Public Health Observatory Local alcohol profiles for England (2010).www.nwph,net/alcohol/lape/
454. Raistrick D, Bradshaw J, Tober G, Weiner J, Healey C. Development of the Leeds dependence questionnaire (LDQ); a questionnaire to measure alcohol and opiate dependence in the context of a treatment evaluation package. Addiction 1994;89:563-72.
455. Stockwell T, Hodgson R, Edwards G, Taylor C, Rankin H. The development of a questionnaire to measure severity of alcohol dependence. Br J Addict Alcohol Other Drugs 1979;74:78-87.

Diagnosis and Clinical Management of Alcohol Use Disorder

456. British National Formulary. No 59 (March). BMI Publishing Group; 2010.
457. Bushe C, Shaw M, Peveler RC. A review of the association between antipsychotic use and hyperprolactinaemia. J Psychopharmacol. 2008;22(Suppl 2):46-55.
458. Carithers RL Jr, Herlong HF, Diehl AM, Shaw, EM, Combes, B, Fallon HJ et al. Methylprednisolone therapy in patients with severe alcoholic hepatitis. N Engl J Med. 1989;110:685-90.
459. Centre for Public Health Excellence at the National Institute for Health and Clinical Excellence, Alcohol-use disorders; preventing the development of hazardous and harmful drinking. (Public Health guideline PH24) 2010.http://guldance.nice.org.uk/PH24.
460. Citrome L, Stroup TS. Schizophrenia, Clinical Antipsychotic Trials of Intervention Effectiveness (CATIE) and number needed to treat: how can CATIE inform clinicians? Int J Clin Pract. 2006;60:933-40.
461. Consensus development conference on antipsychotic drugs and obesity and diabetes. Diabetes Care. 2004;27:595-601.
462. Department of Health. The cost of alcohol harm to the NHS in England an update to the Cabinet Office (2003) study, DH, 2008. www.lho.org,uk/viewResource.aspx?id=13594.
463. Douglas IJ, Smeeth L. Exposure to antipsychotics and risk of stroke: self-controlled case series study. BMJ. 2008;337:a1227.
464. Electronic Medicines Compendium (www.medicines.org.uk).
465. Farah A. Atypicality of atypical antipsychotics. Prim Care Companion J Clin Psychiatry. 2005;7:268-74.
466. Hedges D, Jeppson K, Whitehead P. Antipsychotic medication and seizures: a review. Drugs Today. 2003;39:551-7.
467. Information Centre for Health and Social Care, Statistics on alcohol: England, 2009. www.ic.nhs.uk/statistics-and-data-collections/health-and-lifestyles/alcohol/statlstics-on-alcohol-england-2009%5Bns%5D.
468. Jones PB, Barnes TR, Davies L, Dunn G, Lloyd H, Hayhurst KP, et al. Randomized controlled trial of the effect on quality of life of second- vs first-generation antipsychotic drugs in schizophrenia: Cost Utility of the Latest Antipsychotic Drugs in Schizophrenia. Study (CUtLASS 1). Arch Gen Psychiatry. 2006;63:1079-87.
469. Kesselheim AS, Avorn J. The role of litigation in defining drug risks. JAMA. 2007;297:308-11.
470. Leucht S, Curves C, Arbter D, Engel RR, Li C, Davis JM. Second-generation versus first-generation antipsychotic drugs for schizophrenia: a meta-analysis, Lancet. 2009;373:31-41.
471. Lewis SW, Barnes TR, Davies L, Murray RM, Dunn G, Hayhurst KP, et al. Randomized controlled trial of effect of prescription of clozapine versus other second-generation antipsychotic drugs in resistant schizophrenia. Schizophr Bull. 2006;32:715-23.
472. Lieberman JA, Stroup TS, McEvoy JP, Swartz MS, Rosenheck RA, Perkins DO, et al. Effectiveness of antipsychotic drugs in patients with chronic schizophrenia. N Engl J Med 2005; 353:1209-23.
473. Mackin P. Cardiac side effects of psychiatric drugs. Hum Psychopharmacol. 2008;23(Suppl 1):3-14.
474. National Health Service Business Services Authority. Prescribing review; April-June 2009, antipsychotic drugs. www,nhsbsa.nhs.uk/ PrescriptionServices/945.aspx.

475. National Institute for Health and Clinical Excellence. Alcohol-use disorders: diagnosis, assessment and management of harmful drinking and alcohol dependence, (Clinical guideline) 2011; see http://guidance.nice.org.uk/CG/Wave17/1).
476. National Institute for Health and Clinical Excellence. Alcohol-use disorders: diagnosis and clinical management of alcohol-related physical complications. (Clinical guideline CG100) 2010. http://guidance.nice.org.uk/CG100.
477. Newham JJ, Thomas SH, MacRitchie K, McElhatton PR. McAllister-Williams RH. Birth weight of infants after maternal exposure to typical and atypical antipsychotics: prospective comparison study. Br J Psychiatry. 2008;192:333-7.
478. Osborn DP, Levy G, Nazareth l, Petersen I, Islam A, King MB. Relative risk of cardiovascular and cancer mortality in people with severe mental illness from the United Kingdom's general practice research database. Arch Gen Psychiatry. 2007;64:242-9.
479. Stanniland C, Taylor D. Tolerability of atypical antipsychotics. Drug Saf. 2000;22:195-214.
480. Sullivan JT. Sykora K, Schneiderman J, Naranjo CA, Sellers EM. Assessment of alcohol withdrawal: the revised clinical institute withdrawal assessment for alcohol scale (CIWA-Ar). Br J Addiction. 1989;84:1353-7.
481. Tanne JH. AstraZeneca to pay $198m to patients over diabetes claims. BMJ. 2010;341:c4422.
482. UK Liver Transplant Group. Liver Advisory Group alcohol guidelines:November 2005, www.uktransplant.org.uk/ukt/about_transplants/organ_allocation/pdf/Iiver_advisory_group_alcohol_guidelines-november_2005.pdf.
483. Verdoux H, TournierM, Bégaud B. Antipsychotic prescribing trends: a review of pharmaco-epidemiological studies. Acta Psychiatr Scand. 2010;121:4-10.

Adverse Health Effects of Nonmedical Cannabis Use

484. Abel EL. Marihuana: the first twelve thousand years. New York: Plenum Press; 1980.
485. Advisory Council on the Misuse of Drugs. Cannabis: classification and public health. London: Home Office; 2008. http://drugs.homeoffice.gov.uk/. (accessed June 26, 2008).
486. Ajdacic-Gross V, Lauber C, Warnke I, Haker H, Murray RM, Rossler W. Changing incidence of psychotic disorders among the young in Zurich. Schizophr Res. 2007;95:9-18.
487. Aldington S, Harwood M, Cox B, et al. Cannabis use and risk of lung cancer: a case-control study. Eur Respir J. 2008;31:280-6.
488. Aldington S, Williams M, Nowitz M, et al. Effects of cannabis on pulmonary structure, function and symptoms. Thorax. 2007;62:1058-63.
489. Andréasson S, Engstrom A, Allebeck P, Rydberg U. Cannabis and schizophrenia: a longitudinal study of Swedish conscripts. Lancet. 1987;2:1483-6.
490. Anthony JC, Warner L, Kessler R. Comparative epidemiology of dependence on tobacco, alcohol, controlled substances and inhalants: basic findings from the National Comorbidity Survey. Exp Clin Psychopharmacol. 1994;2:244-68.
491. Anthony JC. The epidemiology of cannabis dependence. In: Roffman RA, Stephens RS (Eds). Cannabis dependence: its nature, consequences and treatment. Cambridge, UK: Cambridge University Press; 2006. pp. 58-105.
492. Arseneault L, Cannon M, Poulton R, Murray R, Caspi A, Moffitt TE. Cannabis use in adolescence and risk for adult psychosis: longitudinal prospective study. BMJ. 2002;325:1212-3.
493. Bachman JG, Wadsworth KN, O'Malley PM, Johnston LD, Schulenberg J. Smoking, drinking, and drug use in young adulthood: the impacts of new freedoms and new responsibilities. Mahwah, NJ: Lawrence Erlbaum; 1997.
494. Beautrais AL, Joyce PR, Mulder RT. Cannabis abuse and serious suicide attempts. Addiction. 1999;94:1155-64.
495. Begg S, Vos T, Barker B, Stanley L, Lopez AD. The burden of disease and injury in Australia 2003. Canberra: Australian Institute of Health and Welfare, 2007. http://www.aihw.gov.au/publications/index.cfm/title/10317. (accessed June 26, 2013).
496. Berthiller J, Straif K, Boniol M, et al. Cannabis smoking and risk of lung cancer in men: a pooled analysis of three studies in Maghreb. J Thorac Oncol. 2008;3:1398-403.
497. Bloch E. Effects of marijuana and cannabinoids on reproduction, endocrine function, development, and chromosomes. In: FehrK, Kalant H (Eds). Cannabis and health hazards. Toronto: Addiction Research Foundation; 1983. pp. 355-432.
498. Block RI, O'Leary DS, Hichwa RD, et al. Cerebellar hypoactivity in frequent marijuana users. Neuroreport. 2000;11:749-53.
499. Block RI, O'Leary DS, Hichwa RD, et al. Effects of frequent marijuana use on memory-related regional cerebral blood flow. Pharmacol Biochem Behav. 2002;72:237-50.
500. Bolla KI, Brown K, Eldreth D, Tate K, Cadet JL. Dose-related neurocognitive effects of marijuana use. Neurology. 2002;59:1337-43.
501. Boydell J, van Os J, Caspi A, et al. Trends in cannabis use prior to first presentation with schizophrenia, in South-East London between 1965 and 1999. Psychol Med. 2006;36:1441-6.
502. Budney AJ, Hughes JR. The cannabis withdrawal syndrome. Curr Opin Psychiatry. 2006;19:233-8.
503. Chang L, Chronicle EP. Functional imaging studies in cannabis users. Neuroscientist. 2007;13:422-32.
504. Day NL, Richardson GA, Goldschmidt L, et al. Effect of prenatal marijuana exposure on the cognitive development of offspring at age three. Neurotoxicol Teratol. 1994;16:169-75.
505. Degenhardt L, Hall WD, Lynskey MT. Testing hypotheses about the relationship between cannabis use and psychosis. Drug Alcohol Depend. 2003;71:37-48.
506. Drummer OH, Gerostamoulos J, Batziris H, et al. The involvement of drugs in drivers of motor vehicles killed in Australian road traffic crashes. Accid Anal Prev. 2004;36:239-48.
507. Dutch National Alcohol and Drug Information System. Treatment demand of cannabis clients in outpatient addiction care in the Netherlands (1994–2001). LADIS Bulletin; 2004.

508. Ellickson P, Bui K, Bell R, McGuigan KA. Does early drug use increase the risk of dropping out of high school?. J Drug Issues. 1998;28:357-80.
509. ElSohly MA. Quarterly report: December 16, 2007 thru March 15, 2008. University, MS: National Center for Natural Products Research, University of Mississippi, 2008. Potency Monitoring Project Report 100.
510. English D, Hulse G, Milne E, Holman C, Bower C. Maternal cannabis use and birth weight: a meta-analysis. Addiction. 1997;92:1553-60.
511. Eyler FD, Behnke M. Early development of infants exposed to drugs prenatally. Clin Perinatol. 1999;26:107-50.
512. Fergusson DM, Boden JM, Horwood LJ. Cannabis use and other illicit drug use: testing the cannabis gateway hypothesis. Addiction. 2006;101:556-69.
513. Fergusson DM, Boden JM, Horwood LJ. The developmental antecedents of illicit drug use: evidence from a 25-year longitudinal study. Drug Alcohol Depend. 2008;96:165-77.
514. Fergusson DM, Boden JM. Cannabis use and later life outcomes. Addiction 2008;103:969-76. Discussion 77-78.
515. Fergusson DM, Horwood LJ, Northstone K. Maternal use of cannabis and pregnancy outcome. Br J Obstet Gynaecol. 2002; 109:21-7.
516. Fergusson DM, Horwood LJ, Swain-Campbell NR. Cannabis dependence and psychotic symptoms in young people. Psychol Med. 2003;33:15-21.
517. Fergusson DM, Horwood LJ. Early onset cannabis use and psychosocial adjustment in young adults. Addiction. 1997;92:279-96.
518. Forrester MB, Merz RD. Risk of selected birth defects with prenatal illicit drug use, Hawaii, 1986—2002. J Toxicol Environ Health A. 2007;70:7-18.
519. Fried PA, Smith AR. A literature review of the consequences of prenatal marihuana exposure: an emerging theme of a deficiency in aspects of executive function. Neurotoxicol Teratol. 2001;23:1-11.
520. Gable RS. Comparison of acute lethal toxicity of commonly abused psychoactive substances. Addiction. 2004;99:686-96.
521. Gardner E. Cannabinoid interaction with brain reward systems. In: Nahas GG, Sutin K, Harvey D, Agurell S (Eds). Marihuana and medicine. Towa, NJ: Humana Press; 1999. pp. 187-205.
522. Gerberich SG, Sidney S, Braun BL, Tekawa IS, Tolan KK, Quesenberry CP. Marijuana use and injury events resulting in hospitalization. Ann Epidemiol. 2003;13:230-7.
523. Goldschmidt L, Day NL, Richardson GA. Effects of prenatal marijuana exposure on child behavior problems at age 10. Neurotoxicol Teratol. 2000;22:325-36.
524. Gottschalk L, Aronow W, Prakash R. Effect of marijuana and placebo-marijuana smoking on psychological state and on psychophysiological and cardiovascular functioning in angina patients. Biol Psychiatry. 1977;12:255-66.
525. Green B, Kavanagh D, Young R. Being stoned: a review of self-reported cannabis effects. Drug Alcohol Rev. 2003;22:453-60.
526. Grotenhermen F, Leson G, Berghaus G, et al. Developing limits for driving under cannabis. Addiction. 2007;102:1910-7.
527. Hall WD, Degenhardt L. Prevalence and correlates of cannabis use in developed and developing countries. Curr Opin Psychiatry. 2007;20:393-7.
528. Hall WD, Lynskey MT. Is cannabis a gateway drug? Testing hypotheses about the relationship between cannabis use and the use of other illicit drugs. Drug Alcohol Rev. 2005;24: 39-48.
529. Hall WD, Pacula RL. Cannabis use and dependence: public health and public policy. Cambridge, UK: Cambridge University Press; 2003.
530. Hashibe M, Morgenstern H, Cui Y, et al. Marijuana use and the risk of lung and upper aerodigestive tract cancers: results of a population-based case-control study. Cancer Epidemiol Biomarkers Prev. 2006;15:1829-34.
531. Hashibe M, Straif K, Tashkin DP, Morgenstern H, Greenland S, Zhang ZF. Epidemiologic review of marijuana use and cancer risk. Alcohol. 2005;35:265-75.
532. Henquet C, Krabbendam L, Spauwen J, et al. Prospective cohort study of cannabis use, predisposition for psychosis, and psychotic symptoms in young people. BMJ. 2004;330:11.
533. Hickman M, Vickerman P, Macleod J, Kirkbride J, Jones PB. Cannabis and schizophrenia: model projections of the impact of the rise in cannabis use on historical and future trends in schizophrenia in England and Wales. Addiction. 2007;102:597-606.
534. Huizink AC, Mulder EJ. Maternal smoking, drinking or cannabis use during pregnancy and neurobehavioral and cognitive functioning in human offspring. Neurosci Biobehav Rev. 2006;30:24-41.
535. Iversen L. The science of marijuana. Oxford: Oxford University Press; 2008.
536. Jones RT. Cardiovascular system effects of marijuana. J Clin Pharmacol. 2002;42:58S-63S.
537. Kandel DB. Stages and pathways of drug involvement: examining the gateway hypothesis. New York: Cambridge University Press; 2002.
538. Laumon B, Gadegbeku B, Martin JL, Biecheler MB. Cannabis intoxication and fatal road crashes in France: population based case-control study. BMJ. 2005;331:1371.
539. Lessem JM, Hopfer CJ, Haberstick BC, et al. Relationship between adolescent marijuana use and young adult illicit drug use. Behav Genet. 2006;36:498-506.
540. Lichtman AH, Martin BR. Cannabinoid tolerance and dependence. Handb Exp Pharmacol. 2005;168:691-717.
541. Lynskey MT, Hall WD. The effects of adolescent cannabis use on educational attainment: a review. Addiction. 2000;96:433-43.
542. Lynskey MT, Heath AC, Bucholz KK, Slutske WS. Escalation of drug use in early-onset cannabis users vs co-twin controls. JAMA. 2003;289:427-33.
543. Macleod J, Oakes R, Copello A, et al. Psychological and social sequelae of cannabis and other illicit drug use by young people: a systematic review of longitudinal, general population studies. Lancet. 2004;363:1579-88.
544. Manzanares J, Corchero J, Romero J, Fernandez-Ruiz JJ, Ramos JA, Fuentes JA. Pharmacological and biochemical interactions

between opioids and cannabinoids. Trends Pharmacol Sci. 1999;20:287-94.

545. McLaren J, Swift W, Dillon P, Allsop S. Cannabis potency and contamination: a review of the literature. Addiction. 2008;103:1100-09.
546. Mehra R, Moore BA, Crothers K, Tetrault J, Fiellin DA. The association between marijuana smoking and lung cancer: a systematic review. Arch Intern Med. 2006;166:1359-67.
547. Mittleman MA, Lewis RA, Maclure M, Sherwood JB, Muller JE. Triggering myocardial infarction by marijuana. Circulation. 2001;103:2805-9.
548. Moir D, Rickert WS, Levasseur G, et al. A comparison of mainstream and side stream marijuana and tobacco cigarette smoke produced under two machine smoking conditions. Chem Res Toxicol. 2008;21:494-502.
549. Moore TH, Zammit S, Lingford-Hughes A, et al. Cannabis use and risk of psychotic or affective mental health outcomes: a systematic review. Lancet. 2007;370:319-28.
550. Morral AR, McCaffrey DF, Paddock SM. Reassessing the marijuana gateway effect. Addiction. 2002;97:1493-504.
551. Mukamal KJ, Maclure M, Muller JE, Mittleman MA. An exploratory prospective study of marijuana use and mortality following acute myocardial infarction. Am Heart J. 2008;155:465-70.
552. Mura P, Kintz P, Ludes B, et al. Comparison of the prevalence of alcohol, cannabis and other drugs between 900 injured drivers and 900 control subjects: results of a French collaborative study. Forensic Sci Int. 2003;133:79-85.
553. Murray RM, Morrison PD, Henquet C, Di Forti M. Cannabis, the mind and society: the hash realities. Nat Rev Neurosci. 2007;8:885-95.
554. Patton GC, Harris JB, Schwartz M, Bowes G. Adolescent suicidal behaviors: a population-based study of risk. Psychol Med. 1997;27:715-24.
555. Pope HG, Gruber AJ, Hudson JI, Huestis MA, Yurgelun-Todd D. Neuropsychological performance in long-term cannabis users. Arch Gen Psychiatry. 2001;58:909-15.
556. Quickfall J, Crockford D. Brain neuroimaging in cannabis use: a review. J Neuropsychiatry Clin Neurosci. 2006;18:318-32.
557. Ramaekers JG, Berghaus G, van Laar M, Drummer OH. Dose related risk of motor vehicle crashes after cannabis use. Drug Alcohol Depend. 2004;73:109-19.
558. Robbe HWJ. Influence of marijuana on driving. PhD thesis, Maastricht: Institute for Human Psychopharmacology, University of Limberg; 1994.
559. Sidney S, Quesenberry CP, Friedman GD, Tekawa IS. Marijuana use and cancer incidence (California, United States). Cancer Causes Control. 1997;8:722-8.
560. Sidney S. Cardiovascular consequences of marijuana use. J Clin Pharmacol. 2002;42:64S-70S.
561. Smiley A. Marijuana: on road and driving simulator studies. In: Kalant H, Corrigall W, Hall WD, Smart R (Eds). The health effects of cannabis. Toronto: Centre for Addiction and Mental Health; 1999. pp. 171-91.
562. Solowij N, Stephens RS, Roffman RA, et al. Cognitive functioning of long-term heavy cannabis users seeking treatment. JAMA. 2002;287:1123-31.
563. Solowij N. Cannabis and cognitive functioning. Cambridge, UK: Cambridge University Press; 1998.
564. Tashkin DP, Baldwin GC, Sarafian T, Dubinett S, Roth MD. Respiratory and immunologic consequences of marijuana smoking. J Clin Pharmacol. 2002;42:71S-81S.
565. Tashkin DP. Effects of cannabis on the respiratory system. In: Kalant H, Corrigall W, Hall WD, Smart R (Eds). The health effects of cannabis. Toronto: Centre for Addiction and Mental Health; 1999. pp. 311-45.
566. Tashkin DP. Smoked marijuana as a cause of lung injury. Monaldi Arch Chest Dis. 2005;63:93-100.
567. Taylor DR, Fergusson DM, Milne BJ, et al. A longitudinal study of the effects of tobacco and cannabis exposure on lung function in young adults. Addiction. 2002;97:1055-61.
568. Tennes K, Aritable N, Blackard C, et al. Marihuana: prenatal and postnatal exposure in the human. In: Pinkert T (Ed). Current research on the consequences of maternal drug abuse. Rockville, MD: US Department of Health and Human Services; 1985. pp. 48-60.
569. Tetrault JM, Crothers K, Moore BA, Mehra R, Concato J, Fiellin DA. Effects of marijuana smoking on pulmonary function and respiratory complications: a systematic review. Arch Intern Med. 2007;167:221-8.
570. UNODC. World drug report 2006. Volume 1: analysis. Vienna: United Nations Office on Drugs and Crime; 2006.
571. UNODC. World drug report 2008. Vienna: United Nations Office on Drugs and Crime; 2007.
572. van Os J, Bak M, Hanssen M, Bijl RV, de Graaf R, Verdoux H. Cannabis use and psychosis: a longitudinal population-based study. Am J Epidemiol. 2002;156:319-27.
573. Wachtel SR, ElSohly MA, Ross SA, Ambre J, de Wit H. Comparison of the subjective effects of Delta(9)-tetrahydrocannabinol and marijuana in humans. Psychopharmacology (Berl). 2002;161:331-9.
574. Wagner FA, Anthony JC. Into the world of illegal drug use: exposure opportunity and other mechanisms linking the use of alcohol, tobacco, marijuana, and cocaine. Am J Epidemiol. 2002;155:918-25.
575. WHO Programme on Substance Abuse. Cannabis: a health perspective and research agenda. Geneva: Division of Mental Health and Prevention of Substance Abuse, World Health Organization, 1997.http://whqlibdoc.who.int/hq/1997/WHO_MSA_PSA_97.4.pdf. (accessed June 26, 2008).
576. Yücel M, Solowij N, Respondek C, et al. Regional brain abnormalities associated with long-term heavy cannabis use. Arch Gen Psychiatry. 2008;65:694-701.
577. Zammit S, Allebeck P, Andréasson S, Lundberg I, Lewis G. Self-reported cannabis use as a risk factor for schizophrenia in Swedish conscripts of 1969: historical cohort study. BMJ. 2002;325:1199-201.

578. Zhang ZF, Morgenstern H, Spitz MR, et al. Marijuana use and increased risk of squamous cell carcinoma of the head and neck.Cancer Epidemiol Biomarkers Prev 1999;8:1071-8. PubMed
579. Zuckerman B, Frank DA, Hingson R, et al. Effects of maternal marijuana and cocaine use on fetal growth. N Engl J Med. 1989;320:762-8.

Tobacco Addiction

580. American Psychiatric Association. Desk Reference to the Diagnostic Criteria from DSM-5. Washington DC; 2013.
581. American Psychiatric Association. Diagnostic and statistical manual of mental disorders, 4th edition. Washington DC: American Psychiatric Association; 1994.
582. American Society of Health-System Pharmacists. AHFS Drug Information. Bethesda: American Society of Health-System Pharmacists American Hospital Formulary Service; 2004.
583. Baker TB, Piper ME, McCarthy DE, et al. Time to first cigarette in the morning as an index of ability to quit smoking: implications for nicotine dependence. Nic Tob Research. 2007;9(suppl 4):s555-70.
584. Balfour DJ. THe neurobiology of tobacco dependence: a preclinical perspective on the role of the dopamine projections to the nucleus accumbens. Nicotine Tob Res. 2004;6:899-912.
585. Benowitz N. Nicotine addiction. Prim Care. 1999;26:611-31.
586. Benowitz NL, Zevin S, Jacob P 3rd. Suppression of nicotine intake nicotine. J Pharamcol Exp Ther. 1998;287:958-62.
587. Benwell ME, Balfour DJ, Birrel CE. Desensitization of the nicotine-induced mesolimbic dopamine responses during constant infusion with nicotine. Br J Pharmacol. 1995;114:454-60.
588. Benwell ME, Balfour DJ. Regional variation in the effects of nicotine on catecholamine overflow in rat brain. Eur J Pharmacol. 1997;325: 13-20.
589. Brandon TH, Tiffany ST, Obremski KM, Baker TB. Post cessation cigarette use: the process of relapse. Addict Behave. 1990;15:105-14.
590. Breslau N, Johnson EO. Predicting smoking cessation and major depression in nicotine-dependent smokers. AM J Public Health. 2000:90:1122-7.
591. Breslau N, Kilbey MM, Andreski P. DSM-III-R nicotine dependence in young adults: prevalence, correlates and associated psychiatric disorders. Addition. 1994;89:743-54.
592. Breslau N, Kilbey MM, Andreski P. Nicotine dependence major depression, and anxiety in young adults. Arch Gen Psychiatry. 1991;48:1069-74.
593. Caggiula AR, Donny EC, Chaudhri N, Perkins KA, Evans-Martin FF, Sved AF. Importance of nonpharmacological factors in nicotine self-administration. Physiol Bheav. 2002;77: 683-7.
594. Caggiula AR, Donny EC, White AR, et al. Cue dependency of nicotine self-administration and smoking. Pharmacol Biochem Behav. 2001;70:515-30.
595. Caggiula AR, Donny EC, White AR, et al. Environmental stimuli promote the acquisition of nicotine self-administration in rats. Psychopharmacology (Berl). 220;163:230-37.
596. Cahill K, Stead LF, Lancaster T. Nicotine receptor partial agonists for smoking cessation. Cochrane Database Syst Rev. 2007;1 CD006103.
597. Centers for Disease Control and Prevention. Cigarette smoking among adults-United States, 2000. MMWR Morb Mortal Wkly Rep. 2002;51:642-5.
598. Chaudhri N, Caggiula AR, Donny EC, Palmatier MI, Liu X, Sved AF. Complex interactions between nicotine and nonpharmacological stimuli reveal multiple roles for nicotine in reinforcement. Psychopharmacology (Berl). 2006;184:353-66.
599. Degenhardt L, Hall W. The relationship between tobacco use, substance-use disorders and mental health: results from the National Survey of Mental Health and Well-being. Nicotine Tob Res. 2001;3:225-34.
600. Donny EC, Chaudhri N, Caggiual AR, et al. Operant responding for a visual reinforce in rats is enhanced by noncontingent nicotine: implications for nicotine self-administration and reinforcement. Psychopharmacology (Berl). 2002;169:68-76.
601. Fagerstrom KO, Schneider NG. Measuring nicotine dependence: a review of the Fagerstrom tolerance questionnaire. J Behav Med. 1989;12:159-82.
602. Fagerstrom KO. Measuring degree of physical dependence to tobacco smoking with reference to individualization of treatment. Addict Behav. 1978;3:235-41.
603. Fiore MC, Hatsukami DK, Baker TB. Effective tobacco dependence treatment. JAMA. 2002;288:1768-71.
604. Fiore MC, Jane CR, Baker TB, et al. Treating tobacco use and dependence 2008 update: clinical guideline. Rockville, MD: US Department of Health and Human Services, Public Health Service; 2008.
605. Fiore MC, Novotny TE, Pierce JP, et al. Methods used to quit smoking in the United States. DO cessation programs help? JAMA. 1990;263:2760-65.
606. Franzon M, Gustavsson G, Korberly H. Effectiveness of over-the-counter nicotine replacement therapy. JAMA. 2002;288:3108.
607. Fryer JD, Lukas RJ. Noncompetitive functional inhabitation at diverse, human nicotinic acetylcholine receptor subtypes by bupropion, phencyclidine, and ibogaine. J Pharmacol Exp Ther 1999;288:88-92.
608. Fu Y, Matta SG, Brower VG, Sharp BM. Norepinephrine secretion in the hypothalamic paraventricular nucleus of rats during unlimited access to self-administered nicotine: an in vivo microdialysis study. J Neurosci. 2001;21:8979-89.
609. Gilbert DG, McCernon FJ, Rabinovich NE, et al. Mood disturbance fails to resolve across 31 days of cigarette abstinence in women. J Consult Clin Psychol. 2002;70:142-52.
610. Glassman AH, Helzer JE, Covery LS. et al. Smoking, smoking cessation, and major depression. JAMA. 1990;264:1546-9.
611. Gonzales D, Rennard SI, Nides M, et al. Varenicline, and alpha4 beta2 nicotinic acetylcholine receptor partial agonist,

vs sustained-release bupropion and placebo for smoking cessation: a randomized controlled trial. JAMA. 2006;296:47-55.
612. Gotti C, Zoli M, Clementi F. Brain nicotinic acetylcholine receptors: native subtypes and their relevance. Trends Pharmacol Sci. 2006;27:482-91.
613. Gourlay SG, Stead LF, Benowitz NL. Clonidine for smoking cessation. Cochrane Database Syst Rev. 2004;3:CD00058.
614. Grant BF, Hasin DS, Chou SP, Stinson FS, Dawson DA. Nicotine dependence and psychiatric disorders in the United State results from the national epidemiologic survey on alcohol and related conditions. Arch Gen Psychiatry. 2004;61:1107-15.
615. Haggstram FM, Chatkin JM, Susenbach-Vaz E, Cesari DH, Fam CF, Fritscher CC. A controlled trial of nortriptyline, Sustained-release bupropion and placebo for smoking cessation: Preliminary results. Pulm Pharmacol Ther. 2006;19:205-9.
616. Hajek P, West R, Foulds J, Nilsson F, Burrows S, Meadow A. Randomized comparative trail of nicotine polacrilex, a transdermal patch, nasal spray, and an inhaler. Arch Intern Med. 1999;159:2033-8.
617. Hall SM, Humfleet GL, Reus VI, Munoz RF, Hartz DT, Maude-Griffin R. Psychological intervention and antidepressant treatment in smoking cessation. Arch Gen Psychiatry. 2002;59:930-6.
618. Haustein KO. Bupropion: Pharmacological and clinical profile in smoking cessation. Int J Clin Pharmacol Ther. 2003;41:56-66.
619. Heatherton TF, Kozlowski LT, Frecker RC, Fagerstrom KO. The Fagerstrom test for nicotine dependence: a revision of the Fagerstrom tolerance questionnaire. Br J Addict. 1991;86:1119-27.
620. Heatherton TF, Kozlowski LT, Frecker RC, Rickert W, Robinson J. Measuring the heaviness of smoking: using self-reported time to the first cigarette of the day and number of cigarettes smoked per day. Br J Addict. 1989;84:791-800.
621. Henningfield JE, Keenan RM, Clarke PBS. Pharmacological aspects of drug dependence: toward an integrated neuro-behavioral approach. In: Schuster CR, Kuhar M (Eds). Handbook of experimental pharmacology. New York: Springer; 1996. pp. 272-314.
622. Henningfield JE, Keenan RM. Nicotine delivery kinetics and abuse liability. J Consult Clin Psychol. 1993;61:743-50.
623. Henningfield JE, Slade J. Tobacco-dependence medications: Public health and regulatory issues. Food Drug Law J. 1998;53(Suppl):75-114.
624. Hughes JR, Gust SW, Keenan RM, Fenwick JW. Effect of dose on nicotine's reinforcing, withdrawal-suppression and self-reported effects. J Pharmacol Exp Ther. 1990;252:1175-83.
625. Hughes JR, Hatsukami DK. The nicotine withdrawal syndrome: a brief review and update. Int J Smoking Cessation. 1992;1:21-6.
626. Hughes JR, Higgins ST, Hatsukami D. Effects of abstinence from tobacco: a critical review. In: Kozlowski LT, Annis H, Cappel HD, et al (Eds). Research advances in alcohol and drug problems. New York: Plenum Press; 1990. pp. 317-98.
627. Hughes JR, Shiffinan S, Callas P, Zhang J. A meta-analysis of the efficacy of over-the counter nicotine replacement. Tob Control. 2003;12:21-7.
628. Hughes JR, Stead LF, Lancaster T. Antidepressants for smoking cessation. Corhrane Database Syst Rev. 2007;1:CD 000031.
629. Hughes JR. Effects of abstinence from tobacco: valid symptoms and time course. Nicotine Tob Res. 2007;9:315-27.
630. Hukkanen J, Jacob P 3rd, Benowitz NL. Metabolism and disposition Kinetics of nicotine. Pharmacol Rev. 2005;57:79-115.
631. Hyman S. Addiction: a disease of learning and memory. Am J Psychiatry. 2005;162:1414-22.
632. John U, Meyer C, Rumpf HJ, Hapke U. Smoking, nicotine dependence and psychiatric comorbidity-a population-based study including smoking cessation after three years. Drug Alcohol Depend. 2004;76:287-95.
633. Jorenby DE, Hays JT, Rigotti NA, et al. Efficacy of varenicline, and alpha5 beta2 nicotinic acetylcholine receptor partial agonist, vs placebo or sustained-release bupropion for smoking cessation: a randomized controlled trial. JAMA. 2006;296:56-63.
634. Jorenby DE, Leischow SJ, Nides MA, et al. A controlled trial of sustained-release bupropion, a nicotine patch, or both for smoking cessation. N Engl J Med. 1000;340:685-91.
635. Joseph AM, Fu SS. Safety issues in pharmacotherapy for smoking in patients with cardiovascular disease. Prog Cardivusc Dis. 2003;45:429-41.
636. Kandel DB, Huang FY, Davies M. Comorbidity between patterns of substance use dependence and psychiatric syndromes. Drug Alcohol Depend. 2001;64:233-41.
637. Killen JD, Fortmann SP. Craving is associated with smoking relapse: findings from three prospective studies. Exp Clin Psychopharmacol. 1997;5:137-42.
638. Lancaster T, Stead LF. Physician advice for smoking cessation. Cochrane Database Syst Rev. 2004;4:CD000165.
639. Lasser K, Boyd JW, Woolhandler S, Himmelstein DU, McCormick D, Bor DH. Smoking and mental illness. JAMA. 2000;284:2606-10.
640. Lerman C, Niaura R. Applying genetic approaches to the treatment of nicotine dependence. Oncogene. 2002;21:|7412-20.
641. Mackay J, Ericksen M, Shafey O. The tobacco atlas, 2nd edition. Atlanta: American Cancer Society; 2006.
642. Mansvelder HD, Keath JR, McGehee DS. Synaptic mechanisms underlie nicotine-induced excitability of brain reward areas. Neuron. 2002;33:905-19.
643. Mansvelder HD, McGehee DS. Long-term potentiating of excitatory inputs to brain reward areas by nicotine. Neuron. 2000;27:349-57.
644. McCarthy DE, Piasecki TM, Fiore MC, Baker TB. Life before and after quitting smoking: an electronic diary study. J Abnorm Psychol. 2006;115:454-66.
645. Munafo M, Clark T, Johnsotone E, Murphy M, Walton R. The genetic basis for smoking behavior: a systematic review and meta-analysis. Nicotine Tob Res. 2004;6:583-97.

646. Nides M, Oncken C, Gonzales D, et al. Smoking cessation with varenicline, a selective alpha4 beta2 nicotinic receptor partial agonist: results form a 7-week, randomized, placebo-and bupropion-controlled trial with 1-year follow-up. Arch Intern Med. 2006;166:1561-8.
647. Office of Population Statistics and Censures. Morbidity statistics from general practice; 4th national study 1991092. OPCS Series MB5/3. London: HM Stationery Office; 1995. pp. 29.
648. Oncken C, Gonzales D, Nides M, et al. Efficacy and safety of the novel selective nicotinic acetylcholine receptor partial agonist, varenicline, for smoking cessation. Arch Intern Med. 2006;166:1571-7.
649. Palmatier MI, Evans-Martin FF, Hoffman A, et al. Dissociating the primary reinforcing and reinforcement-enhancing effects of nicotine using a rat self-administration paradigm with concurrently available drug and environmental reinforces. Psychopharmacology (Berl). 2006;184:391-400.
650. Paterson D, Norberg A. Neuronal nicotinic receptors in the human brain. Prog Neurobiol. 2000;6;75-111.
651. Piasecki TM, Fiore MC, Baker TB. Profiles in discouragement: two studies of variability in the time course of smoking withdrawal symptoms. J Abnorm Psychol. 1998;107:238-51.
652. Piasecki TM, Fiore MC, McCarthy DE, Baker TB. Have we lost our way? The need for dynamic formulations of smoking relapse proneness. Addiction. 2001;97:1093-108.
653. Piasecki TM, Jorenby DE, Smith SS, Fiore MC, Baker TB. Smoking withdrawal dynamics: II. Improved test of withdrawal-relapse relations. J Abnorm Psychol. 2003;112:14-27.
654. Piasecki TM, Jorneby De, Smith SS, Fiore MC, Baker TB. Smoking withdrawal dynamics: I. Abstinence distress in lapsers and abstainers. J Abnorm Psychol. 2003;112:3-13.
655. Piaseki TM, Niaura R, Shadel WG, et al. Smoking withdrawal dynamics in unaided quitters. J Abnorm Psychol. 2000;109: 74-86.
656. Picciotto MR, Corrigall WA. Neuronal systems underlying behaviors related to nicotine addiction: neural circuits and molecular genetics. J Neurosic. 2002;22:3338-41.
657. Pidoplichko VI, DeBiasi M, Williams JT, Dani JA. Nicotine activates and desensitizes midbrain dopamine neurons. Nature 1997; 390: 401-4.
658. Pierce JP, Gilpin EA. Impact of over-the-counter sales on effectiveness of pharmaceutical aids for smoking cessation. JAMA. 2002;288:1260-4.
659. Piper ME, McCarthy DE, Baker TB. Assessing tobacco dependence: a guide to measure evaluation and selection. Nicotine Tob Res. 2006;8:339-51.
660. Rimer B, Orleans C, Keintz M, Cristnzio S, Fleisher L. The older smoker. Status, challenges and opportunities for intervention. Chest. 1990;97:547-53.
661. Rose JE. Nicotine and non-nicotine factors in cigarette addiction. Psychopharmacology (Berl). 2006;184:274-85.
662. Royal College of Physicians of London. Nicotine addiction in Britain: a report of the Tobacco Advisory Group of the Royal College of Physicians. London: Royal College of Physicians of London; 2000.
663. Saccone SF, Hinrichs AL, Saccone NL, et al. Cholinergic nicotinic receptor genes implicated in nicotine dependence association study targeting 348 candidate gens with 3713 SNPs. Hum Mol Genet. 2007;16: 36-49.
664. Schiffer WK, Gerasimov MR, Marsteller DA, et al. Topiramate selectively attenuates nicotine induced increases in monoamine release. Synapse. 2001;42:196-8.
665. Shiffman S, Dresler CM, Hajek P, Gilburt SJ, Target D, Strahs KR. Efficacy of nicotine lozenge for smoking cessation. Arch Intern Med. 2002;162:1267-76.
666. Shiffman S, Gnys M, Richards TJ, Paty JA, Kickcox M, Kassel JD. Temptations to smoke after quitting: a comparison of lapsers and maintainers. Health Psychol. 1996;15:445-61.
667. Silagy C, Lancaster T, Stead L, Mant D, Fowler G. Nicotine Replacement therapy for smoking cessation. J Pharamcol Exp Ther. 2001;117:558-82.
668. Stead LF, Lancaster T, Perera R. Telephone counseling for smoking cessation. Cohrane Database Syst Rev. 2006;3:CD002850.
669. Stead LF. Davis RM. Fiore MC, Hatsukami DK, Raw M, West R. Effectiveness of over-the-counter nicotine replacement therapy. JAMA. 2002;288:3109-10.
670. Sullivan PF, Kendler KS. The genetic epidemiology of smoking. Nicotine Tob Res. 1999;1(Suppl 2):S51-57.
671. Summers KL, Giacobini E. Effects of local and repeated systemic administration of nicotine on extracellular levels of acetylcholine, norepinephrine, dopamine, and serotonin in rat cortex. Neurochem Res. 1995;20:753-9.
672. Task Force on Community Preventive Services. Introducing the guide to community preventive services. Am J Prev Med. 2000;18(Suppl):1-142.
673. Task Force on Community Preventive Services. Tobacco use prevention and control. AM J Prev Med. 2001;20(Suppl):1-88.
674. Tatley M. Bupropion (Zyban) for second-line treatment only. Medsafe, 2001; Prescriber update number 22: 4-8. http://www.medsafe.govt.nz/profs/PUarticles/zyban.htm (accessed July 1, 2012).
675. Taylor T, Lader D, Dryant A, Keyse L, Joloza MT. Smoking-related behavior and attitudes. London: Office for National Statistics; 2005.
676. The Cochrane Collaboration. Cochrane Collaboration Tobacco Addiction Group. http://tobacco.cochrane.org/en/localrevs.html(accessed July 1, 2012).
677. Thompson Healthcare Inc. Physicians' desk reference, 60th edition. Montyale: Thomson PDR; 2006.
678. US Department of Health and Human Services. The health benefits of smoking cessation. A report of the surgeon general. Report number DHHS publication number (CDC) 90-8416. Rockville: Centers for Disease Control, Center for Chronic Disease Prevention and Health Promotion, Office on Smoking and Health; 1990.
679. US Department of Health and Human Services. The health consequences of involuntary exposure to tobacco smoke:

a report of the surgeon general. Atlanta: US Department of Health and Human Services, Centers for Disease Control and Prevention, Coordinating Centre for Health Promotion, National Centre for Chronic Disease Prevention and Health Promotion, Office on Smoking and Health; 2006.

680. US Department of Health and Human Services. The health consequences of smoking: a report of the surgeon general, Atlanta: US Department of Health and Human Services, Centers for Disease Control and Prevention, National Center for Chronic Disease Prevention and Health Promotion, Office on Smoking and Health; 2004.

681. US Department of Health and Human Services. The health consequences of smoking: nicotine and addiction. A report of the surgeon general. Rockville: US Department of Health and Human Services; 1988.

682. Wagena EJ, Knipschild PG, Huibers MJ, Wouters EF, van Schayck CP. Efficacy of bupropion and nortriptyline for smoking cessation among people at risk for or with chronic obstructive pulmonary disease. Arch Intern Med. 2005;165: 2286-92.

683. West R, McNeill A, Raw M. Smoking cessation guidelines for health professionals: an update. Health Education Authority. Thorax 2000; 55: 987-99.

684. West R, Zohu X. Is nicotine replacement therapy for smoking cessation effective in the "real world"? Findings from a prospective multinational cohort study. Thorax. 2007;62:998-1002.

685. WHO. International Classification of disease (ICD-10). Geneva: World Health Organization; 1991.

686. Williams KE, Reeves KR, Billing CB, Pennington AM, Gong J. A double-blind study evaluating the long-term safety of varenicline for smoking cessation. Curr Med Res Opin. 2007;23:193-801.

687. Wonnacott S, Sidhpura N, Balfour DJ. Nicotine: from molecular beta-endorphin neurons to acute and chronic nicotine treatments and following nicotine withdrawal. Life Sci. 1997;61:PL59-66.

688. Wonnacott S, Sidhpura N, Balfour DJ. Nicotine: from molecular mechanisms to behaviour. Curr Opin Pharmacol. 2005;5:53-9.

689. Zevin S, Gourlay SG, Benowitz NL. Clinical pharmacology of nicotine. Clin Dermatol. 1998;16:557-64.

CHAPTER 6 Schizophrenia

Avinash De Souza, Nilesh Shah, Shivanshu Shrivastava, Allen De Souza

6.1 INTRODUCTION AND OVERVIEW

Avinash De Souza, Nilesh Shah

INTRODUCTION

Schizophrenia is a chronic, severe, and disabling brain disease. Approximately 1% of the population develops schizophrenia during their lifetime. Although schizophrenia affects men and women with equal frequency, the disorder often appears earlier in men, usually in the late teens or early twenties, than in women, who are generally affected in the twenties to early thirties. People with schizophrenia often suffer terrifying symptoms such as hearing internal voices not heard by others, or believing that other people are reading their minds, controlling their thoughts, or plotting to harm them. These symptoms may leave them fearful and withdrawn. Their speech and behavior can be so disorganized that they may be incomprehensible or frightening to others. Available treatments can relieve many symptoms, but most people with schizophrenia continue to suffer some symptoms throughout their lives; it has been estimated that no more than one in five individuals recovers completely.

This is a time of hope for people with schizophrenia and their families. Research is gradually leading to new and safer medications and unraveling the complex causes of the disease. Scientists are using many approaches from the study of molecular genetics to the study of populations to learn about schizophrenia. Methods of imaging the brain's structure and function hold the promise of new insights into the disorder.

SCHIZOPHRENIA: THE ILLNESS

Schizophrenia is found all over the world. The severity of the symptoms and long-lasting, chronic pattern of schizophrenia often cause a high degree of disability. Medications and other treatments for schizophrenia, when used regularly and as prescribed, can help reduce and control the distressing symptoms of the illness. However, some people are not greatly helped by available treatments or may prematurely discontinue treatment because of unpleasant side effects or other reasons. Even when treatment is effective, persisting consequences of the illness—lost opportunities, stigma, residual symptoms, and medication side effects—may be very troubling.

The first signs of schizophrenia often appear as confusing, or even shocking, changes in behavior. Coping with the symptoms of schizophrenia can be especially difficult for family members who remember how involved or vivacious a person was before they became ill. The sudden onset of severe psychotic symptoms is referred to as an "acute" phase of schizophrenia. "Psychosis," a common condition in schizophrenia, is a state of mental impairment marked by hallucinations, which are disturbances of sensory perception, and/or delusions, which are false yet strongly held personal beliefs that result from an inability to separate real from unreal experiences. Less obvious symptoms, such as social isolation or withdrawal, or unusual speech, thinking, or behavior, may precede, be seen along with, or follow the psychotic symptoms.

Some people have only one such psychotic episode; others have many episodes during a lifetime, but lead relatively normal lives during the interim periods. However, the individual with "chronic" schizophrenia, or a continuous or recurring pattern of illness, often does not fully recover normal functioning and typically requires long-term treatment, generally including medication, to control the symptoms.

DIAGNOSIS OF SCHIZOPHRENIA

It is important to rule out other illnesses, as sometimes people suffer severe mental symptoms or even psychosis due to undetected underlying medical conditions. For this reason, a medical history should be taken and a physical examination and laboratory tests should be done to rule out other possible causes of the symptoms before concluding that a person has schizophrenia. In addition, since commonly abused drugs may cause symptoms resembling schizophrenia, blood or urine samples from the person can be tested at hospitals or physicians' offices for the presence of these drugs.

At times, it is difficult to tell one mental disorder from another. For instance, some people with symptoms of schizophrenia exhibit prolonged extremes of elated or depressed mood, and it is important to determine whether such a patient has schizophrenia or actually has a manic-depressive (or bipolar) disorder or major depressive disorder. Persons whose symptoms cannot be clearly categorized are sometimes diagnosed as having a "schizoaffective disorder."

Children over the age of five can develop schizophrenia, but it is very rare before adolescence. Although some people who later develop schizophrenia may have seemed different from other children at an early age, the psychotic symptoms of schizophrenia—hallucinations and delusions—are extremely uncommon before adolescence.

CLINICAL FEATURES OF SCHIZOPHRENIA

Distorted Perceptions of Reality

People with schizophrenia may have perceptions of reality that are strikingly different from the reality seen and shared by others around them. Living in a world distorted by hallucinations and delusions, individuals with schizophrenia may feel frightened, anxious, and confused. In part because of the unusual realities they experience, people with schizophrenia may behave very differently at various times. Sometimes they may seem distant, detached, or preoccupied and may even sit as rigidly as a stone, not moving for hours or uttering a sound. Other times they may move about constantly—always occupied, appearing wide-awake, vigilant, and alert.

Hallucinations and Illusions

Hallucinations and illusions are disturbances of perception that are common in people suffering from schizophrenia. Hallucinations are perceptions that occur without connection to an appropriate source. Although hallucinations can occur in any sensory form—auditory (sound), visual (sight), tactile (touch), gustatory (taste), and olfactory (smell)—hearing voices that other people do not hear is the most common type of hallucination in schizophrenia. Voices may describe the patient's activities, carry on a conversation, warn of impending dangers, or even issue orders to the individual. Illusions, on the other hand, occur when a sensory stimulus is present but is incorrectly interpreted by the individual.

Delusions

Delusions are false personal beliefs that are not subject to reason or contradictory evidence and are not explained by a person's usual cultural concepts. Delusions may take on different themes. For example, patients suffering from paranoid-type symptoms—roughly one-third of people with schizophrenia—often have delusions of persecution, or false and irrational beliefs that they are being cheated, harassed, poisoned, or conspired against. These patients may believe that they, or a member of the family or someone close to them, are the focus of this persecution. In addition, delusions of grandeur, in which a person may believe he or she is a famous or important figure, may occur in schizophrenia. Sometimes the delusions experienced by people with schizophrenia are quite bizarre; for instance, believing that a neighbor is controlling their behavior with magnetic waves; that people on television are directing special messages to them; or that their thoughts are being broadcast aloud to others.

Disordered Thinking

Schizophrenia often affects a person's ability to "think straight." Thoughts may come and go rapidly; the person may not be able to concentrate on one thought for very long and may be easily distracted, unable to focus attention. People with schizophrenia may not be able to sort out what is relevant and what is not relevant to a situation. The person may be unable to connect thoughts into logical sequences, with thoughts becoming disorganized and fragmented. This lack of logical continuity of thought, termed "thought disorder," can make conversation very difficult and may contribute to social isolation. If people cannot make sense of what an individual is saying, they are likely to become uncomfortable and tend to leave that person alone.

Emotional Expression

People with schizophrenia often show "blunted" or "flat" affect. This refers to a severe reduction in emotional expressiveness. A person with schizophrenia may not show the signs of normal emotion, perhaps may speak in a monotonous voice, have diminished facial expressions, and appear extremely apathetic. The person may withdraw socially, avoiding contact with others; and when forced to interact, he or she may have nothing to say, reflecting "impoverished thought." Motivation can be greatly decreased, as can interest in or enjoyment of life. In some severe cases, a person can spend entire days doing nothing at all, even neglecting basic hygiene. These problems with emotional expression and motivation, which may be extremely troubling to family members and friends, are symptoms of schizophrenia—not character flaws or personal weaknesses.

Normal Versus Abnormal

At times, normal individuals may feel, think, or act in ways that resemble schizophrenia. Normal people may sometimes be unable to "think straight." They may become extremely anxious, for example, when speaking in front of groups and may feel confused, be unable to pull their thoughts together, and forget what they had intended to say. This is not schizophrenia. At the same time, people with schizophrenia do not always act abnormally. Indeed, some people with the illness can appear completely normal and be perfectly responsible, even while they experience hallucinations or delusions. An individual's behavior may change over time, becoming bizarre if medication is stopped and returning closer to normal when receiving appropriate treatment.

Violence and Aggression

News and entertainment media tend to link mental illness and criminal violence; however, studies indicate that except for those persons with a record of criminal violence before becoming ill, and those with substance abuse or alcohol problems, people with schizophrenia are not especially prone to violence. Most individuals with schizophrenia are not violent; more typically, they are withdrawn and prefer to be left alone. Most violent crimes are not committed by persons with schizophrenia, and most persons with schizophrenia do not commit violent crimes. Substance abuse significantly raises the rate of violence in people with schizophrenia but also in people who do not have any mental illness. People with paranoid and psychotic symptoms, which can become worse if medications are discontinued, may also be at higher risk for violent behavior. When violence does occur, it is most frequently targeted at family members and friends, and more often takes place at home.

Suicide in Schizophrenia

Suicide is a serious danger in people who have schizophrenia. If an individual tries to commit suicide or threatens to do so, professional help should be sought immediately. People with schizophrenia have a higher rate of suicide than the general population. Approximately 10% of people with schizophrenia (especially younger adult males) commit suicide. Unfortunately, the prediction of suicide in people with schizophrenia can be especially difficult.

CAUSATIVE FACTORS IN SCHIZOPHRENIA

There is no known single cause of schizophrenia. Many diseases, such as heart disease, result from an interplay of genetic, behavioral, and other factors; and this may be the case for schizophrenia as well. Scientists do not yet understand all of the factors necessary to produce schizophrenia, but all the tools of modern biomedical research are being used to search for genes, critical moments in brain development, and other factors that may lead to the illness.

Genetics

It has long been known that schizophrenia runs in families. People who have a close relative with schizophrenia are more likely to develop the disorder than are people who have no relatives with the illness. For example, a monozygotic (identical) twin of a person with schizophrenia has the highest risk—40 to 50%—of developing the illness. A child whose parent has schizophrenia has about a 10% chance. By comparison, the risk of schizophrenia in the general population is about 1%. Scientists are studying genetic factors in schizophrenia. It appears likely that multiple genes are involved in creating a predisposition to develop the disorder. In addition, factors such as prenatal difficulties like intrauterine starvation or viral infections, perinatal complications, and various nonspecific stressors, seem to influence the development of schizophrenia. However, it is not yet understood how the genetic predisposition is transmitted, and it cannot yet be accurately predicted whether a given person will or will not develop the disorder. Several regions of the human genome are being investigated to identify genes that may confer susceptibility for schizophrenia. The strongest evidence to date leads to chromosomes 13 and 6 but remains unconfirmed. Identification of specific genes involved in the development of schizophrenia will provide important clues into what goes wrong in the brain to produce and sustain the illness and will guide the development of new and better treatments.

Neurochemical Theories

Basic knowledge about brain chemistry and its link to schizophrenia is expanding rapidly. Neurotransmitters, substances that allow communication between nerve cells, have long been thought to be involved in the development of schizophrenia. It is likely, although not yet certain, that the disorder is associated with some imbalance of the complex, interrelated chemical systems of the brain, perhaps involving the neurotransmitters dopamine and glutamate. This area of research is promising.

Neurobiological Theories

There have been dramatic advances in neuroimaging technology that permit scientists to study brain structure and function in living individuals. Many studies of people with schizophrenia have found abnormalities in brain structure (for example, enlargement of the fluid-filled cavities, called the ventricles, in the interior of the brain, and decreased size of certain brain regions) or function (for example, decreased metabolic activity in certain brain regions). It should be emphasized that these abnormalities are quite subtle and are not characteristic of all people with schizophrenia, nor do they occur only in individuals with this illness. Microscopic studies of brain tissue after death have also shown small changes in distribution or number of brain cells in people with schizophrenia. It appears that many (but probably not all) of these changes are present before an individual becomes ill, and schizophrenia may be, in part, a disorder in development of the brain. Developmental neurobiologists funded by the National Institute of Mental Health (NIMH) have found that schizophrenia may be a developmental disorder resulting when neurons form inappropriate connections during fetal development. These errors may lie dormant until puberty, when changes in the brain that occur normally during this critical stage of maturation interact adversely with the faulty connections. This research has spurred efforts to identify prenatal factors that may have some bearing on the apparent developmental abnormality.

In other studies, investigators using brain-imaging techniques have found evidence of early biochemical changes that may precede the onset of disease symptoms, prompting examination of the neural circuits that are most likely to be involved in producing those symptoms. Meanwhile, scientists working at the molecular level are exploring the genetic basis for abnormalities in brain development and in the neurotransmitter systems regulating brain function.

TREATMENT OF SCHIZOPHRENIA

Since schizophrenia may not be a single condition and its causes are not yet known, current treatment methods are based on both clinical research and experience. These approaches are chosen on the basis of their ability to reduce the symptoms of schizophrenia and to lessen the chances that symptoms will return.

Medications

Antipsychotic medications have been available since the mid-1950s. They have greatly improved the outlook for individual patients. These medications reduce the psychotic symptoms of schizophrenia and usually allow the patient to function more effectively and appropriately. Antipsychotic drugs are the best treatment now available, but they do not "cure" schizophrenia or ensure that there will be no further psychotic episodes. The choice and dosage of medication can be made only by a qualified physician who is well trained in the medical treatment of mental disorders. The dosage of medication is individualized for each patient, since people may vary a great deal in the amount of drug needed to reduce symptoms without producing troublesome side effects.

The large majority of people with schizophrenia show substantial improvement when treated with antipsychotic drugs. Some patients, however, are not helped very much by the medications and a few do not seem to need them. It is difficult to predict which patients will fall into these two groups and to distinguish them from the large majority of patients who do benefit from treatment with antipsychotic drugs.

A number of new antipsychotic drugs (the so-called "atypical antipsychotics") have been introduced since 1990. The first of these, clozapine, has been shown to be more effective than other antipsychotics, although the possibility of severe side effects—in particular, a condition called agranulocytosis (loss of the white blood cells that fight infection)—requires that patients be monitored with blood tests every one or two weeks. Even newer antipsychotic drugs, such as risperidone and olanzapine are safer than the older drugs or clozapine, and they also may be better tolerated. They may or may not treat the illness as well as clozapine, however. Several additional antipsychotics are currently under development.

Antipsychotic drugs are often very effective in treating certain symptoms of schizophrenia, particularly hallucinations and delusions; unfortunately, the drugs may not be as helpful with other symptoms, such as reduced motivation and emotional expressiveness. Indeed, the older antipsychotics (which also went by the name of "neuroleptics"), medicines like haloperidol or chlorpromazine, may even produce side effects that resemble the more difficult to treat symptoms. Often, lowering the dose or switching to a different medicine may reduce these side effects; the newer medicines, including olanzapine, quetiapine, and risperidone, appear less likely to have this problem. Sometimes when people with schizophrenia become depressed, other symptoms can appear to worsen. The symptoms may improve with the addition of an antidepressant medication.

Patients and families sometimes become worried about the antipsychotic medications used to treat schizophrenia. In addition to concern about side effects, they may worry that such drugs could lead to addiction. However, antipsychotic medications do not produce a "high" (euphoria) or addictive behavior in people who take them.

Another misconception about antipsychotic drugs is that they act as a kind of mind control, or a "chemical straitjacket." Antipsychotic drugs used at the appropriate dosage do not "knock out" people or take away their free will. While these medications can be sedating, and while this effect can be useful when treatment is initiated particularly if an individual is quite agitated, the utility of the drugs is not due to sedation but to their ability to diminish the hallucinations, agitation, confusion, and delusions of a psychotic episode. Thus, antipsychotic medications should eventually help an individual with schizophrenia to deal with the world more rationally.

DURATION OF TREATMENT

Antipsychotic medications reduce the risk of future psychotic episodes in patients who have recovered from an acute episode. Even with continued drug treatment, some people who have recovered will suffer relapses. Far higher relapse rates are seen when medication is discontinued. In most cases, it would not be accurate to say that continued drug treatment "prevents" relapses; rather, it reduces their intensity and frequency. The treatment of severe psychotic symptoms generally requires higher dosages than those used for maintenance treatment. If symptoms reappear on a lower dosage, a temporary increase in dosage may prevent a full-blown relapse.

Because relapse of illness is more likely when antipsychotic medications are discontinued or taken irregularly, it is very important that people with schizophrenia work with their doctors and family members to adhere to their treatment plan. Adherence to treatment refers to the degree to which patients follow the treatment plans recommended by their doctors. Good adherence involves taking prescribed medication at the correct dose and proper times each day, attending clinic appointments, and/or carefully following other treatment procedures. Treatment adherence is often difficult for people with schizophrenia, but it can be made easier with the help of several strategies and can lead to improved quality of life.

There are a variety of reasons why people with schizophrenia may not adhere to treatment. Patients may not believe they are ill and may deny the need for medication, or they may have such disorganized thinking that they cannot remember to take their daily doses. Family members or friends may not understand schizophrenia and may inappropriately advise the person with schizophrenia to stop treatment when he or she is feeling better. Physicians, who play an important role in helping their patients adhere to treatment, may neglect to ask patients how often they are taking their medications, or may be unwilling to accommodate a patient's request to change dosages or try a new treatment. Some patients report that side effects of the medications seem worse than the illness itself. Further, substance abuse can interfere with the effectiveness of treatment, leading patients to discontinue medications. When a complicated treatment plan is added to any of these factors, good adherence may become even more challenging.

Fortunately, there are many strategies that patients, doctors, and families can use to improve adherence and prevent worsening of the illness. Some antipsychotic medications, including haloperidol, fluphenazine, perphenazine and others, are available in long-acting injectable forms that eliminate the need to take pills every day. A major goal of current research on treatments for schizophrenia is to develop a wider variety of long-acting antipsychotics, especially the newer agents with milder side effects, which can be delivered through injection. Medication calendars or pill boxes labeled with the days of the week can help patients and caregivers know when medications have or have not been taken. Using electronic timers that beep when medications should be taken, or pairing medication taking with routine daily events like meals, can help patients remember and adhere to their dosing schedule. Engaging family members in observing oral medication taking by patients can help ensure adherence. In addition, through a variety of other methods of adherence monitoring, doctors can identify when pill taking is a problem for their patients and can work with them to make adherence easier. It is important to help motivate patients to continue taking their medications properly.

In addition to any of these adherence strategies, patient and family education about schizophrenia, its symptoms, and the medications being prescribed to treat the disease is an important part of the treatment process and helps support the rationale for good adherence.

SIDE EFFECTS OF PHARMACOTHERAPY

Antipsychotic drugs, like virtually all medications, have unwanted effects along with their beneficial effects. During the early phases of drug treatment, patients may be troubled by side effects such as drowsiness, restlessness, muscle spasms, tremor, dry mouth, or blurring of vision. Most of these can be corrected by lowering the dosage or can be controlled by other medications. Different patients have different treatment responses and side effects to various antipsychotic drugs. A patient may do better with one drug than another.

The long-term side effects of antipsychotic drugs may pose a considerably more serious problem. Tardive dyskinesia (TD) is a disorder characterized by involuntary movements most often affecting the mouth, lips, and tongue, and sometimes the trunk or other parts of the body such as arms and legs. It occurs in about 15–20% of patients who have been receiving the older, "typical" antipsychotic drugs for many years, but TD can also develop in patients who have been treated with these drugs for shorter periods of time. In most cases, the symptoms of TD are mild, and the patient may be unaware of the movements.

Antipsychotic medications developed in recent years all appear to have a much lower risk of producing TD than the older, traditional antipsychotics. The risk is not zero, however, and they can produce side effects of their own such as weight gain. In addition, if given at too high of a dose, the newer medications may lead to problems such as social withdrawal and symptoms resembling Parkinson's disease, a disorder that affects movement. Nevertheless, the newer antipsychotics are a significant advance in treatment, and their optimal use in people with schizophrenia is a subject of much current research.

PSYCHOSOCIAL TREATMENTS

Antipsychotic drugs have proven to be crucial in relieving the psychotic symptoms of schizophrenia—hallucinations, delusions, and incoherence—but are not consistent in relieving the behavioral symptoms of the disorder. Even when patients with schizophrenia are relatively free of psychotic symptoms, many still have extraordinary difficulty with communication, motivation, self-care, and establishing and maintaining relationships with others. Moreover, because patients with schizophrenia frequently become ill during the critical career-forming years of life (e.g., ages 18–35), they are less likely to complete the training required for skilled work. As a result, many with schizophrenia not only suffer thinking and emotional difficulties, but lack social and work skills and experience as well.

It is with these psychological, social, and occupational problems that psychosocial treatments may help most. While psychosocial approaches have limited value for acutely psychotic patients (those who are out of touch with reality or have prominent hallucinations or delusions), they may be useful for patients with less severe symptoms or for patients whose psychotic symptoms are under control. Numerous forms of psychosocial therapy are available for people with schizophrenia, and most focus on improving the patient's social functioning—whether in the hospital or community, at home, or on the job. Some of these approaches are described here. Unfortunately, the availability of different forms of treatment varies greatly from place to place.

REHABILITATION IN SCHIZOPHRENIA

Broadly defined, rehabilitation includes a wide array of nonmedical interventions for those with schizophrenia. Rehabilitation programs emphasize social and vocational training to help patients and former patients overcome difficulties in these areas. Programs may include vocational counseling, job training, problem-solving and money management skills, use of public transportation, and social skills training. These approaches are important for the success of the community-centered treatment of schizophrenia, because they provide discharged patients with the skills necessary to lead productive lives outside the sheltered confines of a mental hospital.

INDIVIDUAL PSYCHOTHERAPY

Individual psychotherapy involves regularly scheduled talks between the patient and a mental health professional such as a psychiatrist, psychologist, psychiatric social worker, or nurse. The sessions may focus on current or past problems, experiences, thoughts, feelings, or relationships. By sharing experiences with a trained empathic person—talking about their world with someone outside it—individuals with schizophrenia may gradually come to understand more about themselves and their problems. They can also learn to sort out the real from the unreal and distorted. Recent studies indicate that supportive, reality-oriented, individual psychotherapy, and cognitive-behavioral approaches that teach coping and problem-solving skills, can be beneficial for outpatients with schizophrenia. However, psychotherapy is not a substitute for antipsychotic medication, and it is most helpful once drug treatment first has relieved a patient's psychotic symptoms.

FAMILY PSYCHOEDUCATION

Very often, patients with schizophrenia are discharged from the hospital into the care of their family; so it is important that family members learn all they can about schizophrenia and understand the difficulties and problems associated with the illness. It is also helpful for family members to learn ways to minimize the patient's chance of relapse—for example, by using different treatment adherence strategies—and to be aware of the various kinds of outpatient and family services available in the period after hospitalization. Family "psychoeducation," which includes teaching various coping strategies and problem-solving skills, may help families deal more effectively with their ill relative and may contribute to an improved outcome for the patient.

SELF-HELP GROUPS AND SUPPORT SYSTEMS

Self-help groups for people and families dealing with schizophrenia are becoming increasingly common. Although not led by a professional therapist, these groups may be therapeutic because members provide continuing mutual support as well as comfort in knowing that they are not alone in the problems they face. Self-help groups may also serve other important functions. Families working together can more effectively serve as advocates for needed research and hospital and community treatment programs. Patients acting as a group rather than individually may be better able to dispel stigma and draw public attention to such abuses as discrimination against the mentally ill. Family and peer support and advocacy groups are very active and provide useful information and assistance for patients and families of patients with schizophrenia and other mental disorders. A list of some of these organizations is included at the end of this document.

A patient's support system may come from several sources, including the family, a professional residential or day program provider, shelter operators, friends or roommates, professional case managers, churches and synagogues, and others. Because many patients live with their families, the following discussion frequently uses the term "family." However, this should not be taken to imply that families ought to be the primary support system.

There are numerous situations in which patients with schizophrenia may need help from people in their family or community. Often, a person with schizophrenia will resist treatment, believing that delusions or hallucinations are real and that psychiatric help is not required. At times, family or friends may need to take an active role in having them seen and evaluated by a professional. The issue of civil rights enters into any attempts to provide treatment. Laws protecting patients from involuntary commitment have become very strict, and families and community organizations may be frustrated in their efforts to see that a severely mentally ill individual gets needed help. These laws vary from State to State; but generally, when people are dangerous to themselves or others due to a mental disorder, the police can assist in getting them an emergency psychiatric evaluation and, if necessary, hospitalization. In some places, staff from a local community mental health center can evaluate an individual's illness at home if he or she will not voluntarily go in for treatment.

Sometimes only the family or others close to the person with schizophrenia will be aware of strange behavior or ideas that the person has expressed. Since patients may not volunteer such information during an examination, family members or friends should ask to speak with the person evaluating the patient so that all relevant information can be taken into account.

Ensuring that a person with schizophrenia continues to get treatment after hospitalization is also important. A patient may discontinue medications or stop going for follow-up treatment, often leading to a return of psychotic symptoms. Encouraging the patient to continue treatment and assisting him or her in the treatment process can positively influence recovery. Without treatment, some people with schizophrenia become so psychotic and disorganized that they cannot care for their basic needs, such as food, clothing, and shelter. All too often, people with severe mental illnesses such as schizophrenia end up on the streets or in jails, where they rarely receive the kinds of treatment they need.

Those close to people with schizophrenia are often unsure of how to respond when patients make statements that seem strange or are clearly false. For the individual with schizophrenia, the bizarre beliefs or hallucinations seem quite real—they are not just "imaginary fantasies." Instead of "going along with" a person's delusions, family members or friends can tell the person that they do not see things the same way or do not agree with his or her conclusions, while acknowledging that things may appear otherwise to the patient.

It may also be useful for those who know the person with schizophrenia well to keep a record of what types of symptoms have appeared, what medications (including dosage) have been taken, and what effects various treatments have had. By knowing what symptoms have been present before, family members may know better what to look for in the future. Families may even be able to identify some "early warning signs" of potential relapses, such as increased withdrawal or changes in sleep patterns, even better and earlier than the patients themselves. Thus, return of psychosis may be detected early and treatment may prevent a full-blown relapse. Also, by knowing which medications have helped and which have caused troublesome side effects in the past, the family can help those treating the patient to find the best treatment more quickly.

In addition to involvement in seeking help, family, friends, and peer groups can provide support and encourage the person with schizophrenia to regain his or her abilities. It is important that goals be attainable, since a patient who feels pressured and/or repeatedly criticized by others will probably experience stress that may lead to a worsening of symptoms. Like anyone else, people with schizophrenia need to know when they are doing things right. A positive approach may be helpful and perhaps more effective in the long run than criticism. This advice applies to everyone who interacts with the person.

PROGNOSIS

The outlook for people with schizophrenia has improved over the last 25 years. Although no totally effective therapy has yet been devised, it is important to remember that many people with the illness improve enough to lead independent, satisfying lives. As we learn more about the causes and treatments of schizophrenia, we should be able to help more patients achieve successful outcomes.

Studies that have followed people with schizophrenia for long periods, from the first episode to old age, reveal that a wide range of outcomes is possible. When large groups of patients are studied, certain factors tend to be associated with a better outcome—for example, a pre-illness history of normal social, school, and work adjustment. However, the current state of knowledge, does not allow for a sufficiently accurate prediction of long-term outcome.

Given the complexity of schizophrenia, the major questions about this disorder—its cause or causes, prevention, and treatment—must be addressed with research. The public should beware of those offering "the cure" for (or "the cause" of) schizophrenia. Such claims can provoke unrealistic expectations that, when unfulfilled, lead to further disappointment. Although progress has been made toward better understanding and treatment of schizophrenia, continued investigation is urgently needed. It is thought that this wide-ranging research effort, including basic studies on the brain, will continue to illuminate processes and principles important for understanding the causes of schizophrenia and for developing more effective treatments.

6.2 SCHIZOPHRENIA: EPIDEMIOLOGY

Avinash De Souza, Nilesh Shah

INTRODUCTION

The epidemiology of schizophrenia has progressed from descriptive accounts to a surge in analytic epidemiologic findings over the last two decades. This chapter reviews the epidemiology of schizophrenia, concentrating on results which are most credible methodologically and consistent across studies, focusing particularly on the most recent developments. We also provide comments about some misconceptions regarding schizophrenia epidemiology, specifically pointing to widespread misinterpretation of evidence regarding some epidemiological aspects of schizophrenia and the disease.

HISTORICAL ASPECTS

The earliest application of an epidemiological method to the investigation of psychoses was the work of a woman physician, Jenny Koller, who examined the aggregation of psychiatric disorders in the families of 284 probands and 370 healthy subjects in the canton of Zürich using a prototype case-control design.[1] Anticipating much later findings of genetic epidemiology, she reported that "the hereditary loading of the healthy subjects is much higher than generally assumed"; that "the strongest loading is that of psychoses and accentuated characters"; and that "the loading in distant relatives is quite low, unless a person at risk is exposed to multiple factors". Kraepelin[2] saw clearly the potential of population research to "throw light on the causes of mental disorder" and advocated comparative studies of the psychoses and personality traits across different cultures. In the first half of the 20th century, epidemiological research into the psychoses took two distinct directions. Whereas the focus of European investigators was primarily on issues of heredity.

North American researchers developed a strong interest in the social ecology of mental illness.[3] Most of the methodological tools of psychiatric epidemiology were developed and applied with considerable success during the four decades between 1910 and 1950.

In a historical analysis, Dohrenwend[4] distinguished 3 periods of epidemiological studies in psychiatry. According to his methodological standards, only the last period, beginning around 1980, has produced valid and transnationally comparable findings. The standards include a precise, operational case definition, the collection of comprehensive data on all "cases" from a sufficiently large, statistically well documented population, symptom assessment by transculturally standardized instruments, and computerized diagnosis independent of the interviewer. The World Health Organization (WHO) "Determinants of Outcome" study[5] was the first to satisfy nearly all of these requirements at each study site in the determination of the incidence of schizophrenia (12 centers, 10 countries). Recently, Thornicroft and Johnson[6] have added a further methodological standard that calls for the assessment of met and unmet needs for care in psychiatric surveys.

DESCRIPTIVE EPIDEMIOLOGY OF SCHIZOPHRENIA

Prevalance Studies

The point prevalence of schizophrenia is the proportion of the population at a point in time that has the disorder. The point prevalence of schizophrenia is about five per thousand in the population. The estimate depends on the age distribution of the population—if persons too young to be at risk are included in the denominator, for example, the estimates will be lower. Table 1 presents findings from areas in which credible estimates of both prevalence and incidence are available.[7] The range in prevalence in Table 1 is from 2.7/1000 to 8.3/1000, and this range would not be much affected if several dozen other studies, available from prior reviews, were included. Lifetime prevalence has been estimated by surveys with examinations by medically trained persons, with resulting estimates not too different from those shown in Table 1.[7]

The majority have produced prevalence estimates in the range 1.4 to 4.6 per 1000 population at risk. However, these are crude prevalence figures which may not be directly comparable due to demographic differences such as age specific mortality and migration. Therefore, the modal prevalence of 1.4–4.6 per 1000 may not reflect the true extent of variation among different populations. Certain populations and groups deviate

Table 1: Prevalence and incidence of Schizophrenia per 1000 population

Area	*Date*	*Prevalence*	*Incidence*
Denmark	1977	2.7	0.12
USA	1972	7	0.7
England	1963	4.4	0.11
Ireland	1986	8.3	0.22
Italy	1989	2.7	0.19
England	1991	5.1	0.21

from the central tendency. Unusually high rates (2–3 times the national or regional rate) have been reported for isolate populations in northern Sweden, several areas in Finland; and for an area in Croatia with high out-migration during the 19th and early 20th century. At the other extreme, a virtual absence of schizophrenia and a relatively high rate of depression has been claimed for the Hutterites in South Dakota, a Protestant sect whose members live in closely-knit endogamous communities sheltered from the outside world.

Low prevalence rates have also been reported for some Pacific island populations but uncertainties about case finding makes the interpretation of such reports problematic. Two carefully planned surveys in Taiwan were separated by 15 years during which major social change had taken place. While the total mental morbidity increased, the prevalence of schizophrenia decreased from 2.1 to 1.4 per 1000. In both surveys, the indigenous Taiwanese had significantly lower rates than the mainland Chinese who had migrated to the island after World War II.[8] The results of the Epidemiologic Catchment Area (ECA) study[9] in the United States which indicate a higher prevalence rate than most other studies, are difficult to interpret. Inconsistencies among the study areas (such as a 13-fold difference in the rates for age group 18–24 across the sites) suggest that the diagnostic procedure, involving the DIS administered by lay interviewers, may have resulted in a number of false positive diagnoses. In the more recent National Comorbidity Survey (NCS), diagnoses of 'nonaffective psychosis' by computer algorithm based on a version of the CIDI were found to agree poorly with clinicians' diagnoses based on telephone re-interviews, resulting in discrepant estimates of the lifetime prevalence of both 'narrowly' and 'broadly' defined psychotic illness.[10]

Incidence Studies

The incidence of schizophrenia is about 0.20/1000/year. The incidences presented are all estimated for one year, making the comparison somewhat tighter. The range in annual incidence in Table 1 is from 0.11/1000/year to 0.70/1000/year. The presentation of prevalence and incidence figures from the same areas in juxtaposition shows that the point prevalence is usually more than ten times the annual incidence, indicating the chronic nature of the disorder. The force of morbidity for schizophrenia peaks in young adulthood. The age of onset varies between men and women, where males tend to have a younger onset.[7] The peak incidence for males and females is in the decade 15–24. The peak for young adults is more marked for males, and the females have a second peak in the years 55–64. Evidence suggests that males have higher lifetime risk of schizophrenia, which is born out in two meta-analysis addressing that issue, showing that males have about 30–40% higher lifetime risk of developing schizophrenia.[11,12]

The incidence rate is a better estimate of the 'force of morbidity' (the probability of disease occurrence at a point in time) in a given population. Its estimation depends on how reliably the point of onset can be determined. Since it is not possible at present to determine the time of onset of any cerebral dysfunction or biochemical lesion underlying schizophrenia, the onset of the disorder is usually defined as the point in time when its clinical manifestations become apparent. The first hospitalization is not a good index of the 'true' onset, due to the variable time lag between the earliest appearance of symptoms and the first admission.[13] A better approximation is provided by the first contact with any psychiatric or general medical service which is accessed by symptomatic individuals for the first time. Studies using a 'broad' definition of schizophrenia (ICD-8 or ICD-9) suggest that rates based on first admissions or first contacts vary about threefold, between 0.17 and 0.54 per 1000 population per year. Studies using restrictive criteria such as the Research Diagnostic Criteria,[14] DSM-III and its successors, or ICD-10 report incidence rates that are two to three times lower than those based on 'broad' criteria.

Up-to-date, the only study which has generated directly comparable incidence data for different populations is the WHO ten-country investigation.[15,16] Incidence rates in the WHO study were estimated from first-in-lifetime contacts with any 'helping agency' (including traditional healers in the developing countries) which were monitored prospectively over a two-year period. Potential cases and key informants were interviewed by clinicians using standardized instruments, and the timing of onset was ascertained for the majority of the patients. In 86% of the 1022 patients the first manifestation of diagnostic symptoms of schizophrenia was within a year of the first contact and, therefore, the first-contact rate was accepted as a reasonable proxy for the onset of psychosis. Two definitions of 'caseness' were used: a 'broad' clinical classification comprising ICD-9 schizophrenia and paranoid psychoses and a restrictive definition including 'nuclear' schizophrenia with Schneiderian first-rank symptoms. The differences between rates for 'broad' schizophrenia (0.16–0.42 per 1000) across the study areas were significant ($p < 0.001$, two-tailed test); however, those for 'nuclear' schizophrenia were not.

ANALYTICAL EPIDEMIOLOGY OF SCHIZOPHRENIA

Onset of the Illness

The onset of schizophrenia is varied. The intensive study of prodrome by Hafner and colleagues[17] suggests onset of negative symptoms tends to occur about five years before the initial psychotic episode, with onset of positive symptoms much closer to the first hospitalization.

Childhood Abnormalities and Schizophrenia

Many long-term follow-up studies, both retrospective and prospective, suggest a variety of signs, symptoms, conditions, and behaviors are associated with raised risk for schizophrenia, but none with such strength or uniqueness as to be useful in prediction. Earlier work on high risk (HR) groups has shown that offspring of schizophrenic parents were more likely to have a lower IQ, poor attention skills, thought disorder-like symptoms, poor social adjustment, and psychiatric symptoms as compared to the offspring of controls. Although several concerns have been raised regarding the generalizability of HR findings to nonfamilial forms of schizophrenia, recent longitudinal studies conducted in the United Kingdom, Sweden, Finland, and New Zealand have provided evidence that individuals with schizophrenia differ from their peers even in early childhood, in a variety of developmental markers, such as the age of attaining developmental milestones, levels of cognitive functioning, educational achievement, neurological and motor development, social competence and psychological disturbances.[18] More recent evidence also suggest the association between low IQ is specific to schizophrenia as it was not found in bipolar disorder. It is noteworthy that there seems to be no common causal paths which link these developmental markers with schizophrenia. The compelling evidence linking an array of childhood developmental abnormalities and schizophrenia is echoing with the hypothesis that schizophrenia is a neurodevelopmental disorder, for which causes may be traced to a defect in the early brain development.[19]

Course of the Illness

The symptomatic course of schizophrenia is varied. Follow-up studies which are not strictly prospective, can be deceptive, because there is a tendency to focus on a residue of chronic cases, making the disorder appear more chronic than it actually is. A study regarding rehospitalization for a cohort of patients with schizophrenia in Denmark revealed that approximately 25% were not rehospitalized even after 15 years. For that subgroup of the cohort with ten hospitalizations, more than 90% are rehospitalized within three years following the tenth episode. While it could be that the occurrence of episodes are reinforcing the illness, (so-called "schubweis (stepwise)" process), or that hospitalization itself is damaging, it seems more likely the cohort is sorting itself into those with tendency for more versus less chronicity of disorder.[20]

Outcome Studies

Predictors of outcome for schizophrenia remain elusive, for the most part. In a review of thirteen prospective studies of course in first onset cohorts, negative symptoms predicted poor outcome in four studies, and gradual onset, typical of negative symptoms as noted above, predicted poor outcome in several studies. There is variation in the course of schizophrenia around the world, with better prognosis in so-called "developing" countries. Those in developing countries are less likely to have been chronically psychotic over the period of follow-up, and more likely to have no residual symptoms after five years, than those in the developed countries. This result remains to be explained. It could be that individuals meeting criteria for schizophrenia in developing countries include a subset destined for better prognosis because of the risk factor structure in those countries—more deaths of compromised fetuses, for example, or a cause connected to good prognosis, such as a parasite which is rare in developed countries. Another interpretation is that the environment of recovery in the developed world is more pernicious, involving harsher economic competition, a greater degree of stigma, and smaller family networks who can share the burden of care for persons with schizophrenia.[21]

Social Variables and Schizophrenia

The course of schizophrenia, from early prodrome through to later outcome, is influenced by social variables, including socioeconomic position and marital status. The individual who eventually is diagnosed with schizophrenia is more likely to be single than others, even as many as 20 years prior to diagnosis, where the relative odds is about 4. The relative odds of being single, as compared to those never diagnosed with schizophrenia, peak at the time of admission, at more than 15, and remain high for decades afterward. The effect is greater for males, possibly because their earlier onset occurs during the years of formation of marriages. Likewise, the individual who eventually is diagnosed with schizophrenia is more likely to be unemployed than others, many years earlier than the first diagnosis of schizophrenia, and many years afterward. Although there is a long literature on the relationship of low socioeconomic position to risk for schizophrenia, it seems likely that the association is due to the effects of insidious onset on the ability of the individual to compete in the job market.[22]

Season of Birth and Schizophrenia

For a long time it has been known that individuals with schizophrenia are more likely to be born in the winter, and the results have been reported from the samples in the Northern and Southern Hemispheres. The relative risk is small, on the order of a 10% increase for those born in the winter versus summer, but it has been replicated many times. One possible explanation is that the mother is passing through the second trimester of her pregnancy in the height of the flu season, and that infections during that period raise risk for schizophrenia in the offspring. Another explanation offered by a recent study suggests that the seasonal effects may increase one's risk of schizophrenia via the interaction with genetic vulnerability.[23]

Obstetric Complications and Schizophrenia

The finding regarding season of birth suggests that something about pregnancy and birth might be awry in individuals who later develop schizophrenia. There have been case-control studies available for decades on this issue, but the generally positive findings were clouded by the possibility that the mother's recall was biased. In the last fifteen years there have been many studies reporting a relative odds of about two for those with one or another sort of birth complication, and several meta-analyses on this topic exist. Later analyses have begun to specify the individual type of birth complication, with the hope of elucidating the causal mechanism. A recent meta-analytic review of this literature categorizes the types of birth complications as complications of pregnancy (bleeding, diabetes, rhesus incompatibility, pre-eclampsia), abnormal fetal growth and development (low birthweight, congenital malformations, reduced head circumference), and complications of delivery (uterine atony, asphyxia, emergency Cesarean section).[24] The review concludes that the investigations into specific mechanisms need to move now from the epidemiological perspective to include a combination of disciplines and approaches. The complications variously suggest as a possible cause malnutrition, extreme prematurity and hypoxia or ischemia.[25]

Maternal Age and Schizophrenia

The role of advanced parental age in relation to a higher risk of schizophrenia was first proposed in the mid-20th century, and has gained extensive scientific attention in recent years. However, subsequent investigations showed inconsistent findings and it was argued that observed maternal age-associated higher risk in schizophrenia might be largely confounded by raised paternal age. Recently, several population-based epidemiological studies in Demark, Israel, Sweden, and the United States have provided stronger evidence as to the role of paternal age in schizophrenia. A population-based birth cohort study from in Israel found that the relative risk of schizophrenia rose monotonically in each 5-year group of paternal age. Additionally, once paternal age is statistically adjusted, maternal age no longer is a significant predictor of schizophrenia. The evidence from one nested case-control study indicates that the paternal age-related excess in the risk of schizophrenia is generally greater in females. In addition, current population-based cohort research tends to support that advancing paternal age-related increased risk of schizophrenia only appears significant among those without family history, indicating the possibility of accumulation of de novo mutations in paternal sperm.[25]

Infections and Schizophrenia

A series of ecologic studies suggest that persons whose mothers were in their second trimester of pregnancy during a flu epidemic have higher risk for schizophrenia. Infection during pregnancy as a risk factor is consistent with the neurodevelopmental theory of schizophrenia. Later studies, which are more convincing, include individual assessment of infection, either via comparison of antibodies in adults with schizophrenia versus normal individuals, or, even more convincing, prospective studies in which the infection can be determined to have occurred during the pregnancy. There is consistent evidence that individuals with antibodies to *Toxoplasmosis gondii* have higher prevalence of schizophrenia. One study suggests a relative risk of 5.2 for individuals with documented infection by the *Rubella virus* during fetal development. Another prospective study found higher risk for psychosis in individuals whose mothers had higher levels of antibodies to herpes simplex virus.[26]

Schizophrenia and Immunity

A relatively small but consistent literature indicates that persons with schizophrenia have unusual resistance or susceptibility to autoimmune diseases. Studies have consistently shown that individuals with schizophrenia are somehow less likely to have rheumatoid arthritis. While it could be that medications for schizophrenia are protective for rheumatoid arthritis in some unknown way, some of the studies were conducted prior to the era in which neuroleptic medications were available. It could be that other physiologic consequences of schizophrenia are protective, or it could be that a single gene raises risk for the one disorder and protects for the other. Other autoimmune disorders have been linked to schizophrenia, including thyroid disorders, type 1 diabetes and celiac disease. Currently the evidence is strongest for thyroid disorders and celiac disease. The results linking schizophrenia to autoimmune disease are paralleled by the clinical and laboratory study of autoimmune processes in schizophrenia. There are apparently abnormalities of the immune system in schizophrenia, but it is not clear whether these are causal or a consequence of schizophrenia or its treatment. It is possible that a single weakness in the immune system in those with schizophrenia explains both the data on infections and the results on autoimmune disorders, but this remains to be proven.[27]

Schizophrenia and Ethnic Groups

Ethnic status is a relatively easy to identify characteristic of an individual which indicates a shared history with others. Markers of ethnic status include race, country of origin, and religion. Country of origin has proven to be a consistent risk factor for schizophrenia in the United Kingdom and the Netherlands. In the United Kingdom, those immigrating from Africa or the Caribbean, and their second generation offspring, have rates of schizophrenia up to ten times higher than those in the general population. Since immigrant groups who do not have black skin do not have higher rates, and since the second generation is affected, it is unlikely to be the stresses of immigration. Since rates in the countries of origin are not elevated it is unlikely to be a genetic difference between races. The cause appears to be the psychological conditions associated with being Black in England, or being from Surinam in Holland. It could be discrimination, or a more subtle form of difficulty associated with planning one's life when the future is as uncertain as it is for racial groups at the structural bottom of society.[28]

Cannabis and Schizophrenia

There are numerous case control studies showing that persons with schizophrenia are more likely to have taken, or be using, cannabis. Recently there have been prospective studies in Sweden, the Netherlands, New Zealand, and Israel, showing higher risk ranging from 2 to as high as 25. It could be that individuals in the premorbid phase of schizophrenia are responding to initial, mild symptoms of schizophrenia by using drugs, even though these studies have attempted to control for premorbid conditions. On the other hand, it could be that cannabis precipitates, or even causes, an episode of schizophrenia.[29]

Schizophrenia and Urbanization

The relative risk is about 2–4 times higher for those born in urban areas. The difficulty is identifying the plausible biological process associated with urban residence. It could include differences in the physical environment, such as the higher concentration of lead in the soil and air in cities; differences in the cultural environment, such as the expectation to leave the family of origin and define a new life plan, differences in birth practices, such as breastfeeding, crowding which might permit spread of infections, discussed below, differences in the manner in which animals are, or are not, brought into the household and a host of other factors.[30]

Epilepsy and Schizophrenia

In a record-linkage study merging data from two Danish registers, researchers found highly significant associations between a diagnosis of epilepsy and a subsequent diagnosis of any nonorganic, nonaffective psychosis (OR 2.30). The association was particularly strong for psychomotor epilepsy and any psychosis in men (OR 5.07) and for psychomotor epilepsy and schizophrenia in men (OR 2.56). The study supports the notion that epilepsy, and in particular temporal lobe epilepsy, is a risk factor for nonaffective psychosis including schizophrenia.[31]

Urban Birth and Schizophrenia

Urban environments have been thought to increase the incidence of psychosis either by directly contributing to causation (the "breeder" hypothesis) or by attracting vulnerable individuals (the "drift" hypothesis). There has been a recent revival of interest in the "urban factor". Authors analysed all first admissions for schizophrenia and other psychoses in Holland between 1942 and 1978 by place of birth and found a statistically significant, linear relationship between size of urban areas and incidence rates of schizophrenia, affective psychoses and other psychoses. The size of this effect tended to increase in successive birth cohorts. However, no distinction could be made between effects attributable to urban birth (i.e. to a factor operating pre- or perinatally) and effects attributable to urban residence (i.e. to factors operating during postnatal development). Although the suspected "urban risk factor" is more likely to be ecological rather than genetic, a broad range of possibilities related either to the physical environment or to lifestyle and social factors need to be considered.[32]

ASSESSMENT METHODS IN SCHIZOPHRENIA EPIDEMIOLOGY

To a greater extent than studies of other complex diseases, the epidemiological investigation of schizophrenia encounters serious methodological problems at the level of case finding and ascertainment. First, the criteria defining schizophrenia depend critically on the ability to elicit and interpret self-reports of subjective experience; the prerequisite clinical skills cannot be easily translated into simple tools for case finding in the field. Secondly, no biological test or psychometric trait marker of the liability to schizophrenia is yet available for use in population screening. Thirdly, schizophrenia is a low-incidence and low prevalence disorder and population-based case finding through door-to-door interviewing is costly.[33]

In the 1980s great hopes for epidemiology were pinned on the development of explicit diagnostic criteria, incorporated in the DSM-III (APA1980) and its successors, and, a few years later, the ICD-10 (WHO 1992). Two types of assessment instruments were developed and linked to the new diagnostic criteria. The NIMH Diagnostic Interview Schedule, DIS and the related WHO/ADAMHA Composite International Diagnostic Interview, CIDI are fully structured interviews targeting the DSM-IIIR and ICD-10 criteria. They are sometimes referred to as "verbatim" interviews, because the interviewer is required to read out to the respondent each word in the interview without deviations from the script. The interviewer makes no judgements about the presence or absence of psychopathology; rather, the interviewer records the judgements of the respondent. Lay interviewers with no clinical skills can be trained to administer the DIS or the CIDI in about a week. The advantage of these interview protocols is that they are inexpensive and have been shown to be reliable. However, their validity for the identification of psychotic symptoms is problematic. Reliance on self-report leads inevitably to emphasis on symptoms at the expense of signs;

but for schizophrenia, signs like flat affect, odd behavior, speech disorder and apathy may be critical for a correct diagnosis. Therefore, the capacity of the new "verbatim" instruments for valid detection of psychotic disorders in community respondents is limited.[34]

Semistructured clinical interviews such as the 10th edition of the Present State Examination (PSE), now incorporated in the Schedules for Clinical Assessment in Neuropsychiatry, SCAN, cover a broad range of psychopathology and require clinical skills to elicit data that can be processed by ICD-10 and DSM-IV diagnostic algorithms. The SCAN and similar interviews are suitable as second-stage diagnostic instruments but there is a clear need for a relatively simple and psychometrically sound screening procedure for case finding of schizophrenia in field surveys, as the available candidates for first-stage screen (DIS and CIDI) have not been successful.[35]

CONCLUSION AND FUTURE RESEARCH AGENDAS

Epidemiological evidence now supports the conclusion that schizophrenia occurs universally and has similar manifestations and age and gender patterns in different populations. However, the extent and nature of the genetic, neurodevelopmental and environmental contributions to its etiology remain elusive. Epidemiological research in the past decade has mapped areas where potential clues might be found. Resolving, one way or another, contentious issues such as seasonality of births, the role of viral or obstetric developmental lesions, the excess incidence in second-generation migrants, and the possible decline in incidence, is a clear priority for the next few years. In the longer term, the research strategies which hold the best promise for new insights are likely to focus primarily on the population distribution and behavioral effects of potential risk factors and markers suggested by biological and genetic research rather than designs based on limited clinical samples. It is increasingly probable that the developmental antecedents and risk factors implicated in schizophrenia are not restricted to the diagnostic categories of DSM-IV and ICD-10 but underlie a broader spectrum of morbidity. Should this be the case, a prospect for epidemiological research would be to study the population distribution of "correlated phenotypes" such as neurocognitive deficits or other quantitative traits associated with the liability to psychosis.

The epidemiology of schizophrenia is still faced with a series of unsolved methodological problems, making conclusive interpretations and meaningful comparisons difficult. Among these problems are the definition of the diagnosis by conventional criteria, the variability of illness courses despite the similarity of psychopathological symptoms, and the heterogeneity of the study populations. The difficulties resulting from non representative study populations or from a failure to check the findings against alternative interpretations are reflected in the controversy produced by the reports of decreasing first-admission rates for schizophrenia from the mid-1960s to the 1980s in some regions. Equally controversial issues are the similarity or difference of age at onset in men and women, the association between social class and the morbidity risk, and the distinction of empirical subtypes of schizophrenia.

It is increasingly clear that the referents of the concept of schizophrenia reside in fundamental aspects of the organization of the human brain, cognition and social communication. Until recently, these ideas have not been accessible to empirical research. Neuroscience is at present making inroads into this complex field. In due time, this may provide the basis for a molecular epidemiology of the psychoses as predisposing genotypes identified by quantitative traits or association studies. It would, therefore, be premature to engage in grand theory building about the nature and causes of schizophrenia; instead, we should aim to enlarge the scope and improve the quality of the knowledge base that would allow psychiatric research to draw on the new concepts and tools emerging in neuroscience, genetics and evolutionary biology.

6.3 SCHIZOPHRENIA: NEUROBIOLOGY

Avinash De Souza, Nilesh Shah

INTRODUCTION

Schizophrenia is a devastating mental illness that affects 1% of the world population. The disease usually manifests itself in early adulthood with hallucinations, delusions and disorganized thought and behavior. In addition, most patients suffer from cognitive impairments and a subset of patients with schizophrenia also present enduring negative symptoms (for example poverty of thought and speech, loss of motivation and affect). There is evidence that negative symptoms develop prior to positive symptoms, thus children who eventually develop schizophrenia show disturbances in attention and social behavior before overt psychosis. Several risk factors including genetic vulnerability, environmental influences and developmental issues have been identified for this heterogeneous disease. Population studies, including twin and family studies indicate that schizophrenia is highly heritable and probably due to a synergistic interaction of multiple genes and environmental factors. Neuropathological studies have shown anomalies (often subtle) in many different brain areas including cerebral cortex, thalamus, basal ganglia, limbic regions and the cerebellum. Finally, several neurotransmitter systems are likely to be affected in schizophrenia including dopamine, glutamate, GABA and serotonin.[36]

Neurochemical investigation has played a major role in the search for the cause of schizophrenia. Initial research strategies involved the direct measurement of neurochemical substances in biological fluids. Subsequently, indirect measures of brain biochemistry including pituitary hormones and responses to pharmacologic probes were examined. Recent advances in *in vivo* functional neuroimaging, biochemical neuropathology, and molecular genetics have extended the scope of clinical neurochemical studies. The historical emphasis on the dopamine neurotransmitter system has subsided in the wake of the demonstrated limitations of the dopamine hypothesis of schizophrenia and increased evidence for the role of other neurotransmitters in the pathophysiology of schizophrenia as well as their interactions with dopamine neural systems.[37] In this chapter, the authors reviewed significant recently published neurochemical and neuroendocrine studies of schizophrenia in the context of previous work and found an extensive but fragmentary body of data which provides neither consistent nor conclusive evidence for any specific etiologic theory. Aspects of the disease and methodological limitations that may account for this as well as future research strategies are discussed.

NEUROCHEMICAL ABNORMALITIES IN SCHIZOPHRENIA

Dopamine and Schizophrenia

The crucial role of Dopamine (DA) in the pathophysiology of schizophrenia was based on early observations that DA agonists can induce paranoid schizophreniform psychosis and that neuroleptics inhibit dopaminergic activity. The DA hypothesis of schizophrenia proposes that schizophrenia is a manifestation of a hyperdopaminergic state and was clearly stated as early as 1967 by Van Rossum who wrote that when the hypothesis of dopamine blockade by neuroleptic agents can be further substantiated it may result in better understanding the pathophysiology of schizophrenia. Overstimulation of dopamine receptors may have etiologic significance. Since its earliest conception this hypothesis has been only partially supported, has had obvious limitations, and subsequently has undergone multiple revisions. Some of the more recent proposals include evidence from preclinical and clinical studies that could support a hypodopaminergic state in certain schizophrenia symptom syndromes.[38,39]

Weinberger has proposed a neurodevelopmental model for schizophrenia in which increased subcortical DA activity is caused by diminished inhibitory effects of hypoactive DA afferent projections from the prefrontal cortex. Carlsson proposed that there may be a thalamic filter that is indirectly modulated by mesostriatal DA that regulates arousal and emotional tone. Schizophrenic psychosis may occur when the filter opens and arousal increases. Meltzer proposed that a functional change in the DA system is either a precondition for schizophrenia or that alterations in DA function may alleviate schizophrenia. He noted that clozapine both blocks D2 receptors as well as preserving and perhaps even increasing DA activity in areas of the brain and increasing DA turnover (probably related to D1 activity). Reynolds on the other hand, emphasized the heterogeneity of schizophrenia, suggesting that the DA hypothesis applies not to schizophrenia as a whole but to "neuroleptic responsive psychoses" with a more generalized cortical neuronal deficit occurring in treatment-resistant patients with primary negative symptoms. He also posited that increased DA function may be caused by a primary abnormality in another neurochemical system.[40,41]

Heritch hypothesized that DA turnover may be reduced secondary to a deficiency of DA release and dysregulated due to a disruption of feedback mechanisms. Davis in his review and reconceptualization of DA in schizophrenia, suggested that schizophrenia is characterized by hypodopaminergia in mesocortical neurons and hyperdopaminergia in mesolimbic neurons. Finally, drawing primarily on postmortem and preclinical studies, researchers proposed that the delusions of paranoid schizophrenia are caused by DA hyperactivity of CA1 hippocampal neurons. Clearly no consensus exists about DA's role in schizophrenia, in part because the nature and results of studies have been inconsistent and the illness itself appears to be heterogeneous. The situation has become even more complex since the discovery of different DA receptor subtypes that may interact with each other and the development of atypical compounds with mechanisms of action different from those of classic antipsychotic drugs.[42,43]

The limitations of the evidence and the explanatory power of the DA hypothesis of schizophrenia have long been apparent. One of the biggest limitations is the lack of direct evidence of increased DA neuronal activity in clinical studies. Cerebrospinal fluid (CSF) studies of DA metabolites have not produced convincing results, and postmortem studies that have found differences between schizophrenia subjects and controls have found abnormalities in different regions and are either inconsistent or subject to the confounding effects of neuroleptic treatment. *In vivo* positron emission tomography (PET) studies of D2 receptors have also provided conflicting results. Previous clinical neurochemical investigations failed to find clear evidence of DA abnormalities. Perhaps this is the reason why in recent years there have been few studies of DA in schizophrenia and of the difference between the CSF level of the DA metabolite homovanillic acid (HVA) in schizophrenia subjects and controls. However, plasma HVA (pHVA) has been studied extensively.[44,45]

Clearly pHVA is influenced by multiple variables that may affect the strength of the relationship between pHVA and psychopathology, treatment response, and outcome; these variables include gender, diet, activity, prior treatment exposure, duration of drug-free period, patient population (acute vs. chronic), renal clearance and diurnal variation. It is important to remember that the peripheral nervous system is the primary contributor of pHVA; only 17% of pHVA originates in the brain. Despite these limitations pHVA remains the most reliable and least invasive method available to evaluate central DA activity.[46]

Serotonin and Schizophrenia

Next to dopamine (DA), serotonin (5-HT) and norepinephrine (NE) have historically been the neurotransmitters most often implicated in schizophrenia. The predominant pharmacologic property of psychotomimetic compounds typified by lysergic acid diethylamide (LSD) is their affinity for 5-HT receptors. 5-HT receptors are distributed in brain regions believed to be important in mediating behavioral functions, including the frontal cortex. Moreover, atypical antipsychotic drugs bind to 5-HT2 receptors. Renewed interest in the 5-HT system has been stimulated recently by the development of a specific class of atypical antipsychotic drugs that have potent activity at 5-HT receptors. Compounds such as clozapine and risperidone have unique clinical properties that some investigators have attributed to their combined effects on the DA and 5-HT system. However, as with DA, direct neurochemical evidence of 5-HT system dysfunction is lacking.[47,48]

In recent years, a limited number of studies have examined 5-HT in patients with schizophrenia. They found 5-HT to be lower in schizophrenia patients with suicidal behavior than in nonsuicidal schizophrenia patients and control subjects. Hyperserotonemia (> 2 standard deviations [SD] from control mean) was found in 39% of the schizophrenia sample and was associated with chronic illness course. They concluded that schizophrenia may involve a progressive disturbance in the central 5-HT system. They found that schizophrenia subjects had higher 5-HT levels than depressed and control subjects. The 5-HT levels were highest in the paranoid schizophrenia and psychotic depression subgroups. The only finding about MAO activity was that females had higher levels. There have also been several reports of behavioral response to m-chlorophenylpiperazine (m-CPP), a selective 5-HT receptor agonist.[49,50]

The lack of a valid peripheral marker for CNS serotonergic activity, as pHVA is believed to be for DA, is an impediment to 5-HT research in schizophrenia. Plasma 5-hydroxyindoleacetic acid (5-HLAA), the major metabolite of DA, has not been examined in schizophrenia largely because it is believed that extensive peripheral contributions from the gastrointestinal tract would render it uninformative. The cloning of genes that code for 5-HT receptor subtypes provide an important strategy for future investigation of 5-HT.[51]

Norepinephrine and Schizophrenia

Beginning with the hypothesis of Stein and Wise, several investigators have postulated that NE plays an important role in the pathophysiology of schizophrenia. The bases for these claims derive from the relationship of the synthetic pathways of DA and NE, empirical data on noradrenergic measures in other neuropsychiatric disease, and experimentally demonstrated interactions between DA and NE systems in the CNS. However, despite the theoretical promise, we found few clinical studies that clearly demonstrated abnormal measures of NE activity in patients with schizophrenia. Researchers have concluded that NE systems played an important role in the mediation of acute psychosis and were dysregulated in a state dependent fashion during periods of exacerbation. Although these data are far from conclusive, they are consistent with the hypothesized involvement of NE in the pathophysiology of schizophrenia. The data indicate that central noradrenergic neurons (like DA neurons) may be suppressed by antipsychotic drug treatment and activated upon drug withdrawal and immediately before symptom exacerbations. Note that the atypical antipsychotic clozapine has been shown to have potent effects on the noradrenergic system, which is believed by some investigators to be critical to its unique clinical properties.[52,53]

Gamma-aminobutyric Acid (GABA) and Schizophrenia

Gamma-aminobutyric Acid, the most abundant inhibitory neurotransmitter in the brain, has long been hypothesized to have a role in the pathophysiology of schizophrenia. Previous studies of postmortem brain tissue and CSF have described abnormalities (primarily reduction) in GABA neuronal activity in schizophrenia. However, the results have been neither consistent nor free of potential confounding effects, such as antipsychotic drug treatment. Moreover, GABA neuronal function is closely linked to DA and glutamatergic systems, two neurotransmitters of great significance in current conceptions of neuropsychiatric disease mechanisms. Recently, GABA receptor subtypes have been identified and genes that code for the receptor subunits have been cloned. Thus, one would expect GABAergic function to be a fruitful area of investigation in schizophrenia. However, we could only find a few studies of GABA in schizophrenia conducted in the last 5 years, and these were indirect neurochemical investigations. Interestingly, the lowest GABA uptake-site binding was found in the left hippocampus and correlated inversely with DA concentration in the amygdala. The authors speculated that a reduction of the inhibitory effects of GABA neurons (via GABA or colocalized cholecystokinin [CCK]) could lead to increased DA activity in mesiotemporal structures. Perhaps the enthusiasm for investigating GABA in schizophrenia has been limited by methodological difficulties such as its biochemical assay and the lack of peripheral measures. The GABA strategy for treatment of schizophrenia (as well as tardive dyskinesia [TD]) has been largely unsuccessful; the main therapeutic application for GABAergic compounds is in seizure disorders. Nevertheless, further investigation of GABA in schizophrenia is warranted. GABA probably will not provide a "single-bullet" explanation to the pathophysiology of schizophrenia, but it could be involved in the disease through its interactions with other aminergic and peptidergic neurotransmitters.[54,55]

Glutamate and Schizophrenia

In the last few years there has been a burgeoning interest in EAA and their role in schizophrenia. Although the involvement of glutamate was proposed over a decade ago, significant interest developed only after the nature and function of the glutamatergic system and its receptor subtypes were identified. Of specific importance was the understanding of the role of glutamate neurotransmission in the induction of long-term potentiation (LTP), the physiologic process believed to be central in learning and memory. Moreover, phencyclidine (PCP), a potent psychotogenic drug that causes symptoms similar to those of schizophrenia and led to the development of an etiologic hypothesis of schizophrenia, was found to be a noncompetitive antagonist of N-methyl-D-aspartic acid (NMDA)-mediated neurotransmission. Added impetus came from studies that linked neurotoxicity to various pathologic conditions including epilepsy, cerebrovascular ischemia, Huntington's disease, and other neuropsychiatric disorders.[56]

In the wake of these developments the topic has been reviewed frequently, and at least five different theoretical models have been proposed that relate glutamate dysfunction to schizophrenia. These models include the following: (1) Activation of DA receptors on corticofugal glutamatergic nerve terminals (which inhibit glutamate release) that may lead to deficient glutamatergic neurotransmission; (2) Decreased activation of NMDA receptors located on DA nerve terminals that inhibits DA release and may cause increased DA release; (3) Glutamate and DA independently modulate GABA-mediated inhibition of the excitatory thalamocortical pathway. This pathway is an important component of the corticostriatothalamocortical circuit that gates sensory input to the cortex; (4) Abnormal genetic regulation of NMDA receptors leading to a persistence of immature forms into adulthood may lead to the development of schizophrenic symptoms; and (5) Disturbance in the normal development of cortical glutamatergic neurons leads to increased innervation of the frontal cortex.[57,58]

Surprisingly, however, there has been a dearth of actual data related to glutamate activity in schizophrenia. Other than four earlier studies of CSF glutamate levels, we could find only one direct clinical neurochemical investigation in schizophrenia. In addition, several postmortem studies have provided some interesting, though inconsistent, results. Several investigators have reported decreased glutamate binding in medial temporal cortical areas of postmortem tissue of schizophrenia patients.[59]

NEUROPEPTIDE ABNORMALITIES IN SCHIZOPHRENIA

Cholecystokinin and Schizophrenia

Early studies focused on the use of behaviorally active neuropeptides as treatment agents but found they had little clinical efficacy. Clinical neurochemical studies of peptides have consisted largely of measurements of CSF concentrations of different neuropeptides and yielded conflicting results. Attention was focused on CCK when Hokfelt reported that it coexisted with DA in a subset of mesencephalic DA neurons. Current research into the interaction between DA and CCK indicates that they interact at both the presynaptic and postsynaptic levels in the nucleus accumbens.[60]

Recently cholecystokinin (CCK) mRNA has also been shown to coexist in DA cells in the ventral mesencephalon of a human with schizophrenia. CCK has been found to display many characteristics of a neurotransmitter or neuromodulator. In clinical studies, basal levels of CSF CCK were reduced in drug-free schizophrenia patients in comparison to controls, and the rapidity of response to haloperidol was inversely related to baseline CSF CCK levels. Earlier studies of schizophrenia and control subjects had found increased, decreased, or no difference in CSF CCK and increased, decreased, or no difference in postmortem brains. Most of the studies of the efficacy of CCK peptides in the treatment of schizophrenia, including the most recent double-blind crossover study of CCK-8, found no significant antipsychotic effect.[61]

CCK has also been shown to have potent excitatory effects on DA cells and potentiate DA-mediated behaviors, and it has therefore been proposed that CCK antagonists instead of agonists could have antipsychotic actions. Clinical studies with apomorphine and other CCK antagonists may be warranted.[62]

Neurotensin and Schizophrenia

Another neuropeptide, neurotensin (NT), has been shown to interact with DA in physiological, anatomical, and behavioral studies. It is colocalized with DA in hypothalamic and midbrain neurons and mimics many of the actions of antipsychotic drugs when administered centrally. Acute and chronic haloperidol treatment increases NT concentrations in the nucleus accumbens and caudate nucleus, whereas clozapine, interestingly, leads to an increase of NT in the nucleus accumbens but not the caudate. Changes in NT concentration appear to be specific to schizophrenia since no differences in CSF NT concentration have been found in patients with other disorders, including depression, Alzheimer's disease, anorexia-bulimia, or premenstrual syndrome. Lower levels of CSF NT in schizophrenia patients have been noted while low CSF NT was associated with therapeutic response to antipsychotic drug treatment. Greater knowledge about NT actions and pathology in schizophrenia may lead to improved understanding of schizophrenia and improved insight for the development of new pharmacologic agents.[63]

Other Neuropeptides and Schizophrenia

Other neuropeptides have recently been studied, including substance P (SP), dynorphin A, neuropeptide Y (NY), peptide YY (PYY), and somatostatin. SP is present in the substantia nigra, striatum, hypothalamus, spinal cord, caudate, olfactory tubercle, and frontal cortex and interacts with the DA system. Chronic treatment with haloperidol, pimozide, or fluphenazine, but not clozapine or sulpiride, decreases SP concentrations in the substantia nigra but not the striatum or hypothalamus. Measurements of SP in postmortem brains have been inconsistent. Studies have found increased CSF NY in drug free schizophrenia patients as compared to controls or no difference in CSF NY between schizophrenia or control subjects. CSF NY was found to be decreased with age and duration of illness and in association with abnormalities on computed tomography (CT) scan.[64]

Somatostatin is distributed abundantly throughout the CNS, with high concentrations in subcortical regions and cortex. Somatostatin stimulates DA release from the striatum and DA in turn stimulates somatostatin release from various regions. It also increases the turnover of DA, NE, 5-HT, and acetylcholine; stimulates 5-HT release; inhibits acetylcholine release; both stimulates and inhibits NE release; is inhibited by GABA; and is stimulated by acetylcholine. Clinical studies have demonstrated abnormalities of the somatostatin neurons in various neuropsychiatric disorders such as depression, Alzheimer's disease, Parkinson's disease, vascular dementia, and multiple sclerosis. Postmortem studies of patients with schizophrenia have found decreased somatostatin concentrations in the hippocampus and frontal cortex.[65]

The results of CSF studies of somatostatin have been less consistent. Recent studies of somatostatin in schizophrenia have found that CSF somatostatin was significantly decreased in chronic schizophrenia subjects with moderate cognitive impairment. These results are consistent with other studies that have found decreased levels, especially in those neuropsychiatric diseases that include cognitive impairment. Given the preclinical evidence for the interaction between the DA and somatostatin systems, the localization of somatostatin in regions critical in the pathophysiology of schizophrenia (prefrontal cortex, striatum, amygdala, and nucleus accumbens), and some clinical data that suggest a functional interaction between somatostatin, DA, and psychopathology, there has been little current investigation. Somatostatin, NT, CCK, and SP have thus all been reported to interact with DA, and abnormalities of these and other neuropeptides (NY, PYY, dynorphin A) have been found in schizophrenia. Since direct evidence of DA abnormalities in schizophrenia is lacking, future studies of neuropeptides that may modulate DA neuronal activity are warranted.[66]

Phospholipids and Schizophrenia

Several investigators have previously hypothesized that schizophrenia may involve abnormalities in the composition and structure of neuronal membranes. Early studies of membrane phospholipid pathology in schizophrenia patients found increased phosphatidylserine (PS), decreased phosphatidylcholine (PC) and phosphatidylethanolamine (PE), and altered anisotropy, reflecting fluidity of the plasma membrane phospholipid bilayer. This research has prompted further studies to replicate these findings. In recent years, there has been continued interest in this area of research and other phospholipid abnormalities have been identified.[67]

Phospholipase A2 (PLA2) is a key enzyme in the metabolism of phospholipids that is concentrated in neuronal membranes and plays an essential role in establishing and maintaining membrane structure. Two recent studies examined PLA2 activity in schizophrenia patients with differing results. In one, patients, had increased PLA2 activity that decreased with treatment. This abnormality appeared to be specific for schizophrenia subjects as no difference was found between nonschizophrenia psychiatric patients and controls. Methodological differences, such as cell culture technique, or subject differences, such as medication status, may account for the discrepant results.[68]

Other studies of phospholipids have involved the measurement of prostaglandins precursors, the essential fatty acids (EFA), and plasma phospholipids. There are two series of EFAs derived from different dietary sources, and both appear to be involved with the DA system. The n-6 EFAs have been shown to influence the amount of DA release from the caudate in response to electrical shock, and both n-6 and n-3 EFAs may be involved in presynaptic receptor control of DA release. Three studies have found abnormalities in EFAs in platelets of schizophrenia patients, although the results have not been entirely consistent. Thus, abnormalities have been found in the fatty acid composition of plasma phospholipids in schizophrenia patients with perhaps the most consistent finding across the studies being a reduction of linoleic acid. Another aspect of phospholipid metabolism and function that has been investigated is the platelet phosphoinositide (PI) system. PIs are membrane phospholipids that are hydrolyzed to the second messengers diacylglycerol (AG) and inositol triphosphate (IP3) following activation of certain receptors.[69]

There is also some evidence to indicate that D2 receptor stimulation indirectly suppresses PI hydrolysis, which, if true, would suggest that hyperdopaminergia in schizophrenia may be related to decreased PI turnover. Findings of phospholipid abnormalities in schizophrenia are also consistent with a recent study of membrane phospholipids and high energy phosphate metabolism by *in vivo* phosphorous 31 nuclear magnetic resonance spectroscopy. First-episode, drug-naive schizophrenia patients had significantly decreased levels of phosphomonoesters and inorganic orthophosphate and increased levels of phosphodiesters and adenosine triphosphate in the dorsal prefrontal cortex as compared to healthy controls, suggestive of functional hypoactivity in this region. The alterations in membrane phospholipid metabolism suggested a role for neuronal membrane development in the pathophysiology of schizophrenia, especially since their sample consisted of never medicated first-episode patients. Phospholipids may thus represent a window into the intracellular events that may be related to the pathophysiology of schizophrenia.[70]

Psychoneuroendocrinology and Schizophrenia

The psychoneuroendocrine strategy for research in neuropsychiatric disorders is based on the unique anatomic relationship of the pituitary gland to the hypothalamus and CNS. Pituitary hormone secretion is predominantly regulated by neurochemical mechanisms. Thus, examination of the secretory patterns of pituitary hormones enables investigators to measure indirectly the neurochemical activity of specific brain structures involved in a given hormone's regulation. The specific anatomic level, that is, pituitary, hypothalamic, or suprahypothalamic, can be determined through the use of pharmacologic probes, for example, releasing factors, and neurotransmitter agonists and antagonists. Following the inception of this approach, numerous neuroendocrine studies of schizophrenia were performed. Enthusiasm for this strategy has waned somewhat in recent years due to its failure to produce clear-cut pathophysiologic findings. Although neuroendocrine investigations are waning, this continues to be an active and potentially fruitful area.[71]

Growth Hormone and Schizophrenia

Of the various pituitary and peripheral endocrine hormones, Prolactin (PRL) and growth hormone have been studied most extensively. This is primarily due to the fact that DA is the major neurotransmitter involved in their regulation. In the case of PRL, DA is secreted into the portal vein and acts as a tonic inhibitor of lactotrophic cell secretion. Thus, enhanced DA levels or receptor sensitivity could be expected to produce diminished PRL secretion. GH, on the other hand, is physically stimulated by DA input to the arcuate nucleus of the hypothalamus, which in turn secretes GH releasing factor and suppression of somatostatin to the anterior pituitary. Because DA drives down relatively low basal concentrations of PRL but stimulates GH, the latter has been more productively investigated.[72]

Various abnormalities in GH secretion have been extensively described in a large number of studies. These studies included differences between schizophrenia patients and control subjects in basal levels, 24-hour and diurnal secretory patterns, and responses to stimulation with pharmacologic agents. Most studies in schizophrenia have involved hypothalamic pituitary axis-mediated GH responses to pharmacologic challenges. Apomorphine is one of the DA agonists most frequently used, since the increment of GH following drug administration is mediated by DA receptors and is blocked by antipsychotic drugs. Past studies have varied greatly in many respects including drug-free period, chronicity of illness, and age, weight, and sex of the patient samples. Furthermore, an increased GH response was associated with greater severity of thought disorder. There was also an association at the trend level between increased GH response at or shortly before the time of relapse. GH response was also related to positive symptoms.[73]

Two other DA agonists that have been used as pharmacologic probes of GH are bromocriptine and methylphenidate. Methylphenidate is an indirect-acting DA agonist that can activate psychotic symptoms in some schizophrenia patients. Past studies found decreased GH response to methylphenidate but GH response to methylphenidate did not distinguish schizophrenia from nonschizophrenia patients, although basal GH and peak GH response was correlated with psychopathology in the schizophrenia patients.[74]

Growth hormone releasing factor (GHRF) stimulates GH release from somatotropin cells and can be used to characterize the anatomic level of GH dysregulation in schizophrenia. Exogenous GHRF stimulates the pituitary directly, thereby allowing evaluation of pituitary function. There have been three recent reports of GH response to GHRF in schizophrenia but none had a placebo-controlled design and all had a small sample size. Consistent with other studies, all found basal GH did not differentiate schizophrenia subjects from controls or patients with major depression. Neuroendocrine challenges evaluating GH response have assessed other neurotransmitter systems besides DA in schizophrenia. These results, in particular, need to be considered preliminary since there have been few such studies and no replications. Finally, GH response to serotonergic agents has been used to determine serotonergic dysfunction in schizophrenia. Authors used fenfluramine, which acts primarily by increasing 5-HT release and blocking 5-HT uptake, and got different results than those who used the precursor amino acid L-tryptophan, which acts by increasing 5-HT synthesis.[75]

These studies have used alterations in GH, either of basal levels or in response to pharmacologic challenges, to assess the role and pathology of different neurotransmitter systems in schizophrenia. Overall, the subtle alterations of basal GH, the normal response to GHRH (in two of three studies), and abnormalities of GH response to various agents suggest a suprapituitary abnormality. It seems likely that more than one neurotransmitter system is involved since GH response to dopaminergic, serotonergic, GABAergic, and noradrenergic agents have been abnormal or have been correlated with psychopathology or treatment response. Still, given the differences observed between acute and chronic patients and between neuroleptic free and medicated patients, the role of patient characteristics must be carefully considered.[76]

Prolactin Responses in Schizophrenia

PRL levels in schizophrenia could be used to predict global outcome. Researchers found a weak correlation between PRL level and clinical response to haloperidol in the 5–20 mg/day dosage range. However, this relationship was much stronger for the 5 mg dosage group. Thus, they concluded that PRL levels may be helpful in determining the lowest effective dosage. Plasma PRL levels above 30 ng/mL were not associated with a significant increase in response. PRL levels may be correlated with clinical response to antipsychotic drugs as long as the dose is low enough to remain below the PRL "ceiling" and on the linear slope of the dose-response curve. In related studies that illustrate the potential interaction between drug treatment and pathophysiology, authors have examined PRL response to an acute parenteral administration of haloperidol in stable outpatient schizophrenia subjects before their assignment to continued maintenance treatment with standard or low doses of fluphenazine decanoate. They found that lower peak PRL responses to haloperidol were associated with an increased risk of relapse and suggested that blunted PRL response may reflect upregulation of D2 receptors in the anterior pituitary and is a neuroendocrine analog of the process that underlies the development of TD in the striatum.[77,78]

Thyroid Releasing Hormone and Schizophrenia

Disturbances of the hypothalamic-pituitary-thyroid (HPT) axis have been demonstrated in some psychiatric disorders, particularly in patients with affective illnesses. There have been relatively few studies evaluating this axis in schizophrenia, although a few previous studies have described some abnormalities. The thyroid releasing hormone (TRH) test has been the main method used to evaluate the HPT function in schizophrenia and has been widely used to examine the HPT axis in patients with MDD. No significant differences were found between basal or peak TSH in schizophrenia patients compared to control subjects.[79]

Also, in an attempt to evaluate the relationship between affective illness and TRH response, authors found that schizophrenia patients with a family history of affective disorder had significantly lower TSH responses than those with a family history of schizophrenia. Those studies that examined correlations between clinical variables and psychopathology did not find any association with abnormalities on the TRH test. Most of these studies were conducted in patients receiving neuroleptic treatment at the time of testing and although some did evaluate drug-free and drug treated patients separately, the relatively small sample sizes may have limited their findings. Further studies using larger samples controlled for medication status are needed. Furthermore, a closer look at schizoaffective and schizophrenia patients with family history of affective illness is warranted since abnormalities on the TRH tests may differentiate them.[80]

Oxytocin and Schizophrenia

Bujanow suggested for the first time the possibility of oxytocin as an anti-schizophrenic hormone. Normal startle (Pulse) is usually suppressed if preceded by a weaker stimulus (pre-pulse). In schizophrenia this normal prepulse inhibition (PPI) is impaired. Subcutaneous injections of oxytocin in doses of 0.04 to 1 mg/kg restored PPI that has been reduced by the NMDA antagonist dizocilpine. In a study using oxytocin knockout mice greater PPI deficits were noted. PPI is disrupted by apomorphine, amphetamine and phencyclidine, all of which are implicated in schizophrenia. Rats treated with antipsychotics have elevated levels of oxytocin. Elevated levels of oxytocin were recorded in schizophrenia but in some cases decreased levels were also noted.[81]

Chronic administration of the psychotomimetic phencyclidine caused social deficits and decreased oxytocin finding in the hypothalamus but increased oxytocin binding in central amygdala. Oxytocin administration into central amygdale reversed the social deficits. Recently authors administered daily intranasal spray of oxytocin in a placebo controlled double blind crossover study in schizophrenia patients having residual symptoms who were undergoing maintenance treatment with antipsychotic drugs. They noted highly significant improvement in symptoms as measured by Positive and Negative Symptoms Scale (PANSS) and Clinical Global Impression (CGI) scale. Further, they noted that oxytocin was well tolerated and produced minimal side effects. Further studies however are warranted in this area.[82]

NEUROIMAGING FINDINGS

Structural Neuroimaging and Schizophrenia

Structural imaging methodologies have proven to be powerful tools enabling the recognition of fundamental brain abnormalities in schizophrenia. To date, these include evidence for widespread deficits in cortical gray matter volumes, regional reductions in heteromodal association cortex and temporolimbic structures, and nonspecific increases in ventricular size, thereby implicating dysfunction of neural circuits involving cortical, thalamic, basal ganglia, and limbic structures in the pathogenesis of the illness. Presumably, the identified patterns of regional change are related to characteristic symptoms of the disorder, although there are still no consistently demonstrated clinicopathologic correlates. The emerging evidence that affected neocortical regions comprise components of the heteromodal neocortical association network may provide a framework for further investigating the otherwise elusive brain structure-function relationships. Furthermore, the converging role of heteromodal regions in both the expression of neuroanatomic gender differences and in normal cerebral asymmetries suggests that disruption of these cortical areas in schizophrenia may be important to the clinical expression of the disease, including clinical differences between men and women with schizophrenia. The continued development of techniques for investigating the brain will ensure that structural neuroimaging will remain a strong contender in helping to address questions related to the origin and mechanism of brain alterations in schizophrenia.[83]

Prior to the advent of MRI, brain abnormalities in schizophrenia were based on crude measurements such as measuring the volume of plaster casts from postmortem brains, and pneumoencephalographic studies, both of which were used to measure ventricular size. The latter studies were quite invasive as they involved pushing air into the brain cavity. Many of these studies, nonetheless, along with CT studies, described above, showed enlarged ventricles in the brains of patients with schizophrenia. MRI studies of schizophrenia have also observed ventricular enlargement in schizophrenia, with approximately 80% of MRI studies reporting this enlargement. Enlarged lateral ventricles, however, are not pathognomonic of schizophrenia, as they are also observed in hydrocephalus, Alzheimer's disease, and other neurodegenerative diseases where brain is replaced by CSF. MRI findings in schizophrenia are relatively similar in terms of the percentage of studies showing abnormalities. More specifically, it was observed that 80% of the studies revealed enlarged lateral ventricles, 73% revealed enlarged third ventricles, and there was a preferential involvement of medial temporal lobe structures (74%) that included amygdala, hippocampus, parahippocampal gyrus, and neocortical temporal lobe structures, i.e. superior temporal gyrus (100% if gray and white matter were differentiated), and moderate evidence for frontal lobe involvement (59% of studies), most notably prefrontal cortex and orbitofrontal cortex. Other brain regions involved, and reported in this earlier review, included parietal lobe abnormalities (60% of studies), particularly inferior parietal lobule, which includes supramarginal gyrus and angular gyrus. Other findings included subcortical abnormalities, including cavum septum pellucidum (92% of studies), basal ganglia (68% of studies), corpus callosum (63% of studies), thalamus (42% of studies), and cerebellum (31% of studies). These numbers have not changed appreciably with the increase in MRI studies since 2001, but they do highlight the fact that there are multiple focal brain regions that are abnormal in schizophrenia, which are not necessarily proximal but which may nonetheless be involved in brain circuits that are abnormal in schizophrenia.[84,85]

Functional Neuroimaging and Schizophrenia

One of the fundamental goals in understanding schizophrenia is linking the observable symptoms to the underlying unobservable pathophysiology. Given recent advances in medical imaging, researchers are increasingly investigating brain-behavior relationships to better understand the neural substrates of negative, positive, and disorganization symptoms in schizophrenia. There have been 28 task-related functional magnetic resonance imaging studies in schizophrenia that have found meaningful small to moderate associations between specific symptom dimensions and regional brain activity. Negative symptoms were related to the functioning of the ventrolateral prefrontal cortex and ventral striatum. Positive symptoms, particularly persecutory ideation, were related to functioning of the medial prefrontal cortex, amygdala, and hippocampus/parahippocampal region. Disorganization symptoms, although less frequently evaluated, were related to functioning of the dorsolateral prefrontal cortex. Surprisingly, no symptom domain had a consistent relationship with the middle or superior temporal regions. While a number of adaptations in experimental design and reporting standards can facilitate this work, current neuroimaging approaches appear to provide a number of consistent links between the manifest symptoms of schizophrenia and brain dysfunction.[86,87]

Diffusion Tensor Imaging and Schizophrenia

Both postmortem and neuroimaging studies have contributed significantly to what we know about the brain and schizophrenia. MRI studies of volumetric reduction in several brain regions in schizophrenia have confirmed early speculations that the brain is disordered in schizophrenia. There is also a growing body of evidence suggesting that a disturbance in connectivity between different brain regions, rather than abnormalities within the separate regions themselves, are responsible for the clinical symptoms and cognitive dysfunctions observed in this disorder. Thus an interest in white matter fiber tracts, subserving anatomical connections between distant, as well as proximal, brain regions, is emerging. This interest coincides with the recent advent of diffusion tensor imaging (DTI), which makes it possible to evaluate the organization and coherence of white matter fiber tracts. This is an important advance as conventional MRI techniques are insensitive to fiber tract direction and organization, and have not consistently demonstrated white matter abnormalities. DTI may, therefore, provide important new information about neural circuitry, and it is increasingly being used in neuroimaging studies of psychopathological disorders. Of note, in the past five years 18 DTI studies in schizophrenia have been published, most describing white matter abnormalities.[88,89]

Spect and Pet Studies

Over the last ten years, several positron emission tomography (PET) and single photon computerized tomography (SPECT) studies of the dopamine (DA) system in patients with schizophrenia were performed to test the hypothesis that DA hyperactivity is associated with this illness. There have 15 brain imaging studies comparing indices of DA function in drug naive or drug free patients with schizophrenia and healthy controls: 13 studies included measurement of DA D2 receptors density, 2 studies compared amphetamine-induced DA release, and 2 studies measured DOPA decarboxylase activity, an enzyme involved in DA synthesis. Analysis of the studies revealed that, compared to healthy controls, patients with schizophrenia present a significant but mild elevation of D2 receptor density parameters and a significant larger variability of these indices. Studies performed with radiolabeled butyrophenones detected a larger increase in D2 receptor density parameters than studies performed with other radioligands, such as benzamides. Studies of presynaptic activity revealed an increase in DA transmission response to amphetamine challenge, and an increase in DOPA decarboxylase activity. Together, these data are compatible with both pre- and postsynaptic alterations of DA transmission in schizophrenia. Future studies should aim at a better characterization of these alterations, and at defining their role in the pathophysiology of the illness.[90,91]

Neuropathology of Schizophrenia

Despite a hundred years' research, the neuropathology of schizophrenia remains obscure. However, neither can the null hypothesis be sustained—that it is a 'functional' psychosis, a disorder with no structural basis. A number of abnormalities have been identified and confirmed by meta-analysis, including ventricular enlargement and decreased cerebral (cortical and hippocampal) volume. These are characteristic of schizophrenia as a whole, rather than being restricted to a subtype, and are present in first-episode, unmedicated patients. There is considerable evidence for preferential involvement of the temporal lobe and moderate evidence for an alteration in normal cerebral asymmetries. There are several candidates for the histological and molecular correlates of the macroscopic features. The probable proximal explanation for decreased cortical volume is reduced neuropil and neuronal size, rather than a loss of neurons. These morphometric changes are in turn suggestive of alterations in synaptic, dendritic and axonal organization, a view supported by immunocytochemical and ultrastructural findings.[92]

Pathology in subcortical structures is not well established, apart from dorsal thalamic nuclei, which are smaller and contain fewer neurons. Other cytoarchitectural features of schizophrenia which are often discussed, notably entorhinal cortex heterotopias and hippocampal neuronal disarray, remain to be studied. Functional imaging data indicate that the pathophysiology of schizophrenia reflects aberrant activity in, and integration of, the components of distributed circuits involving the prefrontal cortex, hippocampus and certain subcortical structures. It is hypothesized that the neuropathological features represent the anatomical substrate of these functional abnormalities in neural connectivity. Investigation of this proposal is a goal of current neuropathological studies, which must also seek (i) to establish which of the recent histological findings are robust and cardinal, and (ii) to define the relationship of the pathological phenotype with the clinical syndrome, its neurochemistry and its pathogenesis.[93,94]

CONCLUSION

Schizophrenia is a common and debilitating illness, characterized by chronic psychotic symptoms and psychosocial impairment that exact considerable human and economic costs. Although studied extensively from a clinical, psychological, biological and genetic perspective, our expanding knowledge of schizophrenia provides only an incomplete understanding of this complex disorder. Recent advances in neuroscience have allowed the confirmation or refutation of earlier findings in schizophrenia, and permit useful comparisons between the different levels of organization from which the illness has been studied. Schizophrenia is defined as a clinical syndrome that may include a collection of diseases that share a common presentation. A neurodevelopmental rather than degenerative process has received more empirical support as a general explanation of the pathophysiology, although simple dichotomies are not particularly helpful in such a complicated disease.

Structural brain changes are present *in vivo* and postmortem, with both histopathological and imaging studies in overall agreement that the temporal and frontal lobes of the cerebral cortex are the most affected. Functional imaging, neuropsychological testing and clinical observation are also generally consistent in demonstrating deficits in cognitive ability that correlate with abnormalities in the areas of the brain with structural abnormalities. The dopamine and other neurotransmitter systems are certainly involved in the treatment or modulation of psychotic symptoms. These broad findings represent the distillation of a large body of disparate data, but firm and specific findings are sparse, and much about schizophrenia remains unknown.

6.4 SCHIZOPHRENIA: GENETICS

Avinash De Souza, Nilesh Shah

INTRODUCTION

The schizophrenias are common disorders with a lifetime prevalence of 0.85–1.0% in most populations. Because we know that genes are largely responsible for the disorder therefore at least 0.85% of the population have inherited disease alleles for schizophrenia. Although there are weaknesses in applying classical behavior genetic methods in human populations. The strength of the molecular genetic evidence has proven that schizophrenia is extremely heterogeneous with many different gene loci involved. Another level of complexity is the obvious allelic and haplotypic heterogeneity with respect to disease alleles. The mode of transmission cannot be determined in the presence of this extreme heterogeneity. The first few etiological base pair changes affecting the *DISC1*, *PCM1* and *SYN2* genes causing schizophrenia have now been reported. For the first time, it has become clear that multiple chromosomal deletions and duplications are responsible for a sizable proportion of the genetic susceptibility to schizophrenia.[95]

Striking overlap for some of these deletion and duplication mutations has been found between epilepsy and schizophrenia and their existence explains a well established clinical comorbidity. Pharmacogenomic strategies for the design of new drug treatments have finally become of great importance because of the identification of etiological base changes. The effects of these changes will dictate how new drugs must be designed either by targeting the pathogenetic systems that are implicated by genetics but also by pointing to what type and directionality of effect is needed by agonist or antagonist or other types of drugs.[96]

FAMILY GENETIC STUDIES IN SCHIZOPHRENIA

Observations of the familial recurrence of schizophrenia cannot be interpreted as providing evidence for the relative importance of cultural, family environment and unique (specific) nonfamilial environmental factors compared to the effects of genes unless the results of several behavior genetic approaches are considered together and compared. The accurate determination of recurrence in relatives is dependent on accurate diagnosis. An important finding is that the diagnosis of schizophrenia is more stable within individuals than is bipolar disorder which is often misdiagnosed as schizophrenia in young males. Authors have found that 92.5% of schizophrenics had a stable diagnosis over a 30–40 year period whereas only 78.3% of bipolar cases had stable diagnoses. This will mean that more cases of bipolar disorder are likely to be incorrectly identified as cases of schizophrenia than vice versa. All family twin and adoption studies have observed that the incidence of the illness in the relatives of schizophrenic probands is considerably greater than in suitable family or population controls.[97]

Given that we now know that schizophrenia is extraordinarily heterogeneous, an important clinical question is to ask to what extent different subtypes of schizophrenia can recur within the same families. Family studies have shown that, within a family, shared genotypes can give rise to clinical diversity within the schizophrenia spectrum. The corollary to this is that clinical heterogeneity does not imply underlying genetic heterogeneity. Although there is little evidence for the proband schizophrenia subtype to breed true other work has suggested a tendency towards homotypia within families with the paranoid and hebephrenic subtypes. Some families have been reported with multiple cases of catatonic schizophrenia. Others have put forward the idea that the hebephrenic form of schizophrenia may be more heritable than the paranoid variety. Tsuang and Winokur have proposed that there is a catatonic-hebephrenic-paranoid continuum of illness with the catatonic type being the most advanced and severe form.[98]

Kendler and others showed that the risk in all interviewed relatives of schizophrenic probands the risk was 6.5% for schizophrenia, 6.8% for schizoaffective disorder and 6.9% for schizotypal personality disorder, 5.1% for nonaffective psychoses, 2.8% for psychotic affective illness and 0.6% for nonpsychotic affective illness. This makes a total of 23.6% of relatives with severe psychiatric disorder. These were very much higher risks than those found for controls. Individuals with schizophrenia were found to have 75% reduced fertility.

The risk for schizophrenia in the parents of probands was much less than that found in siblings indicating partial or incomplete penetrance. These studies also show that the schizophrenia found in these families did not have any strong familial relationship with bipolar affective disorder.[99]

More recently in a meta-analysis of 39 family studies of the first degree relatives of bipolar probands there was no significant increase the rate of schizophrenia compared to control families. In the first degree relatives of probands with schizophrenia there was a small but significant increase in the rate of bipolar disorder compared to controls. This can be explained by assortative mating for schizophrenia and bipolar disorder in the parental generation, i.e. "marrying in" of a family with one disorder to another family with the other disorder. Alternatively misdiagnosis could explain the increased rate of bipolar disorder in the families of a schizophrenic proband with the predicted effect being that a young male bipolar may have been incorrectly designated as being schizophrenic when in fact the illness was a severe mania with schizoaffective symptoms.[100]

GENETIC ASPECTS OF GENDER AND SCHIZOPHRENIA

Until recently it was generally accepted that the prevalence of schizophrenia in males as opposed to females was equal. Some studies have evidence that schizophrenia is commoner in males. Such effects are sometimes called age distribution or decade of birth effects. Kendler and Walsh reviewed twin and family studies before 1995 in order to identify sex effects in the recurrence of schizophrenia in the siblings of schizophrenic probands. They comment that the early twin studies found greater concordance in female/female MZ pairs. The later twin studies showed higher concordances for male/male pairs. The DZ concordances by sex showed no consistent result. Some family studies have found risk of the disease in first-degree relatives to be greater for female probands than for male probands. Family studies which used personal interviews also found significantly less risk of recurrence in the relatives of males than females. Therefore the difference in female and male rates of schizophrenia cannot logically be attributed to the greater rates of in utero or perinatal trauma known to occur in males rather than females.[101]

Given that the X chromosome is the largest human chromosome, it is entirely feasible that there are X-linked semi-dominant or recessive gene susceptibilities to schizophrenia or that genes on this chromosome may increase penetrance for autosomal schizophrenia susceptibility genes in males. A German research group has also found evidence for excess same sex concordance. It seems likely that there have been samples that truly show an excess of same sex concordance but it is uncertain whether this is due to sampling bias or sex chromosome epistatic effects. If the X chromosome does carry susceptibility genes for schizophrenia then this would indeed produce a slight excess of both female/female as well as male/male affected sibling pairs.[102]

STUDIES ON GENETIC ANTICIPATION

Age of onset variation is known to be an important consequence of underlying genetic pathology. It appears to be a well defined variable, but it is easy to introduce selection biases in study samples and valid conclusions may be elusive. Correlations in age at onset between relatives can be used to predict risk to relatives at a given age. An early age at onset was associated with higher risk of illness in siblings and nieces/nephews but not in children. They found that age of onset is correlated between twins. In the Roscommon schizophrenia family study, age of onset was earlier in hebephrenic and catatonic subtypes compared to the later onset paranoid schizophrenic subtype.[103]

The relationship between age of onset in parental and offspring generations and genetic effects has been of great interest since the discovery of gene mutations with trinucleotide repeat insertions, causing diseases such as Huntington's chorea and other neurological disorders. Genomic imprinting which is an epigenetic effect on gene expression, attributed to methylation and other processes during gametogenesis, has been found to differentially alter the expression of genetic diseases in the offspring of transmitting fathers as opposed to transmitting mothers. Authors have reviewed the field and thought it was genuine effect. Although some evidence for trinucleotide repeat gene association with schizophrenia was found by a review and other studies, it was concluded that this type of mutation was not often the cause of anticipation or the cause of a subtype of schizophrenia.[104]

TWIN GENETIC STUDIES IN SCHIZOPHRENIA

The most important assumption of the twin method is that monozygotic (MZ) twins have the same genotype and dizygotic (DZ) twins have on average only 50% of their genes in common while environmental factors in MZ and DZ twins are constant. In fact the special case of twinning may make the assumption of equal environmental effects in families of MZ and DZ twin pairs questionable. Another complication of the twin method is that twins may have different in utero environments such as transfusion syndrome or be monochorionic or dichorionic. However, if one accepts that the twin method has no major flaws then for disorders with a genetic component, there should be greater concordance in monozygotic twins than in dizygotic pairs. This has been found to be true in twin studies of schizophrenia and the MZ:DZ concordance ratio is consistently in excess of 3:1. Some of the earlier twin studies suffered from methodological deficiencies, the most important being selection bias, poor zygosity determination, lack of operational diagnostic criteria and lack of age correction. The earlier twin studies showed higher MZ concordances than the more recent twin studies. Population register twin studies tend to show lower MZ concordance than do twins ascertained through consecutive admissions to hospitals.[105]

If the equal-environments assumption of the twin method is invalid for schizophrenia, then shared family environment factors may cause a more similar clinical picture in MZ twins compared to DZ twins even though there is no genetic effect. This could be particularly powerful in monozygotic twins by virtue of shared placental circulation, greater psychological identification with each other and perhaps by their capacity to evoke similar responses by virtue of their physical similarity. Schizotypal personality disorders were found to be more common among the biological relatives of schizophrenic probands but histrionic personality disorders were less common than among relatives of the control probands. Odd speech, inappropriate affect, odd behavior and excessive social anxiety, were significantly more common among the relatives of schizophrenic probands.[106]

If it is accepted that the twin method is a valid approach for the investigation of schizophrenia then estimates made by authors by combining all the available twin study data, suggests that the variance contributed by the family environment in the susceptibility to develop schizophrenia is less than 1.00%. This does not preclude a role for the family in influencing readmission rates and affecting overall prognosis as described in theories concerning expressed emotion in schizophrenia families.[107]

A more sensitive method of demonstrating structural brain changes, cognitive and neurophysiological deficits in schizophrenia is through the use of an MZ twin as a control. This method also controls for age and for polygenic background effects. CT studies performed with this design show consistent increases in ventricle brain ratio in schizophrenia, and MRI studies document reductions in temporal lobe structures as well. Family history of psychosis, history of substance abuse and history of postnatal cerebral trauma were not related to degree of neurological impairment in the ill or healthy cotwins. In the same sample McNeil investigated obstetric complications (OCs) during pregnancy, labor and the neonatal period. Significant differences in OC rates were found in discordant pairs compared to normal control pairs. Labor complications were more frequent in discordant than concordant pairs. OC rates were equal in affected compared to healthy discordant twins. Trauma at the time of labor and delivery and especially prolonged labor appear to be of importance for brain structure anomalies associated within pairs of discordant for schizophrenia.[108]

Sophisticated measurements of brain morphometry can be made with magnetic resonance imaging (MRI). Authors have described reduced temporal lobe volume as well as reduced temporal lobe grey matter in schizophrenia. Another group found whole brain volume to be strongly genetic in MZ and DZ twins with schizophrenia. Variation in hippocampal and ventricular volumes within discordant monozygotic pairs was observed. Hippocampal volumes of probands were smaller than those of their nonschizophrenic MZ and DZ co-twins and healthy twins. Hippocampal volumes of unaffected co-twins were smaller than those of healthy twins, but those of unaffected MZ and DZ co-twins were similar. Significant decreases over time in whole brain and frontal and temporal lobe volumes were found in patients with schizophrenia and their unaffected co-twins compared with control twins. Bivariate genetic models showed additive genetic effects on progressive whole brain changes in schizophrenics as well as genetic effects on frontal lobe and temporal lobe volume changes.[109]

A review and meta-analysis of functional MRI in case control studies, in twins and in cases with family controls found that vulnerability to psychosis was associated with medium to large effect sizes when prefrontal activation was contrasted with that in controls. Relatives of patients affected with psychosis, the co-twins of patients and subjects with an "at risk mental state" shared similar neurocognitive abnormalities. The prefrontal and anterior cingulate cortex, the basal ganglia, hippocampus and cerebellum were most affected. Authors have studied language lateralization and found that it was decreased in discordant twin pairs compared with the healthy twin pairs. They concluded that decreased language lateralization constitutes a genetic predisposition to schizophrenia.[110]

Clearly within pair differences need an explanation and the recent finding of genomic imprinting differences within MZ twin pairs as reflected in differential methylation effects on DNA is a ready explanation. Such effects could combine with other random stochastic processes or in utero biological effects to produce discordance. Such pleiotropy is found for all disease mutations and is not specific to schizophrenia and does not necessarily point to psychosocial environmental effects.[111]

ADOPTION STUDIES IN SCHIZOPHRENIA

Adoption and cross-fostering studies can clarify the respective contributions of the genes and environment because they are more clearly separated than in the twin method. A potential drawback is that the biological parents of adopted children are known to be more deviant with a higher rate of psychiatric disorder, alcoholism and criminality than ordinary parents. Adopting parents are usually carefully screened and it is possible that there is a process of selective placement such that children offered for adoption are placed in homes where the adoptive parents have similar problems to those occurring in the biological parents. In addition one might expect to find a generalized increase in psychiatric disorder in adopted children who are used as controls.[112]

The most well known studies come from a Danish-American collaboration which used the Danish National Adoption register. The studies have been conducted on a Copenhagen sample, then on provincial samples and finally combined into a national sample. All the studies have shown that the adopted-away children of schizophrenics had a significantly higher risk of developing schizophrenia, or schizotypal disorder and related conditions, than the adopted-away children of controls. Most of the children were born before the first episode of illness in the parent and about a third of the schizophrenic parents were male thus weakening arguments that the schizophrenia may have been caused by early mother-child interaction or by an intrauterine event. The data obtained found an increased incidence of schizophrenia and related disorders in the biological relatives of schizophrenics who had been adopted (20.3%) compared to the incidence in adoptive relatives and relatives of controls (5.8%). The data was reanalyzed using DSM III criteria and an incidence of 13.5% incidence for schizophrenia or schizotypal personality in the biological relatives of schizophrenics was found compared with 1.5% in the controls. In the combined national sample of Copenhagen and provincial adoptees, authors commented that chronic schizophrenia in adoptees was found exclusively in the biological relatives of schizophrenics and that the overall prevalence of schizophrenia in adoptees was 10 times greater than the rate in the biological relatives of controls.[113]

SEGREGATION ANALYSIS STUDIES IN SCHIZOPHRENIA

Twin and family data have been used to show that between 66% and 93% of the variance in the etiology of schizophrenia may be genetic in origin. It has been estimated the contribution from the common or family environment to be less than 1% and the family effect to be about 19%. Research suggests that stochastic processes may be partly responsible for the nonfamilial or specific environmental source of etiological variance. Henderson also points out that the specific environmental variance contains an error term, thus potentially diluting the amount of true specific environmental variance in schizophrenia. Nevertheless, the specific environmental component may include a proportion of schizophrenia being due to viral infection, obstetric complications or other nongenetic causes of brain disorder, but it could be argued that the data as a whole shows that the bulk of the schizophrenias are genetic in origin.[114] The fact that so much heterogeneity in the genetic etiology of schizophrenia has been detected implies that all previous attempts to model the genetic transmission of schizophrenia have been flawed.

GENETIC LINKAGE AND ASSOCIATION STUDIES

Considerable effort has been focused on genetic linkage analysis of schizophrenia employing biological markers. This approach must take into account the complication of heterogeneity of linkage in which a number of susceptibility genes localized to different chromosomes, may contribute on their own or in conjunction with other mutant genes to the development of schizophrenia. An attractive strategy in linkage and association studies is to begin work by concentrating on areas where there is an a priori reason for suspecting involvement between marker and disease.[115]

Three approaches to this have been adopted. One has been to investigate favored loci implicated by cytogenetic abnormalities. A second approach is to simply study relevant genes such as neurobiological enzymes, peptides and receptors. The third approach is to detect functional variations in proteins through the identification of genetic variation at the DNA level relevant to the functioning of the resultant protein. Many analysts have tested hypothetical models for transmission for schizophrenia and have predicted the size of family samples needed to detect heterogeneity. Some have argued that schizophrenia is caused by several genes each contributing susceptibility.[116]

Two-trait-locus, two-marker-locus linkage analysis provides much more linkage information than standard one-trait-locus, one-marker-locus methods, even when locus heterogeneity is present. It was found that one-locus models which test for heterogeneity provide as much information as the two-trait-locus methods. The sibling pair method of linkage analysis which has the advantage of not needing to specify a mode of transmission has been developed considerably.[117]

Early attempts at linkage studies in schizophrenia were hampered by the small number of potential markers, usually protein markers, available and their relatively low degree of polymorphism. Thus most studies were largely uninformative. Early studies of association and linkage between the HLA genes and schizophrenia produce consistently negative results with the exception of association between HLA A9 and paranoid schizophrenia. This has been put into reverse with several genome wide association studies now implicating at least three distinct regions between the major histocompatibility regions.[118]

The first evidence for a positive locus of determination score with genetic linkage markers was claimed when investigating a chromosome 5 region implicated by a cytogenetic abnormality. This cytogenetic abnormality was reported from Canada in a Chinese man and his nephew both suffering from schizophrenia, facial dysmorphism and other abnormalities. An area of trisomy on chromosome 5 was found. Linkage studies using probes localized to the chromosomal area 5q11-5q13 were undertaken in five Icelandic and two British families. The results were analyzed using a variety of diagnostic classifications for schizophrenia and its associated disorders. Genetic association studies in the 5q11-13 region have since implicated the Kinesin Interacting Factor 2A (*KIF2A*) gene in susceptibility to schizophrenia.The evidence implicating the more distal region of chromosome 5 at 5q33 is derived from four independent linkage studies reporting lod scores above 3.00. The human *5HT1a* gene has been localized by linkage to the 5q11-13 region 213 and has therefore been excluded in the linkage studies testing the chromosome 5q11-13 linkage hypothesis for schizophrenia.[119]

Evidence from linkage analysis in families that there is a susceptibility locus for schizophrenia on chromosome 6p22.3 has been provided by several groups. However other research groups were unable to detect the presence of this locus in other family samples. Confirmed evidence for linkage at the 6p22.3 locus was followed up with allelic association studies using the family based methods. In general the potential for confounding of linkage with association is most likely when a family sample has already shown linkage to the markers for which there is apparent evidence for association and when the most common alleles and haplotypes appear to be showing association. In the case of the original report of allelic association between *DTNBP1* gene and schizophrenia the same family sample was already known to show good evidence for linkage.[120]

Researchers have studied the role and distribution of dysbindin in brains from schizophrenics and controls. Dysbindin mRNA levels in the frontal cortex, temporal cortex, hippocampus, caudate, putamen, nucleus accumbens, amygdala, thalamus, and midbrain were significantly reduced in schizophrenic brains. In the midbrain there was a reduction of dysbindin in patients, but this was not statistically significant. Significant genotype dependent differences in cortical levels of dysbindin were also observed.[121] Another effect of over expressing dysbindin was an increase in the phosphorylation of AKT1, a gene that itself has been associated with schizophrenia. The trace amine receptor 4 (TRAR4) on 6q has been implicated in a case control association study.[122]

A genome scan reported linkage between schizophrenia and markers on chromosome 22q12-13. They mention that the candidate gene responsible for metachromatic leukodystrophy and rare cases of psychosis (aryl sulphatase), was localized to this region. In a collaborative analysis in a larger sample from five laboratories this linkage could not be confirmed assuming either homogeneity or heterogeneity. The genetic deletion syndrome, velo-cardio-facial (Di George) syndrome, is known to be associated with psychosis in rare cases. The deletions which may include one copy of the catechol-o-methyl transferase (COMT) gene on chromosome 22q11 are likely to be responsible.[123]

NEUROTRANSMITTER RECEPTOR GENES IN SCHIZOPHRENIA

The dopamine neuroreceptor genes which have recently been cloned are of interest because they are known to be one of the sites of action of many antipsychotic drugs. Authors found a significant allelic association between schizophrenia and a rare Ser311Cys mutation in an exon of the *DRD2* gene compared to controls. The effect was most marked in positive family history cases. Researchers have used linkage analysis to exclude a major etiological role for the D4 receptor gene localized near the telomere of chromosome 11p while others have excluded linkage at the DRD5 locus on chromosome 4. After finding a positive locus near the GABA-A locus found a C6G nucleotide transversion at codon 396 predicting a histidine to glutamine substitution in 3 of 86 unrelated schizophrenic cases. This variant showed a recombination with schizophrenia in an affected person within an apparently linked family.[124,125]

CYTOGENETICS IN SCHIZOPHRENIA

Linkage markers mapping to a favored locus, implicated by familial genetic disease associations with schizophrenia and at cytogenetic abnormalities in rare cases of schizophrenia, have been used to choose markers in linkage studies of schizophrenia. Cytogenetic abnormalities reported in combination with schizophrenic psychoses include fragile sites, deletions, pericentric inversions, trisomies and acentric fragments. Many different genetic deletions and duplications, also known as copy number variants have recently been found to contribute to the genetic etiology of schizophrenia. In some samples, between 10% and 20% of cases were found to be positive for these types of mutation. By contrast the yield of positive results from MRI or CT scans is negligible except perhaps in late onset schizophrenic psychoses. This suggests that clinical investigation with microarrays to detect copy number variants will be a much more productive clinical investigation than MRI scans both for diagnosis and a pointer to more personalized drug and behavioral treatments.[126]

The new concept of a "genomic disorder" has been defined as a genetic disease caused by an alteration in DNA copy number consisting of chromosomal deletions and duplications. These phenomena can now be detected systematically whereas previously only very few had been detected. The first CNVs to be detected which could aid diagnosis of schizophrenia were the deletions and duplications on chromosome 22q11.2 found in cases of velo-cardio-facial syndrome (VCFS). These were difficult to detect but proof that schizophrenia being a genomic as well as genetic disorder has recently emerged from scientific papers from several large consortia of schizophrenia researchers. These research groups used microarray technology in which one million lengths of human DNA have been interrogated by hybridization to detect deletions and duplications across the whole genome.[127]

CONCLUSION

The presence of a strong genetic predisposition is by far the most well confirmed etiological effect in schizophrenia. Life events as a precipitating factor are no longer believed enough for anyone to actually carry out further research in this area. Any environmental such effects are very likely to be an epiphenomena of the genes rather having any causal effect. Attention has now shifted towards methlyation and other epigenetic effects to explain the obvious variable penetrance and pleiotropism of the genetic pathology and variation in clinical symptoms. Despite many genes having been implicated the identification of clinical subtypes of schizophrenia is still in its infancy. DNA sequencing of mutations will lead the way here and these will lead to treatments based on individual genetic tests. Molecular genetic methods have also sought to elucidate the mode of action of antipsychotic drugs and have begun to show that many genes and their resultant mRNAs show altered expression in response to antipsychotics. Genetic variation in specific genes will soon be found to correlate with prognosis and treatment response and new less toxic drugs can be created with this information.

Despite decades of research effort, our understanding of the genesis of schizophrenia remains an enigma. The methods used for mapping susceptibility genes have progressed enormously over the past several years. The genome-wide studies have pointed to the role of both common variants as well as rare variants in schizophrenia susceptibility. Furthermore, the number of total susceptibility variants for schizophrenia may be in the order of thousands. Considering the low effect size observed for the associated SNPs the sample size required for replicating these associations with adequate power would theoretically be up to 100,000 each of cases and controls.

The effect of environmental factors, including maternal infection (serological evidence of influenza infection during pregnancy), and recreational drug use/abuse should also be taken into account when conducting association studies in schizophrenia. Cannabis usage is an important risk factor aggravating psychosis, and preonset cannabis use hastens the onset of prodromal symptoms as well as fully developed psychosis. These and likely other environmental factors need to be considered in the design of future genetic studies. Furthermore, epigenetic changes, including both DNA methylation and histone acetylation, have also been suggested to play an important role in development of major psychoses. These epigenetic mechanisms can be influenced by environmental effects such as stress (cortisol) and hormonal factors. Thus we need a comprehensive systems biology approach to incorporate the effect of genetic and nongenetic factors to understand the genesis of schizophrenia and related disorders.

At this juncture in the research effort, investigations of schizophrenia have demonstrated that genetic factors indeed have an important role to play in its genesis. However, to progress further we need better phenotypic classification of our patients. A major area of development in this regard is the steady advance of neuroimaging technology. We now can have phenotypes of the volume of the dorsal lateral prefrontal cortex, or the connectivity between different brain regions. It should be the case that more accurate study of the target organ in schizophrenia research, that is the brain, will lead to more objective and reliable associations with genetic variants. Also, the methods to capture the complete variability of the genome (as well as the epigenome) will add to the comprehensiveness of the measurement of DNA based information. Furthermore, a concerted effort is needed to understand the biology (the annotation) of the disease-associated genes. These genes will help us in identifying novel targets for drug development and thereby improve the efficacy of the treatment. The discovery of genetic factors also leads to the consideration of whether or not it is useful to perform genetic testing in a clinical setting.

Most regulatory authorities agree that genetic testing for schizophrenia is premature at this stage, given the small odds ratios and inconsistent replications reviewed above. Until some as-yet unknown approach is achieved to combine large numbers of small effect genes into meaningful prediction algorithms, we are likely facing many more years of research before acceptable testing for risk is possible. Through the continued efforts of careful investigation in genetics of schizophrenia that embrace the nuances of phenotype and the latest technological developments, the field has an excellent chance to solve the etiologic puzzle of this enigmatic disorder.

6.5 SCHIZOPHRENIA: FROM PSYCHODYNAMICS TO NEURODYNAMICS

Avinash De Souza, Shivanshu Shrivastava, Nilesh Shah

INTRODUCTION

Schizophrenia is one of the most devastating disorders among all the mental illnesses. The onset can be early, the course insidious and outcome often fatal. Indeed it is truly difficult to imagine a disorder as this, where in the simplest of senses, one is truly "losing one's mind". In fact the idea of being controlled by alien forces, losing the ability to control one's body, hearing voices that no one else can hear—all sounds so bizarre to a nonpsychiatrist. That was also why probably Thomas Szasz termed it as a creation of psychiatrists themselves, to propagate their own field.

The presence of schizophrenia has probably been known. in the ancient civilizations of the Romans, Greeks, Latins, Egyptians and closer home, mention has often been made in ayurvedic medicine. There has been a paradigm shift in the belief of causation of schizophrenia. The initial beliefs were a supernatural attribution to heresy to idiocy. This was followed by the genesis of theorists who believed that a clash of ideas and unfulfilled wishes gave rise to a state of conflict—and these formed the psychodynamic theories of the disorder. Now there is more focus on neurostructure and neurochemistry—these have formulated the neurodynamic theories. In short, from software, the attention has now been shifted to the hardware involved in the illness.

HISTORY

The first documented case in history was none other than by Freud himself, that of Daniel Paul Schreber in 1911. This heralded the onset of the first clearly documented psychodynamic theory. Schreber had written his autobiography. In this he clearly stated the progression of his symptoms. He had started initially with hypochondriacal thoughts. This lead to a state of heightened perplexity and confusion—the classical 'apocalypse'. He then experienced what one can best describe today as the typical catatonic features. He had an ongoing personality change throughout. Finally, he developed the positive symptoms of psychosis-especially grandiose and paranoid delusions. One can see thus how closely this resembles a case one would probably see in one's clinic even today.

The ***psychodynamic models*** thus developed as *classical, interpersonal* and *object-relations models*. These were followed ***family models***. The final shift was attributed to the ***neurodynamic models*** with the advent of biological, adoption studies, stress-diathesis and vulnerability-stress hypothesis. The amalgamation of all these led to the ***biopsychosocial model***.

Today, though the psychodynamic models have their credibility, it is largely the neurodynamic theories which are note popular.

CLASSICAL PSYCHOANALYTIC MODELS

There are three analysts who one must mention here:

1. Sigmund Freud
2. Paul Federn
3. Heinz Hartmann.

Sigmund Freud

True to the rest of explanations offered by him, Freud states that schizophrenia is also a state generated due to internal conflicts.

This can he explained by the structural model of the mind. The *id* is the storehouse of primary impulses of the mind, like sexual and aggressive. This is the primitive mind and is entirely unconscious. On the other hand the superego is that which is largely learned. It symbolizes the rules, regulations and values inherited from parents and society at large. It is mostly also in the unconscious. Its presence is felt through guilt and shame. The ego is the middleman. It is the agent between the id and superego. The ego is very complex, and its development is slow and long. One of the most important functions of the ego is the formation of defense mechanisms. These are activated by anxiety—as a response to the danger signal generated by the internal conflicts.

It is indeed remarkable that Freud, with such less experience with schizophrenics was the first to give a solid explanation for the disease process. He described the causation of schizophrenia due to 2 reasons:

1. The conflict-defense model
2. The deficit or deficiency model.

Conflict-defense Model

The structural model of the mind is the same as that offered for neurotic disorders—i.e. a conflict—leading to an anxiety—leading to defense. The difference between the psychotic and neurotic disorders is more quantitative and not qualitative. The regression is to an earlier stage of development where fixation or arrest occurred prior to the oedipal stage. i.e. before the development of an integrated ego. This further explains why psychoanalysis as a treatment does not really work with schizophrenics, as the arrest is prior to ego development. The primary defenses used here are denial and projection. Here due to denial of the unfulfilled wish, there is projection onto the 'object'. This is classically described in the explanation for latent homosexual impulses:

I love him" t A man's impulse).
"I don't love him" (Denial) hence, "I hate him".
He hates and hence persecutes me" (Protection).

Thus the person develops an entire delusional system based on such conflicts. This can be extrapolated to any case where ambivalence towards any love object exists.

Deficit or Deficiency Model

Here the defense mechanisms do not come into play. Due to the existing conflict, there is a withdrawal of libidinal energy into the self. This energy, now directed towards the self, leads to the grandiosity seen or primary narcissism. This continuous process of withdrawal leads to a break from reality. This leads to a diversion of the libidinal impulses away from the real world and towards internalized, fantasized objects. Thence emerge the positive symptoms of schizophrenia. viz., delusions and hallucinations.

Unfortunately Freud himself was not able to explain the gap between his two theories. Why some people use one model and why some use the other? This led to a lot of controversy and enabled Freud's detractors to divert focus away from his theories.

Paul Federn

Federn was Freud's contemporary. He however differed largely in his views from Freud. He believed that one could use psychoanalysis on schizophrenics. He was the one who studied the ego in more detail. He believed that the ego developed at such a high level of consciousness that it developed its own "feeling", i.e., that of the "self" or "I". Hence, probably, originated the use of the term 'ego', as it is used in common parlance today; and not strictly in the psychodynamic sense. Now Federn believed that the ego exhibited boundaries—both internal and external. When the internal boundary was transgressed it leads to internal regression to an earlier stage of development. The external boundary could be intact—in which case the person can function well in the world despite presence of symptoms; whilst when the external boundary is broken, the person stops functioning even with others, i.e. there is overall decline in functioning.

Again, the feasibility of such a model is questionable. However; Federn is surely credited with the conceptualization of the psychology of "self".

Heinz Hartmann

Hartmann essentially expanded Freud's theory on the ego. He described the ego to have many more functions than described by Freud which included memory, perception, intellect, thinking, attention, judgment, object relations and reality testing to name a few. He believed there was a premorbid ego, and one that developed after the onset of the illness. Due to the illness, there is regression to the primary ego state. This ego, due to the generated conflicts, perceives narcissistic injury to it and responds to this with aggressive impulses. This he explained with the use of defenses—initially intellectualization and sublimation, followed by denial and projection. He believed that the ego was a dynamic system, which constantly expanded its horizon, to adapt to the. Stresses faced by the individual. It is when this dynamic equilibrium gets upset, that the above mechanisms act and lead to schizophrenia.

Hartmann was the First to clearly explain aggression in psychotic patients. He also laid the foundation for many concepts, which later went on to form the neurodynamic theories.

INTERPERSONAL MODEL

The interpersonal model was described by Harry Stack Sullivan. According to this model, man is a social being who depends on his development largely on the interaction with his environment, and society at large. In Freudian psychodynamics, the id impulses are primary, and subsequently modified by the ego and superego. In Sullivanian psychodynamics, the self is a product of the existing world.

He described the first relationship to be that of a mother and child. They initially exist as a symbiotic dyad. Gradually the self separates to realize the mother as an independent entity. It is at this crucial stage that the process of pathological development can start. In case of an over-anxious mother, the child forms a template (something like that seen in the reduplication of the DNA), for the anxiety to develop. In fact, he believed that schizophrenia was an outcome of the struggle that the child faces due to early exposure to anxiety.

The child, who is trying to establish a *'self system'* of equilibrium, now faces three states: *the good me* (low anxiety), *the bad me* (high anxiety) and *the not me* (apocalyptic anxiety of schizophrenia). During adolescence especially, due to the introduction of previously alien sexual drives, the state of anxiety heightens and reaches abnormal proportions. This is when florid psychotic symptoms develop. The remission occurs during the process of reorganization of the self into the pre-existing state of equilibrium. Sullivan thus believed the schizophrenic process to thus begin as an external one (with the mother) and subsequently get internalized.

The world of psychiatry accepts Sullivan's views as the first description of human psychology and its application in this disease process.

OBJECT-RELATIONS MODEL

The object-relations analysts were along similar lines as Sullivan, however were viewing this as a parallel school of thought at the time. The chief contenders of this school were:

- Melanie Klein
- WD Fairburn
- Margaret Mahler
- Ping-Nie Pao.

Melanie Klein

She attributed the importance of love and hate in all relationships. She described the concept of the self as in context to others, and this was termed as *'internal object relations'*. During development, one uses the defenses of splitting and projective identification for adaptation and healthy development of these internal object relations. However, the same defenses used in adults could have disastrous outcomes.

She went on to describe two positions in infancy—the paranoid position and the depressive position. In the paranoid position, the individual splits the 'hate' or bad experiences, and projects them onto others who thus appear to be persecutory.

The infant thus develops with a pre-existing substrate for the genesis of schizophrenia. It then responds to stresses, especially in adolescence, by going to either of the above positions, and obviously in schizophrenics regresses to the paranoid position.

WD Fairburn

Fairburn again believed that human contact was the basis of development, even if that contact was not pleasant. According to him, the absence or a mother during the stage of the paranoid position, gave rise to ambivalent feelings towards love. Hence the schizoid thinking of 'to love or not' developed, and these feelings surfaced during periods of stress, usually the first time being during adolescence. He perceived schizophrenia to be at the extreme end of the schizoid spectrum.

Margaret Mahler

She is credited for mainly describing the stages of development, viz., autism, symbiosis and separation-individuation. Autism is the early infantile stage where the infant largely resides in his or her own fantasy world. The symbiotic relationship is one set up with the mother and child during the early formative years. It is during the last phase of development, the separation-individuation phase of adolescence, in which the stress may become over whelming, and there is a regression to the earlier stage of autism and fantasy.

Ping-Nie Pao

He was the first to describe the onset of psychosis due to either a stressful situation (acute) or due genetic loading (chronic). He believed that abnormal development due to mixed signals emanating from a mother, acting upon a child with a pre-existing vulnerable constitution, lead to distress.

There was an attempt to neutralize this distress and in the process was born the state he called 'organismic panic'. The ego tries to correct this and reintegrate the individual, only to yield symptoms such as delusions, hallucinations and an altered personality. As one can see, Pao successfully attributed possible involvement at all levels—self (constitution), mother (object relations), and biology (genes).

MODEL ON FAMILY DYNAMICS

These models might as well be comparable to the object-relations theory, except for the fact that instead or individual, the relations between all the members of the family come into play.

These theories originated during the World War II, wherein a systematic study of schizophrenic patients revealed that the process extended beyond the individual. Often, a pattern emerged, whereby it was seen that the family transactions, either as dyads or triads or tetrads etc. were faulty. It was thus that the term schizophrenic family originated.

The following were the contributors for the family dynamics theory:

- Fromm
- Bateson and Jackson
- R Lidz and T Lidz
- Wynne and Singer
- Vaughn and Leff and Brown.

Fromm

Fromm-Reichmann first described the theory of a 'schizophrenogenic mother'. According to this theory, the presence of a cold, indifferent and non-reactive mother lead to poor development of socially adaptive behavior in children. This further led to development of poor social skills and abnormal communication. Ultimately a pattern of schizophrenic behavior gradually emerged in these children.

Bateson and Jackson

They explained what is now called the double bind theory' Gregory Bateson and Donald Jackson studied that often in families with a schizophrenic patient, the parents might be giving the children conflicting messages. When a child receives two messages of opposite meanings, it leads to a double bind. The inability to interpret this difference leads to a feeling of guilt. Subsequently, the child may have ambivalent feelings which if generated would lead to an altered pattern of thinking. For, example a mother telling her child 'You do not love me enough' and at the same time indicating that hugging, kissing or showing any form of affection was not acceptable. This kind of a conflict leads to ambivalent feelings in the child and a subsequent schizoid thinking pattern.

R Lidz and T Lidz

They described the theories of 'marital schism' and 'marital skew'.

Schism, as the name suggests, indicates a dichotomous or extreme pattern of existence. Basically, two individuals who do not get along with each other, have completely contrasting views and ideas, yet stay under the same roof. These individuals, as parents, could send conflicting messages to their offspring, and be a fertile ground to yield a schizophrenic mind.

This pattern is often seen in countries like ours, where arranged marriages bring together contrasting individuals, bound together by marriage.

Skew, on the other hand, as in statistics, is an extreme form, or at the extreme end of deviation. In this case there is a chronic disagreement within an outwardly calm family. Here, one parent usually does not fulfill the parental role. As a result, a single parent dominates, and the child subsequently assumes the parent role. There is over-dependence, and ambiguity regarding family boundaries and individual responsibilities. This leads to a lot of confusion and conflict in the child, thus again generating schizophrenic thinking patterns.

Wynne and Singer

They described the 'family communications model'. Here, there are basically two types of communications between families:

1. Amorphous
2. Fragmented

1. *Amorphous*: Here there is vague and indefinite communication. The parents themselves lack concrete ideas and emotions. Their thoughts are ill-defined, The communication between the members thus is not definitive. This probably leads to more of loosening of thoughts and formal thought disorder.
2. *Fragmented*: Here there is poor integration of language and disruption of phrases. The meaning to be conveyed does not get across to the different members. In short the communication is often conflict-laden. The Lidz' were more often able to reduplicate their findings as compared to any of the other theorists. They compared communication between families of neurotic patients and psychotic patients. They found that where the families had both parents with high communication skills the chances were of developing normal and neurotic offspring; in families with both parents having poor communication skills the chances were of developing offspring with schizophrenia; and in families with one parent having good skills and the other having poor skills, the chances of either were 50-50.

Vaughn and Leff

They described a very powerful tool in today's view of the prognosis of a schizophrenic patient; a concept which is called 'expressed emotions'. Here the attitude of the family towards an affected individual can lead to further relapses and a poorer prognosis.

There are in all 5 emotions described:

1. Hostility
2. Criticism
3. Over-involvement
4. Guilt induction
5. Intrusiveness.

Of these the first 3 are found to predict high relapse rates within the first 9 months itself. A structured interview using the 5 scale "Camberwell Family Interview" can be used during the inpatient stay to explore these areas. This phenomenon is seen transculturally, even in India, and accepted worldwide.

Families can be classified as those with 'high EE' and those with 'low-EE'. The data suggests that families with high EE require a contact of 35 hours only, between affected patient and family. These individuals are usually in day-care centers and half-way homes.

NEURODYNAMIC THEORIES

There are four theories as mentioned below:

1. Biological or neuronal network model
2. Adoption studies
3. Stress-diathesis model
4. Vulnerabilty-stress model

Biological or Neuronal Network Model

This states that it is basically an erroneous development in neuroanatomy that yields to aberrant connections with the gray matter. This leads to generation of various pathological symptoms of schizophrenia. We would reach a better understanding if the following concepts are understood

- *Parallel processing model*: The neurons in the cerebral cortex exist by the multiple connections with each other. There are existing synaptic connections between these neurons. Hence from one neuron, multiple connections can go to other neurons, via the synapses; and vice-versa. This sets up a 'neuronal pool' of network. There exist at a given time many such networks simultaneously in the brain, setting up what is called the 'parallel processing'. Thus various inputs can be assimilated at a given time, and stored at different points. This is where the memory circuits come into play. The hippocampus forms the storehouse of memory. Now retrieval of memory occurs in perceiving a cue. This triggers of the neuronal circuitry to get back the stored memory from the hippocampus. Let us understand with an example: A person looking for a building on the street, assimilates a variety of inputs. He sees a bank opposite the building, a lady walking in red, the street lights, boys playing in the park, the buildings around, and the color and dimensions of the particular building that he was looking for. These various bits of information fire thousands of neurons arid set up many parallel memory circuits. These are stored as various hits of information to be used later if required. Now if asked by someone else about the building, the person concerned will give landmarks that he retrieves from his memory, and hence accurately reduplicate his experience. Now let us say that this neuronal pool misfires. Instead of retrieving information only from this memory circuit, it also retrieves memories from other circuits simultaneously. The resultant would be a chaotic response which would lead to disordered thinking, and what now hypothesized as the neuronal basis for delusions and hallucinations. The explanation offered by Freud for dreams, and the mechanism of free association is based on the parallel network model here, the use of condensation, displacement and symbolization, would attribute different values to different memories.

- *Parasitic memories*: Along with formation of memory circuits that are formed from self-experiences, at times there are spurious memories which develop, i.e. these form de-novo. Here, there is storage of an unrelated event, or perception of the same. According to certain theories of physics, detailed explanation which is beyond the explanation of this book there is a certain principle called 'attractor dynamics'. Here, each memory has a certain energy level. Depending on the existing energy fluxes there are signals set up whereby these memories get attracted to various circuits. These may get drawn into circuits not originally attached to them and form something called 'parasitic memories', i.e. they are unwanted and add to the circuit. It is just like parasitic memories that contribute to the vague and often bizarre symptoms of schizophrenia.
- *Aberrant brain circuitry*: The formation of neuronal plates and synapses itself may be faulty. These may occur in a pre-existing faulty brain, thereby implying that the brain development in utero is in itself erroneous. On the other hand, some of the research states that the brain at birth is non-schizophrenic. During development, with the input from the environment, and certain experiences; or perhaps an inherent latency to form faulty circuits, the brain starts forming erroneous connections. Another aspect is the 'pruning' of synapses. When there is either an increase or decrease in the synaptic pruning, this can lead to alteration in the memory storage and retrieval. The generation of hallucinations, is attributed synaptic pruning, as it seen not only in schizophrenia, but also in dementia and other organic states, where paining has been studied in more detail.

Adoption Studies

The most classical genotype model studied was the Finnish Adoption Model done by Pekka Tienari et al. Here the genetic loading was studied, along with environmental contribution. Basically, the groups studied were of 3 types, divided as follows:

1. Progeny of an affected schizophrenic in an adopted family wherein the environment was relatively stress-free.
2. Progeny of an affected schizophrenic in an adopted family with a stressful environment, viz., abnormal communication, emotional over-involvement, etc.
3. Progeny of an unaffected individual in an adopted family with a stressful environment, viz., abnormal communication, emotional over-involvement, etc.

Of all the groups studied, it was found that children group (ii) had the maximum chances of developing schizophrenia. Group (i) though having an obvious genetic vulnerability, adapted due to a healthy environment. Similarly group (iii) having a healthy genetic make-up, did not succumb, but could cope up with the ongoing stresses. This study was a landmark in suggesting that both genes and an unhealthy environment contribute to the full-blown schizophrenic syndrome.

Stress-diathesis Model

This may also be termed as the nature-nurture model. The pioneers of this model are:

- Sandor Rado
- Paul Meehl
- *Sandor Rado*: According to Rada, there is an inherited factor in the genesis of schizophrenia which constitutes the genotype. When this genotype interacts with the environment, it gives rise to a phenotype called as 'schizotype'. This schizotype has often aberrant cognitive processes and a deviant style of communication with family members. However, most important is the symptom of 'anhedonia' or the inability to feel any pleasure. When this schizotype is exposed to a relatively stable environment, he remains a well-compensated but none-the-less schizoid or schizotypal personality. When this person is exposed to a stressful environment, then this schizotype manifests as delusions, hallucinations and bizarre behavior.
- *Paul Meehl*: Meehl believed that it was the faulty neural development that was inherited as a phenotypic trait. This manifested as 'schizotaxia' or the inherent ability to develop the illness. When this schizotaxic individual interacted with an asocial environment, s/he tended to develop faulty cognitive processing. S/he thus in turn tended to become ambivalent, anhedonic, and averse to human relations. These theories further corroborated the contribution of a stressful environment, in the genesis of schizophrenia.

Vulnerability-stress Model

Vulnerability may be defined as 'the inherited tendency towards developing schizophrenia'. At best it is a trait, which is present premorbidly. However, it is unique, in that it is not a fixed trait. It is dynamic, and its characteristics and contribution in the illness process may change from time to time, and with each ensuing episode. Vulnerability, although lamely genetic, may also add an acquired component during the antenatal or postnatal period. It may or may not be contributed to by birth order, season and social environment.

The following are the most common vulnerabilities seen in schizophrenia:

- Cognitive deficits which lead to an inability to filter her out information. As a result there is excessive storage of unrequired information which adds to the schizophrenic process
- Actual deficits in neuronal connections and neurophysiology, leading to the inability in the censoring or filtering mechanism as mentioned above
- Poor social skills development. It reflects an inability to communicate, have eye to eye contact and set tip meaningful relationships
- Poor psychological development and excessive use of few defenses like denial, splitting and projection.

The other side of the coin is the added stress apart from family environment. Here there is a contribution of social networking and class. Often a crowding of schizophrenic patients in the lower social classes is a norm. It is hypothesized that schizophrenia leads to aberrant cognitive and social skills. As a result of this the patients communicates less and less with the surrounding people, both at work and otherwise. She gradually becomes a recluse, or socially isolated, At such a time his/her work may suffer, due to incompetence, and she may suffer a downfall economically too. This leads such a patient to leave from the existing set-up, to a cheaper and mere down-market place of residence, and probably a less-skilled occupation. This forms a vicious cycle and has been termed as the 'social drift hypothesis.' Thus when a vulnerable person is exposed to stress as shown above, each time it leads to an episode of acute on chronic stress. This will give rise to the various exacerbations and relapses seen in schizophrenia.

The above theories all explained their point of view in their own domain alone. Let us view the merit end demerits of each.

Classical Psychoanalytical Theories

Merits: Now more of historic importance in understanding symptomatology and probable doctor-patient relationships.

Demerits: Widely criticized due to:

- Studies are hypotheses. Reproducibility and hence validity and accuracy are low
- The views on child development have come a long way. It is no longer accepted that children are underdeveloped as hypothesized. In such a case then the terms like paranoid position and autism etc. become redundant.
- The main underlying feature is the presence of a traumatic event to trigger the process. These theories do not explain about people, who without devastating trauma, still develop schizophrenia.
- These theories do not explain the latency between a childhood traumatic event, and the development of the disorder much later.

Family Dynamics Models Merits

Merits: These highlighted the importance of involvement of the family members in contributing to the illness process. Features like 'expressed emotions' and poor familial communication are accepted and studied even today.

Demerits: These have also been criticized due to:

- Do not explain why aberrant family interactions do not affect all members equally. In the same dysfunctional family, all siblings do not develop the full syndrome. Some may even be normal. Today this is explained on the genetic basis of incomplete penetrance
- These are not reproducible
- They are not causative in schizophrenia. At best they may facilitate the disease process.

Neurodynamic Models

Merits: Represents a paradigm shift from focus on 'software' in the previous theories to 'hardware' in the new ones. These are the first theories to elaborate on a tangible aspect of the illness—altered anatomy and physiology.

Thus, they have a propensity to be more reproducible and research-oriented. They may also find more support in the non-psychiatric medical fraternity, who would have tendency more towards evidence-based medicine.

Demerits

- Still it the infant stage of development. Requires thorough researching and validation
- Entirely ignore the core aspects of psychological schools, like inherent personality traits, infant and childhood experiences, environmental interactions, etc.

Keeping in mind the complete inability of any one single model to explain the genesis of schizophrenia, today a little contribution of all schools of thought is accepted. This heralded the next model of thought.

6.6 SCHIZOPHRENIA: CLINICAL FEATURES

Avinash De Souza, Allen De Souza, Nilesh Shah

INTRODUCTION

Schizophrenia is a psychotic illness that produces an array of disturbances within the domains of thought, perception, affect and volition. It is one of the most difficult psychiatric syndromes to define and describe. This is because many divergent concepts have been held in different countries and by different psychiatrists. The importance of accurate diagnosis is underscored by emerging evidence that early detection and prompt pharmacologic intervention may improve the long-term prognosis of the illness. However, schizophrenia still remains a diagnosis or exclusion because none of its clinical features are pathognomonic.

Origin of the concept of the word "schizophrenia—is less than 200 years old. The illness itself is generally believed to have accompanied mankind since the beginning of time. Written documents that identify schizophrenia can be traced to old pharaonic Egypt, as far back as the second millennium before Christ. The disease was first identified as a discrete mental illness by Dr Emil Kraepelin, a German physician in 1887. He was the first to classify the mental disorders into different categories. Kraepelin used the term "dementia praecox" (a term First used by psychiatrist Benedict A Morel) for individuals who had symptoms that we now associate with schizophrenia. He was the first to make a distinction in the psychotic disorders and manic depression. Kraepelin believed that dementia praecox was primarily a disease of the brain, and particularly a form of dementia. Kraepelin named the disorder 'dementia praecox" (early dementia) to distinguish it from other forms of dementia (such as Alzheimer's disease) which typically occur late in life. He divided it into four subtypes—simple, marked by slow social decline concomitant with apathy and social withdrawal; paranoid, with its attendant fear and 'persecutory" delusions; hebephrenic and catatonic, characterized by a poverty of movement and expression.

The Swiss psychiatrist, Eugen Bleuler, coined the term "schizophrenia" in 1911. He was also the first to describe the symptoms as "positive" or "negative." Bleuler changed the name to schizophrenia as it was obvious that Kraepelin's name was misleading as the illness was not a dementia (it did not always lead to mental deterioration) and could sometimes occur late as well as 'early in life'. The word "schizophrenia" comes from the Greek roots schizo (split) and phrene (mind) to describe the fragmented thinking of people with the disorder. His term was not meant to convey the idea of split or multiple personality, a common misunderstanding by the public at large. Bleuler defined schizophrenia with his four "A's", referring to the blunted affect (diminished emotional response to stimuli); loosening of associations (by which he meant a disordered pattern of thought, inferring a cognitive deficit), ambivalence (an apparent inability to make decisions, again suggesting a deficit of the integration and processing of incident and retrieved information) a rid Autism (a Loss of awareness of external events, and a preoccupation with the self and one's own thoughts). These were fundamental symptoms, and accessory symptoms in Bleuler's view were hallucinations, delusions, catatonia and abnormal behaviors. Without knowing the exact causes of these diseases, scientists can only base their classifications on the observation that some symptoms tend to occur together.

Ernst Kretschmer compiled data to suggest that schizophrenia occurred more in people with asthenic or dysplastic body types and pyknic body types were more likely to have bipolar disorders. Harry Sullivan emphasized social isolation as a cause and a symptom or schizophrenia. Gabriel Langfeldt gave a bipartite classification with true schizophrenia which had a poor prognosis and schizophrenia like psychosis (or schizophreniform states) which had a good prognosis.

Kurt Schneider tried to make the diagnosis more reliable by identifying a group of symptoms characteristic of schizophrenia, but rarely found in other disorders. Some of these symptoms have now been included in the diagnostic criteria for schizophrenia in DSM-IV and (CD-10. First rank symptoms are auditory hallucinations (hearing thoughts spoken aloud, hearing voices referring to himself/herself, made in the third person and auditory hallucinations in the form of a commentary), thought withdrawal, insertion and interruption, thought broadcasting, somatic hallucinations, delusional perception and feelings or actions experienced as made or influenced by external agents. Second rank symptoms these symptoms could be used for diagnosis if a patient did not show any first rank symptoms include other disorders of perception, sudden delusional ideas, perplexity, depressive and euphoric mood changes and feelings of emotional impoverishment.

CLASSIFICATION

By the 1960s, there were wide divergences in the criteria for diagnosis of schizophrenia. In Europe, Schneider's criteria were employed, while in USA psychodynamic processes were used, leading to more cases and also higher admission rate in USA. There are different classifications which may agree on the core symptomatology that make-up the syndrome of schizophrenia, but differ in terms of duration of the features.

Some of these are:

CATEGO: A computer program designed to process data from a standard interview called the Present Status Examination. It is a 12-point diagnostic system and the cut-off is determined by the examiner.

Feigner's criteria (1972) were developed in St Louis to identify patients with a poor prognosis. They include 6 months duration for diagnosis along with risk factors like (family history, marital status, age of onset, drug history for inclusion). These criteria have been used in research.

Research diagnostic criteria (RDC developed from Feigner's by Spitzer in 1978): The criteria for diagnosis are taken as 2 weeks as compared to 6 months in Feigners criteria.

DSM IV: According to the Diagnostic and Statistical Manual for Psychiatric Disorders—Fourth Edition (DSM-IV), the diagnosis of schizophrenia is based on a constellation of signs and symptoms that are present for a sufficient length of time, are not caused by an another medical disorder or substance, and cause significant impairment in role functioning.

DSM-IV-TR CRITERIA FOR SCHIZOPHRENIA

a. *Characteristic symptoms*: Two (or more) of the following, each present for a significant portion of time during a 1-month period (or less if successfully treated):
   1. Delusions
   2. Hallucinations
   3. Disorganized speech (e.g. frequent derailment or in-coherence)
   4. Grossly disorganized or catatonic behavior
   5. Negative symptoms, i.e. affective flattening, alogia or avolition.

   Note: Only one criterion A symptom is required if delusions are bizarre or hallucinations consist of a voice keeping up a running commentary on the person's behavior or thoughts or two or more voices are conversing with each other.
b. *Social/occupational dysfunction*: For a significant portion of the time since the onset of the disturbance, one or more major areas of functioning, such as work, interpersonal relations, or self-care, are markedly below the level achieved before the onset (or when the onset is in child-hood or adolescence, failure to achieve expected level of interpersonal, academic, or occupational achievement).
c. *Duration*: Continuous signs of the disturbance persist for at least 6 months. This 6-month period must include at least 1 month of symptoms (or less if successfully treated) that meet criterion A (i.e. active-phase symptoms) and may include periods of prodromal or residual symptoms. During these prodromal or residual periods, the signs of the disturbance may be manifested by only negative symptoms or two or more symptoms listed in criterion A present in an attenuated form (e.g. odd beliefs. unusual perceptual experiences).
d. *Schizoaffective and mood disorder exclusion*: Schizoaffective disorder and mood disorder with psychotic features have been ruled out because either (1) no major depressive, manic or mixed episodes have occurred concurrently with the active-phase symptoms; or (2) if mood episodes have occurred during active-phase symptoms; their total duration has been brief relative to the duration of the active and residual periods.
e. *Substance/general medical condition exclusion*: The disturbance is not due to the direct physiologic effects of a substance (e.g. a drug of abuse, a medication) or a general medical condition.
f. *Relationship to a pervasive developmental disorder*: If there is a history of autistic disorder or another pervasive developmental disorder, the additional diagnosis of schizophrenia is made only if prominent delusions or hallucinations are also present for at least a month (or less if successfully treated).

Paranoid type: A type of schizophrenia in which the following criteria are met:
- Preoccupation with one or more delusions or frequent auditory hallucinations.
- *None of the following is prominent:* Disorganized speech, disorganized or catatonic behavior, or flat or inappropriate affect.

Catatonic type: A type of schizophrenia in which the clinical picture is dominated by at least two of the following:
- Motoric immobility as evidenced by catalepsy (including waxy flexibility) or stupor.
- Excessive motor activity (that is apparently purposeless and not influenced by external stimuli).
- Extreme negativism (an apparently motiveless resistance to all instructions or maintenance of a rigid posture against attempts to be moved) or mutism.
- Peculiarities of voluntary movement as evidenced by posturing (voluntary assumption of inappropriate or bizarre postures), stereotyped movements, prominent mannerisms, or prominent grimacing.
- Echolalia or echopraxia.

Disorganized type: A type or schizophrenia in which the following criteria are met:
- Disorganized speech
- Disorganized behavior
- Flat or inappropriate affect
- The criteria are not met for catatonic type.

Undifferentiated type: A type of schizophrenia in which symptoms that meet Criterion A are present, but the criteria are not met for the paranoid, disorganized, or catatonic type.

Residual type: A type of schizophrenia in which the following criteria are met:

- Absence of prominent delusions, hallucinations, disorganized speech, and grossly disorganized or catatonic behavior.
- There is continuing evidence of the disturbance, as indicated by the presence of negative symptoms or two or more symptoms listed in Criterion A for Schizophrenia, present in an attenuated form (e.g. odd beliefs, unusual perceptual experiences).

ICD 10 CRITERIA FOR SCHIZOPHRENIA

The 1CD 10 guidelines compiled by the WHO (1993) uses die code F20.xy for schizophrenia, where x denotes subtype and y denotes course of illness. The normal requirement for a diagnosis of schizophrenia is that a minimum of one very clear symptom (and usually two or more if less clear-cut) belonging to any one of the groups listed as (a) to (d) below, or symptoms from at least two of the groups referred to as (e) to (h), should have been clearly present for most of the time during a period of 1 month or more. Conditions meeting such symptomatic requirements but of duration less than 1 month (whether treated or not) should be diagnosed in the first instance as acute schizophrenia-like psychotic disorder and are classified as schizophrenia if the symptoms persist for longer periods.

- Thought echo, thought insertion or withdrawal, and thought broadcasting
- Delusions of control, influence, or passivity, clearly referred to body or limb movements or specific thoughts, actions, or sensations, delusional perception
- Hallucinatory voices giving a running commentary on the patient's behavior, or discussing the patient among themselves, or other types of hallucinatory voices coming from some part of the body
- Persistent delusions of other kinds that are culturally inappropriate and completely impossible, such as religious or political identity, or superhuman powers and abilities (e.g. being able to control the weather, or being in communication with aliens from another world)
- Persistent hallucinations in any modality, when accompanied either by fleeting or half-formed delusions without clear affective content, or by persistent over valued ideas, or when occurring every day for weeks or months on end
- Breaks or interpolations in the train of thought, resulting in incoherence or irrelevant speech, or neologisms
- Catatonic behavior, such as excitement, posturing, or Waxy flexibility, negativism, mutism and stupor
- "Negative" symptoms such as marked apathy, paucity of speech, and blunting or incongruity of emotional responses, usually resulting in social withdrawal and lowering of social performance: it must be clear that these are not due to depression or to neuroleptic medication
- A significant and consistent change in the overall quality of some aspects of personal behavior, manifest as loss of interest, aimlessness, idleness, a self-absorbed attitude, and social withdrawal.

DSM-5 DIAGNOSTIC CRITERIA FOR SCHIZOPHRENIA

Two changes were made to DSM-IV Criterion A for schizophrenia. The first change is the elimination of the special attribution of bizarre delusions and Schneiderian first-rank auditory hallucinations (e.g. two or more voices conversing). In DSM-IV, only one such symptom was needed to meet the diagnostic requirement for Criterion A, instead of two of the other listed symptoms. This special attribution was removed due to the nonspecificity of Schneiderian symptoms and the poor reliability in distinguishing bizarre from nonbizarre delusions. Therefore, in DSM-5, two Criterion A symptoms are required for any diagnosis of schizophrenia. The second change is the addition of a requirement in Criterion A that the individual must have at least one of these three symptoms: delusions, hallucinations, and disorganized speech. At least one of these core "positive symptoms" is necessary for a reliable diagnosis of schizophrenia.

The DSM-IV subtypes of schizophrenia (i.e. paranoid, disorganized, catatonic, undifferentiated, and residual types) are eliminated due to their limited diagnostic stability, low reliability, and poor validity. These subtypes also have not been shown to exhibit distinctive patterns of treatment response or longitudinal course. Instead, a dimensional approach to rating severity for the core symptoms of schizophrenia is included in Section III to capture the important heterogeneity in symptom type and severity expressed across individuals with psychotic disorders.

DSM-5 Diagnostic criteria for schizophrenia

295.90 (F20.9)

a. Two (or more) of the following, each present for a significant portion of time during a 1-month period (or less if successfully treated). At least one of these must be (1), (2), or (3):
   1. Delusions.
   2. Hallucinations.
   3. Disorganized speech (e.g. frequent derailment or incoherence).
   4. Grossly disorganized or catatonic behavior.
   5. Negative symptoms (i.e. diminished emotional expression or avolition).
b. For a significant portion of the time since the onset of the disturbance, level of functioning in one or more major areas, such as work, interpersonal relations, or self-care, is markedly below the level achieved prior to the onset (or when the onset is in childhood or adolescence, there is failure to achieve expected level of interpersonal, academic, or occupational functioning).

Contd...

Contd...

c. Continuous signs of the disturbance persist for at least 6 months. This 6-month period must include at least 1 month of symptoms (or less if successfully treated) that meet Criterion A (i.e. active-phase symptoms) and may include periods of prodromal or residual symptoms. During these prodromal or residual periods, the signs of the disturbance may be manifested by only negative symptoms or by two or more symptoms listed in Criterion A present in an attenuated form (e.g. odd beliefs, unusual perceptual experiences).
d. Schizoaffective disorder and depressive or bipolar disorder with psychotic features have been ruled out because either (1) no major depressive or manic episodes have occurred concurrently with the active-phase symptoms, or (2) if mood episodes have occurred during active-phase symptoms, they have been present for a minority of the total duration of the active and residual periods of the illness.
e. The disturbance is not attributable to the physiological effects of a substance (e.g. a drug of abuse, a medication) or another medical condition.
f. If there is a history of autism spectrum disorder or a communication disorder of childhood onset, the additional diagnosis of schizophrenia is made only if prominent delusions or hallucinations, in addition to the other required symptoms of schizophrenia, are also present for at least 1 month (or less if successfully treated).

Specify if:

The following course specifiers are only to be used after a 1-year duration of the disorder and if they are not in contradiction to the diagnostic course criteria.

First episode, currently in acute episode: First manifestation of the disorder meeting the defining diagnostic symptom and time criteria. An *acute episode* is a time period in which the symptom criteria are fulfilled.

First episode, currently in partial remission: Partial remission is a period of time during which an improvement after a previous episode is maintained and in which the defining criteria of the disorder are only partially fulfilled.

First episode, currently in full remission: Full remission is a period of time after a previous episode during which no disorder-specific symptoms are present.

Multiple episodes, currently in acute episode: Multiple episodes may be determined after a minimum of two episodes (i.e. after a first episode, a remission and a minimum of one relapse).

Multiple episodes, currently in partial remission

Multiple episodes, currently in full remission continuous: Symptoms fulfilling the diagnostic symptom criteria of the disorder are remaining for the majority of the illness course, with subthreshold symptom periods being very brief relative to the overall course.

Unspecified specify if:

With catatonia (refer to the criteria for catatonia associated with another mental disorder).

Coding note: Use additional code 293.89 (F06.1) catatonia associated with schizophrenia to indicate the presence of the comorbid catatonia.

Specify current severity:

Severity is rated by a quantitative assessment of the primary symptoms of psychosis, including delusions, hallucinations, disorganized speech, abnormal psychomotor behavior, and negative symptoms. Each of these symptoms may be rated for its current severity (most severe in the last 7 days) on a 5-point scale ranging from 0 (not present) to 4 (present and severe) (See Clinician-Rated Dimensions of Psychosis Symptom Severity in the Chapter "Assessment Measures" in Section III of DSM-5).

Note: Diagnosis of schizophrenia can be made without using this severity specifier.

SCHIZOPHRENIA SUBTYPES

Catatonia: Catatonic symptoms occur in two forms: inhibited or stuporous and excited catatonia. The hallucinations, and thought disturbances occur, but are less obvious.

- *Stuporous type*: They show a marked decrease in any spontaneous movements or activity. They may be mute, unresponsive and show symptoms like negativism, echopraxia, automatic obedience (details in Table 2). Stupor may change to a state of uncontrolled motor activity and excitement.
- *Excited type*: They are in a state of extreme psychomotor excitation. They often require physical and medical control, because the dangerous excitation can cause them to injure themselves or others, or collapse from extreme exhaustion.
- *Periodic catatonia*: This is a rare form of catatonia described by Gjessing in 1938, which has a periodic recurrence and appears to be due to shift in the nitrogen balance.

In the past, catatonic schizophrenia tended to have an earlier age of onset, chronic course and poor outcome, but today it seems to have the best prognosis with ECTs and medication. Isolated catatonic symptoms are found in other subtypes of schizophrenia, and in medical illnesses like frontal lobe tumors, diencephalic disorder, basal ganglia lesion, metabolic disturbances and toxic reactions. Catatonic symptoms are being observed less commonly than 50 years ago. The possible explanations are improvement in the social environment where patients are treated, use of more effective biological treatments, or possibly less awareness of the symptoms as before, or recognition of organic syndromes better than before which also lead to catatonic symptoms.

Paranoid: They have a later and more acute onset and run a more remitting course with a better outcome. Kraepelin was the first to identify a paranoid subtype, which is characterized by one or more delusion and/or frequent hallucination. Paranoid patients show hostility, suspiciousness and anxiety but less regression as compared to other subtypes.

Disorganized: As the name implies, this subtype's predominant feature is disorganization of the thought processes. As a rule, hallucinations and delusions are less pronounced, although there may be some evidence of these symptoms. These people may have significant impairments in their ability to maintain the activities of daily living. Even the more routine

Table 2: Stuporous type features

Mutism	Echopraxia
Negativism	Automatic obedience
Posturing	Waxy flexibility
Echolalia	Psychological pillow

tasks, such as dressing, bathing or brushing teeth, can be significantly impaired or lost. Often, there is impairment in the emotional processes of the individual. Disorganized patients are usually active but in an aimless, nonconstructive manner. Incongruous grinning and grimacing are common. The patients' behavior is sometimes described as silly or fatuous.

Undifferentiated: The undifferentiated subtype is diagnosed when patients have symptoms of schizophrenia that are not sufficiently formed or specific enough to permit classification of the illness into one of the other subtypes.

Residual: A form of schizophrenia that is characterized by a previous diagnoses of schizophrenia but no longer having any of the prominent psychotic symptoms. There are some remaining symptoms of the disorder however, such as eccentric behavior emotional blunting, illogical thinking, or social withdrawal. In the residual type of schizophrenia, the patient has had at least one episode of schizophrenia. If delusions or hallucinations are present they are not prominent, and are not accompanied by strong affect.

Type I and Type II: The first model that linked psychopathology to neuropathology was proposed by Crow. He designated these dimensions as type I and type II. Type I was characterized by positive symptoms, sudden onset, good premorbid functioning, good prognosis, and a normal brain structure with dopamine hyperactivity. Type II schizophrenia was characterized by insidious onset, negative symptoms. poor premorbid functioning, poor prognosis with probable drug resistance, and structural abnormalities of the brain. Other subgroupings outlined on this have been positive and negative type or nondeficit and deficit form of schizophrenia. A large number of scales are now used to measure positive and negative symptoms especially to show the efficacy of newer antipsychotics on both the symptoms. According to Andreasen, positive symptoms include disordered thinking, delusions, hallucinations and bizarre behavior. Negative symptoms are affective flattening, impaired attention, avolition, apathy, anhedonia, asociality and alogia. Factors like medication, depression, and institutionalization simulate negative symptoms, and must be distinguished from the core negative symptoms of schizophrenia. Today this classification appears to be an oversimplification of the relationship between symptoms and neuropathology, but it provided a major stimulus to investigation of the enduring deficits.

More recently, this simple binary division has been considered inadequate and three dimensions of psychopathology have been proposed:

- *Psychotic dimension (like positive symptoms):* Delusions and hallucinations
- *Disorganized dimension:* Disorganized speech or behavior, or inappropriate affect
- *Negative dimension (like negative symptoms):* Affective flattening and alogia.

Other Terms and Related Syndromes

Simple deteriorative disorder (simple schizophrenia): This is an uncommon disorder in which there is an insidious but progressive development of oddities of conduct, social and occupation decline. Delusions and hallucinations are not evident, and the disorder is less obviously psychotic than the hebephrenic, paranoid, and catatonic subtypes of schizophrenia. The characteristic "negative" features of residual schizophrenia (e.g. blunting of affect, loss of volition) develop without being preceded by any overt psychotic symptoms. With increasing social impoverishment, vagrancy may ensue and the individual may then become self-absorbed, idle, and aimless.

Postpsychotic depression (Postschizophrenic depression): A depressive episode, which may be prolonged, arising in the aftermath of a schizophrenic illness. Some schizophrenic symptoms must still be present but no longer dominate the clinical picture. It is uncertain, and immaterial to the diagnosis, to what extent the depressive symptoms have merely been uncovered by the resolution on of earlier psychotic symptoms (rather than being a new development) or are an intrinsic part of schizophrenia rather than a psychological reaction to it. They are rarely sufficiently severe or extensive to meet criteria for a severe depressive episode, and it is often difficult to decide which of the patient's symptoms are due to depression and which to neuroleptic medication or to the impaired volition and affective flattening of schizophrenia itself. This depressive disorder is associated with an increased risk of suicide.

Residual schizophrenia: A chronic stage in the development of a schizophrenic disorder in which there has been a clear progression from an early stage (comprising one or more episodes with psychotic symptoms meeting the general criteria for schizophrenia described above) to a later stage characterized by long-term, though not necessarily irreversible, "negative" symptoms.

These include psychomotor slowing, underactivity, blunting of affect, passivity and lack of initiative, poverty of quantity or content of speech, eye contact, voice modulation, arid posture, poor self-care and social performance.

Bouffée délirante: This is an historic and unique French diagnostic term for a short-lived psychosis. The Bouffée délirante reactions are sudden attacks of brief duration with paranoid delusions and concomitant hallucinations, typically precipitated by an intense fear of magical persecution through sorcery or witchcraft. They are also characterized by confusional state, polymorphous symptoms and by highly emotionalized behavior and, amnesia after the attack. In its symptomatology, the Bouffée délirante is reminiscent of the transient psychotic reactions (because remission is within 3 months even without treatment) occurring in the early phases of industrialization and mass-urbanization in 19th century Europe; described under such names as folie hystérique in Paris and amentia transitoria in Vienna and "emotional psychosis" by Swiss psychiatrists. Transient psychotic reactions are of particular interest to comparative cultural psychiatry because they are interwoven with culturally validated beliefs in sorcery and witchcraft which persist even after the traditional resources of protection from, the, assumed persecution by magical or supernatural powers, are no longer available as a consequence of westernization and urbanization.

Schizophreniform states: It was first applied by Langfeldt (1961) to good prognosis cases, and involved acute onset, clouding of consciousness, depressive and hysterical features and a precipitating factor. DSM-IV uses the term to describe a condition similar to schizophrenia but lasting less than 6 months.

PHENOMENA OF SCHIZOPHRENIA

The diagnosis of schizophrenia cannot be made entirely on the basis of observation, logical reasoning, or objective reasoning. The evaluation should take into account the main symptoms, premorbid personality, genetic history, social environment and any precipitating factors. The clinical features embrace a diverse range of disturbance of thought, perception, emotion, cognition and motor activity.

Disorder of Thought

Any classification on the disorder of thinking is bound to be arbitrary. For the sake of discussion, we divide thought disorders of stream (or flow), content, form and possession.

Disorder of Stream of Thought

Flight of ideas: In flight of ideas the patient's thought and conversation move quickly from one topic to another so that one train of thought is not completed before another one appears. Here the thoughts follow each other rapidly and the associations and sequence of the train of thoughts is by verbal associations, proverbs, clang associations (two words with a similar sound), punning (same word with a different meaning). With the eight comes accelerated pressure of speech. Flight of ideas are mostly seen in manic patients.

Thought block and poverty of speech: There is a sudden arrest in the train of thought leaving a blank. Lack of spontaneous speech and brevity of replies is also seen in schizophrenia.

Content of thought delusions: They are false firm unshakeable beliefs that cannot be corrected by reasoning and are idiosyncratic for the patient (i.e. riot pan of the patient's sociocultural and educational environment). Delusions are further divided into primary (autochthonous) and secondary delusions depending on their origins. Primary delusions arise suddenly, from unaccountable origins, whereas secondary delusions arise from some morbid experience and are common in chronic schizophrenics.

Content of delusions: Delusional content is dependent on the sociocultural background, as well as the type of illness. Delusions of persecution, reference, jealousy, love, bizarre thoughts are common in schizophrenia, whereas delusions of grandeur are seen in mania. Delusions of guilt, ill health, nihilism (belief that is part of the body is not functioning) are more common in psychotic depression. Schizophrenic patients may exhibit delusional memories, which are circumstances, which the patient is convinced, they had experienced in the past. Sometimes the patient may attribute a new meaning to a normally perceived object, and this gives a two memberedness to the feature. This is called as delusional perception (e.g. when the patient's brother picked up a pen from the table, he immediately realized that he was accusing the patient of being a homosexual). Strongly held beliefs which dominate person's decisions but nondelusional in their intensity are called overvalued ideas.

Origin of delusions: According to Freud delusions are present because of latent homosexuality. According to Schneider delusional experiences present as a delusional mood wherein a patient knows that something is happening around him, followed by a delusional perception and sudden delusional idea (primary delusion). Similarly Conrad divided the delusional processes into phases called as trema (patient is anxious and may be similar to delusional mood), epiphany (sudden revelation), apocalypse and terminal where the person becomes vegetable-like disorders of content of thought also preoccupations, obsessions, compulsions, phobias, hypochondriacal symptoms and specific antisocial urges that are not the core features of schizophrenia.

Form of Thought

One of the problems lies in the variety of manifestations of disordered form of thought, and it is difficult to tease out the essential elements. Some of the manifestations are:

- Tangentiality—responses that are off the point, but not completely unrelated.
- Perseveration is the persistent and inappropriate repetition of the same thoughts. Thus, in response to a series of simple questions, the person may give the correct answer to the first question but continue to give the

same answer inappropriately to subsequent questions. Perseveration also occurs in dementia.
- Loosening of associations denotes a loss of the normal structure of thinking. Speech becomes incomprehensible as the logical relations between words or sentences is lost. Loosening of associations occurs most often in schizophrenia. Loosening of associations can take several forms.
- Knight's move or derailment refers to a transition between one topic and another, either mid-sentence or between sentences, with no logical connection between the two and no evidence of such links that are found in flight of ideas. When this abnormality is extreme then it can disrupt not only the connection between sentences and phrases, but also the finer grammatical structure of speech. It is then called word salad.
- Verbigeration is when sounds, words or phrases are repeated in a senseless way. It is a type or stereotypy. One effect of loosening of associations is called vorbeireden or talking past the point. The patient seems to get near to the point but never quite reaches it.
- Neologisms—use or new expressions or words to express a concept.
- Metonyms—unusual use of words (hand shoe instead of glove).
- Loss of abstract attitude—this was described by Kurt Goldstein who described concretization of thought as typical of schizophrenia thinking. Asking interpretation of proverb can often bring out this defect; the patient gives the literal meaning of it. The patient may also have idiosyncrasies of logic, which appears to reflect a private logic or autistic logic.
- Overinclusion—Norman Cameron identified this feature; patients with schizophrenia tend to include many irrelevant items in their ideational and verbal behavior. This can explain loosening of association. It usually develops within the setting of a delusional mood and is due to impairment of the filtering process that inhibits irrelevant external and internal sensations. The lack of adequate connection between two thoughts is called asyndesis.

Possession of Thought

Patients with delusions about the possession or thought can be affected in several ways: Those with delusions about thought insertion believe their thoughts have been implanted by an outside agency. This is different from a person who has obsessional thoughts because, no matter how unpleasant the thoughts are, they realize they are their own. The patient with delusion of thought insertion will not accept that the thoughts he possesses originate from his own mind. Patients with delusions of thought withdrawal believe that thoughts have been taken out of their mind. This delusion usually accompanies thought blocking. In delusions of thought broadcasting the patient believes that other people in some way know his unspoken thoughts. Some people believe their thoughts can be heard by other people (Gedankenlautwerden). All three of these symptoms occur more commonly in schizophrenia.

Disorder of Affect

Although disorder of thinking and perception are distinctive, disorders of affect are also a major component of the condition:
- *Blunted or 'restricted affect':* It is a failure to express feelings verbally or nonverbally with no animation of facial expression or voice inflection. It is seen in more than 60% of acute schizophrenics.
- *Incongruous affect*: The affect is inconsistent with the circumstances. A schizophrenic may laugh while describing a death of a loved one. This is common in chronic patients. It happens due to the inability to recognise emotional cues in others.
- *Anhedonia*: It is the inability of the patient to experience pleasure.
- Emotional sensitivity—which is a hypersensitivity to rejection.

Disorder of Volition

This can be seen as weakened volition (lack of spontaneous motor activity), disjointed volition (overactive but in a non coal directed manner), catatonic symptoms, possession of thought leading to motor activity and violent behavior.

Disorder of Perception (Hallucinations and Other Phenomena)

Hallucinations or perceptions in the absence of external stimuli are prominent among the core symptoms of schizophrenia. They may occur in any sensory modality, but most commonly are auditory or hearing voices in the absence of anyone really being there. The auditory hallucinations may be unstructured (hearing nonspecific noise) or structured (hearing voices). The structured hallucinations may be in the third person (two or more voices discussing the patient in the third person) or second person (speaking directly to the patient). The voices can be critical, commanding, derogatory or comforting. Many patients hear their own thoughts spoken out aloud (echo de pensee or thought echo). In schizophrenia hallucinations in other modalities do occur, but are less common. Visual hallucinations are often associated with organic psychosis, but are seen in severe or chronic schizophrenia. Tactile, olfactory, gustatory or somatic hallucinations are also known to be present in schizophrenia.

Some special kinds of hallucinations also seen in schizophrenia are:
- *Functional hallucinations:* A stimulus causes the hallucination, but it is experienced as well as the

hallucination (the clock ticked and she heard the voice of God).

- *Reflex hallucinations:* A type of synesthesia, where a stimulus in one sensory field, produces hallucination in another (a patient attributed the pain in her head to a sneeze she heard).
- *Extracampine hallucination:* Hallucination outside the limits of the sensory field (hearing voices in Mumbai when he knows he is in Delhi). Sometimes other perceptual disturbances like sensory distortions (e.g. micropsia objects appear reduced in size, hyperesthesia, unnatural intensity of color) or deja vu (person feels he has encountered the situation before) may also occur.

Cognitive Disturbances

Patients with chronic schizophrenia also have deficits in cognitive functions, such as memory, learning, and attention. The major cognitive impairments are in the realm of executive functioning, which includes inability to select appropriate responses, problem solving, to retain and organize information and do multitasks simultaneously. Attentional deficits like impairment of selective attention with ability to sustain attention are also noticed. Patients complain that they are bombarded with more stimuli than they can interpret, leading to misinterpretation (delusions confusion (hallucinations) or retreat to safety (negative symptom). Concepts of reality monitoring (distinguishing between imagined and real events) and attribution of thoughts and feelings to oneself are also defective. Working memory (ability to hold stimuli for a short time, and then use it to solve cognitive and behavioral tasks, e.g. dialling a phone number after holding in the memory for a short time) is quite impaired in schizophrenia Stroop test, WAIS, trail making test, Wisconsin card-sorting test along with neuroimaging are widely used for assessment of cognitive deficits. Efforts are being made to classify patients on the basis of cognition and functional outcome or by deficits in the various areas. For example, patients classified as manifesting cortical deficits evidenced reduced temporal lobe gray matter and hypometabolism, and patients classified as subcortical had enlarged ventricles. More the cognitive deficits, worse is the functional outcome and lesser is the benefit from rehabilitation programs. Trials are showing that patients receiving newer medications show small to moderate improvements in several cognitive domains and in global indices of cognitive functioning. Finally use of cognitive enhancers and cognitive remediation strategies might lead to better functional outcome in these patients.

Assessment in Schizophrenia

Apart from the criteria and symptoms discussed above, experienced clinicians speak of the precox feeling (failure to emotionally connect with the patient), although the reliability of this approach is questionable. The prepsychotic personality must also be evaluated although the etiology is multifactorial. Premorbid schizoid traits may be noticed in 25% of patients. Poor premorbid adjustment is shown to correlate with early onset, poor prognosis, negative symptoms and cognitive deficits. Some patients may show a neglected personal appearance, with poor regard for appropriate social norms. There are psychological tests that are more or less compatible with the diagnosis of schizophrenia and make the diagnosis more or less probable. The test batteries used are; Rorschach test, MMPI 2, Brief Psychiatric Rating Scale (Overall and Gorham 1962), Scale for the Assessment of Negative Symptoms (SANS—Andeasen, 1982). Positive and Negative Syndrome-Scale (PANSS; Kay 1991). These scales are used for measuring clinical change overall severity of the illness, and change in severity of individual symptoms and valid assessment of diagnosis especially for research purposes.

Dimensions of Schizophrenia

It is a long-standing debate about the boundaries of schizophrenia with regard to related illnesses. Depression and excitation can occur in schizophrenia, conversely, schizophrenic syndromes can occur in affective psychosis. A family history of schizophrenia in affective disorders and vice versa indicates a spectrum extending from affective psychosis to schizoaffective disorder to schizophrenia. However, differences do extend across causes. Phenomenology, pathophysiology and course of the illnesses. Phenomenological overlap between obsessive compulsive disorder (OCD) and schizophrenia have led to suggestions that OCD may exist on the same continuum. Prevalence of OCD is also higher amongst schizophrenics than general population. Other schizophrenia spectrum disorders with nonschizophrenic diagnosis include schizotypal/schizoid paranoid personality disorder, schizophreniform disorder and delusional disorder.

Differential Diagnosis of Schizophrenia

The diagnosis of schizophrenia should often be thought of as a disorder of exclusion because none of its features arc pathognomic. It remains a clinical diagnosis on historical information, careful mental status examination and a physical examination. One should exclude medical conditions, substance misuse causing psychosis. A major task is also separating schizophrenia from other psychiatric illnesses. Some of the conditions that can mislead the diagnosis are shown in Table 3.

Course of schizophrenia the clinical course and outcome has been studied and debated since Kraepelin first described dementia praecox as chronic and progressive.

The onset of schizophrenia ranges from acute to subacute to insidious. An acute onset generally follows a stressful experience, and is sudden in its appearance. In subacute and insidious, there is a prodromal phase lasting for weeks to years, progressing to preoccupation, social withdrawal before

Table 3: Differential diagnosis of Schizophrenia

Psychiatric illnesses	*Others*
BPAD	Anatomic lesions
Schizoaffective disorder	Metabolic illnesses
Delusional disorder	Endocrine disorders
Schizotypal personality disorder	Infectious illnesses
Paranoid schizoid personality disorder	• Miscellaneous disorders • Vitamin deficiency

overt psychosis appears. These individuals show a childhood pattern of being shy or hostile, awkward motor activities, poor school performance and introspection. In a minority of patients there is complete recovery after the first episode). Longitudinal studies indicate that 20–30% run an episodic course with minor disabilities between episodes. The rate of complete recovery is 12–32%. 20–25% achieve partial remission and 5–10% suffer from serious and persisting symptoms. The period between the first onset of symptoms and the initiation of treatment (duration of untreated psychosis) has been known to correlate with increased time to remission and poor response to treatment. Another hypothesis is that behavioral or pharmacological intervention prior to the onset of psychotic symptoms can delay or prevent the onset of schizophrenia.

The factors that prevent relapses include maintenance antipsychotic medication, supportive social environment with absence of expressed emotions. With a good follow-up therapy, only 10–15% of patients in remission relapse within a year as compared to 60–70% without follow-up. The long-term outcome can show the time scale for improvement to be several decades. Data from many studies show that about 57% of patients followed over a mean period of 27 years showed either recovery or significant improvement. Thus, schizophrenia is not invariably a chronic deteriorating disorder. The course of illness according to ICD 10 is continuous, episodic with progressive deficit, episodic with stable deficit, episodic remittent, incomplete or complete remission. DSM-IV classifies the longitudinal course after 1 year has elapsed since the onset of active symptoms. It is divided as episodic with interepisode residual symptoms, episodic with no interepisode residual symptoms, continuous, single episode in partial remission, and single episode with full remission and unspecified.

CONCLUSION

Schizophrenia undermines the fundamental aspects of personality. It erodes the ability to initiate and organize self-directed mental activity. The illness follows a course in which hallucinations, delusions and florid disorganization of thought are superimposed upon more subtle disorders in the initiation and organization of thought and behavior.

6.7 SCHIZOPHRENIA: SOMATIC TREATMENT

Avinash De Souza, Nilesh Shah

INTRODUCTION

It was not until recently that science has been able to find any kind of effective treatment for schizophrenia, and even though now there appears to be some understanding of the etiology, neurobiology, and treatment of it, in each of these areas, all that is still up for debate, and perhaps further research will find that present understanding is either correct or woefully lacking. Though neuroleptic medicine had begun in the 1950s with chlorpromazine haloperidol and clozapine, there had been fatal agranulocytosis associated with clozapine, while chlorpromazine and haloperidol had severe side effect profiles that made socialized life for the schizophrenic a near impossibility. Successful treatment of schizophrenia, therefore, depends upon a life-long regimen of both drug and psychosocial, support therapies.

While the medication helps control the psychosis associated with schizophrenia, it cannot help the person find a job, learn to be effective in social relationships, increase the individual's coping skills, and help them learn to communicate and work well with others. Poverty, homelessness, and unemployment are often associated with this disorder, but they do not have to be. If the individual finds appropriate treatment and sticks with it, a person with schizophrenia can lead a happy and successful life. But the initial recovery from the first symptoms of schizophrenia can be an extremely lonely experience. Individuals coping with the onset of schizophrenia for the first time in their lives require all the support that their families, friends, and communities can provide. A sudden stopping of treatment will most often lead to a relapse of the symptoms associated with schizophrenia and then a gradual recovery as treatment is reinstated. The introduction of second-generation antipsychotics and cognitive therapies for schizophrenia over the past two decades generated considerable optimism about possibilities for recovery. In view of our improved understanding of the etiology and pathophysiology of schizophrenia, there is an opportunity to develop prevention strategies and treatments based on this enhanced knowledge.

HISTORY OF SCHIZOPHRENIA TREATMENT

Antipsychotic drugs for the treatment of schizophrenia arrived in the clinic in the fifties of the previous century. Until the early fifties, the treatment of schizophrenia was very limited and usually confined to either inducing a condition of shock with for instance cardiazol, insulin or electrical current, or cutting the connections between the frontal cortex and the deeper brain regions. The general idea behind the shock treatment was that the brain needed to be reset. The synthesis of chlorpromazine (4560RP) in 1950 and its subsequent use in schizophrenic patients by Hamon and Delay and Deniker and their colleagues in 1952, marked the beginning of a revolution in the treatment of schizophrenia. Chlorpromazine was the first chemical compound which was able to selectively reduce hallucinations and delusions. Its pharmacologic characteristic of dopamine receptor blockade was linked to its antipsychotic action. Several different chemical families of neuroleptics were identified, developed, and introduced in the next two decades. Additional phenothiazines like fluphenazine, trifluoperazine and thioridazine were introduced onto the market in the 1950s.

In addition, especially in Europe the butyrophenone haloperidol and its close analogs, and the thioxanthenes such as thiothixene, flupenthixol and chlorprothixene became equally popular in the treatment of schizophrenia.

This widespread use of antipsychotic drugs led to a rapid decline in the number of inpatients in psychiatric institutions, but, at the same time, also led to the realization that antipsychotics have several important side effect, most notably the extrapyramidal side effects (EPS, parkinsonism, dystonia and akathisia) and in 1961 the prevalence of EPS was estimated at almost 40%. In addition, at the end of 1950 antipsychotic induced tardive dyskinesia also reported. After this early productivity, drug discovery almost stopped in the area of schizophrenia therapeutics for about 15 years. After 1978 until the approval of clozapine for psychosis in 1990, no new antipsychotic drugs were brought before the United States (US) Food and Drug Administration (FDA). The fact that this drug was an effective antipsychotic although devoid of inducing EPS, earned it the title of an "atypical antipsychotic". After report on drug induced agranulocytosis in Finland, clozapine was withdrawn from the market in 1977, only under strict conditions in 1990, after a landmark study showed its superiority over chlorpromazine. Its unique clinical profile led to an intensified search for new antipsychotics that, like clozapine, would lack EPS but unlike clozapine, would also lack the risk of agranulocytosis. Thus, after a dry spell in the 1970s and 1980s (with only one or two novel antipsychotics being approved in two decades), the 1990s saw the introduction of risperidone (FDA approval in 1993), olanzapine (1996) and quetiapine (1997), followed by ziprasidone (2001) and aripiprazole (2002). In addition, three additional antipsychotics were approved by the FDA in 2009: iloperidone, asenapine and paliperidone palmitate (which is the 9-OH derivative of risperidone) and lurasidone was approved by the FDA in October, 2010.

CLASSIFICATION OF ANTIPSYCHOTICS

a. First generation antipsychotics (FGAs)

1. *Phenothiazines*
   - (a) *Aliphatic side chain:* Chlorpromazine, chlorproethazine, cyamemazine, levomepromazine, promazine, triflupromazine.
   - (b) *Piperidine side chain:* Mesoridazine, piperacetazine, pipoptiazine, propericiazine, sulforidazine, thioridazine.
   - (c) *Piperazine side chain:* Fluphenazine, acetophenazine, butaperazine, dixyrazine, perazine, perphenazine, prochlorperazine, thiopropazate, thioproperazine, trifluoperazine.
2. *Butyrophenones*: Haloperidol, benperidol, blonanserin, bromperidol, droperidol, fluanisone, melperone, moperone, pipamperone, timiperone, trifluperidol.
3. *Thioxanthenes*: Thiothixene, chlorprothixene, clopenthixol, flupenthixol, zuclopenthixol.
4. *Dihydroindolones*: Molindone, oxypertine.
5. *Dibenzoxazepines*: Loxapine, clotiapine.
6. *Diphenylbutylpiperidines*: Pimozide, fluspirilene, penfluridol.
7. *Benzamides*: Sulpiride, nemonapride, sultopride, tiapride.
8. *Iminodibenzyl*: Clocapramine, mosapramine.

b. Second generation antipsychotics (SGAs)

1. *Benzo (diaze- or thiaze-) pines*: Asenapine, Clozapine, Olanzapine, Quetiapine, Zotepine.
2. *Indolones and diones*: Aripiprazole, iloperidone, paliperidone, perospirone, risperidone, sertindole, ziprasidone.
3. *Benzamide*: Amisulpride.

MECHANISM OF ACTION OF ANTIPSYCHOTIC THERAPY

All antipsychotic drugs tend to block D2 receptors in the dopamine pathways of the brain. This means that dopamine released in these pathways has less effect. Excess release of dopamine in the mesolimbic pathway has been linked to psychotic experiences. It is the blockade of dopamine receptors in this pathway that is thought to control psychotic experiences. Typical antipsychotics are not particularly selective and also block dopamine receptors in the mesocortical pathway, tuberoinfundibular pathway, and the nigrostriatal pathway. Blocking D2 receptors in these other pathways is thought to produce some of the unwanted side effects that the typical antipsychotics can produce.

Atypical antipsychotic drugs have a similar blocking effect on D2 receptors. Some also block or partially block serotonin receptors (particularly 5HT2A, C and 5HT1A receptors). The additional effects on serotonin receptors may be why some of them can benefit the "negative symptoms" of schizophrenia. Parkinsonism and extrapyramidal effects occur with antipsychotics which have a high affinity for D2 and which are, therefore, tightly bound to D2. Clozapine and quetiapine have a low affinity for D2, and, being readily displaced by endogenous dopamine, do not give rise to extrapyramidal effects. Because the loosely bound antipsychotics dissociate from D2 more rapidly.

SIDE EFFECTS OF ANTIPSYCHOTIC DRUGS

Antipsychotics are associated with a range of side effects. Extrapyramidal reactions include acute dystonias, akathisia, parkinsonism (rigidity and tremor), tardive dyskinesia, tachycardia, hypotension, impotence, lethargy, seizures, intense dreams or nightmares, and hyperprolactinemia. In "healthy" individuals without psychosis, doses of antipsychotics can produce the negative symptoms (e.g. emotional and motivational difficulties) associated with schizophrenia. Antipsychotics, particularly atypicals, appear to cause diabetes mellitus and fatal diabetic ketoacidosis. Antipsychotics may cause pancreatitis. The atypical antipsychotics (especially olanzapine and clozapine) seem to (due to occupancy of the histamine receptor) cause weight gain more commonly than the typical antipsychotics.

Antipsychotics increase the likelihood of a fatal heart attack, with the risk of death increasing with dose and the length of time on the drug. Clozapine also has a risk of inducing agranulocytosis, a potentially dangerous reduction in the number of white blood cells in the body. Because of this risk, patients prescribed clozapine may need to have regular blood checks to catch the condition early if it does occur, so the patient is in no danger. One of the more serious of these side effects is tardive dyskinesia, in which the sufferer may show repetitive, involuntary, purposeless movements. A potentially serious side effect of many antipsychotics is that they tend to lower an individual's seizure threshold. Chlorpromazine and clozapine, in particular, have a relatively high seizurogenic potential. Dysphoria, Drug-induced parkinsonism due to dopamine D2 receptor blockade may mimic idiopathic parkinsonism.

Sexual dysfunction, which may rarely continue after withdrawal, similar to post-SSRI sexual dysfunction (PSSD). The breasts may enlarge and discharge milk, in both men and women due to abnormally-high levels of prolactin in the blood. Prolactin secretion in the pituitary is normally suppressed by dopamine. Drugs that block the effects of dopamine at the pituitary or deplete dopamine stores in the brain may cause the pituitary to secrete prolactin. There is a possibility that the risk of tardive dyskinesia can be reduced by combining the antipsychotics with diphenhydramine or benzatropine, although this remains to be established. Central nervous system damage is also associated with irreversible tardive akathisia and/or tardive dysphrenia.

The second-generation antipsychotics, also commonly known as atypical antipsychotics, are among the most significant medicines developed in the past decade for the treatment of mental disorders such as schizophrenia, schizoaffective disorder, and mania. These agents are atypical because they are significantly different, both in structure and pharmacology, from the older, typical antipsychotic medications. Having multiple mechanisms of action in the brain, the second-generation antipsychotics have wider applications than just for the treatment the "positive" symptoms of psychosis (e.g. hallucinations, delusions, bizarre behavior, disorganized speech). These medicines have proven to be highly effective for treating negative symptoms of schizophrenia, which are characterized by emotional and social withdrawal, flat affect, lack of spontaneity, inability to feel pleasure, attention impairment, and other restrictions in thought, speech, and behavior. Thus, most clinicians view second-generation antipsychotics not merely as antipsychotic medications but also as psychotropic agents, which are effective in treating a wide spectrum of mental disorders. In addition to blocking the dopamine D2 receptor, most antipsychotics, and especially the SGAs also inhibit a large number of other receptors, including other dopaminergic (D1, D3 or D4), serotonergic (especially 5-HT2A and 5-HT2C), adrenergic (mainly a1) and histaminergic (especially H1). Most of these receptors have been linked to side effects like weight gain (5-HT2C and H1), drowsiness (H1), sexual dysfunction (5-HT2) and orthostatic hypotension. On the other hand, it has also been hypothesized that the 5-HT2A receptor blockade might be beneficial with respect to the negative and/or cognitive symptoms of schizophrenia as well as to a reduced risk for EPS.

COMPARATIVE EFFECTIVENESS OF ANTIPSYCHOTICS IN THE TREATMENT OF SCHIZOPHRENIA

The broad objectives of treatment are to reduce the mortality and morbidity of the disorder by decreasing the frequency and severity of episodes of psychotic exacerbation and improving the functional capacity and quality of lives of the individuals afflicted with the illness. In the past decade, second-generation antipsychotics have essentially replaced the older, conventional antipsychotics. The primary reason for this is that the second-generation antipsychotics are much better tolerated than their older counterparts. The second-generation agents are associated with a substantially lower risk of EPS and tardive dyskinesia (TD). EPS are acute-onset movement disorders characterized by muscular rigidity, tremors, shuffling movement, restlessness, and muscle spasms resulting in abnormal posture. TD is a delayed-onset condition that consists of abnormal involuntary movements usually involving the tongue and mouth and sometimes the arms and trunk. EPS and TD are substantial risks with conventional antipsychotics. Patients frequently cannot, and will not, tolerate the side effects of antipsychotics, and this becomes problematic if long-term treatment is needed. With their more favorable side effect profile, the newer antipsychotics are better tolerated, and patients are more likely to take them consistently.

The other distinguishing advantage of the second-generation antipsychotics is that they are superior in treating negative symptoms. In areas of the brain where emotion and cognition are affected by the balance of serotonin and dopamine, the dual action of the second-generation agents resets this important balance when it has been altered. In patients with mental disorders such as schizophrenia, the balance of these neurotransmitters is disturbed, and patients may manifest negative symptoms. Clozapine, the first so-called atypical or subsequently labeled "second-generation" antipsychotic (SGA), was introduced into clinical practice in the late 1960s. It does not cause EPS or tardive dyskinesia. Its other adverse effects, however, have substantially limited its utilization and agranulocytosis kept it out of most parts of the world until the 1990s. The fact that it was found to be more effective than FGAs in treatment-refractory patients and in reducing suicidality, 30 and was devoid of significant short-term and long-term motor side-effects led to optimism that better antipsychotic treatments for schizophrenia were possible.

All current antipsychotic therapies have been developed on the half-century old platform of dopamine D2 receptor antagonism. The potent serotonin 5HT-2A antagonism characteristic of the more recently developed so-called second-generation antipsychotic agents is associated with a lower risk of neuromotor side effects (EPS and tardive dyskinesia). In view of the therapeutic limitations of these approaches, a range of other molecular and cellular strategies are being evaluated in schizophrenia. In addition to other dopamine and serotonin receptors, a variety of glutamatergic, cholinergic, GABAergic, neuropeptidergic, cannabinoid, and non-neurotransmitter receptor targets are also being studied in the treatment of schizophrenia.

LONG ACTING INJECTABLE ANTIPSYCHOTICS

Importance of extended release delivery systems to antipsychotics: Antipsychotic drugs have revolutionized the therapy and management of schizophrenia. However, patient compliance rates are very poor due to the nature of the disease and troublesome side effects, and are major causes of symptom recurrence. Although some new antipsychotic agents have been marketed to offer broader efficacy with much reduced side effect profiles, the drug delivery systems for antipsychotics are still in the stage of conventional dosage forms, such as tablets, capsules and solutions, and need to be dosed at the frequency of 2–4 times daily. Doubtless novel drug delivery systems, such as sustained and controlled release systems, will be useful for antipsychotics. They should reduce the frequency of dosing enhance drug bioavailability and improve patient compliance.

CONCLUSION

To conclude, the pharmacological treatment of schizophrenia has improved markedly since the introduction of oral conventional antipsychotic drugs. Second-generation 'atypical' antipsychotics then combined efficacy that is as good as that of conventional agents with improved safety and tolerability. Most recently, the first long-acting, injectable formulation of a second-generation antipsychotic has been developed. These formulations should optimize efficacy, tolerability and compliance among patients with chronic schizophrenia who require long-term therapy and have the potential to become the standard treatment in this group of individuals. There is now new research going into the treatment of schizophrenia. The inevitable result of that is that, whether with the current class of atypical neuroleptics, newer medications, or other treatment modalities, there will eventually be a safe and effective way of dealing with schizophrenia.

6.8 SCHIZOPHRENIA: PSYCHOSOCIAL TREATMENTS

Avinash De Souza, Nilesh Shah

INTRODUCTION

Schizophrenia is an illness with many faces, affecting at various times an individual's capacity for thought, emotion, and social discourse. Although currently available treatments cannot cure this disorder, it is widely recognized that medical and psychosocial therapies can contribute to symptomatic and functional recovery. Psychotropic medications have the greatest effects on symptoms such as hallucinations and delusions, but have less impact on social and instrumental deficits. As a result, even individuals who respond well to pharmacotherapy are at risk for interpersonal distress, chronic unemployment, and a diminished quality of life. Psychosocial treatments, which targets problems of social adaptation and role functioning in schizophrenia, represents an essential ingredient in a coordinated, comprehensive, bio-behavioral approach to treatment.[128]

Psychosocial treatment methods have evolved over the past three decades to address the social and instrumental impairments common among people with schizophrenia. The efficacy of behavioral interventions has been evaluated many times, with a general consensus that learning-based therapies provide benefits to schizophrenia patients beyond the benefits obtained through pharmacotherapy alone.

SOCIAL SKILLS TRAINING IN SCHIZOPHRENIA

Psychosocial skills training procedures are rooted in operant conditioning and social learning theory and represent a highly interactive, structured, systematic, and educational approach to therapy. Instructional methods vary considerably, depending on the content areas of the training program (e.g. conversational vs symptom management skills), but most interventions emphasize an incremental approach to skills acquisition. Complex target behaviors are broken down into constituent elements, microbehaviors are organized into a hierarchy of responses, and components are introduced to patients in a graded manner. Skills trainers use active teaching methods such as didactic instruction, modeling, behavior rehearsal, coaching of desired responses, corrective feedback, contingent social reinforcement, and homework assignments to facilitate the acquisition of new competencies. To counteract schizophrenia patients' attentional, memory, and abstraction impairments, learning material is presented slowly and repetitively in small "chunks" that contain numerous reviews and positive reinforcement. Patients are taught to perform component cognitive and behavioral responses sequentially, gradually combining simpler behaviors into more complex reactions.[129]

These methods have been applied in both individual and group formats to improve schizophrenia patients self-care, social, and independent living skills in hospital, clinic, and residential settings. In addition, behavioral learning principles used in skills training—such as shaping, modeling, behavioral rehearsal, prompting, reinforcement, and in vivo homework assignments—have been used effectively in teaching communication and problem-solving skills to families of patients with schizophrenia or bipolar disorder. The application of skills training techniques to family therapy has been the most widely validated method of psychosocial intervention for reducing stress-related relapse.[130]

The conclusions derived from these interventions are remarkably consistent and can be summarized as follows: (1) Patients with schizophrenia can be taught a wide range of social and instrumental competencies, ranging from simple behaviors, such as gazing and reciprocity during conversations, to more complex behaviors, such as assertiveness, conversational skills, and medication self-management; (2) Social skills training has a positive effect on patients' perceptions of themselves as more assertive and less socially anxious after treatment. Skills training has only a moderate impact, however, on psychiatric symptoms, relapse, and rehospitalization; (3) Skills training appears to result in a "gradient of generalization", with treatment effects generalizing well to measures and settings similar to training situations, but less consistently to novel environments.[131]

Data supporting the efficacy of psychosocial skills training continue to accumulate. Such programs should remain as elements of best practices guidelines and treatment recommendations for schizophrenia. Findings expand our knowledge base concerning where, how, and by whom these interventions can be applied to improve the social and instrumental functioning of schizophrenia patients. Unanswered questions remain, but cautious optimism is warranted regarding the further development of clinically effective psychosocial skills training methods. Future directions for psychosocial skills training include integration of assertive case management with skills training interventions, combining skills training procedures with other psychosocial treatments such as vocational rehabilitation and supported housing, and using in vivo training in community settings, with natural caregivers, to create opportunities, encouragement, and reinforcement for the use of coping abilities in everyday life. It must be determined whether the cognitive process improvements noted hold up over time, are maintained in environments outside of the inpatient treatment setting, and can be replicated by others. Finally, motivation and compliance-enhancing strategies deserve further study in psychosocial skills training investigations, particularly those interventions which emphasize collaborative partnerships between consumers of mental health services and those who serve them.[132]

COGNITIVE TRAINING IN SCHIZOPHRENIA

Schizophrenia is generally viewed as a neurodevelopmental cognitive disorder characterized by relatively stable neuropsychological deficits. These deficits include impaired preattentive abilities, attention, memory, learning, conceptualization, organization, planning, self-monitoring, and flexibility of thinking. Neurocognitive impairment has been reported to predict functional outcome in patients with schizophrenia and, in a recent meta-analysis, was shown to explain 20 to 60% of the variance in measured outcomes. Cognitive deficits are thought to play a central role in the social disability and other problems in daily living experienced by patients with schizophrenia. Certain cognitive features, such as perseveration, also have been associated with persistence of delusional beliefs. Furthermore, cognitive impairment appears to be associated with negative symptoms of schizophrenia, which are socially and vocationally incapacitating to the patients as well as bothersome to their caregivers. Finally, impaired cognition may be a "rate-limiting factor" in the success of psychosocial interventions for schizophrenia (e.g. work rehabilitation and social skills training). Thus, amelioration of neurocognitive deficits has been posited to be an important treatment goal in schizophrenia.[133]

A number of investigators have pursued non-pharmacological means of improving residual cognitive and functional deficits in patients with schizophrenia. In the six decades since Goldstein wrote, "We have to attack the disease underlying schizophrenic symptoms by physical and psychological ways," research on "psychological ways" to treat schizophrenia has advanced considerably. The recent Surgeon General's Report on Mental Health emphasizes the combination of pharmacological and psychosocial interventions for increased treatment benefit in schizophrenia. Evidence-based practice guidelines for psychosocial treatment of schizophrenia include psychosocial treatments such as social skills training, cognitive/cognitive-behavioral therapy and vocational rehabilitation as indicated by a number of recent empirical articles and reviews. Literature on cognitive training (CT) in schizophrenia has been reviewed in recent publications as well. It should be noted that cognitive therapy, which focuses on modification of maladaptive beliefs and schemas, is distinguished from cognitive training, which aims to improve neurocognitive abilities such as memory, learning, attention, and executive functioning.[134]

It may be concluded that there are effective elements of computer-assisted CT, automated and strategy-oriented practice CT, and environmental adaptation CT. There is no compelling evidence that the cognitive impairments that characterize schizophrenia can be eliminated by any available treatment. Indeed, few would suggest that short-term CT can permanently resolve long-standing neuropsychological deficits in any population. There is evidence that CT, whether computer-assisted or not, can yield some positive effects in terms of cognitive performance, psychiatric symptoms, and everyday functioning, but it is not known whether these effects are sustainable. Although the question of the mechanism of action underlying the effects of CT has not been empirically investigated, we believe that the primary mechanism is probably compensatory. Both the interventions and the issues related to generalization and maintenance of treatment gains are different.[135]

For example, an environmental approach may foster maintenance as long as the environmental supports are in place, but generalization may be limited. Internal compensatory strategies may be easier to generalize in the short-term but more difficult to maintain over time if people fail to initiate in the real world the strategies they learned during the intervention. CT efforts should focus on improving everyday functioning via compensatory strategies or overlearning of tasks, rather than restoring cognitive abilities *per se*. Given the positive findings of the task practice approaches (whether computer, assisted or not) and the encouraging findings regarding environmental adaptations, clinicians may consider using these tools in appropriate settings while awaiting more definitive research. Another possibility is that CT may be useful in conjunction with other interventions, to maximize learning in, for example, social skills training or vocational rehabilitation.[136]

Adequate sample sizes are needed, based on anticipated effect sizes for different outcome measures. Research on more representative samples of patients with schizophrenia, including women, ethnic minorities, and older patients, would improve the generalizability of findings. Both standard care and attention/training placebo control conditions should be employed. Controlling for type of antipsychotic drug treatment (e.g. conventional vs atypical agents) will be an important advance in this literature; drug treatments could also be investigated as predictors of response to CT. CT manuals should be developed to enhance fidelity of treatment. Outcome measures should include assessments of cognitive performance, psychiatric symptoms, and everyday functioning. Furthermore, these assessments should be carried out longitudinally to (1) establish whether there are clinically meaningful lasting effects of CT, and (2) investigate the mechanisms of action underlying these effects (e.g. to test mediators of the relationship between changes in cognition and changes in everyday functioning).[137]

Establishing which patients benefit from CT, which ones do not, and what costs are associated with CT will be important in the dissemination of CT as a clinical treatment for schizophrenia. Examination of subgroups of patients (e.g. based on demographic variables, severity and chronicity of disease and associated disability, disease subtype, current medication type, and cognitive deficit profile) will allow for better matching of treatment to the individual patient. Regarding cost-of-treatment issues, establishing the efficacy of group-based CT treatments may increase the value of CT in the managed care environment. Theoretically driven research that attempts to delineate restorative, compensatory, or environmental adaptation effects will be helpful in determining which component works in CT for schizophrenia. Acceptance of a common nomenclature (e.g. restorative, compensatory, environmental) and theoretical background may also allow this field to move forward more quickly.[138]

ASSERTIVE COMMUNITY TREATMENT

Systems of care serving persons with schizophrenia should include a program of assertive community treatment (ACT). This intervention should be provided to individuals who are at risk for repeated hospitalizations or have recent homelessness. The key elements of ACT include a multidisciplinary team including a medication prescriber, a shared caseload among team members, direct service provision by team members, a high frequency of patient contact, low patient-to-staff ratios, and outreach to patients in the community. ACT has been found to significantly reduce hospitalizations and homelessness among individuals with schizophrenia. ACT has recently been adapted for forensic populations with the goal of reducing recidivism and promoting engagement in treatment. Modifications to ACT include the addition of a probation officer to the treatment team and, in some cases, the addition of residential housing and addiction treatment services. Evidence for the effectiveness of ACT among individuals with mental illness who also have a criminal background remains mixed, with limited evidence for reduced arrests and days spent in hospital or jail, as well as reduced rates of substance use. Nonetheless, heterogeneity of these ACT adaptations and high levels of study attrition preclude a recommendation for ACT among forensic, mentally ill populations.[139]

SUPPORTED EMPLOYMENT

Any person with schizophrenia who has the goal of employment should be offered supported employment to assist them in both obtaining and maintaining competitive employment. The key elements of supported employment include individually tailored job development, rapid job search, availability of ongoing job supports, and integration of vocational and mental health services. The major components of supported employment are competitive employment in the community, rapid search for a job rather than prolonged pre-employment preparation, integration of employment and mental health services, an emphasis on client preference and choice regarding jobs, and the availability of ongoing job supports. There is clear evidence that employment outcomes are better when there is greater fidelity to the supported employment model (i.e. more of these components are in place). While greater integration of mental health services and vocational services is associated with better outcomes, the individual effectiveness of the other elements of supported employment has not been demonstrated. Thus, it is recommended that supported employment programs make every effort to incorporate all aspects of this treatment model. Despite firm evidence for supported employment as compared with other approaches to vocational rehabilitation, long-term job retention and economic self-sufficiency have not been clearly demonstrated by supported employment. To address these limitations, there has been increased interest in studying methods for enhancing outcomes by augmenting vocational services with interventions such as cognitive remediation, social skills training, and cognitive behavioral therapy (CBT).[140]

TOKEN ECONOMY INTERVENTIONS

Systems of care that deliver long-term inpatient or residential care should provide a behavioral intervention based on social learning principles for patients in these settings in order to improve their personal hygiene, social interactions, and other adaptive behaviors. The key elements of this intervention, often referred to as a token economy, are contingent positive reinforcement for clearly defined target behaviors, an individualized treatment approach, and the avoidance of punishing consequences. The intervention should be delivered in the context of a safe treatment environment that provides patient access to basic amenities, evidence-based pharmacological treatment, and the full range of other recommended psychosocial interventions. The existing literature also does not address the extent to which social learning approaches may benefit patients who are receiving other evidence-based psychosocial and pharmacological interventions. Behavioral interventions based on social learning principles that are developed for specific problem behaviors and that are less comprehensive than the token economy may also be effective; such interventions may also be applied in noninstitutional or in short-stay settings. Implementation of a token economy or related behavioral program should take into account practitioner attitudes and possible misconceptions of the token economy and the principles of social learning on which it is based.[141]

FAMILY INTERVENTIONS

Persons with schizophrenia who have ongoing contact with their families, including relatives and significant others, should be offered a family intervention that lasts at least 6–9 months. Interventions that last 6–9 months have been found to significantly reduce rates of relapse and rehospitalization. Though not as consistently observed, research has found other benefits for patients and families, such as increased medication adherence, reduced psychiatric symptoms, and reduced levels of perceived stress for patients. Family members have also been found to have lower levels of burden and distress and improved family relationships. Key elements of effective family interventions include illness education, crisis intervention, emotional support, and training in how to cope with illness symptoms and related problems. The selection of a family intervention should be guided by collaborative decision-making among the patient, family, and clinician. In addition, a family intervention that is shorter than 6 months but that is at least 4 sessions in length should be offered to persons with schizophrenia who have ongoing contact with their families, including relatives and significant others, and for whom a longer intervention is not feasible or acceptable. Characteristics of the briefer interventions include education, training, and support. Possible benefits for patients include reduced psychiatric symptoms, improved treatment adherence, improved functional and vocational status, and greater satisfaction with treatment. Positive family outcomes include reduced family burden and increased satisfaction with family relationships.[142]

In terms of positive outcomes for family members, family members involved in the family psychoeducation condition reported greater knowledge of schizophrenia and improved family relationships compared with those in the control condition. Overall, the evidence for the effectiveness of a 6–9 month family psychoeducation intervention for reduction of relapse and other outcomes among patients who have not had a recent illness exacerbation is not nearly as strong as the evidence for 6–9 month family psychoeducation for individuals who have had a recent illness exacerbation. Family psychoeducation interventions that are shorter than 6 months (but at minimum 4 sessions) have been shown to contribute to positive patient and family outcomes among both individuals who are psychiatrically stable and those who have had a recent relapse. Notably, these studies show benefit among a range of outcomes, though no single patient outcome is observed in all or the majority of studies. Also, over half of these interventions are designed for family members only and do not include patients in the treatment sessions. However, briefer interventions that include the patient have also been tested. The inclusion of family members only permits families to participate in a program during circumstances when the patient is uninterested or unwilling to participate.[143]

PSYCHOSOCIAL WEIGHT MANAGEMENT

Individuals with schizophrenia who are overweight (body mass index [BMI] = 25.0–29.9) or obese (BMI 30.0) should be offered a psychosocial weight loss intervention that is at least 3 months in duration to promote weight loss. The key elements of psychosocial interventions for weight loss include psychoeducation focused on nutritional counseling, caloric expenditure, and portion control; behavioral self-management including goal setting; regular weighins; self-monitoring of daily food and activity levels; and dietary and physical activity modifications. Despite the preponderance of positive findings, marked variability regarding intervention techniques, materials, settings, intensity, and duration warrant limited interpretation of the current body of evidence. Additional limitations of the evidence include small sample sizes across most of the studies and difficulties with participant retention. Furthermore, there is limited evidence for sustainability of weight loss. While the evidence for interventions for weight loss is strong enough to warrant a recommendation, the current state of the literature exploring psychosocial interventions for the prevention of weight gain among individuals with schizophrenia is not substantial enough to warrant a formal recommendation at this time.[144]

INTERVENTIONS TO INCREASE COMPLIANCE

Nonadherence to prescribed antipsychotic medication regimens is a considerable problem among people with schizophrenia and is associated with psychotic relapse, hospitalization, and other adverse outcomes. A variety of strategies that specifically target medication adherence have been tested in RCTs. Research provides only mixed support for educational approaches. Behavioral tailoring approaches have the most promise as demonstrated by small trials on narrowly defined populations. The provision of environmental supports for medication adherence also has promise. However, at this point, there is insufficient evidence to recommend any specific intervention to promote adherence to antipsychotic medications among persons with schizophrenia.[145]

CONCLUSION

Recent changes in the conceptualization of recovery have pointed to the possibility that psychosocial treatments could again come to play a significant role in the treatment of persons with schizophrenia. In particular we have suggested psychosocial treatments could address two interrelated facets of self-experience personal narrative and the capacity for metacognition and potentially set the stage for the achievement of an enhanced the quality-of-life. We have suggested that with the attainment of a richer personal understanding and greater capacity to think about thinking, individuals with schizophrenia may feel sufficiently empowered and able to envision a realistically hopeful future, and to plan out courses of action likely to lead to goal attainment. With a fuller multidimensional and storied account of one's own strengths and weaknesses, and with a greater ability to reason about one's own internal states, it seems likely that persons could make more reasoned and less impulsive decisions in the face of adversity. In contrast to symptom or problem focused approaches, addressing these larger facets of self-experience might enable persons to flexibly formulate more courses of action in response to a greater range of challenges and to weather general threats to self-esteem, all leading to sustained wellness and the experience on the part of the persons with schizophrenia that they themselves are shaping a meaningful life for themselves in an individualized, self-determined and holistic manner.

6.9 SCHIZOPHRENIA: ROLE OF PSYCHOTHERAPY

Avinash De Souza, Nilesh Shah

INTRODUCTION

The effectiveness of antipsychotic medication has made it central to the treatment of schizophrenia. However, there is an increasing acknowledgment that pharmacological treatment on its own is rarely sufficient for the best outcome in this disabling condition. The final element in the re-evaluation of the treatment of schizophrenia is that there has been a change in perception of psychological interventions, such that they are now recognized as an important component of a comprehensive therapeutic approach.

Antipsychotic drugs have a limited impact on the negative symptoms of schizophrenia, and thus, do not contribute to the development of the skills necessary for successful transition back into the community. There is, thus, a clear requirement for the development of new approaches if the wide ranging needs of people with schizophrenia are to be met. This emphasis is new. In comparison to those channelled into pharmacological interventions, relatively few resources have been spent on evaluating and developing other treatments.[146]

INDIVIDUAL PSYCHOTHERAPY FOR SCHIZOPHRENIA

In the early decades of the 20th century schizophrenia was viewed as unbeatable. "Organic" psychiatry as represented by Emil Kraepelin saw schizophrenic personality disintegration as an inevitable product of neurological deterioration. Following Freud, most psychoanalysts considered dementia praecox to be a "narcissistic neurosis," where transference and analytic treatment were impossible. The diagnosis of dementia praecox most often led to therapeutic nihilism and recommendation of lifelong institutional care.[146]

Frieda Fromm-Reichmann's Principles of Intensive Psychotherapy (1950) was the first systematic elaboration of what became known as intensive psychodynamic psychotherapy. The predecessors of ego and self-psychology, "interpersonal psychiatry" and "psychodynamic psychotherapy," became dominant paradigms in American psychiatry in the 1940s, 1950s, and 1960s. The goal of intensive, or investigative, psychotherapy is alleviation of the patient's emotional difficulties and elimination of symptoms. This is accomplished by undertaking a thorough scrutiny of the patient's life history, reviewing in close detail the realities of the patient's current relationships and life situation and understanding the historical roots and current ramifications of maladaptive interpersonal patterns as reflected in the doctor-patient relationship and in daily life. This process is expected to result in modification of maladaptive interpersonal patterns and personality growth.[147]

The literature on intensive psychotherapy emphasizes the influence of the environment in the etiology of schizophrenia. Characteristic difficulties among patients with schizophrenia are said to include (1) a basic mistrust and expectation of harm from others; (2) a marked ambivalence in relationships, with oscillations between longing for merger based on intolerance of loneliness and withdrawal and isolation based on terror of closeness; and (3) weak or absent ego boundaries with resulting difficulty differentiating one's own thoughts and impulses from those of others. The central conflict of schizophrenia patients was described as "that of a small child dependent on a person by whom he feels persecuted and who is, in his opinion, unstable and uncertain". This position was thought to represent the patient's conviction concerning the nature of human relationships. "Process" refers to expected developments in the doctor-patient relationship as it evolves over time.[148]

"Transference" is the manner in which the perception of others in the present is shaded or distorted by important past relationships. It is thought of as a natural, but often unconscious, aspect of all human relationships. Examining transference in the doctor-patient relationship is a major task in investigative (as opposed to supportive) psychotherapy—this examination is expected to be useful in allowing the patient to better understand his or her current difficulties and respond more realistically to people in his or her current life. "Countertransference" refers to all of the therapist's thoughts and feelings about the patient. Some of these are distortions arising from the therapist's past, but others derive from current interaction with the patient. Feelings that arise in work with schizophrenia patients can be particularly intense and may include discouragement, fear, worthlessness, guilt, rage, envy, or lust. In view of this, awareness of countertransference and the ability through introspection to understand its sources are crucial functions for the psychotherapist. In the tradition of investigative psychotherapy, countertransference also serves as a source of information about the patient's state of mind, and as an indicator for understanding how others typically react and respond to the patient.[149]

Successful management of countertransference allows the therapist to create a "holding" or "containing" relationship with the patient that is postulated to be central to the action of psychotherapy. The literature on intensive psychotherapy describes interventions that correspond to different phases of therapy: (1) establishing a relationship with the patient, (2) elucidating the patient's experience, (3) tolerating mobilized transference and countertransference, (4) integrating the patient's experiences into an expanded perspective of the self, and (5) working through. The accomplishment of earlier tasks allows greater attention to be paid to subsequent ones.[150]

Establishing a relationship with a schizophrenia patient can be challenging. Therapist attributes seen as important are an interest in and capacity to tolerate intense affect, dependency, and ambiguous communication. Basic respect for the patient is a prerequisite. Aloofness, rigidity, and critical pomposity are especially discouraged. The psychotherapist should be flexible, creative, and willing to admit when he or she is wrong. Frequency of visits can range from one to five per week, and free association is discouraged as aggravating disorganization and thought disorder. Within bounds, a reasonable degree of self-disclosure on the therapist's part can help counter distortions by allowing the patient to get a fix on the therapist as a person. A relationship should be sought on the patient's terms. If the initial encounters are traversed successfully, a background feeling of security and predictability will increasingly characterize the therapy. Semrad viewed the three core tasks of psychotherapy as helping the patient acknowledge, bear, and put into perspective his feelings and painful life experiences. Acknowledging the patient's feelings and painful experiences becomes pertinent once a relationship has been established. Acknowledging requires elucidating affects, employing strategies such as listening, narrowing the focus, seeking concrete detail, acknowledging feelings (especially loss, anger, and sadness), and naming or labeling affects. The therapist conveys to the patient that experiencing emotions will neither overwhelm the patient nor hurt others.[151]

Examining the patient's day-to-day life in detail will allow the therapist to develop a more vivid picture of the patient's difficulties, frustrations, and characteristic reactions to others. If successful, therapist and patient will share a common language with which to communicate about the latter's difficulties. Tolerating affects, transference, and countertransference corresponds to Semrad's concept of "bearing" painful feelings. Simply stated, patients experience themselves being accepted, negative emotions and all, and, learning from the therapist's example, become better able to accept unwanted aspects of themselves. Thus, the patient's identification with the therapist and his or her functioning is seen as a major factor in the therapeutic action of psychotherapy. Broadening patients' understanding of themselves and their situation corresponds to the third part of Semrad's triad: helping patients put into perspective their painful affects, life experiences, and maladaptive solutions. Thus, providing insight is another way in which psychotherapy is thought to be useful, complementing identification with the therapist. Integrating the patient's experience entails a change in therapeutic relationship and enlists interpretation as its major technical tool.[152]

Emotional insight, gained by direct experience in the doctor-patient relationship, is emphasized. This derives from interpretations pointing out the transferential nature of the patient's feelings toward the doctor, including their origin in the patient's past experience and their inappropriate application in the patient's current everyday life. If traversed successfully, this phase of therapy will leave patients with a more accepting and complex view of themselves experiencing the full range of human emotions. The patient will recognize that continued progress depends on willingness to attempt new solutions, both inside and outside of treatment. With improvement in psychosis and maturation of the patient's nonpsychotic personality, the phase of integrating evolves into the last phase of working through. The patient becomes better able to help the therapist perform his or her functions and eventually becomes capable of performing these functions independently.[153]

SUPPORTIVE PSYCHOTHERAPY IN SCHIZOPHRENIA

Supportive psychotherapy has been favored by biologically and pharmacologically-oriented clinicians. In theory and technique it is grounded in the medical model where the patient is seen as suffering from an organically-based illness requiring treatment from a physician. As described by Talcot Parsons, the medical model implies essential elements of expected behavior for both the physician and patient. These elements define the physician's and patient's roles, relationship, and responsibilities. The physician's role is characterized by four key qualities: (1) universalistic, (2) functionally specific, (3) affectively neutral, and (4) collectivity oriented. The universalistic norm requires the physician to treat all patients alike according to scientific and medical standards. The role is functionally specific in that the physician is seen as a specialist in health and disease and is expected to limit attention to circumscribed medical matters. Affective neutrality prevents the doctor from entering too sympathetically into the patient's situation; this allows for steadfastness of judgment and the exercise of emotional control. Finally, collectivity orientation, as opposed to self-orientation, demands that the doctor treat the patient according to the patient's needs and the health standards of the community.[154]

The role of the patient, like the role of the physician, is defined by expected behavior that involves both rights and obligations. First, the person who is ill is exempt from normal social responsibilities and excused from customary obligations so he or she may attend to the process of getting well. A second right is exemption from responsibility for illness—the illness is not considered the patient's fault, and the patient has the right to receive care. At the same time, the patient has the obligation to want to get well, to obtain technically competent help, and to cooperate with treatment. In contrast to the ambitious aim of personality change associated with the intensive therapy tradition, the short- and long-term goals of supportive psychotherapy are comparatively modest. They include the following: (1) relief from the immediate crisis or direct reduction of acute disequilibrium, (2) removal of symptoms to premorbid levels, (3) re-establishment of psychic homeostasis through a strengthening of defenses, (4) sealing over psychotic experiences and conflicts, (5) the circumscribed fostering of adaptation, and (6) mobilization and preservation of healthy aspects of the patient to enable optimal functioning and minimize the impact of persistent deficits. Supportive therapy uses the physician-patient relationship to create a background of adequate clinical care to support the prescription of effective pharmacological interventions. Functional or social recovery, rather than personality change, is the primary aim of treatment. The overall technical approach of supportive psychotherapy is one of pragmatism in which the physician, based on medical and psychiatric expertise, helps the patient interpret and adapt to reality.[155]

As such, the therapist employs techniques that include defining reality, offering direct reassurance, giving advice on current problems of living, urging modification of expectations, and actively organizing the environment for patients who cannot do so themselves. To help stabilize the patient's environment, the therapist often maintains close contact with the patient's family or others providing treatment and may intervene on the patient's behalf with family, employers, and social agencies. Eliciting and tracking symptomatology and targeting symptoms for psychopharmacological intervention is a major focus for the supportive psychotherapist. Psychopathology is interpreted in a medical context as the unwanted emergence of signs of illness. The basic content of psychotherapy focuses on teaching and relearning—the patient is educated regarding the nature of the illness, taught to monitor symptoms, and act promptly to suppress his or her exacerbation. The therapist fosters positive transference as a benign authority; positive feelings are regarded as real. Negative transference is avoided. The therapist may become active in helping the patient learn new ways of adapting and may use or prescribe cognitive, behavioral, or social skill training techniques.[156]

COGNITIVE BEHAVIOR THERAPY AND SCHIZOPHRENIA

Cognitive behavioral treatments are at a relatively early stage of development. There are few trials, and patient numbers in the trials tend to be small. This inevitably restricts the conclusions that can be drawn. However, despite the limited number of trials, the treatments have been implemented in a wide range of settings. Our analyses demonstrated that cognitive behavior therapy was effective in improving mental state on measures of 'important improvement', both during treatment and at follow-up. On continuous measures, this effect is only visible at follow-up. The finding of a positive impact of cognitive behavior therapy (CBT) on mental state is not surprising, as CBT tackles the underlying cognitions hypothesized to be inextricably linked to mental state. However, why positive effects on continuous measures of mental state are only apparent at follow-up is less clear.[157]

Our analyses do suggest that cognitive behavioral interventions for schizophrenia offer a potentially effective treatment. The results from the early trials are promising despite their small numbers. Nevertheless, in comparison, for example with most trials of antipsychotic medication, they provide reasonably good follow-up data over extended periods. The positive results of the meta-analysis can, therefore, be taken as confirming the promise of cognitive behavioral treatment in schizophrenia. Much work is needed to refine the treatment in terms of identifying the most effective components and the best methods for delivering it. However, given that many people continue to suffer from symptoms and difficulties despite extensive pharmacological and service-based interventions, it is important that efforts are made to develop CBT. If its promise is confirmed it should be made more generally available in secondary care mental health services, thereby offering a greater choice of psychosocial interventions for sufferers and their carers. While the interventions all met the criteria for CBT and would be recognizable to those trained in the technique, there was considerable variation in the nature and duration of treatment provided.[158]

Although the evidence available from the current trials is limited, there is some suggestion that longer-term treatments are associated with a better outcome. This is evident from the increased effect over time of CBT on mental state. The majority of the studies also concentrate on outpatients with chronic disorders. At this stage in the development of CBT, there is a need for further research that address several issues. The first area for consideration is the range of outcomes. As stated above, there is a need for a robust measure of relapse, applied with consistency across studies. In addition the impact of CBT should be measured not only on the target symptoms (usually hallucinations and delusions) but also on mental state generally and affective state in particular. As with family interventions, the impact of duration and frequency of treatment should be the focus of further research. The results are likely to have considerable implications for the future availability of CBT, in particular whether it remains a treatment for relatively few patients provided by highly trained specialists or becomes more widely available. Little is known about the patient populations that might benefit most from CBT.[159]

The majority of interventions have focused on chronic or treatment resistant schizophrenia. The lack of effect on relapse rates can be understood in this context: the patients are chronically symptomatic, so improvement is an appropriate measure, while relapse generally is not. It is clear, however, that more needs to be understood of the effect of CBT at different stages of the illness and on different presenting symptoms. In patients prone to relapse and recovery, the use of CBT to reduce relapse should be investigated. In part, the answers to these questions will lie in a better understanding of the process of change in treatment.[160]

CURRENT PSYCHOTHERAPY RESEARCH IN SCHIZOPHRENIA

One of the first clinicians to advocate for individual psychotherapy for people with schizophrenia was Carl Jung (1907/1960), who treated many hospitalized patients at the Burghölzli Hospital in the early part of the 20th century. Jung noted that many people with schizophrenia are amenable to therapy, but that caution must be used because under certain conditions, therapy could cause an increase in symptoms. Moreover, with the growth of psychoanalysis, and Freud's (1957) claim that persons with schizophrenia could not benefit from psychoanalysis due an inability on their part to form deep attachments with others, psychotherapy for schizophrenia was virtually nonexistent by the middle of the 20th century. Around that time, however, psychoanalysts such as Fromm-Reichmann (1954), Searles (1965), Sullivan (1962) and Knight (1946) all contended that meaningful intimate bonds with persons with schizophrenia emerged in therapy, and that those bonds could be the basis of a movement towards health.[161]

One of the key studies, referred to as the Boston Psychotherapy Study, randomly assigned over 160 adults with schizophrenia to receive exploratory insight-oriented therapy or a reality-based supportive psychotherapy. Despite extensive training of therapists, methodological sophistication, and careful selection of an appropriate sample, results revealed a drop rate of just over 40% at six months and a drop rate of nearly 70% at two years, in addition to little therapeutic benefit from insight-oriented therapy. A later reanalysis of the data suggested some improvements in negative symptoms among participants assigned to the more skilled therapists. Beyond the finding which suggests two in five persons with schizophrenia are not interested in psychotherapy, at least in the forms offered in the Boston study, evolving scientific research dealt an even more fatal blow to psychotherapy around this same point in time. Empirical research failed to support the etiological theories that were the basis for psychoanalytic psychotherapy of schizophrenia. While some were claiming that psychotherapy alone was the way to address the faulty family dynamics that purportedly caused psychosis, research indicated that schizophrenia was instead a genetically-influenced, neurobiological brain disorder which involves the distortion of basic human experience, and that its etiology was unrelated to unhealthy family dynamics.[162]

Chadwick (2006) developed Person-Based Cognitive Therapy (PBCT) for distressing psychosis, in an effort to move from a symptom-focused to a person-focused therapy. PBCT integrates cognitive theory and therapy, mindfulness, Rogerian principles, and a Vygotskian social-developmental perspective which stresses language as a socially available tool which persons use to make meaning of daily activity. This approach uses cognitive and experiential techniques for working with negative self-schemata and developing positive self-schemata, and for promoting self-acceptance and metacognition. Interest has also increased in using a modified form of psychoanalytic therapy for people with schizophrenia.[163]

Proposed treatment approaches vary somewhat, but all seem to agree on the following principles: (1) psychotherapy with people with schizophrenia is possible; (2) the classic psychoanalytic approach, including free association and lying on the couch with the therapist out of sight, is contraindicated; (3) the present should be emphasized over the past; (4) interpretations should only be used with caution; (5) goals of therapy should include fostering the experience of the self and the therapist as two separate people that share a relationship, stabilization of ego boundaries and identity, and the integration of the psychotic experience; (6) the frequency of sessions should range between 1 and 3 sessions a week and therapy should last for at least two years; and (7) therapists who work with people with schizophrenia need to have a high level of frustration tolerance, and not have a need to derive narcissistic gratification from the patient's effort or progress. Some evidence suggests that such an approach can be helpful, at least for people who are more clinically stable at the outset of treatment. Results reported thus far suggest that both the integrated psychosocial treatment and the supportive psychodynamic psychotherapy may lead to better overall functional outcomes after one year of treatment.[164,165]

FUTURE RESEARCH INTO THE PSYCHOTHERAPY FOR SCHIZOPHRENIA

First, with future general empirical support for these procedures it will have to be determined what would assist clinical settings to implement such a form of psychotherapy. Another set of practical issues to be addressed will also pertain to what forms of training and supervision are necessary to support them. For instance, what sorts of staff can learn and implement these procedures, and what staff and environmental variables determine whether the intervention is implemented faithfully? Second, on a more theoretical note, while we have focused on self-experience as a meaningful domain of recovery in its own right, changes in this domain are likely to lead to changes in other domains of recovery. With new procedures and assessments of changes in self-experience, it may be possible to empirically examine the kinds of reciprocal relationships that exist between changes in the capacities for metacognition and the richness personal narrative with changes in functional assessments of work, interpersonal and community function. Such research would not only be of theoretical import in terms of conceptualizing the process of recovery but also to might help to develop and refine new treatments. Ultimately, such a program of research could be capable of exploring whether the kinds of psychotherapy described above have an effect on more internal and subjective constructs linked to recovery such as the extent to which one feels one is more in control of one's choices, self-esteem, involvement in one's own recovery process, and feeling that one's life has meaning.[166]

Consistent with this, as has been long noted, participation in a range of rehabilitative activities may reshape how one makes meaning of one's life both in the immediate and larger narrative sense. Thus, it seems important to study the psychotherapeutic effects of currently employed rehabilitative and other evidence-based methods which stress the benefits of natural supports. Does the acquisition of skills and the development of natural supports in other evidenced-based programs have similar or different effects on personal narrative, cognition and social skills as psychotherapy? Such research may point to a way to further enhance the effects of these interventions with regard to narrative and metacognition. It may also point to important developments with regards to the interface of psychotherapy and other interventions and some promising avenues for synergistic combinations of interventions. For example, might not cognitive rehabilitation (to improve cognitive flexibility), for instance augment the possible impact of a recovery-oriented psychotherapy leading to greater degree of improvement in the subjective domains of recovery?[167]

Similarly, given findings on the multiple positive effects and meanings of work for people with schizophrenia, might not supported employment help generate beliefs and feelings about the self that can be further explored and integrated with other aspects of personal narrative in psychotherapy. Finally, future research is also needed to address for whom such forms of psychotherapy might be most useful. For instance are these interventions better suited for persons who are earlier vs later on in their illness? Intuitively, given that persons early in the their illness have many difficult things to make sense of (i.e. the meaning of the psychotic episode in their life trajectory, whether it is an obstacle to overcome or evidence of inevitable decline, whether life dreams will be pursued or abandoned, etc.), and many troublesome decisions to reach, a therapy that addressed issues of narrative and metacognition might be uniquely useful. Of note, as suggested in one recent review, the usefulness of more symptom focused cognitive interventions is still a matter of debate.[168]

CONCLUSION

Recent changes in the conceptualization of recovery have pointed to the possibility that psychotherapy could again come to play a significant role in the treatment of persons with schizophrenia. To explore this issue we have summarized literature on the history of psychotherapy for schizophrenia and discussed whether impoverished self experience in schizophrenia, a potent barrier to recovery, could be targeted by psychotherapy. In particular we have suggested psychotherapy could address two interrelated facets of self-experience personal narrative and the capacity for metacognition and potentially set the stage for the achievement of an enhanced the quality-of-life.

In contrast to symptom or problem focused approaches, addressing these larger facets of self-experience might enable persons to flexibly formulate more courses of action in response to a greater range of challenges and to weather general threats to self-esteem, all leading to sustained wellness and the experience on the part of the persons with schizophrenia that they themselves are shaping a meaningful life for themselves in an individualized, self-determined and holistic manner. Regarding future research we have suggested that these possibilities point to the need to develop carefully defined and testable integrative psychotherapeutic methods, tools for tracking change in self-experience over time and explorations of the potential psychotherapeutic impact of existing rehabilitative practices and the synergistic combination of psychotherapy with other practices.

6.10 TREATMENT RESISTANT SCHIZOPHRENIA

Avinash De Souza, Nilesh Shah

INTRODUCTION

The concept of treatment-resistant schizophrenia was associated with the development of antipsychotic drugs. Although previous attempts had been made, the first definition acknowledged in the scientific literature, was linked to the development of an antipsychotic drug, clozapine. A study carried out in 1988 by Kane defined "treatment-resistance" and indicated clozapine as the gold-standard treatment for these patients. This recommendation remains in the clinical guidelines. It is a dichotomous definition of response/no response. Other dimensional definitions, such as by Brenner appeared later and were more applicable to daily practice. The leverage effect of psychotherapeutic and psychosocial interventions has been successively integrated with antipsychotic drugs and resilience to stress factors in the overall response. This has finally led to an integrated biopsychosocial approach and a multilevel assessment of treatment response. There has also been progress in the knowledge of the pathology. Other researchers have pointed out the variability in the clinical course of schizophrenia after a first episode, with regard to different factors that influence both the clinical course and response to treatment. One of the most significant among those referred to is duration of untreated psychosis, which may be related to the severity of the disease and be a marker that determines its course. This evolution reflects changes in the way treatment-resistance is conceptualized, and ranges from dichotomy to dimensionality. Concepts such as remission, much closer to the idea of recovery, had already been developed in the 21st century. Even though this concept was used in the literature, in light of recent advances it has been taken up again with a new meaning.

DEFINITIONS AND CONCEPT OF TREATMENT RESISTANT SCHIZOPHRENIA

At the beginning of the 20th century, since there were no drugs to control symptoms, the criteria of no response were based on the need to be housed in an asylum. The criteria of the time were based on the quality of personal and social functioning. With the development of drugs in the 1970s, certain quantitative criteria were included, but the idea of functioning remained: chronic hospitalization for more than 2 years was one of the criteria for defining a case as treatment-resistant. Other factors which could influence hospitalization and were not symptoms in themselves, were not taken into account. Another criterion used was the persistence of positive symptoms of schizophrenia, despite appropriate antipsychotic treatment. At this time, the difference between chronicity and drug treatment-resistance did not exist as such.

At the beginning of the 1980s, some researchers, attempted to define "treatment-resistance" by introducing pharmacology into the definition. During this period, Deniker et al. also defined "treatment-resistance" as the maintenance of symptoms for 2 years, with standard doses of antipsychotic drugs for 6 months. However, it was following research with clozapine by Kane in 1988, that the definitions of "treatment-resistance" and "treatment-refractoriness" were systemized and scientifically validated, and criteria were applied to different studies. The definition, based on criteria, arose from a pharmacological need, to prove the effectiveness of clozapine on this type of patient and to have it licensed for use on treatment-resistant schizophrenia. In this multicenter study, Kane established the criteria, currently still in use with some changes, for the duration of the treatment needed, the number of failed pharmacological tests, and the necessary pharmacological doses, spurred by evidence that with doses of chlorpromazine 400 mg/day, 80–90% of the dopaminergic receptors were already blocked. These more or less restrictive criteria are currently used in their application: a more restrictive definition for research purposes, another less restrictive one for developing antipsychotic drugs, and another that is more broadly defined being clinically and practically relevant. This difference in criteria is important since discrepancies arise when it comes to quantifying resistance to treatment. The definition by Kane, as well as the previous ones, dichotomously assess response/no response and are discordant with observations in clinical practice, making the definitions incomplete.

KANE'S CRITERIA FOR TREATMENT RESISTANT SCHIZOPHRENIA

- Treatment with different classes of antipsychotics at equal doses of 1000 mg/day of chlorpromazine for at least 3 periods of 6 weeks in the last 5 years without significant clinical improvement.
- Reduction of at least 20% on the BPRS scale, score > 35 points on the BPRS scale after treatment, CGI score > 3 after treatment with 60 mg/day of haloperidol for 6 weeks.

- BPRS score > 45. Score > 2 on BPRS items of conceptual disorganization, unusual thoughts, hallucinatory behavior and mistrust. CGI score > 4.

KANE'S MODIFIED CRITERIA FOR TREATMENT RESISTANT SCHIZOPHRENIA

- Treatment with different classes of antipsychotics at equal doses of 400 to 600 mg/day of chlorpromazine for at least 2 periods of 6 weeks in the last 5 years without significant clinical improvement.
- Reduction of at least 20% on the BPRS scale, score > 35 points on the BPRS scale after treatment, CGI score > 3 after treatment with 60 mg/day of haloperidol for 6 weeks.
- BPRS score > 45. Score > 2 on BPRS items of conceptual disorganization, unusual thoughts, hallucinatory behavior and mistrust. CGI score > 4.

BRENNER'S CRITERIA FOR TREATMENT RESISTANT SCHIZOPHRENIA

- *Level 1: Clinical remission*—No need for a formal rehabilitation program—Rapid response to antipsychotics at recommended doses. Patient may show anhedonia or another negative symptom. CGI normal and score < 2 on BPRS. Good functional level without supervision.
- *Level 2: Partial remission*—No need for a formal rehabilitation program—Rapid reduction of psychotic symptoms. Mild signs of residual psychotic symptoms. CGI 2. None of the BPRS scale items are < 3.
- *Level 3: Light resistance*—Need for a rehabilitation program—Slight or incomplete reduction of symptoms with positive and negative residual symptoms. Alteration of social or personal functioning in at least two areas and requiring occasional supervision. No more than one item with a score < 4 on the BPRS.
- *Level 4: Moderate resistance*—Need for a rehabilitation program—Reduction of symptoms but with a clear persistence of them, affecting six or more areas of social and personal functioning and requiring frequent supervision. CGI 4. A score of 4 or 2 BPRS items. A BPRS score > 45 on the 18-item version and 60 on the 24-item version.
- *Level 5: Severe resistance*—Need for a continuous strategy, individual and oriented toward attempts with atypical antipsychotics and adjuvant treatment. Reduction of symptoms but with a clear persistence of them, affecting six or more areas of social and personal functioning and requiring frequent supervision. CGI 5. A score of 5 on 1 BPRS item of > 4 on 3 items. A total BPRS > 50 on the 18-item version and 67 on the 24-item version.
- *Level 6: Refractoriness*—Longer-term hospitalization with pharmacological and psychosocial attempts. Reduction of mild or nondemonstrable symptoms and persistence of positive and negative symptoms with marked alteration in all areas of social and personal functioning. CGI 6. A score of 6 on 1 BPRS item or of > 5 on 2 items. Total BPRS score of > 5 per level.
- *Level 7: Severe refractoriness*—Longer-term hospitalization with pharmacological and psychosocial attempts. No reduction of symptoms with many positive and negative symptoms associated with behavioral alterations. All areas of social and personal functioning have deteriorated, requiring constant supervision. CGI 7. A score of 7 on 1 BPRS item. Total score of > 5 per level.

MELTZER CRITERIA FOR TREATMENT RESISTANT SCHIZOPHRENIA

Meltzer in 1992 set forth the idea from Brenner. He proposed to assess treatment-resistance according to different parameters: psychopathology, cognitive function, extrapyramidal functions, social functioning, independence and work functioning, quality of life, reinstatement, dependences, cost of the illness, as well as treatment. His criteria are less strict and more useful in clinical practice. The way treatment-resistance is currently defined, is based on previous ideas and is reflected in treatment algorithms in various clinical guides. According to the current definition, schizophrenia is considered an illness in which, besides the existence of acute symptoms, there is a deterioration of the premorbid state. Clinical guides indicate the need to assess adherence to treatment and that this treatment be appropriate, to re-examine the diagnosis, substance abuse and psychosocial stressors, as well as the use of cognitive behavioral and psychosocial therapies, before considering a patient as treatment-resistant, and to propose treatment algorithms.

CONCEPT OF TREATMENT RESISTANT SCHIZOPHRENIA

What has typically been called resistance to antipsychotic treatment is nowadays a fundamental healthcare challenge. It involves deterioration in social adjustment, reduction in the capacity to access rehabilitation programs, and high healthcare costs. Even with overall treatment today, many patients experience variable and fluctuating remission of positive and negative symptoms. In spite of a reduced number of chronic inpatients, this hampers adaptation to the demands of daily life: studies, work, family, partner, social relations, etc. If we perform a historical assessment of the knowledge acquired on the treatment and clinical course of schizophrenia, we arrive at several conclusions. One is heterogeneity in response, and that we are indeed well aware of many factors on which this heterogeneity depends; i.e.

comorbidity, therapeutic noncompliance, factors deriving from the individual metabolism itself, abuse of other substances, and lack of psychosocial support. In many cases, we do not know why some patients receiving overall treatment show partial and fluctuating remission of symptoms, with a negative impact on meeting their objectives. We arrive at another conclusion if we review historical milestones in antipsychotic psychopharmacology, one of the main engines for progress. We find ourselves in a period of stagnation, interrupted by the appearance of different depot formulations of known antipsychotic drugs such as risperidone, olanzapine and paliperidone, which facilitate adherence, the main factor in relapse. However, something else is needed, other than new drugs, for the challenges we face today: negative symptoms, cognitive and social functioning. We must consider what has historically been postulated and what Lieberman and Kopelowicz articulated, speaking of psychiatric advances not only in terms of drugs, but also in rehabilitation and community services, as a stimulus to achieve recovery and restore patients' baseline functioning.

In the clinical practice of today, treatment-resistance cannot be categorically evaluated according to response, or lack thereof, to drug treatment. Setting forth Andreasen's ideas on the concept of remission, we are closer to operational dimensional models that integrate the idea of continuum, and we speak of a lack of sufficient response. We believe that this concept should be more inclusive in its current vision of treatment-resistant schizophrenia, since it could contribute a notion of continuum with response levels up to recovery of premorbid functioning, with regard to the individual's life expectations. Furthermore, it takes up the ideas of Brenner and Meltzer by integrating different pharmacological approaches, without denying the importance of drugs, while hoping for advances in research on procognitive compounds, antipsychotic drugs, etc. which will mark new therapeutic milestones.

MANAGEMENT OF TREATMENT RESISTANT SCHIZOPHRENIA

Many individuals with schizophrenia respond well to antipsychotic medication, although there are many patients for whom initial treatment is insufficient. For patients who do not respond to initial treatments, there are several strategies to guide further treatment. Treatment algorithms, provide guidelines that can help to identify initial tactics that one can try after the first approaches are unsuccessful. Clozapine, which will be discussed in further detail, remains the primary medication for treatment-resistant schizophrenia. Data on other existing medications, sometimes at higher doses than typically used or in combination polypharmacy, continue to be described in the literature. There is also an increasing evidence base for new adjunctive medications to be used in conjunction with antipsychotics. Nonpharmacological treatments including brain stimulation and different forms of psychotherapy also will be discussed both on their own and in conjunction with pharmacotherapy.

CLOZAPINE IN TREATMENT-RESISTANT SCHIZOPHRENIA

Clozapine has been the treatment of choice in treatment-refractory schizophrenia for more than 20 years. Clozapine was first discovered decades earlier; however, limited understanding of its risks and complications initially limited its use. In the United States, it was only available on a compassionate use basis for those with severe tardive dyskinesia, significant treatment resistance, or sensitivity to extrapyramidal side effects. Currently, clozapine is generally considered only for use in patients with treatment-refractory schizophrenia, although some would argue that it should be considered for use earlier in the course of illness, particularly for those who do not immediately respond to a second-generation antipsychotic. The rationale for reserving clozapine for patients with refractory disease is generally based on its more serious side effect profile. Although management strategies are available for many of these side effects; nonetheless, other medications are more easily tolerated. All patients prescribed clozapine must be entered into a national registry for monitoring. Adherence to the prescribed regimen is also essential, because missing the medication for as few as 2 days requires retitration. The most serious risk from using clozapine is for agranulocytosis. Other black box warnings include seizures, myocarditis, hypotension, and the ubiquitous warning for all antipsychotics of the increased risk of mortality in elderly individuals. Pulmonary embolism and bowel perforation are also dangerous risks for patients on clozapine. Less serious, but nevertheless difficult, side effects include sialorrhea and fatigue. The rates of agranulocytosis have dropped significantly since aggressive hematological monitoring and slow-dose titrations have been part of the practice of prescribing clozapine. Full dosing and monitoring instructions are available in the package insert and through the clozapine registry. The greatest risk of agranulocytosis is in the first 3 months of treatment.

Metabolic side effects continue to be difficult to manage. Weight gain, dyslipidemia, and risk for diabetes are all seen frequently with clozapine use. It is important to encourage active participation from the patient's primary care provider with respect to managing many of these metabolic effects, particularly if clozapine is uniquely suited to ameliorating their psychotic symptoms. Fortunately, treatments are available for many of the metabolic side effects, although it would still be preferable to have medications that were effective in treating psychosis without these risks. Long-term consequences of metabolic side effects can affect overall life expectancy if not properly managed. There are some patients for whom clozapine is not an option or for whom it is ineffective. In that case, the art of psychopharmacology comes into play, although there are some data to guide treatments with other agents.

MANAGEMENT IN CLOZAPINE POOR RESPONDERS

Initial psychopharmacological strategies at this point include consideration of either polypharmacy with other antipsychotics or with nonantipsychotic medications. Other possibilities are to use a higher dose of a single antipsychotic. Looking at antipsychotic polypharmacy, there are reports of several different combinations, both with and without clozapine. Given that clozapine is typically used in treatment-resistant schizophrenia, combinations of medications that include clozapine are often tried if clozapine monotherapy is unsuccessful. Sometimes the addition of another agent can help to lower the dose of clozapine and potentially help with lowering the side effect burden. Most reports describe combining clozapine with aripiprazole. Although case reports have suggested benefits from aripiprazole, further studies need to be done to establish its efficacy as an adjunctive agent to clozapine. Risperidone has also shown only limited benefit when added to clozapine. If combining antipsychotic medications is not possible or ineffective, there are several agents worthy of consideration as other augmenting agents. Although none of these are specifically approved for use in schizophrenia, there are various amounts of data to support their use. Several reports recently have indicated benefit for adding lamotrigine to antipsychotic treatment. Lamotrigine decreases glutamate release and increases gamma-aminobutyric acid (GABA) release and, when given with clozapine, has shown enhanced diminution of locomotor activity in rats treated with phencyclidine, a common animal measure of potential antipsychotic efficacy. However, several small trials have failed to demonstrate a statistically significant result in the primary outcome measures. In a recent meta-analysis, the data from these small trials was aggregated for enhanced power to detect a difference between placebo augmentation and lamotrigine augmentation in patients who still had residual symptoms despite treatment with clozapine. With the use of rigorous meta-analysis methodology, it was shown that there was a potential benefit with the addition of lamotrigine in these patients. Benefit was only shown for lamotrigine as an augmenting agent to clozapine, leading to speculation that the glutamatergic properties of lamotrigine may be uniquely suited to working with clozapine. The number needed to treat for this study was four, meaning that a benefit on the PANSS score was seen in one of every four patients treated. Although longer trials are still needed to confirm the effect, lamotrigine may be worth considering in those with schizophrenia that is most refractory to antipsychotic medication.

In addition to lamotrigine, other agents have been studied in conjunction with antipsychotics for treatment resistant schizophrenia. Topiramate, similar to lamotrigine, also affects glutamatergic transmission. Valproate has also never been established as an effective adjunctive agent in long-term treatment of schizophrenia, although benefits in short-term potentiation of treatment have been seen in one study. Modafinil also showed a limited effect in treating refractory negative symptoms. Although it did not reach statistical significance on the primary outcome measure of the SANS, it was well tolerated without positive symptom exacerbation. Antidepressants have long been considered possible augmenting agents, particularly for targeting negative symptoms. Some initial studies were promising as well, However, although a benefit may be seen in targeting depressive symptoms, which are a frequent comorbidity of schizophrenia, current evidence does not show a benefit of treating negative symptoms with an SSRIs. Benzodiazepines are also frequently used as adjunctive agents in schizophrenia. In acute situations, the sedative effects of benzodiazepines can be useful. However, there is limited evidence for overall symptom improvement with benzodiazepines as long-term adjunctive agents. Further clinical trials are needed to fully appreciate the impact of benzodiazepines, but, according to a Cochrane review, there is insufficient evidence to support their long-term use. Using a higher dose of an antipsychotic is a reasonable strategy for management in some patients. The mechanism for such treatment is often unclear, because dopamine receptors are typically saturated at conventional doses, but individuality in treatment response can be difficult to predict. Many case reports are available for successful high-dose treatment with different antipsychotic medications.

Adherence to a medication regimen is essential for successful pharmacotherapy. Patients who are unable to maintain their medication regimen are at a greater risk of relapse, hospitalization, and poor functional outcomes. The more times that a patient discontinues his or her medication, the more difficult treatment becomes in the future and the greater the chance for becoming treatment refractory. Many patients have difficulty in organizing and managing a daily medication regimen. Although simplifying the regimen to using daily instead of multiple daily doses is a start, for many patients, a depot medication is the most parsimonious treatment. There are currently depot preparations for three second-generation antipsychotics: risperidone, paliperidone and olanzapine. These join FGAs haloperidol and fluphenazine as appropriate choices for maintenance therapy. In all cases, patients must be able to demonstrate that they can tolerate an oral dose of medication before starting the long-acting injectable preparation. The switch from oral to depot medication is generally well tolerated.

ELECTROCONVULSIVE THERAPY AND BRAIN STIMULATION

Increasingly, nonpharmacological treatments are gaining attention and compelling data for their use are being generated. Most notably, brain stimulation methods are showing promise for treatment for many patients. These methods, including ECT and especially rTMS, are becoming safer and easier to administer. Although ECT has been used to treat schizophrenia for decades, there is limited data to support its use. A Cochrane systematic review recently concluded that ECT could be effective in those patients who do not respond to treatment with antipsychotic medications, particularly those who need especially rapid treatment. ECT has been shown to be better than sham treatment, although benefits from ECT have not been shown to persist after treatment is concluded, necessitating maintenance treatment for continuation of benefits.

Transcranial magnetic stimulation was recently approved for treatment of major depressive disorder, but currently does not have an indication for treatment of schizophrenia. Unlike ECT, there is greater ability to specify treatment location with rTMS. Transcranial magnetic stimulation is also more easily tolerated and only rarely induces a seizure when properly administered. Treatment for depression typically involves rapid transcranial magnetic stimulation, which serves to enhance excitability in the brain. Schizophrenia treatments have been both rapid and slow wave. Treatments targeting auditory hallucinations have largely been focused on the temporoparietal cortex, whereas treatments targeting negative symptoms have largely used rapid-wave rTMS aimed to the prefrontal cortex (PFC). As in depression, the PFC has been an initial target of the magnet. Initial studies were small and often confounded by difficulties with blinding the sham treatment. In a meta-analysis of several small studies, rTMS was shown to be beneficial in alleviating treatment-resistant auditory hallucinations, although the benefit was not seen in overall measures of positive symptoms. In general, the safety profile of rTMS was reassuring, and treatment was not limited by complications. Decreased auditory hallucinations were also found in a recent randomized, sham-controlled trial of rTMS in the bilateral temporoparietal area. This study showed the same improvement on auditory hallucinations but not general improvements in psychopathology. Transcranial magnetic stimulation has been studied for treatment of negative symptoms, although with limited success. In a meta-analysis, rTMS was seen to have a benefit on negative symptoms in initial, uncontrolled studies, but the effect diminished for controlled trials. Further work needs to be done to more thoroughly study the potential for this therapy to improve otherwise recalcitrant symptoms. Indeed, researchers will need to focus on stimulating other areas besides the PFC because negative symptoms may arise from other parts of the brain, including the anterior cingulate, cerebellum, occipital cortex, and posterior cortical parietal cortex.

CONCLUSION

Multimodal treatment with medication and psychotherapy is the standard of care in most other psychiatric disorders, and schizophrenia should be no exception. Several models of psychotherapy continue to demonstrate efficacy for the treatment of core schizophrenia symptoms. Cognitive behavioral therapy (CBT) is the most thoroughly studied treatment modality, and there are data to support its usage in several domains of illness including both positive and negative symptoms. In addition, CBT can be helpful in enhancing patient adherence to the overall treatment regimen and patient insight. A recent post-hoc analysis demonstrated a benefit of CBT on suicidal ideation as well. Although the benefits may wane after treatment stops, there are profound improvements in the short-term, and some benefits such as with insight, can be seen even 1 year after treatment. The benefits of CBT are more likely to persist than other more benign comparison interventions, such as "befriending" or general supportive care, in which subjects are given the same social benefits of having a therapist to see, but without a specific or targeted intervention. In a study looking at insight, subjects were randomly assigned to CBT or treatment as usual. The CBT group was able to better relabel psychotic symptoms and to understand their need for treatment. There was no difference between the groups with respect to insight into having an illness. Although improvements can be seen with respect to insight, delusions remain difficult to address. However, general psychopathology has been shown to improve, as measured by PANSS score, even in patients who are refractory to clozapine treatment. An initial benefit was seen in quality of life as well, although that did not persist at a 6-month follow-up. General psychopathology improvements were maintained after 6 months, however, in comparison with a befriending comparator group. The inclusion of psychosocial treatments in comprehensive care of the person with schizophrenia is important.

6.11 SCHIZOPHRENIA: PSYCHOSOCIAL REHABILITATION

Avinash De Souza, Nilesh Shah

INTRODUCTION

Enjoying good family relations, a healthy lifestyle, or having a satisfying job ... these are not just a collection of rehabilitation goals but are what most people aspire to. All too often, schizophrenia profoundly disrupts these expectations—social isolation is a daily reality for most people with psychotic disorders. The majority of people with psychotic disorders have lost essential life roles that normally provide self-esteem and meaning. Eighty-four percent are separated, divorced, widowed or single; 85% are reliant on welfare benefits; 72% do not have a regular occupation; and 45% live in institutions, hostels, supported housing or crisis shelters, or are homeless. A psychotic episode also affects those involved with the person affected. The bewildering and distressing symptoms, admission to hospital and administration of medication, combined with lack of understanding, cause significant trauma for all involved. It is crucial that managing people with schizophrenia include integrated rehabilitation services that respond promptly and appropriately to the needs of the individual and the family. Ideally, rehabilitation services should include: psychological treatments (e.g. cognitive behavior therapy), if appropriate; education about the illness and how to cope with symptoms and the effects of disability; family therapy; support for carers; psychosocial rehabilitation; accommodation and employment support; specific skills development; assistance to link into community resources; and help to learn how best to manage and come to terms with the illness. These all take time, and hinge on the presence and efficient coordination of committed teams.

PSYCHOEDUCATION

After a first episode of schizophrenia, the doctor needs to investigate what happened and allow the patient to express the confusion and anger that is commonly felt. The doctor needs to reassure the patient that schizophrenia is not "the end of the world", but a medical condition that can be treated and is experienced by other people as well. It should not be assumed that a person who has been given a diagnosis of schizophrenia will understand what it is. Furthermore, people are affected by the community's lack of understanding and stigma about the illness, and may be reluctant to accept the term "schizophrenia" if they associate it with a "split personality" or other false stereotypes of mental illness that are widely prevalent in the community. Be aware that management is likely to be more effective if the patient understands the diagnosis and the reasons for treatment. Do not assume that because someone has been diagnosed with a mental illness he or she understands the illness.

FAMILY MANAGEMENT

Family members and other carers need to be recognized for the role they play in helping maintain a patient's mental health and need to be included in the overall rehabilitation plan. It is also important that they receive education, support and training in how best to support the patient. As people tend to respond positively to recommendations made by their psychiatrist, it is important for psychiatrists to know of and refer people to support organizations, as well as to generic carer support provided by the Carers Association. Family group therapy, when available, may substantially reduce symptoms and frequency of episodes in the patient, as well as improving the mental health of the entire family. Listen to family members and include them in the "treatment team" whenever appropriate. Inform families about support organizations. Refer families to a group therapy program if available.

WORK AND OCCUPATIONAL MANAGEMENT

Employment reintegrates people back into the community, provides an independent income and a sense of identity, and fills an empty day with purpose and activity. Unpaid voluntary work can also help fulfil this role. The workplace needs to be more accommodating to the unique demands of psychiatric disability. For people with schizophrenia, a major barrier to coping with a job is their understandable reluctance to disclose the illness. This increases the sense of pressure at work and also denies them the right to their equivalent of "ramps and lifts" for people with a physical disability. It is important to encourage people to become active by linking in with local resources. Without these community links, support services run the risk of becoming miniversions of the old psychiatric institutions: the individual does not get to access community resources, and the community does not have the opportunity to engage with and include people with a mental illness. Local neighborhood houses, leisure centers, training centers, employment programs, volunteer options and local clubs should all be part of the life plan, so that support services are seen clearly to assist people to reintegrate into society rather than act as a substitute for it.

Encourage realistic consideration of work and practical steps in preparation for it, such as enrolment at a day program and referral to a Disability Employment Support agency. Be aware that any meaningful occupation, such as unpaid volunteer work, can give people a social role, as well an opportunity to engage with the community and prepare for the challenges of entering the paid workforce.

SOCIAL SKILLS TRAINING

Although neuroleptic drugs undoubtedly extend periods of remission, they do not prevent relapse and are associated with disturbing side effects. Perhaps the greatest limitation of an exclusive reliance on drug therapy is its inability to impart new instrumental role behaviors and interpersonal skills with consequent improvements in patients' quality of life. As Strauss and Carpenter have indicated, premorbid levels of behaviors and skills are important predictors of subsequent social adjustment, clinical outcome, and quality of interpersonal life for the schizophrenic patient. Furthermore, many schizophrenic patients are socially isolated and do not become part of a natural social network that might assist them in coping with social demands. The only natural network of which they may be a part is their families; unfortunately, not only may certain family interactional patterns increase the probability of relapse, but patients often lack the skills to cope with stressful interpersonal interactions. Within the past 10–15 years, two therapies have been developed that hold promise for increasing both the performance of instrumental role behaviors and the development and maintenance of appropriate social behaviors. Both therapies have a behavioral perspective and use techniques such as shaping, positive and negative reinforcement, prompting, modeling, and behavior rehearsal. One therapy, the token economy, has been used primarily with inpatients to increase instrumental role behaviors.

The second therapy, variously labeled assertiveness training, personal effectiveness training, structured learning therapy, and social skills training, has been used with both inpatients and outpatients to increase a broad spectrum of behaviors labeled social skills. The purpose of this article is to review the current state of social skills training for chronic psychiatric patients. First to be summarized will be the conceptual definitions of social skills that have been proposed by several authors. Studies of social skills training will then be reviewed in terms of their methods of evaluation, results, and methodological shortcomings. An expanded conceptual definition will be presented, along with a brief description of a training method that flows directly from this expanded definition. Unfortunately, diagnostic practices in the social skills research literature are rather lax, and this review cannot be focused solely on the effects of training with schizophrenic patients.

Implicit in the choice of a particular method of training and evaluating social skills is a conceptual definition of social skills. Different conceptual definitions result in different methods of training and evaluation, but only a few authors have explicitly defined what they mean by social skills. A common basis for all definitions, of course, is an interpersonal context consisting of the patient, who is the focus of the definitions, and at least one other person. There are four major elements of most definitions of social skills: (1) The patient's internal state—his feelings, his attitudes, and his perceptions of the interpersonal context; (2) The topography of the patient's behaviors—the rate of behaviors such as eye contact, hand gestures, body posture, speech disfluencies, voice volume, and latency of verbal response; (3) The outcome of the interaction as reflected in the achievement of the patient's goals; (4) The outcome of the interaction as reflected in the attitudes, feelings, behaviors, and goals of the other participants. There is considerable variation in the comprehensiveness of the few definitions that have been used by different investigators.

COGNITIVE REMEDIATION

Cognitive remediation is often provided in conjunction with vocational programs for its congruency in treatment focus. Researchers demonstrated that improvement of cognitive functions was related to improvement of vocational functions. Models of rehabilitation for people with chronic psychiatric illness that emphasize community living have been long since established. Representative models include Assertive Community Treatment, Choose-Get-Keep model and Intensive Psychiatric Rehabilitation Treatment. These rehabilitation programs emphasize a multidisciplinary approach, skills acquisition, independent living, consumer advocacy and behavioral intervention in combination with pharmaceutical treatment. They often offer cognitive remediation as a part of their services, as the overall goal of the rehabilitation model for independent living is congruent with the rehabilitation philosophy of cognitive remediation.

The features of the models of cognitive remediation vary, depending on their treatment context and theoretical foundation. While some models emphasize drill practice of isolated cognitive skills, others are offered in conjunction with vocational training. However, it is becoming more common for cognitive remediation to be offered with or as a part of vocational rehabilitation program. The movement toward the inclusion of a vocational approach is consistent with the deinstitutionalization of psychiatry. Originally developed for the rehabilitation of brain injury, cognitive remediation needed to be tailored to address the unique characteristics of schizophrenia. The central characteristics of schizophrenia associated with the induction of cognitive remediation included the issue of motivation and social functions. Avolition is a prominent symptom of schizophrenia and interferes with the treatment compliance. Impairments in social function is another characteristic of schizophrenia. Therefore, a model of cognitive remediation that addresses impairments in motivation and social function is expected to best serve the needs of people with schizophrenia.

Researchers have examined different areas of functions associated with cognitive remediation and cognitive functions. Although social function as an expansive concept has been associated with cognitive functions in the past, this section further categorizes social functions into independent living skills, vocational skills, social problem-solving, social behavior and general social function. Scales relevant to each area are listed as potential outcome measures for cognitive remediation. Enhanced independent living skills have been associated with the increase of cognitive functions. Measures for independent living skills consist of surveys. Surveys are either self-reported or reported by a third party such as the patient's family and/or treatment staff (e.g. Life Skills Profile). Some scales that measure social function as an overarching domain such as the Social Functioning Scale also include subscales for independent living skills. Enhanced vocational skills have been associated with an increase of cognitive functions. Vocational skills have traditionally been measured by scales (e.g. Social Adjustment Scale, Work Behavior Inventory), or more indirectly by vocational goals attainment or vocational status at the completion of cognitive remediation. It should be noted that systematic measures of vocational skills target basic job skills and employment readiness such as punctuality and greetings, and not specific vocational skills such as typing. The attainment of basic job skills such as punctuality and greetings are related to improvement in cognitive functions. It should be noted that impairments in social problem-solving have been viewed as the central features of symptoms of schizophrenia. It has been indicated that enhanced social problem-solving is associated with the increase of cognitive functions. Social problem solving skills are measured by surveys, or by behavior rating. Behavior rating involves analysis of role-play behaviors (Assessment of Interpersonal Problem-Solving Skills, Social Problem-Solving Assessment Battery) and responses to stories involving hypothetical social problems (Means-Ends Problem Solving Procedure).

VOCATIONAL REHABILITATION

A series of principles has emerged from the research literature on heterogeneous groups of people with severe mental illness, and there is some consensus among experts about what works well for notable proportions of people. Many of these principles are borrowed from the field of multidisability vocational rehabilitation, and others have emerged from efforts to meet the unique needs of people with psychiatric disabilities. In this section, we review these principles and cite research supporting them to provide the reader with a general understanding of currently endorsed best practices in vocational rehabilitation. The first principle is use of situational assessment in the evaluation of vocational skills and potential. Situational assessment is the longitudinal observation and rating of job behaviors and attitudes in actual or simulated work environments by a trained evaluator. This approach takes into account the fact that accurate assessment of people with serious mental illness may be complicated by medication side effects, symptomatology, and cognitive impairments that accompany many types of mental illness. Since people with psychiatric disorders perform differently in different environments, situation-specific assessment is preferred over traditional psychiatric assessments, or traditional vocational assessments designed for people with physical disabilities or mental retardation.

The second principle involves offering clients competitive or supported employment rather than sheltered or unpaid work. Enactment of this principle means that clients are rehabilitated by being placed and trained in community jobs in integrated settings, earning minimum wage or above. Wehman and associates demonstrated convincingly that employment outcomes were significantly better for severely disabled individuals, including those with mental illness and mental retardation, when clients were rehabilitated through community placement into jobs at or above minimum wage in socially integrated settings. This followed a long line of research in the 1960s and 1970s suggesting the ineffectiveness of in-hospital work programs and segregated sheltered workshops for psychiatrically disabled populations. Competitive employment appears to offer several rehabilitative advantages over sheltered or volunteer work. Work skills training that occurs in integrated environments alongside nondisabled coworkers offers clients positive role-modeling opportunities Several surveys of people with psychiatric disabilities have shown that employment at or above minimum wage is preferred and offers obvious economic advantages to clients. The place-then-train approach provides on-the-job training that allows workers to learn skills in the same environments in which they will use them and helps prevent "transfer of training" difficulties, which can occur when skills are applied in different settings.

The third principle involves rapid placement into paid community employment versus undergoing a lengthy prevocational training period. This principle acknowledges the importance of swiftly placing clients into community jobs to avoid the demoralization that can accompany lengthy periods of job training and evaluation.

A fourth principle involves the availability of ongoing vocational support appropriate to the individual's needs and situation. The continuous availability of vocational support following job placement is a hallmark of the supported employment model. The idea is that the relapsing and remitting nature of severe mental illness means that clients should not be completely terminated from vocational supports upon attainment of a job; the challenge is to avoid over- or underserving successfully employed clients. Yet another principle is tailoring job development and support to the client's individual preferences. To some extent this principle grew out of a reaction against one size fits-all approaches in some service delivery models of vocational rehabilitation in which clients have little say over the nature of the jobs they are offered and the level of intrusiveness of the job support they receive. Instead, research shows that clients have better outcomes when their services are designed to coincide with their preferences.

One final principle involves explicit acknowledgment and planning regarding how changes in clients' work status can alter their disability income and associated health care coverage. This principle addresses potential economic disincentives to achieving certain levels of paid employment. Such disincentives are inherent in the way disability entitlements are structured. While this research has yet to answer many questions about the relationship between disability payments and employment activity, it has highlighted to service providers the importance of benefits counseling and planning. To summarize, at the end of the 20th century there is a body of research evidence to guide clinical practice in the vocational rehabilitation of people with severe mental illness. The foregoing set of service delivery principles appears repeatedly in published reviews on this topic, with slight variations. We know more about vocational outcomes than ever before; however, we have far less specific knowledge about schizophrenia and vocational rehabilitation as well as whether and how to tailor services for people with this diagnosis. To some extent, this is due to the relative recency of this field of research, which largely followed inauguration of the neuroleptic drug treatment era. This gap also results from an assumption widely held in the field of psychiatric vocational rehabilitation that diagnosis is not a central or even important factor in the ways services are designed and configured. For many years now, the field of psychiatric disability has largely ignored clients' diagnoses in favor of attending to their functional impairments and how these impede rehabilitation success. To address this uneven emphasis, we now turn to research exploring the nature of the direct or indirect relationships between diagnosis and vocational outcome.

6.12 SCHIZOPHRENIA: THE INDIAN SCENARIO

Avinash De Souza, Nilesh Shah

INTRODUCTION

Schizophrenia is a heterogeneous syndrome characterized by perturbations of language, perception, thinking, social activity, affect, and volition. There are no pathognomonic features. The syndrome commonly begins in late adolescence, has an insidious (and less commonly acute) onset, and, classically, a poor outcome, progressing from social withdrawal and perceptual distortions to a state of chronic delusions and hallucinations. In this chapter, we review the factors that influence the outcome of schizophrenia and certain aspects of schizophrenia research in India.

OUTCOME ASPECTS OF SCHIZOPHRENIA IN INDIA

In developing countries around 90% of people with schizophrenia remain untreated. But the outcome of schizophrenia appears to be better in low and middle-income countries. There are several factors that may influence the outcome like employment, marital status, family support, etc. Our aim of the study is to find out the factors that may affect the outcome of schizophrenia in developing in comparison with developed countries. Sex differences in the risk of a particular disorder can yield important clues regarding its pathogenesis. The evidence for a sex difference in the risk of schizophrenia is inconclusive. Although sex difference is not a significant factor in schizophrenia, it has been observed that the clinical remission and recovery is higher in female rather than male. Physical and mental fitness plays a very important role in case of employment. People with schizophrenia in low- and middle-income countries are more likely to be employed than their Western counterparts. Moreover, among untreated Indian people with schizophrenia almost one-third was employed. Generally, high employment rates (up to 75%) have been found in India. These rates of employment are markedly higher than those in similar populations in high income countries.

It has been mentioned earlier around 90% schizophrenic patient remain untreated in developing countries whereas their remission appears to be better, this is probably due employment. When a schizophrenic patient involved in a job he comes in contact with social surroundings and routine work; which helps to lead a normal life. In low- and middle-income countries, social bonding is very strong and work place colleagues are very cooperative. Even study proves that workplace colleagues are found to be generally supportive in low- and middle-income countries. In low- and middle-income countries society plays a very important role in case of marriage. In these countries, marriage considered as a social identity for a person. In developing countries, marriage is an once-in-a-lifetime event and is associated with a high degree of social approval. The sociocultural factors determining marriage and its maintenance are vastly different from those in Western societies. Marital state can be considered an outcome measure, as its maintenance depends on stability and functioning of both partners. Schizophrenia manifests maximally at a marriageable age (i.e. around the 20s). So the marriage rate of schizophrenic patient in developing countries is much higher than that of developed countries. This is because in developing countries schizophrenic patients live with their partners and share their views and feelings. This mental support helps them to lead a normal life and also affect their outcome. Patients, whose marriages have broken down, in addition to the stress of their mental illness, face hostility from family members and rejection by society. This can be a significant contributing factor to outcome in traditional societies.

Family and social support plays vital role in the outcome of schizophrenia. Recent studies propose that supportive and favorable attitudes among family members and the community contribute to the improved outcomes. In low- and middle-incoming countries, majority of people stay in joint families. Schizophrenic patients from these families primarily stay at home as the numbers of family members are large. Since they stay in a family surrounding and get sufficient care from the members, their outcome accelerated in low- and middle-incoming countries. Migration, urbanization, changes in family structure and social support networks, plus the increase in economic insecurity and widening social inequalities which are evident in low- and middle-income countries will change the social support available for people with schizophrenia and influence their outcome.

A significant delay in seeking treatment for people with schizophrenia has been observed in low- and middle-income countries. The reason behind that may be ignorance, superstition and misconceptions of illness. However, recent studies have shown that very few people still named supernatural factors alone as a cause of schizophrenia. In a study of Indian patients, supernatural cause was named by only 12% of families with a member with schizophrenia. Burden of care is related to the different sociocultural factors of a country. As in low- and middle-income countries, the majority of patients stay with their caregivers. So the burden is somewhat higher in low- and middle-income countries compared to the Western countries. In a study it has been found that, there are six areas of burden these are financial, family routine, leisure, interaction, effect on physical health and effect on mental health. In addition, inability to care for others, unpredictable behavior of the patient and dissatisfaction with the help from health care professional also be considered as burden. Some family members leave their ill relatives in psychiatric hospital for long-time but in that case, the outcome follows negative trend. Study shows that caregiver burden decreases with a reduction in the patient's symptoms and improving drug adherence. Reduction of family burden is associated with better outcome and social functioning.

Studies from the West have shown that the duration of untreated psychosis (DUP) is associated with poorer outcome; with the relationship being strongest in the initial months of psychosis. This is particularly relevant in low- and middle-income (LAMI) countries where a significant number of patients come late for treatment. Reasons for this include lack of awareness, a strong belief in magical or religious causes, poor accessibility to health care systems and lack of community care. Nonadherence to prescribed antipsychotic medications places patients with schizophrenia at a greatly increased risk of illness exacerbation and re-hospitalization. The cost of treatment is an impediment to care and subsidized antipsychotic medication would improve the access to treatment and the outcome of psychotic illness in LAMI countries.

INDIAN ASPECTS OF FAMILY INTERVENTIONS IN SCHIZOPHRENIA

Indian families have never been excluded from treatment of the mentally ill; rather, they have always functioned as partners in their care. Some cross-cultural comparisons have suggested that there are significant differences in the social circumstances of Asian patients and their Western counterparts. Moreover, the close knit composition of Asian families also ensures a somewhat greater involvement of families in all aspects of the care of those with mental illness. These differences have led some authors to question the need for structured family-interventions for Asian patients with schizophrenia and their families. These critics have pointed out that the concept of formal family interventions is a foreign one, based on the notion of expressed emotions (EE), which itself is of doubtful relevance in non-Western cultures. Asian families are already more involved in care, and are generally more tolerant and supportive of the patient, which could account for the better outcome of the disorder observed in this part of the world. Finally, such detractors also contend that structured family interventions are costly, time-consuming and labor-intensive, which makes them unsuitable for Asian countries, where trained personnel and mental-health services are scarce.

The construct of EE and its association with relapse has played a central role in the evolution of family-interventions for schizophrenia. These interventions were originally developed to employ a number of different strategies to reduce high levels of EE, thereby preventing relapses of schizophrenia. Unfortunately, the hypothesis that reduction in EE was the crucial process-variable accounting for the success of family-interventions was not borne out by subsequent research. The use of the EE typology to identify families in need of help also proved to have distinct disadvantages in clinical and service settings. Moreover, family-interventions appeared to be equally effective in both high EE and low EE families. Accordingly, alternative theories, which incorporate other elements of family-interventions as potential variables mediating the positive effects of family interventions among Asian families, need to be examined. Such process-variables could include stress-reduction, attitudinal change among relatives leading to more adaptive appraisals, and improved coping by relatives. Other cultural processes could also be assessed to determine whether they contribute to the usefulness of family-interventions.

A variety of family-intervention models and strategies have been developed and empirically tested in the West. Two of the major models are referred to as the behavioral family management model, and the family psychoeducational model. The former involves education about the illness, as well as structured training in problem solving and effective communication skills, whereas the latter places emphasis on developing a therapeutic alliance with the family, providing education and ongoing support, teaching techniques to reduce stress, and identifying and intervening early at times of relapse. These strategies have been used as a part of both group and individual treatment programmes. Another set of strategies, referred to as the family education models, consist of brief educational interventions, either led by professionals or peers, which focus on affected family members rather than patients. A subset of the family education model is the consultation model, in which individual families meet periodically with a professional involved in the patient's treatment, to receive information, advice or support according to their needs. Although some forms of family intervention have been studied more often than others, there is no compelling evidence to suggest the superiority of any particular approach over others. The evidence clearly indicates that relatively simple and inexpensive forms of these interventions, which place emphasis on ongoing contact and medication compliance while offering emotional and practical support, are more likely to succeed in the Asian context. Finally, family-interventions also have to be tailored to the background and needs of the families, to enhance their acceptability, and positively influence the readiness of families to participate in such interventions.

RECOVERY IN INDIAN PATIENTS WITH SCHIZOPHRENIA

For a long-time, the future for patients with schizophrenia was a life-long sentence to a chronic illness with no hope of recovery. Treatment goals were compliance with medications, reduction of hospital admissions, and adjustment to a chronic illness. By the 1990's, patients and families were repudiating those goals and advocating for recovery, the same treatment goal held for patients with medical illnesses. Now, recovery is accepted as the desired outcome of psychiatric treatment. The goals of recovery are for patients to return to a meaningful social role, develop relationships, re-claim a sense of self-identity, and become participating members of the community. The process of recovery involves changes that patients make—keeping hope alive; accepting the need to be actively involved in promoting healing; developing self-confidence, courage and responsibility; finding a new meaning or purpose in life; and rebuilding social connectedness by taking on new roles in relationships, work, and the community. The process of recovery also involves factors external to the patient such as mental health care providers' attitudes of compassion, respect, and belief in patients' ability to achieve healing and the provision of recovery-oriented services. Recovery-oriented services include management of patients' symptoms and distress, meeting patients' needs, promoting rehabilitation, and protecting patients' rights and personal safety.

Comprehensive treatment programs such as Assertive Community Treatment (ACT) that promote the goal of recovery have been found to reduce the hallucinations, delusions, and depression experienced by patients with schizophrenia but are less effective in reducing the problems related to impairment of functioning—deficits in self-care, academic difficulties, inability to work, problems with social interactions, and inability to develop and maintain intimate relationships. Patients' residual impaired functioning often leads to unmet needs with greater impairment of functioning linked with higher rates of unmet needs.

UNMET NEEDS AMONG PATIENTS WITH SCHIZOPHRENIA

Basic survival needs: Food, clothing, housing, transportation, finances, and personal safety. Among patients with severe mental illnesses such as schizophrenia, needs for food and clothing are not often reported as unmet. For example, only 7% of patients with severe mental illness reported an unmet need for food in the study. Patients may live at home or in supervised housing where food and clothing may be provided for them and some may obtain food and clothing from soup kitchens or drop-in centers. The need for appropriate housing was found to be unmet for 46% of patients with schizophrenia. Similarly, transportation is a frequently occurring unmet need. Financial resources are often not adequate to live on. Researchers reported that 27% of patients with schizophrenia living in the community identified financial problems, lack of sufficient funds to get by. For over 30 years, researchers have described the unmet need of patients with schizophrenia for personal safety, safety from abuse and victimization with others reporting victimization rates of 25% to 38%, 12 times the rate for the general population.

HEALTH CARE NEEDS IN SCHIZOPHRENIA

In comparison to the general population, patients with schizophrenia have more health problems and a 20% shorter life span. About 50% have at least one medical condition such as diabetes, obesity, chronic obstructive pulmonary disease, cardiovascular disease, or HIV infection. They also have more dental and eye problems than the general population. However, despite this increased vulnerability, they are less likely to receive preventive care and needed dental care than the general population. Social connectedness, the reciprocal relationships that individuals have with others, provides support and a sense of belonging and is associated with health and well-being. Social connectedness develops from the roles that individuals play in life as partners, friends, teammates, workers, and participants in community and spiritual activities. Among patients with schizophrenia, social connectedness has been found to be a strong predictor of positive response to treatment and patients believe that social connectedness is a key factor in promoting recovery.

Many authors have described the lack of friends among patients with severe mental illness. For example, among patients with severe mental illness who belonged to the National Alliance for the Mentally Ill (NAMI), 62% identified an unmet need for a friend. In describing the effect of lack of friendship among patients with severe mental illness, Wheaton says that it is the sense of isolation, the loneliness, and the lack of someone to talk with that is most troublesome. More than half of patients with severe mental illness describe problems with loneliness in comparison to one-third of the general population. Recently, authors reported that 42% of patients with schizophrenia living in the community identified loneliness as a problem. Role in life is often associated with employment, filling the role of a worker and co-worker. Unfortunately, among patients with schizophrenia, unemployment is high with a rate of 72.9%. Patients with severe mental illness believe that work enables them to have pride in themselves, to develop coping strategies for managing psychotic symptoms so that they can work, and to re-establish a sense of identity. They believe that work promotes recovery.

A sense of meaning or purpose to life encompasses both spirituality and religiousness and is associated with a sense of well-being. Patients with schizophrenia describe religion as being an important part of their daily life; and, they often use religion to cope with the symptoms of their illness and with daily problems. The role that a sense of meaning or purpose plays in recovery is related to its ability to facilitate a reconstruction of a sense of self-identity and to build social connectedness.

CONCLUSION

There is a further need for Indian researchers to meaningfully engage themselves in schizophrenia research. Phenomenology, clinical and psychosocial variables in schizophrenia are the main strengths of Indian research which has to now move over to neurobiology, cognition and genetics. Significant contribution has been made by Indian researchers in the field of prognosis, course and outcome of schizophrenia that has caught the awareness of the whole world fuelling debate whether or not outcome is genuinely better in the Indian context. Operational research and psychosocial intervention researches are still lagging behind and our talented researchers need to make a move in these areas. We also need to have sound psychopharmacological research to enable us to decipher which of the drugs best aids recover in the Indian context. We also need to have further research in the psychotherapy of schizophrenia and group based as well as community and rehabilitative interventions which is lacking in India. India has a huge clinical patient base and immense clinical experience in the management of schizophrenia though the research base today lags far behind.

REFERENCES

Schizophrenia: Epidemiology

1. Koller J. Beitrag zur Erblichkeitsstatistik der Geisteskranken im Canton Zürich; Vergleichung derselben mit der erblichen Belastung gesunder Menschen durch Geistesstörungen u. dergl. Arch Psychiatr. 1895;27:269-94.
2. Kraepelin E. Vergleichende Psychiatrie. Ztbl. Nervenheilk Psychiat. 27:433-7.
3. Faris REL, Dunham HW. Mental disorders in urban areas: an ecological study of schizophrenia and other psychoses. Chicago University Press, Chicago; 1939.
4. Dohrenwend BP, Levav I, Shrout PE, Schwartz S, Naveh G, Link BG, Skodol AE, Stueve A. Socioeconomic status and psychiatric disorders: the causation-selection issue. Science. 1992;255 (5047):946-52.
5. WHO. Schizophrenia. An international follow-up study. Wiley, Chichester; 1979.
6. Waldo MC. Schizophrenia in Kosrae, Micronesia: prevalence, gender ratios, and clinical symptomatology. Schizophr Res. 1999;35:175-81.
7. Eaton WW. Epidemiology of schizophrenia. Epidemiologic reviews. 1985;7:105-26.
8. Eaton WW. Update on the epidemiology of schizophrenia. Epidemiologic reviews. 1991;13:320-8.
9. Sartorius N, Jablensky A, Korten A, Ernberg G, Anker M, Cooper JE, Day R. Early manifestations and first-contact incidence of schizophrenia in different cultures. A preliminary report on the initial evaluation phase of the WHO Collaborative

Study on determinants of outcome of severe mental disorders. Psychological medicine. 1986;16(4):909-28.
10. Munk-Jorgensen P. First-admission rates and marital status of schizophrenics. Acta Psychiatr Scand. 1987;76:210-6.
11. McGrath J, Saha S, Welham J, El Saadi O, MacCauley C, Chant D. A systematic review of the incidence of schizophrenia: the distribution of rates and the influence of sex, urbanicity, migrant status and methodology. BMC medicine. 2004;2:13.
12. Aleman A, Kahn RS, Selten JP. Sex differences in the risk of schizophrenia: evidence from metaanalysis. Arch Gen Psychiatry. 2003;60(6):565-71.
13. Eaton, W. Evidence for universality and uniformity of schizophrenia around the world: assessment and implications. Darmstadt: Steinkopf; 1999.
14. Kendler KS, Gallagher TJ, Abelson JM, Kessler RC. Lifetime prevalence, demographic risk factors, and diagnostic validity of nonaffective psychosis as assessed in a US community sample. The National Comorbidity Survey. Arch Gen Psychiatry. 1996; 53:1022-31.
15. Kendler KS, Diehl SR. The genetics of schizophrenia: a current, genetic-epidemiologic perspective. Schizophr Bull. 1993;19: 261-85.
16. Hafner H, Maurer K, Loffler W. Onset and prodromal phase as determinants of the course. In: Gattaz WF, Hafner H (Eds). Search for the Causes of Schizophrenia: Vol IV—Balance of the Century. Darmstadt: Steinkopf Springer; 1999.pp.35-58.
17. Niemi LT, Suvisaari JM, Tuulio-Henriksson A, Lonnqvist JK. Childhood developmental abnormalities in schizophrenia: evidence from high-risk studies. Schizophr Res. 2003;60(2-3): 239-58.
18. Jones P, Rodgers B, Murray R, Marmot M. Child development risk factors for adult schizophrenia in the British 1946 birth cohort. Lancet. 1994;344(8934):1398-402.
19. Cannon TD, Rosso IM, Bearden CE, Sanchez LE, Hadley T. A prospective cohort study of neurodevelopmental processes in the genesis and epigenesis of schizophrenia. Dev Psychopathol. 1999;11(3):467-85.
20. Malmberg A, Lewis G, David A, Allebeck P. Premorbid adjustment and personality in people with schizophrenia. Br J Psychiatry. 1998;172:308-13.
21. Jones PB, Tarrant CJ. Specificity of developmental precursors to schizophrenia and affective disorders. Schizophr Res. 1999;39(2):121-5.
22. Torrey EF, Miller J, Rawlings R, Yolken RH. Seasonality of births in schizophrenia and bipolar disorder: a review of the literature. Schizophr Res. 1997;28(1):1-38.
23. Davies G, Welham J, Chant D, Torrey EF, McGrath J. A systematic review and meta-analysis of Northern Hemisphere season of birth studies in schizophrenia. Schizophr Bull. 2003;29(3): 587-93.
24. Geddes JR, Verdoux H, Takei N, Lawrie SM, Bovet P, Eagles JM, Heun R, McCreadie RG, McNeil TF, O'Callaghan E, Stober G, Willinger U, Murray RM. Schizophrenia and complications of pregnancy and labor: an individual patient data meta-analysis. Schizophr Bull. 1999;25(3):413-23.
25. Geddes JR, Lawrie SM. Obstetric complications and schizophrenia: a meta-analysis. Br J Psychiatry. 1995;167(6): 786-93.
26. Dalman C, Allebeck P, Cullberg J, Grunewald C, Koster M. Obstetric complications and the risk of schizophrenia: a longitudinal study of a national birth cohort. Arch Gen Psychiatry. 1999;56(3):234-40.
27. Yolken RH, Torrey EF. Viruses, schizophrenia, and bipolar disorder. Clin Microbiol Rev. 1995;8(1):131-45.
28. Leao TS, Sundquist J, Frank G, Johansson LM, Johansson SE, Sundquist K. Incidence of schizophrenia or other psychoses in first- and second-generation immigrants: a national cohort study. J Nerv Ment Disease. 2006;194(1): 27-33.
29. Hall W, Degenhardt L. Cannabis use and psychosis: a review of clinical and epidemiological evidence. Aust NZ J Psychiatry. 2000;34(1):26-34.
30. Eaton WW. Residence, social class, and schizophrenia. J Health Soc Behav. 1974;15(4):289-99.
31. Marcelis M, Navarro-Mateu F, Murray R, Selten JP, Van Os J. Urbanization and psychosis: a study of 1942-1978 birth cohorts in The Netherlands. Psychol Med. 1998;28(4):871-79.
32. McGrath JJ. Myths and plain truths about schizophrenia epidemiology—the NAPE lecture 2004. Acta Psychiatr Scand. 2005;111(1):4-11.
33. Hafner H, An der Haiden W. Epidemiology of schizophrenia. Can J Psychiatry. 1997;42:139-51.
34. Messias M, Chen CU, Eaton WW. Epidemiology of schizophrenia: review of findings and myths. Psychiatr Clin North Am. 2007;30(3):323-38.
35. Jablensky A. Epidemiology of schizophrenia: the global burden of disease and disability. Eur Arch Psychiatry Clin Neurosci. 2000;250:274-85.

Schizophrenia: Neurobiology

36. Howes OD, Fusar-Poli P, Bloomfield M, Selvaraj S, McGuire P. From the prodrome to chronic schizophrenia: the neurobiology underlying psychotic symptoms and cognitive impairments. Curr Pharm Des. 2012;18(4):459-65.
37. Butler T, Weisholtz D, Isenberg N, Harding E, Epstein J, Stern E, Silbersweig D. Neuroimaging of frontal-limbic dysfunction in schizophrenia and epilepsy-related psychosis: toward a convergent neurobiology. Epilepsy Behav. 2012;23(2): 113-22.
38. Dean B. Neurochemistry of schizophrenia: the contribution of neuroimaging postmortem pathology and neurochemistry in schizophrenia. Curr Top Med Chem. 2012;12(21):2375-92.
39. Masana M, Santana N, Artigas F, Bortolozzi A. Dopamine neurotransmission and atypical antipsychotics in prefrontal cortex: a critical review. Curr Top Med Chem. 2012;12(21):2357-74.

40. Boyd KN, Maliman RB. Dopamine receptor signaling and current and future antipsychotic drugs. Handb Exp Pharmacol. 2012;212:53-86.
41. Kuepper R, Skinbjerg M, Abi-Dargham A. The dopamine dysfunction in schizophrenia revisited: new insights into topography and course. Handb Exp Pharmacol. 2012;212:1-26.
42. Tritsch NX, Sabatini BL. Dopaminergic modulation of synaptic transmission in cortex and striatum. Neuron. 2012;76(1):33-50.
43. Eyles D, Feldon J, Meyer U. Schizophrenia: do all roads lead to dopamine or is this where they start? Evidence from two epidemiologically informed developmental rodent models. Transl Psychiatry. 2012;21:e81.
44. Shen LH, Liao MH, Tseng YC. Recent advances in imaging of dopaminergic neurons for evaluation of neuropsychiatric disorders. J Biomed Biotechnol. 2012;259349: Epub.
45. Yin DM, Chen YJ, Sathyamurthy A, Xiong WC, Mei L. Synaptic dysfunction in schizophrenia. Adv Exp Med Biol. 2012;970: 493-516.
46. Lodge DJ, Grace AA. Hippocampal dysregulation of dopamine system function and the pathophysiology of schizophrenia. Trends Pharmacol Sci. 2011;32(9):507-13.
47. Meltzer HY, Massey BW, Horiguchi M. Serotonin receptors as targets for drugs useful to treat psychosis and cognitive impairment in schizophrenia. Curr Pharm Biotechnol. 2012; 13(8):1572-86.
48. Puig MV, Gulledge MT. Serotonin and prefrontal cortex function: neurons, networks and circuits. Mol Neurobiol. 2011; 44(3):449-64.
49. Pytliak M, Vargová V, Mechírová V, Felšöci M. Serotonin receptors—from molecular biology to clinical applications. Physiol Res. 2011;60(1):15-25.
50. Geyer MA, Vollenweider FX. Serotonin research : contributions to understanding psychoses. Trends Pharmacol Sci. 2008;29(9): 445-53.
51. Richtand NM, McNamara RK. Serotonin and dopamine interactions in psychosis prevention. Prog Brain Res. 2008;172: 141-53.
52. Yamamato K, Hornykiewicz O. Proposal for nor-adrenaline hypothesis for schizophrenia. Prog Neuropsychopharmacol Biol Psychiatry. 2004;28(5):913-22.
53. Carlsson A, Hansson LO, Waters N, Carlsson ML. Neurotransmitter aberrations in schizophrenia: new perspectives and therapeutic implications. Life Sci. 1997;61(2):75-94.
54. Stan AD, Lewis DA. Altered cortical GABA neurotransmission in schizophrenia: insights into novel therapeutic strategies. Curr Pharm Biotechnol. 2012;13(8):1557-62.
55. Guidotti A, Auta J, Chen Y, Davis JM, Dong E, Gavin DP, Grayson DR, Matrisciano F, Pinna G, Satta R, Sharma RP, Tremolizzo L, Tueting P. Epigenetic GABAergic targets in schizophrenia and bipolar disorder. Neuropharmacology. 2011;60(7-8):1007-16.
56. Coyle JT, Basu A, Benneyworth M, Balu D, Konopaske G. Glutamatergic synaptic dysregulation in schizophrenia: therapeutic implications. Handb Exp Pharmacol. 2012;213: 267-95.
57. Rotaru DC, Lewis DA, Gonzalez-Burgos G. The role of glutamatergic inputs onto parvalbumin-positive interneurons: relevance for schizophrenia. Rev Neurosci. 2012;23(1):97-109.
58. de Bartolomeis A, Sarappa C, Magara S, Iasevoli F. Targeting glutamate system for novel antipsychotic approaches: relevance for residual psychotic symptoms and treatment resistant schizophrenia. Eur J Pharmacol. 2012;682(1-3):1-11.
59. Gonzalez-Burgos D, Lewis DA. NMDA receptor hypofunction, parvalbumin-positive neurons, and cortical gamma oscillations in schizophrenia. Schizophr Bull. 2012;38(5): 950-7.
60. Bourin M, Malinge M, Vasar E, Bradwejn J. Two faces of cholecystokinin: anxiety and schizophrenia. Fundam Clin Pharmacol. 1996;10(2):116-26.
61. Weinberger DR. The biological basis of schizophrenia: new directions. J Clin Psychiatry. 1997;58(suppl 10):22-7.
62. Bachus SE, Hyde TM, Herman MM, Egan MF, Kleinman JE. Abnormal cholecystokinin mRNA levels in entorhinal cortex of schizophrenics. J Psychiatr Res. 1997;31(2):233-56.
63. Boules M, Shaw A, Fredrickson P, Richelson E. Neurotensin agonists: potential in the treatment of schizophrenia. CNS Drugs. 2007;21(1):13-23.
64. Eaton K, Sallee FR, Sah R. Relevance of neuropeptide Y (NPY) in psychiatry. Curr Top Med Chem. 2007;7(17):1645-59.
65. Ramírez M, Prieto I, Vives F, de Gasparo M, Alba F. Neuropeptides, neuropeptidases and brain asymmetry. Curr Protein Pept Sci. 2004;28(6):595-610.
66. Holsboer F. The role of peptide supplements in the treatment of psychiatric disorders. J Neural Transm. 2003;64:17-34.
67. Schaeffer EL, Gattaz WF, Eckert GP. Alterations of brain membranes in schizophrenia: impact of phospholipase A(2). Curr Top Med Chem. 2012;12(21):2314-23.
68. Kidd PM. Omega-3 DHA and EPA for cognition, behavior, and mood: clinical findings and structural-functional synergies with cell membrane phospholipids. Altern Med Rev. 2007; 12(3):207-27.
69. Du Bois TM, Deng C, Huang XF. Membrane phospholipid compositions, alterations in neurotransmitter systems in schizophrenia. Prog Neuropsychopharmcol Biol Psychiatry. 2005;29(6):878-89.
70. Yao JK, Van Kammen DP. Membrane phospholipids and cytokine interactions in schizophrenia. Int Rev Neurobiol. 2004;59:297-326.
71. Marx CE, Leiberman JA. Psychoneuroendocrinoogy of schizophrenia. Psychiatr Clin North Am. 1998;21(2):413-34.
72. Skare SS, Dysken MW, Billington CJ. A review of the GHRH stimulation test in schizophrenia. Biol Psychiatry. 1994;36(4): 249-65.
73. Garver DL. Neuroendocrine findings in schizophrenia. Endocrinol Metab Clin North Am. 1998;17(1):103-9.
74. Lal S. Apomorphine in the elevation of dopaminergic function in man. Prog Neuropsychopharmacol Biol Psychiatry. 1988; 12(2):117-64.

75. Garver DL. Neuroendocrine findings in schizophrenias. Neurol Clin. 1988;17(1):103-9.
76. Sternberg DE. Biological tests in psychiatry. Psychiatr Clin North Am. 1984;7(3):639-50.
77. Walters J, Jones I. Clinical questions and uncertainty—prolactin measurement in patients with schizophrenia and bipolar disorder. J Psychopharmacol. 2008;22(suppl 2):82-9.
78. Kohen D, Wildgust HJ. The evolution of hyperprolactinemia as an entity in schizophrenia patients. J Psychopharmacol. 2008; 22(suppl 2):6-11.
79. Santos NC, Costa P, Ruano D, Macedo A, Soares MJ, Valente J, Pereira AT, Azevedo MH, Palha JA. Revisiting thyroid hormones in schizophrenia. J Thyroid Res. 2012;569147:ePub.
80. Palha JA, Goodman AB. Thyroid hormones and retinoids: a possible link between genes and environment in schizophrenia. Brain Res Rev. 2006;51(1):61-71.
81. Meyer-Lindenberg A, Domes G, Kirsch P, Heinrichs M. Oxytocin and vasopressin in the human brain: social neuropeptides for translational medicine. Nat Rev Neurosci. 2011;12(9):524-38.
82. Marazziti D, Catena Dell'osso M. The role of oxytocin in neuropsychiatric disorders. Curr Med Chem. 2008;15(7): 698-704.
83. Fitzsimmons J, Kubicki M, Shenton ME. Review of functional and anatomical brain connectivity findings in schizophrenia. Curr Opin Psychiatry. 2013;26(2):172-87.
84. Shenton ME, Whitford TJ, Kubicki M. Structural neuroimaging in schizophrenia: from methods to insights to treatments. Dialogues Clin Neurosci. 2010;12(3):317-32.
85. Olabi B, Ellison-Wright I, McIntosh AM, Wood SJ, Bullmore E, Lawrie SM. Are there progressive brain changes in schizophrenia? A meta-analysis of structural magnetic resonance imaging studies. Biol Psychiatry. 2011;70(1):88-96.
86. Arbabshirani MR, Kiehl KA, Pearlson GD, Calhoun VD. Classification of schizophrenia patients based on resting-state functional network connectivity. Front Neurosci. 2013;30(7): 133-56.
87. van den Heuvel MP, Hulshoff Pol HE. Exploring the brain network: a review on resting-state fMRI functional connectivity. Eur Neuropsychopharmacol. 2010;20(8):519-34.
88. Kuswanto CN, Teh I, Lee TS, Sim K. Diffusion tensor imaging findings of white matter changes in first episode schizophrenia: a systematic review. Clin Psychopharmacol Neurosci. 2012; 10(1):13-24.
89. Kyriakopoulos M, Frangou S. Recent diffusion tensor imaging findings in early stages of schizophrenia. Curr Opin Psychiatry. 2009;22(2):169-76.
90. Gunther W. MRI-SPECT and PET-EEG findings on brain dysfunction in schizophrenia. Prog Neuropsychopharmacol Biol Psychiatry. 1992;16(4):445-62.
91. Erritzoe D, Talbot P, Frankle WG, Abi-Dargham A. Positron emission tomography and single photon emission CT molecular imaging in schizophrenia. Neuroimaging Clin N Am. 2003;13(3):817-32.
92. Harrison PJ. The neuropathology of schizophrenia. A critical review of the data and their interpretation. Brain. 1999;122: 533-44.
93. Irtani S. The neuropathology of schizophrenia: a mini review. Neuropathology. 2007;27(6):604-9.
94. Irtani S. Neuropathology of schizophrenia from a new perspective. Brain Nerve. 2007;59(6):605-616.

Schizophrenia: Genetics

95. Barch DM. Neuropsychological abnormalities in schizophrenia and mood disorders: similarities and differences. Curr Psychiatry Rep. 2009;11(4):313-9.
96. Fornito C, Yucel M, Pantelis C. Reconciling neuroimaging and neuropathological findings in schizophrenia and bipolar disorder. Curr Opin Psychiatry. 2009;22(3):312-9.
97. Watson D, Naragon-Kainey K. On the specificity of positive emotional dysfunction in psychopathology: evidence from the mood and anxiety disorders and schizophrenia/schizotypy. Clin Psychol Rev. 2010;30(7):839-48.
98. Heckers S. Bleuler and the neurobiology of schizophrenia. Schizophr Bull. 2011;37(6):1131-6.
99. Tandon R. The nosology of schizophrenia: towards DSM-5 and ICD 11. Psychiatr Clin North Am. 2012;35(3):557-69.
100. Stanghellini G, Fusar-Poli P. The vulnerability to schizophrenia mainstream research paradigms and phenomenological directions. Curr Pharm Des. 2012;18(4):338-45.
101. Kaiser S, Heekeren K, Simon JJ. The negative symptoms of schizophrenia: category or continnum. Psychopathology. 2011;44(6):345-53.
102. Keshavan MS, Nasrallah HA, Tandon R. Schizophrenia, "Just the Facts" 6. Moving ahead with the schizophrenia concept: from the elephant to the mouse. Schizophr Res. 2011;127(1-3): 3-13.
103. Urfer-Parnas A, Mortensen EL, Parnas J. Core of schizophrenia: estrangement, dementia or neurocognitive disorder? Psychopathology. 2010;45(5):300-11.
104. Torey FF, Davis JM. Adjunct treatments for schizophrenia and bipolar disorder: what to try when you are out of ideas. Clin Schizophr Relat Psychoses. 2012;5(4):208-16.
105. Harvey PD, Heaton RK, Carpenter WT Jr, Green MF, Gold JM, Schoenbaum M. Diagnosis of schizophrenia: consistency across information sources and stability of the condition. Schizophr Res. 2012;140(1-3):9-14.
106. Tiwari AK, Zai CC, Müller DJ, Kennedy JL. Genetics of schizophrenia: where are we now and what do we do next. Dialogues Clin Neurosci. 2010;12(3):289-303.
107. Williams HJ, Owen MJ, O'Donovan MC. Schizophrenia genetics: new insights and new approaches. Br Med Bull. 2009; 91:61-74.
108. Lin PI, Mitchell BD. Approaches for unraveling the joint genetic determinants of schizophrenia and bipolar disorder. Schizophr Bull. 2008;34(4):791-7.

109. Kaur T, Cadenhead KS. Treatment implications of the schizophrenia prodrome. Curr Top Behav Neurosci. 2010;4: 97-121.
110. Stahl SM, Morrissette DA, Citrome L, Saklad SR, Cummings MA, Meyer JM, O' Day JA, Dardashti LJ, Warburton KD. Meta-guidelines for the management of patients with schizophrenia. CNS Spectr. 2013;18(3):150-62.
111. Gejman PV, Sanders AR, Duan J. The role of genetics in the etiology of schizophrenia. Psychiatr Clin North Am. 2010;33(1): 35-66.
112. Barnett JH, Smoller JW. The genetics of bipolar disorder. Neuroscience. 2009;164(1):331-43.
113. Goes FS, Sanders LL, Potash JB. The genetics of psychotic bipolar disorder. Curr Psychiatry Rep. 2008;10(2):178-89.
114. Bramon E, Sham PC. The common genetic liability between schizophrenia and bipolar disorder: a review. Curr Psychiatry Rep. 2001;3(4):332-7.
115. Tsuang MT, Lyons MJ, Faraone SV. Problems of diagnoses in family studies. J Psychiatr Res. 1987;21(4):391-9.
116. Janson LB, Parnas J. Competing definitions of schizophrenia: what can be learnt from polydiagnostic studies. Schizophr Bull. 2007;33(5):1178-200.
117. Allan CL, Cardno AG. McGuffin P. Schizophrenia: from genes to phenes to disease. Curr Psychiatr Rep. 2008;10(4):339-43.
118. Farmer A, Elkin A, McGuffin P. The genetics of bipolar affective disorder. Curr Opin Psychiatry. 2007;20(1):8-12.
119. Shih RA, Belmonte PL, Zandi PP. A review of the evidence from family, twin and adoption studies for a genetic contribution to adult psychiatric disorders. Int Rev Psychiatry. 2004;16(4): 260-83.
120. Hosák L, Silhan P, Hosáková J. Genome-wide association studies in schizophrenia, and potential etiological and functional implications of their results. Acta Medica. 2012; 55(1):3-11.
121. Mowry BJ, Gratten J. The emerging spectrum of allelic variation in schizophrenia: current evidence and strategies for the identification and functional characterization of common and rare variants. Mol Psychiatry. 2013;18(1):38-52.
122. Adida M, Azorin JM, Fakra E, Belzeaux R, Kaladjian A, Pomietto P, Corréard N. Schizophrenia and/or bipolar disorder: neurobiological endophenotypes. Encephale. 2012;38(suppl 3): S98-102.
123. White T, Gottesman I. Brain connectivity and gyrification as endophenotypes for schizophrenia: weight of the evidence. Curr Top Med Chem. 2012;12(21):2393-403.
124. Nenadic I, Gaser C, Sauer H. Heterogeneity of brain structural variation and the structural imaging endophenotypes in schizophrenia. Neuropsychobiology. 2012;66(1):44-9.
125. Nasrallah H, Tandon R, Keshavan M. Beyond the facts in schizophrenia: closing the gaps in diagnosis, pathophysiology, and treatment. Epidemiol Psychiatr Sci. 2011;20(4):317-27.
126. Luck SJ, Mathalon DH, O'Donnell BF, Hämäläinen MS, Spencer KM, Javitt DC, Uhlhaas PJ. A roadmap for the development and validation of event-related potential biomarkers in schizophrenia research. Biol Psychiatry. 2011;70(1):28-34.
127. Amann LC, Gandal MJ, Halene TB, Ehrlichman RS, White SL, McCarren HS, Siegel SJ. Mouse behavioural endophenotypes for schizophrenia. Brain Res Bull. 2010;83(3-4):347-66.

Schizophrenia: Psychosocial Treatments

128. Drake RE, Essock SM, Bond GR. Implementing evidence-based practices for people with schizophrenia. Schizophr Bull. 2009;35:704-13.
129. Bustillo J, Lauriello J, Horan W, Keith S. The psychosocial treatment of schizophrenia: an update. Am J Psychiatry. 2001; 158:163-75.
130. Wallace CJ, Tauber R. Supplementing supported employment with workplace skills training. Psychiatr Serv. 2004;55:513-5.
131. Dilk MN, Bond GR. Meta-analytic evaluation of skills training research for individuals with severe mental illness. J Consult Clin Psychol. 1996;64:1337-46.
132. Kurtz MM, Mueser KT. A meta-analysis of controlled research on social skills training for schizophrenia. J Consult Clin Psychol. 2008;76:491-504.
133. Heaton RK, Gladsjo JA, Palmer B, Kuck J, Marcotte TD, Jeste DV. The stability and course of neuropsychological deficits in schizophrenia. Arch Gen Psychiatry. 2001;58:24-32.
134. Heinssen RK, Liberman RP, Kopelowicz A. Psychosocial skills training for schizophrenia: Lessons from the laboratory. Schizophr Bull. 2000;26(1):21-46.
135. Hermanutz M, Gestrich J. Computer-assisted attention training in schizophrenics. Eur Arch Psychiatr Clin Neurosci. 1991;240: 282-7.
136. Herz MI, Lamberti JS, Mintz J, Scott R, O'Dell SP, McCartan L, Nix G. A program for relapse prevention in schizophrenia: A controlled study. Arch Gen Psychiatry. 2000;57: 277-83.
137. Huxley NA, Rendall M, Sederer L. Psychosocial treatments in schizophrenia: A review of the past 20 years. J Nerv Mental Disease. 2000;188:187-201.
138. Hyde TM, Nawroz S, Goldberg TE, Bigelow LB, Strong D, Weinberger DR, Kleinman JE. Is there cognitive decline in schizophrenia? A cross-sectional study. Br J Psychiatry. 1994; 164:494-500.
139. Nelson G, Aubrey T, Lafrance A. A review of the literature on the effectiveness of housing and support, assertive community treatment, and intensive case management interventions for persons with mental illness who have been homeless. Am J Orthopsychiatry. 2007;77:350-61.
140. Becker DR, Xie H, McHugo GJ, Halliday J, Martinez RA. What predicts supported employment program outcomes? Community Ment Health J. 2006;42:303-13.
141. Glynn SM. Token economy approaches for psychiatric patients: progress and pitfalls over 25 years. Behav Modif. 1990; 14:383-407.

142. Mari JJ, Streiner DL. An overview of family interventions and relapse on schizophrenia: meta-analysis of research findings. Psychol Med. 1994;24:565-78.
143. Pilling S, Bebbington P, Kuipers E, et al. Psychological treatments in schizophrenia: I. Meta-analysis of family intervention and cognitive behaviour therapy. Psychol Med. 2002;32:763-82.
144. Weber M, Wyne K. A cognitive/behavioral group intervention for weight loss in patients treated with atypical antipsychotics. Schizophr Res. 2006;83:95-101.
145. Swanson AJ, Pantalon MV, Cohen KR. Motivational interviewing and treatment adherence among psychiatric and dually diagnosed patients. J Nerv Ment Dis. 1999;187:630-5.

Schizophrenia: Role of Psychotherapy

146. Fenton WS. Evolving perspectives on individual psychotherapy for schizophrenia. Schizophr Bull. 2000;26(1):47-72.
147. Albus M. Clinical courses of schizophrenia. Psychopathology. 2012;45(Suppl 1):S31-35.
148. Roder V, Mueller DR, Schmidt SJ. Effectiveness of integrated psychological therapy (IPT) for schizophrenia patients: a research update. Schizophr Bull. 2011;37(Suppl 2):S71-9.
149. Kern RS, Glynn SM, Horan WP, Marder SR. Psychosocial treatments to promote functional recovery in schizophrenia. Schizophr Bull. 2009;35(2):347-61.
150. Patterson TL, Leeuwenkamp OR. Adjunctive psychosocial therapies for the treatment of schizophrenia. Schizophr Res. 2008;100(1-3):108-19.
151. Gibbs PL. The primacy of psychoanalytic intervention in recovery from the psychoses and schizophrenias. J Am Acad Psychoanal Dyn Psychiatry. 2007;35(2):287-312.
152. Kocmur M. Psychotherapeutic approaches in the management of schizophrenia. Neuro Endocrinol Lett. 2007;28(Suppl 1): 135-45.
153. Spaulding W, Notling J. Psychotherapy for schizophrenia in the year 2030: prognosis and prognostication. Schizophr Bull. 2006;32(Suppl 1):S94-105.
154. Buckley LA, Pettit T, Adams CE. Supportive psychotherapy for schizophrenia. Cochrane Database Syst Rev. 2007;18(3): CD004716.
155. Motlova L. Schizophrenia and the family. Neuro Endocrinol Lett. 2007;28(Suppl 1):147-59.
156. Dickerson FB, Lehman AF. Evidence-based psychotherapy for schizophrenia. J Nerv Ment Disease. 2006;194(1):3-9.
157. Saperstein AM, Kurtz MM. Current trends in the study of cognitive remediation for schizophrenia. Can J Psychiatry. 2013;58(6):311-8.
158. Rector NA, Beck AT. Cognitive behaviour therapy for schizophrenia: an empirical review. J Nerv Ment Disease. 2012; 200(10):832-9.
159. Sivec HJ, Montesano VL. Cognitive behavioural therapy for psychosis in clinical practice. Psychotherapy (Chic). 2012; 49(2):258-70.
160. Tarier N. Cognitive behaviour therapy for schizophrenia and psychosis: current status and future directions. Clin Schizophr Relat Psychoses. 2010;4(3):176-84.
161. Brus M, Novakovic B, Friedberg A. Psychotherapy for schizophrenia: a review of the modalities and their evidence base. Psychodyn Psychiatry. 2012;40(4):609-16.
162. Shean GD. Recent developments in the psychosocial treatments for patients with schizophrenia. Expert Rev Neurother. 2007; 7(7):817-27.
163. Hogarty GE, Kornblith SJ, Greenwald D. Personal Therapy: a disorder-relevant psychotherapy for schizophrenia. Schizophr Bull. 1995;21:379-93.
164. Tarrier N, Yusupoff L, Kinney C, McCarthy E, Gledhill A, Haddock G, Morris J. Randomised controlled trial of intensive cognitive behaviour therapy for patients with chronic schizophrenia. BMJ. 1998;317:303-7.
165. Kuipers E, Fowler D, Garety P, Chisholm D, Freeman D, Dunn G, Bebbington P, Hadley C. London–East Anglia randomized controlled trial of cognitive-behavioural therapy for psychosis. Br J Psychiatry. 1998;173:61-8.
166. Lehman AF, Carpenter WT, Goldman HH. Treatment outcomes in schizophrenia: implications for practice, policy and research. Schizophr Bull. 1995;21:669-76.
167. Coursey RD, Keller AB, Farrell EW. Individual psychotherapy and persons with serious mental illness: the client's perspective. Schizophr Bull. 1995;21:283-301.
168. Eells TD. Psychotherapy for schizophrenia. J Psychother Pract Res. 2000;9(4):249-55.

SUGGESTED READING

Introduction and Overview

1. Bromet EJ, Fennig S. Epidemiology and natural history of schizophrenia. Biol Psychiatry. 1999;46:871-81.
2. Chen YR, Swann AC, Burt DB. Stability of diagnosis in schizophrenia. Am J Psychiatry. 1996;153:682-6.
3. Diagnostic and Statistical Manual of Mental Disorders. 4th edition, text revision. Washington, D.C.: American Psychiatric Association, 2000.pp.297-343.
4. Freedman R. Schizophrenia. New Engl J Med. 2003;349:1738-49.
5. Geddes J, Freemantle N, Harrison P, Bebbington P. Atypical antipsychotics in the treatment of schizophrenia: systematic overview and metaregression analysis. BMJ. 2000;321: 1371-6.
6. Glick ID, Suppes T, DeBattista C, Hu RJ, Marder S. Psychopharmacologic treatment strategies for depression, bipolar disorder, and schizophrenia. Ann Intern Med. 2001;134:47-60.
7. Goodman LS, Gilman A, Hardman JG, Limbird LE. Goodman and Gilman's the Pharmacological Basis of Therapeutics. 10th edition. New York, N.Y.: McGraw-Hill, 2001.pp.500-6.
8. Lewis DA, Lieberman JA. Catching up on schizophrenia: natural history and neurobiology. Neuron. 2000;28:325-34.

9. Mortensen PB, Pedersen CB, Westergaard T, Wohlfahrt J, Ewald H, Mors O, et al. Effects of family history and place and season of birth on the risk of schizophrenia. N Engl J Med. 1999;340:603-8.

Schizophrenia: From Psychodynamics to Neuro-dynamics

10. Bateson G, Jackson D, Haley J, et al. Towards a theory of schizophrenia. Behav Sci. 1956;1:251-64.
11. Brown GW, Birley MT, Wing JK. Influence of the family life on the course schizophrenic disorders: a replication. Br J Psychiatry. 1972;121:241-58.
12. Engel GA. The need for a new medical model: a challenge for biomedicine. Science. 1977;96:129.
13. Federn P. Ego Psychology and the Psychoses. Basic Books, New York, 1952.
14. Feinberg I. Schizophrenia: caused by fault in programmed synaptic elimination during adolescence? J Psychiatr Res. 1982;4:319.
15. Freud S. The Interpretation of Dreams. In: Standard Edition of the Complete Psychological Works of Sigmund Freud, vol. 5. Hogarth Press. London,1953.
16. Freud S. On the history of the psychoanalytic movement. In: Standard Edition of the Complete Psychological Works of Sigmund Freud, vol.14. Hogarth Press, London, 1957.
17. Freud S. Psychoanalytic notes on an autobiographical account of a case of paranoia (dementia paranoides). In: Standard Edition of the Complete Psychological work of Sigmund Freud, vol. 12. Flogarth Press, London, 1958.
18. Fromm-Rein-imam Notes on the development of treatment of schizophrenia by psychoanalytic psychotherapy. Psychiatry. 1948;11:263-73.
19. Greenberg JR, Mitchell SA. Object Relations in Psychoanalytic Theory. Harvard University Press, Cambride, MA, 1983.
20. Hoffman RE. Computer simulations of neural information processing and the schizophrenia/mania dichotomy. Arch Gen Psychiatry. 1987;44:178.
21. Hoffman RE, Dobscha SB. Cortical pruning and the development of SC 3: A computer model. Schizophr Bull. 1989;15:477.
22. Hoffman RE, McGlashan TH. Parallel distributed processing and the emergence of schizophrenic symptoms. Schizophr Bull. 1993;19:119.
23. Hopfield JJ. Neural networks and physical systems with emergent collective computational abilities. Proc N atl Acad Sci USA. 1982;79:2554.
24. Jaspers K. General Psychopathology. Grume and Stratton, New York, 1959.
25. Lichtenberg JD. Pan's Theory Origins and future directions. In: Feirisilver DB (Ed), Towards a Comprehensive. Model for Schizophrenic Disorders. Analytic Press, Hillsdale, NJ, 1986.
26. Lidz T. Schizophrenia and the Family. International Universities Press, New York, 1965.
27. McGlashan TH, Hoffman RE. Schizophrenia: Psychodynamic to Neurodynamic Theories. In: Freedman AM, Kaplan HI. (Eds). Comprehensive Textbook of Psychiatry 2nd edn. Baltimore: Williams & Wilkins. 1999;6:851-60.
28. Meehl PE. Toward an integrated theory of schizotaxia, schizotypy, and schizophrenia. J Pers Disord. 1990;4:1.
29. Mesulam MM. Large-scale neuro-cognitive networks and distributed processing for attention, language and memory. Ann Neurol. 1990;28:567.
30. Padmavati R. Schizophrenia: Role of Family. In: Vyas JN, Ahuja N. (Ed). Textbok of Postgraduate Psychiatry 2nd edn. New Delhi: Jaypee Brothers Medical Publishers. 1999;72:7: 172-5.
31. Pao PN. Schizophrenic Disorders. International University Press, New York, 1979.
32. Segal H. Introduction to the work of Melanie Klein. Basic Books, New York, 1973.
33. Spring B, Zubin J. Vulnerability to schizophrenic episodes and their prevention in adults. In: Albee GW, Joffee JM (Eds). Primary Prevention in Psychopathology: The Issues, vol. 1. University Press of New Englnd, Hanover, NH, 1977.
34. Sullivan HS. Clinical Studies in Psychiatry. Norton, New 29, York. 1956.
35. Tienari P, Sorry A, Lahti I, Narala M1, Wahlberg KE, Ronkko T, Pohjola J, Moring J. The Finnish adoptive family study or schizophrenia, Yale J Biol Med. 1985;58:227.
36. Vaughn CE, Leff JP. Pattern of emotional response in relatives of schizophrenic patients. Schizophr Bull. 1981;7: 43-4.
37. Wig NN, Menon DK, Bedi H, et al. Expressed emotions and schizophrenia in north India. I. Cross-cultural transfer of ratings of relatives expressed emotions. Br Psychiatry. 1987; 156-9.
38. Wynne LC, Singer M. Thought disorder and family relations of schizophrenics: II. Classification of forms of thinking Arch Gen Psychiatry. 1963;9:199.

Schizophrenia: Clinical Features

39. Adler CM, Strakowski SM. Boundaries of schizophrenia. In: PF Buckley (Eds). The Psychiatric Clinic of North America WB Saunders Company, Philadelphia. 2003; vol.1(1):2-23.
40. American Psychiatric Association. Desk reference to the Diagnostic Criteria from DSM-5. Washington DC; 2013.
41. American Psychiatric Association. Diagnostic and Statistical Manual of Mental Disorders. DSM-IV, 4th edition. Washington (DC): American Psychiatric Association; 1994.
42. Andreasen NC. The diagnosis of schizophrenia. Schizophrenia Bulletin. 1987;13:9.
43. Black DW, Andreasen NC, Schizophrenia, schizophreniform disorder, and delusional (paranoid) disorders. In: Hales RE, Yudofsky SC (Eds). Essentials of Clinical Psychiatry. 3rd edition, Washington, DC: American Psychiatric Press, 1999; pp.233-73.

44. Damn P, Murray RM. Neurological soft signs in first-episode psychosis: a systematic review. The British Journal of Psychiatry. 2002;181:s50-s7.
45. David AS. The clinical neuropsychology of schizophrenia, In: MG Gelder, et al. (Eds). New Oxford Textbook of Psychiatry Oxford University Press, UK, 2003. pp. 576-9.
46. Falloon LRH. Early intervention for first episodes of schizophrenia: a preliminary exploration. Psychiatry. 1992;55: 4-15.
47. Fenton WS, McGlashsan Tit. Natural history of schizophrenia subtypes I; longitudinal study of paranoid, hebephrenic and undifferentiated schizophrenia. Archives of General Psychiatrist. 1991;48:969-77.
48. Ganguly R, Brar JS, Chengappa KNR. Mitogen stimulated interleukin 2 production in never medicated, first episode schizophrenic patients. Archives of General Psychiatry. 1995; 52:668-72.
50. Gelder M, Mayou R, Cowen P. Schizophrenia and schizophrenia like disorders. In Shorter Oxford Textbook of Psychiatry—PLTI 11, 4th edition. Oxford University Press, UK; 2002. pp. 327-79.
51. Gupta S, Rajaprabhakaran R, Arndt S, et al. Premorbid adjustment as a predictor of phenomenological and Neurobiological Indices of Schizophrenia Research. 1995;16: 189-97.
52. Hamilton M. Disorders of thought and speech. In Fish's Clinical Psychopathology, 2nd edition, Vergese Publishing House, Mumbai; 1985. pp.37-62.
53. Hamilton NI. Disorders of perception. In Fish's clinical Psychopathology, 2nd edition, Vergese Publishing House, Mumbai; 1985. pp.16-36.
54. Harvey PD, Bowie CR. Cognitive Functioning in Schizophrenia. Current Psychosis and Therapeutics Reports. 2003;1:22-7.
55. Hoffman RAF, McGlashan TH. Parallel distributed processing and the emergence of schizophrenic symptoms. Schizophrenia Bulletin. 1993;19:119-40.
56. Kendler KS, McGuire M, Greunberg AM, et al. Outcome and family study of the subtypes of schizophrenia in West of Ireland. American Journal of Psychiatry. 1994;151:849-56.
57. Kraepelin E. Textbook of Psychiatry, 7th edition (translated, AR Diefendorf) London; Macmillan, 1907.
58. Liddle PF. Schizophrenia—Clinical Picture. In: Stein G, Wilkinson. Seminars in General Adult Psychiatry. Bell and Bain. Glasgow. 1998;(vol 1):pp.272-320.
59. Meynert T. Amentia, die VerwirrtheK. Jahrbuch der Psychiatric (Vienna). 1889;9:1-112.
60. National electronic library for health. Simple schizophrenia. Updated on 21-10-2004. lutpliwww.nefralaorai page viewasp?c= 11)&didaa138 I &fc=001002025.
61. Neylan TC, Va Kammen DP, Kelley ME, et al. Sleep in schizophrenic patients on and off haloperidol therapy: clinically stable versus relapsed patients. Archives of General Psychiatry. 1992;49:643-9.
62. Robert C, Lehmann HE. Schizophrenia: Clinical Features. In: Sadock BJ, Sadock VA (Eds). Kaplan and Sadocks Comprehensive Textbook of Psychiatry. 7th edition, Lippincott. Williams and Wilkins Philadelphia. 2000;(Vol. 1):1169-99.
63. Schizophrenia: From Wikipedia, the free encyclopedia http://en.wikipedia.org /wiki/Schizophrenia#References.
64. World Health Organization. The ICD 10 classification of mental and behavioural disorders—clinical description arid diagnostic guidelines. World Health Organisation, Geneva; 1992.
65. World Health Organization. The International Pi-lot Study of Geneva; WHO 1973.

Schizophrenia: Somatic Treatment

66. Ayd Jr FJ. A survey of drug-induced extrapyramidal reactions. JAMA. 1961;175:1054-60.
67. Carlsson A, Lindquist M. Effect of chlorpromazine and haloperidol on formation of 3-methoxytyramine and normetanephrine in mouse brain. Acta Pharmacol Toxicol. 1963;20:140-4.
68. Cheng YH, Illum L, Davis SS. Schizophrenia and drug delivery systems. J Drug Target. 2000;8(2):107-17.
69. Geddes J, Freemantle N, Harrison P, Bebbington P. Atypical antipsychotics in the treatment of schizophrenia: systematic overview and meta-regression analysis. BMJ. 2000;321(7273): 1371-6.
70. Grunder G, Hippius H, Carlsson A. The 'atypicality' of antipsychotics: A concept re-examined and re-defined. Nat Rev Drug Discov. 2010;8.
71. Idanpaan-Hiekkila J, Alhave E, Olkinuora M, Plava I. Agranulocytosis during treatment with clozapine. Eur J Clin Pharmacol. 1977;11:193-8.
72. Konopaske GT, Dorph-Petersen KA, Sweet RA. Effect of chronic antipsychotic exposure on astrocyte and oligodendrocyte numbers in macaque monkeys. Biol Psychiatry. 2008;63(8): 759-65.
73. Lieberman JA. Effectiveness of antipsychotic drugs in patients with chronic schizophrenia: efficacy, safety and cost outcomes of CATIE and other trials. J Clin Psychiatry. 2007;68(2):04.
74. Mathews M, Muzina DJ. Atypical antipsychotics: new drugs, new challenges. Clev Clin J Med. 2007;74(8):597-606.
75. McEvoy JP, Lieberman JA, Perkins DO, et al. Efficacy and tolerability of olanzapine, quetiapine, and risperidone in the treatment of early psychosis: a randomized, double-blind 52-week comparison. Am J Psychiatry. 2007;164(7):1050-60.
76. Morrens M, Hulstijn W, Sabbe B. Psychomotor slowing in schizophrenia. Schizophr Bull. 2007;33(4):1038-53.
77. Murphy BP, Chung YC, Park TW, McGorry PD. Pharmacological treatment of primary negative symptoms in schizophrenia: a systematic review. Schizophr Res. 2006;88(3):5-25.
78. Newcomer JW. Metabolic considerations in the use of antipsychotic medications: a review of recent evidence. J Clin Psychiatry. 2007;68(Suppl 1):20-7.

79. Peuskens J, De Hert M, Jones M. The clinical value of risperidone and olanzapine: a meta-analysis of efficacy and safety. Int J Psychiatry Clin Pract. 2001;5:179-87.
80. Schultz SH, North SW, Shields CG. Schizophrenia: a review. Am Fam Physician. 2007;75(12):1821-9.
81. Shen WW. A history of antipsychotic drug development. Compr Psychiatry. 1999;40:407-14.

Treatment Resistant Schizophrenia

82. Agid O, Kapur S, Remington G. Emerging drugs for schizophrenia. Expert Opin Emerg Drugs. 2008;13:479-95.
83. Andreasen NC, Carpenter Jr WT, Kane JM, Lasser RA, Marder SR, Weinberger DR. Remission in schizophrenia: proposed criteria and rationale for consensus. Am J Psychiatry. 2005;162:441e9.
84. Barnes TR, McEvedy CJ, Nelson HE. Management of treatment resistant schizophrenia unresponsive to clozapine. Br J Psychiatry Suppl. 1996;(31):31-40.
85. Borgio JG, Bressan RA, Barbosa Neto JB, Daltio CS. Refractory schizophrenia: a neglected clinical problem. Rev Bras Psiquiat. 2007;29:292-3.
86. Brenner HD, Dencker SJ, Goldstein MJ, Hubbard JW, Keegan DL, Kruger G, Kulhanek F, et al. Defining treatment refractoriness in schizophrenia. Schizophr Bull. 1990;16:551e65.
87. Carpenter WT, Koenig JI. The evolution of drug development in schizophrenia: past issues and future opportunities. Neuropsychopharmacology. 2008;33: 2061e79.
88. Cervera Enguix S, Seva Fernández A. Pharmacological treatment resistant schizophrenia. Actas Esp Psiquiatr. 2006; 34(1):48-54.
89. Conley RR, Buchanan RW. Evaluation of treatment resistant schizophrenia. Schizophr Res. 1997;23(4):663-7.
90. Conley RR, Kelly DR. Management of treatment resistance in schizophrenia. Biol Psychiatry. 2001;50:898e911.
91. Kane JM, Marder SR. Psychopharmacologic treatment of schizophrenia. Schizophr Bull. 1993;19:287-302.
92. Meltzer HY. Defining treatment refractoriness in schizophrenia. Schizophr Bull. 1990;16:563-5.
93. Meltzer HY. Treatment of the neuroleptic-nonresponsive schizophrenic patient. Schizophr Bull. 1992;18(3):515-42.
94. Mitelman SA, Buchsbaum MS. Very poor outcome schizophrenia: clinical and neuroimaging aspects. Int Rev Psychiatry. 2007;19(4):345-57.
95. Pantelis C, Barnes TR. Drug strategies and treatment-resistant schizophrenia. Aust N Z J Psychiatry. 1996;30:20-37.
96. Peuskens J. The evolving definition of treatment resistance. J Clin Psychiatry. 1999;60 (Suppl 12):4-8.
97. Williams L, Newton G, Roberts K, Finlayson S, Brabbins C. Clozapine-resistant schizophrenia: a positive approach. Br J Psychiatry. 2002;181:184-7.

Schizophrenia: Psychosocial Rehabilitation

98. Anthony WA, Rogers ES, Cohen M, Davies R. Relationships between psychiatric symptomatology, work skills, and future vocational performance. Psychiatric Services. 1995;46:353-8.
99. Black BJ. Work as Therapy for the Mentally Ill. New York, NY: Altro Institute for Rehabilitation Studies; 1986.
100. Bond GR, Drake R, Mueser K, Becker D. An update on supported employment for persons with severe mental illness. Psychiatric Services. 1997;48:335-46.
101. Cook JA, Razzano L. Vocational rehabilitation for persons with schizophrenia: recent research and implications for practice. Schizophr Bull. 2000;26(1):87-103.
102. Flexor RW, Solomon P. Psychiatric Rehabilitation in Practice. Boston, MA: Andover Medical Publishers; 1993.
103. Medalia A, Herlands T, Baginsky C. Cognitive remediation in the supportive housing setting. Psychiatr Serv. 2003;54: 1219-20.
104. Medalia A, Revheim N, Casey M. The remediation of problem-solving skills in schizophrenia. Schizophr Bull. 2001;27:259-67.
105. Medalia A, Revheim N, Herlands T. Remediation of cognitive deficits in psychiatric patients: a clinician' s manual. New York: Montefiore Medical Center Press; 2002.
106. Stein L. Innovations in Mental Health Services. San Francisco, CA: Jossey-Bass; 1992.
107. Wykes T, Reeder CL, Corner J, William SC, Eberitt, B. The effects of neurocognitive remediation on executive processing in patients with schizophrenia. Schizophr Bull. 1999;25:291-307.
108. Yamashita C, Mizuno M, Nemoto T, Kashima H. Social cognitive problem-solving in schizophrenia: associations with fluency and verbal memory. Psychiatr Res. 2005;134:123-9.
109. Zanello A, Perrig L, Huguelet, P. Cognitive functions related to interpersonal problem-solving skills in schizophrenia patients compared with healthy subjects. Psychiatry Res. 2006;142:67-78.

Schizophrenia: The Indian Scenario

110. Barrowclough C. Issues in the dissemination of family intervention for psychosis. World Psychiatry. 2003;2:31-2.
111. Bustillo J, Lauriello J, Horan W, Keith S. The psychosocial treatment of schizophrenia: an update. Am J Psychiatry. 2001; 158:163-75.
112. Chakrabarti S. Impact of schizophrenia on the family: the Indian perspective. In: Kulhara P, Avasthi A, Grover S, editors. Schizophrenia: the Indian Scene. Chandigarh: Department of Psychiatry PGIMER; 2010.pp.215-62.
113. Cheng AT. Expressed emotion: a cross-culturally valid concept? Br J Psychiatry. 2002;181:466-7.
114. Dixon L, Adams C, Lucksted A. Update on family psycho-education for schizophrenia. Schizophr Bull. 2000;26:5-20.

115. Dixon LB, Lehman AF. Family interventions for schizophrenia. Schizophr Bull. 1995;21:631-43.
116. Falloon IR. Family interventions for mental disorders: efficacy and effectiveness. World Psychiatry. 2003;2:20-8.
117. Knight BG, Sayegh P. Cultural values and caregiving: the updated sociocultural stress and coping model. J Gerontol B Psychol Sci Soc Sci. 2010;65B:5-13.
118. Leggatt M. Families and mental health workers: the need for partnership. World Psychiatry. 2002;1:52-4.
119. Mojtabai R, Nicholson RA, Carpenter BN. Role of psychosocial treatments in management of schizophrenia: a meta-analytic review of controlled outcome studies. Schizophr Bull. 1998;24: 569-87.
120. Murthy RS. Family interventions and empowerment as an approach to enhance mental health resources in developing countries. World Psychiatry. 2003;2:35-7.
121. Paranthaman V, Satnam K, Lim JL, Amar-Singh HSS, Sararaks S, Nafiza MN, Ranjit K, Asmah ZA. Effective implementation of a structured psychoeducation programme among caregivers of patients with schizophrenia in the community. Asian J Psychiatry. 2010;3:206-12.
122. Pharoah F, Mari J, Rathbone J, Wong W. Family intervention for schizophrenia. Cochrane Database Syst Rev. 2010;CD000088.
123. Pilling S, Bebbington P, Kuipers E, Garety P, Geddes J, Orbach G, Morgan C. Psychological treatments in schizophrenia: I. Meta-analysis of family intervention and cognitive behaviour therapy. Psychol Med. 2002;32:763-82.
124. Setty K, Jagannathan A, Rajaram P. Challenges in measuring efficacy of psychoeducation for caregivers of Indian patients with schizophrenia. Acta Psychiatr Scand. 2010;122:516.
125. Shankar R, Rao K. From burden to empowerment: the journey of family caregivers in India. In: Sartorius N, Leff J, Lopez Ibor JJ, Okasha A, editors. Families and mental disorders. Chichester: John Wiley and Sons Ltd.; 2005.pp.259-90.
126. Smith J, Birchwood M. Relatives and patients as partners in the management of schizophrenia. The development of a service model. Br J Psychiatry. 1990;156:654-60.
127. Xia J, Merinder LB, Belgamwar MR. Psychoeducation for schizophrenia. Cochrane Database Syst Rev. 2011;CD002831.

CHAPTER 7

Mood Disorders

JN Vyas, Dinesh Tyagi, Ashok Singhal, Neena Bohra, NK Bohra, RK Solanki, BK Singh, Ajit Avasthi, Sandeep Grover, Alkananda Dutt, Baljit Singh Saluja, SK Pandey, Manoj Dhungana

7.1 EPIDEMIOLOGY AND CLASSIFICATION

JN Vyas, Dinesh Tyagi

The term 'mood disorders' groups together a number of clinical conditions whose common and essential feature is a disturbance of mood, accompanied by related cognitive, psychomotor, psychophysiological, and interpersonal difficulties.

Although human experience includes a variety of emotions such as fear, anger, pleasure and surprise, the clinical conditions considered under the mood disorders include depression and mania.

Mood refers to an internal emotional state of individual, while *affect* is the external expression of internal emotional content. As critical pathology in depression and mania is one of mood and not of affect, affective disorders of DSM-III[1] have been now described as mood disorders in DSM-III-R,[2] DSM-IV[3] and DSM-5

NORMAL VERSUS PATHOLOGICAL MOOD

Normal person experiences a wide range of moods such as feelings of sadness, disappointment, frustration, cheerfulness, hopefulness, confidence; hence the differentiation between normal and one needing clinical attention and therapeutic intervention is necessary. Mood may be recognized as pathological by virtue of its intensity, pervasiveness, persistence, and interference with usual social and physiological functioning.

A number of features distinguish clinically ill patients from those with normal mood. In addition to disturbance of mood, the psychopathological state involves a combination of the following features:

- Impairments of body functioning indicated by disturbances in sleep, appetite, sexual interest, and autonomic nervous system and gastrointestinal activity.
- Reduced desire and ability to perform the usual, expected social roles in the family, at work, in marriage, or in school.
- Suicidal thoughts or acts.
- Disturbances in reality testing, manifested in delusions, hallucinations, or confusion.

On the other level, normal mood such as depression is adaptive as it serves a signal function. It alerts the mother or other members of social group that one of its helpless members, the infant, is in potential danger. That is especially true during the acquisition of cognitive, perceptual, motor and social skills. Alerted protectors can rally resources for nurturance, support and protection, and thus promote biological survival.

HISTORICAL ASPECTS

Depression has been recorded since antiquity. The Old Testament story of King Saul describes a depressive syndrome, as does the story of Ajax's suicide in Homer's Iliad. Hippocrates used the term *mania* and *melancholia* to describe mental disturbances. Aulus Cornelius described melancholia as a depression caused by black bile in 30 AD. In 1686, Bonet described a mental illness called maniacomelancholicus.

Jules Falret described patients who became depressed and elated in a cyclic fashion (*la foliecirculare*) in 1854. Jules Baillarger described the condition *folie a double forme*, in which the patient became deeply depressed and fell into a stuporous state from which he would eventually recover.

Karl Ludwig Kahlbaum made similar observations about mania and melancholia in 1882. He felt that these episodes were different stages of the same disease process, which he called *cyclothymia*.

Emil Kraepelin (1856–1926) made painstaking observations of patients and described a number of mood disorders, including mania, melancholia, recurrent depression, and mild mood swings. In 1921, he concluded that all of these mood disorders are identical in certain ways. He called the underlying illness '*manic depressive illness*'. This formulation of a single, underlying disorder with varied clinical manifestations was widely accepted for several decades.

Kraepelin's notion of a single mood disorder with varied clinical manifestations did not withstand the scrutiny of clinicians in the 1930s and 1940s. By the mid-1950s, it was suggested that some individuals suffered only from depression, while others suffered from cyclic disorder that Kraepelin had described as *manic depression*. The illness, that began after menopause in women and during late adulthood in men, came to be known as involutional melancholia and has since come to be viewed as a variant form of mood disorders.

Karl Abraham (1877–1925) accepted Kraepelin's notion of a single mood illness. In his description of 6 patients, he presented a psychodynamic picture of mood illness, which emphasizes the role of loss in precipitating a mood episode and the element of regression in the clinical presentation.

Sigmund Freud[4] (1856–1939) emphasized the importance of loss in depression. Instead of remaining angry with the lost individual, the anger is turned inward by the depressed person. Freud felt that this phenomenon accounted for the typical findings of guilt, lowered self-esteem, self-reproach, and suicidal ideation. He did not explain all depressions in this manner, however he clearly stated that some depression is psychogenic in origin (i.e. precipitated by loss) and, in other cases biologically determined.

Freud conceptualized two different types of depression. Depression was classified as either endogenous (i.e. biologically determined) or exogenous (i.e. precipitated by loss). It was felt that those patients who develop severe depression in the face of some acute precipitant suffer from a different disorder than those without recent loss in their histories. Many advocated a different treatment for the two groups. Psychotherapy with a focus on reactions to the acute precipitant was advocated for exogenous or reactive depression while medication, electroconvulsive therapy (ECT), or both were prescribed for endogenous depression. This interpretation of depression was accepted well into the 1970s.

The proposal to divide manic depressive illness into separate bipolar (alternating mania and depression) and unipolar (recurrent depression or recurrent mania psychoses) were first brought forward by Leonhard [5] (1959), but it was Angst[6] (1966) who first produced convincing evidence in support of the division. Perris[7] (1968) was able to show that bipolar illness started on an average fifteen years earlier than depression and recurred more frequently.

Venkoba Rao,[8] in a study of 101 endogenous depressives, could not find statistically significant differences in unipolar or bipolar illness but Singh and Aggarwal[9] and Aggarwal[10] reported significant differences in the two groups.

Research, which began in the 1950s, was triggered by a serendipitous observation made in hypertensive patients treated with the then new drug, reserpine. Many of these patients developed severe depression. It was soon realized that alterations in central nervous system biogenic amine functioning (which reserpine caused) altered mood. Since that discovery, much of the research on mood disorders, especially depression, has focused on neurotransmitters and brain pathways.

As research proceeded, controversy about the endogenous and exogenous classification of depression grew with recognition of the clinical similarities between the two groups of depressed patients and laboratory studies.

Manic depression illness, which does not distinguish between the groups, led to the current categorization. It is now felt that presence and absence of a precipitant is less important diagnostically and therapeutically than the signs and symptoms of depression and their severity.

EPIDEMIOLOGY

Major depressive disorder is more prevalent than bipolar disorders.

Incidence and Prevalence

Studies in Great Britain, the United States, and the Scandinavian countries indicate that the risk of developing these severe disorders, ranges from 0.6 to 25.0% over the course of lifetime. Lifetime risk for bipolar disorder ranges from 0.6 to 2% in both men and women. Life-time risk for major depression ranges from 2 to 25%. Most authorities agree that an accurate figure is in the range of 10–15%. It is about 10% in men and 20% in women.

Major Depression and Dysthymia

Prevalence rates of Major Depression and Dysthymia in selected third generation epidemiological surveys have been consistently found 1.5–2.5 times higher in women than in men; for example, in the German study (Jacobi, et al. 2004) the prevalence of any depressive 12-month-diagnosis in women is 14% vs 7.5% in men. Prevalence rates for major depression and dysthymia in these surveys vary widely across countries and, in particular, very low rates of major depression have been reported in studies conducted in Eastern Asian nations. Sociodemographic differences (e.g. discrepancies in the distribution of marital status) or cross-cultural variations (e.g. different social acceptability of the expression of emotions) could explain the discrepancies between the results. Also variability of instruments and design used in these studies can account for differences. For example, the clinicians in the Sesto Fiorentino Study diagnosed 'depressive disorder NOS' significantly more frequently than is reported in studies based on a different methodology; this might explain lower rates of major depression (9.5% vs 13–17% lifetime prevalence in other recent studies).

Roughly 20–40% of unipolar depressive cases are assigned dysthymia as a diagnosis (3–6% lifetime prevalence over most studies). Studies are generally concordant in pointing out that major depression and dysthymia frequently coexist, a disorder sometimes referred to as 'double depression'. The lifetime prevalence of double depression has been reported to range between 1.5% and 2.5%. Data from most cross-sectional community surveys suggest that the prevalence of major depression is increasing in successive generations born after World War II. (Kessler et al. 2003). However, studies relying on single retrospective interviews may be biased by methodological factors such as recall bias increasing with age. Long-term longitudinal follow-up surveys are a much more reliable source of information about this topic; however, available evidence from such studies is limited and inconsistent and, therefore, this issue remains open to debate.

Bipolar Disorders

Prevalence rates of bipolar disorders in selected third generation epidemiological surveys reflect that rates in women and men are roughly the same (lifetime 1–2% in most studies). The differences between lifetime and current (12-month) rates are smaller than in unipolar depressions; this could indirectly indicate a higher chronicity. It has to be mentioned that in this overview bipolar I and bipolar II disorders are lumped together, but most by far of the epidemiological studies on bipolar illness have examined bipolar I disorder.

Risk Factors

Sex

The incidence of bipolar disorder is similar in men and women (1:1.22) while major depressive disorder is diagnosed about two times more often in women as in men. Some investigators have speculated that this difference reflects a bias on the part of clinicians in diagnosing depression more readily in women. In general, women tend to be more emotionally expressive than men and, therefore, they display sadness or unhappiness more easily than men. Recognition of depression in men is often difficult. Investigators have pointed to the higher incidence of substance abuse among men and have identified it as a 'depressive equivalent' or masked depression.

But apart from the social bias or different diagnostic practices, the real reasons for higher incidence of major depression among women may include such factors as child birth, hormonal disturbances, and varying stress.

Age

A large majority of bipolar patients have their first illness around the age of 30 years while major depressive episode occurs around the age of about 40 years. However, this difference could in part be explained by the fact that manics tend to come for treatment early in the course of their illness as compared to depressives and secondarily, even a single episode of mania is taken as bipolar disorder.

Race

The prevalence of mood disorder does not differ from race to race. However, there is a tendency among the clinician to underdiagnose mood disorder and overdiagnose schizophrenia in patients who belong to a different raciocultural background.

Marital Status

In general, unipolar depression occurs more often in widowers, divorced or separated individuals or in persons who have impaired interpersonal relationships. Similarly, bipolar disorder is more commonly seen in divorced and single individuals than amongst the married persons.[11-13]

Social and Cultural Factors

There is no correlation between social class and mood disorder, although some studies show that unipolar depression is more common in lower socioeconomic group and bipolar disorder in higher socioeconomic group. In general, mood disorder is equally common in urban and rural areas.

Religion

Bipolar disorder is more common in religious communities (e.g. the old order Amish), but there appears to be no correlation between religion and unipolar depression.

Family History

Patients with bipolar disorders have a significantly higher risk of having first degree relatives with mood disorders than do those with major depression.

Life Events

In unipolar depression, negative life events are often present before the onset but in bipolar disorder the relationship with life events is unknown.

Cyclothymia and Dysthymia

Data on the incidence and prevalence of these disorders is limited. The one year prevalence rates for dysthymia were found to be between 4.5% and 10.5% and for cyclothymia to be less than 1%.

As in major depressive disorder, dysthymia is reported to be more common in women than in men in a ratio of two or three to one. However, data are not available regarding ratio of men and women for cyclothymia. No differences in the occurrence of either dysthymia or cyclothymia have been identified, among the various socioeconomic groups. Dysthymic disorder is more common among unmarried and young persons and in persons with low incomes. Moreover, dysthymic disorder frequently coexists with other mental disorders, especially major depressive disorder, anxiety disorders, substance abuse and probably borderline personality disorder.

CLASSIFICATION

Numerous classification systems for the mood disorders have been proposed. Broadly these may be divided into two groups: those used in clinical practice and those used primarily in research.

Classifications Used in Clinical Practice

International Classification of Diseases, tenth version (ICD-10)[14] and Diagnostic and Statistical Manual of mental disorders, fourth version (DSM-IV)[3] are used in clinical practice. The ICD-10 consists of an official coding system [Clinical Descriptions and Diagnostic Guidelines (CDDG)] and other related clinical and research documents and instruments. It is the official classification system used in throughout the world.

ICD-10 Classification (CDDG)

In ICD-10, categories F30-F39 describe the mood (affective) disorders. The various categories include:

- Manic episode (hypomania, mania with psychotic symptoms, mania without psychotic symptoms).
- Bipolar affective disorder (current episode hypomanic, manic with psychotic symptoms, mania without psychotic symptoms, mild or moderate depression, with or without somatic symptoms, severe depression, with or without psychotic symptoms.
- Mild or moderate depressive episode (with or without somatic symptoms), severe depressive episode (with or without psychotic symptoms).
- Recurrent depressive disorder.
- Persistent mood disorders (cyclothymia, other persistent mood disorders).
- Other single mood disorders (mixed affective episode)
- Other recurrent mood disorders (recurrent brief depressive disorders).

DSM-IV Classification

In DSM-IV,[3] in the mood disorders, the current state of major depressive disorder or bipolar I disorder is coded in fifth digit as mild, moderate, severe without psychotic features, severe with psychotic features, in partial remission, in full remission, and unspecified.

The various categories include:

- Depressive disorders
  - Major depressive disorder (single episode or recurrent)
  - Dysthymic disorder
  - Depressive disorder NOS
- Bipolar disorders
  - Bipolar I disorder (Single manic episode, or the most recent episode hypomanic, manic, mixed, depressed, or unspecified)
  - Bipolar II disorder
  - Cyclothymic disorder
  - Bipolar disorder NOS
- Mood disorder due to a general medical condition
- Substance related mood disorder.

DSM-5[21] CLASSIFICATION: HIGHLIGHT OF CHANGES MADE FROM DSM-IV

Bipolar and Related Disorders

- *Bipolar disorders:* To enhance the accuracy of diagnosis and facilitate earlier detection in clinical settings, criterion A for manic and hypomanic episodes now includes an emphasis on changes in activity and energy as well as mood. The DSM-IV diagnosis of bipolar I disorder, mixed episode, requiring that the individual simultaneously meet full criteria for both mania and major depressive episode, has been removed. Instead, a new specifier, "with mixed features," has been added that can be applied to episodes of mania or hypomania when depressive features are present, and to episodes of depression in the context of major depressive disorder or bipolar disorder when features of mania/hypomania are present.

  Other specified bipolar and related disorder: DSM-5 allows the specification of particular conditions for other specified bipolar and related disorder, including categorization for individuals with a past history of a major depressive disorder who meet all criteria for hypomania except the duration criterion (i.e. at least 4 consecutive days). A second condition constituting another specified bipolar and related disorder is that too few symptoms of hypomania are present to meet criteria for the full bipolar II syndrome, although the duration is sufficient at 4 or more days.

  Anxious distress specifier: In the chapter on bipolar and related disorders and the chapter on depressive disorders, a specifier for anxious distress is delineated. This specifier is intended to identify patients with anxiety symptoms that are not part of the bipolar diagnostic criteria.
- *Depressive disorders:* DSM-5 contains several new depressive disorders, including disruptive mood

dysregulation disorder and premenstrual dysphoric disorder. To address concerns about potential overdiagnosis and overtreatment of bipolar disorder in children, a new diagnosis, disruptive mood dysregulation disorder, is included for children up to age 18 years who exhibit persistent irritability and frequent episodes of extreme behavioral dyscontrol. Based on strong scientific evidence, premenstrual dysphoric disorder has been moved from DSM-IV Appendix B, "Criteria Sets and Axes Provided for Further Study," to the main body of DSM-5. Finally, DSM-5 conceptualizes chronic forms of depression in a somewhat modified way. What was referred to as dysthymia in DSM-IV now falls under the category of persistent depressive disorder, which includes both chronic major depressive disorder and the previous dysthymic disorder. An inability to find scientifically meaningful differences between these two conditions led to their combination with specifiers included to identify different pathways to the diagnosis and to provide continuity with DSM-IV.

Major depressive disorder: Neither the core criterion symptoms applied to the diagnosis of major depressive episode nor the requisite duration of at least 2 weeks has changed from DSM-IV. Criterion A for a major depressive episode in DSM-5 is identical to that of DSM-IV, as is the requirement for clinically significant distress or impairment in social, occupational, or other important areas of life, although this is now listed as Criterion B rather than Criterion C. The coexistence within a major depressive episode of at least three manic symptoms (insufficient to satisfy criteria for a manic episode) is now acknowledged by the specifier "with mixed features." The presence of mixed features in an episode of major depressive disorder in creases the likelihood that the illness exists in a bipolar spectrum; however, if the individual concerned has never met criteria for a manic or hypomanic episode, the diagnosis of major depressive disorder is retained.

Bereavement exclusion: In DSM-IV, there was an exclusion criterion for a major depressive episode that was applied to depressive symptoms lasting less than 2 months following the death of a loved one (i.e. the bereavement exclusion). This exclusion is omitted in DSM-5 for several reasons. The first is to remove the implication that bereavement typically lasts only 2 months when both physicians and grief counselors recognize that the duration is more commonly 1–2 years. Second, bereavement is recognized as a severe psychosocial stressor that can precipitate a major depressive episode in a vulnerable individual, generally beginning soon after the loss. When major depressive disorder occurs in the context of bereavement, it adds an additional risk for suffering, feelings of worthlessness, suicidal ideation, poorer somatic health, worse interpersonal and work functioning, and an increased risk for persistent complex bereavement disorder, which is now described with explicit criteria in Conditions for Further Study in DSM-5 Section III. Third, bereavement-related major depression is most likely to occur in individuals with past personal and family histories of major depressive episodes. It is genetically influenced and is associated with similar personality characteristics, patterns of comorbidity, and risks of chronicity and/or recurrence as non-bereavement-related major depressive episodes. Finally, the depressive symptoms associated with bereavement-related depression respond to the same psychosocial and medication treatments as nonbereavement-related depression. In the criteria for major depressive disorder, a detailed footnote has replaced the more simplistic DSM-IV exclusion to aid clinicians in making the critical distinction between the symptoms characteristic of bereavement and those of a major depressive episode. Thus, although most people experiencing the loss of a loved one experience bereavement without developing a major depressive episode, evidence does not support the separation of loss of a loved one from other stressors in terms of its likelihood of precipitating a major depressive episode or the relative likelihood that the symptoms will remit spontaneously.

Specifiers for depressive disorders: Suicidality represents a critical concern in psychiatry. Thus, the clinician is given guidance on assessment of suicidal thinking, plans, and the presence of other risk factors in order to make a determination of the prominence of suicide prevention in treatment planning for a given individual. A new specifier to indicate the presence of mixed symptoms has been added across both the bipolar and the depressive disorders, allowing for the possibility of manic features in individuals with a diagnosis of unipolar depression. A substantial body of research conducted over the last two decades points to the importance of anxiety as relevant to prognosis and treatment decision making. The "with anxious distress" specifier gives the clinician an opportunity to rate the severity of anxious distress in all individuals with bipolar or depressive disorders.

CLASSIFICATION USED IN RESEARCH

The various classifications used in research include the following:

- *St. Louis or Feighner criteria:* These criteria developed by Feighner et al.[16] in 1972, are based on a distinction between 'primary' and 'secondary' depression as the central theme. This distinction is drawn on the basis of natural history and antecedents of the disorder in a patient. When depression occurs in a patient with history of any other pre-existing psychiatric illness, it is termed as 'secondary' depression; depression in the absence of such a history is 'primary'. Although this system has considerable value in research, it has not yet been validated.

- *CATEGO:* CATEGO is based on the 9th version of the present state examination (PSE) developed by Wing, et al.[17] in 1974. Although PSE is a reliable and popular instrument, CATEGO classification of depression has not found much enthusiasm for its use among researchers.

  CATEGO describes three classes of depression, namely:
  1. Class DT (or depressive psychosis).
  2. Class R (or retarded depression).
  3. Class N (or neurotic depression).

  It also describes four syndromes of depression, namely depressive delusions and hallucinations, simple depression, special symptoms of depression, and other symptoms of depression.
- *Research diagnostic criteria (RDC):* Developed by Spitzer, Endicott and Robins,[18] RDC lists the various diagnostic categories of depression under two broad headings, namely major depressive disorder and minor depressive disorder, on the basis of severity of symptomatology. Although the major depressive disorder has about 12 subtypes, they are not mutually exclusive. The minor depressive disorder has two subtypes.

  The RDC follows endogenous-reactive, psychotic-neurotic distinction in the classification of depression. It is a precursor to the DSM-III, DSM-III-R and DSM-IV systems, and the resemblance is obvious. It has been extensively used in research in the past.
- *Leonhard's system:* Leonhard[19] has divided the mood (and depressive) disorders into two types, namely unipolar and bipolar disorders. Patients with unipolar disorder have repeated episodes of depression without any manic episodes, whereas patients with bipolar disorder have episodes of both depression and mania.

  A number of studies have supported this distinction. Despite being a very useful research tool, several problems have become apparent, some of which are listed below:
  - A number of manic patients (up to 28%) have episodes of recurrent mania without any episodes of depression (called as *unipolar mania*). Attempts are being made to find out whether they form a separate subtype.
  - The definition and subtyping of unipolar depression is unclear. It is also not clear how many episodes of depression a patient should have, before being labelled as *unipolar depression.*
- *Winokur's familial system:* Winokur[20] has classified unipolar primary depression into the following categories:
  - *Familial pure depressive disease* (FPDD), where these is a family history of depression.
  - *Depressive spectrum disease,* where there is a family history of alcoholism or sociopathy but no family history of depression.
  - *Sporadic depressive disease,* where there is no history of depression, alcoholism or sociopathy.
- *Other systems:* Both DSM-IV and ICD-10 (DCR-Diagnostic Criteria for Research) are also used for research. The above-mentioned systems of classification are also used to classify mania. In addition, Emil Kraepelin's classification of mania into four subtypes is still of considerable clinical interest.[21] He divided mania into following subtypes:
  - *Hypomania*: This is a mild, sometimes long lasting condition, characterized by predominant euphoria, overactivity and disinhibition.
  - *Acute mania*: This is a severe condition, with grandiose delusions, labile mood and occasionally incoherent speech.
  - *Delusional mania*: This condition is characterized by less excitement, more persistent grandiose delusions, and occasional hallucinations.
  - *Delirious mania*: This is characterized by over-activity, labile mood (varying from excitement to depression), variable delusions, hallucinations, and disorientation of time and place.

Another useful classification of mania is into 'primary' subtype, which is a functional psychosis, and 'secondary' subtype, which arises from organic causes. For example, mania can be brought about by antidepressant drug treatment. Secondary mania has also been reported during treatment with amphetamines, corticosteroids, cyclosporines, L-dopa, and isoniazid (INH). It is a rare complication of thyrotoxicosis, and acute and chronic organic mental disorders. Depression can also be similarly classified.

7.2 ETIOLOGY

Ashok Singhal

The causal basis for mood disorders is not known. The causative factors can be divided into biological factors, genetic factors and psychosocial factors. However, these three realms interact among themselves, for example, psychosocial and genetic factors can affect biological factors; biological and psychosocial factors can affect gene expression; and biological and genetic factors can affect the response of a person to psychosocial factors.

BIOLOGICAL FACTORS

In 1921, Emil Kraepelin speculated that mood disorders were due to biological factors. He considered psychological factors to be coincidental. He hypothesized that some inner control mechanism was accelerated or decelerated in mania and depression respectively.

Since then the nature of biological contribution has been examined by use of the techniques of neurochemistry, psychopharmacology, neuroendocrinology and neurophysiology. The development made with regards to neurobiological understanding of mood disorders has been a logical sequence and not just accidental,[22] as depicted in Flow chart 1.

Biochemical Aspects

A number of biochemical aspects have been postulated which include:

- Catecholamine hypothesis,
- Serotonin hypothesis,
- Adrenergic cholinergic balance hypothesis,
- Serotonin norepinephrine dichotomy,
- Opioid hypothesis
- Receptor down-regulation hypothesis
- GABA hypothesis.

Catecholamine Hypothesis

Probably, this is the most widely known and acknowledged of all biological explanations of mood regulation and its disorders.[23]

Flow chart 1: Neurobiological basis of mood disorders: A logical development[22]

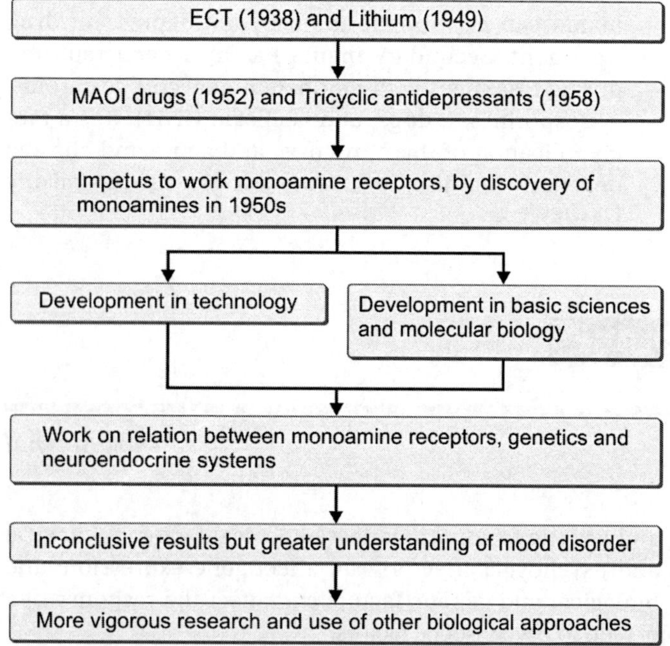

According to this hypothesis, the activity of catecholamines (norepinephrine and dopamine) is too high or low. Elevated levels are associated with mania and diminished levels with depression.

- *Norepinephrine (NE):* When the catecholamine hypothesis of mood disorder was originally proposed,[23] noradrenaline was considered to be the neurotransmitter most likely to be involved.
  - *Neurochemical studies:* Manic patients as a group tend to have higher urinary MHPG (3-methoxy-4-hydroxy-phenylglycol) levels than depressed patients and they consistently demonstrate higher urinary MHPG as compared to depressed patients.[24]

    Plasma MHPG is elevated in manic phases and falls slowly to normal after remission.[25,26]

    Platelet monoamine oxidase (MAO) is found within normal range and, during repeated episodes of mania, there is no change in levels; however, when elevated it is attributed to treatment with lithium.[27-29]

    Plasma levels of cAMP are raised in mania and low in depression. Plasma levels of cAMP in mania fall during treatment with neuroleptic drugs or lithium.[30-32] Beta receptor activity on lymphocytes, as measured by ligand binding or by the cAMP response to isoprenaline, is reduced in mania.[33,34]

    Cerebrospinal fluid (CSF) MHPG has been shown to be higher in mania as compared to depressive illness, but not higher as compared to normal controls.[24] Higher CSF norepinephrine (NE) levels are observed in manic patients than in the majority of neurological controls or depressed patients; however, anxious-depressed patients have similarly raised NE.[35] CSF dopamine β-hydroxylase (enzyme converting DA to NE) is lower in mania but cyclic AMP levels are normal in mania.[36,37]

    The role of NE in depression is evidenced by the correlation between down regulation of β-adrenergic receptors and the clinical antidepressant response. Reduction in the activity of presynaptic β-2 adrenergic receptors, leading to decreased NE is seen among depressive patients. The effect may in part be due to effect of these receptors on serotonergic neurons.
  - *Pharmacological studies*

    Drugs enhancing NE neurotransmission: The majority of antidepressant drugs block the receptor of NE from the synaptic cleft into the presynaptic neurone (some also block reuptake of 5HT, and at least one blocks the DA reuptake).[38]

    Mania is precipitated by monoamine reuptake inhibitors, the overall risk being estimated at 9%. Young depressives receiving clomipramine are more susceptible to switching into mania.[39]

    Psychostimulants (e.g. amphetamine), which can also precipitate mania, also increase catecholamine levels from presynaptic neurons into the synaptic cleft.

Drugs decreasing NE neurotransmission: Fusaric acid inhibits the enzyme DBH (dopamine β-hydroxylase), that converts dopamine to NE, leading to decrease in synthesis of NE and consequently in its level of neurotransmission.[40] Clonidine, an antihypertensive agent, reduces NE neurotransmission by a direct agonist action on the presynaptic receptors and causes amelioration of manic symptoms. On the other hand, its abrupt withdrawal is followed by onset of mania within a few days.[41,42]

Propranolol, a β-receptor blocker, possesses antimanic activity and relapse of symptoms occur when propranolol is stopped.[43] Desipramine, which is almost a purely noradrenergic drug, is clinically effective as antidepressant.

- *Dopamine:* Several studies have suggested that overactivity of dopamine (DA) pathways may play an important role in the pathogenesis of mania.[27,37,38]
  - *Neurochemical studies:* The activity of dopamine pathways has been studied by measuring the levels in the CSF of the major metabolite of DA, namely homovanillic acid (HVA). CSF HVA (as measured by mass spectrophotometry) is elevated in mania and that level falls to normal when the symptoms abate following treatment with lithium. Similarly, slow increase in CSF HVA was noted in a patient during the switch from depression to mania.
  - *Pharmacological studies*

    Drugs enhancing DA neurotransmission: L-DOPA, a precursor of dopamine, when administered to persons with a past history of manic episode, enhances dopamine synthesis within brain and precipitate mania. Amphetamine precipitates manic episode in persons with a history of bipolar illness by causing release of newly synthesized DA from presynaptic neurons (also causes simultaneous release of NE, but its effect is less significant). Dopamine receptor agonists, piribedil and bromocriptine, precipitate mania in patients suffering from bipolar depression.

    Drugs that increase dopamine concentrations, e.g. tyrosine, amphetamine, and bupropion reduce the symptoms of depression.

    Drugs reducing dopamine neurotransmission: Alpha-methyl-paratyrosine (AMPT) inhibits tyrosine hydroxylase, the rate limiting enzyme in the synthesis of DA. Manic patients, given AMPT, show clinically significant improvement. The various antipsychotic drugs (chlorpromazine, haloperidol and pimozide) have dopamine receptor blocking action, which has been shown to be more effective than lithium in acutely disturbed manic patients.[24,44]

    Drugs that reduce dopamine concentrations, e.g. reserpine, and diseases that reduce dopamine concent-rations (e.g. Parkinson's disease) are associated with depressive symptoms.
  - *Neuroanatomical studies:* Two recent theories regarding dopamine and depression are that the mesolimbic dopamine pathways may be dysfunctional in depression and that the D_1 receptor may be hypoactive in depression.[45]

Serotonin Hypothesis

It has been hypothesized that there may be an underlying deficiency in serotonin activity in both mania and depression.[24,46,47]

- *Neurochemical studies:* Most studies have found normal or reduced CSF levels of 5-HIAA, a primary metabolite of serotonin, in manic patients. But this finding is controversial. Elevated levels of DMT (dimethyltryptamine, a monoamine) were found in urine of 50% of manic patients.
- *Pharmacological studies:* Administration of L-tryptophan, which is a precursor of serotonin, is shown to be as effective as chlorpromazine, but the results are controversial.

  With the huge effect that the serotonin specific reuptake inhibitors (SSRIs), e.g. fluoxetine, have made in the treatment of depression, serotonin has become the biogenic amine neurotransmitter that is most commonly associated with depression. Besides the fact that SSRIs and other serotonergic antidepressants are effective in treatment of depression, other types of data indicate that serotonin is involved in pathophysiology of depression Biochemically, there are abnormalities in tryptophan metabolism in depression. Presumptive decrease in brain serotonin can precipitate depression in recovered patients, and platelet 5-HT receptors are increased in depression.

  Some depressed patients have abnormal neuro-endocrine responses, e.g. growth hormone, prolactin and ACTH, to challenges with serotonergic agents.

  It is perhaps consistent with the decrease in serotonin receptors after long-term exposure to antidepressants that a decrease in the number of serotonin reuptake sites (assessed by the binding of H_3-imipramine) and an increased concentration of serotonin have been found at postmortem in the brains of suicide victims.

Adrenergic Cholinergic Balance Hypothesis[48,49]

This hypothesis suggests that affect may represent a balance between cholinergic and catecholamine neurotransmitter activity in those areas of brain which represent mood, with depression being a disease of cholinergic predominance and mania being a disease of adrenergic predominance.[48]

Several anticatecholamine drugs (such as propranolol, α-methyl dopa and reserpine), which can cause depression, have central and peripheral cholinomimetic as well as anti-adrenergic properties. Such pharmacological evidence supports the adrenergic-cholinergic balance hypothesis. Another convincing evidence comes from the observation that physostigmine, a centrally active cholinesterase inhibitor, causes a dramatic but brief reduction in the manic and hypomanic symptoms of bipolar patients. Physostigmine is also found to cause a depressed mood, probably by shifting this balance to a cholinergic predominance. The induction of depressed mood has also been observed in subjects receiving acetylcholine precursors, such as deanol, lecithin and choline. Some studies have shown that REM latency, an acetylcholine sensitive sleep parameter, is decreased by administration of acetylcholine and increased by adrenergic agents; and is decreased in depression and increased in mania.

Serotonin-norepinephrine Dichotomy Hypothesis

The dichotomy hypothesis is based primarily on the psychopharmacological bridge strategy. The first subtype is associated with decreased brain norepinephrine and the second subtype with decreased brain 5-HT activity. According to this hypothesis, whether a given tricyclic antidepressant exerts its influence in a given patient is determined by whether the patient has a noradrenergic or serotonergic depression as measured by the presence of low or high levels of CSF MHPG. Amitriptyline is postulated to work primarily on the serotonergic depression while imipramine works on the noradrenergic depression. Although this hypothesis has much popular appeal, recent studies have not been particularly supportive of it, and most antidepressants have been found to have both central adrenergic as well as serotonergic effect.

Opioid Hypothesis

This hypothesis suggests that the central opioid mechanisms control the expression of mood. Also, depression represents a decrease and mania represents an increase in the brain natural opioid activity. Positive evidence is derived from the use of agonist strategy in which β-endorphins are given intravenously or into CSF. This can cause a mania-like syndrome, as well as a switch from depression to mania in bipolar patients. But, there is evidence against this hypothesis which includes the observation that the opioid agonist methadone does not activate mania or alleviate depression, and that CSF opioid levels are normal in depression.

Receptor Down-regulation Hypothesis

An important discovery in the support of this hypothesis was the presence of noradrenergic subsensitivity in animals following antidepressant drug administration which was linked to a decrease in the number of β-adrenergic receptor sites. This change in sensitivity to NE, associated with decrease in the number of β-adrenergic receptor, has been termed as *down-regulation* of receptors.

In recent years, in patients of mood disorder, cultured lymphoblasts and fibroblasts have been shown to have down-regulated β-receptors, in contrast to nonmood disordered relatives and unrelated control subjects. This alteration is probably due to inherent chromosomal factors in the affected patients.

GABA Hypothesis of Mania[50,51]

The GABA is an inhibitory neurotransmitter, deficiency of whose activity has been postulated to contribute to the etiology of psychotic states, especially mania. The anticonvulsant valproate inhibits the degradation of GABA and is reported to produce improvement in acute mania and to be effective in prophylaxis of bipolar disorder, a finding which is consistent with the above hypothesis.

Neuroendocrinal Aspects

Various neuroendocrinal changes are associated with mood disorders and are as follows:

- *Hypothalamic-pituitary-adrenal axis (HPA axis):* This axis has been extensively studied in mood disorders. Neurons in the paraventricular nucleus release corticotropin releasing hormone (CRH), which stimulates the release of adrenocorticotropic hormone (ACTH) from the pituitary. ACTH in turn, stimulates the release of cortisol from the adrenal cortex. The cortisol feedback on the loop works through at least two mechanisms, a *fast feedback mechanism*, sensitive to the rate of cortisol concentration increase, operates through the cortisol receptors on the hippocampus and results in a decreased release of ACTH; and a *slow feedback mechanism*, sensitive to the steady state cortisol concentration, is thought to operate through pituitary and adrenal receptors.

  Midnight levels of cortisol are high in patients of mood disorder as compared to normal controls. About 50% of the patients of mood disorder (especially depressives) manifest a decreased suppression of cortisol secretion after administration of dexamethasone.

  Dexamethasone suppression test (DST): Under normal conditions, the administration of dexamethasone, a potent synthetic steroid, suppresses the production and release of cortisol from the adrenal gland, by engaging the inhibitory feedback systems of the HPA axis. The presence of this excess synthetic steroid shuts off the hypothalamic production of CRF, thus causing a decrease in the secretion of ACTH from pituitary and then of cortisol output from the adrenal glands. Application of the DST in patients with major depression reveals a more subtle disturbance in depressed patients than that noted in patients with Cushing's disease who have complete nonsuppression of cortisol.

The standardized methodology for DST, suggested by Carrol et al.[52] is to administer 1 mg of dexamethasone orally at 11 PM in the night and to determine the plasma cortisol levels at 8 am, 4 pm and 11 PM. Plasma cortisol level above 5 μg/dL (known as nonsuppression) is considered abnormal (i.e. positive).

The DST can be used to follow the response of a depressed person to treatment. Normalization of DST, however, is not an indication to stop antidepressant treatment, because the DST may normalize before the depression resolves.

Some evidence indicates that patients with a positive DST result (especially > 10 μg/dL) will have a good response to somatic treatment, such as ECT or antidepressant therapy.[53] The sensitivity of DST is considered to be 45% in major depressive disorders and 70% in major depressive episode with psychotic features. The specificity is 90% as compared with controls and 77% as compared with other psychiatric diagnoses. False positive results on DST can be caused by Cushing's disease, pregnancy, estrogens (high doses), severe weight loss, drugs (e.g. phenytoin, barbiturates, carbamazepine, meprobamate, and methyldopa), diabetes mellitus (uncontrolled), high grade fever, dehydration, and acute alcohol withdrawal. False negative results on DST can occur in Addison's disease, hypopituitarism, steroid treatment, and high doses of benzodiazepines.

- *Hypothalamic-pituitary-thyroid axis (HPT axis):* The axis is a complex and highly integrated network. The hypothalamic peptide TRH causes the release of thyroid stimulating hormone (TSH) from pituitary, which in turn regulates the production of thyroid hormones, L-thyroxine (T_4) and L-triiodothyronine (T_3). The thyroid hormones exert a feedback control over the HPT axis. Studies show lesser release of TSH after TRH infusion in depressed patients (30–40%) as compared to normal controls. There are some studies that show improvement in depressed patients following administration of thyroid hormone.

  Thyrotropin releasing hormone test (TRH test): TRH, a hypothalamic tripeptide, is carried via the hypophyseal portal system to the anterior pituitary, where it stimulates the release of TSH. Release of TRH is influenced by input from limbic and other brain areas, as well as by circulating levels of thyroid hormones.

  The standard procedure for the TRH test is as follows. After an overnight fast, 500 mg of TRH is given in the morning by intravenous push over 30 seconds. Blood samples are taken, for measurements of TSH by RIA (radioimmunoassay), from the indwelling catheter at baseline (pre-TRH push), and at regular 15 minutes intervals up to 90 minutes after the administration of TRH. The maximal TSH increment from baseline is calculated, or delta (δ) TSH is calculated by subtracting the baseline TSH from peak TSH levels. A δ-TSH of less than 5–7 mg/mL is considered abnormal. The TRH test can be done on both inpatients and outpatients, is safe, and has only mild and short lived side effects (e.g. nausea, headache, urge to urinate). The factors that can influence the TSH response include thyroid hormone abnormalities, other endocrine disorder, hepatic or renal failure, advanced age, weight loss, alcohol intoxication or withdrawal, and treatment with steroids, estrogens, phenytoin, carbamazepine or lithium.
- *Hypothalamic-pituitary-growth hormone axis (HPGH axis):* As the HPGH axis is very complex, the findings in mood disorder patients have been, in general, confusing and contradictory. CSF levels of somatostatin (a growth hormone release inhibiting factor) have been reported to be decreased in depressed patients but are normal in manics. There is also an abnormal positive GH (growth hormone) response to TRH in depressed patients. Normally, TRH releases TSH and prolactin only, and not GH.
- *Hypothalamic-pituitary-prolactin axis (HPP axis):* The results of the studies of prolactin in depressed patients have been generally inconclusive. Normal base-line prolactin concentration is observed in depressed patients in daytime while the nocturnal secretion is altered. A decreased prolactin response to L-tryptophan in patients of endogenous depression raises the possibility of a defect in the serotonergic control of prolactin secretion. Circulation prolactin levels were usually within normal range in untreated manics, whereas the levels rise with a time course during treatment with pimozide.[54]
- *Melatonin:* Melatonin is a methylated indole secreted from the pineal gland. Its secretion is stimulated by nonadrenergic receptors. It is secreted at night under the influence of endogenous circadian rhythm. The nocturnal melatonin secretion is decreased in depression and increased in mania. Low melatonin syndrome of depression was postulated by Friis[55] and Venkoba Rao.[56] In a series of eight endogenous depressives, Venkoba Rao[56] reported a symptom profile associated with low urinary melatonin levels. More than a dozen studies report a low melatonin level, although some noted no change or even an elevated level.[57]
- *Insulin-tolerance test (ITT):* Up to 44% of the bipolar patients and 60% of the unipolar depressed patients have blunted ITT, even after recovery from the depressive episode.
- *Vasopressin:* It has been proposed that central vasopressin function is augmented in mania and is decreased in depression.[58]

Psychoimmunological Aspects

Some studies show that depression can interfere with immunological competence. Severely depressed patients have reduced *in vitro* lymphocyte response to mitogen stimulation. Other immunological changes in depressed patients include fewer natural killer T-cell lymphocytes, fewer T-suppressor cells (which regulate the antibody production), and fewer circulating lymphocytes, especially in unipolar depressed patients).

Neurophysiological Aspects

Sleep Abnormalities

Sleep electroencephalograms (EEGs) of many depressed persons show abnormalities.[59] The common abnormalities are delayed sleep onset, shortened rapid eye movement (REM) latency (the time between falling asleep and the first REM period), an increased length of first REM period, and abnormal delta sleep. Manic patients show a reduction in REM sleep.

Kindling

Kindling is the electrophysiological process in which repeated sub-threshold stimulation of a neuron eventually generates an action potential. At the organ level, repeated sub-threshold stimulation of an area of the brain results in seizure. The clinical observation that anticonvulsants (e.g. carbamazepine and valproic acid) are useful in treatment of mood disorders,[60] particularly in bipolar I disorder, has given rise to theory that pathophysiology of mood disorder may involve kindling in the temporal lobes.

Skin Conductance

Skin conductance, a measure of central arousal, was found to be raised in mania.

Brain Imaging Studies

Though less consistent, structural brain imaging studies with computed tomography (CT) and magnetic resonance imaging (MRI) have provided the following data. A significant set of bipolar I disorder patients (predominantly male) have enlarged cerebral ventricles. Ventricular enlargement is much less common in patients with depression; however depressed patients with psychotic features tend to have enlarged cerebral ventricles. MRI studies have revealed smaller caudate nucleus and smaller frontal lobes than do control subjects, and depressed patients also have abnormal hippocampal T_1 relaxation times, compared with control subjects.[61,62]

Functional brain imaging studies, like positron emission tomography (PET) and single photon emission computed tomography (SPECT) have shown decreased blood flow in the affected cerebral cortex in general and frontal cortex in particular. Magnetic resonance spectroscopy (MRS) studies have shown involvement of an abnormal regulation of membrane phospholipid metabolism in pathophysiology of mood disorder. Brain concentrations of lithium are about 40% of the plasma concentrations after about one week of treatment.

Neuroanatomical Considerations

Neuroanatomical hypotheses of mood disorder involve pathology of the limbic system, the basal ganglia, and the hypothalamus. Dysfunction of hypothalamus is suggested by the depressed patient's alteration in sleep, appetite, and sexual behavior, and by the biological changes in endocrine, immunological and chronobiological measures. The depressed patient's stooped posture, motor slowness, and minor cognitive impairment are similar to the signs seen in disorders of basal ganglia, such as Parkinson's disease and other subcortical dementias.

Chronobiological (Circadian Rhythms)

The abnormalities of sleep architecture in depression, and the transient clinical improvement in depression that is associated with sleep deprivation, have led to theories that depression reflects an abnormal regulation of circadian rhythms. Some experimental studies with animals indicate that many of the standard antidepressant treatments are effective in chaining the setting of internal biological clocks (i.e. endogenous *zeitgebers*).

Genetic Studies

The role of genetic factors in etiology of mood disorders has been studied by twin studies, adoption studies, and family studies. Twin and adoption studies provide evidence as to whether vulnerability to a disorder has a genetic component or not, while family studies suggest the degree to which the disorder is familial and speculates on the mode of genetic transmission. The evidence for heritability of bipolar mood disorder is stronger than for unipolar mood disorder. If one parent has bipolar mood disorder, there is 27% chance that a child will have mood disorder. If both parents have bipolar mood disorder, there is 50–70% chance that a child will have mood disorder.

Twin Studies

Several studies, both prospective and retrospective, have reported clear differences between the monozygotic (MZ) twins (about 65%) and the dizygotic (DZ) twins (about 15%). Twin studies have shown a concordance rate of 0.67 for bipolar disorder in MZ twins and 0.20 for bipolar disorder in DZ twins. The concordance for bipolar disorders is higher than that reported for unipolar disorders. The morbidity risk in relatives rises with concordance (full concordant twins, 14.5%; partially concordant twins, 8%; and discordant twins, 5.6%).

Adoption Studies

It has been shown that the difference between adoptive and biological relatives of mood disorder patients is not significant, but the difference between the biological relatives of mood disorder patients and those of normal controls is significant.

Family Studies

The relatives of both bipolar and unipolar disorder patients have higher prevalence rates than relatives of normal controls. Major depression is the most frequent mood disorder found in families of both unipolar and bipolar patients. Prevalence rates in first degree relatives of mood disorders are: 25% in bipolar disorder, 20% in unipolar disorder, 37% in schizo-affective disorder, and only 7% in normal controls. Thus, there is a greater morbidity risk for mood disorder in first degree relatives of bipolar as compared to unipolar patients.

Modes of transmission

- Single major locus transmission (either autosomal or X-linked) has not been accepted as the genetic hypothesis underlying mood disorders.
- The multifactorial hypothesis proposes a linear combination of genetic and environmental factors, each making a contribution. The liability threshold model uses forms of mood disorder as threshold determinants with bipolar I → bipolar II → unipolar disorder representing a descending ladder of vulnerability.

However, according to Turner and King,[63] there are at least two genetically distinct forms of bipolar disorders, one with a dominant single gene in which there is no father to son transmission and which might be X-linked, and the other depending on a single dominant gene with a locus on the P_Z region of chromosome number 6 distal to the HLA focus. Studies on the genetic markers, i.e. ABO locus, HLA loci, X chromosome, and autosomal gene, are in progress. No definitive relationship has been established, yet.

The application of molecular genetic techniques, particularly restriction fragment length polymorphism (RFLP) to the study of bipolar mood disorders has recently led to an important discovery. A dominant gene located on the short arm of the chromosome number 11 has been found to confer a strong predisposition to bipolar mood disorder. This gene may be involved in the regulation of tyrosine hydroxylase, a rate limiting enzyme in the synthesis of catecholamines. This data is consistent with the notion that bipolar mood disorders represent a heterogeneous group of disorders.

Genetic studies, beside helping in finding the etiology, provide important information which can be effectively utilized in genetic counseling and clinical work. Such information may include the following:

- *Risk to offsprings*
  Both parents ill: 50–75% risk
  One parent ill: 25–27% risk
- Unipolar patients with family history of bipolar disorder are more likely to show good response to lithium.
- Early detection in the offspring may be effected, and counseling and guidance can be given to patients and relatives.
- Marriage counseling can be provided.

Indian Studies

The discussion till now has centered around reports from western countries in relation to biological etiology of mood disorders. Only a few workers in India have attempted biochemical research, especially in mood disorders. Venkoba Rao et al.[64] Sethi et al.[65] and Varma et al.[66] have reported an increase in the adrenal cortical activity during study of HPA axis in depressed patients.

Boral et al.[67] reported lower levels of T_3 and T_4 in depressives and higher levels in manics, in a study of thyroid functions in bipolar patients. Verghese et al.[68] reported that plasma cortisol was increased in depressed patients but the normal diurnal variation and DST was not disturbed. Tiwari et al.[69] studied serum anticholinesterase activity in depressives and noted significant increase of enzyme activity.

PSYCHOSOCIAL THEORIES

Life Events and Environmental Stress

Many depressed patients attribute their depression to stressful life events. The relationship between life events and depression is difficult to study and some social psychiatrist still doubt whether life events can cause depression.[70] Any person who is depressed for any reason will tend to over-report the preceding life events in an attempt to give a meaningful explanation for the depression. However, long standing clinical observation has replicated that stressful life events more often precede the first episodes of mood disorders than the subsequent episodes. One theory proposes that stress that accompanies the first episode results in long lasting changes in the biology of the brain. The association has been reported for both major depressive disorder and bipolar patients. The life event most often associated with the later development of depression is the loss of a parent before the age of 11 years. The environmental stressor most often associated with the onset of an episode of depression is the loss of a spouse. Moreover, the degree of psychopathology in the family may affect the rate of recovery, the return of symptoms, and the patient's postrecovery adjustment.

Premorbid Personality Factors

No single personality trait or type has been established as being uniquely predisposing to depression. There are certain personality characteristics, such as lack of energy, breakdown under stress, introversion, insecurity, tendency to worry, dependency, and obsessionality, which are thought by some to be more frequent in the premorbid personality of depressed patients. No particular personality disorder is associated with the later development of bipolar disorder; however, dysthymic disorder and cyclothymic disorder are probably more often associated with the later development of bipolar disorder.

Psychoanalytic and Other Theories

Freud's essay, 'Mourning and Melancholia',[71] forms the basis of most psychoanalytic views of depression. Freud saw mourning as the reluctant but progressive detachment of libido from an object or person who was no longer able to receive it.

Karl Abraham[72] thought that the episodes of manifest illness are precipitated by the loss of a libidinal object, eventuating in regressive process in which the ego retreats from its mature functioning state to the one in which the infantile trauma of the oral sadistic stage of libidinal development dominates because of the fixation process in early childhood.

Melanie Klein[73] developed the concept of oral ambivalence and introjection that are to be found in mourning and melancholia, and further described the 'depressive position' to which a patient with depression is thought to regress. Klein regarded mania as a set of defensive operations designed to idealize others, deny any aggression or destructiveness toward others, and restore the lost love objects.

Adolf Meyer[74] believed depression to be the person's reaction to a disturbing life experiencing such as the loss of a loved one, a financial setback, or unemployment.

According to Karen Horney, the child raised by rejecting parents develops feeling of loneliness and insecurity. The child needs to be loved and fears criticism and rejection, and thus is susceptible to feelings of helplessness and depression.

According to Beck,[75] depression results from faulty cognition. He discussed a *cognitive triad,* consisting of:

1. Perceiving oneself as defective and inadequate.
2. Perceiving the world as demanding and punishing.
3. Expecting failure, defeat and hardship.

Bowlby saw the disorder of the mother-infant attachment bond as the paradigm of depression. Sullivan believed that adverse interaction between a person and his psychosocial environment is critical to the development of psychiatric disorders, including depression.

7.3 DIAGNOSTIC CRITERIA, CLINICAL FEATURES AND MANAGEMENT OF MOOD DISORDER, DYSTHYMIC AND CYCLOTHYMIC DISORDERS

JN Vyas, Dinesh Tyagi

DIAGNOSTIC CRITERIA

Major Depressive Disorder

DSM-IV requires the presence of at least five of the following symptoms (in addition to either depressed mood, or loss of interest or pleasure) to have been present during the same 2 week period and it should represent a change from the previous functioning.

These symptoms (which should be present nearly everyday) include depressed mood (present most of the day, nearly everyday, either subjectively or objectively), markedly diminished interest/pleasure in almost all activities (present most of the day, nearly everyday, either subjectively or objectively), significant weight loss or weight gain, or decrease or increase in appetite, insomnia or hypersomnia, psychomotor agitation or retardation, fatigue or loss of energy, feelings of worthlessness or excessive or inappropriate guilt, diminished ability to think or concentrate, or indecisiveness, recurrent thoughts of death, recurrent suicidal ideation or a suicide attempt. The symptoms cause clinically significant distress or impairment in social, occupational or other important areas of functioning.

The symptoms should not due to direct physiological effects of substance or a general medical condition. The symptoms should not be better accounted for by simple, uncomplicated bereavement.

Certain specifiers have been mentioned in the category of major depressive disorder in DSM-IV. These include the following:

- *Mild*: In this category, few (if any) symptoms in excess of those required to make the diagnosis are present. There is only minor impairment in occupational or social functioning.

- *Moderate*: Symptoms and/or functional impairment are between mild and severe.
- *Severe without psychotic features*: Several symptoms in excess of those required to make the diagnosis are present, and symptoms interfere markedly with occupational or social functioning.
- *With psychotic features*: The presence of psychotic features (delusions or hallucinations) in major depressive disorder reflects a more severe disease and is a poor prognostic indicator. If possible, it should be further specified whether the psychotic features are *mood-congruent* (delusions/hallucinations, whose content is entirely consistent with typical depressive themes, like inadequacy, guilt, disease, death, or nihilism) or *mood-incongruent* (delusions/hallucinations, whose content is not consistent with typical depressive themes, e.g. persecutory delusions, thought insertion, thought broadcasting, and delusions of control).
- *In partial remission.*
- *In full remission*: During the past 2 months, no significant signs or symptoms of the disturbance are present.

Clinicians and researchers had dichotomized the major depressive disorder along a psychotic continuum. A review of the literature, comparing psychotic with nonpsychotic major depressive disorder, indicates that the two conditions may be distinct in their pathogenesis. One difference is that bipolar I disorder is more common in the families of probands with psychotic depression than in the families of probands with nonpsychotic depression.

Although mood disordered patients with mood-congruent psychotic symptoms have a psychotic type of mood disorder, the patients with mood-incongruent psychotic symptoms have been variously typed as having schizoaffective disorder, or a subtype of schizophrenia, or some completely distinct diagnostic entity. Although the classification of these mood-incongruent patients remains controversial, the weight of the research data and the guidelines in DSM-IV indicate that one should classify such patients as having a psychotic mood disorder.

Psychotic features are generally a sign of a poor prognosis for patients with mood disorders. The following other factors have been associated with a poor prognosis: long duration of episodes, temporal dissociation between the mood disorder and psychotic symptoms, and a poor premorbid history of social adjustment. The patients with psychotic symptoms may also require antipsychotic drugs, ECT or lithium, in addition to antidepressants, to obtain clinical improvement.

DSM-IV differentiates the first episode of major depressive disorder from major depressive disorder (recurrent). The differentiation between patients, who have a single episode or who have two or more episodes of major depressive disorder, appears justified because of the uncertain course of the patients who have just one episode. Patients who are experiencing at least their second episode of depression are classified as having major depressive disorder, recurrent.

DSM-IV requires that distinct episodes of depression be separated by at least a two-month period during which the patient has no significant symptoms of depression. If this period is less than 2 months, the new symptoms are regarded as a part of the earlier episode rather than specifying a fresh episode.

It appears that the DSM-IV diagnostic criteria for major depressive disorder define a heterogeneous group of disorders. In several studies, one-fourth to one half of the patients of major depressive disorder were later re-classified as having a different psychiatric disorder. Depressed patients with more depressive symptoms are more likely to have stable diagnoses over time and are more likely to have mood disorder relatives than are depressed patients with bipolar I disorder and with bipolar II disorder. Recent diagnostic criteria for major depressive disorder is just launched in 2013 which is given below:

DSM-5 Diagnostic criteria for major depressive disorder

a. Five (or more) of the following symptoms have been present during the same 2-week period and represent a change from previous functioning; at least one of the symptoms is either (1) depressed mood or (2) loss of interest or pleasure.
   Note: Do not include symptoms that are clearly attributable to another medical condition.
   1. Depressed mood most of the day, nearly everyday, as indicated by either subjective report (e.g. feels sad, empty, hopeless) or observation made by others (e.g. appears tearful).
      (*Note*: In children and adolescents, can be irritable mood.)
   2. Markedly diminished interest or pleasure in all, or almost all, activities most of the day, nearly everyday (as indicated by either subjective account or observation).
   3. Significant weight loss when not dieting or weight gain (e.g. a change of more than 5% of body weight in a month), or decrease or increase in appetite nearly everyday.
      (*Note*: In children, consider failure to make expected weight gain.)
   4. Insomnia or hypersomnia nearly everyday.
   5. Psychomotor agitation or retardation nearly everyday (observable by others, not merely subjective feelings of restlessness or being slowed down).
   6. Fatigue or loss of energy nearly everyday.
   7. Feelings of worthlessness or excessive or inappropriate guilt (which may be delusional) nearly everyday (not merely self-reproach or guilt about being sick).
   8. Diminished ability to think or concentrate, or indecisiveness, nearly everyday (either by subjective account or as observed by others).
   9. Recurrent thoughts of death (not just fear of dying), recurrent suicidal ideation without a specific plan, or a suicide attempt or a specific plan for committing suicide.

Contd...

Contd...

b. The symptoms cause clinically significant distress or impairment in social, occupational, or other important areas of functioning.
c. The episode is not attributable to the physiological effects of a substance or to another medical condition.
Note: Criteria A~C represent a major depressive episode.
Note: Responses to a significant loss (e.g. bereavement, financial ruin, losses from a natural disaster, a serious medical illness or disability) may include the feelings of intense sadness, rumination about the loss, insomnia, poor appetite, and weight loss noted in Criterion A, which may resemble a depressive episode.
Although such symptoms may be understandable or considered appropriate to the loss, the presence of a major depressive episode in addition to the normal response to a significant loss should also be carefully considered. This decision inevitably requires the exercise of clinical judgment based on the individual's history and the cultural norms for the expression of distress in the context of loss.
d. The occurrence of the major depressive episode is not better explained by schizoaffective disorder, schizophrenia, schizophreniform disorder, delusional disorder, or other specified and unspecified schizophrenia spectrum and other psychotic disorders.
e. There has never been a manic episode or a hypomanic episode.
Note: This exclusion does not apply if all of the manic-like or hypomanic-like episodes are substance-induced or are attributable to the physiological effects of another medical condition.
- *Severity/course*
- Mild
- Moderate
- Severe
- With psychotic features
- In partial remission
- In full remission
- Unspecified

Specify:
- With anxious distress
- With mixed features
- With melancholic features
- With atypical features
- With mood-congruent psychotic features
- With mood-incongruent psychotic features
- With catatonia
- With peripartum onset
- With seasonal pattern (recurrent episode only)

Bipolar Disorder

For a diagnosis of bipolar I disorder, single manic episode, DSM-IV requires the presence of a distinct period of abnormally and persistently elevated, expansive, or irritable mood, lasting at least a week (or requiring hospitalization). For the second or subsequent episodes of mania, a diagnosis of bipolar I disorder, recurrent should be made, with the most recent episode being specified (e.g. most recent episode—manic hypomanic, mixed, depressed, or unspecified).

Just like for major depressive disorder, in DSM-IV, the episodes of mania are considered distinct if they are separated by at least two months without significant symptoms of mania or hypomania.

DSM-IV also describes the diagnostic criteria for bipolar II disorder, as characterized by the presence during the course of the disorder of depression episodes and hypomanic episodes (i.e. episodes of manic symptoms that do not quite meet the diagnostic criteria for a full manic syndrome).

DSM-IV specifically states that manic episodes that are clearly precipitated by antidepressant treatment (either drug treatment or electroconvulsive therapy) are not indicative of bipolar I disorder.

In DSM-III-R, mixed episodes of bipolar disorder were defined as either rapidly alternative depressive and manic states, or as the concurrent presence of depressive and manic symptoms. DSM-IV reclassifies the rapidly alternating condition as a course specifier (*with rapid cycling*). Mixed episode is diagnosed in those bipolar I disorder patients in whom the full criteria for a major depressive episode (except for duration) and the full criteria for a manic episode are met concurrently, everyday at least for a one week period.

Like for major depressive episode, the most recent episode can be further specified as with or without psychotic features (mood congruent or mood incongruent).

Cross-sectional Symptoms Features and Course Specifiers

DSM-IV defines three additional specifiers (symptoms features) that can be used to describe patients with various mood disorders. Two of the cross-sectional specifiers (melancholic features and atypical features) are limited to the description of major depressive episodes, while the third cross-sectional specifier (catatonic features) can be applied to the description of either depressive or manic episodes.

- *With melancholic features*: It requires the presence of loss of interest in almost all activities or lack of reactivity to usually pleasurable stimuli, with at least three of the following symptoms. These include qualitatively distinct depressed mood, early morning worsening of mood, early morning awakening, marked psychomotor retardation or agitation, marked anorexia or loss of weight, and excessive or inappropriate guilt.
- *With atypical features*: This requires the preservation of the reactivity of mood, along with at least two of the following symptoms. These include significant weight gain or increase in appetite, hypersomnia, 'leaden paralysis', and interpersonal rejection sensitivity (long-standing).

The classical atypical features, however, are overeating and oversleeping. However, the significance of atypical features remains controversial, as does their preferential treatment response to monoamine oxidase inhibitors. In addition to major depressive disorder, the atypical feature specifier can also be applied to dysthymic disorder in DSM-IV.

- *With catatonic features*: Catatonia is a syndrome or symptom complex that can be present in a number of psychiatric disorders. DSM-IV requires the presence of at least two of the following to be present for the specifier 'with catatonic features' to be applied. These include catalepsy (including waxy flexibility) or stupor, motoric excitement, marked negativism or mutism, echolalia or echopraxia, and presence of posturing, stereotypies, prominent mannerisms, or prominent grimacing.

The catatonic signs and symptoms can be seen in catatonic schizophrenia, major depressive disorder (often with psychotic features), mania (often with nongoal directed excitement), and medical and neurological disorders.

In addition, DSM-IV includes criteria for four distinct course specifiers for mood disorders:

- *With rapid cycling:* This is restricted to bipolar I disorder and bipolar II disorder. At least 4 episodes of a mood disturbance in the previous 12 months should have occurred that meet the criteria for a major depressive, manic, mixed, or hypomanic episode. Episodes should be demarcated by either partial or full remission for at least 2 months or a switch to an episode of opposite polarity (e.g. major depressive episode to manic episode).
- *With seasonal pattern:* This can be applied to the bipolar I disorder, bipolar II disorder and major depressive disorder, recurrent. There should be a regular temporal relationship between the onset of major depressive episodes and a particular time of the year (e.g. during winter), excluding the obvious effect of any seasonal-related stressors. Full remission (or a change in polarity from depression to mania/hypomania) should also occur at a characteristic time of the year. Two major depressive episodes should have occurred in the last 2 years that demonstrate the temporal seasonal relationship. Seasonal major depressive episodes should substantially outnumber any nonseasonal major depressive episodes.
- *With postpartum onset*: This can be applied to major depressive or manic episodes in bipolar I disorder, bipolar II disorder, major depressive disorder and brief psychotic disorder. The onset of episode should have occurred within 4 weeks postpartum.
- *Chronic specifier*: If the most recent depressive episode in bipolar I disorder, bipolar II disorder, or major depressive disorder lasts for at least 2 years, it is specified as chronic. DSM-5 Criteria for Bipolar and Related disorder.

DSM-5 Diagnostic criteria for bipolar I disorder

For a diagnosis of bipolar I disorder, it is necessary to meet the following criteria for a manic episode. The manic episode may have been preceded by and may be followed by hypomanic or major depressive episodes.

Contd...

Contd...

Manic Episode

a. A distinct period of abnormally and persistently elevated, expansive, or irritable mood and abnormally and persistently increased goal-directed activity or energy, lasting at least 1 week and present most of the day, nearly everyday (or any duration if hospitalization is necessary).
b. During the period of mood disturbance and increased energy or activity, three (or more) of the following symptoms (four if the mood is only irritable) are present to a significant degree and represent a noticeable change from usual behavior:
   1. Inflated self-esteem or grandiosity.
   2. Decreased need for sleep (e.g. feels rested after only 3 hours of sleep).
   3. More talkative than usual or pressure to keep talking.
   4. Flight of ideas or subjective experience that thoughts are racing.
   5. Distractibility (i.e. attention too easily drawn to unimportant or irrelevant external stimuli), as reported or observed.
   6. Increase in goal-directed activity (either socially, at work or school, or sexually) or psychomotor agitation (i.e. purposeless nongoal-directed activity).
   7. Excessive involvement in activities that have a high potential for painful consequences (e.g. engaging in unrestrained buying sprees, sexual indiscretions, or foolish business investments).
c. The mood disturbance is sufficiently severe to cause marked impairment in social or occupational functioning or to necessitate hospitalization to prevent harm to self or others, or there are psychotic features.
d. The episode is not attributable to the physiological effects of a substance (e.g. a drug of abuse, a medication, other treatment) or to another medical condition.

   Note: A full manic episode that emerges during antidepressant treatment (e.g. medication, electroconvulsive therapy) but persists at a fully syndromal level beyond the physiological effect of that treatment is sufficient evidence for a manic episode and, therefore, a bipolar I diagnosis.

   Note: Criteria A–D constitute a manic episode. At least one lifetime manic episode is required for the diagnosis of bipolar I disorder.

Hypomanic Episode

a. A distinct period of abnormally and persistently elevated, expansive, or irritable mood and abnormally and persistently increased activity or energy, lasting at least 4 consecutive days and present most of the day, nearly everyday.
b. During the period of mood disturbance and increased energy and activity, three (or more) of the following symptoms (four if the mood is only irritable) have persisted, represent a noticeable change from usual behavior, and have been present to a significant degree:
   1. Inflated self-esteem or grandiosity.
   2. Decreased need for sleep (e.g. feels rested after only 3 hours of sleep).
   3. More talkative than usual or pressure to keep talking.
   4. Flight of ideas or subjective experience that thoughts are racing.

Contd...

Contd...

5. Distractibility (i.e. attention too easily drawn to unimportant or irrelevant external stimuli), as reported or observed.
6. Increase in goal-directed activity (either socially, at work or school, or sexually) or psychomotor agitation.
7. Excessive involvement in activities that have a high potential for painful consequences (e.g. engaging in unrestrained buying sprees, sexual indiscretions, or foolish business investments).

c. The episode is associated with an unequivocal change in functioning that is uncharacteristic of the individual when not symptomatic.

d. The disturbance in mood and the change in functioning are observable by others.

e. The episode is not severe enough to cause marked impairment in social or occupational functioning or to necessitate hospitalization.
If there are psychotic features, the episode is, by definition, manic.

f. The episode is not attributable to the physiological effects of a substance (e.g. a drug of abuse, a medication, other treatment).
Note: A full hypomanic episode that emerges during antidepressant treatment (e.g. medication, electroconvulsive therapy) but persists at a fully syndromal level beyond the physiological effect of that treatment is sufficient evidence for a hypomanic episode diagnosis. However, caution is indicated so that one or two symptoms (particularly increased irritability, edginess, or agitation following antidepressant use) are not taken as sufficient for diagnosis of a hypomanic episode, nor necessarily indicative of a bipolar diathesis.
Note: Criteria A–F constitute a hypomanic episode. Hypomanic episodes are common in bipolar I disorder but are not required for the diagnosis of bipolar I disorder.

Major Depressive Episode

a. Five (or more) of the following symptoms have been present during the same 2-week period and represent a change from previous functioning; at least one of the symptoms is either (1) depressed mood or (2) loss of interest or pleasure.
Note: Do not include symptoms that are clearly attributable to another medical condition.
1. Depressed mood most of the day, nearly everyday, as indicated by either subjective report (e.g. feels sad, empty, or hopeless) or observation made by others (e.g. appears tearful). (*Note*: In children and adolescents, can be irritable mood.)
2. Markedly diminished interest or pleasure in all, or almost all, activities most of the day, nearly everyday (as indicated by either subjective account or observation),
3. Significant weight loss when not dieting or weight gain (e.g. a change of more than 5% of body weight in a month), or decrease or increase in appetite nearly everyday. (*Note:* In children, consider failure to make expected weight gain.)
4. Insomnia or hypersomnia nearly everyday.
5. Psychomotor agitation or retardation nearly everyday (observable by others; not merely subjective feelings of restlessness or being slowed down).
6. Fatigue or loss of energy nearly everyday.

Contd...

Contd...

7. Feelings of worthlessness or excessive or inappropriate guilt (which may be delusional) nearly everyday (not merely self-reproach or guilt about being sick).
8. Diminished ability to think or concentrate, or indecisiveness, nearly everyday (either by subjective account or as observed by others).
9. Recurrent thoughts of death (not just fear of dying), recurrent suicidal ideation without a specific plan, or a suicide attempt or a specific plan for committing suicide.

b. The symptoms cause clinically significant distress or impairment in social, occupational, or other important areas of functioning.

c. The episode is not attributable to the physiological effects of a substance or another medical condition.
Note: Criteria A–C constitute a major depressive episode. Major depressive episodes are common in bipolar I disorder but are not required for the diagnosis of bipolar I disorder. *Note:* Responses to a significant loss (e.g. bereavement, financial ruin, losses from a natural disaster, a serious medical illness or disability) may include the feelings of intense sadness, rumination about the loss, insomnia, poor appetite, and weight loss noted in Criterion A, which may resemble a depressive episode. Although such symptoms may be understandable or considered appropriate to the loss, the presence of a major depressive episode in addition to the normal response to a significant loss should also be carefully considered. This decision inevitably requires the exercise of clinical judgment based on the individual's history and the cultural norms for the expression of distress in the context of loss.

DSM-5 Diagnostic criteria for bipolar I disorder

a. Criteria have been met for at least one manic episode (Criteria A–D under "Manic Episode" above).
b. The occurrence of the manic and major depressive episode(s) is not better explained by schizoaffective disorder, schizophrenia, schizophreniform disorder, delusional disorder, or other specified or unspecified schizophrenia spectrum and other psychotic disorder.

DSM-5 Criteria for bipolar II disorder

296.89 (F31.81)

For a diagnosis of bipolar II disorder, it is necessary to meet the following criteria for a current or past hypomanic episode and the following criteria for a current or past major depressive episode:

Hypomanic Episode

a. A distinct period of abnormally and persistently elevated, expansive, or irritable mood and abnormally and persistently increased activity or energy, lasting at least 4 consecutive days and present most of the day, nearly everyday.
b. During the period of mood disturbance and increased energy and activity, three (or more) of the following symptoms have persisted (four if the mood is only irritable), represent a noticeable change from usual behavior, and have been present to a significant degree:
1. Inflated self-esteem or grandiosity.
2. Decreased need for sleep (e.g. feels rested after only 3 hours of sleep)..

Contd...

Contd...

3. More talkative than usual or pressure to keep talking.
4. Flight of ideas or subjective experience that thoughts are racing.
5. Distractibility (i.e. attention too easily drawn to unimportant or irrelevant external stimuli), as reported or observed.
6. Increase in goal-directed activity (either socially, at work or school, or sexually) or psychomotor agitation.
7. Excessive involvement in activities that have a high potential for painful consequences (e.g. engaging in unrestrained buying sprees, sexual indiscretions, or foolish business investments)

c. The episode is associated with an unequivocal change in functioning that is uncharacteristic of the individual when not symptomatic.
d. The disturbance in mood and the change in functioning are observable by others.
e. The episode is not severe enough to cause marked impairment in social or occupational functioning or to necessitate hospitalization.
   If there are psychotic features, the episode is, by definition, manic.
f. The episode is not attributable to the physiological effects of a substance (e.g. a drug of abuse, a medication or other treatment).
   Note: A full hypomanic episode that emerges during antidepressant treatment (e.g. medication, electroconvulsive therapy) but persists at a fully syndromal level beyond the physiological effect of that treatment is sufficient evidence for a hypomanic episode diagnosis.
   However, caution is indicated so that one or two symptoms (particularly increased irritability, edginess, or agitation following antidepressant use) are not taken as sufficient for diagnosis of a hypomanic episode, nor necessarily indicative of a bipolar diathesis.

Major Depressive Episode

a. Five (or more) of the following symptoms have been present during the same 2-week period and represent a change from previous functioning; at least one of the symptoms is either (1) depressed mood or (2) loss of interest or pleasure. *Note*: Do not include symptoms that are clearly attributable to a medical condition.
   1. Depressed mood most of the day, nearly everyday, as indicated by either subjective report (e.g. feels sad, empty, or hopeless) or observation made by others (e.g. appears tearful). (*Note*: In children and adolescents, can be irritable mood.)
   2. Markedly diminished interest or pleasure in all, or almost all, activities most of the day, nearly everyday (as indicated by either subjective account or observation).
   3. Significant weight loss when not dieting or weight gain (e.g. a change of more than 5% of body weight in a month), or decrease or increase in appetite nearly everyday.
      (*Note*: In children, consider failure to make expected weight gain.)
   4. Insomnia or hypersomnia nearly everyday.

Contd...

Contd...

   5. Psychomotor agitation or retardation nearly everyday (observable by others; not merely subjective feelings of restlessness or being slowed down).
   6. Fatigue or loss of energy nearly everyday.
   7. Feelings of worthlessness or excessive or inappropriate guilt (which may be delusional) nearly everyday (not merely self-reproach or guilt about being sick).
   8. Diminished ability to think or concentrate, or indecisiveness, nearly everyday (either by subjective account or as observed by others).
   9. Recurrent thoughts of death (not just fear of dying), recurrent suicidal ideation without a specific plan, a suicide attempt, or a specific plan for committing suicide.

b. The symptoms cause clinically significant distress or impairment in social, occupational, or other important areas of functioning.
c. The episode is not attributable to the physiological effects of a substance or another medical condition.
   Note: Criteria A–C above constitute a major depressive episode.
   Note: Responses to a significant loss (e.g. bereavement, financial ruin, losses from a natural disaster, a serious medical illness or disability) may include the feelings of intense sadness, rumination about the loss, insomnia, poor appetite, and weight loss noted in Criterion A, which may resemble a depressive episode. Although such symptoms may be understandable or considered appropriate to the loss, the presence of a major depressive episode in addition to the normal response to a significant loss should be carefully considered. This decision inevitably requires the exercise of clinical judgment based on the individual's history and the cultural norms for the expression of distress in the context of loss.

DSM-5 Bipolar II disorder

a. Criteria have been met for at least one hypomanic episode (Criteria A–F under "Hypomanic Episode" above) and at least one major depressive episode (Criteria A–C under "Major Depressive Episode" above).,
b. There has never been a manic episode.
c. The occurrence of the hypomanic episode(s) and major depressive episode(s) is not better explained by schizoaffective disorder, schizophrenia, schizophreniform disorder, delusional disorder, or other specified or unspecified schizophrenia spectrum and other psychotic disorder.
d. The symptoms of depression or the unpredictability caused by frequent alternation between periods of depression and hypomania causes clinically significant distress or impairment in social, occupational, or other important areas of functioning.

Specify current or most recent episode:

- Hypomanic
- Depressed

Specify if:

- With anxious distress
- With mixed features
- With rapid cycling
- With mood-congruent psychotic features

Contd...

Contd...

- With mood-incongruent psychotic features
- With catatonia.
- Coding note: Use additional code
- 293.89 (F06.1).
- With peripartum onset
- With seasonal pattern: Applies only to the pattern of major depressive episodes.
- Specify course if full criteria for a mood episode are not currently met:
- In partial remission
- In full remission

Specify severity if full criteria for a mood episode are currently met:

- Mild
- Moderate
- Severe

CLINICAL FEATURES

Major Depression

A change of affect is regarded as the central clinical feature of the mood disorders. In case of mania, the mood is elevated and is described as euphoric, whereas in depression, the mood is often depressed. The depressed mood, loss of interest, guilt and suicide are among the important symptoms of depression.

- *Depressed mood:* It is always present in a mild or severe form. In its mildest form, the patient experiences a flattening of affect, and as the depression increases, the patient is more miserable and unhappy. He becomes preoccupied with gloomy thoughts and tends to look on the dark side of things. Some patients can conceal this mood change from other people, at least for short periods. The patient may try to hide his low mood during the clinical interview, making it more difficult for the clinician to detect depression.
- *Loss of interest:* Loss of interest and an inability to enjoy (anhedonia) are frequent, though not always complained of spontaneously. The patient shows no enthusiasm for daily activities and hobbies, that he would normally enjoy otherwise. He feels no zest for living and no pleasure in everyday things.
- *Anxiety:* It is also frequent, though not invariable, in moderately severe depression. Patients feel tense, unable to relax, with difficulty in concentration and lack of attention. The anxiety is usually accompanied by somatic symptoms like dryness of mouth, palpitations, indigestion, sweating, headache and giddiness.
- *Insomnia:* Sleep disturbance in depressive disorder is of several kinds, the most characteristic of which is early morning awakening. However, delay in falling asleep and waking during the night also occur. Early morning awakening occurs 2–3 hours before the patient's usual time of waking up; he does not fall asleep again, but lies awake feeling unrefreshed and often restless and agitated. The patient thinks about the coming day with pessimism and broods about the past failures, pondering gloomily about the future. It is this combination of early morning awakening with 'depressive thinking' that is important in diagnosis. In some depressed patients, hypersomnia rather than early morning awakening may occur, but they still report that the sleep was not refreshing.
- *Suicide:* Suicidal thoughts are commonly present in depressive patients and they vary from mild to severe in intensity. Usually, the symptom develops slowly. The risk of suicide is greater in men, older women, and those living alone. The risk of suicide must always be considered once a diagnosis of depressive illness has been made, and particularly so if there has been an attempt in a previous or present episode.
- *Guilt:* The guilt feeling in depression varies from culture to culture, and it often does not appear in patients from African and Asian cultures, whereas in Europe and the USA, about three in four patients exhibit guilt to some degree. The underlying guilt is basically a feeling of inadequacy.
- *Somatic symptoms:* Some somatic symptoms are characteristic of depression and may even come to dominate the clinical picture. The patient feels a general loss of energy, quickly becomes tired and completely exhausted, has vague fleeting aches in the muscles and complains of headaches.

  The gastrointestinal symptoms are very common, like decrease in appetite, loss of interest in food, dryness of mouth, and constipation. The patient will lose weight, if he does not eat enough. Hypochondriasis is one of the less common symptoms, in which the patient is convinced of the possibility of presence of a disease, generally serious or even fatal. When this symptom is severe, it may attain delusional intensity.

  Loss of libido occurs early in the development of depressive illness. Men may complain of difficulty with erections, of an inability to ejaculate and finally of complete impotence. Among women, amenorrhea and loss of sexual interest is common.
- *Retardation:* Psychomotor retardation is frequent. The retarded patient walks and acts slowly. There is a slowness or difficulty in thinking, accompanied by a poverty of ideas, This leads to lack of concentration and indecisiveness. In severe forms, the patients' activity is diminished, the voice fades, and the speech becomes an indistinct mumble and finally ceases, leading to mutism.
- *Agitation:* It is a state of restlessness which is experienced by the patient as an inability to relax. The patient is restless and anxious, when it is mild, and seems to be plucking at his fingers and making restless movements of his legs. When agitation is severe, he cannot sit for any length of time, but paces up and down.
- *Diurnal variation of symptoms:* A diurnal variation of symptoms has long been recognized as a typical symptom

of depressive illness and is often present in endogenous depression as an early morning worsening of mood.

- *Panic attacks:* The symptoms of panic are varied and appear suddenly. The patient complains of palpitations, breathlessness, pain in the chest, feeling dizzy, fainting, trembling, choking and sweating, with a sense of impending doom.
- *Uncommon symptoms:* Vague and ill-defined paranoid ideas may be present; obsessional thoughts or even compulsive rituals can occur. Depersonalization and derealization have also been associated with depressive illness. Instead of losing appetite, some patients overeat. Psychotic symptoms have already been discussed.

Mania

- *Mood:* The central features of mania are elevated mood, increased activity, and self-important ideas. When the mood is elevated, the patient seems cheerful and optimistic. However, some patients are irritable rather than euphoric, and this irritability can easily turn to anger. The patients are cheerful, feel well, and enjoy life and all routine activities. The euphoric mood is volatile and can quickly change at the slightest frustration in to anger, resentment and hostility.
- *Thought:* In 'flight of ideas', the patient's thoughts and conversation move quickly from one topic to another, so that one train of thought is not completed before another appears. The characteristics of flight of ideas are preservation of the ordinary logical sequence of ideas, using two words with similar sound (clang associations), or a same word with a second meaning (punning), rhyming, and responding to distracting cues from the immediate environment.

  Expansive ideas are common. The patient believes that his ideas are original, his opinions important and his work of outstanding quality. Many patients become extravagant, spending more than they can afford, buying expensive things and taking reckless decisions.

  Grandiose delusions are quite often seen in manic patients. The patient may believe that he is a religious prophet or destined to advise statesmen about great issues. At times, delusions are persecutory, the patient believing that people are conspiring against him because of his special importance. Delusions of reference and passivity feelings also occur. Schneiderian first rank symptoms (SFRS) have been reported in 10–20% of manic patients. Neither the delusions nor the SFRS last long; most disappear or change in content with in days.
- *Speech:* The patients talk loudly, quickly and too much. The speech is full of jokes, rhymes and puns, and often it is grandiose in manner.
- *Activity:* Manic patients are overactive; sometimes, persistent overactivity leads to physical exhaustion. Manic patients start many activities but leave them unfinished as new ones catch their fancy.
- *Sleep:* Sleep is often reduced with a decrease in the need to sleep. The patient awakes early, feeling lively and energetic; often he gets up and busies himself noisily, to the surprise of other people.
- *Appetite:* Appetite is increased and food may be taken greedily with little attention to the conventional manner of eating.
- *Libido:* Sexual desires are increased and behavior may be disinhibited.
- *Appearance:* The patient's clothing often reflects his prevailing mood in its bright colors and ill-assorted choice of garments. When the condition is more severe, the patient's appearance is often untidy and dishevelled.
- *Insight:* Insight is invariably impaired. The patient may see no reason why his grandiose plans should be restrained or his extravagant expenditure curtailed. He seldom thinks of himself as ill or in need of treatment.

Bipolar and Unipolar Disorders

The major mood disorders are of two types: unipolar and bipolar. In the unipolar type, there are recurrent episodes of depression while in bipolar type, there are recurrent episodes of depression and mania. In a third variety, there are recurrent episodes of mania only, However, this type is regarded as a form of bipolar disorder.

At least two distinct types of bipolar disorder are recognized. The *type I bipolar disorder* is characterized by episodes of mania (severe enough to require hospitalization) and major depression; while *type II bipolar disorder* is characterized by episodes of hypomania (not requiring hospitalization) and major depression. Some workers recognize two more subtypes, one of which is a *type III bipolar disorder*, in which there are episodes of only major depression. Although mania or hypomania are not present, these patients either have a family history of bipolar mood disorder, or develop hypomania or mania on treatment with tricyclic antidepressants. The fourth type, called *bipolar (others)*, encompasses all other remaining forms of bipolar disorder.

The mean age of onset of bipolar disorder is 29 years for men and 34.5 years for women, while for unipolar disorder, it is 51 and 47.5 years, respectively. The episode of the illness, called a *phase*, lasts for an average of 6–12 months. The duration of the phases tends to increase with successive phases, especially for the unipolar disorder.

The duration of the cycle tends to decrease with each successive episode or phase. This decrease is about 20% in the unipolars and about 10% in the bipolars. A prolonged follow-up is needed to determine the number of phases experienced by a particular patient over a lifetime. The antidepressant treatment does not shorten the length of an episode but does lower the amplitude of symptomatology. Lithium lowers the risk of recurrence, reduces the duration of episodes as well as their amplitude, and lengthens the cycle.

MANAGEMENT

MAJOR DEPRESSIVE DISORDER

Each patient treated for major depression requires an individually tailored therapeutic program. Other mental disorders, including alcohol and substance abuse and dependence, and general medical comorbidities must be assessed and treated accordingly. The presence and degree of suicidal ideation/behaviors is an important factor in the choice and intensity of treatment.

A decision is made regarding whether the patient must be treated on an outdoor patient basis, hospitalized or kept in partial hospitalization. Hospitalization may be indicated for patients who lack the capacity to cooperate with treatment, for patients who lack the capacity to cooperate with treatment, are at risk for suicide or other violent behavior, lack psychosocial supports, require detoxification for withdrawal, have other psychiatric or general medical problems that make outpatient treatment unsafe, or are judged to need a hospital environment to safely receive the treatment that is required.

The aim of treatment is to effect and to maintain improvement. The treatment consists of an *acute phase*, during which remission is induced, a *continuation phase*, during which remission is preserved, and a *maintenance phase*, during which the susceptible patient is protected against the recurrence of subsequent depressive episodes.

The therapeutic armamentarium consists of a variety of psychotherapeutic approaches, pharmacotherapy, and electroconvulsive therapy. The various interventions may be used alone or in combinations.

Psychotherapeutic Approaches

The approach most congruent with the patient's condition must be chosen.

- *Supportive psychotherapy:* This consists of a number of complex activities such as:
  - Trusting doctor-patient relationship is established by gaining confidence of the patient and information is gathered in an empathic way.
  - Vigilance is maintained regarding destructive impulses directed towards self or others and an explanation of the symptoms is discussed.
  - Ongoing education, knowledge and feedback is provided regarding patient's illness, prognosis and treatment.
  - Patient is discouraged from instituting major life changes that are predictive of depressive state.
  - Patient's moral is improves by provoking and strengthening expectations of help and hopefulness, realistic, tangible and attainable goals are set, and patient is guided regarding daily schedules and appointments.
- *Psychodynamic psychotherapy and psychoanalysis*: Psychodynamically, depression is a product of relationship with a lost object, resulting in repressed self-directed rage, increased self-criticism and self-destructive impulses.

  Factors contributing to the success of a psychodynamic modality include motivation, capacity for insight, psychological mindedness, capacity to form relationship, mild to moderate illness, and a stable environment.

  Factors which are important include psychological vulnerability, dependency on external sources to maintain self-esteem, and early lack of love, conflicts related to guilt based on harsh conscience, and repressed ego ideals.

  These conflicts engender in the depressed individual self-punitiveness, self-rejection, depleted self-esteem and overt depressive manifestations. The therapy is mainly insight-oriented.
- *Brief therapy:* Brief psychodynamic psychotherapy may be used in the acute phase treatment of depression, especially as an adjunct to pharmacological treatment. The efficacy of brief therapy in the continuation or maintenance phase is not known.
- *Interpersonal therapy:* Interpersonal therapy seeks to recognize and explore depressive precipitants that involve interpersonal losses, role disputes and transitions, social isolation, or deficits in social skills.

  Interpersonal therapy alone is effective in reducing the depressive symptoms in the acute phase of nonmelancholic major depressive episode of less severity. It is especially effective in ameliorating vocational and social aspects of the patient's dysfunction.

  Interpersonal therapy during the maintenance phase can have a useful effect, especially for patients with recent psychosocial conflicts or with work or marital difficulties.
- *Behavior therapy:* Behavior therapy, based on social learning theory, involves activity scheduling, self-control therapy, social skills training, and problem solving.

  Behavior therapy has been reported to be effective in acute treatment of patients with mild to moderately severe depression, especially when combined with drug treatment. The utility of behavior therapy in continuation and maintenance phase treatment has not been subjected to control studies.
- *Marital therapy and family therapy:* Marital and family therapy may reduce depressive symptoms and the risk of relapse in patients with marital and family problems. Marital and family problems may be a consequence of depression but may also increase vulnerability to depression. The therapy includes psychoeducational and strategic marital therapy approaches.

- *Cognitive behavior therapy:* Beck's cognitive therapy was developed for treatment of depression, and was later extended to anxiety disorder and phobias. The cognitive approach to psychotherapy maintains that irrational beliefs and distorted attitudes toward the self, the environment, and the future perpetuate depressive affect and that these may be reversed through cognitive-behavior therapy.

  Such ideas persist even in the presence of contradictory evidence because the patients typically engage in self-defeating and self-fulfilling behaviors in which they selectively perceive the world as harmful while overlooking evidence to the contrary. Other distortions used include overgeneralization, magnification, and absolutistic ('all or none') thinking. In Beck's cognitive therapy, patients are not persuaded to change their beliefs by debate as in *rational emotive therapy* of Ellis; rather they encourage themselves through experiments that allow them to disconfirm their beliefs.

  Beck's cognitive therapy is standardized and brief (15–20 interviews), and is characterized by highly specific learning experiences. Each session consists of a review of reactions to and results of the previous session, planning, specific tasks, and assignment of homework.

  Initially, the patient is assigned reading material on coping with depression and written self-reports (a weekly activity schedule to chart the behaviors, a 'mastery and pleasure schedule' to rank degree of significance and accomplishment).

  Later, assertiveness training, role playing, and cognitive rehearsal (modeling and practice through dramatization or imagination) enable the patient to actively master specific scenarios, which serve as models for real-life achievement.

  The following specialized techniques are used in the problem areas or 'targets': scheduled activity, graded task assignment, masterly and pleasure ratings, cognitive reappraisal alternative explanations for negative experiences, cognitive rehearsal, and homework assignments.

  The effectiveness of Beck's cognitive therapy is under intensive study. At present, most of the studies indict that Beck's cognitive therapy is effective in relieving depression.

Pharmacotherapy

Most depressions are self-limiting cyclic disorders and the pharmacotherapy aims at decreasing the cycle duration, widening the intercycle period, and stabilizing the mood entirely. The success of pharmacotherapy in depression rests on the right diagnosis, right drug, right dosage and right duration of treatment. All the four factors together lead to a right outcome; 70–85% of depressives can lead a normal life.

Drugs currently used in the treatment of depression include:

- *Tricyclic antidepressants*: Imipramine, desipramine, clomipramine, amitriptyline, nortriptyline, doxepin, dothiepin
- *Second generation heterocyclic antidepressants*: trazodone, Maprotiline, mianserin, buproprion, amoxapine
- *MAO inhibitors (monoamine oxidase inhibitors)*: Phenelzine, isocarboxazid, tranylcypromine and moclobemide
- *Selective serotonin reuptake inhibitors*: Fluoxetine, fluvoxamine, paroxetine, sertraline
- Lithium
- *Anticonvulsants*: Carbamazepine, valproic acid divalproex sodium
- Stimulants.

The rate of response to antidepressants is reported to be as high as 60–70%. Patients may show some improvement by the first week, but may not fully respond before 4–6 weeks. As the rate of response is equal for all antidepressant drugs, the choice is based on the sideeffect profile of the drug, specific factors in the patient's psychiatric and medical history, family history of psychiatric disorders, and response to specific treatments.

Side effects are common with tricyclic antidepressants, and include the following:

- *Anticholinergic*: Dry mouth, constipation, epigastric distress, urinary retention, blurred vision, palpitation, sedation, dizziness, and a sense of over-medication, especially with amitriptyline.
- Fine tremors are relatively common. The seizure threshold is lowered and fits may be precipitated, especially in children. Amoxapine has a greater propensity for seizures, while desipramine is safer in this regard.
- Postural hypotension can occur, especially is older patients; is less severe with desipramine.
- Cardiac arrhythmias, especially in patients with ischemic heart disease, may be responsible for sudden death in some patients. AV block, and QT lengthening can also occur.
- Rashes and jaundice due to hypersensitivity are rare.
- *Weight gain*: tricyclic antidepressants, MAOIs, and lithium, all have the capacity to induce weight gain. Bupropion and fluoxetine may cause some degree of appetite and weight loss, which is usually transient.
- *Sexual dysfunctions*, like loss of erectile or ejaculatory function in man, and loss of libido and anorgasmia in both sexes, may be complications with virtually any antidepressant; these side effect appear to be most common with fluoxetine and probably sertraline, and to be least common with bupropion. Trazodone has been reported to induce priapism, which may result in impotence.

- *Insomnia and anxiety*: Fluoxetine, desipramine and bupropion any precipitate/exacerbate anxiety and sleep disturbances in some patients.
- Some patients may switch to hypomania or mania. Probably this reflects underlying bipolar illness, with the other pole being unmasked with antidepressant.

The antidepressants are usually begun in lower dosage, and then slowly raised as tolerated, until a presumably therapeutic dose is reached. The rate of increase and total daily dose vary from individual to individual. Older adults generally require lower doses than to younger adults. Antidepressant, especially tricyclics, are potentially lethal in overdose. Ingestion of a 10 day supply of a tricyclic agent, administered at a dose of 200 mg/day, is often lethal. Hence, early on in the treatment, it is prudent to dispense only small quantities of antidepressant medication.

Patients treated for a first episode of uncomplicated depression, who exhibit a satisfactory response to an antidepressant agent, should continue to receive a full therapeutic dose of that agent for at least 16–20 weeks after achieving full remission. The first 8 weeks after symptom resolution is a period of particularly high vulnerability to relapse. Specific forms of psychotherapy may be used to attenuate stresses and conflicts, which might re-exacerbate the depressive disorder.

Electroconvulsive Therapy

Electroconvulsive therapy (ECT) is a safe, economic, and efficacious therapy with no absolute contraindications, if used judiciously. Myocardial infarction, cardiac arrhythmias, and intracranial space occupying lesions are relative contraindications. The side effects of ECT are mostly cognitive. The treatment is associated with a transient postictal confusional stage and with a period of anterograde and retrograde amnesia, which typically resolves within weeks after cessation of treatment. Occasionally, however, it may take months to resolve.

To minimize the cognitive impairment, ECT may be applied unilaterally on the nondominant hemisphere. But if the initial six treatments are unsatisfactory in uplifting depression, bilateral electrode placement must be used.

ECT should be considered as an initial treatment for severe major depression, when it presents with psychotic features, catatonic stupor, severe suicidality, or for refusal to eat/drink. ECT is also used as initial treatment in conditions, where rapid antidepressant response is required, or in patients who have previously shown a preferential response to this treatment modality.

Maintenance Treatment

Fifty to eighty 5% of major depressive episode patients have another episode within two to three years. Factors predisposing to recurrence include the frequency and severity of past episodes, the efficiency and side effects of continuation treatment, persistence of dysthymic symptoms after recovery from a depressive episode, presence of additional nonaffective psychiatric diagnosis, presence of a chronic general medical condition, and prior history of multiple episodes of depression.

The therapeutic options for maintenance treatment include the various antidepressants and lithium. A reasonable strategy is to continue the antidepressant medication at the full dose used to exert the initial therapeutic effect, until this is well tolerated.

Tapering, rather than abrupt discontinuation, is generally recommended because of the risk of cholinergic rebound with some medications. Patients who are unresponsive to antidepressants and lithium maintenance, or do not tolerate it, may be maintained with periodic ECT. *Maintenance ECT* is usually administered monthly; though if insufficient, may be given at more frequent intervals.

Interpersonal psychotherapy during the maintenance phase may be effective in lengthening the interepisode interval in some less severely ill patients not receiving medication.

Medication Refractory Depression

Twenty to thirty percent of patients with major depressive disorder do not show satisfactory response to antidepressants. Adequate treatment for at least 6–8 weeks is necessary before concluding that a patient is not responsive to a particular medication.

The causes for inadequate response may be faulty diagnosis, inadequate treatment, or failure to diagnose and treat the coexisting general medical and/or psychiatric disorders, and other complicating psychosocial factors.

The treatment consists of the following options:

- Diagnosis to be reviewed, along with search for any contributing, or coexisting factor, e.g. psychosocial stressors, medical disorder, or substance use disorder
- *Addition of an adjunct to the antidepressant*: Lithium is the drug primarily used as an adjunct. It is reported to be useful in over 50% of the antidepressant non-responders and is usually well tolerated. Thyroid hormone supplementation, even in euthyroid patients, may also increase the effectiveness of antidepressant treatment, in a dose of 25 mg/day of triiodothyronine (T_3), increased to 50 mg/day in a week
- *Simultaneous use of multiple antidepressants*: Antidepressant co-administration usually consists of the use of multiple non-MAOI antidepressants. Fluoxetine or MAOIs may also be co-administered with the tricyclics. The combined use of MAOIs and other antidepressants may lead to serious untoward reactions, characterized by delirium, hyper-reflexia, hypertonia, and myoclonus

- *Electroconvulsive therapy*: Approximately 50% of medication resistant patients exhibit a satisfactory response to ECT. Lithium should be discontinued before initiation of ECT, as it has been shown to prolong postictal delirium and recovery from neuromuscular blockade
- *Anticonvulsants*: Carbamazepine and valproic acid have demonstrated some benefit in the treatment of medication-resistant depression. Lithium may also increase the antidepressant effectiveness of carbamazepine.

Clinical Features Influencing Treatment

Choice of Treatment

- *Anxious and agitated depressions*: Sedating antidepressants (amitriptyline, doxepin, clomipramine, trazodone). The benzodiazepine, alprazolam, is an alternative, with combined antidepressant-anxiolytic properties.
- *Withdrawn with motor retardation*: Stimulating antidepressants (imipramine, fluoxetine); low doses of flupenthixol (neuroleptic).
- *Elderly*: Anticholinergic and cardiovascular complications are to be avoided (doxepin, mianserin, trazodone, fluoxetine).
- *Presence of seizures*: Trazodone; ECT is not contraindicated
- *Depression with psychotic features*: Antidepressant with a neuroleptic. Amoxapine, an antidepressant with antipsychotic properties may be used alone. Lithium augmentation is helpful in some cases refractory to combined antidepressant neuroleptic treatment.
- *Severity*: Patients with mild depression may be treated with psychotherapy alone or with a combination of medication and psychotherapy. In moderate and severe depression, ECT plays a greater role as a primary treatment.
- *Prior episode of mania or hypomania*: Increases the likelihood of a switching to another manic or hypomanic episode during treatment or there may be precipitation of rapid cycling between depression and mania. Tricyclics should not be given and lithium should be instituted, preferably alone.
- *Depression with atypical features*: Tricyclics yield response rate of only 35–50% in patients with atypical depression; in contrast, MAOIs yield response rates of 55-75%. Fluoxetine, sertraline and bupropion may be used with considerable success.
- *Alcohol and/or substance abuse or dependence*: A patient with substance use disorder is more likely to require hospitalization, more likely to attempt suicide, and less likely to comply with treatment. It is advisable to detoxify such a patient before initiating antidepressant therapy. A positive family history of depression, history of depression preceding alcohol or other substance abuse, or a history of major depression during periods of sobriety raises the likelihood that the patients would benefit from antidepressant treatment.
- *Depression with obsessive-compulsive features*: (clomipramine, fluoxetine, sertraline).
- *Concurrent general medical condition*:
  - *Asthma*: MAOIs should be avoided.
  - *Cardiac disease*: Tricyclics should be avoided. bupropion, fluoxetine, sertraline, trazodone, mianserin and ECT appears to be safe. Patient must be monitored for emergence of cardiac symptoms, orthostatic blood pressure decrement, and EKG changes (as conduction defect, prolonged Q-T interval)
  - *Dementia*: Bupropion, fluoxetine, sertraline, trazodone, desipramine or nortriptyline. Patient is particularly susceptible to toxic effect of muscarinic blockade on attention and memory.
  - *Glaucoma*: May be treated with antidepressants, but their intraocular pressure is monitored during antidepressant treatment
  - *Obstructive uropathy*: Fluoxetine, sertraline, bupropion and desipramine).
  - *Parkinson's disease*: Bupropion.

Summary of NICE guidelines for treatment of depression

- Antidepressants are not recommended as first-line treatment in recent-onset, mild depression; active monitoring, individual guided self-help, CBT or exercise are preferred
- Antidepressants are recommended for the treatment of moderate to severe depression and for dysthymia
- When an antidepressant is prescribed, a generic SSRI is recommended
- All patients should be informed about the withdrawal (discontinuation) effects of antidepressants
- For severe depression, a combination of an antidepressant and CBT is recommended
- For treatment-resistant depression recommended strategies include augmentation with lithium, an antipsychotic or a second antidepressant
- Patients with two prior episodes and functional impairment should be treated for at least 2 years
- The use of ECT is supported in severe and treatment-resistant depression.

Medical and Healthcare Products Regulatory Agency/ Committee on Safety of Medicines Expert Working Group on SSRIs[2] summary

- Use the lowest possible dose
- Monitor closely in early stages for restlessness, agitation and suicidality. This is particularly important in young people (< 30 years)
- Doses should be tapered gradually on stopping
- Venlafaxine use was originally restricted but this guidance has now been reversed (venlafaxine is probably not cardiotoxic) but has a less favourable profile in overdose than SSRIs.[3,4]

Contd...

Contd...

References

1. National Institute for Health and Clinical Excellence. Depression: the treatment and management of depression in adults (update).CG90. 2009. http://www.nice.org.uk/
2. Committee on Safety of Medicines. Report of the CSM expert working group on the safety of selective serotonin reuptake inhibitor antidepressants. 2004. http://www.mhra.gov.uk
3. Taylor D et al. Volte-face on venlafaxine – reasons and reflections. J Psychopharmacol 2006;20:597–601.
4. Taylor D. Venlafaxine and cardiovascular toxicity. BMJ 2010; 340:327

BIPOLAR DISORDER

The specific goals of treatment are to decrease the frequency, severity, and psychosocial consequences of episodes, and to improve psychosocial functioning between episodes.

The available options include psychiatric management, pharmacological treatment and electroconvulsive therapy.

Psychiatric Management

The general goals of management are to asses and treat acute exacerbations, prevent recurrences, improve interepisode functioning, and provide assistance, insight, and support to patient and family.

The specific goals of psychiatric management include establishing and maintaining a therapeutic alliance, monitoring the patient's psychiatric status, providing education regarding their illness, prognosis and treatment, enhancing treatment compliance (causes for poor complacence include denial of illness, reluctance to give up the experience of mania), promoting regular patterns of activity and wakefulness, promoting understanding of an adaptation to the psychosocial effects of bipolar disorder, identifying new episodes early, and reducing the morbidity and sequelae of bipolar disorder.

Psychiatric management should be an on-going basis. Different interventions will be needed at different times, as the patient experiences episodes of the illness, and as the family develops and grows on the ability to respond adaptively to the demands of the illness.

Pharmacological Treatments

Medications are effective in the treatment of acute episodes, as well as in the prevention of future episodes. Medications which may be used in treatment of bipolar patients include mood stabilizers, antimanic agents and antidepressants, adjunctive medications, and new or atypical medications.

Three *mood stabilizers* currently available are lithium, valporate, and carbamazepine. Traditionally, lithium has been the primary pharmacological treatment for patients with bipolar disorder.

Lithium is effective in the acute treatment of manic and depressive episodes and in the prevention of recurrent manic and depressive episodes. In addition, lithium has been reported to decrease the mood instability and plagues many patients between episodes.

Lithium, valproate and carbamazepine are discussed in Chapter 7.8.

The combination of carbamazepine and lithium may be particularly effective for some patients, although it appears to increase their risk of developing an acute confusional state. During combined treatment, it is important to minimize the dose of other medications, such as neuroleptics, anticholinergics, benzodiazepines, otherwise an acute confusional state may develop.

Neuroleptics have a role in the treatment of acute mania, at least initially, in the highly agitated or psychotic patients alone or in conjunction with mood stabilizers, providing relief till the effects of mood stabilizers emerges. In fact, benzodiazepines are frequently as effective as neuroleptics for adjunctive treatment of mania, yet do not pose a risk of extrapyramidal symptoms or tardive dyskinesia.

Use of neuroleptics, either intermittently or long-term in conjunction with other mood stabilizing agents, may be necessary in those patients whose psychotic symptoms have inadequately responsed to the standard mood stabilizing agents.

Benzodiazepines are effective, in place of or in conjunction with a neuroleptic, in sedating the acutely agitated manic patients, while waiting for the effects of other primary mood stabilizing agents to become evident. Lorazepam is particularly useful due to its good absorption after intramuscular injection. Patients with anxiety and/or insomnia may benefit from the adjunctive use of a benzodiazepine.

Two cautions are necessary while using benzodiazepines: benzodiazepines have the potential to cause either dysphoria or disinhibition, and they can produce dependence, and in patients with comorbid substance use disorder can induce a relapse of another substance use disorder.

Antidepressants, like tricyclics, MAOIs, fluoxetine and bupropion have some efficiency in treatment of bipolar depressed patients. However, studies are few and inconclusive. Further, their use has been associated with the development of rapid cycling and mixed affective states. So, their use is recommended in acute and prophylactic treatment, if bipolar patients continue to develop depression despite optimal doses of mood stabilizers. Patients should receive the lowest effective for the shortest time necessary.

Novel and Adjunctive Pharmacological Treatment

Alternatively, calcium channel blockers, thyroid hormones, clozapine, psychostimulants, light therapy, and sleep manipulation may be used in the treatment of various phases of bipolar disorder. Thyroid hormones (T_3 and T_4) may have mood stabilizing effects in patients with rapid cycling bipolar disorder, regardless of thyroid status, usually when used adjunctively with other mood stabilizing agents. Thyroxine may be used in high doses initially (150–400 mg/day), with an increase in dose to an endpoint of 50% above normal in the free thyroxine index.

Atypical antipsychotic agent, clozapine, may have mood stabilizing as well as antipsychotic effects in bipolar patients with psychotic features, including those with rapid cycling and mixed episodes, with an additional advantage of not being associated with neurological side effects, like akathisia, parkinsonism or tardive dyskinesia, but it may have serious side effects, such as seizures and potentially fatal leukopenia.

Other drugs evaluated in treatment of acute mania include cholinergic drugs, serotonergic agents (fenfluramine, methysergide, and L-tryptophan), α-2 adrenergic agonist, clonidine. These have, however, not produced promising results.

Electroconvulsive Therapy

In acute mania, ECT is rapidly effective in up to 80% of patients. The recommended frequency is three treatments per week. ECT is typically not considered as a first-line treatment for manic episodes, as majority of patients exhibit acute response to mood stabilizing medication and majority of patients treated with ECT are likely to be resistant to conventional antimanic pharmacological agents.

ECT should be considered as a first-line of treatment in cases of manic delirium, in presence of pregnancy (when lithium and carbamazepine are relatively contraindicated), neuroleptic malignant syndrome, catatonia, and comorbid medical disorder with acute bipolar depression.

ECT is the most effective antidepressant treatment available and should be considered as a primary treatment in bipolar depression whenever a rapid response is necessary or when pharmacological interventions are contrai-ndicated (e.g. in pregnancy).

ECT, like antidepressants, may provoke hypomania or mania. Patients receiving lithium during ECT may be at higher risk for delirium and status epileptics. Benzodiazepines raise the seizure threshold and reduce the duration of seizures, and thus may impair the efficacy of ECT. Anticonvulsants may interfere with the production or duration of seizures.

Psychotherapeutic Treatment

The goals of psychotherapeutic treatment are to reduce distress and improve the patient's functioning between episodes to decrease the frequencies of future episodes.

Although psychotherapeutic treatments are discussed here as separate entities, they can also be use in clinical practice in combination.

Inpatient family interventions has brief sessions and integrates psychoeducational approach. The goals include accepting the reality of illness, identifying precipitating stressors, and likely future stressors inside and outside family, planning strategies, and bringing about the patient's family to accept the need for continued treatment after hospital discharge.

Behavioral family management includes psychoeducation, communication skills training, and problem solving skills training. Cognitive behavioral treatment aims at educating the patient regarding bipolar disorder and its treatment, and teach cognitive behavioral skills for coping with psychosocial stressors and attendant problems.

Specific psychotherapies for depressive episode may be used as discussed already. Specific psychotherapy for manic episode consists of reducing external stimulation, which may help calm the manic patient. Thus, a quiet room with few distractions may be desirable. A regular schedule of meetings with the patient may be helpful.

Substance use disorders and personality disorders often complicate the course of bipolar disorder. Group therapy may help certain patients to address such issues as adherence to a treatment plan, adaptation to a chronic illness, regulation of self-esteem and management of marital as well as other psychosocial issues.

Summary of recommended drug choice for the treatment of bipolar depression (Maudsley guideline)

1st Choice: Quetiapine (extensive evidence-based; antimanic; prophylactic effect)
2nd Choice: Lithium, Valproate*
3rd Choice: Lamotrigine (add to mood stabilizers)
4th Choice: Antidepressant + mood stabilizer or antipsychotic (olanzapine + fluoxetine best supported combination).

Summary of NICE Guidance for prophylaxis in bipolar disorder

- Lithium, olanzapine or valproate as first-line prophylactic agents (quetiapine and aripiprazole can now be added to this list, valproate is now second-line)
- Treatment for at least 2 years (longer in high-risk patients)
- Antidepressants (SSRIs are preferred) may be used in combination with a mood-stabilizer to treat acute episodes of depression but should not be routinely used for prophylaxis
- Chronic or recurrent depression may be treated with an SSRI or CBT in combination with a mood stabilizer or quetiapine or lamotrigine
- Combined lithium and valproate for the prophylaxis of rapid cycling illness.

Rapid-cycling bipolar affective disorder (Maudsley Guidance)

Step 1: Withdraw antidepressants
Step 2: Evaluate possible precipitants (e.g. alcohol, thyroid dysfunction, external stressors)
Step 3: Optimise mood-stabilizer treatment (using plasma level) Consider combining mood-stabilisers, e.g. lithium + valproate Lithium may be relatively less effective but this is not certain

Contd...

Contd...

Step 4: Consider other (usually adjunct) treatment options: (alphabetical order, preferred next treatments in bold)
Aripiprazole (15–30 mg/day)
Clozapine (usual doses)
Lamotrigine (up to 225 mg/day)
Levetiracetam (up to 2000 mg/day)
Nimodipine (180 mg/day)
Olanzapine (usual doses)
Quetiapine (300–600 mg/day)
Risperidone (up to 6 mg/day)
Thyroxine (150–400 μg/day)]
Topiramate (up to 300 mg/day)
Choice of drug is determined by patient factors—few comparative efficacy data to guide choice at this stage.
Quetiapine probably has best supporting data and may be considered treatment of choice. Conversely, supporting data for Levetiracetam, Nimodipine, Thyroxine and Topiramate are rather limited
* Note that valproate is teratogenic and should not be routinely used in women of childbearing age

DYSTHYMIC AND CYCLOTHYMIC DISORDERS

DYSTHYMIC DISORDER

Dysthymia is a concept introduced in DSM-III[76] to replace and subsume depressive neurosis, neurasthenia, and other mild chronic depressions. The diagnosis of *depressive neurosis* was the most common psychiatric diagnosis in the 1970s. The term depressive neurosis implies a maladaptive repetitive pattern of thinking and behavior that results in depression. Patients described as depressive neurosis are often anxious, obsessive and prone to somatization. However, dysthymia implies a temperamental dysphoria, i.e. an inborn tendency to experience a depressed mood. Dysthymia is defined as a chronic, less severe, depression usually with an insidious onset. The symptoms of dysthymia in DSM-III-R[77] overlap with those of major depressive disorder, including excessive guilt, difficulty in concentration and loss of interest; also included are symptoms that are not a part of major depression, such as feelings of pessimism, low self-esteem, low energy, irritability, and decreased productivity. This low grade depression must be present for two years for a diagnosis to be made. The ICD-10[78] criteria for dysthymia are very similar to those reported in DSM-IV,[79] including the length of illness. As compared with ICD-10 major depression, ICD-10 dysthymia requires a total of four symptoms as opposed to seven.

Epidemiology

The dysthymic disorder is a common disorder among the general population, affecting 3 to 4% of all patients.[80-82] The one year prevalence rate of dysthymia of 0.5%, is fairly constant throughout adulthood. Dysthymias are well represented across adulthood, with a substantial decrease after the age of 65 and relatively high prevalence among young adolescents. Dysthymic disorder is more common in women, unmarried persons and in lower income group.

The comorbid psychiatric diagnoses include major depressive disorder, anxiety disorders, substance abuse, and probably, borderline personality disorder.

Many believe that early onset dysthymia (age less than 21 years) is the only 'true' dysthymia.[83] Individuals with early onset dysthymia resemble patients with major depression and they have a higher life-time rate of double depression, anxiety disorder, treatment, sleeping behavior, familial depression and chronic depression. However, another study[84] did not find any differences in the type of onset, cognitive styles, coping styles or symptoms, between early and late onset dysthymia.

Etiology

Both biological and psychosocial factors have been implicated in the etiology of dysthymic disorder.

Biological Factors

The biological basis for the symptoms of dysthymic disorder is similar to that of major depressive disorder. However, basis for the underlying pathophysiology is probably different between the two.

Neuroendocrine studies: Adrenal and thyroid axes have been studied in cases of dysthymic disorder. The majority of patients with the disorder do not show abnormalities on dexamethasone suppression test (DST) as compared with the patients with major depression. More patients with dysthymic disorder show abnormalities on thyroid axis as compared to normal controls, and these abnormalities probably represent a trait variable that is associated with chronic illness.

Sleep studies: Sleep studies show similarities to findings observed in major depressive disorder and these include decreased REM latency and increased REM density in the first part of sleep.[85]

Psychological Factors

Psychodynamic theories posit that the disorder results from faulty personality and ego development, culminating in difficulty in adopting to adolescence and young adulthood.

According to Karl Abraham, conflicts of depression center on oral and anal-sadistic traits. Reaction formation is the major defence mechanism used. Low self-esteem, anhedonia and introversion are often associated with the depressive character.

According to Freud, depression can be caused by an interpersonal disappointment early in life that leads to threatened losses in adult life, that trigger depression.

According to cognitive theory, a disparity between real and fantasized situations leads to diminished self-esteem and sense of helplessness.

Diagnosis and Clinical Features

The diagnosis of dysthymic disorder may be made by the criteria as specified in DSM-IV.[79] These include depressed mood for most of the day, for more days that not, as indicated either by subjective account or observation by others, for at least 2 years (during which the person should never be without symptoms for more than 2 months at one time). However, in children, the mood can be irritable and duration must be at least one year.

The presence, while depressed, of two (or more) of the following is required. These include poor appetite or overeating, insomnia or hypersomnia, low energy or fatigue, low self-esteem, poor concentration or difficulty making decisions, and feelings of hopelessness. The symptoms cause clinically significant distress or impairment in social, occupational, or other important areas of functioning.

Of course, no major depressive episode should have been present during the first 2 year of the disturbance, and there should never be a manic, mixed, or hypomanic episode, and criteria should never have been met for cyclothymic disorder.[79] Exclusion criteria include presence of a chronic psychotic disorder (e.g. schizophrenia or delusional disorder). The symptoms should not due to a substance use disorder or a general medical condition.

The course is specified as *early onset* (if onset occurs before age of 21 years) and *late onset* (if onset occurs at the age of 21 years or later). If atypical features are present for the recent 2 years, it is specified *with atypical features*.

The clinical features of dysthymic disorder include its chronic course, milder forms of depressive symptoms, rather than episodic severe symptoms in major depressive disorder. The symptoms may have diurnal variation and the symptoms include feeling of sadness, 'blues,' feeling down in dumps or low, and a lack of interest in the daily activities. The patients may be nihilistic, brooding, demanding and complaining.

The other symptoms are generally changes in appetite and sleep pattern, low self-esteem, loss of energy, psychomotor retardation, decreased sexual drive, and obsessive preoccupation with health matters. Divorce, unemployment, and social problems are often reasons for seeking psychiatrist help.

The comorbid psychiatric diagnoses include major depressive disorder and substance-related disorder. A combination of major depression superimposed on dysthymia, has been termed as *double depression*.[86,87] In comparison with patients with major depression alone, fewer patients recover over time, and of those more relapse. The treatment of patients with double depression should be directed towards both disorders.

DSM-5 Diagnostic criteria for persistent depressive disorder (Dysthymia)

300.4 (F34.1)

This disorder represents a consolidation of DSM-IV-defined chronic major depressive disorder and dysthymic disorder.

a. Depressed mood for most of the day, for more days than not, as indicated by either subjective account or observation by others, for at least 2 years.
   Note: In children and adolescents, mood can be irritable and duration must be at least 1 year.
b. Presence, while depressed, of two (or more) of the following:
   1. Poor appetite or overeating.
   2. Insomnia or hypersomnia.
   3. Low energy or fatigue.
   4. Low self-esteem.
   5. Poor concentration or difficulty making decisions.
   6. Feelings of hopelessness.
c. During the 2-year period (1 year for children or adolescents) of the disturbance, the individual has never been without the symptoms in Criteria A and B for more than 2 months at a time.
d. Criteria for a major depressive disorder may be continuously present for 2 years.
e. There has never been a manic episode or a hypomanic episode, and criteria have never been met for cyclothymic disorder.
f. The disturbance is not better explained by a persistent schizoaffective disorder, schizophrenia, delusional disorder, or other specified or unspecified schizophrenia spectrum and other psychotic disorder.
g. The symptoms are not attributable to the physiological effects of a substance (e.g. a drug of abuse, a medication) or another medical condition (e.g. hypothyroidism).
h. The symptoms cause clinically significant distress or impairment in social, occupational, or other important areas of functioning.
   Note: Because the criteria for a major depressive episode include four symptoms that are absent from the symptom list for persistent depressive disorder (dysthymia), a very limited number of individuals will have depressive symptoms that have persisted longer than 2 years but will not meet criteria for persistent depressive disorder. If full criteria for a major depressive episode have been met at some point during the current episode of illness, they should be given a diagnosis of major depressive disorder. Otherwise, a diagnosis of other specified depressive disorder or unspecified depressive disorder is warranted.

Specify if:
- With anxious distress
- With mixed features
- With melancholic features
- With atypical features
- With mood-congruent psychotic features
- With mood-incongruent psychotic features
- With peripartum onset

Specify if:
- In partial remission
- In full remission

Contd...

Contd...

Specify if:
- **Early onset:** If onset is before age 21 years.
- **Late onset:** If onset is at age 21 years or older.

Specify if (for most recent 2 years of persistent depressive disorder):
- **With pure dysthymic syndrome:** Full criteria for a major depressive episode have not been met in at least the preceding 2 years.
- **With persistent major depressive episode:** Full criteria for a major depressive episode have been met throughout the preceding 2-year period.
- **With intermittent major depressive episodes, with current episode:** Full criteria for a major depressive episode are currently met, but there have been periods of at least 8 weeks in at least the preceding 2 years with symptoms below the threshold for a full major depressive episode.
- **With intermittent major depressive episodes, without current episode:** Full criteria for a major depressive episode are not currently met, but there has been one or more major depressive episodes in at least the preceding 2 years.

Specify current severity:
- Mild
- Moderate
- Severe

DIFFERENTIAL DIAGNOSIS

Minor depressive disorder and brief depressive disorder (recurrent) come in the differential diagnosis of dysthymic disorder.

Symptoms of *minor depressive disorder* are less severe than that of major depression, and unlike dysthymic disorder, they are characterized by discrete episodes. *Recurrent brief disorder* patients have symptoms suggestive of major depression but of brief duration (less than 2 weeks). Both minor depressive disorder and recurrent brief disorder patients have euthymic mood in between the episodes, while patients of dysthymic disorder have virtually no normal mood throughout the duration.

Course and Prognosis

Dysthymic patients generally run a chronic course and many of them progress to major depressive disorder, bipolar II disorder, and a few to bipolar I disorder.

About 10–15% of dysthymic disorder patients are in remission one year after the initial diagnosis. About 25% of all dysthymic disorder patients never attain a complete recovery.[88]

Treatment

The treatment modalities used to treat dysthymic disorder patients include pharmacotherapy and psychotherapy, mainly cognitive and behavioral.

Pharmacotherapy

A few studies, evaluating the efficacy of antidepressant drugs, show mixed results. The tricyclic antidepressants, like mianserin, dothiepin, and imipramine, are more effective than placebo during six weeks of treatment.[89-91] On the other hand, other tricyclics, like doxepin, amitriptyline, and desipramine, are not better than placebo.[92-94]

Monoamine oxidase inhibitor, phenelzine, was found to be more effective than isocarboxazid, which is not better than placebo. Phenelzine is also superior to imipramine in reducing the symptoms of dysthymia during a six weeks treatment period.[95-97]

The newer antidepressants, like serotonin specific reuptake inhibitors (SSRIs) and bupropion have been beneficial in treatment and may become a treatment of choice for dysthymic disorder patients.[98-99]

Psychotherapy

- *Cognitive therapy:* Cognitive therapy is based on the assumptions that negative cognitions apparent during depressive episodes are manifestations of basic beliefs that have been activated by stress.[100] Cognitive therapy is brief, structured treatment, designed to alter the dysfunctional beliefs and negative automatic thoughts typical of depression. A combination of behavioral (activity scheduling, graded task assignment) and cognitive techniques (identification, evaluation and modification of negative automatic thoughts) is used.
- *Behavior therapy:* Several different techniques comprise the behavioral treatment. *Social skills training* has been most widely used for depression. In this treatment, depression is seen as a consequence of insufficient reinforcement, which can result from deficit in social skills. Social skills training, therefore, attempts to correct the behavioral deficits associated with depression, including the inability of patients to obtain social reinforcement from others and the tendency to induce a negative affect in others.
- *Interpersonal psychotherapy (IPT):* Interpersonal psychotherapy has been developed for the treatment of longer duration and for different populations.[101,102] IPT is based on the assumption that the precipitating cause of depression usually occur in an interpersonal context. It generally focuses on the patient's immediate social context, and attempts to intervene in the symptoms formation and social functioning problems associated with depression, rather than enduring aspects of personality.

The combination of pharmacotherapy and either cognitive or behavior therapy may be the most effective treatment of the disorder.

CYCLOTHYMIC DISORDER

Cyclothymic disorder is symptomatically a mild form of bipolar disorder. It is characterized by episodes of hypomania and episodes of mild depression. The history of cyclothymic disorder is based to some extent on the observations of Emil Kraepelin and Kurt Schneider, that one-third to two-thirds of patients with mood disorders exhibit personality disorders. Irritable personality, as described by Kraepelin, has simultaneous presence of manic and depressive personalities.[103]

Epidemiology

The lifetime prevalence of cyclothymic disorder is estimated to be about 1% in general population. Majority of patients have onset in young adulthood, and it is more common in women than in men. Borderline personality disorder frequently coexists with cyclothymic disorder.[104]

Etiology

The biological and psychosocial factors strongly support the assumption that cyclothymic disorder is conceptualized as mood disorder.

Biological Factors

About one-third of all cyclothymic patients have positive family history for bipolar I disorder; conversely, the prevalence of cyclothymic disorder in the relatives of bipolar I disorder patients is much higher than is the prevalence of cyclothymic disorder in relatives of patients with other mental disorders and mentally healthy persons.

Psychosocial Factors

According to Freud, the cyclothymic state is the ego's attempt to overcome a harsh and punitive superego. Hypomania is frequently triggered by a profound interpersonal loss and denial is used as a major defensemechanism. Hypomania may also be associated with an unconscious fantasy that the lost object has been restored.

Diagnosis and Clinical Features

The diagnosis of cyclothymic disorder may be made according to DSM-IV[79] criteria. These include the presence of numerous periods with hypomanic symptoms and numerous periods with depressive symptoms insufficient to meet the criteria for a major depressive episode, lasting for at least 2 years (during which the person should never be without symptoms for more than 2 months at one time). In children and adolescents, the duration requirement is only 1 year.

No major depressive episode, manic episode or mixed episode should have been present during the first 2 years of disturbance. The exclusion criteria include the presence of schizoaffective disorder, schizophreniform disorder, delusional disorder or psychotic disorder, not otherwise specified.

The symptoms should not due to physiological effects of a substance or a general medical condition, and the symptoms should cause clinically significant distress or impairment in social, occupational or other important areas of functioning.

The clinical features are that of minor depressive episode, hypomanic episode, or mixed and irritable picture. The patients generally consult the psychiatrist during the depressive phase of illness. The patient often feels a lack of control on mood, and rapid and abrupt change in mood cause marked distress. The patients may present with marital difficulties and unprovoked disagreement with friends, family or co-workers.

Substance abuse, if any, is usually secondary to attempts of self-medication (alcohol, benzodiazepines and marijuana) or to achieve further stimulation (with cocaine, amphetamines, and hallucinogens).

DSM-5 Diagnostic criteria for cyclothymic disorder[105]

301.13 (F34.0)

a. For at least 2 years (at least 1 year in children and adolescents) there have been numerous periods with hypomanic symptoms that do not meet criteria for a hypomanic episode and numerous periods with depressive symptoms that do not meet criteria for a major depressive episode.
b. During the above 2-year period (1 year in children and adolescents), the hypomanic and depressive periods have been present for at least half the time and the individual has not been without the symptoms for more than 2 months at a time.
c. Criteria for a major depressive, manic, or hypomanic episode have never been met.
d. The symptoms in Criterion A are not better explained by schizoaffective disorder, schizophrenia, schizophreniform disorder, delusional disorder, or other specified or unspecified schizophrenia spectrum and other psychotic disorder.
e. The symptoms are not attributable to the physiological effects of a substance (e.g. a drug of abuse, a medication) or another medical condition (e.g. hyperthyroidism).
f. The symptoms cause clinically significant distress or impairment in social, occupational, or other important areas of functioning.

Specify if:
- With anxious distress

Differential Diagnosis

Differential diagnosis of cyclothymic disorder includes possible medical and substance-related causes of depression and mania, and personality disorders (border-line, antisocial, histrionic or narcissistic). Attention deficit hyperactivity disorder may be difficult to differentiate in cases of children and young adolescents.

Course and Prognosis

Patients with adaptive coping strategy have better outcomes. About 33% of cyclothymic patients go on to have a major mood disorder, most often bipolar II disorder.

Treatment

Biological Treatment

Mood stabilizers are the treatment of choice for patients with cyclothymic disorder. Lithium, carbamazepine and valproate, all may be used in dosage similar to those used in bipolar I disorder. Approximately half of the patients, when treated with antidepressants during depressive phase, switch to mania. Hence, antidepressants must be used with caution in patients with cyclothymic disorder.

Psychosocial Treatment

The psychotherapy for these patients is intended towards increasing the patients' awareness of their diagnosis and helping them develop coping mechanisms for their mood swings. Because of the long-term nature of cyclothymic disorder, patients often require life-long treatment. Family and group therapies may be supportive, educational and therapeutic for the patients and their families.

7.4 GENETICS OF BIPOLAR DISORDER

JN Vyas

BIPOLAR DISORDER GENETICS: ORIENTATION

Bipolar disorder (also known as manic-depressive illness) is an episodic recurrent pathological mood disturbance that ranges from extreme elation or mania to severe depression, and is usually accompanied by disturbances in thinking and behavior, and often by psychotic features (delusions and hallucinations). Diagnostic tests do not yet exist and the bipolar disorder phenotype is defined solely according to clinical features. Several clinical subtypes are recognised, including: bipolar disorder type I (full manic episodes); bipolar disorder type II (no full manic episodes and only milder hypomanic episodes); and bipolar type schizoaffective disorder (a form of recurrent mood and psychotic illness in which manic episodes occur together with schizophrenia-like psychotic symptoms). Furthermore, many people who experience depression and only mild or short-lived hypomanic episodes that do not quite meet the threshold criteria for a diagnosis of bipolar disorder type I or II are diagnosed as having unipolar depression.

The pathogenesis of bipolar disorder is not well understood. Compelling evidence for a substantial genetic contribution to risk, together with the availability of research devices that enable detection of susceptibility genes for common familial disorders, has provided psychiatry with an unprecedented opportunity to identify the biological systems that are involved in illness.

CLASSICAL GENETIC EPIDEMIOLOGY

Inherited factors are known to be important in bipolar disorder. In patients with established disease, a family history of mood or psychotic illness is common. Furthermore, a family history of bipolar disorder is an important clinical predictor of a likely bipolar course in a patient who presents with one or more episodes of depression even before their first personal episode of mood elevation. Consistent with these clinical observations, classical genetic epidemiological research with family, twin, and, to a lesser extent, adoption studies, has produced overwhelming evidence that genes affect predisposition to bipolar disorder. The risk of mood disorder diminishes as the genetic relatedness to a bipolar disorder proband decreases.[106] Owing to variations in study designs, populations analysed, and diagnostic definitions used, much caution is needed in the interpretation of risk data. Indicative figures for the lifetime risks of narrowly defined bipolar disorder in relatives of a bipolar proband are: unrelated member of the general population 0.5–1.5%; first degree relative 5–10% (corresponding to λS [relative risk in a sibling of a proband compared with risk in the general population] of roughly 8); and monozygotic co-twin 40–70% (corresponding to λMZ of about 60).[106] Estimates of heritability from twin studies are high—e.g. 89% in a recent hospital register study of 67 twin pairs in the UK[107] and 93% in a population register study of 19124 same-sex twin pairs in Finland.[108] The high heritability estimates and high monozygotic concordance rate are convincing indicators of the importance of genetic factors affecting bipolar disorder susceptibility. However, the fact that monozygotic concordance (40–70%) is substantially less than 100% shows that genes alone are not the whole story.

In addition to being at increased risk of typical bipolar disorder, relatives of bipolar probands are at increased risk of a range of related psychiatric phenotypes, including recurrent unipolar depression and schizoaffective illness.[109] However, despite some studies showing an overlap in familial risk between bipolar disorder and schizophrenia[110] the totality of the family study data has, for a long-time, been interpreted[109] incorrectly[111] as showing an absence of important shared genetic risk between bipolar disorder and schizophrenia. The error probably resulted from a combination of inadequate sample sizes and methodological biases. However, in the largest family study done so far,[112] investigators showed, with a Swedish population register, that although the cross-disorder risk is lower than the same-disorder risk, partial overlap exists in familial genetic susceptibility for bipolar disorder and schizophrenia. This study provides strong evidence that some susceptibility genes confer a general susceptibility to both bipolar disorder and schizophrenia, whereas others are specific to one disorder or the other. Similar methodology has also shown partial overlap in familial genetic susceptibility for bipolar disorder and autism.[113] Clinically, it is important to remember that the first degree relative of a bipolar proband is actually more likely to meet diagnostic criteria for recurrent unipolar depression than for any other diagnosis, including bipolar disorder. However, the relative risk (i.e. the risk in that family compared with the general population) for recurrent unipolar depression is substantially lower than for bipolar disorder because of the greater lifetime risk of recurrent unipolar depression than of bipolar disorder in the general population.[114]

The overlapping risks across psychiatric phenotypes represent partly shared genetic susceptibility and motivate cross-disorder analyses that use molecular genetic research to inform understanding of the nosological relation between diagnostic entities.[115]

WHAT MECHANISMS OF INHERITANCE DO WE EXPECT?

Experienced clinicians know that the familial transmission of bipolar disorder does not follow any of the simple mendelian patterns of inheritance (i.e. the pattern for one major gene). Mathematical modeling analyses show that bipolar disorder cannot be accounted for by one, or a collection of, rare highly penetrant susceptibility genes, and provides other constraints (e.g. number of loci and manner of interactions) on the types of genetic model that are possible.[116] Population genetics theory predicts that susceptibility alleles will have a range of effect sizes (from small to large) and frequencies (from rare to common).[117] Furthermore, in addition to variation at individual nucleotide bases in DNA sequences, several other known mechanisms can contribute to inherited risk for illness, including structural genomic variation (e.g. copy number variants)[118] dynamic mutation (e.g. expanding trinucleotide repeats), mitochondrial DNA variation, or epigenetic variation.[106] All these mechanisms have been suggested and considered as contributors to bipolar disorder. The evidence obtained so far supports common DNA base changes and rare copy number variants as contributors to bipolar disorder risk. The role of rare DNA base changes has not yet been tested comprehensively.

The association between genotype and phenotype for psychiatric disorders is clearly complex. Reductionist thinking has no place[119] and to think of any case as being either genetic or environmental, or to talk about a gene for bipolar disorder, makes no sense.[120] The key point is that most cases of bipolar disorder involve the interplay of several genes or more complex genetic mechanisms, together with the effects of nongenetic (environmental) risk factors and stochastic factors.[121,122]

LINKAGE FINDINGS IN BIPOLAR DISORDER

During the 1990s in particular, many systematic genome screens were done in samples ranging from large, densely affected pedigrees in genetic isolates to large numbers of affected sibling pairs. No consistent or compelling positive findings were recorded.[123] The largest and most recent linkage analysis[124] was an international collaboration study of 972 pedigrees multiply affected by bipolar disorder, again without strong positive findings. These results allow us to conclude that no locus of large effect is involved in the genetic etiology of bipolar disorder for most people. However, in some rare individuals or families, a single gene of large effect might be the major determinant of risk of bipolar disorder in that family.

ASSOCIATION STUDY FINDINGS

Hundreds of candidate gene association studies of bipolar disorder have been done in the past two decades. Most of these genes were defined as candidates on the basis of biological theories from pharmacological observations or secondary to abnormalities recorded in postmortem human brain tissue from patients. Although the results of these studies are inconsistent, with no compelling support for any candidate,[125] details about many of these, including those of biologically plausible candidates such as *BDNF* and *COMT*, are available in published reviews.[123] The many genes studied probably represent poor candidate choices because of our inadequate understanding of the underlying biology. Other contributing factors vary, and include poor gene coverage by the polymorphisms studied and small sample sizes that were powered insufficiently to detect modest effects. Overall, the candidate gene approach has not delivered robust positive findings. However, the absence of a genetic association signal does not rule out the gene's protein product from a role in disease pathogenesis (Panel 1).

Panel 1: A genetic association—what does it mean?

- The robust and replicable genetic association findings reported in this review are important steps on a long path to an understanding of the mechanisms of pathogenesis. Importantly, effect sizes are small (typical odds ratios of 1·1–1·2 correspond to a 10–20% increase of risk for a carrier of a risk allele compared with an individual without such an allele) and, for the risk alleles identified to date, no clear biological mechanism of affecting risk has been found. In many cases, the allele is probably a correlated proxy for the true risk allele (through a process known as linkage disequilibrium, in which chunks of DNA tend to be inherited as a piece over many generations). In most cases, the mechanism is thought to be the effect of gene expression rather than protein sequence. Confirmation of involvement of a particular gene in pathogenesis needs convergence with nongenetic methods of study.
- Although robust genetic association shows involvement of the protein product in disease pathogenesis, the reverse is not true. A protein might show no genetic variation associated with disease risk and yet be central to pathogenesis. This situation could arise, for example, if a gene was of such biological importance that it was under strong evolutionary pressure for conservation but could be affected by an environmental precipitant of illness.

Development of the technology to simultaneously genotype hundreds of thousands of single nucleotide polymorphisms in thousands of people and the positional information about the sites of almost all common single nucleotide polymorphisms in many populations has allowed for progressively more informative and powerful genome-wide association studies. These studies have the advantage of being unbiased, by contrast with previous biologically driven theories. A major limitation is that they are not well powered to detect rare variation (even that of large effect). The theoretical underpinnings of genome-wide association studies and the specific implications for psychiatric disease are discussed in recent reviews.[126–129]

Genome-wide association studies have enabled substantial progress in the discovery of robust and replicable genetic findings about the etiology of several major psychiatric disorders, including bipolar disorder. Importantly, these results meet community standards in human genetics for significance and replication (Panel 2).[130] The bipolar disorder genome-wide association studies story is similar to that for most other complex genetic disorders.[127] The initial studies did not find convincing signals,[131,132] even though the best combined signal that implicated a calcium channel subunit now seems to be the most widely supported in subsequent more powerful studies. Table 1 lists published bipolar disorder genome-wide association studies, in which all samples are of European origin. Genome-wide significant loci were identified in the largest studies and in the replication and stage 2 samples. The first small study that used pooled genotyping reported a genome-wide significant association with *DGKH* that has not since been replicated in subsequent larger studies.[133] Subsequently, Ferreira and colleagues[134] identified the region of *ANK3* (encoding ankyrin 3) and *CACNA1C* (encoding the alpha subunit of the L-type calcium channel). A third study reported an association with *NCAN* (encoding neurocan),[135] whereas investigators of other studies did not report genome-wide significant loci.[136,137,141] The Psychiatric Genome-Wide Association Study Consortium Bipolar Disorder Working Group (PGC-BD) reported results from the largest study done

Table 1: Genome-wide association studies of bipolar disorder in European-origin samples

	Primary or stage 1		*GWS stage 1?*	*Replication or stage 2**		*GWS stage 2?*
	Cases	*Controls*		*Cases*	*Controls*	
Wellcome trust case control Consortium (2007)[131]	1868	2938	No	–	–	NA
Baum, et al. (2008)[133 †]	461	563	No	772	876	Yes
Sklar, et al. (2008)[132]	1461	2008	No	–	–	NA
Ferreira, et al. (2008)[134]	1098	1267	No	4387	6209	Yes
Cichon, et al. (2011)[135]	682	1300	No	8441	35362	Yes
Scott, et al. (2009)[136]	2076	1676	No	3683	14507	No
Smith, et al. (2009)[137‡]	1003	1033	No	–	–	NA
PGC-BD (2011)[138]	7481	9250	Yes	11974	51792	Yes
Hamshere, et al. (2012)[119]	–	–	NA	2504	2878	Yes
Green, et al. (2012)[140]	1218	2913	No	8699	12163	Yes

* Replication and stage 2 samples often tested only a subset of the most associated single nucleotide polymorphisms in the larger sample.
† Pooled genotyping only.
‡ Study included genome-wide association study in 345 African–American patients.
Abbreviations: GWS, genome-wide significant; NA, not applicable.

so far.[138] Genotype data were assembled from 11 samples and a combined analysis of 16, 731 samples and 46, 912 replication samples identified two genome-wide significant loci: *CACNA1C* and a new locus, *ODZ4* (encoding a human homologue of the *Drosophila* pair-rule gene *ten-m* [*odz4*]). Of note, strong evidence of association (but not genome-wide significant) was reported by Scott and colleauges[136] in the region of *NEK4-ITIH1-ITIH3* on chromosome 3; this region was shown to be genome-wide significant in follow-up studies of schizophrenia and had a replication p value less than 0·05 for bipolar disorder in an independent sample.[139]

Panel 2: Significance levels in genome-wide association studies

A stringent and well-accepted criterion for genome-wide significance takes into account the total number of independent single nucleotide polymorphisms tested (about 1 million), and thus the p value should be equal to or less than 5 × 10–8.25 Since most common variant loci have modest effect sizes (<1·5 fold), then the power to detect loci with stringent thresholds that adjust for the total genome-wide testing burden is low. Thus, although many groups began by using their own samples, they rapidly proceeded to replication of the best loci through collaboration with other groups. This idea can easily be appreciated from Table 1, which shows that most of the primary or stage 1 samples did not detect associated loci, but that after either replication or stage 2 or large meta-analysis, several loci were convincingly associated.

As has been the case for other genetically complex disorders,[127,128] strong evidence suggests that an increase in the bipolar disorder sample sizes will enable the identification of additional loci. In the replication portion of the PGC-BD study,[138] 34 of the most associated single nucleotide polymorphisms were tested in an additional 4496 cases and 42, 422 controls:[136] of these single nucleotide polymorphisms had a signal in the same direction of effect as the original (p = 3·8 × 10 – 7). However, not all loci were replicated independently, especially two significant loci in the stage 1 samples, *ANK3* and *SYNE1*. Although the initial strong findings could have been false positives, the lack of replication might well represent the so-called winner's curse whereby the true effect sizes are smaller than estimated and larger samples are needed for replication.[142] For susceptibility variants of modest effect, it can be expected that as true findings approach genome-wide significance through accumulation of new datasets, wobble occurs about the genome-wide significant threshold. For a true finding, the overall trend should be towards increasing statistical significance, as has subsequently been seen for *SYNE1*, which exceeds genome-wide significance in the largest available meta-analysis.[139] Similarly, recent meta-analyses of a new sample with the PGC-BD sample show genome-wide significant association at two additional loci (Table 2).[140] In Table 2, we use a significance threshold of p < 5 × 10 – 8. Most associations with this level of significance are secure, but some might ultimately prove not to be. The genes closest to each locus are listed in the table, but aetiological variants are generally unknown, and some of the associations probably do not change the function of the designated genes (e.g. *ITIH3-ITIH4* and *PBRM1* are within the same region of chromosome 3p21.1, where several correlated single nucleotide polymorphisms span many genes).

The genome-wide association study analyses described above focus on separate testing of each polymorphism for significant association. An alternative approach is to undertake an analysis that aggregates all potential risk variants and makes en masse comparisons between cases and

Table 2: Genome-wide significant association in European-origin samples for bipolar disorder

	Single nucleotide polymorphism	*Study*	*p value*	*Odds ratio*	*Nearest gene(s)*
BD	rs12576775	PGC-BD[138]	4.4×10^{-8}	1.14	ODZ4
BD	rs4765913	PGC-BD, et al.[138]	1.5×10^{-8}	1.14	CACNA1C
BD	rs1064395	Cichon, et al.[135]	2.1×10^{-9}	1.17	NCAN
BD	rs7296288	Green, et al.[140]	9.0×10^{-9}	0.90	RHEBL1, DHH
BD	rs3818253	Green, et al.[140]	3.9×10^{-8}	1.16	TRPC4AP
BD	rs9371601	Green, et al.[143]	2.9×10^{-8}	1.10	SYNE1
BD + SZ	rs1344706	O'Donovan, et al.[144]	4.1×10^{-13}	1.11	ZNF804A
BD + SZ	rs2239547	PGC SZ[145]	7.8×10^{-9}	1.12	ITIH3-ITIH4
BD + SZ	rs10994359	PGC SZ[145]	2.4×10^{-8}	1.22	ANK3
BD + SZ	rs4765905	PGC SZ[145]	7.0×10^{-9}	1.11	CACNA1C
BD + SZ	rs4583255	Steinberg, et al.[146]	6.6×10^{-11}	1.08	MAPK3
BD + RUD	rs2251219	McMahon, et al.[147]	3.63×10^{-9}	0.87	PBRM1

Here significance threshold p < 5 × 10 – 8 has used. Odds ratio refers to the risk of bipolar disorder conferred by each risk allele at the locus.
Abbreviations: BD, bipolar disorder; PGC-BD, Psychiatric Genome-Wide Association Study Consortium Bipolar Disorder Working Group; PGC SZ, Schizophrenia Psychiatric Genome-Wide Association Study Consortium; SZ, schizophrenia; RUD, recurrent unipolar depression.

controls. Risk variants that have effects sizes that cannot be detected individually can be aggregated and thus identified. With such an approach, the PGC-BD group provided direct evidence for a polygenic component in bipolar disorder ($p < 10 - 8$).[138] This method has previously shown a polygenic component in schizophrenia risk.[149] These polygenic analyses are consistent with the presence of many (hundreds or thousands) common susceptibility variants of weak effect. Early estimates suggest that common variation tagged by single nucleotide polymorphisms can explain roughly 20 to 30% of the heritability estimated from family and twin studies.[149,150]

Another approach to analysis of genome-wide association study data is to focus on whether genetic association signals tend to cluster in particular biologically meaningful patterns (e.g. those representing specific biochemical pathways, functions, or subcellular localisations). The main advantage is to test the overall effect of a pathway by considering all the genes involved. This approach should have more power than the testing of one single nucleotide polymorphism at a time, and addresses the biological question of greatest relevance for disease pathogenesis. Such pathway analysis in the PGC-BD sample showed substantial enrichment in the gene ontology category of voltage gated calcium channel activity (gene ontology: 0015270). Three calcium channel subunits were included in this category: *CACNA1C*, *CACNA1D*, and *CACNB3*. The first two genes encode the major L-type alpha subunits found in the brain, which is of great interest, in view of the published literature regarding the role of ion channels in bipolar disorder; the mood-stabilizing effects of ion channel modulating drugs (e.g. verapamil and diltiazem); and the specific treatment literature suggesting direct efficacy of L-type calcium channel blockers in bipolar disorder.[151]

Pathway analysis strongly suggests that several biological pathways are involved in bipolar disorder pathogenesis[152] and larger samples will provide increasing power to delineate those that are most relevant for genetic susceptibility. For other disorders, insight into pathways often needed 20 to 30 individual loci to be in hand—an essential mass not yet reached for bipolar disorder. Insights can also be gained through consideration of the known biology of genes affected by individual robust association.

Chromosomal abnormalities are known to increase the risk for major psychiatric illness.[153] Case and family reports have been published of chromosome abnormalities in association with bipolar spectrum illness,[154] including the velocardiofacial syndrome deletion on chromosome 22q11[155] and the Prader-Willi syndrome maternal uniparental disomy on chromosome 15q11-q13.[156] The copy number variants (mentioned earlier) are a common cause of genetic variation in humans[118] and can confer risk of neuropsychiatric phenotypes, including autism and schizophrenia.[128,157] The estimated effect sizes for these rare variants are substantially larger than for the single nucleotide polymorphism associations discussed earlier. The role of copy number variants in bipolar disorder has been less well-studied and remains somewhat controversial: some studies report increased rates whereas others do not.[157,158] Only one specific copy number variant (3q29) is reported to have an effect size larger than 5 for bipolar disorder, although in a study of 185 proband—parent trios, investigators found a rate of *denovo* copy number variants that was 4·8-fold higher than that in controls and was similar to that recorded in schizophrenia.[159] Overall, the association of rare copy number variants is substantially less prominent for bipolar disorder than for schizophrenia and seems to be more likely to occur in early-onset cases.[159-163]

A lower copy number variant contribution in bipolar disorder than in schizophrenia could help to explain the generally higher level of cognitive functioning and less persistence of impairment seen in bipolar disorder than in schizophrenia.[162,164] Recent studies have shown distinct bipolar disorder subgroups with cognitive impairments similar to schizophrenia,[165] which suggests the potential benefit of more detailed phenotypic refinement in analyses.

PHENOTYPIC ISSUES

A major weakness of present research is that the clinical phenotype definitions remain rooted in diagnostic concepts from the late 19th century.[166,167] The definitions in use define highly heritable clinical entities, as measured in the family and twin studies discussed earlier, which allows the application of genetic methods. However, we can expect substantial overlaps of genetic susceptibility across, and substantial heterogeneity within, diagnostic categories. Many clinical phenotype variables show intrafamilial correlation within families who are multiply affected by bipolar disorder, and are, therefore, relevant in genetic studies. These variables include lifetime occurrence of psychosis, age at onset, lifetime occurrence of panic episodes, and lifetime occurrence of alcohol misuse, among others.[123] These variables suggest the potential importance of more sophisticated approaches to phenotype that go beyond simple case-control status and consider clinical covariates (dimensional or categorical and preferably extended phenotype measurements, including neurocognitive and imaging information). An example of such an approach is the replicated finding that variation within genes encoding γ-aminobutyric-acid (GABA), a receptor subunits is associated with susceptibility to bipolar-type schizoaffective disorder.[168,169] GABA-A receptors are neuronal ion channels, the function of which is modulated by GABA, so this finding contributes to the emerging evidence that ion channels are important in the pathogenesis of bipolar disorder. Other studies of phenotypic aspects, such as clinical symptom dimensions and categories, are beginning to emerge. These studies include those of negative mood delusions, mood incongruent psychotic symptoms, suicidality, and temperament, and although some have reported signals that just achieve genome-wide significance, they should be interpreted with caution.[170–173] These studies are necessarily smaller in size than the case-control meta-analyses discussed earlier and are hampered by low statistical power and difficulties in finding replication samples, since detailed phenotyping is not widely available in many of the genome-wide association study samples used so far. Maximisation of the power and consistency of these analyses is the rationale for the Cross Disorders Phenotype analyses of PGC.[115,174]

Recent genetic studies have been important in exploring nosological associations between mood and psychotic illness.[167,175] Perhaps surprisingly, cross-disorder analyses that have used available genome-wide association study data for adult mood and psychotic phenotypes have shown greater evidence of overlapping susceptibility between bipolar disorder and schizophrenia than between bipolar disorder and recurrent unipolar depression.[174] Genome-wide association study data have consistently showed overlapping susceptibility loci for bipolar disorder and schizophrenia. Overlap in both specific genetic vulnerability loci[176,177] and in polygenic background[149] have been reported. Large-scale genome-wide association studies have found strengthened signals that are also genome-wide significant when results from schizophrenia and bipolar disorder for *ZNF804A, ITIH3-ITIH4, ANK3, CACNA1C,* and *MAPK3* are combined. The polygenic score profile defined with use of a schizophrenia case-control sample statistically significantly discriminated between cases and controls in two independent bipolar disorder samples. These findings indicate a large molecular overlap in vulnerability alleles for the two disorders. The strength of these observations differs from earlier indications from linkage and candidate gene studies[123] because of the large samples sizes, statistical significance, and replication status of the results. For recurrent unipolar depression, studies in twins suggest that some genes affect susceptibility to both bipolar disorder and recurrent unipolar depression.[4] With some exceptions[147,178] this finding has not been prominent in molecular studies until now. However, findings for recurrent unipolar depression[179] are constrained by the types and numbers of samples used, and with the analysis of larger (and perhaps phenotypically more severe) recurrent unipolar depression samples, the molecular evidence might increase. However, these types of findings clearly have important implications for understanding the biological association between psychiatric phenotypes and will help in progress towards the goal of moving psychiatric diagnostic classification to firmer, data-driven biological foundations.[174,175,180]

CLINICAL RISK PREDICTION

The most likely scenario for bipolar disorder predictive testing is the use of several individual risk alleles together with an overall measure of polygenic risk.[181] Clinically useful tests would have great potential to improve outcomes. People at high risk could be offered lifestyle advice and could benefit from prompt and accurate diagnosis if illness develops, with early introduction of the most appropriate treatments. Physicians working in the psychiatry of intellectual disability are already very familiar with the inclusion of genetic investigation within the clinical assessment when appropriate. As knowledge develops, other areas of psychiatry should be willing to embrace new technologies if they are shown to be clinically beneficial.

Whatever the future developments are, we should remember that the presence of a positive family history in a close relative is still the strongest predictor of risk of bipolar disorder available to the clinician.

Panel 3: Top research priorities

- Use genetics to obtain an unbiased catalogue of the biological pathways of greatest importance for susceptibility to bipolar disorder
- Develop clinically usefully composite genetic tests that can help to predict risk and guide management
- Use knowledge of genetic risk to stratify research samples to enhance power in studies of environmental risk factors and episode triggers
- Follow-up genetic findings with imaging and psychological methods to move biological understanding closer to the mental experiences of patients
- Use molecular genetics, together with other methods of basic and clinical neuroscience, to inform development of diagnostic classifications that relate more closely to the normal and abnormal workings of the brain

CONCLUSION

A range of genetic and nongenetic research approaches (Panel 3) is needed to help us better understand the major biological, psychological, and social processes that contribute to bipolar disorder and other psychiatric illness. Together with these complementary research approaches, the ongoing major investments of time and money in molecular genetic studies of psychiatric disorders have the potential to identify pathways involved in illness and to help psychiatry move towards approaches to diagnosis and treatment that are grounded in a better understanding of pathogenesis. Such progress would help to revolutionize clinical psychiatry, and would be of great benefit to patients.

7.5 BIPOLAR DISORDER: DIAGNOSIS, CHALLENGES AND FUTURE DIRECTION

JN Vyas

BIPOLAR DISORDER DEFINITIONS

The origins of the categorical approach to psychiatric illness lie in the classic work of the founders of modern psychiatry, such as Emil Kraepelin. Kraepelin proposed a dichotomy between psychiatric illnesses characterized by regularly recurring episodes of notable changes in affect; and illnesses characterized by abnormal cognitions, beliefs, and experiences (i.e. psychotic symptoms), which usually manifested in early adulthood and persisted throughout life.[182-187] Kraepelin referred to the first category as "manic—depressive psychosis", including illnesses that we now refer to as affective disorders (e.g. bipolar disorder), and the second as "dementia praecox" (premature dementia), encompassing diseases that we now refer to as psychotic disorders (e.g. schizophrenia). The term bipolar was first used in 1957 by Leonhard[188] for disorders comprising both manic and depressive symptoms. In 1980, the name bipolar disorder was adopted by the Diagnostic and Statistical Manual for Mental Disorders (DSM) to replace the term manic depression.

In present classification systems, bipolar disorder now refers to a group of affective disorders in which patients experience episodes of depression, characterized by low mood and related symptoms (e.g. loss of pleasure and reduced energy), and episodes of either mania, characterized by elated or irritable mood or both, and related symptoms such as increased energy and reduced need for sleep, or hypomania, whose symptoms are less severe or less protracted than are those of mania. The fourth edition of the American Psychiatric Association's Diagnostic and Statistical Manual of Mental Disorders (DSM-IV)[189] contains four main subtypes of bipolar disorder: bipolar disorder type I (episodes of depression and at least one episode of full-blown mania); bipolar disorder type II (several protracted episodes of depression and at least one hypomanic episode but no manic episodes); cyclothymic disorder (many periods of hypomanic and depressive symptoms, in which the depressive symptoms do not meet the criteria for depressive episodes); and bipolar disorder not otherwise specified (depressive and hypomanic-like symptoms and episodes that might alternate rapidly, but do not meet the full diagnostic criteria for any of the aforementioned illnesses; Panel 4). The tenth edition of the International Classification of Diseases (ICD-10)[190] does not discriminate between bipolar disorder types I and II. ICD-10 also requires two discrete mood episodes, at least one of which must be manic or hypomanic, for a bipolar disorder diagnosis. However, in DSM-IV, one episode of mania (or mixed mood), or one episode of hypomania plus one major depressive episode, is sufficient for a diagnosis.

Panel 4: Bipolar disorder subtypes

Diagnostic and Statistical Manual for Mental Disorders 4th edition (DSM-IV) criteria

- Bipolar disorder type I
  - At least one episode of full-blown mania or mixed episode (manic and depressive symptoms). Usually has at least one depressive episode
- Bipolar disorder type II
  - Several protracted depressive episodes and at least one hypomanic episode, but no manic episodes
- Cyclothymic disorder
  - Several periods of hypomanic and depressive symptoms. Depressive symptoms do not meet criteria for depressive episodes
- Bipolar disorder not otherwise specified
  - Depressive and hypomanic-like symptoms and episodes that might alternate rapidly, but do not meet the full diagnostic criteria for any of the above disorders

International Classification of Diseases 10th edition (ICD-10) criteria: differences from DSM-IV

- ICD-10 does not discriminate between bipolar disorder types I and II
- ICD-10 requires two discrete mood episodes, at least one of which must be manic, for a bipolar disorder diagnosis. In DSM-IV, one episode of mania (or mixed mood), or one episode of hypomania plus a major depressive episode, suffice for a BD diagnosis

WHY IS BIPOLAR DISORDER SO DIFFICULT TO DIAGNOSE ACCURATELY?

Bipolar disorder types I and II are especially difficult to diagnose accurately in clinical practice, particularly in their early stages. Only 20% of patients with bipolar disorder who are experiencing a depressive episode are diagnosed with the disorder within the first year of seeking treatment,[5] and the mean delay between illness onset and diagnosis is 5 to 10 years.[191] A major reason for the difficult diagnosis is the challenge of differentiating bipolar disorder type I or II from unipolar depression—an illness characterized by recurrent depressive episodes—especially in patients who present during a depressive episode and in those with no clear history of mania or hypomania.[185,186] Unipolar depression is reportedly the most frequent misdiagnosis in patients with bipolar disorder,[186] especially in bipolar disorder type

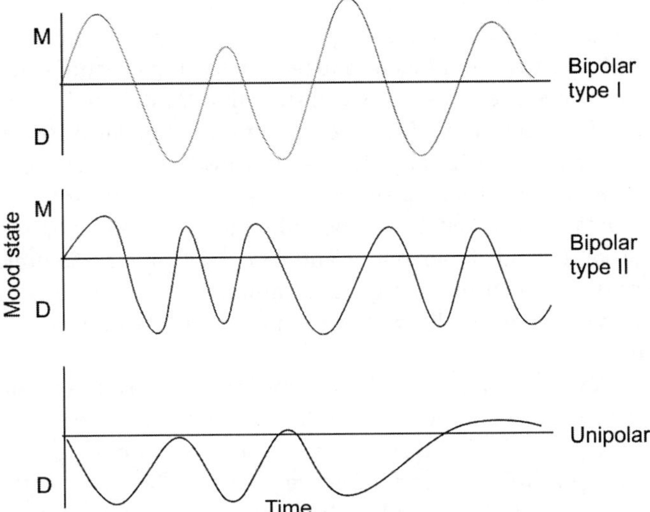

Fig. 1: Mood changes over time in bipolar disorder type I, bipolar disorder II , and recurrent unipolar depressive disorder
Abbreviation: M, mania; m, hypomania; D, depression

II, because patients with this illness, by definition, never experience an episode of mania (Fig. 1).

Another reason for the difficulty in distinction of bipolar disorder type I or II from unipolar depression is that the prevalence of depressive symptoms is higher than that of hypomanic or manic symptoms during the course of bipolar disorder type I or II, and these disorders often start with a depressive episode. People with bipolar disorder type II in particular spend much of their lives in a depressed state,[186,192-194] and more time in depressive than hypomanic or manic episodes, which compounds the diagnostic problem. For example, in two studies, people with bipolar disorder type I experienced hypomanic or manic symptoms only 9% of the time (9% of follow-up weeks),[195] and individuals with bipolar disorder type II experienced hypomanic symptoms only 1% of the time (1% of follow-up weeks).[196] Patients with bipolar disorder type II seek treatment for depressive symptoms much more frequently than they do for hypomanic or manic symptoms, and often do not recognize the consequences of, and thus fail to seek help for, the latter symptoms, which makes identification and treatment of these symptoms by clinicians especially difficult.

Mixed mood episodes, which are characterized by the presence of both depressive and hypomanic or manic symptoms, or a rapid alternation of the three symptom types, are being increasingly recognized as more common in people with bipolar disorder than was previously thought.[197] This idea challenges the traditional view of bipolar disorder as a group of illnesses characterized by discrete depressive, hypomanic, or manic episodes. The identification of hypomanic and manic symptoms in bipolar disorder patients with a history of mixed episodes is made even more difficult, especially for less experienced clinicians, by both the reporting bias towards depressive symptoms and the absence of discrete hypomanic or manic episodes in these patients. Furthermore, increasing evidence suggests that subthreshold symptoms of bipolar disorder (i.e. depressive-like, hypomanic-like, or manic-like symptoms that do not meet diagnostic thresholds for depressive, hypomanic, manic, or mixed episodes) in patients with bipolar disorder are associated with shorter time to future relapse into full-blown illness episodes than in patients without such subthreshold symptoms.[198] This finding emphasizes the significance of the effects of subthreshold symptoms of bipolar disorder on the future disease course.

In parallel, increasing evidence suggests that many patients diagnosed with unipolar depression might actually have a misdiagnosed bipolar disorder subtype. For example, in patients with a unipolar depression diagnosis, the 11-year rate for conversion to bipolar disorder type II is 9%,[199] and the 5-year rate for development of a manic or hypomanic episode is 20%.[200] Furthermore, results from antidepressant treatment trials for patients with unipolar depression indicate that up to two-thirds of these patients do not respond to first-line antidepressants, a third do not achieve full remission from symptoms after four treatments, and the rate of depression recurrence is very high, even in those who achieve remission after treatment with antidepressants.[201,202]

Together, these studies suggest that the boundary between bipolar disorder, particularly type II, and unipolar depression is not clear cut (Panel 5), and that many people with treatment-resistant unipolar depression could have undiagnosed bipolar disorder.[203] Misdiagnosis of bipolar disorder type I or II as unipolar depression has many potentially deleterious consequences, including prescription of inappropriate drugs, such as antidepressants in the absence of a mood-stabilizing drug, which might lead to switching to mania, and, ultimately, poor clinical and functional outcome and high healthcare costs.[204-207] Accurate diagnosis of bipolar disorder in its early stages, ideally before the first episode of hypomania or mania, or when there is no clear history of hypomania or mania, could, therefore, help to prevent the long-term detrimental effects of misdiagnosis.

Panel 5: Challenges and clinical strategies in the diagnosis of bipolar disorder

Reasons for the difficulty in bipolar disorder diagnosis

- Diagnostic criteria for depressive episodes: are identical in bipolar disorder and unipolar depression. Bipolar disorder is thus often misdiagnosed as unipolar depression.
- Many different bipolar disorder subtypes exist. Bipolar disorder type II is especially difficult to distinguish from unipolar depression, because of frequent depressive episodes and the absence of full-blown mania.
- Depressive symptoms are common in bipolar disorder and their prevalence is higher than that of hypomanic or manic symptoms.
- Mixed mood episodes are more common than was previously thought in bipolar disorder. These episodes might obscure detection of mania and hypomania, in view of the reporting bias towards depressive symptoms in people with bipolar disorder seeking treatment.

Contd...

Contd...

- Subthreshold symptoms of hypomania are common in unipolar depression. These symptoms might be more common than was previously thought; they are present in 30–55% of people during a depressive episode and are common in unipolar depression. At least a subset of patients with treatment-resistant unipolar depression might have misdiagnosed bipolar disorder.

Clinical Strategies to Improve Bipolar Disorder Diagnosis

- Additional clinical rating scales help to detect subthreshold hypomanic symptoms in depressed people
- In DSM-5, diagnostic criteria for bipolar disorder now include both changes in mood and changes in activity or energy; the mixed mood episode definition has been changed to acknowledge the coexistence of up to three manic symptoms within a major depressive episode; and short duration hypomania is now acknowledged. Diagnostic criteria in ICD-11 will be standardized
- Careful assessment for previous mania or hypomania should be done in all depressed patients, alongside collateral information from carers.

Dimensional Approaches to Definitions of Affective Disorders

- In the spectrum approach, clinical measures of dimensions of lifetime affective pathology are assessed, including manic and depressive symptoms, traits, and lifestyles that comprise both fully syndromal and subthreshold mood disturbances[237]
- Multidimensional Assessment of Thymic States assesses state-like emotional reactivity[238,239]
- Research Domain Criteria propose a reclassification of psychiatric disorders on the basis of domains of information processing that include dimensions of underlying pathophysiological processes, rather than by phenomenological observations.[240]

Clinical Strategies to Improve Diagnosis of Bipolar Disorder in Depressed Patients

Several changes have been recommended for the bipolar disorder section in DSM-5. First, bipolar disorder and related disorders have their own chapter. Second, the diagnostic criteria for bipolar disorder now include both changes in mood and changes in activity or energy. Previously, the diagnosis of a mixed mood episode required a patient to simultaneously meet the full criteria for both mania and major depression. A new specifier with mixed features has replaced the earlier criteria, and thus acknowledges the coexistence of up to three manic symptoms within a major depressive episode. Other amendments that acknowledge short duration hypomania will now be included in section III of DSM-5 as a mental health condition requiring further study. The recent DSM-5 field trials indicate good test—retest reliability of adult bipolar disorder type I,[208] suggesting that DSM-5 could be a positive step towards improved accuracy of bipolar disorder diagnosis. Additionally, DSM-5 acknowledges that more dimensional measures should be used in research settings for the measurement of psychopathology and to better define the continuum of both manic and depressive bipolar features. Efforts are also underway to harmonize the definitions of many psychiatric illnesses in the new ICD-11 with those in DSM-5.[209]

New self-administered and clinician-administered rating scales have been developed to help improve early detection of clinical features suggestive of a bipolar disorder diagnosis in people with a history of depressive episodes who might otherwise be diagnosed with unipolar depression. These clinical features include subthreshold hypomania, recurrence of mood episodes, and a positive family history of bipolar disorder. Examples of these rating scales include the Bipolar Inventory Symptoms Scale,[210] the Screening Assessment of Depression Polarity,[211] the Hypomania Checklist,[212] and the Probabilistic Approach for Bipolar Depression.[213] Finally, careful assessment for previous mania or hypomania in all depressed patients, combined with collateral information from carers, can help to improve the diagnostic accuracy of bipolar disorder.

Biological Approaches to Identification of Bipolar Disorder: Use of Neuroimaging to Identify Neural Circuit Biomarkers of the Disease

The aforementioned approaches could detect clinical features suggestive of a bipolar disorder diagnosis that might have otherwise been undetected during standard clinical assessment (Panel 5). However, these clinical approaches alone cannot identify objective biomarkers that represent the underlying pathophysiologic processes that vary between bipolar disorder and unipolar depression. The identification of such biomarkers could provide biological measures to inform diagnosis of bipolar disorder in the context of a depressive episode and, perhaps even more importantly, provide biological targets for personalised treatment and for the development of new interventions for bipolar disorder depression. More studies are emphasizing the importance of genetic factors that confer susceptibility to the disorder.[214] Neuroimaging techniques, through analysis of abnormalities in white matter connectivity, abnormalities in grey matter, and functional abnormalities in neural circuitry subserving cognitive and emotional processes that might be aberrant in bipolar disorder and unipolar depression, show particular promise to help identify neural circuit biomarkers that could aid diagnosis of, and provide treatment targets for, bipolar disorder.[215]

A suitable focus for analysis in neuroimaging studies of bipolar disorder and unipolar depression is the neural circuitry that supports emotion and reward processing, and emotion regulation, since these are key processes that are abnormal in all affective disorders. These neural circuitries include subcortical systems involved in emotion and reward processing (e.g. amygdala and ventral striatum); ventromedial and dorsomedial prefrontal and anterior cingulate cortical regions with roles in automatic or implicit regulation of emotion; and lateral prefrontal cortical systems (e.g. ventrolateral prefrontal and dorsolateral prefrontal cortices) implicated in cognitive control and voluntary or explicit top-down regulation of emotion.[216,217] Patterns of mainly raised subcortical activity and reduced prefrontal cortical activity during emotion processing in depressed patients with bipolar disorder and unipolar depression have been increasingly reported,[218] which suggests that functional impairments in top-down emotion regulation circuitry are present across these illnesses.

Neural Circuitry Abnormalities that Differentiate Bipolar Disorder Depression from Unipolar Depression

Surprisingly, the extent to which functional and structural abnormalities in emotion, reward, and emotion regulation neural circuitries can distinguish bipolar disorder from unipolar depression has not been well studied.[218] Thus, whether objective neuroimaging biomarkers can be identified in these circuitries to distinguish these illnesses is unclear.

Nevertheless, some evidence from a few neuroimaging studies comparing patients with bipolar disorder (predominantly type I) depression versus those with unipolar depression, suggests that some neuroimaging measures could help to distinguish the two disorders, at least in patients experiencing a depressive episode. For example, more substantial abnormalities in white matter connecting key prefrontal and subcortical neural regions in emotion processing and regulation neural circuitry,[219,220] and more white matter hyperintensities,[221] are reported in depressed patients with bipolar disorder than in those with unipolar depression. In parallel, findings from functional neuroimaging studies indicate differential patterns of amygdala activity and prefrontal cortical—amygdala connectivity during emotion processing[222] and emotion regulation in bipolar and unipolar depression,[222-225] suggesting either different underlying pathophysiological processes, or varying magnitudes of similar pathophysiological processes, in these disorders.

More neuroimaging studies are clearly needed to compare patients with different bipolar disorder depression subtypes versus those with unipolar depression, since almost no such studies have made these comparisons. Existing neuroimaging studies of bipolar versus unipolar depression have several limitations. For example, many of these studies included bipolar disorder depressed and unipolar depressed groups that were not well matched in terms of illness duration and prescribed drugs, which are potentially confounding factors on neuroimaging measures.[219,222,224,226] In view of the many limitations of existing clinical measures for accurate and early diagnosis of bipolar disorder, especially for patients in a depressive episode, objective biomarkers of bipolar disorder must be identified to improve functional and clinical outcomes for people with the disease. Neuroimaging approaches are at least starting to show promise as methods to help the identification of such biomarkers. Large-scale replication and prospective longitudinal studies are the next stage for this research pathway.

Innovative Approaches to the Study of Bipolar Disorder and Unipolar Depression

Dimensional Approaches

The clinical challenges in differentiation between bipolar disorder and unipolar depression have led to substantial debate about the phenomenological and pathophysiological associations between them. Discussion continues about whether these illnesses might be better represented as an affective disorders continuum, with variable expressions of vulnerability to hypomania or mania contributing to different phenotypes and various types of recurrent illness.[227-231] For example, recent reanalyses of two epidemiological studies, the Early Developmental Stages of Psychopathology study[232] and the National Comorbidity Survey Replication study,[233] showed that the bipolar disorder—unipolar depression dichotomy might be questionable, since hypomanic syndromes that do not meet DSM-IV criteria for bipolar disorder type II are present in about 40% of patients with recurrent unipolar depression.

Similar findings of high rates of hypomania in patients who had otherwise received a unipolar depression diagnosis have been reported in other studies. For example, in the BRIDGE study,[234,235] investigators reported that 16·1% of depressed patients with unipolar depression actually met criteria for either bipolar disorder type I or type II. Furthermore, when the strict DSM-IV criteria for bipolar disorder (manic episode) were relaxed to include increased activity or energy (i.e. removal of the sole emphasis on changes in mood), and the duration cutoff for hypomanic symptoms was reduced, the percentage of people meeting criteria for type I or II bipolar disorder increased to 47%. Similarly, in a UK study, investigators reported that 17% of adults with a diagnosis of unipolar depression endorsed subthreshold hypomania.[236]

In view of these difficulties in categorization of bipolar disorder and unipolar depression, some studies have now adopted dimensional criteria, such as the spectrum approach,[227] in which clinical measures of dimensions of lifetime affective pathology are assessed. These measures focus on manic and depressive symptoms, traits, and lifestyles that characterize the temperamental affective dysregulations that comprise both fully syndromal and subthreshold mood disturbances.[237] With the MOODS-SR (a series of self-report rating scales assessing lifetime spectra of affective symptoms), patients with unipolar depression were shown to present with many hypomanic or manic symptoms, although fewer than those reported by patients with bipolar disorder type I.[227] Another example of a dimensional approach to the study of affective disorders is the Multidimensional Assessment of Thymic States,[238,239] a scale that assesses state-like emotional reactivity in people with bipolar disorder.

These dimensional approaches also parallel the approach advocated by the Research Domain Criteria (RDoC) of the US National Institute of Mental Health, which proposes that psychiatric illnesses should be reclassified on the basis of information processing domains (including dimensions of underlying pathophysiological processes) rather than phenomenological observations.[240] The rationale is that these dimensional measures might be more closely linked to biomarkers of pathophysiologic processes in various psychiatric illnesses than are conventional categories of disorders such as bipolar disorder and unipolar depression.

Adoption of a dimensional approach to the study of affective disorders (Panel 5) could, therefore, potentially redefine bipolarity in terms of different underlying pathophysiological processes, including abnormalities in neural circuitry supporting emotion and reward processing, and emotion regulation. Recent neuroimaging studies have begun to use such approaches in the study of bipolar disorder and unipolar depression. In one study, investigators reported that increased right amygdala activity in response to happy emotional faces in depressed patients with unipolar depression was associated with more MOODS subthreshold manic symptoms experienced throughout life.[241] Importantly, this study was the first to show that even within the unipolar depression diagnostic category, a range of activity in key neural regions important for processing emotional stimuli, especially positive emotional stimuli, seems to exist, and is associated with the extent of subthreshold manic symptoms. In another study, investigators reported a positive correlation between activity in the ventral striatum (a key region for reward processing) during reward anticipation, and reward sensitivity in patients with bipolar disorder type I, bipolar disorder type II, and healthy people.[242] This finding not only emphasizes how a specific dimensional personality trait—reward sensitivity—is associated with activity in underlying reward circuitry, but also shows that this positive association is applicable to different diagnostic categories, and thus supports the RDoC approach.

PATTERN RECOGNITION APPROACHES AND NEUROIMAGING

Pattern recognition approaches are an example of machine learning—a branch of artificial intelligence that develops algorithms to allow computers to automatically learn and recognize complex patterns and to use large amounts of data to make intelligent decisions. Pattern recognition approaches have been used to classify patterns of neural activity elicited by sensory or cognitive processes[243]—i.e. so-called mind-reading devices to predict an individual's brain state. These approaches are now being applied in the clinic to classify groups of patients on the basis of neuroimaging data[244,245] and, therefore, have enormous potential to help classify patients with different affective disorders into diagnostic categories. In recent studies, investigators used combinations of pattern recognition approaches and various neuroimaging techniques to discriminate among bipolar disorder type I depressed, unipolar depressed, and healthy people on the basis of whole brain activity in response to emotional and neutral faces;[246] to distinguish healthy adolescents who are at high genetic risk for future bipolar disorder (because they have a parent with the disorder) from their healthy, low-risk counterparts;[247] and to classify patients as bipolar disorder type I depressed versus unipolar depressed on the basis of patterns of resting blood flow in the anterior cingulate cortex.[248] However, because of the dimensional approach that is being advocated, an important new development in the application of pattern recognition approaches to neuroimaging studies is their ability to place a patient at a point along a dimensional behavioral scale, on the basis of their patterns of neuroimaging data.[249] This exciting development has huge potential to integrate dimensional and individualized approaches to the identification of biomarkers of affective pathology that might cut across conventionally defined diagnostic categories of illness.

INTEGRATIVE BIOLOGICAL SYSTEMS APPROACHES

To move beyond a focus on one unit of measurement can ultimately yield patterns of biomarkers representing pathology at several biological measurement levels,[250] which has been emphasized in the National Institute of Mental Health RDoC, which could encompass genetic, molecular, cellular, neural circuitry, and behavioral measures. Integration across these scales could thus yield different biosignatures that represent dimensions of underlying pathophysiological processes in bipolar disorder and other affective disorders.

A key example of this idea is the integration of peripheral measures of oxidative stress and measures of white matter pathology in bipolar disorder. Oxidative stress is defined as an imbalance between oxidant—antioxidant systems that can ultimately lead to oxidative damage to protein, lipids, and DNA.[251] Increasing evidence suggests that oxidative stress could be implicated in the pathophysiology of mood disorders, particularly bipolar disorder type I.[252,253] Oxidative stress can be detected peripherally by analysis of serum measures of this factor. For example, abnormally high serum amounts of oxidative damage to lipids, proteins, and DNA have been recorded in people with bipolar disorder.[254–257] Additional evidence is available from postmortem brain studies of raised amounts of lipid oxidative stress in the anterior cingulate cortex,[258] and of a specific mitochondrial oxidative cascade enzymal impairment in the prefrontal cortex, probably leading to increased protein oxidation, in patients with bipolar disorder.[259]

In an integrated analysis of peripheral measures of oxidative stress and white matter integrity in bipolar disorder, investigators showed both substantially reduced integrity (reduced fractional anisotropy) of major white matter tracts, mainly in the prefrontal cortex, and substantially increased serum measures of lipid oxidative stress, in patients with bipolar disorder compared with healthy people.[257] Furthermore, these measures correlated significantly and variance in serum measures of lipid oxidation explained nearly 60% of the variance in fractional anisotropy in these tracts. These results are similar to other findings of lower densities of oligodendroglial and glial cells in the prefrontal cortex of patients with bipolar disorder than in healthy people,[260,261] and suggest that lipid oxidative stress could be a pathophysiological mechanism that underlies white matter abnormalities in bipolar disorder. These findings thereby draw attention to the potential of a combination of neuroimaging measures and serum markers of affective disorder pathology, which are also expressed at the neural circuit level, to elucidate pathophysiologic processes. This elucidation would help to identify biosignatures of dimensions of affective disorder pathology that might be applicable to a range of different affective disorders. Ultimately, this integrative approach has the potential to redefine bipolar disorder and all illnesses across the affective disorders spectrum in terms of new, neurobiologically established subgroups based on these biosignatures.

CONCLUSION

Recent evidence from field trials indicates that DSM-5 criteria might help to increase the accuracy of bipolar disorder type I diagnosis, one reason for which could be the less stringent criteria for mixed episodes. However, bipolar disorder, and bipolar disorder type II in particular, remains difficult to diagnose accurately in clinical practice, largely because of its frequent misdiagnosis as unipolar depression in depressed patients, since the diagnostic criteria for depressive episodes are identical for the two disorders. This challenge is compounded by higher prevalence of depressive than hypomanic or manic symptoms in bipolar disorder, and high rates of subthreshold manic symptoms in people diagnosed with unipolar depression. Although clinical approaches to improve the diagnosis of bipolar disorder include rating scales designed to detect subthreshold hypomanic or manic symptoms, these approaches alone cannot identify objective biomarkers that represent underlying pathophysiological processes. Promising findings from studies with different neuroimaging modalities indicate that neuroimaging measures might help to identify biomarkers to differentiate bipolar disorder from unipolar depression. However, the difficulty in identification of a clear boundary between the two disorders suggests that they might be better represented as an affective disorders continuum, with variable expressions of bipolarity representing dimensions of underlying pathophysiologic processes. Neuroimaging studies are starting to adopt this approach. Furthermore, exciting new combinations of neuroimaging and pattern recognition approaches have potential to identify individual patterns of neural circuitry structure and function that can help to both classify a patient into different categories, and place an individual at a point on a behavioral scale. Moving forward, however, the use of biological measurements across genetic, molecular, cellular, neural circuitry, and behavioral levels is imperative to yield patterns of biomarkers (biosignatures) that represent dimensions of underlying pathophysiological processes in bipolar disorder and other affective disorders. Ultimately, this integrative approach has the greatest potential to identify biological targets for personalized treatment and new treatment developments for all such illnesses (Panel 6).

Panel 6: Priority unanswered questions for the diagnosis of bipolar disorder

- Can objective biomarkers be identified to discriminate between bipolar disorder and unipolar depression, and between bipolar disorder subtypes?
- Do biomarkers exist that represent dimensions of pathology that cut across different diagnostic categories in the affective disorders spectrum?
- Can an integrated biological systems approach identify biosignatures, which comprise biomarkers of affective disorders at different biological levels (e.g. genes, cells, and neural circuitries)?
- Can individual biomarkers and biosignatures be identified to improve diagnosis of, and treatment options for, affective disorders in clinical practice?

7.6 TREATMENT OF BIPOLAR DISORDERS

Neena Bohra, NK Bohra

INTRODUCTION

Bipolar disorders types I and II affect about 2% of the world's population, with subthreshold forms of the disorder affecting another 2%.[262,263] Even with treatment, about 37% of patients relapse into depression or mania within 1 year; and 60% within 2 years.[264] In the STEP-BD cohort (n=1469), 58% of patients with bipolar disorder types I and II achieved recovery, but 49% had recurrences in a 2-year interval; twice as many of these recurrences were of depressive polarity (marked by sad mood, loss of interests, or fatigue) rather than of manic polarity (marked by elevated mood, grandiosity, and decreased need of sleep).[265] After initial onset, patients with bipolar disorder have residual depressive symptoms for about a third of the weeks of their lives.[266,267] Patients also experience psychotic symptoms, impaired functioning, compromised quality of life, and stigma.[268,269]

Treatment of bipolar disorder conventionally focuses on acute stabilization, in which the goal is to bring a patient with mania or depression to a symptomatic recovery with euthymic (stable) mood; and on maintenance, in which the goals are relapse prevention, reduction of subthreshold symptoms, and enhanced social and occupational functioning. Treatment of both phases of the illness can be complex, because the same treatments that alleviate depression can cause mania, hypomania, or rapid cycling (defined as four or more episodes in 12 months), and the treatments that reduce mania might cause rebound depressive episodes.[271-290]

TREATMENT OF MANIA

The pioneering trials of lithium and chlorpromazine were done in the 1970s and were followed by a focus on antiepileptics (e.g. valproate and carbamazepine) in the 1980s and 1990s. Few trials directly assessing the comparative efficacy of different second-generation antipsychotics exist but a mixed treatments meta-analysis compared 13 agents studied in 68 randomized controlled trials (16073 participants).[270] This review found substantial and clinically important differences in terms of both efficacy and tolerability between agents. Antipsychotic drugs seem to be better than anticonvulsants and lithium in the treatment of manic episodes, Olanzapine, risperidone, and haloperidol seem to have the best profile of presently available agents.[270] Therefore, antipsychotic agents will often be the appropriate short-term clinical treatment, although a drug with better long-term evidence of efficacy such as 'lithium' might be preferred when continued drug therapy is planned.

TREATMENT OF BIPOLAR DEPRESSION

The treatment of bipolar depression is a major challenge, with few treatments of proven efficacy and, in particular, substantial controversy about the role of antidepressant drugs. Authors of guidelines and consensus statements on this topic often ponder why antidepressants are so commonly used despite the scarce evidence for efficacy.[291-293] Until recently, after the Work of Emil Kraepelin, bipolar depressive episodes were deemed phenomenologically and biologically similar to unipolar depressive episodes. Even as late as the 1990s, inclusion and exclusion criteria in clinical trials of antidepressants in patients with depressive disorder did not usually either select or stratify according to polarity. Earlier trials suggested that when given with antimanic treatment, selective serotonin reuptake inhibitor antidepressants were more effective and no more likely to induce mania than placebo, and were less likely to induce mania than tricyclic antidepressants.[293] In 2007, a large trial found no benefit associated with the addition of paroxetine or bupropion to a mood stabilizer;[294] another reported that paroxetine was no better at achieving a durable recovery than placebo.[295]

A recent updated meta-analysis of antidepressants in polar depression reported a pooled effect no different from placebo (relative risk [RR] of response 1-17, 95% CI 0.82–1.57) with statistically significant heterogeneity.[296] Meta-analyses in patients with bipolar disorder have grouped antidepressant drugs together as one class, despite the observed statistically significant heterogeneity and the evidence in patients with unipolar disorder that antidepressant agents vary to a clinically significant degree in both efficacy and tolerability.[297] Therefore, to conclude that no antidepressant agent is effective in bipolar depression is probably premature, although the emerging evidence suggests that paroxetine is ineffective.

The antiepileptic drug lamotrigine was investigated in patients with bipolar depression after a clinical benefit was seen after treatment with the drug in patients with bipolar disorder.[298] A meta-analysis of individual patient-level data from five trials of lamotrigine in bipolar depression reported a modest treatment effect; however, no one trial showed statistically significant benefits of treatment with lamotrigine in comparison with placebo. Thus, the place of lamotrigine in acute treatment remains uncertain.[299]

Atypical antipsychotics have been investigated in bipolar depression with variable results.[300] Treatment with quetiapine leads to more symptomatic improvement in patients with bipolar depression than do placebo, paroxetine, and lithium.[300] Some evidence exists of a reduced risk of recurrence in patients who respond to acute-phase treatment and continue quetiapine rather than switch to placebo; thus, continuation could be of benefit in patients who can tolerate the drug's adverse effects, including sedation and weight gain.[301] The reasonably fast onset of action of quetiapine is clinically useful because it provides clinicians and patients with a treatment that can be initiated early in the course of a worsening depression in the same way that antipsychotics are used for emerging manic symptoms. Combined olanzapine and fluoxetine leads to more symptomatic improvement than does olanzapine or placebo alone, which could suggest that fluoxetine is an effective treatment of acute bipolar depression or that the combination of fluoxetine and olanzapine synergistic.[302]

So far, the investigation of atypical antipsychotic drugs has been instructive for both clinical and methodological reasons. Quetiapine and olanzapine-fluoxetine combination have regulatory approval for bipolar depression in some countries and are included as first-line recommendations in recent guidelines. Emerging evidence suggests that lurasidone might also be efficacious, whereas aripiprazole does not seem to be so.[300,303] The transdiagnostic benefits of a drug like quetiapine, which is antipsychotic, antimanic, and antidepressant in both unipolar and bipolar depression, emphasizes the importance of the investigation of treatment effects across conventional diagnostic boundaries.[270,301,304] However, this nonspecificity and scarcity of convincing evidence of long-term disease modification by known mechanisms suggests that the effects are mediated by short-term alleviation of symptoms. Nonetheless, because bipolar depression is very difficult to treat, this relief is often useful for patients and clinicians. Further combinations of atypical antipsychotics with selective serotonin-reuptake inhibitors, or with agents that have medium-term to long-term effects on depression (e.g. lamotrigine) are often used in clinical practice and warrant investigation in clinical trials.

Up to a third of patients with bipolar disorder do not respond to treatments in naturalistic studies;[265,266,268] these figures probably underestimate the proportion of treatment-resistant patients with depression in clinical practice. Even patients who receive adequate pharmacotherapy have lengthy and debilitating periods of subthreshold depressive symptoms after major episodes, Longitudinal studies estimate that patients with bipolar disorder type l spend as many as 3 weeks depressed for every 1 week (hypo) manic; the ratio in bipolar disorder type Il is 37:1.[266,305] Subthreshold depressive symptoms are associated with social and occupational impairment,[306] and increased psychosocial impairment is prospectively associated with earlier recurrences.[307,308]

Very little evidence exists of effective strategies for patients who do not respond to first-line treatments. A recent review of strategies reported just seven small trials; one each for ketamine, pramipexole, lamotrigine, and risperidone, and two each for modafinil and electroconvulsive therapy,[309] Therefore, recommendations in clinical practice guidelines for treatment-resistant bipolar depression are still often based on extrapolation from the evidence on augmentation and switching strategies in bipolar major depression. This situation might lead to an underestimation of the attendant risks of treatment-emergent hypomania or mania in patients with bipolar disorder.

LONG-TERM MAINTENANCE TREATMENT

Lithium, introduced by John Cade in 1949, remains the best established long-term treatment for bipolar disorder.[310] Although the metal has been in clinical use for more than 50 years, the most convincing evidence of long-term efficacy comes from randomized clinical trials in which lithium was included as an active comparator.[311] A meta-analysis of five placebo-controlled lithium maintenance trials (n = 770) showed that lithium reduces the risk of manic relapses by 38% (RR 0.62, 95% CI 0-50-0-84) and depressive relapse by 28% (0.72, 0.40-0.95).[312] Lithium is the only known anti-suicidal treatment with randomized evidence of a reduction in the risk of suicide of more than 50%.[313] However, the benefits of lithium are restricted by adverse effects and a low therapeutic index.[52] Although little evidence exists of a clinically substantial reduction in renal function in most patients, the risk of end-stage renal failure remains unclear. The risk of congenital malformations in the babies of mothers who have taken lithium during pregnancy is uncertain, but probably lower than previously thought. The balance of risks should be considered before lithium is withdrawn during pregnancy. In addition to known effects of lithium on the thyroid, the risk of hyperparathyroidism is increased and calcium concentrations should be checked before and during treatment.[313]

The limitations of lithium mean that alternatives are often needed for long-term treatment. A pooled analysis of two randomized lamotrigine versus placebo trials reported a 36% reduction for lamotrigine in the risk of relapse over 18 months.[314] Despite the dramatic increase in the use of valproate in the past two decades,[315] placebo controlled evidence for valproate in long-term prevention remains scarce.[316] Moreover, the BALANCE trial found that lithium was better than valproate in the prevention of mood episodes (RR O.71, 95% CI 0. 51–1. 00), but a combined analysis finds heterogeneity between studies. Combination treatment with lithium (plus valproate is better than treatment with valproate monotherapy (0.59, 0.42–0.83).[317]

Because antipsychotics are the most potent treatments in acute mania,[270] in many clinical situations, it will seem reasonable to continue them after remission from the acute episode.[291] However, there are few long-term trials, most use enrichment designs, and none have the same degree of independent replication of efficacy as lithium. Thus, the role of antipsychotics as long-term mood stabilizers remains uncertain.

PSYCHOSOCIAL TREATMENTS FOR BIPOLAR DISORDER

Treatment guidelines increasingly suggest that optimum management of bipolar disorder needs integration of pharmacotherapy with targeted psychotherapy.[291,318] A recent randomized trial in Denmark has shown clinical benefits from this approach.[319] Psychological approaches build on evidence that psychosocial stressors, including excessive family discord or distress, negative life events, or events that disrupt sleep and wake rhythms or accelerate goal attainment are associated with relapses and worsening symptomatic states.[284] The main goals of adjunctive psychotherapy for bipolar disorder include the education of patients, and when possible, caregivers, about strategies for the management of stress, the identification and intervention of early signs of recurrence, and how to keep regular lifestyle (e.g. sleep and exercise) habits (Panel 7).[320] Moreover, in View of the high rate of nonadherence to drug treatments (up to 60% after acute episodes[288]), psychosocial treatments emphasize consistency with pharmacotherapy.

Panel 7: Common objectives of psychosocial interventions for bipolar disorder

- Improve ability to identify and intervene early with warning signs of recurrences
- Increase acceptance of the illness
- Enhance adherence with drug regimens
- Enhance ability to cope with environmental stressors associated with symptoms
- Stabilize sleep and wake rhythms and other daily routines
- Re-engage with social, familial, and occupational roles
- Enhance family relationships and communication
- Reduce drug or alcohol misuse.

Evidence-based models of psychotherapy[321-341] include cognitive-behavioral therapy family-focused therapy interpersonal and social rhythm therapy group psychoeducation, and systematic care management. Although these models have common objectives, their methods, assumptions, and structure differ substantially.[320,342-345]

ADJUNCTIVE PSYCHOTHERAPY IN ACUTE TREATMENT

Patients in acute manic episodes are not likely to respond well to intensive psychotherapy because of insufficient insight or rejection of help.[346] Some trials have examined whether psychotherapy enhances remission from acute depression.[347] The STEP-BD study compared up to 30 sessions of family-focused therapy, interpersonal and social rhythm therapy, or cognitive-behavioral therapy (i.e. intensive treatment) with a brief psychoeducational therapy (three individual sessions) for 293 patients with acute depression who also received mood stabilizers. Over 1 year, patients in intensive therapy recovered more rapidly (hazard ratio [HR] 1.47, 95% CI 1.08-2.0) and were more likely to be clinically well (1.58, 1.17-2.13) in any study month than those in brief treatment.[322] Effects extended to relationship functioning and life satisfaction.[323] No differences emerged between the three intensive modalities in symptoms or psychosocial functioning over 1 year. Interestingly, patients with depression in STEP-BD who were treated with mood stabilizers and randomly assigned to adjunctive antidepressant treatment did not recover faster than patients who were assigned to adjunctive placebo treatment.[249] Therefore, psychosocial treatment might be a more effective adjunct to mood stabilizers than antidepressants after a bipolar depressive episode.

ADJUNCTIVE PSYCHOTHERAPY IN LONG-TERM MAINTENANCE

Most studies of psychotherapy for bipolar disorder are maintenance trials in which patients receive standard drugs and either an experimental psychosocial intervention or usual care (e.g. brief treatment or a supportive treatment of equal frequency and duration). A meta-analysis of eight maintenance psychotherapy trials, which included family individual, and group treatment trials, yielded effect sizes ranging from an odds ratio (OR) of 0.57 (95% CI 0.39–0.82) for reductions in any type of mood relapse to 1.2 (0.3–2.1) for enhanced social functioning.[348] A second meta-analysis often trials showed an overall RR of 0:74 (0.64–0.85) for mood relapse.[349]

FAMILY-FOCUSED THERAPY

Family-focused therapy is based on the frequently replicated association between criticism and hostility in caregivers (so-called expressed emotion) and an increased likelihood of relapse in mood disorders and schizophrenia.[286] Family-focused therapy involves the patient and caregivers (parents or spouse) in up to 21 sessions of psychoeducation, communication skills training, and problem-solving skills training.[350] Two randomized controlled trials including symptomatic patients with bipolar I and II found that, in the 1 to 2 years after a manic, mixed, or depressive episode, patients with bipolar disorder who received family-focused therapy and pharmacotherapy had 30 to 35% lower rates of relapse and rehospitalization and less severe symptoms than did patients in case management[289] or equally intensive individual treatment.[324] Two randomized controlled trials in pediatric populations-one in adolescents (aged 12–18 years) with bipolar disorder[325] and one in children and adolescents (aged 9–17 years) with depression or hypomania with a first degree relative with bipolar disorder[326] found that children and adolescents who received family-focused therapy and pharmacotherapy recovered more rapidly from depressive episodes (HR 0.37–0.54) than did children and adolescents in brief psychoeducation and pharmacotherapy.

The education of caregivers about bipolar disorder might translate into benefits for patients, even if patients do not attend educational sessions. In one randomized controlled trial,[329] remitted patients whose relatives attended psychoeducation groups had longer intervals (before manic and hypomanic episodes than did those whose relatives did not attend groups. In a second trial,[327] patients whose caregivers attended 12–15 family education sessions showed significant decreases in symptoms of depression, especially if caregivers also showed mood improvement. Thus, adjunctive family interventions have the potential to lengthen periods of stability and alleviate residual symptoms in maintenance care. However; differences in treatment preferences, cultural factors (e.g. willingness to disclose in front of others), and family structure (e.g. parental vs spousal) might affect the Willingness of patients or caregivers to participate family-based treatment.

COGNITIVE-BEHAVIORAL THERAPY

Cognitive-behavioral therapy presumes that recurrences of mood disorder are determined by pessimistic thinking in response to life events and core dysfunctional beliefs about the self the world, and the future.[351] Cognitive-behavioral therapy to treat depression has been adapted for patients with bipolar disorder with recognition that manic episodes are often associated with excessively optimistic thinking.[332] One randomized controlled trial[319] reported that patients who received 12–14 sessions of cognitive-behavioral therapy were less likely to have depressive episodes and had better social functioning than patients in routine care for 30 months, However; an effectiveness trial (n = 252) comparing cognitive-behavioral therapy with treatment as usual in five UK community care centers found no advantage for cognitive-behavioral therapy over 18 months, except among patients with fewer than 12 previous episodes.[334]

INTERPERSONAL AND SOCIAL RHYTHM THERAPY

Substantial evidence exists that mood instability in bipolar disorder is related to changes in circadian rhythms.[281] The relation between sleep and mood disturbances seem to be bidirectional. Polymorphisms in CLOCK genes are related to circadian mood fluctuations and recurrences in bipolar disorder.[352] In one promising animal model,[353] mice with mutations in CLOCK genes behaved in ways that resembled manic behavior in people (e.g. increases in activity and decreased sleep); these behaviors were reversed upon treatment with lithium.

Interpersonal social rhythm therapy, an adaptation of the interpersonal psychotherapy for depression, uses a problem-solving approach to interpersonal problems by encouraging patients to maintain and regulate daily routines and sleep and wake rhythms.[282] In a large (n = 175) randomized clinical trial,[282] acutely manic, mixed, or depressed patients with bipolar I disorder were assigned to weekly interpersonal and social rhythm therapy or to equally intensive clinical management, both with pharmacotherapy. After acute stabilization, random assignment was done again (interpersonal and social rhythm therapy vs clinical management) and treatment continued for a 2-year maintenance phase. No differences in time-to-recovery between the groups during acute stabilization were recorded. However, patients who received interpersonal and social rhythm therapy in the acute phase had longer times to recurrence and better vocational functioning in the maintenance phase than did patients who received clinical management during the acute phase. Moreover, the effects of interpersonal and social rhythm therapy in the delay of recurrences were most pronounced in patients who had been able to stabilize their daily or nightly routines during acute treatment.[282] Thus, to help patients to stabilize their sleep and wake rhythms after an acute episode might have downstream effects on the prevention of future mood instability.

GROUP PSYCHOEDUCATION

In view of the many patients who could benefit from psychoeducation, group approaches following a predesigned curriculum have been proposed. The Barcelona approach[339] emphasizes awareness of illness, treatment adherence, early detection of recurrences, and sleep and wake regularity, In a trial of patients with bipolar disorder types I and II in the euthymic phase of illness, patients were randomly assigned to pharmacotherapy and 21 sessions of structured group psychoeducation or 21 sessions of an unstructured support group. After 5 years, patients who had received the structured groups had fewer relapses and were ill for less time than those who had been in the unstructured group.[290,339]

FUNCTIONAL REMEDIATION

Functional remediation treatment emphasizes patients' cognitive functioning through exercises for memory, attention, problem solving, reasoning, and organization. In a ten-site randomized clinical trial in Spain,[340] 268 euthymic patients who had moderate to severe psychosocial impairment were assigned to 21 weekly group sessions of functional remediation, 21 sessions of standard group psychoeducation, or treatment as usual. Patients in functional remediation showed greater changes in occupational and social functioning than did those treated as usual, but differed only slightly from patients in the standard psychoeducation groups. No differential effects of functional remediation were recorded for neurocognitive or clinical change variables.

SYSTEMATIC CARE MANAGEMENT

Two research groups have examined collaborative care programs that combine protocol-driven pharmacotherapy, group psychoeducation, and intensive patient monitoring by a nurse care manager importantly, these studies were done in managed healthcare cooperatives in the USA and included large patient samples with systematic follow-up. In trials at a group health cooperative (n = 441)[343] and in 11 Veterans Administration sites (n = 306),[344] patients were randomly assigned to systematic care or usual care. Although neither study showed reductions in relapses, patients in systematic care had fewer weeks in manic episodes than did those in usual care. In the Veterans Administration study patients in collaborative care also had improved social functioning and quality of life over 2 years. Cost-effectiveness analyses suggested that the care programmes saved money despite their greater intensity of follow-up.[343,344]

FUTURE DIRECTIONS

Advances in the pharmacological treatment of bipolar disorder have come mainly from the repurposing of drugs used in other neuropsychiatric disorders, and do not target the mood instability that characterizes the disorder.[345-354] Dopamine antagonism seems to be a potential target for antimanic treatments, but the scarce convincing evidence that increasing serotonergic transmission improves symptoms in bipolar depression shows the need for development of bipolar-specific validated targets for novel treatments. Existing treatments (especially lithium) and the gradual emergence of insights into the neurobiology of the disorder provide potential targets. Opportunities should increase with the implementation of new methods such as the use of induced pluripotential stem cells to provide *in vitro* models of neural systems,[355] the identification of genetic and epigenetic factors,[356,357] and the use of optogenetics to develop more precise animal models,[358] Meanwhile, faced with the neurobiological complexity of the disorder, present approaches to drug discovery and repurposing will need to use existing targets in addition to any novel targets such as oxidative damage.[278]

Following-up leads emerging from insights into the underlying neurobiology is already producing promising results. For example, after evidence of dysfunction in the N-methyl-D-aspartate-receptor complex in the glutamatergic system in bipolar disorder, two crossover trials found that infusion of the N-methyl-D-aspartate antagonist ketamine produced rapid alleviation of depressive symptoms in bipolar depression. These findings open a new approach to drug development and provide insights into the neurobiology of the disorder. The recent identification of the failed stroke treatment antioxidant ebselen as a potential lithium mimetic-obtained from screening of 450 compounds from the National Institutes of Health Clinical Collection—is an elegant and comprehensive approach using several targets, which now needs clinical evaluation.[359]

Acceleration of the development of novel treatments needs improved validation strategies for preclinical targets and the development of innovative biomarkers and intermediate outcomes for use in early-phase clinical trials.[360] Validation strategies might include neuroimaging, cognitive or biochemical measures, and molecular genetic studies. Moreover, a more deeply characterized picture of the core clinical phenotype is urgently needed. The emerging picture of the course of bipolar disorder is one of chronic mood instability rather than discrete episodes of mania and depression.[361,362] Early detection of treatment effects on short-term mood instability could provide the much needed intermediate outcomes for early-phase trials and experimental medicine. For example, clarification of the mechanisms by which different mood stabilizers and atypical antipsychotics affect sleep and circadian rhythms and their relation with daily mood fluctuations is likely to help with the treatment selection for individual patients. Conventional episode-based maintenance designs are likely to be inefficient, especially for early-phase therapeutic development.

Substantial progress has been made in the past decade in understanding of the role of psychotherapy in bipolar disorder. All existing forms of psychotherapy for bipolar disorder include psychoeducation, although which didactic ingredients lead to the most clinical change is not clear (panel). The next generation of psychotherapy studies will need to systematically assess mediators in the pathways from treatments to changes in illness course. The identification of mechanisms of change, e.g. regulation of sleep and wake rhythms, reductions in family conflict, consistency of adherence to drugs, or the ability to intervene early with prodromal symptoms-might lead to the development of briefer treatments with more durable effects.[363] The identification of mediators might be enhanced by controlled dismantling designs that test the effects of psychotherapies with and without the components believed to induce change. Further identification of psychological processes underlying mood instability such as the role of imagery in increasing anxiety and mood instability, might lead to more focused psychological interventions.[364]

Drug and psychotherapy trials have largely proceeded independently of one another. Specifically, drug studies have not examined the effects of psychotropic agents on psychosocial variables (e.g. a patient's ability to regulate emotions in response to life events), nor have psychotherapy studies analyzed changes in presumed biological mechanisms (e.g. degree of amygdala activation in emotional challenge paradigms[365]). Pragmatic trials that examine the interactive effects of psychotropic drugs and psychotherapy in maintenance treatment would help to move the field forward. For example, a trial in which patients with bipolar disorder in the depressive phase of illness are initially treated with quetiapine or lithium or both, and then randomly assigned to continued pharmacotherapy with adjunctive psychotherapy versus adjunctive antidepressants, could help to define effective algorithms for bipolar depression.

As the genetic and phenotypic characteristics of children who are predisposed to adult bipolar disorder are identified,[366] the focus of treatment research may change to early intervention. One small randomized trial found that family-focused therapy was more effective than usual care in the treatment of hypomanic and depressive symptoms in young people (aged 9–17 years) with a first-degree bipolar relative.[326] Whether early pharmacological or psychosocial interventions for prodromal youth can help to delay or prevent the transition to bipolar disorder types I or II in adulthood will be crucial to investigate in this decade.

Innovations in service provision often focus on the early detection of manic and depressive symptoms.[319,343,344] In our opinion, early detection combined with helpful self management and targeted psychosocial and drug treatment promises substantial benefits. To be economically sustainable, psychosocial protocols need to be standardized for settings that serve large numbers of patients and have few resources for clinician training. The addition of web-based interactive protocols that track mood and sleep cycles and provide real-time information to providers, such as our OXTEXT program based on mood monitoring, might enhance this effort.[363,364]

7.7 BIPOLAR DISORDER: FOCUS ON BIPOLAR II DISORDERS AND MIXED DEPRESSION

JN Vyas

Bipolar disorder is defined by recurrent periods of highs and lows of mood, thinking, and activity, of varying severity, duration, and frequency, including combinations of manic or hypomanic and depressive symptoms in the same episode (the mixed states). This Seminar focuses more on bipolar II disorder than on bipolar I disorder, because the former is much understudied, and because recent advances in this area are mainly to do with bipolar II and related disorders (the bipolar spectrum).

KRAEPELIN'S CONCEPT OF MOOD DISORDERS

Kraepelin's description of manic-depressive insanity in 1913 comprised almost all currently defined mood disorders, without categorical boundaries between subtypes. Manic-depressive insanity was described in terms of excitement of inhibition (increase or decrease) of three basic domains: mood, thinking, and activity. Of these three, all the domains could move in the same direction, leading to episodes of manic, hypomanic, or depressive states; or the domains could move in opposite directions, leading to the mixed states, which were defined as combinations of manic or hypomanic and depressive symptoms in the same episode. Mania could be diagnosed even if mood was decreased, if thinking and activity were increased. The main components of the concept of manic-depressive insanity were the recurrent, episodic course, including episodes of opposite polarity (i.e. recurrent mania or hypomania and depression); and of one polarity (e.g. recurrent depression); mixture of opposite-polarity symptoms in the same episode (the mixed states); mood temperaments (persistent traits); family history of mood disorder; and young age at onset (Table 3).

Kraepelin's approach to the basic symptoms of mood disorders is the opposite of the approach of the current most commonly used diagnostic system, the diagnostic and statistical manual of mental disorders, fourth edition, text revision (DSM-IV-TR). This manual sets mood change, i.e. elevated or irritable mood in mania/hypomania, low mood in depression as the core feature (criterion A) of mood disorders. However, no sound evidence supports this approach. In the WHO International Classification Diseases (ICD)-10 Classification of Mental and Behavioral Disorders, overactivity is given the same priority as mood change. Recently, overactivity (increased goal directed activity, listed in DSM-IV-TR as criterion B symptom of mania or hypomania) has been upgraded to the same level of priority as mood change in recent studies.

Kraepelin described mania as a psychotic, excited state necessitating hospital admission. Hypomania was described

Table 3: Kraepelin's manic, hypomanic, depressive, and mixed states (episodes)

	Mood	*Thinking*	*Activity*
Mania/Hypomania	Increased	Increased	Increased
Depression	Decreased	Decreased	Decreased
Mixed states (manic and depressive) concurrent, opposite polarity symptoms	Increased or decreased	Increased or decreased	Increased or decreased

as having different levels of severity; and often did not require hospitalization. Disordered thinking in hypomania included creative thinking (more goal-directed, structured planning, more brilliant ideas), crowded thoughts (nonstop thinking), racing thoughts (speedy thinking), and flight of ideas (quick, disconnected thinking). In overactivity, functioning was frequently increased, but could also be decreased (although less than in mania), according to the degree of thinking disorder. Kraepelin, who studied patients in hospital, could not see the milder hypomanic states frequently found in the community. These milder hypomanic states, which often improve functioning, were described by Hecker in outpatient private practice as cyclothymia (similar to the DSM-IV-TR definition of bipolar 2 disorder), and by Falret as circular insanity.

Kraepelin's description of mixed states supported his unitary concept of mood disorders: if symptoms of opposite polarity could be present in the same episode, then mania or hypomania and depression could not be distinct categorical disorders. The mixed states described by Kraepelin were mainly seen in patients, and Hecker described milder depressive and hypomanic mixed states in outpatients. Kraepelin's description of manic-depressive insanity included the fundamental states-temperaments (persistent traits) defined by the same symptoms of the manic, hypomanic, and depressive states and temperaments. The cyclothymic temperament (defined by frequent upswings and downswings of mood, thinking and behavior) was, according to Kraepelin, the main root of manic-depressive insanity.

DSM-IV-TR CLASSIFICATION OF MOOD DISORDERS

In DSM IV-TR, mood disorders are categorically divided into bipolar disorders and depressive disorders. The basic feature distinguishing these groups is mania and hypomania, which is present in bipolar disorders, but absent in depressive disorders. According to Kraepelin, the recurrent course, rather than polarity, was probably the core feature of manic-depressive insanity. The symptoms of mania and hypomania are similar in DSM-IV-TR, except for increased severity of symptoms and present of psychosis in mania.

This list of symptoms, the prioritization of mood change, and the minimum duration of episodes specified, are consensus-based, not evidence-based. The criterion separating mania and hypomania, i.e. marked impairment of functioning in mania is an unclear boundary that can lead to misclassification. Recent findings have challenged these criteria and suggested different groupings of bipolar disorders and depressive disorders, according to the continuation of spectrum concept.

The distinction between bipolar I and II disorders in DSM-IV-TR is mainly based on findings that followed the criteria of Robins and Guzefor diagnostic validity (clinical picture, delimitation, course including diagnostic ability, family history, biology).

CLINICAL PICTURE AND DELIMITATION

Many differences exist between mania, which defines bipolar I disorder, and hypomania, which defines bipolar disorder. Psychosis often occurs in mania, but never in hypomania. Mania markedly impairs functioning, whereas hypomania often improves functioning, or less common causes mild impairment. Mania often requires hospital admission, whereas hypomania, by definition, never does. Mania usually has a longer duration than hypomania (months rather than weeks).

Thought disorders all of which involve mental overactivity, differ between mania, which is associated with flight of ideas (speedy, disconnected thinking plus nonstop talking), and hypomania, in which the severity of thinking disorder can vary between creative thinking, crowded thoughts, racing thoughts, and infrequently flight of ideas. The marked difference in functioning between mania and hypomania is partly related to differences in thinking: hypomania often includes creative and quick thinking that leads to increased goal directed activities, or behavioral overactivity; whereas mania is associated with speedy, disconnected ideas, leading to aimless overactivity.

Critical evaluation of actions also differs: hypomania can include moderate risk-taking behavior, mania includes severe risk taking behavior. That hypomania is not simply mild version of mania is shown by differences in symptom structure. Mania has many defining factors or dimensions of symptoms, whereas hypomania has two to three factors, according to the sample studied (one factor dominated by elevated mood, one dominated by mental and behavioral over activity, and one dominated by irritable risky behaviors). Differences between the sexes are also noted: in bipolar I disorder, female and male patients are equally common whereas more female than male patients are seen in bipolar II disorders.

Course

Long-term follow-up studies have shown high diagnostic stability of bipolar I and II disorders, i.e. patients who present with one type rarely go on to develop the other. The course differs: bipolar I disorder is more likely than bipolar II to include manic or hypomanic episodes and symptoms, whereas bipolar II disorder is more likely to include depressive episodes and symptoms.

Family History

The type of bipolar disorder is likely to run in families, e.g. bipolar I is more common than bipolar II in relatives of probands with bipolar I, and vice versa.

Biology

Pharmacological treatment differs somewhat between bipolar I and II disorders. In bipolar I disorder, complex drug combinations are needed to reach some stability, and antidepressants can induce or facilitate switching from depression to mania or hypomania. In bipolar II disorder, the risk of such switching caused by antidepressants is lower, and mood stabilizing agents may be less necessary, depression is more common than hypomania in this condtion. However, drug treatment of bipolar II disorder is much understudied compared with that of bipolar.

Despite these differences, several lines of evidence (some of which result from different interpretations of the findings mentioned above) question the division between bipolar I and II disorders (Panel 8). The findings that support a distinction between the two seem to be stronger than those that suggest a grading or continuum. The findings of Ghaemi and Baldessarini and Goodwin and colleagues seem to support a distinction between bipolar I and II disorders, and to support a mixed concept of the spectrum, including distinct disorders, with bipolar I disorder and major depressive disorder as extreme poles and, in the middle, a series of overlapping disorders bipolar signs. This concept of spectrum is partly different from Angsts and Akiskal and colleagues continuum or spectrum concept, which includes partial overlap of mood disorders (including depressive disorders).

RESHAPING OF BIPOLAR II DISORDER

The blurring of the boundaries between bipolar disorders and depressive disorders is mainly based on changes in the definition of bipolar II disorder and on the reemergence of the concept of mixed depression. DSM-IV-TR criteria for bipolar II disorder require the presence of recurrent depressive and hypomanic episodes. Similarly, DSM-5 criteria for bipolar also requires at least one hypomanic episode and atleast one major depressive episode (below).

DSM-5 Diagnostic criteria for bipolar II disorder

296.89 (F31.81)

For a diagnosis of bipolar II disorder, it is necessary to meet the following criteria for a current or past hypomanic episode and the following criteria for a current or past major depressive episode:

Hypomanic episode

a. A distinct period of abnormally and persistently elevated, expansive, or irritable mood and abnormally and persistently increased activity or energy, lasting at least 4 consecutive days and present most of the day, nearly everyday.
b. During the period of mood disturbance and increased energy and activity, three (or more) of the following symptoms have persisted (four if the mood is only irritable), represent a noticeable change from usual behavior, and have been present to a significant degree:
   1. Inflated self-esteem or grandiosity.

Contd...

Contd...

   2. Decreased need for sleep (e.g. feels rested after only 3 hours of sleep).
   3. More talkative than usual or pressure to keep talking.
   4. Flight of ideas or subjective experience that thoughts are racing.
   5. Distractibility (i.e. attention too easily drawn to unimportant or irrelevant external stimuli), as reported or observed.
   6. Increase in goal-directed activity (either socially, at work or school, or sexually) or psychomotor agitation.
   7. Excessive involvement in activities that have a high potential for painful consequences (e.g. engaging in unrestrained buying sprees, sexual indiscretions, or foolish business investments).
c. The episode is associated with an unequivocal change in functioning that is uncharacteristic of the individual when not symptomatic.
d. The disturbance in mood and the change in functioning are observable by others.
e. The episode is not severe enough to cause marked impairment in social or occupational functioning or to necessitate hospitalization. If there are psychotic features, the episode is, by definition, manic.
f. The episode is not attributable to the physiological effects of a substance (e.g. a drug of abuse, a medication or other treatment).
   Note: A full hypomanic episode that emerges during antidepressant treatment (e.g. medication, electroconvulsive therapy) but persists at a fully syndromal level beyond the physiological effect of that treatment is sufficient evidence for a hypomanic episode diagnosis. However, caution is indicated so that one or two symptoms (particularly increased irritability, edginess, or agitation following antidepressant use) are not taken as sufficient for diagnosis of a hypomanic episode, nor necessarily indicative of a bipolar diathesis.

Major depressive episode

a. Five (or more) of the following symptoms have been present during the same 2-week period and represent a change from previous functioning; at least one of the symptoms is either (1) depressed mood or (2) loss of interest or pleasure.
   Note: Do not include symptoms that are clearly attributable to a medical condition.
   1. Depressed mood most of the day, nearly everyday, as indicated by either subjective report (e.g. feels sad, empty, or hopeless) or observation made by others (e.g. appears tearful).
      (*Note:* In children and adolescents, can be irritable mood.)
   2. Markedly diminished interest or pleasure in all, or almost all, activities most of the day, nearly everyday (as indicated by either subjective account or observation).
   3. Significant weight loss when not dieting or weight gain (e.g. a change of more than 5% of body weight in a month), or decrease or increase in appetite nearly everyday. (*Note:* In children, consider failure to make expected weight gain.)
   4. Insomnia or hypersomnia nearly everyday.
   5. Psychomotor agitation or retardation nearly everyday (observable by others; not merely subjective feelings of restlessness or being slowed down).
   6. Fatigue or loss of energy nearly everyday.

Contd...

Contd...

7. Feelings of worthlessness or excessive or inappropriate guilt (which may be delusional) nearly everyday (not merely self-reproach or guilt about being sick).
8. Diminished ability to think or concentrate, or indecisiveness, nearly everyday (either by subjective account or as observed by others).
9. Recurrent thoughts of death (not just fear of dying), recurrent suicidal ideation without a specific plan, a suicide attempt, or a specific plan for committing suicide.

b. The symptoms cause clinically significant distress or impairment in social, occupational, or other important areas of functioning.
c. The episode is not attributable to the physiological effects of a substance or another medical condition.
Note: Criteria A–C above constitute a major depressive episode.
Note: Responses to a significant loss (e.g. bereavement, financial ruin, losses from a natural disaster, a serious medical illness or disability) may include the feelings of intense sadness, rumination about the loss, insomnia, poor appetite, and weight loss noted in Criterion A, which may resemble a depressive episode. Although such symptoms may be understandable or considered appropriate to the loss, the presence of a major depressive episode in addition to the normal response to a significant loss should be carefully considered. This decision inevitably requires the exercise of clinical judgment based on the individual's history and the cultural norms for the expression of distress in the context of loss.

DSM-5 Bipolar II disorder

a. Criteria have been met for at least one hypomanic episode (Criteria A–F under "Hypomanic Episode" above) and at least one major depressive episode (Criteria A–C under "Major Depressive Episode" above),
b. There has never been a manic episode.
c. The occurrence of the hypomanic episode(s) and major depressive episode(s) is not better explained by schizoaffective disorder, schizophrenia, schizophreniform disorder, delusional disorder, or other specified or unspecified schizophrenia spectrum and other psychotic disorder.
d. The symptoms of depression or the unpredictability caused by frequent alternation between periods of depression and hypomania causes clinically significant distress or impairment in social, occupational, or other important areas of functioning.

Specify current or most recent episode:
- Hypomanic
- Depressed

Specify if:
- With anxious distress
- With mixed features
- With rapid cycling
- With mood-congruent psychotic features
- With mood-incongruent psychotic features
- With catatonia.

Coding note: Use additional code 293.89 (F06.1).
- With peripartum onset
- With seasonal pattern: Applies only to the pattern of major depressive episodes.

Contd...

Contd...

Specify course if full criteria for a mood episode are not currently met:
- In partial remission
- In full remission

Specify severity if full criteria for a mood episode are currently met:
- Mild
- Moderate
- Severe

Panel 8: Lines of evidence supporting a continuum between bipolar I and bipolar II disorder

- Similar age at onset
- Same core feature of overactivity in mania and hypomania
- Bipolar I and II have long-term diagnostic stability, but hypomania is frequently present in the course of bipolar I
- *Family history:* More likely for relatives to have the same type of disorder as probands than different type (therefore, distinct disorders); but bipolar II not uncommon in relatives of bipolar I probands; bipolar I more common in relatives of bipolar I probands than in controls; major depressive disorder most common mood disorder in relatives of bipolar I and II probands
- *Grading of symptoms:* Syndromal and subsyndromal depressions more common in bipolar II than in bipolar I, syndromal and subsyndromal mania and hypomania more common in bipolar I
- Grading of the switching to mania/hypomania during antidepressants (lower in bipolar II)
- *Clinical picture of depression:* Similar atypical symptoms (e.g. over-sleeping, over-eating) and psychomotor changes
- Manic and hypomanic symptoms predicting onset of both bipolar I and II

DSM-IV-TR reports a lifetime community prevalence of 5% for bipolar II disorder. More recently, better designed studies than those used to inform this manual have shown a much higher lifetime community prevalence of bipolar II and bipolar spectrum disorders, similar to that of depressive disorders: 0–2.4% for bipolar I disorder, 0.3–4.8% for bipolar II disorder, 0.5–6.3% for cyclothymic disorder, and 0.8–13.5% (5% is the most likely value) for bipolar spectrum. Among depressed outpatients with bipolar II disorder, bipolar spectrum, or major depressive disorder, about 50% have been found to be bipolar II disorder, compared with that reported in older studies, is related to several advances. Use of semistructured interviews by trained clinicians, rather than the previous use of fully structured interviews by lay interviewers: the yes or no structured questions, and the absence of clinical evaluation in structured interviewing could lead to underdiagnosis of bipolar II disorder, and misdiagnosis as major depressive disorder. Reduction of minimum duration of hypomania required to diagnose bipolar II disorder of 2 days (evidence-based), instead of the 4-day cutoff used by DSM-IV-TR (consensus-based), bypassing the stem question of the structured clinical interview for DSM-IV to assess history of hypomania. This question requires the patient to remember periods of elevated or irritable mood, but many individuals with bipolar II disorder give a negative response, because they see these periods as normal mood fluctuations, or, if the wording of the question includes "much more than usual", as a severe disorder, which is often denied, shift in focus of investigation for history of hypomania from mood change to overactivity (increased goal directed activities), an observable behavior that is easier to remember than mood change, and frequently aids memories of a concurrent mood change.

Findings of several clinical and psychometric studies. Suggest that over-activity is the core feature of hypomania, lending support to its upgrading to the same priority level as mood change in the diagnosis of hypomania. Instead, however, DSM-IV-TR states that elevated mood is the "prototypical" symptom of hypomania, misleading clinicians into believing that hypomania cannot be diagnosed if elevated mood is absent. Overactivity, more than usual working hours, social life, sexual activity, travels, spending, brilliant ideas, and plans can increase functioning if the concurrent mental overactivity is connected (as often happens), or can reduce functioning if mental over activity is racing too much, leading to disconnection of ideas, or if it is focused more on risky behaviors. Bipolar II disorder and cyclothymic temperament (defined by high instability of mood, thinking and behavior) can occur at the same time. Suicidality, substance abuse, and risky behaviors are more common when these conditions occur together, and this combination increases the instability of bipolar II disorder, easily leading to its misdiagnosis as borderline personality disorder, which is highly unstable.

BIPOLAR II DISORDER COMPARED WITH MAJOR DEPRESSIVE DISORDER

The basic, distinguishing features of bipolar II disorder compared with major depressive disorder are lower age at onset, more recurrence, more bipolar (types I and II) family history, more atypical depressions (including symptoms such as overeating and over-sleeping), and more mixed depression. Mixed depression, which is a key component of the continuum concept of mood disorders, might have important effects on treatment for depression.

MIXED DEPRESSION (DEPRESSIVE MIXED STATES)

Sporadic reports on mixed depression before the year 2000 went almost unnoticed. By strictly following the DSM-IV structured clinical interview, mixed depression cannot be diagnosed in bipolar II and major depressive disorders, because this method does not allow assessment of hypomanic symptoms in major depressive episodes. In DSM-IV-TR, only bipolar I mixed state can be diagnosed, which requires the co-occurrence of full mania and major depressive episode.

Mixed depression is defined by the combination of depression (major depressive episode) and noneuphoric, usually subsyndromal, manic or hypomanic symptoms (Panel 9). It is present in bipolar I and II disorders, and in major depressive disorders. It is most studied in bipolar II and major depressive disorders. Intradepressive manic or hypomanic symptoms may start spontaneously during depression (i.e. manic/hypomanic symptoms are independent episode), or can be related to cycling between mania or hypomania and depression (a transition state, believed by Kraepelin to be the cause of most mixed states). The manic or hypomanic symptoms of mixed depression can also be induced or worsened by antidepressants.

Panel 9: Suggested diagnostic criteria for mixed depression

- A major depressive episode according to DSM-IV-TR
- Two to three or more concurrent DSM-IV-TR manic/hypomanic symptoms
- Transition state during cycling between mania/hypomania and depression
- Independent episode (i.e. unrelated to cycling)
- With psychomotor agitation (agitated depression)
- Antidepressant associated
- In bipolar I disorder
- In bipolar II disorder
- In major depressive disorder.

Mixed depression has a moderate diagnostic stability, which does not support a categorical distinction. Compared with nonmixed depression, it is more common in bipolar disorders, and is more associated with family history of bipolar disorders, lower age at onset, longer duration, worse outcome, and poorer response to treatments. These differences might aid its subtyping.

Definition

Few studies have included samples of untreated mood disorders, allowing the study of spontaneous onset intra-depression manic or hypomanic symptoms. Several definitions of mixed depression have been suggested. Some of which require a cutoff of at least two to three intradepression manic/hypomanic symptoms, and some of which require specific manic/hypomanic symptoms, such as psychomotor agitation (agitated depression). At present, the definition that requires a cutoff of three symptoms is the most validated.

The diagnostic validity of agitated depression, a diagnosis not included in DSM-III and DSM-IV but frequently used in clinical practice, has been tested. Agitated depression was often found to be mixed and bipolar. These findings question the diagnostic validity of the definition and suggest that agitated depression is probably a more mixed variant of mixed depression.

Frequency

Frequency of mixed depression in bipolar I, bipolar II, and major depressive disorders ranges between 20% and 70%

depending on setting, interview methods, instruments used to assess intradepression manic or hypomanic symptoms, prevalence of bipolar disorders compared with major depressive disorder, whether individuals have been treated or not, and definitions used. It is more common in bipolar I and II disorders than in major depressive disorder, but is not uncommon in major depressive disorder (around 30% of outpatients with the condition may have mixed depression).

MANIC AND HYPOMANIC SYMPTOMS AND BIPOLAR NATURE

The most common manic and hypomanic symptoms of mixed depression, which are more severe in bipolar I than in bipolar II and major depressive disorders, are irritability, mental overactivity (flight of ideas, racing thoughts, crowded thoughts, creative thinking), and behavioral overactivity (psychomotor agitation and increased talkativeness), which represent the condition "manic foundation", according to Kraepelin. Manic and hypomanic symptoms listed in DSM-IV-TR include those (such as irritability and psychomotor agitation) that are present in many axis 1 disorders especially anxiety disorders, which are common in mixed depression and in axis 2 (personality) disorders. Whether a correlation exists between psychomotor agitation and anxiety in unclear. Irritability, psychomotor agitation, and racing or crowded thoughts are more likely to be bipolar than nonbipolar in samples of individuals with mood disorders. The bipolar nature of these symptoms is supported, in individuals with mood disorders, by a family history of bipolar disorders. Kraepelin included these symptoms among the basic symptoms of the manic and hypomanic states. However, these symptoms are unlikely to have a bipolar nature when present in nonmood axis 1 disorders. The same reasoning could be applied to psychotic symptoms, which are present in many axis 1 disorders (including mood disorders), but are the stem criterion for diagnosis of psychotic disorders.

A Categorical Definition

A categorical definition of mixed depression is questionable, following Kendell and Jablensky's method based on finding a bi-modal distribution, because the distribution of intradepression hypomanic symptoms between bipolar II disorder and major depressive disorder is not bi-modal, the distribution of lifetime manic or hypomanic symptoms between bipolar I disorder and major depressive disorder is not bi-modal, and the distribution of depressive and manic symptoms of mania is not bi-modal. Furthermore, a proportional relation exists between intradepression hypomanic symptoms and the degree of bipolar family history in bipolar II and major depressive disorders, which should not be found in distinct disorders. For clinicians, however, categories are more useful than dimensions, and a cutoff in the dimensions of mixed depression that defines the need for treatment has to be found. Some investigators have tested definitions of two to three intradepressive manic and hypomanic symptoms in pharmacological studies, and found that the presence of these two to three symptoms increased the risk fo switching to mania or hypomania in bipolar I and II depression treated by antidepressants (Panel 10).

Panel 10: Lines of evidence supporting the bipolar nature of mixed depression

- More common in bipolar I and II disorders than in MDD
- Family history of bipolar disorders
- Dose-response relationship between intradepression hypomanic symptoms and bipolar family history loading
- "Manic/hypomanic/excitement" factor present in MDD
- Factor structure of intradepression hypomanic symptoms similar to factor structure of intradepression hypomania.
- Intradepression full hypomania.
- Mixed MDD closer to bipolar disorder than to nonmixed MDD on bipolar validators
- MDD shifting to bipolar disorder more likely to have mixed depresssion.
- Mixed depression, compared with nonmixed depression, more likely to switch to mania/hypomania with anti-depressants
- Worsening by antidepressants
- MDD Major depressive disorder.

Implications

From a clinical practice point of view, mixed depression has important implications. Depression should be systematically assessed for concurrent manic or hypomanic symptoms, which, if present, should lead to a careful probing for history of mania or hypomania. Antidepressant treatment of mixed depression should be cautious, because antidepressants alone (i.e. not protected by mood stabilizing agents) can worsen intra depression manic and hypomanic symptoms such as racing thoughts and psychomotor agitation, sometimes leading to suicidal behavior. Switching of depression to mania or hypomania while taking antidepressants might be more likely in mixed than in nonmixed depression. The US Food and Drug Administration (FDA), in its recent warning on antidepressants, has listed among possible precursors of occasional suicidality related to antidepressants and several features of mixed depression are such as irritability, psychomotor agitation, and bipolarity. Mixed depression is associated with a higher risk of suicidality than is nonmixed depression. Intradepression psychomotor agitation and racing or crowded thoughts are independent predictors of suicidal ideas, and mixed depression is often present in individuals before suicide attempts. Therefore, the suicidality sometimes related to antidepressants is probably not caused by the antidepressants, but by clinicians using only antidepressant, if necessary. Controlled trials are needed to provide more evidence, but are almost impossible to do in view of the FDA warning. Therefore, retrospective, naturalistic, and reanalysis studies are the only available source of information about treatment of mixed depression. The current, limited evidence seems to lend support to the use of mood stabilizers alone or with antidepressants for treatment of mixed depression.

BIPOLAR DISORDERS IN CHILDREN AND ADOLESCENTS

Perhaps the most advanced studies about bipolar disorders are those that have been done in children and adolescents. These findings might increase insight into the onset and mechanisms of the disease, and lead to treatments that prevent development of adult bipolar disorders.

Prevalence of bipolar disorders in children (mainly bipolar II disorder and bipolar spectrum) can be around 6% in community samples, and in 2–15% in clinical samples. Bipolar disorders in children are often mixed, and very rapid cycling. Mania and hypomania, which are much more common than depression, are often brief (less than minimum duration specified by DSM-IV-TR) and highly recurrent. Course and outcome of childhood or adolescent bipolar disorders are more severe than in adult-onset bipolar disorders. Likelihood family history of bipolar disorder is high, and is greater than in adult-onset bipolar disorders. Mixed mania and mixed depression are common. Irritability is not a distinguishing feature of these mixed states, which have a worse course and outcome than in adults i.e. more recurrences, more impairment, and greater severity. Psychosis, suicidality, anxiety disorders, substance abuse, antisocial behavior and attention-deficit hyperactivity disorder (ADHD) frequently co-occur in bipolar disorders of this age group. Continuous mood lability, irritability, and temper outbursts are also a common state, not meeting any DSM-IV-TR criteria. Differential diagnosis between bipolar disorders and ADHD is based on classic manic and hypomanic symptoms such as elevated mood, grandiosity, and racing thoughts, and on family history of bipolar disorder, because irritability, hyperactivity and short attention span are present in both disorders. Misdiagnosis of bipolar disorder as ADHD and major depressive disorder is common, leading to the use of stimulants and antidepressants, which might worsen the course instead of mood stabilizing agents.

CONTINUUM OR SPECTRUM CONCEPT OF MOOD DISORDERS

The DSM-IV-TR classification of mood disorders is based on the concept of unipolar-bipolar division, which took the place of Kraepelin's unitary view in the 1960s. According to the unipolar-bipolar division concept, unipolar depressive disorders and bipolar disorders are distinct, categorical disorders, separated by clear boundaries. The division of mood disorders was based on differences seen with several diagnostic validators. Compared with unipolar depression, bipolar disorder (at that time only bipolar I was diagnosed), was found to have, apart from mania, the following distinguishing features: sex (female as common as male in bipolar I, female more common than male in unipolar depression); age at onset (often younger than 30 years in bipolar I disorder, often older in unipolar depression); number of episodes (greater in bipolar I disorder); clinical picture of depression (psychomotor retardation and hypersomnia in bipolar I disorder, psychomotor agitation and insomnia in unipolar depression); and family history (mania common in relatives of bipolar I disorder probands, uncommon in relatives of unipolar depression probands). An important limitation of this division is that bipolar II disorder, which seems to be the link between bipolar and depressive disorders, was not included in this classification. Increasingly, evidence supports instead a return to Kraepelin's unitary concept of mood disorders. The continuum (also known as spectrum or dimensional) concept of mood disorders includes disorders ranging from bipolar I and II to recurrent major depressive disorder and minor depressive disorder. Research on bipolar spectrum disorders in children and adolescents has added further support to the concept. The continuum of mood disorders is based on several lines of evidence summarized in Panel 11.

Panel 11: Lines of evidence supporting continuum of mood disorders

- Grading of severity, duration, and frequency of mood episodes
- Mixture of depressive and manic/hypomanic symptoms in the same episode the mixed states)
- Lack of bimodality in manic/hypomanic symptoms in or between bipolar disorder and MDD
- Correlation between manic/hypomanic symptoms and depressive symptoms
- Dose-response relation between intradepression hypomanic symptoms and bipolar family history (i.e. the higher the number/score of intradepression hypomanic symptoms, the higher the bipolar family history (i.e. the higher the number/score of intradepression hypomanic symptoms, the higher the bipolar family history loading)
- No bimodality of age at onset between bipolar disorder and MDD
- No bimodality of temperamental instability between bipolar disorder and MDD
- Many MDD shifting to bipolar disorder in the long-term
- Bipolar signs common in MDD (such as bipolar family history, young age at onset, many recurrences, lifetime and intradepressive manic/hypomanic symptoms)
- Manic/hypomanic symptoms predicting onset of bipolar disorder and MDD
- Residual manic symptoms predicting depressive recurrences in bipolar disorder.

Treatment Findings

The treatment of mood disorders is not discussed in detail in this Seminar; the focus will be on the pharmacological and psychotherapeutic evidence supporting and not supporting the continuum concept.

Response to antidepressants and antibipolar agents can be seen as a proxy of the biology of mood disorders. A similar response by patients with supposedly different disorders to these drugs might support the continuum concept, whereas differing responses might support the division of mood disorders. Since antidepressants are the gold standard of treatment in depressive disorders, where as lithium is the gold standard of treatment for bipolar disorders, the basic test is the assessment of the efficacy of lithium in depressive disorders, and of antidepressants in bipolar disorders. Randomized double blind, placebo-controlled trials can show the best evidence of efficacy, but these trials are limited by the selection of individuals not representative of usual clinical practice. Naturalistic studies of effectiveness in usual clinical practice are more useful, if designed to reduce biases.

ANTIDEPRESSANTS IN BIPOLAR AND DEPRESSIVE DISORDERS

Evidence for the efficacy and effectiveness of antidepressants in acute bipolar depression is mixed, or do not induce switching is uncertain. In depressive disorders, antidepressants do not seem to increase switching more than placebo. If antidepressants facilitated switching in bipolar disorders much more than in depressive disorders, the concept of a continuum would not be supported.

Some evidence suggests that antidepressants might increase the number of recurrences (manic and depressive episodes) in bipolar disorders, including rapid cycling, which is defined as four or more episodes per year (mainly depressive, and mainly in bipolar II disorder). However, the evidence for this pattern is weak. Kraepelins reported a spontaneous increase of recurrences related in ageing in a subgroup of patients with manic depressive insanity. Evidence showing that antidepressants increased recurrences in major depressive disorder. Prevention of recurrences of bipolar (mainly bipolar II) depression by antidepressants, if any, is weak. Antidepressants are not effective and can actually worsen acute mania and hypomania, and can induce, rather than prevent episodes of mania and hypomania.

LITHIUM IN BIPOLAR DISORDERS IN DEPRESSIVE DISORDERS

In acute bipolar (mainly bipolar I) depression, lithium seems to be effetive and no other lithium seems to be more effective. In acute major depressive disorder, the efficacy of lithium, if any, is lower than in bipolar disorder. Cycling and switching can be prevented by lithium. Lithium can prevent recurrences in bipolar disorders (more effective in mania than depression in bipolar I, as effective in depression as in hypomania in bipolar II) and in depressive disorders, and might be as effective as antidepressants in preventing recurrences in MDD.Lithium is effective in treatment of acute mania and hypomania and in prevention of mania and hypomania. The drug has been surpassed (in clinical use, but not in efficacy) by many modern mood, stabilizing agents, such has valproic acid, carbamazepine, neuroleptics (first-generation antipsychotics), and second generation antipsychotics such as olanzapine, risperidone, ziprasidone, quetiapine, and aripiprazole. These agents are effective in acute mania and hypomania, but less effective or ineffective in prevention of bipolar I depression. Only quetiapine seems effective in acute bipolar I and II depression, but more replications in naturalistic settings are needed. Evidence for efficacy of lamotrigine in acute treatment and prevention of depression in bipolar I and II disorders is not strong (negative, unpublished studies have been done), and the drug has little or no effect against mania. It has not been formally tested in major depressive disorder. The combination of olanzapine and fluoxetine seems effective in bipolar I depression, but replication studies are needed.

PSYCHOLOGICAL INTERVENTIONS

Cognitive behavioral therapy is effective in nonpsychotic major depressive disorder. Bipolar I and II depression are associated with more behavioral symptoms (e.g. Loss of energy, hypersomnia) than cognitive symptoms (e.g. Low self-esteem) compared with major depressive disorder. Variants of cognitive behavioral therapy that are more focused on behavioral change, seems as effective in major depressive disorder as in bipolar depression. Efficacy of cognitive behavioral therapy and interpersonal social rhythm therapy is assessed on the basis of effects on symptoms and recurrences.

SUMMARY OF TREATMENT FINDINGS

The effects of antidepressants and lithium in bipolar disorders and in depressive disorders seem to have more differences than similarities, contradicting the idea of a continuum of mood disorders. However, treatment of bipolar II disorder is understudied. The risk of switching to hypomania by use of antidepressants seems lower in bipolar II than in bipolar I disorder, and lithium seems effective in preventing recurrences in major depressive disorder without bipolar signs are the extreme poles of the mood spectrum, differences in treatment responses are more likely to be noted than similarities. However, bipolar II is a disorder positioned between these extremes, and its pharmacotherapy could add important evidence in support of or contradicting, the continuum concept. Prevention of recurrences in bipolar II disorder and major depressive disorder by lithium seems to be preliminary pharmacological evidence in support of a continuum of mood disorders, but several pharmacological data seem to support the opposite view.

CONCLUSION

Bipolar disorders, especially bipolar II and the related bipolar spectrum disorders, are much more common that previously reported, and treatment of bipolar II disorder and bipolar spectrum disorders is much understudied. Controlled pharmacological studies are greatly needed, and should stratify samples taking into account the frequently mixed profile of bipolar disorders.

7.8 BIPOLAR DISORDER: A FOCUS ON DEPRESSION

JN Vyas, RK Solanki

CLINICAL PROBLEM

Bipolar disorder, a medical illness with substantial morbidity and mortality, is characterized by episodic recurrent mania or hypomania and major depression.[367] The hallmark of bipolar disorder is at least one episode of mania (bipolar I disorder) or hypomania (bipolar II disorder) (Table 4).[368] The greater severity of the elevated mood and the associated functional disability distinguish bipolar I mania (which is characterized by psychosis, the need for urgent care or hospitalization, or marked impairment) from bipolar II hypomania. In contrast to patients with mania, patients with hypomania infrequently seek evaluation unless a bipolar diagnosis is already established and there is concern regarding progression of the illness (i.e. becoming manic). Whereas the older term "manic-depressive illness" implied a depressive episode after each episode of mania, many patients present with one or more episodes of major depression before the first manic or hypomanic episode that defines bipolar disorder. The diagnostic criteria for an episode of major depression in bipolar disorder are the same as the criteria for unipolar major depressive disorder (Table 4).

Table 4: Key diagnostic criteria distinguishing bipolar I disorder from bipolar II disorder.

Manic episode (Bipolar I disorder)	*Hypomanic episode (Bipolar II disorder)*
Distinct period during which there is an abnormally and persistently elevated, expansive, or irritable mood lasting at least 15 week (or less if hospitalization is required)	Distinct period during which there is an abnormally and persistently elevated, expansive, or irritable mood lasting at least 4 days
Must be accompanied by at least three of the following symptoms (four if mood is only irritable): inflated self-esteem or grandiosity, decreased need for sleep, pressured speech, racing thoughts, distractibility, increased involvement in goal-directed activity or psychomotor agitation, excessive involvement in pleasurable activities with a high potential for painful consequences.	Must be accompanied by at least three of the following symptoms (four if mood is only irritable): inflated self-esteem or grandiosity, decreased need for sleep, pressured speech, racing thoughts, distractibility, increased involvement in goal-directed activity or psychomotor agitation, excessive involvement in pleasurable activities with a high potential for painful consequences
Symptoms do not meet criteria for a mixed episode	Hypomanic episodes must be clearly different from the person's usual nondepressed mood, and there must be a clear change in functioning that is not characteristics of the persons usual functioning
Disturbance must be sufficiently severe to cause marked impairment in social or occupational functioning or to require hospitalization, or it is characterized by the presence of psychotic features	Changes in mood and functioning must be observable by others. In contrast to a manic episode, a hypomanic episode is not severe enough to cause marked impairment to social or occupational functioning or to require hospitalization, and there are no psychotic features
Symptoms not due to direct physiological effect of medication, general medical condition, or substance abuse	Symptoms not due to direct physiological effect of medication general medical condition, or substance abuse
* Criteria from American Psychiatry Association[2]	

In a US study,[369] the lifetime prevalence rate of bipolar disorder was 4.5% (1.0% for bipolar 1 disorder, 1.1% for bipolar II disorder, and 2.4% for manic and depressive symptoms that did not meet all the diagnostic criteria for bipolar I or bipolar II disorder). Bipolar disorder is associated with premature death and is among the leading causes of disability in the developed world in people 15–44 years of age.[370] The rate of completed suicide is approximately 5% among patients who have never been hospitalized, but it is as high as 25% early in the course of the illness.[371,372] The illness is frequently associated with other coexisting conditions, most commonly anxiety disorders and substance use disorders.[373,374] These disorders are associated with an increased risk of suicidal ideation and of mood switches from depression to mania.[375,376]

Although the severity of mania is evident, most disability associated with bipolar disorder occurs in the depressive phase. In one study, there were significantly more work days lost per ill worker per year among patients with bipolar disorder than among those with unipolar major depression: the difference was driven primarily by recurrent depression, not mania.[377] Depressive episodes and low-level (i.e. subsyndromal) symptoms of depression typically last longer than manic episodes and low level symptoms of mania. In the National Institute of Mental Health's Collaborative Depression Study involving patients with bipolar I disorder who were followed for more than 12 years, patients were symptomatic almost 50% of the time; depressive symptoms occurred about one third of the time; manic symptoms occurred about 10% of the time, and mixed symptoms occurred about 6% of the time.[378] Low-level symptoms of depression are also associated with functional disability[379] and subsequent depressive relapse.[380,381]

DSM-5 Diagnostic criteria manic episode (bipolar I disorder)

a. A distinct period of abnormally and persistently elevated, expansive, or irritable mood and abnormally and persistently increased goal-directed activity or energy, lasting at least 1 week and present most of the day, nearly everyday (or any duration if hospitalization is necessary).
b. During the period of mood disturbance and increased energy or activity, three (or more) of the following symptoms (four if the mood is only irritable) are present to a significant degree and represent a noticeable change from usual behavior:
   1. Inflated self-esteem or grandiosity.
   2. Decreased need for sleep (e.g. feels rested after only 3 hours of sleep).
   3. More talkative than usual or pressure to keep talking.
   4. Flight of ideas or subjective experience that thoughts are racing.
   5. Distractibility (i.e. attention too easily drawn to unimportant or irrelevant external stimuli), as reported or observed.
   6. Increase in goal-directed activity (either socially, at work or school, or sexually) or psychomotor agitation (i.e. purposeless nongoal-directed activity).

Contd...

Contd...

   7. Excessive involvement in activities that have a high potential for painful consequences (e.g. engaging in unrestrained buying sprees, sexual indiscretions, or foolish business investments).
c. The mood disturbance is sufficiently severe to cause marked impairment in social or occupational functioning or to necessitate hospitalization to prevent harm to self or others, or there are psychotic features.
d. The episode is not attributable to the physiological effects of a substance (e.g. a drug of abuse, a medication, other treatment) or to another medical condition.
   Note: A full manic episode that emerges during antidepressant treatment (e.g. medication, electroconvulsive therapy) but persists at a fully syndromal level beyond the physiological effect of that treatment is sufficient evidence for a manic episode and, therefore, a bipolar I diagnosis.
   Note: Criteria A–D constitute a manic episode. At least one lifetime manic episode is required for the diagnosis of bipolar I disorder.

DSM-5 Diagnostic criteria for hypomanic episode (Bipolar II)

a. A distinct period of abnormally and persistently elevated, expansive, or irritable mood and abnormally and persistently increased activity or energy, lasting at least 4 consecutive days and present most of the day, nearly everyday.
b. During the period of mood disturbance and increased energy and activity, three (or more) of the following symptoms have persisted (four if the mood is only irritable), represent a noticeable change from usual behavior, and have been present to a significant degree:
   1. Inflated self-esteem or grandiosity.
   2. Decreased need for sleep (e.g. feels rested after only 3 hours of sleep).
   3. More talkative than usual or pressure to keep talking.
   4. Flight of ideas or subjective experience that thoughts are racing.
   5. Distractibility (i.e. attention too easily drawn to unimportant or irrelevant external stimuli), as reported or observed.
   6. Increase in goal-directed activity (either socially, at work or school, or sexually) or psychomotor agitation.
   7. Excessive involvement in activities that have a high potential for painful consequences (e.g. engaging in unrestrained buying sprees, sexual indiscretions, or foolish business investments).
c. The episode is associated with an unequivocal change in functioning that is uncharacteristic of the individual when not symptomatic.
d. The disturbance in mood and the change in functioning are observable by others.
e. The episode is not severe enough to cause marked impairment in social or occupational functioning or to necessitate hospitalization. If there are psychotic features, the episode is, by definition, manic.
f. The episode is not attributable to the physiological effects of a substance (e.g. a drug of abuse, a medication or other treatment).

Contd...

Contd...

Note: A full hypomanic episode that emerges during antidepressant treatment (e.g. medication, electroconvulsive therapy) but persists at a fully syndromal level beyond the physiological effect of that treatment is sufficient evidence for a hypomanic episode diagnosis. However, caution is indicated so that one or two symptoms (particularly increased irritability, edginess, or agitation following antidepressant use) are not taken as sufficient for diagnosis of a hypomanic episode, nor necessarily indicative of a bipolar diathesis.

STRATEGIES AND EVIDENCE

Diagnosis and Assessment

The initial evaluation of a patient presenting with depressed mood should include screening for alcohol and drug use, assessment of suicidality, personal and family psychiatric history, and a physical examination and laboratory testing as indicated to rule out additional medical problems that may be contributing to symptoms. A meeting with significant others or family member may be helpful in obtaining additional information, particularly regarding the severity of symptoms. A family history of bipolar disorder, the onset of symptoms before 25 years of age, and more frequent episodes with a shorter duration (i.e. <6 months) increase the likelihood of a diagnosis of bipolar depression rather than unipolar depression.[1] Some, but not all, studies have also suggested that hypersomnia and hyperphagia are more common in bipolar depression, whereas insomnia (specifically early morning awakening) and reduced appetite are more typical of unipolar depression.[367]

In conjunction with the clinical assessment, the Mood Disorder Questionnaire is a useful screening instrument for bipolar disorder in patients presenting with depression. This questionnaire includes 13 yes-or-no questions regarding symptoms that are typically associated with mania[382,383]: a "yes" answer to 7 or more questions about symptoms occurring concurrently and associated with at least moderate disability is considered a positive screening result. The Mood Disorder Questionnaire has been validated both in patients in outpatient psychiatric clinic and in the general population. However, recent studies have shown false positive rates between 15% and 30%, reflecting the overlap of symptoms of bipolar disorder with those of conditions such as attention-deficit disorder, eating disorders, substance-use disorder, post-traumatic stress disorder, and borderline personality disorder.[384,385]

MANAGEMENT

FDA-approved Treatments for Bipolar Depression

Although depression is more frequent than mania as a manifestation of bipolar disorder, medications for mania have been studied much more extensively. For acute mania, the Food and Drug Administration (FDA) has approved 10 treatments: one typical antipsychotic agent, lithium, two antiepileptic agents, and six atypical antipsychotic agents. In contrast, there are only two FDA-approved treatments for bipolar depression—quetiapine and a combination of olanzapine and fluoxetine. Quetiapine and olanzapine are among several medications broadly defined as mood stabilizers, on the basis of their efficacy in treating acute mania or depression and in maintaining a clinical response without precipitating a switch to the alternate phase of the illness.

Four 8 week, placebo-controlled trials,[386-389] involving a total of 2593 subjects with bipolar I or bipolar II disorder, have demonstrated the efficacy of quetiapine monotherapy (at a dose of 300 mg or 600 mg) in treating bipolar depression. As compared with placebo, quetiapine resulted in a greater decrease from baseline to 8 weeks in the primary outcome measure (the score on the Montgomery and Asberg Depression Rating Scale (MADRS), which ranges from 0 to 60, with higher scores indicating a greater severity of depressive symptoms), a higher rate of response (defined as a 50% reduction in symptoms), and a higher rate of symptom remission (MADRS score, 12 or lower). Outcomes associated with the 300 mg or 600 mg doses were similar. Two of the trials also included active comparison drugs: lithium[388] or the serotonin reuptake inhibitor paraoxetine.[389] As compared with these other agents, quetiapine (at a dose of 300 mg or 600 mg daily) resulted in a greater decrease from baseline to 8 weeks in the MADRS score, higher rates of response and remission (except remission in the comparison of the 300 mg dose with paroxetine[389]), and a reduced rate of a switch to mania or hypomania (3.1% vs 10.7% with paroxetine and 8.9% with placebo).

In another 8 weeks, randomized trial, involving 833 patients with bipolar I disorder, a combination of olanzapine (mean daily dose, 7.4 mg) and fluoxetine (mean daily dose, 39.3 mg) and olanzapine monotherapy (mean dose, 9.7 mg daily) were both superior to placebo in improving depression scores[390]; the overall decrease in the MADRS score was significantly greater with the olanzapine-fluoxetine combination than with olanzapine monotherapy. The rate of a switch to mania did not differ significantly between the drug combination (6.4%) and placebo (6.7%). Major concerns regarding both quetiapine and the olanzapine-fluoxetine combination are weight gain, with the associated risk of diabetes, and the risk of tardive dyskinesia. Although the risk of tardive dyskinesia cannot be estimated from these short-term trials, other data have indicated that the risk associated with atypical antipsychotic agents is significantly lower than the risk associated with typical (first-generation) antipsychotic agents (e.g. the risk associated with haloperidol is estimated to be 3–5% per year of exposure).[391]

The antidepressant effect reported for quetiapine and olanzapine-fluoxetine does not appear to be generalizable to other atypical antipsychotics. Using the same primary outcome measure, two double-blind, placebo-controlled trials involving a total of 749 patients with bipolar I disorder showed no significant antidepressant effect of aripiprazole, an agent approved for the treatment of mania and for maintenance therapy (i.e. prevention of manic, mixed, or depressive episodes).[392] Similarly, in 6 weeks randomized trials, ziprasidone, another agent approved for mania and maintenance, was no more effective than placebo in reducing depressive symptoms when used either as monotherapy or adjunctive therapy (Table 5).[393]

Table 5: Treatments for bipolar disorder

Drug class and agent	*Dose*	*Research of approval*				*Side effects and warnings*
		Depression	Mania	Mixed Symptoms	Maintenance Therapy	
Atypical antipsychotic agent						Warnings for increased risk of death among elderly patients with dementia-related psychosis, neuroleptic malignant syndrome, tardive dyskinesia, hyperglycemia or diabetes, and seizures
Aripiprazole ↑	For acute mania or maintenance therapy, 15–30 mg/day	Controlled studies do not support use as mono therapy	FDA-approved	FDA-approved	FDA-approved	Extrapyramidal side effects, somnolence, and tremor
Asenapine ↑	For acute mania, 10 mg twice daily sublingually		FDA - approved	FDA-approved		Extrapyramidal side effects, weight gain, somnolence, and dizziness
Olanzapine ↑	For acute mania, 10–20 mg/day; for maintenance therapy, 5–20 mg/day	Controlled study supports use as monotherapy	FDA-approved	FDA-approved	FDA-approved	Extrapyramidal side effects; weight gain, dry mouth, dizziness, tremor, and gastrointestinal side effects; additional warnings for hyperlipidemia and hyperprolactinemia
Quetiapine and quetiapine, extended release ↑‡	For acute mania or maintenance therapy, 400–800 mg/day, for depression, 300–600 mg/day	FDA-approved	FDA approved	FDA-approved	FDA-approved	Extrapyramidal side effects, weight gain, dry mouth, fatigue and gastrointestinal side effects; additional warning for hyperlipidemia
Risperidone Oral ↑ Intramuscular∫	For acute mania, 1–6 mg/day 25 mg every 2 week		FDA-approved	FDA-approved	FDA-approved	Extrapyramidal side effects, somnolence, and gastrointestinal side effects: additional warning for hyperprolactinemia
Ziprasidone‡	For acute mania or maintenance therapy, 80–120 mg/day	Controlled studies do not support use as adjunct or monotherapy	FDA-approved	FDA-approved	FDA-approved	Extrapyramidal side effects, somnolence, dizziness, asthenia, abnormal vision, and vomiting: additional warnings for QT prolongation and rash
Olanzapine-fluoxetine combination	6–12 mg and 25–50 mg once a day	FDA-approved				Fluoxetine associated with increased risk of suicidal thoughts and actions among some children, teenagers, and young adults
Antiepileptic drug						
Carbamazepine, extended release	For acute mania, 400–1600 mg in divided doses twice daily		FDA-approved	FDA-approved		Dizziness, somnolence, and co-ordination problems; warnings for serious rash, including Stevens-Johnson syndrome and toxic epidermal necrolysis, agranulocytosis, suicidal ideation, teratogenicity, and aplastic anemia

Contd...

Contd...

Drug class and agent	*Dose*	*Research of approval*				*Side effects and warnings*
Divalproex sodium, delayed or extended release	For acute mania, 25mg/kg/day, with dose adjusted to obtain clinical response (85–125 mcg/mL)	Meta-analysis supports use as monotherapy	FDA-approved	FDA-approved		Somnolence, gastrointestinal side effects, and dizziness; warnings for hepatotoxicity, pancreatitis, teratogenicity, thrombocytopenia, suicidal ideation, hyperammonemia, and hyperammonemic encephalopathy
Lamotrigine	Maintenance dose, 200–400 mg once a day	Meta-analysis supports use as monotherapy			FDA-approved	Headache, somnolence, nausea, fatigue, and insomnia; warnings for serious rash (including Stevens-Johnson syndrome and toxic epidermal necrolysis), hypersensitivity reaction, suicidal ideation, and aseptic meningitis
Lithium	For acute mania, gradually increase dose to obtain clinical response (0.8–1.2 mmol/liter)		FDA-approved		FDA-approved	Renal and thyroid dysfunction (baseline and periodic monitoring of renal and thyroid function recommended): lithium toxicity closely related to serum lithium levels.

Abbreviation: FDA, Food and Drug Administration.
† This agent is indicated as both monotherapy and an adjunct to lithium or divalproex sodium for manic or mixed symptoms.
‡ This agent is indicated only as an adjunct to lithium or divalproex sodium for maintenance (i.e. prevention of manic, mixed, hypomanic, or depressive episodes).
∫ This agent is indicated as both monotherapy and an adjunct to lithium or divalproex sodium for maintenance therapy (i.e. prevention of manic, mixed, hypomanic or depressive episodes).

ANTIEPILEPTIC DRUGS

Lamotrigine, an FDA-approved drug for the maintenance treatment of bipolar 1 disorder,[394] has been suggested to have an additional antidepressant effect. A 7-week, randomized, double-blind, placebo controlled trial of 200 mg of lamotrigine in 195 patients with bipolar I disorder showed significant decreases in scores on several depression rating scales.[395] Four subsequent placebo-controlled trials with varying inclusion criteria (patients with bipolar I disorder, bipolar II disorder, or both), trial duration (7–10 weeks), and dosing regimens (fixed dose, 50 mg vs 200 mg; flexible dose, 100–400 mg) showed no significant benefit of lamotrigine. However, a recent meta-analysis[396] of all five trials (a total of 1072 patients) suggested a modest benefit of lamotrigine as assessed by a 50% or greater decrease in the MADRAS score (relative risk, 1.22; 95% confidence interval (CI), 1.06–1.41; number needed to treat, 13) or the score on the Hamilton Rating Scale for Depression (relative risk, 1.27; 95% CI, 1.09 to 1.47; number needed to treat, 11). Remission rates were not significantly different as measured by the Hamilton Rating Scale, but they were slightly higher among patients who received lamotrigine, as measures by the MADRS; a prespecified sub-group analysis revealed a greater treatment effect in patients with severe depression.

Other data have also provided support for the use of lamotrigine in patients with bipolar depression. In an 8-week, randomized, a placebo-controlled trial involving 124 outpatients with bipolar I or bipolar II disorder who were receiving lithium maintenance therapy, adjunctive therapy with 200 mg of lamotrigine resulted in greater improvement in the MADRS score and a higher response rate, as compared with placebo (51.6% vs 31%).[397] A small, randomized, crossover trial involving 31 patients with refractory depression compared 6 weeks courses of lamotrigine, gabapentin, and placebo.[398] This trial showed that the percentage of patients whose depressive symptoms were much or very much improved was significantly greater with lamotrigine (52%) than with gabapentin (26%) or placebo (23%).

Divalproex sodium, which is approved for acute mania, has also been studied as monotherapy for bipolar depression. In a meta-analysis of four small, short-term, placebo-controlled trials involving 142 patients with bipolar I or II disorder,[399] divalproex monotherapy resulted in a significantly higher likelihood of clinical response and remission than placebo.

ANTIDEPRESSANT DRUGS

Despite a paucity of data to guide their use in patients with bipolar depression, antidepressant drugs are commonly prescribed. In a prescription database study involving more than 7500 patients, 50% of all initial treatment prescriptions for bipolar disorder were for antidepressant monotherapy.[400]

With the exception of fluoxetine, which is approved in combination with olanzapine for bipolar depression, all FDA-approved antidepressants are indicated only for unipolar depression: patients with a history of bipolar disorder were excluded from all registration trials.

Paroxetine is the selective serotonin-reuptake inhibitor (SSRI) that has been most rigorously studied in patients with bipolar depression,[389,401,402] and available efficacy data provide little support for its widespread use. As noted above, a randomized trial comparing paroxetine with quetiapine suggested that paroxetine was less effective in improving depression scores and was more likely to cause a switch to mania or hypomania.[389] In a randomized, placebo-controlled trial assessing adjunctive therapy with paroxetine (mean dose, 32.6 mg) or imipramine (mean dose, 166.7 mg) in patients with bipolar depression who were receiving lithium maintenance therapy, neither paroxetine nor imipramine was superior to placebo in reducing depressive symptoms at 10 weeks,[401] Finally, in a longer (26 weeks) trial in which 366 patients with bipolar I or bipolar II disorder who were receiving a mood stabilizer were randomly assigned to adjunctive antidepressant therapy (paroxetine or bupropion) or placebo,[402] there were no significant differences among groups in the rates of durable recovery, defined as 8 consecutive weeks of euthymia without a switch to mania or hypomania.

A meta-analysis of 15 randomized, double blind trials comparing short-term antidepressant treatment (up to 4 months) with either placebo or an active comparison drug in 2373 patients with bipolar I or II disorder likewise showed no major benefit of antidepressant therapy.[403] Six of these trials, involving 1469 patients, were placebo-controlled trials evaluating fluoxetine, paroxetine, imipramine, and bupropion, more than two thirds of the participants were receiving mood-stabilizing therapy. Although the definitions of outcomes varied among the studies, pooled analyses showed nonsignificant benefits of antidepressant therapy over placebo in the rates of response (relative risk, 1.18; 95% CI, 0.99–1.4; P = 0.06) and remission (relative risk, 1.20; 95% CI, 0.98–1.47; P = 0.096). Pooled analyses of data from more than 1000 of these patients suggested that antidepressant treatment did not increase the risk of a switch to mania or hypomania. In a smaller analysis comparing the antidepressants sertraline (an SSRI), bupropion, venlafaxine, and desipramine (a tricyclic antidepressant), the tricyclic antidepressant and venlafaxine were associated with higher rates of a switch to mania or hypomania than the other agents (desipramine, 43%; venlafaxine, 15%; sertraline, 7%; and bupropion, 5%).[404]

A meta-analysis of seven trials involved 350 patients with bipolar I or bipolar II disorder who were randomly assigned for at least 6 months to any type of antidepressant with or without a mood stabilizer or to placebo with or without a mood stabilizer. This study showed that antidepressant therapy reduced the risk of recurrent depression (relative risk, 0.73; 95% CI, 0.55–0.97) but increased the risk of a switch to a hypomanic or manic episode (relative risk, 1.72; 95% CI, 1.23–2.41).[405] Antidepressants may result in better outcomes in bipolar II disorder.[406] In a randomized trial of maintenance therapy in patients with bipolar II disorder, 81 patients with an initial response to open-label fluoxetine monotherapy were randomly assigned to continued treatment with fluoxetine, a change to treatment with lithium, or placebo for 50 weeks. The time to relapse or recurrence of depression, the primary outcome, was significantly longer with fluoxetine (250 days) than with lithium (156 days) or placebo (187 days). The risk of a switch to a hypomanic episode was no greater with fluoxetine (10.7%) or lithium (7.7%) than with placebo (18.5%).

PSYCHOTHERAPY

As compared with major depressive disorder, there has been little systematic evaluation of psychotherapy in patients with bipolar depression. The largest comparative trial of psychotherapy randomly assigned 293 outpatients with bipolar I or bipolar II disorder who were receiving medication to one of three forms of intensive psychotherapy (family-focused, interpersonal, or cognitive behavioral therapy) weekly or every other week up to 30 sessions, or to general psychoeducation for 3 sessions.[407] At 1 year, rates of recovery, defined as no more than one or two moderate symptoms of depression for at least 8 weeks, were significantly higher in the intensive-psychotherapy groups than in the group of patients who received general education (64% for the three psychotherapy groups combined vs 52%).

AREAS OF UNCERTAINTY

More research is needed to determine which patients with bipolar depression might benefit from short-term or long-term antidepressant therapy without an undue risk of a switch to mania. Whereas more than 40% of subjects in one study retrospectively reported a switch to a manic or hypomanic episode within 12 weeks after starting an antidepressant at any time in their lives,[408] controlled clinical trials have suggested a much lower rate, prospectively confirmed (i.e. by rating scale assessment).[389] However, patients with bipolar I disorder who are enrolled in trials of antidepressant monotherapy are carefully selected, and the risk of a switch to mania in these study populations may be substantially lower than the risk in clinical practice. In addition to tricyclic antidepressants[403] and possibly venlafaxine,[403,408] several clinical factors (e.g. whether the patient has bipolar I or bipolar II disorder and the lack of a mood stabilizer) have been associated with an increased risk of a switch to mania, and this risk should be taken into account in considering the risk-benefit ratio of antidepressants.[409]

A short-term, placebo-controlled trial showed the efficacy of modafinil, an agent approved to increase wakefulness in patients with certain sleep disorders, in bipolar depression.[410] Pramipexole, a partial dopamine-receptor subtype 2 and dopamine-receptor subtype 3 agonist approved for Parkinson's disease,[411,412] was also effective in improving symptoms of depression in two small, short-term trails (one involving patients with bipolar I disorder and the other involving patients with bipolar II disorder), although psychotic mania developed in one patient with bipolar I disorder after active treatment. More data are needed to determine the role of these agents in practice.

GUIDELINES

Guidelines for the treatment of bipolar depression are currently being revised by the American Psychiatric Association. The guidelines of the International Society for Bipolar Disorders recommend any of the following agents as first-line therapy for bipolar depression: quetiapine, lamotrigine, or lithium monotherapy; olanzapine with an SSRI (i.e. fluoxetine or another SSRI): and lithium or divalproex with an SSRI or bupropion.[413] These guidelines antedate the trials showing the superiority of quetiapine over lithium or paroxetine.

CONCLUSION AND RECOMMENDATIONS

Although both the fluoxetine-olanzapine combination and quetiapine are FDA-approved for bipolar depression, it is recommended the initiation of treatment with quetiapine (at a dose of 300 mg daily), given the amount of evidence that supports that use of this agent.[414] Monitoring is warranted for somnolence, an elevation in the glucose level, weight gain, and tardive dyskinesia (although the risk of tardive dyskinesia is considered to be low). If quetiapine is poorly tolerated or if there is no change in depressive symptoms, lamotrigine (with a gradual increase to a dose of 200 mg) would be reasonable second-line intervention. Usually antidepressant monotherapy would not be recommended. If antidepressant cotherapy is use, careful monitoring is required for suicidal ideation and a switch to mania or hypomania during treatment.

7.9 MECHANISM OF DISEASE: MAJOR DEPRESSIVE DISORDER

RK Solanki

Depression is related to the normal emotions of sadness and bereavement, but it does not remit when the external cause of these emotions dissipates, and it is disproportionate to their cause. Classic several states of depression often have no external precipitating cause. It is difficult, however, to draw clear distinctions between depression with and those without psychosocial precipitating events. The diagnosis of major depressive disorder requires a distinct change of mood, characterized by sadness or irritability and accompanied by at least several psychophysiological change, such as disturbances in sleep, appetite, or sexual desire; constipation; loss of the ability to experience pleasure in work or with friends; crying; suicidal thoughts; and slowing of speech and action. These changes must last a minimum of 2 weeks and interfere considerably with work and family relations. On the basis of this broad definition, the lifetime incidence of depression in the United States is more than 12% in men and 20% in woman. Some have advocated a much narrower definition of severe depression, which they call melancholia or vital depression.

A small percentage of patients with major depression have had or will have manic episodes consisting of hyperactivity, euphoria, and increase in pleasure seeking. Although some pathogenetic mechanisms in these cases and in cases of major depressive disorder overlap, a history of mania defines a distinct illness termed bipolar disorder.

Depression is a heterogeneous disorder with a highly variable course, an inconsistent response to treatment, and no established mechanism. This review presents the major current approaches to understanding the biologic mechanisms of major depression.

GENETICS

Studies comparing concordance rates for major depression between monozygotic and dizygotic twins suggest a heritability of about 37%, which is much lower than the heritability of bipolar disorder or schizophrenia. Some aspects of the normal personality, such as avoidance of harm, anxiousness, and pessimism, are also partly heritable. Kendler, et al. argued that although depression is due in part to heritable depression-prone personality traits, it is also the result of heritable factors that are independent of personality. Early-onset, severe, and recurrent depression may have a higher heritability than other forms of depression. It is clear from studies of families that major depression is not caused by any single gene but is a disease with complex genetic features. Studies of pedigrees with multiple cases of major depression have identified chromosomal regions with linkage to the disorder, and some of these loci have been replicated in more than one study, although no single chromosomal region has been replicated in every family study of genetic linkage in depression. Holmans, et al. found evidence of linkage of recurrent, early-onset depression to chromosome 15q25-q26, but the population attributable risk was small.

No specific molecular risk factor has been reliably identified. One common polymorphic variant of the serotonin-transporter-linked polymorphic region (5-HTTLPR), which affects the promoter of the serotonin-transporter gene, causes reduced uptake of the neurotransmitter serotonin into the presynaptic cells in the brain. Some studies have shown that this polymorphism confers a predisposition to depression, but it also confers a predisposition to an anxious and pessimistic personality. Brain imaging reveals functional differences in emotion-related areas of the brain among carriers of the different common polymorphisms of 5-HTTLPR, although a direct relation to depression is unclear. In a large, prospective epidemiologic study, Caspi et al. found that 5-HTTLPR predicted depression only in association with defined life stresses. Some environmental factors could confer a predisposition to depression by affecting the genome epigenetically-for example, increased maternal care in rodents causes an epigenetic change in the promoter region of the glucocorticoid-receptor gene.

MONOAMINE-DEFICIENCY HYPOTHESIS

The noradrenergic and serotonergic systems originate deep in the brain and fan out over almost the entire brain, suggesting a system capable of modulating many areas of feeling, thinking, and behaving. The early antidepressants blocked the reuptake of norepinephrine and serotonin by the presynaptic neuron. The immediate effects of this pharmacologic action are to increase the availability of norepinephrine and serotonin in the synapse and to increase stimulation of the postsynaptic neuron. Inhibitors of the enzyme monoamine oxidase were also discovered to have antidepressant properties. This enzyme catabolizes norepinephrine and serotonin in their respective presynaptic neurons, and such inhibition could be expected to increase the availability of neurotransmitters. These discoveries led to a major theory of depression known as the monoamine-deficiency hypothesis. Numerous studies of norepinephrine and serotonin metabolites in plasma, urine, and cerebrospinal fluid, as well as postmortem studies of the brains of patients with depression, have yet to identify the purported deficiency reliably. However, a newly discovered form of the enzyme tryptophan hydroxylase, designated TPH-2, specific to the brain and could explain why previous postmortem studies of total enzyme activity did not show differences in tryptophan hydroxylase activity between patients with depression and controls. A recent positron-emission tomographic study using a ligand for brain monoamine oxidase showed a 30% increase of the enzyme in a subgroup of patients with depression. A study measuring differences in monoamine metabolites between the internal jugular vein and the brachial artery showed lower production by the brain of norepinephrine metabolites in patients with depression than in controls. The monoamine-deficiency hypothesis continues to stimulate research whenever a new technical window into the brain is opened.

Serotonin and norepinephrine can be depleted experimentally in humans by oral treatments. A drink containing all amino acids except tryptophan stimulates the liver to synthesize proteins and rapidly depletes the plasma (and therefore the brain) of tryptophan. Tryptophan is rate-limiting for serotonin synthesis is the brain. Such oral tryptophan depletion does not induce depression in healthy subjects but will cause a relapse of depression in patients who have been successfully treated with a serotonin-reuptake inhibitor. Similarly, α-methyl paratyrosine inhibits tyrosine hydroxylase, the rate-limiting step in catecholamine synthesis. Treatment with α-methyl paratyrosine does not induce depression in normal subjects but will induce a relapse in patients who have been treated successfully with a norepinephrine-reuptake inhibitor.These findings suggest that norepinephrine and serotonin have critical roles in the mechanisms of these treatments of depression but that additional neurochemical factors are necessary to cause depression.

Because direct measurements of monoamine neurotransmission did not yield definitive findings in relation to depression, the downstream effects of monoamine neurotransmission were explored. The serotonin-1B receptor is located presynaptically and regulates the release of serotonin by feedback inhibition. Postmortem studies show that the levels of p11, a protein that enhances the efficiency of serotonin-1B receptor signaling, are decreased in the brains of patients with depression. The serotonin-1A receptor is located both presynaptically and postsynaptically to regulate serotonin function. The receptor can be evaluated in patients with depression by injecting specific agonists and measuring specific neuroendocrine responses, such as elevation of the prolactin level. Result suggest that the sensitivity of this receptor is reduced in patients with depression. The α_2-noradrenergic receptor, which is usually presynaptic, modulates norepinephrine release by feedback inhibition. Heightened receptor sensitivity has been described in patients with depression, which is consistent with reduced norepinephrine release.

It is conceivable that the second-messenger systems for serotonergic and noradrenergic neurotransmission malfunction in depression, and for this reason the phosphatidylinositol and cyclic AMP second-messenger systems have been extensively evaluated. Reduce inositol levels have been found in postmortem studies of the brains of persons who have died by suicide and in magnetic resonance spectroscopic studies of the frontal cortex in patients with depression. A blunted cyclic AMP response to stimulation was found in postmortem studies of the brains of patients with depression. These reductions in second-messenger function may impair neurotransmitter function even without changes in monoamine levels or receptor number. These data indirectly support elaborations of the original monoamine-deficiency hypothesis of depression.

G-proteins that mediate signaling between receptors and second-manager systems have also been investigated in patients with depression, both in postmortem studies of the brain and in studies of peripheral-blood cells. Although these systems are clearly affected, no consistent picture has emerged because they are numerous forms of G-proteins that vary in different areas of the brain. The cyclic AMP response element-binding protein (CREB) is a transcription factor affected by cyclic AMP in the cell. In an animal model of depression, rats with overexpression of CREB in the dentate gyrus behaved similarly to rats treated with antidepressants, but the opposite effect was found when CREB was overexpressed in the nucleus accumbens. Thus, the role of CREB in depression in specific to the region of the brain. Most but not all studies show that long-term treatment with antidepressants stimulates CREB function, possibly depending on the type of drug and the dosage. Levels of CREB and phosphor-CREB were reduced in postmortem studies of the cortexes of patients who had a major depressive disorder and had not taken antidepressants, as compared with controls. Many studies of second-messenger systems and transcription factors in depression were inspired by the belief that it takes several weeks before antidepressants treatment has an effect; consequently, the studies were designed to detect time-dependent biochemical changes in the cell. New meta-analyses suggest that antidepressant effects begin rapidly, however, thereby supporting the classic monoamine-deficiency hypothesis.

A strong point of the monoamine theory has been its predictive power. Almost every compound that has been synthesized for the purpose of inhibiting norepinephrine or serotonin reuptake has been proved to be a clinically effective antidepressant. A behavioral model of depression has been developed in which a rodent is placed in a glass cylinder filled with water, the sheer wall offering no chance of escape. The animal struggles for a while and then floats passively (the forced swim test). A single prior injection of antidepressant increases the struggling time; results in this model have excellent predictive validity for new for antidepressants. Other animals models have been developed by selective breeding of rates for depression-like behavior, and these genetically susceptible rodents also have a response to antidepressants. Still other models that can be studied biochemically induce depression with the use of long-term mild stress or learned helplessness. However, no animal model of depression captures the periodic change of behavior into and out of depression that is seen in patients with depression.

Molecular techniques such as gene knockout partially support the monoamine theory of depression. The serotonin-reuptake-transporter knockout mouse is excessively anxious and characterized by increased immobility in the forced swim test, This effects is similar to that of the low-activity polymorphic variant of the serotonin receptor on human personality but is the opposite of the expected effects of serotonin-reuptake-inhibitor antidepressants. However, this inconsistency could be explained by the difference between a chronic monoamine abnormality during brain developmant and the hypothesized acute monoamine depletion in an adult with depression.

The effects of stimulants on mood indirectly support the monoamine-deficiency hypothesis of depression and show that mood can be altered rapidly. Cocaine and amphetamines are powerful releasers of monoamine into the synapse as well as inhibitors of reuptake. Their mood-elevating effects are immediate, but in patients with severe depression they have often been reported to cause agitation rather than relief of depression. This finding could reflect the ability of these stimulants to deplete the presynapse of monoamine and thus cause a "crash" into depression. Recent studies support the theory that an acute response to a single dose of amphetamine predicts a patient's longer-term response to monoamine-reuptake inhibitors.

The role of dopamine deficiency in depression is suggested by the frequency of depression in patients with Parkinson's disease and the effect of reserpine, which depletes serotonin, norepinephrine, and dopamine, causing a hypoactive state in animals. The antidepressant agent bupropion inhibits the reuptake of dopamine. Some direct dopamine-receptor agonists, such as pramipexole, have been reported to be efficacious in the treatment of depression, even though they were developed for Parkinson's disease.

A major liability of the monoamine-deficiency hypothesis is its derivation from the mechanism of currently available antidepressants. Approximately two-thirds of patients have a clinical response to these agents, whereas one-third have a response to placebo. Perhaps the mechanism of depression is not related to monoamines in two of three cases.

STRESS, THE HYPOTHALAMIC-PITUITARY-ADRENAL AXIS AND GROWTH FACTORS

Stress is perceived by the cortex of the brain and transmitted to the hypothalamus, where corticotrophin-releasing hormone (CRH) is released into pituitary receptors. This stimulus results in the secretion of corticotrophin into plasma, stimulation of corticotrophin receptors in the adrenal cortex, and release of cortisol into the blood. Hypothalamic cortisol receptors respond by decreasing CRH production to maintain homeostasis.

There is considerable evidence that cortisol and its central releasing factor, CRH are involved in depression. Patients with depression may have elevated cortisol levels in plasma, elevated CRH levels in cerebrospinal fluid, and increased levels of CRH messenger RNA and protein in limbic brain regions. In studies using dexamethasone to evaluate the sensitivity of the hypothalamus to feedback signals for the shutdown of CRH release, the normal cortisol-suppression response is absent in about half of the most severely depressed patients. Antidepressant-induced clinical remission is accompanied by reversal of some of these abnormalities.

Adults with a history of physical or sexual abuse as children have increased levels of CRH in cerebrospinal fluid. Adult rodents that were separated from their mothers of abused as pups show increased immobility in the forced swim test, which is reversed by antidepressant treatment. Mice with region-specific knockout of the glucocorticoid receptor at an adult age have increased activity of the hypothalamic-pituitary-adrenal axis and increased immobility in the forced swim test, both of which are reversed by antidepressants. Increased levels of monoamine in the synapse affect the hypothalamic-pituitary-adrenal axis and reverse some of the long-term effects of stress. It is possible that antidepressants relieve depression by reducing the secondary stress caused by a painfully dispirited mood rather than by directly elevating mood. An antistress mechanism could explain the general usefulness of antidepressants for a wide variety of psychiatric conditions, including panic disorder, post-traumatic stress disorder, bulimia, premenstrual syndrome, and obsessive-compulsive disorder. CRH-receptor antagonists show antidepressant activity in animals models, but the results of large clinical trials have been disappointing. A compound that blocks the glucocorticoid receptor has been reported has been reported to be efficacious in depression, but only the most severe and psychotic type.

A single test for the cortisol level in blood does not contribute to the diagnosis of depression, since levels of cortisol vary markedly in a circadian rhythm and because the overlap between values in patients and those in controls is considerable. Mild stress induced in the laboratory, such as stress associated with mental arithmetic calculations or simulated public speaking, results in greater changes in plasma cortisol levels than most reported differences between the values in patients with depression and those in controls.It is possible that chronic mild elevations of cortisol, especially at night, when cortisol levels in normal subjects are very low, have a pathogenic role in depression. It is also possible that peripheral cortisol elevations are only a reflection of central disturbances in CRH signaling, which mediate the effects of environmental stress on mood. A major liability of the hypothalamic-pituitary-adrenal axis theory of depression is the difficulty of defining the relationship of stress to depressive episode, whereas a larger proportion have a recurrent or even chronic course. Various types of acute stress, early childhood trauma, or long-term psychosocial problems may be involved and may lead to different responses of the stress system. Stress may be causative in some cases and secondary to depressed mood in others.

Severe stress in rodents does not necessarily model the common stresses of childhood. The association of abuse in childhood with psychopathologic disorders, including depression, in adulthood could be due to common factors linking family perpetrators of abuse & their victims, including not only shared genes but also a shared environment of poverty poor nutrition and poor parental care. Depression is not uncommon in people with no psychosocial risk factors. Most patents treated for depression have no evidence of hypothalamic-pituitary-adrenal dysfunction, just as most such patients have no direct evidence of brain monoamine deficiency.

The classic teaching is that neurons do not divide in the adult mammalian brain, but studies have shown that neurogenesis occurs in several areas of the brain, especially the hippocampus. Neurogenesis is more prominent in rodents than in primates, and some have questioned whether it occurs in the human cortex. Elevated levels of glucocorticoids can reduce neurogenesis, and this has been suggested as a mechanism for the decreased size of the hippocampus on magnetic resonance images of the brain in many patients with depression. In postmortem studies of patients with depression, cell loss in the subgenual prefrontal cortex, atrophy in the dorsolateral prefrontal cortex and the orbitofrontal cortex, and increased numbers of cells in the hypothalamus and the dorsal raphe nucleus have been reported. These effects resemble the atrophic changes in the brain in patients with Cushing's disease and in rodents treated with glucocorticoids.However, cortisol elevations in depression are much lower than in Cushing disease.

Restraint in a small container induces stress in rodents, suppressing neurogenesis, and this effect is countered by antidepressant treatment. Antidepressants also enhance neurogenesis in nonhuman primates. Santarelli et al. irradiated the hippocampus in mice and abolished neurogenesis. They found that the radiation also abolished the ability of the animals to respond behaviorally to antidepressant treatment in the forced swim test, but this phenomenon does not occur in every mouse strain studied. Henn and Vollmayr summarized other studies providing evidence that decreased neurogenesis is a result of stress and anxiety but may not be behaviorally relevant. The relevance of animals models of neurogenesis to clinical studies of depression has been questioned by analogy with studies of neuroprotection strategies in stroke, for which numerous findings in animal models have not been replicated in human studies.

Brain-derived neurotrophic factor (BDNF), a neurotrophic peptide, is critical for axonal growth, neuronal survival, and synaptic plasticity, and its levels are affected by stress and cortisol. A postmortem study of patients with depression who had committed suicide showed that BDNF was reduced in the hippocampus. Antidepressant drugs and electroconvulsive therapy upregulate BDNF and other neurotrophic and growth factors; a single bilateral infusion of BDNF into the dentate gyrus has antidepressant like effects. One study showed that the hippocampal was smaller than normal in patients with depression who carried a met166 BDNF allete. In an animal model of depression, epigenetic histone methylation mediated down-regulation of BDNF transcripts and antidepressant treatment reversed this effects. These studies suggest that BDNF is the link among stress, neurogenesis, and hippocample atrophy in depression. However, a genetic association of the BDNF val166met polymorphism with depression has not been replicated is most studies, and BDNF may be related not only to depression but to multiple psychiatric disorders and BDNF-knockout mice behaviors unrelated to depression. Reduced BDNF levels in the peripheral blood of patients with depression seem to derive almost entirely from blood platelets, and many artifacts must, therefore, be considered in interpreting these findings. Inflammation in the brain and some neurotoxins increase brain BDNF levels, suggesting that the actions of BDNF are not uniformly therapeutic. Castren has proposed that antidepressant treatments may increase synaptic sprouting and allow the brain to use input from the environment more effectively to recover from depression. This hypothesis highlights the role that cognition may play in depression and suggest that biochemical mechanisms may be nonspecific.

Strong epidemiologic data point to an association between major depressive disorder and increased cardiovascular morbidity and mortality. In many patients, cardiovascular disorders precede depression, and in others, depression precedes the cardiovascular disorder. Both n-3 fatty acid deficiency and elevated plasma homocysteine levels have been implicated in cardiovascular disease and in depression. Elevated cortisol levels in depression could increase the risk of coronary artery disease, since cortisol increases visceral fat. Antidepressant treatment increases the survival rate among patients who become depressed after coronary occlusion. Endothelial-cell signaling plays a crucial role in brain neurogenesis and these cells secrete BDNF; thus, both depression and cardiovascular disease could be examples of an endothelial disorder. Signs of inflammatory processes have been described in major depression and in cardiovascular disease. Some data suggest that exercise has protective or therapeutic effects in depression. Rodent models support this possibility.

OTHER POSSIBLE MECHANISMS

Many other mechanisms has been proposed which have also been implicated in psychiatric and neurologic disorders other than depression. Since the components of the brain are highly interconnected, it is not difficult to find possible integrative frame-works between two or more of the various theories. Testing the theories in a manner that can reject the null hypothesis has been more difficult. Research in depression has sometimes been sequentially imitative of dominant ideas in related fields, such as neurogenesis, glutamate neurotransmission, and nicotinic receptors, instead of progressing on its own path.

SUMMARY

It would be appealing to attempt to categorize depression in terms of monoamine-depletion forms that are perhaps related to genes coding for enzymes involved in neurotransmission and cortisol-related forms that are characterized by a more long-term course, hippocampus atrophy, and history of psychosocial stress. However, the clinical data do not fall into such neat categories, since monoamine-based antidepressants are most effective in patents with several depressions when cortisol levels remain high after the administration of dexamethasone.

Major depressive disorder is likely to have a numbers of causes. Middle-aged or elderly patients presenting with depression may have a disorder related to cardiovascular disease and originating from endothelial dysfunction. Patients in their late teens or early 20s who have severe depression may have important genetic risk factors and a high-risk of manic episodes. In patients with an anxious and depressive personality, depression may be due to genetically determined personality factors or adverse childhood experiences.

Avoidance of premature closure on any one scientific theory of the mechanism of depression will best serve the search for new, more effective treatments. It is likely that the pathogenesis of acute depression is different from that of recurrent or chronic depression which is characterized by long-term declines in function and cognition. Mood can be elevated (by stimulants, by brain stimulation, or by ketamine) or depressed (by monoamine depletion in recovered patients) for short periods, but longer-term improvement may require reduction of the abnormal glucocorticoid function induced by stress or increases in brain neurotrophic factors.

7.10 MAJOR DEPRESSIVE DISORDER: NEW CLINICAL, NEUROBIOLOGICAL AND TREATMENT PERSPECTIVE

JN Vyas

EPIDEMIOLOGY, COMORBIDITY AND DIAGNOSIS

Worldwide, depression is a seriously disabling public health problem of very high prevalence. Major depressive disorder has a 12-month prevalence of 6.6% and a lifetime prevalence of 16.2%, is twice as common in women as in men, and causes considerable impairment. Age of onset distributions suggest that depression is prevalent for the entire lifespan. The disorder not only produces decrements in health that are equivalent to those of other chronic diseases (e.g. angina, arthritis, asthma, and diabetes), but also worsens mean health scores substantially more when comorbid with these diseases, than when the diseases occur alone.

Overdetection and underdetection are important factors that should be considered to ensure the appropriate diagnosis and management of clinical depression. Although a meta-analysis concluded that general practitioners correctly exclude depression in most individuals who are not depressed, overdetections (false positives) can outnumber missed cases. The presence of anxiety with depression can increase difficulties in diagnosis. Some researchers have argued that the establishment of anxious depression as a specific diagnosis would substantially improve identification of depression in primary care settings, and such a category has been proposed for the 11th revision of the international classification of diseases (ICD-11). In up to 40% of patients, major depression is associated with lifetime occurrences of isolated manic or hypomanic symptoms that do not cluster in a way that is consistent with a diagnosis of hypomania. Furthermore, such symptoms can be concurrent with syndromal-level major depressive disorder. Further investigation is needed to examine the treatment and prognosis of major depression that is associated either concurrently or at other points in the patient's history with hypomanic symptoms.

Major depressive disorder was assumed to precede generalized anxiety disorder until a 32-year prospective follow-up study challenged this notion. Indeed, the reverse pattern seems to be frequently present, and the combination of generalized anxiety disorder and major depression might represent an additional burden. Social anxiety disorder (social phobia) is now also regarded as an important and consistent risk factor for the development of severe depression. Furthermore, comorbid personality disorder seems to confer a worse prognosis and poorer treatment response than does major depression alone. Some of the risk factors for the metabolic syndrome (e.g. obesity), might also increase the risk of depression and, in turn, depression increases the risk for development of obesity. These two-way relations might be the reason for the increased association between depression and coronary artery disease.

Kendler and colleagues have shown a major relation between depression and coronary artery disease, mainly in acute states. A high severity of depression within several weeks of admission to hospital for an acute coronary syndrome, or an inadequate treatment response in depression, can double cardiac mortality in 6–7 years of follow-up. Studies examining depression and anxiety as predictors of 2-year cardiac events in patients with stable coronary artery disease have shown a high likelihood of major adverse cardiac events in those with depression. These results have led to the recommendation that all patients with coronary artery disease be screened for depression; however; this recommendation is somewhat controversial. Studies of the relation between depression and diabetes have led to new conclusions, e.g. that clinical depression is associated with a 65% increased risk of diabetes in elderly people. Major and minor depressions seem to be implicated in this relation. These studies emphasize the importance of identification and treatment of depression in the physically ill.

ADVANCES IN NEUROBIOLOGY

Genetic Studies

Genetic, molecular, and neuroimaging studies continue to contribute to advances in our understanding of the neurobiological basis of major depressive disorder. However, the extent to which findings from neurobiological studies can help improve the clinical and functional outcome of individuals with the disorder is still uncertain. Thus, in the past 5 years, neurobiological research of depression has become two-tiered to; (1) understand the pathophysiology of the illness; and (2) identify the neurobiological measures for guiding treatment choice.

The identification of single candidate genes associated with major depression has been difficult because of the likelihood that complex psychiatric illnesses are under polygenic influence and are associated with interactions between genetic variants and environmental exposures. One approach has been to go beyond the conventional focus on monoamines in the search for a genetic association. For example, major depressive disorder has been associated with polymorphisms in the glucocorticoid receptor gene NR3C1, the monoamine oxidase A gene,the gene for glycogen synthase kinase-3β (which has a key role in the phosphorylation and regulation of metabolic enzymes and many transcription factors), and a group-2 metabotropic glutamate receptor gene (GRM3). Success has been greater in the identification of candidate genes that are associated with known biological mechanisms and metabolic pathways for antidepressant drugs and, that in turn, can help predict the response from antidepressant treatment.

Many studies have focused on the functional insertion-deletion promoter variant (serotonin transporter-linked polymorphic region [5HTTLPR]) in the serotonin transporter gene (SLC6A4). A meta-analysis showed two associations, first between the 5HTTLPR long allele and increased response to selective serotonin reuptake inhibitor (SSRI) antidepressant drugs (although not to nortriptyline), and reduced side-effects to SSRls; and second between the 5HTTLPR short allele and increased paroxetine-induced, but decreased mirtazapine-induced adverse effects. Several single-nucleotide polymorphism (SNPs) in the gene for the serotonin type-2a receptor are associated with outcomes of SSRl treatment.

Studiesof candidate genes associated with other biological mechanisms have emphasized associations between glutamatergic genes (e.g. GR1K4) and citalopram response and adverse effects; between the Met allele of the functional Val/Met polymorphism (rs6265) in brain-derived neurotrophic factor (BDNF) and SSRI response; and between several other BDNF SNPs and desipramine response. Genetic variation in FKBP5—a protein that helps to regulate cortisol binding to the glucocorticoid receptor is associated with antidepressant response; whereas genetic variants in TREK1—a potassium channel mediating SSRI mechanism of action—are associated with nonresponse to several antidepressants. Genetic variation in the catechol-O-methyltransferase (COMT) gene, which alters COMT activity, is associated with response to treatment with several antidepressants.

Genome-wide association studies further suggest that effectiveness of antidepressants can be predicted by genetic markers other than traditional candidate genes. These genes include those for the corticotrophin-releasing hormone (CRH) receptor-1 (CRHR1) and CRH binding protein (CRHBP), which predict SSRI response in anxious depression, and genes for uronyl-2 sulphotransferase and interleukin-11, which predict response to nortriptyline and escitalopram oxalate, respectively.

Molecular Studies

At least three main categories of peripheral hormone-type factors, for which genetic variants are associated with major depressive disorder, are implicated in the pathophysiology of the illness: (1) neurotrophic factors and other growth factors, including BDNF, vascular endothelial growth factor, and insulin-like growth factor-1; (2) proinflammatory cytokines, including interleukin-1β interleukin-6, and tumor necrosis factor-α; and (3) impaired regulation of the hypothalamic-pituitary-adrenocortical (HPA) axis. For example, serum BDNF is decreased in individuals with major depression, and antidepressant treatment reverses this decrease.

The secretion and production of proinflammatory cytokines are increased in individuals who are stressed and depressed, and, in major depression, antidepressant drugs can return concentrations of these cytokines to normal or suppress their synthesis. Impaired regulation of the HPA axis in an acute episode of depression has long been documented, and published work has indicated attenuation of neuroendocrine response to the combined dexamethasone-corticotrophin-releasing hormone test—a sensitive measure of altered regulation of the HPA system—during antidepressant treatment.

Neuroimaging Studies

Neural systems that are important to understand major depressive disorder include those that support emotion processing, reward seeking, and regulate emotion, all of which are dysfunctional in the disorder. These systems include subcortical systems involved in emotion and reward processing (e.g. amygdala, ventral striatum); medial prefrontal and anterior cingulate cortical regions involved in processing emotion and automatic or implicit regulation of emotion; and lateral prefrontal cortical systems (e.g. ventrolateral prefrontal cortex and dorsolateral prefrontal cortex) involved in cognitive control and voluntary or effortful regulation of emotion. These systems can be conceptualized as a medial prefrontal-limbic network, including amygdala, anterior cingulated cortex, and medial prefrontal cortex that is modulated by serotonin neurotransmission, and a reward network centred on ventral striatum and interconnected orbitofrontal and medial prefrontal cortices that is modulated by dopamine (Fig. 2).

Neuroimaging studies of major depressive disorder have provided evidence for specific functional abnormalities in these neural systems in adults. Converging findings from these studies suggest abnormally increased amygdala, ventral striatal, and medial prefrontal cortex activity, mostly to negative emotional stimuli, such as fearful faces. Abnormally reduced ventral striatal activity to positive emotional stimuli, and during receipt and anticipation of reward in adults and adolescents with depression have also been reported. These findings support a bias of attention towards negative emotional stimuli, and away from positive emotional and reward-related stimuli in individuals with major depression. Further studies are needed to examine

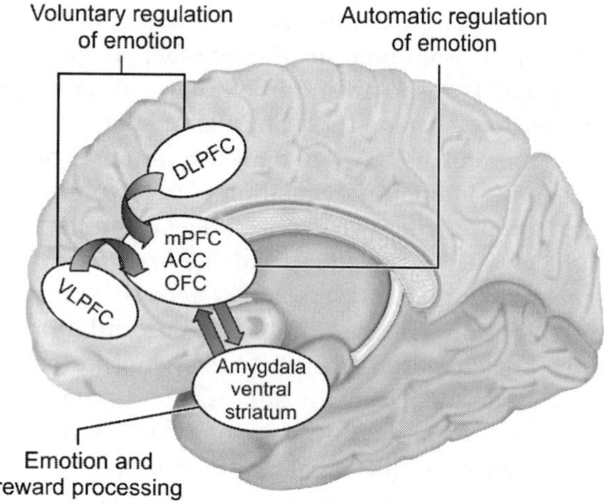

Fig. 2: Neural systems of relevance to major depressive disorder

Key neural regions implicated in emotion and reward processing, and voluntary and automatic emotions are shown superimposed on a gray scale depiction of the human brain.

Abbreviations: DLPFC, dorsolateral prefrontal cortex; mPFC, medial prefrontal cortex; ACC, anterior cingulate cortex; OFC, orbitofrontal cortex; VLPFC, ventrolateral prefrontal cortex.

neural activity in the prefrontal cortical regions that are implicated in voluntary and implicit regulation of emotion. These functional neuroimaging studies are complemented by increased findings suggesting reductions in grey matter in key regions of these neural systems (including amygdala), age-related decreases in volume of the anterior cingulate cortex, and post-mortem findings indicating neural-cell and glial-cell pathology in prefrontal cortical regions.

Additional evidence for abnormalities in neural systems for emotion and reward processing and regulation of emotion in major depressive disorder has come from neuroimaging studies of emotion processing, which used measures of functional connectivity, including effective connectivity, i.e. the effect that activity in one region exerts over that in another. For example, one study reported abnormal-inverse effective connectivity in medial prefrontal cortical-amygdala during emotion labeling of happy faces in individuals with major depression, These findings suggest abnormally increased top-down regulation of the amygdala by medial prefrontal cortex in these individuals, which again suggests a bias away from attendance to positive emotional stimuli.

Other studies have applied diffusion tensor imaging, which uses measures of the diffusivity of water in different direction—either parallel or perpendicular to the direction of white-matter fibers-to construct whole-brain measures of patterns of white-matter connectivity between different neural regions. Findings from these studies, have shown abnormal prefrontal corticosubcortical white-matter connectivity between regions supporting emotion regulation in adults with depression.

Examination of brain activity during rest can provide valuable insights into how the brain functions during self-reflection, which could be abnormal in individuals with major depression. Studies have provided evidence for a malfunction of the default mode network. This network includes several midline regions, including the inferior (ventral) part of the medial prefrontal cortex (vmPFC). Anterior parts of this network (e.g. vmPFC) are involved in self-referential processing and tend to deactivate during cognitive tasks as cognitive resources are redirected. The normal decrease in vmPFC activity during difficult tasks might indicate intact emotional gating and, conversely, absence of this deactivation might indicate impaired gating. Findings from analysis of task-independent deactivations suggest an abnormality of the default mode network in vmPFC in major depressive disorder. A method to examine resting-state-related neural activity is measurement of the correlation of low-frequency blood oxygen level-dependent temporal fluctuations (LFBF) in steady-state functional MRI data between different neural regions. One study showed that individuals with depression had increased resting-state connectivity in medial prefrontal cortex regions in the default mode network, including the anterior cingulated cortex and the vmPFC.

A meta-analysis of several neuroimaging studies of major depressive disorder identified two neural systems of importance to the illness. One network that centered on the dorsolateral prefrontal cortex and more dorsal regions of the anterior cingulate cortex, but that also included other regions implicated in cognitive control, was characterized by reduced activity in the resting state, which returned to normal with treatment. A second network, centerd on medial prefrontal cortex and subcortical regions, was hyperactive to emotional stimuli in the depressed state, but returned to normal after antidepressant treatment. This meta-analysis provides further evidence of increased activity in neural systems supporting emotion processing (amygdala and medial prefrontal cortex), and reduced activity in neural systems supporting regulation of emotion (e.g. dorsolateral prefrontal cortex).

Neuroimaging studies have also examined neural predictors of outcome and neuroimaging measures that change with response to different antidepressant treatments. These studies have focused mainly on the role of the serotonergically-mediated medial prefrontal-limbic network. In major depression, SSRI drugs modulate emotion-induced activity in this network, and response to SSRIs is predicted by activity in this region. LFBF correlations between subcortical regions and the anterior cingulate cortex can also increase after SSRI treatment in individuals with depression. However, less is known about the effects of non-serotonergic drugs on the medial prefrontal-limbic network, and the extent to which pretreatment activity in this region predicts subsequent response to nonserotonergic antidepressants needs to be examined. Desynchronization of the anterior cingulate cortex, and its functional connectivity with the amygdala predicts rapid antidepressant response to ketamine, but response to cognitive behavioral therapy is predicted by reduced medial prefrontal activity, and increased amygdala activation. Response to deep-brain stimulation correlates with reduced activity in ventral (subgenual) regions of the anterior cingulate cortex, and increased metabolism in ventral striatum.

INTEGRATION OF MEASURES

Studies examining a combination of genetic, molecular, and neuroimaging measures to identify relations among genes, molecules, neural systems, and behavior in major depressive disorder could increase our understanding of the underlying pathophysiological processes and prediction of treatment response. Relations between genetic variation in neutrophic factors, and variation in concentrations of these factors, such as BDNF and vascular endothelial growth factor, and structural and functional variation in neural regions supporting mood regulation and associated behaviors and neurocognitive function, are well documented. This variation might in turn reduce the ability to respond to treatments dependent on intact neurocognition, such as cognitive behavioral therapy.

Reports have emphasized associations between genetic variation in function of the HPA axis, genetic variation between—and variation in concentrations of inflammatory cytokines, and functional and structural variation in key neural regions supporting mood regulation. Studies have also indicated how neuroimaging techniques can be applied to diagnosis and how specific neuroimaging measures might help to distinguish major depressive disorder from bipolar depression. In turn, these measures can facilitate early diagnosis and can inform treatment choice. Computerized machine learning and techniques for pattern recognition in combination with neuroimaging techniques can be used to classify individuals, case-by-case, into diagnostic groups on the basis of neuroimaging measures.

ADVANCES IN TREATMENT

Depression-specific Psychotherapies

Pharmacotherapy and manual—driven depression-specific psychotherapy are both effective treatments for unipolar depression, either as monotherapies, or in combination. Although similar results are reported for depression-specific psychotherapy in primary-care samples, fewer published works are available in this area than in psychiatric samples. These studies suggest that interpersonal psychotherapy alone, or in combination with pharmacotherapy, is effective for the acute treatment of depression.

In a clinical trial of inpatients with depression, response rates of patients receiving a combination of interpersonal psychotherapy (modified for inpatients) and pharmacotherapy were higher than those of patients receiving pharmacotherapy alone. The effects of acute interpersonal psychotherapy can be sustained even after remission. Similarly, several trials in the USA and Europe continue to support the acute efficacy of cognitive therapy and its usefulness as an intervention to achieve full remission and reduce the risk of recurrence. Research has also indicated that cognitive behavioral therapy can be effectively implemented in non-traditional ways, e.g. via telephone and the internet-that accommodate the unique needs of primary care practice. A randomized clinical trial comparing cognitive behavioral therapy and interpersonal psychotherapy in participants with major depression found that, on average, the treatments were equally effective. However, for a subset of patients with severe depression (Montgomery-Asberg Depression Rating Scale [MADRS] score >30), those allocated to cognitive behavior therapy had a greater percentage improvement in MADRS score and also had a greater likelihood of response than did those receiving interpersonal psychotherapy. No difference between the two treatments was noted for individuals with melancholic depression. For patients with three or more previous depressive episodes, mindfulness-based cognitive therapy has an additive benefit to usual care. Problem-solving therapy might be as effective as alternative psychotherapies and pharmacotherapies for the treatment of depression, and more effective than control treatments, and might be particularly well-suited for use in primary care.

Antidepressant Pharmacotherapy

Antidepressants were the most commonly prescribed class of drugs in office-based and hospital outpatient-based medical practice in 2005. The Table 6 lists the antidepressants that have been approved by the US Food and Drug Administration (FDA), and the proposed mechanisms of action for the various classes of antidepressants. A complete assessment of their use can be found in the American Psychiatric Association guide lines for depression.

The results of the sequenced treatment alternatives to relieve depression (STAR*D) study which was the largest depression study ever done outside the pharmaceutical industry—have been reported. This study was a practical clinical trial with broad inclusion criteria, resulting in a highly representative sample of the US population. Undertaken in both psychiatric and primary care settings, STAR*D used up to four successive treatment steps, including a switch to and augmentation with additional drug or cognitive therapy in an equipoise randomization design. The goal was for full remission, rather than just response. Remission rates in steps one to four were disappointing at 36.8%, 30.6%, 13.7%, and 13.0%, respectively with a cumulative remission rate of 67% after all four steps. These rates were low compared With efficacy trials of antidepressants, which suggests that, in actual

Table 6: Antidepressants approved by the FDA

	Drugs	*Proposed mechanism of action*
Selective serotonin reuptake inhibitors	Citalopram, escitalopram, fluoxetine, fluvoxamine, paroxetine, sertraline	Selectively inhibits the reuptake of serotonin
Tricyclic antidepressants	Amitriptyline, desipramine, doxepin, imipramine, maprotiline, nortriptyline, protriptyline, trimipramine	Nonselectively inhibits the reuptake of monoamines, including serotonin, dopamine, and norepinephrine
Norepinephrine-dopamine reuptake inhibitor	Bupropion	Inhibits the reuptake of norepinephrine and dopamine
Serotonin modulator	Nefazodone, trazodone	Primarily antagonizes 5-HT_2 receptors
Serotonin-norepinephrine reuptake inhibitors	Desvenlafaxine, duloxetine, venlafaxine	Inhibits the reuptake of serotonin and norepinephrine
Noradrenergic and specific serotonergic modulator	Mirtazapine	Primary antagonizes α_2- and 5-HT_2 receptors
Serotonin reuptake inhibitor and 5-HT_1A-receptor partial agonist	Vilazodone	Potently and selectively inhibits serotonin reuptake and acts as a partial agonist at the 5-HT_1A receptor
MAO inhibitors	Isocarboxazid, phenelzine, tranylcypromine, selegiline	Nonselectively inhibits enzymes (MAO-A and MAO-B) involved in the breakdown of monoamines, including serotonin, dopamine, and norepinephrine MAO-B selective inhibitor

practice, most patients need several sequential treatment steps to achieve remission. The STAR*D trial showed no clear advantage of one strategy of drug over another for patients who did not achieve remission after one or more acute treatments. Furthermore, because there was no placebo control in this hybrid (efficacy-effectiveness) trial, there is no way to know whether any of the strategies were better than maintenance of the original treatment for an additional period. Too few patients received psychotherapy, either as an augmentation or a switch strategy to make firm conclusions about its role. Neither sociodemographic nor clinical (anxious, atypical, and melancholic) features moderated the effect of various switching options after the first nonsuccessful attempt at acute treatment. No differences in outcomes were found between primary care and psychiatric settings in the first two stages of acute treatment, suggesting that primary care physicians can be reasonable providers of care for patients with less complex depression.

Although switching of antidepressants is a common strategy for management of depression, whether effectiveness can be improved remains controversial. Many combination treatment trials of antidepressant drugs or antidepressant and antipsychotic combinations have been done, but caution is warranted for the recommendation of such combinations as first-step treatments. One review also emphasizes the discrepancy between practice patterns and evidence for combination therapy. Lithium carbonate continues to be used as an augmentation strategy, and second-generation antipsychotics have been intensively studied. Drugs recommended for treatment-resistant depression are aripiprazole, quetiapine fumurate, and the combination of olanzapine with fluoxetine.

The notion of sequential combinations of pharmacotherapy or psychotherapy represents a shift in the treatment of mood disorders. Such two-stage approaches are based on awareness that one treatment strategy alone is unlikely to treat the varied symptoms of depression. Because the switch to a different treatment is dependent on the patient's response to the first treatment, reassessment of design and methodological approaches is needed.

Treatment of Psychotic Depression

Patients with psychotic depression (presence of delusions or hallucinations) are often difficult to treat and need several interventions. Although new pharmacological strategies are being tested, electroconvulsive therapy is important as a frequently used and effective treatment. Antipsychotics and antidepressants are being used more often to treat psychotic depression. In two studies, the combination of an antidepressant with an antipsychotic showed greater efficacy than did the antidepressant alone.

DRUG DEVELOPMENT

In the past 5 years, several strategies have been developed to improve depression outcomes, including the use of new compounds and several older drugs. An example is a report showing the benefit of ademetionine (S-adenosyl methionine [SAMe]) augmentation in major depressive disorder. One strategy focuses on the use of N-methyl-D-aspartate glutamate-receptor antagonists providing the promise of rapid antidepressant action, including clinically significant effects from one dose that were sustained for up to 1 week.

Another study has suggested the use of repeated dose intravenous ketamine for the acute treatment of treatment-resistant depression although the effect of glutamate on depression in promising, this has not necessarily been the case for other novel pharmacological mechanisms. The failures of CRF1 antagonist compounds and substance-P antagonists have continually been noted. Another advance is the introduction of agomelatine—a melatonin (MT1 and MT2) agonist and a 5-HT2C-receptor antagonist. Agomelatine has shown a generally favorable tolerability it for patients who do not respond to existing pharmacotherapies, or who cannot tolerate their side-effects. Placebo-controlled research provides evidence for the effectiveness of agomelatine as both an acute and a continuation treatment for major depression.

SUICIDE RISK WITH SSRIs

The safety of SSRIs has been debated because of their potential association with suicidal ideation and behavior as noted from studies of adolescents with depression. Some work suggests that adults treated with antidepressant drugs, including SSRIs, are no more likely to attempt or complete suicide than those not treated with an antidepressant. However, other research suggests a reduced risk of suicide attempt in adults after start of SSRI treatment, particularly with sertraline, and in men. In 2, 26, 866 male veterans with depression, rates of suicide attempt were lower after the start of SSRI treatment than before, and compared with treatment with other antidepressants or no antidepressant. Similarly a study of county-level data in the USA showed that a decrease in suicide rate was associated with SSRIs when prescribed in combination with non-SSRIs or non-tricyclic antidepressants. Despite these findings, caution is needed against strong conclusions being made on the basis of limited ecological analyses.

SAFETY IN PREGNANCY

Data before 2000 provided weak evidence for an association between SSRIs and major fetal malformation. Since then, data have shown that paroxetine might be associated with major malformations, especially cardiac defects. Some evidence is available of an association between a neonatal behavioral syndrome and exposure to SSRIs in utero during the last trimester. This syndrome can be managed with supportive treatment in a special-care nursery. Presence of persistent pulmonary hypertension in the neonate can also be associated with SSRIs taken late in pregnancy. Infants with continuous exposure to mother's depression and continuous exposure to SSRIs throughout gestation were more likely to be born preterm than were infants with partial or no exposure. Guidelines suggest that SSRIs should be used with caution during pregnancy, and that paroxetine be avoided.

STATUS OF NEW SOMATIC TREATMENTS

Although deep brain stimulation is still in the early investigational stages and not approved by the FDA or the European Medicines Agency, it is promising as a treatment for treatment-resistant depression. In deep brain stimulation, electrodes are implanted bilaterally in the brain and are connected to an internal pulse generator. This procedure is fully reversible and the stimulation it provides can be adjusted on the basis of the patient's needs. The treatment might exert its effect by modulating neurotransmission in the cortico-striatal-thalamic-cortical circuit. Work has shown the antidepressant effect of deep brain stimulation when used within the subgenual cingulate white matter (Cg25WM), the nucleus accumbens, the subcollosal cingulated gyrus, and the ventral capsule or ventral stiatum. This treatment has also been discussed for use in the anterior limb of the internal capsule, globus pallidus internus, inferior thalamic peduncle, rostral cingulated cortex, and lateral haenula. Although deep brain stimulation seems to be well tolerated, the possibility of suicide should be monitored. One study notes that although stable remission can be achieved with deep brain stimulation, the affective instability induced by the treatment merits specific attention.

Transcranial magnetic stimulation (TMS) has been approved by the FDA for the treatment of major depressive disorder, especially for those who have not responded to a course of one antidepressant drug. Although this treatment is regarded as safe and well-tolerated, seizures can be a rare side-effect. TMS produces a magnetic field around the brain; the left and right dorsolateral prefrontal cortex (DLPFC) are common target areas for TMS in depression. Several meta-analyses support the use of DLPFC TMS or repetitive TMS to treat depression, because they were more effective than placebo. Some studies suggest that the sizes of these effects are comparable to treatment with antidepressants; however, the sizes are moderate and repetitive TMS seems to be less effective than electro-convulsive therapy. A multisite sham-controlled study of repetitive TMS, which included an open-label extension for patients who did not improve, provided the opportunity to examine predictors of acute outcome, In this sample, low degree of previous drug resistance in the current episode, short duration of current episode, absence of anxiety disorder, high severity of baseline depression, and female sex, were associated with improved outcome in one or both parts of this trial.

7.11 DEPRESSION IN ELDERLY

BK Singh

SUMMARY

In elderly people depression mainly affects those with chronic medical illnesses and cognitive impairment, causes suffering, family disruption, and disability, worsens the outcomes of many medical illness, and increases mortality. Aging-related and disease-related processes, including arteriosclerosis and inflammatory, endocrine, and immune changes compromise the integrity of frontostriatal pathways, the amygdala, and the hippocampus, and increase vulnerability to depression. Heredity factors might also play a part. Psychosocial adversity-economic impoverishment, disability, isolation, relocation, caregiving, and bereavement-contributes to physiological changes, further increasing susceptibility to depression or triggering depression in already vulnerable elderly individuals. Treatment with antidepressants is well tolerated by elderly people and is, overall, as effective as in young adults. Evidence-based guidelines for prevention of new episodes of depression are available as are care-delivery systems the increase the likelihood of diagnosis, and improve the treatment of, late-life depression.

Late-life depression refers to depressive syndromes defined in the American Psychiatric Association's Diagnostic and Statistical Manual (DSM-IV) and in the International Classification of Diseases (ICD-10) that arise in adults older than age 65 years. In old age, depressive syndromes often affect people with chronic medical illnesses, cognitive impairment, or disability. Beyond personal suffering and family disruption, disorders and promotes disability. Although progress has been made in characterizing the presentation of late-life depression and in improving its treatment, it continues to have detrimental consequences.

DIAGNOSIS

For a diagnosis of major depression to be made, DSM-IV and ICD-10 state that either depressed mood or loss of interest or pleasure must be present (Panel 12). Although not part of the diagnostic criteria, late-life major depression is often associated with peripheral body changes and cognitive impairment. Changes to the body include hypercortisolemia, increased abdominal fat, decreased bone density, and increased risk for type 2 diabetes and hypertension. Non-demented elderly people with major depression often have difficulties with concentration, speed of mental processing, and executive function. These deficits improve, but do not completely resolve, after remission of late-life depression.

Psychotic depression is diagnosed in patients with major depression who have delusions or hallucinations. The themes of depressive delusions are guilt, hypochondriasis, nihilism, persecution, and sometimes jealousy.

Dysthymic disorder is a syndrome of depression of mild or moderate severity that lasts at least 2 years (Panel 12). Minor depression (Panel 12) in elderly people is associated with functional disability and about 25% of patients develop major depression within 2 years. In very elderly patients,a long subsyndromal phase of up to 3 years can precede major depression.

Panel 12: Classification and diagnosis of geriatric depression disorders

Major depressive disorder

Five of the following symptoms must be present: depressed mood, diminished interest, loss of pleasure in all or almost all activities, weight loss or gain (more than 5% of body weight), insomnia or hypersomnia, psychomotor agitation or retardation, fatigue, feelings of worthlessness or inappropriate guilt, reduced ability to concentrate, recurrent thoughts of death or suicide.

At least one of the symptoms must be either depressed mood or diminished interest or pleasure. The syndrome should last at least 2 weeks, lead to distress or function impairment, and not be a direct effect of substance use, a medical condition, or bereavement.

Minor depressive disorder

At least two but fewer than five of the symptoms of major depressive disorder must be present.

The syndrome should last at least 2 weeks, lead to distress or functional impairment, and not be a direct effect of substance use, a medical condition, or bereavement.

This diagnosis can only be made in patients without a history of major depression, dysthymia, bipolar, or psychotic disorders.

Dysthymic disorder

Sad mood for more days than not accompanied by another two symptoms of major depressive disorder.

Bipolar I disorder (most recent episode depressed)

Individuals meet criteria for major depressive disorder and have a history of at least one manic episode or a mixed episode.

Adjustment disorder with depressed mood

Individuals who develop depressed mood, tearfulness, or hopelessness within 3 months of the occurrence of a stressor.

The syndrome should lead to great distress or disability, and should subside within 6 months of the removal of the stressor.

Bereavement is not considered a stressor for an adjustment disorder.

Depression is also sometimes a phase of bipolar disorder. Bipolar disorder I (most recent episode depressed) is diagnosed in patients with major depression who have a history of at least one manic or mixed episodes. Elderly patients with bipolar disease have severe and disabling episodes, increased mortality compared with their peers, and are high users of mental health and other medical services.

MEDICAL COMORBIDITY

Late-life depressive syndromes often arise in the context of medical and neurological disorders. The diagnosis of depression due to a general medical condition is given when depressed mood or anhedonia occur in patients already diagnosed with an illness that is associated with depression (Panel 13). About a quarter of individuals who have a myocardial infarction or who are undergoing cardiac catheterization have major depression, and another 25% have minor depression. Approximately half of patients with coronary heart disease and major depression will have had at least one previous episode of major depression, and 50% of those with major depression at the time of cardiac catheterization remain depressed a year after the procedure. The greater the overall medical burden, the higher the risk of depression. Furthermore, some postulate that stress, major depression, and medical illness are reciprocally linked-stress promotes adaptation (allostasis), but when mediators of the stress response are not inhibited (allostatic state) immunity is impaired, arteriosclerosis promoted, and obesity, demineralization, and atrophy of brain cells arise. Allostatic load, expressed as increased adrenocortical activity, raised concentrations of insulin growth factor (IGF)-1, and initiation of the inflammatory response, has been documented in patients with major depression.

Panel 13: Geriatric depression syndromes associated with medical disorder and drug use

Depression due to a general medical condition
Patients who develop sad mood or diminished interest or pleasure in all or almost all activities and have a medical condition physiologically related to depression:
Viral infection
Endocrinopathy-hypothyroidism, hyperthyroidism, hypoparathyroidism, hyperparathyroidism, hypoadrenocorticism, hyperadrenocorticism, Cushing's disease.
Malignant disease-leukemia, lymphoma, pancreatic cancer.
Cerebrovascular disease-lacunar infarcts, stroke, vascular dementia
Myocardial infarction
Metabolic disorder-B_{12} deficiency, malnutrition

Symptoms or syndromes of depression are often present in individuals with dementia. The point prevalence of major depression is about 17% in patients with Alzheimer's diseaseand is even higher in those with subcortical dementias. The US National Institute of Mental Health has developed provisional criteria for the diagnosis of depression individuals with Alzheimer's disease (Panel 14) to help doctors to identify the problem and to promote research in to the disorder. Symptoms or syndromes of depression often proceed cognitive decline, and dementia, with elderly individuals who have major depression and cognitive impairment likely to develop dementia within a few years of onset of depression. Depression in early life is also a possible risk factor for disorders of dementia. Major depression with onset more than 10 year before the diagnosis of dementia, and lifetime history of depression is associated with increased risk for Alzheimer's disease.

Depression exacerbates the outcome of medical illnesses. In one study, elderly individuals with depression were almost four times more likely than abuse without depression to die within 4 months of a myocardial infarction. Platelet aggregation is raised in this group of patients, suggesting that depression increases the risk for cardiovascular disease. Elderly people with depressive symptomatology have poor T-cell responses to mitogens and high concentrations of plasma interleukin, which is indicative of inflammatory activity that might increase the risk for bone resorption. Nevertheless, late-life depression remains under-recognized and undertreated.

Panel 14: Provisional diagnostic criteria for depression in patients with Alzheimer's disease

Clinically significant depressive symptoms
Three or more depressive symptoms during the same 2-week period, representing a change from previous functioning.
At least one of the symptoms must be either depressed mood or decreased positive affect or pleasure. Other depressive symptoms are: clinically significant depressed mood, e.g. depressed, sad, hopeless, discouraged, tearful; decreased positive affect or pleasure in response to social contacts and usual activities; social isolation or withdrawal; disruption in appetite; disruption in sleep; psychomotor changes, e.g. agitation or retardation; irritability; fatigue or loss of energy; feelings of worthlessness, hopelessness, or excessive or inappropriate guilt; recurrent thoughts of death, suicidal ideation, plan or attempt.
Symptoms should not be a result of dementia symptoms, e.g. loss of weight due to difficulties with food intake.
Depression should not be part of idiopathic depression, other mental disorders, a medical condition, or medication use. Disease related changes in the development of depression. However, methodological and conceptual concerns limit their importance.

PSYCHOSOCIAL ADVERSITY

Low economic status, poor physical health, disability, social isolation, and relocation often lead to an adjustment disorder with depressed mood or trigger more severe depressive syndromes than previously present (Panel 12). It is noteworthy, however, that although forced relocation has a negative effect on both morbidity and mortality, voluntary decisions to move to an institution acceptable to the individual can have a beneficial effect.

Additionally, caregivers of elderly disabled individuals are twice as likely as noncaregivers to develop symptoms of depression. This proportion might be even higher, however, since male caregivers and African-American caregivers under-report symptoms of depression. Depressive symptomatology is most likely to develop during long-term caregiving. Additional predisposing factors are a care recipient with behavioral problems and receipt of limited help from others. After placement of the elderly individual in a nursing home, a quarter of caregivers develop symptoms of depression, which remain relatively unchanged overtime in women but worsen in men.

SUBSTANCE-INDUCED DEPRESSION

Patients who develop sad mood or diminished interest or pleasure in all or almost all activities within a month of substance intoxication or withdrawal or medication use causally related to the depression:

Methyldopa	Benzodiazepines	Propranolol
Reserpine	Steroids	Anti-Parkinsonian drugs
β-blockers	Cimetidine,Clonidine	Hydralazine
Estrogens	Progesterone	Tamoxifen
Vinblastine	Vincristine	Dextropropoxyphene

During the first year of bereavement, 10–20% of surviving spouses develop symptoms of depression, which generally persist if left untreated. Elderly individuals are less likely to become depressed than younger adults during the first months of widowhood, but rates of major depression are similar in all ages by the end of the second year. The prevalence of major depression continues to increases during the second year of bereavement, by the end of which 14% of bereaved individuals have major depression, compared with 1–4% of the elderly population in general.

Finally, some psychological traits confer vulnerability to depression (Flow chart 2). Neuroticism, for example, predicted persistence of depression in primary-care patients in one study, even after severity of depression was controlled for. Furthermore, in elderly individuals with major depression, pessimistic thinking predicts sucidal ideation a year later. Elderly people who committed suicide were, however, less open experience than both younger people who committed suicide and controls.

LATE-ONSET DEPRESSION

Late-onset major depression a large subgroup of patients with neurological abnormalities. Although some disagreement exists, generally, when compared with elderly individuals with early-onset major depression, individuals with late-onset major depression have a less frequent family history of mood disorders, a higher prevalence of disorders of dementia, a larger impairment in neuropsychological tests, a higher rate of dementia development on follow-up, more neurosensory hearing impairment, a greater enlargement in lateral brain ventricles, and more white-matter hyperintensities.

Flow chart 2: Model of late-life depression

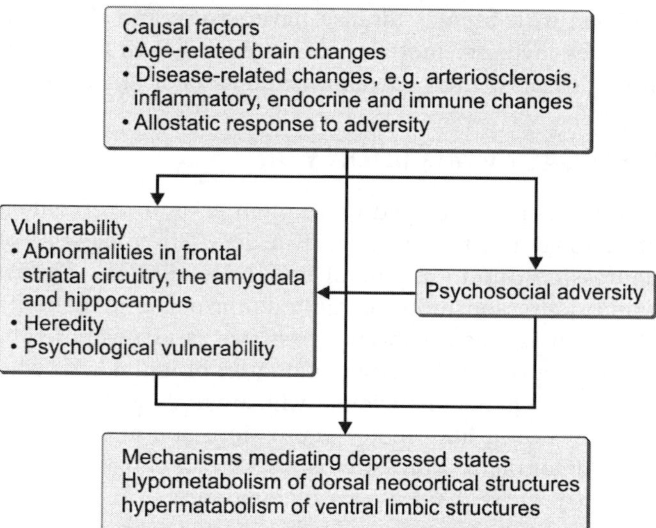

The study of late-onset depression has generated mechanistic hypotheses on the role of aging-related and disease-related changes in the development of depression. However, methodological and conceptual concerns limit their importance. Methodologically, onset of depression is difficult to identify, especially when mild. Conceptually, neurological changes could contribute to a late-life episode irrespective of other depressive episodes in early life. Moreover, early-onset depression might be a risk factor for late-life depression by contributing to brain abnormalities that predispose to depression. One such mechanism involves stress-related hormones leading to a reduction of neurotropic factor secretion, and ultimately a decrease in neurogenesis at the dentate nucleus of the hippocampus .

DEPRESSION WITH REVERSIBLE DEMENTIA

Some elderly individuals develop dementia during episodes of depression that subsides after remission of depression (pseudodementia). Most of these patients have late-onset major depression. Furthermore, a large proportion of those with reversible dementia are left with some form of cognitive impairment after remission of depression, and about 40% develop irreversible dementia within 3 years of follow-up. Thus, reversible dementia is often an early manifestation of a more permanent disorder and constitutes an indication for diagnostic work-up aimed at the identification of treatable dementia.

DEPRESSION-EXECUTABLE DYSFUNCTION SYNDROME

This syndrome has been conceptualized as major depression with prominent frontostriatal dysfunction, and is characterized by psychomotor retardation, reduced interest in activities, impaired instrumental activities of daily living, and limited insight and vegetative signs. Patients with depression and executive dysfunction often have a poor, slow, and unstable response to antidepressants and require careful treatment planning and follow-up. The depression-executable dysfunction syndrome can act as a model for studies of drugs to target neurotransmitters of frontostriatal networks, including dopamine, acetylcholine, and opioids.

VASCULAR DEPRESSION

Cerebrovascular disease might predispose, precipitate, or perpetuate some late-life depressive syndromes. This notion is based on the comorbidity of depressive syndromes with cerebrovascular lesions and cerebrovascular risk factors and on the fact that depression often develops after a stroke. Elderly people with vascular depression have greater disability and cognitive impairment than those who are depressed but do not have vascular stigmata. Verbal fluency and object naming are the most impaired cognitive functions in patients with this form of depression. Affected individuals have more apathy, retardation, and lack of insight, and less agitation and guilt than do elderly individuals who are depressed without vascular risk factors. The vascular depression hypothesis generated hypotheses of clinical important. Drugs used for the prevention of cerebrovascular disease might, for example, reduce the risk for vascular depression. Furthermore, antidepressants that promote ischemic recovery, e.g. dopamine or norepinephrine enhancing agents-might be favored in vascular depression and antidepressants that inhibit ischemic recovery, e.g. α adrenergic blocking agents-are best avoided.

SUICIDE

Suicide is almost twice as frequent in elderly individuals than in the general population. Rates of suicide in elderly individuals are raised almost exclusively in white men. Among those who attempt suicide, elderly people are most likely to die. Depressive syndromes are present in 80% of people aged older than 74 years who commit suicide. Major depression is a risk factor for suicide as is substance abuse. Minor depression, dysthymic disorder, psychotic disorders, and anxiety disorders also raise the risk of suicide. Mood disorders constitute an independent risk factor for suicide in elderly people, whereas physical illness and disability increase suicide risk, but their effect is mediated by depression. Disruption of social ties is associated with late-life suicide independently of depression, especially in individuals with a rigid, anxious, and obsessive personality. Availability of firearms doubles the risk of suicide in elderly people.

Suicidal ideation decreases with aging, but if older people have suicidal thoughts they are at a higher risk of actually committing suicide than younger people. Suicidal ideation is closely associated with severity of depression and previous serious attempts could predict the course of suicidal ideation. During follow-up, contemporaneous severity of depression was the most important determinant of suicidal ideation overtime. These observations can be used to identify elderly people with depression who are at high risk of committing suicide.

EPIDEMIOLOGY

About 1–4% of the general elderly population has major depression, equivalent to an incidence of 0.15% per year. Twice as many women as men are affected. Both the prevalence and the incidence of major depression double after age 70 to 85 years. Similarly, the number of old people is rising and, possibly, because the proportion of elderly individuals with this illness is increasing.

Minor depression has a prevalence of 4–13%. Dysthymic disorder, characterized by low-intensity symptoms of depression that last 2 years or longer, occurs in about 2% of elderly people. An elderly person is as likely or slightly less likely to have clinically significant symptoms of depression than someone who is middle-aged (prevalence 8–16%), but a very old person is particularly prone to this disorder. An increase in disability and cognitive impairment, a fall in socioeconomic status, and the high proportion of women who survive their partner's death might explain this pattern.

The prevalence of late-life depressive syndromes is higher in medical settings than in the community, 10–12% of patients admitted to hospital have major depression, whereas the prevalence among primary-care patients is 6-9%. Additionally, 6% of primary-care patients have minor depression and 10% subsyndromal depression. However, more than half of patients with less severe types of depression remain depressed a year later. The prevalence of major depression among individuals who live in nursing homes is 12 to 14% though 17 to 35% of those in long-term care have minor depression or clinically significant symptoms of depression.

PATHOPHYSIOLOGY

Dorsal neocortical structures are hypometabolic and ventral limbic structures are hypermetabolic during depressed states. Similar changes arise in experimentally induced sadness, but are quickly reversed when stimuli are removed. The persistence of the changes in depressed patients suggests that additional biological factors predispose to depression and sustain depressive symptoms.

Frontostriatal pathways in the brain mediate positive affect-guided anticipation, and abnormalities might result in an inability to anticipate incentives, thus predisposing to depression. The left medial orbitofrontal cortex is activated in response to reward and the right orbitofrontal cortex in response to punishment. Furthermore, the anterior cingulated gyrus has connections to brain structures, subserving functions often impaired in depression. The perigenual cingulated assesses conflicts between current function and information with motivational consequences. The dorsal cingulated monitors competing responses and modulates attention and executive functions in collaboration with the dorsolateral cortex.

Frontostriatal dysfunction could predispose to late-life depression. Executive dysfunction, a clinical expression of frontostriatal abnormalities, is common in late-life depression and persists after improvement of mood-related symptoms. Additionally, subcortical disorders that compromise frontostriatal pathways are often complicated by depression and executive dysfunction. Low volumes of frontostriatal structures have been documented in late-life depression, as have hyperintensities in subcortical structures and their frontal connections. Macromolecular abnormalities in the genu and splenium of the corpus callosum, the right caudate nucleus, and the putamen are seen in elderly people with depression. Reduction in glia of the subgenual anterior cingulate and abnormalities in neurons of the dorsolateral cortex have also been observed in depressed patients.

Frontostriatal dysfunction affects the presentation and course of late-life major depression, increasing executive dysfunction and psychomotor retardation and resulting in greater feeling of apathy. Executive dysfunction generally results in a slow, poor, and unstable response to antidepressants. White-matter and poor outcomes of late-life depression. Hypometabolism of the anterior cingulated was reported in treatment-resistant major depression, while hypermetabolism arose in depressed patients with favorable treatment response. Increased left frontal error negative wave amplitude after a response inhibition task, a function mediated by the anterior cingulated, predicts limited or slow change of major depression in elderly individuals treated with citalopram.

Abnormalities of the amygdala might predispose to depression. The amygdala mediates emotions in response to aversive stimuli and signals to centers responsible for coping behavior and autonomic activity. Age-related changes associated with attenuation of emotional perception could contribute to depressed or pathetic states. Stroke and subcortical disorders can damage the connections between the amygdala, the medial dorsal thalamic nucleus, and the orbital and medial prefrontal cortex, predisposing to depression. Additionally, hypercortisolemia, which arises during chronic medical illnesses, is associated with increased activity of the amygdala, leading to release of cortisol and depression.

During their first episode of major depression, patients have larger amygdala, volumes than those with recurrent depression or healthy controls. Increased activity in this part of the brain is associated with symptoms of depression and negative emotions, and might be a result of its inadequate inhibition by prefrontal centers. Increased activity of the amygdala combined with inadequate cortical modulation of its emotional output probably contribute to depressive symptoms.

Hippocampal abnormalities could also predispose to depression, since the volume of this structure is reduced during a first episode of major depression. However some disagree with this theory. Nevertheless, a reduction in the volume of the hippocampus is correlated with lifetime duration of depression. Moreover, a decline in hippocampal volume has been documented after a first episode of major depression even in patients who received antidepressants.

Hippocampal abnormalities are relevant to the elderly population, since this structure is particularly vulnerable to aging and aging-related changes. Moreover, the CA1 hippocampal region and the subiculum are vulnerable to ischemia and to hypercortisolemia, resulting from stress and chronic medical illness .

HEREDITY

In addition to changes in brain structures, hereditary factors could predispose to late-life depressive syndromes. In community-residing elderly twins, heredity accounted for 18% of the variation in depressive symptoms. Elderly people who are depressed are, however, less likely to have a depressed. Personal or family history of a depressive disorder affects the incidence of depression after stroke as much, if not more, than the site of vascular lesion.

Genetic markers for late-life depression have not been identified. However, results of studies done in twins suggest an association between the serotonin 2A receptor gene promoter A/A genotype and depression in elderly men, but not in elderly women. The serotonin reuptake transporter gene was not associated with depression in elderly twins. Presence of the allele E4 of apolipoprotein-E is a risk factor for Alzheimer's disease and for cerebrovascular disease, which are conditions associated with late-life depression. However, most investigators noted no association between E4 and late-life depression. Genes associated with increased risk for cerebrovascular lesions might increased vulnerability to depression. Patients with late-onset major depression had a higher frequency of the C677T mutation of the enzyme methylene tetrahydrofolate reductase than healthy elderly individuals. These findings suggest that genetic predisposition to late-life major depression is mediated by vascular lesions.

PREVENTION

There is a hypothesis that positive mental health can be enhanced if people believe they have the ability to act in a way that will result in achievement of their goals. As such, elderly individuals with chronic medical illnesses at risk for depression who receive instruction on body-mind relations, relaxation techniques, cognitive restructuring, problem solving, communication, and behavioral management of insomnia, nutrition, and exercise, have increased self-efficacy and reduced symptoms of depression, anxiety, pain, and insomnia. Other approaches to primary prevention include lowering of the risk of vascular depression-through control of hypertension, hyperlipidemia, and concentrations of plasma hornocysteine -use of antidepressants in patients at risk for depression because of medical comorbidity, e.g. macular degeneration threatening complete blindness —education of elderly people about the treatment options available, and reduction of the stigma of depression to increase the number of elderly individuals who seek and adhere to treatment. The findings of secondary prevention studies indicate that antidepressants and psychotherapy alone or in combination reduce the risk for relapse and recurrence of late-life depression in elderly patients who have previously remitted. A shared-care intervention was more effective than usual care in reducing symptoms of depression in old people living in self-care units and hostels. The intervention consisted of multidisciplinary consultation and collaboration, training of family doctors and other health-care workers in detection and management of depression, and provision of education and activity programs for residents. Finally, the results of tertiary prevention studies show that comprehensive clinical management aimed at the symptoms of depression can reduce suicidal ideation and perhaps the risk of suicide.

MANAGEMENT

The aims of treatment are to reduce the symptoms of depression, to prevent suicidal ideation, relapse, or recurrence of symptoms to improve cognitive and functional status, and to help patients develop the skills needed to cope with their disability or psychosocial adversity if appropriate. Behavioral rehabilitation should be combined with antidepressant treatment to improve function as depressive syndromes subside.

Treatment planning should start with an assessment that focuses on identification of any intake of the drugs or presence of illnesses that predispose to depression. Treatment of the underlying illness or removal of offending drugs in necessary, but is often not enough to achieve remission of depression. Antidepressants, psychotherapy, or both, are also generally needed. The combination is the preferred treatment option for late-life major depression. Pharmacotherapy or psychotherapy alone are, however, acceptable alternatives in major depression of mild severity. Electroconvulsive therapy should be considered if patients do not respond to treatment with antidepressants, have severe depression with suicide risk, are likely to die because of lack of nutrition and fluids, or are psychotic.

Antidepressants are as effective when given to elderly individuals as they are when given to younger adults. Selective serotonin reuptake inhibitors (SSRIs) and serotonin-norepinephrine reuptake inhibitors (SNRIs) are the antidepressants of choice, followed by bupropion and mirtazapine. Although the initial doses of SSRIs and SNRIs given to elderly individuals should be low, the final doses should be similar to those used in young adults. Nortriptyline followed by desipramine are reasonable alternatives to SSRIs in severe late-life depression. Amitriptyline, imipramine, doxepin, amoxapine, maprotilene, trazodone, tranylcypromine, and isocarboxazide should be avoided.

For late-life depression initiated by a stressor psychotherapy alone or psychotherapy combined with an antidepressant is recommended. Minor depression in late life is more likely to respond to nonspecific supportive interventions than other forms of depression. Watchful waiting for at least 2 weeks is appropriate in minor depression. However, if symptoms persist for longer than 2–3 months, a combination of SSRI plus psychotherapy is the treatment of choice, though drug treatment alone or psychotherapy alone are reasonable alternatives.

Cognitive-behavioral therapy, supportive psychotherapy, problem-solving therapy, and interpersonal therapy are the preferred psychotherapies for elderly people with depression. Cognitive therapy approaches are as effective in elderly individuals as they are in younger adults. Psychoeducation can help patients and their families with treatment adherence.

Appropriate doses of an antidepressant should be given for at least 4 weeks before the drug is judged ineffective and a different class is tried. If a patient's response to an antidepressant is poor, a higher dose should be tried. If there is no further improvement, use of an augmenting agent should be considered. If the initial antidepressant was an SSRI, bupropion, lithium, or nortriptyline can be added. If the patient was initially treated with bupropion an SSRI or lithium might help. Electroconvulsive therapy is an option at option at any step if the patient worsens.

In late-life psychotic depression, combinations of antidepressants (SSRIs or venlafaxine) and atypical neuroleptics (except clozapine) are recommended. Electroconvulsive therapy should either be considered as a first choice in psychotic depression or be used if combination drug treatment is ineffective.

Late-life depression is a recurring disorder. In one study, 90% of elderly individuals with major depression in remission had a recurrence within 3 years when maintained on placebo, whereas those maintained on nortriptyline and interpersonal psychotherapy had a recurrence rate of 20% and 43% recurred among those who receive nortriptyline and medication clinic visits. For maintenance, antidepressants should be used at the same doses as for treatment. In patients who have a single severe episode of depression, antidepressant drug treatment should continue for at least 1 year. Patients with three lifetime episodes should receive maintenance treatment for longer than 3 years. In patients with psychotic depression who achieve remission after treatment with an antidepressant and an antipsychotic, the general recommendation is that the antipsychotic drug be continued for 6 months. For patients who do not respond to antidepressants but for whom electroconvulsive therapy was effective, continuation or maintenance therapy should consist of an antidepressant not yet tried by the patient and a mood stabilizer. Continuation or maintenance electroconvulsive therapy is another option.

CARE DELIVERY

Most elderly individuals who are depressed are treated in primary-care settings. However, primary-care doctors rarely diagnose depression and, when they do, often provide inappropriate treatment. Barriers to adequate diagnosis and treatment include doctors' reluctance to discuss emotional problems, time constraints, and medical comorbidity, complicating diagnosis and competing for clinical attention. Perceived stigma contributes to patients' reluctance to initiate psychiatric treatment. Furthermore, disability, cognitive impairment, and complex medication regimes undermine treatment adherence.

Several service-delivery models can improve the treatment of depression in primary care-namely, training of primary-care doctors, introduction of computer-driven clinical decision support, and integration of the management of depression with the care of other medical illnesses. Collaborative care, involving primary-care doctors and on-site specialists in mental health enhances quality of care and improves the outcomes of depression.

OUTLOOK

Late-life depressive disorders often arise in the context of psychosocial adversity, chronic medical diseases, and disability, and besides suffering and family disruption worsen medical outcomes. Although ageing and disease-related brain abnormalities that predispose to late-life depression have been identified, a direct lesion-depression association is unlikely. Behavioral abnormalities are subserved by high-level interactive and redundant neural systems. When damaged, these systems can cause diverse behavioral abnormalities. Personal or family history of psychiatric disorders, overall medical burden, disability, and psychosocial adversity are other factors that contribute to depression. Moreover, acquired behavioral skills could moderate or avert depressive symptoms. Finally, the patient's own environmental ecosystem can impede or facilitate the development of symptoms and syndromes of depression, depending on whether it can compensate for the lost functions. Cognitive impairment and disability that accompany late-life depression are becoming the focus of pharmacological and nonpharmacological interventions.

7.12 MEDICAL TREATMENT OF DEPRESSION

JN Vyas

Recurrent episodes of major depression, which is a common and serious illness, are called major depressive disorder; depressive episodes that occur in conjunction with manic episodes are called bipolar disorder. Major depressive disorder accounts for 4.4% of the total overall global disease burden, a contribution similar to that of ischemic heart disease or diarrheal diseases.[415] The prevalence of major depressive disorder in the United States is 5.4–8.9%[416] and of bipolar disorder, 1.7–3.7%[417] and the prevalances in other countries is almost similar. Major depression affects 5-13% of medical outpatients,[418] yet is often undiagnosed and untreated.[419,420] Moreover, it is often undertreated when correctly diagnosed.[420]

The demographics of depression are impressive. Among persons both with major depressive disorder and bipolar disorder, 75–85% have recurrent episodes.[421,422] In addition, 10–30% of persons with a major depressive episode recover incompletely and have persistent, residual depressive symptoms, or dysthymia, a disorder with symptoms that are similar to those of major depression but last longer and are milder.[422,423] Patients who have diabetes, epilepsy, or ischemic heart disease with concomitant major depression have poorer outcomes than do those without depression.[424,425] The risk of death from suicide, accidents, heart disease, respiratory disorders, and stroke is higher among the depressed.[426,427] Effective treatment of depression may reduce mortality or improve the outcome after acute myocardial infarction[428] or stroke[429] and lower the risk of suicide.[430]

PATHOPHYSIOLOGICAL FEATURES OF DEPRESSION

The clinical picture of depression varies from one major depressive episode to another in any given patient. This suggests that major depression, despite its various symptom profiles, may have a common underlying cause. If so, the clinically evident symptom profiles may result from differing patterns of neurotransmitter abnormalities in various brain regions.[431] Consonant with such hypotheses, a host of deficiencies in serotonin, norepinephrine, dopamine, γ-aminobutyric acid (GABA), and peptide neurotransmitters or trophic factors such as brain derived neurotrophic factor, somatostatin, and thyroid related hormones—have been proposed as contributing to depresssion.[432] Furthermore, overactivity in still other neurotransmitter systems involving acetylcholine, corticotropin releasing factor, and substance P are thought to be implicated in depression.[432] Although no specific abnormalities in genes that control neurotransmitter or hormonal synthesis or release have been identified with certainty, both major depressive disorder and bipolar disorder are clearly heritable.[433] How a genetic predisposition interacts with adverse early life experience alter brain development and lead to major depression remains unclear.

Genes and stress are hypothesized to alter neuron size and the extent of neuronal processes, the production of new neurons, and neural repair in major depression. Elevated cortisol levels, which characterize some moderate to severe depressive states, may be associated with a reduction in hippocampal volume, which appears to be proportional to the duration of untreated depression.[434] This process has been linked to a loss of neurons similar to that mediated by corticosteroids in animal models of stress[435] and as suggested by magnetic resonance imaging studies that have reported lower levels of N-acetyl aspartate, a neuronal marker, in depression.[436]

Major depression in response to stressful situations has been reported as more common among persons harboring a variant in the proximal 5′ regulatory region of the gene encoding the serotonin transporter protein (5HTT) (the target of selective serotonin reuptake inhibitors [SSRIs]) that modifies promoter activity. This variant, in the 5HTT gene-linked promoter region (5HTTLPR), modifies promoter activity and is associated with lower transcriptional efficiency of the 5HTT gene, ultimately leading to fewer copies of the messenger RNA encoding the serotonin transporter protein.[437] This lower expressing variant may be associated with the amygdala mediated hyper-responsiveness of young children to frightened or frightening faces that can facilitate encoding of painful memories, leading to stress sensitivity in adulthood.[438] This variant is also associated with a reduction of serotonin function in response to maternal deprivation in nonhuman primates, an effect that persists into adulthood.[439] An induced functional deficiency of the 5HTT protein that is confined to the early postnatal period in mice results in altered behavior when they are grown, indicating possible changes in brain development that affect adult behavior.[440]

Brain imaging has identified numerous regions of altered structure or activity in the brain during major depression, suggesting disordered neurocircuitry in a variety of structures, such as the anterior and posterior cingulate cortex; the ventral, medial, and dorsolateral prefrontal cortex; the insula; the ventral striatum; the hippocampus; the medial thalamus; the amygdala; and the brainstem.[431] These brain areas regulate emotional, cognitive, autonomic, sleep, and stress response behaviors that are impaired in mood disorders. Studies with the use of positron emission tomography (PET) indicate a decrease in serotonin transporters as well as altered post-synaptic serotonin receptor binding in many of the same brain regions, suggesting altered circuitry congruent with serotonin system abnormalities.[441]

DIAGNOSIS OF A MAJOR DEPRESSIVE EPISODE

Diagnosis of major depression is based on standard clinical criteria such as those published by the American Psychiatric Association.[442] The criteria for the diagnosis of an episode include at least two weeks of depressed mood, loss of interest, or diminished sense of pleasure plus four of seven other features that are sufficient to cause clinically important psychological or physical distress or functional impairment. These features include a weight change of 5% or more in one month or a persistent change in appetite, insomnia or hypersomnia on most days, changes in psychomotor state, fatigue, feelings of guilt and worthlessness, diminished concentration and decisiveness, and suicidal ideation or a suicide attempt. First or "early" depressive episodes are often milder than are episodes of returning depression, and an earlier age at onset generally predicts a more severe course.[443] It is thought that early diagnosis and treatment may mitigate adverse effects of depression on education, career, and relationships.

It is important to note that secondary depression that is similar to a primary mood disorder may be triggered by serious physical illness such as cancer, stroke, demyelinating diseases, epilepsy, or even marked anemia. Conversely, major depression may be missed when patients present to primary care physicians with predominantly somatic symptoms, including pain.[444] Typically, symptoms such as anorexia, weight loss, constipation, disturbed sleep, anergia, loss of libido, vague aches and pains, and deficiencies in memory and concentration may result in a missed diagnosis, particularly if the patient does not spontaneously report low mood or other psychological symptoms, such as guilt, hopelessness, anxiety, suicidal ideation, or prior suicide attempts. Delusions of guilt and somatic illness complicate up to 14% of major depressive episodes, especially postpartum depression.[445] For DSM-5 diagnostic criteria of major depressive disorder, refer Chapter 7.3.

Depressive episodes in bipolar disorder may be similar to those in major depressive disorder or may present as part of a mixed state characterized by distressing combinations of depression and mania or hypomania (irritability, racing thoughts, anxiety, suicidal thoughts, and aggressive impulses). Patients with bipolar disorder who present with a depressive episode may be misdiagnosed as having major depressive disorder because they may often underreport hypomanic and manic symptoms, perceiving such features to be closer to well-being than illness. A family history of bipolar disorder can assist in making the correct diagnosis.

Antidepressant Medications

About half of moderate to severe episodes of depression will improve with antidepressant treatment.[446] Classes of antidepressant agents are defined by their mechanism of action. Many agents with effective antidepressant action amplify serotonin or norepinephrine signaling by inhibiting reuptake at the synaptic cleft. The several classes of drugs include SSRIs, norepinephrine reuptake inhibitors, and dual action agents that inhibit uptake of serotonin and norepinephrine. Monoamine oxidase inhibitors (MAOIs) inhibit monoamine degradation by monoamine oxidase A or B. Other antidepressant agents antagonize α2-adrenergic autoreceptors with a resultant increase in the release of norepinephrine, antagonize 5-hydroxytryptamine2A (5HT2A) receptors, or both.

Selective Serotonin Reuptake Inhibitors

Clinical trials have shown little difference in efficacy or tolerability among various available selective serotonin reuptake inhibitors (SSRIs)[446–448] or between SSRIs and other classes of antidepressants.[446,449–452] However, some specific differences should be noted.

The active metabolite of fluoxetine has a half-life that is longer than that of other SSRIs, which permits once daily dosing and thereby reduces the effect of missed doses and mitigates the SSRI discontinuation syndrome. However, fluoxetine should be used with caution in patients with bipolar disorder or a family history of bipolar disorder, because an active metabolite persists for weeks and may aggravate the manic state in the event of a switch from depression to mania. At higher doses, paroxetine and sertraline also block dopamine reuptake, which may contribute to their antidepressant action.

The SSRIs can be helpful in patients who do not have a response to tricyclic antidepressants, an older class of drugs, and appear to be better tolerated with lower rates of discontinuation[446,450,451,453] and fewer cardiovascular effects.[453] Although tricyclic antidepressants may have greater efficacy than SSRIs in severe major depressive disorder or depression with melancholic features, they are less effective than SSRIs for bipolar depression, since they can trigger mania or hypomania.[454] SSRIs appear to be less effective than either tricyclic antidepressants or selective norepinephrine reuptake inhibitors for depression in which physical symptoms or pain is prominent.[455] The SSRI fluoxetine is the only antidepressant that has consistently been shown to be effective in children and adolescents,[456] and SSRIs may be superior to selective norepinephrine reuptake inhibitors in young adults (18–24 years of age),[457] although they are more likely to trigger mania in children.[458]

NOREPINEPHRINE REUPTAKE INHIBITORS

Nortriptyline, maprotiline, and desipramine are tricyclic norepinephrine reuptake inhibitors with anticholinergic effects.[459] Reboxetine is a selective norepinephrine reuptake inhibitor with an effectiveness similar to that of tricyclic antidepressants and SSRIs.[446]

DUAL-ACTION ANTIDEPRESSANTS

Serotonin-norepinephrine reuptake inhibitors such as venlafaxine, and duloxetine block monoamine transporters more selectively than tricyclic antidepressants and without the cardiac conduction effects that can occur with tricyclic agents.[446] Some tricyclics (imipramine and amitriptyline) inhibit both serotonin and norepinephrine reuptake. The dual-action antidepressant venlafaxine appears to demonstrate superior efficacy and higher rates of remission in severe depression as compared with either SSRIs such as fluoxetine or tricyclic antidepressants.[460-462] The efficacy of duloxetine is similar to that of the SSRI paroxetine.[463] Venlafaxine and duloxetine are effective for the treatment of chronic pain[464] and diabetic neuropathic pain, respectively,[465] as well as pain occurring as part of primary or secondary depression.[466,467] Bupropion, which inhibits both norepinephrine and dopamine reuptake, has no direct action on the serotonin system and is generally similar in efficacy to tricyclic antidepressants[446] and SSRIs.[468] Bupropion is associated with less nausea, diarrhea, somnolence, and sexual dysfunction than are SSRIs[468] and constitutes an effective alternative, or adjunctive therapy, for patients who do not have a response to SSRIs.[469,470]

Monoamine Oxidase Inhibitors

Older, irreversible monoamine oxidase inhibitors (MAOIs) nonselectively block MAO A and B isoenzymes and have an antidepressant efficacy similar to that of tricyclic antidepressants. However, MAOIs are not first line drugs because patients who receive them must adhere to a low tyramine diet to prevent hypertensive crisis and because MAOIs carry greater drug interaction risks than do other medications. MAOIs appear to be superior to tricyclic agents for people with depression characterized by extreme fatigue or extreme psychological sensitivity to rejection or failed relationships.[471] MAOIs are also useful for treating patients who do not have a response to tricyclic antidepressants.[472] The reversible selective MAO A inhibitor moclobemide and MAO B selective inhibitor, selegiline, have a greater safety margin than do SSRIs but similar efficacy.[473,474] A selegiline transdermal patch is under consideration by the Food and Drug Administration (FDA).

OTHER ANTIDEPRESSANTS AND NEW THERAPIES

Mirtazapine enhances the release of norepinephrine by blocking α2-adrenergic autoreceptors as well as serotonin 5HT2A and 5HT3 receptors and histamine H1 receptors. Its efficacy is similar to that of tricyclic antidepressants and SSRIs,[475] and it is less likely to have sexual and sleep related side effects.[476,477]

Nefazodone, which blocks the 5HT2A serotonin receptor and serotonin reuptake, has an antidepressant efficacy similar to that of SSRIs but with a lower likelihood of sexual dysfunction and sleep related side effects.[478,479] Nefazodone appears to be useful in postpartum depression,[480] severe depression,[481] and treatment resistant major depression with anxiety.[482]

New antidepressive treatments currently being evaluated include vagal nerve stimulation, rapid transcranial magnetic stimulation, mifepristone (a glucocorticoid antagonist for treatment of delusional depression), and substance P antagonists. Other targets for future agents include neuropeptide Y, vasopressin V1b, N-methyl-D-aspartate, nicotinic cholinergic, delta opiate, cannabinoid, dopamine D1, cytokine, and corticotropin releasing factor 1 receptors, as well as GABA, intracellular messenger systems, and transcription, neuroprotective, and neurogenic factors.

Augmenting and Adjunctive Medications

Various medications used in conjunction with other antidepressants may help to augment the effect of antidepressants. They can also target different components of patients' symptoms (such as delusions) or help to prevent a switch into mania Table 7.

Table 7: Augmenting of adjunctive drugs

Drug	*Starting dose*	*Standard dose*			*Main side effects*			*Other*
	Mg/day		*Weight gain*	*Lethargy*	*Ataxia*	*Nausea*	*Tremor*	
Mood stablizers Lithium	600–900	450–1500	Severe	Mild	Non or mild	Moderate	Severe	Polyuria, fatigue, hypothyroidism, cognitive defects, acne, headache, worsens psoriasis
Lamotrigine (Lamictal)	25	50–300	Mild	Moderate	Moderate	Moderate	None or mild	Dizziness, headache, insomnia, severe skin reactions (3.t, Steven-Johnson syndrome
Valproic acid (Depakene) of diavalproex (Depakote)	15 per kg of body weight	Up to 60 kg of body weight	Moderate	Moderate	Moderate	Moderate	Severe	Headache, overain
			Weight gain	Sedation	Diabetes or Lipid increase	Tardive dyskinesia	Hypotension	
Antipsychotic agents								
Typical								
Chlorpromazine (Thorazine)	25	75–200	Moderate	Severe	None or Mild	Severe	Mild	EPS sinus tachycardia
Haloperidol (Haldol)	2–6	10–20	None or Mild	None or Mild	Severe	Severe	Mild	EPS, akathisia, sinus tachycardia

Contd...

Contd...

Drug	Starting dose	Standard dose			Main side effects			Other
	Mg/day		Weight gain	Lethargy	Ataxia	Nausea	Tremor	
Clozapine (Clozanil)	25	300–400	Severe	Severe	Moderate	None or Mild	Severe	Low white-cell count
Olazapine (Zyprexa)	5	10–20	Severe	Mild	Moderate	Mild	Mild	EPS, hepatic effects, dizziness
Risperidone (Risperdal)	1–2	4–6	Mild	Mild	None or Mild	Mild	Mild	EPS, insomnia, agitation, CVA in dementia
Quetiapine (Seroquel)	50	300–600	Mild	Mild	Mild	Mild	Moderate	Somnolence dizziness, dyspepsia
Aripiprazole (Ability)	10–15	15–30	Mild	Mild	Mild	Moderate	Moderate	EPS, insomnia, agitation, anxiety
Ziprasidone	40–80	80–160	None or Mild	Mild	None or Mild	Mild	Mild	EPS, constipation, fatigue, insomnia, QT prolongation
Thyroid supplement								
Thyroxin (Synthroid)	0.05	0.05–0.1	NA	NA	NA	NA	NA	None if thyroid function is monitored

Mood Stabilizers

Lithium is an antimanic agent and, as a mood stabilizer, prevents the recurrence of mania or depression. It may be superior to placebo for bipolar depression but not for major depression.[483] Lithium is an effective augmenting agent, and the condition of roughly half the patients who do not have a response to a single antidepressant improves when lithium is added.[484,485]

The anticonvulsant lamotrigine reduces glutamatergic activity and has been used as an augmenting agent in major depressive disorder[486] and for treating and preventing depressive relapse in bipolar disorder.[487] Lamotrigine can induce severe skin reactions, including the Stevens-Johnson syndrome and toxic epidermal necrolysis, although gradual dose titration appears to reduce the risk.

Other mood stabilizers, including the anticonvulsants valproic acid, divalproex, and carbamazepine, are used to treat mania in bipolar disorder. Divalproex or valproate may prevent a recurrence of bipolar depression.[488]

Antipsychotic Agents

Typical antipsychotic agents (e.g. chlorpromazine, fluphenazine, and haloperidol) block the dopamine D2 receptor, whereas "atypical" antipsychotic agents (e.g. clozapine, olanzapine, risperidone, quetiapine, ziprasidone, and aripiprazole) act as 5HT2A antagonists. Antipsychotic drugs are combined with antidepressants to treat depression with psychotic features.[489,490] Atypical antipsychotic drugs are also used for treatment resistant major depression[491] and bipolar depression.[492]

Although atypical antipsychotic drugs have a more favorable side effect profile with respect to Parkinsonism, akathisia, and tardive dyskinesia, some develop other risks, such as drug-induced arrhythmia, diabetes, weight gain, and hyperlipidemia.[493,494]

Overall Therapeutic Strategy

Patients who present with the complex, variable clinical picture of major depressive disorder and bipolar disorder may require a multimodal approach that includes pharmacotherapy, education, and psychotherapy. Treatment requires the monitoring of clinical responses, including suicidal ideation or behavior and side effects. To encourage adherence to therapy, education of both patients and their families must emphasize the fact that the effects of antidepressant medication take time. The average treatment duration for an episode is six months, and there is a high risk of future episodes; thus, both patients and their families must be made aware of these facts. The treatment plan should take into account the patient's previous treatment outcomes, the mood disorder subtype, the severity of the current episode of depression, the risk of suicide, coexisting psychiatric and somatic conditions, nonpsychiatric medications, and psychosocial stressors.[459] There are three phases of treatment: the acute, continuation, and maintenance phases.

Acute Phase

The treatment goal in the acute phase is remission—the induction of a state with minimal symptoms—in which the criteria for a major depressive episode have abated and marked improvement in psychosocial functioning has occurred, on the basis of reports from the patient and the patient's family.[495-497] Hospitalization is needed if symptoms are severe (dehydration, delusions, and psychomotor agitation) and there is a risk of suicide (previous suicide attempts or current plan for suicide).

Antidepressants are the treatment of choice for moderate to severe episodes of depression. Since most antidepressants that are used for major depressive disorder have similar effectiveness, the choice of medication depends on depressive symptoms (psychotic or suicidal), the history of responses to medication (including that of first degree relatives), medication tolerability, adverse effects, and the likelihood of adherence. Other considerations are concurrent medical conditions, use of nonpsychiatric drugs, and cost of medication.

The SSRIs and other newer antidepressant drugs with a greater safety margin constitute first line medications for moderate to severe depression, particularly for outpatients, for patients treated by primary care physicians, and for patients with cardiovascular disease.[459,498] Depression in persons 65 years of age or older generally requires relatively low doses of antidepressants,[499] and SSRIs appear to be preferable to nonselective norepinephrine reuptake inhibitors, such as tricyclic antidepressants, because of the lower risk of anticholinergic and cardiovascular side effects.[453]

The acute treatment phase usually lasts 6 to 10 weeks. The patient should be evaluated weekly or twice monthly by the treating physician until substantial improvement is achieved. Doses should be low initially and gradually increased, depending on the clinical response and side effects. The decision to increase the dose, change the medication, or add another medication should be done accordingly. Outpatients at risk for suicide should not be given large supplies of antidepressant drugs that could be lethal in the case of an overdose.

Monitoring Treatment Response

The response of patients to treatment requires systematic monitoring. A practical set of criteria include nonresponse, a decrease in baseline severity of 25% or less; partial response, a 26 to 49% decrease in baseline severity; partial remission, a 50% or greater decrease in baseline severity (residual symptoms); and remission, an absence of symptoms. Options for the evaluation of the response include rating scales and the global judgment of the treating clinician on the basis of patient and family reports. The best predictors of outcome are improvements in anhedonia (loss of pleasure), psychomotor retardation, and loss of interest, which are assessed by asking questions that go beyond "depressed mood." Suicidal ideation or risk of suicide, pessimism, guilt, and other changes in cognition may take longer to improve than vegetative symptoms, such as alterations in sleep or appetite.[500] If initial treatment is not tolerated or the response is unsatisfactory (<50% improvement), a change in medication or approach is indicated. Thirty to fifty percent of patients have substantial residual symptoms after adequate first line treatment.[501] If there has been no improvement after four weeks of treatment with an adequate dose of a given medication, the ultimate response is almost certainly going to be inadequate.[502]

Among patients receiving the same dose of a given drug, blood levels may vary by as much as a factor of 20 because of individual variations in drug metabolism. Such variations are caused by genetic differences, the effects of drugs on liver enzymes, and the effects of aging. Before medications are switched, consideration should be given to the diagnosis, the medication dose, and adherence to the drug regimen. Coexisting medical conditions, alcoholism, substance use disorder, or the use of nonpsychiatric medications such as beta blockers may also underlie treatment failures.

Nonresponse to medication requires a treatment change. Switching to an antidepressant from a different pharmacologic class minimizes polypharmacy and reduces the risk of adverse drug interactions and side effects seen with combinations of similar drugs. The disadvantage of switching agents may be the loss of a possible partial response from the initial drug and a delay in the onset of antidepressant action from the second. The initial medication may need to be tapered to avoid symptoms of discontinuation, such as nausea, headache, and sensory changes. Switching from irreversible MAOIs to most other agents requires a minimum drug free period of two weeks.

Switching to a new antidepressant from the same pharmacologic class is one option. Patients who do not have a response to one SSRI have a 40–70% chance of having a response to a second SSRI.[503] Another approach is the use of two antidepressants from different classes with complementary mechanisms of action to avoid loss of a partial response to the first medication. This approach increases the risk of drug interactions and new side effects, as well as the cost of treatment.

Augmenting antidepressant medication with other agents, so called augmenting agents, that may enhance antidepressant efficacy avoids the transition from the first to the second antidepressant and builds on partial remission. Lithium is a first line augmenting agent.[504] Two to four weeks of lithium treatment are needed before the response can be assessed. Lamotrigine is an effective augmenting agent for patients who do not have an adequate response to fluoxetine.[72] Antipsychotic agents may augment the response in nonpsychotic major depression.[505] Thyroid supplements have been advocated even in the absence of clinical hypothyroidism for the purpose of enhancing antidepressant action. Modafinil is a stimulant and as an adjunct may alleviate residual sleepiness and fatigue.[506]

Mood disorders with delusions or hallucinations respond better to an antidepressant-antipsychotic combination than to either alone.[507] Some patients with this constellation of symptoms will require electroconvulsive therapy (ECT), and almost all must be treated initially as inpatients.

Benzodiazepines are used as an adjunct for anxiety and insomnia in 30–60% of cases, and in that group improve response and reduce the frequency of treatment discontinuation.[508] However, the drugs cause sedation, psychomotor and cognitive impairment, memory loss, and dependence and withdrawal syndromes and are associated with increased rates of falls, fractures, traffic accidents, and death among the elderly.[509,510] The adjunctive use of benzodiazepines should be of limited duration to avoid dependence, and these drugs should be used with caution in the elderly and those with a history of alcohol or drug abuse or dependency.

Continuation Phase

The continuation phase of treatment, generally lasting six to nine months after the induction of remission, aims to eliminate residual symptoms, restore the prior level of functioning, and prevent recurrence or early relapse. Residual symptoms (partial remission) are strong predictors of recurrence, early relapse, or a more chronic future course.[511] Treatment should continue until such symptoms have resolved. Episodes lasting more than 6 months and psychotic depression require a longer continuation phase, up to 12 months.[502] The same medications and doses used to achieve relief in the acute phase are used during the continuation phase.[459]

Discontinuation of Treatment

If there is no recurrence or relapse during continuation therapy, gradual discontinuation may be planned for most patients after at least six months of treatment. Early discontinuation is associated with a 77% higher risk of relapse as compared with continuation treatment.[512] The tapering of medication over several weeks also permits detection of returning symptoms that require reinstitution of a full medication dose for another 3 to 6 months. It also minimizes the discontinuation syndrome, which otherwise may last days or longer and consists of physical symptoms of imbalance, gastrointestinal and influenza like symptoms, and sensory and sleep disturbances, as well as psychological symptoms such as anxiety, agitation, crying spells, and irritability.[513] The discontinuation syndrome is sometimes called the withdrawal syndrome, erroneously implying drug dependence.

Maintenance Phase

Maintenance treatment for 12 to 36 months reduces the risk of recurrence by two thirds.[514] This approach is indicated for patients with episodes that occur yearly, who have impairment because of mild residual symptoms, who have chronic major depression or dysthymia, or who have extremely severe episodes with a high risk of suicide.[422,459,511] The duration of maintenance treatment will depend on the natural history of the illness and may be prolonged or indefinite in the case of recurrent illness.

The first choice of medication for the maintenance phase is the antidepressant that brought about remission.[459] Lithium has no advantage over antidepressants for prophylaxis[483] but may reduce the risk of suicide independently of its effect on mood.[515] Tricyclic antidepressants, SSRIs, MAOIs, and the newer antidepressants (mirtazepine and venlafaxine) all help to prevent recurrence.[483,515-518] Medication tolerability is particularly important during the maintenance phase, because it affects patients' adherence to treatment. Stable patients should see a psychopharmacologist at intervals of 3 to 6 months while they are receiving medication. It is important to monitor adherence and breakthrough symptoms so that problems are detected early. Patient and family education reduces treatment attrition and improves the outcome.

Nonpharmacologic Therapies

Electroconvulsive Therapy

Remission rates with electroconvulsive therapy (ECT) are 60–80% in severe major depressive disorder,[519] though lower success rates are reported in community settings.[520] The maximum response is typically achieved within three weeks. ECT can be a first line treatment for patients who have severe major depressive disorder with psychotic features, psychomotor retardation, or medication resistance.[45] ECT offers rapid relief for patients who are suicidal or pregnant.[45] A course of ECT usually consists of 6 to 12 treatments, rarely exceeds 20 treatments, and is administered 2 or 3 times a week, preferably by an experienced psychiatrist. Side effects include transient postictal confusion and anterograde and retrograde memory impairment; the latter generally improves in days or weeks.[521] After ECT, it is important to start prophylactic treatment with an antidepressant medication combined with an augmenting medication such as lithium, because the relapse rate is more than 50%.[522]

Psychotherapy

Brief, structured psychotherapy techniques—such as cognitive behavioral therapy, interpersonal therapy, and certain problem-solving therapies—appear to be effective in acute phase treatment and to delay relapse during continuation treatment of mild to moderately severe depression.[459,523,524] Psychotherapy can be a first line therapy for mild depression but not for severe depression, particularly psychotic and bipolar forms, unless used in combination with pharmacology.[459,525] A combination of pharmacotherapy and psychotherapy may improve the treatment response, reduce the risk of a relapse, enhance the quality of life, and increase adherence to pharmacotherapy.[526] Psychotherapy should be considered when substantial psychosocial stressors, interpersonal difficulties, or coexisting developmental or personality disorders are present.

SPECIAL PATIENT POPULATIONS

Patients with Bipolar Disorder

Depression in bipolar disorder carries the risk of a switch into mania.[527,528] Mood stabilizers with antidepressant properties, such as lithium and lamotrigine, help prevent mania, hypomania, and mixed or rapid cycling states[529,530] and are recommended as initial treatments of bipolar depression.[517] For severe bipolar depression, a combination of an antidepressant (an SSRI or bupropion) and a mood stabilizer should be considered from the outset.[454,531,532] The atypical antipsychotic drugs olanzapine and risperidone have antidepressant and antimanic effects[533] but are more effective when combined with an antidepressant.[534] The American Psychiatric Association recommends maintenance treatment after a single manic episode.[517]

Children and Adolescents

Fluoxetine is the only antidepressant with demonstrated efficacy in childhood and adolescent depression;[456] other SSRIs, tricyclic agents, and other new generation antidepressants have not been shown to be effective for depression in this age group.[535] Fluoxetine is the only SSRI currently approved for pediatric use.

Rates of spontaneously reported suicidal ideation and suicide attempts have been higher among depressed children and adolescents receiving antidepressants than among those receiving placebo in controlled clinical trials, but no differences were noted on weekly ratings of suicidality. This possible risk needs to be weighed against the risk of untreated depression, the most common cause of suicide in youth.[536]

Pregnant Women

Antidepressant medication should be considered for pregnant women in whom a moderately severe major depressive disorder develops spontaneously, as well as for those at high risk for recurrence if their medication is discontinued.[459] Risks and benefits vary greatly among patients.

SUMMARY

Major depression and bipolar disorder are generally recurrent episodic disorders. Antidepressant and adjunctive medications can successfully treat depression and prevent future episodes.

Future challenges include the identification of antidepressants that act more quickly than those currently available, which take 6 to 8 weeks to achieve remission or substantial improvement, and that do not require continuation and maintenance treatment. A biologic classification system of subtypes of major depression is needed to facilitate the selection of the best antidepressant for each patient.

7.13 DYSTHYMIA: CONCEPTUAL EVOLUTION AND CURRENT STATUS

Ajit Avasthi, Sandeep Grover, Alkananda Dutt, Baljit Singh Saluja

INTRODUCTION

The word dysthymia has its roots in the Greek word of the same name which literally means "being of bad mood" and is still used in Modern Greek with exactly the same meaning. Dysthymia as a psychiatric disorder saw a number of modifications and changes over the years, at times being dropped from the psychiatric nosology altogether. However, the 1970's and 1980's saw a resurgence of interest in the subsyndromal affective disorders, most notably by Akiskal[537] and coworkers which led to the reintroduction of the term.

This chapter will try to trace the origins of the concept of dysthymia and then review its development across the years. This is essential to appreciate today's questions—whether dysthymia can be better accounted for as a personality disorder or as an affective disorder. This will be followed by a review of etiopathogenesis, impact on patient and caregiver and management strategies.

DEVELOPMENT OF THE CONCEPT

1. *Before the 19th century:* Melancholic temperament has been of great importance in human sciences even before the times of Hippocrates. The humoral theory proposed black bile as the cause of melancholia.
2. *The early 19th century:* Carl Freidrich Flemming[538] (1797-1880) was the first psychiatrist to talk of dysthymia. He distinguished between anoesia: disorders of intellect; dysthymia: disorders of mood; mania: disorders of both intellect and mood. Kahlbaum[539] (1863) distinguished between total and partial disorders of the soul. He subdivided partial disorders into disorders of mood: dysthymia; disorders of intelligence: paranoia; and disorders of will: diastrephia.

   Kraepelin[540] is known for his pioneering work in psychiatric nosology. His dichotomy of dementia praecox and manic-depressive insanity permanently changed psychiatric nosology. Kraepelin dropped dysthymia, but retained cyclothymia to describe mild forms or a predisposition (constitution) for manic depressive insanity. Interestingly, though Kraepelin did not retain the term dysthymia, he gave a vivid description of its psychopathology, which is identical to those described in contemporary work and would certainly fulfill the criteria for dysthymic disorder in DSM-IV.
3. *1900–1970:* The term dysthymia played a minor role in the 20th century until the late 1970's. A few authors like Kahn[538] (1928) and Leonhard[538] (1968) included the term in their psychopathic personalities to describe persons who suffered chronically from disturbed or irritable mood. With the increasing influence of the psychodynamic school of psychiatry in the first half of 20th century, the diagnosis of neurotic depression assumed greater importance and soon overshadowed dysthymia. However, before going on to discuss depressive neurosis, a brief description of another precursor of dysthymia, the depressive personality, is warranted.

Depressive Personality

The depressive personality also has a rich theoretical and clinical tradition and workers belonging to very diverse schools of psychiatric thought have described it.

According to Kraepelin,[540] "The depressive temperament is characterized by a permanent gloomy emotional stress in all experiences of life". He considered the depressive temperament as one of the manic-depressive "fundamental states". Kretschmer[541] expressed a similar view in his book "Physique and Character". He described several hereditary affective personality types including the depressive temperament. Due to the influence of psychodynamic psychiatry, the depressive temperament of the German phenomenologist gave way to the developmentally rooted depressive character which focused largely on premorbid personality traits—oral (passive-dependent) and anal (obsessional)—that predisposed to depression.

Kahn[538] (1928) described an enduring depressive character characterized by persistent low self-esteem, helplessness, chronic guilt and dependent relatedness. The patients of depressive personality were supposed to internalize their conflicts which led to self torture and self defeat in the absence of provoked retaliation from others. Phillips et al.[542] in their review of depressive personality argued that though the disorder's proposed clinical features were fairly consistent, most of the writings were theoretical and clinical rather than empirical in nature. Most of the studies were limited by methodological problems such as lack of comparison groups, lack of standardized diagnostic criteria, etc. On the other hand, they suggested that some of the empirical evidence was sufficient to sustain interest and further study was required for the development of an inclusive set of descriptive characteristics.

The early versions of the diagnostic and statistical manual (DSM) of the American Psychiatric Association had no clear description of the depressive personality. Neurasthenic neurosis of DSM-II[543] would seem closely related to the depressive personality. As quoted, "It differs from depressive neurosis in the moderateness of depression and chronicity of its course".

The research diagnostic criteria (RDC)[544] replaced depressive neurosis with three categories: (unipolar) major depressive disorder, minor depressive disorder, and intermittent depressive disorder. Minor depressive disorder could be brief as well as chronic (2 years or longer). In chronic minor depression, mood was consistently depressed (although with fewer symptoms than chronic major depression) while in intermittent depressive disorder, depressed mood could fluctuate, with periods of normal mood lasting from several hours to several days. Intermittent depressive disorder corresponded with the concept of depressive personality or temperament. The RDC categories of chronic minor and intermittent depressive disorders were the predecessors of dysthymic disorder introduced by the DSM-III in 1980,[545] which merged the two. Although the DSM-IIIR[546] added course modifiers of primary (dysphoria resulting from an affective condition) versus secondary (dysphoria resulting from a nonaffective condition) and early versus late (after 21 years of age) onset, it was criticized for its emphasis on somatic symptoms and failure to capture the broader syndrome of cognitive and interpersonal traits emphasized by the concept of depressive temperament or personality.[547] Based on such arguments, the DSM-IV[548] work group on personality disorders considered a proposal for a depressive personality disorder diagnosis under personality disorders-NOS[549,550] and included the proposed criteria in the appendix for further study. This proposed criteria set added cognitive items like low self-esteem, pessimism, guilt, and brooding.

The depressive personality disorder category captures a more fluctuating course of the constellation of depressive traits, that is, a pattern that although characteristic of an individual over long periods, may be more variable in its presence and intensity compared to dysthymia. Secondly depressed mood is not considered as a core feature of depressive personality as in dysthymia. The findings from DSM-IV field trial[551] suggest that the DSM-III-R, DSM-IV, or DSM-IV appendix criteria fail to capture a large proportion of individuals who report lifelong depressive traits thereby giving impetus for its separate existence.

ICD-10[552] (Table 8) however subsumes depressive personality disorder under dysthymia.

Depressive Neurosis

A neurosis is a chronic and recurrent nonpsychotic disorder, characterized mainly by anxiety that is experienced or expressed directly or altered through defense mechanisms. Depressive neurosis as defined in DSM-II[543] was manifested by an excessive reaction of depression to an internal conflict or to an identifiable event such as loss of a loved object or cherished possession.

Neurotic depression was a response to environmental difficulties, occurred in a patient with a prior history of neurotic personality manifestations, was not transmitted by genetic factors, was unaccompanied by the absence of insight, psychotic thought processes, retardation, sleeplessness, or other major bodily-physiological or biochemical changes and responded to psychotherapy.[553]

In the endogenous depressions, on the other hand, the converse of the above factors holds true. The symptoms of depressive neurosis include depressed mood, emptiness, helplessness, loss of confidence and initiative, loneliness, regretful preoccupations, problems at work or difficulty with aggressive strivings, anxiety, anger and guilt; apathy, low level of functioning, presence of one or two 'somatic' symptoms and frequent bodily complaints.

Amongst the affective disorders the nosological status of neurotic depression remained uncertain and controversial. A study by Klerman[554] et al. highlighted the lack of clarity and precision as to the range of phenomena to be subsumed by the nosological class and vagueness as to the criteria for the diagnosis. A number of different meanings for neurotic depression were identified. Neurotic depressions were less socially incapacitating; caused mild level of social dysfunction; were nonpsychotic; did not present with endogenous symptoms; followed a stressful event that was usually, but not exclusively, psychosocial in nature; were the consequences of long standing maladaptive personality pattern; were a result of unconscious conflicts, according to the psychoanalytic theory.

Patients received a diagnosis of neurotic depression based on any or all the above criteria; and implications as to the etiology, clinical course, response to treatment, family history, psychosocial aspects and other relevant variables were unknown.

Akiskal[537] et al. in a 3–4 year prospective follow-up study found that most of the patients diagnosed as 'situational', 'reactive' or 'neurotic' depression were found to be suffering from nonaffective disorders. The major contention was that neurotic depression did not constitute a discrete nosological entity. It seemed that diagnostically and prognostically heterogeneous groups of depressed patients were being lumped into 'neurotic depression'. DSM III[545] included it in dysthymia while ICD-9[555] retained the depressive neurosis category under the neurotic disorders, changing the name to neurotic depression.

Other Nosological Precursors

Hysteroid dysphoria[556] was characterized by frequent repeated, usually short-lived depressive reactions characterized by a loss of self esteem and atypical depressive features, with the normal state characterized by histrionic features.

Chronic minor depression[544] was characterized by depressed mood for at least two years with no clear onset and overlapped with the traditional category of neurotic depression.

By 1980, a number of studies found that the term neurotic depression had multiple meanings, lacked diagnostic specificity and was vague in terms of its defining criteria.

This led to an abandonment of the term neurotic depression because of a lack of clarity, and the obsolete term dysthymia was then resurrected and included in the official nosological systems (DSM-III, 1980[545]).

Thus, the nosological precursors of dysthymic disorder were depressive temperament, depressive character, depressive personality, neurotic depression, hysteroid dysphoria and chronic minor depression. Its essential defining characteristics were chronicity (depressive manifestations for at least two years in adults and 1 year in children and adolescents), subsyndromal intensity, absence of affective delusions and hallucinations and absence of hypomanic or manic swings. The onset was insidious or at least 2 months after recovery from a major depressive episode. The DSM-III dysthymic disorder itself suffered from several problems such as severity, age at onset, type of onset and relationship to personality disorders.[557] Some of the problems were addressed and the criteria were modified in the subsequent editions of the DSM (DSM-III R[546] and DSM-IV[548]).

CURRENT STATUS

The need for the dysthymic construct arose because of the existence of a large number of patients with fluctuating, intermittent or chronic depression in both treatment and community settings.

The basic pattern of depression in these patients is one of low grade symptomatology which begins insidiously, in most cases before the age of 25 years and lasts for at least 2 years (1 year in children).

The early and (onset < 21 years) late onset (onset > 21 years) distinction made by DSM IV[548] (Table 8) is not universally accepted. Although there is no evidence suggesting any difference in the frequency of symptoms in these 2 groups, patients with early-onset dysthymia were more frequently females, single, having longer duration of illness, history of major depression, social phobia, panic disorder and conversion disorder as compared to those with late onset. On the other hand, patients with late-onset disease were more likely to report at least one stressful event in the year preceding the onset of dysthymia and history of generalized anxiety disorder, substance abuse and somatization disorder.[558]

Criteria for Dysthymia

ICD-10 (1992) (WHO): The ICD-10 field trials showed a low reliability coefficient (0.36) for dysthymia. This was related to the difficulty in differentiating dysthymia from mild, recurrent mild and other degrees of recurrent depression and anxiety symptoms.[559] The ICD-10 clinical guidelines proposed two year duration of depression of mood, rarely severe enough to fulfill the criteria for recurrent depressive disorder of mild to moderate severity.

DSM-IV (1994):[548] To fulfill the criteria of dysthymic disorder in DSM-IV, two out of six criteria are required. However, DSM-IV (unlike ICD-10) disallows any major depressive episode during the first two years of illness, in which case it is diagnosed as MDD-chronic or in partial remission.

Two major questions have been raised about dysthymia: Whether it is better conceptualized as a personality disorder or an affective disorder, and its distinction from major depressive disorder (MDD). Validity studies of dysthymia[560,561] lend convincing evidence to the concept of dysthymia being an affective disorder than a personality disorder.

The second question has implications for clinical practice. Major depressive disorder and dysthymic disorder are differentiated on the basis of severity, chronicity and persistence. The cardinal feature of dysthymia is chronically depressed mood for two years and two of additional six

Table 8: Comparison of ICD-10 and DSM-IV

DSM-IV	*ICD-10*
• Disallows any MDD during the first two years of illness (diagnosed as MDD-chronic or in partial remission). In children and adolescents mood can be irritable and duration is 1 year • During the 2 year period (1 year for children and adolescents) the person has never been without symptoms for more than 2 months at a time • No significant sign or symptom of previous depressive episode present for at least 2 months prior to onset of dysthymia	Mild MDD can occur particularly at the onset of the disorder
DSM-IV criteria: 2 out of 6 symptoms • Poor appetite/overeating • Insomnia or hypersomnia • Low energy/fatigue • Low self-esteem • Poor concentration or difficulty in making decisions • Feelings of hopelessness	**ICD-10 research criteria:** 3 out of 11 • Reduced energy/activity • Insomnia • Loss of self confidence or feelings of inadequacy • Difficulty in concentrating • Frequent tearfulness • Loss of interest in enjoyment of sex and other pleasurable activities • Feeling of hopelessness or despair • A perceived inability to cope with routine responsibility of everyday life • Pessimism about future or brooding over the past • Social withdrawal • Reduced talkativeness
Research appendix criteria: 3 out of 9 symptoms • Low self-esteem or confidence or feelings of inadequacy • Feelings of pessimism/despair/hopelessness • Generalized loss of interest or pleasure social withdrawal • Chronic fatigue/tiredness • Feelings of guilt, brooding about the past subjective feelings of irritability or excessive anger • Decreased activity, effectiveness or productivity • Difficulty in thinking reflected by poor concentration, poor memory or indecisiveness	

symptoms, while for MDD it is depressed mood for at least two weeks with four of additional nine symptoms.

However, depressed mood as defined in dysthymia and MDD is identical and there is nothing inherently different about the quality or even intensity of the depressed mood itself. Choosing between a diagnosis of dysthymic disorder and MDD can be difficult as the two disorders have common symptoms in their definitions and the differences between them in onset, duration, persistence and severity are often difficult to evaluate. There has been controversy over which symptoms best define dysthymic disorder. Dysthymic disorder might be characterized more by cognitive symptoms and less by vegetative symptoms than is the case for MDD[562] and this list has been proposed in appendix B of DSM-IV to encourage research and for additional confirming evidence before incorporating them. Dysthymic disorder is also associated with greater comorbidity,[563,564] a higher rate of dysthymia in first-degree relatives[565] *(Klein et al, 1995)*, and greater childhood adversity[566] as compared to nonchronic forms of major depressive disorder.

It must be recognized that the division between major depressive disorder and dysthymia may be somewhat artificial. major depressive disorder and dysthymia may be waxing and waning course of a single depressive disorder. Not surprisingly many individuals of dysthymia go on to develop MDD (10% over the next year).

Additionally an appreciable minority of individuals with either major depressive disorder and dysthymia go on to develop manic or hypomanic episodes.

Rating scales like hamilton depression rating scale (HDRS), the montgomery depression rating scale (MADRS) and the cornell dysthymia rating scale (CDRS),[567] a 20-item clinician-rated inventory are useful. CDRS and the HDRS have high concurrent validity but the CDRS has better content validity than the HDRS in dysthymic population.[568]

DSM-5 Diagnostic criteria for persistent depressive disorder (dysthymia)

300.4 (F34.1)

This disorder represents a consolidation of DSM-IV-defined chronic major depressive disorder and dysthymic disorder.

a. Depressed mood for most of the day, for more days than not, as indicated by either subjective account or observation by others, for at least 2 years.
   Note: In children and adolescents, mood can be irritable and duration must be at least 1 year.
b. Presence, while depressed, of two (or more) of the following:
   1. Poor appetite or overeating.
   2. Insomnia or hypersomnia.
   3. Low energy or fatigue.
   4. Low self-esteem.
   5. Poor concentration or difficulty making decisions.
   6. Feelings of hopelessness.
c. During the 2-year period (1 year for children or adolescents) of the disturbance, the individual has never been without the symptoms in Criteria A and B for more than 2 months at a time.

Contd...

Contd...

d. Criteria for a major depressive disorder may be continuously present for 2 years.
e. There has never been a manic episode or a hypomanic episode, and criteria have never been met for cyclothymic disorder.
f. The disturbance is not better explained by a persistent schizoaffective disorder, schizophrenia, delusional disorder, or other specified or unspecified schizophrenia spectrum and other psychotic disorder.
g. The symptoms are not attributable to the physiological effects of a substance (e.g. a drug of abuse, a medication) or another medical condition (e.g. hypothyroidism).
h. The symptoms cause clinically significant distress or impairment in social, occupational, or other important areas of functioning.
   Note: Because the criteria for a major depressive episode include four symptoms that are absent from the symptom list for persistent depressive disorder (dysthymia), a very limited number of individuals will have depressive symptoms that have persisted longer than 2 years but will not meet criteria for persistent depressive disorder. If full criteria for a major depressive episode have been met at some point during the current episode of illness, they should be given a diagnosis of major depressive disorder. Otherwise, a diagnosis of other specified depressive disorder or unspecified depressive disorder is warranted.

Specify if:
With anxious distress
With mixed features
With melancholic features
With atypical features
With mood-congruent psychotic features
With mood-incongruent psychotic features
With peripartum onset

Specify if:
In partial remission
In full remission

Specify if:
Early onset: If onset is before age 21 years.
Late onset: If onset is at age 21 years or older.
Specify if (for most recent 2 years of persistent depressive disorder):
With pure dysthymic syndrome: Full criteria for a major depressive episodes have not been met in at least the preceding 2 years.
With persistent major depressive episode: Full criteria for a major depressive episode have been met throughout the preceding 2-year-period.
With intermittent major depressive episodes, with current episode: Full criteria for a major depressive episode are currently met, but there have been periods of at least 8 weeks in at least the preceding 2 years with symptoms below the threshold for a full major depressive episode.
With intermittent major depressive episodes, without current episode: Full criteria for a major depressive episode are not currently met, but there has been one or more major depressive episodes in at least the preceding 2 years.

Specify current severity:
Mild
Moderate
Severe

NEUROBIOLOGY

Genetic: Patients with dysthymia have elevated rates of the disorder in first-degree relatives as compared with relatives of nonpsychiatrically ill control subjects.[565] Higher rates of dysthymia have been noted among relatives of pure dysthymics and of double depressives, than among relatives of major depressive probands and normal controls.[569] However, a twin study failed to show a monozygotic-dizygotic difference in the rates of dysthymia.[570] Hence, at present it can be concluded that the shared or family environment may contribute more to the etiology of dysthymia than to major depression.

Neurochemical

The neurochemical alterations in dysthymia have not been studied well and preliminary evidence suggests that the changes are not necessarily in the same direction as are seen in major depression. The blunted TSH response to TRH administration has not been noted among late-onset dysthymics, whereas early-onset dysthymics report a higher rate of dexamethasone nonsuppression and a blunted TSH response.[571] Heightened baseline levels of plasma corticotrophin releasing hormone (CRH) and cortisol similar to major depression has been demonstrated in some[572] but all studies have not replicated such findings in subjects of dysthymia[573] (Ravindran, et al. 1996). Adrenocorticotrophin releasing hormone (ACTH) response to CRH challenge after pretreatment with dexamethasone was significantly enhanced in major depression but not in dysthymia in a small study.[574] Hence, the evidence points towards absence of abnormal dexamethasone suppression tests in dysthymia unlike major depressive disorder suggesting that dysthymia might actually be associated with hypocortisol response.[575,576] In patients with dysthymia reduced levels of plasma norepinephrine with modest changes following exercise coupled with elevated platelet and free Serotonin are suggestive of altered adrenal responsivity to environmental challenges, as well as heightened sympathetic tone.[577] Lower urinary 5-hydroxyindoleacetic acid levels (5-HIAA) were observed prior to treatment among treatment responders relative to nonresponders, and the reduced level in responders normalized following treatment.[575] The efficacy of low dose amisulpride (acts as D2 agonist) in dysthymia suggests that dopamine may play a role in dysthymia.[578]

Neuroanatomy

A recent fMRI study in dysthymia patients showed significantly reduced activation in the dorsolateral prefrontal cortex compared to controls, a finding similar to patients with depressive disorder. The dysthymic patients also exhibited increased activation in the amygdala, anterior cingulate and insula compared to controls and these differences were more evident when processing negative than positive images. The increased activity in the insula, seen in dysthymia patients are similar to patients suffering from major depression. However, the paradoxical increase in activation of anterior cingulate in dysthymia as compared to major depressive disorder may be due to the chronic course of dysthymia. Hence, it is hypothesized that some neural regions may be a common substrate for depressive disorders in general while others may relate specifically to symptom characteristics and the chronic course of dysthymia.[579]

Sleep

Sleep architecture (reduced total sleep time, sleep latency, morning wake time and sleep efficiency) in patients with dysthymia is very similar to major depressive disorder which is consistent with the notion that the two disorders are variants of the same illness.[580,581]

Psychosocial Factors and Stressors in Dysthymia

Dysthymia, like major depression, may be provoked by chronic uncontrollable stressor as suggested by studies reporting higher incidence of major depression and dysthymia among adults who acted as care-givers for a spouse with a progressive dementia (care-giving itself is a profound stressor), as compared to matched controls.[582] Individuals with dysthymia demonstrate altered stress perception, coping styles, reduced perceived daily positive or uplifting events relative to controls.[573,583]

COMORBIDITY

Nearly all anxiety disorders may be comorbid with dysthymia, the most common being panic disorder, generalized anxiety disorder, phobic states[584] like social phobia and agoraphobia. Others include obsessive-compulsive syndrome, binge eating, neurasthenia and benzodiazepine abuse. In terms of physical comorbidity, studies have shown that long-term depression is associated with more cardiac and respiratory syndromes and "other pain" disorders but not with backache and headache as compared to episodic depression.[585]

IMPACT ON PATIENT AND CAREGIVER

The disability of these patients stems from the long standing nature of the symptoms. However, these patients seek medical attention quite late and it is often seen that patients with dysthymia often seek help when their depression is accentuated to such an extent that it meets the criteria for major depressive disorder, the so-called double depressive picture.[586] It is also suggested that long standing sub-affective symptoms can distort character formation and lead to interpersonal difficulties and can serve as a breeding ground for other neurotic developments including social phobia and avoidant patterns.[560]

Significant disability and impairment in quality of life, social support and marital adjustment have been seen in patients with dysthymia when compared to normal/medically ill controls. Wells[587] et al. found that the disability of these patients, both in terms of suffering (or pain) and functional impairment, was worse than for most commonly encountered physical conditions in medical practice. One study from India showed that patients of dysthymia were comparable on quality of life and marital adjustment with patients suffering from recurrent depressive disorder. Duration of illness and severity of depression are important correlates, particularly for impaired quality of life and disability levels.[588]

DIFFERENTIAL DIAGNOSIS

Dysthymia must be differentiated from major depressive disorder and other subthreshold depressive disorders. The most important basis for this differentiation is severity (number of symptoms) of symptoms and duration of symptoms.

Major depressive disorder: It is more severe than dysthymia and tends to last for a shorter period of time. According to DSM-IV major depressive disorder is diagnosed only when 5 out of 9 criteria are fulfilled for at least 2 weeks.

Subsyndromal symptoms of depression (SSD): Although it is similar to dysthymia in not meeting the criteria of major depression (at least two or more current depressive symptoms, present everyday for most or all of the time), but differs from dysthymia on the basis of shorter duration of symptoms (of at least 2 weeks). Again unlike dysthymia it may be a manifestation of the residual symptoms of major depression.

Double depression: Here 2 years of dysthymia is followed by a major depressive episode.

Recurrent brief depression: Presence of the major depressive syndrome according to DSM-IV symptom criteria (five of nine symptoms) with brief duration (less than 2 weeks) usually lasting 1–3 days with frequent recurrences (at least monthly over previous 12 months).

Minor depressive disorder (MDD): It is included in the appendix of DSM-IV and is characterized by presence of at least 2 but less than 5 symptoms of depression, one of which is either depressed mood or anhedonia, present every or nearly everyday for 2 weeks.

Mixed anxiety depressive disorder (MADD): According to DSM-IV it is characterized by dysphoria for at least 1 month combined with other depressive and anxiety symptoms that are subthreshold for both primary affective and anxiety disorder. ICD-10 defines MADD by presence of mild or moderate anxiety and depression, with at least temporary occurrence of vegetative symptoms not fulfilling the criteria of an anxiety disorder or a depressive episode.

Depressive symptoms associated with chronic psychotic disorders: Occurs exclusively during the psychotic disturbance.

Mood disorder due to a general medical condition: Requires the presence of an etiologic general medical condition.

Substance-induced mood disorder: It is due to the direct physiologic effects of a substance.

Bipolar disorder, cyclothymic disorder: It is characterized by manic or mixed episodes or hypomanic periods in addition to depressive periods.[589]

TREATMENT

Pharmacotherapy

The relatively recent identification of dysthymia as a discrete entity has been the main reason for the relatively late application of pharmacotherapeutic approaches. Prior to the recognition of dysthymia as primarily an affective disorder, benzodiazepines were commonly prescribed to control the associated anxiety; however, depressive symptoms did not show sustained improvement and anxiolytics were often overprescribed. However, over the years some data has accumulated with regard to efficacy of antidepressants in the treatment of dysthymia. In a cochrane review of 29 trials comparing drugs with placebo, 17 reported data for the main outcome measure of interest, i.e. the changes on Clinical global impression (CGI) scale and/or final score reduction of at least 50% on the hamilton depression scale (HAM-D) and absence of sufficient symptoms to meet diagnostic criteria for dysthymic disorder at the end of the trial. The review concluded that tricyclic antidepressants, selective serotonin reuptake inhibitors, monoamine oxidase inhibitors, sulpiride, amineptine and ritanserin are effective in the treatment of dysthymia with no major differences between or within drug classes. However, the tricyclic antidepressants were found to be more likely to produce side-effects and dropouts. However the authors pointed out that the quality of the studies was poor, as some important information had been omitted like design of the studies, analysis and generalizability.[590]

Open-label studies with bupropion SR (maximum dose 400 mg/day), citalopram (mean dose = 37.3 mg), mirtazapine, venlafaxine, duloxetine and amisulpride have also shown that these agents are effective and well tolerated in dysthymia.[591-596] Newer agents like acetyl L carnitine have also been shown to as effective as and better tolerated than amisulpride.[597]

The long term studies ranging from 6 months to 12 months have shown promising results with antidepressants like trazodone, phenelzine, imipramine and desipramine. The long term studies suggest that a continuation phase treatment of 9 to 12 months confers ongoing wellness.[598-601]

Treatment Strategy

Data shows good treatment response with standard doses of most classes of antidepressant medication like selective serotonin reuptake inhibitors (SSRIs), tricyclic antidepressants, monoamine oxidase inhibitors in the treatment of dysthymic disorder. Although data is limited, no one class of antidepressants is superior to another. Further studies in subjects with double depression show that they also respond to these agents.[602]

Many of the principles of treatment for dysthymic disorder match those for major depression with a few exceptions. Because dysthymic disorder is less severe, patients may be less likely to tolerate significant side effects. Therefore, an SSRI may be the more favored initial medication started at low doses which is gradually increased. Further, if there is a risk of overdose due to suicidal ideation which is common in chronic depression, SSRls, bupropion, venlafaxine and nefazdone are safer than TCAs. Studies suggest that adequate doses of medications are required for relatively long periods of time (12 weeks) to show a response rate.[603] Education of the patient regarding side effects and response time is essential. If response to one drug is suboptimal, the patient may be changed to an alternative medicine of a different class. Patients with dysthymic disorder may be treatment refractory, hence may require high doses or trials of several different medications until an effective agent is found. If tricyclics are used, they should be dispensed in small quantities.

The length of treatment required is not known. Some authors suggest that approximately 50% of patients will suffer a recurrence if treatment is discontinued after years. Patients should be considered candidates for maintenance therapy if they have recurrent major depression episodes superimposed on dysthymic disorder, have had severe life threatening episodes of major depression, have suffered from chronic suicidal ideation or relapse immediately after extended treatment.

Psychotherapy

As described above for most part of the 20th century, chronic depression was considered a temperamental or character disorder. Its treatment of choice was psychotherapy but such chronic depressions were considered to have a poor prognosis. Yet, psychotherapy for dysthymia should not be abandoned. The limitations of antidepressant medication as well as the treatment preference of patients and therapists argue for the development of effective psychotherapeutic interventions.

Psychodynamic Psychotherapy and Psychoanalysis

The psychoanalytic literature in recent decades is relatively meager regarding depression in general and dysthymia in particular. Although long-term psychodynamic therapy continues to be frequently prescribed for dysthymic patients there is no evidence that either short or long-term psychodynamic treatment benefits such patients.[604]

Cognitive-behavioral Therapy

Cognitive-behavioral therapy is a structured, time-limited psychotherapy developed by Beck and colleagues. The focus of cognitive behavior therapy (CBT) is the automatic negative thoughts that depressed patients report about themselves, their situations and their future. Through rational discussions with their therapists and written and behavioral homework assignments patients learn to modify irrationally negative thoughts.[605] As they do, depression improves. Several cognitive approaches have been tested in dysthymic patients. Some of these approaches are skills-training oriented psychoeducational approach, combined activity scheduling, social competence training and cognitive restructuring including cognitive behavioral therapy of Beck. In summary, there have been several cognitive behavioral approaches in dysthymia. Most of the studies have been limited by small groups with varying outcome measures. Even if the results have not been dramatic, they still do suggest that some dysthymic patients respond to cognitive therapies. In one of the studies, McCullough described 10 patients with DSM-III dysthymic disorder by treated on the basis of his manual based cognitive-behavioral analysis system of psychotherapy, entailing 14-44 weekly sessions. All patients reached termination criteria and nine patients remained in remission 2 years later.[606]

Interpersonal Therapy

Interpersonal therapy (IPT), like cognitive-behavioral therapy, is a time limited, manual-based psychotherapy that has demonstrated efficacy in controlled clinical trials for outpatient major depression and an increasing range of other diagnoses. The therapist helps the patient recognize links between mood and current interpersonal experiences focusing the therapy on one of four interpersonal problem areas: grief, role disputes, role transitions, or interpersonal deficits. Interpersonal approaches have been suggested for treating dysthymia keeping in mind the relationship difficulties such patients tend to suffer.[607]

Pharmacotherapy versus Psychotherapy

A 16 weeks randomized trial of 94 subjects treated with either interpersonal psychotherapy (IPT), brief supportive psychotherapy (BSP), sertraline, or sertraline plus IPT showed better response and remission with sertraline compared to psychotherapy alone. However the study did not provide any follow-up data.[608] In another study, all three treatments were reasonably effective in the long term 18 months follow-up after 6 months of acute phase treatment. Sertraline or combination of sertraline with IPT was more effective than IPT alone. Out of these, the combination treatment was associated with less health and social service costs over 2 years.[609] A meta-analysis including 5 dysthymia studies showed a small but significant advantage for medications over psychotherapy in the treatment of dysthymia. However, duration for which psychotherapy was offered in these trials might have been inadequate.[610]

Recommendations for Psychotherapy

Psychotherapy can be used for both control of symptoms and prevention of relapse, when drug therapy is only producing either a partial response or none at all. Common indications for psychotherapy include marked social and interpersonal disability and enduring coping problematic skills to assist in self-management of symptoms and problems. Thus it can be concluded that for dysthymia, psychosocial therapies should be used in combination with antidepressants rather than alone.

Predictors of Response to Treatment

The factors associated with poor response to pharmacotherapy and psychological treatments in dysthymia are lower-levels of education, high neuroticism, more severe medical illness and being an older female.[611,612] According to one study younger, ethnic minority patients and patients with personality disorders may be at increased risk of dropping out from treatment while combination treatments may increase treatment retention.[612] Understanding self and illness mechanisms, enhanced flexibility of thinking, and change from avoidance coping to approach coping and a helpful relationship with the health care provider are predictors of remission in dysthymia.[613]

Course and Outcome

Dysthymia tend to have a protracted course associated with high risk of relapse. The relapses take a variety of forms and are not limited to dysthymia.[614] Majority of patients with dysthymia ultimately experience a major depressive episode.[615]

CONCLUSION

The original view of dysthymia as a neurotic personality disorder has given way to the modern view of dysthymia as a chronic subaffective disorder that may proceed to the severity of major depressive disorder. Similarly, the earlier view that such long-term neurotic patients cannot be treated is now much less widely held. Although pharmacotherapy is the mainstay of treatment in dysthymic disorder, it should not be administered in isolation but as part of a global treatment strategy.

7.14 RECENT DEVELOPMENT AND CURRENT CONTROVERSIES IN DEPRESSION

JN Vyas, SK Pandey

Compared with other medical diagnoses, depression is very common. It occurs twice as frequently in women as in men, can begin at any age, but has its average age of onset in the mid-20s.[616] Lifetime prevalence estimates for major depressive disorder (Panel 15) in the community range from 15% to 17% (95% CI),[616] 12-month prevalence from 6% to 7% (US national comorbidity replication: n = 9090).[616,618]

Major depressive disorder impairs the ability to function, leading to role impairment in well over 50% of patients.[617] Role impairment is likely to be direct corollary of depressed mood.[619,620] Effective treatment is therefore of the essence. Unfortunately, only 46–57% (95% CI) of the 12-month cases in the USA were receiving health care treatment for major depressive disorder, and only 18–25% were adequately treated.[617] In a European community survey (n = 5993), 25–38% of men and 21–30% of women interviewed and classified as having major depressive disorder used any health services in the past 12 months for their depression. This percentage rose to only 35–49% of those with severe major depressive disorder.[621] Any discussion of the epidemic rise in prescriptions of antidepressants together with popular skepticism towards antidepressants treatments has to be considered against this background. Depression is especially common in many nonpsychiatric medical settings, such as

Panel 15: ICD-10 criteria for depression[618]

Depressive episode
At least two weeks of: depressed mood, loss of interest and enjoyment, reduced energy, increased fatigability, diminished activity, reduced concentration and attention, reduced self esteem and self-confidence, ideas of guilt and unworthiness, bleak view of the future, ideas or acts of self-harm, disturbed sleep, diminished appetite.

Mild depression
Two of depressed mood, loss of interest and enjoyment, reduced energy, and two others. Patient will not cease to function completely.

Moderate depression
Two of depressed mood, loss of interest and enjoyment, reduced energy, and at least three others, some at marked intensity. Considerable difficulty functioning.

Severe depression
Three of depressed mood, loss of interest and enjoyment, reduced energy, and at least four others, some of severe intensity, plus considerable distress and agitation, or psychomotor retardation; sometimes with psychotic symptoms, such as hallucinations or delusions.

Dysthymia
Depression of mood which is never or only very rarely severe enough to fulfill the criteria for recurrent depressive disorder, mild or moderate severity.

inpatients wards, in chronically ill patients and during the recovery from acute medical illness.[617]

A crucial aspect of the epidemiology of major depression is the increased mortality associated with this condition. A recent meta-analysis of 25 studies with 1.3–16 years' follow-up of over 100 000 individuals reported an overall relative risk of dying between 1.58 and 2.07 (95% CI) compared with people who are not depressed.[622] The relative risk in subclinical depression was not substantially smaller than in clinical depression. The analysis did not examine potential confounders, such as chronic illness or lifestyle. The mechanism of increased mortality is therefore not clear. A major contribution to increased mortality in depression will come from the risk of suicide in this patient group. Traditionally, lifetime risk (i.e. proportionate mortality: the percentage of the dead who died by suicide during follow-up) is reported between 15% and 19%.[623,624] This figure is likely to be inflated, especially if the period of follow-up, typically after an acute episode in hospital, carries a higher risk of suicide than periods further removed from the index episode.[625]

Another modifying factor is the diagnostic: system early versions of the diagnostic and statistical manual of mental disorders (DSM), for example, drew the boundaries of depression much narrower than DSM III or IV, which include many milder forms of the illness. A recent review[625] took account of the treatment setting of patients and identified a clear hierarchy of risks, with estimates of lifetime prevalence of suicide being highest in suicidal inpatients (8–6%), lower in other inpatients (4%), and lowest amongst outpatients with affective disorder (2–2%). Even with these revised figures the risk of suicide rises over background levels from four-fold in depressed outpatients to 16 fold in patients with affective disorders admitted because of suicidal risk.[625]

A sixth of people in the community will have major depressive disorder during their lifetime. Only between a quarter and half of patients will be in contact with the health services for their depression. In half the cases, the illness is incapacitating, leading to role impairment at work or at home. The risk of premature death is increased, in part because of a greater risk of suicide.

CAUSES AND ASSOCIATIONS

Genetics and Pharmacogenetics

There is no doubt that genetic factors have an important role in the etiology of depression. Heritability has been estimated from twin studies as 31–42%, with a substantial contribution of environmental effects unique to individuals (including measurement error) of 58–67%.[626] Depression with recurrent episodes and possibly early onset may be associated with greater familial aggregation.[626]

Traditional genetic linkage studies and candidate gene methods have been used with fairly limited success in major depression.[627] Genetic models of etiology generally assume a large number of genes with relatively small contributions to liability. Advances in high-throughput genotyping and microarray techniques have made it more feasible to identify genes with small effect sizes.[627] Of special clinical interest are those studies that are based on pathophysiological notions (candidate genes), and in particular those that examine the probability of patients to respond to particular treatments.

Brain-derived neurotrophic factor may have a central role in the effectiveness of antidepressants, but there is no firm evidence association of its alleles with major depressive disorder.[628-630] Monoamine oxidase A is involved in the metabolism of catecholamines and is the target of one group of antidepressants, the monoamine oxidase inhibitors. Certain monoamine oxidase A gene promoter polymorphisms are found in subgroups of patients with major depression; they are by no means specific to depression, but also occur in patients with anxiety.[631,632] The catechol-O-methyltransferase (another catecholamine metabolising enzyme) Val108/158Met polymorphism has been intensively investigated in psychotic disorders, but has also been associated with treatment response to mirtazepine, but not paroxetine, in major depression.[633] Human tryptophan hydroxylase-2 (hTPH2) is involved in the synthesis of serotonin. The theory that it is the rate limiting step of serotonin synthesis is supported by the occasional success of the augmentation of antidepressants with tryptophan.[634] A single nucleotide polymorphism in its gene with roughly 80% loss function is associated with major depression, but not with bipolar illness.[635]

The most frequently examined candidate gene codes for the serotonin transporter, which is the drug target of serotonin reuptake inhibitors, such as fluoxetine. A 44-bp insertion or deletion results in a long (1) and a short(s) variant of this gene; the s-variant is associated with a two-fold decreased expression and transport activity *in vitro*. Individuals in an epidemiological sample with one or two copies of the short allele of the serotonin transporter promoter polymorphism showed more depressive symptoms, diagnosable depression, and tendency to commit suicide in relation to stressful life events that individuals homozygous for the long allele.[636] Unfortunately, two subsequent twin studies were not concordant in lending support to this result.[637,638] The importance of the s-variant of the gene for stress susceptibility is supported by an increased amygdala response to stimuli of threat during a functional MRI study and an increased prefrontal response to an error processing task in healthy volunteers.[639,640] The association of serotonin transporter alleles with hippocampal size is more complex and seems to be related to age of onset.[641,642] Patients with two alleles of the 1-variant generally show a better clinical response to serotonin reuptake inbibitors in studies of mainly white patients.[643,644] The other serotonin transporter polymorphism described has a variable number of tandem repeats (9, 10, and 12 copies) located in intron 2 of the gene. There may be a better response rate in 12/12, as opposed to 10/12 patients, but this improved rate has only been shown in Asian studies.[643,644] A recent search for pharmacokinetic effects of CYP2D6 and CYP2C19 alleles suggested that for 14 of 20 investigated antidepressants, at least a doubling of the dose would be needed in extensive metabolizers. This variation in effects does strengthen the argument for antidepressant plasma monitoring in depression resistant to treatment.[643] Although promising and fascinating, the prospective practical application of such genetic and pharmacogenetic information is still some time away.

Heritability of depression has been estimated to range from 30 to 40%. Because of its pattern of inheritance, but also because of heterogeneity of clinical samples, no genes of major effect have been identified. A multitude of genes with small effects are likely to be identified, which will be related to certain aspects of genetic vulnerability to depression and will work alongside or interact with environmental factors.

Changes in Cognitive Performance

Most people now accept that major depressive disorder is associated with cognitive impairment. Episodic memory seems to be the main aspect of cognitive functioning that is vulnerable to the negative effects of depression.[645-647] Temporal lobe lesions typically disrupt episodic memory. Since hippocampal atrophy has been shown in patients with major depressive disorder,[648] impaired episodic memory functions in depression might be associated with dysfunction of the hippocampus.[629,650]

Factors that can affect episodic memory in depressive disorders are depression subtype, severity, and age. In one study, major depression and mixed anxiety-depressive disorder were associated with greater impairments than dysthymia, whereas in minor depression cognitive performance was unaffected.[647] In another study,[651] the number of depressive episodes was associated with verbal memory deficits, which could be an indication of sensitization to the effect of depression with progressive cerebral dysfunction and anatomical changes.[649,652]

Further, psychomotor slowing and executive functioning-namely mental flexibility and attention-functioning are impaired in people with depressive disorders.[647,650,652-654] Equally, updating of content i.e. working memory, set-shifting, and inhibition processes are impaired in depressed patients compared with controls.[654] Psychomotor symptoms have been commonly associated with depressive episodes.[655] Since there is no objective evidence that psychomotor retardation is present in dysthymic patients this sign could be used to differentiate between dysthymia and major depressive disorder.[656]

The presence of cognitive abnormalities in some depressed patients is generally accepted now. From a practical point of view, they may interfere with activities of daily life, such as driving or working, but also with attempts to recruit cognitive processes for therapeutic purposes.

In Vivo Anatomical and Functional Brain Changes

Most people now accept that hippocampal size measured by MRI is reduced in patients with unipolar major depressive disorder.[657,658] There is some discussion, however, about the clinical correlates of this change. Duration of illness, repeated episodes, treatment resistance (all partly overlapping) and previous abuse might be associated with hippocampal change.[649,652-659] Hippocampal atrophy has also been described in victims of abuse and of battle-induced post-traumatic stress disorder.[660-663] Findings of animal studies suggest that increased glucocorticoid levels lead to impaired neurogenesis excitotoxic damage or reduced levels of key neurotrophins in the hippocampus.[664,665] Of particular interest of the clinician, however, is that antidepressants can reverse these changes and that blocking hippocampal neurogenesis by irradiation can prevent the action of antidepressants in behavioral animal models of depression.[666-669]

Furthermore, hippocampal atrophy might be associated with cognitive impairment, in particular for episodic memory.[649-670] In the absence of larger longitudinal studies of depressed patients, whether the changes observed in hippocampus in cross-sectional studies are in fact the result of depression and stress (as postulated above), or whether they are the cause of certain clinical characteristics of the illness in the patients affected-such as treatment resistance or frequent relapses-remains to be resolved.[649]

Functional MRI (fMRI) is the method of choice to examine brain-behavior relations. Anterior cingulate, orbitofrontal cortex, dorsolateral cortex, striatum, and medial temporal lobe have repeatedly been reported as abnormal in functional and structural imaging studies of depressed patients.[671-625] In healthy human beings and animals, the ventromedial prefrontal region is associated with emotional experience,[676,677] and the dorsolateral region with cognitive and motor function.[678,679] Findings of neuroimaging studies of mood disorder tend to show abnormally increased activity in emotion-related brain regions and underactivity in cognition-related regions.[623-675,680] Neurosurgery for treatment-resistant mood disorder (a very rarely used procedure) has long targeted the ventromedial prefrontal region, excluding the dorsolateral region, since dorsolateral lesions cause cognitive deficits. Recently, ventromedial prefrontal overactivity was reported to predict response to a neurosurgical procedure for treatment-resistant mood disorder.[681]

As discussed above, major depressive disorder is characterized not only by depressed mood, but also by a substantial impairment of cognitive function. Lateral orbitofrontal cortex is activated in healthy individuals undertaking a verbal fluency task. In depressive illness, impaired verbal fluency is associated with attenuated activation in this brain region.[682] During a spatial working memory task done with gradually increasing task difficulty (n-back task), reduction in task accuracy in depressed patients was related to abnormally increased ventromedial performance in depression.[683] Although not specifically described in these studies, increased activity of the ventromedial emotion-related prefrontal region is often associated with underactivity of the cognitive processing region, and vice-versa.[684]

Many studies of depressive illness have focused on affective response, though such paradigms always include some cognitive component. Decreased rostromedial prefrontal and hippocampal activation, and increased temporal lobe activity in depression were shown in a cognitive picture-caption paradigm to generate an affective response.[685] These changes suggest that in depressive illness the decrease in rostromedial with impairment of positive affect, and the increase in temporal lobe activity with enhanced negative affect. This anatomical dissociation between positive and negative affective response might be related to abnormality in behavioral reward and inhibition systems proposed on the basis of many studies in animals.[676,686] and early deep-brain electrical recording in humans.[687]

A robust finding in neuropsychological studies of depressive illness is a bias towards processing mood-congruent information. By contrast with healthy people, depressed patients show a facilitation of response to stimuli with a negative emotional tone. Studies of abnormal emotional bias have the advantage that they explicitly link mood and cognition in a way that can be related to cognitive-behavioral theories of depressive illness and treatment. In an emotional go/no-go task, patients had attenuated neural responses to emotional targets in the subgenual anterior cingulated and posterior orbitofrontal cortices, and raised responses to sad targets in the rostral anterior cingulated and medial prefrontal cortex.[688] Elliott and colleagues[688] concluded that the orbito-medial prefrontal region has a distinct role in mediating mood-congruent information processing biases in depressive illness. In a study of the neural response to facial expression, a systematic alteration in neuronal activity was associated with such bias in regions that included the parahippocampal gyrus and amygdala.[689] Surguladze and colleagues[689] suggested that this bias could be linked to the negative cognitions and social dysfunction that arise in depressive illness. Depressed individuals characteristically engage in long-term elaborative cognitive processing of emotional information. Using a mathematical, artificial neural network model of attentional biases in depressive illness, Siegle and colleagues[690] made a formal prediction of brain response to positive, negative, and neutral stimuli. They tested these predictions with two emotional processing tasks, and reported that, as predicted, depressed individuals had abnormally sustained amygdala activity in response to affectively negative words, which was related to self-reported rumination.[690]

Formal mathematical models are increasingly used to predict brain activity.[691] Models of emotional learning have been established from extensive work in animals and more recent replicated imaging work on healthy people. Emotional learning involves adaptation and is associated with neural predictive error signals. Mathematical models can describe both the signals and behavior. The hypothesis that depressive illness is a disorder of emotional learning associated with abnormal error signals was tested with a gambling task.[691] Consistent with the prediction, patients had abnormally increased error signals in various limbic brain regions. The results are consistent with cognitive-behavioral theories of depressive illness, neural plasticity theories of antidepressant action, and successful neurosurgical interventions.[691,692]

Recent electrophysiological studies of depressive illness might have direct links to quantitative models of brain function. Of particular interest is the error related negativity (ERN) signal, which is a negative deflection in averaged electroencephalogram (EEG) recordings that peaks about 100 ms after participants make an incorrect response in speeded time-response tasks.[693,694] The onset of this potential precedes the erroneous response, suggesting that the cognitive system knew about the error as it was being made.[694] This signal is sometimes referred to as the response ERN, to distinguish it from another signal, the feedback ERN, which peaks later at 250 ms, and is a response to actual feedback information that the behavior was incorrect. The neural generators of these signals are in the anterior cingulated,[695,696] a structure repeatedly reported as abnormal in functional and structural neuroimaging studies of depressive illness.[674] The ERN has been suggested to be not only an indication of the registering of an error or conflict, but also of the affective consequences of expectancy violations-in particular aversive emotions including anxiety.[697]

Various experimental studies in healthy participants appear to lend support of these theories. For example, people with high trait anxiety have increase ERN,[693,698] and acute alcohol intoxication decreases the ERN.[699] In clinical studies, patients with obsessive-compulsive disorder who were tested with a speeded reaction-time task showed an ERN with substantially raised amplitude.[700] Gehring and colleagues[700] linked this to abnormal behavioral learning mechanisms and aversive emotional experience. In a more recent study, patients with major depressive disorder undertook a signal detection task with continuous feedback that signaled monetary reward. Compared with controls, patients showed a reduced ERN, and the investigators suggested that this reduction indicated under activity of central reward pathways.[701] The same group then replicated this finding with a go/no-go task.[702] Since the ERN could arise as a consequence of phasic decreases in activity of the predictive error signals discussed previously,[703] these findings accord with the idea that depressive illness is a disorder of emotional learning.[692]

The general understanding of depression has evolved from a vague notion of mood and emotion to a differentiated understanding about how emotional and motivational changes interact with information processing in patients' brains. This progress has helped to localize the anatomical structures and neuronal systems underlying depressive symptoms, and at the same time has provided us with a fuller understanding of the real obstacles that depressed patients struggle against.

TREATMENTS

Efficacy of Psychological Treatments

Cognitive behavioral therapy is a psychological treatment which was first formalized in the late 1970s.[704] The main premise is that depressive symptoms arise from dysfunctional beliefs and thought processes as a result of early learning experiences. These beliefs lie dormant for a number of years, but are activated by a situation or an even that has a specific meaning for the individual.[705] Schema focused work tries to directly address this premise; by definition, a schema is a cognitive structure embedded in long-term memory that has been acquired over a lifetime of learning. At best, this information has been stored to allow a person to perceive and understand. For many patients though, identifying and challenging negative automatic thoughts is the main focus of treatment.

Several studies have shown the advantage of cognitive-behavioral therapy over other psychological therapies and placebo and equivalence to treatment as usual (i.e. antidepressant medication) in the treatment of unipolar depression.[706,707] In a primary care setting, cognitive-behavioral therapy and nondirective counseling were both significantly more effective than usual family doctor care at 4 months' follow-up. However, there was no longer a significant difference between these three treatments at 12 months.[708] Not all research has lent support to the use of cognitive-behavioral therapy over other therapies in the treatment of depression. A study of patients treated with fluoxetine dose increase alone or in combination with cognitive-behavioral therapy examined the frequency of residual depressive symptoms during the continuation phase.[709] The combination of cognitive-behavioral therapy with fluoxetine had equal efficacy to fluoxetine alone. In a further study, pharmacotherapy had an advantage over cognitive-behavioral therapy, which tended to be larger in patients with chronic depression.[710] Research looking at the advantages of combining antidepressants with psychotherapy has been equivocal.[711]

Evidence that cognitive-behavioral therapy reduces rates of relapse and recurrence in unibipolar depression has accumulated.[712,713] Although the evidence from these studies is strong, the duration of this preventive effect after the discontinuation of cognitive-behavioral therapy is unclear. In one study the researchers concluded that the effect of cognitive-behavioral therapy in reduction of relapse and recurrence persists for many years, with the effects being lost fully between 3 and 4 years after cessation of the treatment.[714] In a review[715] of the long-term effectiveness of cognitive-behavioral therapy in major depressive disorder. Hensley and colleagues concluded that the evidence lends support to the long-term effectiveness of CBT over tricyclic antidepressants alone. This conclusion, however, should be treated tentatively since only five trials between 1981 and 1992 were included. Thus, we need further studies into the prevention of recurrence with cognitive-behavioral therapy.

Klerman and Wiesmann developed interpersonal therapy in the early 1980s,[716] which is based on the premise that depression occurs in a social and interpersonal context. Interpersonal therapy focuses mainly on present rather than past relationships and on interpersonal rather than intra-psychic processes.

Even though the content of interpersonal therapy differs from that of behavioral and cognitive therapies, treatment outcomes for depression are broadly similar.[717] The recently published National (English and Welsh) Institute of Clinical Excellence (NICE) guidelines on the treatment of depression agree with this finding by stating that there is insufficient evidence to determine whether there is a clinically significant difference between psychotherapies such as interpersonal therapy and cognitive-behavioral therapy on reducing depressive symptoms. Furthermore, they suggest that there is some evidence implying that there is no clinically significant difference between interpersonal therapy and antidepressants on reducing depressive symptoms as measured by the Hamilton rating scale for depression.[718]

There is a dearth of systematic reviews and randomized controlled trials (RCTs) on interpersonal therapy in the recurrence and relapse prevention of unipolar depression. However, a sequential treatment strategy in women with recurrent major depression was investigated to look at the efficacy of adding antidepressant medication (imipramine) to interpersonal therapy in those who did not remit with such treatment alone.[719] The study found that in the absence of remission, adding antidepressant pharmacotherapy to interpersonal therapy could be highly effective, enabling a number of individuals to achieve a full remission from depressive symptoms.[719] A similar study was conducted with dysthymic patients in a primary care setting.[720] The findings were similar to the previous study since the researchers showed that interpersonal therapy plus antidepressant medication (sertraline) was effective in reducing symptoms. However, there was no significant difference between sertraline alone and sertraline plus interpersonal therapy, and these two treatment conditions were more effective than interpersonal therapy alone at 6 months' follow-up. This was also the case at 2 years follow-up.

Additionally, there has been some research on maintenance interpersonal therapy. Maintenance interpersonal therapy employs the same techniques as the standard version, but its main goal is the prevention of recurrence and it is seen more as a long term rather than an acute intervention.[721] The little research that has been compiled on maintenance treatment has concentrated on depression in later life. The findings may be transferable to those suffering with depression between the ages of 18 years to 65 years (mid-life depression). Reynolds and collegues[722] compared medication (nortriptyline) and interpersonal therapy as maintenance therapies for recurrent depression in older adults. They noted that for the treatment of recurrent depression, medication or IPT were better than placebo and clinic visits in prevention of recurrence. Furthermore, the combination of nortriptyline with IPT was the optimum treatment condition.

Problem solving therapy is a cognitive-behavioral approach. The main goal of the treatment is to alter the problematic nature of the current situation, the patients' reaction to such situations, or to achieve both these goals.[723] It works on the premise that by teaching problem solving skills one is able to improve their ability to cope with life stresses.[724] In a primary care based study, problem solving therapy was an effective treatment for patients with major depression and the improvement in mood was maintained over a 52 week follow-up.[725] Furthermore, the combination of this treatment with antidepressant medication (paroxetine or fluvoxamine) was no more effective than either treatment alone. In a community study of the prevention of depression, the participants were randomly assigned to either the problem solving therapy or group psychoeducation.[726] Outcomes were positive for both treatment groups at 6 months' follow-up. However, patients that were assigned to problem solving were less likely to report depressive symptoms.

In a study of remission rates and the correlates of remission of minor depression with problem solving therapy in adult and older adult patients, this treatment as well as paroxetine showed greater effectiveness over placebo plus clinical management.[727] Women, younger patients, and those with lower baseline severity of depression were more likely to achieve remission, independent of whether they had been treated with paroxetine, problem solving therapy, or placebo.[728] Furthermore, problem solving therapy seemed less suitable for patients whose minor depression had arisen as a result of more chronic life and health problems.[728]

Thus, problem solving therapy does have fairly strong support for the treatment of depressive disorders. There is, however, a need for further research, since that done has focused mainly on either dysthymia or minor depression and has been done in a primary-care setting. To further enhance the effectiveness of this treatment it would be worthwhile comparing it with other psychological therapies such as cognitive-behavioral therapy and interpersonal therapy.

Although all three treatments seem to be psychotherapies of choice when treating depression, there are other psychotherapies such as behavior therapy, psychodynamic psychotherapy, and nondirective conseling, to name but a few. However, there are few randomized controlled trials to endorse the efficacy and effectiveness of these treatments in primary care and research settings. An interesting meta-analysis looked at the effects of cognitive-behavioral therapy versus other psychotherapies in the treatment of depression.[729] Psychotherapies were divided into bona fide, i.e. those that have been developed with the specific intention of treating depression and nonbona fide versus CBT. There was no advantage of cognitive-behavioral therapy for depression, and all bona fide psychological treatments were equally effective.[728]

Psychotherapies are now generally recommended as treatment of milder depression or as an adjunct to antidepressant drugs in more severe illness. For obvious reasons their evidence base is thinner than that for antidepressant drugs. There is no evidence for a better rationale of any particular psychotherapy, since several approaches with different underlying assumptions seem to be equally efficacious.

Medication in Depression

In a review of antidepressant treatments, NICE went well beyond guidelines published by the American Psychiatric Association[731] by coming to the conclusion that antidepressants are not recommended for the initial treatment of mild depression, because the risk benefit ratio is poor. Instead it advocates psychosocial treatment or some form of psychotherapy.[718] In moderate to severe depression, antidepressants are recommended, though preferably in combination with psychotherapy.[718] Apart from a small evidence base, there are some practical problems with the implementation of these recommendations, since mood-related cognitive impairment and poor motivation could make psychotherapeutic treatment of depressed patients difficult. Very little evidence exists for the treatment of depression in the context of alcohol and drug dependence, although this is frequent and important comorbidity. The lack of availability of adequately trained psychotherapists is another obstacle.

The NICE recommendations are representative of a trend in public perception, which seems to run ahead of contemporary clinical practice: Although data on effectiveness have been the prime criterion for deciding on treatment recommendations in the past, risks of side-effects and patients' choice are increasingly taking their place next to treatment effectiveness.[730-732] This change in emphasis explains the NICE recommendation for mild depression, as well as the institution of working groups, and enquiries on the treatment of depression children and adults by the US Food and Drug Administration, the US Congress,[733] and the UK Medicines and Healthcare products Regulatory Agency.[734] Antidepressant drugs of choice are, in the first instance, serotonin reuptake inhibitors, such as fluoxetine, paroxetine, fluvoxamine, citalopram, and sertraline.[718] The main risks that have been associated with serotonin reuptake inhibitors are treatment-emergent suicidal behavior and withdrawal symptoms, especially in children and adolescents.[734] Since side-effects are not the primary outcome measure in most drug trials, their recording and reporting tends to be poor. Some potential drug effects, such as suicide, are so rare that drug trials are of necessity underpowered to find any effects. The absence of comprehensive and reliable evidence for risks,[734] perceived industrial interests of clinicians[735,736] as well as publication bias, which is well known to any author of systematic reviews, have in some quarters eroded public faith in the drug treatment of depression and its regulation.[732,737,738]

The most serious risk associated with depression is increased mortality, especially that due to suicide. Experimental studies of suicide risk or prevention *per se* are virtually impossible, because of the very low period prevalence of suicide during clinical studies, even in depressed patients. Indirect methods, such as meta-analyses and epidemiological studies provide some lower level evidence.[739,740] Proxy measures of suicide, such as suicidal behavior, deliberate self harm, or reported suicidal thoughts are more frequent and can be examined instead, as long as they are treated as only one of many risk factors for actual suicide.[741,742] Any intervention that is associated with greater frequency of suicidal thoughts is therefore not necessarily linked to an actual increase in suicides, because suicidal thoughts might in any one case not be the decisive risk fator.[734,741,744] Clinical lore suggests that suicidal risk increases early during treatment, because recovery takes place in degrees, with energy and motivation for example improving before mood. Although there is some evidence of increased suicidal behavior in the early stages of treatment,[135] this does not seem to be linked to a particular drug or class of antidepressant.[126,133,136] The relative risk of finding serotonin reuptake inhibitors at post mortem after self-poisoning is actually smaller than for other antidepressants, presumably because of their lower toxicity in overdose.[745] Post-hoc studies of patients treated in clinical practice have confirmed that there is no increased risk of suicidal behavior with serotonin reuptake inhibitor-withdrawal symptoms seems mainly to be about semantics. There is no doubt that withdrawal symptoms occur after stopping SRIs and other antidepressants. The neologism discontinuation symptoms essentially mean the same as withdrawal symptoms, without having any association with addiction. Withdrawal symptoms are, of course, a common, but by no means a sufficient criterion to define drug dependence or addiction.[734] Withdrawal symptoms occur particularly, but not exclusively, on withdrawal from paroxetine and venlafaxine. An unexpected and rare symptom is the experience of electric shock sensations, often localized to the head and limbs. With increasing numbers of pregnant mothers going through pregnancy on serotonin reuptake inhibitors, the occasional occurrence of withdrawal in neonates needs to be considered.[746] There is no evidence that antidepressants cause actual addiction.[734]

Drug treatments remain the mainstay of antidepressant therapy. Recent moral panics about suicidal effects of dependence-including potential of antidepressants have tilted the balance of publicly perceived risk against them, but both their effectiveness and their ready availability make them the likely choice for most patients.

Physical Treatments in Depression

Transcranial magnetic stimulation has recently received much publicity, both as an interesting method to investigate neuronal function *in vivo* in humans and as a potential treatment method to supplement or even to replace drug treatment and electroconvulsive treatment in depression.[747] It has great potential as a noninvasive investigative method, especially if combined with imaging methods. Transcranial magnetic stimulation is able to disturb neuronal activity in a way that allows for the examination of causality, rather than generating associations, as most imaging methods do. Combined with neuroimaging, the spatial distribution of such stimulated neuronal networks can be mapped. After initial enthusiasm about its treatment potential, the current assessment is more sober. The forest plot of controlled trials in depression indicates a secular trend with more recent trials showing smaller effect sizes.[747-776]

This pattern might be partly due to the choice of treatment-resistant and drug treated patients, but also to inadequate blinding to placebo. The most commonly used placebo condition is to tilt the coil by 45° away from the scalp, a method that may result in some cortical stimulation or in a different perception of surface stimulation of scalp muscles and skin by the patient. Most studies have focused on high frequency (10–20 Hz) stimulation of the left or low frequency (1 Hz) stimulation of the right dorsolateral prefrontal cortex. There is no good evidence that these are the only coil positions and stimulation frequencies with antidepressant effects, although several neuroimaging studies during such stimulation protocols have shown changes in brain activity and neurotransmitter binding that seem relevant to depressive symptoms.[777-779] The development of new stimulation protocols, such as θ burst stimulation[778,780] could lead to more effective treatment protocols, but in the meantime transcranial magnetic stimulation remains as experimental treatment modality.

A potential, but rare side-effect of transcranial magnetic stimulation, especially at higher frequencies and intensities, is the induction of seizures.[781] Because of the actual difficulty of inducing seizures reliably with transcranial magnetic stimulation, attempts to replace electric induction of seizures for electroconvulsive therapy (ECT) with this treatment are fairly recent.[782-785] A major advantage of magnetic over electric seizure induction is that the magnetic field can penetrate scalp and skull without hindrance, whereas the electric current used for ECT is impeded by the resistance of surface structures and the brain, requiring the stimulation of various extracranial and intracranial structures before a seizure can be induced. Magnetic seizure therapy is, therefore, likely to lead to less unnecessary stimulation resulting in fewer side-effects such as memory impairment.[782]

Electroconvulsive Therapy

Despite public and profession misgivings, ECT remains the most effective treatment for depression, especially if it presents with psychotic symptoms, such as delusions and hallucinations.[786,787] Apart from the risk of general anesthetic, the main objection to ECT has been its liability to cause memory impairment. Research on cognitive functioning after ECT has been far from comprehensive and is complicated by the improvement of cognition due to the alleviation of depressive symptoms. A recent robust study examined the effects of ECT on episodic memory and noted that the anterograde amnesic effects of ECT were greater for knowledge about the world—i.e. impersonal memory, than for autobiographical memory—i.e. personal memory.[188] In a systematic review and meta-analysis,[786] the UK ECT Review group stated that data relating to cognitive impairment consisted mostly of temporary anterograde and retrograde amnesia.[786] Furthermore, the method ECT used in the treatment of depression was linked to the degree of cognitive impairment produced. For example, bilateral ECT produces greater impairment than unilateral ECT, and higher energy treatment produces greater impairment than lower energy.[789] The effects of ECT are short-lived so patients are likely to require follow-on pharmacological therapy.[790] Further research into the long-term cognitive effects of ECT is recommended as there is a dearth of randomized controlled trials researching this area.[786]

The role of neurosurgery in the management of patients highly resistant to treatment and its invasive nature make future randomized controlled studies unlikely. Vagal nerve stimulation has been proposed as a treatment in drug-resistant and ECT-resistant depressed patients, but the evidence for its effectiveness is as yet inconclusive.[789] Deep brain stimulation as a currently experimental treatment might offer an intervention similar to neurosurgery, which is both reversible and amenable to within-participant placebo control. Six patients with severe refractory depressive disorder, who had failed to respond to antidepressant, psychotherapeutic, and electroconvulsive therapies were treated in an open study, in which electrodes were implanted in the white matter tracts immediately lateral to the subgenual anterior cingulate.[791] Striking and sustained remission of depression was reported in four of the six patients. Furthermore, PET images showed a pronounced reduction in locally abnormally increased subgenual cerebral metabolism, as well as changes in downstream cortical and limbic sites. The authors[791] concluded that disrupting focal pathological activity in the subgenual region using deep brain stimulation could effectively reverse symptoms in depression that is otherwise resistant to treatment.

Other recent studies have reported the results of deep brain stimulation for refractory obsessive-compulsive and anxiety disorders. Based on studies of internal capsulotomy for these disorders,[792] four patients with treatment refractory severe obsessive-compulsive disorder were reported in an open study. The patients had electrodes implanted in the anterior limbs of the internal capsule.[793] This stimulation had beneficial effects in three patients, with one having an especially striking result. For this one patient, the investigator then did a double-blind trial with video assessment and six independent assessors. The findings of the more rigorous double-blind assessment supported the conclusions of the initial less detailed open study assessment; during deep brain stimulation the patient had a pronounced increase in ratings of social contact, communication, flow of ideas, assertiveness and mobility, a decrease in doubt, and no change in sustained attention.[793]

On the basis of this and other work, an open study investigated treatment of refractory obsessive-compulsive disorder and anxiety disorders with deep brain stimulation of the anatomically adjacent shell of the nucleus accumbens.[794] A good reduction in symptom severity was reported in three of four patients. Additionally, PET images of one patient during stimulation showed a change in brain metabolism as a result of the stimulation.[792-794] shows the locations of these procedures.

Of the physical treatments only ECT is in regular clinical use. Transcranial magnetic stimulation, magnetic seizure therapy and vagal nerve stimulation offer hope of treatment that is potentially less invasive or liable to generate memory impairment. Neurosurgery for mental disorders is reserved for very few highly treatment-resistant patients, whereas deep brain stimulation may be able to emulate some of its effects with the opportunity for blind and randomized assessment, as well as reversibility of its effects.

7.15 TREATMENT RESISTANT DEPRESSION

Manoj Dhungana

Approximately 32–35 million adults in the United States have an episode of major depression sometime during their lifetime, and many of them do not respond to initial treatment.[795] The results of an analysis undertaken by Fava and Davidson[796] suggest that between 29% and 46% of depressed patients fail to respond fully to antidepressant treatment of adequate dose and duration; about 15% of patients fail to respond to multiple treatment trials.[797] Fagiolini and Kupfer[798] have suggested that patients with treatment-resistant depression (TRD) may represent a biologically unique subtype of depressed patients. Unfortunately, the chances for full recovery diminish the longer a patient remains depressed—a fact that lends a sense of urgency for appropriate therapy.[799]

MANAGEMENT STRATEGIES

Before discussing the effectiveness of individual agents in TRD, it is important to review recent evidence regarding the principles of using these agents to maximize the chance of a response.[800-803] The standard strategy for managing patients who are depressed includes an adequate clinical trial; when the response is unsatisfactory, the clinician's options are:

- Switch to another antidepressant
- Combine a second antidepressant with the first
- Add a second drug that is not approved as an antidepressant
- Start psychotherapy.

Antidepressants can be grouped into 6 major categories: tricyclic antidepressants (TCAs), SSRIs, serotonin norepinephrine reuptake inhibitors (SNRIs), monoamine oxidase inhibitors (MAOIs), serotonin neurotransmitter (5-HT2)-receptor antagonists (e.g. nefazodone, trazodone), and novel agents (e.g. mirtazapine, bupropion). If a patient fails to respond to one antidepressant class, it makes sense (at least conceptually) to switch to another, although most guidelines acknowledge that 2 failed trials of SSRIs may be justifiable before switching classes.[801,802] When examining switching studies, be certain that the reason for switching was a failure to respond to an adequate antidepressant trial rather than a lack of tolerability, as these are fundamentally different issues.

Switching

The concept of switching classes of antidepressants is only as valid as the theoretical basis by which the antidepressants are grouped. As noted, some treatment guidelines allow 2 SSRI trials before switching classes. For example, in a study by Thase and colleagues,[804] 58 patients failed a trial of fluoxetine; however, there was a 76% response rate to citalopram among completers. Although this study was not blinded, it is interesting that citalopram (which is believed to be the most selective of the SSRIs) was effective when another SSRI was not. It is hoped that as our knowledge of the mechanism of action of antidepressants grows more sophisticated, methods of classifying these agents will evolve to better guide clinicians in switching and combination strategies.

The clinical trial data on switching are surprisingly sparse—a recent meta-analysis identified only 4 randomized controlled trials.[805] These trials include data from level 2 of the STAR*D study in which patients who were switched from citalopram to sertraline, venlafaxine XR, or bupropion SR showed remission rates of 27%, 25%, and 26% (respectively) based on the Quick Inventory of Depressive Symptomatology, Self-Report (QIDS-SR-16).[806] The meta-analysis found a modest but statistically significant advantage in switching from SSRIs to nonSSRIs. Of the 5 comparisons, 3 used venlafaxine, which is predominately a serotonergic agent (the serotonin-norepinephrine Ki ratio is 30), although it is classified as an SNRI. This may account for the relative lack of separation. One wonders if duloxetine, with a Ki ratio of 9 and relatively greater noradrenergic potency, might show greater separation.[807] However, only one open-label switching study with duloxetine has been published to date.[808]

In switching antidepressants, 2 pharmacokinetic issues are important:

- Drugs with potent cytochrome P-450 (CYP450) effects—particularly fluoxetine (because of its long half-life)—may produce toxic levels of medications taken concurrently, such as TCAs that are also metabolized by these systems. (This effect is even more of an issue with combinations.)

- Antidepressants that are associated with discontinuation symptoms (e.g. paroxetine, venlafaxine, duloxetine) may produce discontinuation syndromes when stopped that can be erroneously attributed to adverse effects of the new drug, particularly if the new drug does not possess a significant degree of serotonin reuptake inhibition.

What we need are agents with novel mechanisms of action. Some of these agents, such as agomelatine, are relatively far along in the clinical trial process with human subjects. Others, such as amibegron and sipatrigine, have been shown to be efficacious only in animal models of depression and their benefit is therefore highly speculative.[809-811] Some of the drugs have been tried as augmentation agents as well (e.g. riluzole). Agents such as pramipexole, memantine, riluzole, and ketoconazole are already available in the United States.

Proposed mechanisms of action vary widely, but 2 development strategies are generating a great deal of activity:

- Agents are being developed that affect corticosteroid function at various levels. (Glucocorticoids have figured prominently in recent theories as major agents in stress-induced neuronal injury and cell death leading to depression.[812])
- Compounds are being developed that induce the synthesis of brain-derived neurotrophic factor (BDNF), particularly through their effects on glutamate receptors.

In a sense, these two strategies are related: it has been proposed that BDNF acts as a modulator of neuronal repair and even neurogenesis in response to cortisol-induced brain injury. The findings with ketamine are particularly exciting. A recent study reported that ketamine, through its activity as an N-methyl-D-aspartate (NMDA)-receptor antagonist, increases synaptic glutamate and therefore stimulates a-amino-3-hydroxy-5-methyl-4-isoxazolepropionic acid (AMPA) receptors (both NMDA and AMPA receptors are subtypes of glutamate receptors).[813] AMPA potentiators are known to induce BDNF production more rapidly than current antidepressants.[814] It has been hypothesized that a more rapid induction of BDNF would lead to a faster onset of antidepressant action. In a study by Zarate and colleagues,[815] the onset of the antidepressant effect of ketamine occurred within 2 hours. Unfortunately, the drug must be given by intravenous infusion, but because the effect persisted for 7 days, ketamine treatment may be useful if given as a series.

Another NMDA-receptor antagonist now available in the United States is memantine (FDA-approved for Alzheimer disease). Memantine was shown to be effective in an open-label study in major depression. In a double-blind, randomized trial it showed comparable effects to escitalopram in patients with major depression and alcohol dependence.[816,817] However memantine failed to separate from placebo in a double-blind, placebo-controlled study in major depression.[818] The less robust antidepressant properties of memantine when compared with those of ketamine may be due to differing NMDA receptor binding properties between the two compounds.[815]

Combining Agents

In this category, there are two similar strategies: (1) combination, that is, combining 2 FDA-approved antidepressants with presumably complementary mechanisms of action; and (2) augmentation, in which a drug not approved as an antidepressant is used with an FDA-approved antidepressant. Such pairings can be used either at the beginning of therapy to speed the response (an accelerator strategy) or to improve the overall response, thereby enhancing the odds of achieving remission. As noted, when combining agents, one must be aware of possible CYP450-based pharmacokinetic interactions or other pharmacological interactions, such as the risk of serotonin syndrome when an SSRI is combined with an MAOI.

Combination strategies. Of the two strategies, the addition of a second antidepressant is the more intuitively obvious. Randomized controlled trials have supported the superior efficacy of a TCA/SSRI combination, as well as a mirtazapine/SSRI combination; open studies have done the same for TCA/MAOI and SSRI/bupropion combinations.[819] A positive retrospective chart review of ten patients treated with a combination of duloxetine and bupropion has also been published.[820]

These findings raise the question of whether combining antidepressants is superior to switching. For example, an open-label, nonrandomized study by Lam and colleagues[821] found that when 61 patients who were taking citalopram or bupropion SR for TRD were either switched to the other drug or given the combination, the combination group showed statistically greater rates of response and remission. At a minimum, combination treatments ensure that a partial response to the first agent will not be lost.

Augmentation strategies: If the switching and combination literature is conspicuous by its paucity, the augmentation literature is abundant—but the quality of evidence varies tremendously and the reader must maintain a "buyer beware" approach. One recent review concluded that although studies of augmentation were abundant, many were underpowered and uncontrolled.[822] Several comprehensive reviews have been published.[822-825]

Evaluation strategies have been suggested to assess the quality of evidence.[822,826] In general, augmentation strategies are recommended in the event of a partial response to an antidepressant. Switching is preferred in the event of a nonresponse.[819] One of the few studies to examine this issue systematically found numerically higher response rates among partial responders compared with nonresponders when lithium or desipramine was added to fluoxetine, but these differences were not statistically significant.[827] Although the amount and quality of evidence about the agents in category A is meaningful, the differentiation of groups B and C is somewhat arbitrary. The presumed mechanism of action of augmentation agents varies tremendously and is generally believed to complement the action of the primary antidepressant in some predictable theoretical manner. Questions remain about the validity of our current classification systems for grouping augmentation agents—an issue of crucial importance for clinicians who need to pair them with antidepressants for maximum benefit.

Lithium, the classic augmentation agent, has been the subject of the greatest number of studies. A recent meta-analysis identified 10 randomized, placebo-controlled trials, all of which were relatively small (the largest included 61 subjects).[828] The authors of these studies concluded that lithium was significantly more effective than placebo. The vast majority of the studies with lithium did not include SSRIs but instead used TCAs. Remission rates from level 3 of the STAR*D trial using lithium as an augmentation agent with citalopram were only 13.2% (measured by QIDS-SR), whereas T3 augmentation remission rates at this same step were 24.7%.[829] Although these differences were not statistically different, there was a significantly higher dropout rate in the lithium group.

As with lithium, a recent review concluded that the trial data that support the efficacy of T3 augmentation are of better quality with TCAs than with SSRIs.[826] Although it has been reported that approximately 50% of patients with unipolar depression given thyroid augmentation show a response, a pooled analysis of 4 randomized double-blind studies of T3 augmentation revealed nonsignificant effects, but the results of 1 of the 4 studies may have accounted for this finding.[830,831]

By contrast to these relatively small studies with classical augmentation agents, there are a number of large, randomized, placebo-controlled trials of atypical antipsychotics in nonpsychotic, unipolar depression in combination with antidepressants. These studies culminated in the first-ever FDA approval of an agent specifically for antidepressant augmentation—aripiprazole. In their meta-analysis, Papakostas and colleagues[832] conclude that the results support the utility of atypical augmentation, even in the absence of double-blind, placebo-controlled trials with aripiprazole (now available) and ziprasidone. Virtually all of the studies to date of atypical augmentation have been conducted with SSRIs, although there are reports that aripiprazole was effective with bupropion, tranylcypromine, and mirtazapine.[833-835]

The study of tranylcypromine (an MAOI) with aripiprazole suggests the need for cautious use of some combinations. As noted in the package insert, tranylcypromine should not be coadministered with dibenzazepine-related entities because of the risk of severe interactions, including hypertensive crises and seizures.[836] Some of the atypical antipsychotics (e.g. aripiprazole, ziprasidone) have a high affinity at the 5-HT1A-receptor; agents such as buspirone, which also binds at this receptor site, are not recommended for use with MAOIs. Ziprasidone also has a similar potency to imipramine in terms of blocking norepinephrine and serotonin reuptake (imipramine is al-so relatively contraindicated with MAOIs).[837] There is a report of 5 patients treated safely with risperidone and MAOIs, and another of 12 patients exposed to olanzapine with the selegiline patch.[838,839]

In general, the effective dosage of atypical antipsychotics in this role seems to be lower than that used in psychosis. Data on the long-term risks in depressed patients, including tardive dyskinesia and metabolic syndrome, are urgently needed. The recent FDA approval of quetiapine as monotherapy in bipolar depression raises questions as to whether some of the atypical antipsychotics may be effective (and perhaps better tolerated) when given as a single agent for unipolar TRD.

In regard to the value of switching atypicals, if one agent fails, is it worth attempting trials of another? There are limited data that show that switching to another atypical is worthwhile.[840,841] However, results from randomized controlled trials are still needed.

SUMMARY

Each of the agents is most effective when used for augmentation purposes. The quality of the evidence varies widely, particularly in the second and third categories of the table. For example, in a pooled analysis, estrogen was effective when added to sertraline in a group of depressed women over 60 years; however, the total sample size was only 127.[842] There are small, positive, double-blind studies for agents such as testosterone, L-tryptophan, and omega-3-fatty acids.[843-845] In the case of pindolol, there are negative studies as well, and in a recent review, the evidence supporting its efficacy was rated as a "C" (the lowest rating).[822,826]

Open-label reports for buspirone were positive, but 2 randomized controlled trials were negative.[846,847] Buspirone was used as an augmentation agent for citalopram in level 2 of STAR*D: remission rates were 33% by the QIDS-SR compared to 39% with bupropion at the same stage. Although the remission rates between the 2 drugs did not differ significantly, the bupropion group had a significantly greater reduction in depression scores.[848]

Despite reports that suggest the efficacy of lamotrigine, this agent did not separate significantly from placebo in the only large, multicenter, double-blind, placebo-controlled trial to date.[849] Modafinil, used in 2 randomized, placebo-controlled trials did not show significant placebo separation on most mood-scale scores, but it did reduce sleepiness and fatigue.[850,851]

The unfortunate reality is that conducting large, double-blind, placebo-controlled trials is extremely expensive and time consuming. Definitive evidence of the efficacy of these agents is likely to accrue slowly. Negative studies may not prove that a drug is ineffective because of factors such as high placebo response rates, or the more subtle reality that there may be meaningful subgroups of patients with TRD that we are currently unable to identify.

7.16 COGNITIVE BEHAVIOR THERAPY FOR DEPRESSION

JN Vyas

BACKGROUND

Cognitive-behavioral therapy (CBT) is a term that encompasses numerous specific treatment approaches for various psychiatric disorders. As the name suggests, cognitive-behavioral treatments incorporate both cognitive and behavioral strategies. With regard to depression, CBT refers to the use of both cognitive restructuring and the behavioral strategy of activity scheduling or behavioral activation.

Cognitive-behavioral approaches to the treatment of depression stem from early behavioral treatments that emerged in the 1960s and 1970s. Among the most prominent was Lewinsohn et al's behavioral treatment for depression.[852] Lewinsohn proposed that depression resulted from deficient response contingent positive reinforcement, which he reported was a function of the following 3 factors:[853]

1. Individual differences in what is experienced as reinforcing.
2. The availability in the individual's environment of potentially reinforcing events.
3. The skill level needed to obtain reinforcement.

For example, if someone found conversing with others to be reinforcing, had other individuals available with whom to converse, and possessed the social skills needed to engage one of those individuals in conversation, then he or she could experience positive reinforcement. Lewinsohn's treatment, therefore, aimed to increase depressed individuals' ability to obtain response-contingent positive reinforcement and therefore improve their mood; he did this by having them identify and engage in events they described as having been, or potentially being, pleasurable and addressing skills deficits that may preclude them from obtaining the desired reinforcement from identified pleasant events. Numerous depression treatments that included activity scheduling emerged during the 1970s and 1980s.[852,854-857]

Although early versions of activity scheduling primarily focused on increasing mood-related pleasant events, Beck incorporated a form of activity scheduling into his cognitive therapy for depression, aimed at increasing both pleasant events and providing a sense of accomplishment or mastery (e.g. working on a resume, completing a school assignment).[858] Following a component analysis of cognitive therapy that found this activity scheduling component to be as effective as the full treatment package,[859] interest in behavioral treatments for depression increased, leading to modern approaches called behavioral activation (BA) treatments.

Modern BA approaches are based on the same principles as early versions of activity scheduling but incorporate more sophisticated strategies for identifying activity assignments and addressing barriers to their completion.[860,861] Several meta-analyses have examined studies of activity scheduling and BA approaches over the past several decades and have provided substantial empirical support for these approaches.[862-863]

During the 1970s, cognitive treatments for depression began to gain in popularity and empirical support, with the most well-known being Beck et al's cognitive therapy for depression.[858] Cognitive therapy is based on the fundamental assumptions that (1) cognitive activity affects behavior, (2) cognitive activity can be monitored and changed, and (3) cognitive changes can lead to desired behavioral changes.[865] Cognitive therapy emphasizes the need to change cognitions in order to achieve improvements in mood and behavior. As mentioned above, Beck's cognitive therapy for depression includes activity scheduling treatment strategies adapted from earlier behavioral interventions but also includes cognitive strategies such as cognitive restructuring that were designed to directly challenge and change maladaptive thoughts.

Although behavioral approaches typically do not include any direct attempts to change cognitions (but attempt to indirectly do so through changes in behavior), cognitive therapy does directly attempt to change behavior but does so for the ultimate goal of changing cognitions in order to reduce depressive symptoms. Therefore, at times, such approaches may be called either cognitive therapy or CBT, with both incorporating behavioral and cognitive interventions.

Within the CBT model, individuals with depression are viewed as exhibiting the "cognitive triad" of depression, which includes a negative view of themselves, a negative view of their environment, and a negative view of their future.[866] Related to the cognitive triad, depressed patients are believed to exhibit numerous cognitive distortions that maintain these negative beliefs.[858] Examples of these distortions include all-or-nothing thinking (i.e. viewing things in black and white categories), overgeneralization (i.e. assuming one negative event constitutes a pattern of never-ending negative events), and fortune telling (i.e. making negative predictions about the future that are often inaccurate or negatively biased).[867] Within Beck's model, negative automatic thoughts and distortions in thinking are hypothesized as stemming from problematic schemas, which are cognitive structures that influence how information is interpreted and recalled.[858,868] Schemas are often targeted in the later phases of treatment, whereas behavioral strategies and efforts to elicit and test automatic thoughts are implemented earlier in treatment.[866] Elaboration of specific treatment strategies is presented below.

INDICATIONS

Individual and group-based CBT is recognized in the most recent American Psychiatric Association Guidelines for the treatment of major depressive disorder as an effective and evidence based treatment for depression.[869] When used, it should be integrated into the overall care that the patient is receiving (i.e. communication is needed between the treating therapist and the prescribing psychiatrist or primary care physician).

The use of CBT for a particular patient is often based on patient preference, severity of depression, and ability of the patient to gain access to the treatment. The use of CBT as a stand-alone treatment is recommended for patients with mild-to-moderate major depressive disorder and should also be considered for women who are pregnant, wish to become pregnant, or are actively breastfeeding. It should also be made available for patients that express a preference to use CBT.

A combination of antidepressant medication and psychotherapy such as CBT is recommended for individuals with moderate-to-severe major depressive disorder or for teens with major depressive disorder in order to reduce the risk of relapse.[869,870] According to the American Psychiatric Association guidelines, CBT combined with pharmacotherapy is also considered first-line treatment in patients with more severe, chronic, or complex presentations of depression.[869]

CONTRAINDICATIONS

CBT has been used clinically in almost every imaginable patient population. No evidence-based exclusion criteria for the use of CBT for depression have been established. Many studies of CBT typically exclude individuals with specific characteristics due to beliefs that these characteristics could lead to less improvement in symptoms over the course of treatment. Typical exclusion criteria include an alcohol or other substance disorder, a psychotic disorder, organic brain syndrome, and mental retardation, with many studies also specifying that participants have major depressive disorder in the absence of suicide risk. More research on this issue is needed; many believe that individuals with these characteristics may still benefit from CBT for depression.

PREVENTION OF COMPLICATION

The support of family members and friends can assist with treatment by helping remind and encourage patients to complete important aspects of treatment such as attending therapy sessions, taking psychiatric medications (if prescribed), and completing therapy assignments. They may also be active participants in some of the activity scheduling assignments. Further, family members may be asked to attend therapy sessions in order to gain information about depression and CBT and to learn specific ways in which they can support or assist the patient.

APPROACH CONSIDERATIONS

CBT for depression begins with a focus on symptom reduction through behavioral techniques and cognitive techniques designed to identify and challenge negative automatic thoughts. Once significant symptom reduction has occurred, individuals practicing Beck's version of cognitive therapy may then shift to a schema-focused phase for the purpose of relapse prevention. During this phase of treatment, the goal is to identify and replace dysfunctional schemas that are thought to enhance vulnerability to depressive episodes.

BEHAVIORAL STRATEGIES

Behavioral strategies are often used in the beginning of CBT for depression. Individuals with depression often engage in significant avoidance and a corresponding decrease in activity level. For instance, many individuals with depression find themselves spending more time in bed and less time engaging in social activities, household tasks, work or school-related activities, and, at times, important hygiene behaviors. Martell and colleagues conceptualize this process with their "3 circles" model, which demonstrates how negative life events lead to depressed mood and other negative emotional responses, which then leads to avoidance behaviors, creating a negative cycle in which depressive symptoms may worsen.[860]

BEHAVIORAL ACTIVATION MODEL OF DEPRESSION[860]

To counteract this, behavioral strategies are used in order to decrease avoidance and increase engagement in the types of activities demonstrated to help alleviate depressive symptoms (i.e. activities associated with pleasure and mastery or accomplishment). Within the model presented in the image above, this involves replacing the avoidance patterns with activation behaviors, which then stops the negative cycle of depression and works to improve mood. These behavioral strategies are especially recommended for patients presenting to treatment who are passive, experiencing anhedonia, are socially withdrawn, and have difficulty concentrating for long periods of time.

Activities are often assigned using a graded approach in which initial assigned activities are less complex and difficult, with more difficult activities being assigned gradually over the course of treatment as the patient becomes more active. For example, a patient with mild-to-moderate depression may be given initial activity assignments of going to a party (pleasurable activity) and spending 20 minutes on a report for work (accomplishment/mastery activity). For patients with moderate-to-severe depression, initial assignments would be less difficult or complex, such as reading a book for 10 minutes (pleasurable activity) and making their bed (accomplishment/mastery activity). The important point is to meet the patient at their current level of functioning based on their depressive symptoms and gradually work to increase engagement in more complex activities.

To assist with activity scheduling, therapists often assign an activity rating form on which patients maintain a record of their activities over the course of each day and provide ratings on a 0-10 scale for how much pleasure and mastery they experienced with each completed activity.

COMPLETED DAILY ACTIVITY MONITORING SHEET

This is often useful data that can serve to counteract patients' beliefs that they are unable to experience joy or gain a sense of accomplishment from any activities, and can help determine specific types of activities to assign in the future that are likely to lead to feelings of pleasure and mastery. To assist with completion of assigned activities, patients may be asked to engage in imaginal rehearsal (sometimes termed cognitive rehearsal), in which they imagine themselves engaging in various activities in order to identify obstacles to experiencing a sense of pleasure or mastery from those events.[858] This enables the therapist and patient to then problem-solve obstacles and increase the chances of assigned activities leading to desired outcomes.

Additional behavioral strategies may be incorporated to assist with other specific problems the patient may experience that influence their depressive symptoms. For instance, patients may be taught specific techniques for improving sleep if they experience significant sleep difficulties. In addition, patients with social skills deficits may require additional treatment focused on their specific skills deficits in order to improve their ability to successfully complete activity scheduling assignments and gain the desired sense of pleasure or mastery from these. Examples of techniques for skills deficits include social skills training, assertiveness training, and strategies targeting communication skills. Therapists may ask patients to engage in in-session role playing in order to practice more effective social skills.

INITIAL COGNITIVE STRATEGIES

The primary cognitive techniques involve eliciting the patient's automatic thoughts, testing these thoughts, and identifying core schemas that influence how the patient views the world. Automatic thoughts are defined as "thoughts that intervene between outside events and the individual's emotional reactions to them."[866] Automatic thoughts tend to occur frequently and to not be noticed by the individual and are therefore often accepted as true without evaluation. For individuals with depression, these automatic thoughts tend to be negative thoughts in line with the cognitive triad and therefore maintain and worsen depressive symptoms. Examples of negative automatic thoughts related to depression may include thoughts such as "I am a worthless person," "nobody likes me," and "I will never get better."

The initial focus is on eliciting automatic thoughts and teaching patients to recognize these thoughts when they occur. One method for doing this is for the therapist to question the patient regarding thoughts that occurred in response to various events. Role playing may also be used to recreate previous events and assess different thoughts the patient experiences throughout the interaction. When eliciting automatic thoughts, the patient is also taught to pay attention to changes in their mood that occur following automatic thoughts, in order to learn about the relationship between their automatic thoughts and their emotions. To assist with this process, patients are often asked to keep a thought record on which they list emotions and automatic thoughts that coincide with distressing situations that occur between therapy sessions. This thought record can then be reviewed during the next therapy session.[866]

When the therapist and patient are able to identify automatic thoughts as they occur, the next step is to challenge these negative automatic thoughts. To do this, the patient is taught to complete additional columns on the thought record. The full thought record often includes columns for describing distressing situations, describing the emotions and negative automatic thoughts that occur in response to these situations, rating their initial belief in the negative automatic thought, generating alternative rational responses to the situation, rating the extent to which they believe the rational alternatives, and finally, indicating which emotions they felt in response to this modified belief.

The thorough record can be individualized to challenge cognitive distortions specific to the patient, with the primary goal being to examine evidence for and against their negative thoughts and determine alternative explanations that are more realistic and less likely to lead to depressed mood, for examples of cognitive distortions frequently endorsed by individuals with depression.[867]

COGNITIVE DISTORTIONS

To challenge a negative automatic thought such as "nobody likes me," the patient may be asked a question such as "what evidence do you have that nobody likes you?" Subsequent questions evaluate each piece of evidence provided to determine whether that piece of evidence directly supports the hypothesis that nobody likes the patient. Typically, individuals with depression do not have much evidence to support their negative beliefs but tend to misinterpret available cues in a manner that maintains or worsens their depressed mood.

Another method for evaluating negative automatic thoughts is to have the patient complete behavioral tests. In order to do this effectively, the patient must agree that the thought is indeed testable and could potentially be modified. If the patient is not yet at this point, further discussion regarding the patient's maladaptive thoughts and symptoms of depression is needed. In addition to having the patient agree that a specific negative thought is testable, the behavior must completed is well defined and that the patient and therapist agree as to what the behavior entails.

Finally, following the behavioral test, the patient is to record conclusions regarding how the behavior went and how it related to their negative thought, and these conclusions are then reviewed by the therapist and patient together.[871] These conclusions are often recorded on the thought record. An example of a behavioral test may involve having a patient with the negative thought, "nobody wants to spend time with me" agree to try calling 10 specific individuals to ask them to get together in the near future and record how many of the 10 agree. The therapist and patient discuss what the patient should say on the phone, when to try calling, and other aspects of the assignment in order to increase chances of success. During the next session, the patient and therapist review the results and discuss how the results relate to the hypothesis that nobody wants to spend time with the patient.

CHANGING MALADAPTIVE SCHEMAS

As mentioned above, once the patient has experienced benefit from the first phase of treatment and experienced significant reductions in their depressive symptoms, CBT may shift to a focus on changing core schemas in order to prevent relapse. This phase of treatment may not be used by CBT therapists not following Beck's specific cognitive therapy protocol.[858]

Schemas are thought to be more difficult to change than negative automatic thoughts and are viewed as stemming from earlier events that occurred in the patient's development. This schema-focused phase places more emphasis on developmental patterns, interpersonal relationships (including the patient-therapist relationship), and emotional/experiential exercises.[866]

The schema-focused phase begins with assessment of the patient's history in order to identify potential schemas as well as provision of education about schemas and how they influence individuals. Once this initial assessment and education phase is completed, efforts to change maladaptive schemas are introduced. The strategies for doing this are often similar to those used in the first phase of treatment (e.g. activity scheduling, cognitive restructuring), but they focus on longstanding patterns in which situations are repeatedly interpreted in a specific manner due to the maladaptive schemas.

OTHER ASPECTS

In addition to the specific treatment strategies reviewed above, CBT also has a specific style and organization. In addition, in contrast with earlier psychodynamic approaches to treatment that tended to involve several years of therapy, CBT approaches are time-limited in nature. For instance, many CBT treatments are designed to be implemented over the course of approximately 12–16 sessions, depending on the severity of symptoms and other specific characteristics of the patient.

CBT approaches emphasize the need for a collaborative therapist-patient relationship in which the therapist and patient work together and adapt a cooperative attitude. This is captured by the focus on jointly determining goals for therapy, such that both the patient and the therapist have input regarding which goals to focus on throughout treatment, the priority of those goals over the course of therapy, and even the goals for each specific session. This is done through the process of setting an agenda. Most CBT therapists begin each session by outlining the agenda for that session and ask for input from the patient regarding items they would like to add to the agenda. This collaborative relationship also includes regular feedback to the patient regarding how they are doing and a rationale for each treatment intervention, such that the patient feels fully informed regarding his or her treatment.[866]

A specific aspect of this collaborative relationship is termed collaborative empiricism. Collaborative empiricism involves having the patient and therapist act as a team set out to investigate and evaluate hypotheses regarding the patient's automatic thoughts and maladaptive schemas in a scientific manner.[858]

Finally, assigning homework between sessions is an important aspect of CBT. Specific homework assignments depend on the phase of treatment and the patient's specific symptoms but often include activity scheduling assignments as well as assignments to regularly complete the thought record and challenge automatic thoughts as they occur.

LONG-TERM MONITORING

As mentioned above, CBT is a time-limited treatment. Following the termination of therapy, however, patients may seek additional follow-up if they notice symptoms returning. If this occurs, patients are encouraged to follow-up with their psychiatrist or primary care physician, or they can directly refer themselves back to their CBT provider if symptoms worsen following treatment discontinuation. At times, therapists may provide "booster" sessions in which CBT strategies are reviewed and specific symptoms may be targeted without the need for resuming weekly therapy sessions.

PATIENT EDUCATION

Patients interested in receiving CBT for depression should be educated about depression treatment by clinicians involved in their care. Topics to be addressed include the following:

- Basic strategies involved in CBT for depression
- Data on the effectiveness of CBT (alone and in combination with medication)
- Anticipated number of sessions or length of stay
- Alternatives to CBT for the treatment of depression
- Ways in which family members and friends can provide support.

FUTURE DIRECTIONS

Many researchers and clinicians are examining ways to make CBT more accessible and cost-effective. One method for doing this is through the use of computerized interventions. These computerized interventions typically present CBT principles in a series of lessons, often with assigned homework and supplementary information.

A meta-analysis by Andrews et al. found that computerized CBT programs targeting 4 disorders, including major depressive disorder, led to significantly greater symptom improvement than a control group and comparable improvement to face-to-face CBT.[872] Andrews et al. also found that most participants completed all lessons and rated the program as being satisfactory. In addition, the National Institute for Health and Clinical Excellence (NICE) in the United Kingdom has endorsed the use of a computerized CBT program titled "Beating the Blues" for individuals with depression and anxiety.[873] Many different computerized CBT programs have been developed for the treatment of depression, and additional research is needed to determine their efficacy.

In addition to full computerized CBT programs, individuals have started to create smartphone applications that include CBT principles and can be used in conjunction with CBT sessions. Many individuals, not just mental health professionals, can create CBT smartphone applications, thus consulting with treatment providers before using any of these programs is essential. Further, this is a fairly recent development, thus more research examining the efficacy of these application is needed.

MEDICATION SUMMARY

As described above, CBT is often used in depression as standalone treatment in mild-to-moderate depression or in combination with other treatments such as medication in more severe depression. Several meta-analyses of studies of the combination of psychotherapy and pharmacotherapy for patients with depression have documented an advantage of the combination treatment compared with either treatment alone.[874-877] This advantage may be particularly pronounced in patients with chronic depression or severe recurrent depression and hospitalized patients.

Combination treatment theoretically adds the unique advantages of both treatment modalities. Pharmacotherapy may provide earlier symptomatic relief and psychotherapy may provide longer lasting symptomatic improvement.[878] CBT can be used to target anxiety and procrastination and can help the patient adhere to more of a schedule, all of which can enhance medication adherence. A Cochrane review showed that adding CBT to a medication regiment improved adherence to the medication and decrease the incidence of hospitalization.[879] CBT can do this by eliciting and modifying maladaptive cognitions about pharmacotherapy such as "if I take a drug I'm weak" or "I'm always the one to get side effects."

Behavioral methods such as reminder systems and pairing medications with routine activities can also enhance adherence. Medications can enhance the therapy by augmenting concentration, sleep, energy or other functions needed to obtain full benefits from psychotherapy.

Risks of combination therapy include medications that interfere with learning and memory, which may make CBT less effective. Medication may also lead to "premature" relief of symptoms, which might reduce motivation to continue in psychotherapy. Evidence does not suggest whether particular antidepressants or classes of antidepressants "combine better" with CBT.

REFERENCES

Epidemiology and Classification

1. American Psychiatric Association. Diagnostic and Statistical Manual of Mental Disorders, 3rd edition, Washington DC: American Psychiatric Association; 1980.
2. American Psychiatric Association. Diagnostic and Statistical Manual of Mental Disorders, 3rd edition, Rev. Washington DC: American Psychiatric Association; 1987.
3. American Psychiatric Association. Diagnostic and Statistical Manual of Mental Disorders, 4th edition, Washington DC: American Psychiatric Association; 1994.
4. Freud S. Mourning and Melancholia. Standard Edition of the Complete Psychological Works of Sigmund Freud. Vol. 14. London: Hogarth; 1957. pp.243-58.
5. Leonhard K. Aufterlung der endogemespsychosen, 2nd edition, Berlin: Springer Verlag; 1959.
6. Augst J. ZurAtiologic and nesologic endogenes depressiv espsychosen. Berlin: Springer Verlag; 1966.

7. Perris C. Genetic transmission of depressive psychoses.Acta Psychiatr Scand. 1968;203(Suppl.):45-52.
8. Venkoba Rao A. Unipolar and bipolar depression: Are they different? Indian J Psychiatry. 1974;16:189.
9. Singh G, Aggarwal ML. A family and genetic study of unipolar and bipolar affective disorders. In: Venkoba Rao A, Pathavi Devi S (Eds). Depressive Illness. New Delhi: ICMR; 1980. p. 89.
10. Aggarwal ML. A study of clinical manifestation of primary affective illness in patients and their relatives. MD (Psychiatry) Thesis, Panjab University, Patiala; 1977.
11. Aggarwal ML, Singh G. Sociodemographic variables in unipolar and bipolar illness. Indian J Psychiatry. 1982;24: 155-8.
12. Brodie HKH, Left ML. Bipolar depression: A comparative patient characteristic. Am J Psychiatry. 1971;127:1036.
13. Winokur G, Clyton PJ, Rikih T, Manic Depression Illness. St Louis: CV Mosby; 1969.
14. World Health Organization. International Classification of Diseases, 10th edition, Geneva: World Health Organization; 1992.
15. American Psychiatric Association. Desk Reference to the Diagnostic Criteria from DSM-5. Washington DC; 2013.
16. Feighner JP, Robins E, Guze SB, et al. Diagnostic criteria for use in psychiatric research. Arch Gen Psychiatry. 1972;26:56-73.
17. Wing JK, Cooper JE, Suntorius N, et al. The Measurements and Classification of Psychiatric Symptoms. London: Cambridge University Press; 1974.
18. Spitzer RL, Endicott J, Robins E. Research Diagnostic Criteria for a Selected Group of Functional Disorder. New York: Biometric Research, Institute of Psychiatry. 1978.
19. Leonhard K. The Classification of Endogenous Psychosis, 5th edition, New York: Irrigation; 1979.
20. Winokour G. Unipolar depression: It is divisible into automomous subtypes. Arch Gen Psychiatry. 1979;36:47-52.
21. Hamilton M. Mood disorders: Clinical features. In: Kaplan HI, Sadock BJ (Eds). Comprehensive Textbook of Psychiatry, 5th edition, Baltimore: Williams and Wilkins; 1989.

Etiology

22. Sethi BB, Chaturvedi PK, Tiwari SC. Biologic basis of depressive disorders. Continuing Medical Education Program Booklets. Indian Psychiatric Society. 1988;7. pp.22-36.
23. Schildkraut JJ. Catecholamine hypothesis of affective disorders. N Engl J Med. 1965;281:302-38.
24. Post RM. Biochemical theories of mania. In: Belmaker RH, van Praag HM. (Eds). Mania. Lancaster: MTP; 1980. pp. 217-65.
25. Halans AE. Plasma 3-methoxy-4-hydroxy-phenyl-glycol in manic psychosis. Am J Psychiatry. 1978;135:493-4.
26. Halan AE, Demet E. Noradrenaline metabolism in manic depressive patient. Lancet. 1980;1:670.
27. Belmaker RH, Ebbeson K, Ebstein R, et al. Platelet monoamine oxidase in schizophrenia and manic-depressive illness. Br J Psychiatry. 1976;126:227-32.
28. Friedman L, Shopsin B, Sathanthan G, et al. Blood platelet monoamine oxidase activity in psychiatric patients. Am J Psychiatry. 1974;131:1392-4.
29. Murphy DL, Wyatt RJ. Enzyme studies in major psychiatric disorders. In: Friedmann DX. (Ed). Biology of the Major Psychosis: A Comparative Analysis. New York: Raven Press; 1975. pp. 289-96.
30. Arato M, Rihmer Z, Felszeghy K. Reduced plasma cyclic AMP level during prophylactic lithium treatment in patients with affective disorder. Biol Psychiatry. 1980;15:319-22.
31. Lybouras E, Garelis E, Varson E, et al. Pysical activity and plasma cyclic monophosphate levels in manic depressive patients and healthy adults. Am J Psychiatry. 1979;136:540-2.
32. Lybouras E, Varson E, Garelis E, et al. Plama cyclic AMP in manic depressive illness. Acta Psychiatr Scand. 1978;57:447-53.
33. Extein I, Tallman J, Smith CC, et al. Changes in lymphocyle β-adrenergic receptors in depression and mania. Psychiatr Res. 1979;2:191-7.
34. Pandey AN, Dysken MW, Garver DL, et al. Beta adrenergic function in affective illness. Am J Psychiatry. 1979;163:675-8.
35. Post RM, Goodwin FK. Approaches to brain amines in psychiatric patients: A revaluation of cerebrospinal fluid studies. In: Inverson LL, Inverson SD, Snyder S (Eds). Handbook of Psychopharmacology. New York: Plenum; 1978. pp. 147-85.
36. Lerner P, Goodwin K, et al. Dopamine β-hydroxylase in the cerebrospinal fluid of psychiatric patient. Biol Psychiatry. 1978; 13:L685-94.
37. Post RM, Cramer H, Goodwin F. Cyclic AMP in cerebrospinal fluid of manic and depressive patients. Psychol Med. 1977;7: 599-605.
38. Bunney WE. Psychopharmacology of switch process in affective illness. In: Lipton MA, Dimascia A, Killan KF (Eds). Psychopharmacology: A Generation of Progress. New York: Raven Press; 1978. pp. 1249-59.
39. van Scheyan JD, van Kammen DP. Clomipramine induced mania in unipolar depression. Arch Gen Psychiatry. 1979;36: 560-5.
40. Sock RL, Goodwin FK. Inhibition of dopamine-β-hydroxylase in manic patients. Arch Gen Psychiatry. 1974;31:649-54.
41. Jouvent R, Lecrufier Y, Pueeh A, et al. Antimanic effect of clonidine. Am J Psychiatry. 1980;137:1275-6.
42. Tollefson GD. Hyperadrenergic hypomania consequent to abrupt cessation of clonidine. Clin Psychopharmacol. 1981; 193-5.
43. Rackensperger W, Fritsch W, Schwartz D, et al. The effect of the beta adrenergic blocking agent propranolol in mania. Arch Psychiatr Nervenkr; 1976;222:223-43.
44. Cookson JC. Oestrogens, dopamine and mood. Br J Psychiatry. 1981;139:365-6.
45. Kapoor S, Mann JJ. Role of the dopaminergic system in depression. Biol Psychiatry. 1992;32:1.
46. Coldeco H, Hazard S, Morganda, et al. Clinical and biochemical aspects of depressive disorders II. Transmitter/receptor theories. Synapse. 1991;9:251.

47. Van Praag HM. Amine hypothesis of affective disorders. In: Inverson LL, Inverson SD, Synder SH. (Eds). Handbook of Psychopharmacology. New York: Plenum; 1978. pp. 187-298.
48. Janowsky DS, Elyousuf MK, Davis JM, et al. A cholinergic-adrenergic hypothesis of mania and depression. Lancet. 1972; 2: 632-5.
49. Davis KL, Hollister CE, Liversy J, et al. CSF anticholinesterase in neuropsychiatric disorders. Psychopharma (Berlin). 1979;63: 155-9.
50. Enrich HM, Zersgen D, Kissling W, et al. The therapeutic effect of valproate in mania. Am J Psychiatry. 1981;138:256.
51. Enrich HM, Zerseen D, Kissling W, et al. One possible role of GABA in mania. Adv Biochem Psychopharmacol. 1981;26: 257-96.
52. Carroll BJ, Feinberg NT, Gerden JF, et al. A specific laboratory test for the diagnosis of melancholia. Arch Gen Psychiatry. 1981;38:15-23.
53. Gastpar M, Gilsdorf V, Abou-Aleh MT, et al. Clinical correlates of response to CRF: The dexamethasone suppression test in depression. A world health organization collaborative study. J Affect Disord. 1992;26:17.
54. Cookson JC, Silverstone T, Ress LT. Plasma prolactine and growth hormone levels in manic patients treated with pimozide Br J Psychiatry. 1982;140:280-6.
55. Fris JB. Melatonin in Depressive Disorders. Karolinska Institute. Department of Psychiatry, Stockholm, Sweden, 1983.
56. VenkobaRao A. Depression, cognitive disorder and melatonin profile. Ann Nat Acad Med Sci (India). 1988;25:41-9.
57. Nair VNP, Sharma M. Neurochemical and receptor theories of depression. Psychiatr J Univ Ottawa. 1989;14:328-41.
58. Godl PW, Goodwin FK. Vasopressin in affective illness. Lancet. 1978;1:1233-6.
59. Kupfer DJ, Ehless CL, Fanke, et al. EEG sleep profiles and recurrent depression. Biol Psychiatry. 1991;30:641.
60. Keck PE, Mcelroy SL, Nemeroff CB. Anticonvulsants in the treatment of bipolar disorder. J Neuropsychiatr Clin Neuro. 1992;4:395.
61. Ciffet CE, Wiskinson WE, Weiner RD, et al. Quantitative cerebral anatomy in depression: A controlled magnetic resonance imaging study. Arch Gen Psychiatry. 1993;50:7.
62. Krishnan KRR, Boyko OB, McDonald W, et al. Magnetic resonance imaging of caudate nuclei in depression. Arch Gen Psychiatry. 1992;49:553-57.
63. Turner WJ, King S. Two genetically distinct forms of bipolar affective disorder. Biol Psyciatry. 1979;21:271.
64. Venkoba Rao A, Parvathi Devi, Muthayya NM. A report on eosinophilic response as a measure of adrenocortical function in depressive illness. Indian J Psychiatry. 1967;9:157.
65. Sethi N, Sethi BB. Plasma cortisol: Its estimation in depressed and nondepressed patients. Indian J Psychiatry. 1971;13:83.
66. Varma VK, et al. Biochemistry of depressive illness: An evaluation of the present status. In: Venkoba Rao A, Parvathi Devi (Eds). Depressive Illness. New Delhi: ICMR, 1980.
67. Boral GC, et al. Thyroid functions in manic depressive psychosis. Indian J Psychiatry. 1979;21:271.
68. Verghese A, Mathew J, Mathai T, et al. Plasma cortisol in depressive illness. Indian J Psychiatry. 1973;15:72.
69. Tiwari SC, et al. Serum acetylcholinesterase activity in schizophrenic and depressive subjects. Indian J Psychiatry. 1982;24:291.
70. Tennant C, Bebbington P. The social causation of depression: A critique of the work of Brom and his colleagues. Psychol Med. 1978;8:565-75.
71. Freud S. Mourning and Melancholia; 1917. pp. 237-60.
72. Abraham K. A short study of development of the libido. In: Selected Papers on Psychoanalysis. New York: basic Books; 1953. p. 418.
73. Klein M. A contribution to the psychogenesis of manic-depressive illness. In: Contributions to Psychoanalysis. London: Hogarth Press, 1934.
74. Meyer A. Psychobiology: A Science of Man. Springfield: Charles C Thomas, 1957.
75. Beck AT. Cognitive Therapy and the Emotional Disorder. New York: International University Press, 1976.

Dysthymic and Cyclothymic Disorders

76. American Psychiatric Association. Diagnostic and Statistical Manual of Mental Disorders, 3rd edition, Washington DC: APA, 1980.
77. American Psychiatric Association. Diagnostic and Statistical Manual of Mental Disorder, 3rd edition, Rev. Washington DC: APA, 1987.
78. World Health Organization. The ICD Classification of Mental and Behavioural Disorders. Geneva: WHO, 1992.
79. American Psychiatric Association. Diagnostic and Statistical Manual of Mental Disorders, 4th edition, Washington DC: APA, 1994.
80. Weissman MM, Bruce ML, Lead, et al. Affective disorders. In: Psychiatric Disorders in America. The Epidemiologic Catchment Area Study. New York, Free Press; 1991, pp. 53-80.
81. Anqst J. Epidemiology of depression. Psychopharmacology 1992;106:571-4.
82. Wittchen HU, Essan, et al. Life time and six-month prevalence of mental disorders, in the Munich follow-up study. European Arch Psychiatr Clin Neuro Sci. 1992;241:247-58.
83. Klien DN, Taylor EB, Dickstein S, et al. The early late onset distinction in DSM-III- R dysthymia. J Affect Dis 1988;14: 25-33.
84. McCullough JP, Braith JA, Chapman RC, et al. Comparison of early and late onset dysthymia. J Nerv Ment Dis 1990;78: 577-81.
85. Howland RH, Thase ME. Biological studies of dysthymia. Biol Psychiatry 1991;30:283-304.
86. Keller MB. Depression: A long term illness. Br J Psychiatry 1994;165(Suppl 26):9-15.

87. Keller MB, Shapiro RW. "Double depression": Superimposition of acute depressive episodes on chronic depressive disorders. Am J Psychiatry 1992;139:438-42.
88. Keller MB, Lavori PW, Endicott J, et al. "Double Depression": Two year follow up. Am J Psychiatry 1983;140:689-94.
89. Guy W, Ban TA, Schaffer JD. Differential treatment responsiveness among mildly depressed patients. In: Clayton PJ, Barett JE (Eds). Treatment of Depression: Old Controversies and New Approaches. New York: Raven Press; 1983. pp. 229-36.
90. Kocsis JH, Frances AJ, Voss C, et al. Imipramine treatment for chronic depression. Arch Gen Psychiatry 1988;45:253-7.
91. Tyrer P, Seive Wright N, Murphy S, et al. The Nottingham study of neurotic disorder: Comparison of drug and pharmacological treatments. Lancet 1998;2:235-40.
92. Stewart JW, Quitkin FM, Liebowitz MR, et al. Efficacy of desipramine in depressed outpatients: Response according to Research Diagnostic Criteria diagnosis and severity of illness. Arch Gen Psychiatry 1983;40:202-7.
93. Paykel ES, Freeling P, Hollyman JA, et al. Predictors of therapeutic benefit from amitriptyline in mild depression as general practice placebo controlled trial. J Affect Dis 1988;14: 83-95.
94. Waring EM, Chamberlaine CH, McCrank EW, et al. Dysthymia: A randomized study of cognitive marital therapy and antidepressants, 1988.
95. Davidson JR, Giller EL, Zisook S, et al. An efficacy study of isocarboxazid and placebo in depression and its relationship to depressive nosology. Arch Gen Psychiatry 1988;45:120-7.
96. Harrison W, Rabtrin J, Steward JW, et al. Phenelzine for chronic depression: A study of continuation treatment. J Clin Psychiatry 1986;47:346-2.
97. Vallejo J, Gasto C, Catalan R, et al. Double blind study of imipramine versus phenelzine in melancholia and dysthymic disorder. Br J Psychiatry 1986;151:639-42.
98. Hellerstain DJ, Yanowitch P, Rosenthal J, et al. A randomized double blind study of fluoxetine versus palcebo in the treatment of dysthymia. Am J Psychiatry 1993;150:1169.
99. Howland RH. Pharmacotherapy of dysthymia: A review. J Clin Psychopharmacol 1991;11:833.
100. Beck AJ. Cognitive Therapy and the Emotional Disorders. New York: International Universities Press, 1976.
101. Klerman GL, Weissman MM. International psychotherapy. In: Paykel ES (Ed). Handbook of Affective Disorders, 2nd edition, London: Churchill Livingstone; 1992. pp. 501-10.
102. Klerman GL, Weissman MM. New Applications of Interpersonal Psychotherapy. Washington DC: APPI, 1993.
103. Howland RH, Thase ME. A comprehensive review of cyclothymic disorder. J Nerv Ment Dis; 1993.181-485.
104. Levitt AJ, Joffe RT, Ennis J, et al. The prevalence of cyclothymia in borderline personality disorder. J Clin Psychiatry 1990;51: 335.
105. American Psychiatric Association. Desk Reference to the Diagnostic Criteria from DSM-5. Washington DC, 2013.

Genetics of Bipolar Disorder

106. Craddock N, Jones I. Genetics of bipolar disorder. J Med Genet. 1999;36:585-94.
107. McGuffin P, Rijsdijk F, Andrew M, et al. The heritability of bipolar affective disorder and the genetic relationship to unipolar depression. Arch Gen Psychiatry. 2003;60:497-502.
108. Kieseppa T, Partonen T, Haukka J, et al. High concordance of bipolar I disorder in a nationwide sample of twins. Am J Psychiatry. 2004;161:1814-21.
109. Tsuang MT, Faraone SV. The genetics of mood disorders. Baltimore: The Johns Hopkins University Press, 1990.
110. Tsuang MT, Winokur G, Crowe RR. Morbidity risks of schizophrenia and affective disorders among first degree relatives of patients with schizophrenia, mania, depression and surgical conditions. Br J Psychiatry. 1980;137:497-504.
111. Van Snellenberg JX, de Candia T. Meta-analytic evidence for familial coaggregation of schizophrenia and bipolar disorder. Arch Gen Psychiatry. 2009;66:748-55.
112. Lichtenstein P, Yip BH, Björk C, et al. Common genetic determinants of schizophrenia and bipolar disorder in Swedish families: a population-based study. Lancet. 2009;373:234-9.
113. Sullivan PF, Magnusson C, Reichenberg A, et al. Family history of schizophrenia and bipolar disorder as risk factors for autism. Arch Gen Psychiatry. 2012;69:1099-103.
114. McGuffin P, Katz R. The genetics of depression and manic-depressive disorder. Br J Psychiatry. 1989;155:294-304.
115. Cross-Disorder Phenotype Group of the Psychiatric GWAS Consortium Craddock N, Kendler K, Neale M, et al. Dissecting the phenotype in genome-wide association studies of psychiatric illness. Br J Psychiatry. 2009;195:97-9.
116. Craddock N, Khodel V, Van Eerdewegh P, et al. Mathematical limits of multilocus models: the genetic transmission of bipolar disorder. Am J Hum Genet. 1995;57:690-702.
117. Wang WY, Barratt BJ, Clayton DG, Todd JA. Genome-wide association studies: theoretical and practical concerns. Nat Rev Genet. 2005;6:109-18.
118. McCarroll SA, Altshuler DM. Copy-number variation and association studies of human disease. Nat Genet. 2007;39 (7 Suppl):S37-S42.
119. Craddock N, O'Donovan MC, Owen MJ. Phenotypic and genetic complexity of psychosis. Invited commentary on ... Schizophrenia: a common disease caused by multiple rare alleles. Br J Psychiatry. 2007;190:200-3.
120. Kendler KS. Reflections on the relationship between psychiatric genetics and psychiatric nosology. Am J Psychiatry. 2006;163:1138-46.
121. Chanock SJ, Manolio T, Boehnke M, et al. NCI-NHGRI Working Group on Replication in Association Studies. Replicating genotype-phenotype associations. Nature. 2007;447:655-60.
122. McCarthy MI, Abecasis GR, Cardon LR, et al. Genome-wide association studies for complex traits: consensus, uncertainty and challenges. Nat Rev Genet. 2008;9:356-69.

123. Craddock N, Sklar P. Genetics of bipolar disorder: successful start to a long journey. Trends Genet. 2009;25:99-105.
124. Badner JA, Koller D, Foroud T, et al. Genome-wide linkage analysis of 972 bipolar pedigrees using single-nucleotide polymorphisms. Mol Psychiatry. 2012;17:818-26.
125. Seifuddin F, Mahon PB, Judy J, et al. Meta-analysis of genetic association studies on bipolar disorder. Am J Med Genet B Neuropsychiatr Genet. 2012;159B:508-18.
126. Psychiatric GWAS Consortium Coordinating Committee Cichon S, Craddock N, et al. Genomewide association studies: history, rationale, and prospects for psychiatric disorders. Am J Psychiatry. 2009;166:540-56.
127. Craddock N, O'Donovan MC, Owen MJ. Genome-wide association studies in psychiatry: lessons from early studies of non-psychiatric and psychiatric phenotypes. Mol Psychiatry. 2008;13:649-53.
128. Sullivan PF, Daly MJ, O'Donovan M. Genetic architectures of psychiatric disorders: the emerging picture and its implications. Nat Rev Genet. 2012;13:537-51.
129. Corvin A, Craddock N, Sullivan PF. Genome-wide association studies: a primer. Psychol Med. 2010;40:1063-77.
130. Pe'er I, Yelensky R, Altshuler D, Daly MJ. Estimation of the multiple testing burden for genomewide association studies of nearly all common variants. Genet Epidemiol. 2008;32:381-5.
131. Wellcome Trust Case Control Consortium. Genome-wide association study of 14 000 cases of seven common diseases and 3,000 shared controls. Nature. 2007;447:661-78.
132. Sklar P, Smoller JW, Fan J, et al. Whole-genome association study of bipolar disorder. Mol Psychiatry. 2008;13:558-69.
133. Baum AE, Akula N, Cabanero M, et al. A genome-wide association study implicates diacylglycerol kinase eta (DGKH) and several other genes in the etiology of bipolar disorder. Mol Psychiatry. 2008;13:197-207.
134. Ferreira MA, O'Donovan MC, Meng YA, et al. Collaborative genome-wide association analysis supports a role for ANK3 and CACNA1C in bipolar disorder. Nat Genet. 2008;40: 1056-8.
135. Cichon S, Muhleisen TW, Degenhardt FA, et al. Genome-wide association study identifies genetic variation in neurocan as a susceptibility factor for bipolar disorder. Am J Hum Genet. 2011;88:372-81.
136. Scott LJ, Muglia P, Kong XQ, et al. Genome-wide association and meta-analysis of bipolar disorder in individuals of European ancestry. Proc Natl Acad Sci USA. 2009;106:7501-6.
137. Smith EN, Bloss CS, Badner JA, et al. Genome-wide association study of bipolar disorder in European American and African American individuals. Mol Psychiatry. 2009;14:755-63.
138. Psychiatric GWAS Consortium Bipolar Disorder Working Group. Large-scale genome-wide association analysis of bipolar disorder identifies a new susceptibility locus near ODZ4. Nat Genet. 2011;43:977-83.
139. Hamshere ML, Walters JT, Smith R, et al. Genome-wide significant associations in schizophrenia to ITIH3/4, CACNA1C and SDCCAG8, and extensive replication of associations reported by the Schizophrenia PGC. Mol Psychiatry. 201210.1038/mp.2012.67.published online May 22.
140. Green EK, Hamshere M, Forty L, et al. Replication of bipolar disorder susceptibility alleles and identification of two novel genome-wide significant associations in a new bipolar disorder case-control sample. Mol Psychiatry 201210.1038/mp.2012.142.published online Oct 16.
141. Smith EN, Koller DL, Panganiban C, et al. Genome-wide association of bipolar disorder suggests an enrichment of replicable associations in regions near genes. PLoS Genet. 2011;7:e1002134.
142. Xiao R, Boehnke M. Quantifying and correcting for the winner's curse in genetic association studies. Genet Epidemiol. 2009;33:453-62.
143. Green EK, Grozeva D, Forty L, et al. Association at SYNE1 in both bipolar disorder and recurrent major depression. Mol Psychiatry 201210.1038/mp.2012.48. published online May 8.
144. O'Donovan MC, Craddock N, Norton N, et al. Identification of loci associated with schizophrenia by genome-wide association and follow-up. Nat Genet. 2008;40:1053-5.
145. Schizophrenia Psychiatric Genome-Wide Association Study (GWAS) Consortium. Genome-wide association study identifies five new schizophrenia loci. Nat Genet. 2011;43:969-76.
146. Steinberg S, de Jong S, Mattheisen M, et al. Common variant at 16p11.2 conferring risk of psychosis. Mol Psychiatry 201210.1038/mp.2012.157. published online Nov 20.
147. McMahon FJ, Akula N, Schulze TG, et al. Meta-analysis of genome-wide association data identifies a risk locus for major mood disorders on 3p21.1. Nat Genet. 2010;42:128-31.
148. Chen DT, Jiang X, Akula N, et al. Genome-wide association study meta-analysis of European and Asian-ancestry samples identifies three novel loci associated with bipolar disorder. Mol Psychiatry. 2013;18:195-205.
149. Purcell SM, Wray NR, et al. International Schizophrenia Consortium. Common polygenic variation contributes to risk of schizophrenia and bipolar disorder. Nature. 2009;460:748-52.
150. Lee SH, Wray NR, Goddard ME, Visscher PM. Estimating missing heritability for disease from genome-wide association studies. Am J Hum Genet. 2011;88:294-305.
151. Casamassima F, Hay AC, Benedetti A, Lattanzi L, Cassano GB, Perlis RH. L-type calcium channels and psychiatric disorders: a brief review. Am J Med Genet B Neuropsychiatr Genet. 2010; 153B:1373-90.
152. Holmans P, Green EK, Pahwa JS, et al. Gene ontology analysis of GWA study data sets provides insights into the biology of bipolar disorder. Am J Hum Genet. 2009;85:13-24.
153. Miro X, Meier S, Dreisow ML, et al. Studies in humans and mice implicate neurocan in the etiology of mania. Am J Psychiatry. 2012;169:982-90.
154. Craddock N, Owen M. Chromosomal aberrations and bipolar affective disorder. Br J Psychiatry. 1994;164:507-12.
155. Papolos DF, Faedda GL, Veit S, et al. Bipolar spectrum disorders in patients diagnosed with velocardiofacial syndrome: does a

hemizygous deletion of chromosome 22q11 result in bipolar affective disorder? Am J Psychiatry. 1996;153:1541-7.

156. Soni S, Whittington J, Holland AJ, et al. The phenomenology and diagnosis of psychiatric illness in people with Prader-Willi syndrome. Psychol Med. 2008;38:1-10.
157. Malhotra D, Sebat J. CNVs: harbingers of a rare variant revolution in psychiatric genetics. Cell. 2012;148:1223-41.
158. Olsen L, Hansen T, Djurovic S, et al. Copy number variations in affective disorders and meta-analysis. Psychiatr Genet. 2011;21: 319-22.
159. Malhotra D, McCarthy S, Michaelson JJ, et al. High frequencies of de novo CNVs in bipolar disorder and schizophrenia. Neuron. 2011;72:951-63.
160. Van Den Bossche MJ, Johnstone M, Strazisar M, et al. Rare copy number variants in neuropsychiatric disorders: Specific phenotype or not? Am J Med Genet B Neuropsychiatr Genet. 2012;159B:812-22.
161. Bergen SE, O'Dushlaine CT, Ripke S, et al. Genome-wide association study in a Swedish population yields support for greater CNV and MHC involvement in schizophrenia compared with bipolar disorder. Mol Psychiatry. 2012;17:880-6.
162. Grozeva D, Kirov G, Ivanov D, et al. Rare copy number variants: a point of rarity in genetic risk for bipolar disorder and schizophrenia. Arch Gen Psychiatry. 2010;67:318-27.
163. Zhang D, Cheng L, Qian Y, et al. Singleton deletions throughout the genome increase risk of bipolar disorder. Mol Psychiatry. 2009;14:376-80.
164. Owen MJ, O'Donovan MC, Thapar A, Craddock N. Neurodevelopmental hypothesis of schizophrenia. Br J Psychiatry. 2011;198:173-5.
165. Burdick KE, Goldberg TE, Cornblatt BA, et al. The MATRICS consensus cognitive battery in patients with bipolar I disorder. Neuropsychopharmacology. 2011;36:1587-92.
166. Kraepelin E. Manic-depressive insanity and paranoia. Edinburgh: Livingstone, 1919.
167. Craddock N, Owen MJ. The beginning of the end for the Kraepelinian dichotomy. Br J Psychiatry. 2005;186:364-6.
168. Craddock N, Jones L, Jones IR, et al. Strong genetic evidence for a selective influence of GABA-A receptors on a component of the bipolar disorder phenotype. Mol Psychiatry. 2010;15: 146-53.
169. Breuer R, Hamshere ML, Strohmaier J, et al. Independent evidence for the selective influence of GABA(A) receptors on one component of the bipolar disorder phenotype. Mol Psychiatry. 2011;16:587-9.
170. Goes FS, Hamshere ML, Seifuddin F, et al. Genome-wide association of mood-incongruent psychotic bipolar disorder. Transl Psychiatry. 2012;2:e180.
171. Greenwood TA, Bipolar Genome Study (BiGS) ConsortiumKelsoe JR. Genome-wide association study of irritable vs. elated mania suggests genetic differences between clinical subtypes of bipolar disorder. PLoS One. 2013;8: e53804.
172. Meier S, Mattheisen M, Vassos E, et al. Genome-wide significant association between a 'negative mood delusions' dimension in bipolar disorder and genetic variation on chromosome 3q26.1. Transl Psychiatry. 2012;2:e165.
173. Perlis RH, Huang J, Purcell S, et al. Genome-wide association study of suicide attempts in mood disorder patients. Am J Psychiatry. 2010;167:1499-507.
174. Cross-Disorder Group of the Psychiatric Genome-Wide Association Study Consortium. Identification of risk loci with shared effects on five major psychiatric disorders: a genome-wide analysis. Lancet. 201310.1016/S0140-6736(12)62129-1. published online Feb 28.
175. Craddock N, Owen MJ. The Kraepelinian dichotomy—going, going... but still not gone. Br J Psychiatry. 2010;196:92-95.
176. Moskvina V, Craddock N, Holmans P, et al. Genome-wide analyses of genome-wide association data sets: evidence for multiple common risk alleles for schizophrenia and bipolar disorder and for overlap in genetic risk. Mol Psychiatry. 2009;14:252-60.
177. Williams HJ, Craddock N, Russo G, et al. Most genome-wide significant susceptibility loci for schizophrenia and bipolar disorder reported to date cross-traditional diagnostic boundaries. Hum Mol Genet. 2011;20:387-91.
178. Green EK, Grozeva D, Jones I, et al. The bipolar disorder risk allele at CACNA1C also confers risk of recurrent major depression and of schizophrenia. Mol Psychiatry. 2010;15: 1016-22.
179. Major Depressive Disorder Working Group of the Psychiatric GWAS Consortium. A mega-analysis of genome-wide association studies for major depressive disorder. Mol Psychiatry 201210.1038/mp.2012.21. published online Apr 3.
180. Hyman SE. Genome-sequencing anniversary. The meaning of the Human Genome Project for neuropsychiatric disorders. Science. 2011;331:1026.
181. Brennand KJ, Gage FH. Modeling psychiatric disorders through reprogramming. Dis Model Mech. 2012;5:26-32.

Bipolar Disorder: Diagnosis, Challenges and Future Direction

182. Craddock N, Owen MJ. The beginning of the end for the Kraepelinian dichotomy. Br J Psychiatry. 2005;186:364-6.
183. WHO. The global burden of disease: 2004 update. Geneva: World Health Organization, 2008.
184. Lozano R, Naghavi M, Foreman K, et al. Global and regional mortality from 235 causes of death for 20 age groups in 1990 and 2010: a systematic analysis for the Global Burden of Disease Study 2010. Lancet. 2012;380:2095-128.
185. Goodwin FK, Jamison KR, Ghaemi SN. Manic-depressive illness: bipolar disorders and recurrent depression. New York: Oxford University Press, 2007.
186. Hirschfeld RM, Lewis L, Vornik LA. Perceptions and impact of bipolar disorder: how far have we really come? Results of

the national depressive and manic-depressive association 2000 survey of individuals with bipolar disorder. J Clin Psychiatry. 2003;64:161-74.

187. Kraepelin E. Manic-depressive insanity and paranoia. New York: E & S Livingstone, 1921.
188. Leonhard K, Beckmann H. Classification of endogenous psychoses and their differential etiology. New York: Springer, 1999.
189. American Psychiatric Association. Diagnostic criteria from DSM-IV-TR. Washington: American Psychiatric Association, 2000.
190. WHO. The ICD-10 classification of mental and behavioural disorders: diagnostic criteria for research. Geneva: World Health Organization, 1993.
191. Baldessarini RJ, Tondo L, Baethge CJ, Lepri B, Bratti IM. Effects of treatment latency on response to maintenance treatment in manic-depressive disorders. Bipolar Disord. 2007;9:386-93.
192. Ghaemi SN, Ko JY, Goodwin FK. "Cade's disease" and beyond: misdiagnosis, antidepressant use, and a proposed definition for bipolar spectrum disorder. Can J Psychiatry. 2002;47:125-34.
193. Lish JD, Dime-Meenan S, Whybrow PC, Price RA, Hirschfeld RM. The National Depressive and Manic-depressive Association (DMDA) survey of bipolar members. J Affect Disord. 1994;31:281-94.
194. Manning JS. Bipolar disorder in primary care. J Fam Pract. 2003 (Suppl): S6-S9.
195. Judd LL, Akiskal HS, Schettler PJ, et al. The long-term natural history of the weekly symptomatic status of bipolar I disorder. Arch Gen Psychiatry. 2002;59:530-7.
196. Judd LL, Akiskal HS, Schettler PJ, et al. A prospective investigation of the natural history of the long-term weekly symptomatic status of bipolar II disorder. Arch Gen Psychiatry. 2003;60:261-9.
197. Marneros A. Origin and development of concepts of bipolar mixed states. J Affect Disord. 2001;67:229-240.
198. DeDios C, Ezquiaga E, Agud JL, et al. Subthreshold symptoms and time to relapse/recurrence in a community cohort of bipolar disorder outpatients. J Affect Disord. 2012;143:160-5.
199. Akiskal HS, Maser JD, Zeller PJ, et al. Switching from 'unipolar' to bipolar II. An 11-year prospective study of clinical and temperamental predictors in 559 patients. Arch Gen Psychiatry. 1995;52:114-23.
200. Goldberg JF, Harrow M, Whiteside JE. Risk for bipolar illness in patients initially hospitalized for unipolar depression. Am J Psychiatry. 2001;158:1265-70.
201. Trivedi MH, Rush AJ, Wisniewski SR, et al. Evaluation of outcomes with citalopram for depression using measurement-based care in STAR*D: implications for clinical practice. Am J Psychiatry. 2006;163:28-40.
202. Rush AJ, Trivedi MH, Wisniewski SR, et al. Acute and longer-term outcomes in depressed outpatients requiring one or several treatment steps: a STAR*D report. Am J Psychiatry. 2006;163:1905-17.
203. Correa R, Akiskal H, Gilmer W, Nierenberg AA, Trivedi M, Zisook S. Is unrecognized bipolar disorder a frequent contributor to apparent treatment resistant depression? J Affect Disord. 2010;127:10-8.
204. Valenti M, Pacchiarotti I, Bonnin CM, et al. Risk factors for antidepressant-related switch to mania. J Clin Psychiatry. 2012;73:e271-6.
205. Baldessarini RJ, Salvatore P, Khalsa HM, et al. Morbidity in 303 first-episode bipolar I disorder patients. Bipolar Disord. 2010;12:264-70.
206. Hirschfeld RM, Lewis L, Vornik LA. Perceptions and impact of bipolar disorder: how far have we really come? Results of the national depressive and manic-depressive association. 2000 survey of individuals with bipolar disorder. J Clin Psychiatry. 2003;64:161-74.
207. Goodwin GM. Bipolar depression and treatment with antidepressants. Br J Psychiatry. 2012;200:5-6.
208. Regier D, Narrow W, Clarke D, et al. DSM-5 field trials in the United States and Canada, part II: test-retest reliability of selected categorical disorders. Am J Psychiatry. 2013;170:59-70.
209. First MB. Harmonisation of ICD-11 and DSM-5: opportunities and challenges. Br J Psychiatry. 2009;195:382-90.
210. Bowden CL, Singh V, Thompson P, et al. Development of the Bipolar Inventory of Symptoms Scale. Acta Psychiatr Scand. 2007;116:189-94.
211. Solomon DA, Leon AC, Maser JD, et al. Distinguishing bipolar major depression from unipolar major depression with the screening assessment of depression-polarity (SAD-P). J Clin Psychiatry. 2006;67:434-42.
212. Angst J, Adolfsson R, Benazzi F, et al. The HCL-32: towards a self-assessment tool for hypomanic symptoms in outpatients. J Affect Disord. 2005;88:217-33.
213. Mitchell PB, Goodwin GM, Johnson GF, Hirschfeld RMA. Diagnostic guidelines for bipolar depression: a probabilistic approach. Bipolar Disord. 2008;10:144-52.
214. Craddock N, Sklar P. Genetics of bipolar disorder. Lancet. 2013;381:1654-62.
215. Phillips ML, Vieta E. Identifying functional neuroimaging biomarkers of bipolar disorder: toward DSM-5. Schizophr Bull. 2007;33:893-904.
216. Phillips ML, Ladouceur CD, Drevets WC. A neural model of voluntary and automatic emotion regulation: implications for understanding the pathophysiology and neurodevelopment of bipolar disorder. Mol Psychiatry. 2008;13:833-57.
217. Kupfer DJ, Frank E, Phillips ML. Major depressive disorder: new clinical, neurobiological, and treatment perspectives. Lancet. 2012;379:1045-55.
218. de Almeida JR, Phillips ML. Distinguishing between unipolar depression and bipolar depression: current and future clinical and neuroimaging perspectives. Biol Psychiatry. 2013;73:111-8.
219. Versace A, Almeida JR, Quevedo K, et al. Right orbitofrontal corticolimbic and left corticocortical white matter connectivity

differentiate bipolar and unipolar depression. Biol Psychiatry. 2010;68:560-7.

220. Macritchie KAN, Lloyd AJ, Bastin ME, et al. White matter microstructural abnormalities in euthymic bipolar disorder. Br J Psychiatry. 2010;196:52-8.
221. Silverstone T, McPherson H, Li Q, Doyle T. Deep white matter hyperintensities in patients with bipolar depression, unipolar depression and age-matched control subjects. Bipolar Disord. 2003;5:53-7.
222. Almeida JR, Versace A, Mechelli A, et al. Abnormal amygdala-prefrontal effective connectivity to happy faces differentiates bipolar from major depression. Biol Psychiatry. 2009;66:451-9.
223. Almeida JR, Versace A, Hassel S, Kupfer DJ, Phillips ML. Elevated amygdala activity to sad facial expressions: a state marker of bipolar but not unipolar depression. Biol Psychiatry. 2010;67:414-21.
224. Taylor, Clark L, Furey ML, Williams GB, Sahakian BJ, Drevets WC. Neural basis of abnormal response to negative feedback in unmedicated mood disorders. Neuroimage. 2008;42:1118-26.
225. Bertocci MA, Bebko GM, Mullin BC, et al. Abnormal anterior cingulate cortical activity during emotional n-back task performance distinguishes bipolar from unipolar depressed females. Psychol Med. 2012;42:1417-28.
226. Benedetti F, Absinta M, Rocca MA, et al. Tract-specific white matter structural disruption in patients with bipolar disorder. Bipolar Disord. 2011;13:414-24.
227. Cassano GB, Rucci P, Frank E, et al. The mood spectrum in unipolar and bipolar disorder: arguments for a unitary approach. Am J Psychiatry. 2004;161:1264-9.
228. Biondi M, Picardi A, Pasquini M, Gaetano P, Pancheri P. Dimensional psychopathology of depression: detection of an 'activation' dimension in unipolar depressed outpatients. J Affect Disord. 2005;84:133-9.
229. Akiskal HS, Mallya G. Criteria for the "soft" bipolar spectrum: treatment implications. Psychopharmacol Bull. 1987;23:68-73.
230. Angst J. The bipolar spectrum. Br J Psychiatry. 2007;190:189-91.
231. Vieta E, Phillips ML. Deconstructing bipolar disorder: a critical review of its diagnostic validity and a proposal for DSM-5 and ICD-11. Schizophr Bull. 2007;33:886-92.
232. Zimmermann P, Bruckl T, Nocon A, et al. Heterogeneity of DSM-IV major depressive disorder as a consequence of subthreshold bipolarity. Arch Gen Psychiatry. 2009;66:1341-52.
233. Angst J, Cui L, Swendsen J, et al. Major depressive disorder with subthreshold bipolarity in the National Comorbidity Survey Replication. Am J Psychiatry. 2010;167:1194-201.
234. Angst J, Azorin JM, Bowden CL, et al. Prevalence and characteristics of undiagnosed bipolar disorders in patients with a major depressive episode: the BRIDGE study. Arch Gen Psychiatry. 2011;68:791-8.
235. Angst J, Gamma A, Bowden CL, et al. Diagnostic criteria for bipolarity based on an international sample of 5635 patients with DSM-IV major depressive episodes. Eur Arch Psychiatry Clin Neurosci. 2012;262:3-11.
236. Forty L, Smith D, Jones L, et al. Identifying hypomanic features in major depressive disorder using the hypomania checklist (HCL-32). J Affect Disord. 2009;114:68-73.
237. Cassano GB, Mula M, Rucci P, et al. The structure of lifetime manic—hypomanic spectrum. J Affect Disord. 2009;112:59-70.
238. Henry C, M'Bailara K, Mathieu F, Poinsot R, Falissard B. Construction and validation of a dimensional scale exploring mood disorders: MAThyS (Multidimensional Assessment of Thymic States). BMC Psychiatry. 2008;8:82.
239. Henry C, M'Bailara K, Poinsot R, et al. Evidence for two types of bipolar depression using a dimensional approach. Psychother Psychosom. 2007;76:325-31.
240. Insel T, Cuthbert B, Garvey M, et al. Research domain criteria (RDoC): toward a new classification framework for research on mental disorders. Am J Psychiatry. 2010;167:748-51.
241. Fournier JC, Keener MT, Mullin BC, et al. Heterogeneity of amygdala response in major depressive disorder: the impact of lifetime subthreshold mania. Psychol Med. 2013;43:293-302.
242. Caseras X, Lawrence NS, Murphy K, Wise RG, Phillips ML. Ventral striatum activity in response to reward: differences between bipolar I and II disorders. Am J Psychiatry. 2013; published online Apr 5. DOI:10.1176/appi.ajp.2012.12020169.
243. Haynes JD, Rees G. Decoding mental states from brain activity in humans. Nat Rev Neurosci. 2006;7:523-34.
244. Koutsouleris N, Meisenzahl EM, Davatzikos C, et al. Use of neuroanatomical pattern classification to identify subjects in at-risk mental states of psychosis and predict disease transition. Arch Gen Psychiatry. 2009;66:700-12.
245. Nouretdinov I, Costafreda SG, Gammerman A, et al. Machine learning classification with confidence: application of transductive conformal predictors to MRI-based diagnostic and prognostic markers in depression. Neuroimage. 2011;56:809-13.
246. Mourão-Miranda J, Almeida JR, Hassel S, et al. Pattern recognition analyses of brain activation elicited by happy and neutral faces in unipolar and bipolar depression. Bipolar Disord. 2012;14:451-60.
247. Mourão-Miranda J, Oliveira L, Ladouceur CD, et al. Pattern recognition and functional neuroimaging help to discriminate healthy adolescents at risk for mood disorders from low risk adolescents. PLoS One. 2012;7:e29482.
248. Almeida JRC, Mourão-Miranda J, Aizenstein HJ, et al. Pattern recognition on anterior cingulate cortex blood flow classifies depressed females with bipolar vs. unipolar depression. Br J Psychiatry (in press).
249. Cohen JR, Asarnow RF, Sabb FW, et al. Decoding continuous variables from neuroimaging data: basic and clinical applications. Front Neurosci. 2011;5:75.
250. McIntosh AM. Toward a systems biology of mood disorder. Biol Psychiatry. 2013;73:107-8.
251. Halliwell B, Gutteridge JMC. Free radicals in biology and medicine. New York: Oxford University Press, 2007.
252. Young LT. Is bipolar disorder a mitochondrial disease?. J Psychiatry Neurosci. 2007;32:160-1.

253. Andreazza AC, Kauer-Sant'anna M, Frey BN, et al. Oxidative stress markers in bipolar disorder: a meta-analysis. J Affect Disord. 2008;111:135-44.
254. Andreazza AC, Cassini C, Rosa AR, et al. Serum S100B and antioxidant enzymes in bipolar patients. J Psychiatr Res. 2007;41:523-9.
255. Yumru M, Savas HA, Kalenderoglu A, Bulut M, Celik H, Erel O. Oxidative imbalance in bipolar disorder subtypes: a comparative study. Prog Neuropsychopharmacol Biol Psychiatry. 2009;33:1070-4.
256. Magalhaes PV, Dean OM, Bush AI, et al. N-acetyl cysteine add-on treatment for bipolar II disorder: a subgroup analysis of a randomized placebo-controlled trial. J Affect Disord. 2011;129:317-20.
257. Versace A, Andreazza AC, Young LT, et al. Elevated serum measures of lipid peroxidation and abnormal prefrontal white matter in euthymic bipolar adults: toward peripheral biomarkers of bipolar disorder. Mol Psychiatry 201310.1038/mp.2012.188.published online Jan 29.
258. Wang JF, Shao L, Sun X, Young LT. Increased oxidative stress in the anterior cingulate cortex of subjects with bipolar disorder and schizophrenia. Bipolar Disord. 2009;11:523-9.
259. Andreazza AC, Shao L, Wang JF, Young LT. Mitochondrial complex I activity and oxidative damage to mitochondrial proteins in the prefrontal cortex of patients with bipolar disorder. Arch Gen Psychiatry. 2010;67:360-8.
260. Rajkowska G, Halaris A, Selemon LD. Reductions in neuronal and glial density characterize the dorsolateral prefrontal cortex in bipolar disorder. Biol Psychiatry. 2001;49:741-52.
261. Tkachev D, Mimmack ML, Ryan MM, et al. Oligodendrocyte dysfunction in schizophrenia and bipolar disorder. Lancet. 2003;362:798-805.

Treatment of Bipolar Disorders

262. Merikangas KR, Akiskal HS, Angst J, et al. Lifetime and 12-month prevalence of bipolar spectrum disorder in the National comorbidity Survey replication. Arch Gen Psychiatry. 2007;64:543-52.
263. Merikangas KR, Jin R, He JP, et al. Prevalence and correlates of bipolar spectrum disorder in the world mental health survey initiative. Arch Gen Psychiatry. 2011;68:241-51.
264. Gitlin MJ, Swendsen J, Heller TL, Hammen C. Relapse and impairment in bipolar disorder. Am J Psychiatry. 1995;152:1635-40.
265. Perlis RH, Ostacher MJ, Patel JK, et al. Predictors of recurrence in bipolar disorder: primary outcomes from the Systematic Treatment Enhancement Program for Bipolar Disorder (STEP-BD). Am J Psychiatry. 2006;163:217-4.
266. Judd LL, Akiskal HS, Schettler PJ, et al. The long-term natural history of the weekly symptomatic status of bipolar I disorder. Arch Gen Psychiatry. 2002;59:530-2.
267. Dilsaver SC. An estimate of the minimum economic burden of bipolar I and II disorders in the United States:2009. J Affect Disord. 2011;129:79-83.
268. Judd LL, Akiskal HS, Schettler PJ, et al. Psychosocial disability in the course of bipolar I and II disorders: a prospective, comparative, longitudinal study Arch Gen Psychiatry. 2005;62:1322-30.
269. Michalak E, Livingston JD, Hole R, Suto M, Hal S, Haddock C. 'It's something that I manage but it is not who I am': reflections on internalized stigma in individuals with bipolar disorder: Chronic Illn. 2011;7:209-24.
270. Cipriani A, Barbui C, Salanti G, et al. Comparative efficacy and acceptability of antimanic drugs in acute mania: a multiple-treatments meta-analysis. Lancet. 2011;378:1306-15.
271. Cousins DA, Butts K, Young AH. The role of dopamine in bipolar disorder. Bipolar Disord. 2009;11:787-806.
272. Stockmeier CA. Involvement of serotonin in depression: evidence from postmortem and imaging studies of serotonin receptors and the serotonin transporter. J Psychiatr Res. 2003;37:357-73.
273. Diazgranados N, Ibrahim L, Brutsche NE, et al. A randomized add-on trial of an N-methyl-D-aspartate antagonist in treatment-resistant bipolar depression. Arch Gen Psychiatry. 2010;67:793-802.
274. Zarate CA Jr, Brutsche NE, Ibrahim L, et al. Replication of ketamine's antidepressant efficacy in bipolar depression: a randomized controlled add-on trial. Biol Psychiatry. 2012;71:939-46.
275. Li x, Frye MA, Shelton RC. Review of pharmacological treatment in mood disorders and future directions for drug development. Neuropsychopharmacol. 2012;37:77-101.
276. Harwood AJ. Lithium and bipolar mood disorder: the inositol-depletion hypothesis revisited. Mol Psychiatry. 2005;10:117-26.
277. Agam O, Shamir A, Shaltiel G. Greenberg ML. Myo-inositol-1-phosphate (MIP) synthase: a possible new target for antibipolar drugs. Bipolar Disord. 2002:4(Suppl 1):15-20.
278. Andreazza AC, Young LT. The neurobiology of bipolar disorder; identifying targets for specific agents and synergies for combination treatment. Int J Neuropsychopharmacol. 2013;1:1-14.
279. Newberg AR, Catapano LA. Zarate CA, Manji HK. Neurobiology of bipolar disorder. Expert Rev Neurother. 2008;8:93-110.
280. Strakowski SM, Adler CM, Almeida J, et al. The functional neuroanatomy of bipolar disorder: a consensus model. Bipolar Disord. 2012;14:313-25.
281. Harvey AG. Sleep and circadian functioning;critical mechanisms in the mood disorders? Ann Rev Clin Psychol. 2011;7:297-319.
282. Frank E, Kupfer DJ, Thase ME, et al. Two-year outcomes for interpersonal and social rhythm therapy in individuals with bipolar I disorder. Arch Gen Psychiatry. 2005;62:996-1004.
283. Malkoff-Schwartz S, Frank E, Anderson B, et al. Stressful life events and social rhythm disruption in the onset of manic and depressive bipolar episodes: a preliminary investigation. Arch Gen Psychiatry. 1998;55:702-07.
284. Miklowitz DJ, Johnson SL. Social and familial risk factors in bipolar disorder: basic processes and relevant interventions. Clin Psychol Sci. 2000;16:281-96.

285. Johnson SL, Cuellar A, Ruggero C, et al. Life events as predictors of mania and depression in bipolar I disorder. J Abnorm Psychol. 2008;117:268-77.
286. Hooley JM. Expressed emotion and relapse of psychopathology Ann Rev Clin Psychol. 2007;3:329-52.
287. Simoneau TL, Miklowitz DJ, Richards JA, Saleem R, George EL. Bipolar disorder and family communication: effects of a psychoeducational treatment program. J Aborm Psychol. 1999;108:588-97.
288. Strakowski SM, Keck PE, McElroy SL, et al. Twelve-month outcome after a first hospitalization for affective psychosis. Arch Gen Psychiatry. 1998;55:49-55.
289. Miklowitz DJ, George EL, Richards JA, Simoneau TL, Suddath RL. A randomized study of family-focused psychoeducation and pharmacotherapy in the outpatient management of bipolar disorder. Arch Gen Psychiatry. 2003;60:904-12.
290. Colom F, Vieta E, Martinez-Aran A, et al. A randomized trial on the efficacy of group psychoeducation in the prophylaxis of bipolar disorder: a five year follow-up. Br J Psychiatry. 2009;194:260-5.
291. Yatham LN, Kennedy SH, Parikh SV, et al. Canadian Network for Mood and Anxiety Treatments (CAN MAT) and International Society for Bipolar Disorders (IISBD) collaborative update of CANMAT guidelines for the management of patients with bipolar disorder: update. 2011. Bipolar Disord. 2013;15:1-14.
292. Gijsman HJ, Geddes JR, Rendell JM, Nolen WA, Goodwin GM. Antidepressants for bipolar depression: a systematic review of randomised controlled trials. Am J Psychiatry. 2004;161:1517-47.
293. Frye MA, Ha K, Kanba S, et al. International consensus group on depression prevention in bipolar disorder. J Clin Psychiatry. 2011;72:1295-310.
294. Sachs GS, Nierenberg AA, Calabrese JR, et al. Effectiveness of adjunctive antidepressant treatment for bipolar depression. N Engl J Med. 2007;356:1711-22.
295. McElroy SL, Weisler RH, Chang W, et al. A double-blind, placebo-controlled study of quetiapine and paroxetine as monotherapy in adults with bipolar depression (EMBOLDEN II). J Clin Psychiatry. 2010;71:163-74.
296. Sidor MM, MacQueen GM. An update on antidepressant use in bipolar depression. Curr Psychiatry Rap. 2012;14:696-704.
297. Cipriani A, Furukawa TA, Salanti G, et al. Comparative efficacy and acceptability of 12 new-generation antidepressants: a multiple-treatments meta-analysis. Lancet. 2009;373:746-58.
298. Weisler RH, Calabrese JR, Bowden CL, Ascher JA, DeVeaugh-Geiss J, Evoniuk G. Discovery and development of lamotrigine for bipolar disorder a story of serendipity clinical observations, risk taking, and persistence. J Affect Disord. 2008;108:1-9.
299. Geddes IR, Calabrese IR, Goodwin GM. lamotrigine for treatment of bipolar depression: an independent meta-analysis and meta-regression of individual patient data from five randomised trials. Br J Psychiatry. 2009;194:4-9.
300. De Fruyt J, Deschepper E, Audenaert K, et al. Second generation antipsychotics in the treatment of bipolar depression: a systematic review and meta-analysis. J Psychopharmacol. 2012;26:603-17.
301. Weisler RH, Nolen WA, Neijber A, Hellqvist A, Paulsson B. Continuation of quetiapine versus switching to placebo or lithium for maintenance treatment of bipolar I disorder (Trial 144: a randomized controlled study). J Clip Psychiatry. 2011;72:1452-64.
302. Tohen M, Vieta E, Calabrese J, et al. Efficacy of olanzapine and olanzapine-fluoxetine combination in the treatment of bipolar I depression. Arch Gen Psychiatry. 2003;60:1079-88.
303. Loebel A, Cucchiaro J, Silva R, et al. Lurasidone monotherapy for the treatment of bipolar I depression: results of a 6-week, double-blind, placebo-controlled study. Philadelphia, PA: American Psychiatric Association, 2012.
304. Weisler RH, Montgomery SA, Earley WR, Szamosi J, Lazarus A. Efficacy of extended release quetiapine fumarate monotherapy in patients with major depressive disorder; a pooled analysis of two 6-week, double-blind, placebo-controlled studies. Int Clin Psychopharmacol. 2012;27:27-39.
305. Judd LL, Akiskal HS, Schettler PJ, et al. A prospective investigation of the natural history of the long-term weekly symptomatic status of bipolar II disorder. Arch Gen Psychiatry. 2003;60:261-69.
306. Altshuler LL, Post RM, Black DO, et al. Subsyndromal depressive symptoms are associated with functional impairment in patients with bipolar disorder: results of a large, multisite study. J Clin Psychiatry. 2006;67:1551-60.
307. Weinstock LM, Miller IW, Functional impairment as a predictor of short-term symptom course in bipolar I disorder. Bipolar Disord. 2008;10:437-42.
308. Weinstock LM, Miller IW. Psychosocial predictors of mood symptoms 1 year after acute phase treatment of bipolar I disorder. Comp Psychiatry. 2010;51:497-503.
309. Sienaert P, Lambrichts L, Dols A, De FJ. Evidence-based treatment strategies for treatment-resistant bipolar depression: a systematic review. Bipolar Disord. 2013;15:61-9.
310. Cade JFJ. Lithium salts in the treatment of psychotic excitement. Med J Aust. 1949;36:349-52.
311. Geddes IR, Burgess S, Hawton K, Jamison K, Goodwin GM. Long-term lithium therapy for bipolar disorder: systematic review and meta-analysis of randomized controlled trials. Am J Psychiatry. 2004;161:217-22.
312. Cipriani A, Pretty H, Hawton K, Geddes JR. Lithium in the prevention of suicidal behaviour and all-cause mortality in patients with mood disorders: a systematic review of randomised trials. Am J Psychiatry. 2005;162: 1805-19.
313. McKnight RF, Adida M, Budge K, Stockton S, Goodwin GM, Geddes IR. Lithium toxicity profile: a systematic review and meta-analysis. Lancet. 2012;379:721-8.
314. Goodwin GM, Bowden CL, Calabrese JR, et al. A pooled analysis of 2 placebo-controlled 18-month trials of lamotrigine and lithium maintenance in bipolar I disorder. J Clin Psychiatry. 2004;65:432-41.

315. Hayes J, Prah P, Nazareth I, et al. Prescribing trends in bipolar disorder cohort study in the United Kingdom THIN primary care database 1995;2009. PLoS One 2011;6: e28725.
316. Macritchie KA, Geddes JR, Scott J, Haslam DR, Goodwin GM. Valproic acid, valproate and divalproex in the maintenance treatment of bipolar disorder. Cochrane Database Syst Rsv. 2001;3: CD003196.
317. Geddes JR, Goodwin GM, Rendell J, et al. Lithium plus valproate combination therapy versus monotherapy for relapse prevention in bipolar I disorder (BALANCE): a randomised open-label trial, Lancet. 2010;375:385-95.
318. Goodwin GM, and Consensus Group of the British Association for Psychopharmacology Evidence-based guidelines for treating bipolar disorder: Revised second edition-recommendations from the British Association for Psychopharmacology. J Psychopharmacol. 2009;23;346-88.
319. Kessing LV, Hansen HV, Hvenegaard A, et al. Treatment in a specialised out-patient mood disorder clinic v standard out-patient treatment in the early course of bipolar disorder: randomised clinical trial. Br J Psychiatr. 2013;202:212-9.
320. Miklowitz DJ, Scott J. Psychosocial treatments for bipolar disorder: Cost-effectiveness, mediating mechanisms, and future directions. Bipolar Disord. 2009;11:110-22.
321. Miklowitz DJ, Otto MW, Frank E, et al. Psychosocial treatments for bipolar depression: a 1-year randomized trial from the Systematic Treatment Enhancement Program. Arch Gm Psychiatry. 2007;64:419-27.
322. Miklowitz DJ, Otto MW, Frank E, et al. Intensive psychosocial intervention enhances functioning in patients with bipolar depression: results from a 9-month randomized controlled trial. Am J Psychiatry. 2007;164:1-8.
323. Clarkin JF, Carpenter D, Hull J, Wilner P, Glick I. Effects of psychoeducational intervention for married patients with bipolar disorder and their spouses. Psychiatr Serv. 1998;49:531-3.
324. Rea MM, Tompson MC, Miklowitz DJ, Goldstein MI, Hwang S, Mintz J. Family-focused treatment versus individual treatment for bipolar disorder: results of a randomized clinical trial. J Consult Clin Psychol. 2003;71:482-92.
325. Miklowitz DJ, Axelson DA, Birmaher B, et al. Family-focused treatment for adolescents with bipolar disorder: results of a 2-year randomized trial, Arch Gen Psychiatry. 2008;65: 1053-61.
326. Miklowitz DJ, Schneck CD, Singh MK, et al. Early intervention for symptomatic youth at risk for bipolar disorder: a randomized trial of family-focused therapy. J Am Acad Child Adol Psychiatry. 2013;52:121-31.
327. Perlick D, Miklowitz DJ, Lopez N, et al. Family-focused treatment for caregivers or' patients with bipolar disorder Bipolar Disord. 2010;12:627-37.
328. Miller JW Keitner GI, Ryan CE, Uebelacker LA, Johnson SL, Solomon DA. Family treatment for bipolar disorder: family impairment by treatment interactions. J Clin Psychiatry. 2008;69:732-40.
329. Reinares M, Colom F, Sanchez-Moreno J, et al. Impact of caregiver group psychoeducation on the course and outcome of bipolar patients in remission: a randomized controlled trial. Bipolar Disord. 2008;10:511-19.
330. Fristad MA, Verducci JS, Walters K, Young ME. Impact of multifamily psychoeducational psychotherapy in treating children aged 8 to 12 years with mood disorders. Arch Gen Psychiatry. 2009;66:1013-21.
331. Cochran SD. Preventing medical noncompliance in the outpatient treatment of bipolar affective disorders. J Cons Clin Psychol. 1984;52:873-8.
332. Lam DH, Hayward P, Watkins ER, Wright K, Sham P. Relapse prevention in patients with bipolar disorder: cognitive therapy outcome alter 2 years. Am J Psychiatry. 2005;162:324-9.
333. Ball JR, Mitchell PB, Corry JC, Skillecorn A, Smith M, Malhi GS. A randomized controlled trial of cognitive therapy for bipolar disorder: focus on long-term change. J Clin Psychiatry. 2006;67:277-86.
334. Scott J, Paykel E, Morriss R, et al. Cognitive behaviour therapy for severe and recurrent bipolar disorders: a randomised controlled trial. Br J Psychiatry. 2006;188:313-20.
335. Zaretsky A, Lancee W, Miller C, Harris A, Parikh SV. In cognitive-behavioural therapy more effective than psychoeducation in bipolar disorder? Can J Psychiatry. 2008;53:441-8.
336. Parikh SV, Zaretsky A, Beaulieu S, et al. A randomized controlled trial of psychoeducation or cognitive-behavioral therapy in bipolar disorder: a Canadian Network for Mood and Anxiety treatments [CANMAT] study. J Clin Psychiatry. 2012;73;803-10.
337. Meyer TD, Hautzinger M. Cognitive behaviour therapy and supportive therapy for bipolar disorders: relapse rates for treatment period and 2-year follow-up. Psychol Med. 2012;42:1429-39.
338. Swartz HA, Frank E, Cheng Y, A randomized pilot study of psychotherapy and quetiapine for the acute treatment of bipolar II depression. Bipolar Disord. 2012;14:211-6.
339. Colom F, Vieta E, Martinez-Aran A, et al. A randomized trial on the efficacy of group psychoeducation in the prophylaxis of recurrences in bipolar patients whose disease is in remission. Arch Gen Psychiatry. 2003;60:402-07.
340. Torrent C, del Mar Bonnin C, Martinez-Aran A, et al. Efficacy of functional remediation in bipolar disorder: a multicentre randomized controlled study. Am J Psychiatry 2013;published online March 20. DOI:10.1176/appi.ajp.2012.12070971.
341. Weiss RD, Griffin ML, Kolodziej ME, et al. A randomized trial of integrated group therapy versus group drug counseling for patients with bipolar disorder and substance dependence. Am J Psychiatry. 2007;164:100-07.
342. Perry A, Tarrier N, Morriss R, McCarthy E, Limb K. Randomised controlled trial of efficacy of teaching patients with bipolar disorder to identity early symptoms of relapse and obtain treatment. BM J1999;318:149-53.
343. Simon GE, Ludman EJ, Bauer MS, Unutzer J, Operskalski B. Long-term effectiveness and cost of a systematic care program for bipolar disorder. Arch Gen Psychiatry. 2006;63:500-08.

344. Bauer MS, McBride L, Williford WO, et al. Collaborative care for bipolar disorder: Part II. lmpact on clinical outcome, function, and costs. Psychiatr Serv. 2006:57:937-45.
345. Miklowitz DJ, Goodwin GM, Bauer M, Geddes JR. Common and specific elements of psychosocial treatments for bipolar disorder: a survey of clinicians participating in randomized trials. J Psychiatr Pract. 2008;14:77-85.
346. Anderson IM, Haddad PM, Scott J. Bipolar disorder: BMJ. 2012;345: e8508.
347. Miklowitz DJ. Adjunctive psychotherapy for bipolar disorder: state of the evidence. Am J Psychiatry. 2008;165:1408-19.
348. Scott J, Colona FEV. A meta-analysis of relapse rates with adjunctive psychological therapies compared to usual psychiatric treatment for bipolar disorders. Int J Neuropsychopharmacol. 2007;10:123-9.
349. Lam DH, Burbeck R, Wright K, Filling S. Psychological therapies in bipolar disorder;the effect of illness history on relapse prevention-a systematic review. Bipolar Disord. 2009;11:474-82.
350. Miklowitz DJ. Bipolar disorder;a family-focused treatment approach (2nd edition). New York: Guilford Press, 2008.
351. Beck AT, Rush AJ, Shaw BF, Emery G, Cognitive therapy of depression. New York: Guilford Press, 1937.
352. Benedetti F, Serretti A, Colombo C, et al. Influence of CLOCK gene polymorphism on circadian mood fluctuation and illness recurrence in bipolar depression. Am J Mod Geri B;Neuropsychiatr Gen. 2003;123:23-6.
353. Roybal K, Theobold D, Graham A, et al. Mania-like behavior induced by disruption of CLOCK. Proc Natl Acad Sci USA. 2007;104:6406-11.
354. Scott J, Colom F. Popova E, et al. Long-term mental health resource utilization and cost of care following group psychoeducational or unstructured group support for bipolar disorders: a cost-benefit analysis. J Clin Psychiatry. 2009;70:378-86.
355. Grskovic M, Javaherian A, Strulovici B, Daley GQ. Induced pluripotent stem cells-opportunities for disease modelling and drug discovery. Nat Rev Drug Discov. 2011;10:915-29.
356. Cross-Disorder Group of the Psychiatric Genomics Consortium. Identification of risk loci with shared effects on five major psychiatric disorders: a genome-wide analysis Lower 2013;published online Feb 27 DOI:10.1016/S0140-6736(12)62129-1.
357. Arrowsmith CH, Bountra C, Fish PV, Lee K, Schapira M. Epigenetic protein families: s new frontier for drug discovery. Nat Rev Drug Discov. 2012;11:384-400.
358. Tye KM, Deisseroth K. Optogenetic investigation of neural circuits underlying brain disease in animal models. Nor Rev Neurosci. 2012;13:251-66.
359. Singh N, Halliday AC, Thomas JM, et al. A safe lithium mimetic for bipolar disorder. Nat Commun. 2013;4:1332.
360. Gelenberg AJ, Thase Me, Meyer RE, et al. The history and current state of antidepressant clinical trial designs: call to action for proof-of-concept studies. J Clin Psychiatry. 2008;69;1513-28.
361. Bopp JM, Miklowitz DJ, Goodwin GM, Stevens W Rendell JM, Geddes IR. The longitudinal course of bipolar disorder as revealed through weekly text-messaging. Bipolar Disord. 2010;12:327-34.
362. Miklowitz DJ, Price J, Holmes EA, et al. Facilitated integrated mood management (FIMM) for adults with bipolar disorder. Bipolar Disord. 2012;14:185-97.
363. Hollon SD, Munoz RF, Barlow DH, et al. Psychosocial intervention development for the prevention and treatment of depression;Promoting innovation and increasing access. Biol Psychiatr. 2002;52:610-30.
364. Holmes EA, Geddes JR, Colom F, Goodwin GM. Mental imagery as an emotional amplifier: Application so bipolar disorder: Behav Res Ther. 2008:46:1251-8.
365. Phillips ML, Kupfer MJ. Bipolar disorder diagnosis: challenges and future directions. Lancet. 2013;381:1663-71.
366. Birmaher B, Axelson D, Goldstein B, et al. Four-year longitudinal course of children and adolescents with bipolar spectrum disorders: the Course end Outcome of Bipolar Youth (COBY) Study. Am J Psychiatry. 2009;166:795-804.

Bipolar Disorder: A Focus on Depression

367. Goodwin FK, Jamison KR. Manic-depressive illness: bipolar disorders and recurrent depression. 2nd edition. New York: Oxford University Press, 2007.
368. Diagnostic and statistical manual of mental disorders, 4th edition. rev.: DSM-IV-R. Washington, DC: American Psychiatric Association, 2000.
369. Merikangas KE, Akiskal HS, Angst J, et al. Lifetime and 12-month prevalence of bipolar spectrum disorder in the National Comorbidity Survey replication. Arch Gen Psychiatry. 2007;64:543-52.
370. Murray CJ, Lopz AD. Alternative projections of mortality and disability by cause 1990-2020: Global Burden of Disease Study. Lancet. 1997;349:1498-504.
371. Tondo L, Isacsson G, Baldessarini R. Suicidal behaviour in bipolar disorder: risk and preventions. CNS Drugs. 2003;17:491-511.
372. Inskip HM, Harris EC, Barraclough B. Lifetime risk of suicide for affective disorder, alcoholism and schizophrenia. Br J Psychiatry. 1998:172:35-7.
373. Frye MA, ALtshuler LL, McElroy SL, et al. Gender differences in prevalence, risk, and clinical correlates of alcoholism comorbidity in bipolar disorder. AM J Psychiatry. 2003;160:883-9.
374. Simon NM, Otto MW, Wisniewski SR, et al. Anxiety disorder comorbidity in bipolar disorder patients: data from the first 500 participants in the Systematic Treatment Enhancement Program for Bipolar Disorder (STEP-BD). Am J Psychiatry. 2004;161:222-9.
375. Simon NM, Zalta AK, Otto MW, et al. The association of comorbid anxiety disorders with suicide attempts and suicidal ideation in outpatients with bipolar disorder. Am J psychiatry Res. 2007;41:225-64.

376. Ostacher MJ, Perlis RH, Nierenberg AA, et al. Impact of substance use disorders on recovery form episodes of depression in bipolar disorder patients: prospective data form the Systematic Treatment Enhancement Program for Bipolar Disorder (STEP-BD). Am J Psychiatry. 2010;168:289-97.
377. Kessler RC, Akiskal HS, Ames M, et al. Prevalence and effects of mood disorder on work performance in a nationally representative sample of U.S. works. Am J Psychiatry. 2006;163:1561-8.
378. Judd LL, Akiskal HS, Schettler PJ, et al. The long-term natural history of the weekly symptomatic status of bipolar I disorder. Arch Gen Psychiatry. 2002;59:530-7.
379. Altshuler LL, Gitlin MJ, Mintz J, Leight KL, Frye MA. Subsyndromal depressions associated with functional impairment in patients with bipoar disorder. J Clin Psychiatry. 2002;62:807-11.
380. Perlis RH, Ostacher MJ, Patel JK, et al. Predictors of recurrence in bipolar disorder: primary outcomes from the Systematic Treatment Enhancement Program for Bipolar Disorder (STEP-BD). Am J Psychiatry. 2006;163:217-24.
381. Frye MA. Yatham LN, Calabrese JR, et al. Incidence and time course of subsyndromal symptoms in patients with bipolar I disorder: an evaluation of 2 placebo-controlled maintenance trials. J Clin Psychiatry. 2006;67:1721-8.
382. Hirschfeld Rm, Williams JB, Spitzer RL, et al. Development and validation of a screening instrument for bipolar spectrum disorder: the Mood Disorder Questionnaire. Am J Psychiatry. 2000;11:1873-5.
383. Hirschfeld RM, Holzer C. Calabrese JR, et al. Validity of the Mood Disorder Questionnaire: a general population study. Am J Psychiatry. 2003;160:178-80.
384. Zimmerman M, Galione JN, Cheminski I, Young D, Dalrymple K. Psychiatric diagnoses in patients who screen positive on the Mood disorder Questionnaire: implications for using the scale as a case-finding instrument for bipolar disorder. Psychiatry Res, 2010.
385. Zimmerman M, Galione JN, Ruggero CJ, et al. Screening for bipolar disorder and finding borderline personality disorder. J Clin Psychiatry. 2010;71:1212-7.
386. Calabrese JR, Keck PE Jr, Macfadden W, et al. A randomized, double-blind, placebo-controlled trial of quetiapine in the treatment of bipolar I or II depression. Am J Psychiatry. 2005;162:1351-60.
387. Thase ME, Macfadden , Weisler RH, et al. Efficacy of quetiapine monotherapy in bipolar I and II depression: a double-blind, placebo-controlled study (the BOLDER II study). J Clin Psychopharmacol. 2006;26:600-9. [Erratum, J Clin Psychopharmacol. 2007;27:51.]
388. Young AH, McElroy SL, Baure M, et al. A double-blind, placebo-controlled study of quetiapine and lithium monotherapy in adults in the acute phase of bipolar depression (EMBOLDEN I). J Clin Psychiatry. 2010;71:150-62.
389. McElroy SL, Weisler RH, Change W, et al. A double-blind, placebo-controlled study of quetiapine and paroxetine monotherapy in adults with bipolar depression (EMBOLDEN II). J Clin Psychiatry. 2010;71:163-74.
390. Tohen M, Vietal E, Calabrese J, et al. Efficacy of olanzapine and olanzapine-fluoxetine combination in the treatment of bipolar I depression. Arch Gen Psychiatry. 2003;60:1079-88. (Erratum, Arch Gen Psychiatry. 2004;61;176.]
391. Kane Jm. Tardive dyskinesia circa 2006. Am J Psychiatry. 2006;163:1316-8.
392. Thase ME, Jonas A, Khan A, et al. Aripiprazole monotherapy in nonpsychotic bipolar I depression: results of 2 randomized, placebo-controlled studies. J Clin Psychopharmacol. 2008;28:13-20 [Erratum, J Clin Psychopharmacol. 2009;29:38.]
393. Clinical Trials.gov home page. (http://www.clinicaltrials.gov).
394. Goodwin GM, Bowden CL, Calabrese JR, et al. A pooled analysis of 2 placebo-controlled 18 month trials of lamotrigine and lithlum maintenance in bipolar I disorder. J Clin Psychiatry. 2004;65:432-41.
395. Calabrese JR, Bowden Cl, Sachs GS, Ascher JA, Monaghan E, Rudd GD, A double-blind placebo-controlled study of lamotrigine monotherapy in our patients with bipolar I depression. J Clin Psychiatry. 1999;60:79-88.
396. Geddes JR, Calabrese JR, Good win GM, Lamotrigine for treatment of bipolar depression: independent meta-analysis and meat-regression of individual patient data from five randomized trials. Br. J Psychiatry. 2009;194:4-9.
397. Van der Loss ML, Mulder PG, Hartong EG, et al. Efficacy and safety of lamotrigine as add-on treatment to lithium in bipolar depression: a multicenter, double blind, placebo-controlled trail. J Clin Psychiatry. 2009;70:2223-31.
398. Frye MA, Ketter TA, Kimbrell TA, et al. A placebo-controlled study of lamotrigine and gabapentin monotherapy in refractory mood disorders. J Clin Psychopharmacol. 2000;20:607-14.
399. Bond BJ, Lam RW, Yatham LN. Divalproex sodium versus placebo in the treatment of acute bipolar depression: a systematic review and meta-analysis, J Affect Disorder. 2010;124:228-34.
400. Baldessarini RJ, Leahy L, Arcona S, Gause D, Zhang W, Hennen J. Patterns of psychotropic drug prescription for U.S. patients with diagnoses of bipolar disorders. Psychiatr Serv. 2007;58:85-91.
401. Nemeroff CB, Evans DL, Gyulai L, et al. Double-blind, placebo-controlled comparison of imipramine and paroxetine in the treatment of bipolar depression. Am J Psychiatry. 2001;158:906-12.
402. Sachs GS, Nierenberg AA, Calabrese JR, et al. Effectiveness of adjunctive antidepressant treatment for bipolar depression. N Eng J Med. 2007;356:171-22.
403. Sidor MM, MacQueen Gm. Antidepressants for acute treatment of bipolar depression: a systematic review and meta analysis. J Clin Psychiatry, 2010.
404. Ghaemi SN, Wingo AP, Filkowski MA, Baldessarini Rj. Long-term antidepressant treatment in bipolar disorder: meta-analyses of benefits and risks. Acta Psychiatr Scand. 2008;118:347-56.

405. Amsterdam JD, Shults J. Efficacy and safety of long-term fluoxetine versus lithium monotherapy of bipolar II disorder: a randomized, double-blind, placebo-substitution study. Am J Psychiatry. 2001;167:792-800.
406. Miklowitz DJ, Otto MW, Frank E, et al. Psychosocial treatment for bipolar depression: a 1-year randomized trial from the Systematic Treatment Enhancement Program. Arc Gen psychiatry. 2007;64:419-26.
407. Truman CJ, Goldberg JF, Ghaemi SN, et al. Self-reported history of manic/hypomanic switch associated with antidepressant use: data from the systematic treatment Enhancement Program for Bipolar Disorder (STEP-BD). J Clin Psychiatry. 2007;68:1472-9.
408. Vieta E, Martinez-Aran A. Goikolea JM, et al. A randomized trail comparing paroxetine and venlafaxine in the treatment of bipolar depressed patients taking mood stabilizers. J Clin Psychiatry. 2002;63:508-12.
409. Frye MA, Helleman G. McElroy SL, et al. Correlates of treatment-emergent mania associated with antidepressant treatment in bipolar depression. Am J Psychiatry. 2009;166:164-72.
410. Frye MA, Grunze H, Suppes T, et al. A placebo-controlled evaluation of adjunctive modafinil in the treatment of bipolar depression. Am J Psychiatry. 2007:164:1242-9.
411. Goldberg JF, Burkick Ke, Endick DJ. Preliminary randomized, double-blind, placebo-controlled trail of pramipexole added to mood stabilizers for treatment resistant bipolar depression. Am J Psychiatry. 2004;161:564-6.
412. Zarate CA Jr, Payne JL, Singh J, et al. Pramipexole for bipolar II depression: a placebo-controlled proof of concept study. Biol Psychiatry. 2004;56:54-60.
413. Yatham LN, Kennedy SH, Schaffer A, et al. Canadian Network for Mood and Anxiety Treatment (CANMAT) and International Society for Bipolar Disorders (ISBD) collaborative update of CANMAT guidelines for the management of patients with bipolar disorder: update 2009. Bipolar Disord. 2009;11:225-55.
414. American Psychiatric Association. Desk Reference to the Diagnostic Criteria from DSM-5. Washington DC, 2013.

Medical Treatment of Depression

415. The world health report 2002—reducing risks, promoting healthy life. Geneva: World Health Organization, 2002.
416. Narrow WE, Rae DS, Robins LN, Regier DA. Revised prevalence estimates of mental disorders in the United States: using a clinical significance criterion to reconcile 2 surveys' estimates. Arch Gen Psychiatry. 2002;59:11-51-23.
417. Kessler RC, McGonagle KA, Zhao S, et al. Lifetime and 12-month prevalence of DSM-IIIR psychiatric disorders in the United States: results from the National Comorbidity Survey. Arch Gen Psychiatry. 1994;51:8-19.
418. Coyne JC, FechnerBates S, Schwenk TL. Prevalence, nature, and comorbidity of depressive disorders in primary care. Gen Hosp Psychiatry. 1994;16:267-76.
419. Hirschfeld RMA, Keller MB, Panico S, et al. The National Depressive and Manic-Depressive Association consensus statement on the undertreatment of depression. JAMA. 1997;277:333-40.
420. Goldman LS, Nielsen NH, Champion HC. Awareness, diagnosis, and treatment of depression. J Gen Intern Med. 1999;14:569-80.
421. Mueller TI, Leon AC, Keller MB, et al. Recurrence after recovery from major depressive disorder during 15 years of observational follow-up. Am J Psychiatry. 1999;156:1000-6.
422. Keller MB, Lavori PW, Rice J, Coryell W, Hirschfeld RM. The persistent risk of chronicity in recurrent episodes of nonbipolar major depressive disorder: a prospective followup. Am J Psychiatry. 1986;143:2-28.
423. Judd LL, Akiskal HS, Maser JD, et al. A prospective 12-year study of subsyndromal and syndromal depressive symptoms in unipolar major depressive disorders. Arch Gen Psychiatry. 1998;55:694-700.
424. Ciechanowski PS, Katon WJ, Russo JE. Depression and diabetes: impact of depressive symptoms on adherence, function, and costs. Arch Intern Med. 2000;160:3278-85.
425. Jiang W, Krishnan RR, O'Connor CM. Depression and heart disease: evidence of a link, and its therapeutic implications. CNS Drugs. 2002;16:111-27.
426. Angst F, Stassen HH, Clayton PJ, Angst J. Mortality of patients with mood disorders: follow-up over 34-38 years. J Affect Disord. 2002;68:167-81.
427. Stark C, Hall D, O'Brien F, Smith H. Suicide after discharge from psychiatric hospitals in Scotland. BMJ. 1995;311:1368-69.
428. Taylor CB, Youngblood ME, Catellier D, et al. Effects of antidepressant medication on morbidity and mortality in depressed patients after myocardial infarction. Arch Gen Psychiatry. 2005;62:792-8.
429. Jorge RE, Robinson RG, Arndt S, Starkstein S. Mortality and poststroke depression: a placebo-controlled trial of antidepressants. Am J Psychiatry. 2003;160:1823-9.
430. Gibbons RD, Hur K, Bhaumik DK, Mann JJ. The relationship between antidepressant medication use and rate of suicide. Arch Gen Psychiatry. 2005;62:165-72.
431. Milak MS, Parsey RV, Keilp J, Oquendo MA, Malone KM, Mann JJ. Neuroanatomic correlates of psychopathologic components of major depressive disorder. Arch Gen Psychiatry. 2005;62:397-408.
432. Mann JJ, Currier D, Quiroz J, Manji HK. Neurobiology of severe mood and anxiety disorders. In: Siegel GJ, Albers RW, Brady S, Price D (Eds). Basic neurochemistry: molecular, cellular and medical aspects, 7th edition. San Diego. 2005;178-86.
433. Kendler KS, Davis CG, Kessler RC. The familial aggregation of common psychiatric and substance use disorders in the National Comorbidity Survey: a family history study. Br J Psychiatry. 1997;170:541-8.
434. Sheline YI, Gado MH, Kraemer HC. Untreated depression and hippocampal volume loss. Am J Psychiatry. 2003;160:1516-8.

435. McEwen BS. Effects of adverse experiences for brain structure and function. Biol Psychiatry. 2000;48:721-31.
436. Bertolino A, Frye M, Callicott JH, et al. Neuronal pathology in the hippocampal area of patients with bipolar disorder: a study with proton magnetic resonance spectroscopic imaging. Biol Psychiatry. 2003;53:906-13.
437. Caspi A, Sugden K, Moffitt TE, et al. Influence of life stress on depression: moderation by a polymorphism in the 5HTT gene. Science. 2003;301:386-9.
438. Hariri AR, Drabant EM, Munoz KE, et al. A susceptibility gene for affective disorders and the response of the human amygdala. Arch Gen Psychiatry. 2005;62:146-52.
439. Bennett AJ, Lesch KP, Heils A, et al. Early experience and serotonin transporter gene variation interact to influence primate CNS function. Mol Psychiatry. 2002;7:118-22.
440. Ansorge MS, Zhou M, Lira A, Hen R, Gingrich JA. Earlylife blockade of the 5HT transporter alters emotional behavior in adult mice. Science. 2004;306:879-81.
441. Parsey RV, Hastings RS, Oquendo MA, et al. [11C]McN5652 binding to the serotonin transporter in human brain: lower binding during a major depressive episode. Am J Psychiatry. 2006;163:48–57.
442. Diagnostic and statistical manual for mental disorders, 4th edtion: DSM-IV. Washington, DC: American Psychiatric Association,. 1994.
443. Zisook S, Rush AJ, Albala A, et al. Factors that differentiate early vs. later onset of major depression disorder. Psychiatry Res. 2004;129:127-40.
444. Kroenke K, Spitzer RL, Williams JB, et al. Physical symptoms in primary care: predictors of psychiatric disorders and functional impairment. Arch Fam Med. 1994;3:774-9.
445. Johnson J, Horwath E, Weissman MM. The validity of major depression with psychotic features based on a community study. Arch Gen Psychiatry. 1991;48:1075-81.
446. Treatment of depression—newer pharmacotherapies. Evidence report/technology assessment no. 7. Washington, DC: Agency for Health Care Policy and Research, March. 1999.
447. Kroenke K, West SL, Swindle R, et al. Similar effectiveness of paroxetine, fluoxetine, and sertraline in primary care: a randomized trial. JAMA. 2001;286:2947-55.
448. Stahl SM. Placebo-controlled comparison of the selective serotonin reuptake inhibitors citalopram and sertraline. Biol Psychiatry. 2000;48:894-901.
449. Geddes JR, Freemantle N, Mason J, Eccles MP, Boynton J. SSRIs versus other antidepressants for depressive disorder. Cochrane Database Syst Rev. 2000;2:CD00185.
450. MacGillivray S, Arroll B, Hatcher S, et al. Efficacy and tolerability of selective serotonin reuptake inhibitors compared with tricyclic antidepressants in depression treated in primary care: systematic review and metaanalysis. BMJ. 2003;326:1014.
451. Anderson IM. Selective serotonin reuptake inhibitors versus tricyclic antidepressants: a meta-analysis of efficacy and tolerability. J Affect Disord. 2000;58:19-36.
452. Simon GE, VonKorff M, Heiligenstein JH, et al. Initial antidepressant choice in primary care: effectiveness and cost of fluoxetine vs. tricyclic antidepressants. JAMA. 1996;275: 1897-902.
453. Peretti S, Judge R, Hindmarch I. Safety and tolerability considerations: tricyclic antidepressants vs. selective serotonin reuptake inhibitors. Acta Psychiatr Scand Suppl. 2000;403:17-25.
454. Gijsman HJ, Geddes JR, Rendell JM, Nolen WA, Goodwin GM. Antidepressants for bipolar depression: a systematic review of randomized, controlled trials. Am J Psychiatry. 2004;161:1537-47.
455. Briley M. Clinical experience with dual action antidepressants in different chronic pain syndromes. Hum Psychopharmacol. 2004;19:-Suppl 1:S21-5.
456. Treatment for Adolescents with Depression Study (TADS) Team. Fluoxetine, cognitive-behavioral therapy, and their combination for adolescents with depression: Treatment for Adolescents with Depression Study (TADS) randomized controlled trial. JAMA. 2004;292:807-20.
457. Mulder RT, Watkins WG, Joyce PR, Luty SE. Age may affect response to antidepressants with serotonergic and noradrenergic actions. J Affect Disord. 2003;76:143-9.
458. Martin A, Young C, Leckman JF, Mukonoweshuro C, Rosenheck R, Leslie D. Age effects on antidepressant induced manic conversion. Arch Pediar Adolesc Med. 2004;158:773-80.
459. American Psychiatric Association. Practice guideline for the treatment of patients with major depressive disorder (revision). Am J Psychiatry. 2000;157 (Suppl):145.
460. Stahl SM, Entsuah R, Rudolph RL. Comparative efficacy between venlafaxine and SSRIs: a pooled analysis of patients with depression. Biol Psychiatry. 2002;52:1166-74.
461. Thase ME, Entsuah AR, Rudolph RL. Remission rates during treatment with venlafaxine or selective serotonin reuptake inhibitors. Br J Psychiatry. 2001;178:234-41.
462. Smith D, Dempster C, Glanville J, Freemantle N, Anderson I. Efficacy and tolerability of venlafaxine compared with selective serotonin reuptake inhibitors and other antidepressants: a metaanalysis. Br J Psychiatry. 2002;180:396-404.
463. Detke MJ, Wiltse CG, Mallinckrodt CH, McNamara RK, Demitrack MA, Bitter I. Duloxetine in the acute and long-term treatment of major depressive disorder: a placebo and paroxetine-controlled trial. Eur Neuropsychopharmacol. 2004;14:457-70.
464. Rowbotham MC, Goli V, Kunz NR, Lei D. Venlafaxine extended release in the treatment of painful diabetic neuropathy: a doubleblind, placebo-controlled study. Pain. 2004;110:697706. [Erratum, Pain. 2005;113:2-48.]
465. Goldstein DJ, Lu Y, Detke MJ, Lee TC, Iyengar S. Duloxetine vs. placebo in patients with painful diabetic neuropathy. Pain. 2005;116:109-18.
466. Goldstein DJ, Lu Y, Detke MJ, Wiltse C, Mallinckrodt C, Demitrack MA. Duloxetine in the treatment of depression: a

doubleblind placebo-controlled comparison with paroxetine. J Clin Psychopharmacol. 2004;24:389-99.
467. Brannan SK, Mallinckrodt CH, Brown EB, Wohlreich MM, Watkin JG, Schatzberg AF. Duloxetine 60 mg once daily in the treatment of painful physical symptoms in patients with major depressive disorder. J Psychiatr Res. 2005;39:43-53.
468. Nieuwstraten CE, Dolovich LR. Bupropion versus selective serotonin reuptake inhibitors for treatment of depression. Ann Pharmacother. 2001;35:1608-13.
469. Fava M, Papakostas GI, Petersen T, et al. Switching to bupropion in fluoxetine resistant major depressive disorder. Ann Clin Psychiatry. 2003;15:17-22.
470. DeBattista C, Solvason HB, Poirier J, Kendrick E, Schatzberg AF. A prospective trial of bupropion SR augmentation of partial and nonresponders to serotonergic antidepressants. J Clin Psychopharmacol. 2003;23:27-30.
471. Quitkin FM, Stewart JW, McGrath PJ, et al. Columbia atypical depression: a subgroup of depressives with better response to MAOI than to tricyclic antidepressants or placebo. Br J Psychiatry Suppl. 1993;21:30-4.
472. Thase ME, Mallinger AG, McKnight D, Himmelhoch JM. Treatment of imipramine resistant recurrent depression. IV. A doubleblind crossover study of tranylcypromine for anergic bipolar depression. Am J Psychiatry. 1992;149:195-8.
473. LotufoNeto F, Trivedi M, Thase ME. Meta-analysis of the reversible inhibitors of monoamine oxidase type A moclobemide and brofaromine for the treatment of depression. Neuropsychopharmacology. 1999;20:226-47.
474.Wecker L, James S, Copeland N, Pacheco MA. Transdermal selegiline: targeted effects on monoamine oxidases in the brain. Biol Psychiatry. 2003;54:1099-104.
475. Montejo AL, Llorca G, Izquierdo JA, RicoVillademoros F. Incidence of sexual dysfunction associated with antidepressant agents: a prospective multicenter study of 1022 outpatients. J Clin Psychiatry. 2001;62:(Suppl 3):10-21.
476. Guelfi JD, Ansseau M, Timmerman L, Korsgaard S. Mirtazapine versus venlafaxine in hospitalized severely depressed patients with melancholic features. J Clin Psychopharmacol. 2001;21:425-31.
477. Feiger A, Kiev A, Shrivastava RK, Wisselink PG, Wilcox CS. Nefazodone versus sertraline in outpatients with major depression: focus on efficacy, tolerability, and effects on sexual function and satisfaction. J Clin Psychiatry. 1996;57 (Suppl 2):53-62.
478. Rush AJ, Armitage R, Gillin JC, et al. Comparative effects of nefazodone and fluoxetine on sleep in outpatients with major depressive disorder. Biol Psychiatry. 1998;44:3-14.
479. Suri R, Burt VK, Altshuler LL. Nefazodone for the treatment of postpartum depression. Arch Women Ment Health. 2005;8:55-56. [Cross-Ref][Medline].
480. Feighner J, Targum SD, Bennett ME, et al. A double blind, placebo-controlled trial of nefazodone in the treatment of patients hospitalized for major depression. J Clin Psychiatry. 1998;59:246-53.
481. Taylor FB, Prather MR. The efficacy of nefazodone augmentation for treatment resistant depression with anxiety symptoms or anxiety disorder. Depress Anxiety. 2003;18:83-8.
482. Goodwin FK, Jamison KR. Manicdepressive illness. New York: Oxford University Press,. 1990.
483. Bauer M, Dopfmer S. Lithium augmentation in treatment resistant depression: metaanalysis of placebo-controlled studies. J Clin Psychopharmacol. 1999;19:427-34.
484. de Montigny C. Lithium addition in treatment-resistant depression. Int Clin Psychopharmacol. 1994;9 (Suppl 2):31-5.
485. Barbosa L, Berk M, Vorster M. A doubleblind, randomized, placebo-controlled trial of augmentation with lamotrigine or placebo in patients concomitantly treated with fluoxetine for resistant major depressive episodes. J Clin Psychiatry. 2003;64:403-7.
486. Yatham LN. Newer anticonvulsants in the treatment of bipolar disorder. J Clin Psychiatry. 2004;65 (Suppl 10):28-35.
487. Bowden CL, Calabrese JR, McElroy SL, et al. A randomized, placebo-controlled 12 month trial of divalproex and lithium in treatment of outpatients with bipolar I disorder. Arch Gen Psychiatry. 2000;57:481-9.
488. Masan PS. Atypical antipsychotics in the treatment of affective symptoms: a review. Ann Clin Psychiatry. 2004;16:313.
489. Rothschild AJ, Williamson DJ, Tohen MF, et al. A double-blind, randomized study of olanzapine and olanzapine/fluoxetine combination for major depression with psychotic features. J Clin Psychopharmacol. 2004;24:365-73.
490. Kennedy SH, Lam RW. Enhancing outcomes in the management of treatment resistant depresssion: a focus on atypical antipsychotics. Bipolar Disord. 2003;5 (Suppl 2):36-47.
491. Keck PE Jr. Bipolar depression: a new role for atypical antipsychotics? Bipolar Disord. 2005;7 (Suppl 4):34-40.
492. Cohen D. Atypical antipsychotics and new onset diabetes mellitus: an overview of the literature. Pharmacopsychiatry. 2004;37:111.
493. Ananth J, Parameswaran S, Gunatilake S. Side effects of atypical antipsychotic drugs. Curr Pharm Des. 2004;10:2219-29.
494. Trivedi MH, Rush AJ, Crismon ML, et al. Clinical results for patients with major depressive disorder in the Texas Medication Algorithm Project. Arch Gen Psychiatry. 2004;61:669-80.
495. Adli M, Berghofer A, Linden M, et al. Effectiveness and feasibility of a standardized stepwise drug treatment regimen algorithm for inpatients with depressive disorders: results of a 2 year observational algorithm study. J Clin Psychiatry. 2002;63:782-90.
496. Hawley CJ, Pattinson HA, Quick SJ, et al. A protocol for the pharmacologic treatment of major depression: a field test of a potential prototype. J Affect Disord. 1998;47:8796-9.
497. Swenson JR, O'Connor CM, Barton D, et al. Influence of depression and effect of treatment with sertraline on quality of life after hospitalization for acute coronary syndrome. Am J Cardiol. 2003;92:1271-6.
498. Katona C. Managing depression and anxiety in the elderly patient. Eur Neuropsychopharmacol. 2000;10 (Suppl 4): S427-S432.

499. Greco T, Eckert G, Kroenke K. The outcome of physical symptoms with treatment of depression. J Gen Intern Med. 2004;19:813-8.
500. Amsterdam JD, Maislin G, Potter L. Fluoxetine efficacy in treatment resistant depression. Prog Neuropsychopharmacol Biol Psychiatry. 1994;18:243-61.
501. Rush AJ, Kupfer DJ. Strategies and tactics in the treatment of depression. In: Gabbard GO (Ed). Treatment of psychiatric disorders. 3rd edition. Washington, DC: American Psychiatric Press;. 2001. pp. 141-739.
502. Thase ME, Rush AJ. When at first you don't succeed: sequential strategies for antidepressant nonresponders. J Clin Psychiatry. 1997;58 (Suppl 13):23-9.
503. Bauer M, Forsthoff A, Baethge C, et al. Lithium augmentation therapy in refractory depression update. 2002. Eur Arch Psychiatry Clin Neurosci. 2003;253:132-9.
504. Shelton RC, Tollefson GD, Tohen M, et al. A novel augmentation strategy for treating resistant major depression. Am J Psychiatry. 2001;158:131-4.
505. Demyttenaere K, De Fruyt J, Stahl SM. The many faces of fatigue in major depressive disorder. Int J Neuropsychopharmacol. 2005;8:93-105.
506. Spiker DG, Weiss JC, Dealy RS, et al. The pharmacological treatment of delusional depression. Am J Psychiatry. 1985;142:430-6.
507. Furukawa TA, Streiner DL, Young LT. Is antidepressant benzodiazepine combination therapy clinically more useful? A metaanalytic study. J Affect Disord. 2001;65:173-7.
508. Vinkers DJ, Gussekloo J, van der Mast RC, Zitman FG, Westendorp RG. Benzodiazepine use and risk of mortality in individuals aged 85 years or older. JAMA. 2003;290:2942-3
509. Hemmelgarn B, Suissa S, Huang A, Boivin JF, Pinard G. Benzodiazepine use and the risk of motor vehicle crash in the elderly. JAMA. 1997;278:27-31.
510. Judd LL, Paulus MJ, Schettler PJ, et al. Does incomplete recovery from first life time major depressive episode herald a chronic course of illness? Am J Psychiatry. 2000;157:1501-4.
511. Melfi CA, Chawla AJ, Croghan TW, Hanna MP, Kennedy S, Sredl K. The effects of adherence to antidepressant treatment guidelines on relapse and recurrence of depression. Arch Gen Psychiatry. 1998;55:1128-32.
512. Schatzberg AF, Haddad P, Kaplan EM, et al. Serotonin reuptake inhibitor discontinuation syndrome: a hypothetical definition. J Clin Psychiatry. 1997;58 (Suppl 7):5-10.
513. Geddes JR, Carney SM, Davies C, et al. Relapse prevention with antidepressant drug treatment in depressive disorders: a systematic review. Lancet. 2003;361:653-61.
514. Thies Flechtner K, Muller Oerlinghausen B, Seibert W, Walther A, Greil W. Effect of prophylactic treatment on suicide risk in patients with major affective disorders: data from a randomized prospective trial. Pharmacopsychiatry. 1996;29:103-7.
515. Montgomery SA, Reimitz PE, Zivkov M. Mirtazapine versus amitriptyline in the long-term treatment of depression: a doubleblind placebo-controlled study. Int Clin Psychopharmacol. 1998;13:63-73. [ISI][Medline].
516. Simon JS, Aguiar LM, Kunz NR, Lei D. Extended release venlafaxine in relapse prevention for patients with major depressive disorder. J Psychiatr Res. 2004;38:249-57. [Erratum, J Psychiatr Res. 2004;38:451.]
517. Prien RF, Kupfer DJ, Mansky PA, et al. Drug therapy in the prevention of recurrences in unipolar and bipolar affective disorders: report of the NIMH Collaborative Study Group comparing lithium carbonate, imipramine, and a lithium carbonate imipramine combination. Arch Gen Psychiatry. 1984;41:1096-104.
518. UK ECT Review Group. Efficacy and safety of electroconvulsive therapy in depressive disorders: a systematic review and metaanalysis. Lancet. 2003;361:799-808.
519. Prudic J, Olfson M, Marcus SC, Fuller RB, Sackeim HA. Effectiveness of electroconvulsive therapy in community settings. Biol Psychiatry. 2004;55:301-12.
520. Nobler MS, Sackeim HA. Electroconvulsive therapy. In: Helmchen H, Henn F, Lauter H, Sartorius C (Eds). Contemporary psychiatry. Heidelberg, Germany: Springer,. 2001:425-34.
521. Sackeim HA, Haskett RF, Mulsant BH, et al. Continuation pharmacotherapy in the prevention of relapse following electroconvulsive therapy: a randomized controlled trial. JAMA. 2001;285:1299-307.
522. Reynolds CF III, Frank E, Perel JM, et al. Nortriptyline and interpersonal psychotherapy as maintenance therapies for recurrent major depression: a randomized controlled trial in patients older than 59 years. JAMA. 1999;281:39-45.
523. DeRubeis RJ, Gelfand LA, Tang TZ, Simons AD. Medications versus cognitive behavior therapy for severely depressed outpatients: megaanalysis of four randomized comparisons. Am J Psychiatry. 1999;156:1007-13.
524. Practice guideline for the treatment of patients with bipolar disorder (revision). Am J Psychiatry. 2002;159 (Suppl):150.
525. Pampallona S, Bollini P, Tibaldi G, Kupelnick B, Munizza C. Combined pharmacotherapy and psychological treatment for depression: a systematic review. Arch Gen Psychiatry. 2004;61:714-9.
526. Belmaker RH. Bipolar disorder. N Engl J Med. 2004;351:476-86.
527. Keck PE Jr, Perlis RH, Otto MW, Carpenter D, Ross R, Docherty JP. Treatment of bipolar disorder. 2004. Expert consensus guideline series. Minneapolis: McGrawHill Healthcare Information,. 2004.
528. Henry C, Sorbara F, Lacoste J, Gindre C, Leboyer M. Antidepressant induced mania in bipolar patients: identification of risk factors. J Clin Psychiatry. 2001;62:249-55.
529. Bottlender R, Rudolf D, Strauss A, Moller HJ. Mood stabilisers reduce the risk of developing antidepressant induced maniform states in acute treatment of bipolar I depressed patients. J Affect Disord. 2001;63:79-83.
530. Peet M. Induction of mania with selective serotonin reuptake inhibitors and tricyclic antidepressants. Br J Psychiatry. 1994;164:549-50.
531. Tohen M, Jacobs TG, Grundy SL, et al. Efficacy of olanzapine in acute bipolar mania: a double blind, placebo-controlled

study. Arch Gen Psychiatry. 2000;57:841-9. [Erratum, Arch Gen Psychiatry. 2002;59:91.]

532. Tohen M, Vieta E, Calabrese J, et al. Efficacy of olanzapine and olanzapinefluoxetine combination in the treatment of bipolar I depression. Arch Gen Psychiatry. 2003;60:1079-88. [Erratum, Arch Gen Psychiatry. 2004;61:176.]
533. Keller MB, Ryan ND, Strober M, et al. Efficacy of paroxetine in the treatment of adolescent major depression: a randomized, controlled trial. J Am Acad Child Adolesc Psychiatry. 2001;40:762-72. [CrossRef][ISI][Medline].
534. Olfson M, Shaffer D, Marcus SC, Greenberg T. Relationship between antidepressant medication treatment and suicide in adolescents. Arch Gen Psychiatry. 2003;60:978-82.
535. Wisner KL, Gelenberg AJ, Leonard H, Zarin D, Frank E. Pharmacologic treatment of depression during pregnancy. JAMA. 1999;282:1264-9.
536. Misri S, Burgmann A, Kostaras D. Are SSRIs safe for pregnant and breastfeeding women? Can Fam Physician. 2000;46:631-3.

Dysthymia: Conceptual Evolution and Current Status

537. Akiskal HS, Bitar AH, Puzantian YR, Rosenthal TL, Parks WW. The nosological status of neurotic depression. Arch Gen Psychiatry. 1978;35:756-66.
538. Brieger RP, Marneros A. Dysthymia and cyclothymia: historical origins and contemporary development. J Affect Disord. 1997;45:117-26.
539. Kahlbaum KL. Die Gruppirune der psychischen krankheiten und die Eintheitung der See len sterungen. A W Kafemann Danzig, 1863.
540. Kraepelin E. Manic depressive Insanity. In: Barclay RM, Robertson GM, (Eds). Edinburgh: Livingstone, 1921.
541. Krestschmer E. Physique and Character-translated by Miller E.London, Kegan Paul, Trench, Trubner and Co, 1936.
542. Phillips KA, Gunderson JG, Hirschfeld RM, Smith LE. A review of the depressive personality. Am J Psychiatry. 1990;147:830-7.
543. American Psychiatric Association. Diagnostic and Slatistical Manual of Mental Disorders, 2nd edn, Washington DC: APA, 1968.
544. Spitzer RL, Endicott J, Robins E. Research diagnostic criteria: Rationale and reliability. Arch Gen Psychiatry. 1978;35:773-82.
545. American Psychiatric Association. Diagnostic and Statistical Manual of Mental Disorders, 3rd edn, Washington DC: APA, 1980.
546. American Psychiatric Association. Diagnostic and Statistical Manual of Mental Disorders, 3rd edn, R Washington DC: APA, 1987.
547. Shea MT, Hirschfeld RMA. Chronic mood disorders and depressive personality. Psychitr Clins of North Am. 1996;19: 103 -20.
548. American Psychiatric Association. Diagnostic and Statistical Manual of Mental Disorders, 4th edn, Washington DC: APA, 1994.
549. Hirschfeld RMA, Holzer CE. Depressive personality disorder: Clinical implications. J Clin Psychiatry. 1994;55:10-7.
550. Phillips KA, Hirschfeld RMA, Shea MT, et al. Depressive personality disorder: Perspectives for DSM-IV. Journal of Personality Disorders. 1993;3:30-42.
551. Keller MB, Klein DN, Hirschfeld RMA, et al. DSM-IV mood disorders field trial investigation results. Am J Psychiatry. 1995;152:843-9.
552. World Health Organization. International Classification of Diseases. 10th revision Geneva: World Health Organization, 1992.
553. Nemiah JC. Depressive neurosis. In: Kaplan and Sadock (Eds). Comprehensive Textbook of Psychiatry, 2nd edition, Baltimore. Williams and Wilkins; 1975. pp. 1225-64.
554. Klerman GL, Endictott J, Spitzer R. Neurotic depressions: A systematic analysis of multiple criteria and meanings. Am J Psychiatry. 1979;136:57-61.
555. World Health Organization. International Classification of Diseases. 9th revision Geneva: World Health Organization, 1977.
556. Klein DF, Davis JM. The diagnosis of affective disorders. In Diagnosis and Treatment of Psychiatric Disorders. Baltimore, Williams and Wilkins, 1965.
557. Kocsis JH, Francis AJ. A critical discussion of DSM-III Dysthymic disorder. Am J Psychiatry. 1987;144:1534-42.
558. Barzega G, Maina G, Venturello S, Bogetto F. Dysthymic disorder: clinical characteristics in relation to age at onset Journal of Affective Disorders. 2001;66:39-46.
559. Sartorious N, Kaelber CT, Cooper lE, Roper MT, Rae DS, Galbinet W, et al. Progress towards achieving a common language in Psychiatry. Arch Gen Psychiatry. 1993;50: 115-24.
560. Akiskal H. Dysthymia: Clinical and external validity. Acta Psychiatr Scand. 1994;89:s19-s23.
561. WPA Dysthymia Working Group. Dysthymia in clinical practice. Br J Psychiatry. 1995;166:174-83.
562. Klein DN, Kocsis JH, McCullough JP, Holzer III CE, Hirschfeld RMA, Keller MB. Symptomatology in dysthymic and major depressive disorder. Psychiatr Clin North Am. 1996;19:41-53.
563. Markowitz JC. Comorbidity of dysthymic disorder. In: Kocsis JH, Klein DN (Eds). Diagnosis and Treatment of Chronic Depressaion, Guilford Press, New York; 1995. pp. 41-57.
564. Pepper CM, Klein DN, Anderson RL, Riso LP, Ouimette PC, Lizardi H. DSM-III-R Axis II comorbidity in dysthymia and major depression. Am J Psychiatry. 1995;152:239-47.
565. Klein DN, Riso LP, Donaldson SK, Schwartz JE, Anderson RL, Crosby Ouimette P, Lizardi H, Aronson TA. Family study of early-onset dysthymia: mood and personality disorders in relatives of outpatients with dysthymia. Arch Gen Psychiatry. 1995;52:487-96.
566. Lizardi H, Klein DN, Ouimette PC, Riso LP, Anderson RL, Donaldson SK. Reports of the childhood home environment in early-onset dysthymia and episodic major depression. J Abnorm Psychol. 1995;104:132-9.

567. Mason BJ, Kocsis JH, Leon AC, et al. Measurement of severity and treatment response in dysthymia. Psychiatric Ann. 1993;23:625-31.
568. Hellerstein DJ, Batchelder ST, Lee A, Borisovskaya M. Rating dysthymia: an assessment of the construct and content validity of the Cornell Dysthymia Rating Scale Journal of Affective Disorders. 2002;71:85-96.
569. Donaldson SK, Klein DN, Riso LP, Schwartz JE. Comorbidity between dysthymic and major depressive disorders: a family study analysis. J Affect Disord. 1997;42:103-11.
570. Lyons MJ, Eisen SA, Goldberg J, True W, Lin N, Meyer JM, et al. A registry-based twin study of depression in men. Archives of General Psychiatry. 1998;55:468-72.
571. Szadoczky E, Sazekas I, Rihmer Z, Arato M. The role of psychosocial and biological variables in separating chronic and nonchronic major depression and early-late onset dysthymia. J Affect Disord. 1994;32:1-11.
572. Catalan R, Gallart JM, Castellanos JM, Galard R. Plasma corticotropin-releasing factor in depressive disorders. Biol Psychiatry. 1998;44:15-20.
573. Ravindran AV, Griffiths J, Merali Z, Anisman H. Primary dysthymia: a study of several psychosocial, endocrine and immune correlates. J Affect Disord. 1996;40:73-84.
574. Oshima A, Yamashita S, Owashi T Murata T, Tadokoro C, Miyaoka H, Kamijima K, Higuchi T. The differential ACTH responses to combined dexamethasone/CRH administration in major depressive and dysthymic disorders. Journal of Psychiatric Research. 2000;34:325-8.
575. Ravindran AV, Bialik RJ, Lapierre YD. Primary early onset dysthymia, biochemical correlates of the therapeutic response to fluoxetine:1. Platelet monoamine oxidase and the dexamethasone suppression test. J Affect Disord. 1994;31:111-7.
576. Ravindran AV, Merali Z, Anisman H. Dysthymia: a biological perspective. In: Licinio J, Bolis CL, Gold P (Eds). Dysthymia: From Clinical Neuroscience to Treatment. World Health Organization: Geneva; 1997. pp. 21-44.
577. Lechin F, van der Dijs B, Orozco B, Lechin AE. Plasma neurotransmitters, blood pressure, and heart rate during supine resting, orthostasis, and moderate exercise in dysthymic depressed patients. Biol Psychiatry. 1994;37:884-91.
578. Lecrubier Y, Boyer P, Turjanski S, Rein W. The Amisulpride Study Group. Amisulpride versus imipramine and placebo in dysthymia and major depression. J Affect Disord. 1997;43:95-103.
579. Ravindran AV, Smith A, Cameron C, Bhatla R, Cameron I, Georgescu TM, Hogan MJ. Toward a functional neuroanatomy of dysthymia: A functional magnetic resonance imaging study. J Affect Disord. 2009 article in press doi:10.1016/j.jad.2009.03.009.
580. Akiskal HS, Judd LL, Gillin C, Lemmi H. Subthreshold depressions: clinical and polysomnographic validation of dysthymic, residual and masked forms. J Affect Disord. 1997;45:53-63.
581. Arriaga F, Cavaglia F, Matospires A, Lara E, Paiva T. EEG sleep characteristics in dysthymia and major depressive disorder. Neuropsychobiology. 1995;32:128-31.
582. Dura JR, Stukenberg KW, Kiecolt-Glaser JK. Chronic stress and depressive disorder in older adults. J Abn Psychol. 1990;99:284-90.
583. Ravindran A, Griffiths J, Waddell C, Anisman H. Stressful life events and coping styles in dysthymia and major depressive disorder: variations associated with alleviation of symptoms following pharmacotherapy. Prog Neuro-Psychopharmacol Biol Psychiatry. 1995;19:637-53.
584. Angst J, Sellaro R, Merikangas KR. Depressive Spectrum Diagnoses Comp. Psychiatry. 2000;41:s39-s47.
585. Angst J, Gamma A, Rössler W, Ajdacic V, Klein DN. Long-term depression versus episodic major depression: Results from the prospective Zurich study of a community sample. J Affect Disord. 2009;115:112-21.
586. Keller MB, Shapiro RW. 'Double depression': Super imposition of acute depressive episodes on chronic depressive disorders. Am J Psychiatry. 1982;139:438-42.
587. Wells KB, Stewart A, Hays RD, et al. The functioning and well-being of depressed patients: results from the Medical Outcomes Study. J Am Med Assoc. 1989;262:914-9.
588. Subodh BN, Avasthi A, Chakrabarti S. Psychosocial impact of dysthymia: A study among married patients J Affect Disord. 2008;109:199-204.
589. First MB, Donovan S, Frances A. Nosology of chronic mood disorders. Psychiatr Clins North Am. 1996;19:29-39.
590. Silva de Lima M, Moncrieff J, Soares B. Drugs versus placebo for dysthymia. Cochrane Database of Systematic Reviews 2005, Issue 2. Art. No.: CD001130. DOI:10.1002/14651858.CD001130.
591. Hellerstein DJ, Batchelder S, Kreditor D, Fedak M. Bupropion sustained-release for the treatment of dysthymic disorder: an open-label study J Clin Psychopharmacol. 2001;21:325-94.
592. Dunner DL, Hendrickson HE, Bea C, Budech CB, O'Connor E. Dysthymic disorder: Treatment with mirtazapine Dep and Anx. 1999;10:68-72.
593. Dunner DL, Hendricksen HE, Bea CBudech CB, Friedman SD. Dysthymic disorder: Treatment with citalopram Dep and Anx. 2002;15:18-22.
594. Ravindran V, Charbonneau Y, Zaharia, Al-Zaid K, Wiens A, Anisman H. Efficacy and tolerability of venlafaxine in the treatment of primary dysthymia J Psychiatry Neurosci. 1998;23:288-92.
595. Koran LM, Aboujaoude EN, Gamel NN. Duloxetine treatment of dysthymia and double depression: an open-label trial. J Clin Psychiatry. 2007;68:761-5.
596. Amore M, Jori MC. Faster response on amisulpride 50 mg versus sertraline 50-100 mg in patients with dysthymia or double depression: a randomized, double-blind, parallel group study. Int Clin Psychopharmacol. 2001;16:317-24.
597. Zanardi R, Smeraldi E. A double-blind, randomised, controlled clinical trial of acetyl-L-carnitine vs. amisulpride in the treatment of dysthymia. European Neuropsychopharmacology. 2006;16:281-7.

598. Fabre LF, Feighner JP. Long-term therapy for depression with trazodone. J Clin Psychiatry. 1983;44:17-21.
599. Harrison W, Rabkin J, Stewart JW, McGrath PJ, Tricarna E, Quitkin F. Phenelzine for chronic depression: A study of continuation treatment. J Clin Psychiatry. 1986;47:346-9.
600. Kocsis JB, Sutton EM, Frances AJ. Long-terms follow up of chronic depression treated with imipramine. J Clin Psychiatry. 1991;52:56-9.
601. Friedman RA, Markowitz JC, Parides M, Gniwesch L, Kocsis JH. Six months of desipramine for dysthymia: can dysthymic patients achieve normal social functioning? Journal of Affective Disorders. 1999;54:283-6.
602. Yonkers KA, Clark RH, Trivedi MH. The psychopharmacological treatment of non-major mood disorders. In Rush AJ eds, Mood disorders. Systematic medication management. Karger. 1997. pp. 146-67.
603. Thase ME, Fava M, Halbreich U, Koran L, Davidson J, Rosenbaum J, et al. A placebo-controlled, randomized clinical trial comparing sertraline and imipramine for the treatment of dysthymia. Arch Gen Psychiatry. 1996;53:777-84.
604. Markowitz Je. Psychotherapy of dysthymia. Am J Psychiatry. 1994;151:1114-21.
605. Beck AT, Rush RJ, Shaw BF, Emery G. Cognitive therapy of depression. New York, Guildford Press, 1979.
606. McCullough JP. Psychotherapy for dysthymia: A naturalistic study of ten patients. Journal of Nervous and Mental Disease. 1991;179:734-40.
607. Klerman GL, Weissman MM, Rousansaville BJ, Chevron ES. Interpersonal psychotherapy of depression. New York, Basic Books; 1984.
608. Markowitz JC, Kocsis JH, Bleiberg KL, Christos PJ, Sacks M. A comparative trial of psychotherapy and pharmacotherapy for pure dysthymic patients J Affect Disord. 2005;89:167-75.
609. Brown G, Steiner M, Roberts J, Gafni A, Byrne C, Dunn E, Bell B, Mills M, Chalklin L, Wallik D, Kraemer J. Sertraline and/or interpersonal psychotherapy for patients with dysthymic disorder in primary care:6-month comparison with longitudinal 2-year follow-up of effectiveness and costs. J Affect Disord. 2002;68:317-30.
610. Imel ZE, Malterera MB, McKaya KM, Wampold BE. A meta-analysis of psychotherapy and medication in unipolar depression and dysthymia J Affect Disord. 2008;110:197-206.
611. Katon W, Russo J, Frank E, Barrett J, Williams JW Jr, Oxman T, Sullivan M, Cornell J. Predictors of nonresponse to treatment in primary care patients with dysthymia Gen Hosp Psychiatry. 2002;24:20-7.
612. McFarland BR, Klein DN. Mental health service use by patients with dysthymic disorder: treatment use and dropout in a 7 1/2-year naturalistic follow-up study Compr Psychiatry. 2005;46:246-53.
613. Svanborg C, Bäärnhielm S, Wistedt AÅ, Lützen K. Helpful and hindering factors for remission in dysthymia and panic disorder at 9-year follow-up: A mixed methods study BMC Psychiatry. 2008, 8:52doi:10.1186/1471-244X-8-52.
614. Klein DN, Shankman SA, Rose S. Ten-year prospective follow-up study of the naturalistic course of dysthymic disorder and double depression. Am J Psychiatry. 2006;163:872-80.
615. Klein DN, Schwartz JE, Rose S, Leader JB. Five-year course and outcome of dysthymic disorder: A prospective, naturalistic follow-up study. Am J Psychiatry. 2000;157:931-9.

Recent Development and Current Controversies in Depression

616. American Psychiatric Association, Diagnostic and statistical manual of mental disorders, 4th edition. Washington, DC: American Psychiatric Association, 1994.
617. Kessler RC, Berglund P, Demler O, et al. The epidemiology of major depressive disorder: results from the national comorbidity survey replication (NCS-R), JAMA. 2003;289:3095-105.
618. WHO, The ICD-10 classification of mental and behavioural disorders: clinical description and diagnostic guidelines (CDDG). Geneva: World Health Organization, 1992.
619. Spijker J, Graff R, Bijl RV, Beekman AT, Ormel J, Nolen WA. Functional disability and depression in the general population. Results from the Netherlands mental health survey and incidence study (NEMESIS). Acta Psychiatr Scand. 2004;110:208-14.
620. Ormel J, Oldehinkel AJ, Nolen WA, Vollebergh W. Psychosocial disability before, during, and after a major depressive episode: a 3-wave population-based study of state, scar, and trait effects. Arch Gen Psychiatry. 2004;61:387-92.
621. Hamalainan J, Isometsa E, Laukkala T, et al. Use of health services for major depressive episode in Finland. J Affect Disord. 2004;79:105-12.
622. Cuijpers P, Smit F. Excess mortality in depression: a meta-analysis of community studies. J Affect Disord. 2002;72:227-36.
623. Guze SB, Robins E. Suicide and primary affective disorders. Br J Psychiatry. 1970;117:437-8.
624. Goodwin FK, Neale MC, Kedler KS. Genetic epidemiology of major depression: review and meta-analysis. Am J Psychiatry. 2000;157:1552-62.
625. Bostwick JM, Pankratz VS. Affective disorders and suicide risk: a re-examination. Am J Psychiatry. 2000;157:1925-32.
626. Sullivan PF, Neale MC, Kendler KS. Genetic epidemiology of major depression: review and meta-analysis. Am J Psychiatry. 2000;157:1552-62.
627. Hong CJ, Tsai SJ. The genomic approaches to major depression. Curr Pharmacogenom. 2003;1:67-74.
628. Schumacher J, Jama RA, Becker T, et al. Evidence for a relationship between genetic variants at the brain-derived neurotrophic factor (BDNF) locus and major depression. Biol Psychiatry. 2005;58:307-14.
629. Tsai SJ, Cheng CY, Yu YW, Chen TJ, Hong CJ. Association study of a brain-derived neurotrophic-factor genetic polymorphism and major depressive disorders, symptomatology, and antidepressant response. Am J Med Genet B Neuropsychiatr Genet. 2003;123:19-22.

630. Hong CJ, Huo SJ, Yen FC, Tung CL, Pan GM, Tsai SJ. Association study of a brain-derived neurotrophic-factor genetic polymorphism and mood disorders, age of onset and suicidal behavior. Neuropsychobiology. 2003;48:186-9.
631. Schulze TG, Muller DJ, Krauss H, et al. Association between a functional polymorphism in the monoamine oxidase A gene promotor and major depressive disorder. Am J Med Genet. 2003;96:801-3.
632. Du L, Bakish D, Ravindran A, Hrdina PD. MAO-A gene polymorphisms are associated with major depression and sleep disturbance in males. Neuroreport. 2004;15:2097-101.
633. Szegedi A, Rujescu D, Tadic A, et al. The catechol-O-methyltransferase Val108/158Met polymorphism affects short-term treatment response to mirtazapine, but not to paroxetine in major depression. Pharmacogenomics J. 2005;5:49-53.
634. Nelson JC. Augmentation strategies in depression 2000. J Clin Psychiatry 2000;61 (Suppl 2):13-9.
635. Zhang X, Gainetdinov RR, Beulieu JM, et al. Loss-of-function mutation in tryptophan hydroxylase-2 identified in unipolar major depression. Neuron. 2005;45:11-6.
636. Caspi A, Sugden K, Moffitt TE, et al. Influence of life stress on depression: moderation by a polymorphism in the 5-HTT gene science. 2003;301:386-9.
637. Gillespie NA, Whitfield JB, Willams B, Heath AC, Martin NG. The relationship between stressful life events, the serotonin transporter (5-HTTLPR) genotype and major depression. Psychol Med. 2004;35:101-11.
638. Kendler KS, Kuhn JW, Vittum J, Prescott CA, Riley B. The interaction of stressful life events and a serotonin transporter polymorphism in the prediction of episodes of major depression: a replication. Arch Gen Psychiatry. 2005;62:529-35.
639. Hariri AR, Mattay VS, Tessitore A, et al. Serotonin transporter genetic variation and the response of the human amygdala. Science. 2002;297:400-3.
640. Fallgatter AJ, Herrmann MJ, Roemmler J, et al. Allelic variation of serotonin transporter function modulates the brain electrical response for error processing. Neuropsychopharmacology. 2004;29:1506-11.
641. Frodl T, Meisenzahl EM, Zill P, et al. Reduced hippocampal volumes associated with the long variant of the serotonin transporter polymorphism in major depression. Arch Gen Psychiatry. 2004;61:177-83.
642. Taylor WD, Steffens DC, Payne ME, et al. Influence of serotonin transporter promoter region polymorphisms on hippocampal volumes in late-life depression. Arch Gen Psychiatry. 2005;62:537-44.
643. Kirchheiner J, Nickchen K, Bauer M, et al. Pharmacogenetics of antidepressants and antipsychotics: the contribution of allelic variations to the phenotype of drug response. Mol Psychiatry. 2004;9:433-41.
644. Smits KM, Smits LJ, Schouten JS, Stelma FF, Nelemans P, Prins MH. Influence of SERTPR and Stin2 in the serotonin transporter gene on the effect of selective serotonin reuptake inhibitors in depression: a systematic review. Mol Psychiatry. 2004;9:433-41.
645. Ilsley JE, Moffoot AP, O'Carroll RE, An analysis of memory dysfunction major depression. J Affect Disord. 1995;35:1-9.
646. Sweeney JA, Kmiec JA, Kuper DJ. Neuropsychologic impairments in bipolar and unipolar mood disorders on the CANTAB neurocognitive battery. Biol Psychiatry. 2000;48:674-84.
647. Airaksinen E, Larsson M, Lundberg I, Forsell Y. Cognitive functions in depressive disorders: evidence from a population based study. Psychol Med. 2004;34:83-91.
648. Sheline YI, Wang PW, Gado MH, Csernansky JG, Vannier MW. Hippocampal atrophy in recurrent major depression. Proc Natl Acad Sci USA. 1996;93:3908-13.
649. Shah PHJ, Ebmeier KP, Glabus MF, Goodwin GM. Cortical grey matter reductions associated with treatment-resistant chronic unipolar depression. Controlled magnetic resonance imaging study Br J Psychiatry. 1998;172:527-32.
650. Austin MP, Mitchell P, Goodwin GM. Cognitive deficits in depression: possible implications for functional neuropathology. Br J Psychiatry. 2001;178:200-6.
651. Fossati P, Harvey PO, Le Bastard G, Ergis AM, Jouvent R, Allilaire JF. Verbal memory performance of patients with a first recurrent depression. J Psychiatr Res. 2004;38:137-44.
652. Fossati P, Coyette F, Ergis AM, Allilaire JF. Influence of age and depression. J Affect Disorde. 2002;68:261-71.
653. Porter RJ, Gallagher P, Thompson JM, Young AH. Neurocognitive impairment in drug-free patients with major depressive disorder. Br J Psychiatry. 2003;182:214-20.
654. Harvey PO, Le Bastard G, Pochon JB, et al. Executive functions and updating of the contents of working memory in unipolar depression. J Psychiatr Res. 2004;38:567-76.
655. Sobin C, Sackeim HA. Psychomotor symptoms of depression. Am J Psychiatry. 1997;154:4-17.
656. Pier MP, Hulstijn W, Sabbe BG. No psychomotor slowing in fine motor tasks in dysthymia. J Affect Disrd. 2004;83:109-20.
657. Videbech P, Ravnkilde B. Hippocampal volume and depression: a meta-analysis of MRI studies. Am J Psychiatry. 2004;161:1957-66.
658. Campbell S, Marriott M, Nahmias C, MacQueen GM. Lower hippocampal volume in patients suffering from depression: a meta-analysis. Am J Psychiatry. 2004;161:598-607.
659. Shah PJ, Glabus MF, Goodwin GM, Ebmeier KP. Chronic treatment-resistant depression and right fronto-striatal atrophy. Br J Psychiatry. 2002;180:434-40.
660. Bremner JD, Randall P, Scott TM, et al. MRI-based measurement of hippocampal volume in patient swith combat-related posttraumatic stress disorder. Am J Psychiatry. 1995;152:973-81.
661. Bermner JD, Randall P, Vermetten E, et al. Magnetic resonance imaging-based measurement of hippocampal volume in posttraumatic stress disorder related to childhood physical and sexual abuse-a preliminary report. Biol Psychiatry. 1997;41:23-32.
662. Gurvits TV, Shenton ME, Hokama H, et al. Magnetic resonance imaging study of hippocampal volume in chronic, combat-related posttraumatic stress disorder. Biol Psychiatry. 1996;40:1091-9.

663. Stein MB, Koverola C, Hanna C, Torchia MG, McClarty B. Hippocampal volume in women victimized by childhood sexual abuse. Psychol Med. 1997;27:951-9.
664. Campbell S, Macqueen G. The role of the hippocampus in the pathophysiology of major depression. J Psychiatry Neurosci. 2004;29:417-26.
665. Fuchs E, Czeh B, Kole MH, Micheaelis T, Lucassen PJ. Alterations of neuroplasticity in depression: the hippocampus and beyond. Eur Neuropsycho-pharmacol. 2004;14 (Supp 5):S481-90.
666. Fuchs E, Czeh B, Flugge G. Examining novel concepts of the pathophysiology of depression in the chronic psychosocial stress paradigm in tree shrews. Behav Pharmacol. 2004;15: 315-25.
667. McEwen BS, Chattarji S. Molecular mechanisms of neuroplasticity and pharmacological implications: the example of tianeptine. Eur Neuropsychopharmacol. 2004;14 (Suppl 5):S497-502.
668. Duman RS. Depression: a case of neuronal life and death? Biol Psychiatry. 2004;56:140-5.
669. Reid IC, Steward CA. How antidepressants work: new perspectives on the pathophysiology of depressive disorder. Br J Psychiatry. 2001;178:299-303.
670. Squire LR. Memory and the hippocampus: a synthesis from findings with rats, monkeys, and humans. Psychol Rev. 1992;99:191-231.
671. Ebert D, Ebmeier KP. The role of the cingulated gyrus in depression: from functional anatomy to neurochemistry. Biol Psychiatry. 1996;39:1044-50.
672. Drevets WC. Neuroimaging studies of mood disorders. Biol Psychiatry. 2000;48:813-29.
673. Mayberg HS. Modulating dysfunctional limbic-cortical circuits in depression: towards development of brain-based algorithms for diagnosis and optimized treatment. In: Frackowiak RS, Jones T, (Eds). Imaging neuroscience: clinical frontiers for diagnosis and management. Oxford: Oxford University Press; 2003. pp. 193-207.
674. Ebmeier KP, Kronhaus D. Brain imaging and mood disorders. In: D'haenen H, den Boer JA, Willner P, (Eds). Biological psychiatry. London: John Wiley and Sons, 2002.
675. Steele JD, Lawrie SM. Neuroimaging In: Johnstone EC, Lawrie SM, (Eds). Edinburgh companion to psychiatric studies. Edinburgh: Churchill Livingstone, 2004.
676. Rolls ET. The brain and emotion. Oxford: Oxford University Press, 1999.
677. Steele JD, Lawrie SM. Segregation of cognitive and emotional function in the prefrontal cortex: a stereotactic meta-analysis. Neuroimage. 2004;21:868-75.
678. Vogt BA, Finch DM, Olson CR. Functional heterogeneity in cingulated cortex: the anterior executive and posterior evaluative regions. Cereb Cortex. 1992;2:435-43.
679. Fuster JM. The prefrontal cortex. New York: Lippincott-Raven, 1997.
680. Drevets WC. Functional anatomical abnormalities in limbic and prefrontal cortical structures in major depression In: Uylings HBM, Van Eden CG, De Bruin JPC, Feenstra MGP, Pennartz CMA, (Eds). Progress in brain research. London: Elsevier Science, 2000.
681. Dougherty DD, Weiss AP, Cosgrove GR, et al. Cerebral metabolic correlates as potential predictors of response to anterior cingulatormy for treatment of major depression. J Neurosurg. 2003;99:1010-7.
682. Okada G, Oamoto Y, Morinobu S, Yamawaki S, Yokota N. Attenuated left prefrontal activation during a verbal fluency task in patients with depression. Neuropsychobiology. 2003;48:21-6.
683. Pochon JB, Levy R, Fossati P, et al. The neural system that bridges reward and cognition in humans: an fMRI study. Proc Natl Acad Sci USA. 2002;99:5669-74.
684. Drevets WC, Raichle ME. Reciprocal suppression of regional cerebral blood flow during emotional versus higher cognitive processes: implications for interactions between emotion and cognition. Cogn Emotion. 1998;12:353-85.
685. Kumari V, Mitterschiffthaler MT, Teasdale JD, et al. Neural abnormalities during cognitive generation of affect in treatment resistant depression. Biol Psychiatry. 2003;54:777-91.
686. Gray JA, McNaughton N. The neuropsychology of anxiety: an inquiry into the functions of the septo-hippocampal system, 2nd edn, Oxford: Oxford University Press, 2000.
687. Heath RG. Correlation of brain function with emotional behavior. Biol Psychiatry. 1976;11:463-80.
688. Elliott R, Rubinsztein JS, Sahakian BJ, Dolan RJ. The neural basis of mood-congruent processing biases in depression. Arch Gen Psychiatry. 2002;59:597-604.
689. Surguladze S, Brammer MJ, Keedwell P, et al. A differential pattern of neural response toward sad versus happy facial expressions in major depressive disorder. Biol Psychiatry. 2005;57:201-9.
690. Siegle GJ, Steinhauer SR, Thase ME, Stenger VA, Carter CS. Can't shake that feeling:event-related fMRI assessment of sustained amygdala activity in response to emotional information in depressed individuals. Biol Psychiatry. 2002;51:693-707.
691. Steele JD, Meyer M, Ebmeier KP. Neural predictive error signal correlates with depressive illness severity in a game paradigm. Neuroimage. 2004;23:269-80.
692. Steele JD. Depressive illness and emotional learning. Curr Med Imaging Rev. 2005;1:157-76.
693. Luu P, Collins P, Tucker DM. Mood, personality, and self-monitoring: negative affect and emotionality in relation to frontal lobe mechanisms of error monitoring. J Exp Psychol Gen. 2000;129:43-60.
694. Holroud CB, Nieuwenhuis S, Mars RB, Coles MG. Anterior cingulated cortex, selection for action, and error processing. In: Posner MJ, (Ed). Cognitive neuroscience of attention. London: Guildford Press, 2004.
695. Holroyd CB, Nieuwenhuis S, Yeung N, et al. Dorsal anterior cingulated cortex shows fMRI response to internal and external error signals. Nat Neurosci. 2004;7:497-8.
696. Luu P, Tucker DM, Derryberry D, Reed M, Poulsen C. Electrophysiological responses to errors and feedback in the process of action regulation. Psychol Sci. 2003;14:47-53.

697. Luu P, Pederson SM. The anterior cingulated cortex, regulating actions in context. In: Posner MJ, (Ed). Cognitive neuroscience of attention. London: Guildford Press, 2004.
698. Hajcak G, McDonald N, Simons RF. Anxiety and error-related brain activity. Biol Psychol. 2003;64:77-90.
699. Holroyd CB, Yeung N. Alcohol and error processing. Trends Neurosci. 2003;26:402-4.
700. Gehring WJ, Himle J, Nisenson LG. Action-monitoring dysfunction in obsessive-compulsive disorder. Psychol Sci. 2000;11:1-6.
701. Ruchsow M, Hermberger B, Wiesend C, Gron G, Spitzer M, Kiefer M. The effect of erroneous responses on response monitoring in patients with major depressive disorder: a study with event-related potentials. Psychophysiology. 2004;41:833-40.
702. Ruchsow M, Hernberger B, Wiesend C, Gron G, Spitzer M, Kiefer M. Error processing in major depressive disorder: evidence from event-related potentials. J Psychiatr Res 2005; published online May 6, DOI:10.1016/j-jpsychites.2005.02.002.
703. Holroyds CB, Coles MG. The neural basis of human error processing: reinforcement learning, dopamine, and the error related negativity. Psychol Rev. 2002;109:679-709.
704. Beck AT, Rush AJ, Shaw BF, Emery G. Cognitive therapy of depression: a treatment manual. New York: Gulford Press. 1979.
705. Scott J. Cognitive therapy for depression. Br Med Bull. 2001;57:101-13.
706. Thase ME, Friedman ES, Berman SR, et al. Is cognitive behavior therapy just a 'nonspecific' intervention for depression? A retrospective comparison of consecutive cohorts treated with cognitive behavior therapy or supportive counseling and pill placebo. J Affect Disord. 1998;49:59-72.
707. Gloaguen V, Cottraux J, Cuchert M, Blackburn IM. A meta-analysis of the effects of cognitive therapy in depressed patients. J Affect Disord. 1998;49:59-72.
708. King M, Sibbald B, Ward E, et al. Randomised controlled trial of non-directive counseling, cognitive-behaviour therapy and usual general practitioner care in the management of depression as well as mixed anxiety and depression in primary care. Health Technol Assess. 2000;4:1-83.
709. Perlis RH, Nierenberg AA, Alpert JE, et al. Effects of adding cognitive therapy to fluoxetine dose increase on risk of relapse and residual depressive symptoms in continuation treatment of major depressive disorder. J Clin Psychopharmacol. 2002;22:474-80.
710. Thase ME, Friedman ES, Fasiczka AL, et al. Treatment of men with major depression: a comparison of sequential cohorts treated with either cognitive-behavioral therapy or newer generation antidepressants. J Clin Psychiatry. 2000;61:466-72.
711. de Jonghe F, Hendricksen M, van Aalst G, et al. Psychotherapy alone and combined with pharmacotherapy in the treatment of depression. Br J Psychiatry 2004;185:37-45.
712. Paykel ES, Scott J, Tesdale JD, et al. Prevention of relapse in residual depression by cognitive therapy: a controlled trial. Arch Gen Psychiatry. 1999;56:829-35.
713. Teasdale JD, Segal ZV, Williams JM, Ridgeway VA, Soulsby JM, Lau MA. Prevention of relapse/recurrence in major depression by mindfulness-based cognitive therapy. J Consult Clin Psychol. 2000;68:615-23.
714. Paykel ES, Scott J, Cornwall PL, et al. Duration of relapse prevention after cognitive therapy in residual depression: follow-up of controlled trial. Psychol Med. 2005;35:59-68.
715. Hensley PL, Nadiga D, Uhlenhuth EH. Long-term effectiveness of cognitive therapy in major depressive disorder. Depress Anxiety. 2004;20:1-7.
716. Kleman GL, Weismann NM, Rounsaville BJ, Chevron ES. Interpersonal psychotherapy of depression. New York: Basic Books, 1984.
717. Barkham M, Hardy GE. Counselling and interpersonal therapies for depression: towards securing an evidence-base, Br Med Bull. 2001;57:115-32.
718. NICE, Depression: management of depression in primary and secondary care. Clinical Guidance 23. London: National Institute for Clinical Excellence, 2004.
719. Frank E, Grochocinski VJ, Spanier CA, et al. Interpersonal psychotherapy and antidepressant medication: evaluation of a sequential treatment strategy in women with recurrent major depression. J Clin Psychiatry. 2000;61:51-7.
720. Browne G, Steiner M, Roberts J, et al. Sertraline and/or interpersonal psychotherapy for patients with dysthymic disorder in primary care:6-month comparison with longitudinal 2-year follow-up of effectiveness and costs. J Affect Disord. 2002;68:317-30.
721. Frank E, Thase ME. Natural history and preventive treatment of recurrent mood disorders. Annu Rev Med. 1999;50:453-68.
722. Reynolds CF 3rd, Frank E, Perel JM, et al. Nortriptyline and interpersonal psychotherapy as maintenance therapies for recurrent major depression: a randomized controlled trial in patients older than 59 years. JAMA. 1999;281:39-45.
723. Nezu AM. Problem solving and behavior therapy revisited. Behavior Therapy. 2004;35:1-33.
724. Nezu AM, Nezu CM. Problem solving therapy. J Psychother Integr. 2001;11:187-205.
725. Mynors-Wallis LM, Gath DH, Day A, Baker F. Randomised controlled trial of problem solving treatment, antidepressant medication, and combined treatment for major depression in primary care. BMJ. 2000;320:26-30.
726. Dowrick C, Dunn G, Ayuso-Mateos JL, et al. Problem solving treatment and group psychoeducation for depression: multi-centre randomized controlled trial. Outcomes of Depression International Network (ODIN) Group. BMJ. 2000;321:1450-4.
727. Barrett JE, Williams JW Jr, Oxman TE, et al. Treatment of dysthymia and minor depression in primary care: a randomized trial in patients aged 18 to 59 years. J Fam Pract. 2001;50:405-12.
728. Frank E, Rucci P, Katon W, et al. Correlates of remission in primary care patients treated for minor depression. Gen Hosp Psychiatry. 2002;24:12-9.
729. Wampold BE, Minami T, Baskin TW, Callen Tierney S. A meta-(re)analysis of the effects of cognitive therapy versus other therapies for depression. J Affect Disord. 2002;68:159-65.

730. Nutt DJ. Death and dependence: current controversies over the selective serotonin reuptake inhibitors. J Psychopharmacol. 2003;17:355-64.
731. Walsh MT, Dinan TG. Selective serotonin reuptake inhibitors and violence: a review of the available evidence. Acta Psychiatr Scand. 2001;104:84-91.
732. Herxheimer A, Mintzes B. Antidepressants and adverse effects in young patients: uncovering the evidence. CMAJ. 2004;170:487-9.
733. Committee on Energy and Commerce. FDA's role in protecting the public health: examining FDA's review of safety of efficacy concerns in anti-depressant use by children. Hearing before the subcommittee on oversight and investigations of the committee on energy and commerce. Washington. DC: House of representatives. One Hundred Eighth Congress, Second Session, 2004.
734. Weller IVD, Ashby D, Brook R, et al. Report of the committee on Safety of Medicines expert working group on the safety of selective serotonin reuptake inhibitor antidepressants. London: Medicines and Healthcare products Regulatory Agency, 2004.
735. Davidoff F, DeAngelis CD, Drazen JM, et al. Sponsorship, authorship, and accountability. Lancet. 2001;358:854-6.
736. Fava GA. Conflict of interest in psychopharmacology: can Dr Jekyll still control Mr Hyde? Psychiather Psychosom. 2004;73:1-4.
737. Whittington CJ, Kendall T, Fonagy P, Cottrell D, Cotgrove A, Boddington E. Selective serotonin reuptake inhibitors in childhood depression: systematic review of published versus unpublished data. Lancet. 2004;363:1341-5.
738. Wohlfarth T, Lekkerkerker F, van Zwieten B. Use of selective serotonin reuptake inhibitors in childhood depression. Lancet. 2004;364:659-60.
739. Gibbons RD, Hur K, Bhaumik DK, Mann JJ. The relationship between antidepressant medication use and rate of suicide. Arch Gen Psychiatry. 2005;62:165-72.
740. Grunebaum MF, Ellis SP, Li S, Oquendo MA, Mann JJ. Antidepressants and suicide risk in the United States, 1985-1999. J Clin Psychiatry. 2004;65:1456-62.
741. Gunnell D, Saperia J, Ashby D. Selective serotonin reuptake inhibitors (SSRIs) and suicide in adults: meta-analysis of drug company data from placebo controlled, randomized controlled trials submitted to the MHRA's safety review. BMJ. 2005;330:385.
742. Fergusson D, Doucette S, Glass KC, et al. Association between suicide attempts and selective serotonin reuptake inhibitors: systematic review of randomized controlled trials. BMJ. 2005;330:396.
743. Jick H, Kaye JA, Jick SS. Antidepressants and the risk of suicidal behaviours. JAMA. 2004;292:338-43.
744. Martinez C, Rietbrock S, Wise L, et al. Antidepressant treatment and the risk of fatal and non-fatal self harm in first episode depression: nested case-control study. BMJ. 2005;330: 389.
745. Isacsson G, Holmgren P, Ahlner J. Selective serotonin reuptake inhibitor antidepressants and the risk of suicide : a controlled forensic database study of 14,857 suicides. Acta Psychiatr Scand. 2005;111:286-90.
746. Sanz EJ, De-las-Cuevas C, Kiuru A, Bate A, Edwards R. Selective serotonin reuptake inhibitors in pregnant women and neonatal withdrawal syndrome: a database analysis. Lancet. 2005;365:482-7.
747. Burt T, Lisanby SH, Sackeim HA. Neuropsychiatric applications of transcranial magnetic stimulation: a meta-analysis. Int J Neuropsychopharmacol. 2002;5:73-103.
748. Pascual-Leone A, Rubio B, Pallardo F, Catala MD. Rapid-rate transcranial magnetic stimulation of left dorsolateral prefrontal cortex in drug-resistant depression. Lancet. 1996;348:233-7.
749. George MS, Wassermann EM, Kimbrell TA, et al. Mood improvement following daily left prefrontal repetitive transcranial magnetic stimulation in the treatment of medication-resistant depression: a placebo controlled crossover trial. Am J Psychiatry. 1997;154:1752-6.
750. Avery DH, Claypoole K, Robinson L, et al. Repetitive transcranial magnetic stimulation in the treatment of medication-resistant depression: preliminary data. J Nerv Ment Dis. 1999;18:114-7.
751. Kimbrell Ta, Little JT, Dunn RT, et al. Frequency dependence of antidepressant response to left prefrontal repetitive transcranial magnetic stimulation (rTMS) as a function of baseline cerebral glucose metabolism. Biol Psychiatry. 1999;46:1603-13.
752. Klein E, Kreinin I, Chistyakov A, et al. Therapeutic efficacy of right prefrontal slow repetitive transcranial magnetic stimulation in major depression: a double-blind controlled study. Arch Gen Psychiatry. 1999;56:315-20.
753. Loo C, Mitchell P, Sachdev P, Mc Darmont B, Parker G, Gandevia S. Double-blind controlled investigation of transcranial magnetic stimulation for the treatment of resistant major depression. Am J Psychiatry. 1999;156:946-8.
754. Padberg F, Zwanzger P, Thoma H, et al. Repetitive transcranial magnetic stimulation (rTMS) in pharmacotherapy-refractory major depression: comparative study of fast, slow and sham rTMS. Psychiatry Res. 1999;88:163-71.
755. Stikhina N, Lyskov EB, Lomarev MP, Aleksanian ZA, Mihailov VO, Medvedev SV. [Transcranial magnetic stimulation neurotic depression]. Zh Nevrol Psikhiatr Im SS Korsakova. 1999;99:26-9.
756. Berman RM, Narasimhan M, Sanacora G, et al. A randomized clinical trial of repetitive transcranial magnetic stimulation in the treatment of major depression. Biol Psychiatry. 2000;47:332-7.
757. Eschweiler GW, Wegerer C, Schlotter W, et al. Left prefrontal activation predicts therapeutic effects of repetitive transcranial magnetic stimulation (rTMS) in major depression. Psychiatry Res. 2000;99:161-72.
758. George MS, Nahas Z, Molloy M, et al. A controlled trial of daily left prefrontal cortex TMS for treating depression. Biol psychiatry. 2000;48:962-70.
759. Garcia-Toro M, Pascual-Leone A, Romera M, et al. Prefrontal repetitive transcranial magnetic stimulation as add on

treatment in depression. J Neurol Neurosurg Psychiatry. 2001;71:546-8.

760. Lisanby SH, Pascual-Leone A, Sampson SM, Boylan LS, Burt T, Sackeim HA. Augmentation of sertraline antidepressant treatment with transcranial magnetic stimulation. Biol psychiatry. 2001;49:81S-S.
761. Manes F, Jorge R, Morcuende M, Yamada T, Paradiso S, Robinson RG. A controlled study of repetitive transcranial magnetic stimulation as a treatment of depression in the elderly. Int Psychogeriatr. 2001;13:225-31.
762. Boutros NN, Gueorguieva R, Hoffman RE, Oren DA, Feingold A, Berman RM. Lack of a therapeutic effect of a 2-week sub-threshold transcranial magnetic stimulation course for treatment resistant depression. Psychol Med. 2003;33:33-40.
763. Padberg F, Zwanzger P, Keck ME, et al. Repetitive transcranial magnetic stimulation (rTMS) in major depression: relation between efficacy and stimulation intensity. Neuropsychopharmacology. 2002;27:638-45.
764. Loo CK, Mitchell PB, Croker VM, et al. Double-blind controlled investigation of bilateral prefrontal transcranial magnetic stimulation for the treatment of resistant major depression. Psychol Med. 2003;33:33-40.
765. Nahas Z, Kozel FA, Li X, Anderson B, George MS. Left prefrontal transcranial magnetic stimulation (TMS) treatment of depression in bipolar affective disorder: a plot study of acute safety and efficacy. Bipolar Disord. 2003;5:40-7.
766. 159.Herwig U, Lampe Y, Juengling FD, et al. Add-on rTMS for treatment of depression: a pilot study using stereotaxic coil-navigation according to PET data. J Psychiatr Res. 2003;37:267-75.
767. Hoeppner J, Schulz M, Irmisch G, Mau R, Schlafke D, Richter J. Antidepressant efficacy of two different rTMS procedures. High frequency over left versus low frequency over right prefrontal cortex compared with sham stimulatin. Eur Arch Psychiatry Clin Neurosci. 2003;253:103-9.
768. Fitzgerald PB, Brown TL, Marston NA, Daskalakis ZJ, De Castella A, Kulkarni J. Transcranial magnetic stimulation in the treatment of depression: a double-blind, sham controlled "add on" trial. J Neurol Neurosurg Psychiatry. 2004;75:320-2.
769. Haussmann A, Kemmler G, Walpoth M, et al. No benefit derived from repetitive transcranial magnetic stimulation in depression: a prospective, single centre, randomized, double blind, sham controlled "add on" trial. J Neurol Neurosurg Psychiatry. 2004;75:320-2.
770. Jorge RE, Robinson RG, Tateno A, et al. Repetitive transcranial magnetic stimulation as treatment of poststroke depression: a preliminary study. Biol Psychiatry. 2004;55:398-405.
771. Holtzheimer PE 3rd, Russo J, Claypoole KH, Roy-Byrne P, Avery DH. Shorter duration of depressive episode may predict response to repetitive transcranial magnetic stimulation. Depress Anxiety. 2004;19:24-9.
772. Kuffmann CD, Cheema MA, Miller BE. Slow right prefrontal transcranial magnetic stimulation as a treatment for medication-resistant depression: a double-blind, placebo-controlled study. Depress Anxiety. 2004;19:59-62.
773. Mosimann UP, Schmitt W, Greenberg BD, et al. Repetitive transcranial magnetic stimulation: a putative add-on treatment for major depression in elderly patients. Psychiatry Res. 2004;126:123-33.
774. Poulet E, Brunelin J, Boeuve C, et al. Repetitive transcranial magnetic stimulation does not potentiate antidepressant treatment. Eur Psychiatry. 2004;19:382-3.
775. Koerselman F, Laman DM, van Dujin H, van Duijin MA. Willems MA. A 3-month, follow-up, randomized, placebo controlled study of repetitive transcranial magnetic stimulation in depression. J Clin Psychiatry. 2004;65:1323-8.
776. Dunlap WP, Cortnia JM, Vaslow JB. Burke MJ. Meta-analysis of experiments with matched groups or repeated measures designs. Psychol Methods. 1996;1:170-7.
777. Shahahan PM, Glabus MF, Steele JD, et al. Left dorso-lateral repetitive transcranial magnetic stimulation affects cortical excitability and functional connectivity, but does not impair cognition in major depression. Prog Neuropsychopharmacol Biol Psychiatry. 2002;26:945-54.
778. Strafella AP, Paus T, Fraraccio M, Dagher A. Straiatal dopamine release induced by repetitive transcranial magnetic stimulation of the human motor cortex. Brain. 2003;126:2609-15.
779. Keck ME, Welt T, Muller MB, et al. Repetitive transcranial magnetic stimulation increases the release of dopamine in the mesolimbic and mesostriatal system. Neuropharmacology. 2002;43:101-9.
780. Huang YZ, Edwards MJ, Rounis E, Bhatia KP, Rothwell JC. Theta burst stimulation of the human motor cortex. Nueron. 2005;45:201-6.
781. Wassermann EM. Risk and safety of repetitive transcranial magnetic stimulation: report and suggested guidelines from the international workshop on the safety of repetitive transcranial magnetic stimulation, 1996.
782. Lisanby SH, Luber B, Schlaepfer TE, Sackeim HA. Safety and feasibility of magnetic seizure therapy (MST) in major depression: randomized within-subject comparison with electroconvulsive therapy. Neuropsychopharmacology. 2003;28:1852-65.
783. Dwork AJ, Arango V, Underwood M, et al. Absence of histological lesions in primate models of ECT and magnetic seizure therapy. Am J Psychiatry. 2004;161:576-8.
784. Kosel M, Frick G, Lisanby SH, Fisch HU, Schlaepfer TE. Magnetic seizure therapy improves mood in refractory major depression. Neuropsychopharmacology. 2003;28:2045-8.
785. Lisanby SH, Moscrip T, Morales O, Luber B, Schroeder C, Sackeim HA. Neurophysiological characterization of magnetic seizure therapy (MST) in non-human primates. Suppl Clin Neurophysiol. 2003;56:81-99.
786. UK ECT Review Group. Efficacy and safety of electroconvulsive therapy in depressive disorders: a systematic review and meta-analysis. Lancet. 2003;361:799-808.

787. NICE. Technology appraisal guidance 59: electroconvulsive treatment, technology appraisal guidances. London: National Institute for Clinical Excellence, 2003.
788. Lisanby SH, Maddox JH, Prudic J, Devanand DP, Sackeim HA. The effects of electroconvulsive therapy on memory of autobiographical and public events. Arch Gen Psychiatry. 2000;57:581-90.
789. Greenberg RM, Kellner CH. Electroconvulsive therapy: a selected review. Am J Geriatr Psychiatry. 2005;13:268-81.
790. Sackeim HA, Haskett RF, Mulsant BH, et al. Continuation pharmacotherapy in the prevention of relapse following electroconvulsive therapy: a randomized controlled trial. JAMA. 2001;285:1299-307.
791. Mayberg HS, Lozano AM, Voon V, et al. Deep brain stimulation for treatment-resistant depression. Neuron. 2005;45:651-60.
792. CRAG Working Group. Neurosurgery for mental disorder (J23187/96). Edinburgh: HM Stationery Office Scotland, 1996.
793. Nuttin B, Cosyns P, Demeulemeester H, Gybels J, Meyerson B. Electrical stimulation in anterior limbs of internal capsules in patients with obsessive-compulsive disorder. Lancet. 1999;354:1526.
794. Sturm V, Lenartz D, Koulousakis A, et al. The nucleus accumbens: a target for deep brain stimulation obsessive-compulsive and anxiety-disorders. J Chem Neuroanat. 2003;26:293-9.

Treatment Resistant Depression

795. Kessler RC, Berglund P, Demler O, et al. The epidemiology of major depressive disorder. results from the National Comorbidity Survey replication (NCS-R). JAMA. 2003;289:3095-105.
796. Fava M, Davidson KG. Definition and epidemiology of treatment-resistant depression. Psychiatr Clin North Am. 1996;19:179-200.
797. Berlim MT, Turecki G. Definition, assessment and staging of treatment-resistant refractory major depression: a review of current concepts and methods. Can J Psychiatry. 2007;52:46-54.
798. Fagiolini A, Kupfer DJ. Is treatment-resistant depression a unique subtype of depression? Biol Psychiatry. 2003;53:640-8.
799. Keller MB, Shapiro RW, Lavori PW, Wolfe N. Recovery in major depression disorder: analysis with the life table and regression models. Arch Gen Psychiatry. 1982;39:905-10.
800. Bauer M, Bschor T, Pfennig A, et al. World Federation of Societies of Biological Psychiatry (WFSBP) Guidelines for Biological Treatment of Unipolar Depressive Disorders in Primary Care. World J Biol Psychiatry. 2007;8:67-104.
801. Crismon ML, Trivedi M, Pigott TA, et al. The Texas Medication Algorithm Project: report of the Texas Consensus Conference Panel on Medication Treatment of Major Depressive Disorder. J Clin Psychiatry. 1999;60:142-56.
802. Kennedy SH, Lam RW, Cohen NL, et al. Clinical guidelines for the treatment of depressive disorders IV. Medications and other biological treatments. Can J Psychiatry. 2001;46(suppl 1):38S-58S.
803. American Psychiatric Association. Practice guidelines for the treatment of patients with major depressive disorder (revision). Am J Psychiatry. 2000;157(Suppl 4):1-45.
804. Thase ME, Feighner JP, Lydiard RB. Citalopram treatment of fluoxetine nonresponders. J Clin Psychiatry. 2001;62:683-7.
805. Papakostas GI, Fava M, Thase ME. Treatment of SSRI-resistant depression: A meta-analysis comparing within-versus across-class switches. Biol Psychiatry. 2008;63:699-704.
806. Rush AJ, Trivedi MH, Wisniewski SR, et al. Bupropion-SR, sertraline, or venlafaxine-XR after failure of SSRIs for depression. N Engl J Med. 2006;354:1231-42.
807. Koch S, Hemrick-Luecke SK, Thompson LK, et al. Comparison of effects of dual transporter inhibitors on monoamine transporters and extracellular levels in rats. Neuropharmacology. 2003;45:935-44.
808. Karp JF, Whyte EM, Lenze EJ, et al. Rescue pharmacotherapy with duloxetine for selective serotonin reuptake inhibitor nonresponders in late-life depression: outcome and tolerability. J Clin Psychiatry. 2008;69:457-63.
809. Norman TR, Burrows GD. Emerging treatments for major depression. Expert Rev Neurotherapeutics. 2007;7:203-13.
810. Overstreet DH, Stemmelin J, Griebel G. Confirmation of antidepressant potential of the selective β3 adrenoreceptor agonist amibegron in an animal model of depression. Pharmacol Biochem Behav. 2008;89:623-6.
811. Tsai SJ. Sipatrigine could have therapeutic potential for major depression and bipolar depression through antagonism of the two-pore-domain K+ channel TREK-1. Med Hypotheses. 2008;70:548-50.
812. Krishnan V, Nestler EJ. The molecular neurobiology of depression. Nature. 2008;455:894-902.
813. Maeng S, Zarate CA Jr, Du J, et al. Cellular mechanisms underlying the antidepressant effects of ketamine: role of a-amino-3-hydroxy-5-methylisoxazole-4-proprionic acid receptors. Biol Psychiatry. 2008;63:349-52.
814. Skolnick P. AMPA receptors: a target for novel antidepressants? Biol Psychiatry. 2008;63:347-8.
815. Zarate CA, Singh JB, Carlson PJ, et al. A randomized trial of an N-methyl-d-aspartate antagonist in treatment-resistant major depression. Arch Gen Psychiatry. 2006;63:856-64.
816. Ferguson JM, Shingleton RN. An open-label, flexible-dose study of memantine in major depressive disorder. Clin Neuropharmacolgy. 2007;30:136-44.
817. Muhonen LH, Lönngvist J, Juva K, Alho H. Double-blind, randomized comparison of memantine and escitalopram for the treatment of major depressive disorder comorbid with alcohol dependence. J Clin Psychiatry. 2008;69:392-9.
818. Zarate CA, Singh JB, Quiroz JA, et al. A double-blind placebo-controlled study of memantine in the treatment of major depression. Am J Psychiatry. 2006;163:153-5.
819. Berlim MT, Fleck MP, Turecki G. Current trends in the assessment and somatic treatment of resistant/refractory major depression: an overview. Ann Med. 2008;40: 149-59.

820. Papkostas GI, Worthington JJ, Iosifescu DV, et al. The combination of duloxetine and bupropion for treatment-resistant major depressive disorder. Depress Anxiety. 2006;23:178-81.
821. Lam RW, Hossie H, Solomons K, Yatham LN. Citalopram and bupropion SR: combining versus switching in patients with treatment-resistant depression. J Clin Psychiatry. 2004;65:337-40.
822. Barowsky J, Schwartz TL. Part 1: An evidence-based approach to augmentation and combination strategies for treatment-resistant depression. Psychiatry. 2006;3:42-61.
823. Carvalho AF, Cavalcante JL, Castelo MS, Lima MC. Augmentation strategies for treatment-resistant depression: a literature review. J Clin Pharm Ther. 2007;32:415-28.
824. DeBattista C, Lembke A. Update on augmentation of antidepressant response in resistant depression. Curr Psychiatry Rep. 2005;7:435-40.
825. Nierenberg AA, Katz J, Fava M. A critical overview of the pharmacologic management of treatment-resistant depression. Psychiatr Clin North Am. 2007;30:13-29.
826. Thase ME. Pharmacologic strategies for treatment-resistant depression. Psychiatr Ann. 2005;35:970-8.
827. Fava M, Alpert J, Nierenberg A, et al. Double-blind study of high-dose fluoxetine versus lithium or desipramine augmentation of fluoxetine in partial responders and nonresponders to fluoxetine. J Clin Psychopharmacol. 2002;22:379-87.
828. Crossley NA, Bauer M. Acceleration and augmentation of antidepressants with lithium for depressive disorders: two meta-analyses of randomized, placebo-controlled trials. J Clin Psychiatry. 2007;68:935-40.
829. Gaynes BN, Rush AJ, Trivedi MH, et al. The STAR*D study: treating depression in the real world. Cleve Clin J Med. 2008;75:57-66.
830. Joffe RT, Sokolov ST. Thyroid hormone treatment of primary unipolar depression: a review. Int J Neuro-psychopharmacol. 2000;3:143-7.
831. Aronson R, Offman HJ, Joffe RT, Naylor CD. Triiodothyronine augmentation in the treatment of refractory depression. A meta-analysis. Arch Gen Psychiatry. 1996;53:842-8.
832. Papakostas GI, Shelton RC, Smith J, Fava M. Augmentation of antidepressants with atypical antipsychotics for treatment-resistant major depressive disorder: a meta-analysis. J Clin Psychiatry. 2007;68:826-31.
833. Sokolski KN. Adjunctive aripiprazole for bupropion-resistant major depression. Ann Pharmacother. 2008;42:1124-9.
834. Goforth HW, Carroll BT. Aripiprazole augmentation of tranylcypromine in treatment-resistant major depression. J Clin Psychopharmacol. 2007;27:216-7.
835. Schüle C, Baghai TC, Eser D, et al. Mirtazapine monontherapy versus combination therapy with mirtazapine and aripiprazole in depressed patients without psychotic features: a 4-week open-label parallel-group study. World J Biol Psychiatry. 2007;8:112-22.
836. Physicians' Desk Reference, 61st edn, Montvale, NJ: Thompson PDR; 2007. pp. 1527-9.
837. Schmidt AW, Lebel LA, Johnson CG, et al. The novel antipsychotic ziprasidone has a unique human receptor binding profile compared to other agents. Soc Neurosci Abstr. 1998;24:2177.
838. Stoll AL, Haura G. Tranylcypromine plus risperidone for treatment-refractory major depression. J Clin Psychopharmacol. 2000;20:495-6.
839. Azzaro AJ, Ziemniak J, Kemper E, et al. Selegiline transdermal system: an examination of the potential for CYP450-dependent pharmacokinetic interactions with 3 psychotropic medications. J Clin Pharmacol. 2007;47:146-58.
840. Barbee JG, Conrad EJ, Jamhour NJ. The effectiveness of olanzapine, risperidone, quetiapine, and ziprasidone as augmentation agents in treatment-resistant major depressive disorder. J Clin Psychiatry. 2004;65:975-81.
841. Barbee JG, Conrad EJ, Jamhour NJ. Aripiprazole augmentation in treatment-resistant depression. Ann Clin Psychiatry. 2004;16:189-94.
842. Schneider LS, Small GW, Clary CM. Estrogen replacement therapy and antidepressant response to sertraline in older depressed women. Am J Geriatr Psychiatry. 2001;9:393-9.
843. Pope HG Jr, Cohane GH, Kanayama G, et al. Testosterone gel supplementation for men with refractory depression. A randomized, placebo-controlled trial. Am J Psychiatry. 2003;160:105-11.
844. Levitan RD, Shen JH, Jindal R, et al. Preliminary randomized double-blind placebo-controlled trial of tryptophan combined with fluoxetine to treat major depressive disorder: antidepressant and hypnotic effects. J Psychiatry Neurosci. 2000;25:337-46.
845. Nemets B, Stahl Z, Belmaker RH. Addition of omega-3 fatty acid to maintenance medication treatment for recurrent unipolar depressive disorder. Am J Psychiatry. 2002;159:477-9.
846. Appelberg BG, Syvälahti EK, Koskinen TE, et al. Patients with severe depression may benefit from buspirone augmentation of selective serotonin reuptake inhibitors: results from a placebo-controlled, randomized, double-blind, placebo wash-in study. J Clin Psychiatry. 2001;62:448-52.
847. Landén M, Björling G, Agren H, Fahlén T. A randomized, double-blind placebo-controlled trial of buspirone in combination with an SSRI in patients with treatment-refractory depression. J Clin Psychiatry. 1998;59:664-8.
848. Trivedi MH, Fava M, Wisniewski SR, et al. Medication augmentation after the failure of SSRIs for depression. N Eng J Med. 2006;354:1243-52.
849. Barbee JG, Jamhour NJ, Stewart JS, et al. Lamotrigine as an antidepressant augmentation agent in treatment refractory unipolar depression. Presented at: Annual Meeting of the American Psychiatric Association; May 19-24, 2007; San Diego.
850. DeBattista C, Doghramji K, Menza MA, et al. Adjunct modafinil for the short-term treatment of fatigue and sleepiness in patients

with major depressive disorder: a preliminary double-blind, placebo-controlled study. J Clin Psychiatry. 2003;64:1057-64.

851. Fava M, Thase ME, DeBattista C. A multicenter, placebo-controlled study of modafanil augmentation in partial responders to selective serotonin reuptake inhibitors with persistent fatigue and sleepiness. J Clin Psychiatry. 2005;66:85-93.

Cognitive Behavior Therapy for Depression

852. Lewinsohn PM, Biglan T, Zeiss, A. Behavioral treatment of depression. In: Davidson P (Ed). Behavioral management of anxiety, depression, and pain. New York: Brunner/Mazel; 1976.

853. Lewinsohn, PM. A behavioral approach to depression. In: Friedman RJ, MM Katz (Eds). The Psychology of Depression: Contemporary Theory and Research. New York: Wiley; 1974. pp. 157-85.

854. Gallagher D, Thompson, LW. Depression in the elderly. A Behavioral Treatment Manual. University of Los Angeles, Southern California Press; 1981.

855. Lewinsohn PM, Weinstein MS, Alper T. A behavioral approach to the group treatment of depressed persons: a methodological contribution. J Clin Psychol. 1970;26(4):525-32.

856. McLean PD. Decision-making in the behavioral management of depression. In: Davidson PO (Ed). Behavioral management of anxiety, depression, and pain. New York: Brunner/Mazel; 1976.

857. Zeiss AM, Lewinsohn PM, Munoz RF. Nonspecific improvement effects in depression using interpersonal skills training, pleasant activity schedules, or cognitive training. J Consult Clin Psychol. 1979;47(3):427-39.

858. Beck AT, Rush AJ, Shaw BF, Emery G. Cognitive therapy of depression. New York: Guilford Press; 1979.

859. Jacobson NS, Dobson KS, Truax PA, Addis ME, Koerner K, Gollan JK. A component analysis of cognitive-behavioral treatment for depression. J Consult Clin Psychol. 1996;64(2):295-304.

860. Martell CR, Addis, ME, Jacobson NS. Depression in Context: Strategies for Guided Action. New York: Norton; 2001.

861. Lejuez CW, Hopko DR, Hopko SD. A brief behavioral activation treatment for depression. Treatment manual. Behav Modif. 2001;25(2):255-86.

862. Cuijpers P, van Straten A, Warmerdam L. Behavioral activation treatments of depression: a meta-analysis. Clin Psychol Rev. 2007;27(3):318-26.

863. Ekers D, Richards D, Gilbody S. A meta-analysis of randomized trials of behavioural treatment of depression. Psychol Med. 2008;38(5):611-23.

864. Mazzucchelli T, Kane R, Rees, C. Behavioral activation treatments for adults: A meta-analysis and review. Clinical Psychology: Science and Practice, 5; 2009. pp. 291-313.

865. Dobson KS, Dozois, DJS. Historical and philosophical bases of the cognitive-behavioral therapies. In: Dobson K (Ed). Handbook of Cognitive-Behavioral Therapies. 3rd Edition, New York: Guilford Press; 2009.

866. Young JE, Weinberger AD, Beck AT. Cognitive therapy for depression. In: Barlow DH (Ed). Clinical Handbook of Psychological Disorders: A Step-by-step Treatment Manual, 3rd edition. New York: Guilford Press; 2001. pp. 264-308.

867. Kuyken W, Beck AT. Cognitive therapy. In: Freeman C, Power M (Eds). Handbook of Evidence-based Psychotherapies: A Guide for Research and Practice. Chichester: Wiley; 2007. pp. 15-39.

868. Beck AT, Freeman A. Associates Cognitive therapy of personality disorders. New York: Guilford Press; 1990.

869. American Psychiatric Association. Treatment of patients with major depressive disorder. American Psychiatric Association Practice Guidelines. 3rd edition; 2010.

870. March J, Silva S, Petrycki S, Curry J, Wells K, Fairbank J. Fluoxetine, cognitive-behavioral therapy, and their combination for adolescents with depression: Treatment for Adolescents with Depression Study (TADS) randomized controlled trial. JAMA. 2004;292(7):807-20.

871. Dobson KS, Hamilton KE. Cognitive restructuring: Behavioral tests of negative cognitions. In: W O'Donohue JE, Fisher SC Hayes (Eds). Cognitive behavior therapy: Applying empirically supported techniques in your practice. Hoboken. NJ: John Wiley & Sons, Inc; 2003. pp. 84-8.

872. Andrews G, Cuijpers P, Craske MG, McEvoy P, Titov N. Computer therapy for the anxiety and depressive disorders is effective, acceptable and practical health care: a meta-analysis. PLoS One. 2010;5(10):e13196.

873. Pittaway S, Cupitt C, Palmer D, et al. Comparative, clinical feasibility study of three tools for delivery of cognitive behavioural therapy for mild to moderate depression and anxiety provided on a self-help basis. Ment Health Fam Med. 2009;6(3):145-54.

874. Keller MB, McCullough JP, Klein DN, Arnow B, Dunner DL, Gelenberg AJ. A comparison of nefazodone, the cognitive behavioral-analysis system of psychotherapy, and their combination for the treatment of chronic depression. N Engl J Med. 2000;342(20):1462-70.

875. de Maat S, Dekker J, Schoevers R, et al. Short psychodynamic supportive psychotherapy, antidepressants, and their combination in the treatment of major depression: a mega-analysis based on three randomized clinical trials. Depress Anxiety. 2008;25(7):565-74.

876. Pampallona S, Bollini P, Tibaldi G, Kupelnick B, Munizza C. Combined pharmacotherapy and psychological treatment for depression: a systematic review. Arch Gen Psychiatry. 2004;61(7):714-9.

877. Thase ME, Greenhouse JB, Frank E, et al. Treatment of major depression with psychotherapy or psychotherapy-pharmacotherapy combinations. Arch Gen Psychiatry. 1997;54(11):1009-15.

878. Hollon SD, Jarrett RB, Nierenberg AA, Thase ME, Trivedi M, Rush AJ. Psychotherapy and medication in the treatment

of adult and geriatric depression: which monotherapy or combined treatment?. J Clin Psychiatry. 2005;66(4):455-68.
879. Haynes RB, Yao X, Degani A, et al. Interventions to enhance medication adherence. Cochrane Database Syst Rev. 2005;(4): CD000011.

SUGGESTED READING

Diagnostic Criteria, Clinical Features and Management of Mood Disorder, Dysthymic and Cyclothymic Disorders

1. American Psychiatric Association. Desk Reference to the Diagnostic Criteria from DSM-5. Washington DC; 2013.
2. American Psychiatric Association. Diagnostic and Statistical Manual, 4th edition, Washington DC: American Psychiatric Association, 1994.
3. Amsterdam JD. Refractory Depression. New York: Raven Press, 1991.
4. Arana GW, Hyman SE. Handbook of Psychiatric Drug Therapy, 2nd edition, Boston: Little, Brown, 1991.
5. Beck AT. Cognitive Therapy and Emotional Disorder. New York: International University Press, 1976.
6. Biel MG, Peselow E, M Mulcare et al. Continuation versus discontinuation of lithium in recurrent bipolar illness: a naturalistic study. Bipolar Disord. 2007;9:435–42.
7. Bowden CL, et al. A randomized, placebo-controlled 12-month trial of divalproex and lithium in treatment of outpatients with bipolar I disorder. Divalproex Maintenance Study Group. Arch Gen Psychiatry. 2000;57:481-9.
8. Cipriani A, et al. Lithium in the prevention of suicidal behavior and all-cause mortality in patients with mood disorders: a systematic review of randomized trials. Am J Psychiatry. 2005;162:1805-19.
9. Cookson J. Side effects of antidepressants. Br J Psychiatry. 1993;163(Suppl 20):20-4.
10. DiMascio A, Weissman MM, Prusolff BA, et al. Differential symptom reduction by drug and psychotherapy in acute depression. Arch Gen Psychiatry, 1979;36:1450-6.
11. et Taylor D, et al. The Maudsley. Prescribing Guidelines in psychiatry. Wiley-Blackwell, 2012
12. Frazer A. Antidepressants. J Clin Psychiatry. 1997.
13. Geddes JR, et al. Long-term lithium therapy for bipolar disorder: systematic review and meta-analysis of randomized controlled trials. Am J Psychiatry 2004;161:217-22.
14. Hartong EG, et al. Prophylactic efficacy of lithium versus carbamazepine in treatment-naïve bipolar patients. J Clin Psychiatry. 2003;64:144-51.
15. Karasu TB. Towards a clinical model of psychotherapy for depression. I. Systemic comparison of three psychotherapies. Am J Psychiatry 1990;147:133-45.
16. Kessing LV, et al. Suicide risk in patients treated with lithium. Arch Gen Psychiatry. 2005;62:860-6.
17. Klerman GL, Weissman MM, Rounsavilla BJ, et al. Interpersonal Psychotherapy of Depression. New York: Basic Books, 1984.
18. Leonhard BE. Biochemical aspects of therapy-resistant depression. Br J Psychiatry 1988;152:453-9.
19. Macritchie KA, et al. Valproic acid, valproate and divalproex in the maintenance treatment of bipolar disorder. Cochrane Database Syst Rev. 2001;CD003196.
20. National Institute for Health and Clinical Excellence. Bipolar disorder. The Management of bipolar disorder in adults, children and adolescents, in primary and secondary care. Clinical Guidance 38. http://www .nice.org.uk. 2006 .
21. Perlis RH, et al. Predictors of recurrence in bipolar disorder: primary outcomes from the Systematic Treatment Enhancement Program for Bipolar Disorder (STEP-BD). Am J Psychiatry 2006;163:217-24.
22. Preskon SH, Burke M. Somatic therapy for major depressive disorder: Selection of an antidepressant. J Clin Psychiatry. 1992;53(Suppl 9):10.
23. Sambunasis A, et al. Development of new antidepressants. J Clin Psychiatry, 1996.
24. Smith LA, et al. Effectiveness of mood stabilizers and antipsychotics in the maintenance phase of bipolar disorder: a systematic review of randomized controlled trials. Bipolar Disord. 2007;9:394-412.
25. Taylor, et al. The Maudsley. Prescribing Guidelines in Psychiatry. Wiley-Blackwell, 2012.
26. Thasse M. Maintenance treatment of recurrent affective disorder. Current Opinion in Psychiatry 1993;6:16-21.
27. Tohen M, et al. Olanzapine versus divalproex sodium for the treatment of acute mania and maintenance of remission: a 47-week study. Am J Psychiatry. 2003;160:1263-71.
28. Vyas JN. Mood disorders. In: Vyas JN, Ahuja N. (Eds). Post-graduate Psychiatry. New Delhi: Churchill Livingstone, 1992.
29. Wexler BE, Cicchetti DV. The outpatient treatment of depression: Implications of outcome research for clinical practice. J NervMent Dis. 1992;180:277.
30. Young AH, et al. Lithium in maintenance therapy for bipolar disorder. J Psychopharmacol. 2006;20:17-22.
31. Young AH, et al. Lithium in mood disorders: increasing evidence base, declining use? Br J Psychiatry. 2007;191:474–6.

Bipolar Disorder: Focus on Bipolar II Disorders and Mixed Depression

32. Akiskal 115, Benazzi F. Toward a clinical delineation of dysphoric hypomania-operational and conceptual dilemmas. Bipolar Disord. 2005;7:456-64.
33. Akiskal HS, Akiskal KK, Lancrenon S, et al. Validating the bipolar spectrum in the French national EPIDEP study: overview of phenomenology and relative prevalence of its clinical prototypes J Affect Disord. 2006;96:197-205.
34. Akiskal HS, Azorin JM, Hantouche EG. Proposed multidimensional structure of mania: beyond the euphoric-dysphoric dichotomy. J Affect Disord. 2003;73:7-18.

35. Akiskal HS, Benazzi F, Perugi G, Rihmer Z. Agitated "unipolar" depression re-conceptualized as a depressive mixed state: implications for the antidepressant-suicide controversy. J Affect Disord. 2005;85:245-58.
36. Akiskal HS, Benazzi F. Family history validation of the bipolar nature of depressive mixed states. J Affect Disord. 2003;73:113-22.
37. Akiskal HS, Benazzi F. Optimizing the detection of bipolar II disorder in outpatient private practice: toward a systematization of clinical diagnostic wisdom. J Clin Psychiatry. 2005;66:914-21.
38. Akiskal HS, Benazzi F. The DSM-IV and ICD to categories of recurrent [major] depressive and bipolar and bipolar II disorders evidence that they lie on a dimensional spectrum. J Affect Disord. 2006;92:45-54.
39. Akiskal HS, Hantouche E.g. Allilaite JF. Bipolar II with and without cyclothymic temperament "dark": and "sunny" expressions of soft bipolarity J Affect Disord. 2003;73:49-57.
40. Akiskal HS, Maser JD, Zeller PJ, et al. Switching from 'unipolar' to bipolar II. An II-year prospective study of clinical and temperamental predictors in 559 patients. Arch Gen Psychiatry. 1995;52:114-23.
41. Akiskal HS. Demystifying borderline personality: critique of the concept and unorthodox reflections on its natural kinship with the bipolar spectrum. Acta Psychiatr Scand. 2004;110:401-07.
42. Altshuler L, Suppes T, Black D, et al. Impact of antidepressant discontinuation after acute bipolar depression permission on rates of depressive relapse at 1 year follow up. Am J Psychiatry. 2001;160:1252-62.
43. Altshuler LL, Suppes T, Black DO, et al. Lower switch rate in depressed patients with bipolar II than bipolar I disorder treated adjunctively with second-generation antidepressants. Am J Psychiatry. 2006;163:113-5.
44. American Psychiatric Association. Desk Reference to the Diagnostic Criteria from DSM-5. Washington DC, 2013.
45. American Psychiatric Association. Diagnostic and statistical manual of mental disorders, 4th edition, text revision (DSM-IV-TR).
46. Angst J, Cassano G. The mood spectrum: improving the diagnosis of bipolar disorder. Bipolar Disorder. 2005;7(Suppl 4):4-12.
47. Angst J, Gamma A, Benazzi F, Ajdacic V, Fich D, Rossler W. Toward a re-definition of subthreshold bipolarity: epidemiology and proposed criteria for bipolar-II, minor bipolar disorders and hypomania. J Affect Disord. 2003;73:7-18.
48. Angst J. Sellaro R, Stassen HH, Gamma A. Diagnostic conversion from depression to bipolar disorders: results of a long-term prospective study of hospital admissions. J Affect Disord. 2005;84:149-57.
49. Angst J. Switch from depression to mania- a record study over decades between 1920 and 1982. Psychopathology. 1985;18:140-54.
50. Augst J, Adolfsoon R, Benazzi I, et al. The HCL-32: towards a self-assessment tool for hypomanic symptoms in outpatients. J Affect Disord. 2005;88:217-33.
51. Augst J. The emerging epidemiology of hypomania and bipolar II disorder. J Affect Disord. 1998;50:141-51.
52. Axelson D, Birmaher B, Strober M, et al. Phenomenology of children and adolescents with bipolar spectrum disorders. Arch Gen Psychiatry. 2006;63:1139-48.
53. Balazs J, Benazzi F, Rihmer Z, Rihmer A, Akiskal KK, Akiskal HS. The close link between suicide attempts and mixed (bipolar) depression: implications for suicide prevention. J Affect Disord. 2006;91:133-8.
54. Baldessarini R. Pompili M, Tondo L. Suicidal risk in antidepressant drug trial. Arch Gen Psychiatry. 2006;63:246-8.
55. Baldessarini RJ. Tondo L, Hennen J. Viguera AC. Is lithium still worth using? An update of selected recent research. Harv Rev Psychiatry. 2002;10:59-75.
56. Bauer MS, Crits-Christoph P, Ball WA. et al. Independent assessment of manic and depressive symptoms by self-rating scale. Characteristics and implications for the study of mania. Arch Gen Psychiatry. 1991;48:807-12.
57. Bauer MS, Simon GF, Ludinan F, Unutzer J. " Bipolarity" in bipolar disorder: distribution of manic and depressive symptoms in a treated population. Br J Psychiatry. 2005;187:87-8.
58. Bauer MS, Wisnlewski SR, Manageell LB, et al. For the STEP-BD Investigators. Are antidepressants associated with new-onset suicidality in bipolar disorder? A prospective study of participants in the systematic treatment enhancement program for bipolar disorder (STEP-BD) J Clin Psychiatry. 2006;67:48-55.
59. Benazzi E. Testing new diagnostic criteria for hypomania Ann Clin Psychiatry (in press).
60. Benazzi F, A comparison of the age of onset of bipolar I and bipolar II outpatients. J Affect Disord. 1999;54:249-54.
61. Benazzi F, Akiskal H. The duration of hypomania in bipolar-II disorder in private practice methodology and validation. J Affect Disord. 2006;96:189-96.
62. Benazzi F, Akiskal HS. Biphasic course in bipolar II outpatients Baillarger and Falret in hospitalized patients in 1854 J Affect Disord. 2006;96:183-7.
63. Benazzi F, Akiskal HS. Clinical and factor analytic-validation of depressive mixed states: a report from the Ravenna-San Diego collaboration. Curr Opin Psychiatry. 2003;16 (Suppl 2):571-8.
64. Benazzi F, Akiskal HS. Refining the evaluation of bipolar II: beyond the strict SCID-CV guidelines for hypomania. J Affect Disord. 2003;73:33-8.
65. Benazzi F. Borderline personality bipolar spectrum relationship Prog Neuropsychopharmacol Biol Psychiatry. 2006;30:68-74.
66. Benazzi F. Challenging the unipolar-bipolar division: does mixed depression bridge the gap? Prog Neuropsychopharmacol Biol Psychopharmacol Biol Psychiatry. 2007;31:97-103.
67. Benazzi F. Diagnosis of bipolar II disorder: a comparison of structured versus semistructured interviews. Prog Neuropsychopharmacol Biol Psychiatry. 2003;73:33-8.
68. Benazzi F. Suicidal ideation and depressive mixed states. Psychother Psychowom. 2005;74:61-2.

69. benazzi F. A continuity between bipolar II depression and major depressive disorder? Prog Neuropsychopharmacol Biol Psychiatry. 2006;30:1043-50.
70. Benazzi F. Agitated depression: a valid depression subtype? Prog Neuropsychopharmacol Biol Psychiatry. 2004;28:1279-85.
71. Benazzi F. Antidepressant-induced or clinician-induced sudcidality in depression? Am J Psychiatry. 2006;163:1644.
72. Benazzi F. Antidepressants-associated hypomania in outpatient depression: a 203 case study in private practice. J Affect Disord. 1997;46:71-7.
73. Benazzi F. Atypical depression and its relation to bipolar spectrum. In: Marneros A, Goodwin F (Eds). Bipolar Disorders. Cambridge: Cambridge University Press,. 2005;46:159-66.
74. Benazzi F. Bipolar family history of the hypomanic symptoms and dimensions of mixed depression. Compr Psychiatry. 2005;46:399-404.
75. Benazzi F. Bipolar II depressive mixed state: finding a useful definition. Compr Psychiatry. 2003;44:21-7.
76. Benazzi F. Bipolar II disorder and major depressive disorder: continuity or discontinuity? World J Biol Psychiatry. 2004;4:166-71.
77. Benazzi F. Bipolar II disorder family history using the family history screen: findings and clinical implications. Compr Psychiatry. 2004;45:77-82.
78. Benazzi F. Bipolar II disorder: current issues in diagnosis and management. Psychiatric Times. 2006;9:26-9.
79. Benazzi F. Challenging DSM-IV criteria for hypomania: diagnosing based on number of no priority symptoms. Fur Psychiatry. 2007;22:99-103.
80. Benazzi F. Depressive mixed states unipolar and bipolar II. Eur Arch Psychiatry Clin Neurosci. 2000;250:249-53.
81. Benazzi F. Does age at onset support a dimensional relationship between bipolar II disorder and major depressive disorder? World J Biol Psychiatry (in press).
82. Benazzi F. Does temperamental instability support a continuity between bipolar II disorder and major depressive disorder? Eur Psychiatry. 2006;21:274-79.
83. Benazzi F. Factor structure of recalled DSM-IV hypomanic symptoms of bipolar II disorder. Compr Psychiatry. 2004;45:441-6.
84. Benazzi F. Family history validation of a definition of mixed depression Compr Psychiatry Clin Neurosci. 2005;46:159-66.
85. Benazzi F. Is overactivity the core feature of hypomania in bipolar ? Psychopathology. 2007;73:49-57.
86. Benazzi F. Is there a continuity between bipolar and depressive disorders? Psychother Psychosom. 2007;76:70-6.
87. Benazzi F. Mixed states in bipolar II disorder: should full hypomania always be required? Psychiatry Res. 2004;127:247-57.
88. Benazzi F. Mood patterns and classification in bipolar disorder. Curr Opin Psychiatry. 2006;19:1-8.
89. Benazzi F. Prevalence of bipolar II disorder in outpatient depression: a. 203-case study in private practice. J Affect Disord. 1997;43:163-6.
90. Benazzi F. The problem of the treatment of bipolar-II depression. Bipolar Disord. 2004;6:440-41.
91. Benazzi F. Unipolar depression with racing thoughts: a bipolar spectrum disorder? Psychiatry Clin Neurosci. 2005;59:570-5.
92. Benazzi F. Which could be a clinically useful definition of depressive mixed state? Prog Neuropsychopharmacol Biol Psychiatry. 2002;26:1105-11.
93. Biondi M, Picardi A, Pasquini M, Gaetano P, Pancheri P. Dimensional psychopathology of depression: detection of an "activation" dimension in unipolar depressed outpatients. J Affect Disord. 2005;84:133-9.
94. Birmaher B, Axelson D, Strober M, et al. Clinical course of children and adolescents with bipolar spectrum disorders Arch Gen Psychiatry. 2006;63:75-81.
95. Bottlender R, Sato T, Kleindienst N, Strausz A, Moller HJ. Mixed depressive features predict maniform switch during treatment of depression in bipolar I disorder. J Affect Disord. 2004;78:149-52.
96. Brown FB, McElroy SL, Keck PE Jr. et al. A 7-week, randomized, double-blind trial of olanzapine/fluoxetine combination versus lamotrigine in the treatment of bipolar I depression. J Clin Psychiatry. 2006;67:1025-33.
97. Calabrese JR, Bowden CL, Sachs G, et al. for the Lamictal 605 Study Group A placebo-controlled 18-month trial of lamotrigine and lithium maintenance treatment in recently depresses patients with bipolar I disorder. J Clin Psychiatry. 2003;64:1013-24.
98. Calabrese JR, Keck PE, Jr. Macfadden W, et al. A randomized, double-blind. Placebo-controlled trial of quetiapine in the treatment of bipolar I or II depression Am J Psychiatry. 2005;162:1351-60.
99. Calabrese JR, Suppes T, Bowden CL, et al. for the Lamictal 614 Study Group. A double-blind, placebo-controlled, prophylaxis study of lamotrigine in rapid cycling bipolar disorder. J Clin Psychiatry. 2000;61:841-50.
100. Cassano GB, Frank E, Miniati M, Rucci P, et al. Conceptual underpinnings and empirical support for the mood spectrum Psychiatr Clin North Am. 2002;25:699-712.
101. Cassano GB, Rucci P, Frank E, et al. The mood spectrum in unipolar and bipolar disorder: arguments for a unitary approach. Am J Psychiatry. 2004;161:1264-9.
102. Cassidy F, Forest K, Murry E, Carroll BJ. A factor analysis of the signs and symptoms of mania. Arch Gen Psychiatry. 1998;55:27-32.
103. Chun BJ, Dunner DL. A review of antidepressant induced hypomania in major depression: suggestions for DSM-5. Bipolar Disord. 2004;6:32-42.
104. Coppen A, Lithium in unipolar depression and the prevention of suicide. J Clin Psychiatry. 2000;61 (suppl 9):52-56.
105. Coyell W, Endicott J, Master JD, Keller MB, Leon AC, Akiskal HS. Long-term stability of polarity distinctions in the affective disorders. Am J psychiatry. 1995;152:185-90.
106. DeBattista C, Soloman A, Arnow B, Kendrick E, Tilston J, Schatzberg AF. The efficacy of divalproex sodium in the

treatment of agitation associated with major depression. J Clin Psychopharmacol. 2005;25:476-9.
107. Dikcos DG, Wickham II, McDonald C, et al. Distribution of symptom dimensions across Kraepelinian divisions. Br J Psychiatry. 2006;189:346-53.
108. Dilsaver SC, Benazzi F, Akiskal HS. Mixed states: the most common outpatient presentation of bipolar depressed adolescents? Psychopathology. 2005;38:268-72.
109. Dilsaver SC, Chen YR, Shoaib AM, Swann AC. Phenomenology of mania: evidence for distinct depressed, dysphoric, and euphoric presentations. Am J Psychiatry. 1999;156:426-30.
110. Duffy A, Grof P, Robertson C, Akla M, The implications of genetics studies of major mood disorders for clinical practice. J Clin Psychiatry. 2000;61:630-2.
111. El-Mallakh Rs, Karippot A, Ghaemi SN. Antidepressants in bipolar depression. In: El-Mallakh Rs, Ghaemi SN, eds. Bipolar depression Washington DC American Psychiatric Publishing; 2006. pp. 167-81.
112. Faedda GL, Baldessarini RJ, Golvinsky IP, Austin NB, Pediatric bipolar disorder: phenomenology and course of illness. Bipolar Disord. 2004;6:305-13.
113. First MB, Spitzer RL, Gibbon M, Williams JBW. Structured clinical interview for DSM-IV axis I disorders-clinician version (SCID-CV). Washington. DC American Psychiatric Press, 1997.
114. Frank E, Kupfer DJ. Thase ME, et al. Two-year outcomes for interpersonal and social rhythm therapy in individuals with bipolar I disorder Arch Gen psychiatry. 2005;62:996-1004.
115. Frye MA, McElroy SL, Hellemann G, et al. Clinical correlates associated with antidepressant-related mania. Toronto: Programme and abstracts of the American Psychiatric Association Annual Meeting. 2006;(abstr NR215).
116. Geller B, Tillman R, Bolhofner K, Zimerman B, Strauss NA, Kaufmann P. Controlled, blindly rated, direct-interview family study of a prepubertal and early-adolescent bipolar I disorder phenotype: morbid risk, age at onset, and comorbidity Anh Gen psychiatry. 2006;63:1130-8.
117. Gershon ES, Hamovit J, Guroff JJ, et al. A family study of schizoaffective, bipolar I, bipolar II, unipolar, and normal control probands. Arch Gen Psychiatry. 1982;39:1157-67.
118. Ghaemi SN, Baldessarini RJ. The manic-depressive spectrum and mood stabilization: Krapelin's ghost. Psychiater Psychorum. 2007;76:65-9.
119. Ghaemi SN, Ko JY, Goodwin FK. "Code's disease" and beyond: misdiagnosis, antidepressant use, and a proposed definition for bipolar spectrum disorder. Can J Psychiatry. 2002;47:125-34.
120. Ghaemi SN, Hsu DJ, Soldani F, Goodwin FK. Antidepressants in bipolar disorder: the case for caution. Bipolar Disorder: the case for caution. Bipolar Disord. 2003;5:421-33.
121. Ghaemi SN. Re-evaluating concepts of depression: the bipolar spectrum. Toronto: Abstract of the Symposium New Vistas in Treatmetn-Resistant Depression of the American Psychiatric Association Annual Meeting, 2006.
122. Gijsman HJ, Geddes JR, Rendell JM, Nolen WA, Goodwin GM. Antidepressants for bipolar depression: a systematic review of randomized, controlled trials Am J Psychiatry. 2004;161:1537-47.
123. Goldberg JF, Harrow M, Whiteside JE. Risk for bipolar illness in patients initially hospitalized for unipolar depression. Am J Psychiatry. 2001;158:1265-70.
124. Goldberg JF, Truman CJ. Fordis J, Wisniewski S, Thase ME, Sachs GS. Antidepressant use during mixed states: naturalistic outcome data from the STEP-1000. Neuropsychopharmacology. 2004;29: S144 (abstr).
125. Goodwin FK, Jamison KR. Manic depressive illness New York Oxford University Press, 1990.
126. Goodwin GM, Bowden CL, Calabrese JR, et al. A pooled analysis of 2 placebo controlled 18 month trials of lamotrigine and lithium maintenance in bipolar I disorder. J Clin Psychiatry. 2004;65:432-41.
127. Gyulai L, Bowden CL, McElroy SL, et al. Maintenance efficacy of divalproex in the prevention of bipolar depression. Neuropsychopharmacology. 2003;28:1174-82.
128. Hantouche E, Akiskal HS, Lancrenon S, et al. Systematic clinical methodology for validating bipolar-II disorder: data in mid-stream from a French national multisite study (EPIDEP). J Affect Disord. 1998;50:163-73.
129. Hantouche FG, Angst J, Akiskal HS. Factor structure of hypomania: interrelationships with cyclothymia and the soft bipolar spectrum. J Affect Disord. 2003;73:39-47.
130. Hawton K, Sutton L, Haw C, Sinclair J, Harriss L. Suicide and attempted suicide in bipolar disorder: a systematic review of risk factors. J Clin Psychiatry. 2005;66:693-704.
131. Heun R, Maler W. The distinction of bipolar II disorder from bipolar I and recurrent unipolar depression: results of a controlled family study. Acta Psychiatr Scand. 1993;87:279-84.
132. Houston JP, Ahl J, Meyers, AL, Kaiser CJ. Tohen M, Baldessarini RJ. Reduced suicidal ideation in bipolar I disorder mixed-episode patients in a placebo-controlled trial of olanzapine combined with lithium of valproate. J Clin Psychiatry. 2006;67:1246-52.
133. Joyce PR, Doughty CJ, Wells JE, et al. Affective disorders in the first-degree relatives of bipolar porbands: results from the South Island Bipolar Study. Compr Psychiatry. 2004;45:168-74.
134. Judd II, Akishka HS, Schettler PJ, et al. The long term natural history of the weekly symptomatic status of bipolar I disorder. American Psychiatry. 2002;50:510-2.
135. Judd LL, Akiskal HS, Schettler PJ, et al. A prospective investigation of the natural history of the long term weekly symptomatic status of bipolar II disorders. Arch Gen Psychiatry. 2003;60:261-9.
136. Judd LL, Akiskal HS. The prevalence and disability of bipolar spectrum disorders in the US population to analysis of the BCA database taking into account subthreshold cases. J Affect Disord. 2003;73:123-31.
137. Kendell R, Jablensky A. Distinguishing between the validity and utility of psychiatric diagnoses. Am J Psychiatry. 2003;160:4-12.
138. Kessler RC, Berglund P, Demler O, Jin R, Merikangas KR, Walters EE. Lifetime prevalence and age-of-onset distributions

of DSM-IV disorders in the National Comorbidity Survey Replication. Arch Gen Psychiatry. 2005;62:593-602.

139. Koukopoulos A. Ewald Hecker's description of cyclothymia as a cyclical mood disorder: its relevance to the modern concept of bipolar II. J Affect Disord. 2003;74:199-205.
140. Koukopoulos A. The primacy of mania. In: Akiskal HS, Tohen M, eds Bipolar psychopharmacology: Chichester: John Wiley and Sons; 2006. pp. 169-92.
141. Koukopoulos K, Sani G, Albert MJ. Minnai GP. Koukopoulos AE. Agitated depression: spontaneous and induced. In: Marneros A, Goodwin F (Eds). Bipolar disorders. Cambridge: Cambridge University Press; 2005. pp. 157-86.
142. Krabbendam L, Myin-Germeys L, De Graaf R, et al. Dimensions of depression, mania and psychosis in the general population. Psychol Med. 2004;34:1-10.
143. Kraepelin F, Martin depressive insanity and paramola. Edinburgh: Livingstone F & S, 1921.
144. Lam DH, Watkins ER, Hayward P, et al. A randomized controlled study of cognitive therapy for relapse prevention for bipolar affective disorder, outcome of the first year. Arch Gen psychiatry. 2003;60:145-52.
145. Levrich GS, Altshuler LL, Frye MA, et al. Risk of switch in mood polarity to hypomania or mania inpatients with bipolar depression during acute and continuation trials of venlafaxine, sertraline, and bupropion as adjuncts to mood stabilizers. Am J Psychiatry. 2006;163:232-9.
146. Mackinnon DF, Potash JB, McMahon FJ, Simpson SG, Raymond Depaulo J, Jr. Zandi PP, for the National Institutes of Mental Health Bipolar Disorder Genetics Initiative. Rapid mood switching and suicidality in familial bipolar disorder. Bipolar Disord. 2006;7:411-48.
147. Maj M, Pirozzi R, Magliano L, Bartoli L. Agitated depression in bipolar I disorder: prevalence, phenomenology, and outcome. Am J Psychiatry. 2003;160:2134-40.
148. Maj M, Pirozzi R, Magliano L, Fiorillo A, Bartoli L. Agitated 'unipolar' major depression: prevalence, phenomenology, and outcome. J Clin Psychiatry. 2006;67:712-9.
149. Mammen OK, Pilkonts PA, Chengappa KN, Kupfer DJ. Anger attacks in bipolar depression predictors and response to citalopram added to mood stabilizers J Clin Psychiatry. 2004;65:627-44.
150. Mantere O, Suominen K, Lep-arhaki S, Valtonen A, Arvilommi P, Isometsa F. The clinical characteristics of DSM-IV bipolar I and II disorders: baseline findings from the Jorvi Bipolar Study (JOBS). Bipolar Disord. 2004;6:395-405.
151. McMabon FJ. Stine OC, Chase GA, Meyers DA, Simpson SG, DePaulo JR Jt. Influence of clinical subtype, sex and lineality on age at onset of major affective disorder in a family sample. Am J Psychiatry. 1994;151:210-5.
152. Mitchell PB, Malhi GS. Bipolar depression: phenomenological overview and clinical characteristics. Bipolar Disord. 2004;6:530-9.
153. Moller HJ, Grunze H, Broich K. Do recent efficacy data on the drug treatment of acute bipolar depression support the position that drugs other than antidepressants are the treatment of choice? A conceptual review. Eur Arch Psychiatry Clin Neurosci. 2006;256:1-15.
154. Perlis RH, Ostacher MJ, Patel JK, et al. Predictors of recurrence in bipolar disorder: primary outcomes from the Systematic Treatment Enhancement Program for Bipolar Disorder (STEP-BD). Am J psychiatry. 2006;163:217-24.
155. Perugi G, Akiskal HS, Micheli C, Toni C, Madaro D. Clinical characterization. J Affect Disord. 2001;67:105-14.
156. Perugi G, Toni C, Travierso MC, Akiskal HS. The role of cyclothymia in atypical depression: toward a data-based reconceptualization of borderline-bipolar II connection. J Affect Disord. 2003;73:87-98.
157. Post RM, Levrich GS, Nolen WA, et al. for the Stanley Foundation Bipolar Network. A re-evaluation of the role of antidepressants in the treatment of bipolar depression: data from the Stanley Foundation Bipolar Network. Bipolar Disord. 2003;5: 196-406.
158. Regeer FJ, Krabberndam L, de Graaf R, ten Have M, Nolen WA, van Os J. A prospective study of the transition rates of subthreshold (hypo) mania and depression in the general population. Psychol Mol. 2006;36:619-27.
159. Robins F, Guze SB. Establishment of diagnostic validity in psychiatric illness: its application to schizophrenia. Am J Psychiatry. 1970;126:983-7.
160. Rybakowski JK, Suwalska A, Lojko D, Rymaszewska J, Kienjna A. Bipolar mood disorders among Polish psychiatric outpatients treated for major depression. J Affect Disord. 2005;84:141-7.
161. Sachs G. Treatment of acute depression bipolar disorder. In Ketter TA, (Ed). Advances in the treatment of bipolar disorder. Washington, DC: American psychiatric Publishing; 2005. pp. 57-109.
162. Sato T, Bottlender R, Kleind-ienst N, Moller HJ. Irritable psychomotor elation in depressed inpatients: a factor validation of mixed depression. J Affect Disord. 2005;84:187-96.
163. Sato T, Bottlender R, Sievers M, Schroter A, Kleindienst N, Moller HJ. Evaluating the inter-episode stability of depressive mixed states. J Affect Disord. 2004;8:103-13.
164. Sato T, Bottlender R, Schroter A, Moller HJ. Frequency of manic symptoms during a depressive episode and unipolar "depressive mixed state" as bipolar spectrum. Acta Psychiatr Scand. 2003;107:268-74.
165. Sedler MJ. Falret's discovery: the origin of the concept of bipolar affective illness. Am J Psychiatry. 1983;140:1127-33.
166. Serretti A, Olgati L. Profiles of "manic" symptoms in bipolar I, bipolar II and major depressive disorders. J Affect Disord. 2005;84:159-66.
167. Simpson SG, McMahon IJ, Mc Innis MG, et al. Diagnosis reliability of bipolar II diagnosis. Arch Gen Psychiatry. 2002;59:736-40.
168. Smith DJ, Harrison N, Muir W, Blackwood DHR. The high prevalence of bipolar spectrum disorders in young adults with recurrent depression: toward an innovative diagnostic framework. J Affect Disord. 2005;84:167-78.

169. Suppes T, McElroy St., Altshuler LL, et al. Mixed hypomania in 908 patients with bipolar disorder evaluated prospectively in the Stanley Bipolar Treatment Network: a gender-specific phenomenon. Arch Gen Psychiatry. 2005;62:1089-96.
170. Swann AC Janicak PL, Calabrese JR, et al. Structure of mania: depressive irritable and psychotics clusters with different retrospectively assessed course patterns of illness in randomized clinical trial participants J Affect Disord. 2001:67:124-32.
171. Thase ME, MacFadden W, Weisler RH, et al. for the BOLDER II Study Group. Efficacy of quetiapine monotherapy in bipolar I and II depression a double blind, placebo controlled study (the BOLDER II study) J Clin Psychopharmacol. 2006;26:600-09.
172. Tohen M, Chengappa KN, Suppes T, et al. Relapse prevention in bipolar I disorder. 18 month comparison of olanzapine plus mood stabilizer v mood stabilizer alone. Br J Psychiatry. 2004;184:337-45.
173. Tohen M, Ketter Ta, Zarate CA, et al. Olanzapine versus divalproex sodium for the treatment of acute mania and maintenance of remission: a 47-week study. Am J Psychiatry. 2003;160:1263-71.
174. Tohen M, Vieta E, Calabrese J. et al. Efficacy of olanzapine and olanzapine-fluoxetine combination in the treatment of bipolar I depression. Arch Gen Psychatry. 2003;60:1079-88.
175. US Food and Drug Administration Center for Drug Evaluation and Research. Labeling change request letter for antidepressant medication. http://www.fda.gov//cder/drug/antidepressants/SSRIlabelChange.htm (accessed Sep 18, 2011).
176. Vieta F, Reinares M, Bourgeois ML. Bipolar I and bipolar II: a dichotomy? In: Marrneros A, goddwin F (eds). Bipolar disorders. Cambridge: Camb-ridge University Press; 2005. pp. 88-108.
177. WHO. The ICD-10 classification of mental and behavioural disorders. Geneva: World Health Organization, 1992.
178. Winokur G, Tsuang MT. The natural history of mania, depression, and schizophrenia. Washington, DC: American Psychiatric Press,1996.
179. Yatham LN. Diagnonosis and management of patients with bipolar II disorder. J Clin Psychiatry. 2005;66 (Suppl 1):13-7.
180. Zomberg GL, Pope HG Jr. Treatment of depression in bipolar disorder: new directions for research. J Clin Psychopharmacol. 1993;13:197-408.

Mechanism of Disease: Major Depressive Disorder

181. Airan RD, Meltzer LA, Roy M, Gong Y, Chan H, Deisseroth K. High-speed imaging reveals neurophysiological links to behavior in an animal model of depression. Science. 2007;317:819-23.
182. Angelucci F, Brene S, Mathe AA. BDNF in Schizophrenia, depression and corresponding animal models. Mol Psychiatry. 2005;10:345-52.
183. Ansorge MS, Zhou M, Lira A, Hen R, Gingrich JA. Early-life blockade of the 5-HT transporter alters emotional behavior in adult mice. Science. 2004;306:879-81.
184. Avissar S, Nechamkin Y, Roitman G, Schreiber G. Reduced G protein functions and immunoreactive levels in mononuclear leukocytes of patients with depression. AM J Psychiatry. 1997;154:211-7.
185. Barbon A, Popoli M, La Via L, et al. Regulation of editing and expression of glutamate alpha-amino-propionic-acid (AMPA)/kainite receptor by antidepressant drugs. Biol Psychiatry. 2006;59:713-20.
186. Bauer M, Heinz A, Whybrow PC. Thyroid hormones, serotonin and mood: of synergy and significance in the adult brain. Mol Psychiatry. 2002;7:140-56.
187. Beasley CL, Honer WG, Bergamann K, Falkai P, Lutjohann D, Bayer TA. Reductions in cholesterol cortex in mood disorders. Bipolar Disord. 2005;7:449-55.
188. Belmark RH. Bipolar disorder. N Engl J Med 2004;351:476-86.
189. Bersudsky Y, Shaldubina A, Agam G, Berry GT, Belmaker H. Homozygote inositol transporter knockout mice show a lithium-like phenotype. Bipolar Disord (in press).
190. Bhagwagar Z, Wylexinska M, Jezzard P, et al. Reduction in occipital cortex gamma-aminobutyric acid concentrations in medication-free recovered unipolar depressed and bipolar subjects. Biol Psychiatry. 2007;61:806-12.
191. Bhansali P, Dunning J, Singer SE, David L, Schmauss C. Early life stress alters adult serotonin 2C receptor pre-mRNA editing and expression of the alpha subunit of the heterotrimeric G-protein G q. J Neurosci. 2007;27:1467-73.
192. Bhardwaj RD, Curtis MA, Spalding KL, et al. Neurogenesis in humans is restricted to development. Proc Natl Acad Sci USA. 2006;103:12564-8.
193. Blendy JA. The role of CREB in depression and antidepressant treatment. Boil Psychiatry. 2006:59:1144-50.
194. Bouchard TJ Jr. Genes, environment, and personality. Science.1994:264;1700-1.
195. Boyle Mp, Brewer JA, Funatsu M, et al. Acquired deficit of forebrain glucocorticoid receptor produces depression-like changes in adrenal axis regulation and behavior. Proc Natl Acad Sci USA. 2005;102:473-8.
196. Brambilla P, Perez J, Barale F, Schettini G, Soares JC. GABAergic dysfunction in mood disorders. Mol Psychiatry. 2003;8:715,721-37.
197. Brown ES, Varghese FP, McEwen BS. Association of depression with medical illness: does cortisol play a role? Bio Psychiatry. 2004;55:1-9.
198. Bunney WE, Bunney BG. Molecular clock genes in man and lower animals: possible implications for circadian abnormalities in depression. Neuropsychopharmacology. 2000;22:335-45.
199. Burke HM, Davis MC, Otte C, Mohr DC. Depression and cortisol response to psychological stress: a meta-analysis. Psychoneuroendocrinology. 2005;30:846-56.

200. Carroll BJ, Cassidy F, Naftolowitz D, et al. Pathophysiology of hypercortisolism in depression. Acta Psychiatr Scand Suppl. 2007;433:90-103.
201. Cases O, Seif I, Grimsby J, et al. Aggressive behavior and altered amounts of brain serotonin and norepinephrine in mice lacking MAOA. Science. 1995;268:1763-6.
202. Caspi A, Sugden K, Moffitt TE, et al. Influence of life stress on depression: moderation by a polymorphism in the 5-HTT gene. Science. 2003;301:386-9.
203. Castren is mood chemistry? Nat Rev Neurosci. 2005;6:641-6
204. Chang A, Li PP, Warsh JJ, cAMP signal transduction abnormalities in the pathophysiology of mood disorder: contribution from postmortem barin studies. In: Agam G, Everall IP, Belmaker RH, (Eds). The postmortem brain in psychiatry research boston: Kluwer Academic; 2002. pp. 341-62.
205. Chen B, Dowlatashahi D, MacQueen GM, Wang JF, Youg LT. Increased hippocampal BDNF immunoreactivity in subjects treated with antidepressant medication. Bio Psychiatry. 2001;50:260-5.
206. Choudary PV, Molnar M, Evans SJ, et al. Altered cortical glutamatergic and GABAergic single transmission with glial involvement in depression. Proc Natl Acad Sci USA. 2005;102:15653-8.
207. Conti AC, Cryan JF, Dalvi A, Lucki I, Blendy JA. cAMP response element-binding protein is essential for the upregulation of brain-derived neurotrophic factor transcription, but not the behavioral or endocrine response top antidepressant drugs. J Neurosci. 2002;22:3262-8.
208. Cooper-Kazaz R, Apter JT, Cohen R, et al. Combind treatment with sertraline and liothyronine in major depression: a randomized, double-blind, placebo-controlled trial. Arch Gen Psychiatry. 2007;64:679-88.
209. Coupland NJ, Ogilive CJ, Hegadoren KM, Seres P, Hanstock CC, Allen PS. Decreased prefrontal myoinositol in major depressive disorder. Biol Psychiatry. 2005;57:1526-34.
210. Cryns K, Shamir A, Van Acker N, et al. IMPA1 is essential for embryonic development and lithium-like pilocarpine sensitivity. Neuropsyhopharmacology (in press).
211. Dantzer R, Wollman E, Vitkovic L, Yirmiya R. Cytokines and depression: for tuitous or causative association? Mol Psychiatry. 1999;4:328-32.
212. de Pablos RM, Villaran RF, Arguelles S, et al. Stress increases vulnerability to inflammation in the rate prefrontal cortex. J Neurosci. 2005:6:241-6.
213. Desoza LA, Ladiwala U, Daniel SM, Agashe S, Vaidya RA, Vaidya VA. Thyroid hormone regulates hippocampal neurogenesis in the adult rat brain. Mol Cell Nwurosci. 2005;29:414-26.
214. Dziedzicka-wasylewska M, Faron-Gorecka A, Kusmider M, et al. Effect of antidepressant drugs in mice lacking the norepinephrine transporter. Neuropsycho-Pharmacology. 2006;31:2424-32.
215. Einat H, Kronfeld-Schor N, Eilam D. Sand rats see the light: short photoperiod induces a depression-like response in a diurnal rodent. Behav Brain Res. 2006;173:153-7.
216. Flores BH, Kenna H, Keller J, Solvason HB, Schatzberg AF. Clinical and biological effect of mifepristone treatment for psychotic depression. Neuropsychopharmacology. 2006;31:628-36.
217. Folstein M, Liu T, Peter I, et al. The homocysteine hypothesis of depression Am J Psychiatry. 2007;164:861-7 [Erratum, Am J Psychiatry. 2007;164:1123]
218. Frodl T, Schule C, Schmitt G, et al. Association of the brain-derived neurotrophic factor Val66Met Polymorphism with reduced hippocampal volumes in major depression. Arch Gen Psychiatry. 2007;64:410-6.
219. George MS, Belmaker RH (Eds). Transcranial magnetic stimulation in clinical psychiatry. Washington, DS: American Psychiatry Publishing, 2007.
220. Gershon AA, Vishne T, Grunhaus L. Dopamine D2-like receptors and the antidepressant response. Biol Psychiatry. 2007;61:145-53.
221. Gingrich JA. Mutational analysis of the serotonergic system: recent findings using knockout mice. Curr Drug Targets CNS Neurol Disord. 2002;1:449-65.
222. Goshen I, Kreisel T, Ben-Menachem-Zidon O, et al. Brain interleukin-1 mediates chronic stress-induced depression in mice via adrenocortical activation and hippocampal neurogenesis suppression. Mol Psychiatry (in press).
223. Hasler G, Neumeister A, van der Veen JW, et al. Normal prefrontal gamma-aminobutyric acid levels in remitted depressed subjects determined by proton magnetic resonance spectroscopy. Biol Psychiatry. 2005;58:869-73.
224. Hasler G, van der Veen JW, Tumonis T, Meyers N, Shan J, Drevets WC. Tumonis T, Meyers N, Shen J, Drevets WC. Reduced prefrontal glutamate/glutamine and gamma-aminobutyric acid levels in major depression determined using proton magnetic resonance spectroscopy. Arch Gen Psychiatry. 2007;64:193-200.
225. Hasting RS, Parsey RV, Oquendo MA, Arango V, Mann JJ. Volumetric analysis of the prefrontal cortex, amygdale, and hippocampus in major depression. Neuropsychopharmacology. 2004;29:952-9.
226. Hedlund PB, Huitron-resendiz S, Henriksen SJ, Sutcliffe JG. 5-HT7 receptor inhibition and inactivation induce antidepressant-like behavior and sleep pattern. Biol Psychiatry. 2005;58:831-7.
227. Heldt SA, Stanek L, Chhatwal JP. Ressler KJ. Hippocampus-specific deletion of PDNF in adult mice impairs spatial memory and extinction of aversive memories. Mol Psychiatry. 2007;12:656-70.
228. Henn FA, Vollmayr B. Neurogenesis and depression: etiology or epiphenomenon? Biol Psychiatry. 2004;56:146-50.
229. Hines LM, Hoffman PL, Bhave S, et al. A sex-specific role of type VII adenylyl cyclase in depression. J Neurosci. 2006;26:12609-19.
230. Holick KA, Lee DC, Hen R, Dulaw SC. Behavioral effects of chronic fluoxetine in BALB/CJ mice do not require adult hippocampal neurogenesis or the serotonin 1A receptor. Neuro pychopharmacology (in press).

231. Holman P, Weiss Man MM, Zubenko GS, et al. Genetics of recurrent early-onset major depression (Gen RED): final genome scan report. Am J Psychiatry 2007;164:248-58.
232. Holsboer F. The corticosteroid receptor hypothesis of depression. Neuropsychopharmacology. 2000;23:477-501.
233. Janowsky DS, Overstreet DH. Cholinergic-muscarinic dysfunction in mood disorders. In: Soares JC, Young AH (Eds). Bipolar disorders: basic mechanisms and therapeutic implications, 2nd edn, New York: Informa Healthcare; 2007. pp. 67-88.
234. Johansson C, Willeit M, Smedh C, et al. Circadian clock-related polymorphisms in seasonal affective disorder and their relevance to diurnal preference. Neuropsychopharmacology. 2003;28:734-9.
235. Kable JW, Murrin LC, Bylund DB. In vivo gene modification elucidates subtype-specific function of alpha (2)-adrenergic receptors. J Pharmacol Exp Ther. 2000;293:1-7.
236. Karege F, Bondolfi G, Gervasoni N, Schwald M, Aubry JM, Bertschy G. Low brain-derived neurophic factor (BDNF) levels in serum of depressed patients probably results from lowered platelet BDNF release unrelated to platelet reactivity. Bio Psychiatry. 2005;57:1068-72.
237. Kendlar KS, Gentz M Gardner CO, Pedersen NL. A Swedish national twin study of Lifetime major depression. Am J Psychiatry 2006;163:109-14.
238. Kendler KS, Bulik CM, Silberg J, Hettema JM, Myers J, Prescott CA. Childhood sexual abuse and adult psychiatric and substance use disorders in women: an epidemiological and cotwin control analysis. Arch Gen Psychiatry. 2000;57:953-9.
239. Kendler KS, Gardner CO, Prscott CA. Clinical characteristics of major depression that predict risk of depression in relatives. Arch Gen Psychiatry. 1999;56:322.[Erratum, Arch Gen Psychiatry. 2000;57:94-5].
240. Kennedy SE, Koeppe RA, Young EA, Zubieta JK. Dysregulation of endogenous opioid emotion regulation circuitry in major depression in women. Arch Gen Psychiatry. 2006;63:1199-208.
241. Kessler RC, Berglund P, Demler O, et al. The epidemiology of major depressive disorder: results from the National Comorbidity Survey Replication (NCS-R). JAMA 2003;289:3095-105.
242. kozlovsky N, Matar MA, Kalplan Z, Kolter M, Zohar J, Cohen H. Long-term down-regulation of BDNF mRNA in rat hippocampal CA1 subregion correlates with PTSD-like behavioural tress response. Int J Neuropsychopharmacol. 2007;10:741-58.
243. Krege F, vaudan G, Schwald M, Perroud N, La Harpe R, Neurotrophin levels in postmortem brains of suicide victims and the effects of antemortem diagnosis and psychotropic drugs. Brain Res Mol Brain Res. 2005;136:29-37.
244. Lambert G, Johansson M, Agren H, Friberg P. Reduced brain norepinephrine and dopamine release in treatment-refractory depressive illness: evidence in support of the catecholamine hypothesis of mood disorders. Arch Gen Psychiatry. 2000;57(8):787-93.
245. Lee R, Geracioti TD JR, Kasckow JW, Coccaro EF. Childhood trauma and personality disorder: positive correlation with adult CSF corticotropin-releasing factor concentrations. Am J Psychiatry. 2005;162:995-7.
246. Lesch KP, Bengel D, Heils A, et al. Association of anxiety-related traits with a polymorphism in the serotonin transporter gene regulatory region. Science. 1996;274:1527-31.
247. Lesch KP, Greenberg BD, Highley JD, Benett A, Murphy DL. Serotonin transporter, personality, and behavior: toward a dissection of gene-gene and gene-environment interaction. In: Benjamin J, Ebstein RP, Belmaker RH, (Eds). Molecular genetics and the human personality. Ash ingon, DC: American Psychiatry publishing; 2002. pp. 109-35.
248. Lesperance F, Frasure-smith N, Koszycki D, et al. Effects of citalopram and interpersonal psychotherapy on depression in patients with coronary artery disease: the Canadian Cardiac Randomized Evaluation of Antidepressant and Psychotherapy Efficacy (CREATE) trial. JAMA. 2007;297:367-79.[Erratum, JAMA. 2007;298:40].
249. Leway AJ, Lafler BJ, Emens JS, Bauer VK. The circadian basis of winter depression. Proc Natl Acad Sci USA. 2006;103:7414-9.
250. Lopez-Rodriguez F. Kim J, Poland RE. Total sleep deprivation decreases immobility in the forced-swim test. Neuropsychopharmacology. 2004;29:1105-11.
251. Louis C, Cohen C, depoortere R, Griebel G. Antidepressant-like effects of the corticotrophin-releasing factor 1 receptor antagonist, SSR125543, and the vasopressin 1b receptor antagonist, SSR149415, in a DRL-72s Schedule in the rat. Neuropsychopharmacology. 2006;31:2180-7.
252. Lyons WE, Mamounas LA, Ricaurte GA, et al. Brain-derived neurotrophic factor-deficient mice develop aggressiveness and hyperphagia in conjunction with brain serotonergic abnormalities. Proc Natl Acad Sci USA. 1999;96:15239-44.
253. MacMaster FP, Russell A, Mirza Y, et al. Pituitary volume in treatment-naïve pediatric major depressive disorder. Biol Psychiatry. 2006;60:862-6.
254. MacQueen GM, Campbell S, MCEwen BS, et al. Course of illness, hippocampal function and hippocampal volume in major depression. Proc Natl Acad Sci USA. 2003;100:1387-92.
255. Mann JJ. The medical management of depression, N Engl J Med. 2005;353:1819-34.
256. Mayberg HS, Lozano AM, Voon V, et al. Deep brain stimulation for treatment resistant depression. Neuron. 2005;45:651-60.
257. McEwen BS. Protective and damaging effects of stress mediators, N Engl J Med. 1998;338:171-9.
258. Merali Z, Du L, Hrdina P, et al. Dysregulation in the suicide brain: mRNA expression of corticotropin-releasing hormone receptor and GAGA(A) receptor subunits in frontal cortical brain region. J Neurosci. 2004;24:1478-85.
259. Meyer JH, ginovart N, Boovariwala A, et al. Elevated monoamine oxide A levels in the brain: an explanation for

the monomine imbalance of major depression. Arch Gen Psychiatry. 2000;57:787-93.

260. Milak MS, Parsey RV, Keilp J, Oquendo MA, Malone KM, Mann JJ. Neuroanatomic correlates of psychopathology components of major depressive disorder. Arch Gen Psychiatry. 2005;62:397-408.
261. Monteggia LM, Luikart B, Barrot M, et al. Brain-derived neurotrophic factor conditional knockouts show gender differences in depression-related behaviors. Biol Psychiatry. 2007;61:187-97.
262. Muller N, Schwarz MJ, Dehning S, et al. The cyclooxygenase-2 inhibitor depression: results of a double-blind, randomized, placebo controlled, add-on pilot study to reboxetine. Mol Psychiatry. 2006;11:680-4.
263. Nabkasorn C, Miyai N, Sootmongkol A, et al. Effects of Physical exercise on depression, neuroendocrine stress hormones and physiological fitness in adolescent females with depressive symptoms. Eur J Public Health. 2006;16:179-84.
264. Nmets B, Stahl Z, Belmaker RH. Addition of omega-3 fatty acid to maintenance medication treatment for recurrent unipolar depressive disorder. AM J Psychiatry. 2002;159:477-9.
265. Ordway GA, Schenk J, Stockmeier CA, May W, Klimek V. Elevated agonist binding to alpha2-adrenoceptors in the locus coeruleus in major depression. Bio Psychiatry. 2003;53:315-23.
266. Overstreet DH, friendman E, Mathe AA, yadid G. The flinders sensitive line rat: a selectively bred putative animal model of depression. Neurosci Biobehav Rev. 2005;29:739-59.
267. Peel P, Roberts I, Sena E, et al. Comparison of treatment effects between animal experiments and clinical trials: systematic review. BMJ. 2007;334:197.
268. Perera TD, Coplan JD, Lisanby SH, et al. Antidepressant-induced neurogenesis in the hippocampus of adult nonhuman primates. J Neuro Sci. 2007;27:4894-901.
269. pezawas L, meyer-lindenberg A, Drabant EM, et al. 5-HTTLPR polymorphism impacts human cingulated-amygdala interactions: a genetic susceptibility mechanism for depression. Nat neurosci. 2005;8:828-34.
270. Pitchot W, Hansenne M, Pinto E, Reggers J, Fuchs S, Ansseau M. 5-Hydroxy-tryptamine 1A receptors, major depression, and suicidal behavior, Bio-Psychiatry. 2005;58:854-8.
271. Pizzagalli DA, Oakes TR, Fox AS, et al. Functional but not structural subgenual prefrontal cortex abnormalities in melancholia. Mol Psychiatry. 2004;29:952-9.
272. Popik P, Kozela E, Krawczyk M. Nicotine and nicotinic receptor antagonists potentiate the antidepressant-like effects of imipramine and cicalopram. Br J Pharmacol. 2003;139:1196-202.
273. Potter GG, Blackwell AD, McQuoid DR, et al. Prefrontal white matter lesions and prefrontal task impersistence in depressed and nondepressed elders. Neuropsychopharmacology. 2007;32:2135-42.
274. Rajkowska G. Postmortem studies in mood disorders indicate altered numbers of neurons and glial cells. Bio Psychiatry. 2000;48:766-77.
275. Rajlowska G, O'Dwyer G, Teleki Z, Stockmeier CA, Miguel-Hidalgo JJ. GABAergic neurons immunoreactive for calcium binding proteins are reduced in the prefrontal cortex in major depression. Neuropsychopharmacology. 2007;32:471-82.
276. Rakic P, Neurogenesis in adult primate neocortex: an evaluation of the evidence. Nat Rev Neurosci. 2002;3:65-71.
277. Reagan LP, Rosell DR, wood GE, et al. Chromic restraint stress up-regulates GLT-1 mRNA and protein expression in the rat hippocampus: reversal by tianeptine. Proc Natl Acad Sci USA. 2004;101:2179-84.
278. Ruhe HG, Mason NS, Schene AH. Mood is indirectly related to serotonin, norepinephrine and dopamine levels in humans: a meta-analysis of monoamine depletion studies. Mol Psychiatry. 2007;12:331-59.
279. Sanacora G, Guerguieva R, Epperson CN, et al. Subtype-specific alterations of gamma-aminobutyric acid and glutamate in patients with major depression. Arch Gen Psychiatry. 2004;61:705-13.
280. Santerelli L, Saxe M, Gross C, et al. Requirement of hippocampal neurogenesis for the behavioral effects of antidepressants. Science. 2003;301:805-9.
281. Sapolsky RM. Glucocorticoids and hippocampal atrophy in neuropsychiatric disorders. Arch Gen Psychiatry. 2000;57:925-35.
282. Schmidt PJ, Daly RC, bloch M, et al. Dehydroepiandrosterone monotherapy in midlife-onset major and minor depression. Arch Gen Psychiatry. 2005;62:154-62.
283. Schramm NL, McDonald MP, Limbird LE. The alpha (2a)-adrenergic receptor plays a protective role in mouse behavioral models of depression and anxiety. J Neurosci. 2001;21:4875-82.
284. Seeman P, Ko F, Tallerico T. Dopamine receptor contribution to the action of PC, LSD and ketamine psychotomimetics. Mol Psychiatry. 2005;10:877-83.
285. Shimon H, Agam G, Belmaker RH, Hyde TM, Kleinman JE. Reduced frontal cortex inositol levels in postmortem brain of suicide victims and patients with bipolar disorder. Am J Psychiatry. 1997;154:1148-50.
286. Shirayama Y, Chen AC, Nakagawa S, Russell DS, Duman RS Brain-derived neurotrophic factor produces antidepressant effects in behavioral models of depression. J Neurosci. 2002;22:3251-61.
287. Shytle RD, Silver AA, Lukas RJ, Newman MB, Sheehan DV, sanberg PR. Nicotinic acetylcholine receptor as targets for antidepressants. Mol Psychiatry. 2002;7:525-35.
288. Spalletta G, Bossu P, Ciaramella A, Bria P, Caltagirone C, Robinson RG. The etiology of poststroke depression: a review of the literature and a new hypothesis involving inflammatory cytokines. Mol Psychiatry. 2006;11:984-91.
289. Strome EM, Wheler GH, Higley JD, Loriaux DL, suomi SJ, Doudet DJ, Intracerebroventricular corticotrophin-releasing factor increases limbic glucose metabolism and has social context-dependent behavioral effects in nonhuman primates. Proc Natl Acad Sci USA. 2002;99:15749-54.

290. Strous RD, Maayan R, Lapidus R, et al. Dehydroepiandrosterone augmentation in the management of negative, depressive, and anxiety symptoms in schizophrenia. Arch Gen Psychiatry. 2003;60:133-41.

291. Sullivan GM, Mann JJ, Oquendo MA, Lo ES, Cooper TB, Gorman JM. Low cerebrospinal fluid transthyretin levels in depression: correlations with suicidal ideation and low serotonin function. Biol Psychiatry. 2006;60:500-6.

292. Sullivan PF, Neale MC, Kendle KS. Genetic epidemiology of major depression: review and meta-analysis. AM J Psychiatry 2000;157:1552-62.

293. Svenningsson P, Chergui K, Rachleff I, et al. Alteration in 5-HT1B receptor function by p11 depression-like states science. 2006;311:77-80.

294. Taylor CB, Youngblood ME, Catellier D, et al. Effects of antidepressant medication on morbidity and mortality in depressed patients after myocardial infarction. Arch Gen Psychiatry. 2005;62:792-8.

295. Taylor MJ, Freemantle N, Geddes JR, Bhagwagar Z. Early onset of selective serotonin reuptake inhibitor antidepressant action:systematic review and meta-analysis. Ach Gen Psychiatry. 2006;63:1217-23.

296. Torregrossa MM, Jutkiewicz EM, Mosberg HI, Balboni G, Watson SJ, Woods JH. Peptidic delta opioid receptor agonists produce antidepressant-like effects in the forced swim test and regulate BDNF mRNA expression in rats. Brain Res. 2006;1069:172-81.

297. Tremblay LK, Naranjo CA, Cardenas L, Herrmann N, Busto UE. Probing brain reward system function in major depressive disorder: altered response to dextro-amphetamine. Arch Gen Psychiatry. 2002;59:409-16.

298. Tsankova NM, Berton O, Renthal W, Kumar A, Neve RL, Nestler EJ. Sustained Hippocampal chromatin regulation in a mouse model of depression and antidepressant action. Nat Neurosci. 2006;9:519-25.

299. Valdizan EM, Gutierrez O, Pazos A. Adenylate cyclase activity in postmortem brain of suicide subjects: reduced response to beta-adrenergic stimulation. Bio Psychiatry. 2003;54:1457-64.

300. Van Praag H, Kempermann G, Gage FH. Running increase cell proliferation and neurogenesis in the adult mouse dentate gyrus. Nat Neuroci. 1999;2:266-70.

301. Van Praag H. Monoamine precursors in depression: present state and prospects. In: Zohar J, Belmaker RH, (Eds.) Treating resistant depression. New York: PMA Publishing; 1987. pp. 279-306.

302. Wakefield JC, Schmitz MF, First MB, Horvitz AV. Extending the bereavement exclusion for major depression to other losses: evidence from the National Comorbidity Survey. Arch Gen Psychiatry 2007;64:433-40.

303. Warner-Schmidt JL, Duman RS. VEGF is an essential mediator of the neurogenic and behavioral actions of antidepressants. Proc Natl Acad Sci USA. 2007;104:4647-52.

304. weaver IC, Cervoni N, Champagne FA, et al. Epigenetic Programming by maternal behavior. Nat Neurosci. 2004;7:847-54.

305. Weber MM, Emrich HM. Current and historical concepts of opiate treatment in psychiatry disorders. Int Clin Psychopharmacol. 1988;3:255-66.

306. Weisstaub NV, Zhou M, Lira A, et al. Cortical 5-HT2A receptor signaling modulates anxiety-like behaviors in mice. Science. 2006;313:536-40.

307. Zarate CA Jr, Singh JB, Carlson PJ, et al. A randomized trial of an N-methyl-D-aspartate antagonist in treatment-resistant major depression. Arch Gen Psychiatry. 2006;63:856-64.

308. Zhang X, Beaulieu JM, sotnikova TD, Gainetdinow RR, Caron MG. Tryptophan hydroxylas-2 identified in unipolar manor depression. Neuron. 2005;45:11-6.

309. Zhang X, Gainetdinow RR, Beaulieu JM, et al. Loss of funtion mutation in tryptophan hydroxylase-2 identified in unipolar major depression. Neuron. 2005;45:11-6.

Major Depressive Disorder: New Clinical, Neurobiological and Treatment Perspective

310. Aan het Rot M, Collins KA, Murrough JW, et al. Safety and efficacy of repeated-dose intravenous ketamine for treatment-resistant depression. Biol Psychiatry. 2010;67:139-45.

311. Akiskal HS, Pinto O. The soft bipolar spectrum: footnotes to Kraepelin on the interface of hypomania, temperament and depression. In: Marneros A, Angst J (Eds). Bipolar disorders:100 years after manic-depressive insanity. Dorderecht, Netherlands: Kluwer Academic; 2000:37-62.

312. Almeida JR, Versace A, Hassel S, Kupfer DJ, Phillips ML. Elevated amygdala activity to sad facial expressions: a state marker of bipolar but not unipolar depression. Biol Psychiatry. 2010;67:414-21.

313. Almeida JR, Versace A, Mechelli A, et al. Abnormal amygdala-prefrontal effective connectivity to happy faces differentiates bipolar from major depression. Biol Psychiatry. 2009;66:451-9.

314. American Psychiatric Association. Practice guideline for the treatment of patients with major depressive disorder, 3rd edn.http://www.psychiatryonline.com/pracGuide/pracGuideTopic_7.aspx. (accessed Feb 26, 2013).

315. Anand A, Li Y, Wang Y, et al. Antidepressant effect on connectivity of the mood-regulating circuit: an FMRI study. Neuropsychopharmacology. 2005;30:1334-44.

316. Anand A, Li Y, Wang Y, Gardner K, Lowe MJ. Reciprocal effects of antidepressant treatment on activity and connectivity of the mood regulating circuit: an FMRI study. J Neuropsychiatry Clin Neurosci. 2007;19:274-82.

317. Bauer M, Adli M, Bschor T, et al. Lithium's emerging role in the treatment of refractory major depressive episodes: augmentation of antidepressants. Neuropsychobiology. 2010;62:36-42.

318. Baune BT, Dannlowski U, Domschke K, et al. The interleukin 1 beta (IL1B) gene is associated with failure to achieve remission and impaired emotion processing in major depression. Biol Psychiatry. 2010;67:543-9.

319. Baune BT, Hohoff C, Berger K, et al. Association of the COMT val158met variant with antidepressant treatment

response in major depression. Neuropsychopharmacology. 2008;33:924-32.

320. Beesdo K, Bittner A, Pine DS, et al. Incidence of social anxiety disorder and the consistent risk for secondary depression in the first three decades of life. Arch Gen Psychiatry. 2007;64: 903-12.
321. Bell AC, D'Zurilla TJ. Problem-solving therapy for depression: a meta-analysis. Clin Psychol Rev. 2009;29:348-53.
322. Benazzi F. Bipolar disorder—focus on bipolar II disorder and mixed depression. Lancet. 2007;369:935-45.
323. Bertolino A, Arciero G, Rubino V, et al. Variation of human amygdala response during threatening stimuli as a function of 5' HTTLPR genotype and personality style. Biol Psychiatry. 2005;57:1517-25.
324. Bewernick BH, Hurlemann R, Matusch A, et al. Nucleus accumbens deep brain stimulation decreases ratings of depression and anxiety in treatment-resistant depression. Biol Psychiatry. 2010;67:110-6.
325. Binder EB, Owens MJ, Liu W, et al. Association of polymorphisms in genes regulating the corticotropin-releasing factor system with antidepressant treatment response. Arch Gen Psychiatry. 2010;67:369-79.
326. Binder EB, Salyakina D, Lichtner P, et al. Polymorphisms in FKBP5 are associated with increased recurrence of depressive episodes and rapid response to antidepressant treatment. Nat Genet. 2004;36:1319-25.
327. Binder EB. The role of FKBP5, a co-chaperone of the glucocorticoid receptor in the pathogenesis and therapy of affective and anxiety disorders. Psychoneuroendocrinology. 2009;34(suppl): S186-S195.
328. Blumberg HP, Wang F, Chepenik LG, et al. Influence of vascular endothelial growth factor variation on human hippocampus morphology. Biol Psychiatry. 2008;64:901-3.
329. Bortolotti B, Menchetti M, Bellini F, Montaguti MB, Berardi D. Psychological interventions for major depression in primary care: a meta-analytic review of randomized controlled trials. Gen Hosp Psychiatry. 2008;30:293-302.
330. Brunoni AR, Lopes M, Fregni F. A systematic review and meta-analysis of clinical studies on major depression and BDNF levels: implications for the role of neuroplasticity in depression. Int J Neuropsychopharmacol. 2008;11:1169-80.
331. Brustolim D, Ribeiro-dos-Santos R, Kast RE, Altschuler EL, Soares MB. A new chapter opens in anti-inflammatory treatments: the antidepressant bupropion lowers production of tumor necrosis factor-alpha and interferon-gamma in mice. Int Immunopharmacol. 2006;6:903-7.
332. Bschor T, Baethge C. No evidence for switching the antidepressant: systematic review and meta-analysis of RCTs of a common therapeutic strategy. Acta Psychiatr Scand. 2010;121:174-9.
333. Campayo A, de Jonge P, Roy JF, Saz P, et al for the ZARADEMP Project. Depressive disorder and incident diabetes mellitus: the effect of characteristics of depression. Am J Psychiatry2010;167:580-8.
334. Cassano GB, Rucci P, Frank E, et al. The mood spectrum in unipolar and bipolar disorder: arguments for a unitary approach. Am J Psychiatry. 2004;161:1264-9.
335. Connolly KR, Thase ME. If at first you don't succeed: a review of the evidence for antidepressant augmentation, combination and switching strategies. Drugs. 2011;71:43-64.
336. Craddock RC, Holtzheimer PE, Hu XP, Mayberg HS. Disease state prediction from resting state functional connectivity. Magn Reson Med. 2009;62:1619-28.
337. Cuijpers P, Dekker J, Hollon SD, Andersson G. Adding psychotherapy to pharmacotherapy in the treatment of depressive disorders in adults: a meta-analysis. J Clin Psychiatry. 2009;70:1219-29.
338. Cuijpers P, van Straten A, van Oppen P, Andersson G. Are psychological and pharmacologic interventions equally effective in the treatment of adult depressive disorders? A meta-analysis of comparative studies. J Clin Psychiatry. 2008;69:1675-85.
339. Dannlowski U, Ohrmann P, Bauer J, et al. Amygdala reactivity to masked negative faces is associated with automatic judgmental bias in major depression: a 3 T fMRI study. J Psychiatry Neurosci. 2007;32:423-9.
340. Dantzer R, O'Connor JC, Freund GG, Johnson RW, Kelley KW. From inflammation to sickness and depression: when the immune system subjugates the brain. Nat Rev Neurosci. 2008;9:46-56.
341. Das-Munshi J, Goldberg D, Bebbington PE, et al. Public health significance of mixed anxiety and depression: beyond current classification. Br J Psychiatry. 2008;192:171-7.
342. Dell'osso B, Altamura AC. Augmentative transcranial magnetic stimulation (TMS) combined with brain navigation in drug-resistant rapid cycling bipolar depression: a case report of acute and maintenance efficacy. World J Biol Psychiatry. 2009;10:673-6.
343. Dillon DG, Bogdan R, Fagerness J, Holmes AJ, Perlis RH, Pizzagalli DA. Variation in TREK1 gene linked to depression-resistant phenotype is associated with potentiated neural responses to rewards in humans. Hum Brain Mapp. 2010;31:210-21.
344. Dotson VM, Davatzikos C, Kraut MA, Resnick SM. Depressive symptoms and brain volumes in older adults: a longitudinal magnetic resonance imaging study. J Psychiatry Neurosci. 2009;34:367-75.
345. Ebmeier KP, Donaghey C, Steele JD. Recent developments and current controversies in depression. Lancet. 2006;367:153-67.
346. Epstein J, Pan H, Kocsis JH, et al. Lack of ventral striatal response to positive stimuli in depressed versus normal subjects. Am J Psychiatry. 2006;163:1784-90.
347. Erickson KI, Prakash RS, Voss MW, et al. Brain-derived neurotrophic factor is associated with age-related decline in hippocampal volume. J Neurosci. 2010;30:5368-75.
348. Fales CL, Barch DM, Rundle MM, et al. Altered emotional interference processing in affective and cognitive-control brain circuitry in major depression. Biol Psychiatry. 2008;63:377-84.

349. Fan M, Liu B, Jiang T, Jiang X, Zhao H, Zhang J. Meta-analysis of the association between the monoamine oxidase-A gene and mood disorders. Psychiatr Genet. 2010;20:1-7.
350. Fitzgerald PB, Laird AR, Maller J, Daskalakis ZJ. A meta-analytic study of changes in brain activation in depression. Hum Brain Mapp. 2008;29:683-95.
351. Forbes EE, Hariri AR, Martin SL, et al. Altered striatal activation predicting real-world positive affect in adolescent major depressive disorder. Am J Psychiatry. 2009;166:64-73.
352. Frank E, Kupfer DJ, Buysse DJ, et al. Randomized trial of weekly, twice-monthly, and monthly interpersonal psychotherapy as maintenance treatment for women with recurrent depression. Am J Psychiatry. 2007;164:761-7.
353. Frasure-Smith N, Lespérance F. Depression and anxiety as predictors of 2-year cardiac events in patients with stable coronary artery disease. Arch Gen Psychiatry. 2009;65:62-71.
354. Fu CH, Mourao-Miranda J, Costafreda SG, et al. Pattern classification of sad facial processing: toward the development of neurobiological markers in depression. Biol Psychiatry. 2008;63:656-62.
355. Gaiteri C, Guilloux JP, Lewis DA, Sibille E. Altered gene synchrony suggests a combined hormone-mediated dysregulated state in major depression. PLoS One. 2010;5: e9970.
356. Gaynes BN, Warden D, Trivedi MH, Wisniewski SR, Fava M, Rush AJ. What did STAR*D teach us? Results from a large-scale, practical, clinical trial for patients with depression. Psychiatr Serv. 2009;60:1439-45.
357. Ghosh A, Hellewell JS. A review of the efficacy and tolerability of agomelatine in the treatment of major depression. Expert Opin Investig Drugs. 2007;16:1999-2004.
358. Giacobbe P, Kennedy SH. Deep brain stimulation for treatment-resistant depression: a psychiatric perspective. Curr Psychiatry Rep. 2006;8:437-44.
359. Gibbons RD, Brown CH, Hur K, Marcus SM, Bhaumik DK, Mann JJ. Relationship between antidepressants and suicide attempts: an analysis of the Veterans Health Administration data sets. Am J Psychiatry. 2007;164:1044-9.
360. Gibbons RD, Hur K, Bhaumik DK, Mann JJ. The relationship between antidepressant medication use and rate of suicide. Arch Gen Psychiatry. 2005;62:165-72.
361. Glassman AH, Bigger JT, Gaffney M. Psychiatric characteristics associated with long-term mortality among 361 patients having an acute coronary syndrome and major depression: seven-year follow-up of SADHART participants. Arch Gen Psychiatry. 2009;66:1022-9.
362. Goldberg D. The detection and treatment of depression in the physically ill. World Psychiatry. 2010;9:16-20.
363. Goodwin GM, Emsley R, Rembry S, Rouillon F for the Agomelatine Study Group. Agomelatine prevents relapse in patients with major depressive disorder without evidence of a discontinuation syndrome: a 24-week randomized, double-blind, placebo-controlled trial. J Clin Psychiatry. 2009;70:1128-37.
364. Greicius MD, Flores BH, Menon V, et al. Resting-state functional connectivity in major depression: abnormally increased contributions from subgenual cingulate cortex and thalamus. Biol Psychiatry. 2007;62:429-37.
365. Gusnard DA, Akbudak E, Shulman GL, Raichle ME. Medial prefrontal cortex and self-referential mental activity: relation to a default mode of brain function. Proc Natl Acad Sci USA. 2001;98:4259-64.
366. Hariri AR, Drabant EM, Munoz KE, et al. A susceptibility gene for affective disorders and the response of the human amygdala. Arch Gen Psychiatry. 2005;62:146-52.
367. Harrison NA, Brydon L, Walker C, Gray MA, Steptoe A, Critchley HD. Inflammation causes mood changes through alterations in subgenual cingulate activity and mesolimbic connectivity. Biol Psychiatry. 2009;66:407-414.
368. Heinz A, Smolka MN, Braus DF, et al. Serotonin transporter genotype (5-HTTLPR): effects of neutral and undefined conditions on amygdala activation. Biol Psychiatry. 2007;61:1011-4.
369. Hollon SD, DeRubeis RJ, Shelton RC, et al. Prevention of relapse following cognitive therapy vs medications in moderate to severe depression. Arch Gen Psychiatry. 2005;62:417-22.
370. Holsboer F. The corticosteroid receptor hypothesis of depression. Neuropsychopharmacology. 2000;23: 477-501.
371. Horstmann S, Lucae S, Menke A, et al. Polymorphisms in GRIK4, HTR2A, and FKBP5 show interactive effects in predicting remission to antidepressant treatment. Neuropsychopharmacology. 2010;35:727-40.
372. Huezo-Diaz P, Uher R, Smith R, et al. Moderation of antidepressant response by the serotonin transporter gene. Br J Psychiatry. 2009;195:30-38.
373. Ising M, Horstmann S, Kloiber S, et al. Combined dexamethasone/corticotropin releasing hormone test predicts treatment response in major depression—a potential biomarker?. Biol Psychiatry. 2007;62:47-54.
374. Joffe RT, Gatt JM, Kemp AH, et al. Brain derived neurotrophic factor Val66Met polymorphism, the five factor model of personality and hippocampal volume: implications for depressive illness. Hum Brain Mapp. 2009;30:1246-56.
375. Kato M, Serretti A. Review and meta-analysis of antidepressant pharmacogenetic findings in major depressive disorder. Mol Psychiatry. 2010;15:473-500.
376. Keedwell PA, Andrew C, Williams SC, Brammer MJ, Phillips ML. A double dissociation of ventromedial prefrontal cortical responses to sad and happy stimuli in depressed and healthy individuals. Biol Psychiatry. 2005;58:495-503.
377. Kendler KS, Gardner CO, Fiske A, Gatz M. Major depression and coronary artery disease in the Swedish twin registry: phenotypic, genetic, and environmental sources of comorbidity. Arch Gen Psychiatry. 2009;66:857-63.
378. Kessler D, Lewis G, Kaur S, et al. Therapist-delivered Internet psychotherapy for depression in primary care: a randomised controlled trial. Lancet. 2009;374:628-34.

379. Kessler RC, Angermeyer M, Anthony JC, et al. Lifetime prevalence and age-of-onset distributions of mental disorders in the World Health Organization's World Mental Health Survey Initiative. World Psychiatry. 2007;6:168-76.
380. Kessler RC, Berglund P, Demler O, et al for the National Comobordity Survey Replication. The epidemiology of major depressive disorder: results from the National Comorbidity Survey Replication (NCS-R). JAMA. 2003;289: 3095-105.
381. Kim DR, Pesiridou A, O'Reardon JP. Transcranial magnetic stimulation in the treatment of psychiatric disorders. Curr Psychiatry Rep. 2009;11:447-52.
382. Kopell BH, Greenberg B, Rezai AR. Deep brain stimulation for psychiatric disorders. J Clin Neurophysiol. 2004;21:51-67.
383. Kronenberg G, Tebartz van Elst L, Regen F, Deuschle M, Heuser I, Colla M. Reduced amygdala volume in newly admitted psychiatric in-patients with unipolar major depression. J Psychiatr Res. 2009;43:1112-7.
384. Krystal JH. N-methyl-D-aspartate glutamate receptor antagonists and the promise of rapid-acting antidepressants. Arch Gen Psychiatry. 2010;67:1110-1.
385. Kuhn J, Gründler TO, Lenartz D, Sturm V, Klosterkötter J, Huff W. Deep brain stimulation for psychiatric disorders. Dtsch Arztebl Int. 2010;107:105-13.
386. Laje G, Paddock S, Manji H, et al. Genetic markers of suicidal ideation emerging during citalopram treatment of major depression. Am J Psychiatry. 2007;164:1530-8.
387. Lekman M, Laje G, Charney D, et al. The FKBP5-gene in depression and treatment response—an association study in the Sequenced Treatment Alternatives to Relieve Depression (STAR*D) Cohort. Biol Psychiatry. 2008;63:1103-10.
388. Li L, Ma N, Li Z, et al. Prefrontal white matter abnormalities in young adult with major depressive disorder: a diffusion tensor imaging study. Brain Res. 2007;1168:124-8.
389. Licinio J, Dong C, Wong ML. Novel sequence variations in the brain-derived neurotrophic factor gene and association with major depression and antidepressant treatment response. Arch Gen Psychiatry. 2009;66:488-97.
390. Lisanby SH, Husain MM, Rosenquist PB, et al. Daily left prefrontal repetitive transcranial magnetic stimulation in the acute treatment of major depression: clinical predictors of outcome in a multisite, randomized controlled clinical trial. Neuropsychopharmacology. 2009;34:522-34.
391. Liu Z, Zhu F, Wang G, et al. Association study of corticotropin-releasing hormone receptor 1 gene polymorphisms and antidepressant response in major depressive disorders. Neuroscience Lett. 2007;414:155-8.
392. Lozano AM, Mayberg HS, Giacobbe P, Hamani C, Craddock RC, Kennedy SH. Subcallosal cingulate gyrus deep brain stimulation for treatment-resistant depression. Biol Psychiatry. 2008;64:461-7.
393. Luppino FS, de Wit LM, Bouvy PF, et al. Overweight, obesity, and depression: a systematic review and meta-analysis of longitudinal studies. Arch Gen Psychiatry. 2010;67:220-9.
394. Luty SE, Carter JD, McKenzie JM, et al. Randomised controlled trial of interpersonal psychotherapy and cognitive-behavioural therapy for depression. Br J Psychiatry. 2007;190:496-502.
395. Lyketsos CG. Depression and diabetes: more on what the relationship might be. Am J Psychiatry. 2010;167:496-7.
396. Malone DA, Dougherty DD, Rezai AR, et al. Deep brain stimulation of the ventral capsule/ventral striatum for treatment-resistant depression. Biol Psychiatry. 2009;65:267-75.
397. Mayberg HS, Lozano AM, Voon V, et al. Deep brain stimulation for treatment-resistant depression. Neuron. 2005;45:651-60.
398. McMahon FJ, Buervenich S, Charney D, et al. Variation in the gene encoding the serotonin 2A receptor is associated with outcome of antidepressant treatment. Am J Hum Genet. 2006;78:804-14.
399. Medicines and Healthcare Products Regulatory Agency. MHRA update on the risks of birth defects in babies born to mothers taking paroxetine—q&a.http://www.mhra.gov.uk/home/groups/pl-p/documents/websiteresources/con2022700.pdf. (accessed July 8, 2013).
400. Meyers BS, Flint AJ, Rothschild AJ, et al (for the STOP-PD Group). A double-blind randomized controlled trial of olanzapine plus sertraline vs olanzapine plus placebo for psychotic depression: the study of pharmacotherapy of psychotic depression (STOP-PD). Arch Gen Psychiatry. 2009;66:838-47.
401. Michels R. Personality disorders in the depressed: seeing clearly through blue lenses. Am J Psychiatry. 2010;167:487-8.
402. Mitchell AJ, Vaze A, Rao S. Clinical diagnosis of depression in primary care: a meta-analysis. Lancet. 2009;374:609-19.
403. Mitka M. Routine depression screening advised for patients with coronary heart disease. JAMA. 2008;300:2356-7.
404. Moffitt TE, Harrington H, Caspi A, et al. Depression and generalized anxiety disorder: cumulative and sequential comorbidity in a birth cohort followed prospectively to age 32 years. Arch Gen Psychiatry. 2007;64:651-60.
405. Moses-Kolko EL, Bogen D, Perel J, et al. Neonatal signs after late in utero exposure to serotonin reuptake inhibitors: literature review and implications for clinical applications. JAMA. 2005;293:2372-83.
406. Moussavi S, Chatterji S, Verdes E, Tandon A, Patel V, Ustun B. Depression, chronic diseases, and decrements in health: results from the World Health Surveys. Lancet. 2007;370:851-8.
407. Murphy GM, Hollander SB, Rodrigues HE, Kremer C, Schatzberg AF. Effects of the serotonin transporter gene promoter polymorphism on mirtazapine and paroxetine efficacy and adverse events in geriatric major depression. Arch Gen Psychiatry. 2004;61:1163-9.
408. Nelson JC. S-adenosyl methionine (SAMe) augmentation in major depressive disorder. Am J Psychiatry. 2010;167:889-91.
409. Olfson M, Marcus SC, Shaffer D. Antidepressant drug therapy and suicide in severely depressed children and adults: a case-control study. Arch Gen Psychiatry. 2006;63:865-72.
410. Olfson M, Marcus SC. A case-control study of antidepressants and attempted suicide during early phase treatment of major depressive episodes. J Clin Psychiatry 69:425-32.

411. Olfson M, Marcus SC. National patterns in antidepressant medication treatment. Arch Gen Psychiatry. 2009;66:848-56.
412. Olié JP, Kasper S. Efficacy of agomelatine, a MT1/MT2 receptor agonist with 5-HT2C antagonistic properties, in major depressive disorder. Int J Neuropsychopharmacol. 2007;10:661-73.
413. Paddock S, Laje G, Charney D, et al. Association of GRIK4 with outcome of antidepressant treatment in the STAR*D cohort. Am J Psychiatry. 2007;164:1181-8.
414. Papakostas GI, Mischoulon D, Shyu I, Alpert JE, Fava M. S-adenosyl methionine (SAMe) augmentation of serotonin reuptake inhibitors for antidepressant nonresponders with major depressive disorder: a double-blind, randomized clinical trial. Am J Psychiatry. 2010;167:942-8.
415. Papakostas GI, Shelton RC, Smith J, Fava M. Augmentation of antidepressants with atypical antipsychotic medications for treatment-resistant major depressive disorder: a meta-analysis. J Clin Psychiatry. 2007;68:826-31.
416. Perlis RH, Fijal B, Adams DH, et al. Variation in catechol-O-methyltransferase is associated with duloxetine response in a clinical trial for major depressive disorder. Biol Psychiatry. 2009;65:785-91.
417. Perlis RH, Laje G, Smoller JW, Fava M, Rush AJ, McMahon FJ. Genetic and clinical predictors of sexual dysfunction in citalopram-treated depressed patients. Neuropsychopharmacology. 2009;34:1819-28.
418. Perlis RH, Moorjani P, Fagerness J, et al. Pharmacogenetic analysis of genes implicated in rodent models of antidepressant response: association of TREK1 and treatment resistance in the STAR(*)D study. Neuropsychopharmacology. 2008;33:2810-19.
419. Pezawas L, Meyer-Lindenberg A, Goldman AL, et al. Evidence of biologic epistasis between BDNF and SLC6A4 and implications for depression. Mol Psychiatry. 2008;13:709-16.
420. Phillips ML, Ladouceur CD, Drevets WC. A neural model of voluntary and automatic emotion regulation: implications for understanding the pathophysiology and neurodevelopment of bipolar disorder. Mol Psychiatry. 2008;13:833-57.
421. Pizzagalli DA, Holmes AJ, Dillon DG, et al. Reduced caudate and nucleus accumbens response to rewards in unmedicated individuals with major depressive disorder. Am J Psychiatry. 2009;166:702-10.
422. Pizzagalli DA. Frontocingulate dysfunction in depression: toward biomarkers of treatment response. Neuropsychopharmacology. 2011;36:183-206.
423. Raison CL, Borisov AS, Majer M, et al. Activation of central nervous system inflammatory pathways by interferon-alpha: relationship to monoamines and depression. Biol Psychiatry. 2009;65:296-303.
424. Rajkowska G, O'Dwyer G, Teleki Z, Stockmeier CA, Miguel-Hidalgo JJ. GABAergic neurons immunoreactive for calcium binding proteins are reduced in the prefrontal cortex in major depression. Neuropsychopharmacology. 2007;32:471-82.
425. Rush AJ, Fava M, Wisniewski SR, et al for the STAR*D Investigators Group. Sequenced treatment alternatives to relieve depression (STAR*D): rationale and design. Control Clin Trials. 2004;25:119-42.
426. Rush AJ, Trivedi MH, Wisniewski SR, et al. Acute and longer-term outcomes in depressed outpatients requiring one or several treatment steps: a STAR*D report. Am J Psychiatry. 2006;163:1905-17.
427. Rush AJ. Combining antidepressant medications: a good idea? Am J Psychiatry. 2010;167:241-3.
428. Salvadore G, Cornwell BR, Sambataro F, et al. Anterior cingulate desynchronization and functional connectivity with the amygdala during a working memory task predict rapid antidepressant response to ketamine. Neuropsychopharmacology. 2010;35:1415-22.
429. Schlaepfer TE, Cohen MX, Frick C, et al. Deep brain stimulation to reward circuitry alleviates anhedonia in refractory major depression. Neuropsychopharmacology. 2008;33:368-77.
430. Schneck CD. Mixed depression: the importance of rediscovering subtypes of mixed mood states. Am J Psychiatry. 2009;166:127-30.
431. Schramm E, van Calker D, Dykierek P, et al. An intensive treatment program of interpersonal psychotherapy plus pharmacotherapy for depressed inpatients: acute and long-term results. Am J Psychiatry. 2007;164:768-77.
432. Schreuders B, van Marwijk H, Smit J, Rijmen F, Stalman W, van Oppen P. Primary care patients with mental health problems: outcome of a randomised clinical trial. Br J Gen Pract. 2009;57:886-91.
433. Schultz W. Behavioral dopamine signals. Trends Neurosci. 2007;30:203-10.
434. Sen S, Duman R, Sanacora G. Serum brain-derived neurotrophic factor, depression, and antidepressant medications: meta-analyses and implications. Biol Psychiatry. 2008;64:527-32.
435. Serretti A, Kato M, De Ronchi D, Kinoshita T. Meta-analysis of serotonin transporter gene promoter polymorphism (5-HTTLPR) association with selective serotonin reuptake inhibitor efficacy in depressed patients. Mol Psychiatry. 2007;12:247-57.
436. Shyn SI, Hamilton SP. The genetics of major depression: moving beyond the monoamine hypothesis. Psychiatr Clin North Am. 2010;33:125-40.
437. Siegle GJ, Carter CS, Thase ME. Use of FMRI to predict recovery from unipolar depression with cognitive behavior therapy. Am J Psychiatry. 2006;163:735-8.
438. Simon GE, Ludman EJ, Rutter CM. Incremental benefit and cost of telephone care management and telephone psychotherapy for depression in primary care. Arch Gen Psychiatry. 2009;66:1081-9.
439. Slotema CW, Blom JD, Hoek HW, Sommer IE. Should we expand the toolbox of psychiatric treatment methods to include Repetitive Transcranial Magnetic Stimulation (rTMS)? A meta-analysis of the efficacy of rTMS in psychiatric disorders. J Clin Psychiatry. 2010;71:873-84.
440. Soliman F, Glatt CE, Bath KG, et al. A genetic variant BDNF polymorphism alters extinction learning in both mouse and human. Science. 2010;327:863-6.

441. Stahl SM, Fava M, Trivedi MH, Caputo A, Shah A, Post A. Agomelatine in the treatment of major depressive disorder: an 8-week, multicenter, randomized, placebo-controlled trial. J Clin Psychiatry. 2010;71:616-26.
442. Surguladze S, Brammer MJ, Keedwell P, et al. A differential pattern of neural response toward sad versus happy facial expressions in major depressive disorder. Biol Psychiatry. 2005;57:201-9.
443. Thase ME, Friedman ES, Biggs MM, et al. Cognitive therapy versus medication in augmentation and switch strategies as second-step treatments: a STAR*D report. Am J Psychiatry. 2007;164:739-52.
444. Thombs BD, de Jonge P, Coyne JC, et al. Depression screening and patient outcomes in cardiovascular care: a systematic review. JAMA. 2008;300:2161-71.
445. Tomba E, Fava GA. The sequential combination of pharmacotherapy and psychotherapy in mood disorders. J Contemp Psycho. 39:101–9.
446. Tsunoka T, Kishi T, Ikeda M, et al. Association analysis of group II metabotropic glutamate receptor genes (GRM2 and GRM3) with mood disorders and fluvoxamine response in a Japanese population. Prog NeuroPsychopharmacol Biol Psychiatry. 2009;33:875-9.
447. Tuccori M, Testi A, Antonioli L, et al. Safety concerns associated with the use of serotonin reuptake inhibitors and other serotonergic/noradrenergic antidepressants during pregnancy: a review. Clin Ther. 2009;31:1426-53.
448. Tyrer P. Are general practitioners really unable to diagnose depression?. Lancet. 2009;374:589-90.
449. Uher R, Perroud N, Ng MY, et al. Genome-wide pharmacogenetics of antidepressant response in the GENDEP project. Am J Psychiatry. 2010;167:555-64.
450. Uher R. The role of genetic variation in the causation of mental illness: an evolution-informed framework. Mol Psychiatry. 2009;14:1072-82.
451. US Food and Drug Administration. Public health advisory: paroxetine.http://www.fda.gov/Drugs/DrugSafety/PostmarketDrugSafetyInformationforPatientsandProviders/DrugSafetyInformationforHeathcareProfessionals/PublicHealthAdvisories/ucm051731.htm. (accessed July 8, 2013).
452. van Rossum EF, Binder EB, Majer M, et al. Polymorphisms of the glucocorticoid receptor gene and major depression. Biol Psychiatry. 2006;59:681-8.
453. Versace A, Almeida JR, Quevedo K, et al. Right orbitofrontal corticolimbic and left corticocortical white matter connectivity differentiate bipolar and unipolar depression. Biol Psychiatry. 2010;68:560-7.
454. Vittengl JR, Clark LA, Jarrett RB. Continuation-phase cognitive therapy's effects on remission and recovery from depression. J Consult Clin Psychol. 2009;77:367-71.
455. Ward HE, Hwynn N, Okun MS. Update on deep brain stimulation for neuropsychiatric disorders. Neurobiol Dis. 2010;38:346-53.
456. Wijkstra J, Burger H, van den Broek WW, et al. Treatment of unipolar psychotic depression: a randomized, double-blind study comparing imipramine, venlafaxine, and venlafaxine plus quetiapine. Acta Psychiatr Scand. 2010;121:190-200.
457. Wilkie MJ, Smith G, Day RK, et al. Polymorphisms in the SLC6A4 and HTR2A genes influence treatment outcome following antidepressant therapy. Pharmacogenomics J. 2009;9: 61-70.
458. Wisner KL, Sit DK, Hanusa BH, et al. Major depression and antidepressant treatment: impact on pregnancy and neonatal outcomes. Am J Psychiatry. 2009;166:557-66.
459. Wolf NJ, Hopko DR. Psychosocial and pharmacological interventions for depressed adults in primary care: a critical review. Clin Psychol Rev. 2008;28:131-61.
460. Yoon HK, Kim YK. Association between glycogen synthase kinase-3β gene polymorphisms and major depression and suicidal behavior in a Korean population. Prog NeuroPscyhopharmacol Biol Psychiatry. 2010;34:331-4.
461. Zarate CA, Singh JB, Carlson PJ, et al. A randomized trial of an N-methyl-D-aspartate antagonist in treatment-resistant major depression. Arch Gen Psychiatry. 2006;63:856-64.
462. Zobel A, Jessen F, von Widdern O, et al. Unipolar depression and hippocampal volume: impact of DNA sequence variants of the glucocorticoid receptor gene. Am J Med Genet B Neuropsychiatr Genet. 2008;147B:836-43.

Depression in Elderly

463. Aledxopoulos GS. Late-life mood disorder. In: Sadavoy J, Jarvik LF, Grossberg GT, Meyers BS (Eds). Comprehensive textbook of geriatric psychiatry, 3rd edition. New York: WW Norton and Company; 2004. pp. 609-53.
464. Alexopoulos GS, Borson S, Cuthbert BN, et al. Assessment of late-life depression. Biol Psychiatry. 2002;31:164-74.
465. Alexopoulos GS, Bruce ML, Hull J, Kakuma T. Clinical determinants of suicidal ideation and behaviour in geriatric depression. Arch Gen Psychiatry. 1999;56:1048-53.
466. Alexopoulos GS, Clinical and Goldfinger SM, Kaufmann CA (Eds). American psychiatric press review of psychiatry. Washi-ngton: American Psychiatric Press; 1990. pp. 249-62.
467. Alexopoulos GS, Katz IR, Bruce ML, et al. Remisssioni in geriatric primary care patients: a report form the PROSPECT Study. Am J psychiatry. 2005;162:718-25.
468. Alexopoulos GS, Katz IR, Reynolds CF, Carpenter D, Docherty JP. The expert consensus guideline series: pharmacotherapy of depressive disorders in older patients. Postgrad Med Special Report. 2001;October:1-86.
469. Alexopoulos GS, Kiosses DN, Choi SJ, Murphy CF, Lim KO. Frontal white matter microstructure and treatment response of late-life depression: a preliminary study. Am J Psychiatry. 2002;159:1929-32.
470. Alexopoulos GS, Kiosses DN, Klimstra S, Kalayam B, Bruce ML. Clinical presentation of the 'depression executive dysfunction syndrome' of late life. Am J Geriatr Psychiatry. 2002;10:98-102.
471. Alexopoulos GS, Klosses DN, Murphy C, Heo M. Executive dysfunction, heart disease burden, and remission of geriatric depression. Neuro-psychopharmacology. 2004;29:2278-84.

472. Alexopoulos GS, Lerner DM, Salzman C. Treatment of depression with tricyclic antidepressants, monoamine oxidase inhibitors, and psychostimulants. In: Salzman C (Ed). Clinical geriatric psychopharmacology, 4th edition, Philadelphia: Lippinocott, Williams and Wilkins; 2005. pp. 233-303.
473. Alexopoulos GS, Meyers BS, Young RC, Campbell S, Sibersweig D, Charlson M. The "vascular depression" hypothesis. Arch Gen Psychiatry. 1997;54:15-22.
474. Alexopoulos GS, Meyers BS, Young RC, et al. Executive dysfunction and long-term outcomes of geriatric depression. Arch Gen Psychiatry. 2000;57:285-90.
475. Alexopoulos GS, Meyers BS, Young RC, Kakuma T, Silbersweig D, Charlson M. Clinically defined vascular depression. Am J Psychiatry. 1997;154:562-65.
476. Alexopoulos GS, Meyers BS, Young RC, Mattis S, Kakuma T. The course of geriatric depression with "reversible dementia": a controlled study. Am J Psychiatry. 1993;150:1693-9.
477. Alexopoulos GS, PROSPECT group, Interventions for depressed elderly primary care patients. Int J Geriatr Psychiatry. 2001;16:553-59.
478. Alexopoulos GS, Young RC, Meyers BS. Geriatric depression: age of onset and dementia. Biol Psychiatry. 1993;34:141-5.
479. Alexopoulos GS, Young RC, Shindlendecker R. Brain computed tomography in geriatric depression and primary degenerative dementia. Biol Psychiatry. 1992;31:591-9.
480. Alexopoulos GS. Frontostriatal and libic dysfunction late-life depression. Am J Psychiatry. 2002;10:687-95.
481. Alexopoulos GS. New concepts for prevention and treatment of latelife depression. Am J Psychiatry. 2001;158:835-8.
482. Alexpoulos GS, Buckwalter K, Olin J, Martinez R, Wainscott C, Krishnan KR. Comorbidity of late-life depression: an opportunity for research in mechanisms and treatment. Biol Psychiatry. 2002;31:543-58.
483. Alzenstein HJ, Nebes RD, Meltzer CC, et al. The relation of White Matter Hyperintensities to implicit learning in healthy older adults. Int J Geriatr Psychiatry. 2002;17:664-69.
484. Anstey K, Brodaty H. Antidepressants and the elderly: double-blind trials. 1987-1992. Int J Geriatr Psychiatry. 1995;10:265-79.
485. Armer J. Elderly relocation to a congregate setting: factors influencing adjustment. Issues Ment Health Nurs. 1993;14:157-72.
486. Ballmaier M, Toga AW, Blanton RE, et al. Anterior cingulated, gyres rectus, and orbitofrontal abnormalities in elderly depressed patients: an MRI-based parcellation of the prefrontal cortex. Am J Psychiatry. 2004;161:99-108.
487. Bartels SJ, Forester B, Miles KM, et al. Mental health service use by elderly patients with bipolar disorder and unipolar major depression. Am J Geriatr Psychiatry. 2000;8:160-6.
488. Batels SJ, Dums AR, Oxman TE, et al. Evidence-based practices in geriatric mental health care: an overview of systematic reviews and meta-analysis. Psychiatr Clin North Am. 2003;26:971-90.
489. Baumgarten M, Battista R, Infante-Rivard C, Hanley J, Becker R, Gauthier S. The psychological and physical health of family members caring for an elderly person with dementia. J Clin Epidemiol. 1991;45:61-70.
490. Beautrais AL. A case control study of suicide and attempted suicide Life Threat Behav. 2002;2:1-9.
491. Berger AK, Small BJ, Forsell Y, Winblab B, Backman L, Preclinical symptoms of major depression in the very old age: a prospective longitudinal study. Am J Psychiatry. 1999;156:1239-41.
492. Blazer D, Hughes DC, George LK. The epidemiology of depression in an elderly community population. Gerontologist. 1987;27:281-7.
493. Blazer D. Psychiatry and the oldest old. 157;1915-24.
494. Blazer DG, Burchett BG, Fillenbaum GG. ApoE e4 and low cholesterol as risk factors in a biracial elderly community sample Am J Geriatr Psychiatry. 2002;10:515-20.
495. Blazer DG, Self-efficacy and depression in late life: a primary prevention proposal. Aging Ment Health. 2002;6:315-24.
496. Blazer DG. Depression in late life: review and commentary. J Gerontol Med Sci. 2003;56A:249-65.
497. Boradty H, Luscombe G, Parker G, et al. Early and late onset depression in old age: different aetiologies, same phenomenology. J Affect Disord. 2001;66:225-36.
498. Borwn ES, Varghese FP, McEwen BS. Association of depression with medical illness: does cortisol play a role? Biol Psychiatry. 2004;55:1-9.
499. Bruce ML, Ten Have TR, Reynolds III CF, et al. Reducing suicidal ideation and depressive symptoms in depressed older primary care patients: a randomized controlled trial. JAMA. 2004;291:1081-91.
500. Bush G, Luu P, Posner MI. Cogitive and emotional influences in anterior cingulated cortex. Trends Cogn Sci. 2000;4:215-22.
501. Butters MA, Becker JT, Nebes RD, et al. Changes in cognitive functioning following treatment of late-life depression. Am J Psychiatry. 2000;157:949-54.
502. Butters MA, Bhalla RK, Mulsant BH, et al. Executive functioning, illness course, and relapse/recurrence in continuation and maintenance treatment of late-life depression. Is there a relationship? Am J Geriatr Psychiatry. 2004;12:387-94.
503. Callahan CM, Nienaber NA, Hendri HC, Tierney WM. Depression of elderly outpatients: primary care physicians' attitudes and practice patterns. J Gen Intern Med. 1992;7:26-31.
504. Campbell S, Marriott M, Nahmias C, MacQueen GM. Lower hippocampal volume in patients suffering from depression: a meta-analysis. Am J Psychiatry. 2004;161:598-607.
505. Carney RM, Freedland KE. Depression, mortality, and medical morbidity in patients with coronary heart disease. Biol Psychiatry. 2003;54:241-57.
506. Casten JR, Rovner BW, Tasman W. Age-related macular degeneration and depression: a review of recent research. Curm Opin Ophthalmol. 2004;15:181-3.
507. Charney DS, Reynolds CF 3rd, Lewis L, et al. Depression and Bipolar Support Alliance consensus statement on the unmet needs in diagnosis and treatment of mood disorders in late life.
508. Clyburn LD, Stones MJ. Hajistrovropoulos T, Tuokko H. Predicting caregiver burden and depression in Alzheimer's disease. J Gerotol I Psychol Sci Soc Sci. 2000;55: S2-13.

509. Collins CE, Stommel M, Wang S, Given CW. Caregiving transitions changes in depression among family caregivers in relatives with dementia. Nurs Res. 1994;43:220-5.
510. Conwell Y, Duberstein PR, Caine ED. Risk factors for suicide in later life. Biol psychiatry. 2002;31:193-204.
511. Conwell Y, Duberstein PR, Hermann J, Forbes N, Caine ED. Age differences in behaviours leading to completed suicide. Am J Geriatr Psychiatry. 1998;6:122-26.
512. Conwell Y, Duberstein PR, Hermann JH, Caine ED. Relationship of age and axis I diagnoses in victims of completed suicide: a psychological autopsy study. Am J Psychiatry. 1996;153:1001-8.
513. Conwell Y, Nelson JC, Kim KM, Majure CM, Depression in late life: age of onset as marker of a subtype. J Affect Disord. 1989;17:189-95.
514. Cramer JA, Rosenheck R. Compliance with medication regimes for mental and physical disorders. Psychiatr Serv. 1998;49:196-201.
515. Davidson RJ. Toward a biology of personality and emotion. Ann NY Acad Sci. 2001;935:191-207.
516. Devanand DP, Sano M, Tang MX, et al. Depressed mood and the incidence of Alzheimer's disease in the elderly living in the community. Arch Gen Psychiatry. 1996;53:175-82.
517. Draper BM, Koschera A, Do older people receive equitable private psychiatric service provision under Medicine? Aust N Z J Psychiatry. 2001;35:626-30.
518. Drevets WC, Prefrontal cortical-amygdalar metabolism in major depression Ann N Y Acad Sci. 1999;877:614-37.
519. Drevets WC. Neuroimaging abnormalities in the amygdala in mood disorders. Ann N Y Acad Sci. 2003;985:420-44.
520. Duberstein PR. Openess to experience and completed suicide across the second half of life. Int Psychogeriatrics. 1995;7:183-98.
521. Duman RS, Heninger GR, Nestler EJ. A molecular and cellular theory of depression. Arch Gen Psychiatry. 1997;54:597-606.
522. Elderkin-Thompson V, Kumar A, Bilker WB, et al. Neuropsychological deficits among patients with late-onset minor and major depression. Arch Clin Neuropsychol Neuropsychol. 2003;18:319-49.
523. Erickson K, Drevets W, Schulkin J. Glucocorticoid regulation of diverse cognitive functions in normal and pathological emotional states. Neurosci Biobehav Rev. 2003;27:233-46.
524. Farran CJ, Miller BH, Kaufman JE, Davis L. Race, finding meaning and caregiver distress. J Aging Health. 1997;9:316-33.
525. Frod T, Meisenzahl E, Zetzsche T, Born C, Groll C, Jager M. Hippocampal changes in patients with a first episode of major depression. Am J Psychiatry. 2002;159:1112-8.
526. Frod T, Meisenzhl EM, Zesche T, et al. Larger Amygdala volumes in first depressive episode and compared to recurrent major depression and healthy control subjects. Biol Psychiatry. 2003;53:338-44.
527. Gallo JJ, Anthony JC, Muthen BO. Age differences in the symptoms of depression: a latent trait analysis. J Gerontol B Psychol Sci Soc Sci. 1994;49:251-64.
528. Gatz M, Pedersen N, Plomin R, Nesselrade J, McClearn G. Importance of shared genes and shared environments for symptoms of depression older adults. J Abnorm Psychol. 1992;101:701-8.
529. Gilbody S, Whitty P, Grimshaw J, Thomas R. Educational and organizational interventions to improve the management of depression in primary care: a systematic review. JAMA. 2003;289:3145-51.
530. Greenwald BS, Kramer-Ginsberg E. Age of onset in geriatric depression: relationship to clinical variables. J Affect Disord. 1988;15:61-8.
531. Harman JS, Mulsant BH, Kelleher KJ, Schulberg HC, Kupfer DJ, Reynolds III CF, Narrowing the gap in the treatment of depression. Int J Geriatr Psychiatry. 2001;31:239-53.
532. Harman JS. Kelleher KJ, Reynolds CF, Pincus HA. Out of pocket healthcare expenditures of older adults with depression. J Am Geriatr Soc. 2004;31:809-13.
533. Hickie J, Scott E, Mitchell P, Wilhelm K, Austin MP, Bennett B. Subcortical hyperintensities on magnetic resonance imaging: clinical correlates and prognostic significance in patients with severe depression. Biol Psychiatry. 1995;37:151-60.
534. Hickie J, Scott E, Naismith S, et al. Late-onset depression: genetic, vascular, and clinical contributions. Psychol Med. 2001;31:1403-12.
535. Jacoby RJ, Levy R, Computed tomography in the elderly, 3: affective disorder. Br J Psychiatry. 1980;136:270-75.
536. Janson M, Gatz M, Berg S, et al. Association between depressed mood in the elderly and a 2-HTR2A gene variant. Am J Med Genet. 2003;120:79-84.
537. Jorm AF. History of depression as a risk factor for dementia: an updated review. Aust N Z J Psychiatry. 2001;35:776-81.
538. Kalayam B, Alexopoulos G, Prefrontal dysfunction and treatment response in geriatric depression. Arch Gen Psychiatry. 1999;56:713-8.
539. Kalayam B, Alexopoulos GS, Left frontal error negativity and symptom improvement in geriatric depression: a preliminary study. Am J Psychiatry. 2003;160:2054-60.
540. Kalayam B, Meyers BS, Kakuma T, et al. Age of onset of geriatric depression and sensorimotor hearing deficits. Biol Psychiatry. 1995;38:649-58.
541. Katon W, Lin E, Von Korff M, et al. The predictors of persistence of depression primary care. J Affect Disord. 1994;31:81-90.
542. Koder DA, Brodaty H, Anstey KH. Cognitive therapy for depression in the elderly. Int J Geriatr Psychiatry. 1996;11:97-107.
543. Kral VA, Emery OB. Long-term follow-up of depressive pseudodementia of the aged. Can J Psychiatry. 1989;34:445-6.
544. Krishnan KRR, Hays JC, Blazer DG. MRI-defined vascular depression. Am J Psychiatry. 1997;154:497-500.
545. Krishnan KRR. Biological risk factors in late life depression. Biol Psychiatry. 2002;31:185-92.
546. Kuller L, Shemanski L, Manolio T. Relationship between ApoE, MRI findings, and cognitive function in the Cardiovascular Health Study. Stroke. 1998;29:388-98.
547. Kumar A, Gupta RC, Thomas MA, Alger J, Wyckoff N, Hwang S, Biophysical changes in normal-appearing white matter and subcortical nuclei in late-life major depression detected using magnetization transfer. Psychiatry Res. 2004;130:131-40.

548. Ledoux J, Emotional memory: in search of systems and synapses. Ann NY Acad Sci. 1993;702:149-57.
549. Llewelly-Jones RH, Baikie KA, Smithers H, Cohen J, Snowdon J, Tennant CC. Multifaceted shared care intervention for late life depression in residential care: randomized controlled trial. BMJ. 1999;319:676-82.
550. Lockwood KA, Alexopoulos GS, van Gorp WG. Executive dysfunction in geriatric depression. Am J Psychiatry. 2002;159:1119-26.
551. Luber MP, Meyers BS, Williams-Russo PG, et al. Depression and service utilization in elderly primary care patients. Am J Geriatr Psychiatry. 2001;9:169-76.
552. Lynch TR, Johnson CS, Mendelson T, Robins CJ, Krishnan RK, Blazer DG, New onset and remission of suicidal ideation among a depressed adult sample. J Affect Disord. 1999;56:49-54.
553. Lyness J, Caine E, King D, Conwell Y, Duberstein P, Cox C. Depressive disorders and symptoms in older primary care patients. Am J Geriatr Psychiatry. 2002;10:275-82.
554. Lyness JM, Cox C, Curry J, Conwell Y, King DA, Caine ED. Older age and the underreporting of depressive symptoms. J Am Geriatr Soc. 1995;43:216-21.
555. Lyness JM, King DA, Cox C, Yoediono Z, Caine ED. The importance of subsyndromal depression in older primary care patients: prevalence and associated functional disability. J Am Geriatr Soc. 1999;47:757-58.
556. MacQeen GM, Macdonand K, Amano S, Joffe RT, Nahmias C, Young LT. Course of illness, hippocampal function and hippocampal volume in major depression. Proc Natl Acad Sci USA. 2003;100:1387-92.
557. Mayberg H. Depression and frontol-subcortical circuits: focus on prefrontal-limbic interactions. In: Lichter DC, Cummings JL (Eds). Frontal-subcortical circuits in psychiatric and neurological disorders. New York: The Guilford Press; 2001. pp. 177-206.
558. McEwan BS. Mood disorders and allostatic load. Biol Psychiatry. 2003;54:200-7.
559. Michelson D, Stratakis C, Hill L. Bone mineral density in women with depression. N Engl Med. 1996;335:1176-81.
560. Miller DB, O'Callghan JP, Effects. Effects of aging and stress on hippocampal structure and function. Metabolism. 2003;31:17-31.
561. Minino AM, Arias E, Kochanek KD, Murphy SL, Smith BL. Daths: final data for 2000. Natl Vital Stat Rep. 2002;50:1-119.
562. Morris PL, Robinson RG, Raphael B, Samuels J, Molloy P. The relationship between risk factors for affective disorder and poststroke depression in hospitalized stroke patients. Aust N Z J Psychiatry. 1992;26:208-17.
563. Murphy CF, Alexopoulos GS. Longitudinal association of initiation/perseveration and severity of geriatric depression. Am J Geriatr Psychiatry. 2003;11:1-7.
564. Murphy SL, Deaths: final data for. 1998. Natl Vital Stat Rep. 2000;48:1-105.
565. Nebes Rd, Pollock BG, Houck PR, et al. Persistence of cognitive impairment in geriatric patients following antidepressant treatment a randomized, double-blind clinical trial with nortriptyline and paroxetine. J Psychiatr Res. 2003;37: 99-108.
566. NIH Consensus Conference. Diagnosis and treatment of depression in late life. JAMA. 1992;268.
567. O'Brien J, Ames D, Chiu E, Schweitzer I, Desmond P, Tress B. Severe deep white matter lesions and outcome in elderly patients with major depressive disorder: follow-up study. BMJ. 1998;317:982-84.
568. O'Doherty J, Krigelbach ML, Rolls ET, Hornak J, Andrews C. Abstract reward and punishment representations in the human orbitofrontal cortex. Nat Neurosci. 2001;4:95-102.
569. Olin JT, Schneider LS, Kat IR, et al. Provisional diagnostic criteria for depression of Alzheimer's disease. Am J Geriatr Psychaitry. 2002;10:125-8.
570. Ongur D, Drevets WC, Price JL. Glial reduction in the subgenual prefrontal cortex in mood disorders. Proc Natl Acad Sci USA. 1998;95:13920-95.
571. Oxman TE, Barrett JE, Barrett J, Gerber P. Symptomatology of late-life minor depression among primary care patients. Psychosomatics. 1990;31:174-80.
572. Oxman TE, Hull JG. Social support and treatment response in older depressed primary care patients. J Gerontol B Psychol Sci Soc Sci. 2001;56:35-45.
573. Palsson S, Ostling S, Skoog I. The incidence of first onset depression in a population followed from the age of 70 to 85. Psychol Med. 2001;31:1159-68.
574. Rajkowska G, Miguel-Hidalgo JJ, Wei J, et al. Morphometric evidence for neuronal and glial prefrontal cell pathology in major depression. Biol Psychiatry. 1999;45:1085-98.
575. Reynolds CF, Frank E, Perel JM, et al. Nortriptyline and interpersonal psychotherapy as maintenance therapies for recurrent major depression: a randomized controlled trial in patients older than 59 years. JAMA. 1999;281:39-45.
576. Robinson RG, Poststroke depression: prevalence, diagnosis, treatment, and disease prevention. Biol Psychiatry. 2003;54: 376-87.
577. Roeloffs C, Sherbourne C, Unutzer J, Fink A, Tang L, Wells KB. Stigma and depression among primary care patients. Gen Hosp Psychiatry. 2003;25:311-5.
578. Romanelli J, Fauerbach J, Buch D, Ziegelstein R. The significance of depression in older patients after myocardial infarction. J Am Geriatr Soc. 2002;50:817-22.
579. Rybarczyk B, Marco G, Dela Cruz M, Laridos S, Comparing mind body wellness interventions for older adults with chronic illness: classroom versus home instruction. Behav Med. 1999;24:181-90.
580. Sackeim HA. Haskett RF, Mulsant BH, et al. Continuation pharmacotherapy in the prevention of relapse following electroconvulsive therapy. JAMA. 2001;285:1299-307.
581. Sajetovic M, Vernon L, Semple W. Clinical characteristics and health resource use of men and women veterans with serious mental illness. Psych Serv. 1997;48:1461-3.
582. Salzman C, Small GW. Treatment of depression with new antidepressants. In: Salzman C (Ed). Clinical geriatric

psychopharmacology, 4th edition. Philadelphia: Lippincott, Williams and Wilkins; 2005. pp. 305-33.
583. Salzman C, wong E, Wright CB. Drugs and ECT treatment of depression in the elderly, 1996-2001: a literature review. Biol Psychiatry. 2002;31:265-85.
584. Saunders A, Hulette C, Welsh-Bohmer K. Sensitivity, and predictive value of apolipoprotein-E genotyping for sporadic Alzheimer's disease. Lancet. 1996;348:90-3.
585. Schulberg HC, Katon W, Simon GE. Rush AJ. Treating major depression in primary care practice: an update of the Agency for Health Care Policy and Research Practice Guidelines. Arch Geriatr Psychiatry. 1998;55:1121-27.
586. Schulz R, Wiliamson G. A 2-year longitudinal study of depression among Alzheimer's caregivers. Psychol Aging. 1991;6:569-70.
587. Sheline Y. 3D MRI studies of neuroanatomic changes in unipolar depression: the role of stress and medical comorbidity. Biol Psychiatry. 2000;48:791-800.
588. Sheline Y. Neuroimagign studies of mood disorder effects on the brain. Biol Psychiatry. 2003;54:331-8.
589. Shulman KI, Tohen M, Satlin A, Gopinath M, Kalunian D. Mania compared with unipolar depression in old age. Am J Psychiatry. 1993;149:341-5.
590. Sirey JA, Bruce ML, Alexopoulos GS, et al. Perceived stigma as a predictor of treatment discontinuation in young and older outpatients with depression. Am J Psychiatry. 2001;158:479-81.
591. Sirey JA, Bruce ML, Alexopoulos GS. The treatment initiation program: an intervention to improve depression outcomes in older adults. Am J Psychiatry. 2005;162:184-6.
592. Sobin C, Sacheim HA. Psychomotor symptoms of depression. Am J Psychiatry. 1997;154:4-17.
593. Stimpson S, Baldwin RC, Jackson A, Burns AS. Is subcortical disease associated with poor response to antidepressants? Neurological, neuropsychological and neuroradiological findings in late-life depression. Psychol Med. 1998;28:1015-26.
594. Teresi J, Abranms R, Holmes D, Ramirez M, Eimicke J. Prevalence of depression and depression recognition in nursing homes. Soc Psychiatry Psychiatr Epidemiol. 2001:36:613-29.
595. Unutzer J, Katon W, Callahan CM, et al. Depression treatment in a sample of 1801 depressed older adults in primary care. J Am Geriatr Soc. 2003;51:505-14.
596. Van Duijn CM, Clayton DG, Chandra V, et al. Interaction between genetic and environmental risk factors for Alzheimer's disease: a reanalysis of case-control studies. Genet Epidemiol. 1994;11:539-51.
597. Waern M, Runeson BS, Allebeck P, et al. Mental disorders in elderly suicides: a case control study. Am J Psychiatry. 2002;159:450-55.
598. Wells KB, Sherbourne C, Schoenbaum M, et al. Impact of disseminating quality improvement programs for depression in managed primary care: a randomized controlled trials. JAMA. 2000;283:212-20.
599. West CG, Reed DM, Gildengorin GL. Can money buy happiness? Depressive symptoms in an affluent older population. J Am Geriatr Soc. 1998;46:49-57.
600. Whyte E, Pollock BG, Wagner W, et al. Influence of serotonin transporter linked region polymorphism on platelet activation in geriatric depression. Am J Psychiatry. 2001;158:2074-6.
601. Wiener P, Alexopoulos GS, Kakuma T, Meyers BS, Rosendhal E, Chester J. The limits of history taking in geriatric depression. Am J Geriatr Psychiatry. 1997;5:116-25.
602. Wilson KC, Chen R, Taylor S, McCracken CF, Copelad JR, Socio-economic deprivation and the prevalene and prediction of depression in older community residents. Br J Psychiatry. 1999;175:549-53.
603. Wragg RE, Jeste DV. Overview of depression and psychosis in Alzheimer's disease. Am J Psychiatry. 1989;146:577-89.
604. Yaffe K, Blackwell T, Gore R, Sands L, Reus V, Browner WS. Depressive symptoms and cognitive decline in non-demented elderly: a prospective study. Rch Gen Psychiatry. 1999;56:425-30.
605. Young RC. Bipolar disorders, In: Roose S, Sackeim HA (Eds). Phenomenology of late life in affective disorders. Oxford: Oxford University Press; 2003. pp. 34-48.
606. Zisook S, Schuchter SR, Sledge R, Diagnostic and treatment considerations in depression associated with late-life bereavement. Diagnosis and treatment of depression in late life: results of the NIH consensus development conference. Washington: American Psychiatric Press; 1994. pp. 419-35.

Recent Development and Current Controversies in Depression

607. Aben I, Verthey F, Strik J, Lousberg R, Lodder J, Honig A. A comparative study into the one year cumulative incidence of depression after stroke and myocardial infraction. J Neurol Neurosurg Psychiatry. 2003;74:581-5.
608. APA. Practice guideline for the treatment of patients with major depressive disorder, 2nd edn, Arlington, VA: American Psychiatric Association, 2000.
609. D'Zurilla TJ, Chang EC, Nottingham EJ 4th, Faccini L. Social problem-solving deficits and hopelessness, depression, and suicidal risk in college students and psychiatric inpatients. J Clin Psychol. 1998;54:1091-107.
610. D'Zurilla TJ, Goldfried MR. Problem solving and behavior modification. J Abnorm Psychol. 1971;78:(1):107-26.
611. Damasio AR. Descarte's error: emotion, reason and the human brain. London: Papermac, 1994.
612. Daw ND, Kakade S, Dayan P. Opponent interactions between serotonin and dopamine. Neural Netw. 2002;15:603-16.
613. Groves DA, Brown VJ. Vagal nerve stimulation: a review of its applications and potential mechanisms that mediate its clinical effects. Neurosci Biobehav Rev. 2005;29:493-500.
614. Kringelbach ML, Rolls ET. The functional neuroanatomy of the human orbitofrontal cortex: evidence from neuroimaging and neuropsychology. Prog. Neurobiol. 2004;72:341-72.
615. Matthews K, Eljamel MS. Status of neurosurgery for mental disorder in Scotland. Selective literature review and over-review of current clinical activity. Br J Psychiatry. 2003;182: 404-11.

616. Newcombe R. The lesion in stereotactic subcaudate tractotomy. Br J Psychiatry. 1975;126:478-81.
617. Owens DC, McKenna PJ, Davenport R. Clinical assessment: interviewing and examination. In: Johnstone EC, Owens DC, Lawrie SM, Sharpe M, Freeman CPL (Eds). Companion to psychiatric studies. Edinburgh: Churchill Livingstone, 2004.
618. Paulus W. Toward establishing a therapeutic window for rTMS by theta burst stimulation. Neuron. 2005;45:181-3.
619. Rose EJ, simonotto E, Ebmeier KP. Limbic over-activity in depression during preserved performance on the n-back task. Neuroimage. 2006;29:203-15.
620. Sackett DL, Richardson WS, Rosenberg W, Haynes RB. Evidence-based medicine: how to practice and teach EBM. London: Churchill Livingstone, 1998.
621. Yerevanian BI, Koek RJ, Feusner JD, Hwang S, Mintz J. Antidepressants and suicidal behaviour in unipolar depression. Acta Psychiatr Scand. 2004;110:452-8.

Treatment Resistant Depression

622. Berman RM, Marcus RN, Swanink R, et al. The efficacy and safety of aripiprazole as adjunctive therapy in major depressive disorder: a multicenter, randomized, double-blind, placebo-controlled study. J Clin Psychiatry. 2007;68:843-53.
623. Binneman B, Feltner D, Kolluri S, et al. A 6-week randomized placebo-controlled trial of CP-316, 311 (a selective CRH1 antagonist) in the treatment of major depression. Am J Psychiatry. 2008;165:617-20.
624. Carpenter LL, Milosavljevic N, Schechter JM, et al. Augmentation with open-label atomoxetine for partial or nonresponse to antidepressants. J Clin Psychiatry. 2005;66:1234-8.
625. Dunner DL, Amsterdam JD, Shelton RC, et al. Efficacy and tolerability of adjunctive ziprasidone in treatment-resistant depression: a randomized, open-label, pilot study. J Clin Psychiatry. 2007;68:1071-7.
626. Fava M, Rush AJ, Alpert JE, et al. Difference in treatment outcomes in outpatients with anxious versus nonanxious depression: a STAR*D report. Am J Psychiatry. 2008;165:342-51.
627. Mahmoud RA, Pandina GJ, Turkoz I, et al. Risperidone for treatment-refractory major depressive disorder. A randomized trial. Ann Intern Med. 2007;147:593-602.
628. Marcus RN, McQuade RD, Carson WH, et al. The efficacy and safety of aripiprazole as adjunctive therapy in major depressive disorder. A second multicenter, randomized, double-blind placebo-controlled study. J Clin Psychopharmacol. 2008;28:156-65.
629. Müller N, Schwarz MJ, Dehning S, et al. The cyclooxygenase—2 inhibitor celecoxib has therapeutic effects in major depression: results of a double-blind, randomized, placebo controlled, add-on pilot study to reboxetine. Mol Psychiatry. 2006;11:680-4.
630. Pilhatsch MK, Burghardt R, Wandinger KP, et al. Augmentation with atomoxetine in treatment-resistant depression with psychotic features. A case report. Pharmacopsychiatry. 2006;39:79-80.
631. Roitman S, Green T, Osher Y, et al. Creatine monohydrate in resistant depression: a preliminary study. Bipolar Disord. 2007;9:754-8.
632. Rush AJ, Trivedi MH, Wisniewski SR, et al. Acute and longer-term outcomes in depressed outpatients requiring one or several treatment steps: a STAR*D report. Am J Psychiatry. 2006;163:1905-17.
633. Sanacora G, Kendell SF, Levin Y, et al. Preliminary evidence of riluzole efficacy in antidepressant-treated patients with residual depressive symptoms. Biol Psychiatry. 2007;61:822-5.
634. Trivedi MH, Rush AJ, Wisniewski SR, et al. Evaluations of outcomes with citalopram for depression using measurement-based care in STAR*D: implications for clinical practice. Am J Psychiatry. 2006;163:28-40.
635. Zarate CA Jr, Payne JL, Quiroz J, et al. An open-label trial of riluzole in patients with treatment-resistant major depression. Am J Psychiatry. 2004;161:171-4.

Cognitive Behavior Therapy for Depression

636. Butler AC, Chapman JE, Forman EM, Beck AT. The empirical status of cognitive-behavioral therapy: a review of meta-analyses. Clin Psychol Rev. 2006;26(1):17-31.
637. Clark DA, Beck AT, Alford BA. Scientific foundations of cognitive theory and therapy of depression. New York: Wiley; 1999.
638. DeRubeis RJ, Crits-Christoph P. Empirically supported individual and group psychological treatments for adult mental disorders. J Consult Clin Psychol. 1998;66(1):37-52.
639. Dobson KS. A meta-analysis of the efficacy of cognitive therapy for depression. J Consult Clin Psychol. 1989;57(3):414-9.
640. Gloaguen V, Cottraux J, Cucherat M, Blackburn IM. A meta-analysis of the effects of cognitive therapy in depressed patients. J Affect Disord. 1998;49(1):59-72.
641. Kanter JW, Bowe, WM, Baruch, DE, Busch, et al. Behavioral Activation. In: Pringer DW, Beevers C, Rubin A (Eds). Treatment of Depression in Youth and Adults. Hoboken, NJ: John Wiley and Sons; 2011. pp. 113-182.
642. Murphy GE, Simons AD, Wetzel RD, Lustman PJ. Cognitive therapy and pharmacotherapy. Singly and together in the treatment of depression. Arch Gen Psychiatry. 1984;41(1):33-41.
643. National Institute for Clinical Excellence. Computerised cognitive behaviour therapy for depression and anxiety: Review of Technology Appraisal 51. Available at http://www.nice.org.uk/nicemedia/pdf/TA097guidance.pdf.
644. Robinson LA, Berman JS, Neimeyer RA. Psychotherapy for the treatment of depression: a comprehensive review of controlled outcome research. Psychol Bull. 1990;108(1):30-49.
645. Task Force on Promotion and Dissemination of Psychological Procedures. A report to the Division 12 Board. Washington DC: American Psychological Association, 1993.

CHAPTER

8

Delusional Disorders

Niraj Ahuja, B Reddy

"In practice, psychiatrists often examine a patient who has nothing but delusions. Such patients have no marked depressive symptomatology, although they may be unhappy. They are not euphoric though they may be grandiose as a natural response to the delusion. They are neither blunted nor inappropriate in affect. Their mind is clear,..." without disturbances of sensorium and "... they are not incoherent. What they have is simply a delusion, nothing more, nothing less."[1] This apparently simplistic, though largely accurate, description of paranoid disorders by George Winokur is in sharp contrast to the often confusing historical evolution of the concept of delusional (paranoid) disorders.

HISTORY AND EVOLUTION OF THE CONCEPT

In the pre-Hippocratic era, the word *paranoia* apparently denoted what later came to be known as insanity. The term has its origin in two Greek words, *para* (meaning beside) and *noos* (meaning the mind, or the intellect).[2] Thus paranoia connoted 'the mind beside itself'.

Hippocrates used the term paranoia for delirium caused by high fever, while others employed it to denote a variety of mental states like dementia and madness.[3] Thereafter, the term fell into disuse for centuries in the medical literature, though it persisted in the lay usage as a synonym for 'folly' or 'thinking amiss'.

Credit is usually given to Vogel[4] for reintroducing the term in medicine in 1764, but it was Heinroth[5] who described the condition in some detail in 1818. According to him, the delusional states were 'disorders of intellect' (*Verruktheit*) not fundamentally involving the other faculties of mind like feeling and will. He, however, recognized that some admixture was usually present.

In 1838, Jean-Étienne Dominique Esquirol,[6] a French psychiatrist, coined the term 'monomania' (*monomanie intellectuelle*), a condition with delusions but no defect in logical reasoning and behavior. Karl Kahlbaum,[7] in 1863, described chronic and fixed delusions of persecution and grandeur under the term paranoia. He referred to this condition as partial insanity that affects the intellect alone. Paranoia was placed among a group of disorders that were called as 'primary' or 'original', meaning that the clinical picture would remain essentially unchanged during the patient's lifetime. Thus, paranoia was distinguished from a second group of 'general' or 'complex' disorders which passed through four stages, with delusions similar to those occurring in paranoia seen sometimes in the stage preceding the final, fourth stage of dementia.

In 1845, Wilhelm Griesinger described paranoia as a condition that occurred secondary to a preceding disorder of feeling (affect). Two decades later, however, he changed his viewpoint and considered delusions as a primary mental disorder, independent of mood disorders.[8] Magnan[2] in 1880s, classified these disorders into two types: one affecting the previously healthy persons at an adult age (*delire chroniquea evolution systematique*), and the other affecting persons in whom hereditary predisposition and mental degeneration predominate (*delire systematises des degeneres*). In 1893, he described four stages of the first type, namely, incubation, persecution, grandeur, and finally dementia.[2] This description had a great influence on the German and Scandinavian evolution of the concept of paranoia.

Emil Kraepelin[9] recognized three types of paranoid psychoses. Within the rubric of dementia praecox, he divided the *dementia paranoides* (the first type) into a *gravis* and a *mitis*form; the former accompanied by disintegration of the mental process and the latter being a milder illness with a better prognosis. Then he segregated the *paraphrenias* (the second type, characterized by systematized hallucinatory forms not leading to deterioration) from dementia praecox. The third type, *paranoia*, was described as a state of completely systematized delusions occurring in the absence of hallucinations, a condition so rare that years may pass between cases.

He stressed on "...the insidious development of a permanent and unshakable delusional system resulting from internal causes, which is accompanied by perfect preservation of clear and orderly thinking, willing and acting."[9]

He regarded paranoia as a psychogenic disorder, in the same group of disorders as hysteria."[10] He classified delusions into the following types:[11]

1. Delusions of persecution
2. Delusions of jealousy
3. Delusions of grandeur, which were further subdivided into four subtypes (eroticism, high descent, inventors, and prophets and saints).

He also considered creation of another subtype for hypochondriacal delusions; however, he felt that these delusions occurred rarely and did not merit a separate category.[11]

Wilhelm Mayer,[12] following up Kraepelin's original paraphrenic patients, found that 40% of them showed obvious signs of dementia praecox within a few years. Further, these patients could not be clinically differentiated from those who remained paraphrenic. A family history of schizophrenia was found in some of Mayer's own paraphrenic patients. According to him, paraphrenia as a disease entity could not be sharply differentiated from schizophrenia.[13]

Karl Kolle described 66 paranoiac patients including 19 (i.e. all) of Kraepelin's own paranoiac patients." In 62 of these patients, primary delusions (which were presumed to be characteristic of schizophrenia) were found to be present. He also found an increased incidence of schizophrenia in the first degree relatives of these patients.[13] As a result of Mayer's study, Kraepelin readmitted paraphrenia into the dementia praecox group. Kolle, however, maintained that the same should be done with paranoia.[14]

Eugen Bleuler[15] broadened the concept of paranoia to also include hallucinations as clinical features. He said that the disorder did not necessarily end in deterioration, and that it could begin later in life. According to him, paranoia was primarily a disorder of intellect and not of the affect.[16] He considered pure paranoia to be a rare condition that did not warrant a separate diagnostic category.[17] He suggested that schizophrenia must be considered as a differential diagnosis in every case of paranoia.

As early as 1896, Sigmund Freud described[18] a case of paranoid psychosis which he interpreted as a 'defense psychosis'. The development of the psychotic process was regarded as a gradual impairment of the defense against self-reproach that persisted in coming into the conscious awareness, but was now relegated to the surroundings in the form of delusions, by the mechanism of '*projection*'. His ideas evolved over the next decade and a half, culminating in 1911 in his description[19] of the famous 'Schreber case' that formed the basis of his theories on paranoia. Freud never saw the patient and based his theory on the autobiography of Daniel Paul Schreber, a distinguished jurist. Although Schreber also described hallucinations among his experiences, he was given a label of paranoia by Freud. Schreber's delusions were interpreted by Freud as an outward projection of his own emotionally ambivalent, latent homosexual attraction to his father. The ego's self-defense against the homosexual tendencies, according to Freud consisted of denial and then projection into the surroundings as delusions. Thus, delusions were thought to be a part of the healing process rather than that of the disorder itself[2] (This theory is discussed in more detail under etiology). Freud's theories on paranoia are controversial but have nonetheless received much attention.

Gaupp,[20] Kretschmer's teacher, made an intensive study of another case, Wagner, a mass murderer who killed his own wife, four children and eight other people, as a part of a careful plan to avenge himself on his supposed enemies. From Wagner's diaries and examination of his mental state, he concluded that Wagner suffered from paranoia. He also attempted to recognize the development of the 'first delusion' as a psychogenic reaction. This was merely a confirmation of the work of other German scientists like Margulies, Friedman, Bonhoeffer and Birnbaum, who believed that psychogenic trauma can act as a precipitating factor for certain types of paranoid psychoses.[2]

Ernst Kretschmer[21] emphasized that paranoia should not be recognized as a disease entity but as a psychogenic reaction occurring in certain 'sensitive' personalities, characterized by susceptibility, vulnerability, and tendency to a depressive and pessimistic outlook. He believed that psychosis is provoked by the interaction of 'paranoid prone personality' and a 'key experience'. The morbid development does not begin until the individual, with his constitutional and mental background, comes up against a special event or situation (the key experience). The prognosis of such patients was good and they did not develop schizophrenic regression.[8]

The Scandinavian psychiatrists[2] group the paranoid disorders and schizophreniform psychoses (as defined by Langfeldt) together under the concept of reactive psychosis. According to Jaspers,[22] reactive psychoses should fulfill the following criteria of 'genuine reactions', namely:

- Intensity of the traumatic experience as an adequate explanation for the patient's breakdown;
- Causation;
- Purpose of the reaction (e.g. in prison psychoses);
- The requirement that the content of the psychosis should reflect the nature of the traumatic experience; and
- Course, and termination of the psychosis upon liquidation of the traumatic experience. However, such attempts in practice have failed.'

Nils Retterstol[23] followed up 334 consecutive first admission patients with paranoid delusions, excluding affective disorders and organic brain syndrome. He divided his patients into four groups:

1. Paranoid psychosis with affective symptoms, where the delusions appear comprehensible considering the affective state.
2. 'Paranoiac psychosis' with systematized firmly knit delusions not accompanied by affective or schizophrenic symptoms (similar to Kraepelin's concept of paranoia).

3. Paranoid psychosis without affective symptoms where delusions are not directly comprehensible on the background of the affective state and there is no schizophrenic symptom or schizophrenia like course.
4. Schizophreniform psychosis (Langfeldt's definition).[24]

In France, chronic delusional psychoses are divided[25] into non-progressive chronic delusional psychoses (including the various forms of paranoia) and progressive deteriorating form (paranoid schizophrenia). The earlier French literature on paranoia is often confusing as the term *delire* was used for the description of both delirium and dementia. *Bouffee delirante*, a French term, is probably equivalent to acute reactive paranoid psychoses in the Scandinavian nomenclature.

The term *paranoid* always had a slightly different meaning in Britain and the rest of Europe. Paranoid meant 'persecuted' to the majority of British psychiatrists whereas in the rest of Europe it seems to have meant being subject to systematized delusions. However, even now the term paranoia is often used by lay persons and professionals to mean any type of suspiciousness.

The eclectic theories of Adolf Meyer,[26] in addition to Freudian psychoanalytic thought, shaped much of the concept of paranoia in the 1970s and 1980s. Meyer emphasized the importance of constitutional and psychogenic factors in the understanding of paranoid psychoses.

COMPARATIVE NOSOLOGIC VIEWPOINTS

DSM-I[27] defined 'paranoid reactions' as conditions showing persistent delusions of persecutory or grandiose type, with emotional responses and behavior consistent with the delusions, and generally without hallucinations. There were two subtypes: *paranoia*, a chronic disorder with systematized delusions, which was believed to be extremely rare; and a *paranoid state*, a disorder of short duration with less systematized delusions. The schizophrenic reaction, paranoid type, included those patients with schizophrenic characteristics and paranoid delusions. The paranoid personality was thought to contain many traits of schizoid personality with a conspicuous tendency toward suspiciousness, envy and jealousy.

DSM-II[28] separated paranoia and involutional paranoid state from schizophrenia of the paranoid type and paranoid personality, cautioning that there was disagreement over whether they should be separated at all.

DSM-III[29] also separated paranoid disorders from schizophrenia-paranoid subtype and paranoid personality disorder, stressing on the imprecise boundaries of the two categories. Here, paranoid disorders included paranoia, shared paranoid disorder, acute paranoid disorder and a residual category, atypical paranoid disorder. To make a diagnosis of paranoid disorder, either persecutory delusions or delusions of jealousy were required.

ICD-9[30] classified paranoid disorders under the category of 'paranoid states' with subtypes of paranoid state-simple; paranoia; paraphrenia; induced psychosis; other paranoid states, and unspecified types. Two other subtypes, acute paranoid reaction and psychogenic paranoid psychosis were placed under 'other non-organic psychosis', while schizophrenia of paranoid type and paranoid disorder were separately classified. The delusions in paranoia, according to ICD-9, are mostly of grandeur, persecution or somatic types.

George Winokur,[31] in 1977, proposed a set of criteria for what he termed as *delusional disorder* or paranoia. The inclusion criteria were the presence of nonbizarre delusions for any period of time and that the delusions had to be related to events that are possible, however implausible. Exclusion criteria include the presence of an affective or organic disorder, age more than 60 years at the time of onset, the presence of bizarre or fantastic delusions, inappropriate or markedly flat (frozen face) affect, and hallucinations.

Kendler,[32] in 1980, proposed three changes in Winokur's criteria. Firstly, the delusions had to be present for at least 2 weeks before a diagnosis could be made. Secondly, thought disorder was included as an exclusion criterion. Thirdly, Kendler proposed a division of delusional disorder into two types, following the work of Werner,[33] namely:

1. Simple delusional disorder, in which hallucinations are absent.
2. Hallucinatory delusional disorder, in which hallucinations of any kind except those described by Schneider as indicative of schizophrenia (i.e. thought echo, voices commenting, and voices discussing the patient) are present.

DSM-III-R[34] classification of delusional disorders borrowed the Kraepelinian concept to a large extent. As the term 'paranoid' (disorder) meant different things to different people, it was dropped (though it appeared in brackets), and replaced by the term delusional disorder. Since the central feature of these disorders is the presence of delusions, this term was more apt and descriptive.

DSM-III-R defined the disorder more broadly, to include delusional themes beyond persecutory delusions. The predominant delusional theme determined the subtype diagnoses that included the erotomanic, grandiose, jealous, persecutory, somatic and unspecified types. A duration criterion of 1 month was specified. Shared paranoid disorder was renamed as 'induced psychotic disorder' and placed under the category of 'psychotic disorders not elsewhere classified'. As the delusional content can be varied in this condition, this change was made.

The only differences in the DSM-III-R subtypes and Kraepelin's subtypes of paranoia are that[11]

1. Kraepelin considered erotomania to be a subtype of the delusion of grandeur (DSM-III-R classified it separately from grandiose subtype); and

2. Kraepelin stopped short of including the hypochondriacal delusion because of its rarity (DSM-III-R includes it as a separate subtype, somatic type).

In DSM-IV,[35] the term paranoid disorders has been removed completely. The definition of delusion, however, remains the same. A new subtype of 'mixed category' has been added. Induced psychotic disorder has been appropriately renamed 'shared psychotic disorder' to avoid reference to any presumed cause.

ICD-10[36] defines these disorders under the principal category of 'persistent delusional disorders' (F22), wherein the delusions must be present for at least 3 months and be clearly personal rather than subcultural. The various subtypes are not clearly specified. Induced delusional disorder has been included as a principal category (F24) in the same rubric as persistent delusional disorders.

In DSM-5, delusional disorder is kept under schizophrenia spectrum and other psychotic disorders. The diagnostic criteria is given below. Comparative features of DSM-III-R, DSM-IV, and ICD-10 delusional disorder are given in Table 1.

DSM-5 Diagnostic Criteria for Delusional Disorder
297.1 (F22)
A. The presence of one (or more) delusions with a duration of 1 month or longer. B. Criterion A for schizophrenia has never been met. **Note:** Hallucinations, if present, are not prominent and are related to the delusional theme (e.g. the sensation of being infested with insects associated with delusions of infestation). C. Apart from the impact of the delusion(s) or its ramifications, functioning is not markedly impaired, and behavior is not obviously bizarre or odd. D. If manic or major depressive episodes have occurred, these have been brief relative to the duration of the delusional periods. E. The disturbance is not attributable to the physiological effects of a substance or another medical condition and is not better explained by another mental disorder, such as body dysmorphic disorder or obsessive-compulsive disorder.
Specify whether: **Erotomanic type:** This subtype applies when the central theme of the delusion is that another person is in love with the individual.
Grandiose type: This subtype applies when the central theme of the delusion is the conviction of having some great (but unrecognized) talent or insight or having made some important discovery.
Jealous type: This subtype applies when the central theme of the individual's delusion is that his/her spouse or lover is unfaithful.
Persecutory type: This subtype applies when the central theme of the delusion involves the individual's belief that he/she is being conspired against, cheated, spied on, followed, poisoned or drugged, maliciously maligned, harassed, or obstructed in the pursuit of long-term goals.
Somatic type: This subtype applies when the central theme of the delusion involves bodily functions or sensations.
Mixed type: This subtype applies when rio one delusional theme predominates.
Unspecified type: This subtype applies when the dominant delusional belief cannot be clearly determined or is not described in the specific types (e.g. referential delusions without a prominent persecutory or grandiose component).
Specify if: **With bizarre content:** Delusions are deemed bizarre if they are clearly implausible, not understandable, and not derived from ordinary life experiences (e.g. an individual's belief that a stranger has removed his/her internal organs and replaced them with someone else's organs without leaving any wounds or scars).
Specify if: The following course specifiers are only to be used after a 1-year duration of the disorder: **First episode, currently in acute episode:** First manifestation of the disorder meeting the defining diagnostic symptom and time criteria. An *acute episode* is a time period in which the symptom criteria are fulfilled. **First episode, currently in partial remission:** *Partial remission* is a time period during which an improvement after a previous episode is maintained and in which the defining criteria of the disorder are only partially fulfilled. **First episode, currently in full remission:** *Full remission* is a period of time after a previous episode during which no disorder specific symptoms are present. **Multiple episodes, currently in acute episode** **Multiple episodes, currently in partial remission** **Multiple episodes, currently in full remission** **Continuous:** Symptoms fulfilling the diagnostic symptom criteria of the disorder are remaining for the majority of the illness course, with subthreshold symptom periods being very brief relative to the overall course.
Unspecified
Specify current severity: Severity is rated by a quantitative assessment of the primary symptoms of psychosis, including delusions, hallucinations, disorganized speech, abnormal psychomotor behavior, and negative symptoms. Each of these symptoms may be rated for its current severity (most severe in the last 7 days) on a 5-point scale ranging from 0 (not present) to 4 (present and severe). (See Clinician-Rated Dimensions of Psychosis Symptom Severity in the chapter "Assessment Measures" in Section III of DSM-5.)
Note: Diagnosis of delusional disorder can be made without using this severity specifier.

EPIDEMIOLOGY

The epidemiological studies of delusional disorders are fraught with many difficulties. Firstly, the patient is often reluctant to seek help.[37] The basic clinical symptoms of suspiciousness, mistrust and lack of insight prevent a realistic estimate of the disorder to be made. The task is made even more difficult by the fact that these patients often have no other symptoms other than delusions that make them look different from rest of the population.[1] The patients' relatives regard them merely as odd or eccentric, and seldom see the need for treatment.[25]

Table 1: Comparison of DSM-III-R, DSM-IV, and ICD-10 delusional disorders

	DSM-III-R	*DSM-IV*	*ICD-10*
Term used	Delusional (paranoid) disorders	Delusional disorders	Persistent delusional disorders
Duration hallucinations	1 month auditory/visual	1 month tactile/ olfactory	3 months auditory
Subtypes	Erotomanic, grandiose, jealous, persecutory, somatic, unspecified	Erotomanic, grandiose, jealous, persecutory, somatic, unspecified and mixed	Not specified
Others	Induced psychotic disorder	Shared psychotic disorder	Induced delusional disorder

Secondly, the definition and classification of delusional disorders is far from clear and has been changing over the last few decades. According to Bleuler,[15] the concept of delusional (paranoid) disorders provided a splendid example of how psychiatrists working with unclear classifications can be lost in a bottomless sea. The epidemiological studies available are based on different diagnostic criteria and classifications. Thus the figures are not directly comparable, though they provide useful general indicators.

Thirdly, the boundary between normal paranoid tendencies and delusional disorders is hazy. Normal people may also harbor irrational beliefs, without sufficient supporting evidence. According to Cameron,[38] it is essential in normal day-to-day life to use perceptions that reveal only fragments of objects, bits of others' speech and actions, drawing inferences regarding others' intent based on a sketchy knowledge of their background. It is not surprising in such a setting of ample potential uncertainty that suspiciousness and mistrust sometimes develop in otherwise normal individuals. This may be particularly accentuated in the setting of disaster or catastrophic stress. The problem of differentiation between normal paranoid ideation and paranoid (delusional) disorder can, however, be surmounted by rigid application of diagnostic criteria.[38]

Generally, delusional disorders are thought to be relatively uncommon, whereas paranoid symptomatology is widely prevalent in a variety of medical and psychiatric disorders. Among a group of 400 patients with paranoid symptoms, Miller[39] found nearly 10% to have paranoid disorder. Among the rest, 38% were paranoid schizophrenics, nearly 16% had senile or 'arteriosclerotic' psychosis, and 9% were suffering from manic depressive illness.

Retterstol,[23,40,41] using a broader concept of paranoid psychosis as reactive psychosis, found that nearly 12% of all patients admitted to the University psychiatric clinic at Oslo during a 5-year period had delusional symptoms. These patients were classified into the four groups described earlier. Out of the 334 patients with paranoid symptoms, only 26 were diagnosed as suffering from paranoia, amounting to less than 0.8% of all admissions during this period.

In a chart review of all the patients admitted during a 10-month period to the psychiatric unit of the University of Chicago hospitals and clinics, Freedman and Schwab[42] found paranoid symptomatology in 40% of 264 patients. However, only 4 (about 1.5%) were diagnosed as having a paranoid state while 32 (nearly 12%) had paranoid schizophrenia.

Winokur[1] while conducting a computerized search of all admissions to the psychiatric hospital of the University of Iowa over a 50-year period, found even lower figures for paranoid disorders. Only 93 patients were diagnosed as suffering from paranoia out of a total of 21,000 patients, giving a figure of about 0.4%. Using stricter criteria, the figure came down to 0.1%. He concluded that delusional disorder is relatively uncommon disorder for a psychiatrist to see, though it does exist, nevertheless.

According to most estimates, the incidence and prevalence of delusional disorder is about 0.7–3.0 per 100,000 and about 0.03% respectively, while the lifetime morbidity risk is between 0.05 and 0.1%.[34] The delusional disorders account for approximately 1 to 2% of all inpatient psychiatric admissions. The age at onset is usually 35–45, with a range from 18–80. The sex ratio for males to females is 0.85.[43]

Although no causal relationships have been determined, it has been suggested that the prevalence of delusional disorders is more in the following groups of people:[37]

- Single, separated or divorced individuals.
- Low socioeconomic status, and socially and educationally disadvantaged people.
- Socially isolated individuals.
- Immigrants.

The male:female sex ratio reported in delusional disorders in the various studies is widely varying. While Kraepelin[10] (70:30) and Winokur[1] (70:30) suggest that these disorders are more common in females, others like Arana,[37] Kendler[44] (46:54), and Rimon, et al.[45] (47.5:52.5) suggest the reverse. DSM-IV35 reports no major gender differences in these disorders, except that the jealous type is more common in men.

ETIOLOGY

It is well known that delusions occur in a wide variety of medical and psychiatric disorders, in addition to delusional disorders. Any theory that explains delusions in delusional disorders must do so for other disorders too.[3] Not only that, the content and type of paranoid phenomenology is strikingly repetitious with a relatively short list of types despite a wide range of diseases in which it occurs.[3] Though there are many theories and hypotheses to account for delusions, hard empirical evidence to support them is lacking. Thus with so many uncertainties, conclusions regarding the etiological basis of delusional disorders must be guarded.

The various etiological models can be discussed under the following headings:

A. Biological theories,
B. Psychological theories, and
C. Psychosocial theories.

Biological Theories

Pathology

Cummings et al.[46] using psychopathological consequences of neurological diseases, proposed that delusions occur in diseases involving the limbic system, particularly the temporal lobe structures and the caudate nuclei. He hypothesized that limbic dysfunction leads to misinterpretation of the environment and inappropriate perception of threat.

Lo et al.[47] found organic delusional disorder patients to have significant neurological problems (e.g. stroke, head injury) and hyperthyroidism among others. CT lesions, though common, were nonspecific, without any laterality of brain lesions. Delusions also occur more frequently in certain disorders, e.g. complex partial seizures, migraine, Alzheimer's dementia, Huntington's chorea, parkinsonism, subdural hematoma (see differential diagnosis).

However at present, there is insufficient data to suggest that biological factors are causative in delusional disorders.

Biochemistry

Cummings et al.[46] reported that diseases characterized by excessive dopaminergic activity or reduced cholinergic activity carry a heightened risk of delusion formation.

Genetics

At the beginning of the twentieth century, it was emphasized that constitutional heritable factors were important in the genesis of paranoia.[37] Though the last few decades has seen a tremendous amount of work in the field of schizophrenia and mood disorders, scant attention has been paid to the genetic research in delusional disorders.

From the genetic perspective it is said that delusional disorders bear little relationship to schizophrenia and mood disorders.[48]

According to DSM-IV35, there is a lack of consensus about the familial pattern of this disorder. There is limited evidence to suggest that avoidant and paranoid personality disorders may be especially common among first degree biological relatives of individuals with delusional disorders.

Psychobiological Mechanisms

In 1942, de Clerambault suggested that chronic delusions resulted from 'abnormal neurological events' like infections, intoxications, lesions, and other forms of damage. These abnormal events lead to what he called as 'automatisms', e.g. hallucinations, thought 'arrest', bizarre tactile and kinesthetic sensations, attentional disturbances, feelings of familiarity, false recognition, and a constant parade of memories. Such 'automatisms' puzzle the patient and demand explanation. The explanations take the form of delusions, providing relief from the puzzlement and distress. It is this relief that works against the abandonment of the explanatory delusions.[3]

Maher also conceptualizes delusions as explanations for anomalous experiences arising in the environment or nervous system (central or peripheral). Just as normal beliefs and scientific hypotheses are formed to explain the experiences, delusions too are formed in a similar manner. The content of the delusions is drawn from the present or past circumstances of the patient.[3] Since hallucinations do not occur in delusional disorders by definition, and sensory impairment and neurological dysfunction have not been consistently found in all patients, it is not clear how relevant this theory is in the explanation of delusional disorders.

Information Processing Theory

Ellis and Young[49] have tried to explain the delusional misidentification syndromes using the information processing model.[50] Impairment in face processing, like recognition and identity, has been quoted as the pathology in Capgras syndrome, Fregoli's syndrome and intermetamorphosis. The evidence for this model comes from the patients with prosopagnosia. As the two conditions are not directly related, this model stands on shaky grounds.[49] It may be that both prosopagnosia and Capgras syndrome represent abnormalities of visual perception occurring at different stages of this neurophysiological process.[49]

Spitzer[51] has proposed a neurocomputational approach where acute delusions are proposed to be the result of increased activity of neuromodulators (e.g. dopamine, norepinephrine) which leads to activation of neural networks in higher order cognitive function. The result is a tendency to attach significance to ordinary, insignificant things or events.

Similarly, chronic delusions are said to be a result of altered neuromodulatory state, which in turn modifies neuroplasticity (the likelihood of change), which distorts 'cortical maps' representing views, attitudes and biases to environmental clues. As distorted cortical maps are difficult to change back to normal, these delusions are relatively stable and do not respond well to treatment.[51]

Psychological Theories

Psychodynamic Mechanisms

Freud described projection[18] as the main defense mechanism in paranoia, in 1896. In 1911, he published the 'Psychoanalytic Notes'[19] upon the autobiographical account of Schreber, a jurist, who had suffered two episodes of psychiatric illness, one in 1884–85 and the other in 1893. The Freudian theory of paranoia, based on the analysis of this autobiographical narrative, explains the various delusions as follows:

- *Delusions of persecution*: The unconscious homosexual impulses ('I love him') are defended against by denial and reaction formation ('I do not love him' and 'I hate him'). However, this hate is still unacceptable at the conscious level. Therefore by projection, it becomes 'He hates me'. In a full-blown paranoid state, this hate is further elaborated into persecution ('I am persecuted by him'). The patient is then able to rationalize his anger by consciously hating those persons who he 'thinks' (perceives) hate him.
- *Delusions of love* (*erotomanic delusions*): Here again the unconscious homosexual impulses ('I, a man, love him') are defended against by denial and displacement ('I do not love him' and 'I love her'), and then are transformed through projection ('She loves me').
- *Delusions of jealousy*: The unconscious homosexual impulses, here, are guarded against by denial ('I love him' changed to 'I do not love him') and displacement ('She, the spouse, loves him'). The man, whom the paranoiac suspects his spouse of loving, is the man toward whom he feels homosexually attracted.
- *Delusions of grandeur* (*grandiosity*): In this case, the unwanted, unconscious homosexual impulses ('I love him') are defended against by denial ('I do not love him'), followed by generalization ('I love no one'). Later, this is elaborated into 'I love only myself'.

These apparently far-fetched dynamic explanations of unconscious homosexuality are the same in the female patient, as in the male patient, in the classical psychoanalytic theory.[3] However, whether homosexuality is the central theme in paranoia (delusional disorders) has been a matter of great controversy. Experimental evidence has tended to negate this hypothesis or has been equivocal. Psychoanalysts are quick to point out that this homosexuality is 'latent' and not 'manifest', and therefore not available for experimentation. Still, this hypothesis seems really implausible in a majority of patients. For one, the persons who persecute a paranoiac are not always known to him. Also, these hypotheses do not satisfactorily account for the persistence of delusions, once they are formed.[3]

Nevertheless, Freud's contributions to the understanding of delusional disorders are substantial, particularly his concept of projection and his view that developmental childhood experiences may influence the content of delusions.[3]

Cameron[38] has described in detail the process of encapsulation of persecutory delusions by elaboration. At first the patient finds malicious intent in trivial and unrelated actions of real persons in the surrounding environment. All these persons are then collectively perceived as organized into a 'community of plotters'. This group or community of plotters is further elaborated by inclusion of imagined people or groups like CID or Mafia. Finally, the paranoiac ascribes motives to these real and imagined persons or groups, which are together known as *pseudocommunity organization* or a *paranoid pseudocommunity*.

The pseudocommunity gives the paranoiac an opportunity to bind together his projected fears to justify his hostile aggression, gives him a tangible target, and also encapsulates his delusional system so that he can keep in touch with the real people and have normal social interactions outside the arena of his delusional system.

In another attempt to find the etiological life experience that leads to the development of delusional disorder, Klein and Horowitz[52] studied 80 paranoid patients. They theorized that the paranoiac fails in childhood in the development of the '*basic trust*', which is the cornerstone for future adult relationships. He faces difficulties in establishing a warm and trusting relationship with the parenting figures who are unable to help the paranoiac as a child in dealing with day-to-day disappointments. Thus, he soon develops an attitude that the environment is consistently hostile and becomes hypersensitive to imagined slights. All his relationships become characterized by a lack of trust. The paranoiac's hypersensitivity causes the significant others to avoid him, and that reaction tends to amplify his hostile and suspicious attitude. Intolerant of critical comments himself, he readily criticizes others.[52]

Finally, psychosis is precipitated as a defense against the feelings of rejection and inadequacy. The inferiority feelings are replaced by grandiose delusions, while the feelings of inadequacy give way to delusions of love and erotomanic delusions.[25]

Several other dynamic explanations have been put forward, which include superego projection, genital conflicts, over-determined goals, faulty maternal identification, infantile sadomasochism, unresolved primal scene fantasies, among others. However, it must be kept in mind that all these explanations are hypothetical and currently lack experimental validation.

Cognitive Behavioral Theory

Tarrier et al.[53] have provided a cognitive-behavioral formulation of non-psychotic morbid jealousy, following

Beck's formulation for depression. Although it is not at present applicable to delusions of jealousy, it provides an important new method to view the possible origin of ideas of jealousy.

Psychosocial Theories

Childhood Experiences or Losses

It has been theorized that loses or adverse experiences in early childhood make a person prone to the development of delusional disorder in later life.

In a retrospective study of 80 paranoid patients,[52] conducted in an American State hospital, it was found that 28 patients had lost one or both parents, had stepparents, or came from broken homes. In addition, the overall family picture was gloomy. 57 patients had parents who were 'cruel' or indulged in child abuse, 63 patients described recurrent inter-parental conflicts leading to a constant state of alarm, 15 patients remembered being subject to pampering and indulgent parental attitudes, while 18 others had 'demandingly' perfectionistic and over-moralizing parents who had rigid views of what is right and what is wrong. Many others described parents who abused alcohol, were psychotic, or were markedly unreliable.

Bonner,[54] Johanson,[55] and Retterstol[40] corroborated these findings of Klein and Horowitz[52] in separate studies. Retterstol,[40] in his Norwegian studies, found an early parental loss (death or separation) in 20% of patients, an extremely insecure childhood in 12% and poor relationships with parents in 50% of the patients.

Although these studies paint a sinister and dismal picture of the childhood of paranoid patients, it must be remembered that these studies are retrospective in nature. Similar studies have been reported in the patients of depression, schizophrenia and other psychiatric disorders. Therefore, if such factors are etiological they must exert a non-specific effect toward the genesis of delusional disorders.

Premorbid Personality Traits

It has been believed that these patients have always been, even premorbidly, generally very anxious, tense, fearful and insecure. The excessive anxiety is discharged in the form of overactivity, chronic anger and/or aggression.[38]

Among the traits, which are thought to be characteristic of the premorbid personality, are suspiciousness, mistrust in others, secretiveness, seclusiveness, constant ideas of reference, and unwarranted hostility. All these traits hinder the development of satisfactory interpersonal relationships. Whatever genuinely close and reciprocal relationships exist are limited to a very few, and even these ties are vulnerable. It is said that the paranoiac has learned early in life that affection is not returned;[38] therefore, he uses reaction formation as an ego defense mechanism against regression, dependency needs, and feelings of affection. The paranoiac, thus, saves himself from rejection by turning his positive feelings into negative ones.[2]

There is often difficulty in confiding in others as they expect people to be unpredictable and untrustworthy. However, despite a tendency toward solitary rumination, they may hide behind a 'brittle' facade of superficial give-and-take. Such people are believed to be relatively incompetent in everyday situation of cooperation and competition, because they are besieged with constant tensions regarding mutual understandings, misinterpretations and self-referential ideation.[38]

Their aggression is rarely aimless; it is nearly always 'reaction sensitive'. There is an exceptional readiness to over-react with counter aggression, to whatever is personally misconceived as a threat to the vulnerable 'security system'. According to Cameron,[38] "it is only when, in the face of exceptional stress, their self-reference focuses upon a particular theme, or singles out certain individuals who seem banded together (to form a pseudocommunity), that a threat of decompensation (to psychosis) looms".

The above description of the paranoid personality traits, of patients with paranoid personality disorder, is based on Freudian psychoanalytic theory. However it is not borne out in the routine clinical practice. According to Forrest,[56] the personality factors present premorbidly in patients of delusional disorder include 'sensitive' personality traits (of Schneider), hysterical and psychopathic personality traits, and obsessional rigidity. Only a few patients reported homosexuality and the concept of latent homosexuality was found to be vague.

According to DSM-IV35, patients with paranoid, schizoid, or avoidant personality disorders may be more likely to develop delusional disorders.

Precipitating Factors

As described earlier, Kretschmer[21] believed that paranoid psychosis is provoked in 'sensitive' personalities by a '*key experience*' that acts as a precipitating factor. Rettersol[2] believes that this key experience is always an event that provokes the individual's insecurity. The greater the impact on the personality, the more purely paranoid will be the resultant clinical picture. This vulnerability is heightened with increasing age; the delusional symptomatology is particularly common in the elderly.

The precipitating factors (or key experiences) can be divided into three main groups,[2] in addition to a miscellaneous group.

- *Sex life and marriage*: One of the most common precipitating factors are traumas associated with the sexual sphere. Instead of the more popularly known homosexual pattern, sexual maladjustment along with the uncertainty about one's own sexuality is more characteristic.[57] Marital and sexual problems are frequent, with the incidence of marriage being far lower than in the general population. In a Norwegian study,[41] it was found that paranoid psychoses were precipitated by sexual problems in nearly 38% of the patients (34% of the males and 44% of the females). Open conflicts with the sexual partner were fairly commonly reported.

In the light of the impairment in interpersonal relationships, it is not difficult to believe that close involvement needed for a sexual relationship, and for marriage, may represent a provocation leading to frustration, anger and hostility. Whether such a stressor can actually precipitate a delusional disorder is merely conjectural.

- *Social isolation*: Apart from the trauma, the common key experiences include events that tend to isolate the individual making him feel like an outsider, either by making him unpopular within his own group, or by removing him to strange and novel surroundings which accentuate his feelings of insecurity. Cameron[58] listed seven situations that favor the development of delusional disorders. These include situations that lead to:
  - Social isolation,
  - Increased expectation of receiving sadistic treatment (from others),
  - Increased distrust and suspicion,
  - Increased envy and jealousy,
  - Lowered self-esteem,
  - A person seeing his own defects in others, and
  - Increased potential for rumination over probable meanings and motivations.

This theoretical construct is exemplified by an increased prevalence of delusional disorders in the migrant, minority, and immigrant groups.

In his now classic study, Allers described the development of persecutory psychosis in prisoners of war (*Allers' syndrome*), placing considerable emphasis on linguistic isolation.[2] Schneider, on the other hand, attributed the psychosis to the totally strange environment with which the individual cannot cope.[2]

A higher incidence of paranoid symptomatology and paranoid psychosis was found by Odegaard,[59] Eitinger[60] (5 times higher incidence as compared with the normal population), and Retterstol.[2] While a change in the environment, either cross-country or inland, can predispose to paranoid (mostly persecutory) symptoms, a return to the original environment frequently leads to disappearance of these symptoms.

- *Somatic illnesses*: Paranoid symptomatology is frequently seen in sensory defects (like impaired hearing or deafness) and following surgical procedures (especially on abdominal and sexual organs).[2]
- *Other factors*: In women, paranoid psychosis can be precipitated by childbirth and breastfeeding, whereas newly established fatherhood can provoke psychosis in immature and insecure men, who thus lose 'their role as their wife's child'.[61] Loss of close supporting figures and interpersonal conflicts in the family, at work and with neighbors can precipitate delusional disorder in predisposed individuals.

CLINICAL FEATURES

The essential feature of delusional disorders is the presence of persistent nonbizarre delusions, not explained by other psychotic disorders. The presence of hallucinations is debated but the general consensus is that transient perceptual disturbances in any modality may be present, usually related to the delusional theme. Thought process is always preserved, and emotional responses and behavior are generally intact. Restlessness and agitation, or even violence may be present.

Swanson et al.[62] have described seven features of paranoid thinking; a combination of any of these are present in paranoid disorder. These features are:

- Projective thinking,
- Suspiciousness,
- Viewing the world as a hostile place,
- Fear of loss of autonomy and control,
- Feeling of self as a central point of events,
- Grandiosity, and
- Delusions.

The delusional disorders can be divided into the following types:

Persecutory Type

(*Earlier names*: Querulous paranoia, Litigious paranoia, Paranoia persecutorica)

This is one of the most common types, accounting for nearly 35% (52%, if litigious and law related delusions are included) of all delusional disorders in clinical practice[1]. The core feature is the presence of delusion(s) of persecution. The delusions are usually systematically elaborated and seem logical and coherent. In some cases, the formation of paranoid pseudocommunity may be evident. The patient's functioning is often satisfactory beyond the realm of the delusional system. Their tendency to be guarded and evasive regarding the delusional area(s) further enhance the apparent normality of these patients.

The paranoid concern may cause these patients to use the legal system as a vehicle to retaliate against their perceived enemies with determination and vindictiveness. They may get involved in repeated court hearings in which they become angry and hostile toward the judges. This condition is called *litigious paranoia.*

Kraft-Ebbing[63] studied patients with querulant delusions who often indulge in multiple claims and complaints lodged against the civic authorities. This querulous or quibbling tendency does not reach delusional proportions, and therefore has been termed as *intermediate paranoia*.

Jealous Type

(*Earlier names*: Conjugal paranoia, Othello syndrome, Delirepassionel, Jealous husband syndrome)

Schaefer[2] first described this type of paranoid psychosis in 1879. Later, Mairet detailed three subdivisions:[64] hyperesthetic jealousy, jealous monomania and delusional jealousy. Henry Ey, however, described a simple dichotomy of delusions of jealousy and emotionally jealous reactions[64] (occurring in some abnormal personalities).

The central theme of the disorder is a delusion of spouse's infidelity and a preoccupation with this delusion. Persecutory delusions may at times be associated (e.g. the spouse is plotting against him, trying to kill him, etc.). The onset is usually sudden, occurring with a minor criticism of the spouse. It gradually progresses from suspiciousness to frank delusions of infidelity. If delusions extend to involve others, they are only in relation to the spouse.

The delusions are often associated with confirmatory behavior pattern wherein spouse's belongings (diaries, clothes, etc.) are extensively searched to substantiate his belief.[53] To confirm the delusions, patients often demand confession from spouse, culminating in spouse abuse, homicide or suicide. If the spouse confesses to soothe the patient, matters only become worse. Though abuse may be recurrent, it is usually a well-kept family secret. Separation and divorce are commonly found in this disorder. The patient may learn to avoid jealousy-provoking situations[53] (e.g. presence of perceived rivals of same sex). Presence of constant jealousy disrupts the patient's social, occupational, interpersonal, and sexual functioning.

It is of interest to note that Cobb and Marks[65] have compared jealousy to obsessive compulsive disorder in that some patients with this disorder present with jealous thoughts as ruminations and checking for evidence of infidelity as compulsive rituals. But, probably this theory is applicable to ideas of jealousy occurring in neurotic and personality disorders, and not to psychotic disorders where delusions of jealousy are present.

Delusions of jealousy commonly occur in other disorders like alcohol and drug dependence, schizophrenia, mood disorders, epilepsy and organic mental disorders. This syndrome is called as *morbid jealousy* (other names are pathological jealousy, sexual jealousy, erotic jealousy, psychotic jealousy, and symptomatic jealousy). Paranoid symptomatology is particularly common during alcohol intoxication, alcohol withdrawal, and as a complication of chronic alcoholism.

Delusions related to conjugal themes accounted for 38% of all delusional disorders in Winoker's study.[1] The disorder is more common in males.

Erotomanic Type

(*Earlier names*: De Clerambault's syndrome, Les psychosis passionelles, Erotomania, Old maid's insanity, Nymphomania, Furor uterinus, Amor insanus, Erotic melancholy).

Descriptions of erotomania are seen in the writings of Hippocrates, Plutarch, Galen and other physicians of seventeenth century. Emil Kraepelin[11] gave the first systematic account of the disorder as a subtype of paranoia. In fact the DSM-IV classification is very similar to that given by Kraepelin. However, the credit for the first description is given to G. de Clerambault[66] who divided the syndrome into two categories:

1. Pure cases, where delusion appears suddenly, unaccompanied by a generalized psychotic process, and
2. Secondary cases, where delusion appears slowly and is only one manifestation of a disorganized, deteriorating course; most commonly seen in paranoid schizophrenia.

Clinically, the syndrome is characterized by an elaborate, systematized delusion that the patient is loved passionately by another person. The object allegedly uses covert and furtive means to signal his or her love. The patient is usually a woman, though not always, coming from a modest background (thus the name, *Old maid's insanity*), while the object is often an older man belonging to higher socioeconomic status and is often either married or otherwise unavailable.

Although the patient usually has had a very casual, if any, contact with the object, she describes in elaborate detail the evidence for her belief. She usually insists that the object was the first one to solicit her love. The cited evidence usually takes the form of meaningful glances, telepathic communication, messages passed through newspapers, and other similar covert methods. Although in some instances the patient may reject the 'professed' love, more commonly she falls in love herself.

The object often reacts to the news with shock, denying it vigorously. Despite the denial, the patient shows the phenomenon of '*paradoxical conduct*'.[11] All such denials by the object are taken as the secret affirmation of her belief, explaining that these were meant to misguide others or to test her love.

The syndrome is believed to occur most often in "individuals of defective sexual life, not much inclined to copulation, sometimes in old maids who have never had an opportunity of marrying,[67]" suggesting extreme sexual frustration as the cause. The typical premorbid personality is characterized by socially empty, lonely and withdrawn life pattern. The patient usually belongs to lower socioeconomic status, is often notably unattractive, and has a poor sexual history, The object of desire, in contrast, is almost always superior in looks, status and authority. Thus, by the presence of the erotomanic delusion, the patient feels herself pulled out of obscurity and singled out especially for the object's attention and love. It has been theorized that the erotomanic delusion provides narcissistic gratification when life cruelly fails in such an attempt. Here, love is a defense against low self-esteem and severe narcissistic injury.[25]

Men make up only a minority (perhaps 20–30%) of all patients of erotomania but they are over-represented in the forensic population. They are often more aggressive in their pursuit of love.[11]

Erotomanicdelusions can also occur in schizophrenia[68] (most commonly paranoid schizophrenia), schizoaffective disorder,[68] bipolar disorder,[68] and organic mental disorder.[3]

The erotomanic delusion usually persists for years and may necessitate hospitalization or legal action to prevent harassment or injury to the object by the insistent patient.[11]

Somatic Type

(*Earlier names*: Monosymptomatic hypochondriacal psychosis or MHP, Paranoia Somatica)

This disorder is characterized by a single, hypochondriacal delusional system distinct from the personality.[69] The delusions may sometimes be associated with tactile or olfactory hallucinations, or illusional misperceptions. The following subtypes are usually described:[70]

Delusional Infestation

(*Earlier names*: Ekbom's syndrome, Delusional parasitosis)

This condition is characterized by the delusion of being infested by parasites. It was first described by Ekbom[71] in 1938 and has been subsequently called by many misnomers such as acrophobia, parasitophobia, somatopsychic schizophrenia, cenesthopathic hypochondriacal schizophrenia, progressive somatic schizophrenia, hypochondriacal paraphrenia, chronic tactile hallucinosis and tactile delusional hallucinosis.

Dermatologists, infectious disease specialists and general physicians see this condition more often than do psychiatrists.[72] Demographic profile reveals a female preponderance,[73] with an onset in late middle age, and no past history of psychiatric contact.[74]

The clinical features include vivid descriptions of crawling, itching, biting, burning, swarming and jumping on the skin surface or below the skin.[75] Multiple etiological explanations of delusional infestation are proposed. Of the organic factors, dermatological conditions, systemic diseases and neurologic diseases are implicated.[76] It may sometimes be seen in cases of schizophrenia.

Delusional Halitosis

(*Earlier names*: Olfactory reference syndrome, Delusional bromosis, Olfactory delusional state, Chronic olfactory paranoid state/syndrome)

This disorder has been described differently by various authors. While some describe it as a syndrome characterized by the delusion of emitting a foul body odor,[77] others describe it as a conviction of having foul breath.[75] The delusions often lead to counter-phobic rituals and social withdrawal. This condition is more prevalent in young, single, males in the absence of past psychiatric treatment. It has earlier been called by a misnomer, *autodysesmophobia*.

Delusional Dysmorphophobia

(*Earlier name*: Beauty hypochondria)

Here the patient is preoccupied with a supposed defect in appearance, of being ugly or misshapen in some way. Morselli first defined the term dysmorphophobia in 1986 as a symptom.[78] Though dysmorphophobia is an overvalued idea, it can reach delusional proportions and then it becomes a delusional disorder.

It usually begins in adolescence and occurs with equal frequency in both genders. Virtually any part of the body can be the focus of concern, but the delusion is usually centered on facial features, hair, genitals, and breasts. In affected women, the common concerns are regarding shape and size of breasts, and loss of hair. The affected males are usually concerned with penile size, shape and deviation of the axis. However, in both sexes, the predominant delusions relate to facial features. There may be associated delusions of reference and repetitive behaviors such as mirror checking, skin picking, etc. The patients may approach plastic surgeons for reconstructive surgical procedures.

Miscellaneous Disorders

In addition to the above three classical disorders, many other delusional presentations are possible. These can include a persistent complaint of abnormal dental bite, spreading infectious diseases, or contracting venereal disease. Some patients with anorexia nervosa, chronic pain, transsexualism and pseudocyesis seem to have delusional features.

Induced delusional disorder occurs in close relatives in about 20 to 25% of all cases of delusional disorder of the somatic type.[79] Hypochondriacal delusions are also seen in other disorders such as schizophrenia, severe depressive disorder, late paraphrenia, organic mental disorder and substance abuse (e.g. cocaine, amphetamines, methylphenidate).[79] It is also seen in vitamin B_{12} and folic acid deficiency states, renal failure, diabetes mellitus and hypothyroidism.[80] Delusional halitosis may also be seen in complex partial seizures.

Grandiose Type

(*Earlier names*: Megalomania, Ambitious paranoia, Negative paranoia, Folie des grandeurs)

A central feature of delusions of grandeur or grandiosity characterizes this disorder. Delusions of grandeur are less common than delusions of persecution but are much more intractable. Some of the common forms of delusions seen clinically are based on the patient's social, educational, cultural and economic background. Thus, the patient may firmly believe himself to be a saint, a god, or goddess, a political or religious leader, the Prime Minister or President of the country, a scientist, a prophet, or a millionaire. He may be preoccupied with matters of universal peace or destruction, being the 'chosenone', being born for a special purpose, or of changing the world. Patients with political and/or religious delusions may have a tremendous need to free themselves of hostile aggression.[25]

Since, in this disorder, the delusions are concerned with matters favorable to the patient rather than with those that are unfavorable, it has also been called as *negative paranoia*. Praise, protection and defense instead of persecution, accusation and offense characterize the delusional content. It is believed that psychodynamically these delusions 'represent a regression to the narcissistic feelings of omnipotence of early childhood, in which feelings of undenied and undiminished powers predominated'.[25]

Shared Psychotic Disorder

(*Earlier names*: Induced psychotic disorder, Shared paranoid disorder, Folie a deux, Double insanity, Folieinduite, Infectious insanity, Mystic paranoia, Influenced psychosis, Collective insanity, Reciprocal insanity, Familial mental infection, Psychic infection, Psychosis of association)

The essential feature is a delusional system that develops in an individual who is involved in a close relationship with another person who already has a psychotic disorder with prominent delusions. The content of delusions is usually within the realm of possibility and often based on common past experiences of both persons.[3] The transfer of delusions occurs between two people who are closely associated for a long-time and typically live together in relative social isolation. If the relationship is interrupted, the delusions usually diminish or disappear. The relationship is usually intrafamilial, common dyads being sister-sister, husband-wife, mother-child, brother-brother, brother-sister, father-child[81] (in that order).

When the number of people involved is two, as is often the case, it is called *folie a deux*. Involvement of three (*trios*), four (*quatre*), five (*cinq*), many members (*beaucoup*), and the whole family (*folie a famille*) has also been reported.

Most of the cases are limited to paranoid and depressive psychotic features; however, pure depressive forms are rare.[4] The syndrome is more common among women.

The disorder can be divided into four clinical subtypes:[4]

1. *Imposed Psychotic Disorder (Folie imposee):* Lasegue and Falret in 1877, first described this disorder. This is the most common type seen in clinical practice. The individual who first has the delusion (*primary case*) is chronically ill and a more influential member of a close relationship with a more suggestible person (*secondary case*) who develops the delusion. The secondary case is usually less intelligent, passive, gullible and lacking in self-esteem. Other associated factors are old age, sensory impairment, cerebrovascular disease and alcohol abuse. Separation of the individuals results in disappearance of the delusions in the secondary case.[4]
2. *Simultaneous psychotic disorder (Folie simultanee):* Regis first described it in 1880. Here, two people become psychotic simultaneously and share the same delusion.[4]
3. *Communicated psychotic disorder (Folie communiquee):* Marandon de Montyel first described this disorder in 1881. The delusions of the primary case are taken over by the secondary case who then works them into his own delusional system, often with elaboration.[4] Separation of the two patients does not result in recovery of the secondary case.
4. *Induced psychotic disorder (Folie induite):* Lehmann first described this disorder in 1885. The important difference here is that the secondary case already has a psychiatric disorder before coming in contact with the primary case. He just adds on the delusions of the primary case to his own symptoms.[4] Separation of the two cases does not result in recovery of the second case.

Acute Paranoid Disorders

(*Earlier name*: Acute paranoid reaction)

On rare occasions, delusional disorders may be precipitated by a stressor and entirely clear within a 6-month period. These cases would be classified under 'acute paranoid disorder' in DSM-III but in DSM-III-R and DSM-IV these would be placed under 'psychotic disorder not otherwise specified'.

In ICD-10, this condition is covered under 'other acute predominantly delusional psychotic disorders'. However, the delusions should not persist for more than 3 months. Acute paranoid disorder can be precipitated by sudden changes in environment, such as imprisonment, immigration, military induction, college enrollment, war or sudden separation from the family.

The subtypes usually described are:

- Prison psychosis.[82,83]
- Delusional disorders in immigrants and refugees.[84,85]
- Culture-bound delusional disorders.[86]

Late Paraphrenia

(*Earlier names*: Senile paraphrenia, Involutional paraphrenia, Paranoia senilis)

Kraepelin[10] described paraphrenia as a state that is intermediate between paranoia and paranoid schizophrenia, developing later in life and being milder than dementia praecox (schizophrenia). However, Mayer[12] found, as

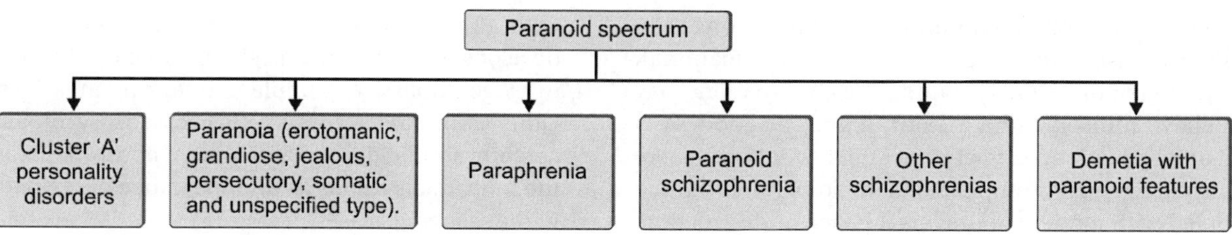

Fig. 1: The paranoid spectrum

described earlier, that nearly 40% of all paraphrenic patients later develop schizophrenia.

Roth[87] coined the term 'late paraphrenia' in 1955 to describe delusional disorders of elderly in whom signs of 'organic dementia', sustained confusion or primary affective illness could not explain the symptomatology, and whose outcome was much better in respect of mortality than senile and arteriosclerotic dementias.[8]

Kay and Roth[88] found 10% of all geriatric (aged 60 or more) psychiatric admissions to have late paraphrenia. The average age of onset was 70 years with a female preponderance (7:1). These patients lived alone, with few surviving relations and many (40%) had significant hearing impairment. Abnormal premorbid personalities with paranoid and schizoid traits were often found.

Almeida and colleagues[89] studied 47 patients with late paraphrenia and found a wide range of delusions, frequent among them being persecutory and referential. 38% had some form of hallucinations, while thought disorder and affective disturbances were uncommon. Females with hearing impairment were reported to be at high risk. Neurological soft signs indicating brain disease were associated more often with the development of psychotic symptoms in late life.[90,91]

Hallucinations of all kinds may be seen, such as elementary auditory hallucinations, hearing voices, and olfactory and visual hallucinations.[92] Memory, intelligence and judgement regarding matters not concerned with the paranoid symptoms are usually intact. They are prone to develop malnutrition and dehydration due to decreased intake of food and water, as they frequently believe that they are being poisoned.[92]

Herbert and Jacobson[93] considered late paraphrenia to be an illness essentially belonging to the group of schizophrenias, but one that is modified by age and other factors. The prognosis was poor with a chronic course.

Many authors believe that late paraphrenia is a heterogenous entity consisting of many subtypes.[13,94,95] Hence, the term was dropped from the official classificatory system of DSM-III and DSM-IV. It, however, remains as an inclusion term under delusional disorder in ICD-10.

Paranoid Spectrum Concept

Considering the wide spectrum of paranoid symptomatology, it is rational to conceptualize them on a continuum with paranoid personality on one end and paranoid schizophrenia on the other end.[17]

Alistair Munro[96] has provided a comprehensive schema of the spectrum (Fig. 1).

Delusional Misidentification Syndromes

Ever since the publication of the seminal paper by Capgras and Reboul-Lachaux,[97] nearly a dozen different misidentification syndromes[98] have been reported in the psychiatric and neurological literature. The delusional misidentification syndromes can be broadly classified into Capgras' delusion, Fregoli's delusion, delusion of intermetamorphosis and delusion of subjective doubles.[99]

Capgras' Delusion

The Capgras' delusion refers to the existence of unseen doubles. The first patient described by Capgras and Reboul-Lachaux was a 53-year-old woman who displayed what they called as '*I'illusion des sosies*', a delusional belief that people she knew had been replaced by identical doubles. The patient herself used the word 'sosies', the French word for 'doubles'. It derives from Plutus' play 'Amphitryon', which draws upon the Greek mythology of Zeus and Mercury impersonating as Amphitryon and his servant Sosia, so as to seduce their respective wives. In addition to believing that her husband and children had been replaced by doubles, the woman also claimed later that police and neighbors too had been similarly duplicated as a part of the plot to steal her property and inheritance. She also believed that there existed doubles of her own self.

The patients with Capgras delusion feel that those who have been changed look more or less exactly like the original except for small differences in appearance. According to Berson,[100] three preconditions must exist before the delusion will appear. These are:

- A psychotic state,
- A marked paranoid tendency, and
- Pathological splitting of internalized object representation.

In some variants of Capgras' delusion, objects or animals are believed to be changed which parallels agnosias specific to objects and prosopagnosia specific to faces. Signer[101] reported 315 cases from literature, the majority of whom had a diagnosis of schizophrenia.

Some investigators have found evidence for a biological basis of Capgras' syndrome in the form of brain lesions, poisoning or some exogenous factor. Two thirds of Capgras' patients had abnormal cranial CT scans.[102]

Capgras' delusion has been described in paranoid disorder, paranoid schizophrenia, mood disorder, alcoholism, borderline personality disorder and post-partum disorders. About one-fifth of the patients have organic psychotic reactions.[3] Cases have also been described following metrizamidemyelography, an overdose of a bronchodilator, diabetes and even ECT.[49] Since the delusion can occur in a variety of disorders, it is better termed as *Capgras' symptom.*

Capgras' syndrome has been linked to reduplicative paramnesia (of Pick). Reduplicative paramnesia consists of selective reduplication of places, persons, time, events, objects, parts of the body or even self. A combination of bilateral frontal and right hemisphere damage is implicated in both disorders.[103] Kapur[104] et al. have reported the dissociable nature of the two conditions.

Similarly, a link has been suggested between Capgras' syndrome and prosopagnosia. However, the Capgras' patients are not prosopagnosic as they continue to recognize without any apparent difficulty the doubles who have replaced their near ones.[49]

Fregoli's Delusion

Courbon and Fail[105] were the first to describe Fregoli's syndrome in 1927. They named the condition after the famous Italian actor and mimic, Leopoldo Fregoli. Their patient was a 27-years-old female who developed the idea that actresses in the theater were disguising themselves to look completely different in order to persecute her.

In Fregoli, the belief is that certain unfamiliar person or people may in reality be another familiar person in disguise, in order to influence the patient's behavior.[99] Here it is just the personality that changes, the physical appearance of the unfamiliar person remaining unaltered, in contrast to Capgras' delusion where the physical appearance of the familiar person is changed to 'largely' the same as the original (imposter) but personality is thought to be quite different. Hence, Fregoli's is described as 'hyperidentification' whereas Capgras' is described as 'hypoidentification'.[49]

Intermetamorphosis

Courbon and Tusques first described this syndrome in 1932.[106] They described a patient who saw another person looking like her son and husband altering his appearance to look exactly like the neighbor. Here there is simultaneous alteration in both the appearance and personality. Though rare, this condition has been reported in paranoid schizophrenia, temporal lobe epilepsy and in cases of bilateral cortical atrophy.[49]

Subjective Doubles Delusion (or Autoscopic Type)

Christodoulou[107] gave the detailed description of subjective doubles delusion (also called as Doppelganger, autoscopy or heautoscopy). The patients report that there are doubles of them elsewhere or perceive others as being themselves. The existing doubles carry out independent actions.

Fish[108] described autoscopy as phantom mirror image, i.e. a perceptual phenomenon, in which the patient sees himself and knows that it is he. In addition to a visual hallucination, kinesthetic and somatic sensations are also present. The organic states often associated with autoscopy are epilepsy and focal lesions affecting the parieto-occipital region and toxic infective states affecting the basal regions of the brain. It is also found in cases of drug and alcohol dependence.

Another type of this delusion is a belief that others are in fact the same person as subject, but at various ages, thereby appearing differently.

Silva and Leong[109] defined several reverse forms of delusional misidentification syndromes. In these forms the patients believe that their own identity is altered. These include *reverse subjective doubles* (a belief in psychological but not physical changes in identity), *reverse intermetamorphosis* (a belief in psychological as well as physical changes in identity), *reverse Fregoli* (a belief in physical but not psychological changes in identity), and *reverse Capgras*[110] (a belief in self as a psychological imposter, inhabiting a body that is not recognized as his/her own).

Delusional misidentification syndromes have recently been classified according to several parameters[110] (e.g. etiology, denial or affirmation of familiarity, recognition of altered identity, and manner of alteration).

DIFFERENTIAL DIAGNOSIS

Paranoid or delusional symptoms commonly occur in a wide variety of psychiatric and medical conditions. As delusional disorders are uncommon, considering other diagnoses is very logical. The following clinical points are often helpful in differential diagnosis.

- Age of onset
- Mode of onset
- Premorbid personality traits
- Course of the illness
- Associated symptomatology: psychiatric and medical
- Signs of physical illness
- Impairment of higher mental or cognitive functions
- Response to the antipsychotic drug treatment.

A detailed psychiatric and medical history, general and systemic physical examination, and mental status examination are essential in every patient with delusional symptomatology. Appropriate laboratory tests (e.g. drug screens) and psychological tests should be performed, whenever indicated.

Organic Delusional Disorder

The most common causes of 'organic delusional disorder' are drug intoxication and dependence (e.g. amphetamines, cocaine, steroids and L-dopa), and alcohol dependence (e.g. pathological jealousy). These organic delusional disorders are characterized by prominent delusions in the absence of any cognitive deficit. Other important causes like hypothyroidism, Cushing's disease and Addison's disease should also be kept in mind.

Although the presentation as organic delusional disorder is the most common, paranoid symptoms or delusions can also appear in dementia (the second commonest cause) and delirium. Other common disorders which can present with organic delusions include Huntington's chorea, parkinsonism, migraine, complex partial seizures, subdural hematoma, subarachnoid hemorrhage, narcolepsy, multiple sclerosis, acute intermittent porphyria, sex chromosome disorders, vitamin B deficiency, electrolyte imbalance and infections (especially AIDS, and syphilis).

The following points are important indicators of the organic basis of delusional disorders.

- Disturbances of higher mental or cognitive functions, like consciousness, orientation, memory, attention and concentration.[25]
- Rapid fluctuations of clinical features.[25]
- Abrupt onset, especially in the absence of a stressor and particularly in the elderly.[3]

Substance-induced Psychotic Disorder

Drug intoxications are particularly of relevance because abused drugs such as amphetamines and cocaine as well as over-the-counter drugs such as sympathomimetics and prescribed drugs like steroids and L-dopa can cause psychotic disorders with delusions.

Schizophrenia

The delusions in schizophrenia are bizarre, affect is blunted or incongruous, thought and perceptual disorders are usually present, personality is disorganized (though less so in paranoid subtype), contact with reality is grossly disturbed, role functioning is often significantly impaired, family history of schizophrenia may be present, and the onset occurs usually early in life.

Major Depression

The delusions occurring in 'major depression with psychotic features' are often mood congruent, e.g. delusions of guilt, worthlessness, hopelessness, nihilism, disease and death. However, mood incongruent delusions may also occur sometimes. These delusions usually begin after the classical symptoms of depression have set in.

Mania

Delusions of grandeur may be present in both delusional disorder-grandiose type and mania. Delusions of love may also occur in both the conditions. At times, persecutory delusions may be seen in mania, but they are usually secondary to grandiose delusions. The presence of elated mood, cyclic nature of illness, associated manic symptomatology, family history of bipolar disorder, and history of good response to lithium or carbamazepine can differentiate mania from delusional disorder.

Obsessive Compulsive Disorder

Severe forms of this disorder should be considered as a differential diagnosis for delusional disorder.

Somatoform Disorders

Severe forms of body dysmorphic disorder may be difficult to distinguish from delusional disorder.

Paranoid Personality Disorders

In this personality disorder, delusions are absent though other paranoid symptomatology may be present. Over-valued ideas may be present along with pervasive and long-standing suspiciousness. Schizoid and schizotypal personality disorders may at times be the differential diagnoses to be considered.

Normal Aging

It must be remembered that paranoid symptoms commonly occur in the elderly. Probably several factors contribute to this development, e.g. social isolation, lack of stimulating partner, loss of hearing and/or vision, the aging process itself, and medical illness(es).

However, major depression, late paraphrenia and dementia should be ruled out first before labeling the condition as a senile paranoid change.

PSYCHOLOGICAL TESTS

Although not diagnostic by themselves, psychological tests can on occasion provide useful help in differentiation of delusional disorders from other psychiatric disorders. The paranoiac is usually guarded, tense, hesitant and suspicious of anything he does not understand. Therefore, it is important that the examiner establishes a good rapport with the patient before proceeding with the administration of psychological tests.

Intelligence Tests

It is best to begin with the administration of intelligence tests like WAIS-R. These tests are neutral in contrast to the projective tests that provoke strong emotions. Although it is strongly believed that paranoiacs are very intelligent, it is not usually true in the clinical setting. A majority of these patients have average or sub-average intelligence.

On WAIS-R, a paranoiac usually scores higher on the verbal scale as compared with the performance scale. Scores on the similarities and the picture arrangement subtests are usually lower than on the vocabulary subtests. Wide variation between the various subtest scores may occur, indicating the underlying mistrust, suspiciousness, and test anxiety.[25]

Projective Techniques

Rorschach Test

Paranoid symptomatology is evaluated on this test in the following manner:

- Patient's test behavior (e.g. guardedness, evasiveness, suspiciousness, darting eyes, alertness for examiner's comments, hostility).
- Evaluation of the content of the patient's responses of the cards (e.g. emphasis on seeing eyes, faces, masks, confusion in gender identity, homosexual content).
- Other responses (e.g. card rejection, limited number of total responses, prolonged reaction time for response on certain cards, low score on color response, high movement score).

Thematic Apperception Test

This may help by showing themes of manipulations, critical comments and observations, sexual distortions, and 'moralizing', which keep recurring.[25]

Sach's Sentence Completion Test

This simple test usually helps in identifying the areas of conflict.

Draw A Person Test

Although of little significance, this easily administered test may show rigidity of posture, gender confusion, emphasis on drawing eyes and ears, and a hostile stance of the drawn person.

Neuropsychological Assessment

The neuropsychological test batteries may help detect the evidence of underlying brain function abnormalities and help in the diagnosis of symptomatic or secondary delusional disorders. The Bender-Gestalt (BG) test can be more easily used for the same purpose, though it is less sensitive.

Minnesota Multiphasic Personality Inventory (MMPI)

The scale 6 or Pa (paranoia) scale of MMPI is used to identify paranoid symptomatology. Extremely high (>75) or low (<35) T scores are suggestive of frank paranoid or psychotic behavior, whereas moderately high T scores indicate paranoid personality traits.

COURSE AND OUTCOME

The age of onset of delusional disorders is generally in the middle or late adult life but it can begin in adolescence too. The pattern of course is different in acute (presenting within 6 months of onset) and chronic forms (illness duration more than 6 months).

In the acute forms, the onset is in the fourth decade and nearly 50% of patients recover fully, about 37% have a relapsing course and about 10% go on to a chronic illness.[111] The chronic form begins in early fifth decade and two-thirds have an acute onset. About 53% of these cases were well at follow up, 10% were better and 31% remained unchanged.[111]

The persecutory type is the most common having a more chronic, waxing and waning course. The jealous type has a more favorable outcome. Severe impairment or change in personality is rarely seen and most patients live a normal life span.

Thus, the prognosis and outcome in delusional disorders is not as poor as is generally believed. The outcome is even better if treatment is provided early in the course of the disorder. For example, nearly 75–80% of all patients of delusional disorder of somatic type show marked improvement on treatment with pimozide.[79] The prognostic factors are discussed in Table 2.

MANAGEMENT

Treating a patient with delusional disorder is often difficult as he lacks insight, is suspicious of the therapist's motive(s), may express hostility, refuse medication, may include the therapist in his paranoid pseudocommunity and usually has to be forced into treatment involuntarily. An effective therapeutic therapist-patient relationship is fundamental for success in management. The therapist must work to decrease the

Table 2: Prognostic factors in delusional disorders

	Variables	*Good prognostic factors*	*Poor prognostic factors*
1.	Age of onset	Early (<30 years)	Late
2.	Mode of onset	Acute	Chronic
3.	Precipitating factors	Present	No stressor
4.	Sex	Female	Male
5.	Marital status	Married	Unmarried
6.	Duration of hospitalization	Less than 6 months	Longer duration before psychosis
7.	Diagnosis	Reactive paranoid psychosis	Absence of reactive factors
8.	Content of delusions	Persecutory, Jealousy	Grandeur, reference somatic, primary delusions, delusions of influence, thought broadcast
9.	Systematization of delusions	Poor systematization	Good systematization
10.	Associated depressed mood	Present	Absent
11.	Hallucinations	Absent	Present
12.	Emotional contact	Good	Poor
13.	Response to treatment with antipsychotics	Good	Poor

patient's anxiety and fear, and should exude 'nonpossessive' warmth. The aim is to establish a two-way communication.

Psychopharmacological Treatment

Antipsychotics are the drugs of choice in treatment of delusional disorders. However due to rarity of the disorder, controlled studies are lacking. Choice of a particular antipsychotic depends on previous response to the drug, age, general physical condition and side effect profile of the drug.

In acutely agitated or delusional patients, use of a parenteral antipsychotic (e.g. haloperidol, alone or with a benzodiazepine like lorazepam or diazepam) is advocated. Once agitation is controlled, oral medication may be given. In cases where compliance is poor, parenteral depot neuroleptics may be used (fluphenazinedecanoate or haloperidol decanoate).

Some investigators have reported beneficial response in the delusional disorder-somatic type with pimozide in doses of 2–10 mg/day (with or without antiparkinsonian medication). Improvement is also reported in other subtypes of delusional disorders like erotomania and pathological jealousy. When depressive symptoms are prominent, a trial of combined antidepressant and antipsychotic treatment is worthwhile.[112] Serotonin specific reuptake inhibitors have also been used in some cases.

In non-responsive cases, trials of lithium, carbamazepine, or a combination of both have been advocated.

Hospitalization

Although a patient with delusional disorder is best managed on an outpatient basis, admission in a hospital setting may be necessary, if:

- Patient is a serious threat to himself (suicidal) or to others (homicidal).
- Patient reacts to his delusions in such a way that it prevents adequate social functioning.
- Patient shows poor treatment compliance.
- Patient shows poor impulse control.

When indicated, the hospital stay should be as short as feasible. The aim of hospitalization is not the complete remission of the delusions, but to ensure adequate and satisfactory social functioning. After discharge, the management should continue on an outpatient basis, preferably with the same therapist who was treating in the hospital setting.[2]

Electroconvulsive Therapy

This is not the first line of management in delusional disorders. However, it should be used when secondary depression is present, or when paranoid symptomatology is secondary to psychotic depression, or when antipsychotics fail to control the agitation in delusional disorder.

Psychotherapy

A combination of supportive psychotherapeutic techniques is usually advocated. The basis of effective psychotherapy is the establishment of a trusting therapist-patient relationship. It must be remembered that it is not the delusion that needs treatment, but the frightened patient.[37]

The therapist should try not to oppose the patient's delusional belief but at the same time he should not agree with the patient's convictions. The patient should be guided into therapy by focusing on his other symptoms like sleep impairment, anxiety or any non-delusional somatic symptoms.

The aim of the therapy is to strengthen the patient's ego, move ego defense mechanisms to handle anxiety and agitation, and adjustment to reach a satisfactory social, interpersonal and occupational equilibrium despite the presence of delusions.

As a general rule, insight oriented psychotherapy is usually contraindicated in delusional disorders. During the acute stage, any kind of confrontation with the patient is harmful and should be avoided.

Patients with paranoid symptomatology do not do well in group therapy settings due to their extreme sensitivity and suspiciousness. They are liable to misinterpret well-intentioned statements and may react with undue rage.

Cognitive Therapy

Cognitive approaches have been tried to reduce delusional thinking through modification of the belief itself.[114] Unlike noncognitive behavioral approaches that center attention on reduction of verbal behavior, like talking about the delusion, this strategy seeks a more lasting and clinically meaningful intervention by focusing on the reasoning or the reality testing of the deluded patient. The techniques used here include distancing, homework and exploration of emotions associated with the various delusions.[115] The effectiveness of cognitive and behavior therapies has not been studied enough to justify recommendation. Nevertheless they are promising enough to continue assessment.

REFERENCES

1. Winokur G. Delusional disorder (Paranoia). In: Spitzer RL, Klein DF (Eds). Critical Issues in Psychiatric Diagnosis. New York: Raven Press; 1978. pp. 109-21.
2. Retterstol N. Paranoid disorders. In: Helzer JE, Guze SB. Eds. Psychiatry. Vol. II. Psychoses, affective disorders, and dementia. New York: Basic; 1986. pp. 245-63.
3. Manschreck TC. Delusional (paranoid) disorders. In: Kaplan HI, Sadock BJ (Eds). Comprehensive Textbook of Psychiatry, 6th edition. Vol. 1. Baltimore: Williams and Wilkins; 1995. pp. 1031-48.
4. Hinsie LE, Campbell RJ. Psychiatric Dictionary, 4th edition. New York: Oxford University Press; 1970.
5. Heinroth JCA. Lehrbuch der Strorungen des Seelenlebens. Leipzig: Vogel; 1818.
6. Esquirol E. Des Maladies Mentales. Vol. I and II. Paris: Bailliere; 1838.
7. Kahlbaum K. Die Gruppirung der Psychiscfon Krankheiten. Danzig: Kafemann; 1863.
8. Tanna VL. Paranoid states: A selected review. Compr Psychiatry. 1974;15:453-70.
9. Kraepelin E. Psychiatrie: EinLehrbuch fur Studierende and Aertzte. 8 Aufl. Leipzig: Barth; 1919.
10. Kraepelin E. Manic-depressive Insanity and Paranoia. Edinburgh: Livingstone; 1921.
11. Segal JH. Erotomania revisited: From Kraepelin to DSM-III-R. Am J Psychiatry. 1989;146:1261-6.
12. Mayer W. Uberparaphrenepsychosen. Z GesNeurol Psychiatry. 1921;71:187.
13. Hamilton M (Ed). Fish's Schizophrenia. 2nd edition. Bristol: John Wright; 1976. pp. 89-101.
14. Berner P, Gabriel E., Schanda H. Nonschizophrenic paranoid syndromes. Schiz Bull. 1980;6:627-32.
15. Bleuler E. Dementia Praecox or The Group of Schizophrenias. New York: International Universities Press; 1950.
16. Bleuler E. Affectivitat, Suggestibilitat, Paranoia. Halle: Marhold; 1906.
17. Kumar S. Overview of paranoid disorders. In: Ramachandran V, Palaniappan V, Shah LP. Eds. Continuing Medical Education Programme Booklet. Vol. 3. Madras: Indian Psychiatric Society; 1983. pp. 69-78.
18. Freud S. Further remarks on the defenseneuro-psychoses (1986). In: Collected Papers. Vol. 1. London: Hogarth Press; 1959.
19. Freud S. Psychoanalytical notes upon an autobiographical account of a case of paranoia (dementia paranoides) (1911). In. Collected Papers. Vol. 3. London: Hogarth Press; 1950.
20. Gaupp R. The scientific significance of the case of Ernst Wagner (1914). In: Hirsch SR, Shepherd M (Eds). Themes and Variations in European Psychiatry; 1974. pp. 121-33.
21. Kretschmer E. Der Sensitive Bezeihungswahn. (1927). Reprinted and translated. In: Hirsch SR, Shepherd M (Eds). Themes and Variations in European Psychiatry; 1974.
22. Jaspers K. General Psychopathology. Hoenig J., Hamilton MW. Transl. Chicago: University of Chicago Press; 1963, pp. 383-93.
23. Retterstol N. Paranoid psychosis: The stability of nosologic categories illustrated by a personal follow up investigation. Br J Psychiatry. 1966;114:553-62.
24. Langfeldt G. The schizophreniform states: A catamnestic study based on individual re-examination. Copenhagen: Munksgaard; 1939.
25. Walker JI, Brodie HKH. In: Kaplan HI, Sadock BJ. Eds. Comprehensive Textbook of Psychiatry, 3rd edition. Vol. II. Baltimore: Williams and Wilkins; 1980. pp. 1288-300.
26. Meyer A. Treatment of paranoia and paranoid states. In: White WA, Jeleffe SE (Eds). Modern Treatment of Nervous and Mental diseases. Vol. 1. Philadelphia: Lea and Febinger; 1913. pp. 614.
27. American Psychiatric Association. Diagnostic and Statistical Manual of Mental Disorders, 1st edition. Washington DC: American Psychiatric Association; 1952.
28. American Psychiatric Association. Diagnostic and Statistical Manual of Mental Disorders, 2nd edition. Washington DC: American Psychiatric Association; 1968.
29. American Psychiatric Association. Diagnostic and Statistical Manual of Mental Disorders, 3rd edition. Washington DC: American Psychiatric Association; 1980.
30. World Health Organization. International Classification of Diseases (ICD-9). Chapter V. Mental Disorders. Geneva: World Health Organization; 1978.

31. Winokur G. Delusional disorder (paranoia). Compr Psychiatry. 1977;18:511-21.
32. Kendler KS. The nosologic validity of paranoia (simple delusional disorder). Arch Gen Psychiatry. 1980;37:699-706.
33. Werner C. Die Paranoia. Stuttgart: Verlag; 1891.
34. American Psychiatric Association. Diagnostic and Statistical Manual of Mental Disorders, 3rd edition. Rev. Washington DC: American Psychiatric Association; 1987.
35. American Psychiatric Association. Diagnostic and Statistical Manual of Mental Disorders, 4th edition. Washington DC: American Psychiatric Association; 1994.
36. World Health Organization. The ICD-10 Classification of Mental and Behavioural Disorders. Geneva: World Health Organization; 1993.
37. Arana JD. Paranoid psychoses. In: Balis GU, Wurmser L, McDaniel E (Eds). Clinical Psychopathology: The Psychiatric Foundations of Medicine. Vol. 4. Boston: Butterworths; 1978. pp. 157-78.
38. Cameron NA. Paranoid conditions and paranoia. In: Arieti S, Brody EB (Eds). American Handbook of Psychiatry. Vol. 3. Adult Clinical Psychiatry, 2nd edition. New York: Basic; 1974. pp. 676-93.
39. Miller C. The paranoid syndrome. Arch Neurol Psychiatry. 1941;49:953-61.
40. Rettersol N. Paranoid and Paranoiac Psychoses. Springfield: Charles C Thomas; 1966.
41. Rettersol N. Prognosis in Paranoid Psychoses. Springfield: Charles C Thomas; 1970.
42. Freedman R, Schwab PJ. Paranoid symptoms in patients in a general hospital psychiatry unit: Implications for diagnosis and treatment. Arch Gen Psychiatry. 1977;35:965.
43. Kendler KS. Demography of paranoid psychosis (delusional disorder). Arch Gen Psychiatry. 1982;39:890.
44. Kendler KS, Tsuang MT. Nosology of paranoid schizophrenia and paranoid psychoses. Schiz Bull. 1981;7:594-610.
45. Rimon R, Stenback A, Achte K. A sociopsychiatric study of paranoid psychoses. Acta Psychiatr Scand. 1964;40(Suppl. 180):335-47.
46. Cummings J. Organic delusions: phenomenology, anatomical correlation, and review. Br J Psychiatry. 1985;146:184.
47. Lo Y, Tsai SJ, Chang JP, et al. Organic delusional disorder in psychiatric inpatients: comparision with delusional disorder. Acta Psychiatr Scand. 1997;95:161-3.
48. Kendler KS, Davies KL. The genetics and biochemistry of paranoid schizophrenia and other paranoid psychoses. Schiz Bull. 1981;7:689-709.
49. Ellis HD, Young AW. Accounting for delusional misidentifications. Br J Psychiatry. 1990;157:239-48.
50. Bruce V, Young A. Understanding face recognition. Br J Psychol. 1986;77:305-27.
51. Spitzer M. A neurocomputational approach to delusions. Compr Psychiatry. 1995;36:83-105.
52. Klein HR, Horowitz WA. Psychosexual factors in paranoid phenomena. Am J Psychiatry. 1949;105:697.
53. Tarrier N, Beckett R, Harwood S, et al. Morbid jealousy: A review and cognitive-behavioral formulation. Br J Psychiatry. 1990;157:319-26.
54. Bonner H. The problem of diagnosis in paranoid disorders. Am J Psychiatry. 1951;107:677.
55. Johanson E. Mild paranoia. Acta Psychiatr Scand. 1964; 177(Suppl).
56. Forrest AD. Schizophrenia, schizophreniform and paranoid psychosis. In: Forrest AD, Afflect JW, Zealley AK (Eds). Companion to Psychiatric Studies, 2nd edition. Edinburgh: Churchill Livingstone; 1978. pp. 438-58.
57. Arieti S. Interpretation of schizophrenia. New York: Brunner; 1955.
58. Cameron NA. Personality development and psychopathology. Boston: Houghton Mifflin; 1963.
59. Odegaard O. Emigration and insanity. Acta Psychiatr Scand. 1932;4(Suppl).
60. Eitinger L. The symptomatology of mental disease among refugees in Norway. J Ment Sci. 1960;106:947.
61. Retterstol N. Paranoid psychoses associated with impending or newly established fatherhood. Acta Psychiatr Scand. 1968; 44:51.
62. Swanson DW, Bohnert PJ, Smith JA. The Paranoid. Boston: Little Brown; 1970.
63. Gelder M, Gath D, Mayou R. Oxford Textbook of Psychiatry, 2nd edition. Oxford: Oxford University Press; 1989. pp. 324-44.
64. Shepherd M. Morbid jealousy: Some clinical and social aspects of a psychiatric symptom. J Ment Sci. 1961;107:687-704.
65. Cobb J, Marks I. Morbid jealousy featuring as obsessive compulsive neurosis: reatment by behavioral psychotherapy. Br J Psychiatry. 1979;134:301-5.
66. de Clerambault G. Les Psychosis Passionales. (1921). In: Oeuvre Psyciatrique. Paris: Presses Universities de France; 1942.
67. Enoch MD, Trethowan WH. Uncommon Psychiatric Syndromes. Chicago: Year Book; 1979.
68. Rudden M, Sweeney J, Frances A. Diagnosis and clinical course of erotomanic and other delusional patients. Am J Psychiatry. 1990;147:625-8.
69. Munro A. Monosymptomatichypochondriacal psychosis. Br J Hosp Med. 1980;24:34-8.
70. Munro A. Monosymtomatichypochondriacal psychosis: A diagnostic checklist based on 50 cases of the disorder. Can J Psychiatry. 1982;27:374-6.
71. Ekbom KA. Der praesenile Dermatozoenwahn. Acta Psychiat Neurol. 1938;13:227-59.
72. Wykoff RF. Delusions of parasitosis: A review. Rev Infect Dis. 1987;9:433-7.
73. Bishop ER. An olfactory reference syndrome: Monosymptomatic hypochondriasis. J Clin Psychiatry. 1980;41:57-9.
74. Andrews E, Bellard J, Walter-Ryan W. Monosymptomatic hypochondriacal psychosis manifesting as delusions of infestation: Case studies of treatment with haloperidol. J Clin Psychiatry. 1986;47:188-90.

75. Baker PB, Cook BL, Winokur G. Delusional infestation, the interface of delusions and hallucinations. Psychiatr Clin N Am. 1995;18:345-62.
76. Berrios G. Delusional parasitosis and physical disease. Compr Psychiatry. 1985;26:395-403.
77. Pryse-Phillips W. An olfactory reference syndrome. Acta Psychiatr Scand. 1971;47:484-509.
78. Birtchnell SA. Dysmorphophobia: A centenary discussion. Br J Psychiatry; 1988;153(Suppl. 2):41-3.
79. Munro A. Monosymptomatichypochondriacal psychosis. Br J Psychiatry. 1988;153(Suppl. 2):37-40.
80. Reilly TM. Delusional infestation. Br J Psychiatry; 1988; 153(Suppl. 2):44-6.
81. Gralnick A. Folie a deux: The psychosis of association. Psychiatr Q. 1942;16:230.
82. Faergeman P. Psychogenic Psychoses. London: Butterworths; 1963.
83. Slater E, Roth M (Eds). Clinical Psychiatry. New Delhi: JP Brothers; 1985.
84. Eitinger L. The incidence of mental disease among refugees in Norway. J Ment Sci. 1959;105:326-38.
85. Mezey A. Personal background, emigration and mental disorder in Hungarian refugees. J Ment Sci. 1960;106:618-27.
86. Mezzich JE, Lin KM. Acute and transient psychotic disorders and culture-bound syndromes. In: Kaplan HI, Sadock BJ (Eds). Comprehensive Textbook of Psychiatry, 6th edition. Vol. 1. Baltimore: Williams and Wilkins; 1995. pp. 1049-59.
87. Roth M. The natural history of mental disorder in old age. J Ment Sci. 1955;101:281-301.
88. Kay DWK, Roth M. Environmental and hereditary factors in the schizophrenia of old age ('late paraphrenia') and their bearing on the general problem of causation in schizophrenia. J Ment Sci. 1961;107:649-86.
89. Almeida OP, Howard RJ, Levy R, et al. Psychotic states arising in late life (late paraphrenia) Psychopathology and nosology. Br J Psychiatry. 1995;166:205-14.
90. Almeida OP, Howard RJ, Levy R, et al. Psychotic states arising in late life (late paraphrenia) The role of risk factors. Br J Psychiatry. 1995;166:215-28.
91. Almeida OP, Howard RJ, Levy R, et al. Clinical and cognitive diversity of psychotic states arising in late life (late paraphrenia). Psychol Med. 1995;25:699-714.
92. Fish F. Senile schizophrenia. J Ment Sci. 1960;106:938-46.
93. Herbert M, Jacobson S. Late paraphrenia. Br J Psychiatry. 1967; 113:461-9.
94. Howard R, Almeida O, Levy R. Phenomenology, demography and diagnosis in late paraphrenia. Psychol Med. 1994;24: 397-410.
95. Post F. Persistent persecutory states of the elderly. Oxford: Pergamon; 1966.
96. Munro A. The classification of delusional disorders. Psychiatr Clin N Am. 1995;18:199-212.
97. Capgras J, Reboul-Lachaux J. L'illusion des 'sosies' dans un delire systematise chronique. Bulletin de la Societes Clinique de Medecine Mentale. 1923;11:6-16.
98. DePaw KW, Szulecka TK. Dangerous Delusions: Violence and the misidentification syndromes. Br J Psychiatry. 1988;152: 91-6.
99. Ellis HD, Luaute JP, Retterstol N. Delusional misidentification syndromes. Psychopathology. 1994;27:117-20.
100. Berson RJ. Capgras' syndrome. Am J Psychiatry. 1983;140: 969-78.
101. Kiriakos R, Ananth J. Review of 13 cases of Capgras syndrome. Am J Psychiatry. 1980;137:1605-7.
102. Joseph AB. Focal central nervous system abnormalities in patients with misidentification syndromes. Bibliotheca Psychiatrica. 1986;164:68-79.
103. Alexander MP, Stuss DT, Benson DF. Capgras syndrome: A reduplicative phenomenon. Neurology. 1979;29:334-9.
104. Kapur N, Turner A, King C. Reduplicative paramnesia: Possible anatomical and neuropsychological mechanisms. J Neurol Neurosurg Psychiatry. 1988;51:579-81.
105. Courbon P, Fail G. Illusion of Fregoli syndrome and schizophrenia. Societes Clinique de Medecine Mentale; 1927.
106. Courbon P, Tusques J. Illusionsd'intermetamorphose et de charme. Annales Medico-Psychologiques. 1932;14:401-6.
107. Christodoulou GN. Syndrome of subjective doubles. Am J Psychiatry. 1978;135:249-51.
108. Fish F. In: Hamilton M (Ed). Fish's Clinical Psychopathology, 2nd edition. Bristol: John Wright; 1976.
109. Silva JA, Leong GB. The Capgras syndrome in paranoid schizophrenia. Psychopathology. 1992;25:147-53.
110. Pauw KW. Delusional misidentification: A plea for an agreed terminology and classification. Psychopathology. 1994;27: 123-9.
111. Berrios GE, Kan Chung-Sing. A conceptual and quantitative analysis of 178 historical cases of dysmorphophobia. Acta Psychiatr Scand. 1996;94:1-7.
112. Jorgensen P, Aagaard J. Clinical predictors of course and outcome in delusional psychosis. Acta Psychiatr Scand. 1988; 77:332-7.
113. Fernando N. Monosymptomatic hypochondriasis treated with a tricyclic antidepressant. Br J Psychiatry. 1988;152:851-2.
114. Alford BA, Beck AT. Cognitive therapy of delusional beliefs. Behav Res Ther. 1994;32:369.
115. Chadwick PD, Lowe CF. A cognitive approach to measuring and modifying delusion. Behav Res Ther. 1994;32:355-68.
116. American Psychiatric Association. Desk Reference to the Diagnostic Criteria from DSM-5. Washington DC. 2013.

CHAPTER 9

Other Psychotic Disorders

Jayesh Ranjan

The history of psychosis is the history of psychiatry. More than 150 years after its establishment as an independent scientific discipline in German universities, psychiatry is still dominated by conflicts among contrasting schools of thought, as to the true essence of the major metal disorders and by debates among clinicians on the correct interpretations and definitions of terms currently used.

An additional disturbing characteristic is the tendency among research workers to follow the circular pathway postulated for Medicine by Francis Bacon in the 17th century, and to come back again and again to old positions.

Examples of this tendency can be seen in the revival of a Kraepelinian conception of the boundaries of the endogenous psychoses and in a renewed interest in Zeller's and Griesinger's concept of *unitary psychoses.*

Schizophrenia or affective psychosis may each be defined broadly or narrowly. When schizophrenia is broadly defined, affective psychosis and other functional psychoses are less frequently diagnosed. Conversely narrowing the definition of schizophrenia increases the pool and heterogeneity of affective psychoses, and increases interest in other functional psychoses.

HISTORICAL DEVELOPMENT OF THE CONCEPT OF PSYCHOSIS

The concept of psychosis, as we know it, dates only from the late 19th century. It was formed out of the remnants of three ancient categories, namely insanity, alienation and dementia. At the beginning of the 19th century, 'insanity' as a concept encompassed all manner of delusional states accompanied by personality and behavioral disorganization. Whereas 'alienation' referred to affections of mind, in opposition to those of the brain. 'Dementia' referred to a variety of states of psychological dilapidation, whether related to chronic insanity or to brain damage. The word *psychosis* was allowed during the second half of the 19th century to displace old terms such as madness, *folie, pazzia, locura* and *wahnsinn.*

During the first half of the 19th century, *neuroses* included an enormous class of diseases, including present day neuroses, all the 'insanities', most neurological conditions and many other medical disorders. Their definitory features were absence of fever and disorder of the 'general' function of the central nervous system. Hence, the neuroses were considered during this period as 'organic' affections, whilst the psychoses simply referred to psychological experiential states.

The two terms underwent major changes in meaning during the 19th century. By 1900 AD., the membership of the class *neuroses* had been drastically reduced and its a few members redefined as 'psychological' disorders. In contradistinction to this, the *psychoses* came to encompass an ever-growing class of disorders whose common denominator was the claim that they were 'organic' in the nature.

The final factor in the shaping of the new concept of the psychosis was the adoption of the term itself. The Austrian physician von Feuchtersleben, in 1847, named it as "those conditions which we usually call, in a more restricted sense, mental derangement, psychoses".

In German psychiatry, the singular of the term, *psychose* referred to the psychological meaning and the plural, *psychosen* to the insanities themselves.

Not everyone accepted that it was possible to classify these phenomena. Some suggested that there was only one form of insanity and that its varied manifestations depended upon individual characteristics and environmental co-factor; the concept of the *unitary psychoses* (*einheitspsychose*).

The debate between unitarians and classificators did not last long. By the end of the 19th century, it was no longer a question whether classification was possible but along what lines.

Two different classificatory systems vied for supremacy during this period and, in the end, Wernicke was the loser; not necessarily because his ideas were wrong, but because of his untimely death. Had he lived longer, Psychiatry and, most certainly, the classification of the functional psychoses might have been very different today.

But, Kraepelin[1-3] was the victor and in his scheme of things, the number of the insanities were drastically reduced to two:

1. Dementia precox, and
2. Manic depressive insanity.

Since then, two important problems have been under permanent discussion with in Psychiatry. The first concerns what limits are to be drawn between these two forms of psychoses, and the second concerns the question whether the whole field of so-called functional or nonorganic psychoses could be covered by these two disease concepts, or perhaps combinations of them.

Most psychiatrists will agree that a considerable number of psychoses occur, which do not naturally fit in to Kraepelin's two forms, and which nosologically probably have very little, if anything at all, in common with schizophrenia or manic depressive disorder. The expression '*third psychosis*' has been applied to these.

Even Kraepelin himself admitted some doubt about the classification of mixed psychoses (*mischpsychosen*), which shared features of dementia precox and manic depressive insanity. Kraepelin postulated that mixed psychoses had to be due to the simultaneous occurrence in one and the same patient, of a family loading with both dementia precox and manic depressive insanity.

Bleuler[4] also discussed the occurrence of mixed psychoses, when describing the differential diagnosis of both manic depressive insanity and schizophrenia, and admitted some uncertainty as to the correct classification of recurrent psychotic motility disorders.

Kretschmer's theories of a relationship between body build, temperament and mental illness opened the way to new hypotheses, according to which the pathoplastic influence of constitutional factors comprising the physical constitution and the premorbid personality characteristics was alleged to explain the occurrence of *'legierung'* or the *intermediary psychoses.*

Mayer-Gross[5] found the hypothesis of mixture of body build and personality disposition venturesome and rather unconvincing for explaining the occurrence of mixed psychoses. He was also critical of the hypothesis of a double hereditary loading. However, he admitted that a definite answer to the question to the nature of the mixed psychoses was not yet available.

Schneider, in differentiating between schizophrenia and affective psychoses, described 'cases-in-between', in which the diagnoses of schizophrenia or affective psychoses can both be made with equally strong arguments.

SOME HISTORICAL CONCEPTS

Bouffées Délirantes

In 1880, in France, Magnan[6] described the acute transient psychoses under the term, '*Bouffées délirantes polymorphes des degeneres*'. The classical description of the transitory delusional states was given in 1886, by Magnan's pupil Legrain.[7]

The French psychiatric school, even after the incorporation into its nosology of the Kraepelinian dementia precox, and later of the Bleulerian schizophrenia, has retained until the present day the category, *bouffées délirante,* as an independent mental disorder.[8]

The modern day diagnostic criteria for *bouffées délirante,* according to Pichot[9] are:

- *Age of onset*: Approximately between 20 and 40 years.
- *Onset*: Acute, without and prior psychiatric history (other than identical episodes).
- *No chronicity*: Active phases fade away completely in several weeks or months, possibly recurring under the same form, the patient remaining devoid of all abnormality in the interval.
- Characteristic symptoms include all of the following:
  - Delusions and/or hallucinations of any type.
  - Depersonalization/derealization and/or confusion.
  - Depression and/or elation.
  - Symptoms varying from day-to-day, even from hour-to-hour.
- Not caused due to any organic mental disorder, alcoholism or drug abuse.

Reactive Psychosis

The term *psychogenic* was probably first used by the German psychiatrist, Robert Sommer[10] in his '*Textbook of Psychiatry*', in the year 1894. The first two psychiatrists to give clear and exhaustive descriptions of *psychogenic psychoses* were Karl Jaspers[11,12] in Germany and August Wimmer[13] in Denmark.

In 1913, in the first edition of his famous '*General Psychopathology*', Jaspers gave the following criteria for determining the reactive nature of the psychosis:

- The onset of the illness must have a clear temporal relationship to a precipitating stress, which must be adequate.
- There must be meaning for the reaction; it should serve as a defense, a wish fulfilment or as an escape.
- The contents of the reaction must reflect the stress in a meaningful way.
- The abnormal reaction comes to an end when the primary cause for the reaction is removed.

The first monograph on the psychogenic psychoses under the name of *psychogenic mental disease* was written by August Wimmer in 1916. His definition of psychogenic psychoses was very similar to that of Jaspers. The term was later replaced in Denmark by *psychogenic psychoses,* under the influence of Faergeman's book,[14,15] in Norway by *constitutional psychosis* and, finally generally, by *reactive psychosis,* which is used today by the whole Scandinavian school.

Following the investigation of Wimmer, there was a considerable lag before Faergeman's investigation. The patients originally diagnosed by Wimmer, as having psychogenic psychoses, were followed up by Faergeman 15 to 25 years after their index admission. In the follow-up, it is reported that only 50% of the patients could the considered confirmed cases of psychogenic psychoses.

In his review, Slater[16,17] offers the opinion that the low confirmation rate reported by Faergeman was clear evidence against psychogenic psychoses representing a valid diagnostic category. Slater does not indicate what diagnosis he presumes for the cases, which were confirmed. In his follow-up study of patients with psychogenic psychoses, Faergeman[15] reports that a clear association with emotional trauma improves the prognosis.

Welner and Stromgren[18] report a follow-up of 106 patients with schizophreniform psychoses. Of these, 72 were found to follow a benign course. In 40% of those which followed a benign course, "the psychological and temporal relationship between the commencement of the psychosis and mental trauma or stress was so clear, that it would be far fetched to deny that psychogenesis played a role." Somatic precipitants were considered significant in another 10% of the cases following a benign course. Eitinger et al.[19] in following up 154 cases of schizophrenic and schizophreniform psychoses, note that the *schizophreniform psychoses* "often have a directly precipitating factor", but do not mention the frequency with which this observation was made. Retterstol,[20,21] reporting on a follow-up of patients with reactive paranoid psychoses and paranoid schizophrenia, finds that precipitating factors occur more often in the reactive group.

Noreik[22] indicates that 'acute psychic traumata' occur more frequently in verified reactive psychoses than in schizophrenia. Further, 56% of the patients originally diagnosed as having reactive psychoses had a schizophrenic course.

Each of these investigations emphasized similar clinical features for reactive psychoses. Among patients who recover, affective features are common, mood is often depressed, the onset in acute, and affect and personality are preserved. A clear relationship to an emotional trauma is an extremely common feature.

For the analysis of the predisposition to reactive psychosis, family studies have been performed by Faergeman in Denmark, Langfeldt[23,24] in Norway, Labhardt[25] in Switzerland, McCabe[26-28] in Denmark, and Shapiro[29] in Denmark. The results suggest that a predisposition for psychogenic reactions may be inherited but that the occurrence of severe mental stress decides whether on this background, a psychogenic psychosis will arise.

According to Winokur[30] "*reactive psychoses* are different from schizophrenia and affective disorders on a clinical basis as well as on an etiological basis. The presence of precipitating events and systematic family study, as well as clinical differences would lend support to the view of the *third psychosis*".

According to McCabe, the features usually identified with reactive psychosis are: acute onset in association with a precipitating stress; affective features not associated with endogenous depression; nonschizoid premorbid personality; absence of autism; preservation of affect; and brief duration of illness. Genetic studies of such patients reveal an absence of schizophrenic heredity, but a variable association with the affective disorders. He concluded at the end of his study on reactive psychosis: "the author believes that evidence from previous studies and the current study is sufficient to justify considering reactive psychosis to be a third functional psychosis after manic depressive psychosis and schizophrenia".

According to Andersen and Laerum's study,[31] "the psychogenic/reactive psychosis is a psychiatric disorder with a good prognosis as to subsequent psychiatric illness." Stephens et al.[32,33] found that compared to *systematic schizophrenics,* the reactive patients had: (i) a more acute onset, (ii) more precipitating stress, (iii) more affective symptoms, (iv) more confusion, (v) less affective blunting, (vi) a better premorbid adjustment, ((vii) less premorbid schizoid traits, (viii) fewer schizophrenic relatives, and (ix) a much more favorable long term outcome.

Stromgren[34] summarized in the following words, "first, the reactive psychoses seem to be nosologically quite different from the other large groups of functional psychoses, i.e. schizophrenia and major affective disorder. Genetic studies have shown this quite clearly. Second, the course of these disorders differs from that of the other functional psychoses. They do not become chronic, like so many schizophrenias and they do not relapse nearly as frequently as the affective disorder".

Munoz et al.[35] feel that "the criteria proposed for the DSM-III-R do not facilitate the diagnosis of *brief reactive psychosis* but perhaps make it even more confusing", while Jauch and Carpenter,[36,37] in their review of the subject, felt that, "the DSM-III and DSM-III-R criteria for brief reactive psychosis change the original concept of this disorder in a manner so restrictive, as to virtually eliminate the diagnosis". Further they argue that the operational criteria of the DSM-III-R do not enhance the study of this putative disease entity but rather thwart this goal by restricting the diagnosis so severely that too few cases will be found to test the third psychosis hypothesis. So, they suggested revised criteria that will retain the essential features of the traditional concept while defining explicit criteria in the style of the DSM-III-R.

Jorgensen and Mortensen,[38] in their study, found that "using mortality as an index of outcome, first admitted patients with reactive psychosis have as poor as outcome as patients with the endogenous psychoses, i.e. schizophrenia and manic depressive psychosis, and thus an excess mortality risk compared with that of the population in general. Reactive depressed patients have even a higher relative mortality risk than endogenous depressed patients".

Thus, from a practical viewpoint, the proper diagnosis of reactive psychosis as distinct from the functional psychoses has important therapeutic and prognostic implications.[39]

Reactive Psychosis: An Indian Perspective

An ancient Indian medical text, *Sushruta Samhita*[40] describes a type of insanity borne out of grief, *shokaja*. Insanity due to psychological stressors manifested itself with incoherent speech and singing and laughing in a a stupid fashion. The treatment of insanity caused by grief included removal of the cause of grief. It is interesting to note that features of 'incoherence and singing and laughing in a stupid fashion' are similar to the DSM-III *brief reactive psychosis* features of 'emotional turmoil and incoherence or loosening of association'.[41,42] Thus, in *Sushruta Samhita*, the role of psychological as well physical factors in causing insanity was recognized and forms the basis of classification. The separation of conditions caused by psychological stress (such as grief) from those caused by toxins and biological factors is similar to modern day separation of reactive from endogenous, or organic from functional psychosis.

Kapur and Pandurangi,[43] in a comparative study of reactive psychosis and acute psychosis without precipitating stress, concluded that the two groups differed markedly on several dimensions. The reactive psychotics has more hysterical and affective features, more vulnerable personality, higher stress experience in their life prior to illness, and relatively better prognosis compared to the acute psychotics. Reactive psychosis was more akin to affective psychosis, and acute psychosis more akin to schizophrenia.

Chavan and Kulhara[44] concluded that in India, most of the patients diagnosed to have reactive psychosis have a mixed clinical picture of disturbance of affect, thinking and perception. Further, life stresses do have a pivotal role in the genesis of reactive psychosis.

Schizophreniform Psychosis

The concept of 'schizophreniform state' was developed by Langfeldt[24] in 1939, in Norway. He observed that some schizophrenics were not influenced by electroshock therapy, whereas other patients, with an apparently similar clinical picture, were improved or even cured. He proposed, for the cases with a good therapeutic prognosis, the term *schizophreniform states*. He suggested later that the schizophreniform states were in many points clinically different from the therapy resistant 'true' or 'process' schizophrenias. According to Langfeldt, the distinctive features of the schizophreniform psychoses were an acute onset, most often in relation to a precipitating stressful event, the presence of confusion during the acute episode, a pyknic body build, absence of schizoid personality traits, cyclothymic temperament, depressive symptoms, self reference tendencies, incoherence, and catatonic and pathoplastic features. The concept of *schizophreniform psychosis,* as defined by Langfeldt proved to have good predictive validity, as shown in repeated studies by both Scandinavian authors and research workers in other countries.[18,19,33,45-48]

Coryell and Tsuang,[49] in their study, found that the outcome ratings for schizophreniform disorder fell between those for affective disorder and those for schizophrenia. Furthermore, schizophreniform probands had patterns of family psychopathology that resembled those for schizophrenic probands more than those for affective disorders probands. The family history data, therefore, echo the results of follow-up in that schizophreniform disorder resembled schizophrenia more than primary affective disorder.

On the other hand, Fogelson et al.[50] from their study, concluded that the schizophreniform patients did not differ importantly from patients with affective disorders but differed markedly from schizophrenic patients in past psychiatric history, family history, acute treatment response, short-term course and dexamethasone suppression test results. The findings suggest that *schizophreniform disorder*, as defined by DSM-III, may not be a valid entity separate from affective disorder and that acuteness of onset, even in the absence of affective symptoms, implies the presence of affective disorder.

Langfeldt[51] proposed five different types of psychoses to be classified as *schizophreniform psychoses*: (i) preponderantly endogenically conditioned (constitutional) form, (ii) neurosis like, psychogenically more comprehensible cases, (iii) symptomatic and other predominantly exogenically (infectiogenic, traumatogenic, psychogenic) precipitated psychoses, (iv) cases belonging to the manic depressive group of psychoses, and (v) real atypical schizophrenias. He observed that "psychoses that I would diagnose as schizophreniform psychosis have been described with new names, such as schizoaffective psychoses, oneirophrenia, brief reactive psychoses, atypical schizophrenias and others". Further, "the DSM-III definition has nothing to do with the psychiatric states described in my papers".

Kendler et al.[52,53] suggested that schizophreniform disorder belongs within the '*schizophrenia spectrum.*' Beiser et al.[54] (1988) in their study, suggested "several features that, at initial examination, differentiate schizophreniform disorder from schizophrenia, such as higher DSM-III Axis V ratings, lack of flattened affect and better rapport with the examiner."

Guldberg et al.[55] found no correlation between the presence of two or more good prognostic features and favorable outcome. Confusion, disorientation, or perplexity at the height of the psychotic episode was the only feature consistently associated with a favorable outcome in their sample. They concluded that the introduction of good prognostic features of schizophreniform disorder by DSM -III-R has been done, without due consideration to the methodological problems of prediction research.

Bergem et al.[56] reclassified Langfeldt's cases of schizophreniform psychoses, according to the ICD-9 and DSM-III-R diagnostic systems. Most of the schizophreniform psychoses did not appear 'schizophrenia-like 'at all, but turned out to be mainly affective disorder. Those included in Langfeldt's diagnosis of 'schizophreniform psychoses' were found to be too heterogeneous to validate the existence of this syndrome.

Schizoaffective Psychosis

The term 'schizoaffective' was introduced in 1933 by the American psychiatrist J Kasanin.[57] He gave a synthetic description of *schizoaffective psychosis,* which can be summarized into four points:

1. The patients are between 20 and 30 and in excellent physical health. The personality is not very much different from the general run of people in the community, and the social and industrial adjustment is normal.
2. There is a definite and specific environmental stress.
3. There is a very sudden onset in a setting of emotional turmoil, with a distortion of the outside world and presence of false sensory impressions in some cases. The symptomatology is made up of a blending of schizophrenic and affective symptoms. Absence of passivity and of withdrawal are good prognostic features.
4. The psychosis lasts a few months and is followed by a recovery.

The official American history of schizoaffective psychosis can be followed in the successive editions of the Diagnostic and Statistical Manual of Mental Disorders (DSM's) of the American Psychiatric Association.[58] DSM-I describes among the *schizophrenic reactions*, the *schizoaffective type*. But, the criteria are at variance with Kasanin's original descriptions. No mention is made of sudden onset, shortness of episode or of complete recovery. On the contrary, evolution toward a (probably) chronic schizophrenic state is stressed as being usual. In DSM-II,[59] the definition has became very brief and non-committal, "patients showing a mixture of schizophrenic symptoms and pronounced elation and depression".

The DSM-III draft included a special category, schizo-affective disorders, completely distinct from schizophrenic disorders. It also stated that "the term schizoaffective has been used in many different ways.....at the present time, there is a controversy as to whether this disorder represents a variant of affective disorder, or schizophrenia, or a third independent nosological entity, or part of a continuum between pure affective disorder and pure schizophrenia". The separate listing was justified by "the accumulated evidence that individuals with a mixture of affective and schizophrenic symptoms, as compared with individuals diagnosed as having schizophrenia, have a better prognosis, a tendency towards acute onset and resolution, more likely recovery to premorbid level of functioning, and an absence of an increase of prevalence of schizophrenia among family members".

Two years later, in the printed edition of the DSM-III,[60] the category had practically disappeared. Though it formally retained a category called schizoaffective disorder, it was without diagnostic criteria and was considered as a residual class. In DSM-III-R,[61] this category has specified diagnostic criteria. The approach taken emphasizes the temporal relationship of schizophrenic and mood symptoms.

Currently, it is common for the clinical diagnosis of schizoaffective disorder to require both affective and schizophrenic symptoms, combined with a minimum duration.[62-73] Despite the impression of catalogued precision, which some of these definitions give and certain themes which recur among them, a number of them have been shown not to select the same group of patients.

In 1979, Brockington and Leff[74] reported the results of an objective comparison for some of these criteria. They tested the validity of eight different sets of criteria for schizoaffective disorder, including the CATEGO system,[75] Kendell's[76] criteria, Kasanin's criteria, Stephen's criteria for 'good prognosis schizophrenia', the study criteria of Welner,[63,64] and Spitzer's RDC for schizoaffective disorders.[62] The researchers found a very low level of concordance between the eight different definitions of schizoaffective disorder, compared with criteria for schizophrenia and affective disorder. The authors concluded that it is highly unlikely that the diagnostic concept of schizoaffective disorder currently in use corresponds to anything coherent in nature. Later research by Brockington et al.[77,78] further undermined the concept of schizoaffective disorder. Their study of 32 patients, meeting criteria for '*schizomanic psychosis,*' led them to conclude that, in terms of response to lithium treatment and overall outcome, most of their patients could be reclassified as manic.

Kolb[79] and Lehman[80] state that schizoaffective psychosis is a subtype of schizophrenia, although Lehman recognizes that there is controversy regarding this. Detre and Jarecki[81] strongly admonish against considering the so-called schizoaffective reactions as a separate entity distinct from schizophrenia. Klein and Davis[82] contend that the illness of schizoaffective patients is closely allied to manic depressive psychosis, while admitting that the dividing line between manic depressive illness and schizophrenia is unclear.

Redlich and Freedman[83] describe schizoaffective psychosis as a hybrid or border state, and not as a classical schizophrenic subtype. Beck's[84] position is analogous. He sees a spectrum of psychoses with manic depressive illness at one end and schizophrenia at the other, with schizoaffective psychosis being intermediary. A similar idea is espoused by Fish,[46,85] who believes that there exists a group of psychoses in which the symptoms clearly exceed manic depressive illness, yet recovery ensues.

Batcheldor[86] believes that the term schizoaffective is often a misnomer. Slater and Roth[17] state that a careful diagnostic evaluation in the supposed schizoaffective cases will lead to a rediagnosis either of schizophrenia or of affective disorder.

Procci,[87] in a survey of the literature on schizoaffective psychosis, concluded that while the term 'schizoaffective' as commonly used probably describes a heterogenous group of psychosis, considerable evidence supports the hypothesis that at least a subgroup of these psychoses has a definite relationship to the major affective disorder Tsuang,[71] in his study, suggests that schizoaffective disorder is genetically heterogenous, with at least two subtypes, one a variant of affective disorder and the other a variant of schizophrenia. Pope et al.[88] found that, while the diagnostic separation of schizophrenia from schizoaffective disorder and manic disorder appears to be valid, the diagnostic separation of schizoaffective disorder from manic disorder does not appear to be valid as judged by available criteria.

Gershon et al.[89] have presented family data which supports the idea that schizoaffective disorder, bipolar illness, unipolar illness and normality are points on a continuum of vulnerability. Singh and Sachdeva[90] reported that their findings do not support the generally held view of schizoaffective disorders being a subtype of schizophrenia. On the contrary, they suggested that these patients are in fact suffering from a primary affective disorder. Winokur[91] interpreted his data as not favoring either psychotic unipolar or psychotic bipolar illness, or schizo-affective disorder being considered autonomous.

Tsuang and Simpson[72] pointed out that the divergence of research findings in this field should be largely ascribed to be differences in the diagnostic criteria used for patient selection by the various authors and to the intrinsic heterogeneity of schizoaffective syndrome.

Maj and Perris[92] presented a classification of schizo-affective disorder for the research purposes. Tsuang and Marneros[73] pointed to the need for continued research to validate the core concept of schizoaffective disorder. Similarly, Pichot[9] said that the time has come to investigate with presently available techniques, its existence, its homogeneity and its limits.

Kendell's[76] view is that for the time being, they should be classified separately. Berner and Lenz's[93] findings stress the importance of differentiating between bipolar and unipolar affective disorders, and of subsequently applying a similar subdivision to schizoaffective conditions.

According to Angst,[94] two main factors which distinguish schizoaffective disorders from affective disorders, are a much earlier age of onset and probably an outcome intermediate between affective disorders and schizophrenia. Rudin[95] concluded that, from a genetic point of view, the schizoaffective (atypical) psychoses are clearly heterogenous.

As Meltzer[96] points out, current studies on the biology of schizoaffective psychoses are clearly preliminary in nature. Some of the findings that Meltzer reports as common in both the schizoaffective and the affective disorders are, abnormalities in platelet 5-HT uptake, CSF tryptophan, plasma tryptophan and 5-HIAA levels following a tryptophan load, TRH induced increase in TSH, clonidine induced increase in growth hormone, nonsuppression of DST, and absence of exaggerated increases in growth hormone following apomorphine. Some findings appear to suggest a closer similarity between schizoaffective and schizophrenic psychoses, like CSF NE, clonidine induced decrease in plasma MHPG, platelet 5-HT content and PGE-1 stimulated adenylate cyclase activity.

Some biological abnormalities are common in all three types of psychoses, namely low urinary MHPG, elevated CSF GABA, and increased plasma CK activity. Some parameters have distinctive values in the schizoaffective patients, like number of platelet a-2 adrenergic receptors and MEMA.

Marneros and Tsuang,[97,98] in their book on schizo-affective psychoses, concluded that the essential condition for precise definitions, symptomatological homogeneity and reliability of factors and findings, is the correct application of the rules of descriptive psychopathology.

According to Williams and McGlashan,[99] the schizo-affective psychosis is closer to schizophrenia than to affective disorder. McGlashan and Williams[100,101] compared three schizoaffective subtypes, namely manic, bipolar and depressive, across multiple baseline (demographic, premorbid, morbid) and long-term outcome dimensions. Their results failed to support the validity of such subtyping in schizoaffective disorder.

According to Levinson and Levitt,[102] family, clinical and treatment studies suggest that RDC's mainly affective subtype of schizoaffective mania is a variant of psychotic bipolar disorder. Limited available data suggest that the family schizophrenic subtype has poorer prognosis and includes cases more closely related to schizophrenia. In Opjordsmoen[103] study, the outcome in the schizoaffective disorder-depressive type was between that of the major depressive disorder and schizophrenia, but closer to major depressive disorder.

According to McGlashan and Williams.[101] two dimensions regularly predicted better outcome in schizoaffective psychosis; these are better developed premorbid instrumental skills and fewer typically schizophrenic symptoms. While Vega and Gutierrez,[104] in their study, concluded that the schizoaffective disorder, as defined by ICD-9 and RDC criteria, represents a heterogenous group as regards premorbid personality, DSM-III diagnosis, the presence or absence of inter-episodic psychotic symptoms, and hyperthymic episodes.

Cycloid Psychosis

Cycloid psychosis is a diagnostic concept, which has evolved gradually over the last 100 years, mainly in Germany and Scandinavia. It denotes a group of heritable, endogenous psychoses which are acute, recurrent and benign, and whose symptomatology is neither typically schizophrenic nor typically affective, but polymorphic. According to Fish,[85] the concept has a curious origin in the mid 19th century idea of 'degeneration' or hereditary mental illness. The roots of the concept of endogenous cycloid psychosis can be easily traced back to the work of Augustin Morel, and to his Darwinian conception of degeneration. Magnan,[6] inspired by Morel, was first to describe the syndrome of 'bouffee delirantes' in successive generations of degenerate families.

The concept of *degenerative psychosis* won acceptance in Germany and several workers published papers on it;

Bonhoeffer[105] and Birnbaum on 'degenerative phantasten,' Schroder[106] on 'autochthonen degenerative psychosis,' and Binswanger on 'classification of degenerative psychoses.'

Wernicke,[107] whose textbook first appeared in 1894, never accepted the 'two entities principles' of Kraepelin, and held on to a more differentiated view of the nosology of the psychoses. He introduced the concept of the *motility psychoses*, which were particularly associated with menstruation and childbirth, and which could exist in hyperkinetic, akinetic or cyclic forms. He died in 1905, but his ideas were continued by Kleist,[108] who wrote about motility psychosesin 1911, namely revelation and confusion psychoses and autochthonous degeneration psychoses. In 1926, he united the motility and confusion psychoses into an entity roughly equivalent to the degeneration psychoses, called the *cycloid psychoses* or 'zykloide psychosen.'

Leonhard[109] classified the endogenous psychoses into five main groups: (i) Unipolar psychoses, (ii) Manic depressive disease, (iii) Cycloid psychoses, (iv) Unsystematic schizophrenias, and (v) Systematic schizophrenias. To Kleist's cycloid psychosis, Leonard added a third group, the *anxiety elation psychoses*. Thus, the three subtypes of cycloid psychosis were:

1. The 'Anxiety-Happiness-Ecstasy' psychosis,
2. The 'Excited-Inhibited Confusion' psychosis, and
3. The 'Hyperkinetic-Akinetic Motility' psychosis.

The three subtypes of cycloid psychosis are conceived by Leonhard[110,111] as being bipolar disorders. But, the concept of bipolarity does not completely correspond to the same characteristic of the manic depressive psychosis. In fact, bipolar manifestation in patients suffering from cycloid psychosis occur more frequently within one and the same episode than as distinct episodes, as it is the case with mania and depression. Common to all three forms is the fact that they show a phasic course, followed by complete recovery, and that they run in families with high degree of homogeneity. The patients do not show peculiar premorbid personality characteristics. They occur more frequently in women than in men, and the mean age at onset being around 30 years.

Perris[112,113] developed the diagnosis of cycloid psychosis in two ways. First, he provided operational definition similar to the Research Diagnostic Criteria. His other contribution has been to change the diagnostic emphasis somewhat. Although, the symptoms emphasized by Leohard are still used, the main accent is placed on three cardinal features, namely the presence of confusion, the polymorphic symptomatology and the acute onset.

Cutting et al.[114] used Perris's definition in their study of 2500 admissions to the Maudsley professorial unit from 1955 to 1964. They found that cycloids were 3% of all admissions and 8% of psychotic admissions. Cycloid psychosis was the fourth most common psychotic diagnosis in the series, after depressive psychosis (18%), schizophrenia (16%), and organic conditions (10%); thus, it was more common than mania (5%). The characteristic features of cycloid psychosis were a female predominance and a remittent course. The cycloid group resembled the conventional groups in some respects, but differences from schizophrenic, affective and, to a lesser extent, schizoaffective groups were also striking.

Perris and Brockington[112] gave the following diagnostic criteria for cycloid psychosis:

- An acute psychotic condition, not related to the administration or the abuse of any drug or to brain injury, occurring for the first time in subjects in the age range 15 to 50 years.
- The condition has a sudden onset, with a rapid change from a state of health to a full blown psychotic condition within a few hours or, at most, a very few days.
- At least four of the following must be present:
  - Confusion of some degree, mostly expressed as perplexity or puzzlement.
  - Mood incongruent delusions of any kind, most often with a persecutory content.
  - Hallucinatory experience of any kind, often related to themes of death.
  - An overwhelming, frightening experience of anxiety, not bound to particular situations or circumstances (pan anxiety).
  - Deep feelings of happiness or ecstasy, most often with a religious coloring.
  - Motility disturbances of an akinetic or hyperkinetic type, which are mostly expressional.
  - A particular concern with death.
  - Mood swings in the background and not so pronounced to justify a diagnosis of affective disorder.
- There is no fixed symptomatological combination; on the contrary, the symptomatology may change frequently during the episode and shows a bipolar characteristic.

Brockington et al.[115,116] found that overall about 10% of the psychotic patients were diagnosed as cycloids. There was a poor concordance between cycloid and schizoaffective psychosis. Further more, there was a negligible overlap between cycloid and manic depressive psychosis. He came to the conclusion that the cycloids had an exceptionally good prognosis, much better than schizophrenia and at least as good as manic depressive patients, but their clinical picture did not correspond to the group of patients diagnosed as suffering from bipolar affective disorder.

In Perris's[69] opinion, the causes of cycloid psychosis have yet to be explored and this exploration can only be unbiased, if the concept is clearly defined and classified independently of other concepts.

Hysterical Psychosis

Hysterical psychosis was a popular term in United States and Europe during the early part of this century. Central to the concept of hysterical psychosis is a presumed interaction between environmental trauma and personality defect, the two varying in degree in a complementary fashion.

Hollender and Hirsch,[117] in their review of literature, concluded that "*hysterical psychosis* is marked by a sudden and dramatic onset, temporally related to a profoundly upsetting event or circumstance. Its manifestations include hallucinations, delusions, depersonalization and grossly unusual behavior. Thought disorders, when they occur, are usually sharply circumscribed and very transient. Affectivity, if altered, is changed in the direction to volatility and not flatness. The acute episode seldom lasts longer than one to three weeks, and the eruption is sealed off, so that there is practically no residue. Hysterical psychosis is encountered most commonly in persons referred to as hysterical characters or personalities, when faced by trying life situations or problems".

Langness[118] feels that, while the term *hysterical psychosis* appears to have been used in the literature on crosscultural psychopathology partly because of nosological difficulties, it may describe a widely distributed type of abnormal behavior. Prinquet[119] framed the hysterical psychosis in terms similar to Hollender and Hirsch.

In 1969, Hollender and Hirsch[120] revised their original findings, delineating three different types of hysterical psychoses.

Group I: Culturally sanctioned behavior, e.g. Latah, Amok, Neginegi, Whitiko.
Group II: Appropriation of psychotic behavior.
Group III: True psychosis.

Wig and Narang[121] observed that hysterical psychosis is not uncommon in Indian culture, where conversion hysteria symptoms are frequent and pleaded that hysterical psychosis should be viewed separately from schizophrenia. In Richman and White's[122] view, the hysterical psychosis, like conversion reaction, can be an alternative when repression fails and this choice of illness can be best understood in the family context. Siomopoulos[123] suggested that hysterical psychosis could be considered as a regression to the specific form of thought activity involved in children's play. Martin[124] found that women, who have hysterical personality structures and have disturbed marriages, are prone to hysterical psychosis.

Spiegel and Fink[125] provide additional evidence supporting the validity of the concept of a hysterical psychosis, while Bishop and Holt described their own version of *Pseudopsychosis.*

According to Kuruvilla and Sitalakshmi,[126] hysterical psychosis is characterized by acute onset, often following the occurrence of an emotionally disturbing event, absence of any characteristic thought disturbance, emotional volatility and good prognosis. Even though physical methods of treatment, like drugs and ECT, had to be used in many patients to control the acute disturbance, psychotherapy and family therapy were found to be essential for the abatement of presenting symptoms as well as prevention of their recurrences.

Gift, et al.[127] systematically applied Hollender and Hirsch's criteria for hysterical psychosis to a representative sample of 217 patients and found that no patients met all of these criteria. Therefore, they questioned the clinical utility of the concept of hysterical psychosis.

Atypical Psychosis

The impact of German psychiatry has been noticeable in Japan, where the hypotheses of Kleist and Leonhard have been integrated in the genetic research by Mitsuda,[128] Mitsuda and Fukuda, Kurosawa,[129] and Hatotani and Nomura.[130] According to the family studies by Mitsuda, atypical psychoses are to be regarded as separate from both schizophrenia and manic depressive psychosis and from the epileptic psychosis.

However, the concept of atypical psychosis is not used consistently by all Japanese authors. In fact, whereas the description given by Kurosawa, in his genetic study, largely corresponds to that of Leonhard's cycloid psychosis, the term *atypical psychosis,* as used by Mitsuda and Hatotani, seems to be much more comprehensive. It encompasses any psychopathological manifestation that is not regarded in Japan as typical of schizophrenia or manic depressive psychosis.

On the other hand, Mitsuda in one of his later papers stressed that the pathology of typical schizophrenia is that of the personality, whereas that of the atypical psychosis is a pathology of consciousness. Tsuang[70] concluded that the atypical schizophrenia differed remarkably from schizophrenia and most closely resembled the bipolar affective disorder. Singh and Sachdev,[131] in a clinical and follow up study of atypical psychoses, suggested that the cases showing admixture of schizophrenic and affective symptoms are probably a variant of affective disorders, although a possibility of their being a third independent psychosis can not be ruled out.

Menuck et al.[132] in their review of literature concerning *remitting atypical psychoses*, concluded that a recognizable syndrome of non-organic remitting psychosis has been described under a variety of labels, including schizoaffective psychosis, hysterical psychosis, bouffee delirante, reactive (psychogenic) psychosis, cycloid psychosis, brief reactive psychosis, schizophreniform disorder and atypical psychosis. These diverse labels all denote a syndrome of benign psychotic disturbance with brief duration and remitting outcome, that is often associated with premorbid personality problems, sudden onset after external stress, and a long-term pattern of recurrences. In some respects, the syndrome is consistent with one or more subtypes of psychotic disorders not elsewhere classified in DSM-IV, but none of those categories provides a satisfactory fit for the clinical picture that has been described. They proposed an independent category of psychotic illness called *remitting atypical psychosis* to denote the symptoms and longitudinal features that define the syndrome and demarcate it from others, while leaving open considerations about specific etiologic factors and psychopathologic characteristics that require further investigations.

Episodic Psychosis

According to Monroe,[133] the episodic behavioral disorder due to a limbic ictus can be differentiated from schizophrenia as rigorously defined in DSM-III. The acute mode of onset and the remitting course are the most useful differentiating features between schizophrenia and the episodic disorder. The presence of toxic or other organic symptoms, including clouding of sensorium, illusions, visual hallucinations, *forme fruste* of epilepsy, childhood history of minimal brain dysfunction, or attentional deficits, and soft neurological signs aid in differentiating the episodic disorders from manic and depressive episodes. The crucial symptoms of the episodes disorders are precipitous onset, intense affects, intermittent course and symptoms free intervals. In conclusion, Monroe stated that the episodic disorders are offered as a heuristically valuable concept for integrating many of the atypical psychoses.

Monroe[134] reviewed the data which supports the concept of a limbic ictus as an etiological mechanism in many patients with diagnoses of atypical psychoses.

According to Tucker et al.[135] the remarkable similarity of phenomenology of complex partial seizures, to what has been described as atypical or episodic psychosis, provides a possible theoretical link to the etiology of atypical psychosis.

Acute Schizophrenia/Acute Psychosis

Bleuler, in 1924, introduced the term *acute schizophrenia*, which arose from his observation that individuals with an acute onset of typical schizophrenic symptoms, did not necessarily have had deteriorating course, as had been suggested by Kraepelin, and that nearly 25% remitted. He admitted that in acute psychosis, there remains nothing to be done but to make a diagnosis of schizophrenia in those cases, which present with the symptoms of schizophrenia. This point of view was accepted by most of International Psychiatry and was reflected in the description of *acute schizophrenic episode* in ICD-9.

Rennie[136] had found that psychoses, which start with an acute onset, have a good prognosis and last only for a short time. Lambo[137] mentioned that high emotional lability was a special feature of the psychotic conditions with acute onset, which he had come across in Nigeria. In India, Wig and Singh[138] pointed to the 'acute psychosis of uncertain origin,' as being different from the clear cut manic depressive or schizophrenic psychoses and, apart from the acute onset, were characterized by florid symptomatology and good prognosis.

Taylor et al.[139] in their study, concluded that many patients receiving the diagnosis of acute schizophrenia actually suffer from an affective illness and rarely satisfy rigorous criteria for schizophrenia. While Singh and Sachdev[140] disputed the officially held view of ICD-8 and ICD-9 that acute schizophrenic episode was a subtype of schizophrenia. They found that it was not only different from schizophrenia but also from pure cases of manic depressive insanity in many respects. Hence, they suggested that these cases were probably suffering from a third psychosis, which on grounds of clinical features, response to treatment, family history and course of illness, tended to fall in between the cases of true schizophrenia and manic depressive illness.

Indian Council of Medical Research[141] conducted a collaborative study on the phenomenology and natural history of acute psychosis involving four centres in 1989. The study included 323 cases of acute psychosis, which were followed for a minimum of one year. Acute psychotic patients constituted 9% of all psychotic patients attending the facility for the first time. The most common presenting symptoms of such patients were ideas of reference, delusions of persecution, irritability, agitation or excitement, overactivity and inappropriate or bizarre behavior. Presence of anxiety, depression and hostile irritability was also seen in a fair number of cases. Primary schizophrenic thought disorder or voices speaking to the patients were uncommon. Majority of the patients were in the age group of 21 to 30 years, with equal distribution of males and females. Presence of psychological stress was seen in half of the cases and, in another 20% cases, there was some additional physiological or somatic stress. The onset of illness was very acute. It was less than 48 hours in over half the cases. Majority of the patients had a normal premorbid personality (74%). The clinical presentation of acute psychotic Illness included three main categories of patients: (i) approximately 25% were, both at initial contact and at 1 year follow-up, confirmed by CATEGO performance to be cases of schizophrenia, (ii) 25% were found to be cases of manic depressive psychosis, and (iii) remaining 50% cases, in whom there were no clear cut symptoms of schizophrenia or primary affective disorder, constituted the third group of *acute psychosis*, not before recognized as a separate group. These patients differed on the basis of their clinical picture, normal premorbid personality, absence of family history of mental illness and an excellent recovery rate of 85%.

Miscellaneous Terms

Luther Bell,[142] in 1849, described 40 cases of acute 'mania'; 30 of these terminated fatally and ten ended in full recovery. These patients had an acute onset and a good premorbid adjustment. When ill, they became poorly oriented, suspicious of being poisoned and would 'stand until exhausted'; yet ten cases recovered. Although Bell gave no name to the illness, over the years the syndrome became known as *Bell's mania*. Osler,[143] in 1893, referred to it as an almost invariably fatal disease, characterized by 'the wildest hallucinations' and stereotypy.

In 1861, Griesinger[144] described a syndrome entitled 'melancholia with stupor'. These patients showed depersonalization, dissociation of thoughts, hallucinations and delusions; yet they recovered. Prominent in their history were acute onset, visibly depressed affect, catatonia, confusion, and concern with dying.

The very next year, in 1862, Bucknill and Tuke[145] pointed out that 'acute dementia' was often benign and appeared to be similar to what Baillarger had called 'melancolie avec stupeur', and that many acute dementias were in reality, states of 'profound melancholy'.

Four decades later, Kaepelin[1-3] said the same thing. He recognized that stupors of the sort already mentioned, occurred both in his 'katatonia' and in 'circular depression'. He associated the former with a very poor prognosis and the latter with complete recovery between episodes. In the stupors which remitted, he noted flight of ideas, thoughts of death, confusion, and what he called 'divertability'. He noted that the same patients exhibited symptoms typical of his 'dementia precox'. He called this group '*mixed conditions of maniacal depressive insanity*'.

In 1910, Dunton[146] described psychoses that had a dementia precox picture, but had a cyclic or intermittent initial course of illness. Deterioration did ultimately occur in these cases. In 1913, George Kirby[147] noted that "many benign and recurrent psychoses did not fit into the manic depressive formula". He then went on to comment upon "the catatonic syndrome and its relation to manic depressive insanity". In patients with good premorbid personality, he described a stuporous, cataleptic psychosis, with an acute onset, occurring in relation to an object loss and accompanied by ideas of dying.

In 1920, Edward Kempf[148] devised another euphemism for recovered schizophrenics, '*homosexual panic*'. He described his syndrome as frequently associated with catatonia and accompanied by confusion. The onset was sudden, and both depression and concern with dying were manifest. He described a good prognosis for the given episode. To complicate the picture further, the panic has been referred to as '*Kempf's disease*'.

In 1921, August Hoch[149] presented 37 cases of '*benign stupors*: a new manic depressive reaction type'. His description of these cases (catatonia, flattened affect and loose associations) is indistinguishable from that of acute catatonic excitement. The affect was depressed, the onset was acute and the sensorium was confused. Almost all cases showed concern with dying, the symbolism of the symptoms was often clear and related to a precipitating stress. Several of his cases had a manic depressive heredity and all his cases went on to recover.

Hoch's cases were subjected to follow-up by Rachlin[150] in 1933, who challenged the concept of benign stupors as part of manic depressive disease. He stated that a large percentage of patients had ultimately deteriorated. After publication of his work, Hoch's eponym was generally abandoned.

Bleuler,[4] in the fourth edition of his textbook (1924), stated, 'one class of the psychoses shows itself as a morbid reaction to an affective experience as a *hysterical twilight state* to a jilting on the part of the beloved (reactive psychoses, situation psychoses). Although, resembling acute schizophrenia, Bleuler thought his 'remitting hysterical twilight state' was unrelated to the disorder.

In 1938, Gjessing[151] tried to separate a group of recoverable schizophrenics by a metabolic disturbance. *Periodic catatonia* or *Gjessing's syndrome* was characterized by stupor, acute and periodic onset, and recovery.

In 1929, Kasanin and Kaufman[152] were probably the first to refer to 'reactive psychosis of adolescence'. Keiser,[153] and Warren and Cameron,[154] also described the same picture.

In 1947, Adland[155] summarized the vast literature on the '*acute exhaustive psychoses*'. In his own cases, Adland described the familiar syndrome of confusion, acute onset, good premorbid adjustment, concern with death and symptomatology suggestive of the affective psychosis.

In 1940, Kant[156] described '*recovered schizophrenics*' as having more bipolar affectives than schizophrenics among their relatives, pyknic physique, psychogenic precipitant of psychotic episodes, acute or subacute onset, duration of several months, complete recovery, clouding of consciousness, psychotic experience, ideas of reference and auditory hallucinations.

In 1924, Mayer Gross described psychotic states in which a dream-like change of consciousness was present and called these '*oneroid states*'. These were characterized by good premorbid adjustment, and atypical course and often a heredity with a heavy admixture of manic depressive illness.

Meduna and McCulloch[157] grouped together all acute schizophrenic clinical pictures in which clouding of consciousness occurred and called them '*oneirophrenia*'. They claimed that an anti-insulin factor was present in the blood of these patients.

In Switzerland, the term '*schizophrenie-ahnliche emotions psychosen*', which was coined by Staehelin[158] (1947), had been used for cases which are quite similar to subgroups of the Scandinavian psychogenic psychoses. A large material of these psychoses has been described in an excellent monograph by Labhardt (1963).[25]

Fernandes (1957) proposed the comprehensive term of '*holodysphrenias*' to indicate provisionally recurrent acute psychotic conditions, characterized by confusion and by a polymorphous symptomatology. Goas (1968) presented his own comprehensive classification of '*marginal psychoses*'.

In 1963, Vaillant[159] suggested that *acute schizoaffective psychosis*, as defined by Kasanin was a more appropriate diagnosis for patients who recover from schizophrenic thought disorder, than terms like 'adolescent turmoil', 'schizophreniform state' or 'reactive psychosis'. Further, he stated that there seems no justification in separating 'remitting schizophrenia' from the broader classification of 'the group of schizophrenias'. He[160] fitted 16 eponyms used in history for schizophrenia-like psychoses, which recovered/remitted, into one diagnostic bed. He remarked that, although their inventors felt they were defining new ground, the schizophrenia-like psychoses have had much in common.

Robins and Guze[161] concluded that 'good prognosis schizophrenia' was not mild schizophrenia but a different illness. According to Fowler et al.[162] the family studies do not validate 'good prognosis schizophrenia' as schizo-phrenia and suggested that most good prognosis cases were variants of affective disorder. Similarly, McCabe et al.[26] demonstrated a close clinical relationship between good prognosis schizophrenia and the affective disorders. McCabe[28] came to the conclusion that the patients ordinarily given the diagnoses of acute schizophrenic episode and/or schizoaffective schizophrenia may be more appropriately diagnosed as having either affective disorder or reactive psychosis.

According to Stevens,[163] a high incidence of brief schizophrenia-like psychosis in Africa and other parts of the developing world has been repeatedly documented, by many psychiatrists working in these regions.[164-168]

COMMON FACTORS

The factors common to most of the above concepts are:

- Acute onset, often in the face of a precipitating environmental stress.
- Early age of onset, between 20 and 40 years.
- Marked emotional turmoil.
- Good premorbid functioning, with good social and vocational adjustment.
- No evidence of emotional withdrawal.
- Brief duration of the psychotic illness.
- No family history of schizophrenia.
- Presence of a family history of mood disorder.
- Good outcome, with preservation of social and vocational functioning.

CURRENT CLASSIFICATION

ICD-10

In ICD-10,[169] the category F20-F29 deals with *'schizophrenia, schizotypal and delusional disorders'*. The diagnosis of schizophrenia depends upon the presence of typical delusions, hallucinations or other symptoms, and a minimum duration of 1 month is specified.

ICD-10 has introduced a new category of F23 *'acute and transient psychotic disorders'*. It admits that "systematic clinical information, that would provide definitive guidance on the classification of acute psychotic disorders is not yet available, and the limited data and clinical tradition, that must therefore be used instead, do not give rise to concepts that can be clearly defined and separated from each other".

The order of priority used is (i) an acute onset (within 2 weeks) as the defining feature of the whole group, (ii) the presence of typical syndromes, and (iii) the presence of associated acute stress.

The acute onset is defined as a change from a state without psychotic features, to a clearly abnormal psychotic state, within a period of 2 weeks or less. The abrupt onset is defined as that occurring within 48 hours or less. It admits that "the nomenclature of these acute disorders is as uncertain as their nosological status, but an attempt has been made to use simple and familiar terms".

In the diagnostic guidelines, the manic (F30) or depressive (F32) episodes are excluded, and so is the 'organic causation' and 'obvious intoxication by drugs or alcohol'.

There are various subdivisions of the *acute psychosis*. In the inclusion terms are mentioned, bouffée délirante, cycloid psychosis, acute (undifferentiated) schizophrenia, brief schizophreniform disorder, brief schizophreniform psychosis, oneirophrenia, schizophrenic reaction, paranoid reaction, psychogenic paranoid psychosis and brief reactive psychosis.

ICD-10 was in dilemma whether to put schizoaffective disorder in block F20-29 (schizophrenia, schizotypal and delusional disorders) or in F30-39 (mood disorders). It finally decided to put it in F20-29, influenced by feedback from field trials of its 1987 draft,[170] which favored its retention among schizophrenia and delusional disorders. The diagnostic guidelines mentions that, "a diagnosis of schizoaffective disorder should be made only when both definite schizophrenic and definite affective symptoms are prominent simultaneously, or within a few days of each other, within the same episode of illness".

Its inclusion terms include both schizoaffective psychosis and schizophreniform psychosis. Others included are cyclic schizophrenia and mixed schizophrenic and affective psychosis.

The term 'schizophreniform' has not been used for a defined disorder in this classification, because "it has been applied to several different clinical concepts over the last few decades and is associated with various mixtures of characteristics".

The 'schizotypal disorder' (F21) "is not recommended for general use because it is not clearly demarcated, either from simple schizophrenia or from schizoid or paranoid personality disorder".

DSM-IV

In DSM-IV,[171] all the disorders characterized by having psychotic symptoms as the defining feature are classified under the heading *"schizophrenia and other psychotic disorders"*.

In DSM-IV, schizophrenia is a disturbance that lasts for at least 6 months and includes at least 1 month of active phase symptoms, while schizophreniform disorder is characterized by a symptomatic presentation that is equivalent to schizophrenia, except for its duration (i.e. the disturbance lasts from 1–6 months) and the absence of a requirement that there be a decline in functioning.

Schizoaffective disorder has been defined as a disturbance, in which a mood episode and the active phase symptoms of schizophrenia occur together, and were preceded, or are followed, by at least 2 weeks of delusions or hallucinations without prominent mood symptoms.

Delusional disorder is characterized by at least 1 month of nonbizarre delusions, without other active phase symptoms of schizophrenia. Brief psychotic disorder is a psychotic disturbance, that lasts more than 1 day and remits by 1 month. Shared psychotic disorder is a rare entity.

The category, psychotic disorder, not otherwise specified (NOS), includes psychotic symptomatology about which there is inadequate information to make a specific diagnosis, or contradictory information, or they do not meet the criteria for any specific psychotic disorder.

DSM-5 DIAGNOSTIC CRITERIA[172]

Recently DSM-5 criteria made change the heading od DSM-IV *"schizophrenia and other psychotic disorder"* to Schizophrenia spectrum and other psychotic disorder under which following disorder are included:

- Schizotypal (personality) disorder
- Delusional disorder
- Brief psychotic disorder
- Schizophreniform disorder
- Schizophrenia
- Schizoaffective disorder
- Substance/medication-induced psychotic disorder
- Psychotic disorder due to another medical condition
- Catatonia
- Catatonic disorder due to another medical condition
- Unspecified catatonia
- Other specified schizophrenia spectrum and other psychotic disorder
- Unspecified schizophrenia spectrum and other psychotic disorder.

EPIDEMIOLOGY

As the very concepts have been disputed in the past as well as in the present (e.g. differences among ICD-10 and DSM-IV), there is no reliable data regarding incidence, prevalence or course. There has been very few studies and most of them contradict each other, to be able to come to a firm conclusion.

TREATMENT

The treatment of other psychotic disorders is empirical and depends upon the conceptual orientation of the clinician. The commonly used medicines are antipsychotics, antidepressants, lithium, carbamazepine and sodium valproate in different combinations, doses and length of time. Electroconvulsive therapy may also be used for recalcitrant patients. As in other aspects, the researchers do not agree with each other even on the treatment aspects.

In acute psychosis, the treatment of choice is anti-psychotics. In acute phase, injectables may be used and, subsequently, the patient is put on oral antipsychotics, and is maintained on lowest possible doses of antipsychotic for a minimum period of 6 months. If the psychotic symptoms persist for more than 6 moths, the diagnosis may have to be reconsidered.

In schizoaffective disorder, manic type, the drug of choice is antipsychotic, in combination with lithium (or carbamazepine or sodium valproate). Antipsychotics are gradually tapered down and the patient is maintained on the mood stabiliser for varying length of time, depending upon the past history.

In schizoaffective disorder, depressed type, a combination of antipsychotics and antidepressants is used. Antipsychotics are tapered down to the minimum dose possible without relapse. The treatment duration depends upon the past history. In refractory cases, ECT is used with good response.

In schizophreniform disorder, the drug of choice is antipsychotics. If the symptoms persists for more than 6 months, the diagnosis is changed to schizophrenia and managed as such.

Similarly, brief psychotic disorder is treated with anti-psychotics and, if the symptoms persists for more than 1 month, the diagnosis is reconsidered.

In these disorders, apart from medicines, supportive psychotherapy, family counseling, support to family and stress management also play an important role in the management.

CULTURE BOUND SYNDROMES

Cultural factors play an important role in the manifestation of psychotic illness. There is a cultural bias in interpreting the official nosological system. Most of the official diagnostic systems are based on western nosological concepts and criterias, which are sometimes difficult to apply cross-culturally, especially in non-western societies.

In folk nosological systems in traditional societies, there are descriptions of specific patterns of aberrant behavior, which are difficult to place in a specific category in the official diagnostic system of ICD-10 or DSM-IV. Earlier in western literature, they were called *'cultural and ethnic psychoses and neuroses'* or *'atypical and exotic psychotic syndromes'*. Currently, they are known as *'culture bound syndromes'*.

CONCLUSION

Until our knowledge of basic neurosciences and causes of mental illness improves, the very concepts of schizophrenia and other psychotic disorders will remain debatable. Therefore, we should concentrate on researches in basic neurosciences, genetics, epidemiology and other fields, using well-defined criterias in standard, internationally accepted classification systems.

REFERENCES

1. Kraepelin E. Clinical Psychiatry. Ed. Johnstone T. New York: William Wood, 1913.
2. Kraepelin E. Dementia Praecox. Edinburgh: ES Livingstone, 1919.
3. Kraepelin E. Manic Depressive Insanity and Paranoia. Robertson GM. Edinburgh (Eds): ES Livingstone; 1921.
4. Bleuler E. Textbook of Psychiatry. Transl. Brill AA. IV German (Eds). New York: MacMillan; 1924.
5. Mayer Gross W. Selbstschilderungen der Verwirrtheit. Berlin: Julius Springer; 1924.
6. Magnan V. Lecons Cliniques, 2nd edition, Paris: Bataille; 1893.
7. Legrain M. Du delire Chez les degeneres. Librairie Deshaze et Liscroshier, Paris; 1886.
8. Pichot P. The diagnosis and classification of mental disorders in French speaking countries: Background, current views and comparison with other nomenclatures. Psychol Med. 1982;12: 475-92.
9. Pichot P. A Comparison of Different National Concepts of Schizoaffective Psychoses. Berlin: Springer; 1986.
10. Sommer R. Daignostic der Geisteskrankheiten. Vienna: Urban and Schwarzeberg; 1984.
11. Jaspers K. Allgemeine Psychopathologie. Berlin: Springer; 1913.
12. Jaspers K. (1913). Allgemeine Psychopathologic. General Psychopathology. Transl. Hoenig J, Hamilton MW. Manchester: Manchester University Press; 1963.
13. Wimmer A. Psykogene Sindssygdomsformer (Psychogenic forms of mental dirorders) in St. Hans Hospital (1816-1916). Copen-hagen: Jubilee Publication; 1916. pp. 85-216.
14. Faergeman PM. De psykogene psychoser belyst gennem Kata mnestiske undersogelser. Munksgaard, Copenhagen; 1945.
15. Faergeman PM. 'Psychogenic psychoses'. London: Butterworths; 1963.
16. Slater E. Distinguishing the effect of heredity and environment. Int J Psychiatry. 1967;3:416-7.
17. Slater E, Roth M, Mayer Gross. Clinical Psychiatry, 3rd edition. Baltimore: Williams and Wilkins; 1969.
18. Welner J, Stromgren E. Clinical and genetic studies on benign schizophreniform psychoses based on a follow up. Acta Psychiatr Scand. 1958;33:377-99.
19. Eitinger L, Laane C, Langfeldt G. The prognostic value of the clinical picture and the therapeutic value of physical treatment in schizophrenia and the schizophreniform states. Acta Psychiatr Scand. 1958;33;33-53.
20. Retterstol N. Paranoid and Paranoiac Psychoses. Thomas: Springfield; 1966.
21. Retterstol N. Prognosis in Paranoid Psychoses. Oslo: Universitets for laget; 1970.
22. Noreik K. Follow up and classification of functional psychoses, with special references to reactive psychoses. Olso, Universitets for laget; 1970.
23. Langfeldt G. The prognosis in schizophrenia and the factors influencing the course of the disease. A Katamnestic study, including individual re-examination in 1936. Copenhagen, Munksgaard; 1937.
24. Langfeldt G. The Schizophreniform States. Ed. Milferd H. London: Oxford University Press; 1939.
25. Labhardt F. Die Schizophrenieahnlichen Emotionpsychosen. Berlin: Springer; 1963.
26. McCabe MS, Fowler RC, Cadoret RJ, et al. Symptom differences in schizophrenia with good and poor prognosis. Am J Psychiatry. 1972;128:1239.
27. McCabe MS. Reactive psychoses: A clinical and genetic investigation. Acta Psychiatr Scand Supplementum 259, Munksgaard, Copenhagen; 1975.
28. McCabe MS. Reactive psychoses and schizophrenia with good prognosis. Arch Gen Psychiatry. 1976;33:571.
29. Shapiro RW. A twin study of non endogenous depression. Copenhagen, Munksgaard; 1970.
30. Winokur G. Preface. In: McCabe MS. Reactive Psychosis. Acta Psychiatr Scand Supplementum 259, Copenhagen, Munksgaard; 1975.
31. Andersen J, Laerum H. Psychogenic psychoses. Acta Psychiatr Scand. 1980;62:331-42.
32. Stephens JH, Shaffer JW, Carpenter WR. Reactive psychoses. J Nerv Ment Dis. 1982;170:657-63.
33. Stephens JH, Adtrup C, Mangrum JC. Prognostic factors in recovered and deteriorated schizophrenics. Am J Psychiatry. 1966;122:1116-21.
34. Stromgren E. Reactive (psychogenic) psychoses and their relations to schizoaffective psychoses. In: Marneros A, Tsuang MT (Eds). Schizoaffective Psychoses. Berlin: Springer Verlag; 1986.
35. Munoz RA, Admado H, Hyatt S. Brief reactive psychosis. J Clin Psychiatry. 1987;48:324-27.
36. Jauch DA, Carpenter WT Jr. Reactive psychosis. I. Does the Pre-DSM-III concept define a third psychosis? J Nerv Ment Dis. 1988;176:72-81.
37. Jauch DA, Carpenter WT Jr. Reactive Psychosis. II. Does DSM-III-R define a third psychosis. J Nerv Ment Dis. 1988;176:82-6.
38. Jorgensen P, Mortensen PB. Reactive psychosis and mortality. Acta Psychiatr Scand. 1990;81:277-9.
39. Ungvari GS, Hantz PM. Reactive psychosis among elderly people. Acta Psychiatr Scand. 1990;82:141-4.
40. Sushruta Samhita, 3rd edition, Transl. Bhishagratna KK. Vol. III. Varanasi: Chowkhamba Sanskrit Series; 1981.
41. Haldipur CV. Madness in ancient India: Concept of insanity in Charaka Samhita (First century AD). Compr Psychiatry. 1984; 25:335-44.
42. Haldipur CV. Psychiatric nosology and taxonomy in ancient India. Acta Psychiatr Scand. 1989;80:148-50.
43. Kapur RL, Pandurangi AK. A comparative study of reactive psychosis and acute psychosis without precipitating stress. Br J Psychiatry. 1979;35:544-50.

44. Chavan BS, Kulhara P. A clinical study of reactive psychosis. Acta Psychiatr Scand. 1988;78:712-5.
45. Holmoboe R, Astrup C. A follow up study of 255 patients with acute shcizophrenia and schizophreniform psychoses. Acta Psychiatr Scand. 1957;Suppl.:115.
46. Fish FJ. Schizophrenia. Baltimore: Williams and Wilkins; 1962.
47. Achte KA. On prognosis and rehabilitation in schizophrenic and paranoid psychoses. Acta Psychiatr Scand. 1967;Suppl.: 196.
48. Astrup C, Noreik K. Functional psychoses: Diagnostic and prognostic models. Springfield, Thomas; 1966.
49. Coryell W, Tsuang MT. DSM-III schizophreniform disorder. Arch Gen Psychiatry. 1982;32:66-9.
50. Fogelson DL, Cohen BM, Pope HG. A study of DSM-III schizophreniform disorders. Am J Psychiatry. 1982;39: 1281-5.
51. Langfeldt G. Definition of "schizophreniform psychoses." Am J Psychiatry. 1982;139:703.
52. Kendler KS, Gruenberg AM, Tsuang MT. Psychiatric illness in the first degree relatives of schizophrenic and surgical control patients. Arch Gen Psychiatry. 1985;42:770-9.
53. Kendler KS, Gruenberg AM, Tsuang MT. A DSM-III family study of non-schizophrenic psychotic disorders. Am J Psychiatry. 1986;143:1098-105.
54. Beiser M, Fleming JAE, Iacono WG, et al. Refining the diagnosis of schizophreniform disorder. Am J Psychiatry. 1988;145: 695-700.
55. Guldberg CA, Dahl AA, Hansen H, et al. Predictive value of the four good prognositc features in DSM-II-R schizophreniform disorder. Acta Psychiatr Scand. 1990;82:23-5.
56. Bergem ALM, Dahl AA, Guldberg C, et al. Langfeldt's schizophreniform psychoses fifty years later. Br J Psychiatry. 1990;157:351-4.
57. Kasanin J. The acute schizoaffective psychoses. Am J Psychiatry. 1933;13:97-126.
58. American Psychiatric Association. Diagnostic and Statistical Manual of Mental Disorders. Washington: American Psychiatric Association; 1952.
59. American Psychiatric Association. Diagnostic and Statistical Manual of Mental disorders, 2nd edition, Washington: American Psychiatric Association; 1968.
60. American Psychiatric Association. Diagnostic and Statistical Manual of Mental disorders, 3rd edition, Washington: American Psychiatric Association; 1980.
61. American Psychiatric Association. Diagnostic and Statistical Manual of Mental disorders, 3rd edition, Rev. Washington: American Psychiatric Association; 1987.
62. Spitzer RL, Endicott J, Robins E. Research diagnostic criteria: Rationale and reliability. Arch Gen Psychiatry. 1978;35:773-82.
63. Welner A, Croughan JL, Rohins E. The group of schizoaffective and related psychoses: Critique, record, follow up and family studies. Arch Gen Psychiatry. 1974;31:628.
64. Welner A, Croughan J, Fishman R, et al. The group of schizoaffective and related psychoses: A follow up study. Compr Psychiatry. 1977;18:413-22.
65. Kendell RE, Gourley J. The clinical distinction between affective psychoses and schizophrenia.Br J Psychiatry. 1970; 117:261-6.
66. Angst J, Felder W, Lohmeyer B. Schizoaffective disorders. I. Results of a genetic investigation. J Affect Dis. 1979;1:139-53.
67. Meddlewicz J, Linkowski P, Wilmotte J. Relationthip between schizoaffective illness and affective disorders or schizophrenia. J Affect Dis. 1980;2:289-302.
68. Perris C. A study of bipolar (Manic depressive) and unipolar recurrent depressive psychoses. Acta Psychiatr Scand. 1966; Suppl.:194.
69. Perris C. The case for the independence of cycloid psychotic disorder from the schizoaffective disorders. In: Marneros A, Tsuang MT Eds. Schizoaffective Psychoses. Berlin: Springer Verlag; 1986.
70. Tsuang MT, Dempsey GM, Rausher F. A Study of atypical schizophrenia: Comparison with schizophrenia and affective disorder by sec, age of admission, precipitant, outcome and family history. Arch Gen Psychiatry. 1976;33:1157-60.
71. Tsuang MT. Schizoaffective disorder: Dead or alive? Arch Gen Psychiatry. 1979;36;633.
72. Tsuang MT, Simpson JC. Schizoaffective disorder: Concept and reality. Schizophr Bull. 1984;10:14-25.
73. Tsuang MT, Marneros A. Schizoaffective psychosis: Questions and directions. In: Marneros A, Tsuang MT (Eds). Schizoaffective Psychoses. Berlin: Springer Verlag; 1986.
74. Brockington IF, Leff JR. Schizoaffective psychosis: Definition and incidence. Psychol Med. 1979;9:91-9.
75. Wing JK, Cooper JE, Sartorius N. The measurement and classification of psychiatric symptoms. London: Cambridge University Press; 1974.
76. Kendell RE. The relationship of schizoaffective illnesses to schizophrenic and affective disorders. In: Marneros A, Tsuang MT (Eds). Schizoaffective Psychoses. Berlin: Springer Verlag; 1986.
77. Brockington IF, Wainwright S, Kendell RE. Manic patients with schizophrenic or paranoid symptoms. Psychol Med. 1980;10: 73-83.
78. Brockington IF, Kendell RE, Wainwright S. Depressed patients with schizophrenic or paranoid symptoms. Psychol Med. 1980; 10:665-75.
79. Kolb LC. Modern Clinical Psychiatry, 8th edition, Philadelphia: WB Saunders; 1973.
80. Lehman H. Schizophrenia: Clinical features. In: Freedman AM, Kaplan HI, Sadock JB, Eds. Comprehensive Textbook of Psychiatry, 2nd edition, Baltimore: Williams and Wilkins; 1975. pp. 890-923.
81. Detre TP, Jarecki HB. Modern Psychiatric Treatment. Philadelphia: JB Lippincott; 1971.
82. Klein DF, Davis JM. Diagnosis and Drug Treatment of Psychiatric Disorders. Baltimore: Williams and Wilkins; 1969.
83. Redlich FC, Freedman DX. The Theory and Practice of Psychiatry. New York: Basic Books; 1966.
84. Beck AT. Depression: Causes and Treatment. Philadelphia: University of Pennsylvania Press; 1967.

85. Fish FJ. The cycloid psychoses. Compr Psychiatry. 1964;5: 155-69.
86. Batcheldor IRC. Hendersen and Gllespie's Textbook of Psychiatry. London: Oxford University Press; 1969.
87. Procci WR. Schizoaffective psychosis: Fact or fiction? Arch Gen Psychiatry. 1976;33:1167-78.
88. Pope HG, Lipinski JF, Cohen BM, et al. Schizoaffective disorder: An invalid diagnosis? Am J Psychiatry. 1980;137:921.
89. Gershon E, Hamovit J, Curoff J. A family history of schizoaffective, bipolar I, bipolar II, unipolar and normal control probands. Arch Gen Psychiatry. 1982;39:1157-67.
90. Singh G, Sachdeva JS. Schizoaffective psychoses: Are they schizophrenic? Indian J Psychiatry. 1982;24:42-8.
91. Winokur G. Psychosis in bipolar and unipolar affective illness with special reference to schizoaffective disorder. Br J Psychiatry. 1984;145:236-42.
92. Maj M, Perris C. An approach to the diagnosis and classification of schizoaffective disorder for research purposes. Acta Psychiat Scand. 1985;72:405-13.
93. Berner P, Lenz G. Definitions of schizoaffective psychosis: Mutual concordance and relationship to schizophrenia and affective disorder. In: Marneros A, Tsuang MT (Eds). Schizoaffective Psychoses. Berlin: Springer Verlag; 1986.
94. Angst J. The course of schizoaffective disorders. In: Marneros A, Tsuang MT (Eds). Schizoaffective psychoses. Berlin: Springer Verlag; 1986.
95. Rudinzerbin E. Schizoaffective and other atypical psychoses: The genetical aspect. In: Marneros A, Tsuang MT (Eds). Schizoaffective psychoses. Berlin: Springer Verlag; 1986.
96. Meltzer HY. Biological studies of the nosology of the major psychoses: A status report on the schizoaffective disorders. In: Marneros A, Tsuang MT (Eds). Schizoaffective psychoses. Berlin: Springer Verlag; 1986.
97. Marneros A, Tsuang MT. Schizoaffective Psychoses. Berlin, Springer-Verlag; 1986.
98. Marneros A, Tsuang MT. Schizoaffective disorders: Present level and future perspectives. In: Marneros A, Tsuang MT (Eds). Schizoaffective Psychoses. Berlin: Springer Verlag; 1986.
99. Williams PV, McGlashan TH. Schizoaffective psychosis: I comparative long term outcome. Arch Gen Psychiatry. 1987; 44:130.
100. McGlashan TH, Williams PV. Schizoaffective psychosis. II. Manic, bipolar and depressive subtypes. Arch Gen Psychiatry. 1987;44:138.
101. McGlashan TH, Williams PV. Predicting outcome in schizoaffective psychosis. J Nerv Ment Dis. 1990;178:518-20.
102. Levinson DF, Levitt MEM. Schizoaffective mania reconsidered. Am J Psychiatry. 1987;155:415.
103. Opjordsmoen S. Long term course and outcome in unipolar affective and schizoaffective psychoses. Acta Psychiatr Scand. 1989;79:317-26.
104. Vega JM del RIO, Gutierrez JL Ayuso. Course of schizoaffective psychosis: A retrospective study. Acta Psychiatr Scand. 1990; 81:534-7.
105. Bonhoeffer K. Klinischer Beitrag zur hehre von den degenerations psychoses. Marhold: Halle; 1907.
106. Schroder P. Degeneratives irresein und degenerations psychosen. Z Gesamte Neurol Psychiatry. 1920;60:119-26.
107. Wernicke C. Grundriss der Psychiatric in Klinischen Vork Surgen. Thieme: Leipzig; 1894.
108. Kleist K. Uber zykloride degeneration-psychosen, besonders Verwirrtheits. Arch Psychiatry. 1926;78:100-15.
109. Leonhard K. Auffeilung der endogenen Psychosen. 1st-4th. Akademic Jena (Ed), 1957-1969.
110. Leonhard K. Cycloid psychoses: Endogenous psychoses which are neither schizophrenia nor manic depressive. J Ment Sci. 1961;107:632-48.
111. Leonhard K. The Classification of Endogenous Psychoses, 5th edition. New York: Irvington Publishers; 1979.
112. Perris C, Brockington IF. Cycloid psychoses and their relation to the major psychoses. In: Perris C, Struwe D, Janson B (Eds). Biological Psychiatry. Amsterdam: Elsevier; 1981. pp. 447-50.
113. Perris C. A study of cycloid psychoses. Acta Psychiatr Scand. 1974;Suppl.:253.
114. Cutting JC, Clare AW, Mann AH. Cycloid psychosis and investigation of the diagnostic concept. Psychol Med. 1978;8: 637-48.
115. Brockington IF, Perris C, Kendell RE. The course and outcome of cycloid psychosis. Psychol Med. 1982;12:97-105.
116. Brockington IF, Perris C, Meltzer HY. Cycloid psychoses: Diagnosis and heuristic value. J Nerv Ment Dis. 1982;170: 651-6.
117. Hollender MH, Hirsch SJ. Hysterical psychosis. Am J Psychiatry. 1964;120:1066-74.
118. Langness LL. Hysterical psychosis: The cross-cultural evidence. Am J Psychiatry. 1967;124:143-52.
119. Prinquet G. A propos d'un cas de psychose hysterique. Nouv Presse Med. 1977;6:441-3.
120. Hirsch SJ, Hollender MH. Hysterical psychosis: Clarification of the concept. Am J Psychiatry. 1969;125:909-15.
121. Wig NN, Narang RL. Hysterical psychosis. Indian J Psychiatry. 1969;11:93.
122. Richman J, White H. A family view of hysterical psychosis. Am J Psychiatry. 1970;127:280.
123. Siomopoulos V. Hysterical psychosis: Psychopathological aspects. Br J Psychol. 1971;44:95.
124. Martin PA. Dynamic considerations of the hysterical psychosis. Am J Psychiatry. 1971;128:745.
125. Binswanger O. Die klinische stellung der degeneration psychosen. Schweiz Arch Psychiatr Neurol. 1928;83:299-325.
126. Kuruvilla K, Sitalakshmi N. Hysterical psychosis. Indian J Psychiatry. 1982;24:352-9.
127. Gift TE, Strauss JS, Young Y. Hysterical psychosis: An empirical approach. Am J Psychiatry. 1985;142:345-7.
128. Mitsuda H. The concept of atypical psychosis from the aspect of clinical genetics. Acta Psychiatr Scand. 1965;41:372.
129. Kurosawa R. Untersuchung der atypischen endogenen psychosen. Psychiatr Neurol Med Psychol. 1961;13:364-70.

130. Hatotani N, Nomura J. Neurobiology of Periodic Psychoses. Tokyo: Igaku-Shoin; 1983.
131. Singh G, Sachdev JS. A clinical and follow up study of atypical psychosis. Indian J Psychiatry. 1980;22;167-72.
132. Menuck M, Legault S, Schmidt P, et al. The nosologic status of remitting atypical psychoses. Compr Psychiatr. 1989;39; 53-73.
133. Monroe RR. DSM III style diagnoses of the episodic disorders. J Nerv Ment Dis. 1982;170:664.
134. Monroe RR. Limbic ictus and atypical psychoses. J Nerv Ment Dis. 1982;170:711.
135. Tucker GJ, Price TRP, Johnson VB, et al. Phenomenology of temporal lobe dysfunction: A link to atypical psychosis: A series of cases. J Nerv Ment Dis. 1986;174:348.
136. Rennie TAC. Follow up study of 500 patients with schizophrenia admitted to the hospital from 1913 to 1923. Arch Neurol Psychiatry. 1939;42:277.
137. Lambo TA. Schizophrenia and borderline states. In: Reuck AVS, Porter R (Eds). Transcultural Psychiatry. Ciba Foundation Symposium. London: Churchill; 1965.
138. Wig NN, Singh G. A proposed classification of psychiatric disorders for use in India. Indian J Psychiatry. 1967;9:158.
139. Taylor MA, Gaztznaga P, Abrams R. Manic-depressive illness and acute schizophrenia: A clinical, family history and treatment response study. Am J Psychiatry. 1974; 131:678.
140. Singh G, Sachdev JS. Acute schizophrenic episodes: Are they schizophrenic? Indian J Psychiatry. 1982;24:42-8.
141. Indian Council of Medical Research. Collaborative Study on the Phenomenology and Natural History of Acute Psychosis. New Delhi: ICMR; 1989.
142. Bell LV. On a new form of disease. Am J Insanity. 1849;6:97-127.
143. Osler W. The Principles and Practice of Medicine. New York: Appleton; 1893.
144. Griesinger W. Mental Pathology and Therapeutics. II German Ed. London: New Sydenham Society; 1867.
145. Bucknill JC, Tuke DH. Psychological Medicine. London: John Churchill; 1862.
146. Dunton WR. The cyclic forms of dementia praecox. Am J Insanity. 1910;66:465-76.
147. Kirby GH. The catatonic syndrome and its relation to manic depressive insanity. J Nerv Ment Dis. 1913;40:694-704.
148. Kempf EJ. Psychopathology. St. Louis: Mosby; 1920.
149. Hoch A. Benign stupors: A study of a new manic depressive reaction type. New York: MacMillan; 1921.
150. Rachlin HL. A follow up study of Hoch's benign stupor cases. Am J Psychiatry. 1935;92:531-58.
151. Gjessing R. Disturbances of somatic functions in catatonia with a period course, and their compensation. J Ment Sci. 1938;84: 608-21.
152. Kasanin J, Kaufman MR. A study of the functional psychoses in childhood. Am J Psychiatry. 1929;9:307-84.
153. Keiser S. Severe reactive states and schizophrenia in adolescent girls. Nerv Child. 1944;4:17-25.
154. Warren W, Cameron K. Reactive psychosis in adolescence. J Ment Sci. 1950;96:448-57.
155. Adland ML. Review, case studies, therapy, and interpretation of the acute exhaustive psychoses. Psychiat Quart. 1947;21:38-69.
156. Kant O. Types and analyses of the clinical pictures of recovered schizophrenics. Psychiat Quart. 1940;14:676-700.
157. Meduna LJ. Oneirophrenia. Urbana; 1950.
158. Staehelin JE. Zur Grage dev Emotion psychosen. Bull Schweiz Akad Med Wiss. 1947;2:121-30.
159. Vaillant GE. The natural history of the remitting schizophrenias. Am J Psychiatry. 1963;120:367.
160. Vaillant GE. An historical review of the remitting schizophrenias. J Nerv Ment Dis. 1964;138:48.
161. Robins E, Guze SB. Establishment of diagnostic validity in psychiatric illness: Its application to schizophrenia. Am J Psychitry. 1970;126:107.
162. Fowler RC, McCabe MS, Cadoret RJ, et al. The validity of good prognosis schizophrenia. Arch Gen Psychiatry. 1972;26;182.
163. Stevens J. Brief psychoses: Do they contribute to the good prognosis and equal prevalence of schizophrenia in developing countries? Br J Psychiatry. 1987;151:393-6.
164. Dembovitz N. Psychiatry amongst west African troops. J Roy Army Med Corps. 1945;84:70-4.
165. Carothers JC. The African Mind in Health and Disease: A Study of Ethnopsychiatry. Geneva: World Health Organisation; 1953.
166. Jillek WG, Jilek Aall L. Transient psychoses in Africans. Psychiatr Clin. 1970;3:337-64.
167. German CA. Aspects of clinical psychiatry in sub-Saharan Africa. Br J Psychiatry. 1972;121:291-303.
168. Leighton AH, Lambo TA, Hughes CC, et al. Psychiatric Disorder Among the Yoruba. Ithaca: Cornell University Press; 1963.
169. World Health Organisation. The ICD-10 Classification of Mental and Behavioural Disorders. Geneva: WHO; 1992.
170. World Health Organisation. ICD-10, 1990 Draft of Chapter V. Mental and Behavioural Disorders. Geneva: WHO; 1990.
171. American Psychiatric Association. Diagnostic and Statistical Manual of Mental Disorders, 4th edition, Washington DC: American Psychiatric Association; 1994.
172. American Psychiatric Association. Desk Reference to the Diagnostic Criteria from DSM-5. Washington DC, 2013.

CHAPTER 10

Anxiety Disorders: Overview

Dinesh Tyagi

10.1 GENERAL ASPECTS OF ANXIETY DISORDER

Anxiety disorders are the most prevalent mental disorders in the general population. Nearly 35 million peoples are affected in united states and more in other countries. The patient with anxiety or a panic state is a common problem in the emergency department worldwide. Usually, these patients have chief complaints of somatic distress, such as chest pain or dyspnea. Once the anxious patient has been found to have no medical illness, he is often considered to have been fully evaluated and efforts are made to discharge the patient from emergency room, perhaps with the reassurance that nothing is really wrong. Unfortunately, clinicians may dismiss symptoms of endogenous anxiety as 'hysterical', failing to realize that, patient with these symptoms are suffering from an exceedingly unpleasant state and that they have treatable a psychophysiological disorder. Patients with chronic anxiety disorder may develop a pattern of frequent emergency room visits. Such patients evoke strong negative responses among clinicians if they request specific doses of anti-anxiety medications.

Till the later part of nineteenth century, anxiety disorders were conspicuously missing from the classification of psychiatric disorders. This was because at that time the classification were mainly concerned with the patients seen in psychiatric hospitals. Henry Maudsley,[1] in his influential book, 'The Pathology of Mind', describes the panic attack occurring in association with melancholia. He wrote about *melancholic panic* as follows: "the attack often comes on quite suddenly. The convulsive panic is preceded by an anomalous and alarming sensation of distress about the region of the stomach or of the heart... accompanied by an indescribable terror and feeling of helplessness".

Beard, in 1869, introduced the term *neurasthenia,* when lesser degrees of anxiety were grouped with minor depressive disorders.[2] Further, Hecker (1893) observed that half of his neurasthenia patients suffered from panic attack, either in specific circumstances or spontaneously, and he gave a clear account of anxiety attacks describing palpitations, rapid breathing, dizziness, sweating and frequency of micturition.[3] The first step in identifying anxiety disorder was taken by Westphal in 1871, who described the syndrome of *agoraphobia.*[4] At that time, it appeared that the word 'anxiety' was derived from the mistranslation of Freud's word for fear (*angst*). In 1895, Freud separated anxiety disorders from neurasthenia and suggested the name *anxiety neurosis.*[5] He included in the syndrome simple phobia, agoraphobia, generalized anxiety and panic attacks. At that time, cases, which are now called as panic disorders without agoraphobia, were recognized but regarded as cardiac and not anxiety disorders. They were called as *'irritable heart'* by da costa (1871) and subsequently referred to as *'da costa syndrome'*, 'disorderly action of heart', or 'effort syndrome'.[6]

The modern classification of anxiety disorders is controversial, which is reflected in DSM-III. However,[7] this controversy has been resolved up to some extent in ICD-10 and DSM-IV.[8]

ICD-10 has divided the anxiety disorders mainly into two categories, i.e. phobic disorders and other anxiety disorders, and each is further subdivided into three groups. The three phobic disorders are agoraphobia, social phobia and specific phobia. The three subgroups of other anxiety disorders are panic disorder, generalized anxiety disorder (GAD), and mixed anxiety and depressive disorder. ICD-10 does not include obsessive-compulsive disorder (OCD) under the group of anxiety disorders. Gelder,[9] very recently, reviewed the classification of anxiety disorders and pointed out that there is no strong reason to separate patients with panic attacks into a distinct nosological group of 'panic disorder' and there is even less justification for dividing agoraphobia into two groups, one with and one without panic attacks. However, Okasa et al.[10] have carried out a study with the purpose to find evidence from descriptive, psychodemographic, clinical, psycho-metric and biological investigations that supports the validation of panic disorder and GAD as independent identities. He concluded that panic disorder exists as an independent diagnostic category.[10-12]

In DSM-5,[13] OCD, PTSD and acute stress disorder and adjustment disorder are separated from anxiety disorder. OCD is kept under Obsessive-Compulsive and Related Disorders and rest are kept under Trauma- and Stressor-Related Disorders.

ANXIETY: NORMAL OR PATHOLOGICAL

Anxiety is commonly experienced by virtually all humans. Anxiety is an alerting signal; it warns of threat, external or internal, and it is probably life saving, more than once in a life time.[11] Anxiety initiates person to take necessary steps to prevent the threat, or at least lessen its consequences, e.g. getting down to hard word to prepare for examination. Since it is beneficial for a person to respond with anxiety in certain threatening situations, one can speak of normal anxiety in contrast to abnormal or pathological anxiety.

Pathological anxiety, on the other hand, is an inappropriate response to a given stimulus, by virtue of either its intensity or duration. The complete absence of anxiety is just as pathological as excessive anxiety. Anxiety has an inverted 'U-shaped relationship' with performance, as demonstrated by well known *Yerkes-Dodson law*. In Yerkes-Dodson law, it is seen that at very low level of anxiety, the performance is poor. Each increment of anxiety produces equivalent increment in performance. This can be regarded as normal or healthy anxiety. Then, there is a phase where performance has reached its maximum and any increase in anxiety does not improve the performance any further. At this stage, the subject may in fact begin having the symptoms of anxiety, although symptoms produced at this stage do not affect performance. The anxiety, at this point, acts as a secondary reinforcer, often leading to behaviors that reduce the anxiety level. Later on, any minor increase in anxiety causes deterioration in performance, which may in turn produce more anxiety. However, there are a number of other factors which influence the anxiety response to a given stimulus, indicating individual vulnerability in such responses.

ETIOLOGY

Psychological Theories

Psychoanalytic Theories

Freud, in his book 'Inhibitions, Symptoms and Anxiety' (1926), proposed that anxiety is a signal to the ego to take defensive action against the 'pressure' from within. If anxiety rises above the low level of intensity characteristic of its function as a signal, it may emerge with all the fury of a panic attack. Ideally, the use of *repression* alone results in a restoration of psychological equilibrium without symptom formation, because effective repression completely contains the drives and their associated affects and fantasies, rendering them unconscious. If repression is unsuccessful as a defense, other defense mechanisms (such as conversion, displacement and regression) may result in symptom formation, thus producing picture of classic neurotic disorders such as hysteria, phobia and OCD.

Within psycho analytic theory, anxiety is seen as falling into four major categories. *Id or impulse anxiety* is related to the primitive, diffuse discomforts of infants when they feel overwhelmed with needs and stimuli over which their helpless state provides no control. *Separation anxiety* occurs in somewhat older but still preoedipal children, who fear the loss of love or even abandonment by their parents, if they fail to control and direct their impulses in conformity with their parents' standards and demands. *Castration anxiety* of adult reflects the castration fantasies of oedipal child, in relation to child's developing sexual impulses. *Superego anxiety* is the direct result of the final development of superego that marks the passing of the oedipus complex and the prepubertal period of latency.

The various personality theories differ regarding establishing the sources and the nature of anxiety. Otto Rank, e.g. traced the genesis of all anxiety back to the '*trauma of birth*'. Harry Stack Sullivan emphasized the early relationship between the mother and child, and the transmission of mother's anxiety to her infant. Regardless of the school of psychoanalysis, however, the treatment of anxiety disorders by psychoanalytical methods usually involves long-term, insight-oriented psychotherapy or psychoanalysis directed toward the formation of a transference, which allows the re-working of the development problem and the resolution of the neurotic symptoms.

Behavioral Theories

Behavioral theories propose that anxiety is a conditioned response to specific environmental stimuli. In a model example of classic conditioning, a person who does not have any food allergies may become sick after eating contaminated seafood in a restaurant. Subsequent exposures to seafood may cause that person to feel sick. Through generalization, such a person may come to distrust all food prepared by others. As an alternative causal possibility, the person may learn to have an internal response of anxiety, imitating the anxiety responses of his parents (*social learning theory*). In either case, treatment is usually with some form of desensitization by repeated exposure to the anxiogenic stimulus, coupled with cognitive psychotherapeutic approaches.

Recently, the proponents of behavioral theories have shown increasing interest in cognitive approaches to conceptualizing and treating anxiety disorders. The cognitive concept of non-phobic anxiety states that faulty, distorted or counterproductive thinking patterns accompany or precede maladaptive behaviors and emotional disorders. According to one model, patients suffering from anxiety disorders tend to overestimate the degree of danger and the probability of harm in a given situation, and tend to underestimate their abilities to cope with perceived threats to their physical or psychological well-being. The patients with panic disorder, according to this model, often have thoughts of loss of control and fears of dying, that follow inexplicable physiological sensations (such as palpitations, tachycardia and light-headedness).

Existential Theories

There is no specific identifiable stimulus for a chronic anxious feeling. The central concept of existential theories is the persons' awareness of a profound nothingness in their lives, which may be more profoundly discomforting than an acceptance of their inevitable death. Anxiety is the person's response to that void of existence and meaning.

Biological Theories

Preclinical studies with animal models of anxiety, growing knowledge regarding basic neuroscience, and the actions of psychotherapeutic drugs have led to the development of biological theories of anxiety disorders. There are two poles of thought; one posits that biological changes reflect psychological conflicts, and other posits that biological changes precede psychological conflicts. Both situations may exist in a specific person, and a range of biologically based sensitivities may exist among person with the symptoms of anxiety disorders.

ANS

Stimulation of the autonomic nervous system causes cardiovascular, respiratory and gastrointestinal symptoms. These peripheral manifestations of anxiety are neither peculiar to anxiety disorders nor necessarily correlated with the subjective experience of anxiety. In early 20th century, Cannon demonstrated that cats exposed to barking dogs exhibited behavioral and physiological signs of fear that are associated with adrenal release of norepinephrine.

The James Lange theory states that subjective anxiety is a response to peripheral phenomena. It is now generally thought that central nervous system anxiety precedes the peripheral manifestations of anxiety, except when a specific peripheral cause is present, e.g. pheochromocytoma. Some anxiety disorder patients, especially those with panic disorder, have autonomic nervous systems that exhibit increase sympathetic tone, adapt slowly to repeated stimuli, and respond excessively to moderate stimuli.

Neurotransmitters

Based on animal studies and responses to drug treatments, these neurotransmitters have been implicated in the genesis of anxiety disorders.

Norepinephrine

Anxiety disorder patients have a poorly regulated noradrenergic system, that has occasional bursts of locus ceruleus. Cell bodies of the NE system are localized to the locus ceruleus, from where axons project to cerebral cortex, limbic system, brain stem, and spinal cord. Experiments in primates have demonstrated that stimulation of the locus ceruleus produces a fear response in animals and that ablation of the same area inhibits or completely blocks the ability of the animals to form a fear response.

Human studies have found that, in patients with panic disorder, α-adrenergic agonists (e.g. isoproterenol) and α2-adrenergic antagonists (e.g. yohimbine) can produce frequent and severe panic attacks. Conversely clonidine, an adrenergic agonist, reduces anxiety symptoms in some experimental and therapeutic situations. A less consistent finding is that patients with anxiety disorders, particularly panic disorder, have elevated cerebrospinal fluid or urinary levels of the noradrenergic metabolite, 3-methoxy-4-hydroxyphenyl-glycol (MHPG).

Serotonin

Observations regarding the role of serotonin are contradictory. On the one hand, chlorimipramine (serotonergic antidepressant) and buspirone ($5HT_{1A}$ receptor agonist) are beneficial in the treatment of anxiety disorders. On the other hand, m-chlorophenylpiperazine (MCPP) and fenfluramine (which cause release of serotonin), serotonergic hallucinogens and stimulants (e.g. lysergic acid diethylamide or LSD), and 3, 4-methylenedioxymethamphetamine (MDMA) are associated with development of both acute and chronic anxiety disorders.

The cell bodies of most of the serotonergic neurons are located in the raphe nuclei in the rostral brain stem and project to the cerebral cortex, limbic system (especially hippocampus and amygdala) and hypothalamus.

GABA (Gamma amino butyric acid)

There is inconclusive evidence regarding the role of GABA in anxiety disorders. The effectiveness of benzodiazepines, which enhance the activity of GABA at the GABA-A receptor, in the treatment of some anxiety disorders, and occurrence of panic attacks in panic disorder patients by flumazenil (a benzodiazepine antagonist) are suggestive of the role of GABA in the genesis of anxiety disorder, at least in some patients.

Aplysia

A neurotransmitter model for anxiety disorder is based on the study of *aplysia californica*, a sea snail that reacts to danger by moving away, withdrawing into its shell, and decreasing its feeding behavior. Those behaviors can be classically conditioned, so that the snail responds to a neutral stimulus as if it were a dangerous stimulus. The snail can also be sensitized by random shocks, so that it exhibits a flight response in absence of real danger. Parallels have previously been drawn between classical conditioning and human phobic anxiety. The classically conditioned aplysia shows measurable changes in presynaptic facilitation, resulting in the release of increased amounts of neurotransmitter. Although the sea snail is a simple animal, the experiment shows a novel approach to the complex neurochemical processes potentially involved in anxiety disorders in humans.

Brain Imaging Studies

Some patients with anxiety disorders have demonstrable cerebral pathology which may be causally relevant to their anxiety symptoms. This has been interpreted from the findings of enlarged cerebral ventricles and specific defects in the right temporal lobe (not the left hemisphere) in structural brain studies by computed tomography (CT) and magnetic resonance imaging (MRI). One study has correlated even the increase in size of ventricle to the length of time the patients had been taking benzodiazepines.

Similarly, functional brain imaging studies, e.g. positron emission tomography (PET), single photon emission tomography (SPECT), and electroencephalography (EEG) of anxiety disorder patients have variously reported abnormalities in frontal cortex, occipital and temporal areas, and parahippocampal gyrus.

Genetic Studies

Genetic studies have produced solid data that at least some genetic component contributes to the development of anxiety disorders. Almost half of all patients with panic disorders (although not too high) also indicate a higher frequency of the illness in first degree relatives of affected patients than in the relatives of non-affected persons. Although adoption studies with anxiety disorders have not been reported, data from twin registers also support the hypothesis that anxiety disorders are at least partially genetically determined.

Neuroanatomical Considerations

The focus of neuroanatomical consideration lies on the limbic system and cerebral cortex. Limbic system contains a high concentration of GABA receptors along, with receiving noradrenergic and serotonergic innervation. Ablation and stimulation studies in non-human primates have also implicated limbic system in the generation of anxiety and fear responses. Two areas of limbic system have received special attention; Cingulate gyrus has been implicated in the pathophysiology of OCD, and increased activity of the septo-hippocampal pathway has been shown to lead to anxiety.

The frontal cerebral cortex is connected with parahippocampal region, cingulate gyrus and hypothalamus. There, it may be related to the production of anxiety disorders. The temporal cortex has also been implicated as a pathophysiological site in anxiety disorder. That association is based in part on the similarity in clinical presentation and electrophysiology between some patients with temporal lobe epilepsy and patients with OCD.

CLASSIFICATION

According to DSM-IV,[12] anxiety disorders are classified as follows:

- Panic disorder without agoraphobia.
- Panic disorder with agoraphobia.
- Agoraphobia without history of panic disorder.
- Specific phobia.
- Social phobia.
- Obsessive compulsive disorder.
- Post-traumatic stress disorder.
- Acute stress disorder.
- Generalized anxiety disorder.
- Anxiety disorder due to a general medical condition; Substance induced anxiety disorder.
- Anxiety disorder NOS.

In the ICD-108, anxiety disorders have been included under the broad group of 'neurotic, stress-related and somatoform disorders'. These have further subdivided as follows:

- *Phobic anxiety disorders*
  - Agoraphobia
    - Without panic disorder
    - With panic disorders
  - Social phobias
  - Specific (isolated) phobias
  - Other phobic anxiety disorders
  - Phobic anxiety disorder, unspecified.
- *Other anxiety disorders*
  - Panic disorder (episodic paroxysmal anxiety)
  - Generalized anxiety disorder
  - Mixed anxiety and depressive disorders
  - Other mixed anxiety disorders
  - Other specified anxiety disorders
  - Anxiety disorder, unspecified.

DSM-5[13] Classification	
According to DSM-IV,[12] anxiety disorders are classified as follows:	
1.	Separation anxiety disorder
2.	Selective mutism
3.	Specific phobia
4.	Social anxiety disorder (social phobia)
5.	Panic disorder
6.	Agoraphobia
7.	Generalized anxiety disorder
8.	Substance/medication-induced anxiety disorder
9.	Anxiety disorder due to another medical condition
10.	Other specified anxiety disorder
11.	Unspecified anxiety disorder
Note: In DSM-5,[13] OCD, PTSD and acute stress disorder and adjustment disorder are separated from anxiety disorder. OCD is kept under Obsessive-Compulsive and Related Disorders and rest are kept under Trauma- and Stressor-related Disorders.	

10.2 PANIC DISORDERS

Panic disorder is characterized by the spontaneous, unexpected occurrence of panic attacks. Panic attacks are relatively short lived (usually <1 hour) periods of anxiety or fear, which are accompanied by somatic symptoms like palpitations and tachypnea.

EPIDEMIOLOGY

Epidemiological studies show lifetime prevalence of 1.5–2%, and up to 35% of the population experiences at least one panic attack during their lifetime.[14] Women are two to three times more likely to be affected than are males. There is bimodal age distribution; the early one in the age group of 15–24 years for both males and females, and the later mode occurs in the age group of 45–54 years. The persons with low educational achievement suffer more with panic attacks. Though panic disorder has been reported to occur in children and adolescents, it is probably underdiagnosed in them.

ETIOLOGY

Biological Factors

A range of findings have emerged from the research regarding the biological basis of panic disorder. One interpretation is that the symptoms of panic disorder can result in a range of biological abnormalities in brain structure and brain function. The greatest amount of work has been done in area of using biological stimulants to induce panic attacks in patients with panic disorder. The various means by which panic attacks can be provoked in experimental situations are listed below in Table 1.

These and other studies have resulted in hypotheses implicating both peripheral and central nervous system

Table 1: Provocation of panic attacks	
Some challenge paradigms (possible mechanisms)	
1.	Lactate (pH and pCO_2 changes)
2.	Bicarbonate (pH and pCO_2 changes)
3.	Hypercapnia with 5% or 35% CO_2 (pCO_2 changes)
4.	Hyperventilation (pCO_2 changes)
5.	Caffeine (Adenosine, benzodiazepine receptors)
6.	Noradrenergic agents like isoprenaline and noradrenaline (NE)
7.	Yohimbine (NE, 5-HT)
8.	Tricyclic antidepressants (NE, 5-HT)
9.	Clomipramine (5-HT)
10.	mCPP (5-HT receptor stimulation)
11.	Benzodiazepine receptor agents like FG 7142 (inverse agonist) and flumazenil (antagonist) (Benzodiazepine/GABA receptor)
12.	Cholecystokinin (CNS/peripheral action)
13.	Hypoglycemia (Peripheral autonomic activation)
14.	Cognitive (Catastrophic misinterpretation)

dysregulation in the pathophysiology of panic disorder. The automatic nervous systems of some panic disorder patients have been reported to exhibit increased sympathetic tone, to adapt slowly to repeated stimuli, and to respond excessively to moderate stimuli. Studies of neural endocrine status disorder patients have reported several abnormalities, although the studies have been inconsistent in their findings.

The major neurotransmitter systems, that have been implicated, are those for norepinephrine, serotonin, and gamma-amino-butyric acid (GABA). Evidence for a noradrenergic contribution to panic disorder comes from a number of sources, including challenge tests with selective drugs such as yohimbine, clonidine, noradrenaline and isoprenaline. Yohimbine is an $\alpha 2$ receptor antagonist, which can cause anxiety in normal subjects. It activates noradrenergic neurons in the central nervous system (CNS) and increases the firing rate of locus ceruleus. Directly enhancing noradrenergic function by infusing adrenaline, noradrenaline or the selective α-agonists (isoprenaline) has been claimed to provoke panic attacks. Clonidine acts at central $\alpha 2$-adrenoceptor to decrease all firing of the locus ceruleus, reduce sympathetic outflow, and decrease anxiety. Clonidine has been used to treat panic disorder with some success. Studies have demonstrated a subsensitivity of post-synaptic brain $\alpha 2$ adrenoceptors and failure of mechanisms, controlling activity of locus ceruleus. Such a failure of control leads to excessive swings in activity, which leads to paroxysmal central and peripheral activation, and thus panic attacks. Evidence of the role of serotonergic neurotransmitter system comes from the anxiogenic effect of single dose of m-CPP (a 5-HT agonist) in patients with panic disorder.

The biological data has led to a focus on the brain stem (locus ceruleus and median raphe nucleus), the limbic system (possibly responsible for the generation of anticipatory anxiety) and the prefrontal cortex (possibly responsible for the generation of phobic avoidance). Structural brain imaging studies (e.g. MRI) in panic disorder patients have implicated pathology in the temporal lobes, particularly the hippocampus. For example, one MRI study reported abnormalities, particularly cortical atrophy, in the right temporal lobe of panic disorder patients. Functional brain imaging studies (e.g. PET) have implicated a dysregulation of cerebral blood flow. Specifically, anxiety disorders and panic attacks are associated with cerebral vasoconstriction, which may result in CNS symptoms, such as dizziness, and in PNS symptoms that may be induced by hyperventilation and hypocapnia. Most functional brain imaging studies have used a specific panic inducing substance (e.g. lactate, caffeine or yohimbine), in combination with PET or single photon emission tomography (SPECT), to assess the effects of the panic inducing substance and the induced panic attack in cerebral blood flow.

Recent research has almost completely removed any clinical significance or relevance to the association between mitral valve prolapse and a panic disorder. Mitral valve prolapse is a heterogenous syndrome, consisting of the prolapse of one of the mitral valve leaflets, resulting in a mid-systolic click on cardiac auscultation. Research studies have found that the prevalence of panic disorder in patients with mitral valve prolapse is no different from the prevalence of panic disorder in patients without mitral valve prolapse.

Genetic Factors

Although the number of well-controlled studies of the genetic basis of panic disorder and agoraphobia is small, the data suggests that the disorders have a distinct genetic component. In addition, some data indicates that panic disorder with agoraphobia is a severe form of panic disorder without agoraphobia and is, thus more likely to be inherited. Various studies have found a four-fold to eight-fold increase in the rise for panic disorder among first degree relations of panic disorder patients as compared with first degree relatives of other psychiatric patients. The studies have generally reported that monozygotic twins are more likely to be concordant for panic disorders than are dizygotic twins.

Psychosocial Factors

Both cognitive-behavioral and psychoanalytic theories have been used to explain the pathogenesis of panic disorder and agoraphobia. The success of cognitive behavioral approaches to the treatment of these disorders may add credence to the cognitive behavioral theories.

Cognitive Behavioral Theories

Behavioral theories posit that anxiety is a learned response, either from modeling parental behavior or through the process of classical conditioning. In a classic conditioning approach to panic disorder and agoraphobia, a noxious stimulus (e.g. a panic attack) that occurs with a neutral stimulus (e.g. a bus ride) can result in the avoidance of the neutral stimulus. Other behavioral theories posit a linkage between the sensation of minor somatic symptoms (e.g. palpitations) and the generation of a complete panic attack. Although cognitive behavioral theories can help explain the development of agoraphobia or an increase in the number of severity of panic attacks, they do not explain the occurrence of the first unprovoked and unexpected panic attack that an affected patient can experience.

Psychoanalytic Theories

Psychoanalytic theories conceptualize panic attacks as resulting from an unsuccessful defense against anxiety provoking impulses. What was previously a mild signal anxiety, becomes an overwhelming feeling of apprehension, complete with somatic symptoms.

Many patients describe panic attacks as coming out of the blue as though no psychological factors was involved, but the psychodynamic exploration frequently reveals a clear psychological trigger for the panic attack. Although panic attacks are correlated neurophysiologically with the locus ceruleus, the onset of panic is related to environmental or psychological factors. Patients with panic disorder have a higher incidence of stressful life events, particularly loss, as compared with controls in the months before the onset of panic disorder. Moreover, the patients typically experience greater distress about life events than do controls.

The hypothesis, that stressful psychological events produce neurophysiological changes in panic disorder, finds support from a study of female twins. The research findings revealed that panic disorder was strongly associated with parental separation as well as parental death before the age of 17 years. Separation from the mother early in life was clearly more likely to result in panic disorder than was paternal separation in the cohort of 1018 pairs of female twins. Further support for psychological mechanism in panic disorder can be inferred from a study of panic disorder patients, who were successfully treated with cognitive therapy. Before the therapy, the patients responded to lactate infusion with a panic attack. After successful cognitive therapy, lactate infusion no longer resulted in a panic attack.

The research indicates that the cause of panic attacks is likely to involve the unconscious meaning of stressful events and that the pathogenesis of the panic attacks may be related to neurophysiological factors triggered by psychological reactions. Psychodynamic clinicians should always do a thorough investigation of the possible trigger mechanisms, whenever a diagnostic assessment is being performed on a patient with panic disorder.[15]

CLINICAL FEATURES

The first panic attack is often completely spontaneous, although panic attacks occasionally follow excitement, physical exertion, sexual activity, or moderate emotional trauma. The attack often begins with a 10-minute period of rapidly increasing symptoms. The major mental symptoms are external fear and a sense of impending death and doom. Patients are usually not able to name the source of their fear. The patients may feel confused and have problem in concentrating. The physical signs often include tachycardia, palpitations, dyspnea and sweating. Patients often try to leave whatever situation they are in, to seek help. The attack generally lasts 20–30 minutes and rarely more than 1 hour.

A formal mental status examination during a panic attack may reveal ruminations, difficulty in speaking and an impaired memory. Patients may experience depression or depersonalization during an attack. The symptoms may disappear quickly or gradually. Between the episodes, patients may have anticipatory anxiety about having another attack. Somatic concerns of death from a cardiac or respiratory problem may be the major focus of patients' attention during panic attack. Patients may believe that the symptoms of palpitations and pain in the chest indicate that they are about to die. As many as 20% of such patients actually have syncopal episodes during a panic attack.

The patients may present to emergency rooms as young (in 20s), physically healthy persons, who nevertheless insist that they are about to die from a heart attack. Rather than immediately diagnosing hypochondriasis, the physician should consider a diagnosis of panic disorder. The hyperventilation and CO_2 inhalation may induce the panic attacks. Panic patients are more sensitive into the anxiogenic effect of CO_2 than controls, and CO_2 is a more potent anxiogenic stimulus than room-air hyperventilation.[16]

Associated Symptoms

Sometimes, depressive symptoms are present in panic disorder and a large proportion of individuals with panic disorder report suicidal ideation.[17] Thirty-one percent of patients with panic disorder report suicide ideation in the past year, while 18% patients report suicidal attempts at other times in their lives. Individuals with panic disorder have a significantly higher rate of associated gastrointestinal symptoms, including those typically associated with irritable bowel syndrome, such as abdominal pain, diarrhea or constipation, and abdominal bloating, as compared to the patients with other or no psychiatric disorder.

Agoraphobia

Agoraphobic patients rigidly avoid situations in which it would be difficult to obtain help. They prefer to be accompanied by a friend or a family member in such places as busy streets, crowded stores, closed-in places (such as tunnels, bridges and elevators), and closed-in vehicles (such as subways, buses and aeroplanes). The patients may insist that they be accompanied every time they leave the house. The behavior may result in marital discord, which may be misdiagnosed as a primary problem. Severely affected patients may simply refuse to leave the house. Particularly before a correct diagnosis is made, the patients may be terrified that they are going crazy.

DIAGNOSTIC CRITERIA

DSM-IV does not specify a minimum number of panic attacks or a time frame but does require that at least one attack be followed by at least a month long period of concern about having another panic attack or about the implications of attack or a significant change in behavior, while previous diagnostic criteria like RDC, ICD and DSM-III-R have used the minimum of panic attack to be 6. 3 and 4 attacks respectively, within a specified time period of 6 weeks, 3 weeks and 4 weeks.

Here, the criteria given by DSM IV[18] are described. Panic disorder is characterized by a discrete period of intense fear or discomfort, in which four (or more) of the following symptoms develop abruptly and reached a peak within 10 minutes. These symptoms include palpitations, pounding heart, or accelerated heart rate; sweating, trembling or shaking; sensations of shortness of breath or smothering; feeling of choking; chest pain or discomfort; nausea or abdominal distress; feeling dizzy, unsteady, light-headed or faint; derealization, or depersonalization; fear of losing control of going crazy; fear of dying; paresthesias; and chills or hot flushes.[18]

In DSM-IV[18], agoraphobia is characterized by anxiety about being in places or situations from which escape might be difficult or in which help may not be available in the event of having an unexpected or situationally predisposed panic attack or panic like symptoms. Agoraphobic fears typically involve characteristic cluster of situations that include being outside the home alone, being in a crowd or standing in a line, being on bridge and travelling in bus, train or automobile.[18] The situations are avoided (e.g. travel is restricted) or else are endured with marked distress or with anxiety about having a panic attack or panic like symptoms, or require the presence of a companion.

DSM-IV[18] specifies that both for panic disorder and agoraphobia, the anxiety or phobic avoidance should not be not better accounted for by another mental disorder such as social phobia, specific phobia, OCD, post-traumatic stress disorder, or separating anxiety disorder.

DSM-5 Diagnostic criteria for agoraphobia 300.22 (F40.00)
A. Marked fear or anxiety about two (or more) of the following five situations: 1. Using public transportation (e.g. automobiles, buses, trains, ships and planes). 2. Being in open spaces (e.g. parking lots, marketplaces and bridges). 3. Being in enclosed places (e.g. shops, theaters and cinemas). 4. Standing in line or being in a crowd. 5. Being outside of the home alone.
B. The individual fears or avoids these situations because of thoughts that escape might be difficult or help might not be available in the event of developing panic-like symptoms or other incapacitating or embarrassing symptoms (e.g. fear of falling in the elderly; fear of incontinence).
C. The agoraphobic situations almost always provoke fear or anxiety.
D. The agoraphobic situations are actively avoided, require the presence of a companion, or are endured with intense fear or anxiety
E. The fear or anxiety is out of proportion to the actual danger posed by the agoraphobic situations and to the sociocultural context.

Contd...

Contd...

F. The fear, anxiety, or avoidance is persistent, typically lasting for 6 months or more.
G. The fear, anxiety, or avoidance causes clinically significant distress or impairment in social, occupational, or other important areas of functioning.
H. If another medical condition (e.g. inflammatory bowel disease, Parkinson's disease) is present, the fear, anxiety, or avoidance is clearly excessive.
I. The fear, anxiety, or avoidance is not better explained by the symptoms of another mental disorder, e.g. the symptoms are not confined to specific phobia, situational type; do not involve only social situations (as in social anxiety disorder); and are not related exclusively to obsessions (as in OCD), perceived defects or flaws in physical appearance (as in body dysmorphic disorder), reminders of traumatic events (as in post-traumatic stress disorder), or fear of separation (as in separation anxiety disorder).
Note: Agoraphobia is diagnosed irrespective of the presence of panic disorder. If an individual's presentation meets criteria for panic disorder and agoraphobia, both diagnoses should be assigned.

DSM-5 Criteria for panic disorder 300.01 (F41.0)
A. Recurrent unexpected panic attacks. A panic attack is an abrupt surge of intense fear or intense discomfort that reaches a peak within minutes, and during which time four (or more) of the following symptoms occur:
Note: The abrupt surge can occur from a calm state or an anxious state. 1. Palpitations, pounding heart, or accelerated heart rate. 2. Sweating. 3. Trembling or shaking. 4. Sensations of shortness of breath or smothering. 5. Feelings of choking. 6. Chest pain or discomfort. 7. Nausea or abdominal distress. 8. Feeling dizzy, unsteady, light-headed, or faint. 9. Chills or heat sensations. 10. Paresthesias (numbness or tingling sensations). 11. Derealization (feelings of unreality) or depersonalization (being detached from oneself). 12. Fear of losing control or "going crazy." 13. Fear of dying.
Note: Culture-specific symptoms (e.g. tinnitus, neck soreness, headache, uncontrollable screaming or crying) may be seen. Such symptoms should not count as one of the four required symptoms.
B. At least one of the attacks has been followed by 1 month (or more) of one or both of the following: 1. Persistent concern or worry about additional panic attacks or their consequences (e.g. losing control, having a heart attack, "going crazy"). 2. A significant maladaptive change in behavior related to the attacks (e.g. behaviors designed to avoid having panic attacks, such as avoidance of exercise or unfamiliar situations).

Contd...

Contd...

C. The disturbance is not attributable to the physiological effects of a substance (e.g. a drug of abuse, a medication) or another medical condition (e.g. hyperthyroidism, cardiopulmonary disorders).
D. The disturbance is not better explained by another mental disorder (e.g. the panic attacks do not occur only in response to feared social situations, as in social anxiety disorder; in response to circumscribed phobic objects or situations, as in specific phobia; in response to obsessions, as in OCD; in response to reminders of traumatic events, as in post-traumatic stress disorder; or in response to separation from attachment figures, as in separation anxiety disorder).

DSM-5 Criteria for panic attack specifier
Note: Symptoms are presented for the purpose of identifying a panic attack; however, panic attack is not a mental disorder and cannot be coded. Panic attacks can occur in the context of any anxiety disorder as well as other mental disorders (e.g. depressive disorders, post-traumatic stress disorder, substance use disorders) and some medical conditions (e.g. cardiac, respiratory, vestibular, gastrointestinal). When the presence of a panic attack is identified, it should be noted as a specifier (e.g. "post-traumatic stress disorder with panic attacks"). For panic disorder, the presence of panic attack is contained within the riteria for the disorder and panic attack is not used as a specifier.
An abrupt surge of intense fear or intense discomfort that reaches a peak within minutes, and during which time four (or more) of the following symptoms occur:
Note: The abrupt surge can occur from a calm state or an anxious state.
1. Palpitations, pounding heart, or accelerated heart rate. 2. Sweating. 3. Trembling or shaking. 4. Sensations of shortness of breath or smothering. 5. Feelings of choking. 6. Chest pain or discomfort. 7. Nausea or abdominal distress. 8. Feeling dizzy, unsteady, light-headed, or faint. 9. Chills or heat sensations. 10. Paresthesias (numbness or tingling sensations). 11. Derealization (feelings of unreality) or depersonalization (being detached from oneself). 12. Fear of losing control or "going crazy." 13. Fear of dying.
Note: Culture-specific symptoms (e.g. tinnitus, neck soreness, headache, uncontrollable screaming or crying) may be seen. Such symptoms should not count as one of the four required symptoms.

DIFFERENTIAL DIAGNOSIS

The differential diagnosis includes both psychiatric and medical disorders.

The psychiatric differential diagnoses include malingering, somatoform disorder, post-traumatic stress disorder, hypochondriasis, depressive disorders, depersonalization disorder and schizophrenia.

Unexpected panic attacks are the hallmark of panic disorder. Differential diagnosis from social phobia and specific phobia depends on the fear of getting a panic attack in panic disorder, while in phobias there is fear of specific situation or social speaking.

The medical differential diagnoses include disorders mentioned in Table 2.

COURSE AND PROGNOSIS

Panic disorder usually has its onset during the late adolescence or early childhood. It is generally a chronic disorder, with 30–40% of patients seeming to be symptom free at long term follow-up, about 50% having symptoms that are mild enough not to affect their lives significantly, and about 10–20% continuing to have significant symptoms.

About 40–80% of patients develop depression, with an associated risk of suicide. Alcohol and other substance dependence occur in about 20–40% of all patients and OCD may also develop. Patients with good premorbid functioning and a brief duration of symptoms tend to have good prognosis.

MANAGEMENT

The two most effective treatments of panic disorder are pharmacotherapy and cognitive behavior therapy.

Pharmacotherapy

Tricyclic and Tetracyclic Drugs

Among tricyclic drugs, imipramine and clomipramine are effective in the treatment of panic disorder, but a problem in clinical experience is that patients report an initial increase in tension and arousal.[19,20] Clark et al.[21] observed that this could be avoided by using a small initial dose, followed by gradual increments as also suggested by Fyer and Sandberg.[19] Clomipramine and imipramine are initiated at low dosages (10 mg/day) and titrated slowly upwards at first by 10 mg at definite intervals of every 2–3 days. If the low dosages are well tolerated, then increments can be made more rapidly, in 25 mg/day at intervals of every 2–3 days. Panic disorder patients need full dosages of clomipramine or imipramine, and generally require a long-time to respond, usually 8–12 weeks, rather than 6 to 8 weeks as for depression.

Other tricyclic drugs are also effective. Nortriptyline may be used because this drug is associated with fewer adverse effects.

Table 2: Medical differential diagnosis of panic disorder

I.	*Cardiovascular disorders*: Angina, hypertension, hyperactive α-adrenergic state, mitral valve prolapse, myocardial infarction, paradoxical atrial tachycardia
II.	*Neurological disorders*: Cerebrovascular diseases, epilepsy, Huntington's disease, infections, Meniere's disease, migraine, multiple sclerosis, transient ischemic attack, tumors, Wilson's disease, temporal arteritis
III.	*Endocrine disorders*: Addison's disease, carcinoid syndrome, Cushing's syndrome, diabetes, hyperthyroidism, hypoglycemia, hypoparathyroidism, menopausal disorders, pheochromocytoma, premenstrual syndrome.
IV.	*Drug intoxication*: Amphetamines, amyl nitrite, anti-cholinergics, cocaine, hallucinogens, marijuana, nicotine, theophylline
V.	*Drug withdrawal*: Alcohol, antihypertensives, opioids, sedative-hypnotics
VI.	*Other conditions*: Pulmonary conditions (like asthma, hyperventilation, and pulmonary embolus), anemia, CRF, anaphylaxis, B_{12} deficiency, electrolyte disturbance, heavy metal poisoning, systemic infections, systemic lupus erythematosus, temporal arteritis, uremia.

MAO Inhibitors

Phenelzine and tranylcypromine are effective in anti-depressant dosages, when given for 8–12 weeks. They have the additional benefit of not causing over-stimulation as an initial side effect, as seen with tricyclics.

All selective serotonin reuptake inhibitors (SSRIs) are shown to be effective, such as fluoxetine, paroxetine, sertraline, fluvoxamine and clomipramine, but over-stimulation in initial stages of treatment can be a problem, so dosages must be titrated slowly.

Benzodiazepines

Benzodiazepines are quickly effective (onset of action in 1–2 hours), but dependence, cognitive impairment and abuse are a few of the problems associated with their use. The most commonly effective dosages are 4–6 mg of alprazolam. Alprazolam blocks the CO_2-provoked panic in patients of panic disorders.[22] The problem of dependence may be countered by slow tapering of alprazolam. Though there is dependence, however, tolerance does not develop to the anti-panic effects of alprazolam.

Clonazepam and lorazepam have been also shown to be effective.

Duration of Pharmacotherapy

Once effective, pharmacotherapy should generally be continued for 8–12 months. Thirty to ninety percent of the successfully treated panic disorder patients relapse, when their medication is discontinued.

Cognitive and Behavioral Therapies

Cognitive procedures help patients identify and change misinterpretations of bodily sensations and substitute them with more realistic interpretations (e.g. explaining to patients that panic attacks are time limited and not life-threatening). Behavioral procedures include inducing feared situations (by hyperventilation), focusing attention on the body, or reading words representing the feared situations, in order to demonstrate passible causes of patient's symptoms, and stopping safety behaviors (such as holding onto solid objects when feeling dizzy), in order to help patients disconfirm their negative predictions about consequences of their symptoms.[23,24]

Applied relaxation techniques, like that of Herbert Benson's relaxation training and the one devised by Ost[25] are commonly used. In Ost's procedure, the patients are taught to identify the early signs of panic and relax rapidly. As panic attacks can occur in any situation, the training consists of a series of stages, in which patients are taught to relax more and more quickly while performing the everyday activities, such as walking and shopping. Homework assignments include twice-daily relaxation practice.

One direct approach to control panic attacks is to train patients how to control the urge to hyperventilate by respiratory training, since hyperventilation associated with panic attacks is probably related to some symptoms, such as dizziness, faintness.

Psychosocial therapies, such as family therapy and insight oriented psychotherapy, can also be of benefit in the treatment of panic disorder.

Choice of Therapy

Combined cognitive behavior therapy and pharmacotherapy are more effective then either therapy alone. However, cognitive therapy is superior to both applied relaxation and imipramine.[23]

Cognitive therapy, administered in parallel with alprazolam maintenance and taper, is effective in preventive relapse after drug discontinuation.[26,27]

In a comprehensive treatment program, initial pharmacotherapy should use alprazolam for its quick onset, with slow titration of tricyclic or other anti-depressants, and then tapering of alprazolam, with application of cognitive behavior therapy to prevent relapse.

10.3 GENERALIZED ANXIETY DISORDERS

Generalized anxiety disorder (GAD), one of the anxiety states described in DSM-III, was a relatively new diagnostic entity in DSM-III.[28] It was conceptualized as a residual diagnostic category for those patients who did not meet the criteria for other diagnosis, but were characterized by apprehensive expectation or chronic worry focused on multiple life situations.

DSM-III-R[29] revised the diagnostic criteria for GAD, which had its own key features like excessive and/or unrealistic worry with associated symptoms criteria requiring at least six of 18 symptoms from three clusters, namely motor tension, autonomic hyperactivity, and vigilance and scanning. GAD is defined in DSM-IV[30] as excessive and pervasive worry, accompanied by a variety of somatic symptoms that causes significant impairment in social or occupational functioning or marked distress in the patient. DSM-IV eliminates the DSM-III-R category of 'overanxious disorder of childhood,' to include them in the diagnostic criteria for GAD.

EPIDEMIOLOGY

Generalized anxiety disorder is a common condition. However, with the restrictive criteria of DSM-III-R and DSM-IV, generalized disorder may be found less often now than when DSM-III criteria were used. Reasonable estimates for 1 year prevalence of anxiety disorder range from 3% to 8%. GAD, along with phobic disorders, account for the most anxiety in late life.[31] Six-month prevalence of GAD in persons over 65 years of age is about 2%, with the highest rate in black females in US.[32]

Studies reveal high rates of psychiatric comorbidity in GAD.[33] Nearly 42% of patients experience at least one major depressive episode during their life time.

ETIOLOGY

Both biological and psychosocial factors have been implicated, probably both working together.

Biological Factors

Neurotransmitter Systems

Gamma aminobutyric acid (GABA) and serotonin neuro-transmitters systems are the focus of current biological research efforts. Benzodiazepines' anti-anxiety effect (benzodiazepine receptor agonist) and flumazenil (a benzodiazepine receptor antagonist) and b carbolines' (benzodiazepine receptor reverse agonist) anxiety-inducing. effect favors the role of GABA in etiology of anxiety. Efficacy of buspirone ($5HT_{1A}$ receptor agonist) as an anti-anxiety agent gives rise to the hypothesis that the regulation of the serotonergic system in GAD is abnormal.

Norepinephrine, glutamate, and cholecystokinin are the other neurotransmitter systems that are at the focus of current research. Subsensitivity of $\alpha 2$ adrenergic receptors, as indicated by the blunted release of growth hormone after clonidine infusion, may be a factor responsible for the genesis of GAD.

Neuroanatomical and Brain Imaging Studies

Researchers have focused on the occipital lobe, which has the highest concentration of benzodiazepine receptors. The other brain areas that have been hypothesized to be involved in GAD are basal ganglia, limbic system and frontal cortex.

Brain imaging studies, like positron emission tomography (PET) have reported a lower metabolic rate in basal ganglia and white matter in GAD patients as compared to normal controls.[34]

Genetic Studies

About 25% of the first degree relatives of patients with GAD are also affected. Studies conducted recently also state that GAD is a moderately familial disorder with a heritability calculated to be around 30%. The male relatives are likely to have an alcohol use disorder. Some twin studies record a concordance rate of 50% in monozygotic twins and 15% in dizygotic twins.[35,36]

EEG Studies

A variety of EEG abnormalities have been observed. Sleep EEG studies have reported increased sleep discontinuity, decreased delta sleep, decreased stage I sleep and reduced rapid eye movement sleep.

Psychosocial Factors

Cognitive Behavioral Theory

This theory hypothesizes that patients with GAD are responding to incorrectly and inaccurately perceived dangers. The inaccuracy is generated by selective attention to negative details in the environment, by distortions in information processing, and by an excessively negative view of one's own ability to cope.

Psychoanalytic Theory

The psychoanalytic theory hypothesizes that anxiety is a symptom of the unresolved unconscious conflicts. The psychological theory of anxiety was first presented by Sigmund Freud in 1909, with his description of 'little Hans.' Earlier, Freud had conceptualized anxiety as having a physiological basis.

A hierarchy of anxieties is related to the various developmental levels. At the most primitive level, anxiety may relate to the fear of annihilation or fusion with another person. At a more mature level of development, anxiety is related to separation from a love object. At a still more mature level, anxiety is connected to the loss of love from an important object. *Castration anxiety* is related to the oedipal phase of development and is considered one of the highest levels of anxiety. *Superego anxiety*, the fear of disappointing one's own ideals and values (derived from internalized parents), is the most mature form of anxiety.

Environmental Factors

With the increasing emphasis placed on the biological etiology of anxiety, the importance of environmental factors on the onset of anxiety symptoms must not be overlooked. This is especially true for GAD. One study conducted to assess the role of stressful life events in the onset of GAD reported that both men and women experienced one or more unexpected, negative, but important life event before the onset of GAD.

DIAGNOSIS

Despite the fact that the diagnostic reliability of GAD is lower than that of other anxiety disorders, the factors constituting diagnostic criteria for GAD have been found to be reliable. Several studies have shown that the content and presence of spheres of worry involved in GAD can be identified reliably.[37-40] Although GAD has been retained as a diagnosis in DSM IV, researchers should be aware that there are a number of unresolved issues surrounding the empirical basis of diagnosis. The difficulties include the problems with diagnostic unreliability, shown by recent studies using the DSM-III-R criteria. It is possible that DSM-IV definitions may improve reliability, but there is no evidence yet that this will happen.

The second most important issue related to the DSM-IV diagnosis of GAD is the high rate of comorbidity. The future research will have to focus on this area of research. One recent study conducted to test the validity of GAD as an independent diagnostic category and to evaluate the prevalence and type of other psychiatric disorders co-existing with GAD, concluded that 23% patients have comorbid diagnosis of social phobia and 21% have simple phobia. However, 42% of the patients did not exhibit any other associated psychiatric diagnosis. The results of this study show that GAD occurs independently, as well as there is equally high rate of comorbidity.[33]

DSM-IV[30] has specified the diagnostic criteria for the diagnosis of GAD. These are excessive anxiety and worry, occurring more days than not for at least 6 months, about a number of events or activities. The person finds it difficult to control the worry. The anxiety and worry are associated with at least three of the following six symptoms (with at least some symptoms present for more days than not for the past 6 months). However, only one item is required in children.

These symptoms include restlessness or feeling keyed up or on edge, being easily fatigued, difficulty concentrating or mind going blank, irritability, muscle tension, and sleep disturbance (difficulty falling or staying asleep, or restless unsatisfying sleep).[30]

The anxiety should not be confined merely to the other Axis I psychiatric disorders (e.g. mood disorder, psychotic disorder, social phobia, OCD, separation anxiety disorder, anorexia nervosa, somatization disorder, hypochondriasis, or post-traumatic stress disorder), substance use disorder (intoxication or withdrawal), or a general medical condition (e.g. hyperthyroidism).

DSM-5 Diagnostic criteria for generalized anxiety disorder 300.02 (F41.1)
A. Excessive anxiety and worry (apprehensive expectation), occurring more days than not for at least 6 months, about a number of events or activities (such as work or school performance).
B. The individual finds it difficult to control the worry.
C. The anxiety and worry are associated with three (or more) of the following six symptoms (with at least some symptoms having been present for more days than not for the past 6 months):
Note: Only one item is required in children.
1. Restlessness or feeling keyed up or on edge. 2. Being easily fatigued. 3. Difficulty concentrating or mind going blank. 4. Irritability. 5. Muscle tension. 6. Sleep disturbance (difficulty falling or staying asleep, or restless, unsatisfying sleep).
D. The anxiety, worry, or physical symptoms cause clinically significant distress or impairment in social, occupational, or other important areas of functioning.
E. The disturbance is not attributable to the physiological effects of a substance (e.g. a drug of abuse, a medication) or another medical condition (e.g. hyperthyroidism).
F. The disturbance is not better explained by another mental disorder (e.g. anxiety or worry about having panic attacks in panic disorder, negative evaluation in social anxiety disorder (social phobia), contamination or other obsessions in OCD, separation from attachment figures in separation anxiety disorder, reminders of traumatic events in post-traumatic stress disorder, gaining weight in anorexia nervosa, physical complaints in somatic symptom disorder, perceived appearance flaws in body dysmorphic disorder, having a serious illness in illness anxiety disorder, or the content of delusional beliefs in schizophrenia or delusional disorder).

DIFFERENTIAL DIAGNOSIS

All the medical disorders that may cause anxiety must be included in the differential diagnosis. Routine blood chemistry tests, EKG, and thyroid function tests are necessary. Caffeine intoxication, stimulant abuse, alcohol withdrawal, and sedative, hypnotic, or anxiolytic withdrawal must be ruled out. The history and mental status examination must explore the diagnostic possibility of panic disorder, phobic disorder and OCD. Distinguishing GAD from major depressive disorder and dysthymic disorder can at times be difficult, in fact the disorders frequently coexist. Other diagnostic possibilities are adjustment disorder with anxiety, hypochondriasis, adult attention deficit hyperactivity disorder, somatization disorder, and personality disorders.

The presence of autonomic, cardiovascular, and respiratory hyperarousal is an important marker of anxiety.[41,42] The discriminating ability of cognitive symptoms including threat-related thoughts, worry and subjective anxiety indicates that the cognitive component of anxiety should be considered when attempting a differential diagnosis with depressive disorders.[43]

COURSE AND PROGNOSIS

The clinical course and the prognosis of disorder is difficult to predict. However, the patients with GAD almost universally have other comorbid disorders,[44] most likely to have at least one other anxiety disorder or major depressive disorder at intake,[45] have earlier age at onset, and have the worst emotional health rating.

MANAGEMENT

Psychotherapy

The major psychotherapeutic approaches to GAD are cognitive behavioral, supportive and insight-oriented therapies.

Cognitive Behavior Therapy

Cognitive behavior therapy seems to have both short and long term efficacy. The cognitive approaches directly address the patient's hypothesized cognitive distortions, and the behavioral approaches address the somatic symptoms directly.

Cognitive therapy is likely to be more effective than psychodynamic psychotherapy with chronically anxious patients and 8–10 sessions have been found to be of comparable efficacy to 16–20 sessions.

The major behavioral techniques used are relaxation, biofeedback, meditation and Yoga. For relaxation, Jacobson's procedure[46] needs mention, in addition to Benson's and Ost's procedures mentioned in Chapter 10.2. Patients are taught to tense the muscles in one portion of the body and then they are instructed to relax each muscle individually and to discriminate the subtle proprioceptive sensation that accompanies muscle tension. Patients are taught to recognize very low levels of muscle tension, so that they can perceive every day levels of tension. They are further asked to relax without deliberate tension at all. The yogic relaxation techniques include the various *yoga-asanas,* such as *sukhasna, talasna, yoga mudra, nispandbhav* and *savasna.*

In a comparison study between progressive relaxation and yoga, it was observed that the yogic techniques produced greater motivation to practice than progressive relaxation.[47]

Meditation

Patanjali, an Indian Philosopher, advocates the practice of meditation to combat anxiety. According to Patanjali, an individual's thoughts and behavior tend to depend on the environmental feedback.[48] Every action of an individual results in a feedback from the environment. Positive feed back is reassuring, while negative feedback induces a subjective feeling of inadequacy and anxiety. Anxiety reduces the attention span and increases distractibility; such a state adversely affects the personal and occupational efficiency, thus reinforcing the negative feedback and a subjective feeling of unpleasantness is then generated. This would in turn, aggravate psychological and physiological symptoms of anxiety. This cycle then self-perpetuates. This preoccupation with environmental feedback contributes to the psychological and physiological symptoms of anxiety.

Meditation is defined as "a family of techniques which have in common a conscious attempt to focus attention in a non-analytical way, and attempt not to dwell on discursive ruminating thoughts."

The therapy aims at learning to focus attention on chosen imagery and to learn not to dwell upon discursive thoughts. Patients are helped to select an appealing, everlasting and unchanging mental image. They are asked to assume a comfortable, supine posture and concentrate on the chosen imagery, while regulating breathing. They are informed that concentration would be intercepted by various thoughts and that a voluntary effort is to be made to exclude these discursive thoughts and to focus attention on the chosen imagery. With practice, the ability, to discard discursive thoughts and retain concentration on the chosen imagery, improves. Over a period of time, this ability is noticed in daily life situations.

In a recent study,[49] meditation was found to be as effective as pharmacotherapy in controlling symptoms of anxiety. It is in fact superior in altering the trait anxiety. Meditation is easy to learn and is a cost-effective therapy. It has a distinct edge over pharmacotherapy in that it does not have the associated problem of habit formation, withdrawal effects, overdosage or other undesirable effects.[50]

Preliminary data indicates that the combination of cognitive and behavioral approaches is more effective than either technique used alone.

Supportive Psychotherapy

Supportive therapy offers patients of GAD reassurance and comfort, although its long term efficacy is doubtful.[51]

Insight-oriented Psychotherapy

It focuses on uncovering the unconscious conflicts and identifying ego strengths. The efficacy of insight-oriented psychotherapy for generalized anxiety disorder is reported, but large controlled studies are lacking.

Pharmacotherapy

Benzodiazepines

Benzodiazepines are among the most widely prescribed agents in the world.[52] They have been the drugs of choice for GAD. Benzodiazepines can be prescribed on an as needed basis, so that patients take a rapidly acting benzodiazepine when they feel particularly anxious. The alternative approach is to prescribe benzodiazepine for a limited period, during which psychosocial therapeutic approaches are implemented.

Several problems are associated with the use of benzodiazepines in generalized anxiety disorder. About 25 to 30% of all patients fail to respond, and tolerance and dependence may occur. Some patients also experience impaired alertness while taking drugs. The decision to initiate benzodiazepines treatment should be specific regarding patients' diagnosis, the specific target symptoms, and the duration of treatment. Treatment for most anxiety conditions lasts for 2–6 weeks, followed by 1 or 2 weeks of tapering of the drug before it is discontinued.[52]

The drug should begin at the low end of its therapeutic range and then increased to achieve a therapeutic response. The use of intermediate half-life benzodiazepines (8–15 hours) is better than long half-life benzodiazepines, and divided doses prevent the development of adverse effects associated with high peak plasma levels. The results show that alprazolam is as effective as diazepam, but drowsiness is less often reported.[53]

Buspirone

Buspirone is most likely effective in 60 to 80% of patients with GAD.[54] It is more effective in reducing the cognitive symptoms of GAD than in reducing the somatic symptoms. Its effects take 2–3 weeks to become evident and it does not produce cognitive and psycho-motor adverse effects. Muscle relaxation and sense of wellbeing, as seen with benzodiazepines, is not reported.

Absence of tolerance, dependence and withdrawal symptoms may make it the first line drug in the treatment of GAD, but buspirone is not an effective treatment for the benzodiazepine withdrawal syndrome.

Alpidem

This is an imidiazo-(1,2-a)-pyridine molecule that shows anxiolytic activity comparable with that of established benzodiazepines, without causing any significant sedative effects, myorelaxation, or impairment of motor function.[55,56] In humans, it is best tolerated up to doses of 300 mg. In situational and chronic anxiety, it is of comparable efficacy to benzodiazepines (such as lorazepam and diazepam), while being safer.[57] No withdrawal or rebound symptoms were observed in anxious patients when alpidem was abruptly discontinued after 6–12 months of continuous therapy. Alpidem may be a valid alternative to the current benzodiazepine anxiolytic therapy because it produces fewer and weaker withdrawal symptoms than alprazolam and is better tolerated.

Other Drugs

If treatment with buspirone or a benzodiazepine is not effective (or not completely effective), treatment with a tricyclic drug or a β-adrenergic antagonist (e.g. propranolol) can be considered. The tricyclic drugs have been proved to be effective in the treatment of anxiety. β-adrenergic antagonists are limited to the treatment of peripheral manifestations of anxiety and anticipatory anxiety. Alternatively, benzodiazepines, in combination with buspirone or other anxiolytics, may be used.

REFERENCES

General Aspects of Anxiety Disorder

1. Maudsley H. The Pathology of Mind. London: MacMillan; 1879.
2. Beard G. Neurasthenia or nervous exhaustion. Boston Med Surg J. 1969;3:217-22.
3. Hacker E. Ueberlavire and abortive angstzustandsbei Neurasthewie. Zentralblah fur nerverheilfunde. 1893;4: 565-72.
4. Westphal C. Die agoraphobe, eineneuro pathologischeer-schenung. Archiv fur psychiatric and nervenbrankheiton. 1871;3:138-61.
5. Freud S. On the ground for detaching a particular syndrome from neurasthenia under the description 'anxiety neurosis'. In: Standard Edition of the Sigmund Freud. Vol. 3. London: Hogarth Press; 1895. p. 90.
6. Da Costa JM. On irritable heart: A clinical study of a form of functional cardiac disorder and its consequences. Am J Med Sci. 1871;61:17-52.

7. American Psychiatric Association. Diagnostic and Statistical Manual. III Ed. Washington DC: American Psychiatric Association; 1980.
8. WHO. International Classification of Diseseas: Mental and Related Behavioral Disorders. Chapter V. Geneva: World Health Organization; 1992.
9. Cohen ME, et al. The high familial incidence of neurocirculatory asthenia (anxiety neurosis). Am J Hum Genet. 1951;3: 126.
10. Gelder M. The clarification of anxiety disorder. Br J Psychiatry. 1989;154 (Suppl.):28-32.
10. Okasa A, et al. Panic disorder: An overlapping or independent entity. Br J Psychiatry. 1994;164:818-25.
11. Freedman AM, Kaplan HI (Eds). Comprehensive Textbook of Psychiatry. Baltimore: Williams and Wilkins; 1967. p. 858.
12. American Psychiatric Association. Diagnostic and Statistical Manual. IV Ed. Washington DC: American Psychiatric Association; 1994.
13. American Psychiatric Association. Desk Reference to the Diagnostic Criteria from DSM-5™. Washington DC: American Psychiatric Association; 2013.

Panic Disorders

14. Eaton WW, Kessler RC, et al. Panic and panic disorder in the United States. Am J Psychiatry. 1994;151:413-28.
15. Shear MK, Cooper AM, Klerman GL, et al. A psychodynamic model of panic disorders. Am J Psychiatry. 1993;150:859.
16. Gorman JM, Papp LA, et al. Anxiogenic effects of CO_2 and hyperventilation in patients with panic disorders. Am J Psychiatry. 1994;151:547-53.
17. Co BJ, Direnfeld DM, Swinson RP, et al. Suicidal ideation and Suicidal attempts in panic disorder and social phobia. Am J Psychiatry. 1994;151:882-7.
18. American Psychiatric Association. Diagnostic and Statistical Manual. IV Ed. Washington DC: American Psychiatric Association; 1994.
19. Fyer AJ, Sandberg DP. Pharmacological treatment of panic disorder. In: Frances AJ, Hales RE (Eds). Review of Psychiatry. New York: American Psychiatric Press; 1988.
20. Nutt DJ, Glur P. Clinical pharmacology of anxiolytics and antidepressants: A psychopharmacological perspective. Pharmacol Ther. 1989;44:309-34.
21. Clark DM, Salkovski PM, et al. A comparison of cognitive therapy: Applied relaxation and imipramine is the treatment of panic disorder. Br J Psychiatry. 1994;164:759-69.
22. Sanderson WC, Asnis GM, et al. Alprazolam blockade of CO_2 provoked panic in patients with panic disorder: Am J Psychiatry. 1994;151:1220-22.
23. Clark DM. Anxiety states: Panic and generalized anxiety. In: Hawton K, Salkovskis P, Kirb J, et al. (Eds). Cognitive Behavior Therapy for Psychiatric Problems: A Practical Guide. Oxford: Oxford University Press; 1994. pp. 52-96.
24. Salkovski PM, Clark DM. Cognitive therapy for panic disorder. J Cognitive Psychother. 1991;5:215-26.
25. Ost LG. Applied relaxation: Description of a coping technique and review of controlled studies. Behav Res Ther. 1991;25:397-410.
26. Spiegel DA, Bruce TJ, Gregg SF, et al. Does cognitive behavior therapy assist slow-taper alprazolan discontinuation in panic disorder. Am J Psychiatry. 1994;151:876-81.
27. American Psychiatric Association. Desk Reference to the Diagnostic Criteria from DSM-5. Washington DC; 2013.

Generalized Anxiety Disorders

28. American Psychiatric Association. Diagnostic and Statistical Manual. III Ed. Washington DC: American Psychiatric Association; 1980.
29. American Psychiatric Association. Diagnostic and Statistical Manual. III Ed. Rev. Washington DC: American Psychiatric Association; 1987.
30. American Psychiatric Association. Diagnostic and Statistical Manual. IV Ed. Washington DC: American Psychiatric Association; 1994.
31. Flint AJ. Epidemiology and comorbidity of anxiety disorders in elderly. Am J Psychiatry. 1994;151:640-49.
32. Blazes D, et al. The epidemiology of anxiety disorders: An age comparison. In: Salzman C, Lebowitz B. Anxiety in the Elderly: Treatment and Research. New York: Springer; 1991.
33. Brawman-Mintzer O, et al. Psychiatric comorbidity in patients with generalized anxiety disorder. Am J Psychiatry. 1993; 150:1216-8.
34. Wu JC, et al. PET in generalized anxiety disorder. Biol Psychiatry; 1991.
35. Kendler KS, et al. Major depression and generalized anxiety disorder: Same genes, (partly) different environments. Arch Gen Psychiatry. 1992;49:716.
36. Kendler KS, et al. Generalized anxiety disorder in women: A population based twin study. Arch Gen Psychiatry. 1992;49: 267.
37. Sanderson WC, et al. A description of patients diagnosed with DSM-III-R generalized anxiety diorder. J Nerv Ment Dis. 1990; 178:588-91.
38. Barlow DH, et al. The diagnosis of generalized anxiety disorder: Development, current status, and future directions. In: Ropee RM, Barlow DH (Eds). Chronic Anxiety, GAD and Mixed Anxiety Depression. New York: Guilford Press; 1991.
39. Borkovec TD, Shodick RN, Hopkins M. The nature of normal and pathological worry. In: Ropee RM, Barlow DH (Eds). Chronic Anxiety, GAD and Mixed Anxiety Depression. New York: Guilford Press; 1991.
40. Craske MG, et al. Qualitative dimensions of worry in DSM-III-R generalized anxiety disorder subjects and non-anxious controls. Behav Res Ther. 1989;27:397-402.
41. Hoehn, Sonic R, Mcleod DR. Generalized anxiety disorder. Psychiatr Clin N Am. 1985.pp.873-88.

42. Clark LA, Watson D. Tripartite model of anxiety and depression: Psychometric evidence and taxonomic implications. J Abnor Psychol. 1991;100:316-36.
43. Beck AT, Emery G. Anxiety disorders and phobias: A cognitive perspective. New York: Basic books; 1985.
44. Brawman-Mintzer O, et al. Somatic symptoms in GAD with and without comorbid psychiatric disorders. Am J Psychiatry. 1994;151:930-32.
45. Psychiatric morbidity in panic disorder and generalized anxiety disorder. Am J Psychiatry. 1993;150:600-07.
46. Jacobson E. Self operation as control: Foundation for progressive relaxation. Illinois: Thomas, Springfield; 1964.
47. Sahasi G, et al. Comparative study of progressive relaxation and Yogic techniques of relaxation in the management of anxiety neurosis. Indian J Psychiatry. 1991;33:27-32.
48. Vivekananda Swami. Patanjali's Yoga Sutra (Aphonisms) in Raja Yoga. Calcutta: Advaita Ashram; 1966. pp. 123-236.
49. Vahia VN, et al. Efficacy of meditation in generalized anxiety disorder. Indian J Psychiatry. 1993;35:87-91.
50. Shapiro DH. Overview: Clinical and physiological comparison of meditation with other self control strategies in meditation. In: Shapiro DH, Walsh RN (Eds). Classic and contemporary perspectives. New York Academy; 1988.pp.5-12.
51. Frank JD. The psychotherapy of anxiety. In: Grinspoon L (Ed). Psychiatry Update. Vol. III. Washington DC: American Psychiatric Press; 1984. pp. 418-26.
52. American Psychiatric Association (APA). Task Force Report on Benzodiazepine Dependence, Toxicity and Abuse. Washington DC: APA; 1990.
53. Shah LP, et al. Comparative evaluation of alprazolam and diazepam in the treatment of anxiety: A double blind multicenter study. Indian J Psychiatry. 1990;33:126-30.
54. Gammans RE, et al. Use of buspirone in patients with GAD and coexisting depressive symptoms: A meta-analysis of eight randomized, controlled studies. Neuropsychobiology. 1992;25:193.
55. Dimsdale M, et al. Alpidem. Drugs of the Future. 1988;13: 106-9.
56. Bianchetti G, et al. Pharmacokinetic profile of alpidem: A new anxiolytic in healthy volunteers. Proceedings of the Third European Congress of Biopharmaceutics and Pharmacokinetics, 1987, Friburg, Abstract no. 339.
57. Morselli PL. On the therapecutic action of alpidem in anxiety disorders: An overview of the European data. Pharmacopsychiatry. 1990;23:129-34.

SUGGESTED READING

1. American Psychiatric Association. Desk Reference to the Diagnostic Criteria from DSM-5. Washington DC; 2013.
2. Berger A, Dukes E, Wittchen HU, Morlock R, Edelsberg J, Oster G. Patterns of healthcare utilization in patients with generalized anxiety disorder in general practice in Germany. Eur J Psychrary. 2009;23:90-100.
3. Culpepper L. Generalized anxiety disorder and medical illness. J Clin Psychiatry. 2009;70(suppl 2):20-4.
4. Kessler RC, Ormel J, Demler O, Stang PE. Comorbid mental disorders account for the role impairment of commonly occurring chronic physical disorders: results horn the National Comorbidity Survey. J Occup Environ Med. 2003;45: 1257-66.
5. Nisenson LG, Pepper CM, Schwenk TL, Coyne JC. The nature and prevalence of anxiety disorders in primary care. Gen Hosp Psychiatry. 1998;20:21-8.
6. Shin LM, Liberzon l. The neurocircuitry of fear, stress, and anxiety disorders Neuropsychopharmacolagy. 2008;35: 169-91.
7. Strawn JR, Bitter SM, Weber WA, Chu WJ, Whitsel RM, Adler C, et al. Neurocircuitry of Generalized Anxiety Disorder in Adolescents, a pilot functional neuroimaging and functional connectivity study. Depress Anxiety 2012; published online 24 May.

CHAPTER 11

Generalized Anxiety Disorder: Diagnosis and Treatment

JN Vyas, Deyashini Lahiri Tikka, Jayati Simlai

Generalized anxiety disorder (GAD) is a common psychiatric disorder, with lifetime prevalence varying from 2 to 7%. It is a chronic disorder characterized by uncontrollable worry and apprehension, associated with various physiological symptoms like disturbed sleep, muscle tension, and impaired concentration. The disorder leads to impaired socio-occupational functioning, and it is commonly comorbid with other anxiety disorders, and poses an increased risk for suicide as well.[1] GAD is commonly underdiagnosed because of predominant physical symptoms and stigma associated with mental illnesses. However, GAD has many evidence-based treatment options. This chapter reviews current understanding about the diagnosis and various treatment options—both biological and psychological, available for GAD.

WHAT IS GENERALIZED ANXIETY DISORDER?

Generalized anxiety disorder (GAD) is characterized by excessive worry and restlessness, insomnia, and muscle tension, which are symptoms of physiological arousal. To meet Diagnostic and Statistical Manual of Mental Disorders, fifth edition (DSM-5)[2] criteria for the disorder, patients must have excessive and difficult to control anxiety for at least 6 months and about different settings. For example, anxiety confined to personal safety concerns should not be qualified as under GAD. In addition to this excessive worry across various situations, patients must have at least three physiological symptoms such as restlessness, fatigue, muscle tension, etc. (see box one next page). Moreover, these symptoms must not have been caused by another psychiatric disorder like depression or medical disorder like hypertension, or by the use of drugs, and they must cause serious distress or impairment for the clinical diagnosis to be made. The ICD (International classification of diseases) (10th revision)[3] description of GAD contains slightly different description of symptoms. It focuses on physiological arousal such as trembling, sweating, palpitations, dizziness and does not require symptoms to be present for six months. It defines GAD as anxiety that is generalized and persistent, and hence, not restricted to particular environmental circumstances (it is free-floating). The predominant symptoms may be variable but include physiological complaints such as persistent nervousness, trembling, muscular tensions, etc. Because most clinical trials use DSM-criteria, we will focus on GAD as defined by the DSM classificatory system, so that the reader can best evaluate the treatment trial data.

WHO GETS GENERALIZED ANXIETY DISORDER?

The lifetime prevalence was determined to be 5.7% in a sample from the United States, a similar rate to that found in other countries. The highest prevalence (7.7%) occurred in the 45–59 year age range. There is a skewed gender distribution with prevalence being less in men (4%) than women (7%). Other social predictors have been identified as having a marital status of separated, widowed or divorced and an employment status of being unemployed or being a homemaker.[4] In a study of children followed into adulthood, low socioeconomic status, childhood maltreatment, internalizing problems, and conduct problems in childhood were risk factors. GAD has been shown frequently been associated with serious disability and below standard quality of life. In an international study of disability caused by mental illness, 3–8% of people with GAD had moderate to severe occupational role impairment, with an average of 6.3 days a month of missed work or loss of role functioning.[5]

HOW IS GENERALIZED ANXIETY DISORDER DIAGNOSED?

The disorder is not very well-recognized in primary care. Primary care physicians have been found to be correctly recognizing and diagnosing GAD only 34% of the time.[6] Part of the problem may be the misdiagnosis of anxiety as depression. In one study in primary care settings, only about one-fourth of the patients with pure anxiety were diagnosed with anxiety, compared with 65% of those with pure depressions.[7] In other work, researchers examined patients who had been given a false positive diagnosis of depression: 27% of these patients had an anxiety disorder instead.[8]

In addition, a focus on somatic symptoms may distract patient and doctors from the psychological symptoms; it is known that patients with symptoms requiring a diagnosis GAD seek primary care consultation more often than the general population. A study of healthcare utilization patterns found that such patients visited primary care an average of 5.6 more times a year than age and sex matched controls without anxiety or depression.[9] Patients presenting with GAD also have higher rates of medical conditions. Associations have been found between GAD and increased rates of pain and gastrointestinal, cardiovascular, endocrine, and respiratory conditions.[10] Abnormal neural processing of emotional stimuli has been hypothesized as an underpinning pathophysiology of GAD, but this area is poorly understood and research has been minimal.

To improve detection and treatment, the International Consensus Group on Depression developed a consensus statement on GAD. It recommends asking two screening questions, one about being bothered by feeling worried, tense, or anxious most of the time in the past four weeks and another on whether one is feeling frequently tense, irritable, and having trouble sleeping.[11] However, it is not known how sensitive or specific these questions are.

DSM-5 diagnostic criteria is given below:

DSM-5 Diagnostic criteria for generalized anxiety disorder 300.02 (F41.1)
A. Excessive anxiety and worry (apprehensive expectation), occurring more days than not for at least 6 months, about a number of events or activities (such as work or school performance).
B. The individual finds it difficult to control the worry.
C. The anxiety and worry are associated with three (or more) of the following six symptoms (with at least some symptoms having been present for more days than not for the past 6 months): 1. Restlessness or feeling keyed up or on edge. 2. Being easily fatigued. 3. Difficulty concentrating or mind-going blank. 4. Irritability. 5. Muscle tension. 6. Sleep disturbance (difficulty falling or staying asleep, or restless, unsatisfying sleep). *Note:* Only one item is required in children.
D. The anxiety, worry, or physical symptoms cause clinically significant distress or impairment in social, occupational, or other important areas of functioning.
E. The disturbance is not attributable to the physiological effects of a substance (e.g. a drug of abuse, a medication) or another medical condition (e.g. hyperthyroidism).
F. The disturbance is not better explained by another mental disorder (e.g. anxiety or worry about having panic attacks in panic disorder, negative evaluation in social anxiety disorder (social phobia), contamination or other obsessions in obsessive-compulsive disorder, separation from attachment figures in separation anxiety disorder, reminders of traumatic events in post-traumatic stress disorder, gaining weight in anorexia nervosa, physical complaints in somatic symptom disorder, perceived appearance flaws in body dysmorphic disorder, having a serious illness in illness anxiety disorder, or the content of delusional beliefs in schizophrenia or delusional disorder).

Contd...

Contd...

DOES GENERALIZED ANXIETY DISORDER OCCUR WITH OTHER DISORDERS?

Psychiatric comorbidity is common in GAD-29-62% of patients are estimated to have major depression.[5,7] Other common comorbidities are social anxiety disorder (3.14%) and alcohol misuse (3.8%). Unfortunately, patients who also have comorbid psychiatric disorders are more impaired and have a less successful response to treatment than those with GAD alone.[12] The high comorbidity (and symptom overlap) with depression has led to a conceptual uncertainty of whether GAD is distinct from depression. However, symptoms unique to GAD-such as worry, differential response to benzodiazepines (not effective for depression), different patterns of rapid eye movement (REM) sleep disturbance, and opposing patterns of response to emotional stimuli in the laboratory (relative insensitivity in depression and hyperactivity in GAD)-support it being a distinct disorder.[13,14] When making a diagnosis in a patient with current depression, symptoms that overlap with depression—such as restlessness, difficulty concentrating, and sleep disturbance—cannot be used in the diagnosis of GAD. Ultimately, however, distinguishing between GAD and GAD with comorbidities should not overly concern the clinician because many treatment strategies are the same.

Although they are distinct disorders, the presence of GAD predisposes to the subsequent development of major depression. One large prospective study of adolescents and adults found that GAD increased the odds of developing depression within four years 4.5-fold.[15] Interestingly, drug treatment for GAD significantly lowers the risk of developing major depression.[16]

WHAT IS KNOWN ABOUT THE CAUSES?

A complex gene-environmental interaction plays a role in the development of GAD. Data from family and twin studies suggests that GAD has a modest heritability (0.32, compared with 0.43 for panic disorder).[17] More recently, a genetic association study of 1059 Spanish primary care attendees found that a polymorphic variation in the serotonin (5HT) 1-A receptor gene was associated with the common dual diagnostic presentation of GAD and major depression.[18] The above meta-analysis also found that environmental experiences are significantly associated with GAD, highlighting the importance of environmental stressors as a risk factor.

WHAT ARE THE TREATMENT OPTIONS?

Treatment options include psychological therapies and drugs. Psychological therapies include cognitive behavioral therapy (CBT), behavioral therapy relaxation response training, and mindfulness meditation training. Of these, CBT is the most well studied and commonly used. Drugs include antidepressants, notably the serotonin reuptake inhibitors as first-line agents, benzodiazepines, and the anticonvulsant pregabalin. NICE—National Institute for Health and Clinical Excellence treatment guidelines recommend treating patients with active substance dependence (different from nonharmful substance misuse) before starting treatment. Unfortunately, it is unclear whether psychotherapy or drugs should be tried first, with some studies showing a benefit of CBT over drugs,[19] and others showing a benefit of drugs, such as sertraline, over CBT.[20] The decision should be made after a discussion with the patient, during which the patients values, attitudes, beliefs, preferences, and resources are reviewed. Furthermore, it is unclear whether the combination of drugs and psychotherapy is better than using one strategy alone.

WHAT PSYCHOSOCIAL TREATMENTS CAN BE USED?

Several types of psychotherapy have been used, with varying levels of empirical support. For anxiety disorders, CBT—a time limited symptom focused treatment is the most well-studied and highly utilized. Several well-conducted meta-analyses have shown significant benefit of CBT compared with control groups,[21-23] and NICE guidelines recommend CBT as first-line treatment.

This technique traditionally combines cognitive therapy-which focuses on monitoring thoughts and understanding self-perpetuated cognitive distortions, habitual thought patterns, and subsequent behaviors with behavioral therapy, which aims to expose the patient to feared experiences (originally, phobias). In GAD, targeted cognitions might, for example, be negative interpretations of emotionally neutral events, which can be systematically evaluated and questioned. Patients with GAD are more likely to see neutral stimuli as potentially threatening than those without an anxiety disorder,[24,25] so automatic anxious thought patterns can be reduced by evaluating thoughts and impressions more objectively. Behavioral therapy is more difficult in GAD than with simple phobias, because worry-based anxiety triggers for GAD are more difficult to target, more diffuse, and often shift. One approach has been to use exposure techniques to focus attention on the worries, which themselves may be serving as avoidance against more distressing emotions, such as anger or grief.[26,27]

Cognitive behavioral therapy (CBT) is usually provided by a specially trained psychotherapist on an individual basis, with 6–12 sessions of one hour's duration as standard. Some studies suggest that CBT can be delivered over the internet, but how it compares to office-based CBT is unclear. There is also preliminary evidence that internet-based CBT administered by a nonclinician may be effective, although only one randomized controlled trial has been published to date and it was not tested against standard CBT.[28]

Several other psychotherapeutic approaches can be combined with CBT. For example, relaxation response training, in the form of progressive muscle relaxation or diaphragmatic breathing, has been added to CBT or used alone. Two small to medium sized randomized controlled studies comparing cognitive therapy alone with relaxation training alone found that they both significantly and equally reduce anxiety symptoms in GAD.[29,30] New cognitive therapy uses similar techniques to those of old cognitive therapy technique (working to correct automatic or distorted thinking) but also tackles about worrying itself—for example, thoughts that the worrying will become uncontrollable or will cause negative consequences for the patient. The therapy focuses instead on changing beliefs about worry and guides patients away from a force on attempts to control the worry.[31]

Two newer psychotherapies have recently been introduced for the treatment of GAD; both share a theoretical framework with CBT but include mindfulness training. Mindfulness was originally introduced in mental health treatment settings through meditation training strategies, such as mindfulness-based stress reduction.[32] Mindfulness teaches participants to increase awareness of present moment experiences, such as thoughts and emotions, without judgment or striving to make the experience last or disappear. One of these newer psychotherapies, which have support from a small but well-conducted randomized controlled trial, is acceptance-based behavioral therapy. This therapy focuses on accepting problems rather than striving for immediate change, and uses-mindfulness to help patient foster a compassionate and nonjudgmental awareness of their experiences (which promotes clearer decision making) and a focus on present moment experiences rather than worries.[33] Emotion regulation therapy also uses mindfulness training but focuses on addressing deficits in regulating emotions through additional techniques.[34] The use of mindfulness meditation training for GAD is validated by a recent small randomized controlled trial, which found significant benefits compared with an active control class.[35]

Traditional psychodynamic psychotherapy has been less well-studied in GAD, possibly because of methodological challenges in studying a longer duration and less focused treatment where duration/direction varies greatlyamong individuals. More recently, short-term psychodynamic psychotherapy was compared with CBT in a group of 57 patients with GAD as part of a randomized controlled trial.[36] Both treatments showed significant decreases in anxiety symptoms and no intertreatment difference on the primary outcome measure.

Although not a treatment for GAD by itself, education on sleep hygiene can be useful in primary care settings given the prominence of sleep disturbance in this disorder. It is sometimes used with CBT to ensure the best possible sleep efficiency and quality. Advice includes going to bed and waking up at the same time each day, eliminating alcohol after 6 pm, and getting out of bed if unable to fall asleep, to avoid negative associations with the bed environment.[37] In addition, although not widely studied in GAD, physical exercise decreased anxiety symptoms.[38] Lastly, self-help books or manuals may be useful, according to a meta-analysis that included six randomized controlled trials; two of them showed a benefit over a waiting list control.[39]

WHEN SHOULD DRUGS BE PRESCRIBED?

In 2011, NICE issued treatment guidelines outlining an algorithm for the treatment of GAD. It recommended drug treatment if symptoms cause marked functional impairment. This was defined as self-reported socio-occupational, academic and leisure functioning; higher scores on screening instruments such as the seven item "GAD-7";[40] or persistence of symptoms despite psychoeducation and low intensity psychological intervention (such as self-help and psychoeducational groups). Currently, there is no clear time frame for exactly when drugs should be considered. One large open label study examining the duration of "untreated" GAD (no drug treatment) found that treatment (antidepressants) was more successful when started within one year, suggesting that drugs should be offered within one year of persistent symptoms. This treatment effect was not found with benzodiazepines.[41]

WHICH DRUGS ARE EFFECTIVE?

Antidepressants

Antidepressants have well-documented efficacy in treating patients with GAD, regardless of the presence of comorbid depression.[41] Treatment efficacy is measured by clinical response (defined in most studies as >50% reduction from baseline in HAM-A (Hamilton rating scale- for anxiety) score or remission (defined as reaching a final HAM-A score of '7').

Selective serotonin reuptake inhibitors (SSRIs) and serotonin-norepinephrine reuptake inhibitors (SNRIs) are considered first-line pharmacological options for treatment, largely because of their combined efficacy tolerability, and safety profile. Response and remission rates have been known to vary across different studies. A recent systematic review in 2012, of 50 studies attempted to clarify the expected clinical response and remission rates for GAD treated by drugs. It is reported that the probability of a response with first-line therapy is 67.7%, compared with 50.5% for second-line therapy.[42] Remission rates for first-line therapy averaged 39.7%, but insufficient data were available in the reviewed studies on remission for second-line therapy. "Second-line therapy" in this study was diverse, including benzodiazepines, buspirone, and pregabalin, which limited the predictive value for this arm of the treatment. One review suggests that, although it is difficult to make individualized treatment response predictions, response to antidepressants is less likely if there is no evidence of an effect within four weeks.[43] Others have suggested that a minimum trial period should be eight weeks or more, because 44% of patients with another anxiety disorder who did not respond to an SSRI at four weeks responded by 12 weeks.[44]

The SSRI, sertraline, is recommended by NICE[41] as the initial treatment for GAD. This recommendation is based on its cost effectiveness (it is available as a generic). We are unaware of any head to head trial demonstrating an efficacy advantage for sertraline over other SSRIs or SNRls for GAD, However, known clinical advantages of sertraline include its minimal drug-drug interactions (making it preferable to fluoxetine, paroxetine, and fluvoxamine), the lack of associated electrocardiographic changes (compared with citalopram), and its lower risk of symptoms on discontinuation compared with paroxetine and venlafaxine.

If no effect is seen after a four to eight week trial of an SSRI, consider switching to another SSRI or to the SNRI class of antidepressants. However, if a partial effect is seen at four weeks, it is worth waiting until eight weeks because the effect of SSRIs can continue to increase during this period. The SNRIs—venlafaxine and duloxetine, can also be considered as first-line pharmacological options for treating GAD. Both are licensed in the UK for this indication; their efficacy has been confirmed in many randomized controlled studies of adult outpatients with GAD.[43] A large randomized controlled study of venlafaxine for GAD in primary care setting patients with and without comorbid depression found a significant reduction in anxiety scores for both depressed and non-depressed venlafaxine treated groups (a net decrease of 2.1 points) compared with placebo.[45] Another large double blind randomized placebo-controlled study examining the efficacy/tolerability of another SNRI, duloxetine for the treatment of GAD found that duloxetine (at 60 and 120 mg/day) was beneficial, as measured by a significantly reduction in anxiety scores compared with the placebo group. Patients treated with duloxetine also had greater functional improvements as measured by scores on the Sheehan disability scale.[46]

Other Drugs

Pregabalin is an anticonvulsant and antineuralgic agent commonly prescribed for diabetic peripheral neuropathy and postherpetic neuralgia. Since 2000, several randomized controlled studies have investigated the efficacy of pregabalin in the treatment of GAD.[47] NICE guidance suggests that pregabalin be offered as an initial treatment option for patients with GAD who cannot tolerate SSRIs or SNRIs.[41] Similar to benzodiazepines, pregabalin has a rapid onset of action, with anxiolytic action occurring within one week of starting treatment. Sedation, headache, dizziness and dryness of mouth are some of the most common side effects of this drug.[47] Although, pregabalin is generally not considered habit forming, there have been case reports of misuse and symptoms on withdrawal. Sudden discontinuation of pregabalin and other anticonvulsants has been associated with an acute confusional state, with reversible vasogenic edema of the splenium of the corpus callosum.[42-48] Gabapentin, another anticonvulsant drug often used for neuropathic pain, has also been used off label for the treatment of GAD, although evidence favors its use only for social anxiety.[49]

For the short-term treatment of GAD, benzodiazepines have a confirmed efficacy profile.[43] Because of their habit forming potential and the availability of alternative nonhabit forming drugs, NICE guidance recommends that they are to be used in the treatment of GAD, only for a short-term course required for crisis intervention.[41] Moreover, unwanted side effects (including sedation and psychomotor impairment) and the potential for withdrawal symptoms (necessitating a gradual discontinuation of treatment) limit their suitability. Short acting benzodiazepines such as alprazolam may lead to rebound anxiety, which can inadvertently promote long-term use. Benzodiazepines (ideally longer acting ones like clonazepam) are mainly recommended as short-term treatment for acute anxiety. They can also be used as an initial adjunct to antidepressants given the delayed onset of action of these drugs and the ability of benzodiazepines to attenuate some of the initial side effects of SSRIs and SNRIs.[43]

Buspirone is a nonbenzodiazepine anxiolytic that is effective in treating GAD.[50] The comparative efficacy of buspirone with other antidepressants or pregabalin is unclear, given the current lack of head to head trials.[51] Comparison studies of buspirone versus benzodiazepines have mixed results, although buspirone being less effective in patients who were recently treated with benzodiazepines.[52] The advantage of this drug over benzodiazepines is its lack of sedation, withdrawal symptoms, and physical or physiological dependence.[50] A period of two to four weeks or more is typically needed for eliciting a response.[41]

Placebo has been used as the main comparator in most studies, and few head to head clinical studies exist. Thus, little is known about the comparable efficacy of the drugs used to treat GAD. A recent systematic review that pooled data from 27 randomized controlled trials of various drugs found a possible response and remission advantage for fluoxetine compared with all other treatments tested (benzodiazepines, buspirone, and quetiapine were not included).[43] More head to head studies are needed. Augmentation pharmacotherapy for GAD is another area that requires further study.

Unlicensed Treatments Used in Refractory GAD

If patients do not improve despite the use of treatments of adequate duration, consider unlicensed treatments as a possible next step. Unlicensed treatments should be initiated only by a specialist.

Recently, there is an increased interest use of second generation antipsychotics, both as monotherapy and as an augmentation strategy because only a minority of patients with GAD achieve remission despite current treatments. A recent systematic review and meta-analysis looked at augmentation and monotherapy with newer antipsychotics in the treatment of GAD.[53] The study reviewed five separate randomized placebo-controlled augmentation studies (total of 912 patients), which failed to show a significant clinical advantage for second generation antipsychotics over placebo. Moreover, augmentation was associated adverse effects that lead to a higher dropout rate. The same review found more promising results with studies of second generation antipsychotic monotherapy. Four randomized placebo-controlled monotherapy studies (total of 1383 patients) showed significant efficacy of quetiapine monotherapy (up to 150 mg/day) over placebo. As with the augmentation studies, patients treated with quetiapine had an increased risk of all cause discontinuation and weight gain.[53] Currently, antipsychotics should not be offered as an initial treatment option for GAD.[51]

HOW LONG DRUGS BE CONTINUED?

If a particular drug is effective, the optimal treatment duration is generally one year, given the lower relapse rate for patients who continue on pharmacotherapy versus placebo.[51] Treatment should also be continued for several months because an extended course of treatment increases the chances of remission while reducing the likelihood of relapse.[41] This observation is supported by double blind randomized controlled trials that found better response and remission rates when the initial eight weeks treatment course was extended to six months.[43]

WHEN SHOULD BE INVESTIGATED?

Generalized anxiety disorder (GAD) is more than just excessive worrying, and it is often a chronic disorder. In a group of older people with GAD who still remained symptomatic, the mean total duration spent with illness has been shown to be 37 years.[54] However, when successfully treated, the disorder can remit. Follow-up studies on GAD patients, most of whom received treatment, find that majority of the patients had been symptom free for at least one year at the time of follow-up.[55] The course of GAD was longer in patients with comorbid depressive episodes or substance dependence.[56]

Healthcare professionals should consider how long the worries have been present, whether they span several different topics of concern, and whether they are associated with the physical symptoms listed above. Physical examinations and laboratory testing can help rule-out medical causes of anxiety or the physical symptoms associated with GAD. The possibility of thyroid dysfunction, hypoglycemia, hyperparathyroidism, arrhythmias, chronic obstructive pulmonary disease, seizure disorder, and more rarely pheochromocytoma should be investigated.

Investigate effects related to sympathomimetic, Beta adrenergic agonists, corticosteroids, thyroid hormone, and other drugs along with possible effects of substance use (such as CNS stimulants—caffeine, amphetamines, etc.) and withdrawal from CNS depressants (such as alcohol, sedative hypnotics, etc.). When not associated with other disorders, GAD can often be treated successfully in primary care with the first-line drugs listed above or with referral to psychotherapy. Primary care providers can also successfully advise patients with sleep difficulties on sleep hygiene and teach some of the simple CBT skills.[39] However, in the presence of comorbid major depression, alcohol or substance use disorders, or any other anxiety disorders, referral to a psychiatrist may be indicated.

SUMMARY POINTS

- Substantial distress and disability is associated with GAD
- GAD is often comorbid with other medical and psychiatric disorders
- Antidepressants, such as SSRIs, are generally considered first-line pharmacological options
- Psychotherapy and other psychosocial treatments are also effective in managing GAD
- Preventive approaches are crucial as GAD increases the risk of major depression in its course.

GAD: Summary of NICE Guidelines

Psychological mode of management is more effective than pharmacological therapy and should be used as first-line where possible. Details of the types of therapy recommended and their duration can be found in the NICE guidelines.

- Pharmacological therapy is also effective. Most evidence supports the use of the SSRIs.
- Benzodiazepines' use beyond 2–4 weeks is discouraged.
- SSRI should be used as first-line.
- Self-help (based on CBT principles) should be encouraged.

REFERENCES

1. Nepon J, Belik SL, Bolton J, Sareen J. The relationship between anxiety disorders and suicide attempts: findings from the national epidemiologic survey on alcohol and related conditions. Depress Anxiety. 2010;27:791-8.
2. American Psychiatric Association. Desk Reference to the Diagnostic Criteria from DSM-5. Washington DC:APA. 2013:18.
3. World Health Organization. The ICD-10 classification of mental and behavioral disorders: Diagnostic criteria for research. Geneva: World Health Organization; 1992.
4. Kessler RC, Berglund P, Demler O, Jin R, Merikangas KR, Walters EE. Lifetime prevalence and age-of-onset distributions of DSM-IV disorders in the national comorbidity survey replication. Arch Gen Psychiatry. 2005;62:593-602.
5. Wittchen HU, Zhao S, Kessler RC, Eaton WW, DSM-III-R generalized anxiety disorder in the national comorbidity survey. Arch Gen Psychiatry. 1994;51:355-64.
6. Ormel J, Vonkorff M, Ustun TB, Pini S, Korten A, Oldehinkel T. Common mental disorders and disability across cultures. Results from the WHO Collaborative Study on Psychological Problems in General Health Care. JAMA. 1994;272:1741-8.
7. Wittchen HU, Kessler RC, Beesdo K, Krause P, Hofler M, Hoyer J. Generalized anxiety and depression in primary care: prevalence, recognition, and management. J Clin Psychiatry. 2002;63(Suppl 8):24-34.
8. Ormel J, Koeter MW, van den Brink W, van de Willige G. Recognition, management, and course of anxiety and depression in general practice. Arch Gen Psychiatry. 1991; 48:700-6.
9. Nisenson LG, Pepper CM, Schwenk TL, Coyne JC. The nature and prevalence of anxiety disorders in primary care. Gen Hosp Psychiatry. 1998;20:21-8.
10. Culpepper L. Generalized anxiety disorder and medical illness. J Clin Psychiatry. 2009;70(Suppl 2):20-4.
11. Ballenger JC, Davidson IR, Lecrubier Y, Nutt DJ, Borkovec TD, Rickels K, et al. Consensus statement on generalized anxiety disorder from the International Consensus Group on Depression and Anxiety. J Clin Psychiatry. 2001;62(Suppl 11): 53-8.
12. Olfson M, Fireman B, Weissman MM, Leon AC, Sheehan DV Kathol RG, et al. Mental disorders and disability among patients in a primary care group practice. Am J Psychiatry. 1997;154:1734-40.
13. Hettema JM. The nosologic relationship between generalized anxiety disorder and major depression. Depress Anxiety. 2008; 25:300-16.
14. Mennin DS, Heimberg RG, Fresco DM, Ritter MR. Is generalized anxiety disorder an anxiety or mood disorder? Considering multiple factors as we ponder the fate of GAD. Depress Anxiety. 2008;25:289-99.

15. Bittner A, Goodwin RD, Wittchen HU, Beesdo K, Holfer M, Lieo R. What characteristics of primary anxiety disorders predict subsequent major depressive disorder? Clin Psychiatry. 2004; 65:618-26; quiz 730.
16. Goodwin RD, Gorman IM. Psychopharmacologic treatment of generalized anxiety disorder and the risk of major depression. Am J Psychiatry. 2002;159:1935-7.
17. Hettema JM, Neale MC, Kendler KS. A review and meta-analysis of the genetic epidemiology of anxiety disorders. Am J Psychiatry. 2001;158:1568-78.
18. Molina E, Cervilla J, Rivera M, Torres F, Bellon JA, Moreno B, et al. Polymorphic variation at the serotonin 1-A receptor gene is associated with comorbid depression and generalized anxiety. Psychiatr Genet. 2011;21:195-201.
19. Power KG, Simpson RI, Swanson V, Wallace LA, Feistner ATC, Sharp D. A controlled comparison of cognitive-behaviour therapy, diazepam, and placebo, alone and in combination, for the treatment of generalised anxiety disorder. J Anxirty Disord. 1990;4:267-92.
20. Schuurmans J, Comijs H, Emmelkamp PM, Gandy CM, Weijnen l, van den Hout M, et al. A randomized, controlled trial of the effectiveness of cognitive-behavioral therapy and sertraline versus a waitlist control group for anxiety disorders in older adults Am J Geriatr Psychiatry. 2006;14:255-63.
21. Mitte K. Meta-analysis of cognitive-behavioral treatments for generalized anxiety disorder: a comparison with pharmacotherapy. Psychol Bull. 2005;131:785-95.
22. Hofmann SG, Smits JA. Cognitive behavioral therapy for adult anxiety disorders—a meta-analysis of randomized placebo-controlled trials. J Clin Psychiatry. 2008;69:621-32.
23. Hunot V, Churchill R, Silva de Lima M, Teixeira V. Psychological therapies for generalised anxiety disorder. Cochrane Database Syst Rev. 2007;1:CD001848.
24. Aikins DE, Craske MG. Cognitive theories of generalized anxiety disorder. Psychiatr Clin North Am. 2001;24:57-74.
25. Mathews A, Richards A, Eysenck M. Interpretation of homophones related to threat in anxiety states. J Abnorm Psychol. 1989;98:31-4.
26. Borkovec TD, Whisman MA. Psychosocial treatment for generalized anxiety disorder. In: Mavissakalian MR, Prien RF (Eds). Long-term treatments of anxiety disorders. American Psychiatric Press; 1996: pp. 171-99.
27. Borkovec TD, Newman MG, Castonguay LG. Cognitive-behavioral therapy for generalized anxiety disorder with integrations from interpersonal and experiential therapies. CNS Spectr. 2003;8:382-9.
28. Robinson E, Titov N, Andrews G, Mclntyre K, Schwencke G, Solley K. Internet treatment for generalized anxiety disorder: a randomized controlled trial comparing clinician vs. technician assistance. PLoS One2010;5:e10942.
29. Ost LG, Breitholtz E. Applied relaxation vs. cognitive therapy in the treatment of generalized anxiety disorder. Behav Res Ther. 2000;38:777-90.
30. Arntz A. Cognitive therapy versus applied relaxation as treatment of generalized anxiety disorder, Behav Res Ther. 2003;41:633-46.
31. Hoyer J, Gloster AT. Psychotherapy for generalized anxiety disorder: don't worry, it works! Psychiatr Clin North Am. 2009;32:629-40.
32. Nyklícek I, Kuijpers KF. Effects of mindfulness-based stress reduction intervention on psychological well-being and quality of life: is increased mindfulness indeed the mechanism? Ann Behav Med. 2008;35:331-40.
33. Larzelere MM, Jones GN. Stress and health. Prim Care. 2008;35:839-56.
34. Gratz KL, Weiss NH, Tull MT. Examining Emotion Regulation as an Outcome, Mechanism, or Target of Psychological Treatments. Curr Opin Psychol. 2015;3:85-90.
35. Asmaee Majid S, Seghatoleslam T, Homan H, Akhvast A, Habil H. Effect of mindfulness based stress management on reduction of generalized anxiety disorder. Iran J Public Health. 2012;41:24-8.
36. Salzer S, Winkelbach C, Leweke F, Leibing E, Leichsenring F. Long-term effects of short-term psychodynamic psychotherapy and cognitive-behavioural therapy in generalized anxiety disorder: 12-month follow-up. Can J Psychiatry. 2011;56:503-8.
37. Gellis LA, Lichstein KL. Sleep hygiene practices of good and poor sleepers in the United States: an internet-based study. Behav Ther. 2009;40:1-9.
38. Bartley CA, Hay M, Bloch MH. Meta-analysis: aerobic exercise for the treatment of anxiety disorders. Prog Neuropsychopharmacol Biol Psychiatry. 2013;45:34-9.
39. van Boeijen CA, van Balkom AJ, van Oppen P, Blankenstein N, Cherpanath A, van Dyck R. Efficacy of self-help manuals for anxiety disorders in primary care: a systematic review. Fam Pract. 2005;22:192-6.
40. Spitzer RL, Kroenke K, Williams JB, Löwe B. A brief measure for assessing generalized anxiety disorder: the GAD-7. Arch Intern Med. 2006;166:1092-7.
41. Kendall T, Cape J, Chan M, Taylor C. Guideline Development Group. Management of generalised anxiety disorder in adults: summary of NICE guidance. BMJ. 2011;342:c7460.
42. Baldwin DS, Allgulander C, Bandelow B, Ferre F, Pallanti S. An international survey of reported prescribing practice in the treatment of patients with generalised anxiety disorder. World J Biol Psychiatry. 2012;13:510-6.
43. Baldwin D, Woods R, Lawson R, Taylor D. Efficacy of drug treatments for generalised anxiety disorder: systematic review and meta-analysis. BMJ. 2011;342:d1199.
44. Davidson JR, Zhang W, Connor KM, Ji J, Jobson K, Lecrubier Y, McFarlane AC, Newport DJ, Nutt DJ, Osser DN, Stein DJ, Stowe ZN, et al. A psychopharmacological treatment algorithm for generalised anxiety disorder (GAD). J Psychopharmacol. 2010;24:3-26.
45. Lenox-Smith AJ, Reynolds A. A double-blind, randomised, placebo-controlled study of venlafaxine XL in patients with

generalised anxiety disorder in primary care. Br J Gen Pract. 2003;53:772-7.

46. Gale CK, Millichamp J. Generalised anxiety disorder. BMJ Clin Evid. 2011;2:1002.
47. Montgomery SA. Pregabalin for the treatment of generalised anxiety disorder. Expert Opin Pharmacother. 2006;7: 2139-54.
48. Garcia-Monco JC1, Cortina IE, Ferreira E, Martínez A, Ruiz L, Cabrera A, Beldarrain MG. Reversible splenial lesion syndrome (RESLES): what's in a name? J Neuroimaging. 2011;21:e1-14.
49. Van Ameringen M, Mancini C, Pipe B, Bennett M. Antiepileptic drugs in the treatment of anxiety disorders: role in therapy. Drugs. 2004;64:2199-220.
50. Loane C, Politis M. Buspirone: what is it all about? Brain Res. 2012;1461:111-8.
51. Bandelow B1, Zohar J, Hollander E, Kasper S, Möller HJ. WFSBP Task Force on Treatment Guidelines for Anxiety, Obsessive-Compulsive and Post-Traumatic Stress Disorders. World Federation of Societies of Biological Psychiatry (WFSBP) guidelines for the pharmacological treatment of anxiety, obsessive-compulsive and post-traumatic stress disorders- first revision. World J Biol Psychiatry. 2008;9: 248-312.
52. Huh J, Goebert D, Takeshita J, Lu BY, Kang M. Treatment of generalized anxiety disorder: a comprehensive review of the literature for psychopharmacologic alternatives to newer antidepressants and benzodiazepines. Prim Care Companion CNS Disord. 2011;13.
53. Hershenberg R, Gros DF, Brawman-Mintzer O. Role of atypical antipsychotics in the treatment of generalized anxiety disorder. CNS Drugs. 2014;28:519-33.
54. Miloyan B, Pachana NA. Clinical significance of worry and physical symptoms in late-life generalized anxiety disorder. Int J Geriatr Psychiatry. 2015;6:78.
55. Sibrava NJ, Beard C, Bjornsson AS, Moitra E, Weisberg RB, Keller MB. Two-year course of generalized anxiety disorder, social anxiety disorder, and panic disorder in a longitudinal sample of African American adults. J Consult Clin Psychol. 2013;81:1052-62.
56. Locke AB, Kirst N, Shultz CG. Diagnosis and management of generalized anxiety disorder and panic disorder in adults. Am Fam Physician. 2015;91:617-24.

CHAPTER

12 Obsessive-Compulsive Disorder

Christoday RJ Khess, Roshan V Khanande, Bhoomika Sachacher, Summant Khanna

INTRODUCTION

Obsessive-compulsive disorder (OCD) is a commonly reported, chronic, and debilitating disorder characterized by obsessions and/or compulsions which are ego dystonic, intrusive and purposeless, and imparts significant distress not only to the suffering individual but also to his family. OCD, traditionally, was considered a disorder without any treatment but, research in last few decades have unrivalled mysteries of epidemiological, pathophysiological and pharmacotherapeutic aspects of the disorder.[1]

After 1980s, various studies started reporting response to serotonergic medications in OCD. On one hand clomipramine a tricyclic antidepressant (TCA) with serotonergic properties was found to be promising, and on the other, nonserotonergic TCAs were ineffective in OCD. Over the years, research has revealed that OCD seems to have a very specific profile as compared to other psychiatric disorders. Its specific response to serotonergic drugs has set in motion various researches in the areas of pathophysiology of OCD and related disorders.[2]

There is strong evidence suggesting genetic basis for OCD[3] which has led to search in the area endophenotype, cognitive and electrophysiological.

CLINICAL FEATURES

Obsessive-compulsive disorder (OCD) is a disorder with varied and unique symptomatology. The affected individual can have both obsessions and/or compulsions. Obsessions are thoughts, images, or impulses which are repetitive, intrusive, and disturbing to the individual, who considers them purposeless. Obsessions are often disagreeable and raise an individual's anxiety. Whereas compulsions are acts, mental and/or behavioral, in response to the obsessions performed to reduce anxiety. Opposition in carrying out compulsion increases anxiety. Usually the individual is made to perform compulsions against his/her will. The individual usually realizes that both obsessions and compulsions are ego dystonic. Obsessions or compulsions that cause great distress, are time consuming (more than 1 hour/day), and/or significantly hinder regular day-to-day activities. During the course of the disorder, at some juncture, the affected individual must have recognized the obsessions and compulsions were excessive and/or purposeless, not necessarily during current visit or presentation. This norm is inapplicable to children as they may not possess the cognitive ability to understand what is happening with them. If during current presentation resistance, anxiety for obsessions and/or compulsions is absent, the diagnosis could be referred to as OCD with poor insight.

Nearly three-fourth of the affected individuals report both obsessions and compulsions. The symptoms may change over the course of the disorder. OCD can present itself with different symptoms—checking, religious, sexual or dirt-contamination obsessions, and washing, ordering or counting compulsions.

The most common clinical presentation is obsessional doubt of contamination by dirt or germs. An affected individual owing to his doubt feels that his hands, clothes or his belongings are contaminated, and would never be satisfied by cleaning them as per common societal ways.

The second common clinical presentation is obsessional doubt along with compulsive checking. This behavior of the affected individual can have range of presentation from checking door locks multiple times to driving past a same site repeatedly to see whether they have hurt someone.

Obsessive-compulsive disorder (OCD) in some individuals can present with intrusive thoughts and/or images of some sexual or violent act. These sexual images can be blasphemous. Often it is seen that the affected individual avoids stimulus that might arouse such images/thoughts. In these individuals, mental compulsions are frequently reported.

At times it is seen that patients take long hours to perform an act, or asking family members to answer a question numerous times in a particular way as per their satisfaction in an never ending effort to get 'just right' result. This is to get things done just the way they want it to—'just right phenomenon'. An example, a patient repeatedly asks same question to her mother in order to receive exactly the same answer with respect to words used and the tone of the voice.

The greatest agony to the individuals suffering with OCD is the perceived irrationality of the symptoms on one hand, and the unsurpassable desire to yield to these symptoms on the other.

Research has indicated that some obsessions and compulsions tend to co-occur. There are five main dimensions commonly seen:[4]

1. Obsessions for considering himself/herself accountable for failing to prevent or causing harm; reassurance-seeking and checking compulsions.
2. Obsessions for symmetry, ordering and counting rituals.
3. Obsessional doubt of contamination, and washing and cleaning compulsions.
4. Obsessions concerning sex, violence, and religion which are disgusting for the sufferer.
5. Hoarding obsessions which are related to taking possession of and retaining objects, and collecting compulsions.

Relevance of these five dimensions across ages, from childhood through adulthood, has been backed by recent research.[5-7]

OBSESSIVE-COMPULSIVE DISORDER AND ITS RELATIONSHIP WITH SCHIZOPHRENIA

Obsessive-compulsive disorder (OCD) symptoms are almost reported in 25% of the patients with schizophrenia. And among them nearly 15% fulfil diagnostic criterion for OCD. OCD symptoms can be a part of schizophrenia prodrome; associated symptom of presentation; or drug induced (antipsychotics). Presence of OCD in the patients with schizophrenia is considered to be poor prognostic factor. Prospective follow-up studies have demonstrated diagnostic stability of this entity. When patients with schizophrenia present with OCD they tend to respond to unique combination of antipsychotic and serotonin reuptake inhibitors. All the research till date backs the existence of a new diagnostic category, 'Schizo-Obsessive', which might be of clinical utility in future.[2]

PREVALENCE, DEMOGRAPHIC FEATURES, AND COMORBIDITY

When compared with other anxiety or mood disorders, the individuals with OCD are less likely to get married, remain unemployed, and experience dysfunction at social and occupational levels.[8] OCD has a lifetime prevalence rate of 2–3%.[9] However, in child and adolescent population it is reported to be more common in boys as compared to girls.[10] Similar trend is not seen in adult population. The disorder usually starts gradually, often following stressors. It tends to run a chronic course if not treated.[11,12] The symptoms usually start appearing during late adolescence or early adulthood, even though it can start in childhood or late adulthood.[13] Clinical presentation of the disorder in children is no different from adults.[1]

Obsessive-compulsive disorder (OCD) has been reported and identified in many different ethnic groups all over world.[14] Across nations the prevalence rate differ which at times difficult to explain. Some of the reasons cited are obvious cultural differences and freeness with which a suffering individual can seek medical help without getting stigmatized. Some of the main features of OCD are reported consistently over time and, region; for example, obsessions about breaking inviolable social rules and beliefs, mainly related to aggression and sexual behavior.[15,16] But, culture is strong enough a factor to affect content of obsessions and compulsive behavior.[17] For an example, blasphemous thoughts and images, compulsive praying would be more common in ethnic groups than less religious groups because of obvious cultural influence in the earlier.[18]

At least 50% of people with OCD suffer from one other psychological illness—a comorbid anxiety disorder, most commonly (e.g. phobias) or depressive disorder.[18,19] 20–30% of OCD patients report current or past history of tics.[1] Substance abuse and dependence, especially alcohol is found to be more common among OCD patients than general population.[8]

ETIOLOGY

Neurochemistry and Neuroanatomy

Historically response to serotonin reuptake inhibitors in OCD has been a proof for serotonin system dysfunction in the disorder.[20] Moreover, serotonin system abnormality is considered to be cause for not only OCD but also for many other psychiatric disorders. And that brings us to the difficult to answer question, which part of serotonin system dysfunction is responsible for OCD and why it represents such a diverse symptomatology. Hypersensitivity of postsynaptic serotonin receptors has been associated with obsessive-compulsive disorder as per major research findings.[21] Serotonin transporter (5-HTT) gene and serotonin receptor (5HT2A) gene dysfunction has been reported,[22] however, the research lacks consistent findings.[23] Research in OCD has also implicated dysfunctional glutamate system responsible for its debilitating symptoms.[24] Preliminary research have tentatively named few of the responsible genes—Sapap[25,26] and SLC1A1[27-29] in the disorder. Dopamine system has also been researched with inconclusive findings.[30]

Some of the brain areas, the orbitostriatal area including the caudate nucleus and the dorsolateral prefrontal cortex has been repeatedly shown to be of major influence in governing few of the cognitive processes such as response inhibition and planning. In OCD, similar cognitive faculties have been found impaired.[31] Moreover, a recently conducted meta-analysis of brain imaging in adults has pointed towards abnormal functioning of the orbital cortex and the caudate nucleus in individuals with obsessive-compulsive symptoms.[32] Similar results have also been found for studies on children.[33] Some of the studies have also reported white matter abnormalities in frontal region in individuals with OCD which is consistent with the frontal lobe dysfunction hypothesis for OCD.[34,35] Figure 1 illustrate the orbitosubcortical circuits those connecting regions of the brain related with OCD symptoms. Over activity of the direct pathway is thought to be associated with obsessive-compulsive symptoms.

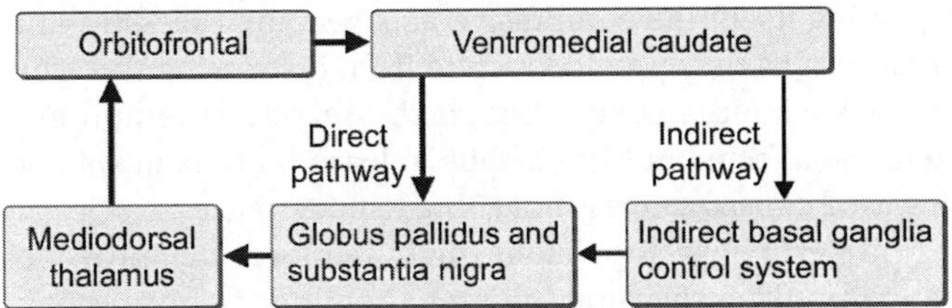

Fig. 1: Direct (thick arrows) and indirect (thin arrows) pathways connecting neuroanatomical structures related to the symptoms of obsessive-compulsive disorder

Genetic Factors

First-degree family members of individuals with OCD are more likely to suffer from OCD as compared to normal controls.[36] 27–47% of variance in score on measures of obsessive-compulsive symptoms is attributed to genetic factors as suggested by twin studies on adult OCD patients.[37,38] The rest 53–73% of the variance is thought to be because of environment factors. In studies conducted on children the variance due to genetic factors increases to 45–65%.[38] No gender difference exists in heritability of childhood-onset OCD and adult onset OCD.[39,40]

Autoimmunity

A set of clinical conditions called pediatric autoimmune neuropsychiatry disorders associated with streptococcal infection (PANDAS) is associated childhood-onset OCD.[41] Basal ganglia inflammation is suppose to be the reason for obsessive-compulsive symptoms in these cases. For few of such cases, obsessive-compulsive symptoms may respond to antibiotic treatment if identified early in the course of the illness.[42] But, infection associated OCD accounts for not more than 10% of early-onset OCD patients,[43] hinting towards multiple other possible causes for the disorder.

Biological Models

Obsessive-compulsive disorder (OCD) phenomenology can have varied presentations which raises the question whether we can imagine single model explaining causality for OCD, or whether different presentations require seemingly varied explanations. Indeed, separate models might be thought of to encompass different phenomenological presentations of OCD, as all the OCD presentations can never be explained by direct pathway over activity (Fig. 1) or frontal lobe dysfunction. Empirical studies have provided some support for biological models, but it fails to clarify why one patient with OCD develops obsession for dirt and contamination, and another suffers from repetitive blasphemous thoughts. Individual differences in learning might be of certain value in development of array of obsessive-compulsive symptoms in individuals with putative biological abnormalities. If environmental influence is one of the determining factors in the presentation of OCD symptomatology, then biological models deciphering OCD needs reshaping, taking into account the interplay between biological systems and environment.[32,37]

Cognitive and Behavioral Models

Of the existing psychological models of obsessive-compulsive disorder, empirical support is for the cognitive-behavioral approach, which proposes dysfunctional beliefs as the root cause for development of obsessions and compulsions, and the strength with which it is held determine the risk of developing obsessions and compulsions.[44-46] At the center for this models is the well-established finding that most people in the general population experience unwanted cognitive intrusions (unpleasant thoughts that intrude into consciousness).[47] These cognitive intrusions have been found similar to obsessions experienced by patients with OCD.

For example, cognitive intrusions might consist of thoughts of killing one's family or useless thoughts of blurting out obscenities to people in authority. Studies have indicated that these everyday intrusions are highly unacceptable or immoral, personally important, or poses a risk for which an individual with OCD considers himself/herself personally liable.[48,49] For example, if we consider the despised, invasive image of stabbing one's child with a vegetable knife. Cognitive intrusion such as this would be considered as pointless incidents with no associated danger by most people. As per cognitive behavioral model if an individual assigns excessive importance to it, and takes undue responsibility for such cognitive intrusion, it evolves into an obsession: "Harboring images of stabbing my child is indication of my deranged mental state; I might kill my child". Now one such unnecessary thought is given excessive importance, the individual would try to reduce associated anxiety by resisting the thought or would try to change it with a different nonunpleasant one. This gives rise to compulsions.

According to this view, compulsive rituals are product of attempts to remove intrusions and to stop any perceived harmful consequences from happening. As per cognitive-behavioral model these are building blocks for vicious cycle repeating itself; the compulsive acts become excessive and persistent as they provide respite from distressing thoughts and associated anxiety, though the respite is temporary. Here the affected individual fails to learn that the unwanted despised consequence is not going to materialize.

Interestingly compulsions might reinforce the intrusion, i.e. compulsion by functioning as reminder of obsession. For example, washing hands (compulsion) might just work as a reminder—"oh! My hands are dirty". Similarly, when an individual tries to distract himself by replacing intrusive thought with another; the replacement thought can become reminder of the initial intrusive thought. For an individual with OCD repeated completion of compulsive acts gives rise to the belief that execution of the compulsive act prevents the dreaded consequence from happening and which intern feed the perceived responsibility to perform compulsions to prevent harmful consequences. Figure 2 depicts the cognitive-behavioral model of OCD.

The cognitive-behavioral model gives the liberty to attend to individual specific intrusive images, thoughts, impulses and behavior along with their learning experiences. So, this model is able to explain, to some extent, the diversity in the presentation of the disorder. To quote an example, a person who takes his religion seriously would be disgusted on experiencing blasphemous thoughts and would definitely be at greater risk for developing religious obsessions than a person who does not take his faith seriously. Cross-sectional, experimental, and prospective studies have supported cognitive-behavioral approach.[48,49] But, this approach fails to explain all the presentations of OCD, as research have shown that some of the individuals with OCD score at par with the unaffected individuals on scales measuring such appraisals and beliefs.[50] As both biological and cognitive-behavioral models of OCD, to some extent, have succeeded in explaining OCD symptomatology, a theoretical approaches taking both the models into consideration is needed.[51]

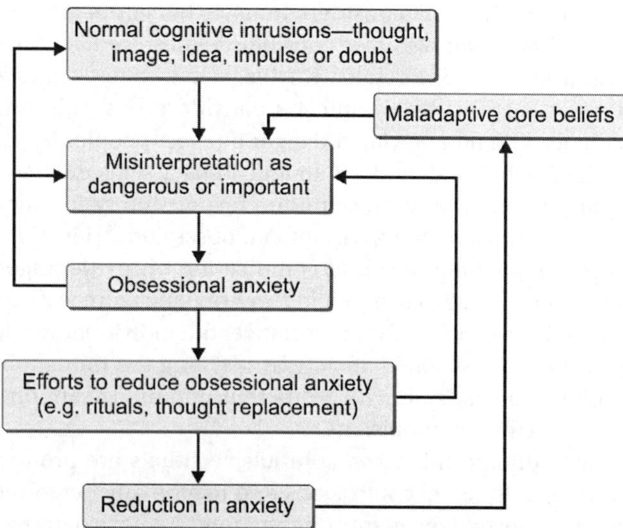

Fig. 2: Cognitive-behavioral model of OCD

Classification Controversies

There is a debate over whether OCD should be classified separately as it is there in DSM-5 or it should be classified as an anxiety disorder along with others of that group.[50] Its classification under obsessive-compulsive-related disorders in DSM-5 does not mean that the patients with OCD are not anxious, however it implies that OCD has more in common with obsessive-compulsive-related disorders than anxiety disorders. This school of thought also asserts similarity at the level of circuits and neurotransmitters, comorbidity, inheritance, and response to treatments.[52]

The other side of argument differs significantly from the just stated one on both empirical and conceptual understanding of OCD.[53] Supporters of the category-obsessive-compulsive-related disorders suggest that OCD and related disorders share similar type of symptoms, for example, repetitive behavior.

As per some researchers comorbidities presenting with OCD does not support a different category.[54,55] This group of researchers stress the fact that OCD usually presents itself with mood and anxiety disorders.[56]

The opponents of obsessive-compulsive-related disorders category express their concern regarding phenomenological difference between repetitive behavior in OCD and impulse control disorders. In OCD repetitive behavior is for reducing anxiety and the repetitive behavior of trichotillomania is for pleasure-seeking.[57] They also oppose the idea entertaining any relation between OCD and related disorders concerning neurobiological correlates,[58,59] genetic transmission,[52] and response to psychological or pharmacological treatment.[60-62]

Treatment

Pharmacotherapy

Response to treatment in OCD started with serotonin reuptake inhibitors (SRIs) clomipramine. In comparison to other less potent SRIs clomipramine has been found effective in OCD.[63-65]

As per a meta-analysis effective pharmacotherapy for OCD includes SRI such as clomipramine and some selective serotonin reuptake inhibitors (SSRIs).[66] The mean effect size for OCD symptoms in 18 randomized-controlled trials studied for SRI was 0.91. This is a large effect size as per comprehensive OCD pharmacotherapy meta-analysis.[66] Yet, even after adequate trial most of the initial responders showed residual symptoms. Relapse after discontinuation of medication was almost inevitable. It varied from medication to medication. It was modest 24% for sertraline,[67] and ranged from 31% to 89% for clomipramine.[68,69] These values are much higher than the 12% relapse after completion of exposure response prevention therapy.[70] Most of the patients do respond to medications but often the improvement is short lasting with lingering residual symptoms.

Meta-analysis of pharmacotherapy of pediatric OCD, mainly for four SSRIs (fluvoxamine, paroxetine, sertraline, and fluoxetine) together with clomipramine,[71] as expected, revealed that the treatment was better than placebo. However, with mean effect size of 0.46, pharmacotherapy was modestly effective. Most of the patients responded partially to the medications.

Other Pharmacological Treatment Approaches

Addition of atypical antipsychotics (risperidone or quetiapine) to SRI treatment has been found effective in treating OCD in patients with personal or family history of tic disorder.[72] Highly potent typical antipsychotics (haloperidol or pimozide) when added to SSRI treatment have shown effectiveness in reducing OCD symptoms.[73] As per a meta-analysis of OCD pharmacotherapy studies patients having residual symptoms even after 3-month treatment with SSRIs at maximal tolerated dose showed significant improvement with addition of an antipsychotic medication.[74]

Glutamate system dysregulation in OCD has been reported in recent years. Riluzole an antiglutamateric agents has been tried in treatment of OCD with modest effect on OCD symptoms.[75,76]

Psychological Treatments

Various modes of psychological intervention have been tried in treating OCD. Some of the cognitive behavioral techniques used are thought stopping, flooding, aversive conditioning, desensitization and, exposure and response prevention. Cognitive behavioral approaches are one of the most promising psychological treatment modalities and tend to show long lasting effects.[77] Even neuroimaging studies have reported similar changes in cerebral metabolism in the patients treated by behavioral therapies as compared to pharmacotherapy.[78]

In exposure and response prevention, exposure implies repeated systematic exposure to anxiety provoking stimulus and response prevention demands stopping the anxiety reducing compulsive behaviors and rituals. For example, an individual harboring dirt and contamination obsessions is made to face situations where he feels exposed to dirt, provoking anxiety, and at the same time he is not allowed to perform washing behavior, i.e. compulsive behavior. The purpose of exposure and response prevention is all about provoking anxiety and making patient understand that it is not going to last forever; once it starts, it has to come down. Exposure and response prevention also impart patients with confidence to face and bare anxiety. It also serves as a meaningful tool to correct the faulty cognition—if (obsessions) not acted upon bad things will happen.[79,80]

In thought stopping the individual is taught to say 'stop' or apply aversive stimulus to self when faced with obsessional thoughts. He can even imagine a signpost reading 'stop' or change the image to something which is nonanxiety provoking.

The only psychological treatment gaining empirical support in treating OCD is exposure and response prevention, a form of cognitive-behavioral therapy.[79] whoever, along with ERP supportive psychotherapy might be helpful in improving adjustment and functionality. Family therapy has a definite place in the management of patients facing marital problems.[81]

Studied using Yale Brown obsessive-compulsive scale (Y-BOCS)[82] have repeatedly shown the effectiveness of ERP over other forms of psychotherapy and placebos.[83-87] These findings have also been validated by large effect size seen in Meta-analyses for trials of ERP in adults [88-90] and children.[91,92] Though effective, ERP induces severe anxiety in the recipients resulting into as high as 25% drop out rate.[93] If the research has to be believed the ERP has lasting therapeutic effects, even up to 2 years.[79]

Pharmacotherapy versus Exposure and Response Prevention

Study conducted by Foa[86] compared ERP with clomipramine monotherapy, the combination of clomipramine and ERP, and placebo. EPR managed to reduce Y-BOCS[82] scores by 55%, where clomipramine monotherapy alone managed 31% reduction in Y-BOCS scores. Surprisingly, the combination of clomipramine and ERP worked better, reducing Y-BOCS scores by 58%. The combination therapy was found to be effective than clomipramine monotherapy, but slightly less effective than ERP alone. All the treatment modalities were found to be better than placebo as per Y-BOCS scores.

On the whole, findings from randomized controlled trials speak volumes about the effectiveness of ERP in reducing OCD symptoms.

Surgery and Deep Brain Stimulation

Surgical interventions are often retained for OCD patients who have been refractory to both pharmacological and psychological treatments. Surgical procedures are planned at targeting tracts connecting different areas of brain involved in production of OCD symptoms.[94] Surgical targets are areas such as anterior cingulotomy, subcaudate tractotomy, limbic leucotomy and anterior capsulotomy. Nevertheless, individual safety and effectiveness of such invasive procedures remains a big issue; research in the areas of noninvasive treatment modalities is gaining pace in recent years.[94] Basal ganglia stimulation called deep brain stimulation by surgically placed electrodes have shown promising results to start with;

the safety and efficacy of such a specific intervention poses a difficult question.[95] A portable, easy to administer and non-invasive brain stimulation technique- Repetitive Transcranial Magnetic Stimulation (RTMS), which alters electrical activity of the brain by placing external electromagnet over particular area of the scalp approximated to a particular brain region has shown promise in treating OCD. Still not yet studied thoroughly, initial reports testing its effectiveness in OCD are not promising.[96]

CONCLUSION

From considered to be demonic possession in 15th century, OCD and psychiatry have come a long way. Jean Dominique Esquirol in the early part of 20th century described a disorder similar to OCD, he called it monomania. From virtually no remedy to current research in its treatment a lot has happened since we started using clomipramine in 1980s for OCD. Search for its etiology has brought forward various models and theories, none explaining it holistically however, it has helped us in understanding the elusive disorder. SRIs are now main stay of treatment in OCD. Drugs like sertraline, fluoxetine, fluvoxamine, paroxetine, clomipramine have been found effective in treating OCD. Cognitive and behavioral therapy has emerged as one of the most promising modalities available. ERP along with pharmacotherapy has gained support as the most effective approach for OCD treatment. Research has branched out in the areas of pediatric OCD (POCD) and obsessive-compulsive-related disorders. As the pool of symptoms remains constant for different age groups, the approach in treating POCD follows that of adult OCD. The classification change for OCD in DSM-5 has hardly affected its treatment approach.

With the turn of the century, in the past decade or so, even new modes of treating OCD have come-up. From psychosurgery to deep brain stimulation, from ECT to RTMS, the available treatment tools have become more sophisticated and less harmful to the patients. The range of drugs available to clinicians treating OCD is like never before. The future looks promising.

From no treatment to difficult to treat, OCD still remains a challenge for the clinicians and researchers alike. Current and future research will pave the way for better treatment for the patients with OCD.

REFERENCES

1. American Psychiatric Association. Diagnostic and statistical manual of mental disorders, 4th edition. Washington, DC; 2000.
2. OTP Zohar J, Fostich L, Juven-Wetzler E. Obsessive-compulsive disorder. In: Gelder MC, Andreasen NC, Lopez-Ibor Jr. JJ, Geddes JR (Eds). New Oxford Textbook of Psychiatry, Oxford University Press, New York; 2011.pp.765-73.
3. Hanna GL, Himle JA, Curtis GC, et al. A family study of obsessive-compulsive disorder with pediatric probands. Am J Med Genet B Neuropsychiatr Genet. 2005;134:13-9.
4. McKay D, Abramowitz J, Calamari J, et al. A critical evaluation of obsessive-compulsive disorder subtypes: symptoms versus mechanisms. Clin Psychol Rev. 2004;24:283-313.
5. Mataix-Cols D, Rosario-Campos M, Leckman J. A multi-dimensional model of obsessive-compulsive disorder. Am J Psychiatry. 2005;162;228-38.
6. Stewart SE, Rosario MC, Baer L, et al. Four-factor structure of obsessive-compulsive disorder symptoms in children, adolescents, and adult. J Am Acad Child Adolesc Psychiatry. 2008;47:763-72.
7. Abramowitz J, Wheaton M, Storch A. The status of hoarding as a symptom of obsessive-compulsive disorder. Behav Res Ther. 2008;46:1026-33.
8. Torres A, Prince M, Bebbington P, et al. Obsessive-compulsive disorder, prevalence, comorbidity, impact, and help-seeking in the British National Psychiatric Comorbidity Survey of 2000. Am J Psychiatr. 2006;163:1978-85.
9. Kessler R, Berglund P, Demler O, Jin R, Walters E. Lifetime prevalence and age-of-onset distributions of DSM-IV disorders in the National Comorbidity Survery Replication. Arch Gen Psychiarty. 2005;62:593-602.
10. Geller D. Obsessive-compulsive and spectrum disorders in children and adolescents. Psychiatr Clin North Am. 2006;29: 353-70.
11. Mataix-Cols D, Rauch S, Baer I, et al. Symptom stability in adult obsessive-compulsive disorder: data form a naturalistic two-year follow-up study. Am J Psychiatry. 2002;159:263-68.
12. Stewart S, Geller D, Jenike M, et al. Long-term outcome of pediatric obsessive-compulsive disorder: a meta-analysis and qualitative review of the literature. Acta Psychiatr Scand. 2004; 110:4-13.
13. Heyman I, Formbonne E, Simmons H, Ford T, Meltzer H, Goodman R. Prevalence of obsessive-compulsive disorder in the British nationwide survey of child mental health. Int Rev Psychiatry. 2003;15:178-84.
14. Fontenelle LF, Mendlowicz MV, Versiani M. The descriptive epidemiology of obsessive-compulsive disorder. Prog Neuropsychopharmacol Biol Psychiatry. 2006;30:327-37.
15. Spitzer M, Sigmund D. The phenomenology of obsessive-compulsive disorder. Int Rev Psychiatry. 1997;9:7-14.
16. Alvarenga PG, Hounie Ag, Mercadante MT, Miguel EC, Concicao M. Obsessive-compulsive disorder. A historical overview. In: Storch E, Geffken GR, Murphy TK (Eds). Handbook of child and adolescent obsessive-compulsive disorder. Mahwah, NJ: Erlbaum; 2007.pp.1-15.
17. Pallanti S. Transcultural observations of obsessive-compulsive disorder. Am J Psychiatry. 2008;165:169-70.
18. Vishne T, Misgav S, Bunzel ME. Psychiatric disorders related to menstrual bleeding among an ultra-orthodox population: case series and literature review. Int J Soc Psychiatry. 2008;54: 219-24.

19. Steketee G, Barlow D. Obsessive-compulsive disorder. In: Barlow DH (Ed). Anxiety and its disorders. 2nd edition. New York Guilford; 2002. pp. 516-50.
20. Lozez-Ibor M. Research on obsessive-compulsive disorder. Curr Opin Psychiatry. 2003;16 (Suppl 2):S85-S91.
21. Gross R, Sasson Y, Chopra M, Zohar J. Biological models of obsessive-compulsive disorder. The serotonin hypothesis. In: Swinson RP, Antony MM, Rachman S, Richter MA (Eds). Obsessive-compulsive disorder: theory, research, and treatment, New York: Guilford; 1998.pp.141-53.
22. Greenberg B, Banjamin J, Martin J, et al. Delayed obsessive-compulsive disorder symptom exacerbation after a single dose of serotonin antagonist in fluoxetine-treated but not untreated patients. Psychopharmacology. 2000;140:434-44.
23. Saiz P, Garcia-Portilla M, Prango C, et al. Association study between obsessive-compulsive disorder and serotonin candidate genes. Prog Neuropsychopharmacol Biol Psychiatry. 2008;32:765-70.
24. Griest JH, Jefferson JW, Kobak KA, Katzelnick DJ, Serilin RC. Efficacy and tolerability of serotonin transport inhibitors in obsessive-compulsive disorder. A meta-analysis. Arch Gen Psychiatry. 1995;52:53-60.
25. Chakrabatry K, Bhattacharyya S, Christopher R, Khanna S. Glutamatergic dysfunction in OCD. Neuropsychopharmacology. 2005;30:1735-40.
26. Welch JM, Lu J, Rodriguiz RM, et al. Cortico-striatal synaptic defects and OCD-like behaviours in Sapap3-mutant mice. Nature. 2007:448:894-900.
27. Arnold PD, Sicard T, Burroughs E, RIchter MA, Kennedy JL. Glutamate transporter gene *SLC1A1* Associated with obsessive-compulsive disorder. Arch Gen Psychiatry. 2006;63: 769-76.
28. Dickel DE, Veenstra-Vander Weele J, Cox NJ, et al. Association testing of the positional and functional candidate gene *SLC1A1/EAAC1* in early-onset obsessive-compulsive disorder. Arch Gen Psychiatry. 2006;63:778-85.
29. Stewart SE, Fagerness JA, Platko J, et al. Association of the *SLC1A1* glutamate transporter gene and obsessive-compulsive disorder. Am J Med Genet B Neuropsychiatr Genet. 2007;144B: 1027-33.
30. Camarena B, Loyzaga C, Aguilar A, Weissbecker K, Nicolini H. Association study between the dopamine receptor D-sub-4 gene and obsessive-compulsive disorder. Eur Neuropsychopharmacology. 2007;17:406-09.
31. Rauch S, Whalen P, Dougherty D, Jenike M. Neurobiologic models of obsessive-compulsive disorder. In: Jenike MA, Baer L, Minichiello WE (Eds). Obsessive-compulsive disorders: practical management. St Louis, MoM Mosby; 1998. pp. 222-53.
32. Whiteside S, Port J, Abramowitz J. A meat-analysis of functional neuromaging in obsessive-compulsive disorder. Psychiatr Res Neuroimag. 2004;132:69-79.
33. MacMaster FP, O'Neill J, Rosenberg DR. Brain imaging in pediatric obsessive-compulsive disorder. J Am Acad Child Adolesc Psychiatry. 2008;47:1262-72.
34. Menzies L, Williams GB, Chamberlain SR, et al. White matter abnormalities in patients with obsessive compulsive disorder and their first-degree relatives, AM J Psychiatry. 2008;32:1221-6.
35. Nakamae K, Narumoto J, Shibata K, et al. Alteration of fractional anisotropy and apparent diffusion coefficient in Prog Neuropsychopharmacol Biol Psychiatry. 2008;32:1221-6.
36. Hettema J, Neale M, Kendler K. A review and meta-analysis of the genetic epidemiology of anxiety disorders. Am J Psychiatry. 2001;158:1568-78.
37. Van Grootheest D, Cath D, Deekman A, Boomsma D. Genetic and environmental influences on obsessive-compulsive symptoms in adults: population-based twin-family study. Psychol Med. 2007;37:1635-44.
38. Van Grootheest DS, Cath DC, Beekman AT, Boomsma DI. Twin studies on obsessive-compulsive disorder: a review. Twin Res Human Genet. 2005;8:450-8.
39. Rosario-Campos MC, Leckman JF, Curi M, et al. A family study of early-onset obsessive-compulsive disorder. Am J Med Genet B Neuropsychiatr Genet. 2005;136B;92-97.
40. Nestadt G, Samuels J, Riddle M, et al. A family study of obsessive-compulsive disorder. Arch Gen Psychiatry. 2000;57: 358-63.
41. da Rocha FF, Correa H, Teixeira AL. Obsessive-compulsive disorder and immunology: a review. Prog Neuropsychopharm Biol Psychiatry. 2008;32:1139-46.
42. Swedo S. Genetics of childhood disorders: XXXIII. Autoimmunity, part 6: poststreptococcal autoimmunity. J Am Acad Child Adolesc Psychiatry. 2001;40:1479-82.
43. Trifiletti R, Packard A. Immune mechanisms in pediatric neuropsychiatric disorders: Tourette's syndrome, OCD, and PANDAS. Child Adolesc Psychiatr Clin N Am. 1999;8:767-75.
44. Rachman S. A cognitive theory of obsessions. Behav Res Ther. 1997;35:793-802.
45. Rachman S. A cognitive theory of obsessions: elaborations. Behav Res Ther. 1998;36:385-401.
46. Salkovskis P. Obsessional-compulsive problems: a cognitive-behavioral analysis. Behav Res Ther. 1985;23:571-83.
47. Gibbs N. Nonclinical populations in research on obsessive-compulsive disorder. Clin Psychol Rev. 1996;16:729-73.
48. Abramowitz J, Khandker M, Nelson C, Deacon B, Rygwall R. The role of cognitive factors in the pathogenesis of obsessions and compulsions; a prospective study. Behav Res Ther. 2006;44: 1361-74.
49. Abramowitz J. Nelson C, Rygwall R, Khandker M. The cognitive mediation of obsessive-compulsive symptoms: a longitudinal study. J Anxiety Disord. 2007;21:91-104.
50. Taylor S, Abramowitz JS, McKay D, et al. Do dysfunctional beliefs play a role in all types of obsessive-compulsive disorder? J Anxiety Disord. 2005;20:85-97.
51. Abramowitz JS. Understanding and treating obsessive-compulsive disorder: a cognitive-behavioral approach. Mahwah, NJ: Erlbaum; 2006.
52. Hollander E, Braun A, SImeon D. Should OCD leave the anxiety disorders in DSM-5? The case for obsessive compulsive-related disorders. Depress Anxiety. 2008;25:317-29.

53. Storch E, Abramowitz J, Goodman W. Where does obsessive-compulsive disorder belong in DSM-5? Depress Anxiety. 2008;25:336-47.
54. Bienvenu O, Samuels J, Riddle M, et al. The relationship of obsessive-compulsive disorder to possible spectrum disorders: results from a family study. Biol Psychiatry. 2000;48:287-93.
55. Jaisoorya T, Teddy Y, Srinath S. The relationship of obsessive compulsive disorder and affective disorder in the family study. Biol Psychiatry. Biol Psychiatry. 2005;58:429-34.
56. Nestadt G, Samuels J, Riddle M, et al. The relationship between obsessive-compulsive disorder and anxiety and affective disorders: results from the Johns Hopkins OCD Family Study. Psychol Med. 2001;31:481-7.
57. Grant J, Potenza M. Impulse control disorders: Clinical characteristics and pharmacological management. Ann Clin Psychiatry. 2004;16:27-34.
58. O'Sullivan R, Rauch S, Brieter H. Reduced basal ganglia volumes in trichotillomania measured via morphometric MRI. Biol Psychiatry. 1997;42:39-45.
59. Stein D, Coetzer R, Lee M. Magnetic resonance brain imaging in women with obsessive-compulsive disorder and trichotillomania. Psychiatr Res. 1997;74:177-82.
60. Christenson G, Mackenzie T, Mitchell J, Callies A. A placebo-controlled, double-blind crossover study of fluoxetine in trichotillomania. Am J Psychiatry. 1991;148:1566-71.
61. Ninan P, Rothbaum B, Marsteller F, Kinght B, Eccard M. A placebo-controlled trial of cognitive-behavioral therapy and clomipramine in trichotillomania. J Clin Psychiatry. 2000;61: 47-50.
62. Van Minnen A, Hoogduin K, Keijsers G, Hellenbrand I, Hendriks G. Treatment of trichotillomania with behavioural therapy of Fluoxetine: a randomized, waiting-list controlled study. Arch Gen Psychiatry. 2003;60:517-22.
63. OTP 7 Zohar J, Insel T. Obsessive-Compulsive disorder: psychobiological approaches to diagnosis, treatment, and pathophysiology. Biol Psychiatry. 1987;22:667-87.
64. OTP 8 Gooman WK, Price LH, Delgado PL, et al. Specificity of serotonin reuptake inhibitors in the treatment of obsessive-compulsive disorder: comparison of Fluvoxamine and desipramine. Arch Gen Psychiatry. 1990;47:577-85.
65. OTP 9 Leonard H, Swedo SE, Lenane MC, et al. A double blind desipramine substitution during long term clomipramine treatment in children and adolescents with obsessive-compulsive disorder. Arch Gen Psychiatry; 1999;48:922-7.
66. Eddy KT, Dutra L, Bradley R, Westen DA. A multidimensional meta-analysis of psychotherapy and pharmacotherapy for obsessive-compulsive disorder. Clin Psychol Rev. 2004;24: 1011-30.
67. Koran L, Hanna G, Hollander E, Nestadt G, Simpson H. Practice guideline for the treatment of patients with obsessive-compulsive disorder. Am J Psychiatry. 2007;164(Suppl 7): 5-53.
68. Ravizza L, Barzega G, Bellino S, Bogetta F, Maina G. Drug treatment of obsessive compulsive disorder long term trial with clomipramine and selective serotonin reuptake inhibitors. Psychopharmacol Bull. 1996;32:167-73.
69. Pato M, Zohar-Kadouch R, ZOhar J, Murphy D. Return of symptoms after discontinuation of clomipramine in patients with obsessive-compulsive disorder. Am J Psychiatry. 1988; 145:1521-5.
70. Simpson H, Liebowitz M, Foa E, et al. Post-treatment effects of exposure therapy and clomipramine in obsessive-compulsive disorder. Depress Anxiety. 2004;19:225-33.
71. Geller DA, Biederman J, Stewart SE, et al. Which SSRI? A meta-analysis of pharmacotherapy trials in pediatric obsessive-compulsive disorder. AM J Psychiatry. 2003;160:1919-28.
72. OTP 53 Mundo E, Richter MA, Zai G, et al. 5HT1D beta receptor gene implicated in the pathogenesis of obsessive-compulsive disorder: further evidence from a family-based association study. Mol Psychiatry. 2002;7:805-9.
73. OTP 73 McDougle J, Goodman, WK, Price LH, et al. Neuroleptic addition in Fluvoxamine refractory obsessive-compulsive disorder. AM J Psychiatry. 1990;147:652-4.
74. Bloch M, Landeros-Weisenberger A, Kelmendi B, Coric V, Bracken M, Leckman J. A systematic review: antipsychotic augmentation with treatment refractory obsessive-compulsive disorder. Mol Psychiatry. 2006;11:622-32.
75. Coric V, Taskiran S, Pittenger C, et al. Riluzole augmentation in treatment-resistant obsessive-compulsive disorder: an open-label trail. Biol Psychiatry. 2005;58:424-8.
76. Grant P, Lougee L, Hirschtritt M, Swedo SE. An open-label trial of riluzole, a glutamate antagonist, in children with treatment-resistant obsessive-complsive disorder. J Child Adolesc Psychopharmacol. 2007:17:761-7.
77. OTP 76 Van Balkom AJLM, De Haan E, Van Oppen P et al. Cognitive and behavioural therapies alone versus in combination with Fluvoxamine in the treatment of obsessive-compulsive disorder. The Journal of Nervous and Mental Disease. 1998;186:492-9.
78. OTP 79 Schwartz JM, Stoessel PW, Baxter LR Jr., et al. Systematic in the cerebral glucose metabolism rate after successful behavioural modification treatment of OCD. Arch Gen Psychiatry. 1996;53:109-13.
79. Abramowitz J. The psychological treatment of obsessive-compulsive disorder. Can J Psychiatry. 2006;51:407-16.
80. Abramowitz J, Taylor S, McKay D. Exposure-based treatment for obsessive-compulsive disorder. In: Steketee G (Ed). New York: Oxford University Press, in press.
81. McKay D, Taylor S, Abramowitz Js. Obsessive compulsive disorder. In: McKay D, Abramowitz Js, Taylor S (Eds). Cognitive behaviour therapy for refractory cases: turning failure into success. Washington, DC: American Psychological Association, in press.
82. Goodman W, Price L, Rasmussen S, Mazure C, Delgado P, Heninger G, Charney D. The Yale-Brown obsessive compulsive scale: validity. Arch Gen Psychiatry. 1989:46:1012-6.
83. Fals-Stewart W, Marks A, Schafer J. A comparison of behavioral group therapy and individual behavior therapy in treating

obsessive-compulsive disorder. J Nerv Ment Disord. 1993;181: 189-93.

84. Lindsay M, Crino R, Andrews G. Controlled trail of exposure and response prevention in obsessive-compulsive disorder. Br J Psychiatry. 1997;171:135-9.
85. Van Balkom A, De Haan E, Van Oppen P, Spinhoven P, Hoogduin K, Van Dyck R. Cognitive and behavioral therapies alone versus in combination with fluvoxamine in the treatment of obsessive compulsive disorder. J Nerv Ment Disord. 1998; 186:492-9.
86. Foa E, Liebowitz M, Kozak M, et al. Randomized, placebo-controlled trail of exposure and ritual prevention, clomipramine, and their combination in the treatment of obsessive-compulsive disorder. Am J Psychiatry. 2006;162:151-61.
87. Nakatani E, Nakagawa A, Nakao T, et al. A randomized trial of Japanese patients with obsessive-compulsive disorder: effectiveness of behavior therapy and fluvoxamine. Psychother Psychosom. 2005;74:269-76.
88. Abramowitz J, Franklin M, Foa E. Empirical status of cognitive-behavioral therapy for obsessive-compulsive disorder: a meta-analytic review. Rom J Cogn Behav Psychother. 2002;2:89-104.
89. van Balkom AJLM, van Oppen P, Vermeulen AWA, van Dyck R, Nauta MCE, Vorst HCM. A meta-analysis on the treatment of obsessive-compulsive disorder: a comparison of antidepressants, behavior therapy, and cognitive therapy. Clin Psychol Rev. 1994;14:359-81.
90. Abramowitz J. Effectiveness of psychological and pharmacological treatments for obsessive-compulsive disorder; a quantitative review. J Consult Clin Psychol. 1997; 65:44-52.
91. Abramowitz J, Whiteside S, Deacon B. The effectiveness of treatment for pediatric obsessive-compulsive disorder: a meta-analysis. Behav Ther. 2005;36:55-63.
92. Watson HJ, Rees CS. Meta-analysis of randomized controlled treatment trials for pediatric obsessive-compulsive disorder. J Child Psychol Psychiatry. 2008;49:489-98.
93. Franklin M, Abramowitz J, Foa E, Kozak M, Levitt J. Effectiveness of exposure and ritual prevention for obsessive-compulsive disorder: randomized compared with nonrandomized samples. J Consult Clin Psychol. 2000;68:594-602.
94. Aouizerate B, Rotge J-Y, Martin-Guehl C, et al. A systematic review of psychosurgical treatments for obsessive-compulsive disorder: does deep brain stimulation represent the future trend in psychosurgery? Clin Neuropsychiatry. 2006;3: 391-403.
95. Kopell B, Greenberg B. Anatomy and physiology of the baal ganglia implications for DBS in psychiatry. Neurosci Biobehav Rev. 2008;32:408-22.
96. Sachdev PS, Loo CK, Mitchell PB, McFarquhar TF, Malhi GS. Repetitive transcranial magnetic stimulation for the treatment of obsessive compulsive disorder a double-blind controlled investigation. Psychol Med. 2007;37:1645-9.

CHAPTER 13

Phobic Disorders

Ashok Singhal

Phobia is a persistent avoidance behavior secondary to irrational fear of a specific object, activity or situation. Marks[1] has defined phobia on the following four criteria:

1. The fear is out of proportion to the demands of the situation.
2. It cannot be explained or reasoned away.
3. It is beyond voluntary control.
4. The fear leads to an avoidance of the feared situation.

Either the presence or anticipation of the phobic entity results in severe distress in the affected person, who recognizes that the fear is excessive. Nevertheless, the phobic reaction results in a disruption of the person's ability to function in life.

Phobias are very common mental disorders seen in the general population. Approximately, 5–10% of the population is affected with phobias. Phobias are often responsive to treatment with cognitive and behavioral psychotherapies, and to treatment with specific pharmacotherapies. Therefore, they must be recognized, otherwise they can lead to psychiatric complications, like major depressive disorder, other anxiety disorder or substance related disorders, especially alcohol use disorders.

The fourth edition of the Diagnostic and Statistical Manual of Mental disorders (DSM-IV)[2] includes three types of phobic disorders: agoraphobia, specific phobia and social phobia. The tenth version of the International classification of diseases (ICD-10),[3] includes phobic anxiety disorders (F40) under the broad group of neurotic, stress related and somatoform disorders, with agoraphobia (with and without, panic disorder), social phobias and specific (isolated) phobias as the sub-categories. In addition, the sub-categories of other phobic anxiety disorders and phobic anxiety disorder (unspecified) are also included here.

EPIDEMIOLOGY

Phobias are one of the common mental disorders in United States, with an estimated 5–10% population being affected. The life time prevalence of agoraphobia ranges from 0.6 to 6%. In community samples, half of the agoraphobic patients have panic disorder. Specific phobia is the most common mental disorder among women and the second most common in men. The six month prevalence being 5–10% and the females suffering twice as compared to males. The six months prevalence for social phobia is about 2–3%.

The typical age of onset of phobias is usually in childhood and adolescence.[4,5] The age of onset is earliest in animal phobias, intermediate in social phobias and latest in agoraphobia.

Patients with agoraphobia consistently have the highest rate of comorbidity, and animal and situational phobias the lowest, while social phobias intermediate.[4,6,7] Life-time major comorbid disorders are present in 69% of subjects with social phobia. Patients with social phobia have an increased rate of suicidal ideation, financial dependency and having sought medical treatment.[8]

ETIOLOGY

Behavioral Factors

Stimulus Response Model

Watson's formulation from his experiences with little Albert, an infant having fear of rats and rabbits that were induced by scientific experiments of two psychologists, used techniques that had successfully induced conditioned responses in laboratory animals. These involved the traditional Pavlovian stimulus response model of the conditioned response to account for the creation of phobia.[9] That is, anxiety is aroused by a naturally frightening stimulus that occurs in contiguity with a second inherently neutral stimulus. As a result of the contiguity, especially when the two stimuli are paired on several occasions, the originally neutral stimulus takes on the capacity to arouse anxiety by itself. The neutral stimulus, therefore, becomes a conditioned stimulus for anxiety production.

Operant Conditioning Theory

In the classic stimulus response theory, the conditioned stimulus gradually loses its potency to arouse a response, if it is not reinforced by a periodic repetition of the unconditioned stimulus. In the phobic symptoms, the attenuation of the response to the phobic stimulus (that is deconditioning of stimulus) does not occur. The symptom may last for years without any apparent external reinforcement. The operant conditioning theory provides a model to explain that phenomenon. According to it, anxiety is a drive that motivates the organism to do what it can, to obviate the painful affect. In the course of its random behavior, the organism learns that certain actions enable it to avoid the anxiety-provoking stimulus. Those avoidance patterns remain stable for long periods of time, as a result of the reinforcement they receive from their capacity to diminish activity.

Psychoanalytic Theories

Sigmund Freud presented a formulation of phobic neurosis. According to the psychoanalytic theory, the major function of anxiety is a signal to the ego, that a forbidden unconscious drive is pushing for conscious expression, thus altering the ego to strengthen and marshal its defenses against the threatening instinctual force.

In social and specific phobia, the conflict is regarding sexual arousal, leading to castration anxiety. When repression fails to be entirely successful, the ego must call on auxiliary defenses. These defenses in social and specific phobia are of displacement, symbolization and avoidance. In agoraphobia, it is the separation anxiety playing a central role. Clinical observations show that anxiety associated with phobias has a variety of sources and colorings.

Genetic-environmental Factors

Phobic disorders illustrate the interaction between genetic constitutional diathesis and environmental stressors. Recent studies suggest that the subtypes of phobias can be placed along an etiologic continuum. At one end of this continuum lies agoraphobia, which has the latest age at onset, the highest rate of comorbidity, the highest heritability, the highest loading on the environmental common factor, the least specific environmental influences, and the lowest loading on the genetic common factor.

At the other end of this continuum lie the simple phobias (animal and situational) which have the earliest age at onset, the lowest rate of comorbidity, the lowest heritability, the lowest loading on environmental influences, and the highest loading as the common genetic factor. On nearly all of these measures, social phobia lies intermediate between agoraphobia and the simple phobia.[4] In simple phobias, pathogenic environmental experiences are usually highly specific (e.g. being locked in a dark closet, bitten by a snake, nearly falling out of a window, etc.).[10] When these individual specific traumatic experiences act on the constitutionally predisposed children having specific temperament (known as behavioral inhibition to the unfamiliar), a picture of full-blown phobia is created.

CLINICAL FEATURES AND DIAGNOSTIC CRITERIA

Agoraphobia

Agoraphobic patients rigidly avoid situations in which it would be difficult to obtain help. They prefer to be accompanied by a friend or a family member in such places as busy streets, crowded stores, closed-in spaces (such as tunnels, bridges, subways and elevators), and closed-in vehicles (such as buses and airplanes). The patients may insist that they be accompanied every time they leave the house. This behavior may result in marital discord, which may be misdiagnosed as the primary problem. Severely affected patients may simply refuse to leave the house. Particularly before a correct diagnosis is made, patients may be terrified that they are going crazy. Psychosocial consequences of agoraphobia, in addition to marital discord, can include time lost from work, financial difficulties related to the loss of work, and alcohol and other substance abuse. But, agoraphobic patients have significantly better adjustment in most areas of social functioning, especially related to interpersonal contact, work leisure activities and sexual life.

According to DSM-IV, agoraphobia is not a codable disorder. Disorder in which the agoraphobia occurs (e.g. panic disorder with agoraphobia or agoraphobia without history of panic disorder) is specified. DSM-IV conceptualizes[2] agoraphobia as anxiety about being in places or situations from which escape might be difficult (or embarrassing) or in which help may not be available in the event of having an unexpected (or situationally predisposed) panic attack or panic like symptoms. Agoraphobic fears typically involve characteristic clusters of situations that include being outside house alone, being in a crowd or standing in a line, being on a bridge, and travelling in a bus, train or automobile.

The situations are then avoided or are endured with marked distress or with anxiety about having a panic attack or panic like symptoms. The resulting anxiety may necessitate the presence of a companion. The symptoms should not better accounted for by another psychiatric disorder (e.g. social phobia, specific phobia, obsessive compulsive disorders, post-traumatic stress disorder or separation anxiety disorder).

DSM-5 Diagnostic criteria for agoraphobia 300.22 (F40.00)
A. Marked fear or anxiety about two (or more) of the following five situations: 1. Using public transportation (e.g. automobiles, buses, trains, ships, planes). 2. Being in open spaces (e.g. parking lots, marketplaces, bridges). 3. Being in enclosed places (e.g. shops, theaters, cinemas). 4. Standing in line or being in a crowd. 5. Being outside of the home alone.
B. The individual fears or avoids these situations because of thoughts that escape might be difficult or help might not be available in the event of developing panic-like symptoms or other incapacitating or embarrassing symptoms (e.g. fear of falling in the elderly; fear of incontinence).
C. The agoraphobic situations almost always provoke fear or anxiety.
D. The agoraphobic situations are actively avoided, require the presence of a companion, or are endured with intense fear or anxiety.
E. The fear or anxiety is out of proportion to the actual danger posed by the agoraphobic situations and to the sociocultural context.
F. The fear, anxiety, or avoidance is persistent, typically lasting for 6 months or more.
G. The fear, anxiety, or avoidance causes clinically significant distress or impairment in social, occupational, or other important areas of functioning.
H. If another medical condition (e.g. inflammatory bowel disease, Parkinson's disease) is present, the fear, anxiety, or avoidance is clearly excessive.
I. The fear, anxiety, or avoidance is not better explained by the symptoms of another mental disorder—for example, the symptoms are not confined to specific phobia, situational type; do not involve only social situations (as in social anxiety disorder); and are not related exclusively to obsessions (as in obsessive-compulsive disorder), perceived defects or flaws in physical appearance (as in body dysmorphic disorder), reminders of traumatic events (as in post-traumatic stress disorder), or fear of separation (as in separation anxiety disorder).
Note: Agoraphobia is diagnosed irrespective of the presence of panic disorder. If an individual's presentation meets criteria for panic disorder and agoraphobia, both diagnoses should be assigned.

Specific Phobia

In DSM-III-R, this was known as simple phobia, but as the name simple does not allow the occurrence of panic attacks, which are common in these patients, DSM-IV uses the term specific phobias. DSM-IV includes distinctive types of specific phobia, for example, animal type, natural environmental type (for example, storms), blood/injection/injury type, situational type (for example, cars), and other types (for specific phobia that do not fit into previous four types). The natural environmental type is the most common in children under 10 years old and the situational type in the early 20s. The blood/injection/injury type of specific phobia is particularly likely to affect many members and generation of family. Space phobia is a recently reported type in which patients are afraid of falling when there is no nearby support, such as a wall or a chair.

The patients seeking treatment help are often different from untreated groups. The treated individuals report more phobias involving dogs and cats, elevators, and transportation; most have multiple phobias,, and many experience panic attacks in the context of their phobias. The untreated individuals typically report only one phobia, which is often related to blood-injury and is seldom complicated by panic symptoms.[11]

Alexithymia (difficulty identifying and describing subjective feelings, a paucity of fantasies determined by feelings and impulses) is reported by less proportion of specific phobias (12.5%) in comparison to panic disorder patients (46.7%).[12]

According to DSM-IV, specific phobia is characterized[2] by marked and persistent fear that is excessive or unreasonable, cued by the presence (or anticipation) of a specific object or situation (e.g. flying, heights, animals). Exposure to the phobic stimulus almost invariably provokes an immediate anxiety response, which may take the form of a situationally bound or situationally predisposed panic attack. The person recognizes that the fear is excessive or unreasonable, except in children. The phobic situation is then avoided, or endured with intense anxiety or distress. The avoidance, anxious anticipation, or distress in the feared situation interferes significantly with the person's normal occupational, social or interpersonal functioning, or there is marked distress about having the phobia. The symptoms should not better accounted for the another psychiatric disorder (such as obsessive-compulsive disorder, post-traumatic stress disorder, separation anxiety disorder, social phobia, panic disorder with agoraphobia or agoraphobia without history of panic disorder).

DSM-5 Criteria for specific phobia
A. Marked fear or anxiety about a specific object or situation (e.g. flying, heights, animals, receiving an injection, seeing blood). **Note:** In children, the fear or anxiety may be expressed by crying, tantrums, freezing, or clinging.
B. The phobic object or situation almost always provokes immediate fear or anxiety.
C. The phobic object or situation is actively avoided or endured with intense fear or anxiety.
D. The fear or anxiety is out of proportion to the actual danger posed by the specific object or situation and to the sociocultural context.

Contd...

Contd...

E. The fear, anxiety, or avoidance is persistent, typically lasting for 6 months or more.
F. The fear, anxiety, or avoidance causes clinically significant distress or impairment in social, occupational, or other important areas of functioning.
G. The disturbance is not better explained by the symptoms of another mental disorder, including fear, anxiety, and avoidance of situations associated with panic-like symptoms or other incapacitating symptoms (as in agoraphobia); objects or situations related to obsessions (as in obsessive-compulsive disorder); reminders of traumatic events (as in post-traumatic stress disorder); separation from home or attachment figures (as in separation anxiety disorder); or social situations (as in social anxiety disorder).
Specify if: Code-based on the phobic stimulus: 300.29 (F40.218) Animal (e.g. spiders, insects, dogs) 300.29 (F40.228) Natural environment (e.g. heights, storms, water) 300.29 (F40.23x) Blood-injection-injury (e.g. needles, invasive medical procedures).
Coding note: Select specific ICD-10-CM code as follows: F40.230 fear of blood; F40.231 fear of injections and transfusions; F40.232 fear of other medical care; or F40.233 fear of injury. 300.29 (F40.248) Situational (e.g. airplanes, elevators, enclosed places) 300.29 (F40.298) Other (e.g. situations that may lead to choking or vomiting; in children, e.g. loud sounds or costumed characters).
Coding note. When more than one phobic stimulus is present, code all ICD-10-CM codes that apply (e.g. for fear of snakes and flying, F40.218 specific phobia, animal, and F40.248 specific phobia, situational).

Social Phobia

DSM-IV2 adds a type of social phobia, generalized type that may be of use in the prediction of course, prognosis, and treatment response. DSM-IV excludes a diagnosis of social phobia when the symptoms are a result of social avoidance stemming from embarrassment about another psychiatric or non-psychiatric medical condition. The common social situations generating anxiety in a descending order are speaking to a large audience (i.e. public speaking) (55+), speaking to a small group of familiar peoples (24.9%), dealing with people in authority (23.3%), attending social gatherings (14.5%), speaking to strangers or meeting new people (13.7%) and eating (7.1%) or writing (5.1%) in front of the others.[13]

Social phobia and panic disorder may coexist in many cases, and the presence of social phobia may be associated with a higher morbid risk for major depression in this population.[14] Rates of social phobia are highest among women and persons who are younger (age, 18–29 years), less educated, single, and of lower socioeconomic class. Lifetime major comorbid disorders are present in 69% of subjects with social phobia and usually have onset after social phobia.[8] Symptoms associated with social phobia usually involve blushing, muscle twitching, and anxiety about scrutiny.

According to DSM-IV, social phobia is characterized[2] by a marked and persistent fear of one or more social or performance situations in which the person is exposed to unfamiliar people or to possible scrutiny by others. The individual fears that he/she will act in a way (or show anxiety symptoms) that will be humiliating or embarrassing. Exposure to the feared social situation almost invariably provokes anxiety, which may take the form of a situationally bound or situationally predisposed panic attack. The person recognizes that the fear is excessive or unreasonable, except in children. The feared social or performance situations are avoided, or endured with intense anxiety or distress. The avoidance, anxious anticipation, or distress in the feared situation interferes significantly with the person's normal occupational, social or interpersonal functioning, or there is marked distress about having the phobia. The fear or avoidance is not due to the direct physiological effects of a substance or a general medical condition, and is not better accounted for by another psychiatric disorder (e.g. panic disorder with or without agoraphobia, separation anxiety disorder, body dysmorphic disorder, pervasive developmental disorder or schizoid personality disorder).

DSM-5 Diagnostic criteria for social anxiety disorder (Social Phobia) 300.23 (F40.10)
A. Marked fear or anxiety about one or more social situations in which the individual is exposed to possible scrutiny by others. Examples include social interactions (e.g. having a conversation, meeting unfamiliar people), being observed (e.g. eating or drinking), and performing in front of others (e.g. giving a speech). **Note:** In children, the anxiety must occur in peer settings and not just during interactions with adults.
B. The individual fears that he/she will act in a way or show anxiety symptoms that will be negatively evaluated (i.e. will be humiliating or embarrassing; will lead to rejection or offend others).
C. The social situations almost always provoke fear or anxiety. **Note:** In children, the fear or anxiety may be expressed by crying, tantrums, freezing, clinging, shrinking, or failing to speak in social situations.
D. The social situations are avoided or endured with intense fear or anxiety.
E. The fear or anxiety is out of proportion to the actual threat posed by the social situation and to the sociocultural context.
F. The fear, anxiety, or avoidance is persistent, typically lasting for 6 months or more.
G. The fear, anxiety, or avoidance causes clinically significant distress or impairment in social, occupational, or other important areas of functioning.

Contd...

Contd...

H. The fear, anxiety, or avoidance is not attributable to the physiological effects of a substance (e.g. a drug of abuse, a medication) or another medical condition.
I. The fear, anxiety, or avoidance is not better explained by the symptoms of another mental disorder, such as panic disorder, body dysmorphic disorder, or autism spectrum disorder.
J. If another medical condition (e.g. Parkinson's disease, obesity, disfigurement from burns or injury) is present, the fear, anxiety, or avoidance is clearly unrelated or is excessive.
Specify if: *Performance only:* If the fear is restricted to speaking or performing in public.

DIFFERENTIAL DIAGNOSIS

Common for Social and Specific Phobia

- Appropriate fear and normal shyness
- Nonpsychiatric medical conditions (Central nervous system tumors, cerebrovascular disease)
- Use of substances like hallucinogens and sympathomimetics
- Schizophrenia
- Panic disorder
- Agoraphobia.

Specific Phobia

- Hypochondriasis
- Obsessive compulsive disorder
- Paranoid personality disorder.

Social Phobia

- Major depressive disorder
- Schizoid personality disorder.

Agoraphobia

- All medical conditions causing anxiety or depression
- Major depressive disorder
- Schizophrenia
- Paranoid personality disorder
- Avoidance personality disorder
- Dependent personality disorder.

COURSE AND PROGNOSIS

Agoraphobia without a history of panic disorder is often incapacitating and chronic. Depressive disorders and alcohol dependence often complicate the course of agoraphobia. As social phobia and specific phobia are relatively new diagnoses, little is known about their course and prognosis. However, due to high rate of comorbidity and impairment in person's ability to function the affected patient may have financial dependence on others as adults and varying degrees of impairment in their social lives. The development of associated substance related disorders can also adversely affect the course and the prognosis of the disorders.

TREATMENT

Psychotherapy, cognitive-behavior therapy and pharmacotherapy all have been used to treat phobic disorders.

Psychotherapy

Insight-oriented psychotherapy is the superior to psychoanalytic psychotherapy. Insight-oriented psychotherapy enables the patient to understand the origin of the phobia, the phenomena of secondary gain and the role of resistance, and enables the patient to seek healthy ways of dealing with anxiety provoking stimuli.

Cognitive-behavior therapy and various techniques of behavior therapy like desensitization, flooding and social skill training are used. Desensitization is carried out entirely in imagination and geared around the hierarchy of anxiety provoking situations whereas in flooding most therapeutic effect is concentrated at the top of hierarchy. The therapist teaches the patient various techniques to deal with the anxiety, including relaxation, breathing control and cognitive approaches to situation.

Social skill training includes such methods as modeling and role-playing. All the three types of behavior therapies are useful in the treatment. Different studies showing slightly superiority to different therapies.[14-17]

The key aspects of successful behavior therapy are: (1) The patient's commitment to treatment, (2) Clearly identified problems and objectives, and (3) Available alternative strategies for copying with the patient's feelings. In the special situation of blood/injection/injury phobia, some therapists recommend patients to tense their bodies during the exposure to help avoid possibility of fainting from vasovagal reaction to phobic stimulation.

Cognitive-behavioral treatment of social phobia includes imaginal exposure, in which patients visualize their own participation in phobic events, performance based exposure in which patients enacted simulated phobic situations during sessions, cognitive restructuring, in which patients' cognitions experienced during exposure situation and home work assignments involving confrontation of environmental events. Most patient gain significantly and improvement is maintained at 3 months and 6 months.[19] Desensitization, flooding and social skill training are also used as behavioral techniques with equal efficacy.[17,18]

Pharmacotherapy

For generalized type or social phobia, phenelzine, tranylcypromine, clonazepam, alprazolam, moclobemide and (possibly) serotonin reuptake inhibitors have been found useful.[20-28] Phenelzine is superior to atenolol and somewhat more than moclobemide.[26] Dosages of these drugs parallel those for their use in depressive disorders. Patients treated with phenelzine are nonimproved on measure of work and social disability.[27,28]

The treatment of social phobia associated with performance situation frequently involves use of b-adrenergic antagonists atenolol and propranolol. Both cognitive behavioral and pharmacotherapy are effective treatments.[29-34] Both pharmacotherapy and psychotherapy can be associated with marked cognitive and behavioral changes, but no single treatment can yet be designated as most effective.[28]

REFERENCES

1. Marks IM. Fears, Phobias and Rituals. New York: Academic Press; 1987.
2. American Psychiatric Association. Diagnostic and statistical Manual of Mental Disorder, 4th edition. Washington: American Psychiatric Press; 1994.
3. WHO. International Classification of Mental and Behavioural Disorders, 10th edition, Geneva: World Health Organization; 1992.
4. Kendler, et al. Epidemiology of phobias in women. Arch Gen Psychiatry. 1992;49:273-81.
5. Burke CB, et al. Age at onset of selected mental disorders in five community populations. Arch Gen Psychiatry. 1990;47: 511-8.
6. Schapira K, et al. Phobias and affective illness Br J Psychiatry. 1970;117:25-32.
7. Boyd JH, et al. Exclusion criteria of DSM-III-R study of co-occurrence of hierarchy-free syndromes. Arch Gen Psychiatry. 1984;41:983-9.
8. Schneider, et al. Social phobia: comorbidity and morbidity in an epidemiological sample. Arch Gen Psychiatry. 1992;49: 282-8.
9. Watson JB, et al. Conditioned emotional reactions. J Exp Psychol. 1920;3:1-14.
10. Ost LG, et al. Acquisition of phobias and anxiety response patterns in clinical patients. Behav Res Ther. 1981;19:439-47.
11. Chapman TF, et al. A comparison of treated and untreated simple phobia. Am J Psychiatry. 1993;150:816-8.
12. Parker JDA, et al. Alexithymia in panic disorder and simple phobia: A comparative study. Am J Psychiatry. 1993;150:1105-7.
13. Stein MB, et al. Setting diagnostic threshold for social phobia: considerations from a community survey of social anxiety. Am J Psychiatry. 1994;151:408-12.
14. Stein MB, et al. Social phobic symptoms in patients with panic disorder: practical and theoretical implications. Am J Psychiatry. 1989;146:235-8.
15. Gelder MG, et al. Specific and non-specific factors in behaviour therapy. Br J Psychiatry. 1973;123:445-62.
16. Marks IM. Behavioral treatment of phobic and obsessive-compulsive disorders. In: Hersen M, Eister RM, Miller PM (Eds). Progress in Behaviour Modification. New York: Academic Press, Vol. 1, 66-143.
17. Shaw P. A comparison of three behaviour therapies on the treatment of social phobias. Br J Psychiatry. 1979;134:620-3.
18. Hussain MZ. Desensitization and flooding (implosion) in the treatment of phobias. Am J Psychiatry. 1971;127:1509-14.
19. Gorman JM, et al. Treatment of social phobia with atenolol. J ClinPsychopharm. 1985;5:298-301.
20. Heimberg RG, et al. Treatment of social phobia by exposure, cognitive restructuring and home work assignments.
21. Liebowitz MR, et al. Social phobia: review of a neglected anxiety disorder. Arch Gen Psychiatry. 1985;42:729-36.
22. Lydiard RB, et al. Alprazolam in the treatment of social phobia. J Clin Psychiatry. 1988;49:17-9.
23. Mountjoy CQ, et al. A clinical trial of phenelzine in anxiety depressive and phobic neuroses. Br J Psychiatry. 1977;131: 486-92.
24. Munjack DJ, et al. Clonazepam in the treatment of social phobia: a pilot study. J Clin Psychiatry. 1990;51(Suppl):35-40.
25. Van AM, et al. Fluoxetine efficacy in social phobia. J Clin Psychiatry. 1993:54:27.
26. Gelenter ES, et al. Cognitive-behavioral and pharmacological treatment of social phobia: A controlled study. Arch Gen Psychiatry. 1991;48:938-45.
27. Liebowitz MR, et al. Phenelzine vs. atenolol in social phobia. Arch Gen Psychiatry. 1992;49:290-300.
28. Versiani M, et al. Pharmacotherapy of social phobia. A controlled study with moclobemide and phenelzine. Br J Psychiatry. 1992;161:353-60.
29. Marks IM, Gelder MG. Different ages of onset in varieties of phobias. Am J Psychiatry. 1966;123:218-21.
30. Schneier FR. Clinical practice. Social anxiety disorder. N Engl J Med. 2006;355:1029-36.
31. Cox BJ, Fleet C, Stein MB. Self-criticism and social phobia in the US National Comorbidity Survey. J Affect Disord. 2004; 82:227-34.
32. Vythilingum B, Stein DJ, Soifer S. Is "shy bladder syndrome" a subtype of social anxiety disorder? A survey of people with paruresis. Depress Anxiety. 2002;16:84-7.
33. Ruscio AM, Brown TA, Chiu WT, Sareen J, Stein MB, Kessler RC. Social fears and social phobia in the USA: results from the National Comorbidity Survey Replication. Psychol Med. 2008;35:15-28.
34. American Psychiatric Association. Desk Reference to the Diagnostic Criteria from DSM-5. Washington DC; 2013.

CHAPTER

14

Panic Disorder

JN Vyas, Sandeep M, Jayati Simlai

INTRODUCTION

Panic disorder first emerged as a diagnostic entity only 25 years ago with the publication of the Diagnostic and Statistical Manual of Mental Disorder (DSM-III).[1] However, accounts of a clinically similar syndrome characterized by paroxysmal autonomic nervous system arousal, catastrophic cognitions and profound fatigue have appeared much earlier (e.g. Da Costa's soldiers heart,[2] Wheeler's neurocirculatory asthenia,[3] and Lewis's effort syndrome).[4] The military contexts in which these syndromes developed, implied a prominent role for stress and trauma, suggesting a possible overlap with post-traumatic stress disorder, another anxiety illness that often includes panic attacks. Panic disorder has been the most intensively studies during the past 25 years, has advanced our understanding of the psychology and neurobiology of anxiety, and has helped dispel the notion that anxiety is a trivial problem (i.e. affecting worried yet well individuals) not needing definitive treatment.

DIAGNOSIS AND DIFFERENTIAL DIAGNOSIS

The descriptions of panic disorder differ slightly between DSM-III,[1] DSM-III R,[5] and DSM-IV,[6] but the essential elements of the syndrome are consistent with the International Classification of Diseases (ICD-10) description. Currently, diagnosis requires the presence of recurrent panic attacks, along with any of the following: worry about the possibility of future attacks, development of phobic avoidance, i.e. staying away from places or situations in which the individual fears could elicit a panic attack, where escape of obtaining help in the event of an attack would be unlikely or difficult (e.g. sitting in a crowded movie theater, driving on a bridge), or any other change in behavior due to the attacks (e.g. visits to the emergency room or doctor because of concerns about undiagnosed medical illness).[6] Panic attacks are sudden and sometimes unexpected paroxysmal bursts of severe anxiety, accompanied by several physical symptoms (e.g. cardiorespiratory, gastrointestinal, autonomic or otoneurological). Such attacks are often striking in their initial presentations, affect the individual's function, and could be progressively disabling, especially if complicated by agoraphobia (an extreme form of phobic avoidance).

Controversy continues about the nosological status of agoraphobia without panic attacks, which is infrequent in clinical setting.[7] Agoraphobia precedes the onset of panic in almost the third of people with panic disorder, suggesting that not all agoraphobia is a consequence of panic.[8] Moreover, some instances of agoraphobia without panic attacks might be causally distinct from agoraphobia with panic attacks, indicating the development of agoraphobic behavior in response to a physical illness (e.g. vestibular disease, postural instability due to Parkinson's disease) that impairs an individual's sense of competence of safety in doing everyday activities.[9]

Not all panic attacks are suggestive of panic disorder. The same physical and cognitive symptom constellation can occur in individuals with specific phobias when exposed to the feared stimulus (e.g. heights, snakes, spiders) or in those with social phobia when faced with situations where they might be scrutinized. The difference in such situation is that individual is keenly aware of the source of their fearful sensations, whereas in panic disorder, these same types of sensations are unprovoked, unexplained, and often occur out of the blue. Panic attack can also take place in people with post-traumatic stress disorder, for whom exposure to reminders of a traumatic event can trigger attacks and can be especially difficult to discern as such, unless a careful history of previous traumatic experiences is recorded.

DSM-5 Criteria for panic disorder 300.01 (F41.0)
A. Recurrent unexpected panic attacks. A panic attack is an abrupt surge of intense fear or intense discomfort that reaches a peak within minutes, and during which time four (or more) of the following symptoms occur:
Note: The abrupt surge can occur from a calm state or an anxious state.

Contd...

Contd...

1. Palpitations, pounding heart, or accelerated heart rate. 2. Sweating. 3. Trembling or shaking. 4. Sensations of shortness of breath or smothering. 5. Feelings of choking. 6. Chest pain or discomfort. 7. Nausea or abdominal distress. 8. Feeling dizzy, unsteady, light-headed, or faint. 9. Chills or heat sensations. 10. Paresthesias (numbness or tingling sensations). 11. Derealization (feelings of unreality) or depersonalization (being detached from oneself). 12. Fear of losing control or "going crazy." 13. Fear of dying.
Note: Culture-specific symptoms (e.g. tinnitus, neck soreness, headache, uncontrollable screaming or crying) may be seen. Such symptoms should not count as one of the four required symptoms.
B. At least one of the attacks has been followed by 1 month (or more) of one or both of the following: 1. Persistent concern or worry about additional panic attacks or their consequences (e.g. losing control, having a heart attack, "going crazy"). 2. A significant maladaptive change in behavior related to the attacks (e.g. behaviors designed to avoid having panic attacks, such as avoidance of exercise or unfamiliar situations).
C. The disturbance is not attributable to the physiological effects of a substance (e.g. a drug of abuse, a medication) or another medical condition (e.g. hyperthyroidism, cardiopulmonary disorders).
D. The disturbance is not better explained by another mental disorder (e.g. the panic attacks do not occur only in response to feared social situations, as in social anxiety disorder; in response to circumscribed phobic objects or situations, as in specific phobia; in response to obsessions, as in obsessive-compulsive disorder; in response to reminders of traumatic events, as in post-traumatic stress disorder; or in response to separation from attachment figures, as in separation anxiety disorder).

DSM-5 Criteria for panic attack specifier
Note: Symptoms are presented for the purpose of identifying a panic attack; however, panic attack is not a mental disorder and cannot be coded. Panic attacks can occur in the context of any anxiety disorder as well as other mental disorders (e.g. depressive disorders, post-traumatic stress disorder, substance use disorders) and some medical conditions (e.g. cardiac, respiratory, vestibular, gastrointestinal). When the presence of a panic attack is identified, it should be noted as a specifier (e.g. "post-traumatic stress disorder with panic attacks"). For panic disorder, the presence of panic attack is contained within the criteria for the disorder and panic attack is not used as a specifier. An abrupt surge of intense fear or intense discomfort that reaches a peak within minutes, and during which time four (or more) of the following symptoms occur:
Note: The abrupt surge can occur from a calm state or an anxious state.

Contd...

Contd...

1. Palpitations, pounding heart, or accelerated heart rate. 2. Sweating. 3. Trembling or shaking. 4. Sensations of shortness of breath or smothering. 5. Feelings of choking. 6. Chest pain or discomfort. 7. Nausea or abdominal distress. 8. Feeling dizzy, unsteady, light-headed, or faint. 9. Chills or heat sensations. 10. Paresthesias (numbness or tingling sensations). 11. Derealization (feelings of unreality) or depersonalization (being detached from oneself). 12. Fear of losing control or "going crazy." 13. Fear of dying.
Note: Culture-specific symptoms (e.g. tinnitus, neck soreness, headache, uncontrollable screaming or crying) may be seen. Such symptoms should not count as one of the four required symptoms.

Panic disorder mimics many medical conditions. Therefore, patients often have increased use of healthcare visits, procedures, and laboratory test.[10,11] Panic attacks can also be a symptom of common conditions such as hyperthyroidism, caffeine and stimulant use (e.g. cocaine, methamphetamine), and occasionally in disorders such as pheochromocytoma or partial complex seizures. The comorbidity of cardiovascular (e.g. paroxysmal atria tachycardia, mitral-valve), respiratory (e.g. asthma and chronic obstructive pulmonary disease), and ontological (e.g. Meniere's disease) disorder rises with panic disorder but these conditions are rarely a direct cause of panic attacks.[12]

EPIDEMIOLOGY

National Comorbidity Survey-Replication (NCS-R) reports prevalence estimates of 2.7% at 12 months and 4.7% during lifetime for panic disorders.[13,14] These rates are higher than those reported in the original NCS publication,[15-19] in the older Epidemiological Catchment Area (ECA) study,[16] and in a complication of cross-national surveys done at the same time as the ECA study.[20] Some investigators have suggested a trend of increasing prevalence over the past two decades,[21] however, the varying prevalence in these contemporaneous international data strongly indicate differences in the diagnostic methodology and variations in the diagnostic criteria. Despite variability in prevalence, studies across cultures[15,16,20] consistently show an excess of panic disorder in females, modal age of onset in late adolescence or early adulthood, and strong associations with both agoraphobia and major depression. Some evidence of a lower prevalence in older individuals could suggest decreasing severity[22] to the level of subclinical values which may possibly be due to age-related changes in key brain regions mediating anxiety responses.[23]

Panic disorder rarely occurs in clinical settings without other psychopathological comorbidity. Other axis I psychiatric disorders, especially major depression,[15] bipolar illness,[24] other anxiety disorders,[25] and possibly alcohol abuse have been reported with increased occurrences of panic disorder.[26] Panic could be the main illness in terms of temporal precedence in many circumstances. However, panic might also be secondary and be seen as a severity maker of the comorbid illness.[27] In children and adolescents, the disease tends to have a chronic course and often comorbid with other anxiety, mood and disruptive disorders.[28] Data suggest that childhood panic,[29] as well as its possible precursor, behavioral inhibition[30] (which is also a risk factor for social anxiety disorder), are more common in the offspring of parents with panic disorder. Separation anxiety is specific to childhood panic and does not reliably develop into adult panic. It is also more common in children who have parents with panic disorder than those who do not.[31]

Reports[32] indicate association between panic disorder and increased risk of lifetime suicide attempts. Subsequent analyses and studies[33] have attributed this association to the comorbid conditions accompanying panic disorder, such as major depression, borderline personality, or alcohol abuse. An analysis of the NCS dataset suggest that, although the association between lifetime panic disorder and lifetime suicide attempts is eliminated after controlling for other factors, more recent (12-month) disease remains significantly related to more recent (12-month) suicide attempts, even when comorbidity and history of childhood abuse are accounted for.[34] Furthermore, data from a prospective population-based survey in Netherlands show strong association between panic disorder and suicidal ideation as well as suicide attempts, even after adjustment for affective comorbidity and other suicide risk factors.[35] These observations indicate that clinicians should be vigilant to the probability that their patients with panic disorder could be at an increased risk for suicide.

Attempts have been made to define subtypes of panic disorder on the basis of prominence of distinct symptoms clusters (e.g. dizziness, dyspnea). However, these have not shown consistent results.[36] Panic disorder occurring predominantly during sleep seems to share many characteristics with daytime illness and has a similar response to treatment.[37] The course and outcome of panic disorder is consistent with decade-old reports emphasizing on the chronicity of anxiety disorder. Only 30% of patients remit without subsequent relapse in a few years, although a similar proportion (35%) show notable improvement, albeit with a waxing and waning course.[38,39] However, one study showed that naturalistic prognosis in panic disorder, especially in the absence of agoraphobia, is better than that of generalized and social anxiety disorders that tend to be much more chronic.[40] The number of individuals with continued poor response in the study could be related to low community rates of receiving evidence-based treatment and many patients receiving inappropriate or inadequate treatment.[41]

Many epidemiological studies have investigated risk factors for panic disorder. A stress-diathesis model is commonly used to explain the genesis and maintenance of the disorder, as in case of many psychiatric conditions. Twin studies suggest heritability of about 40%, with contributions for common (i.e. familial) environmental effects (<10%) and unique environmental effects (>50%).[42] Data have suggested that early life trauma or maltreatment[43] along with an anxious temperament that is characterized by neuroticism[44] and anxiety sensitivity[45] is an important risk factor. Stressful life events probably contribute to the onset as well as maintenance of the disorder.[46,47] Cigarette smoking and nicotine dependence in adolescence have been implicated as risk factors for later onset of panic disorder. The cause of this association, however, has been questioned.[48]

CAUSE AND PATHOLOGICAL CHANGE

Genetic Susceptibility

Similar to other psychiatric disorders,[49] panic disorder is thought to be complex with many genes conferring vulnerability through unknown pathways. Panic might exist in many distinct genetic forms, each with a different set of genes. It could also exist in many distinct genetic forms, each with a different set of genes. It may also exist in one form with an underlying set of genes that reflect a broad vulnerability, the panic and anxiety. Evidence for a specific type of panic disorder associated with bladder problems (possibly urinary interstitial cystitis)[50] that is linked to locus q32-33 on chromosome 13 is available.[51] An association study[52] has also related this same chromosomal region to panic disorder, irrespective of associated features. A subtype of bipolar illness, associated with panic attacks has been linked to a locus on chromosome 18[53] and might show clinical difference from other forms of bipolar illness (i.e. rapid mood switching).[54] These findings are neither consistent nor robust and; the exact genes, gene products, or functions related to the genetic regions implicated in both these phenotypes of panic disorder, remain unknown. Finally, a genome-wide scan of an Icelandic cohort revealed linkage on chromosome 9q31.[51-56] This chromosome has also been linked to cigarette smoking.[57] This common region is notable because of the previously reported association between teenage smoking and adult risk of panic disorder.[48,58] This could constitute another possible phenotype of the disorder.

Other studies have focused on genes seemingly having a functional importance in anxiety pathophysiology. A genome-wide scan[59] implicated regions on chromosome 1. This finding is consistent with QTL (quantitative trait loci) studies linking anxiety to this locus in both healthy human beings and mice[60] and to chromosome 11p at a marker for the cholecystokinin-B (CCK-B) receptor gene. This is consistent with the known ability of CCK to precipitate panic attacks in some individuals with panic disorder.[61] However, not all studies have shown an association between the *CCK-B* gene and the disorder.[62] Finally, both association[63] and linkage[64] studies have implicated the adenosine 2A receptor gene in panic disorder as consistent with the anxiogenic effects of caffeine (a known antagonist of this receptor) and with the finding that allelic variations in the gene have been associated with caffeine-induced anxiety.[65]

Association studies show that genes in neurotransmitter systems which are thought to be associated with fear and anxiety (e.g. norepinephrine and serotonin) have produced inconsistent, often nonreplicated results. The most consistent data implicate the gene *22q11* for catechol-o-methyl-transferase (COMT) that codes for the enzyme responsible for norepinephrine metabolism. Linkage[66] and association studies[67] have implicated this region of chromosome 22. By contrast, two association studies have failed to link the norepinephrine transporter to panic disorder.[68] Most studies of serotonin-related genes have been negative. Including the serotonin-transporter-promoter region previously linked to anxiety states in general,[69] the serotonin 1A receptor,[70] and the serotonin 2C receptor.[70] Only one study has shown an association between the serotonin 2A receptor gene and panic disorder.[70]

Of these negative studies, several have compared panic disorder with and without agoraphobia and have shown some positive but inconsistent findings for the agoraphobia subgroup. These investigations have been restrictive due to lack of enough knowledge about the pathophysiology of panic disorder, and about the most heritable phenotypes of the illness. The failure to replicate genetic associations, however, is not a problem for panic disorder only. It shows inherent difficulties in the extant association approaches to complex genetic diseases.[71,72] Genome-wide association methods[72] will be used to study panic disorder further complemented by the scrutiny of gene-environment interaction.

Neurobiological Process

Ferris Pitt's observed that hyperosmolar sodium lactate provoked panic attacks in patients with panic disorder but not in controls.[73] Since then, several compounds with disparate mechanisms of action (e.g. caffeine, isoproterenol, yohimbine, carbon dioxide, and CCK) have shown abilities to provoke panic in patients but not in controls (and in some instances, not in patients with other anxiety or mood disorder without panic attacks).[74] Though these approaches have not improved biological understanding of panic, many of these findings can now be subsumed by more general cognitive-behavioral theories of panic disorder or the current neural systems models for panic disorder that emphasise amygdale and related structures as part of a dysfunctional anxiety assessment and response system (Fig. 1).[75]

Changes in these neural circuits of patients with panic disorder include: reduced volumes in amygdala,[76] temporal lobe;[77] lowered amounts of creatine and phosphocreatine metabolites in the medial temporal lobe;[78] and decreased cerebral glucose metabolism in amygdale, hippocampus, thalamus, and brain-stem areas.[79] Reduced orbitofrontal blood flow that predicts panic response to doxapram,[80] a respiratory stimulant, accords with the breaking action of this area on amygdale activity. Many of these findings are not specific to panic disorder, and co-occur in various combinations in other anxiety disorders such as social anxiety and post-traumatic stress disorder.[81]

Finally, several[82,83] but not all[84] studies have shown reductions in benzodiazepine-receptor density in peri-hippocampal and amygdale areas. These findings are consistent with the evidence that patients with panic disorder are less sensitive to the effects of infused benzodiazepines,[85] have lower concentrations of cortical γ-aminobutyric acid (GABA) at baseline,[86] and show smaller decreases in cortical GABA in response to benzodiazepine challenge,[87] compared with controls. One study,[88] consistent with animal knockout models of this same receptor resulting in pathological anxiety and changes in GABA,[89] showed reductions in 5HT1A receptor concentrations. These findings establish a link with the two neurochemical systems that mediate the effects of the two major classes of antipanic drugs (i.e. serotonin-reuptake-inhibitor [SSRI] antidepressants and benzodiazepines).

Psychopathological Process

Psychosocial Risk Factors

There are factors that increase the salience of bodily sensations and are central to the onset of panic disorder. One such factor is anxiety sensitivity.[90] Anxiety may cause deleterious physical, social, and psychological consequences that extend beyond any immediate physical discomfort experienced during a panic attack. In a study, anxiety sensitivity index values predicted the onset of panic attacks in adolescents,[91] university students,[92] and community sample groups,[93] and also predicted spontaneous panic attacks and worry during 5 weeks of basic military training,[94] even after history of panic attacks and trait anxiety were controlled for.[94] Study found that anxiety sensitivity accounted less for the variance in panic disorder onset than neuroticism, or proneness to have negative emotions in general.

Anxiety sensitivity could be acquired insidiously from various sources such as lifetime of direct aversive experiences (i.e. personal history of severe illness or injury), vicarious observations (i.e. severe illnesses or death among family members), informational transmissions (i.e. parental warnings),[95] or parental reinforcement of attention to somatic symptoms and parent modeling of distressed reactions to bodily sensations.[96,97] Finally, panic attacks themselves increase anxiety sensitivity.[98,99] The peak in prevalence

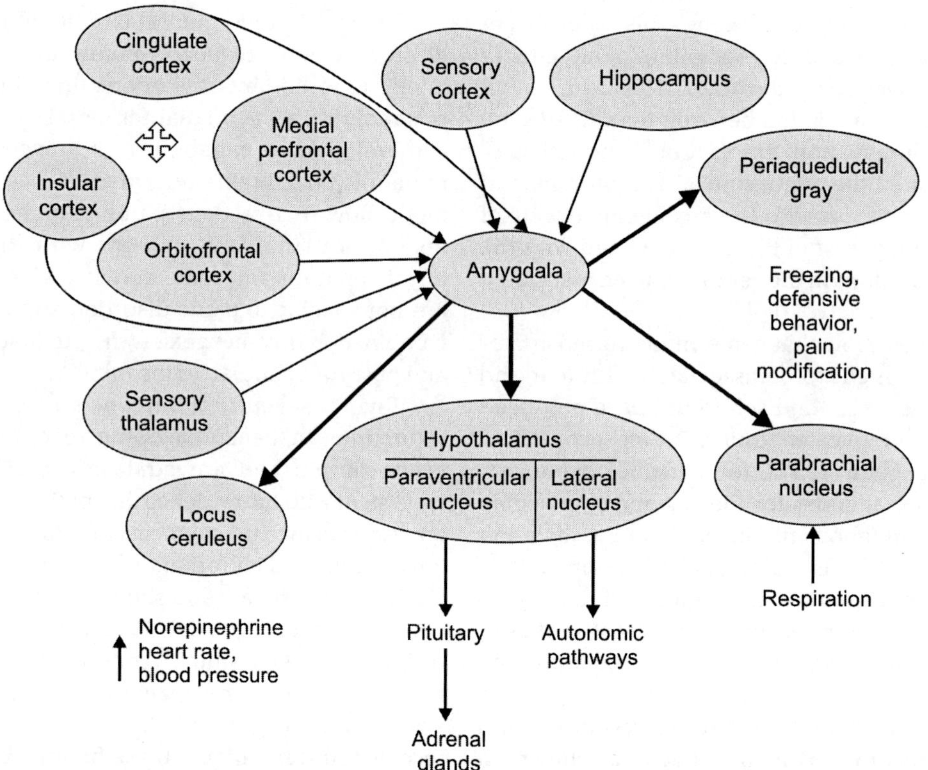

Fig. 1: Proposed neural circuitry of panic: The amygdale has an important role as an anxiety way station. It mediates incoming stimuli from the environment (thalamus and sensory cortex) and stores experience (frontal cortex and hippocampus (thick arrows), which affects anxiety and panic by stimulating various brain areas responsible for key panic symptoms (thin arrow). The periaqueductal gray in the midbrain is especially important for medicating panic-anxiety. Drug treatments can target all parts of this system, affecting amygdale and frontal-lobe interpretation of stimuli, or output effects. Cognitive-behavioral treatment affects the medial prefrontal cortex which is known to inhibit input to the amygdale by using a breaking action

between ages 15 years and 19 years possibly occurs due to added salience of bodily cues at this stage of psychosocial development characterized by sexual development and hormonal changes.[100]

Maintenance of Panic

After initial panic attacks, acute fear of fear develops that is attributed to two factors. The first factor is interceptive conditioning, i.e. conditioned fear of internal cues (e.g. raised heart rate) which occurs when early somatic components of the anxiety response cause pronounced bursts of panic anxiety.[101] In this model, slight changes in bodily functions that patients may or may not be conscious of[102,103] can elicit conditioned fear and panic as a result of previous pairings with the fear of panic.[101,104] This could contribute to the unexpected quality of panic.[103] Such changes in bodily function might result from subclinical cardiorespiratory or vestibular dysfunction. However, it is unknown whether the interoceptive conditioning model can be tested or not.

The second factor that can operate subconsciously (Fig. 2)[101] is catastrophic misappraisals of bodily sensations (e.g. imminent death or loss of control).[105] Functional neuroimaging data suggest that a specific brain region, the insular cortex, could mediate heightened anxiety sensitivity. Insular cortex activation is associated with some bodily awareness,[106] besides monitoring the heartbeat. Activation of this region during risky decision-making correlates with both neuroticism and harm avoidance[107] and; anticipation of emotionally aversive stimuli activates the right insular cortex.[108] These data herald much closer ties between the psychological and biological theories of panic disorder.

TREATMENT

Pharmacotherapy

In 1964, Donald Klein first described the efficacy of tricyclic antidepressant imipramine for blocking panic attacks.[109] Since then, many studies have recorded the efficacy of most antidepressants in panic disorder. Benzodiazepines are another effective class of medications currently available while other treatments with theoretically relevant mechanisms of action (e.g. corticotropin-releasing-factors receptor-1 antagonists) are still in development.

The aim of pharmacotherapy, besides preventing the occurrence of panic attacks; is also to reduce or eliminate

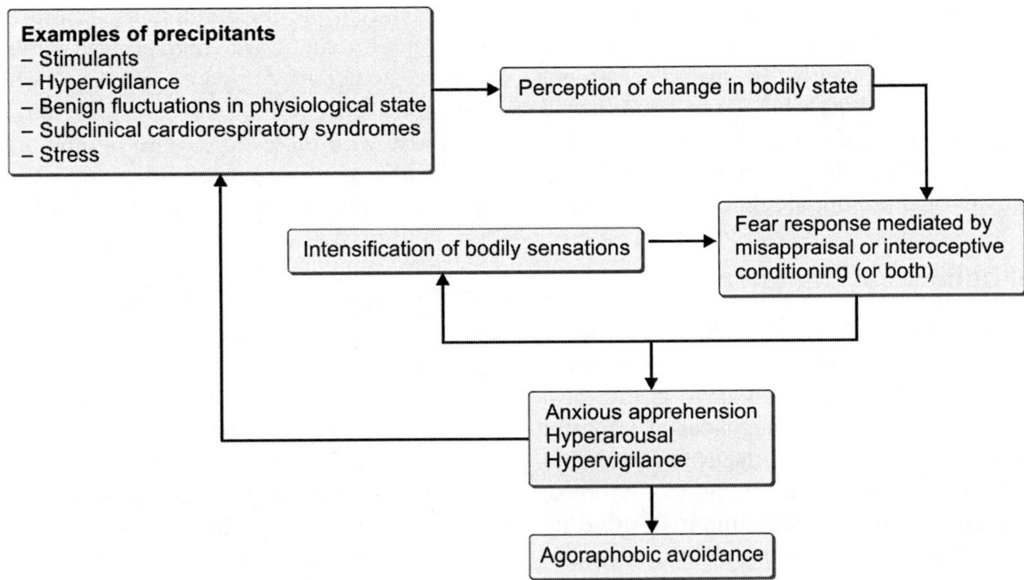

Fig. 2: Cognitive factors that initiate and maintain panic attacks

associated anticipatory anxiety, phobic avoidance, and other symptoms of comorbid conditions such as major depression. Currently, SSRIs are the preferred treatment for panic disorder. Positive placebo-controlled, randomized trials support the efficacy of six different drugs—fluoxetine, fluvoxamine, sertraline, paroxetine, citalopram, and escitalopram.[110] Meta-analyses and reviews[111-114] focusing on many of these agents have reported medium to large effect sizes compared with placebo. Though many trials have examined and confirmed longer-term efficacy of up to 1 year, most of these trials have been short-term.[115] These compounds are also effective for associated mood and other anxiety disorders. Therapeutic response in panic disorder is a class effect, which is common to all the SSRIs, with no evidence of differential efficacy within the class. Although relevant differences exist in drug interactions, side-effect profiles, and half-life; differences in cost due to availability of the generic forms of these substances (fluoxetine, paroxetine, sertraline, and citalopram being currently available in the USA) are probably more important.

Placebo-controlled trials[116] also support the efficacy for an extended-release form of venlafaxine in panic disorder. Either efficacy findings are absent (e.g. for duloxetine, mirtazapine, nefazodone) or evidence indicates a low efficacy (e.g. for trazodone,[117] bupropion)[118] for other second-generation antidepressants. The older class of tricyclic antidepressants, although associated with more side-effects,[113] includes drugs that are less expensive and similarly effective than newer classes of antidepressants. Many studies indicate efficacy for imipramine, desipramine, clomipramine, nortriptyline, and amitriptyline,[110] and six older pre-DSM-III studies[110] show efficacy of monoamine oxidase (MAO) inhibitors in the phobic anxiety of panic-like symptoms. These compounds, especially MAO inhibitors, may be useful in treatment-refractory patients.

Benzodiazepines are very effective against panic disorder. They work rapidly (within days to 1 week), are better tolerated than the very tolerable SSRIs, and have many generic versions available.[119] However, they are restricted by their narrow range of efficacy across disorders (panic disorder, generalized anxiety disorder, and social anxiety disorders; but not obsessive-compulsive disorder, post-traumatic stress disorder, or major depression), and the risk of abuse. Since many patients do not respond fully to SSRIs, the co-prescription of benzodiazepines to anxious patients treated with antidepressants is quite common.[119] Although guidelines from the UK National Institute of Clinical Excellence (NICE)[120] suggest that long-term use of benzodiazepines is contraindicated, many North American psychiatrists still think of long-term treatment benefits to patients.[121] Adjuvant treatment with a benzodiazepine can also be given to achieve a rapid reduction in panic attacks during the several weeks needed for an SSRI to take effect.[122] No controlled data strongly supports anecdotal reports of the efficacy of various anticonvulsant drugs for panic disorder. Controlled studies have also failed to support the efficacy of buspirone[123] and β-blockers.[124]

Many studies clearly show that discontinuation of medication results in relapse in a substantial proportion of patients (25–50% recorded within 6 months).[110] Additionally, SSRIs, serotonin–noradrenaline-reuptake inhibitors (SNRIs), tricyclic antidepressants (TCAs), and benzodiazepines are associated with a time-limited withdrawal syndrome (much worse for benzodiazepines),[125] which could be an interceptive stimulus that promotes panic disorder relapse.

Yet, no placebo-controlled studies have been done to validate the effectiveness of switching agents within or between antidepressant classes in patients who do not respond to treatment. Also, there is dearth of studies on the effectiveness of augmenting SSRIs with benzodiazepines, other antidepressants, or atypical neuroleptic substances in patients who respond partly. Cognitive-behavioral treatment (CBT) could be used for individuals who do not respond well to pharmacotherapy. Two controlled studies have shown that paroxetine is more effective than placebo in nonresponders to CBT[126] and in augmenting the antipanic effects of brief CBT.[127]

Psychological-behavioral Treatment

Cognitive-behavioral treatment (CBT) is the most widely studied and validated psychotherapeutic treatment for panic disorder. It is effective both, individually or in group. Two large meta-analyses reported large effect sizes of 1.55 and 0.90.[128] CBT for panic disorder is found effective in comorbid conditions as well.[129] Although the nature of evidence is robust, such approaches are underused in USA, compared with drug treatment.[130] Despite increasing interest in CBT for anxiety and depression in the UK,[131] similar underuse exists in the UK.[132] Low rates of use are probably due to: public unfamiliarity with the nature and efficacy of CBT relative to medications; restricted access to special mental-health treatment and professionals familiar with efficacy and delivery of CBT; and little training with CBT for many mental-health professionals who currently treat patients with panic disorder.

Cognitive-behavioral treatment (CBT) is based on both the interoceptive conditioning and cognitive theories. The two major forms of CBT developed for panic disorder have been Barlow and Caske's panic control treatment and the interoceptive exposure to feared bodily sensations (e.g. palpitations, dyspnea, and dizziness). In vivo exposure to feared situations (e.g. unfamiliar areas, driving), is useful to obtain corrective information that disproves fearful misappraisals and to lessen fear responding. Retraining of breathing to help patients cope with their panic and anxiety has been found to be unnecessary.[133] Several studies[134] indicate the effectiveness of applied relaxation that incorporates exposure to feared stimuli. Delivery of CBT by alternative routes such as computers and the internet might also be effective.[135]

Other psychotherapeutic treatments often used by clinicians for panic disorder are not as well supported by rigorous empirical study as is CBT. These include insight-oriented therapies, hypnosis, relaxation training without exposure, stress management, and eye-movement desensitization and reprocessing (EMDR) therapy.

Comparative and Combination Treatments

A meta-analysis[136] of 21 randomized trials that included more than 1700 patients with panic disorder (with or without agoraphobia) clearly showed that combined treatment with antidepressants and psychotherapy (behavior, CBT, and other) was more effective than antidepressants alone [relative risk 1.24 (95% CI 1.92–1.52)] and psychotherapy alone [1.16 (1.03–1.20)] in the acute phase.[136] After treatment was discontinued, patients who had received combined treatment continued to benefit compared with those who had received medication only [1.61(1.02–1.30)] but did not do better than those who received psychotherapy only [0.96 (0.79–1.16)]. Although the analysis did not show heterogeneity in psychotherapies, relative risks differed among them. CBT seemed to be the most effective (combined treatment was not significantly better than CBT alone). Although two large trials[137,138] suggested that, after discontinuing medication, patients who had received medication with CBT actually fared worse than those who received CBT only. These provocative findings need further replication. A large study examining the effects of CBT combined with benzodiazepines[138] showed similar but marginal advantages of the combination treatment in the acute phase. Another meta-analytic data[139] which compared the effects of 1 year of clomipramine and psychodynamic therapy, with clomipramine only; found that patients receiving the combination treatment had improved outcomes at 6 months after treatment was discontinued.

As seen in NICE guidelines,[120] CBT effects are generally more durable than those of medication after discontinuation. Meta-analysis show that cognitive-behavioral treatments yield large effect size (averaging over all dependent variables; mean 0.88–0.90) than antidepressants (0.40–0.55) or benzodiazepines (0.40), even-though patient samples might not be the same across all the studies in the meta-analyses.[113,140] Thus, the evidence base is not yet mature enough to yield firm recommendations on whether most patient with panic disorder should begin with medication, CBT, or combination treatment.[141] However, inclusion of CBT at some point during treatment will probably enhance long-term wellbeing.

Summary of NICE Guidelines for the Treatment of Panic Disorder

- Psychological therapy is more effective than pharmacological therapy and should be used as first-line where possible. Details of the types of therapy recommended and their duration can be found in the NICE guidelines.
- Pharmacological therapy is also effective. Most evidence supports the use of the SSRIs.
- Benzodiazepines should not be used.
- A SSRI should be used as first-line. If SSRIs are contra-indicated or there is no response, imipramine or clomipramine can be used.
- Self-help (based on CBT principles) should be encouraged.

Challenges for Treatment Delivery

Most patients with panic disorder are treated in the primary-care setting[10] and this is not surprising since the physical symptoms of panic disorder may drive patients to seek care for what they perceive to be a physical ailment.[10] Difficulties in the diagnosis of panic disorder in this setting argue for possible primary care, even if the effects of comorbid physical and depressive illnesses are accounted for.[142] However, given the quality of primary care given to patients with panic disorder (and other anxiety disorders) only 19–40% of patients are estimated to receive the minimum standards accepted for evidence-based treatment.[130,143] In addition to difficulties pertaining to detection and diagnosis, many other barriers to care exist that include uncertainty about where to seek help, insufficient organization of primary care to treat chronic disease, and problems with insurance coverage and concerns about cost of care (especially in the USA).[142]

New approaches are needed to overcome these barriers and improve the delivery of health care for patients with panic disorder.[144] Some models of care have emphasized the role of primary-care physician along with the support from a mental-health provider to deliver medications ($p = 0.42–0.69$),[145] managing care in general,[146] or provide CBT specifically adapted for the setting. This approach has been shown to be effective (0.23–0.51).[147,148] Other promising approaches that could supplement the care provided by primary-care physicians, or might be used alone for some patients, include self-help treatments for which computer (internet-based) delivery approaches are being proposed.[149]

PREVENTION

Since the onset of panic disorder is highest in adolescence, prevention efforts could be best directed during or before this critical developmental period. In a study[150] individuals with panic attacks visiting the emergency room with panic attacks were assigned to 1-hour's contact with the clinician from whom they received reassurance or exposure instruction. Compared with controls, the exposure group improved on all measures of anxiety and panic after 6 months. Since 40% of the sample group already met the criteria for panic disorder; this investigation was thus, not a pure prevention study. In another study,[151] students with at least one panic attack in the past year and moderate anxiety sensitivity were put on either a wait list group or a 5-hour cognitive-behavioral workshop group.[148] 8 months later, 13.6% of controls developed panic disorder, compared with only 1.8% of individuals in the workshop group. It is thus, indicated that increased research directed towards methods for detection and identification of individuals at risk for panic disorder would be crucial.

REFERENCES

1. American Psychiatric Association. Diagnostic and statistical manual of mental disorders, 3rd edition. Washington, DC: American Psychiatric Association; 1980. pp. 230-32.
2. Wooley CF. Jacob Mendez DaCosta: medical teacher, clinician, and clinical investigator. Am J Cardiol. 1982;50:1145-8.
3. Wheeler EO, White PD, et al. Neurocirculatory asthenia, anxiety neurosis, effort syndrome, neurasthenia; a 20-year follow-up study of 173 patients. J Am Med Assoc. 1950;142:878-89.
4. Nixon PG. The grey area of effort syndrome and hyperventilation: form Thomas Lewis to today. J R Coll Physicians Lond. 1993;27: 377-83.
5. American Psychiatric Association. Diagnostic and statistical manual of mental disorders, 3rd edition revised. Washington, DC: American Psychiatric Association; 1987. pp. 235-40.
6. American Psychiatric Association, DSM-IV diagnostic and statistical manual of mental disorders, 4th edition. Washington, DC: American Psychiatric Association; 1994.
7. Wittchen HU, Reed V, Kesslar RC. The relationship of agoraphobia and panic in a community sample of adolescents and young adults. Arch Gen Psychiatry. 1998;55:1017-24.
8. Bienvenu OJ, Onyike CU, Stein MB, et al. Agoraphobia in adults: incidence and longitudinal relationship with panic. Br J Psychiatry. 2006;188:432-8.
9. Lang AJ, Stein MB. Anxiety disorders. How to recognize and treat the medical symptoms of emotional illness. Geriatrics. 2001;56:24-7.
10. Roy-Byrne PP, Stein MB, Russo J, et al. Panic disorder in the primary care setting: comorbidity, disability, service utilization, and treatment. J Clin Psychiatry. 1999;60:492-9.
11. Katon W. Panic disorder and somatization. Review of 55 cases. Am J Med. 1984;77:101-6.
12. Simon NM, Fischmann D. The implications of medical and psychiatric comorbidity with panic disorder. J Clin Psychiatry. 2005;66(Suppl 4):815.
13. Kessler RC, Chiu WT, Demler O, Merikangas KR, Walters EE. Prevalence, severity, and comorbidity of 12-month DSM-IV disorders in the National Comorbidity Sruvey Replication. Arch Gen Psychiatry. 2005;62:617-27.
14. Kessler RC, Berglund P, Demler O, Jin R, Merlkangas KR, Walters EE. Lifetime prevalence and age-of-onset distributions of DSM-IV disorders in the National Comorbidity Survey Replication. Arch Gen Psychiatry. 2005;62:593-602.
15. Kessler R, Stang P. Wittchen H, Ustum B, Roy-Byrne P, Walters E. Lifetime panic-depression comorbidity in the National Comorbidity Survey. Arch Gen Psychiatry. 1998;55:801-8.
16. Eaton WW, Anthony JC, Romanoski A, et al. Onset and recovery form panic disorder in the Baltimore Epidemiologic Catchment Area follow-up. Br J Psychiarty. 1998;173:501-7.
17. Bromet EJ, Gluzman SF, Paniotto VI, et al. Epidemiology of psychiatric and alcohol disorders in Ukraine: findings from the Ukraine World Mental Health survey: Soc Psychiatry Epidemiol. 2005;40:681-90.
18. Kawakarrn N, Takeshima T, Ono Y, et al. Twelve-month prevalence, severity, and treatment of common mental disorders in communities in Japan: preliminary finding from the World Mental Health Japan Survey 2002-2003. Psychiatry Clin Neurosci. 2005;59:441-52.

19. Good win Rd, Faravelli C, Rosi S, et al. The epidemiology of panic disorder and agoraphobia in Europe. Eur Neuropsychopharmacol. 2005;15:435-43.
20. Weissman MM, Bland RC, Canion GJ, et al. The cross-national epidemiology of panic disorder. Arch Gen Psychiatry. 1997;54:305-9.
21. Goodwin RD. The prevalence of panic attacks in the United States: 1980 to 1995. J Clin Epidemiol. 2003;56:914-6.
22. Sheikh JI, Swales PJ, Carlson EB, Lindley SE. Aging and panic disorder, phenomenology, comorbidity, and risk factors. Am J Geriatr Psychiatry. 2004;12:102-9.
23. Charney DS, Woods SW, Krystal JH, Nagy LM, Heninger GR. Noradrenergic neuronal dysregulation in panic disorder the effects of intravenous yohimbine and clonidine in panic disorder patients. Acta Psychiatry Scand. 1992;86:273-82.
24. Goodwin RD, Hoven CW. Bipolar-panic comorbidity in the general population: prevalence and associated morbidity. J After Disord. 2002;70:27-33.
25. Goisman RM, Goldenberg I, Visile RG, Keler MB. Comorbidity of anxiety disorders in a multicentre anxiety study. Compr Psychiatry. 1995;36:303-11.
26. Zimmermann P, Wittchen HU, Hofler M, Pfister H, Kessler RC, Lieb R. Primary anxiety disorders and the development of subsequent alcohol use disorders: a 4-year community study of adolescents and young adults. Psychol Med. 2003;33:1211-22.
27. Kessler RC, Stang PE, Wittchne HU, Ustum TB, Roy-Byrne PP, Walters EE. Lifetime panic-depression comorbidity in the National Comorbidity Survey. 1998;55:801-8.
28. Biederman J, Faraone SV, Marrs A, et al. Panic disorder and agoraphobia in consecutively referred children and adolescents. J. Am Acad Child Adolesc Psychiatry. 1997;36:214-23.
29. Biederman J, Petty C, Faraone SV, et al. Parental predictors of pediatric panic disorder/agoraphobia: a controlled study in high-risk offspring. Anxiety. 2005;22:114-23.
30. Rosenbaum JF, Biederman J, Hirshfeld-Becker DR, et al. A controlled study of behavioral inhibition in children of parents with panic disorder and depression. Am J Psychiatry. 2000; 157:2002-10.
31. Aschenbrand SG, Kendall PC, Webb A, Safford SM, Plannery-Schroeder E. Is childhood separation anxiety disorder a predictor of adult panic disorder and agoraphobia? A seven-year longitudinal study. J Am Acad Child Adolesc Psychiatry. 2003;42:1478-85.
32. Weissman MM, Klerman GL, Markowitz JS, Ouellette R. Suicidal ideation and suicide attempts in panic disorder and attacks. N Engl J Med. 1989;321:1209-14.
33. Vickers K, McNally RJ. Panic disorder and suicide attempt in the National Comorbidity Survey. J Abnorm Psychl. 2004;113:582-91.
34. Goodwin RD, Roy-Byrne P. Panic and suicidal ideation and suicide attempts: result from a National Comorbidity Survey. Depress Anxiety. 2006;23:124-32.
35. Sareen J, Cox BJ, Afifi TO, et al. Anxiety disorders and risk for suicidal ideation and suicide attempts: a population-based longitudinal study. Arch Gen Psychiatry. 2005;62:1249-52.
36. Goodwin RD, Hamilton SP, Milne BJ, Pine DS. Generalizability and correlates of clinically derived panic subtypes in the population. Depress Anxiety. 2002;15:69-74.
37. Craske MG, Lang AJ, Mystkowski JL, Zucker BG, Bystritsky A, Yan-Go F. Does nocturnal panic represent a more severe form of panic disorder? J Nerv Ment Dis. 2002;190:611-8.
38. Katsching H, Amering M. The long-term course of panic disorder and its predictors. J Clin Psychopharmacol. 1998;18: 6-11S.
39. Roy-Byrne PP, Cowley DS. Curse and outcome in panic disorder: a review of recent follow-up studies. Anxiety. 1995;1:151-60.
40. Bruce SE, Yonkers KA, Otto MW, et al. Influence of psychiatric comorbidity on recovery and recurrence in generalized anxiety disorder, social phobia, and panic disorder: a 12-year prospective study. Am J Psychiatry. 2005;162:1179-87.
41. Wang PS, Berglund P, Kessler RC. Recent care of common mental disorders in the United States: Prevalence and conformance with evidence-based recommendations. J Gen Intern Med. 2005;15:284-92.
42. Hettema JM, Neale MC, Kendler KS. A review and meta-analysis of the genetic epidemiology of anxiety disorders. Am J Psychiatry. 2001;158:1568-78.
43. Stein MB, Wlaker JR, Anderson G, et al. Childhood physical and sexual abuse in patients with anxiety disorders and in a community sample. Am J Psychiatry. 1996;153:275-7.
44. Roth M. Agoraphobia, panic disorder and generalized anxiety disorder: some implications of recent advances. Psychilatr Dev. 1984;2:31-52.
45. McNally RJ. Anxiety sensitivity and panic disorder. Biol Psychiatry. 2002;52:938-46.
46. Watanabe A, Nakao K, Tokuyama M, Takeda M. Prediction of first episode of panic attack among white-collar workers. Psychiatry Clin Neurosci. 2005;59:119-26.
47. Roy-Byrne PP, Geraci M, Uhde TW. Life events and the onset of panic disorder. Am J Psychiatry. 1986;143:142-7.
48. Isensee B, Wittchen HU, Stein MB, Hofler M, Lieb R. Smoking increases the risk or panic; findings from a prospective community study. Arch Gen Psychiatry. 2003;60: 692-700.
49. Kendler KS. "A gene for ....": the nature of gene action in psychiatric disorders. Am J Psychiatry. 2005;162:1243-52.
50. Weissman MM, Gross R, Fyer A, et al. Interstitial cystitis and panic disorder: a potential genetic syndrome. Arch Gen Psychiatry. 2004;61:273-9.
51. Hamilton SP, Fyer AJ, Durner M, et al. Further genetic evidence for a panic disorder syndrome mapping to chromosome 13q. Proc Natl Acad Sci USA. 2003;100:2550-5.
52. Schumacher J, Abou Jamra R, Becker T, et al. Investigation of the DAOA/G30 locus in panic disorder. Mol Psychiatry. 2005; 10:428-9.
53. MacKinnon DF, Xu J, McMahon FJ, et al. Bipolar disorder and panic disorder in families: an analysis of chromosome 18 data. Am J Psychiatry. 1998;155:829-31.
54. MacKinnon DF, Zandi PP, Gershon ES, Numberger JI Jr, DePaulo JR Jr. Association of rapid mood switching with panic

disorder and familial panic risk in familial bipolar disorder. Am J Psychiatry. 2003;160:1696-8.

55. MacKinnon DF, Zandi PP, Copper J, et al. Comorbid bipolar disorder and panic disorder in families with a high prevalence of bipolar disorder. Am J Psychiatry. 2002;159:30-5.
56. Thorgeirsson TE, Oskarsson H, Desnica N, et al. Anxiety with panic disorder linked to chromosome 9q in iceland. Am J Psychiatry. 2003;72:1221-30.
57. Gelernter J, Liu X, Hesselbrock V, Page GP, Goddard A, Zhang H. Results of a genomewide linkage scan: support for chromosomes 9 and 11 loci increasing risk for cigarette smoking. Am J Med Genet B Neuropsychiatr Genet. 2004;128: 9410-1.
58. Breslau N, Klein DF. Smoking and panic attacks: and epidemiologic investigation. Arch Gen Psychiatry. 1999;56: 114-7.
59. Gelernter J, Benovicini K, Page G, et al. Linkage genome scan for loci predisposing to panic disorder or agoraphobia. Am J Med Genet. 2001;105:548-57.
60. Fullerton J, Cubin M, Tiwari H, et al. Linkage analysis of extremely discordant and concordant sibling pairs identifies quantitative-trait loci that influence variation in the human personality trait neuroticism. Am J Med Genet. 2003;72:879-90.
61. van Megen HJ, Westenberg HG, Den Bore JA, Khan RS. The panic-including properties of the cholecystokinin tetrapeptide CCK4 in patients with panic disorder. Eur Neuropsychopharmacol. 1996;6:187-94.
62. Hamilton SP, Slager SL, Helleby L, et al. No association or linkage between polymorphisms in the genes encoding cholecystokinin and cholecystokinin B receptor and panic disorder. Mal Psychiatry. 2001;6:59-65.
63. Deckert J, Nothen MM, Franke P, et al. Systematic mutation screening and association study of the A1 and A2a adenosine receptor genes in panic disorder suggest a contribution of the A2a gene to the development of disease. Mol Psychiatry. 1998;3:81-5.
64. Hamilton SP, Slager SL, De Leon AB, et al. Evidence for genetic linkage between a polymorphism in the adenosine 2A receptor and panic disorder. Neuropsychopharmacology. 2004;29: 558-65.
65. Alsene K, Deckert J, Sand P, de Wit H. Association between A2a receptor gene polymorphisms and caffeine-induced anxiety. Neuropsychopharmacology. 2003;28:1694-702.
66. Hamilton SP, Slager SL, Heminan GA, et al. Evidence for a susceptibility locus for panic disorder near the catechol-O-methyltransferase gene on chromosome 22. Bio Psychiatry. 2002;51:591-601.
67. Domschke K, Freitag CM, Kuhlenbaumer G, et al. Association of the functional V158M catechol-O-Methyl-transferase polymorphism with panic disorder in women. Int J Neuropsychopharmacol. 2004;7:183-8.
68. Lee YJ, Hohoff C, Domschke K, et al. Norepinephrine transporter (NET) promoter and 5'-UTR polymorphisms: association analysis in panic disorder. Neutosci Lett. 2005;377: 40-3.
69. Sand P, Lesch KP, Catalano M, et al. Polymorphic MAO-A and 5-HT-transporter genes: analysis of interactions in panic disorder. World J Biol Psychiatry. 2000;1:147-50.
70. Inada Y, Yoneda H, Koh J, et al. Positive association between panic disorder and polymorphism of the serotonin 2A receptor gene. Psychiatry Res. 2003;118:25-31.
71. Ioannidis JP, Trikalinos TA, Ntzani EE. Contopoulos-Ioannidis DG. Genetic associations in large versus small studies: an empirical assessment. Lancet. 2003;361:567-71.
72. Hirschhorn JN, Daily MJ. Genome-wide association studies for common diseases and complex traits. Nat Rev Genet. 2005;6: 9510-8.
73. Pitts FN Jr, McClure JN Jr. Lactate metabolism in anxiety neurosis. N Engl J Med. 1967;277:1329-36.
74. Krystal JH, Deutsch DN, Charney DS. The biological basis of panic disorder. J Clin Psychiatry. 1996;57(Suppl 10):23-31.
75. Gorman JM, Kent JM, Sullivan GM, Coplan JD, Neuroanatomical hypothesis of panic disorder, revised. Am J Psychiatry. 2000;157:193-505.
76. Massana G, Serra-Grabulosa JM, Salgado-Pineda P, et al. Amygdalar atrophy in panic disorder patients detected by volumetric magnetic resonance imaging. Neuroimage. 2003; 19:80-90.
77. Uchida RR, Del-Ben CM, Santos AC, et al. Decreased left temporal lobe volume of panic patients measured by magnetic resonance imaging. Braz J Med Biol Res. 2003;36:925-9.
78. Massana G, Gasto C, Junque C, et al. Reduced levels of creatine in the right medial temporal love region of panic disorder patients detected with (1)H magnetic resonance spectroscopy. Neuroimage. 2002;16:836-42.
79. Sakai Y, Kumano H, Nishikawa M, et al. Cerebral glucose metabolism associated with a fear network in panic disorder. Neuroreport. 2005;16:927-31.
80. Kent JM, Coplan JD, Mawlawi O, et al. Prediction of panic response to a respiratory stimulant by reduced orbitofrontal cerebral blood flow in panic disorder. Am J Psychiatry. 2005; 162:1379-81.
81. Kent JM, Rauch SL. Neurocircuitry of anxiety disorders. Curr Psychiatry Rep. 2003;5:266-73.
82. Bremner JD, Innis RB, White T, et al. SPECT [I-123] iomazenil measurement of the benzodiazepine receptor in panic disorder. Biol Psychiatry. 2000;47:96-106.
83. Malizia AL, Conningham VJ, Bell CJ, Liddle PF, Jones T, Nutt DJ. Decreased brain GABA (A)-Benzodiazepine receptor binding in panic disorder: preliminary results form a quantitative PET study. Arch Gen Psychiatry. 1998;55:715-20.
84. Brandt CA, Meller J, Keweloh L, et al. Increased benzodiazepine receptor density in the prefrontal cortex in patients with panic disorder. J Neutal Transm. 1998;105:1325-33.
85. Roy-Byrne PP, Cowley DS, Greenblatt DJ, Shader RJ, Hommer D. Reduced benzodiazepine sensitivity in panic disorder. Arch Gen Psychiatry. 1990;47:534-8.
86. Goddard AW, Mason GF, Almai A, et al. Reductions in occipital cortex GABA levels in panic disorder detected with 1h-magnetic resonance spectroscopy. Arch Gen Psychiatry. 2001;58:556-61.

87. Goddard AW, Mason GF, Appel M, et al. Impaired GABA neuronal response to acute benzodiazepine administration in panic disorder. Am J Psychiatry. 2004;161:2186-93.
88. Neumeister A, Bain E, Negent AC, et al. Reduced serotonin type 1A receptor binding in a panic disorder. J Neurosci. 2004; 24:589-91.
89. Sibille E, Pavilids C, Benke D, Toth M. Genetic inactivation of the Serotonin (1A) receptor in mice results in downregulation of major GABA(A) receptor binding, and benzodiazepine-resistant anxiety. J Neurosci. 2000;20:2758-65.
90. Reiss S. Pavlovian conditioning and human fear: an expectancy model. Behavior Therapy. 1980;11:380-96.
91. Hayward C, Killen JD, Kraemer HC, Taylor CB. Predictors of panic attacks in adolescents. J Am Acad Child Adolesc Psychiatry. 2000;39:207-14.
92. Maller RG, Reiss S. Anxiety sensitivity in 1984 and panic attacks in 1987. J Annxiety Disorders. 1992;6:241-7.
93. Ehlers A. A 1-year prospective study of panic attacks: clinical course and factors associated with maintenance. J Abnorm Psychol. 1995;104:164-72.
94. Schmidt NB, Lerew DR, Jackson RJ. The role of anxiety sensitivity in the pathogenesis of panic prospective evaluation of spontaneous panic attack during acute stress. J Abnorm Psychol. 1997;106:335-64.
95. Craske MG, Rowe MK, Nocturnal panic. Clin Psychol Sci Pract. 1997;4:153-74.
96. Watt MC, Stewart SH. Anxiety sensitivity mediates the relationship between childhood learning experiences and elevated hypochondriacal concerns in young adulthood. J Psychosom Res. 2000;49:107-18.
97. Watt MC, Stewart SH, Cox BJ. A retrospective study of the learning history origins of anxiety sensitivity. Behav Res Ther. 1998;36:505-25.
98. Schmidt NB, Lerew DR, Joiner TE Jr. Prospective evaluation of the etiology of anxiety sensitivity: test of a scar model Behav Res Ther. 2000;38:1083-95.
99. Weems CF, Hayward C, Killen J, Taylor CB. A longitudinal investigation of anxiety sensitivity in adolescence. J Abnorm Psychol. 2002;111:471-7.
100. Buchanan CM, Eccles JS, Becker JB. Are adolescents the victims of raging hormones: evidence for activational effects of hormones on moods and behavior at adolescence. Psychol Bull. 1992;111:62-107.
101. Bouton ME, Mineka S, Barlow DH. A modern learning therapy perspective on the etiology of panic disorder. Psychol Rev. 2001;108:4-32.
102. Block RI, Ghoneim MM, Fowles DC, Kumar V, Pathak D. Effects of a subanesthetic concentration of nitrous oxide on establishment, elicitation, and semantic and phonemic generalization of classically conditioned skin conductance response, Pharmacal Biochem Behav. 1987;28:7-14.
103. Craske MG, Lang AJ, Rowe M, et al. Presleep attributions about arousal during sleep: nocturnal panic. J Abnorm Psychol. 2002;111:53-62.
104. Barlow DH. Anxiety and its disorders: the nature and treatment of anxiety and panic. New York, NY: Guilford Press; 1998.
105. Clark DM. A cognitive approach to panic. Behav Res Ther. 1986; 24:461-70.
106. Critchley HD, Wiens S, Rotshtein P, Ohman A, Dolan RJ. Neural systems supporting interceptive awareness. Nat Neurosci. 2004;7:189-95.
107. Paulus MP, Rogalsky C, Simmons A, Feinstein JS, Stein MB. Increased activation in the right insula during risk-taking decision making is related to harm avoidance and neuroticism. Neuroimage. 2003;19:1439-48.
108. Simmons A, Matthews SC, Stein MB, Paulus MP. Anticipation of emotionally aversive visual stimuli activates right insula. Neuroreport. 2004;15:2261-5.
109. Klein DF. Delineation of two drug-responsive anxiety syndromes. Psychopharmacologia. 1964;17:397-408.
110. Roy-Byrne PP, Cowley D. Pharmacologic treatments for panic disorder, generalized anxiety disorder, specific phobia and social anxiety disorders. In: PEN, Gorman J (Eds). A guide to treatments that work. New York: Oxford University Press; 2002. pp. 337-65.
111. Otto MW, Tuby KS, Gould RA, McLean RY, Pollack MH. An effect-size analysis of the relative efficacy and tolerability of serotonin selective reuptake inhibitors for panic disorder. Am J Psychiatry. 2001;158:1989-92.
112. Boyer W. Serotonin uptake inhibitors are superior to imipramine and alprazolam in alleviating panic attacks: a meta-analysis. Int Clin Psychopharmacol. 1995;10:45-9.
113. Bakker A, van Balkom AJ, Spinhoven P. SSRIs vs TCAs in the treatment of panic disorder: a meta-analysis. Acta Psychiatr Scand. 2002;106:163-7.
114. Matte K. A meta-analysis of the efficacy of psycho-and pharmacotherapy in panic disorder with and without agoraphobia. J Affect Disord. 2005;88:27-45.
115. Pollack MH, Allgulander C, Bandelow B, et al. WCA recommendations for the long-term treatment of panic disorder. CNS Spectrums. 2003;8:17-30.
116. Bradwejn J, Ahokas A, Stein DJ, Salinas E, Emilien G, Whitaker T. Venlafaxine extended-release capsules in panic disorder: Flexible-dose, double-blind, placebo-controlled study. Br J Psychiatry. 2005;187:352-9.
117. Charney DS, Woods SW, Goodman WK, et al. Drug treatment of panic disorder: the comparative efficacy of imipramine, alprazolam, and trazodone. J Clin Psychiatry. 1986;47:580-6.
118. Sheehan DV, Davidson J, Manschreck T, Van Wyck Fleet J. Lack of efficacy of a new antidepressant (bupropion) in the treatment of panic disorder with phobias. J Clin Psychopharmacol. 1983; 3:28-31.
119. Bruce SE, Vasile RG, Goisman RM, et al. Are Benzodiazepines still the medication of choice for patients with panic disorder with or without agoraphobia? Am J Psychiatry. 2003;160: 1432-8.
120. NICF NCG. Anxiety: management of anxiety (panic disorder, with or without agoraphobia, and generalized anxiety disorder)

in adults in primary, secondary and community care. London: National Collaborating Center for primary care; 2004.

121. American Psychiatric Association. Practice guideline for the treatment of patients with panic disorder. Work Group on Panic Disorder. American Psychiatric Association. Am J Psychiatry. 1998;155(Suppl):1-34.
122. Goddard AW, Brouette T, Almai A, Jetty P, Woods SW, Charney D. Early coadministration of clonazepam with sertraline for panic disorder. Arch Gen Psychiatry. 2001;58:681-6.
123. Sheehan DV, Raj AB, Harnett-Sheehan K, Soto S, Knap E. The relative efficacy of high-dose buspirone and alprazolam in the treatment of panic disorder: a double-blind placebo-controlled study. Acta Psychiatr Scand. 1993;88:1-11.
124. Noyse R Jr. ANderson DJ, Clancy J. et al. Diazepam and propranolol in panic disorder and agoraphobia. Arch Gen Psychiatry. 1984;41:287-92.
125. Rickels K, Schweizer E, Weiss S, Zavodnick S. Maintenance drug treatment for panic disorder. II Short - and long-term outcome after drug taper. Arch Gen Psychiatry. 1993;50:61-8.
126. Kampaman M, Keijseres GPJ, Hoogduin CAL, Hendriks G-J. A randomized double-blind, placebo-controlled study of the effects of adjunctive paroxetine in panic disorder patients unsuccessfully treated with cognitive-behavioral therapy alone. J Clin Psychiatry. 2002;63:772-7.
127. Stein MB, Norton GR, Walker JR, Chartier MJ, Graham R. Do SSRIs enhance the efficacy of very brief cognitive behavioral therapy for panic disorder? A pilot study. Psychiart Res. 2000; 94:191-200.
128. Westen D, Morrison K. A multidimensional meta-analysis of treatments of depression, panic, and generalized anxiety disorder: an empirical examination of the status of empirically supported therapies. J Consult Clin Psychol. 2001;69:875-99.
129. Tsao JCI, Mystkowski J, Zucker B, Craske MG. Effects of cognitive-behavioral therapy for panic disorder on comorbid conditions: Replication and extension. Behav Ther. 2002;33: 439-509.
130. Young AS, Klap R, Sherbouren CD, Wells KB. The quality of care for depressive and anxiety disorders in the Unites States. Arch Gen Psychiatry. 2001;58:55-61.
131. Bower P, Gilbody S. Stepped care in psychological therapies: access, effectiveness and efficiency. Narrative literature review. Br J Psychiatry. 2005;186:11-7.
132. Bebbington PE, Brugha TS, Meltzer H, et al. Neurotic disorders and the receipt of psychiatric treatment. Psychol Med. 2000;30: 1369-76.
133. de Beurs E, Lange A, Van Dyck R, Koele P. Respiratory training prior to exposure in vivo in the treatment of panic disorder with agoraphobia: efficacy and predictors of outcome. Aust N Z J Psychiatry. 1995;29:104-13.
134. Arntz A, van den Hout M. Psychological treatments of panic disorder without agoraphobia: cognitive therapy versus applied relaxation. Behav Res Ther. 1996;34:113-21.
135. Carlbring P, Nilsson-Ihrfelt E, Waara J, et al. Treatment of panic disorder live therapy vs self-help via the internet. Behave Res Ther. 2005;43:132-3.
136. Furukawa TA, Watanabe N, Churchill R. Psychotherapy plus antidepressant for panic disorder with or without agoraphobia: systematic review, Br. J Psychiatry. 2006;188:305-12.
137. Barlow DH, Gorman JM, Shear MK, Woods SW. Cognitive-behavioral therapy imipramine, or their combination of panic disorder a randomized controlled trail. JAMA. 2000;283: 2529-36.
138. Marks IM, Swinson RP, Basoglu M, et al. Alprazolam and exposure alone and combined in panic disorder with agoraphobia. A controlled study in London and Toronto. Br J Psychiatry. 1993;162:776-86.
139. Wiborg IM, Dahl AA. Does brief dynamic psychotherapy reduce the relapse care of panic disorder? Arch Gen Psychiatry. 1996:53:689-94.
140. Gould RA, Otto M, Pollack M. A meta-analysis of treatment outcome for panic disorder. Clin psycho Review. 1995;15: 819-44.
141. Roy-Byme PP, Katon W, Gewley DS. et al. Panic disorder in primary care: biopsychosocial differences between recognized and unrecognized patients. Gen Hosp Psychiatry. 2000;22: 405-11.
142. Pignone MP, Gaynes BN, Rushton JL, et al. Screening for depression in adults: a summary of the evidence for the US Preventive Services Task Force. Ann Intern Med. 2002;136: 765-76.
143. Stein MB, Gaynes BN, Rushton JL, et al. Quality of care for primary care patients with anxiety disorders. Am J Psychiatry. 2004;161:2230-7.
144. Craske MG, Edlund MJ, Sullivan G, et al. Perceived unmet need for mental health treatment and barriers to care among patients with panic disorder. Psychiatr Serv. 2005;56: 988-94.
145. Roy-Byrne PP, Katon WJ, Cowley DS, Russo J. A randomized trial of collaborative care for patients with panic disorder in primary care. Arch Gen Psychiatry. 2001;58:869-76.
146. Rollman BL, Belnap BH, Reynolds CF, Schulberg HC, Shear MK. A contemporary protocol to assist primary care physicians in the treatment of panic and generalized anxiety disorders. Gen Hosp Psychiatry. 2003;25:74-82.
147. Roy-Byrne PP, Craske MG, Stein MB, et al. A randomized effectiveness trail of cognitive-behavioral therapy and medication for primary care panic disorder. Arch Gen Psychiatry. 2005;62:290-8.
148. Katon W, Russo J, Sherbourne C, et al. Incremental cost-effectiveness of a collaborative care intervention of panic disorder. Psychol Med. 2006;36:353-63.
149. Proudfoot J, Ryden C, Everitt B, et al. Clinical efficacy of computerize cognitive-behavioral therapy for anxiety and depression in primary care; randomized controlled trial. Br J Psychiatry. 2004;185:46-54.
150. Swinson RP, soulios C, Cox Bj, Kuch K. Brief treatment of emergency room patients with panic attacks. Am J Psychiatry. 1992;149:944-6.
151. Gardenswarz C, Craske MG. Prevention of panic disorder. Behav Ther. 2001;32:725-37.

CHAPTER 15

Social Anxiety Disorders

JN Vyas, Bhoomika Sachacher, Roshan V Khanande, Jayati Simlai

INTRODUCTION

Most commonly reported psychiatric problems in the society are anxiety related. About 18% of the population suffer from some form of anxiety disorder on yearly basis.[1] These disorders are classified as phobic (anxiety) disorder in Diagnostic and Statistical Manual of Mental Disorders V (DSM-V)[2] and International Classification of Disease 10 (ICD-10).[3] Social anxiety disorder (SAD) was differentiated from other forms of anxiety disorders by researchers nearly 40 years ago.[4] Social phobia is another terminology for SAD in the literature. Individual suffering with SAD feel fearful in social situations and more often than not avoid them just to evade anticipated scrutiny. The faulty cognition in facing such situations is—they feel they might be humiliated in front of everyone. In some of the individuals the concern would be such that they might even avoid close relatives and friends, and would rarely appear in public gatherings with utmost discomfort. The field of medical science has started to understand the impact of this disorder on general population. With recent advances in understanding SAD, it has become very much treatable.[5,6]

Usually these individuals are uncomfortable in meeting unknown people. They usually keep quit in unfamiliar settings. In such situations, they often feel emotionally overwhelmed and exhibit physical symptoms such as tremors, sweating and difficulty in concentration. It is not that they do not crave for social relations, but they avoid it as they fear they would not be liked or would be considered boring. They lack in confidence and often exhibit self-critical attitude.[7] Similarly they avoid any situations where contact with strangers and expressing public opinion is required. A rare type of SAD called as paruresis or shy bladder syndrome has also been described where irrational fear of urinating in public bathrooms is present. Individuals with Social anxiety disorder often present with depression in clinical settings.[8]

A subtype, generalized social anxiety disorder, is included in DSM-V classification. As per recent research there is minimal evidence for diagnosing distinct subtypes on the basis of extent and kind of fear.[9] However, it gives an added advantage to the clinicians to express multiple fears and pervasive nature of the disorder in some of the patients.[10] The fears in generalized type usually extend beyond the levels of normally expressed concerns. It (generalized SAD) is said to affect half of the societal cases affecting from SAD and most approaching for consultation; it remains one of the gravest disorders among anxiety disorders.[10-12]

EPIDEMIOLOGY

As per replication of National Comorbidity Survey SAD's yearly prevalence rate was 7.1% in the community with a lifetime prevalence rate of 12.1%. A higher percentage of females reported symptoms of SAD.[1,9] With some methodological differences (higher threshold for symptoms than required for the DSM-IV diagnosis) the National Epidemiologic Survey on Alcohol and Related Conditions places 12-month prevalence at 2.8% and lifetime at 5.0%, respectively.[13]

Not only USA but also other western and westernized (Israel) countries report similar rates.[14] Some of the countries with exceptionally different culture (Iran[15]) have reported SAD in there population, but at much lower rates. Similarly lower rates have also been reported from Asian countries.[16]

Social anxiety disorder (SAD) usually starts at very young age, with generalize type appearing as early as childhood.[17] However, both adults and adolescents had a similar prevalence of SAD (6–8%) in one of the studies.[18] SAD is one of the most universal reasons for school refusal and dropouts, and it is not unusual to see the disorder take a chronic course.[17,19,20] As it is with other anxiety disorders and depression, SAD is often presents itself along with physical illnesses. Up to 3 to 7% patients with SAD report at primary health care centers.[21,22] Its presence seriously affects functioning and quality of life. This results into financial loss because of the disability and poor performance at work.[21-24]

Behavioral inhibition, one of the heritable temperamental traits, is commonly reported predisposing factor for SAD.[25] Generalized type of SAD, as per research, runs in the family with moderate heritability of 2 to 6%. Twin studies confirm the role of genetic factors in susceptibility to SAD.[26-29] Moreover, to back these findings, it is seen that the rates of childhood abuse and psychosocial misfortune in children having this disorder are no different from general population.[17]

Diagnosis and Evaluation

Usually the patients with SAD come across as soft spoken; they often talk to the point using minimal words. Eye contact is poorly maintained. They almost never come out with their problems on their own because they feel they might not be taken seriously. At the same time expressing it to an unwelcoming stranger (examiner) makes them uncomfortable.[30] These are the obvious difficulties faced by the patients and it affects patient-mental health professional relationship. A skilled professional who suspects the disorder in the client, probably should start by asking "Is it difficult for you to meet strangers in a social gathering". This line of questioning might lead to a proper interview and diagnosis. Self-rating tools can be used to screen social SAD among adults (Table 1).[31-35] Screening for children by clinician administered questioners is also available.[36]

The biggest criticism for the current classification and understanding of SAD is whether anxiety and shyness can be explained on the basis of normal variation in human behavior and personality,[37] and equally important is whether mental health professionals are wrongly labeling extreme anxiety with a diagnosis. Only a handful of children with shyness go on to exhibit SAD in adulthood; similarly only half the number of affected individuals report anxiety problems in childhood.[38,39] In other words it also means, it is not imperative that SAD roots from shyness. SAD—a manmade disorder—is one more profound criticism haunting the stability of this category of diagnosis. Some factions of society claim that the disorder is created just to benefit drug manufacturing companies. But, on the flip side, it is evident that SAD impacts public health as per days of work lost[40] and quality of life.[41] However, the process of tagging a condition as pathological must be thought over.[42]

Differential Diagnosis

A person being shy is not something new as per personality aspects and temperaments go, but if this attribute is affecting the functioning of the individual, and that individual finds it distressing, then a diagnosis of SAD can be considered. For this disorder to be diagnosed, as it has been discussed previously, a clinician with a keen eye is needed. If not carefully interviewed, the diagnosis is often missed.

It is not easy to differentiate SAD from panic disorder and agoraphobia. Usually it is seen that they present together. However, with the help of a good interview, specifically asking for reasons for the anxiety symptoms, one can reach the diagnosis. Patients suffering from panic disorder and/or agoraphobia often cannot explain their symptoms or for that matter reasons for it. But, one affected with SAD knows the problem well.[43]

Anxiety disorders and depressive disorder tend to coexist, but they cannot be equated. Staying away from friends and family for brief periods of depression can be explained on the basis of low mood, than anxiety. Keeping this in mind depression can easily be distinguished from SAD.[44] As obsessive compulsive disorder (OCD) is an anxiety disorder conceptually; it can present itself with social anxiety. The best way to set them apart for a clinician is to elicit whether public avoidance is because of obsessions and/or compulsions.[45-47] In case of eating disorders it is imperative to see whether the social escapism is for core symptoms of the disorder or due to associated comorbid SAD.[48]

In dysmorphophobia, i.e. body dysmorphic disorder (BDD) the escaping of social situation is for overvalued ideas about one's body parts and facial features. If carefully interviewed, this can easily be found out. Coexistence of SAD and BDD is not uncommon.[49] Substance abuse is commonly reported problem among patients suffering from anxiety disorders; they consume it to lessen the anxiety.[50]

Starting from childhood and running a chronic course, SAD remains one of the close differential diagnoses of anxious avoidant personality disorder. Nearly all (40–90%) the patients with social anxiety disorder are diagnosed with anxious avoidant personality disorder,[51,52] and these

Table 1: Screening instruments for social anxiety disorder in adults

Tools	*Format*	*Comments*
Anxiety and Depression Detector (ADD)[31]	5-item self-report	Sensitive to major depression and other anxiety disorders but not social anxiety disorder
Generalized Anxiety Disorder-7(GAD-7)[22]	7-item self-report	Sensitive to anxiety disorder but not specific for social anxiety disorder
Liebowitz Social Anxiety Scale (LSAS)[32]	24-item self-report	Sensitive and specific for social anxiety disorder, including generalized subtype
Social Interaction Anxiety Scale (SIAS)[33]	20-item self-report	Preliminary evidence of usefulness for screening
Social Phobia Inventory (SPIN)[34]	17-item self-report	Sensitive and specific for social anxiety disorder
Mini-Social Phobia Inventory (Mini-SPIN)[35]	3-item self-report	Very brief yet sensitive and specific for generalized social anxiety disorder

two terms are often used interchangeably in the literature. However, extreme form of generalized SAD can be labeled with anxious avoidant personality disorder, just to reflect upon its severity.[53]

Children presenting with autism frequently have anxiety in unfamiliar situations. But, stereotypical behavior and language problems along with poor eye contact make its differentiation easy from anxiety in SAD.[54] Children with selective mutism more often than not have SAD which completely seizes them in social gatherings.[55,56,17]

Some other psychiatric disorders may look like social anxiety disorder on face value. Patients with schizophrenia exhibit social fears, but it is the persecution part which makes them escape social situations than fear of humiliation in public. Bipolar affective disorder not infrequently presents with social anxiety disorder.[47]

A few physical disorders, for their associated body damaging capacity, render an individual unappealing. From acne to severe burn scars can make a person anxious in societal gatherings. Intentionally diagnosing such cases will definitely help in managing their anxiety.[57,58,6]

The pictographic view of the above discussion is shown in Figure 1.

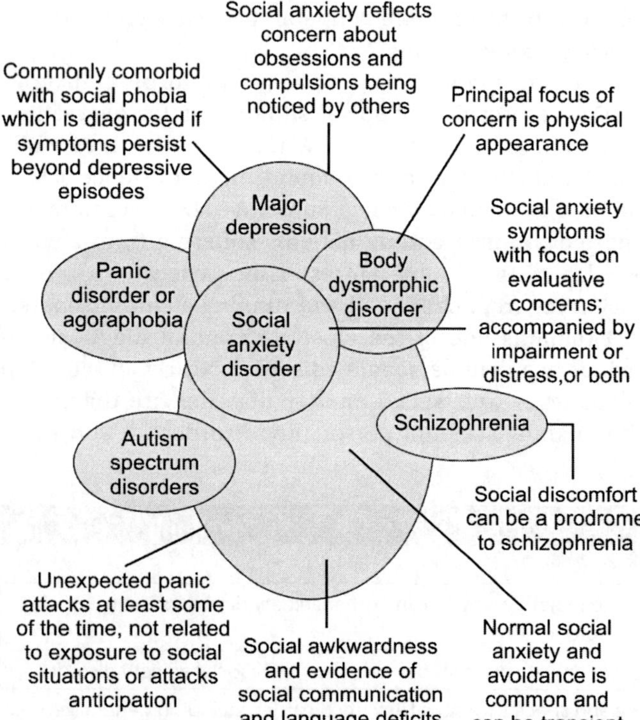

Fig. 1: Conditions that commonly overlap with social anxiety disorder (social phobia) and might be considered in the differential diagnosis of an individual with social anxiety symptoms

Causes and Pathogenesis

Decades of research has given us glimpse of the possible causes of SAD. Few of the heritable behavioral underpinnings such as inhibition in initiating any behavior have been found associated with anxiety spectrum disorders and not specifically for any particular disorder.[25,29] Research in the field of genetics has come up with chromosome 16, proximate to norepinephrine transporter, which is thought to be associated with SAD.[59] Low levels of extraversion has classically been described as a psychodynamic part associated with anxiety disorders. It has been found related to a functional character at β-adrenergic receptor (ADRB1) gene[60,61] and with single nucleotide polymorphisms (SNPs) within catechol-O-methyl-transferase (COMT) gene in females.[62]

Behavioral inhibition, an attribute, has been related to corticotrophin releasing hormone (CRH) gene by a group of researchers.[63] A type of polymorphism—5HTTLPR—at serotonin transporter gene has also been found related to shyness commonly seen in anxiety disorders.[64,65] Similar findings have also been reported in animal studies for *RGS2* gene.[66] Research into neuroimaging has documented activation of amygdale and insula to exposure of faces portraying various emotions. SAD's association with glutamic acid decarboxylase 1 (GAD1) gene has also been reported.[67]

Research conducted till date reveals a lot of things, but it also projects a lot many questions. Autism and SAD overlap significantly for a single symptom—anxiety; a counterpart of behavioral inhibition. Studying comparing genome of families with both the disorders will pave way in the search for gene governing the trait; behavioral inhibition.[27] Now is the time to move beyond candidate gene studies, scanning the whole genome through genome wide association approaches.[68]

In patients with Parkinson's disease having striatal dopamine deficiency, SAD is commonly detected.[69] Similarly, striatal dopamine dysfunction has been seen by dopamine receptor positon emission tomography (PET) studies in patients with generalized SAD[70,71] with reduced activation in the left caudate during a functional task, highlighting the role of striatal dysfunction in this disorder.[72]

Functional studies have pointed out the role of amygdala in response to fear.[73] The level of its activation corresponds with the severity of SAD.[74] A similar association could be found between activation of both insular cortices and anxiety disorders[75] and anxious individuals who were not patients.[76] Children with behavioral inhibition when grow up into adults also have increased activation of amygdala to new faces[77] which is reduced/absent in patients with William's syndrome who lack social fear.[78] The results from various other neuroimaging studies have been given in Table 2.[79-83]

Within the neurocircuitry, the corticolimbic and corticostriatal tracts are commonly involved in SAD.[84]

Table 2: Summary of neuroimaging studies in social anxiety disorder

Studies	*Findings*
Proton (1H) MRS	Increased glutamate in anterior cingulate cortex versus healthy controls[79]
PET rCBF	Increased amygdale blood flow during public speaking in patients versus healthy controls. Reduction in amygdale blood flow with cognitive behavioral therapy or pharmacological treatment[80]
PET receptor density with specific ligands	Reduced striatal dopamine reuptake site density in patients.[71] Low striatal dopamine D2 receptor binding potential in patients.[70] Reduced serotonin-1A (5-HT1A) binding potential in amygdale, anterior cingulate, and insula in patients[81]
Functional MRI	Increased amygdale activation in patients during emotional face processing.[74,82] Increased anterior cingulate activation in patients during disgust face processing.[83] Reduced striatal (left caudate activation) activation in patients during implicit sequence learning[72]

The abnormalities described in the amygdala and insula have been shown to normalize by pharmacotherapy or psychotherapy.[80,85] Serotonin dysfunction has been implicated[86] with some of the variants causing its depletion leading to loss of beneficial effect provided by antidepressants.[87] Some of the nuero-endocrine hormones (e.g. oxytocin and vasopressin)[88] involved in regulation of emotions such as trust, rejection and fear[89,90] have also been found to be beneficial paving the way for new treatment options.

Treatment

Both medications and cognitive behavior therapy (CBT) are effective interventions for SAD.[91,92] Further, when both were compared against each other, pharmacotherapy was shown to bring about a rapid improvement while the effects of CBT were shown to be long lasting.[93,94] Though the guidelines pitch for either of the two modalities as the first-line of treatment,[95] their combination has not been found to be beneficial than either alone.[96,97] Thus, the preference of one treatment over the other, or the use of combined treatment rests upon clinical judgment, e.g. preference to pharmacotherapy in an extremely anxious patient or who is not able to follow the instructions of the therapy. A novel glutamatergic agent D—cycloserine has been shown to be a potent augmenting agent for psychotherapy in social phobia,[98] paving way for more mechanism-oriented treatments for SAD.

Table 3: Data on SSRIs/SNRIs for SAD

SSRI/SNRI	*Dose (mg/ day)*	*Number of patients*	*Response rate for drug*	*Response rate for placebo*
Citalopram[85]	40	36	50%	8%
Escitalopram[101,102]	5–20	1028	54–71%	39–50%
Fluvoxamine[103-105]	50–300	422	43–48%	7–44%
Fluoxetine[92,106]	20–60	108	40–51%	30–32%
Paroxetine[101,107-110]	20–50	2188	55–72%	8–50%
Sertraline[96,111-113]	50–200	616	40–53%	9–29%
Venlafaxine[108,114-116]	75–225	1547	44–69%	30–36%

Monoamine oxidase inhibitors were one of the earliest agents found to be efficacious in generalized SAD,[99] but their use has markedly decreased due to the need for dietary restrictions and associated adverse effects. Though the reversible inhibitors of monoamine oxidase A (RIM A) such as moclobemide were devoid of these limitations, its use has largely been restricted due to lack of approval in countries such as USA or absence of benefit in short-term trials. Another class of drugs which have received less attention are the benzodiazepines (alprazolam or clonazepam) for fear of their dependence potential.[93,100]

With respect to pharmacotherapy, both the selective serotonin reuptake inhibitors (SSRIs) and selective serotonin—norepinephrine reuptake inhibitors (SNRIs) have proved their worth making them the first choice of treatment.[101-116] The outcome in most of the studies was measured using the Liebowitz Social Anxiety Scale.[117] Their details have been provided in Table 3.

Among both the groups of drugs, results with use of fluoxetine have not been consistent.[106] In a meta-analysis, both the group of drugs were comparable to their use in depression or medications used in general medicine.[108,118] The dose response curve for these drugs is flat[107,114] and so some patients might respond to higher doses or might respond only by week 12.[100] Though the relapse rates with the use of escitalopram, paroxetine, sertraline (4–14%) have been lower when compared to placebo (36–39%),[119-121] treatment should be continued for at least 12 months after the acute management of symptoms. It would be prudent to add CBT in long-term treatment that might help in tapering and removing the drug after response but more data is awaited on this contention. Most of the multicenter trials have been conducted in tertiary care centers with the aim of gaining approval for the use of drugs in this disorder, however, their use in SAD has been found to be cost effective.[122] Similarly, predictability studies on the response to drugs are lacking but some studies have shown that length of treatment was a predictor of response to paroxetine[110] whereas S/S variant of SLC6A4 promoter polymorphism 5HTTLPR was predictive of poor response to

SSRIs.[123] Studies in children and adolescents are lacking with some finding fluvoxamine[124] and paroxetine[125] to be safe and effective[126] in SAD though monitoring for suicidal ideation in this population is pertinent.[127] Studies comparing the intraclass drugs or interclass drugs are negligible, however, it has been noted that serotonergic reuptake blockade rather than noradrenergic reuptake blockade is essential for the response in SAD.[123]

As already discussed CBT also forms the first-line of management for SAD. The module is based on the relationship between dysfunctional beliefs and avoidance behavior.[83] The components of a successful therapy should include:[128]

- Psychoeducation
- Relaxation exercises
- Social skills training
- Imaginal and in vivo exposure
- Cognitive restructuring.

However, the inclusion of which of the above components, crucial for the success of therapy remains controversial,[129] though inclusion of cognitive component has been found to be essential. Further, evidence for individual therapy is more compelling than group therapy[130] but its usefulness in real world settings is yet to be proven.[131] The beneficial role of CBT for children and adolescents with SAD has been proven[17] with a potential role for prevention[132] in the presence of risk factors such as behavioral inhibition.

In the absence of response to first-line agents, there is preliminary support for the use of benzodiazepines[133] and pindolol[134] with SSRIs. Some other agents such as mirtazapine,[135] gabapentin,[136] and pregabalin[137] have been found useful in treating SAD. The atypical antipsychotics have been used in some treatment resistant anxiety disorders[138] but their use in SAD is yet to be established. Again, drug refractory patients can benefit from psychotherapy as an augmenting agent but data remains inconclusive.

CONCLUSION

Though the field of social anxiety disorder (SAD) has witnessed significant headways, there is a compelling need to generate search for underlying endophenotypes as the field of neuroscience is rapidly expanding. Long-term studies are required in real life context to establish the effectiveness of available therapies. As many patients remain undiagnosed and untreated for year's altogether, efforts are needed to cater to early identification and effective utilization of health care services to reduce the burden due to this disorder.

REFERENCES

1. Kessler RC, Chiu WT, Demler O, Walters EE. Prevalence, severity, and comorbidity of 12-month DSM-IV disorders in the National Comorbidity Survey Replication. Arch Gen Psychiatry. 2005;62:617.
2. American Psychiatry Association. Diagnostic & statistical manual for mental disorder (DSM), 4th edition. Washington, DC; American Psychiatry Press, Inc; 1994.
3. WHO. International Statistical Classification of Diseases and Related Health Problems, 10th Revision. World Health Organization, 2007. *http://www.who.int/classifications/apps/icd/icd10online/* (accessed Oct 15,2011).
4. Marks IM, Gelder MG. Different ages of onset in varieties of phobias. Am J Psychiatry. 1966;123:218-21.
5. Stein MB. How shy is too shy? Lancet. 1996;347:1131-2.
6. Schneier FR. Clinical practice. Social anxiety disorder. N Engl J Med. 2006;355:1029-36.
7. Cox BJ, Fleet C, Stein MB. Self-criticism and social phobia in the US National Comorbidity Survey. J Affect Disord. 2004;82:227-34.
8. Vythilingum B, Stein DJ, Soifer S. Is "shy bladder syndrome" a subtype of social anxiety disorder? A survey of people with paruresis. Depress Anxiety. 2002;16:84-7.
9. Ruscio AM, Brown TA, Chiu WT, et al. Social fears and social phobia in the USA: results from the National Comorbidity Survey Replication. Psychol Med 2008;35:15-28.
10. Kessler RC, Stein MB, Berglund PA. Social phobia subtypes in the National Comorbidity Survey. Am J Psychiatry. 1998;155: 613-9. 11.
11. Katzelnick DJ. Kobak KA, Deleire T, et al. Impact of generalized social anxiety disorder in managed care. Am J Psychiatry. 2001;158:1999-2007.
12. Stein MB, Walker JR, Forde DR. Public-speaking fears in a community sample: Prevalence, impact on functioning and diagnostic classification. Arch Gen Psychiatry. 1996;53: 169-74.
13. Grant BF, Hasin DS, Blanco C, et al. The epidemiology of social anxiety disorder in the United States: results from the National Epidemiologic Survey on Alcohol and Related Conditions. J Clin Psychiatry. 2005;66:1351-61.
14. Iancu I, Levin J, Hermesh H, et al. Social phobia symptoms: prevalence, sociodemographic correlates, and overlap with specific phobia symptoms. Compr Psychiatry. 2006;47: 399-405.
15. Mohammadi MR, Ghanizadeh A, Mohammadi M, Mesgarpour B. Prevalence of social phobia and its comorbidity with psychiatric disorders in Iran. Depress Anxiety. 2006;23:405-11.
16. Matsunaga H, Kiriike N, Matsui T, Iwasaki Y, Stein DJ. Taijin Kyofusho: a form of social anxiety disorder that responds to serotonin reuptake inhibitors? Int J Neuropsychopharmacol. 2001;4:231-7.
17. Chacira DA, Stein MB. Childhood social anxiety disorder: from understanding to treatment. Child Adolesc Psychiatry Clin N Am. 2005;14:797-818.
18. Chavira DA, Stein MB, Bailey K, Stein MT. Child anxiety in primary care: prevalent but untreated. Depress Anxiety. 2005; 20:155-64.
19. Stein MB, Kean Y. Disability and quality of life in social phobia. Am J Psychiatry. 2000;157:1606-13.

20. Cairney J, McCabe L, Veldhuizen S, Corna LM, Streiner D. Herrmann N. Epidemiology of social phobia in later life. Am J Geriatr Psychiatry. 2007;15:224-33.
21. Kroenke K, Spitzer RL, Williams JB, Monahan PO, Lowe B. Anxiety disorder in primary care: prevalence, impairment, comorbidity, and detection. Ann Intern Med. 2007;146: 317-25.
22. Sareen J, Jacobi F, Cox BJ, Belik SL, Clara I, Stein MB. Disability and poor quality of life associated with comorbid anxiety disorders and physical conditions. Arch Intern Med. 2006; 166:2109-16.
23. Stein MB, Roy-Byrne PP, Craske MG, et al. Functional impact and health utility of anxiety disorders in primary care outpatients. Med Care. 2005;43:1164-70.
24. Wang PS, Lane M, Olfson M, Pincus HA, Wells KB, Kessler RC. Twelve-month use of mental health services in the United States: results from the National Comorbidity Survey Replication. Arch Gen Psychiatry. 2005;62:629-40.
25. Hirshfeld-Becker DR, Biderman J, Henin A, et al. Behavioural inhibition in preschool children at risk is a specific predictor of middle childhood social anxiety: a five-year follow-up. J Dev Behav Pediatr. 2007;164:1714-21.
26. Stein MB, Chartier MJ, Hazen AL, Kozak MV, Tancer ME, Lander S, et al. A direct-interview family study of generalized social phobia. Am J Psychiatry. 1998;155:90-7.
27. Stein MB, Gelernter J, Smoller JW. Genetic aspects of social anxiety and related traits. In: Bandelow B, Stien DJ (Eds). Social anxiety disorder, more than shyness. New York: Marcel Dekker; 2004. pp. 197-214.
28. Stein MB, Jang KL, Livesley WJ. Heritability of social-anxiety related concerns and personality characteristics: a twin study. J Nerv Ment Dis. 2002;190:219-24.
29. Bienvenu OJ, Hetterna JM, Neale MC, Prescott CA, Kendler KS. Low extraversion and high neuroticism as indices of genetic and environmental risk for social phobia, agoraphobia, and animal phobia. Am J Psychiatry. 2007;164:1714-21.
30. Roy-Byrne PP, Stein M B. Social anxiety in primary care: hidden in plain view? Gen Hosp Psychiatry. 2005;27:155-7.
31. Means-Christensen AJ, Sherbourne CD, Roy-Byrne PP, Craske MG, Stein MB. Using five questions to screen for five common mental disorders in primary care: diagnostic accuracy of the Anxiety and Depression Detector. Gen Hosp Psychiatry. 2006;28:108-18.
32. Mennin DS, Fresco DM, Heimberg RG, Schneier FR, Davies SO, Liebowitz MR. Screening for social anxiety disorder: in the clinical setting: using the Liebowitz Social Anxiety Scale. J Anxiety Disord. 2002;16:661-73.
33. Rodebaugh TL, Woods CM, Heimberg RG, Liebowitz MR. Schneier FR. The factor structure and screening utility of the social interaction anxiety scale. Psychol Assess. 2006;18:231-7.
34. Connor KM, Davidson JR, Churchill LE, Sherwood A, Foa EB, Weisler RH. Psychometric properties of the Social Phobia Inventory (SPIN): a new self-rating scale. Br J Psychiatry. 2000; 176:379-86.
35. Connor K, Kobak KA, Churchil E, Katzelnick DJ, Davidson JRT. Mini-SPIN: a brief screening assessment for generalized social anxiety disorder. Depress Anxiety. 2001;14:137-40.
36. Bailey KA, Chavira DA, Stein MT, Stein MB. Brief measures to screen for social phobia in primary care pediatrics. J Pediatr Psychol. 2006;31:512-21.
37. Wakefield JC, Horwitz AV, Schmitz MF. Are we overpathologizing the socially anxious? Social phobia from a harmful dysfunction perspective. Can J Psychiatry. 2005;50:317-9.
38. Cooper PJ, Eke M. Childhood shyness and maternal social phobia: a community study. Br J Psychiatry. 1999;174:439-43.
39. Cox BJ, MacPherson PS, Enns MW. Psychiatric correlates of childhood shyness in a nationally representative sample. Behav Res Ther. 2005;43:1019-27.
40. Alonso J, Angermeyer MC, Bernert S, et al. Disability and quality of life impact of mental disorders in Europe: results from the European Study of the Epidemiology of Mental Disorders (ESEMeD) project. Acta Psychiatr Scand Suppl. 2004;420:38-46.
41. Saarni SJ, Suvisaari J, Sintonen H, et al. Impact of psychiatric disorders on health-related quality of life. Br J Psychiatry. 2007;190:326-32.
42. Stein DJ. Philosophy and the DSM-III. Compr Psychiatry. 1991; 32:404-15.
43. Roy-Byrne PP, Craske MG, Stein MB. Panic disorder. Lancet. 2006;368:1023-32.
44. Rush AJ, Zimmerman M, Wisniewski SR, et al. Comorbid psychiatric disorders in depressed outpatients: demographic and clinical features. J Affect Disord. 2005;87:43-55.
45. Beesdo K, Bittner A, Pine DS, et al. Incidence of social anxiety disorder and the consistent risk for secondary depression in the first three decades of life. Arch Gen Psychiatry. 2007;64:903-12.
46. Pallanti S, Quercioli L, Hollander E. Social anxiety in outpatients with schizophrenia: a relevant cause of disability. Am J Psychiatry. 2004;161:53-8.
47. Simon NM, Otto MW, Wisniewski SR, et al. Anxiety disorder comorbidity in bipolar disorder patients: data from the first 500 participants in the Systematic Treatment Enhancement Program for Bipolar Disorder (STEP-BD). Am J Psychiatry. 2004;161:2222-9.
48. Kaye WH, Bulik CM, Thornton L, Barbarich N, Masters K. Comorbidity of anxiety disorders with anorexia and bulimia nervosa. Am J Psychiatry. 2004;161:2215-21.
49. Coles ME, Phillips KA, Menard W, et al. Body dysmorphic disorder and social phobia: cross-sectional and prospective data. Depress Anxiety. 2006;23:26-33.
50. Sareen J, Chartier M, Paulus MP, Stein MB. Illicit drug use and anxiety disorders: findings from two community surveys. Psychiatry Res. 2006;142:11-7.
51. Shea MT, Stout RL, Yen S, et al. Associations in the course of personality disorder and axis I disorders over time. J Abnorm Psychol. 2004;113:499-508.
52. Grant BF, Hasin DS, Stinson FS, et al. Co-occurrence of 12-month mood and anxiety disorders and personality

disorders in the US: results from the national epidemiologic survey on alcohol and related conditions. J Psychiatry Res. 2005;39:1-9.
53. Massion AO, Dyck I, Shea MT, Phillips KA, Warshaw MG, Keller MB. Personality disorders and time to remission in generalized anxiety disorder, social phobia, and panic disorder. Arch Gen Psychiatry. 2002;59:434-40.
54. Baron-Cohen S, Belmonte MK. Autism: a window onto the developmental of the social and the analytic brain. Ann Rev Neurosci. 2005;28:109-26.
55. Cohan SL, Price JM, Stein MB. Suffering in silence: why a developmental psychopathology perspective on selective mutism is needed. J Dev Behav Pediatr. 2006;27:341-55.
56. Chavira DA, Shipon-Blum E, Hitchcock C, Cohan S, Stein MB. Selective mutism and social anxiety disorder, all in the family? J Am Aced Child Adolesc Psychiatry. 2007;46:1464-72.
57. Schneier FR, Barnes LF, Albert SM, Louis ED. Characteristics of social phobia among persons with essential tremor. J Clin Psychiatry. 2001;62:367-72.
58. Stein MB, Baird A, Walker JR. Social phobia in adults with stuttering. Am J Psychiatry. 1996;153:278-80.
59. Gelernter J, Page GP, Stein MB, Woods SW. Genome-wide linkage scan for loci predisposing to social phobia: evidence for a chromosome 16 risk locus. Am J Psychiatry. 2004;161: 59-66.
60. Stein MB, Chartier MJ, Lizak MV, Jang KL. Familial aggregation of anxiety-related quantitative traits in generalized social phobia: Clues to understanding "disorder" heritability? Am J Med Genet. 2001;105:79-83.
61. Stein MB, Schork NJ, Gelernter J. A polymorphism of the beta (1)-adrenergic receptor is associated with low extraversion. Biol Psychiatry. 2004;56:217-24.
62. Stein MB, Fallin MD. Schork NJ, Gelernter J. COMT Polymorphisms and anxiety-related personality traits. Neuropsychopharmacology. 2005;30:2092-102.
63. Smoller JW, Yam Aki LH. Fagerness JA, et al. The corticotropin-releasing horm one gene and behavioral inhibition in children at risk for panic disorder. Biol Psychiatry. 2005;57:1485-92.
64. Arbelle S, Benhamin J, Golin M, Kremer I, Belmaker RH, Ebstein RP. Relation of shyness in grade school children to the genotype for the long form of the serotonin transporter promoter region polymorphism. Am J Psychiatry. 2003;160:671-6.
65. Rattaglia M, Ogliari A. Zanoni A, et al. Influence of the serotonin transporter promoter gene and shyness on children's cerebral responses to facial expressions. Arch Gen Psychiatry. 2005;62:85-94.
66. Smoller JW, Paulus MP, Fagerness JA, et al. RSG2 influences anxiety-related temperament, personality and brain function. Arch Gen Psychiatry. 2008;65:298-308.
67. Hettema JM, Neale MC, Myers JM, Prescott CA, Kendler KS. A population-based twin study of the relationship between neuroticism and internalizing disorder. Am J Psychiatry. 2006; 163:857-64.
68. Papassotiropoulos A, Stephan DA, Huentelman MJ, et al. Common Kibra alleles are associated with human memory performance. Science. 2006;314:475-8.
69. Stein MB, Heuser IJ, Juncos JL, Uhde TW. Anxiety disorders in patients with Parkinson's disease. Am J Psychiatry. 1990;147:217-20.
70. Schneier FR, Liebowitz MR, Abi-Dargham A, Zea-Ponce Y, Lin S-H, Laruelle M. Low dopamine D2 receptor binding potential in social phobia. Am J Psychiatry. 2000;157:457-9.
71. Tiihonen J, Kuikka J, Bergstrom K, Lepola U, Koponen H. Leinonen E. Dopamine reuptake site densities in patients with social phobia. Am J Peychiatry. 1997;154:239-42.
72. Sareen J, Campbell DW, Leslie WD, et al. Striatal function in generalized social phobia: a functional magnetic resonance imaging study. Biol Psychiatry. 2007;61:396-404.
73. Etkin A, Wager TD. Functional neuroimaging of anxiety: a meta-analysis of emotional processing in PTSD, social anxiety disorder, and specific phobia. Am J Psychiatry. 2007; 164:1476-88.
74. Phan KL, Fitzgerald DA, Nathan PJ, Tancer ME. Association between amygdala hyperactivity to harsh faces and severity of social anxiety in generalized social phobia. Biol Psychiatry. 2006;59:424-9.
75. Paulus MP, Stein M B. An insular view of anxiety. Biol Psychiatry. 2006;60:383-7.
76. Stein MB, Simmons A, Feinstein JS, Paulus MP. Increased amygdala and insula activation during emotion processing in anxiety-prone subjects. Am J Psychiatry. 2007;164:318-27.
77. Schwartz CE, Wright CI, Shin LM, Kagan J, Rauch SL. Inhibited and uninhibited infants "grown up": adult amygdala response to novelty. Science. 2003;300:1952-3.
78. Meyer-Lindenberg A, Hariri AR, M unoz KE, et al. Neural correlates of genetically abnormal social cognition in Williams syndrome. Nat Neurosci. 2005;8:991-3.
79. Phan KL, Fiezgerald DA, Cortese BM, Seraji-Bozorgzad N, Tancer ME, Moore GJ. Anterior cingulate neurochemistry in social anxiety disorder: 1H-MRS at 4 Tesla. Neuro Report. 2005;16:183-6.
80. Furmark T, Tillfors M, Marteinsdottir I, et al. Common changes in cerebral blood flow in patients with social phobia treated with citalopram or cognitive-behavioral therapy. Arch Gen Psychiatry. 2002;59:425-33.
81. Lanzenberger RR, Mitterhauser M, Spindelegger C, et al. Reduced serotonin-1A receptor binding in social phobia. Biol Psychiatry. 2007;61:1081-9.
82. Stein MB, Goldin PR, Sareen J, Zorrilla LT, Brown GG. Increased amygdale activation to angry and contemptuous faces in generalized social phobia. Arch Gen Psychiatry. 2002;59: 1027-34.
83. Amir N, Klumpp H, Elias J, Bedwell JS, Yanasak N, Miller LS. Increased activation of the anterior cingulate cortex during processing of disgust faces in individuals with social phobia Biol Psychiatry. 2005;57:975-81.

84. Rapee RM, Spence SH. The etiology of social phobia empirical evidence and an initial model. Clin Psychol Rev. 2004;24:737-67.
85. Furmark T, Appel L, M ichelgard A, et al. Cerebral blood flow changes after treatment of social phobia with the neurokinin-1 antagonist GR205171, citalopram, or placebo. Biol Psychiatry. 2005;58:132-42.
86. Hariri AR, Drabant EM, Weinberger DR. Imaging genetics: perspective from studies of genetically driven variation in serotonin function and corticolimbic affective processing. Biol Psychiatry. 2006;59:888-97.
87. Argyropoulos SV, Hood SD, Adrover M, et al. Tryptophan depletion reverses the therapeutic effect of selective serotonin reuptake inhibitors in social anxiety disorder. Biol Psychiatry. 2004;56:503-9.
88. Bartz JA, Hollander E. The neuroscience of affiliation: forging links between basic and clinical research on neuropeptides and social behavior. Horm Behav. 2006;50:518-28.
89. Kosfeld M, Heinrichs M, Zak PJ, Fischbacher U, Fehr E. Oxytocin increases trust in humans. Nature. 2005;435:673-6.
90. Kirsch P, Esslinger C, Chan Q, et al. Oxytocin modulates neural circuitry for social cognition and fear in humans. J Neutosci. 2005;25:11489-93.
91. Fedoroff IC, Taylor S. Psychological and pharmacological treatments of social phobia: a meta-analysis. J Clin Psychopharmacol. 2001;21:311-24.
92. Stein DJ, Ipser JC, Balkom AJ. Pharmacotherapy for social phobia. Cochrane Database Syst Rev. 2004;4:CD001206.
93. Gelernter CS, Uhde TW, Cimbolic P, et al. Cognitive-behavioral and Pharmacological treatments of social Phobia: a controlled study. Arch Gen Psychiatry. 1991;48:938-45.
94. Heimberg RG, Liebowitz MR, Hope DA, et al. Cognitive behavioural group therapy vs phenelzine therapy for social phobia: 12-week outcome. Arch Gen Psychiatry. 1998;55:1133-41.
95. Swinson RP, Antony MM, Bleau PB, et al. Clinical practice guidelines: management of anxiety disorders. Can J Psychiatry. 2006;51(Suppl 2):1-92.
96. Blomhoff S, Haug TT, Hellstrom K, et al. Randomized controlled general practice trial of sertraline, exposure therapy and combined treatment in generalized social phobia. Br J Psychiatry. 2011;179:23-30.
97. Davidson JR, Foa EB, Huppert JD, et al. Fluoxetine, comprehensive cognitive behavioural therapy, and placebo in generalized social phobia. Arch Gen Psychiatry. 2004;61:1005-13.
98. Hofmann SG, Meuret AE, Smits JA, et al. Augmentation of exposure therapy with D-cycloserine for social anxiety disorder. Arch Gen Psychiatry. 2006;63:298-304.
99. Liebowitz M R, Schneier FR, Campeas R, et al. Phenelzine vs atenolol in social phobia. Arch Gen Psychiatry. 1992;49:290-300.
100. Davidson JRT, Potts NL, Richichi E, Krishnan KR. Treatment of social phobia with clonazepam and placebo. J Clin Psychopharm. 1993;13:423-8.
101. Lader M, Stender K, Burger V, Nil R. Efficacy and tolerability of escitalopram in 12-and 24-week treatment of social anxiety disorder: randomized, double-blind placebo-controlled, fixed-dose study. Depress Anxiety. 2004;19:241-8.
102. Kasper S, Stein DJ, Loft H, Nil R. Escitalopram in the treatment of social anxiety disorder: randomized, placebo-controlled, flexible-dosage study. Br J Psychiatry. 2005;186:222-6.
103. Van Vliet IM, den Boer JA, Westenberg HGM. Psychopharmacological treatment of social phobia; a double-blind placebo-controlled study with fluvoxamine. Psychopharmacology. 1994;115:128-34.
104. Stein MB, Fyer AJ, Dacison JRT, Pollack MH, Wiita B. Fluvoxamine in social phobia (social anxiety disorder): a double-blind, placebo-controlled clinical study. Am J Psychiatry. 1999;156:756-60.
105. Westenberg HG, Stein DJ, Yang H, Li D. Barbato LM. A double-blind, placebo-controlled study of controlled release fluvoxamine for the treatment of generalized social anxiety disorder. J Clin Psychopharmacol. 2004;24:49-55.
106. Kobak KA, Greist JH, Jefferson JW, Katzelnick DJ. Fluoxetine in social phobia: a double-blind, placebo-controlled pilot sturdy. J Clin Psychopharmacol. 2002;22:257-62.
107. Liebowitz MB, Stein MB, Tancer ME, Carpenter D, Oakes R, Pitts CD. A randomized, double-blind, fixed-dose comparison of paroxetine and placebo in the treatment of generalized social anxiety disorder. J Clin Psychiatry. 2002;63:66-74.
108. Liebowitz MR, Gelenberg AJ, Munjack D. Venlafaxine extended release vs placebo and paroxetine in social anxiety disorder. Arch Gen Psychiatry. 2005;62:190-8.
109. Stein MB, Liebowitz MR, Lydiard RB, Bushnell W, Gergel IP. Paroxetine treatment of generalized social anxiety disorder (social phobia): a randomized controlled trial. JAMA. 1998;280:708-13.
110. Stein DJ, Stein MB, Pitts CD, Kumar R, Hunter B. Predictors of response to pharmacotherapy in social anxiety disorder: an analysis of 3 placebo-controlled paroxetine trials. J Clin Psychiatry. 2002;63:152-5.
111. Katzelnick DJ, Kobak Kalaiya, Greist JH, Jefferson JW, Mantle JM, Serlin RC. Sertraline for social phobia: a double-blind, placebo-controlled crossover study. Am J Psychiatry. 1995;152:1368-71.
112. Van Ameringen M, Lane RM. Walker JR, et al. Sertraline treatment of generalized social phobia: A 20-week, double-blind, placebo-controlled study. Am J Psychiatry. 2001;158:275-81.
113. Liebowitz MR, DeMartinis NA, Weihs K, et al. Efficacy of sertraline in severe generalized social anxiety disorder: results of a double-blind, placebo-controlled study. J Clin Psychiatry. 2013;64:785-92.
114. Stein MB, Pollack MH, Bystritsky A, Kelsey JE, Mangano RM. Efficacy of low and higher dose extended-release venlafaxine in generalized social anxiety disorder: a 6-month randomized controlled trial. Psychopharmacology (Berl). 2005;177:280-8.

115. Rickels K, Mangano R, Khan A. A double-blind, placebo-controlled study of a flexible dose of venlafaxine ER in adult outpatients with generalized social anxiety disorder. J Clin Psychopharmacol. 2004;24:488-96.
116. Liebowitz MR, Mangano RM, Bradwejn J, Asnis G. A randomized controlled trail of venlafaxine extended release in generalized social anxiety disorder. J Clin Psychiatry. 2005;66:238-47.
117. Heimberg RG, Horner KJ, Juster HR, et al. Psychometric properties of the Liebowitz Social Anxiety Scale. Psychol Med. 1999;29:199-212.
118. ven der Linden G, stein DJ, ven Balkom AJ. The efficacy of the selective serotonin reuptake inhibitors for social anxiety disorder (social phobia): A meta-analysis of randomized controlled trails. Int Clin Psychopharm. 2000;15(Suppl 2): S15-23.
119. Stein DJ, Versiani M, Hair T , Kumar R. Efficacy of paroxetine for relapse prevention in social anxiety disorder : a 24-week study. Arch Gen Psychiatry. 2012;59:1111-87.
120. Montgomery SA, Nil R, Durr-Pal N, Loft H, Boulenger JP. A 24-week randomized, double-blind, placebo-controlled study of escitalopram for the prevention of generalized social anxiety disorder. J Clin Psychiatry. 2005;66:1270-8.
121. Walker JR, Van Ameringen MA, Swinson R, et al. Prevention of relapse in generalized social phobia: results of a 24-week study in responders to 20 weeks sertraline treatment. J Clin Psychopharm. 2000;20:636-44.
122. Issakidis C, Sanderson K, Corry J, Andrews G, Labslay H. Modelling the population cost-effectiveness of current and evidence-based optimal treatment for anxiety disorder. Psychol Med. 2004;34:19-35.
123. Stein MB, Seeat S, Gelernter J. Serotonin transporter gene promoter polymorphism predicts SSRI response in generalized social anxiety disorder. Psychopharmacology (Berl). 2006; 187:68-72.
124. The Research Unit on Pediatric Psychopharmacology Anxiety Study Group, Fluvoxamine for the treatment of anxiety disorders in children and adolescents. N Engl J Med. 2001;344: 1279-85.
125. Wagner KD, Berard R, Stein MB, et al. A multicenter, randomized, double-blind, placebo-controlled trial of paroxetine in children and adolescents with social disorder. Arch Gen Psychiatry. 2004;61:1153-62.
126. Bridge JA, Iyengar S, Salary CB, Barbe RP, Birmaher B, Pincus HA, et al. Clinical response and risk for reported suicidal ideation and suicide attempts in pediatric antidepressant treatment: a meta-analysis of randomized controlled trials. JAMA. 2007;297:1683-96.
127. Jick H, Kaye JA, Jick SS. Antidepressants and the risk of suicidal behaviors. JAMA. 2004;292:338-43.
128. Huppert JD, Roth DA, Foa EB. Cognitive-behavioral treatment of social phobia: new advances. Curr Psychiatry Rep. 2003;5:289-96.
129. Clark DM, Ehlers A, Hackmann A, et al. Cognitive therapy versus exposure and applied relaxation in social phobia: A randomized controlled trial. J Consult Clin Psychol. 2006;74:568-78.
130. Mortberg E, Clark DM, Sundin O, Aberg WA. Intensive group cognitive treatment and individual cognitive therapy vs treatment as usual in social phobia: a randomized controlled trial. Acta Psychiatr Scand. 2007;115:142-54.
131. Gaston JE, Abbott MJ, Rapee RM, Neary SA. Do empirically supported treatments generalize to private practice? A benchmark study of a cognitive-behavioural group treatment programme for social phobia. Br J Clin Psychol. 2006;45: 33-48.
132. Donovan CL, Spence SH. Prevention of childhood anxiety disorders. Clin Psychol Rev. 2000;20:509-31.
133. Seedat S, Stein MB. Double-blind, placebo-controlled assessment of combined clonazepam with paroxetine compared with paroxetine monotherapy for generalized social anxiety disorder. J Clin Psychiatry. 2004;65:244-8.
134. Stein MB, Sareen J, Hami S, Chao J. Pindolol potentiator of paroxetine for generalized social phobia: a double-blind, placebo-controlled, crossover study. Am J Psychiatry. 2001;158:1727.
135. Muehlbacher M, Nickel MK, Nickel C, Kettler C, Lahmann C, Pedrosa GF, et al. Mirtazapine treatment of social phobia in woman: a randomized, double-blind, placebo-controlled study. J Clin Psychopharmacol. 2005;25:580-3.
136. Pande AC, Feltner DE, Jefferson JW, et al. Efficacy of the novel anxiolytic pregabalin in social anxiety disorder: a placebo-controlled, multicenter study. J Clin Psychopharmacol. 2004;24:141-9.
137. Pande AC, Davidson JR, Jefferson JW, et al. Treatment of social phobia with: gabapentin: a placebo-controlled study. J Clin Psychopharmacol. 1999;19:341-8.
138. Pollack MH, Simon NM, Zalta AK, et al. Olanzapine augmentation of fluoxetine for refractory generalized anxiety disorder: a placebo-controlled study. Biol Psychiatry. 2014;59:211-5.

CHAPTER 16 Adjustment Disorders and Bereavement

Shree Ram Ghimire

16.1 ADJUSTMENT DISORDER

INTRODUCTION

Adjustment disorder refers to the psychological reactions arising in relation to adapting to new circumstance. Such circumstances include divorce and separation, a major change of work and abode such as transition from school to university, or migration, or birth of handicapped child, etc.

The ICD-10[1] and DSM-IV[2] define adjustment disorders as transient states of distress and emotional disturbance, which arise in the course of adapting to a significant life change, stressful life event, serious physical illness, or possibility of serious illness.

The stressor may involve only the individual, or may also affect their wider community. Individual predisposition plays a greater role in the risk of occurrence of adjustment disorders than it does in the other reactions to stressful events, such as post-traumatic stress disorder, but it is assumed that the condition would not have arisen without the stressor. ICD-10 defines the stressor as "not of an unusual or catastrophic type."

Adjustment disorder is sometimes criticized as "medicalizing of problems of living,"[3] because there is an indistinct separation between the condition and normal reactions to stress.[4] However, most studies have shown that adjustment disorder is a distinct psychiatric condition. DSM-IV does not allow a diagnosis of adjustment disorder to be made if the disturbance meets the criteria for a different psychiatric condition, or if the disturbance is an exacerbation of a pre-existing psychiatric condition or personality disorder. The symptoms can include depressed mood, anxiety, worry, a feeling of inability to cope, plan ahead, or continue in the present situation, and a degree of difficulty in day-to-day living. The individual may feel liable to dramatic behavior or outbursts of violence.[5,6]

ICD-10 DIAGNOSTIC CRITERIA VERSUS DSM-IV-TR DIAGNOSTIC CRITERIA

ICD-10 states the stressor is "not of an unusual or catastrophic type". DSM-IV states that the symptoms are "clinically significant as evidenced by; marked distress in excess of what would be expected from exposure to the stressor; or, significant impairment in social or occupational functioning." ICD-10 and DSM-IV both require that the onset is within 3 months of the occurrence of the stressful event or life change, but ICD-10 adds that the onset is usually within 1 month. ICD-10 states that the duration of symptoms does not usually exceed 6 months (except in the case of "prolonged depressive reaction", which is a specific type of adjustment disorder). DSM-IV states that the symptoms must resolve within 6 months of the termination of the stressor, unless the stressor is chronic or has enduring consequences.

By convention, the normal reaction to bereavement is not diagnosed as an adjustment disorder. However, both ICD-10 and DSM-IV allow grief to be diagnosed as an adjustment disorder if it is of an abnormal type, or if it lasts longer than 6 months. As described above, the criteria in ICD-10 and DSM-IV are slightly different. The same individual may or may not be diagnosed with adjustment disorder, depending upon which classification system is used.

Both the ICD-10 and DSM-IV sub-types of adjustment disorder depend on the profile of symptoms which an individual experiences. However, it should be noted that although the overall condition of adjustment disorder is valid, separating the disorder into sub-categories may be of no benefit.[7] Some changes have been made in DSM-5. Adjustment disorder is kept under trauma and stressor-related disorders.

Controversies and Dilemmas

A diagnosis of adjustment disorder raises a number of dilemmas. The first is the distinction from normal reactions to stress, a separation that is important so as not to pathologize the day-to-day travails of life. There is nothing to assist the clinician in making this distinction except that ICD-10 requires both functional impairment and symptoms to make the diagnosis, while DSM requires symptoms or impairment. Thus, ICD is more stringent and has a higher threshold than DSM. Arguably, a decision on whether a reaction is pathological should take account of a number of factors, including:[7]

- Cultural differences in the expression of emotion
- Individual circumstances (e.g. the loss of a job may render a person homeless, which is appropriately associated with high levels of distress)
- The mere fact of visiting a doctor or being referred to a mental health professional should not inevitably be regarded as indicative of disorder
- The level of functional impairment as a result of the symptoms (ICD-10 only).

The second dilemma is the differentiation of adjustment disorder from other Axis I disorders, such as generalized anxiety disorder (GAD) and major depressive disorder (MDD).[3] Simply on the basis of symptom numbers and duration of more than 2 weeks, adjustment disorder would be relabeled as MDD after the time threshold has been crossed, even though the onset of symptoms was temporally close to the stressor. Thus, a young woman with children who had received a diagnosis of stage IV cancer 3 weeks earlier and now has low mood, is not sleeping, is unable to get pleasure from life, has recurrent thoughts of dying, and has poor concentration might variously be thought to be experiencing an appropriate reaction, an adjustment disorder, or MDD. Examples such as this highlight the need for continued monitoring.

Ordinarily, one would expect the symptoms to resolve when the stressor diminished or was removed. At other times, notwithstanding the persistence of the stressor or its ramifications, the person adapts. A diagnostic conundrum arises, however, when the symptoms and the stressor persist in tandem—is the appropriate diagnosis chronic adjustment disorder, MDD, or appropriate sadness? In general, normal reactions to events resolve quickly and do not persist, hence the time frames specified in DSM-IV and ICD-10.[8] A further reason for monitoring is that the symptoms may represent a disorder, such as evolving MDD that emerges more clearly over time.

Another controversy stems from the sub-syndromal nature of adjustment disorder. It may be that allowing MDD to override a diagnosis of adjustment disorder is a clinical mistake, since there is little to distinguish one from the other in terms of symptoms, although the course of each is different.[2] In addition, doing so is illogical because the diagnosis of MDD is cross-sectional and is based on symptom numbers and duration; the course of adjustment disorder is longitudinal and is based on etiology and duration. Thus, MDD and adjustment disorder represent conceptually different, non-overlapping dimensions.

This suggests that the current diagnostic system based on symptom thresholds is limited and that in DSM-5, more emphasis should be placed on the specific symptom clusters and their quality. Moreover, the longitudinal course of adjustment disorder should receive more attention. Since, currently, a diagnosis of adjustment disorder cannot be made when the threshold for another condition is met, it is regarded as a subsyndromal rather than a full Axis I disorder. However, its clinical importance may be such that it should be accorded full syndromal status with its own diagnostic criteria.[7]

Epidemiology

There is little information regarding the prevalence of adjustment disorder in the community. In US psychiatric clinics, 2.3% of patients present with adjustment disorder.[8] A study of US, Canadian, and Australian general hospitals showed that 12% of patients develop the condition,[9] probably in the context of reaction to a diagnosis of serious physical illness.

The overall prevalence of adjustment disorder in military settings is unknown. However, in a survey of seventy-eight Sri Lankan Air Force personnel referred to psychiatric services, one quarter had a diagnosis of adjustment disorder, one quarter were classified as having other stress-related symptoms, and one half had one of a number of other psychiatric diagnoses.[10] This study used DSM-IV diagnostic criteria, but because psychiatric conditions are influenced by sociocultural factors, the results may not be generally applicable to other populations.

Etiology

Role of Identifiable Stressors

A diagnosis of adjustment disorder requires the identification of a stressful event. Thus individuals must have undergone a stressful event to be considered as having adjustment disorder. Stressors may be single: job loss, divorce, etc. or multiple such as death of person important to patient that coincides with patient's own physical illness and loss of job. It may be recurrent such as seasonal business difficulties or continuous, e.g. chronic illness or poverty.[3]

Sometimes it occurs in group or community settings and stressors affect several persons: e.g. natural disaster, racial, social or religious persecution, etc. Stressor in specific developmental stages are:[6]

- Beginning school
- Leaving home
- Getting married

- Becoming parent
- Failing to achieve occupational goal
- Child leaving home
- Retiring.

However, stress and psychiatric disorder in the military are not always related to combat exposure in UK. The majority of personnel in the above study were not deployed in war zones at the time of the onset of their symptoms,[10] so their stress was not likely to be related to combat.

Vulnerability

Individuals have different vulnerability to adjustment disorder depending on their personal and background characteristics. Not all individuals undergoing similar stress develop the condition. Research concluded that the following factors are associated with adjustment disorder. Higher educational level appears to protect against psychological distress.[11] The evidence for marriage being a protective factor is conflicting.[11]

Association of Factors

It should be remembered that just because there is an association between a factor and adjustment disorder, there may not be a causal link, or the link may be reversed. For instance, people with a tendency toward adjustment disorder might be less likely to be married or achieve high education because their adjustment disorder interferes with their ability in relationships or at school, rather than because single status or low education confers vulnerability to adjustment disorder.

In a naval population, being conscripted as opposed to enlisted increased the risk of psychological problems related to stress and adjustment.[11] The link between personality disorder and adjustment disorder is unclear. Although personality disorder may increase the risk of development of adjustment disorder, patients with adjustment disorder are less likely to have a co-existing personality disorder than patients with depression.[12] These three studies involve civilian populations in Ireland, Italy and Norway.

Childhood factors have been implicated; a controlling mother and an abusive father are associated with an increased risk of adjustment disorder,[13] as is an over-protective mother.[14] Personal factors of high neuroticism and low extraversion may be associated with adjustment disorder.[14] However, in both these studies,[11,14] the subjects were conscripts and the findings may not be applicable to enlisted men.

Psychodynamic Factors

Many psychoanalytic researchers pointed out the same stress can produce a range of responses in various persons. Sigmund Freud was interested in why the stresses of ordinary life produce illness in some and not in others and pointed out the role of constitutional factors (i.e. interacting with a person's life experiences to produce fixation).[6,15]

Role of mother and rearing environment in a person's has also shown the later capacity to cope stress. Deprived need and support in childhood lead to decrease tolerance capacity of stress in later life. Each child develops a unique set of defense mechanisms to deal with stressful events. Some children have less mature defensive constellations than others because of greater amount of trauma. This disadvantage may cause them as adults to react with substantially impaired functioning with stressors.

Clinical Features

Adjustment disorder is diagnosed when an individual develops psychiatric symptoms in the course of adjusting to new circumstances. There is a mixture of symptoms which can include:

- *Psychological symptoms:* These include depression, anxiety, worry, poor concentration and irritability
- *Physical symptoms:* These include palpitations, rapid breathing, diarrhea and tremor
- *Behavioral disturbances:* These can consist of aggression, deliberate self-harm, abuse of alcohol, drug misuse, social difficulties, and occupational problems.[3]

The symptoms arise gradually after a stressful event, and usually occur within 1 month of it. The disorder rarely lasts longer than 6 months.

Individuals suffering from adjustment disorder will have difficulties in social and occupational functioning; work and relationships may suffer due to ongoing distress or poor concentration. However, these difficulties will be limited and may not impair their daily life to a significant degree.[11] Examples of such stressful events include relationship break-up, unemployment, occupational dispute, bereavement, illness and other major changes.

The stressful event does not have to be of an exceptional severity, unlike in the condition post-traumatic stress disorder (PTSD). Personal vulnerability in response to stress is said to play a greater role in the development of adjustment disorder, than in the development of other stress-related psychiatric conditions (such as PTSD).[1,2] However, there is limited evidence to confirm or refute this.[5]

Structured Diagnostic and Screening Instruments

Structured interviews are frequently considered the gold standard in psychiatric research because they eliminate the subjective element of the diagnostic process; however, for purposes of diagnosing adjustment disorder, there are problems. Some of the most widely used structured interviews in research, such as the Clinical Interview Schedule and the Composite International Diagnostic Interview, fail to include adjustment disorder.[14,16] Others, such as SCID, SCAN, and the Mini International Neuropsychiatric Interview, include adjustment disorder but regard it as a subsyndromal diagnosis. This commonly leads to adjustment disorder being ignored or conflated with and subsumed by MDD (Major depressive disorder).[11] Screening instruments have likewise met with little success in distinguishing between adjustment disorder and MDD. The Zung Depression Scale, the One-Question Interview, the Impact Thermometer, and the Hospital Anxiety and Depression Scale, although helpful in identifying possible mood disorders, are of little use in differentiating adjustment disorder from MDD.[17,18]

Diagnosis

The presence of a stressor is central to the diagnosis of adjustment disorder, and this is the consideration that most sets adjustment disorder apart from other disorders in DSM-IV and ICD-10. This makes adjustment disorder similar to PTSD and to acute stress disorder, which also require a stressor—the symptoms would not have developed if there had been no stressor. This differs from MDD, which does not require a stressor, although many episodes of MDD are preceded by a life event.

Adjustment disorder is more strongly associated with marital problems and less with family-related or occupational stressors than MDD.[19] Clinically, this is unlikely to be helpful because the types of events are not specific and even traumatic events can trigger adjustment disorder as well as PTSD.

Symptoms are important to any clinical diagnosis, but they are not sufficiently specific to allow a distinction to be made between adjustment disorder and MDD.[20,21] While neither of the classifications specifies the symptoms required for a diagnosis of adjustment disorder, there are some symptoms that may be indicative of adjustment disorder. Yates and colleagues[22] found that diurnal mood variation, the loss of mood reactivity, a distinct quality to the mood, and a family history of MDD were predictive of a diagnosis of MDD rather than adjustment disorder. Further studies are needed to demonstrate whether these symptoms have sufficient specificity.

The mood state of those with adjustment disorder often depends on the cognitive presence of the stressor so that immediate impairment of mood is observed when the stressor is discussed, with more obvious mood recovery when the patient is distracted. Thus, removing the person from the stressful situation will lead to a reduction in symptoms that would otherwise persist.

Because of the limitations in the criteria for diagnosing adjustment disorder, the diagnosis is based on the presence of a precipitating stressor and on a clinical evaluation of the likelihood of symptom resolution on removal of the stressor. For those exposed to stressors long-term, the diagnosis of adjustment disorder is less clear because this type of exposure can be associated with MDD, GAD, or adjustment disorder.[19,21]

ICD-10[1] Diagnostic Criteria

- Experience of an identifiable psychosocial stressor, not of an unusual or catastrophic type, within 1 month of the onset of symptoms.
- Symptoms or behavior disturbance of types found in any of the affective disorders (except for delusions and hallucinations), any disorders in neurotic, stress related and somatoform disorders and conduct disorders, so long as the criteria of an individual disorder are not fulfilled. Symptoms may be variable in both form and severity.

  Predominant features of symptoms may be further specified:
  - A transient mild depressive state of a duration not exceeding 1 month.
  - *Prolonged depressive reaction:* A mild depressive state occurring in response to a prolonged exposure to a stressful situation but of a duration not exceeding 2 years.
  - *Mixed anxiety and depressive reaction:* Both anxiety and depressive symptoms are prominent, but at levels no greater than specified in mixed anxiety and depressive disorder or other mixed anxiety disorders.
  - *Adjustment disorder with predominant disturbance of other emotions:* The symptoms are usually of several types of emotion, such as anxiety, depression, worry, tensions and anger. Symptoms of anxiety and depression may meet the criteria for mixed anxiety and depressive disorder or other mixed anxiety disorders, but they are not so predominant that other more specific depressive or anxiety disorders can be diagnosed.[23]

    This category should also be used for reactions in children in which regressive behavior such as bedwetting or thumb-sucking are also present.
  - *Adjustment disorder with predominant disturbance of conduct:* The main disturbance is one involving conduct, e.g. an adolescent grief reaction resulting in aggressive or dissocial behavior.
  - *Adjustment disorder with mixed disturbance of emotions and conduct:* Both emotional symptoms and disturbances of conduct are prominent features.
  - Adjustment disorder with other specified predominant symptoms
- Except in prolonged depressive reaction, the symptoms do not persist for more than 6 months after the cessation of stress or its consequences.

DSM-IV-TR[2] Diagnostic Criteria

- The development of emotional or behavioral symptoms in response to an identifiable stressor(s) occurring within 3 months of the onset of the stressor(s).
- These symptoms or behaviors are clinically significant as evidenced by either of the following:

- Marked distress that is in excess of what would be expected from exposure to the stressor
- Significant impairment in social or occupational or academic functioning

- The stress-related disturbance does not meet the criteria for another specific Axis I disorder and is not merely an exacerbation of a pre-existing Axis I or Axis II disorder.
- The symptoms do not represent bereavement.
- Once the stressor or its consequences have terminated, the symptoms do not persist for more than an additional 6 months.

Specify if:

Acute: if the disturbance lasts less than 6 months.

Chronic: if the disturbance lasts for 6 months or longer.

Subtypes in DSM-IV are given below. The disorders are specified as "acute" if lasting less than 6 months, or "chronic" if the disturbance persists for longer than 6 months in the presence of a long-lasting stressor.

- Adjustment disorder with depressed mood
- Adjustment disorder with anxiety
- Adjustment disorder with mixed anxiety and depressed mood
- Adjustment disorder with disturbance of conduct
- Adjustment disorder with mixed disturbance of emotions and conduct
- Unspecified adjustment disorder.

DSM-5 Criteria for adjustment disorder	
A.	The development of emotional or behavioral symptoms in response to an identifiable stressor(s) occurring within 3 months of the onset of the stressor(s).
B.	These symptoms or behaviors are clinically significant, as evidenced by one or both of the following: 1. Marked distress that is out of proportion to the severity or intensity of the stressor, taking into account the external context and the cultural factors that might influence symptom severity and presentation. 2. Significant impairment in social, occupational, or other important areas of functioning.
C.	The stress-related disturbance does not meet the criteria for another mental disorder and is not merely an exacerbation of a pre-existing mental disorder.
D.	The symptoms do not represent normal bereavement.
E.	Once the stressor or its consequences have terminated, the symptoms do not persist for more than an additional 6 months.
Specify whether: **309.0 (F43.21) With depressed mood:** Low mood, tearfulness, or feelings of hopelessness are predominant. **309.24 (F43.22) With anxiety:** Nervousness, worry, jitteriness, or separation anxiety is predominant. **309.28 (F43.23) With mixed anxiety and depressed mood:** A combination of depression and anxiety is predominant. **309.3 (F43.24) With disturbance of conduct:** Disturbance of conduct is predominant. **309.4 (F43.25) With mixed disturbance of emotions and conduct:** Both emotional symptoms (e.g. depression, anxiety) and a disturbance of conduct are predominant. **309.9 (F43.20) Unspecified:** For maladaptive reactions that are not classifiable as one of the specific subtypes of adjustment disorder.	

Differential Diagnosis

Depending on the predominant symptoms, the differential diagnosis may be MDD, GAD, or evolving MDD. When the person exhibits behavioral disturbance such as self-harm or anger, borderline personality disorder must be excluded. For those who have experienced a traumatic event, PTSD must be considered; however, PTSD does not develop in all persons who have been exposed to a traumatic event, and therefore adjustment disorder may be a more appropriate diagnosis. Unlike most other disorders in DSM, adjustment disorder must be distinguished from a normal homeostatic reaction to stress. Failure to consider this could lead to normal distress being miscategorized as a psychiatric disorder.[24]

Course and Prognosis

The condition usually arises within 1 month of a stressful event, and resolves within 6 months. It is rare for adjustment disorder to become long-term. There is a high rate of return to work by 6 months;[9] only rarely do they become long-term. There are no studies investigating the effectiveness of treatment.

In a study of over two thousand US naval personnel,[5] adjustment disorder was found to be less severe and less disabling than other psychiatric conditions in terms of shorter illnesses, better subsequent return to effective work and fewer and shorter hospital admissions. A study of children in the US with adjustment disorder[20] showed an average duration of the condition of 7 months and a recovery rate of 97%. In a study of Sri Lankan Air Force personnel,[10] four-fifths of patients with adjustment disorder returned to work within 6 months. These studies are likely to be of some relevance to this discussion, although once again it should be stressed the data are unlikely to have exact equivalence to UK populations.

In one US study,[15] five years after diagnosis 79% of adult patients were well, although 8% of them had experienced a relapse of symptoms. Of the remaining 21% who were unwell, most had gone on to develop depression or alcohol problems. Other studies of civilian populations have found less than 18% of individuals develop long-term adjustment disorder.[7,19]

Regarding the risk of suicide, some work has shown that 2% of patients with adjustment disorder commit suicide during the following 5 years.[21] Although this is higher than the suicide risk in the general population, it is substantially lower than for other forms of psychiatric disorder. Some research suggests that if the stressor continues (for example, continued ill-health or financial stress), the adjustment disorder can become long-term. Adjustment disorders can resolve without medical intervention.[6]

Treatment

Treatment of adjustment disorder includes:
- Psychotherapeutic interventions
- Psychopharmacologic intervention
- Nontraditional approaches.

Psychotherapeutic Intervention[22]

Psychotherapeutic intervention is the treatment of choice in adjustment disorder. It includes:

- *Psychoanalytic and psychodynamic approaches:* There are numerous viewpoints from which psychological disturbances can be modeled in the effort to create treatment approaches. Historically, psychoanalytic and psychodynamic approaches have taken a leading role in the interpretation of behavior and emotion. In this view, individuals with adjustment disorder struggle unsuccessfully with effects of a stressor that most would manage more adaptively. Different forms of stress, difficult as they are to quantify, affect individuals in markedly different ways. Each individual has coping skills and mechanisms, some of which are used out of habit. Patients accommodate more easily to currently unmanageable stress when a history of similar difficulties is brought to light. Such a history can be examined in the transference, where perceptions of the relationship between the patient and the therapist are contaminated by attributes from prior relationships despite therapeutic neutrality. As therapy unfolds, the therapist becomes a target for misdirected anger and resentment, which is pointed out and examined as a means of exploring the problem. The work of therapy is to help the patient recognize and understand the unconscious struggle that arises when the pursuit of pleasure and relief from irritants (the pleasure principle) stands in the way of grasping reality (the reality principle), as pursued within the transference relationship.[25,27]

  Trauma or loss may be perceived as an assault on a strongly developed self-perception, too noxious to be accessible to grief-coping mechanisms. Inflated perceptions of the self and unreasonable expectations of others are usually strongly guarded secrets. In analytic treatment, transference may contain the perception that the therapist is a harbinger of these demands. The overburdening super-ego (internal conscience) can then be revealed as the true aggressor, alleviating the exaggerated sense of the loss. Although the loss remains a reality, its importance then diminishes to a more acceptable level. Being able to project the cause of discomfort away from inappropriate self-blame onto a realistic outside agent will relieve the patient's sense of responsibility for the loss. For example, irrational guilt can arise over having been away on a trivial errand when a parent dies of cancer. The patient, after expressing a feeling that even the therapist blames him/her, is able to examine the need to accept cancer as the cause of loss.

  Other, briefer types of therapies are encouraged in the current managed care environment. Although good comparison studies are lacking, certain individuals will probably do as well with briefer approaches. Psychodynamic, crisis-focused, time-limited psychotherapies require careful patient selection based on strong past interpersonal relationships, good pre-morbid functioning, and the absence of personality disorder. Some authors limit the use of these more confrontational techniques to situations in which there is a circumscribed focus, high motivation and capacity for insight, and a powerful degree of involvement in the interview. The time-structure of this technique is set out clearly at the beginning, with planned termination emphasized and treated as a new stressor to be managed throughout. Goals must be defined clearly. For example, self-deprecating patients may perceive parents as simultaneously irreproachable yet harsh and over-demanding. Such patients may have recurrent, severe (but brief) emotional similarities to maladaptive but customary rules of relationships from childhood. Such therapy allows recognition of relationship patterns without focusing primarily on the transference. Brief dynamic therapy has been shown to be effective compared to other therapies.[25-27]
- *Cognitive-behavioral approaches:* It provides the patient with tools for the recognition and modification of maladaptive beliefs regarding the stressor and the patient's ability to cope with it. Adjustment disorders can be addressed in this way because the importance of the stressor is often unrealistically overestimated in the patient's perception. In a cognitive-behavioral therapy the patient learns to recognize connections between emotions and maladaptive perceptions or beliefs, and then learns to challenge those beliefs. Cognitive-behavioral therapy has demonstrated utility in occupational health. It has been successfully used in telepsychiatry for adjustment disorders in patients with cancer.[25-27]
- *Interpersonal psychotherapy:* Some clinicians prefer interpersonal therapy, especially for patients who have chronic medical illness or HIV infection. Many patients with severe medical illness shun intrapsychic introspection and benefit more from a psycho-educational approach. This is true for many adolescents. Discussion remains in a here-and-now about the sick role,

which is a complicated balance of needs, independence, and becoming a more or less willing target for the caring of other individuals. Open discussions ensure about who does what for whom in which way, and about how the illness and its consequences will affect the self and others. The modeling of coping mechanisms can be helpful. Humor can be effective, if introduced carefully. Death and dying become more approachable. These individuals often benefit from a reframing of problems from an interpersonal perspective and welcome discussions of ways to change dysfunctional behavior. The therapist may be able to address issues inaccessible to a medical-surgical team. The patient may be reluctant to seem ungrateful to, and fearful of losing a relationship with, the primary care physician. Such a patient may regard the medical caregiver's purpose as one that provides medical treatment alone.

- *Supportive therapy:* It is sometimes erroneously written off as hand-holding and comforting, whereas "real therapy" involves confrontation, analysis, and intellectualization. Supportive therapy interventions have the goal of shoring up inadequate defense mechanisms. Intervention gently guides the individual to a verbalization of emotions regarding the stress. Communication, relaxation and anger control (e.g. "counting to 10") are emphasized. In an acute crisis involving loss, or in medical settings where new information brings acute distress, a skilled supportive intervention can be eminently appropriate and effective.[7,25-27]
- *Family therapy:* It is often recommended. It can be among the most effective approaches to alleviating adjustment disorder by identifying the role that family plays in promoting a maladaptive coping response. However, some families are ill – prepared to participate in treatment for the "identified" patient. In family sessions, lines of support can be examined and re-established by skilful work to minimize distortions, blame and isolation.[7,27,28]
- *Crisis intervention:* It is short-term treatment aimed at helping persons with to resolve the stressful situation quickly by supportive techniques, suggestion and reassurance.[7,15]
  - Environmental modification
  - Even hospitalization if necessary

Frequency and length of visit for crisis support vary according to patient's need (daily sessions or 2–3 times/day).[25]

Psychopharmacological Intervention

The use of medication for adjustment disorder is still controversial since no studies have assessed the efficacy of pharmacological intervention.[4] Drug treatment is advisable if it evolves into major psychiatric illness.[3,6] Small doses of anxiolytics or antidepressants may be appropriate in case of dysphoria remains profound despite several session of psychological treatment. Psychological intervention combined with benzodiazepines for patient with severe life stresses. TCAs or buspirone is preferable in place of benzodiazepines for adjustment disorder patients with current or past alcohol use because of risk of dependence. Antipsychotics may be used if there are signs of decompensation or impending psychosis. Recently, SSRIs have been used to augment psychotherapy.[28]

Nontraditional Approaches

Nontraditional approaches such as relaxation techniques, yoga, massage, progressive muscle relaxation reported as helpful in some cases. Acupuncture has been used to treat adjustment disorders, but result is unclear.[27]

Treatment Guidelines Recommendation

There is little in the way of formal guidelines for the treatment of adjustment disorders but the British Association for psychopharmacology consensus statement recommends that antidepressants are avoided and education support and simple problem solving are recommended.[25]

16.2 BEREAVEMENT

INTRODUCTION

Bereavement is the state of loss resulting from death of a loved person; the time period following a loss. The other two terms which resembles to bereavement are grief and mourning. Grief is the strong, complex involuntary emotional and behavioral response to bereavement. Mourning is the process of adaptation; public rituals associated with bereavement. The system of classification does not make these distinctions in consistent ways.

In ICD-10,[29] bereavement is coded approximately as Z63.4, that is as one of the 'factors influencing health status and contact with health services'. In DSM-IV,[30] bereavement is coded as a 'condition that may be the focus of clinical attention', thus the term is used to denote the response to bereavement rather than the event itself. ICD-10 codes grief under adjustment disorder, but uses term grief reaction.

EPIDEMIOLOGY

Considering the ubiquity of bereavement, the consequences of grief are of global importance. Incidence rates for pathological grief are not available; estimates of prevalence vary from 14 to 34%, based primarily on sample drawn from the United State and Europe. In geographical areas prone to natural disasters and places engaged in active military conflict these rates will obviously rise significantly in line with death rates, and in such cases particular attention should be paid to the concurrent trauma that will have accompanied the loss. Overall, at the age of 65 years, over 50% of women and 10% of men have been bereaved at least once and at the age of 85 years, 80% of women and 40% of men have been bereaved at least once.[32]

PHENOMENOLOGY

Bereavement reactions include intense feeling states, invoke a variety of coping strategies, and lead to alterations in interpersonal relationships, biopsychosocial functioning, self-esteem, and world view that can last indefinitevely.[31]

Manifestation of grief reflect individual's:
- Personality
- Previous life experience
- Past psychological history
- Significance of loss
- Nature of bereaved's relationship
- Intercurrent life events health and other resources.

Recent research has shown sequential peaks of the reactive phenomena: disbelief, yearning, anger and depression, which bereaved people are usually describe as sadness. Grief may be precipitant of depression in those with pre-existing or bereavement related vulnerabilities and the differentiation of normal and more pathological forms of grief from depression is important clinically. Intense grief and peaks of distress identified above do not usually continue beyond the first 4–6 months. Continue of acute grief beyond this time suggests the possibility of pathological response, as do other risk indicators, although some phenomena may continue intermittently for many years. The studies suggested that the intensity of grief among adult is likely to be greatest for the death of a child, then spouse, or partner, then parent.[32]

Biological Perspectives

Grief is both a physiological and emotional response. During acute grief, person may suffer disruption of biological rhythms. Grief is also accompanied by impaired immune functioning, i.e. decreased lymphocyte proliferation and impaired functioning of natural killer cells. Whether the immune changes are clinically significant has not been established, but the mortality rate for widowers following the death of spouse is higher than that in the general population. Widowers appear to be risk longer than widows.[31]

Sequence of Phases

The bereaved are believed to transition through a sequence of phases. These phases are not rigidly demarcated, rather they merge gradually one into the other.[33,34]
- Initial numbness, sense of unreality
- Waves of distress occur as bereaved suffers intense pining, yearning
- Disorganization emerges as loneliness sets in
- Reorganization, recovery, personal growth and creativity.

Phase I: Shock (Minutes, Days, Weeks)

- Numbness, throat tightness and crying
- Sighing, searching behavior and abdominal emptiness
- Sense of unreality
- Denial, disbelief.

Phase II: Preoccupation with Deceased (Weeks, Months)

- Anger, sadness, insomnia and anorexia
- Restless, agitated
- Weakness, fatigue
- Guilt, dreams, thoughts of dead
- Illusion, vivid imagery
- Experience of presence
- Anhedonia, introversion
- Aimless and a motivated
- Hallucination of dead person voice.

Phase III: Resolution (Months, Years)

- Have grieved
- Return to work
- Resume old roles
- Acquire new roles, re-experience pleasure
- Seek companionship and love of others.

According to Bowlby, there are 4 stages of bereavement:[33]

1. Stage I (early phase of acute despair)
   - Numbness and protest
2. Stage II
   - Phase of intense yearning and searching for the person who has died.
3. Stage III
   - Phase of disorganization and despair, the reality of loss begin to shrinking
4. Stage IV
   - Phase of reorganization

Psychodynamics

Sigmund Freud (1917) wrote in Mourning and Melancholia that normal grief (mourning) results from the withdrawal of the libido from its attachment to the lost object. In normal mourning, the loss is clearly and unambivalently, perceived, and person who died is eventually, through the grief work, internalized as a loving and loved object. In abnormal grief, the lost object is not given up but is incorporated in the survivor's psyche as an object infused with negative feelings.[33,34]

These negative feelings toward the deceased person are experienced as part of the self, and survivor become depressed, has low self-esteem, feels worthless and become self-accusatory, with possible expectations of punishment.

Freud distinguish between mourning and melancholia is still considered valid, i.e. an exaggerated loss of self-esteem is not part normal grieving.[33,34]

Bereavement during Childhood

Children may display minimal grief at the time of death and experience the full effect of loss later. Grieving children may not withdraw and dwell on person who died but, anger or misbehavior may be displayed rather than sadness.

Children often play death games as a way of working out their feelings and anxieties. Children less than 2 years of age may show loss of speech or diffuse distress, where as children less than 5 years may show eating, sleeping and bowel bladder dysfunction. School age children may become phobic, hypochondriacal, withdrawn, and have decrease school performance.[33]

Bereavement during Adolescence

In adolescence, symptoms ranging from behavioral problems, somatic symptoms and erratic mood. Boys may become delinquent and girls may turn to sexual pattern for comfort. Behavior disturbances and depression are common in all age groups but rate of depressive episodes in adolescence is higher than adulthood.[34]

Bereavement during Adulthood

No data exists on which type of loss is associated with most severe reactions. Death of spouse is often ranked as most stressful life events. Some argued that losing a child is even more profound. The death of sibling and parent loss is comparatively mild. Grief appears most intense for the mother in late perinatal losses rather than miscarriages and often re-experience during subsequent pregnancy. Sudden infant death syndrome is particularly problematic in that the death is sudden and unexpected. Parents may experience extra guilt or blame each other, often resulting in marital difficulties. The elderly face more losses than individuals at other phases of life cycle, and intense loneliness may be lasting memorial to those who have died.[34]

Psychiatric Comorbidity

Acute bereavement is associated with an increased risk for a range of psychiatric disorders, including major depression, panic disorder, generalized anxiety disorder (GAD), and post-traumatic stress disorder (PSTD). Any of these may occur: Comorbidity with pathological grief, when between 17% and 13% will also meet criteria for major depression, 13% panic disorder, 39% GAD, and 9% PTSD. However, these figures should be treated with caution since the criteria for pathological and the timing and consistency of assessment can greatly affect the results. What is clear though, is that the rate of co-morbidity following bereavement is significant, with estimates suggesting more than half of the bereaved suffer from two disorders. Hence, having diagnosed one disorder in the bereaved patient (be it psychiatric or pathological grief,) the clinician should be particularly alert to the possible presence of additional, complicating disorders. It is unclear whether this co-morbidity is best conceived as the presence of one disorder predisposing the patient to additional pathology, or simply the presence of two coexisting disorders whose symptoms may or may not aggravate each other. Whichever, it is essential that both domains of symptoms are separately monitored and, to the extent that it differs, treatment for both disorders is given.

Primary Complication

If intense symptoms last longer than 6 months, then it is called "chronic grief", or sometimes "complicated grief". If depression develops, the rate is nine times higher than in general population, and is also sometimes called "complicated" grief. Now term "bereavement-related depression" is used which is less long-lasting than chronic grief. Chronic grief is more predictive of overall functioning, depression of mental health status.

Mortality

Much evidence shows that the bereaved in general (irrespective of whether a pathological response develops) are at greater risk of dying themselves than would be expected given mortality rates in the population at large. Mortality is elevated by a factor of two to three, applying nor only to spousal loss, but also to parental, sibling, and child loss. These findings have proved robust across cultures and generations. The point of highest risk is the weeks and months immediately following the loss, although the data suggest it remains elected for several years. This evidence should alert the clinician to pay particular attention to all forms of presenting grief, whether normal or pathological.

Within a bereaved population additional factors moderate this mortality risk, although. Thus, the younger bereaved are at a higher relative risk of death themselves than the older, as are widowers compared to windows (although remarriage selectively reduces the risk in widowers). The cause of bereavement is also important, mortality risk being particularly elevated for bereavements involving suicide, accidents, liver cirrhosis, and heart disease.

Hard evidence concerning the underlying reason for reduced longevity following bereavement is scarce, but factors both directly and indirectly related to the loss may be involved. For example, psychological consequences such as the loss of the will to live might directly lead to increased suicides and carelessness. Indirectly, the change in lifestyle necessitated by bereavement may lead to the adoption of health-impairing behaviors (neglect of diet, exercise, general well being) or may create psychological stress, which in turn could have serious negative consequences for health.

Differentiating Bereavement and Depression

Bereavement	*MDD*
Symptoms may meet syndromal criteria for depression but survivor rarely has morbid feelings of guilt and worthlessness, suicidal ideation or psychomotor retardation	Any symptoms as defined by DSM-IV-TR
Dysphoria often triggered by thoughts or reminders of the deceased	Dysphoria often autonomous and independent of thoughts or reminders of the deceased
Onset within first 2 months of bereavement	Onset at any time
Duration of depressive symptoms <2 months	Depression often become chronic, intermittent, or episodic
Functional impairment is transient and mild	Clinically significant distress or impairment
No family or past personal history of major depressive disorder	Family or past personal history of major depressive disorder

Treatment

Normal grief will resolve spontaneously over time. Treatment options for pathological grief fall into the categories of pharmacology, psychotherapies, cognitive/behavioral therapies, and self-help often be obtained by the prudent combination of drugs with psychological treatment. In practice, individual circumstance and the local availability of treatment will inevitably impose restrictions.[36]

Pharmacology Treatment

Pharmacological treatment is usually not recommended. Drug treatment cannot remove the distress of normal grief but may be needed in some circumstances. Anxiolytics and hypontics may be needed to restore sleep or relieve anxiety. Antidepressants may be needed if criteria for depressive disorder is met.[35]

The few studies available looking specifically at drug treatment following bereavement suggest that both tricyclic antidepressants and selective serotonin-reuptake inhibitors (SSRIs) may provide effective relief of symptoms. The tricyclics appear to be more confined in their effects, influencing primarily depressive symptoms, whereas the SSRIs have the additional advantage of more tolerable side-effects, as well as being safer in overdose. Individual circumstances, side-effect profiles, and any known personal or family history of response to treatment can act as a guide in the selection of therapy. However, SSRIs are found more effective than tricyclics.[36]

Psychological Treatment

Counseling

The bereaved person needs to talk about the loss, to express feelings of sadness, guilt, or anger, and to understand the normal course of grieving.[37]

Psychotherapies

Neither there is evidence nor practical to provide psychotherapy to all bereaved persons. For abnormal grief, psychotherapy has shown some effectiveness. Psychodynamic forms of psychotherapy tend to be favoured nowadays over those of a psychoanalytical persuasion. The former center around the developing relationships between therapist and client; and focus on the ongoing change in the presenting psychological processes observed in the client. Current opinion suggests that this form of psychotherapy may yield more on a re-evaluation of personal history as the means to personal change.

Psychotherapies that have been used specifically to treat the bereaved include crisis intervention and brief dynamic psychotherapy.[37] One study of crisis intervention psychotherapy, given immediately after the loss, lasted for several months and involved reviewing aspects of the lost relationship within the context of the psychodynamic relationship. A significant reduction in symptoms was noted. Only a marginal symptom improvement was found By contrast, in a study of a psychodynamic therapy starting several months after the loss.[38]

Cognitive-behavioral Therapies

Cognitive-behavior therapy (CBT) is a popular form of treatment for many psychological disorders. It combines behavioral techniques such as relaxation and exposure, with cognitive restructuring in which the patient is encouraged to identify and alter maladaptive styles of thinking that are thought to maintain ongoing psychological distress. While there is no data specifically considering the efficacy of this treatment for bereavement, it is likely to confer similar benefits to those noted elsewhere. In relation to separation anxiety disorder, which could be considered as a childhood analog of pathological grief, a 60% recovery to normal functioning has been reported, sustained over a follow-up year.[39]

Exclusively behavioral techniques have also been used. These involve exposure to feared or avoided stimuli in order to produce habituation, and may also incorporate relaxation techniques to aid this process. Guided mourning and trauma desensitization are two such treatment. Both appear to selectively reduce somatic and avoidance symptoms, having less of an effect on depressive symptoms and preoccupation with the deceased.

Support Groups

Sharing experiences with othersrecently bereaved people can share grief, obtain practical advice, and discuss way of coping. Self-help groups should not be overlooked as a possible supplement to treatment, either to aid transition following successful treatment, or in a preventive capacity. Some evidence suggests that with appropriately trained group leaders, benefit conferred may be equivalent to some of the more formal treatments discussed above.[40]

Prognosis

Pathologic grief responses may be chronic and unremitting without medical intervention, and a prolonged course of 2 years or more is likely where symptoms persist beyond the first year. In the case of normal grief, most of the acute symptoms of mourning may be exported to dissipate within several months to a year, but some level of emotional involvement may persist indefinitely. Those at higher risk of a pathological grief response may include the young, women, those who suffer multiple losses, and those who have suffered childhood loss. The risk is increased following sudden, unexpected, violent, or suicidal death, an ambivalent or insecure relationship to the deceased ('attachment disturbance') also schizoid personality. Finally, transient features displayed in an individual, such as the inability to accept an imminent death, or severe distress during a terminal illness, increase that individual's risk for pathological grief.[41,42]

Prevention

Primary measures fall largely in the domain of social policy, such as gun control, safe driving practice, or healthy living styles. These can directly reduce deaths due to unnatural causes. However, the clinician may also play a role by moderating the impact of death, particularly when it is sudden or unexpected. This would include allowing ample time to be spent with a dying or indeed a deceased patient in a quiet and supportive atmosphere which can enable associated others to more effectively assimilate their loss.

Secondary prevention might include screening bereaved population at high risk. At the level of the individual this would include, maintaining contact, monitoring progress, and providing early intervention where appropriate.

Tertiary prevention, to moderate the extent of disability, can be implemented by considering appropriate medium- to long-term treatment. Patients may well present late in the course of pathological grief, prompted intervention is preferable, an appropriate selection from the treatment options discussed above is skill likely to confer some benefit.

REFERENCES

Adjustment Disorder

1. World Health Organization. International statistical classification of diseases and related health problems, 10th revision. WHO, Geneva; 1992.
2. American Psychiatric Association. Diagnostic and statistical manual of mental disorders, 4th edition. American Psychiatric Association, Washington, DC; 1994.
3. Casey P. Adult adjustment disorder: a review of its current diagnostic status. J Psychiatr Pract. 2001;7:32-40.
4. Casey P, Dowrick C, Wilkinson G. Adjustment disorders; fault line in the psychiatric glossary. Br J Psychiatry. 2001;179: 479-81.
5. Gelder MG, Andreasen NC, Lopez-Ibor JJ, Geddes JR. New Oxford Textbook of Psychiatry, Oxford University Press, 2nd edition., Vol. 1, 2009.
6. Sadock BJ, Sadock VA, Ruiz P. Kaplan and Sadock's Comprehensive Textbook of Psychiatry, 9th edition., Lippincott Williams & Wilkins; 2009.
7. Baumeister H, Maercker A, Casey P. Adjustment disorder with depressed mood: a critique of its DSM-IV and ICD-10 conceptualisations and recommendations for the future. Psychopathology. 2009;42:139-47.
8. Strain JJ, Diefenbacher A. The adjustment disorders: the conundrums of the diagnoses. Compr Psychiatry. 2008;49: 121-30.

9. Strain J, Smith G, Hammer J, et al. Adjustment disorder; a multi-site study of its utilization and interventions in the consultation-liaison psychiatry setting. Gen Hosp Psychiatry. 1998;20:139-49.
10. Perera H, Suveendran T, Mariestella A. Profile of psychiatric disorders in the Sri Lanka Air Force and the outcome at 6 months. Mil Med. 2004;169:396-9.
11. Casey P, Maracy M, Kelly BD, et al. Can adjustment disorder and depressive episode be distinguished? Results from ODIN. J Affect Disord. 2006;92:291-7.
12. Lung F, Lee F, Shu B. The relationship between life adjustment and parental bonding in military personnel with adjustment disorder in Taiwan. Mil Med. 2002;167:678-82.
13. Giotakos O, Konstantakopoulos G. Parenting received in childhood and early separation anxiety in male conscripts with adjustment disorder. Mil Med. 2002;167:28-33.
14. Lewis G, Pelosi AJ, Araya R, Dunn G. Measuring psychiatric disorder in the community: a standardized assessment for use by lay interviewers. Psychol Med. 1992;22:465-86.
15. Sadock BJ, Sadock VA. Kaplan and Sadock's Synopsis of Psychiatry, Behavioral Sciences/Clinical Psychiatry, 10th edition., Lippincott Williams & Wilkins; 2007.
16. Kessler RC, Ustun TB. The World Mental Health (WMH) Survey Initiative Version of the World Health Organization (WHO) Composite International Diagnostic Interview (CIDI). Int J Methods Psychiatr Res. 2004;13:93-121.
17. Gawronski I, Privette G. Empathy and reactive depression. Psychol Rep. 1997;80(3, pt 1):1043-9.
18. Akizuki N, Akechi T, Nakanishi T, et al. Development of a brief screening interview for adjustment disorder and major depression in patients with cancer. Cancer. 2003;97:2605-13.
19. Despland JN, Monod L, Ferrero F. Clinical relevance of adjustment disorder in DSM-III-R and DSM-IV. Compr Psychiatry. 1995;36:454-60.
20. Taggart C, O'Grady J, Stevenson M, et al. Accuracy of diagnosis at routine psychiatric assessment in patients presenting to an accident and emergency department. Gen Hosp Psychiatry. 2006;28:330-35.
21. Shear MK, Greeno C, Kang J, et al. Diagnosis of nonpsychotic patients in community clinics. Am J Psychiatry. 2000;157:581-7.
22. González-Jaimes EI, Turnbull-Plaza B. Selection of psychotherapeutic treatment for adjustment disorder with depressive mood due to acute myocardial infarction. Arch Med Res. 2003;34:298-304.
23. Parker G. Beyond major depression. Psychol Med. 2005;35: 467-74.
24. Maj M. Are we able to differentiate between true mental disorders and homeostatic reactions to adverse life events. Psychother Psychosom. 2007;76:257-9.
25. Tyrer P, Silk KR. Cambridge Textbook of Effective Treatment in Psychiatry. Cambridge University Press; 2008. pp. 588-91.
26. Vyas, JN, et al. Essential of Postgraduate psychiatry. Paras Medical Publisher. Vol. I and II. 2005.
27. Ebert MH, Loosen PT, Nurcombe B, Leckman JF. Current diagnosis & treatment. Psychiatry, Tata McGraw-Hill Edition 2nd edition. 2010.
28. Olfson M, Marcus SC. National patterns in antidepressant medication treatment. Arch Gen Psychiatry. 2009;66: 848-56.

Bereavement

29. World Health Organization. International statistical classification of diseases and related health problems, 10th revision. WHO, Geneva; 1992.
30. American Psychiatric Association. Diagnostic and statistical manual of mental disorders, 4th edition. American Psychiatric Association, Washington, DC; 1994.
31. Gelder MG, Andreasen NC, Lopez-Ibor JJ, Geddes JR. New Oxford Textbook of Psychiatry, Oxford University Press, 2nd edition., Vol. 1. 2009.
32. Maciejewski PK, Zhang B, Block SD, et al. An empirical examination of the stage theory of grief. The Journal of American Medical Association. 2007;297:716-23.
33. Sadock BJ, Sadock VA, Ruiz P. Kaplan and Sadock's Comprehensive Textbook of Psychiatry, 9th edition, Lippincott Williams & Wilkins, 2009.
34. Sadock BJ, Sadock VA. Kaplan & Sadock's Synopsis of Psychiatry, Behavioral Sciences/Clinical Psychiatry, 10th edition., Lippincott Williams & Wilkins, 2007.
35. Cook AS. Ethical Issues in Bereavement Research: an overview. Death Studies. 1995;19:103-22.
36. Forte, et al. Bereavement Care interventions: a systematic review. BMC Palliative Care. 2004;3:3.
37. Hynson JL. Research with bereaved parents: a question of how not why. Palliative Medicine. 2006;20:805-11.
38. Stroebe M. Bereavement Research: methodological issues and ethical concerns. Palliative Medicine. 2003;17:235-40.
39. Report on Bereavement and Grief Research. Center for the Advancement of Health. Death Studies. 2004;28: 491-575.
40. Richardson & Balaswamy. Men with active church involvement had more negative, less positive affect; poor relationships or selection issue?. 2001.
41. Vyas JN, et al. Essential of Postgraduate psychiatry. Paras Medical Publisher. Vol. I and II; 2005.
42. American Psychiatric Association. Desk Reference to the Diagnostic Criteria from DSM-5. Washington DC, 2013.

CHAPTER 17

Acute Stress Reaction

Shree Ram Ghimire

INTRODUCTION

Any stressful life events can cause severe psychological symptoms, including anxiety, feelings of derealization and depersonalization, and hyper-arousal.

Acute stress reaction is a transient disorder of significant severity which develops in an individual without any other apparent mental disorder in response to exceptional physical and/or mental stress and which usually subsides within hours or days.[1]

Acute stress reactions was recognized by the International Classification of Diseases (ICD-6) in 1948. Early reactions to exceptionally stressful life events are diagnosed as acute stress reaction in ICD-10[2] which is kept under 'Reactions to severe stress, and adjustment disorders'. DSM-IV[3] in 1994 recognized acute trauma reactions by introducing the new diagnosis of acute stress disorder into the anxiety disorders section. The diagnoses of acute stress reactions in ICD-10 and of acute stress disorder in DSM-IV have similarities in that they are caused by extreme stress and have some overlap in symptom patterns but difference in underlying concepts.

EPIDEMIOLOGY

Incidence

Rates in the population are unknown. Little research has been done till date to demonstrate what proportion of people develop acute stress reactions to severe stress. In a study of accident survivors, 14% experienced a response pattern characterized by derealization, and a further 17% exhibited strong anxiety or dysphoria.[4]

The incidence of acute stress disorder is 13–14% in motor vehicle accident survivors, 19% in assault victims, and 33% in witnesses of a mass shooting.[1]

ETIOLOGY

Many kinds of events can provoke an acute response to stress, for instance motor accidents, fire, an event that involves actual or threatened injury such as a physical assault or rape, or sudden discovery of serious illness, natural catastrophe, unusually sudden and threatening change in social position etc. Not all people exposed to the same stressful situation develop the same degree of response. This variation suggests that difference in constitution, previous experience, and coping styles may play a part in etiology.[5]

Acute stress reaction describes a transient disturbance and there are no specific theories of acute stress reactions as defined in ICD-10. However both psychological and biological theories have attempted to explain the symptoms of acute stress disorder. They overlap largely with theories of PTSD.[1]

PSYCHOLOGICAL THEORIES

The psychological mechanism that has received the most attention in relation to acute stress disorder is dissociation, as reflected in the DSM-IV criteria. It has been argued that dissociation minimizes the adverse emotional consequences of trauma by restricting awareness of the experience to avoid overwhelming fear and loss of control. Dissociation is thought to prevent recovery because it prevents the integration of the traumatic experience into existing schemas and it prevents the full activation of the trauma memory which is thought to be necessary for its modification. In line with these hypotheses, dissociation during or immediately after a traumatic event predicts PTSD.[1]

Psychological theories of acute stress disorder and PTSD focus on personal meaning of the trauma and its consequences, and characteristic of trauma memory. Several hypotheses about the problems in memory that are responsible for the characteristic re-experiencing symptoms have been suggested.[1]

Psychological models of post-trauma reactions concur that successful adaptation to trauma involves integration of corrective information, and any strategies that minimize this process will contribute to subsequent PTSD. Moreover, the excessive use of such avoidant strategies (e.g. trying not to think about the trauma, efforts to push intrusive memories out of one's mind, ruminating about how the trauma could have been avoided) prevents recovery.[1]

BIOLOGICAL THEORIES

Biological model has focused on fear conditioning and progressive neuronal sensitization in the weeks after trauma. Specifically, when a traumatic event (unconditioned stimulus) occurs, people typically respond with fear (unconditioned response). It is argued that the strong fear elicited by the trauma will lead to strong associative conditioning between the fear and the stimuli surrounding the trauma. As reminders of trauma occur (conditioned stimuli), people then respond with fear reactions (conditioned response).[1]

It has been hypothesized that extreme sympathetic arousal at the time of a traumatic events may result in the release of stress neurochemicals including norepinephrine and epinephrine into the cortex, mediating an overconsolidation of trauma memories. Thus sensitization occurs as a result of repetitive activation by trauma reminders and re-experiencing symptoms, elevating sensitivity of limbic networks, and that as the time progresses, these responses become increasingly conditioned to trauma related stimuli.[1]

CLINICAL FEATURES

According to ICD-10,[2] acute stress reactions are transient reactions to exceptional physical and/or mental stress. There is great variation in symptoms but typically they include an initial stage of a 'daze', including narrowing of attention, inability to comprehend stimuli, and disorientation. This state is followed by a rapidly changing picture of symptoms which may include withdrawal from the surrounding situation, flight reactions, panic anxiety and autonomic hyper-arousal (sweating, palpitation, tremor), depression, anger, or despair. Here the symptoms usually begin to diminish after 24–48 hours and should be minimal after about 3 days.

According to DSM-IV,[3] acute stress disorder is only diagnosed if the psychological symptoms persist for more than 2 days. Dissociative symptoms dominate the symptom pattern and given priority. Dissociation refers to a disruption of the usually integrated feelings of consciousness, memory, identity, or perception of the environment. Symptoms include a subjective sense of numbing or detachment, reduced awareness of surroundings, derealization, depersonalization, or dissociative amnesia. In addition, patients with acute stress disorder experience symptoms that are typical of PTSD, namely re-experiencing aspects of the event, avoidance of reminders of the event, and hyperarousal symptoms. Acute stress disorder is seen in DSM-IV as a precursor of PTSD. If the re-experiencing, avoidance, and hyperarousal symptoms persist for more than 4 weeks, PTSD is diagnosed.

CLASSIFICATION

ICD-10[2] classifies acute stress reactions (F43.0) among the reactions to severe stress and adjustment disorders (F43) that are primarily caused by stressful events. DSM-IV[3] classifies acute stress disorder (308.3) among the anxiety disorders, like PTSD. DSM-5 made some changes and it is kept under trauma and stressor related disorders.

DIAGNOSIS[2,3]

The main diagnostic criteria for acute stress reactions (ICD-10) and acute stress disorder (DSM-IV) are compared in Table 1.

STRESSOR CRITERION

Both ICD-10 and DSM-IV require that acute stress responses must occur in the immediate after an exceptionally stressful event. ICD-10 uses a broad concept of what qualifies as an 'exceptional mental or physical stressor'. This includes stressors that would be regarded as traumatic (e.g. rape, criminal assault, natural catastrophe) as well as unusually sudden changes in the social position and/or network of the individual (e.g. domestic fire or multiple bereavement).

In contrast, DSM-IV uses a narrow definition of stressors that lead to acute stress disorder, which is identical to the stressor criterion of PTSD. It requires (a) that the traumatic event must have involved actual or threatened death or serious injury, or a threat to the physical integrity of self or others, and (b) that the person's response to the traumatic event must have involved intense fear, helplessness, or horror (or disorganized or agitated behavior in children).

SYMPTOM PATTERNS

The diagnostic criteria for acute stress reactions (ICD-10) and acute stress disorder (DSM-IV) overlap, in that they include symptoms of dissociation, anxiety, and hyperarousal. DSM-IV puts a much greater emphasis on dissociation, requiring a minimum of three of the dissociative symptoms specified in Criterion B. According to ICD-10, any combination of a minimum of four symptoms of generalized anxiety disorder (specified in Criterion C) would be sufficient to establish the diagnosis of acute stress reaction. In addition, DSM-IV, but not ICD-10, requires the individual to have at least one re-experiencing symptom, to show marked avoidance of reminders of the trauma, and to experience significant distress or impairment of functioning.

In contrast to DSM-IV, ICD-10 distinguishes between mild, moderate, and severe forms of acute stress reactions on the basis of additional symptoms (Criterion C,

Table 1: Comparison of the criteria for acute stress reaction (ICD–10) and acute stress disorder (DSM–IV)

Acute stress reaction (ICD–10 research diagnostic criteria)		*Acute stress disorder (DSM – IV)*
Stressor	Exposure to exceptional mental or physical stress	1. Exposure to event involving actual or threatened death or serious injury to self or others 2. Experience of fear, helplessness, or horror
Symptoms	*Criterion C*: Symptoms of gereralized anxiety disorder (at least 4 symptoms) Palpitations, sweating trembling, dry mouth, difficulty breathing, choking, chest pain, nausea, dizziness, derealization or depersonalization, fear of losing control, fear of dying, hot flushes, numbness or tingling, muscle tension, restlessness, keyed up, difficulty concentrating, irritability, difficulty getting to sleep *Criterion C*: Additional symptoms to determine severity Social withdrawal, narrowed attention, disorientation, aggression, hopelessness, overactivity, excessive grief	*Criterion B*: Dissociation (at least 3 symptoms) Numbing, reduced awareness, derealization, depersonalization, dissociative amnesia *Criterion C*: Re-experiencing (at least one symptoms) Recurrent images, thoughts, dreams, illusions, flashbacks, reliving, distress on exposure *Criterion D*: Marked avoidance Avoidance of thoughts, feelings, conversions, activities, place, people associated with the trauma *Criterion E*: Marked anxiety or increased arousal Difficulty sleeping, irritability, poor concentration, hypervigilance, exaggerated startle response, motor restlessness *Criterion F*: Clinically significant distress or impairment in functioning
Time from trauma	Onset within 1 hour	Onset within 4 weeks; lasts for at least 2 days
Time course	Transient; symptoms begin to diminish within 48 hours	May result in post-traumatic stress disorder
Relationship to post-traumatic stress disorder	Alternative diagnosis	Precursor
Diagnostic group	Reactions to severe stress	Anxiety disorder
Exclusion criteria	No other concurrent (within last 3 months) mental or behavioral disorder, except for generalized anxiety disorder or personality disorder	1. Not due to effects of a substance or general medical condition 2. Not better accounted for by brief psychotic disorder 3. Not merely exacerbation of pre-existing Axis I or Axis II disorder

additional symptoms) such as social withdrawal, hopelessness, or excessive grief. A mild severity is said when none of these symptoms are present, moderate when two are reported, and severe when four are reported or when there is dissociative stupor.

Time Course of Symptoms

To meet the criteria of acute stress reaction (ICD-10), symptoms must be manifest within 1 hour of the stressor (Criterion B) and begins to diminish after no more than 48 hours for an enduring stressor (Criterion D).

Similarly the diagnostic criteria for acute stress disorder (DSM-IV) require that the disturbance must last for minimum of 2 days and a maximum of 4 weeks post-trauma, after which a diagnosis of PTSD can be considered.

DSM-5 Diagnostic criteria for acute stress disorder 308.3 (F43.0)

A. Exposure to actual or threatened death, serious injury, or sexual violation in one (or more) of the following ways:
   1. Directly experiencing the traumatic event(s).
   2. Witnessing, in person, the event(s) as it occurred to others.
   3. Learning that the event(s) occurred to a close family member or close friend. *Note*: In cases of actual or threatened death of a family member or friend, the event(s) must have been violent or accidental.
   4. Experiencing repeated or extreme exposure to aversive details of the traumatic event(s) (e.g. first responders collecting human remains, police officers repeatedly exposed to details of child abuse).

Note: This does not apply to exposure through electronic media, television, movies, or pictures, unless this exposure is work related.

Contd...

Contd...

B. Presence of nine (or more) of the following symptoms from any of the five categories of intrusion, negative mood, dissociation, Trauma- and Stressor-Related Disorders avoidance, and arousal, beginning or worsening after the traumatic event(s) occurred: **Intrusion symptoms** 1. Recurrent, involuntary, and intrusive distressing memories of the traumatic event(s). *Note*: In children, repetitive play may occur in which themes or aspects of the traumatic event(s) are expressed. 2. Recurrent distressing dreams in which the content and/or affect of the dream are related to the event(s). *Note*: In children, there may be frightening dreams without recognizable content. 3. Dissociative reactions (e.g. flashbacks) in which the individual feels or acts as if the traumatic event(s) were recurring. (Such reactions may occur on a continuum, with the most extreme expression being a complete loss of awareness of present surroundings) *Note*: In children, trauma-specific reenactment may occur in play. 4. Intense or prolonged psychological distress or marked physiological reactions in response to internal or external cues that symbolize or resemble an aspect of the traumatic event(s). **Negative mood** 5. Persistent inability to experience positive emotions (e.g. inability to experience happiness, satisfaction, or loving feelings). **Dissociative symptoms** 6. An altered sense of the reality of one's surroundings or oneself (e.g. seeing oneself from another's perspective, being in a daze, time slowing). 7. Inability to remember an important aspect of the traumatic event(s) (typically due to dissociative amnesia and not to other factors such as head injury, alcohol, or drugs). **Avoidance symptoms** 8. Efforts to avoid distressing memories, thoughts, or feelings about or closely associated with the traumatic event(s). 9. Efforts to avoid external reminders (people, places, conversations, activities, objects, situations) that arouse distressing memories, thoughts, or feelings about or closely associated with the traumatic event(s). **Arousal symptoms** 10. Sleep disturbance (e.g. difficulty falling or staying asleep, restless sleep). 11. Irritable behavior and angry outbursts (with little or no provocation), typically expressed as verbal or physical aggression toward people or objects. 12. Hypervigilance. 13. Problems with concentration. 14. Exaggerate
C. Duration of the disturbance (symptoms in Criterion B) is 3 days to 1 month after trauma exposure.
Note: Symptoms typically begin immediately after the trauma, but persistence for at least 3 days and up to a month is needed to meet disorder criteria.

Contd...

Contd...

D. The disturbance causes clinically significant distress or impairment in social, occupational, or other important areas of functioning.
E. The disturbance is not attributable to the physiological effects of a substance (e.g. medication or alcohol) or another medical condition (e.g. mild traumatic brain injury) and is not better explained by brief psychotic disorder.

Assessment Instruments

There are no established standardized assessment instruments for transient acute stress reactions (ICD-10). However, there are three clinician-administered and one self-report measure of acute stress disorder (DSM-IV) available.[1]

- *Acute stress disorder interview*: This structured clinical interview establishes the presence or absence of 19 symptoms of acute stress disorder. The sum of the symptoms scored as being present indicates acute stress disorder severity. This measure has very good internal consistency, and, with clinician-based diagnoses as the criterion, very good sensitivity (91%) and specificity (93%). Test–retest reliability is strong.
- *Structured clinical interview for DSM-IV (SCID)*: The SCID interview indexes the presence, absence, or subthreshold presence of each acute stress disorder symptom specified in DSM-IV. An advantage of employing this interview is that it provides a comprehensive assessment of the differential diagnoses and comorbid disorders that can be present in trauma populations.
- *Stanford acute stress reaction questionnaire*: It is the self-report inventory that asks patients to rate the frequency of a range of dissociative, intrusive, somatic anxiety, hyperarousal, attention disturbance, and sleep disturbance symptoms. It can be employed as a measure of the severity of symptoms, but does not allow the diagnosis of acute stress disorder to be established as it has not yet been validated against clinician diagnosis.
- *Acute stress disorder scale*: This self-report scale is scored on 5-point scale that reflects degree of severity of 19 acute stress disorder symptoms. It possess good sensitivity and specificity (95% and 83%).

Differential Diagnoses

- *Post-traumatic stress disorder*: PTSD is conceptualized as an alternative diagnosis of acute stress reactions in ICD-10. The definitions of acute stress reaction and PTSD differ in terms of the stressor criterion (exceptionally stressful life event vs exceptionally threatening or catastrophic event), the time course (symptoms start to diminish within 48 hours versus no time limit), and symptom pattern (PTSD, but not acute stress reaction, includes involuntary re-experiencing the traumatic event).

In contrast, acute stress disorder can be distinguished from PTSD by the time-frame covered by the diagnosis in DSM-IV. Acute stress disorder refers to the period from 2 days to 1 month post-trauma, after which a diagnosis of PTSD can be considered. The primary difference between the symptom criteria for acute stress disorder and PTSD in DSM-IV is the former's emphasis on dissociative reactions.

- *Adjustment disorder*: It covers a wide range of emotional or behavioral symptoms indicative of distress, which are judged to be out of proportion to the stressor experienced. This broad coverage can be contrasted with (1) the specific set of symptoms described by the acute stress disorder and acute stress reaction criteria, and (2) the stipulation that the stressor involves both a threat to life and a subjective response of fear for the acute stress disorder and an exceptional stressor in the case of acute stress reaction.
- *Brain injury*: Most of acute stress disorder symptoms overlap with symptoms of brain injury including reduced awareness, depersonalization, derealization, irritability, and concentration difficulties. While results from neuropsychological and neurological investigations may assist in the differential diagnosis, there appear to be a group of individuals with a mild head injury for whom there are no known tools to differentiate whether the disturbance is due to brain injury or acute stress disorder, or whether both are present.
- *Brief psychotic disorder*: It should be considered when there is one or more psychotic symptoms present after experiencing an extreme stressor.
- *Dissociative disorders*: Given the emphasis on dissociative symptoms in acute stress disorder, it needs to be distinguished from dissociative amnesia and depersonalization disorder. The criteria for these diagnoses stipulate that if the amnesia or depersonalization can be accounted for by acute stress disorder then a dissociative disorder cannot be diagnosed.

Predictors of Acute Stress Disorder

Little is known about predictors of acute stress reactions. A history of psychiatric disorder, depressive and dissociative symptoms prior to the traumatic event, and previous trauma predict acute stress disorder.

TREATMENT

Psychological Treatments

Debriefing[1,4]

After a major incident, counseling has often taken the form which is known as debriefing or Critical incident stress debriefing (CISD). It is a widely practised intervention that has the goal of promoting adaptation to traumatic events.

Debriefing is generally conducted in a group within 24–72 hours of the trauma. However, these parameters have been modified to permit more flexible interventions.

Mitchell proposes that debriefing comprises seven phases[6]:

1. An initial outline of the purpose and benefits of debriefing.
2. The fact phase, in which participants relate what happened to them.
3. A thought phase, in which participants relate their initial thoughts after the critical incident.
4. A feeling phase, which requires participants to focus on the worst aspects of the incident and engage in their emotional reactions to the incident.
5. An assessment phase, in which participants are trained to note their physical, cognitive, emotional, and behavioural symptoms.
6. An education phase, which provides information about stress responses and ways to manage them.
7. The re-entry phase, in which the information given is summarized and referral information offered.

These phases may take 1–5 hours, and are usually co-ordinated by a trained mental health professional. Despite its widespread use, very few controlled trials have been conducted. A Cochrane review of randomized controlled studies of individual debriefing found that although participants usually found the intervention useful, debriefing did not prevent the onset of PTSD nor reduce psychological distress as compared to control.

Cognitive Behavior Therapy

Cognitive behavioral interventions are found effective in the treatment of PTSD.[7] It was supported by the result of two randomized controlled studies of rape victims and road traffic accident survivors. It suggests a brief five-session version of this treatment is effective in acute stress disorder and prevents the development of chronic post-trauma reactions. Treatment involved the following:

1. Education about trauma reactions.
2. Progressive muscle relaxation.
3. Prolonged exposure.
4. Cognitive restructuring of fear-related beliefs.
5. Graded *in vivo* exposure.

Cognitive behavioral therapy was found to be effective and superior to other psychological therapies in preventing chronic PTSD.[8]

Psychopharmacological Treatment

There is little study regarding pharmacological intervention for the treatment of acute stress reaction/disorder. Case studies report on the utility of tricyclic antidepressants, but no or even harmful effects of benzodiazepines. Research on PTSD suggests that selective serotonin-reuptake inhibitors (SSRIs) are the best pharmacological treatment for persistent reactions to traumatic stress.[8]

There is increase interest in pharmacological intervention in the acute phase following trauma/stress that may prevent the development of PTSD symptoms.[9] A pilot study was done to prevent PTSD using propranolol with in 6 hours of trauma exposure. The study revealed that there is no difference in symptoms immediately as compared to placebo, however it reduced PTSD 3 months later.[10] This approach is based on evidence that propranolol abolishes the epinephrine enhancement for fear conditioning. Other pilot study used high dose of hydrocortisol in medical patients in an intensive environment had beneficial effect on subsequent PTSD symptoms.[9]

Selection of Treatment Plan

Initially treatment should be focused on ensuring trauma survivors' safety and security, providing support and practical assistance and encourage them to use their social support.

Short-term hypnotics medication or long-term use of antidepressants should be considered for the management of significant sleep disturbance in the acute phase after trauma. If symptoms persists for 2 weeks or longer, treatment may be indicated. However, patients with low symptoms severity have a good chance of recovering without intervention.

For those with more severe acute stress disorder symptoms, a course of cognitive-behavioral treatment may be considered. It is not provided within 2 weeks of trauma exposure. If the patient is offered cognitive-behavioral treatment, therapists need to be aware that avoidance is a hallmark symptom of acute stress disorder and may reduce the likelihood that an individual will attend treatment sessions regularly. Flexible treatment procedures (e.g. initial contacts by telephone, scheduling sessions around the patient's preferences) and discussions about the ambivalence toward treatment may be helpful. Therapists need to be knowledgeable about the conditions surrounding the traumatic event and be sensitive to the particular socio-cultural background of the patient, which will affect the personal meaning of the event.[7,8]

Since there is lack of randomized controlled trial, so pharmacological treatment cannot be considered a front-line treatment for acute stress disorder, but research on PTSD suggests that selective serotonin reuptake inhibitors may be helpful.[8]

Preventive Measures[1]

Early identification of highly symptomatic individuals with acute stress disorder and providing a cognitive-behavioral intervention from approximately 2 weeks post-trauma may reduce the risk of later PTSD. Moreover, additional preventive methods have been explored that prepare individuals 'at risk' (e.g. emergency services and military personnel) for experiencing trauma so as to enhance their coping strategies and reduce the risk of them developing longer term symptomatology. Individuals at high risk of experiencing a trauma need to provide training to remain calm, evaluate the situation objectively, to not identify with victims, to utilize social supports, and to express emotional reactions have all been found to be associated with better coping after the trauma.[11,12]

REFERENCES

1. Gelder MG, Andreasen NC, Lopez-Ibor JJ, Geddes JR. 2009, New Oxford Textbook of Psychiatry, Oxford University Press, 2nd edn., Vol. 1.
2. World Health Organization. International statistical classification of diseases and related health problems, 10th revision. WHO, Geneva; 1992.
3. American Psychiatric Association. Diagnostic and statistical manual of mental disorders (4th edn). American Psychiatric Association, Washington, DC; 1994.
4. Schnyder U, Malt UF. Acute stress response patterns to accidental injuries. Journal of Psychosomatic Research. 1998; 45:419-24.
5. Sadock BJ, Sadock VA, Ruiz P. Kaplan & Sadock's Comprehensive Textbook of Psychiatry, 9th edition. Lippincott Williams & Wilkins; 2009.
6. Bryant RA, Moulds ML, Guthrie RM, et al. The additive benefits of hypnosis and cognitive behavioral therapy in treating acute stress disorder. Journal of Consulting and Clinical Psychology. 2005;73:334-40.
7. Australian Centre for Post Traumatic Mental Health. Australian guideline for the treatment of acute distress disorder and post traumatic stress disorder; 2007.
8. National Institute of Clinical Excellence. Clinical guideline 26: Post Traumatic Stress Disorder: Management of PTSD in adults and children in primary and secondary care; 2005.
9. Pitman RK, Delahanty DL. Conceptually driven pharmacologic approaches to acute trauma. CNS spectrums. 2005;10: 99-106.
10. Vaiva G, et al. Immediate treatment with propranolol decrease posttraumatic stress disorder two months after trauma. Biology Psychiatry. 2003;54:947-9.
11. Sadock BJ, Sadock VA (Eds). Kaplan and Sadock's Synopsis of Psychiatry, Behavioral Sciences/Clinical Psychiatry, 10th edn., Lippincott Williams and Wilkins. 2007. pp. 579-633.
12. American Psychiatric Association. Desk Reference to the Diagnostic Criteria from DSM-5. Washington DC; 2013.

CHAPTER 18

Post-traumatic Stress Disorder

Shree Ram Ghimire

INTRODUCTION

Disasters, both natural and man-made, affect millions of people around the world every year. Natural disasters (e.g. earthquakes and hurricanes) and man-made disasters (e.g. traffic accidents, acts of terrorism and wars) can cause mental trauma with long-lasting consequences.[1,2] The impact of a mass disaster or man-made trauma on the individual is a composite of two major elements: the catastrophic event itself and the vulnerability of those people affected by the event. These traumatic events can lead to severe psychological disturbance.

It was found that the long-standing psychological problems of many war veterans, especially Vietnam veterans, that changed this view and convinced clinicians and researchers that even people with sound personalities can develop clinically significant psychological symptoms if they are exposed to horrific stressors. This prompted the introduction of post-traumatic stress disorder (PTSD) as a diagnostic category in DSM-III.[3] It was thus recognized that traumatic events such as combat, rape, man-made or natural disasters give rise to a characteristic pattern of psychological symptoms. The diagnostic criteria specified the experience of a traumatic event as a necessary condition for the diagnosis. ICD-10 emphasized the causal role of traumatic stressors in producing psychological dysfunction even more clearly, in that a specific group of disorders, 'reaction to severe stress, and adjustment disorders', was created. These disorders are thought to arise always as a direct consequence of the acute severe stress or continued trauma. The stressful event is the primary and overriding causal factor, and the disorder would not have occurred without its impact.[4]

EPIDEMIOLOGY

Most of the available epidemiological data so far stem mainly from studies conducted in the United States. It remains to be investigated whether these data replicate in other countries. Some researchers who have examined gender differences suggest that females are more likely than males to develop PSTD.[5,6] A possible explanation for this is the specific reactions that result from feminine characteristics to a traumatic event. Additionally, there are previous studies that have associated old age with an increased risk of developing PTSD. However, a recent study has suggested contradictory results.[5]

The first Gulf war and more recent wars in Iraq and Afghanistan have built on the earlier body of work with Vietnam war veterans and there is marked variation of prevalence rate of PTSD from 2 to 70%.[7] But studied found the similar pattern of illness (PTSD and depression) among marked exposure in Iraq and Afghanistan.[8]

Breslau et al.[9] estimated that 6 to 7% of the US population is exposed to disaster or trauma every year. The prevalence of PTSD ranged from 3.0 to 34.3% in Taiwan after the 1999 earthquake, it was approximately 25% in Turkey after the 1999 earthquake, and it was reported as 74% in Armenia after the 1988 earthquake.[1] In a systemic review of the literature, Andrews, et al. found that delayed-onset PTSD in the absence of any prior symptoms was rare, whereas delayed onset that represented exacerbations or reactivations of prior symptoms accounted for, on average, 38.2% and 15.3% of military and civilian cases of PTSD, respectively.[10] Women are at least twice as likely to develop PTSD in response to a traumatic event than men. This enhanced risk is not explained by differences in the type of traumatic event. The estimated lifetime prevalence for women is approximately 10 to 12%, and for men 5 to 6%.[11]

PTSD with Psychiatric Comorbidity

The majority of the research provides evidence of psychological sequelae that includes PTSD, major depressive episodes, sleep disorder, anxiety, somatization and substance abuse such as alcohol after disasters. Furthermore, major depressive episodes and PTSD are the most common disaster-related psychiatric diagnoses and are strongly associated with one another.[12] In the study by Kessler et al. 88.3% of the men and 78.1% of the women with PTSD had comorbid psychiatric diagnoses.[13] Individuals confronted with disasters or major stressors exhibit greater psychological impairment and are more vulnerable to psychiatric diseases. The incidence of PTSD is higher than that of other major depressive episodes in the majority of the studies.[1] Higher co-morbidity has been found with combat-related PTSD. Such co-morbidity includes drug and alcohol abuse, antisocial personality disorder, somatization disorder, and depression, and it is particularly prevalent when determined from an historical perspective. PTSD can be triggered by a variety of traumatic events and is strongly associated with all other examined mental disorders.[14] For example, the combination of PTSD and panic and phobic disorders is an important predictor for PTSD chronicity. Furthermore, the rate of psychopathology is higher in post-disaster groups than in either the same groups prior to trauma or in control groups.[13]

ETIOLOGY

Risk Factors of PTSD

Researchers who study risk factors for PTSD have identified aspects of traumatic stressors, psychological factors, biological factors psychiatric symptoms, and post-trauma social resource factors as important factors that contribute to the development of the disorder.

Psychological Processes[11,13]

Mower's two-factor conditioning theory of phobias has been applied to PTSD. It is suggested that through Pavlovian classical conditioning, stimuli that were present at the time of the trauma (unconditioned stimulus) become associated with fear and arousal responses. Subsequently the conditioned stimuli trigger similar (conditioned) responses when presented on their own. Through stimulus generalization and higher-order conditioning, a wide variety of stimuli become triggers of distress in the aftermath of trauma. Naturally, the person try to avoid the conditioned stimuli and the associated distress. The avoidance behavior is negatively reinforced (operant or instrumental conditioning) because it leads to reduction in psychological and physical discomfort. In long-term, however, avoidance prevents extinction of conditioned fear responses to reminders of traumatic event, and thus maintains the problem.

Characteristics of the Traumatic Stressor

Stressors of human design such as rape and violent assault are usually more pathogenic than either accidental trauma or natural disaster. Sudden unexpected, and life-threatening events are especially pathogenic.[11] 65% of the men and 46% of the women who had been raped met PTSD criteria in the Kessler et al. study. Accidents, witnessing death or injury, and fire or natural disasters were associated with relatively low lifetime PTSD rates of less than 10%.[11]

Biological Factors

Neuroendocrine data provide evidence of insufficient glucocorticoid signaling in stress related neuropsychiatric disorders, while Nutt[15] has suggested that individuals develop PTSD due to neuroendocrine dysregulation. Furthermore, impaired feedback regulation of relevant stress responses, especially immune activation/inflammation, may, in turn, contribute to stress-related pathology that includes alterations in behavior, insulin sensitivity, bone metabolism, and acquired immune responses.[16]

Because the hypothalamic-pituitary gland-adrenal axis (HPA) regulates hormone reactions during stress, PTSD severity seems to decrease when individuals exposed to traumatic events experience decreased stress levels. It was found from study that more positive soft neurological signs in PTSD participants than in participants who experienced similar trauma but did not develop PTSD. Many trauma victims complain of memory impairment, such as difficulty remembering daily activities, frequent compulsive recall of the traumatic event in detail, memory gaps, island-like memory, difficulties with declarative memory, and intrusive memories. Anderson et al.[10] used functional magnetic resonance imaging (fMRI) to identify the neural systems involved in keeping unwanted memories out of one's awareness. Controlling unwanted memories is associated with increased dorsolateral prefrontal activation (DLPF), reduced hippocampal activation, and impaired retention of those memories. Both prefrontal cortical and right hippocampal activations predicted the magnitude of forgetting. These results confirm the existence of an active forgetting process and establish a neurobiological model for guiding inquiry into motivated forgetting. Some studies have found an increased levels of thyroid hormones in patients with PTSD. These correlated with the severity of hyperarousal symptoms.[13]

Veterans with PTSD show enhanced levels of corticotrophin-releasing factor (CRF) in their cerebrospinal fluid compared to normal controls. Intraventricular administration of CRF has been shown to lead to enhanced plasma adrenaline and noradrenaline concentrations and anxiety and fear-related behaviors in animals, and it is thus thought that the enhanced CRF levels could cause these symptoms in PTSD patients. The dopaminergic, γ-aminobutyric acid, and *N*-methyl-D-aspartate (NMDA) systems have also been implicated in PTSD, but the evidence for these hypotheses is sparse at this stage.

Genetic Factors

There are still gaps in the understanding of the genetic underpinnings of PTSD. For example, while Stein et al.[17]

have found moderate hereditary factors in individuals with PTSD symptoms, no single gene that causes PTSD has been identified. Twin studies have found a higher concordance of PTSD among monozygotic than dizygotic twins. There is also an increased prevalence of psychiatric disorders, especially anxiety disorders, affective disorders, sociopathy, and/or substance abuse, among family members of people with PTSD.

Research on Vietnam found that the rate of PTSD was 16.8% in cotwins who had served in Vietnam war and 5% in their co-twins who had served else where. Subsequent study shown that monozygotic twins were more concordant for combat exposure than dizygotic twins.[11]

Post-trauma Social Resource Factors

Inadequate social support after the trauma adds to the risk of developing PTSD. Not surprisingly, higher levels of post-disaster life events are also related to the risk of developing PTSD. Similarly, social stressors such as economic or marital issues or a disruption of one's daily life, including relocation, the death of an intimate partner, or other significant loss problems are associated with a greater risk for developing PTSD.[1]

Neuroimaging[11,13]

Magnetic resonance imaging studies have shown a reduced hippocampal volume in veterans and women with a history of childhood sexual abuse. This line of research was prompted by animal studies showing that high levels of cortisol seen during stress are associated with damage to the hippocampus. Disturbances of hippocampal function may lead to enhanced reactivity to stimulation, and may be involved in the deficits in autobiographical memory observed in PTSD patients. It remains unclear whether the decreased hippocampal volume is a risk factor for the development of PTSD or a consequence of chronic PTSD.

It has been suggested that PTSD is characterized by dysfunctions in the amygdalae or the areas that project to them (the hippocampus, septum, and prefrontal cortex), leading to problems in the extinction of fear responses to reminders of the traumatic event. Animal studies established that conditioned fear responses could only be extinguished if the cortex was intact. Consistent with possible deficits in cortical control, positron emission tomography studies have shown a relative decrease in middle temporal blood flow (and several adjacent medial prefrontal areas) in patients with PTSD relative to controls when they imagined the traumatic event or were presented with reminders of it. The middle temporal cortex plays a role in the extinction of fear through inhibition of amygdala function. At the same time, PTSD patients showed increased blood flow in the limbic regions (parahippocampus and cingulate).

Hypothesis for PTSD

Hobfoll's conservation of resources (COR) model has been well supported by previous studies on natural disasters. According to Hobfoll's conservation of resources stress theory resource loss is an important determinant of individual stress and physical and mental health, including PTSD[2]. Brewin et al.[18] also found that the effect sizes of all risk factors were modest. Factors operating during or after the trauma (e.g. trauma severity, lack of social support, and additional life stress), however, had somewhat stronger effects than did pretrauma factors. Consequently, multiple risk factors constitute a network that results in psychiatric illness. According to Hobfoll's[2] conservation of resources theory, resource loss is an important determinant of individual stress and physical and mental health, including PTSD. Our hypothesis states that an individual reaches a sub-threshold of psychiatric illness and then develops the illness due to a decreasing availability of resources, an accumulation of risk factors, and/or a major stressful event. Furthermore, unresolved, sub-clinical psychiatric symptoms caused by a disaster or major life event may increase a survivor's sensitivity to future stresses. When faced with stress, frustration (e.g. life events), or traumatic events (e.g. brain damage or deprivation of internal or external resources) individuals, either suddenly or gradually, become more vulnerable to psychiatric impairment and diseases such as PTSD. An individual might reach a sub-threshold of PTSD and then develop the illness due to a decreased availability of resources, an accumulation of risk factors (personality traits, poor social interactions, etc.) or a major stressful event. Furthermore, unresolved, subclinical psychiatric symptoms caused by a disaster may increase a survivor's sensitivity to future stresses. Other factors that tend to increase an individual's vulnerability to psychiatric problems include brain damage, heredity, personality traits, life events, and social interactions.[1,2]

CLINICAL FEATURES

The most characteristic symptoms of PTSD are the re-experiencing symptoms. Patients involuntarily re-experience aspects of the traumatic event in a very vivid and distressing way. This includes: flashbacks in which the person acts or feels as if the event were recurring; nightmares; and intrusive images or other sensory impressions from the event. Despite vivid memory fragments, intentional recall of the event is often poor and disorganized, and some patients have amnesia for parts of the event.[13] Reminders of the trauma arouse intense distress and/or physiological reactions and are consequently avoided, including conversations about the event. Patients try to push memories of the event out of their mind and avoid thinking about the event in detail, particularly about its worst moments. On the other hand, many ruminate excessively about questions that prevent them from coming to terms with the event, for example about why the event happened to them, about how it could have been prevented, or about how they could take revenge.[3]

The emotional state of patient ranges from intense fear, anger, sadness, guilt, or shame to emotional numbness. Patient often describe feeling detached from other people and give up previously significant activities. Various symptoms of hyperarousal include hypervigilance, exaggerated startle responses, irritability, difficulty concentrating, and sleep problems are common.[11,13]

CLASSIFICATION

ICD-10[4] classifies PTSD (F43.1) among the reactions to severe stress and adjustment disorders (F43) that are primarily caused by stressful events. DSM-IV[19] classifies PTSD (309.81) among the anxiety disorders because symptom patterns, psychophysiological responses, family studies, and the efficacy of exposure treatment and serotonergic drugs suggested a relationship with other anxiety disorders. However, some of the symptoms would also suggest a relationship with dissociative disorders (e.g. amnesia) or depression (e.g. loss of interest).[3]

DSM-5 diagnostic criteria has made some change and PTSD is kept under trauma and stressor related disorders. Other changes are specific to criteria which is given below.

DIAGNOSIS

Diagnostic Criteria in ICD-10 and DSM-IV

Comparison of the diagnostic criteria of ICD-10[4] and DSM-IV[9] as well as ICD-10 research diagnostic criteria are included in Table 1. The diagnostic systems agree on the core symptoms

Table 1: Diagnostic criteria for PTSD in ICD-10[4] and DSM- IV[9]

ICD-10 diagnostic guidelines	*ICD-10 research diagnostic criteria*	*DSM-IV criteria*
Stressor criterion 1. Event or situation of exceptionally threatening or catastrophic nature 2. Likely to cause pervasive distress in almost anyone	a. 1. Event or situation of exceptionally threatening or catastrophic nature 2. Likely to cause pervasive distress in almost anyone	a. 1. The person experienced, witnessed or was confronted with an event or events that involved actual or threatened death or serious injury, or a threat to the physical integrity of self or others 2. The person's response involved intense fear, helplessness, or horror (or disorganized or agitated behavior in children
Symptom criteria		
Necessary symptoms	*Necessary symptoms*	*Necessary symptoms*
1. Repetitive intrusive recollection or re-enactment of the event in memories, daytime imagery, or dreams **Other typical symptoms** 2. Sense of 'numbness' and emotional blunting, detachment from others, unresponsiveness to surroundings, anhedonia 3. Avoidance of activities and situations reminiscent of trauma **Common symptoms** 4. Autonomic hyper-arousal with insomnia 5. Anxiety and depression **Rare symptoms** 6. Dramatic acute bursts of fear, panic, or aggression triggered by reminders	b. Persistent remembering or 'reliving' of the stressor in intrusive 'flashback', vivid memories, or recurring dreams, and in experiencing distress when exposed to circumstances resembling or associated with the stressor c. Actual or preferred avoidance of circumstances resembling or associated with the stressor which was not present before exposure to the stressor d. 1. Inability to recall, either partially or completely, some important aspects or the period of exposure to the stressor 2. Persistent symptoms of increased psychological sensitivity and arousal (not present before exposure to stressor), shown by any two of the following: a. Difficulty in falling or staying asleep b. Irritability or outbursts of anger c. Difficulty in concentrating d. Hypervigilance e. Exaggerated startle response	b. The traumatic event is persistently re-experienced in one (or more) of the following ways: 1. Recurrent and intrusive distressing recollections of the events, including images, thoughts, or perceptions (or repetitive play in which the themes or aspects of the trauma are expressed in children) 2. Recurrent distressing dreams of the event (or frightening dreams without recognizable content in children) 3. Acting or feeling as if the traumatic event were recurring (or trauma-specific re-enactment in children) 4. Intense psychological distress at exposure to internal or external cues that symbolize or resemble an aspect of the traumatic event 5. Psychological reactivity at exposure to internal or external cues that symbolize or resemble an aspect of the traumatic event

Contd...

Contd...

ICD-10 diagnostic guidelines	*ICD-10 research diagnostic criteria*	*DSM-IV criteria*
		c. Persistent avoidance of stimuli associated with the trauma and numbing of general responsiveness (not present before trauma), as indicated by three (or more) of the following: 1. Efforts to avoid thoughts, feelings, or conversations associated with the trauma 2. Efforts to avoid activities, places, or people that arouse recollections of the trauma 3. Inability to recall an important aspect of the trauma 4. Markedly diminished interest or participation in significant activities 5. Feeling of department or estrangement from others 6. Restricted range of affect 7. Sense of foreshortened future
		d. Persistent symptoms of increased arousal (not present before the trauma), as indicated by two (or more) of the following: 1. Difficulty falling or staying asleep 2. Irritability or outbursts of anger 3. Difficulty concentrating 4. Hypervigilance 5. Exaggerated startle response
Time frame Symptoms should usually arise within 6 months of the traumatic event	Symptoms should usually arise within 6 months of the traumatic event	Symptoms present for at least 1 month
Disability criterion N/A	N/A	The disturbance causes clinically significant distress or impairment in social, occupational, or important areas of functioning

of PTSD, i.e. re-experiencing, avoidance, emotional numbing, and hyper-arousal but differ in the weight assigned to them.

DSM-IV puts a stronger emphasis on the avoidance/numbing cluster of symptoms by requiring a minimum of three of these symptoms. Although emotional numbing is listed prominently in the ICD-10 diagnostic guidelines, it was not included in the ICD-10 research diagnostic criteria. As a consequence, patients that meet ICD-10 criteria may not fulfill the criteria for a DSM-IV PTSD diagnosis if they have too few of the numbing symptoms. They would be diagnosed as having an adjustment disorder according to DSM-IV. The ICD-10 research diagnostic criteria require the patient to either suffer from psychogenic amnesia or hyperarousal symptoms. Thus, in contrast to DSM-IV, a patient could be diagnosed as having PTSD in the absence of hyperarousal symptoms if amnesia is present.[11,13]

DSM-IV states two additional criteria that are not included in ICD-10. First, it requires a minimum symptom duration of 1 month because acute stress disorder would be diagnosed before 4 weeks have elapsed. Second, it requires that the symptoms cause significant distress or impaired functioning. Thus, although the diagnostic systems largely agree on the type of symptoms that characterize PTSD, DSM-IV criteria are stricter.[11,13]

DSM-5 Diagnostic criteria for PTSD 309.81 (F43.10)[20]
Post-traumatic Stress Disorder
Note: The following criteria apply to adults, adolescents, and children older than 6 years. For children 6 years and younger, see corresponding criteria below. A. Exposure to actual or threatened death, serious injury, or sexual violence in one (or more) of the following ways: 1. Directly experiencing the traumatic event(s). 2. Witnessing, in person, the event(s) as it occurred to others. 3. Learning that the traumatic event(s) occurred to a close family member or close friend. In cases of actual or threatened death of a family member or friend, the event(s) must have been violent or accidental. 4. Experiencing repeated or extreme exposure to aversive details of the traumatic event(s) (e.g. first responders collecting human remains; police officers repeatedly exposed to details of child abuse).

Contd...

Contd...

Note: Criterion A4 does not apply to exposure through electronic media, television, movies, or pictures, unless this exposure is work related.

B. Presence of one (or more) of the following intrusion symptoms associated with the traumatic event(s), beginning after the traumatic event(s) occurred:
   1. Recurrent, involuntary, and intrusive distressing memories of the traumatic event(s).
      Note: In children older than 6 years, repetitive play may occur in which themes or aspects of the traumatic event(s) are expressed.
   2. Recurrent distressing dreams in which the content and/or affect of the dream are related to the traumatic event(s).
      Note: In children, there may be frightening dreams without recognizable content.
   3. Dissociative reactions (e.g. flashbacks) in which the individual feels or acts as if the traumatic event(s) were recurring (such reactions may occur on a continuum, with the most extreme expression being a complete loss of awareness of present surroundings).
      Note: In children, trauma-specific reenactment may occur in play.
   4. Intense or prolonged psychological distress at exposure to internal or external cues that symbolize or resemble an aspect of the traumatic event(s).
   5. Marked physiological reactions to internal or external cues that symbolize or resemble an aspect of the traumatic event(s).

C. Persistent avoidance of stimuli associated with the traumatic event(s), beginning after the traumatic event(s) occurred, as evidenced by one or both of the following:
   1. Avoidance of or efforts to avoid distressing memories, thoughts, or feelings about or closely associated with the traumatic event(s).
   2. Avoidance of or efforts to avoid external reminders (people, places, conversations, activities, objects, situations) that Posttraumatic Stress Disorder 145 arouse distressing memories, thoughts, or feelings about or closely associated with the traumatic event(s).

D. Negative alterations in cognitions and mood associated with the traumatic event(s), beginning or worsening after the traumatic event(s) occurred, as evidenced by two (or more) of the following:
   1. Inability to remember an important aspect of the traumatic event(s) (typically due to dissociative amnesia and not to other factors such as head injury, alcohol, or drugs).
   2. Persistent and exaggerated negative beliefs or expectations about oneself, others, or the world (e.g. "I am bad," "No one can be trusted," "The world is completely dangerous," "My whole nervous system is permanently ruined").
   3. Persistent, distorted cognitions about the cause or consequences of the traumatic event(s) that lead the individual to blame himself/herself or others.
   4. Persistent negative emotional state (e.g. fear, horror, anger, guilt, or shame).

Contd...

Contd...

   5. Markedly diminished interest or participation in significant activities.
   6. Feelings of detachment or estrangement from others.
   7. Persistent inability to experience positive emotions (e.g. inability to experience happiness, satisfaction, or loving feelings).

E. Marked alterations in arousal and reactivity associated with the traumatic event(s), beginning or worsening after the traumatic event(s) occurred, as evidenced by two (or more) of the following:
   1. Irritable behavior and angry outbursts (with little or no provocation) typically expressed as verbal or physical aggression toward people or objects.
   2. Reckless or self-destructive behavior.
   3. Hypervigilance.
   4. Exaggerated startle response.
   5. Problems with concentration.
   6. Sleep disturbance (e.g. difficulty falling or staying asleep or restless sleep).

F. Duration of the disturbance (Criteria B, C, D, and E) is more than 1 month.

G. The disturbance causes clinically significant distress or impairment in social, occupational, or other important areas of functioning.

H. The disturbance is not attributable to the physiological effects of a substance (e.g. medication, alcohol) or another medical condition.

Specify whether:

With dissociative symptoms: The individual's symptoms meet the criteria for post-traumatic stress disorder, and in addition, in response to the stressor, the individual experiences persistent or recurrent symptoms of either of the following:

1. *Depersonalization:* Persistent or recurrent experiences of feeling detached from, and as if one were an outside observer of, one's mental processes or body (e.g. feeling as though one were in a dream; feeling a sense of unreality of self or body or of time moving slowly).
2. *Derealization:* Persistent or recurrent experiences of unreality of surroundings (e.g. the world around the individual is experienced as unreal, dreamlike, distant, or distorted).

Note: To use this subtype, the dissociative symptoms must not be attributable to the physiological effects of a substance (e.g. blackouts, behavior during alcohol intoxication) or another medical condition (e.g. complex partial seizures).

Specify if:

With delayed expression: If the full diagnostic criteria are not met until at least 6 months after the event (although the onset and expression of some symptoms may be immediate).

Post-traumatic Stress Disorder for Children 6 Years and Younger

A. In children 6 years and younger, exposure to actual or threatened death, serious injury, or sexual violence in one (or more) of the following ways:
   1. Directly experiencing the traumatic event(s).
   2. Witnessing, in person, the event(s) as it occurred to others, especially primary caregivers.

Contd...

Contd...

Note: Witnessing does not include events that are witnessed only in electronic media, television, movies, or pictures. Post-traumatic stress disorder 147

3. Learning that the traumatic event(s) occurred to a parent or caregiving figure.

B. Presence of one (or more) of the following intrusion symptoms associated with the traumatic event(s), beginning after the traumatic event(s) occurred:
   1. Recurrent, involuntary, and intrusive distressing memories of the traumatic event(s).
      Note: Spontaneous and intrusive memories may not necessarily appear distressing and may be expressed as play re-enactment.
   2. Recurrent distressing dreams in which the content and/or affect of the dream are related to the traumatic event(s).
      Note: It may not be possible to ascertain that the frightening content is related to the traumatic event.
   3. Dissociative reactions (e.g. flashbacks) in which the child feels or acts as if the traumatic event(s) were recurring (such reactions may occur on a continuum, with the most extreme expression being a complete loss of awareness of present surroundings). Such trauma-specific re-enactment may occur in play.
   4. Intense or prolonged psychological distress at exposure to internal or external cues that symbolize or resemble an aspect of the traumatic event(s).
   5. Marked physiological reactions to reminders of the traumatic event(s).

C. One (or more) of the following symptoms, representing either persistent avoidance of stimuli associated with the traumatic event(s) or negative alterations in cognitions and mood associated with the traumatic event(s), must be present, beginning after the event(s) or worsening after the event(s):
   Persistent avoidance of stimuli
   1. Avoidance of or efforts to avoid activities, places, or physical reminders that arouse recollections of the traumatic event(s).
   2. Avoidance of or efforts to avoid people, conversations, or interpersonal situations that arouse recollections of the traumatic event(s).

   Negative alterations in cognitions
   1. Substantially increased frequency of negative emotional states (e.g. fear, guilt, sadness, shame, confusion).
   2. Markedly diminished interest or participation in significant activities, including constriction of play.
   3. Socially withdrawn behavior.
   4. Persistent reduction in expression of positive emotions.

D. Alterations in arousal and reactivity associated with the traumatic event(s), beginning or worsening after the traumatic event(s) occurred, as evidenced by two (or more) of the following:
   1. Irritable behavior and angry outbursts (with little or no provocation) typically expressed as verbal or physical aggression toward people or objects (including extreme temper tantrums).
   2. Hypervigilance.

Contd...

Contd...

   3. Exaggerated startle response.
   4. Problems with concentration.
   5. Sleep disturbance (e.g. difficulty falling or staying asleep or restless sleep).

E. The duration of the disturbance is more than 1 month.

F. The disturbance causes clinically significant distress or impairment in relationships with parents, siblings, peers, or other caregivers or with school behavior.

G. The disturbance is not attributable to the physiological effects of a substance (e.g. medication or alcohol) or another medical condition.

Specify whether:

With dissociative symptoms: The individual's symptoms meet the criteria for post-traumatic stress disorder, and the individual experiences persistent or recurrent symptoms of either of the following:

1. *Depersonalization*: Persistent or recurrent experiences of feeling detached from, and as if one were an outside observer of, one's mental processes or body (e.g. feeling as though one were in a dream; feeling a sense of unreality of self or body or of time moving slowly).
2. *Derealization*: Persistent or recurrent experiences of unreality of surroundings (e.g. the world around the individual is experienced as unreal, dreamlike, distant, or distorted).

Note: To use this subtype, the dissociative symptoms must not be attributable to the physiological effects of a substance (e.g. blackouts) or another medical condition (e.g. complex partial seizures).

Specify if:

With delayed expression: If the full diagnostic criteria are not met until at least 6 months after the event (although the onset and expression of some symptoms may be immediate).

Differential Diagnoses[11,13] (Table 2)

PTSD symptoms may overlap with symptoms of number of other disorders. Distinguishing features include the following: the type of stressor (adjustment disorders, enduring personality change) the symptom pattern (adjustment disorders, enduring personality change) the duration of the symptoms (acute stress disorder, acute stress reaction) the question of whether the avoidance, numbing, and hyper-arousal symptoms were present before the traumatic event occurred (other anxiety or depressive disorders) the nature of the intrusive cognitions and perceptual disturbances (obsessive-compulsive disorder, psychotic symptoms, substance-induced symptoms).

Prolonged repeated trauma, such as captivity or repeated childhood sexual abuse, may lead to a more complex pattern of symptoms, 'complex PTSD', that is characterized by somatization, dissociation, affect dysregulation, poor impulse control, self-destructive behavior, and pathological patterns of relationships. It was debated whether to include a

Table 2: Differential diagnosis

ICD-10 diagnostic guideline	*ICD-10 research diagnostic criteria*	*DSM-IV Criteria*
Differential diagnoses		
1. Acute stress reaction F43.0 (immediate reaction in the first 3 days after event)	Same as ICD-10 diagnostic guidelines	1. Acute stress disorder (duration of up to 4 weeks)
2. Enduring personality change after a catastrophic experience F62.0 (present for at least 2 years, only after extreme and prolonged stress)		2. Adjustment disorder (less severe stressor or different symptom pattern)
3. Adjustment disorder (less severe stressor or different symptom pattern)		3. Mood disorder or other anxiety disorder (symptoms of avoidance, numbing, or hyperausal present before exposure to the stressor)
4. Other anxiety or depressive disorders (absence of traumatic stressor or symptoms precedes stressor)		4. Other disorders with intrusive thoughts or perceptual disturbances (e.g. obsessive-compulsive disorder, schizophrenia, other psychotic disorders, substance-induced disorders)

category 'disorders of extreme stress not otherwise specified' (DESNOS) into DSM-IV to accommodate these cases, but the decision was not to include it. In ICD-10, the diagnosis 'enduring personality changes after catastrophic experience' covers such long-standing consequences of enduring trauma. Furthermore, it is currently being debated whether an additional diagnostic category 'traumatic grief' should be included into the psychiatric classification system.

The differential diagnosis is important but, notwithstanding, PTSD is unlikely to occur in isolation. Psychiatry comorbidity is the rule rather than exception. It should be explore accordingly.

Assessment Instruments[11,13]

Several semi-structured interviews assess the DSM-IV criteria for PTSD. The Structured Clinical Interview for DSM-IV (SCID) allows one to establish the diagnosis of PTSD. The Clinician Administered PTSD Scale (CAPS) and the Anxiety Disorders Interview Schedule for DSM-IV (ADIS-IV) provide measures of symptom severity as well as establishing the diagnosis of PTSD.

The most widely used self-report measure of PTSD symptoms used to be the Impact of Event Scale. The original scale contained two scales, an intrusion and an avoidance scale. It has recently been expanded to include an additional hyperarousal scale (IES-R). The IES-R does not cover all the symptoms of PTSD specified in DSM-IV. This is why new measures that are modelled on the DSM-IV criteria are now commonly used in research studies, for example the Post-traumatic Stress Diagnostic Scale.

Partial PTSD

Several studies have found substantial levels of distress and disability for traumatized people who met some, but not all, of the PTSD criteria specified in DSM-IV. These people may be at greater risk of developing the full PTSD syndrome than people with fewer symptoms.[11]

Course and Prognosis

Immediately following traumatic exposure mixed symptoms begins to develop in vast majority of PTSD cases. Delayed onset is found in a minority (11% or less) of the cases. A series of prospective longitudinal studies suggest that a large proportion of people who initially develop PTSD recover within the first year after a traumatic event. Across different studies, it can be estimated that about 50% of those with initial PTSD symptoms will recover during the first year. Long-term outcome depends on initial symptom severity. People with high initial PTSD severity were more likely to remain symptomatic at follow-up than those with low initial symptom severity.[11,13]

The substantial rate of initial recovery does not imply, however, that PTSD in general has a good prognosis. A substantial proportion of traumatized individuals will suffer long-standing morbidity after a traumatic event. Retrospective studies suggest that about one-third of people who develop PTSD after a traumatic event will not recover for many years.[11]

FACTORS AFFECTING RECOVERY FROM TRAUMA

Recovery Environment

Recovery is facilitated by social support and the absence of negative responses from others after the event. Further stressful or traumatic life events impede recovery from PTSD. This includes the stress caused by long-lasting negative effects of the event on health and personal appearance, financial difficulties, disruptions in everyday life etc.

Psychological Processes

Excessively negative appraisals of the traumatic event impede. If individuals interpret their initial PTSD symptoms as signs that they are going mad or losing control, or as signs of a permanent change for the worse, they are less likely to recover. If individuals engage in behaviors or cognitive coping styles that prevent them from 'working through' and accepting the trauma, they are less likely to recover. Such maladaptive behaviors include avoidance, not talking about the experience, safety behaviors, denial, thought suppression and rumination.

Treatment of PTSD

Several psychological and pharmacological treatments are effective in PTSD.

Psychological Treatments

Psychological treatment is the first choice in PTSD and lead to large improvement shown by clinical study. Not all psychological treatments are equally effective in treating PTSD. Trauma focused cognitive-behavioral therapy (CBT) and eye movement desensitization and reprocessing were superior to stress management and other measures.[20,21]

TRAUMA-FOCUSED PSYCHOLOGICAL TREATMENT

Cognitive-behavioral Therapy

Cognitive-behavioral treatments are effective in the treatment of PTSD. This includes an element of psychoeducation about common reaction to trauma that normalizes the symptoms. All versions of CBT include some form of education about the symptoms of PTSD and treatment rationales. Common reactions to trauma are explained to normalize the patient's PTSD symptoms. The therapists explains the necessity of confronting the memory of the traumatic event and of giving up behaviors that maintain the problem such as avoidance and safety behaviors.[13,21,22]

Exposure

Exposure treatment for PTSD comprises two components. In imaginal exposure, patients are asked to relive the traumatic event in their imagination, including their thoughts and feelings at the time. This is repeated until the reliving no longer evokes high levels of distress. In vivo exposure involves confronting (safe) situations that patients avoid because they remind them of the trauma (e.g. going to the site of the traumatic event, driving again after a road traffic accident). Exposure is repeated until the patient no longer responds with high levels of distress. There are probably several mechanisms for the efficacy of exposure treatment. First, patients realize that exposure does not lead to a feared outcome (e.g. going to the site of an accident will not mean that another accident will happen; thinking about the trauma will not make them go mad) and thus helps in correcting dysfunctional beliefs about danger of the world and the meaning of PTSD symptoms. Second, the repeated reliving of the event helps them to create an organized memory and facilitates the distinction that intrusive thoughts and images are memories rather than something happening right now.

Exposure treatment is superior to supportive psychotherapy and relaxation treatment. Whereas exposure treatment is effective in the majority of cases, a minority of patients become worse). In particular, exposure treatment does not appear suitable for patients whose traumatic memories are about being perpetrators rather than victims. It may also have limits in treating survivors of complex and prolonged traumatic events such as torture, war, or captivity.[13,21,22]

Cognitive Therapy

Cognitive therapy identifies and modifies excessively negative appraisals of the traumatic event and/or its sequelae. Methods include discussion of the evidence for and against the appraisals, identification of thinking errors, challenging of appraisals with behavioral tests, and imagery modification. Recent studies have shown that cognitive therapy is effective on its own, without additional exposure treatment.[13,21,22]

Eye-movement Desensitization Reprocessing

It helps patient process their traumatic memory and think more positively about their experience. The patient is instructed to focus on a trauma-related image and its accompanying feelings, sensations, and thoughts, while visually tracking the therapist's fingers as they move back and forth in front of the patient's eyes. After a set of approximately 24 eye movements, cognitive and emotional reactions are discussed with the therapist. Coping statements are also introduced while the scene is being imagined. A series of studies have established that eye-movement desensitization reprocessing is effective, at least for self-rated PTSD symptoms.[13,21,22]

Other Psychological Treatments[13,21,22]

Stress Management (Stress Inoculation)

The goal of this treatment is to teach the patient a set of skills that will help them cope with stress. It includes relaxation training, training in slow abdominal breathing, thought stopping of unwanted thoughts, assertiveness training, and training in positive thinking. Stress management is more effective than supportive psychotherapy but less effective than trauma focused treatment.

Psychodynamic Therapy

Psychodynamic based approaches is thought to help the patient reengage normal mechanisms of adaptation. The treatment focuses on understanding the meaning of the traumatic event in the context of the patient's previous experiences, personality, and attitudes. The goal of the treatment is to work through and resolve an unconscious conflict which the traumatic event is thought to have provoked. The treatment strategy includes exploratory insight oriented, supportive or directive activity.

Hypnotherapy

In this therapy, the patient is given instructions to induce a state of highly focused attention, a reduced awareness of peripheral stimuli, and a heightened suggestibility. The goal of this treatment is to enhance control over trauma-related emotional distress and hyperarousal symptoms and to facilitate the recollection of details of the traumatic event.

Supportive Therapy

It is non-directive and non-advisery. Here patients are encouraged to explore their thoughts, feelings and behavior to cope more effectively and talking relevant actions.

Pharmacological Treatments

Although recent guidelines (NICE) recommended trauma focused psychological treatments as the first line treatments for PTSD, they also point out the role of medication. A Cochrane review found an advantage of medication over placebo with the response rate of 59.1 and 38.5% respectively. The indications for medication according to NICE guidelines include patient choice, severe ongoing threat, too depressed patient or unstable to engage in psychological treatment, and failure to respond to psychological treatment.[21]

Selective Serotonin-reuptake Inhibitors (SSRIs)

SSRIs have been most widely studied and are recommended as first line medication choice for PTSD from recent Cochrane review.[23] Among the SSRIs Paroxetine has received the most consistent support from its efficacy. SSRIs are an attractive choice because they reduce alcohol consumption; a relevant finding given the high comorbidity of PTSD with substance abuse or dependency.

Monoamine Oxidase Inhibitors (MAOIs)

Phenelzine has shown good effects on re-experiencing symptoms and insomnia, but weak effects on avoidance, numbing, and hyper-arousal symptoms. Thus, there is some evidence MAOIs such as phenelzine may be useful in the treatment of PTSD, but cannot be considered among the first-choice treatments because of the risks of hypertensive crisis and the necessary dietary restrictions.

Tricyclic Antidepressants

There is some evidence for the efficacy of tricyclic antidepressants especially amitriptyline in the treatment of PTSD.[23]

Mirtazapine

It is a noradrenergic and specific serotonergic antidepressant, has shown effectiveness in initial trials has been recommended as one of the treatment options for PTSD.[22,23]

Benzodiazepines

Although benzodiazepines may show some effects on insomnia, irritability, and general anxiety and arousal symptoms, they do not appear to be effective in the treatment of PTSD. They do not affect the re-experiencing, avoidance, and numbing symptoms.[22,23]

Choice of Treatment[22,23]

The best treatment options of PTSD to date are cognitive-behavioral treatments and SSRIs. Effect sizes of these treatments are comparable. Psychological treatments have the advantage of lower drop-out rates. The meta-analysis found that, across studies, 14% of the patients dropped out of psychological treatments, compared with 36% for the SSRIs. An additional advantage of cognitive-behavioral treatments is their established long-term effectiveness.

Treatment gains are maintained during follow-up. In contrast, long-term follow-up studies are lacking for pharmacological treatments, so that it is not known whether treatment-effects are maintained when medications are withdrawn or when they are continued for long periods. The advantage of SSRIs compared to cognitive-behavioral treatment is that they are more readily available.

Recent expert consensus guidelines concluded that cognitive-behavioral treatments are the treatment of choice for PTSD. For very severe or special cases (e.g. geriatric patients) the combination of these psychological treatments with pharmacotherapy is recommended as an alternative to psychological treatment alone.

Special considerations may apply to subgroups of PTSD patients. The efficacy of psychological treatments in patients with comorbid substance dependence remains to be established. It has been suggested that SSRIs are particularly useful for these patients, but controlled trials are lacking.

REFERENCES

1. Chou FH, Su TT, Chou P, Ou-Yang WC, Lu MK, Chien IC. Survey of Psychiatric Disorders in a Taiwan Village Population Six Months after a Major Earthquake. J Formosan Med Association. 2005;104: 308-17.
2. Chou FH, Wu HC, Chou P, Su CY, Tsai KY, Chao SS, et al. Epidemiologic Psychiatric Studies on Postdisaster Impact among Chi-Chi Earthquake Survivors in Yu-Chi, Taiwan. Psychiatry Clin Neurosci. 2007;61: 370-78.
3. Gelder M, Harrison Paul, Cowen P. Shorter Oxford Textbook of Psychiatry, Oxford University Press; 2010; 5th edn.
4. World Health Organization. International statistical classification of diseases and related health problems, 10th revision. WHO, Geneva; 1992.
5. Lazaratou H, Paparrigopoulos T, Galanos G, Psarros C, Dikeos D, Soldatos C. The psychological impact of a catastrophic earthquake: a retrospective study 50 years after the event. J Nerv Ment Dis. 2008;196:340-44.
6. Johnson H, Thompson A. The development and maintenance of post-traumatic stress disorder (PTSD) in civilian adult survivors of war trauma and torture: a review. Clin Psychol Rev. 2008;28:36-47.
7. Ikin JF, Sim MR, Creamer MC, et al. War related psychological stressors and risk of psychological disorders in Australian veterans of 1991 Gulf war, Br J Psychiatry. 2004;185:116-26.
8. Miliken CS, Auchterlonie JL, Hoge CW. Longitudinal assessment of mental health problems among active and reserve component soilders returning from the Iraq war, JAMA. 2007;298:2141-3.
9. Breslau N, Davis GC, Andreski P, Peterson E. Traumatic events and post-traumatic stress disorder in an urban population of young adults. Arch Gen Psychiatry. 1991;48:216-22.
10. Anderson MC, Ochsner KN, Kuhl B, Cooper J, Robertson E, Gabrieli SW, et al. Neural systems underlying the suppression of unwanted memories. Science. 2004;303:232-5.
11. Sadock BJ, Sadock VA, Ruiz P. Kaplan & Sadock's Comprehensive Textbook of Psychiatry, 9th edn., Lippincott Williams & Wilkins; 2009.
12. Goenjian AK, Steinberg AM, Najarian LM, Fairbanks LA, Tashjian M, Pynoos RS. Prospective study of posttraumatic stress, anxiety, and depressive reactions after earthquake and political violence. Am J Psychiatry. 2000;157: 911-6.
13. Gelder MG, Andreasen NC, Lopez-Ibor JJ, Geddes JR. New Oxford Textbook of Psychiatry, Oxford University Press; 2009; 2nd edn., Vol. 1.
14. Brady KT, Killeen TK, Brewerton T, Lucerini S. Comorbidity of psychiatric disorders and posttraumatic stress disorder. J Clin Psychiatry. 2000;61(Suppl)7: 22-32.
15. Nutt DJ. The psychobiology of posttraumatic stress disorder. J Clin Psychiatry. 2000;61(Suppl): 24-9; discussion 30-2.
16. Raison CL, Miller AH. When not enough is too much: the role of insufficient glucocorticoid signaling in the pathophysiology of stress-related disorders. Am J Psychiatry. 2003;160:1554-65.
17. Stein MB, Jang KL, Taylor S, Vernon PA, Livesley WJ. Genetic and environmental influences on trauma exposure and posttraumatic stress disorder symptoms: a twin study. Am J Psychiatry. 2002;159:1675-81.
18. Brewin CR, Andrews B, Valentine JD. Meta-analysis of risk factors for posttraumatic stress disorder in trauma-exposed adults. J Consult Clin Psychol. 2000;68:748-66.
19. American Psychiatric Association. Diagnostic and statistical manual of mental disorders (4th edn). American Psychiatric Association, Washington, DC; 1994.
20. American Psychiatric Association. Desk Reference to the Diagnostic Criteria from DSM-5. Washington DC; 2013.
21. National Institute of Clinical Excellence. Clinical guideline 26: Post Traumatic Stress Disorder: Management of PTSD in adults and children, 2005.
22. Australian Centre for Post Traumatic Mental Health. Australian guideline for the treatment of acute distress disorder and post traumatic stress disorder; 2007.
23. Stein DJ, Ipser JC Seedat S. Pharmacotherapy for posttraumatic stress disorder(PTSD), The Cochrane Database of Systemic Reviews, The Cochrane Library, 2. 2007.

SUGGESTED READING

1. American Psychiatric Association. Anxiety Disorders. In: Diagnostic and Statistical Manual of Mental Disorders, Fourth Edition, Text Revision, DSM-VI-TR. Washington, DC: American Psychiatric Association; 2000.pp.463-8.
2. American Psychiatric Association. High Percentage of Youth in the US Report Symptoms of Posttraumatic Stress and Other Disorders [press release]. Washington, DC: American Psychiatric Association; 2003.
3. Bandelow B. Defining response and remission in anxiety disorders: toward an integrated approach. CNS Spectr. 2006; 11(10 Suppl 12):21-8 [Medline].
4. Becker-Lausen E, Sanders B, Chinsky JM. Mediation of abusive childhood experiences: depression, dissociation, and negative life outcomes. Am J Orthopsychiatry. 1995;65(4):560-73 [Medline].
5. Bisson JI, Ehlers A, Matthews R, et al. Psychological treatments for chronic post-traumatic stress disorder. Systematic review and meta-analysis. Br J Psychiatry. 2007;190:97-104 [Medline].
6. Bremner JD. Neuroimaging in posttraumatic stress disorder and other stress-related disorders. Neuroimaging Clin N Am. 2007;17(4):523-38, ix [Medline].
7. Bronson D, Franco K, Budur K. Posttraumatic stress disorder in primary care patients. Compr Ther. Winter 2007;33(4):208-15 [Medline].
8. Brunet A, Orr SP, Tremblay J, et al. Effect of post-retrieval propranolol on psychophysiologic responding during subsequent script-driven traumatic imagery in post-traumatic stress disorder. J Psychiatr Res. 2008;42(6):503-6 [Medline].

9. Connor KM, Davidson JR. Further psychometric assessment of the TOP-8: a brief interview-based measure of PTSD. Depress Anxiety. 1999;9(3):135-7 [Medline].
10. Connor KM, Sutherland SM, Tupler LA, et al. Fluoxetine in post-traumatic stress disorder. Randomised, double-blind study. Br J Psychiatry. 1999;175:17-22 [Medline].
11. Davis LL, Frazier EC, Williford RB, Newell JM. Long-term pharmacotherapy for post-traumatic stress disorder. CNS Drugs. 2006;20(6):465-76 [Medline].
12. de Quervain DJ, Margraf J. Glucocorticoids for the treatment of post-traumatic stress disorder and phobias: a novel therapeutic approach. Eur J Pharmacol. 2008;583(2-3):365-71 [Medline].
13. Deykin EY. Posttraumatic Stress Disorder in Childhood and Adolescence: A Review. 1999. Medscape Mental Health [online]. Available at http://medscape.com.
14. Dickie EW, Brunet A, Akerib V, Armony JL. An fMRI investigation of memory encoding in PTSD: influence of symptom severity. Neuropsychologia. 2008;46(5):1522-31 [Medline].
15. Fiszman A, Mendlowicz MV, Marques-Portella C, et al. Peritraumatic tonic immobility predicts a poor response to pharmacological treatment in victims of urban violence with PTSD. J Affect Disord. 2008;107(1-3):193-7 [Medline].
16. Germain A, Shear MK, Hall M, Buysse DJ. Effects of a brief behavioral treatment for PTSD-related sleep disturbances: a pilot study. Behav Res Ther. 2007;45(3):627-32 [Medline].
17. Grinage BD. Diagnosis and management of post-traumatic stress disorder. Am Fam Physician. 2003;68(12):2401-8 [Medline].
18. Hamilton A. Diagnosis and rating of anxiety. Br J Psychiatry. 1969;Special Publication 3:76-9.
19. Hamilton M. Development of a rating scale for primary depressive illness. Br J Soc Clin Psychol. 1967;6(4):278-96 [Medline].
20. Hogberg G, Pagani M, Sundin O, et al. Treatment of post-traumatic stress disorder with eye movement desensitization and reprocessing: outcome is stable in 35-month follow-up. Psychiatry Res. 2008;159(1-2):101-8 [Medline].
21. Hoge CW, Auchterlonie JL, Milliken CS. Mental health problems, use of mental health services, and attrition from military service after returning from deployment to Iraq or Afghanistan. JAMA. 2006;295(9):1023-32 [Medline].
22. Hoge CW, Castro CA, Messer SC, et al. Combat duty in Iraq and Afghanistan, mental health problems, and barriers to care. N Engl J Med. 2004;351(1):13-22 [Medline].
23. Hoge CW, Clark JC, Castro CA. Commentary: women in combat and the risk of post-traumatic stress disorder and depression. Int J Epidemiol. 2007;36(2):327-9 [Medline].
24. Johnson H, Thompson A. The development and maintenance of post-traumatic stress disorder (PTSD) in civilian adult survivors of war trauma and torture: a review. Clin Psychol Rev. 2008;28(1):36-47. [Medline].
25. Kasai K, Yamasue H, Gilbertson MW, et al. Evidence for acquired pregenual anterior cingulate gray matter loss from a twin study of combat-related posttraumatic stress disorder. Biol Psychiatry. 2008;63(6):550-6 [Medline].
26. Krahe B, Scheinberger-Olwig R, Waizenhofer E, Kolpin S. Childhood sexual abuse and revictimization in adolescence. Child Abuse Negl. 1999;23(4):383-94 [Medline].
27. Lambert MT. Aripiprazole in the management of post-traumatic stress disorder symptoms in returning Global War on Terrorism veterans. Int Clin Psychopharmacol. 2006;21(3):185-7 [Medline].
28. Litz BT, Engel CC, Bryant RA, Papa A. A randomized, controlled proof-of-concept trial of an Internet-based, therapist-assisted self-management treatment for posttraumatic stress disorder. Am J Psychiatry. 2007;164(11):1676-83 [Medline].
29. Marshall RD, Pierce D. Implications of recent findings in posttraumatic stress disorder and the role of pharmacotherapy. Harv Rev Psychiatry. 2000;7(5):247-56 [Medline].
30. Medina J. Stress, PTSD and the Hippocampus. Presented at: 16th Annual US Psychiatric and Mental Health Congress. Orlando, Fla; November 6-9, 2003. Tape available at: http://www.psychcongress.com/tapes.html. Continuing Medical Education Inc.
31. Milad MR, Orr SP, Lasko NB, et al. Presence and acquired origin of reduced recall for fear extinction in PTSD: results of a twin study. J Psychiatr Res. 2008;42(7):515-20 [Medline].
32. National Institute of Mental Health. Facts about Post-Traumatic Stress Disorder. NIH Publication No. OM-99 4157 (Revised). Bethesda, MD: National Institutes of Health; 2001. [Full Text].
33. National Institute of Mental Health. Helping Children and Adolescents Cope with Violence and Disasters. NIH Publication No. 01-3518. Bethesda, Md: National Institute of Mental Health; 2001 [Full Text].
34. Olsson KA, Kenardy JA, De Young AC, Spence SH. Predicting children's post-traumatic stress symptoms following hospitalization for accidental injury: combining the Child Trauma Screening Questionnaire and heart rate. J Anxiety Disord. 2008;22(8):1447-53 [Medline].
35. Raskind MA, Peskind ER, Hoff DJ, et al. A parallel group placebo controlled study of prazosin for trauma nightmares and sleep disturbance in combat veterans with post-traumatic stress disorder. Biol Psychiatry. 2007;61(8):928-34 [Medline].
36. Risser HJ, Hetzel-Riggin MD, Thomsen CJ, McCanne TR. PTSD as a mediator of sexual revictimization: the role of reexperiencing, avoidance, and arousal symptoms. J Trauma Stress. 2006;19(5):687-98 [Medline].
37. Rodriguez BF, Weisberg RB, Pagano ME, Machan JT, Culpepper L, Keller MB. Mental health treatment received by primary care patients with posttraumatic stress disorder. J Clin Psychiatry. 2003;64(10):1230-6 [Medline].

38. Rona RJ, Fear NT, Hull L, Wessely S. Women in novel occupational roles: mental health trends in the UK Armed Forces. Int J Epidemiol. 2007;36(2):319-26 [Medline].
39. Schwartz AC, Bradley R, Penza KM, et al. Pain medication use among patients with posttraumatic stress disorder. Psychosomatics. 2006;47(2):136-42 [Medline].
40. Sheehan DV, Harnett-Sheehan K, Raj BA. The measurement of disability. Int Clin Psychopharmacol. 1996;11 Suppl 3:89-95 [Medline].
41. Smith ME. Bilateral hippocampal volume reduction in adults with post-traumatic stress disorder: a meta-analysis of structural MRI studies. Hippocampus. 2005;15(6): 798-807 [Medline].
42. Sonne SC, Back SE, Diaz Zuniga C, et al. Gender differences in individuals with comorbid alcohol dependence and post-traumatic stress disorder. Am J Addict. 2003;12(5): 412-23 [Medline].
43. Stoudemire A. Clinical Psychiatry for Medical Students. 2nd edn. Philadelphia, Pa: JB Lippincott; 1994.pp.260-5.
44. Yehuda R, McFarlane AC. Conflict between current knowledge about posttraumatic stress disorder and its original conceptual basis. Am J Psychiatry. 1995;152(12): 1705-13 [Medline].
45. Yehuda R, Spertus I, Golier J. Relationship between childhood traumatic experiences and PTSD in adults. Rev Psychiatry. 2001;20(1):117-58.

CHAPTER 19

Psychosomatic Medicine and Somatoform Disorder

Avinash De Souza, RK Chadda

19.1 PSYCHOSOMATIC MEDICINE—CONCEPT

Avinash De Souza

CONCEPT OF STRESS

The term stress has a varied history in view of its changing meaning and usage throughout the centuries. Stress, used as a noun, probably originated as a form of distress and was used to denote hardship, adversity and sometimes to describe forces or pressures applied to a person for purposes of compulsion or extortion. The word stress has been applied to external forces or stimuli as well as to the effects of such on the organism and sometimes to the point of interaction between them. In biology and medicine the term stress is of comparatively recent introduction and has been variously applied to external stimuli as well as their effects on the organism. Anything may be considered a stress if it threatens the biological integrity of the organism, whether directly by its physical or chemical properties or indirectly because of its symbolic meaning. In general medicine and psychiatry the term stress is commonly used to denote various psychosocial situations which tend to produce disorganization of behavior, including physical and mental illnesses. Responses of different individuals to potentially stressful psychosocial situations show considerable variation. The response may be apt and adaptive or it may be inept or maladaptive, the latter sometimes taking the form of physical or mental illness. The precise relationships between the psychosocial situations which are potentially stressful and their effects on the organism on the one hand, and the various stressor agents and their effects on the organism on the other, require further research for their elucidation.[1,2]

A convenient definition of stress would be any stimulus or change in the external or internal environment which disturbs homeostasis and which, under certain conditions, can result in illness. The terms stress and stressor are really abstractions and are only meaningful in relation to their effects on the organism and it might be better to use stress adjectivally as suggested in reactions to stress, namely: (1) The forces, stimuli, changes, conditions or situations which are stressful. (2) The processes whereby produce their effects on the organism. (3) The changes in the organism resulting from including behavioral, emotional, physiological, biochemical and structural changes.[3]

CONCEPT OF PSYCHOSOMATIC DISORDER

Psychosomatic disorder is a term for those physical illnesses in which psychogenic as well as physiogenic factors are etiologically important. I am including under this rubric only those disorders in which emotional and other psychogenic factors play a predisposing or precipitating role, demonstrable clinically or experimentally. In the majority of disorders so defined, genetic and constitutional factors are also important. The consideration of the role of stress in the genesis of psychosomatic disorders brings us into the complicated field of etiology. Theoretically there are innumerable possible causes which may be considered in relation to any event including illness. In medicine it is clearly unprofitable to consider all possible causes in illnesses as only some will be relevant in clinical practice and therefore the problem resolves itself into a search for factors in the environment or in the individual which are relevant and causal. As physicians we are particularly interested in the extent to which these forces can be controlled or modified. Some causes will be essential, without which a disease cannot develop, but there will be other factors which will have as much claim to be a cause as they determine the actual manifestation of the essential cause as a disease.[4]

STRESS IN THE ETIOLOGY OF PSYCHOSOMATIC DISEASES

In considering the role of stress in the etiology of psychosomatic disorders it is first necessary to establish a statistically significant temporal relationship between the occurrence of stress and the manifestations of the disorder and then to determine whether the stress comes under the category of essential causes or sufficient causes. During recent decades a number of theories alleging specificity in psychosomatic relationships have been postulated and greatly elaborated. Specific factors in the environment and in the individual have been claimed to be causally relevant in the development of psychosomatic disorders; for example, French and Alexander claimed that the asthmatic attack occurs when there is a separation or a threat of separation from the mother; Miller and Baruch describe specific parental attitudes in the etiology of asthma in children; Lidz and Whitehorn report specificity in the type of psychosocial stress at the onset of thyrotoxicosis, namely a break of important interpersonal relationships; Wittkower relates outbreaks of urticaria to a loss or threatened loss of love; Lindemann stresses the importance of bereavement and grief reactions in ulcerative colitis and so on. Specificity in attitudes in various life situations for different psychosomatic disorders is reported by Grace and Graham; specificity of personality type or profile for each psychosomatic disorder is put forward by Flanders Dunbar and Halliday.[5,6]

Others claim that specificity of emotional changes and physiological concomitants occurs in different psychosomatic disorders. Theories of specificity relate largely to a specificity of stimulus which allegedly produces specific psychophysiological responses and specific psychosomatic disorders. In all ages and in both sexes, a diversity of stressful life situations was found, with no evidence of any specificity for each particular disorder. Some of the stresses were sudden, occurring at a definite point in time, e.g. bereavement, accidents and illnesses to a loved person and various traumatic experiences of the patient. Other stresses operated over a longer period of time; such as family and marital difficulties, work and financial problems, sex conflicts and a variety of miscellaneous conflict situations. The type of psychosocial situation which is potentially stressful and relevant in development of psychosomatic disorders varies according to the age of the individual. In asthmatic children, parental lack, faulty parental attitudes, particularly those of rejection, overprotection or perfectionism are especially important, whereas in elderly asthmatic patients, stresses arising from adjustment difficulties following retirement or death of a spouse were found to be of particular importance.[7]

The types of life situation associated with the occurrence of attacks during the course of the illness were similar to those associated with the onset. All varieties of stressful situation were found in each disorder with no evidence of specificity of life situation in the precipitation of attacks during the illness. The life situations relevant in this connection were varied and do not lend themselves readily to classification but the following constituted the main groups: (1) Bereavement of a loved person. (2) Threat to a loved person by illness or accident or other cause. (3) Marital and family problems. (4) Work and financial problems. (5) Conflicts relating to individual needs, including sex drives, ambitions, prestige, status. We therefore find no evidence of any specificity in the type of stressful life situations, either at the onset or in association with the occurrence of attacks during the course of the illness. The common factor appears to be that which is perceived by the individual as a threat to security in its widest sense.[8]

EMOTIONS AND PSYCHOSOMATIC DISEASES

The study of correlations between stressful life situations or emotional changes and attacks is facilitated when the manifestations of the illness occur at a definite point in time and are readily observable by the investigator, as in asthma, vasomotor rhinitis, hay fever and urticaria/angioneurotic cedema. In the case of peptic ulcer and thyrotoxicosis it is less easy to study such relationships. It will be seen that emotional changes can precipitate attacks in from one-third to three-quarters of patients but that other precipitants operate also in the majority of patients. It was found that a variety of emotions could precipitate attacks or produce exacerbations in every disorder and there was no evidence at all of any specificity of emotional change for this disorder. In fact many different kinds of emotional change were found to be capable of precipitating attacks in all disorders, the most common being anxiety, anger, resentment, hostility, humiliation, depression and sometimes even joy and elation. The suppression or bottling up of emotions was found to be more important than the type of emotion experienced. There was, however, a tendency for certain traits of personality to be significantly higher in some psychosomatic disorders than their corresponding control groups, particularly the following: anxious, sensitive, obsessional, meticulous. These tended to be higher in all psychosomatic disorders rather than to be specifically related to any particular condition.[9]

MULTIFACTORIAL CAUSATION AND THEIR INTER-RELATIONSHIPS

This brings us to the interrelationships of different etiological factors in certain psychosomatic disorders. We have noted that plurality of causal factors is the general rule in psychosomatic disorders. In asthma, vasomotor rhinitis and urticaria, for example, there is clinical and experimental evidence that allergy, infections, physical agents and emotional factors can exert summative effects in producing manifestations of these disorders.

The onset is sometimes due to a combination of stress with allergy or infection. Similarly the response to allergens is influenced by the patient's emotional state and by infections which also are facilitated by certain emotional changes. Emotional states which precipitate attacks of these disorders are mediated by the parasympathetic (cholinergic) pathways. The local tissue changes in vascularity, swelling and glandular secretion due to cholinergic activity have additive effects with some tissue changes produced by allergens and mediated by histamine and infections. Clusters of illnesses could be identified in many individuals, the majority of such clusters tending to occur when the individual perceives his life situation to be unsatisfactory, over-demanding, or a threat to security, or with failure to satisfy important personal needs. This applied to all forms of illness, medical, surgical and psychiatric. These findings indicate that the term psychosomatic is applicable to a greater range of diseases than formerly believed.[10,11]

19.2 SOMATOFORM DISORDERS

RK Chadda

Somatoform disorders as a diagnostic group have a very short history going back to 1980, when the term was introduced in the scientific literature by the American Psychiatric Association in the third edition of its Diagnostic and Statistical Manual of Mental Disorders (DSM III),[12] though some of the disorders included in the group are known since centuries. World Health Organization's ICD-9 did not have this diagnostic category but it was included in the ICD-10 in 1992.[13]

The various disorders included in the group share the central characteristic of having physical symptoms without organic basis as the presenting feature. The physical symptoms suggest a physical illness (hence somatoform) for which there are no demonstrable organic findings or known physiologic mechanisms but there is positive evidence, or a strong presumption, that the symptoms are linked to psychological factors or conflicts.[14] These include somatization disorder, conversion disorder, hypochondriasis, psychogenic pain disorder, body dysmorphic disorder (dysmorphophobia), somatoform autonomic dysfunction and undifferentiated somatoform disorder.

HISTORY

In 1900 BC, Kahn in Medical Papyrus described 'hysteria' as a number of maladies supposedly caused by wandering of the uterus. Hippocrates in Greek era and Galen in Roman era defined 'hysteria' as a disorder of women, attributed to the movements of uterus (Greek, hysteria-uterus) and caused by sexual abstinence. Hypochondriasis was described as symptoms due to disturbance of viscera below the diaphragm. In middle ages, Heinrich, Kramer and Springier attributed hysteria and related illnesses to the possession by evil forces.[14]

Sydenham, in 1682, stated that hysteria could mimic almost all known physical diseases and described hypochondriasis as the masculine version of hysteria in females. In 1859, Briquet gave systematic and clearer clinical definition of hysteria and classified the symptoms in 8 minor categories. Falret, in 19th century, opined that hypochondriacs have a morbid preoccupation with bodily functions and insistence that they suffer from a serious illness. Later Breuer, in 1895, stressed on the role of unconscious memories of emotionally traumatic events in the production of hysterical symptoms. Freud, in earlier part of his work, described the mechanism of conversion and fixation at oedipal phase for hysteria, and defined hypochondriasis as an actual neurosis in which somatic factors play prominent causal role.

Janet described dissociation as the basis for hysteria in 1907. Savill and Putell also provided clinical descriptions of hysterical patients (the present day 'somatization' patients). A clearer clinical definition of hypochondriasis, consisting of 5 criteria, was given by Gillespie in 1928.[14] Kenyon[15] viewed hypochondriasis always as a part of another syndrome, mostly an affective one. In 1968, hypochondriasis was for the first time included as an official diagnosis in DSM-II.[16]

Whitloch (1967) and Ludwig (1972) provided neurophysiological bases of hysteria as corticofugal inhibition of afferent stimulation at the level of reticular activating system (RAS).[17] Celani emphasized the role of cultural, social and interpersonal influences in hysteria, while Barr and Abennathy gave behavioral basis of hysterical symptoms, conceptualizing the symptoms as an adaptation to the frustrating life experiences.[18] In 1980, a new category of somatoform disorder included in DSM-III.[12]

Brown and Vaillant[19] presented the concept of repressed hostility as the etiology of hypochondriasis. Barsky and Klerman[20] emphasized the role of perceptual and cognitive anomalies in hypochondriasis. Hollender, and Ford and Foulks viewed that conversion disorders were forms of nonverbal communication using somatic language.[14,18] The category of somatoform disorder gained worldwide acceptance by its inclusion in the World Health Organization's 10th edition of International Classification of Diseases (ICD-10) in 1992.[2] DSM-IV has further refined the category of somatoform disorders.[21]

Recently, the World Health Organization has also initiated a multicentric international study on somatoform disorders in 11 countries including India, Brazil, USA, Italy and Zimbabwe.[22] Analysis of a part of Indian data has revealed association of some life events like going on pleasure trip/pilgrimage, marriage of daughter/dependent son, trouble with neighbors, robbery/theft and change of sleep habits with somatoform disorders.[23]

NOSOLOGICAL ISSUES AND RELATED CONTROVERSIES

Inclusion of the category of somatoform disorders in DSM-III was an attempt to bring together a group of disorders known since long by different names as distinct diagnostic entities into a more discrete category. However, except for somatization disorder, which has been extensively studied for diagnostic stability and validity,[24-28] the other somatoform diagnoses are just nonspecific symptom clusters that cannot be properly operationalized and rarely occur in pure forms. Each of these disorders has arisen in a different school of psychiatric thought. The concept of conversion disorder is basically a psychodynamic one, whereas somatization disorder is a result of phenomenological and descriptive research. The pain disorder has achieved recognition primarily because of its clinical significance.

Out of the various somatoform disorders, conversion disorder and hypochondriasis have been traditionally grouped under neuroses, whereas somatization disorder was considered a type or variant of hysteria. Psychogenic pain disorder (pain disorder in DSM-IV) has also gained a honorable position, as earlier it was put in miscellaneous group in various classifications. DSM-III-R and DSM-IV have also included the categories of undifferentiated somatoform disorder and body dysmorphic disorder in an attempt to be more specific. ICD-10 differs from DSM-IV in not including the categories of conversion disorder in somatoform disorders. Another important diagnosis, neurasthenia (chronic fatigue syndrome) does not find place in somatoform disorders, though its presentation is predominantly somatic.

Similarly, in case of certain culture bound syndromes like Koro and Dhat syndrome, the presentation is predominantly somatic, and therefore, there is a cause to include these under somatoform disorders.[29-31] Some beginning has been made in this direction in ICD-10 by including such disorders under other unspecified neurotic disorders.[2] The duration criteria of 6 months for somatoform pain disorder and undifferentiated somatoform disorder in DSM-IV result in too many NOS diagnoses in clinical practice.[32-34] Such duration criteria are of more utility in the research settings rather than in clinical practice.[33]

Hysteria, another disorder with frequent somatic presentation, has been extensively studied in this century. Traditionally, based on its psychodynamic origin and clinical presentation, it was recognized to be of two types: conversion and dissociation types. But, its diagnostic stability and validity has not been established. In the famous follow-up study by Slater averaging 9 years, the diagnosis remained stable only in 25% of patients.[35,36] But, the term 'hysteria' has been used in literature in so many ways: as a pejorative adjective to describe the highly colorful behavior (mostly in women); for conversion symptoms; for dissociation states; Briquet hysteria; a pathologic personality type; and phobic disorder-anxiety hysteria. This has caused a great confusion.[37]

DSM III, by abandoning the term and by organizing various such disorders in a systematic way, tried to clear this dilemma. But, it perhaps overshot the mark by sharply separating conversion disorders from dissociation disorders, ignoring the central and common role that the mechanism of dissociation plays in both the disorders.[1] However, ICD-10 has included both the conditions under 'neurotic disorders' as a single distinct category separate from somatoform disorders.[13] Somatization disorder, which was earlier known as Briquet's hysteria or syndrome, and was traditionally described as a presentation of hysteria, has been given a special status, thanks to the extensive and systematic studies of the disorder by St. Louis group.[24,38-42]

Like hysteria, the term 'hypochondriasis' has also been used in literature in a number of ways. The hypochondriacal symptoms are mostly a part of clinical picture of some other psychiatric illness, so much so that DSM-I did not assign it an official diagnostic label. Kenyon,[15] in his extensive work of 500 patients with hypochondriacal symptoms, concluded that hypochondriasis is always a part of another syndrome, most commonly an affective one. However, DSM-II assigned it an official diagnostic status[16] and ICD-9 included it as a separate diagnostic category under neuroses.[43] In DSM-III, DSM-IV and ICD-10, it was grouped under somatoform disorders. Since hypochondriasis is usually a chronic disorder, another term 'transient hypochondriasis' has been described in recent literature, which is a transient reaction to stress. Being transient, it is less than 6 months in duration, and therefore in the classification systems it would be included in somatoform disorders NOS.[44,45]

Pain with no organic basis is another symptom, which has puzzled the psychiatrists as well as physicians. It is quite difficult to establish the role of psychological factors in all patients with chronic idiopathic pain. The category of psychogenic pain disorder in DSM-III required a positive evidence of a psychological etiology (either primary or secondary gain) to differentiate it from pain of organic origin, a finding, which is often lacking and has a poor reliability and validity. Because of this limitation, its name was changed to somatoform pain disorder in DSM-III-R,[46] in which a positive evidence of psychogenicity was not necessary for the diagnosis. DSM-IV has even dropped the word somatoform and labels the category as 'pain disorder'. ICD-10 keeps the

Table 1: Classification of somatoform disorders

DSM-IV	*ICD-10*
Somatization disorder	Somatization disorder
Conversion disorder	Hypochondriacal disorder
Hypochondriasis	Somatoform autonomic dysfunction
Pain disorder	Persistent somatoform pain disorder
Body dysmorphic disorder	Other somatoform disorders
Undifferentiated	Somatoform disorder, unspecified
Somatoform disorder	
Somatoform disorder NOS	

DSM-5 Classification of somatic symptom and related disorders

- Somatic symptom disorder
- Illness anxiety disorder
- Conversion disorder (Functional neurological symptom disorder)
- Psychological factors affecting other medical conditions
- Factitious disorder
- Other specified somatic symptom and related disorder
- Unspecified somatic symptom and related disorder

category under the label of 'persistent somatoform pain disorder'.

Body dysmorphic disorder (dysmorphophobia in DSM-III) is another category, which after being classified in miscellaneous groups for long, was put under a formal diagnostic group in DSM-III. The disorder, however, has been included under hypochondriasis in ICD-10.

Two new disorders, which have been included in somatoform disorders in the current classificatory systems, are undifferentiated somatoform disorder (in DSM-III-R, DSM IV and ICD-10) and somatoform autonomic dysfunction (in ICD-10). Nosological aspects of these disorders are not clear, as not much data is available about these disorders.

The various disorders included under somatoform disorders in ICD-10 are shown in Table 1.

In DSM-5, somatoform disorders are now referred to as somatic symptom and related disorders. Diagnosis of somatisation disorder, hypochondriasis, pain disorder and undifferentiated somatoform disorder have been removed.

SOMATIZATION DISORDER

Somatization disorder is characterized by presence of recurrent and multiple, frequently changing somatic complaints of several years duration, for which medical attention has been sought, but these apparently are not due to any physical disorder. The disorder usually begins in early adult life and runs a chronic but fluctuating course (DSM-IV). ICD-10 puts a minimum duration of 2 years before the disorder is diagnosed. It is an equivalent of the disorder described by Briquet way back in 1859.

Epidemiology

Lifetime prevalence in females varies from 0.2% to 2% and is less than 0.2% in men. The disorder is more common in the less educated, the poor and those from lower occupational groups.[21] Prevalence of the disorder has often been underestimated in studies relying on interviews by nonphysicians. This may account for the low prevalence estimates of the disorder in large scale interviews, which used non-physician interviewers.[47] Though initially thought to be almost nonexistent in men, it is now documented to exist in men and have similar characteristics as in women except for the sex specific symptoms. Low prevalence in men may be due to men reporting lesser number of symptoms than women and the somatization spectrum consisting of antisocial personality in men.[48,49]

Though somatization disorder is not so common, subsyndromal somatization illness, which includes lesser number of physical symptoms, are much more common.[48,50] There are also reports of the disorder reported in HIV negative men indulging in high risk behavior.[51] A multicenter international study, being done by WHO in 14 countries, has found ICD-10 defined somatization disorder to be uncommon in primary care settings. However, the frequency of unexplained somatic symptoms did not vary geographically or with level of economic development.[50]

Etiology

The exact etiology is not known. Probably multiple factors are at work, which include contributions by genetic and environmental factors, and some defects in neurophysiological functions like information processing.

Familial Factors

The role of familial factors is well established in the etiogenesis of somatization disorder. It has been found that the risk to develop the disorder is 10–20% in female first-degree relatives of probands with somatization disorder, whereas the male relatives show an increased risk of antisocial personality and alcoholism.[27,52-54] However, somatization in men is probably heterogeneous in character. Cloninger et al.[53] could not find any familial association in male somatizers.

Genetic factors, environmental factors, or both can cause the familial aggregation. An adoption study of somatoform disorders done in Sweden[55-57] has established the role of both genetic and environmental factors in the genesis of somatization disorder. There is also evidence for genetic relationship between attention deficit disorder with hyperactivity in children and Briquet syndrome.[58,59] Tendency to somatize has been linked to emotional closeness in families, family togetherness in health matters and to anomalies in children's social relationships. Family modeling and reinforcement of illness behavior may also play an important role.[60]

Neurophysiological Basis

Patients with Briquet syndrome have been found to have low pain threshold.[61] Some abnormalities in information processing system have also been reported, like distractibility, difficulty in differentiating between target and non-target stimuli, and impaired verbal communication.[62-66] This leads to inability to habituate to repetitive stimuli. Flor-Henry et al.[65] found that Briquet syndrome patients, when compared with normal controls, have a bilateral and symmetrical pattern of frontal lobe impairment. They also have bilateral, but principally nondominant (right sided) posterior temporal deficits. This peculiar pattern of information processing explains many of their clinical features. The distractibility and impaired differentiating ability leads to vague nonspecific labels for various experiences, and unclear and incomplete statements of ideas and feelings, and distortion of new information to fit earlier preconceptions. Selective attention also increases the perception of somatic sensations, which increases with conditioning.[65]

Evoked potential studies have reported large N_1 amplitudes in somatization disorder patients, suggesting a disturbed capacity to filter out trivial afferent stimuli.[67,68] Similarly, increased P_1N_1 amplitude change as a function of stimulus intensity in patients with somatization disorder suggest an enhanced CNS response to sensory input.[66] Mismatch negativity (MMN), another EP parameter has been reported to be smaller, suggesting that somatizers probably respond more similarly than the normals to relevant and irrelevant stimuli.[69] Loss of stimulus discrimination, self regulation and cognitive integration of experience appear to be in background of tendency to somatize.[70]

Sociocultural Factors

Sociocultural factors are also responsible for the somatizing tendency. It has been documented that the tendency to perceive and report distress in psychological or somatic terms is influenced by various social and cultural factors, including the degree of stigma associated with particular symptoms. Qualitative analysis has shown that somatic symptoms, even of psychogenic origin, are less socially disadvantageous than psychological symptoms like of depression.[71] Negative mood states are also the most consistent predictors of later physical symptom reports.[72] Sometimes, somatization symptoms may be attributed to a normal or non-pathological vaginal discharge in women as a part of deeply ingrained sociocultural belief.[73]

Clinical Presentation

The patients present with multiple somatic complaints of several years duration, which are recurrent and frequently changing. There is a long and complicated medical history, during which numerous medical diagnoses have been entertained and many negative investigations or fruitless operations might have been carried out. Symptoms may refer to any part of the body, but common ones are gastrointestinal symptoms (e.g. abdominal pain, bowel problems, nausea, vomiting, belching, regurgitation, etc.), pain in the various body parts (extremities, back, joints, etc.), conversion symptoms (pseudoseizures, fainting, incoordination, loss of voice, difficulty in swallowing, etc.), symptoms referring to cardiopulmonary system (pain chest, palpitation, etc.), and sexual and menstrual disturbances.

One recent Indian study has reported the sufferers to be predominantly married women from low-income group, with onset in teens. The majority presented with gastrointestinal symptoms as a cluster, and pain in extremities and back pain individually. Headache was an important part of diagnostic symptomatology.[74] There are some recent reports of higher occurrence of somatization symptoms like headache and other forms of pain on left side suggesting right hemispheric involvement.[75]

The patients have often marked anxiety and depression, and are severely disabled and incapacitated due to their illness. Interpersonal problems are frequently present. Histrionic personality traits are common. Due to frequent use of medications, there is always possibility of drug abuse or dependence. History is usually vague, imprecise, inconsistent and disorganized. The patients often describe their complaints in a dramatic, emotional and exaggerated fashion, using vivid and colorful language.

In DSM-5, diagnosis of somatisation disorder is removed.

Management

Management of somatization disorder patients is quite difficult because there is no definite therapy and the patients usually have very high expectations, especially about the symptoms removal and a high tendency to change their doctor frequently. Goals of treatment include reduced frequency and severity of physical complaints, improvement in social adjustment and reduction in the cost and frequency of medical treatment.

The first step is the establishment of rapport and an empathic relation with a single physician based on trust and confidence. For this, the patient needs be told that it is necessary to see him or her at least a few times to know and understand his illness due to its long duration, and

DSM-5 Criteria of somatic symptom disorder 300.82 (F45.1)

A. One or more somatic symptoms that are distressing or result in significant disruption of daily life.
B. Excessive thoughts, feelings, or behaviors related to the somatic symptoms or associated health concerns as manifested by at least one of the following:
   1. Disproportionate and persistent thoughts about the seriousness of one's symptoms.
   2. Persistently high level of anxiety about health or symptoms.
   3. Excessive time and energy devoted to these symptoms or health concerns.
C. Although any one somatic symptom may not be continuously present, the state of being symptomatic is persistent (typically more than 6 months).

Specify if:
With predominant pain (previously pain disorder): This specifier is for individuals whose somatic symptoms predominantly involve pain.

Specify if:
Persistent: A persistent course is characterized by severe symptoms, marked impairment, and long duration (more than 6 months).
Specify current severity:
Mild: Only one of the symptoms specified in Criterion B is fulfilled.
Moderate: Two or more of the symptoms specified in Criterion B are fulfilled.
Severe: Two or more of the symptoms specified in Criterion B are fulfilled, plus there are multiple somatic complaints (or one very severe somatic symptom).

for reviewing his medical history and prior diagnostic evaluations. This usually helps in developing the relationship. The next step is to explain the patient that he is suffering from somatization disorder. He should be told that it is a real disorder, which leads to the type of symptoms the patient has got. This reassures the patient that his illness has been understood and diagnosed.

Management can be outlined as adherence to a few treatment modalities. Limit the number of doctors the patient is seeing. The patient may be seen by his family doctor, which may be aided by liaison with a psychiatrist, especially if psychosocial problems are prominent. Avoid unnecessary diagnostic evaluations. The investigations should be based on objective evidence and not on subjective complaints. Prescription of medication should be kept at minimum. Antianxiety drugs or antidepressants may be used whenever indicated. Some patients with history of attention deficit disorder in childhood show good response to stimulants (amphetamines, pemoline, etc.).

Due to limited interpersonal and social skills, the patients have difficulties in dealing with the various stressful interpersonal problems, which lead to anxiety or depressive symptoms and also precipitate their physical symptoms. Their information processing deficits make it difficult for them to recognize the relationship between their physical complaints and social problems. Eclectic supportive psychotherapy with emotional tone is quite helpful. These problems can be lessened using simple behavioral management techniques. Firm limits need to be exercised on excessive or manipulative demands of the patients guided by the principles outlined above.[76] Gask et al.[77] suggest a three stage retribution model for management of somatization, consisting of encouraging patients to re-attribute their symptoms and relate then to psychosocial problems. The stages consist of feeling understood, changing the agenda and making a link. The physician should show minimal interest in physical complaints and more in personal and social problems. Relaxation techniques can be used in such a situation.

Contact with family members is important because the somatization disorder patients are often poor observers. The family members can confirm and add to information, and can also assist in maintaining compliance. This can alert the treating physician to the emerging social problems, doctor shopping, medication abuse or noncompliance with therapy.

Morrison[78] has summarized the management of somatization disorder in ABCs as follows:

- Accommodate initially to forge rapport.
- Behavior modification (ignore symptoms, praise for improved behavior).
- Confrontation later about effects of behavior style.
- Decrease drugs gradually with praise for reduction.
- Educate about course and meaning of illness.
- Family involvement to give information and help with treatment.
- Guilt should be assuaged in physicians, who may blame themselves, when patients do not improve.
- Hospitalize only for serious suicide risk, substance abuse or other extreme behavior.
- Intercurrent depression should be treated conservatively.

CONVERSION DISORDER (FUNCTIONAL NEUROLOGICAL SYMPTOM DISORDER)

Conversion disorder, the most well investigated and the most common of all the somatoform disorders, is characterized by an alteration or loss of some physical function, which is a result of a psychological conflict or need.[79] Symptoms are not intentionally produced and cannot be explained by any physical disorder or known pathophysiological mechanism. The disorder has been historically, as well as in ICD-9, known as hysterical neurosis, conversion type or conversion hysteria. Though DSM IV has included it under somatoform disorders, ICD-10 categorizes it along with dissociation disorders. Nosological studies comparing ICD-9 and DSM III have found conversion disorder to be the most prominent diagnostic category amongst ICD-9 diagnosed hysteria cases.[80]

Epidemiology

Incidence and prevalence of conversion symptoms is uncertain, because vast majority of such symptoms remit spontaneously without treatment.[81] Reported rates of conversion disorder have varied widely, ranging from 11/100,000 to 300/100,000 in general population samples.[21] Lifetime prevalence of conversion symptoms varies from 25% to 30%, whereas prevalence among general hospital inpatients needing psychiatric consultation has been reported between 5% and 16%.[48,81,82] Nearly 10% of general hospital psychiatric unit attendees have been reported to suffer from hysteria diagnosed on ICD-9.[83,84] However, psychiatrists see very few patients of conversion disorders, with annual incidence of such patients seen by psychiatrists as low as 0.01 to 0.02%.[48,81,82] Twenty-five percent have a past history of conversion symptoms.[80] Sometimes, hysterical symptoms occur in epidemic form, called as 'mass hysteria'.[85,86]

It is often said that the incidence of conversion symptoms is declining in the developed countries.[37,48,87] Such trends have also now being reported from the developing countries but this finding is still controversial.[88,89]

Conversion disorder is 2–5 times more common in women than in men and more prevalent in persons from low education, low economic and rural backgrounds.

Etiology

There are three theories of origin of conversion symptoms: psychodynamic, interpersonal and neurophysiological.

Psychodynamic Theories

Psychodynamics hypothesizes that the hysterical symptoms occur from failure of mental forces to integrate mental functions, because of which certain functions escape from active central control. Freud attributed the conversion symptoms to an unconscious intrapsychic conflict. This conflict occurs between an instinctual impulse (aggressive or sexual) and the prohibitions against its expression. The anxiety of unconscious intrapsychic conflict is converted into somatic symptom, and the mechanism is called conversion. The symptom allows partial expression of the impulse in a disguised way so that the person is not confronted by the unacceptable impulses. The resultant reduction in psychological distress and anxiety is called primary gain. The symptom is the symbolic expression of unconscious conflict. However, in practice it is very difficult or impossible to evaluate the symptoms in brief consultations. Social learning, suggestion or a model[37] often influences the choice of symptoms.

Neurophysiological Mechanisms

These patients perhaps suffer from excessive cortical arousal, which causes reactive inhibition of signals at synapses in sensorymotor pathways by way of negative feedback relationship between the cerebral cortex and the brainstem reticular formation. This explains the diminished awareness of bodily sensations in some conversion disorder patients.[90] This also explains the precipitation of symptoms by stress, reduction of anxiety following appearance of symptoms and effectiveness of amobarbital infusion and other sedatives in symptom remission.[91-93] The increased susceptibility of certain individuals, like those with histrionic, dependent or antisocial personality traits, and others has also been explained on neurophysiological basis. Probably, some of them have low sedation threshold, dominant cerebral hemisphere dysfunction or have suffered from frontal lobe trauma or impairment.[65]

Most patients have bilateral symptoms.[94] But when the symptoms are unilateral, left side is usually affected. This phenomenon is more common in women and is probably a direct consequence of brain neural organization.[65,75,95]

Interpersonal Theory

The conversion symptoms serve the purpose of nonverbal interpersonal communication of the stress or suffering and also function as nonverbal means of controlling or manipulating others. An emotionally charged feeling or idea, blacked from expression by personal or cultural restraints is expressed in form of the conversion symptom. Patients with more frequently recurring conversion symptoms have been reported to have significantly higher number of problems in their private lives.[96]

Clinical Presentation

The most common conversion symptoms are sensory or motor symptoms suggesting a neurological illness. Common sensory symptoms are anesthesia, paresthesia, tunnel vision, blindness, etc. Common motor symptoms include paralysis, paresis, abnormal movements, pseudoseizures, gait disturbances, aphonia, dyskinesia, etc. The symptoms do not correspond to neuroanatomic distribution. To make a definite diagnosis of conversion disorder, there should be a temporal relation between the symptom and a significant psychosocial stressor.

Traditionally, identification of the conflict, symbolic nature of the symptom, primary gain, secondary gain and la belle indifference have been described as the characteristics of conversion symptoms, but these have limited diagnostic validity. Complete resolution of symptoms by suggestion, hypnosis or intravenous amobarbital is helpful in distinguishing conversion symptoms from physical disorders.[93] But, partial improvement may lead to missing the diagnosis of physical disorders.[97,98]

Three to 11 years follow-up studies have revealed that 13–60% of all hospitalized patients receiving the diagnosis of conversion symptoms subsequently develop an organic illness, which was actually responsible for the earlier symptoms.[25,99] A majority (74%) of the patients of hysteria after a follow up of 5–8 years had no symptoms or were better than before in two of Indian studies.[100,101] The most reliable predictor of symptom being a functional one is the previous history of conversion symptoms or unexplained physical symptoms.[35,40,91,98] One 29 year follow-up study found that one third of patients later developed psychotic illness.[48]

DSM-5 Diagnostic disorder of conversion disorder (Functional neurological symptom disorder)[158]

A. One or more symptoms of altered voluntary motor or sensory function.
B. Clinical findings provide evidence of incompatibility between the symptom and recognized neurological or medical conditions.
C. The symptom or deficit is not better explained by another medical or mental disorder.
D. The symptom or deficit causes clinically significant distress or impairment in social, occupational, or other important areas of functioning or warrants medical evaluation.

Coding note: The ICD-9-CM code for conversion disorder is 300.11, which is assigned regardless of the symptom type. The ICD-10-CM code depends on the symptom type (see below).

Specify symptom type:
(F44.4) with weakness or paralysis
(F44.4) with abnormal movement (e.g. tremor, dystonic movement, myoclonus, gait disorder)
(F44.4) with swallowing symptoms
(F44.4) with speech symptom (e.g. dysphonia, slurred speech)
(F44.5) with attacks or seizures
(F44.6) with anesthesia or sensory loss
(F44.6) with special sensory symptom (e.g. visual, olfactory, or hearing disturbance)
(F44.7) with mixed symptoms

Specify if:
Acute episode: Symptoms present for less than 6 months.
Persistent: Symptoms occurring for 6 months or more.

Specify if:
With psychological stressor (specify stressor)
Without psychological stressor

Management

The management is in two phases:

1. Symptom removal.
2. Recognition and coping with the psychosocial stresses provoking the symptoms.

1. *Symptom Removal*: Prompt elimination of the symptom is important to prevent the secondary gains from reinforcing it and making it chronic. The patient should not be told that there is nothing wrong, but should be reassured that the symptom is going to disappear quickly and completely. After detailed examination, a suggestion may even be made that it has already started improving. Mild sedation, relaxation exercises, hypnosis and anxiolytics may be used at this stage and are quite effective.[93] If there is no response, amobarbital or pentothal interview may be used, which has both diagnostic and therapeutic value. During the interview, it may be suggested that the medication will lead to symptom remission and patient should be asked to recall the circumstances preceding the onset of symptoms. Often the removal of symptom is accompanied by recall of the precipitating stress.[97] Parenteral lorazepam sometimes is followed by improvement. Medication may reduce anxiety and play a facilitative role in psychotherapy process.[48]
2. *Dealing with psychosocial stresses*: If the precipitating stress is transient or is unlikely to recur and there is no significant psychopathology, this phase of treatment is brief. If the stress is persistent or there is significant psychopathology, insight-oriented psychotherapy or dynamic therapy is to be used. In recent years, briefer and more directive forms of psychotherapies have also been used to treat conversion disorders. A nonconfrontational approach is encouraged.

In addition, secondary gain should be cut to minimum, using environmental manipulation. The family should be told to encourage the patient's autonomy, self-sufficiency and independence, and to discourage the sick role.

HYPOCHONDRIASIS

Hypochondriasis is characterized by a preoccupation with fear of having or developing a serious physical illness. The fear is often a result of unrealistic interpretation of physical signs or sensations as evidence of disease. The disorder is often chronic, with symptoms present for months or years. Hypochondriacal symptoms frequently occur in other psychiatric disorders like depression, schizophrenia, other somatoform disorders and anxiety disorders. In hypochondriasis or hypochondriacal disorder, the hypochondriacal symptoms are the primary symptom.

Epidemiology

The prevalence of hypochondriasis in general population is not known. The prevalence in general medical setting is reported to be 4–9%. The disorder affects both sexes equally or may be slightly predominant in men. The peak age of onset is probably between 20 and 30, though it may occur at any age. However, it rarely presents for the first time after 50.[21] One recent study put the one-year prevalence in general population at 4.5%.[102]

Etiology

There are three theories of origin of hypochondriasis, namely psychodynamic theory, sociocultural theory, and neuropsychological theory.

Dynamic Theory

The dynamic theory describes hypochondriasis as an alternate channel to deflect sexual, aggressive or oral drives or an ego defense against guilt and low esteem or a sign of excessive self concern. The aggressive and hostile wishes towards others are transformed into physical complaints through repression or displacement. Freud explained it as a withdrawal of sexual libido from external objects, which is reinvested as narcissistic libido and eventually overflows into actual somatic changes.[14]

The hypochondriacal symptoms have also been viewed as an expression of pregenital wishes for caring, nurturance, attention, sympathy and physical contact. Others have described it as a defense against low self-esteem, guilt and a sense of innate badness.[103-105]

Sociocultural Theory

Hypochondriasis has also been visualized as a learned social behavior, serving the purpose of nonverbal interpersonal communication. The behavior shows that as if being a patient is their sole avocation and the patient's full time vocation.[106-109] The behavior was learned because of its success in past in eliciting caretaking and in securing the other secondary gains of the sick role. They may have assumed the sick role initially as a result of an accident, injury or medical illness or by modeling themselves after someone, who successfully used the sick role.[109] The sick role serves to convey about their distress and disability to others, serving nonverbal communication.[108]

Neuropsychological Theory

According to this theory, hypochondriasis is the result of an underlying perceptual or cognitive abnormality. The patients amplify and augment normal bodily sensations and perceive them as more noxious and intense than does the person, who is not hypochondriacal. They have constitutionally lower thresholds and tolerance for physical discomfort.[110-112] They misinterpret normal bodily sensations, physiological functions, the trivial symptoms of every day life and the somatic symptoms of emotional arousal by misattributing them to a serious disease process. Recently, it has been reported that, though the hypochondriacal patients are more sensitive to normal physiological sensations and minor bodily parameters than the nonhypochondriacs, objective parameters like ability to discriminate between two factual bodily signals do not confirm it.[113-115] They are also probably constitutionally predisposed to thinking and perceiving in concrete and physical terms rather than in emotional and subjective terms.[20,113]

Clinical Presentation

The patient usually presents with a detailed and exhaustive history of multiple complaints and explanations for the symptoms. Often he has a full file of medical records, has consulted a number of doctors and undergone a variety of diagnostic procedures. The interview is a monologue rather than a dialogue. The patient believes that he has a serious disease, which has not yet been diagnosed and he can not be persuaded to the contrary.

The most common complaints are pain and symptoms referable to gastrointestinal and cardiovascular systems. The symptoms usually run a chronic, waxing and waning course. Often the patient comes with a detailed pathophysiological model explaining his symptoms.

The hypochondriacs are profoundly preoccupied with their bodies and their health status. They keep on scrutinizing their body functioning, always preoccupied with their body appearance, functional limitations and health considerations. They often complain of abnormal body sensations, disturbed body functions or anatomical deviations suggesting disease.[116-118]

Recently, there has been interest in an entity called transient hypochondriasis. It refers to hypochondriacal symptoms lasting for short periods, and is seen particularly following life stresses or during recovery from medical illnesses.[44] Interestingly medical students, when first subjected to the stress of caring for gravely ill patients, frequently experience transient hypochondriasis.[119,120]

In DSM-5, diagnosis of hypochondriasis have been removed.

Management

Hypochondriacs are one of the most difficult patients to treat. Like somatization disorder, most of these patients are seen in primary care settings and can be managed by general physicians. Since hypochondriacs are clinging, demanding and harboring unrealistic expectations, their relations with doctors are often strained and unsatisfactory. Their doctor shopping behavior also elicits negative reaction from the treating physician. For the treatment to be successful, regular contact with a single doctor is very important.

Basic principles of treatment can be outlined as:

- Treatment by a single physician, with whom the patient feels confident.
- Supportive approach and regularly scheduled visits, that are not on as needed basis or based on development of new or exacerbation of existing symptoms.
- Avoidance of hospitalizations, diagnostic procedures and medications with abuse potential.
- Focussing on symptoms and brief examination in initial visit to facilitate rapport development and gradually concentrating on social or interpersonal problems.

The physician's approach should be of care rather than of cure. The patient should be helped in learning to cope with and tolerate their symptoms and to live with them as adaptively as possible, rather than to remove them. Regular scheduled visits ensure the patient that his or her complaints have been understood and are being taken seriously by the doctor. Trying to give these patients an insight into psychosocial or psychodynamic origin of symptoms is generally not helpful. It is always better to offer them an alternative explanation for symptoms, a model of dysfunction rather than of a structural abnormality. Suggestion about disturbance in perceptual function and cognitive interpretation of body functioning may be given.[121,122]

Selected patients respond to supportive psychotherapy. Group psychotherapy has also been found useful. Good psychotherapy outcomes are associated with illness of less than 3 years duration, absence of severe personality disorder and possibly higher social class.[122]

Drugs do not have any role in primary hypochondriasis. But, if there are significant anxiety or depressive symptoms, corresponding drugs may be used.

PAIN DISORDER

Pain disorder (persistent somatoform pain disorder in ICD-10) is characterized by presence of severe and prolonged pain for which there is no adequate medical explanation. DSM-III-R adapted the term somatoform in preference to psychogenic, since the term psychogenic infers that some positive evidence of psychological etiology should be present to make the diagnosis, which is usually lacking in such patients. Williams and Spitzer[123] suggested the term idiopathic to replace psychogenic, but DSM-III-R identified the category as somatoform pain disorder. It is presumed that psychological factors are important in causation, even though evidence for them might not be readily apparent in each case.

Epidemiology

The exact prevalence of pain disorder is not known, because diagnostic criteria have been frequently changing. One recently done community survey puts one-year prevalence at 0.6%.[123] However, it is quite common. Forty to fifty percent of patients, who present with nonspecific pain abdomen, have symptoms attributed primarily to psychiatric factors.[123-126] Similarly, a wide range of psychopathology has been found in patients with chronic pelvic pain and other pains.[127-129] In patients with chest pain undergoing elective coronary angiography, 10–20% cases are found to have pain of psychogenic or idiopathic origin.[130,131]

The disorder is more common in women, about twice more than in men. The peak age of onset is in fourth and fifth decades.

Etiology

There are 4 ways of understanding genesis of somatoform pain disorder: psychodynamic, behavioral, interpersonal and neurophysiological.

Psychodynamic Theory

Pain in these patients serves the purpose of punishment and atonement for unconscious guilt. Their childhood histories are marked by physical abuse, use of pain as punishment and emotional distance from parents. They have also difficulties in expressing anger. Certain authors have noticed high frequency of histories of childhood neglect and abuse, distorted self-image and interpersonal difficulties in these patients.[127,129,132]

Behavioral Theory

Pain related behavior might also be learnt by operant and classical conditioning. The pain related behaviors include grimacing, complaining, lying down, taking analgesics and staying away from work. Such behaviors are learnt, when pain occurs for the first time and are reinforced by increased attention from friends and relatives, and relief from carrying out undesirable activities such as hard physical labor and sexual obligations. Pleasurable effects of analgesics, when given for pain and possibility of monetary gain from litigation or compensation, further reinforce these behaviors. Classical conditioning occurs when certain neutral objects and settings begin to evoke pain-related behavior by their association with pain, such as patient's bed room or his work place. Pain may act as a defense against emotional distress from achievement, either in academic work or in sports.[123,133]

Interpersonal Theory

Pain serves as nonverbal interpersonal communication and may be used for manipulation or gaining advantage in interpersonal relationships. This phenomenon has also been referred to as pain games or painsmenship. Sometimes, pain may be maintained in the patient, when it is psychologically important to the other family members to do this. This is also called tertiary gain. Prior social models and cultural attitudes may also predispose certain individuals to develop chronic pain related behavior.[48,123]

Neurophysiological Theory

Serotonin has been implicated in pain disorder since it has an inhibiting effect on pain perception and is probably the neurotransmitter of the descending inhibitory pathways that arise in the raphe nucleus of the medulla. Endorphins and serotonin metabolism are decreased in cerebrospinal fluid of chronic pain patients.[134] Patients with somatoform pain syndromes have higher autonomic and muscle activity as compared to controls. There is dysfunction of corticofugal inhibitory system resulting in insufficient inhibition of the afferent stimulation, which results in amplification of heightened arousal to somatic sensory input (pain).[135] Substance P, another neurotransmitter, is also involved in altering the pain threshold.[48]

Clinical Presentation

The patient presents with preoccupation with continuous and severe pain, which defies any medical explanation. The pain may involve any body area. A number of somatoform pain syndromes, depending on the area involved, have been described in literature like somatoform facial pain syndrome, somatoform headache syndrome, somatoform abdominal pain syndrome, somatoform pelvic pain syndrome and somatoform chest pain syndrome.[124-131] Women tend to complain of pain in the face, abdomen of genital region, whereas men usually complain of pain in the back of chest.[124]

The pain is usually constant and does not vary from day to day or week to week. The pain is often inconsistent with neurological innervation of the affected area, but may sometimes mimic the pain distribution of a known disease. In some cases, patient's symptoms appear to have psychological significance, for example, mimicking those of some near dear one but clear evidence of psychological etiology in form of primary or secondary gain is absent in many cases.[136]

The patients often display a lifestyle, which can be described as the disease of the D's:[137]

- Dramatic display in describing the painful experience
- Disuse and degeneration of various body functions as consequences of the pain related behavior
- Drug misuse and doctor shopping
- Dependency, passivity and learned helplessness, which lead to demoralization and depression
- Disability, pain-contingent financial compensation or desire for compensation through litigation and disability claims.

Alexithymia is also reported to be common in these patients. Depressive symptoms are a very common accompaniment. Major depression can be diagnosed in 25–30% of somatoform pain patients.[129,138]

Determination of pain being of psychogenic origin has always been attached with controversies. Even when clinicians attempt to rate the etiology of chronic pain on an organic–nonorganic continuum based on comprehensive diagnostic data, the agreement among different raters is at best moderate.[18,124,136-138]

In DSM-5, diagnosis of pain disorder have been removed.

Management

The most important thing in management is that it should be emphasized to the patient that his pain is real and not imaginary, but psychological factors are important whether as cause or consequence, and treatment needs to be taken in that direction. Because multiple factors are usually operative in the patient, a multidisciplinary approach using psychotherapeutic, behavioral and psychopharmacological principles is needed.[128,136-138]

The goal of treatment is to replace pain-related behavior with normal activity and to counteract the D's by:

- Controlling drug misuse
- Decreasing subjective pain intensity
- Increasing activities of daily living
- Teaching competent coping skills to deal with impairment and suffering, and
- Providing vocational evaluation and rehabilitation.

The treatment modalities include the following:

Drugs

The broad principles can be outlined as follows:

- Because of the misuse and dependency risks, antianxiety drugs and sedatives should not be prescribed.
- If analgesics are needed, aspirin and nonsteroid anti-inflammatory drugs should be used.
- Antidepressants such as amitriptyline, imipramine, doxepin and phenelzine have been found effective, even when depressive symptoms are not prominent, and sometimes provide pain relief at dosage lesser than those required to treat depression. If there is no response after 6 weeks of an adequate dose, another agent should be tried before concluding that antidepressants are not effective. Whether antidepressants reduce pain by their antidepressant action or have independent direct analgesic effect (on serotonergic inhibitory pain pathways) remains unclear.[48,123,128]
- Anticonvulsants such as, phenytoin, carbamazepine, and clonazepam are effective in treating neuropathic and neuralgic pain, at least for short periods.
- No drug should be prescribed on 'as needed' basis. Time contingent prescriptions are less likely to lead to drug misuse through conditioning.

Behavioral Interventions

A wide variety of behavioral techniques like behavior modification (using principles of operant conditioning to discourage pain related behavior, and to shape and reinforce new health related behaviors), relaxation training, cognitive therapy and graduated exercise program may be used. The family and other figures important to patient may be involved in management. They should be explained the importance of normal activities of daily living and range of physical activity, which can be carried out by the patient without risk.[137]

Any statement of disability from the physician, whether to the patient, the family, employers, lawyers or the others should be objectively documented, not based on subjective complaint alone. It should always be time-limited rather than indefinite.[138]

In recent years, biofeedback has been found moderately helpful in some cases, especially in migraine, myofascial pain and muscle tension states (such as tension headaches).[123,128]

Psychotherapeutic Intervention

Traditional psychotherapeutic interventions do not have much role in somatoform pain disorder patients. However, family therapy and group therapy, along with supportive psychotherapy in combination with other treatments, bring about beneficial results. The focus should be on exploring how pain is being used as an aid in interpersonal communication and role it plays in patient's daily life.

Pain Clinics and Pain Control Programs

In recent years, a number of such facilities have come up. These usually have a multidisciplinary team consisting of physicians, psychologists, anesthesiologists, physiotherapists and occupational therapists. About 70% of patients, who go through such programs, show improvement.[138]

BODY DYSMORPHIC DISORDER OR DYSMOSRPHOPHOBIA

Body dysmorphic disorder or dysmorphophobia is characterized by preoccupation with some imagined defect in appearance in a normal appearing person or a grossly excessive concern about a slight physical anomaly. The belief is not of delusional intensity. According to DSM-IV, the diagnosis is not made if symptoms are seen exclusively during the course of anorexia nervosa or trans-sexualism. The disorder is included under hypo-chondriasis in ICD-10.

The term dysmorphophobia was dropped in DSM-III-R and DSM-IV, since it gives false impression of the illness being a phobia. Body dysmorphic disorder has traditionally been described as a form of monosymptomatic hypochondriasis, along with delusions of parasitosis and delusions of bromosis (olfactory reference syndrome). The latter two disorders are usually representative of a psychotic rather than somatoform disorder.[139-145]

Epidemiology

Recently one community survey done in Italy found one-year prevalence as 0.7%.[137] The exact prevalence is not known. It is a rare disorder. Dermatologists, plastic surgeons and internists usually see the patients. Two percent of patients coming to plastic surgeons for cosmetic purposes are found to suffer from body dysmorphic disorder. The onset usually occurs in adolescent or young adulthood and it takes some years before the patient presents to the psychiatrist.[142-145]

Etiology

Not much is known about the etiology of body dysmorphic disorder. According to psychodynamic theory, these patients invest a particular body part with a high level of unconscious meaning that can be traced to an event during an earlier stage of psychosexual development. Important defense mechanisms are repression, dissociation, distortion, symbolization and projection. In some patients, the symptoms are a part of some other disorder such as schizophrenia, mood disorder, obsessive compulsive disorder or severe personally disorder.[139,141,143,144]

Clinical Presentation

The patients present with some imaginary defects in their bodily appearance, mostly of face, nose, hair, breasts or genitalia. They may attach excessive significance of facial wrinkles and minor scar marks, and feel more distressed in social situations. Secondary symptoms like anxiety, insomnia and depression are often present.

Most patients indulge in excessive and repetitive behaviors such as mirror checking, skin picking and reassurance seeking. Premorbidly, these patients often have schizoid or obsessional traits.

The patients resist psychiatric referral and psychiatric treatment, and keep on consulting plastic surgeons and dermatologists, and requesting for cosmetic surgery or related treatments. Follow-up studies have revealed the presence of severe personality disorder and schizophrenia.[140,142,145-147]

Management

These patients are very difficult to treat, as they refuse psychiatric referral and treatment. Symptoms have been reported to respond to pimozide, other antipsychotics, tricyclic antidepressants and monoamine oxidase inhibitors. There are some recent reports of good response to selective serotonin uptake inhibitors like clomipramine and fluoxetine. However, most patients retain some concern about their problem, but are able to lead more normal lives, because the distress is lessened significantly. Long-term treatment is required, since relapses after discontinuation of medication are quite common. Cognitive behavioral strategies, using exposure and response prevention, may be helpful.[148,149]

UNDIFFERENTIATED SOMATOFORM DISORDER

Undifferentiated somatoform disorder was introduced as a residual entity in DSM-III in 1987, to accommodate the patients with subsyndromal somatization disorder, i.e. patients presenting with lesser number of symptoms or duration required for the diagnosis of somatization disorder. The entity has been retained in DSM-IV and has also been included in ICD-10. The diagnosis is made when one or more physical symptoms (e.g. fatigue, loss of appetite, urinary or gastrointestinal complaints), without an adequate medical explanation, are present for a minimum duration of 6 months (ICD-10 does not specify any duration for making a diagnosis). The symptoms should not occur only in the course of any other major psychiatric disorder or another somatoform disorder. There is either a single symptom or several circumscribed symptoms. Anxiety and depressive symptoms are a frequent accompaniment.

This category was included in DSM-III-R since patients with multiple physical symptoms of functional origin are very common in clinical practice and most of such patients do not have adequate number of symptoms sufficient for the diagnosis of somatization disorder. In fact, a number of workers advocated for inclusion of abridged definition of somatization disorder in DSM-IV, i.e. a disorder which requires presence of lesser number of symptoms out of the somatization disorder symptoms checklist, also named as somatization syndrome.[47,48,150-153] The patients suffer significant psychosocial dysfunction, and are at elevated risk for self-reported disease burden, negative perception of their health. They also have comorbid depression and generalized anxiety disorder, and disability.[50,153,154]

The disorder is less disabling than somatization disorder and has a better prognosis than somatization disorder.

Epidemiology

Undifferentiated somatoform disorder is much more common than somatization disorder, with a 30 times higher prevalence. Life-time prevalence is estimated at 4–11%[48] and one-year prevalence of 13.8% was reported recently from Italy.[137] It is more common in women and in those from lower socioeconomic groups.

Etiology

The etiological theories are similar to those of somatization disorder.

Course and Prognosis

The course is likely to be chronic and relapsing. However, being a recently introduced diagnostic category, long-term follow-up studies are lacking.

Management

The management is on similar lines as in somatization disorder.

SOMATOFORM AUTONOMIC DYSFUNCTION

This is a new diagnostic category introduced in ICD-10, and does not find place in DSM IV. The disorder is characterized by symptoms relating to organs or systems under autonomic innervation and control, e.g. cardiovascular, gastrointestinal and respiratory systems and other historical syndromes like cardiac neurosis, psychogenic hyperventilation and hiccough, gastric neurosis and nervous diarrhea. Symptoms may be of two types: one, characterized by complaints based upon objective signs of autonomic arousal (such as palpitations, sweating, flushing and tremors); and the other, characterized by more idiosyncratic, subjective and nonspecific symptoms (such as sensations of fleeting aches and pains, burning, heaviness, tightness and sensations of being bloated or distended). The patient is quite distressed and preoccupied with the possibility of a serious disorder as a result of a significant structural or physiological disturbance to explain the symptoms. Symptoms do not respond to repeated reassurance or explanations.[13,155-156]

The disorder is likely to be common, especially in non-psychiatric settings. Being a new entity, no epidemiological data is available. Differential diagnoses include generalized anxiety disorder, depression, somatization disorder and undifferentiated somatoform disorder. Physical causes should be excluded.

SOMATOFORM DISORDER NOT OTHERWISE SPECIFIED

This is a residual category for somatoform disorders, which do not meet the criteria for any other somatoform disorder or adjustment disorder with physical complaints. For example, a patient having hypochondriacal symptoms or pain of idiopathic origin or an illness involving nonstress related physical complaints of less than six months duration, will be included here. Similarly, patients who fear that they have symptoms of AIDS, although they had no contact or exposure to a putative carrier, can be classified in this category.

SOMATOFORM DISORDERS: FUTURE DIRECTIONS

Somatoform disorders, as a diagnostic group, is still in infancy and large amount of research is needed to establish the diagnostic stability of individual disorders and rationale for keeping such heterogenous disorders together. A beginning has been made. A recent study on genetics of somatoform disorders by Torgerson[157] found a higher concordance in monozygotic (29%) than in dizygotic twins (10%). Interestingly all the concordant pairs consisted of partners with two different somatoform disorders, which points towards nosologic similarity of disorders. However, there is need for studies with bigger samples. Research is needed in the etiology, nosology, diagnostic stability on long-term follow-up, and treatment of these disorders.

Epidemiological studies with special emphasis on newly formed categories, such as undifferentiated somatoform disorders, are required. In community and clinic samples, a large number of patients do not fit into any formal diagnostic category and are placed under NOS categories, e.g. transient hypochondriacal, transient pain and transient somatization phenomenon, whose status needs to be clarified. World Health Organization is doing a multinational study on somatoform disorders in 11 countries, results of which would also throw light on the diagnostic stability, etiogenesis, and prognosis of the various somatoform disorders in different cultures. Most of the entities being relatively new, genetic, neurophysiological and long-term follow-up studies are required in the field, which would also be helpful in devising standardized treatment modalities for this very common group of disorders. Research is also needed in understanding the neurophysiological basis of symptoms, which may help in developing biological treatments for various somatoform disorders.

REFERENCES

Psychosomatic Medicine—Concept

1. Kiecolt-Glaser JK, McGuire L, Robles TF, Glaser R. Psychoneuroimmunology and psychosomatic medicine: back to the future. Psychosom Med. 2002;64(1):15-28.
2. Figueira ML, Ouakinin S. From psychosomatic to psychological medicine: what's the future? Curr Opin Psychiatry. 2008;21(4):412-6.
3. Novack DH, Cameron O, Epel E, Ader R, Waldstein SR, Levenstein S, Antoni MH, Wainer AR. Psychosomatic medicine: the scientific foundation of the biopsychosocial model. Acad Psychiatry. 2007;31(5):388-401.
4. Lane RD, Waldstein SR, Critchley HD, Derbyshire SW, Drossman DA, Wager TD, Schneiderman N, Chesney MA, Jennings JR, Lovallo WR, Rose RM, Thayer JF, Cameron OG. The rebirth of neuroscience in psychosomatic medicine, Part II: clinical applications and implications for research. Psychosom Med. 2009;17(2):135-51.
5. Lipowski ZJ. Psychosomatic medicine: past and present. Part II—current state. Can J Psychiatry. 1986;31(1):8-13.
6. Leigh R, Reiser MF. Major trends in psychosomatic medicine. The psychiatrist's evolving role in medicine. Ann Intern Med. 1977;87(2):233-9.
7. Smith GC. From psychosomatic medicine to consultation liaison psychiatry. Med J Aust. 1993;159(11-12):745-50.
8. Fava GA, Wise TN, Molnar G, Zielezny M. The medical-psychiatric unit: a novel psychosomatic approach. Psychother Psychosom. 1985;43(4):194-201.
9. von Rad M, Sellschopp A. The integrated psychosomatic inpatient unit. A new approach to hospital medical care. Psychother Psychosom. 1987;48(1-4):101-9.
10. Pontzen W. 10 years of the psychosomatic department at a general hospital—retrospect and perspectives. Psychother Psychosom. 1990;40(9-10):346-55.
11. Miller G, Chen E, Cole SW. Health psychology: developing biologically plausible models linking the social world and physical health. Annu Rev Psychol. 2009;60:501-24.

Somatoform Disorders

12. American Psychiatric Association. Diagnostic and Statistical Manual of Mental Disorders, 3rd edition. Washington: American Psychiatric Association; 1980.
13. World Health Organization. The ICD-10 Classification of Mental and Behavioural Disorders: Clinical Descriptions and Diagnostic Guidelines. Geneva: World Health Organization; 1992.
14. Nemiah JC. Somatoform disorders. In: Kaplan HI, Freedman AM, Sadock BJ (Eds). Comprehensive Textbook of Psychiatry. 3rd edition. Baltimore: Williams & Wilkins; 1980.pp.1525-43.
15. Kenyon FE. Hypochondriasis: A clinical study. Br J Psychiatry, 1964;110:478-88.
16. American Psychiatric Association. Diagnostic and Statistical Manual of Mental Disorders, 2nd edition. Washington: American Psychiatric Association; 1968.
17. Ludwig AM. Hysteria: A neurobiological theory. Arch Gen Psychiatry. 1972;27:771-86.
18. Cloninger CR. Somatoform and dissociative disorders. In: Winokur G, Clayton P (Eds). The Medical Basis of Psychiatry. Philadelphia: WB Saunders; 1986.
19. Brown HN, Vaillant GE. Hypochondriasis. Arch Intern Med. 1981;141:723-6.
20. Barsky A, Kiemran G. Overview: Hypochondriasis, bodily complaints, and somatic styles. Am J Psychiatry. 1983;140:273-83.
21. American Psychiatric Association. Diagnostic and Statistical Manual of Mental Disorders. 4th edition. Washington: American Psychiatric Association; 1994.
22. Janca A, Burke Jr JD, Isaac M, et al. The World Health Organization Somatoform Disorders Schedule. A Preliminary report on design and reliability. Eur Psychiatry. 1995;10:373-8.
23. Chandrashekhar CR, Reddy V, Isaac MK. Life events and somatoform disorders. Indian J Psychiatry. 1997;39:166-72.
24. Perley KN, Guze SB. Hysteria: the stability and usefulness of clinical criteria. N Engl J Med. 1962;266:421-6.
25. Guze SB. The diagnosis of hysteria: What are we trying to do? Am J Psychiatry. 1967;124:491.
26. Cloninger CR, Guze SB. Psychiatric illness and female criminality: The role of sociopathy and hysteria in the antisocial women. Am J Psychiatry. 1970;127:303-11.
27. Woerner PI, Guze SB. A family and marital study of hysteria. Br J Psychiatry. 1968;114:161-8.
28. Guze SB, Cloninger CR, Martin RL, et al. A follow-up and family study of Briquet's syndrome. Br J Psychiatry. 1986;149:17-23.

29. Bernstein RL, Gaw AC. Koro: a proposed classification for DSM IV. Am J Psychiatry. 1990;147:1670-4.
30. Chadda RK. Dhat syndrome. Is it a distinct clinical entity? A study of illness behaviour characteristics. Acta Psychiatr Scand. 1995;91:136-9.
31. Chaudhary AN. Analysis of clinical profile of 101 koro patients. Indian J Soc Psychiatry. 1992;8:67-70.
32. Chadda RK, Bhatia MS, Shome S. Physical symptoms in psychiatric practice: diagnostic uncertainties and clinical characteristics. Indian J Psychiatry. 1991;33:200-5.
33. Chadda RK. DSM-III-R diagnoses in psychiatric patients with physical symptoms. Indian J Soc Psychiatry. 1992;8:74.
34. Mayou R. Somatisation. Psychother Psychosm. 1993;59:69-83.
35. Slater ETO. Diagnosis of hysteria. Br Med J. 1965;1:1395-9.
36. Slater E, Glithero E. A follow-up study of patients diagnosed as suffering from hysteria. J Psychosom Res. 1965;9:9-13.
37. Chodoff P. The diagnosis of hysteria: An overview. Am J Psychiatry. 1974;131:1073-8.
38. Guze SB, Perley MJ. Observations on the natural history of hysteria. Am J Psychiatry. 1963;119:960-5.
39. Guze SB. The role of follow-up studies: their contribution to diagnostic classification as applied to hysteria. Seminars Psychiatry. 1970;2:392-402.
40. Guze SB, Woodruff RA Jr, Clayton PJ. Sex, age and diagnosis of hysteria (Briquet's syndrome). Am J Psychiatry. 1973;129:745-8.
41. Guze SB, Woodruff RA Jr, Clayton PJ. A study of conversion symptoms in psychiatric outpatients. Am J Psychiatry. 1971;127:643-6.
42. Woodruff RA, Clayton PJ, Guze SB. Hysteria: Studies of diagnosis, outcome and prevalence. JAMA. 1971;215:425-8.
43. World Health Organization. Mental disorders: Glossary and Guide to Their Classification in Accordance with the Ninth Revision of the International Classification of Diseases. Geneva: World Health Organization; 1978.
44. Barsky AJ, Wyshak G, Klerman GL. Transient hypochondriasis. Arch Gen Psychiatry. 1990;47:746-52.
45. Kellner R. Psychosomatic syndromes, somatization and somatoform disorders. Psychother Psychosom. 1994;61:4-24.
46. American Psychiatric Association. Diagnostic and Statistical Manual of Mental Disorders, 3rd edition. Revised. Washington: World Health Organization; 1987.
47. Cloninger CR. Somatoform and dissociative disorders. In: Winokur G, Clayton PJ (Eds). The Medical Basis of Psychiatry. 2nd edition. Philedelphia: WB Saunders; 1994.pp.169-92.
48. Guggenheim FG, Smith GR. Somatoform disorders. In: Kaplan HI, Sadock BJ (Eds). Comprehensive Textbook of Psychiatry, 6th edition. Baltimore: Williams and Wilkins; 1995. pp.1251-70.
49. Golding JM, Smith GR Jr, Kashner TM. Does somatization disorder occur in men? Clinical characteristics of women and men with multiple unexplained somatic symptoms. Arch Gen Psychiatry. 1991;48:231-5.
50. Gureja O, Simon GE, Ustun TB, et al. Somatization in cross-cultural perspective: A World Health Organization study in primary care. Am J Psychiatry. 1997;154:989-95.
51. Chandra PC, Ravi C. Somatization disorder in HIV seronegative men: A report of three cases. Indian J Psychiatry. 1995;37:41-42.
52. Cloninger CR, Reich T, Guze SB. The multi-factorial model of disease transmission: III. Familial relationship between sociopathy and hysteria (Briquet's syndrome). Br J Psychiatry. 1975;127:11-22.
53. Cloninger CR, Martin RL, Guze SB, et al. A prospective follow-up and family study of somatization in men and women. Am J Psychiatry. 1986;143:873-8.
54. Coryell W. A blind family hisotry of Briquet's syndrome. Further validation of the diagnosis. Arch Gen Psychiatry. 1980;37:1266-9.
55. Cloninger CR, Sigvardsson S, von Knorring AL, et al. An adoption study of somatoform disorders. II. Identification of two discrete somatoform disorders. Arch Gen Psychiatry. 1984;41:863-71.
56. Bohman M, Cloninger CR, von Knorring AL, et al. An adoption study of somatoform disorders. III. Cross fostering analysis and genetic relationship to alcoholism and criminality. Arch Gen Psychiatry. 1984;41:872-8.
57. Sigvardsson S, von Knorring AL, Bohman M, et al. An adoption study of somatoform disorders. I. The relationship of somatization to psychiatric disability. Arch Gen Psychiatry. 1984;41:853-9.
58. Cantwell D. Psychiatric illness in the families of hyperactive children. Arch Gen Psychiatry. 1972;27:414-7.
59. Morrison JR, Stewart MA. The psychiatric status of the legal families of adopted hyperactive children. Arch Gen Psychiatry. 1973;28:888-91.
60. Garralda ME. Somatization in children. J Child Psychol Psychiatry. 1996;37:13-33.
61. Bianchi GN. Patterns of hypochondriasis: A principal component analysis. Br J Psychiatry. 1973;122:541-8.
62. Ludwig AM. Hysteria: A neurophysiological theory. Arch Gen Psychiatry. 1972;27:771-86.
63. Bendefeldt F, Miller LL, Ludwig AM. Cognitive hysteria. Arch Gen Psychiatry. 1976;33:1250-4.
64. Almgren PE, Nordgren L, Skantze H. A retrospective study of operationally defined hysterics. Br J Psychiatry. 1978;132:670-3.
65. Flor-Henry P, Fromm-Auch D, Tapper M, et al. A neuro-psychological study of the stable syndrome of hysteria. Biol Psychiatry. 1981;16:601-26.
66. James L, Gordon E, Kraiuhin C, et al. Augmentation of auditory evoked potentials in somatization disorder. J Psychosom Res. 1990;24:155-63.
67. Gordon E, Kraiuhin C, Kelly P, et al. A neurophysiological study of somatization disorder. Compr Psychiatry. 1986;27:295-301.
68. Gordon E, Kraiuhin C, Meares R, et al. Auditory evoked response potentials in somatization disorder. J Psychiatric Res. 1986;20:237-48.
69. James L, Gordon E, Kraiuhin C, et al. Selective attention and auditory event related potentials in somatization disorder. Compr Psychiatry. 1989;30:84-9.
70. van der Kolk BA, Pelcovitz D, Roth D, et al. Dissociation, somatization, and affect dysregulation: The complexity of adaptation of trauma. Am J Psychiatry. 1996;153 (7 suppl):83-93.

71. Raguram R, Weiss MG, Channabasavanna SM, et al. Stigma, depression, and somatization in South India. Am J Psychiatry. 1996;153:1043-9.
72. Leventhal EA, Hansell S, Diefenbach M, et al. Negative affect and self report of physical symptoms: Two longitudinal studies of older adults. Health Psychol. 1996;15:193-9.
73. Chaturvedi SK, Chandra PS, Isaac MK, et al. Somatization misattributed to non-pathological vaginal discharge. J Psychosom Res. 1993;37:575-9.
74. Harihara G, Ramakrishan AN, Mathrubootham N. A study of somatization disorder in an industrial hospital. Indian J Psychiatry. 1993;35:200-2.
75. Min SK, Lee BO. Laterality in somatisation. Psychosom Med. 1997;59:236-40.
76. Murphy GE. The clinical management of hysteria. JAMA. 1982;247:2559-64.
77. Gask L, Goldberg D, Porter R, et al. The treatment of somatization: Evaluation of a teaching package with general practice trainees. J Psychosom Res. 1989;33:697-703.
78. Morrison J. Managing somatization disorder. Disease A Month. 1991;36:537-91.
79. Bass C, Benjamin S. The management of chronic somatisaton. Br J Psychiatry. 1993;162:472-80.
80. Saxena S, Pachauri R, Wig NN. DSM III diagnostic categories for ICD-9 hysteria: A study of 103 cases. Indian J Psychiatry. 1986;28:47-50.
81. McKegney FP. The incidence and characteristics of patients with conversion reactions: I. A general hospital consultation service sample. Am J Psychiatry. 1967;124:542-5.
82. Ziegler FJ, Imbolden JB, Meyer E. Contemporary conversion reactions: A clinical study. Am J Psychiatry. 1960;116:901-9.
83. Subramanian D, Subramanian K, Devaky MN, et al. A clinical study of 276 patients diagnosed as suffering from hysteria. Indian J Psychiatry. 1980;22:63-8.
84. Vyas JN, Bhardwaj PK. A study of hysteria: An analysis of 304 patients. Indian J Psychiatry. 1977;19:71-3.
85. Ali-Gombe A, Guthrie E, McDermott N. Mass hysteria: One syndrome or two. Br J Psychiatry. 1996;168:633-5.
86. Stefansson JG, Messina JA, Meyerowitz S. Hysterical neurosis, conversion type: Clinical and epidemiological considerations. Acta Psychiatr Scand. 1976;53:110-38.
87. Stephens JH, Kemp M. On some aspects of hysteria. A clinical study. J Nerv Ment Dis. 1962;134:305.
88. Nandi DN, Banerjee G, Nandi S, et. al. Is hysteria on the wane? A community survey in West Bengal, India. Br J Psychiatry. 1992;160:87-91.
89. Lal R, Biswas C, Chaudhary K. The changing profile of hysteria. Indian J Psychiatry. 1991;33:118-22.
90. Behrman J, Levy R. Neurophysiological studies on patients with hysterical disturbances of vision. J Psychosom Res. 1970;14:187-94.
91. Raskin M, Talbott JA, Meyerson AT. Diagnosis of conversion reactions: Predictive value of psychiatric criteria. JAMA. 1966;197:102-6.
92. Lader M. The psychophysiology of hysteria. In: Roy A (Ed). Hysteria. New York: John Wiley; 1982.pp.81-7.
93. Frumkin LB, Ward NG, Grim PS. A possible cerebral mechanism for the clearing of psychogenic symptoms with amobarbital. Biol Psychiatry. 1981;16:687-6091.
94. Moldofsky H, England RS. Facilitation of somatosensory average—evoked potentials in hysterical anesthesia and pain. Arch Gen Psychiatry. 1975;32:193-7.
95. Merskey H, Watson GD. The lateralisation of pain. Pain. 1979;7:271-80.
96. Gunther V, Mayr-Graft A, Miller C, et al. A comparative study of psychological aspects of recurring and non-recurring aphonias. Eur Arch Otorhinolaryngol. 1996;253:240-4.
97. Watson CG, Buranen C. The frequency and identification of false positive conversion reactions. J Nerv Ment Dis. 1979;167: 243-7.
98. Gatfield PD, Guze SB. Prognosis and differential diagnosis of conversion reactions (A follow-up study). Dis Nerv Sys. 1962;23:1-8.
99. Hafeiz HB. Hysterical conversion: a prognostic study. Br J Psychiatry. 1980;136:548-51.
100. Wig NN, Mangalwadhe K, Bedi H, et al. A follow-up study of hysteria. Indian J Psychiatry. 1982;24:120-5.
101. Chandrasekaran R, Goswami U, Sivakumar U, et al. Hysterical neurosis—a follow-up study. Acta Psychiatr Scand. 1994;89:78-80.
102. Faravelli C, Salvatori S, Galassi F, et al. Epidemiology of somatoform disorders: a community survey in Florence. Soc Psychiatry Psychiatr Epidemiol. 1997;32:24-29.
103. Sullivan HS. The Interpersonal Theory of Psychiatry. New York: WW Morton; 1953.
104. McCranie EJ. Hypochondriacal neurosis. Psychosomatics. 1979;20:11-15.
105. Kellner R. Somatization and Hypochondriasis. New York: Praeger-Greenwood; 1986.
106. Pilowskly I. From conversion hysteria to somatization to abnormal illness behaviour. Editorial. J Psychosom Res. 1996;40:345-50.
107. Pilowsky I. The diagnosis of abnormal illness behaviour. Aust NZ J Psychiatry. 1971;5:136-8.
108. Pilowsky I. Aspects of abnormal illness behaviour. Indian J Psychiatry. 1993;35:145-50.
109. Wooley SC, Blackwell B, Winget C. A learning theory model of chronic illness behaviour: theory, treatment and research. Psychosom Med. 1978;40:379-401.
110. Barsky A. Patients who amplify bodily sensations. Ann Intern Med. 1977;91:63-70.
111. Robbins JM, Kirmayer LJ. Transient and persistent hypochondriacal worry in primary care. Psychol Med. 1996; 26:575-89.
112. Mayou R. The nature of bodily symptoms. Br J Psychiatry. 1976;129:55-60.
113. Barsky A, Wyshak G. Hypochondriasis and somatosensory amplification. Br J Psychiatry. 1990;157:404-9.
114. Haenen MA, Schmidt AJM, Schoenmakers M, et al. Tactual sensitivity in hypochondriasis. Psychother Psychosom. 1997; 66:128-32.
115. Barsky AJ. Amplification, somatizaton and somatoform disorders. Psychosomatics. 1992;33:28-34.

116. Warwick HMC, Salkovskis PM. Hypochondriasis. Behav Res Ther. 1990;28:105-17.
117. Kellner R. Functional somatic symptoms and hypochondriasis. Arch Gen Psychiatry. 1985;42:821-33.
118. Idzorek S. A functional classification of hypochondriasis with specific recommendations for treatment. South Med J. 1975;68:1326-32.
119. Wood SM, Natterson J, Silverman S. Medical students disease: Hypochondriasis in medical students. J Med Education. 1966;41:785-90.
120. Kellner R, Wiggin RG, Pathak D. Hypochondriacal fears and beliefs in medical and law students. Arch Gen Psychiatry. 1986;43:487-9.
121. Kellner R. Psychotherapeutic strategies in hypochondriasis. Am J Psychotherapy. 1982;36:146-57.
122. Kellner R. Prognosis of treated hypochondriasis. Acta Psychiatr Scand. 1983;67:69-79.
123. Williams JEW, Spitzer RL. Idiopathic pain disorder: A critique to pain prone behaviour and proposal for a revision of the DSM-III category psychogenic pain disorder. J Nerv Ment Dis. 1982;170:410-9.
124. Stoudmire GA, Sandhu J. Psychogenic/idiopathic pain syndromes. Gen Hosp Psychiatry. 1987;9:79-86.
125. Woodhouse CRJ, Bochner S. Chronic abdominal pain: A surgical or psychiatric symptom? Br J Psychiatry. 1979;66:348-9.
126. Sarfeh IJ. Abdominal pain of unknown origin. Am J Surgery. 1976;132:22-25.
127. Grose RJ, Doerr N, Caldirola D, et al. Borderline syndrome and incest in pelvic pain patients. Int J Psychiatry Med. 1981;10:79-86.
128. Feinmann C, Harris M, Cawley R. Psychogenic facial pain: Presentation and treatment. Br Med J. 1984;228:436-8.
129. Hodgkins AD, Wastson JP. Psychiatric morbidity and illness behaviour in women with chronic pelvic pain. J Psychosom Res. 1994;38:3-9.
130. Mayou R. Atypical chest pain. J Psychosom Res. 1989;33:393-406.
131. Cormier LE, Katon W, Russo J, et al. Chest pain with negative cardiac diagnostic studies. J Nerv Ment Dis. 1988;176: 351-8.
132. Tinling DC, Klein RF. Psychogenic pain and aggression: The syndrome of solitary hunter. Psychosomatic Med. 1966;28: 738-47.
133. Szer IS. Musculoskeletal pain syndromes that affect adolescents. Arch Pediatr Adolesc Med. 1996;150:740-7.
134. von Knorring L, Almay BGL, Johansson F, et al. Endorphins in CSF of chronic pain patients, in relation to augmenting—reducing response in visual averaged evoked response. Neuropsychobiology. 1979;5:322-6.
135. Miller L. Neuropsychological concepts of somatoform disorders. Int J Psychiatry Med. 1984;14:31-46.
136. Klimes I, Mayou RA, Pearce MJ, et al. Psychological treatment for atypical non-cardiac chest pain. Psychol Med. 1990;20:605-11.
137. Philips HC. The effects of behavioural treatment on chronic pain. Beh Res Therapy. 1987;25:365-77.
138. Koopmans GI, Meeuwesen L, Huyse FJ, et al. Effects of psychiatric consultation on medical consumption in medical outpatients with low back pain. Gen Hosp Psychiatry. 1996;18:145-54.
139. Munro A, Stewart M. Body dysmorphic disorder and the DSM-IV: The demise of dysmorphophobia. Can J Psychiatry. 1991;36:91-96.
140. Hollander E, Cohen LJ, Simeon D. Body dysmorphic disorder. Psychiatr Annals. 1993;23:359-64.
141. Brady KT, Austin L, Lydiard RB. Body dysmorphic disorder: The relationship to obsessive compulsive disorder. J Nerv Ment Dis. 1990;178:538-40.
142. Phillips KA. Body dysmorphic disorder: The distress of imagined ugliness. Am J Psychiatry. 1991;148:1135-9.
143. Brawman-Mintzer O, Lydiard RB, Phillips KA, et al. Body dysmorphic disorder in patients with anxiety disorders and major depression. Am J Psychiatry. 1995;152:1665-7.
144. Phillips KA, McElroy SL. Insight, overvalued ideation, and delusional thinking in body dysmorphic disorder. J Nerv Ment Dis. 1993;181:699-702.
145. Phillips KA, McElroy SL, Keck PE Jr, et al. Body dysmorphic disorder: 30 cases of imagined ugliness. Am J Psychiatry. 1993;150:302-8.
146. Connoly FH, Gipson M. Dysmorphophobia—a long term study. Br J Psychiatry. 1978:132:568-70.
147. Andreasen NC, Bardch J. Dysmorphophobia: Symptom or disease. Am J Psychiatry. 1977;134:673-6.
148. Hollander E, Liebowitz MR, Winchel R, et al. Treatment of body dysmorphic disorder with serotonin reuptake blockers. Am J Psychiatry. 1989;146:768-70.
149. Phillips KA. Body dysmorphic disorder: Diagnosis and treatment of imagined illness. J Clin Psychiatry. 1996;57 (Suppl 8): 61-64.
150. Escobar JL, Ribio-Stipec M, Canino G, et al. Somatic Symptom Index (SSI): A new and abridged somatization construct. J Nerv Ment Dis. 1989;177:140-6.
151. Katon W, Lin E, von Korff M, et al. Somatization: A spectrum of severity. Am J Psychiatry. 1991;148:34-40.
152. Fink P. Somatization—beyond symptom count. Editorial. J Psychosom Res. 1996;40:7-10.
153. Portegijs PJ, vander Horst FG, Proot IM, et al. Somatization in frequent attenders of general practice. Soc Psychiatry Psychiatr Epidemol. 1996;31:29-37.
154. Chadda RK, Bhatia MS, Shome S, et al. Psychosocial dysfunction in somatising patients. Br J Psychiatry. 1993;163:510-3.
155. Barsky AJ, Delamater BA, Clancy SA, et al. Somatised psychiatric disorder presenting as palpitation. Arch Intern Med. 1996;156:1102-8.
156. Labott SM, Preisman RC, Torosian T, et al. Screening for somatizing patients in the pulmonary subspeciality clinic. Psychosomatics. 1996;37:327-38.
157. Togerson S. Genetics of somatoform disorders. Arch Gen Psychiatry. 1986;43:502-5.
158. American Psychiatric Association. Desk Reference to the Diagnostic Criteria from DSM-5. Washington DC; 2013.

CHAPTER

20 Dissociative Disorders

Niraj Ahuja, Sudhir Hebbar

CONCEPT OF HYSTERIA

In recent years, hysteria has stood out among medical concepts for the sheer volume of discussion among professional historians, philosophers, sociologists, feminists, literature specialists, and others.[1] Slater[2] said that 'it is generally agreed that no one has yet framed a satisfactory definition of 'hysteria'; but it is usually claimed that it can be recognized when met with'. Hysteria has been called the 'mocking bird of nosology' by Johnson (1849) and 'that strange disease' by Gowers (1885).[2]

The word hysteria has been used in so many contexts that it no longer has any one meaning. These various contexts include the following:[3,4]

- Impulsive, uncontrolled behavior (impulse dyscontrol)
- Manipulative, dramatic, exhibitionistic, emotional and/or seductive behavior (histrionic or hysterical personality traits)
- Absence of objective signs of an organic illness
- Presence of multiple vague somatic symptoms, especially in a female patient (somatization disorder or Briquet's hysteria)
- Hypochondriasis
- Any mental illness
- Presence of certain symptoms which are not explainable in the context of present organic illness (functional overlay, conversion symptoms)
- Difficult patient; poor doctor-patient communication
- 'Sick' role or 'abnormal illness behavior'
- Psychosomatic disorders
- Malingering
- Psychosexual dysfunctions
- Even to describe certain brief psychotic conditions[5] (hysterical psychosis)
- To describe 'infectious' spread of certain culturally sanctioned behaviors (epidemic or mass hysteria)[5,6]
- Presence of dissociative states, in absence of organic factors
- The term *anxiety hysteria* to indicate phobic disorders[5]
- As a pejorative term of opprobrium and disgrace.[7]

This list is not exhaustive. Therefore it is not surprising that the word hysteria has been removed from DSM-IV[8] as well as ICD-10[9]. The term has been replaced in ICD-10 by 'dissociative (conversion) disorders.'[9] However, in DSM-IV, both conversion and dissociative disorders are still listed separately.[8]

Although hysteria has been variously defined in the past and although the nature of the diagnosis of hysteria has been repeatedly criticized,[10,11] dissociation and conversion have always been prominent features of hysteria.

HISTORICAL PERSPECTIVE AND THE CONCEPTS OF DISSOCIATION AND CONVERSION

Patients who present with unexplained physical symptoms (functional somatic symptoms) haunted the physicians from the dawn of the civilization till our times. The presentation varies from transient single symptom to multiple changing symptoms with multisystemic involvement. Probably, the physicians easily recognized the later type as a separate disorder.

The history of 'simulation' of neurologic diseases dates back to 1900 BC in Egypt.[12] The Egyptian physicians thought hysterical symptoms to be due to upward mobility of the uterus in the abdomen, probably because such dramatic symptoms were more common in females. Hippocratic physicians used this concept and coined the term *hysteria* ('hystera' in Greek means uterus). The boundaries of this diagnosis were not clear and hence other physicians used different terms for similar problems. In fact, Hippocrates writes on difficulties in differential diagnosis of hysterical seizures and true seizures ('the sacred disease').

Both possession syndrome (described as *rakshasapraha*) and pseudoseizures (described as *grahi,* and differentiated from true seizures called as *apasmara*) find a mention in the mental disorders detailed in *Atharvaveda*, the ancient Indian Vedic Text.[13]

Galen (130-200 AD) defined hysteria as a complex, incurable disease with an unknown physical cause. He located the seat of the disorder in the cerebellum, which he defined as 'the seat of carnal love.'[14,15] In the Middle ages, hysteria was often confused with demonic possession and therapeutic interventions were largely limited to eradication of the demons by various barbaric means, including stoning to death and burning at stake. These are detailed in the *Malleus Maleficarum*, written by two Dominician monks, Heinrich Kramer and James Sprenger.

Thomas Sydenham (1624-1689) called the male counterpart of the female hysteric, a hypochondriac. William Cullen (1712-1790) used the word *neurosis* to mean diseases that are not accompanied by fever or other localized pathology. He believed that neurosis was due to decay in the nervous system. He accurately described the autonomic symptoms (anxiety symptoms). The misconception of Greeks regarding uterine origins of hysteria was replaced by another misconception by Villermay (1816),[16] that the most frequent causes of hysteria were deprivation of the pleasures of love, griefs connected with this passion and disorders of menstruation.

Out of the confusion created by the multiple changing complaints the credit, of description of the disorder and validating it with course and family history, goes to Paul Briquet (1796-1881), a French psychiatrist who described hysteria (now known as Briquet's syndrome or somatization disorder)[12] in 1859. He noted that this condition had an early onset, was polysymptomatic, tended to be familial, was more common in females and had a poor prognosis. Later, giving more importance to fatigue and nerve exhaustion, George Beard (1839-1883) coined the term *neurasthenia*.

John Ferriar (1795),[17] an English physician, used the word *conversion* for the changing physical symptoms, some of which ended fatally (especially when treated[18]), but some of which remained benign. Interestingly, the term *conversio* was earlier employed in the Middle Ages to refer to the development of 'suffocation of womb' into other diseases following a 'crisis.'[18,19]

The earliest description of multiple personality disorder is attributed to Paracelsus in 17th century, who observed a woman whose secondary personality 'stole' her money.[20] Carlson[21] attributes the 1st reports of both dissociative amnesia and multiple personality disorder in America to Benjamin Rush. However, the first well-described case of MPD was Mary Raynolds by Dr. SL Mitchell[22,23] in 1815, followed by a second case in Bavaria[22] in 1828. Subsequently, several fictional and actual accounts of MPD followed in the literature. Some celebrated ones include *The Strange Case of Dr. Jekyll and Mr. Hyde,*[24] Christine Beauchamp,[25] *Three Faces of Eve,*[26] and *Sybil* (a girl who presented with 16 separate personalities, two of which were men).[27]

Jean Martin Charcot (1825-1893), a French Neurologist, was conducting studies on hysteria (probably patients who had pseudoneurological symptoms) at the well-known La Salpetriere in Paris. He was using hypnosis and suggestions to correct the weakness of nervous system seen in these patients. He viewed 'hysteria' as a hereditary degenerative disease because these patients could be easily hypnotized[28] (unlike Bernheim at Nancy Hospital, who thought that hypnotizability is a normal phenomenon). Patients under the influence of posthypnotic suggestion performed complex tasks without any conscious memory of the actions, suggesting presence of an unconscious that contained thoughts and feelings capable of influencing a person without his knowledge.[21] He classified hysteria in to 2 types: convulsive and nonconvulsive.[29]

Under Charcot's influence, a young philosophy student, Pierre Janet (1889), started using hypnosis on his patients and elaborately described several hysterical cases.[30,31] He coined the word *dissociation* ('*desagregationmentale*'), which meant that the conscious mental elements (like memory, sensation, and volition) become unconscious because of the deficiency of mental energy (a model of 'idea-complexes existing outside of consciousness'). Once unconscious, these cognitive processes appeared to be able to create altered states of consciousness, paralyses, amnesias, fugues, and multiple personality. These could be reintegrated back to the consciousness by hypnosis to return the patient to normalcy.

Later Morton Prince (1906), an American neuro-psychiatrist, wrote a book '*The dissociation of personality*' describing multiple personality disorder.[22,25] He proposed a theory of *co-consciousness*, in which different conscious states exist in a person without his awareness, as his attention is not focused on them.[21]

Breuer[32] described a model of '*hypnoid states*' in which ideas that were registered in an altered state of consciousness became unavailable to the person in his normal conscious state.[21] He noted the importance of autohypnosis in creating the altered state of consciousness into which the dissociated ideas are registered.

Sigmund Freud, who was also working with hysterical patients along with Josef Breuer,[32] also used the term *conversion* in a different context, meaning somatic transformation of the traumatic effect. This was a temporary relief, because the repressed ideas still remained unconscious which Freud thought were childhood traumatic memories (usually sexual trauma, either real or imagined).[33] Although, Freud used the term *repression* to depict the phenomenon of ideas kept out of consciousness, the model described was really that of *dissociation.*[21] Freud conceptualized *dissociation* as an active process, warding off ('banning of') painful affects from conscious awareness,[34] in sharp contrast to the passive process of co-consciousness described by Prince.

Ferenczi redefined the term *conversion* as a transformation of a genital impulse only, which was couched in 'a peculiar symbolic language termed as the hysterical idiom.'[35,36] On the other hand, Fairbairn[37] simplified the definition of conversion as 'the substitution of a bodily state for a personal problem.'

Lord Brain (1963) made two important contributions to the concept of hysteria.[38] Firstly, he assigned a central position to dissociation in the production of hysterical symptoms, a concept recently adopted by ICD-10 for its classification.[8] Secondly, he described the possibility of co-existence of hysteria with other physical disorders (e.g. epilepsy, organic brain disease) and psychiatric disorders (like anxiety, depression, and even mental subnormality). He described the merits of describing the condition as a hysterical 'reaction' instead of as a disease.[2,38]

Slater,[2] (a Neurologist) in his now famous article, dissuaded the clinicians against the use of hysteria as a diagnosis, both theoretically and practically. He said that 'the diagnosis of hysteria is a disguise for ignorance and a fertile source of clinical error. It is in fact not only a delusion but also a snare.' However, Sir Aubrey Lewis countered this statement with a comment that 'hysteria tends to outlive its obituarists.'[39]

Chodoff (1974) emphasized how the nosological status of hysteria had became fragmented and clearly defined three main meanings:[40,41]

1. Briquet's hysteria,
2. Conversion hysteria, and
3. Histrionic personality.

These meanings (along with the concept of dissociative disorders) became components of classification in DSM-III, as somatization disorder, conversion disorder, histrionic personality disorder and dissociative disorder.

EPIDEMIOLOGY

Until recently dissociative disorders were thought be extremely uncommon. However, there is increasing evidence that they are actually more common than it was once believed.[42]

In the various reports from psychiatric clinics from India and elsewhere, hysteria constitutes 6–15% of the all the OPD diagnoses[43-51] and about 14–20% of all neurotic patients.[43,51] Females usually outnumber males,[45-49,52-54] but in children the percentage may be similar.[55] The onset usually occurs after 5 years of age[56-58] and the average age of onset is 10–25 years.[45,47,49,53,59] The majority of Indian patients are married[45-47,53,60] and have a lower educational level.[45,46,53,60]

In developing countries, neurology clinics diagnose conversion disorders with 1% frequency.[61] In general population, especially in female population, the lifetime occurrence of conversion symptoms (not disorder) may be as high as 33%.[62] In psychiatric patients, 24% reported unexplained neurological symptoms, dubbed as conversion symptoms.[63] Conversion symptoms are seen all across the life span but are more commonly seen in children and young adults. Stefansson et al. (1976) reported an annual incidence of conversion reactions of 22/100,000 in Monroe county (New York) and 11/100,000 in Iceland.[64]

Both dissociation and conversion symptoms are more prevalent in the military population, particularly during combat, where they are more common in men and have a later age of onset.[65-67] The estimates of prevalence of 'hysteria' have varied from 1% to 30% in military or neurological hospitals, depending on whether hysteria was the primary diagnosis or whether associated 'hysterical symptoms' were included too.[61,68,69] Saha and Dutta,[16] in 1942, reported that during the World War II in Bengal, hysteria appeared to be second only to malaria in incidence. In Indian soldiers (Military Hospital, Delhi, 1944), hysteria was preponderant among the various types of 'nervous' disorders encountered.[15] More than 50% of these 370 cases had 'fits'; there were also cases of aphonia (12), deafness (11), paralysis (10), blindness (7), and amnesia (25).

Dissociative (and conversion) disorders constitute 2.3–13% of all psychiatry OPD cases.[45,51,53,70-73] Conversion symptoms are found more frequently as compared to dissociative symptoms.[49,55] Among the dissociative disorders, dissociative convulsions (nonepileptic seizures) are most common,[52,70,75,78] followed by trance and possession states,[70,75] amnesia,[75] and fugue states.[71,74,75] A few cases of multiple personality disorder have also been reported from India.[76,77] Possession states constitute 10 to 12% of the cases of hysteria.[70,71,75] One study[75] has identified 10% cases of amnesia and 6% cases of fugue, but some other studies,[70,78] have reported none of these cases. According to some authors, atypical dissociative disorders are the most common presentations of dissociative (conversion) disorders in Indian patients.[70,71,78]

Saxe et al. (1993) found 15% of 110 psychiatric inpatients in a US psychiatric hospital to be suffering from dissociative disorders, out of which 4% had multiple personality disorder.[79] DSM-IV[8] reports a prevalence rate of 0.01 to 0.3% for conversion disorders and 0.2% for dissociative fugue in the general population.

Recently, there has been an exponential rise in the number of cases of MPD from the North America.[42,80,81] More than 1,000 cases have been documented. Surprisingly, there is no such trend on the other side of Atlantic. Therefore, some researchers feel that MPD is an extremely rare disorder while others point out that it is mostly unrecognized and underdiagnosed. In Modestin' study (1992), just 3 psychiatrists (less than 0.5% of the total surveyed) contributed 128 of the 221 MPD cases.[82] Thig-pen and Cleckley (1984), who wrote '*The Three Faces of Eve*' (1957),[26] commented that they received hundreds of referrals of patients thought to be suffering from MPD in 30 years, out of which only one case had undeniable multiple personality disorder.[83]

In developing and developed countries, the prevalence of both dissociation and conversion disorders may be falling and instead the prevalence of depression may be increasing.[48,84] Nandi et al. (1992) found a marked decline in the prevalence of hysteria (both conversion and dissociation) in the two rural areas in West Bengal (India); after a period of 10 years in one area (from 16.9/1000 to 4.6/1000) and after 15 years in the other area (from 32.3/1000 to 2.05/1000).[85] The total mental morbidity, however, did not change in that period, and the decline in hysteria was counterbalanced by an increase in the prevalence of depression.

There are studies that looked at childhood hysterical disorders. Early studies[72,86] have focused on the prevalence and sociodemographic characteristics rather than on the clinical features. Some studies[52,54] have included pain and other visceral symptoms that make comparison with current categories impossible. In one study,[52] 69.2% of children exhibited neurotic traits prior to the onset of the illness, while 26.9% had a past history of hysteria. Raju et al. (1969) found that hysteria constituted 2.7% of all children seen in the CGC of a general hospital.[87] Uma and Kapur (1987) found 20% of cases of hysteria in children presented with brief unresponsiveness, while 34% had abnormal motor movements.[55]

CLASSIFICATION

DSM-I separated dissociative reactions from conversion reactions.[88] The dissociative reactions included amnesia, stupor, fugue, somnambulism, dream states, and depersonalization. DSM-II regrouped the conversion and dissociative categories as 2 subtypes under the single category of hysterical neurosis.[89]

DSM-III made a major change in the classification of hysteria by splitting the term into somatoform disorders (including conversion disorders) and dissociative disorders, and removing the term hysteria from the nomenclature.[90] Dissociative disorders in DSM-III included psychogenic amnesia, psychogenic fugue, multiple personality, depersonalization disorder, and atypical dissociative disorders. Somnambulism was removed from dissociative disorders and classified under sleepwalking disorders (disorders of infancy and childhood).

This practice was continued in DSM-III-R.[91] However, the name psychogenic amnesia was changed to dissociative amnesia, psychogenic fugue to dissociative fugue, and multiple personality to multiple personality disorder. DSM-IV[8] adapted the classification from DSM-III-R without many changes. However, the name multiple personality disorder was changed to dissociative identity disorder.

Recently, ICD-10 too made significant changes in the classification of hysteria by removing the word hysteria.[9] However, unlike DSM-IV, ICD-10 has retained the conversion and dissociative disorders under the single rubric of dissociative disorders. The term conversion appears at certain places, only in brackets. ICD-10 has also included a category of *organic dissociative disorder* under organic mental disorders, without describing it in detail.[9]

It has been suggested that both conversion and dissociative disorder share a common underlying psychogenic mechanism, though whether it is conversion[5] or dissociation[71,92,93] is debatable. Also, considerable overlapping of conversion disorders and dissociation disorders (15–29%) has been reported in the patient populations.[71,92,94] One study found 91% comorbidity of dissociative disorders in patients of pseudoseizures.[95] Therefore, it seems logical to place both conversion disorders and dissociation disorders under a common diagnostic entry.[8,96]

DSM-5 Diagnostic criteria for dissociative disorder

The new Diagnostic and Statistical Manual of Mental Disorders, 5th Edition (DSM-5) has a number of changes to dissociative disorders, including dissociative identity disorder. It outlines some of the major changes to these conditions.

According to the American Psychiatric Association (APA), the publisher of the DSM-5, the major changes to this category of disorders includes:
- Derealization is included in the name and symptom structure of what previously was called depersonalization disorder. The disorder is now called depersonalization/derealization disorder (that's a mouthful!)
- Dissociative fugue is now a specifier of dissociative amnesia — rather than as a separate diagnosis
- Diagnostic criteria for dissociative identity disorder have been updated
- Symptoms of disruption of identity may now be reported, as well as observed
- Gaps in the recall of events may occur for everyday events—not just traumatic events
- Experiences of pathological possession in some cultures are included in the description of identity disruption

Dissociative Identity Disorder (DID) In DSM-5

Dissociative identity disorder (DID)—also known by some by its very old name, multiple personality disorder—undergoes some changes to its diagnostic criteria. According to the APA, Criterion A has been "expanded to include certain possession-form phenomena and functional neurological symptoms to account for more diverse presentations of the disorder."
The first criterion also now specifically states that transitions in identity may be observable by others or self-reported. Last, according to Criterion B, individuals with dissociative identity disorder may now have recurrent gaps in recall for everyday events, not just for traumatic experiences.

CLINICAL FEATURES

Conversion Disorder

The following clinical features characterize conversion disorder:

- Presence of symptoms or deficits affecting motor or sensory function, suggesting a medical or neurological disorder

- Sudden onset
- Development of symptoms or deficits, usually in the presence of significant psychosocial stressor(s)
- A clear temporal relationship between stressor and development or exacerbation of symptoms
- The symptoms are not intentionally produced orfeigned
- There is usually a 'secondary gain' (although this is not required by DSM-IV or ICD-10 for a diagnosis of conversion disorder to be made)
- Detailed physical examination and investigations do not reveal any medical (or neurological) disorder or substance use disorder that can explain the symptoms adequately
- The symptom may have a 'symbolic' relationship with the stressor/conflict.

There are usually two types of disturbances in conversion disorder, voluntary motor and sensory. Autonomic nervous system is typically not involved, except when voluntary musculature is involved, e.g. vomiting, globus hystericus.

In DSM-5 Conversion disorder is also given new name as functional neurological symptom disorder.

DSM-5 Diagnostic disorder of conversion disorder (Functional Neurological Symptom Disorder)
A. One or more symptoms of altered voluntary motor or sensory function. B. Clinical findings provide evidence of incompatibility between the symptom and recognized neurological or medical conditions. C. The symptom or deficit is not better explained by another medical or mental disorder. D. The symptom or deficit causes clinically significant distress or impairment in social, occupational, or other important areas of functioning or warrants medical evaluation.
Coding note: The ICD-9-CM code for conversion disorder is 300.11, which is assigned regardless of the symptom type. The ICD-10-CM code depends on the symptom type (see below).
Specify symptom type: **(F44.4) With weakness or paralysis** **(F44.4) With abnormal movement** (e.g. tremor, dystonic movement, myoclonus, gait disorder) **(F44.4) With swallowing symptoms** **(F44.4) With speech symptom** (e.g. dysphonia, slurred speech) **(F44.5) With attacks or seizures** **(F44.6) With anesthesia or sensory loss** **(F44.6) With special sensory symptom** (e.g. visual, olfactory, or hearing disturbance) **(F44.7) With mixed symptoms**
Specify if: **Acute episode:** Symptoms present for less than 6 months. **Persistent:** Symptoms occurring for 6 months or more.
Specify if: **With psychological stressor** *(specify stressor)* **Without psychological stressor**

In DSM-IV,[8] conversion disorder is further sub-classified into conversion disorder with motor symptom or deficit, conversion disorder with sensory symptom or deficit, conversion disorder with seizures or convulsions, and conversion disorder with mixed presentation. As mentioned earlier in ICD-10, conversion disorder is subsumed under '*dissociative disorders of movement and sensation*', a subtype under '*dissociative (conversion) disorders*'. It is further classified into dissociative motor disorders, dissociative anesthesia and sensory loss, and dissociative convulsions.[9]

Dissociative Motor Disorders

The motor disturbance usually involves either loss (complete or partial) of the ability to perform voluntary movement (including loss of speech, producing aphonia) or abnormal movements. The 'paralysis' may be a monoplegia, paraplegia or quadriplegia. Classically, the symptom distribution is according to the patient's knowledge of the nervous system. The examination shows normal or voluntarily increased tone and normal deep tendon reflexes. The patient may drag the affected limb rather swing it, as is seen in true hemiplegia. However, a prolonged 'paralysis' may lead to the development of contractures. Patients with conversion aphonia are able to produce simple sounds, are able to cough and may sometimes be able to whisper.

The 'abnormal movements' (also called as psychogenic movement disorders)[97] range from tremors, choreiform movements, dystoniatics, parkinsonism, hemiballismus, gait disturbances, to convulsive movements. These movements either occur or increase when attention is directed towards them, and may disappear when patient is watched unobserved. These movements do not fit the 'typical' clinical picture of the abnormal involuntary movement disorders. The gait disturbance (*astasia abasia*, a name given by Paul Blocq in 1888) is usually characterized by a wide-based, staggering, jerky, dramatic and irregular gait, with exaggerated body movements and an inability to stand (*astasia*) or walk (*abasia*).[98] Rarely, the patient may present with *camptocormia* (or hysterical bentback),[99] characterized by a frontal flexion of the vertebral column with passive dropping of both arms and a variable degree of genuflexion, producing a simian appearance.

Differential diagnosis with neurological disorders is particularly important in 'dissociative movement disorders', as 6–30% of these patients are subsequently found to have a medical illness that can account for their symptoms. This is especially true for idiopathic dystonia,[61] in which 25–52% of patients are initially misdiagnosed as suffering from a psychiatric disorder.[100,101] The presence of '*sensory tricks*' may be valuable in diagnosis of dystonia.[97] Fahn and Williams (1988) have defined four levels of certainty for the diagnosis of 'psychogenic dystonia', which can be applied to all types of movement disorders.[102] Even astasia abasia may have an underlying organic cause.[103]

Sensory (Dissociative) Anesthesia and Sensory Loss

The sensory disturbance is exemplified by a 'glove and stocking' anesthesia (absence of all sensations with an abrupt boundary, not conforming with the distribution of dermatomes, and usually limiting at wrists and ankles), hemianesthesias, blindness or contracted visual fields ('tubular vision'), and deafness (rare[104]). The detailed examination usually shows absence of objective signs of the particular illness and the disturbance is usually based on patient's knowledge of that illness.

Sensory disturbances are inconsistent with the anatomic patterns expected. Often all sensory modalities (like touch, pain, temperature and position sense) are affected at the same level.[28] In conversion disorder, the loss of vibration sense maintains a strict midline separation in spite of the fact that vibrations can be perceived on the other side through bone conduction.[28] However, this is not a foolproof test.[61]

A patient with bilateral conversion blindness is able to go about his way reasonably well and does not injure himself by walking into obstacles. In unilateral conversion blindness, the pupillary reflex of the affected eye is normal. A normal visual evoked potential (VEP) study in a patient presenting with sever monocular or binocular visual loss with a normal neuro-ophthalmological examination excludes any major organic pathology and favors a diagnosis of conversion disorder or malingering.[105] Conversion blindness should be differentiated from Anton's syndrome.

Mixed presentations with both sensory and motor symptoms are quite common. When sensory or motor symptoms are encountered, conditions like myasthenia gravis, multiple sclerosis, degenerative disorders of brain, movement disorders, connective disorders, and porphyria should be considered. The electrodiagnostic examination (EDX) is a useful procedure in the investigation of conversion motor and sensory symptoms. It usually consists of nerve conduction studies (NCS), needle electrode examination (NEE), special studies consisting of H-reflex and F-waves.[106] However, many of the findings in conversion disorders are also seen in upper motor neuron (UMN) lesions.

Dissociative Convulsions

Dissociative convulsions were earlier known as 'hysterical fits' or pseudoseizures. Since at least the 17th century, authors have described episodes that superficially resemble epileptic seizures but are not of epileptic origin.[107,108] Most authors have used the word 'hysterical' to describe these seizures, but later the term '*pseudoseizure*' was used to refer to these seizures.[109] Other terms, that have been used to describe them, include hysteroepilepsy, psychogenic seizures, hysterical pseudoseizures, pseudoepileptic seizures,[110] nonepileptic attack disorders[111] and *nonepileptic seizures* (NES).[112]

Convulsive movements and/or a partial loss of consciousness characterize these disorders (However, ICD-10 specifies that sudden, unexpected spasmodic movements, *not* followed by loss of consciousness characterize dissociative convulsions). Nonepileptic seizures (NES) are one of the most common dissociative symptoms in India (and other developing countries) and tend to present with a mixture of both dissociative and conversion symptoms.[46]

The NES can sometimes take the form of a brief lasting stupor or 'faint-like' attacks. A recent study from Iowa[7] reports that the unresponsive behavior in the absence of motor manifestations was the most common of ictal presentation. Indian authors have called these unresponsive disorders as *simple dissociative disorder*[70,113] or *brief dissociative stupor.*[78] This condition has been reported to be the most common form of NES, is mainly seen in females, and is frequently associated with panic symptoms.[78] It appears that NES resemble complex partial seizures more than generalized tonic clonic seizures.

There are several other causes of nonepileptic seizures, e.g. malingering, factitious disorders, secondary to major depression, but dissociative convulsions account for the most of these. Differentiation of true seizures from NES at times may be difficult or impossible because of several reasons.

Co-occurrence of both true seizures and NES is also fairly common (5–30%).[108,114,115] One of the famous examples of co-existence of true seizures and NES is described in the famous literary work, 'The Brothers Karamazov'. The true seizure acts as a model for NES. NES occurring in the patients with true seizures are often well controlled by anticonvulsant therapy. There is evidence that the development of NES can be facilitated by anticonvulsant toxicity or even by adequate dosage of anticonvulsants necessary for proper control of seizures.[69] Psychological stress is important in the precipitation of both the seizure types.

There are several studies that have quantitatively compared the phenomenological features of NES and epileptic seizures. There appears to be agreement regarding the increased length and high degree of vocalization in NES. Epileptic vocalization, if present, is often monotonous. Posturing of the upper extremity in abduction appears to be more common in epilepsy. Other wide variety of features, including self-reported emotional distress before the onset of seizure, failed to differentiate between these conditions. The 'gold standard' for diagnosis is a simultaneous video-telemetric EEG study,[108,114,115] documenting spontaneous and provoked episodes that are termed typical by experienced professional observers.

Differential diagnosis with true seizures is important. The main differentiating points between epileptic seizures and dissociative convulsions are listed in Table 1.

Table 1: Epileptic seizures vs dissociative convulsions

	Clinical points	*Epileptic seizures*	*Dissociative convulsions*
1.	Clinical pattern of events	Stereotyped, known clinical patterns (however, bizarre complex automatisms may occur in frontal lobe complex partial seizures)	Absence of any established clinical pattern. Purposive body movements occur
2.	Place of occurrence	Anywhere	Usually indoors or at safe places
3.	Warning	Both prodrome and aura are stereotyped	Variable; variable somatic symptoms
4.	Time of day	Anytime. Can occur during sleep	Usually never occur during sleep
5.	Tongue bite	Usually present; usually on lateral aspect of tongue	Usually absent. Cheek and lip bite may be present; tip of tongue may be rarely bitten
6.	Incontinence of urine and feces	Can occur	Very rare
7.	Injury	Can occur	Very rare. If occurs, it is minor or may be accidental
8.	Speech	No verbalization during the seizure; monotonous, repetitive speech in supplementary motor area seizures; vocalization may occur in postictal phase	Verbalization may occur during the fit; may be emotionally charged
9.	Facial expression	Trismus in tonic phase; symmetrical twitching in clonic phase of generalized tonic clonic seizures	Emotional expressions may be seen
10.	Duration	Usually about 70 sec. (Shorter)	20–800 sec. (Prolonged)
11.	Head turning	Unilateral	Side to side turning may occur
12.	Eye gaze	Staring, if eyes are open	Avoidant gaze, may resist eye opening
13.	Pupillary reaction to light	Absent; usually dilated pupils	Present
14.	Corneal reflexes	Absent	Present
15.	Cyanosis	May be present	Absent
16.	Amnesia	Complete or partial	Often partial
17.	Neurological signs	Present, e.g. upgoing plantars	Absent
18.	Postictal confusion	Present	Absent
19.	Stress	Present in 25%	Present much more often
20.	EEG or Video-telemetry study	Usually abnormal during the seizure; postictal slowing may last for a few hours	Usually normal; a burst of muscle artifact may be present
21.	Serum prolactin	Increased to more than 1000 IU/mL 15–20 more than 500 IU/mL minutes after a generalized seizure; back to normal levels in 1 hour	Usually normal or not

In addition to generalized tonic clonic seizures, other important differential diagnoses include other episodic disorders, like syncope, panic disorders, reflex epilepsy, dissociative fugues, paroxysmal choreo-athetosis,[110] kinesigenic or non-kinesigenic dyskinesias, akinetic seizures, emotionally induced epilepsy, and startle induced myoclonus (leading to falls).

Diverse manifestations of CPS (complex partial seizures), which might arise from temporal or frontal lobe, and seizures arising from prefrontal lobes or frontal motor association cortex can induce bilateral movements even in the preserved consciousness. They present more difficulties in differential diagnosis as compared to generalized tonic clonic seizures. Complex partial seizures are usually brief (lasting a few minutes; however, CPS status can last longer and cause difficulties in diagnosis) and stereotyped. Careful enquiry regarding the presence of automatisms and blank, staring expression on the face has to be made from a 'good' informant who has observed the episodes.

There is a high degree of comorbidity with NES,[95,116] including depression, true seizures, somatoform disorders, personality disorders, post traumatic stress disorder, other anxiety disorders, child abuse, and high dissociation scores. Patients with 'pseudoseizure status'[117] or 'pseudostatus epilepticus'[118] often have severe affective imbalances, disturbed impulse control and repeated deliberate self-harm.[117]

Dissociative Disorder

The following clinical features characterize these disorders:

- Disturbance in the normally integrated functions of consciousness, identity, memory and/or perception of the environment.
- Onset is usually sudden (though not always) and the disturbance is usually temporary. Recovery often is abrupt.
- A precipitating stress is not uncommonly found before the onset of the disorder. There is a clear temporal relationship between the stressor and the onset of the illness.
- A 'secondary gain' resulting from the development of symptoms may be found (although this is not required by DSM-IV or ICD-10 for a diagnosis of dissociative disorder to be made).
- Detailed physical examination and investigations do not reveal any evidence of a physical disorder that can explain the symptoms present.

In DSM-IV,[8] dissociative disorder is further sub-classified in to dissociative amnesia, dissociative fugue, dissociative identity disorder, depersonalization disorder, and dissociative disorder not otherwise specified. Dissociative trance disorder is described in DSM-IV[8] under the 'criteria sets and axes provided for further study'. In ICD-10, dissociative disorder[9] is subsumed under 'dissociative (conversion) disorders'. It is further classified into dissociative amnesia, dissociative fugue, dissociative stupor, trance and possession disorders, and other dissociative disorders (including multiple personality disorder). Depersonalization-derealization syndrome is not classified under dissociative disorders in ICD-10; instead, it is classified under other neurotic disorders along with neurasthenia.

The common clinical types are described in Table 1.

Dissociative Amnesia

This is the most common clinical type of dissociative disorder seen in the Western countries. It occurs mostly in the adolescents and young adults, affecting more women than men, except in war. Dissociative amnesia is characterized by a sudden amnesia (either partial or complete) for recent events, particularly concerning stressful or traumatic life events. The amnesia cannot be explained by everyday forgetfulness and there is no evidence of an underlying medical illness. Most often, dissociative amnesia follows a traumatic or stressful life situation. Sometimes, imagined stressors or expression of 'forbidden' impulses may also precipitate the onset of amnesia.

This amnesia is of four types:

1. *Circumscribed or localized amnesia*: This is the most common type. There is an inability to recall all the personal events during a circumscribed period of time (usually for a few hours), frequently corresponding with the presence of the stressor.
2. *Selective or systematized amnesia*: This less common type is similar to circumscribed amnesia but there is an inability to recall only some selective personal events during that period while some other events during the same period may be recalled.
3. *Continuous amnesia*: In this rare type, there is an inability to recall all personal events following the stressful event, till the present time.
4. *Generalized amnesia*: In this very rare type, there is an inability to recall the personal events of the whole life, in the face of a stressful life event.[119] Later, it may make way for a more localized amnesia.

During the amnesic period, there may be slight clouding of consciousness. In the postamnesic period, the awareness of disturbance of memory is present. Some patients are disturbed about the memory disturbance but others appear unconcerned. Most cases recover spontaneously and long-term impairment is usually minimal. However, recurrences are known, particularly when faced with stressful life situations. In addition to stressor, the predisposing factors for dissociative amnesia include depressed mood, alcohol or drug use, head injury, and a history of seizures.

Dissociative amnesia is usually limited to a disturbance of recall of personal memories and does not interfere with the ability for new learning as well as of completing complicated mental tasks during the interview. The amnesia is limited to personal, episodic memory (involving personal events) but does not implicate public, episodic memory (involving public events).[120]

'Organic' amnesia includes defective memory for both personal and public memories; a temporal gradient in memory loss is usually seen. TGA (*transient global amnesia*) is an important differential diagnosis for dissociative amnesia and is characterized by brief episodes of repeated questioning, anterograde amnesia and confusion, in the absence of loss of personal identity, occurring usually in the 7th or 8th decade of life. TGA may be a manifestation of TIA (transient ischemic attacks) affecting midline limbic structures or of complex partial seizures (called sometimes as *transient epileptic amnesia*).[120,121] About 14–33% of cases of TGA are preceded by the presence of stressful life events.[122,123]

The other important differential diagnoses include *complex partial seizures* (EEG and the characteristic clinical picture may be helpful in diagnosis), alcohol or other substance-induced *amnestic disorder* or blackouts (history of alcohol and other drug dependence present), *postconcussional amnesia* (retrograde amnesia; history of head injury present), and *malingering* (immediate psychosocial benefit may be evident). The other dissociative disorders (Table 2) and *post-traumatic stress disorder* (PTSD) should also be considered in the differential diagnosis.

Table 2: Differential diagnosis of dissociative amnesia

Disorder	*Amnesia*	*Loss of personal identity*	*Wandering away*	*Assumption of a new identity*	*Alternating personalities*
Dissociative amnesia	Yes	May occur	No	No	No
Dissociative fugue	Yes	Yes	Yes	May occur	No
Multiple personality disorder	Yes	Yes	Usually No	Yes	Yes
Trance and possession disorder	Yes	Yes	No	Yes	No

Dissociative Fugue

Dissociative fugue is characterized by episodes of unexpected, yet organized wandering away from home, office or places of usual everyday social activities. During the episode, the person usually adopts a new identity[91] (or is confused about his identity[7]) with complete amnesia for the earlier life. The onset is usually sudden, often in the presence of severe stress. The termination too is abrupt and is followed by amnesia (either partial or complete) for the episode, but with recovery of memories of the life before the onset of fugue state.

The characteristic feature is the assumption of a purposeful new identity (though not always present), with an absence of awareness of amnesia. The behavior in dissociative fugue is more purposeful and integrated than that occurring in patients with dissociative amnesia, but the new identity is less complete and does not alternate with the original as in multiple personality disorder.

Most instances of dissociative fugue occur during wars, natural disasters or severe personal stress. In addition to stressor(s), the predisposing factors include depression, alcohol or drug use, head injury, histrionic personality disorder, and a history of seizures.

Dissociative fugue states should be differentiated from fugue states seen in complex partial seizures. Fugues seen in complex partial seizures usually last for minutes to hours, and may commonly be associated with automatisms. There is no assumption of a new identity; confusion or disorientation is present during the episode and usually there is no precipitating stress. Sometimes, 'dissociative' fugue (and even multiple personality) can be seen in the interictal period of patients of temporal lobe epilepsy.[124] Prolonged ambulatory behavior occurring in epilepsy, which is not amenable to recall, has been called as *poriomania*.[125]

Dissociative fugue, on the other hand, lasts for several days and the behavior during the fugue appears to be well organized and more orderly. At the end of the dissociative fugue, the person is usually well preserved, has maintained basic self-care (e.g. has eaten) and maintained simple social interaction with strangers (e.g. buying tickets or petrol, ordering food, asking directions).[9] Whereas, in the case of 'epileptic fugue', the person is often dirty, disheveled and neglected.[126] Here again, the amnesia is limited to personal, episodic memory (involving personal events) but does not implicate public, episodic memory (involving public events).[120]

Other differential diagnoses include schizophrenia, mania (purposeful travel associated with grandiose ideas/ delusions and other manic symptoms), dementia (aimless wandering), depression (a depressive component is common in a great majority of fugues; sometimes a suicidal impulse is transformed into an impulse to wander[126]) and malingering. The other dissociative disorders (*see* Table 2) and somnambulism (wandering during sleep) should also be considered in the differential diagnosis of dissociative fugue.

Multiple Personality (Dissociative Identity) Disorder

In multiple personality disorder (MPD), the person is dominated by two or more distinct personalities, of which only one is being manifest at one time. These personalities are usually different, at times even opposing. Each personality has a full range of higher mental functions, and performs complex behavior patterns. Usually one personality is not aware of the existence of the other(s), i.e. there are amnesic barriers between the personalities. The number of personalities reported ranges from 2 to more than 100, with nearly half of the reported cases presenting with 10 or less personalities.[7] The patient may complain of time lapses ('losing periods of time') or being accused of misdeeds that he does not recall having committed.[21,22] Both the onset and termination of control of the each personality is sudden.

Multiple personality disorder is often considered the most severe of all dissociative disorders[127-129] and is often linked to intense childhood trauma (like incest and childhood abuse).[130-132] The diagnosis is usually made in the early adulthood or rarely in adolescence. The first dissociative experience usually occurs several years before the proper diagnosis is made. More than 90% of the cases seen in the clinic population are women, while men with multiple personality disorder are more often seen in the criminal justice population.

Hallucinatory experiences, even Schneiderian First Rank Symptoms, are frequently reported. Therefore, the diagnosis may be mistaken for schizophrenia. Substance abuse or dependence, borderline personality disorder, somatization disorder, and post-traumatic stress disorder are frequent comorbid conditions. Suicidal attempts are not uncommon in multiple personality disorder.

Multiple personality disorder should be differentiated from *borderline personality disorder* (BPD), both of which are often comorbid.[133] In BPD, self is poorly formed but multiple identities are not found, and significant amnesic gaps are also not seen. However, dissociative phenomena are rather common in borderline personality disorder.[133] Other differential diagnoses include *trance and possession disorder* (in multiple personality disorder, each personality is a separate, complete, and complex entity with full range of functions, unlike in trance and possession disorders), *schizophrenia* (as mentioned above), *complex partial seizures* (rarely, as distinct personalities are unusual in complex partial seizures) and *malingering* (e.g. the famous case of Kenneth Bianchi, the Californian 'Hillside Strangler', who faked multiple personality and hypnosis to avoid death penalty and fooled many expert psychiatrists and psychologists[5,80]).

The diagnosis of MPD has been critiqued on several grounds, like:

- Vague and over-inclusive diagnostic criteria.[134]
- Recent, sudden rise in the number of cases reported[81] from North America and very few cases reported from rest of the World.
- Dramatization and popularization of the concept of MPD by the media.
- Exposure to malpractice risk.[5,81,135]
- *Issue of child abuse*:[81] Some studies report severe childhood trauma (usually sexual) in more than 90% of patients of multiple personality disorder. However, it has been suggested that therapists do not uncover historical truth (objective facts and details of a life story) but aid in producing narrative truth (which is a re-evaluation of the past in the light of present-day experience, as well as a product of the patient-therapist communication).[81] Some authors[135,136] have suggested that there is a 'false memory syndrome' in which therapist suggests to patients events that never actually occurred.
- Possibly iatrogenic,[22,78,89] with a possible role of treating physician in causation and/or shaping the course of illness by use of hypnosis (patients of multiple personality disorder have excellent hypnotizability) or suggestion.[81,137]
- Encouragement of regressive and 'nonresponsible' behavior during therapy,[81] by using techniques such as 'internal group therapy' (of asking alter personalities to talk to each other),[138] 'bulletin board' (of asking personalities to postmessages to each other),[139] and 'mapping the system.'[139]

Under ICD-10[9], multiple personality disorder is classified under 'other dissociative disorders', signifying that the disorder may be less common in clinical practice worldwide (with the exception of North America) as compared to trance and possession disorders.[77] Varma et al. (1981) speculated that the higher prevalence of MPD in the West may be related to social approval of role playing,[140] while a higher prevalence of possession disorders in India may be related to religious beliefs in polytheism and reincarnation. On the other hand, Adityanjee et al. (1989) discussed regarding the possibility of the majority of cases of multiple personality disorder in India having been diagnosed as possession syndrome.[77]

Both disorders are described as 'parallel dissociative disorders' and the differences in the clinical presentations explained on the basis of pathoplastic influences of the prevailing culture. Others have also described dissociative trance disorder in the developing countries as being similar to dissociative identity disorder in the West.[141,142]

Trance and Possession Disorders

In trance disorders, there is usually a temporary, marked constriction of consciousness with selective focusing on stimuli, loss of usual sense of personal identity (without replacement with a new identity), sometimes with repetitive motor behavior and speech. Response to environmental stimuli may be variable. Vocalizations or repetition of words may be seen.

If a new identity (usually a spirit, ghost, deity, divine power, or some other person) takes over the control of person's personality during the episodes, the condition is called as possession disorder. The voice and behavior may appear like that of the 'possessed spirit.'[143] Usually the person is aware of the existence of the other (i.e. 'possessor'), unlike in multiple personality disorder. In DSM-IV,[8] these disorders are called as dissociative trance disorder and placed under the category of 'dissociative disorder NOS (not otherwise specified)'. In appendix, DSM-IV[8] describes research criteria for diagnosis of 'dissociative trance disorder', similar to 'trance and possession disorders' in ICD-10.

These disorders are very commonly seen in India and certain African countries, where a belief in the supernatural forces is very widely prevailing. Therefore, it is extremely important to ensure that the disorder being diagnosed is not merely a culturally sanctioned behavior. It must be 'unwanted and troublesome, occurring outside, or being a prolongation of, similar states in religious or other culturally acceptable situations.'[9] In fact many patients with possession symptoms do not come for treatment, as these symptoms are often considered culturally permitted ways of expressing distress.[144,145] In India, a significant number of patents of trance and possession disorders usually first reach the 'faith healers' and it is only when the faith healers' efforts fail to ameliorate the condition, the patients seek psychiatric help.[145] The 'possessed' individual may even be accorded respect by the community, particularly in the rural areas.[53] There are instances of possession states being utilized to treat psychiatric patients (mainly neurotics) by faith healers.[145]

In different cultures, finer manifestations may vary and sometimes constitute culture bound syndromes (like pibloktoq, whitigo, latah, bebainan, and voodoo). It has been pointed out that multiple personality (or dissociative identity) disorder and possession disorder share commonalties, suggesting that multiple personality disorder may be a culture bound syndrome in the American context.

Yap (1960) divided the state of possession into three degrees:[146,147]

1. *First degree or complete*: There is clouding of consciousness, anesthesia to pain, a changed demeanor and change of voice, impossibility of recalling the patient to reality, and subsequent amnesia.
2. *Second degree or partial*: There is mild clouding of consciousness, partial anesthesia, and no change in voice or demeanor, while there is possibility of recalling the patient to reality and partial amnesia is subsequently present.
3. *Third degree or histrionic*: There is absence of clouding of consciousness and anesthesia, and no change in voice or demeanor. There is possibility of immediate recall to reality. There may be mannerisms like giggling, and other attention seeking behaviors.

Another traditional way of classification of possession states is to divide them in to two types:[148]

1. The *somnambulic state*, in which there is unawareness of consciousness of self and the later, there is amnesia for the events during the episode.
2. The *lucid state*, in which awareness of both self and the 'intruder' remains.

Possession symptom may also be seen in *mania* (differential diagnosis from delusion of grandiosity is important), *depression, schizophrenia* (differential diagnosis from delusion of control, 'made phenomenon', and thought alienation is important), and *obsessive compulsive disorder.*[145]

Dissociative Stupor

Dissociative stupor is characterized by an absence (akinesis) or marked diminution (hypokinesis) of voluntary movements and speech (mutism), in the presence of normal or relatively preserved conscious awareness (some degree of responsiveness to light, noise and touch, normal muscle tone, normal breathing, and often limited coordinated eye movements).[8] The onset is sudden and usually related to a stressful life event, unlike manic and depressive stupor, which develop more slowly.[5]

The differentiation of 'organic' and dissociative stupor is made on the basis of antecedent medical and psychiatric history, the mode of onset, detailed physical and neurological examination, with observation of the patient over a period of lime. Apparently purposeful eye movements, variation in symptomatology over time, abrupt changes in motor behavior and last minute responses may mislead the physician in diagnosing dissociative stupor instead of organic stupor. The features that help in differential diagnosis are summarized in Table 3. The differential diagnosis includes *nonconvulsive status* (complex partial status or absence

Table 3: Organic stupor vs dissociative stupor

	Features	*Organic stupor*	*Dissociative stupor*
1.	Previous psychiatric illness	Usually absent	Usually present
2.	Previous medical illness	Usually present	Usually absent
3.	Previous episodes of stupor	10%	24–33%
4.	Precipitating stressor	Usually absent	Usually present
5.	Course	Longer	Usually shorter, generally recover within 7 days
6.	Frequency	More common	Uncommon (3.5% of all stupor cases)
7.	Blepharospasm	Absent	May be present
8.	Menace reflex	Absent	Present
9.	Oculocephalic reflex (Doll's head eye phenomenon)	Present	Absent
10.	Henry and Woodruff's sign	Absent	Present
11.	Roving, eye movements	May be present	Absent
12.	Protective response	Absent	Present
13.	Sympathetic overactivity	Usually absent	Usually present
14.	Resistance to eye opening	Absent	Usually present
15.	Preservation of ability to help feeding and eliminative functions	Usually absent	May be present
16.	Meaningful posture and facial expressions	Absent	May be present
17.	Urinary/fecal incontinence	Usually present	Unlikely
18.	Abnormal EEG	More likely	Less likely
19.	Oculovestibular reflex	Absent	Present
20.	Pentothal (or amytal) interview	Low dose increases stupor and neurological signs develop	High dose increases alertness and mental status examination may be possible
21.	Mortality	35%	0–3%

status), *akineticmutism*, other causes of *coma*, and *catatonic stupor*.

Miscellaneous Dissociative Disorders

Discussed here are several disorders that have in the past been associated with hysteria, conversion disorders, and dissociative disorders.

Atypical or unspecified dissociative disorders: Several studies from India have found that 80–90% of the patients with dissociative disorders are classified under atypical or unspecified dissociative disorders.

Saxena (1987) criticized DSM-III criteria for dissociative disorders on its inability to classify Indian patients[113] and proposed the categories of simple dissociative disorder and possession disorder.[71] The criteria given by him for possession disorder are based on the criteria given by Yap for possession disorder. Saxena[71] reported that 80% of the patients diagnosed as dissociative hysteria had simple dissociative disorder and 10% had possession attacks. 6% of patients had psychogenic fugue and rest had depersonalization disorder.

Alexander (1997) proposed a new category called brief dissociative stupor (BDS)[78] to account for the majority of their patients who suffered from brief unresponsiveness. These patients could not be diagnosed as dissociative convulsions, as the criteria[8] require the presence of sudden and spasmodic movements for the diagnosis to be made. BDS was supposed to differ from SDD[113] by the absence of motor symptoms. However, Saxena (1987) specified that accompanying motor movements need not be present in every patient with SDD.[113]

Instead of including the new categories of SDD[113] or BDS,[78] it may be better if ICD-10 (or ICD-11 in future) widened the scope of dissociative convulsions by including brief periods of unconsciousness too. The category can be renamed simply as *dissociative seizures* or *dissociative nonepileptic seizures*.[78]

Ganser syndrome and hysterical pseudodementia: Ganser syndrome was originally reported to be common in prison inmates. It has been variously classified as a factitious disorder or as a dissociative disorder (not otherwise specified). The characteristic feature is *vorbeireden* (also called as Ganser response, Ganser symptom, 'approximate answers', or 'answering past the point'). The answers are inaccurate but show that the person understands the nature of question asked. For example, when shown a red pen, the patient calls it blue. In addition, there may be disturbances of consciousness, amnesia for the episode, hallucinations, and motor or sensory deficits similar to those seen in conversion disorders. There may be spontaneous recovery in some cases.

Ganser syndrome is frequently associated with other dissociative symptomatology like amnesia, fugue, conversion symptoms, and perceptual disturbances.[148] Although Ganser syndrome is uncommon, Ganser symptom is found in a variety of psychiatric (and even organic brain) disorders.[126] Although most authors equate Ganser syndrome with hysterical pseudodementia, others think differently.[126] Severe forms of hysterical pseudodementia have been described as *hysterical infantilism* or *hysterical puerilism*. In this extremely rare condition, the patient regresses to the helpless state of infancy, losing the ability to walk and talk, making inarticulate noises and wetting his bed.[126]

Mass hysteria (Synonyms: epidemic hysteria, communicable hysteria): Epidemics of frenzy behavior in women have been well-recognized in history. For example, dancing manias of Middle Ages may be manifestations of epidemic hysteria. Hecker (1867) reported examples of nuns mewing and biting like cats, which spread from convent to convent.[149]

The cases occur mostly in females of younger age and children. Schools, functions or sports events are the usual situations where it tends to occur. Usually the group cohesion is be high and the group will be under some stress. The index case is often of a 'high status'. Spread occurs in the peer group through audio-visual 'transmission'. Outsiders from the group are usually not affected. Mass fainting and over-breathing are common forms, while nausea, abdominal pain and headache the uncommon forms.

Sirois (1974) classified epidemic (mass) hysteria into five types:[150]

1. Sudden onset - explosive type,
2. Explosive with identifiable prodromal struggle,
3. Cumulative outbreak type,
4. Rebound outbreak, and
5. Large diffuse outbreak with slow transmission of symptoms.

Recently, Wessely (1987) suggested[151] that mass hysteria could be divided into two syndromes: '*mass anxiety hysteria*' and '*mass motor hysteria*'. The mass anxiety hysteria is characterized by episodes of acute anxiety (abdominal pain, chest tightness, dizziness, fainting, headache, hyperventilation, nausea and palpitations), occurs mostly in school children, evidence of prior tension is absent and the spread is rapid by visual contact. Separation of children retards the spread rapidly. On the other hand, the *mass motor hysteria* occurs in any age group, prior tension is present, presents with 'conversion symptoms', the spread is gradual (weeks to months) and the prognosis is guarded. Overlap between these two forms is also seen.[152]

In India, epidemics of possession states have been described during outbreaks of measles and chicken pox.[153] Nandi et al. (1985) have described[154] a case of persistent mass (motor) hysteria, emphasizing the need for early intervention, while Narayanan and Mahal (1977) have described 6 cases occurring within a family.[155]

Combat hysteria: Also called as War neurosis or shell-shock, combat hysteria is particularly common during wars, the classical cases being described ever since World War I. The common symptoms described were paralysis (usually paraplegia), blindness and mutism. The symptoms show a tendency to spread 'infectiously', very much like in mass hysteria, from soldier to soldier.

It affected soldiers across all barriers of intelligence, levels of bravery, and background, showing that severe stress can be a great leveler for causation of conversion and dissociative symptoms.

Hysterical psychoses: Hysterical psychosis is discussed in the chapter on 'other psychotic disorders'.

Culture bound syndromes: Some culture bound syndromes (called as culture-specific disorders in ICD-10)[8] may be mistaken for dissociative fugue states (e.g. pibloktoq or Arctic hysteria, and amok) or trance and possession disorders (latah, windigo, zar possession, voodoo, and ufufuyane or saka). These conditions are characterized by a trance like state, with increased or decreased activity, potentially dangerous behavior in the form of running or fleeing, marked suggestibility, and resulting exhaustion, sleep and amnesia for the episode.[7,8]

Organic hysteria: A category of organic dissociative disorder has been included under 'organic mental disorders' in ICD-10, without being described in detail.[8] It includes all cases of dissociative (conversion) disorders, in which there is an evidence of an organic etiology (the category of 'other mental disorders due to brain damage and dysfunction and to physical disease'). Some reports of organic dissociative disorder (fugue states)[156,157] have appeared in literature.

Post-traumatic stress disorder: Post-traumatic stress disorder (PTSD) patients often reports dissociative symptoms and a dissociative subtype of PTSD has been suggested.[158] Self-reports of dissociation during a disaster were a significant predictor of later PTSD.[159] Koopman et al. (1994) suggested that dissociation might be adaptive during and immediately following a traumatic event.[160] However, the chronic use of dissociative mechanisms as a means of dealing with the trauma may lead to a failure to process trauma cognitively and emotionally, and therefore, result in more severe PTSD.

Depersonalization derealization syndrome: Depersonalization disorder is classified under 'dissociative disorders' in DSM-IV while it comes under 'other neurotic disorders' in ICD-10. Janet (1903), in his book 'Obsessions and Psychasthenia', considered that hyperactivity of memory in a setting of narrowed consciousness was the essential factor in causation of depersonalization.[161] Schilder described depersonalization as a state in which the individual feels himself changed throughout in comparison with his former state.[162] For describing alienation of the outer world, Mapother coined the term '*derealization*'.

Depersonalization is characterized by an alteration in the perception or experience of self, so that the feeling of one's own reality is temporarily changed or lost. The patient recognizes that things have not really changed but appear 'as-if' as changed. The changes are noticed in body, self, emotions, and activity. Essentially all the aspects of personality appear to have changed and the experience involves feeling lifeless, automatic and remote (like an automaton). The affected person often describes observing his own actions like an observer. Depersonalization is often accompanied by derealization, which is an alteration in the perception or experience of external world, so that the feeling of reality of external world is temporarily changed.

Both depersonalization and derealization occur in many other disorders, like primary psychiatric disorders (panic disorder, agoraphobia, dysthymia, depressive episode, and schizophrenia), neurological and organic mental disorders (complex partial seizures, migraine, cerebral tumors and substance use disorder), and even normal subjects (boredom, sensory deprivation, and fatigue). Therefore, the term depersonalization disorder should be used only when other disorders have been ruled out. Because of high comorbidity with anxiety disorders, a syndrome of *phobic anxiety depersonalization* has been described in literature. *Primary depersonalization* is a rare entity which is resistant to treatment and traces a fluctuating course.

DSM-5

Major changes in dissociative disorders in DSM-5 include the following: (1) derealization is included in the name and symptom structure of what previously was called depersonalization disorder and is now called depersonalization/derealization disorder, (2) dissociative fugue is now a specifier of dissociative amnesia rather than a separate diagnosis, and (3) the criteria for dissociative identity disorder have been changed to indicate that symptoms of disruption of identity may be reported as well as observed, and that gaps in the recall of events may occur for everyday and not just traumatic events. Also, experiences of pathological possession in some cultures are included in the description of identity disruption.

Dissociative Identity Disorder

Several changes to the criteria for dissociative identity disorder have been made in DSM-5. First, Criterion A has been expanded to include certain possession-form phenomena and functional neurological symptoms to account for more diverse presentations of the disorder. Second, Criterion A now specifically states that transitions in identity may be observable by others or self-reported. Third, according to

Criterion B, individuals with dissociative identity disorder may have recurrent gaps in recall for everyday events, not just for traumatic experiences. Other text modifications clarify the nature and course of identity disruptions.

ETIOLOGY

The causal theories of dissociative (conversion) disorders are predominantly of the following types:

Psychological Theories

Psychodynamic Theory

According to Freud,[33] important defense mechanisms involved in the formation of conversion symptoms are repression, dissociation, conversion, symbolization and identification. Repressed materials are sexual or aggressive conflicts arising during oedipal phase of development. Under the influence of a stressor, repression fails partly or completely, leading to the formation of a conversion or dissociation symptom. Freud believed hysterical patients to be fixated at the phallic-genital phase of psychosexual development. Regression to the phallic stage accounts for the infantile character of the hysteric's sexuality. In hysteria, more than any other neurotic disorder, the 'Oedipal complex' is considered the core problem in the psychoanalytic theory.[163]

Thus, unpleasant repressed material is converted to somatic symptom leading to relief of anxiety, in conversion. This is called as the 'primary gain' and because of this relief from anxiety, patient is theorized to have the '*la belle indifference*' in spite of having a serious physical symptom. According to this theory, the conversion symptom adopted will have a symbolic meaning, which represents the childhood conflict. Sometimes, the conversion symptoms arise out of identification with a significant individual, often someone whom the patient associates with loss and has also experienced such symptoms (*conversion model*).

Dissociative symptomatology has received scant attention from psychoanalysis. In dissociative disorders, amnesia is seen as a result of repression (which is more massive, primitive, and pervasive than in any other neurotic disorder[163]) of unacceptable thought and wishes, which if conscious, would cause distress. Fisher and Josephs (1949), Luparello (1970), and Rapaport (1967) later modified the Freudian model to consider amnesia as a result of patient's regression to an altered state of consciousness as a compromise formation to solve a painful internal psychic conflict.[21] In this model, the patient with dissociative fugue could both express prohibited feelings and impulses (i.e. are not repressed) and simultaneously deny authorship of them.[21]

Jung (1902) approached the problem of possession from a teleological angle. He felt that possession represented the idealized image of the person struggling to be born. His later formulations (1921) of personal unconscious and collective unconscious suggest the division of possession cases into two categories: those produced by dead relatives and those possessed by culture-heroes and gods.[145]

Hypnosis, Dissociation and Suggestibility

Any discussion of dissociation will be incomplete without discussion of its relation with hypnosis and suggestibility. Dissociation can be described as a structured separation of mental processes (e.g. perceptions, conation, emotions, memories, and identity) that are ordinarily integrated in and accessible to conscious awareness.[164] About 90% of general population has some degree of hypnotizability, while 10% are profoundly so.[20] The patient with innately high hypnotizability, when faced with stressor,[20,164] unwittingly uses autohypnosis and enters an altered state of consciousness, suggesting to self. The dissociative amnesia, fugue[21] or identity disorder[80] is the result of the posthypnotic state. The trance state induced during hypnosis may sometimes result in secondary personalities and cause amnesia in the primary personality. The power of suggestion is best exemplified in the phenomenon of voodoo death.

Babibski (1908)[15] coined the word 'pithiatism' maintaining that everything that is hysterical may be caused by and removed by 'forced suggestion', at least temporarily. On the other hand, both Kraepelin and Bleuler distinguished between the fragmentation or molecular dissociation of schizophrenia and the block or molar dissociation characteristic of hysteria.[15]

The key dysfunction in dissociative disorders is a loss of the unitary state of self and consciousness. However, Hilgard (1986), in his neodissociation theory,[165] proposed that 'the unity of consciousness is illusory' and that a spectrum of dissociation is inherent in normal mental function. He said that mental functions, both receptive and active, may be regulated by multiple and overlapping control systems that are not always accessible to the conscious mind.

Learning and Behavioral Theories

Symptom of an illness that has been experienced earlier may appear again through classical conditioning when challenged with a stressor. Development of the symptom brings about psychological relief (from 'dysphoric affect'[166]) by avoidance of stress and is thus secondarily reinforced. So, once that symptom is produced, the external reinforcements will lead to chronicity of the symptom through the operant conditioning. Reinforcement can occur because of reduced responsibility, increased attention due to sick role, etc. These are called '*secondary gains*'.

Wolpe (1958) divides reactions to noxious situations or conflicts in to two types:[167] *anxiety reactions* involving the autonomic nervous system and *nonanxiety reactions* involving the sensory, motor and cognitive reaction systems of the individual. He proposes that the second reaction predominates in hysteria. The central feature of hysterical reaction, according to him, is conditioning of neurotic reactions other than anxiety, in conditions of stress. 'Hysterics' only show a low-intensity anxiety reaction in stress situations, which makes other nonanxiety reactions more likely. These nonanxiety reactions (which include inhibition of particular sensory, motor, or cognitive processes) then become conditioned.

Dollard and Miller (1950) suggest two possible sources of hysterical symptoms.[168] The first is organic (earlier experience of organic/medical symptoms/disease) and the second is a model (whose symptoms are copied). They also acknowledge other sources of symptoms, though. Whatever the source, once symptoms occur, they sharply reduce anxiety. This decrease in anxiety produces further relief from responsibilities and reinforces the symptoms. The decrease in anxiety may also produce la belle indifference.

Abnormal Illness Behavior and Care-eliciting Behavior

Immature and dependent individuals, according to this theory, use conversion symptoms to effect a dependency adaptation and to obtain attention.[28] Helplessness arising out of conversion symptoms can be used to control family members and members of the treating team.

Biological Theories

Neurophysiological and Neuropsychological Theories

The preponderance of left-sided symptoms in hysteria, especially in women, gives clues towards the probable nondominant hemisphere defect. Studies have indicated instability of right hemispheric organization in women. Since conversion is more common in women, the above fact adds to the possibility of involvement of right hemisphere in conversion disorder. Also a strong association of conversion disorders with depression again points towards a non-dominant involvement.[169]

Ludwig (1972) proposed a neurobiological model[170] regarding hysteria as a dysfunction of attention, vigilance and recent memory due to increased corticofugal inhibition of afferent stimulation at the level of brain stem reticular formation. Hypochondriasis is presumed to be just the reverse, related to decreased corticofugal inhibition of afferent stimulation. The symptoms in hysteria can be caused by an excessive cortical arousal that sets off negative feedback loops between the cerebral cortex and brainstem reticular formation. Elevated levels of corticofugal output, in turn, inhibits the patient's awareness of body sensation, which in some conversion disorder patients may explain the observed sensory deficit.[170,171]

Neuropsychological testing has revealed impaired vigilance, attention and short-term memory in patients with conversion disorder, along with imprecise verbal communications and subtle affective incongruity. A recent study[172] found evidence of subtle neuropsychological deficits on WAIS-R (on memory/distractibility factor) in patients of multiple personality disorder and other dissociative disorder patients. Localizing studies using Halstead-Reitan battery revealed dysfunction of both hemispheres, with a greater dysfunction of the nondominant hemisphere.[173]

In a study of evoked potentials[174] in patients with 'hysterical' anesthesia, two underlying mechanisms, consisting of a lowering of peripheral receptor sensitivity and a central mechanism of inhibition along different pathways, were suggested.

In patients of post-traumatic stress disorder with dissociative symptoms (so-called dissociative subtype of PTSD),[158] there is a suppression of autonomic physiological responses even when the subject reports feeling subjectively aroused and upset (lack of association between affect and physical reactivity).

Stress-diathesis Model

Mayer-Gross, Janet,[31] and Breuer proposed an inborn neurological susceptibility of entering altered states of consciousness in response to intense stimuli.[21] The patient is then unable to recall in his normal state experiences that were registered during the altered or hypnoid states, something similar to 'state dependent learning'. Butler et al (1996) suggest that innately high hypnotizability may be a diathesis for pathological dissociative states, particularly under conditions of acute traumatic stress.[164]

Severe psychosocial stress (usually of a sexual nature, though not always) in early childhood may lead to early splits in the personality either through dissociation or autohypnosis, and thus to a vulnerability to use dissociation to deal with later life stressors.[21]

Kendell (1974)[3] and Smith (1978)[175] have proposed similar models in which symptoms develop as a response to emotional stress or conflict when a series of environmental, biological and personal predisposing (vulnerability) factors are present within the individual or as a part of the current life situation. These factors include illness-rewarding situation (when the advantages of being sick outweigh those of health) and individual variables (e.g. female gender, younger age, hysterical personality traits, suggestibility, a tendency to dissociate, availability of model(s) of illness, etc.).[110]

Genetic Theories

There is an increased likelihood of conversion disorder in the first-degree relatives of patients of conversion disorder. Increased risk of conversion disorder in monozygotic but not dizygotic twin pairs has been reported.[7] An increased prevalence of hysteria is also seen in the first-degree relatives of male sociopaths and also increased alcoholism among the first-degree relatives. Several studies have found that multiple personality disorder is more common in the first-degree relatives with the disorder as compared with normal population.[93]

Ljungberg (1957)[176] found heterogeneity of psychiatric illness in family members of patients with conversion symptoms. Sociopathy in fathers appears to be particularly associated with the development of hysteria in delinquent and sociopathic girls. Hyperactive children appear to carry an increased risk of delinquency, sociopathy and hysteria.

State Dependent Learning

It has been observed even in normal individuals that learning is often contextual-dependent or state-dependent.[131] So, information that is learned during a particular behavior (e.g. being in the classroom), a pharmacological state (e.g. while drinking alcohol), or a mood state (profound sadness) is often recalled more easily while re-experiencing the original state. It has been suggested that the amnesia seen in dissociative disorders may be due to the memory of a traumatic event being laid down during the stressful event. As the emotional state is so out of ordinary for the affected person that it is difficult for the person to remember the information learned during such a state.[126,177]

Other Biological Theories

The biological basis of dissociative (conversion) disorders is far from proven. Some long-term studies[2] have found that up to 80% of patients, diagnosed as 'hysteria', were later found to have physical illnesses. However, replications of such studies have not found such high figures, as discussed above. But, it still seems that organic brain disease facilitates the use of hysterical mechanisms.[110]

Cerebral blood flow patterns in a single-case study of multiple personality disorder[178] showed right temporal hyperperfusion following transition between alter personalities. Imaging studies done by Flor-Henry (1981) emphasized[173] that there is hypofunction of the dominant hemisphere systems, with a consequent dysfunctional overactivity of nondominant hemisphere, and impaired interhemispheric communication.

Conversion symptoms are frequently seen in patients of epilepsy and it may at times be difficult to differentiate between true and pseudoseizures. Similarly, 'conversion-release' symptoms are seen in some cerebral cortex lesions. Temporal lobe abnormalities, multiple sclerosis, and head injury[126,171] have been suggested to predispose to conversion symptoms.[179] Soft neurological signs are also found more commonly in patients of 'hysteria.'[171] Similarly, dissociative states have been regarded as atypical and often chronic varieties of complex partial seizures of temporal lobe origin.[124]

Several studies have found a lateralization to the non-dominant hemisphere in right handed individuals suffering from conversion disorders.[180-184]

Sociocultural Theories

A Form of Communication

It has been proposed that conversion symptom is a form of communication through body language when overt expression of emotions is blocked.[185] In cultures where psychological symptoms are stigmatized, the distress may be communicated by body language.[185,186] The patient may learn to communicate helplessness by hysterical symptoms, thereby avoiding aggressive impulses and facilitating an environment in which attention and support are gained.[187] Therefore, caregivers' providing unnecessary attention can further reinforce hysterical symptoms.

Engel (1970) suggested[188] that conversion symptoms have four unconsciously determined aims. These are:

1. To permit expression of the forbidden wish in a disguised manner,
2. To achieve punishment through suffering for having such a wish,
3. To remove the person from a threatening life situation, and
4. To provide a new mode of relating to others, the sick role.

Szasz (1961) described[189] hysteria as a form of primitive communication or protolanguage, a kind of double bind charade not clearly comprehended by the patient who manifests it or by the doctor to whom it is directed and who has the task of decoding it. He declared that hysteria was not really an illness at all.

Social Role Model

Kirshner (1973) described[190] dissociative amnesia as a well-defined 'social role', which the patient uses to protect himself from social responsibility and/or criticism. Parsons (1951) described[191] the concept of 'sick role' and the secondary gains associated with it, some of which may underlie the causation of dissociative (conversion) disorders. Adoption of sick-role may be easier when faced with stress than assuming responsibility for handling life situations.

Ethological and Anthropological Perspectives

According to Kretschmer, most forms of hysteria emanate from two instinctive, protective and adaptive mechanisms that we share with the other animals.[192,193] These are allesthetic displays designed to alter the behavior of other animals. These are:

- The *violent motor reaction* (or *instinctual flurry*) characterized by uncoordinated frantic attempts to flee when face with external danger. Examples are a bird in a closed room, a person who cannot swim thrown in water, and people in a crowd at the time of a catastrophe. In hysteria, the danger is instead internal (fantasized or imagined) and the striving to get away from danger is not under conscious control. Examples of 'hysterical reactions' arising out of violent motor reaction include fugue states, convulsive movements, violent emotional attacks with subsequent amnesia, and tremors.
- The *sham-death reflex* (also called as *immobilization reflex* or death feint or playing possum). In animals, this reflex is very useful, as death-feint makes prey unattractive to predator for hunting. Peromyscus (the deer mouse), for example, maintains in a small proportion of its population a gene for convulsing if shaken, which helps reduce risk from predators.[194,195] In hysteria, nonconvulsive seizures, paralyses, blindness, deafness and analgesia were ascribed to sham-death reflex by Kretschmer.

Ludwig (1972) proposed,[170] as an extension of Kretschmer's theory[193] and writings of Hughlings Jackson,[196] another instinctive mechanism of an ability to react in progressively more primitive ways when confronted with danger (regression). This type of regressive activity contributes to a posture of helplessness and defense-lessness which wards off 'attack' (like in sham-death reflex) from members of the same species.

However, these adaptive behaviors are usually transient (unlike dissociative disorders) and do not explain dissociative (conversion) disorders adequately.

Assortative Mating

There appears to be a pattern of assortative mating between hysterical women and sociopathic men. Sociopathy is increased in husbands of hysterical women and hysteria is increased in the wives of sociopathic men.

Iatrogenic

The issue of iatrogenesis in the etiology of multiple personality disorder has already been discussed.

Eclectic Theories

Kluft (1988) has suggested an eclectic model for the development of dissociative disorders, particularly multiple personality disorder.[148] This model provides for 4 factors, which need to be present before the disorder can manifest in an individual. Factor 1 is the biological potential for dissociation or hypnotizability. Factor 2 is the life experience that traumatically overwhelms adaptive capacities of the child's ego, thereby mobilizing the dissociative ones. Factor 3 is the shaping influences and substrates that determine the form taken by the dissociative disorder. Factor 4 is the inadequate provision of stimulus barriers and restorative experiences by significant others.

DIAGNOSIS

Diagnosis is not merely based on the absence of objective signs of physical illness, although it is very important to exclude an underlying or associated physical illness, as well as other primary psychiatric disorders. It is important to remember that absence of physical findings applies universally to a stage in the development of all diseases.[2] Also, physical findings that appear nonrelevant at first may assume significance later.[2]

Presence of positive points in history and examination should be present, before a diagnosis of dissociative (conversion) disorders can be made. These positive points are the characteristic clinical features listed previously. As dissociative (conversion) disorders and physical illness can be co-existing, a detailed clinical examination is absolutely essential. If dissociative (conversion) symptoms appear for the first time in an elderly person, especially in a male more than 40 years old, a strong suspicion of underlying physical or major psychiatric illness should be kept in mind.

Issue of Positive Signs

Charcot emphasized the value of physical stigmata of 'hysteria' and later Henry Head[197] popularized the positive signs of hysteria, like tunnel vision, discrete anesthetic patches, astasia-abasia, Hoover test, preserved cough in hysterical aphonia, and hemianesthesia sharply separated at the midline. The central component of the clinical rules described by Head was that the physician should try to discover the normally preserved functional (physiological) capacities underlying the superficial appearance of incapacity. However, he did not give any criteria for distinguishing the 'hysteric' from a normal individual.[2] In addition to positive signs, hysterofrenic areas (areas on body, which when pressed, abort the hysterical episode, usually convulsive in nature) and hysterogenic areas (areas on body, e.g. a hyperesthetic spot, which when pressed can induce a hysterical episode) were also described.[15]

Unfortunately, these positive signs can also be seen in neurological patients. Gould et al. (1986) applied the (so-called) positive signs of hysteria to 30 consecutive neurological admissions (25 of which had acute strokes).[17] These signs (7 in number) included secondary gain, *la belle indifference*, nonanatomic sensory loss, midline split of pain or vibratory stimulation, changing boundaries for hypalgesia, give away weakness, and history of hypochondriasis. All 30 patients showed at least one out of 7 features, most exhibited more than one feature and one patient had all 7 signs. So, it is apparent that hysteria is easily misdiagnosed (overdiagnosed) if the 'positive criteria' are taken to be pathognomonic.

Issue of Stressor

ICD-10 DCR (Diagnostic criteria for research)[9] specifies that there should be convincing associations in time between the onset of symptoms of the disorder and 'stressful (life) events, problems, or needs'. However, in clinical studies, the presence of stressor is found in only 37–69% of cases.[53,55,75,198] It is also important to remember that stressful events occur all the time in the lives of normal individuals. In fact, stressor may focus attention on the early symptoms of cerebral tumors and other medical disorders.[126,199] So, the severity and temporal correlation of stressor(s) with the onset of symptoms should be clearly delineated, whenever present.

Issue of La Belle Indifference

The early French literature described *la belle indifference*,[31] that is a lack of appropriate concern towards the symptoms, despite the apparent severity of disability produced. It was argued[166] that because anxiety is converted into somatic symptoms or repressed, the conscious anxiety is 'warded off', presenting clinically as '*la belle indifference*'. Although earlier thought to be a hallmark of dissociative (conversion) disorders, it is now known to be present even in physical illnesses. Also, it is not always present in dissociative (conversion) disorders.[49,183] In fact, several patients with conversion disorder describe their symptoms with embellishments and elaboration.

In fact, Lader and Sartorius[200] found that a majority of patients with conversion disorder were highly aroused and anxious, as compared to normal controls or even patients with phobic or anxiety states. Katoch et al. (1994) also found considerable anxiety levels in patients with conversion disorders, dissociative disorders, and a group with both diagnoses.[94]

Issue of Secondary Gain

The gains from dissociative and conversion disorders can be multiple and not mutually exclusive.[5] These may include:

- Relief from the unpleasant conflicts and associated anxiety (primary gain).
- Attention seeking or gain of sympathy from significant others, by adopting a sick-role (secondary gain).
- Relief from responsibilities and duties (secondary gain).
- Manipulations of personal relationships (secondary gain).
- Symbolic expression of an emotionally laden idea (secondary gain).
- Alleviation of guilt through suffering (secondary gain).
- Significant others may derive gains because of patient's illness, thereby reinforcing the continuation of symptoms (tertiary gain).

In DSM-III-R, the introductory paragraph refers to the importance of secondary gain but the diagnostic criteria have removed secondary gain from the list. Both DSM-IV and ICD-10 specifically do not require secondary gain in the diagnostic criteria.

Issue of Premorbid Personality

Premorbid histrionic personality traits are often present, although a personality disorder is less common[49,61,183,201,202] despite claims to the contrary.[203] The comorbid personality disorders include passive-aggressive, dependent, avoidant, borderline, and antisocial, in addition to the histrionic type.[66,95,201,202,204] 66% of patients in one study[53] had features of extraversion in the personality.

Issue of False Positive Diagnosis

False positive diagnoses of conversion disorder have been substantiated in the literature.[2] A recent review[205] states that there is a significant increase in the rates of false positive 'conversion reactions' and mixed picture cases ('hysterical overlays') with neurological and psychiatric components. One study[206] found a false positive rate of 25% at a 10-year follow-up. False positive diagnosis is very likely if importance is given only to the symptom and attention is not given to the underlying physical or psychiatric morbidity. The false positivity is further confounded by the presence of significant comorbidity of medical disorders.[183]

Some of the diagnostic difficulties (diagnostic snares) include idiopathic dystonia,[198] dopa-responsive dystonia (a type of childhood dystonia, presenting with bizarre gait, unexpected falls, and gait dystonia),[97] myasthenic syndrome (Lambert-Eaton syndrome), blepharospasm,[61] primary orthostatic tremor,[61] multiple sclerosis,[126,207] apraxias,[198] paroxysmal choreoathetosis, reflex epilepsy, porphyrias,[126] subdural hematoma,[169] early manifestations of AIDS,[169] paroxysmal hemicrania,[6] and thoracic outlet syndrome,[6] among many others.

It is also likely that these false positive diagnoses are made more often in women, homosexual men, psychiatrically patients, patients presenting plausible psychogenic explanations for their illnesses, and patients with unusual movement disorders.[16] It is almost 'axiomatic to view with great suspicion' hysterical symptoms that make their first appearance only in middle life.[126]

Issue of Impaired Sexuality

Freud explained conversion and dissociation symptoms as the consequence of unconscious sexual conflict(s). Although Purtell et al.[208] found significant evidence of sexual disturbance in their sample of 50 patients with hysteria (86% sexual indifference, 73% lack of sexual pleasure, 98% some sexual symptom), other studies[54,202] have failed to find such a robust correlation. It seems stressors of all kinds, including (but not exclusively) sexual ones, may occur before the onset of dissociative disorders. Sometimes, even physical illnesses (e.g. fever) may serve as precipitating stressors.[145]

Miscellaneous Issues

The conversion and dissociative symptoms on several occasions are modeled on the similar symptoms observed in some other individual with whom the patient identifies.

Lazare (1981) has discussed the usefulness of 10 criteria for the diagnosis.[73] According to him, the criteria with greater validity are somatization (3+), associated psychopathology (2+), presence of a model for symptoms (2+), and emotional stress before the onset of symptoms (1+). Traditional symptoms like symbolic meaning, secondary gain, hysterical personality, and la belle indifference were regarded as having no validity. A recent study has tried to validate these criteria further.[183]

Marsden (1986) described 6 rules of hysteria.[61] These rules specify that those with hysterical symptoms usually do not have histrionic personalities, are unlikely to conform to Briquet's syndrome, may well have underlying recognized or unrecognized physical or psychiatric illness, require further neurological and psychiatric exploration, and may well be exhibiting abnormal illness behavior.

OUTCOME AND PROGNOSIS

Since at no time the definition of dissociation disorders, conversion disorders, and hysteria were uniform, the outcome studies suffer from the differences in the sample selected. Outcome also depends upon the setting in which the study was conducted. However, it is well known that chronicity of symptoms leads to intractable disability.

Earlier follow-up studies of patients presenting to neurologists or general physicians reveal that 50–70% of cases with 'hysteria' develop diagnosable neurological disorders within the next few years.[2,61,171,202,209-211]

However, recent studies have reported a much lower prevalence (0–15%) of organicity at follow-up.[44,75,198,207] Several reasons have been ascribed for these revised lower figures. For example, in Slater's study,[2,209] the patients were older (mean age 39 years), with a higher percentage of males (33%), and only a third saw a psychiatrist before a diagnosis of hysteria was made by a neurologist.[207]

Thus, it would seem that a diagnosis of hysteria, when made in a psychiatric hospital or clinic (by a psychiatrist), does have some validity and remains uniform over a period of time.[5] Interestingly patients, who initially present to psychiatrists, are later found be suffering from alcohol dependence, personality disorders, depression and/or schizophrenia.[61,64,204,205,212]

The death rate from suicide and fatal neuromedical illnesses is significantly increased in the follow-up studies of patients presenting with conversion symptoms. This implies that the physician[2,64] must regard the conversion as well as dissociation symptoms seriously.

Older studies[176,209,211,213] indicate that the prognosis for different conversion symptoms differs and changes in symptoms over time are also seen.[205] About 25–50% remain symptomatic at follow-up. Several studies[46,116,176,213] have studied NES (nonepileptic seizures) and more than 20–50% of patients continued to have NES on follow-up. One study from Sudan[48] concluded that symptoms such as motor disturbances and aphonia had favorable prognosis but 'fits' (NES) had a poor outcome.[48]

One study[214] followed up patients with dissociative identity disorder over 2 years and found marked improvement in the symptoms and integration of the personality.

Wig, et al. (1982) suggested that patients presenting initially with monosymptomatic conversion symptoms had a better outcome.[46] Ford and Folks (1985) also suggested that most presentations of conversion hysteria might be expected to enjoy rapid symptom recovery.[186] Several other studies[46,48,53,75,198,213] have reported complete improvement of symptoms in 59–84%, particularly so if the improvement occurs in the initial period in hospital.[198] When conversion symptoms persist for several years, the disorder tends to resemble somatization disorder.[207]

Some studies[75,207] have also pointed out that the presence of premorbid hysterical personality disorder is a bad prognostic feature, while the presence of affective symptoms predicted a better outcome.[207] Other prognostic factors like presence of precipitating factor, better premorbid health, and type of symptoms did not make any difference in the outcome.

An older study[215] found a close association of hysteria with depression. 30% of their patients with conversion has depression while 28% of a group of depressive patients had conversion symptoms. Similarly, 58% of women (as compared with 10% of normal controls) reported depression in another study.[208] Other studies have also found significant comorbidity of depression with dissociative and conversion disorders.[40,216-218] Other comorbid disorders in addition to depression include borderline personality disorder, post-traumatic stress disorder, substance dependence or abuse[79] and somatization disorders.[219]

INVESTIGATIONS

Dissociative Experience Scale

The dissociative experience scale (DES)[220,221] is a self-report measure that requires subjects to indicate the frequency of 28 dissociative experiences, which are considered key aspects of the dissociation construct. These include[23] autobiographical amnesia, depersonalization, derealization, absorption, identity alteration, and gaps in the continuity of awareness. Similar events occurring under the influence of drugs and alcohol are excluded. The scale yields item, subscale, and total scores, which range from 0 to 100. Total scores are calculated by averaging the 28 item scores.[23] DES has been found to possess very good reliability and validity, and has a very good inter-rater and test-retest reliability. In a study,[79] 15% of general psychiatric inpatients were found to have a score of above 25 on DES, and all of these patients met DSM-III criteria for a dissociative disorder.

Elevated levels of DES scores are found in eating disorders, borderline personality disorder, somatization disorder, post-traumatic stress disorder, multiple personality disorder, other dissociative disorders, and about 5% of the general population.

Questionnaire of Experiences of Dissociation

Questionnaire of experiences of dissociation (QED) is a 26 item, true-false questionnaire[222] with a possible score between 0 and 26. A Hindi translation is also available.[94]

Dissociative Disorders Interview Schedule

The dissociative disorders interview schedule (DDIS) consists of 131 structured interview items,[223] based on DSM-IV.

Miscellaneous Scales

The other scales that have been used for the assessment of dissociative/conversion/hysterical symptoms include hysteroid-obsessoid questionnaire (HOQ),[224] somatoform dissociation questionnaire (SDQ-20),[225] peritraumatic dissociation index (for assessing dissociative symptoms in PTSD),[158] dissociation questionnaire (DIS-Q),[226] child dissociative checklist (CDC),[227] and autobiographical memory interview (AMI).[228]

Psychometry

MMPI (Minnesota Multiphasic Personality Inventory) shows elevated scores on hysteria and hypochondriasis scales, with lower depression scores (called as a conversion V pattern). However, this is neither invariable nor essential.[169] Similarly, classical signs have been described on Rorschach test like *erlebnistypus*or *extratensive balance* (EB), few M (movement) responses, labile use of color responses (CF+C>FC), crude W responses, among many others. However, projective tests are not diagnostic in dissociative or conversion disorders.

MANAGEMENT

It has been said that, "hysteria imposes a test on our professional skills."[6] The management of dissociative and conversion disorders involves a comprehensive medical, psychiatric and psychosocial evaluation of the patient. A thorough initial medical and neurological assessment is also crucial. Relevant investigations (like urinary drug screen to rule out drug use, EEG to rule out complex partial seizures, IQ testing to rule out borderline intellectual functioning) should be done whenever indicated. The possibility of dissociative or conversion symptoms superimposed on neurological or medical disorders, or other psychiatric disorders must always be considered. Attempt should be made to identify the patient's psychosocial stressors, coping abilities to handle stressful life situations, as well as secondary gains, if any.

The treatment usually consists of two parts: early treatment directed towards symptom removal, and long-term treatment directed towards resolution of conflicts and prevention of further episodes.

Psychotherapy

The cornerstones of successful therapy include establishment of rapport and therapeutic alliance. It is often useful to communicate to the patient that he is responding to the stresses in life. The therapist tries to help the patient be aware of his tendency to use dissociation and amnesia to deal with painful conflicts, and understand and accept his individual conflicts so they can be integrated into the primary personality.[21] Focusing of attention on the patient rather than on the symptoms can often help in decreasing or abolishing the symptoms. Strong suggestion for return to normalcy[48,213] and amplification of suggestion (with hypnosis, free-association, intravenous amobarbital or thiopentone, or intravenous diazepam) can often facilitate the rapid dissolution of symptoms.

As the symptoms begin to subside, patient may sometimes manifest depressive features or other conversion or dissociative features (called as *symptom substitution*). Occasionally, distress may be expressed by deliberate self-harm, damage to property, or demanding histrionic behavior. In such a condition, consistent limit setting may be essential for continuation of psychotherapy. Regularity of follow-up visits after discharge is important so that the patient does not need to 'produce' a symptom to visit the therapist.[229]

Problem-solving techniques and stress management techniques are important adjuncts of long-term successful therapy. Cognitive behavioral therapy (CBT) is often found not to be useful, as a majority of the patients of dissociative disorder are not cognitively oriented.[229] CBT techniques have, however, been applied successfully in the treatment of dissociative symptoms associated with trauma.[230] Direct confrontational approaches should be best avoided, as they only exacerbate repression and defensiveness.

Several options have been described for the treatment of multiple personality disorder. They include waiting for spontaneous resolution, attempting a resurgence of the main personality, focusing on the healthiest personality, treating each personality separately, and attempting a forced integration or fusion.[231,232] Although achievement of integration of personalities is considered desirable, all that can be achieved in some cases is a reasonable degree of conflict-free collaboration between the personalities.

Behavior Therapy

Typically, the therapist focuses on the current manifest behavior itself rather on its distant historical associations.[233]

Since patients with dissociative and conversion disorders are attention seeking and their symptoms increase with focus of attention, the symptoms should be ignored;[213] the patients not conferred a sick-role; and any improvement should be encouraged by providing more attention and giving praise.

Since these patients are also very suggestible, they respond quickly to above mentioned methods, and a consistently firm attitude. However, any confrontational approach towards the patient should be avoided. It is also very important that all members of the treating team should adopt such an approach.

When there is a sudden, acute symptom, its prompt removal may prevent habituation and future disability. This may be achieved by one of the following methods:

- *Aversion therapy* for unwanted behavior has been employed in resistant cases, using liquor ammonia, aversive Faradic stimulation,[48,234] pressure just above eyeballs, tragus of ear or over sternum, and closing the nose and mouth. But, the use of aversion as a mode of therapy should be decried as it tends to get over-used, may harm the patient, violates the basic human rights of the patient, and lends a wrong mental picture of the patient in the physician's mind, that of a 'manipulator' needing punishment.
- *Morrison's behavior modification technique*[235] involves selective attention (or inattention) and verbal rewards. This approach should be followed only after careful exclusion of any underlying physical illness (by clinical examination and completion of requisite investigations).
- The other behavioral techniques employed in the treatment include modeling, shaping, extinction (of symptomatic behavior), relaxation methods, systematic exposure (for anxiety-linked behavior) and operant conditioning (using reinforcements).[233]

Freud (1893) suggested that symptom removal does not cure hysteria and symptom substitution occurs ["You must not imagine that very much has been gained by this (symptomatic cure) for the therapeutics of hysteria"]. Eysenck and Beech (1971) countered that "cure the symptom (or rather the totality of symptoms...) and you have cured the disease."[236] Several studies[48,233] have suggested that symptom substitution is not common with the use of behavior therapy for symptom removal.

Abreaction

Abreaction is bringing to conscious awareness, thoughts, affects and memories for the first time, with or without the use of drugs. This may be achieved by:

- Hypnosis
- Free association, or
- Drugs, like intravenous barbiturates like thiopentone (Pentothal), amobarbital (Amytal), ketamine, diazepam, methylphenidate, or methamphetamine (methedrine).

The aim of abreaction with IV amobarbital or thiopentone is, both, to make the conflicts conscious and to make the patient more suggestible to therapist's advice. It is best to begin with neutral topics and to approach affect-laden or traumatic material gradually. Once the conflicts have become conscious and the associated affects have been released, the conversion/dissociative symptom disappears. Contraindications of the amytal/pentothal interview include history of porphyria, hypersensitivity to barbiturates, or substance-use disorder, presence of severe cardiac, hepatic or renal disease, and compromised respiratory function or airway obstruction.

However, psychiatrists have cautioned against the use of such techniques (particularly hypnosis) as they may foster further dissociative states and may encourage further separation of alter selves (in multiple personality disorder).[231] The patients treated with such techniques may perceive the therapist as sanctioning the dissociative states.[21]

Psychoanalysis and Psychodynamic Psychotherapy

Long-term insight-oriented psychotherapy (either psychoanalysis or psychoanalytical psychotherapy) is chosen not on the basis of conversion/dissociative symptoms but on the total personality structure of the patient. Some patients respond remarkably well. The total length of therapy may be five years or more. Shorter, expressive-supportive psychodynamic psychotherapy and brief, active psychodynamic psychotherapy have been used for treatment of dissociative disorders (e.g. multiple personality disorder) and conversion disorders.[147,237,238]

Drug Therapy

Drug treatment has a very limited role in dissociative (conversion) disorders (apart from the use of IV thiopentone, amytal or diazepam in abreaction and suggestion). Few patients have disabling symptoms and may need short-term benzodiazepines. As substance use disorder (often iatrogenic) is not an uncommon comorbid condition, care must taken in prescribing benzodiazepines. Associated depression (or more commonly, depression emerging after recovery) may need treatment with antidepressants. Antipsychotics may be indicated in patients presenting with hysterical psychosis and some patients of multiple personality disorder with persistent auditory hallucinations. However, most patients do not require drug treatment.

Placebo effect, although used sometimes in dissociative (conversion) disorders for diagnostic and treatment purposes, does not prove the diagnosis. Several other reasons exist for the placebo effect, like suggestibility, hypnotizability, and doctor-patient relationship.

Hospitalization

Admission to the inpatient setting can be helpful, if the symptoms are disabling or alarming to the family. A short-term admission (with a nongratifying restricted routine) can remove the patient from the stressful situation, demonstrate to the patient and significant others that the matter is important but will not elicit the kind of attention patient wants, and lead to the resolution of the trauma. Secondary gains must be minimized.

Family and Marital Therapy

Working simultaneously with the patient's family (and spouse, if married) is an important component of the management. Direct communication with the family members will also reduce the opportunities for manipulation and misunderstanding.

Group Therapy

These patients respond favorably to group therapies wherein the patients learn to confront each other with the relationship of stressors with symptoms, thereby reducing the demands on the therapist.[239] Participation in a group setting may diminish the patient's sense of loneliness, make available a secure place to discuss traumatic matter(s) that patients without dissociative disorder may not be able to tolerate, to study interpersonal relationships, to develop more functional interactions, and learn more about coping mechanisms. However, patients in a group may also develop profound pathologic transferences to one another and/or the treating therapist, learn new symptoms, and intensify their attention-seeking behavior by striving to be the sickest.[240]

Miscellaneous Therapies

Sometimes, in patients with treatment-resistant conversion symptoms, prokaletic therapy[241-243] and paradoxical therapy[110] have been found to be useful. Other techniques include providing inexact interpretations and environmental manipulation (e.g. isolation of individual members in mass hysteria; alteration of stress causing conditions at home).

REFERENCES

1. Micale M. Hysteria and its historiography: the future perspective. History of Psychiatry. 1990;1:33-124.
2. Slater E. Diagnosis of hysteria. Br Med J. 1965;1(5447):1395-9.
3. Kendell RE. A new look at hysteria. Medicine. 1974;30: 1780-2.
4. Ahuja N. Neurotic, stress-related and somatoform disorders. A Short Textbook of Psychiatry, 3rd edition. New Delhi: Jaypee Brothers Medical Publishers; 1995. pp. 85-91.
5. Freeman CPL. Neurotic disorders. In: Kendell RE, Zealley AK (Eds). Companion To Psychiatric Studies. 5th edition. Edinburgh: Churchill Livingstone; 1993. pp. 485-524.
6. Merskey H. The importance of hysteria. Br J Psychiatry. 1986; 149:23-8.
7. Cummings JL. Clinical Neuropsychiatry. Orlando: Grune and Stratton; 1985.
8. American Psychiatric Association. Diagnostic and Statistical Manual of Mental Disorders, 4th edition. Washington DC: APPI; 1994.
9. World Health Organization. The ICD-10 Classification of Mental and Behavioral Disorders: Diagnostic Criteria for Research. Geneva: WHO; 1992.
10. Guze SB. The diagnosis of hysteria: What are we trying to do? Am J Psychiatry. 1967;124:491-8.
11. Hyler SE, Spitzer RL. Hysteria split asunder. Am J Psychiatry. 1978;135:1500-04.
12. Veith I. Hysteria: The History of a Disease. Chicago: Univ of Chicago Press;1965.
13. Balodhi JP, Roy Chowdhury J. Psychiatric concepts in Atharvaveda: A review. Indian J Psychiatry. 1986;28:65-7.
14. Ahuja N. History of Psychiatry. In: Vyas JN, Ahuja N (Eds). Postgraduate Psychiatry. New Delhi: BI Chuchill Livingstone; 1992.
15. Harriman PL. Modern Psychology. New Jersey: Littlefield, Adams; 1963.
16. Abse DW. Hysteria and Related Mental Disorders: An Approach to Psychological Medicine, 2nd edition. Littleton: Wright-PSG; 1987.
17. Gould R, Miller BL, Goldberg MA, et al. The validity of hysterical signs and symptoms. J Nerv Ment Dis. 1986;174:593-7.
18. Mace CJ. Hysterical conversion, 1st edition. A history. Br J Psychiatry. 1992;161:369-77.
19. Jacquart D, Thomasset C. Sexuality and Medicine in Middle Ages. Trans. Adamson M. London: Polity Press.
20. Bliss EL. Multiple personality, Allied Disorders, and Hypnosis. New York: Oxford; 1986.
21. Gilmore MM, Kaufman C. Dissociative disorders. In: Michels R, Cavenar JO, Brodie HKH, et al (Eds). Psychiatry. Vol. 1, Chap. 39. New York: Lippincott; 1985. pp. 1-12.

22. Greaves GB. Multiple personality 165 years after Mary Reynolds. J Nerv Ment Dis. 1980;168:577-96.
23. Putnam FW, Carlson EB, Ross CA, et al. Patterns of dissociation in clinical and non-clinical samples. J Nerv Ment Dis. 1996; 184:673-9.
24. Stevenson RL. The Strange Case of Dr. Jekyll and Mr. Hyde (1877). Public Domain. Several editions.
25. Prince M. Dissociation of a Personality. New York: Longmans, Green and Co., 1906.
26. Thigpen CH, Cleckley H. The Three Faces of Eve. New York: McGraw Hill; 1957.
27. Schreiber FR. Sybil. Chicago: Regnery; 1973.
28. Viederman M. Somatoform and factitious disorders. In: Michels R, Cavenar JO, Brodie HKH, et al (Eds). Psychiatry. Vol. 1, Chap. 35. New York: Lippincott; 1985. pp. 1-20.
29. Abse DW. Hysterical conversion and dissociative syndromes and the hysterical character. In: Arieti S (Ed). American Handbook of Psychiatry, 2nd edition. New York: Basic Books; 1974. pp. 155-94.
30. Janet P. L'Automatism Psychologique. Paris: Felix Alcan; 1889.
31. Janet P. The Major Symptoms of Hysteria. New York: Macmillan; 1907.
32. Breuer J, Freud S. Studies on Hysteria (1893-1895): Complete Psychological Works. Standard Ed. Vol. 2. London: Hogarth Press; 1955.
33. Freud S. A disturbance of memory on the acropolis. In: Strachey J (Ed). The Complete Psychological Works of Sigmund Freud. London: Hogarth Press; 1964.
34. Freud S. Lecture quoted. In: Strachey J (Ed). The Complete Psychological Works of Sigmund Freud. London: Hogarth Press; 1962.
35. Ferenczi S (1919). The phenomenon of hysterical materialization. Further Contributions to the Theory and Technique of Psychoanalysis. New York: Brunner/Mazel; 1950. pp. 89-104.
36. Mace CJ. Hysterical conversion, 2nd edition. A critique. Br J Psychiatry. 1992;161:378-89.
37. Fairbairn WRD. Observations on the nature of hysterical states. Br J Med Psychol. 1954;27:105-25.
38. Brain WR. The concept of hysteria in the time of William Harvey.Proc Roy Soc Med. 1963;56:317-24.
39. Lewis A. The survival of hysteria. Psychol Med. 1975;5:9-12.
40. Wilson-Barnett J, Trimble MR. An investigation of hysteria using the illness behavior questionnaire. Br J Psychiatry. 1985; 146:601-8.
41. Chodoff P. The diagnosis of hysteria: An overview. Am J Psychiatry. 1974;131:1073-8.
42. Ross CA. Epidemiology of Multiple personality disorder and dissociation. Psychiatr Clin North Am. 1991;14:503-17.
43. Dutta Ray S, Mathur SB. Pattern of hysteria observed at psychiatric clinic, Irwin Hospital, Delhi. Indian J Psychiatry. 1966;8:32.
44. Bhattacharya DD, Bhardwaj P. Reassessment of Perley-Guze criteria for the diagnosis of hysteria: A study based on 304 Indian patients. Indian J Psychiatry. 1977;19:38-42.
45. Bagadia VN, Sastri PC, Shah LP. A prospective study of demographic factors of 192 cases of hysteria. Indian J Psychiatry. 1973;15(2):179-86.
46. Wig NN, Mangalwedhe K, Bedi H, et al. A follow-up study of hysteria. Indian J Psychiatry. 1982;24(2):120-5.
47. Vyas JN, Bhardwaj PK, Sharma KK. Aversion therapy in hysterical fits. Indian J Psychiatry. 1977;19(4):27-30.
48. Hafeiz HB. Hysterical conversion: A prognostic study. Br J Psychiatry. 1980;136:548-51.
49. Hafeiz HB. Clinical aspects of hysteria. Acta Psychiatr Scand. 1986;73:676-80.
50. Singh G. A clinical psychological study of hysteria. Indian J Psychiatry. 1968;10:84.
51. Khanna BC, Wig NN, Varma VK. General hospital psychiatric clinic: An epidemiological study. Indian J Psychiatry. 1974; 16(3):211-20.
52. Trivedi JK, Singh H, Sinha PK. A clinical study of hysteria in children and adolescents.Ind J Psychiatry. 1982;24:70-4.
53. Subramanian D, Subramaniam K, Devaky MN, et al. A clinical study of 276 patients diagnosed as suffering from hysteria. Indian J Psychiatry. 1980;22:63-8.
54. Somasundaram O, Raghavan GV, Krishan G. Hysteria in children and adolescents. Indian J Psychiatry. 1974;16:274.
55. Uma H, Kapur M. A retrospective study of hysteria in a child guidance clinic. Indian J Psychiatry. 1987;29:283-6.
56. Rock NL. Conversion reactions in childhood: A clinical study of childhood neurosis. J Am Acad Child Psychol. 1971;10:65-93.
57. Goodyer I. Hysterical conversion reactions in childhood. J Child Psychol Psychiat. 1981;22:179.
58. Robins E, O'Neal P. Clinical features in childhood with a note on prognosis. The Nervous Child. 1953;10:246-71.
59. Marfatia JC. Psychiatric problems of children. Bombay: Popular Prakashan; 1971.
60. Mathur KK. Hysterical reactions in a section of Indian soldiers. Indian J Psychiatry. 1975;17:179.
61. Marsden CD. Hysteria: A neurologist's view. Psychol Med. 1986;16:277-88.
62. Farley J, Woodruff RA, Guze SB. The prevalence of hysteria and conversion symptoms. Br J Psychiatry. 1968;114:1121-5.
63. Woodruff RA, Clayton PJ, Guze SB. Hysteria: AN evaluation of special diagnostic criteria by the study of randomly selected psychiatry clinic patients. Br J Psychiatry. 1969;115:1243-8.
64. Stefansson JG, Messina JS, Meyerowitz S. Hysterical neurosis, conversion type: Clinical and epidemiological considerations. Acta Psychiatr Scand. 1976;53:119-38.
65. Robins E, Purtell JJ, Cohen ME. Hysteria in men. N Engl J Med. 1952;246:677-85.
66. Parfitt DN, Gall CM. Psychogenic amnesia: The refusal to remember. J Ment Sci. 1944;90:511.
67. Kanzer M. Amnesia: A statistical study. Am J Psychiatry. 1939; 96:711-6.
68. Weinstein EA, Eck RA, Lyerly OG. Conversion hysteria in Appalachia. Psychiatry. 1969;32:334-41.
69. Trimble MR. Neuropsychiatry. Chichester: Wiley; 1981.

70. Das PS, Saxena S. Classification of dissociative states in DSM-III-R and ICD-10 (1989 draft). A study of Indian out-patients. Br J Psychiatry. 1991;159:425-7.
71. Saxena S, Prasad KVSR. DSM-III subclassification of dissociative disorders applied to psychiatry outpatients in India. Am J Psychiatry. 1989;146:261-7.
72. Lal N, Sethi BB, Tandon AK, et al. Child guidance clinic in a psychiatric hospital. Indian J Paed. 1976;43:59.
73. Lazare A. Conversion symptoms. N Engl J Med. 1981;305:745-8.
74. Nagaraja J. Hysterical twilight and fugue states in early adolescence. Indian J Psychiatry. 1969;11:46.
75. Chandrasekaran R, Goswami U, Sivakumar V, et al. Hysterical neurosis: A follow-up study. Acta Psychiatr Scand. 1994;89:174-9.
76. Alexander VK. A case study of multiple personality. J Abnorm Soc Psychol. 1956;52:272-6.
77. Adityanjee, Raju GSP, Khandelwal SK. Current Status of multiple personality disorder in India. Am J Psychiatry. 1989;146:1607-10.
78. Alexander PJ, Joseph S, Das A. Limited utility of ICD-10 and DSM-IV classification of dissociative and conversion disorders in India. Acta Psychiatr Scand. 1997;95:177-82.
79. Saxe GN, van der Kolk BA, Berkowitz R, et al. Dissociative disorders in psychiatric inpatients. Am J Psychiatry. 1993;150:1037-42.
80. Fahy TA. The diagnosis of multiple personality disorder: A critical review. Br J Psychiatry. 1988;153:597-606.
81. Piper A Jr. Multiple personality disorder. Br J Psychiatry. 1994;164:600-12.
82. Modestin J. Multiple personality disorder in Switzerland. Am J Psychiatry. 1992;149:88-92.
83. Thigpen CH, Cleckley HM. On the incidence of multiple personality disorder: A brief communication. Int J Clin Exp Hypn. 1984;32:63-6.
84. Stefanis C, Markidis M, Christodoulou G. Observations on the evolution of the hysterical symptomatology. Br J Psychiatry. 1976;128:269-75.
85. Nandi DN, Banerjee G, Nandi S, et al. Is hysteria on the wane? A community survey in West Bengal, India. Br J Psychiatry. 1992;160:87-91.
86. Manchanda M, Manchanda R. Neuroses in children: Epidemiological aspects. Indian J Psychiatry. 1978;20:161-5.
87. Raju VB, Sundaravalli N, Somasundaram O, et al. Neurotic disorders in children. Indian Paed. 1969;6:296.
88. American Psychiatric Association. Diagnostic and Statistical Manual of Mental Disorders, 1st edition. Washington DC: APPI; 1952.
89. American Psychiatric Association. Diagnostic and Statistical Manual of Mental Disorders, 2nd edition. Washington DC: APPI; 1968.
90. American Psychiatric Association. Diagnostic and Statistical Manual of Mental Disorders, 3rd edition. Washington DC: APPI, 1980.
91. American Psychiatric Association. Diagnostic and Statistical Manual of Mental Disorders, 3rd edition. Rev. Washington DC: APPI; 1987.
92. Saxena S, Pachauri R, Wig NN. DSM-III diagnostic categories for ICD-9 hysteria: A study on 103 cases. Indian J Psychiatry. 1986;28:47-9.
93. Nemiah JC. Dissociative disorders. In: Kaplan HI, Sadock BJ (Eds). Comprehensive Textbook of Psychiatry, 6th edition. Baltimore: Williams and Wilkins; 1995. pp. 1281-94.
94. Katoch V, Jhingan HP, Saxena S. Level of anxiety and dissociation in patients with conversion and dissociative disorders. Indian J Psychiatry. 1994;36:67-9.
95. Bowman ES, Markand ON. Psychodynamics and psychiatric diagnoses of pseudoseizure subjects. Am J Psychiatry. 1996;153:57-63.
96. Nemiah JC. Dissociation. Conversion, and Somatization. In: Tasman A, Goldfinger SM (Eds). American Psychiatric Press Review of Psychiatry. Vol. 10, Washington DC: APPI; 1991. pp. 248-60.
97. Marjama J, Troster AI, Koller WC. Psychogenic movement disorders. Neurol Clin. 1995;13(2):283-97.
98. Keane JR. Hysterical gait disorders: 60 cases. Neurology. 1989;39:586-9.
99. Perez-Sales P. Camptocormia. Br J Psychiatry. 1990;157:765-7.
100. Cooper IS, Cullinan T, Riklan M. The natural history of dystonia. Adv Neurol. 1976;14:157-69.
101. Eldrige R, Riklan M, Cooper IS. The limited role of psychotherapy in torsion dystonia: Experiences with 44 cases. JAMA. 1969;210:705-8.
102. Fahn S, Williams D. Psychogenic dystonia. Adv Neurol. 1988;50:431-55.
103. Lafforgue P, Toussirot E, Bille F, et al. Astasia-abasia revealing a primary Sjögren's syndrome. Clin Rheum. 1993;12:261-4.
104. Wolf M, Birger M, Ben Shoshan J, et al. Conversion deafness. Ann Oto Rhin Laryng. 1993;102:349-52.
105. Rover J, Bach M. Pattern electroretinogram plus visual evoked potential: A decisive test in patients suspected of malingering. Doc Ophthalmol. 1987;66:245-51.
106. Wilbourn AJ. The electrodiagnostic examination with hysteria-conversion reaction and malingering. Neurol Clin. 1995;13(2):385-404.
107. Glaser G. Epilepsy, hysteria and possession. J Nerv Ment Dis. 1978;166:268-74.
108. King DW, Gallagher BB, Murvin AJ, et al. Pseudoseizures: Diagnostic evaluation. Neurology. 1982;32:18-23.
109. Liske E, Forster F. Pseudoseizures: A problem in the diagnosis and management of epileptic patients. Neurology. 1964;14:41-9.
110. Fenton GW. Epilepsy and hysteria. Br J Psychiatry. 1986;149:28-37.
111. Betts TA. Pseudoseizures: Seizures that are not epilepsy. Lancet. 1990;336:163-4.
112. Trimble MR. Pseudoseizures. Neurol Clin. 1986;4(3):531-48.
113. Saxena S. Simple dissociative disorder: A subcategory in DSM-III-R? Am J Psychiatry. 1987;144:524-5.

114. Lesser RP. Psychogenic seizures. Neurology. 1986:27:923-9.
115. VenkatRamani S, Quesney LF, Olson D, et al. Diagnosis of hysterical seizures in epileptic patients. Am J Psychiatry. 1980; 137:705-9.
116. Lempert T, Schmidt D. Natural history and outcome of psychogenic seizures: A clinical study in 50 patients. J Neurol. 1990;237:35-8.
117. Rechlin T, Loew TH, Joraschky P. Pseudoseizure status. J Psychosom Res. 1997;42:495-8.
118. Wilner AN, Brean PR. Status epilepticus and pseudostatus epilepticus. Seizure. 1993;2:257-60.
119. Sengupta SN, Jena S, Saxena S. Generalized dissociative amnesia. Aust NZ J Psychiatry. 1993;27:699-700.
120. Kapur N. Amnesia in relation to fugue states: Distinguishing a neurological from a psychogenic basis. Br J Psychiatry. 1991; 159:872-7.
121. Kopelman MD, Panayiotopoulos CP, Lewis P. Transient epileptic amnesia differentiated from psychogenic 'fugue': Neuropsy-chological, EEG, and PET findings. J Neurol Neurosurg Psychiatry. 1994;57:1002-4.
122. Miller JW, Peterson RC, Metter EJ, et al. Transient global amnesia: Clinical characteristics and prognosis. Neurology. 1987;37:733-7.
123. Hodges JR, Ward CD. Observations during transient global amnesia: A behavioural nd neuropsychological study of 5 cases. Brain. 1989;112:595-620.
124. Schenk L, Bear D. Multiple personality and related dissociative phenomenon in patients with temporal lobe epilepsy. Am J Psychiatry. 1981;138:1311-6.
125. Mayeux R, Alexander MP, Benson DF, et al. Poriomania. Neurology. 1979;29:1616-9.
126. Lishman WA. Organic Psychiatry: The Psychological Consequences of Cerebral Disorder. Oxford: Blackwell; 1998.
127. Coons PM. Dissociative identity disorder not otherwise specified: A clinical investigation of 50 cases with suggestions for typology and treatment. Dissociation. 1992;5:187-95.
128. Ross CA, Anderson G, Fraser G, et al. Differentiating multiple personality disorder and dissociative disorder NOS. Dissociation. 1992;5:87-90.
129. Boon S, Draijer N. Multiple Personality in the Netherlands. Amsterdam: Swets and Zeitlinger; 1993.
130. Kluft RP (Ed). Childhood Antecedents of Multiple Personality Disorder. Washington DC: APPI; 1985.
131. Putnam FW, Guroff JJ, Silberman EK, et al. The clinical phenomenology of multiple personality disorder: Review of 100 recent cases. J Clin Psy. 1986;47:285-93.
132. Ross CA. Dissociative Identity Disorder: Diagnosis, Clinical Features, and Treatment of Multiple Personality, 2nd edition. New York: John Wiley; 1997.
133. Shearer SL. Dissociative phenomena in women with borderline personality disorder. Am J Psychiatry. 1994;151:1324-8.
134. Mezzich JE, Fabrega H, Coffman GA, et al. DSM-III disorders in a large sample of psychiatric patients: frequency and specificity of diagnoses. Am J Psychiatry. 1989;146:212-9.
135. Loftus EF. Creating false memories. Sci Am; 1997. pp. 70-75.
136. Loftus EF, Garry M, Feldman J. Forgetting sexual trauma: What does it mean when 38% forget? J Consult Clin Psychol. 1994;62: 1177-81.
137. American Medical Association Council on Scientific Affairs. Scientific status of refreshing recollection by the use of hypnosis. JAMA. 1985;253:1918-23.
138. Caul D. Group and videotape techniques for multiple personality disorder. Psychiat Ann. 1984;14:43-50.
139. Putnam FW. Diagnosis and Treatment of Multiple Personality Disorder. New York: Guilford; 1989.
140. Varma VK, Bouri M, Wig NN. Multiple personality in India: Comparison with hysterical possession state. Am J Psychother. 1981;35:113-20.
141. Castillo RJ. Spirit possession in South Asia: Dissociation or hysteria? Part 2. Case histories. Culture Med Psychiatry. 1994; 18:141-62.
142. Ferracuti S, Sacco R, Lazzari R. Dissociative trance disorder: Clinical and Rorschach findings in ten persons reporting demon possession and treated by exorcism. J Personal Assess. 1996;66:525-39.
143. Osterreich TK. Possession: Demonical and other. New York: University Books.
144. Kiev A. Spirit possession in Haiti. Am J Psychiatry. 1961;118:133.
145. Teja JS, Khanna BC, Subramanyam TS. Possession states in Indian patients. Ind J Psychiatry. 1970;12:71-8.
146. Yap PH. The possession syndrome: A comparison of Hong Kong and French findings. J Ment Sci. 1960;106:114.
147. Kluft RP. The post-unification treatment of multiple personality disorder: First findings. Am J Psychother. 1988;42:212-28.
148. Kluft RP. The dissociative disorders. In: Talbott JA, Hales RE, Yudofsky SC (Eds). The American Psychiatric Press Textbook of Psychiatry. Washington DC: APPI; 1988.
149. Rosen G. Madness in Society. London: Routledge, Kegan and Paul; 1968.
150. Sirois F. Epidemic hysteria. Acta Psychiatr Scand. 1974; 252(Suppl).
151. Wessely S. Mass hysteria: two syndromes? Psychol Med. 1987; 17:109-20.
152. Ali-Gombe A, Guthrie E, McDermott N. Mass hysteria: One syndrome or two. Br J Psychiatry. 1996;168:633-5.
153. Varma LP, Srivastav DK, Sahay RN. Possession syndrome. Indian J Psychiatry. 1970;12:58-70.
154. Nandi D, Banerjee G, Bera S, et al. Contagious hysteria in a West Bengal village. Am J Psychother. 1985;39: 247-52.
155. Narayanan HS, Mahal AS. A clinical report of epidemic hysteria in six members of a family. Indian J Psychiatry. 1977;19(3): 39-42.
156. Good MI. Organic dissociative syndrome associated with antimigraine pharmacotherapy. Can J Psychiatry. 1991;36: 597-9.
157. Reither AM, Stoudemire A. Psychogenic fugue states: A review. South Med J. 1988;81:568-71.

158. Griffin MG, Resick PA, Mechanic MB. Objective assessment of peritraumatic dissociation: Psychophysiological indicators. Am J Psychiatry. 1997;154:1081-8.
159. Holen A. The North Sea oil rig disaster. In: Wilson JP, Raphael B (Eds). International Handbook of Traumatic Stress Syndromes. New York: Plenum; 1993.
160. Koopman C, Classen C, Spiegel D. Predictors of posttraumatic stress symptoms among survivors among survivors of the Oakland/Berkeley, Calif, firestorm. Am J Psychiatry. 1994;151: 888-94.
161. Janet P. Les Obsessions et la psychasthenie. Paris: Felix Alcan; 1903.
162. Schilder P. The Image and Appearance of the Human Body. New York: International Universities Press; 1950.
163. Buss AH. Psychopathology. New York: John Wiley; 1966.
164. Butler LD, Duran REF, Jasiukaitis, et al. Hypnotizability and traumatic experience: A diathesis-stress model of dissociative symptomatology. Am J Psychiatry. 1996;153(Suppl):S42-S63.
165. Hilgard ER. Divided Consciousness: Multiple Controls in Human Thought and Action. New York: Wiley; 1986.
166. Zeigler FJ, Jolla LA, Imboden JB. Contemporary conversion reaction, 2nd edition: A conceptual model. Arch Gen Psychiatry. 1962;6:279-87.
167. Wolpe J. Psychotherapy by Reciprocal Inhibition. Stanford: Stanford University Press; 1958.
168. Dollard J, Miller NE. Personality and psychotherapy. New York: McGraw-Hill; 1950.
169. Guggenheim FG, Smith GR. Somatoform disorders. In: Kaplan HI, Sadock BJ. Comprehensive Textbook of Psychiatry, 6th edition. Baltimore: Williams and Wilkins; 1995. pp. 1251-70.
170. Ludwig AM. Hysteria: A neurobiological theory. Arch Gen Psychiatry. 1972;27:771-7.
171. Whitlock FA. The etiology of hysteria. Acta Psychiatr Scand 1967;43:144-62.
172. Rossini ED, Schwartz DR, Braun BG. Intellectual functioning of inpatients with dissociative identity disorder and dissociative disorder not otherwise specified: Cognitive and neuropsychological aspects. J Nerv Ment Dis. 1996;184:289-94.
173. Flor-Henry P, Fromm Auch D, Tapper M, et al. A neuropsychological study of the stable syndrome of hysteria. Biol Psychiatry. 1981;16:601-26.
174. Levy R, Muskin J. Somatosensory evoked potentials in patients with hysterical anesthesia. J Psychosom Res. 1973;17:81.
175. Smith AC. Hysteria. In: Rawd E, Hudson B (Eds). Current Themes in Psychiatry. London: Macmillan; 1978.
176. Ljungberg L. Hysteria: A clinical, prognostic and genetic study. Acta Psychiatr Neurol Scand. 1957;32:(Suppl 112):1-162.
177. Kopelman MD. Amnesia: Organic and psychogenic. Br J Psychiatry. 1987;150:428-42.
178. Mathews RJ, Jack RA, West WS. Regional blood flow in a patient with multiple personality. Am J Psychiatry. 1985;142:504-5.
179. Pincus J. Hysteria. Chichester: John Wiley; 1982.
180. Galin D, Diamond R, Graff D. Lateralization of conversion symptoms: More frequent on the left. Am J Psychiatry. 1977; 134:578-80.
181. Bishop ER, Mobley MC, Forr WE. Lateralization of conversion symptoms. Compr Psychiatry. 1978;19:393-6.
182. Stern DB. Handedness and the lateral distribution of conversion reactions. J Nerv Ment Dis. 1977;164:122-8.
183. Sharma P, Chaturvedi SK. Conversion disorder revisited. Acta Psychiatrica Scand. 1995;92:301-4.
184. Weintroub MI. Hysterical conversion symptoms: A clinical guide to diagnosis and treatment. New York: SP Medical; 1983.
185. Hollender MH. Conversion hysteria: A post-Freudian re-interpretation of 19th century psychosocial data. Arch Gen Psychiatry. 1972;26:311-4.
186. Ford CV, Folks DG. Conversion disorders: An overview. Psychosomatics. 1985;26:371-83.
187. Celani D. An interpersonal approach to hysteria. Am J Psychiatry. 1976;133:1414-8.
188. Engel GL. Conversion symptoms. In: MacBryde CM, Blacklow RS (Eds). Signs and Symptoms, 5th edition. London: Pitman Medical; 1970. pp. 650-68.
189. Szasz TS. The Myth of Mental Illness: Foundations of a Theory of Personal Conduct. New York: Harper and Row; 1961.
190. Kirshner LA. Dissociative reaction: An historical review and clinical study. Acta Psychiatr Scand. 1973;49:696-711.
191. Parsons T. The Social System. New York: Free Press; 1951.
192. Kretschmer E. Hysteria. Transl. Batz OH. New York: Nervous and Mental Disease Publishing Co., 1926.
193. Kretschmer E. Hysteria, Reflex and Instinct. Transl. Baskin V & W. London: Peter Owen; 1961.
194. Taylor DC. Hysteria, play-acting and courage. Br J Psychiatry. 1986;149:37-41.
195. Chance MRA, Russell WMS. Protean displays: A form of all aesthetic behavior. Proc Zoo Soc London 1959;132:65-70 Cited in Taylor DC (1986).
196. Jackson HD. The selected writings of Hughlings Jackson. Vol. I & Vol. II, New York: Basic Books; 1958.
197. Head H. The diagnosis of hysteria. Br Med J. 1922;1:827-9.
198. Couprie W, Wijdicks EFM, Rooijmans HGM, et al. Outcome of conversion disorder: A follow-up study. J Neurol Neurosurg Psychiatry. 1995;58:750-2.
199. Chambers WR. Neurosurgical conditions masquerading as psychiatric diseases. Am J Psychiatry. 1955;112:387-9.
200. Lader M, Sartorius N. Anxiety in patients with hysterical conversion symptoms. J Neurol Neurosurg Psychiat. 1968;31: 490-5.
201. Chodoff P, Lyons H. Hysteria, the hysterical personality and 'hysterical' conversion. Am J Psychiatry. 1958;114:734-40.
202. Merskey H, Trimble M. Personality, sexual adjustment and brain lesions in patients with conversion symptoms. Am J Psychiatry. 1979;136:179-82.
203. De Alarcon R. Hysteria and the hysterical personality: How come one without the other? Psychiatr Quart. 1973;47: 258-75.
204. Guze SB, Woodruff RA, Clayton PJ. A study of conversion symptoms in psychiatric outpatients. Am J Psychiatry. 1971; 128:643-6.

205. Boffeli TJ, Guze SB. The simulation of neurologic disease. Psychiatr Clin North Am. 1992;15(2):301-10.
206. Watson CG, Buranen C. The frequency and identification of false positive conversion reactions. J Nerv Ment Dis. 1979;167: 243-7.
207. Mace CJ, Trimble MR. Ten-year prognosis of conversion disorder. Br J Psychiatry. 1996;169:282-8.
208. Purtell JJ, Robins E, Cohen ME. Observations on clinical aspects of hysteria: A quantitative study of 50 hysteria patients and 156 control subjects. JAMA. 1951;146:902-9.
209. Slater E, Glithero E. A follow-up of patients diagnosed as suffering from 'hysteria.' J Psychosom Res. 1965;9:9-13.
210. Merskey H, Buhrich NA. Hysteria and organic brain disease. Br J Med Psychol. 1975;48:359-66.
211. Gatfield PD, Guze SB. Prognostic and differential diagnosis of conversion reactions: A follow-up study. Dis Nerv Sys. 1962;23: 623-31.
212. Zeigler FJ, Imbolden JB, Meyer E. Contemporary conversion reactions: A clinical study. Am J Psychiatry. 1960;116: 901-10.
213. Carter AB. The prognosis of certain hysterical symptoms. Br Med J. 1949;1(4615):1076-9.
214. Ellason JW, Ross CA. Two-year follow-up of inpatients with dissociative identity disorder. Am J Psychiatry. 1997;154:832-9.
215. Zeigler FJ, Imboden JB, Rodgers DA. Contemporary conversion reaction, 3rd edition: Diagnostic considerations. JAMA. 1963; 186:307.
216. Roy A. Hysteria. J Psychosom Res. 1980;24:53-6.
217. Ellason JW, Ross CA, Fuchs DL. Lifetime axis I and II comorbidity, and childhood trauma history in dissociative identity disorder. Psychiatry. 1996;78:707-16.
218. Klerman GL. In: Roy A (Ed). Hysteria. Chichester: Wiley; 1982.
219. Saxe GN, Chinman G, Berkowitz R, et al. Somatization in patients with dissociative disorders. Am J Psychiatry. 1994;151: 1329-34.
220. Bernstein EM, Putnam FW. Development, reliability and validity of a dissociation scale. J Nerv Ment Dis. 1986;174: 727-35.
221. Carlson EB, Putnam FW. An update on the dissociative experiences scale. Dissociation. 1993;6:16-27.
222. Riley KC. Measurement of dissociation. J Nerv Ment Dis. 1988; 176:449-50.
223. Ross CA, Heber S, Norton GR, et al. The Dissociative Disorders Interview Schedule: A structured interview. Dissociation. 1989; 2:169-89.
224. Caine TN, Hope K. Manual of Hysteroid-obsessoid questionnaire. London: University of London Press; 1967.
225. Nijenhuis ERS, Spinhoven P, van Dyck R, et al. The development and psychometric characteristics of the somatoform dissociation questionnaire (SDQ-20). J Nerv Ment Dis. 1996; 184:688-94.
226. Vanderlinden J, van Dyck R, Vandereycken W, et al. The dissociation questionnaire: Development and characteristics of a new self-reporting questionnaire. Clin Psychol Psychother. 1993;1:21-7.
227. Putnam FW, Helmers K, Trickett PK. Development, reliability and validity of a child dissociative scale. Child Abuse and Neglect. 1993;17:731-41.
228. Kopelman MD. The autobiographical memory interview (AMI) in organic and psychogenic amnesia. Memory. 1994;2:211-35.
229. Murphy GE. The clinical management of hysteria. JAMA. 1982; 18:2559-64.
230. Kennerley H. Cognitive therapy of dissociative symptoms associated with trauma. Br J Clin Psychol. 1996;35:325-40.
231. Bowers M, Brecher S. The emergence of multiple personality in the course of hypnotic investigation. In J Clin Exp Hypn. 1955; 3:188-99.
232. Bradsma J, Ludwig A. A case of multiple personality: Diagnosis and therapy. Int J Clin Exp Hypn. 1974;22:216-33.
233. Bird J. The behavioral treatment of hysteria. Br J Psychiatry. 1979;134:129-37.
234. Vyas JN, Bhardwaj PK. A study of hysteria: An analysis of 304 patients. Indian J Psychiatry. 1977;19(4):71-4.
235. Morrison JR. Management of Briquet's syndrome (hysteria). West J Med. 1978;128:482-7.
236. Eysenck HS, Beech HR. Counter-conditioning and related methods in behavior therapy. In: Bergin EE, Garfield SL (Eds). Handbook of Psychotherapy and Behavior Change. New York: Wiley; 1971.
237. Putnam FW, Loewenstein RJ. Treatment of multiple personality disorder: A survey of current practices. Am J Psychiatry. 1993; 150:1048-52.
238. Viederman M. Metaphor and meaning in conversion disorder: a brief, active therapy. Psychosom Med. 1995;57:403-9.
239. Valko RJ. Group therapy with patients of hysteria. Dis Nerv Sys. 1976;37:484-7.
240. Jacobson JL, Jacobson AM. Psychiatric Secrets. New Delhi: Jaypee Brothers; 1996.
241. Kraupl-Taylor F. Prokaletic measures derived from psycho-analytic technique. Br J Psychiatry. 1869;115:407-19.
242. Neeleman J, Mann AH. Treatment of hysterical aphonia with hypnosis and prokaletic therapy. Br J Psychiatry. 1993;163:816-9.
243. American Psychiatric Association. Desk Reference to the Diagnostic Criteria from DSM-5. Washington DC; 2013.

CHAPTER

21 Malingering and Factitious Disorders

Sandeep Grover, Munish Agarwal, Ajit Avasthi

INTRODUCTION

Diagnosing, distinguishing and managing malingering, factitious disorder and dissociative states can be very important clinical challenge. All these disorders have certain commonalities and important distinguishing features. Malingering can best be conceptualized a focus of clinical attention rather than as a psychopathological condition in itself. Although any medical condition may be faked, malingering of psychiatric disorders is perhaps commoner than previously considered and is particularly difficult to detect. Factitious disorder thought to lie somewhere in between malingering and dissociative disorder as there is intentional production of the symptoms and absence of any obvious external motive and the desire to produce symptom arises subconsciously. In the dissociative states patient presents with symptoms, for which there is no tangible external motivation and the symptoms are produced unconsciously. The dissociative disorders are understood as a disturbance in the organization of identity, memory, perception, or consciousness.

Malingering

Malingering is not considered to be a medical or psychiatric diagnosis. However, physicians or psychiatrists may encounter such subjects in their routine practice or may be called upon to evaluate them as part of medicolegal proceedings. Although any disorder may be simulated, malingerers particularly favor psychiatric disorders as these are difficult to identify objectively. The commonly seen malingered psychiatric symptoms are mental retardation or mental deficiency, dementia or cognitive disorders, amnesia, psychosis which may include hallucinations or delusions or both, post-traumatic residual symptoms. Besides the motivations of feigning symptoms for external incentives, the motive behind feigning of psychiatric symptoms can be getting disability or social benefits, claim compensation after any accidental injury, settle scores with hated employer, etc.

Prevalence

It is estimated that the prevalence of malingering among mental health patients is around 1% in civilian clinical practice and 5% is the military context. The rates of malingering psychological symptoms following personal injury vary from 1–50%. As expected, in a medicolegal setting, the prevalence is reported to be between 10% and 20%, which is higher than in other conditions and may be spuriously inflated due to the adversarial nature of such evaluation (Hickling et al., 1999). Malingering has been reported across all age groups including children.

Definition as Per Current Nosology

Malingering is defined in DSM-IVTR as the intentional production of false or grossly exaggerated physical or psychological symptoms, motivated by external incentives such as avoiding military duty, avoiding work, obtaining principal compensation, evading criminal prosecution or obtaining drugs (American Psychiatric Association, 2000). It further mentions that, under some circumstances, it may represent adaptive behaviour.

Historical and Conceptual Issues

Malingering has been said to be synonymous with faking, lying and fraud and these have been integral parts of human behavior since the earliest times. Lying seems to extend across a spectrum with normal behavior at one end, malingering at the other end and personality disorders, somatoform disorders and factitious disorders in between. Descriptions of feigned madness appear in the Bible. The earliest scientific reference to malingering can be found in “On Feigned Disease and the detection of them” by Galen in 2nd century AD and the first notable American text on the subject was Theodore Beck’s ‘Elements of Medial Jurisprudence’. In the 20th century, one of the earliest landmark studies in this field was carried out by Rosenhan (1973), entitled “On being sane in an insane place” which highlighted the difficulties in detecting malingering of mental illness. Thereafter, over the past 4th decades, there has been a renewed interest in this area, which may be due to an increasing awareness and proliferation of knowledge about various psychiatric disorders.

Conceptually malingering has been understood as a disease and as an adaptive response. From the disease point of view, those with psychoanalytic background consider it to be an arrest of development at an early phase and it reflects an ineffectual attempt to keep other symptoms under control. Studies have also shown some evidence in favor of this conceptualization, in that those malingering an illness actually turnout to be ill, when followed over a course of time. However, such studies are few and contemporary literature has pointed out that the disease model is flawed because it perceives a breakdown between conscious and unconscious psychological defense mechanisms, which is not evident in all cases. Moreover, most of these subjects miraculously recover from their symptoms after termination of litigation. So, currently malingering is not considered to be either a disease or indicative of a disease. However, an overlap between psychopathology and malingering may still occur, and is important to identify. According to the adaptative response model malingering represents an adaptation to hostile circumstances. According to this model there are two broad dimensions in malingering, i.e. cost-benefit analysis and adversarial setting. Malingerers perceive the environment in 'adversarial and risky' terms and malingering is seen as a behavior, which maximizes the chances for success in such a situation. Although this model may account for a small percentage of malingerers, it has been criticized for its failure to account for those who malinger purely for profit. On the other hand, this model is preferred by some, as it seems to be minimally pejorative.

The DSM concept of malingering is the most recently proposed one and is widely accepted as being the ultimate among the above concepts. However, the DSM concept of malingering is in stark contrast to the above two models. It relies on specific objective criteria for its definition rather than theoretical constructs. It lists malingering as an additional condition that may be a focus of clinical attention. It is suggested that malingering should be suspected when there is a medicolegal context of presentation; discrepancy between subjective complaints and objective findings; lack of co-operation during diagnostic evaluation and treatment; and antisocial personality disorder.

Out of the four criteria given in DSM, the criteria of discrepancy between subjective complaints and objective findings has been suggested as being the most reliable of all four criteria with empirical support. According to one study, discrepancies between subjective complaints and objective findings were absent only in 6.0% of malingerers in contrast to 74.5% of control subjects (non-malingering, psychiatric inpatients). However, some of the researchers argues that the DSM approach to malingering is that of a "criminological" model and is vague, binary, unsupported by research, moralistic and should be abandoned.

Subtyping of Malingering

Malingering may be *pure or partial* and *positive or negative.* Pure malingering implies false production of non-existent symptoms while partial malingering implies exaggeration of pre-existing symptoms. Positive malingering implies that the subject is feigning the symptoms of an illness while negative malingering implies that the subject is hiding or misreporting the symptoms. Data tampering, staging of false events, false imputation and misattribution of symptoms are also mentioned as being subtypes of malingering varying in the degree of intentionality, symptom exaggeration and actual impairment. Staging events means carefully planning, orchestrating and executing events, which might result later in an injury or an explanation for a feigned disability. Data tampering involves altering diagnostic instruments, data or record, so as to influence the results of an examination or test. False imputation involves ascribing actual symptoms to a cause consciously understood to have no relation to the symptoms and misattribution implies ascribing actual symptom to a cause erroneously believed to have given rise to them. It may, however, involve unconscious processes and may not always be a part of malingering.

Assessment of Malingering

Malingering should be suspected in situations involving atypical, bizarre or absurd presentation in the context of external motives, when there are criminal cases related to competency or criminal responsibility, when there is marked discrepancy between subjective complaints and objective findings, or there is lack of co-operation during diagnostic evaluation and presence of antisocial personality disorder. DSM-IV particularly cautions clinicians and researchers to rule out malingering when issues of compensation apply in order to prevent a false rise in the post-traumatic stress disorder database (Rosen, 2006). As there is no single test, which can confirm that a subject is malingering, once it is suspected, a systematic approach incorporating all the clues should be employed.

Steps to be followed while evaluation includes:

Interview

Interview with the patient: This should be long, detailed, gruelling and as early as possible after the event in question. It is difficult for the malingerer to maintain guard for protracted periods of time. The subject may be asked leading questions about a different illness to see how they respond to it. An elaborate 5-step 'Cross Examination Clinical Interview' should include: listen, tag, confront, solve and approve. The first step involves asking open-ended questions and encouraging elaboration, not giving any clues to the suspicion held by the examiner. Tagging implies double-checking the subject's story for accuracy, clarification and identifying rehearsed statements, inconsistencies, excessive details and attitude. In the confrontation phase, the subject's inconsistencies are pointed out by juxtaposing contradictions in a questioning but non-threatening manner. Thereafter, a process of yes or no questioning is initiated and kept up despite resistance by the patient. Finally, disclosure is greeted by approval of the subject's decision to take steps toward recovery. The central emphasis during the whole interview is on maintaining an alliance with the subject while taking the position of an adversary to his lie but not to him.

Interview of collateral sources: This may serve to refute or confirm the patient's information or provide additional information.

Review of records of prior functioning: Records of prior functioning at the work place may be reviewed to confirm or refute any evidence of claimed disability. Any history of substance abuse, psychiatric illness or antisocial acts will increase the suspicion of malingering.

Observation

Important points need to be noted both during the interview with the subject and across time and situations.

Observation during interview situation: Verbal behavior, facial expressions and bodily gestures may provide important clues. Subjects who are lying tend to speak in high-pitched voices; make frequent grammatical errors and also hesitate and pause during interviews more than genuine subjects. Their pauses may be filled with non-informative fillers such as "uh, er. Ah". However, changes in pitch and volume are less reliable indicators of deception. Gestures and facial expression are less apt to be rehearsed since facial muscles are under both voluntary and involuntary control. In addition, false affects are 'deliberate'; 'prolonged' and lack the usual 'crescendo-decrescendo" of natural affects. The quality of a false smile also differs from a genuine one as it is asymmetric; usually involving only the lower face. With respect to specific emotions, "anger" and "surprise" can be more readily feigned as compared to the other emotions. The timing of affective display may be either early or late as compared to normal subjects. Some changes associated with emotions viz. "blanching" or "flushing" are difficult to feign for obvious reasons. Body movements are less frequently monitored by a malingerer and are a good source of leakage. In a malingerer, illustrators, i.e. gestures that accompany speech are used less frequently; emblems, i.e. gestures that communicate a specific meaning in a specific culture, may be discordant with the spoken language, and manipulators, i.e. movements involving self-grooming, scratching, pulling, rubbing another body part and use of props viz. a pen, are distinctly prolonged and frequently repeated by the subject.

Longitudinal Observation: Observational methods to confirm suspicion of malingering may involve controlled environment observation, i.e. clinical observation of behaviors in an in-patient unit and real world surveillance. This is most advantageous when physical disabilities are claimed and involves covert observations and video recordings of the claimant. Due to inherent stress in attempting to maintain deception for 24 hours a day; there is often a breakdown of the discipline required, thus providing an opportunity for detection of the same.

Psychological Tests

In a quest to ensure objectivity, various psychological tests have been used as an aid to detect malingering. However, it is important to note that these are not necessary, as none has been found to be definitive, but can be a useful adjunct to support this diagnosis. These may only be considered as supportive indicator that can be put up as corroborating evidence to establishing the diagnosis of malingering. Nevertheless, when used an examiner is likely to detect malingering on these tests because malingerers do not known when to start faking; they fail on simple items but may pass the difficult ones and will have patterns of error different from those with a genuine impairment and cannot gear their responses to the reported level of impairment. The most commonly used instruments are Minnesota Multiphasic Personality Inventory, Structured Interview of Reported Symptoms, personality assessment inventory, structured inventory of malingered symptomatology and Rorschach test. Some of these instruments have been developed with particular attention to the response style of the subjects and this constitutes their strength in detecting fake responses.

Other scales like M-Test, Wildman symptom checklist, Trauma Symptom Inventory, Mississippi Scale for Combat-Related PTSD, Morel Emotional Numbing Test for PTSD have been investigated for the detection of malingered PTSD. However, results have not been encouraging.

Factitious Disorder

Factitious disorder is one of the most unique and challenging phenomena in clinical practice. It involves efforts to garner gratification intrinsic to the sick role through the simulation, exaggeration, aggravation or induction of physical or psychological signs and symptoms. In this role, sick individuals are excused from social responsibility, are expected to perceive their condition as undesirable, lack voluntary control over it and are therefore not considered at fault, and are expected to seek help medical help in ameliorating or curing the condition. Usually, the patient's primary goal is to receive medical, surgical, or psychiatric care to gratify some unconscious psychological needs. Factitious disorders with physical signs and symptoms have been described quite frequently, in the form of factitious hematuria, hemoptysis, torsion dystonia, feculent urine, self-mutilation, pulmonary manifestations, dermatitis artefacta, fever of unknown origin, renal stones, hypoglycemia, diarrhea, and anemia. In neurological practice, seizures and paralysis are probably the most commonly feigned diseases.

Factitious disorders with psychological presentation are most frequently seen in conjunction with physical complaints. When manifestations of factitious disorder consist of psychological symptoms only, the subject exhibits peregrination, antisocial behavior and lack of intimate and sustained relationship. Factitious disorders with symptoms of depression, bereavement, post-traumatic stress disorder, alcohol dependence and psychosis have been described in the past.

Definition as Per Current Nosology

According to *Diagnostic and Statistical Manual of Mental Disorders*, Fourth Edition, Text Revision (DSM-IV-TR), for a diagnosis of factitious disorder to be entertained, a person must be intentionally producing illness; his or her motivation is to occupy the sick role, and there must not be external incentives for the behavior. Although DSM is clear that no external incentives can be present to meet the criteria for the diagnosis, it is rarely the case that there is absolutely no secondary gain for a patient (as the sick role automatically conveys some external benefits such as release from usual duties). In practice, clinicians will often diagnose patients with factitious disorder in the presence of some external gain as long as the external benefits do not appear to be a major motivation for the production of symptoms. At the same time it is important to remember that some patients blur the distinction between factitious disorder and malingering, as they appear to be motivated both by seeking the sick role and by powerful external motivations.

DSM further sub-classifies factitious disorder depending on the predominant symptoms into predominantly physical, psychological, or a combination of both.

International classification of Disorder 10th edition (ICD-10), classifies factitious disorder under "other disorders of adult personality and behavior," under "intentional production or feigning of symptoms or disabilities either physical or psychological (factitious disorder)- F68.1."

DSM-5 Criteria for Factitious Disorder 300.19 (F68.10)

Factitious Disorder Imposed on Self

A. Falsification of physical or psychological signs or symptoms, or induction of injury or disease, associated with identified deception.
B. The individual presents himself or herself to others as ill, impaired, or injured.
C. The deceptive behavior is evident even in the absence of obvious external rewards.
D. The behavior is not better explained by another mental disorder, such as delusional disorder or another psychotic disorder.

Specify: Single episode
Recurrent episodes (two or more events of falsification of illness and/or induction of injury)

Factitious Disorder Imposed on Another (Previously Factitious Disorder by Proxy)

A. Falsification of physical or psychological signs or symptoms, or induction of injury or disease, in another, associated with identified deception.
B. The individual presents another individual (victim) to others as ill, impaired, or injured.
C. The deceptive behavior is evident even in the absence of obvious external rewards.
D. The behavior is not better explained by another mental disorder, such as delusional disorder or another psychotic disorder.

Note: The perpetrator, not the victim, receives this diagnosis.

Specify: Single episode
Recurrent episodes (two or more events of falsification of illness and/or induction of injury)

Prevalence

Because of its nature, it is difficult to estimate the incidence and prevalence rates of factitious disorder in the general population. Hence, the estimates are limited to inpatient populations only. There has been steady increase in the number of case reports of Munchausen's syndrome. The prevalence estimates of the cases vary widely because of the secretive nature of the illness and it largely depends upon case reports and small studies. One study reported an incidence rate of 0.8 % at a tertiary medical center on the basis of patients being referred for psychiatric consultations. The prevalence rate of factitious disorder in medical and psychiatric inpatient setting has varied from 0.5 to 5%.

Conceptual Issues

Its history extends many centuries and has been mentioned in both professional and lay literature. However, the term factitious disorder was used for the first time by Hector Gavin in 1838, though he mentions his source as *"Cyclopedia of Practical Medicine."* In 1951, Richard Asher used the term to describe five cases, in which subjects travelled to multiple hospitals giving dramatic description of illness and seeking medical attention, which he described as cases of Munchausen's syndrome.

No specific etiology could be found for factitious disorder. Factitious disorder has been found to be more common in subjects associated with medical profession. Certain subjects have history of suffering from a serious illness in childhood or their caregivers having an illness during their childhood. Family history of factitious disorder has been found to be a risk factor. Certain personality traits like dissocial, histrionic and borderline personality traits are found to be more common in patients with patients with factitious disorder and they are found to have emotionally deprived or abusive childhood. It has also been reported that patients with factitious disorder usually have a poor sense of identity, poor sexual adjustment, poor frustration tolerance, strong dependency needs and narcissism. A strong association with substance abuse has also been reported.

Etiological theories have been suggested, Karl Jaspers had suggested in his book General Psychopathology that once person starts with it, he tries to run away from reality to the existence of self-deception and self-surrender to factitious disorder. Asher (1951) described that individual want to deceive everyone and lying as he has to lie.

Etiologically, factitious disorder serves the function of meeting patients' psychological needs. One of these needs could be gaining a sense of control and mastery over some traumatic childhood illness through factitious signs and symptoms. Another common theme is masochism, where patients feel a compulsion to suffer and seek self-punishment as atonement for various forbidden emotions and wishes, such as sexual excitement or anger. A third common psychological factor in factitious disorder is that of dependency gratification. Many factitious disorder patients experienced significant deprivation in childhood. Hence, factitious disorder may be a way to have their unfulfilled dependency needs met in a socially sanctioned medical setting. Some authors have also attributed factitious disorder to a need to feel superior to authority figures, which is gratified by being able to deceive the therapist. The behaviorists view factitious disorder as a coping mechanism learned and reinforced in childhood.

How to Distinguish These Disorders

It is very important and challenging to distinguish these disorders from one another and a true medical/surgical disorder. Malingering and factitious disorder have similar features of conscious intentional production of signs and symptoms of a disease. However, in malingering the goal is to achieve some external incentives such as financial compensation, avoidance of military duty, evasion of criminal prosecution, avoiding work, obtaining financial compensation or obtaining drugs. Patients with malingering are frequently uncooperative for diagnostic evaluation and in complying with the prescribed treatment regimen. But problems in diagnosis always remain and sometimes it appears to be a mixed up puzzle. A patient might malinger to obtain tangible gains associated with sick role but might still enjoy the nurturing and care that such a role provides. Though, similar to malingering in terms of conscious intentional production of signs and symptoms of a disease, factitious disorder differs from malingering in term of motivation to produce symptoms, which is adoption of the 'sick-role' rather than the attainment of a tangible external gain. Usually, the patient's primary goal is to receive medical, surgical, or psychiatric care to gratify some unconscious psychological needs. The symptom production in factitious disorder may involve simulation, exaggeration, aggravation or induction of physical or psychological signs and symptoms. Compared to malingering, patients with factitious disorder would be cooperative for diagnostic evaluation and in complying with the prescribed treatment. Somatoform and dissociative disorders are characterized by the presence of somatic complaints or dissociative symptoms that have no demonstrable peripheral organ disorder, psychological disturbances and the magnified health concerns not under the conscious control of the patient. In contrast with malingering, these disorders have a distinctive symptom profile and absence of a clear external incentive. In conversion disorder, as in malingering, objective signs cannot account for the subjective experience and differentiation between the two can be very arduous. However, certain factors which may point toward malingering are that malingerers are more likely to be suspicious and uncooperative; they may try to avoid diagnostic evaluations and refuse treatment; they may refuse employment opportunities designed to circumvent their disabilities and are less likely to have historical gaps and inaccuracies in their account. Rather, they may provide detailed descriptions of the events, which reportedly precipitated their symptoms. Further patients with malingering often have associated antisocial traits, like history of acting out, previous lawsuits, difficulty with law enforcement agencies. Observing patients when they think they are not being observed gives a clue to the diagnosis (e.g. the conversion patient with paralysis will remain paralyzed whereas a patient with malingering may move their limbs). However it is also important to remember that some of the patients with somatization or dissociative disorders are often suspected to be malingerers, not only by their relatives or their workmates, but also by doctors who are not familiar with psychiatric disorders. When such is the case, the clinician should address the relatives and workmates and should try to explain the underlying issues as part of the clinical management of the case.

Apart from the above, malingering of a certain disorder or symptoms might co-exist with another actual disorder, which should not be ignored. Cases of partial malingering, where underlying symptoms are exaggerated also need to be differentiated from cases of pure malingering.

Management

Malingering: As malingering is not considered to be a diagnosis, management does not imply the kind of measures utilized for the treatment of psychiatric illnesses. However, certain guidelines have been suggested for the physicians or psychiatrists who are convinced that the subject examined by them have malingering. Careful and detailed documentation supporting the diagnosis should be done, as the diagnosis of malingering carries a definitive risk for the clinician. Consultations to other medical specialists should be avoided because such referrals only perpetuate malingering. The patient should not be accused directly of faking an illness as hostility, breakdown of the doctor-patient relationship, lawsuit against the doctor, and, rarely, violence may result. The more advisable approach is to confront the person indirectly by remarking that the objective findings do not meet the physician's objective criteria for diagnosis and the person who is malingering should be given the opportunity to save face. Despite all this, the subject may still continue to malinger the symptoms and the likelihood of success with such approaches is inversely related to the rewards for the malingering behavior.

Factitious disorder: Patients with factitious disorder present a challenging treatment problem. The treatment of factitious disorder should aim at minimizing the damage done by the disorder to both the patient's own health and the health care system, and to help patients recover from the same. The most important thing in management of these cases is to secure an enduring and stable patient-therapist relationship, which can be achieved by being non-confrontational and reframing the manifestation as a "cry for help". Use of supportive, face-saving techniques may help a patient to accept appropriate treatment. Some authors have proposed "contract conference" approach for these patients in whom the therapist emphasizes on the need for the patient to express him/herself in the common language of difficult relationships, feelings and problems in the living instead of the language of illness. Another important issue in management involves therapist's own counter-transference reactions. Discussing the same with superiors or colleagues often leads to avoidance of ineffective management. Predictors of favorable response to treatment include the presence of an underlying treatable psychiatric condition such as depression, anxiety, substance abuse or conversion symptoms, the absence of borderline or antisocial personality traits, good psychosocial supports, and the ability to form a therapeutic alliance with a therapist, characterized by the capacity to establish and maintain rapport, accept confrontation, and comply with treatment recommendations.

CONCLUSION

Malingering is best conceptualized as a condition which is focus of clinical attention rather than as a psychopathological condition in itself. It is important to remember that any medical condition may be faked; however, malingering of psychiatric disorders is perhaps commoner than previously considered and is particularly difficult to detect. Factitious disorder is classified as a disorder in which symptoms are produced unconsciously and the motivation is to assume a sick role. Both of these conditions require high index of suspicion and an accepting therapeutic environment for improvement.

SUGGESTED READING

1. American Psychiatric Association. Desk Reference to the Diagnostic Criteria from DSM-V. Washington DC, 2013.
2. Bhugra D. Psychiatric Munchausen's syndrome. Literature review with case reports. Acta Psychiatrica Scandinavica, 1988;77:497-503.
3. Cunnien AJ. Psychiatric and medical syndromes associated with deception. In: Rogers R (Ed). Clinical assessment of malingering and deception, 2nd edition. New York: Guilford press; 1997.pp.169-207.
4. Eisendrath SJ, Feder A. Current overview of factitious disorder. In: The spectrum of factitious disorder. Feldman MD & Eisendrath SJ (Eds). American Psychiatric Press, Washington DC, 1996.
5. Feldman MD, Ford CV. Factitious disorder. In: Comprehensive textbook of Psychiatry, 7th edition. Sadock BJ & Sadock VA (Eds). Philadelphia, Lippincott Williams and Wilkins. 2000.pp 1533-43.
6. Hall HV, Pritchard DA. Detecting malingering and deception: Forensic distortion analysis, 2nd edition. Sanford, Florida: DC Press; 2000.
7. Hay GG. Feigned Psychosis - A review of the Simulation of mental illness. British Journal of Psychiatry. 1983;143:8-10.
8. Huffman JC, Stern TA. The diagnosis and treatment of Munchausen's syndrome. General hospital Psychiatry. 2003;25:358-63.
9. Knoll J, Resnick PJ. The detection of malingered post-traumatic stress disorder. Psychiatr Clin North Am. 2006;29:629-47.
10. Lipian MS, Mills MJ. In: Sadock BJ, Sadock VA (Eds). Comprehensive textbook of psychiatry, 7th edition. Philadelphia: Lippincott Williams and Wilkins. 2000. pp.1898-908.
11. Lipian MS, Mills MJ. Malingering. In: Comprehensive textbook of Psychiatry, 7th edition. Sadock BJ & Sadock VA (Eds). Philadelphia, Lippincott Williams and Wilkins, 2.
12. Lo Piccolo CJ, Goodkin K, Baldewicz T. Current issues in the diagnosis and management of malingering. Ann Med. 1999;31:166-74.
13. Mills MJ, Lipian MS. Malingering. In: Sadock BJ, Sadock VA (Eds). Comprehensive textbook of psychiatry, 8th edition. Philadelphia: Lippincott Williams and Wilkins. 2005. pp.2247-58.
14. Singh J, Avasthi A, Grover S. Malingering of psychiatric disorders: A review. German Journal of Psychiatry. 2007;10:126-32.
15. Spivak A, Eisendrath SJ. Factitious disorder. In: Encyclopedia of the neurological Sciences, Elsevier Science (USA), 2003.
16. Wildman RW, Wildman RW. The detection of malingering. Psychol Rep. 1999;84:386-8.
17. Wiley SD. Deception and detection in psychiatric diagnosis. Psychiatr Clin North Am. 1998;21:869-73.

CHAPTER

22 Psychosomatic Disorders

JN Vyas, VS Chadha

INTRODUCTION

In the 19th century, it was widely accepted that psychological factors can play an important part in the etiology of physical illness. It is significant that the 27th World Health Assembly, held in May 1974, endorsed a holistic and ecological approach to medical research, practice, and training.[1] The participants urged all nations to support research on the role of psychological factors in health and disease. They contended that these factors can precipitate and counteract physical and mental illness, and are thus crucially important in the prevention and management of all disease. This historical resolution indicated the traditional psychosomatic viewpoint.

The knowledge of these developments is not prevalent; confusion about the current state of psychosomatic medicine is widespread. Some psychiatrists and physicians view psychosomatic medicine as an improbable hybrid of clinical thinking, physiological speculation and psychoanalytic theory,[2] or as a doctrine of well-meaning but ill-defined humanism.[3]

Psychosomatic affection is defined as a bodily disorder whose nature can be appreciated only when emotional disturbances (i.e. psychological happenings) are investigated, in addition to physical disturbances (i.e. somatic happenings). Psychosomatic theory holds that emotional changes in human beings are accompanied by psychological changes and that if these emotional changes are persistent or frequent, then pathological physical factors can help to maintain or aggravate the disease, or to trigger relapses. It is also assumed that physical conditions induced in this way will improve if the psychological disturbance improves, either spontaneously or as a result of psychological treatment.

Psychosomatic medicine has three interrelated facts that jointly define its scope: (a) it is a scientific discipline concerned with the study of the biological, psychological and social determinants of health and disease, (b) it is a set of postulates and guidelines embodying a holistic approach to the practice of medicine, and (c) it encompasses consultation-liaison psychiatry.[4]

This tripartite definition includes both the scientific and clinical aspects of the field which have always been its integral constituents.[5] As a scientific discipline, psychosomatic medicine has focused on the reciprocal relationship between psychological and physiological variables and has attempted to correlate them with specified conditions and changes in the person's social environment. To do so, it has had to simultaneously employ research methods, explanatory concepts, and languages belonging to three distinct levels of abstraction—social, psychological and physiological. A complementary task has involved the study of the influence of specified physiological variables on psychological functioning, in all of its principal aspects: information processing, motivation, emotions, and psychomotor behavior, both normal and abnormal.

To achieve a comprehensive knowledge of people, it is necessary to study them as individual mind-body complexes, ceaselessly interacting with the social and physical environment in which they are embedded. Thus, the psychosomatic conception of man is integrative, holistic and dynamic. Psychosomatic medicine advocates a unified concept of health and disease.[4]

HISTORICAL OVERVIEW

In primitive society, it was believed that disease is caused by spiritual means; the evil spirit that enters and affects the total being must be liberated by exorcism or trepanation. In Leydon, Professor of Medicine, Gaub stated that "the reason why a sound body becomes ill, or an ailing body recovers, very often lies in the mind". Contrariwise, the body can frequently both beget mental illness and heal its offspring.[6] Tuke[7] compiled a vast body of observations and anecdotes recorded in the medical literature pertaining to the influence of the mind on the body in health and disease.

In the 19th century, the stage was set for psychosomatic medicine to emerge from the background of philosophy and medical folklore. The term '*psychosomatic*' was first used by Johann Christian Heinroth in 1818, with regard to insomnia. The 'specificity of attitude' hypothesis by Grace and Grahams specifies that there is an association with each psychosomatic disease of a specific attitude towards the life events that precipitate the first appearance of or later exacerbation of the disease. For many years, the field followed the two major directions:

1. Psychophysiological theory (or theory of psychological stress).
2. Psychodynamic (or psychoanalytic) theory.

In the twentieth century, Freud's psychoanalytic formulations emphasized the role of psychic determinism in somatic conversion reaction. The early concepts are limited to major hysterical conversions. With transference and counter-transference, Freud pulled the doctor-patient relationship out of the religious framework of hope and faith, and into an intellectually understandable dynamism. He redignified the investigation of the emotions as a separate study and pointed to their relationship with the soma, continuing where the Greeks and Romans had left off. Subsequently, Alexander differentiated conversion reaction from psychosomatic diseases.[8]

According to Alexander,[9] a patient, with vulnerability of a specific organ or somatic system and a characteristic psychodynamic constellation, develops the corresponding diseases when the turn of events in his life occurs to mobilize his earlier established central conflicts, breaking down his primary defenses against them. This means that if the precipitating external environmental stimuli never occur, the patient may, in spite of the presence of predisposing emotional pattern and of organ vulnerability, never develop the disease.[9] Wolff[10] used objective laboratory tests to correlate life stress to physiological responses and found that if the physiological change is prolonged it may lead to structural changes. Margolive, on the other hand, recommended the correlation of unconscious conflicts with physiological responses.

Selye[11] stated that due to stress, there is development of a general adaptation syndrome, in which the physiological reaction is induced by adrenal cortical hormones. Mahl[12] questioned whether any specific conflict is associated with ulcer formation, which may result from any conflict, conscious or unconscious, external or internal. This is so because the important factor is chronic anxiety, and not the nature of conflict.

CLASSIFICATION

The concept of psychosomatic medicine was included in DSM-I (1952) as 'psychosomatic disorders' and in DSM-II (1968) as 'psychophysiological: autonomic and visceral disorders'; while after much debate, in DSM-III-R, it was redesignated as 'psychological factors affecting physical conditions'.[13]

In DSM-IV, psychosomatic disorders are renamed as 'psychological factors affecting medical conditions'. The diagnostic criteria in DSM-IV specify that psychological factors affect the medical condition adversely in one of various ways. The essential component is that "the psychological factors have affected the course of general medical condition as shown by close temporal association between the development or exacerbation of, or delayed recovery from, a general medical condition". The psychological factors may include mental disorders (e.g. major depressive disorder), psychological symptoms (e.g. anxiety, depressive symptoms), personality trait or coping style (e.g. pathological denial of the need for surgery), maladaptive health behaviors (e.g. stress related exacerbation of ulcer), and other unspecified psychological factors (e.g. interpersonal or cultural factors).

The important change in DSM-IV from DSM-III-R is that DSM-IV allows the clinician to specify the psychological factors that affect the medical condition of a patient. Psychologically meaningful environmental stimuli were related to physical disorder temporally in DSM-III-R. DSM-IV's emphasis on psychological factors includes a wide range of psychological stimuli, e.g. maladaptive health behaviors, and personality traits.

The DSM-IV classification specifically excludes the following categories from psychosomatic disorders:

- Psychiatric disorders presenting with physical symptomatology (e.g. conversion disorder).
- Somatization disorders and hypochondriasis, in which the physical symptoms are not due to a physical disorder.
- Physical complaints that are usually associated with major psychiatric disorders (e.g. depression).
- Physical complaints associated with substance use disorders (e.g. cough in a patient with nicotine dependence).

In ICD-10, the disorders called as 'psychosomatic' can be found under category F45 (somatoform disorders), F50 (eating disorders), F52 (sexual dysfunction) and F54 (psychological or behavioral factors associated with disorders or diseases classified elsewhere). The category F54 should be used to record the presence of psychological or behavioral factors thought to have played a major part in the etiology of physical disorders which can be classified elsewhere in ICD-10.

CURRENT STATUS OF PSYCHOSOMATIC THEORY

The influence of psychoanalysis on psychosomatic medicine has gradually diminished over the last two decades. It has proven difficult to validate the proposed primacy of unconscious psychological factors in the pathogenesis of these disorders. Alexander's specificity theory still has a few adherents and attempts to validate it have continued. Other psychoanalytical concepts like conversion, somatization, physiological regression, repressed affects and psychogenesis, continue to be used by some workers to account for the various psychosomatic disorders.

The current psychosomatic theory has also been influenced by general systems theory; somatic function and behavior; notions of psychophysiological reasons; specificity and activation; theory of operant conditioning and self-concept of visceral functions; hypothesis of object loss as an antecedent of disease; and by concepts of psychosocial stress, cognitive appraisal and meaning, individual susceptibility to disease, adaptation, coping and feedback.

Family interaction and disruptions, occupational conditions and relationships, urbanization, poverty, migration, and rapidly changing value system and lifestyles are some of the social variables which have an impact on the psychophysiological functioning. Such hypotheses have complemented, not supplanted, the traditional, psychodynamic and psychophysiological approaches.[6] As Dubos[14] reminds us, "the understanding and control of disease requires that body-mind complex be studied in its relation to external environment".

Another major shift in focus is shown in the current concern with conscious emotions and cognitive processes, and their anatomical substrates and physiological concomitants. These psychological variables are more easily quantified than the unconscious ones.

The following lines of evidence have been used to support the presumed importance of psychological variables in the production of psychosomatic disorders:

- Occurrence of repeated episodes following emotional stress (e.g. bronchial asthma precipitated by separation anxiety).
- Presence of characteristic personality types in certain diseases (e.g. oral dependence related conflicts in ulcer patients; suppressed anger in rheumatoid arthritis patients; type A personality in patients of coronary artery disease).
- Conditionability of attacks due to stimuli of nonbiological origin (e.g. allergy to roses precipitating an asthmatic attack in the presence of an artificial rose).
- Demonstration of individual physiological stereotyped response to the various stimuli in the environment.
- Conditionability of some autonomic nervous system responses.
- Patients of different psychosomatic disorders express characteristic attitudes; the experimental production of appropriate physiological changes through the hypnotic inculcation of these attitudes has been demonstrated.

Although the concept of psychosomatic disease, as a conditioned response to specific psychological conflict or stress is attractive, there are some problems. First, there is no evidence to support the belief that the sustained emotional and physiological reactions induced by conflict can produce specific disease in individuals. Second, there is no evidence that patients with specific psychosomatic disorders display more unique conflicts or different personality configurations than do appropriate control groups, or even if they do, whether these conflicts or personality configurations represent an antecedent or a consequence of the illness. Third, these disorders are unlikely to occur in persons who are not already biologically predisposed.[15]

The importance of stress and psychological factors as causative factors does not prove their role in worsening of these diseases, since higher cortical influences may induce widespread physiological and endocrinal responses through actions on the hypothalamus and limbic system. These changes may be sufficient to alter the internal milieu, so that the situation becomes more conducive to the development or accentuation of symptoms in susceptible individuals. It can be said in a different way that a major, complex interaction takes place among three major components:

1. An acquired or innate biological susceptibility to a particular disease.
2. The exposure of the individual to a sustained period of potential 'stress'.
3. A particular psychological configuration permitting interpretation of the nonspecific situation as threatening and, hence, stressful.

THEORETICAL CONCEPTS AND FORMULATIONS

Psychosomatic hypotheses are attempting to answer some deceptively simple questions, like why does a person respond to particular social situations and specific life events with a given pattern of psychological and physiological changes; through which pathways and mechanisms do symbolic stimuli bring about changes in susceptibility to somatic illness; which psychological variables may help predict when an individual will become ill and what illness he will develop; which kind of social situations and events are most likely to predispose to and precipitate illness in a given person or group; which behavior, attitudes and social conditions are more conducive to health and to adaptive coping with illness; and what are the psychological characteristics of people who most readily become ill or complain of bodily symptoms or both?

Answers to these questions are needed to advance control over disease and suffering because the main goal is to identify those psychosocial variables which increase the susceptibility to illness as well as those which enhance resistance and adaptive coping. Such information is needed as a basis for psychological measures that will help to ameliorate diseases causing chronic disability and/or premature death. There is evidence that this goal may be achieved by modifying specific behaviors, attitudes, emotional responses and improving social supports.

MODELS OF PSYCHOSOMATIC MEDICINE

There is ample evidence in the literature suggesting the role of psychological and physiological processes in the genesis of psychosomatic diseases. The major question is how to explain the interplay of these processes. This explanation has been attempted through various models, which include the following:

Concomitant Effects

One of the models of concomitant effects agrees to the meaningful relationship of psychological and physiological processes but it disagrees that this relationship is causal. It explains these concurrences as a result of their being joint consequences of other preceding factors, usually biological in nature.[13] Another concomitant model stresses upon the complexity of events that are experienced psychologically. Life events have multiple stimulus components, some of which may act directly on physiological systems, whereas others have primary psychological effects. There is no reason to believe that when multiple stimulus properties impinge, they are clearly divided into physiological systems and psychological experiences; but certainly once an event occurs, this will simultaneously act upon psychological and physiological processes.[13]

Somatopsychic Causation

This model explains that when concurrence arises, there is a sequence which proceeds from body to mind; psychological changes are understood as reactions to biological events, or in other words, psychological effects may secondarily produce the physiologically changes.

Psychosomatic Specificity

As recently revised,[16] this concept pertains to the probability that a person will respond to a given stimulus situation with a predictable set of psychological and physiological changes. Such a prediction must be based on the following three sets of variables:

1. It depends upon the nature, the intensity and the duration of the stimulus situation. If stimulus evokes similar responses, then one talks of stimulus response specificity or stereotypy.
2. *Individual response specificity*: The enduring psychological and physiological response characteristics of the person in having individual differences in response to same type of stimulus. Factors like life events, personality, genetic factors, developmental history, past exposure to illness, attitudes and operant conditioning have all been invoked to account for individual response specificity.
3. The current psychophysiological state of the person, current emotional state, fatigue, level and pattern of autonomic arousal, presence of physical illness and state of consciousness are some of the variables subsumed under this category. This concept highlights the current attempts to study the interaction of multiple variables influencing psychophysiological functioning in health and disease. Hawkins[17] discussed the present status of personality and behavior patterns as markers in psychosomatic medicine, as well as the possible relationship of personality profiles to genetic factors, developmental issues, psychological conflicts and other approaches to psychophysiological disorder.

Psychosocial Stress

The stress model also accepts the psychosomatic sequence, but rejects the idea that specific psychological factors are involved. It suggests that the initiating factor is stress which arises from noxious psychological experiences leading to physiological changes, which in turn have effect on an organ predisposed by genetic defects and past damage.

Reiser,[18] in an extension of the above model, suggested that the physiological changes that have occurred due to stress, act on the brain as a target organ which then affects its integrative functions. He also stated that psychological processes would be simultaneously causing ego functions to become more primitive, with a breakdown of defenses. Because of its focus on internal mechanisms, in terms of both predispositions and stress, Weiner[19] has classified this model as 'internal loop transduction'.

Individual Susceptibility to Disease

Psychosomatic theories of etiology can be broadly divided into two categories: (i) specificity, and (ii) generality. Both assert that social and psychological variables contribute to morbidity. However, they differ with regard to the proposed nature of pathogenesis. The specificity theory postulates that specific psychosocial factors like somatic disorders, and unconscious conflicts over sexual, dependent or holistic strivings contribute to specific or individual susceptibility to disease. A well-known example of the proposed specificity is the relationship between type A behavior pattern and the development of coronary artery disease and its complications.[20]

The generality theory holds that a wide range of life events may increase the probability that the person will become ill. According to Lipowski, the generality and specificity theories complement each other neatly. The former theories have identified conditions in a person's life whose occurrence increases the probability of imminent disease; while the later theories allow a measure of prediction of which events are potentially hazardous for a given person or class of people sharing one or more psychological characteristics, and which illness is most likely to follow exposure to such events. The analysis of temporal course of psychosomatic syndromes shows that the previous history strongly determined the occurrence of psychosomatic syndromes in the future.[21]

PATHOGENESIS OF DISEASE

It is rather difficult to say when the symptom of a disease begins. Morton Reiser[22] has indicated the importance of recognizing three major phases in the development of any disease. The initial phase exists before any evidence of disease onset, when the main concern is with the predisposing factors. The second stage is initiation of the state of illness, when the interest centers on the precipitating forces and mechanisms. The third stage is its course, when the focus is on factors that influence the further development, disappearance or recurrence of the illness. Reiser[22] makes the key point that the factors operating at any stage are likely to be different from those at others.

Predisposing Factors

The predisposing factors are those which lead to a capacity for developing a specific disease, e.g. anatomical, physiological, chemical and psychological factors. Although these may represent normal variations, they play a major role in determining why certain individuals develop a disease.

Early experience factors have been demonstrated to alter the brain anatomy, neurotransmitters and level of hormones, later stress responses, in addition to conditioning CNS pathways. Mirsky[23] has suggested a mechanism in which a somatic predisposition could lead to ulcer formation as well as the specificity findings. Even if psychological factors predispose to disease, it is unlikely that they act alone.

Precipitating Factors

Among the individuals who have predisposing factors, all do not develop disease. There are three psychosomatic explanations which may be responsible for the factor which initiates the active disease:

- Specific conflict
- Loss and bereavement
- Stress and coping.

Concurrent Factors

Observations have revealed that recurrences of somatic illness often lead to stressful life events, intensified conflict and emotional distress, and vice-versa. Therefore, interventions should be properly directed to alleviate both psychic and somatic stress. Conceptually, however, untangling the sequence is crucial. Only if a psychological factor is said to be antecedent can it be causal. However, this issue remains central to the assertions of specificity theory regarding the initiation of disease, because these were based on psychological observations in already ill persons. Only prospective studies initiated before the onset of disease can begin to clarify the direction of that causal sequence.[6]

GASTROINTESTINAL DISORDERS

It is not surprising that mouth is considered as the organizing focus of all subsequent maturational processes. Digestion, from the incorporation of food substances (nutriment) at one opening to elimination of waste from the other, is basic to life sustenance and thus to the life cycle. It was logical and reasonable that psychoanalytic theory invested in the significance of symbolism, fantasy and the impact of emotional experience as it centered on first the mouth and then the anus. Also, not surprising is that the psychological processes would be described as incorporation, introjection and projection; terms as appropriate to gastroenterological function as to defenses of ego.

The gut as a responder to and communicator of feeling is as old as human language. Contemporary idioms describe anxiety as 'butterflies in the stomach', anger as 'unable to stomach him', disgust as 'making one want to throw up', fear as 'crapping in my pants', and depression as 'food does not interest me'. The psychologically and medically naive refer to being 'down in the mouth' when vengeful, and 'having a gut feeling' when intuitively responsive to subtle external and emotional cues.

The researchers[25] were careful to avoid unilinear explanations as they studied a wide range of affects, behaviors, interpersonal relations, gastric secretions and other physiological responses of the gut mucosa. The results reflect a complex reactive and developmental process in which object relations, affective states, physical behavior and physiological functions are all interrelated. It appears that genesis of early object relations includes as assimilative process, largely orally organized and the stomach participates as if the intention is also to take objects into it. In human research, physiological to psychological variables have made remarkable progress to interrelate towards more multilinear models. Even as etiology and pathogenesis remains obscure, efforts at treatment have shown beneficial results. The discovery that what was once considered under involuntary nervous system control is capable of conscious influence has opened up new areas of therapeutic interventions based on learning and behavior therapies; psychotherapy continues to produce positive results.

Aphthous stomatitis, gingivitis, dental caries, drymouth, hypersalivation and 'burning mouth' are observed in association with mood disorder, but how emotional factors takes part in etiology is still not clear. Other psychosomatic conditions of upper GIT include rumination, esophageal dysfunction, hyperemesis gravidarum, nausea and vomiting, peptic ulcer disease and pylorospasm. Anorexia nervosa and bulimia nervosa are poorly understood eating disorders with serious systemic consequences which occur without any detectable organic lesion of the gastrointestinal system.[24,25]

Engel[25] considered that anorexia, bulimia and globushystericus all may represent various forms of conversion disorder, while another study suggested hyperemesis gravidarum to be a specific form of somatization, a somatic response to dysphoric mood caused by a combination of increased stress and inadequate social support.[25]

Peptic Ulcer

This condition is characterized by a circumscribed ulceration of mucous membrane of the stomach or duodenum, penetrating to the muscularis mucosa, and occurring in areas exposed to gastric acid and pepsin.

The absolute prevalence of duodenal ulcer is not known but is estimated approximately to be 6–16%, with a 3:1 male predominance. Duodenal ulcer has a peak incidence in men between 45 and 55, whereas gastric ulcer occurs about 10 years later. The emotional factors are believed to be more relevant to the incidence of duodenal than to gastric ulcer.

Alexander[9] hypothesized that chronic frustration of intense dependency needs results in a characteristic unconscious conflict. This conflict pertains to intense dependent oral, receptive longing to be cared for and loved. This causes a chronic regressive unconscious hunger and anger which, by persistent vagal hyperactivity, leads to gastric acid hypersecretion, and ulcer formation may result.

Stress and anxiety caused by nonspecific conflicts may produce gastric hyperacidity and hypersecretion of pepsin, resulting in an ulcer. Peptic ulcers have been diagnosed in all personality types.

To support these theories, Takeuchi and others[26] investigated the influence of stress on gastric acid and duodenal HCO_3 secretion in rats, and determined whether duodenal ulcers develop in rats under stress conditions, in the absence or presence of acid hypersecretion caused by histamine. They found exposure of rats to stress decreases duodenal HCO_3^- secretion and increases the susceptibility of the mucosa to acid emptied from stomach, thereby inducing duodenal ulcers if acid hypersecretion is also present. Feldman et al.[27] have found a strong association among stressful life events, psychosocial factors and peptic ulcer disease.

Irritable Bowel Syndrome

It is a prototype of functional gastrointestinal disorders. Also named as spastic colon, mucous colitis or nervous stomach, it is considered a benign, noninflammatory, nonprogressive and chronic disease. It is characterized by constipation and diarrhea in regular, intermittent or alternating patterns, with or without pain. There are no clear pathognomonic features or laboratory findings. This disturbance of GIT motility is believed to be highly responsive to psychosocial stress or emotional perturbation.

Epidemiologically, this syndrome is two to three times more common in women, can occur as early as childhood or adolescence and as late as middle age, and is more prevalent in developing countries.

Irritable bowel syndrome is characterized by an abnormal increase in gut motility of more than 3 cycles per minute. Other hypotheses suggest excessive parasympathetic stimulation of the bowel; neural and hormonal idiosyncrasies of the bowel wall tonus in response to substances like cholecystokinin and pentagastrin; and variations in the intraluminal pressure affecting the stool habit, consistency and movement. Fiber deficiency is also thought to increase intraluminal pressure, which is the basis for increased dietary bulk as treatment. One hypothesis suggests that exposure to early attitudes, beliefs and family behaviors regarding functions of the alimentary tract, whether at the intake or the outlet ends, is responsible for conditioning a learned response to bowel function.[6]

The key issue is not to fulfil an accomplishment to a key dependency figure. Essentially frustrated dependency stimulates oral aggressive feelings, producing guilt and anxiety, and resulting in restitution of the 'gifting of diarrhea'. With regard to colitis, George Engel described a pathological mother-child relationship resulting in the feeling of hopelessness-helplessness and a 'giving up-given up' complex.[24,25]

Personality traits of these patients are orderliness, punctuality, cleanliness, greediness, rigidity, obsessive-compulsiveness and other characteristics associated with the psychoanalytic concept of an anal personality. Early psychoanalytic research suggested that conflicts concerning giving, receiving and aggression accompanied symptoms of diarrhea and constipation. Constipation was seen as withholding by stubborn or stingy individuals, whereas diarrhea suggested unconscious aggressive and deprecatory urges. On MMPI, these IBS patients scored higher than normal on scales of hypochondriasis, hysteria and depression, but these factors did not influence motor or electric activity.[28]

Ulcerative Colitis

It is a chronic inflammatory ulcerative disease of colon and is usually associated with bloody diarrhea, familial incidence and genetic factors are significant.

Research studies show a predominance of compulsive personality traits characterized by neat, orderly, punctual hyper-intellectual, timid and anger-inhibition traits.

CARDIOVASCULAR SYSTEM

Some researchers in the field of psychosomatic disorders of CVS speculate that there can be deleterious effects of emotions on CVS, although these effects resemble the effects of physical stress.

Physical effort and emotional arousal may increase myocardial irritability, heart failure or ischemia. As several investigators have described, emotional stress and emotion-laden life events frequently precede such cardiac events as congestive heart failure and sudden death.

Threatening arrhythmias such as ventricular tachycardia and ventricular fibrillation, as well as increases in premature ventricular beats, occur due to emotional upset and anxiety.

The efficacy of b-adrenergic agents in protecting against emotionally induced arrhythmias emphasizes the role of peripheral adrenergic neurotransmitters.

Considerable data has accumulated, however, implicating the central neural mechanisms as initiators or triggers of sympathetic arousal, while the role of parasympathetic nervous system is less evident, although an intact vagus nerve, along with both stellate ganglia, appears necessary for ventricular fibrillation to be centrally activated in a normal heart.

Vasovagal syncope, a parasympathetic response to emotional stimuli causing bradycardia, hypotension, and syncope, is a typical response to acute emotional arousal.

The following are the main psychosomatic cardiovascular diseases.

Coronary Artery Disease

Coronary artery disease causes myocardial ischemia and is characterized by episodic subcordial pain, discomfort or pressure. It is usually precipitated by exertion or stress. The major postulated psychosocial risk factors for the development of CAD are:

- Type A behavior pattern
- Occupational or marital dissatisfaction
- Status incongruity
- Work overload
- Disturbing emotions of anxiety and depression.

The personality of CAD patients is often aggressive-compulsive type with a tendency to work long hours and to seize authority. Freidman[29] defined type A and type B personalities. Type A personalities are action-oriented individuals who struggle to achieve poorly defined goals by means of competitive hostility. There are two major criteria for diagnosis: (i) time urgency, and (ii) excessive competitiveness and hostility. Other characteristics are aggressiveness, competitiveness, ambitiousness, drive for success, restlessness, impatience, devotion to work, a subjective sense of time urgency, abruptness of speech and gestures, and tendency to hostility. On the other hand, type B personalities are relaxed, less aggressive and tend to strive less vigorously to achieve their goals. Type A personalities have increased amounts of low density lipoprotein, serum cholesterol, triglycerides and 17-hydroxycorticosteroids, and are more prone to develop this disease.

Hostility and unexpressed anger are the critical variables in the composite of factors said to be coronary prone. To modify or reduce the type A behavior, the combination of patient education and behavior modification like progressive relaxation, autosuggestion, hypnosis, meditation and biofeedback produce good results;[29] this whole method is called as 'cardiac stress management program'. It is aimed at two objectives:

1. Stress management training.
2. Change of habitual behavior.

Stress management training involves teaching the person how to relax and identify situations inducing stress responses in him, and controlling the stimuli evoking such responses and the responses themselves. The type A person is helped to learn to make changes in daily routine and to avoid persons and situations that induce in him competitiveness, time pressure, achievement motivation and hostility. Type a behavior can be modified by counseling to protect against the recurrence of a coronary event possibly because the patient fears another event and is thus more cooperative. However, multiple risk factor intervention trial (MRFIT) showed no relationship between type A pattern and mortality or morbidity from coronary artery disease.[30,31]

Essential Hypertension

It is a multi-causal disorder of homeostasis. If defined as a blood pressure of 160/95 mm Hg or greater, hypertension afflicts 18% of adult population, with a cut-off of 140/90 mm Hg which is a reasonable threshold for caution.

Psychological, social, environmental as well as life events have major role in the etiology of hypertension.

The person at risk for hypertension has personality traits of compliance and congeniality, longing for approval, and anger which is not expressed openly; there is much inhibited rage. This dilemma derives from childhood experience with parents towards whom anger could not be expressed, without real or imagined loss of love and security. The desire to please, in tandem with an antagonistic battle-ready stance is felt. When chronic stress occurs in a generally predisposed compulsive personality, who has repressed and suppressed rage, hypertension may result.

The relation of stress and hypertension is well established. In a relatively nonspecific way, stress produces sympathetically mediated vasoconstriction and other responses in persons predisposed to hypertension. The notion of an autonomic response specificity in some, leading to enduring changes secondary to stress induced autonomic arousal, has received laboratory support.

Anger, suppressed hostility and anxiety have been associated with hypertension and may be associated with a higher risk of established hypertension in borderline hypertensive subjects. More intense anger is associated with more blood pressure in borderline hypertensives. In a comprehensive social, psychiatric and medical survey, a significant relationship was found between hypertension and neuroticism.[32,33]

Essential hypertension may not be a homogeneous disorder, occurring in various forms differing in etiopathogenesis. Researchers have shown that normotensive persons with a family history of hypertension have more risk for developing essential hypertension. In a study, Jorgensen et al.[34] compared two subgroups; the family history positive subjects, who were characterized by denial and unwillingness to admit neurotic feelings or aggressiveness, showed exaggerated blood pressure reactivity to other experimental tasks.

Another study[35] found that there is a widespread psychological difference between high renin and low renin patients who are hypertensive. High renin hypertensives are emotionally labile because of excessive activity of the sympathetic nervous system. Thus, high renin patients may show a greater response to b-adrenergic blocking agents than do low renin patients.[35]

RESPIRATORY DISORDERS

Breath Holding

This condition often begins in a few month old child and usually disappears at 4–5 years of age. It is usually a state provoked by parental anger. The child, during cry, holds his breath at the end of expiration and becomes cyanosed and apneic, sometimes progressing to loss of consciousness. But it differs from epilepsy, because it is a transient condition unlike prolonged postictal unconsciousness. Breath holding disappears as child grows up or finds other ways to manifest his autonomy.

Hyperventilation

These patients breathe rapidly and deeply for several minutes, feel light-headed and faint, due to cerebral vasoconstriction and respiratory alkalosis. Other symptoms like carpopedal spasm and paresthesias may prevail. These episodes are recurrent and subsequent episodes are as frightening as the initial one. It is best understood as a manifestation of anxiety or panic attacks.

It should be differentiated from medical disorders, e.g. pathology of brain stem, metabolic disorder (e.g. diabetic coma), cardiopulmonary disease (e.g. pulmonary embolism), poisoning, epilepsy, bronchial asthma, acute porphyria, Meniere's disease, and pheochromocytoma; as well as psychiatric disorders, e.g. anxiety and panic attacks, acute stress reaction, adjustment disorder, hysteria, borderline or histrionic personality disorder, phobic or obsessive disorders and psychotic disorders like paranoid, depressive and schizophreniform disorders.

Psychopathology of hyperventilation can be explained on the basis that this type of illness and autonomic function irregularities are an immediate response to conditions of acute fear. Usually, the patient complains that there is something wrong with his chest or heart. It means that the anxiety is focused on body, on a vital organ. It can be understood in varying instances like, for example persons, in a situation in which they cannot manage when they think they should, may accept that a physical problem is actually what is preventing them from achieving ('I would if I could'). Psychic reality is more complex usually; the reported stress may not be really the source of anxiety that it seems to be.

Bronchial Asthma

Asthma is a Greek word which means 'difficult breathing'. It is chronic, recurrent obstructive disease of the bronchial airways which tends to respond to various stimuli by bronchial constriction, edema and excessive secretion. Allergic factors, infections, and acute and chronic stress all combine to produce the disease. The rate and depth of respiration may be changed voluntarily and may correlate with different emotional states; such changes may become aggravated and prolonged.

In consideration of psychopathology, no specific personality type has been identified though excessive dependency needs are commonly found. The psychological pattern of conflicts and defenses that Alexander proposed for asthma can be described as 'a suppressed cry for the mother'. There is a basic conflict between attachment to the mother, the desire to communicate with her, crying as a call to the mother in childhood period, or confiding in a trusted person as an adult figure of the same impulses, and opposed to it, the fear of rejection by the mother who is threatened by the emergence of the child's striving towards maturation and independence.

In this hypothesis, the mother is expected to be ambivalent and unpredictable. The child restrains and suppresses calling or crying for the mother. Later in life, the wish to confide and the fear of rejection at occasions disturbs communications and inhibits the use of the respiratory function, mainly the expiration, for verbal communication. According to Alexander, 'an asthmatic attack can be understood as an inhibition of the expiratory act for communication, either by crying or confession'. This view is most comprehensive but criticized in that how these symbolic factors can interact with physiology.

The respiratory function in general is highly sensitive to emotions. In asthmatic patients, there was a modest lowering of airway conductance and significantly less elevation of urinary epinephrine and of plasma free fatty acids than in the normals.

It may be that a gradient of adrenal medullary responsiveness exists in asthmatics. For these asthmatic patients, with a low epinephrine response, a stress would not provide the homeostatic protection of an epinephrine rise against smooth muscle constriction or against potential mast cell degranulation. A hypnotic therapy or relaxation technique is an effective treatment for adult asthmatics who are moderately to highly susceptible to hypnosis.[36]

EATING DISORDERS

Obesity

It can be defined from Bray's normogram for obtaining body mass index (BMI) based on height and weight. Here, overweight is defined as a body mass index of more than 30 kg per square meter, which is roughly 20% above the upper limit for weight on the metropolitan life tables.[6]

There is a familial predisposition to obesity; in addition, early developmental factors can be seen in childhood obesity. The obese children have an increased number of fat cells (hyperplastic obesity) which predisposes them to adult obesity. However, if obesity occurs for the first time in adult life, it is usually of hypertrophic type (increase in fat cell size). Obesity also tends to limit the physical activity, which further aggravates the condition.

Psychological factors are important in hyperphagic (overeating) obesity while emotional disturbances are usually evident in all obese persons. They experience body image disparagement and intense hatefulness towards their own body. This disturbed body image makes them avoid seeing the mirror, making social contacts and engaging in activities. If obese persons undergo psychotherapeutic sessions, they can change their self-image even before they learn to control the eating. Psychological conflict reflects the view that obesity may sometimes be a consequence of schizophrenic or bipolar illness.

The important concepts in the psychoanalytic drive theory include oral fixation, oral regression and over-valuation of food. Conflicts over the satisfaction of libidinal and aggressive needs through sucking or biting are felt to be related to food distastes and idiosyncrasies, as well as specific character traits and abnormalities. These personality traits are excessive optimism or pessimism, greed demandingness, dependence and impatience.

Bruch[37] divided her obese patients in three groups:

1. Patients without significant psychological factors.
2. Patients whose obesity was interwoven with the whole personality development (developmental obesity).
3. Patients who became obese as a reaction to some traumatic life event (reactive obesity).

In reactive obesity, the patients are usually mature and eat more when they are worried, tense or anxious due to some traumatic event like death of a family member, loss of a love object, separation from home. These patients have difficulty with aggressive feelings, and tend to become depressed and overeat in response to aggression and other undesirable emotions.

Developmental obesity usually develops in adolescence, due to psychological factors. These persons have serious adjustment problems, whereas inactivity and overeating become integral parts of their personal development. They fail to achieve a sense of ownership of their body or sense of themselves as active participants in the outcome of their life. Their initiative and autonomy appear poorly developed.

Anorexia Nervosa

It is one of the few psychiatric disorders that may have poor prognosis or an unremitting course. It occurs more commonly in women. The disorder is characterized by disturbance of body image and an intense fear of gaining weight, leading to peculiar patterns of food-handling and weight loss. In females, amenorrhea usually develops.

MUSCULOSKELETAL DISORDERS

Rheumatoid Arthritis

It is a musculoskeletal disorder characterized by pain caused by inflammatory process involving joints. It is a chronic disorder and has significant hereditary allergic, immunological and psychological etiological factors. The chronicity of this disease, along with resultant crippling deformities and loss of productivity, contributes to psychiatric disabilities.

Certain clinical findings are consistent with nervous system involvement in rheumatoid arthritis. Joints are innervated by corpuscular mechanoreceptors and plexus, and by the free endings of small unmyelinated, sensory afferent nerve fibers. Such fibers contain neuropeptide P which is responsible for transmission of pain signals. The effect of substance P on the functions of synoviocytes in rheumatoid arthritis was tested by measuring PGE_2 (prostaglandin E_2) and collagenase production.

Substance P increased PGE_2 release in a dose-dependent manner and led to proliferation of synoviocytes. The augmentation of collagenase release, also linked to substance P, may stimulate cartilage loss and lesions in the adjacent bone, whereas enhanced PGE_2 release may be a signal to perpetuate inflammatory process. These observations define a specific pathway by which nervous system derived peptide substance P could contribute to pathogenesis of rheumatoid arthritis.[38]

Stress predisposes patients to rheumatoid arthritis as well as to other autoimmune diseases. The arthritic feels restrained, tied down and confined, because these persons were earlier very active physically. They often have repressed rage about the inhibition of their muscle function, which aggravates their stiffness and immobility.

The psychological factors play an important role in a subform of this disorder where onset is sudden and there is no family history of rheumatoid arthritis. In this form, the course is usually intermittent, exacerbated when the similar life situations recur. There is an increasing evidence that emotionally traumatic life events frequently precede the initial symptoms of rheumatoid arthritis and precipitate its onset.[38]

Gupta et al.[39] demonstrated that rheumatic pain modulation disorder (RPMD) could be a variant of depression, as both are associated with mood dysphoria, fatigue, and sleep abnormalities. Physical problems during sleep had more alpha (7-11.5Hz) activity in non-REM sleep while dysthymic patients had deeper sleep. The sleep disturbance of fibrositis can be corrected by tricyclic drugs and phenothiazines, and by exercise.[40]

Low Backache

It is felt in lower lumbosacral and sacroiliac regions. The physician should be alert to take the history of trauma, ruptured intervertebral disc, congenital defects of lower spine, or ligamentous or muscle strain followed by severe disabling pain. Very often, the patient will report that the pain was initiated at the time of psychological stress.[41] In addition, the patient's reaction to the pain is disproportionately emotional, with excessive anxiety and depression. Furthermore, the distribution of the pain rarely follows a normal neuroanatomic path.

NEUROLOGICAL DISORDERS

Headaches

Headaches are the most common neurological symptoms in a medical clinic. The majority of headaches are not associated with significant organic disease. Many persons are susceptible to headaches at times of emotional stress. Moreover, some psychiatric diseases, like anxiety and depression, present with headache as a common symptom.

Psychological stress usually exacerbates headaches, whether the primary cause is physical or psychological. Psychosomatic headache is sometimes differentiated from psychogenic headache. In patients with psychogenic headache, the pain symbolises psychological conflicts, and the symptoms are mediated through the voluntary sensory or motor nervous system. In contrast, psychosomatic headaches are defined as autonomic responses to conscious or unconscious conflicts and are not symbolic in nature. The two main psychosomatic headaches are:

1. Migraine (vascular headaches).
2. Tension headache (muscular contraction).

1. *Migraine headache*: It is a paroxysmal disorder characterized by recurrent headaches with or without visual and gastric disturbances. They are probably caused by functional disturbances in the circulation of cranium. These patients have a family history of similar disorder in two-third of cases. The personality of these patients is usually obsessive with overly controlled and suppressed anger. Genetically predisposed to such type of headaches, they develop symptoms under severe nonspecific emotional stress. Drugs, along with psychotherapy and biofeedback behavioral technique, may be helpful in decreasing the symptoms.
2. *Tension headache*: Due to any traumatic event or emotional stress, there is a contraction of head and neck muscles, which over several hours may constrict the blood vessels and result in ischemia. A dull aching pain starts suboccipitally and spreads over the head. The scalp may be tender and a feeling like a tightening band develops. In contrast with migraine, the headache is usually bilateral and not associated with prodromal symptoms, nausea and vomiting.

The onset of tension headache usually occurs on the weekend or in the early evening, when the person wants to relax but the familial and personal pressures are equal to or greater than those at work. Anxiety and depression are usually associated with this disorder. Type A personality individuals are particularly prone to this disorder.

Electromyogram biofeedback technique, relaxation therapy, medication or other changes in the pressured life style may provide symptomatic relief for these patients.

SKIN DISORDERS

Psychosomatic skin disorders include a variety of abnormal skin sensations and disorders, in which emotional factors are etiologically important.

A variety of mechanisms have been postulated for the etiological factors in psychogenic skin diseases. These range from the classical Freudian ideas of hysterical conversion mechanism to the ideas of skin as an infantile preverbal means of communicating emotions which is brought back into operation at times of regression or is repeatedly utilized by those who have failed physically or psychologically to develop the language to express feelings or the emotional outlet.[42]

A review[42] of psychosomatic aspects of dermatology classified psychocutaneous diseases, on the basis of treatment approach, into three categories:

1. Conditions that are strictly psychological in origin.
2. Conditions in which strong psychogenic factors are relevant, e.g. chronic urticaria and hyperhidrosis.

3. Conditions that are dependent on genetic and environment factors but in which the course of disease is substantially affected by stress, e.g. psoriasis, atopic dermatitis and recurrent herpes simplex.

Eller[43] described a fourth category, i.e. skin disorders that are likely to affect the psyche, e.g. those associated with disfigurement, chronic pain, or itching.

According to Kolbenzer, the first category (strictly psychological in origin) includes:

- Dermatitis artefacta, which may be defined as any form of self-inflicted skin injury in which the patient denies producing the lesions.
- Delusional parasitosis, in which patients have an erroneous but unshakable belief that their skin is infested by parasites.
- Dermatological nondisease, which is a common disorder of cutaneous body image in which the patient presents with dermatological complaints but with no significant skin pathology on examination.

In a study of these patients, Sheppard[42] advised that early recognition and intervention is important. It is an important area where close liaison between psychiatrists and dermatologists is essential. Some important disorders are discussed here.

Generalized Pruritus

It denotes that no organic cause, but emotional conflicts has been established for its occurrence. Itching caused by 'itching dermatoses' like scabies and pediculosis should be differentiated from internal disorders, e.g. nephritis, leukemia, and food allergy.

Psychological factors which are believed to be important include repressed anger and repressed anxiety. Whenever these persons consciously (or preconsciously) experience anger or anxiety, they scratch themselves, often violently. These patients have need for affection, and frustration of this need elicits aggressiveness that is inhibited. The rubbing of skin provides a substitute gratification of frustrated needs, and scratching represents aggression turned against the self.

Localized Pruritus

The two important types are:

1. *Pruritus ani*: It is a distressing complaint which interferes with job and social as well as familial activity. After detailed investigation and psychological assessment, it is often found that personality deviations precede this condition.
2. *Pruritus vulvae*: In some patients, scratching and rubbing gives a feeling of pleasure. They realize that it is a symbolic form of masturbation though the pleasure element is often repressed. On detailed evaluation, it is often found that there is evidence of sexual frustration that is intensified at the time of pruritus.

Hyperhidrosis

The sweat secretion is increased by fear, rage and tension. Emotional sweating appears primarily on sole, palm and axillae, while thermal sweating occurs on forehead, neck and trunk. Under prolonged emotional stress, excessive sweating (hyperhidrosis) may lead to skin changes like rashes and blisters. This is viewed as an anxiety phenomenon mediated by the autonomic nervous system. It must be differentiated from drug-induced hyperhidrosis.

Shelly and Shelley[44] demonstrated a new form of stress-induced urticaria, known as adrenergic urticaria. It should be differentiated from cholinergic urticaria. Cholinergic urticaria is induced by stress, heat or emotion. It appears as a small papule in the center of a large, bright red flare of axon-mediated vasodilation. It represents a unique response to ACTH mediated by the autonomic nervous system, while adrenergic urticaria is caused by a unique response to noradrenaline. It can be distinguished from cholinergic urticaria in that the primary urticarial papule is surrounded by a halo of balanced constricted skin. The adrenergic urticarial lesion appears to be ultimately mediated by histamine, as shown by the mast cell degranulation. Retesting of patients currently diagnosed as cholinergic urticaria, despite a negative acetylcholine skin test, is recommended since they may actually have adrenergic urticaria. Propranolol seems to be the specific treatment for this condition.[43-45]

ENDOCRINAL AND METABOLIC DISORDERS

Endocrinal system is the regulatory system which controls differences in the various body mechanisms through release of the various chemical substances. There is interrelationship between the central nervous system and the endocrinal system which is evident from the main role performed by the hypothalamus where the autonomic and endocrinal systems are integrated, and through the various trophic peptides it regulates the peripheral endocrinal activity. In addition, these peripheral hormones provide feedback on neurons in the pituitary and brain, leading to regulation of further release of these hormones and the function of brain, too. Therefore, brain becomes a site of action for the various hormones and, in addition, a regulator of hormonal action.

The hypothalamus and diencephalon are the two main sites which coordinate the endocrinal-neuronal interaction and have behavioral significance.

Hyperthyroidism

It is a syndrome characterized by biochemical and psychological changes, which in turn occur because of the chronic endogenous or exogenous excess of thyroid hormone.

It has been seen that in a few genetically predisposed individuals, stress is usually associated with the onset of hyperthyroidism when the regulatory mechanisms break down, resulting in premature stimulation of the body's psychophysiological defenses and thyrotoxicosis usually results.

According to the psychoanalytic theory, hyperthyroid patients, in their childhood, have unusual attachment and dependence on one parent, usually mother, and any threat to mother's approval or affection becomes intolerable. These patients in childhood lack adequate support because of economic crisis, death or divorce of parent(s), or due to multiple siblings. This constant threat to the security in early life results in premature and unsuccessful attempts to identify with an adult object. Moreover, this leads to early stress and over-utilization of endocrinal system and further frustration of childhood dependence cravings. Because of this failure, the patients always strive towards premature self-sufficiency and try to dominate over others with smothering attention and affection. They also develop defenses against repetition of same unbearable feelings of rejection and isolation that occurred in childhood.

Diabetes Mellitus

It is a metabolic disorder in which hereditary factors are etiologically important.

If the onset is acute, it is usually associated with emotional stress which disturbs the homeostatic balance in predisposed patients. The main psychological factors which seem significant are those which provoke the feelings of frustration, loneliness and dejection. Diabetic patients, who are supposed to maintain dietary control, often become depressed and dejected. They overeat or overdrink self-destructively and cause loss of control of diabetes. This is more common in juvenile diabetics. A few psychological traits like oral, dependent, maternal, attention seeking and passivity are commonly seen in diabetic patients.

Although it is assumed that 'stress' can raise the blood glucose levels in normal as well as diabetic subjects, Kemmer et al.[46] did not find any change in the blood glucose level in diabetic patients under stress. This may be because of the individual differences in subjects, their personality and the nature of stressor used.

Disorders Associated with Female Endocrine Functions

- *Premenstrual syndrome (PMS)*: It is characterized by cyclic, subjective changes in mood and general sense of physical and psychological wellbeing related to the menstrual cycle. Psychological stress plays an important role in its pathogenesis, along with other social and biological factors. The symptoms usually start post-ovulation, gradually increase and become maximum just about 4–5 days before the menstrual period. It has been recently hypothesized that excessive exposure to and subsequent abrupt withdrawal of endogenous opiate peptides, which fluctuate under the influence of gonadal steroids due to anxiety, fear and tension, may contribute to the onset. An increase in prostaglandins secreted by the uterine musculature is responsible for the severe pain.
- *Late luteal phase dysphoric disorder (LLPDD)*: This disorder occurs in late thirties and produces more distress than PMS. According to DSM-IV, it is characterized by emotional and behavioral symptoms that interfere with the social and occupational functioning. The symptoms appear in the last week of luteal phase of the cycle and remit within few days after onset of the follicular phase.

  The most commonly experienced symptom is affective lability (e.g. sudden episodes of tearfulness, sadness or irritability, anger and tension); feeling of depression may be accompanied by deliberate self-harm ideation, decreased energy and feeling of fatigue. Anorexia or craving for carbohydrate foods, irregular sleep, weight gain, joint and muscular pains, headaches, breast tenderness and a feeling of being bloated may also be present.

  This disorder should be differentiated from dysmenorrhea, depression and panic attacks. According to DSM-IV, dysmenorrhea is characterized by symptoms that occur with menses, whereas in LLPDD the onset of symptoms is premenstrual. The diagnosis of LLPDD should not be made if the symptoms preceding the menses are limited to pain and physical discomfort. Depression and panic attacks can be differentiated from LLPDD, because these disorders do not remit regularly with the onset of menses.
- *Menopausal distress*: This physiological state occurs about 1 year after the cessation of periods in the mean age group of 51.4 years. It can also occur after bilateral oophorectomy. The 'involutional period' refers to the advancing age, while 'climacteric' refers to the involution of the ovaries.

  Many psychological symptoms have been attributed to menopause including anxiety, fatigue, tension, emotional lability, irritability, depression, dizziness and insomnia. Physical signs and symptoms include night sweats, flushes and hot flashes. There are changes in the calcium and lipid metabolism due to low levels of estrogens and these may be associated with postmenopausal problems like osteoporosis and coronary atherosclerosis. The effects of osteoporosis on mood may be indirectly moderated through its influence on androgen production.

  Psychosocial factors play an important role in the clinical presentation. Women, who have previously experienced psychological difficulties, such as low self-esteem and low life satisfaction, are likely to be vulnerable to these problems during menopause. Women who have invested heavily in child bearing and child rearing activities are most likely to suffer distress during the postmenopausal period. Concerns about aging, loss of child bearing capacity and changes in appearance may be focused on the social and symbolic significance attached to the physical changes of menopause.

- *Idiopathic amenorrhea*: Cessation of normal menstrual cycle in nonpregnant, premenopausal women, in the absence of organic causes, is termed as idiopathic amenorrhea. Disturbed menses or delayed menses is a well-known response of a healthy woman to stress.

After exclusion, the diagnosis can be made by identifying possible primary psychogenic causes like anorexia nervosa and pseudocyesis. Other conditions may include massive obesity and in some cases excessive running or jogging. Organic causes which should be excluded are diseases of pituitary and drug-induced (reserpine and chlorpromazine) amenorrhea, which is almost always accompanied by galactorrhea and increased levels of prolactin. Psychotherapy may be helpful in restoring regular menses.

Sexuality and mood: Adler et al.[47] studied the relationship between mood, sexuality and hormone levels, and found that breast feeding women appear to be more likely to experience loss of sexual interest. The only striking relationship is that a fall in the sexual desire or interest is somehow causally related to the low levels of testosterone and androstenedione.

The postpartum period is one of major change and the mother has to adjust to the impact of her new child as well as to her altered physical state. Sexual activity declines during pregnancy and does not immediately return to pre-pregnancy levels after delivery. Many factors can affect mood and sexuality, including the hormonal levels. There are changes in the hormonal status after birth once the placenta is delivered, as well as changes later that appear to be due to breast feeding. Lactating women have high levels of prolactin and low levels of estrogen and progesterone. Conversely, nonbreast feeding women usually return to normal ovarian cyclicity, 6–15 weeks after delivery.

IMMUNE DISORDERS

There is evidence of a relationship among psychosocial factors, immune function and ill-health. The psychosocial processes, including life experiences and personality state and traits influence the brain, thereby encouraging the suppression of immune activity.

The endocrine system is highly influenced by life experiences and psychological states, and it has a significant effect on immune responses. A wide variety of stressors associated with emotional changes induce classical stress response within the organism and release ACTH, followed by a release of corticosteroids. These steroids have been found to alter the various immune responses and usually suppress, but occasionally may enhance, the immune response.

The effects of a single stress on the hypothalamopituitary-adrenal axis are well established, but the effects of repeated stressors (chronic stress) are less clear. Young et al.[48] found that the cells of actually stressed animals showed less, while the chronically stressed animals showed more, secretion of ACTH and b-endorphin in response to stimulation of CRF and AVP. It could be due to a change in the availability of releasable material, change in sensitivity of steroid negative feedback or changes in sensitivity to corticotropin-releasing factors (CRF) and arginine vasopressin (AVP). This differential release was not reflected in the differences in plasma levels of both peptides. Both in acutely and chronically stressed animals, plasma levels of corticosteroids were equally elevated.

- *Stress and immunity*: There is much evidence that stressful events may affect the body's resistance to infections and malignant diseases. Recent research indicates that such effects may be mediated through immune system. Stress related changes in the percentages of total T-lymphocytes, helper T-cells and suppressor T-cells were significantly lower in value as compared to baseline.[49] Immunological changes were not immediately associated with an increase in illness in a young and healthy subject. Such changes might have important consequences in individuals whose health is already impaired.

There is accumulating evidence that anxiety and depressed mood are related to a number of changes in the immune system. In a study, Arnetz, et al.[50] revealed that chronic unemployment produces a decrease in lymphocyte reactivity to phytohemagglutinin (PHA) and purified protein derivative (PPD). But recently, much attention has been given to the changes in cell mediated immune function that occurs in persons during distressing life experiences. There are two other indicators of immune function (natural killer cell activity and measure of T-cell subpopulation) which can increase understanding of the effects of psychological process on immune function.[51]

Psychological stresses appear to have a role in the regulation of natural killer cell activity. Impairment of such activity has been found in depressed, anxious and lonely people. The natural killer cell activity was found to be significantly lower in women undergoing major life changes, such as bereavement, than in subjects with few life changes.[51]

- *Cancer*: Studies are available in the literature which suggest a relationship between life events and malignancy. It has been reported that life experiences, particularly separation and loss of loved object, frequently precede the onset of various neoplasms, including cancer of cervix, leukemia and lymphoma. In contrast, several studies have found no relationship of such type.

Various studies have tried to correlate personality traits with susceptibility to cancer. Patients of lung cancer have been reported to be less able to discharge emotions than patients without cancer. Other studies reported that these patients excessively used the defenses of denial and repression.

The recent information of the immunological aspects of cancer raises the possibility that psychological influences are important in the mediation of immunological mechanisms in the susceptibility and course of neoplastic diseases. Stress has been associated with alteration of humoral and cellular immune mechanisms in experimental studies. Factors determining the effects of stress on the immune system and tumour growth include stress chronicity, timing, intensity and controllability.

Recent data from Shauit et al.[52] suggests that exposure to stress can cause release of opioid peptides from central and peripheral sites and cause analgesia. This also indicates that stressors different only by small amount could have very different neurochemical and hormonal consequences.

There is growing evidence that opioid peptides are involved in the immune system, e.g. opioid peptides enhance the cytotoxic activity of natural killer cells, and opiate agonists and antagonists have been related in tumor development. However, it is not clear whether opiates and opioid peptides act directly or indirectly on immune function. When the effects of opioid and nonopioid stress, and morphine on tumor growth were tested, the opioid, but not the nonopioid, form of foot shock stress given before tumor implantation had reduced median survival time and percent survival, as compared with nonstressed controls. Thus, it is likely that opioids are involved in the effect of stress on tumor growth. The tumor enhancing effect of the opioid stress was blocked by naltrexone and was mimicked by morphine.

MANAGEMENT

The psychosomatic approach is more than what has been called the bedside manner or medical art, more than the magnetic influence of the physician's or psychiatrist's personality on the patient, filling him with trust and confidence. It is based on specific knowledge of the emotional factors or stressors or reaction to life events operating in each and every case, and of those physiological mechanisms by which emotional factors influence the disease process. Only with this knowledge can psychotherapy be intelligently coordinated with somatic measures. A general knowledge of pathology, both psychological and somatic, is the primary requirement before starting the treatment or management of these disorders.

The most persistent error or misconception in this field is the belief that if emotional etiology in a case has been established, medical management becomes unnecessary and patients can be turned over to a psychiatrist. Progress in modern era consists specifically in the cooperation of the psychiatrist and nonpsychiatric personnel, both in diagnosis and in treatment. For example, a case of peptic ulcer requires first the remedy of this local lesion. Such a patient requires medical care, dietary management, pharmacological treatment, sometimes surgery, and psychotherapy aimed at the specific emotional factors of etiological significance. This is a long-term project and must be coordinated with the rest of medical management.

The first step is to arrive at a psychosomatic diagnosis. The psychosocial evaluation beyond the psychiatric history, social history, medical history and mental status examination should concentrate on the stimuli affecting the physical condition. These stimuli may include stress, home environment, or losses. These emotional conflicts, which the patients could not resolve, often have a disturbing influence upon vegetative functions. This is usually how the somatic symptoms make their first appearance. These first symptoms may appear in infancy, in the latency period or during adolescence. They seldom manifest themselves for the first time in adulthood. Careful study of these precursory, often transitory, symptoms in the earlier age periods shows that they develop during times of emotional stress and disappear with the relief of emotional tension, only to recur whenever new conflict situations arise under the vicissitudes of life.

A comparison of the emotional constellation during these different stages helps to establish the patient's typical pattern. For example, in a peptic ulcer patient, it is not unusual to find out any GIT disturbance in childhood when the first time the patient was forced to combat with his dependency needs, e.g. eating problems during the weaning period, nervous vomiting during the school going period, strenuous preparation for examination or on promotion to first job in adult life. So, these types of continued exposure to stress are responsible for such symptoms. Without a careful history and examination, it is not possible to study such precursors and their manifestations.[53]

Management of these disorders requires close collaboration with the primary physician or psychiatrist, with an emphasis on the doctor-patient relationship. There are two important points to remember:

1. The success of psychiatric intervention depends on how well the patient understands and accepts the psychological component of the illness and the rationale for its treatment.
2. The physician should know how to interpret the patient's recollections in the framework of his emotional development which can usually be reconstructed with great accuracy from history. This reconstruction requires a thorough knowledge of psychodynamics.

Alexithymic (lack of words to describe feelings) patients may respond better to pharmacologic or behavioral interventions.

Somatic Treatment

The psychopharmacological agents can only be useful if there is an underlying psychiatric disorder, like depression and anxiety. The pharmacological agents would not serve as a substitute for interaction with the primary physician, however.[54]

Psychosocial Treatment

After a somatic and personality diagnosis and clearly understanding the psychodynamics of emotional development, a treatment plan can be formulated. The acute or immediate care measures have preference over the long-range psychotherapeutic measures aimed at the basic etiologic factors.

As already seen, stress can cause serious complications. Thus, it needs to be reduced with coping mechanisms, which include relaxation training, hypnosis, biofeedback and systematic desensitization. The impact of stressor can sometimes be reduced, if a person has control over the stressor. Some people are better than others at coping with stressors. The more successful copers are said to have the following characteristics:[55]

- They seek information about how to deal with the problem and the availability of alternatives.
- They are prone to take direct action to reduce the effect of stressors.
- They are flexible in trying to cope, first trying one measure and then another.
- They try not to deal with the stressor through impulsive actions.
- They use cognitive mechanisms to deal with the stressor, such as reappraisal of the situation.

In psychosocial treatment, it is not possible to make fixed rules for psychotherapeutic intervention. The psychosomatic problems cannot be divided into physical and mental for treatment purposes; they must be treated in their totality. So, medical care and psychotherapy can be carried out simultaneously.

In other cases, psychotherapy must be postponed until the physiological disturbances are improved with the help of medical management. It is important to realize that penetrating psychotherapeutic measures which attack the fundamental emotional factors are apt to lead to transient increases of emotional tension, and may thus precipitate exacerbations of somatic symptoms. The psychotherapist or psychiatrist tries to re-expose the patient's ego to the original conflict situation. The expert psychotherapist will do so only gradually, constantly gauging the ego's capacity to deal with the conflict. Otherwise, transitory conflicts arise and may exacerbate somatic complaints. So, close cooperation between medical management and psychotherapeutic management is needed.

Psychosocial treatment is often beneficial if tailored to the stimuli affecting the physical condition. Some important therapies are:

- *Individual psychotherapy*: The most important factor is the development of strong doctor-patient relationship or bond of faith and belief. The exploratory or supportive individual psychotherapy can be beneficial when neurotic or personality factors make the subject or individual vulnerable to psychological stimuli.
- *Family therapy*: It is beneficial only when familial, interpersonal and other issues are influencing the course of the physical disease.
- Behavior therapy.
- Primary relaxation training.
- Biofeedback.

  These three therapies (c, d, e) need long-term therapeutic validation. These psychotherapeutic measures may be helpful in treatment of eating disorders, mild essential hypertension, skin disorders, pain syndromes and tension headaches.
- *Hypnosis and self-hypnotic training*: It has been reported to be useful in the treatment of pain, asthma, some gastro-intestinal disorders and some skin disorders.

Treatment of Specific Disorders

The treatment of psychosomatic disorders related to systems and individual disease is briefly discussed below:

- *Essential hypertension*: If the patient is settled on antihypertensive drugs and has a good compliance, he improves when he feels permitted to express his pent-up, hostile impulses during the interview or is encouraged to a greater extent of self-assertion in occupational situations or in relation to his family. The analysis of guilt feelings and dependent needs in these cases contributes greatly to the patient's ability to express his self-assertive tendencies with greater freedom and to find suitable outlets for his tension.

  Supportive psychotherapy and behavioral approaches (e.g. relaxation, mediation and biofeedback) have been reported to be useful in treatment.[56]
- *Coronary artery disease*: Medical management for occlusion and pain should be supportive and reassuring, with some psychological emphasis on the alleviation of psychic stress, compulsivity and tension.
- *Bronchial asthma*: Some asthmatic children improve if separated from mother. These patients should be treated jointly by physicians, allergists and psychiatrists. The asthmatic attack may be relieved by giving the patient an opportunity to 'confess' his repressed ego-alien tendencies in a few psychotherapeutic sessions. All standard psychotherapeutic approaches are used; individual, group, behavioral and hypnotic.[57]
- *Hyperventilation syndrome*: Proper education or training is required so that the patient can understand how these symptoms are evoked by hyperventilation, so that the patient may avoid these precipitating symptoms consciously.[58]
- *Peptic ulcer*: Apart from medical treatment (cimetidine or ranitidine or famotidine and antacids), dietary control is indicated in the ulcer management. The patient gets relief from acute symptoms within a few sessions if he is given legitimate outlets for passive dependent desire. The physician may order the patient in an authoritative

manner to go on a vacation, thus giving him an acceptable excuse for relaxation. Another approach is to give outlet in the transference situation for the patient's dependent needs. This can be achieved by analyzing the guilt and pride which are the emotional factors responsible for the repression of passive dependent longings or aggressive demanding attitudes.

Psychotherapy is directed towards the patient's dependency conflict. Biofeedback and relaxation techniques may be more beneficial.[59]

- *Ulcerative colitis*: Medical treatment consists of nonspecific supportive medical measures, such as anticholinergics and antidiarrheal agents. Bismuth containing medications have a specific role in the management of diarrhea.

  Supportive psychotherapy is indicated during the acute phase of colitis, with more interpretative psychotherapy during the more quiescent periods. In this disease, the weakness of the ego of these patients leads to a tendency to paranoid projection. Some patients suffer from borderline psychosis. Therefore, it is important for the therapist to gauge how far he can go in burdening the ego with uncovered repressed impulses.

  In many cases, superficial supportive psychotherapy is useful in relieving symptoms whereas deep, penetrating therapy may lead to an exacerbation of the illness or may precipitate a psychotic episode. In supportive therapy, the physician must be aware of the fundamental conflict situation in order to assume the right approach. In many cases, helping the patient loosen his conflict over his regressive tendencies and allowing him to repudiate responsibilities without guilt feelings may stabilize the intestinal tract. This does not mean that the personality problem has been resolved. The organic disease, however, may be controlled by these relatively simple psychotherapeutic measures.[60]
- *Obesity*: It may be controlled through dietary limitation and reduction of caloric intake. Supportive psychotherapy and biofeedback behavior modification may be useful for anxiety and depression associated with over-eating and dieting.
- *Rheumatoid arthritis*: In these cases, rest and exercise is very useful along with supportive psychotherapy, especially in acute cases. The physician's knowledge of the specific emotional factors may be helpful in hastening remissions. If the patient can express his resentment in conjunction with useful service to others, his symptoms are often relieved. The environmental conditions can often be manipulated and rendered suitable for draining hostile impulses through acceptable media.[61]
- *Low backache*: The treatment should be conservative. Analgesics, anxiolytics, rest and simple exercises are advised. Supportive psychotherapy regarding the precipitating emotional trauma, relaxation technique or biofeedback mechanism are often helpful. Patients should be encouraged to return to their usual activities as soon as possible.
- *Headaches*: During the prodromal phase of migraine, ergotamine tartrate and analgesics are helpful. Prophylactic use of propranolol or dilantin is advocated if the headaches are frequent. Psychotherapy to diminish stress and biofeedback mechanism have proved useful.
- *Tension headaches*: These may be treated by anxiolytic drugs, muscle relaxants and massage or heat application to the head and neck. If there is underlying depression, antidepressants can be used. Supportive psychotherapy, biofeedback, behavior therapy, relaxation, meditation, changes in pressured life style and learning to avoid or better cope with tension are the most effective long-term management approaches.[55]
- *Hyperthyroidism*: Antithyroid medication sometimes along with anxiolytics and supportive psychotherapy is used. Crisis intervention may be useful in acute phase.
- *Diabetes mellitus*: Supportive psychotherapy may play an important role in order to achieve cooperation in the medical management. Supportive therapy should encourage diabetics to lead as normal a life as possible, with the recognition that they have a chronic but manageable disease.
- *PMS and LLPDD*: The symptoms of both diseases are treated conservatively. Water retention, which accounts for a bloating feeling, weight gain and edema may be relieved by diuretics, hormones and salt restriction. Pain responds to analgesics, preferably acetaminophen which does not interfere with the clotting mechanism as compared to aspirin.

  Mental manifestations (fatigue, lassitude and general malaise) respond to small doses of amphetamines, which appear to act synergistically with analgesics to relieve pain.[58] It is important to make the individuals aware that PMS represents a recurring syndrome that can be anticipated. Psychotherapy may be helpful. Rarely, psychotic symptoms appear in LLPDD that respond to antipsychotic medication.
- *Menopausal distress*: Treatment programs must be individualized. Postclimacteric women may be asymptomatic, may have estrogen deprivation or may manifest estrogen excess (dysfunctional uterine bleeding). Exercise, diet and symptomatic treatment are helpful in reducing physical discomfort.

  Psychological distress should be evaluated and treated primarily by appropriate psychotherapeutic and sociotherapeutic approaches.[58] Psychotherapy should include an exploration of the life stage and the meaning of age and sexual life of patient. Individual should be encouraged to live a normal life and accept the truth that menopause is a natural life event. Patients should be advised to develop new activities, interests, and gratifications.

- *Idiopathic amenorrhea*: Psychotherapy may be the only useful measure in restoring regular menses. It helps to determine its cause and help get rid off these symptoms.

REFERENCES

1. World Health Organization. Technical Discussion of World Health Assembly. Geneva: WHO, 1974.
2. Shepherd M. Book Review. Hillow (Ed). Modern Trends in Psychosomatic Medicine. J Neuro Neurosurg Psychiatry. 1971; 34:207.
3. Lipowski ZJ. Psychosom Med. 1974;1:175.
4. Lipowski ZJ. Review of consultation psychiatry and psychosomatic medicine: Theoretical issues. Psychosom Med. 1968;30:422.
5. Wittkower ED. Historical perspective of contemporary psychosomatic medicine. Int J Psychol Med. 1970;5:309-19.
6. Lipowski ZJ. Psychosomatic medicine in the seventies: An overview. Am J Psychiatry 1977.
7. Tuke DH. Illustrations of the Influence of the Mind upon Body in Health and Disease. London: Church; 1872.
8. Alexander F. Psychosomatic Medicine. New York: Norton; 1950.
9. Alexander F, French T, Pollack GH. Psychosomatic Specificity: Experimental Study and Results. Chicago: University of Chicago Press; 1968.
10. Wolf S, Wolff HG. Human Gastric Function: New York: Oxford University Press; 1943.
11. Selye H. The physiology and pathology of exposure to stress. Acta Montreal; 1950.
12. Mahl GG. The effect of chronic fear in gastric secretion. Psychosom Med. 1949;11:30.
13. Kaplan JI, Sadock BJ. Comprehensive Textbook of Psychiatry. 5th edition. Baltimore: Williams and Wilkins; 1989.
14. Dubos R. Man, Medicine and Environment. New York: Ican Library, 1968.
15. Ludwig AM. Principles of Clinical Psychiatry, 2nd edition; 1986. pp. 518-20.
16. Roessler R, Engel BT. The current status of the concepts of physiological response specificity and activation. Int J Psychiatry Med. 1974;5:359-66.
17. Hawkins DR. Specificity revisited: Personality profile and behavioral issues. Psychother Psychosom. 1982;38:54-63.
18. Reiser MF. Mind, Brain, Body: Towards a Convergence of Psychoanalysis and Neurobiology. New York: Basic Books; 1984.
19. Weiner H. Psychobiology and Human Disease. New York: Elsevier; 1977.
20. Friedman IN, Rosenman RH. Type A Behavior and Your Heart. New York: Alfred A Knopf; 1974.
21. Binder JA. Prospective epidemiological study of psychosomatic and psychiatric syndromes in young adults.Psychother Psychosom. 1982;38:128-40.
22. Reiser MF. Changing theoretical concepts in psychosomatic medicine. In: Arieti S (Ed). American Handbook of Psychiatry. 5th edition. Vol. 4. New York: Basic Books; 1977. p. 117.
23. Mirsky IA. Physiologic, psychologic and social determinants in the etiology of duodenal ulcer. Am J Dig Dis. 1958;3:285.
24. Kaplan HI, Sadock BJ. Synopsis of Psychiatry, 5th edition. Baltimore: Williams and Wilkins; 1988. pp. 412.
25. Engel GL, Psychological aspects of gastrointestinal disorders. In: Reiser MF. (Ed). American Handbook of Psychiatry. 2nd edition. Vol. 4. New York: Basic Books; 1975. p. 653.
26. Takeuchi K, Furukawa O, Okabe S. Induction of duoedenal ulcers in rats under water immersion stress conditions: Influence of stress on gastric acid and duodenal alkaline secretion. Gastroenterology. 1986,91:554-63.
27. Feldman M, Walker P, Green JL, et al. Life events stress and psychosocial factors in men with ulcer disease: A multidimensional case controlled study.
28. Meghkinpour WPH, Hochler F. The effect of stress on colon motor and electrical activity in irritable bowel syndrome. Psychosom Med. 1985;47:139-49.
29. Friedman M, Thoresen CE, Gill JJ, et al. Feasibility of altering type A behavior pattern after myocardial infarction: Recurrent coronary prevention project study methods, baseline results and preliminary findings. Circulation. 1982;66:83.
30. Shekelle RB, Hulley SB, Neeton JD, et al. The MRFIT Behavior pattern study. II. Type A behavior and incidence of coronary heart disease. Am J Epidemiol. 1985;122:559-70.
31. Gill JJ, Price VA, Friedman M, et al. Reduction in Type A behavior in healthy middle aged American military officers. Am Heart J. 1985;110:503-14.
32. Elk R, Mashes. Hypertension in the aged: Psychosocial and psychiatric concomitants in colored community. S Africa Med J. 1985;67:1046-9.
33. Schnieden RH, Egan BM, Johnson EH, et al. Psychosom Med. 1986;48:242-8.
34. Jorgensen RS, Housten BH. Family history of hypertension: Personality patterns and borderline hypertension. Psychosom Med. 1986;48:242-8.
35. Thailer SA, Friedman R, Hirshfield GA, et al. Psychologic differences between high, normal and low renin hypertension. Psychosom Med. 1985;47:294-7.
36. Ewer TC, Stewarts DE. Improvement in bronchial hyperresponsiveness in patients with moderate asthma after treatment with a hypnotic technique: A randomized controlled trial. Br Med J. 1986;293:1129-32.
37. Bruch H. Eating Disorders. New York: Basic Books; 1973.
38. Lotz M, Carson DA, Vaushan JH. Rheumatoid synoviocytes: Pathway in pathogenesis of arthritis. Science. 1987;235: 893-5.
39. Gupta MA, Moldofsky H. Dysthymic disorder and rheumatic pain modulation disorder (fibrositis syndrome): A comparison of symptoms and sleep physiology. Can J Psychiatry. 1986;31: 608-16.

40. Daniel HH, Lourie FRS, Meltzer HJ, et al. The Year Book of Psychiatry and Applied Mental Health; 1988. p. 257.
41. Rimon R, Zaokso RL. Life stress and rheumatoid arthritis: Fifteen year follow-up study. Psychiatrica Fennia. 1984;15: 91-7.
42. Sheppard NP, Loughlin SO, Malone JP. Psychogenic skin disease: A review of 35 cases. Br J Psychiatry. 1986;149: 636-43.
43. Eller JJ. Skin disorder and the psychecutis. 1974;13:395-416.
44. Shelly WB, Shelley ED. Adrenergic urticaria: A new form of stress-induced hives. Lancet. 1985;2:1013-33.
45. Weiner H, Freedman DX, Lourie RS. The Year Book of Psychiatry and Applied Mental Health, 1987.
46. Kemmer FW, Bisping R, Steingruber HJ, et al. Psychological stress and metabolic control in patients with type I diabetes mellitus. N Engl J Med. 1986;314:1078-84.
47. Adler EM, Cook A, Davidson D, et al. Hormones, mood and sexuality in lactating women. Br J Psychiatry. 1986;148: 74-9.
48. Young EA, Ali H. CRF stimulation of adreno-corticotropin and b-endorphin release effects of acute and chronic stress. Am J Psychiatry. 1985;117:23-30.
49. Ronald G, Glaser JK, Stout JC, et al. Stress and related impairment in collector immunity. Psychiatr Res. 1985;16: 223-39.
50. Ametz BB, Petrini WB, Bremner SO, et al. Immune function in unemployed women. Psychosom Med. 1987;49:3-12.
51. Irwin M, Daniels M, Bloom ET, et al. Life events, depressive symptoms and immune function. Am J Psychiatry. 1987;144: 437-41.
52. Shauit J, Teman GW, Martin FC, et al. Stress, opioid peptides, the immune system and cancer. J Immunol. 1985;135: 8345-75.
53. Alexander F. Psychosomatic Medicine: Its principles and applications. Therapy. 1952;263:271.
54. Flaherty JA, Chanon RA, Davis JM. Psychiatric Diagnosis and Therapy: Psychological Factors Affecting Physical Illness. Lange; 1989. pp. 210-12.
55. Morgan CT, King RA, Weizz JR, et al. Introduction to Psychology; 1989. pp. 326-8.
56. Wise TN. "Update on consultation-liaison psychiatry (psychosomatic medicine)". Curr Opin Psychiatry. 2008;21(2): 196-200.
57. Levenson, James L. (2006) Essentials of Psychosomatic Medicine. American Psychiatric Press Inc. ISBN 978-1-58562-246-7.
58. Nurdeen Deuraseh, Mansor Abu Talib. "Mental health in Islamic medical tradition", The International Medical Journal. 2005;4(2):76-9.
59. Asaad, G. Psychosomatic Disorders: Theoretical and Clinical Aspects. Brunner-Mazel. 1996;129-130. ISBN 978-0-87630-803-5.
60. Erwin, Edward. The Freud Encyclopedia: Theory. Therapy and Culture. Routledge. 2002;245-6. ISBN 978-0-415-93677-4.
61. Sarno, John. The Divided Mind. Regan Books; 2006. ISBN 0-06-085178-3.

CHAPTER

23

Chronic Fatigue Syndrome

Rakesh Lal

Chronic fatigue syndrome (CFS) is the term that is generally accepted by scientists and mostly by clinicians for the range of complaints that patients commonly refer to as myalgic encephalomyelitis (ME) or chronic fatigue and immune dysfunction syndrome. CFS is characterized by persistent and unexplained fatigue resulting in severe impairment in daily functioning. Sporadic CFS-like cases and epidemics were described first in the 19th and 20th centuries, but interest in CFS increased in the early 1980s with the advent of ME, a term that had been introduced 30 years earlier for an epidemic of neurological symptoms among staff at the Royal Free Hospital in London, UK.

In the illness ME, apart from neurological symptoms, chronic fatigue was a main symptom. Initially, comparisons with neurasthenia were made, and a possible role of viruses and other microorganisms was examined. In the absence of a recognizable cause, ME was referred to as a psychiatric disorder or a 20th century illness. Controversial views about the dichotomy of organic versus functional were presented. Since then, practitioners have disagreed on whether the illness really exists. Researchers, practitioners, and patients have not been able to agree on the name (ME or CFS), on case definitions, on the acceptability of diagnosing CFS as an illness, on the absence of underlying pathophysiology and the need to continue research in somatic causes, or on the effectiveness of cognitive behavior therapy (CBT). All these issues are discussed here, including those of epidemiology, clinical manifestations, and management of CFS. We also look forward to future studies resulting from a few promising hypotheses.

Definitions

The first studies of CFS were limited by the lack of proper diagnostic features and definitions. From 1988 onwards, several case definitions of CFS were developed. In 1994, a consensus was reached on a revised case definition from the US Centers for Disease Control and Prevention (Panel 1). The importance of criteria on non-specific accompanying symptoms has been questioned, since the number of additional symptoms depends strongly on the assessment method used and no differences have been found in fatigue severity between patients whose disease met the criteria and those whose disease did not. The CFS of groups of patients who met the case definitions but had different symptom severities. Also, heterogeneity has been found within samples of patients with chronic fatigue. Between 2000 and 2002, international experts joined forces and identified ambiguities in the case definition for CFS. Guidelines for systematic and uniform case ascertainment and specific instruments for classification were developed to resolve ambiguities. In 2003, another case definition was proposed in an attempt to exclude psychiatric cases. Although they differ, all case definitions select severely fatigued groups of patients. Since CFS is neither a distinct nosological disorder nor a discrete diagnostic entity, the main purpose of a case definition is to identify patients who are at the tail end of the dimension fatiguing illness. The most widely supported scientific case definition is the 1994 definition from the US Centers for Disease Control and Prevention, which is now considered the standard.

One thing the scientists agreed on naming the illness CFS, whereas patients and practitioners preferred ME. Patients were reluctant to use CFS, because in the WHO 1992 classification, neurasthenia, which was associated with CFS, was linked to psychiatry and postiviral fatigue syndrome (benign myalgic encephalomyelitis) was linked to neurology, although the descriptions of the two disorders were identical. During the past few years, the UK collaborating center of the WHO Guide to Mental Health in Primary Care unified CFS and ME in a single psychiatric code. However, the WHO did not permit dual classification of the same disorder; ME remained classified as a neurological disorder and patients' organizations adopted the name CFS/ME.

To resolve the difficulties related to the definition of CFS, the consensus criteria should be validated by study of cohorts of patients with the disorder in several countries in the near future.

Epidemiology and Prognosis

The difficulties with definition have affected the results of epidemiological studies. Prevalence varies widely. For this reason, only studies using the 1994 case definition of the Centers for Disease Control and Prevention have been reviewed. Two US community based CFS studies found prevalences among adults of 0.23% and 0.42%; the rates were higher in women, members of minority groups, and people with lower educational attainment and occupational status. A prospective primary-care study in the UK found a CFS rate of 2.6%. After exclusion of patients with comorbid psychological disorders, the prevalence is 0.50%, a rate similar to those in the community-based studies, which did not exclude such cases. The reason why rates from the two countries differ is not clear. Two studies have found incidences of 0.18% and 0.37%, which seem high. However, owing to differences in study methods, they cannot be compared with the prevalences mentioned above. The estimated prevalence of CFS is much lower among children and adolescents than among adults.

A recent systematic review of the prognosis of CFS showed that full recovery without treatment is rare. Most prognostic studies were done in specialist centers with a bias towards severe cases. The duration of follow-up of prognostic studies ranged from 1 year to 5 years. The median recovery rate was 5% (range 0 to 31%) and the median improvement rate 39.5% (range 8 to 63%). A better outcome was predicted by less severe fatigue at baseline and the patient's not attributing the illness to physical causes, whereas psychiatric disorder predicted poorer outcomes.

Demographic data show that in most studies 75% or more of patients with CFS are female. The mean age at onset of CFS is between 29 years and 35 years. The mean illness duration ranges from 3 years to 9 years.

Few reliable and valid epidemiological data on CFS are available. Future epidemiological studies should focus on both the incidence and prevalence of CFS in the general population.

Panel 1: 1994 case definition for CFS from US Centers for Disease Control and Prevention characterized by persistent or relapsing unexplained chronic fatigue

- Fatigue lasts for at least 6 months
- Fatigue is of new or definite onset
- Fatigue is not the result of an organic disease or disease of continuing exertion
- Fatigue is not alleviated by rest
- Fatigue results in a substantial reduction in previous occupational, educational, social, and personal activities
- Four or more of the following symptoms, concurrently present for $\geq$ 6 months: impaired memory or concentration, sore throat, tender cervical or axillary lymph nodes, muscle pain, pain in several joints, new headaches, unrefreshing sleep, or malaise after exertion
- Exclusion criteria
- Medical condition explained fatigue
- Major depressive disorder (psychotic features) or bipolar disorder
- Anorexia nervosa, bulimia nervosa
- Alcohol or substance abuse
- Severe obesity

Clinical Manifestations

The main complaint of patients with CFS is persistent severe fatigue, but most have many concomitant symptoms and, in some, complaints of pain and cognitive dysfunction are just as prominent as the fatigue. Unprompted, patients mention an average of eight complaints and report symptoms of myalgia, impaired memory or concentration, gastrointestinal problems, headaches, and pain in muscles or several joints. Dizziness, nausea, anorexia, and night sweats are also reported. Many patients, especially those presenting to tertiary care, report an acute onset of symptoms after an infectious illness. In nearly all cases, the symptoms have resulted in substantial reduction in previous degree of occupational, educational, social, and personal activities. Symptom characteristics differ between individuals diagnosed as having CFS and those with CFS in the general population. In the general population, the onset of fatigue is gradual in most individuals with CFS. Patients with tender lymph nodes and a sore throat were more likely to see a physician than those without these symptoms and might be over-represented in clinic-based studies.

Etiology

Many studies have investigated the etiology and pathogenesis of CFS. More than half of the CFS studies between 1980 and 1995 concentrated on the physical etiology of CFS, with a slight shift towards psychological and psychiatric research in the next few years. Many somatic and psychosocial hypotheses on the etiology of CFS have been explored. Explanations for CFS were sought in viral infections, immune dysfunction, neuroendocrine responses, dysfunction of the central nervous system, muscle structure, exercise capacity, sleep patterns, genetic constitution, personality, and (neuro) psychological processes. Although several studies found abnormalities, only a few were diagnosed in large groups of patients with CFS and were independently confirmed in well controlled studies, an exception being the subtle changes in the hypothalamopituitary-adrenal axis. The etiology and pathogenesis are generally believed to be multifactorial. Distinction between categories of predisposing, precipitating, and perpetuating factors is useful for understanding of this complex disorder. The assumption is that one or more factors of each of these categories is conditional but insufficient for development of CFS.

Precipitating Factors

Acute physical or psychological stress might trigger the onset of CFS. Three-quarters of patients with the disorder have reported an infection, such as a cold, flulike illness, or infectious mononucleosis, as the trigger. A causal relation has been found between infectious mononucleosis and chronic fatigue. High rates of chronic fatigue after Q fever and Lyme disease have been found. However, no differences have been found in load of Epstein-Barr virus and immunological reactivity between individuals who developed CFS and those who did not. Precipitating somatic events such as serious injuries, surgery, pregnancy, or labor, which are reported as the onset of CFS by patients, have not been studied systematically. Psychological stress as a trigger of CFS has also been studied. Serious life events, such as the loss of a loved one or a job, and other stressful situations have been found to precipitate the disorder.

Perpetuating Factors

Once CFS has developed, several maintaining factors can impede recovery. Psychological processes seem to be involved in the perpetuation of complaints in patients with CFS. These processes involve ideas or cognitions of patients about complaints and behavioral factors such as persistent avoidance of activities associated with an increase in symptoms. A strong belief in a physical cause of the illness, a strong focus on bodily sensations, and a poor sense of control over complaints contribute to an increase in fatigue severity and functional impairment. In a study of monozygotic twins discordant for CFS, the affected twins used more avoidance strategies than their non-fatigued co-twins. Inactivity of patients with CFS is caused by perceptions and expectations rather than by physical fitness. In CFS, discrepancies between perceived and actual cognitive performance have been found. A similar perception problem has been found for sleep disturbance. Twin studies have contributed particularly to evidence on the difference between perception and actual functioning of patients with CFS.

Other perpetuating CFS factors that have been identified are social processes ranging from solicitous behavior to lack of social support. Illness perceptions and illness behavior can be reinforced by people in the patient's environment, such as a partner or family. Practitioners can contribute to the persistence of CFS by continuously encouraging unnecessary medical diagnostic procedures, by persistently suggesting psychological causes, or by not acknowledging CFS as a diagnosis, thus causing communication problems. Apart from the many disadvantages, long-lasting illness can also have more desirable consequences, such as care, attention, disengagement, or even financial benefits, which might also be considered perpetuating factors.

Pathophysiology

The nature of the underlying pathophysiology of CFS remains unclear. Many biological mechanisms have been hypothesized. Abnormalities in the central nervous system and immune system have been extensively studied. Evidence of discrete neuroendocrine abnormalities has been found. Neuroendocrine challenge tests have found a lower than normal cortisol response to increased corticotropin concentrations and upregulation of the serotonergic system. Studies of neuroendocrine function in patients with CFS have found no evidence for uniform dysfunction of the hypothalamopituitary-adrenal axis or stress hormones. Increasing evidence points to acquired neuroendocrine dysregulations in patients with CFS. Evidence for immunological dysfunction is not consistent. Many studies, some of which were not well controlled for nonspecific stress effects, focused on cytokines and shifts in T-lymphocyte subsets and had variable results. The studies in monozygotic twins discordant for CFS have not provided support for immunological abnormalities. Nevertheless, at the tissue level, cytokines such as interleukin-6 might have an important role in CFS, because they are also involved in the stress response and are crucial inducers of sickness behavior, which is characterised by avoidance behavior, apathy, sleepiness, impaired memory and concentration, anorexia, mild fever, and increased sensitivity for pain.

The role of RNase L molecule in the type 1 interferon pathway is unclear. No specific pattern of cerebral abnormalities in patients with CFS has been found. Functional MRI studies in patients with CFS have shown that various areas in the brain are activated during erroneous performance in a motor imagery task, which suggests a motivational disturbance. Two studies have also found a reduction in the volume of gray matter in patients with CFS, but independent confirmation is needed.

Abnormalities of the neuroendocrine and central nervous systems alone are not sufficient to explain the symptoms of CFS. More complex interactions between regulating systems are assumed to be at work and seem to involve the central nervous system, the immune system, and hormonal regulation systems.

Diagnosis and Management

Guidelines for clinical management of CFS have received much less attention than those for its definition. Although CFS protocols have been developed, clinicians still express difficulty in diagnosing the disorder. Apart from having to cope with the definition difficulties, they also have to deal with patients who can present their complaints of severe fatigue in different ways. Some patients simply wonder what is going on, whereas others diagnose CFS/ME themselves, which can lead to irritation on the doctor's part, especially if he or she is uncertain or skeptical about the CFS diagnosis or even contests it. Some patients have been searching for a diagnosis for a long time. This diversity of presentations challenges the management skills of general practitioners and specialists. In all cases, the first step in the symptom specific history is to gain insight into the patient's expectations and objectives. Many patients with CFS attribute symptoms to somatic factors, which cause them to expect too much of diagnostic tests. Some might have a hidden agenda involving insurance issues and invalidity-benefit claims. Identification of these issues and expectations at an early stage makes communication more transparent and prevents the doctor and patient from taking up entrenched positions. In a survey of patients with CFS, two-thirds were dissatisfied with the quality of medical care and pointed out the need for better communication and more on productivity costs and use a longer period of follow-up.

The Future

Although adherents of biopsychosocial and pathological CFS models have made steps towards agreement on definition and diagnosis, some of the patients' organizations seem to share the opinion that the success of CBT confirms the bias that CFS has a psychogenic cause. This argument reinforces the old model in which diseases or complaints are considered as either somatic or psychiatric in origin. In modern medicine, the biopsychosocial approach should guarantee that both facts are attended to. The use of a phychological CFS model does not, preclude neurobiological components. Until recently, studies on biological or psychological CFS mechanisms were directed at one feature of the illness and not at the integral syndrome. Pathophysiological research should follow two strategies. The first consists of distinguishing CFS from other disorders. The characteristics and pathophysiology of chronic fatigue in, for example, neurological disorders (multiple sclerosis, neuromuscular disorders, after stroke), in or after cancer, and in chronic inflammatory disorders such as rheumatoid arthritis, should be compared with those in CFS. The other strategy consists of investigating the similarities and dissimilarities in functional somatic syndromes. Modern neurosciences offer some explanatory models, which might bridge the gap between somatic and psychological models that might show both similarities and differences.

The challenge is to find out what is wrong in the molecular interplay at the level of the central nervous system. In the brain, hormones such as corticotropin-releasing factor, corticotropin, and cortisol interact with cytokines (such as interleukins 6 and 1) and neuropeptides (such as serotonin and dopamine). In this network of molecules, receptors are also modulated. Techniques such as bioimaging and proteomic strategies, and perhaps a systems biology approach should be applied to try to elucidate such complicated interactions.

In other models, chronic and severe disturbance of homeostatic mechanisms is supposed to be the basis for deregulating systems in functional somatic syndromes. Psychobiological responses to extreme stress have been identified and related to resilience or vulnerability. Like fibromyalgia, CFS could be conceptualized as a stress disorder, in which adverse life experiences, stress regulation, and pain-processing mechanisms are highly inter-related. Psychobiological sensitization mechanisms might be related to functional somatic syndromes. During chronic stress, the central nervous system, especially the limbic system, is supposed to increase sensitization. In this setting other areas of the central nervous system lose control and contribute to increases in symptoms and avoidance behavior.

Another important question is whether CFS is a homogeneous or heterogeneous disorder. Various researchers have called for investigations of subgroups by features such as chronicity, immunology, activity and neurobiology.

Mechanisms of Improvement

How a psychological treatment such as CBT contributes to physical improvement is not yet known. What elements in CBT are essential for recovery? Do cognitive and behavioral interventions need equal attention? Is graded exposure to exercise or increased physiological fitness essential for recovery? A recent randomized controlled trial has found that the treatment effect of graded exercise therapy (GET) is mediated by a decrease in symptom focusing rather than an increase in fitness. This finding is remarkable, since increased activity was assumed to be necessary for recovery. Studies on the process of change during CBT are necessary for the best treatment to be achieved. Perception seems to have a more central role than exercise. Since cortisol is related to cognitive appraisal, in which perception is the first step, CBT studies should pay more attention to changes in neuroendocrine functions as outcome measures. The important question is whether neuroendocrine and immunological abnormalities are reversible, for example after successful CBT, or do these abnormalities predict a negative outcome of CBT? There is some evidence that neuroendocrine abnormalities revert with successful CBT.

Tailor-made Treatment

Once we know more about the elements in CBT that cause the main improvements in specific groups of patients with CFS, more efficient and less expensive treatments can be developed. GET with low numbers of individual treatment sessions and telephone follow-up calls has shown promising results for patients without strong illness beliefs or concurrent emotional difficulties. Cooperation with patients' support groups has been suggested as a way to spread evidence based advice among patients with CFS. For some patients, group CBT might be more efficient by combining patients' support and evidence-based interventions. However, group therapy for CFS also has disadvantages. It can lead to reinforcement of dysfunctional behavior or resistance against psychotherapy. Furthermore, individualized CBT is more difficult to achieve for each patient in a group. When more knowledge is available about processes involved in improvement, research into CBT and GET might focus on tailor-made treatment with variable intensity or forms. Internet therapy or self-help better education of doctors in the diagnosis and management of their illness.

A thorough history, a meticulous physical examination, a mental status examination, and a minimum array of laboratory tests are necessary. Laboratory investigation is meant only to detect other disorders, not to find out whether a patient has CFS. Assessment of fatigue severity and functional impairment in the history of the patient remains difficult. If there is doubt about symptom severity or disability, brief questionnaire assessment might be considered to optimize the process of diagnosis. The diagnostic value of the accompanying symptom criteria in the case definition still has to be proven in a clinical setting. In the absence of sufficient symptom severity or disability for the diagnosis of CFS, appropriate acknowledgment of the patients' symptoms and suffering by the doctor prevents patients from radicalizing disease opinions. Diagnosis of CFS alone is not sufficient. Education of the patient should include an explanation of the illness model, information about effective treatments, and motivation for therapy. More attention to these factors in the education of doctors is essential.

Treatment

Systematic reviews have investigated the effectiveness of several CFS treatments. CBT and GET are the only interventions found to be beneficial. The subtle changes found in the hypothalamopituitary-adrenal axis have led to two randomized controlled trials, on the basis of which the researchers have not concluded that steroids are the treatment of choice. For immunological interventions such as immunoglobulin, the evidence has been inconclusive. There has also been insufficient evidence of the effectiveness of pharmacological, supplementary, complementary, and other interventions. The conclusions from these reviews have not been refuted as yet.

The model of perpetuating factors in CFS, which shows causal relations between both cognitive and behavioral factors and CFS symptoms, has been a promising starting point for elaboration on CBT. This therapy is a general form of psychotherapy directed at changing condition-related cognitions and behaviors. CBT for depression has not been effective for patients with CFS. This lack of efficacy is not surprising, since there are clear differences between depressed patients with CFS and patients with major depression. Central CBT components for CFS include explanation of the etiological model, motivation for CBT, challenging and changing of fatigue-related cognitions, achievement and maintenance of a basic amount of physical activity, gradual increase in physical activity, and planning work rehabilitation or rehabilitation in other personal activities. CBT teaches patients with CFS how to acquire control over symptoms. In several randomized controlled trials, CBT for CFS has been compared with standard medical care and other treatments, such as immunotherapy, relaxation therapy, and support groups. The same has been done for GET. CBT for CFS is based on a behavioral model of avoidance and always includes a graded activity programme. GET is based on a physiological model of deconditioning and has no intention of explicitly treating cognitions. In a few GET studies, cognitions to encourage graded exercise have been modified. CBT is generally a more complex treatment than GET, which might explain why CBT studies show better improvement rates (around 70%) than those with GET (around 55%). A treatment advocated by patients is pacing, which is lifestyle management allowing optimum adaptation to the illness, including an appropriate balance of rest and activity. A current study in the UK is comparing pacing with CBT and GET, but no evidence for this treatment is available as yet.

Most CBT studies strive for rehabilitation of patients with CFS. The study had cure of CFS as its explicit goal of therapy. Cure has been defined as disappearance of symptoms and functional impairment, ability to return to work and to undertake other activities, no longer interpreting everyday bodily signs as indicating CFS, and letting go of the label "CFS patient". As in other chronic diseases, the meaning of cure varies tremendously among patients. At the beginning of CBT, recovery seems vague and unattainable for most patients. Therapists should broaden the patient's vision to a future life as a healthy person. A personal goal can never be achieved if it not aimed for. By striving for rehabilitation only, therapists might deprive patients with CFS of a potential cure.

Lasting benefits of CBT recovery or improvement have been shown by significant differences between the original groups of two randomized controlled trials at 2-year and 5-year follow-up. However, not all patients benefit from CBT or GET. Predictors of poor treatment outcome were membership of a self-help group, receipt of a sickness benefit, claiming a disability-related benefit, low sense of control, a strong focus on symptoms, and a pervasively passive activity pattern. Duration of illness, surprisingly, did not predict treatment outcome. Most CBT/GET studies had samples of patients with median duration of illness of about 5 years. If CBT were offered to patients at an earlier stage of the illness, medical and societal costs might be substantially reduced.

Economic analysis of CBT and GET for patients with CFS and chronic fatigue have shown that the cost of therapy was higher than that of usual care, but the outcome was better. For more accurate estimation of the cost-effectiveness of CBT in patients with CFS, future research should focus instruction might be useful for some patients. Similarly, more insight into the neurobiology of CFS might lead to a new drug treatment, which might be used separately or in combination with CBT.

SUGGESTED READING

1. Afari N, Buchwald D. Chronic fatigue syndrome: a review. Am J Psychiatry. 2003;160:221-36.
2. Afari N, Schmaling K, Herrell R, Ashton S, Goldberg J, Buchwald DS. Coping strategies in twins with chronic fatigue and chronic fatigue syndrome. J Psychosom Res. 2000;48:547-54.
3. Afari N, Van Der Meer J, Bleijenberg G, Buchwald D. chronic fatigue syndrome in practice. Psychiatr Ann. 2005;35:350-60.
4. Ball N, Buchwald DS, Schmidt D, Goldberg J, Ashton S, Armitage R. Monozygotic twins discordant for chronic fatigue syndrome objective measures of sleep. J Psychosom Res. 2004;56:207-12.
5. Barsky AJ, Borus JF. Functional somatic syndromes. Ann Intern Med 1999;130:910-21.
6. Bazelmans E, Bleijenberg G, van der Meer JWM, Folgering H. Is physical deconditioning a perpetuating factor in chronic fatigue syndrome? Psychol Med. 2001;31:107-14.
7. Bazelmans E, Prins JB, Lulofs R, van der Meer JWM, Bleijenberg G. Cognitive behavior group therapy for chronic fatigue syndrome: a non-randomised waiting list controlled study. Psychother Psychosom. 2005;74:218-24.
8. Bell EJ, McCartney RA. A study of coxsackie B virus infections, 1972-1983. J Hyg. 1984;93:197-203.
9. Bentall RP, Powell P, Nye FJ, Edwards RHT. Predictors of response to treatment for chronic fatigue syndrome. Br J Psychiatry. 2002;181:248-52.
10. Blacker CV, Greenwood DT, Wesnes KA, et al. Effect of galantamine hydrobromide in chronic fatigue syndrome: a randomized controlled trial. JAMA. 2004;292:1195-204.
11. Bleijenberg G, Vercoulen JHMM, van der Meer JWM. How important are symptom criteria in the definition of CFS? J Intern Med. 2004;256:268-9.
12. Bleijenberg G. Chronic fatigue and chronic fatigue syndrome in the general population. Health Qual Life Outcome. 2003;1:52.
13. Blockmans D, Persoons P, van Houdenhove B, Lejeune M, Bobbaers H. Combination therapy with hydrocortisone and fludrocortisone does not improve symptoms in chronic fatigue syndrome: a randomized place-controlled, double-blind, crossover study. Am J Med. 2003;114:736-41.
14. Bonner D, Ron M, Chalder T, Butler S, Wessely S. Chronic fatigue syndrome: a follow-up study. J Neurol Neurosurg Psychiatry. 1994;57:617-21.
15. Brace MJ, Scott SM, McCauley E, et al. Family reinforcement of illness behaviour: a comparison of adolescents with chronic fatigue syndrome, jurvenile arthritis and healthy controls. J Dev Behav Pediatr. 2000;21:332-9.
16. Brouwers FM, van der Werf S, Bleijenberg G, van der Zee L, van der Meer JWM. The effect of a polynutrient supplement on fatigue and physical activity of patients with chronic fatigue syndrome: a double-blind randomized controlled trial. QJM. 2002;95:677-83.
17. Buchwald D, Herrell R, Ashton S, Belcourt M, Schmaling K, Goldberg J. A twin study of chronic fatigue: Psychosom Med. 2001;63:936-43.
18. Buchwald D, Sullivan JL, Komaroff AL. Frequency of "chronic active Epstein-Barr virus infection" in a general medical practice. JAMA. 1987;257:2303-07.
19. Buchwald DS, Rea TD, Katon WJ, et al. Acute infectious mononucleosis: characteristics of patients who report failure to recover. Am J Med. 2000;109:531-7.
20. Butler JA, Chalder T, Wessely S. Causal attribution for somatic sensations in patients with chronic fatigue syndrome and their partners. Psychol Med. 2001;31:97-105.
21. Butler S, Chalder T, Ron M, Wessely S. Cognitive behaviour therapy in chronic fatigue syndrome. J Neurol Neurosurg Psychiatry. 1991;54:153-8.
22. Byrne E. Idiopathic chronic fatigue and myalgia syndrome (myalgic encephalomyelitis): some thoughts on nomenclature and etiology. Med J Aust. 1988;148:80-2.
23. Cairns R, Hotopf M. A syntematic review describing the prognosis of chronic fatigue syndrome. Occup Med. 2005;55:20-31.
24. Capuron L, Gumnick JF, Musselman DL, et al. Neurobehavioral effects of interferon-alpha in cacer patients: phenomenology and paroxetine responsiveness of symptom dimensions. Neuropsychopharmacology. 2002;26:643-52.
25. Carruthers BM, Jain AK, De Meirleir KL, et al. Myalgic encephalomyelitis/chronic fatigue syndrome: clinical working case definition, diagnostic and treatment protocols. J Chronic Fatigue Syndr. 2003;11:7-115.
26. Chalder T, Goodman R, Wessely S, Hotopf M, Meltzer H, Epidemiology of chronic fatgue syndrome and self reported myalgic encephalomyelitis in 5-15 years old: cross sectional study. BMJ. 2003;327:654-5.
27. Charney DS. Psychobiological mechanisms of resilience and vulnerability: implications for successful adaptation to extreme stress. Am J Psychiatry. 2004;161:195-216.

28. Chaudhare A, Bechan PO. Fatigue in neurological disorders. Lancet. 2004; 363:978-88.
29. Clark C, Buchwald D, Maclutyre A, Sharpe M, Wessely S. Chronic fatigue syndrome: a step towards agreement. Lancet. 2002;359:97-8.
30. Clarke JN, James S. The radicalized self: the impact on the self of the contested nature of the diagnosis of chronic fatigue syndrome. Soc Sci Med. 2003;1387-95.
31. Cleare AJ, Heap E, Malhi GS, Wessely S, O'keane V, Miell J, Lowdose hydrocortisone in chronic fatigue syndrome: a randomized crossover trial. Lancet. 1999;353:455-8.
32. Cleare AJ. The HPA axis and the genesis of chronic fatigue syndrome. Trends Endocrinol Metabol. 2004;15:55-9.
33. Cleare AJ. The neuroendocrinology of chronic fatigue syndrome. Endocr Rev. 2003;24:236-52.
34. Cleare AJ. The neuroendocrinology of chronic fatigue syndrome. Endocr Abst. 2003;5:S35.
35. David A, Wessely S, Chronic fatigue, ME, and ICD-10, Lancet. 1993;342:1247-48.
36. David AS, Wessely S, Pelosi AJ. Postviral fatigue syndrome: time for a new approach. BMJ. 1988;296:696-9.
37. de Becker P, McGregor N, de Meirleir K, Possible triggers and mode of onset of chronic fatigue syndrome. J Chronic Fatigue Syndr. 2002;10:3-18.
38. de Lange FP, Kalkman JS, Bleijenberg G, et al. Neural correlates of the chronic fatigue syndrome: an FMRI study. Hrain. 2004; 127:1948-57.
39. de Lange FP, Kalkman JS, Bleijenberg G, Hagoort P, Van Der Meer JWM, Toni I. Grey matter gvolume reductopn in chronic fatigue syndrome. Neuroimage (in press).
40. de Meirleir K, Bisbal C, Campine I, et al. 37 kda 2-5A binding protein as a potential biochemical marker for chronic fatigue syndrome. Am J Med. 2000;108:99-105.
41. Deale A, Chalder T, Marks I, Wessely S. Cognitive behaviour therapy for chronic fatigue syndrome: a randomized controlled trial. Am J Psychiatry. 1997;154:408-14.
42. Deale A, Husain K, Chalder T, Wessely S. Long-term outcome of cognitive behaviour therapy versus relaxation therapy for chronic fatigue syndrome: a 5-year follow-up study. Am J Psychiatry. 2001;158:2038-42.
43. Deale A, Wesselu S. Patients perceptions of medical care in chronic fatigue syndrome. Soc Sci Med. 2001;52:1859-64.
44. Edmonds M, McGuire H, Price J. Exercise therapy for chronic fatigue syndrome. Cochrane Database Syst Rev. 2004;3:CD003200.
45. Eriksen HR, Ursin H. Subjective health complaints, sensitization, and sustained cognitive activation (stress). J Psychosom Res. 2004;56:445-8.
46. Friedberg F, Krupp LB. A comparison of cognitive behavioral therapy in chronic fatigue syndrome. Clin Infect Dis. 1994;18 (Suppl 1):105-9.
47. Fukuda K, Stratus SE, Hickie I, et al. The chronic fatigue syndrome: a comprehensive approach to its definition and study. Ann Intern Med. 1994;121:953-9.
48. Fulcher KY, White PD. Randomised controlled trial of graded exercise in patients with chronic fatigue syndrome: BMJ. 1997;314:1647-52.
49. Gaab J, Engert V, Heitz V, Schad T, Schurmeyer TH, Ehlert U. Association between neuroendocrine response to insulin tolerance test and patient characteristics in chronic fatigue syndrome. J Psychosom Res. 2004;56:419-24.
50. Gow JW, Simpson K, Bechan PO, Chaudhuri A, Mc Kay IC, Behan WM. Antiviral pathway activation in patients with chronic fatigue syndrome and acute infection. Clin Infect Dis. 2001;33:2080-1.
51. Hatcher S, House A. Life events, difficulties and dilemmas in the onset of chronic fatigue syndrome: a case-control study. Psychol Med. 2003;33:1185-92.
52. Heijmans JWM. Coping and adaptive outcome in chronic fatigue syndrome importance of illness cognitions. J Psychosom Res. 1998;45:39-51.
53. Hickie I, Bennett B, LIoyd A, Health A, Martin N. Complex genetic and environmental relationships between psychological distress, fatigue and immune functioning: a twin. Psychol Med. 1999;29:269-77.
54. Hickie I, Kirk K, Martin N. Unique genetic and environmental determinants of prolonged fatigue: a twin study. Psychol Med. 1999;29:259-68.
55. Holmes GP, Kaplan JE, Gantz NM, et al. Chronic fatigue syndrome: a working case definition. Ann Intern Med. 1988;108:378-9.
56. Hoogveld S, Prins J, de Jong L, et al. Persoonlijkheidskenmerken en het chronisch vermoeidheidssyndroom: een literatuuroverzicht (Personality characteristics and the chronic fatigue syndrome: a review of the literature). Gelragstherapie. 2001;34:275-305.
57. Hotopf M, wessely S. Stress in the workplace: unfinished business. J Psychosom Res. 1997;43:1-6.
58. Jason IA, Richman JA, Rademaker AW, et al. A community-based study of chronic fatigue syndrome. Arch Intern Med. 1999;159:2129-37.
59. Jason LA, Corradi K, Torres-Harding S, Taylor RR, King C. Chronic fatigue syndrome: the need for subtypes. Neuropsych Rev. 2005;15:29-58.
60. Jones J, Nisenbaum R, Solomon L, Reyes M, Reeves WC. Chronic fatigue syndrome and other fatiguing illnesses in adolescents: a population based study. J Adolesc Health. 2004;35:34-40.
61. Jordan KM, Landis DA, Downey MC, Osterman SL, Thrm AE, Jason IA. Chronic fatigue syndrome in children and adolescents: a review. J Adolesc Health. 1998;22:4-18.
62. Joyce J, Hotopf M, Wessely S. The prognosis of chronic fatigue and chronic fatigue syndrome: a systematic review. QJM. 1997;90:223-33.
63. Kelley KW, Bluthe RM, Dantzer R, et al. Cytokine-induced sickness behaviour: mechanisms and implications. Trends Neurosci. 2002;25:154-9.
64. Kennedy G, Abbot NC, Spence V, Underwood C, Belch JJ. The specificity of the CDC-1994 criteria for chronic fatigue

syndrome: comparison of health status in three groups of patients who fulfil the criteria. Ann Epidemiol. 2004;14:95-100.

65. King C, Jason LA. Improving the diagnostic criteria and procedures for chronic fatigue syndrome. Biol Psychol. 2005;68:87-106.
66. Komaroff AL, Fagioli LR, Geiger AM, et al. An examination of the working case definition of chronic fatigue syndrome. Am J Med. 1996;100:56-64.
67. Konsman JP, Parnet P, Dantzer R. Cytokine-induced sickness behaviour: mechanisms and implications. Trends Neurosci. 2002;25:154-9.
68. Lawrie SM, Mander DN, Geddes JR, Pelosi AJ. A population-based incidence study of chronic fatigue. Psychol Med. 1997;27:343-53.
69. LIoyd AR, Hickie I, Boughton CR, Spencer O, Wakefield D. Prevalence of chronic fatigue syndrome in an Australian population. Med J Aust. 1990;153:522-8.
70. LIoyd AR, Hickie I, Brockman A, et al. Immunologic and psychologic therapy for patients with chronic fatigue syndrome: a double-blind, placebo-controlled trial. Am J Med. 1993;94:197-203.
71. LIoyd AR. Postinfective fatigue. In: Jason LA, Fennell PA, Taylor RR (Eds). Handbook of chronic fatigue syndrome. Hoboken, New Jersey: John Wiley & Sons; 2003. pp. 108-23.
72. Lyall M, Peakman M, Wessely S. A systematic review and critical evaluation of the immunology of chronic fatigue syndrome. J Psychosom Res. 2003;55:79-90.
73. Mahurin RK, Clapoole KH, Goldberg JH, Arguelles L, Ashton S, Buchwald D. Cognitive processing in monozygotic twins discordant for chronic fatigue syndrome. Neuropsychology. 2004;18:232-9.
74. McCrone P, Ridsdale L, Darbishire L, Seed P. Cost-effictiveness of cognitive behavioural therapy, graded exercise and usual care for patients with chronic fatigue in primary care. Psychol Med. 2004;34:991-9.
75. McKenzie R, O'fallon A, Dale J, et al. Low-dose hydrocortisone for treatment of chronic fatigue syndrome: a randomized controlled trial. JAMA. 1998;280:1061-6.
76. Melamed BG. Family systems perspective. In: Jason LA, Fennell PA, Taylor RR (Eds). Handbook of chronic fatigue syndrome. Hoboken, New Jersey: John Wiley & Sons; 2003. pp. 192-201.
77. Metzger FA, Denny DR. Perception of cognitive performance in patients with chronic fatigue syndrome. Ann Behav Med. 2002;24:106-12.
78. Michiels V, Cluydts R. Neuropsychological functioning in chronic fatigue syndrome: a review. Acta psychiatr scand. 2001;103:84-93.
79. Moss-Morris R, Petrie KJ, Weinman J. Functioning in chronic fatigue syndrome: do illness perceptions play a regulatory role? Br J Health Psychol. 1996;1:15-25.
80. Moss-Morris R, Sharon C, Tobin R, Baldi JC. A randomized controlled trial of patient education to encourage graded exercise in chronic fatigue syndrome: outcomes and mechanisms of change. J Health Psychol. 2005;10:245-59.
81. Nijs J, de Meirleir K, Meeus M, Mc Gregor NR, Englebienne P. chronic fatigue syndrome: intracellular immune deregulations as apossible etiology for abnormal exercise response. Med Hypothess. 2004;62:759-65.
82. Nisenbaum R, Jones J, Unger E, Reyes M, Reeves W. A population-based study of the clinical course of chronic fatigue syndrome. Health Qual Life Outcomes. 2003;1:49.
83. Okada T, Tanaka M, Kuratsune G, Watanabe Y, Sadato N. Mechanisms underlying fatigue: a coxel-based morphometric study of chronic fatigue syndrome. BMC Neurol. 20034;4:14.
84. Olson LG, Ambrogetti A, Sutherland DC. A pilot randomized controlled trial of dexamphetamine in patient with chronic fatigue syndrome. Psychosomatics. 2003;44:38-43.
85. Page LA, Wessely S. Medically unexplained symptoms. exacerbating factors in the doctor-patient encounter. J R Soc Med. 2003;96:223-7.
86. Petrie K, Moss-Morris R, Weinman J. The impact of catastrophic beliefs on functioning in chronic fatigue syndrome. J Psychosom Res. 1995;39:31-7.
87. Powell P, Bentall RP, Nye FJ, Edwards RHT, Randomised controlled trial of patient education to encourage graded exercise in chronic fatigue syndrome. BMJ. 2001;322:1-5.
88. Powell P, Bentall RP, Nye FJ, Edwards RHT. Patient education to encourage graded exercise in chronic fatigue syndrome: 2-year follow-up of randomized controlled trial. Br J Psychiatry. 2004;184:142-6.
89. Powell R, Dolan r, Wessely S. Attributions and self-esteem in depression and chronic fatigue syndromes. J Psychosom Res. 1990;34:665-73.
90. Price JR, Couper J. Cognitive behaviour therapy for adults with chronic fatigue syndrome. Cochrane Database Syst Rev. 2002; 2:cd 001027.
91. Prins JB, Bleijenberg G, Bazelmans E, et al. Cognitive behaviour therapy for chronic fatigue syndrome: a multicentre randomized controlled trial. Lancet. 2001;357:841-7.
92. Prins JB, Bleijenberg G, de Boo Th M, van der Meer JWM. Cognitive behaviour therapy for chronic fatigue syndrome: correspondence, authors' reply. Lancet. 2001;358:240-1.
93. Prins JB, Bleijenberg G, Klein Rouweler E, van der Meer JWM. Psychiatric disorders among patients with chronic fatigue syndrome in a randomized controlled trial for the effectiveness of cognitive behaviour therapy. Br J Psychiatr. 2005;187:184-5.
94. Prins JB, Bleijenberg G, Klein Rouweler E, Van Weel C, Van Der Meer J WM. Doctor-patient relationship in primary care of chronic fatigue syndrome: perspectives of the doctor and the patient. J Chronic Fatigue Syndr. 2007; 7:3-15.
95. Prins JB, Bleijenberg G, van der Meer JWM. Chronic fatigue syndrome and myalgic encephalomyelitis. Lancet. 2002;359:1699.
96. Prins JB, Bos I, Servaes P, et al. Social support and the persistence of complaints in chronic fatigue syndrome. Psychother Psychosom. 2004;73:174-82.
97. Prins JB, Elving l, Koning H, Bleijenberg G, Van Der Meer JWM. Diagnosing chronic fatigue syndrome: comparison of

a protocol and computerized questionnaires, N J Med. 2003; 61:29-35.
98. Reeves WC, LIoyd A, Vernon SD, et al. Identification of ambiguities in the 1994 chronic fatigue syndrome research case definition and recommendations for solution. BMC Health Serv Res. 2003;3:25.
99. Reid S, Chalder T, Cleare A, Hotopf M, Wessely S. Extracts from "clinical Evidence": chronic fatigue syndrome. BMJ. 2000; 320:292-6.
100. Reyes M, Nisenbaum R, Hoaglin DC, et al. Prevalence and incidence of chronic fatigue syndrome in Wichita, Kansas. Arc Intern Med. 2003;163:1530-6.
101. Sabath DE, Barcy S, Koelle DM, Zeh J, Ashton S, Buchwald D. Cellular immunity in monozygotic twins discordant for chronic fatigue syndrome. J Infect Dis. 2002;185:828-32.
102. Salit IE, Precipitating factors for the chronic fatigue syndrome. J Psychiatr Res. 1997;31:59-65.
103. Schluederberg A, Straus SE, Peterson P, et al. Chronic fatigue syndrome research: definition and medical outcome assessment. Ann Intern Med. 1992;117:325-31.
104. Schmaling KB, Smith WR, Buchwald DS. Significant other responses are associated with fatigue and functional status among patients with chronic fatigue syndrome. Psychosom Med. 2000;62:444-50.
105. Severens JL, Prins JB, van der Wilt GJ, van der Meer JWM, Bleijenberg G. Cost effectiveness analysis of cognitive behaviour therapy for patients with chronic fatigue syndrome. QJM. 2004;97:153-61.
106. Sharpe M, Hawton K, Simkin S, et al. Cognitive therapy for chronic fatigue syndrome: a randomized controlled trial. BMJ. 1996;312:22-6.
107. Sharpe M. Medically unexplained symptoms and syndromes. Clin Med. 2002;2:501-4.
108. Sharpe MC, Archard LC, Banatvala JE, et al. A report-chronic fatigue syndrome: guidelines for research. JR Soc Med. 1991;84:118-21.
109. Shorter E, From paralysis to fatigue: a history of psychosomatic illness in the modern era. New York: NY Free Press, 1992.
110. Smith J, Fritz EL, Kerr JR, Cleare AJ, Wessely S, Mattey DI. Association of chronic fatigue syndrome with human leucocyte antigen class II alleles. J Clin Pathol. 2005;58:860-63.
111. Solomon L, Nisenbaum R, Reyes M, Papanicolaou DA, Reeves WC. Functional status of persons with chronic fatigue syndrome in the Wichita, Kansas, population. Health Qual Life Outcome. 2003;1:48.
112. Solomon L, Reeves WC. Factors influences the diagnosis of chronic fatigue syndrome. Arch Intern Med. 2004;164:2241-45.
113. Stanley I, Salmon P, Peters S. Doctors and social epidemics: the problem of persistent unexplained physical symptoms, including chronic fatigue. Br J Gen Pract. 2002;52:355-6.
114. Stulemeijer M, de Jong LWAM, Fiselier TJF, Hoogveld SWB, Bleijenberg G. Cognitive behaviour therapy for adolescents with chronic fatigue syndrome: a randomized controlled trial. BMJ. 2005;330:14.
115. Surawy C, Hackmann A, Hawton K, et al. Chronic fatigue syndrome: a cognitive approach. Behav Res Ther. 1995;33: 535-44.
116. Swanink CMA, van der Meer JWM, Vercoulen JHHM, et al. Epstein-Barr virus (EBV) and the chronic fatigue syndrome: normal virus load in blood and normal immunologic reactivity in the EBV regression assay. Clin Infect Dis. 1995;20:1390-92.
117. Swanink CMA, Vercoulen JHHM, Bazelmans E, et al. Viral antibodies in chronic fatigue syndrome. Clin Infect Dis. 1995;21:708-09.
118. Swanink CMA, Vercoulen JHHM, Bleijenberg G, Fennis JFM, Galama JMD, van der Meer JWM. Chronic fatigue syndrome: a clinical and laboratory study with a well-matched control group. J Intern Med. 1995;237:499-506.
119. Theorell T, Blomkvist V, Lindh G, Evengard B, Critical life events, infections, and symptoms during the year preceding chronic fatigue syndrome (CFS): an examination of CFS patients and subjects with a nonspecific life crisis. Psychosom Med. 1999;61:304-10.
120. van der Greef J, Stroobant P, van der Heijden R. The role of analytical sciences in medical systems biology. Curr Opin Chen Biol. 2004;8:559-65.
121. van Houdenhove B, Egle UT. Fibromyalgia: a stress disorder? Putting pieces of the biopsychosocial puzzle together. Psychother Psychosom. 2004;5:267-75.
122. Vercoulen JHMM, Bazelmans E, Swanink CMA, et al. The prevalence of neuropsychological impairment in chronic fatigue syndrome. J Clin Exp Neuropsychol. 1998;20:144-56.
123. Vercoulen JHMM, Swanink CMA, Fennis JFM, Galama JMD, van der Meer JWM, Bleijenberg G. Dimensional assessment of chronic fatigue syndrome. J Psychosom Res. 1994;38:388-92.
124. Vercoulen JHMM, Swanink CMA, Galama JMD, et al. The persistence of fatigue in chronic fatigue syndrome and multiple sclerosis: the development of a model. J Psychosom Res. 1998;45:507-17.
125. Vercoulen JHMM, Swanink CMA, Zitman FG, et al. A randomized, double-blind, placebo-controlled study of fluoxetime in chronic fatigue syndrome. Lancen. 1996;347:858-61.
126. Viner R, Hotopf M. Childhood predictors of self-reported chronic fatigue syndrome/myalgic encephalomyelitis in adults: national birth cohort study. BMJ. 2004;329:941.
127. Vollmer CU. Acute sickness behaviour: an immune system-to-brain communication? Psychol Med. 2001;31:761-7.
128. Wallman KE, Morton AR, Goodman C, Grove R, Guilfoyle AM. Randomised controlled trial of graded exercise in chronic fatigue syndrome. Med J Aust. 2004;180:444-8.
129. Watson NF, Jacobsen C, Goldberg J, Kapur V, Buchwald D. Subjective and objective sleepiness in monozygotic twins discordant for chronic fatigue syndrome. Sleep. 2004;27:973-7.
130. Watson NF, Kapur V, Arguelles LM, et al. Comparison of subjective and objective measures of insomnia in monozygotic twins discordant for chronic fatigue syndrome. Sleep. 2003;26:324-8.

131. Wealtherley-Jones E, Nicholl JP, Thomas KJ, et al. A randomized, controlled, triple-blind trial of the efficacy of homeopathic treatment for chronic fatigue syndrome. J Psychosom Res. 2004;56:189-97.
132. Wearden AJ, Morriss RK , Mullis R, et al. Randomised, double-blind, placebo-cotrolled treatment trial of fluoxetine and graded exercise for chronic fatigue syndrome. Br J Psychiatry. 1998;172:485-90.
133. Wessely S, Chalder T, Hirsch S, Wallace P, Wright D. The prevalence and morbidity of chronic fatigue and chronic fatigue syndrome: a prospective primary care study. Am J Public Health. 1997;87:1449-55.
134. Wessely S, Hotopf M, Sharpe M, Chronic fatigue and its syndromes. Oxford: Oxford University Press,1998.
135. Wessely S, Nimnuan C, Sharpe M. Functional somatic syndromes: one or many? Lancet. 1999;354:936-9.
136. Wessely S, Old wine in new bottles: neurasthenia and 'ME.' Psychol Med. 1990;20:35-53.
137. Wessely S, White PD. There is only one functional somatic syndrome. Br J Psychiatry. 2004;185:95-6.
138. White PD, Thomas JM, Kangro Ho, et al. Predictions and associations of fatigue syndromes and mood disorders that occur after infection mononucleosis. Lancet. 2001;358: 1946-54.
139. White PD. What causes chronic fatigue syndrome? BMJ. 2004;329:928-9.
140. Whiting P, Bagnall A, Sowden A, Cornell J, Mulrow C, Ramirez G. Interventions for the treatment and management of chronic fatigue syndrome: a systematic review. JAMA. 2001;286: 1360- 8.
141. Wilson A, Hickie I, Hadzi-Pavlovic D, et al. What is chronic fatigue syndrome? Heterogeneity within an international multicenter study. Aust N Z J Psychiatry. 2001;35:520-7.
142. Working group on CFS/ME (Chronic Fatigue Syndrome/MYalgic Encephalomyelitis). Report to the Chief Medical Officer of an idependent working group. Available at: http://www.dh.gov.uk/Publications And Statistics/Publications/Publications Policy And Guidance/PublicationsPAmpG Browsable Document/fs/en?CONTENT_ID=4095249&chk=jVPh3V (accessed Aug 1, 2005).
143. Zachrisson O, Regland B, Jahreskog M, Jonsson M, Kron M, Gottries CG. Treatment with staphylococcus toxoid in fibromyalgia/chronic fatigue syndrome—a randomized controlled trial. Eur J Pain. 2002;6:455-66.

CHAPTER 24

Personality Disorders

Sumant Khanna, Balati W

Personality consists of ingrained, pervasive, enduring and habitual ways of psychological functioning, that characterize one's style (Millon, 1987). It is a tightly interrelated organization of attitudes, perceptions, habits, emotions and behaviors that characterize a person's distinctive way of relating to others and to himself.

Personality is defined in the second edition of the WHO Lexicon of Psychiatric and Mental Health Terms as "The ingrained patterns of thought, feeling and behavior characterizing an individual's unique lifestyle and mode of adaptation and resulting from constitutional factor, development, and social experience".

Personality traits are defined as enduring patterns of perceiving; relating and thinking about the environment and oneself that are exhibited in a wide range of important social and personal contexts. However, personality is not just a collection of traits or predispositions, it also involves the ways in which the mind processes the input, i.e. it is synthesizing and integrative functions include recognition of motivations.

Personality disorders (PDs) according to DSM-IV (American psychiatric association 1994), are patterns of inflexible and maladaptive personality traits that cause subjective distress, significant impairment in social or occupational functioning or both. These traits must also deviate markedly from the culturally expected and accepted range, or norm, and this deviation must be manifested in more that one of the areas: cognition, affectivity, control over impulses and need gratification, and ways of relating to others.

Personality disorders according to ICD-10 guidelines "deeply ingrained and enduring behavior patterns, manifesting themselves as inflexible responses to a broad range of personal social situations. They represent either extreme of significant deviations from the way the average individual in a given culture perceives, thinks, feel and particularly relates to others. Such behavior patterns tend to be stable and to encompass multiple domains of behavior and psychological functioning. They are frequently, but not always, associated with various degrees of subjective distress and problems in social functioning and performance".

Personality Disorder Defined

It has several features which taken together identify the group of illness we refer to as PDs.

They are:

1. *Early onset*: It must manifest itself in adolescence or early adulthood.
2. *Stable and persistent*: It should be consistent over a period of time. Even though individual symptoms come and go, the severity may wax and wane, the basic behavior, syndrome and style remains.
3. *Pervasive*: It should not be restricted to any one kind of situation and must affect behavior across a variety of domains such as work, family and recreation.
4. *Interpersonal focus*: It is defined and expressed primarily in an interpersonal context.
5. *Impairment*: It must cause impairment that crosses the line from an abnormal or undesirable personality to a psychiatric disorder.

The distinction between personality disorder and mental disorder is valuable in everyday clinical practice, but is not always easy to make. Central to the concept in the duration of the abnormal behavior, if the person has previously behaved normally and then behaves abnormally, he is said to have a mental disorder, if the person has always behaved abnormally, he is said to have a personality disorder. The distinction is usually easy when behavior changes quickly (acute manic episode), but difficult when behavior changes slowly (schizophrenia). Impairment and pervasiveness of disorder is what makes it a mental disorder, whereas interpersonal nature, stability and persistence of the disorder make it personality disorder.

SIGNIFICANCE OF PERSONALITY DISORDERS

Personality disorders do, by definition, cause significant problems for those who have them and it becomes important for all the clinicians to identify personality disorders in their patients. Persons with these disorders often suffer and their relationship with others, are problematic. They have difficulty responding flexibly and adaptively to the environment and to the changes and demands of life, and they lack resilience when under stress. Instead, their usual ways of responding tend to perpetuate and intensify their difficulties. However, these individuals are often oblivious to the fact that their personality causes them problems, and they may instead blame others for their difficulties or even deny that they have any problems at all.

Personality disorders are costly to the society. Individuals with personality disorders frequently have considerable difficulty in their family, academic, occupational and other roles. They have elevated rates of separation, divorce, child custody proceedings, unemployment, homelessness (Caton et al, 1994), and perpetration of child abuse (Dinwiddie & Bucholz 1993). They also have increased rates of accidents (McDonald and Davey 1996), emergency department visits, medical hospitalization (Reich et al, 1989), violence, including homicide (Miller et al, 1993, Raine 1993), self injurious behavior (Hillbrand et al, 1994), attempted suicide and completed suicide (Brent et al, 1994), Hawton et al, 1993). There are well-established relations between personality and crime (70–80% of criminals have PDs), alcoholism (60–70% of alcoholics have PDs) and drug abuse (70-90% of drug abusers have PDs).

When co-morbid Axis I disorders (psychotic and neurotic disorders) are being treated, the presence of personality disorders need to be identified and treated as they often affect the prognosis and outcome of these disorders. Patients with depressive disorders, panic disorders and obsessive compulsive disorder often respond less well to pharmacotherapy when have a co-morbid personality disorder.

HISTORY

Personality type and disorders have been described for thousands of years, as evidenced by Hippocrates description of four temperaments—the pessimistic, melancholic, the overly optimistic Sanguine, the irritable choleric and the apathetic phlegmatic. It is interesting that the early Greeks theory that these temperaments were determined by the relative proportion of the four bodily humors (Black bile, yellow bile, blood and phlegm, respectively) is reflected in current attempts to discover biogenetic bases of personality.

In the beginning of the 19th century French Psychiatrist Pinel described "manie sans delire" (delire, a French term for delusion) and applied this term to patients who were prone to outburst or rage and violence but were not deluded. Presumably this group of patients included not only those who would now be regarded as having Antisocial personality disorder, but also those who were mentally ill but not deluded, e.g. some with mania. Referring to Pines' manie sans delire, J C Pritchard in 1835 suggested a new term "moral insanity" which he defined as "a morbid perversion of natural feelings, afflictions, inclinations, temper, habits, moral dispositions and natural impulses without any remarkable disorder or defect of the intellect or knowing and reasoning faculties and particularly without any insane illusion or hallucination". Although this description included the violent patient described by Pinel, Pritchard clearly had a wider group in mind, since he added a propensity to there is sometimes a feature of moral insanity and sometimes it is its leading if not sole characteristic.

In the late 1800s more specific personality types were described, e.g. Janet and Freud described the psychological traits associated with hysteria, the forerunner of histrionic personality disorder. Subsequently within the framework of early psychoanalytic instinct theory, Abraham proposed that arrests at the three psychosexual stages of childhood development—the oral, anal and phallic phases, led to the development of the dependent, obsessive compulsive and hysterical character types respectively. However, this view changed as early instinct theory and the subsequent ego-psychological model of psychoanalytic theory were gradually supplanted by object relations theory, which proposes that personality is shaped largely by the child early parental relationships. In this framework, dependent personality traits derive from parental deprivation, obsessive-compulsive traits from control struggles with parental figures, and hysterical traits in part from parental seduction and competition. The borderline and narcissistic personality disorder concepts also developed out of the object relations framework.

Personality types were described by Kraeplin (1921) and Kretschmer (1925), from a quite different prospect. They described in terms of Spectrum concept-according to them personality types are biogenetically related variants of the paranoid and affective psychoses (which would be now be considered as Axis-l disorders). Kraeplin described antisocial type, excitable, unstable, eccentric, liars, swindlers and quarrelsome. These early spectrum personality types were forerunners of the current paranoid, schizotypal, cyclothymic, and depressive personality disorders. Schneider a German phenomenologist, defines abnormal personalities in a statistical sense. He considered personality disorders to represent socially deviant and extreme variants of normally occurring personality traits. Some of these are psychopathic personalities who as a result of their abnormality, suffer or make others suffer. He developed the first comprehensive system of personality disorder categories, which provided the template for many of those contained in lCD-l0 and DSM-IV.

MODELS OF PERSONALITY

Personality disorders are studied based on two types of model, categorical and dimensional.

Categorical Models

Categorical models consider discontinuous personality categories. This type of model is used in DSM-IV and ICD-10, because of the need for a specific diagnostic. The categorization of the illness is based on the symptom and on their etiopathology, and says nothing about the nature of the disorders themselves. In the case of personality disorders, the categorization does not affirm or deny that they are disorders or illnesses, nor does it indicate where the symptoms differ from non-morbid behavior patterns. The better a personality disorder in understood an the more biological correlations are found in it, the more likely it is to be transferred from Axis II to Axis-I of DSM-IV. Epileptic personality, depressive personality, cyclothymic personality and even schizothymic personality disorders are now classified as Axis I disorders.

Dimensional Model

Dimensional model is based on the concept of trait or disposition. Jung was the fist person who made important contribution of the dimensional model. Traits are dimensions along which persons can be classifies, These models are based on the supposition that We all share the personality structure, differing only in the various combinations of trait The main problem is to define the number of dimensions that define personality and to establish whether or not these traits are universal. Eysenck identified three basic personality types, extraversion-introversion, neuroticism, and psychoticism, each including many levels of traits. Establishing correlations between the dimension and biological, cultural and genetic factors solves the problem.

Cloninger (1987) has attempted to overcome the dichotomy between—dimensional and categorical models by using four temperamental dimensions (novelty seeking, harm avoidance, reward dependence and persistence) which are lifelong and stable, and three character dimensions (self direction, co-operation and self-transcendence) which are variable and susceptible to environmental and development.

The five-factor model, based on factorial studies and individual differences has been widely accepted. It comprises the personality dimensions openness, conscientiousness, extraversion, agreeableness and neuroticism.

CLASSIFICATION OF PERSONALITY DISORDERS

Before considering ways of classifying the abnormal personalities, it is important to realize that any category in any classification scheme represented and ideal type, which few patients fit exactly. To quote Schneider "Any clinician would be greatly embarrassed if asked to classify into appropriate types the psychopaths (that is abnormal personalities) encountered in any one year", there are only a few cases in which one of the characteristic types of description or combination can be applied without further qualification. Human beings resist precise measurement and, unlike the phenomena of disease, abnormal individuals cannot be classified neatly in the manner of clinical diagnoses. The consequence is that many abnormal personalities fulfill criteria for more that one of the personality disorders listed in the system of classifications.

Personality disorders are grouped into three clusters in DSM-IV. Cluster A, the odd or eccentric, covers the paranoid, schizoid and schizotypal personality disorder, Cluster B, the dramatic, emotional, or eccentric covers borderline, histrionic, narcissistic and antisocial personality disorder. Cluster C, the anxious or fearful includes avoidant, dependent and obsessive compulsive personality disorder. Another category called personality disorder not otherwise specified, which includes passive aggressive personality disorder and depressive personality disorder. People with those disorders seem anxious or fearful. Many people exhibit traits that are not limited to a single personality disorder, when a patient meets the criteria for more than one personality disorder clinicians should diagnose each.

Another way of classifying personality disorders is using dimensional or categorical models. Each of the two approaches has specific advantages and disadvantages. For example, the dimensional model, with it is potential use of many personality descriptions and its ability to assess the degree to which traits are present, may more comprehensively cover problematic traits. It does not confine clinicians to the use of a limited number of categories. In addition, most of the traits embodied by the Axis-II criteria can be found in less self-extreme form in psychiatrically healthy people. The categorical model, however better reflects how clinicians think—that is in terms of pathological syndromes that a person have or does not have. The use of categorical model makes it possible for clinician succinctly to summarize patients difficulties and facilitates communication among them.

The main drawback of this approach are represented by the difficulty of classifying patients who are at the boundary of different categories or who do not meet the diagnostic criteria for any specific personality disorder, but who still have significant pathology. Although DSM-IV is based primarily on the categorical model, it also incorporates a dimensional approach to some extent, in that it encourages clinicians to identify problematic traits that are subthreshold for any particular diagnoses.

Table 1: Mature and immature personality disorders

Mature personality disorder	*Immature personality disorder*
Anankastic (obsessive compulsive)	Antisocial (dissocial)
	Borderline (impulsive)
Paranoid	Histrionic
Schizoid (and schizotypal)	Dependent
Anxious (avoidant)	Narcissistic

Tyrer and Seivewright (1988), studying personality disorder with regards to age, described two groups immature personality disorders which improves over time and mature personality disorders that tend to persist into late middle or old age (Table 1).

As shown in Table 2, there is a specific correspondence between ICD-10 and DSM-IV for seven categories of personality disorders namely paranoid, schizoid, dissocial/ antisocial, histrionic, anankastic/obsessive compulsive, anxious/avoidant and dependent personality disorders. For three categories, there are differences in the nomenclature between the two systems, in particular ICD-10 uses the term 'anankastic' instead of 'obsessive compulsive', in order to avoid erroneous implication in inevitable link between this type of personality and GCD. ICD-10 also uses the term 'dissocial' in order to prevent any possible connotation of stigmatization and the term 'anxious' instead of 'avoidant'. Moreover, while DSM-IV classifies borderline personality disorder as a specific category, ICD-10 includes it as subcategory of emotionally unstable personality disorder.

Narcissistic and passive-aggressive personality disorder (present in DSM-IV) are included in ICD-10 under the category of "other specific personality disorders". Finally while DSM-IV includes schizotypal personality disorder as a personality disorder, ICD-10 classifies it is in the overall group of "schizophrenia schizotypal and delusional disorder" to highlight the contiguity between this disorder and schizophrenia disorders; as shown by genetic and clinical studies. DSM-IV has the category 'personality disorders not otherwise specified', while ICD-10 has the category 'other specific personality disorders'. Both DSM-IV and ICD-10 have opted for polythetic approach to diagnosis, in which no single criterion is absolutely required, although a certain minimum number of criteria are needed for the diagnosis. Implicit in this system is an assumption that individual patients for the diagnosis. Implicit perfect examples of a given personality disorder but rather the individuals approximate to the prototype to a greater or lesser extent.

Table 2: Comparison of classification of personality disorders in ICD-10 and DSM-IV

ICD-10	*DSM-IV*
Paranoid PD Schizoid PD Dissocial PD	Paranoid PD Schizoid PD Antisocial PD
Emotionally unstable PD	
a. Impulsive type b. Borderline type	a. Nil b. Borderline PD
Histrionic PD Anankastic PD Anxious avoidant PD Dependent PD Other specific PDs	Histrionic PD Obsessive compulsive PD Avoidant PD Dependent PD Schizotypal PD Narcissistic PD PD NOS

ASSESSMENT OF PERSONALITY DISORDERS

The assessment of Axis Il disorders is in some ways more complex than that of Axis I disorders. It can be difficult to assess multiple domains of experience and behavior (i.e. cognition, affect, intrapsychic experience, inter personal interactions) and to determine that traits are not only distressing, impairing, and of early onset, but also pervasive and enduring. Nonetheless, a personality disorder assessment is essential to the comprehensive evaluation and adequate treatment of all patients. Table 3 shows the main methods currently available for assessing all personality disorders the following points related to these methods need to be mentioned.

The assessment methods described have shown a satisfactory inter rater reliability, while test-retest reliability has not been well established. However, two assessment methods show reasonably good test-retest reliability they are:

1. Personality assessment schedules (PAS) (Tyrer et al, 1983)
2. International personality disorder examination (IPDE) (Loranger et al, 1991)

It is suggested that in the assessment of personality disorders, the stability over time is important, as personality characters tend to be long lasting.

Most of the methods described have been standardized on psychiatric inpatient or outpatient populations, and hence their applicability in community based epidemiological studies in not known.

Some patients with personality disorders are unaware of the traits that reflect their disorder, or they may not perceive them as problematic. This limited self-awareness can interfere with personality disorder assessment, especially if the questions asked have negative or unflattering implications.

Another methodological problem is related to the choice of the person to be interviewed. Many authors argue that besides patients, a key informant should also be interviewed, as many patients may not reply reliable to questions asked about their personality. Moreover there is also a possibility that informant ratings may differ substantially from the patient ones. However, in such cases there arises another problem, i.e. whom to believe in the case of disagreement over ratings, as yet there are no guidelines to solves this issue.

The personality assessment is affected by the presence co-morbid Axis-I disorders (non-personality emotional disorder). Some structured interviews try to correct this by asking the patients about times when they ere not suffering from an Axis-I disorder and the use of informants who have patients over time and without an Axis-I disorder.

In general the agreement between clinician's diagnoses of personality disorders and self-report measures are poor. This may be due to,

Table 3: Assessment method of personality disorders

Name of Method	*Author(s)*	*Method of Assessment*	*No. of Items*	*Time Required (minutes)*
Diagnostic interview for PD (DIPD)	Zanarini	Semi-structured interview with patient using DSM-IIR criteria	101	60–120
International personality disorder examination (IPDE)	Loranger et al	Semi-structured using ICD-10 and DSM-IIIR criteria	157	150
Millon clinical multiaxial inventory (MCMI)	Millon	Self-report by patient using DSM-IIIR criteria	175	20–30
Personality assessment	Tyrer et al	Semi-structured interview with informants using DSM-III-R criteria	24	60
Schedule (PAS) personality diagnostic questionnaire-revised (PDQ-R)	Hyler and Reider	Self-report by patient or informant using DSM-IIIR criteria	152	30
Personality interview with questions II (PIQ-II)	Widger	Semi-structured patient using DSM-III criteria	375	60–120
Schedule for normal and abnormal PD (SNAP)	Clark	Self-report by patient using and DSM-III and dimensional criteria	106	10
Standardized assessment of personality (SAP)	Pilgrim and Mann (1990)	Semi-structured interview with informants using DSM-III-R ICD-10 criteria	NA	10–15
Structured clinical interview for DSM-III-R personality disorder (SCID-II)	Spitzer and Williams	Semi-structured interview with patient using DSM-IIIR criteria	120	60–90
Structured interview for DSM-III PD (SIPD)	Pfohl et al	Semi-structured interview with patient or informant using DSM-III criteria	136	90
Tridimensional personality questionnaire (TPQ)	Cloninger	Self-report by patient	100	20–30
Wisconsin personality inventory (WISPI)	Klein	Self-report by patient using DSM-III criteria	360	20

- Variation in raters (clinician, non-clinician)
- Interview occasions,
- Sources of information (patients or information),
- Availability of historical clinical data,
- Sensitivity to state affects (e.g. depression or anxiety may affect the prevalence of personality disorders using many current assessment methods) and
- Format (e.g. methods that have a dichotomic format (yes/no) may fail to distinguish between sporadic occurrences and enduring patterns of behavior).

Hence Perry (1992) suggested a different approach to assessment, involving an interview with the patient, in which occurrence of both Axis-I and Axis-II disorders during patient's life is assessed.

- Are personality disorder diseases?
- Are personality disorders are devisable from neurosis?

The origin of the current nomenclature of personality is diverse, Concepts like borderline personality disorder and narcissistic personality disorder have psychoanalytical roots, unlike the concept of schizotypal disorder arose out of the Scandinavian studies. Anxious avoidant and anankastic personality disorders have behavioral origins. As a matter of fact, the differentiation of anxious avoidant personality disorder from social phobia is so difficult that many researches and clinicians do not accept this dichotomy. Antisocial personality disorder is based on legal and social moral, and has actually shown a change of criteria because of this over time. Concepts like schizoid and paranoid personality disorder reflect more core phenomenological underpinnings. Realizing that personality disorders have such diverse origins probably constitutes a major part in the lack of their clarity in nomenclature.

Etiology

One of the most interesting and a challenging question with regards to personality disorders is what courses them. There are many studies truing to identify the factors responsible for the occurrence of these personality disorders but none were totally successful in achieving that goal, various hypothesis have been put forward over the years. Earlier it was though that development and environmental factors, such as pathological and inadequate parenting, constitutional or biological factors contributed to the development of personality disorder. It is unlikely that any one single cause will cause the personality disorders. Rather available data suggests that personality disorders result from a complex combination of and interaction between temperament (genetic and other biological factors) and psychological (developmental or environmental) factors.

Genetic factors have been found to play an important role in the development of personality disorders as shown by the family, twin and adoption studies. Among monozygotic twins the concordance for personality disorders were several times higher than that among dizygotic twins. Also according to another study monozygotic twins reared apart are about as similar as monozygotic twins reared together. Coming to personality disorders as such Cluster A personality disorder (paranoid, schizoid and schizotypal) are more common in the biological relatives of schizophrenia patients than among control groups. Cluster B disorder (antisocial, borderline, histrionic and narcissistic) apparently have a genetic base, as antisocial personality disorder is associated with alcohol use disorder. On the other hand, although there is some evidence for a genetic component in borderline personality disorder, the impact of the environment (i.e. development experiences) appears to be more important. The etiology and pathophysiology of the cluster C disorder have undergone little investigation. Of relevance, however, are studies indicating that approximately half the observed variance in personality traits such as neuroticism, introversion and submissiveness can be traced to genetic variation.

Investigation into the fields of Neurobiology as the causes for the personality disorders is rapidly increasing as the alterations in brain structure and function have been shown to be related to deficit like symptoms and increased dopaminergic function to psychotic symptoms in persons with schizotypal personality disorder. Abnormalities in the serotonin system, which appears to mediate behavioral inhibition, have been found in individuals with borderline and antisocial personality disorders. The recent finding, which requires replication, that the amount of the neuroticism is influenced by two alleles of a gene encoding a transporter for serotonin is an example of the groundbreaking work being in this important area.

Increasing numbers of studies of environmental antecedents of personality disorders, such as family, environment and sexual and physical abuse, are substantiating a likely role of for such factors in the development of certain disorders (e.g. Borderline personality disorder). In addition defense mechanisms appear to play an important role in the expression of personality disorder, which are characterized by less mature defense mechanisms such as projection and acting out.

SPECIFIC PERSONALITY DISORDERS: PARANOID PERSONALITY DISORDER

The essential feature of paranoid personality disorder is a pattern of pervasive distrust and suspiciousness of others such that their motives are interpreted as malevolent. This pattern begins by early adulthood and is present in a variety of contexts.

Epidemiology

The prevalence of paranoid personality disorder is 0.5 to 2.5 % of the general population. In the study by Baron, paranoid personality disorder was remarkably more common among relatives of schizophrenia probands (7.3%) than among relatives of control probands (2.7%). Most studies using DSM-IIIR criteria, which have reported high prevalence of personality disorders, have shown that paranoid personality disorder was present in less than 1/4th of patients. In most studies paranoid personality disorder overlapped extensively with schizotypal personality disorder with which it shares diagnostic criteria of paranoid ideation. Familial and genetic studies have showed that paranoid personality disorder shares a stronger familial relationship with Axis-I delusion disorder than with schizophrenia.

Clinical Features

The essential features of paranoid personality disorders are suspiciousness and sensitivity and pervasive distrust. Individuals with this disorder may be constantly on a look out for attempts by others to bet the better of him, to deceive him, or to play tricks on him. Thus, they may question, without justification, the loyalty or trustworthiness of friends or sexual partners, and they are reluctant to confide in others for fear that the information will used against them. They do not make friendship easily and may avoid involvement in-groups, appear guarded, tense, and hypervigilant, and they constantly scan the environment for clues of possible attack, deception, or betrayal. In response to perceived or actual insults or betrayals, these individuals overreact, quickly becoming excessively angry and responding with counterattacking behavior. They are unable to forget such incidents and instead bear long-term grudges against their supposed betrayers Ideas of reference and logically defended delusions are common.

Persons with this disorder effectively restricted and appear to be unemotional. They pride themselves on being rational and objective, but such is not the case.

They Lack warmth and are impressed with and pay close attention to power and rank they express disdain for those who are seen as weak, sickly, impaired or in some way defective. In social situations, people with paranoid personality disorder may appear business-like and efficient, but they often generate fear or conflict in others.

Differential Diagnosis

Paranoid personality disorders can be differentiated from other Axis-I disorders such as paranoid schizophrenia by the absence of hallucinations and formal thought disorder, and

DSM-5 Diagnostic criteria for paranoid personality disorder

a. A pervasive distrust and suspiciousness of others such that their motives are interpreted as malevolent, beginning by early adulthood and present in a variety of contexts, as indicated by four (or more) of the following:
   1. Suspects, without sufficient basis, that others are exploiting, harming, or deceiving him/her.
   2. Is preoccupied with unjustified doubts about the loyalty or trustworthiness of friends or associates.
   3. Is reluctant to confide in others because unwarranted fear that the information will be used maliciously against him/her.
   4. Reads hidden demeaning or threatening meanings into benign remarks or events.
   5. Persistently bears grudges (i.e. is unforgiving of insults, injuries, or slights).
   6. Perceives attack on his or her character or reputation that are not apparent to others and is quick to react angrily or to counterattack.
   7. Has recurrent suspicious, without justification, regarding fidelity of spouse or sexual partner.

b. Does not occur exclusively during the course of Schizophrenia, a mood disorder with psychotic features, or another psychotic disorder and is not due to the direct physiological effects of general medical condition.
Note: If criteria are met prior to the onset of schizophrenia, add "pre-morbid", i.e., "paranoid personality disorder (pre-morbid)".

from delusion disorder by the absence of fixed delusion. It can be distinguished from borderline personality disorder because paranoid patients are rarely capable of overly involved, tumultuous relationships with others. Paranoid patients lack the long history of antisocial behavior of people with antisocial character. People with schizoid personality disorder are withdrawn an aloof and do not have paranoid ideation.

Course and Prognosis

The course of paranoid personality disorder tends to be lifelong in some people while in others it is harbinger of schizophrenia. In still others paranoid traits give way to reaction formation, appropriate concern with morality and altruistic concerns as they mature or as stress diminishes. In general, however, those with paranoid personality disorder have lifelong problems working and living with others. Occupational and martial problems are common.

Treatment

Psychotherapy is the treatment of choice for paranoid personality disorder. Because they mistrust others, they usually avoid psychiatric treatment. If they do seek treatment, the therapist immediately encounters the challenge of engaging them, and keeping them is treatment. Therapists should be unusually respectful, straightforward in dealing with these patients. If a therapist is accused of an inconsistency or fault, honesty and an apology are preferable to a defensive explanation. It is also to avoid and overly warm style, because excessive warmth and expression can exacerbate the patient's paranoid tendencies.

Paranoid patients usually do not do well with group therapy and cognitive-behavior therapy (Turket and Maisto 1985) used to improve social skills and diminishing suspiciousness through role-playing. They tend to resist such approaches because of their suspiciousness and fear of losing control and being criticized. Paranoid patients are profoundly frightened when they fell that those trying to treat them are weak and helpless: therefore therapists should never offer to take control unless they are willing and able to do so.

Pharmacotherapy is useful in dealing with anxiety and agitation, even though they may view such treatment with mistrust. In most cases an anti-anxiety agent such as diazepam is sufficient, but a small doses of an antipsychotic may be necessary to control severe agitation or delusional thinking.

SCHIZOID PERSONALITY DISORDER

Schizoid personality disorder is one of the three odd eccentric personality disorders with phenomenological similarities to schizophrenia, the other two being paranoid and schizotypal personality disorders. Schizoid personality disorder as a trait like variant of schizophrenia was described by Hoch (1910) as the "shut is personality", by Bleuler (1922) as "schizondie", and by Kraeplin (1919) as "autistic personality". The essential features of people with this disorder are a lifelong pattern of social withdrawal, introversion, bland or constricted affect and their discomfort with human interaction.

Epidemiology

The prevalence of schizoid personality disorder is not clearly established, but the disorder may affect 7.5% of the general population. The sex ratio of the disorder is unknown, some studies report a 2:1 male to female ratio. Baron reported a rate 1.6% of schizoid personality disorder among relatives of schizophrenic probands, but no cases among relatives of control probands. In a longitudinal, epidemiological study of adolescents and children using DSM-HR criteria, Bernstein (1990) reported prevalence rate of 1.7% for schizoid personality disorder. When criterion analysis was made with DSM-lllR categories, the only criterion, 'neither desires nor enjoys close relationship', demonstrated high sensitivity and specificity and this was considered prototypal by clinicians.

Clinical Features

People with this disorder are introspective and prone to engage in fantasy rather than to take actions. They appear detached,

DSM-5 Diagnostic criteria for schizoid personality disorder

a. A pervasive pattern of detachment from social relationships and a restricted range of expression of emotions in interpersonal settings, beginnings by early adulthood and present in a variety of contexts, as indicated by four (or more) of the following:
   1. Neither desires nor enjoys close relationships, including being part of the family.
   2. Almost always chooses solitary activities.
   3. Has little, if any, interest in having sexual experiences with another person.
   4. Takes pleasure in few, if any, activities.
   5. Lacks close friends or confidants other than first-degree relatives.
   6. Appears indifferent to the praise or criticism of other.
   7. Shows emotional coldness, detachment or flattened affectivity.

b. Does not occur exclusively during the course of Schizophrenia, a mood disorder with psychotic features, or another psychotic disorder, or a pervasive developmental disorder and is not due to the direct physiological effects of a general medical condition. *Note:* If criteria are met prior to the onset of schizophrenia, add "pre-morbid", i.e. "schizoid personality disorder (pre-morbid)".

aloof, and humorless, and seem incapable of expressing affection or tenderness. They prefer to engage in solitary, often intellectual activities such as computer games, puzzles, and they often create an elaborate fantasy world into which they retreat and which substitutes for relationships with others. As a result, they do not make intimate friendships and remained unmarried. Their sexual lives may exist exclusively in fantasy, and they may postpone mature sexuality indefinitely. Men may not marry because they are unable to achieve intimacy, women may passively agree to marry an aggressive man who wants-the marriage. They show little concern for the opinions of other people and they pursue a lonely course through life.

Although people with this disorder appear self-absorbed and lost in daydreams, they have a normal capacity to recognized reality. Because aggressive acts are rarely included in their repertoire of usual responses, most threats real or imagined, are dealt with by fantasized omnipotence or resignation. They are often seen as aloof yet such people can sometimes conceive, develop, and give to the world genuinely original, creative ideas.

Differential Diagnosis

Schizoid personality disorder patients unlike patients with schizophrenia or schizotypal personality disorder do not have schizophrenic relatives. They differ from schizophrenic patients by exhibiting no thought disorder or delusional thinking. Although characteristics of social isolation and restricted affectivity are common to schizoid, schizotypal, and paranoid personality disorders, schizoid personality disorders can be distinguished from schizotypal personality disorder the lack of cognitive and perceptual distortion, and from paranoid personality disorder by the lack of suspiciousness and paranoid ideation. The social isolation of schizoid personality disorder can be distinguished from that of avoidant personality disorder, which is due to fear of being embarrassed or found inadequate and excessive anticipation of rejection. In contrast people with schizoid personality disorder have a more pervasive detachment and limited desire for social intimacy.

Course and Prognoses

The onset of schizoid personality disorder usually occurs in early childhood. Like all personality disorders, schizoid personality is log lasting, but not necessarily lifelong. The proportion of patients who incur schizophrenia is unknown.

Treatment

Peoplewithschizoidpersonalitydisorderrarelyseektreatment. They do not perceive the formation of any relationship—including a therapeutic relationship, as potentially valuable or beneficial. They may, however, occasionally seek treatment for an associated problem, such as depression, or others may bring them for treatment. Development of an alliance may be difficult and can be facilitated by an interested and caring attitude and an avoidance of early interpretation or confrontation. Some authors have suggested the sue of so-called inanimate bridges, such as writing and artistic productions, to easy the patient into the therapy relationship. Once the trust develops, schizoid patients may with great trepidation, reveal a plethora of fantasies, imaginary friends and fear of unbearable dependence—even of merging with therapist. Incorporation of cognitive-behavioral approaches that encourages gradually increasing social involvement may be of value (Liebowitz et al, 1986). Although many patients may be unwilling to participate in a group, group therapy may also facilitate the development of social skills and relationships.

Pharmacotherapy with small doses of antipsychotics, antidepressants, and psychostimulants has been effective in some patients. Serotonergic agents may make patients less sensitive to rejection.

SCHIZOTYPAL PERSONALITY DISORDER

Schizotypal personality disorder is one of the three "odd eccentric personality disorders with phenomenological similarities to schizophrenia, the other two being paranoid and schizoid personality disorders. Bleulers concept of latent schizophrenia, which consisted of mild or attenuated schizophreniasymptomswithoutdeteriorationintopsychosis, was one of the major clinical forerunners of schizotypal personality disorder. The essential features of people with this disorder are a pervasive pattern of detachment from social relationships and a restricted range of expression of emotions in interpersonal settings.

Epidemiology and Etiology

This disorder occurs in about 3% of the population with the median prevalence rate of 0.6%. The sex ratio is unknown. Schizotypal personality disorder is a schizophrenia-spectrum disorder, i.e. it is related to axis I schizophrenia. Phenomenological, biological, genetic, treatment response, and outcome data support this link.

The publication of Danish adoption studies demonstrated that there appeared to be a broad range of abnormalities, so called schizophrenic spectrum disorders, which were commoner in the biological relatives of schizophrenics, than in the adoptive relatives or controls. Kendler et al (1981), applying DSM-lll definitions of schizophrenia and schizotypal personality disorder to Danish adoption data, showed that rates of schizophrenia and related disorders was 22% in the biological relatives of schizophrenia, when compared to 2% in adoption relatives and control. Gottesman and shields (1972), applying DSM-lll criteria for schizotypal personality disorder and schizophrenia in re-analysis of the classic twin study, produced a higher monozygotic twins to dizygotic twins, concordance ratio than when the diagnoses was restricted to schizophrenia alone. In addition, at least some forms of schizotypal personality disorder involve biological abnormalities characteristic of schizophrenia, e.g. an increased ventricular-brain ratio on computed tomography scan, higher cerebrospinal fluid homovanillic acid concentrations (Siever et al, 1993), impaired smooth pursuit eye movements and impaired performance on tests of executive function and other tests of visual or auditory attention, such as the Wisconsin card sorting test, the backward masking task, the continuous performance task, and sensory gating tests, suggesting altered functioning (Siever et al, 1991; Trant et al, 1995).

These evidences support the inclusion of schizotypal personality disorder in schizophrenia section of Axis-I disorders in ICD-10. However, genetic and epidemiological studies suggest that schizophrenia related personality disorders may be more common manifestations of genotypes predisposing to schizophrenia-related disorders, than chronic schizophrenia itself; i.e. Schizophrenia spectrum may include more individuals with Axis-II than with Axis-I disorders. However, DSM-IV does not acknowledge the concept of spectrum disorders and hence, schizotypal personality disorder is retained in Axis-II disorder. However schizotypal personality disorder does not satisfy criteria for an Axis-II disorder, such as "an enduring constellation of traits that describes as individuals interpersonal, cognitive and affective lifestyle".

One solution to the above problem is to explicitly acknowledge the schizotypal personality disorders on both Axis-l and Axis-ll, introducing the concept of spectrum disorders in the multi-axial system, and to clarify why schizotypal personality disorder is noted in both Axis-l and Axis-ll disorders.

Clinical Features

Schizotypal personality disorders is characterized by social anxiety, inability to make close friendships, eccentric behavior, oddities of speech, inappropriate affect, suspicious, ideas of reference, other odd ideas, and unusual perceptual experiences. These distortions, which are inconsistent with subcultural norms, occur frequently and are an important and pervasive component of the person's experience. These individuals may, e.g. talk to themselves in public, gesture for no apparent reason, or dress in a peculiar or unkempt fashion. Like patients with schizophrenia, those with schizotypal personality disorder may not know their own feelings, yet are exquisitely sensitive to, and aware, of the feelings of others, especially negative affects like anger.

People with this disorder are also socially uncomfortable and isolated, and they have few friends. This isolation is often due to their eccentric cognition and behavior as well as to their lack of desire for relationships, which stems in part from their

DSM-5 Diagnostic criteria for schizotypal personality disorder

a. A pervasive pattern of social and interpersonal deficits marked by acute discomfort with, and reduced capacity for, close relationships as well as by cognitive or perceptual distortion and eccentricities of behavior, beginning by early adulthood and present in a variety of contexts, as indicated by five (or more) of the following:
   1. Ideas of reference (excluding delusions of reference).
   2. Odd beliefs or magical thinking that influences behavior and is inconsistent with subcultural norms (e.g. superstitiousness, belief in clairvoyance, telepathy, or "sixth sense"; in children and adolescents, bizarre fantasies or preoccupations).
   3. Unusual perceptual experiences, including bodily illusions.
   4. Odd thinking and speech (e.g. vague, circumstantial, metaphorical, overlaborate, or stereotyped).
   5. Suspiciousness or paranoid ideation
   6. Inappropriate or constricted affect
   7. Behavior or appearance that is odd, eccentric, or peculiar
   8. Lack of close friends or confidants other than first-degree relatives
   9. Excessive social anxiety that does not diminish with familiarity and tends to be associated with paranoid fears rather than negative judgments about itself
b. Does not occur exclusively during the course of schizophrenia, a mood disorder with psychotic features, another psychotic disorder, or autism spectrum disorder.
   Note: If criteria are met prior to the onset of schizophrenia, add "premorbid", e.g. "schizotypal personality disorder (premorbid")

suspiciousness of others. If they develop a relationship, they tend to remain distant or may even terminate it because of their persistent social anxiety and paranoia. They may show features of borderline personality disorder and indeed, both diagnoses can be made. Under stress, patients with this disorder may decompensate and have psychotic symptoms, but these are usually of brief duration. In severe cases they may present with anhedonia and severe depression.

Differential Diagnosis

Schizotypal personality disorder can be distinguished from schizophrenia by the absence of psychosis, if psychotic symptoms do appear they are brief and fragmentary. Although paranoid and schizoid personality disorders may also be characterized by social detachment and restricted affect, schizotypal personality disorder can be distinguished by the presence of cognitive or perceptual distortions and marked eccentricity of oddness. Some may meet the criteria for both schizotypal and borderline personality disorder.

Course and Prognoses

Retrospective studies have shown that many patients thought to have had schizophrenia actually had schizotypal personality disorder, and according to current clinical thinking the schizotypal is the pre-morbid personality of the patients with schizophrenia. Some however, maintain a stable schizotypal personality throughout their lives and marry and work in spite of their oddities. A long-term study by Thomas Mc-Glashan reported that 10% of people with this disorder eventually committed suicide.

Treatment

Schizotypal personality disorder patients usually avoid treatment because of their social anxiety and paranoia. When they become depressed or psychotic they seek treatment or are brought by their family members. It is difficult to establish a therapeutic alliance with these patients, and they are unlikely to tolerate exploratory techniques that emphasize interpretation or confrontation. A supportive relationship that counters cognitive distortions and ego-boundary problems may be useful. This may involve an educational approach that fosters the development of social skills or encourages risk-taking behavior in social situation. If the patient is willing to participate, cognitive-behavioral therapy and highly structured educational groups with a social skill focus may be helpful.

Pharmacotherapy in the form of low dose antipsychotics (haloperidol) has been useful to ameliorate anxiety and in dealing with psychotic like features and other symptoms of this disorder and can be used in conjunction with psychotherapy. The result of an open label trial (Markovitz et al, 1991) suggested that fluoxetine may also diminish features of schizotypal personality disorders.

AVOIDANT PERSONALITY DISORDER

People with avoidant personality disorder show an extreme sensitivity to rejection and may lead a socially withdrawn life. They are commonly described as having an inferiority complex. In DSM-IV the term "avoidant" is used to denote this kind of personality disorder, whilst in lCD-10 the term 'anxious personality' is preferred, with 'avoidant' as an accepted alternative.

Epidemiology and Etiology

Avoidant personality disorder is common. The prevalence of this disorder is l to 10% of the general population with the median prevalence of 0.7%. Sex ratio and familial pattern of this disorder is not known. Infants classified, as having a timid temperament may be more prone to the disorder than are those high on activity approach scales.

This disorder as suggested by Millon (1981) develops from parental rejection and censure, which may be reinforced by rejecting peers. Psychodynamic theory suggests that avoidant behavior may derive from early life experiences that lead to an exaggerated desire for acceptance or an intolerance to criticism.

Clinical Features

The essential feature of this disorder is hypersensitivity to rejection, with the main personality trait being timidity. They are persistently anxious, ill at ease in company, fearing disapproval, criticism or rejection, and worrying that they will be embarrassed or ridiculed. People with this disorder desires the warmth and security of human companionship, they avoid them because they fear being rejected or humiliated.

Because they are hypervigilant about rejection, they are afraid to speak in public places, or to make requests of others. The refusal of any request leads them to withdraw from and to feel hurt. They often take jobs on the sidelines, and rarely attain much personal achievement or exercise much authority, but seem shy and eager to please. These people are generally unwilling to enter relationships, when they do enter into social situations or relationships, they feel inept and are self-conscious, shy, awkward, and preoccupied with being criticized or rejected. Consequently they often have no close friends or confidants.

Differential Diagnoses

Avoidant personality disorder consists of several traits and behaviors of which the features of performing in situations,

DSM-5 Diagnostic criteria for avoidant personality disorder

A pervasive pattern of social inhibition, feeling of inadequacy, and hypersensitivity to negative evaluation, beginning be early adulthood and present in a variety of contexts, as indicated by four (or more) of the following:

1. Avoids occupational activities that involve significant interpersonal contact because of fears of criticism, disapproval or rejection.
2. Is unwilling to get involved with people unless certain of being liked.
3. Shows restraint within intimate relationships because of the fear of being shamed or ridiculed.
4. Is preoccupied with being criticized or rejected in social situations.
5. Is inhibited in new interpersonal situations because of feeling of inadequacy
6. Views self as socially inept, personality unappealing, or inferior to others.
7. Is unusually reluctant to take personal risks or to engage in any new activities because they may prove embarrassing.

where as avoidant personality disorder is characterized by avoidance of all situations and relationships involving possible rejection or disappointment. Social phobic patients may have a multitude of satisfying social/personal relationships with others, where as avoidant personality disorder is socially withdrawn, has few close relationships, desires them but does riot trust sufficiently to relate closely without assurance of acceptance. Patients with avoidant personality disorder desire social interactions unlike patients with schizoid personality disorder, who wants to be alone. Patients with avoidant personality disorder are not as demanding, irritable or unpredictable, as are those with borderline and histrionic personality disorders. Patients with dependent personality disorder are presumed to have greater fear of being abandoned or unloved than to those with avoidant personality disorder, but the clinical picture may be indistinguishable.

Course and Prognoses

Many people with avoidant personality disorder are able to function in a protected environment. Some marry, have children, and live their lives surrounded only by family members. Should their support system fail, however, they are subjected to depression, anxiety, and anger. There is some evidence that in adults this disorder tends to become less evident or to remit with age.

Treatment

People with avoidant personality disorder, because of their excessive fear of rejection and criticism and their reluctance to form relationships, are difficult to engage in treatment. Psychotherapeutic treatment depends on solidifying an alliance with patients. Engagement in psychotherapy may be facilitated by the therapist's use of supportive techniques, sensitivity to the patient's hypersensitivity, and gentle interpretation of the defensive use of avoidance. They usually respond to all kinds of psychotherapy, including short-term. Long-term and psychoanalytic approaches. But therapists should be cautious when giving assignments to exercise new skills outside therapy; failure may reinforce a patient's already poor self-esteem. Group therapy may help patients understand the effects of their sensitivity to rejection on themselves and others. Assertiveness and social training may increase patient's confidence and willingness to take risks in social situations.

Pharmacotherapy has been used to manage anxiety and depression when they are associated with this disorder. Anxiolytics help patients manage anxiety caused by facing previously avoided situations or trying new behaviors. Some promising studies (Deltito and Stam, 1989, Versiani et al, 1992) suggest that avoidant personality disorder may improve with treatment with mono-oxidase inhibitors or serotonin re-uptake inhibitors.

ANTISOCIAL PERSONALITY DISORDER

Antisocial personality disorder is an inability to confirm to the social norms that ordinarily govern may aspects of people's adolescent and adult behavior. Although characterized by continual antisocial or criminal acts, the disorder is not synonymous with criminality. Recent changes in classification of personality disorder according to abnormal personality traits, rather than abnormal behavior. Longitudinal concept (life-span perspective) has been omitted from the category of ICD, especially the presence of conduct disorder in childhood. However, this is important in terms of prognosis and the ability to differentiate antisocial behavior secondary to other psychiatry conditions in their life. ICD-10 used the term "dissocial" in place of "antisocial" and places more emphasis on personality traits, such as lack of remorse or guilt, callous lack of empathy and failure to accept responsibility for one's action. DSM-IV places more emphasis.

Epidemiology

Antisocial is the most studied personality disorder. The prevalence is 3% in men and 1% in women. It is most common among younger adults, those living in urban areas, and the lower social economic classes. Studies in prison settings have shown high prevalence, varying from 39% to 76%. A familial pattern is present, in that, the disorder is five times more common among first degree relatives of men with the disorder than among the controls.

Clinical Features

The central characteristic features of antisocial personality disorder are a long-standing pattern of socially irresponsible behaviors that reflects a disregard for the rights of others. Lying, truancy, running away from home, thefts, fights, substance abuse, and illegal activities are typical experiences that patients report as beginning in childhood. Patients with this disorder exhibit no anxiety or depression, a lack that may seem grossly incongruous with their situations, although suicide traits and somatic preoccupations may be common. They are extremely manipulative and frequently talk others into participating into schemes for easy ways to make money or to achieve fame or notoriety. These schemes may eventually lead the unwary to financial ruin or social embarrassment or both. Some antisocial persons posses a glibness and charm that can be used to seduce, outwit, and exploit others. They do not tell truth and cannot be trusted to carryout any task or adhere to any conventional standard of morality. Promiscuity, spouse abuse, child abuse, and substance abuse are common habits in there lives.

Etiology

Findings of twin and adoptive studies indicate that genetic factors predispose to development of antisocial personality disorder. Mcguffin and Gottesman (1984) pooled the results of seven studies of adult criminality and five studies of juvenile delinquency. The weighted mean concordance for adult criminality in monozygotic twins is 51% and a dizygotic twins as 22%, suggesting a definite genetic contribution by contrast, for juvenile delinquency there was little difference in monozygotic and dizygotic concordance rates at 87% and 72%, suggesting that juvenile delinquency is almost familial, but probably does not have genetic component. Cloninger (1978) applying a two-threshold model, assume that liability to become criminal is contributed by an additive combination of genetic and environmental factors and those whose liability at some stage certain threshold manifest criminal behavior.

Adoption studies have been more consistent and suggest that family background does play a part but only when there is already a genetic predisposition toward criminality. Guze and Clomnger (14967, 1973–1975), using a multiple threshold model, suggested that somatization disorder (or Briquet syndrome) is a sort of female equivalent of antisocial personality and there is a' high prevalence of antisocial personality disorder among relatives of women diagnosed and having Briquet Syndrome.

Growing evidence indicate that impulsive and aggressive behavior may be mediated by abnormal Serotonin transporter functioning in the brain (Cpccaro et al, 1996). It is clear that even in the absence of genetic vulnerability, the early family life of these persons often posses environmental handicaps in the form of absent, assaultive or inconsistent parenting. Indeed, many family members also have significant action oriented psychopathology such as substance abuse or antisocial personality disorder itself.

DSM-5 Diagnostic criteria for antisocial disorder

a. There is a pervasive pattern of disregard for and avoidant of the rights of others, occurring since age 15 years, as indicated by three (or more) of the following,
    1. Failure to conform to social norms with respect to lawful behaviors as indicated by repeatedly performing acts that are grounds for arrest.
    2. Deceitfulness, as indicated by repeated lying, use of aliases, or conning others for personal profit or pleasure
    3. Impulsivity or failure to plan ahead
    4. Irritability and aggressiveness, as indicated by repeated physical fights or assaults
    5. Reckless disregard for safety of self or others.
    6. Consistent irresponsibility, as indicated by repeated failure to sustain consistent work behavior or honor financial obligations
    7. Lack of remorse, as indicated by being indifferent to or rationalizing having hurt, mistreated, or stolen from another
b. The individual is at least 18 years of age.
c. There is evidence of conduct disorder with onset before age 15 years.
d. The occurrence of antisocial behavior is not exclusively during the course of schizophrenia or bipolar disorder.

Differential Diagnosis

The primary differential diagnosis issue involves narcissistic personality disorder. However, the antisocial person, unlike the narcissistic person, is likely to be reckless and impulsive. In addition, narcissistic individual's explosiveness and disregard for others are attributable to their sense of uniqueness and superiority rather than to desire for materialistic gains. Individuals with histrionic and borderline personality disorders are manipulative who gain nurturance, whereas those with antisocial personality disorder are manipulative to gain profit, power, or some other materialistic gratification.

Course and Prognosis

Once an antisocial personality disorder develops, it runs an unremitting course, with the height of antisocial behavior usually occurring later at adolescence. The prognosis is variable. Longitudinal follow-up studies have shown that the prevalence of the disorder diminishes with the age as these individuals become more aware of the social and interpersonal mal-adaptiveness of their most noxious behavior.

Treatment

It is clinically important to recognize antisocial personality disorder because an uncritical acceptance of these individuals glib or shallow statements of good intentions and collaborations can permit them to have a disruptive influence on treatment teams and other patients. However there is little evidence to suggest that this disorder can be successfully treated by usual psychiatry interventions.

Hospitalization of patients with this disorder for psychotherapy is helpful, as they become more amenable to therapy. Self-help groups and therapeutic community settings are more productive than institutionalization in producing a change. Limit setting, environmental manipulation and assertiveness (openness), while interpreting manipulative behavior are essential.

Pharmacology is used to deal with incapacitating symptoms such as anxiety, range, and depression, but they must used judiciously as these patients are more prone to abuse them. Psycho-stimulants such as methylphenidate may be used if a patient shows the evidence of attention-deficit/hyperactivity disorder.

BORDERLINE PERSONALITY DISORDER

The essential features of borderline personality disorder is a pervasive pattern of instability of interpersonal relationship, self-image, and affects and marked impulsivity that begins by early adulthood and is present in a variety of contexts. People with this disorder stand on the border between neurosis and are characterized by extraordinarily unstable affect, mood, and behavior, object relations and self-image. The disorder has also been called ambulatory schizophrenia, as if personality (Helene Deutsch) pseudo-neurotic schizophrenia (Paul Hoch and Philip Politan) and psychotic character disorder (John Forch). lCD-10 used the term emotionally unstable personality disorder.

Epidemiology

The prevalence of this disorder is 1–2% of general population, twice as common in women as in men. This is the most widely studied personality disorder. Evidence for its validity is growing, and the disorder is now recognized as the most prevalent Axis-II disorder in all kinds of clinical settings, cases of the disorder making up 12–15% of cases of Axis-II disorder (Gunderson 1992)

Psychoanalytic theories have emphasized the importance of early parent child relationship in the etiology of borderline personality disorder. Such reports have emphasized maternal mismanagement of the 2–3 years old child's efforts to become autonomous (Masterson 1972), exaggerated maternal frustration that aggravates the child's anger (Kernberg 1975) and in attention to the child's emotions and attitudes (Alder 1985).

Clinical Features

People with this disorder almost always appear to be in a state of crisis, mood swings are common. They can be argumentative at one moment, depressed at next and later complain of having no feelings. They distort the relationship with others by considering each person to be either all good or all bad. They see people as either nurturing attachments figures or has hateful and sadistic figures who deprive them of security needs and threaten them with abandonment whenever they feel dependent. As a result of this splitting good person is idealized and a bad person is devalued. Shifts of allegiance from one person or group to another are frequent. When patients experience in absence of a sustaining, holding, or caring relationship, dissociative experiences, ideas of reference, or desperate impulsive acts which are shortly lived rather than full blown episodes occur. Their behavior is unpredictable and their achievements are rarely at the level of their abilities.

Because they feel both dependent and hostile, people with this disorder; have tumultuous interpersonal relationships. They can be dependent on those to whom they are close and when they are frustrated can express enormous anger toward their intimate friends. People with this disorder cannot tolerate being alone, and they prefer a frantic search for companionship, no matter how unsatisfactory, to their own company. To assuage loneliness, if only for brief period, they accept a stranger as a friend or behave promiscuously.

DSM-5 Diagnostic criteria for boderline personality disorder

A pervasive pattern of instability of interpersonal relationships, self-image and affects and marked impulsivity beginning by early adulthood and present a variety of contexts, as indicated by five (or more) of the following:

1. Frantic efforts to avoid real or imagined abandonment. (Note: Do not include suicidal or self-mutilating behavior covered in criterion 5.)
2. A pattern of unstable and intense interpersonal relationships characterized by alternating between extremes of idealization and devaluation.
3. Identity disturbance; marked and persistently unstable self-image or sense of self.
4. Impulsivity in at least two areas that potentially self-damaging (e.g. spending, sex, substance abuse, reckless driving, binge eating). (Note: Do not include suicidal or self-mutilating behavior covered in criterion 5.)
5. Recurrent suicidal behavior, gestures, or threats, or self-mutilating behavior.
6. Affective instability due to a marked reactivity of mood (e.g. intense episodic dysphoria, irritability, or anxiety usually lasting a few hours and only rarely more than a few days).
7. Chronic feelings of emptiness
8. Inappropriate, intense anger of difficulty controlling anger (e.g. frequent displays of temper, constant anger, recurrent physical fights)
9. Transient, stress-related paranoid ideation or severe dissociative symptoms.

Differential Diagnosis

Borderline personality disorder is differentiated from schizophrenia by the lack of prolonged psychotic episodes, thought disorder, and other classic schizophrenia signs. People with schizotypal personality disorder show marked peculiarities of thinking, strange ideation and recurrent ideas of reference whereas people with Borderline personality disorder generally has chronic feeling of emptiness and short lived psychotic episodes. Although, borderline patients with antisocial personality disorder, may be reckless and impulsive, their behavior are primarily interpersonally oriented and aimed toward obtaining rather than materialistic gains.

Course and Prognosis

This disorder is fairly stable and patients change little overtime. They show no progression toward schizophrenia but have a high incidence of major depressive disorder. The diagnosis is usually made before the age of 40 years, when patients are attempting to make occupational, marital, and other choices and are unable to deal with the normal stages of life cycle.

Treatment

Psychotherapy has been the ideal treatment of choice for this disorder and it is difficult for the therapist and patients alike. Patients regress easily, act out their impulses, and show labile or fixed negative or positive transparences which are difficult to analyze. Projective identification may also cause counter transference problems when therapist is unaware that patients are unconsciously trying to coerce him or her to act out a particular behavior. Splitting as a defense mechanism causes patients to alternatively love and hate therapists and others in the environment. Behavior therapy is used to control patient's impulses and angry outburst and to reduce their sensitivity to criticism and rejection. They often do well in a hospital setting in which they receive intensive psychotherapy on both individual basis and groups basis.

Antipsychotics have been used anger, hostility and brief psychotic episodes. As they are more prone to develop major depressive disorder, antidepressants find a place. The mono-amino oxidase inhibitors (MAOIs) have been effective in modulating impulsive behavior in some patients. Anticonvulsant such as carbamazepine may improve global functioning in some patients.

HISTRIONIC PERSONALITY DISORDER

The important features of this kind of disorder are self-dramatization, a craving for novelty and excitement, and self-centered approach to personal relationships. The roots of histrionic personality disorder can be traced to cases of hysterical neuroses described by Freud and these cases would be classified with somatization or conversion disorders in the current classificatory systems. Kernberg (1967) attempted to outline those features that distinguishes histrionic personality disorder from related disorders. However, several of these are not represented by current DSM-IIIR or DSM-IV criteria's for histrionic personality disorder. Lazare and colleagues were the first to systematically examine for clustering of traits, by using a 200 item self-report rating scale (Lazare-Klerman Trait Scale, LKTS). A hysterical factor emerged from factor analysis and this strongly resembled the current criterias for histrionic personality disorder (Table 4).

Table 4: Prototype traits for personality disorder

Kernberg	*Lazare et al. (factor analysis)*
Emotional liability	Aggression
Over-involvement (superficial resonance with others)	Emotionality
Dependent and exhibitionistic needs	Oral aggression
Pseudo-hypersexuality	Exhibitionism
Sexual inhibition	Egocentricity
Competitiveness (oedipal rivalry)	Sexual provocativeness
Masochism (strict punitive superego)	Dependence
	Obstinacy

Epidemiology

The prevalence of histrionic personality disorder is 2–3% in the general population. When structured assessment were used in the inpatients and outpatients mental health settings, the prevalence of 10–15% were reported. This disorder is more frequently diagnosed in women than in men. No significant differences were found in terms of race and education, but the prevalence was significantly higher among separated and divorced persons.

Clinical Features

In the normal personality, minor histrionic traits can be socially advantageous. People with such traits make lively engaging company and are popular guests; they do well in amateur dramatics and are entertaining public speakers. They tend to wear their emotions on their sleeves and are easily moved to joy or tears, but their feelings soon pass. When these traits are exaggerated in histrionic personality disorder they become less acceptable. People with this disorder spend an excessive amount of time seeking attention and making themselves attractive. The desire to be found attractive may lead to inappropriately seductive of provocative dress and flirtatious behavior, and the desire for attention may lead

DSM-5 Diagnostic criteria for personality disorder

A pervasive pattern of excessive emotionality and attention seeking, beginning by early adulthood and present in a variety of contexts, as indicated by five (or more) of the following:

1. In uncomfortable in situations in which he/she is not the center of attention.
2. Interaction with others is often characterized by inappropriate sexually seductive or provocative behavior.
3. Displays rapidly shifting and shallow expression of emotions.
4. Consistently uses physical appearances to draw attention to self.
5. Has a style of speech that is excessively impressionistic and lacking in detail.
6. Shows self-dramatization, theatrically and exaggerated expression of emotion.
7. Is suggestible, i.e. easily influenced by others or circumstances.
8. Consider relationships to be intimate than they actually are.

to other flamboyant acts or self-dramatizing behavior. They display temper tantrums, tears and accusations when they are not the center of attention or not receiving praise or approval.

Seductive behavior is common in both sexes. Sexual fantasies about people with whom patients involved are common, but patients are inconsistent about verbalizing these fantasies and may be coy or flirtatious rather than sexually aggressive. In fact these patients have psychosexual dysfunction. Their relationships tend to be superficial, however, and they can be vain, self-absorbed and fickle. Their strong dependence needs make them overtly trusting and gullible. They often present with complaints or depression, somatic problems of unclear origin, and history of disappointing romantic relationships.

Differential Diagnoses

Histrionic personality disorder can be confused with borderline, dependent and narcissistic personality disorder. In borderline personality disorder, suicide attempts, identity diffusion, and brief psychotic episodes are likely. Histrionic individuals are often willing, even eager, to have others make decisions and organize activities for them, however unlike persons with dependent personality disorder, histrionic persons are unihibited and lively companions who willingfully forgot appearing autonomous because they believe this is desired by others. Persons with narcissistic personality disorder also seek attention to sustain their self-esteem but differ in that their self-esteem is characterized by grandiosity, and the attention they crave must be admiring, e.g. unlike the histrionic person, they would be crushed to he described as "cute" as "silly".

Course and Prognoses

People with this disorder are sensation seekers and may get into trouble with the law, abuse substance and act promiscuously. With age, people with histrionic personality disorders have fewer symptoms, but because they lack the energy of earlier years, the differences in number of symptoms may be more apparent than real.

Treatment

Psychoanalytically oriented psychotherapy, weather group or individual, is probably the treatment of choice for histrionic personality disorder. This treatment is directed at increasing patient's awareness of (1) how their self-esteem is maladaptively tied to their ability to attract attention at the expense of developing other skills and (2) how their shallow relationships and emotional experiences reflect unconscious fears of real commitments. Therapists should be aware that the typical idealization and eroticization that such patients bring into treatment are the material for exploration, and thus therapists should be aware of counter tanferential gratification.

Pharmacotherapy can be used to treat adjunctive symptoms such as anxiolytics for anxiety, antidepressants for depression, and antipsychotics for derealization and illusions.

NARCISSISTIC PERSONALITY DISORDER

People with this disorder are characterized by pervasive pattern of grandiosity, need for admiration and lack of empathy that begins by early adulthood and is present in a variety of contexts.

Epidemiology

The prevalence of this disorder range from 2% to 16% in the clinical population and less than 1% in the general population. People with this disorder may impart to their children an unrealistic sense of omnipotence, grandiosity, beauty and talent; thus offspring of such parents may have higher than the usual risk of developing the disorder themselves.

Clinical Features

People with this disorder have grandiose sense of self-importance, they consider themselves special and except special treatment. They sense of entitlement is striking. They handle criticism poorly and may become enraged when someone dares to criticize them, or they may appear completely differently to criticism. People with this disorder want there own way and are frequently ambitious to achieve fame and fortune. They are likely to feel that those with whom they associate need to be special and unique because they see themselves in these terms: thus, they usually wish to be associated with persons, institutions, or possessions that will confirm their sense of superiority. There relationships are fragile and they make furious by their refusal to obey

DSM-5 Diagnostic criteria for narcissistic personality disorder

A pervasive pattern of grandiosity (in fantasy or behavior), need for admiration, and lack of empathy, beginning by early adulthood and present in a variety of context, as indicated by five (or more) of the following:

1. Has a grandiose sense of self-importance (e.g. exaggerate achievements and talents, expects to be recognized as superior without commensurate achievements).
2. Is preoccupied with fantasies of unlimited success, power, brilliance, beauty, or ideal love.
3. Believe that he/she is "special" and unique and can only be understood by, or should associate with, other special or high-status people (or institutions).
4. Requires excessive admiration.
5. Has a sense of entitlement, i.e. unreasonable expectations of especially favourable treatment of automatic compliance with his/her expectations.
6. Is interpersonally exploitative (i.e. takes advantages of others to achieve his/her own ends).
7. Lacks empathy: is unwilling to recognize or identify with feelings and needs for others.
8. Is often envious of others or believes that others are envious of him/her.
9. Shows arrogant, haughty behavior or attitudes.

conventional rules of behavior. They are unable to show empathy and feign sympathy only to achieve their selfish ends. Because of their self-esteem, they are prone to depression.

Differential Diagnosis

Borderline, histrionic and antisocial personality disorders often accompany narcissistic personality disorder so that differential diagnosis is difficult. Patients with narcissistic personality disorders have less anxiety than with those borderline personality disorders: their life tends to be less chaotic, and they are less likely to attempt suicide. Like person with anti-social personality disorder those with narcissistic personality disorder are capable of exploiting others but usually rationalize their behavior on the basis of their specialness of their goals of their virtue, in contrast, antisocial person goals are materialistic, and their rationalizations, if offered are based on view that others would do the same to them. The narcissistic persons excessive pride in achievements, relative constraint in expression of their feelings, disregard for other people's rights and sensitivities help distinguish him/her from persons with histrionic personality disorder.

Course and Prognosis

Narcissistic personality disorder is chronic and difficult to treat. Aging is handled poorly: patient's value, beauties, strength and youthful attributes; to which they claim inappropriately. They may be more vulnerable, to mid life crisis than are other groups.

Treatment

Because the patients must renounce their narcissism to make progress, the treatment of narcissistic personality disorder is difficult. Individual psychodynamic psychotherapy, including psychoanalysis, is the cornerstone of treatment for persons with this disorder. Psychiatrists such as Otta, Kernberg and Heinz Kohut have advocating using psychoanalytic approaches to affect change: but much research is required to validate the diagnosis and to determine the best treatment.

Patients with this disorder tolerate rejection poorly and are prone to depression. Antidepressants especially serotonergic drugs may be useful in treating them. When they present with mood swings, lithium may be used to control them.

OBSESSIVE-COMPULSIVE PERSONALITY DISORDER

The essential features of obsessive-compulsive personality disorder is a preoccupation with orderliness, perfectionism and mental and interpersonal control, at the expense of flexibility, openness, and efficiency. This pattern begins by early adulthood and is present in a variety of contexts. ICD-10 uses the term anankastic personality disorder.

Epidemiology

The median prevalence of this disorder obtained from eight studies was found to be 1.7%. Males have a rate about five times higher than females. This disorder was also more frequent among white, highly educated, married and employed subjects and it was associated with anxiety disorders. The disorder also occurs more frequently in first-degree biological relatives of people with this disorder than in the general population.

Freud hypothesized that the disorder is associated with difficulties in the anal stage of psychosexual development, generally around the age of 2 years, was elaborated on by subsequent psychoanalytic thinkers, such as Karl Abraham and Wilhelm Reich (1933). According to this theory, children's infantile-erotic libidinal impulses conflict with parental attempts to socialize them in particular, to toilet trains them. Although these theories emphasize the importance of children's perception of parental disapproval during toilet training, and of ensuing parent-child control struggles—what Rado (1959) referred to as "the battle of the chamber pot", these factors are not currently considered central to this disorder's etiology. It may be, however, that conflicts arising during toilet training—such as those characteristic of Ericson's (1950) stage of autonomy versus shame—and continuing during other developmental stages do play a role in this disorder's etiology (Perry and Valliant, 1989). In particular, excessive parental control, criticism, and shaming may result in an insecurity that is defended against with perfectionism, orderliness, and an attempt to maintain excessive control.

Clinical Features

People with this disorder are preoccupied with rules, regulations, orderliness, neatness, details and the achievement of perfection. Attention to details is so excessive or time consuming that the point of activity is lost, conscientiousness is so extreme that it causes rigidity and inflexibility, and perfectionism interferes with task completion. And although these individuals tend to work extremely hard, they do so at the expense of leisure activities and relationships. As Shapiro (1965) pointed out, the most characteristic thought of obsessive-compulsive persons is "I should",—a phrase that aptly reflects their severe superego and captures their overly high standards, driveness, and excessive conscientiousness, perfectionism, rigidity, and devotion to work and duties.

These individuals also tend to be overly concerned with control, not over details of their own lives but over their emotions and other people. They have difficulty expressing warm and tender feelings, often using stilted and distant phrasing that reveals little of their in experience. And they may be obstinate and reluctant to delegate tasks or to work with others unless others submit exactly to their way of doing things, which reflects their need for interpersonal controls as well as their fear of making mistakes. Their tendency to doubt and worry also manifests itself in their inability to discard worn-out or worthless objects that might be needed for future catastrophes, and they are miserly toward themselves and others.

DSM-5 Diagnostic criteria for obsessive-Compulsive personality disorder

A pervasive pattern of preoccupations with orderliness, perfectionism, and mental interpersonal control, at the expense of flexibility, openness, and efficiently, beginning by early adulthood and present in a variety of contexts, as indicated by four (or more) of the following:

1. Is preoccupied with details, rules, lists, order, organization, or schedules to the extent that the major point of the activity is lost.
2. Shows perfectionism that interferes with task completion (e.g. is unable to complete a project because his/her own overly strict standards are not met).
3. Is excessively devoted to work and productivity to the exclusion of leisure activities and friendships (not accounted for by obvious economic necessity).
4. Is over-conscientious, scrupulous, and inflexible about matters of morality, ethics, or values (not accounted for by cultural or religious identification).
5. Is unable to discard worn-out or worthless objects even when they have no sentimental value.
6. Is reluctant to delegate tasks or to work with others unless they submit to exactly his/her way of doing things.
7. Adopts a miserly spending style toward both itself and others; money is viewed as something to be hoarded for future catastrophes.
8. Shows rigidity and stubbornness.

Differential Diagnoses

Obsessive-compulsive personality disorder differs from Axis-I obsessive-compulsive disorder in that the later disorder consists of specific repetitive thoughts and ritualistic behavior rather than personality traits. In addition, obsessive compulsive disorder has traditionally been considered ego-dystonic whereas obsessive-compulsive personality disorder has been considered ego-syntonic. These two disorders are sometimes, but not necessarily co-morbid.

Course and Prognosis

The course of obsessive-compulsive personality disorder is variable and unpredictable. From time-to-time, people may develop obsessions or compulsions in the course of their disorder. They may develop obsessions or compulsions in the course of their disorder. They may flourish in position demanding methodical, deductive, or detailed work, but they are vulnerable to unexpected changes, and their personal lives may remain barren. Depressive disorders, especially those of late onset are common.

Treatment

When compared to patients with other personality disorders, those with obsessive-compulsive personality disorder are often unaware of suffering, and they seek treatment on their own. They are often difficult to treat because of their excessive intellectualization and difficulty expressing emotions. However these patients respond well to psychoanalytic psychotherapy. Therapists usually need to relatively active in treatment. They should also avoid being drawn into interesting but affectless discussions that are unlikely to have therapeutic benefits, in their words, rather than intellectualizing with patient, therapists should be identified such as rationalization, isolation, undoing, and reaction formation, should be identified and clarified. Group therapy and behavior therapy offer some advantages. Although patients may resist group treatment because of their need for control, dynamically oriented groups that may focus on feeling may provide insight and increase their comfort with exploring and expressing new affects.

DEPENDENT PERSONALITY DISORDER

People with the dependent personality disorder present with the pervasive and excessive need to be taken care of that leads to submissive and clinging behavior and fears of separation.

This pattern begins by early adulthood and is present in variety of context.

Epidemiology

The prevalence of this disorder 2.5% of all personality disorder diagnosed. The median prevalence rate is 0 7%. Dependent personality disorder is more common in women than in men, also more common in young children than older ones.

Clinical Features

Dependent personality disorder is characterized by excessive need to be cared for by others, which leads to submissive and clinging behavior and excessive fears of separation from others. Because of their low self-esteem and doubt about their effectiveness they avoid positions of responsibility and become anxious if asked to assume a leadership role. Because they feel unable to function without excessive guidance, they got great lengths to maintain the dependant relationships. They may: for example, always agree with those on whom they depend, and they tend to be excessively clinging, submissive, passive and self-sacrificing. If the dependent relationship ends, these individuals feel helpless and fearful. Because they feel incapable of caring of themselves, and they often then indiscriminately find another person with whom to have the relationship, so that they can be provided with direction and nurturance—an unfulfilling or even an abusive relationships may seem better than being their own.

DSM-5 Diagnostic criteria for dependent personality disorder

A pervasive and excessive need to be taken care of that leads to submissive and clinging behavior and fears of separation, beginning by early adulthood and present in a variety of contexts, as indicated by five (or more) of the following:

1. Has difficulty making everyday decisions without an excessive amount of advice and reassurance from others.
2. Needs others to assume responsibility for most areas of his/her life.
3. Has difficulty expressing disagreement with others because of fear of loss of support or approval. (Note: Do not include realistic fears of retribution.)
4. Has difficulty initiating projects or doing things on his/her own (because of a lack of self-confidence in judgment or abilities rather than a lack of motivation or energy)
5. Goes to excessive lengths to obtain nurturance and support from others, to point of volunteering to do things that are unpleasant.
6. Feels uncomfortable or helpless when alone because of exaggerated fears of being unable to care for him- or herself.
7. Urgently seeks another relationship as a source of care and support when a close relationship ends.
8. Is unrealistically preoccupied with fears of being left to take care of him- or herself.

Differential Diagnosis

Many psychiatric disorders present with the traits of dependence, which makes the diagnosis difficult. Dependence is the prominent factor in patients with histrionic and borderline personality disorders, but those with dependent personality disorder usually have a long-term relationship with one person, rather than a series on whom they are dependent, and they do not tend to be overtly manipulative. Although, both avoidant and dependant personality disorders are characterized by low self-esteem, rejection sensitivity, and excessive need for reassurance, person with dependent personality disorder seek out rather than relationship, and they quickly and indiscriminately replace ended relationship instead of further withdrawing from others. Dependant behavior may occur in agoraphobia, but these patients tend to have a high level of overt anxiety and even panic.

Course and Prognosis

Dependent personality disorder patients have impaired occupational functioning because of their lack of ability to act independently and without close supervision. Social relationships are limited to those on whom they can depend, and many suffer physical or mental abuse because they cannot assert themselves. If they lose the dependent relationship they tend to develop a major depressive disorder, but with treatment the prognosis favorable.

Treatment

Patients with dependent personality disorder often enter therapy with complains of depression or anxiety that may be precipitated by the threatened or actual lose of dependant relationship. The treatment of this disorder is often successful. Insight oriented therapies enable patients to understand the antecedents of their behavior, and with the support of a therapist, patients can become more independent, assertive and self-reliant. Behavioral therapy, assertiveness training, family therapy, and group therapy have all been used, its successful outcome in many cases.

A pitfall in treatment may arise when a therapist encourages a patient to change the dynamics of a pathological relationship. At this point patient may become anxious and unable to cooperate in therapy: they may feel torn with complying with the therapist and losing a pathological external relationship. Therapist must show great respect for this patient's feelings of attachment, no matter how pathological these feeling may seem.

Because these patients usually suffer from anxiety and depression, drugs such as benzodiazepines and serotonergic agents have been used to control the symptoms.

Table 5: Medical conditions associated with personality change
Head trauma
Cerebrovascular disease
Cerebral tumors
Epilepsy (particularly complex partial epilepsy)
Huntington's disease
Multiple sclerosis
Endocrine disorders
Heavy metal poisoning (manganese, mercury)
Neurosyphilis
Acquired immune deficiency syndrome (AIDS)

PERSONALITY CHANGE DUE TO GENERAL MEDICAL CONDITION (TABLE 5)

Personality change due to general medical condition is characterized by marked change in personality, style and traits from previous level of functioning. ICD-10 includes this category that consists of personality and behavioral disorder due to brain disease, damage and dysfunction, post-encephalitic syndrome, and post concussional syndrome.

People with personality change due to medical condition have a clear sensorium. Mild disorders of cognitive functions often coexist, but do not amount to intellectual deterioration. They may be inattentive, which may account for disorders of recent memory. With some probing however, patents are likely to recall what they claim to have changes in behavior or personality involving emotional ability and impaired impulse control, who have no history or mental disorder, and whose personality changers occur abruptly or over a relatively brief time.

Management of personality change involves treatment of the underlying organic condition when possible. Psychopharmacological treatment of specific symptoms may be indicated in some cases such as haloperidol for aggression or fluoxetine for depression.

BIBLIOGRAPHY

1. Abraham K. The influence of oral eroticism on character formation, in selected papers on psychoanalysis. Edited by Jones E. London, Hogarth Press; 1927. pp. 393-106.
2. Alder G. Borderline psycopathology and its treatment. New York, Jason Aronson; 1985.
3. American Psychiatric Association. Desk Reference to the Diagnostic Criteria from DSM-5. Washington DC. 2013.
4. American Psychiatric Association: Diagnostic and Statistical Manual 1 Mental disorders. Washington DC, American Psychiatric Association; 1952.
5. American Psychiatric Association: Diagnostic and Statistical Manual: Mental disorders. 3rd edition. revised Washington DC, American Psychiatric Association; 1987
6. American Psychiatric Association: Diagnostic and Statistical Manual: Mental disorders edition revised Washington DC, American Psychiatric Association; 1994
7. American Psychiatric Association: Diagnostic and Statistical Manual Mental disorders. 2nd edition. Washington DC. American Psychiatric Association; 1968.
8. American Psychiatric Association; Diagnostic and Statistical Manual: Mental disorders, 3rd edition. Washington DC, American Psychiatric Association; 1980.
9. Bernstein DP, Useda D, Siever LJ. Paranoid personality disorder: a review of its current status: Journal of personality disorders. 1993;7:53-62.
10. Bleuler E. die Problems der schizodie under Syntonie Zeitschrift fur die gasame, Neurologic and Psychiatric. 1922;78:373-88.
11. Breuer J, Freud S. Studies on hysteria (1893-1895), translated and edited by Strachey J. New York, Basic books; 1957.
12. Carey G, DiLalla DL. Personality and Psychopathology: Genetic perspectives. J Abnorm Psychol. 1994;103:32-43.
13. Cloninger CR. A systematic method for clinical description and classification of personality variants. Arch Gen Psychiatry. 1987;44:573-88.
14. Cooper AM, Ronningstanr E. Narcissistic personality disorder, in American Psychiatric press review of Psychiatry. Tasman A, Riba ME (Eds). Washington DC, American Psychiatric Press. 1992;11:80-7.
15. Costa P, McCrae R. Personality disorders and the five-factor model of personality. Journal of personality disorders. 1990; 4:362-71.
16. Cowdry RW, Gardner DL. Pharmacotherapy of borderline personality disorder: alprazolam, carbamazepine, trifluperazine and tranylcypromine. Arch Gen Psychiatry. 1988;45:111-9.
17. Erikson EH. Childhood and society New York, WW Norton; 1950.
18. Fenichel O. The psychoanalytic Theory of the neurosis. New York, WW Norton; 1945.
19. Frances A. Categorical and dimensional systems of personality diagnosis: a comparison. Compr Psychiatry. 1982;23:516-27.
20. Freud S. Character and anal eroticism (1908), in Collected Papers, Vol 2 London, Hogarth Press; 1924. pp. 45-50.
21. Goldberg DC, Schulz C, Schulz PM, et al. Borderline and schizotypal personality disorders treated with low dose thiothexene vs. placebo. Arch Gen Psychiatry. 1986;43:680-6.
22. Grove WM, Eckert ED, Heston L, et al. Heritability of substances abuse and antisocial behavior: a study of monozygotic twins reared apart. Biol Psychiatry. 1990;27:1293-304.
23. Gunderson JG. Diagnostic controversies, in American Psychiatric Press Review of Psychiatry. Tasman A, Riba M (Eds). Washington DC, American Psychiatric Press. 1992;11:9-24.
24. Gunderson JG. Borderline personality disorder. Washington DC, American Psychiatric Press; 1984.
25. Hare RD, Hard SD, Harpur TJ. Psychopathy and the DSM-IV criteria for antisocial personality disorder. J Abnorm Psychol. 1991;100:391-8.

26. Hirschfeld RMA, Shea MT, Wiese R. Dependent personality disorder: perspectives for DSM-IV. Journal of Personality Disorders. 1991;5:135-49.
27. Janet P. The Mental State of Hystericals: A study of Mental Stigmata and Mental Accidents Translated by Corson CR. New York, Putnam; 1901.
28. Jones M. The therapeutic community—A new treatment in psychiatry, New York, Basic Books; 1953.
29. Kalus O, Bemstein DP, Siever LJ. Schizoid personality disorder: a review of its current status. Journal of personality disorders; 1993;7:43-52.
30. Kendler KS, Gruenberg AM. Genetic relationship between paranoid personality disorder and the "schizophrenic spectrum" disorder. Am J Psychiatry. 1982;139:1185-6.
31. Kernberg OF. Borderline Conditions and Pathological Narcissism, New York, Jason Aronson; 1975.
32. Kindler KS, McGuire M, Gruenberg AM, et al. The Roscommon Family study; III schizophrenia—related personality in relatives. Arch Gen Psychiatry. 1993;50:781-8.
33. Klein DN. Depressive personality; reliability, validity and relationship to dysthymia. J Abnorm Psychol. 1990;99:412-21.
34. Klein M. Wisconsin personality Inventory-Revised Madison, WI, University of Wisconsin; 1990.
35. Kraeplin E. Dementia Precox and paraphreina, Edinburg, ED and S Livingstone.
36. Lazare A, Klerman G, Artmor D. Oral, obsessive and hysterical personality patterns: replications of factor analysis in an independent sample. J Psychiatr Res. 1970;7:275-9.
37. Lesch KP, Bengel D, Hells A. Association of anxiety-related traits with polymorphism in the serotonin transporter gene regulatory region, Science. 1996;274:1527-31.
38. Liebowitz MR, Stone MH, Turker lD. Treatment of personality disorders, in psychiatry Update: American Psychiatric Association Annual Review, Vol 5. Fraces AJ, Hales RE (Eds). Washington.
39. Loranger AW. Personality Disorders Examination (PDE) Manual, Yonkers, NY, DV Communications; 1988.
40. Millon T. Avoidant personality disorder: a brief review of issues and data. Journal of Personality Disorders. 1991;5: 353-362.
41. Millon T. disorders of personality-DSM-III: Axis-ll New York, Wiley; 1981.
42. Millon T. Millon Clinical multiaxial inventory-ll Manual, Minnetonka MN, National computer system; 1987.
43. Ogata SN, Silk KR, Goddrich S, et al. Childhood sexual and physical abuse in adult patients with borderline personality disorder. Am Psychiatry. 1990;147:1008-13.
44. Paris J. Personality Disorders a biophysical model. Journal of personality disorders. 1993;7:255-64.
45. Perry JC, Vailant GE. Personality disorders, in Comprehensive Textbook of Psychiatry, 5th edition. Kaplan Hl, Sadock BJ, Baltimore MD (Eds). Williams & Wilkins; 1989;2: 1352-87.
46. Pfohl B, Blum N. Obsessive-compulsive personality disorder; a review of a available data and recommendations for DSM-lV. Journal of personality Disorders. 1991;5:363-75.
47. Pfohl B. Histrionic personality disorder; a review of available data and recommendations for DSM-lV. Journal of Personality Disorders. 1991;5:150-66.
48. Phillips KA, Gunderson JG, Hirschfeld RMA, et al. A review of the depressive personality. Am J Psychiatry. 1990;147:830-7.
49. Pritchard JC. A Treatise on Insanity. London, Sherwood, Gilbert and Piper, 1835.
50. Rado S. Schizotypal organization; preliminary report on a clinical study of schizophrenia, in Psychoanalysis and behaviour. New York, Grune & Stratton; 1956. pp. 1-10.
51. Reiss D, Hetherington EM, Plomin R, et al. Genetic questions for environmental studies differential parenting and psychopathology in adolescence. Arch Gen Psychiatry. 1995; 52:925-36.
52. Schneider K. Die Psychopathischen Personlichkeiten, Vienna, Deuticke; 1923.
53. Schneider K. Psychopathic Personalities, Springfield, II, Charles C Thomas; 1958.
54. Siever LJ, Amin F, Coccaro EF, et al. CSF Hoinovanillic acid in schizotypal disorders, Am J Psychiatry. 1991;148; 1647-58.
55. Siever LJ, Davis KL. A psychobiological perspective on the personality disorders. Am J Psychiatry. 1991;148:1647-58.
56. Spitzer RL, Williams JBW, Gibbon M, et al. Structured clinical Interview for DSM-lll R (SCID), Washington DC, American Psychiatric Press; 1990.
57. Torgerson S, Onstad S, Skre I, et al. "True" schizotypal personality disorder, a study of co-twins and relatives of schizophrenia probands. Am J Psychiatry. 1993;150:1661-7.
58. Valliant GE. Ego Mechanisms of Defense; A guide for clinicians and Researchers, Washington DC, American Psychiatric Press; 1992.
59. Valliant GR. Ego Mechanisms of Defense and Personality Psychopathology. J Abnorm Psychol. 1994;103:44-50.
60. Weissman MM. The epidemiology of personality disorders: 1 1990 update. Journal of Personality Disorders. 1993;7:44-62.
61. Widiger TA, Corbin EM, Millon T. Antisocial personality disorder, in American Psychiatric Press Review of Psychiatry. Tasman A, Riba ME, (Eds). Washington DC. American Sychiatric Press. 1992;11:63-79.
62. Widiger TA. Personality disorder dimensional model proposal for DSM-IV. Journal of Personality Disorders. 1991;5:386-98.
63. Widiger TA. Personality Interview Questions-II. Lexington, KY, University of Kentucky; 1987.
64. World Health Organization: International Statistical Classification of Diseases and Related Health Problems, 10th Revision. Geneva, World Health Organization; 1992.
65. Zanarini MC, Frankenburg FR, Chauncey DL, et al. The Diagnostic Interview for Personality Disorders: inter-rater and test-retest reliability. Compr Psychiatry. 1987;28:467-80.

CHAPTER

25 Normal Human Sexuality and Sexual Disorders

TS Sathyanarayana Rao, Abhinav Tandon

ANATOMY AND PHYSIOLOGY

The genetic, neuroanatomical and neurochemical aspects of sexual functioning are as important to human sexuality as psychological and social factors.

In males, it includes the external genitalia (penis, scrotum, testes, epididymis, part of the vas deferens), the internal components (vas deferens, ejaculatory duct and prostate gland). As per Masters and Johnson, size of the penis varies from 7 to 11 cm in the flaccid state to 14–18 cm in the erect state. Concern with the size of the penis has been found to be very common in men. 'Penis' is derived from Latin which means "to hang"; it has been called 'the executive organ of sexuality' by Freud. The penis may be circumscribed either surgically for a medical reason or as part of the religious belief in Muslims and Jews.

Sexual desire is mediated by emotions originating from the limbic system. Activation of amygdala can lead to penile erection, sensations of extreme pleasure and sexual feelings. Amygdala is known to produce sex specific behaviors. Sexual stimulation from visual stimuli is found to have greater activation of amygdala in males when compared to females. An increased density of enkephalins and opiate receptors gives amygdala the ability to produce feelings of pleasure and motivate individuals for pleasure seeking behavior.[1-3]

Brainstem exerts excitatory and inhibitory influence over sexual impulses from the spinal cord. Ejaculation is the forceful expulsion of semen and seminal fluid from the epididymis, vas deferens, seminal vesicles and prostate into the urethra. Normal antegrade ejaculation includes three steps: emission (under sympathetic control; T10-L2), ejection (under parasympathetic control; S2-4) and orgasm (occurs due to cerebral processing of sensory stimuli from pudendal nerve).[4]

In females, vulva forms the external genitalia and includes the mons pubis, major and minor lips, clitoris, glans, vaginal orifice, vestibule of vagina. The internal system includes part of the vagina, uterus, Fallopian tubes and ovaries. Masters and Johnson have described the clitoris as the primary female sexual organ. Thrusting of the penis stimulates the clitoris via traction on the minor lips and leads to orgasm. Ernst Grefenberg in 1950 described an area of around 0.5–1 cm in the anterior wall of vagina surrounding the female urethra, known as G spot; it is considered equivalent of prostate in males. Stimulation of this area is highly pleasurable and leads to orgasm in females.

Nerves from the autonomic nervous system (ANS) innervate the sexual organs; parasympathetic nerves (S2,3,4) mediate reflex erections and a thoracolumbar sympathetic system mediates psychological impulses. Both sympathetic and parasympathetic systems mediate are involved in relaxing cavernosal smooth muscles which is aided by nitric oxide (NO). In females the sympathetic system causes contraction of smooth muscles of vagina, urethra and uterus during orgasm. The ANS is influenced by external events like stress and also by biological mediators (internal events) of sexual functioning.

Erection involves dopamine (increases), serotonin (minimal change), norepinephrine (decreased activity at α and increased activity at β) and modulation of acetylcholine. Dopamine antagonists cause erectile dysfunction whereas dopamine agonists enhance erection and libido. Alpha 1-blockade may lead to priapism and Beta-blockade may lead to impotence.[5] Multiple neurotransmitters like dopamine, norepinephrine, serotonin, acetylcholine, oxytocin, GABA (gamma amino butyric acid) and nitric oxide are involved in ejaculation.[6] Dopamine promotes seminal emission and ejaculation whereas serotonin is inhibitory. During ejaculation and orgasm there is increased activity of norepinephrine at α1-receptors. Alpha 1-blockers may lead to impaired ejaculation and serotonergic agents may impair impotence.[5] It has been hypothesized that men with premature ejaculation have hyposensitivity of 5-HT2C and/or hypersensitivity of 5-HT1A receptors.[7,8] Dopamine promotes sexual desire and arousal. Serotonin through inhibition of dopamine and norepinephrine, has a negative impact on desire and arousal phases of the cycle. Therefore, the serotonergic system, may contribute to various sexual problems across the sexual response cycle.

Testosterone is associated with libido in both men and women; in men it is inversely related to stress and lifestyle factors with highest levels seen in the morning (normal range 270–1100 ng/dL). Estrogen, testosterone and progesterone promote sexual desire; oxytocin enhances sexual activity in both sexes and promotes orgasm. Prolactin inhibits arousal; androgens are said to increase libido in females but this still needs further confirmation.

SEXUAL RESPONSE CYCLE

Masters and Johnson[9] proposed the four phase model of human sexual response which can be abbreviated as the 'EPOR Model'.

E-Excitation: Somatic and psychogenic stimuli lead to increasing sexual tension and subjective sense of pleasure.

P-Plateau: Intensified sexual tension and sexual pleasure

O-Orgasmic: Involuntary pleasurable climax; peaking of sexual pleasure with release of sexual tension.

R-Resolution: A sense of well being and relaxation; men have a refractory period for subsequent orgasm whereas women can have multiple orgasms.

With subsequent research by Robinson and Helen Kaplan, the above model got modified into the DEOR model. Here 'D' stands for the 'Desire phase' which is influenced by sexual drive and fantasies and is the conscious desire to have sex.[10] The 'Plateau phase' has been merged with the 'Excitation phase' as it is considered to be the final stage of the 'Excitation phase'.[11] The 'Desire phase' depends on the psychological makeup and is influenced by the biological characteristics of the individual. The 'Excitation phase' begins with psychological or physiological (or both) stimulation and leads to penile tumescence and enlargement of testes in males and vaginal lubrication, hard clitoris, formation of orgasmic platform (vagina becomes barrel shaped with constriction in outer 1/3rd), thickening of labia minora, increase in breast size in females and nipple erection in both sexes. There is increase in heart rate, respiratory rate and blood pressure. In the 'Orgasmic phase', sexual pleasure peaks and there is rhythmic contraction of perineal muscles and reproductive organs; inevitable ejaculation triggers orgasm in males whereas in females there are involuntary contractions of uterus and lower third of vagina.

Resolution phase is characterized by disengorgement of blood from the genital organs; following orgasm a general feeling of well-being and muscular relaxation occur (resolution is rapid following orgasm). However, if orgasm does not occur, resolution may take up to 6 hours and may be associated with irritability.

SEXUALITY AND PSYCHOSEXUALITY

Sexuality depicts the sexual functions, activities, attitudes and orientations of an individual.[12] According to Levine (1989), an adult's sexuality has seven components: gender identity, orientation, intention, desire, arousal, orgasm and emotional satisfaction. It is determined by the biological, sociocultural and environmental factors affecting an individual. The experiences of an individual during development and relationships help in forming various aspects of the personality and sexuality of an individual. The term 'psychosexual' is used to describe personality development, as shaped by the sexuality of an individual. It is used in a much broader sense and is not synonymous to libido as described by Freud.

In the Oxford dictionary, 'sex' refers to male or female based on reproductive functions and biological characteristics of an individual. However, 'gender' refers to the public lived role as male or female, typically used with reference to social and cultural differences rather than biological ones; gender identity refers to the social identity of the individual.[13] The affective symptoms of discontent with one's designated birth sex, which arise as a result of gender identity of an individual are referred to as gender dysphoria. Gender identity starts developing at 18 months age and is firmly established before 3 years age. This is primarily determined by anatomical sex (biological sex) by the presence of genitals (phenotype), genetic factor (genotype) and early upbringing. Sexual desire has three interactive components: (1) Sexual drive-biological component; (2) Sexual motivation-psychological component; and (3) Sexual wish-social component.[14]

Masturbation: It is a form of stimulation which leads to sexual pleasure and lasts throughout one's lifetime; it acts as a precursor for object related sexual behavior. Though masturbation has been condemned by culture and protectors of various religions, no scientific evidence exists that masturbation leads to ill-health. It forms part of healthy psychosexual development. Genital self-stimulation is often observed in toddlers at around 1.5 years of age. Masturbation acts as a method of self-stimulation and release of sexual tension in teenagers; in adults it acts as a method of sexual satisfaction when intercourse with a partner is unsatisfactory or when the partner is unavailable. In the 1960s, Masters and Johnson described the various methods of masturbation; in women stimulation of shaft of clitoris has been preferred. It needs professional advice and treatment only when it becomes compulsive. As per Kinsey (1940), all men and approximately 3/4th women masturbate at sometime during their lives.

Sexual development through the life span: In Freud's words, child development lays the foundation for adult

Table 1: Phase of life and etiology of sexual dysfunction

Phase of life	*Etiology of sexual dysfunction*
Adolescence	Difficulty consolidating the sexual identity
Young adult	Psychological conflict in giving and receiving sexual pleasure; difficulty integrating sex as part of a healthy relationship
Middle life	Difficulty in maintaining intimacy
Old age	Failure in maintaining healthy sexual functioning due to age related biological changes and cultural issues

sexual behavior. Appropriate parent-child interaction and relationship lays the foundation for a healthy sexual development. The normal tasks of sexual development at different phases of life may provide a clinician with an insight into the age related sexual dysfunctions (Table 1).[14]

Sexuality depends on four interrelated psychosexual factors as mentioned below.

- *Sexual identity* is formed by a person's biological sexual characteristics, genital and secondary sex characteristics.
- *Gender identity* is a person's sense of being male or female. It is firmly established by the age of 2 or 3 years.
- *Sexual orientation* is determined, depending on the object of a person's sexual impulses: heterosexual, homosexual, or bisexual. The overwhelming majority of people have a heterosexual orientation.
- *Sexual behavior* "includes desire, fantasies, pursuit of partners, autoeroticism, and all the activities engaged into express and gratify sexual needs." Normal sexual behavior brings pleasure to both partners; it is devoid of inappropriate feelings of guilt or anxiety and is not compulsive.[15]

SEXUAL DISORDERS

DSM-5 (Diagnostic and Statistical Manual of Mental Disorders 5th Edition) released in May 2013 defines Sexual Dysfunctions as "a heterogeneous group of disorders that are typically characterized by a clinically significant" disturbance in a person's ability to respond sexually or to sexual pleasure."[13] Subtypes include Lifelong vs acquired and generalized vs situational. Also (i) partner's and individual vulnerability factors (ii) relationship factors (iii) psychiatric comorbidity (iv) cultural and (v) general medical factors need to be considered.[13]

Classically, sexual inadequacy refers to some specific disruption of the 'Sexual Response Cycle, (as described by Masters and Johnson in 1970).[9,16] A client centered approach is considered to be more appropriate; that is to say a sexual problem is said to be present when an individual goes to a clinician and reports some problem with his/her sexual functioning. It should be remembered that sexual dysfunctions do not follow all or none phenomenon; rather sexual problems like many other psychiatric problems occurs on a continuum. Sexual inadequacies need to be differentiated from Gender identity disorders and paraphilias.

Epidemiology

Studying the epidemiology of sexual dysfunctions becomes difficult as the frequency of reporting and seeking help varies; the reason for the same ranges from availability of sexual health care center, knowledge and attitude about the problem, to the social and cultural upbringing of the individual. Variability in reported prevalence can also be attributed to variations in how sexual problems are defined and the methodology used to assess distress associated with the problem.

Masters and Johnson in 1970 reported that 50% of all Americans have sexual problems sometime during their life.[9,16] The prevalence of sexual dysfunctions has been reported to be high, affecting 43% women and 31% men.[17] It has been estimated that 20% of the total population have hypoactive sexual desire disorder and is more commonly seen in women.[15] In 1978, a study conducted by Frank has documented sexual dissatisfaction in 5th of women and 3rd of the men. In 2004 the 'Committee on Epidemiology/ Risk Factors for Sexual Dysfunction' with international collaboration among four countries has reported the incidence of erectile dysfunction as 25–30 cases/1000 person years. Around 40–45% of adult women and 20–30% of adult men have at least one sexual dysfunction. The prevalence of ED increases with age; it is 1–9%:<40 years, 2–9% and 20–30%: in 40–59 years age group, 20–40%: 60–69 years age group: and 50–75% in the 7th and 8th decade. Prevalence rates for ejaculatory dysfunction range from 9% to 31%.[18]

A study conducted at Chandigarh, India by Natera, Wig and Verma in 1977, found sexual problems in 10% of males attending psychiatry and medical out patient department (OPD). A study done by TSS Rao and Darshan MS in Suttur village in South India found that among those above 60 years of age and sexually active, 43.5% of the male subjects had male erectile dysfunction, 10.9% male premature ejaculation, 0.77% male hypoactive sexual desire disorder and 0.38% male anorgasmia. Among females the prevalence of female arousal dysfunction was found to be 28%, female hypoactive sexual desire disorder 16%, female anorgasmia 20% and female dyspareunia in 8% of the female subjects.[19] TSS Rao in 2003 reported that 6% of the males had sought psychiatric help primarily for sexual problems in a tertiary care teaching Hospital at Mysore in South India.[20-22] A 2-year-retrospective study conducted at a general hospital and a private psychiatry OPD at Mysore by the TSS Rao revealed that 50% of the patients had Dhat syndrome with poor follow-up at the health care facility. In 1972, Bagadia and his colleagues studied 258 male out patients in a teaching hospital setting and found the most common disorders to be: anxiety associated with nocturnal emission (65%) and passing semen in urine (47%): in the unmarried group. Impotence (48%), premature ejaculation (34%) and passing semen in urine (47%) were common in the married group. In 2007, Kar and Koola conducted a postal survey on English speaking south Indian women and found that 28.6% of women had orgasmic difficulties. Around 40% of women reported to have never masturbated. In 2008, Kendurkar and his colleagues retrospectively assessed 1242 individuals attending a marriage and sex clinic from 1979 to 2005 through their medical records and found premature ejaculation to be the most common complaint followed by male erectile problems and Dhat syndrome.[23] A cross-sectional survey conducted on 149 married women attending a medical outpatient clinic, by Singh and colleagues in 2009, found female sexual dysfunction in 73.2% women, with 77.2% having desire disorder, 91.3% arousal disorder, 96.6% inadequate lubrication, 86.6% orgasmic dysfunction, 81.2% dissatisfied, 64.4% having pain disorder.[24]

Etiology

Human sexual response is a complex phenomenon and involves biological, interpersonal, social and cultural factors. Generally speaking, sexual dysfunctions are multi-factorial in etiology. In addition to the lifelong/acquired and generalized/situational subtypes, DSM-5 mentions five factors which play their part either individually or in combination in sexual dysfunction. These include:

- *Partner factors*: Partner's health particularly sexual health.
- *Relationship factors*: Poor communication and intimacy; discrepancy in desire.
- *Individual vulnerability factors*: History of sexual abuse, psychiatric comorbidity, stressors, performance anxiety leading to excitement inhibition.
- *Cultural and religious factors*: Attitude toward sexuality.
- Medical factors

DSM-5 highlights the point that a sexual dysfunction diagnosis is not made if the problem is better explained by a non-sexual mental disorder, stressor, substance use or a

Table 2: Etiology of sexual disorders

Sexual disorder/clinical feature	*Etiology*
Disorder of desire/arousal: Female sexual interest[#]/arousal disorder and male hypoactive sexual desire disorder[#]	Low arousal in females associated with thyroid problems, arthritis, irritable bowel disease *Drugs*: Antihypertensives, psychotropics, dopamine blockers, alcohol Androgen deficiency
Disorder of desire: Compulsive sexual behaviors	Psychogenic (obsessive-compulsive sexuality, sex impulsivity)
Disorder of arousal: Erectile disorder[#]	Systemic diseases, vascular insufficiency, neurological disorders, androgen deficiency, hypertension); *Drugs*: Antihypertensives, anticholinergics, psychotropics, digoxin, cigarette smoking, substance abuse, estrogens
Disorders of orgasm	
Premature (early) ejaculation-lifelong/acquired[#]	Prostatic disease, increased central dopaminergic activity, increased penile sensitivity Drugs
Delayed ejaculation[#]	Spinal cord lesions *Drugs*: Antihypertensives, antidepressants, antipsychotics, alcohol
Female orgasmic disorder[#]/male orgasmic disorder	CNS disease, Parkinson's disease *Drugs*: SSRIs*, TCAs*[2], substance abuse
Absent ejaculation (anejaculation)	*Neural*: Spinal cord injury, colorectal surgery, diabetes *Drugs*: Antihypertensives, psychotropics, alcohol Androgen deficiency
Postejaculation pain	Psychogenic
Failure of detumescence: Priapism (primary or secondary)	Structural penile disease, Peyronie's disease; idiopathic (primary); Secondary-hematological disorders: leukemia, infiltrative: amyloidosis *Inflammatory:* Mumps Neurological disorders; Tumors
Others	
Genito-pelvic pain/penetration disorder[#]	Associated with reduced sexual desire and interest General medical factors Perimenopausal

[#]Mentioned in DSM-5
*Selective serotonin reuptake inhibitors
*[2]Tricyclic antidepressants

general medical condition. Table 2 details the etiology of sexual disorders.[13,25-31]

General Medical Causes

They could be cardiovascular (hypertension, atherosclerosis, peyronie's disease), neurological (cauda-equina syndrome, spinal cord lesions, peripheral neuropathy), pulmonary disorders (chronic obstructive pulmonary disease, asthma), renal disorders, liver disorders, infections, malignancies, endocrinal disorders, surgical procedures, traumatic causes, Iatrogenic (drugs and the local causes involving both the sexes. Sexual dysfunctions caused by some of the routinely used drugs are mentioned in Table 3.[25,26,32]

Drugs Commonly Associated with Sexual Dysfunction

Antihypertensives particularly diuretics, sympatholytics (central agents-methyldopa, clonidine, nonselective beta-blockers) may lead to erectile dysfunction (ED) and decreased libido.

Antipsychotics act as dopamine antagonists, also block adrenergic and cholinergic receptors and many lead to prolactin elevation leading to sexual dysfunction. Chlorpromazine, trifluperazine and thioridazine cause erectile dysfunction (haloperidol may also lead to ED) and retrograde ejaculation and hence orgasm without ejaculation. Second generation antipsychotics like quetiapine and aripriprazole have minimal sexual side effects perhaps due to there prolactin sparing effect. Clozapine, ziprasidone and olanzapine have minimal effect on prolactin levels but agranulocytosis risk due to clozapine is a major limitation for its frequent use.[33] When hyperprolactinemia occurs during treatment and is associated with menstrual or sexual dysfunction, consideration should be given to changing the patient's medication to a prolactin-sparing agent.[34] Sexual dysfunction as a side-effect of first generation antipsychotics, in schizophrenics, can be reduced by shifting them to second generation antipsychotics.[35] 30–90% patients on selective serotonin reuptake inhibitors (SSRIs) develop sexual side effects. Kennedy and colleagues studied 134 patients with major depressive disorder and found that 40% of men and 50% of women reported reduced sexual interest, whereas 40–50% of the total patients reported reduced arousal.[36-39] For treating SSRI induced sexual dysfunction, a number of strategies may be tried. These include: allowing tolerance to develop (which is not common), reducing the current dose (but the therapeutic effect may decrease), drug holidays (this may however lead to noncompliance and side effects due to abrupt discontinuation).[40-42]

Shifting to other antidepressants like bupropion, mirtazapine and nefazodone which have little risk of sexual dysfunction may be helpful, but the symptoms of primary psychiatric disorder may again surface up. A 8-week double blind trial of paroxetine (20 mg/day) vs duloxetine (20–60 mg twice/day) revealed that duloxetine is associated with less sexual side effects on parameters of drive, arousal and orgasm.[43] Mirtazapine in higher doses (more than 30 mg/day) has a more favorable sexual functioning profile when compared with higher doses of sertraline (more than 100 mg/day).[44] Gepirone differs from SSRIs in only affecting the 5HT(1A) receptors. It has been shown to improve sexual functioning in women and all domains of sexual functioning in men, independent of its antidepressant or anxiolytic effect.[45] Gepirone has also been reported to have efficacy in the treatment of hypoactive sexual desire disorder in depressed and possibly in nondepressed women, independent of the antidepressant effect.[46]

Sildenafil may be used as and when required if other factors are favorable.[38,39,41,47,48] Tricyclic antidepressants (TCAs) and selective serotonin reuptake inhibitors (SSRIs) may cause erectile dysfunction. Fluoxetine and multicyclic antidepressants may cause anorgasmia, which may be reduced by serotonergic antagonist cyprohepatidine; however it is to be remembered that cyprohepatidine may cause anticholinergic crisis.[49,50] Clomipramine may increase sex drive in some individuals. Lithium may reduce excessive sexual drive in manic state; it may impair erection. Antihistamines decrease sexual functioning by their anticholinergic property. Stimulants like methylphenidate and amphetamines increase libido by elevating dopamine and norepinephrine levels; however long term use decreases desire and erection.[5]

Psychogenic causes include sociocultural, individual and relationship factors. Individuals may develop an idea that 'sex

Table 3: Drugs most commonly associated with sexual dysfunction

Type of sexual dysfunction	*Drug*
Erectile dysfunction	Antihypertensives Antipsychotics Antidepressants Antiandrogenic (Digoxin, Histamine H_2 receptor blockers *Others*: Alcohol, ketoconazole, phenobarbital, phenytoin
Decreased libido	Antihypertensives Psychotropics (Tricyclic antidepressants Benzodiazepines Antiandrogenic (digoxin, histamine H_2 receptor blockers *Others*: Alcohol, ketoconazole, niacin, phenobarbital, phenytoin
Ejaculatory dysfunction	Alpha blockers, SSRIs
Multiple phases of sexual function	Antipsychotics, Monoamine oxidase inhibitors

is dirty' and it is only for reproduction and not for pleasure. Trauma in early adolescence and hasty sexual encounters can have a predominant negative impact on the sexuality of an individual. Individuals may develop performance anxiety due to self-imposed high standards. Monitoring one's own sexual expertise and myths particularly concerning semen, masturbation, menstruation can have a negative impact. (Flow chart 1).

Flow chart 1: Sexual dysfunction due to psychogenic causes

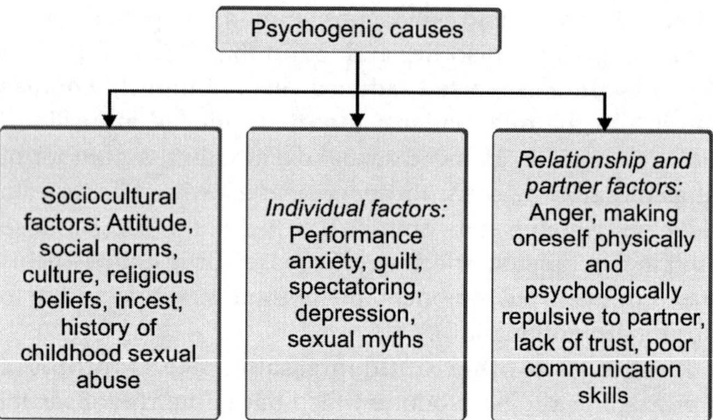

DIAGNOSTIC EVALUATION

While taking a sexual history the clinicians should make the patient comfortable with adequate privacy. Maintaining confidentiality is of utmost importance and the clinicians should inform the patient regarding the same. Both the clinician and the patient should be comfortable with the language in which the patient is interviewed. Developing rapport, being empathic and non-judgmental are important and a physical examination is a must in all the cases.[27] Differences in socioeconomic level, age, gender and culture between the clinician and the patient can be barriers toward adequate history taking.[57] When we address sexuality related issues we are opening a window to the patient's psyche. This gives us information regarding the individual's capacity to be psychologically intimate, love and be loved and give and receive pleasure.[58]

Patient's current complaint, duration, associated symptoms, mode of onset, frequency and severity of the problem should be noted; whether the problem is generalized or situational, life-long or acquired needs to be enquired into. Enquire regarding sexual practices, fantasies and goals,

Common sexual dysfunctions or inadequacies

DSM-5 (Diagnostic and statistical manual of mental disorders 5th edition)	*ICD-10 (International classification of mental and behavioral disorders 10th edition)*
Female sexual interest/arousal disorder# Significantly reduced or absence of sexual interest or arousal manifested by any 3 of the following: (1) Reduced interest (2) Absent/reduced erotic thoughts (3) Absent/reduced initiation of sexual activity or no response to partner's attempt to initiate the same (4) Absent/Reduced sexual excitement (5) Absent/reduced response to erotic cues (6) Absent/reduced genital or nongenital sensations during sexual activity. Symptoms 4–6 are present:* **Male hypoactive sexual desire disorder**# Persistently deficient sexual thoughts or fantasies and desire for sexual activity. The symptoms are present for a minimum period of 6 months and cause significant distress.[13] The judgment of deficiency or absence is made by the clinician, taking into account the factors that affect sexual functioning such as age and the context of the person's life.	**Lack or loss of sexual desire** (Includes hypoactive sexual desire disorder) Loss of sexual desire is the principal problem and is not secondary to other sexual difficulties like erectile dysfunction; here initiation of sexual activity is diminished **Sexual aversion and lack of sexual enjoyment** In sexual aversion the idea of sexual interaction is associated with strong negative emotions and the fear associated leads to avoidance of sexual activity In some cases, sexual responses may occur normally with orgasm but pleasure is lacking, which leads to lack of enjoyment
Erectile disorder# Marked difficulty in obtaining or maintaining an erection during sexual activity or marked decrease in erectile rigidity:*	**Sexual dysfunction not caused by organic disorder or disease** **Failure of genital response** (Includes female sexual arousal disorder; male erectile disorder; psychogenic impotence) **Male erectile disorder**: Problem in developing or sustaining erection suitable for satisfactory intercourse. In females, vaginal dryness can be a result of infection, estrogen deficiency or psychogenic
Delayed ejaculation:# Marked delay, infrequent or absence of ejaculation:*	
Premature (Early) ejaculation# Persistent ejaculation occurring within 1 minute of vaginal penetration and before the individual wishes:* This diagnosis may be applied in cases of nonvaginal sexual activities.	**Premature ejaculation** The inability to hold ejaculation for sufficient time, for both partners to enjoy sexual interaction; mostly psychogenic If erection requires prolonged stimulation the time duration between adequate erection and ejaculation is shortened: delayed erection

Contd...

Contd...

Female orgasmic disorder[#] Marked delay, infrequent, reduced intensity or absence of orgasm:* [#]All the above sexual dysfunctions mentioned in DSM-5 can be further classified as (1) Lifelong vs acquired (2) Generalized vs Situational (3) Mild, Moderate or Severe	**F52.3 Orgasmic dysfunction** (Includes Inhibited Orgasm: male/ female and Psychogenic anorgasmy) This may be psychological or organic. It is more common in women.
Genito-Pelvic Pain/Penetration Disorder Persistent any of the following symptoms: (1) Difficulty in vaginal penetration (2) Significant pain during vaginal intercourse/penetration (3) Fear/anxiety related to point 2. (4) Significant contraction of pelvic floor muscles during vaginal penetration attempt. The symptoms are present for a minimum period of 6 months and cause significant distress[13] Genito-pelvic pain disorder can be further classified into (1) Lifelong vs Acquired and (2) Mild, moderate or severe	**Nonorganic vaginismus** Spasm of the muscles surrounding the vagina, making penile entry impossible or painful. **Nonorganic dyspareunia** Pain during sexual intercourse in males or females. **Excessive sexual drive** (Includes Nymphomania, satyriasis) Seen in males or females during teenage or adulthood. When associated with an affective disorder the primary mood disorder should be quoted.
Other sexual dysfunctions mentioned in DSM-5 **Substance/medication induced sexual dysfunction** **Other specified sexual dysfunction** **Unspecified sexual dysfunction** For making any of the above diagnosis as per DSM-5, a nonsexual mental disorder, substance abuse/general medical cause leading to sexual dysfunction and severe relationship distress should be ruled out.[13]	**Other sexual dysfunction, not caused by organic disorder or disease** **Unspecified sexual dysfunction, not caused by organic disorder or disease**
*On almost all or greater than 75% occasions of sexual activity with a partner (in identified situations or, if generalized, in all situations), and without the individual desiring delay. The symptoms are present for a minimum period of 6 months and cause significant distress.[2]	**DHAT syndrome** This term has been used to refer to a culture bound syndrome of sexual dysfunction. It is seen in India and the subcontinent, as a mixture of neurotic features of asthenia, anxiety, depression, phobia and hypochondria is in patients, who are usually young and attribute the myriad of symptoms to loss of semen, in nocturnal emission, 'bad dreams', semenuria, masturbation or sexual intercourse. As the misplaced fear and ignorance are the core features of this syndrome, treatment primarily involves sex education and counseling.[51-53]

Note: Masters & Johnson defined a person as 'premature ejaculator ' if he cannot control his ejaculatory process for a sufficient length of time during intravaginal containment to satisfy his partner in atleast 50% of their coital connections.
Premature ejaculation has been recognized in majority of cases as psychogenic, secondary to anxiety, conditioned by early sexual experiences, guilt and hostility towards the partner.[54-56]

intimacy issues with partner, and relationship problems affecting the current sexual functioning. Ask regarding any other associated factors aggravating the current problem and life stressors if any. Past sexual history, mode of gaining information regarding sexual functioning, history of first sexual activity, history regarding masturbation, sexual orientation and past history of sexual abuse need to be noted. Also note any guilt associated with sexual self-stimulation, premarital and extramarital sexual activities, live-in relationships.

The development of sexual identity through childhood and the effect of family members, family environment and other significant individuals and past life events on the sexuality of the individual should be discussed. Both recent and past sexual history should be covered. The effect of children, professional commitments and extramarital or premarital relationships if any, on the sexual life of the couple needs discussion. It is necessary to understand relationship difficulties among the couple, whether partner is sympathetic or asympathetic toward the problem, their expectation and motivation for treatment.[59] High risk sexual behaviors should be enquired into. Females are usually reluctant to express their sexual problems more so in the Indian context. Enquire regarding the sexual equilibrium established; sexual equilibrium is formed by the interaction of individual's identity, desire arousal, orgasmic and attainment characteristics. A partner's displeasure or lack of satisfaction may alter this equilibrium and make the individual sexually dysfunctional.

Men with erectile dysfunction may have normal libido and ejaculatory function. Usually, psychogenic potency problems begin suddenly, are situation specific and are accompanied by normal nocturnal and early morning tumescence. However, organic erectile dysfunction starts gradually, presents consistently and there would be loss of early morning erections. The differentiating features between organic and psychogenic sexual dysfunction are highlighted in Tables 4 and 5.

Laboratory studies should include blood tests for complete blood count, blood urea, serum creatinine, lipid profile, blood sugar, urine analysis, thyroid function and other endocrinal and other tests as required. Nocturnal penile tumescence, intracavernous pharmacologic injection using a vasodilating agent like papaverine, phentolamine and prostaglandin E1, Duplex color ultrasonography, dynamic infusion pharmacocavernosometry and cavernosography, pharmacologic pelvic penile angiography are the other tests in some selected cases.[60,61] Differentiating features between psychogenic and organic sexual dysfunctions are given in Table 4.[62] Differentiating features between psychogenic and organic erectile dysfunction are given in Table 5.[30,31] Areas to be covered in History taking of sexual disorders is given in Table 6.[63]

MANAGEMENT OF SEXUAL INADEQUACIES

Organic illness needs to be ruled out. A detailed history should be taken to identify various psychological, social and relationship factors affecting the current problem. It is important here to note that even if an organic illness is present which is affecting the sexual functioning, associated other factors aggravating the problem are likely to be present. However, in actual practice psychological and other pharmacological therapies are often required for the management (Flow chart 2).

Sex therapy as it is referred to today is essentially a modified form of the original therapy as founded by Masters and Johnson in 1970. The individual psychotherapies were the most common intervention for sexual dysfunction before 1970. However the 'new' sex therapy essentially followed a brief, problem focused, directed and behavioral approach. The classic psychodynamic theories stressed on the early developmental conflicts as the core issue for sexual dysfunction. Hence resolution of these conflicts would lead to acceptance of sexual impulses to the ego and resolution of the problem. The 'new' sex therapy focused on relief of

Table 4: Differentiating features between psychogenic and organic sexual dysfunction**

Characteristics	*Organic*	*Psychogenic*
Age	Older	Younger
Onset	Gradual (except trauma or surgery)	Acute
Circumstances	Global	Situational
Symptom course	Consistent or progressive	Intermittent
Desire	Normal	Decreased
Organic risks	Present	Absent, variable
Partner problem	Secondary	At onset
Anxiety and fear	Secondary	Primary

**Adopted from Clinical Practice Guidelines for Management of Sexual Dysfunctions published by Indian Psychiatric Society (2006)[61]

Table 5: Differentiating features between psychogenic and organic erectile dysfunction**

Parameters	*Psychogenic*	*Organic*
Onset of disorder	Situational with defined onset (onset associated with specific emotional event)	Insidious
Precipitating event	Psychogenic condition	Debilitating disease, vascular insufficiency or CNS abnormality, penile trauma or interfering drugs
Erectile function before intromission	May be present	Usually absent except in patients with pelvic steal phenomenon
Erectile function after intromission	Variable with different partners	Usually absent
Erectile response to other sexual stimuli	Usually present	Usually absent
Nocturnal or morning erections	Initially present and full, lost in long standing dysfunction	Absent or reduced in frequency and intensity
Course of disorder	Episodic or transient loss of erection	Persistent and progressive erectile dysfunction
Associated ejaculatory disorder	Premature ejaculation and intermittent loss of ejaculation	Retrograde or absent ejaculation
Nocturnal Penile tumescence Total time Circumferential change Penile-brachial index (PBI) Bulbocavernosus reflex latency	 >90–80 min/night .2 cm >0.70 <35 sec	 <60 min/night 2 cm <0.60 >40 sec

**Adopted from Clinical Practice Guidelines for Management of Sexual Dysfunctions published by Indian Psychiatric Society (2006)[61]

Table 6: History taking for sexual disorders

Identification	*Including age, sex, education, profession, relationship status, sexual orientation, religion, social class, current stressors*
Current sexual functioning	Type of sexual problem; onset, course, duration, aggravating and relieving factors; generalized or situational; with a particular partner only (if multiple partners +) Frequency of sexual activity; description of sexual interaction including foreplay, communication and after play. Enquire regarding desire, arousal and orgasm Biological, psychological, interpersonal and cultural factors influencing the current sexual problem
Past sexual history: Development of sexuality of the individual from childhood to being an adult	Family attitude toward sex; family environment and parental attitudes affecting sexuality in childhood; obtaining information/misinformation about sex in childhood; childhood sex activities *Clarify regarding three components of sexual identity:* Gender identity, orientation and intention Adolescent sexual development-masturbation, experiences related to any sexual interaction. Adult sexual activities: premarital and post marriage (frequency of sexual interaction, first experience, masturbation, conflict with spouse) Sexual equilibrium
Other issues	Sexual abuse, chronic illness, paraphilic disorder, gender identity dysphoria, psychiatric history (anxiety, depression), substance abuse Expectations from treatment

Flow chart 2: Causes and management of sexual problems (Adopted from Elizabeth Stanley)

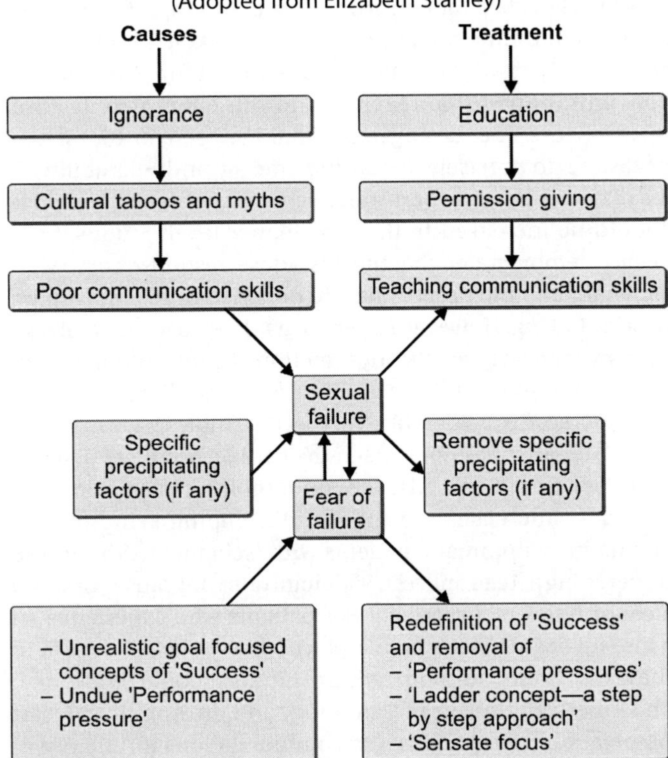

immediate symptoms and acted as a bridge between the traditional psychoanalytic and the more recent contemporary behavioral approaches. Here the therapist would move to the psychodynamic approaches only if the initial behavioral techniques did not produce symptom relief.

As elaborated by Masters and Johnson in 1970, sex therapy (dual sex therapy) ideally includes involvement of both the patient and the partner for satisfactory outcome. Information regarding anatomy and physiology of sexual function is explained and any myths or doubts are cleared through counseling the couple as a male-female pair of co-therapists. Therapy should emphasize that there is no use blaming one's partner or oneself, that sex is a mutual act between two individuals, and it is not something a man does to a woman or woman to a man. It can be a form of interpersonal communication at a highly intimate level; enhanced social communication benefits the relationship.[64] Educating the couple, improved communication, heightening sensory awareness, and sensate focus exercises are taught to the couple. Behavioral exercises include nondemand pleasuring or sensate focus, to allow the individual to re-experience pleasure without any pressure of performance or self-monitoring (spectatoring).

The assessment and treatment need to be tailored depending upon one's setting, profession, specialty and most important of all, the type of the problem encountered in the client, wherein different approaches may be helpful.

BEHAVIORAL TECHNIQUES

Sexual dysfunction is considered as a maladaptive behavior by behavioral therapists. Using a hierarchy of anxiety provoking sexual interactions the client systematically desensitized.

Different approaches include Masters and Johnson's approach, Kaplan's approach and the PLISSIT MODEL with some variations in the treatment process. Annon (1974) proposed a graded intervention popularly called as PLISSIT MODEL wherein the individual letters stand for: P: Permission giving, LI: Limited information, SS: Specific suggestion and IT: Intensive sex therapy.

Permission giving: In the first phase the client is assured that their thoughts, feelings, fantasies and behaviors are normal till they are not affecting the partner in a negative manner. In

'Limited Information' phase the client is given information related to his or her sexual problem. In 'Specific Suggestion' behavioral exercises like start-stop technique, 'sensate focus' are taught and home-work assignments are given. These help in improved communication between the couple and in learning new arousal behaviors. Intensive therapy is considered if the first three fail. Here insight oriented and psychosexual approaches are taken to make the client aware of their feelings.[65-68]

Sex therapy involves primarily Sensitization, desensitization techniques.[59] The general principles are applicable to majority of the inadequacies encountered in clinical practice. The major guide-lines to be followed are: (1) Educating the couple (2) Setting the framework for the therapy (3) Proscribe sex (4) Sensate focus exercises (5) Systematic sensitization and desensitization:

1. The couple is advised to talk on issues bothering them in a nonjudgmental way, encourage partners to see, hear and understand each other 's perception and teach verbal and nonverbal communication skills,[69] in general and during sexual activity in particular.
2. Inform ground rules of the therapy, dispel negative and sensational images of sex therapy and allow the couple to recognize and take responsibility for much of their treatment. The treatment has to be tailored towards the couple which acts as a marital unit, focusing in particular on the problems associated with the marital unit.[5]
3. To take off performance anxiety and pressure.
4. These are structured exercises, about 3–5 sessions assigned between the visits. Help couple recognize that sexual activity is not limited to sexual intercourse and that 'Pleasuring' and 'Receiving Pleasure' can be enjoyable without being regarded as foreplay or a preliminary to sexual intercourse. Slow progress from nondemanding pleasure, i.e. pleasing to explore one's own feelings about the experience from non-genital area to breasts and then to penile pleasuring.[70] Various stimulation methods are taught and the couple is advised to try different intercourse positions which may not necessarily lead to completion of sexual intercourse. One of these stimulation methods is, using fantasies for stimulation, to avoid obsessive concerns termed 'spectatoring'.[15]
5. 'Start-Stop Sensitization' technique used for premature ejaculation is one of the most common and useful techniques under this heading. Here one partner provides manual stimulation to the other and is stopped at a signal from him when orgasm becomes imminent. Repeating this activity for certain duration of time, leads to some degree of control over ejaculation. Further the partners are advised to should then try intra vaginal containment, usually in Female Superior Position. Partners should increase the rhythmic movements until the man gives the signal to stop. After a pause and they should repeat he act. With repeated attempts, the partners learn how to prolong the pleasure of intercourse while containing the urge to ejaculate.[71] Similar desensitizing and sensitizing techniques are utilized in treating psychogenic erectile and orgasmic dysfunctions in men and arousal and orgasmic dysfunctions in women. In women, with progressive stimulation of clitoral and other genital areas by partner, arousal is experienced without demand or pressure of intercourse.

PHARMACOTHERAPY FOR SEXUAL DYSFUNCTION

Nitric Oxide Enhancers

These drugs improve inflow of blood into the penis and improve erection. First drug developed in this class was **sildenafil citrate**. It acts on the nitric oxide mechanism by blocking PDE-5 (Phosphodiesterase-5) enzyme. It is the first approved non-surgical treatment for erectile dysfunction and was approved by US Food and Drug Administration (US-FDA) in 1998 for prescription sale. It is rapidly absorbed after oral administration and has to be taken 1 hour before sexual activity which is the time required for peak plasma concentrations to be reached and the effect may last for up to 4 hours. The starting dose should be used on atleast four occasions to precisely access the efficacy and tolerability. If a satisfactory sexual performance is not achieved, the dose should be increased to the next higher level. Studies have clearly demonstrated that there is a dose-response curve with sildenafil and the best results are obtained upto a maximum dose of 100 mg. However, sildenafil has been used as a salvage therapy for severe erectile dysfunction at a maximum dose of 200 mg, but the incidence of side effects and discontinuation rates increase considerably. Very recent studies have reported that sildenafil does not worsen the cardiac profile of patients with ischemic heart disease, undergoing stress exercises. Sildenafil increases the time to developing symptoms of angina in symptomatic patients with ischemic heart disease undergoing a treadmill test. Sildenafil does not cause coronary steal or reflex tachycardia.[72] For patients who experience an acute myocardial ischemia and who have taken sildenafil in the last 24 hours, administration of nitrates should be avoided. The American College of Cardiology and the American Heart Association have published recommendations for the use of sildenafil in patients with cardiac risk. Sildenafil should be used with caution in individuals maintained on multiple antihypertensive drugs.[73]

Adverse effects with sildenafil are dose dependent. Common adverse effects are headache (most common), flushing, rhinitis and visual disturbance changes in the perception of color, hue or brightness. The adverse effects are usually mild and transient, lasting a few minutes to a few hours after drug administration. It is contraindicated in patients on concurrent organic nitrates. This is because it potentiates the hypotensive action of such drugs through its effects on nitric oxide/c-GMP mechanisms.[73] It should be used with caution in persons with anatomical deformities of the penis (e.g. angulation, cavernosal fibrosis, peyronie's disease), and in patients at risk for priapism (e.g. patients with sickle cell anemia, multiple myeloma, leukemia, bleeding disorders, retinitis pigmentosa). Rare side effect reported is Nonarteritic Ischemic Optic Neuropathy (NAION).

Vardenafil is given in a dose of 5–20 mg. It has mild side effects like headache, dyspepsia, body aches, nausea, dizziness and increased muscle enzyme creatine kinase. Individuals with blood cell disorders like sickle cell anemia are at risk of developing priapism. It should not be taken by people taking nitrates, as it can cause severe hypotension. People with QT prolongation and those on alpha-blockers should avoid vardenafil.

Tadalafil has much longer duration of action (36 hours). The clearance is reduced in the elderly, in patients with severe renal insufficiency and in those with liver disease. It is effective irrespective of the etiology of the erectile dysfunction. Patients who have benefited are those who have had erectile dysfunction due to psychogenic causes, spinal cord injury, diabetes mellitus and prostate surgery. Patients also benefit irrespective of age or baseline severity of erectile dysfunction. The magnitude of the benefit however varies. This means it does not produce a magic erection; rather it improves the strength of the erection, the duration of the erection, and the number of occasions on which the erection is satisfactory.

Oral phentolamine and apomorphine are helpful as potency enhancers in minimal erectile dysfunction.[15] *Apomorphine* effects are mediated through the autonomic nervous system causing arterial vasodilation and has dopamine receptor stimulating effect.[74,75] Phentolamine decreases sympathetic stimulation and relaxes corporeal smooth muscle.[15]

Smooth muscle relaxants like papaverine, phentolamine, phenoxybenzamine are used in ICIVAD (Intracavernosal injection of vasoactive drugs) techniques for ED; Prostaglandin E (Alprostadil) through injection or through intraurethral insertion is an effective agent for ED.[15,76-78]

Nitric oxide beads injected into the penis have been shown to improve erectile function in animal studies and is likely to be studied on humans in near future.[79]

A topical cream containing three vasoactive agents: aminophylline, isosorbide dinitrate and co-dergocrine mesylate with or without alprostadil is helpful in ED. An alprostadil cream and vaginally applied phentolamine are helpful for female sexual arousal disorder.

Yohimbine is a central α-2 adrenoreceptor blocker and increases sympathetic drive. Its effectiveness is doubtful in ED.

Horny Goat weed (Epimedium) has been used as a traditional remedy for ED in China.

Trazodone, an antidepressant acts by inhibiting serotonin uptake and also by influencing α adrenergic and dopaminergic function. Results are inconsistent in erectile disorders.[80,81]

Table 7: Pharmacotherapeutic agents used in premature ejaculation

Oral therapies	*Recommended dose*
Tricyclic antidepressant Clomipramine	 25–50 mg/day or 25 mg 4–24 hours before intercourse
Selective Serotonin Reuptake Inhibitors (SSRIs) Fluoxetine Paroxetine Sertraline Dapoxetine	 5–20 mg/ day 10–40 mg/day or 20 mg 3–4 hours preintercourse 25–200 mg/day or 50 mg 4–8 hours before intercourse 30–60 mg 1–3 hours before intercourse
Topical therapies	Dose
Lidocaine/prilocaine cream	Lidocaine 2.5% 20–30 min pre-intercourse

Pharmacotherapy for premature ejaculation: These have been outlined in Table 7.[82]

Hormonal therapies: Testosterone is definitively effective only in case of hypogonadism. It can increase the desire but has no effect on erectile functioning. Female low sex drive and anorgasmia can be tried under careful monitoring.

Hormone Replacement Therapy (HRT) with estrogen in case of menopausal women as vaginal function, particularly lubrication is determined by them.

Hyperprolactinemia is treated by administration of dopaminergic drugs like bromocriptine.

Naltrexone, an opiate antagonist, can antagonize the inhibition of sexual functions.[83]

Aswagandha, Shathavari, Korean red ginseng are helpful in enhancing sexual functioning in both males and females.

Aswagandha (Indian ginseng) enhances sexual desire in men. *Shathavari* (*Asparagus racemosus*), a creeper which grows in low jungle areas throughout India is considered to be the women's equivalent to *Ashwagandha* and enhances female sexual functioning.

Some of the traditional herbal medicines used in medieval Persia, have been shown to be helpful in ED by relatively recent research. These include ginger (*Zingiber officinale*), almond (*Amygdalus communis*), spice commonly known as '*grains of paradise; melegueta pepper*' (*Aframomum melegueta*), and certain *brassica* species and seed of garden cress (*Lepidium spp*).[84-89] Saffron (30 mg/day) has been shown to improve sexual function (arousal, lubrication and pain domain) in females with SSRI induced sexual dysfunction.[90] Snacking on pistachio nuts, 100 g/day for 3 weeks, has been shown to improve erectile dysfunction.[91]

In some selected cases when psychotherapy, behavior techniques and drugs fail or seen to be not very effective, vacuum devises, injections and implants, vibrators are found to be relatively effective. Ultimately, the success of sex therapy depends on a host of factors. Therapy duration ranges from 6 weeks to more than a year in occasional cases. Sexual dysfunctions respond to treatment better compared to gender identify disorders and paraphilias, which are very resistant to therapy. More than half of the cases of erectile dysfunction and almost all the cases of premature ejaculation respond to combination of therapies.

Gender Identity Disorders

Gender identity refers to the expression of gender identify toward oneself and others.

Dual role transvestism: The subject wishes to lead a double role, spending part of his time as a male and part as a female.

Gender identity disorder of childhood: Is listed in ICD-10 while DSM-5 has used the term "Gender Dysphoria" (instead of Gender Identity Disorder used in DSM-IV) with different sets of criteria for children and adolescents/adults.[13] Individuals with gender dysphoria have a significant incongruence between the gender they have been assigned at birth (natal gender) and their expressed gender and there is a strong desire to be of the other gender or insistence that one belongs to the other gender.

Intersexuality: Develops where there was ambiguity at birth regarding child's external genitalia. Androgen sensitivity syndrome or congenital adrenal hyperplasia are the examples.

Sexual maturation disorder: Here the person suffers from uncertainty about his/her gender identity or sexual orientation which causes anxiety or depression.

Transexualism: It is a gender identity disorder characterized by a persistent belief to be of the opposite sex. A male transsexual believes that he will grow up to be woman and lose his genitals. A female transsexual tends to present masculine appearance and behavior. These individuals are characterized by behavior of cross dressing before the age of 4 years in 75% of the individuals. No specific factor has been established conclusively. Early upbringing, lack of proper parental identification etc. are the causes. Treatment involves psychotherapy, behavior modification, family therapy and in some selected cases sexual reassignment surgery.

Paraphilias (Sexual Deviations or Perversions)/ Paraphilic Disorders

The term 'paraphilia' is derived from the Greek words "para" which means next to and "philia" meaning love. DSM-5 describes term "paraphilia" as "any intense and persistent sexual interest other than sexual interest in genital stimulation or preparatory fondling with phenotypically normal, physically mature, consenting human partners".[13]

DSM-5 has further described Paraphilic Disorders as disorders based on (1) anomalous activity preferences further subdivided into (i) courtship disorders (voyeuristic disorder, exhibitionistic disorder and frotteuristic disorder) and (ii) algolagnic disorders which involve pain and suffering (sexual masochism disorder and sexual sadism disorder) (2) anomalous target preferences: (i) toward humans (pedophilic disorder) and (ii) directed elsewhere (fetishistic disorder and transvestic disorder).[13]

These are rare and occur mostly in men. They are characterized by recurrent intense sexual urges and sexually arousing fantasies generally involving either nonhuman objects, the suffering or humiliation of oneself or one's partner or children or other nonconsenting persons. For the paraphilic patient, the imagery is persistent, the fantasies evoked are necessary for erotic arousal, for the relief from non-erotic tension and for sexual excitement and orgasm. Many paraphilics feel no distress and represent an impairment in the capacity for reciprocal affectionate sexual activity. Though increased incidence of criminality is known with extra Y chromosome, no known genetic or biological factors have been implicated in its etiology. Only upbringing, problems in mother-child relationship etc. have been implicated. History of being sexually abused as children is common among these groups.

1. *Fetishism:* Sexual arousal is produced by nonliving objects such as women's clothing.
2. *Transvestism:* Must dress in women's clothes in order to become sexually aroused.
3. *Frotteurism:* Sexually arousing urges to touch or rub against a nonconsenting person, usually in a crowded setting where detection can be avoided. Common in men 15–25 years age.
4. *Pedophilia:* Sexual activity or fantasy involves prepubertal children of either sex.
5. *Exhibitionism:* Recurrent and intense sexual arousal from the exposure of one's genitals to unsuspecting persons either in fantasies causing significant distress or in behavior with a nonconsenting person; seen usually in psychologically immature men.
6. *Voyeurism:* Urges and fantasies about seeing unsuspecting people naked, in the act of disrobing or having sex, usually heterosexual in nature and is commonly referred as 'Peeping Tom'. It excludes watching pornography or normal sexual play in which individuals being watched

are willing. DSM-5 gives a minimum duration of 6 months for a diagnosis to be made. Voyeuristic acts are most common law breaking sexual behaviors.

7. *Masochism and Sadism:* Achievement of sexual pleasure and intense sexual arousal only through physical pain or suffering of self (masochism) or others (sadism).
8. *Bestiality or Zoophilia:* Sex with animals in the presence of other natural sexual outlets.
9. *Homosexuality:* is the sexual relationship between the persons of the same sex. It is no more considered a sexual deviation. This is a disorder when it is the dominant, significant and persistent mode of sexual relationship for that person and causes significant distress to the individual and is called ego-dystonic homosexuality. ICD-10 recognizes this as a category when sexual development and orientation are problematic to the individual. Five percent of all males and 2% of all female are reported to be homosexual. A whole spectrum of biological and social causes has been implicated in its causation.

The treatment of gender identity disorders and paraphilias are difficult and time consuming, often needs professional intervention. The basic guidelines are:

1. To decrease deviant sexual arousal
2. To develop heterosexual arousal
3. To develop skills or social interaction with members of the opposite sex
4. To provide training in assertiveness
5. To provide training in empathy
6. To attain sexual knowledge
7. To treat sexual dysfunction with the marital unit.

Freud's theory of sexuality has remained the basis of the psychoanalytic understanding of sexual deviance. During the 20th century psychoanalysis by Freud remained the main treatment option for sexual deviations. However, Freud also realized that perversions were due to a combination of biological and developmental factors.[92-94] The initial treatment approach of sexual deviations was formed in the late 19th century when in 1892 surgical castration was done for a patient with neuralgic pain of the testis with hypersexuality.[95] In the 20th century surgical castration remained the method of treatment for sex offenders, in United States and some European countries.[96] Surgical castration was legally reintroduced for sex offenders in certain US states in 1996 and thereafter.[97] Biological treatments include use of estrogens in 1940s (has feminizing side effects), luteinizing hormone releasing hormone (anti-libido medication which replaced estrogens in 1960s), cyproterone acetate (oral and depot) and medroxyprogesterone acetate (drug of choice in US). Other drugs which may have some beneficial effect include SSRIs, psychotrophic medications which reduce libido, thioridazine, clomipramine and lithium. Drugs as and when required depending upon the associated symptoms are helpful.

Cognitive behavior therapy (CBT): Core beliefs of an individual leads to formation of intermediate beliefs and conditional assumptions and then negative automatic thoughts. Associated cognitive errors may be systematic thinking errors, information processing biases, dichotomous or polarized thinking, and other cognitive errors like arbitrary inference, selective abstraction, emotional reasoning, disqualifying the positive, overgeneralization or catastrophization. Therapy begins with working on automatic thoughts and then dealing with distorted beliefs.

Relapse prevention techniques, like avoiding situations which generate unacceptable desires are helpful. In "covert sensitization" the undesirable sexual impulse is paired with an unpleasant stimulus. In orgasmic conditioning the patient is reconditioned to a more acceptable stimulus by, initially masturbating to his/her undesirable sexual impulse and concentrating on a more acceptable fantasy, just before orgasm.[98]

Social skills training is done simultaneously as many of these patients lack the ability to develop relationships. Sexual education, developing intimacy and how to converse with others is taught.

Twelve step programs similar to alcoholics anonymous which includes cognitive restructuring and social support to the patient and reliance on spiritual "higher power".[98] Group therapy is helpful to break through denial and help the patient in accepting his/her paraphilia.

DSM-5 Diagnostic and Statistical Manual of Mental Disorders 5th Edition[13]

Sexual Dysfunctions
302.74 (F52.32) Delayed Ejaculation
302.72 (F52.21) Erectile Disorder
302.73 (F52.31) Female Orgasmic Disorder
302.72 (F52.22) Female Sexual Interest/Arousal Disorder
302.76 (F52.6) Genito-Pelvic Pain/Penetration Disorder
302.71 (F52.0) Male Hypoactive Sexual Desire Disorder
302.75 (F52.4) Premature (Early) Ejaculation
___ (___)# Substance/ Medication induced Sexual Dysfunction
302.79 (F52.8) Other Specified Sexual Dysfunction
302.70 (F52.9) Unspecified Sexual Dysfunction

Gender Dysphoria
___ (___)# Gender Dysphoria
302.6 (F64.2) Gender Dysphoria in Children
302.85 (F64.1) Gender Dysphoria in Adolescents and Adults
302.6 (F64.8) Other Specified Gender Dysphoria
302.6 (F64.9) Unspecified Gender Dysphoria

Paraphilic Disorders
302.82 (F65.3) Voyeuristic Disorder
302.4 (F65.2) Exhibitionistic Disorder
302.89 (F65.81) Frotteuristic Disorder
302.83 (F65.51) Sexual Masochism Disorder
302.84 (F65.52) Sexual Sadism Disorder
302.2 (F65.4) Pedophilic Disorder
302.81 (F65.0) Fetishistic Disorder
302.3 (F65.1) Transvestic Disorder
302.89 (F65.89) Other Specified Paraphilic Disorder
302.9 (F65.9) Unspecified Paraphilic Disorder

Contd...

Contd...

#There are no corresponding DSM IV TR and ICD-10 codes.

ICD-10- WHO (World Health Organization) Classification[44]

F52: Sexual dysfunctions, not caused by organic disorder or disease

F52.0 Lack or loss of sexual drive
F52.1 Sexual aversion and lack of sexual enjoyment
F52.2 Failure of genital response
F52.3 Orgasmic dysfunction
F52.4 Premature ejaculation
F52.5 Non-organic vaginismus
F52.6 Non-organic dyspareunia
F52.7 Excessive sexual drive
F52.8 Other sexual dysfunctions not caused by organic disorders or disease.
F52.9 Unspecified sexual dysfunction, not caused by organic disorder or disease.

F64: Gender Identity Disorders

F65: Disorders of Sexual Preference (Includes Paraphilias)

F66: Psychological and behavioral disorders associated with sexual development and orientation

F66.0 Sexual maturation disorder
F66.1 Ego dystonic sexual orientation
F66.2 Sexual relationship disorder
F66.8 Other psychosexual development disorders
F66.9 Psychosexual development disorders-unspecified

REFERENCES

1. Georgiadis J, Holstege G. Human Brain activation during stimulation of the Penis. Journal of Comparative Neurology. 2005;493:33-8.
2. Hamann S, Herman R, Nolan C, Wallen K. Men, Women differ in amygdala response to visual sexual stimuli. Nature Neuroscience. 2004;7(4):325-6.
3. Zimmer C. The Brain: Where Does Sex Live in the Brain? From Top to Bottom. Discover Magazine October 2009 Issue.
4. Rowland D, McMahon CG, et al. Disorders of orgasm and ejaculation in men. The journal of sexual Medicine. 2010;7(2):1668-86.
5. Sadock BJ, Sadock VA. Human Sexuality. In: Kaplan and Sadock's Synopsis of Psychiatry: Behavioral Sciences/Clinical Psychiatry. 10th Edition. Lippincott Williams & Wilkins 2007;21:680-717.
6. McMahon CG, Abdo C, Incrocci L, et al. Disorders of orgasm and ejaculation in men. J Sex Med. 2004;1:58-65.
7. Waldinger MD. The neurobiological approach to premature ejaculation. J Urol. 2002;168:2359-67.
8. Waldinger MD, Olivier B. Animal models of premature and retarded ejaculation. World J Urol. 2005;23:115-8.
9. Masters WH, Johnson VE. Human sexual response. Little, Brown, Boston, MA. 1966.
10. Kaplan H. Disorders of sexual desire. Simon and Schuster New York; 1979.
11. Robinson P. The modernization of sex. Cornell University Press, Ithaca, NY; 1976.
12. Prakash O, Rao TSS. Sexuality research in India: An update. Indian J Psychiatry. 2010;52 (Suppl 1):S260-3.
13. Diagnostic and Statistical Manual of Mental Disorders: DSM-5. American Psychiatric Publishing Washington DC 2013; 5th edition. 423-460,685-706.
14. Levine SB. Sexual Disorders. In: Tasman A, Kay J, Lieberman JA (Eds). Psychiatry. 2nd edition. John Wiley and Sons Ltd. 2003;1471-1500.
15. Sadock VA. Normal Human Sexuality and Sexual Dysfunctions. In: Sadock BJ, Sadock VA, Ruiz P (Eds). Kaplan and Sadock's Comprehensive Textbook of Psychiatry, 9th edition. Lippincott Williams and Wilkins 2009;18.1a:2027-59.
16. Masters WH, Johnson V. Human Sexual Inadequecy. Churchill, London 1970.
17. Laumann EO, Gagnon JH, Michael RT, Michael S. The social organization of sexuality: sexual practices in the United States. Chicago: University of Chicago Press 1994.
18. Fugl-Meyer KS, Lewis RW, Bosch R. Definitions, classification, and epidemiology of sexual dysfunction. In: Lue T, Giuliano F, Khoury S, Montorsi F, Rosen R (Eds). Sexual medicine volume 1: sexual dysfunction in men health publications. United Kingdom 2004:1-36.
19. Rao TSS, Darshan MS. Sexual disorders among elderly. An epidemiological study in South Indian rural population. Indian Association of Social Psychiatry: Dr GC Boral Award [In Press]
20. Rao TSS, Rao SV, Marutham P, Anand MS, Guph MR, Chandrashekhar BM. A study of sexual concerns in the general population. Sexuality in new millennium. 14th World Congress of Sexology. Editrice Compositeri, Italy 2000:89-91.
21. Rao TSS, Rao VS Arif M, Rajendra PN. Sexual problems in medical practice: a study on its prevalence in an out patient setting. Indian Journal of Psychiatry 1997;39(Suppl):53.
22. Rao TSS, Rao VS, Guptha AR, et al. A study on desire disorders in women. Indian Journal of Psychiatry 2003;45(Suppl):86.
23. Kendurkar A, Kaur B, Agarwal AK, Singh H, Agarwal V. Profile of adult patients attending a marriage and sex clinic in India. Int J Soc Psychiatry. 2008;54:486-93.
24. Singh JC, Tharyan P, Kekre NS, Singh G, Gopalkrishnan G. Prevalence and risk factors for female sexual dysfunction in women attending a medical clinic in South India. J Postgrad Med. 2009;55:113-20.
25. Butcher J. ABC of sexual health Female sexual problems I: Loss of desire—what about the fun? BMJ. 1999;318:41-3.
26. Butcher J. ABC of sexual health Female sexual problems II: Sexual pain and sexual fears Josie Butcher. BMJ. 1999;318:110-2.
27. Fazio L, Brock G. Erectile dysfunction: management update. CMAJ. 2004;170:1429-37.
28. Levine LA, Kloner RA. Importance of asking questions about erectile dysfunction. Am J Cardiol. 2000;86:1210-13.
29. Levine LA. Diagnosis and Treatment of Erectile Dysfunction. Am J Med. 2000;109:3S-12S.
30. Ralph D, McNicholas T. UK management guidelines for erectile dysfunction. BMJ. 2000;321:499-503.
31. Swerdloff RS, Kandeel FR. In: Textbook of Internal Medicine, Lippincott Co. 1992.

32. Crenshaw TL, Goldberg TL. Sexual Pharmacology. Drug that affect sexual functioning. W W Norton and Company. New York. 1996.
33. Cutler AJ. Sexual dysfunction and antipsychotic treatment. Psychoneuroendocrinology. 2003;28(Suppl 1):69-82.
34. Ucok AL, Gaebel W. Side effects of atypical antipsychotics:a brief overview. World Psychiatry. 2008;7(1):58-62.
35. Mahmoud A, Hayhurst KP, Drake RJ, Lewis SW. Second generation antipsychotics improve sexual dysfunction in schizophrenia: A randomized controlled trial. Schizophrenia Research and Treatment 2011; Article ID 596898, 6 pages http://dx.doi.org/10.1155/2011/596898
36. Kennedy SH, Dickens SE, Eisfeld BS, Bagby RM. Sexual dysfunction before antidepressant therapy in major depression. J Affect Disord. 1999;56:201-8.
37. Clayton AH, Pradko JF, Croft HA, et al. Prevalence of sexual dysfunction among newer antidepressants. J Clin Psychiatry. 2002;63:357-66.
38. Ferguson JM. The effects of antidepressants on sexual functioning in depressed patients: a review. J Clin Psychiatry 2001;62(Suppl 3):22-34.
39. Rosen RC, Lane RM, Menza M. Effects of SSRIs on sexual function: a critical review. J Clin Psychopharmacol. 1999;19:67-85.
40. Montejo-Gonzalez AL, Llorca G, Izquierdo JA, et al. SSRI-induced sexual dysfunction: fluoxetine, paroxetine, sertraline, and fluvoxamine in a prospective, multicenter, and descriptive clinical study of 344 patients. J Sex Marital Ther. 1997;23:176-94.
41. Ashton AK, Rosen RC. Accommodation to serotonin reuptake inhibitor-induced sexual dysfunction. J Sex Marital Ther 1998;24:191-2.
42. Rothschild AJ. Selective serotonin reuptake inhibitor-induced sexual dysfunction: efficacy of a drug holiday. Am J Psychiatry 1995;152:1514-6.
43. Brannon SK, Detke MJ, Wang F, Mallinckrodt CH, Tran PV, Delgado PL. Comparison of sexual functioning in patients receiving duloxetine or paroxetine: acute and long-term data. Program and abstracts of the American Psychiatric Association 156th Annual Meeting; 17-22, 2003; San Francisco, California. Abstract NR477.
44. Vester-Blokland ED, Van der Flier S. Sexual functioning of patients with major depression treated with mirtazapine orally disintegrating tablet or sertraline. Program and abstracts of the American Psychiatric Association 156th Annual Meeting; San Francisco, California. Abstract NR494; 2003. pp.17-22.
45. Fabre LF, Clayton AH, Smith LC, Goldstein I, Derogatis LR. The effect of gepirone-ER in the treatment of sexual dysfunction in depressed men. J Sex Med. 2012;9(3):821-9.
46. Fabre LF, Brown CS, Smith LC, Derogatis LR. Gepirone-ER treatment of hypoactive sexual desire disorder (HSDD) associated with depression in women. J Sex Med. 2011;8(5): 1411-9. doi: 10.1111/j.1743-6109.2011.02216.x. Epub 2011.
47. Kavoussi RJ, Segraves RT, Hughes AR, Ascher JA, Johnston JA. Double-blind comparison of bupropion sustained release and sertraline in depressed outpatients. J Clin Psychiatry. 1997;58:532-7.
48. Gelenberg AJ, McGahuey C, Laukes C, et al. Mirtazapine substitution in SSRI-induced sexual dysfunction. J Clin Psychiatry. 2000;61:356-60.
49. Sovner R. Treatment of tricyclic antidepressant induced orgasmic inhibition with cyprohepatidine. Journal of Clinical Psychopharmacology. 1984;4:169.
50. Pontius EB. Case report of an anticholinergic crisis associated with cyproheptadine treatment of desipramine induced anorgasmia. Journal of Clinical Psychopharmacology. 1988;8:230.
51. Chadda RK. Dhat syndromes: is it a distinct clinical entity? A study of illness behaviour characteristics. Acta Psychiatr Scand. 1995;91:136-9.
52. Behere PB, Natraj GS. Dhat syndrome: the phenomenology of a culture bound sex neurosis of the orient. Indian Journal of Psychiatry. 1984;26:76-8.
53. Gregoire A. ABC of sexual health: assessing and managing male sexual problems. BMJ. 1999;318:315-7.
54. American Urological Association. Premature ejaculation. Guidelines for pharmacological management of premature ejaculation; 2003.
55. American Urological Association. Guidelines for pharmacological management of premature ejaculation 2004.
56. Bhatia MS, Malik SC. Dhat syndrome—a useful diagnostic entity in Indian culture. Br JPsychiatry 1991;159:691-5.
57. Friedman CR. Reproductive psychiatry and sexuality. In: Kupfer DJ, Horner MS, et al. (Eds). Thase ME, Travis MJ, Semple D, Smyth R, Burns J, Darjee R, McIntosh A (Eds). Oxford American Handbook of Psychiatry. Oxford University Press. 2008. pp. 493-532.
58. Levine SB. Sexuality in mid-life. New York: Plenum; 1998.
59. Hengeveld MW. Erectile disorder: A psychosexological review. In: Jonas U, Thon WF, Stief CG (Eds). Erectile dysfunction. Berlin: Springer-Verlag 1991. pp.14-22.
60. Feldman HA, Goldstein I, Hatzichristou DG, Krane RJ, McKinlay JB. Impotence and its medical and psychosocial correlates: results of the Massachusetts Male Aging Study. J Urol. 1994;151:54-61.
61. Avasthi A, Rao TSS, Grover S, Biswas P, Kumar S. Clinical practice guidelines for management of sexual dysfuntions. In: Gautham S, Avasthi A. Clinical practice guidelines for management of substance abuse disorders, sexual dysfunctions and sleep disorders editors. Published by Indian Psychiatric Society, 2006. pp. 144-32.
62. Hawton K. Sexual dysfunctions. In: Cognitive Behaviour Therapy for Psychiatric Problems. A Practical Guide (Eds: K Hawton, P M Salkovskis, J Kirk, D M Clerk). Oxford University Press, New York; 1989.
63. Tiefer L, Schuetz-Mueller D. Psychological issues in diagnosis and treatement of erectile disorders. Psy Clin North Am. 1995; 22:767-73.
64. Avasthi A, Banerjee ST. Guidebook on sex education. Marital and Psychosexual Clinic, Department of Psychiatry, PGIMER, Chandigarh, 2002.

65. Hogan, Douglas R. The effectiveness of sex therapy: A review of literature. In: LoPicolo Joseph and LoPicolo Leslie (Eds). Handbook of sex therapy. New York: Plenum Press; 1978. pp. 57-84.
66. Annon, Jack S. The behavioral treatment of sexual problems: Brief Therapy New York Harper & Row 1976.
67. Kaplan HS. The new sex therapy: Active treatment of sexual dysfunctions. New York: Brunner/Mazel 1974.
68. Hawton K. The behavioral treatment of sexual dysfunction. British J Psychiatry. 1982;140:94-101.
69. Meuleman EJ, Diemont WL. Investigation of erectile dysfunction. Diagnostic testing for vascular factors in erectile dysfunction. Urol Clin North Am. 1995;22:803-19.
70. American Urological Association. Erectile Dysfunction Clinical Guidelines Panel. Treatment of Organic Clinical Practice Guidelines; 1996.
71. Guiliano F, Jardin A, Gingell CJ. Sildenafil (VIAGRA), an oral treatment for erectile dysfunction: a 1-year, open label extension study. British Journal of Urology; 1997;80:93.
72. Fox KM, Thadani U, Patrick TS, et al. Sildenafil citrate does not reduce exercise tolerance in men with erectile dysfunction and chronic stable angina. Eur Heart J. 2003;24(24):2206-12.
73. Cheitlin MD, Hutter AM, Brindis RG, et al. Use of Sildenafil in patients with Cardiovascular Disease(ACC/AHA Expert Consensus Document) Circulation. 1999;99:168-77. Available at: *http://circ.ahajournals.org/content/99/1/168.full*
74. Van Ahlen H, Piechota HJ, Kias HJ, Brennemann W, Klingmuller D. Opiate antagonistsin erectile dysfunction: a possible new treatmentoption? Results of a pilot study with Naltrexone. European Urology. 1995;28:246-50.
75. Padma-Nathan H. Efficacy and tolerability of Tadalafil, a novel phosphodiesterase 5 inhibitor in treatment of erectile dysfunction. American Journal of Cardiology. 2003; 92:19M-25M.
76. Bella AJ, Brock GB. Intracavernous Pharmacotherapy for erectile dysfunction. Endocrine. 2004;23:149-55.
77. Fink HA, MacDonald R, Rutks IR, Wilt TJ. Trazodone for erectile dysfunction: a systemic review and meta-analysis. British Journal of Urology International. 2003;92:441-6.
78. World Health Organization. ICD-10 classification of mental and behavioural disorders: Diagnostic criteria for Research. World health organization, Geneva; 1993.
79. Soni S, Song S, West J, Khera M. Nitric Oxide-Releasing Polymeric Microspheres Improve Diabetes-Related Erectile Dysfunction. Journal of Sexual Medicine; 2013.
80. Costa P. Multidimensional nature of Apomorphine SL (Ixense) therapy. International Journal of Impotence Research 2003;15(Supp 2):S13-S15.
81. Dula E, Keating W, Siami RF, et al. Efficacy and safety of fixed-dose and dose optimization regimens of sublingual Apomorphine versus placebo in men with erectile dysfunction. The Apomorphine Study Group. Urology. 2000;56:130-5.
82. Chen J, Mabjeesh NJ, Matkzin H, Greenstein A. Efficacy of sildenafil as adjuvant therapy to selective serotonin reuptake inhibitor in alleviating premature ejaculation. Urology. 2003;61:197-200.
83. Linet OI, Ogrinc FG. Efficacy and safety of intracavernosal alprostadil in men with erectile dysfunction. The Alprostadil Study Group, New England Journal of Medicine. 1996;334:873-7.
84. Ghadiri MK, Gorji A. Review of Impotence: Natural remedies for impotence in medieval Persia. International Journal of Impotence Research. 2004;16:80-3.
85. Shelly TE, McInnis DO. Exposure to ginger root oil enhances mating success of irradiated, mass-reared males of Mediterranean fruit fly (Diptera: Tephritidae). J Econ Entomol 2001;94:1413-8.
86. Qureshi S, Shah AH, Tariq M, Ageel AM. Studies on herbal aphrodisiacs used in Arab system of medicine. Am J Chin Med. 1989;17:57-63.
87. Kamtchouing P, et al. Effects of Aframomum melegueta and Piper guineenseon sexual behaviour of male rats. Behav Pharmacol. 2002;13:243-7.
88. Gonzales GF et al. Effect of Lepidium meyenii (Maca), a root with aphrodisiac and fertility-enhancing properties, on serum reproductive hormone levels in adult healthy men. J Endocrinol 2003;176:163-8.
89. Zheng BL, et al. Effect of a lipidic extract from Lepidium meyenii on sexual behavior in mice and rats. Urology. 2000;55:598-602.
90. Kashani L, Raisi F, Saroukhani S, et al. Saffron for treatment of fluoxetine-induced sexual dysfunction in women: Randomized double-blind placebo-controlled study. Hum Psychopharmacol Clin Exp. 2012;28(1):54-60.
91. Aldemir M, Okulu E, Neselioglu S, Erel O, Kayigil O. Pistachio diet improves erectile function parameters and serum lipid profiles in patients with erectile dysfunction. Int J Impot Res. 2011;23(1):32-8.
92. Freud S. Three essays on the theory of sexuality. In: Complete psychological works of Sigmund Freud. Standard Edition. Vol. 7. London: Hogarth Press 1905/1953.
93. Rosen I. Sexual deviation. 3rd ed. Oxford: Oxford University Press 1997.
94. Thibaut F, La Barra FD, Gordon H, Cosyns P, Bradford JMW and the WFSBP Task Force on Sexual Disorders. GUIDELINES: The World Federation of Societies of Biological Psychiatry (WFSBP): Guidelines for the biological treatment of paraphilias. The World Journal of Biological Psychiatry. 2010;11:604-55.
95. Sturup GK. Castration: the total treatment. Int Psychiatry Clin. 1972;8:175-95.
96. Bremer J. Asexualization: a follow-up study of 244 cases. New York: MacMillan Co, 1959.
97. Weinberger LE, Sreenivasan S, Garrick T, Osran H. The impact of surgical castration on sexual recidivism risk among sexually violent predatory offenders. J Am Acad Psychiatry Law. 2005;33:16-36.
98. Krueger RB, Kaplan MS. Behavioral and psychopharmacological treatment of the paraphilic and hypersexual disorders. J Psychiatr Pract. 2002;8(1):21-32.

CHAPTER 26

Sleep Disorders

RK Solanki, Nikhil Jain

Sleep is one of the cardinal symptoms in psychiatry and indeed in medicine as a whole. A good knowledge about the various aspects of sleep is essential for every student of psychiatry.

Normal sleep: Behaviorally, sleep is a reversible state of reduced awareness of and responsiveness to the environment. Sleep is postulated to serve many functions:[1]

- Physical and psychological restoration and recovery,
- Energy conservation,
- Memory consolidation,
- Discharge of emotions,
- Brain growth, and other various biological functions including maintenance of immune systems.

Micro-structure of sleep and memory consolidation: Recent literature suggests the importance of the first half of the night for declarative memory consolidation originates from sleep spindles and slow electroencephalogram (EEG) oscillations. These distinct polysomnographic phenomena characterizing sleep microstructure show a decrease as aging progresses.[2]

Based on physiological parameters observed on EEG, electro-oculogram (EOG) and electromyogram (EMG), sleep has been classified in Rapid eye movement (REM) and non-rapid eye movement (NREM) sleep.[3] Continuous recording of the above mentioned electro-physiologic parameters is called polysomnography.

NREM sleep: It is divided into four stages of increasing depth.

- Stage I occurs at sleep onset or following arousal from another stage of sleep. The EEG is low voltage with mixed frequencies and reduced alpha activity compared with the awake state. Vertex sharp waves are seen in the EEG and slow rolling eye movements occur. This stage represents 4–5% of the main sleep period.
- Stage II contains more slow activity, and sleep spindles and K complexes are seen. It accounts for 45–55% of overnight sleep.
- Stage III (4–6% of total sleep time) contains yet more slow EEG activity.
- Stage IV is characterized by the slowest activity and constitutes 12–15% of sleep.

The combination of Stages III and IV is called slow-wave sleep (SWS) or delta sleep. This is considered to be the deepest form of sleep from which awakening is particularly difficult. The arousal disorders (confusional arousals, sleep walking, and sleep terrors) arise from SWS.

REM sleep: It is also called paradoxical sleep because brain metabolism is highest in this stage of sleep.

- There is a low voltage, mixed frequency, non-alpha EEG
- Spontaneous rapid eye movements are seen
- Electromyogram activity is virtually absent
- Heart rate, blood pressure, and respiration are all variable
- Body temperature regulation ceases temporarily
- Penile and clitoral tumescence occurs.

REM sleep usually takes up 20–25% of total sleep time. Most dreams, including nightmares, occur in REM sleep.

Sleep architecture: Sleep cycles consisting of about 80 minutes of NREM sleep followed by about 10 minutes of REM sleep are repeated 3–6 times every night. As the night progresses, the duration of REM sleep increases. The timing of sleep is regulated by a circadian 'clock' in the suprachiasmatic nucleus of the hypothalamus. Without an environmental cue to time of day, the duration of the endogenous 'free running' sleep–wake cycle in humans has generally been considered to be about 25 hours. From an early age the individual's sleep–wake rhythm has to synchronize with the 24-hour day-night rhythm. The main environmental cues by which this is achieved ('entrainment') is sunlight, but social cues, such as meal times and social activities, are also important, as well as ambient temperature or noise level, and internal body signals such as hunger, temperature, and hormonal changes.

Changes in the sleep pattern occur with change in age. In essence, with advancing age, the total sleep time and the time spent in NREM sleep decreases.

ASSESSMENT OF SLEEP PROBLEMS[4,5]

Sleep History

Routinely, all patients should be asked the following screening questions.
- Do you sleep long enough or well enough?
- Are you very sleepy during the day?
- Is your sleep disturbed at night?

Ideally, the history should be corroborated by the bed partner.

If the answer to any of these enquiries is positive, a detailed sleep history is required covering the following points about the sleep problem:
- Precise nature of the sleep complaint, its onset, development, and current patterns
- Medical or psychological factors initiating or maintaining the sleep problem
- Patterns of occurrence of the symptoms—aggravating or relieving factors, week-days compared with weekends, or work compared with holiday periods
- Effects on mood, work and social life
- Past and present treatments for sleep problems and their effects
- Past and present medication or other treatments for other illness or disorder.

Breathing difficulties and nocturia should receive special attention amongst medical complaints for obvious reasons. Past treatment history for medical and psychiatric illness should also be enquired.

Sleep Diary

Maintenance of a systematic recording using a standardized format of daily sleep pattern avoids the bias or distortion of retrospective generalizations. It is generally maintained for a period of 2 weeks.

Times of going to bed, getting to sleep, awake periods during the night, final awakening, and getting up are recorded. Estimates of total sleep time, sleep efficiency (proportion of time in bed the patient is actually asleep), and number of awakenings are made from the recorded data.

The occurrence and nature of night-time episodes of disturbed Behavior, daytime events including sleepiness can also be recorded.

Previously unrecognized patterns of occurrence of these sleep phenomena may become apparent including temporal patterns, shift of the sleep phase, or relationships to stressful events or other factors.

Videography and actigraphy: Video recordings can be very useful in the parasomnias, sometimes revealing a very different clinical picture than that provided in the clinic. Video recording using mobile phone systems can be useful alternative where admission to hospital is not feasible. Similarly, monitoring of body movements by means of wrist-watch-like devices (actigraphy) can be used at home, if necessary.

Polysomnography

Physiological sleep studies are necessary for diagnosis in only the minority of sleep disorders. A new addition in this field is the development of home based polysomnography.

Basic polysomnography comprises of the recording of an EEG, an EOG, and an electromyogram. Basic measures obtained from this information are as follows:
- *Sleep continuity:* Total time in bed (TIB); total sleep time (TST); total time awake; number of awakenings; sleep efficiency (TIB/TST × 100).
- *NREM measures:* Actual and percentage time in Stages I–IV; total SWS.
- *REM measures:* REM latency; actual and percentage time in REM sleep; total REM sleep.

Polysomnography can be supplemented by studying respiratory variables, use of additional EEG channels (to rule out epilepsy), EMG of anterior tibialis (to rule out PLMS)

Recently, analysis of heart rate variability during sleep is emerging as important clinical and prognostic markers of autonomic cardiovascular control.

Multiple sleep latency test (MLST): The multiple sleep latency test uses basic polysomnography variables to quantify the degree of daytime sleepiness by measuring the time a patient takes to fall asleep during five opportunities to do so during the day. In adults a mean sleep latency of 5 minutes or less indicates pathological sleepiness (usually of organic origin); 5–10 minutes is a gray area which usually includes excessive sleepiness associated with primary psychiatric disorder; while longer than 10 minutes is normal. These values do not apply to children, whose sleep tendency varies with age.

GENERAL APPROACH TO THE MANAGEMENT OF SLEEP DISORDERS[6,7]

Educating the patient about the problem and dispelling myths goes a long way in the management of sleep disorders. Encouraging good sleep hygiene is very important. The principles of sleep hygiene are enlisted below:

Sleep Hygiene

- Control of environmental factors (noise, light, temperature)
- Use of distractions from the day's stresses (reading, watching television, listening to music, having a warm bath)
- Avoidance of caffeine-containing drinks after about 4 pm
- Not smoking at least for an hour before bed

- Regular exercise (not late at night)
- Warm milk at bedtime
- Avoidance of naps during the day
- Learning to set aside a time during the day to reflect on problems and stresses
- Go to bed only when sleepy
- Avoid other activities (with the exception of sex) whilst in bed
- If sleep does not occur, do not remain in bed for more than 10 to 20 minutes, get up and go to another room (without turning on all the lights), returning to bed only when sleepy
- Establish a regular time to get up, with no more than 1 hour's variation (even at weekends and during holidays).

If possible, the treatment of underlying cause should be treated.

Provision of safe sleeping environment, in case of parasomniaa should be attempted.

Behavioral approaches for insomnia include:

- Positive association
- Modification of inappropriate Behavior
- Sleep consolidation.

Chronobiological approaches:

- Light therapy
- Sleep phase rescheduling.

Medications: These are highly overused in practise and should be used with caution. They should only be used to treat insomnia when it is severe, disabling, or subjecting the individual to extreme distress. Ideally hypnotics should be used as short-term adjuncts to other forms of therapy and prolonged administration should be avoided. Choices include: benzodiazepines, zopiclone/zolpidem, chloral hydrate, and sedating antidepressants (e.g. trazodone).

Melatonin is often used in sleep disturbances associated with circadian rhythm disturbances. Stimulants are used in hypersomnia conditions.

SLEEP DISORDERS

Based on the international classification of sleep disorders (revised), 1997;[8] sleep disorders can be broadly classified into:

1. Dyssomnias: (a) extrinsic sleep disorders, (b) intrinsic sleep disorders, (c) circadian rhythm sleep disorders
2. Parasomnias: (a) arousal disorder, (b) sleep-wake transition disorder, (c) parasomnia associated with REM sleep
3. Sleep disorders associated with mental, neurological or other medical disorders.

Dyssomnia

Insomnia-persistent problems (at least 3 days/weeks for 1 month) falling asleep, maintaining sleep, or poor quality of sleep qualifies as clinically important insomnia. Individuals are often preoccupied and excessively concerned with their sleep problems, distressed by them, and social or occupational functioning is affected.[9] The causes of insomnia may be classified as follows:

Intrinsic

- *Psychophysiological insomnia:* A Behavioral disorder in which patients are preoccupied with a perceived inability to sleep adequately at night. Such patients become hyperaroused by their own efforts to sleep or by the sleep environment, and the insomnia becomes a conditioned or learned response. Patients may be able to fall asleep more easily at unscheduled times (when not trying) or outside the home environment. Sleep hygiene and correction of counter-productive hyper-arousal Behavior correction forms the mainstay of treatment.
- *Sleep apnea:* Respiratory dysfunction during sleep is a common, serious cause of excessive daytime somnolence as well as of disturbed nocturnal sleep. Episodes of cessation/reduction of breathing lasting 10 to 50 seconds occur many times in the night. These episodes may be due to either an occlusion of the airway (obstructive sleep apnea), absence of respiratory effort (central sleep apnea), or a combination of these factors (mixed sleep apnea). Failure to recognize and treat these conditions appropriately may lead to impairment of daytime alertness, increased risk of sleep-related motor vehicle accidents, hypertension and other serious cardiovascular complications, and increased mortality.[10] Sleep apnea is particularly prevalent in overweight men and in the elderly, yet it is estimated to remain undiagnosed in 80–90% of affected individuals. Management includes continuous positive airways pressure (CPAP), bi-level positive airways pressure (BiPAP) or corrective surgery like nasal reconstruction, tonsillectomy, etc.
- *Periodic limb movement disorder:* It consists of periodic episodes of repetitive, stereotyped limb movements. It may be a feature in up to 15% of patients with insomnia. Movements are usually reported by the bed partner. It is associated with daytime somnolence. Polysomnography may aid diagnosis. Treatment consists of reassurance and judicious use of hypnotics.
- *Restless leg syndrome:* It is associated with unpleasant, often painful sensations in the legs, particularly on sleep onset, which significantly interfere with the ability to get to sleep.[11] It is usually idiopathic or familial. The condition is exacerbated by caffeine, fatigue, or stress.

This condition is associated with periodic limb movement syndrome, pregnancy, uraemia, rheumatoid arthritis, iron deficiency anemia, folate deficiency, hypothyroidism, poliomyelitis, peripheral neuropathy (e.g. diabetes), chronic myelopathy, Parkinson's disease, drug-related (e.g. antidepressants; phenothiazines; lithium; calcium channel blockers; withdrawal from barbiturates, other sedatives and opiates).

Management consists of: General movement (walking, stamping) or stimulation of the legs (rubbing, squeezing, hot showers, hot packs, ointments). The symptoms of Restless leg syndrome respond well to dopaminergic drugs (e.g. pramipexole 0.25–0.5 mg q8PM or ropinirole 0.5–4 mg q8PM), which are the treatments of choice.

Extrinsic

- *Inadequate sleep hygiene:* Clinically significant disruption of the normal sleep-wake schedule can occur due to a wide range of daily living activities (e.g. level of coffee consumption, frequent late nights). This disruption is inconsistent with the maintenance of good quality sleep and full daytime alertness.
- *Management:* Understand the contribution of each factor and take steps to eliminate or minimize their effects.
- *Adjustment disorder:* sleep is often disrupted in adjustment disorder. A stressor can often be identified.
- *Substance abuse:* a wide range of psychoactive substances can cause sleep disturbances.
- Others include altitude insomnia, environmental insomnia, food allergy insomnia, etc.

Circadian Rhythm Sleep Disorders

A subset of patients presenting with either insomnia or hypersomnia may have a disorder of sleep timing rather than sleep generation. The symptoms reflect the influence of the underlying circadian pacemaker on sleep-wake function. Thus, effective therapeutic approaches should aim to entrain the oscillator at an appropriate phase.[12]

- *Jet lag disorder:* Trans-meridian air travel is often associated with excessive daytime sleepiness, sleep onset insomnia, and frequent arousals from sleep, particularly in the latter half of the night. Gastrointestinal discomfort is common. The syndrome is transient, typically lasting 2–14 days depending on the number of time zones crossed, the direction of travel, and the traveller's age and phase-shifting capacity. Travellers who spend more time outdoors reportedly adapt more quickly than those who remain in rooms, presumably due to brighter light exposure. Avoidance of antecedent sleep loss and obtaining nap sleep on the afternoon prior to overnight travel greatly reduce the difficulty of extended wakefulness. Laboratory studies suggest that sub milligram doses of the pineal hormonemelatonin can enhance sleep efficiency, but only if taken when endogenous melatonin concentrations are low (i.e. during biologic daytime), and that melatonin may induce phase shifts in human rhythms.
- In addition to jet lag associated with travel across time zones, many patients report a behavioral pattern that has been termed social jet lag, in which their bedtimes and wake times on weekends or days off occur 4–8 hours later than they do during the week. This recurrent displacement of the timing of the sleep-wake cycle is common in adolescents and young adults and is associated with sleep onset insomnia, poorer academic performance, increased risk of depressive symptoms, and excessive daytime sleepiness.
- *Shift-work disorder (SWD):*[13,14] Shift work involving work at various times in the night and day is increasingly common in the modern society. This results in both sleep loss and misalignment of the circadian rhythm with respect to the sleep-wake cycle. Sleep deprivation, increased length of time awake prior to work, and misalignment of circadian phase produce decreased alertness and performance, increased reaction time, and increased risk of performance lapses, thereby resulting in greater safety hazards among night workers and other sleep-deprived individuals. Sleep disturbance nearly doubles the risk of a fatal work accident. Additional problems include higher rates of breast, colorectal, and prostate cancer and of cardiac, gastrointestinal, and reproductive disorders in long-term night-shift workers. Recently, the World Health Organization has added night-shift work to its list of probable carcinogens.

From 5–10% of individuals scheduled to work at night or in the early morning hours have much greater than average difficulties remaining awake during night work and sleeping during the day; these individuals are diagnosed with chronic and severe SWD. Patients with this disorder have a level of excessive sleepiness during night work and insomnia during day sleep that the physician judges to be clinically significant; the condition is associated with an increased risk of sleep-related accidents and with some of the illnesses associated with night-shift work. Patients with chronic and severe SWD are profoundly sleepy at night. In fact, their sleep latencies during night work average just 2 minutes, comparable to mean sleep latency durations of patients with narcolepsy or severe daytime sleep apnea.

Management: Caffeine is frequently used to promote wakefulness, but its efficacy in the disorder is dubious. Postural changes, exercise, and strategic placement of nap opportunities can sometimes temporarily reduce the risk of fatigue-related performance lapses. Properly timed exposure to bright light can facilitate rapid adaptation to night-shift work.

While many techniques (e.g. light treatment) used to facilitate adaptation to night-shift work may help patients with this disorder, modafinil is the only therapeutic intervention that has ever been evaluated as a treatment for this specific patient population.

General measures include education and designing the shifts in such a way that: (1) exposure to night work,

(2) the frequency of shift rotation so that shifts do not rotate more than once every 2–3 weeks, (3) the number of consecutive night shifts, and (4) the duration of night shifts are minimized. Adequate rest should be ensured between shifts.

- *Delayed sleep phase disorder:* It is characterized by (1) reported sleep onset and wake times intractably later than desired, (2) actual sleep times at nearly the same clock hours daily, and (3) essentially normal all-night polysomnography except for delayed sleep onset. Patients exhibit an abnormally delayed endogenous circadian phase, with the temperature minimum during the constant routine occurring later than normal. This delayed phase could be due to (1) an abnormally long, genetically determined intrinsic period of the endogenous circadian pacemaker; (2) an abnormally reduced phase-advancing capacity of the pacemaker; (3) a slower rate of buildup of homeostatic sleep drive during wakefulness; or (4) an irregular prior sleep-wake schedule, characterized by frequent nights when the patient chooses to remain awake well past midnight (for social, school, or work reasons). In most cases, it is difficult to distinguish among these factors, since patients with an abnormally long intrinsic period are more likely to "choose" such late-night activities because they are unable to sleep at that time. Patients tend to be young adults. This self-perpetuating condition can persist for years and does not usually respond to attempts to re-establish normal bedtime hours. Treatment methods involving bright-light phototherapy during the morning hours or melatonin administration in the evening hours show promise in these patients, although the relapse rate is high.
- *Advanced sleep phase disorder (ASPD):* This is the converse of the delayed sleep phase syndrome. Most commonly, this syndrome occurs in older people, 15% of whom report that they cannot sleep past 5 AM, with twice that number complaining that they wake-up too early at least several times per week. Patients with ASPD experience excessive daytime sleepiness during the evening hours, when they have great difficulty remaining awake, even in social settings. Typically, patients awaken from 3 to 5 AM each day, often several hours before their desired wake times. In addition to age-related ASPD, an early-onset familial variant of this condition has also been reported. Patients with ASPD may benefit from bright-light phototherapy during the evening hours, designed to reset the circadian pacemaker to a later hour.
- *Non-24-H sleep-wake disorder:* This condition can occur when the synchronizing input (i.e. the light-dark cycle) from the environment to the circadian pacemaker is compromised (as in many blind people with no light perception) or when the maximal phase-advancing capacity of the circadian pacemaker is not adequate to accommodate the difference between the 24-hour geophysical day and the intrinsic period of the pacemaker in the patient. Alternatively, patients' self-selected exposure to artificial light may drive the circadian pacemaker to a greater than 24-hour schedule. Affected patients are not able to maintain a stable phase relationship between the output of the pacemaker and the 24-hour day. Such patients typically present with an incremental pattern of successive delays in sleep propensity, progressing in and out of phase with local time. When the patient's endogenous circadian rhythms are out of phase with the local environment, insomnia coexists with excessive daytime sleepiness. Conversely, when the endogenous circadian rhythms are in phase with the local environment, symptoms remit. The intervals between symptomatic periods may last several weeks to several months. Blind individuals unable to perceive light are particularly susceptible to this disorder, although it can occur in sighted patients. Nightly low-dose (0.5 mg) melatonin administration has been reported to improve sleep and, in some cases, to induce synchronization of the circadian pacemaker.

Medical implications of circadian rhythmicity: Prominent circadian variations have been reported in the incidence of acute myocardial infarction, sudden cardiac death, and stroke. Platelet aggregability is increased in the early morning hours, coincident with the peak incidence of these cardiovascular events. Misalignment of circadian phase, such as occurs during night-shift work, induces insulin resistance and higher glucose levels in response to a standard meal. Blood pressure of night workers with sleep apnea is higher than that of day workers. A better understanding of the possible role of circadian rhythmicity in the acute destabilization of a chronic condition such as atherosclerotic disease could improve the understanding of its pathophysiology.[14]

Excessive Daytime Sleepiness

Narcolepsy: Narcolepsy is both a disorder of the ability to sustain wakefulness voluntarily and a disorder of REM sleep regulation. The classic "narcolepsy tetrad" consists of excessive daytime somnolence plus three specific symptoms related to an intrusion of REM sleep characteristics (e.g. muscle atonia, vivid dream imagery) into the transition between wakefulness and sleep: (1) sudden weakness or loss of muscle tone without loss of consciousness, often elicited by emotion (cataplexy); (2) hallucinations at sleep onset (hypnagogic hallucinations) or upon awakening (hypnopompic hallucinations); and (3) muscle paralysis upon awakening (sleep paralysis). Symptoms of narcolepsy typically begin in the second decade, although the onset ranges from ages 5–50 years. Once established, the disease is chronic without remissions. Narcolepsy is now known to be related to hypocretin deficiency. Secondary forms of narcolepsy have been described (e.g. after head trauma). Objective verification of excessive daytime somnolence, typically with Multiple Sleep Latency Test (MSLT) <8 minutes, is an essential if nonspecific diagnostic feature. Other conditions that cause excessive sleepiness, such as sleep apnea or chronic sleep deprivation, must be rigorously excluded. The other objective diagnostic feature of narcolepsy is the presence of REM sleep in at least two of the naps during the MSLT. Abnormal regulation of REM sleep is also manifested by the appearance of REM sleep immediately or within minutes after sleep onset in 50% of narcoleptic patients, a rarity in unaffected individuals maintaining a conventional sleep-wake schedule.

The treatment of narcolepsy is symptomatic.[15] Somnolence is treated with wake-promoting therapeutics. Modafinil is now the drug of choice, principally because it is associated with fewer side effects than older stimulants and has a long half-life; 200–400 mg is given as a single daily dose. Older drugs such as methylphenidate (10 mg bid to 20 mg qid) or dextroamphetamine (10 mg bid) are still used as alternatives, particularly in refractory patients.

Treatment of the REM-related phenomena of cataplexy, hypnagogic hallucinations, and sleep paralysis requires the potent REM sleep suppression produced by antidepressant medications. The tricyclic antidepressants [e.g. protriptyline (10–40 mg/day) and clomipramine (25–50 mg/day)] and the selective serotonin reuptake inhibitors (SSRIs) [e.g. fluoxetine (10–20 mg/day)] are commonly used for this purpose. Efficacy of the antidepressants is limited largely by anticholinergic side effects (tricyclics) and by sleep disturbance and sexual dysfunction (SSRIs). Alternately, gamma hydroxybutyrate (GHB), given at bedtime, and 4 hour later, is effective in reducing daytime cataplectic episodes. Adequate nocturnal sleep time and planned daytime naps (when possible) are important preventive measures.

Other causes of excessive daytime somnolence:
- Kleine-Levin syndrome
- Menstrual related hypersomnia
- Post traumatic hypersomnia
- Insufficient sleep syndrome
- Idiopathic hypersomnia.

Parasomnias

Parasomnias are defined as undesirable physical phenomena accompanying sleep that involve skeletal muscle activity and/or autonomic nervous system changes. Parasomnias can be objectively diagnosed by means of polysomnography, and can be successfully treated.[16,17]

The often "bizarre" nature of the parasomnias frequently leads them to being misdiagnosed and mistreated as other psychiatric disorders; particularly if they appear temporally related to stressful situations. Rarely there may be forensic implications, where there is a history of sleep-related violence.

The International Classification of Sleep Disorders (Revised) classification of parasomnias (according to stage of sleep):

Arousal disorders (disorders of non-REM sleep)
- Confusional arousals
- Sleep walking
- Sleep terrors

Sleep-wake transition disorders
- Rhythmic movement disorder
- Sleep starts
- Sleep talking
- Nocturnal leg cramps

Parasomnias usually associated with REM sleep
- Nightmares
- Sleep paralysis
- Impaired sleep-related penile erections
- Sleep-related painful erections
- REM sleep-related sinus arrest
- REM sleep Behavior disorder.

Other parasomnias
- Sleep bruxism
- Sleep enuresis
- Sleep-related abnormal swallowing syndrome
- Nocturnal paroxysmal dystonia
- Sudden unexplained nocturnal death syndrome
- Primary snoring
- Infant sleep apnoea
- Congenital central hypoventilation syndrome
- Sudden infant death syndrome
- Benign neonatal sleep myoclonus
- Other parasomnia not otherwise stated.

Arousal Disorders (of non-REM Sleep)

Confusional Arousals (Sleep Drunkenness)

Clinical features: Confusion during and following arousals from sleep, most typically from deep sleep in the first part of the night. Individuals appear disoriented, incoherent, hesitant and slow, but may walk about, get dressed, and even perform complex motor Behaviors. Violence, assault, and even homicide may occur (rare). Planning or premeditation is not possible.

Polysomnography: Arousal out of SWS, usually in the 1st third of the night.

Prevalence: Almost universal in young children (before aged 5 years), become less common in older childhood. Fairly rare in adulthood, usually occurring in the context of sleep deprivation, exacerbated by alcohol or other depressant drugs.

Associated disorders: Sleep apnea syndromes, narcolepsy, idiopathic hypersomnia and encephalopathy.

Differential diagnosis: Acute confusional states, sleep terrors (evident autonomic arousal), somnambulism (usually docile, not aggressive when challenged), and REM sleep Behavior disorder.

Management

- Prevent the patient from falling into deep, prolonged SWS by avoiding of sleep deprivation
- Restrict use of alcohol and other sedatives
- Sleep hygiene measures.

Sleepwalking (Somnambulism)

Clinical features: Complex, automatic Behaviors (automatisms) (e.g. aimless wandering, attempting to dress or undress, carrying objects, eating, urinating in unusual places, and, rarely, driving a car) can occur. Such episodes are of variable duration and usually occur 15–120 minutes following sleep onset. Eyes are usually wide open and talk is incoherent with communication usually impossible. Injury may occur (e.g. falling down the stairs, exiting through a window). Activity never appears intentional or planned, and only rarely aggressive Behavior occurs. The person is usually easily returned to bed, falls back into normal sleep, and has no recollection of the episode the following morning. If awakened during the episode, the patient may appear confused and disoriented.

Polysomnography: Light, non-REM sleep, with episodes sometimes preceded by hypersynchrony of generalized (non-epileptic) high-voltage delta waves.

Prevalence: Common in childhood and less common in adults. Familial forms do occur. Precipitants are similar to confusional arousals.

Management

- Reassurance
- Protect the patient from coming to harm (e.g. closing windows, locking doors, sleeping downstairs)
- Relaxation techniques and minimization of stressors
- Sleep hygiene measures
- Avoidance of sleep deprivation
- In high risk patients, small doses of benzodiazepine may be indicated.

Sleep Terrors (Parvor Nocturnes, Incubus)

Clinical features: Sudden awakening with loud terrified screaming and marked autonomic arousal. Sometimes frenzied activity occurs, which may lead to injury. Episodes usually last for a few minutes, with evident increase in muscle tone and resistance to physical contact. If wakened, the individual appears confused and incoherent, but soon falls asleep, wakening the next morning with no memory of the event.

Polysomnography: Abrupt wakening out of Stage 3 or 4 sleep is seen on EEG, with generation of alpha activity, usually in the 1st third of the night. Partial arousals out of SWS, occurring up to 10–15 times in one night, are also seen even when a full episode is not recorded.

Management

- Reassurance
- Protect the patient from coming to harm
- Relaxation techniques and minimisation of stressors
- Sleep hygiene measures
- Avoidance of sleep deprivation
- In high risk patients, small doses of benzodiazepine may be indicated.

Sleep-wake Transition Disorders

Rhythmic Movement Disorder

Clinical features: Stereotyped, repetitive movements involving large muscles, usually of the head and neck, typically immediately prior to sleep, sustained into light sleep.

Polysomnography: Rhythmic movement artifacts during light non-REM sleep, without evidence of epileptiform activity.

Associated problems: Developmental problems/psycho-pathology (older children).

Management

- Reassurance
- Low dose benzodiazepine may be indicated in extreme cases.

Sleep Starts (Hypnic Jerks)

Clinical features: Occur at sleep onset and presents as sudden abrupt contractions of muscle groups, usually the legs, but sometimes also involving the arms, neck, or even the entire body. When wakened by jerks, an individual may have the feeling of falling in space. Sometimes this feeling is so intense and frightening that it can lead to fear of going to sleep with subsequent sleep-onset difficulties.

Polysomnography: Occasional vertex waves, associated with muscular contraction.

Differential diagnosis:
- Nocturnal myoclonic jerks (with evident epileptiform activity on EEG)
- Fragmentary myoclonus (during non-REM sleep)
- PLMS (often associated with restless legs syndrome).

Management: Treatment usually unnecessary. If there is significant interference with sleep, general measures (e.g. avoidance of stimulants such as caffeine, nicotine) or low-dose clonazepam at night is indicated.

Sleep Talking (Somniloquy)

Clinical features: The common uttering of words or sounds during sleep, without subjective awareness, and speech generally devoid of meaning.

Polysomnography: Brief partial arousal during non-REM sleep is usually seen on EEG in about 60% of cases. Less commonly, somniloquy may occur during REM sleep, if it is related to dream content or in association with another disorder of REM sleep.

Associated disorders: Confusional arousals, sleep terrors, REM sleep Behavior disorder.

Management: Unless the problem is leading to disruption of sleep in a bed partner, or is a secondary symptom of other sleep pathology, treatment is rarely necessary.

Nocturnal Leg Cramps

Clinical features: Sensations of painful muscular tightness or tension, in the calf (or the foot), occurring during sleep, which awaken the sufferer.

Associated problems: Excessive muscular activity, dehydration, diabetes, arthritis, pregnancy, and Parkinson's disease.

Differential diagnosis:
- Periodic leg movements of sleep (painless)
- Muscle spasm due to spasticity following stroke
- Other neurological causes of muscle spasticity.

Management: Treatment is required only in severe cases. Palliative measures (heat, massage, muscle stretching) are often useful. Quinine sulphate (325 mg) may be of some value.

Disorders Associated with REM Sleep[18]

Nightmares

Clinical features: Frightening dreams that usually awaken the sleeper from REM sleep, without associated confusion.

Polysomnography: Increased REM density, lasting about 10 minutes, terminated by an awakening, usually in the 2nd half-of the night.

Differential diagnosis:
- Sleep terrors
- REM sleep Behavior disorder
- Nocturnal panic attacks.

Management: Treatment is usually unnecessary. General measures include avoidance of stress and principles of sleep hygiene.

Sleep Paralysis

Clinical features: It is a frightening experience of being unable to perform voluntary movements either at sleep onset (hypnagogic) or awakening (hypnopompic).

Polysomnography: Atonia in peripheral muscles (as in REM sleep) despite desynchronised EEG with eye movements and blinking (i.e. awake). H-reflex activity is also abolished during an episode (as in REM sleep).

Differential diagnosis:
- Narcolepsy
- Periodic hypokalemia.

Management: Sleep hygiene esp. avoidance of sleep deprivation, may help to prevent episodes. Persistent problems may respond to REM-suppressant medication (e.g. clomipramine 25 mg or an SSRI).

REM Sleep Behavior Disorder (RSBD)

Clinical features: Vivid, intense, violent dreams (reported as nightmares), dream-enacting Behaviors (verbal and motor), sleep injury (of self and bed partner), general sleep disruption.

Polysomnography: Elevated submental EMG tone and/or excessive phasic submental/limb EMG twitching during REM sleep, in the absence of EEG epileptiform activity.

Associated disorders: Fifty percent of cases are associated with neurological disorders, usually degenerative (e.g. Parkinson's disease), and narcolepsy. A full neurological examination should be performed. It is rarely associated with other psychiatric disorders, but may be induced or aggravated by psychiatric drugs (e.g. TCAs, MAOIs, high-dose SSRIs, SNRIs), cessation/misuse of REM-suppressing agents (e.g. alcohol, amphetamine, cocaine), or severe stress related to traumatic experiences.

Differential diagnosis:
- Sleepwalking
- Sleep terrors

- Nocturnal dissociative disorders
- Nocturnal epilepsy
- Obstructive sleep apnea
- Intoxication
- Malingering.

Management: Ensure a safe sleeping environment. Eliminate any factors that might be inducing or aggravating the condition. If symptoms persist and are problematic, clonazepam is the treatment of choice, effectively controlling both Behaviors and dreams.

Insomnia Due to General Medical Conditions[14]

A number of medical conditions are associated with disruptions of sleep. The association is frequently nonspecific, e.g. sleep disruption due to chronic pain from rheumatologic disorders. Attention to this association is important in that sleep-associated symptoms are often the presenting or most bothersome complaint. Treatment of the underlying medical problem is the most useful approach. Sleep disruption can also result from the use of medications such as glucocorticoids.

Sleep Disorders Related to Psychiatric Disorders[19]

Although it is unusual for psychiatric patients to present with a primary sleep disorder, it is not uncommon for psychiatrists to have to deal with secondary problems of insomnia or hypersomnia, in the context of a primary psychiatric disorder, or as a consequence of medication. Equally, sleep deprivation may have its own psychological consequences, or may precipitate the onset of a psychiatric illness, particularly a manic episode.

Major Affective Disorders

Alterations in sleep are central symptoms in the mood disorders. Initial insomnia, frequent waking (for often prolonged periods), early morning waking, vivid or disturbing dreams, daytime fatigue are frequently seen in major depressive disorder. Occasionally, hypersomnia may be a feature in atypical cases, bipolar affective disorder, and seasonal affective disorder. Episodes of mania may be characterized by marked insomnia and a decreased need for sleep. Sleep architecture is also disturbed in depression.

Most antidepressants are REM-suppressant and may exacerbate underlying primary sleep disorders either on commencement or cessation.

Anxiety Disorders

Anxiety disorders commonly disrupt the normal sleep pattern leading to insomnia, which may be triggered by an acute stressful event. Symptoms include: initial insomnia, frequent waking, reduced total sleep time, and early morning waking.

Panic disorder (nocturnal) attacks may occur with associated intense fear, feelings of impending doom, autonomic arousal, somatic symptoms, and fear of going to sleep (leading to avoidance Behavior that may present as insomnia).

Schizophrenia

Patients with schizophrenia demonstrate increased nocturnal wakefulness and daytime somnolence. It is often difficult to disentangle the effects of medication, active positive symptoms, persistent negative symptoms, and disorganized Behavior.

Dementia

Normal aging is associated with increased sleep latency, reduced total sleep time, loss of SWS, frequent arousals leading to fragmentation of nocturnal sleep, and an increase in daytime napping.

Some sleep disorders (e.g. sleep apnea syndromes, PLMS) occur more frequently in the elderly population.

Dementia generally causes further increases in sleep latency, further reductions in total sleep time, and increased fragmentation of nocturnal sleep, in proportion to the severity of the illness.

Disorders of normal circadian rhythm are also commonly seen, with a characteristic "sundown syndrome" of confusion and agitation at bedtime.

Effects of Psychiatric Medication on Sleep

Antidepressants

Sedating: TCAs are usually sedative due to their anticholinergic effects.

Tetracyclic antidepressants (maprotiline, mianserin) and trazodone also have marked sedating properties, although these are less related to their anticholinergic properties and may be due to their 5HT2 and histamine antagonism properties shared by some of the newer antidepressants (e.g. nefazodone, mirtazepine).

Alerting: MAOIs, SSRIs, NARIs (reboxetine), DARIs (bupropion), SNRIs (venlafaxine) all tend to have alerting effects which may, be useful in the treatment of hypersomnolence.

Mood-stabilizing Drugs

Lithium tends to be mildly sedating. Carbamazepine may cause drowsiness at the start of treatment or when the dose is being increased, but this is usually a transient effect. Sodium valproate is less sedative than carbamazepine, with only mild effects on sleep.

Antipsychotic Drugs

Most antipsychotics cause drowsiness and impaired performance. There is a great degree of variability even within groups of antipsychotics. Chlorpromazine and clozapine cause marked sedation while aripriprazole is activating.

Benzodiazepines and Associated Hypnotics

By definition, benzodiazepines and barbiturates are sedating. Problems arise due to REM rebound on discontinuation, tolerance to the beneficial hypnotic effects after long-term use, and problems of dependence. Newer hypnotics, such as zopiclone and zolpidem, share the sleep-enhancing properties of the benzodiazepines, but may be less likely to cause rebound or dependence.

Psychostimulant Drugs

Although very useful in the treatment of hypersomnia (particularly in narcolepsy), ADHD, and to suppress appetite, this group of drugs all tend to cause insomnia with fragmented sleep due to frequent awakenings (e.g. dexamphetamine, methylphenidate, methamphetamine, mazinol, pemoline, and modafinil) and should not be taken in the evening. Cessation, with the notable exception of modafinil, leads to increases in total sleep time and REM rebound.

Changes in DSM-5[20,21]

Sleep disorders related to another mental disorder and sleep disorder related to a general medical condition have been removed from DSM-5, to emphasize that an individual has a sleep disorder warranting independent clinical attention, in addition to any medical and mental disorders that are also present. It is also an acknowledgement of the bidirectional and interactive effects between sleep disorders and coexisting medical and mental disorders. It moves away from making causal attributions between coexisting disorders.

The diagnosis of primary insomnia has been renamed insomnia disorder to avoid the differentiation of primary and secondary insomnia. DSM-5 also distinguishes narcolepsy, which is now known to be associated with hypocretin deficiency, from other forms of hypersomnolence. These changes are a reflection of advancement in neurobiological and genetic understanding of the disorder. Developmental criteria and text are integrated where existing science and considerations of clinical utility support such integration.

Breathing-related Sleep Disorders

In DSM-5, breathing-related sleep disorders are divided into three relatively distinct disorders: obstructive sleep apnea hypopnea, central sleep apnea, and sleep-related hypoventilation.

Circadian Rhythm Sleep-wake Disorders

The subtypes of circadian rhythm sleep-wake disorders have been expanded to include advanced sleep phase syndrome, irregular sleep-wake type, and non-24-hour sleep-wake type, whereas the jet lag type has been removed.

Rapid Eye Movement Sleep Behavior Disorder and Restless Legs Syndrome

The use of DSM-IV "not otherwise specified" diagnoses has been reduced by designating rapid eye movement sleep behavior disorder and restless legs syndrome as independent disorders.

DSM-5 Diagnostic criteria for sleep-wake disorders

Insomnia Disorder

780.52 (G47.00)

a. A predominant complaint of dissatisfaction with sleep quantity or quality, associated with one (or more) of the following symptoms:
   1. Difficulty initiating sleep (In children, this may manifest as difficulty initiating sleep without caregiver intervention).
   2. Difficulty maintaining sleep, characterized by frequent awakenings or problems returning to sleep after awakenings. (In children, this may manifest as difficulty returning to sleep without caregiver intervention).
   3. Early-morning awakening with inability to return to sleep.
b. The sleep disturbance causes clinically significant distress or impairment in social, occupational, educational, academic, behavioral, or other important areas of functioning.
c. The sleep difficulty occurs at least 3 nights per week.
d. The sleep difficulty is present for at least 3 months.
e. The sleep difficulty occurs despite adequate opportunity for sleep.
f. The insomnia is not better explained by and does not occur exclusively during the course of another sleep-wake disorder (e.g. narcolepsy, a breathing-related sleep disorder, a circadian rhythm sleep-wake disorder, a parasomnia).
g. The insomnia is not attributable to the physiological effects of a substance (e.g. a drug of abuse, a medication).
h. Coexisting mental disorders and medical conditions do not adequately explain the predominant complaint of insomnia.

Specify if:

With non-sleep disorder mental comorbidity, including substance
use disorders

With other medical comorbidity

Contd...

Contd...

With other sleep disorder
Coding note: The code 780.52 (G47.00) applies to all three specifiers. Code also the relevant associated mental disorder, medical condition, or other sleep disorder immediately after the code for insomnia disorder in order to indicate the association.

Specify if:
Episodic: Symptoms last at least 1 month but less than 3 months.
Persistent: Symptoms last 3 months or longer.
Recurrent: Two (or more) episodes within the space of 1 year.
Note: Acute and short-term insomnia (i.e. symptoms lasting less than 3 months but otherwise meeting ail criteria with regard to frequency, intensity, distress, and/or impairment) should be coded as an other specified insomnia disorder.

Hypersomnolence Disorder
780.54 (G47.10)

a. Self-reported excessive sleepiness (hypersomnolence) despite a main sleep period lasting at least 7 hours, with at least one of the following symptoms:
   1. Recurrent periods of sleep or lapses into sleep within the same day.
   2. A prolonged main sleep episode of more than 9 hours per day that is non restorative (i.e. unrefreshing).
   3. Difficulty being fully awake after abrupt awakening.
b. The hypersomnolence occurs at least three times per week, for at least 3 months.
c. The hypersomnolence is accompanied by significant distress or impairment in cognitive, social, occupational, or other important areas of functioning.
d. The hypersomnolence is not better explained by and does not occur exclusively during the course of another sleep disorder (e.g. narcolepsy, breathing-related sleep disorder, circadian rhythm sleep-wake disorder, or a parasomnia).
e. The hypersomnolence is not attributable to the physiological effects of a substance (e.g. a drug of abuse, a medication).
f. Coexisting mental and medical disorders do not adequately explain the predominant complaint of hypersomnolence.

Specify if:
With mental disorder, including substance use disorders
With medical condition
With another sleep disorder
Coding note: The code 780.54 (G47.10) applies to all three specifiers. Code also the relevant associated mental disorder, medical condition, or other sleep disorder immediately after the code for hypersomnolence disorder in order to indicate the association.

Specify if:
Acute: Duration of less than 1 month.
Subacute: Duration of 1–3 months.
Persistent: Duration of more than 3 months.

Specify current severity:
Specify severity based on degree of difficulty maintaining daytime alertness as manifested by the occurrence of multiple attacks of irresistible sleepiness within any given day occurring, e.g. while sedentary, driving, visiting with friends, or working.

Contd...

Contd...

Mild: Difficulty maintaining daytime alertness 1–2 days/week.
Moderate: Difficulty maintaining daytime alertness 3 days/week.
Severe: Difficulty maintaining daytime alertness 5–7 days/week.

Narcolepsy

a. Recurrent periods of an irrepressible need to sleep, lapsing into sleep, or napping occurring within the same day. These must have been occurring at least three times per week over the past 3 months.
b. The presence of at least one of the following:
   1. Episodes of cataplexy, defined as either (a) or (b), occurring at least a few times per month:
      a. In individuals with long-standing disease, brief (seconds to minutes) episodes of sudden bilateral loss of muscle tone with maintained consciousness that are precipitated by laughter or joking.
      b. In children or in individuals within 6 months of onset, spontaneous grimaces or jaw-opening episodes with tongue thrusting or a global hypotonia, without any obvious emotional triggers.
   2. Hypocretin deficiency, as measured using cerebrospinal fluid (CSF) hypocretin-1 immunoreactivity values (less than or equal to one-third of values obtained in healthy subjects tested using the same assay, or less than or equal to 110 pg/mL). Low CSF levels of hypocretin-1 must not be observed in the context of acute brain injury, inflammation, or infection.
   3. Nocturnal sleep polysomnography showing rapid eye movement (REM) sleep latency less than or equal to 15 minutes, or a multiple sleep latency test showing a mean sleep latency less than or equal to 8 minutes and two or more sleep-onset REM periods.

Specify whether:
347.00 (G47.419) Narcolepsy without cataplexy but with hypocretin deficiency: Criterion B requirements of low CSF hypocretin-1 levels and positive polysomnography/multiple sleep latencytest are met, but no cataplexy is present (Criterion B1 not met).

347.01 (G47.411) Narcolepsy with cataplexy but without hypocretin deficiency: In this rare subtype (less than 5% of narcolepsy cases), Criterion B requirements of cataplexy and positive polysomnography/multiple sleep latency test are met, but CSF hypocretin-1 levels are normal (Criterion B2 not met).

347.00 (G47.419) Autosomal dominant cerebellar ataxia, deafness, and narcolepsy: This subtype is caused by exon 21 DNA (cytosine-5)-methyltransferase-1 mutations and is characterized by late-onset (age 30–40 years) narcolepsy (with low or intermediate CSF hypocretin-1 levels), deafness, cerebellar ataxia, and eventually dementia.

347.00 (G47.419) Autosomal dominant narcolepsy, obesity, and type 2 diabetes: Narcolepsy, obesity, and type 2 diabetes and low CSF hypocretin-1 levels have been described in rare cases and are associated with a mutation in the myelin oligodendrocyte glycoprotein gene.

347.10 (G47.429) Narcolepsy secondary to another medical condition: This subtype is for narcolepsy that develops secondary to medical conditions that cause infectious (e.g. Whipple's disease, sarcoidosis), traumatic, or tumoral destruction of hypocretin neurons.

Contd...

Contd...

Coding note (for ICD-9-CM code 347.10 only): Code first the underlying medical condition (e.g. 040.2 Whipple's disease; 347.10 narcolepsy secondary to Whipple's disease).

Specify current severity:

Mild: Infrequent cataplexy (less than once per week), need for naps only once or twice per day, and less disturbed nocturnal sleep.

Moderate: Cataplexy once daily or every few days, disturbed nocturnal sleep, and need for multiple naps daily.

Severe: Drug-resistant cataplexy with multiple attacks daily, nearly constant sleepiness, and disturbed nocturnal sleep (i.e., movements, insomnia, and vivid dreaming).

DSM-5 Diagnostic criteria for breathing-related sleep disorders

Obstructive Sleep Apnea Hypopnea
327.23 (G47.33)

a. Either (1) or (2):
   1. Evidence by polysomnography of at least five obstructive apneas or hypopneas per hour of sleep and either of the following sleep symptoms:
   a. Nocturnal breathing disturbances: snoring, snorting/gasping, or breathing pauses during sleep.
   b. Daytime sleepiness, fatigue, or unrefreshing sleep despite sufficient opportunities to sleep that is not better explained by another mental disorder (including a sleep disorder) and is not attributable to another medical condition.
   2. Evidence by polysomnography of 15 or more obstructive apneas and/or hypopneas per hour of sleep regardless of accompanying symptoms.

Specify current severity:

Mild: Apnea hypopnea index is less than 15.

Moderate: Apnea hypopnea index is 15–30.

Severe: Apnea hypopnea index is greater than 30.

Central Sleep Apnea

a. Evidence by polysomnography of five or more central apneas per hour of sleep.
b. The disorder is not better explained by another current sleep disorder.

Specify whether:

327.21 (G47.31) Idiopathic central sleep apnea: Characterized by repeated episodes of apneas and hypopneas during sleep caused by variability in respiratory effort but without evidence of airway obstruction.

786.04 (R06.3) Cheyne-Stokes breathing: A pattern of periodic crescendo-decrescendo variation in tidal volume that results in central apneas and hypopneas at a frequency of at least five events per hour, accompanied by frequent arousal.

780.57 (G47.37) Central sleep apnea comorbid with opioid use: The pathogenesis of this subtype is attributed to the effects of opioids on the respiratory rhythm generators in the medulla as well as the differential effects on hypoxic versus hypercapnic respiratory drive.

Contd...

Contd...

Coding note (for 780.57 [G47.37] code only): When an opioid use disorder is present, first code the opioid use disorder: 305.50 (F11.10) mild opioid use disorder or 304.00 (F11.20) moderate or severe opioid use disorder; then code 780.57 (G47.37) central sleep apnea comorbid with opioid use. When an opioid use disorder is not present (e.g. after a one-time heavy use of the substance), code only 780.57 (G47.37) central sleep apnea comorbid with opioid use.

Specify current severity:

Severity of central sleep apnea is graded according to the frequency of the breathing disturbances as well as the extent of associated oxygen desaturation and sleep fragmentation that occur as a consequence of repetitive respiratory disturbances.

DSM-5 Diagnostic criteria for parasomnias

DSM-5 Diagnostic Criteria for Non-Rapid Eye Movement Sleep Arousal Disorder

a. Recurrent episodes of incomplete awakening from sleep, usually occurring during the first third of the major sleep episode, accompanied by either one of the following:
   1. **Sleep walking:** Repeated episodes of rising from bed during sleep and walking about. While sleep walking, the individual has a blank, starring face; is relatively unresponsive to the efforts of others to communicate with him/her, and can be awakened only with great difficulty.
   2. **Sleep Terrors:** Recurrent episodes of abrupt terror accuses from sleep, usually beginning with a panicky scream. There is intense fear and signs of autonomic arousal, such as mydriasis, tachycardia, rapid breathing, and sweating, during each episode. There is relative unresponsiveness to efforts of others to comfort the individual during the episodes.
b. No or little (e.g. only a single visual scene) dream imagery is recalled.
c. Amnesia for the episodes is present.
d. The episodes cause clinically significant distress or impairment in social, occupational, or other important areas of functioning.
e. The disturbance is not attributable to the physiological effects of a substance (e.g. a drug of abuse, a medication)
f. Coexisting mental and medical disorders do not explain the episodes of sleep walking or sleep terrors.

Coding note: For ICD-9-CM, code 307.46 for all subtypes. For ICD-10-CM, code is based on subtype.

Specify whether:

307.46 (F51.3) Sleepwalking type

Specify if:

With sleep-related eating

With sleep-related sexual behavior (sexsomnia)

307.46 (F51.5) Sleep terror type

DSM-5 Diagnostic Criteria for Nightmare Disorder 307.47 (F51.5)

a. Repeated occurrences of extended, extremely dysphoric, and well-remembered dreams that usually involve efforts to avoid threats to survival, security, or physical integrity and that generally occur during the second half of the major sleep episode.

Contd...

Contd...

b. On awakening from the dysphoric dreams, the individual rapidly becomes oriented and alert.
c. The sleep disturbance causes clinically significant distress or impairment in social, occupational, or other important areas of functioning.
d. The nightmare symptoms are not attributable to the physiological effects of a substance (e.g. a drug of abuse, a medication).
e. Coexisting mental and medical disorders do not adequately explain the predominant complaint of dysphoric dreams.

Specify if:
During sleep onset

Specify if:
With associated non-sleep disorder, including substance use disorders
With associated other medical condition
With associated other sleep disorder
Coding note: The code 307.47 (F51.5) applies to all three specifiers. Code also the relevant associated mental disorder, medical condition, or other sleep disorder immediately after the code for nightmare disorder in order to indicate the association.

Specify if:
Acute: Duration of period of nightmares is 1 month or less.
Subacute: Duration of period of nightmares is greater than 1 month but less than 6 months.
Persistent: Duration of period of nightmare is 6 months or greater.

Specify current severity:
Severity can be rated by the frequency with which the nightmares occur.
Mild: Less than one episode per week on average.
Moderate: One or more episodes per week but less than nightly.
Severe: Episodes nightly.

DSM-5 Diagnostic Criteria for Rapid Eye Movement Sleep Behavior Disorder 327.42 (G47.52)

a. Repeated episodes of arousal during sleep associated with vocalization and/or complex motor behaviors.
b. These behaviors arise during rapid eye movement (REM) sleep and therefore usually occur more than 90 minutes after sleep onset, are more frequent during the later portions of the sleep period, and uncommonly occur during day time naps.
c. Upon awakening from these episodes, the individual is completely awake, alert, and not confused or disoriented.
d. Either of the following:
   1. REM sleep without atonia on polysomnographic recording.
   2. A history suggestive of REM sleep behaviors disorder and an established synucleinopathy diagnosis (e.g. Parkinson's disease, multiple system atrophy).
e. The behaviors cause clinically significant distress or impairment in social, occupational, or other important areas of functioning (which may include injury to self or the bed partner.
f. The disturbance is not attributable to the physiological effects of a substance (e.g. a drug of abuse, a medication) or another medical condition.
g. Coexisting mental and medical disorders do not explain the episodes.

Contd...

Contd...

DSM-5 Diagnostic Criteria for Restless Legs Syndrome 333.94 (G25.81)

a. An urge to move the legs, usually accompanied by or in response to uncomfortable and unpleasant sensations in the legs, characterized by all of the following:
   1. The urge to move the legs begins or worsens during periods of rest or inactivity.
   2. The urge to move the legs is partially or totally relieved by movement.
   3. The urge to move the legs is worse in the evening or at night than during the day, or occurs only in the evening or at night.
b. The symptoms in Criterion A occur at least three times per week and have persisted for at least 3 months.
c. The symptoms in Criterion A are accompanied by significant distress or impairment in social, occupational, educational, academic, behavioral, or other important areas of functioning.
d. The symptoms in Criterion A are not attributable to another mental disorder or medical condition (e.g. arthritis, leg edema, peripheral ischemia, leg cramps) and are not better explained by a behavioral condition (e.g. positional discomfort, habitual foot tapping).
e. The symptoms are not attributable to the physiological effects of a drug of abuse or medication (e.g. akathisia).

DSM-5 Diagnostic Criteria for Substance/Medication-Induced Sleep Disorder

a. A prominent and severe disturbance in sleep.
b. There is evidence from the history, physical examination, or laboratory findings of both (1) and (2):
   1. The symptoms in Criterion A developed during or soon after substance intoxication or after withdrawal from or exposure to a medication.
   2. The involved substance/medication is capable of producing the symptoms in Criterion A.
c. The disturbance is not better explained by a sleep disorder that is not substance/medication-induced. Such evidence of an independent sleep disorder could include the following:
   The symptoms precede the onset of the substance/medication use: the symptoms persist for a substantial period of time (e.g. about 1 month) after the cessation of acute withdrawal or severe intoxication; or there is other evidence suggesting the existence of an independent non-substance/medication-induced sleep disorder (e.g. a history of recurrent non-substance/medication-related episodes).
d. The disturbance does not occur exclusively during the course of a delirium.
e. The disturbance causes clinically significant distress or impairment in social, occupational, or other important areas of functioning.

Specify whether:
Insomnia type: Characterized by difficulty falling asleep or maintaining sleep, frequent nocturnal awakenings, or non -restorative sleep.
Daytime sleepiness type: Characterized by predominant complaint of excessive sleepiness/fatigue during waking hours or, less commonly, a long sleep period.
Parasomnia type: Characterized by abnormal behavioral events during sleep.

Contd...

Contd...

Mixed type: Characterized by a substance/medication-induced sleep problem characterized by multiple types of sleep symptoms, but no symptom clearly predominates.

Specify if:
(See Table 1 in the chapter "Substance-Related and Addictive Disorders" for diagnoses associated with substance class):
With onset during intoxication: This specifier should be used if criteria are met for intoxication with the substance/medication and symptoms developed during the intoxication period.
With onset during discontinuation/withdrawal: This specifier should be used if criteria are met for discontinuation/withdrawal from the substance/medication and symptoms developed during, or shortly after, discontinuation of the substance/medication.

REFERENCES

1. Horne J. Why we sleep? Oxford University Press: 1988.
2. Ferini-Strambi L, Galbiati A, Marelli S. Sleep Microstructure and Memory Function. Front Neurol. 2013;4.
3. Rechtschaffen A, Kales A. A Manual of Standardized Terminology, Techniques and Scoring System for Sleep Stages of Human Subjects. US Government Printing Office, Public Health Service: Washington DC; 1968.
4. Principles and practice of sleep medicine, 2nd edn. Saunders, Philadelphia, PA.
5. Morin C. Insomnia: psychological assessment and management. Guilford Press: New York; 1993.
6. Stores G, et al. Sleep-Wake Disorders. New Oxford Textbook of Psychiatry; 2000.
7. Katz M, Shapiro C. ABC of sleep disorder. Dreams and medical illness. BMJ. 1993;306: 993-5.
8. International classification of sleep disorders, revised: diagnostic and coding manual. Rochester; 1997.
9. Doghramji K. The evaluation and management of insomnia. Clin Chest Med. 2010; 31.
10. Cartwright R. Obstructive sleep apnea: A sleep disorder with major effects on health. Dis Mon. 2001;47:109-47.
11. Hening W. Restless legs syndrome: the most common and least diagnosed sleep disorder. Sleep Med. 2004;5:429-3.
12. Kanathur N, Harrington J, Lee-Chiong TJ. Circadian rhythm sleep disorders. Clin Chest Med. 2010;31:319-25.
13. Schwartz J, Roth T. Shift work sleep disorder: burden of illness and approaches to management. Drugs. 2006;66:2357-70.
14. Czeisler C. Sleep disorders. Harrison's Principles of Internal Medicine.
15. Ahmed I, Thorpy M. Clinical features, diagnosis and treatment of narcolepsy. Clin Chest Med. 2010;31.
16. Tinuper P, Bisulli F, Provini F. The parasomnias: mechanisms and treatment. Epilepsia. 2012;53(Suppl):12-9.
17. Yamadera H. The topics of sleep disorder: concerning sleep-wake rhythm disorder. J Nippon Med Sch. 2001;68:344-8.
18. Arnulf I. REM sleep behavior disorder: motor manifestations and pathophysiology. Mov Disord. 2012;27:667-89.
19. Oxford Handbook of Psychiatry. Oxford University Press; 2005.
20. Grohol J. DSM-5 Changes: Sleep-Wake Disorders. Psych Central. *http://pro.psychcentral.com/2013/dsm-5-changes-sleep-wake-disorders/004414.html*
21. American Psychiatric Association. Desk Reference to the Diagnostic Criteria from DSM-5. Washington DC; 2013.

CHAPTER 27

Chronic Insomnia

BS Bhogle, SN Ali, Asha Krishnan, Christoday RJ Khess

INTRODUCTION

Insomnia is a common complaint that can present independently or comorbidly with another medical disorder (e.g. pain) or psychiatric disorder (e.g. depression). Insomnia is the most prevalent sleep disorder and affects large proportions of the population on a situational, recurrent, or persistent basis. It carries a heavy burden for both patients and the healthcare system as evidenced by its effect on quality of life, and on psychological, occupational, and economic domains.[1-4] Insomnia is often unrecognized and untreated because of barriers to assessment and management.

CLINICAL PRESENTATION AND ENDINGS

Insomnia is characterized by subjective complaints about dissatisfaction with sleep quality or duration, difficulty in night or too early in the morning, or non-restorative or falling asleep at bedtime, waking up in the middle of the poor quality sleep. Insomnia also includes subjective reports of daytime symptoms such as fatigue or low energy, difficulties with cognitive functions (e.g. attention, concentration, and memory), and mood disturbances (e.g. irritability, dysphoria), all of which can produce functional impairments and are often the primary concerns that prompt patients to seek treatment.[5-8]

Polysomnographic assessment can show objective sleep impairments (e.g. longer sleep latencies, reduced sleep time), but severity does not always match the patients complaint of poor sleep. The cortex is more active in people with insomnia than in good sleepers, both around sleep onset and during non-rapid eye movement sleep;[9] this is consistent with the general state of hyperarousal in people with insomnia. For daytime symptoms, assessment of neurobehavioral performance with objective tests shows selective performance deficits (e.g. attention, memory) in individuals with primary insomnia.[10,11] Nonetheless, most patients perceive their global functioning as greatly impaired. The patients appraisal of sleep and daytime functioning is crucial since a diagnosis of insomnia is based on clinical symptoms rather than on objective laboratory findings.

EPIDEMIOLOGY

Prevalence

About 25% of adults are dissatisfied with their sleep, 10–15% report symptoms of insomnia associated with daytime consequences, and 6–10% meet criteria for an insomnia disorder.[8,12-14] Insomnia is one of the most prevalent complaints in primary care;[15-17] complaints increase with age and are twice as prevalent in women as in men.[8,12]

Comorbidity

A high rate of comorbidity exists between chronic insomnia and medical and psychiatric disorders.[13-18] In the 2002 US National Health Interview Survey,[18] individuals with insomnia were more than five times [odds ratio (OR) 5.64, 99% CI 5.07–6.29] as likely to present anxiety or depression, and more than twice (OR 2.24, 99% CI 1.60–3.14) as likely to present congestive heart failures as individuals without insomnia (Panel 1). Likewise, the US National Comorbidity Survey[13] showed that insomnia was frequently comorbid with anxiety, mood, impulse-control, and substance misuse disorders (median OR 3.4, IQR 2.8–3.9). A strong association between sleep disturbances and pain has been reported.[19] Although insomnia has traditionally been conceptualized as a symptom of another disorder longitudinal suggest that it can be a risk factor for new onset psychiatric disorders, most notably depression, anxiety and substance misuse disorders.[20,21] Findings from one study showed that individuals with insomnia were four times more likely to develop new major depression over the next 3.5 years than were individuals without insomnia; risks to develop anxiety and substance misuse disorders were twice and seven times higher respectively.[21] Jansson-Frojmark and colleagues[22] reported a bidirectional relation between insomnia and anxiety, and depression. Insomnia and fatigue are the most common residual symptoms in patients treated for depression[23,24] and increase the risk of relapse for future depressive episodes.[25]

Panel 1: Assessment of insomnia (adapted from Schutte-Rodin[46]) complaint

Symptoms
- Difficulty falling asleep
- Number and duration of nocturnal awakenings
- Early morning awakening
- Nonrestorative sleep

Onset
- Gradual or abrupt
- Circumstances (e.g. changes in health, stressors, drugs)

Duration
Days, weeks, months, years

Severity
Frequency, intensity, effect on daytime functioning

Course
- Acute, episodic, persistent
- Precipitants and perpetuating factors (e.g. stress, pain, illness)
- Previous treatments and response

Presleep conditions
- Presleep activities (including before bedtime and in bed)
- Bedroom environment
- Psychological state before bedtime (e.g. worries about sleep, thoughts and emotions)

Sleep-wake schedule
- Bedtime and time needed to fall asleep
- Wake-up time end time out of bed
- Regularity of schedule (weekdays and weekends)
- Behaviors during nocturnal arousals (e.g. use of toilet, eating or drinking)

Daytime function
- Sleepiness versus fatigue*
- Cognitive functions; mood disturbances (Panel 2)
- Daytime activities including exercise; regularity of schedule

Drug and substance use
- Over-the-counter agents
- Prescription drugs
- Recreational drugs including alcohol, tobacco, and caffeine

Other sleep-related symptoms
- Respiratory (e.g. snoring, witnessed apneas, waking gasping for breath)
- Motor (e.g. restless legs, kicking/twitching during sleep, sleepwalking)
- Other medical (e.g. pain, reflux, urinary frequency)

Medical history and examination, psychiatric history and examination, sleep log or diary (at least 2 weeks)
Polysomnography

*Only in cases of suspected sleep apnea, movement disorder, or parasomnia.

COURSE AND PROGNOSIS

Insomnia can be a situational, recurrent, or persistent problem. Acute insomnia is often associated with life events or sleep schedule changes (e.g. jet lag or shift work) and usually remits once the precipitating event has subsided.[26] For some individuals, sleep disturbance can persist even after the initial cause has disappeared. Insomnia can follow an intermittent course, with recurrent episodes of sleep difficulties associated with stressful events. Even in persistent insomnia, night-to-night variability in sleep is often reported, with an occasional good night's sleep intertwined with periods of disrupted sleep.[27]

Results of longitudinal studies show that nearly 70% of individuals with insomnia at baseline continue to report insomnia 1 year later, and 50% still have insomnia up to 3 years later.[28-30] The prognosis of untreated insomnia is not well documented; however, chronic insomnia raises the risks for depression,[21,28] hypertension,[31] and possibly mortality in older adults.[32,33] These associations reinforce the need to identify and treat insomnia early to prevent chronicity and morbidity.

The course do insomnia is best understood by considering three types of contributing factors.[34] Predisposing factors increase vulnerability to insomnia, e.g. age, sex, hyperarousability, anxiety-prone personality family or personal history of insomnia, and genetic factors, such as the presence of the short allele of the serotonin transporter gene.[35] Sleep disturbances are more likely to arise in such individuals when exposed to stressful life events (e.g. illness, separation) or to less severe but more chronic daily struggles (e.g. occupational stress). Whereas most individuals resume normal sleep patterns after the triggering event has disappeared, some continue experiencing persistent sleep difficulties. Factors such as irregular sleep scheduling and the fear of not sleeping feed into and perpetuate the insomnia. Since psychological and behavioral factors are involved in perpetuation of insomnia, need to be targeted in treatment.

PATHOPHYSIOLOGICAL MECHANISMS

Definitive pathophysiological mechanisms have not been identified, although several neurobiological abnormalities are associated with insomnia. Patients with insomnia show increased activation of the autonomic nervous system, as evidenced by sleep-related elevations in heart rate and heart rate variability, metabolic rate, body temperature, activity of the hypothalamic-pituitary-adrenal axis activity, and norepinephrine secretion.[36,37] In one study, night-time blood pressure was higher in patients with insomnia than in controls.[38]

Changes in brain activity consistent with hyperarousal occur in insomnia.[36,37] Spectral analyses of electroencephalogram power during sleep show increased activity in faster frequencies (beta and gamma) which are thought to be associated with increased cognitive activity. Slow wave sleep is generally decreased compared with age-matched controls,[39] but this finding has not been reported consistently.[37] PET studies show raised brain glucose metabolism in sleep and waking, and smaller sleep-related reductions in brain glucose metabolism in wake-promoting regions.[40]

Individuals with insomnia are more likely to have a family history of the disorder,[41] which suggests a genetic vulnerability, a common environmental factor, or a learned component. Abnormalities related to sleep-wake regulatory genes have not yet been identified in insomnia.

Most studies investigating the role of hyperarousal in insomnia are correlational and thus the reported abnormalities could be the result of insomnia, associated sleep loss, or comorbidities such as depression. For example, patients with insomnia show reduced gray matter volume in the led orbitofrontal cortex and hippocampus,[42,43] and a greater frequency of the short allele of 5-HTTLPR (the 5' regulatory region of serotonin transporter gene);[35] these markers have also been reported in depression. Further studies are needed to clarify the role of arousal in the pathogenesis of insomnia and its specific genetic and neurobiological mechanisms.

ASSESSMENT AND DIAGNOSIS

In view of the high prevalence and substantial morbidities of insomnia, patients should routinely be asked about sleep problems by health-care providers.[44,45] Patients who report difficulty sleeping should be questioned about the specific symptoms of insomnia, and their frequency and severity (Panel 1). Although no standardized quantitative definitions for insomnia exist, several criteria are suggested; average reported sleep latency of more than 30 minutes, wakefulness after sleep onset of more than 30 minutes, sleep efficiency of less than 85% or total sleep time of less than 6.5 hours.[46] A key element for the diagnosis of insomnia is the presence of distress or daytime consequences, or both. Individuals who complain about inability to sleep at night but without daytime impairment might merely be short sleepers.

Daily sleep diaries are helpful to obtain an accurate report of the sleep-complaint over time; these should include bedtime and time arising from bed, time to fall asleep, number and duration of awakenings during the night, time of final awakening in the morning, and daytime naps.[46] Although polysomnography is the gold standard for measuring sleep, this test is not routinely indicated in the assessment of insomnia, except in cases of suspected sleep apnea or sleep-related movement disorders, or when violent or potentially self-injurious behavior occurs during sleep,[47] or for patients who are treatment resistant.

Patients with chronic insomnia should be screened for comorbid disorders that might be contributory, such as psychiatric illnesses and medical problems. Insomnia can be a symptom of other sleep disorders, including sleep apnea, sleep related movement disorders, and circadian rhythm disorders. For example, findings of a review of studies into the comorbidity of insomnia and sleep apnea showed that 29–67% of older adults with insomnia (n = 674 across three studies) have obstructive sleep apnea with an apnea-hypopnea index greater than five.[48] Treatment of apnea can improve sleep, whereas many hypnotic drugs can worsen sleep apnea. Panel 2 lists common disorders that present with insomnia.

Use of prescription, over-the-counter (OTC) or recreational drugs frequently contributes to sleep disturbance; these include stimulants, antidepressants, methylxanthines, decongestants, diuretics, corticosteroids, and anti-hypertensives. Patients often use alcohol to induce sleep. However, alcohol can cause sleep disruption during the latter part of the night when blood alcohol concentrations drop. Long-term use of alcohol can lead to chronic insomnia that might not fully resolve with abstinence. Recreational drugs can contribute to insomnia related to use (stimulants) or upon withdrawal (sedatives).

Two of the main nosology for diagnosis are the International Classification of Sleep Disorders: Diagnostic and Coding Manual 2nd edition (ICSD-2) (Panel 3),[5] and the Diagnostic and Statistical Manual of Mental Disorders (DSM) 4th edition (Panel 4), with the 5th edition expected in 2013.[49] The ICSD-2 states that acute or adjustment insomnia is associated with an identifiable stressor, remits when the stressor is removed, and lasts no more than 3 months, Insomnia of at least a month's duration is deemed chronic

Panel 2: Disorders that present with symptoms of insomnia

Circadian Rhythm Disorders

- Inability to sleep at the desired time, hut able to sleep at other times.
- *Delayed sleep phase:* Difficulty falling asleep until several hours after desired bedtime, with difficulty waking up on time for school or work. Common in young adults.
- *Advanced sleep phase:* Difficulty staying up until desired bedtime, accompanied by early morning awakening. More common in elderly people.
- *Shift work sleep disorder:* Difficulty sleeping at scheduled time and difficulty maintaining alertness while working. Usually seen with night shift or rotating shift work.

Sleep apnea

- Complaints of fragmented or nonrestorative sleep; daytime sleepiness can also be present.
- *History of apnea symptoms:* Snoring, witnessed apneas, waking choking or gasping, morning headaches, nocturia, fatigue or sleepiness. More common in men and those with obesity, crowded upper airway, hypertension, diabetes.

Restless legs

Uncomfortable sensation that occurs during rest, usually worst at night, and relieved by movement. Can lead to great difficulty falling asleep and staying asleep.

Psychiatric disorders

Insomnia is often associated with anxiety and mood disorders but can be present with any psychiatric disorder. Insomnia usually worsens when psychiatric disorder is more symptomatic. All patients with chronic insomnia should be screened for psychiatric disorders.

Panel 3: Criteria for diagnosis of insomnia (ICSD-2)[5]

a. One or more of the following symptoms;
   - Difficulty initiating sleep
   - Difficulty maintaining sleep
   - Waking up too early
   - Nonrestorative sleep I
b. Sleep difficulty occurs despite adequate opportunity for sleep
c. At least one of the following daytime symptoms related to the night-time sleep difficulty reported:
   - Fatigue or malaise
   - Attention, concentration, or memory impairment
   - Social or vocational dysfunction or poor school performance
   - Mood disturbance or irritability
   - Daytime sleepiness
   - Motivation or energy or initiative reduction
   - Proneness for errors or accidents
   - Tension headaches or gastrointestinal symptoms, or both
   - Concerns or worries about sleep

A+B+C defines insomnia

and is diagnosed on the basis of its presumed causes, either primary or comorbid with other conditions. In comorbid insomnia, disorders or substances contribute to the insomnia[50] and the insomnia is severe enough to cause distress or require specific treatment, separate from treatment for the primary disorder.[5] The DSM-5 proposes to use the same criteria to define insomnia as DSM-IV and the ICSD-2, but does not have separate categories for insomnias with presumed underlying causes. Furthermore, the sleep disturbance needs to be present at least 3 nights per week for at least 3 months to meet criteria as a chronic insomnia disorder.[49]

COGNITIVE BEHAVIORAL THERAPY

Rationale and Indication

Cognitive behavioral therapy (CBT) for insomnia is a brief, sleep focused, multimodal intervention that includes psychological and behavioral procedures such as sleep restriction, stimulus control, relaxation, cognitive strategies and education about sleep hygiene (Panel 5).[51,52] These therapies can be used singly, although a combined, approach is preferred because several dimensions of includes a behavioral (stimulus control, sleep restriction relaxation) component combined with a cognitive and an educational (sleep hygiene) component. The objective of CBT is to change factors that perpetuate insomnia, including behavioral factors (poor sleep habits, irregular sleep schedules), psychological factors (unrealistic expectations, worry, unhelpful beliefs), and physiological factors (mental and somatic tension, hyperarousal). The main CBT indications include persistent insomnia, primary or comorbid, and insomnia in young and older adults. Caution is advised for use of sleep restriction, which could produce daytime sleepiness or exacerbate mania in a bipolar patient. Evidence of daytime sleepiness should prompt a warning against driving or operating dangerous machinery.

Evidence for Efficacy

The 2005 US National Institutes of Health state-of-the-science conference on insomnia concluded that only two treatment modalities [CBT and benzodiazepine receptor agonists (BzRAs)] had adequate evidence to support their use in the management of chronic insomnia.[3] Evidence from meta-analyses[53-55] and systematic reviews[56-60] suggest that CBT produces moderate to large effect sizes for sleep onset latency (range from 0.41–1.05) and sleep quality (0.94–1.14), and small to moderate effect sizes for the number of awakenings (0.25–0.83), duration of awakenings (0.61–1.03), and total sleep time (0.15–0.49), 70–80% of patients achieve a therapeutic response, whereas about 40% achieve clinical remission.[61] In terms of symptom reductions, subjective sleep latency and time awake after sleep onset are reduced from an average baseline of 60–70 minutes to about 35 minutes, and total sleep time is increased by 30 minutes, from 6 to 6.5 hours. Evidence that CBT improves fatigue, quality of life, and psychological symptoms is limited.[59,62]

Clinical evidence suggests that behavioral interventions aimed at curtailing time spent in bed are especially effective for improvement of sleep continuity, whereas cognitive strategies are instrumental for reduction of psychological distress[59] and dysfunctional beliefs.[63] Education about sleep hygiene is incorporated in most treatments, but it should be seen as a minimum intervention, since alone it produces little effect on sleep.

Long-term Outcomes

The CBT produces sleep improvements that are sustained over time,[59,64] which is a clear advantage compared with drug treatment. Although interventions that restrict the amount of time spent in bed can yield slight increases (or even a reduction) of sleep time during initial treatment, this situation usually improves with time, with total sleep time often exceeding 6.5 hours at 6-month follow-ups. Even patients who respond well to short-term therapy can be vulnerable to recurrent episodes of insomnia. Long-term, maintenance therapies to prevent or minimize insomnia recurrence need to be developed and assessed.

CBT for Comorbid Insomnia

Patients with a range of medical and psychiatric disorders can benefit from CBT for insomnia.[65] For example, CBT is effective for insomnia associated with chronic pain,[66] fibromyalgia,[67] cancer,[68,69] and various medical conditions in older adults.[70,71] Likewise, treatment of insomnia in the context of co-occurring major depression[72,73] or substance misuse[74] can be helpful.

In a study that examined the effect of augmentation of an antidepressant drug with a brief symptom focused, CBT for insomnia in patients with major depressive disorder, the augmented therapy regimen produced higher remission rates for both depression (62% vs 33% for antidepressant drugs plus placebo) and insomnia (50% vs 8%).[73]

Thus, the presence of a comorbid disorder should not preclude the targeting of insomnia for treatment. Insomnia can be more severe at baseline in patients with comorbid disorders, but the absolute changes on sleep outcomes during treatment are similar to those obtained by patients with primary insomnia. For some conditions, addition of CBT to other treatment regimens or adaptation of CBT to disease specific conditions is necessary; for example, the addition of fatigue management to standard CBT has been helpful for insomnia patients with cancer[69] and traumatic brain injury.[75]

CBT for Older Adults

Insomnia is more prevalent in older adults and is more likely to be associated with other medical disorders. Findings from a meta-analysis[57] showed that treatment effect sizes were similar (moderate to large) for middle-aged and older adults for subjective measures of sleep latency, Wake after sleep onset, and sleep quality. In a systematic review McCurry and colleagues[58] concluded that multimodal CBT and sleep restriction therapy alone met criteria for empirically validated therapies, whereas evidence was insufficient to support cognitive therapy, relaxation, or education about sleep hygiene as stand-alone therapies for insomnia in older adults. Results of some studies show that older adults with comorbid medical or psychological disorders can benefit from sleep-specific treatment.[70,71,76] Rybarczyk and colleagues[71] reported that older adults with chronic obstructive pulmonary disease, osteoarthritis, or coronary artery disease benefited from group CBT as evidenced by improved sleep continuity and satisfaction and enhanced quality of life.

Discontinuation of hypnotic agents can be difficult especially after long-lasting use. A supervised and time limited withdrawal programme can ease discontinuation of hypnotic drugs in long-term users.[77-79] For example, in a study of 76 older adults who had used benzodiazepines for insomnia for nearly 20 years, treatment was effective to reduce the quantity (90% reduction) and frequency (80% reduction) of drug use, and 63% were drug-free within the 10-week intervention.[78] The addition of CBT to supervised drug withdrawal minimized rebound insomnia.

Panel 4: DSM-5 insomnia disorder 307.42[49]

a. The predominant complaint is dissatisfaction with sleep quantity or quality made by the patient (or by a caregiver or family in the case of children or elderly people)
b. Report of one or more of the following symptoms:
   - Difficulty initiating sleep; in children this symptom might be manifested as difficulty initiating sleep without caregiver intervention
   - Difficulty maintaining sleep characterized by frequent awakenings or trouble returning to sleep after awakenings (in children this symptom might be manifested as difficulty returning to sleep without caregiver intervention)
   - Early morning awakening with inability to return to sleep
   - Nonrestorative sleep
   - Persistent resistance to going to bed or bedtime struggles (children)
c. The sleep complaint is accompanied by great distress or impairment in daytime functioning as shown by the report of at least one of the following:
   - Fatigue or low energy
   - Daytime sleepiness
   - Cognitive impairments (e.g. attention, concentration, memory)
   - Mood disturbance (e.g. irritability, dysphoria)
   - Behavioral difficulties (e.g. hyperactivity, impulsivity, aggression)
   - Impaired occupational or academic function
   - Impaired interpersonal/social function
   - Negative effect on caregiver or family functioning (e.g. fatigue sleepiness)
d. The sleep difficulty occurs at least 3 nights per week
e. The sleep difficulty is present for at least 3 months
f. The sleep difficulty occurs despite adequate opportunity for sleep

Duration
- Acute insomnia (<1 month)
- Subchronic insomnia (1–3 months)
- Persistent insomnia (>3 months)

Clinically Comorbid Disorders
- Psychiatric (specify)
- Medical (specify)
- Another (specify)

PRACTICAL CONSIDERATIONS FOR CBT IMPLEMENTATION

The CBT is typically delivered in the context of four to six therapy sessions at weekly intervals, although the number of follow-up visits can vary as a function of insomnia severity, comorbidity, and patient motivation. Acute and milder forms of insomnia might need less time and be manageable in primary care clinics, but more complex cases might need to be handled by behavioral sleep medicine specialists.

CBT is generally well accepted by patients,[80] but barriers to implementation include time and scarce availability of clinicians with CBT skills. Since individual, face-to-face therapy with a sleep specialist is not always feasible, alternative treatment delivery models can improve access to CBT. With training and supervision, nurses can deliver effective CBT for insomnia in primary care settings.[62,68] Group therapy and telephone consultations represent other cost-effective methods.[74,81] Self-help approaches using printed materials[82,83] videos,[84] internet-based programmes[85] are helpful as stand-alone treatments or as additions to professionally

Panel 5: Psychological and behavioral therapies for insomnia[51]

Treatment (level of endorsement)[60]

Stimulus control therapy (standard)

Behavioral recommendations designed to reinforce the association between the bed or bedroom and sleep, and to strengthen a consistent sleep-wake schedule: (a) go to bed only when sleepy; (b) get out of bed when unable to sleep; (c) use the bed for sleep only (no reading, problem-solving in bed), (d) arise at the same time every morning; (e) avoid napping.

Sleep restriction therapy (guideline)

A method that limits the time spent in bed as close as possible to the actual sleep time, thereby producing a mild sleep deprivation, which results in more consolidated sleep. The sleep window is gradually increased throughout a few days or weeks until optimum sleep duration is achieved.

Relaxation training (standard)

Clinical procedures aimed at reduction of somatic tension (e.g. progressive muscle relaxation, autogenic training) or intrusive thoughts (e.g. imagery training, meditation) interfering with sleep, Most relaxation techniques need professional guidance initially and daily practice for a few weeks.

Cognitive therapy (insufficient evidence as single therapy)

Psychotherapeutic method aimed at alleviating excessive worries and revising misconceptions about sleep, insomnia, and daytime consequences. Specific targets include unrealistic sleep expectations, fear of the consequences of insomnia, and misconceptions of the causes of insomnia.

Sleep hygiene education (insufficient evidence as single therapy)

General guidelines about health practices (e.g. diet, exercise, substance use) and environmental factors (e.g. light, noise, temperature) that might promote or interfere with sleep: (a) avoid stimulants (e.g. caffeine, nicotine) for several hours before bedtime; (b) avoid alcohol around bedtime as it fragments sleep during the second half of the night; (c) exercise regularly, it can deepen sleep; (d) do not watch the clock; (e) keep the bedroom environment dark, quiet, and comfortable.

Cognitive behavioral therapy (standard)

A combination of any of the above behavioral (e.g. sleep restriction, stimulus control instructions, relaxation) and cognitive procedures.

administered therapy.[86] Although these different treatment delivery models can ease treatment access, they should be judged in the larger context of a stepped-care approach.[87] Some patients might need little guidance. Whereas others might need more intensive and structured therapy. Ultimately the success of CBT depends on the patients willingness to comply with treatment recommendations. To optimize outcome, follow-up visits are often necessary to monitor progress, address compliance issues, and provide guidance and support.

PHARMACOTHERAPY

Various drugs are used to treat insomnia, including over-the-counter agents (antihistamines, melatonin, and herbal preparations), prescription hypnotic drugs for insomnia (BzRAs, chronobiotic agents, and low-dose doxepin hydrochloride), and other prescription agents not specifically indicated for insomnia (antidepressants, antipsychotics, and anticonvulsants) (Table 1).

For agents not approved by the US Food and Drug Administration (FDA), scarce data exist about efficacy for improvement of sleep, and little or no data exist about improvement of daytime functions or medical outcomes for any prescription drugs. Furthermore, all agents used for promotion of sleep can potentially produce adverse effects, some of them severe, particularly in elderly people.

Over-the-Counter Agents

Antihistamines used as sleep-inducing agents include diphenhydramine or doxylamine succinate, which are often combined with pain-relieving drugs such as paracetamol or ibuprofen. Antihistamines can cause drowsiness but there are few data about their efficacy for insomnia. Side-effects include agitation, anticholinergic effects (e.g. dry mouth, urinary retention), and exacerbation of restless legs syndrome.[88] Tolerance can develop[89] and abrupt. Withdrawal can lead to rebound insomnia.

Melatonin is a hormone produced by the pineal gland that contributes to reinforcement of circadian and seasonal rhythms. Synthetic melatonin is sold as a dietary supplement in the USA, but in some countries it is deemed a prescription drug. Results from studies into the efficacy of melatonin as a hypnotic agent are inconclusive; findings from a meta-analysis showed a reduction in sleep latency of only 7.2 minutes.[90] Some evidence supports use of synthetic melatonin for insomnia related to circadian rhythm disorders such as delayed sleep phase and shin work sleep disorder.[91] Side-effects can include drowsiness, dizziness, headache, nausea, and nightmares.

A range of herbal preparations are used for insomnia, most commonly Valerian. Valerian binds to gamma aminobutyric acid (GABA) type A receptors to improve response to GABA.[92] Results of a meta-analysis showed subjective improvement in sleep quality, although improvement in quantitative measures of sleep has not been shown.[93] Side-effects can include drowsiness dizziness, and allergic reactions.

Hypnotic Agents

Most prescription hypnotic agents act as agonists at the benzodiazepine receptor; these include several benzodiazepines and the structurally distinct BzRAs (Table 1). These agents act by binding to the GABA type A receptor and are effective in promotion of sleep onset. Hypnotic agents with short half-lives (e.g. triazolam, zaleplon, and zolpidem) mainly reduce latency to sleep. Zaleplon, with its ultra-short half-life, can even be used after awakening during the night without substantial risk of daytime effects. Whereas zolpidem is more likely to produce residual effects the next day after middle-of-the-night dosing.[94,95] Agents with longer half-lives are effective in reduction of Wakefulness during sleep,[44] but can lead to hangover and daytime impairment, especially with regular nightly use.[96] Side-effects include sedation cognitive impairment, motor incoordination, ataxia, dizziness, and gastrointestinal upset. Long-term use can lead to dependence or misuse in some individuals. Abrupt discontinuation can lead to transient rebound insomnia, which can be more severe than the initial insomnia disorcler.[97,98] Adverse effects are probably more severe with use of benzodiazepines than with the newer BzRAs.[3]

Chronobiotic agents for insomnia include prolonged-release melatonin and ramelteon. Prolonged-release melatonin is indicated for poor quality sleep in adults aged 55 years or older. Ramelteon, a melatonin receptor agonist, reduces latency to sleep, but does not increase total sleep time. It has no demonstrable misuse potential, does not seem to cause next-day impairment and does not lead to rebound insomnia, by contrast with the benzodiazepines and BzRAs.[98] Ramelteon might help to promote circadian rhythm entrainment at lower doses,[99] although it is not specifically indicated for this aim.

Rare but potentially serious side effects, including abnormal sleep-related behaviors (e.g. eating, driving, or sexual activity during sleep) and severe allergic reactions can occur with use of hypnotic agents.[98,100] Abnormal behaviors during sleep are more likely when hypnotic agents are taken at higher doses or in combination with alcohol or other sedating drugs. A concern for elderly people is whether the use of hypnotic agents could increase the risk of falls; the evidence, however, suggests that both insomnia and use of sedating drugs are associated with increased falls in older adults.[101-104]

A major issue regarding the use of hypnotic agents for chronic insomnia is duration of treatment. Although insomnia is a disorder that often lasts for years or decades, relatively few long term, randomized controlled trials have been done. Results from studies of eszopiclone for 6 months in adults[105] and 12 weeks in elderly patients[106] show continued efficacy with no rebound insomnia. Results of a 24-week study of extended-release zolpidem showed long term efficacy, without evidence of statistically significant tolerance or rebound insomnia or residual day time effects.[107] Ramelteon consistently reduced latency to sleep onset in a 6-month trial in adults with chronic insomnia, without evidence of tolerance, rebound insomnia, or residual daytime effects.[108]

Most studies into the efficacy of hypnotic drugs have been undertaken in patients with primary insomnia, but clinical trials for comorbid insomnia have been done with some of the newer agents. Eszopiclone improves insomnia when given with selective serotonin reuptake inhibitors in patients with either major depression (given fluoxetine) or generalized anxiety disorder (given escitalopram);[109,110] symptoms of depression and anxiety seemed to resolve more quickly in patients receiving eszopiclone than in those given placebo. A trial of extended-release zolpidem with escitalopram showed statistically and clinically significant improvement in insomnia, but no additional reduction of anxiety symptoms, compared with the group given escitalopram and placebo.[111] Hypnotic drugs seemed to decrease symptoms of insomnia in patients with chronic pain but had no consistent effects introduction of pain.[112]

Other Prescription Agents[113-126]

Antidepressants with sedating effects are some of the most commonly prescribed drugs for insomnia although data about efficacy are generally scarce. The doses of antidepressants typically used to induce sleep are substantially less than antidepressant doses. A sedating antidepressant might be appropriate for a patient with insomnia and major depression, either when used at a therapeutic dose or in combination with another blockade of histamine and 5-HT2C receptors.[127,128] Side-effects can be serious and include substantial weight gain, abnormal lipid and glucose regulation, and increased mortality particularly in elderly people. They can exacerbate restless leg syndrome and, possibly, increase rates of parasomnias such as sleep walking and eating during the night.

Choice of Drug

The choice of drug for insomnia treatment should be based on the pharmacological characteristics of the agent (Table 1) and clinical factors related to the patient (Panel 6).[46,129] Drugs with shorter time to peak blood concentration ($\dagger_{max}$) will probably have a more rapid onset of action and aid sleep onset, whereas those with longer half-lives ($t_{1/2}$) can provide better sleep maintenance but have the potential for daytime hangover. Mechanism of action is relevant to explain side-effects; it might have increasing relevance as underlying mechanisms for sleep disorders are identified and better understood (e.g. insomnia clue to a circadian rhythm disorder could benefit from an agent that can synchronise the circadian clock).

Patient-related factors that affect drug choice include nature of insomnia symptoms (sleep initiation vs maintenance), age (doses might need to be lowered for elderly patients), response to previous treatments, and cost. Patients might have disorders that are contraindications for some choices (e.g. benzodiazepines in patients with severe sleep apnea or pulmonary disease), or disorders that make a non-First-line agent more desirable (e.g. a sedating antidepressant in a patient with major depression). Other drugs that are being taken can preclude certain choices (e.g. ramelteon should not be given to patients taking fluvoxamine).

Duration of treatment and frequency of dose depend on the clinical situation. Patients should be reassessed within a month of starting a hypnotic drug and then at intervals of at least every 6 months to assess continued effectiveness and potential side-effects. In general, hypnotic drugs should be used at the lowest effective dose and the need for continued use should be determined by attempts to wean patients from the drug periodically. However, some patients might need and benefit from long-term treatment with hypnotic drugs without pronounced adverse effects. Some patients might need nightly dosing, although intermittent dosing could be sufficient for episodic insomnia and might reduce the risks for tolerance or daytime sedation due to increased drug concentrations of longer-acting agents.

Table 1: Pharmacological treatment for insomnia

	Dones range (mg)	*Dose in elderly people (mg)*	*Half-life(h)*	*Peak plasma concentration (after administration)*	*Side-effects*
Benzodiazepine receptor agonists: benezodiazepines					
Estazolam	1–2	0.5	10–124	2	Dizziness, drowsiness, lightheadedness, ataxia, amnesia, gastrointestinal (GI) symptoms
Flurazepam	15–30	15	47–100	2	As for estazolam
Quazepam	7.5–15	7.5	25–41	1.5	As for estazolam
Temazepam	7.5–30	7.5	6–16	1	As for estazolam
Triazolam	0.25–0.50	0.125–0.250	1.5–5.5	2	As for estazolam
Benzodiazepine receptor agonists: nonbenezodiazepines					
Eszopiclone‡	2–3	1.2	5–6	1	Unpleasant taste, dry mouth, dizziness, drowsiness, amnesia, GI symptoms
Zopiclone‡	3.75–75	7.5	5	>2	As for eszopiclone
Zaleplon	10–20	5–10	1	1	Dizziness, headache, GI symptoms, drowsiness, amnesia
Zolpidem	10	5	2.5	1.6	As for zaleplon
Melatonin receptor agonist					
Melatonin, prolonged release‡	2 (2–2 hours before bedtime and after food)	2	3.5–4	3	Headache, pharyngitis, back pain, asthenia, irritability, nervousness, dizziness, somnolence, abdominal pain, constipation
Ramelteon‡	8	8	1–2.6	0.75	Drowsiness, dizziness, interaction with fluvoxamine
Antidepressants					
Amitriptyline*	50–100	20	10–28 (including the metabilite nortriptyline	4–8	Drowsiness, dizziness, confusion, blurrred vision, dry mouth, constipation, urinary retention, arrhythmias, orthostatic hypotension, weight gain, exacerbation of restless legs, periodic limb movements, or rapid eye movement sleep behavior disorder
Doxepin	75–100	25–50	8–24	2–3	As for amitriptyline
Trimipramine‡	25–200	25–100	11–23	2	As for amitriptyline
Mirtazapine*	15–45	7.5–15	20–40	2	Drowsiness, dizziness, increased appetite, constipation, weight gain
Agomelatine*‡	25–50		1–2	1–2	Can raise liver enzymes; check liver functions prior to initiation and at 6, 12, 24 weeks, and periodically thereafter Nausea, dizziness, headache, somnolence, anxiety, abdominal pain, back pain, interaction with fluvoxamine

Contd...

Contd...

	Dones range (mg)	Dose in elderly people (mg)	Half-life(h)	Peak plasma concentration (after administration)	Side-effects
Trazodone*	150–400	150	7	1	Drowsiness, dizziness, headache, blurred vision, dry mouth, arrhythmias, orthostatic hypotension, priapism
Anticonvulsants*					
Clonazepam	0.25–0.50	0.25	30–40	1–4	Drowsiness, dizziness, ataxia, depression, nervousness, reduced intellectual ability
Gabapentin	300–600	300	5–7	2–4	Drowsiness, dizziness, emotional lability, ataxia, tremor, blurred vision, diplopia, nystagmus, myalgia, peripheral edema
Tiagabine	4–8	4	7–9	0.75	Drowsiness, dizziness, ataxia, tremor, new-onset seizures in patients, without epilepsy, difficulty in concentration or attention, nervousness, asthenia, abdominal pain, diarrhea, nausea
Antipsychotics*					
Olanzapine	5–10	5	21–54	6	Drowsiness, dizziness, tremor, agitation, asthenia, extrapyramidal symptoms, dry mouth, dyspepsia, constipation, orthostatic hypotension, with gain, new-onset diabetes mellitus
Quetiapine	25–200	25	6	15	As for olanzapine

*Not approved for treatment of insomnia by the US Food and Drug Administration. *Not available in European Union.

COMBINED CBT AND DRUG TREATMENT

The CBT and drug treatment can have complementary roles in the management of insomnia. For instance, no single treatment is effective for all forms of insomnia or acceptable to all patients, even in those who respond to treatment, and few reach complete remission. Combined approaches should optimize outcome by taking advantage of the more immediate and potent effects of hypnotic agents and the more sustained effects of behavioral interventions. Comparisons of effect sizes derived from meta-analyses of these two treatment modalities suggest that CBT might have a slight advantage for measures of sleep latency and sleep quality, whereas pharmacotherapy (BZRAS) produces a more favorable outcome on total sleep time.[54,55,130]

Finding from studies that directly contrast the effects of CBT and drug treatment for insomnia[61,64, 131-136] show that these two therapies are effective in the short-term, with drugs producing faster results in the acute (first week) phase of treatment, whereas they are equally effective in the short-term (4–8 weeks). Patients given CBT maintain their improvements with time, whereas those given drugs alone tend to relapse after discontinuation. Combined interventions have a slight advantage compared with single modalities during initial treatment, but this advantage does not always persist with time. Long-term effects are more equivocal with some studies suggesting that a combined intervention produces more sustained benefits than drugs alone,[131,132] whereas others suggest more variability across patients for long-term outcomes.[64,135]

Two studies have examined the effect of sequential therapies. In a small investigation,[133] the best outcome was obtained when CBT was introduced first in the sequence, irrespective of whether it was used alone or with drug treatment. In a larger study of 160 patients with persistent insomnia, a two-stage treatment approach was used to assess the added benefit of drugs to CBT and the effect of different maintenance therapies on long-term outcomes.[61] CBT used singly or combined with drug treatment produced similar rates of treatment responders (60% vs 61%) and remitters (39% vs 44%) after the acute 6-week treatment phase. After the 6-month extended treatment, a higher remission rate was reported for combined therapy than for CBT alone (57% vs 45%) and this higher remission rate was sustained throughout the 24-month follow-ups. In patients initially given combined therapy those who continued with maintenance CBT but discontinued drug treatment during extended therapy achieved better long-term outcomes than those who continued using drugs intermittently. This finding suggests that, although drugs can provide an initial added benefit, discontinuation of drug treatment. While patients are still receiving CBT is the best option.

Panel 6: Guidelines for choice of pharmacotherapy agent

The American Academy of Sleep Medicine clinical guideline for management of insomnia recommends the following sequence of choices for pharmacotherapy[46]

- Short or intermediate-acting benzodiazepine-receptor agonists (BzRA) or Ramelteon. No particular drug recommended; choice should depend on clinical factors.
- Alternative BZRA or ramelteon. Choice based on response to first drug, e.g. if duration of action insufficient, choose an agent with a longer half-life.
- Sedating low-dose antidepressant. For patients with depressive symptoms, treatment failures.
- Combination of BzRA add antidepressant. Combination therapy might improve efficacy while minimizing toxicity by use of agents at lower doses.

A potential explanation of these findings is that behavioral and attitudinal changes are often essential to sustain sleep improvements. Attribution of therapeutic benefits to the hypnotic drug alone, without integration of self-management skills, could place a patient at greater risk for recurrence of insomnia once drug treatment is discontinued. Availability of drugs might undermine a patients efforts and motivation for behavioral changes. Additional research is needed to assess the effects of combined therapies and examine the best methods for their integration.

Evidence for efficacy of other prescription drugs (e.g. tiagabine, pregabalin, quetiapine, olanzapine) is insufficient to recommend their use for primary insomnia, but they could be helpful in patients who have other indications for their use (e.g. chronic pain conditions, psychiatric disorders).

Agents not recommended for use include alcohol, chloral hydrate, and non-barbiturate non-benzodiazepine drugs such as meprobamate because of adverse effects, toxic effects, and risk for misuse and dependence. Antihistamines should be avoided because of their potential for adverse effects and scarce efficacy data. Long-term use of over-the-counter agents such as valerian and melatonin is generally not recommended because of the absence of safety or efficacy data.

CONCLUSION

Insomnia is a prevalent and costly public health problem. It is associated with substantial long-term effects on psychological, occupational, and physical functioning. Despite advances in diagnosis and management, insomnia is still under-recognized and often goes untreated. Although insomnia often presents with a comorbid medical or psychiatric disorder, it usually warrants separate treatment. Two therapeutic options-CBT and approved hypnotic drugs-have adequate evidence from clinical trials to support their use in the management it insomnia. Nonetheless, not all patients respond to these interventions. Important challenges for the future include the need to validate treatment algorithms that would take into account insomnia phenotypes, patient preference, and second line therapies for patients who do not respond to first line treatment. There is also an urgent need for more public education about sleep and broader dissemination of evidence-based therapies for insomnia, and education and training prepare health-practitioners to attend and treat insomnia complaints according to clinical guidelines.

REFERENCES

1. Daley M, Morin CM, LeBlanc M, Gregoire JP, Savard J. The economic burden of insomnia: direct and indirect costs for individuals with insomnia syndrome, insomnia symptoms, and good sleepers. Sleep. 2009;32:55-64.
2. Daley M, Morin CM, LeBlanc M, et al. Insomnia and its relationship to health-care utilization, work absenteeism, productivity and accidents. Sleep Med. 2009;10:427-38.
3. National Institutes of Health. National Institutes of Health state of the science conference statement on manifestations and management of chronic insomnia in adults; 2005. pp.13-5. Sleep 2005;28:1049-57.
4. Sivertsen B, Overland S, Neckelmann D, et al. The long-term effect of insomnia on work disability: the HUNT-2 historical cohort study. Am J Epidemiol. 2006;163:1018-24.
5. American Academy of Sleep Medicine. International classification of sleep disorders: diagnostic and coding manuel, 2nd edition. Westchester: American Academy of Sleep Medicine; 2005.
6. Edinger JD, Bonnet MH, Bootzin RR, et al. for the American Academy of Sleep Medicine Work Group Derivation of research diagnostic criteria for insomnia: report of an American Academy of Sleep Medicine Work Group. Sleep. 2004;27:1567-96.
7. Buysse DJ, Thompson W, Scott J, et al. Daytime symptoms in primary insomnia: a prospective analysis using ecological momentary assessment. Sleep Med. 2007;8:198-208.
8. Morin CM, LeBlanc M, Daley M, Gregoire JP, Merette C. Epidemiology of insomnia: prevalence, self-help treatments, consultations, and determinants of help-seeking behaviors. Sleep Med. 2006;7:123-30.
9. Perlis ML, Smith MT, Andrews PJ, Orff H, Giles DE. Beta/Gamma EEG activity in patients with primary and secondary insomnia and good sleeper controls. Sleep. 2001;24:110-17.
10. Shekleton JA, Rogers NL, Rajaratnam SM. Searching for the daytime impairments of primary insomnia. Sleep Med Rev. 2010;14:47-60.
11. Fortier-Brochu E, Beaulieu-Bonneau S, Ivers H, Morin CM. Insomnia and daytime cognitive performance: a meta-analysis. Sleep Med Rev. 2011;published online May 31. DOI:10.1016/j.smrv.2011.03.008.
12. Ohayon MM. Epidemiology of insomnia: what we know and what we still need to learn. Sleep Med Rev. 2002;6:97-111.
13. Roth T, Jaeger S, Jin R, Kalsekar A, Stang PE, Kessler RC. Sleep problems, comorbid mental disorders, and role functioning in

the national comorbidity survey replication. Biol Psychiatry. 2006;60:1364-71.

14. Ohayon MM, Reynolds CF 3rd. Epidemiological and clinical relevance of insomnia diagnosis algorithms according to the DSM-IV and the International Classification of Sleep Disorders (JCSD). Sleep Med. 2009;10:952-60.
15. Hohagen F, Rink K, Kappler C, et al. Prevalence and treatment of insomnia in general practice. A longitudinal study. Eur Arch Psychiatry Clin Neurosci. 1993;242:329-36.
16. Simon GE, VonKorff M. Prevalence, burden, and treatment of insomnia in primary care. Am Psychiatry. 1997;154:1417-23.
17. Aikens JE, Rouse ME. Help-seeking for insomnia among adult patients in primary care. J Am Board Fam Pract. 2005;18: 257-61.
18. Pearson NI, Johnson LL, Nahin RL. Insomnia, trouble sleeping, and complementary and alternative medicine: analysis of the 2002 national health interview survey data. Arch Intern Med. 2006;166:1775-82.
19. Smith MT, Haythornthwaite JA. How do sleep disturbance and chronic pain inter-relate? Insights from the longitudinal and cognitive-behavioral clinical trials literature. Sleep Med Rev. 2004;8;119-32.
20. Chang PP, Ford DE, Mead LA, Cooper-Patrick L, Klag MJ. Insomnia in young men and subsequent depression. The Johns Hopkins Precursors Study. Am J Epidemiol. 1997; 146:105-14.
21. Breslau N, Roth T, Rosenthal L, Andreski P. Sleep disturbance and psychiatric disorders: a longitudinal epidemiological study of young adults. Biol Psychiatry. 1996;39:411-18.
22. Jansson-Frojmark M, Lindblom K. A bidirectional relationship between anxiety and depression, and insomnia? A prospective study in the general population. J Psychosam Res. 2008; 64:443-49.
23. Nierenberg AA, Husain MM, Wisniewski SR, et al. Residual symptoms after remission of major depressive disorder with citalopram and risk of relapse;a STAR*D report. Psychol Med. 2010;40:41-50.
24. Nierenberg AA, Keefe BR, Leslie VC, et al. Residual symptoms in depressed patients wire respond acutely to fluoxetine. J Clin Psychiatry. 1999;60:221-5.
25. Perlis ML, Giles DE, Buysse DJ, Tu X, Kupfer DJ. Self-reported sleep disturbance as a prodromal symptom in recurrent depression. J Affect Disord. 1997;42:209-12.
26. Bastien CH, Vallieres A, Morin CM. Precipitating factors of insomnia. Behav Sleep Med. 2004;2:50-62.
27. Vallieres A, Ivers H, Bastien CH, Beaulieu-Bonneau S, Morin CM. Variability and predictability in sleep patterns of chronic insomniacs. J Sleep Res. 2005;14:447-53.
28. Buysse DJ, Angst J, Gamma A, Ajdacic V, Eich D, Rossler W. Prevalence, course, and comorbidity of insomnia and depression in young adults. Sleep. 2008;31;473-80.
29. Morphy H, Dunn KM, Lewis M, Boardman HF, Croft PR. Epidemiology of insomnia: a longitudinal study in a UK population. Sleep. 2007;30:274-80.
30. Morin CM, Belanger L, LeBlanc M, et al. The natural history of insomnia: a population-based 3-year longitudinal study. Arch Intern Med. 2009:169:447-53.
31. Suka M, Yeshida K, Sugimori H. Persistent insomnia is a predictor of hypertension in Japanese male workers. J Occup Health. 2003;45:344-50.
32. Dew MA, Hoch CC, Buysse DJ, et al. Healthy older adults' sleep predicts all-cause mortality at 4 to 19 years of follow-up. Psychosom Med. 2003;65:63-73.
33. Vgontzas AN, Liao D, Pejovic S, et al. Insomnia with short sleep duration and mortality: the Penn State cohort. Sleep. 2010;33:115-64.
34. Spielman AJ, Glovinsky PB. The varied nature of insomnia. In: Hauri P (Ed). Case studies in insomnia. New York: Plenum Press; 1991. pp.1-15.
35. Deuschle M, Schredl M, Schilling C, et al. Association between a serotonin transporter length polymorphism and primary insomnia. Sleep. 2010;33:343-47.
36. Bonnet MH, Arand DL. Hyperarousal and insomnia: state of the science. Sleep Med Rev. 2010;14:9-15.
37. Riemann D, Spiegelhalder K, Feige B, et al. The hyperarousal model of insomnia: a review of the concept and its evidence. Sleep Med Rev. 2010;14:19-31.
38. Lanfranchi PA, Pennestri MH, Fradette L, et al. Night-time blood pressure in normotensive subjects with chronic insomnia: implications for cardiovascular risk. Sleep. 2009;32:760-6.
39. Benca RM, Obermeyer WH, Thisted RA, Gillin JC. Sleep and psychiatric disorders. A meta-analysis. Arch Gen Psychiatry. 1992;49:651-68.
40. Nofzinger EA, Buysse DJ, Germain A, Price JC, Miewald JM, Kupfer DJ. Functional neuroimaging evidence for hyperarousal in insomnia. Am J Psychiatry. 2004;161:2126-8.
41. Beaulieu-Bonneau S, LeBlanc M, Merette C, Dauvilliers Y, Morin CM. Family history of insomnia in a population-based sample. Sleep 2007;30:1739-45.
42. Altena E, Vrenken H, Van Der Werf YD, van den Heuvel OA, Van Someren EJ. Reduced orbitofrontal and parietal gray matter in chronic insomnia: a voxel-based morphometric study. Biol Psychiatry. 2010;67:182-5.
43. Riemann D, Voderholzer U, Spiegelhalder K, et al. Chronic insomnia and MRI-measured hippocampal volumes: a pilot study. Sleep. 2007;30:955-8.
44. Benca RM. Diagnosis and treatment of chronic insomnia: a review. Psychiatr Serv. 2005;56:332-43.
45. Chesson A Jr, Hartse K, Anderson WM, et al. Practice parameters for the evaluation of chronic insomnia. An American Academy of Sleep Medicine report. Standards of Practice Committee of the American Academy of Sleep Medicine. Sleep. 2000;23;237-41.
46. Schutte-Rodin S, Broch L, Buysse D, Dorsey C, Sateia M. Clinical guideline for the evaluation and management of chronic insomnia in adults. J Clin Sleep Med. 2008;4:487-504.
47. Littner M, Hirshkowitz M, Kramer M, et al. For the American Academy of Sleep Medicine Standards of Practice Committee.

Practice parameters for using polysomnography to evaluate insomnia: an update. Sleep. 2003;26:754-60.
48. Luyster FS, Buysse DJ, Strollo PJ. Comorbid insomnia and obstructive sleep apnea: challenges for clinical practice and research. J Clin Sleep Med. 2010;6:196-204.
49. American Psychiatric Association. DSM-5 Development. Sleep-wake disorders.*http://www.dsm5.org/proposedrevision/Pages/Sleep-WakeDisorders.aspx.* (accessed Aug 1, 2011).
50. Sateia MJ, Doghramji K, Hauri PJ, Morin CM. Evaluation of chronic insomnia. An American Academy of Sleep Medicine review. Sleep. 2000;23:243-308.
51. Morin CM, Espie CA. Insomnia: a clinical guide to assessment and treatment. New York: Kluwer Academic/Plenum; 2003.
52. Edinger JD, Carney CE. Overcoming insomnia: a cognitive-behavioral therapy approach-therapist guide. New York: Oxford University Press; 2008.
53. Murtagh DR, Greenwood KM. Identifying effective psychological treatments for insomnia: a meta-analysis. J Consult Clin Psychol. 1995;63:79-89.
54. Morin CM, Culbert JP, Schwartz SM. Nonpharmacological interventions for insomnia: a meta-analysis of treatment efficacy. Am J Psychiatry. 1994;151:1172-80.
55. Smith MT, Perlis ML, Park A, et al. Comparative meta-analysis of pharmacotherapy and behavior therapy for persistent insomnia. Am J Psychiatry. 2002;159:5-11.
56. Morin CM, Hauri PJ, Espie CA, Spielman AJ, Buysse DJ, Bootzin RR. Nonpharmacologic treatment of chronic insomnia. An American Academy of Sleep Medicine review. Sleep. 1999;22:1134-56.
57. Irwin MR, Cole JC, Nicassio PM. Comparative meta-analysis of behavioral interventions for insomnia and their efficacy in middle-aged adults and in older adults 55+ years of age. Health Psychol. 2006;25:3-14.
58. McCurry SM, Logsdon RG, Teri L, Vitiello MV. Evidence-based psychological treatments for insomnia in older adults. Psychol Aging. 2007;22:18-27.
59. Morin CM, Bootzin RR, Buysse DJ, et al. Psychological and behavioral treatment of insomnia: update of the recent evidence (1998—2004). Sleep. 2006;29:1398-1414.
60. Morgenthaler T, Kramer M, Alessi C, et al. For the American Academy of Sleep Medicine. Practice parameters for the psychological and behavioral treatment of insomnia: an update. An American academy of sleep medicine report. Sleep. 2006;29:1415-9.
61. Morin CM, Vallieres A, Guay B, et al. Cognitive behavioral therapy, singly and combined with medication, for persistent insomnia: a randomized controlled trial. JAMA. 2009;301: 2005-15.
62. Espie CA, MacMahon KM, Kelly HL, et al. Randomized clinical effectiveness trial of nurse-administered small-group cognitive behavior therapy for persistent insomnia in general practice. Sleep. 2007;30:574-84.
63. Morin CM, Blais F, Savard J. Are changes in beliefs and attitudes about sleep related to sleep improvements in the treatment of insomnia? Behav Res Ther. 2002;40:741-52.
64. Morin CM, Colecchi C, Stone J, Sood R, Brink D. Behavioral and pharmacological therapies for late-life insomnia: a randomized controlled trial. JAMA. 1999;281:991-9.
65. Smith MT, Huang MI, Manber R. Cognitive behavior therapy for chronic insomnia occurring within the context of medical and psychiatric disorders. Clin Psychol Rev. 2005;25:559-92.
66. Currie SR, Wilson KG, Pontefract AJ, deLaplante L. Cognitive-behavioral treatment of insomnia secondary to chronic pain. J Consult Clin Psychol. 2000;68:407-16.
67. Edinger JD, Wohlgemuth WK, Krystal AD, Rice JR. Behavioral insomnia therapy for fibromyalgia patients: a randomized clinical trial. Arch Intern Med. 2005;165:2527-35.
68. Espie CA, Fleming L, Cassidy J, et al. Randomized controlled clinical effectiveness trial of cognitive behavior therapy compared with treatment as usual for persistent insomnia in patients with cancer. J Clin Oncol. 2008;26:4651-8.
69. Savard J, Simard S, Ivers H, Morin CM. Randomized study on the efficacy of cognitive-behavioral therapy for insomnia secondary to breast cancer, part I: sleep and psychological effects. J Clin Oncol. 2005;23:6083-96.
70. Lichstein KL, Wilson NM, Johnson CT. Psychological treatment of secondary insomnia. Psychol Aging. 2000;15:232-40.
71. Rybarczyk B, Stepanski E, Fogg L, Lopez M, Barry P, Davis A. A placebo-controlled test of cognitive-behavioral therapy for comorbid insomnia in older adults. J Consult Clin Psychol. 2005;73:1164-74.
72. Taylor DJ, Lichstein KL, Weinstock J, Sanford S, Temple JR. A pilot study of cognitive-behavioral therapy of insomnia in people with mild depression. Behav Ther. 2007;38:49-57.
73. Manber R, Edinger JD, Gress JL, San Pedro-Salcedo MG, Kuo TF, Kalista T. Cognitive behavioral therapy for insomnia enhances depression outcome in patients with comorbid major depressive disorder and insomnia. Sleep. 2008;31:489-95.
74. Currie SR, Clark S, Hodgins DC, El-Guebaly N. Randomized controlled trial of brief cognitive-behavioural interventions for insomnia in recovering alcoholics. Addiction. 2004;99:1121-32.
75. Ouellet MC, Morin CM. Efficacy of cognitive-behavioral therapy for insomnia associated with traumatic brain injury: a single-case experimental design. Arch Phys Med Rehabil. 2007;88:1581-92.
76. Pallesen S, Nordhus IH, Kvale G, et al. Behavioral treatment of insomnia in older adults: An open clinical trial comparing two interventions. Behav Res Ther. 2003;41:31-48.
77. Morgan K, Dixon S, Mathers N, Thompson J, Tomeny M. Psychological treatment for insomnia in the management of long-term hypnotic drug use: a pragmatic randomised controlled trial. Br J Gen Pract. 2003;53:923-8.
78. Morin CM, Bastien C, Guay B, et al. Randomized clinical trial of supervised tapering and cognitive behavior therapy to facilitate benzodiazepine discontinuation in older adults with chronic insomnia. Am J Psychiatry. 2004;161:332-42.
79. Soeffing JP, Lichstein KL, Nau SD, et al. Psychological treatment of insomnia in hypnotic-dependant older adults. Sleep Med. 2008;9:165-71.

80. Vincent N, Lionberg C. Treatment preference and patient satisfaction in chronic insomnia. Sleep. 2001;24:411-7.
81. Bastien CH, Morin CM, Ouellet MC, Blais FC, Bouchard S. Cognitive-behavioral therapy for insomnia: comparison of individual therapy, group therapy, and telephone consultations. J Consult Clin Psychol. 2004;72:653-9.
82. Belleville G, Guay C, Guay B, Morin CM. Hypnotic taper with or without self-help treatment: a randomized clinical trial. J Consult Clin Psychol. 2007;75:325-35.
83. Mimeault V, Morin CM. Self-help treatment for insomnia: bibliotherapy with and without professional guidance. J Consult Clin Psychol. 1999;67:511-9.
84. Savard J, Villa J, Simard S, Ivers H, Morin CM. Feasibility of a self-help treatment for insomnia comorbid with cancer. Psychooncology. 201010.1002/pon.1818.
85. Ritterband LM, Thorndike FP, Gonder-Frederick LA, et al. Efficacy of an internet-based behavioral intervention for adults with insomnia. Arch Gen Psychiatry. 2009;66:692-8.
86. van Straten A, Cuijpers P. Self-help therapy for insomnia: a meta-analysis. Sleep Med Rev. 2009;13:61-71.
87. Espie CA. "Stepped care": a health technology solution for delivering cognitive behavioral therapy as a first line insomnia treatment. Sleep. 2009;32:1549-58.
88. Hening WA, Allen RP, Chokroverty S, Earley CJ. Restless Legs Syndrome. Philadelphia: Saunders; 2009.
89. Richardson GS, Roehrs TA, Rosenthal L, Koshorek G, Roth T. Tolerance to daytime sedative effects of H1 antihistamines. J Clin Psychopharmacol. 2002;22:511-15.
90. Buscemi N, Vandermeer B, Hooton N, et al. The efficacy and safety of exogenous melatonin for primary sleep disorders. A meta-analysis. J Gen Intern Med. 2005;20:1151-8.
91. Sack RL, Auckley D, Auger RR, et al. For the American Academy of Sleep Medicine. Circadian rhythm sleep disorders: part I, basic principles, shift work and jet lag disorders. An American Academy of Sleep Medicine review. Sleep. 2007;30:1460-83.
92. Benke D, Barberis A, Kopp S, et al. GABA A receptors as in vivo substrate for the anxiolytic action of valerenic acid, a major constituent of valerian root extracts. Neuropharmacology. 2009;56:174-81.
93. Fernandez-San-Martin MI, Masa-Font R, Palacios-Soler L, et al. Effectiveness of Valerian on insomnia: a meta-analysis of randomized placebo-controlled trials. Sleep Med. 2010;11:505-11.
94. Hindmarch I, Patat A, Stanley N, Paty I, Rigney U. Residual effects of zaleplon and zolpidem following middle of the night administration five hours to one hour before awakening. Hum Psychopharmacol. 2001;16:159-67.
95. Zammit GK, Corser B, Doghramji K, et al. Sleep and residual sedation after administration of zaleplon, zolpidem, and placebo during experimental middle-of-the-night awakening. J Clin Sleep Med. 2006;2:417-23.
96. Holbrook AM, Crowther R, Lotter A, Cheng C, King D. Meta-analysis of benzodiazepine use in the treatment of insomnia. CMAJ. 2000;162:225-33.
97. Kales A, Manfredi RL, Vgontzas AN, et al. Rebound insomnia after only brief and intermittent use of rapidly eliminated benzodiazepines. Clin Pharmacol Ther. 1991;49:468-76.
98. Zammit G. Comparative tolerability of newer agents for insomnia. Drug Saf. 2009;32:735-48.
99. Richardson GS, Zee PC, Wang-Weigand S, Rodriguez L, Peng X. Circadian phase-shifting effects of repeated ramelteon administration in healthy adults. J Clin Sleep Med. 2008;4:456-61.
100. Hoque R, Chesson AL. Zolpidem-induced sleepwalking, sleep related eating disorder, and sleep-driving: fluorine-18-fluorodeoxyglucose positron emission tomography analysis, and a literature review of other unexpected clinical effects of zolpidem. J Clin Sleep Med. 2009;5:471-6.
101. Avidan AY, Fries BE, James ML, et al. Insomnia and hypnotic use, recorded in the minimum data set, as predictors of falls and hip fractures in Michigan nursing homes. J Am Geriatr Soc. 2005;53:955-62.
102. Brassington GS, King AC, Bliwise DL. Sleep problems as a risk factor for falls in a sample of community-dwelling adults aged 64-99 years. J Am Geriatr Soc. 2000;48:1234-40.
103. Wang PS, Bohn RL, Glynn RJ, Mogun H, Avorn J. Zolpidem use and hip fractures in older people. J Am Geriatr Soc. 2001;49:1685-90.
104. Mendelson WB. Clinical distinctions between long-acting and short-acting benzodiazepines. J Clin Psychiatry. 1992;53 (Suppl):4-7.
105. Krystal AD, Walsh JK, Laska E, et al. Sustained efficacy of eszopiclone over 6 months of nightly treatment: results of a randomized, double-blind, placebo-controlled study in adults with chronic insomnia. Sleep. 2003;26:793-9.
106. Ancoli-Israel S, Krystal AD, McCall WV, et al. A 12-week, randomized, double-blind, placebo-controlled study evaluating the effect of eszopiclone 2 mg on sleep/wake function in older adults with primary and comorbid insomnia. Sleep. 2010;33:225-34.
107. Krystal AD, Erman M, Zammit GK, Soubrane C, Roth T. Long-term efficacy and safety of zolpidem extended-release 12·5 mg, administered 3 to 7 nights per week for 24 weeks, in patients with chronic primary insomnia: a 6-month, randomized, double-blind, placebo-controlled, parallel-group, multicenter study. Sleep. 2008;31:79-90.
108. Mayer G, Wang-Weigand S, Roth-Schechter B, Lehmann R, Staner C, Partinen M. Efficacy and safety of 6-month nightly ramelteon administration in adults with chronic primary insomnia. Sleep. 2009;32:351-60.
109. Pollack M, Kinrys G, Krystal A, et al. Eszopiclone coadministered with escitalopram in patients with insomnia and comorbid generalized anxiety disorder. Arch Gen Psychiatry. 2008;65:551-62.

110. Fava M, McCall WV, Krystal A, et al. Eszopiclone co-administered with fluoxetine in patients with insomnia coexisting with major depressive disorder. Biol Psychiatry. 2006;59:1052-60.
111. Fava M, Asnis GM, Shrivastava R, et al. Zolpidem extended-release improves sleep and next-day symptoms in comorbid insomnia and generalized anxiety disorder. J Clin Psychopharmacol. 2009;29:222-30.
112. Roehrs TA. Does effective management of sleep disorders improve pain symptoms?. Drugs. 2009;69 (Suppl 2):5-11.
113. Wiegand MH. Antidepressants for the treatment of insomnia: a suitable approach?. Drugs. 2008;68:2411-7.
114. Mayers AG, Baldwin DS. Antidepressants and their effect on sleep. Hum Psychopharmacol. 2005;20:533-59.
115. Ferguson SA, Rajaratnam SM, Dawson D. Melatonin agonists and insomnia. Expert Rev Neurother. 2010;10:305-18.
116. Buscemi N, Vandermeer B, Friesen C, et al. The efficacy and safety of drug treatments for chronic insomnia in adults: a meta-analysis of RCTs. J Gen Intern Med. 2007;22:1335-50.
117. Roth T, Rogowski R, Hull S, et al. Efficacy and safety of doxepin 1 mg, 3 mg, and 6 mg in adults with primary insomnia. Sleep. 2007;30:1555-61.
118. Scharf M, Rogowski R, Hull S, et al. Efficacy and safety of doxepin 1 mg, 3 mg, and 6 mg in elderly patients with primary insomnia: a randomized, double-blind, placebo-controlled crossover study. J Clin Psychiatry. 2008;69:1557-64.
119. Wilson S, Argyropoulos S. Antidepressants and sleep: a qualitative review of the literature. Drugs. 2005;65:927-47.
120. Walsh JK. Enhancement of slow wave sleep: implications for insomnia. J Clin Sleep Med. 2009;5:S27-S32.
121. Roth T, Wright KP, Walsh J. Effect of tiagabine on sleep in elderly subjects with primary insomnia: a randomized, double-blind, placebo-controlled study. Sleep. 2006;29:335-41.
122. Walsh JK, Zammit G, Schweitzer PK, Ondrasik J, Roth T. Tiagabine enhances slow wave sleep and sleep maintenance in primary insomnia. Sleep Med. 2006;7:155-61.
123. Walsh JK, Perlis M, Rosenthal M, Krystal A, Jiang J, Roth T. Tiagabine increases slow-wave sleep in a dose-dependent fashion without affecting traditional efficacy measures in adults with primary insomnia. J Clin Sleep Med. 2006;2:35-41.
124. Montgomery SA, Herman BK, Schweizer E, Mandel FS. The efficacy of pregabalin and benzodiazepines in generalized anxiety disorder presenting with high levels of insomnia. Int Clin Psychopharmacol. 2009;24:214-22.
125. Crofford LJ, Rowbotham MC, Mease PJ, et alfor the Pregabalin 1008—105 Study Group. Pregabalin for the treatment of fibromyalgia syndrome: results of a randomized, double-blind, placebo-controlled trial. Arthritis Rheum. 2005;52:1264-73.
126. Russell IJ, Crofford LJ, Leon T, et al. The effects of pregabalin on sleep disturbance symptoms among individuals with fibromyalgia syndrome. Sleep Med. 2009;10:604-10.
127. Cohrs S. Sleep disturbances in patients with schizophrenia: impact and effect of antipsychotics. CNS Drugs. 2008;22:939-62.
128. Wine JN, Sanda C, Caballero J. Effects of quetiapine on sleep in nonpsychiatric and psychiatric conditions. Ann Pharmacother. 2009;43:707-13.
129. Krystal AD. A compendium of placebo-controlled trials of the risks/benefits of pharmacological treatments for insomnia: the empirical basis for U.S. clinical practice. Sleep Med Rev. 2009;13:265-74.
130. Nowell PD, Mazumdar S, Buysse DJ, Dew MA, Reynolds CF, Kupfer DJ. Benzodiazepines and zolpidem for chronic insomnia: a meta-analysis of treatment efficacy. JAMA. 1997;278:2170-7.
131. Milby JB, Williams V, Hall JN, Khuder S, McGill T, Wooten V. Effectiveness of combined triazolam-behavioral therapy for primary insomnia. Am J Psychiatry. 1993;150:1259-60.
132. McClusky HY, Milby JB, Switzer PK, Williams V, Wooten V. Efficacy of behavioral versus triazolam treatment in persistent sleep-onset insomnia. Am J Psychiatry. 1991;148:121-6.
133. Vallieres A, Morin CM, Guay B. Sequential combinations of drug and cognitive behavioral therapy for chronic insomnia: an exploratory study. Behav Res Ther. 2005;43:1611-30.
134. Sivertsen B, Omvik S, Pallesen S, et al. Cognitive behavioral therapy vs zopiclone for treatment of chronic primary insomnia in older adults: a randomized controlled trial. JAMA. 2006;295:2851-8.
135. Hauri PJ. Can we mix behavioral therapy with hypnotics when treating insomniacs?. Sleep. 1997;20:1111-8.
136. Jacobs GD, Pace-Schott EF, Stickgold R, Otto MW. Cognitive behavior therapy and pharmacotherapy for insomnia: a randomized controlled trial and direct comparison. Arch Intern Med. 2004;164:1888-96.

CHAPTER

28 Eating Disorders

Prabha S Chandra, Santosh K Chaturvedi, AW Jagdeesh

CLASSIFICATION AND DIAGNOSIS

Diagnosis is challenging because diagnostic symptoms and associated behaviors substantially overlap across the range of eating disorders.[1] For example, extreme dietary restraint, binge eating, and overvalued ideas about weight and shape can be present in all forms of eating disorder. Additionally, the subjective interpretation and justification behind diagnostic behaviors is often not clear or is limited by developmental constraints (as in childhood anorexia nervosa), further complicating diagnosis.

In the diagnostic and statistical manual of mental disorders fourth edition (DSM-IV),[2] three broad categories are delineated: anorexia nervosa, bulimia nervosa, and eating disorder not otherwise specified. The international classification of diseases tenth revision (ICD-10) has three categories: anorexia nervosa, bulimia nervosa, and atypical eating disorder.[3] Briefly, anorexia nervosa is characterized by extremely low bodyweight and a fear of its increase; bulimia nervosa comprises repeated binge eating, followed by behaviors to counteract it. The category of eating disorder not otherwise specified encompasses variants of these disorders, but with subthreshold symptoms (e.g. menstruation still present despite clinically significant weight loss, purging without objective binging). Panel 1 shows some key symptoms of eating disorders in general. The weight criteria used for diagnosis need to be adjusted for age,[4] height, sex, and the developmental weight trajectory of the individual.

This panel outlines the most common symptoms of eating disorder. A range of symptoms caused by starvation are also present in anorexia nervosa, which are not all detailed here. All these symptoms are not usually volunteered by the patient and often have to be gently elicited or are noted by informants.

More than 50% of cases in the community fall into the category termed eating disorder not otherwise specified (or atypical).[5] Proposals to reduce the specificity of some of the diagnostic criteria in anorexia nervosa and bulimia nervosa have been made, which would reduce the proportion of cases that fall within the not-otherwise-specified category.[6]

Panel 1: Common symptoms in eating disorders

Behaviors

Restrictive behavior

- Cutting back on amount of food eaten
- Strict rules about eating (e.g. time of day, specific macronutrient content)
- Prolonged fasting (greater than 8 waking hours)
- Ritualized behavior associated with the purchase, preparation, and consumption of food
- Little variety in foods (e.g. extreme vegan diets, avoidance of fat, etc.)
- Avoidance of social eating
- Secret eating
- Social competitiveness around eating

Binge eating

- Eating an amount of food in a discrete time that is considered excessive in view of the situational context (objective)
- Eating an amount of food that is not excessive in view of the context but is considered large by the individual because of associated feelings of loss of control over eating (subjective)

Associated features of binge eating

- Eating more rapidly than normal
- Eating until uncomfortably full
- Eating large amounts when not hungry
- Eating alone because of embarrassment
- Feeling disgusted, depressed, or very guilty because of eating

Purgative behavior

- Self-induced vomiting; spitting
- Misuse of laxatives, diuretics, diet pills, etc.

Excessive exercise

- Intense, highly driven exercising of a compulsive nature
- The drive to exercise is associated with impaired social or physical function, or both

Drinking

- Limited drinking (<0.5 L per day)
- Excess drinking (>1.5 L per day)

Body checking

- Repeated weighing
- Pinching or measuring the size of body parts (e.g. circumference of wrist)
- Repeatedly checking the protrusion of specific bones

Contd...

Contd...

- Checking that specific clothes fit
- Mirror gazing
- Comparison with others' bodies

Body avoidance

- Avoidance of behaviors above (e.g. refusal to weigh, avoidance of mirrors, wearing bulky clothes)

Psychopathology

Body image disturbance

- Weight and shape concerns (e.g. preoccupation with weight, shape, or both)
- Overvaluation of shape and weight in determination of self-worth
- Minimization or denial of symptom severity
- Disturbance in the way body is experienced
- Intense fear of weight gain, even though underweight

Physical symptoms

- Weight loss or failure of growth with associated features of starvation, e.g. amenorrhea
- Absence of at least three consecutive menstrual cycles (women)
- Reduced libido
- Reduction in waking erections (men)
- Reduced beard growth in men
- Sensitivity to cold
- Weakness, fatigue, etc.

Subgroups within obesity with mental or behavioural components, such as binge eating disorder and night eating syndrome, can be delineated.[7]

Binge eating disorder is a subcategory of eating disorder not otherwise specified, and is defined as frequent binge eating distinguished from bulimia nervosa by the absence of recurrent inappropriate compensatory behaviors. Hence binge eating disorder is often associated with obesity. Transition from severe restriction into binge eating behavior is common;[8] however, the reverse process (a shift from binge eating into restriction) is less usual. The criteria for diagnosis of binge eating disorder in DSM-IV appendix B include associated behavioural and affective features,[2] and these criteria have been extensively used in research in the past 15 years. Support is growing for recognition of binge eating disorder as a specific entity[9] on the basis of taxometric analyses,[10] family aggregation studies,[11] treatment response research,[12] and studies of clinical course.[13]

Furthermore, interest is growing in a transdiagnostic approach to eating disorders, both within[14] and outside the category of eating disorders, with proposals for links to the obsessive compulsive and autistic spectrum of disorders[15] and anxiety and mood disorders.[16,17] Several articles present the arguments for diagnostic change in DSM-5.[7,18]

PSYCHIATRIC COMORBIDITY

Comorbidity is the rule rather than the exception for patients with eating disorders.[19,20] Developmental disorders (e.g. those of the autistic spectrum and attention-deficit

DSM-5 Diagnostic criteria for anorexia nervosa

a. Restriction of energy intake relative to requirements, leading to a significantly low body weight in the context of age, sex, developmental trajectory, and physical health. *Significantly low weight* is defined as a weight that is less than minimally normal or, for children and adolescents, less than that minimally expected.
b. Intense fear of gaining weight or of becoming fat, or persistent behavior that interferes with weight gain, even though at a significantly low weight.
c. Disturbance in the way in which one's body weight or shape is experienced, undue influence of body weight or shape on self-evaluation, or persistent lack of recognition of the seriousness of the current low body weight.

Coding note: The ICD-9-CM code for anorexia nervosa is **307.1,** which is assigned regardless of the subtype. The ICD-10-CM code depends on the subtype (see below).

Specify whether:

(F50.01) Restricting type: During the last 3 months, the individual has not engaged in recurrent episodes of binge eating or purging behavior (i.e. self-induced vomiting or the misuse of laxatives, diuretics, or enemas). This subtype describes presentations in which weight loss is accomplished primarily through dieting, fasting, and/or excessive exercise.

(F50.02) Binge-eating/purging type: During the last 3 months, the individual has engaged in recurrent episodes of binge eating or purging behavior (i.e. self-induced vomiting or the misuse of laxatives, diuretics, or enemas).

Specify if:

In partial remission: After full criteria for anorexia nervosa were previously met, Criterion A (low body weight) has not been met for a sustained period, but either Criterion B (intense fear of gaining weight or becoming fat or behavior that interferes with weight gain) or Criterion C (disturbances in self-perception of weight and shape) is still met.

In full remission: After full criteria for anorexia nervosa were previously met, none of the criteria have been met for a sustained period of time.

Specify current severity:

The minimum level of severity is based, for adults, on current body mass index (BMI) (see below) or, for children and adolescents, on BMI percentile. The ranges below are derived from World Health Organization categories for thinness in adults; for children and adolescents, corresponding BMI percentiles should be used. The level of severity may be increased to reflect clinical symptoms, the degree of functional disability, and the need for supervision.

Mild: BMI >17 kg/m^2 **Moderate:** BMI 16–16.99 kg/m^2 **Severe:** BMI 15–15.99 kg/m^2 **Extreme:** BMI <15 kg/m^2

DSM-5 Diagnostic criteria for bulimia nervosa

307.51 (F50.2)

a. Recurrent episodes of binge eating. An episode of binge eating is characterized by both of the following:
   1. Eating, in a discrete period of time (e.g. within any 2-hour period), an amount of food that is definitely larger than what most individuals would eat in a similar period of time under similar circumstances.

Contd...

Contd...

2. A sense of lack of control over eating during the episode (e.g. a feeling that one cannot stop eating or control what or how much one is eating).

b. Recurrent inappropriate compensatory behaviors in order to prevent weight gain, such as self-induced vomiting; misuse of laxatives, diuretics, or other medications; fasting; or excessive exercise.
c. The binge eating and inappropriate compensatory behaviors both occur, on average, at least once a week for 3 months.
d. Self-evaluation is unduly influenced by body shape and weight.
e. The disturbance does not occur exclusively during episodes of anorexia nervosa.

Specify if:
In partial remission: After full criteria for bulimia nervosa were previously met, some, but not all, of the criteria have been met for a sustained period of time.
In full remission: After full criteria for bulimia nervosa were previously met, none of the criteria have been met for a sustained period of time.

Specify current severity:
The minimum level of severity is based on the frequency of inappropriate compensatory behaviors (see below). The level of severity may be increased to reflect other symptoms and the degree of functional disability.
Mild: An average of 1–3 episodes of inappropriate compensatory behaviors per week.
Moderate: An average of 4–7 episodes of inappropriate compensatory behaviors per week.
Severe: An average of 8–13 episodes of inappropriate compensatory behaviors per week.
Extreme: An average of 14 or more episodes of inappropriate compensatory behaviors per week.

DSM-5 Criteria for binge-eating disorder

307.51 (F50.8)

a. Recurrent episodes of binge eating. An episode of binge eating is characterized by both of the following:
   1. Eating, in a discrete period of time (e.g. within any 2-hour period), an amount of food that is definitely larger than what most people would eat in a similar period of time under similar circumstances.
   2. A sense of lack of control over eating during the episode (e.g. a feeling that one cannot stop eating or control what or how much one is eating).
b. The binge-eating episodes are associated with three (or more) of the following:
   1. Eating much more rapidly than normal.
   2. Eating until feeling uncomfortably full.
   3. Eating large amounts of food when not feeling physically hungry.
   4. Eating alone because of feeling embarrassed by how much one is eating.
   5. Feeling disgusted with oneself, depressed, or very guilty afterward.
c. Marked distress regarding binge eating is present.

Contd...

Contd...

d. The binge eating occurs, on average, at least once a week for 3 months.
e. The binge eating is not associated with the recurrent use of inappropriate compensatory behavior as in bulimia nervosa and does not occur exclusively during the course of bulimia nervosa or anorexia nervosa.

Specify if:
In partial remission: After full criteria for binge-eating disorder were previously met, binge eating occurs at an average frequency of less than one episode per week for a sustained period of time.
In full remission: After full criteria for binge-eating disorder were previously met, none of the criteria have been met for a sustained period of time.

Specify current severity:
The minimum level of severity is based on the frequency of episodes of binge eating (see below). The level of severity may be increased to reflect other symptoms and the degree of functional disability.
Mild: 1–3 binge-eating episodes per week.
Moderate: 4–7 binge-eating episodes per week.
Severe: 8–13 binge-eating episodes per week.
Extreme: 14 or more binge-eating episodes per week.

hyperactivity disorder) have been reported to affect about a fifth of patients with anorexia nervosa.[21,22] Moreover, a small proportion of adults with attention-deficit hyperactivity disorder have additional symptoms of eating disorders.[23] Obsessive compulsive traits[24,25] or disorder,[26] and anxiety disorders[27,28] and some borderline traits,[25] have been reported both before and after the onset of eating disorders, and are also diagnosed in family members.[29,30] Bulimia nervosa and binge eating disorder are associated with affective disorders[31,32] and with alcohol[33] or substance[34] misuse.

EPIDEMIOLOGY

Eating disorders and related behaviors are common in young people. Investigators of a study of a large sample of American children aged 9-14 years reported that 7.1% of boys and 13.4% of girls displayed disordered eating behaviors.[35] The pivotal effect on health has led to the inclusion of eating disorders among the priority mental illnesses for children and adolescents identified by WHO.[36] Eating disorders have been reported worldwide both in developed regions and emerging economies such as Brazil and China.[37,38] The lifetime prevalence of eating disorders in adults is about 0.6% for anorexia nervosa, 1% for bulimia nervosa, and 3% for binge eating disorder.[19,20] Women are more affected than are men, and the sex differences in lifetime prevalence in adults could be less substantial than that quoted in standard texts: 0.9% for anorexia nervosa, 1.5% for bulimia nervosa, and 3.5% for binge eating disorder in women; and 0.3%, 0.5%, and 2.0%, respectively, in men.[20] Many people with eating disorders, who were detected in community studies in the USA, do not seek treatment.[20]

PATHOGENESIS

A comprehensive review published in 2004 summarized the risk factors for eating disorders,[39] and a position paper from the Academy of Eating Disorders outlined the evidence supporting these diseases as biologically-based forms of severe mental illnesses.[40] In this section, we draw attention to some present areas of emphasis.

GENETIC FACTORS

The most potent risk factor is female gender. How much this association can be attributed to biological rather than social factors is uncertain. Sexual divergence is less pronounced in binge eating disorder[23] and in prepubertal anorexia nervosa.[41] Twin and family studies suggest that anorexia nervosa, bulimia nervosa, and binge eating disorder are complex genetic diseases, and for each disorder the estimated heritability ranges between 50% and 83%.[11,42,43] Linkage studies have identified loci for anorexia and bulimia nervosa and for associated behavioral traits such as compulsivity.[44–46] About a third of genetic risk for eating disorders and depression,[47] anxiety disorders,[48] and addictive disorders[49] is shared. All the above studies are limited because of low power; however, international collaborations are working at pooling cases and using newer forms of analysis such as genome-wide associations.

BIOLOGICAL FACTORS

Although many of the biological findings in eating disorders can be best understood as results of starvation and disturbed eating behaviors, some are causally linked as risk or maintaining factors. The brain is particularly vulnerable to the consequences of poor nutrition since it uses around 20% of the caloric intake and is especially dependent on glucose. Therefore, poor nutrition has a general effect on brain function in addition to the specific effect on the appetite system. Most eating disorders emerge during adolescence—a vulnerable period of brain reorganization, and malnutrition during this crucial period can negatively affect illness trajectories.

Starvation shrinks the brain and is associated with many behavioral and psychosocial disturbances such as rigidity, emotional dysregulation, and social difficulties.[50] Many symptoms resolve with weight gain and when brain mass is restored.[51] Concentrations of brain-derived neurotrophic factor, a regulator of brain plasticity, in blood are reduced in acute anorexia nervosa,[52] and genetic studies suggest a trait-related disturbance in this system.[53]

The characterization of the central control of appetite[54,55] could improve our understanding of eating disorders. A simplified heuristic is to consider three components. First is the homeostatic system that is centered mainly in the brain stem and hypothalamus, which integrates peripheral metabolic markers with information from the gastrointestinal tract to affect subjective states of hunger, satiety, and autonomic nervous activity. Second is the drive system, with distributed neural circuitry within the mesolimbic cortex and striatum that has afferent inputs from sense organs and neural structures that are implicated in learning and memory. This system registers the reward value associated with food and is involved in the motivation to seek food and eat. Third is the self-regulation system, within which a form of so-called top-down control contextualises appetite within life goals, values, and meaning.

Abnormal changes in all three of these systems have a role in the risk and maintenance of eating disorders. A hypothesis suggests that these disorders could result from pervasive deficits in self-regulatory systems.[56] Furthermore, eating disorder behaviors affect the drive system, as shown by models of binge eating in laboratory rodents for which scientists have replicated the conditions implicated in the increase of binge eating, i.e. food restriction, gastric drainage (an analog of vomiting), stress, and intermittent access to highly palatable food—and produced animals with an addiction to food. The investigators noted that not only did these animals binge eat, but they also showed withdrawal effects. Moreover, they had a propensity to relapse after a time, and cross-tolerance to alcohol and cocaine.[57,58] Underpinning these behavioral changes are alterations in the chemical transmitters (dopamine and opioids). Finally, the response to changes in food intake of the putative homeostatic system could contribute, e.g. anorexia nervosa is often linked to premorbid and familial leanness,[59] whereas the reverse is the case for bulimia nervosa and binge eating disorder.[60]

Brain monoamine function in eating disorders has been studied in the acute state (which can be confounded by illness effects) and after recovery with specific ligands and positron emission tomography. These findings for anorexia nervosa have been synthesized into an explanatory model.[61] 5HT2A receptors are reduced and 5HT1A receptors are increased in both the acute and recovered state, and dopamine receptors (DA2) within the striatum are increased after recovery.[62] Less research has been done into binge eating disorders and bulimia nervosa, but anomalies in the dopamine system could heighten food reward.[63]

Abnormalities in both illness-related (food and body shape) and non-illness-related information processing are detected in eating disorders. An attentional bias is evident toward food and body shape[64] associated with increased activation in distributed neural networks connected with self-regulation and hedonic motivation.[61,65] General problems include difficulties in decision making,[66] abnormal striatal activation by reward,[67,68] reduced flexibility[69] associated with decreased activation in the striatum and associated areas,[70] a bias toward focusing on detail at the expense of seeing the general picture (weak central coherence),[71] problems in social cognition,[72] and dysfunctional emotional regulation.[73] These functional anomalies can maintain eating disorder behaviors. For example, an eye for detail and inflexibility can allow an individual to understand the laws of thermodynamics in relation to energy intake and expenditure and succeed in weight loss, whereas impaired social and emotional regulation could isolate the individual.

ENVIRONMENTAL CONTEXT

The environment shapes the developmental course of the individual beginning at the time of conception. For example, mothers of people who later develop an eating disorder might be more exposed to stress during pregnancy.[74] Birth-related perinatal complications (e.g. cephalohematoma) and premature delivery increase the risk of development of an eating disorder.[75] Epigenetic mechanisms or damage to the brain from hypoxia can also mediate these effects.

In some developed countries, the excess value placed on thinness encourages extreme dieting and weight control practices. Negative comparisons between an individual's body shape and that of the ideal contributes to poor self-esteem.[76] Criticism, teasing, and bullying focused on food, weight, and shape issues specifically increase the risk of developing an eating disorder.[77] The tension between the stigmatization of fatness, idealization of thinness, and easy access to highly palatable foods, perhaps eaten in secret, could lead to weight control behaviors that can have a destabilizing effect on the biology of appetite control. In addition to food-related and weight-related harmful experiences, general adversity (neglect and physical and sexual abuse) also increases the risk of developing an eating disorder.

INTERACTIONS BETWEEN THE ENVIRONMENT AND INDIVIDUAL BIOLOGY

The postpubertal years are a crucial time of vulnerability. Developmental changes of puberty (the hormonal fluxes and synaptic pruning and myelination within the brain), stressful events, and challenges (e.g. changes in social affiliation and ranking) could trigger eating disorder behaviors. The consequent nutritional deficits can induce factors that maintain the illness. These factors have been grouped into four broad domains: the medical effect on the body and brain, the interpersonal effect, the exaggeration of avoidant coping, and obsessive compulsive traits.[78]

TREATMENT

Medical Complications

Although eating disorders can begin in adulthood, the highest incidence is between 10 and 19 years of age,[79] potentially disrupting optimum growth and development. Most pathophysiological complications are reversible with improved nutritional status or remittance of abnormal eating and purging behaviors. However, some physical consequences can be life-threatening, such as electrolyte imbalances (e.g. hypokalemia) due to excessive vomiting or laxative and diuretic misuse. Additionally, nutritional deficiencies increase the risk of cardiac arrhythmias and intercurrent infection. Comprehensive reviews[80,81] and the previous Seminar1 discuss the physical abnormalities of eating disorders in great depth.

Many practice guidelines discuss how to measure and assess medical risk.[82–84] Children and adolescents have less nutritional reserve than do adults, so their risk can rapidly escalate. Body-mass index (BMI) is not a useful index of nutritional compromise for men, children, tall and muscular individuals, and those with water retention. Other comorbid medical disorders also increase vulnerability and might need regular monitoring, such as diabetes mellitus, which can increase risk at any level of BMI. Apart from these caveats, standard forms present a means of giving both personalised and normative feedback on medical risk. (Examples include the Maudsley BMI chart and the Risk Assessment in Eating Disorders). Table 1 shows an abridged set of markers of nutritional and cardiovascular decompensation that signal the need for increased or urgent care. These markers should be considered in the context of the complete clinical picture, expertise of the treating team, and local availability of eating disorder units. Signs of increased medical risk suggest the need for immediate specialist consultation or inpatient treatment, or both, especially in people with a recent, acute onset.

The deficits in anorexia nervosa gradually evolve and are general rather than specific. Therefore, they should be rectified slowly, orally, and with food supplemented with multivitamin and multimineral preparations. In the first phase (3–7 days), a soft diet of about 5–10 kcal/kg per day with thiamine and vitamin B co-strong in small portions throughout the day, and foods with high phosphorus content (e.g. milk-based products) accords with guidelines from the UK National Institute for Health and Clinical Excellence (NICE) describing refeeding of severely undernourished patients, and reduces the risk of refeeding syndrome.[85] On special units with skilled nursing, feeding by tube is rarely necessary. At moderate levels of risk the aim is to produce a weight gain between 250 g and 450 g/week in outpatients, and around 1 kg in those treated in hospital.[83]

Some weight change strategies—such as vomiting or misuse of diuretics, laxatives, or caffeinated and carbonated drinks—can result in underhydration or overhydration and electrolyte imbalance. Acute renal failure can occur in severe cases. Oral replacement is usually the first line of management, but the full clinical diagnosis and level of risk (Table 1) decide the appropriate setting and method of replacement. Persistent hypokalemia can be linked to low

Table 1: An abridged set of markers of nutritional and cardiovascular decompensation that signal the need for increased or urgent care in people with eating disorders

	Moderate risk	*High risk*
Nutrition		
Body-mass index (kg/m²)	<15	<13
Body-mass index centiles	<3rd	<2nd
Weight loss (kg per week)	>0.5	>1.0
Purpuric rash		+
Circulation		
Sytstolic blood pressure (mm Hg)	<90	<80
Diastolic blood pressure (mm Hg)	<60	<50
Postural drop (mm Hg)	>10	>20
Pulse rate (beats per min)	<50	<40
Oxygen saturation (%)	<90%	85%
Extremities		Cyanotic
Musculoskeletal (squate test*)		
Unable to get up without use of arms for balance	+	
Unable to get up without use of arms as leverage		+
Temperature		
Core temperature (°C)	<35	<34.5
Investigations		
FBC, urea, electrolytes (including phosphate), LFT, albumin, creatinine kinase, glucose	Concern if outside normal limits	Potassium <2.5 mmol/L, sodium <130 mmol/L, phosphate <0.5 mmol/L
Electrocardiograph		Prolonged QT interval espically in context of low postassium

+ = present. FBC = full blood count. LFT = liver function test.
* The instructions for the squat test are that the patient squats on her/his haunches and has to stand up without, if possible, using her/his hands.

calcium and magnesium (which also need rectification), or to sustained purging behaviors. Proton-pump inhibitors to inhibit gastric acid secretion reduce metabolic alkalosis and help to conserve potassium.[86] They can also prevent esophageal and tooth damage.

LONG-TERM EFFECTS ON PHYSICAL HEALTH

Some medical consequences of eating disorders can be irreversible or have later repercussions on health, especially those affecting the skeleton, the reproductive system, and the brain. Dental problems, growth retardation, and osteoporosis are some of the long-term problems. Bone loss in lumbar spine, radius, and proximal femur can be detected within a year of illness and progresses to produce fractures, kyphoscoliosis, and chronic pain. Weight gain alone improves bone density, especially if it is sufficient to restore menses. Several treatments have been investigated, including antiresorptive agents, estrogens, insulin growth factor, and calcium supplementation, but none can be recommended on the basis of present evidence.[87]

The fertility and maternity rate of women with anorexia nervosa is reduced; a Swedish study[88] suggested that the rate of fertility was 70% of that in the general population. Infant birthweight is lower in mothers with anorexia nervosa[89] but higher in those with bulimia nervosa.[90] The miscarriage rate for women with bulimia nervosa is higher than for healthy women—those with bulimia nervosa were twice as likely to have two or more miscarriages compared with the general population.[89] Perinatal problems can be increased,[91] and feeding difficulties reducing infant growth have been reported.[92] Infertile and pregnant women should be screened for eating disorders and offered treatment to optimize the wellbeing of their offspring.[82]

PATHWAYS OF CARE

High levels of health-care use are common across all forms of eating disorders.[93] The management of bulimia nervosa and binge eating disorder can be complicated by medical (e.g. diabetes and obesity) and psychiatric (e.g. affective disorders and addictions) comorbidity, but acute medical risk is less of a problem than it is for anorexia nervosa, and care is typically delivered on an outpatient basis in adult services.

NICE guidelines recommended that people with anorexia nervosa should first be offered outpatient treatment[82] and that inpatient care be used for those who do not respond or who present with high risk and little psychosocial resources. Whether inpatient admissions should be short to alleviate acute risk or prolonged to attain full weight restoration (thought to reduce relapse) is controversial.[94] Models of day treatment provide an intermediate service model.[95]

Practice recommendations emphasise the importance of specialized care for the treatment of eating disorders, but such care is not often accessible. Hence, new forms of service delivery (e.g. E-mailing, Text-messaging) with use of treatment directed via mobile phones, the internet, or telemedicine [e.g. cognitive behavioral therapy (CBT) delivered by a therapist via the internet] are being assessed.[96-99] A systematic review[98] of self-help interventions (computerized or manual modelled after empirically validated approaches concluded that with professional oversight (guided self-help) these interventions could have benefit in bulimia nervosa and binge eating disorder, although some uncertainty still remains.[98,100,101]

EVIDENCE-BASED TREATMENTS

Anorexia Nervosa

The evidence base relating to the treatment of anorexia nervosa is meagre.[82] Two main factors contribute to difficulties in trials of treatment for this disease: clinician-instigated protocol withdrawal because of failure to stabilize risk, and patient withdrawal and difficulties in recruitment because of poor acceptability of treatments. Thus, treatment guidelines rely on expert recommendations. These recommendations emphasise the importance of a multidisciplinary approach including medical, nutritional, social, and psychological components.[82-84] Psychotherapy can be delivered individually or with the family. The involvement of families in treatment depends on several factors, e.g. age of the patient, living arrangements, the patient's level of risk and dependence, and the ethos of the treatment team.

For adolescents with anorexia nervosa, family psychotherapy as practised according to the Maudsley method is recommended (Table 2).[102] Six months of treatment can be sufficient unless there is obsessive compulsive comorbidity or non-intact families.[103] Families with extremes of overprotection or criticism have better outcomes in separated family therapy (child and parents seen separately) than in combined family therapy.[104] Parents are

Table 2: Treatments for anorexia nervosa, bulimia nervosa, and binge eating disorder and strength of their empirical support

	Anorexia nervosa		*Bulimia nervosa*		*Binge eating disorder*	
	Evidence	*Effect*	*Evidence*	*Effect*	*Evidence*	*Effect*
Pharmacological treatment						
Antidepressants (acute phase)	Weak	–	Strong	+	Moderate	+
SSRIs	Weak*	–	Strong*	+	Moderate	–/+
TCAs	Weak*	–	Weak*	+	Weak	+
Other classes	..	..	Weak*	–/+	..	..
SNRIs (atomoxetine)	..	..	..	..	Weak	+
Antidepressants (relapse prevention)	Weak*	–/+	Weak	–/+	Weak	–/+
Antipsychotic olanzapine	Weak*	–/+	..	..	..	..
Zinc	Weak*	–/+	..	..	..	..
Drugs for osteoporosis/osteopenia	Weak*	–	..	..	..	..
Anticonvulsant: topiramate	..	..	Weak		Moderate	++
Appetite suppressor: sibutramine	..	..	..	..	Moderate	++
Obesity drug: orlistat	..	..	..	..	Weak	+
Behavioral treatment						
Cognitive behavioral therapy	Weak*	+	Strong*	++	Moderate	+++
Interpersonal psychotherapy	Weak*	+	Moderate	+	Weak	++
Congnitive analytical therapy	Weak	+	..	..	..	..
Dialectrical behavioral therapy	..	..	Weak	+	Weak	+
Psychodynamic therapies	Weak	+	Weak	–/+	..	..
Behavioral therapies	Weak	–/+	Moderate	+	..	..
Family-based therapy (Maudsley)	Moderate*	++	Weak*	+	..	..
Specialist clinical management	Weak*	+	..	..	..	..
Nutritional counseling (alone)	Weak*	–	Weak	–/+	Weak	+
Behavioral weight loss therapy	..	..	..	..	Weak	++
Self-help interventions (GSH/PSH)	..	..	Weak*	+	Weak	+
Mobile/internet/telemedicine	..	..	Weak	–/+	Weak	–/+

SSRIs, Selective serotonin reuptake inhibitors; TCAs, Tricyclic antidepressants; SNRIs, Serotonin-norepinephrine reuptake inhibitors; GSH, Guided self-help; PSH, Pure self-help. Evidence grades; .., Non-existent or not applicable; grades weak/moderate/strong. Beneficial effect (reduction of symptoms or behaviors or maintenance of improvements); .., No randomized controlled trial available; –, No beneficial effect; –/+, Mixed results or still inconsistent results (possible beneficial effect); +, Slight beneficial effect; ++, Moderate beneficial effect; +++, Strong beneficial effect.
* At least one trial included adolescents (<18 years).

distressed and burdened by symptoms and behaviors of eating disorders.[105] These feelings can be alleviated by group educational interventions.[106]

A Cochrane collaboration review (updated in 2008) concluded that the evidence accumulated so far does not lend support to any one particular psychotherapeutic method for adults with anorexia nervosa, although support from a nonspecialist clinician might be less efficacious than might that from a specialist delivering a specific form of psychotherapy.[107]

No strong evidence lends support to drug treatment either in the acute or maintenance phases of the illness.[108,109] A few randomized controlled trials have been done since the last Seminar. The previous expectation that fluoxetine could have a role in prevention of relapse in anorexia nervosa[110] weakened after the negative findings from a large and thorough study.[111] Interest has been renewed in the potential use of atypical antipsychotic drugs to target dopaminergic dysregulation and comorbid features of this disease.[112] The idea is that by reducing distorted cognitions and anxiety symptoms, resistance to weight gain decreases. Initial, small randomized studies[113,114] report decreases in obsessive symptoms and an increased rate of weight gain. Larger trials are necessary, however, to substantiate these benefits and elucidate harms with this drug, such as a potential increase of QTc interval with the risk of cardiac arrhythmias.

Bulimia Nervosa

The evidence base[115] for the original CBT model of bulimia nervosa[116] and its use as the first-line treatment is strong. Although CBT has good acceptability, binge remission rates (cessation of binge eating or purging) at the end of treatments are only 30–40%.[117, 118] An enhanced form of CBT with a broader focus including interpersonal factors, emotional tolerance, perfectionism, and self-esteem did not substantially improve this outcome.[119] Furthermore, combining antidepressants (tricyclics or fluoxetine) with CBT did not significantly add to the effect of CBT alone.[117] Interpersonal therapy is efficacious as a treatment alternative, although it showed a slower response of symptom change than did CBT (similar results to CBT only after 1 year of follow-up).[115,117] Other models of treatment are being considered for use in bulimia nervosa, such as those with a focus on emotional regulation (e.g. dialectical behavior therapy).[120]

Two studies have assessed the role of family-based psychotherapy for adolescent bulimia nervosa.[121,122] One suggested that guided CBT could have advantages compared with family-based treatment in terms of cost and speed of response,[121] whereas the other suggested that family-based treatment had advantages compared with individual supportive therapy.[122]

A 2004 review of treatment for bulimia nervosa and binging included seven trials in which participants with the form of eating disorder not otherwise specified that was similar to bulimia nervosa formed part of the sample.[123] The conclusion from this and from a recent trial[119] is that CBT is as effective for non-specified eating disorder similar to bulimia nervosa as it is for bulimia nervosa itself.

Pharmacotherapy has been recommended in the treatment of bulimia nervosa and binge eating disorder, especially if psychotherapy is either unavailable or unacceptable.[82,83] Evidence from pharmacological trials in bulimia nervosa is strong, and it is increasing in studies of binge eating disorder, but this finding mainly indicates efficacy in the acute stage after short-term treatment. Overall, evidence for long-term effects after medication is scarce. Additionally, pharmacological agents have been mainly tested in adults, and the results might not be generalized to adolescents and children. Moreover, use of antidepressant drugs in children and young people is controversial because of increased suicidal risk.[124]

Three systematic reviews detected strong evidence for the use of antidepressants to treat bulimia nervosa in the short term (around 8 weeks).[115,117,125] However, the pooled effect from one meta-analysis (with eight studies, 901 patients) was judged only moderate for clinical improvement, which was defined as the number of patients with 50% or more reduction of binge eating (57% of patients receiving antidepressants vs 33% receiving placebo), and remission rates with antidepressants were usually less than 20% (similar to placebo).[125] Overall acceptability of antidepressant treatment is low (around 40% dropout rates) when drugs are given alone.[125] Fluoxetine is the main drug tested in trials and approved for use in bulimia nervosa by health regulatory agencies; it is recommended in a dose (60 mg/day) that is higher than is usually necessary to treat depression (20–40 mg/day).[115] There is less evidence of efficacy for other serotonin reuptake inhibitors (citalopram, sertraline, fluvoxamine).[117,126] Whether antidepressant treatment can prevent relapse in bulimia nervosa is not yet known, since the few trials that were done were limited by their high attrition rates.[115,117,127] Topiramate can be effective in reduction of bulimic and purging symptoms, but the safety profile of this drug still needs to be established in this disease.[117,128,129]

BINGE EATING DISORDER

Psychological interventions that have shown efficacy in treatment of bulimia nervosa have also been tested in binge eating disorder with positive results, particularly modified CBT, interpersonal therapy, and dialectical behavior therapy.[130] Large effect sizes in a meta-analysis have been reported for CBT compared with a control for reduction of binge frequency and for binge abstinence.[100] An additional challenge in the treatment of binge eating disorder is weight management, since individuals are often classified as being overweight or obese. So far, psychological interventions for this disorder have not consistently shown clinically relevant weight losses.[100] However, behavioral weight loss treatments have shown a moderate reduction in weight and improvement in binge abstinence.[100] Binge abstinence is an important treatment goal because it has been associated with increased weight loss in both psychological and pharmacological trials.[131,132] A few studies with long-term follow-up suggest that abstinence from bingeing could persist for 12 months[132,133] and 24 months.[134]

Systematic reviews[130] and meta-analyses[100,135] of treatments for binge eating disorder suggest that drug treatments show, at least, a moderate effectiveness in reduction of binge frequencies and promotion of binge remission in the short term, with a remission rate of 48.7% reported with pharmacotherapy (including antidepressants, anticonvulsants, and obesity drugs) compared with 28.5% with placebo.[135] Several guidelines recommend short-term treatment with antidepressants (mainly serotonin reuptake inhibitors) as an alternative first approach to CBT. Although antidepressants are usually effective in reducing binges,[100,135] some studies have reported negative findings,[130,136] and their effect on depressive symptoms and on weight is uncertain.[135,137]

Modest weight loss and binge remission have been reported with drugs approved for use in obesity,[135] such as sibutramine[138,139] and orlistat,[140] and with drugs associated with weight loss, such as topiramate,[141] zonisamide,[142] and atomoxetine.[143] Sibutramine and topiramate have both been tested in multicenter trials and showed binge remission rates greater than with serotonin reuptake inhibitors compared with placebo.[138,139,144] Supplementation of CBT or behavioral weight loss treatments with the obesity drug orlistat[145] or topiramate[144] might increase weight loss.[146] Although these drugs can be considered as part of the available regimen to treat binge eating disorder, the short-term duration of trials (12–24 weeks), high dropout rate, and placebo-response rates restrict the conclusions about their use.[100,130] Additionally, the risk–benefit balance is uncertain since intolerable adverse effects have been reported with some drugs (e.g. zonisamide, topiramate).[117,130,142]

Prognosis

Recovery from anorexia nervosa becomes much less likely the longer that the illness has persisted. This finding contrasts with that of bulimia nervosa, for which the chance of recovery becomes higher the longer the illness duration.[147] A systematic review[148] has compiled data for all outcomes for eating disorders and reported an increased mortality rate for anorexia nervosa (the reported range is wide, varying with case mix and length of follow-up) and persistent psychiatric problems in many cases.

In anorexia nervosa, a young age at onset and short duration of illness was associated with a good outcome, and somatic and psychiatric comorbidity with a poor outcome.[149] This disease disrupts education[150] and vocational functioning, which contributes to difficulties in independent living in 20% of cases up to 10–20 years after the onset of the illness.[88] Less is known about the effect of other eating disorders in this domain of life.

Little research has been done into the long-term outcome of bulimia nervosa and binge eating disorder. Of a cohort of patients with both these diseases admitted for hospital treatment in Germany, a third had an eating disorder diagnosis 12 years later; 36% of patients with binge eating disorder and 3.6% with bulimia nervosa had a BMI greater than 30 kg/m^2.[151]

CONCLUSION

The diagnostic criteria for anorexia nervosa, bulimia nervosa and Binge-eating disorder are made some change in DSM-5.[152] Eating disorders arise from an interaction between environmental events and the biological, and developmental features of the individual. Abnormal eating behaviors produce both medical and psychosocial results. The psychosocial consequences derive partly from the effects of starvation on the brain and can perpetuate the illness. Several treatments and their combinations have been tested for binge eating disorder, with possible efficacy in the short-term. New forms of treatment delivery have also been tested for bulimia nervosa and binge eating disorder with promising results. Progress has been made in treatment of adolescent anorexia nervosa, although not for the adult expression of this disorder.

REFERENCES

1. Fairburn CG, Harrison PJ. Eating disorders. Lancet. 2003;361: 407-16.
2. American Psychiatric Association. Diagnostic and statistical manual of mental disorders. Washington, DC: American Psychiatric Association; 1994.
3. WHO. International statistical classification of diseases and related health problems (ICD-10). Geneva: World Health Orgaganization; 1992.
4. Cole TJ, Flegal KM, Nicholls D, Jackson AA. Body mass index cut offs to define thinness in children and adolescents: international survey. BMJ. 2007;335:194.
5. Fairburn CG, Cooper Z. Thinking afresh about the classification of eating disorders. Int J Eat Disord. 2007;40 (Suppl):S107-S110.
6. Walsh BT, Sysko R. Broad categories for the diagnosis of eating disorders (BCD-ED): an alternative system for classification. Int J Eat Disord. 200910.1002/eat.20722.
7. Marcus MD, Wildes JE. Obesity: is it a mental disorder?. Int J Eat Disord. 200910.1002/eat.20725. published online July 16. PubMed.
8. Eddy KT, Dorer DJ, Franko DL, et al. Diagnostic crossover in anorexia nervosa and bulimia nervosa: implications for DSM-5. Am J Psychiatry. 2008;165:245-50.

9. Wilfley DE, Bishop ME, Wilson GT, Agras WS. Classification of eating disorders: toward DSM-5. Int J Eat Disord. 2007;40 (Suppl): S123-S9.
10. Williamson DA. Does the evidence point to a binge eating phenotype? Comment on Gordon and Wonderlich, et al. (2007). Int J Eat Disord. 2007;40 (Suppl): S72-S5.
11. Javaras KN, Laird NM, Reichborn-Kjennerud T, et al. Familiality and heritability of binge eating disorder: results of a case-control family study and a twin study. Int J Eat Disord. 2008;41:174-9.
12. Wilson GT, Grilo CM, Vitousek KM. Psychological treatment of eating disorders. Am Psychol. 2007;62:199-216.
13. Pope HG, Lalonde JK, Pindyck LJ, et al. Binge eating disorder: a stable syndrome. Am J Psychiatry. 2006;163:2181-3.
14. Fairburn CG, Cooper Z, Shafran R. Cognitive behaviour therapy for eating disorders: a "transdiagnostic" theory and treatment. Behav Res Ther. 2003;41:509-28.
15. Hollander E, Kim S, Khanna S, Pallanti S. Obsessive-compulsive disorder and obsessive-compulsive spectrum disorders: diagnostic and dimensional issues. CNS Spectr. 2007;12:5-13.
16. Pallister E, Waller G. Anxiety in the eating disorders: understanding the overlap. Clin Psychol Rev. 2008;28:366-86.
17. Hudson JI, Pope HG. Genetic epidemiology of eating disorders and co-occurring conditions: the role of endophenotypes. Int J Eat Disord. 2007;40 (Suppl): S76-S8.
18. Thomas JJ, Vartanian LR, Brownell KD. The relationship between eating disorder not otherwise specified (EDNOS) and officially recognized eating disorders: meta-analysis and implications for DSM. Psychol Bull. 2009;135:407-33.
19. Jacobi F, Wittchen HU, Holting C, et al. Prevalence, co-morbidity and correlates of mental disorders in the general population: results from the German Health Interview and Examination Survey (GHS). Psychol Med. 2004;34:597-611.
20. Hudson JI, Hiripi E, Pope HG, Kessler RC. The prevalence and correlates of eating disorders in the National Comorbidity Survey Replication. Biol Psychiatry. 2007;61:348-58.
21. Wentz E, Lacey JH, Waller G, Rastam M, Turk J, Gillberg C. Childhood onset neuropsychiatric disorders in adult eating disorder patients. A pilot study. Eur Child Adolesc Psychiatry. 2005;14:431-7.
22. Gillberg IC, Gillberg C, Rastam M, Johansson M. The cognitive profile of anorexia nervosa: a comparative study including a community-based sample. Compr Psychiatry. 1996;37:23-30.
23. Nazar BP, Pinna CM, Coutinho G, et al. Review of literature of attention-deficit/hyperactivity disorder with comorbid eating disorders. Rev Bras Psiquiatr. 2008;30:384-9.
24. Anderluh MB, Tchanturia K, Rabe-Hesketh S, Treasure J. Childhood obsessive-compulsive personality traits in adult women with eating disorders: defining a broader eating disorder phenotype. Am J Psychiatry. 2003;160:242-7.
25. Lilenfeld LR, Wonderlich S, Riso LP, Crosby R, Mitchell J. Eating disorders and personality: a methodological and empirical review. Clin Psychol Rev. 2006;26:299-320.
26. Halmi KA, Tozzi F, Thornton LM, et al. The relation among perfectionism, obsessive-compulsive personality disorder and obsessive-compulsive disorder in individuals with eating disorders. Int J Eat Disord. 2005;38:371-4.
27. Kaye WH, Bulik CM, Thornton L, Barbarich N, Masters K. Comorbidity of anxiety disorders with anorexia and bulimia nervosa. Am J Psychiatry. 2004;161:2215-21.
28. Godart NT, Flament MF, Curt F, et al. Anxiety disorders in subjects seeking treatment for eating disorders: a DSM-IV controlled study. Psychiatry Res. 2003;117:245-58.
29. Strober M, Freeman R, Lampert C, Diamond J. The association of anxiety disorders and obsessive-compulsive personality disorder with anorexia nervosa: evidence from a family study with discussion of nosological and neurodevelopmental implications. Int J Eat Disord. 2007;40(Suppl):S46-S51.
30. Lilenfeld LR, Kaye WH, Greeno CG, et al. A controlled family study of anorexia nervosa and bulimia nervosa: psychiatric disorders in first-degree relatives and effects of proband comorbidity. Arch Gen Psychiatry. 1998;55:603-10.
31. McElroy SL, Kotwal R, Keck PE. Comorbidity of eating disorders with bipolar disorder and treatment implications. Bipolar Disord. 2006;8:686-95.
32. Mangweth B, Hudson JI, Pope HG, et al. Family study of the aggregation of eating disorders and mood disorders. Psychol Med. 2003;33:1319-23.
33. Gadalla T, Piran N. Co-occurrence of eating disorders and alcohol use disorders in women: a meta analysis. Arch Womens Ment Health. 2007;10:133-40.
34. Calero-Elvira A, Krug I, Davis K, et al. Meta-analysis on drugs in people with eating disorders. Eur Eat Disord Rev. 2009;17:243-59.
35. Neumark-Sztainer D, Hannan PJ. Weight-related behaviors among adolescent girls and boys: results from a national survey. Arch Pediatr Adolesc Med. 2000;154:569-77.
36. WHO (Europe). Mental health of children and adolescents. (Facing the challenges and finding solutions). Geneva: World Health Organization; 2005.
37. Chen H, Jackson T. Prevalence and sociodemographic correlates of eating disorder endorsements among adolescents and young adults from China. Eur Eat Disord Rev. 2008;16: 375-85.
38. de Souza Ferreira JE, da Veiga GV. Eating disorder risk behavior in Brazilian adolescents from low socio-economic level. Appetite. 2008;51:249-55.
39. Jacobi C, Hayward C, de Zwaan M, Kraemer HC, Agras WS. Coming to terms with risk factors for eating disorders: application of risk terminology and suggestions for a general taxonomy. Psychol Bull. 2004;130:19-65.
40. Klump KL, Bulik CM, Kaye WH, Treasure J, Tyson E. Academy for eating disorders position paper: eating disorders are serious mental illnesses. Int J Eat Disord. 2009;42:97-103.
41. Olivry E, Corcos M. Eating disorders. Prepubertal anorexia nervosa. Presse Med. 1999;28:100-2.

42. Bulik CM, Landt MC Slof-Op't, van Furth EF, Sullivan PF. The genetics of anorexia nervosa. Ann Rev Nutr. 2007;27:263-75.
43. Bulik CM, Tozzi F. The genetics of bulimia nervosa. Drugs Today (Barc). 2004;40:741-9.
44. Bacanu SA, Bulik CM, Klump KL, et al. Linkage analysis of anorexia and bulimia nervosa cohorts using selected behavioral phenotypes as quantitative traits or covariates. Am J Med Genet B Neuropsychiatr Genet. 2005;139B:61-8.
45. Bergen AW, Yeager M, Welch R, et al. Candidate gene analysis of the Price Foundation anorexia nervosa affected relative pair dataset. Curr Drug Targets CNS Neurol Disord. 2003;2:41-51.
46. Bulik CM, Devlin B, Bacanu SA, et al. Significant linkage on chromosome 10p in families with bulimia nervosa. Am J Hum Genet. 2003;72:200-7.
47. Wade TD, Bulik CM, Neale M, Kendler KS. Anorexia nervosa and major depression: shared genetic and environmental risk factors. Am J Psychiatry. 2000;157:469-71.
48. Keel PK, Klump KL, Miller KB, McGue M, Iacono WG. Shared transmission of eating disorders and anxiety disorders. Int J Eat Disord. 2005;38:99-105.
49. Baker JH, Mazzeo SE, Kendler KS. Association between broadly defined bulimia nervosa and drug use disorders: common genetic and environmental influences. Int J Eat Disord. 2007;40:673-8.
50. Keys A, Brozek J, Henschel A. The biology of human starvation. Minneapolis: University of Minnesota Press; 1950.
51. Castro-Fornieles J, Bargallo N, Lazaro L, et al. A cross-sectional and follow-up voxel-based morphometric MRI study in adolescent anorexia nervosa. J Psychiatr Res. 2009;43:331-40.
52. Nakazato M, Tchanturia K, Schmidt U, et al. Brain-derived neurotrophic factor (BDNF) and set-shifting in currently ill and recovered anorexia nervosa (AN) patients. Psychol Med. 2009;39:1029-35.
53. Ribases M, Gratacos M, Fernandez-Aranda F, et al. Association of BDNF with restricting anorexia nervosa and minimum body mass index: a family-based association study of eight European populations. Eur J Hum Genet. 2005;13:428-34.
54. Berthoud HR, Morrison C. The brain, appetite, and obesity. Ann Rev Psychol. 2008;59:55-92.
55. Berridge KC. 'Liking' and 'wanting' food rewards: brain substrates and roles in eating disorders. Physiol Behav. 2009;97:537-50.
56. Marsh R, Maia TV, Peterson BS. Functional disturbances within frontostriatal circuits across multiple childhood psychopathologies. Am J Psychiatry. 2009;166:664-74.
57. Avena NM. Examining the addictive-like properties of binge eating using an animal model of sugar dependence. Exp Clin Psychopharmacol. 2007;15:481-91.
58. Boggiano MM, Artiga AI, Pritchett CE, Chandler-Laney PC, Smith ML, Eldridge AJ. High intake of palatable food predicts binge-eating independent of susceptibility to obesity: an animal model of lean vs obese binge-eating and obesity with and without binge-eating. Int J Obes (Lond). 2007;31:1357-67.
59. Hebebrand J, Remschmidt H. Anorexia nervosa viewed as an extreme weight condition: genetic implications. Hum Genet. 1995;95:1-11.
60. Hudson JI, Lalonde JK, Berry JM, et al. Binge-eating disorder as a distinct familial phenotype in obese individuals. Arch Gen Psychiatry. 2006;63:313-9.
61. Kaye WH, Fudge JL, Paulus M. New insights into symptoms and neurocircuit function of anorexia nervosa. Nat Rev Neurosci. 2009;10:573-84.
62. Frank GK, Bailer UF, Henry SE, et al. Increased dopamine D2/D3 receptor binding after recovery from anorexia nervosa measured by positron emission tomography and [(11)C] raclopride. Biol Psychiatry. 2005;58:908-12.
63. Davis C, Patte K, Levitan R, et al. From motivation to behaviour: a model of reward sensitivity, overeating, and food preferences in the risk profile for obesity. Appetite. 2007;48:12-19.
64. Lee M, Shafran R. Information processing biases in eating disorders. Clin Psychol Rev. 2004;24:215-38.
65. Van den Eynde F, Treasure J. Neuroimaging in eating disorders and obesity: implications for research. Child Adolesc Psychiatr Clin N Am. 2009;18:95-115.
66. Liao PC, Uher R, Lawrence N, et al. An examination of decision making in bulimia nervosa. J Clin Exp Neuropsychol. 2009;31:455-61.
67. Wagner A, Aizenstein H, Venkatraman VK, et al. Altered reward processing in women recovered from anorexia nervosa. Am J Psychiatry. 2007;164:1842-9.
68. Wagner A, Aizenstein H, Venkatraman VK, et al. Altered striatal response to reward in bulimia nervosa after recovery. Int J Eat Disord 200910.1002/eat.20699. published online May 11.
69. Roberts ME, Tchanturia K, Stahl D, Southgate L, Treasure J. A systematic review and meta-analysis of set-shifting ability in eating disorders. Psychol Med. 2007;37:1075-84.
70. Zastrow A, Kaiser S, Stippich C, et al. Neural correlates of impaired cognitive-behavioral flexibility in anorexia nervosa. Am J Psychiatry. 2009;166:608-16.
71. Lopez C, Tchanturia K, Stahl D, Treasure J. Central coherence in eating disorders: a systematic review. Psychol Med. 2008;38:1393-404.
72. Zucker NL, Losh M, Bulik CM, et al. Anorexia nervosa and autism spectrum disorders: guided investigation of social cognitive endophenotypes. Psychol Bull. 2007;133:976-1006.
73. Harrison A, Sullivan S, Tchanturia K, Treasure J. Emotion recognition and regulation in anorexia nervosa. Clin Psychol Psychother. 2009;16:348-56.
74. Shoebridge P, Gowers SG. Parental high concern and adolescent-onset anorexia nervosa. A case-control study to investigate direction of causality. Br J Psychiatry. 2000;176:132-7.
75. Favaro A, Tenconi E, Santonastaso P. Perinatal factors and the risk of developing anorexia nervosa and bulimia nervosa. Arch Gen Psychiatry. 2006;63:82-8.

76. Groesz LM, Levine MP, Murnen SK. The effect of experimental presentation of thin media images on body satisfaction: a meta-analytic review. Int J Eat Disord. 2002;31:1-16.
77. Wade TD, Gillespie N, Martin NG. A comparison of early family life events amongst monozygotic twin women with lifetime anorexia nervosa, bulimia nervosa, or major depression. Int J Eat Disord. 2007;40:679-86.
78. Schmidt U, Treasure J. Anorexia nervosa: valued and visible. A cognitive-interpersonal maintenance model and its implications for research and practice. Br J Clin Psychol. 2006;45:1-25.
79. Currin L, Schmidt U, Treasure J, Jick H. Time trends in eating disorder incidence. Br J Psychiatry. 2005;186:132-5.
80. Gowers S, Bryant-Waugh R. Management of child and adolescent eating disorders: the current evidence base and future directions. J Child Psychol Psychiatry. 2004;45:63-83.
81. Williams PM, Goodie J, Motsinger CD. Treating eating disorders in primary care. Am Fam Physician. 2008;77:187-195.
82. National Collaborating Centre for Mental Health. National Clinical Practice Guideline: eating disorders: core interventions in the treatment and management of anorexia nervosa, bulimia nervosa, and related eating disorders. National Institute for Clinical Excellence. *http://www.nice.org.uk/search/guidancesearchresults.* (accessed Oct 27, 2009).
83. American Psychiatric Association. In: Practice guidelines for the treatment of patients with eating disorders. Practice guidelines for the treatment of psychiatric disorders, 3rd edition. Arlington: American Psychiatric Association. 2006: 1097-222.
84. Beumont P, Hay P, Beumont D, et al. Australian and New Zealand clinical practice guidelines for the treatment of anorexia nervosa. Aust N Z J Psychiatry. 2004;38:659-70.
85. National Collaborating Centre for Acute Care. Nutritional support in adults: NICE Clinical Guideline 32. London: National Institute for Health and Clinical Excellence (NICE) NHS, 2006.
86. Eiro M, Katoh T, Watanabe T. Use of a proton-pump inhibitor for metabolic disturbances associated with anorexia nervosa. N Engl J Med. 2002;346:140.
87. Mehler PS, Mackenzie TD. Treatment of osteopenia and osteoporosis in anorexia nervosa: a systematic review of the literature. Int J Eat Disord. 2009;42:195-201.
88. Hjern A, Lindberg L, Lindblad F. Outcome and prognostic factors for adolescent female in-patients with anorexia nervosa: 9- to 14-year follow-up. Br J Psychiatry. 2006;189:428-32.
89. Micali N, Simonoff E, Treasure J. Risk of major adverse perinatal outcomes in women with eating disorders. Br J Psychiatry. 2007;190:255-9.
90. Bulik CM, Von Holle A, Siega-Riz AM, et al. Birth outcomes in women with eating disorders in the Norwegian Mother and Child cohort study (MoBa). Int J Eat Disord. 2009;42:9-18.
91. Sollid CP, Wisborg K, Hjort J, Secher NJ. Eating disorder that was diagnosed before pregnancy and pregnancy outcome. Am J Obstet Gynecol. 2004;190:206-10.
92. Stein A, Woolley H, Cooper S, Winterbottom J, Fairburn CG, Cortina-Borja M. Eating habits and attitudes among 10-year-old children of mothers with eating disorders: longitudinal study. Br J Psychiatry. 2006;189:324-9.
93. Patton GC, Coffey C, Carlin JB, Sanci L, Sawyer S. Prognosis of adolescent partial syndromes of eating disorder. Br J Psychiatry. 2008;192:294-9.
94. Kaplan AS, Walsh BT, Olmsted M, et al. The slippery slope: prediction of successful weight maintenance in anorexia nervosa. Psychol Med. 2009;39:1037-45.
95. Fittig E, Jacobi C, Backmund H, Gerlinghoff M, Wittchen HU. Effectiveness of day hospital treatment for anorexia nervosa and bulimia nervosa. Eur Eat Disord Rev. 2008;16:341-51.
96. Hailey D, Roine R, Ohinmaa A. The effectiveness of telemental health applications: a review. Can J Psychiatry. 2008;53:769-78.
97. Mitchell JE, Crosby RD, Wonderlich SA, et al. A randomized trial comparing the efficacy of cognitive-behavioral therapy for bulimia nervosa delivered via telemedicine versus face-to-face. Behav Res Ther. 2008;46:581-92.
98. Perkins SJ, Murphy R, Schmidt U, Williams C. Self-help and guided self-help for eating disorders. Cochrane Database Syst Rev. 2006;3:CD004191.
99. Robinson P, Serfaty M. Getting better byte by byte: a pilot randomised controlled trial of email therapy for bulimia nervosa and binge eating disorder. Eur Eat Disord Rev. 2008;16: 84-93.
100. Vocks S, Tuschen-Caffier B, Pietrowsky R, Rustenbach SJ, Kersting A, Herpertz S. Meta-analysis of the effectiveness of psychological and pharmacological treatments for binge eating disorder. Int J Eat Disord. 2009;10.1002/eat.20696. published online April 28.
101. Sysko R, Walsh BT. A critical evaluation of the efficacy of self-help interventions for the treatment of bulimia nervosa and binge-eating disorder. Int J Eat Disord. 2008;41:97-112.
102. Keel PK, Haedt A. Evidence-based psychosocial treatments for eating problems and eating disorders. J Clin Child Adolesc Psychol. 2008;37:39-61.
103. Lock J, Agras WS, Bryson S, Kraemer HC. A comparison of short- and long-term family therapy for adolescent anorexia nervosa. J Am Acad Child Adolesc Psychiatry. 2005;44:632-9.
104. Eisler I, Simic M, Russell GF, Dare C. A randomised controlled treatment trial of two forms of family therapy in adolescent anorexia nervosa: a five-year follow-up. J Child Psychol Psychiatry. 2007;48:552-60.
105. Zablana M, Macdonald P, Treasure J. Appraisal of caregiving burden, expressed emotion and psychological distress in families of people with eating disorders: a systematic review. Eur Eat Disord Rev. 2009;17:327-30.
106. Zucker NL, Marcus M, Bulik C. A group parent-training program: a novel approach for eating disorder management. Eat Weight Disord. 2006;11:78-82.
107. Hay PPJ, Bacltchuk J, Byrnes RT, Claudino AM, Ekmejian SS, Yong PY. Individual psychotherapy in the outpatient treatment of adults with anorexia nervosa (review), 2nd edition. Cochrane Database Syst Rev. 2008;1:CD003909.

108. Crow SJ, Mitchell JE, Roerig JD, Steffen K. What potential role is there for medication treatment in anorexia nervosa?. Int J Eat Disord 2009;42:1-8.
109. Claudino AM, Hay P, Lima MS, et al. Antidepressants for anorexia nervosa. Cochrane Database Syst Rev 2006;1:CD004365.
110. Kaye WH, Nagata T, Weltzin TE, et al. Double-blind placebo-controlled administration of fluoxetine in restricting- and restricting-purging-type anorexia nervosa. Biol Psychiatry. 2001;49:644-52.
111. Walsh BT, Kaplan AS, Attia E, et al. Fluoxetine after weight restoration in anorexia nervosa: a randomized controlled trial. JAMA. 2006;295:2605-12.
112. Bosanac P, Norman T, Burrows G, Beumont P. Serotonergic and dopaminergic systems in anorexia nervosa: a role for atypical antipsychotics?. Aust N Z J Psychiatry. 2005;39:146-53.
113. Brambilla F, Garcia CS, Fassino S, et al. Olanzapine therapy in anorexia nervosa: psychobiological effects. Int Clin Psychopharmacol. 2007;22:197-204.
114. Bissada H, Tasca GA, Barber AM, Bradwejn J. Olanzapine in the treatment of low body weight and obsessive thinking in women with anorexia nervosa: a randomized, double-blind, placebo-controlled trial. Am J Psychiatry. 2008;165:1281-8.
115. Shapiro JR, Berkman ND, Brownley KA, et al. Bulimia nervosa treatment: a systematic review of randomized controlled trials. Int J Eat Disord. 2007;40:321-36.
116. Fairburn CG, Marcus MD, Wilson GT. Cognitive-behavioral therapy for binge eating and bulimia nervosa: a comprehensive treatment manual. In: Fairburn CG, Wilson GT (Eds). Binge eating: nature, assessment, and treatment. New York: The Guilford Press, 1993:361-404.
117. Hay PJ, Bacaltchuk J. Bulimia nervosa. Clin Evid (Online). 2008:1009. June 12, pii:
118. Mitchell JE, Agras S, Wonderlich S. Treatment of bulimia nervosa: where are we and where are we going?. Int J Eat Disord. 2007;40:95-101.
119. Fairburn CG, Cooper Z, Doll HA, et al. Transdiagnostic cognitive-behavioral therapy for patients with eating disorders: a two-site trial with 60-week follow-up. Am J Psychiatry. 2009;166:311-9.
120. Chen EY, Matthews L, Allen C, Kuo JR, Linehan MM. Dialectical behavior therapy for clients with binge-eating disorder or bulimia nervosa and borderline personality disorder. Int J Eat Disord. 2008;41:505-12.
121. Schmidt U, Lee S, Beecham J, et al. A randomized controlled trial of family therapy and cognitive behavior therapy guided self-care for adolescents with bulimia nervosa and related disorders. Am J Psychiatry. 2007;164:591-8.
122. Ie GD, Crosby RD, Rathouz PJ, Leventhal BL. A randomized controlled comparison of family-based treatment and supportive psychotherapy for adolescent bulimia nervosa. Arch Gen Psychiatry. 2007;64:1049-56.
123. Hay PJ, Bacaltchuk J, Stefano S. Psychotherapy for bulimia nervosa and binging. Cochrane Database Syst Rev. 2004;3: CD000562.
124. Stone M, Laughren T, Jones ML, et al. Risk of suicidality in clinical trials of antidepressants in adults: analysis of proprietary data submitted to US Food and Drug Administration. BMJ. 2009;339: b2880.
125. Bacaltchuk J, Hay P. Antidepressants versus placebo for people with bulimia nervosa. Cochrane Database Syst Rev. 2003;4. CD003391.
126. Milano W, Siano C, Putrella C, Capasso A. Treatment of bulimia nervosa with fluvoxamine: a randomized controlled trial. Adv Ther. 2005;22:278-83.
127. Romano SJ, Halmi KA, Sarkar NP, Koke SC, Lee JS. A placebo-controlled study of fluoxetine in continued treatment of bulimia nervosa after successful acute fluoxetine treatment. Am J Psychiatry. 2002;159:96-102.
128. Nickel C, Tritt K, Muehlbacher M, et al. Topiramate treatment in bulimia nervosa patients: a randomized, double-blind, placebo-controlled trial. Int J Eat Disord. 2005;38:295-300.
129. Hedges DW, Reimherr FW, Hoopes SP, et al. Treatment of bulimia nervosa with topiramate in a randomized, double-blind, placebo-controlled trial, part 2: improvement in psychiatric measures. J Clin Psychiatry. 2003;64:1449-54.
130. Brownley KA, Berkman ND, Sedway JA, Lohr KN, Bulik CM. Binge eating disorder treatment: a systematic review of randomized controlled trials. Int J Eat Disord. 2007;40:337-48.
131. Devlin MJ, Goldfein JA, Petkova E, et al. Cognitive behavioral therapy and fluoxetine as adjuncts to group behavioral therapy for binge eating disorder. Obes Res. 2005;13:1077-88.
132. Wilfley DE, Welch RR, Stein RI, et al. A randomized comparison of group cognitive-behavioral therapy and group interpersonal psychotherapy for the treatment of overweight individuals with binge-eating disorder. Arch Gen Psychiatry. 2002;59: 713-21.
133. Agras WS, Telch CF, Arnow B, Eldredge K, Marnell M. One-year follow-up of cognitive-behavioral therapy for obese individuals with binge eating disorder. J Consult Clin Psychol. 1997;65:343-7.
134. Devlin MJ, Goldfein JA, Petkova E, Liu L, Walsh BT. Cognitive behavioral therapy and fluoxetine for binge eating disorder: two-year follow-up. Obesity (Silver Spring). 2007;15:1702-1709.
135. Reas DL, Grilo CM. Review and meta-analysis of pharmacotherapy for binge-eating disorder. Obesity (Silver Spring). 2008;16:2024-38.
136. Guerdjikova AI, McElroy SL, Kotwal R, et al. High-dose escitalopram in the treatment of binge-eating disorder with obesity: a placebo-controlled monotherapy trial. Hum Psychopharmacol. 2008;23:1-11.
137. Stefano SC, Bacaltchuk J, Blay SL, Appolinario JC. Antidepressants in short-term treatment of binge eating disorder: systematic review and meta-analysis. Eat Behav. 2008;9:129-36.
138. Appolinario JC, Bacaltchuk J, Sichieri R, et al. A randomized, double-blind, placebo-controlled study of sibutramine in the treatment of binge-eating disorder. Arch Gen Psychiatry. 2003;60:1109-16.

139. Wilfley DE, Crow SJ, Hudson JI, et al. Efficacy of sibutramine for the treatment of binge eating disorder: a randomized multicenter placebo-controlled double-blind study. Am J Psychiatry. 2008;165:51-8.
140. Golay A, Laurent-Jaccard A, Habicht F, et al. Effect of orlistat in obese patients with binge eating disorder. Obes Res. 2005;13:1701-8.
141. McElroy SL, Hudson JI, Capece JA, et al. Topiramate for the treatment of binge eating disorder associated with obesity: a placebo-controlled study. Biol Psychiatry. 2007;61:1039-48.
142. McElroy SL, Kotwal R, Guerdjikova AI, et al. Zonisamide in the treatment of binge eating disorder with obesity: a randomized controlled trial. J Clin Psychiatry. 2006;67:1897-906.
143. McElroy SL, Guerdjikova A, Kotwal R, et al. Atomoxetine in the treatment of binge-eating disorder: a randomized placebo-controlled trial. J Clin Psychiatry. 2007;68:390-8.
144. Claudino AM, de Oliveira IR, Appolinario JC, et al. Double-blind, randomized, placebo-controlled trial of topiramate plus cognitive-behavior therapy in binge-eating disorder. J Clin Psychiatry. 2007;68:1324-32.
145. Grilo CM, Masheb RM, Salant SL. Cognitive behavioral therapy guided self-help and orlistat for the treatment of binge eating disorder: a randomized, double-blind, placebo-controlled trial. Biol Psychiatry. 2005;57:1193-201.
146. Reas DL, Grilo CM. Review and meta-analysis of pharmacotherapy for binge-eating disorder. Obesity (Silver Spring). 2008;16:2024-38.
147. Von HA, Pinheiro AP, Thornton LM, et al. Temporal patterns of recovery across eating disorder subtypes. Aust N Z J Psychiatry. 2008;42:108-17.
148. Berkman ND, Lohr KN, Bulik CM. Outcomes of eating disorders: a systematic review of the literature. Int J Eat Disord. 2007;40:293-309.
149. Papadopoulos FC, Ekbom A, Brandt L, Ekselius L. Excess mortality, causes of death and prognostic factors in anorexia nervosa. Br J Psychiatry. 2009;194:10-17.
150. Byford S, Barrett B, Roberts C, et al. Economic evaluation of a randomised controlled trial for anorexia nervosa in adolescents. Br J Psychiatry. 2007;191:436-40.
151. Fichter MM, Quadflieg N, Hedlund S. Long-term course of binge eating disorder and bulimia nervosa: relevance for nosology and diagnostic criteria. Int J Eat Disord. 2008;41:577-86.
152. American Psychiatric Association. Desk Reference to the Diagnostic Criteria from DSM-5. Washington DC; 2013.

CHAPTER 29

Postpartum Psychiatric Disorders

Neena Bohra, NK Bohra

The traditional view that there are three postpartum psychiatric disorders—the maternity blues, puerperal psychosis, and postnatal depression—is an oversimplification. The range of disorders is wide. This review focuses on those important to general psychiatrists and family practitioners. It does not cover mild disorders that require no treatment (such as the maternity blues), nor grieving over fetal loss, nor rare complications (such as organic psychoses), nor the effect of childbirth on eating disorders or ethanol misuse. It draws attention to gaps in knowledge and research priorities.

POSTPARTUM PSYCHOSES

The sudden onset of psychosis after childbirth has intrigued medical practitioners for centuries. More than 2000 papers have been published. This group of disorders is diverse; including psychogenic and organic psychoses.[1] Only one form is commonly seen in countries with modern obstetric services. This form is generally called puerperal psychosis and takes the form of mania, severe depression (with delusions, confusion, or stupor), or acute polymorphic (cycloid) psychosis. Record-linkage studies[2,3] give an incidence of about one per 1000 births. The claim that this is a "disease in its own right" was disproved long ago by the long-term case studies of Esquirol,[4] and there is now much evidence for a link with manic depressive psychosis.[1] Children, together with abortion[1,5] and menstruation,[6] is one of the triggers of bipolar episodes in susceptible women. Research on these triggers is a promising avenue to a greater understanding of manic depression. Puerperal psychosis has a high and specific heritability.[7] The recurrence rate is about one in four pregnancies. In recurrence rate is about one in four pregnancies. In treatment, haloperidol should be used with caution, because dangerous side-effects including neuroleptics malignant syndrome have been reported.[1,8,9] The newer neuroleptics drugs, such as olanzapine, seem to be safer, although their safety has not yet been proven by treatment trials. Electroconvulsive treatment is useful,[10] and lithium can be effective prophylaxis.[11]

DISORDERS OF THE MOTHER-INFANT RELATIONSHIP

Childbirth presents many challenges to the mother:trauma, sleep deprivation, breastfeeding, adjustments in conjugal and other relationships, and social isolation. However, the central and most important psychological process is development of the relationship with the infant. Disturbances in this process were recognized long ago, when hatred of children[12,13] and child abuse[14] were described. Various terms have been used for these disturbances. "Bonding" is a useful lay term, but neither "bonding" nor "attachment" describes the essential symptom, which is the mother's emotional response to the infant-aversion, hatred, or pathological anger. "Mother-infant interaction" reflects this response and has the advantage that it can be recorded and measured. But the concept of "postnatal depression with impaired mother-infant interaction" is inadequate to encompass such a profound emotional disorder, which can occur without depression.[15] The concept of mother-infant relationship disorder is controversial. It is not recognized in the tenth revision of the International Classification of Diseases (ICD-10) nor the Diagnostic and Statistical Manual IV (DSM-IV). One of the challenges for ICD-11 and DSM-5 is to find a place for these disorders, so that they can be recognized by practitioners and referred for expert treatment. This process will involve a difficult innovation, because "hatred" does not fit comfortably with the concept of disease or illness. If hatred of a rival or political enemy is not an illness, why should a mother's hatred and rejection of an infant be listed as a disease? But medicine has pragmatic rather than logical boundaries, and psychiatry often challenges the definition of disease.

Disorders of the mother-infant relationship are prominent in 10–25% of women referred to psychiatrists after childbirth.[1] At the extreme of rejection of the infant, the mother may try to persuade a family member to take over care permanently or may demand that the baby be adopted. She may try to escape. The most poignant manifestation is the wish that the baby disappear—be stolen or succumb to cot death. Rejection is accompanied in many cases by pathological anger, with shouting, cursing, or screaming at the infant, accompanied by impulses to strike, shake, or smother the child. These disorders are more common, intractable, and serious in their effects than puerperal psychosis. With treatment, they can resolve completely. Without it, there are high risks of child abuse and neglect, long-term impairment of the mother-child relationship, and psychiatric or learning disorders in the children. The effects have been studied indirectly through cohort studies of children born after refused termination of pregnancy.[16,17] For example, a Danish study[18] followed up unwanted children in a cohort of 4269 male births. A combinations and early child rejection carried a risk of violent criminality four times higher than the reference category.

For more direct evidence, there are studies of the effects of "postnatal depression" on the child. Most have not assessed the mother-infant relationship, but Murray and colleagues[19] made brief audio recordings and videotapes of mother-child interaction. They compared 61 mothers in Cambridge, UK, depressed 5–6 weeks after childbirth, with 42 controls. Mother-child interaction was assessed at 2 months, and the children were followed up for 5 years. Cognitive functioning was not affected by maternal depression but was predicted by mother-infant interaction ($r = 0.29$, $p<0.05$). More research should be focused on the effects of these disorders on children's intellectual development and mental health, and their relation to child abuse and neglect.

The diagnosis is facilitated by screening questionnaires,[20,21] which can also be used to chart progress in treatment. An interview, in which 24 probes explore the mother-infant relationship, has been published.[1] Observational data can be obtained in hospital[22,23] or can be used. However, more research is needed to improve our recognition and measurement of these disorders, clarifying the link between symptoms explored by interviews and questionnaires and direct observations of mother-infant interaction.

In management, depression should be treated, even when signs are negligible. The specific psychological treatment is play therapy in various forms,[24] interaction coaching, or baby massage,[25,26] which can be undertaken by nursing staff or psychologists. The aim is to help the mother to enjoy her interactions with the child.

DEPRESSION

Although puerperal melancholia has been recognized for centuries, American research in the 1950s drew attention to the prevalence of milder postpartum depression. A concept of postnatal depression emerged, which has been useful as a lay term. It reduces stigma and enables mothers with various postpartum psychiatric disorders to recognize that they are ill and to seek help. It is a focus for self-help groups and lobbying to improve services.

As a medical concept, however, it is less useful. Unless practitioners appreciate that the concept is merely a rubric, research and clinical practice will be left at a basic level.[27] Patients who score above threshold on screening questionnaires or meet criteria for major depression are heterogeneous: their illnesses include a variety of anxiety, obsessional, and post-traumatic stress disorders, together with depression associated with adversity and primary depression linked to bipolar disorder. A diagnostic concept needs an epidemiological association, indicating the presence of specific causal factors. This association is lacking for postpartum depression. Depression is common in all women, whether infertile, menopausal, pregnant, puerperal, or involved in child-rearing. The rates of depression show little difference between women just after childbirth and other women.[28,29]

Maternal morbidity and mortality are not the only reason why effective action to deal with postpartum depression is necessary. Postpartum depression can have pervasive effects on the family. Although deficits are not universal in depressed mothers,[30] depression can lead to reduced interaction and irritability misdirected at the children.

Depression may be the most frequent psychiatric disorder seen after childbirth. During the past 7 years, the output of publications on this subject has greatly increased.

The diagnosis of postpartum depression is facilitated by the involvement of midwives and health visitors in the puerperium. The Edinburgh postnatal depression scale (EPDS)[31] is widely used and has been translated into many languages. A Norwegian paper reviewed 18 validation studies.[32] The EPDS also measures anxiety[33,34] and could be general screening tool for the whole range of postpartum psychiatric disorders.[35] Other questionnaires used are the general health questionnaire, the Beck depression inventory,[36] and the postpartum depression screening scale.[37]

A positive score on a self-rating questionnaire needs to be followed by an interview clarifying the symptoms of depression and coexisting psychiatric disorders. The wider context must be explored, including the woman's life history, personality, and circumstances; the course of the pregnancy, including parturition and the puerperium; and relationships with partner, other children, family of origin, and, especially, the infant. In addition to diagnosing depression and other disorders, vulnerability factors and the availability of support must be identified.

Treatment is focused on depression and any underlying vulnerability. It will always involve psychotherapy,[38] generally given by hospital and community nurses, health visitors, and lay counselors. It may involve medication or other specific treatments. In pharmaceutical treatment, no drug is clearly superior, but there have been many publications on drug treatment in lactating women, with more than 50 reviews. The most recent is that of Wisner and colleagues[39] and the most detailed is by Spigser and Hagg.[40] The suckling infant is at risk because of the immaturity of body systems: lack of body fat, low plasma protein binding, immature liver and kidney, and undeveloped blood-brain barrier. Nevertheless, few adverse effects have been reported, and the general view is that breastfeeding can continue and that, with the exceptions of nefazodone,[41] doxepin,[42] and fluoxetine,[39] antidepressant agents can be given. To illustrate the safety of sertraline, one study[43] investigated serotonin concentrations in mothers and infants: they fell in the mothers but did not change in the infants, indicating that insufficient drug had reached the infant through breastmilk. Antidepressive drugs should be used cautiously in lactating mothers, and administration after a breastfeed might be helpful.

Gregoire and colleagues[44] researched the effect of 17β-estradiol patches in chronic treatment-resistant postpartum depression. Treatment was beneficial ($p<0.0001$). This study adds to many others, going back 70 years,[45] in support of estrogen's antidepressive properties. By contrast, a controlled prophylactic trial of the progestagen norethisterone enanthate showed increased depression with the drug.[46]

Prevention is important in women with a history of postpartum depression. There is a great opportunity to identify women at risk during their attendance at antenatal clinics. Some have had previous postpartum episodes. Some are already depressed. Others have obvious risk factors such as frictional relationships, social isolation, addiction, or unwanted pregnancy. Another research priority is to find the best way of screening pregnant women. Support from community nurses, voluntary agencies, or groups can begin during pregnancy. If pregnant women are well, all that is necessary is to establish contact, so that a recurrence is diagnosed and treated promptly.

Prophylactic antidepressive drug therapy is rational in women at risk of recurrence, but a double-blind randomized trial showed unexpectedly that nortriptyline did not prevent recurrence in mothers with a history of postpartum depression.[47]

POST-TRAUMATIC STRESS DISORDER

Bydlowski and Raoul-Duval[48] described post-traumatic stress disorder (PTSD) after childbirth in 1978. Long ordeals during labor led to secondary tocophobia, and the recurrence of tension, nightmares, and flashbacks toward the end of the next pregnancy. There are now about 40 publications on this disorder, which has been called the fourth postpartum mental disorder.[49] The stressful experience is pain in most cases, but loss of control and fear of death can be the focus.[50,51] There have been eight quantitative studies.[48,52-58] Case reports suggest that depression, an impaired mother-infant relationship,[59] and sexual dysfunction can result. In Stockholm, half of mothers with a very negative birth experience at their first delivery avoided any further pregnancy.[60] These women should be referred for specific psychological treatment, such as massed practice, which might accelerate accommodation to the traumatic memory.

VARIOUS MORBID PREOCCUPATIONS

Distress about the bodily changes resulting from pregnancy and childbirth are common. Such women complain of weight gain, stretch marks, or scars. They are reluctant to undress in front of their partners, avoid looking at themselves naked, and can even avoid being seen in public.

Conjugal jealousy is another disorder sometimes linked to pregnancy and childbirth. Preoccupying worries about the spouse's fidelity are an understandable reaction to pregnancy changes and the relative quiescence of sexual life. Most publications are case reports.[1] In the unpublished study mentioned above, postpartum morbid jealousy was evident in 5% of women.

Complaints about obstetric management can be preoccupying. They are relatively common after emergency cesarean section.[61] Childbirth is a key experience, and a woman may feel bitter disappointment over delivery perceived as mismanaged. Such feelings can lead to litigation and in some cases preoccupy the woman for weeks or months and interfere with care of the infant. These disorders are sometimes confused with PTSD, but the dominant emotion is ruminative anger not anxiety, and the treatment is different-distraction from the perceived injury and redirection of attention to positive activity. The frequency in the above-mentioned unpublished study was 10%.

ANXIETY DISORDERS SPECIFIC TO THE PUERPERIUM

Several studies have reported the effect of pregnancy on panic disorder. A review of eight studies showed an improvement, but in 44% there was an exacerbation in the postpartum period and in 10% new onset in the puerperium.[62] Recent studies suggest that postpartum anxiety disorders are under-emphasized and are more common than depression.[63,64] There could be a biological basis for some postpartum anxiety. McIvor and colleagues[65] studied the growth-hormone response to apomorphine (a test of dopamine D2 receptor sensitivity) in 14 puerperal women with a history of depression. The greatest increase in receptor sensitivity was found in three greatest increase in receptor sensitivity was found in three women who developed postpartum anxiety disorders.

ICD-10 and DSM-IV give criteria for anxiety disorders as a group, but the focus of anxiety is also important, because it can indicate specific psychological treatment. This issue is a challenge for the next generation of international classifications. De Armond[66] described fear of the newborn infant based on the awesome responsibility of care. Most women are shielded from this fear by family support, but in isolated nuclear families it can be a severe problem. Support from family or nursing staff is all that is required. Fear of cot death can reach a pathological degree.[67] Reproductive losses (e.g. recurrent miscarriage) or infertility of long duration can be an antecedent factor. The main manifestation is nocturnal vigilance. The mother lies awake listening to the infant's breathing, and often checks that he/she is still alive. This fear can last for months and lead to exhausting sleep deprivation. It is not easy to treat. A baby monitor can be useful, as can nights of respite, when another trusted person looks after the infant and the mother sleeps under sedation. Involvement of a panel of mothers who have recovered from this disorder is useful, as in other postpartum disorders. Many mothers are excessively anxious about the health and safety of their children, described as maternity neurosis[68] or maternal separation anxiety.[69] There is some evidence that severe postpartum anxiety has adverse effects on the child, with a high proportion of insecure and disorganized attachments.[70] Drug treatment can be used, but, in lactating women, anxiolytic benzodiazepines should be used with caution. They are well absorbed from the gut, have long half-lives, and are more slowly metabolized by the liver in infants. Lethargy and weight loss have been reported in an infant exposed to diazepam. For this reason, oxazepam has been recommended.[40] A woman with infant-focused anxiety may avoid the infant in a typical phobic reaction.[71] Such women respond well to treatment by desensitization in a mother and baby unit. Many cases of postpartum anxiety disorders require the skills of a clinical psychologist, using relaxation techniques and cognitive therapy.

OBSESSIONS OF CHILD HARM

Obsessions of infanticide were one of the first postpartum disorders to be described,[72] and several recent series have been published.[73-75] The central symptoms is of impulses to attack the child, but the setting is different from the pathological anger that precedes child abuse. The mother is gentle and devoted. She experiences extravagant infanticidal impulses, together with fantasies of the family's horror and grief, causing intense distress and leading to reduced contact with the baby. The content can include child sexual abuse.[76] Classic papers were written by Chapman[77] and Button and Reivich,[78] who found 42 cases among 1317 consecutive consultations. Buttolph and Holland[79] report that 27 of 39 female patients with obsessive-compulsive disorder (OCD) had onset or worsening in pregnancy or after childbirth. Jennings and colleagues[80] interviewed 100 depressed mothers: 21 had repeated thoughts of harming their children and took precautions, and 24 were afraid to be alone with their children. An Italian group[81] studied the triggers of OCD and found that childbirth was the only life event significantly associated with onset. The management involves specific psychological treatment as well as antidepressant therapy. Avoidance of the child should be discouraged, and cuddling and play encouraged, strengthening positive maternal feelings.

SPECIALIST TEAMS

Given the diversity of postpartum mental illness and its risks for infants, there is a case for setting up specialist services for pregnant and puerperal women. In the UK, after the pioneering has been gained, through the concentration of severe cases in mother and baby units. However, in the absence of service evaluation, good clinical practice is based on ideas and innovation, rather than rigorous outcome data. The essence of these services is a multidiscipilinary specialist team, including psychiatrists, psychologists, nurses (probably also nursery nurses), and social workers. The aims are prevention, early diagnosis, and versatile intervention, with the minimum family disruption. Such teams can serve a wide area, taking over the treatment of severe and intractable illness, developing services, training staff, and conducting research. They can provide a trial of mothering in complex cases, and give medicolegal advice. Domiciliary assessment and home treatment are appropriate. A day hospital, with a wide range of interventions—groups, play therapy, motherhood classes, anxiety management, and occupational therapy—has the advantage of putting women with similar disorders in touch with each other, without disrupting family life. If a woman must be admitted to hospital, joint admission of mother and infant has advantage over admission of the mother alone, because it preserves their relationship. Units devoted to postpartum care are probably safer and more effective than general psychiatric wards. A research priority is to investigate the advantages and safety of these units, which have an important role, especially in early diagnosis and prevention. They also need links with pediatric units, social services, and child protection teams to collaborate in the prevention of child abuse. Links with voluntary agencies are important because self-help groups provide much support for depressed and isolated mothers and can collaborate in treatment.[82] There are many specialist services in the UK and Australasia, fewer in European countries, and very few elsewhere.

REFERENCES

1. Brockington IF. Motherhood and mental health. Oxford:Oxford University Press, 1996.
2. Kendell RE, Chalmers JC, Platz C. Epidemiology of puerperal psychoses. Br J Psychiatry. 1987;150:662-73.
3. Terp IM, Mortensen PB. Post-partum psychoses: clinical diagnoses and relative risk of admission after parturition. Br T Psychiatry. 1998;172:521-6.

4. Esquirol JED. Mental maladies. A treatise on insanity. Facsimile of English edition of 1845. New York Hafner. 1965:125-43.
5. David HP, Rasmussen NK, Holst E. Postpartum and postabortion psychotic reactions. Fam Plann Perspect. 1981;13:88-92.
6. Brockington IF. Menstrual psychosis. Arch Women Ment Health. 1998;1:3-13.
7. Jones I, Coyle N, Robertson E, et al. Puerperal psychosis: evidence for familiarity of the puerperal trigger. Mol Psychiatry. 1999;4:S26.
8. Klompenhouwer JL, Puerperal psychosis. PhD thesis: University of Rotterdam, 1992.
9. Price DK, Turnbull GJ, Gregory RP, Stevens DG. Neuroleptic malignant syndrome in a case of postpartum psychosis. Br J Psychiatry. 1989;155:849-52.
10. Reed P, Sermin N, Appleby L, Faragher B. A comparison of clinical response to electroconvulsive therapy in puerperal and non-puerperal psychoses. J Affect Disord. 1999;54:255-60.
11. Stewart DE, Klompenhouwe JL, Kendell RE, Van Hulst A.M. Prophylactic lithium in puerperal psychosis: the experience of three centres. Br J Psychiatry. 1991;158:393-97.
12. Boileau de Castelnau P. Misopedie ou lesion de I'amour de la progeniture. Ann Medico-psychol 1861:3rd series 7:553-68.
13. Oppenheim H. Uber misopadie. Z Gesamte Neurol Psychiatr. 1919;45:1-18.
14. Tardieu A. Etude medicolegale surles services et mauvais traitements exercise sur des enfants. Ann Hygiene. 1860;15: 361-98.
15. Righetti-Veltema M, Conne-Perreard E, Bousquet A, Manzano J. Postpartum depression and mother-infant relationship at 3 months old. T effect Disord. 2002;70:291-306.
16. Kubicka L, Matejcek Z, Bavid HP, et al. Children from unwanted pregnancies in Prague, Czech Republic, revisited at age thirty. Acta Psychiatr Scand. 1995;91:361-9.
17. Myrhman A, Rantakallio P, Isohanni M, Jones P, Partanen U. Unwantedness of a pregnancy and schizophrenia in the child. BR J Psychiatry. 1996;169:637-40.
18. Raine A, Brennan P, Mednick SA. Birth complications combined with early maternal rejection at age 1-year predispose to violent crime at age 18 years. Arch Gen Psychiatry. 1994;51:984-8.
19. Murray L, Hipwell A, Hooper R, et al. The cognitive development of 5-year old children of postnatally depressed mothers. J Child Psychol Psychiatry. 1996;37:927-35.
20. Nagata M, Nagai Y, Sobajima H, et al. Materinity blues and attachment to children in mothers of full-term normal infants. Acta Psychiatr Scand. 2000;101:209-17.
21. Brockington IF, Oates J, George S, et al. A screening questionnaire for mother-infant bonding disorders. Arch Women Ment Health. 2001;3:133-40.
22. Salariya EM, Cater JI. Mother-child relationship: FIRST score. T Adv Nurs. 1984;9:589-95.
23. Hipwell AE, Kumar R. Maternal psychopathology and prediction of outcome based on mother-infant interaction ratings. Br J Psychiartry. 1996;169:655-61.
24. Brockington IF, Brierley E. Rejection of a child by his mother, successfully treated after 3 years. Br J Psychiatry. 1984;145:316-18.
25. Field T, Grizzle N, Scafidi F, et al. Massage therapy for infants of depressed mothers, infant Behav Dev. 1996;19:107-12.
26. Onozawa K, Glover V, Adams D, Modi N, kumar R. Infant massage improves mother-infants interaction for mothers with postnatal depression. J Affect Disord. 2001;63:201-07.
27. Jones HW, Venis JA. Identification and classification of postpartum psychiatric disorders. J Psychosoc Nurs Ment Health Serv. 2001:39:23-30.
28. Cooper PJ, Campbell EA, Day A, Kennerley H, Bond A. Non-psychotic psychiatric disorder after childbirth: a prospective study of prevalence, incidence, course and nature. Br J Psychiatry. 1988;152:799-806.
29. Cox JL, Murray D, Chapman G. A controlled study of the onset, duration and prevalence of postnatal depression. Br J Psychiatry. 1993;163:27-31.
30. Pound A, Puckering C, Cox A, Mills M. The impact of maternal depression on young children. Br J Psyhother. 1988;4:240-52.
31. Cox JL, Holden JM, Sagovsky R. Detection of postnatal depression: development of the 10-item Edinburgh Postnatal Depression Scale. Br J Psychiatry. 1987;150:782-6.
32. Eberhard-Gran M, eskild A, Tambs K, Opjordsmoen S, SAmuelsen SO. Review of validation studies of the Edinburgh Postnatal Depression Scale. Acta Psychiatr Scand. 2001;104: 243-9.
33. Stuart S, Couser G, Schilder K, O'Hara M, Gorman L. Postpartum anxiety and depression:onset and comorbidity in a community sample. J Nerv Ment Dis. 1998;186:420-4.
34. Brouwers ePM, van Baar, AL, POP VJM. Does the Edinburgh Postnatal Depression Scale measure anxiety? J Psychosom Res. 2001;51:659-63.
35. Lappin J. Depressed mood during pregnancy and after childbirth. BMJ. 2001;323:1367.
36. Lee DTS, Yip ASK, Chiu HFK, Leung TYS, Chung TKH. Screening for postnatal depression:are specific instruments madatory? J Affect Dis. 2000;63:233-8.
37. Beck CT, Gable RK. Comparative analysis of the Performance of the Postpartum Depression Screening Scale with two other depression instruments. Nurs Res. 2001;50:242-50.
38. Blum LD. Postpartum depression. N Engl J Med. 2003;348:1294.
39. Wisner KL, Parry BL, Piontek CM. Postpartum depression. N Engl J Med. 2002;347:194-9.
40. Spigset O, hagg S. Excretion of psychotropic drugs into breast milk. CNS Drugs. 1998;9:111-34.
41. Yapp P, Ilett KF, Kristensen JH, et al. Drowsiness and poor feeding in a breast-fed infant:association with nefazodone and its metabolites. Ann Pharmacother. 2000;34:1269-72.
42. Natheson I, Pande H, Alertsen AR. RESpiratory depression caused by N-desmethyldoxepin in breast milk. Lancet. 1985;2:1124.
43. Epperson N, Czarkowski KA, Ward-O'Brien D, et al. Maternal sertraline treatment and serotonin transport in breast-feeding mother infant pairs. Am J Psychiatry. 2001;158:1631-7.

44. Gregpore AJP, Kumar R, Everitt B, Henderson AF, Studd JWW. Transdermal oestrogen for treatment of severe postnatal depression. Lancet. 1996;347:930-3.
45. Sevringhaus EL. The use of folliculin in involutional states. Am J Obstet Gynecol. 1933;25:361-8.
46. Lawrie TA, Hofmeyr GJ, De Jager M, et al. A double blind randomized placebo controlled trial of postnatal norethisterone enanthate:the effect on postnatal depression and serum hormones. Br J Obstet Gynaecol. 1998;105:1082-90.
47. Wisner KL, Perel JM, Peindl KS, Hanusa B, Findling RL, Rapport D. Prevention or recruitment postpartum depression: a randomized clinical trial. J Clin Psychiatry. 2001;62:82-6.
48. Bydlowski M, Raoul-Duval A. Un avatar psychique meconnu de la puerperalite: La nevrose traumatique post-obstetricale. Perspect Psychiatr. 1978;4:321-8.
49. Godfroid IO, Charlot A. Psychiatric du post-partum. Rev Med Brux. 1996;17:22-3.
50. Menage J. Post-traumatic stress disorder in women who have undergone obstetric and/or gynaecological procedures: a consecutive series of 30 cases of PTSD. J Reprod Infant Psychol. 1993;11:221-8.
51. Ryding EL. Investigation of 33 women who demanded a Caesarian section for personal reasons. Acta Obstet Gynecol Psychol. 1993;72:280-85.
52. Wijma K, Soderquist J, Wijma B. Post-traumatic stress disorder after childbirth: a cross sectional study. J Anxiety Disord. 1997;11:587-97.
53. Lyons S. A prospective study of post traumatic stress symptoms one month following childbirth in a group of 42 first time mothers. J Reprod Infant Psychol. 1998;16:91-105.
54. Czarnocka J, Slade P. Prevalence and predictors of post-traumatic stress symptoms following childbirth. Br J Clin Psychol. 2000;39:35-51.
55. Creedy DK, Shochet IM, Horsfall J. Childbirth and the development of acute trauma symptoms: incidence and contributing factors. Birth. 2000;27:104-11.
56. Ayers S, Pickering AD. Do women get post-traumatic stress disorder as a result of childbirth? A prospective study of incidence. Birth. 2001;28:111-18.
57. Pantlen A, Rohde A. Psychische Auswirkungen traumatisch erlebter Entbindungen. Zentralbl Gynakol. 2001;123:42-7.
58. Soet JE, Brack GA, Dilorio C. Psychological trauma during childbirth. Birth. 2003;30:36-46.
59. Kumar R. "Anybody's child": severe disorders of mother-infant bonding. Br J Psychiatry. 1997;171:175-81.
60. Gottvall K, Waldenstrom U. Does a traumatic birth experience have an impact on future reproduction? Br j Obstet Gynaecol. 2002;109:254-60.
61. Ryding EL, Wijma K, Wijma B. Experiences of emergency Caesarean section: a phenomenological study of 53 women. Birth. 1998;25:246-51.
62. Hertzberg T, Wahlbeck K. The impact of pregnancy and puerperium on panic disorder: a review. J Psychosom Obstet Gynecol. 1999;20:59-64.
63. Matthey S, Barnett B, Howie P, Kavanagh DJ. Diagnosing postpartum depression in mothers and fathers: whatever happened to anxiety? J Affect Disord. 2003;74:139-47.
64. Wenzel A, Haugen EN, Jackson LC, Robinson K. Prevalence of generalized anxiety at eight weeks postpartum. Arch Women Ment Health. 2003;6:43-9.
65. McIvor RJ, Davies RA, Wieck A, et al. The growth hormone response to apomorphin at 4 days postpartum in women with a history of major depression. J Affect Disord. 1996;40:131-6.
66. De Armond M. A type of post partum anxiety reaction. Dis Nerv Syst. 1954;15:26-9.
67. Wightman H, Dalal BM. Brockington IF. Pathological fear of cot death. Psychopathology. 1998;31:246-9.
68. Moll L. Die Maternitatsneurose. Win Klin Wochenschr. 1920;33:160-2.
69. Hock E, McBride S, Gnezda MT. Maternal separation anxiety:mother-infant separation from the maternal perspective. Child Dev. 1989;60:793-802.
70. Manassis K, Bradley S, Goldberg S, Hood J, Swinson RP. Attachment to mothers with anxiety disorders and their children. J Am Acad Child Adolesc Psychiatry. 1994;33:1106-13.
71. Sved-Williams AE. Phobic reactions of mothers to their own babies. Aust NZ J Psychiatry. 1992;26:631-8.
72. Woodward J. Autochthonous delusion, 1757. Reproduced in: Hunter R, McAlpine I, (Eds). Three hundred years of psychiatry. Oxford:Oxford University Press. 1963:338-41.
73. Sichel DA, Cohen LS, Dimmock JA, Rosenbaum JF. Postpartum obsessive compulsive disorder: a case series. J Clin Psychiatry. 1993;54:156-59.
74. Williams KE, Koran LM. Obsessive-compulsive disorder in pregnancy, the puerperium and the premenstruum. J Clin Psychiatry. 1997;58:330-4.
75. Wisner KL, Peindl KS, Gigliotti T, Hanusa BH. Obsessions and compulsions in women with postpartum depression. J Clin Psychiatry. 1999;60:176-80.
76. Filer ADJ, Brockington IF. Maternal obsessions of child sexual abuse. Psychopathology. 1996;29:135-8.
77. Chapman AH. Obsessions of infanticide. Arch Gen Psychiatry. 1959;1:12-6.
78. Button JH, Revich RS. Obsession of infanticide: a review of 42 cases. Arch Gen Psychiatry. 1972;27:235-40.
79. Buttolph ML, Holland AD. Obsessive-compulsive disorders in pregnancy and childbirth. In: Jenike MA, Baer L, Minichiello WE (Eds). Obsessive-compulsive disorder:theory and management, 2nd edition. Chicago: Yearbook Medical Publishers. 1990:89-95.
80. Jennings KD, Ross S, Popper S, Elmore M. Thoughts of harming infants in depressed and non-depressed mothers. J Affect Disord. 1999;54:21-8.

81. Maina G, Vaschetto P, Ziero S, Di Lorenzo R, Bogetto F. IL Postpartum come fattore di rischio specifico per l'esordio del disturbo ossessivo-compulsivo: studio clinico controllato. Epidemiol Psichiatr Soc. 2001;10:90-5.
82. Oates M. The development of an integrated community-orientated service for severe postnatal mental illness. In: Kumar R, Brockington IF (Eds). Motherhood and mental illness: causes and consequences. London: Wright. 1988.pp.133-58.

SUGGESTED READING

1. Affonso DD, De AK, Horowitz JA, Mayberry LJ. An international study exploring levels of postpartum depressive symptomatology. J Psychosom Res. 2000;49:207-16.
2. Ainsworth MDS, Bell SM, Stayton DJ. Individual differences in the development of some attachment behaviours. Merrill Palmer Quart. 1972;18:123-43.
3. Appleby L, Mortensen PB, Faragher EB. Suicide and other causes of mortality after post-partum psychiatric admission. Br T Psychiatry. 1998;173:209-11.
4. Appleby L, Warner R, Whitton A, Faragher B. A controlled study of fluoxetine and cognitive-behavioural counseling in the treatment of postnatal depression. BMJ. 1997;314:932-6.
5. Armstrong KL, Franser JA, Dadds MR, Morris J. A randomized, controlled trial of nurse home visiting to vulnerable families with newborns. J Paediatr Child Health. 1999;35:237-44.
6. Baker D, Taylor H. The relation between condition-specific morbidity, social support and material deprivation in pregnancy and early motherhood. Soc Sci Med. 1997;45:1325-36.
7. Bloch M, Schmidt PJ, Danaceau M, et al. Effects of gonadal steroids in women with a history of postpartum depression. Am J Psychiatry. 2000;157:924-30.
8. Brugha TS, Wheatley S, Taub NA, et al. Pragmatic randomized trial of antenatal intervention to prevent post-natal depression by reducing psychosocial risk factors. Psychol Med. 2000;30:1273-81.
9. Chabrol H, Teissedre F, Saint-Jean M, et al. Depistage, prevention et traitment des depressions du postpartum: une etude controlee chez 859 sujets. Encephale. 2002;28:65-70.
10. Chen CH, Tseng YF, Chou FH, Wang SY. Effects of support group intervention in postnatally distressed women: a controlled study in Taiwan. J Psychosom Res. 2000;49:395-9.
11. Cooper PJ, Landman M, Tomlinson M, Molteno C, Swartz L, Murray L. Impact of a mother-infant intervention in an indigent pen urban South African context. Br T Psychiatry. 2002;180:76-80.
12. Cooper PJ, Murray L, Wilson A, Romaniuk H. Controlled trial of the short-and long-term effect of psychological treatment of post-partum depression: 1, impact on maternal mood. Br J Psychiatry. 2003:182:412-19.
13. Dennis CL. The effect of peer support on postpartum depression: a pilot randomized controlled trial. Can J Psychiatry. 2003;48:115-24.
14. Elliott SA, Leverton TJ, Sanjack M, et al. Promoting mental health after childbirth: a controlled trial of primary prevention of postnatal depression. Br J Clin Psychol. 2000;39:223-41.
15. Fisch RZ, Tadmor OP, Dankner R, Diamant YZ. Postnatal depression: a prospective study of its prevalence, incidence and psychosocial determinants in an Israeli sample. J Obstet Gynaecol Res. 1997;23:547-55.
16. Fleming As, Klein E, Corter C. The effects of a social support group on depression, maternal attitudes and behaviors in new mothers. J Child Psychol Psychiatry. 1992;33:685-98.
17. Gissler M, Hemminki E, Lonnqvist J. Suicides after pregnancy in Finland 1987-1994: register linkage study BMT. 1996;313:1431-4.
18. Gordon RE, Gordon KK, Some social-psychiatric aspects of pregnancy and childbearing. J Med Soc NT. 1957;54: 569-72.
19. Gordon RE, Gordon KK. Social factors in the prevention of postpartum emotional problems. Obster Gynecol. 1960;15:433-8.
20. Gurel S, Gurel H. The evaluation of determination of early postpartum low mood: the importance of parity and inter-pregnancy interval. Eru J Obstet Gynecol Reprod Biol. 2000;91:21-4.
21. Hayes BA, Muller R, Bradley BS. Perinatal depression: a randomized controlled trial of an antenatal education intervention for primiparas. Birth. 2001;28:28-35.
22. Holden JM, Sagovsky R, Cox JL. Counselling in a general practice setting:controlled study of a helath visitor intervention of postnatal depression. BMJ. 1989;298:223-6.
23. Honey KL, Bennett P, Morgan M. A brief psycho-educational group intervention for postnatal depression. Br J Clin Psychol. 2002;41:405-09.
24. Kit LK, Janet G, Jegasothy R. Incidence of postnatal depression in Malaysian women. T Obstet Gynaecol Res. 1997;23:85-9.
25. La Vecchia C, Lucchini F, Levi F. Worldwide trends in suicide mortality,1955-89. Acta Psychiatr Scand. 1994;90:53-64.
26. Lavender T, Walkinshaw SA. Can midwives reduce postpartum psychological morbidity? A randomized trial. Birth. 1998;25:215-19.
27. Lee DTS, Yip ASK, Leung TYS, Chung TKH. Identifying women at risk of postnatal depression:prospective longitudinal study. Hong Kong Med J. 2000;6:349-54.
28. Mac Arhur C, Winter HR, Bick DE, et al. Effects of redesigned community postnatal care on womens' health 4 months after birth: a cluster randomized controlled trial. Lancet. 2002;359:378-85.
29. Main TF. Mothers with children in a psychiatric hospital. Lancet. 1958;2:845-7.
30. Misri S, Kostaras X, Fox D, Kostaras D. The impact of partner support in the treatment of postpartum depression. Can J Psychiatry. 2000;45:554-8.
31. Morrell CJ, Spiby H, Stewart P, Walters S, Morgan A. Costs and effectiveness of community postnatal support workers: randomized controlled trial. BMJ. 2000;321:593-8.

32. Murray L, Cooper PJ, Wilson A, Romaniuk H. Controlled trial of the short-and long-term effect of psychological treatment of post-partum outcome. Br J Psychiatry. 2003;182:420-7.
33. Nahas VL, Hillege S, Amasheh N. Postpartum depression: the lived experiences of Middle Eastern migrant women in Australia J Nurse Midwifery. 1999;44:65-74.
34. Naman JM, Andersen MJ, Bor W, O'Callaghan MJ, Williams GM. Postnatal depression: myth and reality:maternal depression before and after the birth of a child. Soc Psychiatry Psychiatr Epidemiol. 2000;35:19-27.
35. Nielsen Forman D, Videbech P, Hedegaard M, Dalby Salvig J, Socher NJ. Postpartum depression:identification of women at risk. Br J Obstet Gynaecol. 2000;107:1210-17.
36. Oates M. Deaths from psychiatric causes. In: Lewis G (Ed). Why mothers die: 5th Report of the Confidential Enquiries into Maternal Deaths in the United Kingdom. London: Royal College of Obstetrics and Gynaecology Press. 2001: 165-87.
37. O'Hara MW, Stuart S, Gorman LL, Wenzel A. Efficacy of interpersonal psychotherapy for postpartum depression. Arch Gen Psychiatry. 2000;57:1039-45.
38. Reid M, Glazener C, Murray GD, Taylor GS. A two-centred pragmatic randomized controlled trial of two interventions of postnatal support. Br J Obstet Gynaecol. 2002;109:1164-70.
39. Small R, Lumley J, Donhue L, Potter A, Waldenstrom U. Randomised controlled trial of midwife-led debriefing to reduce maternal depression after operative childbirth. BMJ. 2000;321:1043-47.
40. Stuchbery M, Matthey S, Barnett B, Postnatal depression and social supports in Vietnamese, Arabic and Anglo-Celtic mothers. Soc Psychiatry Psychiatr Epidemiol. 1998;33:483-90.
41. Treloar SA, Martin NG, Bucholz KK, Madden PAF, Health AC. Genetic influences on post-natal depressive symptoms:findings from an Australian twin sample. Psychol Med. 1999;29:645-54.
42. Tronick E, Als H, Adamson L, Wise S, Braselton TB. The infant's response to entrapment between contradictory messages in face-to-face interaction. T Am. Acad Child Adolesc Psychiatry. 1978;17:1-13.
43. Wendland-Carro J, Piccinini CA, Millar WS. The role of an early intervention on enhancing the quality of mother-infant interaction Child Dev. 1999;70:713-21.
44. Wickberg B, Hwang CP. Counselling of postnatal depression: a controlled study on a population based Swedish sample. J Affect Dis. 1996;39:209-16.
45. Wolman WL, Chalmers B, hofmeyr GJ, Nikodem Vc. Postpartum depression nad companionship in the clinical birth environment: a randomized, controlled study. Am J Obstet Gynecol. 1993;168:1388-93.
46. Yonkers KA, Ramin SM, Rush AJ, et al. Onset and persistence of postpartum depression in an inner city maternal health clinic system. Am J Psychiatry. 2001;158:1856-63.
47. Zlotnick C, Johnson SL, Miller IW, Pearlstein T, Howard M. Postpartum depression in women receiving public assistance:pilot study of an interpersonal-therapy-oriented group intervention. Am J Psychiatry. 2001;158:638-40.

CHAPTER 30

Premenstrual Disorders

Neena Bohra, NK Bohra

INTRODUCTION

Most women of reproductive age have one or more emotional or physical symptom in the premenstrual phase of the menstrual cycle. The symptoms are mild, but 5–8% have moderate to severe symptoms that are associated with substantial distress or functional impairment. In early medical reports about this issue, clinically significant premenstrual symptoms were named premenstrual tension (PMT)[1] or premenstrual syndrome (PSM).[2] The WHO International Classification of Diseases (ICD) includes "premenstrual syndrome" under the heading "Diseases of the Genitourinary Tract". However, like PMS and PMT, this description is not useful for the purpose of clinical diagnostics, drug labeling, or research, since it is not defined by specific criteria, and does not specify severity.

DIAGNOSIS

In the mid-1980s, a multidisciplinary US National Institutes of Health consensus on PMS proposed criteria that were adopted by the Diagnostic and Statistical Manual III (DSM III)[3] to define the severe form of this condition. Originally entitled "late luteal phase dysphoric disorder", it was later renamed "premenstrual dysphoric disorder" (PMDD). The diagnosis of PMDD stipulates (1) the presence of at least five luteal-phase symptoms (Panel 1), at least one of which must be a mood symptoms (i.e. depressed mood, anxiety or tension, affect lability, or persistent anger and irritability); (2) two cycles of daily charting to confirm the timing of symptoms; and (3) evidence of functional impairment. Finally, symptoms must not be the exacerbation of another psychiatric condition.[4]

A problem with the PMDD diagnosis is that many women with clinically significant premenstrual symptoms do not meet full diagnostic criteria; they might not have a prominent mood symptom or the five different symptoms required as a minimum by DSM IV. The American College of Obstetrics and Gynecology (ACOG) has attempted to rectify this situation by defining moderate to severe PMS; the criteria are the presence of at least one psychological or physical symptoms that causes significant impairment and is confirmed by means of prospective ratings.[5]

PREVALENCE

Most studies on the prevalence of premenstrual complaints are based on retrospective reports which, by their nature, can introduce recall bias.[6-12] However, the findings of these studies are consistent with those from the few epidemiological studies that used prospective symptom ratings.[13,14] Findings of prospective and retrospective studies suggest that 5–8% of women with hormonal cycles have moderate to severe symptoms. However, some studies suggest that up to 20% of all women of fertile age have premenstrual complaints that could be regarded as clinically relevant.[15]

Panel 1: Clinical criteria for premenstrual dysphoric disorder
• In most menstrual cycles during the past year, at least five of the following symptoms should have been present for most of the last week of the luteal phase, remitted within a few days after onset of menses, and remained absent in the week after menses. At least one symptom must be 1, 2, 3 or 4: 1. Depressed mood or dysphoria 2. Anxiety or tension 3. Affect lability 4. Irritability 5. Decreased interest in usual activities 6. Concentration difficulties 7. Marked lack of energy 8. Marked change in appetite, overeating, or food cravings 9. Hypersomnia or insomnia 10. Feeling overwhelmed 11. Other physical symptoms, e.g. breast tenderness, bloating
• Symptoms markedly interfere with work, school, social activities, or relationships
• Symptoms are not just an exacerbation of another disorder
• The first three criteria must be confirmed by prospective daily ratings for at least two consecutive menstrual cycles
Adapted from the Diagnostic and Statistical Manual IV (DSM- IV).

DSM-5 Diagnostic criteria: premenstrual dysphoric disorder 625.4 (N94.3)
A. In the majority of menstrual cycles, at least five symptoms must be present in the final week before the onset of menses, start to *improve* within a few days after the onset of menses, and become *minimal* or absent in the week postmenses.
B. One (or more) of the following symptoms must be present: 1. Marked affective lability (e.g. mood swings; feeling suddenly sad or tearful, or increased sensitivity to rejection). 2. Marked irritability or anger or increased interpersonal conflicts. 3. Marked depressed mood, feelings of hopelessness, or self-deprecating thoughts. 4. Marked anxiety, tension, and/or feelings of being keyed up or on edge.
C. One (or more) of the following symptoms must additionally be present, to reach a total of *five* symptoms when combined with symptoms from Criterion B. 1. Decreased interest in usual activities (e.g., work, school, friends, hobbies). 2. Subjective difficulty in concentration. 3. Lethargy, easy fatigability, or marked lack of energy. 4. Marked change in appetite; overeating; or specific food cravings. 5. Hypersomnia or insomnia. 6. A sense of being overwhelmed or out of control. 7. Physical symptoms such as breast tenderness or swelling, joint or muscle pain, a sensation of "bloating," or weight gain.
Note: The symptoms in Criteria A-C must have been met for most menstrual cycles that occurred in the preceding year.
D. The symptoms are associated with clinically significant distress or interference with work, school, usual social activities, or relationships with others (e.g. avoidance of social activities; decreased productivity and efficiency at work, school, or home).
E. The disturbance is not merely an exacerbation of the symptoms of another disorder, such as major depressive disorder, panic disorder, persistent depressive disorder (dysthymia), or a personality disorder (although it may co-occur with any of these disorders).
F. Criterion A should be confirmed by prospective daily ratings during at least two symptomatic cycles. (*Note:* The diagnosis may be made provisionally prior to this confirmation.)
G. The symptoms are not attributable to the physiological effects of a substance (e.g. a drug of abuse, a medication, other treatment) or another medical condition (e.g. hyperthyroidism).

PATTERN OF SYMPTOM EXPRESSION

The length of symptoms expression varies between a few days and 2 weeks. Symptoms often worsen substantially 6 days before, and peak at about 2 days before, menses start.[16,17] Anger and irritability are the most severe complaints and start slightly earlier than other symptoms. It is not uncommon for symptoms to linger into the next menstrual cycle[16-18] but, by definition, there must be a symptom-free interval before ovulation. Typically, women have the some set of symptoms from one cycle to the next.[19]

Several patterns of true or apparent comorbidity can occur in a women with premenstrual symptoms. First, she might have another psychiatric disorder at another point in her life (lifetime comorbidity). Second, she might have an ongoing psychiatric or general medical condition and concurrent premenstrual symptoms that are not part of the co-occurring disorder (concurrent comorbidity). Third, she might have an ongoing psychiatric or general medical condition that becomes worse premenstrually-usually defined as premenstrual exacerbation.[4,20]

Estimates for lifetime comorbidity between PMS and other mood disorders range from 30% to 70%.[12,21-23] This prevalence is higher than one would expect, even taking into consideration that mood disorders are common in women (at least 30% of women have a minor or major depressive disorder at some point in their lives); estimates of comorbidity, however, might be inflated because of an overlap in symptoms. It is notable that the risk of developing perimenopausal depression[24] and postnatal depression[25,26] has been reported to be higher in women who have PMS, leading some to suggest that these different conditions share a vulnerability to change in gonadal steroid concentrations.

Anxiety disorder also occur at a higher rate in women with PMS.[27,28] Women with PMS, like those with panic disorder (but in contrast to those with other mood disorders), have an increased tendency to panic when exposed to panicogenic agents such as lactate and carbon dioxide, suggesting that panic disorder and PMS share certain pathophysiological mechanisms.[27,28]

ETIOLOGY AND PATHOPHYSIOLOGY

Since most women of reproductive age report at least mild premenstrual symptoms, a certain degree of discomfort during the luteal phase should probably be considered physiological rather than pathological. In evolutionary terms,[29] luteal mood change could be remnants of the estrous cycle-related fluctuations in behavior shown by lower species with the original purpose of promoting reproduction: sexual receptivity being increased and aggression decreased when estrogen is high before ovulation.[30-32]

In this context, one should consider the fact that, historically, repeated pregnancies, lactation, or malnourishment led to extended periods of amenorrhea, a situation that has changed by advances in nutrition and with our capacity to control reproduction.[33] The result is that women today have much longer periods of cyclic fluctuations of estrogen and progesterone with associated premenstrual symptoms.[33]

Since the most characteristic feature of PMS is the relation between symptom appearance and menstrual cyclicity, researchers have long suggested that gonadal steroids are involved in the pathophysiology.[1] In line with this notion, symptoms are absent during non-ovulatory cycles,[34] abolished by ovariectomy[35-37] or treatment with ovulation inhibitors,[38-41] and reinstated by administration of exogenous hormones.[42-45]

How changes in sex steroid production provoke luteal symptoms, however, remains to be understood. Many researchers suggest that premenstrual complaints are elicited by the drop in progesterone concentrations in the late luteal phase, and link this to changes in CNS neurotransmitters such as γ-aminobutyric acid (GABA).[46,47]

Moreover, for women in whom the endogenous hormonal cyclicity had been abolished by pretreatment with an agonist of gonadotropin-releasing hormone (GnRH), daily progesterone administration for a month provoked symptoms (with some delay), despite hormone concentrations remaining stable.[45] Also, if a luteal decrease in progesterone was the precipitating factor, administration of progesterone during this phase would be an effective treatment, which it is not.[48] The alternative hypothesis, that symptoms are triggered by the preovulatory peak in estradiol, or by the postovulatory increase in progesterone, or both,[45,49] thus seems more likely. This theory does not explain, however, why symptoms begin with ovulation for some women but late into the luteal phase for others.

The importance of progesterone compared with estrogen in triggering symptoms is equally unclear. Mood change reported by postmenopausal women taking sequential hormone replacement therapy suggests that progesterone, rather than estrogen, is responsible for inducing dysphoria;[42,50] moreover, estrogen exerts an antidepressant effect in women with perimenopausal depression.[51] of note, the days of the cycle during which symptoms are likely to appear are those in which progesterone dominates over estrogen. On the other hand, oestradiol has been reported to be as effective as gestagen in provoking PMS-like complaints,[45] and the estrogen component of hormone replacement therapy can enhance gestagen-induced dysphoria.[52] Moreover, luteal administration of estrogen has been reported to aggravate premenstrual symptoms,[53] and luteal administration of an estrogen antagonist reduces premenstrual mastalgia.[54]

Evidence suggests that woman with and without PMS do not differ with respect to the production of gonadal steroids,[55] indicating that PMS might instead by associated with enhanced responsiveness to normal, fluctuating concentrations of these hormones. In line with this, administration of exogenous gonadal steroids provoked PMS-like symptoms after pretreatment with an ovulation inhibitor in woman with PMS, but not in controls.[45]

Such an enhanced tendency to have dysphoria as a result of the effects of sex steroids on the brain might be heritable, as suggested by twin studies.[56-58] Other possible risk factors for PMS are high body-mass index,[59] stress,[7] and traumatic events.[60]

With respect to hormones other than the sex steroids, thyroid indices are reported to be more variable in woman with PMS than in controls.[61,62] Moreover, as in anxiety and mood disorders, changes in circadian rhythms have been noted in PMS. Some studies thus suggest that the absolute levels of hormones such as melatonin, cortisol, thyroid-stimulating hormone, and prolactin are not altered but that the timing of their excretion might be aberrant in woman with PMS.[63]

CENTRAL NEUROTRANSMISSION IN PREMENSTRUAL SYNDROME

Since mood and behavioral symptoms are key features of PMS, underlying mechanisms must involve the brain. Indeed, sex steroids easily pass the blood-brain barrier, and sex steroid receptors are abundant in many brain regions that regulate emotions and behavior, including the amygdale and the hypothalamus.

The brain neurotransmitter serotonin is implicated in the regulation of mood and behavior, partly because of observations made in preclinical studies, and partly because of the antidepressant and anxiety-reducing effects exerted by serotonin-facilitating drugs in human beings. This notion has also gained support from genetic studies[64,65] and from brain imaging experiments.[66]

The most clear-cut change in rodents exposed to serotonin depletion is an increase in aspects of behavior that are dependent on sex steroids, i.e. aggression and sexual activity, suggesting that a major physiological role for serotonin is to modulate or dampen sex-steroid-driven behavior.[31,67] Consistent with this, reduced libido is probably the most common side-effect of long-term treatment with serotonin reuptake inhibitors (SRIs).[68-73]

The importance of serotonin for the regulation of mood and aggression, and the probable role of serotonin in modulating sex-steroid-driven behavior, suggest that serotonin could be involved in the pathophysiology of PMS. Support for this theory is provided by three sources of evidence. First, premenstrual symptoms are effectively dampened not only by SRIs, but also by other serotonin-enhancing treatments, such as serotonin-releasing agents,[74,75] a serotonin precursor,[76] and a serotonin-receptor agonist.[77] Second, impairment in serotonergic transmission achieved by a tryptophan-free diet,[78] or by treatment with a serotonin-receptor antagonist,[79] provokes symptoms. Third, various indices of serotonergic transmission are reported to be aberrant in woman with PMS.[75,80-89]

Another neurotransmitter that has been linked to PMS in the inhibitory aminoacid GABA. This theory gains support from an imaging study,[90] the fact that some progesterone metabolites interact with GABA A receptor,[46,47] and the observation that woman with PMS seem to differ form controls with respect to the responsiveness of this receptor complex.[91] To what extant woman with PMS have an abnormal production of GABA-A-modulating progesterone metabolites, however, is a matter of controversy,[92-94] and whether modulation of GABA A activity can relieve symptoms is unclear.[95] Moreover, much of the work implicating GABA in the pathophysiology of PMS is based on the assumption that premenstrual complaints are due to progesterone withdrawal, a notion that has been questioned. Notably, there are important interactions between GABAergic and serotonergic neurons;[96,97] a theory implicating GABA in the pathophysiology of PMS, is thus not in conflict with the serotonin hypothesis. Further, several SRIs, which have therapeutic benefit for PMS, also have profound effects on enzymes involved in the production of progesterone metabolites that modulate GABA A receptor.[98,99]

PATHOPHYSIOLOGY OF SOMATIC SYMPTOMS

It remains unclear whether premenstrual somatic symptoms —such as breast tenderness, bloating, and joint and muscle pain-result from reduced tolerance to physical discomfort while in a dysphoric mood state, or are caused by changes in hormone-responsive tissues in the periphery. Studies have failed to confirm fluid retention or breast enlargement in woman reporting these symptoms;[100,101] moreover, treatment aimed at influencing brain neurotransmission, e.g. the SRIs-exerts at least some palliative effect on somatic symptoms. On the other hand, the dopamine D2 receptor agonist, bromocriptine,[102,103] or chasteberry,[104] which lower serum concentrations of prolactin, are effective for the treatment of premenstrual mastalgia, but not for mood symptoms. Likewise, a specific by effect on premenstrual mastalgia could be achieved by luteal administration of danazol[105] or an estrogen-receptor antagonist.[54]

Results of some early studies suggest the involvement of aldosterone[106] or deoxycorticosterone, a progesterone metabolite and aldosterone agonist,[33,106] in the pathophysiology of premenstrual bloating. Given that severe abdominal bloating occurs in the absence of weight gain, any theory related to water retention is, however, called into doubt. Many believe that premenstrual headache, migraine, and epilepsy should not be regarded as part of PMS, but as separate conditions. Notably, SRIs have no effect on premenstrual headache. Painful menstrual, and menopausal symptoms are often confused with PMS,[107] but they are separate and must be clearly distinguished as such in research and in the clinic environment.

TREATMENT

Before pharmacological treatment is considered, the medical history of woman with presumed PMS should be investigated for conditions such as depression, dysthymic disorder, anxiety disorders, and hypothyroidism. Given the possible links between PMS and sexual abuse, as well as with post-traumatic stress disorder,[60] a history that assesses the presence of these factors , as well as domestic violence, should be obtained. Some individuals with anxiety and mood disorders, including PMS, attempt to cope with symptoms by using alcohol or illicit drugs, although these substances can provoke or worsen dysphoria and anxiety. Thus, the possible use of such substances should be addressed during the evaluation.

The diagnosis of PMS (according to ACOG criteria) and PMDD requires daily charting of symptoms over two menstrual cycles; various methods have been developed for this purpose, such as the Daily Record of Severity of Problems.[108] A woman with severe symptoms, however, might not be willing to accept the delay in treatment involved with such recording. However, the benefit for the patient and the clinician is that it enables a clear diagnostic distinction between PMS/PMDD on the one hand, and premenstrual exacerbation of an underlying psychiatric disorder, or a condition with no relation to the menstrual cycle, on the other.

Many treatment regimens have been touted as effective for PMS, but few are supported by clinical evidence. Since effective treatments do not necessarily reduce all symptoms equally, assessing improvement using summary scales that evaluate change in many symptoms could obscure a specific effect on a particular symptom. Given that some medications might work better for particular symptoms, treatment should be individualized according to the symptom profile.

SEROTONIN REUPTAKE INHIBITORS (SRIs)

Many clinical trials evaluating the efficacy of an SRI for the management of PMS/PMDD have shown benfit,[109] the response rate usually being 60–90% for active treatment versus 30–40% for placebo.[110] SRIs that have been shown effective are the serotonergic tricyclic antidepressant clomipramine,[111,112] the selective SRIs citalopram,[113] escitalopram,[114] fluoxetine,[115-120] paroxetine,[121-125] and sertraline,[126-130] and the serotonin and noradrenaline reuptake inhibitor venlafaxine.[131,132] SRIs reduce both mood symptoms and somatic complaints, and they also improve quality of life and social functioning (Table 1).[122,140,141] Many believe that SRIs should be regarded as first-line treatment in PMS patients with severe mood symptoms.[142,143]

SRIs are more effective for PMS than are antidepressants that predominantly affect noradrenergic transmission,[115,121,133] implying that the effect of SRIs in PMS is not merely an antidepressant effect. This notion is also supported by the fact that the beneficial effect of SRIs for PMS begins rapidly, whereas the antidepressant effect is slow in onset. The fast onset of action in PMS renders intermittent treatment, from midcycle to menses, a feasible alternative to continuous therapy.[112,113,119,120,125,127,128,134,144] Data suggest that even

Table 1: Major strategies for treatment of premenstrual syndrome

	Dose	*Most important side-effects*
Serotonin reuptake inhibitors		
Clomipramine[111,112]	50–70 mg daily or for half cycle	Dry mouth, sedation, sexual dysfunction, nausea, jitteriness
Citalopram[114]	20–40 mg daily or for half cycle	Sexual dysfunction, nausea, jitteriness
Escitalopram[114]	10–20 mg daily for half cycle	Sexual dysfunction, nausea, jitteriness
Fluoxetine[115-120]	20–60 mg daily or for half cycle	Sexual dysfunction, nausea, jitteriness
Paroxetine[121,125]	20–30 mg daily or for half cycle	Sexual dysfunction, nausea, jitteriness
Paroxetine-CR[122-124]	12.5–25.0 mg daily or for half cycle	Sexual dysfunction, nausea, jitteriness
Sertraline[126-130,133,134]	50–150 mg daily or for half cycle	Sexual dysfunction, nausea, jitteriness
Venlafaxine[131-132]	50–200 mg daily or for half cycle	Sexual dysfunction, nausea, jitteriness
Hormonal interventions		
Estradiol transdermally,[135] must be combined with oral progestogen intermittently, or intrauterine progestogen Estradiol subcutaneous implant;[136] must be combined with oral progestogen intermittently, or intrauterine progestogen	200 µg estradiol twice weekly via patch; see references for doses of progestogen 100 µg subcutaneous implant of estradiol; see references for doses of progestogens	Skin irritation, oral progestogen can cause PMS-like symptoms (which is unlikely with intrauterine progestogen). Mastalgia, PMS-like symptoms from oral progestogen
GnRH agonists,[38-41] long-term treatment only in rare cases; monitoring bone density and "add-black" estrogen is mandatory; estrogen must be combined with oral progestogen intermittently, intrauterine progestogen, or oral tibolone continuously.[137]	Depended on which GnRH agonist used: see references; also see references for doses of estrogen plus progestogens or tibolone	PMS-like symptoms from oral progestogen
Drospirenone—ethinyl estradiol[138,139]	3 mg drospirenone plus 20 µg ethinyl estradiol for 24 days	Breast pain

briefer periods of active treatment are more effective than placebo.[124,146]

Clinical experience suggests that most but not all woman with PMS prefer intermittent treatment to continuous. SRIs administered intermittently, however, seem less effective for somatic symptoms than for mood symptoms than is continuous treatment.[125]

Side-effects of SRIs are usually mild. Nausea is very common during the first days of treatment, but vanishes after a few days. It usually does not reappear, even when the treatment is intermittent.[125] Reduced libido and anorgasmia are not uncommon, and often persist for the duration of treatment,[69] but are not present during the drug-free intervals of intermittent treatment. SRIs are not addictive, but many individuals experience discontinuation symptoms when they stop medication abruptly.[16] When SRIs are used intermittently, discontinuation symptoms are seldom a problem, suggesting that 2 weeks is too short an exposure period to elicit withdrawal symptoms.[113,117,124]

There is no sharp demarcation between mild PMS and PMDD and that approval of an SRI for PMDD lead to unwarranted medication in mild cases. Additionally, they said, PMDD is a condition that could go on for years, and that long-term trials would be needed to assess long-term tolerability. However, these same arguments could be, but have not been, applied to other long-term condition, such as generalized anxiety disorder, social phobia, and dysthymic disorder—for which SRIs are approved in Europe and for which it is equally true that there is no sharp borderline between mild and severe variants.

OTHER PSYCHOACTIVE DRUGS

Other CNS-acting drugs tested for use in PMS do not seem to be particularly effective. Whereas lithium[147] and nonserotonergic antidepressants[121,133,148] have been completely ineffective, the serotonergic 5HTI1-A agonist buspirone[77,149] exerts weak beneficial effects. For the high-affinity benzodiazepine, alprazolam, efficacy data are conflicting;[95,150-153] alprazolam can, however, be a helpful adjunctive treatment for woman who identify premenstrual insomnia or overwhelming anxiety as important symptoms. Treatment with alprazolam should be monitored carefully because of the risk of dependence, particularly if the individual has a history of substance abuse.

HORMONAL INTERVENTIONS

Given the involvement of sex steroids in the triggering of premenstrual symptoms, many regard treatment that target these hormones as the most rational approach for reducing premenstrual complaints.

The rationale behind the hormonal treatment of PMS is thus not simply to correct a hormonal abnormality, but to interrupt the normal hypothalamus-pituitary-gonadal cyclicity that is triggering the symptoms. This can be achieved by administering a long-acting GnRH agonist.[38-41] There is persuasive evidence that these preparations are extremely effective. They are, however, relatively invasive since they result in a "medical menopause", which is accompanied by typical menopausal symptoms, particularly flushing, as well as a risk of osteoporosis if the therapy is prolonged. These side-effects, entirely due to the estrogen deficiency, can be prevented by estrogen replacement, combined with a gestagen to prevent estrogen-induced endometrial hyperplasia. Whereas some patients report returning symptoms when given gestagens,[44] a meta-analysis suggests that this option is nevertheless often feasible.[41] A promising alternative is to combine a GnRh agonist with continuous administration of tibolone, a synthetic estrogen, progestogen and androgen receptor agonist.[41,154]

Other method to inhibit ovarian cyclicity, such as surgical bilateral oophorectomy (which can be undertaken laparoscopically), also abolish PMS.[35,36,155] As with treatment with long-acting GnRH agonists, oophorectomy requires hormonal add-back with estrogen plus gestagens. If bilateral oophorectomy and hysterectomy are combined, estrogen can be used alone. Surgical therapy tends to be too invasive an approach for most patients with PMS. However, patients who have a separate gynecological disorder requiring hysterectomy usually must consider removal or conservation of the ovaries. Conservation of the ovaries is nearly always advised in younger woman—however, if a patient has debilitating PMS, conservation of the ovaries might be inadvisable, and the patient could request that her ovaries are removed. Although no research evidence is available to support this, administration of a GnRH agonist for 2–3 months before surgery will show the patient the probable effect of removing the ovaries and could inform her decision.

Administration of estrogen at doses that inhibit ovulation[135,137] is one of the simplest ways to effectively abolish PMS symptoms. Oral therapy is not usually advised; instead estrogen administered as a transdermal patch[135] or subcutaneous implant[136,156] has been recommended. Doses are usually higher than are those required for hormone replacement treatment, but lower than for the oral contraceptive pill; for patches, 100, 150, or 200 µg could be necessary. Unless the patient has had a hysterectomy, she will need to be given a progestogen to prevent endometrial hyperplasia. This could result in restimulation of PMS in some patients, unless it is administered within a progesterone-containing levonorgestrel-containing intrauterine system. Although there is clear-cut evidence that estrogen suppresses both ovulation and symptoms, and there is good evidence that the intrauterine system prevents hyperplasia, evidence for the use of this combination as treatment for PMS is limited.[157,158]

Many clinicians use oral contraceptive to manage PMS, but placebo-controlled studies have been few and mostly negative.[159,160] Since woman taking oral contraceptive might have more hormone-related symptoms during the 7 days hormone-free interval than during hormone ingestion,[161] and since shortening of the hormone-free interval reduces such complaints,[162] oral contraceptive with few hormone-free days might also be of value for PMS. In line with this, studies show efficacy of a novel oral contraceptive with a hormone-free interval of 4 rather than 7 days.[138,139] In part, the therapeutic benefit of this oral contraceptive, however, could be a result of the gestagen component, drospirenone, exerting antialdosterone and antiandrogen effects.

The synthetic androgen and gonadotropin inhibitor danazol, when administered at doses that block ovulation, is effective for PMS;[163-165] however, hirsutism and risk of teratogenicity preclude its use as a first-line agent. Danazol administered at low doses in the luteal phase of the cycle only is not effective for the general symptoms of PMS but for the management of mastalgia and with minimal side-effects.[105] Luteal administration of an estrogen receptor antagonists[54] also reduces mastalgia.

OTHER TREATMENTS

Possible alterations in circadian rhythmicity[63] suggest that bright light treatment might be effective for moderate to severe PMS. One controlled study[166] suggests benefit for this intervention, but it is not clear how long the possible therapeutic effects persist.

The aldosterone antagonist spironolactone seems to be effective for symptoms of bloating and breast pain in PMS,[106,167,168] although the link between premenstrual somatic symptoms and water retention is questionable.

Most studies assessing the therapeutic effect of vitamin B6 (pyridoxine) in PMS had several methodological limitations, including lack of prospective ratings. Definitive conclusions regarding efficacy cannot be drawn, but a quantitative review suggested that B6 has benefit over placebo.[169] Calcium supplements could be helpful for woman with PMS,[135] as could Vitex agnus-castus (chasteberry), which is claimed to have antiprolactin effects.[170] The use of evening primrose oil has been popularized but seems to be ineffective.[171] Several studies have assessed the therapeutic benefit of magnesium treatment and some,[172] but not all,[173] have found it effective. However, these studies have been small and are not definitive; moreover, magnesium can be poorly tolerated.

Although books and magazine articles for the lay public have touted the benefit of restricting sugar and eating multiple small meals as management of PMS, there is little support for these strategies. On the other hand, studies of diets that increase the relative intake of complex carbohydrates suggest benefit, which might be due to an enhanced transport of the serotonin precursor tryptophan into the brain, leading to a transient increase in the synthesis of this transmitter.[174,175] Cognitive behavioral therapy[176] and exercise[177] have also has been claimed to be beneficial.

Various other treatments have been assessed in PMS, but cannot yet be regarded as evidence-based because the studies were not controlled, were flawed, or their findings not replicated. The non-steroidal anti-inflammatory medications mefenamic acid[178,179] as well as the opioid receptor blocker naltrexone[180,181] are among these.

REFERENCES

1. Frank R. The hormonal causes of premenstrual tension. Arch Neurol Psychiatry. 1931;26:1053-7.
2. Greene R, Dalton K. The premenstrual syndrome. BMJ. 1953;1:1007-14.
3. American Psychiatric Association. Diagnostic and statistical manual of mental disorders-DSM-III, 3rd edition. Washington DC: American Psychiatric Association; 1980.
4. American Psychiatry Association. Diagnostic and statistical manual of mental disorders-DSM-IV, 4th edition. Washingtion DC: American Psychiatric Association; 1994.
5. ACOG. ACOG practice bulletin: premenstrual syndrome. Int J Gynecol Obstet. 2001;73:183-91.
6. Johnson SR, Machesney C, Bean JA. Epidemiology of premenstrual symptoms in a no clinical sample-I: Prevalence, natural history and help-seeking behavior. J Repro Med. 1988; 33:340-6.
7. Deuster P, Adera T, South-Paul J. Biological, social, and behavioral factors associated with premenstrual syndrome. Arch Flam Med. 1999; 8:122-8.
8. Ramacharan S, Love EJ, Fick GH, Goldfien A. The epidemiology of premenstrual symptoms in a population based sample of 2650 urban women. J Clin Epidemiol. 1992:45:377-81.
9. Woods NF. Most A, Dery GK. Prevalence of premenstrual symptoms. Am J Public Health. 1982;72:1257-67-64.
10. Andersch B, Wendestam C, Hahn L, Ohman R. Premenstrual complaints. Prevalence of premenstrual symptoms in a Swedish urban population. J Psychiatry Obstet Gynaecol. 1986;5:39-49.
11. Angst J, Sellaro R, Merikangas KR, Endicott J. The epidemiology of premenstrual psychological symptoms. Acta Psychiatry Scand. 2001;104:110-6.
12. Wittchan H, Becker E, Liab R, Krause P. Prevalence, incidence and stability of premenstrual dysphoric disorder in the community. Psychol Med. 2002;32:119-32.
13. Rivera-Tovar AD, Frank E. Late luteal phase disorder in young woman. Am J Psychiatry. 1990;147:1634-6.
14. Soares C, Cohen L, Otto M, Harlow B. Characteristics of woman with premenstrual dysphoric disorder (PMDD) who did or did not report history of depression: a preliminary report from the Harvard study of moods and cycles. J Woman's Health Gend Based Med. 2001;10:873-8.
15. Borenstein J, Dean B, Endicott J, et al. Heath and economic impact of the premenstrual syndrome. J Reprod Med. 2003; 48:515-24.
16. Pearlsterin T, Yonkers K, Fayyad R, Gillespie J. Pretreatment pattern of symptom expression in premenstrual dsyphoric disorder. J Affect Disord. 2005;85:275-82.
17. Meaden PM, Hartlage SA, Cook-Kerr J. Timing and severity of symptoms associated with the menstrual cycle in a community-based sample in the Midwestern United States. Psychiatry Res. 2005;134:27-36.
18. Sternfeld B, Swindle R, Chawla A, Long S, Kennedy S. Severity of premenstrual symptoms in a health maintenance organization population. Obstet Gynecol. 2002;99:1014-24.
19. Bloch M, Schmidt PJ, Rubinow DR. Premenstrual syndrome: Evidence for symptom stability across cycles. Am J Psychiatry. 1997;154:1741-6.
20. Steiner M, Born L. Diagnosis and treatment of premenstrual dysphoric disorder: an update. Int Clin Psychopharmacol. 2000;15(Suppl 3):S5-17.
21. Pearlstein TB, Frank E, Ricera-Tovar A, et al. Prevalence of axis I and axis II disorders in woman with late luteal phase dysphoric disorder. J Affect Disord. 1990;20:129-34.
22. Halbreich U, Endicott J. Relationship of dysphoric premenstrual changes to depressive disorder. Acta Psychiatrica Scandinacica. 1985;71:331-8.
23. Mackenzia TB, Wilcox K, Baron H. Lifetime prevalence of psychiatric disorders in woman with premenstrual difficulties. J Affect Disord. 1986;10:15-9.
24. Richards M, Rubinow DR, Daly RC, Schmidt PJ. Premenstrual symptoms and perimenopausal depression. Am J Psychiatry. 2006;163:133-7.
25. Studd JWW, Smith RNJ. Estrogens and depression in woman. Menopause: J North Am Menopause Soc. 1994;1:33-7.
26. Bloch M, Schmidt PJ, Danaceau M, et al. Effects of gonadal steroids in woman with a history of postpartum depression. Am J Psychiatry. 2000;157:924-30.
27. Landen M, Eriksson E. How does premenstrual dysphoric disorder relate to depression and anxiety disordwers? Depress Anxiety. 2003;17:122-9.
28. Yonkers KA. Anxiety symptoms and anxiety disorders: How are they related to premenstrual disorders. J Clin Psychiatry. 1997;58:62-7.
29. Rosseinsky DR, Debonnel PG. An evolutionary theory of premenstrual tension. Lancet. 1974;2:1024.
30. Rapkin AJ, Pollack DB, Raleigh MJ, Stone B, McGuire MT. Menstrual cycle and social behavior in varvet monkeys. Psychoneuroendocrinology. 1995;20:289-97.
31. Ho H-P Olsson M, Westberg L, Melke J, Eriksson E. The serotonin reuptake inhibitor fluoxetine reduces sex steroid-related aggression in female rats: an animal model of

premenstrual irritability? Neuropsychopharmacology. 2001;24: 502-10.
32. Hyde J. Sawyer TF. Estrous cycle fluctuations in aggressiveness of house mice. Horm Behav. 1977;9:290-5.
33. MacDonald PC, Dombroski RA, Casey ML. Recurrent secretion of progesterone in large amounts: An endocrine/metabolic disorder unique to young woman? Endocrine Rev. 1991;12:372-401.
34. Hammarback S, Ekholm UB, Backstrom T. Spontaneous anovulation causing disappearance of cyclical symptoms in woman with the premenstrual syndrome. Acta Endocrinologica. 1991;125:132-7.
35. Casper P, Hearn MT. The effect of hysterectomy and bilateral oophorectomy in woman with severe premenstrual syndrome. Am J Obstet Gynecol. 1990;162:99-105.
36. Casson P, Hahn PM, Van Vugt DA, Reid RL. Lasting response to ovariectomy in severe intractable premenstrual syndrome. Am J Obstet Gynecol. 1990;162:99-105.
37. Cronje WH, Vashisht A, Studd JWW. Hysterectomy and bilateral oophorectomy for severe premenstrual syndrome. Him Reprod. 2004;19:2152-5.
38. Muse KN, Cetel NS, Futterman LA, Yen SSC. The premenstrual syndrome: effects of "medical ovariectomy". N Engl J Med. 1984;311:1345-9.
39. Bancroft J, Boyle H, Warner P, Fraser HM. The use of an LHRH agonist, buserelin, in the long-term management of premenstrual syndromes. Clin Endocrinol. 1987;27:171-82.
40. Hammarback S, Backstrom T. Induced anovulation as treatment of premenstrual tension syndrome: a double-blind cross-over study with GnRH-agonist versus placebo. Acta Obstet Gynecol Scand. 1988;67:159-66.
41. Wyatt KM, Dimmock PW, Ismail KMK, Jones PW, O'Brien PMS. The effectiveness of GnRHa with and without "add-back" therapy in treating premenstrual syndrome: a meta analysis. BJOG: Int J Obsts Gynaecol. 2004;111:585-93.
42. Magos AL, Brewster E, Singh R, et al. The effects of norethisterone in postmenopausal woman on estrogen replacement therapy: a model for the premenstrual syndrome. BJOG. 1986;93:1290-6.
43. Henshaw C, Foreman D, Belcher J, Cox J, O'Brien S. Can one induce premenstrual symptomatology in woman with prior hysterectomy and bilateral oophorectomy? J Psychoson Obstet Gynecol. 1996;17:21-8.
44. Leather AT, Studd JW, Watson NR, Holland EF. The treatment of severe premenstrual syndrome with goserelin with and without "add-back" estrogen therapy: a placebo-controlled study. Gynecol Endocrinol. 1999;13:48-55.
45. Schmidt PJ, Nieman LK, Danaceau MA, Adams LF, Rubinow DR. Differential behavioral effects of gonadal steroids in woman with and in those without premenstrual syndrome. N Engl J Med. 1998;338:209-16.
46. Smith SS, Ruderman Y, Frye C, Homanics G, Yuan M. Steroid withdrawal in the mouse results in anxiogenic effects of 3 alpha, 5 beta-THP: a possible model of premenstrual dysphoric disorder. Psychopharmacology. 2005;29:1-11.
47. Sundstrom Poromaa I, Smith S, Gulinello M. GABA receptor, progesterone and premenstrual dysphoric disorder. Arch Woman Ment Health. 2003;6:23-41.
48. Wyatt K, Dimmock P, Jones P, Obhrai M, O'Brien S. Efficacy of progesterone and progestogens in management of premenstrual syndrome: systematic review. BMJ. 2001;323: 776-81.
49. Schmidt PJ, Nieman LK, Grover GN, et al. Lack of effect of induced menses on symptoms in woman with premenstrual syndrome. N Engl J Med. 1991;324:1174-9.
50. Hammarback S, Backstrom T, Holst J, von Schoultz B, Lyrenas S. Cyclical mood changes as in the premenstrual tension syndrome during sequential estrogen-progestagen posmenopausal replacement therapy. Arch Obstet Gynecol Scand. 1985;64:393-7.
51. Schmidt PJ. Depression, the perimenopause, and estrogen therapy. Am NY Acad Sci. 2005;1052:27-40.
52. Bjorn I, Sundstrom-Poromaa I, Bixo M, et al. Increase of estrogen dose deteriorates mood during progestin phase in sequential hormonal therapy. J Clin Endocrinol Metab. 2003;88:2026-30.
53. Dhar V, Murphy BEP. Double-blind randomized crossover trial of luteal phase estrogens (Premarin) in the premenstrual syndrome (PMS). Psychoneuroendocrinology. 1991;15:489-93.
54. Oksa S, luukkaala T, Maenpaa J. Toremifene for premenstrual mastalgia: randomized, placebo-controlled crossover study. BJOG. 2006;113:713-8.
55. Rubinow D, Schmidt P. The neuroendocrinology of menstrual cycle mood disorders. Ann N Y Acad Sci. 1995;771:648-59.
56. Condon JT. The premenstrual syndrome: A twin study. Br J Psychiatry. 1993;162:481-6.
57. Kendler KS, Karkowski LM, Corey LA, Neale MC. Longitudinal population-based twin study of retrospectively reported premenstrual symptoms and lifetime major depression. Am J Psychiatry. 1998:155:1234-40.
58. Treloar S, Health A, Martin N. Genetic and environmental influences on premenstrual symptoms in Australian twin sample. Psychol Med. 2002;32:25-38.
59. Masho SW, Adera T, South-Paul J. Obesity as a risk factor for premenstrual syndrome. J Psychosom Obstet Gynaecol. 2005;26:33-339.
60. Perkonigg A, Yonkers K, Pfister H, Lieb R, Wittchen HU. Risk Factor for premenstrual dysphoric disorder in a community sample of young women: The role of traumatic events and posttraumatic stress disorder. J Clin Psychiatry. 2004;65: 1314-22.
61. Girdler SS, Pederson CA, Light KC. Thyroid axis function during the menstrual cycle in women with premenstrual syndrome. Psych oneuroendocrinol. 1995;20:395-403.
62. Schmidt PJ, Grover GN, Roy-Byrne PP, et al. Thyroid function in women with premenstrual syndrome. J Clin Endocrinol Metab. 1993;76:671-4.
63. Parry BL, Newton RP. Chronobiological basis of female-specific mood disorders. Neuropsychopharmacology. 2001;25 (Suppl 5): S102-08.

64. Hariri AR, Mattay VS, Tessitore A, et al. Serotonin transporter genetic variation and the response of the human amygdale. Science. 2002;297:400-03.
65. Caspi A, Sugden K, Moffitt TE, et al. Influence of life stress on dépression: Moderation by a polymorphism in the 5-HTT gene. Science. 2003;301:386-9.
66. Parsey RV, Hastings RS, Oquendo MA, et al. Lower serotonin transporter binding potential in the human brain during major depressive episodes. Am J Psychiatry. 2006;163:52-8.
67. Eriksson E, Andersch B, Ho HP, Landen M, Sundblad C. Diagnosis and treatment of premenstrual dysphoria. J Clin Psychiatry. 2002;63 (Suppl 7):16-23.
68. Gregorian RS, Golden KA, Bahce A, et al. Antidepressant-induced sexual dysfunction Ann Phyrmacother. 2002;36: 1577-89.
69. Sundblad C, Wikander I, Andersch B, Erilsson E. A naturalistic study of paroxetine in premenstrual syndrome: efficacy and side effects during ten cycles of treatment. Eur Neuropsychopharmacology. 1997;7:201-6.
70. Carlsson M, Carlsson A. A regional study of sex differences in rat brain serotonin. Prog Neuro-Psychopharmacol Biol Psychiatry. 1988;12:53-61.
71. Hiroi R, McDevitt RA, Neumaier JF. Estrogne selectively increases tryptophan hydroxylase-2 mRNA expression in distinct subregions of rat midbrain raphe nucleus: association between gene expression and anxiety behavior in the open field Biol Psychiatry. 2006;60:288-95.
72. Rubinow DR, Schmidt PJ, Roca CA. Estrogen-serotonin interactions: implications for affective regulation. Biol Psychiatry. 1998;44:839-50.
73. Bethea CL, Lu NZ, Gundlah C, Streicher JM. Diverse actions of ovarian steroids in the serotonin neural system. Front Neuroendocrinol. 2002;23:41-100.
74. Brzezinski AA, Wurtman JJ, Wurtman RJ, Gleason R, Greenfield J, Nader T. d-fenfluramine suppresses the increased calorie and carbohydrate intakes and improves the mood of woman with premenstrual depression. J Am Coll Obstet Gynecol. 1990;76:296-300.
75. Su T-P, Schmidt PJ, Danaceau M, Murphy DL, Rubinow DR. Effect of menstrual cyle phase on neuroendocrine and behavioral responses to the serotonin agonist m-chlorophenylpiperazine in J Clin Endocrinol Metab. 1997;82:1220-8.
76. Steinberg S, Annable L, Young S, Liyanage N. A placebo-controlled clinical trial of L-tryptophan in premenstrual dysphoria. Biol Psychatry. 1999;45:313-20.
77. Landen M, Eriksson O, Sundblad C, Andersch B, Naessen T, Eriksson E. Compounds with affinity for serotonergic receptors in the treatment of premenstrual dysphoria: a comparison of buspirone, nafazodone and placebo. Psychopharmacology. 2001;155:292-8.
78. Menkes DB, Coates DC, Fawcett JP. Acute tryptophan depletion aggravates premenstrual syndrome. J Affect Disord. 1994;32:37-44.
79. Roca C, Schamidt P, Smith M, Danaceau M, Murphy D, Rubinow D. Effects of metergoline on symptoms in woman with premenstrual dysphoric disorder. Am J Psychiatry. 2002;159:1876-81.
80. Bancroft J, Cook A, Davidson D, Bennie J, Goodwin G. Blunting of neuroendocrine responses to infusion of L-tryptophan in woman with perimenstrual mood change. Psychol Med. 1991;21:305-12.
81. Eriksson O, Wall A, Marteiensdottir I, et al. Mood changes correlate to change in brain serotonin precursor trapping in woman with premenstrual dysphoria. Psychiatry Res. 2006;146:107-16.
82. Fitzgerald M, Malone KM, Li S, et al. Blunted serotonergic response to fenfluramine challenge in premenstrual dysphoric disorder. Am J Psychiatry. 1997;154:556-8.
83. Halbreich U, Tworek H. Altered serotonergic activity in woman with dysphoric premenstrual syndromes. Int J Psychiatry Med. 1993;23:1-27.
84. Rojansky N, Halbreich U, Zander K, Barkai A, Goldstein S. Imipramine receptor binding and serotonin uptake in platelets of woman with premenstrual changes. Gynecol Obstet Investing. 1991;31:146-52.
85. Steege JF, Stout AL, Knight BS, Nemeroff CB. Reduced platelet tritium-labeled imipramine binding sites in woman with premenstrual syndrome. Am J Obstet Gynecol. 1992;167: 168-72.
86. Rasgon N, McGurie M, Tanavoli S, Fairbanks L, Rapkin A. Neuroendocrine response to an intravenous L-tryptophan challenge in woman with premenstrual syndrome. Fertil Steril. 2000;73:144-9.
87. Steiner M, LN Y, Coote M, Wilkins A, Lepage P. Serotonergic dysfunction in woman with pure premenstrtual dysphoric disorder: is the fenfluramine challenge test still relevant. Psychiatry Res. 1999;87:107-15.
88. Yatham L, Barry S, Dinan TG. Serotonin receptors, buspirone, and premenstrual syndrome. Lancet. 1989;1:1447-8.
89. Melke J, Westberg L, Landen M, et al. Serotonin transporter gene polymorphisms and platelet [3H] paroxetien binding in premenstrual dysphoria. Psychoneuroendocrinology. 2003;28:446-58.
90. Epperson CN, Haga K, Mason GF, et al. Cortical gamma-aminobutyric acid levels across the menstrual cycle in healthy woman and those with premenstrual dysphoric disorder: A proton magnetic resonance spectroscopy study. Arch Gen Psychiatry. 2002;59:851-8.
91. Sundstrom I, Ashbrook D, Backstrom T. Reduced benzodiazepine sensitivity in patients with premenstrual syndrome: a pilot study. Psychonuroendocrinol. 1997;22:25-38.
92. Schmidt PJ, Purdy RH, Paul SM, Rubinow DR. Circulating levels of anxiolytic steroids in the luteal phase in woman with premenstrual syndrome and in control subjects. J Clin Endocrinol Metab. 1994;79:1256-60.
93. Rapkin AJ, Morgan M, Goldman L, Brann DW, Simone D, Mahesh VB. Progesterone metabolite allopregnanolone

in woman with premenstrual syndrome. Obstet Gynecol. 1997;90:709-14.

94. Girdler S, Straneva P, Light K, Pederson C, Morrow A. Allopregnanolone levels and reactivity to mental stress in premenstrual dysphoric disorder. Biol Psychiatry. 2001;49: 788-97.
95. Schmidt PJ, Grover GN, Rubinow DR. Alprazolam in the treatment of premenstrual syndrome: a double-blind, placebo-controlled trial. Arch Gen Psychiatry. 1993;50:467-73.
96. Bhagwagar Z, Wylezinska M, Taylor M, et al. Increased brain GABA concentrations following acute administration of a selective serotonin reuptake inhibitor. Am J Psychiatry. 2004;161:368-70.
97. Sundstrom I, Backstrom T. Citalopram increases pregnanolone sensitivity in patients with premenstrual syndrome: an open trial. Psychoneuroendcrinology. 1998;23:73-88.
98. Pinna G, Costa E, Guidotti A. Fluoxetine and norfluoxetion stereospecificlly and selectively increase brain neurosteroid content at does that are inactive on 5-HT reuptake Psychopharmacology (Berl). 2006;186:362-72.
99. Griffin LD, Mellon SH. Selective serotonin reuptake inhibitors directly alter activity of neuorsteroidogenic enxymes. Proc Natl Acad Sci USA. 1999;96:13512-7.
100. Faratian B, Gaspar A, O'Brien PM, Johnson IR, Filshie GM, Prescott P. Premenstrual syndrome: weight abdominal swelling, and perceived body image. Am J Obstet Gynecol. 1984;150:200-04.
101. Andersch B, Hahn L, Andersson M, Isaksson B. Body water and weight in patients with premenstrual tension. BJOG. 1978;85:546-50.
102. Andersch B. Bormocriptine and premenstrual symptoms: a survey of double blind trials. Obstet Gynecol Surv. 1983;38: 643-6.
103. Ylostalo P, Kauppila A, Puolakka J, Ronnberg L, Janne O. Bromocriptine and norethisterone in the treatment of premenstrual syndrome. J Am Coll Obstet Gynecol. 1981;58:292-8.
104. Wuttke W, Jarry H, Christoffel V, Spengler B, Seidlova-Wuttke D. Chaste tree (Vitex agnus-custus)—pharmacology and clinical indications. Phytomedicine. 2003;10:348-57.
105. O'Brien P, Abukhalil I. Randomized controlled trial of the management of premenstrual syndrome and premenstrual mastagia using luteal phase-only danazol. Am J Obstet Gynecol. 1999;180:18-23.
106. O'Brien PM, Craven D, Sellby C, Symonds EM. Treatment of premenstrual syndrome by spironolactone. BJOG. 1979;86:142-7.
107. Bancroft J, Rennie D. Perimenstrual depression: its relationship to pain, bleeding, and previous history of depression. Psychosom Med. 1995;57:445-52.
108. Endicott J, Nee J, Harrison W. Daily record of severity of problems (DRSP): reliability and validity. Arch Womens ment Heatlth. 2006;9:41-9.
109. Wyatt KM, Dimmock PW, O'Brien PMS. Selective serotonin reuptake inhibitors for premenstrual syndrome. Cochrane Database of Syst Rev. 2003;3:CD001396.
110. Yonkers KA, Clark RH, Trivedi MH. The psychopharmacological treatment of nonmajor mood disorders. In: Rush AJ (Ed). Mood disorders: systematic medications management-modern problems of pharmacopsychiatry. II series edition. Basel: Karger. 1997.pp.146-66.
111. Sundblad C, Modigh K, Andersch B, Eriksson E. Clomipraine effectively reduces premenstrual irritability and dysphoria: a placebo-controlled trial. Acta Psychiatr Scand. 1992;85:39-47.
112. Sundblad, C, Hedberg MA, Eriksson E. Clomipramine administered during the luteal phase reduces the symptoms of premenstrual syndrome: a placebo-controlled trial. Neuropsychopharmacology. 1993;9:133-45.
113. Wikander I, Sundblad C, Andersch B, et al. Citalopram in premenstrual dysphoria: is intermittent treatment during luteal phase more effective than continuous medication throughout the menstrual cycle? J Clin Psychopharmaocol. 1998;18:390-8.
114. Eriksson E, Nissbrandt H, Sorvik K, et al. Esictalopram in the trestment of premenstrual dysphoric disorder. Eur Neuropsychopharmacol. 2005;15(Suppl 3):S636.
115. Pearlstein TB, Stone AB, Lund SA, et al. Comparison of fluoxetine, buproprion, and placebo in the treatment of premenstrual dysphoric disorder. J Clin Psychopharmacol. 1997;17:261-5.
116. Steiner M, Steinberg S, Stewart D, et al. Fluoxetine in the treatment of premenstrual dysphoria. N Engl J Med. 1995;332: 1529-34.
117. Stone AB, Pearlstein TB, Brown WA. Fluoxetine in the treatment of premenstrual dysphoric disorder. J Clin Psychiatry. 1991;52:290-3.
118. Wood SH, Mortola JF, Chan YF, Moossazadeh F, Yen SSS. Treatment of premenstrual syndrome with fluoxetine: a double-blind, placebo-controlled, crossover study. Obstet Gynecol. 1992;80:339-44.
119. Cohen L, Miner C, Brown E, et al. Premenstrual daily fluoxetine for premenstrual dysphoric disorder: a placebo-controlled, clinical trial using computerized diaries. Obstet Gynecol. 2002;100:435-44.
120. Miner C, Brown E, McCray S, Gonzales J, Wohlreich M. Weekly luteal phase dosing with enteric-coated fluoxetine 90 mg in premenstrual dysphoric disorder: a randomized, double-blind, placebo-controlled clinical trial. Clin Ther. 2002;24:417-33.
121. Eriksson E, Hedberg MA, Andersch B, Sundblad C. The serotonin reuptake inhibitor paroxetine is superior to the noradrenaline reuptake inhibitor maprptiline in the treatment of premenstrual syndrome. Neuropsychopharmacology. 1995;12:167-76.
122. Cohen L, Soares C, Yonkers K, et al. Paroxetine controlled release for premenstrual dysphoric disorder: a double-blind, plecbo-cont rolled trial. Psychosom Med. 2004;66:707-13
123. Steiner M, Hirschberg A, Bergeron R, et al. Luteal phase dosing with paroxetine controlled release (CR) in the treatment of premenstrual dysphoric disorder. Am J Obstet Gynecol. 2005;193:352-60.
124. Yonkers KA, Holthausen GA, Poschman K, Howell HB. Symptom-onset treatment for woman with premenstrual

dysphoric disorder. J Clin Psychopharmacol. 2006;26: 198-202.
125. Landen M, Nissbrandt H, Allgulander C, et al. Placebo-controlled trial comparing intermittent and continuous paroxetine in premenstrual dysphoric disorder. Neuropsychopharmacology. 2007;32:153-61.
126. Freeman E, Rickels K, Sondheimer S, Polansky M. Differential reponse to antidepressants in woman with premenstrual syndrome/premenstrual dysphoric disorder: a randomized controlled trial. Arch Gen Psychiatry. 1999;56:932-9.
127. Halbreich U, Smoller JW. Intermittent luteal phase sertraline treatment of dysphoric premenstrual syndrome. J Clin Psychiatry. 1997;58:399-402.
128. Jermain DM, Preece CK, Sykes RL, Kuehl TJ, Sulak PJ. Luteal phase sertraline treatment for premenstrual dysphoric disorder: results of a double-blind, placebo-controlled crossover study. Arch Fam Med. 1999;8:328-32.
129. Young SA, Hurt PH, Benedek DM, Howard RS. Treatment of premenstrual dysphoric disorder with sertraline during the luteal phase: a randomized, double-blind, placebo-controlled crossover trial. J Clin Psychiatry. 1998;59:76-80.
130. Freeman E, Rickels K, Sondheimer S, Polansky M, Xiao S. Continuous or intermittent dosing with sertraline for patients with severe premenstrual syndrome or premenstrual dysphoric disorder. Am J Psychiatry. 2004;161:343-51.
131. Freeman E, Rickels K, Yonkers K, et al. Venlafaxine in the treatment of premenstrual dysphoric disorder. Obstet Gynecol. 2001;98:737-44.
132. Cohen L, Soares C, Lyster A, Cassano P, Brandes M, Leblanc G. Efficacy and tolerability of premenstrual use of venlafaxine (flexible dose) in the treatment of premenstrual dysphoric disorder. J Clin Psychopharmacol. 2004;24:540-3.
133. Freeman EW, Rickels K, Sondheimer SJ, Polansky M. Differential response to antidepressants in woman with premenstrual syndrome/premenstrual dysphoric disorder: a randomized controlled trial. Arch Gen Psychiatry. 1999;56:932-9.
134. Halbreich U, Bergeron R, Yonkers K, et al. Efficacy of intermittent, luteal phase sertraline treatment of premenstrual dysphoric disorder. Obstet Gynecol. 2002;100:1219-29.
135. Watson NR, Studd JW, Savvas M, Garnett T, Baber RJ. Treatment of severe premenstrual syndrome with oestradiol patches and cyclical aral norethisterone. Lancet. 1989;2:730-32.
136. Magos AL, Brincat M, Studd JW. Treatment of the premenstrual syndrome by subcutaneous estradiol implants and cyclical oral norethisterone: placebo-controlled study. BMJ. 1986;292: 1629-33.
137. Thys-Jacobs S, Starkey P, Bernstein D, Tian J. Calcium carbonate and the premenstrual and menstrual symptoms: Premenstrual Syndrome Study Group. Am J Obstet Gynecol. 1998;179:444-52.
138. Yonkers K, Brown C, Pearlstein T, et al. Efficacy of a new low-dose oral contraceptive with drospirenone in premenstrual dysphoric disorder. Obstet Gynecol 2005;106:492-501.
139. Pearlstein T, Bachmann G, Zacur H, Yonkers K. Treatment of premenstrual dysphoric disorder with a new drospirenone-containing oral contraceptive formulation. Contraception. 2005;72:414-21.
140. Pearlstein T, Halbreich U, Batzar E, et al. Psychosocial functioning in women with premenstrual dysphoric disorder before and after treatment with sertraline or placebo. J Clin Psychiatry. 2000;61:101-9.
141. Steiner M, Brown E, Trzepacz P, et al. Fluoxetine improves functional work capacity in woman with premenstrual dysphoric disorder. Arch Women's Ment Health. 2003;6:71-7.
142. Eriksson E, Endicott J, Andersch B, et al. New perspective on the treatment of premenstrual syndrome and premenstrual dysphoric disorder. Arch Women's Ment Health. 2002;4:111-9.
143. Steiner M, Pearlstein T, Cohen LS, et al. Expert guidelines for the treatment of severe PMS, PMDD, and comorbidities: the role of SSRIs. J Women's Health. 2006;15:57-69.
144. Young SA, Hurt PH, Benedeck DM, Howard RS. Treatment PDD with sertraline during the luteal phase: a randomized, double-blind, placebo controlled crossover trial. J Clin Psychiatry. 1998;59:76-80.
145. Freeman E, Sondheimer S, Sammel M, Ferdousi T, Lin H. A preliminary study of luteal phase versus symptom-onset dosing with escitalopram for premenstrual dysphoric disorder. J Clin Psychiatry. 2005;66:769-73.
146. Steiner M, Romano S, Babcock S, et al. The efficacy of fluoxetine in improving physical symptoms associated with premenstrual dysphoric disorder. Br J Obstet Gynaecol. 2001;108:462-8.
147. Steiner M, Haskett RF, Osmun JN, Carroll BJ. Treatment of premenstrual tension with lithium carbonate. A pilot study. Acta Psychiatry Scand. 1980;61:96-102.
148. Pearlstein TB, Stone AB, Lund SA, et al. Comparison of fluoxetine, bupropion, and placebo in premenstrual dysphoric disorder. J Clin Psychopharmacol. 1997;17:261-6.
149. Rickels K, Freeman E, Sondherimer S. Buspirone in treatment of premenstrual syndrome. Lancet. 1989;4:777.
150. Smith S, Rinehart JS, Ruddock VE, Schiff I. Treatment of premenstrual syndrome with alprazolam: Results of a double-blind, placebo-controlled, randomized crossover clinical trial. Obstet Gynecol. 1987;70:37-43.
151. Harrison WM, Endicott J, Nee J. Treatment of premenstrual dysphoria with alprazolam. Arch Gen Psychiatry. 1990;47: 270-5.
152. Freeman EW, Rickels K, Sondheimer SJ, Polansky M. A double-blind trail of oral progesterone, alpraxolam, and placebo in treatment of severe premenstrual syndrome. JAMA. 1995;274:51-7.
153. Wyatt KM, Dimmock PW, Frischer M, Jones PW, O'Brien SP. Prescribing patterns in premenstrual syndrome. BMC Women Health. 2002;2:4.
154. Di Carlo C, Palomba S, Tommaselli G, Guida M, Sardo ADS, Nappi C. Use of leuprolide acetate plus tibolone in the treatment of severe premenstrual syndrome. Fertil Steril. 2001;75: 380-4.

155. Cronjo W, Studd J. Premenstrual syndrome and premenstrual dysphoric disorder. Prim Care. 2002;29:1-12.
156. Watson NR, Studd JW, Savvas M, Baber RJ. The long-term effects of estradiol implant therapy for the treatment of premenstrual syndrome. Gynecol Endocrinol. 1990;4:99-107.
157. O'Brien P, Abukhalil I, Henshaw C. Premenstrual syndrome. Curr Obstet Gyneacol. 1995;5:30-5.
158. Domoney C, Panny N, Hawkins A, Studd JWW. Treatment of Premenstrual syndrome with transdermal estrogen. Int J Gynaecol Obstet. 2003;83(Suppl 3):37.
159. Bancroft J, Rennie D. The impact of oral contraceptives on the experience of per menstrual mood, clumsiness, food craving and other symptoms. J Psychiatry Res. 1993;37:195-202.
160. Graham CA, Sherwin BB. A prospective treatment study of premenstrual symptoms using a triphasic oral contraceptive. J Psychosom Res. 1992;36:257-66.
161. Sulak P, Scow R, Preece C, Riggs M, Kuehl T. Hormone withdrawal symptoms in oral contraceptive users. Obstet Gynecol. 2000;95:261-6.
162. Sulak P, Kuehl T, Ortiz M, Schull B. Acceptance of altering the standard 21-day/7-day oral contraceptive regimen to delay menses and reduce hormone withdrawal symptoms. Am J Obstet Gynecol. 2002;186:1142-9.
163. Halbreich U, Rojansky N, Palter S. Elimination of ovulation and menstrual cyclicity (with danazol) improves dysphoric premenstrual syndromes. Fertil Steril. 1991;56: 1066-9.
164. Watts JF, Butt WR, Edwards RL. A clinical trial using danazol for the treatment of premenstrual tensiohn. BJOG. 1987; 94:30-4.
165. Hahn PM, Van Vugt DA, Reid RL. A randomized, placebo-controlled, crossover trial of danazol for the treatment of premenstrual syndrome. Psychoneuroendocrinology. 1995;20: 193-9.
166. Lam R, Carter D, Misri S, et al. A controlled study of light therapy in woman with late luteal phase dysphoric disorder. Psychiatry Res. 1999;86:185-92.
167. Vellacott I, Shroff N, Pearce MY, Stratford ME, Akbar FA. A double-blind, placebo-controlled evaluation of spironolactone in the premenstrual syndrome. Curr Med Res Opin. 1987;10:450-6.
168. Aslaksen K, Falk V. Spironolactone in the treatment of premenstrual tension: A double-blind study of spironolactone vs bendroflumethiazide and placebo. Curr Ther Res Clin Exper. 1991;49:120.
169. Wyatt KM, Dimmock PW, Jones PW, Shaughn O'Brien PM. Efficacy of vitamin B-6 in the treatment of premenstrual syndrome: systematic review. BMJ (Clin Res Ed). 1999;318: 1375-81.
170. Schellenberg R. treatment for the premenstrual syndrome with agnus castus fruit extract: prospective, randomized, placebo controlled study. BMJ. 2001;322:134-7.
171. Budeiri D, Li Wan Po A, Dornan JC. Is evening primrose oil of value in the treatment of premenstrual syndrome? Control Clin Trials. 1996;17:60-8.
172. Walker A, De Souza M, Marakis G, et al. Unexpected benefit of sorbitol placebo in Mg intervention study of premenstrual symptoms: implications for choice of placebo in RCTs. Med Hypotheses. 2002;58:213-20.
173. Khine K, Rosenstein DL, Elin RJ, et al. Magnesium (mg) retention and mood effects after intravenous mg infusion in premenstrual dysphoric disorder. Biol Psychiatry. 2006;59: 327-33.
174. Sayegh R, Schiff I, Wurtman J, et al. The effect of a carbohydrate-rich beverage on mood, appetite, and cognitive function in woman with premenstrual syndrome. J Am Coll Obstet Gynecol. 1995;86:520-8.
175. Freeman EW, Stout AL, Endicott J, Spiers P. Treatment of premenstrual syndrome with a carbohydrate-rich beverage. Int J Gynecol Obstet. 2002;77:253-4.
176. Hunter MS, Ussher JM, Browne SJ, et al. A randomized comparison of psychological (cognitive behavior therapy), medical (fluoxetine) and combined treatment for woman with premenstrual dysphoric disorder. J Psychosom Obstet Gynaecol. 2002;23:193-9.
177. Steege JF, Blumenthal JA. The effects of aerobic exercise on premenstrual symptoms in middle-aged woman: a preliminary study. J Psychosom Res. 1993;37:127-33.
178. Mira M, McNeil D, Fraser IS, Vizzard J, Abraham S. Mefenamic acid in the treatment of premenstrual syndrome. J Am Coll Obstet Gynecol. 1986;68:395-8.
179. Facchinetti F, Fioroni L, Sances G, Romano G, Nappi G, Genazzani AR. Naproxen sodium in the treatment of premenstrual symptoms: a placebo-controlled study. Gynecol Obstet Investig. 1989;28:205-8.
180. Chuong CJ, His BP. Effect of naloxone on luteinixing hormone secretion in premenstrual syndrome. Fertil Steril. 1994;61:1039-44.
181. American Psychiatric Association. Desk Reference to the Diagnostic Criteria from DSM-5. Washington DC; 2013.

CHAPTER 31

Abnormal Illness Behavior

Issy Pilowsky

INTRODUCTION

I took my first steps towards formulating the concept of '*Abnormal Illness Behavior*' (AIB) in 1961 when I was working in Sheffield under the mentorship of Erwin Stengel. He had taken the Chair as Foundation Professor in 1957 after a period as a Reader at the Institute of Psychiatry in London. Although his main interest in the 1960s lay in the area of suicide and attempted suicide, he had always retained a fascination with psychobiological phenomena since his days in Vienna, where he trained in the neuropsychiatric and psychoanalytic traditions and was especially influenced by Paul Schilder with whom he had coauthored a paper on 'pain asymbolia', i.e. congenital indifference to pain. Schilder's[1] interest in the body image, and abnormal disorders associated with it, always remained in Stengel's mind, so that when appointed to the Sheffield Chair in a department associated with a general hospital, he responded with his usual creative energy to the challenge presented by patients referred by his medical and surgical colleagues. I joined the department in 1959; in the summer of 1961, after I had expressed a serious interest in research, he handed me his copy of Gillespie's[2] monograph on hypochondria, suggesting that it might be a suitable topic for an MD thesis. I accepted this advice with some trepidation, and the more I read of Gillespie's book, the more worried I became; in particular, I did not see how I was going to measure hypochondriasis. In the end, I decided to construct a questionnaire, which I will discuss later.

At this time I was having helpful discussions with Harold Merskey and Graham Spear, who were both engaged in the study of chronic pain. Together, they later produced a seminal book[3] on psychiatric and psychological aspects of pain, based on their respective doctoral theses.

Apart from developing a questionnaire, I was also conducting a clinical study which involved interviewing and in many cases treating patients who manifested hypochondriacal syndromes. Merskey was conducting a similar study on chronic pain.

As time passed, I noticed that some of Merskey's patients with unexplained chronic pain were finding their way into my study group of hypochondriacal patients, and vice versa; there was clearly an overlap between the two disorders. Merskey[4] eventually came to the main conclusion than these patients suffered from a form of hysteria. At about this time, Slater[5] published a study which he claimed showed that hysteria did not exist. Francis Walshe,[6] an eminent neurologist, at once published an elegant response, asserting that hysteria did exist and calling on neurologists to "justify the concept of hysteria as a nosological entity in its own right".

This controversy led me to wonder what these patients had in common and what distinguished between them.

At this point, the concept of '*illness behavior*' presented itself, formulated by two American medical sociologists, Mechanic and Volkart.[7] They defined *illness behavior* as the various ways in which individuals perceived, evaluated and acted upon symptoms. Exploring this idea led me to the '*sick role*' as described by Talcott Parsons in 1951.[8] After a while, it occurred to me that illness behavior was a useful overarching concept and that hypochondriasis and hysteria could be regarded as abnormal forms. Furthermore, it seemed to me that the sick role concept was important in that it underlined the salience of the doctor's function in the legitimation of illness; the task of clarifying that the individual wishing to adopt this role had fulfilled society's requirement to seek medical help and cooperate with the person qualified to provide it. Resonating with this societal imperative is the clinical criterion for the diagnosis of hypochondriasis, which states that the preoccupation with disease "does not respond to medical reassurance." This makes hypochondriasis quite unusual in medicine, because firstly it assumes the appropriateness of the doctor's functioning as an integral part of the diagnostic process, and secondly, it accepts the patient's "intransigence" as a key criterion.

In the 1969 paper,[9] I described AIB with a focus on the disagreement between patient and doctor over the sick role. In 1978, a more precise definition was presented in the following form (the word 'accurate' was added later):

"*Abnormal Illness Behavior* is an inappropriate or maladaptive mode of experiencing, perceiving, evaluating or responding to one's own state of health which persists despite the fact that a doctor (or other appropriate social agent) has offered an accurate and reasonably lucid explanation of the nature of the person's health status and the appropriate course of management (if any), with provision of adequate opportunity for discussion, clarification and negotiation based on a thorough examination of all parameters of functioning (psychological, social and biological), and taking into account the individual's age, sex, educational and sociocultural background".[10]

The various elements of this definition were later elucidated, with greater detail. Since then, the concept of abnormal illness behavior[11] has increasingly occupied a point of convergence for general medicine, psychiatry, psychology, psychoanalysis, philosophy, economics, sociology, jurisprudence and anthropology, all of which contribute to our understanding of illness and abnormal illness behavior. This was reflected in two conferences on 'Social and Clinical Aspects of Illness Behavior' held in 1984 (Adelaide) and 1985 (Toronto). Papers from the former appeared in *Psychiatric Medicine* and from the latter in one volume edited by McHugh and Vallis. From the doctor's point of view, the challenge resides in having to convince society that a person who refuses to cooperate with an 'appointed agent of society' is entitled to the sick-role, because the refusal itself represents psychopathology and is the symptom of a 'legitimate' illness.

Society's stake in this concept cannot be overestimated, because of its relevance to issues such as health economics, invalid pensions, and worker's compensation. For health services (and for the legal profession, which is so often involved) the concept of an illness characterized by a mistaken belief in the presence of illness is difficult to assimilate. It goes without saying that lurking in the wings is always the spectre of the malingerer.

In the early 1960s in the UK, the issue of worker's compensation did not impinge on my mind to the extent that it does now. Perhaps this was because my research was carried out within a National Health Service. However, in countries such as Australia where health services operate on a fee-for-service basis, there is as great a concern with medical 'over servicing' as there is with fraud. How then does a doctor convince an insurer that he is legitimately treating a patient for a condition in which the latter either thinks he is sick when he isn't, or is sicker than he is supposed to be? Does the doctor adopt the insurer's perspective, abandon professional objectivity, and confront the patients? Some do, but are well advised not to. The few recent case reports in the literature describing patients who have murdered doctors involved situations where the latter took sides in a dispute over compensation or invalidity.

In the 1978 paper entitled '*A general classification of Abnormal Illness Behavior*'[10] the concept of AIB was also extended, and various terms such as 'illness'[8] were more explicitly defined. The paper made clear that illness could not only be abnormally affirmed but also denied, and that the focus could be either a somatic or a psychological condition. A search of the literature revealed examples of all such forms of AIB, although not all were regarded as nosological entities. However, it is interesting to note that it was recently proposed by Strauss et al[12] that the 'Maladaptive Denial of Illness' be included in DSM-IV.

As might be expected, the definition of AIB turned out to be a controversial one: for example, in 1984 the late and sorely missed Heinz Wolff, at a plenary session on AIB during a London meeting of the European Society for Psychosomatic Research, called AIB 'a dangerous idea.' I was grateful to have the opportunity later to convince him that not only was I not offended by his statement (as he thought I might be) but that I agreed with him completely, and that was why I felt that the criteria attaching the AIB label had to be so carefully and precisely delineated.

It is of considerable interest to dwell on the aspect of the definition of AIB which is perceived to be most dangerous. It will be recalled that a key part of the definition ran as follows: "despite the fact that doctor has offered an accurate and reasonably lucid explanation of the nature of the person's health status and the appropriate course of management (if any)". The question repeatedly posed is: "What if the doctor is wrong?" This is indeed a crucial issue. Why, one may wonder, was such a question rarely, if ever, asked about the definition of hypochondriasis before, given that nonresponse of medical reassurance has always been a central criterion? One possible explanation is that this criterion was not very critical in earlier times, because most presentations of AIB to psychiatrists were of clearly psychotic delusions; it was abundantly plain to everyone that the patients' ideas were grossly abnormal. However, in recent decades, psychiatrists have functioned in general hospital and community settings, where patients' ideas about their health are rarely psychotic and the diagnosis is far from clear-cut.

How then do we deal with this challenging question?

Firstly, it should be said that the 'doctor' in the definition is an 'ideal type', a conception used for the purpose of definition since, if we cannot conceive of doctors being 'right' in an opinion, we are hardly able to sustain the idea of hypochondriasis (or any other form of AIB) because it is self-evident that an abnormal or false idea about one's health status can only be validated against the opinion of someone who is qualified to carry out a clinical assessment and arrive at an opinion which can be communicated to a patient.

There is, however, room for compromise: for example, it is reasonable for a 'provisional' or 'tentative' diagnosis of AIB to be made on the basis of the patient's phenomenology, even before the doctor has been able to gather all the information needed to make a confident pronouncement about the patient's state of health. In any event, for the purpose of definitional conciseness, we are oversimplifying a complex interactional process which evolves over time.

A concern of a rather different sort has been articulated, especially by medical sociologists, including David Mechanic [personal communication]. It is that Illness Behavior may come to be regarded as inherently 'abnormal' when, in fact, it refers to an essentially normal and universal human response.

I readily acknowledge that this may be a danger, although I have not yet heard my colleagues describing patients as suffering from 'Illness Behavior.' What I have heard is patients being described as showing abnormal illness behavior when there was insufficient justification for such a statement. Two common errors are: firstly, to use the term AIB simply to describe the presentation of physical complaints where no adequate physical explanation is found, and secondly, to apply the term when patients with physical symptoms manifest anxiety, depression or perhaps even 'unattractive' personality traits.

Thus the term AIB, which I hoped might militate against the inappropriate and pejorative use of labels such as 'hysteric' and 'hypochondriac,' can itself be used as a pejorative term. One can only hope that the more precise definition offered by AIB will at least provide a firmer basis for questioning whether the term is being applied correctly.

Interestingly, there is some evidence that despite the fact that these pejorative labels may be bandied about in ordinary conversation, doctors probably never document such opinions in patients' case notes. Most GPs will, if asked, admit to some anxiety about doing so.

We should also bear in mind that the label AIB concerns diagnosis and classifications: it is discussed in categorical terms as if conditions are either absent or present. We know that this is an artificial approach, albeit useful. In practice, the various forms of illness behavior lie on a continuum and consist of a constellation of features, each of which can vary between and within individuals. The degree of insight is an example of this. From a research point of view, the dimensional perspective is reflected in the Whiteley Index of Hypochondriasis and the Illness Behavior Questionnaire, which are described below.

CLASSIFICATION AND DIAGNOSIS

Since 1969, there have been major developments in the classification of psychiatric illness, foreshadowed by the WHO monograph on the subject written by Erwin Stengel[13] and published in 1960. In this report, he urged the setting up of a pilot study by WHO with the ultimate goal of achieving a generally acceptable basis for psychiatric diagnosis.

DSM-III, DSM-III-R, and DSM-IV

In parallel, the American Psychiatric Association mounted a massive initiative and produced in 1977 a multiaxial criterion-based diagnostic system: the 3rd Diagnostic and Statistical Manual, better known as DSM-III. One of its most important guiding principles was that it be based on clinical phenomenology, i.e. on description rather than on any etiological theory.

Two features of DSM-III are relevant in this context. The first is that an entirely new term sprang full grown from the heads of its creators, 'somatoform disorders.' These were described as psychiatric disorders which present with symptoms which suggest the presence of physical disorder. Among these were to be found conversion disorder, hypochondriasis and for the first time 'psychogenic pain disorder.' 'Somatization disorders' (Briquet's hysteria) were also described. The locus of abnormality varied from condition to condition. In conversion disorder it was the symptom, in hypochondriasis the ideas, and in somatization the behavior (especially care-seeking).

Since then, we have had DSM-III-R and now DSM-IV. In these versions, the diagnosis of hypochondriasis has remained essentially the same, with the lack of response to "medical reassurance" always a key criterion.

The second significant feature of DSM-III, DSM-III-R, and now DSM-IV was that in the case of the somatoform disorders the principle of adhering to descriptive phenomenology only was abandoned, and the assumption of the presence of 'conflicts or other stressors' was considered to be part of the diagnosis of these conditions. For example, the relevant aspects of the criteria for *conversion disorder* read as follows:

Psychological factors are judged to be associated with the symptom or deficit because the initiation or exacerbation of the symptoms or deficit is preceded by conflicts or other stressors.

In the case of *hypochondriasis*, the key criteria are:

- Preoccupation with fears of having, or the idea that one has, a serious disease based on the person's misinterpretation of bodily symptoms; and
- The preoccupation persists despite appropriate medical evaluation and reassurance.

Thus, the nonresponse to reassurance is retained, with the significant addition of the words 'evaluation' and 'appropriate.'

ICD-10

The ICD-10 Classification of Mental and Behavioral Disorders appeared in 1992. This document shows evidence of a somewhat more flexible approach to diagnosis, having no doubt benefited from the development of the response to DSM-III, III-R and IV. For example, in this volume the term 'guidelines' is used rather than 'criteria': the latter are dealt with separately in a volume concerned with research. In general, I cannot help but be impressed by the language of ICD-10 and its sensitivity to the needs of clinicians. The separation into two volumes of 'Clinical Description and Diagnostic Guidelines' and 'Diagnostic Criteria for Research' seems to me to have been a master-stroke.

In a submission to the ICD-10 committee on *somatoform disorders*, I emphasized the need to comment on what might be considered optimal behavior on the part of doctors. The patient's negative attitude to the possibility of psychosocial stressors was also proposed as an important criterion.

The ICD-10 text states:

"Even when the onset and continuation of the symptoms bear a close relationship with unpleasant life events or with difficulties or conflicts, the patient usually resists attempts to discuss the possibility of psychological causation; this may even be the case in the presence of obvious depressive and anxiety symptoms. The degree of understanding, either physical or psychological, that can be achieved about the cause of the symptoms is often disappointing and frustrating for both patient and doctors."

The diagnostic guidelines for *hypochondriasis* in ICD-10 read as follows:

For a definite diagnosis, both of the following should be present:

- A persistent belief in the presence of at least one serious physical illness underlying the presenting symptom or symptoms, even though repeated investigation and examinations have identified no adequate physical explanation, or a persistent preoccupation with a presumed deformity or disfigurement.
- A persistent refusal to accept the advice and reassurance of several different doctors that there is no physical illness or abnormality underlying the symptoms.

The ICD-10 seems to me to be an improvement on what went before, but I believe we could do better by describing some of these guidelines more explicitly from the patient's viewpoint, along the following lines:

- An uncomfortable awareness of bodily events most of the time.
- Fears and concerns about health and disease which are present most of the time.
- An awareness of an inability to accept reassurance from doctors associated with the concern that doctors have not done everything possible to detect disease or are withholding information and/or treatment which could be helpful.
- An awareness of an inability to accept the suggestion that nonphysical, i.e. psychosocial factors may be relevant to one's condition, and marked emotional discomfort when this possibility is raised or pressed. This criterion could replace or be added to the DSM-IV criterion referring to "psychological factors".

The Diagnostic Process in the Clinical Setting

In clinical practice, the diagnosis of AIB emerges from a sequence of interactions during which the patient's inability to negotiate towards and intersubjective understanding of the presenting problem in any other than a somatic way, becomes increasingly apparent. We can divide them albeit artificially, into the following stages:

- Firstly, we have Adaptive Illness Behavior, where the doctor and patient reach agreement at an early stage.
- In a second stage, the doctor needs to explain to the patient that emotions are accompanied by somatic changes; the patient is then able to reattribute the somatic symptoms to psychosocial stressors.
- Finally, we have the stage of Abnormal Illness Behavior, in which the patient cannot accept medical explanations and is preoccupied by an inaccurate view of his health status: this may take the form of phobia, a morbid preoccupation, overvalued idea or a delusion.

The label to be attached will depend on the classification being used and the criteria fulfilled.

QUANTIFYING AIB

As mentioned earlier, in the mid 1960s I constructed a hypochondriasis questionnaire, named the Whiteley Index after the Whiteley Woods Clinic of the Department of Psychiatry in Sheffield, where the work was carried out.[14] A factor analysis revealed three dimensions: disease conviction, illness phobia and somatic awareness. This instrument was constructed because of dissatisfaction with the MMPI Hypochondriasis Scale, which consisted essentially of a symptom list and neglected attitudes to illness. The Whiteley Index was later expanded into the Illness Behavior Questionnaire (IBQ) and applied mainly to the assessment and study of patients attending pain clinics, many of whom met the criteria for a diagnosis of 'somatoform pain disorder' (DSM-IV) or 'persistent somatoform pain disorder' (ICD-10).

The IBQ has subsequently been used in a number of ways:

- As a basis for separating out the dimensions of illness behavior in various clinical populations, with the application of statistical techniques such as principal component analysis and numerical taxonomy.
- To delineate predictors of treatment outcome.
- To delineate predictors of health care utilization.
- As a measure of various aspects of illness behavior in particular clinical populations.

To my knowledge, the questionnaire has been translated into a number of languages including French, Portugese, Spanish, Italian, German, Polish, Norwegian, Swedish, Chinese, Hindi, Serbo-Croat, Greek and Japanese.

A few representative examples of IBQ based research are presented below.

Factor Analytic Studies

Using principal component analysis on the responses of pain clinic patients to the IBQ, the following factors were generated; these formed the basis for seven scales which are now named General (Phobic), Hypochondriasis, Disease

Conviction, Psychological vs. Somatic Functioning, Affective Inhibition, Affective Disturbance, Denial and Irritability.

A discriminant function analysis produced an equation which separated Pain Clinic and General Practice patients. This is now used as a measure of the likelihood of a patient having a somatoform pain disorder.

In a recent replication[15] of the original factor analytic study[9] involving a such larger number of pain clinic patients (over 800), new factors emerged which are of interest but have yet to be evaluated as measures. We have named these new factors interpersonal sensitivity, responsiveness to medical reassurance, insight and biological functions. Completed IBQs of pain clinic patients (over a 10 year period) were most recently analyzed[16] using a numerical taxonomy procedure; two classes emerged which were distinguished by item responses indicating an acceptance or rejection of a psychological viewpoint.

Predicting Response to Treatment and Long-term Outcome

The IBQ has been used to predict response to treatment. Examples include the response to surgical treatment for low back pain (Waddell et al),[17] and the long-term outcome in the chronic fatigue syndrome (CFS).[18] In both cases, the important predictor was the score on the Disease Conviction Scale [either on its own or as part of the Disease Affirmation (second order) Scale]. In the case of the CFS, the Disease Conviction Scale was the only variable significantly correlated with the Global Outcome Rating, the delayed hypersensitivity skin test and the Karnofsky Quality of Life Index. In a previous study by this group,[19] Disease Conviction and Denial were found to be significant characteristics of CFS compared to a GP population. Schweitzer et al[20] have essentially replicated this finding.

In a recent British Medical Journal editorial commenting on the work of Wilson et al,[18] Lawrie and Pelosi[21] called for research to establish whether psychological treatment might have a role in modifying the attitude measured by the Disease Conviction Scale. Recent reports on the treatment of hypochondriasis offer reason for optimism in this regard.[22-24]

Interestingly, the article by Wilson et al[18] evoked a flurry of correspondence reflecting the controversial nature of the topic, but if CFS can be considered an example of a controversial area into which the AIB idea and the IBQ have been drawn, another even more heatedly debated condition was the one named Repetitive Strain Injury (RSI) in Australia, a syndrome encountered in the work place and very similar to 'Writer's Cramp.' Here, compensation was a major issue, and so heated did the argument over the legitimacy of this diagnosis become a few years ago, with claims and counter-claims in the medical and lay press, that at one stage trade unions issued a warning to their members not to accept administration of the MMPI or the IBQ, because psychiatrists were trying to prove that their condition was psychological, i.e. that they were malingering. This was reported on the front page of the highly respected *Sydney Morning Herald*, where examples were given of 'outlandish' questions, all of which were taken from the MMPI, I am happy to say.

Conscious Exaggeration Scale

An attempt has been made to use the IBQ to detect malingering by the development of a 'Conscious Exaggeration Scale.' This strikes me as entirely misguided for a number of reasons which are beyond the scope of this chapter, but should, I think, be fairly obvious.

TREATMENT

A particularly heartening development over the past 25 years has been a change in the attitude to the treatment of AIB in its various manifestations.

Prominent among those who have contributed to these advances are Smith,[25] Goldberg and Bridges (somatization),[26] Warwick and Marks,[27] Kellner,[28] Barsky et al[22] and House[23] (hypochondriasis), and in the pain area, Fordyce,[29] Sternbach,[30] Meichenbaum et al,[31] Turner,[32] Tunks,[33] my colleagues, Bassett,[34] Barrow,[35] Spence,[36] and of course many others.

What is particularly striking is the change in the attitude to the psychological treatment of hypochondriasis and chronic pain, which were previously regarded most pessimistically from a therapeutic viewpoint unless they were secondary to depressive or anxiety disorders. There are doubtless many reasons for the change, but foremost among them must be the presence of psychiatric units in general hospitals actively engaged in consultation liaison activities, and the involvement within the orbit of such units of clinical psychologists, who have contributed their knowledge of cognitive and behavioral psychotherapies so effectively. This has led to the use of so-called cognitive-behavioral therapies, with considerable success, especially when combined with physiotherapy, family therapy, brief psychotherapy, and (especially in chronic pain) antidepressants.[35] In the area of chronic pain, the need for a multidisciplinary approach has been well recognized, leading to the formation of 'Pain Clinics.'

What has emerged from all these activities is the need for flexibility on the part of clinicians wishing to treat abnormal illness behavior of the somatoform type. If purism was ever out of place, it is in the management of somatoform disorders. Equally, if interdisciplinary collaboration was ever essential, it is also essential in the management of these conditions.

The Transition Phase in Treatment

It has become increasingly obvious that all treatments involve a transition phase, during which the patient is helped to make a shift from viewing the illness as purely physical to accepting that psychosocial factors are also worthy of consideration as contributors to the problem. Achieving this transition requires the acquisition of new skills by clinicians and a preparedness to tolerate the blurring of system boundaries.

Lest we imagine this to be a new discovery, we may recall that Freud's management of Elizabeth von R (one of the cases described in *Studies in Hysteria*) proceeded very much along these lines. He describes providing a period of physical therapy before introducing the so-called 'new' treatment to the patient. The transition included electrical stimulation to the patient's painful legs administered by Freud himself "in order to keep in touch with her." And in the case of Frau Emmy von N, he reports: "I ordered her to be given warm baths and I shall massage her whole body twice a day."

It should be emphasized that while the transition to the psychosocial domain is important, it does not entail a complete abandonment of the somatic domain, which must always be kept in mind. Nor does the transition necessarily entail a move from the care of a physician or GP to that of a psychiatrist or psychologist. Any doctor who is trained to detect and deal with psychosocial issues, no matter what the primary diagnosis may be, is able to manage and help these patients.

In 1969, I sent a proof copy of my paper introducing abnormal illness behavior[9] to Sir Francis Walshe, the eminent neurologist who has defended hysteria against Slater's onslaught. He wrote back saying that he liked the idea. I wonder now, in retrospect, whether he really grasped what I was getting at. Heinz Wolf, you will recall, said that it was 'a dangerous' idea. I think he really got the message.

By way of concluding, may I say that it seems that the concept of AIB has now been around long enough for it to be a part of psychiatry's intellectual furniture, virtually taken for granted.

When all is said and done, we know that patients with AIB suffered from their condition; but tragically, the nature of their presentation tends to drive others (including doctors) away from them when they need them most.

Their contribution to Medicine is to force us all to think deeply about the doctor-patient relationship and constantly to review out standards for medical behavior.

REFERENCES

1. Schilder P. The image and appearance of the human body. New York: Kegan Paul; 1950.
2. Gillespie RD. Hypochondria. London: Trench; 1928.
3. Merskey H, Spear FG. Meaning and definition of pain. Pain: Psychological and Psychiatric Aspects. London: Bailliere, Tindall and Cassell; 1967.pp.14–24.
4. Merskey H. The characteristics of persistent pain in psychological illness. J Psychosom Res. 1965;9:291-8.
5. Slater E. Diagnosis of "hysteria". Br Med J. 1965;1:1385-99.
6. Walshe F. Diagnosis of hysteria. Br Med J. 1965;2:1451-4.
7. Mechanic D, Volkart EH. Illness behaviour and medical diagnosis. Health Human Behav. 1960;1:86-94.
8. Parsons T. Social Structure and Personality. London: Collier-Macmillian; 1964.
9. Pilowsky I. Abnormal illness behaviour. Br J Med Psychol. 1969;42:347-51.
10. Pilowsky I. A general classification of abnormal illness behaviour. Br J Med Psychol. 1978;51:131-7.
11. Pilowsky I. Illness behaviour and neuroses. Current Opinion in Psychiatry. 1989;2:217-24.
12. Strauss DH, Spitzer RL, Muskin PR. Maladaptive denial of physical illness: A proposal for DSM-IV. Am J Psychiatry. 1990;147:1168-72.
13. Stengel E. Classification of mental disorders. Bull WHO. 1960;21:601-63.
14. Pilowsky I. Dimensions of hypochondriasis. Br J Psychiatry. 1967;113-89-93.
15. Pilowsky I. Dimensions of illness behaviour as measured by the Illness Behaviour Questionnaire: A replication study. J Psychosom Res. 1993;37:53-62.
16. Pilowsky I, Katsikitis M. A classification of illness behaviour in pain clinic patients. Pain. 1994;57:91-4.
17. Waddell G, Pilowsky I, Bond MR. Clinical assessment and interpretation of abnormal illness behaviour in low back pain. Pain. 1989;39:41-53.
18. Wilson A, Hickie I, Lloyd A, et al. Longitudinal study of outcome of chronic fatigue syndrome. Br M J. 1994;308:756-9.
19. Hickie I, Lloyd A, Wakefield D, et al. The psychiatric status of patients with the chronic fatigue syndrome. Br J Psychiatry. 1990;156:534-40.
20. Schweitzer R, Robertson DL, Kelly B, Whiting J. llness behaviour of patients with chronic fatigue syndrome. J Psychosom Res. 1994;38:41-9.
21. Lawrie SM, Peolosi AJ. Chronic fatigue syndrome: Prevalence and outcome. Br Med J. 1994;308-732-3.
22. Barsky AJ, Geringer E, Wood CA. A cognitive-education treatment for hypochondriasis. Gen Hosp Psychiatry. 1988; 10:322-7.
23. House A. Hypochondriasis and related disorders: Assessment and management of patients referred or a psychiatric opinion. Gen Hosp Psychiatry. 1989;11:156-65.
24. Creed F, Firth D, Timol M, et al. Somatization and illness and illness behaviour in neurology ward. J Psychosom Res. 1990;34:427-37.
25. Smith GR. The epidemiology and treatment of depression when it coexists with somatoform disorders, somatization, or pain. Gen Hosp Psychiatry. 1992;14:265-72.
26. Goldberg DP, Bridges K. Somatic presentations of psychiatric illness in primary care setting. J Psychosom Res. 1988;32: 137-44.
27. Warwick H, Marks IM. Behavioural treatment of illness phobia and hypochondriasis.Br J Psychiatry. 1988;152:239-41.

28. Kellner R. Psychotherapeutic strategies on hypochondriasis: A clinical study. Am J Psychother. 1982;36:146-57.
29. Fordyce WE. Behavioural methods for chronic pain and illness. St Louis: Mosby; 1976.
30. Sternback R. Psychological aspects of chronic pain.Clin Ortho Related Res. 1977;129:155-60.
31. Meichenbaum J, Turk DC, Genest M. Pain and Behavioral Medicine: A Cognitive-Behavioural Perspective. New York: Guilford; 1983.
32. Turner J. Comparison of group progressive-relaxation training and cognitive behavioural group therapy for chronic low back pain. J Consult Clin Psychol. 1982;50:757-65.
33. Solomon P, Tunks E. The role of litigation in predicting disability outcomes in chronic pain patients. Clin J Pain. 1991;7:300-4.
34. Pilowsky I, Bassett DL. Individual dynamic psychotherapy for chornic pain. In: Tunks R (Ed). Chronic Pain: Psychosocial Factors in Rehabilitation. Baltimore: Williams & Wilkins; 1982.
35. Pilowsky I, Barrow CG. A controlled study of psychotherapy and amitriptyline used individually and in combination in the treatment chronic intractable "psychogenic" pain. Pain. 1990;40:3-19.
36. Pilowsky I, Spence ND. Patterns of illness behaviour in patients with intractable pain. J Psychosom Res. 1975;19:279-87.

CHAPTER 32

Consultation Liaison Psychiatry

GC Munjal, Niraj Ahuja

INTRODUCTION

With an emphasis on improving the relationship between medicine and psychiatry, psychiatrists have been under pressure to prove themselves as members of a medical discipline distinct from nonmedical psychology and psychiatric social work. Psychiatry, as a branch of medicine, has been described as searching for an identity of its own as compared to other nonmedical mental health professions.[1-5] Some have professed psychiatry to be in a crisis.[1,6-11]

On the other hand, physicians and surgeons are increasingly becoming aware that one third to two thirds of their patients have significant psychiatric symptomatology which is amenable to treatment by psychiatrists.[11,12] The fact, that psychiatric patients can also present to the medical or surgical units due to antecedent physical illnesses and may need additional care by psychiatrists is being recognized.

These two factors, combined with the movement of psychiatric units from mental asylums to general hospitals in 1920s and 1930s saw the birth of consultation-liaison psychiatry. Availability of newer and medical modes of treatment in 1950s further strengthened the growing base of consultation-liaison psychiatry.

HISTORY OF EVOLUTION OF CONCEPT

Since times immemorial, the intimate relationship between mind and body has been recognized in the field of medicine. The strength of this relationship varied at different points of time in the history of medical psychology. As Moore[2] said "the relationship between psychiatry and medicine has been a long and stormy courtship, with many broken engagements, an occasional annulment and sometimes outright divorce."

In 1818, Heinroth[13] coined the word psychosomatic disorder for insomnia. The use of this term spread to involve those disorders in which emotional and somatic activities influence each other to a significant level. With the influence of persuasive authors like Groddeck, Gama, Dunbar,[14] Ferenczi[14] and Wolff,[15] the concept of psychosomatic disorders gained ground. Franz Alexander's[16] specificity hypothesis and recognition of the seven 'classical' psychosomatic disorders (namely bronchial asthma, ulcerative colitis, peptic ulcer, neurodermatitis, thyrotoxicosis, rheumatoid arthritis and essential hypertension) was readily accepted by the medical profession. Thus, psychosomatics flourished from the 1930s to 1960s and gave an added impetus to the development of consultation-liaison psychiatry.

Two other factors helped strengthen the already growing field of consultation-liaison psychiatry. One was the development of effective methods of treatment, mainly pharmacological, in the 1950s. This enabled the psychiatrists to interact with the physicians more freely in a language that they could understand. Another important factor was the movement of psychiatry departments from the mental hospitals/asylums to the general hospital setting in the 1930s to 1960s. Availability of a consultant psychiatrist in the close vicinity of medical units resulted in more referrals being sent to the psychiatrists. Ever since the development of the close liaison between psychiatry and medicine, consultation-liaison psychiatry has not looked back.

The earliest inpatient ward for the mentally ill in a general hospital was probably opened by Rhazes[17] (865–925 AD), also known as Persian Galen, the physician-in-chief at the Baghdad Hospital. However, this was soon discontinued because of lack of any successful treatment and, the mentally ill were being kept in the asylums the world over. The first so called liaison-psychiatric service in this century was opened in 1902 at Albany Hospital, New York.[18] As early as 1929, Henry[19] suggested guidelines to the consultant psychiatrist who wished to work in collaboration with physicians. The suggestions, even six decades later, are still valid. He recommended that communication should be straightforward and free of jargon, and laid emphasis on careful observation rather than inspired guess-work. He advised flexibility in the application of the theory and the choice of treatment used. By 1987, there were about 850 liaison-psychiatry services in USA alone.[18] Consultation-liaison psychiatry has now become an essential part of medical student training in Europe and America.[20]

In India, the interplay of mind and body is known since antiquity. An ancient Indian medical text, Sushruta Samhita[21] describes a type of insanity borne out of grief, *Shokaja*, which '..... occurs in a person who is frightened by a thief, a king's officer, or his own enemy; or due to the loss of wealth; or bereavement; or disappointment in love....' Another text[22] describes four types of insanity which manifest when mind is afflicted '.... by passion, anger, greed, excitement, fear, attachment, exertion, anxiety or grief' and also caused by 'fierceful battles, destruction of countries, communities and towns....'

As world over, mentally ill were kept in lunatic asylums in India. Till 1905, all lunatic asylums were under the additional charge of the Civil Surgeon. Since then, a new provision was made to keep the mentally ill under the care of an alienist (as psychiatrists were then called). This was the first time that psychiatry was recognized as a specialty in India.[23] Considering this, it is surprising that within 30 years, consultation-liaison psychiatry took its birth in India. In 1933, Dr Girindra Sekhar Bose (1886–1959) opened a psychiatric unit in a general hospital (RG Kar Medical College, Kolkata) for the first time in India.[24] This was followed by the opening of more psychiatric units in general hospital setting in other parts of the country, for example, at JJ Hospital, Mumbai by Dr KK Masani (1938); at Medical College, Kolkata (1939); at KEM College, Bombay by Dr NS Vahia (1947).[23]

By 1982, there were 83 departments of psychiatry in 106 medical colleges in India. In addition, psychiatric units were opening in various general hospitals run by industries (e.g. Bokaro, Baroda, Rourkela etc.), Railways, Army Command (Lucknow, Mumbai, Delhi and Kolkata) and at district level.[23] There was no provision under the Indian Lunacy Act[25] for opening of inpatient wards for the mentally ill in general hospitals. This has been rectified in the new Mental Health Act.[26]

Initially, the medical professionals had reacted adversely to the entry of mental hospital patients in general hospitals,[27] but soon they reconciled with the fact as this change did not cause significant interference in their teaching and research programs, and in fact accorded them the benefit of consulting a psychiatrist for their own difficult patients. It was recognized that there were significant number of cases of organic brain syndromes, psychological overlays on existing medical illnesses[28] and troublesome neurotics in the medical and surgical out-patient and inpatient departments.

It is speculated[29] that the birth of general hospital psychiatry in India was due to the lack of sufficient funds to open more lunatic asylums. These new units needed mobilization of very few resources like a little space in an already functioning hospital and a few mental health professionals to manage the mentally ill. What started as probably an economic necessity has now become a major force in the delivery of mental health care.

The consultation-liaison psychiatry, as it exists today, is not tied to any one philosophy or theoretical viewpoint. Instead, its approach is eclectic, combining the practical application of all psychiatric knowledge, techniques and ideas, the central aim being the care and understanding of patients, the education of the consultee and a better delivery of health care.

BASIC CONCEPTS

Consultation psychiatry has been defined[30] as "an area of clinical psychiatry which includes diagnostic, therapeutic, teaching and research activities of psychiatrists in the non-psychiatric parts of the general hospital". This definition was later modified[31] to include settings other than the hospital, such as nursing homes, doctors' offices, and community health centers.

Consultation-liaison psychiatry is different from the other types of consultation performed by psychiatrists, e.g. in schools, business, court, industry and sports. Such consultation rarely includes a liaison function, and the purpose, techniques and problems are different from those encountered in the medical settings. The medical consultation involves:[32,33]

- Operation in the context of health care delivery, both administratively and conceptually
- Adherence to the psychosomatic approach, an approach that proposes that human health and disease result from an interaction of biological, psychological and social factors,[34] and
- A focus on people whose psychiatric problems are related to physical illness and disability, or who communicate their distress in terms of somatic symptoms.

A consultant is defined[35] in traditional medicine and psychiatry as an advisor to the treating physician on matters of diagnosis, treatment, rehabilitation and similar issues.

Ordinarily the consultant is a specialist whose expert advice is sought by the attending physician or sometimes by the patient. He may or may not see the patient but usually does not take actual charge of the case. Instead, he advises the physician-in-charge, although his advice is *patient-oriented.*

Another type of consultation is *colleague-oriented.*[35] Here the consultant advises, counsels or educates his medical colleagues about a particular area of his expertise. Although the management problems of a specific patient may be addressed to in the course of consultation, the primary focus of the consultation is not a particular patient but the other physician(s).

A third type of consultation is *agency-oriented.* Here the consultant advises, counsels or educates an entire organization of agency under focus.

Thus, consultation psychiatry may refer to any of the above-mentioned types of consultation performed by a psychiatrist. Often, however, it is limited to the activity of the psychiatrist (diagnostic, research, teaching) in the non-psychiatric parts of a general hospital. When used in this sense, it is synonymous with liaison psychiatry.[35]

New Webster's[36] defines liaison (psychiatry) as the connection or cooperative relationship between divisions (psychiatry and other medical specialties) of any organization (general hospital) to ensure concerted action (patient care, education and research). Consultation-liaison psychiatry differs from other branches of psychiatry in the type of patients seen, the milieu in which the psychiatrist functions and the need to work cooperatively with nonpsychiatrist physicians.

The liaison psychiatrist has been compared[37] to a fire inspector while the consultant psychiatrist has been likened to a fire fighter. The liaison psychiatrist tries to prevent damage by pointing out the conditions that can cause fire. The psychiatric consultant is called after the fire has started, when preventive measures have not been applied, have failed or are not available. The consultant psychiatrist focuses on the direct assessment and treatment of patients and families, the liaison psychiatrist focuses on the educational activities directed to the medical team on the psychosocial aspects of medical care.[38] However, the distinction is far from clear. At many times, the one has to function as the other (Table 1).

McKegney[39,40] describes the following four stages in the chronological development of consultation-liaison psychiatry in any health-care system.

1. *No consultation and no liaison*: Here the patient is under the care of general health care system. The psychiatrist is present in the system but there is no interaction, or there is no psychiatrist in the system.
2. *Consultation but no liaison*: Predominantly referral system established for patient care. Minimal education and research.
3. *Consultation and liaison*: Progressively intense liaison teaching activities built on the already growing base of consultations.
4. *Liaison but no consultation*: This is an utopian phase, one of purely liaison psychiatry. Here the psychiatrist does not have patient contact, but works in collaboration with the nonpsychiatrist treatment team.

The primary objective of liaison teaching work is to broaden the medical professionals' expertise in psycho-biosocial spheres, to enable them finally to manage their patients on their own with little teaching help from liaison psychiatrists.

As Strain[41] said "liaison psychiatry is a pedagogic pursuit that attempts to teach medical caretakers... about core issues in medical psychology... with the expectation that in time... other health care workers will provide most of the psychological care for the patients themselves."

REASONS OF CONSULTATION

Lipowski[30,33] gave a general classification for the types of diagnostic situations the consultant-liaison psychiatrist may encounter. These conditions are:

- Psychological presentation of an organic disease, with anxiety or depression possibly masking the underlying disease.
- Psychological complications of an organic disease, for example, delirium as a result of drug withdrawal, alcoholism, open-heart surgery or eye surgery.
- Psychological reaction to an organic disease.
- Psychological results of stress, such as unpleasant affect (anxiety, guilt, hopelessness); pathological affective stages that are long lasting or excessively intense; the use of ego mechanisms of defense against unpleasant affect; the inadequate evaluation and avoidance of

Table 1: Consultation versus liaison psychiatrist

		Consultant psychiatrist	*Liaison psychiatrist*
1.	Site of work	Usually psychiatric unit of a general hospital	A member of nonpsychiatric treatment team (usually high-risk units like ICU, CCU, etc.)
2.	Mode of contact	Usually a referral or a phone call	Meets regularly with the team of physicians. Attends ward rounds and sees patients regularly
3.	Patients seen	Only referred patients	Makes a suggestion about treatment of all patients under the care of nonpsychiatric treatment team. Even when the need of intervention is not apparent to the rest of the team, he can make recommendations
4.	Type of patients seen	Usually violent, disturbing or difficult patients	Usually less disturbing and disturbed than those seen by a consultant psychiatrist
5.	Primary stress	On treatment of acute cases	On prevention and early treatment
6.	Education of health professionals	Occasional	Regular
7.	Nature of advice	Cannot order. Can only make suggestions	Cannot order. Can only make suggestions

external stresses as a possible consequence of defense mechanisms; harmful somatic effects of the psychological concomitants of dysphoric affect which may, for example, bring on anginal pain; and the positive feedback effects of the resulting psychopathology on the original stress.
- Somatic presentation of psychiatric disorders, for example, insomnia, pain, headache and palpitations that may mask depression.
- Psychosomatic disorders, which are actually a fraction of all cases and which Lipowski called a 'misnomer with a vague meaning.'

A much simpler classification of diagnostic situations for consultation-liaison psychiatrists is as follows:
- Organic mental disorders and organic brain syndromes
- Primary psychiatric disorders (mistaken/masked by a medical disorder or symptom)
- Psychological factors affecting physical conditions (including psychosomatic disorders)
- Psychological reaction to medical illnesses/procedures
- Primary psychiatric disorder but antecedent medical illness necessitating admission in medical units.

The first 4 types of this classification include all the 6 types of Lipowski's classification. The fifth type was missing in Lipowski's classification.

The common reasons for referral are:[18,30]
- Suicidal hint, threat, ideation, gesture or attempt
- Diagnostic uncertainty (when there seems no plausible reason for patient's symptoms—either their presence, their persistence or their severity—despite medical/ surgical investigations or treatment)
- Grossly abnormal behavior disturbing the ordered harmony of the ward
- Demanding, hostile, manipulative, difficult patients, or refusal to cooperate or emotionally involved physicians, leading to staff-patient conflict
- Patient seems to have a psychiatric disorder or has a history of one (even though presently there are no problems related to it)
- Psychiatric emergencies (e.g. stupor, catatonia)
- Psychiatric side effects of drugs
- Patient has nowhere to go or does not seem competent to manage on his own
- Patient has asked to see a psychiatrist
- Disposition (convalescence, rehabilitation, continued psychiatric treatment)
- Presence of substance abuse or dependence.

Although the diagnostic categories for which consultation can be sought are far more than those that can be listed, the above categories account for more than two-thirds of all the consultations.

The scope of liaison psychiatry, of course, is much wider and goes beyond the realm of diagnostic categories. Whenever faced with a problem patient (problem for diagnosis or management), the treating physician or surgeon usually consults other physicians (usually specialists/ senior physicians). This tradition is age-old. Although it is well known that medical/surgical patients have a high prevalence of psychosocial problems, psychiatrists are called in much less often for consultation than are other medical or surgical consultants. Even among the various branches of medicine, there is a disparity in the referral rate for psychiatric consultation that does not correlate with independently assessed prevalence of psychiatric morbidity in the various branches.

Various factors have been identified which influence the referral rate. These are:
- Attitude of physicians towards psychiatry and psychiatrists.[40,42]
- Knowledge and awareness of psychiatry by the physician.[40,42]
- Quality of consultation-liaison provided by the psychiatrist.
- Physicians' feeling that psychiatrists have very little to offer for practical management of patients.[40]

  As Nandi said, "knowledge of psychosomatic illness will make no difference in the treatment and unless the psychiatrist.... proves that he would be more successful than the general practitioner for such cases, he will not be consulted".

  Many nonpsychiatrist physicians react differentially to psychiatric patients. According to one study[43] questioning 50 nonpsychiatric physicians about their attitudes to 'psychiatric patients', more than two-thirds showed a different response to these patients when compared 'to other patients'. About 38% of the physicians wanted to avoid them and the rest responded with negative feelings to the apparent threats caused by anxiety, seemingly produced by either rejecting the patient or because of strong empathy caused by the affliction.

  Like many members of the general public, many doctors feel something less than enthusiasm for those patients whose complaints have no apparent physical basis. It is known that only a minority of general practitioners has an active interest in psychiatry. Tolerant indifference, rather than active aversion, is the most usual attitude towards psychiatric patients.[44] These emotions (which include ambivalence, overt or covert hostility, apart from tolerant indifference) of the physicians are often expressed in a joking manner. One of the major tasks of the consultant psychiatrist is to influence their non-psychiatric physician colleagues' attitudes sufficiently to increase effective referrals for psychiatric consultation-liaison.[40] Each referral is an opportunity to modify such negative attitudes.[45]
- Relationship of individual physician with the consultation-liaison psychiatrist.
- Presence of psychiatrist's consulting chamber in close vicinity of the medicine unit.

  Most psychiatrists have limited contact with other physicians and are frequently much less available than

consultants in other specialities.[40] Increased availability of psychiatrists by opening of consultation liaison services can help greatly in the care, of those patients with psychological problems who are admitted in the medical or surgical units of the general hospital.
- Decision to refer is influenced less by the presence or severity of the psychopathology than by such factors as noncompliance, unexplained somatic complaints or disturbing behavior on the part of patients.
- Patient bias against being seen by a psychiatrist plays a role, but may be less of a factor than the consultee factors.
- Physicians consult psychiatrists more often than do surgeons. Many reasons have been given to explain this phenomenon:
  - Physicians are more concerned with the conditions in which psychological factors are important.[46]
  - Physicians have a broader, more psychosomatic approach and have a better orientation to psychiatry than other-nonpsychiatric specialists.[28,47]
  - Surgeons have an increased tolerance to psychiatric symptoms and refer patients only on account of 'major' symptoms or disruptive behavior,[46] probably because they are repeatedly exposed to agitated patients in the postoperative period and thus become used to them.
  - Patients suffering from psychiatric disorders with predominantly bodily symptoms are more likely to get admitted in medical units of the hospital.[28] Chronic organic brain syndrome patients are also more often admitted in the medical units.[28]
  - Surgeons' attention is more closely focused down into specific organs, at a time when the patient is also in the same state of mind.
  - Surgical patients remain in the hospital only half the time as compared to the medical patients, and hence less time is available for psychological symptoms to develop or to be observed, once developed.[46]
  - Surgeons are not only less oriented to psychiatry but are also positively hostile to this discipline.[47]
  - In some hospitals, surgeons consult physicians to decide whether a psychiatric consultation is needed.
- Very few referral requests are received from obstetrics and gynecology units. Although the psychiatric morbidity in obstetrics and gynecology unit patients is relatively high, the low rate of consultation requests is surprising.[28,48] Attempts have been made to explain away this fact on the basis of the gynecologists' acceptance of psychological disturbance, in relation to menstruation, pregnancy and menopause, as often normal.

ROLES OF A CONSULTATION-LIAISON PSYCHIATRIST

The consultation-liaison psychiatrist often performs several of the below-mentioned roles:
- Recognition of the nature of psychosocial problem which is the reason for consultation.
- Complete physical (especially neurological) examination of the patient in the light of psychiatric symptoms (even if the consultee has done it already).
- Assessment of the patient's personality and current psychological state to predict his likely response to medical/surgical investigations/treatment procedures.
- Assessment of any coexisting or new psychiatric disorder.
- Management of psychiatric emergencies (especially suicide).
- Prompt detection of organic brain syndromes and search for underlying etiologies.
- Psychopharmacological, behavioral and psychotherapeutic interventions, where ever appropriate.
- Follow-up on a regular basis.
- Close collaboration with the medical colleagues in evaluation and treatment of the referred patients.
- Education of the nonpsychiatric treatment team about psychiatric symptoms, diagnosis, management techniques, implications of doctor-patient relationships and the patient environment.
- Addressing the staff issues of team development and maintenance, as a liaison psychiatrist. Also addressing the system problems.[40]
- Education of the patients, their relatives, and the nursing and paramedical staff in principles of caring for the patient as a whole rather than treating a disease.[18]
- Research activities relating specifically to psychosocial and psychiatric aspects of medical and surgical specialties,[18] and relating to staff-attitudes and care-giving skills.[40]
- Prevention of dehumanization and depersonalization of medical care.[43]

Glickman[37] said that a consultation-liaison psychiatrist must function at times as an internist, a neurologist, a social worker, a legal expert, a patient advocate, a medicator, a negotiator, a psychopharmacologist and a supportive psychotherapist.

So, the roles a psychiatrist can play in this setting are many and varied, and depend on the degree of liaison developed with the nonpsychiatric treatment team. The greater are the benefits perceived by the team, the greater is the role a consultation-liaison psychiatrist would be asked to play in the health-care delivery system.

ASSESSMENT AND FORMULATION

Every consultation is preceded by a request for consultation by the consultee, who is usually the treating physician/surgeon. Most often the request is made in writing. Certain minimum information is a must in every consultation request or referral form. This includes:
- Name of the patient
- Age

- Sex
- CR no. (Medical record no.)
- Ward no.
- Bed no.
- Date and time of request
- Date of admission
- Consultee's name, designation and unit
- Provisional diagnosis (Primary medical or surgical diagnosis)
- Procedures performed (If any)
- Urgency
- Patient ambulatory or nonambulatory
- Short history
- Reasons for consultation
- Specific goals expected
- Patient and relatives informed about psychiatric consultation
- Signature of consultee.

On receipt of the consultation request, the consultant is obliged to see the patient at the earliest possible. Urgent requests/emergencies should be seen within one to two hours while routine consultations can be seen within one working day. Any unexplained delay can erode the confidence of the consultee in the consultant and can be detrimental to the welfare of the concerned patient.

Routine consultations for ambulatory patients can be seen in the psychiatric clinic itself but a vast majority of referred patients are either nonambulatory or unwilling to visit a psychiatric clinic. Many of these are urgent, emergency referrals. Such patients are best seen at their bedside by a visit to the ward.

Any psychiatric consultation has the following steps:

- Receipt of a consultation-request
- Assessment
- Formulation of diagnosis and treatment plan
- Consultation notes for the treatment-team
- Follow-up visits.

Before assessing the patient, the consultant should read the consultation-request carefully and discuss the case and its problems with the physician/surgeon in-charge. Under ideal conditions, the patient is seen in the presence of his physician[37] as this helps in convincing the latter of the psychiatrist's recommendations, but it is seldom practicable. The consultant should go through the patient's case-file including investigations, temperature, intake/output and weight records, and treatment sheet, in detail. Thus, before approaching the patient, the consultant should be aware of the patient's physical status and the treating team's perception of patient's illness and his behavior in the ward.

The assessment begins with eliciting of the patient's current and past history—both medical and psychiatric. The starting point is usually the patient's presenting complaints before admission or the consultee's current presenting complaint (the reason for consultation). The data is collected from various sources, including the patient, relatives, nursing staff, and treating team and the consultee.

A consultant (or liaison) psychiatrist should always perform a general physical examination, and especially a brief neurological examination. Although the visiting psychiatrist often does not wish to repeat the examination already done by the consultee, it is a mistake not to do so. Many a times relevant clinical findings are missed[49,50] by the treating team either because the patient is 'disturbed', violent or anger-provoking, or because of the belief that once a patient has been labelled as 'psychiatric' by the team, he or she can have no possible physical illness. At other times, new findings have emerged since the team last examined the patient.

The mental status examination is usually ignored. Although the consultant examines the mental status in accordance with his learned pattern, it is often missing from the written record. Its skillful documentation underscores the necessity of mental status examination as a component of a medical work-up.[51] It helps to remove the myth that psychiatrists diagnose cases on their intuition, rather than on signs and symptoms. It not only demonstrates to the consultee that the diagnosis in psychiatry too is syndromal but that the serial mental status examination can chart a patient's progress towards improvement.[37]

Cognitive functions should be examined in every patient referred for consultation. A brief scale like Folstein's mini mental state[52] is usually helpful in a standardized assessment.

The 'written psychiatric consultation' is an official doctor-to-doctor communication, which is the distillation of consultant's assessment of the patient, outlines his suggested treatment plan and answers the questions asked by the consultee about patient's diagnosis and care. It is one universal element of the consultation process.[54]

Often, the consultation notes are written on a separate, printed (and usually, differently colored) consultation form. Even then, it is often difficult for the consultee to trace the consultation notes in a plethora of case notes, progress notes, nurses' notes, investigation reports and other nonpsychiatric consultation notes in the case file. This is circumvented if consultation notes are properly titled[53] as 'Psychiatry referral', 'Psychiatry consultation', 'Psychiatry notes', or 'Psychiatry opinion'. Repeat consultations should be titled 'Psychiatry review', 'Psychiatry work-up' or 'Psychiatry follow-up'.

Next to the title, consultant's designation, date, and time of examination should be recorded. The informants and their reliability should be indicated, next. This should be followed by the presenting complaints, the history of present and past medical and psychiatric illnesses, general physical examination, mental status examination, diagnostic formulation and recommendations made.

There is a difference in opinion on whether the consultant psychiatrist should use technical psychiatric language, or not.[37,54-58] Dean[59] went to the extent of saying that "a psychiatric report... should be completely free from professional jargon... (written) in ordinary language... keeping to a description of the facts and having in mind the subject-person (consultee) as the ultimate reader." Such simplistic views lead to nonmedical impressions regarding psychiatry as a subject, and take for granted the resistance of the consultee in learning psychiatry as a discipline of medicine. This is self-defeating, as one of the major goals of consultation-liaison psychiatry is the education of nonpsychiatric consultees enabling them to understand, diagnose and manage psychiatric problems occurring in medical practice.

The consultant psychiatrist should 'strike a balance between oversimplification and technical obfuscation.'[59] The amount of technical language used should depend on the knowledge of psychiatric jargon by the consultees, potential and opportunity for education, need for diagnostic vis-a-vis descriptive accuracy, tendency to perceive psychiatric diagnoses as pejorative, urgency of clinical situation, and the degree of rapport between the consultant and consultee. "In general, as in all writing, the aim is to be as clear, direct and concise, as possible."[53]

Another important issue is 'how much to write'. The views again vary from one page[58] to six pages,[37] as the optimum. Although detailed history taking and examination is central to a patient's care, an extensively written consultation is perceived by the consultee as superfluous. The consultee, instead of reading the whole notes, will just scan through them before reading the recommendations. Anyway, the 'Recommendations', 'Advice' or 'Treatment plan' is often the first and many times the only part that a consultee consults practically. It is here, he expects to find the solution to his current problem in diagnosing and/or treating the particular patient. He expects to be provided with clear and detailed guidelines in further management, which are practical and not merely theoretical.

The recommendations usually include more than one of the following:

- *Investigations*: Laboratory tests for diagnosis of abnormalities that are primary, contributory, secondary or associated.
- Eliciting more history from more reliable informant or old medical records.
- Psychological testing by clinical psychologists.
- Consultation request to other nonpsychiatric consultants.
- Modification/alteration in consultee's management including change of drugs and drug dosages.
- Management by the consultee using pharmacological, psychotherapeutic, social or situational methods.
- Transfer to inpatient psychiatry unit or involuntary institutionalization.
- Psychotropic medication.
- Psychotherapy—short term/behavioral therapy/abreaction.
- Electroconvulsive therapy.

All recommendations made should be definite and specific. For example, if psychotropic medication is suggested, specific detailed regimen should be written, along with expected therapeutic and side effects. The treatment plan should not oblige the consultee to make decisions about drug dosage and/or duration of therapy.

Lastly, most of the patients should be followed-up by repeat visits, whether or not the consultee has asked for them. During follow-up, it should be determined whether the recommendations were followed. How is the patient's progress and what treatment he requires now? A follow-up is central to patient-care and is a characteristic of good consultation-liaison service. It also provides the consultant with more cooperation and support from the treatment team during future consultations and establishes a rapport between the consultee and the consultant.

The commonly encountered conditions in consultation liaison setting are discussed in the chapters on psychiatric aspects of medical disorders and psychosomatic disorders.

Why Guidelines for Consultation-Liaison Psychiatry?

For hundreds of years, physicians have been aware that psychiatric factors increase the risk for the development and outcomes of physical disorders. Scientific confirmation of these clinical intuitions has been rapidly accumulating. At the basic science level, the field of psychoimmunology has documented that stress and depression can impair immunocompetency.[60] Psychocardiology research suggests that type A behavior, when associated with hostility, imparts higher risk for the development of cardiovascular disease;[61] that ventricular arrhythmias and myocardial ischemia can be induced by stress;[62] and that major depression is associated with exaggerated platelet reactivity, which can increase the chance of ischemic events in patients prone to cardiac and cerebrovascular disease.[63] Clinical research has not only revealed relatively high rates of psychiatric illness in most medical illnesses, but also that the presence of major depression negatively affects the outcome of some illnesses such as myocardial infarction.[64] Furthermore, patients with poststroke depression have a poorer prognosis and lower rates of functional recovery than patients who do are not depressed.[65,66]

Recent reviews have examined the literature on the epidemiology of psychiatric disorders in primary care, the impact of psychological factors on the onset and course of medical illness, intervention studies, and the impact of psychiatric education and training of primary care physicians.[67-70] Research by Wells et al. has documented at length the increased costs associated with comorbid medical–psychiatric illness, the negative impact of psychiatric illness on the functioning of medical patients, and the generally poor quality of psychiatric care in the primary care setting.[71]

In well-conducted studies of patients in health care delivery systems, it has been documented that patients with depression incur twice the costs of nondepressed patients and that the costs associated with management of the depression are only a fraction of these increased expenditures.[72] Even when depression, anxiety, and somatization disorders are recognized by primary care physicians—which occurs in only about 50% of the cases—such recognition does not guarantee appropriate treatment.[73] Involvement of a consulting psychiatrist appears to be critical in improving depressed patient outcomes in the primary care setting. Katon et al. has developed models for co-management between family physicians and psychiatrists as well as educational and training models that have been proven to improve medication compliance and clinical outcomes, compared with "routine" or "usual" care by primary care physicians. In similar efforts, Smith et al. developed models of psychiatric consultation in the identification and management of patients with somatization disorders, with improved patient outcomes and dramatic reductions in medical utilization.[74]

Interventions in hospitalized patients are also effective. Both depression and delirium are associated with increased hospital lengths of stay. Elderly patients with hip fractures who are psychiatrically screened and assessed have a shortened length of stay and have increased rates of home versus institutional placement than hip-fracture patients who do not receive psychiatric intervention.[75] Thus, both clinical quality as well as economic value are improved by psychiatric interventions in many medical–surgical disorders with comorbid psychiatric disorders.

The aforementioned data clearly document that psychological factors affect the development and outcome of comorbid disease states. Furthermore, the high rate of psychiatric illness that exists in both ambulatory, hospital, and long-term care settings is poorly recognized and managed.[76] This situation causes increased financial costs and emotional pain, which often can be decreased by behavioral interventions.

Given that health care delivery systems will continue to discourage specialty referrals such as psychiatry, we need to teach primary care residents and physicians the basic aspects of diagnosis and treatment exists, as well as, actively involve a consulting psychiatrist for more difficult patients. As psychologists, social workers, and nurses will be used for screening and psychotherapy because of lower costs, these individuals need and frequently request similar education in psychiatric diagnosis and psychopharmacology, as do nonpsychiatric physicians.

Because of such cost factors, the psychiatrist has evolved as an expert diagnostician, psychopharmacologic expert, systems coordinator, and consultant/supervisor for complex patients. With a medical heritage and psychiatric expertise, the psychiatric physician is mandatory for any mental health team within a medical setting. It is essential that the psychiatrist be part of such teams.

The Academy of Psychosomatic Medicine, the society for psychiatrists working at the interface between medicine and psychiatry, has developed standards for the training of psychiatric residents in consultation-liaison psychiatry as well as established standards and an accreditation process for fellowship training in the subspecialty.[76] This organization formally examines and certifies fellowship programs in consultation-liaison psychiatry. In "The Academy of Psychosomatic Medicine Practice Guidelines: Psychiatric Consultation in the General Medical Setting," Harold Bronheim, MD, and associates have comprehensively documented the integrated basis for psychiatric consultation and liaison in medical care.

Through these guidelines, the Academy documents the need for expert consultation in the general medical setting; outlines the knowledge base and clinical skills necessary to render quality care; and sets the basic standards for the diagnostic evaluation, psychotherapeutic, and pharmacologic treatment of this patient population.

Why are guidelines necessary?[77] The primary reason is to ensure that patients with psychiatric illness in medical–surgical settings receive the highest possible quality of care. Thus, the guidelines specify the special training, knowledge, and skills required to provide psychiatric consultation for medical patients and their physicians and delineate the appropriate areas of clinical expertise in this process for mental health professionals. Special emphasis is placed on fundamental components of psychiatric assessment (history taking; physical, neurological, and mental states examination; laboratory and neuroradiographic tests) as well as the process of consultation systems analysis. Treatment issues receive special attention as well and emphasize treatment intervention based on a biopsychosocial model. Hence, the intervention recommended should be based on a knowledgeable assessment of the biological/medical aspects of the patient, which may require additional medical testing, change, or adjustment of medications used to treat the patient's medical disorder, as well as specialized psychopharmacology for the medical patient. Special issues in psychotherapy for the medically ill are noted, taking into consideration the need for pragmatic, often shorter, forms of dynamic and cognitively based interventions to address the impact of acute and chronic illness on the patient's emotional equilibrium. The importance of family and social assessment and intervention in the treatment plan is also outlined. The third part of the guidelines discuss special issues such as supervision standards, ethical standards, research issues, and special considerations for medically ill children and adolescents.

These guidelines are not meant as a mandatory set of imposed standards that the psychiatrist must follow. Guidelines are meant to assist the physician in treating the patient; the uniqueness and necessities of each individual clinical situation is paramount. Ideally, guidelines should be based on well-developed scientific evidence such as controlled clinical studies. Because medicine is a continuously evolving field, guidelines by their nature are a hybrid construction from evidence based on scientific investigation and evidence based on consensus opinions from clinicians. The Institute of Medicine has outlined the process of developing guidelines that incorporates these principles.[77] The present guidelines represent such a hybrid, which is based on an extensive examination of the available scientific evidence as well as the consensus opinion not only of the task force but also of the members of the Executive Council of the Academy.

As the primary goals of medicine are the prevention of disease and the promotion of the health and well-being of the patient, we hope these guidelines will help achieve these ends by ensuring excellence in the clinical care of patients with combined medical and psychiatric illness.

REFERENCES

1. Eaten JS Jr, Goldstein LS. Psychiatry in crisis. Am J Psychiatry. 1977;134:642-5.
2. Moore GL. The adult psychiatrist in the medical environment. Am J Psychiatry. 1978;15:13-6.
3. Fink PJ, Field HL. Residency training—a changing scenario. Psychiatric Opinion. 1978;135:413-9.
4. Hackett TP. The psychiatrist: in the mainstream or on the banks of medicine? Am J Psychiatry. 1977;134:432-4.
5. Pardes H. Future needs for psychiatrists and other mental health personnel. Arch Gen Psychiatry. 1979;36:1401-8.
6. Tucker GJ. The coming shortage in psychiatric manpower. Psychiatric Opinion. 1978;15:9-12.
7. Borus JF. Issues critical to the survival of community mental health. Am J Psychiatry. 1978;135:1029-35.
8. Engel GL. Is psychiatry failing in its responsibilities to medicine. Am J Psychiatry. 1972;128:1561-4.
9. Fink PJ, Weinstein SP. Whatever happened to psychiatry? The deprofessionalization of community mental health centres. Am J Psychiatry. 1979;136:406-9.
10. Freedman DX. The almamater is smoking—this is dangerous to your health! Arch Gen Psychiatry. 1976;33:407-10.
11. Von-Ammon Cavanaugh S. The prevalence of emotional and cognitive dysfunction in a general medical population. Gen Hosp Psychiatry. 1983;5:15-24.
12. Nabarro J. Unrecognized psychiatric illness in medical patients. Br Med J. 1984;284:635-6.
13. Heinroth JC. Lehrbuch der Stoerungen des Seelenlebensodor der Seelenstoerungen und ibrerBehandlung. Leipsic: Vogel; 1818.
14. Dunbar F. Emotions and Bodily Changes. New York: Columbia University Press; 1954.
15. Wolf S, Wolff HG. Human Gastric Function. New York: Oxford University Press; 1943.
16. Alexander F. Psychosomatic Medicine—Its Principles and Applications. New York: Norton; 1950.
17. Zilboorg GA. History of Medical Psychology. New York: Norton; 1941.
18. Gomez J. Liaison Psychiatry—Mental Health Problems in the General Hospital. London: Croom Helm; 1987.
19. Henry GW. Some modern aspects of psychiatry in general practice. Am J Psychiatry. 1929;86:481-99.
20. Lipowski ZJ. Psychosomatic Medicine: an overview. In: Hill O (Ed). Modern Trends in Psychosomatic Medicine. London: Butterworths. 1976;3:1-20.
21. ShastriKaviraj. Sushruta Samhita. Varanasi: Chowkhamba Sanskrit Sansthan; 1976.
22. Sharrna RK, Dash VB. Agnivesa's Charaka Samhita. Varanasi: Chowkhamba Sanskrit Sansthan; 1977.
23. Varma LP. History of Psychiatry in India. Continuing Medical Education Programme Booklet. Indian Psychiatric Society. 1982;1:1-14.
24. Sharma SD. History of mental hospitals in Indian subcontinent. Indian J Psychiatry. 1984;26:295-300.
25. Government of India. The Indian Lunacy Act. Act 4 of 1912; 1912.
26. Government of India. Mental Health Act. Act 14 of 1987; 1987.
27. Wig NN. General hospital psychiatric units—right time for evaluation. Indian J Psychiatry. 1978;20:1-9.
28. Wig NN, Shah DK. Psychiatric unit in a general hospital in India: pattern of inpatient referral. J Indian Med Assoc. 1973;60:83-6.
29. Khorana AB. Consultation-liaison Psychiatry. In: Continuing Medical Education Programme Booklet. Indian Psychiatric Society; 1983. pp.91-9.
30. Lipowski ZJ. Review of consultation psychiatry and psychosomatic medicine: I. General principles. Psychosom Med. 1967;29:153-71.
31. Lipowski ZJ. Consultation—liaison Psychiatry: Past, Present and Future. In: Pasnau RO (Ed). Consultation—Liaison Psychiatry. New York: Grune & Stratton; 1975. p.1.
32. Lipowski ZJ. Review of consultation—liaison psychiatry and psychosomatic medicine: III. Psychosom Med. 1968;30: 395-402.
33. Lipowski ZJ. Consultation—liaison psychiatry: An overview. Am J Psychiatry. 1974;131:623-30.
34. Engel GL. The clinical application of the biopsychosocial model. Am J Psychiatry. 1980;137:535-44.
35. Hinsie LE, Campbell PJ. Psychiatric Dictionary. 4th edition. New York: Oxford; 1970.
36. New Webster's Dictionary of the English Language. Delair. 1985, 549.
37. Glickman LS. Theory and Technique. In: Psychiatric Consultation in the General Hospital. New York: Marcel Dekker; 1980. pp.1-52.
38. Pasnau RO. Consultation-liaison psychiatry at the cross-roads: In search of a definition for the 1980's. Hosp Comm Psychiatry. 1982;33:989-95.
39. McKegney FP, Beckhardt RM. Evaluative research in consultation-liaison psychiatry. Gen Hosp Psychiatry. 1982;4: 197-202.

40. McKegney FP. Consultation-liaison psychiatry. In: Kaplan HI, Sadock BJ (Eds). Comprehensive Textbook of Psychiatry. 4th edition. Baltimore: Williams & Wilkins; 1985.
41. Strain JJ. Liaison psychiatry (letter). Am J Psychiatry. 1977;134: 1050-51.
42. Lipowski ZJ, Wolston AD. Liaison psychiatry: Referral patterns and their stability over time. Am J Psychiatry. 1981;138:1608-11.
43. Krakowski AJ. Doctor-doctor relationship—II: Conscious factors influencing the consultation process. Psychosom. 1972; 13:158-64.
44. Hill D. Psychiatry in Medicine. The Rock Gaarling Fellowship. The Nuffield Provincial Hospitals Trust; 1969.
45. Mayou R, Smith EBO. Hospital doctors' management of psychological problems. Br J Psychiatry. 1986;148:194-7.
46. Fleminger JJ, Mallett BL. Psychiatric referrals from medical and surgical wards. J Ment Sci. 1962;108:183-90.
47. Chatterjec SB, Kutty PR. A study of psychiatric referrals in military practice in India. Indian J Psychiatry. 1977;3:32-8.
48. Kenyon FE, Rutter ML. The psychiatrist and the general hospital. Compr Psychiatry. 1963;4:80-9.
49. Leeman C. Diagnostic errors in emergency room medicine: physical illness in patients labeled 'psychiatric' and vice versa. Int J Psychol Med. 1975;6:533.
50. Sarivay SM, Komn LM. Organic disease mistakenly diagnosed as psychiatric. Psychosom. 1977;18:6-11.
51. Langsley DG. The mental status examination. In: Usdin G, Lewis JM (Eds). Psychiatry in General Medical Practice. New York: McGraw-Hill; 1979.
52. Folstein M, Folstein S, Mellugh P. Mini Mental State: A practical method for grading the cognitive state of patients for the clinician. J Psychiatr Res. 1975;12:189-98.
53. Garrick TR, Stotland NL. How to write a psychiatric consultation. Am J Psychiatry. 1982;139:849-55.
54. Engel GL, Green WL Jr, Reichsman F, et al. A graduate and undergraduate teaching program on the psychological aspects of medicine. J Med Educ. 1957;32:859-70.
55. Krakowski AJ. Doctor-doctor relationship. III. A study of feelings influencing the vocation and its tasks. Psychosom. 1973;14:156-61.
56. Kaufman MR. The role of the psychiatrist in the general hospital. Psychiatr Q. 1953;27:367-81.
57. Strain JJ. Psychological Interventions in Medical Practice. New York: Appleton-Century-Crafts; 1978.
58. Schwab JJ. Handbook of Psychiatric Consultation. New York: Appicton-Century-Crofts; 1968.
59. Dean ES. Writing psychiatric reports. Am J Psychiatry. 1963; 119:759-62.
60. Ursin H. Stress, distress, and immunity. Ann NY Acad Sci. 1994; 741:204-11 [Medline]
61. Frasure-Smith N, Lesperance F, Talajic M. The impact of negative emotions on prognosis following myocardial infarction: is it more than depression? Health Psychol. 1995; 14:388-98.
62. Willich SN, MacLure M, Mittleman M, et al. Sudden cardiac death: support for a role of triggering in causation. Circulation. 1993; 87:1442–50 [Abstract]
63. Krantz DS, Kop WJ, Santiago HT, et al. Mental stress as a trigger of myocardial ischemia and infarction. Cardiol Clin. 1996; 14:271-87 [Medline]
64. Lesperance F, Frasure-Smith N, Talajic M. Major depression before and after myocardial infarction: its nature and consequences. Psychosom Med. 1996;58:99-110 [Medline]
65. Ng KC, Chan KL, Straughan PT. A study of poststroke depression in a rehabilitative center. Acta Psychiatr Scand. 1995;92:75-9 [Medline]
66. Robinson RG, Kubos KL, Starr LB. Mood disorder in stroke patients: importance of location of lesion. Brain. 1984;107: 81-93 [Abstract]
67. Schulberg HC, Magruder KM, deGruy F. Major depression in primary medical care practice. Research trends and future priorities. Gen Hosp Psychiatry. 1996;18:395-406 [Medline]
68. Noyes R Jr., Holt CS, Kathol RG. Somatization: diagnosis and management. Arch Fam Med. 1995;4:790–95 [Medline]
69. Peden JG Jr., Lichstein PR. Management strategies for depression in primary care. Am J Med. 1996;101(suppl): 18S-25S.
70. Wells KB, Stewart AL, Hays RD, et al. The functioning and well-being of depressed patients: results from the Medical Outcomes Study. JAMA. 1989;262:914-9 [Medline]
71. Katon W, Von Korff M, Lin E, et al. Collaborative management to achieve treatment guidelines. Impact on depression in primary care. JAMA. 1995;273:1026-31 [Medline]
72. Kirmayer LJ, Robbins JM. Patients who somatize in primary care: a longitudinal study of cognitive and social characteristics. Psychol Med. 1996;26:937-51 [Medline]
73. Smith GR Jr, Rost K, Kashner TM. A trial of the effect of a standardized psychiatric consultation on health outcomes and costs in somatizing patients. Arch Gen Psychiatry. 1995; 52:238-43 [Medline]
74. Levitan SJ, Kornfeld D. Clinical and cost benefits of liaison psychiatry. Am J Psychiatry. 1981;138:790-93 [Abstract]
75. Katon W, Schulberg HC. Epidemiology of depression in primary care. Gen Hosp Psychiatry. 1992;14:237-47 [Medline]
76. Gitlin DF, Schindler BA, Stern TA, et al. Recommended guidelines for consultation-liaison psychiatric training in psychiatry residency programs: a report from the Academy of Psychosomatic Medicine Task Force on Psychiatric Resident Training in Consultation-Liaison Psychiatry. Psychosomatics. 1996; 37:3-11 [Medline]
77. Woolf SH. Practice guidelines: a new reality in medicine. I. Recent developments. Arch Intern Med. 1990;150:1811-8 [Medline]

CHAPTER

33

Psychiatric Aspects of Medical Disorders

Adarsh Tripathi, Shaswat Saxena, (Late) JK Trivedi

INTRODUCTION

Psychiatric symptoms are commonly seen with various physical disorders.[1-10] Mind and body are inseparable.[11] Stress due to physical disorders predisposes to psychiatric symptoms and that due to physical disorders predisposes for various physical disorders. An immunological, biochemical and hormonal reaction to stress is probable explanation of this vicious circular relationship between physical and psychiatric symptoms.[12] Psychiatric problems associated with medical disorders can be classified as:

1. Psychiatric disorders due to general medical condition.
2. Psychiatric disorder comorbid with physical disorder (may be as a reaction to physical disorder).
3. Psychiatric problems arising following treatment of physical disorder, e.g. problems or symptoms arising as side-effects of medications being used in treatment of physical disorder.

Importance of simultaneous presence of physical and psychiatric disorders:

1. It leads to worse outcome of the medical disorder due to non-compliance poor self-care.
2. There is increased mortality with the comorbidity.
3. Simultaneous treatment of the disorders leads to increases chances of drug-drug interaction.

NOSOLOGY AND CLASSIFICATION

International classification of diseases (ICD-10) grouped a range of mental disorders on the basis of their common etiology in cerebral disease, cerebral injury or any other physical disease leading to cerebral dysfunction.

The term organic here reflects that conditions described elsewhere have not got any direct correlation of physical disorder or brain dysfunction with psychiatric symptoms. To diagnose such a case, one requires objective evidence (examination or investigations or typical history) regarding physical disorder with temporal correlation of relationship of psychiatric symptoms with physical disorders (either start of fresh symptoms or exacerbations) and significant improvement of the psychiatric symptom or disorder following improvement of presumed causative physical disorder (ICD-10 DCR).

ICD-10 Classifies other mental disorders due to brain damage and dysfunction and to physical disease as

F06.0 Organic hallucinosis
F06.1 Organic catatonic disorder
F06.2 Organic delusional (schizophrenia-like) disorder
F06.3 Organic mood (affective) disorder
.30 Organic manic disorder
.31 Organic bipolar disorder
.32 Organic depressive disorder
.33 Organic mixed affective disorder
F06.4 Organic anxiety disorder
F06.5 Organic dissociative disorder
F06.6 Organic emotionally labile (asthenic) disorder
F06.7 Mild cognitive disorder
.70 Not associated with a physical disorder
.71 Associated with a physical disorder
F06.8 Other specified mental disorders due to brain damage and dysfunction and to physical disease
F06.9 Unspecified mental disorder due to brain damage and dysfunction and to physical disease

Contrary to DSM-IV which classified the group as mental disorders due to general medical conditions, DSM-5 classifies such disorders as "disorders due to another medical condition" as subtype in each group of psychiatric disorders such as "anxiety disorder due to another medical condition" is classified under anxiety disorders.

There are differences in the nosology of delirium in ICD-10 and DSM-5. Delirium in ICD-10 is classified separately as F05 (delirium, not induced by alcohol and other psychoactive substances) and as subgroup of "Mental and behavioral disorder due to psychoactive substances use (F 10-19)" in withdrawal state (1 × 0.4) and acute intoxication with delirium (1 × 0.03). Whereas, DSM-5 classifies delirium under neurocognitive disorders and describes delirium due to another medical condition as a subtype of it with substance intoxication delirium, substance withdrawal delirium and medication induced delirium.

PSYCHIATRIC ASPECTS OF NEUROLOGICAL DISORDERS

Epilepsy

Psychiatric symptoms are common in patients with epilepsy. The prevalence of epilepsy in the general population is approximately 1% and about 30 to 50% of all epileptic patients have significant psychiatric problems.

Psychiatric symptoms due to epilepsy can be classified as those occurring during ictal, inter-ictal and post-ictal period

Symptoms

Ictal Phenomenon:

1. *Prodromal phase:* Affective symptoms, irritability, dysphoria, apathy and mental dullness are seen.
2. *Auras:* Aversive aura in frontal lobe seizure, paresthesia type aura in parietal lobe seizure, postural movements in seizure arising from medial surface of cerebral hemisphere,visual hallucinations in occipital lobe seizures are seen.
3. *Simple partial seizures:* Symptoms depend upon the focus of discharge and can occur with motor,sensory autonomic or psychic symptoms. Symptoms include focal motor activity,unformed hallucinations and automatism.
4. *Complex partial seizures:* Disturbances in consciousness, unresponsiveness, confusion, memory disturbance and memory impairment are seen. Panoramic memories, illusion of memory, jamais vu are also common.
5. *Absence seizures:* There is brief loss of consciousness when patient loses contact with environment.
6. *Generalized tonic-clonic seizures:* Can present as confusional state, psychotic state or prolonged twilight state.[13]

Postictal Phenomenon: There is forgetfulness for the period of seizure. Headache is common after seizure. Confusion is common postictally and some sort of automatism which may range from purposeless activity to outburst of anger or irritability.[13]

Interictal Phenomenon: Personality disturbances are commonly reported in patients of temporal lobe epilepsy. Changes in personality as viscosity, religiosity, heightened emotional experiences and change in sexual behavior are seen. *Viscosity,* described as over inclusiveness and overinvolved with minor details which are reflected in writing as hypergraphia, is typical finding. These patients are often slow and ponderous. The syndrome of personality disturbance and seizure is commonly known as "Geschwind syndrome".[14]

Alteration in sexual behavior as hyposexuality, hypersexuality and sexual deviations are seen. Hyposexuality has been found to be directly related with seizure activity.

Psychosis: schizophrenia like psychosis is seen in interictal period and is more frequent in temporal lobe epilepsy. It is seen in upto 10 to 30% of patients. Risk factors for psychosis in these patients are early onset of seizures, female gender, complex partial seizure and left sided lesion.

Mood disorders: depression, mania and bipolar disorder are less common than psychosis. These are more common in patients of temporal lobe with origin from non-dominant hemisphere. Suicide is more common among patients of epilepsy.

Parkinson's Disease

Non-motor symptoms in Parkinson's disease (PD): Depression, dementia, psychotic symptoms and impulse control disorders are common in parkinsonism and have major impact on quality of life of patients.[15] These psychiatric comorbidities largely remain unidentified and this often adds to the plight of the debilitate dpatients.[16]

Upto 40% of patients may suffer from depression in Parkinson's disease. It is most common psychiatric complication of PD.[17] It occurs mostly with symptoms of anxiety.[18] Risk of depression correlates with severity of Parkinson's disease and was seen significantly more in patients of Parkinson's with dementia than with Parkinson's disease alone. However, no correlation is seen with depression in PD with duration of illness or age of onset.[19] Depression may arise because of damage to serotonergic and dopaminergic transmissionin Parkinson's patients.[15] An elevated homocysteine levels have been found to be associated with depression and cognitive impairment in Parkinson's disease.[20]

Upto 30% of parkinsonian patients may suffer from psychosis. Visual hallucinations are more common in patients of PD presenting with psychosis. The most important reason behind the same appears to be anti-parkinsonian drugs. Depression and dementia appear to predispose to psychosis in these patients.[21]

Treatment

1. *Depression in Parkinsonism:* One should first exclude any organic cause of depression in PD (like hypothyroidism). Selective serotonin reuptake inhibitors (SSRI) are agent of choice in these patients as tricyclic anti-depressants are associated with increased anti-cholinergic side-effects. Augmentation with pramipexole has been found to be helpful in patients which are not responding to SSRI alone. Electroconvulsive therapy (ECT) is helpful in

patients which are not responding to standard drug regimen.

2. *Psychosis in Parkinsonism:* An organic causes like delirium needs to be ruled out first. Attempt should be made to manage the symptoms without medications by improving the orientation. Minor hallucinatory experiences which are non-impairing should better be avoided and patient should be helped to live with these experiences. A try thereafter can be given to withdraw dopaminergic drugs. Second generation anti-psychotics are preferred treatment for psychosis in these patients and clozapine has got highest efficacy in treating psychosis in Parkinson's disease.[22] ECT should be considered in all resistant cases.

Wilson's Disease

Wilson's disease (WD) is an autosomal recessive disorder of copper metabolism resulting from mutation in genes coding for ATP7B.[23] ATP7B is important for transportation of copper across membranes. The illness generally presents in pediatric and adolescent age group.[24] Psychiatric symptoms may be the presenting symptoms in Wilson's disease, preceding hepatic and neurological signs in upto 20% patients.[25] Upto two-third of the patients of Wilson's disease develop psychiatric symptoms sometime during their illness.[25] Depression, psychosis and cognitive impairment are three most common psychiatric symptoms of Wilson's disease.[16] Suicidal behavior is seen in upto 10% of the patients.[7] Other common feature in WD is personality change which manifests as irritability, impulsivity and emotionality.[26] Cognitive dysfunction is seen in less than quarter of WD patients and is mostly mild. Cognitive dysfunction increases with progress of the disease.[27]

Treatment of Wilson's disease per se, does improve various psychiatric symptoms in WD. Tetrathiomolybdate has been seen to be associated with improvement in both psychiatric and neurological symptoms.[28] D-penicillamine another drug used in WD, however, has been shown to worsen the psychiatric symptoms or precipitate psychiatric symptoms in previously asymptomatic WD patients.[29] There are some evidences of usefulness of atypical anti-psychotics like clozapine and olanzapine in WD.[30,31]

PSYCHIATRIC ASPECTS OF NUTRITIONAL DISORDERS

Psychiatric Aspects of Vitamin B1 Deficiency

Vitamin B1 (Thiamine) is water soluble vitamin required for formation of thiamine pyrophosphate which is essential for intermediary carbohydrate metabolism. Thiamine is also needed by cell membranes to maintain osmotic gradients and neurotransmitter synthesis. Thiamine deficiency may present as wet beriberi (neuropathy with high output congestive cardiac failure), dry beriberi (neuropathy), gastrointestinal beriberi (abdominal pain, vomiting and lactic acidosis),Wernicke's encephalopathy and Korsakoff's syndrome.[32] Thiamine deficiency can also present as psychosis or anxiety symptoms.[33]

Wernicke's Encephalopathy

Wernicke's encephalopathy (WE) described as classic triad of ocular symptoms, mental confusion, and cerebellar is most important neurological complication of thiamine deficiency. The most common cause of Wernicke's syndrome is chronic alcoholism. Cancer, bariatric surgery,[34] hyperemesis gravidarum,[35] starvation, malnutrition, gastrointestinal tract disease[32] and parental nutrition[36] are other important causes of WE. After bariatric surgery the risk of Wernicke's is long lasting though most cases are seen within 6 months of surgery.

The classic triad of Wernicke's is seen in limited number of patients (approx. 10%). The triad is more commonly seen in alcoholic Wernicke's encephalopathy. The symptoms of WE can be described under eight categories: dietary deficiencies (characterized by low body mass index, historically poor thiamine intake), eye signs (ophthalmoplegia, nystagmus and gaze palsy), cerebellar signs (ataxia, past pointing), seizures, frontal lobe dysfunction (difficulty in planning, abstract thinking), amnesia (memory loss), mild memory impairment and altered mental state (confusion, disorientation, impaired attention or coma). Among these broad categories cerebellar signs have got highest sensitivity and seizures have got lowest sensitivity to diagnose WE. The classic triad has got low sensitivity however an addition of dietary deficiency and mild memory impairment to the criteria greatly increase the sensitivity for diagnosis of WE

Neurological lesions in Wernicke's are seen as mammillary body atrophy, cerebellar vermal atrophy, ventricular dilatation and cerebral atrophy. Mammillary bodies are most commonly affected in the disease.[37]

Investigations

1. *Erythrocyte transketolase activity assay:* It is most commonly used to assess blood thiamine levels.
2. High performance liquid chromatography (for direct measurement of thiamine and its phosphate esters in human blood): HPLC is more accurate than erythrocyte transketolase for assessing thiamine levels.
3. *Magnetic resonance imaging (MRI):* Symmetrical lesions are seen in thalamus, mammillary bodies, tectal plate and periaqueductal area. Cytotoxic edema which was found to be reversible was most characteristic feature of WE. MRI findings are seen in approximately two-third of patients.[38] Cytotoxic edema in acute Wernicke's may be

seen as symmetric hypodensity in CT scan and signal intensity alteration in MRI. Thiamine deficiency causes disturbed osmotic gradient maintenance resulting in swelling in intra-extracellular spaces which than presents as edema, spongy degeneration, swelling of capillary endothelial cells and erythrocyte extravagation.[38]

Treatment

Intravenous thiamine (200 mg) three times a day should be administered before any carbohydrate in all patients of suspected or manifested WE. Glucose administration may precipitate WE.[39] A proper diet after then should be given to the patient immediately after injection. Treatment should be continued till there is improvement. It is worth mentioning, that dose required in alcoholics is higher as compared to non-alcoholics and chronic alcoholics may need upto 500 mg thrice a day to show proper improvement.

For people on hunger strike oral thiamine upto 600 mg with a tablespoon of sugar is likely to prevent WE.[10] Prophylactic thiamine injections are also recommended in patients undergoing bariatric surgery as they vomit oral medication.

Korsakoff's Syndrome

Korsakoff's syndrome (KS) is thiamine deficiency induced impairment in memory with relative preservation of other cognitive function.[40] The working memory is most commonly affected in Korsakoff's syndrome. The syndrome generally develops as a sequel to WE and presents when altered consciousness state (confusional state) of WE resolves.

Clinical Features

There is severe anterograde amnesia in KS and patient may not remember recent events or instructions given an hour back. Loss of memory of events that occurred before the onset of disorder is also disturbed. There is relative preservation of procedural memory and patient may perform complex motor tasks.[41]

Changes in mood or apathy may also be seen in the syndrome. Patient may confabulate to make up for memory deficit. However with time the confabulation decreases.[40]

Investigations

Magnetic resonance imaging shows degeneration in thalamic and mammilary body and frontal lobe atrophy.

Prevention

Early treatment of WE can prevent development of KS.

Treatment and Prognosis

Ophthalmoplegia starts improving within hours to weeks of starting therapy and cerebellar signs like nystagmus, ataxia start improving by a week in Wernicke's syndrome. However, residual symptoms of nystagmus and ataxia may be present in upto half of the patients.[42]

Korsakoff's syndrome has worse prognosis and more than two-third of patients are left with residual memory problems. There is a high mortality of upto 20% in Wernicke's–Korsakoff complex. The main reasons of collapse being pulmonary infection decompensated liver disease and irreversible thiamine deficiency.[4]

Psychiatric Aspects of Vitamin B12 Deficiency

Vitamin B12 is a water soluble vitamin, which is a cofactor for synthesis of neurotransmitters particularly dopamine and serotonin.[43] Vitamin B12 deficiency mostly arises because of failure of gastric mucosa to secrete intrinsic factor, which is required for its absorption from terminal intestine. It can present with variety of psychiatric symptoms as these neurotransmitters are involved in regulation of mood and sleep. Vitamin B12 deficiency generally presents with hematological (macrocytic megaloblasticanemia), neurological (peripheral neuropathy, myeloneuropathy, subacute combined degeneration of spinal cord, cerebellar ataxia or occasionally optic atrophy) and psychiatric [mood disorders, delusions, obsessive-compulsive disorder (OCD) or dementia]. Mostly the deficiency presents with a varying combination of symptoms like anemia, neurological and psychiatric symptoms. However in a few cases psychiatric symptoms precede hematological and neurological findings and are presenting symptoms.[44] Various case reports have reported dementia,[45] OCD,[43] organic psychosis,[46] mood disorder[47] as presenting feature of vitamin B12 deficiency in which symptoms improved dramatically after vitamin B12 therapy. However, it has been found that vitamin B12 may improve frontal and language function but may not improve dementia as such.[45] Cochrane review[48] also suggest that there is less evidence to support role of vitamin B12 for improvement of cognition in patients of dementia.

Measurement of serum vitamin B12 levels is essential to reach to a conclusive diagnosis and for assessment of clinical condition then-after. In most cases Intravenous vitamin B12 (1000 μg/day) for 7 days, than vitamin B12 (1000 μg) intramuscularly every week for 1 month and then maintenance intramuscular injections (1000 μg of vitamin B12) for a year are enough for replenishing Vitamin B12. Psychiatric symptoms start improving within a week of initiation of therapy. Neurological symptoms show improvement by 1 month of therapy.[49]

PSYCHIATRIC ASPECTS OF RENAL DISORDERS

Renal dysfunction and psychiatric problems:

1. *Renal dysfunction:* It is becoming increasingly common. The prevalence of renal diseases is increasing fast and is likely to bring it to the epidemic level globally.[1] End stage renal disease has been estimated at around 229 per million in Indian population.[5] End stage renal disease (ESRD) is described as GFR < 15 ml/min/1.73 m^2 and generally needs either transplantation or dialysis.
   Renal dysfunction has been described under five subgroups (K/DOQI guidelines):

Stage 1	GFR >90 mL/min/1.73 m^2 with other evidence of chronic renal failure
Stage 2	Mild impairment; GFR 60-89 ml/min/1.73 m^2 with other evidence of chronic renal failure
Stage 3	Moderate impairment, GFR 30-59 ml/min/1.73 m^2
Stage 4	Severe impairment GFR 15–29 ml/min/1.73 m^2
Stage 5	Established renal failure; GFR< 15 ml/min/1.73 m^2

2. *Psychiatric symptoms in patients of renal dysfunction:* Adjustment problems (anxiety, insomnia, irritability, low mood, etc.) and negative psychological reactions like denial, negative thoughts are extremely common in patients of ESRD. Perceived loss of body function, fear of impending death and perceived dependence on others and machines are most important psychological reactions in patients of dialysis.[50] If unattended these reactions are likely to result in major mood disorders. The most common psychiatric disorder in patients of renal failure is depression.[51] An early age of ESRD, female sex, more than 2 years of dialysis and previous history of depression has been associated with depression in this group of patient.[52] It was also found that low mood, worthlessness, excessive guilt and reduced interest have been found to be helpful in differentiating major depressive disorder from symptoms arising due to dialysis in these patients. Whereas fatigue, insomnia and loss of libido has not been found to be helpful in the dfferentiation.[52] Episodes of depression in ESRD patients are associated with poorer outcome because of poor compliance, nutrition, self-care and comorbidities.

   Other set of symptoms which are common in ESRD are cognitive dysfunctions. They can be subtle or may be part of delirium and uremic encephalopathy. Lower performance on IQ scores has been found to be in patients after dialysis as compared to IQ before dialysis.[53] Delirium may occur as a result of changes in electrolytes associated with ESRD or because of other metabolic changes. Uremic encephalopathy is associated with changes in psychomotor activity, restlessness, cognition, agitation and change in personality.[18]

   Moreover, patients of renal dysfunction may have comorbid psychiatric disorders as bipolar disorder, dementia, psychosis, OCD.

3. *Effect of renal dysfunction on drugs:* Renal dysfunction affects almost every aspect of drug metabolism. Renal dysfunction may be associated with impaired absorption (resulting from altered gastric pH due to uremia , change in gastrin levels and due to vomiting), alteration in distribution (increased extracellular fluid as in edema or decreased volume of distribution as in dehydration/cachexia), metabolism (severe renal dysfunction is generally associated with decreased hepatic metabolism) or excretion (drugs like lithium which are primarily excreted by kidney whereas there are others active metabolites of which are excreted by kidney).

   Not only there is pharmacokinetic effect but pharmacodynamic effect is also evident. It has been seen that there are more treatment emergent side-effects in ESRD patients either because of uremic toxins or due to increased drug translocation toward blood-brain barrier.[54]

4. *Management of psychiatric problems in renal dysfunction:* Psychiatric treatment should be offered to all the patients of renal dysfunction having symptoms suggestive depression, agitation, delirium or psychosis. Cognitive therapy can be offered for management of psychological problems in these patients. Patients who perceive greater fear of losing control of their vital organs are more likely to get more depressed. Cognitive behavior therapy helps in the way illness is perceived and thus is helpful in alleviating depressive symptoms.[55]

   While prescribing psychotropic in renal dysfunction one should consider route of metabolism of drug, anticholinergic effect of drug (it may lead to urinary retention), effect of drug on QT interval, drug-drug interactions and possible specific nephrotoxic effect of any drug. General principles while prescribing psychotropic include :

   1. Starting at a low dose and titrating gradually.
   2. Avoiding depot injections or drugs with longer duration of action.
   3. Choosing a drug which is safer in renal dysfunction.
   4. Choosing a drug with less drug-drug interaction, anti-cholinergic side-effects, less chances to prolong QTc prolongation.

   Use of anti-psychotics in renal dysfunction: Among anti-psychotics haloperidol, aripiprazole and ziprasidone are excreted less than 1% unchanged in urine. Haloperidol is preferred drug (2–6 mg/day) among first generation anti-psychotics. Lesser anticholinergic side effects with haloperidol also favor its use in these patients. Caution though needed for QT prolongation. Chlorpromazine should generally be avoided considering its anti-cholinergic, hypotensive and sedative effects. Sulpiride should be avoided as it is mostly excreted through kidney. Olanzapine, aripiprazole and ziprasidone may be used among second generation antipsychotics. However, experience of using olanzapine is more. Therefore, olanzapine (5 mg/day) is preferred over others. Amisulpiride should be avoided as it has renal excretion mostly. Both risperidone and paliperidone should be used with caution as there active metabolites are excreted through kidney. Clozapine should be used with caution as it may aggravate postural hypotension, diabetes, enuresis and retention. Plasma clearance of quetiapine is reduced and is associated with postural hypotension.[56]

Among mood stabilizers lithium is avoided considering its nephrotoxic effects and possibility to lower glomerular filtration rate. Valproate, carbamazepine and lamotrigine should be used at lower doses initially and then should be gradually increased, monitoring there side-effects. There are case reports of nephritis and tubular necrosis following valproate and carbamazepine.[56]

Among anti-depressants sertraline and citalopram have been suggested among SSRI as safer options and amitriptyline among tricyclic anti-depressants has been found to be useful (less than 2% of amitriptyline is excreted in kidney unchanged). However, while using amitriptyline one should be cautious for its anti-cholinergic side-effects and hypotension.Fluoxetine and paroxetine need cautious use considering long half-life and renal excreted metabolite of former and anti-cholinergic effects of latter.Mirtazapine is mostly excreted unchanged in urine and therefore its renal clearance is reduced.Duloxetine doesnot need dose adjustment till GFR>30mL/min however it is contraindicated for GFR lower than this. Clearance of venlafaxine is decreased and half- life is prolonged in renal impairment. In ESRD sage 50% dose reduction of venlafaxine is advised. Active metabolite of buspirone is excreted through kidney and therefore needs dose reduction in anuria and is contraindicated in severe renal impairment.

Among anti-dementia drugs rivastigmine is considered better choice than others considering it is not excreted unchanged in urine. Clearance of donepezil too is not affected by renal impairment and studies conducted have found similar pharmacokinetics in moderate to severe renal dysfunctions as in healthy controls. Memantine should be started at lower dose and then titrated upwards.

Among benzodiazepines lorazepam is considered reasonable choice in patients of renal dysfunction. Clonazepam too is excreted less than 1% unchanged in urine and does not require any major dosage change. However, caution is needed considering sedation with lorazepam and possible chances of accumulation with clonazepam. Diazepam and chlordiazepoxide should be possibly avoided as they have longer half-lives, whereas nitrazepam needs dose reduction with lower GFR values.

Zaleplon and zopiclone are not preferred as zolpidem's clearance is moderately reduced and zaleplon is not recommended at GFR <20ml/min. Zopiclone on the other hand doesnot accumulate in renal dysfunction. However, it too should be initiated at lower dose and then titrated upwards.[56]

5. Psychiatric drugs causing renal dysfunction: Lithium, commonly used mood stabilizer has been found to be associated with chronic tubule-interstitial nephropathy and thus may predispose to renal failure.

LIVER DYSFUNCTION AND PSYCHIATRIC PROBLEMS

Psychiatric aspects of liver dysfunction:

1. *What is liver dysfunction and its importance:*
   a. Liver dysfunction may present clinically as jaundice, ascitis, hepatomegaly, encephalopathy, palmar erythema, varices etc. or may be assessed by liver function tests by elevated bilirubin, bleeding time, liver enzymes (SGOT, SGPT, ALT or GGT) or decreased albumin levels.
   b. Liver dysfunction is an important aspect of consultation liaison considering most of the psychotropics are metabolised by liver one way or the other.
   c. Secondarily, liver dysfunction may lead to encephalopathy which may mimic psychiatric symptoms.
   d. Thirdly, alcohol abuse or dependence have been closely linked with liver dysfunction and treatment of which is important prevent deteriorating liver functions.
2. Epidemiology; chronic liver disease (CLD) has prevalence of around 15%.[57] The prevalence of non-alcoholic fatty liver disease is gradually increasing and is around 11% as compared to 5% in last century.Whereas, hepatitis infection and alcohol as a cause of liver dysfunction have remained relatively stable.[57] There is increased incidence of liver dysfunction among psychiatric patients.[58]

   Advanced age, female gender, alcoholism, multiple drug use, enzyme inducing drugs, pre-existing liver disease and obesity are risk factors for drug induced liver dysfunction.[59]
3. *Investigations and their interpretations:*
   a. Around 10% population has liver function outside the normal range and around the same percentage of patients who have liver dysfunction have normal liver function tests. However, the absolute values of liver dysfunction don't reflect severity of liver disease. LFT changes less than 2 times normal are not clinically significant generally however; elevations of reference values more than 3 times normal are mostly significant and associated with symptoms. Drug

related hepatotoxicity is mostly a hypersensitivity type of reaction (at times associated with rash and fever) and occurs early in treatment.

b. Mechanism of liver dysfunction due to drugs: Drug induced liver injury (DILI) can present as acute or chronic liver disease. There are two types of hepatotoxicity (DILI) dose dependent and idiosyncratic. Advanced age, female sex, concomitant disease or drugs are known risk factors for liver dysfunction resulting from drugs.[60]
c. What to consider in drug while prescribing: Drugs which have got high hepatic clearance or have very low therapeutic index should be avoided (e.g., lamotrigine). Those drugs which have wide therapeutic index but are metabolized mostly by liver than in that case caution should be exercised in prescribing the drug. If the drug has mostly renal clearance (upto 90%) then it's unlikely that liver dysfunction would affect its levels.
d. *Prescribing drugs in liver dysfunction:* While prescribing drugs in liver dysfunction one should give minimum drugs, at lowest possible dose and should be titrated gradually. Those drugs which are extensively metabolized by liver or are known to be hepatotoxic (e.g. chlorpromazine) should be avoided or are very sedative or constipating should be avoided (these drugs may precipitate encephalopathy). Liver functions should be monitored closely every week and side-effects should be monitored. Psychotherapies are effective and safe alternative to drug treatment in liver dysfunction wherever indicated like exposure and response prevention in liver dysfunction.[59]

Low dose haloperidol or amisulpride among anti-psychotics, lithium among mood stabilizers, lorazepam, oxazepam and temazepam among sedatives and citalopram and paroxetine (titrated gradually after starting at low dose) are preferred drugs in liver dysfunction. It is preferable to measure liver functions before starting any psychotropics.[59]

PSYCHIATRIC ASPECTS OF TUBERCULOSIS

Epidemiology: Tuberculosis, caused by *Mycobacterium tuberculosis*,[61] is one of the leading causes of mortality globally.[62]

Studies have suggested upto 50% of patients suffering from mental disorders, particularly depression and anxiety.[63] Higher psychiatric comorbidity has been reported with severity of tuberculosis[9]particularly drug resistant tuberculosis and prolonged duration of illness.[64] Not only does tuberculosis and its treatment predisposes to psychiatric problems but psychiatric disorders do also increase risk of tuberculosis and treatment failure in patients of tuberculosis.[9] Higher prevalence of alcohol and nicotine use disorders, injectable drug use disorder, diabetes and HIV predispose to tuberculosis.[65] A higher prevalence of psychiatric comorbidity with tuberculosis can be attributed to effect of stress on proliferation of lymphocytes and natural killer cells which can explain recovery from disease or relapse.[66]

Psychiatric symptoms in tuberculosis: Most common psychological reaction following diagnosis of tuberculosis was of anxiety and depression and very few people were hopeful of cure at the time of diagnosis.[67] About a tenth of patients reported suicidal thoughts following diagnosis[68] and it has been proposed that people with perceived stigma and poor self-image are at higher risk of developing mental disorders.[2] Suicides have been reported in chronically ill patients who are abandoned by family.[66]

Various psychiatric problems arising in tuberculosis can be classified as those occurring as a result of tuberculosis (psychiatric disorder due to general medical condition), those occurring as a result of anti-tubercular drugs e.g. isoniazid induced psychosis) and those occurring as a separate comorbidity with tuberculosis.

Treatment with anti-tubercular drugs has been associated with psychiatric symptoms. Isoniazid[69,70] ethionamide, cycloserine and ethambutol have been implicated mostly in it.[9] Isoniazid has been associated with a range of psychiatric symptoms including anxiety, confusion, agitation to frank psychosis. Isoniazid induced psychosis generally presents within a week of starting the drug and is characterized by disorganized behavior, visual hallucinations, restlessness and agitation, aimless wandering. Cycloserine which is second line drug for tuberculosis treatment has been reported to cause impaired functioning, psychotic symptoms or seizures in patients.[9] Ethambutol has been reported to cause disorientation hallucinations after 7 days of treatment.[71] Symptoms are likely to subside once the implicated drug is stopped.[9]

Treatment of various psychiatric disorders in tuberculosis: Selective serotonin reuptake inhibitors (SSRIs) are considered drug of choice for depression in tuberculosis. However, caution and close monitoring is required considering ability of isoniazid to cause monoamine oxidase inhibition and possible chances of serotonin syndrome resulting from interaction of isoniazid and SSRI. Isoniazid inhibits CYP2E1, CYP1A2, CYP2C9, CYP2C19, and CYP3A at varying degrees. Paroxetine which is primarily metabolized by CYP2D6 appears to have least interaction with isoniazid. Rifampicin is a known enzyme inducer and is known to decrease the levels of antidepressants, antipsychotics and benzodiazepines. In drug induced psychosis withdrawing the offending drug improves the symptoms.[58] Pyridoxine which has been shown to improve and prevent isoniazid induced neurological symptoms has not been found to help in ameliorating or preventing psychiatric symptoms.[58]

PSYCHIATRIC ASPECTS OF OTHER RESPIRATORY DISORDERS

A psychic disturbance leads to variation in breathing and vice-versa.[11] The prevalence of physical disorders is more common in child and adolescent group and upto half of patients of anxiety among children might be suffering from physical disorders.[72] Chronic obstructive lung disease, chronic bronchitis and asthma are known to be associated with depression with/without anxiety.[73] Presence of depression in these disorders significantly affects the quality of life of patients in these disorders.[74] Lehrer et al. (2002), suggested various psychological states like sadness, anxiety, stress can affect asthma and rather both asthma and these psychological states do potentiate each other in patients. Hence it has also been suggested that stress management, hypnosis, yoga and biofeedback procedures may be valuable adjuvant in treatment of asthma.

An important consideration remains for substance dependence patient having comorbid respiratory disorders. It has been seen that cannabis dependent patients start having obvious changes in spirometry even at young age and even if cannabis is used for short duration.[75] Similarly, COPD in smokers is associated with higher degree of cigarette dependence, but no greater desire to quit smoking than other smokers.[76]

PSYCHIATRIC ASPECTS OF GASTROINTESTINAL DISORDERS

Irritable bowel syndrome (IBS), which is characterized by chronic abdominal pain, bloating and alteration in bowel habits, is a common gastrointestinal disorder which has got high functional component. It has got high bidirectional comorbidity with physical disorder.[77] Upto one-third patients of OCD have symptoms of irritable bowel syndrome. SSRI may worsen the symptoms of IBS.[78] Improvement of depression or anxiety symptoms leads to improved functioning in these patients. Anxiety disorders have been associated with higher prevalence of peptic ulcer and peptic ulcer patients have perceived more stress life events.[11] A higher prevalence of peptic ulcer is seen in patients of nicotine and alcohol dependence. Serotonergic dysfunction associated with celiac disease has been implicated in high depression in celiac disease patients.[79] Trichobezoar seen in trichotillomania is a rare but known cause of intestinal obstruction.[80] There are case reports of gastric perforation in patients of tricholithobezoar.[81] Psychotropic drugs have been known to affect bowel function mostly causing constipation due to anti-cholinergic affects.

PSYCHIATRIC ASPECTS OF ENDOCRINAL DISORDERS

1. *Cushing's syndrome and Addison's disease:* Major depression may affect upto 50% of patients of Cushing's disease. It is the most common psychiatric comorbidity.[17] Anxiety and irritability commonly occur along with depression in these patients.[82,83] The severity of endocrinal problem has been found to correlate with depression.[84] An association of stressful life events and Cushing's disease onset has been found in pituitary-dependent Cushing's disease.[85] Anti-depressants are not as effective in treatment of depression in these patients as in general population. However, steroid inhibitors (ketoconazole, metyrapone, etc.) have been found to be useful in treatment.[17,86] In patients with severe anxiety benzodiazepines are helpful.[17] Treatment of affective symptoms may be required even after normalization of hormonal levels because of irreversible damage due to long-standing illness. Treatment with antisteroids is indicated to control depressive symptoms before surgical intervention in these patients.[17] Mania and cognitive dysfunction are other psychiatric features of Cushing's disease.[85]

   Addison's disease is associated with depression, disturbance of motivation and behavior. Psychiatric symptoms may be the presenting features in these patients. Rare patients of Addison's have presented with catatonia and self-mutilation.[87] Symptoms are likely to improve with steroid replacement.[88]
2. *Hyperprolactinemia:* Hostility, low mood and irritability commonly occur in patients having hyperprolactinemia. Depression in these patients has shown improvement with bromocriptine rather than with antidepressants.[89]

   Hyperprolactinemia is very common in patients of schizophrenia who are on anti-psychotics (more so with typical antipsychotics). Almost half of those patients who are on antipsychotics (mostly typical and some atypicals like risperidone, paliperidone, amisulpride and zotepine) have hyperprolactinemia. Antipsychotics are the most common cause of hyperprolactinemia in psychiatric patients.[90] Management of hyperprolactinemia in patients on antipsychotics include reducing their dose, choosing an antipsychotic (clozapine, quetiapine, olanzapine, aripiprazole) which has minimal effect on prolactin levels or the judicious use of dopamine agonists like bromcriptine. Symptoms of hyperprolactinemia secondary to antipsychotic medications can be reversed with adjuvant treatment with aripiprazole.[91]

   Hypothyroidism and hyperthyroidism: Hypothyroidism affects mood and cognitive state. Slowed information processing and poor executive functions has been specifically linked with low thyroid hormone levels.[92] Hypothyroidism has been shown to reduce central serotonin activity and thus high serum TSH levels have been found to correlate with depression.[93] Therefore, thyroxin replacement increases central serotonin activity and reverses depressive symptoms in patients.[94] Psychosis in patients of untreated hypothyroidism is also seen which remits with treatment, however its incidence is decreasing due to widespread use of thyroid tests and early intervention in hypothyroidism. Hashimoto encephalopathy, a type of delirium which has associated features of psychosis, seizures and focal neurological signs is a rare complication of hypothyroidism. High antithyroid antibodies are seen in this presumed immunological condition, which responds to corticosteroids.

Subclinical hypothyroidism has been linked with mood disorders and subsyndromal depressive and anxiety symptoms.[8] Subclinical hypothyroidism (elevated thyroid stimulating hormone and normal thyroxin levels) is seen more commonly in elderly particularly women and is shown to predispose to depression, dementia and cognitive impairment.[92]

Major depression particularly associated with anxiety and irritability are most common comorbidity with hyperthyroidism. These symptoms do respond to endocrinal treatment.[95] Psychosis and delirium are also seen in hyperthyroidism. Psychosis occurs more in exophthalmic goiter and delirium in hyperfunctioning adenomatous goiter.

PSYCHIATRIC ASPECTS OF CANCER

Affective and anxiety disorders have been associated with cancer.[96] The frequency of depression is higher in patients undergoing rehabilitation than those undergoing acute care.[96] Almost 25% of cancer patients suffer from depression. Advanced disease, uncontrolled pain, poor physical condition and previous history of depression are risk factors of depression in these patients. Stress related to diagnosis, brain metastasis nutritional deficiencies and endocrinal problems, medications (like corticosteroids, interferons, vincristine, etc.) predispose to depression. Social anxiety disorder is also quite prevalent in cancer patients and should be considered as comorbidity in patients of non-responding depression or if there is any problem of interaction between patient and staff.[6] Radiation phobia, needle phobia and claustrophobia are more commonly seen. Sudden severe anxiety in cancer patients is associated with pulmonary embolism whereas exacerbations of anxiety are associated with SSRI, mirtazapine and venlafaxine are used to improve depression whereas TCAs particularly nortriptyline is used to ameliorate depression and pain symptoms. SSRIs and low dose benzodiazepines are indicated for treatment of anxiety in these patients.

Psychotherapy in cancer patients does help in accepting diagnosis, overcoming the fear, enhancing treatment acceptance, treatment of depression or denial and improving sense of control and reducing distress.

PSYCHIATRIC ASPECTS OF HIV INFECTION

Psychiatric comorbidities in AIDS: psychiatric problems are more common in AIDS patients than among patients suffering from other sexually transmitted diseases.[97] Depression, anxiety, cognitive dysfunction, psychosis are common comorbidities in these patients.[98] Study conducted by Chandra et al. (1996) found depression in about 40% of patients and about 14% were having suicidal thoughts. Suicidal risk increases at the time of disclosure of diagnosis.[99] About a quarter of patients suffer from anxiety or adjustment.[100] Upto half of the patients with advanced HIV infection show some form of cognitive deficits.[101]

HIV associated dementia is seen late stages of HIV illness usually when CD4 count is less than 200/mm^3. Risk factors for HIV associated dementia is high HIV viral Load, older age, anemia, illicit drug use and female sex. Markers for HIV associated dementia are CSF, HIV, RNA, CSF beta microglobulin and prostaglandins. Apathy is an early sign of dementia in AIDS patients and depression in these patients presents as irritable mood and anhedonia rather than as sadness and crying spells. HIV associated dementia is strong risk factor for suicide and is also rapidly progressive. Zidovudine has been found to improve dementia.[102]

Depression in HIV patients has more risk for suicide and needs prompt treatment. Medications should be started at low dosage as these patients are very prone to side effects and should be raised slowly. SSRI, SNRI (venlafaxine) and mirtazapine have been studied and have been found to be affective 70 to 90% of patients. However, drug-srug interaction considering most antiretrovirals being inhibitors of CYP3A4 and ritonavir being inducer at CYP1A2 should be kept in mind while prescribing.[102]

Bipolar disorder is more prevalent among HIV patients. HIV associated mania is seen in patients having CD4 counts less than 100 cells/mm^3. HIV associated mania is generally more chronic than episodic it shows more irritability than elevated mood and is seen with cognitive decline. It is further more important as during mania high-risk behavior is further is increased. Lithium should be avoided considering low safety index and carbamazepine should be avoided as it has high interactions. Valproate is comparatively better choice and olanzapine can be helpful (it increases weight, has less interactions and is associated with less chances of extrapyramidal syndrome).[102]

REFERENCES

1. A Meguid El Nahas, Aminu K Bello;Chronic kidney disease: the global challenge;Lancet. 2005;365:331-40.
2. Deribew A, Tesfaye M, Hailmichael Y, et al. "Common mental disorders in TB/HIV co-infected patients in Ethiopia," BMC Infectious Diseases, vol. 10, article 201, 2010.
3. Aasheim ET. Wernicke encephalopathy after bariatric surgery: a systematic review. Ann Surg. 2008;248:714-20.
4. Adams RD, Victor M. In: Principles of neurology.New York: McGraw-Hill; 1989.pp.821-4.

5. Singh AK, Youssef MKF, Mittal BV, et al. Epidemiology and risk factors of chronic kidney disease in India results from the SEEK study. BMC Nephrology. 2013;14:114.
6. Akechi T, Okuyama T, Sagawa R, Uchida M, Nakaguchi T, Ito Y, Furukawa TA. Social anxiety disorder as a hidden psychiatric comorbidity among cancer patients; Palliat Support Care. 2011;9(1):103-5.
7. Akil M, Brewer GJ. Psychiatric and behavioral abnormalities in Wilson's disease. AdvNeurol. 1995;65:171-8.
8. Almeida C, Brasil MA, Costa AJ, Reis FA, Reuters V, Teixeira P, Ferreira M, Marques AM, Melo BA, Teixeira LB, Buescu A, Vaisman M. Subclinical hypothyroidism: psychiatric disorders and symptoms; Rev Bras Psiquiatr. 2007;29(2):157-9
9. Argiro P, Dionisios B, Georgios M, Athanasios T. Psychiatric Morbidity and Other Factors Affecting Treatment Adherence in Pulmonary Tuberculosis Patient, Tuberculosis Research and Treatment. 2013.
10. Basoglu M, Yetimalar Y, Gurgor N, et al. Neurological complications of prolonged hunger strike. Eur J Neurol. 2006;13:1089-97.
11. Shiv Gautam. Fourth revolution in psychiatry—Addressing comorbidity with chronic physical disorders;Indian J Psychiatry. 2010;52(3):213-19.
12. Caine D, Halliday GM, Kril JJ, Harper CG. Operational criteria for the classification of chronic alcoholics: identification of Wernickes encephalopathy. J Neurol Neurosurg Psychiatry. 1997;62:51-60.
13. Trivedi JK, Abdul Khalid. Chapter on Psychiatric Aspects of Medical Disorders in Textbook of Postgraduate Psychiatry, 2nd edition, Edited by JN Vyas and Neeraj Ahuja, published by Jaypee publishers; 432-50.
14. Benson DF. The Geschwind syndrome; Adv Neurol. 1991;55:411-21.
15. Remy P, Doder M, Lees A, Turjanski N, Brooks D. Depression in Parkinson's disease: loss of dopamine and noradrenaline innervation in the limbic system. Brain. 2005:1314-22.
16. Scheinberg IH, Sternlieb I. Wilson's disease. In: Smith LH Jr, editor. Major Problems in Internal Medicine. Vol. 23. WB Saunders: Philadelphia; 1984.
17. Sonino N, Fava GA. Psychiatric disorders associated with Cushing's syndrome. Epidemiology, pathophysiology and treatment;CNS Drugs. 2001;15(5):361-73.
18. Brown RG, Landau S, Hindle JV, et al. Depression and anxiety related subtypes in Parkinson's disease. J Neurol Neurosurg Psychiatry. 2011;82(7):803-9.
19. Riedel O, Heuser I, Klotsche J, Dodel R, Wittchen HU. GEPAD Study Group. Occurrence risk and structure of depression in Parkinson disease with and without dementia: results from the GEPAD Study; J Geriatr Psychiatry Neurol. 2010;23(1):27-3.
20. O'Suilleabhain PE, Sung V, Hernandez C, et al. Elevated plasma homocysteine level in patients with Parkinson disease: motor, affective, and cognitive associations. Arch. Neurol. 2004;61: 865-8.
21. Giladi N, Treves TA, Paleacu D, Shabtai H, Orlov Y, Kandinov B, et al. Risk factors for dementia, depression and psychosis in long-standing Parkinson's disease. J Neural Transm. 2000;107(1):59-7.
22. Rabey JM. Hallucinations and psychosis in Parkinson's disease.
23. Frydman M, Bonné-Tamir B, Farrer LA, et al. Assignment of the gene for Wilson's disease to chromosome 13: linkage to the esterase D locus. Proc Natl Acad Sci USA. 1985;82(6): 1819-21.
24. Tanzi RE, Petrukhin K, Chernov I, et al. The Wilson disease geneis a copper transporting ATPase with homology to the Menkes disease gene. Nat Genet. 1993;5(4):344-50.
25. Walshe JM, Yealland M. Wilson's disease: The problem of delayed diagnosis. J NeurolNeurosurg Psychiatry. 1992;55: 692-6.
26. Dening TR, Berrios GE. Wilson's disease: psychiatric symptomsin 195 cases. Arch Gen Psychiatry. 1989;46:1126-34.
27. Rathbun JK. Neuropsychological aspects of Wilson's disease. Int J Neurosci. 1996;85(3-4):221-9
28. Brewer GJ, Johnson V, Dick RD, Kluin KJ, Fink JK, Brunberg JA. Treatment of Wilson disease with ammonium tetrathiomolybdate II: Initial therapy in 33 neurologically affected patients and followup with zinc therapy. Arch Neurol. 1996;53(10):1017-25.
29. McDonald LV, Lake CR. Psychosis in an adolescent patient with Wilson's disease: effects of chelation therapy. Psychosom Med. 1995;57:202-4.
30. Krim E, Barroso B. Psychiatric disorders treated with clozapine in a patient with Wilson's disease. Presse Med. 2001;30(15): 73.
31. Chroni E, Lekka NP, Tsibri E, Economou A, Paschalis C. Acute, progressive akinetic-rigid syndrome induced by neuroleptics in a case of Wilson's disease. J Neuropsychiatry ClinNeurosci. 2001;13(4):531-2.
32. Galvin R, Bråthen G, Ivashynka A, Hillbom M, Tanasescu R, Leone MA. EFNS; EFNS guidelines for diagnosis, therapy and prevention of Wernicke encephalopathy; Eur J Neurol. 2010;17(12):1408-18.
33. Sasaki T, Yukizane T, Atsuta H, Ishikawa H, Yoshiike T, Takeuchi T, Oshima K, Yamamoto N, Kurumaji A, Nishikawa T. A case of thiamine deficiency with psychotic symptoms—blood concentration of thiamine and response to therapy; SeishinShinkeigakuZasshi. 2010;112(2):97-110.
34. Singh S, Kumar A. Wernicke encephalopathy after obesity surgery: a systematic review. Neurology. 2007;68:807-11.
35. Togay-Işikay C, Yiğit A, Mutluer N. Wernicke's encephalopathy due to hyperemesis gravidarum: an under-recognised condition. Aust N Z J Obstet Gynaecol. 2001;41(4):453-6.
36. Hahn JS, Berquist W, Alcorn DM, Chamberlain L, Bass D. Wernicke encephalopathy and beriberi during total parenteral nutrition attributable to multivitamin infusion shortage; Pediatrics. 1998;101(1).
37. Harper C. Wernicke's encephalopathy: a more common disease than realised. J Neurol, Neurosurg Psychiatry.1979;42:226-31.

38. Zuccoli G, Pipitone N. Neuroimaging findings in acute Wernickes encephalopathy: review of the literature. AJR Am J Roentgenol. 2009;192:501-8.
39. Sechi G, Serra A. Wernickes encephalopathy: new clinical settings and recent advances in diagnosis and management. Lancet Neurol. 2007;6:442-55.
40. Kopelman MD. The Korsakoff syndrome. Br J Psychiatry. 1995; 166:154-73.
41. Fama R, Pfefferbaum A, Sullivan EV. Visuoperceptual learning in alcoholic Korsakoff syndrome. Alcohol ClinExp Res. 2006;30:680-87.
42. Mancall EL. Nutritional disorders of the nervous system. In: Aminoff MJ, ed. Neurology and general medicine. New York: Churchill Livingstone; 1995.pp.285-301.
43. Maryam V, Nasim V. Obsessive Compulsive Disorder as Early Manifestation of B12 Deficiency. Indian J Psychol Med. 2011;33(2):203-20.
44. Gomez-Bernal GJ, Bernal-Perez M. Vitamin B12 deficiency manifested as mania: A case report. Prim Care Companion. J Clin Psychiatry. 2007;9:23.
45. Eastley R, Wilcock GK, Bucks RS. Vitamin B12 deficiency in dementia and cognitive impairment: the effects of treatment on neuropsychological function. Int J Geriatr Psychiatry. 2000;15(3):226-33.
46. Evans DL, Edelsohn GA, Golden RN. Organic psychosis without anemia or spinal cord symptoms in patients with vitamin B12 deficiency. Am J Psychiatry. 1983;140(2):218-21.
47. Tufan AE, Bilici R, Usta G, Erdoğan A. Mood disorder with mixed, psychotic features due to vitamin B12 deficiency in an adolescent: case report; Child Adolesc Psychiatry Ment Health. 2012;6(1):25. doi:10.1186/1753-2000-6-25.
48. Malouf R, AreosaSastre A. Vitamin B12 for cognition; Cochrane Database Syst Rev. 2003;(3):CD004326.
49. German Jorge Gomez-Bernal, Milagros Bernal-Perez. Vitamin B_{12} deficiency manifested as mania: A case report. Prim Care Companion. J Clin Psychiatry. 2007;9(3):238.
50. De-Nour, AK. Psychotherapy with patients on chronic haemodialysis. British Journal of Psychiatry. 1970;116: 207-15.
51. Chen Y, Wu S, Wang S. Depression in chronic hemodialysed patients. Nephrology. 2003;8:121-6.
52. Craven J, Rodin G, Johnson L. The diagnosis of major depression in renal dialysis patients. Psychosomatic Medicine. 1987;49:482-92.
53. Osberg J, Meares G, McKee D, et al. Intellectual functioning in renal failure and chronic dialysis. Journal of Chronic Disease. 1982;35;445-57.
54. Roger SM, Nour TB, Banil S, Swartz SA. The Use of Psychotropic Drugs in Patients with Impaired Renal Function. Primary Psychiatry. 2008;15(1):73-88.
55. Sensky, T. Psychosomatic aspects of end-stage renal failure. Psychotherapy and Psychosomatics. 1993;59:56-68.
56. David Taylor, Carol Paton, Shitij Kapur. chapter: Use of psychotropics in special population, Renal Impairment. The South London and Maaudsley NHS Foundation Trust and Oxleas NHS Foundation Trust Prescribing Guidelines, 10th edition; published by Informa Healthcare.
57. Younossi ZM, Stepanova M, Afendy M, Fang Y, Younossi Y, Mir H, Srishord M. Changes in the prevalence of the most common causes of chronic liver diseases in the United States from 1988 to 2008; Clin Gastroenterol Hepatol. 2011;9(6): 524-30.
58. Prasad R, Garg R, Verma SK. Isoniazid- and ethambutol-induced psychosis. Ann Thorac Med. 2008;3(4):149-51.
59. David Taylor, Carol Paton, Shitij Kapur. chapter: Use of psychotropics in special population, Liver Impairment.The South London and Maaudsley NHS Foundation Trust and Oxleas NHS Foundation Trust Prescribing Guidelines, 10th edition; published by Informa Healthcare.
60. Stefan Russmann, Gerd A. Kullak-Ublickl and Ignazio Grattagliano: Current Concepts of Mechanisms in Drug-Induced Hepatotoxicity; Current Medicinal Chemistry. 2009; 16:3041-53.
61. TE Herchline, BA Cunha, PS Chavis, et al. Tuberculosis. Medscape Reference, WebMD, Updated: March, 2012.
62. Martin P. "Tuberculosis at the end of the century," MedDigest. 1996;22:10-11.
63. Bender A, Hyman I, Guruge S. "Exploring tuberculosis, mental health, and immigrant health through a syndemic approach," CERIS Final Report, 2011.
64. Panchal SL. "Correlation with duration and depression in TB patients in rural Jaipur district," International Journal of Pharma and Bio Sciences. 2011; 2(2):B.263.
65. Sanchez M, Nicholls T, Currier G. "Risk factors for tuberculosis in the psychiatric emergency department," Emergency Psychiatry, 1998;4:33-4.
66. Kant L, Nagpaul DR. "Psychiatric disorders and illness perceptions in tuberculosis," The Indian Journal of Tuberculosis. 2001;48(2):55-6.
67. Eram U, Khan IA, Tamanna Z, Khan Z, Khaliq N, Abidi AJ. "Patient perception of illness and initial reaction to the diagnosis of tuberculosis," Indian Journal of Community Medicine, vol. 31, no. 3, 2006; pp. 2006-07-2006-09.
68. Rajeswari R, Muniyandi M, Balasubramanian P, Narayanan PR. "Perceptions of tuberculosis patients about their physical, mental and social well-being: a field report from south India," Social Science and Medicine. 2005;60(8):1845-53.
69. Bedi RS. "Isoniazid induced pyrexia and psychosis in a single individual," Indian Journal of Tuberculosis, 1994;41:269-70.
70. Tiwari VK, Verma SM. "Homicide by a tuberculous prisoner possibly having drug induced acute delusional psychosis," Indian Journal of Tuberculosis. 1997;44(2):95-96.
71. Pickles RW, Spelman DW. "Suspected ethambutol-induced mania," Medical Journal of Australia, 1996;164:445-6.

72. Chavira DA, Garland AF, Daley S, Hough R. The impact of medical comorbidity on mental health and functional health outcomes among children with anxiety disorders. J Dev Behav Pediatr. 2008;29:394-402.
73. Brenes GA. Anxiety and chronic obstructive pulmonary disease: Prevalence, impact, and treatment. Psychosom Med. 2003;65:963-70.
74. Wagena EJ, Kant I, van Amelsvoort LG, Wouters EF, van Schayck CP, Swaen GM. Risk of Depression and Anxiety In Employees With Chronic Bronchitis: The Modifying Effect of Cigarette Smoking. Psychosom Med. 2004;66:729-34.
75. Taylor D. Robin, Richie Poulton Terrie E. Moffitt Padmaja Ramankutty and Malcolm R. Sears. The respiratory effects of cannabis dependence in young adults. Addiction. 2000;95(11): 1669-77.
76. Shahab L, Jarvis MJ, Britton J, West R. Prevalence, diagnosis and relation to tobacco dependence of chronic obstructive pulmonary disease in a nationally representative population sample; Thorax. 2006;61(12):1043-7.
77. Tillisch K, Mayer EA. Pain Perception in Irritable Bowel Syndrome. CNS Spectr. 2005;10:877-82.
78. Masand PS, Keuthen NJ, Gupta S, Virk S, Yu-Siao B, Kaplan D. Prevalence of Irritable Bowel Syndrome in Obsessive-Compulsive Disorder. CNS Spectr. 2006;11:21-5.
79. Ciacci C, Iavarone A, Siniscalchi M, Romano R, De Rosa A. Psychological dimensions of celiac disease: Toward an integrated approach. Dig Dis Sci. 2002;47:2082-7.
80. Gaujoux Sébastien, Gaëlle Bach, Joyce Au, Gaëlle Godiris-Petit, Nicolas Munoz-Bongrand, Pierre Cattan, Emile Sarfati. Trichobezoar: A rare cause of bowel obstruction. World J Gastrointest Surg. 2011;3(4):54-55.
81. Valenciano JS, Nonose R, Cruz RB, Tiemi SD, Monteiro FFF, Nascimento EF, et al. Tricholithobezoar causing gastric perforation. Case Rep Gastroenterol. 2012;6(1):26-32.
82. Dorn LD, Burgess ES, Friedman TC, Dubbert B, Gold PW, Chrousos G. The longitudinal course of psychopathology in Cushing's syndrome after correction of hypercortisolism. Journal of Clinical Endocrinology and Metabolism. 1997;82: 912-9.
83. Kelly WF, Kelly MJ, Faragher B. A prospective study of psychiatric and psychological aspects of Cushing's syndrome. Clinical Endocrinology. 1996;45:715-20.
84. Sonino N, Zielezny M, Fava GA, Fallo F, Boscaro M. Risk factors and long-term outcome in pituitary-dependent Cushing's disease. Journal of Clinical Endocrinology and Metabolism. 1996;81:2647-52.
85. Sonino N, Fallo F, Fava GA. Psychosomatic aspects of Cushing's syndrome. Rev EndocrMetabDisord. 2010;11(2):95-104. doi:10.1007/s11154-009-9123-7.
86. Sonino N, Fava GA, Belluardo P, Girelli ME, Boscaro, M. Course of depression in Cushing's syndrome: response to treatment and comparison with Graves' disease. Hormone Research, 1993a;39:202-6.
87. Rebecca E, Anglin P, Michael FM. The Neuropsychiatric Profile of Addison's Disease: Revisiting a Forgotten Phenomenon. The Journal of Neuropsychiatry and Clinical Neurosciences. 2006;18:450-9.
88. Boswell EB, Anfinson TJ, Nemeroff CB. Depression associated with endocrine disorders. In: Robertson MM, Katona CLE (Eds) Depression and Physical Illness, Wiley, Chichester; 1997. pp. 2255-92.
89. Reavley S, Fisher AD, Owen D, Creed FH, Davis JRE. Psychological distress in patients with hyperprolactinemia. Clinical Endocrinology. 1997;47:343-8.
90. Carvalho MM, Góis C. Hyperprolactinemia in mentally ill patients; Acta Med Port. Epub 2012 Feb 20. 2011;24(6): 1005-12.
91. Shim JC, Shin JG, Kelly DL, Jung DU, Seo YS, Liu KH, Shon JH, Conley RR. Adjunctive treatment with dopamine partial agonist, aripiprazole, for antipsychotic-induced hyperprolactinemia: a placebo-controlled trial. Am J Psychiatry. 2007;164(9):1404-10.
92. Davis JD, Stern RA, Flashman LA. Cognitive and neuro-psychiatric aspects of subclinical hypothyroidism: significance in the elderly. Curr Psychiatry Rep. 2003;5(5):384-90.
93. Cleare AJ, McGregor A, O'Keane V. Neuroendocrine evidence for an association between hypothyroidism, reduced central 5-HT activity and depression; Clin Endocrinol (Oxf). 1995;43(6):713-9.
94. Cleare AJ, McGregor A, Chambers SM, Dawling S, O'Keane V. Thyroxine replacement increases central 5-hydroxytryptamine activity and reduces depressive symptoms in hypothyroidism; Neuroendocrinology. 1996;64(1):65-9.
95. Fava GA, Sonino N, Morphy MA. Psychosomatic view of endocrine disorders. Psychotherapy and Psychosomatics. 1993;59:20-33.
96. Härter M, Reuter K, Aschenbrenner A, Schretzmann B, Marschner N, Hasenburg A, Weis J. Psychiatric disorders and associated factors in cancer: results of an interview study with patients in inpatient, rehabilitation and outpatient treatment. Eur J Cancer. 2001;37(11):1385-93.
97. Satapathy R, Muralikrishna N, Babu MA, Vijayagopal M. A study of psychiatric manifestations of physically asymptomatic HIV-1 seropositive individuals. Indian J Psychiatry. 2000;42: 427-33.
98. Jayarajan N, Chandra PS. HIV and mental health: An overview of research from India. Indian J Psychiatry. 2010;52:S269-73.
99. Chandra PS, Krishna VA, Ravi V, Desai A, Puttaram S. HIV related admissions in a psychiatric hospital: A five year profile. Indian J Psychiatry. 1999;41:320-4.
100. Chandra PS, Carey MP, Carey KB, Shalinianant A, Thomas T. Sexual coercion and abuse among women with a severe mental illness in India: An exploratory investigation. Compr Psychiatry. 2003;44:205-12.
101. Yepthomi T, Paul R, Vallabhaneni S, Kumarasamy N, Tate DF, Solomon S, et al. Neurocognitive consequences of HIV in southern India: A preliminary study of clade C virus. J Int Neuropsychol Soc. 2006;12:424-30.
102. Crystal CW, Niccolo D, Della P, Andrew A, Angelino GJ, Treisman M. HIV/AIDS. In: James L (Ed). Textbook of

Psychosomatic Medicine Psychiatric Care of the Medically Ill, 2nd edition. Lavenson published by American Psychiatric Publishing Inc. pp. 637-67.

SUGGESTED READING

1. Brown T, Brown R. Neuropsychiatric consequences of renal failure. Psychosomatics. 1995;36:244-53.
2. Carney RM, Freedland KE, Miller GE, Jaffe AS. Depression as a risk factor for cardiac mortality and morbidity. A review of potential mechanisms. J Psychosom Res. 2002;53:897-902.
3. Chandra PS, Ravi V, Puttaram S, Desai A. HIV and mental illness. Br J Psychiatry. 1996;168:654.
4. Davis JD, Tremont G. Neuropsychiatric aspects of hypothyroidism and treatment reversibility. Minerva Endocrinol. 2007;32(1):49-6.
5. K/DOQI clinical practice guidelines for chronic kidney disease: evaluation, classification, and stratification. Am J Kidney Dis. 2002;39(2 suppl 1):S1-266.
6. Mary Jane Massie, Kimberley Miller. Chapter on Oncology in Textbook of Psychosomatic Medicine Psychiatric Care of the Medically Ill, 2nd Edition; James L (Ed). Lavenson published by American Psychiatric Publishing Inc. p. 525-51.
7. Merims D, Freedman M. Cognitive and behavioural impairment in Parkinson's disease. Int Rev Psychiatry. 2008;20(4):364-73.
8. Parkinsonism RelatDisord. 2009;15 Suppl 4:S105-10.
9. Presne C, Fakhouri F, Noel LH, et al. Lithium-induced nephropathy: Rate of progression and prognostic factors. Kidney Int. 2003;64(2):585-92.
10. Shashwat Saxena, Sujit K Kar, Trivedi JK. Depression in neurological disorders;Indian Journal of Behavioral Sciences. 2012;22(2).
11. Shulman LM, Taback RL, Weiner WJ. Non-recognition of depression and other non-motor symptoms in Parkinson's disease; Parkinsonism and Related Disorders. 2002;8(3):193-7.
12. Thanvi BR, Munshi SK, Vijaykumar N, Lo TC. Neuropsychiatric non-motor aspects of Parkinson's disease. Postgrad. Med J. 2003;79(936):561-5.

CHAPTER

34

Psychiatry in Oncology

Gayatri Saraf, Santosh K Chaturvedi

INTRODUCTION

Psychiatric oncology in its broadest sense deals with the detection and treatment of psychiatric problems in patients who are screened for, diagnosed with, being treated, facing impending death due to cancer or are surviving cancer. Psychiatric oncology as a sub-specialty, focuses on a number of issues, which include the role of life events, stress, and other psychological factors in the causation, maintenance, and prognosis of cancer; psychological and emotional reactions to diagnosis of cancer, its recurrence, metastasis; psychiatric disorders in relation to cancer and its treatment; psychological methods of treatment, and counseling, communicating with cancer patients and their relatives; terminal care and palliative care; study and management of grief and bereavement related to cancer; and staff stress and burnout among professionals treating cancer patients.

Inspite of significant psychological issues in cancer patients, the topic has received scarce clinical and modest research attention at best. It has been demonstrated time and again that most health care professionals are not trained for picking up psychiatric disorders in cancer patients, and hence miss out on even clinically significant causes of morbidity.

CANCER AND MENTAL HEALTH

A majority of the studies have revealed a significant level of psychiatric morbidity among cancer patients. A study conducted on an outpatient cancer population reported 34% to have a clinically significant level of psychological distress, and another study of cancer patients admitted to three centers in USA also revealed similar results.[1,2] In the Indian setting, 38% of cancer patients were found to have identifiable DSM-III-R anxiety or depressive disorder.[3] Earlier studies did not differentiate the psychiatric morbidities related to different types of cancer. Differential effects of other factors like, the impact of the diagnosis, stage of disease and the type of the treatment were also not given due attention in these studies. While in the early stage of the disease it is the impact of the diagnosis and the treatment which have most effects, in advanced disease the physical symptoms and impending death assume importance.

Response to the Diagnosis of Cancer

A diagnosis of cancer is a life-changing event and brings in its wake a plethora of negative feelings such as shock, disbelief, confusion, anger, despair, hopelessness and guilt. The severity of a patient's distress after diagnosis of cancer is the most important predictor of later adjustment disorder. There might be significant guilt about any past wrong doings and sexual transgressions. In India, chronic disease is usually taken as an atonement for past sins (*Karma*). An adjustment disorder is the most common psychiatric diagnosis with reported prevalence from 12.5%[4] to as high as 68%.[2] Majority of the patients have been found to have adjustment disorder mainly with depressed mood, anxious mood and mixed emotional disturbances. A diagnosis of adjustment disorder should be considered when an acute stress response persists in a stereotyped fashion and interferes significantly with functioning.

Depression

Around 20–50% of cancer patients have mental health problems requiring intervention, with atleast 25% meeting the criteria for major depressive disorder or adjustment disorder of the depressive type, which is the most common diagnosis.[5,6] The prevalence of major depression has been reported to be 13–40% in various studies.[2,7,8] The risk of major depression also increases with recurrence, terminal disease and chronic intractable pain. Depression is directly related to the severity of cancer symptoms and leads to reduced optimism about the efficacy of treatment. The risk of suicide is higher in the early stages of coping with cancer. Chronic and sustained depression after diagnosis of cancer, as opposed to reactive depression, is associated with faster progression of cancer and shorter survival.

There are multiple mechanisms that can cause depression in cancer patients. Reactive depression to the diagnosis of cancer can be understood from a psychosocial perspective in that it is caused by distress regarding the diagnosis of cancer and the resulting implications on an individual's life. However, recently other mechanisms have also been elucidated. A *sickness syndrome*[9] has been described in individuals with chronic illness which has signs and symptoms of depression such as anhedonia, fatigue, loss of appetite, sleep and libido, lethargy, cognitive symptoms, psychomotor slowing and weight loss. These symptoms may be understood as stemming from the pathophysiologic alterations caused by cancer, due to paraneoplastic syndromes or by chemo/radiotherapy.[10] These symptoms are also present in depression making differentiation difficult. However, more often than not, major depression in addition, is also accompanied by guilt, depressive cognitions and suicidality.[10] Sickness syndrome can be caused by proinflammatory cytokines that are released after tissue damage and destruction.

Numerous approaches have been used to diagnose depression in patients with cancer. The inclusive approach advocates that neurovegetative symptoms be counted while assessing for depression, whereas in the exclusive approach, these symptoms are not considered.[11] Some suggest a compromise wherein an amalgamation of both approaches can be used depending on the purpose for which depression is being assessed.[12] The inclusive symptoms could be used for clinical purposes as treatment would not differ because often even neurovegetative symptoms of any cause respond favorably to antidepressants. The exclusive approach can be used for research purposes to obtain more specificity in assessment of depression. Regardless of the approach, the general consensus is that treatment of even subsyndromal depression improves quality of life and hence clinicians should keep a low threshold for diagnosis of depression.[13]

Treatment used for cancer such as IL-2 or IFN-α and a variety of other chemotherapeutic agents can also cause depressive symptoms.[14] The prevalence of depression is higher in cancer survivors who have received intense chemotherapeutic exposure in childhood.[15] Oncologic surgery may also increase chances of having depression. In breast cancer patients, patients who had a mastectomy had greater prevalence of depression than those who had breast-conserving surgery.[16] Though the obvious reason for this might be related to more disfigurement caused by mastectomy and resulting body-image concerns, the underlying reason could also be that more radical surgery might induce activation of proinflammatory cytokines which are known to play a causative role in depression (Table 1).[17]

Depression interferes with adherence to medical treatment for cancer[18] and ability to care for oneself and thus might have an effect on disease progression. Depressive symptoms are associated with an increased risk of dying.[19] A depressive coping style has been found to predict decreased survival.

Factors influencing depression
Disease related factors
Recurrence
Site of cancer—More in pancreatic, oropharyngeal, breast carcinomas
Chronic pain
Severe disease
Disability
Metabolic factors : Deranged electrolytes, paraneoplastic syndromes
Patient related factors
Depressive coping style
Less social support
Younger age
Living alone
Economic difficulties
Past psychiatric illness or h/o suicide attempt
Recent losses
Tendency towards pessimism
Iatrogenic causes
Chemotherapy
Disfiguring surgery : e.g Mastectomy > Breast conservation
Colostomies
Diagnostic criteria used
Inclusive >Exclusive

Table 1: Cancer medications that can cause depression
IL-2
IFN-α
Amphotericin-B
Cycloserine
Glucocorticoids
L-asparginase
Leuprolide
Procarbazine
Tamoxifen
Vincristine
Vinblastine

Management of Depression

Pharmacotherapy

Newer antidepressants have an excellent risk-benefit ratio and can be used for isolated symptoms in the absence of a depressive syndrome as well. Also these isolated symptoms can be forerunners for a full blown depressive episode, amount to significant morbidity and respond to antidepressant treatment. Therefore, their treatment can also prevent an episode and improve quality of life in cancer patients. Imipramine, Fluoxetine,[20] Paroxetine,[21] Amitriptyline,[21] Mianserin,[22] Mirtazapine[23] and Desipramine[20] have been found to be effective in treating depression in various studies. Pain can be treated with tricyclics or SNRIs. Mirtazapine has been found to be useful for insomnia and nausea associated with chemotherapy.[24] Fluoxetine,[25] Paroxetine[26] and Venlafaxine[27] are also useful in decreasing hot flashes in patients with cancer.

Electroconvulsive therapy can be considered for cancer patients with severe, life-threatening depression, those with a history of good response to ECT in the past, and for those who are unable to tolerate the side effects of antidepressants or are nonresponsive to antidepressants. Psychotropic medications can also be safely and effectively used in palliative care of the terminally ill cancer patients.

Psychological Treatments

Supportive psychotherapy or cognitive behavior therapy can be employed to facilitate ventilation, enhance coping skills and to correct cognitive errors and maladaptive schemas.

Recent evidence suggests the use of combined pharmacotherapy and psychological therapies for depressive disorders, with no clear benefit of one over the other.

Somatic Complaints

Somatic symptoms in cancer are frequent and contribute to illness behavior. Somatic symptoms could be in the form of pain, fatigue, anorexia, weight loss, reduced energy, lethargy and tremor. They pose a challenge in the diagnosis of depression in cancer patients as they overlap with symptoms of depression.

Somatic symptoms in cancer could be due to emotional disturbances which lower the pain threshold, or they could be due to the underlying pathology itself. It is difficult to determine the exact cause of somatic symptoms when they occur as it could be multifactorial, viz. due to physical, psychological causes, cancer chemotherapy, radiotherapy, a combination of these or idiopathic. Persistence of somatic complaints after recovery from cancer could also be a part of abnormal illness behavior and trying to maintain the sick role. Somatic complaints that have a clear correlation with life events or stress are more likely to be psychogenic in origin, whereas those that are aggravated by disease progression or treatment are likely to have physical causation.[28]

Chronic fatigue has been associated with a poor quality of life (QOL) in cancer patients. Somatic symptoms also associated with poor QOL, more morbidity and complicate treatment decisions. Aggravation of somatic symptoms that are psychological in origin can wrongly lead to more aggressive treatment of cancer and hence, a careful assessment is warranted.

Grief

A grief reaction to the diagnosis of cancer is common and understandable as the person copes with the loss of the previously healthy self, of a particular body part (breast, hair) and resulting disfigurement, of one's role in the society and family, work functioning or impending loss of life.

Anxiety

The word 'cancer' itself can provoke intense anxiety in seemingly normal people. Thus anxiety in the initial stages after the disclosure of having cancer is made can be a normal reaction to the news.

Anxiety symptoms manifest as apprehension about the future and treatment, constant worries of oneself and family members, restlessness, a sense of foreboding, sleep disturbances, inability to relax and misinterpretation of bodily sensations. Post-traumatic stress symptoms such as intrusive recollections, flashbacks, autonomic arousal and avoidance of reminders of cancer may follow diagnosis or unpleasant treatment.

Anxiety in cancer can be considered from multiple viewpoints. Whilst it might be a normal reaction to certain aspects such as cost of treatment, non-response, worries about family members and health, unfinished business, lack of adequate communication by health professionals and uncertainty stemming from the same, etc. pathological anxiety should be recognized and treated.[29] Pathological anxiety is identified by being out of proportion to the level of stress, persists or aggravates if not managed, and cause significant impairment in functioning.[30] Anxiety could be a part of depression and also caused by drugs.

It can have a significant impact on perceived quality of life,[31] increased sensitivity to side-effects of treatment[32] and cancer care.[33]

Factors associated with anxiety in cancer patients
Demographic factors
• Young age
• Female gender
Disease related factors
• Onset of symptoms
• Diagnosis
• Investigations
• Extensive illness
• Recurrence
• Pain
Treatment related factors
• Oncological surgery
• Side effects due to chemo/radiotherapy
• Termination of chemo/radiotherapy cycles
• Medications: Corticosteroids, interferon alpha

Management of Anxiety

Pharmacological: SSRIs, in particularly escitalopram can be used in view of relative safety with regards to drug interactions. Benzodiazepines can be used in the short term for the management of acute anxiety, however, should be avoided over long-term due to the risk of potential for abuse and dependence.

Psychosocial: Cognitive behavior therapy can be used. Mindfulness based therapies such as mindfulness based stress reduction have been tried with encouraging results.[34] Relaxation, guided imagery and systematic desensitisation can also be used.

Psychosexual Dysfunctions

Sexuality and intimacy are altered following mastectomy. Wellisch et al.[35] found that approximately 36% husbands reported that mastectomy had a 'bad' or 'somewhat bad' influence on their sexual relationships. Maguire et al.[36] found that 1 year after the wives' mastectomy 29% husbands reported moderate to severe sexual difficulties.

A review of sexual functioning morbidity estimates for major organ sites, indicates that a large number of cancer patients have problems in sexual functioning. The highest rates are in those patients where the cancer is at a sexual or reproductive body site.[37] The exact prevalence of psychosexual problems is not known among cancer patients, but it is thought to be much more prevalent than expected. Cancer survivors experience rates of sexual dysfunction ranging upto 90%;[37] actual rates may be even higher than reported rates due to widespread reluctance of patients to discuss sexual problems with staff.[38]

Sexual problems among cancer patients usually start acutely, after diagnosis, or treatment. In some cases, such as in prostate cancer or cervical cancers, sexual problems may be the earliest sign of disease. Problems in sexual excitement and arousal are common , orgasmic problems are also quite frequent while in some there may be pain during intercourse.[39,40] Sexual activity and satisfaction is affected by the malignancy, its effect on the health, changes in body image, foul smelling or blood stained discharges from the tumor site, chemotherapy, radiotherapy or surgery. Loss of libido could be due to the above factors, but it could at times be a manifestation of depression associated with cancer. General weakness and cachexia could also contribute to the sexual weakness, and disinclination. Fatigue after the treatment can be very severe and interfere with sexual activity.[39]

Management

General guidelines include treatment medical cause if any, treatment of depression, allaying anxieties and fears related to contagion, pain or, bleeding, and dispelling myths and misconceptions. It is useful to include partner in the treatment. Treatment of specific phase problems include decreasing anxiety and performance fears by discussion and clarification of doubts, non-performance touching should be encouraged to increase intimacy without fears of having sexual contact. Sensate focus exercises which involve non-genital touch and increase arousal and resexualizing the relationship is an important part of treatment. Many couples would have terminated sexual contact and resuming the sexual nature of the relationship plays an important role.

Vaginal lubricant or estrogen cream can also be useful. Sexual alternatives to intercourse such as non-penetrative sex or mutual masturbation may be encouraged whenever there are fears of pain.

Partner support is an important part of treatment as partners are very often unaware of sexual issues. They may also feel left out and isolated during the course of treatment and feel distant from their spouse.

Use of Prosthesis and Dilators: Vaginal Synechiae and stenosis are common problems associated with radiation therapy among woman with uterine cancers which leads to sexual dysfunction and dyspareunia. At the Tata Memorial Hospital, Occupational therapy department, soft washable and reusable vaginal dilators have been used which significantly reduce problems related to sexual intercourse. Women found these self-dilators very useful specially if used early. Penile prosthesis in prostatic cancers and cancer of the penis are increasingly being used and have been reported to be quite effective and useful. These are still not popular and not easily available in the Indian context.

Sleep Disorders

Sleep disturbances are common in cancer patients, but there are few specific data on their prevalence. Sleep problems may be a symptom of cancer itself, part of the stress reaction to having cancer, as sequelae to some other cancer symptom such as pain, or a side effect of cancer treatment. Insomnia is the more common sleep problem, although hypersomnia also occurs. Most insomnias are related either to pain or to psychophysiological factors.

A few studies undertaken in this area have found that sleep disturbance as a symptom is common in cancer patients and the prevalence of sleep disturbances in patients with advanced pancreatic cancer was found to be as high as 54%.[41] In our experience with cancer patients, we have also found that a significant number of patients had insomnia as a major problem, both in the presence and absence of other emotional problems. A few patients with insomnia reported that they were disturbed emotionally because of the sleep problems. It has been found, in a study that patients with lung cancer, rarely complained of sleep disturbance though most of them had a sleep architecture similar to that of insomniacs.[42]

Management

Treatment of sleep disturbances should start with the identification of a specific cause of the problem and one should do a thorough medical and psychological evaluation of the patient; after that behavioural interventions, medications, or psychotherapy may be helpful. When using medications, keep in mind possible complications such as daytime sedation, tolerance, and rebound insomnia.

Anticipatory Nausea and Vomiting

This is a conditioned response that develops through classical conditioning usually before the next chemotherapy cycle, but can also after during and after cycles. It is also associated with higher anxiety.[43]

The conditioned side effects are thought to develop through a classical conditioning.

Management

Behavioral techniques may be designed to:

1. Reduce autonomic arousal and thereby produce a physical state incompatible with the concomitant of nausea and vomiting.
2. Control the cues: Internal cues can be controlled by the autonomic arousal while external cues can be controlled by changing pairing chemotherapy with environmental stimuli.
3. Reduce post-chemotherapy nausea or vomiting, thereby reducing a reliable predictor of anticipatory symptoms.
4. Change cognition or perception concerning chemotherapy, as well as teach self-control and coping strategies.
5. Control anxiety: Low dose benzodiazepines can be used for the same over the short-term.

Relaxation techniques like muscle relaxation, relaxing imagery and hypnosis may also be useful in the treatment of conditioned response to chemotherapy.[44]

Neuropsychiatric Syndromes

The most common organic mental syndrome in cancer patients is delirium.[1] Delirium can be produced either by cancer directly and its treatment or because of associated mental disorder and their treatment. The commonly used drugs which produce delirium are narcotic analgesics like morphine and methadone, sedatives-hypnotics mainly benzodiazepines like diazepam, nitrazepam, alprazolam, drugs with anticholinergic effects and drugs with psychoactive side-effects, digitalis, anti-hypertensives, etc. Delirium and dementia can also be a sequelae to brain metastasis caused by certain tumors. They also arise as a result of autoimmune response to the tumor as a part of paraneoplastic syndromes. Metabolic encephalopathies, organ failure, electrolyte imbalance, nutritional deficiencies, infection and hypoxia are some of the related medical disorders causing delirium.

The recommended management of delirium is quick and aggressive, giving the appropriate medication in the early stages of the disorder. Low dose benzodiazepines and antipsychotics are the drugs of choice. Intravenous route is preferred because it works faster and avoids the need for repeated intramuscular injections.

Distress

Also described as the 6th vital sign, distress in cancer can be multidimensional viz, physical, mental, emotional, spiritual and existential. Other causes of psychological distress among cancer patients include problems due to finances, family worries and spiritual and existential doubts. Unpleasant symptoms due to cancer therapy such as pain, nausea, fatigue are also an important cause of distress and reduced quality of life.

Substance Abuse

Alcohol use is a risk factor for malignancies of gastrointestinal system, head and neck, and the hepatobiliary system. Nicotine use is associated with pulmonary and head and neck cancers. Opioids may be abused for pain relief. Abstinence from alcohol leads to a better prognosis than continuing alcohol use. Patients with comorbid substance require additional help in management of these disorders.

Fear of Cancer Recurrence

Most cancer survivors live in a constant dread about cancer recurrence. This anxiety may be intensified especially during the chemo/radiotherapy termination as the protective cover of chemo/radiotherapy is no longer available and the patient feels exposed to the risk of disease progression.

Personality

Galen observed that women with breast cancer frequently tended to be melancholic. Much has been discussed and written about the 'Cancer prone' personality. Type C personality traits characterized by suppression of emotions, high conformity and tendency to avoid emotional outbursts has been often associated with cancer. Certain personality traits have been found to predispose individuals to cancer, or, when present, are associated with faster progression.[45] These are:

1. Difficulty in expressing emotions
2. Attitude of helplessness/hopelessness

In a study done on medical students, those who had a tendency of emotional expression/acting out were less likely to develop cancer later whereas a group characterized as "Loners" who had difficulties with emotional expression were 16 times more likely to develop cancer.[46] However, there is inconclusive evidence to support these theories and positive findings in this area have not been consistently replicated.[47]

Psychosis

Schizophrenia and other functional psychoses are comparatively less frequent than the other above mentioned disorders but contrary to the earlier beliefs cancer is not rare in schizophrenic patients than in general population. Vinca alkaloids can produce hallucinations.

PSYCHIATRIC DISORDERS RELATED TO DISEASE AND TREATMENTS

1. *Effect of the cancer:* Psychiatric symptoms sometimes occur due to the direct effect of the disease process. Psychiatric symptoms are seen in almost all patients with supratentorial tumors and are the presenting symptoms in 25% of cases.[1] A common presentation of carcinoma of pancreas is with depression.[3] Physiologically active tumors of endocrine glands like thyroid, pituitary and parathyroid can also manifest as psychiatric syndromes. In the advanced stage, cancer can produce psychiatric symptoms by metastasis, and other modes as in paraneoplastic syndrome.
2. *Morbidity associated with treatment modalities:* Differentiation of psychiatric morbidity related to the cancer as such or from treatment is rarely clear. The three forms of treatment available—surgery, chemotherapy and radiotherapy are associated with psychiatric morbidity. Psychiatric morbidity associated with cancer therapies range from 18 to 40%.[48]

Due to Surgery

Surgery often generates fear of the procedure and grief over the lost body parts. Mastectomy is the surgical treatment which has been studied extensively. Anxiety, depression and sexual problems were found in a 'substantial minority' of patients who had undergone this treatment.[36,48] In the study conducted by Maguire et al.[36] women with breast cancer were followed up for 1 year after the surgery. The anxiety symptoms noted were persistent tension, inability to relax, palpitations and panic attacks. Roughly one-third of the patients had sexual problems. They had either stopped intercourse or ceased to enjoy it. Husbands of mastectomy patients also reported sexuality and intimacy as the severely affected areas following the surgery.[35]

Other problems reported in this area were disturbances in the body-image and a feeling of personal inadequacy.[48] Ray[49] reported the persistence of concerns regarding disfigurement for several years after the surgery. Subsequent studies except one[50] confirmed these findings. Though the initial reports blamed mastectomy as the sole cause of the psychiatric morbidity, later studies comparing the psychiatric morbidity of mastectomy patients with patients who had breast conservative surgery revealed that breast conservation did not categorically eliminate psychiatric problems.[51] Anxiety levels, in fact, were found to be a little higher among patients who underwent conservative surgery in the recovery phase. Mastectomy group was different only in the negative body image and experienced more intense and persistent negative feelings about their bodies. Colostomy, laryngectomy and hysterectomy are the other surgical treatments studied in this respect. Colostomy patients have significantly more depression, sexual dysfunctions and other social problems than patients undergoing bowel resection without colostomy.[52,53] Depression, anxiety and disturbances in familial and social relationships have been noted as main problems in laryngectomy patients.[54,55] In a comparison of pre-operative and post-operative laryngeal and oral cancers in India,[55,56] concerns about disease and treatment significantly reduced following laryngectomy, but the concerns about speech and communication were reported by 76% of laryngectomees following surgery. These were then attended to by the speech therapist. Mastectomy, permanent colostomy, maxillofacial surgery and hysterectomy have also been studied well and reported to produce immense psychological impact on patients, like depressive illness, psychosexual problems and social problems (isolation, loneliness, decreased social visits), drinking, and occasionally suicide.

Due to Radiotherapy

Radiation treatment (RT) is associated with highly unpleasant side effects. The side effects include nausea, vomiting and increasing fatigue. A prospective study of patients receiving radiotherapy had shown significant psychiatric problems in first 3 months.[57] Different authors have tried to correlate the psychiatric problems to the common side effects of Radiotherapy.[58] The unpleasant fatigue usually seen in radiotherapy patients had a high correlation with psychiatric morbidity. Radiotherapy has also been reported to cause nausea, a peculiar denerving kind of fatigue, poor psychosocial adjustment, unrealistic expectation about the outcome and non-engagement with the physician.[7] In an prospective study on levels of anxiety and depression in patients receiving radiation treatment in a cancer hospital in India,[59] anxiety and depressive disorders were detected frequently both prior to treatment and later during follow-up. Frequency of anxiety increased significantly after initiating RT, but later reduced during follow-up assessments after a few months.

Due to Chemotherapy

In some of the neoplastic disorders like Wilm's tumor or Hodgkin's disease chemotherapy produces dramatic improvement. But, most often prolongation of life is achieved at the cost of quality of life (QOL). Most of the studies in this area, which judge outcome solely on the basis of survival ignore QOL and psychiatric morbidity. This is a reflected in the result of study which reported the quality of lives of patients receiving multiple chemotherapeutic drugs as unsatisfactory.[60] The psychiatric morbidity related to chemotherapy has been studied extensively in patients with breast cancer. Adjuvant chemotherapy in mastectomy patients was found to be associated with a significant increase in the incidence of depression, anxiety and sexual problems.[61] Hughson[61] found that chemotherapy in patients with breast cancer was associated with greater psychiatric morbidity than radiotherapy. However, in another study,[62] the overall level of psychological distress did not significantly correlate with the physical side effects of treatment. Silberfarb et al.[63] studied two groups of patients with small cell carcinoma of lung receiving different chemotherapeutic agents and found that patients receiving vinca alkaloids had a higher incidence of psychiatric problems. All chemotherapeutic agents can produce organic mental syndromes.

Chemotherapy can produce nausea and vomiting as immediate effects. Though various chemotherapeutic agents vary in this emetogenic potency, almost all have side effects. After an initial episode of nausea and vomiting 15 to 65% of patients develop anticipatory nausea and vomiting.[1] Sometimes, it becomes so severe that they cannot continue treatment. Patients may also develop a conditioned response when exposed to sights and smells reminiscent of chemotherapy experience. Lung cancer patients receiving palliative chemotherapy were found to have fewer depression and communication problems than those receiving no treatment at all.[64] In this case chemotherapy may promote a feeling of optimism. Maguire et al.[65] noted that chemotherapy caused fatigue, nausea and irritability along with adverse effects on the family and/or sexual life. Vinca alkaloids are especially known to cause depression.

PSYCHIATRIC MORBIDITY IN ADVANCED CANCER

Advanced cancer is associated with increased psychiatric morbidity for mainly three reasons:

1. Physical symptoms like pain, nausea, vomiting, and weakness cause emotional distress.
2. Fear of death produces severe emotional distress.
3. Disease process or its spread and metastasis may directly produce psychiatric problems.

In active and advancing disease physical problems become more significant. Bukberg et al.[11] found that depression was associated with increasing levels of physical disability. Cancer pain which becomes severe in advanced stage has concomitant psychiatric morbidity.[66] In the advanced stage of disease the patient is usually aware of the progressive and irreversible nature of cancer. Fear is a common reaction during this stage. Patients are preoccupied with fear of abandonment by doctors, fear of loss of composure, bodily function and dignity and above all fear of death. In addition, the disease process also produces psychiatric problems directly. Brain metastasis can cause clinical symptoms in 10 to 15 % of cases. Lung, breast, kidney and testis are the common primary sites. Non-metastatic neurological complications are also not uncommon. Cancer related medical problems like metabolic encephalopathy, infection, electrolyte imbalances can also produce psychiatric problems like delirium and other organic mental syndromes.

PEDIATRIC MALIGNANCY

Pediatric malignancies often pose special problems. Children often exhibit behavior problems in response to the illness and treatment. Many parents react to the diagnosis with shock.[67,68] Anxiety, grief, hostility, anger, guilt and disbelief are other responses which may be observed in parents. Despite the improvement in medical outlook, most parents display practically identical responses to the diagnosis of cancer,[69,70] implying that for most parents a diagnosis of cancer in their child is still inextricably connected with death.

For parents, learning the diagnosis is the first serious confrontation with the potential death of their child. The initial parental reactions to the diagnosis have a striking resemblance with the emotional and behavioral effects of normal grief at or after the death of a loved one. The term 'anticipatory mourning' is introduced to refer to parental reactions of mourning and grief prior to the final loss. Viewed from the parental perspective, it is generally assumed that anticipatory mourning serves as an adaptive function in case the child dies because the parent relinquishes the attachment to the dying child over time.[71] Parents who had difficulties in accepting the fatal prognosis and as a consequence failed to mourn in anticipation found no relief after the death of the child.[72] From the child's perspective the parental anticipatory mourning can be destructive for the relationship between parents and child. This has been noted in those instances in which the child who was realistically mourned for, lived on.[73] When the child is clinically doing well, the immediate threat of loss becomes remote and parents move from a state of anticipatory mourning to an increased hope for cure. With continued remission, affirmation of life becomes stronger, and most parents whose child was in remission expressed few difficulties and returned to normal life.[74] However, when the child relapses the threat of loss becomes real and the process of anticipatory mourning is relived.[75] Parents find the first relapse worse than the initial diagnosis. Although parents continue to hope, their hope narrows with the progression of disease, finally converging in living on a day-to-day basis.[75]

Instruments Used to Assess for Psychiatric Comorbidity

1. Confusion assessment method[76]—can be used for assessment of delirium in cancer patients.
2. Beck depression inventory[77]—stresses more on mood and cognitive symptoms of depression.
3. Montgomery-Asberg depression rating scale[78]—useful to assess depression in the context of medical illness.
4. Hospital anxiety and depression scale[79]—excludes somatic symptoms of the illness.
5. State-trait anxiety inventory[80]—useful as a screening instrument.
6. General health questionnaire[81]—excludes somatic symptoms of the illness and also useful for screening.
7. Edinburgh depression scale[82]—has been validated to assess for depression in palliative care settings.
8. The coping and concerns checklist[56,83]—has been used to detect common physical and psychosocial problems in patients with cancer.

STRESS-CANCER LINK

A significant association between stressors and progression of cancer has been observed. Studies have found increased stressful life events in the year before the diagnosis of breast cancer and malignant melanoma.[84,85] In breast cancer, stressful events like bereavement, loss of a job were also associated with relapse.[86]

Stress can lead to immunosuppression and increased substance use, which in turn can lead to cancer. It can lead to a decreased ability to repair damaged DNA,[87] thus contributing to tumor formation. Neuroendocrine effects of stress might predispose to tumor progression. Stress hormones can suppress body's natural immune resistance to tumors. Tumor cells might also become more resistant to catabolic actions of cortisol, leading to shunting of more energy toward tumor cells.[88] An association between elevation of glucocorticoids and more rapid tumor growth has been found in animal models.[89]

Depressive symptoms are associated with reduced WBC as well as NK cell counts,[90] and reduced NK cell cytotoxicity.[91] However, inflammatory activation, produced by either cancer or with treatment also predisposes to depression. Raised IL-6 levels have been observed in cancer patients who have depression as compared to those who do not.[92]

Depression leads to a higher 24-hour mean cortisol and a flattened circadian cortisol rhythm. Circadian rhythm of cortisol is also disrupted in breast and ovarian tumors, which is associated with earlier mortality among metastatic breast cancer patients. There is evidence that psychotherapy normalizes cortisol levels. In two separate studies, experiential-existential group therapy[93] and CBT[94] were found to lower cortisol levels in breast cancer patients.

Thus, the link between depression, stress and cancer iss being understood better and soon, this knowledge might have clinical applications in the form of effective treatments for both cancer and depression that target the immune cascade.

Cancer and the Mental Health Professional

"Please don't tell me you know just how I feel—you don't." —Shirley Corder, *Strength Renewed: Meditations for Your Journey Through Breast Cancer.*

Most studies have found the oncologists' ability to detect psychological distress far from satisfactory. This could be due to various reasons. First, the current medical undergraduate and postgraduate training in India does not focus on communication skills and does not equip one to probe into psychological issues when patients express concerns. Second, most of the patient's concerns are taken as a natural reaction to the diagnosis of cancer, which might not always be true. Thirdly, the oncologists themselves work in a very stressful, difficult and physically and emotionally taxing environment where too less doctors see too many patients. This makes it difficult for them to do an in-depth assessment when they encounter psychological issues. Also neurovegetative symptoms of depression are most often, present due to cancer, and hence missed. Identification of psychiatric problems, therefore, is a very necessary prerequisite to their management. Nursing staff in oncology can therefore play a key role in identification of mental health problems, and can then refer patients for further management.

The first and foremost kind of communication skills that medical and paramedical professionals in the field should be armed with is the skill of breaking bad news in a manner that is sensitive, conveys the appropriate information, and imparts a sense of hope in a realistic manner.[95]

Guidelines for breaking bad news

1. Breaking bad news starts with asking questions and assessing the patient's and family's readiness to grasp the information that is being conveyed.
2. An appropriate setting and privacy needs to be ensured.
3. Next, one should find out how much the patient already knows and whether they want any or more information.
4. After making sure that the patient is ready, the session should progress in a way that patient and family have a sense of control over the quantity of new information that is being received.
5. A 'warning shot' or an indication needs to be given at this stage, that something serious has happened, after which information is provided in steps.
6. After informing the diagnosis, it is important to pause, and acknowledge that the news could have shocked or distressed the person.
7. Further concerns or queries are explored and discussed and ventilation is facilitated.
8. Session is summarized and availability for a further session is emphasized.

Collusion in Psycho-oncology

Collusion in health care refers to withholding or not sharing important information on certain aspects of medical diagnosis/investigations with patients/relatives. Collusion may be two-sided. It may be manifested as family members not wanting the health care professional to share some information with the patient, or also they may themselves not share information with the health care team. It may be partial or complete. The 'recovery plot' that is often followed by patients and relatives involves focusing mainly on treatment and recovery, while ignoring issues such as risk of relapses and recurrences, long term prognosis, pain, disability and death. Physicians also unwittingly find themselves becoming a part of this, when it is referred to as 'medical activism.[96] Collusion is also affected by gender and age of the patient and cultural factors. Most western cultures respect autonomy and independence as opposed to Indian culture which is paternalistic and frequent demands from relatives to protect the patient are common. Therefore, collusion manifests differently depending on the sociocultural milieu.

Handling Collusion[96]

1. Acknowledge that collusion exists
2. Identify the same
3. Explore and validate the reasons for collusion, most common one being wanting to protect the patient from distress.
4. Establish the potential emotional and psychological cost of collusion. Once detected, it can lead to mistrust, anger, distress and a sense of having been betrayed. Patient might find it difficult to trust family and treating team further as they may become unsure of what else is being hidden from them. It thus also hinders a healthy therapeutic alliance.
5. The next step is to establish a contract with the relatives that there is no intention of disclosing anything to the patient without the relatives' explicit consent.
6. Explore patient's awareness of the seriousness of his/her medical condition, which is usually underestimated by relatives. In fact, most of the times patients are well aware of their health condition.
7. Assess patient's and relatives' feelings periodically.
8. Pace of handling collusion should be acceptable and tolerable and health professionals should make themselves available whenever needed.
9. Assess for grief, distress and depression and handle them.

Caregiver Burden

A diagnosis of cancer and its subsequent course is a significant stressful life event not only for the patient, but also close relatives of the person. There is recent mounting evidence that highlights the importance of specific psychosocial interventions not only for the patients, but carers as well in order to cope with burden, end-of-life issues and anxiety. Religion, spiritual practices like having faith and trying to find meaning in the caregiving experience, religious and community support are factors that help in coping and positive psychological adjustment among caregivers. Cognitive behavior group therapy[97] and caregiver sleep intervention (CASI)[98] are some specific forms of psychotherapeutic intervention that have been found useful in caregivers.

Palliative and End-of-life Care

In terminally ill patients, confronting the fear of death and death itself is a challenge. And guiding people through this process is a challenge in itself that psycho-oncologists face. It is not just about addressing physical, medical and mental health concerns, but going beyond that and addressing larger issues such as existential concerns, spiritual and religious issues at the end of life.

The word palliation has its roots in the latin word *'palliare'* which means 'to conceal.' This implies that though a dying patient cannot be cured, his suffering can be concealed. According to WHO (2009), palliation is best done in an interdisciplinary team approach and should aim at pain relief, affirmation of dying as a normal process, offering support to patients and families to cope and enhancing quality of life. Answering questions about life and death, coping with grief and spiritual issues also acquire a whole new dimension toward the end-of-life.[56]

Physicians are faced with a lot of ethical and moral dilemmas as patients make requests and even demands for assisted suicide or euthanasia. Psycho-oncologists, at the outset need to be aware of the fact that this could be a manifestation of untreated depression, which should be treated promptly in such cases. A syndrome of demoralization is distinct from depression and consists of a triad of loss of meaning, hopelessness and desire for death.[99] The desire for hastened death (DHD) also arises because of loss of dignity, autonomy and a sense of powerlessness.

The entire topic is fraught with controversies between the medical fraternity and legal system as well as within the fraternity. Some countries have legalized euthanasia. However, regardless of one's moral or ethical stance or laws of the land, a desire for death should be explored from various vantage points, depression and demoralization should be assessed for and ameliorative measures like pain relief, attempts to enhance quality of life should be instituted.

Pharmacotherapy

Haloperidol has emerged as the most effective medication for managing delirium toward the end-of-life. Pain relief and management acquire a lot of importance in palliative care settings as the focus is on symptom relief. Depression and anxiety can be treated symptomatically.

Psychotherapy

Existential therapies help the patient try to make sense of and find meaning in their adverse experiences. Viktor Frankl's logotherapy is one such approach. Another kind of existential therapy is the use of life narrative. In this method, past coping skills and strengths are highlighted and the physical illness is understood as a part of the larger canvass of life. Life review is a similar method which uses various techniques like story-telling, constructing family tree, reminiscing to promote a dignified acceptance of death. Meaning center therapy and dignity therapy has also been used in this group. Dignity therapy, a brief empirically based structured psychotherapy that addresses pride, maintaining dignity and continuity can also be used to address end-of-life concerns.[100]

GENERAL PRINCIPLES OF MANAGEMENT

Cancer is a word, not a sentence.

—John Diamond

Medications

It is very important to take into account potential drug-drug interactions while prescribing psychotropic medications. Prescribing psychotropic is complicated by a plethora of factors such as multiple medications these patients are on including anti-cancer, hypoglycemic agents, analgesics and drugs for comorbid cardiac, hepatic or renal conditions. It is also prudent to keep in mind factors such as cancer cachexia, extremes of age, varied nutritional states, differences in drug metabolism, comorbid substance abuse, debilitation and malnutrition.[101] A temporal correlation between the starting of a particular drug and the beginning of an adverse effect guards a clinician against a possible drug-drug interaction. Some strategies to lessen interactions include choosing a psychotropic with a profile that is least likely to interfere with concurrent medications, reducing the dose of the offending agent, therapeutic drug monitoring and monitoring for adverse effects.

Psychotherapy

Having a life changing diagnosis is not something one is prepared for by life. Being diagnosed with cancer can lead to intense disease and death related dysphoria and anxiety, so much so that a person can feel punished, estranged and isolated. Faced with the ultimate existential concern of death, cancer patients are in the throes of a spiritual and existential crisis right from the time of diagnosis. However, most of the current oncology practice does not focus on helping a person find meaning of the experience, resolve existential concerns, enhance social support and process their emotions. Finding meaning in the experience, making the most of life that is left and relinquishing control over things that cannot be controlled are some positive coping strategies that can be employed. Suppression of emotional expression and avoidance are found to hinder coping with cancer.

Psychological interventions with its emphasis on fostering a positive attitude, helping the patients to comply and cope with the treatment and reducing emotional distress, can in fact compliment the traditional medical treatment. Many of the patients who suffer from cancer related psychiatric problems do not receive any professional help because physicians rarely ask patients about their emotional well-being, and patients are reluctant to disclose their distress.

The types of psychological interventions used in cancer patients are many and diverse, like behavior therapy, cognitive therapy and supportive therapy. The aims of the psychological interventions are: (1) To reduce anxiety, depression and other emotional distresses. (2) To improve the mental adjustment to cancer by imparting a positive attitude. (3) To promote a sense of personal control over cancer and its treatment. (4) To improve patients communications with the spouse or other family members. (5) To encourage the open expression of emotions.

During psychological intervention for cancer related problems, it should be acknowledged that a cancer patient, after all, is a psychologically normal individual under severe stress. Hence, the therapy should be brief and directed toward current problems. There should be also be an active attempt to identify and make use of the personal strengths.

Supportive Therapy

Supportive therapy can be done in individual as well as group setting.

Individual supportive therapy: Here one to one setting helps to develop a relationship of trust so that patient can talk freely. Efforts should be made to reduce denial but maintain hope. Meaningful activities should be encouraged for as long as possible. Simply listening, understanding and sometimes just sitting quietly with the patient were also described as elements of therapy.

Group supportive therapy: Support groups are frequently employed in psychosocial intervention to provide emotional support. Groups of cancer patients, recovered cancer patients, those who have undergone surgery, chemotherapy or radiotherapy, spouses, or family members can be very effective in alleviating distress among participants. Obviously, groups are not the answer for every cancer patient, at the same time there is some evidence to suggest that support groups are associated with better psychosocial adjustment to cancer in some.

The two main functions of supportive therapy are emotional support and provision of information regarding the disease and its treatment. The stress of having cancer and the mode of its treatment create the need for emotional support. The patients also need clear, unambiguous information about the disease and its treatment which should be imparted sensitively.

Both group and individual psychotherapy have been found to have positive effects on depression and anxiety and have also been found in some studies to prolong survival. Supportive-expressive group therapy (SEGT) improved QOL in women with breast cancer, though it did not prolong survival over long-term follow-ups.[102]

Counseling: During counseling the cancer patient, the therapist should be on a look out for 'cues' of emotional distress which are likely to be given out by the patient. The aim is to optimize patient to disclose his distress or facilitate emotional expression. The counseling sessions may achieve three levels. First, in which the patient will give a lot of information about the physical condition, physical symptoms, family or other issues, but not anything about emotions. Second, in which the patient besides giving information about physical aspects may talk about emotional distress, but would not express or show the feelings. The third level, would have not only information about physical and psychological aspects, but it would also have the expression of emotional distress. The therapist should attempt to achieve this third level to be effective in his role.

In patients who have difficulty in expressing the emotions visual imagery or role play may be useful. Ventilation is an effective way of relief when the emotion is elicited. If the emotional expression is maladaptive, it should either be channelized to a positive action or the patient should be taught a safe way of expressing it.

Effectiveness of Psychological Intervention

Patients with early or treatable cancers are different from those with terminal disease and hence it is convenient to discuss the effectiveness of these two groups of patients separately. Regarding patients with early cancer, Weisman et al.[103] reported that patients who received psychological treatment had a better outcome than the untreated control subjects. Both kinds of psychological treatment, the consultation therapy and cognitive skills training were found to be equally effective.

The assumption that all cancer patients need therapy and that any type of therapy is better than no therapy is unjustified. Some patients may actually do worse in treatment than they would have without psychotherapeutic intervention. Worden and Weisman[104] described the three approaches that have been used in this regard. The first advocates providing treatment for everyone. The second suggests waiting to see who gets into serious emotional difficulties before treatment is offered, whereas the third attempts to identify those at high risk and implement preventive measures. They have suggested that high risk patients can be identified by mood, vulnerability, concerns about self and others and problem is coping.

In conclusion, psychiatric oncology has made numerous advances in the understanding of psychiatric disturbances, and care of cancer patients. There have been advances in psychoneuroimmunology, internet and phone based therapies for cancer patients and assessment and addressal of spirituality at the end-of-life. Medical education needs to be tailored to impart communication skills to medical graduates as well as post-graduates specializing in oncology. More randomised and controlled studies in the area are required, with longer follow-up periods and larger samples.

REFERENCES

1. Lederberg MS, Holland JC. Psycho-oncology in Comprehensive Textbook of Psychiatry London: Williams and Wilkins; 1989.
2. Derogatis LR, Morrow GR, Fetting J, Penman D, Piasetsky S, Schmale AM, et al. The prevalence of psychiatric disorders among cancer patients. JAMA. 1983;249(6):751-7.
3. Chaturvedi SK, Chandra P, Channabasavanna SM. Detection of anxiety and depression in cancer patients. NIMHANS Journal. 1994;12:141-4.
4. Mehnert A, Vehling S, Scheffold K, Ladehoff N, Schon G, Wegscheider K, et al. [Prevalence of Adjustment Disorder, Acute and Posttraumatic Stress Disorders as well as Somatoform Disorders in Cancer Patients.] Psychother Psychosom Med Psychol; 2013.
5. Sellick SM, Crooks DL. Depression and cancer: an appraisal of the literature for prevalence, detection, and practice guideline development for psychological interventions. Psycho-oncology. 1999;8(4):315-33.
6. Fallowfield L, Ratcliffe D, Jenkins V, Saul J. Psychiatric morbidity and its recognition by doctors in patients with cancer. Br J Cancer. 2001;84(8):1011-5.
7. Hughes J. Emotional reactions to the diagnosis and treatment of early breast cancer. J Psychosom Res. 1982;26(2):277-83.
8. Naysmith A, Hinton JM, Meredith R, Marks MD, Berry RJ. Surviving malignant disease. Psychological and family aspects. Br J Hosp Med. 1983;30(1):22, 6-7.
9. Kent S, Bluthe RM, Kelley KW, Dantzer R. Sickness behavior as a new target for drug development. Trends Pharmacol Sci. 1992;13(1):24-8.
10. Raison CL, Miller AH. Depression in cancer: new developments regarding diagnosis and treatment. Biol Psychiatry. 2003;54(3): 283-94.

11. Bukberg J, Penman D, Holland JC. Depression in hospitalized cancer patients. Psychosom Med. 1984;46(3):199-212.
12. Cohen-Cole SA, Brown FW, McDaniel JS. Diagnostic assessment of depression in the medically ill. New York: Oxford University Press; 1993.
13. McDaniel JS, Musselman DL, Porter MR, Reed DA, Nemeroff CB. Depression in patients with cancer. Diagnosis, biology, and treatment. Arch Gen Psychiatry. 1995;52(2):89-99.
14. Capuron L, Ravaud A, Dantzer R. Timing and specificity of the cognitive changes induced by interleukin-2 and interferon-alpha treatments in cancer patients. Psychosom Med. 2001;63(3):376-86.
15. Zebrack BJ, Zeltzer LK, Whitton J, Mertens AC, Odom L, Berkow R, et al. Psychological outcomes in long-term survivors of childhood leukemia, Hodgkin's disease, and non-Hodgkin's lymphoma: a report from the Childhood Cancer Survivor Study. Pediatrics. 2002;110(1 Pt 1):42-52.
16. Omne-Ponten M, Holmberg L, Burns T, Adami HO, Bergstrom R. Determinants of the psycho-social outcome after operation for breast cancer. Results of a prospective comparative interview study following mastectomy and breast conservation Psychosocial adjustment after mastectomy and breast-conserving treatment. Eur J Cancer. 1992;28A(6-7):1062-7.
17. Jakeways MS, Mitchell V, Hashim IA, Chadwick SJ, Shenkin A, Green CJ, et al. Metabolic and inflammatory responses after open or laparoscopic cholecystectomy. Br J Surg. 1994;81(1):127-31.
18. Pirl WF, Roth AJ. Diagnosis and treatment of depression in cancer patients. Oncology (Williston Park). 1999;13(9):1293-301; discussion 301-2, 305-6.
19. Stommel M, Given BA, Given CW. Depression and functional status as predictors of death among cancer patients. Cancer. 2002;94(10):2719-27.
20. Holland JC, Romano SJ, Heiligenstein JH, Tepner RG, Wilson MG. A controlled trial of fluoxetine and desipramine in depressed women with advanced cancer. Psychooncology. 1998;7(4):291-300.
21. Pezzella G, Moslinger-Gehmayr R, Contu A. Treatment of depression in patients with breast cancer: a comparison between paroxetine and amitriptyline. Breast Cancer Res Treat. 2001;70(1):1-10.
22. van Heeringen K, Zivkov M. Pharmacological treatment of depression in cancer patients. A placebo-controlled study of mianserin. Br J Psychiatry. 1996;169(4):440-3.
23. Theobald DE, Kirsh KL, Holtsclaw E, Donaghy K, Passik SD. An open-label, crossover trial of mirtazapine (15 and 30 mg) in cancer patients with pain and other distressing symptoms. J Pain Symptom Manage. 2002;23(5):442-7.
24. Kast RE. Mirtazapine may be useful in treating nausea and insomnia of cancer chemotherapy. Support Care Cancer. 2001;9(6):469-70.
25. Loprinzi CL, Sloan JA, Perez EA, Quella SK, Stella PJ, Mailliard JA, et al. Phase III evaluation of fluoxetine for treatment of hot flashes. J Clin Oncol. 2002;20(6):1578-83.
26. Stearns V, Isaacs C, Rowland J, Crawford J, Ellis MJ, Kramer R, et al. A pilot trial assessing the efficacy of paroxetine hydrochloride (Paxil) in controlling hot flashes in breast cancer survivors. Ann Oncol. 2000;11(1):17-22.
27. Loprinzi CL, Kugler JW, Sloan JA, Mailliard JA, LaVasseur BI, Barton DL, et al. Venlafaxine in management of hot flashes in survivors of breast cancer: a randomised controlled trial. Lancet. 2000;356(9247):2059-63.
28. Chaturvedi SK, Peter Maguire G, Somashekar BS. Somatization in cancer. Int Rev Psychiatry. 2006;18(1):49-54.
29. Chaturvedi SK, Uchitomi Y. Psychosocial and Psychiatric Disorders. Clinical Psycho-Oncology: An international perspective; 2012.pp.55-69.
30. Stark DP, House A. Anxiety in cancer patients. Br J Cancer. 2000;83(10):1261-7.
31. Redeker NS, Lev EL, Ruggiero J. Insomnia, fatigue, anxiety, depression, and quality of life of cancer patients undergoing chemotherapy. Sch Inq Nurs Pract. 2000 Winter;14(4):275-90; discussion 91-8.
32. Cameron LD, Leventhal H, Love RR. Trait anxiety, symptom perceptions, and illness-related responses among women with breast cancer in remission during a tamoxifen clinical trial. Health Psychol. 1998;17(5):459-69.
33. Thomas SF, Glynne-Jones R, Chait I, Marks DF. Anxiety in long-term cancer survivors influences the acceptability of planned discharge from follow-up. Psychooncology. 1997;6(3):190-6.
34. Henderson VP, Massion AO, Clemow L, Hurley TG, Druker S, Hebert JR. A randomized controlled trial of mindfulness-based stress reduction for women with early-stage breast cancer receiving radiotherapy. Integr Cancer Ther. 2013;12(5):404-13.
35. Wellisch DK, Jamison KR, Pasnau RO. Psychosocial aspects of mastectomy: II. the man's perspective. Am J Psychiatry. 1978;135(5):543-6.
36. Maguire GP, Lee EG, Bevington DJ, Kuchemann CS, Crabtree RJ, Cornell CE. Psychiatric problems in the first year after mastectomy. Br Med J. 1978;1(6118):963-5.
37. Andersen BL. Sexual functioning morbidity among cancer survivors. Current status and future research directions. Cancer. 1985;55(8):1835-42.
38. Auchincloss SS. Evaluation and management of sexual dysfunction in cancer patients. Current Concepts in Psycho Oncology and AIDS: Memorial Sloan Kettering Cancer Centre; 1987.pp.183-90.
39. Andersen BL, Woods XA, Copeland LJ. Sexual self-schema and sexual morbidity among gynecologic cancer survivors. J Consult Clin Psychol. 1997;65(2):221-9.
40. Anderson BL, Schmuch G. Sexuality and cancer. Atlanta, GA: The Society: American Cancer Society textbook of clinical oncology; 1991.pp.606-16.
41. De Simone GG. Palliation of Pancreatic Cancer. Progress in Pall Care. 1994;2:126-31.
42. Silberfarb PM, Hauri PJ, Oxman TE, Schnurr P. Assessment of sleep in patients with lung cancer and breast cancer. J Clin Oncol. 1993;11(5):997-1004.

43. Ingle RJ, Burish TG, Wallston KA. Conditionability of cancer chemotherapy patients. Oncol Nurs Forum. 1984;11(4):97-102.
44. Burish TG, Carey MP, Krozely MG, Greco FA. Conditioned side effects induced by cancer chemotherapy: prevention through behavioral treatment. J Consult Clin Psychol. 1987;55(1):42-8.
45. Temoshok L. Personality, coping style, emotion and cancer: towards an integrative model. Cancer Surv. 1987;6(3):545-67.
46. Shaffer JW, Graves PL, Swank RT, Pearson TA. Clustering of personality traits in youth and the subsequent development of cancer among physicians. J Behav Med. 1987;10(5):441-7.
47. Wellisch DK, Yager J. Is there a cancer-prone personality? CA Cancer J Clin. 1983;33(3):145-53.
48. Morris T, Greer HS, White P. Psychological and social adjustment to mastectomy: a two-year follow-up study. Cancer. 1977;40(5):2381-7.
49. Ray C. Adjustment to Mastectomy: The Psychological impact of disfigurement. Baltimore, Md: University Park Press; 1978.
50. Battersby C, Armstrong J, Abrahams M. Mastectomy in a large public hospital. Aust NZJ Surg. 1978;48(4):401-4.
51. Schain WS, d'Angelo TM, Dunn ME, Lichter AS, Pierce LJ. Mastectomy versus conservative surgery and radiation therapy. Psychosocial consequences. Cancer. 1994;73(4):1221-8.
52. Devlin HB, Plant JA, Griffin M. Aftermath of surgery for anorectal cancer. Br Med J. 1971;3(5771):413-8.
53. Wirsching M, Druner HU, Herrmann G. Results of psychosocial adjustment to long-term colostomy. Psychother Psychosom. 1975;26(5):245-56.
54. Barton RT. Life after laryngectomy. Laryngoscope. 1965;75(9): 1408-15.
55. Chaturvedi SK, Prasad KMR, Senthilnathan SM, Shenoy A, BS PK. Quality of life of Oral Cancer Patients. New Delhi: MacMillan India, Ltd; 1996.
56. Chaturvedi SK, Shenoy A, Prasad KM, Senthilnathan SM, Premlatha BS. Concerns, coping and quality of life in head and neck cancer patients. Support Care Cancer. 1996;4(3): 186-90.
57. Schmale AH, Morrow GR, Davis A, Illies E, McNally J, Wright G, et al. Pretreatment behavioral profiles associated with subsequent psychosocial adjustment in radiation therapy patients: a prospective study. Int J Psychiatry Med. 1982;12(3):187-95.
58. Holland JC, Rowland J, Lebovits RA. Reaction to cancer treatment. Assessment of emotional response to adjuvant radiotherapy as a guide to planned intervention. Psychiatric Clinics of North America. 1979;2:347-58.
59. Chaturvedi SK, Chandra PS, Channabasavanna SM, Anantha N, Reddy BKM, SS. Levels of anxiety and depression in patients receiving radiotherapy in India. Psycho-Oncology 1996;5:343-6.
60. Morrison JM. The West Midlands co-operative trial of adjuvant chemotherapy for operable breast cancer. Cancer Treat Rev. 1979;6 Suppl:87-90.
61. Hughson AVM, Cooper AF, McArdle CS, Russel AR, Smith DC. Psychiatric morbidity in disease free survivors following radiotherapy and adjuvant chemotherapy for breast cancer: A two year follow up study. British Journal of Surgery. 1980;67:370-6.
62. Meyerowitz BE, Sparks FC, Spears IK. Adjuvant chemotherapy for breast carcinoma: psychosocial implications. Cancer. 1979;43(5):1613-8.
63. Silberfarb PM, Holland JC, Anbar D, Bahna G, Maurer LH, Chahinian AP, et al. Psychological response of patients receiving two drug regimens for lung carcinoma. Am J Psychiatry. 1983;140(1):110-1.
64. Hughes JE. Depressive illness and lung cancer. II. Follow-up of inoperable patients. Eur J Surg Oncol. 1985;11(1):21-4.
65. Maguire GP, Tait A, Brooke M, Thomas C, Howat JM, Sellwood RA, et al. Psychiatric morbidity and physical toxicity associated with adjuvant chemotherapy after mastectomy. Br Med J. 1980;281(6249):1179-80.
66. Chaturvedi S. Psychiatric aspects of pain in cancer patients. Indian Journal of Pain. 1985;1:42-5.
67. Binger CM, Ablin AR, Feuerstein RC, Kushner JH, Zoger S, Mikkelsen C. Childhood leukemia. Emotional impact on patient and family. N Engl J Med. 1969;280(8):414-8.
68. Lansky SB. Childhood leukemia. The child psychiatrist as a member of the oncology team. J Am Acad Child Psychiatry. 1974 Summer;13(3):499-508.
69. Johnson FL, Rudolph LA, Hartmann JR. Helping the family cope with childhood cancer. Psychosomatics. 1979;20(4):241, 5-7, 51.
70. Kagen-Goodheart L. Reentry: living with childhood cancer. Am J Orthopsychiatry. 1977;47(4):651-B.
71. Lowenberg JS. The coping behaviors of fatally ill adolescents and their parents. Nurs Forum. 1970;9(3):269-87.
72. Townes BD, Wold DA, Holmes TH. Parental adjustment to childhood leukemia. J Psychosom Res. 1974;18(1):9-14.
73. Naylor A. Premature mourning and failure to mourn: their relationship to conflict between mothers and intellectually normal children. Am J Orthopsychiatry. 1982;52(4):679-87.
74. Kupst MJ, Schulman JL, Honig G, Maurer H, Morgan E, Fochtman D. Family coping with childhood leukemia: one year after diagnosis. J Pediatr Psychol. 1982;7(2):157-74.
75. Friedman SB, Chodoff P, Mason JW, Hamburg DA. Behavioral Observations on Parents Anticipating the Death of a Child. Pediatrics. 1963;32:610-25.
76. Inouye SK, van Dyck CH, Alessi CA, Balkin S, Siegal AP, Horwitz RI. Clarifying confusion: the confusion assessment method. A new method for detection of delirium. Ann Intern Med. 1990;113(12):941-8.
77. Steer RA, Ball R, Ranieri WF, Beck AT. Dimensions of the Beck Depression Inventory-II in clinically depressed outpatients. J Clin Psychol. 1999;55(1):117-28.
78. Montgomery SA, Asberg M. A new depression scale designed to be sensitive to change. Br J Psychiatry. 1979;134:382-9.

79. Zigmond AS, Snaith RP. The hospital anxiety and depression scale. Acta Psychiatr Scand. 1983;67(6):361-70.
80. Spielberger C. The Manual for the State-Trait Anxiety Inventory. Palo Alto : Consulting Psychological Press. 1983.
81. Goldberg DP, Gater R, Sartorius N, Ustun TB, Piccinelli M, Gureje O, et al. The validity of two versions of the GHQ in the WHO study of mental illness in general health care. Psychol Med. 1997;27(1):191-7.
82. Lloyd-Williams M, Shiels C, Dowrick C. The development of the Brief Edinburgh Depression Scale (BEDS) to screen for depression in patients with advanced cancer. J Affect Disord. 2007;99(1-3):259-64.
83. Chaturvedi SK. Exploration of concerns and role of psychosocial intervention in palliative care--a study from India. Ann Acad Med Singapore. 1994;23(2):256-60.
84. Geyer S. Life events, chronic difficulties and vulnerability factors preceding breast cancer. Soc Sci Med. 1993;37(12):1545-55.
85. Havlik RJ, Vukasin AP, Ariyan S. The impact of stress on the clinical presentation of melanoma. Plast Reconstr Surg. 1992;90(1):57-61; discussion 2-4.
86. Ramirez AJ, Craig TK, Watson JP, Fentiman IS, North WR, Rubens RD. Stress and relapse of breast cancer. BMJ. 1989; 298(6669):291-3.
87. Kiecolt-Glaser JK, Stephens RE, Lipetz PD, Speicher CE, Glaser R. Distress and DNA repair in human lymphocytes. J Behav Med. 1985;8(4):311-20.
88. Romero LM, Raley-Susman KM, Redish DM, Brooke SM, Horner HC, Sapolsky RM. Possible mechanism by which stress accelerates growth of virally derived tumors. Proc Natl Acad Sci U S A. 1992;89(22):11084-7.
89. Rowse GJ, Weinberg J, Bellward GD, Emerman JT. Endocrine mediation of psychosocial stressor effects on mouse mammary tumor growth. Cancer Lett. 1992;65(1):85-93.
90. Andersen BL, Kiecolt-Glaser JK, Glaser R. A biobehavioral model of cancer stress and disease course. Am Psychol. 1994;49(5):389-404.
91. Andersen BL, Farrar WB, Golden-Kreutz D, Kutz LA, MacCallum R, Courtney ME, et al. Stress and immune responses after surgical treatment for regional breast cancer. J Natl Cancer Inst. 1998;90(1):30-6.
92. Musselman DL, Miller AH, Porter MR, Manatunga A, Gao F, Penna S, et al. Higher than normal plasma interleukin-6 concentrations in cancer patients with depression: preliminary findings. Am J Psychiatry. 2001;158(8):1252-7.
93. van der Pompe G, Duivenvoorden HJ, Antoni MH, Visser A, Heijnen CJ. Effectiveness of a short-term group psychotherapy program on endocrine and immune function in breast cancer patients: an exploratory study. J Psychosom Res. 1997;42(5):453-66.
94. Cruess DG, Antoni MH, McGregor BA, Kilbourn KM, Boyers AE, Alferi SM, et al. Cognitive-behavioral stress management reduces serum cortisol by enhancing benefit finding among women being treated for early stage breast cancer. Psychosom Med. 2000;62(3):304-8.
95. Chaturvedi SK, Chandra PS. Breaking bad news-Issues important for psychiatrists. Asian J Psychiatr. 2010;3(2): 87-9.
96. Chaturvedi SK, Loiselle CG, Chandra PS. Communication with relatives and collusion in palliative care: a cross-cultural perspective. Indian J Palliat Care. 2009;15(1):2-9.
97. Cohen M, Kuten A. Cognitive-behavior group intervention for relatives of cancer patients: a controlled study. J Psychosom Res. 2006;61(2):187-96.
98. Carter PA. A brief behavioral sleep intervention for family caregivers of persons with cancer. Cancer Nurs. 2006;29(2): 95-103.
99. Kissane DW, Clarke DM, Street AF. Demoralization syndrome--a relevant psychiatric diagnosis for palliative care. J Palliat Care. 2001 Spring;17(1):12-21.
100. Johns SA. Translating dignity therapy into practice: effects and lessons learned. Omega (Westport). 2013;67(1-2):135-45.
101. Kalash GR. Psychotropic drug metabolism in the cancer patient: clinical aspects of management of potential drug interactions. Psychooncology. 1998;7(4):307-20.
102. Kissane DW, Grabsch B, Clarke DM, Smith GC, Love AW, Bloch S, et al. Supportive-expressive group therapy for women with metastatic breast cancer: survival and psychosocial outcome from a randomized controlled trial. Psychooncology. 2007;16(4):277-86.
103. Weisman A, Worden W, Sobel HJ. Psychological screening and intervention with cancer patients. Massachussets General Hospital Psychiatry, Boston. 1979.
104. Worden JW, Weisman AD. Preventive psychosocial intervention with newly diagnosed cancer patients. Gen Hosp Psychiatry. 1984;6(4):243-9.

Further Reading

1. Chandra P, Chaturvedi SK, Channabasavanna SM. Lecture Notes in Psycho-oncology. NIMHANS. Bangalore, 1996.
2. Chandra PS, Chaturvedi SK (Eds). Psycho-oncology: Current Issues. NIMHANS. Bangalore, 1998.
3. Chaturvedi SK, Kumar, Satheesh. Anil Kumar. Psycho-oncology. In: JN Vyas, Niraj Ahuja (Eds). Textbook of Postgraduate Psychiatry. Jaypee Publishers, New Delhi; 1999;pp.450-64.
4. Chaturvedi SK. Psycho-oncology. In: JN Vyas, N Ahuja (Eds). Recent Advances in Psychiatry. JP Publishers, New Delhi. 1994;1:114-29.
5. Dahale A, Sivasankaran SV, Chaturvedi SK. Depression in oncology. In: Elsevier Update: Psychiatry, Dealing with Depression in Medically Ill Patients. Elsevier. New Delhi; 2012. pp.83-92.
6. Jimmie Holland, Williams Brietbart, PB Jacobsen. Handbook of Psycho-oncology, Oxford University Press, New York, 2nd edn. 2010.
7. Luigi Grassi, Michelle Riba (Eds). Clinical Psycho-Oncology: An International Perspective. Wiley Blackwell, Oxford UK, 2012.

CHAPTER

35 Dermatopsychiatric Disorders

RA Bumb, RD Mehta

INTRODUCTION

Skin has a special place in psychiatry with its responsiveness to emotional stimuli and ability to express emotions such as anger, fear, shame and frustration, and by providing self-esteem, the skin plays an important role in the socialization process, which continues from childhood to adulthood.[1] The relationship between skin and the brain exists due to more than a fact, that the brain, as the center of psychological functions, and the skin, have the same ectodermal origin and are affected by the same hormones and neurotransmitters.[2] Psychodermatology describes an interaction between dermatology and psychiatry and psychology. The incidence of psychiatric disorders among dermatological patients is estimated at about 30–60%.[3] Psychiatry is more focused on the 'internal' nonvisible disease, and dermatology is focused on the 'external' visible disease. Connecting the two disciplines is a complex interplay between neuroendocrine and immune systems that has been described as the NICS, or the neuro-immunocutaneous system. The interaction between nervous system, skin and immunity has been explained by release of mediators from NICS.[4] It has been reported that psychologic stress perturbs epidermal permeability barrier homeostasis, and it may act as precipitant for some inflammatory disorders like atopic dermatitis and psoriasis.[5] Dermatologists have stressed the need for psychiatric consultation in general, and psychological factors may be of particular concern in chronic intractable dermatologic conditions, such as eczema, prurigo and psoriasis.[6,7] Patients with psychocutaneous disorders frequently resist psychiatric referral, and the liaison among primary care physicians, psychiatrists and dermatologists can prove very useful in the management of these conditions. Thus, consideration of psychiatric and psychosocial factors is important both for the management of psychodermatologic disorders and for some aspects of secondary and tertiary prevention of a wide range of dermatologic disorders.[8] Regardless of psychiatric morbidity, skin diseases can greatly affect patients' quality of life.[9] The drugs used in the treatment of dermatological diseases such as steroid and retinoid may lead to psychiatric symptoms.[10] Not surprisingly, a relationship between psychological factors and skin diseases has long been hypothesized. There is a common opinion that many cases of skin disease are caused by psychological stress, or are related to certain personality traits, or represent a complication of a psychiatric disorder. Although the dermatologists awareness of the problem is increasing,[11] co-occurring mental disorders go often unrecognized and are believed to be less frequent than they actually are in many skin conditions. There is a need for a biopsychosocial approach to patients with skin disease.[12,13] Liaison therapy enables multidisciplinary approach with the cooperation of psychiatric and dermatologic terms and simultaneous diagnostic procedures and treatment of patients with psychodermatologic disorders.[14]

Some of the cutaneous stimuli are the basic need in mammals. Skin is the organ of touch, pain, temperature and erogenous stimulus. It has great psychological influence at all the ages. Disfiguring skin lesions influence the development of child, though the attitude of parents, teachers and school mates has a contributory influence over it. The role of dermatologist at this juncture is, in not only to explain and reassure the child but, also to extend the advice to protect the child from ill-advised interference, e.g. in the unnecessary early treatment of cavernous nevus.

As the child approaches puberty, the increased anxiety associated with disfiguring skin lesions hampers the personality development, as well as disappoints them even up to the extent of interfering with development of easy relationship with the peer group and the opposite sex. Some react in form of aggressiveness and become uncooperative, while other children turn introspective and solitary. This behavior is to be dealt with sympathy by dermatologist, taking the psychological impact of disfiguring condition over child's behavior.

It is not possible to specify and generalize the effect of such lesions because of number of factors which affect the ultimate results such as, with caring and affectionate patents and intelligent teachers, the child with disfiguring dermatological lesion may have normal psychological development with successful carrier. The picture can be just upside down with illiterate and ignorant patients and non-considerate teachers. Simultaneously, skin acts as an organ of emotional expression and site for discharge of anxiety. Its color and texture has socio-political impact, even in this ultramodern progressive world where equality for human race is the talk of the age. The skin disorders carry with them exceptionally massive psychological punishment. Talking in terms of psychopathology, skin can be used for the expression of hysterical exhibitionism, for the satisfaction of masochistic impulses and for displaced libidinal discharge.

THE BODY IMAGE

The concept of the body as seen by the patient and dermatologist differs a lot unless the dermatologist has the vision to integrate, even temporarily, with the person who has come to take his help. Our perceiving capabilities of normal body image bear little relation to that of anxious and disturbed patient whose vision of himself and his relationship with the surroundings may be distorted by anxiety, depression and loss of sleep due to itching. In females, the face figures largely in the body image and minor skin problems of this area are a common cause of a condition called as *dermatological non-disease.* Dysmorphophobia stands for patient's excessive preoccupation with a minor complaint that he believes, without reasons, to be conspicuous to others. It is a disorder of body image and may present initially to plastic surgeons and is associated with poor prognosis.

CLASSIFICATION[4,5]

Though it is very cumbersome and overlap always exists, we have tried to systematize the classification of dermatology-psychiatric disorders.

- Primarily psychiatric conditions usually presenting to dermatologist:
  - Delusions of parasitosis
  - Delusions of body image
    - Dysmorphophobia
    - Vulvodynia
    - Glossodynia
    - Solatics
  - Olfactory delusion
  - Phobic states
    - Dirt and bacteria
    - Pigmented lesions
    - Syphilophobia, AIDS-phobia, venereophobia
    - Anorexia nervosa
- Dermatoses primarily emotional in origin
  - Simulated disease (contrived disease)
  - Dermatitis artefacta and factitious cheilitis
  - Neurotic excoriations
  - Trichotillomania and onychotillomania
  - Psychogenic purpura and pathomimicry
  - Secretan's syndrome
  - Autoerythrocyte sensitization syndrome
- Dermatoses aggravated by self-induced trauma
  - Lichen simplex
  - Acne excoriee
  - Prurigo
- Dermatoses due to accentuated physiological responses
  - Blushing
  - Hyperhidrosis
  - Mental sweating
- Dermatoses in which emotional disturbances are precipitating factors
  - Pompholyx
  - Atopic dermatitis in the adult
  - Seborrheic dermatitis
  - Psoriasis
  - Localized or generalized pruritus
  - Alopecia areata
  - Aphthosis
  - Rosacea
  - Urticaria
- Miscellaneous conditions
  - Psychic possession
  - Witchcraft syndrome
  - Habituation to occlusive dressing
  - Sick building syndrome
  - Psychogenic pruritus.

Primarily Psychiatric Conditions Usually Presenting to Dermatologist

Delusions of Parasitosis

It is a condition in which the patient has an unshakable conviction that his skin is infested by parasites. It is different from parasitophobia where there is fear of becoming infested. Illicit exposure to drugs, such as ampheta-mine or cocaine, may cause delusion of parasitosis. It has been described in pellagra,[6] Vitamin B_{12} deficiency,[7] severe renal disease.[8] Sometimes, it is part of a delusion shared with another family member. The patients with delusions of parasitosis fall into the category single, fixed hypochondriacal delusion which is apparently not secondary to another psychiatric disorder.[9]

Most of the patients are intelligent but solitary and eccentric individuals. As it is well said, it is difficult to know where 'eccentricity' ends and 'madness' begins.[10] Delusion of parasitosis may follow a cerebrovascular accident in non-dominant hemisphere. It is, however, important to exclude the possibility of real infestation.

It is seen in a ratio of 1:1 in males:females, below the age of 50 years, but after 50 it becomes 1:3, with women being more common sufferers.

Many of these cases are 'doctor shoppers', always complaining about the incompetence of their medical advisers. Subjective feeling about the condition is that it is a dermatological condition, whereas the medical advisers rightly see them in psychiatric terms.

Symptomatology is usually ill-defined. Some say, that they have the sensation of insect crawling. They describe and draw the insect. There is no obvious skin disease, except scratch marks or excoriations which follow after attempts by patient to extract the parasites. Sometimes, patient may bring small containers (match box, etc.) containing the culprit insects. On microscopy, these offerings turn out to be fragments of skin, hair, or living mites or flies. Purification rituals are established and patients vigorously cleanse their skin and go to great lengths to cleanse the environment. These delusions may be shared between a husband and a wife, and sometimes by all the members of a family.

It is difficult to manage the patients with delusional parasitosis. Pimozide is the drug of choice in delusions of parasitosis, with initial dose of 2 mg/day, which may later be increased.[11] Sulpiride, 200 mg twice daily, is an alternative for non- or poor-responders to pimozide.

Delusions of Body Image

Dermatological Non-disease (Dysmorphophobia)

The term dermatological non-disease was carried to depict the clinical features of patient who are rich in symptoms (specifically in areas important in the body image) but poor in signs of organic dermatological conditions.[12] The most common psychiatric disorder associated with these patients is depression. The symptoms involve three areas: face (including mouth), scalp and genital area. Facial symptoms presented by the patients are excessive redness, blushing, burning sensation, scarring, large pores, greasiness and excessive facial hair. Some of them may complain of orodynia and glossodynia.

Symptoms of scalp may be of burning and excessive hair loss. Peripheral symptoms in males present as discomfort in genital areas, herpes, AIDS like symptoms, excessive redness of scrotum and urethral discharge. The female patients complain of volvodynia, i.e. the burning vulva syndrome. At certain times, discomfort is so severe that patient neither sits nor lies down. Facial and scalp symptoms are common in females, whereas perineal symptoms are more commonly seen in males.

Some of the patients are examples of monosymptomatic hypochondriacal psychosis. These persons are often solitary, unmarried or divorced. They socialize poorly and do not like contact with other people. An obsessional premorbid personality is common. Depression is the most common psychiatric problem associated with dysmorphophobia.[13] In adults or teenagers, it can be the presentation of schizophrenia while in old persons, dementia may be considered. The symptoms appear after emotional marital problems, whereas perineal symptoms in male usually follow imagined or real sexual exposure. There is no evidence of any underlying organic disease.

Patients of dysmorphophobia usually do not respond to placebo, rather they develop nocebo reaction in which, after receiving the placebo they develop the complaints which they attribute to it. The consultation is time consuming with such patients. The same ground has to be gone over again and again. The patient never appreciates normal non-verbal communication from the doctor. The patients ask, re-ask the similar questions which have already been answered again and again in the recent past.

The person with overvalued ideas may respond to superficial psychotherapy. But, the completely deluded with rich symptomatology with high scores on depression inventories show partial response to antidepressants. Reassurance at liaison clinic between psychiatrist and dermatologist may work.

Solatics

It is a phenomenon in which patient suffers from a delusional belief that all the lesions are due to sunlight. It may happen to such an extent that the person ventures out only in moonlit nights.[14]

Olfactory Delusions

Patients with olfactory delusions should be dealt with care because the delusions may drive them to homicide. The patients with delusions that they are passing excessively foul smelling flatus are usually referred to gastroenterologists, who then exclude steatorrhea. Some may complain of excessive bad smell from their axillae, feet or genitalia. Like other dermatological delusional conditions, they are also eccentric and socially isolated. Patients try themselves to get rid of the imaginative odor changing shoes and socks several times a day. Psychotherapy may help in these cases.

Phobic States

Dirt and Bacteria

Certain cases of OCD are phobic about dirt and bacteria, presenting to dermatologist as cases of hand eczema due to repetitive hand washing. Similar presentation may be seen in patients with anorexia nervosa.

Warts

Persons, who are phobic about warts, are afraid of touching anything in the consultation room and hospital. Such persons are found wearing gloves either during day-to-day shopping or daily activities. The sight of warts in certain persons may cause acute panic. The obsessive concerns about warts may reach such proportions that the patients become exhausted and suicidal.

Pigmented Lesions

In western world, due to over-enthusiastic publicity about the early diagnosis of malignant melanoma, people have developed phobia about pigmented lesions. Patient suffering from pigmentary diseases repeatedly consult dermatologists.

Syphilophobia, AIDS phobia and Venereophobia

Patients have overvalued ideas about the possibility of venereal disease. Most of them are young or middle aged people who are suffering from feelings of sexual guilt. Patients may think of having contracted venereal diseases, e.g. AIDS, syphilis or herpes simplex lesions. Surprisingly, the persons who had venreal disease in the past, and are at risk of having it again, don't suffer from venereophobia. The patients are badly disturbed and even the repeated negative serology cannot reassure them. Most of them are early cases of schizophrenia, or anxious, depressed or obsessional personality.[15]

Anorexia Nervosa

These persons have 'phobia' about their body weight[16] and present as cases of pseudojaundice because of raised blood carotene levels, increased lanugo hair, diffuse non-scarring alopecia and calluses on their fingers due to repetitive self-induced vomiting.[17]

Dermatoses Primarily Emotional in Origin

Simulated Disease (Contrived Disease)

In this condition, there is no real disease but patient tries to deceive the doctors by simulating symptoms and signs. These persons develop expertise to manipulate and deceive the treating doctors.[18] As the condition is difficult to diagnose, the patients are put to battery of investigations to rule out any organic pathology.

These simulated diseases come into their own at war time (for invalidity purposes), to extract maximum out of litigation, or when emotional pressure peaks to extremes.

Simulated disease includes mainly body systems. Munchausen's syndrome,[19] factitious pyrexic bruising, bleeding or drug-induced color changes in the skin are the examples. There can be severe self-mutilations, e.g. autocastration seen in persons suffering from schizophrenia.[20] Some cause superficial slashing of extremities; most of the patients are young females with borderline personality disorders[21] or with history of anorexia nervosa, or drug or alcohol abuse.[22]

Dermatitis Artefacta

Young adult females or adolescent girls constitute the group so as to make the female-to-male (F:M) ratio as 7:1. Most of them possess some sort of superficial medical knowledge. The sufferers are of inward looking, self-centerd disposition, with emotional immaturity and restricted interests.[23] Artefactual lesions are precipitated by stress or wide variety of recent events.

Cutaneous artefacts are the lesions only produced or exaggerated by the patient's own action. These form part of a broad spectrum of artefactual disease which can affect any organ and present to any discipline.[24]

The sites commonly involved are easily accessible sites to patient's hand, e.g. face, hands and arms. The lesions are usually bizarre, with irregular rectilinear outlines and geographical pattern, not suggesting any spontaneous process.

The lesions observed depend upon the mode used to inflict the skin. These can be of wide variety, from deep excoriations with finger nails or sharp objects; scarification with knife or broken glass piece; application of caustics, disinfectants and burning with cigarettes. Elastic bands are used to produce edema, ulcers or even bone lesions. Hair is plucked, or cut. More than one person may be involved, in the same family as in the *folie a deux* of two patients with factitious ulcers.[25] In some cases, diagnosis becomes extremely difficult when target tissue is subcutaneous tissue. Chronic panniculitis was observed due to blunt trauma in some patients.[26]

The patients strongly deny the fact that they themselves are inflicting the lesions and it really becomes difficult whether they are truly unconscious of actions performed.

Factitious Cheilitis

In this condition, the patients present with most persistent gross crusting and scaling of lips and nose,[27] consequent to repetitive biting, licking and picking. It is seen in emotionally immature or disturbed patients of both sexes.[28]

Neurotic Excoriations

It is a more common presentation amongst the self-inflicted dermatose. Amazingly, the patients admit having an irresistible desire to gauge and pick at their skin. Middle age females are more commonly affected as compared to males.[29] The patients commonly seem to be under stress or may be depressed.[30] The most frequent character traits are hypersensitivity and lack of self-confidence.[31] Itching may or may not be present and, rarely, the primary skin lesions is seen. Minor irregularities in skin are compulsively scratched and picked, exaggerating them and ultimately a vicious cycle sets in.[32] Few of the patients do it unknowingly, while others enjoy picking off crusts.

The excoriations are less than 1 cm in size which are covered with sanguineous crusts having erythematous edges. Lesions heal with a pale scar with hyperpigmented borders. Pleomorphism is quite evidence at any point of time. Extensors of arm, face, neck and shoulders are commoner sites to be involved.

In such cases, dermatopsychiatric liaison clinic may be helpful in management. Tricyclic antidepressants, doxepine[33] or naltrexone[34] may be used.

Psychogenic Purpura

The minor form of dermatitis artefacta is psychogenic purpura. It occurs by deliberate infliction of bruises.[35] Some consider this condition not to be a separate entity but as autoerythrocyte sensitization (AES).[36] However, it seems that the mechanism is more complex in AES. Though the bruises are produced by patients with same background as those with AES, but they are not accompanied by the same degree of tenderness, and intradermal injection of erythrocytes gives a negative reaction.

Secretan's Syndrome

It is factitious traumatic edema, with or without hemorrhage on dorsa of hands.[37] When the condition is present over forearm and upper arm, it is known as Charcot's *'I edema bleu.'* [38] Hallow history[39] is diagnostic feature, as the patient does not allow the clinician to have a clear impression of the pathogenesis of lesions. Unnatural configuration of lesion should give rise to suspicion of dermatitis artefacta, which can be confirmed by occlusive dressing and close watch during hospital stay when no new lesions would appear. Pemphigoid must be considered while diagnosing suction blisters.[40] Similarly, artefacts over hands or arms must be distinguished from porphyria cutanea tarda, polyarteritis nodosa, fixed drug eruption or hemorrhagic lesions of amyloidosis, before diagnosing a case to be of dermatitis artefacta.

Dermatopsychiatric liaison can be an effective mode of therapy. It should be done with patient alone, as the presence of patient's attendants may not allow revelation of the emotional situation which precipitated the motivation for infliction of lesions. In most of the cases, the lesion is inflicted to draw attention of significant others. If the underlying problem is resolved, the condition improves.

Autoerythrocyte Sensitization (Painful Bruising Syndrome)

It is rare distinctive clinical entity but well recognized due to allergic sensitivity to RBCs in the tissues. Minor extravasation of blood is followed by intense inflammatory reaction.[41,42]

It is almost always seen in women in whom tender bruises arise after trivial trauma or emotional stress. The onset follows accidental or surgical trauma and may be associated with abdominal pain, bleeding from internal organs and neurological symptoms. In one series, 70% of the cases showed psychiatric symptoms.[43] Several emotional disturbances and typical psychological profile are characteristic features.

The typical ecchymotic lesions can be reproduced by the intradermal injection of patient's own RBCs and by phosphatidyl/L-serine.[44] Simpson[45] has emphasized the similarities between AES and stigmatization. A condition, in which self-induced trauma produces a clinical entity similar to autoerythrocyte sensitization, has been termed as purpura factitia.[46]

Recently, plasmapheresis has been used successfully to treat the case of autoerythrocyte sensitization.

Dermatological Pathomimicry

In this condition, the patient causes recurrences or aggravation of already existing diseases, by using different methods. In one series described by Millard,[47] most of the patients were young females. The recurrence or aggravation is brought by taking drugs to which reaction occurs or eating gluten diet when intolerance was known to them. Deterioration of atopic dermatitis was observed after knowingly contacting a horse. Similarly, exposure to sunlight in case of photodermatoses or application of known irritants deliberately, e.g. neomycin and lanolin, may occur. Most of the persons are 'sympathy seekers.'

Trichotillomania

It is a compulsive habit in which person plucks his hair repeatedly. This condition is more common in young female children.[48] Emotional deprivation in the child-parent relationship can induce this habit, which usually replaces thumb sucking. This habit of twisting the hair and then plucking starts gradually and unconsciously, but later on patient admits it. In severe cases, the plucked area involves the whole scalp except margins known as 'tonsure alopecia.'[49] Rarely, hair are plucked from beard, eyebrows, eyelashes, mons pubis and perianal area.[50,51] Behavioral therapy or tranquilizers may help in such cases.

Onychotillomania

Combes[52] considers it to be a habit tic which is closely associated with parasitophobia, where the patient picks off pieces of nail folds and claims those to be parasites. The nail and nail fold left are rough and irregular. Many finger nails are involved. In some cases, manual or chewing damage to nails leads to longitudinal melanonychia. Trauma results in stimulation of the matrix melanocytes.[53] Pimozide has been found to effective in this condition.[54]

Dermatoses Aggravated/Perpetuated by Self-induced Trauma

Lichen Simplex

It is a condition where there is no predisposing skin disorder. Patients with lichen simplex are more readily conditioned to a scratch response to an itch stimulus than are control subjects.[55] In the predisposed subject, emotional tension certainly plays an important role in favoring the development of lichenification and ensuring its perpetuation.[56] The term 'circumscribed neurodermatitis' is often used as synonym for this condition.

Middle aged women are more commonly affected. Easily accessible sites like nape of neck, lower legs, ankles, side of neck, upper thighs, vulva, pubis, scrotum and extensors of forearm are usually involved. Hendy and Munro[57] described lichen simplex of scrotum as a treatable cause of male infertility, which may be due to excessive heat in gonads because of hyperemia and scrotal thickening.

Psychotherapy (aversion therapy), to break the scratching habit, can be used as mode of effective treatment. Sedation and topical steroids under occlusive bandage may also help to prevent the scratching.

Acne Excoriee

Acne plays an important role in patient's emotional well-being.[58] Acne may impair the person's self-esteem and body image.[59] Severe form of acne is seen in persons with considerable anxiety and anger.[60] This condition is usually seen in females. There are two subgroups: (1) patients with primary acne lesions, and (2) patients without lesions. In both groups, the females are in habit of fiddling with their skin, consequently exacerbating the smallest of lesions. There is usually some personality or psychological problem associated with such patients.[61]

Use of tetracycline (1 g/day) for 6 months helps to reduce the number of lesions, in the acne group, whereas in the 'no acne group', trifluoperazine hydrochloride (5–30 mg/day) or pimozide (4 mg/day), with psychotherapy may be beneficial.

Prurigo

It is an intensely pruritic eruption in which there is no identifiable etiological factor.[62] It comprises of heterogenous group of clinical conditions in which, either lesions cause irritation or lesions result from scratching.

Subacute prurigo (acne urticata) and nodular prurigo are the conditions in which mental stress or emotional problems precipitate the conditions.[63] The intensely pruritic lesions involve the cape area, face, scalp, neck, lower trunk and buttocks. Local applications are of little value. PUVA[65] and benoxaprofen[64] may help in some cases. But, a thorough assessment of person's psychological state is a must. Tranquilizers may prove fruitful in some patients.

Dermatoses due to Accentuated Physiological Responses

Blushing

Blushing may be considered normal under some circumstances. But at other times, when frequency and extent becomes excessive, it causes erythrophobia which is a compulsive state related to fear of blushing. It is commonly observed in women.[65] Such patients suffer from emotional difficulties and inhibitions. Hyperthyroidism and carcinoid syndrome must be excluded before labelling the condition to be compulsive in origin. Psychotherapeutic reassurance can be helpful to treat such cases.

Hyperhidrosis

Excessive production of sweat is labelled as hyperhidrosis. Overproduction of sweat may be due to overactivity of one of the three centers: thermoregulatory, mental and gustatory. Besides, there can be change in sweat glands. Pharmacologically active substances acting on glands and abnormal activity of sympathetic pathway between hypothalamus and nerve endings may also cause hyperhidrosis.[66,67] Clinically generalized or symmetrical hyperhidrosis is seen in thermoregulatory overactivity and mental sweating, whereas neurological lesion and gustatory sweating may be asymmetrical or localized.

Mental Sweating

Emotional or mental activity increases sweating on palms, soles, axillae and to lesser extent to groins, and over face. Sometimes, there may be generalized sweating.[68] Deep seated emotional factors may act as trigger.

It can be continuous or phasic. The continuous hyperhidrosis is worse in summer and mental factors are not clear, whereas phasic hyperhidrosis may be precipitated by minor emotional factors and there is nomarked seasonal variation. The palms may be cold and sometimes there is acrocyanosis. The male-to-female (M:F) ratio is same. It begins at puberty and there is positive family history in most of the cases. Reassurance and explanation to the patient about the nature of the disorder is primary requirement. In topical therapy, formalin 1% soaks for feet, glutaraldehyde 10%, aluminium chlorhydrate 20% and aluminium chloride are used. Iontophoresis with tap water or anticholinergic drugs, like glycopyrronium bromide, may be of some use. Propantheline (15 mg thrice daily), sedatives and tranquillizers may be helpful. Sympathectomy for the localized area can be tried. Conventional psychotherapy and behavioral therapy are gaining important role in the treatment of mental hyperhidrosis.

Miscellaneous Conditions

Psychic Possession

This condition is common in the factories where female employees are in abundance. There are reported outbreaks of industrial dermatitis,[69] which were instigated by one worker in other female workers with non-industrial dermatoses. There was no industrial cause observed for epidemic of such dermatoses. The phenomenon observed was similar to that of psychic possession or persuasion in middle ages in Europe. It is more common where compensation and dermatitis are commonly linked.

'Witchcraft' Syndrome

In this condition, an artefact is produced on others by an aggrieved or emotionally disturbed person. One of the interesting exemplary incidences is of a saloon. Several customers developed contact urticaria when owner's daughter applied a rubefacient (benzyl ester of nicotinic acid) while hairdressing. As absorption of this chemical is low in the palms, the patient vented her anger on others' skin rather than hers.[70]

Habituation to Occlusive Dressing

It is observed in elderly male patients, who live a lonely, life. They develop unusual addiction to local medication even when that is no more required for stasis eczema or gravitational ulcers. They insist occlusive therapy to be continued for many years even after the skin has become absolutely normal.[71]

Sick Building Syndrome

Dryness and itching may take a shape of an epidemic amongst the workers of 'sick building', where ventilation and humidity are less than optimum requirement. Berg[72] described a similar condition of facial complaints which can be out of proportion amongst females working at a visual display unit.

Psychogenic Pruritus

One mode to relieve everyday irritation is to scratch a little,[73] like a driver stopping at a red light is invariably found scratching one of the accessible sites. Similarly, all of us develop a habit to scratch a little to relieve the itch we develop from time-to-time in a day. Musaph[73] labels this phenomenon as 'traffic light phenomenon' and explains it as a common method to deal with minor frustrations.

Dermatoses in which Emotions are Precipitating or Perpetuating Factors

Pompholyx

It is a vesicular eczema of the palms and soles which is modified by its special site. It is a non-specific type of reaction provoked by various factors in a person with hereditary predisposition. Emotionally activated palmo-plantar hyperhidrosis[74] is an important etiological factor, besides atopy, active dermatophytosis[75] at other sites, and irritant and allergic dermatitis of various origins.

Clinically, pompholyx presents as crops of clear vesicles which look like deep seated sago-like grains with sensation of heat and severe itching. The typical lesions are present on the palms, soles and sides of fingers. Rest and bland applications help the acute phase and topical steroids have a definite role in subacute and recurrent cases. Most important of all is to remove the precipitating environmental stress, psychotherapy and use of sedatives as and when required.

Atopic Dermatitis

Atopy is a genetically determined disorder where there is an increased tendency to form reaginic IgE antibodies and enhanced susceptibility to develop certain diseases, e.g. asthma, hay fever and atopic dermatitis. In this condition, inherently irritable skin is there, with itching and scratching being amongst the precipitating factors. These are further modified by climatic, immunological and psychological factors.[76,77]

Whilock[78] describes atopic personalities as outwardly calm, seething with suppressed anxieties and frustrations, insecurity, aggression, egotism and above average intelligence. Persistent skin disease throughout infancy and childhood leads to personality changes. Simultaneously, maternal rejection further aggravates the condition. It is seen to be of persistent type with restless temperament.

Clinically in infants, lesions are erythematous and exudative, over cheeks, and cubital and popliteal fossae. The condition is extensively pruritic and infant may develop secondary infection due to constant rubbing and scratching. In adults, the lesions are dry, scaly, erythematous and lichenified. These are intensely pruritic, so much, so that only itching affects patient's attention rather than lesions. Sweating (thermal or emotional in origin) precipitates itching.

Treatment consists of topical steroids, besides psychological and psychopharmacological measures. Dysfunctional relationship between parents and child may worsen the condition.[79] Therapeutic psychological intervention may be beneficial in treating such cases, because extensive literature documents the fact that atopic dermatitis can be aggravated by emotional stress and that, as baseline, patients with atopic dermatitis score high in both trait anxiety and state anxiety. However, the existence of a definable pathological personality in the patient has never been substantiated. So, psychotherapeutic measures, stress management techniques and group therapy may be used as adjuncts to dermatological therapeutics.

Other Eczemas

Nummular and dyshidrotic eczema are also known to be exacerbated by emotional stress.

Nummular eczema, manifests as coin shaped lesions, with erythema and pruritus. Dyshidrotic eczema involves the lateral aspect of fingers and palms. It comprises of tiny vesicular lesions, which coalesce to form pruritic, erythematous eczematoid lesions.

Acne Vulgaris

It is a commonly known as pimples. It is a chronic inflammatory disorder of pilosebaceous units, typically starting at puberty. These manifest clinically as inflammatory papules, pustules, nodules and cysts, and non-inflammatory comedones (white heads and black heads). These lesions are present over face, chest and upper part of back. It is self-limiting disease, vanishing in late teens or early twenties. But, it may persist in to third or fourth decade of life. The commonly observed exacerbating factors are hormonal changes, e.g. premenstrual exacerbation, oral contraceptive pills (particularly high progesterone preparations), greasy comedonogenic skin preparations, and emotional stress.

In one study,[80] 55% of acne patients reported close association of exacerbation of acne lesions with the episodes of emotional stress. As per one hypothesis, aggravation of acne and emotional stress involves the release of certain hormones, such as glucocorticoids and adrenal androgens, which are associated with emotional stress. These hormones facilitate the formation of acne and may induce worsening of pre-existing lesions.

Besides dermatological modalities, patients may show beneficial results with the use of stress management techniques, e.g. biofeedback assisted relaxation and cognitive imagery in reducing the severity of acne.

Alopecia Areata

It is a common non-scarring form of hair loss, in which the hair on scalp or other body sites are lost in circular, oval patchy areas. This condition is not associated with any other cutaneous or systemic manifestations. When there is complete hair loss from entire scalp, it is called as 'alopecia totalis'. In the severe form, when whole of the body hair are lost, it is called 'alopecia universalis'.[81]

Its incidence is equal in males and females, and it can start at any age. Early age of onset, greater extent of involvement, association with other autoimmune diseases, hypertensive parenthood, etc. are poor prognostic signs.

Only 13.3% of patients of alopecia areata had either moderate or major life stresses arising during the year before the onset of first appearance of alopecia patches.

Other studies using scales, that measure non-specific and less catastrophic life stressors, have found increased reporting of stressors from the alopecia areata patients, as compared with general population. More authentic investigations are to needed to clarify this issue.

It is not established that psychiatric intervention, meant for diminishing the psychological stressor to initiate improvement of alopecia areata, may be of any help. However, psychiatric assistance is no doubt helpful in addressing the negative psychological effects of being afflicted with the disfiguring condition.

Urticaria

It is commonly known as *hives* or *nettle rash*. It consists of circumscribed, raised erythematous and pruritic plaques of dermal edema. The lesions usually disappear within 24-48 hours, although the main crop may continue to appear. It can arise as an allergic reaction to various stimuli, including pollen, food, medications, physical trauma, sunlight, cold temperature and water. In most of the cases, particularly chronic cases, the precipitating factors remain unknown, despite extensive, exhaustive questioning and investigations. In this group, emotional factors are frequently thought to play an important role. According to one study, 68% of the patients reported emotional stress to be a triggering factor.

The relation between stress and urticaria has been worked out for one distinct type of urticaria, adrenergic urticaria, in which the patient experiences attacks of urticaria in concurrence with increased plasma levels of adrenaline and noradrenaline. In this rare type of urticaria, the symptoms and signs are reproduced by intradermal injection of adrenaline. Conversely, the condition responds well to β adrenergic blocker, propranolol.

In routine, oral antihistaminics, corticosteroids and mast cell stabilizers (ketotifen and sodium chromoglycate) are used in the treatment of urticaria. Hypnosis, relaxation therapy and doxepine[82] are also used with limited success to treat resistant cases of chronic urticaria.

Localized and Generalized Pruritus

Itching is an individual's perception to various conditions. In general, psoriasis is non-itchy but persons with anxiety neurosis or depressive psychopathology can scratch it vigorously. In most of the cases of dermatological lesions, if present on exposed or accessible sites, the person tends to scratch it irresistibly. It stands true in most of the cases of localized or generalized neurodermatitis, in the beginning, but later on, the itch or scratch cycle goes out of hand. Few patients get an immense feeling of pleasure after scratching and it is thought to be related to release of opioids centrally. Some consider pruritus ani and pruritus vulvae for which no organic cause, like candidiasis, could be specified, as a psychogenic localized form of pruritus.

Itch, has been postulated to be mediated by enkephalins and endorphins in central nervous system, sharing common neurological pathway as that of pain. Centrally, itch can be elicited by morphine which may be resultant of binding of opioid receptors and this binding may mimic physiological binding of enkephalins and endorphins. Opioid antagonists, e.g. naloxone, reduce or stop histamine induced itching. So morphine, which alleviates pain, increases the itching.

Cotterill[12] authenticates that the persons with complaints of generalized pruritus in good number, may suffer from depression if no organic cause can be labelled for.

Seborrheic Dermatitis

It can be simply defined as dermatitis of seborrheic area, i.e. areas rich in sebaceous glands such as face, upper part of chest and interscapular area. Hyper-responsive androgen receptors, at sebaceous glands and pityriosporumovale, are the known etiological factors, but psychological status imparts an important contributory factor. Premenstrual exacerbation of increased sebaceous activity is a common examples of psychogenic factors influencing dermatitis.

Psoriasis

Psoriasis is a genetically determined, inflammatory and proliferative skin disorder manifesting as well-defined erythemo-squamous plaques mainly over extensors. It becomes a cosmetic disability when present over exposed parts. It is found only in genetically predisposed persons (HLA-B14, HLA-B17 and HLA-CW6), with trauma, infection, endocrinal factors, UV radiation, metabolic factors, and certain drugs being known factors. Similarly, stress can also exacerbate psoriasis. It is postulated that psychological stress decreases the will to follow regular therapeutic schedule, leading to further deterioration of the condition.

Cosmetic disability further depresses the patient with prolonged phases of active disease. Thus, a vicious cycle sets in, as anxiety and emotional stress related with disease process itself further deteriorate the prevailing status of the disease.

Besides topical therapy with potent steroids, tar products, dithranol and systemic PUVA therapy, oral retenoic acid derivative (etretinate) and methotrexate, antidepressants and anxiolytics may prove beneficial to achieve prompt remissions.

Rosacea

It is a chronic dermatological condition involving mainly the convexities of face. The characteristic features are erythema, telangiectasia, papules, swelling and pustules. Amongst these features, erythema and telangiectasia are the persistent one, whereas the rest appear with acute episodes of inflammation. The probable hypotheses for etiopathogenesis include psychological factors, besides alimentary, climatic, immunological, infective and pharmacological factors.

The rosacea patients were found to be depressed and 'retiring' because of red rash and flushing. They also develop neuroticism, but a second school of thought finds depression and neuroticism as a result of the disease process rather than being causative.

Aphthosis

In this condition, there is recurrent ulceration of oral mucosa. The role of L-form of bacteria, against which hypersensitivity has been demonstrated by skin test, autoimmunity, streptococcus, and vitamin B_{12}, folic acid and iron deficiency have been postulated as etiological factors. Any form of emotional stress has been found to precipitate the recurrence and may even exacerbate the existing lesions.

CUTANEOUS MANIFESTATIONS OF DRUGS USED IN PSYCHIATRY

Drugs commonly prescribed in psychiatry may give rise to certain cutaneous reactions. Table 1 shows the various dermatological side effects of drugs used in psychiatry.

MANAGEMENT

As we are aware, 'disease' is really a perception of ill health rather than a physical entity. The same degree of organic damage may be translated into different diseases by different persons. In many persons, psoriasis is not associated with itching but in others it may be severely itchy. So, the condition is same but interpretation and perception differ so widely that it becomes a must to understand the language in which the disease process is expressed. Once understood, the key lies with us for understanding the patient's particular concern and appropriate channel of therapeutic communication can be set for.[83]

In diseases, where rapid cure is possible (like diseases of infective origin), there is no great problem in management of such patients. But, where the disease is of unknown etiology or unpredictable duration (like autoimmune diseases), it is likely to assume undue proportions in patient's thought.

Table 1: Dermatological manifestations of psychotropic drugs

Manifestation(s)	*Drugs*
Exanthematous rash	Barbiturates, carbamazepine, imipramine, phenytoin, phenothiazines
Urticaria	Barbiturates, chlordiazepoxide phenytoin, glutethimide, imipramine carbamazepine, trimethadione
Exfoliative dermatitis	Barbiturates, carbamazepine, chlorpromazine, phenytoin, imipramine, lithium, trimethadione
Fixed drug eruption	Barbiturates, chlordiazepoxide, chloral hydrate, meprobamate, temazepam, trifluoperazine, glutethimide, amineptine
Acneform and pustular eruptions	Carbamazepine, lithium
Bullous eruptions	Barbiturates, diazepam, glutethimide nitrazepam
Erythema multiforme	Barbiturates, mianserin, chlordiazepoxide, carbamazepine, trimethadione
Toxic epidermal necrolysis	Barbiturates, carbamazepine, phenytoin
Lichenoidal eruption	Carbamazepine, chlorpromazine phenytoin
Lupus erythematous like syndrome	Barbiturates, chlorpromazine, phenytoin, lithium, carbamazepine
Photosensitivity	Barbiturates, imipramine, chlordiazepoxide, chlorpromazine

Particularly in dermatology, as in other spheres of life, the unknown is feared. The spots of acne are magnified in any mirror. The patient and doctor see two different images. It is the patient rather than the spots that must be treated.

Some element of anxiety or depression can be seen amongst the patients with skin diseases. It may unrelated to their skin diseases but more often plays some part in it or quite frequently may be the reason for its presentation. When the anxiety is reasonable and openly expressed, e.g. fear of cancer, ignorance of prognosis, anxiety about scarring, the patient can be reassured with clear explanation, in easily understandable language. When anxiety is obviously present, but at first denied, it must be elicited by careful intelligent questioning. Persons with fully repressed conflicts, but whose skin lesions are often factitious in nature and leave no doubt about the cause, present the most difficult problems.

Most of the patients with skin diseases respond to sympathetic and receptive methodologies. Visible conditions have disturbing emotional effect, which gets intensified with itching. The treating doctor must have patience, sympathy and insight into human behavior, and should inspire the patient to talk freely. Advice should be given sparingly without expecting it to be always followed up in totality. For chronic dermatological conditions with phases of remission and exacerbation, organic mental disease and endogenous depression, should always be taken into consideration.

Physician's personality has an immense effect on therapy he conducts. Stronger is the personality, often less are the drugs necessary. Similarly, the act of touching a patient with dermatological disease relieves the anxiety of those who have feelings of guilt and ostracism. 'Listening ear', does have equal importance as the 'seeing eyes', when emotional background is to be brought to surface. Tones of voice, transient stammer, hesitancy, or an unguarded or ambiguous remark provide the key to emotional stress. The initial explanations given by a patient are usually cover stories and should not be believed.

In the management, the first aim should be to determine whether any significant emotional condition is present or not; secondly, the reaction is one of anxiety, hysteria or depression. When reached to a conclusion, efforts should be made to reduce the environmental stress and patient's guilt, frustration or aggression should be eased or re-channelled. Hidden fears can be remedied, if these are expressed; anxiety about a child, spouse or parent may be the cause of rudeness; fatigue itself can give rise to stressful condition and the adjustment of household burdens, insistence on holidays or proper periods of rest and the provision of 'emotional bunkers', when the situation cannot be avoided, are matters of common sense and experience of what is feasible. Feelings of guilt, dirtiness and inadequacy, frequently components of depressive state, are more difficult to dispel and require expert help. Obsessional behavior and phobias are beyond superficial counseling.

For proper assessment of domestic and social situation, medical social worker may be required. He may extract information about family relationships and stresses. Relatives may provide help in dealing with the emotional situation. The parents of children with trichotillomania or of adults with artefacts should be approached tactfully, as they often contribute to the causation. Similarly, employers, school teachers and rehabilitation officers may give further information about the stress causing factors. In some patients, a priest's aid may be invaluable.

Three general points are to be taken into consideration. Firstly, the patient may present with a dermatosis which represents only one facet of a complex psychocutaneous situation. It serves its function in expressing the emotional disturbance. If cured, 'too quickly', without attending the underlying emotional condition, the patient may again develop some other less accessible ills. Secondly, try to avoid different opinions and advice regarding etiology and approach to treatment; otherwise, the patient may lose confidence in the doctors. Thirdly, there is a group of patients who do not want to get better. Such persons are skilled at deceiving their doctors, their friends and their spouses. They suffer from 'too good husbands' and 'too kind doctors'. Many of these patients have an histrionic personality. Once recognized, certain principles of management should be followed; even then, the prognosis is not good. The patient has 'too much to lose' by recovering.

Drugs

In the recent past, there is a healthy trend against the overuse of drugs in the management of psychoneurotic patients and some patients may refuse to take them.[84] However, short term therapy with anxiolytics or sedatives may be as helpful to anxious itchy patient as analgesics relieve to those in pain. Sleep deprivation is usually associated; so, hypnotics can be used to restore normal pattern of sleep. Similarly, antihistaminics with sedative side effects can also be used. Some patients may even show good response to placebos while few may develop adverse reactions to these.

Monosymptomatic hypochondriacal syndromes in dermatology like delusions of parasitosis or onychotillomania, pimozide is the drug of choice. Tricyclic antidepressants[85] can be used in frank depressive disorders associated with chronic skin disorders or for patients with symptoms, such as burning or itching but no physical signs for the symptomatology. Some of these drugs act on serotonin metabolism. Doxepine has also an antihistaminic action and can be used in neurotic excoriations also.[86]

Other Measures

The following measures are also used in the management of psychocutaneous disorders with significant emotional components.

Abreactive Techniques

These are rarely used nowadays.

Hypnosis and Relaxation

It has a limited scope in treating psychocutaneous disorders. However, relaxation techniques, some of which approximate to light autohypnotic states, may help the stressed or the agitated. Hertzers[87] study of chronic urticaria shows that patients improve symptomatically, though number of weals remain the same. Similarly, lesions of verruca may disappear with hypnotic therapy.[88]

Biofeedback Techniques

It has been found useful in dyshidrotic eczema[89] and hyperhidrosis.[90] In this technique, patients are given visual or auditory information about the level of particular autonomic function and then to learn some voluntary control over it.

Behavior Therapy

It is used for patients who scratch repeatedly. As per one study,[91] parents were asked to withdraw attention when their ward scratched. The second mode is for the patient to monitor his scratching, and to gain therapist's attention intervals without scratching were required.[92] In cases of atopic eczema, habit reversal therapy is found to be effective.[93]

Group Therapy

In psoriatic patients, group therapy has been found to be effective.[94] In this, a small group of patients meet to discuss their problems with a trained fellow psoriatic and a physician; anxiety, depression and illness behavior are reported to decrease. 'Self-help groups' may also play a similar role.[95]

MISCELLANEOUS ISSUES

Psychiatric Problems Caused by Dermatological Treatment

Systemic glucocorticoid therapy, quite often used by dermatologist, can give rise to depression, hypomania or psychosis. Acyclovir,[96] a commonly prescribed antiviral, has been found to cause psychosis in patients with impaired renal function. Antimalarials, used as systemic sunscreen,[97] and dapsone,[98] the antileprotic, can give rise to psychosis.

Skin Disease in the Mentally Subnormal Patients

Mental deficiency is not a disease in itself but a condition resulting from either inborn or acquired causes. There are number of syndromes in which cutaneous lesions and mental deficiency may be associated with some biochemical defects or chromosomal abnormality.

In most of these cases, the mechanism of cutaneous changes in mental impairment is not well understood. The severity of mental defect and of skin involvement usually run parallel with each other.

Nonspecific Cutaneous Lesions Showing Increased Prevalence in Mental Retardation

Moniliform Hamartoma

Beaded strands of papules on forehead and temples develop at puberty in some mentallly retarded individuals. Its incidence is more amongst negroids than caucasians.

Atypical Keratosis Pilaris

Asymmetrical erythematous follicular papules are seen from base of neck to the lumbar region, in young adults who are mentally retarded.[99] It may represent pityrosporum folliculitis.

Abnormal Hair Patterns

Fusion of eyebrow and lower frontal hair lines has been found in microcephalics. Hypertrichosis of limbs and trunk have been found in mentally retarded.

Atopic Dermatitis

Atopic dermatitis has been found in patients with phenylketonuria and Down's syndrome. Only one patient was found amongst 200 mentally retarded children with atopic dermatitis and low prevalence of eczema was also found.[100]

Traumatic Keratoses and Hypertrichosis

Many mentally retarded individuals develop the habit of biting or chewing the forearm, fingers, lips and hand, when excited or angry. Repeated biting at same site may lead to thickening, hyperpigmentation and hypertrichosis; sometimes, atrophic scarring may be seen. Keratoses in unusual sites may result from repeated adoption of some posture.

Traumatic Alopecia

In mentally subnormal individuals, hair pulling from the frontoparietal area or pubic area may occur. Multiple self-mutilations, including traumatic alopecia, are seen in children with familial sensory neuropathy.

Crusted Scabies

It is seen in mild mental retardation,[101] as they have an increased threshold for scratching.

Bacterial Infections

The high incidence of bacterial infections may be due to low resistance to pyogenic infections and unhygienic habits of mentally subnormal persons. Folliculitis of thighs in children and adolescents of both sexes, chronic suppurated hidradenitis is seen in adolescent boys. Savin[102] has found high incidence of erythroderma.

Mycoses

Amongst mentally retarded, trichophyton infections are quite common. The colonies found are refractory in nature because the antipsychotic drugs reduce the efficacy of griseofulvin, through enzyme induction.

Intertrigo

Intertrigo of genitocrural areas is seen frequently in incontinent, bed ridden patients. Perleche is also complicated by fissuring and secondary infection.

Primary Irritant Dermatitis

The mentally retarded are prone to develop primary irritant dermatitis because of improper use of disinfectants and cleansing agents. It is common amongst patients who are encouraged to carry out simple domestic jobs. Allergic contact dermatitis is uncommon because exposure to potential sensitizing agents is checked.

REFERENCES

1. Domonkos AN. Andrew's Disease of the skin, 6th edition. Philadelphia: WB Saunders C. Pruritus, Cutaneous neuroses and Neurocutaneous dermatoses; 1971.pp.61-76.
2. Koblenzer CS. Psychosomatic concepts in dermatology. Arch Dermatol. 1983;119:501-12 [PubMed].
3. Korabel H, Dudek D, Jaworek A, Wojas-Pelc A. Psychodermatology: Psychological and psychiatrical aspects of aspects of dermatology. Przegl Lek. 2008;65:244-8 [PubMed].
4. Misery L. Neuro-immuno-cutaneous system (NICS) Pathol Biol. 1996;44:867-87 [PubMed].
5. Garg A, Chren MM, Sands LP, Matsui MS, Marenus KD, Feingold KR, et al. Psychological stress perturbs epidermal barrier homeostasis. Arch Dermatol. 2001;137:53-9 [PubMed].
6. Humphreys F, Humphreys MS. Psychiatric morbidity and skin disease: What dermatologists think they see? Br J Dermatol. 1998;139:679-81 [PubMed].
7. Capoore HS, Rowland Payne CM, Goldin D. Does psychological intervention help chronic skin conditions? Postgrad Med J. 1998;74:662-4. [PMC free article] [PubMed].
8. Kieć-Swierczyńska M, Dudek B, Krecisz B, Swierczyńska-Machura D, Dudek W, Garnczarek A, et al. The role of psychological factors and psychiatric disorders in skin diseases. Med Pr. 2006;57:551-5 [PubMed].
9. Finlay AY. Quality of life assessments in dermatology. Semin Cutan Med Surg. 1998;17:291-6 [PubMed].
10. Koo J, Lee CS. Psycotropic agents. In: Koo J (Ed). Comprehensive Dermatologic Drug Therapy, 1st edition. Philadelphia: WB. Saunders Company; 2001.pp.402-22.
11. Millard L. Dermatological practice and psychiatry. Br J Dermatol. 2000;143:920-1 [PubMed].
12. Picardi A, Amerio P, Baliva G, Barbieri C, Teofoli P, Bolli S, et al. Recognition of depressive and anxiety disorders in dermatological outpatients. Acta Derm Venereol. 2004;84: 213-7 [PubMed].
13. Richards HL, Fortune DG, Weidmann A, Sweeney SK, Griffiths CE. Detection of psychological distress in patients with psoriasis: Low consensus between dermatologist and patient. Br J Dermatol. 2004;151:1227-33 [PubMed].

14. Koo J. Skin disorders. In: Kaplan HI, Saduck BJ, (Eds). Comprehensive textbook of psychiatry, 6th edition. Baltimore: Williams and Wilkins; 1995.
15. Oates JK, Gamaz J. Venereophobia. Br J Hosp Med. 1984;31: 435-6.
16. Luck P, Wackerling A. Increased cutaneous vasoreactivity to cold in anorexia nervosa. Clin Sci. 1981;61:559-67.
17. Gupta MA, Gupta AK, Haberman HF. Dermatologic signs in anorexia nervosa and bulimia nervosa. Arch Dermatol. 1987;123:1386-90.
18. Naish JM. Problems of deception in medical practice. Lancet. 1979;ii:139-42.
19. Asher R. Munchausen's syndrome. Lancet. 1951;i:339-41.
20. Simpson MA. Self multilation. Br J Hosp Med. 1976;16:430-38.
21. Schaffer CB, Carroll J, Abramovitz SL. Self mutilation and borderline personality. J Nerv Ment Dis. 1982;170:468-70.
22. Sneddon IB. Simulated disease: Problems in diagnosis and management. J Roy Coll Phys Lond. 1983;17:199-205.
23. Lyell A. Dermatitis artefacte in relation to the syndrome of contrived disease. Clin Exp Dermatol. 1976;1:109-26.
24. Fabisch W. Psychiatric aspects of dermatitis artefacta. Br J Dermatol. 1980;102:29-34.
25. Hubler WR, Hubler WB Sr. Folie a deux factitious ulcers. Arch Dermatol. 1980;116:1303-4.
26. Winkelmann RK, Barker SM. Factitial traumatic panniculitis. J Am Acad Dermatol. 1985;13:988-94.
27. Savage J. Localised crusting as an artefact. Br J Dermatol. 1978;117:338-40.
28. Crotty CP, Dicken CG. Factitious lip crusting. Arch Dermatol. 1981;117:338-40.
29. Nielsen H, Fruensgaard K, Hjortosh A. Controlled neuro-psychological investgation of patients with neurotic excoriations. Psychother Psyohosom. 1980;34:52-61.
30. Fisher BK, Peare KL. Cutis. 1974;14:251.
31. Fruensgaard K. Neurotic excoriations. Int J Dermatol. 1978;17: 761-7.
32. Koblenzer CS. Psychosomatic concepts in dermatology. Arch Derm. 1983;119:501-12.
33. Harris BA, Shertez EF, Flowers FP. Improvement of chronic neurotic excoriations with oral doxepin therapy. Int J Dermatol. 1987;26:541-3.
34. Smith KC, Pittelkow MR. Naltrexone for neurotic excoriations. J Am Acad Derm. 1989;20:860-61.
35. Ratnoff OD. The psychogenic purpuras: a review of autoerythrocyte sensitization, aut sensitization on to DNA, hysterical and factitious bleeding and the reliious stigmata. SeminHematol. 1980;17:192-213.
36. Eagles DW. Skin disorders: Psychological factors affecting physical conditions (psychosomatic disorders). In: Kaplan HI, Sodock BJ (Eds). Comprehensive Texbook of Psychiatry. 6th edition. Baltimore: Williams & Wilkins; 1995.pp.1178-87.
37. Angelini G, Meneghini CL, Vena CA. Secretan's syndrome: An artefact edema of the hand. Contact Dermatitis. 1982;8:345-6.
38. Brunning J, Gibson AG, Perry M. Oedema blue: A reappraisal. Lancet. 1980;i:810-12.
39. Lyell A. Cutaneous artefactual disease. J Am Acad Dermatol. 1979;1:391-407.
40. Dufton P, Griffiths H. Suction blisters mimicking pemphigoid: An unusual case of dermatitis artefacta. Clin Exp Dermatol. 1981;6:163-6.
41. Hersle K, Mobacken H. Autoerythrocyte sensitization syndrome (painful bruising syndrome): Report of two cases and review of the literature. Br J Dermatol. 1969;81:574-87.
42. Ratnoff OD. The psychogenic purpura: A review of autoerythrocyte sensitization autosensitization to DNA, hysterical and factitious bleeding and the religeous stigmata. Semin Hematol. 1980;17:192-213.
43. Hersle K, Mobacken H. Br J Dermatol. 1969;81:574.
44. Agle DP, et al. Psychosoma Med. 1967;29:491.
45. Simpson CJ. The stigmata: Pathology or miracle. Br Med J. 1984;289:1746-8.
46. Stefanini M, Blumgart ET. Purpurafactitia. Arch Dermatol. 1972;106:238-41.
47. Millard LG. Dermatological pathomimcry: A form of patient maladjustment. Lancet. 1984;ii:969-71.
48. Muller SA, Winkelmann RK. Trichotillomania. Arch Dermatol. 1972;105:535-43.
49. Sanderson KV, Hall Smith P. Tonsure trichotillomania. Br J Dermatol. 1970;105:535-43.
50. Jillson OF. Alopecia. II. Trichotillomania (Trichotillohabitus). Cutis. 1983;31:383-6.
51. Mehergan AH. Trichotillomania: A clinicopathological study. Arch Dermatol. 1970;102:129-35.
52. Combes FC, Scott MJ. Onychotillomania. Arch Dermatol Syphil. 1951;63:778-80.
53. Baran R. Nail biting and picking as a possible cause of longitudinal malanonychia: A study of 6 cases. Dermatologica; 181.pp.126-8.
54. Hamann K. Onychotillomania treated with pimozide (Orap). Acta Derma Venereol. 1982;62:364-7.
55. Robertson IM, Jordan JM, Whilock FA. Emotions and skin. III. The conditioning of scratch responses in cases of lichen simplex. Br J Dermatol. 1975;92:4407-12.
56. Cormia FE. Basic concepts in the production and management of psychosomatic deratoses. II. Br J Dermatol. 1951;63:129-51.
57. Hendry WF, Munro DD. "Wash leather scrotum" (scrotal dermatitis): A treatable cause of male infertility. Fertility and Sterility. 1990;53:379-81.
58. Sneddon J, Sneddon I. Acne excoree: A protective device. Clin Exp Dermatol. 1983;8:65-8.
59. Shuster S, Fisher G, Harris E, et al. The effect of skin disease on self image. Br J Dermatol. 1978;99(Suppl. 16):18-9.
60. Wu SF, Kinder BN, Trunnel TN, et al. Role of anxiety and anger in acne patients: A relationship with severity of the disorder. J Am Acad Dermatol. 1988;18:325-33.
61. Schaffer CB, Carroll J, Abramovitz SI. Self mutilation and the borderline personality. J Nerv Ment Dis; 1982;170:468-70.
62. Jorrizo J, Gath S, Smith EB. Prurigo: A clinical review. J Am Accad Dermatol. 1981;4:723-9.

63. Vaatainen N, Hannukesla M, Karvonen J. Local photochemotherapy in nodular prurigo. Acta Derm Venereal. 1974;59:544-7.
64. Hindson C, Lawlor F, Waks H. Treatment of nodular prurigo with benoxaprofen. Br J Dermatol. 1982;107:369.
65. Parkes Weber F. Rare diseases, 2nd edition. London: Staples; 1947.pp.61.
66. Herxheimer A. Gustatory sweating and pilomotion. Br Med J. 1958;i:688-9.
67. Sulzberger HB, Hermann F. The Clinical Significance of Disturbances in the Delivery of Sweat. Springfield: Thomas; 1954.
68. Allen JA, et al. J Physiol. 1973;235:749.
69. Mcguire A. Psychic possession among industrial workers. Lancet. 1978;i:376-8.
70. Bandman HJ, Wahl B. Contact uritcariaartefacta (witchcraft syndrome) Contact Derm. 1983;8:145-6.
71. Liddell K, Cotterill JA. Habituation to occlusive dressings. Lancet. 1973;i:1485-6.
72. Berg M. Facial skin complaints and work at visual display units: Epidemiological clinical and histopathological studies. Acta Dermatol Venereol. 1989;69(Suppl. 150):6-9.
73. Muspah H. Psychogenic pruritus. Semin Dermatol. 1983;2:217-22.
74. Simons RDGP. Eczema of the Hands. 2nd edition. Basel: Karger, 1966.
75. Menne T, Holm NB. Int J Dermatol. 1983;22:22.
76. Hanifen JM. J Am Acad Dermatol. 1982;6:I.
77. Rajaka G. Acta Dermatol Venereol (Stockholm) 1979: Suppl. 92.
78. Whitlock FA. Psychophysiological Aspects of Skin Disease. London: Saunders; 1976.
79. Koblenzer CS, Koblenzer PH. Chronic intractable atropic eczema: Its occurrence as a physical sign of impaired parent child relationship and its psychological developmental arrest; Improvement through parent insight and education. Arch Dermatol. 1988;124:1677-82.
80. Koo John YM, Smith LL. Psychological aspects of acne. Pediatr Dermatol. 1991;8:185.
81. Koo John YM, Pham CT. Psychodermatology. Arch Dermatol. 1992;128:381.
82. Figueiredo A, Riberio CA, Gonacalo M, et al. Mechanism of action of doxepin in the treatment of chronic urticaria. Fundam Clin Pharmacol. 1990.p.147.
83. Sarti MG, Cossidente A. Therapy in psychosomatic dermatology. Clin Dermatol. 1984;2:255-73.
84. Gupta MA, Gupta AK, Haberman HF. Psychotropic drugs in dermatology. J Am Accad Dermatol. 1986;14:633-45.
85. Gupta MA, Gupta AK, Ellis CN. Antidepressant drugs in dermatology. Arch dermatol. 1987;123:647-52.
86. Harris BA, Sheretz EF, Flowers EP. Improvement of chronic neurotic excoriations with doxepin therapy. Int J Dermatol. 1987;26:541-3.
87. Hertzer CL, Lookingbill DP. Effects of relaxation therapy and hypnotizability in chronic urticaria. Arch Dermatol. 1987;123:913-6.
88. Champion RH, Burton JL, Ebling FJG. In: Textbook of Dermatology. IV Ed. Vol 1. Oxford: Blackwell; 1992.
89. Miller RM, Coger RW. Skin conductance conditioning with dyshidrotic eczema patients. Br J Dermatol. 1979;101:435-40.
90. Duller P, Gentry WD. Use of biofeedback in treating chronic hyperhydrosis: A priliminary report. Br J Dermatol. 1980;103:143-6.
91. Allen K, Harris FR. Elimination of a child's excessive scratching by training the mother in reinforcement procedure. Behav Res Ther. 1966;4:79.
92. Catoldo MF, Varni JW, Russo DC, et al. Behaviour therapy techniques in treatment of exfoliative dermatitis. Arch Dermatol. 1980;116:919-22.
93. Noren P, Melin L. The effect of combined topical steroids and habit reversal treatment in patients with atopic dermatitis. Br J Dermatol. 1989;121:359-66.
94. Schutle MB, Cormane RH, Van Dijk E, et al. Group therapy of psoriasis. J Am Acad Dermatol. 1985;12:61-6.
95. Logan RA. Self help groups for patients with chronic skin diseases. Br J Dermatol; 1988.
96. Thomson CR, Goodship THJ, Rodger RSC. Psychiatric side effects of acyclovir in patients with chronic renal failure. Lancet. 1985;ii:385-6.
97. Evans RL, Khalid S, Kinney JL. Antimalarial psychosis revisted. Arch Dermatol. 1984;120:765-7.
98. Daneshmend TK. The neurotoxicity of dapsone: Adverse drug reactions. Acute Poisoning Rev. 1984;3:53-8.
99. Coombs FP, Butterworth T. Atypical keratosis pilaris. Arch Dermatol. 1950;62:305-13.
100. Butterworth T, Wilson M Jr. Incidence of diseases of skin in feeble minded persons. Arch Dermatol Syphiol. 1938;38:203-9.
101. Metaxotou C, Ikkos D, Panagiotopoulou P, et al. A familial X/Y translocation in a boy with ichthyosis, hypogonadism and mental retardation. Clin Genet. 1983;24:380-83.
102. Fried RG, Gupta MA, Gupta AK. Depression and skin disease. Dermatol Clin. 2005;23(4):657-64.

SUGGESTED READING

1. Andresen EM, Malmgren JA, Carter WB, Patrick DL. Screening for depression in well older adults: evaluation of a short form of the CES-D (Center for Epidemiologic Studies Depression Scale). Am J Prev Med. 1994;10(2):77-84.
2. Bell S, Lee C. Perceived stress revisited: the Women's Health Australia project young cohort. Psychol Health Med. 2003;8(3):343-53.
3. Benea V, Muresian D, Manolache L, Robu E, Diaconu J. Stress and atopic dermatitis. Dermatol Psychosom. 2001;220:5-7.
4. Bingefors K, Lindberg M, Isacson D. Self-reported dermatological problems and use of prescribed topical drugs correlate with decreased quality of life: an epidemiological survey. Br J Dermatol. 2002;147(2):285-90.
5. Brown WJ, Bryson L, Byles J, et al. Women's Health Australia: recruitment for a national longitudinal cohort study. Women Health. 1998;28(1):23-40.

6. Brown WJ, Dobson A, Bryson L, Byles J. Women's Health Australia: on the progress of the main cohort studies. J Womens Health Gend Based Med. 1999;8(5):681-8.
7. Chida Y, Hamer M, Steptoe A. A bidirectional relationship between psychosocial factors and atopic disorders: a systematic review and meta-analysis. Psychosom Med. 2008;70(1):102-16.
8. Chiu A, Chon SY, Kimball AB. The response of skin disease to stress: changes in the severity of acne vulgaris as affected by examination stress. Arch Dermatol. 2003;139(7):897-900.
9. Dalgard F, Gieler U, Holm JO, Bjertness E, Hauser S. Self-esteem and body satisfaction among late adolescents with acne: results from a population survey. J Am Acad Dermatol. 2008;59(5):746-51.
10. Dalgard F, Svensson A, Holm JO, Sundby J. Self-reported skin morbidity among adults: associations with quality of life and general health in a Norwegian survey. J Investig Dermatol Symp Proc. 2004;9(2):120-25.
11. Dalgard F, Svensson A, Holm JO, Sundby J. Self-reported skin morbidity in Oslo: associations with sociodemographic factors among adults in a cross-sectional study. Br J Dermatol. 2004;151(2):452-7.
12. Dalgard F, Svensson A, Sundby J, Dalgard O. Self-reported skin morbidity and mental health: a population survey among adults in a Norwegian city. Br J Dermatol. 2005;153(1):145-9.
13. Evers AW, Lu Y, Duller P, van der Valk PG. Kraaimaat FWvan de Kerkhof PC Common burden of chronic skin diseases? contributors to psychological distress in adults with psoriasis and atopic dermatitis. Br J Dermatol. 2005;152(6):1275-81.
14. Hagforsen E, Michaelsson K, Lundgren E, et al. Women with palmoplantar pustulosis have disturbed calcium homeostasis and a high prevalence of diabetes mellitus and psychiatric disorders: a case-control study. Acta Derm Venereol. 2005;85(3):225-32.
15. Hashiro MO, Kumura M. Anxiety, depression and psychosomatic symptoms in patients with atopic dermatitis: comparison with normal controls and among groups of different degrees of severity. J Dermatol Sci. 1997;14(1)63-7.
16. Huerta C, Rivero E, Rodriguez L. Incidence and risk factors for psoriasis in the general population. Arch Dermatol. 2007;143(12):1559-65.
17. Kellett SC, Gawkrodger DJ. The psychological and emotional impact of acne and the effect of treatment with isotretinoin. Br J Dermatol. 1999;140(2):273-82.
18. Kilkenny M, Stathakis V, Hibbert ME, Patton G, Caust J, Bowes G. Acne in Victorian adolescents: associations with age, gender, puberty and psychiatric symptoms. J Paediatr Child Health. 1997;33(5):430-33.
19. King RM, Wilson GV. Use of a diary technique to investigate psychosomatic relations in atopic dermatitis. J Psychosom Res. 1991;35(6):697-706.
20. Koo J, Lebwohl A. Psycho dermatology: the mind and skin connection. Am Fam Physician. 2001;64(11):1873-8.
21. Linnet J, Jemec GB. An assessment of anxiety and dermatology life quality in patients with atopic dermatitis. Br J Dermatol. 1999;140(2)268-72.
22. Magin P, Adams J, Heading G, Pond D, Smith W. The psychological sequelae of acne vulgaris: results of a qualitative study. Can Fam Physician. 2006;52(8):978-9.
23. Magin P, Adams J, Heading G, Pond D, Smith W. The psychological sequelae of psoriasis: results of a qualitative study. Psychol Health Med. 2009;14(2):150-61.
24. Naldi L, Peli L, Parazzini F, Carrel CF. Psoriasis Study Group of the Italian Group for Epidemiological Research in Dermatology, Family history of psoriasis, stressful life events, and recent infectious disease are risk factors for a first episode of acute guttate psoriasis: results of a case-control study. J Am Acad Dermatol. 2001;44(3):433-8.
25. Picardi A, Abeni D. Stressful life events and skin diseases: disentangling evidence from myth. Psychother Psychosom. 2001;70(3):118-36.
26. Sampogna F, Tabolli S, Abeni. DIDI Multipurpose Psoriasis Research on Vital Experiences (IMPROVE) investigators, The impact of changes in clinical severity on psychiatric morbidity in patients with psoriasis: a follow-up study. Br J Dermatol. 2007;157(3):508-13.
27. Saunes M, Smidesang I, Holmen T, Johnsen R. Atopic dermatitis in adolescent boys is associated with greater psychological morbidity compared with girls of the same age: the Young-HUNT study. Br J Dermatol. 2007;156(2): 283-8.
28. Scheier MF, Carver C, Bridges M. Distinguishing optimism from neuroticism (and trait anxiety, self-mastery, and self-esteem): a reevaluation of the life orientation test. J Pers Soc Psychol. 1994;67(6):1063-78.
29. Sherbourne CD, Stewart AL. The MOS social support survey. Soc Sci Med. 1991;32(6):705-14.
30. Taieb A, Finlay A, Myon E. Psoriasis: quality of life according to gender. J Eur Acad Dermatol Venereol. 2004;18786.
31. Twisk JR. Applied Longitudinal Data Analysis for Epidemiology. Cambridge, England: Cambridge University Press; 2003.
32. World Health Organisation Collaborating Centre for Mental Health and Substance Abuse Treatment Protocol Project: Management of Mental Disorders. Vol 1. 3rd edition. Sydney, Australia: World Health Organisation; 2000.

CHAPTER 36

Neuropsychiatric Disorders

JN Vyas

ABSTRACT

Neuropsychiatry is concerned with disorders of affect, cognition, and behavior that arise from overt disorder in cerebral function, or from indirect effects of extracerebral disease.

The clinician needs to have a practical approach to the assessment, investigation, and management of patients manifesting cognitive and behavioral change, and to be aware of the specific cerebral and extracerebral disorders that commonly involve or are accompanied by cognitive or behavioral change.

In the assessment and classification of mental and behavioral disorders it is crucial to: (1) distinguish between acute and chronic disorders, particularly between delirium and dementia; (2) distinguish between cognitive and psychiatric disorder—misdiagnosis of depression presenting as a 'pseudodementia', or of delirium as psychosis, are errors that can have direct consequences for the patient; (3) determine whether cognitive impairment is specific or generalized-specific impairments are more likely to be due to a focal brain lesion; and (4) determine whether any underlying condition is reversible or irreversible.

Acute Cognitive and Behavioral Disturbance

Delirium—can be caused by a very wide range of conditions and needs to be distinguished from acute psychosis, which can be difficult. Features that support the diagnosis of delirium are (1) deficits of attention that may range from distractibility and inability to follow complicated conversations, through an almost complete inability to register information or to concentrate (manifest poor performance on serial subtraction test), progressing in the extreme case to diminished consciousness and coma; (2) attentional difficulties that tend to have a sudden onset and to fluctuate over time; (3) muddled thinking and speech showing considerable perseveration; (4) illusions and hallucinations that tend to include a strong visual component, although auditory hallucinations and misperceptions are common; and (5) delusions are usually simple, persecutory in nature, fluctuating, and transient.

Psychiatric disorders a past history of psychiatric contact or treatment should be sought in all those with behavioral disturbance. In patients with an underlying psychiatric disorder there is usually a background of insidious behavioral disturbance or personality change. Delusions in psychotic disorders tend to be complex, bizarre, and consistently held, visual hallucinations are rare, and marked attentional and memory deficits are not typical.

Alcohol and substance misuse—about one-quarter of all male medical admissions have a current or previous alcohol problem, and such patients are vulnerable to a large number of complications that may precipitate delirium.

Clinical approach—it is necessary to consider a wide range of factors and medical conditions that can both predispose to and precipitate delirium. A history of alcohol and/or illicit substance misuse is of particular importance. Although not always easy, a thorough physical examination with particular attention to the neurological system is essential. A routine screen-including full blood count, electrolyte, and γ-glutamyl transferase (GCT) measurements, liver and thyroid function tests, glucose estimation, and C-reactive protein (CRP)/ erythrocyte sedimentation rate (ESR)—is required, as this might indicate delirium where the diagnosis is in doubt. Infection is implicated in around one-third of hospital inpatients who are delirious, and a midstream urine sample (MSU) and chest radiograph are usually warranted. Relevant history and findings on physical examination determine the need for more specific investigation, e.g. brain CT, lumbar puncture, malarial blood film.

Management—delirium is a medical emergency. Management consists of treating the underlying causes and containment of any behavioral disturbance with general measures in the first instance, including nursing in a bright, simple room with minimal changes in staff and good lighting at night. Where sedation is required, then a regular oral antipsychotic such as haloperidol can be administered.

Chronic and Subacute Cognitive and Behavioral Disturbance

The diagnostic challenges in this group of patients are exemplified by the complex differentiation between dementia and depression or 'depressive pseudodementia.

Dementia-this is a progressive neurodegenerative syndrome involving a pervasive impairment of higher cortical functions resulting from widespread brain pathology. Reversible causes must be excluded. A typical diagnostic screen will include a full blood count, electrolyte and metabolic screen, thyroid screen, vitamin B_{12} and folate levels, syphilis serology, urinalysis, chest radiography, electrocardiography, and CT/MRI brain imaging. In some cases, lumbar puncture, electroencephalography, and (rarely) brain biopsy will be required. Functional brain imaging is likely to assume greater importance in the future.

Focal cognitive disorders—a variety of neuropsychiatric syndromes may arise from regional cerebral impairments diverse cause and may present in the absence of generalized cognitive impairment; frontal lobe, temporal lobe, parietal lobe, and diencephalic syndromes are recognized.

INTRODUCTION

Neuropsychiatry is concerned with disorders of affect, cognition, and behavior that arise from overt disorder in cerebral function, or from indirect effects of extracerebral disease. The term has largely replaced the earlier expression 'organic psychiatry', which originated in the classification of mental disorders as either 'organic' or 'functional' on the basis of the presence or absence of pathological changes in the brain. The latter distinction has become increasingly ambiguous as a result of the development of new methods for detecting abnormal brain pathology and pathophysiology in so-called 'functional' disorders such as depression and schizophrenia. Indeed, the most recent version of the Diagnostic and statistical manual of mental disorders, 4th edition (DSM-IV, American Psychiatric Association) states, 'the term organic mental disorder is no longer used in DSM-IV because it incorrectly implies that 'non-organic' mental disorders do not have a biological basis'. Nevertheless, a creative conflict has always pertained between neurological and psychological theories of behavior and, in the absence of satisfactory alternatives, these terms have retained a place in clinical practice. In part, this serves to demarcate the uneasy and shifting boundary between disorders predominantly diagnosed and managed by physicians and psychiatrists, respectively.

In this chapter, we provide a consideration of practical issues related to the assessment, investigation, and management of patients manifesting cognitive and behavioral change, and we discuss specific cerebral and extracerebral disorders that commonly involve or are accompanied by cognitive or behavioral change. Our intention is to help in the identification of possible diagnoses causing particular behavioral features, and also to alert clinicians to the likely neuropsychiatric sequelae of specific medical disorders.

ASSESSMENT AND DIFFERENTIAL DIAGNOSIS OF PATIENTS WITH COGNITIVE AND BEHAVIORAL CHANGE

The assessment and classification of mental and behavioral disorders is a frequent source of misunderstanding and confusion for clinicians, the process being undermined by the absence of robust clinical and laboratory markers for these conditions. Moreover, the clinical terminology used to describe certain symptoms and signs (such as 'confusion') is often unsatisfactory and unreliable. Although the major systems of classification are broadly similar, they continue to use different terminology: e.g. the World Health Organization's International statistical classification of diseases and health-related problems, 10th revision (ICD-10) retains the term 'organic disorders', whereas DSM-IV uses the broad grouping 'delirium, dementia, amnesic, and other cognitive disorders'. In addition, some of the operational diagnoses may have little validity in assisting the clinician to determine the appropriate investigation and treatment, e.g. the ICD-10 'unspecified organic personality and behavioral disorders due to brain disease, damage and dysfunction'. Kopelman and Fleminger proposed a few principles that should be considered in revising ICD-10 and DSM-IV: the existing classification should be simplified; new syndromes should be incorporated where they have pathological justification; links to other specialist diagnostic classifications should be made; a broader range of 'neuropsychiatric disorders' should be incorporated, including alcohol-related organic disorders, head injury, sleep disorders, and if possible also 'psychogenic syndromes'; progressive, degenerative disorders need to be clearly distinguished from nonprogressive syndromes, and some gradation of severity needs to be built; and finally the definitions need to be concise and accurate. Nevertheless, there is consensus on the essential clinical features of these disorders, and in this section we shall describe their assessment on the basis of a number of core features underpinning the differential diagnosis.

Organic Comorbidity in Psychiatric Disorders

Missing an underlying 'organic' diagnosis remains a continuing concern for clinicians responsible for the assessment and treatment of new cases of an apparent psychiatric disorder. (1) Organic psychotic disorder-debate remains over the degree of investigation appropriate at the onset of psychosis. Patients with cognitive impairment, abnormal neurological signs, atypical illnesses not responding to treatment, or other indications from the history, certainly warrant further investigations. Where appropriate, this should include neuroimaging, electroencephalography, syphilis serology, and other investigations indicated by the clinical picture. (2) Organic mood disorder—a variety of medical conditions are associated with prominent affective disorder. (3) Organic personality disorder—insidious changes in personality may reflect frontal lobe pathology.

Acute versus Chronic Disorder

The differentiation of acute and chronic cognitive disorder essentially determines the boundary between delirium and dementia. This distinction should be apparent from the history and mode of presentation, although difficulties may arise where a clear history is lacking due to disturbed communication or the absence of an adequate informant. However, they can usually be distinguished on the basis that conspicuous impairment of attention is typical of an acute disorder, together with a fluctuating course and prominent perceptual disturbance, but the 'acute vs chronic' disorder—where there is a delirium superimposed on a chronic cognitive disorder—should not be overlooked. Caution is also needed in patients in hospital where protracted periods of delirium exceeding 6 months have been reported.

Cognitive versus Psychiatric Disorder

The distinction between a cognitive and a psychiatric disorder is not always easy. It is important to recognize that an apparent cognitive abnormality may be seen in psychiatric disorders such as schizophrenia and depression. In depression, impairment of memory and concentration together with somatic complaints may lead to a misleading impression of dementia, so-called 'pseudodementia' or 'reversible dementia'. Likewise, the distinction between acute psychotic disorders and delirium can be difficult where both conditions show behavioral disturbance and disturbed communication. The risks associated with the wrongful categorization of delirium as psychosis are high: delirium is a medical emergency with high morbidity and mortality, and it is potentially reversible. Likewise, the attribution of a psychiatric disorder as delirium or dementia bears costs in terms of performing unnecessary investigations and pursuing the wrong therapy in an inappropriate setting, thereby compounding any illness behavior.

Specific versus Generalized Cognitive Impairment

If cognitive impairment is identified, it needs to be determined whether this is generalized to many cognitive functions or affects a specific function such as memory, planning, perception, language, or attention. Identification of a specific impairment, such as the amnesic syndrome, offers important clues as to the aetiology and management, and is more likely to result from a focal brain lesion(as opposed to an extracerebral disorder).

Reversible versus Irreversible

The range of causes for any psychiatric or cognitive impairment needs to be fully assessed. In particular, it is essential that those conditions that can be reversed or arrested should be specifically considered. Also, it is important to note that many of the psychiatric and cognitive disturbances caused by underlying organic conditions have a time window for their reversibility, which is usually only in the early phases of the disease, although recent studies suggest that true reversibility of cognitive impairment in the older patient is actually very uncommon.

Acute Cognitive and Behavioral Disturbance

A wide range of disorders may cause acute emotional and behavioral disturbances (Box 1). One of the most problematic aspects of assessment is the distinction between an acute psychotic episode and delirium. The clinical features of delirium (also known as 'acute organic brain syndrome' or 'acute confusional state') and of the 'functional' psychoses typical of schizophrenia or affective disorder share a number of characteristics. First, both involve a pervasive disruption of thought, cognition, communication, and behavior in the patient, hence presenting particular difficulties in assessment. Second, both conditions may involve abnormalities of perception in the form of hallucinations or illusions; abnormalities of belief in the form of delusions or overvalued ideas; psychomotor abnormalities, including hypo or hyperactivity; disturbance of the sleep-wake cycle; and emotional disturbance encompassing the range from depression to irritability and euphoria. These similarities cause practical difficulties in diagnostic differentiation, and they also hint that an absolute distinction between 'functional' psychosis and 'medical' delirium is probably untenable.

Delirium

A thorough history of the antecedents and onset of any behavioral and mental disturbance, as well as details of any

Box 1: Causes of acute behavioral change

- Delirium
- Alcohol and substance misuse
- Psychosis
- Personality disorder
- Acute stress reaction
- Adjustment disorder
- Depression
- Dissociative disorder
- Malingering

past medical or psychiatric disorder, will yield important clues as to the likelihood of an organic aetiology to behavioral change. A drug history should be sought, in particular regarding use of anticholinergic agents.

The uncooperative or mute patient presents a particular challenge as important historical details may not be forthcoming, such as head injury, substance misuse, foreign travel, diabetes, or other medical disorders. Furthermore, accurately eliciting a mental and cognitive state is problematic, and it is in this group that a history from an informant, ward staff or relatives is especially important. The diagnosis of delirium should be suspected where the history of behavioral disturbance is of recent onset, fluctuating, and there is evidence of deterioration at night. Difficulty in communicating with a patient is frequently the first indication of an underlying delirium.

Older people and general hospital inpatients are particularly vulnerable to delirium and there is an expanding literature advocating prevention through early detection and assertive management of risk factors including dehydration, sensory impairment, immobility, sleep deprivation, and cognitive impairment (Box 2). A prevalence of between 10% and 20% has been identified in hospital inpatients. Any change of environment such as a recent admission to residential care or pre-existing cognitive impairment will heighten this vulnerability. Among inpatients the problem is compounded by inadequate information, impersonal environments, and confusing exposure to a myriad of different professionals. It is common for the diagnosis to be missed where there is no overt agitation or antisocial behavior.

Behavioral changes seen with delirium include irritability, repetitive purposeless movements, and disorganization or difficulty performing routine tasks such as undressing. It is important to recognize that patients may be both overactive and noisy or inactive and slow.

The predominant clinical feature of delirium has been described as 'clouding of consciousness' or 'clouding of the sensorium'. There are no consensus definitions for these terms and they are not clear in practice, but have traditionally been used to describe a combination of orientation, attention, and memory deficits. Consequently, deficits of attention are stressed in diagnostic criteria, which in the delirious patient may range from distractibility and inability to follow complicated conversations, through an almost complete inability to register information or to concentrate, progressing in the extreme case to diminished consciousness and coma. Furthermore, such attentional difficulties tend to have a sudden onset and to fluctuate over time. Thinking tends to be muddled and speech may show considerable perseveration. The illusions and hallucinations associated with delirium tend to include a strong visual component, although auditory hallucinations and misperceptions are common. Delusions are usually simple, persecutory in nature, fluctuating, and transient.

Box 2: Risk factors predisposing to delirium

- Age
- Sensory impairment
- Male
- Cognitive impairment
- Depression
- Immobility
- Dehydration
- Alcohol and substance misuse
- Severity of physical illness
- Postoperative and intensive care

It should be noted that if delirium and cognitive impairment are simply assessed by orientation in time, place, and person, then 'mild' or "early" delirium may be missed, and it is therefore important to use additional tests of concentration and memory. All patients should be screened with a small battery of bedside cognitive tests that include specific tests of concentration such as serial subtractions and an assessment of memory for recent events and new information. The Mini-Mental State Examination (MMSE), is often used, but should be supplemented with a few additional memory and other tests.

PSYCHIATRIC DISORDER

A past history of psychiatric contact or treatment should be sought in all those with behavioral disturbance, as this is an indicator of putative psychiatric causation. In those with an underlying psychiatric disorder there is usually a background of insidious behavioral disturbance or personality change, and this will often become apparent from any informant. Delusions in psychotic disorders tend to be complex, bizarre, and consistently held, but this may not be so in early cases. Visual hallucinations are rare in psychosis. Marked attentional and memory deficits are not typical of psychosis, although more subtle attentional problems and a range of other cognitive deficits may be present. Distractibility as a consequence of internal experiences may give the impression of confusion and attentional impairment, but careful cognitive assessment will usually indicate preserved function.

Delirium in those with Psychiatric Disorder

The diagnosis of delirium is particularly difficult in those with a history of severe psychiatric disorder and/or learning disability. Difficulty in communicating with and examining such patients, who may have baseline cognitive impairment, means that delirium is particularly likely to be overlooked. Patients with severe mental illness will often attend for emergency consultations where the initial impression is of deterioration in their mental state, often coupled with a recent history of failing to comply with prescribed treatment or a disengagement from services provided. It should always be remembered that there is a high rate of undiagnosed physical illnesses in this population, and their risk of delirium is also raised because of serious side effects from psychotropic medication, including neuroleptic malignant syndrome and lithium toxicity that can result in a deteriorating mental state. In addition, other aspects of these patients' behavior place them at risk of physical illness, such as coexisting substance and alcohol dependency.

Alcohol and Substance Misuse

About one-quarter of all male medical admissions have been found to have a current or previous alcohol problem. Such individuals commonly attend accident and emergency departments in a state of withdrawal or intoxication that engender negative attitudes from clinical staff. Often, there is an expectation that the behavioral disturbance is due to intoxication or a withdrawal syndrome, without adequate assessment of any other physical pathology. Alternatively, such patients may attempt to minimize their alcohol and drug history so that the contribution of these to their complaints may not be immediately apparent.

Patients with a history of excessive alcohol consumption are vulnerable to a large number of complications that may precipitate delirium (Box 3) and care is needed to assess all of these possibilities. The onset of hallucinations may be mistakenly labelled as a consequence of delirium tremens without consideration of other 'organic' or 'functional' disorders.

Delirium tremens carries a mortality risk of about 5% and there is a danger that a withdrawal or intoxication syndrome may mask the emergence of other complications of alcohol and substance misuse. A history of recent blackouts or seizures should alert the physician to the possibility of hypoglycaemia or epilepsy. A careful assessment of the mental state is needed to differentiate 'functional' disorders, such as alcoholic hallucinosis, from schizophrenia as treatment of a mental disorder may be overlooked. Physical examination should include a careful assessment for signs of cirrhosis or acute hepatic encephalopathy and Wernicke's encephalopathy should always be considered since it may be seen in up to 3% of all admissions for alcohol complications.

Investigation

It is necessary to consider a wide range of factors and medical conditions that can both predispose to (Box 2) and precipitate (Table 1) delirium. A history of alcohol and/or illicit substance misuse may offer important indicators of etiology. Although not always easy, a thorough physical examination, with particular attention to the neurological system, is essential in the assessment of all patients with acute disturbance. In addition, a routine screen, including full blood count, electrolyte and γ-glutamyltransferase (GGT) measurements, liver and thyroid function tests, glucose estimation, and C-reactive protein (CRP)/erythrocyte sedimentation rate (ESR)—is required, as this might indicate delirium where the diagnosis is in doubt. Infection is implicated in around one-third of hospital inpatients who are delirious, and a midstream urine sample (MSU) and chest radiograph are usually warranted inaddition to routine blood testing in these patients.

Relevant history and findings on physical examination usually guide more specific investigation. Encephalitis and intracerebral hemorrhage sometimes present with acute disturbance and cognitive impairment with no additional abnormalities in the history or clinical examination. An urgent CT or MRI of the head is indicated where the immediate cause of acute cognitive impairment is not apparent or there are focal neurological signs. Appropriate tests for infectious diseases such as malaria, trypanosomiasis, typhoid fever, and typhus will also need to be considered when there is a history of foreign travel. An EEG with evidence of progressive cortical slowing may suggest a delirium and the need for more extensive investigations where the diagnosis is in doubt.

Management

Delirium is a medical emergency and management essentially consists of treating the underlying causes. Containment of any behavioral disturbance should involve general measures in the first instance, rather than psychotropic drug treatment, although sedation is necessary in some cases. Careful and repeated explanation of the diagnosis, investigations, and treatment to the patient and relatives is important. The patient should be nursed in a bright, simple room with minimal changes in staff and good lighting at night to reduce perceptual disturbance. Drugs, especially psychoactive and anticholinergic agents that may exacerbate confusion, should be reduced to a minimum. Where sedation is required,

Box 3: Causes of behavioral disturbance associated with a history of alcohol dependency

- Alcohol intoxication
- Alcohol withdrawal
- Alcoholic blackouts
- Head injury
- Delirium tremens
- Wernicke's encephalopathy
- Intracranial hemorrhage
- Pneumonia
- Tuberculosis
- Hepatic encephalopathy
- Epilepsy
- Hypoglycemia
- Hypomagnesemia
- Withdrawal and other alcohol—related seizures
- Alcoholic hallucinosis

Table 1: Precipitants of delirium

Infection	Pneumonia, urinary tract infection, septicemia, any other infection, e.g. HIV, malaria, encephalitis, etc.
Iatrogenic	Drug toxicity-anticonvulsants, psychotropics, anticholinergics, opiates
Vitamin deficiencies	Thiamine, nicotinic acid, and vitamin B_{12} deficiency
Epileptic	Complex partial seizures, postictal states, petit mal epilepsy
Metabolic	Hypoxia, hypercapnia, electrolyte and acid-base disturbances, liver disease, uremia hypothermia, hyperthermia, and porphyria
Endocrine	Hypoglycemia, hypo- and hyperthyroidism, addisonian crisis, hypo- and hyperparathyroidism, hypopituitarism
Trauma	Head injury, acute post-traumatic psychosis
Vascular	Cerebrovascular accident, subarachnoid hemorrhage, hypertensive encephalopathy
Toxic	Alcohol and drug withdrawal and intoxication, carbon monoxide poisoning

Box 4: Disorders presenting with chronic/subacute cognitive and behavioral disturbance

Cognitive
- Dementia
- Frontal lobe syndrome
- Amnesic disorder

Psychiatric
- Depression
- Schizophrenia
- Dissociative disorder

then a regular oral antipsychotic such as haloperidol can be administered, although the clinician should be alert to the powerful antidopaminergic side effects of these drugs.

Chronic and Subacute Cognitive and Behavioral Disturbance

In the assessment of patients with a more insidious onset of cognitive and psychiatric disturbances there can again be uncertainty as to the relative etiological roles of organic or behavioral factors. This may lead to unnecessary investigations at both considerable expense and discomfort to the patient, with attention diverted from appropriate management. Moreover, failure to consider a treatable cerebral disorder such as a space-occupying lesion may lead to avoidable and irreversible brain damage. Box 4 outlines a list of cognitive and psychiatric disorders that may exhibit evidence of cognitive impairment.

The diagnostic challenges in this group of patients are exemplified by the complex differentiation between dementia and depression or 'depressive pseudodementia,' where there are changes in behavior, mood, intellectual functioning, and cognitive performance. Differentiation is complicated by the fact that depressed mood is a frequent prodrome for an emerging dementia such as Alzheimer's. Furthermore, depression is a common complication or consequence of Alzheimer's and other dementias. It is therefore essential in the clinical setting that the relative contributions of behavioral and pathological factors in any given case are considered, and that assessment includes a thorough physical, neurological, and psychiatric examination.

Table 2: Clinical features of dementia

Behavior	Disorganized, inappropriate, and distractible behavior. Lack of interest and initiative. Personality change, antisocial behavior, sleep disturbance, incontinence. Self-neglect
Mood	Anxiety, agitation, irritability and depression. Lability of mood
Thinking and perception	Delusions, illusions, and hallucinations
Cognition	Disorientation, recent and remote memory impairment, deficits in language; comprehension, production, recognition. Apraxia and agnosia
Insight	Impaired

Dementia

Dementia is a progressive neurodegenerative syndrome involving a pervasive impairment of higher cortical functions resulting from widespread brain pathology, the extent of which is best determined by formal neuropsychological assessment using instruments such as the revised Wechsler Adult Intelligence Scale (WAIS-R or WAIS-III), as well as standard memory and executive tests. The etiology and characteristic clinical features of dementia are summarized in Table 2, and the most important causes are shown in Table 3.

In the investigation of dementia it is essential to' identify or exclude reversible causes: this should therefore include a full blood count, electrolyte and metabolic screen, thyroid screen, vitamin B_{12} and folate levels, syphilis serology, urinalysis, chest radiography, and electrocardiography. Imaging techniques are continually improving and are crucially important in the

Table 3: Causes of dementia

Degenerative	Alzheimer's, cerebrovascular disease, Picks disease, Creutzfeldt-Jakob disease, Parkinson's disease, multiple sclerosis; normal-pressure hydrocephalus
Infection	HIV, neurosyphilis, Whipple's disease
Metabolic	A renal dialysis (aluminum toxicity), liver failure, metachromatic leukodystrophy
Endocrine	Hypothyroidism
Vitamin deficiency	Vitamin B_{12} and folate deficiency, pellagra
Space-occupying	Subdural hemorrhage, tumor
Traumatic	Punch-drunk syndrome
Genetic	Wilson's disease, Huntington's chorea
Autoimmune	SLE, APS
Anoxia	Respiratory failure, cardiac arrest, CO poisoning
Toxic	Alcohol dementia, heavy metal poisoning (lead, arsenic, mercury, and thallium)

Abbreviations: APS, antiphospholipid antibody syndrome; SLE, systemic lupus erythematosus

diagnosis of dementia (see section on 'Focal disorders'). In some cases, EEG and cerebrospinal fluid examination are essential. Brain biopsy can be of additional assistance when justified by the clinical setting. However, one should keep in mind that choosing the appropriate investigation is dependent on the nature of clinical presentation: e.g. any suggestion of sporadic Creutzfeldt-Jakob disease (CJD) would make an EEG essential; focal neurological signs would indicate the need for early neuroimaging to exclude a space-occupying lesion; a known history of HIV infection may warrant a lumbar puncture; evidence of extrapyramidal disturbance should alert the clinician to the possibility of Wilson's disease, necessitating serum copper and ceruloplasmin level investigation and slit lamp examination for Kayser–Fleischer rings.

The presence of a family history of early-onset cognitive impairment may raise the possibility of predictive and diagnostic genetic testing after appropriate counselling. These can be used in Huntington's disease (huntingtin or HTT gene), familial Alzheimer's disease (FAD) (three genes responsible for autosomal dominant FAD have been identified: amyloid precursor protein gene (APP), presenilin 1 (PSENI) gene, and presenilin 2 (PSEN2) gene, as well as in familial frontotemporal dementia (MAPT gene). However, a number of risks to such testing need to be considered, including psychological effects (i.e. depression, plans of suicide), prenatal diagnosis and testing of children, impact on insurances and employment, legal aspects, possible third-party coercion, and an understanding of the test limitations.

Focal Cognitive Disorders

Focal degenerative disorders were described long ago by Pick and others, but little recent attention was given to the reports of focal or lobar atrophy until Mesulam reported about primary progressive aphasia in 1982. A variety of neuropsychiatric syndromes may arise from regional cerebral impairments of diverse cause and may present in the absence of generalized cognitive impairment. However, classifying these syndromes has been difficult and the terminology remains-confusing. Broadly, the frontal variant and temporal lobe variants of frontotemporal dementia have been distinguished, and within the temporal lobe variant-progressive aphasia may be 'fluent' (as in 'semantic dementia') or nonfluent. However, the underlying histopathology has been shown to be very heterogeneous even within these broad lobar variants.

Frontal Lobe Syndromes

Particular neuropsychiatric interest is attached to the consequences of damage to the anterior regions of the brain. These are frequently neurologically 'silent', but they can also result in remarkable alterations in behavior and personality, with preservation of spatial skills as well as cognitive functions such as memory and intelligence. Thus, neuropsychiatric manifestations may be the only signs of frontal brain disease, and psychiatric disturbance may be an impediment to medical management. Two clinical syndromes (which frequently coexist) are recognized. The first is characterized by emotional blunting, lack of empathy, indifference, and loss of initiative and motivation with impoverished speech and communication to the extreme of mutism. The second is characterized by decline in social conduct, loss of social awareness, disinhibition, impulsivity (occasionally with aggression), poor attention and concentration span, and decline in personal hygiene and grooming: in general, such patients are excessively talkative and may confabulate spontaneously. In addition, mental rigidity, fixed ideation, and stereotyped behaviors, including mannerisms or ritualistic preoccupations are common. Both of these syndromes have been subsumed under the term 'dysexecutive syndrome' (also known as 'strategy application disorder'), which attempts a unitary cognitive psychological perspective on the condition. Interesting parallels have been drawn between the clinical frontal lobe syndrome and features of neurological conditions such as Parkinson's disease and psychiatric disorders, such as the negative syndrome in schizophrenia: in both these examples it is thought that impaired dopaminergic neurotransmission in prefrontal brain regions gives rise to the particular symptomatology.

Temporal Lobe Syndromes

A variety of syndromes are recognized following temporal lobe damage depending upon the particular area affected.

Personality disturbance may be seen, although usually with neurological impairments. A particular variant of this is Kluver-Bucy syndrome following bilateral lesions to the medial and lateral temporal lobes: these results in placidity, hyperorality, bulimia, abnormal sexual behavior, and visual agnosia. It is a rare neurobehavioral condition but can be seen in patients with extensive temporal lobe damage as a result of post-traumatic, postinfectious, and degenerative (dementias) disorders.

Hemisphere specific, language dominant temporal lobe lesions may produce aphasia, 'surface' dyslexia, and/or dysgraphia, frequently accompanied by neurological impairments on the contralateral side. Progressive aphasia can be fluent or nonfluent. Nondominant lesions may particularly affect facial, spatial, or autobiographical memory, or may appear to be cognitively 'silent'. There is a recognized association between temporal lobe lesions, particularly those giving rise to epileptic activity, and psychosis, which may bear striking similarities with that seen in schizophrenia or affective disorder. Severe bilateral mediotemporal lobe damage usually gives rise to a profound amnesic syndrome, with an almost complete loss of the ability to learn new material (anterograde amnesia) and a variable degree of retrograde loss of memory. Pathology in the left inferior and lateral temporal gyri can produce severe deficits in semantic memory as seen in progressive fluent aphasia.

Parietal Lobe Syndromes

The parietal lobes play a critical role in numerous cognitive functions such as attention, spatial representation, working memory, mental calculation, eye movements, and the guidance of actions. However, perhaps the main role of the parietal lobes is in determination of what is attended and what is ignored, in the representation of space, and in the aspects of sensorimotor conversions. Balint's syndrome, caused by bilateral parietal damage, is a particularly striking disorder characterized by gaze apraxia, optic ataxia and simultanagnosia. It causes impairment in space representation, while visual processing of basic perceptual features (colour and form) is spared.

Damage to the inferior parietal region may result in a profound neglect, which is thought to be an attentional impairment, not a perceptual deficit, although it can be difficult to fully distinguish between the two. Theories about inferior parietal lobe involvement in attentional processing suggest that either (1) it is involved in the disengagement of attention-patients with unilateral parietal damage have difficulty disengaging spatial lattention from the ipsilesional visual field, making it difficult to direct attention to contralesional stimuli-and/or (2) it participates in the detection of salient items embedded in a rapid sequence of events and in maintaining or controlling attent ionover time.

The posterior parietal cortex plays a critical role in multimodal spatial integration and in the fusion of different coordinates into a unified representation of space.

Hemisphere differences between right and left also appear to be important: right inferior and temporal parietal lobe lesions commonly lead to neglect, whereas damage to the homologous region in the left hemisphere can lead to an apraxic syndrome.

Diencephalic Syndromes

Lesions to the deep midline structures of the thalamus, the anterior nucleus and mamillary bodies as well as the degeneration of key fiber tracts connecting the limbic structures are associated with amnesic syndrome, particularly exemplified by the Wernicke-Korsakoff syndrome. The crucial pathology here is thought to involve neuronal loss, gliosis, and microhemorrhages that produce disruption of complex mammilothalamic circuits. Pathology in the paraventricular and periaqueductal grey matter, and in the frontal lobes is also common. Clinically the condition is characterized by profound anterograde amnesia relative to any generalized cognitive impairment, and is usually associated with disorientation in time. Typically, these patients also perseverate when faced with shifts in the task demands. An interaction between ethanol neurotoxicity and thiamine deficiency has been postulated, contributing to the development of behavioral alterations and cerebral damage. An amnesic syndrome can also be caused by herpes simplex encephalitis, carbon monoxide poisoning, cerebral anoxia, thalamic infarction, subarachnoid hemorrhage, head injury, deep midline space-occupying lesions, or tuberculous meningitis;

Investigation

Cognitive Assessment

Neuropsychological tests require the patient's cooperation and may fail to discriminate reliably between a cognitive and a psychiatric disorder. However, they may furnish important indications of localized cerebral dysfunction, and they assist the clinician in monitoring the (treatment) progress of any cognitive impairment; they give valuable information about daily functioning; and they help in planning rehabilitation and intervention programmes. A wide range of tests is available to evaluate patterns of disability.

Brain Imaging

Also important in investigating suspected neuropsychiatric disorders are brain imaging techniques, the technology and application of which has expanded greatly in recent years. For structural imaging, CT is able to reveal most cerebral lesions, but should nowadays be reserved for the investigation of symptoms of acute onset, where time is of essence and management decisions must be made rapidly. In more insidious, less acute contexts, the structural brain imaging of choice is MRI, which allows both a higher spatial resolution with fine anatomical detail and a choice of endogenous/exogenous tissue contrast modalities, producing greater diagnostic yield. MRI is more sensitive than CT in identifying small vascular lesions or demyelination, but less sensitive in detecting calcified lesions. Sequential estimation of cerebral atrophy and quantitative approaches can facilitate the accurate assessment of disease progression. More sophisticated techniques, such as serial volumetric imaging and voxel compression subtraction, with emphases on a quantitative approach, have been developed to reveal changes overtime. However, the time consuming nature of these procedures prevents their widespread use as diagnostic tools. Diffusion tensorimaging MRI (DTI) can be used to determine the integrity of subcortical fiber tracts in vivo, but is generally restricted to research settings.

The past decade has also seen an enormous expansion in functional brain imaging that allows assessment of brain regional engagement during cognitive processing. Changes in regional cerebral blood flow using positron emission tomography (PET), or in regional hemoglobin oxygenation status using blood oxygenation level dependent (BOLD) functional MRI (fMRI), can be measured during cognitive performance. Magnetic resonance spectroscopy (MRS) allows noninvasive in vivo analysis of neurochemicals and their metabolites, and over the last two decades has been performed in patients with a range of neurological and psychiatric disorders to help understand the underlying pathological mechanisms, to monitor long-term changes with or without drug therapy, and to identify differences between diagnostic groups. More recently, changes in MRS measures have been correlated with cognitive performance in normal populations and in patients with cognitive disorders. Magnetic resonance perfusion (MRP), magnetic resonance diffusion (MRD) weighted imaging, and single photon emission computed tomography (SPECT), can help to identify subtle pathophysiological changes in the brain, before structural changes are present, thereby offering the potential for accurate and early diagnosis. Even though these functional imaging techniques are mainly used in research settings at present, they may well offer clinical value to diagnostic classification in the future.

Neurophysiology

The EEG is frequently employed in the investigation of neuropsychiatric disorder as it is both widely available and a sensitive, if relatively nonspecific, indicator of cerebral dysfunction. Focal abnormalities are characteristic of epilepsy that may, in turn, reflect vascular change. Diffuse slowing (i.e. a shift to lower frequency ranges) is a sensitive indicator of brain dysfunction arising from metabolic and degenerative processes that correlates with the degree of cognitive impairment, although with relatively little specificity. Characteristic EEG changes are associated with Huntington's disease (pronounced flattening of traces), sporadic Creutzfeldt-Jakob disease (repetitive and triphasic spike discharges), and in association with specific drugs. Medial temporal slowing can be suggestive of early Alzheimer's dementia.

ORGANIC COMORBIDITY IN PSYCHIATRIC DISORDERS

Missing an underlying 'organic' diagnosis remains a continuing concern for clinicians responsible for the assessment and treatment of new cases of an apparent psychiatric disorder. The diagnosis of secondary psychotic/affective/personality disorder is used according to DSM-IV if the psychopathology is comparable to that of idiopathic disorder but caused by an organic brain disease. However, in many cases the causal relationship between the organic dysfunction and the psychiatric symptoms remains unclear. Therefore, instead of using the 'organic' diagnosis, the concept of comorbidity is widely used. Table 4 outlines some common brain disorders causing psychiatric disorder.

Organic Psychotic Disorder

Clinical experience and numerous case reports attest to the wide range of disorders that may emerge following the initial diagnosis of a 'functional' psychosis. One follow-up study of a sample of patients with first-episode schizophrenia found that 15 out of 268 had a neurological disorder that appeared relevant to the mental state, with 13 out of these 15 having salient features in the medical history or neurological signs

Table 4: Neuropsychiatric causes of psychiatric disorders

Intracranial disorder	Cerebrovascular stroke, head injury, Parkinson's disease, multiple sclerosis, brain tumor, epilepsy, Huntington's disease, postencephalitic
Endocrine disorder	Hypothyroidism, hyperthyroidism, hyperparathyroidism, hypopituitarism, Addison's disease, Cushing's disease, hypoglycemia, diabetes mellitus
Systemic disorder	Hepatic failure, renal failure, pernicious anemia, rheumatoid arthritis, systemic lupus erythematosus, malignant neoplasia, viral infection (particularly infectious mononucleosis, influenza)
Pharmacological causes	Corticosteroids, estrogens (e.g. Hormone replacement therapy), oral contraceptives, L-DOPA, clonidine, methylphenidate, withdrawal from stimulant agents, e.g. amphetamines

that could have alerted the clinician to the underlying disorder, the two exceptions both having a diagnosis of neurosyphilis. HIV is increasingly prevalent in this population and one recent cohort identified a known diagnosis of HIV in about 6% of the patients, with many subjects not tested. An assessment of risk factors for HIV is therefore required in all the new cases of psychotic disorder. Overall, the literature suggests that the risk of missing underlying medical or neurological disorder is relatively low, provided that a thorough clinical assessment is performed. Some debate remains over the degree of investigation appropriate at the onset of psychosis. Patients with cognitive impairment, abnormal neurological signs, atypical illnesses not responding to treatment, or other indications from the history, certainly warrant further investigations. Where appropriate this should include neuroimaging, electroencephalography, syphilis serology, and other investigations indicated by the clinical picture. Increasingly, neuroimaging provides important information relevant to the management of the particular case, although in the absence of specific indications the identification of treatable neurological disease is low.

Organic Mood Disorder

A variety of medical conditions are associated with prominent affective disorder, including anxiety, elation, and depressive symptoms. In many of these there appears to be a direct relationship between the presence of brain disease and depression, and the latter does not just seem to reflect the disabling social consequences of chronic disease, although the 'psychological reaction' to the disablement may well be an important contributory factor, e.g. there is accumulating evidence suggesting that depression in Parkinson's disease is secondary to the underlying neuroanatomical degeneration, rather than simply a reaction to the psychosocial stress and disability. Furthermore, the severity of depression may correlate with the 'objective' disability or the prognosis of the disorder or cognitive impairment, and in some disorders, such as multiple sclerosis, can be associated with either euphoria or depression, or mood swings between the two extremes.

Organic Personality Disorder

Organic personality disorder is an unhappy term employed in ICD-10 to denote acute or (more typically) insidious changes in personality, defined as a significant alteration in the habitual disposition and behavior of a patient from their premorbid state. The syndrome is well recognized, although often in retrospect, and may often reflect frontal lobe pathology. Most prominently affected is the degree of emotional expression and levels of activity in the absence of pronounced cognitive alterations, except where 'higherlevel' functions such as planning complex actions or anticipation of social and emotional consequences are affected. Table 5 outlines some of the common causes.

Advances in brain imaging have led to a progressive increase in studies focusing on structural markers of human personality. These suggest a relationship between personality change and atrophy, particularly in the frontal lobes, but also in supplementary motor area gray matter, right anterior cingulate cortex, or the whole brain. Functional imaging studies have identified a number of personality traits supposedly associated with alterations in central metabolism, neurotransmitter function, or cerebral blood flow. However, these findings have not yet been closely related to neuropsychiatric symptoms.

Specific Conditions Giving Rise to Neuropsychiatric Symptoms

This section attempts to address two aspects of neuropsychiatric problems associated with medical conditions: (1) to prompt the recognition and exploration of psychiatric abnormality in 'high risk' conditions where such associations are well recognized; and (2) to encourage appropriate medical examination and investigation in the presence of outwardly psychiatric abnormality.

Psychological or psychiatric disorder may become manifest as an adjustment reaction to medical disability, malaise, and handicap, and this can affect not only the patient, but also family members, who often bear the practical burden of care. Psychiatric disorder may also result from a specific compromise of cerebral function, either directly or systemically mediated. For example, postoperative psychiatric disturbance is common and usually the result of infective, metabolic, or drug-induced delirium. However, the circumstances of operation may lead to the precipitation of disorientation in the presence of an insidious dementia, or a withdrawal syndrome in an alcohol-dependent individual. Furthermore, the emotional reaction in response to life-threatening and life-altering circumstances may be profound following major surgery. These factors interact, and the ultimate expression of mental disturbance depends upon a particular patient's premorbid disposition and social circumstances, as well as specific illness factors. Nevertheless, the recognition and specific ascertainment of the presence

Table 5: Causes of 'organic personality disorder

Intracerebral insult	Cerebrovascular stroke, head injury, tumor (frequently frontal/sphenoidal meningioma), abscess, encephalitis (frequently herpes encephalitis, which has a recognized tropism for frontotemporal brain regions), subdural hematomas (chronic)
Neurodegenerative conditions	Huntington's disease, Wilson's disease (hepatolenticular degeneration), Pick's disease, Creutzfeldt-Jakob disease, subcortical dementias

of mental disturbance in certain conditions has profound diagnostic and prognostic importance.

Neurological Disorders

Cerebrovascular Disorders

The psychiatric complications associated with stroke illustrate the relevance of a neuropsychiatric perspective. Early studies recognized distinct emotional reactions associated with cerebral damage. These include the catastrophic reaction (often extreme or disproportionate emotional outburst to small demands), an indifference reaction (associated with fatuous mood, indifference to failures, and unilateral neglect and anosognosia), and pathological laughter/crying reaction (also known rather pejoratively as emotional incontinence', where emotional displays occur seemingly spontaneously or to trivial provocation). The mood consequences of stroke are often disproportionate to the objective disability and it is important to screen for depression and anxiety in the first months after a stroke. The relationship between mood disorder and lesion location has been contentious, although there is an emerging consensus that anterior lesions are more associated with depression.

Cerebral Tumors

Cerebral tumors are frequently associated with neuropsychiatric disability, ranging from understandable reactions to the diagnosis to frank syndromes resulting from impaired brain function. Minor psychological disturbance including anxiety, depression, and occasionally hysterical symptoms may be seen before the medical diagnosis is made, and specific signs of cerebral pathology need to be excluded in this group of patients. The regional syndromes outlined above are notable in cases of primary or secondary cerebral tumors, in particular when the tumor is rapidly progressive or where multiple brain regions are involved with metastases.

The most common adult-onset primary tumor is the ostensibly 'benign' meningioma, which is notoriously slow growing (estimates of growth indicate that at diagnosis it has often been present for some 10 to 15years) and hence cerebral function is only slowly compromised. Coupled with their propensity for a frontal location, in which there may be few frank neurological signs, this can lead to tragic cases where the cause of progressive personality deterioration is missed.

More dramatic impairments of cerebral function are particularlyassociated with rapidly progressive tumors in which raised intracranial pressure, irritative epileptic phenomena, and an overall distortion in brain structure may combine—to produce delirium and dementia.

There can be remote effects of malignant disease on cerebral function: hypercalcemia may present with an acute confusional state or with other psychological/psychiatric manifestations, and some forms of lung carcinoma (in particular) secrete growth factor/endocrine hormones that result in neurodegenerative changes and a dementia-like picture. Furthermore, both episodic and prolonged confusional states have been reported in malignant disease in the absence of a clear metabolic disturbance or focal brain involvement, e.g. in diffuse leptomeningeal disease. Recent studies suggest that cognitive function is an important outcome measure in patients with brain tumors and is an independent prognostic factor in the survival of glioma patients. Moreover, cognitive deterioration may be the first indicator of progressive disease following treatment.

Head Injury

Head injury often leads to impairment in personality, affect, and social/occupational function that is more prominent than the objective dysfunction would suggest. The wide range of neuropsychiatric sequelae recognized after head injury are outlined in Box 5. The most disabling and distressing problems for both patients and carers are often the emotional and behavioral effects and in particular, personality change. This may reflect the vulnerability of the anterior temporal poles, frontal polar regions, and the orbitofrontal cortex to closed head injuries. After traumatic brain injury the risk of suicide increases threefold, with around 15% attempting suicide in the first 5 years after injury.

Impairment of consciousness is characteristic after all but the most mild head injuries and features of delirium are often seen after severe injuries. The period of post-traumatic amnesia represents the time that elapses between the moment of injury and the restoration of continuing memory for everyday events. This remains an important predictor of outcome, correlated with personality change as well as intellectual impairment and neurological disorder. By contrast, memory loss for the events of the trauma itself sometimes appears to protect against the development of post-traumatic stress disorder.

Box 5: Neuropsychiatric consequences of head injury

- Delirium
- Focal cognitive disorder (frontal lobe syndrome, amnestic disorder)
- Global cognitive disorder
- Subdural hematoma
- Post-traumatic epilepsy
- Delusional syndrome and hallucinosis
- Affective syndrome
- Post-traumatic disorder
- Anxiety disorder
- Personality change
- Conversion disorders
- Postconcussional syndrome
- Alcohol misuse

Cognitive impairment following head injury is usually more apparent after a post-traumatic amnesia exceeding 24 hours and testing reveals that Performance IQ is more vulnerable to the effects of trauma than Verbal IQ. Penetrating and localized injuries tend to result in more focal cognitive deficits dependent on the site of injury. Dysexecutive syndrome and anterograde memory impairment are commonly seen. In rare cases head injuries may predispose to Alzheimer's disease.

Personality change is particularly common after severe head injury and frontal lobe damage, including irritability, impatience, apathy and lability of mood. There is also an inability to learn from experience with poor judgement and lack of initiative. Aggression and sexual disinhibition may necessitate high levels of subsequent care and are predicted by early agitation after head injury. Delusional disorders are frequently observed in the early stages of recovery and may reflect the persistence of disordered cognition; mood and anxiety disorders are also often seen. Premorbid alcohol misuse may have predisposed to the trauma and alcohol tolerance can decline markedly after severe injury. Problems with heavy drinking are common in this group, which may reflect poor insight and drinking in response to stressful circumstances. Caution is needed to exclude chronic subdural hematoma and post-traumatic epilepsy before ascribing emotional and behavioral change to a psychiatric diagnosis.

Complex rehabilitation strategies are often needed to manage this group of patients and novel pharmacological managements are being assessed.

Epilepsy

In assessing epilepsy it is important to establish the extent of underlying cerebral damage giving rise to the epileptic discharge, as well as the nature and severity of any cognitive impairment. While compatible with normal intelligence, epilepsy is more common in patients with a learning disability and is related to its severity, presumably as both epilepsy and a learning difficulty arise from underlying cerebral dysfunction. Thus, the capacity of individuals to manage their epilepsy is highly variable and poses an important problem-for management. Furthermore, there can be a relationship between emotional state and epileptic seizures, indicative of an important brain-mind correlation.

The neuropsychiatric consequences of epilepsy are best considered in terms of peri-ictal and interictal disorders, which are outlined in Table 6. This has important implications for management in which the focus should be on optimal control of seizures. Psychotropic medication can decrease the seizure threshold and possible interactions with anticonvulsants should be considered. The S2-D2 (refers to antagonism of atypical antipsychotics at the dopamine type 2 receptor and the serotonin type 2A receptor) or atypical neuroleptics are current first-line treatments for psychosis and are also used in aggression and irritability; olanzapine, risperidone, and quetiapine are particularly recommended. Selective serotonin reuptake inhibitors (SSRIs) are generally agreed to be safe treatments for depression in patients with epilepsy.

Subacute Encephalopathies

A well-recognized manifestation of acute cerebral infection or encephalitis is a dramatic behavioral disturbance that may involve violence and delirium. This is a relatively common diagnostic problem and it is clearly of vital importance to make a correct diagnosis. Of particular note are, firstly, that the particular groups relatively predisposed to the development of encephalitis are alcohol and drug misusers, where attitudes of medical staff may exert a pejorative effect, and secondly, that the disordered behavior may be sufficiently extreme to render medical examination and management difficult.

Herpes simplex encephalitis is particularly implicated in such presentations, perhaps as the most common encephalitis and also because of tropism of the virus to frontal and temporal regions. Damage in these areas may lead to psychosis, abnormalities incognitive or social processing, or a syndrome resembling autism, particularly early in the course of disease. However, these presentations rarely persist in isolation and are less common than paresis or seizures. Furthermore, it is quite common that frontotemporal damage in these patients causes persistent behavioral deficits.

Table 6: Neuropsychiatric complications of epilepsy

Ictal and peri-ictal disorders	
Prodromal states Complex partial seizures	Tension, irritability, and depression may be seen automatisms, distortions of perception, hallucinations, deja vu, unusual disturbances of memory, thinking sudden changes in affect
Interictal disorders non-epileptic seizures cognitive impairment	Seen in about one-third of those attending specialist epilepsy centers. Associated with physical and sexual abuse. This usually reflects underlying brain damage, and developmental consequences of repeated seizures and treatment with anticonvulsants. Associated with duration and frequency of previous seizures
Personality	Probably only related to severe epilepsy where there is underlying brain damage
Schizophrenia-like psychosis	Associated with temporal lobe epilepsy
Depression	Suicide is four times more frequent in epileptics: those with adverse social factors and temporal lobe epilepsy are particularly at risk

Other forms of encephalitis can also produce striking behavioral change, e.g. Epstein-Barr virus may lead to visual metamorphosis ('Alice in Wonderland' syndrome; an unusual syndrome characterized by visual hallucinations and bizarre perceptual distortions of form, size, movement, and color, where objects appear larger or smaller than their actual size, associated with an abnormal sense of time or place), occasionally with persistent complications.

Intracranial Infections

Neurosyphilis

Neurosyphilis can result in several different syndromes from infection of the brain, meninges or spinal cord. While its incidence is still rather low, neurosyphilis has become more common due to an increased prevalence of immunosuppression. The presentation can be subtle, atypical, often monosymptomatic, and it can present with psychiatric symptoms alone. Patients with neurosyphilis may show a normal MRI head scan, or bilateral mesiotemporal T2 hyperintensity, or meningeal thickening. A wide range of neuroimaging findings can resemble those found in herpes simplex encephalitis, mesial temporal sclerosis, leukoaraiosis, normal pressure hydrocephalus, and glioblastoma multiforme. However, neurosyphilis most commonly adopts either a meningeal form (leptomeningeal granulomas that may also occur intra-axially) or avascular form (typically presenting with cortical and subcortical infarcts), which often occur together. CSF findings can vary from positive oligoclonal IgG bands and high IgG index to pleocytosis with or without CSF venereal disease research laboratory test (VDRL). Clinicians should be aware that dementia in young patients with temporal lobe atrophy and/or vascular damage can be caused by syphilis, and therefore these findings necessitate CSF and syphilis testing.

Human Immunodeficiency Virus

Human immunodeficiency virus (HIV) is a neurotropic virus that enters the brain within 2 weeks of initial infection. Combination antiretroviral therapies have changed the course of the illness, but many patients with HIV still show signs of associated neurocognitive dysfunction. The clinical features of HIV-associated neurocognitive impairment are thought to reflect widespread synaptodendritic problems in the fronto-striato-thalamo-cortical circuit. Patients typically have problems with executive functions (e.g. abstraction, processing speed, verbal fluency, decision making and attention) as well as with learning new information. It has also been postulated that prospective memory is particularly affected, i.e. ability to execute a future intention. The severity of cognitive decline can increase with age and in association with high viral loads and reduced $CD4^+$ cell counts, as well as in association with age-related decline in functioning of fronto-striato-thalamo-cortical circuitry. Cognitive impairment can predict mortality, independent of clinical stage or $CD4^+$ cell counts.

There is also an overall increased susceptibility of patients with HIV to develop a major psychiatric disorder: new-onset psychosis is reported in up to 15% and can occur without encephalopathy. The putative involvement of subcortical dopaminergic systems, particularly basal ganglia structures, is supported by high rates of antipsychotic-related extrapyramidal symptoms and neuropathological studies in HIV-infected patients.

Mood disorders are common in patients with HIV and effective treatment may result in considerable health and economic benefits. Depressive disorders are reported among 20–40%; they are commonly unrecognized but respond to appropriate treatment interventions in 80–90% of cases. Mania without pre-existing bipolar disorder or family history is found in 8% of patients in the late stages of disease, typically in the context of dementia and CNS involvement; early in HIV infection, episodes of mania are more commonly related to pre-existing bipolar disorder or family history.

Variant Creutzfeldt–Jakob Disease

Variant Creutzfeldt-Jakob disease (VCID) appears to present in a much younger population (mean age at death is 29 years) than the sporadic variant (mean age at death is 63). Difficulties occur in diagnosis because the early symptoms of VCID are often nonspecific such as anorexia, mild insomnia, apathy, mood swings, and personality changes, and prominent neurological signs are lacking. Neurological examination in the early stages is usually normal but subsequent neurological decline is characterized by progressive ataxia, paraesthesia in legs and face, unusual aches and pains in hands, feet, face and lumbar region, and cognitive impairment. Careful clinical assessment remains the most important element in the early detection of symptomatic disease.

The most useful noninvasive investigation in advanced cases has been MRI imaging, particularly fluid attenuated inversion recovery (FLAIR) sequence. The pulvinar sign (a symmetrical region of signal hyperintensity in the pulvinar nucleus of the thalamus) has been reported to have sensitivity of up to 95% in the appropriate clinical context. EEG generally does not show the typical appearances of sporadic CJD. Definitive diagnosis of vCID is based on neuropathological findings, obtained by brain biopsy, and supplemented by prion protein (PrP) immunohistochemistry and molecular strain typing by Western blotting of human brain tissue. Because PrP immunoreactivity is present in the tonsils of vCJD patients, tonsil biopsy has been proposed as a less invasive alternative to brain biopsy. The WHO published diagnostic criteria for sporadic CJD in 2001, suggesting that neuropathological examination (biopsy) is not mandatory for the confirmation of the diagnosis.

Neurodegenerative Conditions

Multiple Sclerosis

Affective disorders are common in multiple sclerosis (MS) and have been divided into four categories; depressive disorder, bipolar affective disorder, euphoria, and pseudobulbar affect. Both bipolar affective disorder and depression are more common in patients with MS than in the general population, with the lifetime prevalence for the latter being 50%. Euphoria is more common in patients with advanced disease, with a median prevalence of 25%. Pseudobulbar affect is found in about 10% of MS patients.

It is important not to dismiss these symptoms as they all are associated with significant morbidity and mortality. Furthermore, a strong association between affective disorder and cognitive impairment (40–65%) is recognized in MS. Depression can exert particularly adverse effects on the executive component of working memory. Cognitive functions in progressive MS subtypes are likely to decline across time, particularly on tasks requiring concurrent multiple abilities, i.e. visuospatial ability and processing speed or working memory and processing speed. Cognitive impairment in MS may reflect several underlying defects such as lesion severity, changes in neuronal signaling caused by axonal degeneration, and demyelination. Neurotransmitter changes are also recognized, e.g. a decline in choline acetyltransferase activity, and there are a number of studies showing benefits with acetylcholine esterase inhibitors. MS can also occasionally present as a cortical variant alone, with significant psychiatric complaints prior to sensory and motor presentations.

Parkinson's Disease and Movement Disorders

There are four particular aspects of neuropsychiatric disturbance relevant to the consideration of idiopathic and atypical parkinsonian syndromes, including multisystem atrophy:

1. A prodromal period without frank movement disorder is well recognized and may be typified by sleep disturbances, depression, as well as sensory and autonomic dysfunction, possibly reflecting the non-dopaminergic-cell dysfunction. Interestingly, these nonmotor symptoms are also prominent in advanced stages of the disorders.
2. Dopaminergic replacement therapy, whether with cholinergic antagonists, dopamine agonists, or levodopa (L-DOPA), is associated with a substantial incidence of psychosis and delirium. However, the neuronal degeneration of the pedunculopontine nucleus, locus coeruleus, and the dopaminergic raphe nuclei may also play a role.
3. There is a strong association between Parkinson's disease and depression (10–50%), with possibly a more significant biological than purely reactive basis. Depression is characterized by a feeling of guilt, lack of self-esteem, sadness, and remorse.
4. Many patients develop 'diffuse' (extranigrostriatal) Lewy body disease, characterized by a progressive dysexecutive syndrome with impairment of visuospatial abilities and memory against a background of loss of response to dopaminergic drugs.

Particular mention should be made here of the iatrogenic movement disorder attendant upon antipsychotic and antidepressant medication. The mechanisms underlying this drug-induced movement disorder are largely unclear, but drug-induced movement disorders are generally reversible once the medication is removed, suggesting that the drugs produce an interference with neuronal function.

Learning Disability

Although beyond the immediate scope of this chapter, the diverse conditions that give rise to learning disorders have been the subject of intense recent interest. In particular, their strong associations with attention deficit-hyperactivity disorder (ADHD), fetal alcohol syndrome, and autism have underscored a probable neuropsychiatric basis. Interestingly, studies suggest a critical role of the prefrontal cortex and its connections to the parietal cortex and striatum in children with ADHD in divided attention tasks, in inhibiting distraction and prepotent responses, and in maintaining the information 'on line' in working memory. From a neurodevelopmental perspective, attention deficit in children is strongly linked to conduct disorder and may have diverse consequences in adulthood, providing a precursor for some instances of personality disorder, traditionally not viewed in neuropsychiatric terms.

Another relevant area of interest is the concept of behavioral phenotypes, where consistent behavioral abnormalities are associated with distinct genotypic abnormalities. For example, the frequently occurring chromosomal disorders of Down's syndrome, Turner's syndrome and Klinefelter's syndrome have distinct and consistent neuropsychiatric aspects, albeit of variable degree. In Turner's syndrome, overall IQ is variable but distinct difficulties in visuospatial function give rise to large Verbal-Performance IQ deficits.

Extracerebral Disorders

Endocrine Disorders

Endocrine disorder has an important influence on mental function and there are characteristic associations with neuropsychiatric disorder. The use of "routine" blood tests of endocrine function has resulted in the earlier detection of problems, such that florid states are now rarely seen. The focus of clinical interest in this area is upon "preclinical" endocrine dysfunction, the complications arising from the disorder and treatment.

Diabetes Mellitus

The neuropsychiatric aspects of diabetes mellitus (DM), both insulin-dependent (IDDM) and non-insulin-dependent (NIDDM) forms, may be considered in four aspects:

1. The syndrome itself and the constraints of optimal management have a considerable impact on the lives of people with the disorder. The disorder is stigmatizing, especially in the young, and is associated with significant morbidity and mortality. There is a risk of impaired psychological development, personality difficulties and affective disorder. There is clear evidence of a relationship between 'stress', emotional disturbance, and impaired glycemic control, although whether this is mediated directly or indirectly (through neglect of diet and treatment) is unclear.
2. Increased prevalence of psychological disturbance has been reported, particularly with IDDM. Anxiety disorder has been linked to poor glycemic control, which in turn relates to fear of hypoglycemia. IDDM-associated hypoglycemic episodes can also cause frank automatisms.
3. Cognitive dysfunction in diabetic subjects has been recognized since the early 20th century. Both IDDM and NIDDM are associated with slowing of mental speed and diminished mental flexibility and NIDDM is also associated with deficits in actual learning and memory processing. Several studies have shown that the rate of cognitive decline is accelerated in older people with NIDDM. There are several proposed pathophysiological mechanisms linking diabetes to changes in the brain and cognitive decline, including atherosclerosis (macroangiopathy, increased risk of stroke), microvascular disease (microangiopathy, small vessel disease), glucose toxicity (advanced protein glycation and oxidative stress, 'advanced aging'), and insulin mediated changes (increased secretion and decreased break-down of the amyloid). Neuroimaging studies suggest that the appearances of the brain in patients with diabetes resemble that of normal aging, but appear to develop at a younger age than in normal population.
4. The incidence of dementia is higher in people with diabetes compared with the normal population. However, the risk factors and mechanisms underlying the association between diabetes, accelerated cognitive decline, and vascular dementia still need to be identified.

Thyroid Disorder

It is rare for classical presentations of thyroid disease to be missed in clinical practice, but interesting to note that surveys reveal that more than 5% of attendees at psychiatric consultations have an abnormality in thyroid function. While not all of this group would benefit from treatment for thyroid disease, it underscores the insidious nature of thyroid dysfunction. The rule should be to exclude this whenever suspicions are aroused. In particular, hypothyroidism may commonly manifest as apathy, depression, memory impairment, and dementia with prominent cognitive slowing: the condition may be reversible if recognized and treated early, but rarely so in long-lasting cases of hypothyroidism. Neonatal hypothyroidism or 'cretinism' is now rare as a result of routine screening, but this indicates the importance of adequate thyroid function for cerebral development. Occasionally, adult hypothyroidism may be associated with psychosis (most commonly a delirium with-prominent agitation), famously termed 'myxoedema madness'.

Hyperthyroidism is commonly associated with a subjective feeling of tension, irritability, and high arousal. Initially this may be confused with anxiety, but in more severe cases behavior can be frankly disturbed, although the individual concerned generally retains insight. However, it should be noted that studies show no clear association between anxiety or depression and serum concentration of thyroid hormones. In a similar way, no strict relationship has been found between severity of symptoms of hyperthyroidism and degree of elevation in thyroid hormones concentrations. Hypomania is rare but has been reported. Thyroid 'crises' with delirium are occasionally seen following radioiodine treatment.

Both hypothyroidism and hyperthyroidism are common consequences of lithium treatment in bipolar affective disorder. This introduces the possibility of confusing a thyroid disorder with the recurrence of an affective disorder, although it should be effectively excluded by the routine monitoring of lithium treatment.

Hashimoto's encephalopathy is an uncommon condition of presumed autoimmune etiology characterized by the presence of high titres of antithyroid microsomal/peroxidase antibodies. The condition can follow a relapsing and remitting course, with features including confusion, cognitive decline, hallucinations, stroke-like episodes, myoclonus, or seizures. Thyroid function is typically normal. Treatment with corticosteroids is almost always effective.

Cushing's Syndrome

It is estimated that more than 70% of patients with Cushing's syndrome can present psychiatric problems, ranging from anxiety and agitated depression to psychosis. Some degree of psychiatric disturbance frequently persists even after treatment. Furthermore, impairment in anterograde memory and cognition is common and can persist for at least a year after treatment. These effects are associated with a reduction in apparent brain volume, particularly in the hippocampal formation, which have been shown to be only partially reversible after correction of hypercortisolemia. Exogenous steroids have also been shown to reduce hippocampal volume and to impair declarative memory.

Pheochromocytoma

Pheochromocytoma can mimic endocrine, cardiovascular, and neurological, as well as psychiatric conditions. The latter include panic and anxiety disorder, depressive disorder, and substance misuse. Common symptoms include dizziness, tremulousness, palpitations, and the subjective feeling of intense fear, leading to confusion with anxiety and panic attacks. The diagnostic feature is the elevation of blood pressure during an attack, and if such attacks are reported, routine testing for adrenergic metabolites should be conducted. Attacks are occasionally of sufficient intensity to lead to confusion and delirium.

Pituitary Disorder

Panhypopituitarism with consequent adrenal failure produces a characteristic neuropsychiatric picture with apathy, fatigue, weight loss, inability to attend and concentrate, and memory impairment. The disorder may be confused with chronic fatigue, depression, or even dementia, and the weight loss has been confused with anorexia nervosa, although neither appetite disturbance nor distorted body image is usually found. Acromegaly can also result in a rather characteristic apathy and lack of concern, with occasional depression and irritability, perhaps reflecting a degree of global hypopituitarism.

There are two other particular neuropsychiatric issues that arise in consideration of a pituitary disorder. First, cerebral irradiation of pituitary tumors may give rise to collateral damage to adjacent brain structures, and there are reports of memory impairment, perhaps reflecting diencephalic and/or hippocampal damage. Second, endocrine replacement therapy following pituitary ablation maybe suboptimal, indeed replacement of sex steroids is occasionally omitted because of their propensity to release sexual drive, which may be inappropriate.

Gonadal Dysfunction

Contrary to previous beliefs, the menopause is not necessarily associated with psychological problems in healthy women. However, the following risk factors have been associated with affective disturbance: psychiatric problems; poor social, educational, occupational, and health status; stressful life events; high body mass index (BMI); cigarette smoking; as well as negative attitudes toward menopause and aging. Successful treatments for mood disturbance include hormone therapy and psychological interventions, particularly cognitive behavioral therapy. Furthermore, increasing evidence supports the hypothesis that estrogen treatment can have positive effects on cognitive performance in aging. The initiation of estrogen treatment at the time of menopause, or soon after ovariectomy, is considered to provide a window of opportunity for the protection of memory in women. Imaging studies provide evidence of the neuroprotective role of estrogen, particularly on the hippocampal volume in aging, and that it may lose its effectiveness after a specific period of time.

While significant advances have been made in our understanding of the modulatory effects of ovarian hormones on cognition in women, relatively little attention has been directed toward understanding the role of gonadal steroids on the modulation of cognitive functions in men. However, there are some studies which suggest that low premorbid testosterone levels are associated with a higher risk for Alzheimer's disease. Furthermore, it may be that low testosterone has a selective effect on memory consolidation. Preliminary data suggest that replacement therapy can modify the deficits. However, one should note that the adverse effects the low testosterone levels have on mood, arousal, and attention may also indirectly affect higher cognitive functions.

Neuropsychiatric Systemic Lupus Erythematosus (SLE) and Antiphospholipid Antibody Syndrome (APS)

Neuropsychiatric SLE is becoming an increasingly prevalent manifestation of SLE, estimated to affect 14–75% of patients and able to cause chronic irreversible brain injury. The American College of Rheumatology has recently revised its definition of neuropsychiatric SLE, distinguishing 12 types of central neurological involvement. There is no single diagnostic test that is sensitive or specific, hence, the diagnosis depends on the combination of rheumatological examination, immunoserology, and brain imaging as well as psychiatric and neuropsychological tests in the presence of lupus disease activity. Recent neuropsychological investigations suggest that patients with SLE have particularly poor performance on verbal and memory tests. Furthermore, about 10–40% of patients have depression, for which risk factors are thought to include direct brain damage, concomitant neuropsychiatric disorders, steroid administration, and the patient's response to the burden of the disease.

The clinical antiphospholipid antibody syndrome (APS) is found in 30% of patients with SLE or may occur in isolation. It is characterized by venous and arterial thromboses and neurological disease in the presence of antiphospholipid antibodies.

Voltage-gated Potassium Channel Antibody-mediated Syndromes

In the last few years, the role of channelopathies has been recognized in acute or transient neuropsychiatric disorders. Evidence has accumulated that voltage-gated antibody to potassium channels are involved in certain limbic syndromes, and in some patients with subacute onset of unexplained epilepsy. Voltage-gated potassium channel (VGKC) antibodies were initially identified in patients with Isaac's syndrome, which is an acquired syndrome of peripheral nerve hyperexcitability. Patients may present with myokymia and often have hyperhidrosis. Subsequently, two VGKC antibody syndromes have been described with CNS manifestations: limbic encephalitis and Morvan's syndrome. Limbic encephalitis is an inflammatory disorder affecting prominently the mesial temporal lobes and characterized by confusion, disorientation, amnesia, personality change, and seizures. Patients develop acute or subacutememory loss and confusion, progressing over days or weeks to temporal lobe/partial complex epileptic seizures. Cognitive impairment is typically profound, with significant retrograde and anterograde amnesia. MRI usually shows high signal in the hippocampalregion(s). In Morvan's syndrome, the peripheral and the CNS manifestations of the VGKC antibody syndromes coexist, characterized by severe and persistent insomnia, autonomic instability, lability of affect, cognitive impairment, hallucinations, and peripheral hyper-excitability. Patients with limbic encephalitis or Morvan's syndrome may improve spontaneously over time, but this is unusual. Treatment usually consists of immunotherapies similar to those employed for myasthenia gravis and other autoimmune disorders.

FURTHER READING

1. Alper KR, Barry H, Balabanov AJ. Treatment of psychosis, aggression, and irritability in patients with epilepsy. Epilepsy Behav. 2002;3 (Suppl 1):13-8.
2. Arnsten AFT. ADHD and The Prefrontal Cortex. J Pediatrics. 2009;154(5) s1:1-S43.
3. Basson R, Women's sexual function and dysfunction: current uncertainties, future directions - REVIEW. International Journal of Impotence Research. 2008;20:466-78.
4. Biessels GI, et al. Risk of dementia in diabetes mellitus: a systematic review. Lancet Neurol. 2006;5:64-74.
5. Binetti G, et al. Areas of intervention for genetic counselling of dementia: Cross-cultural comparison between Italians and Americans. Patient Educ Couns. 2006;64:285-93.
6. Bourne RS, Tahir TA, Borthwick M, Sampson EL. Drug treatment of delirium: Past, present and future.I Psychoso Res. 2008;65(3):273-82.
7. Brinar VV, Habek M. Dementia and white-matter demyelination in young patient with neurosyphilis. Lancet. 2007;368(9554):2258.
8 Bunevicius R, Velickiene D, Prange AJ Jr. Mood and anxiety disorders in women with treated hyperthyroidism and ophthalmopathy caused by Graves' disease. Gen Hosp Psychiatry. 2005;27:133-9.
9. Burns A, Gallagley A, Byrne I. Delirium. J Neurol Neurosurg Psychiatry. 2004;75:362-367.
10. Cruess DG, et al. Prevalence, diagnosis, and pharmacological treatment of mood disorders in HIV disease, Biol Psychiatry. 2003;54:307-16.
11. Culham JC, Kanwisher NG. Neuroimaging of cognitive functions in human parietal cortex. Curr Opin Neurobiol. 2001;11:157-63.
12. David et al. (2009). Lishman's Organic Psychiatry.4th Ed. Wiley-Blackwell. Dickerson BC, Eichenbaum H (2009). The Episodic Memory System: Neurocircuitry and Disorders. Neuro-psychopharmacology REVIEWS, 1-19. 10.1038/npp.2009.126
13. d'Ydewalle G, Van Damme I. Memory and the Korsakoff syndrome: Not remembering what is remembered. Neuropsychologia. 2007;45:905-20.
14. Eller M, Williams DR. Biological fluid biomarkers in neurodegenerative parkinsonism - Review. Nature Reviews Neurology. 2009;5:561-70.
15. Ekstrand IR, et al. The presence of psychiatric disorders reduces the likelihood of neurologic disease among referrals to a neurology clinic, J Psychosom Res. 2004;57:11-6.
16. Feinstein A. Mood disorder in multiple sclerosis and the effects on cognition. J Neural Sci. 2006;245:63-6.
17. Ferguson SM, Rayport M. Pathogenesis of psychosis in epilepsy. The 'seesaw' theory: myth or reality? Int Rev Neurobiol. 2006;76:45-61.
18. Finberg KE. Mad cow disease in the United States: an update on bovine spongiform encephalopathy and variant Creutzfeldt-Jakob disease. Clin Microbiol Newsl. 2004;26:113-8.
19. Florian Holsboer. How can we realize the promise of personalized antidepressant medicines? Nature Reviews Neuroscience. 2008;9:638-46.
20. Folstein MF, Folstein SE, McHugh PR. 'Mini mental state'. A practical method for grading the cognitive state of patients for the clinician. J Psychiatr Res. 1975;12:189-98.
21. Fong TG, Tulebaev SR, Inouye SK. Delirium in elderly adults: diagnosis, prevention and treatment. Nature Reviews Neurology. 2009;5:210-20.
22. Frackowiak RSI, et al. (Eds). Human brain function. Academic Press Inc; 1997.
23. Giaconne G, Mangieri M, Capobianco R, et al. Tauopathy in human and experimental variant Creutzfeldt-Jakob disease. Neurobiology of Aging. 2008;29(12):240-3.
24. Gotz J, Ittner LM. Animal models of Alzheimer's disease and frontotemporal dementia. Nature Reviews Neuroscience. 2008;9:532-44.
25. Gouveia PA, et al. Disorders in planning and strategy application in frontal lobe lesion patients. Brain Cogn. 2007;63:240-6.
26. Gupta N, de Jonghe J, Schieveld J, Leonard M, Meagher D. Delirium phenomenology: What can we learn from symptoms of delirium. J Psychosomc Res. 2008;65(3):215-22.
27. Harisingani R. Where are the reversible dementias? J Am Geriatr Soc. 2005;53:1066-8.
28. Hebb DO. Man's frontal lobe: a critical review. Arch Neurol Psychiatry. 1945;54:10-24.
29. Hillman CH, Erickson KI, Kramer AF. Be smart, exercise your heart: exercise effects on brain and cognition. Nature Reviews Neuroscience. 2008;9:58-65.
30. Huijbregts SC, et al. Cognitive impairment and decline in different MS subtypes. J Neurol Sci. 2006;245:187-94.
31. Hunter M, Rendall M. Bio-psycho-socio-cultural perspectives on menopause. Best Pract Res Clin Obstet Gynaecol. 2007;21: 261-74.

32. Husain M, Nachev P. Space and the parietal cortex. Trends Cogn Sci. 2007;11:30-6.
33. Hyman SE. A glimmer of light for neuropsychiatric disorders. Nature. 2008;455:890-3.
34. Janowsky JS. Thinking with your gonads: testosterone and cognition. Trends Cogn Sci. 2006;10:77-82.
35. Kanner AM. Depression in epilepsy: a frequently neglected multifaceted disorder. Epilepsy Behav. 2003;4 (Suppl 4): 11-9.
36. Karp G, et al. Syphilis and HIV co-infection - Review article. Eur J Int Med. 2009;20(1):9-13.
37. Kopelman MD. Structured psychiatric interview: psychiatric history and assessment of the mental state. Br J Hosp Med. 1994;52:93-8.
38. Kopelman MD. The Korsakoff syndrome. Br J Psychiatry. 1995;166:154-73.
39. Kopelman MD. Disorders of memory. Brain. 2002;125:2152-90.
40. Kopelman MD, Fleminger S. Experience and perspectives on the classification of organic mental disorders. Psychopathology. 2002;35:76-81.
41. Lee Y-S, Silva AI. The molecular and cellular biology of enhanced cognition. Nature Reviews Neuroscience. 2009;10:126-40.
42. Lipkin WI, Hornig M, Psychotropic viruses. Curr Opin Microbiol. 2004;7:420-5.
43. Mesulam MM. Slowly progressive aphasia without generalized dementia. Ann Neurol. 1982;11:592-98.
44. Michaud L, et al. Delirium: guidelines for general hospitals. J Psychosom Res. 2007;62:371-83.
45. Minden SL, et al. Predictors and outcomes of delirium. Gen Hospital Psychiatry. 2005;27:209-14.
46. Oksenberg JR, Baranzini SE, Sawcer S, Hauser SL. The genetics of multiple sclerosis: SNPs to pathways to pathogenesis -Review. Nature Reviews Genetics. 2008;9:516-26.
47. Okuda DT. Unanticipated demyelinating pathology of the CNS -Review. Nature Reviews Neurology. 2009;5:591-7.
48. Park Y-M, Che H-J, Im C-H, et al. Decreased synchronization and its correlation with symptom severity in Alzheimer's disease. Neurosci Res. 2008;62(2):112-7.
49. Peng F, Hu X, Zhong X, et al. CT and MRI findings in HIV-negative neurosyphilis. Eur J Radiology. 2008;66(1):1-6.
50. Perrin RI, Fagan AM, Holtzman DM. Multimodal techniques for diagnosis and prognosis of Alzheimer's disease. Nature 2009;461:916-22.
51. Pitel AL, Beaunieux H, Guillery Girard B, et al. How do Korsaltoff patients learn new concepts? Neuropsychologia, 2009;47(3):879-86.
52. Ponholzer A, et al. Serum androgen levels and their association to depression and Alzheimer dementia in a cohort of 75-year-old men over 5 years: results of the VITA study - ORIGINAL ARTICLE. International Journal of Importance Research. 2009;21:187-91.
53. Postle BR. Working memory as an emergent property of the mind and brain. Neuroscience. 2006;139:23-38.
54. Rademakers R, Rovelet-Lecrux A. Recent Insights into molecular genetics of dementia. TINS. 2009;32(8):451-61.
55. Rolfson D. The causes of delirium. In: Lindesay I, Rockwood K, Macdonald A (eds) Delirium in the elderly. Oxford University Press, Oxford; 2002. pp. 101-22.
56. Rumboldt Z, Thurnher MM, Gupta RK. Central nervous system infections, Sem Roentgenol. 2007;42:62-91.
57. Rutter M, Taylor E (Eds). Child and adolescent psychiatry, 4th edition.Wiley-Blackwell; 2005.
58. Sacks O. An anthropologist on Mars.Picador, London; 1995.
59. Santosa M, Kovaria E, Hofd PR, et al. The impact of vascular burden on late-life depression - Review. Brain Res Reviews, In Press; 2009.
60. Savage LM, Roland J, Klintsova A. Selective septohippocampal-but not forebrain amygdalar-cholinergic dysfunction in diencephalic amnesia. Brain Res. 2007;1139:210-9.
61. Schwartz JM, Marsh L. The psychiatric perspectives of epilepsy. Psychosomatics. 2000;41:31-8.
62. Silver JM, Yudofsky SC, Hales RE (Eds). Neuropsychiatry of traumatic brain injury. American Psychiatric Press, Washington DC; 1994.
63. Stefanova E, et al. Depression predicts the pattern of cognitive impairment in early Parkinson's disease. J Neurol Sci. 2006;248: 131-7.
64. Stuss DT, Anderson V. The frontal lobes and theory of mind: developmental concepts from adult focal lesion research. Brain Cogn. 2004;55:69-83.
65. Tairyan K, Illes J. Imaging genetics and the power of combined technologies: a perspective from neuroethics. Neuroscience. 2009;164(1):7-15.
66. Taphoorn MJ, Klein M. Cognitive deficits in adult patients with brain tumours. Lancet Neurol. 2004;3:159-68.
67. Turner MS, et al. Qualitatively different memory impairments across frontal lobe subgroups, Neuropsychologia. 2007;45: 1540-52.
68. Vincent A, Lang B, Kleopa KA. Autoimmune channelopathies and related neurological disorders. Neuron. 2006;52:123-38.
69. Von Gunten A, et al. Neural substrates of cognitive and behavioral deficits in atypical Alzheimer's disease. Bruin Res Rev. 2006;51:176-211.
70. Wichowicz HM, Cubala WJ, Slawek J. Wilson's disease associated with delusional disorder. Psychiatry Clin Neurosci. 2006;60:758-60.
71. Whalley LJ, Dick FD, McNeill G. A life-course approach to the aetiology of late-onset dementias. Lancet Neurol. 2006;5:87-96.
72. World Health Organization. The ICD-10 classification of mental and behavioural disorders. World Health Organization. Geneva; 1992.
73. Wright Cl, et al. Neuroanatomical correlates of personality in the elderly. Neuroimage. 2007;35:263-72.
74. Yeap BB. Are declining testosterone levels a major risk factor for ill-health in aging men. REVIEW. Int J Impotence Res. 2009;21:24-36.
75. Zandman-Goddard G, Chapman J, Shoenfeld Y. Autoantibodies involved in neuropsychiatric SLE and antiphospholipid syndrome. Semin Arthritis Rheum. 2007;36:297-315.
76. Zarei M. Clinical characteristics of cortical multiple sclerosis. J Neurol Sci. 2006;245:53-8.

CHAPTER 37

Psychiatric Aspects of Parkinsonism

Andrea-Sylvia Winkler, K Ray Chaudhuri

James Parkinson, in 1817, described "the shaking palsy" consisting of resting tremor, bradykinesia, postural abnormalities and gait propulsion with normal sensation and cognition.[1] Charcot later termed this condition Parkinson's disease (PD) and contrary to Parkinson's observations emphasised that alterations of mental function are a part of the disease process.[2] Over the years, alteration in cognition has become a recognized part of the disease process in PD and cognitive dysfunctions described in PD include psychiatric syndromes such as dementia, depression and acute psychotic disorders, sleep disturbances or any combination of these.[3] This review focuses on the neuropsychiatric aspects of PD and other a kinetic rigid syndromes such as Lewy body dementia (LBD), Alzheimer's disease (AD) or progressive supranuclear palsy (PSP), which clinically mimic PD (Table 1).

Table 1: Syndromes with parkinsonism and psychiatric manifestations

Degenerative	*Infectious disorders*	*Genetic disorders*
Parkinson's disease (PD) Alzheimer's disease (AD) Lewy body dementia (LBD) Multiple system atrophy (MSA) Progressive supranuclear palsy (PSP) Pick's disease Corticobasal degeneration Motor neuron disease (MND)	Autoimmune deficiency syndrome (AIDS) Creutzfeldt-Jakob's disease (CJD) MPTP-intoxication Dementia of the Guam type	Huntington's disease (HD) Wilson's disease (WD) Wilhelmsen-Lynch disease Dentato-rubro-pallido-luysian atrophy (DRPLA)

NEUROANATOMY AND NEUROPHARMACOLOGY

Dopamine is the principle neurotransmitter affected in parkinsonism. Dopamine is chiefly present in the nigrostriatal and mesocortical limbic pathways, and acts through the various dopamine receptors, divided into Dl and D2 like receptors. Each of these contains subtypes, Dl and D5 (Dl like) and D2, D3 and D4 (D2 like). Dl and D2 receptors are principally located in the striatum, nucleus accumbens and olfactory tubercle, and scattered to a lesser extent in the substantia nigra, septum pellucidum, hypothalamus and cerebral cortex. D3, D4 and D5 receptors are more selectively associated with the mesolimbic pathways.[4-6] The importance of the dopamine receptors in relation to mood and behavioral disorders has recently been investigated and it is likely that the mechanism for drug-induced psychotic symptoms in PD may be in part mediated through the dopaminergic system, but other neurotransmitter systems such as the serotonergic pathways are likely to be also involved.[7]

PARKINSONISM AND NEUROPSYCHIATRIC PROBLEMS

Neuropsychiatric problems in parkinsonism can be either primary, due to the underlying degenerative disorder, or secondary to antiparkinsonian medication or fluctuations in motor responses which occur typically in L-dopa-responsive idiopathic PD. These include:

BRADYPHRENIA

Celesia and Wanamaker reported that cognitive dysfunction and neuropsychological deficits may occur in up to 40% of patients with PD without any sign of overt dementia.[3] Formal neuropsychometry may reveal frontal lobe impairment with difficulties in alternate problem solving ability, perseveration and deficits in establishing internal action plans.[8] These cognitive abnormalities can be discovered by subtle and sensitive psychometric testing and might be present in very early stages of the disease. However, it must be emphasized that evaluation of the cognitive status can interfere with motivational and emotional factors as well as motor slowness, and these states might confound the neuropsychological observations.[9] Bradyphrenia is thought to be a psychic equivalent of motor slowness.[10] It represents slowing of motor function but, also in addition, indicates inattention, apathy and the inability to sustain effort for completion of the task at hand in the absence of impairment of consciousness, memory and executive function.[11] The bradyphrenia of parkinsonism or PD does not usually respond to L-dopa treatment. This may suggest that the bradyphrenic element of parkinsonism may not be related principally to the dopaminergic system and some workers have suggested that dysfunction of the locus ceruleus, mediating the noradrenergic pathway, may be implicated.[12]

DEMENTIA

Estimates of prevalence of dementia in PD are highly variable, but generally range from 15% to 20%.[13] Several studies have shown a high incidence of Alzheimer type pathology in Parkinson's disease patients with dementia.[12] Cortical or diffuse Lewy body disease with distribution of Lewy bodies in the cortex as well as in the brainstem is possibly the second commonest cause of dementia overall, and represents a subgroup of Lewy body disease known as Lewy body dementia.[14,15] The typical clinical syndrome of dementia in PD is usually subcortical, characterized by forgetfulness, slowing of thought process, and alteration in mood and personality. There is also decreased ability to manipulate acquired knowledge.[16] It must be noted that there is considerable overlap of clinical and pathological findings with the cortical dementia of Alzheimer's disease.[12]

ANXIETY AND DEPRESSION

Anxiety disorders are common in PD, and Parkinsonism. In PD, anxiety disorders may be found in approximately 40% of patients.[17] This might lead to agitation or panic attacks. There is some controversy as to whether worsening of motor disability is also linked to an increase in anxiety.[17,18] It is clear however that with worsening anxiety state patients may exhibit more fluctuations in motor responses.[17] Furthermore, provocation of anxiety can lead to improvement in ability in some patients, the so-called "kinesia paradoxa".[19]

Symptoms of anxiety or panic attacks may co-exist with depression which is found in up to 60% of patients with PD.[20,21] Depression may be related to the seventy of the disability, but depression may also occur in patients prior to the appearance of motor signs, thus suggesting an endogenous origin.[22] The depressive state may be mild to moderate and is characterized by dysphoria, pessimism, somatic symptoms and, in rare cases, intellectual impairment. Suicidal thoughts occur rarely. The diagnosis of depression in PD is confounded by the presence of vegetative signs of PD which complicate the distinction between reactive and endogenous depression.[23]

A mood disorder, distinct from depression and characterized principally by anxiety, decreased attention span, apathy and/or anhedonia affects many PD patients.[24] Unlike patients with true clinical depression, patients with this mood disorder may not complain of guilt, remorse or sadness and this disorder may not respond to standard anti-depressants.

PSYCHOSIS AND HALLUCINATIONS

Psychosis in PD can be very variable and this may manifest as hallucinations, delusions, confusion, delirium and mania. Virtually all these psychoses are due to medication such as anticholinergic or dopaminergic antiparkinsonian drug therapy. Primary psychosis represents less than 1% of psychiatric complications in PD.[25] The incidence of hallucinations is estimated to be about 20% and is most pronounced with the use of dopamine agonists such as bromocriptine, lisuride, amantadine, selegiline or anti-cholinergic drugs such as benzhexol. L-dopa therapy also may cause hallucinations but there is some evidence to suggest that dopamine agonists have a greater potential for causing hallucinations.[26] A recent study by Goetz, et al. suggests that intravenous administration of large doses of L-dopa may not indeed cause hallucinations in patients who were otherwise having hallucinations on oral antiparkinsonian drugs (oral presentation, PD meeting, London 1997). Apomorphine, a potent Dl and D2 agonist is, however, reported to be less likely to cause hallucinations, a possible underlying mechanism being the antipsychotic moiety piperidine contained in the structure of apomorphine.[27] The earliest sign of psychosis in parkinsonism is often the appearance of restlessness, vivid dreams and nightmares leading to sleep disturbances. Advanced symptoms consist of hallucination, delusion, paranoid ideation and sometimes delirium. Hallucinations are typically visual; they involve family members and non-ferocious animals and are non-threatening and most common at night.[28,29]

DIFFERENTIAL DIAGNOSES

Syndromes with parkinsonism and psychiatric manifestation are listed in Table 1. The main conditions mimicking PD, often complicated by neuropsychiatric problems are discussed briefly.

LEWY BODY DEMENTIA

Lewy body dementia or diffuse Lewy body disease is the major differential diagnosis in a patient with parkinsonism and cognitive deficits or visual hallucinations. In Lewy body dementia, numerous cortical Lewy bodies are found in frontal, temporal and parietal association neocortex. Lewy bodies also occur in the subcortical and brainstem nuclei.[14] There is a considerable degree of overlap with Alzheimer pathology.[30] The central feature of Lewy body dementia, as suggested in the Newcastle criteria, is a progressive cognitive decline with attention, frontal subcortical skills and visuospatial deficits. Memory impairment may not occur in the early stages. Fluctuating deficits of attention, alertness and episodic delirium may be present. Recurrent visual hallucinations are usually well formed and detailed.[31] Further supportive features for the diagnosis of Lewy body dementia are listed in Table 2. It is important to note however that patients with Lewy body dementia may initially respond well to L-dopa treatment and, in the early stages, the condition may be indistinguishable from PD.[32] An accurate antemortem clinical diagnosis of diffuse Lewy body disease or Lewy body dementia is important because there is need for caution with neuroleptic medication in these patients. Patients with Lewy body dementia may have a much greater sensitivity to neuroleptics than Alzheimer's disease patients, with worsening of extrapyramidal symptoms, rapid decline and increased mortality rate.[33]

WILHELMSEN-LYNCH DISEASE

Wilhelmsen-Lynch disease (hereditary frontotemporal dementia) comprises three different phenotypes of parkinsonism with psychiatric features which have been linked to chromosome 17.[34] The disinhibition-dementia-parkinsonism-amyotrophy complex (DDPAC) is characterized by marked personality and behavioral changes associated with parkinsonian features.[35,36] The pallido-ponto-nigral degeneration (PPND) subtype presents with dementia and parkinsonism, and the syndrome of familial progressive subcortical gliosis (FPSG) consists of personality change, extrapyramidal signs and dementia.[37,38]

Table 2: Features supporting the diagnosis of lewy body disease
• Repeated falls
• Syncope
• Transient loss of consciousness
• Systematized delusions
• Hallucinations in other modalities

ALZHEIMER'S DISEASE

As mentioned above, there is an overlap of Alzheimer's disease, PD and Lewy body dementia.[12,14,30] However, the dementia of Alzheimer's type lends to be "cortical" as opposed to "subcortical". Consistent with the pathology the main features of Alzheimer's disease are early, and mostly severe, impairment of memory and focal neurological symptoms, such as dysphasia or dyspraxia. Disturbance of mood may be prominent, but psychotic features are rare in early stages.[39] After some years, parkinsonian features may develop as well as pyramidal signs.[40]

PROGRESSIVE SUPRANUCLEAR PALSY

Progressive supranuclear palsy consists of supranuclear paralysis of external ocular movement, especially in the vertical plane, dysarthria, pseudobulbar palsy, rigidity of the neck and trunk, and dementia of the "subcortical type".[41,42] Memory is not truly impaired but rather the timing mechanism, which enables the memory to function at normal speed. The clinical picture is characterized by "forgetfulness", slowing of thought processes, alteration in mood and personality (depression and euphoria), and decreased ability to manipulate acquired knowledge.[42] The term "subcortical dementia" has also been used to describe cognitive disturbances in Huntington's and Wilson's disease.

TREATMENT

Satisfactory treatment of psychiatric manifestations in parkinsonism involves the exact differentiation of primary and secondary symptoms and, in secondary symptoms, determination of whether these are fluctuation-related or drug-induced. "Off" phase related psychiatric symptoms might respond to treatment of motor symptoms.

Iatrogenic neuropsychiatric symptoms should be treated by a staged reduction of potentially psychotoxic anti-PD drugs. If memory problems are dominant, anticholinergics should be discontinued first, followed by tricyclic antidepressants and amantadine. If confusion is a major symptom, anticholinergic drugs should be stopped first, followed by selegiline, tricyclic antidepressants. amantadine and dopamine agonists. The last step would be the reduction of L-dopa. If agitation or hallucinosis are the major symptoms, selegiline should be discontinued first, then amantadine and followed by dopamine agonists or anticholinergics. If there is still no improvement, L-dopa can be titrated downward.[43]

If psychiatric symptoms are due to a primary neuro-pathological process, counseling is important, followed by judicious administration of anxiolytics, antidepressants or antipsychotics in selected cases.

Anxiety, agitation and panic attacks can be treated with benzodiazepines such as alprazolam 0.5–1 mg three times daily or diazepam 2.5–5 mg four times daily. If benzodiazepines do not prove effective, imipramine or buspirone can be considered.[43]

Patients suffering from primary depression may need treatment with antidepressants.[44] Nortriptyline is a better choice than amitriptyline because of its lower anticholinergic potency.[43] The recommended initial dose lies between 20–40 mg, which can be gradually built up to 100 mg per day. Some selective serotonin reuptake inhibitors, such as fluoxetine, sertraline and paroxetine, have also been used.[43] However, recent reports suggest that these may worsen movement disorders and may precipitate a serotonin syndrome.[45,46] Serotonin reuptake inhibitors have an adverse interaction with selegiline and concurrent use should be avoided.[47] There is some anecdotal evidence that pramipexole, a newly available dopamine agonist, may actually improve a mood disorder, described above, which is different from depression and presents with anxiety, decreased attention span and apathy.[48] These observations will need to be validated by further studies investigating the role of pramipexole in mood disorders in PD.

Drug-induced hallucinations, which cannot be improved by reduction of medications as described above, may well need antipsychotic treatment. However, administration of antipsychotic drugs might be problematic because most of them cause parkinsonism (most neuroleptics are powerful D2 antagonists). Neuroleptics with high affinity to D2 receptors, such as haloperidol or chlorpromazine should be avoided. However sulpiride, which belongs to the same group as haloperidol, can be tried in patients with drug-induced hallucinations. Contrary to other neuroleptics, sulpiride has a biphasic pharmacological effect, blocking D3 receptors up to a dose of 400–500 mg and therefore can be administered in patients with predominantly negative symptoms. At higher doses, blockade of the D2 receptors will lead to aggravation of parkinsonian symptoms.[49] A convenient therapeutic strategy is a slow build-up of sulpiride from 25 mg upwards, with a concomitant increase in L-dopa dose.

Thioridazine is a low potency neuroleptic and, when used at a low dose of 20–30 mg per day, may act preferentially on mesolimbic dopamine receptors and therefore, may not have a major effect on parkinsonian symptoms.[43,50]

Risperidone is a potent 5HT2A and relatively weak D2 dopamine receptor antagonist. However, its absolute affinity to the D2 receptor is similar to that of haloperidol, inducing extrapyramidal side effects, when doses higher than 0.5–1 mg a day are used.[43,54]

Clozapine, an atypical neuroleptic, has a predilection for the D4 and 5HT2/3 receptors and acts preferentially on the mesolimbic D4 receptors. Its affinity toward the D2 receptor increases gradually, when higher doses are used. Based on recent findings, the recommended starting dose is 6.25 mg every night or every other night and increase by 6.25–25 mg every 4–7 days until adequate control of symptoms is achieved or adverse events occur. However, the final dosage of 50–100 mg should not be exceeded. Clozapine may cause agranulocytosis in approximately 2% of patients, therefore weekly FBC controls are needed.[51-54]

Olanzepine, another atypical neuroleptic blocking mainly the D4 receptor at low doses, can also be used to treat psychotic symptoms in PD.[53]

Ondansetron, a selective 5HT3 antagonist, may reduce L-dopa associated psychosis in a dosage of 2–10 mg a day.[55]

Recently, Ellis, et al. showed a reduction in psychiatric side effects when using subcutaneous apomorphine in parkinsonian patients treated with L-dopa.[27] Doses up to 40 mg per 12 hours were effective in reducing neuropsychiatric symptoms while improving motor symptoms. The mechanism of action is unclear. The piperidine moiety, contained in the structure of apomorphine may be antipsychotic itself and apomorphine lacks the serotonergic effect of bromocriptine or the ergolides.[27]

The newly developed D3-agonist, pramipexole acts on pre-synaptic inhibitory dopamine D3 autoreceptors when used at low doses, thus reducing drug-induced psychotic symptoms. However, at higher doses, pramipexole binds preferentially to postsynaptic receptors and can be used for treatment of parkinsonian symptoms.[56]

Currently, efforts are being made to produce selective Dl agonists to treat PD. Animal work suggests that Dl agonists, such as ABT431 may reduce dyskinesia but also provide reduced liability to precipitate neuropsychiatric complications in PD, thought to be secondary to overstimulation of D2 receptors.[57] Recently attention has also been drawn to adenosine receptors, which are co-localized with the D2 mediated indirect striato-pallidal pathway and may enhance its effect.[58] Therefore, development of adenosine antagonists might be of use in the treatment of L-dopa induced psychosis.

DEPRESSION, ANXIETY AND APATHY IN PARKINSON'S DISEASE

Depression is common in Parkinson's disease and is associated with reduced cognitive performance and quality of life. Leentjens recently reviewed new findings and conceptual issues. In a prospective study over 11 years, Hughes, et al. reported that depression and dementia, but not motor symptoms, were associated with increased mortality in Parkinson's disease.[59,60] In a study of 114 Parkinson's disease patients, Weintraub, et al. found that depression and cognitive impairment were associated with impaired functional ability, in addition to psychosis, age, duration of Parkinson's disease, apathy, sleepiness and motor impairment. Nuti, et al.[61] reported major depression in 21% and dysthymia in 19% according to Diagnostic and Statistical Manual of Mental

Disorders (DSM) IV in a convenience sample of 90 Parkinson's disease patients. This is in line with some previous studies, but higher than studies of community-based samples.[62-66] Moreover, they found generalized anxiety disorder in 11% and panic disorder in 30% of patients. Comorbid anxiety and an affective disorder were present in 19%. Major depression and panic disorder was significantly more common in Parkinson's disease than in a control group. Only 13% of this Parkinson's disease group were without a DSM-IV diagnosis.[67]

Lauterbach, et al. administered a semi-structured interview and recorded lifetime and point-prevalence of DSM-III diagnoses in 28 Parkinson's disease and 28 dystonia patients recruited from a tertiary movement disorder clinic. Compared with the dystonia group, Parkinson's disease patients more often had a primary (i.e. occurred before Parkinson's disease) diagnosis of simple phobia and a secondary atypical depression (i.e. more limited, paroxysmal and recurrent than major depression).[68-74]

Treatment

Although there is preliminary evidence suggesting that antidepressants, electroconvulsive therapy (ECT), and even dopamine agonists may improve depression in Parkinson's disease, there is insufficient trial evidence as to the treatment of depression[75] and anxiety in Parkinson's disease patients. The results of a small prospective open-label trial on 10 patients suggest that citalopram improves depression, disability and comorbid anxiety.[76] Repetitive transcranial magnetic stimulation (TMS) is as effective as fluoxetine in the treatment of Parkinson's disease related depression.[77] As has been shown after ECT, TMS may also lead to some improvement of motor symptoms. In contrast to ECT, there are some indications that TMS may even improve some aspects of cognition.[78]

Sexual problems, especially hypoactive but also hyperactive disturbances, are common in Parkinson's disease. In the first study exploring sexual function in Parkinson's disease following STN DBS, small but positive effects were reported. Patients younger than 60 years in particular were more satisfied with their sexuality after a short-term treatment with DBS.[79] Testosterone deficiency is one common cause of sexual dysfunction as well as causing other psychological problems in Parkinson's disease,[80] and was also found to be associated with apathy[81] and executive dysfunction.[82] Thus, replacement of testosterone, which in preliminary studies was associated with improvement of cognition, sexual dysfunction and general well-being, may potentially also improve apathy.[83,84]

RECENT FINDINGS

Many new studies of cognitive impairment and dementia in Parkinson's disease have been published. Cognitive impairment has been demonstrated even during the first 1–2 years after onset of disease.[85-99] Whereas executive and attentional impairment is typical, learning deficits occur early in some patients. Both functional and structural imagings suggest that in addition to fronto-subcortical deficits, temporal and parietal changes occur early as well. In the first large placebo-controlled trial, the cholinesterase inhibitor rivastigmine improved cognition, daily functioning and psychiatric symptoms without worsening of parkinsonism.[100,101] The frequency and characteristics of depression, anxiety and hallucinations have been explored in several studies. Unfortunately, there is still little scientific evidence available to guide the treatment of these important aspects of Parkinson's disease, and adequately designed clinical trials are needed. Although subthalamic stimulation, in addition to improvement of movement, is frequently associated with some affective and cognitive improvement, permanent and significant worsening may occur in some. Future studies should aim at identifying at-risk patients, as well as identifying the optimal pharmacological and stimulation treatments for individual patients.

REFERENCES

1. Parkinson J. An Essay on the Shaking Palsy. London: Sherwood; 1817.
2. Charcot JM, Vulpian A. De la paralysie agitante. Gazette hebdomadaire de lamedecine et de la chirurgie. 1861;8:765-7.
3. Celesia GH, Wanamarker WM. Psychiatric disturbances in Parkinson's disease. Dis Nerv Sys. 1972;33:577-83.
4. Sunahara RK, Seeman P, Van Tol HHM, et al. Dopamine receptors and antipsychotic drug response. Br J Psychiatry. 1993;163(Suppl 22):31-8.
5. Civelli O. Molecular biology of the dopamine receptor subtypes. In: Bloom FE, Kupfer DJ (Eds). Psychopharmacology: The Fourth Generation of Progress. New York: Raven Press; 1995. pp. 155-61.
6. Jenner P. The contribution of dopamine receptor subtypes to the therapeutic actions and side effects of antiparkinsonian drugs. In: Matthew B, Stem MD (Eds). Beyond the Decade of the Brain. Emerging Therapies in Neurologic Disease: Parkinson's, Alzheimer's, Stroke and Epilepsy. Kent: Wells Medical Limited.
7. Factor SA, Molho ES, Podskalny GD, et al. Parkinson's disease: drug induced psychiatric states. Adv Neur. 1995;65:115-38.
8. Poewe W, Ceballos-Baumann AO, Conrad B. Parkinson-Krankheit. In: Conrad B, Ceballos-Baumann AO (Eds). Bewegungsstorungen in der Neurologie. Stuttgart: Thieme Verlag. 1996;30-67.
9. Brown RG, Marsden CD. Cognitive function in Parkinson's disease. Trends Neurosci. 1990;13:29-31.
10. Birkmayer W, Danieiczyk W, Riederer P. Symptoms and side effects in the course of Parkinson's disease. J Neural Trans. 1983;19:185-99.
11. Mayeux R, Stem Y, Sano M, et al. Clinical and biochemical correlates of bradyphrenia in Parkinson's disease. Neurology. 1987;37:1130-34.

12. Caspar P, Gray F. Dementia in idiopathic Parkinson's disease. Acta Neuropathol. 1984;64:43-52.
13. Biggins CA, Boyd JF, Harrop FM, et al. A controlled longitudinal study of dementia m Parkinson's disease. J Neurol Neurosurg Psychiatry. 1992;55:566-71.
14. Pollanaen MS, Dickson DW, Bergeron C. Pathology and biology of the Lewy body. J Neuropathol Exper Neurol. 1993;52:183-91.
15. Den Hartog Jager WA, Bethlem J. The distribution of the Lewy bodies in the central and autonomic nervous system m idiopathic paralysis agitans. J Neurol Neurosurg Psychiatry. 1960;23:283-90.
16. Cummings JL, Benson DF. Subcortical dementia: review of an emerging concept. Arch Neurol. 1984;41:874-9.
17. Stem MB, Heuser IJ, Juncos JL, et al. Anxiety disorders in patients with Parkinson's disease. Am J Psychiatry. 1990;147: 217-20.
18. Siemers ER, Shekhar A, Quaid K, et al. Anxiety and motor performance in Parkinson's disease. Movement Dis. 1993;8: 501-6.
19. Babinski J, Jarkowsky B, Plichet V. Kinesie paradoxale. Mutisme parkinsonian. Rev Neurol. 1921;37:1266-70.
20. Henderson R, Kurlan R, Kersim JM, et al. Preliminary examination of the comorbidity of anxiety and depression in Parkinson's disease. J Neuropsychiat Clin Neurosci. 1992;4: 257-64.
21. Poewe WH. Die Neuropsychologic der Parkinson-Krankhei L. In: Stem GM, Madeja UD, Poewe WH (Eds). Trends in Diagnostik and Therapie des Morbus Parkinson. Berlin: De Gruyter; 1993. pp. 43-9.
22. Mayeux R, Stem Y, Rosen J, et al. Depression, intellectual impairment and Parkinson's disease. Neurology. 1981;31: 645-50.
23. Mayeux R. Depression and dementia in Parkinson's disease. In: Marsden CD, Fahn S (Eds). Movement Disorders. London: Butterworths; 1981. pp. 75-95.
24. Lees AJ, Smith E. Cognitive deficits in the early stages of Parkinson's disease. Brain. 1983;106:257-70.
25. Huber ST, Bomstein RA. Neuropsychological evaluations of Parkinson's disease, in Parkinson's disease: Neurobehavioral Aspects. In: Huber SJ, Cummings JL (Eds). New York: Oxford University Press; 1992. pp. 32-45.
26. Goetz CG, Tanner CM, Klawans HL. Pharmacology of hallucinations induced by long-lerm drug therapy. Am J Psychiatry. 1982;139:494-7.
27. Ellis C, Lemmens G, Parkes JD, et al. Use of apomorphine in parkinsonian patients with neuropsychiatric complications to oral treatment. Parkinsonism and Related Disorders. 1997;3:103-7.
28. Glantz RH, Bielauskuas L, Paleogos N. Behavioral indicators of hallucinosis in levodopa-treated Parkinson's disease, in Parkinson's disease. In: Yahr MD, Bergmaim KJ (Eds). Advances in Neurology Series. New York: Raven Press; 1986. pp. 417-20.
29. Tanner CM. Drug-induced movement disorders, in Extrapyramidal Disorders. In: Vinken PJ, Bruyn GW, Klawans HL (Eds). Handbook of Clinical Neurology. Amsterdam: Elsevier Science; 1986. pp. 185-204.
30. Hansen L. Salmon D, Galasko D, et al. The Lewy body variant of Alzheimer's disease: A clinical and pathologic entity. Neurology. 1990;40:1-8.
31. McKeith I, Galasko D, Kosaka K, et al. Consensus guidelines for the clinical and pathologic diagnosis of dementia with Lewy bodies (DLB): Report of the consortium on DLB international workshop. Neurology. 1990;47:1113-24.
32. Byme EJ, Lennox G, Lowe J, et al. Diffuse Lewy body disease: Clinical features in 15 cases. J Neurol Neurosurg Psychiatry. 1989;52:709-17.
33. McKeith I, Fairbairn A, Perry R, et al. Neuroleptic sensitivity in patients with senile dementia of Lewy body type. Br Med J. 1992;305:673-8.
34. Fahn S, Mayeux R, Rowland LP. A new eponym: Wilhelmsen-Lynch disease. Neurology 1995; 1980 (letter).
35. Wilhelmsen KC, Lynch T, Pavlou E. Localisation of the disinhibition-dementia-Parkinsonism-amyotrophy complex to 17q21-22. Am J Human Genet. 1994;55:1159-65.
36. Lynch T, Sano M, Marder KS, et al. Clinical characteristics of a family with chromosome 17-linked disinhibition-dementia-Parkinsonism-amyotrophy complex. Neurol. 1994;44:1878-84.
37. Wijker M, Wszoiek ZK, Welters ECH, et al. Localisation of the gene for rapidly progressive autosomal dominant Parkinsonism and dementia with pallido-ponto-nigra) degeneration to chromosome 17q2L. Human Molecular Genetics. 1996;5:151-4.
38. Lanska DJ, Cuirier RD, Cohen M. Familial progressive subcortical gliosis. Neurology. 1994;44:1633-43.
39. Sjogren T, Sjogren H, Lindgren AGH. Morbus Alzheimer and Morbus Pick: A genetic, clinical and patho-anatomical study. Acta Psychiatr et Neurol Scand. 1952;82(Suppl):1-152.
40. Pearce J, Miller E. Clinical Aspects of Dementia. London: Bailliere Tindall; 1973.
41. Steele JC, Richardson JC, Olszewski J. Progressive supranuclear palsy. Arch Neurol. 1964;10:333-59.
42. Albert ML, Feldman RG, Willis AL. The subcortical dementia of progressive supranuclear palsy. J Neurol Neurosurg Psychiatry. 1974;37:121-30.
43. Koller WC, Silver DE, Lieberman A. An algorithm for the management of Parkinson's disease. Neurology. 1994;44 (Suppl. 10).
44. Huber SJ, Paulson GW. Management of behavioral symptoms in Parkinson's disease. In: Koller WC, Paulson GE (Eds). Therapy to Parkinson's Disease. New York: Marcel Dekker; 1990.
45. Weiss DM. Serotonin syndrome in Parkinson disease. J Am Board Family Pract. 1995;8:400-02.
46. Sporer KA. The serotonin syndrome: Implicated drugs, pathophysiology, and management. Drug Safety. 1995;13: 94-104.
47. Suchowersky O, deVries JD. Interaction of fluoxetine and selegiline. Can J Psychiatry. 1990;35:571-2.
48. Lieberman A, Ranhosky A, Korts D. Clinical evaluation of pramipexole in advanced Parkinson's disease: Results of

a double-blind, placebo-controlled, parallel-group study. Neurology. 1997;49:162-8.

49. Seeman P, Van Tol HHM. Dopamine receptor pharmacology. Trends Pharma Sci. 1994;15:264-70.
50. Doraiawarny M, Martin W, Metz A, et al. Psychosis in Parkinson's disease: Diagnosis and treatment. Prog Neuropsychopharmacol Biol Psychiatry. 1995;19:835-46.
51. Rich SS, Friedman JH, Ott BR. Risperidone versus clozapine in the treatment of psychosis in six patients with Parkinson's disease and other a kinetic rigid syndromes. J Clin Psychiatry. 1995;56:556-9.
52. Greene P. Use of clozapine in Parkinson's disease. Focus on Parkinson's Disease; 1995. pp.4-8.
53. Meltzer HY. Atypical antipsychotic drugs. In: Bloom FE. Kupfer J (Eds). Psychopharmacology: The Fourth Generation of Progress. New York: Raven Press; 1995. pp.1277-86.
54. Factor SA, Friedman JH. The emerging role of clozapine in the treatment of movement disorders. Movement Dis. 1997;12: 483-96.
55. Zoldan J, Friedberg G, Goldberg SH, et al. Parkinson's disease: Ondansetron for hallucinosis in advanced Parkinson's disease. Lancet. 1993;341:562-3.
56. Camacho-Ochoa M, Walker EL, Evans DL, et al. Rat binding sites for pramipexole: A clinically useful DA-preferring dopamine agonist. Neurosci Letters. 1995;196:97-100.
57. Shiosaki K, Jenner P, Asin KE, et al. ABT-431: The diacetyl prodrug of A-86929, a potent and selective Dl receptor agonist, in vitro characterization and effects in animal models of Parkinson's disease. J Pharma Exper Ther. 1996;276:150-60.
58. Poewe W, Ceballos-Baumann AO, Conrad B. Pathophysiologic der Bewegungsstörungen. In: Com'ad B, Ceballos-Baumann AO (Eds). Bewegungsstörungen in der Neurologic. Stuttgart: Thieme Verlag; 1996. pp.11-29.
59. Cummings JL. Depression and Parkinson's disease: a review. Am J Psychiatry. 1992;149:443-54.
60. Slaughter JR, Slaughter KA, Nichols D, et al. Prevalence, clinical manifestations, etiology, and treatment of depression in Parkinson's disease. J Neuropsychiatry Clin Neurosci. 2001;13:187-96.
61. Leentjens AF. Depression in Parkinson's disease: conceptual issues and clinical challenges. J Geriatr Psychiatry Neurol. 2004;17:120-26.
62. Leentjens AF, Marinus J, Van Hilten JJ, et al. The contribution of somatic symptoms to the diagnosis of depression in Parkinson's disease: a discriminant analytic approach. J Neuropsychiatry Clin Neurosci. 2003;15:74-7.
63. Starkstein SE, Preziosi TJ, Forrester AW, Robinson RG. Specificity of affective and autonomic symptoms of depression in Parkinson's disease. J Neurol Neurosurg Psychiatry. 1990;53:869-73.
64. Marsh L, McDonald WM, Cummings JL, et al. Provisional diagnostic criteria for depression in Parkinson's disease: report of an NINDS/NIMH work group. Mov Disord. 2006;21:148-58.
65. Wermuth L, Sørensen PS, Timm S, et al. Depression in idiopathic Parkinson's disease treated with citalopram: a placebo-controlled trial. Nord J Psychiatry. 1998;52:163-9.
66. Kummer A, Cardoso F, Teixeira AL. Frequency of social phobia and psychometric properties of the Liebowitz social anxiety scale in Parkinson's disease. Mov Disord. 2008;23:1739-43.
67. Pluck GC, Brown RG. Apathy in Parkinson's disease. J Neurol Neurosurg Psychiatry. 2002;73:636-42.
68. Starkstein SE, Mayberg HS, Preziosi TJ, Andrezejewski P, Leiguarda R, Robinson RG. Reliability, validity, and clinical correlates of apathy in Parkinson's disease. J Neuropsychiatry Clin Neurosci. 1992;4:134-9.
69. Kuzis G, Sabe L, Tiberti C, Leiguarda R, Starkstein SE. Cognitive functions in major depression and Parkinson disease. Arch Neurol. 1997;54:982-6.
70. Wertman E, Speedie L, Shemesh Z, et al. Cognitive disturbances in Parkinsonian patients with depression. J Neuropsychiatry Neuropsychol Behav Neurol. 1993;6:31-7.
71. Anguenot A, Loll PY, Neau JP, et al. Depression and Parkinson's disease: study of a series of 135 Parkinson's patients. Can J Neurol Sci. 2002;29:139-46.
72. Tröster AI, Stalp LD, Paolo AM, Fields JA, Koller WC. Neuropsychological impairment in Parkinson's Disease with and without depression. Arch Neurol. 1995;52:1164-9.
73. Sheikh JI, Yesavage JA. Geriatric Depression Scale (GDS): recent evidence and development of a shorter version. In: Brink TL (Ed). Clinical Gerontology: A Guide to Assessment and Intervention. New York, NY: The Haworth Press; 1986:165-73.
74. Weintraub D, Oehlberg KA, Katz IR, Stern MB. Test characteristics of the 15-item geriatric depression scale and Hamilton depression rating scale in Parkinson's disease. Am J Geriatr Psychiatry. 2006;14:169-75.
75. Weintraub D, Saboe K, Stern MB. Effect of age on geriatric depression scale performance in Parkinson's disease. Mov Disord. 2007;22:1331-5.
76. Schrag A, Barone P, Brown RG, et al. Depression rating scales in Parkinson's disease: critique and recommendations. Mov Disord. 2007;22:1077-92.
77. Inzelberg R, Kipervasser S, Korczyn AD. Auditory hallucinations in Parkinson's disease. J Neurol Neurosurg Psychiatry. 1998;64:533-5.
78. Fénelon G, Mahieux F, Huon R, Ziegler M. Hallucinations in Parkinson's disease: prevalence, phenomenology, and risk factors. Brain. 2000;123:733-45.
79. Henderson MJ, Mellers JDC. Psychosis in Parkinson's disease: 'between a rock and a hard place'. Int Rev Psychiatry. 2000;12:319-34.
80. Moskovitz C, Moses H, Klawans HL. Levodopa-induced psychosis: a kindling phenomenon. Am J Psychiatry. 1978;135:669-75.
81. Pappert E, Goetz C, Niederman FG, Raman R, Leurgans S. Hallucinations, sleep fragmentation and altered dream phenomena in Parkinson's disease. Mov Disord. 1999;14: 117-21.

82. Arnulf I, Bonnet AM, Damier P, et al. Hallucinations, REM sleep, and Parkinson's disease: a medical hypothesis. Neurology. 2000;55:281-8.
83. Fernandez HH, Aarsland D, Fénelon G, et al. Scales to assess psychosis in Parkinson's disease: critique and recommendations. Mov Disord. 2008;23:484-500.
84. Ravina B, Marder K, Fernandez HH, et al. Diagnostic criteria for psychosis in Parkinson's disease: report of an NINDS, NIMH work group. Mov Disord. 2007;22:1061-8.
85. Pillon B, Deweer B, Agid Y, Dubois B. Explicit memory in Alzheimer's, Huntington's, and Parkinson's diseases. Arch Neurol. 1993;50:374-9.
86. Turner MA, Moran NF, Kopelman MD. Subcortical dementia. Br J Psychiatry. 2002;180:148-51.
87. Weintraub D, Moberg PJ, Culbertson WC, Duda JE, Stern MB. Evidence for both impaired encoding and retrieval memory profiles in Parkinson's disease. Cogn Behav Neurol. 2004;17:195-200.
88. Filoteo JV, Rilling LM, Cole B, et al. Variable memory profiles in Parkinson's disease. J Clin Exp Neuropsychol. 1997;19:878-88.
89. Cahn-Weiner DA, Grace J, Ott BR, et al. Cognitive and behavioral features discriminate between Alzheimer's and Parkinson's disease. Neuropsychiatry Neuropsychol Behav Neurol. 2002;15:79-87.
90. Bliwise DL, Watts RL, Watts N, Rye DB, Irbe D, Hughes M. Disruptive nocturnal behavior in Parkinson's disease and Alzheimer's disease. J Geriatr Psychiatry Neurol. 1995;8:107-10.
91. Folstein MF, Folstein SE, McHugh PR. "Mini-Mental State": a practical method for grading the cognitive state of patients for the clinician. J Psychiatr Res. 1975;12:189-98.
92. Nazem S, Siderowf A, Duda JE, et al. Montreal cognitive assessment performance in patients with Parkinson's disease with "normal" global cognition by mini-mental state examination Score. J Am Geriatr Soc. 2009;57:304-8.
93. Brandt J, Benedict RHB. The Hopkins Verbal Learning Test-Revised. Odessa, Fla: Psychological Assessment Resources; 2001.
94. Lima CF, Meireles LP, Fonseca R, Castro SL, Gattett C. The Frontal Assessment Battery (FAB) in Parkinson's disease and correlations with formal measures of executive functioning. J Neurol. 2008;255:1756-61.
95. Pagonabarraga J, Kulisevsky J, Llebaria G, García-Sánchez C, Pascual-Sedano B, Gironell A. Parkinson's disease-cognitive rating scale: a new cognitive scale specific for Parkinson's disease. Mov Disord. 2008;23:998-1005.
96. Kalbe E, Calabrese P, Kohn N, et al. Screening for cognitive deficits in Parkinson's disease with the Parkinson neuropsychometric dementia assessment (PANDA) instrument. Parkinsonism Relat Disord. 2008;14:93-101.
97. Emre M, Aarsland D, Brown R, et al. Clinical diagnostic criteria for dementia associated with Parkinson's disease. Mov Disord. 2007;22:1689-1707.
98. Leentjens AFG, Dujardin K, Marsh L, et al. Anxiety rating scales in Parkinson's disease: critique and recommendations. Mov Disord. 2008;23:2004-14.
99. Leentjens AF, Dujardin K, Marsh L, et al. Apathy and anhedonia rating scales in Parkinson's disease: critique and recommendations. Mov Disord. 2008;23:2015-25.
100. Galpern W, Stacy M. Management of impulse control disorders in Parkinson's disease. Curr Treat Options Neurol. 2007;9:189-97.
101. Voon V, Fox SH. Medication-related impulse control and repetitive behaviors in Parkinson disease. Arch Neurol. 2007;64:1089-96.

CHAPTER

38

Seizure Disorder

KK Verma, JN Vyas

38.1 EPILEPSY

KK Verma

Epilepsy is a disorder of the brain characterized by an enduring predisposition to generate epileptic seizures, and epileptogenesis is the development of a neuronal network in which spontaneous seizures occur. Epilepsy affects the whole age range from neonates to elderly people, and has varied causes and manifestations, with many distinct seizure types, several identifiable syndromes, but also much that is poorly classified. There are very many comorbidities that complicate assessment and treatment planning, including learning disabilities, fixed neurological deficits, progressive conditions, psychological and psychiatric problems, and, particularly in the older age group, concomitant medical conditions.

Classification of epileptic seizures and syndromes is continually evolving. The present proposed classification is across five axes that consider seizure types, focal or generalized seizure onset, the syndrome, causation, and associated deficits.[1] Here, we have defined individuals aged 16 years and older as adults. The UK National Institute for Health and Clinical Excellence (NICE) produced in October 2004 detailed evidence based guidelines[2] for the clinical management of individuals with epilepsy (panel). Other guidelines include those of the American Academy of Neurology and the Scottish Intercollegiate Guidelines Network.

Stigma and prejudice mark epilepsy out from the neurological conditions. The past decade has seen considerable progress in epilepsy research, and improvement in public understanding. Much, however, remains to be done, especially for people for whom drugs are ineffective. An important issue that needs urgent attention is the fact that most people with epilepsy live in resource poor countries where the management of epilepsy is inconsistent. There is a great diagnostic gap in large parts of the world because there are too few trained personnel and medical facilities. The WHO-led Global Campaign Against Epilepsy with the active support of the International League Against Epilepsy and International Bureau for Epilepsy (the two major international nongovernmental organizations in epilepsy) is seeking to address these issues.[3,4] Additionally, there is a large treatment gap in resource poor countries, and worldwide, less than 20% of people with the disorder are estimated to be treated at any time.[5,6] However, resolving these difficulties will require tremendous effort and will take time to achieve.

NATIONAL INSTITUTE FOR HEALTH AND CLINICAL EXCELLENCE EPILEPSY GUIDELINES[2]

- Diagnosis should be made urgently by a specialist with an interest in epilepsy
- Electroencephalogram used to support diagnosis when the clinical history suggests it
- Magnetic resonance imaging should be used in people who develop epilepsy as adjusts, in whom focal onset is suspected, or in whom seizures persist
- Seizure types and epilepsy syndrome, cause, and comorbidity should be determined
- Initiation of appropriate treatment recommended by a specialist
- Treatment individualized according to the seizure type, epilepsy syndrome, comedication and comorbidity, individual's lifestyle, and personal preferences
- Individual with epilepsy, and their family, cares, or both, participate in all decisions about their care, taking into account any specific need
- Comprehensive care plans agreed
- Comprehensive provision of information about all aspects of condition
- Regular structured review at least once a year
- Referral back to secondary or tertiary care if epilepsy inadequately controlled pregnancy considered or pregnant
- Antiepileptic drug withdrawal considered.

EPIDEMIOLOGY

The incidence of epilepsy in developed countries is around 50 per 100,000 people per year, and is higher in infants and elderly people.[7-9] Less wealthy people show a higher incidence, for unknown reasons.[10] Poor sanitation, inadequate health delivery systems, and a higher risk of brain infections and infestations could contribute to a higher incidence-usually above 100 per 100,000 people per year in resource poor countries where most people with epilepsy usually do not receive treatment.[8,11] Childhood incidence has fallen over the past three decades in developed countries, which could be a result of adoption of healthier lifestyles by expectant mothers, improved perinatal care, and immunization programmes. A parallel rise in incidence in elderly people could be related to improved survival in people with cerebrovascular disease and cerebral degeneration.[8,12]

The prevalence of epilepsy is between 4 and 10 per 1,000 people per year.[8,9] A few (typically small) studies from isolated geographical areas with unique genetic or environmental factors[8] have shown higher rates. Lifetime prevalence rates are much higher than rates of active epilepsy, even in resource poor countries where most people do not have access to antiepileptics.[8] This difference is mainly explained by the cessation of seizures in most people who develop the disorder, but also partly by increased mortality in epilepsy.[13,14]

Risk factors vary with age and geographical location. Epilepsy associated with head trauma, central nervous system infections, and tumors occurs at any age. Cerebrovascular disease is the most common risk factor in people older than 60 years.[15] Endemic parasitic diseases such as falciparum malaria and neurocysticercosis are probably the most common preventable risks for epilepsy worldwide.[11,16-20] Recently, toxocariasis and onchocerciasis have been suggested as important risk factors.[21,22] Susceptibility to epilepsy could be partly genetically determined. The complex interplay between genetic and environmental factors might underly our incomplete understanding of the population dynamics of the disorder.[11] Additionally, some epileptic syndromes evolve over time. Two examples of this evolution are infantile spasms progressing to Lennox Gastaut syndrome (an especially severe form of epilepsy), and the occurrence of febrile convulsions in an infant leading to the later development of medial temporal lobe epilepsy. From an epidemiological or biological point of view, however, the mechanisms of progression have not yet been fully elucidated and genetic factors are likely to have a role.

In developed countries, more than 60% of patients achieve long-term remission, usually within 5 years of diagnosis; the possibility of remission decreases the longer the epilepsy is active.[8] Predictors of good outcome include earlier age of onset, fewer early seizures,[23,24] and early response to drug treatment.[25] In any individual, outcome response to drug treatment.[25] In any individual, outcome and response to treatment can be inherent to either the condition or to the individual, and seizure control in some can be difficult from the outset.[8,26] In developed countries, the overall good prognosis is often attributed to the widespread use of antiepileptic drugs. In resource poor countries lacking such drugs, however, many patients enter long-term remission, lending support to the suggestion that prognosis is dependent on the cause of the epilepsy and not on drug treatment.[26] Up to a third of people having seizures develop chronic epilepsy.[26] However, up to 20% of patients referred to clinics with refractory epilepsy might have been misdiagnosed, and many more could be helped by optimum treatment.[27] People with chronic epilepsy also have an increased risk of comorbid conditions, including cardiovascular and cerebrovascular disorders, gastrointestinal disorders, fractures, pneumonia, chronic lung diseases, and diabetes.[28]

MORTALITY

People with epilepsy have an increased risk of premature death.[29] Symptomatic epilepsy can reduce life expectancy by up to 18 years.[30] Sudden death, trauma, suicide, pneumonia, and status epilepticus are more common in people who have epilepsy than those without the disorder.[31] Little is known about mortality in resource poor countries, although circumstantial evidence suggests that it is higher than in developed countries, helping to explain the discrepancy between the higher incidence and lower prevalence of active epilepsy in poor countries.[8]

Sudden unexpected death in epilepsy is though to account for at least 500 deaths per year in the UK, and is not fully explained.[32] In people with refractory epilepsy attending specialist clinics, the yearly rate is one per 200. The highest risk is in male teenagers and young adults with convulsive seizures.[33] High seizure frequency and severity are risk factors, and in the highest risk group (i.e., those who have been considered for surgery but declined) the yearly rate is one per 75 individuals.[34] Sleeping unattended is another risk factor.[35,36] The pathophysiological causes of sudden unexplained death in epilepsy is unknown, but cardiac arrhythmias—in particular asystole secondary to seizures have been noted in monitoring studies and might only arise with occasional seizures.[37] Further long-term electrocardiogram (ECG) monitoring studies are needed to identify characteristics that carry a high risk of asystole and indicate prophylactic cardiac pacing.[38]

PATHOPHYSIOLOGY

An epileptic seizure is a transient occurrence of signs, or symptoms, or both, due to abnormal excessive or synchronous activity of a group of neurons leads to the interictal spike, which has a duration of less than 70 ms and is distinct from a seizure.[39] Indeed , the site of interictal spiking can be separate from the zone of seizure onset.

An early view that disruption of the normal balance between excitation and inhibition in the brain results in seizure generation is now thought to be an over simplification. The function of the brain depends on cooperation between disparate networks that is probably mediated through oscillations within these networks. Cortical networks generate oscillations, for which inhibitory neurons,[40] neuronal communication (e.g. synaptic transmission), and intrinsic neuronal properties (e.g. the ability of a neuron to maintain burst firing) are crucial. The occurrence of epileptic activity might be an emergent property of such oscillatory networks.[41]

Transition from normal to epileptiform behavior is probably caused by greater spread and neuronal recruitment secondary to a combination of enhanced connectivity, enhanced excitatory transmission, a failure of inhibitory mechanisms, and change in intrinsic neuronal properties. In studies in man the electro encephalogram (EEG) becomes less chaotic within large areas of cortex before a seizure, suggesting that widespread synchronization is taking place.[42]

In focal epilepsies, focal functional disruption often due to focal pathological changes (e.g. autosomal dominant frontal localized fashion, which then spread by recruitment of other brain areas. The site of the focus and the speed and extent of spread determine the clinical manifestation of the seizure.

Generalized epilepsies result in seizures occurring throughout the cortex because of a generalized lowering of seizure threshold, and are usually genetically determined. Absence seizures are a distinct form of generalized seizure generated by thalamocortical loops.[43] Absences were originally believed to be generated subcortically, by thalamic neurons driving recruitment of neocortical neurons. However, paroxysmal oscillations within thalamocortical loops in absence seizures in rats seem to originate in the somato sensory cortex rather than the thalamus, with synchronization mediated by rapid intracortical propagation of seizure activity.[44] Together with observations of subtle cortical structural abnormalities in some patients with absence seizures,[45] and the potential of focal pathological change in the medial frontal lobe to generate absence like seizures, the distinction between focal and generalized epilepsies has become blurred.

GENETIC BASIS AND CONTRIBUTION

Genetic variation can determine the causes, susceptibility, mechanisms, syndrome, treatment response, prognosis, and consequences of the epilepsies to varying degress. Part of the promise of genetics lies in its power to relate these characteristics of the overall clinical presentation of the individual patient. There has been considerable progression this area.[46,47] Several monogenic Mendelian epipelsies are known, but are generally rare and account for few cases. There can be variation in the genetic causes of a clinically homogeneous syndrome, such as juvenile myoclonic epilepsy,[48,49] and, conversely, different mutations in a single gene can cause various epilepsy syndromes.

Thus different mutations in the gene SCN1A, which encodes a neuronal sodium channel a subunit, underlie a range of epilepsies, from the severe myoclonic epilepsy of infancy to the usually more benign generalized epilepsy with febrile seizures plus,[50,51] which, conversely, might result from mutations in other genes.[52,53]

The present belief that most common epilepsies are complex traits with environmental effects acting on a background of multigenic or oligogenic susceptibility, mediated by common genetic variation especially single nucleotide polymorphisms is largely based on genetic epidemiological studies.[54] Idiopathic generalized epilepsies are emerging as an example of such complex disease causation.[55,56] Relevant genetic variation is usually identified by population genetic association studies of large groupings of well characterized patients whose genotypes are related to their phenotypes. Many such studies of susceptibility and other phenotypic features have been published, but very few have been replicated.[57,58] Evolving methods and larger collaborative studies will reveal single nucleotide polymorphisms and other common genetic variants that confer disease susceptibility.[59]

DIAGNOSIS AND INVESTIGATION

The diagnosis of epilepsy remains clinical and is based on probability after assessment of the whole individual. Misdiagnosis is potentially very damaging. The differential diagnosis must therefore always be carefully considered. In some cases the diagnosis of epilepsy syndrome or seizure types of incorrect, or the events are not due to epilepsy syndrome or seizure types is incorrect, or the events are not due to epilepsy at all, but instead have their basis in a cardiac, psychological, psychiatric, or metabolic disturbance. Such nonepileptic seizures are important to identify since they have distinct causes, treatments, and risks, including the results of inappropriate use of antiepileptic drugs, especially in an emergency setting, and withholding of appropriate therapy.[27]

Sometimes, diagnosis of epilepsy has to be delayed while witness accounts are sought. Video recordings filmed out of hospital are increasingly accessible and form a very useful adjunct, especially when seizures are infrequent. Other investigation will only rarely affect the actual diagnosis of epilepsy, although it can be crucial for establishing the syndromic diagnosis and cause. Good practice is to do an ECG for everyone presenting with possible seizures, especially if the events include loss of awareness and falls. A proportion of such episodes will be due to cardiac arrhythmia indicated, for example, by a prolonged QT interval. In cases of diagnostic uncertainty a full cardiac assessment is appropriate and could reveal a primary cardiovascular cause. For infrequent events with a possible cardiac cause, an implanted ECG loop recorder is an essential diagnostic aid, often leading to specific and effective therapy.[60]

In clinical practice, the hallmark of epilepsy is interctal epileptic activity: spikes, sharp waves, and spike wave discharges. The integration of the clinical description of the seizures, the age and comorbidities of the patient, the EEG patterns, and brain imaging lead to a syndromic diagnosis that conveys prognostic information. Prolonged digital ambulatory and video EEG provide greater temporal samples than a standard 30 minutes EEG and, if seizures are frequent, the realistic possibility of direct observation and recording of habitual seizures. Such information is invaluable in the event of diagnostic uncertainty and if surgical treatment is considered.[61]

The mainstay of elective brain imaging is MRI, which is becoming increasingly available. The quality of MRI has improved greatly over the past decade. There remains a gulf between the sensitivity and specificity of optimum imaging as obtained at a center of excellence, and nonimaging as obtained at a center of excellence, and nonspecialized routine brain MRI.[62,63] Widespread adoption of agreed imaging protocols[64,65] would be an important step forward. In resource—poor countries, access to MRI can be restricted or nonexistent. In this situation, CT might be more accessible and can be used to assess gross pathological changes, but cannot identify most of the subtle changes that commonly underlie epilepsy. MRI is especially important in individuals with refractory partial seizures who would be potential candidates for surgical treatment, and in those with progressive neurological or psychological deficits.[64,65] The sensitivity of MRI in detection of subtle change that could underlie refractory focal epilepsies, such as focal cortical dysplasia, is improving with new MRI acquisition sequences. Diffusion tensor imaging,[66] magnitization transfer imaging,[67] and T2 mapping[68,69] show promise. Tractography can visualize white-matter tracts including connections of eloquent areas[70] and can be used to reduce the risks of surgery.[71]

Automated data analysis is becoming an important adjunct to visual interpretation.[72,73] Voxal based analysis can identify subtle changes in the neocortex over time that are not evident on visual inspection.[74] In some selected patients with temporal lobe epilepsy serial studies have shown a reduction hippocampal volume with time,[75,76] but this is a rare finding.[74] There is an increased risk of focal and diffuse neocortical atrophy developing in all epilepsies, but considerable heterogeneity exists between patients.[74]

Functional MRI (fMRI) of the blood-oxygen-level-dependent (BOLD) contrast is increasingly used to lateralize language before surgery[77,78] and can predict deficits after temporal lobe resection.[79,80] fMRI is removing the need for the carotid amytal test, but caution is required because discrepancies can arise.[81] Impairment of memory after temporal lobe resection, particularly of verbal memory after left anterior temporal lobe resection, is a concern. fMRI can visualize the functional anatomy of memory tasks[82-85] and hence the probable effects of surgery on individuals, assisting decision-making and planning of surgery. The simultaneous recording of EEG and fMRI can visualize the BOLD response to interictal epileptic activity. This emerging technique could assist in identifying targets for surgical treatment.[86,87]

Functional imaging of the brain with isotopes has a clinical rose in assessment of suitability for epilepsy surgery. Objective analyses of single photon emission computed tomography (SPECT) studies of ictal, postictal, and interictal blood flow have shown focal ictal hyperperfusion with surrounding hypoperfusion, followed by hypoperfusion in the focus and then return to the interictal state. SPECT could be useful identification of a possible epileptic focus, particularly when structural imaging is unremarkable, to generate hypotheses that can be tested with intracranial EEG studies,[88] and indicate areas involved in the spread of seizures from the medial temporal lobe.[89] PET imaging with fluorodeoxyglucose might show an area of hypometabolism that, if MRI is normal, could suggest the possible site of seizure onset, which could then be tested with intracranial EEG.[90]

Flumazenil binding to the central benzodiazepine receptor complex with GABA might be abnormal in a more restricted area than is fluorodexyglucose binding, and might provide data that are useful to presurgical assessment when MRI is not definitive.[91] Other tracers that explore the pathogenesis of epilepsies and which could have localizing value include alphamethyl tryptopham[92] and 5HT 1A.[93]

DRUG TREATMENT

Antiepileptic drugs are the mainstay of epilepsy treatment. Nonpharmacological treatments are feasible only in a few selected cases and usually after antiepileptics have failed. Nonpharmacological options include curative surgery, palliative surgical procedures, and the ketogenic diet. The main indications for the ketogenic diet are severe forms of drug resistant epilepsy in pediatric practice.[94,95] Overall, antiepileptic drugs are effective in 60–70% of individuals. The aim of antiepileptic[8] treatment is to control seizures as quickly as possible without adverse effects.[96] Improved seizure control is likely to reduce morbidity and premature mortality associated with continuing seizures, especially convulsive attacks.[11] Further, seizure remission is the major determinant of good quality of life.[97]

Drugs for epilepsy increase inhibition, decrease excitation, or prevent aberrant burst-firing of neurons. Some were discovered empirically through screening programmes of induced seizures in animals without epilepsy. The mechanisms of action are not fully understood and many antiepileptic drugs have multiple actions. The principal mechanisms of present drugs are thought to be enhancement of the inhibitory GABAergic system (e.g. carbamazepine, oxcarbamezepine, lamortrigine and phenytoin).[98] Even within these groups, drugs can have very different modes of action. Benzodiazepines bind to GABAA recepetors, potentiate the response to GABA, and are used in generalized and partial seizures. Tiagabine, on the other hand, inhibits GABA uptake, potentiating GABAA and GABA[8] receptor responses, which pyperpolarize and decrease the excitability of neurons.[98] Although this process suppresses partial seizures, hyperpolarization of thalamocortical cells can results in exacerbation of absences.

Drugs that specifically target glutamate receptors have had little success because of unacceptable side effects, but some useful drugs (e.g. topiramate) might affect glutamatergic transmission. Antiepileptic drugs can act on ion channels that affect neuronal excitability and also for neurotransmitter release. Calcium channels are crucial for cell excitability and also for neurotransmitter release. Ethosuximide might target T type calcium channels, which would explain its specificity for absence seizures. Other drugs (e.g. gabapentin, pregabalin) target presynaptic calcium channels, thus inhibiting neurotransmitter release. Modulation of neurotransmitter release. Modulation of neurotransmitter release might be an effective ways of modifying network excitability. Levetiracetam binds specifically to a presynaptic vescular protein that affects neurotransmitter release.[99] Interest is also growing in the cationic h-channel, which inhibits regenerative dendritic action potentials, since lamotrigine[100] and possibly gabepentin[101] potentiate this current.

Conventionally, antiepileptic drugs are divided into old drugs and new drugs, according to whether or not they were available before the 1990s. Some of these drugs are used as first-line treatment and are selected mainly according to their clinical effectiveness for the epileptic syndrome or seizure type, and for tolerability and individual patients' circumstances.[2,96,101-104] This individualized approach to treatment is recommended in all treatment guidelines.[2,5] Existing NICE guidelines suggest a range of drugs as potential first-line treatments for the different seizure types and epilepsy syndromes that are most likely to be seen in adult practive. New antiepileptic drugs have often been promoted as having advantages over old drugs.[105-107] There is, however, no evidence that new drugs are more effective, although they might be better tolerated, than old drugs. A comparative study of the tolerability and efficacy of two newer drugs, lamotrigine and gabapentin, with carbamazepine, showed no difference in efficacy in elderly people, but the new drugs were better tolerated than the old ones in this age group.[108] A major pragmatic clinical trial (SANAD)[109] comparing newer and older antiepileptic drugs is underway and will report within the next year.

Despite the fact that several new drugs have been licensed in recent times, the principles of epilepsy treatment have not changed much.[96] Antiepileptic treatment is still essentially empirical rather than rational. However, a rational approach to management is warranted, with a clear individualized management plan established at the earliest opportunity. For instanse, women of childbearing potential should not be started on drugs that carry on increased risk of detrimental effects to a fetus unless there is no other choice.[110] In elderly people, who might be taking several drugs for other conditions, drugs that are likely to interact with others should be avoided if possible.

When should treatment should be started in people with few or infrequent seizures? A recurring issue has been whether seizures beget seizures, and therefore whether failure of early treatment leads to chronicity.[26,111]

Recent evidenc shows no difference in the long-term outlook for deferred versus immediate treatment,[104] which justifies the practice of waiting for further events rather than starting treatment immediately after a single seizure. Patients perceived to be at high-risk of recurrence because of a structural abnormality thought to be responsible for the seizure, an abnormal EEG, a preexisting neurological deficit, or an initial high density of seizures, should, however, still be offered antiepileptics at the first opportunity. The same holds true for those who, on understanding the risks of recurrence and the scope and limitations of these drugs wish to take medication to reduce the risk of a further seizure.

Although randomized clinical trials provide useful data for guiding drug treatment, they are of little practical use. The studies are generally short-term and usually do not take into account the heterogeneity of patients in terms of epilepsy syndrome, associated comorbidites, and lifestyle factors that direct advice on individual treatment options.[112] This necessity was recognized by the recent NICE guidelines on the management of epilepsy .[2,113]

Antiepileptic drugs should always be introduced cautiously and the dose stepped-up gradually. Titration of the drug is usually symptorn led, and if seizures are still taking place, the drug should be titrated up to the up to the maximum tolerated dose. If toxic effects occur at any point, the dose should be reduced. If one first-line drug fail then second-line options should be added. Monotherapy is preferable because polytherapy increases the possibilities of poor compliance, drug interactions teratogenicity, and long-term toxic effects. There are, however, some individuals for whom polytherapy cannot be avoided. Consideration has been given to the notion of rational polytherapy, i.e. the use of combinations of drugs with different putative mechanisms of action, aiming at synergy of effect but not of adverse effects.[114] However, apart from some evidence that lamotrigine and sodium valproate might be better in combination that either alone,[115] there is no consistent evidence that synergisms exist between different drugs, and this area needs further investigation.

Despite the existence of many antiepileptic drugs, a third of people who develop epilepsy continue to experience seizure unabated.[26] For most of these individuals, in particular those who are not candidates for curative epilepsy surgery, the only hope for improved seizure control lies with drugs to which they have not been previously exposed. New agents are rapidly being developed and efforts are being directed at disease modification in addition to symptom control.[116]

ADVERSE DRUG EFFECTS

Occasionally, seizures can be aggravated by antiepileptic drugs.[117-120] Before attributing exacerbation of seizures to a drug, alternative explanations need to be excluded, such as natural fluctuation of seizure occurrence, irregular adherence to the prescription, comorbid illness, and development of tolerance.[120] Information on aggravation of seizures is based on anecdotal case reports or case series and should be interpreted cautiously. In practice, the possibility of seizure aggravation should be considered in particular when treating idiopathic generalized epilepsy with drugs that modulate sodium channels and certain GABAergic drugs and consequently, these drugs are best avoided in the initial management of this disorder.[120]

The potential clinical implications of the well-established adverse effects of older antiepileptic drugs on bone metabolism and density[121-124] have generated studies investigating the extent of these problems and associated risk factors. Whether or not this problem is also associated with the newer drugs is yet to be proven. There have been renewed concerns about the potential tertogenicity of sodium valproate.[125-132] Another issue is that sodium valproate exposure *in utero* might impair neuropsychological development, even in children without overt physical malformation.[133,134] Prospective studies are being done in both the UK and the USA to address this issue, and are of great importance because sodium valproate is still one of the most effective drugs, especially for some forms of idiopathic generalized epilepsy.[115,135]

Antiepileptic drugs that interact with hormonal contraceptives usually do so by enhancing clearance of the estrogen component.[136] This potential for contraceptive failure is an important issue in the treatment of women with epilepsy. A different form of interaction with oral contraceptive steroids has been described: levels of lamotrigine are substantially reduced by the estrogen component of oral contraceptives,[137] which has clinical implications because initiation of estrogen contraception could therefore result in recurrence or exacerbation of seizures.

PHARMACOGENETICS AND DRUG RESISTANCE

Pharmacogenetics addresses the effect of genetic variation on drug response and adverse effects. Environmental factors (e.g. alcohol abuse) can partly account for resistance to drugs, but are poorly understood. Major advances in genetic biotechnology make understanding the genetic contribution to varying drug responses a realistic possibility. Little is known of epilepsy pharmacogenetics, apart from the acknowledged effect on phenytoin dosing of variation in the gene encoding the metabolizing enzyme CYP2C9, although pretreatment genotyping of such variation has not found a place in clinical practice.[138] Pharmacogenetics holds the promise of therapy that more closely suits an individual's profile and type of epilepsy. Pharmacogenetics will support, and not supplant, the treating physician, who can place the cost-effective interpretation of data in the individual's clinical and environmental context.

Common variation in the gene SCN1A affects the maximum dose of phenytoin or carbamazepine, which act on the sodium channel subunit encoded by this gene.[118] Although the recorded genotypic variation explained only around 5% of the dose variation seen, the implementation of dosing pharmacogenetics could lead to more effective use of existing specific antiepileptic drugs in patients who are constitutionally suited to them. However, much more research is needed to make use of data on individual genetic variation, to guide drug choice, and to predict dosing and response.

Pharmacoresistance *per se* has received fresh attention:[139] two key hypothesis postulates alteration in drug targets at some stage, leading to poor response to drug treatment.[140] The transporter theory posits that certain multidrug transporters expressed in the brain could reduce antiepileptic drug concentration around neurons in the seizure focus by active export away from neurons, back into capillary lumina. Variation in the gene ABCB1 encoding one such transporter, P glycoprotein, was shown to associate with a phenotype of broad drug resistance.[141] However, a formal replication did not lend support to the original finding.[142] Replication and functional explanation of reported associations are essential before therapy or prognostication can depend on such reports.[143] However, the potential of pharmaco genetics makes such investment worthwhile, since results generated in this way could lead to improved management more quickly than through an understanding of disease susceptibility genetics.

SURGERY

In view of the rapidly diminishing chances of becoming seizure-free after trying three antiepileptic drugs,[141] individuals continuing to have focal seizures should have surgical treatment considered early on. The most common operations are temporal lobe resections, which are cost effective procedures[144] carrying a 60–70% chance of making the individual seizure free[145,146] with improved quality of life.[147] The chance of a good outcome is greatest if the underlying cause is removed, driving research efforts to improve imaging detetion of the cause before operation. If surgical treatment is proposed, localization of the site of seizure onset or critical point in a network, is necessary. This localization is usually accomplished with longlasting scalp video EEG recordings.

If the site of seizure onset is not clear, or if there is discrepancy between data, invasive EEG recordings might be necessary, with depth electrodes placed sterotactically within the brain tissue or subdural strips and grids of electrodes placed on the surface of the brain. This technique has restricted spatial sampling, and the approach needs to be individualized for each patient to test specific hypotheses that can be generated with functional imaging.[148]

Complete seizure control might not be a realistic objective, but useful palliation can still be gained with a cerebral resection or techniques such as corpus callosotomy and multiple subpial transection. Vagal nerve stimulation, by a subcutaneous pulse generator, can also provide palliation when restive surgery is not a viable option.[149] On average, a 50% reduction of seizures can be expected in up to 30–40% of patients, but seizure freedom is seldom seen.[150] Deep brain stimulation is being assessed for refractory epilepsy, and at present there is no consensus about its usefulness. With the heterogeneity of structural and functional networks that might sustain epilepsy, the likelihood of achieving more than palliation through an effect on a final common pathway does not seem probable.

NEW TREATMENT PROSPECTS

There remain difficulties in epilepsy treatment. Treatment should be individualized but remains empirical, and antiepileptic drugs fail for some patients. Despite the success of surgery in the treatment of such refractory focal epilepsy, it is suitable for less than 10% of these patients.[151] Thus, new treatment strategies remain necessary.

Early prediction of seizure could have an enormous effect on the treatment of epilepsy, since it would allow action to be taken to prevent the seizure occurring such an approach is already used in catamenial epilepsy, and by people who have lengthy aura. Use of EEG in predicting seizures is a fast growing technique. Nonlinear analyses of signals can anticipate seizures by several minutes. In practical terms, at present there are limitations of sensitivity and specificity, and the usefulness of this method in clinical is yet to be established.[152-154]

With advances in stem cell science and viral gene expression systems, interest has grown in focal approaches to the treatment of epilepsy.[155] At present, such approaches remain experimental. Focal treatments use two approaches: (1) focal application of drugs, cells or a virus to the epileptogenic zone; (2) focal application to areas that regulate seizure threshold, propagation, or both. The first approach is dependent on identifying where the seizures originate. The advantage over surgery is that tissue destruction can be avoided, and thus this approach could be used in eloquent cortex. If the focus cannot be identified, similar methods could be used to express or release antiepileptic compounds into areas that regulate cortical excitability and seizure threshold.[156]

CONCLUSION

The epilepsies are common, and heterogeneous by virtue of different seizure types, syndromes, causes, comorbidities, and other individual patient factors. Although up to 70% of patients will have their condition controlled with drugs, the remainder continue to have seizures and their negative effects on quality of life, morbidity, and risk of mortality. Surgical treatment is life changing for a small proportion of patients. As genomics and proteomics unfold, the causation of epilepsies will become better understood, and will prompt selection of optimum treatment and development of new treatments. For selected individuals, methods to anticipate seizures and local drug delivery hold promise. Individuals with epilepsy will still need sympathetic, well informed professional advisers to integrate the science with a person's life and thus generate holistic care plans.

38.2 NEWER DRUGS FOR FOCAL EPILEPSY IN ADULTS

JN Vyas

WHAT ARE THE NEWER ANTIEPILEPTIC DRUGS?

Epilepsy is resistant to drug treatment in a third of patients.[157] Driven by this high prevalence of drug resistance, 12 agents have been developed to treat adult epilepsy since the late 1980s. These are often referred to collectively as the "newer" antiepileptic drugs—that is, newer than the established drugs, such as phenobarbital, phenytoin, carbamazepine, sodium valproate, and several benzodiazepines, with phenobarbital having been around for 100 years.[158] In this article we will review the clinical use of (in chronological order of approval in the United Kingdom) lamotrigine, gabapentin, topiramate, oxcarbazepine, levetiracetam, pregabalin, zonisamide, and lacosamide (Table 1).[159]

Table 1: Mechanisms of action, year first licensed, and approved indications for newer antiepileptic drugs discussed in this review for use in adults

Antiepileptic drug (year first licensed)	*Mechanism of action*	*Indications seizure type**	*Add-on therapy*	*Monotherapy*
Lamotrigine (1991)	Blocks fast-inactivated state of sodium channel	Focal, generalized	Yes	Yes
Oxcarbazepine (2000)	Blocks fast-inactivated state of sodium channel	Focal	Yes	Yes
Lacosamide (2008)	Blocks slow-inactivated state of sodium channel	Focal	Yes	
Gabapentin (1993)	Blocks high voltage-activated calcium channel	Focal	Yes	
Pregabalin (2004)	Blocks high voltage-activated calcium channel	Focal	Yes	
Levetiracetam (2000)	Modulates synaptic vesicle protein 2A	Focal, generalized	Yes	Yes
Topiramate (1995)	Various actions on multiple targets	Focal, generalized	Yes	Yes
Zonisamide (2005)	Various actions on multiple targets	Focal	Yes	

*Seizures are broadly classified into focal or generalized on the basis of the mode of onset.[3] Focal (partial) epileptic seizures are conceptualized as originating within networks limited to one hemisphere and may be discretely localized or more widely distributed. Focal seizures may or may not lead to impairment of consciousness or awareness and may evolve to bilateral convulsive seizures (secondarily generalized tonic-clonic seizure). Generalized epileptic seizures are conceptualized as originating at some point within, and rapidly engaging, bilaterally distributed networks. Examples include (primarily) generalized tonic-clonic, absence, myoclonic seizures.

HOW WELL DO THE NEWER ANTIEPILEPTIC DRUGS WORK?

Add-on Therapy

To obtain licensing approval as add-on therapy, all AEDs have to show superior efficacy compared with placebo in double blind randomized controlled trials. In regulatory studies for AEDs, the primary efficacy measure is statistical significance against placebo for responder rate in Europe (defined as a ≥50% reduction in seizure frequency) and median reduction in seizure frequency in the United States.[160] A recent meta-analysis that evaluated the clinical effectiveness and tolerability of the newer AEDs included 62 placebo controlled studies in children and adults in terms of responder and withdrawal rates.[161] Owing to methodological heterogeneity—such as in the range of dosages tested and of treatment durations (8–26 weeks)—and the small differences found, caution is needed in drawing comparisons between these drugs. In addition, the clinical relevance of the responder rate as a useful clinical end point remains questionable. The recent consensus from the International League Against Epilepsy[162] proposes that a treatment's success should be defined by sustained freedom from seizures, as that is the only efficacy outcome consistently associated with improved quality of life (and in the UK the only efficacy outcome that allows a patient to drive legally). Using this measure, another meta-analysis showed that the overall weighted pooled-risk difference in favor of the newer AEDs compared with placebo for freedom from seizures during the limited study periods was only 6% (95% confidence interval 4%–8%; number needed to treat in terms of freedom from seizures, 16).[163]

Monotherapy

Several of the newer AEDs have shown efficacy similar to that of the older drugs (mostly carbamazepine), and sometimes similar to that of each other, for the treatment of new onset focal epilepsy in adults in head to head monotherapy trials and have been approved for this indication in the UK and other European countries.[164] These approved drugs include levetiracetam, lamotrigine, oxcarbazepine, and topiramate and in some countries gabapentin. Seizure-free rates for a year in this highly selective population have increased to about 60% as the design of the studies has evolved.[165]

However, although there is evidence of efficacy under controlled research conditions for these drugs, their clinical effectiveness and cost effectiveness have been poorly studied. The greater overall effectiveness for focal seizures (mostly in terms of better tolerability) of lamotrigine compared with carbamazepine, oxcarbazepine, and gabapentin in the randomised open-label Standard and New Antiepileptic Drugs (SANAD) study of 1,721 patients arguably makes it the drug of first choice in this clinical setting.[166] The SANAD study found that gabapentin had significantly inferior efficacy compared with carbamazepine, and most experts do not recommend gabapentin as initial monotherapy.

HOW SAFE ARE THE NEWER ANTIEPILEPTIC DRUGS?

All AEDs are associated with a range of adverse effects, the main reason for withdrawal in regulatory trials.[161] Many adverse effects were detected only during postmarketing surveillance, and their long-term adverse effects (such as on bone health) are unknown.

Idiosyncratic Reactions

Such reactions are unpredictable adverse effects independent of dosage.[167] The most common of these is rash, which develops in 3–5% of patients taking lamotrigine, zonisamide, or oxcarbazepine but in <1% of those taking topiramate, levetiracetam, gabapentin, or pregabalin.[168] Lamotrigine and oxcarbazepine can rarely lead to Stevens-Johnson syndrome or toxic epidermal necrolysis. Other rare idiosyncratic reactions include hepatitis, pancreatitis, and blood dyscrasias.

Ophthalmic Effects

Rare cases of acute angle-closure glaucoma and myopia have been reported with topiramate.

Neurotoxicity

Typical dose related symptoms including nausea, diplopia, dizziness, headache, tiredness, somnolence, sedation, and ataxia can occur with all AEDs.[169]

Renal Calculi

Topiramate and zonisamide carry a small (1%) risk of symptomatic renal calculi as both drugs inhibit carbonic anhydrase.

Cardiac Effects

Minor prolongation in the PR interval has been observed in clinical studies with lacosamide.

Psychiatric Effects

Topiramate is associated with anorexia, weight loss, word finding difficulties, and neuropsychiatric complications. Behavioral problems, such as agitation, aggression, hostility, psychosis, anxiety, and depression, have been reported in patients treated with levetiracetam. Zonisamide can also produce or exacerbate psychiatric comorbidities, particularly depression.[170] The US Food and Drug Administration analyzed data from 199 placebo controlled trials of 11 AEDs and found an increase in risk of suicidal behavior or ideation among patients receiving them (0.43%) compared with those receiving placebo (0.22%).[171] A community based case-control study in treated epilepsy documented increased risk of suicidal behavior associated with some newer AEDs (such as topiramate, levetiracetam) only in patients with a high risk of depression.[172]

Teratogenicity

Recent data from EURAP, the largest international prospective cohort study of 3909 pregnancies, reported that *in utero* exposure to lamotrigine monotherapy was associated with an overall, dose dependent rate of major fetal malformation at 1 year of age that ranged from 2% (<300 mg/day) to 4.5% (≥300 mg/day). This was less than that with carbamazepine (3.4–8.7%), phenobarbital, (5.4–13.7%) and particularly sodium valproate (5.6–24.2%).[173] The UK pregnancy register reported a rate of major fetal malformation for untreated women with epilepsy (n = 239) of 3.5% (95% confidence interval 1.8–6.8%).[174] Children exposed to lamotrigine *in utero* had similar IQs at age 3 years to those exposed to phenytoin and carbamazepine, which was around 10 percentage points higher than those taking high dose sodium valproate.[175] Data from the US and UK pregnancy registries indicate an increased risk of oral clefts in infants exposed to topiramate monotherapy during the first trimester.[176] Sufficient data for other newer AEDs are lacking, although preliminary experience from the UK pregnancy registry has suggested a low risk of teratogenicity with levetiracetam.[177]

WHAT ARE THE PRECAUTIONS?

Precautions relate to potential adverse effects as discussed above. Examples are outlined as follows:

Rash

Closely monitor patients with a history of allergic rash when introducing an AED as they have an approximate fivefold increased risk of developing another rash.[168] Avoid oxcarbazepine in patients with a history of rash induced by carbamazepine because of a cross sensitivity rate between these drugs of 25–31%.

Cardiac Problems

For patients with a history of cardiac problems, including conduction block, taking drugs known to prolong the PR interval, and for those aged over 65, use lacosamide cautiously and perform electrocardiography before starting treatment and after titration to optimal dosage.

History of Psychiatric Illness

Avoid topiramate, levetiracetam, and zonisamide, or, if essential, use these cautiously.

History of Renal Calculi

Avoid topiramate and zonisamide as they inhibit carbonic anhydrase; advise all patients taking these drugs to avoid dehydration.

Renal Impairment

For patients with renal impairment prescribe lower doses of gabapentin, levetiracetam, and pregabalin as these are predominantly excreted unchanged in the urine.

Interaction with Oral Contraceptives

As oxcarbazepine and topiramate (at daily doses above 200 mg) selectively induce the breakdown of the estrogenic component of oral contraception,[169] patients taking oral contraception need formulations with higher doses (50 µg) of estrogen, with subsequent adjustment of hormones depending on any breakthrough bleeding; other contraceptive measures must be taken until the menstrual pattern has been stable for at least three months. As the estrogenic component of oral contraception significantly increases the metabolism of lamotrigine, the dosage of lamotrigine may need adjustment when starting combined oral contraception (to maintain seizure control) and when stopping the pill (to minimize adverse effects of lamotrigine).[178]

Pregnancy

Limited data are available on the teratogenic risk of the newer AEDs. Counsel women of childbearing potential on pregnancy matters early.[179] Advise them to plan pregnancy, so that any changes to their regimen of AED treatment can be made before conception (because teratogenesis may occur early in the first trimester). Treatment with AEDs should be continued during pregnancy on the basis that seizures, especially convulsive seizures, are more harmful to the mother and fetus than are the drugs themselves; however, treatment should be tapered to a minimal effective dose before pregnancy, if possible to a single AED. Supplemental folic acid is advised (≥400 µg daily) before conception and during pregnancy to reduce the risk of major congenital malformation.[180] Offer prenatal diagnosis using targeted fetal ultrasonography to detect any major structural abnormalities. After delivery, encourage all mothers to breast feed their babies. If the AED dose, particularly that of lamotrigine, has been increased during pregnancy, consider a reduction in dosage after delivery.

Breastfeeding

Lamotrigine can accumulate in the breastfed baby because of slow elimination. However, few data relate to the other newer AEDs. As a general rule, if the baby is noted to be drowsy or sedated, breast feeding should be alternated with bottle feeding or discontinued.

HOW ARE THE NEWER ANTIEPILEPTIC DRUGS TAKEN AND MONITORED?

All the newer AEDs discussed in this article are taken orally. Oxcarbazepine and levetiracetam are available in liquid formulations. Lacosamide is also available as a syrup and by intravenous injection. An intravenous formulation of levetiracetam has been licensed in Europe for patients aged ≥4 years when oral administration is temporarily not feasible.

In general, start newer AEDs at low dosage, with increments over several weeks to establish an effective and tolerable regimen.[169] Some agents, such as gabapentin and levetiracetam, can be started at effective doses with or without rapid titration, whereas others, such as lamotrigine and topiramate, require slow titration to reduce the risk of rash and cognitive impairment, respectively. Slow titration will also facilitate the development of tolerance to sedation and will ensure early detection of potentially serious idiosyncratic reactions.

Once the target dosage has been reached, adjust the dose further on the basis of seizure control and tolerability. Routine measurement of serum concentrations of the newer AEDs is not recommended (and not available in most clinical settings), as they do not correlate well with efficacy or side effects.[181] However, serum concentrations of lamotrigine fall dramatically during pregnancy, in patients who have recently started taking an oral contraceptive containing estrogen, and in women just before the onset of the menses. Lamotrigine monitoring is particularly helpful in guiding dosing during pregnancy.[180] Such monitoring is not available routinely across the UK and is best performed with advice from an epilepsy specialist. Arguably, however, lamotrigine concentrations should be measured before conception, regularly throughout pregnancy, and in the puerperium.[181]

HOW COST EFFECTIVE ARE THE NEWER ANTIEPILEPTIC DRUGS?

Whether the better tolerability and interaction profile of newer AEDs are worth the higher price has been much debated. High quality cost effectiveness studies are lacking. The guidelines from the National Institute for Health and Clinical Excellence (NICE) included cost utility analyses of AEDs and found lamotrigine to be the most cost effective monotherapy (although carbamazepine may be as cost effective).[182] However, such cost utility analyses often do not adequately account for indirect or "hidden" costs such as interactions between drugs and long-term adverse effects. Moreover, generic formulations are becoming available for many of the newer AEDs, thus driving down prescription costs.

HOW DO THE NEWER ANTIEPILEPTIC DRUGS COMPARE WITH THE ESTABLISHED ONES?

Given the limited number of comparative studies, AED treatment for the individual patient is not based entirely on these and depends also on the patient's age, weight, sex, comorbidities, and perceived differences in adverse effects, propensity for interactions, and cost. Owing to the absence of adequate evidence, judgments about treatment choice (in an attempt to be rational) are based on what we think we know about these other factors. Table 2 lists some advantages and disadvantages of the established and newer AEDs.

Choice of Drug in Newly Diagnosed Epilepsy

Based on a systematic review and consideration of clinical benefits, harms, and cost-effectiveness, the updated NICE guidelines recommend offering carbamazepine or lamotrigine as first line treatment to children, young people, and adults with newly diagnosed focal seizures; if these are unsuitable or not tolerated, NICE recommends levetiracetam (if its acquisition cost falls to at least 50% of the value at June 2011), oxcarbazepine, or sodium valproate.[182] The American Academy of Neurology supports starting treatment with the older AEDs and lamotrigine, gabapentin, oxcarbazepine, or topiramate. Choice will depend on individual patients' characteristics.[183] The International League against Epilepsy adopts a stricter classification of evidence, supporting only carbamazepine, phenytoin, and valproic acid as initial monotherapy for partial onset seizures in adults and lamotrigine and gabapentin for older people.[184] On the basis of the double blind, randomized monotherapy study of levetiracetam versus extended release carbamazepine in newly diagnosed epilepsy, which fulfilled the strict criteria of the International League against Epilepsy, levetiracetam can also be recommended for this indication.[9] These differing recommendations may reflect fundamental differences in the purposes of the various guidelines and in the approaches adopted by the groups developing them.

Choice of Drug in Uncontrolled Epilepsy

As very few head to head comparisons of new AEDs exist for the treatment of drug resistant epilepsy, choice remains largely empirical. The increasing number of available agents has encouraged consideration of their different mechanisms of action (Table 1) in optimising their efficacy in combination. The broad spectrum AEDs levetiracetam, topiramate, and zonisamide, which have multiple mechanisms of action, are often chosen in drug resistant epilepsy.[185]

Table 2: Advantages and disadvantages of the established and newer antiepileptic drugs

	Advantages	*Disadvantages*
Older antiepileptic drugs		
Carbamazepine	Cost effective for new onset focal seizures	Dizziness, headache, drowsiness, diplopia, rash, hyponatremia, osteoporosis, enzyme induction, blood dyscrasias
Phenobarbital	Broad spectrum of activity; once daily; cheap	Sedation, behavioral disturbances, hyperactivity, rash, teratogenesis, osteoporosis, folate deficiency, enzyme induction, Dupuytren's contracture
Phenytoin	Once daily; rapid titration; intravenous formulation available; cheap	Headache, dizziness, ataxia, rash, gum hyperplasia, hirsutism, acne, osteoporosis, peripheral neuropathy, enzyme induction, saturation kinetics, cerebellar atrophy
Sodium valproate	Cost-effective for new onset generalized seizures; broad spectrum of activity; rapid titration; few interactions	Nausea, diarrhea, lethargy, drowsiness, weight gain, thrombocytopenia, alopecia, tremor, extrapyramidal symptoms, enzyme inhibition, teratogenesis
Newer antiepileptic drugs		
Gabapentin	Low-risk of allergic reactions; low-risk of drug interaction	Drowsiness, dizziness, ataxia, weight gain, diarrhea, dose adjustment needed in renal impairment
Lacosamide	Low-risk of drug interaction; intravenous formulation available	Dizziness, headache, diplopia, nausea, vomiting, tremor, rash, minor prolongation in the PR interval
Lamotrigine	Cost-effective for new onset focal seizures; broad spectrum; few interactions; better tolerated than older drugs; low-risk of teratogenicity	Headache, insomnia, diplopia, dizziness, ataxia, rash, interacts with combined contraception pill
Levetiracetam	Broad spectrum of activity; intravenous formulation available; low-risk of drug interaction	Somnolence, headache, neuropsychiatric and behavioral effects such as aggression, depression, dose adjustment needed in renal impairment
Oxcarbazepine	Better tolerated than older drugs	Dizziness, nausea, vomiting, headache, drowsiness, rash, hyponatremia, interacts with combined contraception pill
Pregabalin	Low-risk of allergic reactions; low-risk of drug interaction	Dizziness, somnolence, headache, ataxia, weight gain, peripheral edema, sexual dysfunction, dose adjustment needed in renal impairment
Topiramate	Broad spectrum; weight loss in obesity	Dizziness, paraesthesia, somnolence, confusion, fatigue, weight loss, renal stones, neuropsychiatric effects, interacts with combined contraception pill
Zonisamide	Broad spectrum; once daily; weight loss in obesity; low-risk of drug interaction	Anorexia, dizziness, fatigue, nausea, vomiting, weight loss, renal stones, rash, neuropsychiatric effects especially depression

38.3 DIAGNOSIS AND MANAGEMENT OF THE EPILEPSIES IN ADULTS AND CHILDREN: SUMMARY OF UPDATED NICE GUIDANCE

KK Verma

Epilepsy is a common neurological disorder characterized by recurring epileptic seizures; it is not a single diagnosis but is a symptom with many underlying causes, more accurately termed the epilepsies. Antiepileptic drugs (AEDs) to prevent recurrence of seizures form the mainstay of treatment. Diagnosis can be challenging, making accurate prevalence estimates difficult. With a prevalence of active epilepsy of 5–10 cases per 1000,[186] epilepsy has been estimated to affect between 362,000 and 415,000 people in England, but with a further 5 to 30% (up to another 124,500 people) misdiagnosed with epilepsy.[187] Consequently, it is a physician or pediatrician with expertise in epilepsy who should diagnose and manage the condition. The 2004 guideline from the National Institute for Health and Clinical Excellence on the management of the epilepsies in adults and children was recently partially updated with regard to drug management. This article summarizes the main recommendations of the updated version; new recommendations are indicated in parentheses.[3]

RECOMMENDATIONS

The NICE recommendations are based on the best available evidence and explicit consideration of cost-effectiveness. When minimal evidence is available, recommendations are based on the Guideline Development Group's experience and opinion of what constitutes good practice. Evidence levels for the recommendations are given in italic in square brackets.

After a First Seizure

- Children, young people, and adults presenting to an emergency department after a suspected seizure should be screened initially for epilepsy. This should be done by an adult or pediatric physician with onward referral to a specialist when an epileptic seizure is suspected or there is diagnostic doubt. (A specialist is defined in the guidance as either a "medical practitioner with training and expertise in epilepsy" (for adults) or a "pediatrician with training and expertise in epilepsy" (for children and young people).

Diagnosis

- All children, young people, and adults with a suspected seizure of recent onset should be seen urgently (within two weeks) by a specialist. This is to ensure precise and early diagnosis and start of therapy as appropriate to their needs.
- A definite diagnosis of epilepsy may not be possible. If the diagnosis cannot be clearly established, consider further investigations and/or referral to a tertiary epilepsy specialist. Always arrange follow-up. [*Based on the experience and opinion of the GDG*][188]

Investigations

- Children, young people, and adults needing electroencephalography should have the test performed soon (within four weeks) after it has been requested.
- Do 12 lead electrocardiography in adults with suspected epilepsy.
- In children and young people, consider 12 lead electrocardiography in cases of diagnostic uncertainty.
- Magnetic resonance imaging should be the imaging investigation of choice in everyone with epilepsy.
- Magnetic resonance imaging is particularly important in those:
  - Who develop epilepsy before the age of 2 years or in adulthood
  - Who have any suggestion of a focal onset on history, examination, or electroencephalography (unless there is clear evidence of benign focal epilepsy)
  - In whom seizures continue despite first line medication.
- Children, young people, and adults needing magnetic resonance imaging should have it done soon.

General Information about Drug Treatment

- Adopt a consulting style that enables the child, young person, or adult with epilepsy, and their family and/or carers as appropriate, to participate as partners in all decisions about their healthcare and take fully into account their race, culture, and any specific needs.
- Everyone with epilepsy should have a comprehensive care plan that is agreed between the person, their family and/or carers as appropriate, and primary and secondary care providers.
- Individualize the strategy for AED treatment according to the seizure type; epilepsy syndrome; comedication and

comorbidity; the lifestyle of the child, young person, or adult; and the preferences of the person, their family, and/or carers as appropriate.
- If using carbamazepine, offer controlled release preparations (New recommendation).

For specific advice for women and girls of childbearing potential about AEDs, including sodium valproate, see later in this article.

Starting Drug Treatment

- When possible, offer an AED chosen on the basis of the presenting epilepsy syndrome. If the epilepsy syndrome is not clear at presentation, base the decision on the presenting seizure type(s). (New recommendation.) Seen the full version of this article on bmj.com for two tables summarizing the different drug options according to seizure type and syndrome.

First Line Treatment for Newly Diagnosed Focal Seizures

- Offer carbamazepine or lamotrigine as first line treatment. (New recommendation)
- Levetiracetam is not cost-effective at June 2011 unit costs (the estimated cost of a 1500 mg daily dose was £2.74 (€3.30; $4.20) in June 2011).[189] Offer levetiracetam, oxcarbazepine, or sodium valproate (provided the acquisition cost of levetiracetam falls to at least 50% of the June 2011 value documented in the National Health Service Drug Tariff for England and Wales) if carbamazepine and lamotrigine are unsuitable or not tolerated. If the first AED tried is ineffective, offer an alternative from these five AEDs. (New recommendation)
- Consider adjunctive treatment if a second, well tolerated AED is ineffective (New recommendation).[190]

Adjunctive Treatment for Refractory Focal Seizures

- If first line treatments are ineffective or not tolerated, offer carbamazepine, clobazam, gabapentin, lamotrigine, levetiracetam, oxcarbazepine, sodium valproate, or topiramate as adjunctive treatment. (New recommendation).
- If adjunctive treatment is ineffective or not tolerated, discuss with, or refer to, a tertiary epilepsy specialist, who may consider other AEDs: eslicarbazepine acetate, lacosamide, phenobarbital, phenytoin, pregabalin, tiagabine, vigabatrin, and zonisamide. Carefully balance the risks and benefits when using vigabatrin because of the risk of an irreversible effect on visual fields (New recommendation).

First Line Treatment for Newly Diagnosed Generalized Tonic-clonic Seizures

- Offer sodium valproate as first line treatment (New recommendation).
- If sodium valproate is unsuitable, offer lamotrigine. If the person has myoclonic seizures or is suspected of having juvenile myoclonic epilepsy, be aware that lamotrigine may exacerbate myoclonic seizures (New recommendation).
- Consider carbamazepine and oxcarbazepine, but be aware of the risk of exacerbating myoclonic or absence seizures (New recommendation).

Adjunctive Treatment for Generalized Tonic-clonic Seizures

- If first line treatments are ineffective or not tolerated, offer clobazam, lamotrigine, levetiracetam, sodium valproate, or topiramate as adjunctive treatment (New recommendation).
- If myoclonic seizures are absent or if juvenile myoclonic epilepsy is suspected, do not offer carbamazepine, gabapentin, oxcarbazepine, phenytoin, pregabalin, tiagabine, or vigabatrin (New recommendation).

Continuation of Drug Treatment

- Maintain a high level of vigilance for the emergence of adverse effects associated with the drug treatment (such as reduced bone density) and neuropsychiatric problems (as there is a small risk of suicidal thoughts and behavior; available data suggest that this risk applies to all AEDs and may occur as early as a week after starting treatment[5]) (New recommendation).

Ketogenic Diet

- Refer children and young people with epilepsy whose seizures have not responded to appropriate AEDs to a tertiary pediatric epilepsy specialist for consideration of introducing a ketogenic diet (New recommendation).

Prolonged or Repeated Seizures and Convulsive Status Epilepticus

- Only prescribe buccal midazolam or rectal diazepam for use in the community for those who have had a previous episode of prolonged or serial convulsive seizures (New recommendation).
- Administer buccal midazolam as first line treatment in the community. Administer rectal diazepam if preferred or if buccal midazolam is not available. If intravenous

access is already established and resuscitation facilities are available, administer intravenous lorazepam (New recommendation).

Advice for Women and Girls with Epilepsy

- Discuss with women and girls of childbearing potential (including young girls who are likely to need to continue treatment into their childbearing years)—and their parents and/or carers if appropriate—the risk of AEDs causing malformations and possible neurodevelopmental impairments in an unborn child. Assess the risks and benefits of treatment with individual drugs. Data are limited on the risks to the unborn child that are associated with newer drugs. Specifically discuss the risk to the unborn child of continued use of sodium valproate, being aware that higher doses of sodium valproate (>800 mg a day) and multidrug treatment, particularly with sodium valproate, are associated with greater risk (New recommendation).
- Discuss with women and girls taking lamotrigine the evidence that the simultaneous use of any estrogen based contraceptive can result in a significant reduction in lamotrigine levels and loss of seizure control. When starting or stopping these contraceptives, the dose of lamotrigine may need adjustment (New recommendation).

People with Learning Disabilities

- Ensure adequate time for consultation to achieve effective management of epilepsy (New recommendation).
- Do not discriminate against people with learning disabilities; offer the same services, investigations, and treatments to them as to the general population (New recommendation).

Older People with Epilepsy

- Do not discriminate against older people; offer the same services, investigations, and treatments to them as to the general population (New recommendation).
- Pay particular attention to pharmacokinetic and pharmacodynamic problems with multidrug treatment and comorbidity. Consider using lower doses of AEDs, and, if using carbamazepine, offer controlled release carbamazepine preparations (New recommendation).

Review and Referral

- Provide a regular structured review to everyone with epilepsy. In children and young people, conduct the review at least yearly (but this may be reduced to between 3 and 12 months by arrangement) by a specialist. In adults, conduct the review at least yearly by a generalist or a specialist, depending on how well the epilepsy is controlled and/or the presence of specific lifestyle problems (such as sleep pattern, alcohol consumption).

Overcoming Barriers

The Guideline Development Group was aware of concerns about prescribing sodium valproate to girls and women of childbearing age. The updated recommendations offer alternative prescribing options for this group and also provide additional relevant information when considering prescribing antiepileptic drugs to women of childbearing age. The group also wished to ensure that people with learning disabilities and older people had optimal treatment and had the same opportunities as other adults to access treatments and specialist epilepsy services; the group expressed concern that this is not necessarily current practice.

REFERENCES

Epilepsy

1. Engel J Jr. A proposed diagnostic scheme for people with epileptics seizures and with epilepsy: report of the ILAE Task Force on Classification and Terminology. Epilepsia. 2001;42:79-803.
2. NICE, The epilepsics: the diagnosis and management of the epilepsies in adults and chindren in primary and secondary care http://www.nice.org.uk/page.aspx3o=227586 (accessed Mar 16, 2006).
3. De Boer HM. "Out of the shadows": a global campaign against epilepsy. Epilepsia. 2002:43(suppl 6):7-8.
4. Diop AG, De Boer HM, Mandlhate C, et al. The global campaign against epilepsy in Africa. Acta Trop. 2003;87:149-59.
5. Scott RA, Lhatoo SD, Sander JW. The treatment of epilepsy in developing countries: where do we go from here? Bull World Health Organ. 2001;79:344-51.
6. Menardi H, Scott RA, Reis R, et al. The treatment gap in eplilepsy: the current situation and ways forward. Epilepsia. 2001;42:136-49.
7. MacDonald BK, Cockerell OC, Sander JW, et al. The incidence and lifetime prevalence of neurological disorders in a prospective community based study in the UK. Brain. 2000;123:665-76.
8. Sander JW. The epidemiology of epilepsy revisited. Curr Opin Neurol. 2003;16:165-70.
9. Forsgren L, Beghi E, Oun A, et al. The epidemiology of epilepsy in Europe—a systematic review. Eur J Neurol. 2005;12:245-53.
10. Henary DC, Macdonald BK, Everitt A, et al. Socioeconomic variation in incidence of epilepsy: prospective community based study in south east England. BMJ. 2002;325: 1013-6.

11. Sander JW. Infectious agents and epilepsy. In: Knobler S, O'connor S, Lemon SM, Najafi M (Eds). The infectious etiology of chronic diseaes: defining the relationship, enhancing the research and mitigating the effects. Washington: The National Academics Press; 2004. pp. 93-9.
12. Everitt AD, Sander JW, Incidence of epilepsy is now higher in elderly people than children. BMJ; 2002. pp. 316-780.
13. Sander JW, Bell GS, Reducing mortality: an important aim of epilepsy management. J Neurol Neurosurg Psychiatry. 2004;75:349-51.
14. Morgan CL, Kerr MP. Epilepsy and mortality: a record linkage study in a UK population. Epilepsia. 2002;43:1251-5.
15. Granger N, Convers P, Beauchet O, et al. First epileptic seizure in the elderly. Electroclinical and etiological data in 341 patients. Rev Neurol (Paris). 2002;158:1088-95.
16. Carpio A. Neurocysticercosis: an updata. Lancet Infect Dis. 2002;2:751-62.
17. Garcia HH, Gonzalz AE, Evans CA, Gilman RH. For the Cysticercosis Working Group in Peru. Taenia solium cysticercosis. Lancet. 2003;362:547-56.
18. Magiuire JH. Tapeworms and seizures treatment and prevention. N Engl J Med. 2004;350:215-7.
19. Carter JA, Neville BG, White S, et al. Increased prevalence of epilepsy associated with severe faciparum malaria in children. Epilepsia. 2004;45:978-81.
20. Medina MT, Duron RM, Martinez L, et al. Previlence, incidence, and etiology of epilepsies in rural Honduras: the Salama Study. Epilepsia. 2005;46:124-31.
21. Nicoletti A, Bartoloni A, Reggio A, et al. Epilepsy, cysticercosis, and toxocariasis: a population based case control study in rural Bolivia. Neurology. 2002;58:1256-61.
22. Boussinesq M, Pion SD, Demanga N, et al. Relationship between onchocerciasis and epilepsy: a matched case control study in the Mbam Valley, Republic of Cameroon, Trans R Soc Trop Med Hyg. 2002;96:537-41.
23. MacDonald BK, Johnson AL, Goodridge DM, et al. Factors predicting prognosis of epilepsy after presentation with seizures. Ann Nuerol. 2000;48:833-41.
24. Brodie MJ, Kwan P. Staged approach to epilepsy management. Neurology. 2002;58(suppl 5):52-8.
25. Dlugos DJ, Sammel MD, Storm BL, et al. Response to first drug trial predicts outcome in childhood temporal lobel epilepsy. Neuorlogy. 2001;57:2259-64.
26. Kwan P, Sander JW. The natural history of epilepsy: an epidemiological view. J Neurol Neurosurg Psychiatry. 2004;75: 1376-81.
27. Smith D, Defalla BA, Chadwick DW. The misdiagnosis of epilepsy and the management of refractory epilepsy in a specialist clinic. QJM. 1999;92:15-23.
28. Gaitatzis A, Carroll K, Majeed A, et al. The epidemiology of the comorbidity of epilepsy in the general population. Epilepsia. 2004;45:1613-22.
29. Lhatoo SD, Johnson AL, Goodridge DM, et al. Mortality in epilepsy in the first 11 to 14 years after diagnosis: multivariate analysis of a long-term. Prospective, population-based cohort. Ann Nueorl. 2001;49:336-44.
30. Gaitazis A, Jonhso AL, Chadwick DW, et al. Life expectancy in people with newly diagnosed epilepsy. Brain. 2004;127:2427-32.
31. Gaitazis A, Sander JW. The mortality of epilepsy revisited. Epuleptic Disord. 204;6:3-13.
32. Hanna, J, Black, M, Sander JW, et al. Death in the shadows: the national sentinel clinical audit into epilepsy death. London: National Institute for Clinical Excellence; 2002.
33. Nilsson L, Farahmand BY, Persson PG, Thiblin I, Tomson T, Risk factors for sudden unexpected death in epilepsy: a case-control study. Lancel. 1999;353:888-93.
34. Sperling MR, Feldman H, Kinman J, et al. Seizure control and mortality in epilepsy. Ann Neurol. 1999;46:45-50.
35. Opeskin K, Berkovic SF. Risk factors for sudden unexpected death in epilepsy: a controlled prospective study based on coroners cases. Seizure. 2003;12:456-64.
36. Langan Y, Nashef L, Sander JW. Case control study of SUDEP. Neurology. 2005;64:1131-3.
37. Rugg-Gunn FJ, Simister RJ, Squirrell M, Holdright DR, Duncan JS. Cardiac arrhythmias in focal epilepsy: a prospective long-term study. Lancet. 2004;364:2212-9.
38. Fisher RS, van Emde BW, Blume W, et al. Epileptic seizures and epilepsy: definitions proposed by the International League Against Epilepsy (ILAE) and the International Buereau for Epilepsy (IBE). Epilepsia. 2005;46:63:541-67.
39. de Curtis M, Avanzini G. Interictal spikes in focal epileptogenesis. Prog Neurobiol. 2001;63:541-67.
40. Ward LM. Synchronous neural oscillations and cognitive processes. Trends Cogn Sci. 2003;7:553-9.
41. Jefferys JG, Models and mechanisms of experimental epilepsies. Epilepsia. 2003;44(suppl 12):44-50.
42. Litt B, Echauz J. Prediction of epileptic seizures. Lancel Neurol. 2002;1:22-30.
43. McCormick DA, Contreâras D. On the cellular and network bases of epileptic seizures. Ann Rev Physiol. 2001;63:815-46.
44. Meeren H, can Luijteiaar G, Lopes DS, et al. Evolving concepts on the pathophysiology of absence seizures: the cortical focus theory. Arch Neurol. 2005;62:371-6.
45. Woermann FG, Free SL, Koepp Mj, et al. Abnormal cerebral structure in juvenile myclonic epilepsy demonstrated with voxel-based analysis of MRI. Bain. 1999;122:2101-8.
46. Guerrini R. Genetic malformations of the cerebral cortex and epilepsy. Epilepsia. 2005;46(suppl 1):32-57.
47. Gutierrez-Delicado E, Serratosa JM. Genetics of the epilepsies. Curr Opin Neurol. 2004;17:147-53.
48. Cossette P, Liu L, Brisebosis K, et al. Mulatation of GABRA1 in an autosomal dominant form of juvenile myoclonic epilepsy. Nat Genet. 2002;31:184-9.
49. Suzuki T Delgado-Escueta AV, Aguan K, et al. Mutations in EFHC1 cause juvenile myoclonic epilepsy. Nat Genet. 2004; 36:842-9.
50. Kanai K, Hirose S, Oguni H, et al. Effect of localization of missense mutations. In SCN1A on epilepsy phenotype severity. Neurology. 2004;63:329-34.

51. Mulley JC, Scheffer IE, Petrou S, et al. SCN1A mutations and epilepsy. Hum Mutat. 2005;25:535-42.
52. Baulac S, Huberfeld G, Gour-finkel-An I, et al. First genetic evidence of GABA(A) receptor dysfunction in epilepsy: a mutation in the gamma2-subunit gene. Nat Genet. 2001;28:46-8.
53. Bonanni P, Malcarne M, Moro F, et al. Generalized epilepsy with febrile seizures plus (GEFS+): clinical spectrum in seven Italian families unrelated to SCN1A, SCN1B, and GABRG2 gene mutations. Epilepsia. 2004;45:149-58.
54. Anderson E, Berkovic S, Dulac O, et al. ILAE genetics commission conference report: molecular analysis of complex genetic epilepsies. Epilepsia. 2002;43:1262-7.
55. Marini C, Scheffer IE, Crossland KM, et al. Genetic architecture of idiopathic generalized epilepsy: clinical genetic analysis of 55 multiplex families. Epilepsia. 2004;45:467-78.
56. Greenberg DA, Cayanis E, Strug L, et al. Malic enzyme 2 may underlie susceptibility to adolescent onset idiopathic generalized epilepsy. Am J Hum Genet. 2005;76:139-46.
57. Tan NC, Mulley JC, Berkovic SF. Genetic association stidues in epilepsy: "the truth is out there". Epilepsia. 2004;45:1429-42.
58. Carvalleri GI, Lynch JM, Depondt C, et al. Failure to replicate previously reported genetic associations with sporadic temporal lobe epilepsy: where to from here? Brain. 2005;128:1232-40.
59. Ottman R. Analysis of genetically complex epilepsies. Epilepsia. 2005;46(suppl 10)7-14.
60. Zaidi A, Clough P, Cooper P, et al. Misdiagnosis of epilepsy: many seizure like attacks have a cardiovascular cause. J Am Coll Cardiol. 2000;36:181-4.
61. Cascino GD. Video-EEG monitoring in adults. Epilepsia. 2002; 43(suppl 3):80-93.
62. Von Oertzen J, Urbach H, Jung-bluth S, et al. Standard magnetic resonance imaging in inadequate for patients with refractory focal epilepsy. J Neuroal Neurosurg Psychiatry. 2002;73:643-7.
63. Duncan JS. Neuroimaging for epilepsy: quality and not just quantity is important. J Neurol Neurosurg Psychiatry. 2002;73: 612-3.
64. Recommendations for neuroimaging of patients with epilepsy. Commission on Neuroimaging of the International League Against Epilepsy. Epilepsia. 1997;38:1255-6.
65. Berkovic SF, Duncan JS, Barkovich AJ, et al. ILAE neuro imaging commission of persons with refractory epilepsy. Epilepsia. 1998;39:1375-6.
66. Rugg-Gunn FJ, Eriksson SH, Symms MR, et al. Diffusion tensor imaging of cryptogenic and acquired partial epilepsies. Brain. 2001;124:627-68.
67. Rugg-Gunn FJ, Eriksoon SH, Boulby PA, et al. Magetization transfer imaging in focal epilepsy. Neurology. 2003;60:1638-45.
68. Briellmann Rs, Jackson GD, Pell GS, et al. Structural abnormalties remote from the seizure focus: a study using T2 relaxometry at 3 T. Neurology. 2004;63:2303-8.
69. Rugg-Gunn FJ, Boulby PA, Symms MR, et al. Whole-brain T2 mapping demonstrates occult abnormalities in focal epilepsy. Neurology. 2005;64:318-25.
70. Guye M, Parket GJ, Symms M, et al. Combined functional MRI and tractography to demonstrate the connectivity of the human primary motor cortex *in vivo*. Neuroimage. 2003;19: 1349-60.
71. Powell HW, Parket GJ, Alexander DC, et al. MR tractography predicts visual field defects following temporal lobe resection. Neurology. 2005;65:596-9.
72. Antel SB, Collins DL, Bernasconi N, et al. Automated detection of focal cortical dysplasia lesions using computational models of their MRI characteristics and texture analysis. Neuroimage. 2003;19:1748-59.
73. Keller SS, Wilke M, Wieshmann UC, et al. Comparison of standard and optimized voxel-based morphormentry for analysis of brain changes associate with temporal lobe epilepsy. Neuroimage. 2004;23:860-68.
74. Liu RS, Lemieux L, Bell GS, et al. Progressive neocortical damage in epilepsy. Ann Neurol. 2003;53:312-24.
75. Briellmann RS, Berkovic SF, Synegeniotis A, et al. Seizure associated hippocampal volume loss: a longitudinal magnetic resonance study of temporal lobe epilepsy. Ann Neurol. 2002;51:641-4.
76. Fuerst D, Shah J, Shah A, et al. Hippocampal sclerosis is a progressive disorder: a longitudinal volumetric MRI study. Ann Neurol. 2003;53:413-6.
77. Adcock JE, Wise RG, Oxbury JM, et al. Quantiative fMRI assessment of the differences in lateralization of language related brain activation in patients with temporal lobe epilepsy. Neuroimage. 2003;18:423-38.
78. Liegeols F, Connelly A, Cross JH, et al. Language reorganization in children with early-onset lesions of the left hemisphere: an fMRI study. Brain. 2004;127:1229-36.
79. Sabsevitz DS, Swanson SJ, Hammeke TA, et al. Use of preoperative functional neuroimaging to predict language deficits from epilepsy surgery. Neurology. 2003;60:1788-92.
80. Noppeney U, Price CJ, Duncan JS, et al. Reading skills after left anterior temporal lobe resection: an fMRI study. Brain. 2005; 128:1377-85.
81. Woermann FG, Jokeit H, Luerding R, et al. Language lateralization by Wada test and fMRI in 100 patients with epilepsy. Neurology. 2003;61:699-701.
82. Golby AJ, Poldrack RA, Illes J, et al. Memory laterlization in medial temporal lobe epilepsy assessed by functional MR1. Epilepsia. 2002;43:855-63.
83. Richardson MP, Strange BA, Duncan JS, et al. Preserved verbal memory function in left medial temporal pathology involves reorganization of function to right medial temporal lobe. Neuroimage. 2003;20(suppl 1):S112-19.
84. Richardson MP, Strange BA, Thompson PJ, et al. Preoperative verbal memory fMRI predicts postoperative memory decline after left temporal lobe resection. Brain. 2004;127: 2419-26.
85. Rabin ML, Narayan VM, Imberg DY, et al. Functional MRI predicts postsurgical memory following temporal lobectomy. Brain. 2004;127:2286-98.

86. Federico P, Archer JS, Abbott DF, et al. Cortical/subcortical BOLD changes associated with epileptic discharges: an EEG-fMRI study at 3 T. Neurology. 2005;64:1263-6.
87. Kobyashi E, Bagshaw AP, Jansen A, et al. Instrinsic epileptogenicity in polymicrogyric cortex suggested by EEG-fMRI BOLD responss. Neurology. 2005;64:1263-6.
88. Cascino GD, Buchhalter JR, Mullan BP, et al. Ictal SPECT in nonlesional extratemporal epilepsy. Epilepsia. 2004;45(suppl 4):32-4.
89. Van Paesschen W, Dupont P, Van Driel G, et al. SPECT perfusion changes during complex partial seizures in patients with hippocampal sclerosis. Brain. 2003;126:1103-11.
90. Chassoux F, Sermah F, Bouilleret V, et al. Metabolic changes and electro-clinical patterns in mesio-temporal lobe epilepsy: a correlative study. Brain. 2004;127:164-74.
91. Hammers A, Koepp MJ, Richardson MP, et al. Grey and white matter flumazenil binding in neocortical epilepsy with normal MRI, a PET study of 44 patients. Brain. 2003;126:1300-18.
92. Juhasz C, Chugani DC, Muzik O, et al. Alpha-methyl-L-tryptophan PET detects epileptogenic cortex in children with intractable eipilepsy. Neurology. 2003;60:960-68.
93. Merlet I, Ryvlin P, Costes N, et al. Statistical parametric mapping of 5-HT1A receptor binding in temporal lobe epilepsy with hippocampal ictal onset on intracranial EEG. Neuroimage. 2004;22:886-96.
94. Sheth RD, Stafstrom CE, Hsu D. Nonpharmacological treatment options for epilepsy. Semin Pediatr Neurol. 2005;12:106-13.
95. Kossoff EH. More fat and fewer seizures: dietary therapies for epilepsy. Lancet Neurol. 2004;3:415-20
96. Sander JW. The use of antiepileptic drugs-principles and practice. Epilepsia. 2004;45(suppl 6):28-34.
97. Birbeck GL, Hays RD, Cui X, et al. Seizure reduction and quality of life improvements in people with epilepsy. Epilepsia. 2002; 43:535-8.
98. Walker MC, Fisher A, Mechanisms of antiepileptic drugs. In: Shorvon S, Fish DR, Dodson E, Perucca E (Eds). The treatment of epilepsy. Oxford: Blackwells; 2004. pp. 96-119.
99. Lynch BA, Lambeng N, Nocka K, et al. The synaptic vesicle protein SV2A is the binding site for the antiepileptic drug levetiracetam. Proc Natl Acad Sci USA. 2004;101:9861-6.
100. Poolos NP, Migliore M, Johnson D. Pharmacological up-regulation of h-channels reduces the excitability of pyramidal neuron dendrites. Nat Neurosci. 2002;5:767-74.
101. Surges R, Freiman TM, Feuerstein TJ. Gabapentin increases the hyperpolarization-activated cation current l h in rat CA 1 pyramidal cells. Epilepsia. 2003;44:150-6.
102. Walker MC, White HS, Sander JW. Disease modification in partial epilepsy in adults. Lancet Neurol. 2004;3:729-35.
103. McCorry D, Chadwick D, Marson A, Current drug treatment of epilepsy in adults. Lancet Neurol. 2004;3:729-35.
104. Marson A, Jacoby A, Johnson A, et al. Immediate versus deferred antiepileptic drug treatment for early epilepsy and single seizures: a randomized controlled trial. Lancet. 2005; 365:2007-13.
105. Beghi E. Efficacy and tolerability of the new antiepileptic drugs: comparison of two recent guidelines. Lancet. 2005;365: 2007-13.
106. Vazquez B, Monotherapy in epilepsy: role of the newer antiepileptic drugs. Arch Neurol. 2004;61:1361-5.
107. LaRoche SM, Helmers SL. The new antiepileptic drugs: clinical applications. JAMA. 2004;291:615-20.
108. Rowan AJ, Ramsay RE, Collins JF, et al. New onset geriatric epilepsy: a randomized study of gabapentin, lamotrigine, and carbamazepine. Neurology. 2005;64:1868-73.
109. University of Liverpool. SANAD http://www.liv.ac.uk/neuroscience/sanad (accessed Mar 16, 2006).
110. Tomson T, Perucca E, Battino D. Navigating toward fetal and maternal health: the challenge of treating epilepsy in pregnancy. Epilepsia. 2004;45:1171-5.
111. Hauser WA, Lee JR. Do seizures? Prog Brain Res 2002;135: 215-9.
112. Panayiotopoluos CP, Benbadis SR, Covanis A, et al. Efficacy and tolerability of the new antiepileptic drugs I: treatment of new onset epilepsy: report of the Therapeutics and Technology Assessment Subcommittee and Quality Standards Sulxcommittee of the American Academy of Neurology and the American Epilepsy Society. Neurology. 2005;64:172-4.
113. Perucca E. NICE guidance on newer drugs for epilepsy in adults. BMJ. 2004;328:1273-4.
114. Brodie MJ. Medical therapy of epilepsy: when to initiate treatment and when to combine? J Neurol. 2005;252: 125-30.
115. Pisani F, Oteri G, Russo MF, et al. The efficacy of valproate lamotrigine comedicationin refractory complex partial seixures: evidence for a pharmacodynamic interaction. Epilepsia. 1999;40:1141-6.
116. Bialer M, Johannessen SI, Kupferberg HJ, et al. Progress report on new antiepileptic drugs: a summary of the Seventh Eilat Conference (EILAT VII). Epilepsy Res. 2004;61:1-48.
117. Benbadis SR, Tatum WO, Gieron M, Idiopathic generalized epilepsy and choice of antipeileptic drugs. Neurology 2003; 61:1793-5.
118. Perucca E, Gram L, Avanzrni G, et al. Antiepileptic drugs as a cause of worsening seizures. Epilepsia. 1998;39:5-12.
119. Hirsch E, Genton P. Antiepileptic drug induced pharmaco dynamic aggravation of seizures: does valproate have a lower potential? CNS Drugs. 2003;17:633-40.
120. Chaves, J, Sander, JW. Seizure aggravation in idiopathic generalized epilepsies. Epilepsia. 2005;46(suppl 9):133-9.
121. Vestergaard P, Rejnmark L, Mosekilde L. Fracture risk associated with use of antiepileptic drugs. Epilepsia. 2004;45: 1330-37.
122. Ensrud KE, Walczak TS, Blackwell T, et al. Antiepileptic drug use increases rates of bone loss in old women: a prospective study. Neurology. 2004;62:2051-7.
123. Ecevit C, Aydogan A, Kavakli T, et al. Effect of carbamazepine and valproate on bone mineral density. Pediatr Neurol. 2004; 31:279-82.

124. Pack AM, Morrell MJ, Marcus R, et al. Bone mass and turnover in women with epilepsy on antiepileptic drug monotherapy. Ann Neurol. 2005;57:252-7.
125. Vajda F, Lander C, O'Brien T, et al. Australian pregnancy registry of women taking antiepileptic drugs *in utero*, with emphasis on carbamazepine and valproic acid: a nation-wide, population based register study. Acta Paediatr. 2004;93:174-6.
126. Holmos LB, Wyszynski DF, Lieberman E, The AED (antiepileptic drug) pregnancy registry: a 6-year experience. Arch neurol. 2004;61:673-8.
127. Wide K, Winbladh B, Kallen B. Major malformations in infants exposed to antiepileptic drugs *in utero*, with emphasis on carbamezapine and valproic acid: a nation wide, population based register study. Acta Paediatr. 2004;93:174-6.
128. Russel AJ, Craig JJ, Morrison P, et al. UK epilepsy and preganancy group. Epilepsia. 2004;45:1467.
129. Holmes LB, Wyszynski DF. North American antiepileptic drug pregnancy registry. Epilepsia. 2004;45:1465.
130. Artama M, Auvinen A, Raudaskoski T, et al. Antiepileptic drug use of women with epilepsy and congenital malformations in offspring. Neurology. 2005;64:1874-8.
131. Wyszynski DF, Nambisan M, Surve T, et al. Increased rate of major malformations in offspring exposed in valproate during pregnancy. Neurology. 2005;64:961-5.
132. Cunnington M, Tennis P. Lamotrigine and the risk of malformations in pregenency. Neurology. 2005;64:955-60.
133. Adab N, Kini U, Vinten J, et al. The longer term outcome of children born to mothers with epilepsy. J Neurol Neurosurg Psychiatry. 2004;75:1575-83.
134. Vinten J, Adab N, Kini U, et al. Neuropsychological effects of exposure to anticonvulsant medication *in utero*. Neurology. 2005;64:949-54.
135. Nicolson A, Appleton RE, Chadwick DW, et al. The relationship between treatment with valproate, lamotrigine and topiramate and the prognosis of the idiopathic generalized epilepsies. J Neurol Neurosurg Psychiatry. 2004;75:75-9.
136. Patsalos PN, Perucca E. Clinically important drug interactions in epilepsy. General features and interactions between antiepileptic sdrugs. Lancet neurol. 2003;2:347-56.
137. Sabers A, Ohman I, Christensen J, et al. Oral contraceptives reduce lamotrigine plasma levels. Neurology. 2003;61:570-1.
138. Tate SK, Depondt C, Sisodiya SM, et al. Genetic predictors of the maximum doses patients receive during clinical use of the antiepileptic drugs carbamazepine and phenytoin. Proc Natl Acad Sci USA. 2005;102:5507-12.
139. Scmidt D, Loscher W. Drug resistance in epilepsy: putative neurobiologic and clinical mechanisms. Epilepsia. 2005;46: 858-77.
140. Remy S, Gabriel S, Urban BW, et al. A novel mechanism underlying drug resistance in chronic epilepsy. Ann Neurol. 2003;53:469-79.
141. Siddiqui A, Kerb R, Weale ME, et al. Association of multidrug resistance in epilepsy with a polymorphism in the durg transporter gene ABCB1. N Engl J Med. 2003;348: 1422-48.
142. Tan NC, Heron SE, Scheffer IE, et al. Failure to confirm association of a polymorphism in ABCB1 with multidrug resistant epilepsy. Neurology. 2004;63:1090-92.
143. Kwan P, Brodie MJ. Early identification of refractory epilepsy N Engl J Med. 2000;342:314-9.
144. Picot MC. Neveu D, Kahane P, et al. Cost effectiveness of epilepsy surgery in a cohort of patients with medically intractable partial epilepsy preliminery results. Rev Neurol (Paris). 2004;160:5S354-67.
145. Weibe S, Blurne WT, Girin JP, et al. A randomized, controlled trial of surgery for temporallobe epielspy. N Engl J Med. 2001; 345:311-8.
146. Mcintosh AM, Kalnins RM, Mitchell LA, et al. Temporal lobectomy: long-term seizure outcome. Late recurrence and risks for seizure recurrence. Brain. 2004;127:2018-30.
147. Wiebe S, Matijevic S, Eliasziw M, et al. Clinically important change in quality of life in epilepsy. J Neurol Neurosurg Psychiatry. 2002;73:116-20.
148. Thandani VM, Seigel A, Lewis P, et al. Validation of ictal single photon emission computed tomography with depth encep halography and epilepsy surgery. Neurosurg Rev. 2004;27: 27-33.
149. FineSmith RB, Zampella E, Devinsky O, Vagal nerve stimulator: a new approach to medically refractory epilepsy. N J Med. 1999; 96:37-40.
150. Theodore WH, Fisher RS. Brain stimulation for epilepsy. Lancet Neurol. 2004;3:111-8.
151. Lhatoo SD, Solomon JK, McEvoy AW, et al. A prospective study of the requirement for and the provision epilepsy surgery in the United Kingdom. Epilepsia. 2003;44:673-6.
152. Aschenbrenner Scheibe R, Maiwald T, Winterhalder M, et al. How well can epileptic seizures: is there an identifiable preictal period? Clin Neurophysiol. 2005;116:552-8.
153. Jouny CC, Franaszczuk PH, Bergey GK. Signal complexity and synchrony of epeileptic seizures: is there an identifiable preictal period? Clin Neurophysical. 2005;116:552-8.
154. Mormann F, Kreuz T, Rieke C, et al. On the predictability of epileptic seizures. Clin Neurophysiol. 2005;116:569-87.
155. Nilsen KE, cock HR, Focal Treatment for recractory epielspy: hope for the future ? Brain Res Brain Res Rev. 2004;44: 141-53.
156. Stein AG, Eder HG, Blum DE, et al. An automated drug delivery system for focal epilepsy. Epilepsy Res. 2000;39: 10-3-14.

Newer Drugs for Focal Epilepsy in Adults

157. Kwan P, Schachter SC, Brodie MJ. Drug-resistant epilepsy. N Engl J Med. 2011;365:919-26.
158. Brodie MJ. Antiepileptic drug therapy the story so far. Seizure. 2010;19:650-5.

159. Berg AT, Berkovic SF, Brodie MJ, Buchhalter J, Cross JH, van Emde BW, et al. Revised terminology and concepts for organization of seizures and epilepsies: report of the ILAE Commission on Classification and Terminology, 2005-2009. Epilepsia. 2010;51:676-85.
160. Porter RJ, Baulac M, Nohria V. Clinical development of drugs for epilepsy: a review of approaches in the United States and Europe. Epilepsy Res. 2010;89:163-75.
161. Costa J, Fareleira F, Ascencao R, Borges M, Sampaio C, Vaz-Carneiro A. Clinical comparability of the new antiepileptic drugs in refractory partial epilepsy: a systematic review and meta-analysis. Epilepsia. 2011;52:1280-91.
162. Kwan P, Arzimanoglou A, Berg AT, Brodie MJ, Allen HW, Mathern G, et al. Definition of drug resistant epilepsy: consensus proposal by the ad hoc Task Force of the ILAE Commission on Therapeutic Strategies. Epilepsia. 2010;51:1069-77.
163. Beyenburg S, Stavem K, Schmidt D. Placebo-corrected efficacy of modern antiepileptic drugs for refractory epilepsy: systematic review and meta-analysis. Epilepsia. 2010;51(1):7-26.
164. Kwan P, Brodie MJ. Clinical trials of antiepileptic medications in newly diagnosed patients with epilepsy. Neurology. 2003;60(11 suppl 4):S2-12.
165. Brodie MJ, Perucca E, Ryvlin P, Ben-Menachem E, Meencke HJ. Comparison of levetiracetam and controlled-release carbamazepine in newly diagnosed epilepsy. Neurology. 2007;68:402-8.
166. Marson AG, Al-Kharusi AM, Alwaidh M, Appleton R, Baker GA, Chadwick DW, et al. The SANAD study of effectiveness of carbamazepine, gabapentin, lamotrigine, oxcarbazepine, or topiramate for treatment of partial epilepsy: an unblinded randomised controlled trial. Lancet. 2007;369:1000-15.
167. Zaccara G, Franciotta D, Perucca E. Idiosyncratic adverse reactions to antiepileptic drugs. Epilepsia. 2007;48:1223-44.
168. Arif H, Buchsbaum R, Weintraub D, Koyfman S, Salas-Humara C, Bazil CW, et al. Comparison and predictors of rash associated with 15 antiepileptic drugs. Neurology. 2007;68:1701-9.
169. Perucca E, Tomson T. The pharmacological treatment of epilepsy in adults. Lancet Neurol. 2011;10:446-56.
170. Loring DW, Marino S, Meador KJ. Neuropsychological and behavioral effects of antiepilepsy drugs. Neuropsychol Rev. 2007;17:413-25.
171. Food and Drug Administration. Information for healthcare professionals: suicidal behavior and ideation and antiepileptic drugs. www.fda.gov/Drugs/DrugSafety/PostmarketDrugSafetyInformationforPatientsandProviders/ucm100192.htm.
172. Andersohn F, Schade R, Willich SN, Garbe E. Use of antiepileptic drugs in epilepsy and the risk of self-harm or suicidal behavior. Neurology. 2010;75:335-40.
173. Tomson T, Battino D, Bonizzoni E, Craig J, Lindhout D, Sabers A, et al. Dose-dependent risk of malformations with antiepileptic drugs: an analysis of data from the EURAP epilepsy and pregnancy registry. Lancet Neurol. 2011;10:609-17.
174. Morrow J, Russell A, Guthrie E, Parsons L, Robertson I, Waddell R, et al. Malformation risks of antiepileptic drugs in pregnancy: a prospective study from the UK Epilepsy and Pregnancy Register. J Neurol Neurosurg Psychiatry. 2006;77:193-8.
175. Meador KJ, Baker GA, Browning N, Clayton-Smith J, Combs-Cantrell DT, Cohen M, et al. Cognitive function at 3 years of age after fetal exposure to antiepileptic drugs. N Engl J Med. 2009;360:1597-605.
176. Food and Drug Administration. FDA drug safety communication: risk of oral clefts in children born to mothers taking Topamax (topiramate). www.fda.gov/Drugs/DrugSafety/ucm245085.htm.
177. Hunt S, Craig J, Russell A, Guthrie E, Parsons L, Robertson I, et al. Levetiracetam in pregnancy: preliminary experience from the UK Epilepsy and Pregnancy Register. Neurology. 2006;67:1876-9.
178. Dutton C, Foldvary-Schaefer N. Contraception in women with epilepsy: pharmacokinetic interactions, contraceptive options, and management. Int Rev Neurobiol. 2008;83:113-34.
179. Tomson T, Hiilesmaa V. Epilepsy in pregnancy. BMJ. 2007;335:769-73.
180. Harden CL, Pennell PB, Koppel BS, Hovinga CA, Gidal B, Meador KJ, et al. Management issues for women with epilepsy—focus on pregnancy (an evidence-based review): III. Vitamin K, folic acid, blood levels, and breast-feeding: report of the Quality Standards Subcommittee and Therapeutics and Technology Assessment Subcommittee of the American Academy of Neurology and the American Epilepsy Society. Epilepsia. 2009;50:1247-55.
181. Patsalos PN, Berry DJ, Bourgeois BF, Cloyd JC, Glauser TA, Johannessen SI, et al. Antiepileptic drugs—best practice guidelines for therapeutic drug monitoring: a position paper by the subcommission on therapeutic drug monitoring, ILAE Commission on Therapeutic Strategies. Epilepsia. 2008;49:1239-76.
182. National Institute for Health and Clinical Excellence. The epilepsies: the diagnosis and management of the epilepsies in adults and children in primary and secondary care. (Clinical guidance 137.) 2112. http://guidance.nice.org.uk/CG137.
183. French JA, Kanner AM, Bautista J, Abou-Khalil B, Browne T, Harden CL, et al. Efficacy and tolerability of the new antiepileptic drugs, I: Treatment of new-onset epilepsy: report of the TTA and QSS Subcommittees of the American Academy of Neurology and the American Epilepsy Society. Epilepsia. 2004;45:401-9.
184. Glauser T, Ben-Menachem E, Bourgeois B, Cnaan A, Chadwick D, Guerreiro C, et al. ILAE treatment guidelines: evidence-based analysis of antiepileptic drug efficacy and effectiveness as initial monotherapy for epileptic seizures and syndromes. Epilepsia. 2006;47:1094-120.
185. Brodie MJ, Sills GJ. Combining antiepileptic drugs—rational polytherapy? Seizure. 2011;20:369-75.

Diagnosis and Management of the Epilepsies in Adults and Children: Summary of Updated Nice Guidance

186. Clinical Standards Advisory Group. Services for patients with epilepsy. London: Department of Health, 2000. www.dh.gov.uk/en/Publicationsandstatistics/Publications/PublicationsPolicyAndGuidance/DH_4009240.
187. Chowdhury FA, Nashef L, Elwes RD. Misdiagnosis in epilepsy: a review and recognition of diagnostic uncertainty. Eur J Neurology. 2008;15:1034-42.
188. National Institute for Health and Clinical Excellence. The epilepsies: the diagnosis and management of the epilepsies in adults and children in primary and secondary care (update). (Clinical guideline 137.) 2012. http://guidance.nice.org.uk/CG137.
189. National Health Service Drug Tariff for England and Wales. www.ppa.org.uk/ppa/edt_intro.htm.
190. Medicines and Healthcare Products Regulatory Agency. Antiepileptics. 2011. www.mhra.gov.uk/PrintPreview/DefaultSplashPP/CON019574?DynamicListQuery=&DynamicListSortBy=xCreationDate&DynamicListSortOrder=Desc&DynamicListTitle=&PageNumber=1&Title=Antiepileptics%20&ResultCount=10.

CHAPTER 39

Neuropsychiatry

DK Kochar, Shubhakaran, RP Agarwal

39.1 NEUROPSYCHIATRIC MANIFEST RELATED TO MALARIA

DK Kochar, Shubhakaran

INTRODUCTION

Malaria is the most important parasitic disease of human beings. More than 40% of the world's population lives in malaria endemic areas.[1] About 110 million cases are reported each year from over 100 countries, with tropical Africa contributing over 80% of the total cases. The disease is known to be associated with considerable mortality, i.e. 1 million per year.[2] Though there has been a decline in the total number of reported cases from India (2.099 million by 1992 from 6.47 million in 1976), the plasmodium falciparum (PF) cases have registered a significant increase, i.e. from 0.75 million in 1976 to 0.879 million by 1992,[3] extending to new areas covering almost the entire country. It is a common knowledge that gross under-reporting of malaria cases is done in many countries including India, hence the morbidity and mortality figures do not reflect the actual dimensions of the problem of malaria. Probably between 200 and 400 million cases of clinical disease occur each year throughout the world.[4]

Malaria is transmitted by different species of anopheles mosquitoes; *A. stephensi* and *A. culicifacies* are the main vectors in this part of India. The pattern of malaria transmission is changing considerably in different regions due to ecological changes, resulting in altered vector distribution. A remarkable feature of this change is the spring transmission in northern and central parts of India. The situation of malaria in the country has deteriorated rapidly, due to creation of mosquitogenic potential under the impact of developmental activities and adaptation of vector to the atmospheric variations.

Four species of plasmodium are responsible for producing malaria in human beings, i.e. *P. vivax, P. ovale, P. falciparum* and *P. malariae*. However, in India only vivax and falciparum produce the disease. Severe and complicated malaria is mainly produced by *P. falciparum* only and the important syndromes are cerebral malaria, renal failure, jaundice, seizures, ARDS, severe anemia, etc. Cerebral malaria is associated with high mortality as well as neuropsychiatric complications in survivors.[5]

P. falciparum malaria is a potentially fatal infection where progression to severe and complicated disease can be rapid. In low endemicity area, it occurs both in adults and children, whereas in holo- or hyperendemic areas, it is less common in older children and adults due to partial immunity. Non-immune travelers, migrant workers and pregnant women are also equally vulnerable.[5,6]

P. vivax and *P. ovale* infections are generally considered to be benign, except traumatic or spontaneous rupture of spleen, the incidence being very low. There have been many unconvincing case reports of cerebral malaria attributed to *P. vivax*, however coexistent and inapparent mixed infection with PF could not be excluded in these cases. Rarely, life threatening anemia due to *P. vivax* infection has been reported.[5]

PATHOPHYSIOLOGY OF SEVERE FALCIPARUM MALARIA

There are several hypotheses to understand the pathophysiological mechanisms of cerebral malaria.

1. The *sludging hypothesis*: Parasitized erythrocytes stick together in deep vascular bed, resulting in marked reduction in blood flow through the capillary bed.[7]
2. The *permeability hypothesis*: Cerebral edema develops due to increased capillary permeability, resulting in local hemoconcentration and reduced blood flow.[8] The factors responsible for this were considered to be kinins. Toro and Roman[9] suggested that cerebral malaria is a form of disseminated vasculomyelinopathy followed by brain edema, perivascular infiltrates, ring hemorrhages,

perivascular demyelination and gliosis (malarial granuloma) in the late stages. Adding to this catastrophe is the effect of hyperpyrexia leading to degeneration of neurons in the cerebellum, cerebral cortex and basal ganglia.[10]

3. The *mechanical hypothesis*: Parasitized erythrocytes are attached to the endothelial cells lining the small blood vessels, causing a phenomenon called cytoadherence. *P. falciparum* infected red cells also adhere to uninfected red cells to form rosettes, interfering with microcirculatory flow and metabolism in brain, giving rise to cerebral malaria.[11]
4. *Immunological hypothesis*: Though the role of immune mechanism in the pathogenesis of acute cerebral malaria remains unconvincing,[5] it may well be important in delayed cerebellar ataxia (postmalarial) and in chronic processes such as quartan nephropathy and tropical splenomegaly.
5. *Role of cytokines*: Serum tumor necrosis factor (TNF) concentrations are elevated in acute malaria and other parasitic diseases. TNF may mediate some of the clinical features and complications of *falciparum* malaria. It also increases the cytoadherence of parasitized red cells.[12] Interleukins 1, 2, 6 and gamma interferon may also play a role in pathogenesis of malaria.[13]

Thus pathophysiologically, there is sequestration of erythrocytes, containing highly metabolically active parasites in the vascular beds of internal organs, i.e. brain white matter, liver, kidneys, intestines, heart and adipose tissue. Reduction in deformability, cytoadherence and rosetting of parasitized and uninfected red cells are major factors in pathogenesis. Rosetting is more commonly associated with malarial parasites causing cerebral malaria, and increased cytoadherence with other vital organ dysfunction. Malarial parasites induce release of cytokines, initially the tumor necrosis factor (TNF) which plays a central role, followed by interleukin (IL)-1 causing malaise and pyrexia, and subsequently IL-6 and IL-8, the proinflammatory cytokines.[14]

In gross autopsy finding, brain is often edematous and there are associated punctate hemorrhages in white matter in a majority of cases. Pigmentation and infarctions are also seen.[15] Microscopically, white matter shows a gamut of changes, from congestion and plugging of capillaries and smaller blood vessels by parasitized and pigmented RBCs, to perivascular ring or ball hemorrhages, perivascular demyelination, formation of malarial granuloma, glial node and gliosis.[15] Nonspecific changes are mild meningitis and brain edema, which may be marked in children.

NEUROPSYCHIATRIC MANIFESTATION OF MALARIA

The neuropsychiatric manifestations of malaria are due to plugging of smaller vessels of brain, producing local *hypoxia* and edema. The symptomatology thus produced can be broadly classified under three headings:

1. Cerebral malaria, in which the patient is deeply comatose and should fulfil the criteria of WHO definition, i.e. presence of unrousable coma lasting for more than 30 minutes with exclusion of other encephalopathies (especially bacterial meningitis and locally prevalent viral encephalitides) and confirmation of acute *P. falciparum* infection by peripheral blood film examination.[16] Hypoglycemia is to be seriously ruled out, as it also produces clinical picture indistinguishable from cerebral malaria with severe neurological deficit as sequele in survivors.[17,18] The commonly observed neurological sequele in the survivors of cerebral malaria are in the form of hemiplegia, cranial nerve palsies, paraplegia, aphasia, extrapyramidal rigidity, psychosis, myelitides like ALS, cerebellar dysfunction, neuritis, etc.
2. Noncomatose patients with predominantly neuropsychiatric signs and symptoms, like psychosis, cerebellar ataxia, convulsions, extrapyramidal disorders, etc. The postictal unconsciousness should not be confused with cerebral malaria, and if it lasts for more than 30 minutes it should be included under the heading of cerebral malaria. As per WHO, these are not classified under the heading of cerebral malaria but should always be treated on the line of cerebral malaria.[5]
3. Some neuropsychiatric syndromes occur after the patient has become completely well from the acute attack of malaria and, at the time of appearance of neuropsychiatric syndrome, there is no evidence of asexual phase of *P. falciparum* in the blood smear. This is known as *post-malarial neurological syndrome* (PMNS). Criteria for inclusion under this category are recent symptomatic malarial infection with parasites cleared from blood (and in cases of cerebral malaria, full recovery of consciousness), and development of neurological or psychiatric symptoms within two months after the acute illness. The important manifestations are generalized convulsions, delayed cerebellar ataxia, psychosis, tremors, etc.[19]

CLINICAL FEATURES

Cerebral malaria is the most common clinical presentation and cause of death in severe falciparum malaria in many parts of the world and, in some reports, accounting for about 10% of all cases of falciparum malaria admitted to hospital and for 80% of the fatal cases.[20]

In adults, cerebral malaria usually develops after several days of fever and other nonspecific symptoms,[21] but in children, the history is usually less than two days. Cerebral malaria often starts dramatically with a generalized convulsion, followed by persistent unconsciousness. In adults, the level of consciousness is assessed by observing motor and vocal responses to painful stimuli. Neck rigidity and photophobia do not occur, but mild neck stiffness is not uncommon, and neck retraction and opisthotonos may occur in severely ill adults and children.[5]

Cerebral Disorders

Cerebral disorders include acute febrile encephalopathy with coma.[22] Focal signs of cerebral malaria as spastic hemiplegia, paraplegia or/and aphasia may occur. The patient may show alternating spastic and flaccid paralysis. Pronounced paresis occurs in certain patients while others may have only discrete hyper-reflexia and positive pyramidal (Babinski) sign.[23]

Meningeal irritation can occur with headache, vomiting, neck stiffness and positive Kernig's sign.[24] The most common neurological picture is of asymmetrical upper motor neuron lesion. Muscle tone and tendon reflexes are often exaggerated but general reduction in tone and reflexes may also be observed. Ankle and, sometimes, patellar clonus may be elicited and the plantar reflexes are usually extensor. Abdominal reflexes are invariably absent, while forcible jaw closure and teeth grinding (bruxism) are common. The jaw jerk may be brisk and a pout reflex is usually elicited. A grasp reflex is a rare occurrence. The gag reflex is usually preserved.[5]

Convulsions are observed in about half of the adult patients and are more common in children. They are usually generalized but Jacksonian type or persistent focal seizures are also observed.[25]

Various forms of extensor posturing may be observed, including decerebrate and decorticate rigidity. Sustained upward deviation of the eyes, extension of neck, pouting and cyclic periods of stertorous breathing are probably a forme fruste of opisthotonus.[26,27] These signs were seen in both hypoglycemic and normoglycemic patients with cerebral malaria.[17,28]

In adults, corneal and eyelash reflexes are usually intact and pupils are normal. Disorders of conjugate gaze are very common, the usual findings in Thai adults being divergent eyes with normal oculocephalic (Doll's eye) and oculovestibular (caloric) reflexes.[21] Conjugate deviation of the eye to one side and divergent eyes have been observed in African children. Convergence spasm implying an upper brainstem lesion, transient ocular bobbing, horizontal and vertical nystagmus, and sixth nerve palsies have been observed rarely. In some patients, cortical blindness is also noticed.

In our series of 185 adult patients of cerebral malaria, 62 (33.5%) died and 123 (66.5%) survived. Convulsions were present in 40 (21.62%) at the time of admission, besides unconsciousness. After recovery from coma, hemiplegia was present in 3 (2.43%), cerebellar ataxia in 6 (4.87%), aphasia in 5 (4.06%), psychosis in 11 (8.94%), convulsions in 2 (1.62%), extrapyramidal rigidity in 2 (1.62%), extrapyramidal rigidity with trismus in 1 (0.81%), trismus in 2 (1.62%), decerebrate rigidity in 2 (1.62%) and decorticate rigidity in 3 (2.43%).

According to WHO,[5] papilledema is not a feature of cerebral malaria. However, various authors have described it as an important observation of severity of malaria.[29] This had been observed more frequently by Indian authors.[15,30-34] In our series, retinal hemorrhages were observed in about 10% of cases; exudates were rare. In Africa and Thailand, retinal hemorrhages were almost always associated with cerebral malaria.[35] However, in Papua New Guinea, there was no correlation between the presence of retinopathy and severity, or even the species of plasmodium implicated in the infection.[36]

Psychiatric Manifestations

The psychiatric manifestations related to malaria have been best exemplified by the following citation from BMJ:[37]

By all accounts Gladwin Buttle was an outstanding man as he emerges as a true original, someone who left the world different from who he found it and who would have been a welcome dinner guest.

We returned from dinner at the Turf Club to the fifteenth Scottish general hospital (his base) to be told that there was an unconscious man in the operating theater. He had cut his throat in a hotel and had lost a lot of blood. Buttle said, "Give him some O blood, while I find out who he is". After nearly three pints the patient was coming round and getting restless. Buttle returned and said, "Catch your train back to Alexandria; I will takeover". I asked, "Who is he?" He replied, "Orde Wingate". At breakfast next day, there was discussion about how this already near legendary guerrilla fighter had been so depressed that he had cut his throat. A malariologist asked, "Have you looked at a blood film?" It was swarming with malarial parasites. Wingate had cerebral malaria, not atabrine poisoning as others have suggested. Buttle told me recently that he had several talks with Wingate while he recuperated and he was eminently sane; and of course, he was found fit some months later to command four divisions of Allied Chindits, when he was tragically flown into a mountain on the Burmese front".

Acute psychiatric manifestations of malaria may be classified as follows:[23]

1. Neurasthenic syndrome with marked weakness. It occurs either intermittently or in association with fever.
2. Clouding of consciousness up to coma.
3. Malarial psychosis.

Malarial psychosis, described in 1952, is based on the underlying encephalitic process, manifesting paranoid and manic syndromes in the acute stage, whereas depression is a late sequele. Confusional stages, stupor, hallucinatory delirium and loss of memory are well known, and clinical pictures similar to schizophrenic states have also been described. Occasionally, permanent impairment such as personality disturbance, memory and intelligence disorders, and even dementia-like picture may remain in some patients.[38]

Agitation and confusion may develop, as the patient recovers from consciousness and transient paranoid psychosis, delirium, or brief reactive psychosis sometimes follow the acute illness.[33,39,40] Psychiatric manifestations may be the presenting features in patients with acute malaria, especially if there is high fever,[41] and neuropsychiatric complications are more common with the use of chloroquine, mefloquine, mepacrine, phenothiazines and other drugs.[5,42,43] Other factors implicated in malarial psychosis include alcohol, stress associated with life, or military service in tropical countries, and exacerbation of pre-existing functional psychoses.[40,44] In a study conducted by Bajiya and Kochar,[33] psychosis was observed in 11 (8.94%) patients just after recovery from coma, out of 123 survivors of cerebral malaria (out of a total of 185 patients). These patients had not received any psychotropic drugs prior to hospitalization and had no family history of psychosis, and were neurologically and mentally normal before the acute disease.

Nguyen et al.[19] while describing 22 cases of PMNS, had observed psychosis or acute confusional episodes in 15 (68%) patients. Twelve patients had an acute confusional state with clouding of consciousness and inappropriate speech or behavior, six of whom experienced florid visual hallucinations, and two developed a prolonged confusional state following generalized convulsions. Two patients with acute confusional states had periods of classic catatonia with waxy flexibility. Three patients developed acute psychotic symptoms without clouding of consciousness. Of these, two had serious and prolonged persecutory delusions (one attempted suicide), and the other become acutely manic and experienced visual hallucinations.

Malarial psychosis recovers completely by one month in majority of patients, while it may take longer time (up to 3 months) in a few patients.[33,41]

Cerebellar Dysfunctions

Cerebellar signs in acute falciparum malaria have been described since the beginning of this century. It has been reported to occur, both in cerebral malaria as part of a global encephalopathy[39,45,46] and as a selective impairment of cerebellar function in patients who are fully conscious.[39,41,47,48] Cerebellar lesions have been found at autopsy in patients dying of cerebral malaria.[9]

There has been a recent resurgence of reports regarding cerebellar involvement in PF malaria from India and Sri Lanka.[41,46,48-50] The cerebellar signs and symptoms were transient and there was complete neurological recovery.

Senanayake and De Silva[51] have reported the clinical features of 74 patients with delayed cerebellar ataxia (DCA) following falciparum malaria. Similarly, Kocharet et al.[18] have described DCA in 10 patients. According to De Silva et al.[52] and Senanayake and DeSilva,[51] this neurological syndrome is due to a mutant strain of *P. falciparum*, mediated via an immune mechanism.

Extrapyramidal Disorders

Extrapyramidal syndrome in cerebral malaria is a very rare feature and has been reported as late sequele in India and abroad.[53] Tremors, rigidity and choreoathetosis, and lock jaw, all may occur singly or in combination.[15,23,33,54,55] These may also occur during acute illness and without cerebral manifestation,[41] and completely recover after successful treatment.

Subarachnoid Hemorrhage

These are few case reports of subarachnoid hemorrhage from India. Mathuret et al.[56] reported a case of falciparum malaria presenting as subarachnoid hemorrhage, with bleeding from multiple sites due to DIC. In this case, there was thrombocytopenia, as well as a reduction in plasma fibrinogen level. Sharaswal[57] also reported a case of cerebral malaria presenting as subarachnoid hemorrhage.

Spinal Disorders

Myelitides, as well as spinal and cerebrospinal meningitis, have also been observed. The spinal syndrome resembles those of amyotrophic lateral sclerosis, funicular myelosis, spastic spinal paralysis and tabesdorsalis.[23] In cases of simultaneous occurrence of cerebral malaria and spinal disease, the clinical picture may resemble disseminated encephalomyelitis. These symptoms regress after successful treatment with quinine.

Disorders of Peripheral Nervous System

Cranial nerve lesions, polyneuropathy, mononeuritis multiplex, and Guillian-Barre syndrome have been reported, but these are unusual.[58,59] Two cases of vivax malaria with Guillian-Barre type peripheral neuropathy have also been reported by Padmini and Maheshwari.[59]

Neuropsychiatric Sequelae

Neuropsychiatric complications may also persist for a few days to weeks after the patient has recovered from acute illness. In African children, the incidence reported was 10%, especially when the disease was complicated by hypoglycemia.[17,60] In Gambian children, hemiplegia was the most common neurological sequel; cortical blindness, ataxia, behavior disturbances and other focal neurological signs were also seen. Neurological sequele may also be in the form of cranial nerve lesions, extrapyramidal tremors, polyneuropathy, mononeuritis multiplex, Guillian-Barre syndrome and greatly prolonged coma, but these are unusual.[59,61] Among adult patients in Thailand, more than 95% of the survivors lacked even transient neurological sequele.[21]

Bajiya and Kochar[33] observed neurological sequele in 13 (10.5%) of the 123 survivors of acute insult, out of 185 patients of cerebral malaria. They were in the form of psychosis in 5 patients (6.4%), cerebellar ataxia in 4 patients (3.2%), extrapyramidal rigidity in 2 patients (1.62%) and hemiplegia in 2 patients (1.62%). All of them recovered fully at the end of one month, except persistence of psychosis in 3 patients.

Nguyen et al.[19] described postmalarial neurological syndrome (PMNS) in 22 patients, of whom 16 developed during the same admission as the malarial illness; six patients were readmitted after being discharged as clinically well. These were in the form of generalized convulsions in 8 (36%) patients, psychotic or acute confusional episodes in 15 (68%), and tremors in 1 patient. In these patients, PMNS was associated with the use of oral mefloquine.

NEUROPSYCHIATRIC MANIFESTATIONS RELATED TO DRUG THERAPY IN MALARIA

There were many reports of psychiatric manifestations of malaria, both as the presenting feature of an acute attack of malaria and as a sequel to an episode of severe or otherwise uncomplicated malaria.[39,40,43,62-65] Limitations of many of these reports include failure to confirm the diagnosis of malaria, and to exclude antimalarial drugs and other causes of the psychiatric symptoms. Thus mepacrine (quinacrine, atabrine), which was widely used for the treatment of malaria in 1930s and 1940s, chloroquine (which was introduced in the 1950s), and more recently mefloquine, have been reported to cause mental disturbances.[42,43] Chloroquine can cause insomnia, toxic confusional psychosis, personality changes, mania and suicidal impulses.[43] In about 4/1000 users, mefloquine has caused anxiety, restlessness, depression, amnesia, confusion, hallucinations, and psychotic or paranoid reaction.

Neuropsychiatric manifestations were reported by Weinke et al.[42] in users of mefloquine in 12 patients, of which 8 patients used it therapeutically and 4 prophylactically; the incidence being one of 215 therapeutic users, compared with one of 13,000 in the prophylactic group (making the risk of neuropsychiatric reactions after mefloquine treatment 60 times higher than after prophylaxis). These were in the form of acute psychosis, delusion, hyperactivity, major disturbances of sleep-wake rhythm, agitation, confusion, hallucinations, disturbed consciousness, blocked thought process, paranoia, anxiety, seizures with convulsions, depression, vertigo, abnormal neurological coordination, perceptual disorders, blurred vision, and manic behavior. Similarly, neuropsychiatric adverse events were reported in 0.7% of travelers taking mefloquine, compared with 0.09% of those taking proguanil plus chloroquine in a study conducted on 1214 travels by Barrett et al.[66] and Nguyen et al.[19] have found association of PMNS with the use of mefloquine.

39.2 PSYCHIATRIC ASPECTS OF DIABETES MELLITUS AND CARDIOVASCULAR DISEASE

RP Agarwal

INTRODUCTION

Depression, anxiety disorders, dementia, schizophrenia, and bipolar disorder (BD) occur more commonly in diabetes mellitus (DM) patients.[67,68] DM may be involved in the development of the first three conditions.[69] The exact mechanism by which DM may be linked to these conditions is not fully understood.

There appears to be a bidirectional relationship between DM and depression.[70] About 7% of DM cases are thought to be attributed to depression.[71] Depression is associated with a 60% to 65% increased risk of DM.[71,72] Depression, which is postulated to be a state of chronic stress, has been associated with elevated cortisol levels and hypothalamic-pituitary-adrenal axis abnormalities.[73-76] Additionally, depression has been associated with IR.[75,77] Both depression and high cortisol levels are associated with an increased risk of MetS.[78] A possible correlation has been found between a 10-point difference in Beck Depression Inventory score and a 1% (approximate) change in hemoglobin A1C (HbA1C).[79] Depression also is associated with increased severity of diabetic complications.[80]

Central serotonergic function has been linked to both depressive symptomatology and IR.[75] Further, depressed patients are more likely to be unengaged in self-care, noncompliant with dietary and weight-loss recommendations, or physically inactive—all of which can worsen obesity and IR.[76,81] This risk is compounded by medications used to treat depression, which may contribute to weight gain (WG) and obesity and may be associated with increased risk of DM.[70,76,81] Anxiety has been associated with an increase in inflammatory markers in DM patients, and up to 80% of DM patients experience anxiety secondary to their underlying endocrine abnormality.[82,83]

The DM appears to double the risk of dementia.[84] Numerous mechanisms have been proposed to explain this relationship. These include reduced insulin production; increased IR, resulting in peripheral hyperinsulinemia (HI); decreased insulin signaling in the brain, which may be related to increased tau phosphorylation and amyloid-beta (AB) levels (since insulin may interfere with AB breakdown); alterations in early insulin response; and hyperglycemia (HG)-related increased advanced glycation end products and oxidative stress, inflammation, and macrovascular and microvascular injury.[84-88] DM appears to promote the formation of neurofibrillary tangles through involvement of free fatty acids, which are increased in obese patients.[85,88]

Insulin is involved in acetylcholine synthesis.[84] Impaired insulin signaling may be due to neurotoxins known as AB-derived diffusible ligands.[84] IR results in decreased insulin transport across the blood–brain barrier, reducing insulin levels and brain activity.[85] Further, IR has been associated with increased tumor necrosis factor (TNF) levels, which may promote brain accumulation of AB.[85] IR occurs in dementia as well as in MetS.[85] Increased interleukin-6 levels have been found in dementia patients with functional impairment and in DM patients.[89] An alteration in insulin degrading enzyme, which is related to DM development, is associated with impaired degradation of AB protein.[88] Lastly, lower insulin levels in the central nervous system have been associated with increased dementia, brain atrophy, and cognitive impairment.[86]

Increased rates of DM were identified in schizophrenia patients before the advent of antipsychotic medications, indicating that schizophrenia is associated with a state of IR or impaired fasting glucose tolerance.[90] Psychiatric illness has a physiologic impact on carbohydrate metabolism, including effects on cortisol secretion, growth hormone production, and catecholamine secretion.[69] There is a 10% to 15% prevalence of DM among schizophrenia patients, representing a relative risk (RR) of 2 to 3. The prevalence of DM among BD patients is 8% to 17%, representing an RR of 1.5 to 3.[90]

Despite the increased risk of suicide in psychiatric patients, the leading cause of death in patients with schizophrenia or BD is cardiovascular disease (CVD). This is especially true in younger patients, with the risk of CVD and stroke more than two to three times greater than in a nonpsychiatric population.[90] MetS occurs in 37–63% of schizophrenia patients and in 30%–49% of BD patients.[90] Psychotropic medications used for managing mental illness can contribute to the development of MetS.[91] A detailed review of the pharmacologic mechanisms associated with antipsychotic-induced metabolic abnormalities (MAs) recently was published.[92]

The risk factors that contribute to CVD (e.g. lack of insight, poor self-care, smoking, dyslipidemia, HTN, MetS, and visceral or abdominal obesity) also contribute to—or are present in conjunction with—DM.[90] DM is associated with an increased body-mass index (BMI). Obesity constitutes a BMI ≥30 kg/m^2 or a waist circumference (WC) of 102 cm in men or 88 cm in women. In Asian patients, WC of >90 cm in men or 80 cm in women is considered central obesity, as is BMI ≥25 kg/m^2.[93,94] Increased visceral adiposity and development of MetS are greater in schizophrenia patients and BD patients versus nonpsychiatric patients.[95] Among antipsychotic users, younger patients with BMI <25, white patients, and patients experiencing a first episode of schizophrenia appear to be at greatest risk for WG.[95] Other psychotropic classes are associated with WG.[95,96] Recently, selective serotonin reuptake inhibitors have been associated with development of abdominal obesity and hypercholesterolemia, which are elements of MetS. This relationship was not evident in older patients.[97]

DRUG-INDUCED WEIGHT GAIN

Among AAs, clozapine and olanzapine are associated with the greatest WG; quetiapine and risperidone with intermediate WG; and aripiprazole, paliperidone, and ziprasidone with the least WG.[95] Long-term data for paliperidone and iloperidone are lacking; however, based on five 6-week trials in patients with schizophrenia or schizoaffective disorder, paliperidone was associated with a ≥7% increase in body weight (BW) in 6–9% of patients (depending on dose) versus 1–9% of placebo patients.[98] Iloperidone was associated with a ≥7% WG in 12–18% of treated patients (depending on dose) versus 4% of placebo patients. Overall, based on 4- to 6-week trials in schizophrenia patients, iloperidone was associated with a mean WG of 2.1 kg.[99]

There is an FDA class warning regarding these drugs' potential for inducing WG, thereby hastening the onset of or worsening DM.[100] Low-potency conventional antipsychotics (CAs)—e.g., chlorpromazine, mesoridazine, thioridazine—also are associated with WG.[101] Possible mechanisms for psychotropic-related WG include WG secondary to improved mood/affect; increased food cravings; alterations in resting metabolic state; sedation; increased cellular lipogenesis; and changes in neurotransmitters (e.g. 5-HT [serotonin] 1 and 2A/C receptor antagonism) and neuropeptides (e.g. leptin, ghrelin, cytokines such as TNF).[95] Whereas antagonism of muscarinic (M) 3 and 5-HT1A receptors may lead to decreased pancreatic beta-cell responsiveness, 5-HT2A receptor antagonism suppresses glucose uptake into skeletal muscle; both factors appear to contribute to AA-induced HG.[102] Medications with the greatest likelihood of increasing BW also are associated with increased IR and hypertriglyceridemia. Most WG occurs within the first 38–40 weeks after AA therapy is initiated, and WG reaches a plateau by about 9 months.[101]

Additionally, increased levels and patterns of circulating cortisol and catecholamines and immunologic alterations—including altered cytokine expression—that appear to be related to the underlying mental illness place the psychiatric patient at further risk for CVD.[90]

PSYCHIATRIC DRUGS THAT CAUSE GLUCOSE INTOLERANCE (GI) OR DIABETES MELLITUS

Numerous medications have been associated with drug-induced HG.[103] A connection has been found between antipsychotic agents and development of DM.[104,105] Some studies have found a stronger association in patients who are younger or African American; others have reported older age and nonantipsychotic psychotropics as risk factors.[102,105,106] A pattern similar to that for AA-associated WG has been seen for drug-induced DM, with drugs such as clozapine and olanzapine associated with greater risk of glucose abnormalities compared with other agents in the class.[105] HI has been reported in 30–70% of patients receiving clozapine or olanzapine.[107]

Inadequate treatment of MAs in psychiatric patients may be due to lack of knowledge on the part of treating psychiatrists. The Atypical Antipsychotic Therapy and Metabolic Issues National Survey found that only 59% of psychiatrists recognized WG as a potential AE of AAs, and just 51% acknowledged DM as a potential complication of AAs. Even fewer psychiatrists recognized dyslipidemia (22%) or metabolic decompensation—e.g. diabetic ketoacidosis (DKA)—(2%) as possible AEs. However, 85% stated that they had changed a patient's regimen because of concerns about adverse metabolic consequences.[108]

Some cases of AA-induced DM appear to be related to significant WG, but up to one-quarter may not be.[102] This points to the possibility of two different mechanisms that may contribute to drug-induced DM: a direct cellular effect on glucose utilization by blocking glucose transporter protein in cell membranes, and an indirect effect on carbohydrate metabolism via the neuroendocrine system. Antipsychotics may directly contribute to development of DM by altering beta cells' capacity to secrete sufficient insulin.[109]

A review was recently published on postulated mechanisms behind AA-induced DM.[110] Insulin metabolism and carbohydrate regulation may be affected, which may explain the rapid fluctuations in blood glucose (BG) noted in some patients despite the absence of massive WG.[96] AAs may lead directly to production of atherogenic dyslipidemia, which has been associated with IR. In patients who develop dyslipidemia and IR, there may be a rapid increase in fasting TG levels upon therapy initiation and an equally rapid decrease upon discontinuation.[109] Likewise, AAs may induce MAs in the absence of significant WG.[102] AAs, but not CAs, appear to impair the action of insulin on adipocytes, which has a negative impact on the lipid profile.[102]

AAs have been associated with DKA and hyperglycemic hyperosmolar syndrome. It is thought that M3 cholinergic receptor antagonism may play a role in the development of these life-threatening conditions. These conditions occur rapidly upon initiation of antipsychotic therapy, often within the first week.[111] At greatest risk are younger patients, those with a lower BMI, and female patients. Although these conditions can be fatal, especially if the antipsychotic is not withdrawn, they usually resolve upon discontinuation.[109] Positive rechallenge has been noted, however.[111]

MANAGING PSYCHOTROPIC DRUG-ASSOCIATED BLOOD GLUCOSE ALTERATIONS

Various interventions have been tried to help manage the WG and MAs associated with psychotropic medications. A consensus statement has been published on AAs and the development of obesity and DM.[112] Weight checks are recommended at baseline, monthly for the first 3 months, and quarterly thereafter, with additional checks performed at every visit.[112] Lifestyle modifications such as nutritional counseling, behavioral interventions, and increased physical activity are recommended for overweight or obese psychiatric patients taking AAs.[112]

Interventions to prevent WG should be started when a patient's BMI is >25 kg/m^2. Active weight-loss intervention should be undertaken for those with a BMI of 30 kg/m^2; BMI between 25 kg/m^2 and 29.9 kg/m^2 in the presence of two or more risk factors; or WC >88 cm in women or 102 cm in men, along with two or more risk factors (e.g. HTN, dyslipidemia, CVD, DM, sleep apnea). Lifestyle interventions should be tried for 6 months before re-evaluation to determine the need for more aggressive treatment.[95]

Early (i.e. within the first 4–12 weeks of therapy) WG is a predictor of long-term substantial WG, even though WG may plateau around week 40. For most AAs, a clear dose-WG relationship has not been firmly established, although evidence points to a direct correlation for clozapine.[47] Patients with a BMI <25 kg/m^2 appear to be at greater risk for developing WG from AAs.[95]

If additional interventions are desired or if lifestyle interventions alone are unsuccessful, one strategy is to switch to an AA with a lower likelihood of WG.[95,111,113] Care must be exercised, however, since switching antipsychotics carries a risk of loss of symptom control.[90,111] Different strategies have been used for switching, including abrupt discontinuation of the offending agent or gradual tapering followed by slow uptitration of a new drug with a more benign AE profile.[111] The comparison of antipsychotics for metabolic problems study is examining the issue of antipsychotic switching in schizophrenia patients.[114]

Guidelines have been developed for the prevention and treatment of antipsychotic-associated AEs on glucose-insulin homeostasis and lipid metabolism.[107] Adjunctive pharmacotherapeutic agents also have been tried, although none is approved for managing psychotropic-induced WG or MetS. A goal of therapy is to lose 5–10% of initial BW over 3–6 months.[111] Drugs utilized are orlistat, an enteric inhibitor of pancreatic enzymes; sibutramine, a reuptake inhibitor of norepinephrine, serotonin, and dopamine; topiramate, a mood stabilizer/anticonvulsant; H_2 receptor antagonists (i.e., nizatidine, ranitidine, famotidine); amantadine, an antiviral/antiparkinsonian; antidepressants (e.g. fluoxetine, fluvoxamine); phenylpropanolamine, a sympathomimetic; dextroamphetamine, a psychostimulant; rosiglitazone, a thiazolidinedione; modafinil, an analeptic; and metformin.[113,115]

Two recent papers describe these modalities.[113,115] Most trials have enrolled small numbers of patients and have yielded conflicting outcomes, resulting in insufficient support for their use. Results have been somewhat favorable for topiramate, reboxetine, and amantadine, but have been more nebulous for sibutramine and largely negative for H_2 receptor antagonists and fluoxetine.[113]

These drugs are not indicated for the prevention or treatment of psychotropic-induced WG or metabolic disturbances. Diet and exercise are more beneficial than the use of adjunctive pharmacotherapy, which should be reserved for patients who have failed lifestyle modifications alone.[95,113] Of the above mentioned agents, the most promising is metformin, although results are mixed.[102,116]

Metformin, a biguanide hypoglycemic agent, is useful for preventing or delaying the onset of type 2 DM in high-risk patients.[117] Metformin has been used alone, in combination with lifestyle modifications, or with sibutramine. Doses studied have ranged from 500 mg/day to 2,250 mg/day. Patients experiencing metabolic complications secondary to AA therapy who are younger or who are placed on biguanide shortly after initiating antipsychotic therapy appear to benefit most from metformin.[102]

Guidelines for the use of metformin in managing AA-induced WG and glucose-metabolism dysregulation were recently published.[102] A point system was developed in which a score of ≥4 points renders a patient a potential candidate for metformin therapy. The point system is divided into baseline features. These include family history of DM or CVD; current BMI within normal range (18.5–24.9 kg/m^2), but a positive history of overweight or obesity; BMI in the overweight or obese range; presence of HG or GI; and features developing after antipsychotic initiation (including progression of normal baseline BMI to overweight or obese status and new-onset HG or GI).[102] Metformin may be discontinued if no benefit is noted after 6–8 months.[102]

Health outcomes are generally poorer for patients with DM and concomitant psychiatric illness. This is largely attributed to noncompliance with BG monitoring and failure to adhere to pharmacologic and behavioral treatment plans.[69] However, this assumption has been challenged by a study that concluded that glucose control was better in DM patients receiving psychiatric services for schizophrenia than in DM patients without mental illness.[118]

MONITORING PATIENTS

The American Diabetes Association (ADA)—in conjunction with the American Psychiatric Association, the American Association of Clinical Endocrinologists, the North American Association for the Study of Obesity, and the Mount Sinai Conference—has published recommendations for monitoring patients taking antipsychotics.[112,119] When therapy is initiated, the ADA advises monitoring weight and BMI at baseline; at 4, 8, and 12 weeks; and quarterly thereafter. Patients should monitor their weight and track any changes. WG of >5% over baseline may indicate the need to switch to an agent less likely to cause WG. Fasting glucose, lipid levels, and blood pressure (BP) should be monitored at baseline and at 3 months. Thereafter, BG and BP may be monitored yearly and a lipid profile taken every 5 years if they remain within normal limits. If abnormal glucose or lipid levels are present, the patient should undergo further evaluation even if asymptomatic. WC and family or personal history should be determined at baseline and annually thereafter.[112]

The Mount Sinai guidelines recommend monitoring weight, lipid profile, and glycemic status.[119] Patients should be weighed and have their WC determined at baseline or upon change of therapy and at every subsequent visit for the first 6 months. If WG of ≥1 BMI is present or if the WC is >35 inches in women or >40 inches in men, a weight-loss plan should be initiated and a switch to an agent less likely to cause WG should be considered. Patients should be weighed at every visit until their weight has stabilized, and every 3 months thereafter. Patients should self-monitor their weight and report any significant gains to their health care provider.

Patients who already have DM, who present with HG prior to AA initiation, or who need a change of antipsychotic should be referred to a medical provider. In the absence of DM or HG, patients at high risk for glucose abnormalities should test their glucose in 4 months. If the patient is hyperglycemic, a referral is recommended; if not, glucose should be checked annually. Results that call for more frequent BG monitoring include WG of ≥1 BMI unit, fasting BG >110 mg/dL, random BG >200 mg/dL, or HbA1C >6.1%.[119]

If a baseline lipid profile reveals no abnormalities, lipids may be tested every 2 years. If lipids are elevated at baseline or upon a change in therapy, the patient should be referred to a medical provider, or diet and lipid-lowering therapy should be considered. In this population, the lipid profile should be monitored every 6 months if LDL >130 mg/dL.[119] Caution is advised in administering AAs with statins, as cases of rhabdomyolysis have been reported.[111]

Guidelines have indicated that either a fasting glucose or HbA1C may be used for monitoring blood sugar.[117,119] Despite this, monitoring of metabolic profiles in patients taking AAs remains insufficient.[120,121] Another problem the psychiatric patient faces, besides insufficient screening and management of MAs, is the inadequate management of depression.[122]

CONCLUSION

Management of metabolic complications, including DM and MetS, in the psychiatric patient is complex. Pharmacists are uniquely suited to guide patients in this regard, as it has been shown that they can reduce CVD risk, even in DM patients with psychiatric conditions.[123] There is a monitoring gap in clinical practice that the pharmacist can help fill.[120] In patients with severe mental illness, the provision of regularly scheduled psychiatric care may positively impact glycemic control.[124,125] It is important to take a holistic approach to the care of these patients, addressing both their psychiatric and physical health care needs.[126,127] In keeping with this holistic approach, treatment of the underlying psychiatric condition should not be neglected. For example, only about one-quarter of depressed DM patients are appropriately diagnosed and treated for their depression.[122]

It is projected that, by 2020, depression will be the second leading cause of disease worldwide. Depression is especially problematic in older adults, as it complicates the course and outcome of other illnesses.[128] The pharmacist's role is likely to expand as the United States faces an obesity epidemic and an aging population often afflicted with psychiatric conditions such as dementia, depression, and late-onset schizophrenia.

REFERENCES

Neuropsychiatric Manifest Related to Malaria

1. Nosten F, Price RN. New antimalarials: A risk benefit analysis. Drug Safety 1995;12:264-73.
2. Indian College of Physicians. Academic Wing of API. Misra NP. (Ed). Malaria. Technical Report Series II. Bombay: ICP (JAPI); 1996.pp.1-80.
3. Pattanayak S, Sharma VP, Kalra NP, et al. Malaria paradigms in India and control strategies. J Malariol. 1994;31:141-99.
4. World Health Organization. Weekly epidemiological record. 1989;32:241-97.
5. World Health Organization. Division of Control of Tropical Disease. Severe and Complicated Malaria. Trans Roy Soc Trop Hyg. 1990;84(Suppl. 2):1-65.
6. White NJ. Malaria. In: Gorden C (Ed). Manson's Tropical Diseases. 20th edition. London: WB Saunders. 1996.pp.1087-164.
7. Gaskell JF, Miller WL. Studies on malignant malaria in Macadonia. Quart J Med. 1920;13:381-3.
8. Maegreith BG, Fletcher A. The pathogenesis of mammalion malaria. Adv Parasitology. 1972;10:49-75.
9. Toro G, Roman G. Cerebral malaria: A disseminated vasculo-myelinopathy. Arch Neurol. 1978;35:271.
10. Suri ML, Vijayan GP. Neurological sequelae of heat hyperpyrexia. JAPI. 1978;26:203-13.
11. Howard RJ, Gilladogga AD. Molecular studies related to the pathogenesis of cerebral malaria. Blood. 1989;74:2603-18.
12. Scuderi P, Sterling KE, Lam KS, et al. Raised serum levels of tumour necrosis factor in parasitic infections. Lancet 1986;i:1364. Proguanil as antimalarial prophylaxis: Postal and telephone survey of travellers. Br Med J. 1996;12:928-31.
13. Mohanty S, Patel DK, Pati SS, Mishra SK. Adjuvant therapy in cerebral malaria. Indian J Med Res. 2006;124(3):245-60.
14. Anstey NM, Russell B, Yeo TW, Price RN. The pathophysiology of vivax malaria. Trends Parasitol. 2009;25(5):220-7.
15. Crabb BS, Cowman AF. *Plasmodium falciparum* virulence determinants unveiled. Genome Biol. 2002;3(11):REVIEWS1031.
16. Garg RK, Karak B, Misra S. Neurological manifestations of malaria: an update. Neurol India. 1999;47(2):85-91.
17. Taylor TE, Molyneux ME, Wirima JJ, et al. Blood glucose levels in Malawian children before and during the administration of intravenous quinine for severe faciparum malaria. N Engl J Med. 1988;319:1010-47.
18. Kochar DK, Kumawat BL, Kochar SK, et al. Delayed cerebellar ataxia: A complication of plasmodium falciparum malaria. JAPI. 1996;44:686-8.
19. Nguyen Thi HM, Nicholas PJ Day, Ly Van Choung, et al. Post malarial neurological syndrome. Lancet. 1996;348:917-921.
20. Spitz S. Pathology of acute falciparum malaria. Military Med. 1946;99:555-6.
21. Warrell DA. The impact of clinical investigation on two third world diseases: Cerebral malaria and louseborne relapsing fever. In: Saunders KB (Ed). Advanced Medicine. XIX Symposium. London: Pitman Medical; 1983.pp.99-111.
22. Dhamija RM, Bannerjee AK, Venkataraman S. Cerebral malaria. In: Ahuja MMS (Ed). Advances in Clinical Medicine. Vol. 1. New Delhi: BI Churchill Livingstone; 1991.pp.3-27.
23. Vietze G. Malaria and other protozoal diseases. In: Vinken PJ, Bruyn GW (Eds). Handbook of Clinical Neurology. Vol. 37. Infection of Central Nervous System. Amsterdam: North Holland; 1978.pp.143-60.
24. Russel PF, West LS, Manwell RD, et al. Practical Malariology. 2nd edition. London: Oxford University Press; 1963.
25. White NJ, Looareesuwan S, Phillips RE, et al. Single dose phenobarbitone prevents convulsions in cerebral malaria. Lancet. 1988;2:64-6.
26. White NJ, Looareesuwan S. Cerebral malaria. In: Infections of the Nervous System. 1987.pp.118-43.
27. Bradley DJ, Newbold GJ, Warrell DA. Malaria. In: Oxford Textbook of Medicine. 2nd edition. Oxford: Oxford University Press. 1987;5:474.

28. Warrell DA, Looareesuwan S, Warrell MJ. Dexamethasone proves deleterious in cerebral malaria: A double blind trial in 100 comatose patients. N Engl J Med. 1982;306:313-9.
29. Lewallen S, Terrie E, Taylor DO, et al. Ophthalmolgy. 1993;100:857-61.
30. Gopinathan VP, Ganguly SD, Chivukula LK. Cerebral malaria: A clinicopathological study. JAPI. 1986;34:473-5.
31. Gupta A, Malhotra HS, Bombary P. Clinical pattern of complicated malaria in North-West India. JAPI. 1987;35:15 (abstract).
32. Padhiary KN, Padhi PK, Behera GB, et al. Neurological complications of falciparum malaria. JAPI. 1996;44:910-11 (abstract).
33. Bajiya HN, Kochar DK. Incidence and outcome of neurological sequelae in survivors of cerebral malaria. JAPI. 1996;44:679-81.
34. Kochar DK. Personal Communication; 1997.
35. Looareesuwan S, Warrell DA, White NJ, et al. Retinal hemorrhage: A common sign of prognostic significance in cerebral malaria. Am J Trop Med Hyg. 1983;324:911-5.
36. Davis MW. The significance of retinal hemorrhages in cerebral malaria. Am J Trop Med Hyg. 1984;33:1287-8.
37. Br Med J. An editor's view. Stephan Lock. 1984;288:123.
38. Gopinathan VP, Thampi VR, Ganguly SB. Neuropsychiatric manifestation of falciparum malaria. IMA. 1978;78.
39. Anderson WK. Malarial psychoses and neuroses: Their medical, sociological and legal aspects. Oxford Medical Publication; 1927.p.251.
40. Blocker WW, Kasti AJ, Droff RB. The psychiatric manifestations of cerebral malaria. Am J Psychiatry. 1968;125:192.
41. Kochar DK, Shubhakaran, Thanvi I, et al. Neurological manifestations of falciparum malaria. JAPI. 1997 (in press).
42. Weinke T, Trautmann M, Held T et al. Neuropsychiatric side effects after the use of mefloquine. Am J Trop Med Hyg. 1991;45:86-91.
43. Akhtar S, Mukherjee S. Chloroquine induced mania. Int J Psy Med. 1993;23:349-56.
44. Forrester ATW. Malaria and insanity. Lancet. 1920;i:16-17.
45. Illangasekera VLU, DeSilva S. Acute cerebellar syndrome in falciparum malaria. Ceylon Med J 1976;22:130-2.
46. Kochar DK, Kumawat BL. Cerebral malaria of *Plasmodium falciparum* malaria with hypoglycaemia. Lancet. 1996;347: 1549-50.
47. Chadda VS, Mathur MS, Kothari RP. Cerebellar syndrome in malaria. JAPI. 1978;26:445-6.
48. Chitkara AJ, Anand NK, Saini L. Cerebellar syndrome in malaria. Indian Paed. 1984;21:908-10.
49. Senanayke N. Delayed cerebellar ataxia.A new complication of falciparum malaria. Br Med J. 1987;294:1253-4.
50. Desilva HJ, Gamage R, Herath HKN, et al. A self limiting midline cerebellar syndrome: Is falciparum malaria the cause? Tropical Doctor. 1988;18:5-6.
51. Senanayake N, De Silva HJ. Delayed cerebellar ataxia complicating falciparum malaria, a clinical study of 74 patients. J Neurol. 1994;241:456-59.
52. DeSilva HJ, DeSilva NR, Dunuwille A, et al. An epidemiological study of delayed onset cerebellar ataxia complicating falciparum malaria. J Trop Geogr Neurol. 1992;2:181-4.
53. Bhargave RK, Prakash KL, Gauri MN, et al. Extrapyramidal syndromes after antimalarials. JAPI. 1973;2:969-71.
54. Arya TVS, Prasad RN, Bhutani J. Extrapyramidal syndrome in falciparum malaria. JAPI. 1989;37:393-4.
55. Chaudhary HR, Meena SR, Jain D, et al. Extrapyramidal syndrome in cerebral malaria. JAPI. 1992;40:347.
56. Mathur SL, Hakim A, Lodha R, et al. Subarachnoid hemorrhage in falciparum malaria: An unreported presentation. JAPI. 1992;40:348.
57. Sharaswal DK. A case of cerebral malaria presenting as subarachnoid hemorrhage. JAPI. 1994;42:756.
58. Arya TVS, Prasad RN. Faciparum malaria presenting as Guillian-Barre syndrome. Br Med J. 1986;292:1430.
59. Padmini R, Maheshwari MC. P vivax malaria complicated by peripheral neuropathy with electrophysiological studies. JAPI. 1980;28:153-6.
60. Schmutzhard E, Gerstenbrand F. Cerebral malaria in Tanzania: Its epidemiology, clinical symptoms and neurological long term sequelae in the light of 66 cases. Trans Roy Soc Trop Med Hyg. 1984;78:351.
61. Roger H, Boudouresques J. Les polyneuritesdespaludeens. Annales de Medicine. 1938;43:235-48.
62. Arbuse DI. Neuropsychiatric manifestations in malaria.US Navel Med Bull. 1945;45:304-9.
63. Arieti S. Histopatholigic changes in cerebral malaria and their relation to psychotic sequele. Arch Neurol Psychiatr. 1946;56:79-104.
64. Masson CB. Effects of malaria on the nervous system with special reference to the malarial psychosis. Am J Med Sci. 1924;168:334-71.
65. Wintrob RM. Malaria and acute psychotic episode. J Ment Dis. 1973;150:306-15.
66. Barrett PJ, Emmins PD, Clarke PD, et al. Comparison of adverse events associated with use of mefloquine and combination of chloroquineand.

Psychiatric Aspects of Diabetes Mellitus and Cardiovascular Disease

67. Expert Panel on Detection, Evaluation, and Treatment of High Blood Cholesterol in Adults. Executive summary of the Third Report of the National Cholesterol Education Program (NCEP) Expert Panel on Detection, Evaluation, and Treatment of High Blood Cholesterol in Adults (Adult Treatment Panel III). JAMA. 2001;285:2486-97.
68. Newcomer JW. Metabolic syndrome and mental illness. Am J Manag Care. 2007;13(suppl 7):S170-S177.
69. Myers KA, Edwards AL. Diabetic patients with psychiatric illness. Curr Diabetes Rev. 2010;6:222-7.
70. Lyketsos CG. Depression and diabetes: more on what the relationship might be. Am J Psychiatry. 2010;167:496-7.

71. Campayo A, de Jonge P, Roy JF, et al. Depressive disorder and incident diabetes mellitus: the effect of characteristics of depression. Am J Psychiatry. 2010;167:580-8.
72. Mezuk B, Eaton WW, Albrecht S, Golden SH. Depression and type 2 diabetes over the lifespan: a meta-analysis. Diabetes Care. 2008;31:2383-90.
73. Wolkowitz OM, Epel ES, Reus VI. Stress hormone related psychopathology: pathophysiological and treatment implications. World J Biol Psychiatry. 2001;2:115-43.
74. Boyle SH, Surwit RS, Georgiades A, et al. Depressive symptoms, race, and glucose concentrations: the role of cortisol as mediator. Diabetes Care. 2007;30:2484-8.
75. Okamura F, Tashiro A, Utsumi A, et al. Insulin resistance in patients with depression and its changes in the clinical course of depression: a report on three cases using the minimal model analysis. Intern Med. 1999;38:257-60.
76. Golden SH, Williams JE, Ford DE, et al. Depressive symptoms and the risk of type 2 diabetes: the Atherosclerosis Risk in Communities study. Diabetes Care. 2004;27:429-35.
77. Ramasubbu R. Insulin resistance: a metabolic link between depressive disorder and atherosclerotic vascular diseases. Med Hypotheses. 2002;59:537-51.
78. Vogelzangs N, Suthers K, Ferrucci L, et al. Hypercortisolemic depression is associated with the metabolic syndrome in late-life. Psychoneuroendocrinology. 2007;32:151-9.
79. Van Tilburg MAL, McCaskill CC, Lane JD, et al. Depressed mood is a factor in glycemic control in type 1 diabetes. Psychosom Med. 2001;63:551-5.
80. de Groot M, Anderson R, Freedland KE, et al. Association of depression and diabetic complications: a meta-analysis. Psychosom Med. 2001;63:619-30.
81. Brown LC, Majumdar SR, Newman SC, Johnson SA. History of depression increases risk of type 2 diabetes in younger adults. Diabetes Care. 2005;28:1063-7.
82. Brennan AM, Fargnoli JL, Williams CJ, et al. Phobic anxiety is associated with higher serum concentrations of adipokines and cytokines in women with diabetes. Diabetes Care. 2009;32:926-31.
83. Tuncay T, Masabak I, Gok DE, Kutlu M. The relationship between anxiety, coping strategies and characteristics of patients with diabetes. Health QualLife Outcomes. 2008; 6:79.
84. Kroner Z. The relationship between Alzheimer's disease and diabetes: type 3 diabetes? Altern Med Rev. 2009;14:373-9.
85. Craft S. The role of metabolic disorders in Alzheimer disease and vascular dementia: two roads converged. Arch Neurol. 2009;66:300-5.
86. Burns JM, Donnelly JE, Anderson HS, et al. Peripheral insulin and brain structure in early Alzheimer disease. Neurology. 2007;69:1094-104.
87. Rönnemaa E, Zethelius B, Sundelöf J, et al. Glucose metabolism and the risk of Alzheimer's disease and dementia: a population-based 12 year follow-up study in 71-year-old men. Diabetologia. 2009;52:1504-10.
88. Akomolafe A, Beiser A, Meigs JB, et al. Diabetes mellitus and risk of developing Alzheimer disease: results from the Framingham Study. Arch Neurol. 2006;63:1551-5.
89. Zuliani G, Guerra G, Ranzini M, et al. High interleukin-6 plasma levels are associated with functional impairment in older patients with vascular dementia. Int J Geriatr Psychiatry. 2007;22:305-11.
90. Holt RIG, Peveler RC. Diabetes and cardiovascular risk in severe mental illness: a missed opportunity and challenge for the future. Practical Diabetes Int. 2010;27:79-84.
91. Wofford MR, King DS, Harrell TK. Drug induced metabolic syndrome. J Clin Hypertens (Greenwich). 2006;8:114-9.
92. Reynolds GP, Kirk SL. Metabolic side effects of antipsychotic drug treatment—pharmacological mechanisms. Pharmacol Ther. 2010;125:169-79.
93. Tan CE, Ma S, Wai D, et al. Can we apply the National Cholesterol Education Program Adult Treatment Panel definition of the metabolic syndrome to Asians? Diabetes Care. 2004;27:1182-6.
94. Anuurad E, Shiwaku K, Nogi A, et al. The new BMI criteria for Asians by the regional office for the Western Pacific Region of WHO are suitable for screening of overweight to prevent metabolic syndrome in elder Japanese workers. J Occup Health. 2003;45:335-43.
95. Citrome L, Vreeland B. Schizophrenia, obesity, and antipsychotic medications: what can we do? Postgrad Med. 2008;120:18-33.
96. Vieweg WVR, Levy JR, Fredrickson SK, et al. Psychotropic drug considerations in depressed patients with metabolic disturbances. Am J Med. 2008;121:647-55.
97. Raeder MB, Bjelland I, Vollset SE, Steen VM. Obesity, dyslipidemia, and diabetes with selective serotonin reuptake inhibitors: the Hordaland Health Study. J Clin Psychiatry. 2006;67:1974-82.
98. Invega (paliperidone) product information. Titusville, NJ: Ortho-McNeil-Janssen Pharmaceuticals, Inc; 2010.
99. Fanapt (iloperidone) product information. Rockville, MD: Vanda Pharmaceuticals Inc; 2010.
100. FDA Patient Safety News. Warning about hyperglycemia and atypical antipsychotic drugs. June 2004. www.accessdata.fda.gov/scripts/cdrh/cfdocs/psn/transcript.cfm?show=28#4. Accessed June 20, 2010.
101. Newcomer JW. Comparing the safety and efficacy of atypical antipsychotics in psychiatric patients with comorbid medical illnesses. J Clin Psychiatry. 2009;70(suppl 3):30-36.
102. Hasnain M, Vieweg WVR, Fredrickson SK. Metformin for atypical antipsychotic—induced weight gain and glucose metabolism dysregulation: review of the literature and clinical suggestions. CNS Drugs. 2010;24:193-206.
103. Luna B, Feinglos MN. Drug-induced hyperglycemia. JAMA. 2001;286: 1945-8.
104. Lambert MT, Copeland LA, Sampson N, Duffy SA. New-onset type-2 diabetes associated with atypical antipsychotic medications. Prog Neuropsychopharmacol Biol Psychiatry. 2006;30:919-23.

105. Gianfrancesco FD, Grogg AL, Mahmoud RA, et al. Differential effects of risperidone, olanzapine, clozapine, and conventional antipsychotics on type 2 diabetes: findings from a large health plan database. J Clin Psychiatry. 2002;63:920-30.
106. Bailey RK. Atypical psychotropic medications and their adverse effects: a review for the African-American primary care physician. J Natl Med Assoc. 2003;95:137-44.
107. Melkersson KI, Dahl ML, Hulting AL. Guidelines for prevention and treatment of adverse effects of antipsychotic drugs on glucose-insulin homeostasis and lipid metabolism. Psychopharmacology (Berl). 2004;175:1-6.
108. Newcomer JW, Nasrallah HA, Loebel AD. The Atypical Antipsychotic Therapy and Metabolic Issues National Survey: practice patterns and knowledge of psychiatrists. J Clin Psychopharmacol. 2004;24(5 suppl 1):S1-S6.
109. Stahl SM, Mignon L, Meyer JM. Which comes first: atypical antipsychotic treatment or cardiometabolic risk? Acta Psychiatr Scand. 2009;119:171-9.
110. Buchholz S, Morrow AF, Coleman PL. Atypical antipsychotic-induced diabetes mellitus: an update on epidemiology and postulated mechanisms. Int Med J. 2008;38:602-6.
111. Tschoner A, Engl J, Laimer M, et al. Metabolic side effects of antipsychotic medication. Int J Clin Pract. 2007;61:1356-70.
112. American Diabetes Association, American Psychiatric Association, American Association of Clinical Endocrinologists, North American Association for the Study of Obesity. Consensus development conference on antipsychotic drugs and obesity and diabetes. Diabetes Care. 2004;27:596-601.
113. Faulkner G, Cohn TA. Pharmacologic and nonpharmacologic strategies for weight gain and metabolic disturbance in patients treated with antipsychotic medications. Can J Psychiatry. 2006;51:502-11.
114. Stroup TS, McEvoy JP, Swartz MS, et al. Comparison of Antipsychotics for Metabolic Problems (CAMP): a NIMH Schizophrenia Trials Network study. Clin Schizophr Rel Psychoses. 2007;1:69-72.
115. Baptista T, ElFakih Y, Uzcátegui E, et al. Pharmcological management of atypical antipsychotic-induced weight gain. CNS Drugs. 2008;22:477-95.
116. Miller LJ. Management of atypical antipsychotic drug-induced weight gain: focus on metformin. Pharmacotherapy. 2009;29:725-35.
117. American Diabetes Association. Executive summary: standards of medical care in diabetes—2010. Diabetes Care. 2010;33(suppl 1):S4-S10.
118. Dixon LB, Kreyenbuhl JA, Dickerson FB, et al. A comparison of type 2 diabetes outcomes among persons with and without severe mental illnesses. PsychiatrServ. 2004;55: 892-900.
119. Covell NH, Jackson CT, Weissman EM. Health monitoring for patients who have schizophrenia. Summary of the Mount Sinai Conference recommendations. Postgrad Med. 2006 Sept;spec no:20-26.
120. Morrato EH, Newcomer JW, Kamat S, et al. Metabolic screening after the American Diabetes Association's consensus statement on antipsychotic drugs and diabetes. Diabetes Care. 2009;32:1037-42.
121. Nasrallah HA, Meyer JM, Goff DC, et al. Low rates of treatment for hypertension, dyslipidemia and diabetes in schizophrenia: data from the CATIE schizophrenia trial sample at baseline. Schizophr Res. 2006;86:15-22.
122. Rubin RR, Ciechanowski P, Egede LE, et al. Recognizing and treating depression in patients with diabetes. Curr Diabetes Rep. 2004;4:119-25.
123. Taveira TH, Pirraglia PA, Cohen LB, Wu WC. Efficacy of a pharmacist-led cardiovascular risk reduction clinic for diabetic patients with and without mental health conditions. Prev Cardiol. 2008;11:195-200.
124. Dixon LB, Kreyenbuhl A, Dickerson FB, et al. A comparison of type 2 diabetes outcomes among patients with and without severe mental illnesses. Psychiatr Serv. 2004;55:892-900.
125. Copeland LA, Zeber JE, Wang CP, et al. Patterns of primary care and mortality among patients with schizophrenia or diabetes: a cluster analysis approach to the retrospective study of healthcare utilization. BMC Health Serv Res. 2009;9:127.
126. Metabolic and lifestyle issues and severe mental illness—new connections to wellbeing? J Psychopharmacol. 2005;19(suppl 6):118-122.
127. Vreeland B. Treatment decisions in major mental illness: weighing the outcomes. J Clin Psychiatry. 2007;68(suppl 12): 5-11.
128. Chapman DP, Perry GS. Depression as a major component of public health for older adults. Prev Chronic Dis. 2008;5:A22.

FURTHER READING

Neuropsychiatric Manifest Related to Malaria

1. Aleem MA. Epilepsy in malaria. Epilepsia. 2005;46(4):601. Author reply 601-2.
2. Arun Prakash MV, Stein G. Malaria presenting as atypical depression. Br J Psychiatry. 1990;156:594-5.
3. Beare NA, Taylor TE, Harding SP, Lewallen S, Molyneux ME. Malarial retinopathy: a newly established diagnostic sign in severe malaria. Am J Trop Med Hyg. 2006;75(5):790-7.
4. Bhandari K, Bhandari P. Cerebellar syndrome in malaria. Indian Pediatr. 1989;26(10):1037-8.
5. Blocker WW, Kastl AJ, Daroff RB. The psychiatric manifestations of cerebral malaria. Am J Psychiatry. 1968;125:192-6.
6. Carter JA, Neville BG, White S, et al. Increased prevalence of epilepsy associated with severe falciparum malaria in children. Epilepsia. 2004;45(8):978-81.
7. Clark IA, Alleva LM, Mills AC, Cowden WB. Pathogenesis of malaria and clinically similar conditions. Clin Microbiol Rev. 2004;17(3):509-39.
8. Das CJ, Sharma R. Central pontine myelinolysis in a case of cerebral malaria. Br J Radiol. 2007;80(960):e293-e295.

9. Dwarakanath S, Suri A, Mahapatra AK. Spontaneous subdural empyema in falciparum malaria: a case study. J Vector Borne Dis. 2004;41(3-4):80-2.
10. Gall C, Spuler A, Fraunberger P. Subarachnoid hemorrhage in a patient with cerebral malaria. N Engl J Med. 1999;341(8):611-3.
11. Kale VP, Bichile LS, Bajpai S. Falciparum malaria induced retrobulbar neuritis. J Postgrad Med. 2004;50(2):150.
12. Kanjalkar M, Karnad DR, Narayana RV, Shah PU. Guillain-Barre syndrome following malaria. J Infect. 1999;38(1):48-50.
13. Kochar DK, Joshi A, Agarwal N, Shubhkaran, Thanvi I. Hemiparesis: an uncommon complication of falciparum malaria. J Assoc Physicians India. 1999;47(11):1108-9.
14. Kochar DK, Shubhakaran, Kumawat B. Neuropsychiatric manifestations in malaria. J Assoc Physicians India. 1998;46: 886-90.
15. Kochar DK, Shubhakaran, Kumawat BL, et al. Cerebral malaria in Indian adults: a prospective study of 441 patients from Bikaner, northwest India. J Assoc Physicians India. 2002;50:234-41.
16. Lawn SD, Flanagan KL, Wright SG, Doherty TF, Godfrey-Faussett P. Postmalaria neurological syndrome: two cases from the Gambia. Clin Infect Dis. 2003;36(2):e29-e31.
17. Mathur SL, Hakim A, Lodha R, Chowdhry P, Jain R. Subarachnoid hemorrhage in falciparum malaria: an unreported presentation. J Assoc Physicians India. 1992;40(5):348.
18. Maude RJ, Dondorp AM, Abu Sayeed A, Day NP, White NJ, Beare NA. The eye in cerebral malaria: what can it teach us? Trans R Soc Trop Med Hyg. 2009;103(7):661-4.
19. Mishra SK, Newton CR. Diagnosis and management of the neurological complications of falciparum malaria. Nat Rev Neurol. 2009;5(4):189-98.
20. Mishra SK, Pati SS, Mahanta KC, Mohanty S. Rhabdomyolysis in falciparum malaria—a series of twelve cases (five children and seven adults). Trop Doct. 2010;40(2):87-88.
21. Mohapatra MK, Panda BK, Das SP. Cerebellar ataxia in falciparum malaria—a report of two cases. Indian J Malariol. 2000;37(1-2):46-48.
22. Newton CR, Hien TT, White N. Cerebral malaria. J Neurol Neurosurg Psychiatry. 2000;69(4):433-41.
23. Nguyen TH, Day NP, Ly VC, et al. Post-malaria neurological syndrome. Lancet. 1996;348(9032):917-21.
24. Onifade EU, Danesi MA. Acute cerebellar ataxia associated with falciparum malaria in Nigerian patients. Niger Postgrad Med J. 2004;11(2):140-4.
25. Phillips RE, Solomon T. Cerebral malaria in children. Lancet. 1990;336(8727):1355-60.
26. Prendki V, Elzière C, Durand R, et al. Postmalaria neurological Syndrome—two cases in patients of African origin. Am J Trop Med Hyg. 2008;78(5):699-701.
27. Sahoo S, Kumar M, Sinha VK. Chloroquine-induced recurrent psychosis. Am J Ther. 2007;14(4):406-7.
28. Schnorf H, Diserens K, Schnyder H, et al. Corticosteroid-responsive postmalaria encephalopathy characterized by motor aphasia, myoclonus, and postural tremor. Arch Neurol. 1998;55(3):417-20.
29. Sokrab TE, Eltahir A, Idris MN, Hamid M. Guillain-Barré syndrome following acute falciparum malaria. Neurology. 2002;59(8):1281-3.
30. Thapa R, Biswas B. Childhood mefloquine-induced mania and psychosis: a case report. J Child Neurol. 2009;24(8):1008-9.
31. Van Hensbroek MB, Palmer A, Jaffar S, Schneider G, Kwiatkowski D. Residual neurologic sequelae after childhood cerebral malaria. J Pediatr. 1997;131(1 Pt 1):125-9.
32. Waruiru CM, Newton CR, Forster D, et al. Epileptic seizures and malaria in Kenyan children. Trans R Soc Trop Med Hyg. 1996;90(2):152-5.
33. Wijesundere A. Guillain-Barré syndrome in *Plasmodium falciparum* malaria. Postgrad Med J. 1992;68(799):376-7.

CHAPTER

40

Psychiatric Disorders of HIV Infection and AIDS

Prabha S Chandra

INTRODUCTION

The Joint United Nations Programme on HIV/AIDS has estimated that, as of 2004, more than 40 million people worldwide were living with HIV virus type 1.[1] In North America, between 540,000 and 1.6 million adults and children are thought to be infected, and these are predominantly injection drug users and men who have sex with men. Far from over, this pandemic has also seen the number of women infected with HIV increase rapidly across the globe, and women now account for half of all people living with HIV worldwide. However, recent advances in the treatment of this retrovirus have increased the life expectancy of seropositive people, which makes it more likely that clinicians will encounter patients with neuropsychiatric manifestations of the disease.

The most common neurologic manifestations are minor cognitive and motor disorder (MCMD) and HIV-associated dementia (HAD). The most common psychiatric manifestations are depressive spectrum disorders. In both cases, the impact of these syndromes on seropositive patients is significant and appropriate intervention is required, the key to optimal treatment resting with early diagnosis and aggressive treatment. In this paper, we describe the major neuropsychiatric manifestations of HIV spectrum disease and also discuss the diagnosis and treatment of these types of conditions.

NEUROLOGIC MANIFESTATIONS OF HIV INFECTION

The first cases of HIV-related infections were reported in 1981, and the virus was identified 2 years later.[2] Neurologic complications were recognized very early in the epidemic.[3] It is now known that HIV can be isolated from the cerebrospinal fluid (CSF) and can also be found in brain tissue, which suggests that the virus can cross the blood-brain barrier. Sacktor et al.[4] reported that when monotherapy was a mainstay of treatment (between 1990 and 1992), the mean incidence of HAD was 21.1 cases per 1000 person-years, whereas when highly active antiretroviral therapy (HAART) became the norm (between 1996 and 1998), the mean incidence of HAD decreased significantly, to 10.5 cases per 1000 person-years.[4] These authors also noted a concurrent decrease in the incidence of opportunistic central nervous system (CNS) infections for the same observation periods.

Another team of researchers found a decrease in prevalence rates of opportunistic CNS infections over the same period; however, using autopsy data, they found an increase in the prevalence of HIV encephalopathy in the post-HAART years.[5] This would suggest that despite improved therapeutic options and an apparent decrease in neurologic complications, HIV seems to continue to infiltrate the CNS.

The presence and action of HIV in the CNS are now much better understood. HIV crosses the blood-brain barrier by a Trojan-horse-type mechanism using macrophages it infects.[6] Once in the brain, HIV targets and infects glial cells, from which it later secretes neurotoxins that lead to neuronal damage and death.[7] The extent of this neuronal damage is thought to be linked to the level of clinical neurologic deficits. Postmortem neuropathologic examinations of HIV-positive patients have revealed the presence of virus in cortical and subcortical structures, namely the frontal lobes, the subcortical white matter and the basal ganglia.[8,9] Some authors have suggested that the caudate nucleus and the basal ganglia are the primary areas of pathogenesis.[10,11]

The underlying mechanisms leading to neurocognitive impairment are now also better understood.[6] Recent evidence supports a mechanism by which neurotoxins released by periventricular macrophages and microglia trigger cytokine and chemokine release,[12] which in turn leads to modification of synaptic architecture in the cortex.[13-15] It is thought that apoptosis, or programmed cell death, is the most common mechanism resulting in cell loss.[16,17]

People with severe neurocognitive deficits or HAD usually have higher plasma HIV viral load; however, an elevated viral load does not always lead to HAD, and HAD has been documented in the absence of elevated viral load.[7,18,19] Hence, correlates have been identified in the CSF.

Generally, HIV viral loads in the CSF are similar to those in the serum.[20] However, elevation of levels of certain substances in the CSF has been positively correlated with the presence of severe neurocognitive deficits. These substances include β2-microglobulin,[21] neopterin,[22] quinolinic acid[23] and Fas receptors and Fas ligands.[24] The latter finding is interesting since Fas is associated with the execution of apoptotic programs. Nevertheless, these findings currently have no diagnostic value.

Although HIV may remain dormant in the CNS for many years, its mere presence might lead to subtle deficits in cognitive functioning. However, these deficits are not found in all patients, which has led some authors to suggest that peripheral triggers might be involved.[25,26] Much more research is needed before it can be determined which individuals or subgroups of individuals are more vulnerable to neurologic complications.

Neurocognitive deficits are manifestations of both direct and indirect effects of HIV on the CNS.[27] While it is generally agreed that people with advanced disease present with deficits in many cognitive domains,[28-31] there is conflicting evidence regarding whether similar deficits occur in asymptomatic individuals. For example, some investigators have found neuropsychologic deficits in asymptomatic patients,[32-36] whereas others have found similar levels of neurocognitive impairment in seropositive and match-controlled seronegative individuals.[37,38] In a review of 57 studies examining neurologic functioning, the median rate of neuropsychologic impairment based on test performance was 35% for seropositive and 12% for seronegative patients.[39] However, in another review of 36 cross-sectional studies and 9 longitudinal studies, more than half of the studies showed no significant differences in the results of neuropsychologic testing between symptomatic and asymptomatic participants as well as no baseline impairment in seropositive patients.[40] Although methodologic differences might help to explain the discordant findings, research suggests that when deficits are present in asymptomatic patients, they are subtle and limited to fewer cognitive domains.[28,40] When depressive symptoms are also present, psychomotor slowing accompanies verbal memory deficits, whereas when depressive symptoms are absent, only verbal and nonverbal cognitive deficits are evident.[41]

As HIV disease progresses, additional cognitive domains often become impaired. Attention and concentration, as measured by dual task or divided attention paradigms, are decreased.[42,43] The presence of HIV in the frontosubcortical circuitry and its deleterious impact on working memory means that executive function is also affected.[44] Learning and memory, as measured by information retrieval, are also impaired.[31]

The most prominent and common neurocognitive deficit is psychomotor retardation.[7] Cognitive slowing can be seen with or without normal motor function.[29] Thus, HIV-seropositive patients should be assessed for these types of neurocognitive impairments in the presence of subjective or behavioral indications.

DIAGNOSIS AND TREATMENT OF NEUROLOGIC MANIFESTATIONS OF HIV INFECTION

The American Academy of Neurology has put forth diagnostic criteria for HIV-associated MCMD and HAD.[45] Whereas HAD is thought to represent neuronal death, MCMD is thought to be a lesser form of dementia on a continuum of cognitive deficits, representing neuronal dysfunction. The previous expression for this condition, AIDS dementia complex, has been dropped because seropositive patients not presenting with AIDS-defining criteria have presented with dementia.[46]

Both MCMD and HAD are diagnoses of exclusion, and CNS pathology must be ruled out. For example, CNS infectious pathogens or tumors as well as metabolic causes of encephalopathy must be investigated before the cognitive and motor deficits can be attributed to HIV infection. Among the more frequent CNS infections are toxoplasmosis and progressive multifocal leukoencephalopathy, which is caused by the papovavirus, whereas non-Hodgkins CNS lymphoma is the most common cancer associated with neurocognitive changes.[47]

Once opportunistic infections have been ruled out or treated if necessary, there are potentially 2 therapeutic options for neurocognitive deficits: diminish the effects of the virus on the CNS through better control of viral load or develop neuroprotective agents to shield the CNS from HIV-induced virotoxins. Unfortunately, antiretrovirals are not always successful in crossing the blood–brain barrier, but, as evidenced by the decrease in the incidence of HAD with the advent of HAART, they offer good results.[48] There are, in theory, neuroprotective agents against the virotoxins of HIV,[49,50] including pentoxyfilline,[51,52] nimodipine,[53] peptide T, memantine,[53] selegiline[54] and lexipafant.[55] However, supporting evidence is available only for selegiline as a potential therapeutic agent.

Traditional approaches to treating dementia in the course of HIV infection have also shown some success. Psychostimulants have been useful in treating both apathy and cognitive slowing in HAD.[56-58] Dopamine agonists have shown some success as well,[59] but there have been no controlled trials of cholinesterase inhibitors in treating dementia in HIV illness. Similarly, despite anecdotal evidence suggesting some success with agents such as donepezil, placebo-controlled trials have not yet been conducted.

Agitation and psychosis associated with dementia in HIV-infected patients are often treated with mood stabilizers and antipsychotics. In addition, the presence of cognitive slowing may be related to concurrent depressive symptoms. As such, an underlying depressive illness should be ruled out. These concerns are reviewed in the next section, which examines the impact of depression and other psychiatric illnesses on HIV disease and outlines the treatment of these psychiatric disorders.

PSYCHIATRIC MANIFESTATIONS OF HIV INFECTION

Recognizing the psychiatric manifestations of HIV disease can be complicated by the complex biologic, psychologic and social circumstances associated with this illness, and psychiatric symptoms often go unrecognized and untreated.[60] The significance of these findings is magnified by emerging evidence that certain symptoms, such as depression, may be associated with an increase in mortality rate among HIV-seropositive women[61] and with disease progression in HIV-seropositive men.[62] Here, we examine the main psychiatric conditions observed among HIV-seropositive patients, including mood disorders and psychosis.

Depression

Depression is one of the most common psychiatric disorders observed in people infected with HIV. Prevalence rates have shown wide variation, with estimates of between 4% and 22% for HIV-seropositive men and between 2% and 18% for HIV-seropositive women.[63-65] Earlier controlled studies found that the prevalence of major depression and other mood disorders was higher among asymptomatic HIV-seropositive men than in the general population[66,67] but was similar to that of HIV-seronegative gay men.[63,68]

Most prevalence studies have focused on HIV-seropositive men, even though it is estimated that women constitute 50% of new cases of HIV infection worldwide 1 and that women account for more than 16% of all cases of HIV infection in the United States;[69] moreover, women report higher rates of depression than men in the general population.[70] Current estimates of depression among HIV-seropositive women range from 1.9% to 35% in clinical samples[71,72] and from 30% to 60% in community samples.[61,73]

In addition, more recent studies with large sample sizes and controlled study designs have reported that HIV-positive women are at significantly greater risk for major depressive disorder than demographically matched HIV-negative women. Ickovics et al.[61] reported chronic depressive symptoms in 42% and intermittent depressive symptoms in 35% of a sample of 765 HIV-positive women. In a clinical study of 93 HIV-seropositive women and 62 HIV-seronegative women, Morrison et al.[74] found that the prevalence of major depressive disorders was significantly higher among HIV-positive women than among HIV-negative controls (19.4% v. 4.8%).

Whereas depression is increasingly recognized as a cause of increased morbidity and mortality in many chronic medical illnesses, it remains undiagnosed and untreated in the HIV-infected population.[60,75] In the context of HIV infection, the diagnosis of depressive disorders can be even more challenging because many vegetative symptoms of depression (e.g. fatigue, pain, anorexia and insomnia) are observed in many patients throughout the course of their HIV illness, even when depression is not present. However, in both the early and late phases of HIV disease, these symptoms correlate more closely with a mood disorder (when present) than with clinical correlates of infection.[76] The prominence of diminished mood in the morning coupled with anhedonia should alert clinicians to the presence of a major depressive disorder and should help distinguish it from demoralization or an adjustment disorder.[77] Clinical detection of depressive symptoms is even more important given a well-documented decrease in adherence to HAART in the context of depression.[78-80] Fortunately, recent studies have shown that the treatment of depressive symptoms in patients with HIV infection improves psychosocial functioning and quality of life.[81]

Mania

Higher rates of mania have also been noted with progression of HIV infection. In early HIV infection, 1–2% of patients experience manic episodes,[76] which is only slightly higher than the rate in the general population. However, after the onset of AIDS, 4–8% of patients appear to experience mania.[82,83] This increased frequency of mania around the time of onset of AIDS has been closely associated with cognitive changes or dementia and is thought to be a secondary manic syndrome due to HIV infection of the CNS. In a 17-month chart review, among the 8% of patients with manic episodes, counts of helper/inducer lymphocyte (CD3+/CD4+) cells were significantly higher in those with a history of mood disorder, suggesting that mania may be a direct effect of HIV on the CNS.[82] In a case-control study of 19 patients with HIV-associated mania and 57 HIV-seropositive controls, AIDS dementia was significantly more common in patients with mania, which suggests a strong association between HIV neuropathology and manic symptoms.[83] Sometimes referred to as "AIDS mania," this condition is phenomenologically different from the typical manic syndrome of bipolar disorder in both its symptom profile and severity,[76] and it is often characterized by irritability rather than euphoria.

Psychosis

Psychosis is a recognized but—relative to the mood disorders —uncommon psychiatric manifestation of AIDS.[84,85] Even less commonly, antiretroviral therapy may precipitate psychosis. For example, there have been anecdotal reports of psychosis associated with ganciclovir[86,87] and efavirenz.[88] Psychosis was found more frequently in patients with AIDS-related neurocognitive impairments.[69] Using chart reviews,

Navia and Price[89] found that 15% of 46 patients with HAD experienced psychotic symptoms. These findings were supported by data from the San Diego HIV Neurobehavioral Research Center suggesting that HIV-infected patients with psychosis exhibited greater neurocognitive impairments than HIV-positive controls without psychosis.[84]

TREATMENT OF PSYCHIATRIC MANIFESTATIONS OF HIV INFECTION

Although a growing body of evidence supports the importance of treatment of mood disorders in HIV disease, controlled studies of somatic therapies are often lacking in this population, with polypharmacy and drug–drug interactions often presenting as complicating factors.

Tricyclic Antidepressants

Numerous studies have reported the efficacy of tricyclic antidepressants (TCAs) for the treatment of HIV-seropositive patients with depressive disorders.[90,91] Rabkin et al.[92] in a double-blind, randomized, placebo-controlled trial of 97 HIV-seropositive patients, demonstrated the effectiveness of imipramine in the treatment of depression. At 6 weeks of treatment, 74% of the imipramine group and 26% of the placebo group showed improvement of depressive symptoms without changes in CD3+/CD4+ cell counts. It is important to note, however, that more than one-third of the subjects in that study discontinued treatment because of anticholinergic side effects. Elliott et al.[93] using a similar design, compared imipramine, paroxetine and placebo in 75 HIV-positive subjects. The 2 antidepressants were equally efficacious at 6, 8 and 12 weeks and were significantly more efficacious than placebo. Again, attrition due to side effects was 48% with imipramine, 20% with paroxetine and 24% with placebo.

Selective Serotonin Reuptake Inhibitors

As suggested by the Elliott et al. study described above,[93] selective serotonin reuptake inhibitors (SSRIs) are as effective as TCAs in the treatment of depression in HIV-seropositive patients, and they have a more favorable side effect profile. Rabkin et al. in an extension of their TCA study,[92] enrolled HIV-seropositive subjects with depression in whom treatment with imipramine had failed (because of lack of efficacy or intolerability of side effects) in a 12-week open-label trial of fluoxetine.[94] Although the baseline depression severity scores on the Hamilton Rating Scale for Depression (HAM-D) (mean 12.5) were lower than scores for the imipramine trial (mean 15.8), 83% of subjects treated with fluoxetine at 15–60 mg/day exhibited significant reductions in HAM-D scores. Although it did not alter CD3+/CD4+ cell counts, fluoxetine was well tolerated by subjects. In another study, Rabkin et al.[95] used a randomized, placebo-controlled design to compare the efficacy of fluoxetine and placebo for treatment of depression in HIV-seropositive patients. Seventy-four percent of the subjects responded to fluoxetine, whereas 47% responded to placebo, but an intention-to-treat analysis showed that the differences between groups were less remarkable.

Ferrando et al.[96] compared paroxetine, fluoxetine and sertraline in a 6-week open trial in 33 symptomatic HIV-seropositive subjects. Eighty-three percent of the subjects reported improvements in depression and somatic symptoms related to HIV disease. Only 73% of subjects completed the study because of complaints of agitation, anxiety and insomnia at weeks 1 and 3. Because of the limited sample size, no differences in efficacy could be ascertained. In another 6-week trial of paroxetine in 10 HIV-positive patients with major depression, significant improvements in HAM-D scores were noted between weeks 2 and 6.[97] Overall, these studies seem to show that SSRIs are effective in reducing depressive symptoms in HIV-seropositive patients and may be better tolerated than traditional TCAs.

Newer Antidepressant Agents

Recent studies suggest that several of the newer antidepressant agents may be useful for the treatment of depression in HIV-seropositive patients. In an open trial of nefazodone in 15 outpatients, the response rate was 73% and there were few adverse effects.[98] However, reports of nefazodone-induced liver toxicity[99] may be relevant, given that many patients with HIV infection also have hepatitis B and C infection. Mirtazapine has also shown some benefit for patients with HIV infection, promoting weight gain and decreasing nausea; however, its sedating side effects can be problematic. In a recent 6-week open-label, flexible-dose trial of sustained-release buproprion in 20 HIV-seropositive depressed men and women, 12 patients attained remission at a mean dose of 265 mg/day. Fourteen of the patients reported some adverse events, and 5 patients discontinued the study because of side effects (panic attacks, agitation and irritability).[100]

Reboxetine, a selective norepinephrine reuptake inhibitor that is currently marketed in Europe, was studied in an open trial of 20 HIV-seropositive men with depression.[101] At 12 weeks, the 15 patients completing the trial showed at least a 50% reduction in symptoms at a dose of 8 mg/day. The 5 patients who discontinued the study did so because of side effects of insomnia, shivering and sweating. Overall, these open trials of newer antidepressants suggest efficacy similar to that observed in the controlled trials of TCAs and SSRIs, but controlled trials of the newer agents have lacked HIV-seropositive subjects.

Psychostimulants and Novel Agents

Methylphenidate and dextroamphetamine have been used in the treatment of depression in chronic medical illness, and both have been studied in placebo-controlled trials in patients infected with HIV. Fernandez et al.[58] compared treatment response of desipramine and methylphenidate in 15 subjects, with both drugs leading to improvements of 50%. However, the desipramine-treated patients exhibited more side effects including dry mouth, anxiety and insomnia, consistent with previous studies of imipramine.[92,93]

Wagner et al.[102] in an open trial of dextroamphetamine treatment of 24 patients with AIDS and depression who exhibited debilitatingly low energy levels, found a response rate of 75%. Improvements in mood and energy coincided with significant reductions in HAM-D scores, which were noted as early as week 2. Although systematic follow-up evaluations were not available, the treatment effects were maintained over 2 years. A placebo-controlled trial of dextroamphetamine showed a significant improvement in initiative and mood in 73% of depressed patients assigned to the drug and 25% of those receiving placebo.[103] These observations warrant further study.

HIV-associated reductions in testosterone levels have been correlated with changes in mood, appetite and sexual function.[104] Studies examining the effects of testosterone supplementation on depression[104,105] and the adrenal steroid dehydroepiandrosterone[106] have shown promise for improving mood as well as anabolic and androgenic parameters. Exercise may also augment improvement in psychologic and nutritional status in HIV-seropositive patients receiving testosterone therapy.[107]

Mood Stabilizers

Recent studies examining the efficacy of mood stabilizers for the treatment of manic symptoms in HIV-infected patients indicate that AIDS-associated manic states are responsive to available antimanic agents, but patients are more prone to neurocognitive side effects.[108,109] The results of these mainly open trials should be interpreted with caution as they are limited by small sample sizes and other methodologic difficulties.

When mood stabilizers are used to treat HIV-infected patients, knowledge of the metabolic pathways of psychotropic agents and the influence of particular agents on overall drug metabolism is important. For example, carbamazepine may interact with antiretrovirals. As a potent inducer of CYP3A enzymes, carbamazepine may increase the metabolism of protease inhibitors such as indinavir[110] and non-nucleoside reverse transcriptase inhibitors such as delavirdine.[111] Conversely, because ritonavir is a potent enzymatic inhibitor of the CYP3A system that may raise serum levels of carbamazepine, carbamazepine toxicity is possible when these 2 drugs are used together.[112] In addition, medical conditions or treatments occurring during the course of HIV illness, such as hypoalbuminemia or administration of antibiotics, could elevate the free drug concentration of valproic acid.

In a case series of HIV-seropositive gay men, lithium was not well tolerated, and signs and symptoms of toxicity developed in 8 out of 10 patients, 7 of whom needed to stop treatment.[108] Dehydration and fluid shifts associated with diarrhea have also been reported.[90]

Antipsychotic Agents

The use of antipsychotic agents in the treatment of mood disorders and psychotic disorders in HIV-infected patients is less well studied. Reports indicate that HIV-seropositive patients may be more sensitive to the extrapyramidal side effects associated with dopamine receptor antagonists. This may be related to the psychomotor slowing associated with HIV infection.[84] In a case series of 21 patients with psychotic symptoms (12 of whom had mania with psychotic features), risperidone was efficacious and produced fewer side effects than conventional neuroleptics, although some studies have reported increased sensitivity to both older and newer antipsychotic agents.[113] An open-label study using clozapine reported improvements in psychotic symptoms in HIV-infected patients without extrapyramidal symptoms.[114] Clearly, controlled trials are needed in this area.

Psychopharmacology Summary

The studies reviewed above point to the need for more controlled trials of psychopharmacologic agents for psychiatric disorders in people living with HIV, but they also provide support for the efficacy of these agents in the treatment of mood disorders. A recent study by Vitiello et al.[115] however, points out that even when psychiatric disorders are recognized, they may remain untreated. In a study of the prevalence and patterns of use of psychotropic medications, for which these authors used a probability sample of 1561 HIV-seropositive patients with a diagnosis of major depression or dysthymia, only 43% of subjects reported ever receiving antidepressant medication. They also noted that African-American HIV-seropositive patients with depression were less likely to receive antidepressant medications than any other ethnic group. This is especially concerning given that this group is over represented in the HIV-infected population.

In the treatment of HIV-infected patients, strategies similar to those that apply for treatment of psychiatric disorders in the general population should be followed. Knowledge of the metabolic pathways of psychotropic agents as well as the major antiretrovirals are useful because of potential adverse drug–drug interactions. Reassuringly, there are no absolute contraindications specific to this patient population other than an increased sensitivity to side effects, which has been widely reported.[90,116]

The use of nontraditional agents (such as herbal agents) to treat psychiatric symptoms must also be monitored in HIV-seropositive patients. An open-label study revealed that the serum concentration of the protease inhibitor indinavir, metabolized by the 3A4 isoenzyme system, was markedly reduced by the administration of St. John's wort, a 3A4 inducer.[117] This reduction in indinavir levels was significant enough to potentially cause drug resistance and treatment failure. Similar caution should be exercised with concomitant use of alcohol or recreational drugs such as Ecstasy: alcohol can increase the risk for pancreatitis,[118] and Ecstasy has proven nearly fatal in combination with ritonavir.[119]

PSYCHONEUROIMMUNOLOGY OF HIV INFECTION

Despite the development of effective combination antiretroviral therapies for HIV that have lengthened the life expectancy of HIV-infected patients, there continues to be wide variability in the course of HIV disease, specifically in the length of time before diagnosis of AIDS or death. These findings have prompted investigators to look at other factors that might influence the disease, such as stress, depression and other psychosocial factors.

Evidence has been mounting that chronic stress and dysfunctional coping may affect the immune system, exerting potentially harmful effects on cellular immunity,[120-123] but studies assessing the effects of depression on immunity in HIV-positive patients have yielded conflicting results.[124-126] One research group has shown significant effects of stress on cellular immune parameters,[127] and depressive symptoms (especially in the presence of severe stress) were related to declines in several lymphocyte subsets (NK cells and CD16, CD56 and CD8 cytotoxic suppressor cells) over a 2-year period in HIV-seropositive men.[128]

Additional evidence is emerging from longitudinal studies to suggest that depression is associated with disease progression or death in HIV-infected subjects. Among 7 prospective studies with long-term follow-up, 6 studies found that depression was associated with HIV disease progression[62,129,130] and death.[61,131,132] However, no relation was found between baseline depression and progression to AIDS or decline in CD4 lymphocytes in the Multicenter AIDS Cohort Study.[133] Other major longitudinal studies with shorter follow-up periods have shown no relation of stress and depression to changes in CD4 cell counts.[124,125]

While most studies have focused on men, recent data support the negative impact of depressive symptoms on immunity in women. Ickovics et al.[61] have shown that depression among women infected with HIV is associated with HIV disease progression and mortality. Furthermore, depressive symptoms have been shown by another group to be significantly associated with higher counts of activated T cells (CD8+, CD38+, DR+) and higher viral loads, all of which are associated with advancing HIV disease.[134] Major depression was also associated with reductions in NK cell activity.

CONCLUSION

People infected with HIV have a better life expectancy today than in the early days of the epidemic, mostly because of recent advances in antiretroviral therapy. Although the relations among neuropsychiatric symptoms, neuroendocrine peptides and the immune system remain unclear, the emergence of neuropsychiatric complications during HIV infection or AIDS can have serious effects if they are not identified promptly. Whether these complications are due to the direct or indirect effects of HIV on the brain or to the effects of stress and depression, careful diagnosis and treatment are necessary. Continued investigation to elucidate potential causal mechanisms holds the promise of refinement of existing therapies and development of new treatment options.

REFERENCES

1. AIDS epidemic update: December 2004. Geneva: Joint United Nations Programme on HIV/AIDS; World Health Organization; 2004.p.1.
2. Sepkowitz KA. AIDS—the first 20 years. N Engl J Med. 2001;344:1764-72. [Pub Med]
3. Snider WD, Simpson DM, Nielsen S, Gold JW, Metroka CE, Posner JB. Neurological complications of acquired immune deficiency syndrome: analysis of 50 patients. Ann Neurol. 1983;14:403-18. [Pub Med]
4. Sacktor N, Lyles RH, Skolasky R, Kleeberger C, Selnes OA, Miller EN, et al. HIV-associated neurologic disease incidence changes: Multicenter AIDS Cohort Study 1990-1998. Neurology. 2001;56: 257-60. [Pub Med]
5. Neuenburg JK, Brodt HR, Herndier BG, Bickel M, Baccheti P, Price RW, et al. HIV-related neuropathology, 1985 to 1999: rising prevalence of HIV encephalopathy in the era of highly active antiretroviral therapy. J Acquir Immune Defic Syndr. 2002;31:171-7. [Pub Med]
6. Lawrence DM, Major EO. HIV-1 and the brain: connections between HIV-1-associated dementia, neuropathology and neuroimunology. Microbes Infect. 2002;4:301-8. [Pub Med]
7. Clifford DB. AIDS dementia. Med Clin North Am. 2002;86:537-50. [Pub Med]
8. Aylward EH, Henderer JD, McArthur JC, Brettschneider PD, Harris GJ, Barta PE, et al. Reduced basal ganglia volume in HIV-1-associated dementia: results from quantitative neuroimaging. Neurology. 1993;43:2099-104. [Pub Med]
9. Navia BA, Cho ES, Petito CK, Price RW. The AIDS dementia complex: II. Neuropathology. Ann Neurol. 1986;19:525-35. [Pub Med]
10. Aylward EH, Brettschneider PD, McArthur JC, Harris GJ, Schlaepfer TE, Henderer JD, et al. Magnetic resonance imaging measurement of gray matter volume reductions in HIV dementia. Am J Psychiatry. 1995;152:987-94. [Pub Med]
11. van Gorp WG, Mandelkern M, Gee M, Hinkin CH, Stern CE, Paz DK, et al. Cerebral metabolic dysfunction in AIDS: findings in

a sample with and without dementia. J Neuropsychiatry Clin Neurosci. 1992;4:280-7. [Pub Med]

12. Nath A. Human immunodeficiency virus (HIV) proteins in neuropathogenesis of HIV dementia. J Infect Dis. 2002;186(Suppl 2): S193-8. [Pub Med]
13. Sa MJ, Madeira MD, Ruela C, Volk B, Mota-Miranda A, Lecour H, et al. AIDS does not alter the total number of neurons in the hippocampal formation but induces cell atrophy: a stereological study. Acta Neuropathol (Berl). 2000;99:643-53. [Pub Med]
14. Everall IP, Heaton RK, Marcotte TD, Ellis RJ, McCutchan JA, Atkinson JH, et al. Cortical synaptic density is reduced in mild to moderate human immunodeficiency virus neurocognitive disorder. Brain Pathol. 1999;9:209-17. [Pub Med]
15. Masliah E, Heaton RK, Marcotte TD, Ellis RJ, Wiley CA, Mallory M, et al. Dendritic injury is a pathological substrate for human immunodeficiency virus-related cognitive disorders. Ann Neurol. 1997;42:963-72. [Pub Med]
16. Kaul M, Garden GA, Lipton SA. Pathways to neuronal injury and apoptosis in HIV-associated dementia. Nature. 2001;410:988-94. [Pub Med]
17. Thompson KA, McArthur JC, Wesselingh SL. Correlation between neurological progression and astrocyte apoptosis in HIV-associated dementia. Ann Neurol. 2001;49:745-52. [Pub Med]
18. McArthur JC, McClernon DR, Cronin MF, Nance-Sproson TE, Saah AJ, St Clair M, et al. Relationship between human immunodeficiency virus-associated dementia and viral load in cerebrospinal fluid and brain. Ann Neurol. 1997;42:689-98. [Pub Med]
19. Ellis RJ, Hsia K, Spector SA, Nelson JA, Heaton RK, Wallace MR, et al. Cerebrospinal fluid human immunodeficiency virus type 1 RNA levels are elevated in neurocognitively impaired individuals with acquired immunodeficiency syndrome. Ann Neurol. 1997;42:679-88. [Pub Med]
20. Foudraine NA, Hoetelmans RM, Lange JM, de Wolf F, van Benthem BH, Maas JJ, et al. Cerebrospinal-fluid HIV-1 RNA and drug concentrations after treatment with lamivudine plus zidovudine or stavudine. Lancet. 1998;351:1547-51. [Pub Med]
21. Brew BJ, Bhalla RB, Paul M, Sidtis JJ, Keilp JJ, Sadler AE, et al. Cerebrospinal fluid β2-microglobulin in patients with AIDS dementia complex: an expanded series including response to zidovudine treatment. AIDS. 1992;6:461-5. [Pub Med]
22. Brew BJ, Bhalla RB, Paul M, Gallardo H, McArthur JC, Schwartz MK, et al. Cerebrospinal fluid neopterin in human immunodeficiency virus type-1 infection. Ann Neurol. 1990;28:556-60. [Pub Med]
23. Heyes MP, Brew BJ, Martin A, Price RW, Salazar AM, Sidtis JJ, et al. Quinolinic acid in cerebrospinal fluid and serum in HIV-1 infection: relationship to clinical and neurological status. Ann Neurol. 1991;29:202-9. [Pub Med]
24. Sabri F, De Milito A, Pirskanen R, Elovaara I, Hagberg L, Cinque P, et al. Elevated levels of soluble Fas and Fas ligand in cerebrospinal fluid of patients with AIDS dementia complex. J Neuroimmunol. 2001;114:197-206. [Pub Med]
25. Gartner S. AIDS: HIV infection and dementia. Science. 2000;287:602-4. [Pub Med]
26. Pulliam L, Gascon R, Stubblebine M, McGuire D, McGrath MS. Unique monocyte subset in patients with AIDS dementia. Lancet. 1997;349:692-5. [Pub Med]
27. Atkinson JH, Grant I. Natural history of neuropsychiatric manifestations of HIV disease. Psychiatr Clin North Am. 1994;17:17-33. [Pub Med]
28. Heaton RK, Grant I, Butters N, White DA, Kirson D, Atkinson JH, et al. The HNRC 500—neuropsychology of HIV infection at different disease stages. J Int Neuropsychol Soc. 1995;1:231-51. [Pub Med]
29. Llorente AM, Miller EN, D'Elia LF, Selnes OA, Wesch J, Becker JT, et al. Slowed information processing in HIV-1 disease. J Clin Exp Neuropsychol. 1998;20:60-72. [Pub Med]
30. Maj M, Satz P, Janssen R, Zaudig M, Starace F, D'Elia L, et al. WHO Neuropsychiatric AIDS study, cross-sectional phase II. Neuropsychological and neurological findings. Arch Gen Psychiatry. 1994;51:51-61. [Pub Med]
31. Peavy G, Jacobs D, Salmon DP, Butters N, Delis DC, Taylor M, et al. Verbal memory performance of patients with human immunodeficiency virus infection: evidence of subcortical dysfunction. The HNRC Group. J Clin Exp Neuropsychol. 1994;16:508-23. [Pub Med]
32. Bornstein RA, Nasrallah HA, Para MF, Whitacre CC, Fass RJ. Duration of illness and neuropsychological performance in asymptomatic HIV infection. J Neuropsychiatry Clin Neurosci. 1994;6:160-4. [Pub Med]
33. Bornstein RA, Nasrallah HA, Para MF, Whitacre CC, Rosenberg P, Fass RJ, et al. Neuropsychological performance in asymptomatic HIV infection. J Neuropsychiatry Clin Neurosci. 1992;4:386-94. [Pub Med]
34. Marder K, Stern Y, Malouf R, Tang MX, Bell K, Dooneief G, et al. Neurologic and neuropsychological manifestations of human immunodeficiency virus infection in intravenous drug users without acquired immunodeficiency syndrome. Relationship to head injury. Arch Neurol. 1992;49:1169-75. [Pub Med]
35. Marsh NV, McCall DW. Early neuropsychological change in HIV infection. Neuropsychology. 1994;8:44-8. [Pub Med]
36. Wilkie FL, Eisdorfer C, Morgan R, Loewenstein DA, Szapocznick J. Cognition in early human immunodeficiency infection. Arch Neurol. 1990;47:433-40. [Pub Med]
37. Miller EN, Selnes OA, McArthur JC, Satz P, Becker JT, Cohen BA, et al. Neuropsychological performance in HIV-1-infected homosexual men: the Multicenter AIDS Cohort Study (MACS). Neurology. 1990;40:197-203. [Pub Med]
38. McArthur JC, Cohen BA, Selnes OA, Kumar AJ, Cooper K, McArthur JH, et al. Low prevalence of neurological and neuropsychological abnormalities in otherwise healthy HIV-1-infected individuals: results from the Multicenter AIDS Cohort Study. Ann Neurol. 1989;26:601-11. [Pub Med]

39. White DA, Heaton RK, Monsch AU. Neuropsychological studies of asymptomatic human immunodeficiency virus-type-1 infected individuals. The HNRC Group. HIV Neurobehavioral Research Center. J Int Neuropsychol Soc. 1995;1:304-15. [Pub Med]
40. Newman SP, Lunn S, Harrison MJ. Do asymptomatic HIV-seropositive individuals show cognitive deficit? AIDS. 1995;9:1211-20. [Pub Med]
41. van Gorp WG, Hinkin C, Satz P, Miller EN, Weisman J, Holston S, et al. Subtypes of HIV-related neuropsychological functioning: a cluster analysis approach. Neuropsychology. 1993;7:62-72. [Pub Med]
42. Sorenson DJ, Martin EM, Robertson LC. Visual attention in HIV-1 infection. Neuropsychology. 1994;8:424-32. [Pub Med]
43. Hinkin CH, Castellon SA, Hardy D. Dual task performance in HIV-1 infection. J Clin Exp Neuropsychol. 2000;22:16-24. [Pub Med]
44. Castellon SA, Hinkin CH, Wood S, Yarema KT. Apathy, depression, and cognitive performance in HIV-1 infection. J Neuropsychiatry Clin Neurosci. 1998;10:320-9. [Pub Med]
45. Nomenclature and research case definitions for neurologic manifestations of human immunodeficiency virus type-1 (HIV-1) infection. Report of a Working Group of the American Academy of Neurology AIDS Task Force. Neurology. 1991;41:778-85. [Pub Med]
46. Navia BA, Jordan BD, Price RW. The AIDS dementia complex: I. Clinical features. Ann Neurol. 1986;19:517-24. [Pub Med]
47. Bredesen DE, Levy RM, Rosenblum ML. The neurology of human immunodeficiency virus infection. Q J Med. 1988;68:665-77. [Pub Med]
48. Sacktor NC, Lyles RH, Skolasky RL, Anderson DE, McArthur JC, McFarlane G, et al. Combination antiretroviral therapy improves psychomotor speed performance in HIV-seropositive homosexual men. Neurology. 1999;52:1640-6. [Pub Med]
49. Gelbard HA. Neuroprotective strategies for HIV-1-associated neurological disease. Ann N Y Acad Sci. 1999;890:312-3. [Pub Med]
50. Ying Wang J, Peruzzi F, Lassak A, Del Valle L, Radhakrishnan S, Rappaport J, et al. Neuroprotective effects of IGF-I against TNFα-induced neuronal damage in HIV-associated dementia. Virology. 2003;305:66-76. [Pub Med]
51. Peterson PK, Gekker G, Hu S, Schoolov Y, Balfour HH Jr, Chao CC. Microglial cell upregulation of HIV-1 expression in the chronologically infected promonocytic cell line U1: the role of tumor necrosis factor alpha. J Neuroimmunol. 1992;41:81-7. [Pub Med]
52. Wilt SG, Milward E, Zhou JM, Nagasato K, Patton H, Rusten R, et al. *In vitro* evidence for a dual role of tumor necrosis factor-alpha in human immunodeficiency virus type 1 encephalopathy. Ann Neurol. 1995;37:381-94. [Pub Med]
53. Lipton SA. HIV-related neuronal injury: potential therapeutic intervention with calcium channel antagonists and NMDA antagonists. Mol Neurobiol. 1994;8:181-96. [Pub Med]
54. Koutsilieri E, Gotz ME, Sopper S, Sauer U, Demuth M, ter Meulen V, et al. Regulation of glutathione and cell toxicity following exposure to neurotropic substances and human immunodeficiency virus-1 *in vitro*. J Neurovirol. 1997;3:342-9. [Pub Med]
55. Persidsky Y, Limoges J, Rasmussen J, Zheng J, Gearing A, Gendelman HE. Reduction in glial immunity and neuropathology by a PAF antagonist and an MMP and TNFalpha inhibitor in SCID mice with HIV-1 encephalitis. J Neuroimmunol. 2001;114:57-68. [Pub Med]
56. Hinkin CH, Castellon SA, Hardy DJ, Farinpour R, Newton T, Singer E. Methylphenidate improves HIV-1-associated cognitive slowing. J Neuropsychiatry Clin Neurosci. 2001;13:248-54. [Pub Med]
57. Holmes VF, Fernandez F, Levy JK. Psychostimulant response in AIDS-related complex patients. J Clin Psychiatry. 1989;50:5-8. [Pub Med]
58. Fernandez F, Levy JK, Samley HR, Pirozzolo FJ, Lachar D, Crowley J, et al. Effects of methylphenidate in HIV-related depression: a comparative trial with desipramine. Int J Psychiatry Med. 1995;25: 53-67. [Pub Med]
59. Kieburtz KD, Epstein LG, Gelbard HA, Greenamyre JT. Excitotoxicity and dopaminergic dysfunction in the acquired immunodeficiency syndrome dementia complex. Therapeutic implications. Arch Neurol. 1991;48:1281-4. [Pub Med]
60. Evans DL, Staab JP, Petitto JM, Morrison MF, Szuba MP, Ward HE, et al. Depression in the medical setting: biopsychological interactions and treatment considerations. J Clin Psychiatry. 1999;60(Suppl 4):40-55. [Pub Med]
61. Ickovics JR, Hamburger ME, Vlahov D, Schoenbaum EE, Schuman P, Boland RJ, et al. Mortality, CD4 cell count decline, and depressive symptoms among HIV-seropositive women: longitudinal analysis from the HIV Epidemiology Research Study. JAMA. 2001;285:1466-74. [Pub Med]
62. Leserman J, Petitto JM, Gu H, Gaynes BN, Barroso J, Golden RN, et al. Progression to AIDS, a clinical AIDS condition and mortality; psychosocial and physiological predictors. Psychol Med. 2002;32:1059-73. [Pub Med]
63. Atkinson JH, Grant I, Kennedy CJ, Richman DD, Spector SA, McCutchan JA. Prevalence of psychiatric disorders among men infected with human immunodeficiency virus: a controlled study. Arch Gen Psychiatry. 1988;45:859-64. [Pub Med]
64. Perkins DO, Stern RA, Golden RN, Murphy C, Naftolowitz D, Evans DL. Mood disorders in HIV infection: prevalence and risk factors in a non-epicenter of the AIDS epidemic. Am J Psychiatry. 1994;151:233-6. [Pub Med]
65. Stern RA, Singer NG, Silva SG, Rogers HJ, Perkins DO, Hall CD, et al. Neurobehavioral functioning in a nonconfounded group of asymptomatic HIV-seropositive homosexual men. Am J Psychiatry. 1992;149:1099-102. [Pub Med]
66. Smith DK, Moore JS, Warren D, Solomon L, Schuman P, Stein M, et al. The design, participants, and selected early findings of the HIV Epidemiology Research Study. In: O'Leary A, Jemott

LS, (Eds). Women and AIDS: coping and care. New York: Plenum Press; 1996.p.185-206. [Pub Med]

67. Robins LN, Helzer JE, Weissman MM, Orvaschel H, Gruenberg E, Burke JD Jr, et al. Lifetime prevalence of specific psychiatric disorders in three sites. Arch Gen Psychiatry. 1984;41:949-58. [Pub Med]
68. Williams JB, Rabkin JG, Remien RH, Gorman JM, Ehrhardt AA. Multidisciplinary baseline assessment of homosexual men with and without human immunodeficiency virus infection. II: Standardized clinical assessment of current and lifetime psychopathology. Arch Gen Psychiatry. 1991;48:124-30. [Pub Med]
69. Evans DL, Mason KI, Bauer R, Leserman J, Petitto J. Neuropsychiatric manifestations of HIV-1 infection and AIDS. In: Charney D, Coyle J, Davis K, Nemeroff C, (Eds). Psychopharmacology: the fifth generation of progress. New York: Raven Press; 2002.pp.1281-99. [Pub Med]
70. Blazer DG, Kessler RC, McGonagle KA, Swartz MS. The prevalence and distribution of major depression in a national community sample: the National Comorbidity Survey. Am J Psychiatry. 1994;151:979-86. [Pub Med]
71. Boland RJ, Moore J, Schuman P. The longitudinal course of depression in HIV-infected women [abstract]. Psychosomatics. 1999;40:160. [Pub Med]
72. Goggin K, Engelson ES, Rabkin JG, Kotler DP. The relationship of mood, endocrine, and sexual disorders in human immunodeficiency virus positive (HIV+) women: an exploratory study. Psychosom Med. 1998;60:11-6. [Pub Med]
73. Moore J, Schuman P, Schoenbaum E, Boland B, Solomon L, Smith D. Severe adverse life events and depressive symptoms among women with, or at risk for, HIV infection in four cities in the United States of America. AIDS. 1999;13:2459-68. [Pub Med]
74. Morrison MF, Petitto JM, Ten Have T, Gettes DR, Chiappini MS, Weber AL, et al. Depressive and anxiety disorders in women with HIV infection. Am J Psychiatry. 2002;159:789-96. [Pub Med]
75. Evans DL, Charney DS. Mood disorders and medical illness: a major public health problem. Biol Psychiatry. 2003;54:177-80. [Pub Med]
76. Lyketsos CG, Treisman GJ. Mood disorders in HIV infection. Psychiatr Ann. 2001;31:45-50. [Pub Med]
77. Treisman GJ, Angelino AF, Hutton HE. Psychiatric issues in the management of patients with HIV infection. JAMA. 2001;286:2857-64. [Pub Med]
78. Ammassari A, Antinori A, Aloisi MS, Trotta MP, Murri R, Bartoli L, et al. Depressive symptoms, neurocognitive impairment, and adherence to highly active antiretroviral therapy among HIV-infected persons. Psychosomatics. 2004;45:394-402. [Pub Med]
79. Kleeberger CA, Buechner J, Palella F, Detels R, Riddler S, Godfrey R, et al. Changes in adherence to highly active antiretroviral therapy medications in the Multicenter AIDS Cohort Study. AIDS. 2004;18:683-8. [Pub Med]
80. Starace F, Ammassari A, Trotta MP, Murri R, De Longis P, Izzo C, et al. AdICoNA Study Group; NeuroICoNA Study Group. Depression is a risk factor for suboptimal adherence to highly active antiretroviral therapy. J Acquir Immune Defic Syndr. 2002;31(Suppl 3):S136-9. [Pub Med]
81. Elliott AJ, Russo J, Roy-Burne PP. The effect of changes in depression on health related quality of life (HRQoL) in HIV infection. Gen Hosp Psychiatry. 2002;24:43-7. [Pub Med]
82. Lyketsos CG, Hanson AL, Fishman M, Rosenblatt A, McHugh PR, Treisman GJ. Manic syndrome early and late in the course of HIV. Am J Psychiatry. 1993;150:326-7. [Pub Med]
83. Mijch AM, Judd FK, Lyketsos CG, Ellen S, Cockram A. Secondary mania in patients with HIV infection: Are antiretrovirals protective? J Neuropsychiatry Clin Neurosci. 1999;11:475-80. [Pub Med]
84. Sewell DD, Jeste DV, Atkinson JH, Heaton RK, Hesselink JR, Wiley C, et al. HIV-associated psychosis: a study of 20 cases. San Diego HIV Neurobehavioral Research Center Group. Am J Psychiatry. 1994;151:237-42. [Pub Med]
85. de Ronchi D, Faranca I, Forti P, Ravaglia G, Borderi M, Manfredi R, et al. Development of acute psychotic disorders and HIV-1 infection. Int J Psychiatry Med. 2000;30:173-83. [Pub Med]
86. Chen JL, Brocavich JM, Lin AY. Psychiatric disturbances associated with ganciclovir therapy. Ann Pharmacother. 1992;26:193-5. [Pub Med]
87. Hansen BA, Greenberg KS, Richter JA. Ganciclovir-induced psychosis [letter]. N Engl J Med. 1996;335:1397. [Pub Med]
88. De La Garza CL, Paoletti-Duarte S, Garcia-Martin C, Gutierrez-Casares JR. Efavirenz-induced psychosis. AIDS. 2001;15: 1911-2. [Pub Med]
89. Navia BA, Price RW. The acquired immunodeficiency syndrome dementia complex as the presenting or sole manifestation of human immunodeficiency virus infection. Arch Neurol. 1987;44:65-9. [Pub Med]
90. Robinson MJ, Qaqish RB. Practical psychopharmacology in HIV-1 and acquired immunodeficiency syndrome. Psychiatr Clin North Am. 2002;25:149-75. [Pub Med]
91. Wagner GJ, Rabkin JG, Rabkin R. A comparative analysis of standard and alternative antidepressants in the treatment of human immunodeficiency virus patients. Compr Psychiatry. 1996;37:402-8. [Pub Med]
92. Rabkin JG, Rabkin R, Harrison W, Wagner G. Effect of imipramine on mood and enumerative measures of immune status in depressed patients with HIV illness. Am J Psychiatry. 1994;151:516-23. [Pub Med]
93. Elliott AJ, Uldall KK, Bergam K, Russo J, Claypoole K, Roy-Byrne PP. Randomized, placebo-controlled trial of paroxetine versus imipramine in depressed HIV-positive outpatients. Am J Psychiatry. 1998;155:367-72. [Pub Med]
94. Rabkin JG, Rabkin R, Wagner G. Effects of fluoxetine on mood and immune status in depressed patients with HIV illness. J Clin Psychiatry. 1994;55:92-7. [Pub Med]
95. Rabkin JG, Wagner GJ, Rabkin R. Fluoxetine treatment for depression in patients with HIV and AIDS: a randomized,

placebo-controlled trial. Am J Psychiatry. 1999;156:101-7. [Pub Med]

96. Ferrando SJ, Goldman JD, Charness WE. Selective serotonin reuptake inhibitor treatment of depression in symptomatic HIV infection and AIDS: improvements in affective and somatic symptoms. Gen Hosp Psychiatry. 1997;19:89-97. [Pub Med]
97. Grassi B, Gambini O, Garghentini, Lazzarin A, Scarone S. Efficacy of paroxetine for the treatment of depression in the context of HIV infection. Pharmacopsychiatry. 1997;30:70-1. [Pub Med]
98. Elliott AJ, Russo J, Bergam K, Claypoole K, Uldall KK, Roy-Byrne PP. Antidepressant efficacy in HIV-seropositive outpatients with major depressive disorder: an open trial of nefazodone. J Clin Psychiatry. 1999;60:226-31. [Pub Med]
99. Tzimas GN, Dion B, Deschenes M. Early onset, nefazodone-induced fulminant hepatic failure. Am J Gastroenterol. 2003;98:1663-4. [Pub Med]
100. Currier MB, Molina G, Kato M. A prospective trial of sustained-release buproprion for depression in HIV-seropositive and AIDS patients. Psychosomatics. 2003;44:120-5. [Pub Med]
101. Carvalhal AS, de Abreu PB, Spode A, Correa J, Kapczinski F. An open trial of reboxetine in HIV-seropositive outpatients with major depressive disorder. J Clin Psychiatry. 2003;64:421-4. [Pub Med]
102. Wagner GJ, Rabkin JG, Rabkin R. Dextroamphetamine as a treatment for depression and low energy in AIDS patients: a pilot study. J Psychosom Res. 1997;42:407-11. [Pub Med]
103. Wagner GJ, Rabkin R. Effects of dextroamphetamine on depression and fatigue in men with HIV: a double-blind, placebo-controlled trial. J Clin Psychiatry. 2000;61:436-40. [Pub Med]
104. Rabkin JG, Wagner GJ, Rabkin R. A double-blind, placebo-controlled trial of testosterone for HIV-positive men with hypogonadal symptoms. Arch Gen Psychiatry. 2000;57:141-7. [Pub Med]
105. Rabkin JG, Wagner GJ, Rabkin R. Testosterone therapy for human immunodeficiency virus-positive men with and without hypogonadism. J Clin Psychopharmacol. 1999;19:19-27. [Pub Med]
106. Rabkin JG, Ferrando SJ, Wagner GJ, Rabkin R. DHEA treatment for HIV+ patients: effects on mood, androgenic and anabolic parameters. Psychoneuroendocrinology. 2000;25:53-68. [Pub Med]
107. Wagner G, Rabkin J, Rabkin R. Exercise as a mediator of psychological and nutritional effects of testosterone therapy in HIV+ men. Med Sci Sports Exerc. 1998;30:811-7. [Pub Med]
108. Parenti DM, Simon GL, Scheib RG, Meyer WA III, Sztein MB, Paxton H, et al. Effect of lithium carbonate in HIV-infected patients with immune dysfunction. J Acquir Immune Defic Syndr. 1988;1:119-24. [Pub Med]
109. Halman MH, Worth JL, Sanders KM, Renshaw PF, Murray GB. Anticonvulsant use in the treatment of manic syndromes in patients with HIV-1 infection. J Neuropsychiatry Clin Neurosci. 1993;5:430-4. [Pub Med]
110. Hugen PW, Burger DM, Brinkman K, ter Hofstede HJ, Schuurman R, Koopmans PP, et al. Carbamezapine–indinavir interaction causes antiretroviral therapy failure. Ann Pharmacother. 2000;34:465-70. [Pub Med]
111. Tran JQ, Gerber JG, Kerr BM. Delavirdine: clinical pharmacokinetics and drug interactions. Clin Pharmacokinet. 2001;40: 207-26. [Pub Med]
112. Berbel Garcia A, Latorre Ibarra A, Porta Etessam J, Martinez Salio A, Perez Martinez D, Siaz Diaz R, et al. Protease inhibitor-induced carbamezapine toxicity. Clin Neuropharmacol. 2000;23:216-8. [Pub Med]
113. Meyer JM, Marsh J, Simpson G. Differential sensitivities to risperidone and olanzapine in a human immunodeficiency virus patient. Biol Psychiatry. 1998;44:791-4. [Pub Med]
114. Lera G, Zirulnik J. Pilot study with clozapine in patients with HIV-associated psychosis and drug-induced parkinsonism. Mov Disord. 1999;14:128-31. [Pub Med]
115. Vitiello B, Burnam MA, Bing EG, Beckman R, Shapiro MF. Use of psychotropic medications among HIV-infected patients in the United States. Am J Psychiatry. 2003;160:547-54. [Pub Med]
116. Gillenwater DR, McDaniel JS. Rational psychopharmacology for patients with HIV infection and AIDS. Psychiatr Ann. 2001;31:28-36. [Pub Med]
117. Piscitelli SC, Burstein AH, Chaitt D, Alfaro RM, Falloon J. Indinavir concentrations and St. John's wort. Lancet. 2000;355:547-8. [Pub Med]
118. Whitfield RM, Bechtel LM, Starich GH. The impact of ethanol and Marinol/marijuana usage in HIV+/AIDS patients undergoing azidothymidine, azidothymidine/dideoxycytidine or dideoxyinosine therapy. Alcohol Clin Exp Res. 1997;21: 122-7. [Pub Med]
119. Harrington RD, Woodward JA, Hooton TM, Horn JR. Life-threatening interaction between HIV-1 and protease inhibitors and the illicit drugs MDMA and gamma-hydroxybutyrate. Arch Intern Med. 1999;159:2221-4. [Pub Med]
120. Evans DL, Folds JD, Petitto JM, Golden RN, Pedersen CA, Corrigan M, et al. Circulating natural killer cell phenotypes in men and women with major depression: relation to cytotoxic activity and severity of depression. Arch Gen Psychiatry. 1992;49:388-95. [Pub Med]
121. Stein M, Miller AH, Trestman RL. Depression, the immune system and health and illness. Findings in search of meaning. Arch Gen Psychiatry. 1991;48:171-7. [Pub Med]
122. Herbert TB, Cohen S. Stress and immunity in humans: a meta-analytic review. Psychosom Med. 1993;55:364-79. [Pub Med]
123. Herbert TB, Cohen S. Depression and immunity: a meta-analytic review. Psychol Bull. 1993;113:472-86. [Pub Med]
124. Rabkin JG, Williams JB, Remien RH, Goetz R, Kertzner R, Gorman JM. Depression, distress, lymphocyte subsets, and human immnodeficiency virus symptoms on two occasions in HIV positive homosexual men. Arch Gen Psychiatry. 1991;48: 111-9. [Pub Med]
125. Perry S, Fishman B, Jacobsberg L, Frances A. Relationships over 1 year between lymphocyte subsets and psychosocial variables

among adults with infection by human immunodeficiency virus. Arch Gen Psychiatry. 1992;49:396-401. [Pub Med]
126. Zorrilla EP, McKay JR, Luborsky L, Schmidt K. Relation of stressors and depressive symptoms to clinical progression of viral illness. Am J Psychiatry. 1996;153:626-35. [Pub Med]
127. Evans DL, Leserman J, Perkins DO, Stern RA, Murphy C, Tamul K, et al. Stress-associated reductions of cytotoxic T lymphocytes and natural killer cells in asymptomatic HIV infection. Am J Psychiatry. 1995;152:543-50. [Pub Med]
128. Leserman J, Petitto JM, Perkins DO, Folds JD, Golden RN, Evans DL. Severe stress, depressive symptoms, and changes in lymphocyte subsets in human immunodeficiency virus-infected men. A 2-year follow-up study. Arch Gen Psychiatry. 1997;54:279-85. [Pub Med]
129. Page-Shafer K, Delorenze GN, Satariano WA, Winkelstein W Jr. Comorbidity and survival in HIV-infected men in the San Francisco Men's Health Survey. Ann Epidemiol. 1996;6:420-30. [Pub Med]
130. Burack JH, Barrett DC, Stall RD, Chesney MA, Ekstrand ML, Coates TJ. Depressive symptoms and CD4 lymphocyte decline among HIV-infected men. JAMA. 1993;270:2568-73. [Pub Med]
131. Mayne TJ, Vittinghoff E, Chesney MA, Barrett DC, Coates TJ. Depressive affect and survival among gay and bisexual men infected with HIV. Arch Intern Med. 1996;156:2233-8. [Pub Med]
132. Semple SJ, Patterson TL, Straits-Troster K, Atkinson JH, McCutchan JA, Grant I. Social and psychological characteristics of HIV-infected women and gay men. HIV Neurobehavioral Research Center (HNRC) Group. Women Health. 1996;24: 17-41. [Pub Med]
133. Lyketsos CG, Hoover DR, Guccione M, Senterfitt W, Dew MA, Wesch J, et al. Depressive symptoms as predictors of medical outcomes in HIV infection. Multicenter AIDS Cohort Study. JAMA. 1993;270:2563-7. [Pub Med]
134. Evans DL, Ten Have TR, Douglas SD, Gettes DR, Morrison M, Chiappini MS, et al. Association of depression with viral load, CD8 T lymphocytes, and natural killer cells in women with HIV infection. Am J Psychiatry. 2002;159:1752-9. [Pub Med]

CHAPTER 41

Psychiatric Emergencies

Shivananda Jena

Psychiatric emergencies are conditions in which there is alteration in behavior, emotion or thought, presenting in an acute form, needing immediate attention and care. This has become a challenging field in the face of rise in incidence of violence, rape, abuse, addiction and murder in the society. Effective and prompt emergency care in emergency room (ER) not only helps stabilize the emergency conditions but also lessens the burden on routine services.

HISTORY

Community Mental Health Control Act (USA) in 1963 provided that emergency psychiatric treatment be included as one of the five essential services in federally funded community mental health center.[1] This Act led to decline in the census of patients in mental hospitals in the USA.[2] As a result of deinstitutionalization, as well as of the current trend towards briefer period of hospitalization, emergency facilities have assumed a more important role in the management of severely disturbed patients and have often come to represent the 'revolving door', through which such patients are repeatedly channelled into other segments of the mental health services network.[3]

GENERAL APPROACH

Psychiatric emergencies are seen mostly in ER of a hospital, but these can be encountered in any routine psychiatric set up. Psychiatry emergencies do not mean that patients are suffering from only psychiatric disorders. They may present due to medical conditions, or conditions unrelated to medical field, like disaster, rape, violence.

Problems in Emergency Room[4]

Following are some of the common problems encountered in the ER:

- Tense and chaotic atmosphere
- Time constraint
- Impersonal and transient doctor-patient relationship
- Primary physician is not a psychiatrist
- Antipathy feeling towards psychiatrist by emergency staff
- Lack of confidence and faith by relatives of patient in psychiatrists
- Often used by nonemergency cases as an easy way to be in contact with psychiatric services, leading to loss of valuable time
- Often viewed by psychiatrist as a nonrewarding job.

Triage

It is a system often followed in ER to prioritize cases like emergency, acute and nonacute.

Initial Approach[5,6]

The initial approach to a case should be warm, direct and concerned. A quick evaluation to identify the nature of the condition and to institute care on the basis of seriousness is essential. Flow chart 1 serves as a general guideline in the ER.

In case of emergency being managed at an ER of a psychiatric hospital, the case needs to sent to an ER of a general hospital for life threatening medical conditions, as early as possible. Children and adolescents should not preferably be managed in ER of a psychiatric hospital. The emergency staff should have basic knowledge of handling psychiatric emergencies before a psychiatrist on call reaches the ER. Essential psychiatric medicines to manage emergency conditions need to be available. Medicolegal cases need to be registered separately and informed to the police of the locality. Hospital security must be adequate to control violent and dangerous patients. History and clinical findings should be recorded clearly in the emergency file. Instructions to the medical and paramedical staff need to be clear and unambiguous. Patient's condition and plans of management should be explained in simple language to the person(s), who have accompanied the patient. It is to be seen that a case is

Flow chart 1: General guidelines for managing psychiatric emergencies in emergency room (ER)

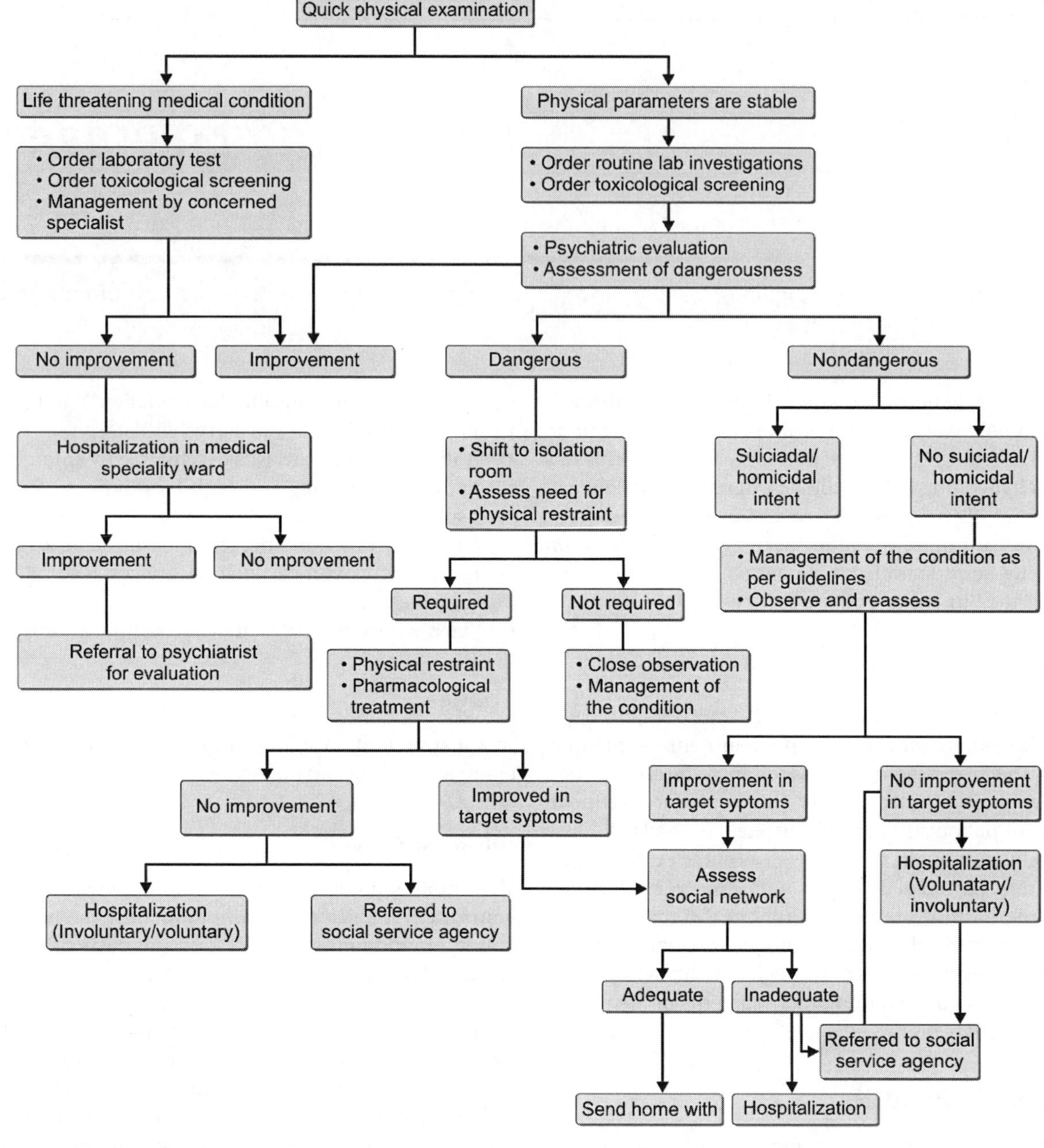

not kept in the ER for more than required time, to give way to other patients coming for treatment. A psychiatric evaluation is modified and tailor-made in order to save time in the decision making. In case of a patient staying in the ER beyond a particular shift, all important information has to be passed on to the team taking over the charge. If possible, old records of patient are retrieved, particularly in cases in which little information is obtained.

Features indicating a possibility of medical illness:

- Acute onset
- Old age
- First episode
- Nonauditory hallucinations
- Disorientation/confusion
- Memory impairment
- Catatonic state
- Neurological symptoms, like unconsciousness, seizures, head injury and visual problems.

Guidelines for effective and quality emergency care:[4]

- Quiet and comfortable room, that insulates both the patient and the therapist from the hectic atmosphere of the ER, with a 'panic button' and an easy access to door.
- Provision of round-the-clock holding unit, that would make unhurried assessment and management possible.

- Staffing arrangements should be made in a manner that ensure the continuity of care and allow for the development of expertise in the delivery of emergency services.
- Regular availability of senior staff for supervision and teaching.

Evaluation approach for emergency psychiatric treatment:[4]
- The nature and availability of support system and capacity of the patient to use it
- Dangerousness
- Psychiatric history and current psychiatric status, including patient's ways of coping with similar stressors previously
- Ability to care for oneself
- Motivation and capacity to participate in the treatment process
- The request(s) of patient and family
- Medical status.

COMMON PSYCHIATRIC EMERGENCIES

Only those emergency conditions not covered elsewhere in this book will be discussed here.

Violence[5,6]

Violence is physical aggression by one person on another. It is important to note that most violent individuals are not psychiatrically ill. Violence is most commonly associated with psychotic disorders, personality disorders (antisocial and paranoid), delirium, drug intoxication or withdrawal, mental retardation, CNS disorders and domestic quarrel. The risk factors for violence include a statement of intent or plan, availability of means of violence, male sex, young age, low socio-economic status, poor social support, past history of violence, poor impulse control and recent stressor(s).

Do's
- Do protect yourself
- Unarm the patient
- Keep the door(s) open
- Keep others near you
- Do restraint if necessary
- Wear white coat and ID card
- Assert authority
- Show concern, establish rapport, and assure the patient.

Don'ts
- Do not keep any potential weapon near the patient
- Do not sit with back to patient
- Do not wear neck tie or jewellery
- Do not keep any provocative family member or friend in the room
- Do not confront
- Do not sit close to the patient.

Management

- Physical restraint, if necessary
- *Pharmacological agents*: Give injection haloperidol (5 mg IM or IV) with or without lorazepam (2 mg IV). Repeat every 2 hours, if necessary
- Hospitalization
- Referral to psychiatric service for further management and follow-up.

Methods of physical restraint
- Use restraint judiciously for the minimum period possible
- Explain to the patient the reason for restraint
- It should be done by trained personnel
- Use leather restraint, if available
- At least five persons are usually required to restraint
- Restraint is done one limb at a time, while the other limbs are held firmly by others
- Restraint in arms are placed in such a way that IM or IV injections can be given easily
- Intoxicated patient should be restrained in the left lateral position
- Assess periodically about removal of restraint
- Remove restraint one limb at a time
- Vitals should be monitored periodically.

Victims of Disaster

Victims of disaster are people, who have survived a sudden, unexpected, overwhelming stress, that is beyond normally expected in life, like earthquake, flood, riots and terrorism. Other victims are relatives of survivors and rescue workers.

Anger, frustration, guilt, numbness and confusion are common features in these people.

Management

1. Treatment of the life threatening physical problems.
2. Crisis intervention:
   i. Sympathetic and flexible attitude toward the victims.
   ii. Victims should be kept in a place together unless somebody is severely disturbed.
   iii. Allow the victims to express their feelings about their experience.
   iv. Provide accurate and responsible information to the victims.
3. Group therapy
4. *Pharmacotherapy*: In selected cases, benzodiazepines are prescribed to reduce anxiety and induce sleep.
5. Referral to psychiatric service, if required.

Grief[5,6]

Grief is a reaction of an individual to a significant loss.

Factors affecting grief reaction:
- Abruptness of loss
- Extent of loss
- Preparation for loss
- Significance of the lost person (object) to the individual
- Past experience of grief
- Cultural background
- Personality traits.

Uncomplicated Grief

The clinical features of uncomplicated grief are sadness, insomnia, poor appetite, loss of interest, guilt and death wish.
Stages
1. Hours to days : Shock and disbelief.
2. Weeks to months : Anger, resentment, depression.
3. Six months to a year : Acceptance of reality.

Management
- Evaluation to find out any primary psychiatric disorder.
- *Crisis intervention*: Patient is encouraged to talk about his feeling concerning the deceased in a private room. Reassurance is given that this is a normal process and will subside on its own. Do not discourage expression of anger or hostility towards either the deceased or the physician.
- *Pharmacotherapy*: Avoid drug treatment, as far as possible. Prescribe night time sedatives on an as-needed (SOS) basis.
- Referral to psychiatric service for primary psychiatric condition, if necessary.

Complicated Grief

It is characterized by suicidality, prolonged functional impairment, marked psychomotor retardation, morbid preoccupation with feelings of worthlessness, or unresolved uncomplicated grief.

Management
- Facilitate grieving process by helping the patient to remember the deceased and the nature of relationship.
- Brief supportive psychotherapy.
- Hospitalization, if required.

Rape Victim[5,6]

Rape is a perpetuation of an act of sexual intercourse with a female against her will and consent.[7]

Phases of psychological difficulties
- *Acute disorganization*: It lasts for several weeks. Self blame, fear of being killed, feeling of degradation and loss of self-esteem, feelings of depersonalization and derealization, recurrent intrusive thoughts, anxiety and depression are commonly seen.
- *Long-term psychological effects*: They take the form of post traumatic stress disorder (PSTD).[8,9]

Management

- Preferably a lady doctor should examine the patient, after obtaining a written consent from her
- Attend to medical conditions, if any
- Give morning after pill to prevent possible pregnancy
- Send samples for STD and HIV infection
- Be supportive, reassuring and nonjudgemental
- Educate about the availability of medical, legal services and rape crisis centers
- Avoid pharmacotherapy as far as possible. Short-term benzodiazepines may be given
- Warn the patient about PSTD, sexual problems, like vaginismus and anorgasmia, which may appear latter
- Referral to a support group for rape victims
- Referral to psychiatric services for further treatment
- Exposure therapy and cognitive therapy are some-times beneficial in presence of PTSD.[10]

Special Populations[11]

Emergency Room Repeaters

Normally, 3% of patients account for about 20% of the psychiatric visits in a given year.

Management
- Make a consistent and unified approach to explore the emergency problem(s) and manage it
- Do not entertain the case, in case of nonemergency.

Young Adult Chronic Patients

These patients are often brought to ER by families because of decompensation following discharge and discontinuation of medication.

Management
- Direct communication with the primary treating team.
- Referral to appropriate program.

Elderly Patients

Elderly patients seek ER services less than their younger counterparts. The most common presenting complaint is peculiar or disturbing behavior for six months or more. The common diagnoses are major depressive disorder, substance abuse and medication side effects.

Management
- Treat the patient's presenting problem
- Family consultation.

Children and Adolescents

Family crisis often precipitates an emergency in this group. Suicide attempts, gestures and ideation occur about twice as often as in an adult emergency population.

Management
- Rapid intervention is needed, focusing on the presenting problem.
- Deal with family issues attributable to emergency.

ETHICAL ISSUES[6]

Confidentiality

Confidentiality concerns the clinician's obligation not to reveal information about the patient to others, without the patient's specific permission to do so.

Exceptions to Confidentiality

- *Emergencies*: In bonafide emergencies, information may be released for the sake of emergency interventions but efforts should be made to obtain the patient's permission.
- *Reportable conditions*: It is mandatory to report certain conditions to the government agencies.
- *Duties to inform third parties*: When a patient makes a threat to seriously harm a specific person and when there is a clear and present danger that patient will carry out the threat, a therapist has an obligation to breach confidentiality and to warn and protect the potential victim.

Involuntary Hospitalization

When a patient is dangerous to self, to others and/or is unable to take care of oneself, an involuntary hospitalization can be considered by the psychiatrist in the ER.

Documentation

The areas commonly neglected by psychiatrists in ER documentation include the following:
- *Disposition*: Clinicians are usually careful to note the data supporting the emergency commitment of a patient but frequently fail to note adequately why a patient was felt to be safe to release. Document should outline the reasoning process regardless of the final disposition.[12]
- *Seclusion, restraint and forced medication*: These are frequently employed in emergencies and frequently not adequately documented. The symptoms and behaviors that justify these measures should be recorded somewhere in the medical chart. Periodic assessments of the need for continuing prolonged seclusion or restraint should be performed.[13,14]

Future Research

Studies have assessed virtually every variable conceivably related to disposition and have frequently found significance. If at all possible, however, a multivariate design should be adopted from the onset to analyze interactions among all variables and identify the key variables that together account for the disposition.[12-15]

REFERENCES

1. Joint Commission on Mental Health and Mental illness. Action for Mental Health. New York: Basic Books; 1961.
2. Slovenko R, Luby E. From moral treatment to railroading out of mental hospital. Bull Am Acad Psychiatry Law. 1974;2:223-36.
3. Johnson J. Psychiatric emergencies in the community. Compr Psychiatry. 1968;10:275-84.
4. Gerson S, Basank E. Psychiatric emergencies: An Overview. Am J Psychiatry. 1980;137:1-11.
5. Kaplan HI, Sadock BJ. Pocket Handbook of Emergency Psychiatric Medicine. New Delhi: BI Publications; 1993.
6. Steven EH. Manual of Psychiatric Emergencies. Boston: Little Brown; 1988.
7. Brownmiller S. Against Our Will: Men, Women and Rape. New York: Simon and Schuster; 1975.
8. Rothbann BO, Fao EB, Murdoch J, et al. A prospective examination of post traumatic stress disorder in rape victims. J Traum Stress. 1992;5:455-75.
9. Lopez G, Piffant G, Seguin A. Psychological treatment of victims of rape. Psychol Med. 1992;24:286-8.
10. Solomon SD, Gerity ET, Muff AM. Effcacy of treatment for post traumatic stress disorder. JAMA. 1992;268:633-8.
11. Fauman BJ. Other psychiatric emergencies. In: Kaplan HI, Sadock BJ. (Eds). Comprehensive Textbook of Psychiatry. Maryland: Williams and Wilkins; 1995.pp.1752-65.
12. Marson DC, McGovern MP, Pomp HC. Psychiatric decision making in the emergency room: A research review. Am J Psychiatry. 1988;145:918-25.
13. American Psychiatric Association. Psychiatric ethics primer. Washington DC. American Psychiatric Publishing Inc; 2001.
14. Montgomery J. Health care law. Oxford University Press. Oxford; 2002.
15. Hope T, Savelescu J, Hendrick J. Medical ethics and law: the core curriculum. Churchil Livingstone, London; 2003.

CHAPTER 42

Human Self-destructive Behavior

KE Sadanandan Unni

Sri Bhagavan uvaca (Bhagavad Gita,[1] Stanza 11)
"asocyan anvasocas tvam prajna-vadams ca bhasase, gat'asun agatasums ca n'anusocanti panditah".
(The Blessed Lord said: "You are moaning for those who should not be moaned for. You speak like a wise man. The truly wise never weep either for the dead or for the living").

(Bhagavad Gita,[1] Stanza 11)
"Na tvevaham jatu nasam, na tvam n'eme jan'ahipah, nac'aiva na bhavisyamah sarve vayam atah param"
(Never was there a time when I did not exist, nor you, nor these rulers of men. Nor shall all of us cease to be hereafter).

(Bhagavad Gita,[1] Stanza 13)
"Dehino' smin yatha dehe kaumaram yauvanam jari, tatha de ha'ntari praptir dhiris tatra na muhyati"
(Even as the attainment of the childhood, youth and old age is to one in this physical life, so is the change to another body—at death—for the embodied soul. Wise men are not unrealistic about this aspect of the soul).

Lord Krishna explains regarding the imperishable or non-destructive nature of life, the '*jeevatma which is a part of paramatma*' in the above manner. Social homeostasis is a dynamic process. Altruism can be the hallmark of eusociality. Eusociality where cooperation and coexistence are passwords, is considered as the most developed form of social life.[2] Non-violent, nondrinking, pacifist, cooperative, coexistent communities, like the Amish in southern Pennsylvania[3] or the '*Cholanaikers*' of northern Kerala are exceptions. Competitive selfishness is the central theme of natural selection.[4] It is a common observation that the social environments in countries around the globe are changing and increasingly becoming competitive. When these changes happen at a fast pace, human beings find it difficult to adapt to the situation.[5] While biological psychiatry highlights heredofamilial and neurochemical basis of suicidal behavior, one has to bear in mind that it is only one aspect of the subject. No scientific investigation has proved whether the biological aspect is the cause of certain mental phenomenon or a consequence of environmental factors which we call as stressors.[6,7]

Many examples of so-called "suicide" in animals are actually extreme cases of territoriality or dispersal mechanisms when population density rises. Lemmings marching into the sea are the unfortunate victims of emigrations in all directions, one of which happens to be the ocean, away from an exploding population. So, in action only, man shares the suicidal tendencies (and completion) with animals like lemmings.[8]

Vidya Sagar in his presidential address (1973) quotes Brock Chisholm, the first Director General of WHO; "the destructive potentialities of man have become so great that his inferiorities, fears, anxieties, hates, aggressive pressures, fanaticism and even increasing devotion and loyalties, which are among the common symptoms of physical, mental and social ill-health, may now constitute a serious threat to the continued existence of a large number of people who previously were far beyond his reach". Chisholm wrote it in 1942. After 55 years we have to add that apart from man's destructive potentiality, self-destructive behavior also has increased.[9]

Human self-destructive behavior has many determinants.[10] In considering animal models for human behavior one cannot propose that similar behaviors necessarily have the same causation in human beings. Even if environmental conditions or the resulting behaviors vary for different species, the biochemical intermediaries may be similar. However, if a simple explanation can account for the production of a particular behavioral syndrome in animals, it can help to structure our thoughts regarding the etiology of the behavior in humans. The ethological aspect of such discussion may help to place human self-destructive behavior in a continuum with that of animals drawing direct parallels may be out of place but we can conclude that humans are not alone in exhibiting self-initiated behaviors that produce self-harm or death.[8]

Human suicidal behavior has always been a source of dread and wonder to mankind. When a person has suicidal ideas he is thinking of preponing his death and undergoing that process, sudden or slow voluntarily. All suicidal people are not death seekers. Some attempt to communicate pain, to reduce isolation, to avoid consequences of social status change, seek revenge and convey a whole lot of other meanings which are essentially individualistic.[11-13]

HISTORICAL, RELIGIOUS, PHILOSOPHICAL AND CULTURAL BACKGROUND

Ramayana and Mahabharata have recorded instances of suicide. When Lord Sri Rama died, there was an epidemic of suicide in Ayodhya. Bhagvad Gita is against self-torture and self-killing. Brahmanical view was that anyone who tries to kill oneself but fails should fast for a stipulated period. Raja Ram Mohan Roy organized agitation against sati. During Vedic and Upanishadic times, apart from sati, death from drowning at the confluence of rivers to achieve '*punya*' (salvation in the next life), the self-destruction for incurable diseases, ascetics undertaking a great journey towards the last years of life (*mahaprasthan*), were allowed. Vedic and Upanishadic period penalized suicide in general but with the above exceptions. Islam asks man and woman to wait for his or her destiny, rather than snatching it from the hands of God. If he does not, he will be depicted as a unfaithful wretch.[14] Some studies have shown that in comparison to Jews and Catholics, the Protestants have a higher rate of suicide. But statistics give only a rough idea of people's psychic life.[15]

Terminologies in Suicidology

Suicide: Killing oneself. To diagnose any death as suicide, there must be evidence that it resulted from the decedent's deliberately initiated action (or inaction) and that the person had a specific intention to cause his or her own death.

Suicide, adolescent: Studies of adolescents who died by suicide indicate that:

- Adolescent suicide is associated with substance abuse more often than with any other psychiatric disorder
- Those with an affective disorder have concomitant affective and nonaffective disorders, more often than do adult suicide victims
- Acute interpersonal conflict is no more prevalent among adolescent suicide victims than among other psychiatrically ill adolescents
- Four of five talked about their suicidal state of mind with others (usually to siblings and friends of the same age) within the week before their suicide
- Only a third of adolescents who died by suicide had ever seen a mental health professional, even once.

Suicide attempt: Life-threatening act requiring medical attention that is committed with a conscious intent to end one's life.

Suicide attempted: Unsuccessful, but potentially lethal action, a risk factor for future completed suicide, and a potential indicator of other biopsychosocial health problems such as alcohol and substance abuse, depres-sion, or adjustment and stress reactions. Attempted suicide is also a morbid health event that results in personal suffering and considerable economic cost.

Suicide cluster: Individuals or groups committing suicide shortly after the suicide(s) of acquaintances or public figures, or after publicity about suicide clusters.

Suicide gesture: Behavior purposefully undertaken by an individual in which the outcome is reasonably likely to be self-harm, in the absence of explicit data suggesting that suicide was not intended.

Suicide gesture/false-positive: Engaging in suicide gestures that do not portend subsequent suicide.

Suicide pact: Agreement or pledge between two or more persons to take their own lives simultaneously.

Suicide, physician-assisted: Death caused by the action(s) of a physician who agreed with the patient's intent to die and acted to directly bring it about.[16]

Consummated suicide: Results when an individual reaches the point of "no return", either because he/she did not receive rapid and effective assistance or because in spite of medical attention, the damage was irreversible.[17]

Risk factor: Risk factor is a characteristic variable or hazard that increases the likelihood of development of adverse outcome, which is measurable and precedes the outcome. Distal risk factor is the threshold that increases the individual risk for later vulnerability to proximal risk factors. This risk factor is the foundation upon which suicide is built up. Distal risk factors are triggering events or precipitants which vary with age and other sociodemographic characteristics, and which are closely and temporally related to the suicide event. Unlike proximal risk factors, these are considered sufficient for suicide to occur. Psychopathology, its heredofamilial contribution, substance abuse, neurochemical factors, and sociofamilial risk factors are distal risk factors. Proximal risk factors act as precipitants or triggering events. These proximal risk factors are more closely related temporally to the suicidal event. When both distal and proximal risk factors co-occur there is greatest occurrence of suicides. Proximal risk factors include pesticides, firearms, stressful life events, medical disorders, availability of prescribed medicines etc.[18]

Correlates of suicide: These can be concomitants and consequences of the adverse outcome. Their relatedness to the causation is low in comparison to the causation.[18]

Double suicide: Two people dying together following a pact. This results from a depressed patient instigating another (cooperator) who is psychiatrically normal. In some cases, the depressed patient may commit homicide before suicide.[14]

Suicide counters: Those factors that inhibit the suicidogenic tendencies are called suicide counters. These can be economic, religious, moral, ethical and social. The environment offers both suicidogenic factors and also those that suppress them; the latter are called suicide counters.[14]

Indirect self-destructive behaviors: These are long drawn out life-shortening, self-defeating, or death-hastening behaviors with varying degree of unconscious motivation for self-destruction. These are covert suicidal behaviors. The social attitude is that the individual is not considered impaired in his judgement, unlike the patient with a overt suicidal behavior. And so, no intervention is thought necessary. Karl Menninger, in 1938, developed the concept of death instinct more comprehensively, which includes the indirect self-destructive behavior also.[16,19]

Definitions

Shneidman's: Human act of self-inflicted, self-intentioned cessation.

Shneidman's revised definition: Suicide is a conscious act of self-induced annihilation, best understood as a multidimensional malaise in a needful individual, who defines an issue for which suicide is perceived as the best solution.[20]

Existential definition: A behavior that seeks and finds solution to an existential problem by making an attempt on the life of the subject.[21]

In 1968, *WHO* defined suicidal act as the injury with varying degrees of lethal intent, and suicide is defined as a suicidal act with fatal outcome.[22]

Diekstra redefined suicide as an act with fatal outcome that is deliberately initiated and performed by the person himself or herself in the knowledge or expectation of its fatal outcome.[23]

Suicidal acts with nonfatal outcome are labeled by *WHO* as either suicide attempts, attempted suicides, parasuicides or acts of deliberate self-harm. Currently, there is growing tendency among experts in this field to broaden the concept of suicide and speak of suicide behaviors instead. In this chapter, the more traditional and accepted conceptual issues on suicide only will be dealt with, while one waits for the new paradigm of suicide behaviors to get consolidated.[23]

Legal definition: For the purpose of establishing the cause of death, suicide is legally defined as the intentional act of self destruction committed by someone knowing what he is doing and knowing the probable consequences of his action. The verdict of suicide should be supported with evidence. It can never be presumed.[24]

Oxford advanced learners' dictionary: It defines suicide as the act of killing oneself intentionally.[25]

MEANINGS OF SUICIDE

Social Meaning of Suicide

Suicide exists in every society. But, it is viewed differently by different societies. It may be seen as a sin (against the Gods) or as a crime (against the law). The ancient Greeks and Romans endorsed suicide in some circumstances, e.g. on behalf of one's country (*harakiri* in Japan) as a means of execution in others, and as in those condoned in *sati*, except among slaves and soldiers, and those who used it to escape the ignominy of law. Attitude towards suicide is dynamic. There is no universal definition of any crime; it changes in and between societies, reflecting functioning of different views of the relationships between the individual, the state and the ruling regime or ideology. It is not clear why a form of behavior will be prohibited through the common law, civil law in another and yet remain as the matter of private morals in the third. Such a prohibition tended to be associated with sexual behavior (homosexuality, adultery and prostitution), but has also included suicide.[24]

Early Christians took recourse to suicide when persecuted for the faiths, until St. Augustine (354-430 AD) declared that it is a sin punishable by eternity of Hell. The established church accepted the new regime's attitude and it remained relevant for many centuries.[24]

Legal Meaning of Suicide

In UK under the code of common law, murder was unlawful ending of human life, even one's own. Self-murder was felony and its attempt a misdemeanor, as early as in the tenth century. It became a crime by 1485, but the term was utilized in the legal language in England only by 1651. Because of the Suicide Act 1961, suicide ceased to be a crime in England and European countries. Since then penalties for suicide, even if possible by law, were not consistently applied in the 17th century. After the French revolution in 1789, attempted suicide ceased to be considered as offence in France. In England by the 18th century, it became a crime of the highest degree.[24]

In India according to section 309 of Indian penal code, "whoever attempts to commit suicide or any act towards the commission of such offence shall be punished with simple imprisonment for a term which may extent to one year or a fine or both". According to the Indian legal system, life of an individual is considered not only valuable to himself but also to the state. Section 309 is reinforced by sections 306 and 304b, the former dealing with the abetment of the commission of suicide, while the latter deals with dowry deaths. Section 304b says that a person shall be deemed to have caused a death of a woman if that woman dies as result of burns or injury within 7 years of her marriage and if before her death she has been subjected to cruelty or harassment by her in-laws in connection with dowry. There are many lacunae in the law of the land concerning suicide: (1) attempted suicide is not punishable if the person took the overdose of poison by mistake or under an intoxicated state: (2) regarding declaration to fast unto death and self-immolation, the Indian law is quite unclear. Allahabad high court (Ram Sundar v State, AIR 1962 Allahabad, 262) has said that people who declare themselves of pursuing such act which are long drawn out processes, can be interrupted at any stage, except the very last. It is also said that even if there was such a declaration by the person it is difficult to be sure that he really intended to persevere to the end.[12] The legal system is basing its views on the intention of the individual for self-destruction of his life. The legal system gathers information to this extent before a judgment is passed.[12]

The views of psychiatrists, psychologists and sociologists on suicide have imparted newer insights in this area for the legal community. In 1971, the Law Commission recommended the abolition of section 309 of IPC. Government of India accepted the recommendation but could not pass the bill in the Lok Sabha in 1979, as the elected body was dissolved and the bill elapsed.[12]

Religion and Suicide

Studies done in the early part of the twentieth century have illustrated that Catholic communities have low suicide rates than Jewish and Protestant communities. There are differences in the concepts based on observations made by the researchers of the beginning of the century and those of the last part of the century regarding the association between religion and suicide.[14]

Neeleman et al.[26] worked on the background idea that there is a negative association between religion and suicide in individuals and countries; it may be mediated by the degree to which suicide is tolerated. Using logistic regression, the association between suicide tolerance and strength of religious belief in 28,085 individuals in nineteen western countries in 1989–90, was done to find out whether the association between suicide tolerance and religious belief in individuals depended on the extent of religious belief in their country. Ecological association between religious variables and suicide rates are stronger for women than for men, stronger for measures of belief than observance and is mediated by tolerance to suicide. In individuals, stronger religious beliefs were associated with lower tolerance to suicide and for men exposure to a religious environment may protect against suicide by reducing its acceptability.[26]

Suicide rates are lower in religious than secular countries. It is not clear whether a negative association between religious and suicidal behavior also applies at the individual level. Neelman's study simultaneously examined individual and contextual issues of a protective factor against suicide.[26]

CLASSIFICATION OF SUICIDE

"*Classer est une necessite. Tout vaut mieux que le chaos.*" (Classifying is a necessity. Order is better than chaos), said Lemperiere Presidente of Symposium on DSM-IV, a nice approach to affective disorders held in Paris on 13th May 1995.[27] Similarly, there are many approaches to the classification of suicide (Table 1).[27]

Sociological Approach and Emile Durkheim's Classification

Emile Durkheim[28] is responsible for the methodological concept and theory of '*sociologism*'. In 1896, Durkheim began publishing *L'Annee sociologique*. Sociologism means study of social facts or social reality. A social fact is any external constraint on the individual and having its own existence independent of individual manifestation. The individual, right from birth, finds readymade laws and customs, rules of conduct, religious beliefs and rituals, language and monetary system that operated as constraints independently of him/her.[29]

Durkheim's[28] was the first major contribution to the study of the problem of suicide made at the end of the last century. According to Durkheim, anomic and egoistic suicides were responsible for the rising suicide rates of Europe. With industrial and scientific development, the family, the state, and the church were not the forces for social integration that they had once been, and nothing had been found to replace them. Suicide, like crime, neurosis and alcoholism, is a factor that measures social pressure and tension. The extremely high rate seen in West Berlin is perhaps the most dramatic manifestation of this principle.[28–30]

Criticism of Durkheim

The critics of Durkheim[18,28-30] wanted to extrapolate his findings to the present day society. The causes of suicide, the risk of suicide in people, the impact of suicide in family and society, etc. do change with time, but no generalization at one period of time can be extrapolated onto any other. But with regard to urbanization, overcrowding and overpopulation, anomic phenomenons do occur.

Table 1: Types of suicide

Characteristics	*Egoistic*	*Altruistic*	*Anomic*	*Fatalistic*
Nature of individual	High isolation, individuation. Individual not strongly integrated to society. Cut off from supportive significant others in society.	Insufficient individuation. Individual excessively integrated to society or group	Experiences violent accusations and counter accusations between self and significant others. Recrimination against life in general is experienced.	Rules and regulations excessively regulate the individual.
Nature of society (Social context)	Within religion.Within family. Within politics.	Specific classes in societies like soldiers, national (harakiri) or religious martyrs (sati).	Prone to sudden social or economic changes, societies in which divorce is common. Societies in which liberal occupations are possible.	Prison communities, cults, slaves, childless married women.
Effect of individual society	Interaction on the individual (effect of personal, social interaction on individual).	Apathy, depression in individual who finds no basis for existence in life. Individuals feel obliged to perform the self-destructive act. Unusual mystical enthusiasm is felt by the individual. Renunciation by the individual appreciated by society. The more the social integration the more the suicide rate.	Balance of persons integration into society is suddenly disturbed leaving the individual without his customary norms of behavior, e.g. during drastic financial failure; in divorced individuals suicide is more common than the married.	Social integration do not protect individuals. The more the social integration the higher the suicide rate.

Understanding of the interpersonal aspects is not the all and end all of suicidology. Individuals are unique and so can be their causes of suicide. The present day technoscience tries to build the image of a standardized man and then applies the rules and regulations concerning this standard man onto others. This also can be wrong. Statistics do help to a certain extent, but not all statistical findings cannot be extrapolated to any individual.

The morphological methods proposed originally by Durkheim, were completely abandoned by him and he concentrated on social facts, the aggregate of which was society. An important characteristic of social facts, namely the pressure exerted on individuals by legal, moral and religious rules and the manner in which these compelled the individuals to act in a certain manner was the main subject matter of his study in suicidology.

Durkheim assumed that his sociologistic theory of suicide is correct and then explained away any contrary data. Death certificates and official statistics cannot be expected to have any significant value in constructing or testing sociological theories of suicide. The more socially integrated an individual is, the more he and his significant others (which can include doctors, coroners and those responsible for deciding the cause of death) will try to avoid having his death categorized as a suicide. The assumption being that suicidal actions have a necessary and sufficient unidimensional meaning throughout the western world. A basic reorientation of sociological work on suicide in the direction of intensive observation, description and analysis of individual cases is required instead of predicting suicide in abstract collective terms like anomie and egoism. Suicidologists should observe the first person accounts of serious suicide attempters than the third person accounts of medical examiners and focus on the subjective meanings of actual suicidal individuals.[18,28,30]

In spite of criticisms of Durkheim, vital statistics continue to be utilized in suicidology research, as there are no other practical alternatives and vital statistics are not that inaccurate.[18,28-30]

Hendin's Classification of Suicide Behavior

Herbert Hendin[31] classified suicides into five different types, depending on how death is viewed, based on variables like the patient's age, beliefs, mental mechanisms, and affectivity.

- *Retaliatory abandonment*: Death is viewed as an act of leaving or abandonment. This concept is derived during childhood. Most often children view the dead person as someone who left voluntarily. Sometimes they view death as a violent act inflicted on the dead. Children who have lost their parents react as though he/they have chosen to abandon them.
- *Retroflexed murder*: Suicide is considered as a murderous rage, which is turning in and which is not repressed. Usually in young, disturbed, and seriously suicidal

patients, suicide can be the outcome of a severe struggle with the overt desire to murder. These patients can be basically aggressive and violent with an overt desire to murder.

- *Reunion*: Death is viewed as a pleasurable act and is incorporated into the fantasy of reunion with parental figures, with life partners, loved ones, and siblings substituting parents whose are already dead and gone. Here, the emphasis is placed on the self-fulfillment which can follow for the suicide in the other world by joining the forefathers or partners.
- *Self-punishment*: Suicidal self-punishment reaction occurs in men over failure at work or failure at fulfilling their duty to the class or country. Some women who have inability to love and look after the child, have a self-expectation and expectation by others that she should feel what she is not feeling. This expectation and their inability in combination produces a self-hatred, with the consequent need for self-punishment. The original emotion may be guilt over aggression and guilt over failure to mother. Desire for self-punishment develops further and this desire gets dissociated from the original emotions.
- *Seeing oneself as already dead*: The equivalent of emotional dying is manifested as strong feelings of detachment, repressed aggression and affectivity which has gone into a frozen state, and is perceived by some patients as their emotional death. Clinical manifestation of this is apathy rather than depression. If such patients attempt suicide, the act rarely changes their mood. They see suicide as a way out, a solution to their torture. Some may see it as the practicing of an act which has already been carried out before.[31]

Schneidman and Farberow's Classification

Schneidman and Farberow[32,33] have classified suicides into four groups:

1. Patients who conceive suicide as a means to better life.
2. Patients who commit suicide as a result of psychosis, with associated delusions and hallucinations.
3. Patients who commit suicide out of revenge against a loved person.
4. Patients who are old and infirm, for whom suicide is said to be a release.

Schneidman[20,33] classifies suicidal behavior into parasuicide and suicide (Table 2).

Classification Based on the Strength of the Suicidal thought and the Determination/ Decision Taken Towards Ending of the Life

Suicide ideator: It can be a wish for death. It can be just a thought that death could have been better than the psychological pain of living with certain situations in life. If episodic or long lasting, it may have a cumulative effect and

Table 2: Suicide and parasuicide

Aspects of behavior	*Suicide*	*Parasuicide*
1. The stimulus of psychological pain suffered by patient	Unendurable quantitatively overwhelming	Endurable to some extent quantitatively not overwhelming
2. The purpose of the behavior	Solution to an overwhelming problem, where no other option is felt worth trying	The patient tries to evoke a response in others who may help him or her to solve a problem
3. The nature of the behavior	Conclusive	Evocative/even provocative
4. The sociological nature of behavior	Autistic to a certain extent	Enacted on an interpersonal stage
5. The target of evocation in the behavior	Self punishment	Punishing a specific other or generalized others
6. Goal of behavior	Cessation of consciousness (stopping life/ genuine wish to die)	Reorder life space and meanwhile decrease discomfort (changing the life/wish for change of their circumstances)
7. Content of thought of the patient	Hopelessness, helplessness, worthlessness	Disconnectedness, disenfranchisement, disenchantedness
8. Subject's attitude	Indecision which is ambivalent or bivalent—to live or to die	Indecision which is trivalent—among the options of living, suffering, dying
9. Cognitive state of the subject	Intellectual and perceptual constriction	Obseional or ruminative painfulness
10. Communication or message of the act	Is one of patient's decision	Is one of patient's unhappiness and cry for help or call for rescue
11. The action per se	Is an escape, or leaving life	Is aimed towards emotional linking and unity with life

may or may not overwhelm the threshold for suicide. It may be expressed much more freely than the similar idea of an attempter or a completer of suicide. It may or may not be serious than the attempter's or completer's idea. It may or may not evolve into attempt or completion.

There are finer differences between attempted suicide and parasuicide (Table 3).

EPIDEMIOLOGICAL APPROACH

Investigating the uneven distribution of suicidal behavior in different populations, and determining which population groups have a greater or lesser rate of suicide, can lead to knowledge about the risk factors and suggest ways in which different factors promote or prevent it. Examining the demographic information that is included in death certificates, by prospective controlled follow-up studies of high risk groups, and by retrospective enquiries about suicide victims (*psychological autopsy*), are the accepted methods.

Epidemiological studies for the identification of suicide risk factors include studying the prevalence and incidence and also the determinants of the suicidal behavior.

Table 3: Attempted suicide and parasuicide

	Attempted suicide	*Parasuicide*
1.	Very definite conscious effort	Less definite conscious effort
2.	Very determined effort, but failed	Less determined effort
3.	Very serious effort, but failed	Less serious
4.	Somehow survival by chance or by a chance intervention	No problem regarding survival
5.	Overlapping populations but distinct from suicide	Does not overlap with suicide, may overlap with attempted suicide
6.	More homogeneous group based on seriousness	Heterogeneous group based on gradations of seriousness and manipulative nature
7.	Genuine wish to die	Wish for change of life circumstances
8.	Can be well planned	Less well planned
9.	Can be secretive	Freely expressed
10.	Can be violent act, a threat to life	Less violent act, may not be a threat to life
11.	Can easily go into consummated suicide for want of proper medical attention or because the injury or lethality is serious	Need not necessarily progress to consummated suicide
12.	Is an event in which there is a failure of conscious effort to end life, pseudosuicide is not a synonym.	Self injury, deliberate self poisoning, deliberate self harm, pseudo-suicide etc are synonyms

Population based psychological autopsy is a powerful tool in verifying fossil hypothesis generated from hospital-based observation study. It gives additional data on completed suicide that are generalizable in the community. Population based samples are unbiased, unlike self-selected clinical samples. Descriptive epidemiological studies informs one about the scope and impact of suicide behavior, whereas analytic epidemiological studies test fossil hypothesis before quantifying sensitive human behavior like suicide. Behavior can be qualitatively analyzed by methods like walking across village, social mapping, case study method, in-depth case study method etc. Qualitative methods provide data which will utilize generate hypothesis. It will also help in understanding the broad patterns of suicidal behavior. In multivariate analysis, the procedure distinguishes risk factors from other characteristics, such as concomitants or consequences of outcome, which are only correlates of suicide behavior and not necessarily risk factors.[34]

Magnitude of the Problem

Everyday thousands of people commit suicide in the world. Approximately one percent of the general population die by suicide. In every country, there are certain areas which are called *suicide sites*. For example, 'suicide point' in Ooty and Kodaikanal (India) and 'Golden Gate Bridge' in San Francisco (USA). Barraclough et al. demonstrated that 93% of individuals of general population, who committed suicide, were suffering from psychiatric disorders prior to the death.[35] Suicide is currently the 9th leading cause of death in the United States; formerly, it was the 8th leading cause. Deaths from human immunodeficiency virus infection has displaced it from the 8th to the 9th position.[36]

The world scenario is illustrated in the Table 4.[23] 4,00,000 people commit suicide every year around the world. Suicide is among the ten leading causes of death for all ages in most of the countries. In some countries, it is among the top three causes of death for people between 15 and 34 years (Table 5).

Table 4: Psychiatric diagnoses in 5,588 cases of suicide

Diagnosis	*N*	*%*
Organic brain syndrome	308	5
Substance abuse	947	16
Schizophrenia	612	10
Affective disorders	1,400	24
Neurotic and personality disorders	1,340	22
Other mental disorders	1,259	21
No diagnosis	137	2
Total	6,003	100

(Adapted from WHO publication 1993 on suicide)[23]

Table 5: Suicide rates in selected countries

(Per 1,00,000 population; all age groups; latest available year)

Suicide rate by sex	*Male*	*Female*	*Both sexes*
Hungary	58.0	20.7	38.6
Sri Lanka	48.8	22.3	35.8
Finland	48.9	11.7	29.8
Switzerland	34.3	11.6	22.7
Belgium	32.0	13.8	22.7
Austria	34.6	11.6	22.6
Denmark	30.0	15.1	22.4
France	29.6	11.1	20.1
Sweden	26.8	10.6	18.6
Czechoslovakia	27.3	8.9	17.9
Germany	24.9	10.7	17.5
Japan	20.6	11.8	16.1
Norway	23.3	8.0	15.5
Poland	23.9	4.4	13.9
Singapore	14.7	11.5	13.1
Canada	20.4	5.2	12.7
USA	19.9	4.8	12.2
Puerto Rico	19.4	2.1	10.5
Uruguay	16.6	4.2	10.3
Netherlands	12.3	7.2	9.7
Portugal	14.9	4.6	9.6
Ireland	14.4	4.7	9.5
UK	12.4	3.6	7.9
Spain	11.6	3.9	7.7
Italy	11.2	4.1	7.5
Thailand	4.5	4.5	5.8
Chile	9.8	1.5	5.6
Venezuela	7.8	1.8	4.8
Greece	5.5	1.5	3.5
Colombia	5.1	1.5	3.3
Mexico	3.9	0.7	2.3

(Adapted from WHO 1993 publication on suicide)[23]

Rates per year as high as 1 suicide per 1,000 population (e.g. Falkland Islands) and 1 suicide per 1,500 population (e.g. Hungary) are reported. Suicide is under-reported by 20% to 100%, according to prevailing beliefs and consequent negative sanctions attached to it in different cultures of the world. Developed and developing countries and countries with quite distinct cultural traditions (e.g. Surinam, Srilanka, Switzerland and Japan) are affected by the social problem. Islamic countries may be exceptional.[36]

Indian Scenario

In India, according to national crime records bureau, suicide is among the top ten causes of death. Suicide is also among the top 3 causes of death in India between 16 and 35 year range. In 1984, around 50,000 people (Fig. 1) (50,571, i.e. 6.8 per lakh) committed suicide. In 1994, around 90,000 people (Fig. 2) (89,195, i.e. 9.9 per lakh) committed suicide (Table 6). Number of suicide attempts are around 10 times than that of the number of suicides. Pondicherry is considered to be currently the highest rate area (7 times the national rate, i.e. 70 per lakh) followed by West Bengal (12,389, i.e. 14% of all suicides). 16% of the people, who commit suicide in these two states, are below 30 years of age. Other high risk areas include Maharashtra, Andhra Pradesh, Karnataka, Tamil Nadu and Kerala.[36] Among the 89,195 cases of suicide 52,752 (59%) were males and 36,443 (41%) were females, making males to female ratio 1.45:1 (Table 7).

Murthy,[38] in a seminar on suicidology in 1993, had pointed out that:

- There was about 10% increase in suicide rate in one year and it has gone up from 6.3% in 1978 to 8% in 1988,
- While the population increase during the period was 25%, the suicide rate increased by 60%,
- Among the cities in India, the suicide rate was least in Calcutta and highest in Bangalore,
- Among the states the highest rate was in Kerala and lowest rate was in Jammu and Kashmir (Table 8), and
- The causes are largely 'social', with only 3.4% attributed to mental illnesses.[37,38] Over the six years from 1988 to 1994, highest suicide rate city status has shifted from Bangalore (previously called as the '*suicide city*' of India) to Pondicherry. Calcutta paradoxically is the city with lowest suicide rate (Table 9).[37,38]

Sociodemographic Pattern

Sex

Men commit suicide more than 3 times as often as do women, a rate that is stable over all ages. Women, on the other hand, are 3 times as likely to attempt suicide as are men (Table 10).

Age

The significance of the mid-life crisis is underscored by suicide rates. Among men, suicides peak after age 45; among women, the greatest number of completed suicides occurs after age 55. Rates of 50 per 100,000 population are found in men age 65 and older; the elderly attempt suicide less often than younger people but are successful more frequently, accounting for 25% of the suicides, although the elderly make up only 10% of the total population. A decline in suicide in men begins between the ages 75 to 85. A peak risk among males is found also in late adolescence, when death by suicide is exceeded only by death attributed to accidents and cancer.

Race

Suicide among whites is recorded at nearly twice the rate as among non-whites, but these figures are increasingly called into question. Among the black, ghetto youth and certain Native American and Alaskan Indian groups, suicide rates greatly exceed the national rate. Two out of every three suicides are white males.

Religion

Historically, suicide rates among Catholic populations have been recorded as lower than rates among Protestants and

Table 6: Causes of suicide in percentage in 1994

Causes	*Percentage*
Debilitating illness	13.5
Quarrel with spouse	5.8
Failed affairs	5.8
Quarrel with parents-in-law	4.9
Insanity	3.5
Poverty	2.2
Property-related dispute	2.2
Failure in examination	2.1
Dowry dispute	1.9
Bankruptcy	1.7
Death of a dear person	1.6
Unemployment	1.5
Fall in social reputation	1.4
Unclear causes	51.9
(Adapted from National Crime Records Bureau, 1984–94)[37]	

Table 7: The means adopted for suicide (in %)

Methods	*1984*	*1994*
Poison	31.4	34.8
Hanging	23.4	23.9
Burning	9.4	11.5
Drowning	14.9	9.4
Railways	5.4	3.9
Jumping	1.1	1.2
Electric wires	0.3	0.9
Sharp material/weapons	0.5	0.8
Sleeping pills	0.3	0.7
Fire arms	0.8	0.7
Other methods	11.7	12.7
(Adapted from National Crime Records Bureau, 1984–94)[37]		

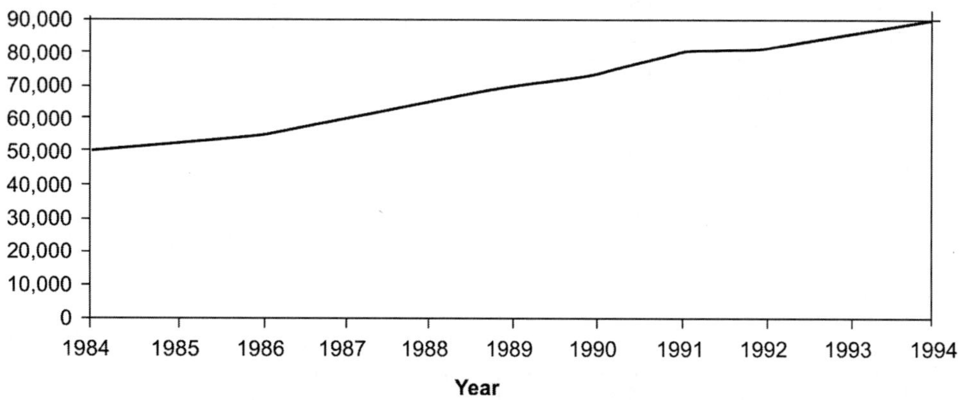

Fig. 1 Total number of suicides, yearwise
(Adapted from National Crime Records Bureau, 1984–94)[37]

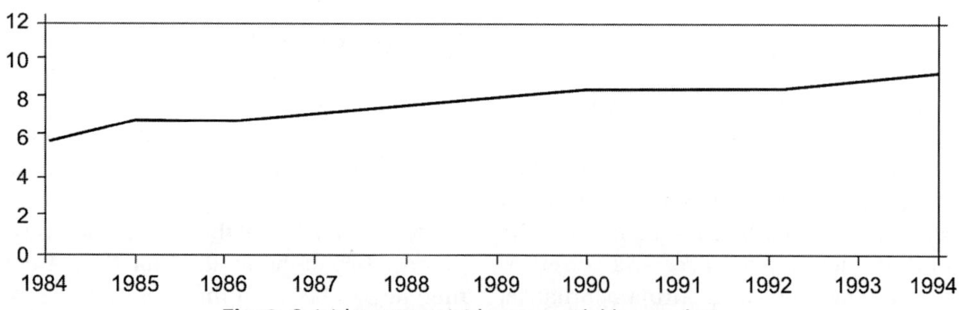

Fig. 2 Suicides rate: suicide per one lakh population
(Adapted from National Crime Records Bureau, 1984–94)[37]

Table 8: Rate of suicide per 100,000 population in India, statewise (1988)

State	*Rate*
Jammu and Kashmir	0.5
Nagaland	0.6
Uttar Pradesh	1.8
Assam	10.1
Goa	12.3
Karnataka	15.6
West Bengal	15.7
Tamil Nadu	17.9
Tripura	21.1
Kerala	24.7
(Adapted from Murthy RS)[38]	

Table 9: Rate of suicide per 100,000 population in India, citywise (1988)

City	*Rate*
Kolkata	3.2
Jaipur	4.4
Kanpur	5.8
Mumbai	6.0
Delhi	6.4
Lucknow	7.8
Ahmedabad	9.1
Nagpur	11.1
Hyderabad	13.0
Pune	15
Chennai	22
Bengaluru	24.6
(Adapted from Murthy RS)[38]	

Jews. It may be that degree of orthodoxy and integration within a religion are a more accurate measure of risk within this category, than is simple institutional religious affiliation.

Marital Status

Marriage, reinforced by children, seems to significantly lessen the risk of suicide. Among married persons, the rate is 11 per 100,000. Single, never-married persons register an overall rate of nearly double the married rate. Previously married persons show sharply higher rates; 24 per 100,000 among the widowed; 40 per 100,000 among divorced persons, with divorced men registering 69 suicides per 100,000 as compared with 18 per 100,000 per divorced women.

Table 10: Incidence of suicide per 100,000 population

State	*1872*	*1972*
Bengal (W Bengal)	2.3	15.9
Bombay Presidency (Maharashtra)	4.73	8.26
Madras Presidency (TN)	7.85	11.30
Central Province (MP)	6.10	7.83
(Adapted from Venkoba Rao A, 1992)[14]		

Health

The relationship of physical health and illness to suicide is both predictable and inconsistent and, in either case, significant. Prior medical care appears to be a negatively correlated risk indicator of suicide; 42% of suicides have had medical attention within 6 months of death. Seventy percent of victims have been affected by one or more active and, for the most part, chronic-illness at the time of death. Among suicide attempts studied, more than one-third of the persons were actively ill at the time of the attempt, and more than 90% of the attempts were influenced by the illness. In both groups, psychosomatic illnesses constituted the majority of diagnoses.

Factors associated with illness and contributing to both suicides and attempts were loss of mobility among persons for whom physical activity was occupationally or recreationally important; disfigurement, particularly among women; and chronic, intractable pain. In addition to the direct effects of illness, the investigators noted the secondary effects of illness-for example, disruption of relationships and loss or required change of occupational status.

Occupation

Among occupational rankings with respect to risk for suicide, physicians have traditionally been considered to stand out, and psychiatrists are considered to be at greatest risk followed by ophthalmologists and anesthesiologists. Special at risk populations are musicians, dentists, law enforcement officers, lawyers, and insurance agents.[33]

SOCIOFAMILIAL APPROACH

This approach should delineate genetic and biological contribution from dysfunctional or abnormal sociofamilial interpersonal interactions towards the suicidee's family pathology. Suicidees' social relation can be divided into 'absent relations' and 'negative relations.'

Absent relations: Loss of parents at an early age.

Absent parents: Disrupted social relations like anomie, etc. and 'negative relations' include suicidogenic relations of bad parenting (parental suicide as a model or child abuse, negative social relations (of cults). The latter group may have an element of altruism in their suicidal behavior.

In 1980, Philip et al.[39,40] demonstrated the contagious nature of the suicide behavior. Sensational newspaper reports have increased rate of suicide, e.g. New York Times publishing suicide reports in 1948 to 1967.

Social stresses can be suicidogenic. Black women are protected against suicide by their social support system despite large family disruptions, clinical depression, and financial depression. House et al. defined stress as "when an individual confronts a situation her usual mode of bravery is not sufficient and the consequence of nonadaptability are serious". Recent life event[41-43] is considered as a change in the external social environment that can be defined approximately. Life crisis is a cluster of life events whose values summed up to 150 life change units or more in one year. The greater the summed up scores of life changes or adaptive requirements, the more the possibility of suicidal completion.[41-43]

PSYCHOLOGICAL APPROACH

Rojtenberg[17] had recently reviewed the psychological approach to suicide.

Freud:[44] The first important psychological insight into suicide came from Freud. In his 1917 paper 'Mourning and Melancholia,' Freud stated that the self-hatred seen in depression originated in anger toward a love object, anger that the person turned back on himself. He regarded suicide as the ultimate form of this phenomenon, and doubted that there would be a suicide without the earlier repressed desire to kill someone else. Freud wrote in 1915 that the unconscious does not believe in its own death. Suicide is a form of self-directed violence.

Zilboorg:[45] He elaborated the importance of unconscious fantasies of immaturity, particularly for suicidal patient. It was an elaboration of Freud's statement that unconscious does not believe in its own death. He expressed that most suicides are committed by persons who were normal prior to the act.

Melanie Klein:[46] She postulated that while the ego tries to kill the bad objects and the id, it simultaneously tries to save the good object by internalizing them and the part of the ego which is identified with them.

Researchers following Klein have considered suicidal act as a psychotic action resulting from defence mechanisms that are responding to persecutory anxieties. To reduce these persecutory anxieties, the suicide victim places an impenetrable barrier between him and the persecutor; beyond that barrier he or she considers that his or her survival will be assured, out of reach of the persecutor. Suicide victim considers that this is the only escape from persecution of the individual by terrorific internal superego images. This fantasy uses mental mechanisms of magic and omnipotence in the belief that suicide act will annihilate the persecutory objects. According to Klein, there are also manic feelings in the suicide victim based on the denial of persons on death. Suicide victim tries to project this persecutory guilt on to his or her objects. This attempt is experienced as a manic triumph over the persecutor.

Alejandro Gomez Ch: This Chilean psychiatrist said that "schizophrenic patients commit suicide because of their illness, and not because of their madness". Schizophrenic patient may commit suicide in a "moment" of improvement. During this period of improvement, the patient perceives the disintegration of his psyche and its social consequences. He becomes exhausted. He becomes sick of his illness. He decides not to go on living with it and commits suicide.[16]

Sergio L Rojtenberg:[17] In his article, 'Suicide: Death as a way out', he concludes that suicide victim values death as an alternative, the only one which will help him/her to stop his/her intense suffering and psychological pain.[17]

Menninger:[19] Menninger says, in committing suicide, the individual kills himself, murders somebody and also fulfills his wish to die. This is called the *Menninger's triad*. Death was considered the only aim of the suicide. This notion is corrected by the psychological interpretation of the meaning of the suicide by experts.

PSYCHIATRIC APPROACH[13,48,59]

Durkheim did not consider mental illness as a cause of suicide.[28] Kraepelin said that one-third of suicide have psychiatric illness,[50] but for Stengel[47] suicidal act successful or unsuccessful may be associated with any clinical psychiatric disorder. To Stengel all fatal acts are suicides and nonfatal self-injury with conscious self-destructive intent is attempted suicide. To Menninger's triad, Stengel added two more dimensions called the *appeal* and the *ordeal*, which arise from urge towards self-preservation.

Suicide attempt complicates and suicide terminates at times almost all forms of mental illness, except mania and anxiety neurosis.[51] Silverman[52] said that depression prior to suicide is probably universal. The follow-up study in western literature reveal that 15% die of suicide among psychotic or neurotic depressives; 10% each from schizophrenia and 5% from psychopathy. Not more than 6–7% were regarded normal among the completed suicides.[53-57]

In their work on depression, Venkoba Rao and Nammalwar[58] recorded suicidal ideas in 48 patients and found history of attempted suicide in 23. Psychiatric profile of 100 suicide attempters studies by Unni et al.[13] between 1992–93, revealed that 47 had definite psychiatric disorders and 43 had no definite psychiatric diagnosis except for the fact that 28 of them had adjustment disorder. There are studies in which suicide among depressive are not reported as frequently as in the Western report. Among the 122 cases of depressives, followed up by Venkoba Rao and Nammalwar for 3–13 years, only 1 committed suicide.[58] Majority of 159 cases of Unni et al.

from South Arcot District of Tamil Nadu, who underwent psychiatric evaluation in a general hospital psychiatric facility in the early 1990s, had some form of depression.[59] Table 11 shows the mortality rates from suicide among depressed as reported by various authors.

BIOLOGICAL ASPECTS OF SUICIDAL BEHAVIOR

Trivedi[49] had reviewed the approach to suicide in biological psychiatry between 1976 and 1990. The first finding of correlation between suicide and low CSF 5-HIAA in depressives with violent methods of suicide attempt, was by Asberg et al. (1976) in Sweden.[47] Out of further 15 studies on patients with recent suicidal attempt, 10 of them demonstrated low CSF 5-HIAA, thus replicating the same finding of Asberg et al.[60,61,63-66,69-71,73] Negative correlation between CSF 5 HIAA and suicidal behavior was reported in the studies done by only 3 groups of authors.[62,67,72] Three other groups of authors found no significant correlation that is no significant difference in the CSF 5 HIAA in suicide attempters.[68,74,75]

The relationship of CSF5-HIAA to suicidality was demonstrated in depression, personality disorders, schizophrenia, alcoholism, adjustment disorders, etc. and also in relation to current writings of suicidology, recent suicide attempts and life time suicide attempts. The findings suggest that low CSF 5-HIAA is correlated to suicide attempts, irrespective of the presence or absence of depression,[2] more strongly to violent attempts than nonviolent attempts, though significantly to both.

Neuroendocrine studies, brainstem studies and genetic studies are the biological approaches based on the medical model of suicide. The biological substrate of suicide is studied by neuroendocrine pharmacochallenge test.

Table 11: Depression and suicide

Authors	*Cases No.*	*Follow-up*	*Dead (No.)*	*Suicide (No.)*	*% Death from suicide (in years)*
Langeludocke	341	40	268	41	15.3
Slater	138	30	59	9	15.3
Lundquist	319	30	119	17	14.3
Seulz	2004	5	492	66	13.4
Stendedt	216	10	42	6	14.3
Pitts and Winokur	56	Death	56	9	16.0
Venkaba Rao and Nammalwar (1977)	122	13	8	1	0.8
-do- (1982)	288	Death	-	3	1.02
(Table adapted from Venkoba Rao A 1992)[14]					

Neuroendocrine Studies

There is evidence for central nervous system serotonergic dysfunction. Some evidence for dopaminergic and LHP target organ axes alterations is also available. These three findings may be related. Valid correlation between CNS function and psychopathology aiming at finding out a marker with predictive value, is the aim of biological approach to suicidology. Neurotransmitter or its metabolite estimation, hormonal measures, receptor density and binding studies, are all traditional methods which may not reflect dynamic neurophysiological processes. Pharmacochallenge is the method for *in vivo* study of targeted neuroendocrine pathways. Pharmacochallenge involve administration of a psychoactive agent and subsequent monitoring of a hormonal response parameter (Table 12).[76-91]

Hierarchical organization of neuroendocrine circuits: Cortical > Subcortical (Limbic) > Hypothalamus> Pituitary body > End organs > Hormones

Weiss and Coccaro[76] in 1997 have summarized the serotonergic challenge studies done between 1984 and 1996. In 1984, Meltzer et al.[77] using the probe 5-HTP (5 hydroxytryptamine) found increased cortisol in suicide attempters of the 40 depressed or manic sample in comparison to healthy controls. Using L-tryptophan, d-fenfluramine, clomipramine, m-chlorophenylpiperazine, buspirone or flesinoxan as probe and using the endocrine variable prolactin, growth hormone or cortisol, no correlation between suicidal variable and the endocrine variable was found in many of the studies.[78,79,81-83,85-87] Decreased cortisol in suicide attempters was found by Pitchot et al.[88] Decreased prolactin in suicide attempters and high lethality suicide attempters were found in for studies using clomipramine or d-fenfluramine.[80,84,87,89,90] Using flesinoxan or d-fenfluramine challenge, decreased cortisol were well correlated with depressed patients having suicide attempt or ideation.[88-90]

Neuroendocrine challenge studies were divided by Mann[91] into transmitter-nonspecific neuroendocrine studies and neurotransmitter-specific neuroendocrine studies. The former implicates limbic-hypothalamic-pituitary-adrenal (LHPA) axis hyperactivity in suicidal behavior. High plasma cortisol and high 17-hydroxy-corticosteroids were both indicative of high suicide risk. The transmitter nonspecific neuroendocrine studies also include pharmacochallenge of the limbic-hypothalamic-pituitary-thyroid (LHPT) axis by using the standard procedure of TRH stimulation test. However definitive the TRH test is, the methodological issues remain and both positive and negative studies utilizing small samples or inadequately specified methods yielding inconclusive results. The positive studies have

Table 12: Pharmacochallenge paradigms

	Pharmacochallenge paradigms	*Yield*
1.	Dexamethasone suppression test	General localization to particular neuroendocrine pathway
2.	Neurotransmitter related pharmacochallenge strategies	Enable study of specific areas of the LHP target organ axes
3.	Pre- and postsynaptic probes (releasing agents, uptake inhibitors, precursors)	Indirect neurotransmitter agonist information conveying endogenous
4.	Direct agonist (serotonin 1a receptor selective agent)	Postsynaptic function at a given receptor subtype[76]

found a connection between suicidality and blunted TSH. The extra usefulness of TRH stimulation test over basal TSH determination methods has been questioned.

Limitations of neuroendocrine research in suicidology

- Many confounding variables present themselves in this research. Pharmacochallenge agents are partially selective and our knowledge of the specific efficacy of the probe and neuroanatomy of a given hormonal response is not complete.
- *Nonchallenge related factors*: Need for placebo correction to contain the pharmacokinetic and pharmacodynamic issues, like exclusion of variance due to nonchallenge related factors like stress of the procedure of challenge and its effects, probes absorption metabolism and distribution, interindividual difference in its handling, and bioavailability mandate the reporting of assays of blood levels of probe. The impact of this variable is proved in DST studies.
- *Interindividual differences*: These are relating to age, gender, weight, and menstrual status. These affects neuroendocrine responses. These are to be minimized in challenge tests.
- *Nonstandardized methodologies and dose response relationships*: Challenge protocols are not standardized. Different probes evaluating the same neuroendocrine circuits have varying properties, making comparison impossible.
- *Ambiguity of the term suicidal*: 'Suicidal' refers to a continuum of heterogeneous and complex phenomena ranging from nonsuicidal thought at one extreme through transient suicidal thought, more continuous intense suicidal ideation, verbal expression of the ideas, gestures and attempts of varied severity, to completed suicide at the extreme. Any, all or some of these can be further subgrouped according to injury or medical lethality, intent and impassivity, and violence of the method. There can be theoretically speaking quite varied relationships between the biological substrate and the varied clinical manifestations.
- *Covariance of depressive illness*: Depressive illness covaries with suicidality. So, it is difficult to separate neuroendocrine aberrations related to depressions from any that are specific to suicidality.[77]

Neuroanatomy of Suicidal Behavior

Arango[92] has summarized the biological alterations in the brain stem of suicidees. Biological abnormalities of brain of persons, who complete or attempt suicide, form some base as to the cause of suicide. Sylvia Plath, the American poet who committed suicide in the year 1963, had several episodes of severe depression.[93] Dr. Trimble on 21-2-97, while delivering the 18th TS Srinivasan endowment lecture in Chennai, illustrated that manic depressions, suicide and mood swing are over-represented among writers; among creative artists, writers are more prone to manic depression. Poetic creativity is linked to the right hemisphere of the brain, which deals with ambiguity, rhythm and metaphor and elements of creative metaphoric language, with emotional coloring and with being mediated by the right cerebral hemisphere.[94]

Locus Coeruleus System (LC)

Norepinephrine (NE) innervation is solely from pigmented LC neurons; these provide innervation throughout the neuraxis including limbic system. At the junction between pons and cerebral peduncles, LC neurons appear in the dorsomedial pons, located bilaterally and symmetrically in the ventrolateral quadrants of central grey. Caudally, it extends up to the rostral-most appearance of motor division of trigeminal nucleus, which is organized in a tubular fashion and reaching 3 to 5 mm caudal to the trochlear nerve decussation. Studies suggest that reduced NE neurotransmission is associated with suicidal behavior.

There is also 23% fewer LC neurons and 38% lower density of LC neurons in suicidees than controls. Reduction is localized to the rostral 2/3rd of the left LC than the right LC. No such laterality is found in the controls. LC length and LC values of suicidees and controls are the same. LC neuron morphometry rostrocaudal difference in normal distribution of neuron size and shape were found within the LC of both suicidees and controls. There were no significant differences in either the size or the shape of neurons in suicidees compared to controls in any region of LC. Females had greater neuronal area and perimeter on the left side of LC in comparison to right side of LC. In males, no such differences were found.

The prefrontal cortex serotonergic function decreases the inhibition on the behavior, which translates the suicidal idea into action in impulsive and violent suicide irrespective of their diagnosis.[92]

Dorsal Raphe Nucleus (DRN)

Approximately 100,000 neurons embedded in the ventral part of the central gray matter of caudal mesencephalon and rostral pons constitute the dorsal raphe nucleus. They are serotonin synthesizing neurons innervating the forebrain with Nissl material; the 5 of its subnuclei, namely ventrolateral, median, dorsal, lateral and caudal. Tissues immunoreacted with an antitryptophan hydroxylase sera actually demonstrate the additional ventral and lateral subnucleus. Their cells are oriented parallel to the midline and their processes extend within the median longitudinal fasciculi. It extends from the anterior pole of the dorsal raphe nucleus to the rostral appearance of median sulcus of fourth ventricle. Caudal to these all dorsal raphe nuclear are neurons on either side of the floor of the fourth ventricle. The serotonergic target cells in the cortex are GABAergic inhibitory neurons. The ascending serotonergic projections include those arising (1) from fine DRN, dorsal, and (2) those arising from DRN, median raphe nucleus. The prefrontal cortex innervation density is in layer I in motor areas, and layer IV in sensory areas, as demonstrated in primates. It may be the same in humans.[92]

In completed suicide, there is reduced 5-HT transporter binding in the prefrontal cortex. It may be due to reduced serotonergic innervation or due to deficient serotonin transporter sites synthesis in the presence of a normal or increased number of serotonergic neurons.

Arango et al.[92] studied the morphometry of 5-HT neurons of DRN (i.e. the total number of 5-HT neurons in DRN and their distribution, neuronal size and shape) and made comparison of the suicidees with controls. Both controls and suicidees exhibit loss of serotonin neurons with increasing age. The demonstration of the alteration of number and density of DRN neurons, as solely due to suicide status may be possible only by stricter designs of controlled studies.

5-HT System

Quantitative postmortem brain tissue studies have revealed neurotransmitter abnormalities in the ventral and lateral prefrontal cortex of the suicide victims. This area is concerned with the behavioral restraint mechanisms. Failure of restraint mechanism may result in suicidal behavior. Morphology and neurochemical studies of dorsal raphe nucleus (5-HT) and locus ceruleus (NE) neurons were studied.

The finding of reduced 5-HT in dorsal and median raphe nucleus and 5-HT in receptor changes in prefrontal cortex in suicide victims may be due to fewer 5-HT synthesizing neurons in the dorsal raphe nucleus of the suicidees. Alterations in the 5-HT neurons in the suicidees may reflect a neurodevelopmental effect of probably genetic origin.

Fenfluramine stimulated prolactin release to test the integrity of 5-HT system showed a blunted response in suicide attempters. In serotonergic function studies in-vivo by using PET and with fenfluramine stimulation, Mann[48,49] found blunted cerebral metabolic response in depressed patients at their prefrontal and temporoparietal cortices, suggesting reduced 5-HT neurotransmission associated with major depression.

Postmortem studies enabling direct examination of brain tissue with high anatomical resolution and quantitative measurement support evidence for serotonergic system abnormalities at the level of brainstem and prefrontal cortex.[92]

Pre- and postsynaptic receptor alterations have been observed in prefrontal cortex in suicidees. This is also consistent with the low serotonergic transmission. Reduced binding to the serotonin transporter is seen in ventral and lateral prefrontal regions, and increased binding to postsynaptic 5-HT_{1A} and 5-HT_{2A} receptors in prefrontal cortex have been found in most studies. Early brainstem serotonergic neuron studies found reduced 5-HT or 5-HIAA in the whole brainstem in suicide victims.[92]

Genetic Studies

Roy et al. (1997) have reviewed the genetic studies pertaining to suicidology.[95-103]

Family Studies

Family studies have shown that suicide can run in families. People who have relatives who died by suicide are at greater risk for suicide.

Serotonergic indices in primates have strong genetic distribution. An altered number of neurons may represent a suicide. The *Ramayana* has details of how Sri Rama suffered from his first episode of depression in his 15th year. Rama's father suffered thrice.[14] Ernest Hemingway's father, brother, sister and himself, and his granddaughter committed suicide. The granddaughter herself felt that the family had inherited alcoholism and suicide.[95]

The questions to be answered by genetic studies are: (i) what is inherited, and (ii) what is the mode of inheritance? Tishler et al.[96] found that 22% of 108 adolescents attempters seen in the emergency services had history of one family member having suicidal behavior. Garfinkel et al.[97] found that in his study of 505 adolescent suicide attempters when compared with youthful controls had a family history of suicidal behavior. Among completed suicides, Shaffer[98] reported that suicidal behavior in a first degree relative had occurred in 7 of 31 youth suicides, 22.6% occurring in England and Wales between 62 and 68. Of the 20 adolescents in Kentucky, Shafii[99] found a significantly high number having a family history suicide, as compared to youths who were controls. In Shaffer's[98] preliminary report on young suicides of New York city, 20 out of 52, 19 years and below age group reported family history of suicide and attempted suicide. Farberow and Simon[100] found 6 out of 100 suicide in Vienna and Los Angeles had a parent who had committed suicide. This is more than 88 times the expected rate.

Robins et al.[101] found that of the 109 suicide attempters, 11% had a family history of suicidal behavior. Pitts and Winokur[102]found 37 out of 748 consecutive cases reporting possible or definite suicide in 1st degree relatives (4.9%). In 25 out of 37 cases, the diagnosis was affective disorder. The familial nature of suicide are reported by Unni[103] and Fakri Dabbagh.[104] But the authors were not sure what was inherited affective disorder or suicidal behavior. Roy et al.[96] reported that violent suicide attempters share a family history of suicide more often than nonviolent suicide attempters. Unni's[104] report of hanging in family members and Dabbagh's[105] report of burning in family members are noteworthy. 123 out of 713 (14%) of Linkowski's[105] depressed patients had a first or second degree relative who committed suicide. He found that a family history of suicide significantly increased the probability of suicide attempt in depressed women, especially the victim of a violent suicide attempt.

Iowa-500 follow-up study of 525 psychiatric patients in comparison to 160 mentally normal appendicectomy patients showed that 30 out of these 685 patients committed suicide during the decade long follow up from 1934-1944. 29 were from the psychiatric patients and only 1 was from the appendicectomy group (5.5% vs 0.6%), thus conclusively proving the association of suicide and psychiatric disorders. Out of 525 patients, 260 were schizophrenics, 100 manics and 225 depressed patients. Egeland and Sussex[106] found only 26 suicides during the 100 years from 1880 to 1980 in the anabaptist, nondrug, nonviolent community of Lancaster county in Southern Pennsylvania; 24 out of 26 suicides had major depression. Three quarters of these 26 suicides cluster together in 4 families of Amish county[3]. In one family, there were 7 suicides and all of them had affective disorder. In a second pedigree also, there was heavy loading of affective disorder; there had been 6 suicides. There were other families with heavy loading of affective disorder but no suicide. Converse is not true. So, familial loading for affective disorder in itself is not a predictor of suicide.

Twin Studies

Monozygotic twins share the same genes but dizygotic twins share only 50% of the genes. In 1967, Haberlandt[107] reviewed 149 sets of twins reported in which one twin had committed suicide. Among the 149 twin pairs, there were 9 monozygotic twin pairs concordant for suicide; there were no dizygotic twin pairs concordant for suicide. Roy et al.[108] studied 35 twins, where one cotwin had committed suicide. They interviewed the living cotwins about their suicidal behavior. They found 10 of 26 living monozygotic cotwins had themselves attempted suicide in comparison to 0 of 9 dizygotic cotwins ($p<0.04$).

Papadimitriou et al.[109] interviewed one relative per subject of his 549 depressed patients; 15 of them had 2 or more first or second degree relatives who had committed suicide. He, however, did not find unilateral pairs of suicide in the family to demonstrate single gene inheritance. Their study is compatible with polygenic inheritance.

Adoption Studies

Danish adoption studies[110,111] demonstrated genetic factors in suicide. Adoptees share their genes but not the subsequent environmental experience with their biological parents. Their '*nature*'aspects are separated from '*nurture*' aspects. Adoptees share their environmental experience with the adopting parents through their but not in their genes. Twin studies show increased suicidal rate in identical twins, regardless of like or different parentage.

SUICIDAL BEHAVIOR IN SPECIAL GROUPS

Children of Prepubertal Age Groups

Pfeffer[112] deals with children and adolescent suicidal behavior along a continuum, with nonicidal behavior at one end, going through suicidal ideation, attempts and suicide.

The child and adolescent suicidal behavior is complex. Pfeffer[112] points out the need to delineate the differences in the behavior during each phase of the child and adolescent development, in a developmental perspective.[113]

Epidemiology

Suicidal behavior in psychiatric prepubertal child patients is higher than the prepubertal children in community. One hundred and one children from psychiatric prepubertal and 101 children from the community were compared for suicidal behavior. In the family groups, 23.8% represented suicidal ideation and 1% attempted suicide, whereas in the latter 10.9% reported suicidal ideation and 1% attempted suicide. Other studies also support that ideation is more common than attempts (Among 40 prepubertal psychiatric outpatient children, 15% some form of suicidal behavior and 3% reported suicidal attempt in history). Suicidal behavior below 5 years is rare. In white nonhispanic male youth, suicide peaks at puberty.

Suicide in 5 to 14 age group is the 6th leading cause of death and in 15 to 24 year olds, it is the 3rd leading cause of death in the United States, accidents and homicide being the first and second. Among nonhispanic 5 to 14 years old boys, committing suicide is the fourth leading cause of death and for girls, it is 6th leading cause of death, and among blacks of this non-hispanic group, suicide is the 8th leading cause of death in the United States. The most common method used is guns and firearms.

Pfeffer's approach to characterization of prepubertal and young adolescent suicidal behavior is based on cognitive maturity (Table 13), emotional expression and behavioral components, apart from familial and extrafamilial factors.

Cognitive Component

Prepubertal children depend on parental and peer support for compensating their immaturity in cognitive development involving self-esteem. Inadequate parenting produces poor self esteem. Self-esteem is a shield against stressful life experiences. Enhancement of self-esteem can be a preventive intervention in prepubertal child suicidology.

Emotional Expression

Anxiety, depression and aggression are the three major emotions associated with prepubertal and young adolescent suicidal behavior. Low mood affects self-esteem, which lead to hopelessness and suicidal ideation and attempt. Prepubertal psychiatrically hospitalized children have increased risk of suicidal behavior. Those of them who have psychotic disorder have a distinct risk of suicide. As substance abuse and alcoholism are not prevalent in the prepubertal and young adolescents, these risk factors are not relevant in these age groups (Table 14).

Presence of a mood disorder contributes to a five fold or four fold higher prevalence of suicide attempt than in children without mood disorder. Suicide attempts took place within mood disorder and not within a disruptive disorder. Low mood in dysthymic and adjustment disorder also increase the risk of suicide. Comorbidity of both mood and disruptive disorder increased suicidal behavior than when mood disorder alone was present.

Table 13: Cognitive components of suicidal behavior in prepubertal children

	Cognitive state	*Consequence of cognitive state*
1.	Prepubertal children have concrete operational level cognitive development	Children appreciate situations in dichotomous ways that lack abstract levels of thinking
2.	They have rigid thinking. Concept of causality, degrees of lethality of attempt and finality of death are not understood fully till age 10	Multiple solutions to problematic situation not possible
3.	Having high feelings of repulsiveness of life (repulsiveness of life) acts as a negative force against living	The degree of mental and physical suffering a child experiences
4.	Have low levels of perception of death and high levels of perception of the attractiveness of death	This persuades the prepubertal children to effect their own death in psychologically overwhelmingly painful situations
5.	No independent problem solving capacity	This produces problems in social adjustment in family, peer and school situations, especially when parental or other external assistance is not provided
6.	Immaturity in coping skills	This produces magnification of hopelessness experienced in stressful situations

Behavioral Components

Impulsive behavior in general is a well correlated risk factor for suicidal behavior. Child suicidal behaviors are provoked by acute events for which child responds with impulsive self-destructive action, most often in the presence of the person with whom adverse interpersonal event happened. Serotonin alterations are implicated in adolescent and adult impulsivity. More studies are required to rule out or confirm the same factor in impulsive behavior of prepubertal children.

Familial and extrafamilial environmental contextual factors also influence prepubertal child's suicidal behavior. Family discord is an important external stress. Parental loss due to separation, death, divorce, war or riots produce a constellation of internal factors in the form of a stressful life event. Parental abuse of children is associated with cognitive distortion, instability, impulsivity, shame, guilt and propensity for suicidal ideation and behavior. Family psychopathological history of suicidal prepubertal children reveals more violence, alcoholism, substance abuse and impulsivity, than non-suicidal prepubertal children. Suicidal prepubertal children have more suicide attempts and suicide among the relatives than nonsuicidal prepubertal children. Failure in social and academic activities in school are a major insult to their sense of self-acceptance, producing acute personal crisis and suicidal behavior. These extrafamilial factors also produce a strain on the cognitive immaturity and inadequate problem solving capacity of prepubertal children.

Prepubertal suicide attempts makes the youngster risky for recurrent attempts. Prepubertal psychiatric inpatient, who attempted suicide, is six times more likely to attempt

Table 14: Prevalence of suicidal behavior in prepubertal children

Psychiatric diagnosis	*Suicidal ideation*	*Suicidal attempt*
Major depressive disorder	65%	17%
Dysthymic disorder	65%	9%
Adjustment disorder with depressive mood	58%	5%
Children without mood disorder	39%	-

Table 15: Characteristics of elderly suicide

Characteristics	Young suicide	Elderly suicide
1. Lethality	Less lethal	Lethal, as a rule
2. Ratio of attempt to completion	200:1	4:1
3. Factors affecting lethality		Frailer subject to acute and chronic diseases; More isolated, probably neglected. Greater determination to die; fewer warnings of suicidal plans, violent/ deadly methods, often, greater planning/ resolve; once initiated, becomes deadly
4. Management	Emphasis on primary and secondary prevention. Identification of risks groups in hospital and community	Emphasis solely on primary prevention. Identification of risks groups in primary care before the suicidal crisis

suicide in adolescence, than the children in the community. Prepubertal psychiatric inpatients with suicidal ideations have four times risk for attempting suicide within ten years than children in general population. Adolescent psychiatric inpatient, who attempts suicide, have significant risk for repeating the act within six months after discharge. Children with major affective disorder are at a higher risk for suicide attempt in adolescence and suicide in young adulthood. Copycat cluster suicide, more common in youth, are reported in 1986 and 1989.[114-119]

Elderly Suicide

Suicide in those over 65 years of age occurs predominantly in men (80%), a third of whom are married and living with their spouse. Almost two-thirds, at the time of suicide, are living with family members or friends. About half explicitly mention thoughts of suicide or of dying in the last 6 months of life, yet their suicide surprises those who knew them. About 10% are terminally ill and 25% have a severe chronic medical illness. Their rate of suicide is 15 times higher for this age group than in the general population The majority (90%) have symptoms of major depression, but only a few have contact with a psychiatrist or a mental health professional. One-fifth of geriatric suicide patients see a physician within 24 hours before their death, and almost half see a physician within a week prior to their suicide (Table 15).[141]

Biological Risks

Twin and adoption studies have not included elderly subjects. Family history of affective illness is less likely with older age of onset of affective disorder. In elderly suicide, genetic predisposition is less of risk factor, but 5-HT, norepinephrine and neuroendocrine systems are most consistently implicated in elderly suicide.

Trait and State Characteristics

Fewer personality disorders can be implicated in elderly suicide than in younger adults and personality disorders as a cause of suicide in the elderly is not established. However, personality traits like timidity, restricted interest, tendency to hypochondriasis and seclusiveness are identified in the elderly suicidees, who become hostile, irritable and difficult to satisfy when confronted with disease. Elderly male suicidees going through a narcissistic crisis induced by aging related changes, with rigid and fiercely independent styles in the face of covert dependency, is a common finding in the elderly. Elderly are methodical, anhedonic and emotionally constricted, with less openness to newer experiences. These can be factors which make them vulnerable for suicidal behavior. Beck has demonstrated that hopelessness is an important factor, apart from past history of attempt in elderly suicidees.[120,121]

Ferrey has observed that, in France also, either people rarely attempt but when they do they really choose the definite methods. He is of the opinion that suicide in the elderly is a barometer for their misery. Between 1977 and 1983, there was a considerable increase in the total number of suicide in France (1977—9,000, 1983—12,000). The toll of suicide was stable between 1950 and 1976, at around 15.5/100,000 population, and in the 1990s it became 20/100,000 population. For the elderly suicides for both sexes, the frequency is more in the rural milieu than in the urban setting. He is of the opinion that the chances for socialization for the elderly, which are available in the cities, are 'suicide counters'. Just like other countries, for the female population, matrimonial status is not a determinant factor with regard to chances of suicide. But the widows commit suicide two times more often than the married women. Suicide rate is high for the widower, for the single unmarried men, for the divorcee and for the married people in the order of recurrence. The fact that the social milieu of cities is protective for the elderly suicidees is an interesting and paradoxical factor in comparison to the cities in India.[122]

Suicide Among Migrant Population

Patel and Gaw[123] reviewed all medicine references on completed suicides from 1966-1994 and psychiatric abstracts in immigrants to USA from Indian Subcontinent (India, Pakistan, Srilanka and Bangladesh) to know the psychosocial factors contributing to suicide in this group. Suicide rates of young women immigrants from the Indian Subcontinent were found higher than those of their male counterparts and of young women in the indigenous population of the countries to which they immigrate. Suicide rate among older men in this group was low. Hanging and poisoning were common in both men and women. Disproportionately higher number of Hindus committed suicide. Family conflict was a precipitating factor and mental illness was cited as a cause. Depression, anxiety and domestic violence might have caused the higher rates. Selective disorders may be underdiagnosed in this population

Fiji has equal number of Indians and indigenous Fijians. Earlier studies with police records have demonstrated racial, regional, age and gender differences in suicidal behavior. Pridmore et al.[124] analyzed hanging and poisoning autopsy reports from 2 different regions. Rates of autopsy were 19.5/100,000 population per year for Indians and 1.53 for Fijians. There were more autopsies in females than males, and percentage of hanging autopsy among the total suicides in Fijian males (1.98) were significantly greater than the females (0.40) Among Indians, there were no significant differences. Hanging remained the preferred method of all groups. The mean age at autopsy was 31.7. There was no difference in the mean ages of the two races, sexes or the regions. Thus, they demonstrate significant racial differences in rates of suicide and influence of age, region and method are not significant.[124]

Paris[125] demonstrated cultural factors in the emergence of borderline personality pathology. Borderline personality disorder (BPD) can be diagnosed in developing countries too, even if reports are more for the western societies. It is likely that this type of pathology is more prevalent in North America and Europe. However, the personality traits and psychological risk factors underlying the borderline personality may also be found in individuals from developing countries. They demonstrated cases in which the borderline pathology emerged only after migration. Social protective factors may be suppressing the development of these traits into the diagnostic personality disorder.[125] Neeleman et al.[126] studied the referral rates amongst different ethnic groups to the inner city deliberate self-harm team over a 6 months period, using native British standard. Indian female ratio were 2.6 times that of whites. Among United Kingdom born Indian females, crude rates were 7.8 times those of UK born white females. Unemployment was associated with 9 times increased referral rate amongst whites and 3 times increased referral rate amongst ethnic minorities. Ethnicity modified the association between unemployment and deliberate self-harm rates.

Maniam[127] studied 40 Indian families, 19 suicides with age, sex and educational level matched 21 controls with the index case of suicide. Among the different variables like income,overcrowding, birth order of index cases of suicide, family history of suicide behavior and mental illness, marital disharmony, alcohol abuse, availability and knowledge of pesticide, talk or behavior of suicide in family members, and experience of significant losses in the past one year. The significant differences were found only for the suicides. More than 75% of birth groups had alcohol related problems. Equal proportion of each group had family history of suicide or mental illness. There were statistically insignificant higher rate of marital disharmony in families of suicide.[127]

INDIRECT SUICIDAL BEHAVIOR

Nandi[9], speaking on aggression in 1985, had pointed out that the method of self-torture for the propitiation of God is practiced in every religion, e.g. the rituals to invoke Lord Shiva ('*Gajan*' rituals in Bengal). The procedure includes fasting, prostrating before place of worship, piercing the tongue with a nail, fire walking, walking on thorns, traversing a specified distance by repeatedly rolling in prostrated body position ('*dandapranam*' in Hindi, '*angaprathakshanam*' in Tamil, and '*Sayanapra-dakshanam*' in Malayalam) are used in the prayer places.

Dharna and hunger strikes are part of political demonstrations with similar qualities.[9] Khandelwal et al.[128] reported autocastration in a patient with a sadness, hopelessness, worthlessness and intense suicidal wishes. There were no features to diagnose schizophrenia or delirium in this 80-year-old patient. The autocastration was done with a serious intent to die. The authors did not know why the old patient chose such a unusual and gruesome method for suicide.

Dermatitis artefacta in an 18-year-old girl as a method of disfiguring herself while her lover denied life partnership, was reported by Unni et al. in 1992. This will come under the category of chronic suicide.[129]

Chandrasekaran et al.[130] described Munchausen syndrome in a 38-year-old male who, on psychological tests, proved to be an emotionally unstable introvert who had unhappy childhood, frustration with parents, his ill-health, feelings of impotency, unwanted marriage and unhappy work environment and preference to take shelter in hospitals and 'remain undiagnosed'. In cases of Munchausen syndrome by proxy, the accompanying mother who invariably is the inducer of the 'lesion/illness' in the child, shares the help seeking characteristic of the suicide attempter, who wishes to change her life circumstances.[131]

The incidence in Madurai city (way back in 1966) and the incidence in North 24 Parganas in West Bengal (in 1990), apart from that of Daspur village (Calcutta, in 1979) and that of Warangal District (in 1993), illustrates that India is a highly suicide prone area. However, the findings from other studies as shown above suggest that suicide prone areas may be patchy in India. Till simultaneous all state level, zonal level and national level epidemiological reports are available, one can infer only to the above extent. Considering the fact that what we have is data based on police records, the unreliability and distortion of information in the available reports cannot be ruled out; there will be intracultural variations in the reports on the population of the police districts.

Table 16 shows that between the 1960 and 1993, the preponderance of the age group (second and third decade) has remained the same. Female preponderance was reported by Ayappan and Jayadev in 1956 and the same continues to be the case in 1961, 1979 and 1990. But the Government of India report in 1976 illustrates male preponderance. This finding is true in the report of authors in 1966, 1980 and 1993. Over-representation of married people, in most of the studies where details are available, is noteworthy. Domestic problems and quarrels, and problems related to employment (including unemployment), examination, love affair and physical illnesses reported in the above studies are according to the age group within the second and third decade (Table 17). Fire arms were never used by any of the subjects in the above studies.[132-144]

Ponnudurai,[144] after reviewing twelve studies on suicidology from different parts of the country, has concluded that second and third decade of life seems to be most susceptible period for Indian suicides. Noteworthy causative factor was strain of the relationship with the significant to others. Marriage appeared to increase the proneness for suicidal behavior. In gradation, poisoning, hanging, drowning and burning were utilized by the suicidees. Mehta et al., Unni et al. and Sudhir kumar et al. have studied suicidal behavior in Pondicherry area.[13,145,146] Major illness, which the patients suffered, was found to be some form of depression and majority of their samples were represented by single unemployed low literate subjects. Mahla et al.[147] have studied the psychopathology of self-immolation in India.

Table 16: Suicidology in India: some findings-incidence[132-144]

Author, Year	*Place*	*Incidence (per 100,000 population)*
Nandi et al. 1979	Kolkata (Chandrakona village)	5.13
Govt. of India Report 1988	–	6.8
Govt. of India Report 1976	–	7.8
Satyavathi and Murti Rao 1961	Bengaluru	8.1
Hegde 1980	North Karnataka: Rural	9.3
Shah 1960	Sourashtra	14.1
Ponnudurai et al. 1990	Chennai	14.14
Sharma and Sawang 1993	Warrangal district: Rural	22.83
Nandi et al. 1979	Kolkata (Daspur village)	28.57
Sukula et al. 1990	Jhansi	29
Ganapati and Venkoba Rao 1966	Madurai	43
Banarjee et al. 1990	North 24 Parganas (West Bengal)	43.4

Venkoba Rao et al.[148] studied 100 female burns cases in Madurai Kamaraj Hospital and reported that only 23% of them had psychiatric disorders; 15% of them had physical illnesses, and 51% had marital interpersonal problems. He utilized psychological autopsy for collection of data and reconstruction of the anatomy of the suicide.

MANAGEMENT OF SUICIDAL BEHAVIOR

Suicidal patients frequent psychiatric emergency services and are subject to recurrent crises in management. It is difficult to identify the suicidal person with definiteness. He is averse to hospitalization and difficult to manage in the outpatient services.

Risk Assessment

Weissman and Jorden (1972) have suggested risk-rescue rating, which is reported to be valuable in determining the patient's lethality, need for psychiatric hospitalization and perhaps overall prognosis. The risk factors include the agent used, impairment of consciousness, toxicity and extent of lesions, reversibility and treatment required. The rescue factors include the location of the attempt, the person initiating the rescue, the probability of discovery, the accessibility to rescue and the delay until discovery.

Risk-rescue rating = risk score/risk score + rescue score

The possible lethality ratings range from 17 (denoting the lowest risk score of 1 and a high rescue score of 5) to 83 (indicating a high risk score of 5 and a low rescue score of 1).[149]

Suicidal Patient in Psychiatric Emergency

In any given casualty service, 0.3% to 1% of all patients constitute suicide attempts. Risk factors cited in the literature include major depression, male sex, alcohol/substance abuse, previous suicide attempts and threats, unmarried or widowed individuals, youth and elderly (bimodal pattern), unemployment (especially recently unemployed), living alone, and chronic illness or chronic pain. Risk factors actually are age related.

Suicide Risk Factors: Ages 13 to 30

Male suicides are predominant. Whites commit suicide more often than blacks. Risk factors include psychiatric

Table 17: Demographic variables, mode and cause[132-144]

Author	*Sex*	*Age group*	*Marital status*	*Mode of suicide*	*Cause of suicide*
Sathyavathi and Murti Rao (Bengaluru) (1961)	Females	II and III decade	Married	-	Domestic problems
Ganapathy and Venkoba Rao (Madurai) (1966)	Males	-do-	-	Poisoning	Failure in exam and love affair in younger age group, poverty, unemployment and physical illness in older age group.
Nandi et al. Chandrakona village (1979) (Kolkata)	Females	-do-	-	Poisoning	Quarrel with spouse
-do- Daspur village (Kolkata)	Females	-do-	-	Poisoning	-do-
Hegde (1980) (North Karnataka-Rural)	Males	-do-	-	Drowning	Quarrel with spouse and in-laws
Ponnudurai and Jayakar (Chennai) (1980)	Males	-do-	Married (in women)	Hanging	Quarrel with spouse (in females)
Ponnudurai et al. (Chennai) (1990)	-	-do-	-	-	-
Shukla et al. (Jhansi) (1990)	Females	-do-	Married	Poisoning	Domestic strife
Banerjee et al. North 24 Parganas (West Bengal) (1990)	Females	-do-	-	-do-	Quarrel with spouse
Sarma and Sawang (Warrangal district rural areas) (1993)	Males	-do-	-	-do-	Physical problems

illness (depression, affective disorders, and substance abuse, including alcohol), positive family history of early-onset affective disorder, and history of previous suicide attempts.[16,34]

Suicide Risk Factors: Ages 30+

Important factors are family history of suicide (suggesting genetic transmission), diagnosis of a major affective disorder (bipolar disorder or recurrent unipolar depression), schizophrenia and alcoholism. Suicide risk is not constant in the clinical course of these disorders. Episodes of acute depressive symptoms, accompanied by feelings of hopelessness, despair, pessimism, and helplessness). Although females are more likely to become depressed than males, males are more prone to suicide, especially alcoholic males. Single, separated, divorced, or widowed status, associated medical illness, lack of support, sudden change in social or economic status and inadequate or no treatment of the associated psychiatric disorder.[16,34]

Goals of Evaluation

Assessment of suicidal thinking (ideas, wishes, motives), suicidal intent (both stated intent and inferred intent), suicidal plans, any deterrents to the attempt (religion/family/fear), reaction to the attempt, future orientation and relevant mental status are to be done at the time of hospitalization and serially after hospitalization.

Hospitalization

Inpatient care is mandatory when a patient expresses the intention to commit suicide and has definite plans and means to do it, when he has uncontrollable suicidal impulses, or is acutely psychotic with suicidal ideation/attempt, when the degree of attempt is severe and the intent to die is marked, when the patient has comorbid substance/alcohol abuse, if he has major depression with or without history of attempts, when outpatient treatment is a failure, and a repeat detailed work-up is warranted.

Basic steps of the management for a person who attempts suicide include maintenance of a supportive, accepting, nonjudgmental attitude, management of the medical or surgical problem created by the attempt, assessment of the patient's mental state, assessment of the patient's feeling and determination of appropriate consultation, admission or discharge.[16,34,149]

Management of Prepubertal Suicidal Patient

Developing trustful atmosphere, diligent and truthful communication, consistent empathic but objective approach of the therapist to the youngster, discussion and demonstration of new coping strategies, and finding out of the actual motivation of the suicidal behavior are some of the different aspects undertaken in the hospital based on a multimodal paradigm. Dynamic, supportive, cognitive and drug therapy are instituted while trying to identify biological basis, if any, of suicidal behavior. Once identified they are treated with more specific psychopharmacological interventions. Parental participation, parental marriage counseling, reorientation of parenting, collaboration with the teacher, collaboration with the local general practitioner or patient's family physician are also important aspects in the treatment of the growing child.

Treatment of Suicidal Children

Treatment approaches in this age group are based on clinical experience. No controlled studies of suicidal children are available. The aim is to decrease the likelihood of self-inflicted injury or death. There is no medication specific to suicidal behavior. Hospitalization for 24 hour monitoring and removing the youngster from stressful situation, psychotherapy to build up a trustful atmosphere for truthful communication, delineation of the motivation for the suicidal act, in a multi model approach form the basis of management of child suicidal behavior. Multimodal approach includes simultaneous use of dynamic, supportive, cognitive psychotherapy, psychopharmacotherapy, apart from treatment of parents and relatives, if they have psychopathology which impairs the youngster's family milieu. Collaboration with school teacher, school psychologists and school guidance counselors, who may interact with youngsters during school hours, is of much help in managing child suicidal behavior.

Prevention

Public health model strategies include developing a method for public to respond to a youth suicidal behavior, training of media personnel to report the incident in less sensational manner, and follow-up monitoring of youngsters who have a family history of suicidal behavior and mood and psychiatric disorders. Legal prevention of weapons used by civilians, like guns and firearms, and spiritual intervention to take care of the spiritual health of the youngster are some of the preventive strategies. Seshadri et al., in their study of attempted suicide in children, reported that the extent of such behavior are difficult to gauge as they are reported as accidental.[112,113,150]

Management of Suicidal Patient with Schizophrenia

Suicidal behavior is considered to be the main cause of premature death in schizophrenia. 10 to 13% of patients with schizophrenia commit suicide, while 20 to 40% of them attempt suicide. According to WHO, 'the risk for suicide in schizophrenia is as great, if not greater, than the risk of suicide associated with affective disorders'. This finding is based on a five year follow-up study of 1065 patients with psychosis. Single and unemployed individuals with schizophrenia are at a higher risk for suicidal behavior than married and employed. Most of the schizophrenic patients are single and unemployed as the illness starts at a very early age before they settle down in employment and marriage. So it is difficult to interpret the findings of these sociodemographic studies.

The assessment of risk factors for suicidal behavior in schizophrenia includes previous attempts, postpsychotic depression, comorbid substance abuse, changes in social functioning, aggression and impulsiveness. In people with schizophrenia, the single best predictor of suicidal behavior is previous attempts. There has been little evidence that psychosis precipitates suicidal behavior. Suicidal behavior is only very rarely precipitated by command hallucinations. Some researchers have found higher rate of depression in schizophrenia patients who are suicide attempters and completers. Others have maintained that there is no difference between schizophrenia patients with and without suicidal behavior. A third group is of the opinion that hopelessness and decreased self-esteem, rather than depressed mood, account for the differences between suicidal and nonsuicidal schizophrenic patients. These depressive symptoms may be a differentiating factor between the suicidal and nonsuicidal schizophrenic patients. In schizophrenia, some researchers have demonstrated increased substance abuse in attempters and completers than the nonsuicidal schizophrenic patients.

Limited social support from the family and recent loss or changes in social structure are found to be associated with increased suicidal behavior in schizophrenia. A period of increased risk for suicidal behavior occurs when patients with schizophrenia are informed that they will not be able to return home to family members. Assessment of social support system and networking are important aspects of suicide prevention in schizophrenia. Suicidal behavior is multi-determined in schizophrenia. Even if the treatment focus is on risk assessment with regard to planfulness, persistence and potential lethality, if one patient with schizophrenia reports hallucinations with suicidal content, treatment should be multifaceted including psychopharmacotherapy, nonpharmacotherapeutic intervention, manipulation of the treatment milieu, hospitalization, improvement of crisis services, and enhancement of family environment and social support network. Management of postpsychotic depression is an important factor in the prevention of suicide in schizophrenic patients. Varghese[151] has pointed out that schizophrenic patients are usually seclusive with regard to their suicidal ideas, often use violent and definite successful methods, and often complete suicide.

Treatment of Suicidal Patients with Affective Disorder

People with bipolar affective disorder, borderline personality disorder and alcohol dependence are at a highest risk among the suicidal patients with affective disorder. There is very strong evidence from controlled trials that mood elevators are more effective than placebo in reducing suicidal ideation. It is less clear that antidepressant medication reduces the risk of suicide attempts. An evaluation of the design of different studies shows that the efficacy of antidepressants in reducing the risk of suicide attempt has not been assessed adequately with a control study. Serotonergic agents may produce a more rapid improvement in suicidal ideation at about two weeks of treatment, relative to other antidepressants. This differential effect disappears by 4 to 6 weeks of treatment. Serotonergic activity is related to the risk of suicide and serious suicide attempts, according to postmortem studies of suicide victims. Altered serotonin function represents a critical biologic substrate forming the basis for understanding the pathogenesis and final common pathway of suicidal thoughts. This may provide a target for future antisuicide pharmacotherapies.

According to Venkoba Rao, all depressives are potential suicidees. Serotonin substrate is also related to aggressive behavior. Suicide risk, once antidepressant therapy is initiated, is at its peak when the patient actually comes out of depression. Before starting the antidepressant therapy the patient is at highest risk, during the period while he goes into a depression. Hospitalization is necessary for higher risk patients, especially during these two stages of the course of their disease. There is some question as to whether raising the threshold for suicidal behavior with a more serotonin-selective agents may protect the patient during the initial period before the antidepressant action of the medication has begun to take hold. A third phase of risk for hospitalized depressed patients is when they are discharged from the hospital. Every effort should be made for close clinical follow-up and interdisciplinary communication between inpatient and outpatient clinicians during the days and weeks following hospital discharge.

Some studies have reported that the rate of suicide per suicide attempts per prescription is much higher with older generation antidepressants like tricyclic antidepressants in comparison to new generation antidepressants. In patients with significant suicidal ideation or a past history of suicidal behavior, new generation antidepressants may be a better choice. The role of electroconvulsive therapy is demonstrated by significantly lower rates for suicide following electroconvulsive therapy than with medication. Understanding the mechanism of action of electroconvulsive therapy may be relevant in understand-ing the brain mechanisms associated with suicidal behavior. Patient, family and public psychoeducation are other strategies for reducing suicidal behavior in affectively ill patients.

The role of mood stabilizers, like lithium, carbamazepine and sodium valproate, is demonstrated in the treatment of suicidal depressives. Their success in the management of explosive symptoms suggest that they may be beneficial in reducing the frequency and intensity of suicidal behavior in bipolar affective disorder. A novel psychotherapy, known as dialectical behavior therapy, is devised specifically targeting suicidal behavior in borderline personality disorders. This, in conjunction with pharmacotherapy for the management of suicidal behavior in depressed borderline personality disorder population, needs further evaluation. Disproportionate suicidality among depressed alcoholics has persuaded researchers to recommend that patients with comorbid depression and alcohol abuse or dependence should be treated with SSRI antidepressants.[152]

Management of Elderly Suicidal Behavior

Management is mainly by prevention, as the suicidal behavior in the elderly is more lethal than in the younger age groups. There are five risk factors contributing to the risk of elderly suicide in an overlapping fashion. These include factors connected with genetics and family history, biology, personality traits, psychiatric disorder and psychosocial milieu. Methods to alleviate the contribution towards the suicide risk by adequate intervention of aging, neurotransmitter and neuroendocrine related systems of neurobiological substrate are central to treatment of suicidal behavior in the elderly. The treatment of psychiatric illness, especially depression (most often single episode unipolar depression), may be of much help in suicide prevention in the elderly. Comorbid substance abuse, if present, is also to be addressed in the treatment of elderly depressives.

Late life depression should be diagnosed early for early intervention. Prevention is by improving the skills of the primary care physician, who is frequently visited by the elderly suicide completor during the weeks prior to his suicidal behavior. Apart from the environmental manipulation to decrease loneliness of the elders, strategies to decrease the elder abuse also should be implemented in the psychoeducational and family intervention of the elderly suicidal patients. This aspect can fill the last days of the elderly with hope and opportunity for sharing of ideas and their ability for acknowledging the respect, love and affection by their younger relatives and friends.[153]

COMPREHENSIVE CASCADE MODEL (FIG. 3)

After referring to Koestler,[154] Shaffer et al.,[98] Wells and Stuart,[116] Farmer and Hirsch[117] and Shafii et al.,[99] Roy et al.,[95,108] Malone et al.,[90] and Mann et al.[91] the comprehensive cascade model of suicide is proposed by the author. Neurobiological[91] and genetic[95] approach enables one to think that the genetic risk factors are available in the child right from the birth, when the zest for life[154] (resistance to misfortune) is at its peak.[115,116] Psychological autopsy method in adolescent suicidology reveals that risk factors are present in childhood.[155-157]

Resistance to misfortune or the zest for the life is a product of the interaction of neurobiological substrate with the environment, which is manifested in the form of adjustment to changing situations, and coping strategies. This is floated in the Y axis and the life events and its cumulative effect are floated in the X axis. At birth in the life space, the zest for life is at its peak and the onslaught of environmental problems are minimum. Each life events triggers a chain of reaction which are manifested as coping skills and adjustments, but at the same time the memory of the life events persists. This may add to a percentage of decrease in the threshold of suicide.[156,157] Havens[155] described suicide as the final common pathway of diverse circumstances, of an in-depth dependence network rather than an isolated cause, a knot of circumstances tightening around a single time and place. Social support and/or professional support can reduce the negative impact of adverse life events on the coping strategies/resources of the individual.

According to Arthur Koestler, organisms are social bodies or *holons*. There are universal characteristic of holons in the holarchic order every holon is possessed of two opposite potentials; an integrative tendency to function as part of the larger whole, and self-assertive tendency to preserve its individual autonomy. Such polarities are reflected as:

Integration ↔ Self-assertion; Partness ↔ Wholeness
Dependence ↔ Autonomy; Centripetal ↔ Centrifugal
Cooperation ↔ Competition; Altruism ↔ Egotism

These are manifestations of eros and thanatos. These are even beyond thanatos. Resistance to misfortune and self-destructive behavior are the extreme manifestation of the polarity in the holons.

Resistance to misfortune is a result of the interaction of the biological matrix of the holon with the environment, and so is his self destructive behavior. Life events interact with this continuum, and produce a cumulative effect, which helps the reduction of the threshold for individual's suicide.

Each life event produces an impact on the continuum and the resistance to misfortune decreases in the individual. Repair mechanisms of the resistance matrix help to tide over a particular life event, and the individual recovers from the impact. Memories of previous life events get extrapolated into the future confrontation of life events, producing a cumulative effect and a reduction of his reserves of resistance to misfortune and threshold for suicide. When the threshold is low, the individuals kill themselves after slight troubles. These slight troubles, or the substantial understandable life events, finally push the individuals to decide upon the plans, and the practice of those plans to their successful completion. Self-esteem, or the estimate man passes on himself, is decisive in his psychological development and motivation. This value judgment of the self by the self, depends on self-confidence, the sense of self-efficacy and self-respect, and the sense of selfworthiness. Fundamental requirement of self-esteem is the preservation of one's will to understand. In suicidal behavior, these aspects are impaired.

This comprehensive cascade theory encompasses the multi-dimensional, interactive, multidetermined nature of suicide, genetic contribution, personality characteristics, temperamental traits and disorders, impact of life events, coping styles, result of coping strategies, adjustments to life situations, course of different impacts, coping styles and adjustments, their cumulative effects towards the decrease of the zest for life, leading to gradual decrease in the threshold for suicidal behavior (Fig. 3). These are taking place in the individual in a dynamic interactive fashion, interaction being between his biological substrate and his social, interpersonal and material milieu. These interactions involve his coping mechanisms, help seeking behavior and the social support extended or otherwise by the society.

In this model, the life event (LE) is conceptualized to be pushing down the individual with regard to his resistance to misfortune in his life space. This downward trend is arrested by social support (SS) and professional support (PS). PS and SS include not only the reduction, control or arrest of suicidal ideas, but also the restriction of access the lethal material. The timeliness of SS and PS will help this downward course to be arrested early. The adequacy of the SS and PS will help arrest the downward trend adequately.

Thus, the life events have a cascading effect on the steady progress of the individual, based on his zest for life, in his life space.

METHODS IN SUICIDOLOGY (FIG. 4)

Psychological autopsies with a systematic sample of intimate individual survivors of completed suicides, case controlled design with completed suicides as cases and known fatal suicide attempters and natural deaths as the control groups,

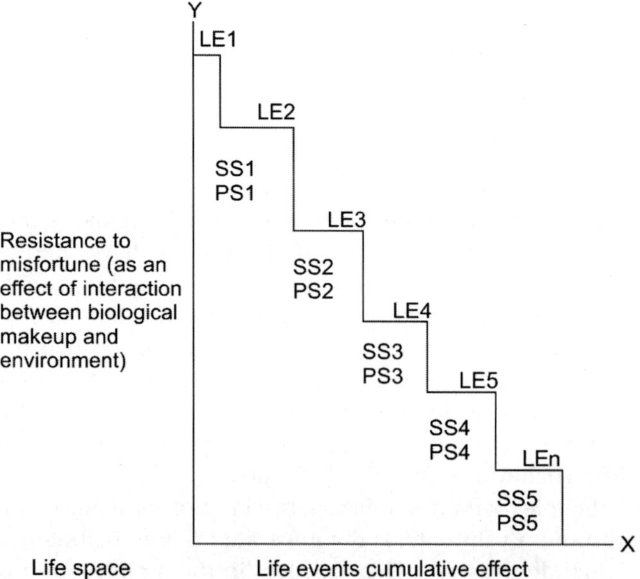

Fig. 3 Comprehensive cascade model
Abbreviations: LE, life event; SS, social support; PS, professional support; Life space, the socioenvironmental milieu

employing sophisticated multivariate statistical analyses, developing a biopsychosocial model of suicide outcome, exploring religious attitudes and behavior and conceiving of suicide developmentally etc were the methods of study used by Maris in suicidology.[18,28,29]

Psychological Autopsy

In-depth study of the suicidee's history prior to the act is called psychological autopsy. The information gathered by this method will enable the researcher to reconstruct the events leading to the suicide behavior and to determine the exact nature of the method used. A discrepancy between dying declaration and information given to the researcher may be noticeable. The psychological autopsy findings are usually compared with the medicolegal autopsy findings. A tally or congruence or otherwise, of these to autopsy findings can reveal many aspects of phenomenon like burns cases in the community. Data gathered by these methods in suicide should be researched, along with the findings of prospective suicides undergoing treatment in hospitals wards. The results may offer clues for suicide prevention.[158]

Postvention[14,159]

This procedure is part of suicide prevention. It is aimed at survivors' welfare. The family welfare or relatives of the suicidee will be left with the social stigma of the family event, the sociofamilial phenomenon's psychological contingence on the family members. This may cause repetition of the act by another family member, when confounded with a stressful situation. Some may be pondering over the idea immediately after the suicide victim's death. This procedure is also aimed at survivor death of a failed suicide attempt. It includes immediate psychotherapeutic intervention (crisis intervention) for resolution of conflicts and planning of treatment of any family member who has grief reaction, mental or physical illness. The therapist should accept the emotional impact of the family member like shock, grief, guilt, depression, or anxiety. Therapist should keep in mind both the nature-nurture paradigms for the management of family members' emotional problems. Research on completed suicide, otherwise confines to protocols on post mortem studies.

The suicidal idea is a contagion. It can be taken up and enacted by children, adolescents or young adults, in children and adolescents especially it can occur on a 'copycat' model. The heredofamilial nature of the suicide is another aspect which the therapist should keep in mind.[14,159]

Measuring Scales Used in Suicidology Research

Some measuring scales used in suicidology research include:

- Brief cognitive rating scale[160]
- International personality disorder examination[161]
- Risk rescue rating scale[162]
- Suicide intent scale[163,164]
- Hopelessness scale[165]
- Montgomery asberg depression rating scale[166]
- Presumptive stressful life events scale.[41]

Problems in the Interpretation of Suicide Literature (Fig. 4)

- Statistics obtained at one point in time may not be valid at a later point in time. Morgan[167] demonstrates the instability of suicide statistics across decades.
- Statistics obtained in one population may not be extrapolated with validity to other populations. For example, considerable differences exist between suicide

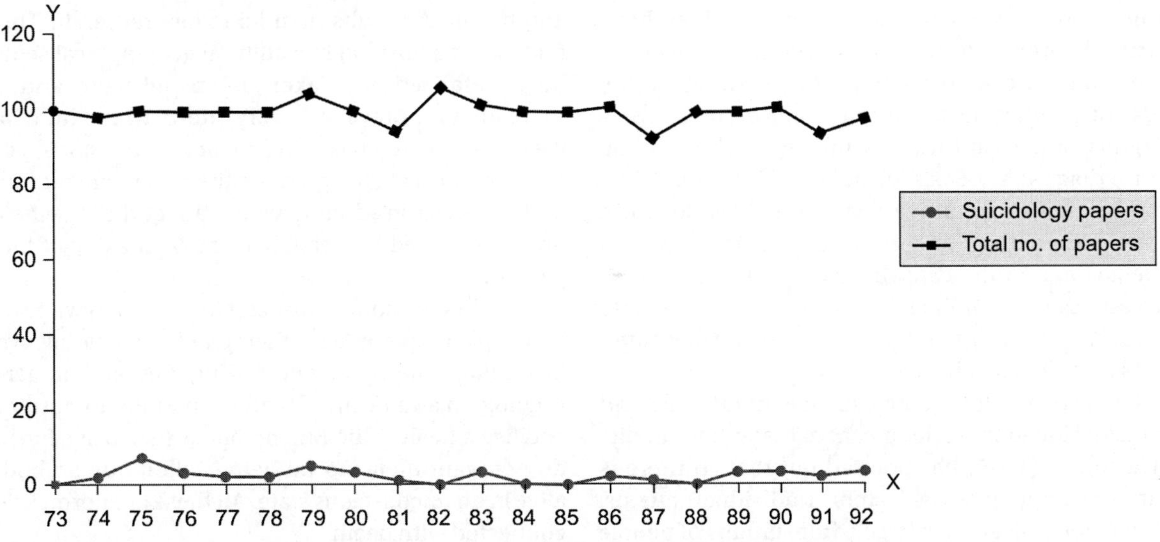

Fig. 4 Layout of research done on suicide per year from 1973–92

attempters in India (Gupta and Singh,[168] Ponnudurai et al.)[169] and Puerto Rico (Fernandez Pol)[170] and Singapore (Hassan).[171]

- Statistics may reflect sampling bias. For example, a series obtained at a general hospital may differ from that at a psychiatric facility, which in turn may differ from that at a suicide prevention organization, whether lay or professional; none of these may be congruent with general population statistics recorded by civic bodies. The last-mentioned set of statistics suffers from the additional liability of poor case identification and deliberate nonreport. Other related difficulties are discussed by Morgan.[167]
- Statistics describing a heterogeneous (in sociodemographic or clinical variables) population (e.g. all suicides and parasuicides) in a given hospital over a given period of time may not be valid for a homogenous population (e.g. depressives, or schizophrenics, or children, or the elderly etc.) as the subsequent sections clarify.[172]

Seshadri and Babu[173] have noted that suicidology deals mainly with a (1) evaluation of previous and current behavior in terms of risk of death, and (2) prediction of possibility of future repetition. Clinical and socioeconomic differences between suicides and attempters is 1:10, as reported by Stengel[174,175] in 1970. Paykel et al.[176] in 1975 have demonstrated that patients with suicidal behavior show four times an incidence of upsetting, threatening life events outside the respondents' control than the subjects of general population.

Seshadri et al. said that there is an ethical paradox of establishing that predictions regarding risk for suicide are accurate. Recording the number of life events will not define the complex personal experiences of the life events and their meaning to the individual who suffered. 43% of the patients do not seek help. A third do, but the general practitioners whom they approach are not equipped with the know-how to deal with them. Another third seek psychiatric help with the general practitioners.

Hawton[177] says 96% of the completed suicides have a psychiatric disorder. So many antecedents for primary prevention constitute a complex problem. A secondary level model or primary intervention could be by attempting to diagnose and treat these DSH patients while having a psychiatric diagnosis. Beck's formulation[165,166] of suicidal behavior is related to cognitive distortion. This does not explain the connecting link between depression and suicidal behavior, and the catalytic agent of hopelessness. The hopelessness scale of Beck is a twenty item true/false statement (1974). Subsequent studies have substantiated hopelessness in suicidal behavior.

Beck et al. also had formulated suicide intent scale and scale for suicidal ideation, scales meant to assess and predict suicide. Hawton[177] (1987) has pointed out that (i) there is difficulty in applying general risk factors to individual patients, (ii) risk factors identification is largely from groups of people who either attempted or completed suicide but not extracted from groups of attempters vs ideators, (iii) the problem of identifying long term risk as against the short term risk, (iv) change of risk factors, i.e. most risk factors are dynamic and not stable, (v) risk factors are not universal, (vi) researchers attempting to demonstrate the efficacy of psychiatric intervention in the 20% help seekers to psychiatrists have not proved the efficacy of the psychiatric intervention. There is a tendency of self-harm to become self-perpetuating. Primary intervention techniques, like counseling services, as a substitute for pharmacotherapy are needed, and (vii) methodological flaws in biological suicide research are listed by Van Prag[178] as:

a. Conceptualizing suicide as disturbed aggression regulation at the exclusion of motivational dynamics,
b. Assuming a correlation between lethality of attempt and lethality of intent,
c. The problem of time lag between a suicide attempt and estimation of biological variables (especially if the latter are state-related),
d. Heterogeneity of suicidal manifestations, and
e. Differentiation of suicidal acts.

Agarwal and Aga[179] had compiled the number of studies per topic in each decade in mental health research in India in an overview.

CONCLUSION

Each individual is unique in this world; even if two of them are monozygotic twins, both are not hundred percent alike. This basic reality is forgotten in the pursuit in research of picturing a standardized man with standardized vulnerability due to genetic or monoamine based biological explanation of causes of suicide. Sociological/community statistics is getting extrapolated into the individual case and the clinical setup. This, and the lack of morphological approach initially envisaged by Durkheim but later not followed, is another of the faults of suicidology research. The clinical findings of a hospital in a cultural geographical setup cannot be generalized and taken as gospel truth and standard phenomenon prevalent everywhere. In the individual case itself, no research has proved whether the suicide came first or the biological change came first; there are many variables and co-occurring factors which affect the threshold for the final undaunted irreversible decision making of the suicidal patient.

We do see peoples' real zest for life, even while terminally ill. People do prepare for their death by handing over power, belongings and by way of retiring. Research in gerontology is going on as a result of man's aspiration to postpone death and live a healthy life But, no one wants to live forever. Many do not want their mortal being called human body to stay alive in an unconscious state. All these are normal viewpoints connected with death.

Anticipation is neurobiologically originating from the frontal lobe. Apart from the capacity of planning, foresight and preparation, the frontal lobes, according to Sutter,[180] has the unique property of anticipation, which may be an area of future research in suicidology. Considering the serotonergic system, the connection between the prefrontal cortex and limbic system, its involvement in the memory, emotion and motivation dysfunction of this system and its consequences on anticipation should be addressed in future research in suicidology. Self-esteem,[181] quality of life, coping strategies, environmental factors (including light-dark span and ambient temperature) are other front line areas of research in suicidology. Primary health care physician have a unique role to play in the prevention of suicide in the elderly. Effect of protective factors and positive factors (suicide counters) in the environment, on the individual, are not clear. This can be defined by future suicidology research.

Regarding substance abuse, Janakiramaiah had commented, "it is high time that both planners and physicians take a comprehensive long-term view of the health care strategy in relation to drug, alcohol, tobacco and related problems in the country."[182] In relation to indirect suicidal behavior or chronic suicide, and its preventive care, this statement is very relevant. If one considers the fact that one fourth of all suicides have alcohol abuse as an associated factor, the relevance of the statement becomes clearer. The neurobiological approach[14,49,67] and the social-community approach[5,38] have got well established in the country. There is an untapped human resource (e.g. the sociologists) with regard to preventive care in suicidology. India, in an intersectoral cooperative approach, with the help of specialists from UNICEF, Central Ministry of welfare and Tata Institute of Social Sciences had declared in Bombay, in 1994 its commitment to family well-being, utilizing the international year of the family as a catalyst.[183]

Kishore et al.[184], in his sample of 122 adolescents from the Delhi area who regularly view cable TV, have demonstrated that the percentage representing suicidal talks are statistically insignificant whereas those showing aggression and violent behavior form a statistically significant group. This study still has a bearing on the concept of contagious nature of suicidal behavior.

Research on elder abuse can throw light on the preventive care that one has to provide for the elderly citizens of the society.[185]

Child friendly schools' initiative and life skills education in schools, including child's homework management, can provide newer areas of research and application in the prevention of suicidal behavior in prepubertal children.[186]

WHO sometimes uses prominent personalities to have a social impact on certain health related messages. In 1995, Nelson Mandela spoke in the following manner, "I call on youth not to take up this deadly addiction. The time has come for governments and countries and individuals to build up a healthy tobacco free world." Contagion can be one of the mechanism of spread of suicidal behavior. The same mechanism via media can be utilized for the spread of ideas of prevention of chronic suicidal behavior like tobacco smoking.[187]

No two patients and no two situations are identical. Clinical complexities in care occur in physical and psychosocial domains, often confounded by the family's views. An ethical framework for clinical decision making is essential to underpin robust management of difficult clinical situations regarding palliative care and care of the terminally ill and also regarding newer clinical areas like physician assisted suicide.[188]

Cooperation between agencies to develop preventive services is growing. *Befrienders international* is doing yeoman service in the field of prevention of suicidal behavior in the community.[189] Developing volunteer action to prevent suicide is an important response of any community.[189-192] But, the impact of this response on the outcome of suicidal behavior of citizens in society is not yet known.[23] The result of such research is not yet known. Such researches are also very difficult to organize. For example, given the nature of work of preventive care codified by organizations like *Befrienders International* with regard to privacy, confidentiality and anonymity guaranted to this subject by the organization.[189-192] Evaluation of effect of suicide prevention centres is either missing or indicates no positive results.[23]

Suicidology, a subject that cuts across the varied topics under psychiatry, is an important area for research in India considering the magnitude of the problem in the country. Agarwal and Aga's overview[179] is highly illustrative of the work that is yet to be done in the field.

Latest Glance to Suicide in India 2013

Traditionally, in western literature risk factors associated with suicide, including suicidal attempts—include young age (15–24 years), female gender, low educational attainment, unemployment, living alone, and history of socioeconomic deprivation.[193] In this section, we examine the demographics of suicide in India.

Age

Although suicide rates were commonly highest among older adult males, rates among young people have been increasing. Young adults are a particularly vulnerable group and currently show the highest rates of suicide the world over. Suicide is responsible for 6% of all deaths among young people.[194] Developed countries show a second peak of increased suicide rate in the elderly (above 60 years).

An Indian study showed that the suicide rate was highest in the 15 to 29 years age group (38 per 100,000 population) followed by the 30 to 44 years group (34 per 100,000 population). The rates of suicide was 18 per 100,000 in those aged 45-59 years and 7 per 100,000 in those aged >60 years.[195] Since these figures are calculated for the general population and not the age-specific "population of interest", the higher risk in youth may reflect a higher representation of youth in the population.

The National Crime Records Bureau report of 2009 shows a similar pattern. Youth in the age group 15 to 29 years accounted for the largest proportion (34.5%) of suicides followed by those in the age group 30 to 44 years (34.2%). Other studies in India also indicate that young adults are at increased risk, with ages 20 to 24 years followed by 25 to 29 years showing the highest rates of suicide in a psychological autopsy study,[197] and the15 to 39 age group identified as the most vulnerable in another study.[198] Two-thirds of women who completed suicide were <25 years.[199,200]

This trend is also seen in attempted suicides. In one study, the mean age of attempters was 25.3 years.[201] Suicidal ideation was also more common in the 16 to 45 years age group in a study of suicidal ideators in a general hospital setting.[202]

Adolescents and Young Adults

Youth is a period of heightened risk of suicide[203] and suicide is a leading cause of death among young people in India. In a study which evaluated the cause of death among those aged 10 to 19 years, in a rural population of 108,000 in south India, suicide accounted for about a quarter of all deaths in males and between 50% and 75% of all deaths in females aged 10 to 19 years. The average suicide rate for girls was 148 per 100,000, and for boys, 58 per 100,000

Among young people, suicidal behavior was found to be associated with female gender, not attending school or college, independent decision making, premarital sex, physical abuse at home, lifetime experience of sexual abuse, and probable common mental disorders.[204] Violence and psychological distress were independently associated with suicidal behavior. Factors associated with gender disadvantage increased vulnerability, particularly in rural women.[204]

Elderly

There is a global trend toward increased suicide in late life, again mainly in men. [205,206] However, in a 5 year study of 6312 suicide attempters, only 47 were above the age of 60 years.[207] The low prevalence of suicide among the elderly in India may be because the aged are well-integrated and respected in the family; children take responsibility for their care. Also, life expectancy in the elderly is lower in India than elsewhere, contributing to the comparatively lower suicide rate.[208]

The ratio of completed suicide to attempted suicide in India is about 1:7 in the elderly, which is double the ratio of 1:15 in lower age groups.[207] This may reflect a poorer ability of the elderly to recover from the bodily insult of a suicide attempt. Although studies from the west implicate social isolation, as defined by 'living along' as a risk factor for suicide among the elderly, an early study speculated that for elderly in India 'family and social integration' were the real determinants of risk, even if they were living by themselves.[209]More recent studies from the west appear to support this position.[210]

Gender

Globally, attempted suicide is commoner in women and completed suicide is commoner in men.[211] In Chinese women, however, the suicide rate is approximately twice that of women elsewhere.[211] Men commonly use more lethal modes and plan the act more meticulously to avoid detection. In contrast, women commonly use less lethal modes, and are more impulsive, less well planned, and more likely to be found and rescued. The male:female suicide ratio is 3.8, 3.9, 4.1, and 3.4 in Australia, Canada, the United States, and the UK, respectively[212] and it is lower in Asian countries.[213]

What are the data for India? Although some Indian studies have found a higher incidence of suicide in men than in women,[195] others have found the contrary.[199] The male:female suicide ratio was 1.78 in India in 2008 and 2009. In children up to age 14 years, the ratio was 1.04; that is, almost equal between the sexes.[196] In young men and women in 1991–1997, the ratio was 1.3, contrasting with the male preponderance in developed countries.[214] The reasons for greater female suicide completion in India may be sociocultural. The common practice of arranged marriages in India result in social and family pressure for the woman to stay married even in an abusive relationship; this may increase the risk of suicide in women.[215] Also, stresses related to dowry demands may drive young brides to suicide.[216]

And what of suicide attempters in India? Although attempted suicide was as high as 1.2 times higher in women relative to men in some studies others studies showed a male predominance, male: female ratio ranging from 1.13:1 to 1.63:1. These differences may be reconciled by an appreciation of social changes in India, with a shift toward nuclear families and the cultural emphasis on the male stereotype which the individual tries to fulfill in vain.[197]

Marital Status

In the West, marriage is generally protective against suicide; this empirical regularity is referred to as the "coefficient of preservation" based on Durkheim's 1897 seminal monograph Le Suicide.[217] Divorced, separated, widowed, and single people are more likely to commit suicide than married people. Persons living alone are at particular risk.[193] This protective effect of marriage was seen more for men than for women and rates of suicide decreased in order from widowers to divorced, single, and married men. Young widowers were at highest risk. Lower rates of suicide among married compared to unmarried women may be explained by sociological theories based on marital status integration and social integration.[218]

Marriage is not a strong protective factor for suicide attempts in developing countries.[219] In 2009, 70.4% of all suicide victims in India were married and 21.9% were unmarried. Divorcees and individuals who were separated accounted for about 3.4%, while widows and widowers comprised 4.3% of the total suicide victims.[196] In individual studies, some show higher attempted suicides among unmarried persons[220] while others show a higher rate among those who are married. Among attempters, men were more likely to be single and women, married.[221] In a general hospital study, no suicide attempter was separated or living alone. Those who were unmarried were living with their extended families. Widowed, separated and divorced individuals were commoner among cases of completed suicide relative to controls in a study of 100 suicide cases.[198]

The quality of marital relationship, emotional warmth, extended family support, and ability to handle stresses related to marriage and child rearing are more important than marital status, per se, but these qualifiers of marital status are difficult to study.

Education

Low intelligence results in a 2-3-fold increased risk of suicide. Possible explanations are that persons with low intelligence are less able to compete for jobs and therefore acquire lower income and social status. They may also be less efficient in coping with stress. Finally, neurodevelopmental vulnerabilities may increase their risk of a psychiatric disorder.[222]

Level of educational attainment is a surrogate marker of intelligence, though drawing conclusions on this premise is problematic when education is not universally available. The NCRB data reveal that 25.3% of suicide victims were educated up to primary level, 23.7% had a middle-school education, 21.4% were illiterate, and 3.1% were graduates or postgraduates.[196] These percentages, however, may reflect the proportion of persons with different educational attainment in India.

In one study of attempted suicide in India, 55.5% were uneducated. In another study, 54% of suicide attempters had received high school education or higher. Women attempting suicide tended to have a lower educational status compared to men.[220] Again, it is hard to interpret these percentages in the absence of information about the educational attainment of the population from which the samples originated.

Family Structure

The sociological theory of suicide emphasizes social integration, a theme reflected in John Donne's "No Man is an Island". People who are well integrated with their families and community have a good support system during crises, protecting them against suicide. Risk factors related to the family include parenting style, family history of mental illness and suicide, and physical and sexual abuse in childhood. "Affectionless control", a parenting style characterized by a combination of low levels of emotional warmth and high levels of parental control or overprotection, is associated with a three-fold increase in the risk of suicidal behavior.[223] Suicide attempters with a history of sexual or physical abuse in childhood show more suicidal behavior and are at a higher risk for mental disturbances in adulthood even after controlling for other contributory factors.[224]

India has witnessed a change in family structure during recent decades, with more people moving out of joint and extended families into nuclear family structures. The effect of this change on suicide rate has not been systematically studied. Varying results in research may tap a secular trend. The majority of suicide attempters were from nuclear families, possibly reflecting the role of social integration, though an earlier study shows that more suicide attempters come from joint families.[225] A study on burns victims found that being in a joint family was a risk factor for dowry deaths.[226] Another study found that family and marital conflict was a major reason for suicide.[201]

Urban vs. Rural Residence

The suicide rate is generally reported to be higher in urban areas because of a variety of stressors related to living and working in cities, including overcrowding and social isolation. In India, during the year 2000, though the suicide rate for the country was 10.8, the rate in urban areas was slightly lower at 9.94.[227] There has since been an increase in urban suicide rates to 11.4% in 2005, around 13% in 2006 and 2007, and 12.1% to 12.5% in 2008 and 2009.[196] Studies in recent years are consistent in this regard: suicide and attempted suicide were more common in persons living in urban areas.

Occupation

There is a fairly strong association between unemployment rates and suicide, but the nature of this association is complex. Unemployment may drive up the suicide risk through factors such as poverty, social deprivation, domestic difficulties, and hopelessness. Furthermore, persons with psychiatric disorders are at higher risk of suicide and are also more likely to be unemployed; this may be a double whammy. Adding to the complexity is recent loss of employment vs long-term unemployment; the former is associated with greater risk.[228] The association between unemployment and suicide may also be more significant for young adults.[229] In India, in one study of suicide attempters, 46% were unemployed. In another study, >50% of patients were employed, 12% were unemployed and some were either students or housewives.

The NCRB data shows that housewives account for 18.6% of total persons committing suicides and for 52.8% of the total female victims. Those involved in farming and agriculture form the next largest group, comprising 11.9% of the total victims followed by those working in the private sector (7.8%) and unemployed (7.5%). and public sector (7.8% and 2.2%, respectively). Students accounted for 5.5% of total suicides while unemployed persons accounted for 5.5% and 7.5%, respectively. Those employed in the public sector (2.2% of total suicides) and government servants (1.3% of total suicides) were the least represented group.[220]

Precipitating Event

The relationship of suicide to negative life events, stress, object loss, and negative interaction needs to be understood in the framework of a model of vulnerability, support, coping, and problem-solving. Rich and Bonner [230]found in a stress-vulnerability model that negative life events and stress accounted for 30% of the variance in suicidal ideation. Indian society, being sociocentric, lays importance on interpersonal relationships. It is therefore unsurprising that marital conflict is the commonest cause of suicide among women, while interpersonal conflict is the commonest cause among men.[199]

Other suicide triggers include physical illness, bankruptcy, illicit relationships, and drug intoxication. An interesting finding, rarely seen in the West, is the high rate of suicide associated with sexual abuse and illegitimate pregnancy. This may be a reflection of cultural taboos related to sexuality in India.

A similar trend is seen for attempted suicide with interpersonal conflict, financial stressors, and educational burden being the most common triggers.[231] Chronic pain and illness is featured as a common reason in some studies.

Studies which measured stressful life events found that approximately 90% of suicide attempters reported negative life events and about 35% experienced stressful life events in the previous 6 months. However, in the absence of a control group, it is hard to interpret the significance of life events. After all, everybody experiences stressful or negative life events.[221]

MOTIVES FOR SUICIDE

A truism in suicide literature is that "not all persons who commit suicide want to die and not all persons who want to die commit suicide". The intentionality and lethality of suicide are important dimensions which describe the motive behind the act. Lethality is a function of the mode of suicide and has already been examined in an earlier section. Motives may go beyond Freud's concept of the 'wish to kill', the 'wish to die' and the 'wish to be killed', and beyond Durkhiem's sociological typology; and may be more complex than just a cry for help. The motive for suicide may be as diverse as a need for identification as in the case of 'copy-cat' suicides (also called the Werther effect) to delusional beliefs as in the case of Klingsor syndrome (genital self-mutilation based on religious delusions).[232]

An Indian study of suicide attempters classified motivation into 'the wish for change' and 'the wish to die' groups and found that the former had low lethality, lack of planning for their attempt, more likelihood of rescue and were not intoxicated during the attempt. The latter group utilized more drastic measures, such as hanging and was more likely to have a psychiatric disorder with comorbid alcoholism.[233]

In India, the top 10 causes or correlates of suicide in 2009 were family problems (23.7%), illness (21%) [including insanity/mental illness (6.7%)], unemployment (1.9%), love affairs (2.9%), drug abuse/addiction (2.3%), failure in examination (1.6%), bankruptcy or sudden change in economic status (2.5%), poverty (2.3%), and dowry dispute (2.3%).[196] The high rates of suicide among persons with mental illness and drug abuse/addiction, though not a measure of intent, are of much concern. Many of the remaining causes [namely, suspected/illicit relation, cancellation/nonsettlement of marriage, not having children (barrenness/impotency), death of a dear one, dowry dispute, divorce, ideological causes/hero worship, illegitimate pregnancy, physical abuse (rape, incest, etc.), poverty, professional/career problem[196] reflect the unique social structure of our society and the social pressures that individuals face.

Studies on suicide notes report that a last wish was mentioned in 30%.[234] Mass suicides are seen as suicide pacts in couples or families[20] rather than as part of religious cults as in western societies. Suicide pacts are rare, accounting for <1% of all suicides, and there is a trend in western literature showing a decrease in rates over the years.[235] Suicide pacts almost always involve people well known to each other, mostly spouses, most of them childless.[236] However, there is an emerging trend for cyber-based internet-facilitated suicide pacts which increasingly involve two or more strangers who meet on the internet and share similar world views. Such cases have been reported in the press, but have not been studied in a scientific manner.

Psychiatric Diagnosis

Mental disorders (particularly depression and alcohol use disorders) are a major risk factor for suicide in Europe and North America; however, in Asian countries impulsiveness plays an important role. It is often reported that rates of psychiatric disorders are higher among suicide completers in developed countries relative to developing countries, though under-diagnosis in developing countries is a possible explanation.

Studies in India show varying results with rates of psychiatric disorders ranging from 9.5 to 24.9%.[237,238] In one psychological autopsy study, 24% of suicides had a psychiatric diagnosis, namely major depressive disorder, bipolar affective disorder, or schizophrenia; substance abuse was prevalent in 18%.[197] In a study of attempted suicide, 11.6% had a psychiatric diagnosis with alcohol dependence followed by depression being the commonest diagnoses; schizophrenia, conduct disorder, and personality disorder comprised the rest. In a psychological autopsy of 100 consecutive suicides in a rural population, 37% had a DSM-III-R psychiatric diagnosis; alcohol dependence (16%) and adjustment disorders (15%) were the commonest diagnoses, and schizophrenia, major depressive episode, and dysthymia constituted a smaller proportion (2% each).[239]

Rates of psychiatric diagnosis as high as 46.7%, 59.7%, 57%and even 93% have been described among suicide attempters.[240] Mood disorders, particularly depressive disorders, were the most common diagnosis followed by alcohol abuse.[240] Neurotic, stress-related, and somatoform disorders were diagnosed in 14.5%.[241]

In a study of patients with major depressive disorder with suicidal ideation, incidence of suicidal attempt was 16.6%, all attempters were <30 years old. Suicidal attempt has also been found to be positively correlated with severity of depression.[242]

Dysthymia underlying suicidal behavior is commoner in India than in the West.[241] In a general hospital study on suicidal ideation, psychiatrically ill patients were overrepresented: 59.74% had depression followed by substance abuse and psychosis in 9.74% each. 9.09% were diagnosed with bipolar disorder and 7.14% constituted a group with neurotic disorders.[202]

In a study of 1560 patients with schizophrenia, the rate of attempted suicide was 4.7%. These patients did not differ in illness duration from patients with depression who had attempted suicide.[243]

Personality Disorders

Multiple suicide attempts of low intentionality and lethality are typically associated with maladaptive coping and impulsivity in personality disorders. The rate of personality disorders among those who attempt suicide in India ranges from 7 to 50% in various studies.[241,243] The most common diagnoses were schizoid, borderline, and antisocial personality disorders.[243]In a study of personality disorder among first attempters, the most common diagnoses were anankastic and histrionic personality disorder.[241] In a 16-PF study of personality, self-immolators were found to lack ego strength, lack frustration tolerance, be emotionally less stable, and be impulsive.[244] The association of impulsivity and marital discord among self-immolators has been frequently reported in Indian[99] and other Asian studies.[245]

Physical Illness

Chronic physical illness, abnormal vaginal discharge, and tobacco use are risk factors for common mental disorders among women in India.[246] A similar pattern is seen among suicide attempters. About one-fifth were found to have a physical illness in one study with dysmenorrhoea being the commonest ailment, followed by peptic ulcer disease; hypertension, bronchial asthma and arthritis comprised the remaining. Pain in the abdominal and pelvic regions has been reported more frequently among attempters.[247] This finding was also reported in Hispanics[248] and Americans.[249]

REFERENCES

1. Swami Tapasyananda. Srimad Bhagavad Gita: The Scripture of Mankind. Transl. Madras: Sri Ramakrishna Math; 1984.
2. Wilson EO. The Insect Societies. Cambridge: Harvard University Press,1971.
3. Egeland J, Sussex J. Suicide and family loading for affective disorders. JAMA. 1985;254:915-8.
4. Wilson EO. Sociobiology: The New Synthesis. Cambridge: Harvard University Press; 1975.
5. Murthy RS. Urbanisation and mental health.Indian J Soc Psychiatry. 1993;9:16-9.
6. Horton R. The crisis in psychiatry. Lancet. 1997;349:965.
7. Katschnig H. Life Events and Psychiatric Disorders: Controversial Issues. Cambridge: Cambridge University Press; 1986.
8. Crawley JN, Sutton ME, Pickar D. Animal models of self-destructive behavior and suicide. Psychiatr Clin N Am. 1985;8: 299-310.
9. Nandi DN. On aggression.Dr. DLN Murthy Rao oration. Indian J Psychiatry. 1985;27:17-33.
10. Roy A. Suicide: A multidetermined act. Psychiatr Clin N Am. 1985;8:243-50.
11. Kreitman N. Suicide and parasuicide. In: Kendell RE, Zeally AK (Eds). Companion to Psychiatric Studies. London: Churchill Livingstone. 1988. pp.459-75.
12. Trivedi JK. Punishing attempted suicide: Anachronism of twentieth century. Editorial. Indian J Psychiatry. 1997;39: 87-9.
13. Unni KES, Rotti SB, Chandrasekaran R. An exploratory study of motivation in suicide attempters. Indian J Psychiatry. 1995;37:169-75.
14. Venkoba Rao A. Suicide. In: Vyas JN, Ahuja N (Eds). Postgraduate Psychiatry. New Delhi: BI Churchill Livingstone; 1992.
15. Jaspers K.General Psychopathology. Manchester: Manchester University Press; 1963.
16. Ayd FJ. Lexicon of Psychiatry, Neurology, and the Neurosciences. New Delhi: BI Waverly; 1995.
17. Rojtenberg SL. Suicide: Death as a way out. World Psychiatry. 1995;3:2-5.
18. Maris RW. Social and familial risk factors in suicidal behavior. Psychiatr Clin N Am. 1997;20:519-50.
19. Menninger K. Man Against Himself. New York: Harcourt, Brace and World; 1938.
20. Shneidman ES. Definition of Suicide. New York: John Wiley; 1985.pp.214-19.

21. Bacchler. Suicides. New York: Basic Books; 1979.
22. World Health Organisation. Prevention of Suicide. Public Health Paper No. 35, Geneva:WHO; 1968.
23. Bertolote JM. Ed. Guidelines for the Primary Prevention of Mental, Neurological and Psychosocial Disorders. IV. Suicide. Geneva: World Health Organisation; 1993.
24. Levey S. Suicide. In: Blueglass R, Bowden P (Eds). Principles and Practice of Forensic Psychiatry. pp. 597-610
25. Hornby AS. Oxford Advanced Learner's Dictionary of Current English. Oxford: Oxford University Press; 1995.
26. Neeleman J, Halpern D, Leon D, Lewis G. Tolerance of suicide, religion and suicide rates: an ecological and individual study in 19 Western countries. Psychol Med. 1997;27:1165-71.
27. Lemperiere T. President. DSM IV une meilleure approche des troubles de l'humeur? Symposium.l'encephale revue de psychiatrie clinique biologique et therapeutique. 1995;21: 1-67.
28. Durkheim E. Le Suicide. Paris: PUF; 1990.
29. Osipova E. Emile Durkheim's sociology. In: Kon IS (Ed). A History of Classical Sociology. Moscow: Progress Publishers; 1989.
30. Douglas JD. The social meaning of suicide. Princeton: Princeton University Press; 1967.
31. Hendin H. Psychotherapy and suicide. Am J Psychother. 1961;35:469-80.
32. Farberow NL, Shneidman E (Eds). The Cry for Help. New York: McGraw Hill; 1961.
33. Kaplan HI, Sadock BJ. Comprehensive Textbook of Psychiatry. III Ed. Baltimore: Williams & Wilkins; 1981.
34. Moscicki EK. Identification of suicide risk factors using epidemiological studies. Psychiatr Clin N Am. 1997;20:499-517.
35. Barraclough B, Bunch J, Nelson B, et al. A hundred cases of suicide: Clinical aspects. Br J Psychiatry. 1974;125:355-73.
36. La Vecchia C, Lucchini F, Levi F. Worldwide trends in suicide mortality; 1955-1989. Acta Psychiatr Scand 1994.
37. National Crime Records Bureau, India; 1984-1994 records.
38. Murthy RS. Suicide prevention: Policies and priorities; Community mental health perspective. Indian J Soc Psychiatry. 1993;9:47-52.
39. Philps DP. The influence of suggestion on suicide. Am Sociol Rev. 1994;39:340.
40. Philips DP, Lesyna K, Paight DJ. Suicide and the media: Research and policy implications. In: Diekstra R, et al (Eds). Assessment and Prevention of Suicide. New York: Guilford Press; 1992. pp. 499.
41. Singh G, Kaur D, Kaur H. Handbook of Presumptive Stressful Life Events Scale. Agra: National Psychological Corporation; 1983.
42. Holmes TH, Rahe RH. The social adjustment rating scale. J Psychosom Res. 1967;11:213.
43. Paykel ES. Stress and life events. In: Davidson L, Linnile M (Eds). Report of the Secy's Task force on youth suicide. Vol.II. Washington: US Govt. Printing Press; 1989. pp.110.
44. Freud S. Mourning and Melancholia. In: Strachey J (Ed) & Transl. Standard Edition of the Complete Works of Sigmund Freud. Vol.14. London: Hogarth Press; 1917. pp.237-58.
45. Zilboorg G. Differential diagnosis of types of suicide. Arch Neur Psychiat. 1936;35:270.
46. Klein M (Ed). Contributions to Psychoanalysis; 1921-1945. London: Hogarth Press; 1948.
47. Stengel E. Suicide and Attempted Suicide. New York: Jason Aronson; 1964.
48. Mann JJ, McBride PA, Malone KM, et al. Blunted serotonin responsivity in depressed inpatients. Neuropsycho pharmacology. 1995;13:53-68.
49. Trivedi JK. Serotonin and its metabolites as biological markers of suicidal behavior. Indian J Psychiatry. 1992;34:174-97.
50. Kraepelin E. Lecturers on Clinical Psychiatry. New York: Wood;1917.
51. Venkoba Rao A. Attempted suicide (parasuicide) and suicide. In: Verghese A, Abraham A. Introduction to Psychiatry. Madras: The Christian Literature Society; 1983.pp.117-21.
52. Silverman C. The Epidemiology of Depression: A review. Am J Psychiatry. 1968;124:883.
53. Robins E, Murphy GE, Wilkinson RH, et al. Some clinical considerations in the prevention of suicide based on a study of 134 successful suicides. Am J Pub Health. 1959;49:888-9.
54. Weissman MM. The Epidemiology of suicide attempts, 1960 to 1971. Arch Gen Psychiatry. 1974;30:737.
55. Pokorny AD. Suicide rates in various psychiatric disorders. J Nerv Ment Dis. 1964;139:499.
56. Silver MA, Behnert MAT, et al. Relation of depression to attempted suicide and seriousness of intent. Arch Gen Psychiatry. 1975;25:573.
57. Kiev A. The Suicidal Patient: Recognition and Management. Chicago: Nelson-Hall; 1977.
58. Venkoba Rao A, Nammalvar N. The course and outcome of depressives in depressive illness. Br J Psychiatry. 1977;130:392.
59. Unni KES, Mani AJ. Psychodemographic profile of suicidal ideators.Indian J Psychiatry. 1996;38:79-85.
60. Asberg M, Traskman I, Thoren P. 5-HIAA in the cerebrospinal fluid: A biochemical suicide predictor? Arch Gen Psychiatry. 1976;33:1193-7.
61. Brown GL, Goodwin FK, Ballenger FC, et al. Aggression in humans correlates with cerebrospinal fluid amine metabolites. Psychiatr Res. 1979;12:131-9.
62. Agren H. Life at risk: Markers of suicidality in depression. Psychiatr Dev. 1983;1:87-104.
63. Traskman L, Tybring G, Asberg M, et al. Cortisol in the CSF of depressed and suicidal patients. Arch Gen Psychiatry. 1980;37: 761-7.
64. Oreland L, Widberg A, Asberg M, et al. Platelet MAO activity and monoamine metabolites in cerebrospinal fluid in depressed and suicidal patients and in healthy controls. Psychiatr Res. 1981;4:21-29.

65. Brown GL, Ebert MH, Goyar PF, et al. Aggression, suicide and serotonin: Relationships to CSF amine metabolites. Am J Psychiatry. 1982;139:741-6.
66. Van Praag HM. Depression, suicide, and the metabolism of serotonin in the brain. J Affect Disord. 1982;4:275-90.
67. Palaniappan V, Ramachandran V, Somasundaram O. Suicide ideation and biogenic amines in depression. Indian J Psychiatry. 1983;25:286-292.
68. Roy-Byrne P, Post RM, Rubinow DR, et al. CSF 5-HIAA and personal and family history of suicide in affectively ill patients: A negative study. Psychiatry Res. 1983;10:263-74.
69. Linnoila M, Virkkunen M, Schelnin M, et al. Low cerebrospinal fluid 5-hydroxyindoleacetic acid concentration differentiates impulsive from nonimpulsive violent behaviour. Life Sci. 1983;33:2609-14.
70. Banki CM, Arato M, Papp Z, et al. Biochemical markers in suicidal patients: Investigations with cerebrospinal fluid amine metabolites and neuroendocrine test. J Affect Disord. 1984;6: 341-50.
71. Ninan PT, van Kammen DP, Schelnin M, et al. CSF 5-hydroxy-indolacetic acid in suicidal schizophrenic patients. Am J Psychiatry. 1984;141:566-9.
72. Lopez-Ibor JJ, Salz-Ruiz J, Perez de los, et al. Biological correlations of suicide and aggressivity in major depressions (with melancholia): 5-hydroxyindoleacetic acid and cortisol in cerebral spinal fluid, dexamethasone suppression test and therapeutic response to 5-hydroxytryptophan. Neuropsychobiologica. 1985;14:67-74.
73. Lidberg L, Tuck JR, Asberg M, et al. Homicide, suicide, and CSF 5-HIAA.Acta Psychiat Scand. 1985;71:230-6.
74. Berrettini WH, Nurunberger JI Jr., Narrow W, et al. Cerebrospinal fluid studies of bipolar patients with and without a history of suicide attempts. Ann NY Acad Sci. 1986;487:197-201.
75. Roy A, Agren H, Linnoila M, et al. Reduced CSF concentrations of homovanillic acid to 5-HIAA ratios in depressed patients: Relationship to suicidal behaviour and DST. Am J Psychiatry. 1986;1539-45.
76. Weiss D, Coccaro EF. Neuroendocrine challenge studies of suicidal behaviour. Psychiatr Clin N Am. 1997;20:563-79.
77. Meltzer HY, Perline R, Tricou BJ, et al. Effects of 5-hydroxy-tryptophan on serum cortisol levels in major affective disorders. II. Relation to suicide, psychosis and depressive symptoms. Arch Gen Psychiatry. 1984;41:379.
78. Cowen PJ, Charig EM. Neuroendocrine responses to intravenous tryptophan in major depression. Arch Gen Psychiatry. 1987;44:958.
79. Lopez-Ibor JJ, Saiz-Ruiz J, Iglesias LM. The fenfluramine challenge test in the affective spectrum: A possible marker of endogeneity and severity. Pharmacopsychiatry. 1988; 21:9.
80. Coccaro EF, Siever LJ, Klar H, et al. Serotonergic studies in patients with affective and personality disorders: Correlates with suicidal and impulsive aggressive behaviour. Arch Gen Psychiatry. 1989;46:587.
81. Golden RN, Gilmore JH, Corrigan MHN, et al. Serotonin, suicide, and aggression: Clinical studies. J Clin Psychiatry. 1991;52(suppl):61.
82. O'Kenae V, Dinen TG. Prolactin and cortisol responses to d-fenfluramine in major depression: Evidence for diminished responsivity of central serotonergic function. Am J Psychiatry. 1991;148:1009.
83. Wetzler S, Kahn RS, Asnis GM, et al. Serotonin receptor sensitivity and aggression. Psychiatry Res. 1991;37:271.
84. Anderson IM, Ware CJ, Da Roza Davis JM, et al. Decreased 5-HT-mediated prolactin release in major depression. Br J Psychiatry. 1992;160:372.
85. Korn ML, Asnis G, Brown SL, et al. Serotinin receptor sensitivity and suicide. Biol Psychiatry. 1992;32:209.
86. Moeller FG, Steinberg JL, Fulton M, et al. A preliminary study with buspirone in major depression. Neuropsychopharmacology. 1994;10:75.
87. Mann JJ, McBride PA, Malone KM, et al. Blunted serotonergic responsivity in depressed inpatients. Neuropsychopharmacology. 1995;13:53.
88. Pitchot W, Ansseau M, Gonzalez Moreno A, et al. The flesinoxan 5-HT_{1A} receptor challenge in major depression and suicidal behavior. Pharmacopsychiatry. 1995;28(suppl):91.
89. Cleare AJ, Murray RM, O'Keane V. Reduced prolactin and cortisol responses to d-fenfluramine in depressed compared to healthy matched control subjects. Neuropsychopharmacology. 1996;14:349.
90. Malone KM, Corbitt EM, Li S, et al. Prolactin response to fenfluramine and suicide attempt lethality in major depression. Br J Psychiatry. 1996;168:324.
91. Mann JJ. Neurobiological models. In: Mann JJ (Ed). Models of Depressive Disorders: Psychological, Biological and Genetic Perspective. New York: Plenum; 1989.
92. Arango V, Underwood MD, Mann JJ. Biologic alterations in the brainstem of suicides.Psychiatr Clin N Am. 1997;20:581-93.
93. Clayton PJ. Suicide. Psychiatr Clin N A. 1985;203-14.
94. Trimble MR. Towards a Neuropsychiatric Theory of Literary Creativity. 18th T.S. Srinivasan Endowment Lecture, Chennai; 1997.
95. Roy A, Rylander G, Sarchiapone M. Genetic studies of suicidal behaviour. Psychiatr Clin N Am. 1997;20:595-611.
96. Tishler C, McKenry P, Morgan K. Adolescent suicide attempts: Some significant factors. Suicide Life Threat Behav. 1981;11: 86-92.
97. Garfinkel B, Froese A, Hood J. Suicide attempts in children and adolescents. Am J Psychiatry. 1982;139:1257-61.
98. Shaffer D. Suicide in childhood and early adolescence. J Child Psychol Psychiatry. 1974;5:275-91.
99. Shafii M, Carrigan S, Whittinghill R, et al. Psychological autopsy of completed suicides in children and adolescents. Am J Psychiatry. 1985;142:1061-4.
100. Farberow N, Simon M. Suicide in Los Angels and Vienna: An intercultural study of two cities. Pub Health Rep. 1969;84: 389-403.

101. Robins E, Schmidt E, O'Neal P. Some interrelations of social factors and clinical diagnosis in attempted suicide. Am J Psychiatry. 1957;114:221-31.
102. Pitts F, Winokur F. Affective disorder. III. Diagnostic correlates and incidence of suicide. J Nerv Ment Dis. 1964;139:176-81.
103. Unni KES. Familial suicide. Indian J Psychiatry. 1996;38:146-7.
104. Dabbagh F. Family suicide. Br J Psychiatry. 1977;130:159-161.
105. Linkowski P, de Maertelae V, Mendlewicz J. Suicidal behavior in major depressive illness. Acta Psychiatr Scand. 1985;72: 233-8.
106. Egeland J, Sussex J. Suicide and family loading for affective disorders. JAMA. 1985;254:915-8.
107. Haberlandt W. Aportacion a la genetica del suicido. Folia Clinica Internationale. 1967;17:319-22.
108. Roy A, Segal N, Sarchiapone M. Attempted suicide among living cotwins of twin suicide victims. Am J Psychiatry. 1995;152: 1075-6.
109. Papadimitriou G, Linkowski P, Delarbre C, et al. Suicide on the paternal and maternal sides of depressed patients with a lifetime history of attempted suicide. Acta Psychiatr Scand. 1991;83:417-9.
110. Wender P, Kety S, Rosenthal D, et al. Psychiatric disorders in the biological and adoptive families of adopted individuals with affective disorder.Arch Gen Psychiatry. 1986;43:923-9.
111. Schulsinger R, Kety S, Rosenthal D, et al. A family study of suicide. In: Schou M, Stromgren E (Eds). Origins, Prevention and Treatment of Affective Disorders. New York: Academic Press; 1979. pp.277-87.
112. Pfeffer CR. Suicidal Behaviour in Children and Adolescents: Causes and Management. In: Lewis M (Ed). Child and Adolescent Psychiatry: A Comprehensive Textbook. Baltimore: William & Wilkins; 1996. pp.666-73.
113. Pfeffer CR. Childhood suicidal behaviour: A developmental perspective. Psychiatr Clin N Am. 1997;20:551-62.
114. Ministry of Welfare, Govt. Of India, Tata Institute of Social Sciences and UNICEF, India. India's Commitment to Family Well-being: An Overview of the Report of the National Seminar on the International Year of the Family,1994. Bombay: Tata Institute of Social Sciences; 1994.
115. Seshadri S, Srinath S, Girimaji S. Deliberate self-harm (attempted suicide) in children. Indian J Psychol Med. 1989;1:13-15.
116. Wells CF, Stuart IR (Eds). Self-Destructive Behaviour in Children and Adolescents. London: Van Nostrand Renhold Company; 1981.
117. Farmer R, Hirsch S. The Suicide Syndrome. London: Croom Helm; 1980.
118. Gispert M, Davis MS, Marsh L, Wheeler K. Predictive factors in repeated suicide attempts by adolescents. Hosp Comm Psychiatry. 1987;38:390-93.
119. Jacobs J. Adolescent Suicide. New York: Wiley Interscience; 1971.
120. Lehmann HE. Recognition and treatment of depression in geriatric patients. In: Ayd FJ Jr (Ed). Clinical Depression: Diagnostic and Therapeutic Challenges. Baltimore: Ayd Medical Communications; 1980.pp.57-69.
121. Conwell Y. Management of suicidal behaviour in the elderly. Psychiatr Clin N Am. 1997;20:667-83.
122. Ferrey G, Le Goues G. Psychopathologie du sujet age. Paris: Masson; 1993.
123. Patel SP, Gaw AC. Suicide among immigrants from the Indian subcontinent: A review. Psychiatr Serv. 1996;47:517-21.
124. Pridmore S, Lawler A, Couper D. Hanging and poisoning autopsies in Fiji. ANZ J Psychiatry. 1996;30:685-7.
125. Paris J. Cultural factors in the emergence of borderline pathology. Psychiatric. 59:185-192.
126. Neeleman J, Jones P, Van Os J, et al. Parasuicide in Camberwell: Ethnic differences. Soc Psychiatry Psychiatric Epidemiol. 1996;31:284-7.
127. Maniam T. Family characteristic suicides in Cameron Highlands : A controlled study. Med J Malaysia. 1994;49:247-51.
128. Khandelwal SK, Varma VK, Gupta R. Auto-castration: Review with a case report. Indian J Psychol Med. 1981;4:119-21.
129. Unni KES, Venugopal, Padmavathy, et al. Review of spurious dermatitis: case study of dermatitis artefacta. The Antiseptic. 91;381-383.
130. Chandra Sekhar K, Bhadrinath P, Venkataramaiah, et al. Munchausen syndrome: Review of literature and a case report. Indian J Psychol Med. 1980;3:101-4.
131. Libow JA, Schrier HA. Three forms of fictitious illness in children: When is it Munchausen syndrome by proxy. Am J Orthopsychiatr. 1986;56:602-11.
132. Government of India. Suicides in India,1964-1972. New Delhi: Government of India; 1976. pp.12-19, 34-37.
133. Aiyappan A, Jayadev CJ. Society in India. Madras: Social Science Publication; 1956.
134. Sathyavathi K, MurtiRao, DLN. A study of suicide in Bangalore. Transactions of All India Institute of Mental Health. 1961;2: 1-19.
135. Ganapathy MN, VenkobaRao A. A study on suicide in Madurai.J Indian Med Assoc. 1966;46:18-23.
136. Nandi DN, Mukherjee SP, Banerjee G, et al. Is suicide preventable by restricting the availability of lethal agents? A rural survey of West Bengal. Indian J Psychiatry. 1979;21:251-5.
137. Nandi DN, Banerjee G, Boral GC. Suicide in West Bengal: A century apart. Indian J Psychiatry. 1978;20:155-60.
138. Hegde RS. Suicide in a rural community of North Karnataka. Indian J Psychiatry. 1980;22:368-70.
139. Ponnudurai R, Jayakar J. Suicide in Madras. Indian J Psychiatry. 1980;2:203-5.
140. Ponnudurai R, Patnaik KA, Sathianathan R, et al. A study on the venues of suicide. Indian J Psychiatry. 1995;37(Suppl.):51.
141. Shukla GD, Verma BL, Mishra DN. Suicide in Jhansi City. Indian J Psychiatry. 1990;32:44-51.
142. Banerjee G, Nandi DN, Nandi S, et al. The vulnerability of Indian women to suicide: A field study. Indian J Psychiatry. 1990;32:305-308.
143. Sarma PG, Sawang DG. Suicides in rural areas of Warangal District. Indian J Behav Sci. 1993;3:79-84.
144. Ponnudurai R. Suicide in India. Indian J Psychol Med. 1996;19: 19-25.

145. Mehta SP, Sharma S, Ramalingam G. Epidemiology of parasuicides in Pondicherry Union Territory from 1975-79. Indian J Prev Soc Med. 1982;13:8-11.
146. Sudhir Kumar CT. A study of psychosocial factors associated with attempted suicide. MD dissertation submitted to the Pondicherry University; 1998.
147. Mahla VP, Bhargava SE, Dogra R, et al. The psychology of self immolation in India. Indian J Psychiatry. 1992;34:108-13.
148. Venkoba Rao A, Mahendran N, Gopalakrishnan C, et al. One hundred female burns cases: A study in suicidology. Indian J Psychiatry. 1989;31:43-50.
149. Mohandas E. Psychiatric emergencies. Indian J Psychol Med. 1996;11-18.
150. Greenhill LL, Waslick B. Management of suicidal behaviour in children and adolescents. Psychiatr Clin N Am. 1997;20: 641-66.
151. Harkavy-Friedman JM, Nelson-E. Management of the suicidal patient with schizophrenia.Psychiatr Clin N Am. 1997;20: 625-40.
152. Malone KM, Haas GL, Sweeney JA, et al. Major depression and the risk of attempted suicide. J Affect Dis. 1995;34:173-85.
153. Conwell Y. Management of suicidal behaviour in the elderly. Psychiatr Clin N Am. 1997;20:667-83.
154. KoestlerA. Janus: A Summing Up. London: Picador, Pan Books; 1979.
155. Havens L. The anatomy of a suicide. NEJM. 1965;272:401-6.
156. Chadda R, Kulhara P. Prevalence of various depressive symptoms in major depressive disorders. Indian J Psychol Med. 1987;10:1-6.
157. Mann JJ, Arango V. Integration of neurobiology and psychopatho-logy in a unified model of suicidal behaviour. J Clin Psychophar-macol. 1992;12(Suppl):2S-7S.
158. Venkoba Rao A. Psychological autopsy.
159. Venkoba Rao A. Post-vention: Madurai experience with suicide survivors. Indian J Psychol Med. 1997;20:6-13.
160. Reisberg B, Schneck MK, Ferris SH, et al. The Brief Cognitive Rating Scale (BCRS): Findings in Primary Degenerative Dementia (PDD). Psychopharmacol Bull. 1983;19:47.
161. Jablensky A, Sartorius N, Hirschfeld RMA, et al. Diagnosis and classification of mental disorders and alcohol and drug related problems: A research agenda for the 1980's. Psychol Med. 1983;13:907-21.
162. Weisman AD, Worden JW. Risk rescue rating in suicide assessment. Arch Gen Psychiatry. 1972;26:553-61.
163. Beck AT, Beck R, Kovacs M. Classification of suicidal behaviours: Quantifying intent and medical lethality. Am J Psychiatry. 1975;132:285-7.
164. Gupta SC, Anand R, Trivedi JK. Development of a suicide intent questionnaire. Indian J Psychiatry. 1983;25:57-62.
165. Beck AT, Weissman A, Lester D, et al. The measurement of pessimism: the hopelessness scale. J Consult Clin Psychol. 1974;42:861-5.
166. Bech P, Malt UF, Dencker SJ, et al. Scales for assessment of diagnosis and severity of mental disorders. Acta Psychiatr Scand. 1993;87(suppl.):37-41.
167. Morgan HG. Deliberate self harm. In: Granville-Grossman K (Ed). Recent Advances in Clinical Psychiatry. IV. London: Churchill Livingstone; 1982.
168. Gupta SC, Singh H. Psychiatric illness in suicide attempters. Indian J Psychiatry. 1981;23:75-8.
169. Ponnudurai R, Jayakar J, Saraswathy M. Attempted suicides in Madras. Indian J Psychiatry. 1986;28:59-62.
170. Fernandez-Pol B. Characteristics of 77 Puerto Ricans who attempted suicide. Am J Psychiatry. 1986;143:1460-63.
171. Hassan R. A Way of Dying. Karachi: Oxford University Press; 1983.
172. Andrande C, Vythilingam M, Channabasavanna SM. Evaluating the suicidal patient: Theoretical and practical aspects in the assessment of risk in India. Indian J Psychol Med. 1989;12: 75-86.
173. Seshadri S, Babu RK. Some psychiatric aspects of deliberate self harm. Indian J Psychol Med. 1988;11:67-71.
174. Stengel E. Suicide and Attempted suicide. Rev Ed. Great Britain: Penguin Books; 1970.
175. Stengel E, Cook NG. Attempted Suicide. London: Chapman & Hall,1958.
176. Paykel ES, Prussof BA, Myers JK. Sucide attempts and recent life events: A controlled comparison. Arch Gen Psychiatry. 1975;32:327-33.
177. Hawton K. Assessment of suicide risk. Br J Psychiatry. 1987;150: 145-153.
178. Van Praag HM, Putchik R, Conte H. The serotonin hypothesis of auto-aggression: Critical appraisal of the evidence. Ann NY Acad Sci. 1986;487:150-67.
179. Agarwal AK, Aga VM. Overview of psychiatric research in India. (1973-1992). Souvenir of the 46th Annual National Conference of Indian Psychiatric Society, 6th to 9th Jan.1994, Madras, pp.1-15.
180. Sutter J. L'anticipation. Paris: Presses Universitaires de France; 1983.
181. Branden N. The Psychopathology of Self-esteem. London: Bentam Books; 1971.
182. Janakiramaiah N. Editorial. Substance related disorders and the health sector response. De-addiction Quarterly (Bangalore, NIMHANS) 1996;2:1.
183. Ministry of Welfare, Govt. Of India, Tata Institute of Social Sciences and UNICEF, India. India's Commitment to Family Well-being: An Overview of the Report of the National Seminar on the International Year of the Family,1994. Bombay: Tata Institute of Social Sciences,1994.
184. Kishore J, Singh A, Grewal I, et al. Risk behaviour and viewing television in an adolescent male population of Delhi. J Mental Health and Human Behaviour. 1997;2:35-39.
185. Vernon MJ, Bennett GCJ. Elder abuse. J Applied Medicine. 1997;615-620.
186. WHO Programme on Mental Health: Life Skills Education in Schools. World Health Organisation,1994.
187. World Health Organisation. Message by Nelson Mandela, President of Republic of South Africa. Tobacco Alert; 1995 July.
188. Finlay I. Difficult decisions in palliative care. J of Applied Medicine. 1997;23:431-434.

189. McKenna P (Ed). Befriending Worldwide. The Newsletter of Befrienders International. 1996;49.
190. Scott V. Director General. Befrienders International. Developing volunteer action to prevent suicide. Personal communication; 1996.
191. Usha V. Founder member and former Director (1992-1997).' Maitreyi'-non-governmental organization for the prevention of suicide, Pondicherry; 1997.
192. Vijayakumar L. Founder member (since 1980), 'Sneha',- non-governmental organisation for the prevention of suicide, Madras; 1996.
193. Schmidtke A, Bille-Brahe U, DeLeo D, Kerkhof A, Bjerke T, Crepet P, et al. Attempted suicide in Europe: Rates, trends and sociodemographic characteristics of suicide attempters during the period 1989-1992. Results of the WHO/EURO Multicentre Study on Parasuicide. Acta Psychiatr Scand. 1996;93:327-38. [PubMed]
194. Patton GC, Coffey C, Sawyer SM, Viner RM, Haller DM, Bose K, et al. Global patterns of mortality in young people: A systematic analysis of population health data. Lancet. 2009;374:881-92. [PubMed]
195. Gururaj G, Isaac MK. Epidemiology of suicides in Bangalore. Bangalore: National Institute of Mental Health and Neuro Sciences; 2001. Report No: Publication No 43.
196. Accidental Deaths and Suicides in India 2007. New Delhi: Ministry of Home Affairs, Government of India; 2009. National Crime Records Bureau.
197. Khan FA, Anand B, Devi MG, Murthy KK. Psychological autopsy of suicide-a cross-sectional study. Indian J Psychiatry. 2005;47:73-8. [PMC free article] [PubMed]197-35.
198. Vijayakumar L, Rajkumar S. Are risk factors for suicide universal? A case-control study in India. Acta Psychiatr Scand. 1999;99:407-11. [PubMed].
199. Banerjee G, Nandi DN, Nandi S, Sarkar S, Boral GC, Ghosh A. The vulnerability of Indian women to suicide a field-study. Indian J Psychiatry. 1990;32:305-8. [PMC free article] [PubMed]
200. Nandi DN, Banerjee G, Boral GC, Chowdhury A, Bose J. Is suicide preventable by restricting the availability of lethal agents? A rural survey of West Bengal. Indian J Psychiatry. 1979;21:251-5.
201. Srivastava MK, Sahoo RN, Ghotekar LH, Dutta S, Danabalan M, Dutta TK, et al. Risk factors associated with attempted suicide: A case control study. Indian J Psychiatry. 2004;46:33-8. [PMC free article] [PubMed].
202. Unni SK, Mani AJ. Suicidal ideators in the psychiatric facility of a general hospital—a psychodemographic profile. Indian J Psychiatry. 1996;38:79-85. [PMC free article] [PubMed].
203. Vijayakumar L, John S, Pirkis J, Whiteford H. Suicide in developing countries (2): Risk factors. Crisis. 2005;26:112-9. [PubMed].
204. Pillai A, Andrews T, Patel V. Violence, psychological distress and the risk of suicidal behaviour in young people in India. Int J Epidemiol. 2009;38:459-69. [PubMed].
205. Crepet P, Caracciolo S, Casoli R, Fabbri D, Florenzano F, Grassi GM, et al. Suicidal behavior in Italy: Data, trends and guidelines for a suicide intervention/prevention policy. Suicide Life Threat Behav. 1991;21:263-78. [PubMed].
206. Adamek ME, Kaplan MS. The growing use of firearms by suicidal older women; 1979-1992: A research note. Suicide Life Threat Behav. 1996;26:71-8. [PubMed].
207. Rao AV, Madhavan T. Depression and suicide behaviour in the aged. Indian J Psychiatry. 1983;25:251-9. [PMC free article] [PubMed].
208. Shukla GD, Verma BL, Mishra DN. Suicide in Jhansi city. Indian J Psychiatry. 1990;32:44-51. [PMC free article] [PubMed].
209. Rao AV. Suicide in the elderly: A report from India. Crisis. 1991;12:33-9. [PubMed].
210. Purcell B, Heisel MJ, Speice J, Franus N, Conwell Y, Duberstein PR. Family connectedness moderates the association between living alone and suicide ideation in a clinical sample of adults 50 years and older. Am J Geriatr Psychiatry. 2011 [PMC free article] [PubMed].
211. Phillips MR, Yang G, Li S, Li Y. Suicide and the unique prevalence pattern of schizophrenia in mainland China: A retrospective observational study. Lancet. 2004;364:1062-8. [PubMed].
212. Desjarlais RE, Good B, Kleinman A. World mental health: Problems and priorities in low-income countries. New York: Oxford University Press;1995. Suicide.
213. Lester D. Suicide in an international perspective. Suicide Life Threat Behav. 1997;27:104-11. [PubMed].
214. Mayer P, Ziaian T. Suicide, gender, and age variations in India. Are women in Indian society protected from suicide? Crisis. 2002;23:98-103. [PubMed].
215. Gururaj G, Isaac MK, Subbakrishna DK, Ranjani R. Risk factors for completed suicides: A case-control study from Bangalore, India. Inj Control Saf Promot. 2004;11:183-91. [PubMed].
216. Kumar V. Poisoning deaths in married women. J Clin Forensic Med. 2004;11:2-5. [PubMed].
217. Durkheim E. Le Suicide: Etude de Sociologie. Paris: Presses Universitaires de France;1897.
218. Cutright P, Stack S, Fernquist R. Marital status integration, suicide disapproval, and societal integration as explanations of marital status differences in female age-specific suicide rates. Suicide Life Threat Behav. 2007;37:715-24. [PubMed].
219. World Report on Violence and Health. Geneva: WHO;2002. WHO.
220. Sudhir Kumar CT, Mohan R, Ranjith G, Chandrasekaran R. Gender differences in medically serious suicide attempts: A study from south India. Psychiatry Res. 2006;144:79-86. [PubMed].

221. Srivastava AS, Kumar R. Suicidal ideation and attempts in patients with major depression: Sociodemographic and clinical variables. Indian J Psychiatry. 2005;47:225-8. [PMC free article] [PubMed].
222. Gunnell D, Magnusson PK, Rasmussen F. Low intelligence test scores in 18 year old men and risk of suicide: Cohort study. BMJ. 2005;330:167. [PMC free article] [PubMed].
223. Martin G, Waite S. Parental bonding and vulnerability to adolescent suicide. Acta Psychiatr Scand. 1994;89:246-54. [PubMed].
224. van Egmond M, Garnefski N, Jonker D, Kerkhof A. The relationship between sexual abuse and female suicidal behavior. Crisis. 1993;14:129-39. [PubMed].
225. Adityanjee DR. Suicide attempts and suicides in India: Cross-cultural aspects. Int J Soc Psychiatry. 1986;32:64-73. [PubMed]
226. Gupta RK, Srivastava AK. Study of fatal burns cases in Kanpur (India) Forensic Sci Int. 1988;37:81-9. [PubMed].
227. Accidental Deaths and Suicides in India. New Delhi: NCRB;2000.
228. A Resource for General Physicians. Geneva: WHO;2000. Preventing Suicide.
229. Pritchard C. Is there a link between suicide in young men and unemployment? A comparison of the UK with other European Community Countries. Br J Psychiatry. 1992;160:750-6. [PubMed].
230. Rich AR, Bonner RL. Concurrent validity of a stress-vulnerability model of suicidal ideation and behavior: A follow-up study. Suicide Life Threat Behav. 1987;17:265-70. [PubMed].
231. Mohanty S, Sahu G, Mohanty MK, Patnaik M. Suicide in India: A four year retrospective study. J Forensic Leg Med. 2007;14:185-9. [PubMed].
232. Bhargava SC, Sethi S, Vohra AK. Klingsor syndrome: A case report. Indian J Psychiatry. 2001;43:349-50. [PMC free article] [PubMed].
233. Unni KE, Rotti SB, Chandrasekaran R. An exploratory study of the motivation in suicide attempters. Indian J Psychiatry. 1995;37:169-75. [PMC free article] [PubMed].
234. Bhatia MS, Verma SK, Murty OP. Suicide notes: Psychological and clinical profile. Int J Psychiatry Med. 2006;36:163-70. [PubMed].
235. Brown M, Barraclough B. Epidemiology of suicide pacts in England and Wales; 1988-92. BMJ. 1997;315:286-7. [PMC free article] [PubMed].
236. Bardale RV, Dixit PG. Dying together: A report of two-suicide pacts and an overview of the phenomenon. Calicut Med J. 2007;5:e6.
237. Rao A. Attempted suicide. Indian J Psychiatry. 1965;7:253-64.
238. Ponnudurai R, Jeyakar J, Saraswathy M. Attempted suicides in Madras. Indian J Psychiatry. 1986;28:59-62. [PMC free article] [PubMed].
239. Manoranjitham SD, Rajkumar AP, Thangadurai P, Prasad J, Jayakaran R, Jacob KS. Risk factors for suicide in rural south India. Br J Psychiatry. 2010;196:26-30. [PubMed]
240. Jain V, Singh H, Gupta SC, Kumar S. A study of hopelessness, suicidal intent and depression in cases of attempted suicide. Indian J Psychiatry. 1999;41:122-30. [PMC free article] [PubMed]
241. Chandrasekaran R, Gnanaseelan J, Sahai A, Swaminathan RP, Perme B. Psychiatric and personality disorders in survivors following their first suicide attempt. Indian J Psychiatry. 2003;45:45-8. [PMC free article] [PubMed].
242. Srivastava S, Kulshreshtha N. Expression of suicidal intent in depressives. Indian J Psychiatry. 2000;42:184-7. [PMC free article] [PubMed].
243. Gupta SC, Singh H, Trivedi JK. Evaluation of suicidal risk in depressives and schizophrenics: A 2-year follow-up study. Indian J Psychiatry. 1992;34:298-310. [PMC free article] [PubMed].
244. Kannapiran T, Haroon AE, Vivekanandan S, Arunagiri S. Personality profiles of self-immolators. Indian J Psychiatry. 1997;39:37-40. [PMC free article] [PubMed].
245. Suk JH, Han CH, Yeon BK. Suicide by burning in Korea. Int J Soc Psychiatry. 1991;37:141-5. [PubMed].
246. Patel V, Kirkwood BR, Pednekar S, Weiss H, Mabey D. Risk factors for common mental disorders in women.Population-based longitudinal study. Br J Psychiatry. 2006;189:547-55. [PubMed].
247. Rao AV. Suicide attempters in Madurai. J Indian Med Assoc. 1971;57:278-83. [PubMed].
248. Magni G, Rigatti-Luchini S, Fracca F, Merskey H. Suicidality in chronic abdominal pain: An analysis of the Hispanic Health and Nutrition Examination Survey (HHANES) Pain. 1998;76:137-44. [PubMed].
249. Smith MT, Edwards RR, Robinson RC, Dworkin RH. Suicidal ideation, plans, and attempts in chronic pain patients: Factors associated with increased risk. Pain. 2004;111:201-8. [PubMed]

SUGGESTED READING

1. Aaron R, Joseph A, Abraham S, Muliyil J, George K, Prasad J, et al. Suicides in young people in rural southern India. Lancet. 2004;363:1117-8. [PubMed]
2. Abraham VJ, Abraham S, Jacob KS. Suicide in the elderly in Kaniyambadi block, Tamil Nadu, south India. Int J Geriatr Psychiatry. 2005;20:953-5. [PubMed]
3. Accidental Deaths and Suicides in India 1990. New Delhi: Ministry of Home Affairs, Government of India; 1992. National Crime Records Bureau.
4. Accidental Deaths and Suicides in India 2006. New Delhi: Ministry of Home Affairs, Government of India; 2008. National Crime Records Bureau.
5. Accidental Deaths and Suicides in India 2007. New Delhi: Ministry of Home Affairs, Government of India; 2009. National Crime Records Bureau.
6. Accidental Deaths and Suicides in India 2008. New Delhi: Ministry of Home Affairs, Government of India;2010. National Crime Records Bureau.

7. Anguiano L, Mayer DK, Piven ML, Rosenstein D. A literature review of suicide in cancer patients. Cancer Nurs. 2012;35:E14-26. [PubMed]
8. Behere PB, Behere AP. Farmers' suicide in Vidarbha region of Maharashtra state: A myth or reality? Indian J Psychiatry. 2008;50:124-7. [PMC free article] [PubMed]
9. Bertolote JM, Fleischmann A. Suicide and psychiatric diagnosis: A worldwide perspective. World Psychiatry. 2002;1:181-5. [PMC free article] [PubMed]
10. Bhatia MS, Aggarwal NK, Aggarwal BB. Psychosocial profile of suicide ideators, attempters and completers in India. Int J Soc Psychiatry. 2000;46:155-63. [PubMed]
11. Bhat M. Vol. 7. Minneapolis, MI, United States: Centre for Population Analysis and Policy, Humphrey Institute of Public Affairs, University of Minnesota; 1991. Mortality from accidents and violence in India and China, Research Report 91-06-1.
12. Bhugra D. Sati: A type of nonpsychiatric suicide. Crisis. 2005;26:73-7. [PubMed]
13. Birbal R, Maharajh HD, Clapperton M, Jarvis J, Ragoonath A, Uppalapati K. Cybersuicide and the adolescent population: Challenges of the future? Int J Adolesc Med Health. 2009;21:151-9. [PubMed]
14. Bose A, Konradsen F, John J, Suganthy P, Muliyil J, Abraham S. Mortality rate and years of life lost from unintentional injury and suicide in south India. Trop Med Int Health. 2006;11:1553-6. [PubMed]
15. Braun W. Sallekhana: The ethicality and legality of religious suicide by starvation in the Jain religious community. Med Law. 2008;27:913-24. [PubMed]
16. Chavan BS, Singh GP, Kaur J, Kochar R. Psychological autopsy of 101 suicide cases from northwest region of India. Indian J Psychiatry. 2008;50:34-8. [PMC free article] [PubMed]
17. Das PP, Grover S, Avasthi A, Chakrabarti S, Malhotra S, Kumar S. Intentional self-harm seen in psychiatric referrals in a tertiary care hospital. Indian J Psychiatry. 2008;50:187-91. [PMC free article] [PubMed]
18. Department of injuries and violence prevention. Noncommunicable Diseases and Mental Health Cluster. Geneva: WHO;2002. WHO. The Injury Chart Book. A graphical overview of the global burden of injuries. http://whqlibdoc.who.int/publications/924156220x.pdf.
19. Department of Mental Health, Social Change and Mental Health. Geneva: WHO;1999. WHO. Figures and facts about suicide 1999. http://whqlibdoc.who.int/hq/1999/WHO_MNH_MBD_99.1.pdf.
20. Diekstra RF. Suicide and the attempted suicide: An international perspective. Acta Psychiatr Scand Suppl. 1989;354:1-24. [PubMed]
21. Elangbam V, Singh AB, Devi KS, Devi LU. Suicidal acts reported at a teaching hospital in manipur. Indian J Community Med. 2009;34:357-8. [PMC free article] [PubMed]
22. Ernst C, Mechawar N, Turecki G. Suicide neurobiology. Prog Neurobiol. 2009;89:315-33. [PubMed]
23. Evans G, Norman L. The Encyclopedia of Suicide. New York, NY: Facts on File;1988. Farberow.
24. Gajalakshmi V, Peto R. Suicide rates in rural Tamil Nadu, south India: Verbal autopsy of 39 000 deaths in 1997-98. Int J Epidemiol. 2007;36:203-7. [PubMed]
25. Gururaj GA, Isaac MK, Latif MA, Abeyasinghe R, Tantipiwatanaskul P. SEA/Ment/118. New Delhi: WHO/SEARO;2001. Suicide prevention- emerging from darkness.
26. Hawton K, van Heeringen K. Suicide. Lancet. 2009;373:1372-81. [PubMed]
27. International Association for Suicide Prevention. World Suicide Prevention Day. Sep 10, [Last cited in 2011]. Available from: http://www.iasp.info/wspd/2011_wspd.php.
28. Isaac M, Elias B, Katz LY, Belik SL, Deane FP, Enns MW, et al. Gatekeeper training as a preventative intervention for suicide: A systematic review. Can J Psychiatry. 2009;54:260-8. [PubMed]
29. Jena S, Sidhartha T. Non-fatal suicidal behaviors in adolescents. Indian J Psychiatry. 2004;46:310-8. [PMC free article] [PubMed]
30. Joseph A, Abraham S, Muliyil JP, George K, Prasad J, Minz S, et al. Evaluation of suicide rates in rural India using verbal autopsies, 1994-9. BMJ. 2003;326:1121-2. [PMC free article] [PubMed]
31. Kandasamy A, Chaturvedi SK, Desai G. Spirituality, distress, depression, anxiety, and quality of life in patients with advanced cancer. Indian J Cancer. 2011;48:55-9. [PubMed]
32. Kar N. Profile of risk factors associated with suicide attempts: A study from Orissa, India. Indian J Psychiatry. 2010;52:48-56. [PMC free article] [PubMed]
33. Khan FA, Anand B, Devi MG, Murthy KK. Psychological autopsy of suicide-a cross-sectional study. Indian J Psychiatry. 2005;47:73-8. [PMC free article] [PubMed]
34. Latha KS, Bhat SM. Suicidal behaviour among terminally ill cancer patients in India. Indian J Psychiatry. 2005;47:79-83. [PMC free article] [PubMed]
35. Lee WJ, Cha ES, Park ES, Kong KA, Yi JH, Son M. Deaths from pesticide poisoning in South Korea: Trends over 10 years. Int Arch Occup Environ Health. 2009;82:365-71. [PubMed]
36. Manoranjitham S, Abraham A, Jacob KS. Towards a national policy to reduce suicide in India. Natl Med J India. 2005;18:118-22. [PubMed]
37. Mendonsa RD, Appaya P. Psychiatric morbidity in outpatients of gynecological oncology clinic in a tertiary care hospital. Indian J Psychiatry. 2010;52:327-32. [PMC free article] [PubMed]
38. Narang RL, Mishra BP, Nitesh M. Attempted suicide in Ludhiana. Indian J Psychiatry. 2000;42:83-7. [PMC free article] [PubMed]
39. Niederkrotenthaler T, Voracek M, Herberth A, Till B, Strauss M, Etzersdorfer E, et al. Media and suicide. Papageno v Werther effect. BMJ. 2010;341:c5841. [PubMed]
40. Nordentoft M. Prevention of suicide and attempted suicide in Denmark.Epidemiological studies of suicide and intervention studies in selected risk groups. Dan Med Bull. 2007;54:306-69. [PubMed]
41. Rajagopal S. Suicide pacts and the internet. BMJ. 2004;329:1298-9. [PMC free article] [PubMed]
42. Ramadas S, Kuttichira P. The development of a guideline and its impact on the media reporting of suicide. Indian J Psychiatry. 2011;53:224-8. [PMC free article] [PubMed]

43. Ruzicka LT. Suicide in countries and areas of the ESCAP region. Asia Pac Popul J. 1998;13:55-74. [PubMed]
44. Saddichha S, Prasad MN, Saxena MK. Attempted suicides in India: A comprehensive look. Arch Suicide Res. 2010;14:56-65. [PubMed]
45. Saddichha S, Vibha P, Saxena MK, Methuku M. Behavioral emergencies in India: A population based epidemiological study. Soc Psychiatry Psychiatr Epidemiol. 2010;45:589-93. [PubMed]
46. Sarkar P, Sattar FA, Gode N, Basannar DR. Failed suicide and deliberate self-harm: A need for specific nomenclature. Indian J Psychiatry. 2006;48:78-83. [PMC free article] [PubMed]
47. Sauvaget C, Ramadas K, Fayette JM, Thomas G, Thara S, Sankaranarayanan R. Completed suicide in adults of rural Kerala: Rates and determinants. Natl Med J India. 2009;22:228-33. [PubMed]
48. Sharma RC. Attempted suicide in Himachal Pradesh. Indian J Psychiatry. 1998;40:50-4. [PMC free article] [PubMed]
49. Soman CR, Safraj S, Kutty VR, Vijayakumar K, Ajayan K. Suicide in south India: A community-based study in Kerala. Indian J Psychiatry. 2009;51:261-4. [PMC free article] [PubMed]
50. Soomro GM. Deliberate self-harm (and attempted suicide) Clin Evid (Online) 2008;2008 [PMC free article] [PubMed]
51. Suresh Kumar PN. An analysis of suicide attempters versus completers in Kerala. Indian J Psychiatry. 2004;46:144-9. [PMC free article] [PubMed]
52. Terao T, Soeda S, Yoshimura R, Nakamura J, Iwata N. Effect of latitude on suicide rates in Japan. Lancet. 2002;360:1892. [PubMed]
53. Thomas K, Chang SS, Gunnell D. Suicide epidemics: The impact of newly emerging methods on overall suicide rates - a time trends study. BMC Public Health. 2011;11:314. [PMC free article] [PubMed]
54. Vijayakumar L, Satheesh-Babu R. Does 'no pesticide' reduce suicides? Int J Soc Psychiatry. 2009;55:401-6. [PubMed]
55. Vijayakumar L, Umamaheswari C, Shujaath Ali ZS, Devaraj P, Kesavan K. Intervention for suicide attempters: A randomized controlled study. Indian J Psychiatry. 2011;53:244-8. [PMC free article] [PubMed]
56. Vijayakumar L. Altruistic suicide in India. Arch Suicide Res. 2004;8:73-80. [PubMed]
57. Vijayakumar L. Suicide prevention: The urgent need in developing countries. World Psychiatry. 2004;3:158-9. [PMC free article] [PubMed]
58. WHO. Suicide prevention (SUPRE) [Last accessed on 2012 Mar 27]. Available from: http://www.who.int/mental_health/prevention/suicide/suicideprevent/en/
59. World Health Organization. Global Burden of Disease. 2004. [Last cited in 2004]. Update. Available from: http://www.who.int/healthinfo/global_burden_disease/GBD_report_2004update_full.pdf.
60. World Health Organization. Suicide rates per 100,000 by country, year and sex. [Last accessed on 2013 Mar 27]. Available from: http://www.who.int/mental_health/prevention/suicide_rates/en/index.html.
61. Yip PS. Charcoal-burning suicides and strategies for prevention. Crisis. 2007;28:21-7.

Textbook of
Postgraduate Psychiatry

Textbook of Postgraduate Psychiatry

Third Edition

Volume 2

Editors

JN Vyas

MBBS DPM MNAMS MAPA (USA) DIPLO WPA

Professor and Head
Department of Psychiatry
National Medical College and Teaching Hospital
Birgunj, Nepal

Former Superintendent
PBM Group of Hospitals, Bikaner and
Psychiatric Center, Jaipur

Former Principal and Controller
SP Medical College and Associated Group of Hospitals, Bikaner

Former Head
Department of Psychiatry, SMS Medical College, Jaipur
Dr SN Medical College, Jodhpur and SP Medical College, Bikaner

Former Head, Department of Psychiatry
Mahatama Gandhi National Institute of Medical Sciences, Jaipur, Rajasthan, India

Former Head, Department of Psychiatry
Universal College of Medical Sciences, Bhairahwa, and
Nepalgunj Medical College, Nepalgunj, Nepal

Shree Ram Ghimire

MBBS (TU) MD (TU) MPH/MHID (Flinders University, Australia)

Consultant Psychiatrist
Transcultural Psychosocial Organization Nepal
Baluwatar, Kathmandu, Nepal

Former Lecturer, Department of Psychiatry
National Medical College and Teaching Hospital, Birgunj, Nepal

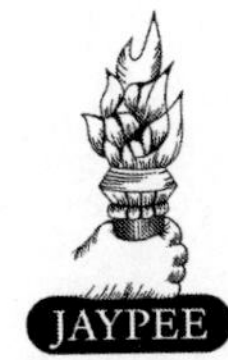

JAYPEE BROTHERS MEDICAL PUBLISHERS
The Health Sciences Publisher
New Delhi | London

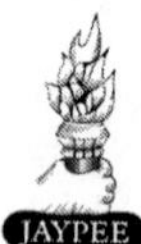

Jaypee Brothers Medical Publishers (P) Ltd

Headquarters
EMCA House
23/23-B, Ansari Road, Daryaganj
New Delhi 110 002, India
Landline: +91-11-23272143, +91-11-23272703
+91-11-23282021, +91-11-23245672
E-mail: jaypee@jaypeebrothers.com

Corporate Office
4838/24, Ansari Road, Daryaganj
New Delhi 110 002, India
Phone: +91-11-43574357
Fax: +91-11-43574314
E-mail: jaypee@jaypeebrothers.com

Overseas Office
J.P. Medical Ltd
83 Victoria Street, London
SW1H 0HW (UK)
Phone: +44 20 3170 8910
E-mail: info@jpmedpub.com

EU GPSR Authorised Representative
Logos Europe, 9 rue Nicolas Poussin
17000, La Rochelle, France
Phone: +33 (0) 6 67 93 73 78
E-mail: contact@logoseurope.eu

Website: www.jaypeebrothers.com
Website: www.jaypeedigital.com

Inquiries for bulk sales may be solicited at: jaypee@jaypeebrothers.com

Inquiries for bulk sales may be solicited at: jaypee@jaypeebrothers.com

Textbook of Postgraduate Psychiatry (2 Volumes)

First Edition : 1992
Second Edition : 1999
Third Edition : **2016**
Reprint: **2026**

ISBN 978-93-5152-910-1

Printed at: Samrat Offset Pvt. Ltd.

Dedicated to

My beloved mother Smt Lal Kaur Devi and father, (Late) Shri KN Vyas and to my grandchildren—Abhishek, Eshita, Om Narain and Hari Narain

– JN Vyas

My beloved parents, brother, sister, wife, children (Smriti, Ritu, Pratik and Aarush), all mentally ill patients and their family members

– Shree Ram Ghimire

Contributors

Abhinav Tandon
Consultant Psychiatrist
Neuropsychiatric Centre
Allahabad, Uttar Pradesh, India

Abhishek Pathak
Senior Resident
Department of Psychiatry
Institute of Medical Sciences
Banaras Hindu University
Varanasi, Uttar Pradesh, India

Adarsh Tripathi
Assistant Professor
Department of Psychiatry
King George's Medical University
Lucknow, Uttar Pradesh, India

A Das
Resident
Department of Psychiatry
Jawaharlal Nehru Medical College
Wardha, Maharashtra, India

Ajit Avasthi
Professor
Department of Psychiatry
Postgraduate Institute of Medical Education and Research (PGIMER)
Chandigarh, India

AK Agarwal
Former Professor and Head
Department of Psychiatry
King George's Medical University
Lucknow, Uttar Pradesh, India

Alakananda Dutt
Senior Resident
Department of Psychiatry
Postgraduate Institute of Medical Education and Research (PGIMER)
Chandigarh, India

Allen De Souza
Research Assistant
Desousa Foundation
Mumbai, Maharashtra, India

A Mulmule
Resident
Department of Psychiatry
Jawaharlal Nehru Medical College
Wardha, Maharashtra, India

AN Basu
Consultant Psychoanalyst
Girindra Sekar Clinic
Kolkata, West Bengal, India

Andrea-Sylvia Winkler
Registrar
King's Healthcare NHS Trust
Mapother House
King's College Hospital
Denmark Hill, London, UK

Anjali Chabbria
Lecturer
Department of Psychological Medicine
Dr RN Cooper Hospital and KEM Group of Hospitals
Mumbai, Maharashtra, India

Anjanik Kumar Ranjan
Senior Resident
Central Institute of Psychiatry
Ranchi, Jharkhand, India

Anushul Khichy
Senior Resident
Central Institute of Psychiatry
Ranchi, Jharkhand, India

Aparna Garg
Assistant Professor
Department of Physiology
Mahatma Gandhi Medical College and Hospital
Jaipur, Rajasthan, India

AP Behere
Consultant (Attending) Child and Adolescent Psychiatrist
Mid Coast Mental Health Centre and Pen Bay Psychiatry
Rockland, Belfast, USA

AP Dadhich
Professor and Head
Department of Pharmacology
Christian Medical College
Ludhiana, Punjab, India

A Prasad
Assistant Professor
Department of Neurology
Institute of Human Behaviour and Allied Sciences, New Delhi, India

A Puri
Formerly Clinical Psychologist
Department of Pediatrics
Postgraduate Institute of Medical Education and Research (PGIMER)
Chandigarh, India

AR Garg
Former Professor and Head
Department of Psychiatry
Jawaharlal Nehru Medical College
Ajmer, Rajasthan, India

Asha Krishnan
Senior Resident
Central Institute of Psychiatry
Ranchi, Jharkhand, India

Ashok Singhal
Assistant Professor
Department of Psychiatry
SP Medical College
Bikaner, Rajasthan, India

Avinash De Souza
Research Associate
Department of Psychiatry
Lokmanya Tilak Municipal Medical College
Mumbai, Maharashtra, India

AW Jagdeesh
Resident
Department of Psychiatry
National Institute of Mental Health and Neurosciences
Bengaluru, Karnataka, India

Baljit Singh Saluja
Department of Psychiatry
Postgraduate Institute of Medical Education and Research
Chandigarh, India

Bhoomika Sachacher
Research Officer
Project HIFAZAT
Regional Technical Training Centre
Ranchi, Jharkhand, India

Bikramaditya Jaiswal
Senior Resident
Central Institute of Psychiatry
Ranchi, Jharkhand, India

BK Singh
Professor and Head
Department of Psychiatry
Patna Medical College and Hospital
Patna, Bihar, India

BN Gangadhar
Professor
Department of Psychiatry
National Institute of Mental Health and Neurosciences
Bengaluru, Karnataka, India

B Reddy
Senior Resident
Department of Psychiatry
Jawaharlal Institute of Postgraduate Medical Education and Research
Puducherry, India

BS Bhogle
Professor and Head
Department of Psychiatry
Medical College
Belgaum, Karnataka, India

BS Chavan
Professor and Head
Department of Psychiatry
Government Medical College
Chandigarh, India

Chittaranjan Andrade
Professor
Department of Psychiatry
National Institute of Mental Health and Neurosciences
Bengaluru, Karnataka, India

Christoday RJ Khess
Director
Professor and Head
Central Institute of Psychiatry
Ranchi, Jharkhand, India

CR Chandrashekar
Additional Professor
Department of Psychiatry
National Institute of Mental Health and Neurosciences
Bengaluru, Karnataka, India

CR Mukundan
Professor and Head
Department of Psychiatry
Neuropsychology Laboratory
National Institute of Mental Health and Neurosciences
Bengaluru, Karnataka, India

Deyashini Lahiri Tikka
Assistant Professor
Department of Clinical Psychology
Central Institute of Psychiatry
Ranchi, Jharkhand, India

Dhanesh K Gupta
Assistant Professor
Department of Psychiatry
All India Institute of Medical Sciences
New Delhi, India

Dilip R Patel
Professor
Department of Pediatrics
Michigan State University
Kalamazoo Center for Medical Studies
Oakland, USA

Dinesh Mohan Das
Senior Resident
Department of Psychiatry
Dr RN Cooper Hospital and
Seth GS Medical College
Mumbai, Maharasthra, India

Dinesh Tyagi
Consultant Psychiatrist
Senior Resident
Department of Psychiatry
Institute of Human Behaviour and Allied Sciences
New Delhi, India

DK Kochar
Professor
Department of Medicine
Neurology Section
SP Medical College
Bikaner, Rajasthan, India

DN Nandi
Consultant Psychiatry
Garindra Sekar Clinic
Kolkata, West Bengal, India

Eesha Sharma
Lecturer
Department of Psychiatry
King George's Medical University
Lucknow, Uttar Pradesh, India

Gayatri Saraf
Post Doctoral Fellow in Consultation Liaison Psychiatry and Senior Resident
Department of Psychiatry
National Institute of Mental Health and Neurosciences
Bengaluru, Karnataka, India

GC Munjal
Formerly Professor and Head
Department of Psychiatry
GB Pant Hospital and
Maulana Azad Medical College
New Delhi, India

Geeta Mehta
Professor and Head
Department of Microbiology
Lady Hardinge Medical College
New Delhi, India

GN Saxena
Principal
Professor of Medicine
Mahtama Gandhi Institute of Medical Sciences
Jaipur, Rajasthan, India

G Prasad Rao
Professor and Head
Department of Psychiatry
Bhaskar Medical College
Director
Schizophrenia and Psychopharmacological Division
Asha Hospital
Hyderabad, Telangana, India

Hemant Vyas
Former Senior Demonstrator
Department of Community Medicine
Mahatma Gandhi Institute of Medical Sciences
Jaipur, Rajasthan, India

Hitesh Khurana
Senior Resident
Department of Psychiatry
Postgraduate Institute of Medical Education and Research
Chandigarh, India

Indira Sharma
President
Indian Psychiatric Society
President
SAARC Psychiatric Foundation
Vice President
Asian Federation of Psychiatric Associations
Professor and Head
Department of Child and Adolescent Psychiatry Unit
Institute of Medical Sciences
Banaras Hindu University
Varanasi, Uttar Pradesh, India

Issy Pilowsky
Professor
Department of Psychiatry
The University of Adelaide
Royal Adelaide Hospital Adelaide
South Australia

Jagadisha Thirthalli
Additional Professor
Department of Psychiatry
National Institute of Mental Health and Neurosciences
Bengaluru, Karnataka, India

Jayati Simlai
Additional Professor and Head
Department of Psychiatry
Ranchi Institute of Neuro-Psychiatry and Allied Sciences
Ranchi, Jharkhand, India

Jayesh Ranjan
Consultant Neuropsychiatrist
Ranchi Mental Hospital
Ranchi, Jharkhand, India

JN Vyas
Professor and Head
Department of Psychiatry
National Medical College and Teaching Hospital
Birgunj, Nepal
Former Superintendent
PBM Group of Hospitals, Bikaner and Psychiatric Center
Jaipur
Former Principal and Controller
SP Medical College and Associated Group of Hospitals
Bikaner
Former Head
Department of Psychiatry
SMS Medical College, Jaipur
Dr SN Medical College, Jodhpur and
SP Medical College
Bikaner
Former Head
Department of Psychiatry
Mahatama Gandhi National Institute of Medical Sciences
Jaipur, Rajasthan, India
Former Head
Department of Psychiatry
Universal College of Medical Sciences
Bhairahwa and
Nepalgunj Medical College
Nepalgunj, Nepal

Johnson Pradeep R
Assistant Professor
Department of Psychiatry
St. John's Medical College Hospital
St. John's National Institute of Health Sciences
Bengaluru, Karnataka, India

Joyita Sinha
Senior Resident
Central Institute of Psychiatry
Ranchi, Jharkhand, India

Jyoti Ahuja
Clinical Psychologist
National Institute of Mental Health and Neurosciences
Bengaluru, Karnataka, India

KA Khurshid
Senior Resident
Department of Psychiatry
All India Institute of Medical Sciences (AIIMS)
New Delhi, India

KE Sadanandan Unni
Assistant Professor
Department of Psychiatry
Jawarhar Lal Institute of Medical Education
Puducherry, India

KK Verma
Assistant Professor
Department of Psychiatry
SP Medical College
Bikaner, Rajasthan, India

K Ray Chaudhuri
Consultant Neurologist and Senior Lecturer
Department of Neurology
King's Healthcare NHS Trust
Mapother House
King's College Hospital
Denmark Hill, London, UK

KS Anand
Associate Professor
Department of Neurology
Institute of Human Behaviour and Allied Sciences
New Delhi, India

Late JK Trivedi
Formerly Professor
Department of Psychiatry
King George's Medical College
Lucknow, Uttar Pradesh, India

Late V Ramachandran
Formerly Professor
Department of Psychiatry
Madras Medical College, Chennai
Formerly Neuropsychiatrist
Institute of Mental Health
Chennai, Tamil Nadu, India

Laura Murray
Clinical Psychologist
Michigan State University
Kalamazoo Center for Medical Studies
Oakland, USA

LN Gupta
Professor
Department of Psychiatry
SMS Medical College
Jaipur, Rajasthan, India

Malavika Kapur
Professor
Department of Psychiatry
National Institute of Mental Health and Neurosciences
Bengaluru, Karnataka, India

Manju Mehta
Additional Professor
Department of Clinical Psychology
All India Institute of Medical Sciences (AIIMS)
New Delhi, India

Manoj Dhungana
Senior Psychiatrist
Former Assistant Professor
Universal Medical College
Bhairahawa, Nepal

Mridula Vyas
Professor and Head
Department of Mathematics
Vivekananda Institute of Technology
Jaipur, Rajasthan, India

M Behere
Psychiatric Social Worker
Department of Psychiatry
Jawaharlal Nehru Medical College
Wardha, Maharashtra, India

Munish Aggarwal
Senior Resident
Department of Psychiatry
Postgraduate Institute of Medical Education and Research (PGIMER)
Chandigarh, India

Naveen Kumar C
Assistant Professor
Department of Psychiatry
National Institute of Mental Health and Neurosciences
Bengaluru, Karnataka, India

Neena Bohra
Former Senior Psychiatrist
Professor
Department of Psychiatry
Lady Hardinge Medical College
New Delhi, India

Neha Singh
Senior Resident
Central Institute of Psychiatry
Ranchi, Jharkhand, India

Nikhil Jain
Senior Resident
Department of Psychiatry
Dr SN Medical College
Jodhpur, Rajasthan, India

Nilesh Shah
Professor and Head
Department of Psychiatry
Lokmanya Tilak Municipal Medical College, Mumbai, Maharashtra, India

Nimesh G Desai
Professor and Head
Department of Psychiatry
Institute of Human Behaviour and Allied Sciences, New Delhi, India

Niraj Ahuja
Assistant Professor
Department of Psychiatry
Jawaharlal Institute of Postgraduate Medical Education and Research
Puducherry, India

NK Bohra
Director
Neuropsychiatric Center
New Delhi, India
Director
Delhi Academy of Practicing Psychaitrists
Former President, Association of Private Psychiatrists of India
Former President of Indian Association of Biological Psychiatry

NK Singh
Professor and Head
Department of Psychiatry
Patna Medical College and Hospital
Patna, Bihar, India

N Parvez
Senior Resident
Central Institute of Psychiatry
Ranchi, Jharkhand, India

N Sanjay Kumar Rao
Royal Edinburgh Hospital
Edinburgh, UK

PB Behere
Director
Research and Development (R&D)
Professor and Head
Department of Psychiatry
Jawaharlal Nehru Medical College
Datta Meghe Institute of Medical Sciences, Wardha, Maharashtra, India
Visiting Professor
University of Chester, UK
Adjunct Faculty, Georgia Southern University, USA

Prabha S Chandra
Professor
Department of Psychiatry
National Institute of Mental Health and Neurosciences
Bengaluru, Karnataka, India

Pramodh Bhardhwaj
Former Professor and Head
Department of Psychiatry
Rabindra Nath Tagore Medical College
Udaipur, Rajasthan, India

Priti Arun
Senior Lecturer
Department of Psychiatry
Government Medical College
Chandigarh, India

PSDV Prasadarao
Assistant Professor
Department of Clinical Psychology
National Institute of Mental Health and Neurosciences
Bengaluru, Karnataka, India

RA Bumb
Professor and Head
Department of Dermatology, Venereology and Leprosy
SP Medical College
Bikaner, Rajasthan, India

Radha Prabhu
Clinical Psychologist
National Institute of Mental Health and Neurosciences
Bengaluru, Karnataka, India

Rajesh Sagar
Assistant Professor
Department of Psychiatry
All India Institute of Medical Sciences
New Delhi, India

Raju Sedhain
Pediatrics Consultant
Mechi Hospital, Jhapa, Nepal

Rakesh Lal
Additional Professor
Department of Psychiatry
All India Institute of Medical Sciences (AIIMS)
New Delhi, India

Raminder Kalra
Tutor
Rajkumari Amrit Kaur
College of Nursing, New Delhi, India

R Chandrasekaran
Professor and Head
Department of Psychiatry
Jawaharlal Institute of Postgraduate Medical Education and Research
Puducherry, India

RC Chowdhary
Professor and Head
Department of Community Medicine
Mahatma Gandhi National Institute of Medical Sciences
Jaipur, Rajasthan, India

RC Jiloha
Professor and Head
Department of Psychiatry
GB Pant Hospital and
Maulana Azad Medical College
New Delhi, India

RD Mehta
Assistant Professor
Department of Dermatology, Venereology and Leprosy
SP Medical College
Bikaner, Rajasthan, India

RK Chadda
Professor
Department of Psychiatry
All India Institute of Medical Sciences
New Delhi, India

RK Solanki
Senior Professor and Head
Department of Psychiatry
Dr SN Medical College
Jodhpur, Rajasthan, India

Roshan V Khanande
Senior Resident
Central Institute of Psychiatry
Ranchi, Jharkhand, India

RP Agarwal
Assistant Professor
Department of Medicine
SP Medical College
Bikaner, Rajasthan, India

Sachchidanand Singh
Senior Resident
Central Institute of Psychiatry
Ranchi, Jharkhand, India

Sai Krishna Tikka
Senior Resident
Central Institute of Psychiatry
Ranchi, Jharkhand, India

Sandeep Grover
Associate Professor
Department of Psychiatry
Postgraduate Institute of Medical
Education and Research
Chandigarh, India

Sandeep M
Senior Resident
Central Institute of Psychiatry
Ranchi, Jharkhand, India

Santosh K Chaturvedi
Professor
Department of Psychiatry
National Institute of Mental Health and
Neurosciences
Bengaluru, Karnataka, India

Sarita Parajuli
Chakrabarti Habi Nursing College
Bhaktapur, Nepal

SC Bhargav
Professor
Department of Psychiatry
Medical College
Rohtak, Haryana, India

SC Gupta
Reader
Department of Psychiatry
King George's Medical College
Lucknow, Uttar Pradesh, India

SC Malik
Formerly Professor and Head
Department of Psychiatry
Lady Hardinge Medical College
New Delhi, India

SC Pradhan
Senior Resident
Institute of Human Behaviour and
Allied Sciences
New Delhi, India

Shashi Kiran
Formerly Assistant Professor
Department of Psychiatry
National Institute of Mental Health and
Neurosciences
Bengaluru, Karnataka, India
Currently Child and Adolescent
Psychiatry Consultant
County Durham and Darlington
Priority Services NHS Trust
Durham, UK

Shaswat Saxena
Senior Resident
Department of Psychiatry
King George's Medical University
Lucknow, Uttar Pradesh, India

Sheela Jain
Associate Professor
Department of Anatomy
SP Medical College
Bikaner, Rajasthan, India

Shivananda Jena
Assistant Professor
Department of Psychiatry
GB Pant Hospital and
Maulana Azad Medical College
New Delhi, India

Shivanshu Shrivastava
Research Assistant and Observer
Department of Psychiatry
Lokmanya Tilak Municipal
Medical College
Mumbai, Maharashtra, India

Shree Ram Ghimire
Consultant Psychiatrist
Transcultural Psychosocial
Organization Nepal
Baluwatar, Kathmandu, Nepal
Former Lecturer
Department of Psychiatry
National Medical College and Teaching
Hospital
Birgunj, Nepal

Shubhakaran
Senior Registrar
SP Medical College
Bikaner, Rajasthan, India

S Kalyanasundaram
Principal and Professor
Department of Psychaitry
The Richmond Fellowship Post
Graduate College for Psychosocial
Rehabilitation
Bengaluru, Karnataka, India

SK Pandey
Senior Psychiatrist
Carewell Family Clinic
Jaipur, Rajasthan, India

SK Verma
Additional Professor
Department of Clinical Psychology
Postgraduate Institute of Medical
Education and Research
Chandigarh, India

SN Ali
Central Institute of Psychiatry
Ranchi, Jharkhand, India

Somnath Sen Gupta
Associate Professor
Department of Psychiatry
Kasturba Medical College and Hospital
Manipal, Karnataka, India

Sourav Khanra
Senior Resident
Central Institute of Psychiatry
Ranchi, Jharkhand, India

SS Nathawat
Former Professor and Head
Department of Psychology
University of Rajasthan
Jaipur, Rajasthan, India

Sudhir Hebbar
Senior Resident
Department of Psychiatry
Jawaharlal Institute of Postgraduate
Medical Education and Research
Puducherry, India

Sudhir Kumar CT
Senior Resident
Department of Psychiatry
National Institute of
Mental Health and Neurosciences
Bengaluru, Karnataka, India

Sujata Malik
Senior Occupational Therapist
Safdarjung Hospital
New Delhi, India

Sumant Khanna
Former Professor
Department of Psychiatry
National Institute of Mental Health and Neurosciences
Bengaluru, Karnataka, India

Sunila Chadda
Professor and Head
Department of Pathology
Dr SN Medical College, Jodhpur
SP Medical College
Bikaner, Rajasthan, India

Suresh Bada Math
Additional Professor
Department of Psychiatry
National Institute of Mental Health and Neurosciences
Bengaluru, Karnataka, India

Swarnali Bose
Clinical Psychologist and Training Co-ordinator
Project HIFAZAT
Regional Technical Training Centre
Ranchi, Jharkhand, India

TS Sathyanarayana Rao
Editor
Indian Journal of Psychiatry
Chief Advisor
Indian Journal of Psychological Medicine, Indian Journal of Geriatric Psychiatry, Indian Journal of Social Psychiatry, Indian Journal of Private Psychiatry, Andhra Pradesh Journal of Psychological Medicine
President Elect
Indian Association for Geriatric Mental Health
Professor
Department of Psychiatry
JSS Medical College and Hospital
Mysuru, Karnataka, India

Uma Joshi
Professor
Department of Physiology
Mahatma Gandhi Institute of Medical Sciences
Jaipur, Rajasthan, India

Umesh S
Senior Resident
Central Institute of Psychiatry
Ranchi, Jharkhand, India

Urvakhsh Mehta
Assistant Professor
Department of Psychiatry
National Institute of Mental Health and Neurosciences
Bengaluru, Karnataka, India

V Balasubramaniam
Department of Neurosurgery
Institute of Medical Sciences
Banaras Hindu University
Varanasi, Uttar Pradesh, India

Varun S Mehta
Senior Resident
Central Institute of Psychiatry
Ranchi, Jharkhand, India

Veena Vyas
Social Scientist
Jaipur, Rajasthan, India

Vijaya S Nathawat
Department of Psychology
University of Rajasthan
Jaipur, Rajasthan, India

V Kumaraiah
Professor and Head
Department of Clinical Psychology
National Institute of Mental Health and Neurosciences
Bengaluru, Karnataka, India

VK Verma
Formerly Professor and Head
Department of Psychiatry
Postgraduate Institute of Medical Education and Research (PGIMER)
Chandigarh, India

VN Vahiya
Professor and Head
Department of Psychiatry
Dr RN Cooper Municipal Medical College and General Hospital
Mumbai, Maharashtra, India

VS Chadda
Former Professor an Head
Department of Medicine
SP Medical College
Bikaner, Rajasthan, India

VS Randhawa
Assistant Professor
Department of Microbiology
Lady Hardinge Medical College
New Delhi, India

W Balati
Department of Psychiatry
National Institute of Mental Health and Neurosciences
Bengaluru, Karnataka, India

Preface to the Third Edition

Textbook of Postgraduate Psychiatry (3rd edition, 2 vols) is assimilated with all modern developments in psychiatry and their effects on clinical practice. It incorporates over 10,000 references with some of the original data on which modern evidence-based medicine depends. There are a few new chapters on clinical epidemiology, genetics in psychiatry, neuropsychiatry, special areas of interest and others. This is a highly readable and comprehensive package of modern psychiatry. It places emphasis on detailed clinical descriptions of both common and rare psychiatric disorders and their places within 10th revision of the International Statistical Classification of Diseases and Related Health Problems (ICD-10), Diagnostic and Statistical Manual of Mental Disorders, 4th Edition (DSM-IV) and Diagnostic and Statistical Manual of Mental Disorders, 5th Edition (DSM-5). Clinical management is given due prominence, with extensive accounts of modern drug management, cognitive therapy, psychosocial approaches and current guidelines such as those published in American Psychiatric Association (APA) and National Institute for Health and Clinical Excellence (NICE). Easy to read with over 400 tables and boxes summarizing information, this is an essential text for trainees studying for their MD (Psychiatry), DNB, DMP and MRC Psychiatry examinations. It is also a best reference book for established practitioners across the world. We hope that readers will welcome this edition with the same spirit with which they liked the previous two editions. We welcome any suggestions for further improvements to be incorporated in future.

JN Vyas
Shree Ram Ghimire

Preface to the First Edition

It has been a long-felt need of the postgraduate resident in psychiatry in India for a textbook that covers this subject matter comprehensively, with up-to-date references, and is in a simple language and easily comprehensible. The 'Western' textbooks are either too lengthy or make difficult reading, or are not comprehensive and integrated, or are not adequately referenced, or lack internal citations in the text. Moreover, they are exorbitantly priced, and do not take note of the psychiatric research done in the Indian subcontinent.

The time was, therefore, ripe for *Textbook of Postgraduate Psychiatry*. It attempts to cover clinical psychiatry and allied subjects comprehensively in a lucid style, making it easily understandable and interesting. It is replete with references and each chapter provides a 'further reading' list. Though comprehensive, it is yet concise, avoiding circumstantial explanations. Indian research work in psychiatry is adequately covered, and it is not merely compiled but cited in the context of world literature on the subject.

Textbook of Postgraduate Psychiatry is addressed primarily to the postgraduate student in psychiatry and allied mental health fields, but it should equally serve as a good source of revision and reference to psychiatrists, who have already completed their training, and to practitioners and clinicians, and other mental health professionals.

Such an exhaustive textbook cannot be justifiably written by one or two authors. The contributors include renowned authorities in the various subspecialties of psychiatry with original work to their credit as well as young, zealous psychiatrists, who are actively involved in academic life. We wish to express our deep appreciation to the contributors who worked with enthusiasm and cooperated fully in the preparation of the textbook.

The preparation of the book was a major endeavor that involved the efforts of several persons, too numerous to be mentioned individually. In particular, we wish to thank *Padma Shree* Dr SR Mehta, Ex-Principal, SMS Medical College, Jaipur, Rajasthan; Dr Rajeshwar Sharma, Ex-Principal, SMS Medical College, Jaipur; Dr GC Munjal, Director-Professor and Head, Department of Psychiatry, GB Pant Hospital and Maulana Azad Medical College, New Delhi; Dr SC Malik, Professor and Head, Department of Psychiatry, SK Hospital and Lady Hardinge Medical College, New Delhi; Dr Neena Bohra, Head, Department of Psychiatry, RML Hospital, New Delhi; and Dr SK Khandelwal, Associate Professor, and Dr K Chandiramani, Assistant Professor, Department of Psychiatry, All India Institute of Medical Sciences (AIIMS), New Delhi, India; for their constructive advice and comments. Dr Pradeep Sharma, Assistant Professor, Department of Psychiatry, SMS Medical College, Jaipur, helped in the initial stages of this project.

We are grateful to the publishers, BI Churchill Livingstone, for their useful suggestions and editorial assistance. We are also thankful to Remson Press for their efficient typesetting and to Ram Printograph, India, for their neat and speedy printing.

Textbook of Postgraduate Psychiatry would not have seen the light of the day without constant encouragement and support from our respective families.

The book must finally be assessed by the reader, for whom it is meant. We intend to revise and update it at regular intervals in the light of newer developments.

We welcome suggestions and critical comments from the reader.

JN Vyas
Niraj Ahuja

Acknowledgments

Textbook of Postgraduate Psychiatry is not the effort of a single hand but of multiple contributors. I am especially thankful to them for their laudable efforts, and I am particularly indebted to Drs Shree Ram Ghimire and Jayati Simlai, whose team stood by me at every step and put in hard labor. I would like to thank all contributors and advisors for their coordination and hard work. I would like to thank Dr Jainuruddin Ansari, Chairman, National Medical College and Teaching Hospital, Birgunj, Nepal; Dr Basuruddin Ansari, Managing Director, National Medical College; Drs SN Hissaria, KN Singh, Mohamad Aslam and Abid Hussain Ansari, for their kind blessing and support. I thank all wellwishers, advisors, and contributors. The outstanding coordination, cooperation and patience of the publisher, M/s Jaypee Brothers Medical Publishers (P) Ltd, New Delhi, India, is always gratefully acknowledged. I would also like to thank my family members including my wife Manju, sons Hemant and Kapil, and daughters-in-law Mridula and Veena for their consistent moral support. Last but not least, I am very much thankful to Drs Sarita Parajuli, Jyoti Dahal, Kiran Dahal and Niranjan Chaudhary for their help in editing the book, without whose contribution, the publication of the book would not have been possible. Readers are the best critics of any book. All creative minds are most welcome to critically analyze the book, and provide their feedback through email us at: *drsrghimire@gmail.com* or *jnvyas2012@gmail.com*. Critical feedback is always appreciated to improve standard of the book.

JN Vyas

Contents

VOLUME 1

SECTION 1
Clinical Examination in Psychiatry and Epidemiology of Mental Disorder

SECTION 2
Organic Mental Disorder and Substance Related Disorders

SECTION 3
Schizophrenia, Other Psychotic Disorders and Mood Disorder

SECTION 4
Anxiety Disorders

SECTION 5
Stress Related Disorders

SECTION 6
Psychosomatic Medicine, Somatoform Disorder, Dissociative Disorder and Other Related Disorders

SECTION 7
Personality Disorder, Sexual Disorder, Sleep Disorder and Eating Disorders

SECTION 8
Pregnancy and Menstruation Related Disorders

SECTION 9
Liaison Psychiatry, Neuropsychiatry, Psychiatric Aspect of Medical Disorders and Other Related Conditions

Section 10
Emergency in Mental Health

VOLUME 2

SECTION 11
Child and Adolescent Psychiatry

SECTION 12
Basic Sciences and Imaging in Psychiatry

SECTION 13
Neuropsychology, Research Methods, Statistics and Genetics in Psychiatry

SECTION 14
Biological Therapies

SECTION 15
Psychological Methods of Treatment

SECTION 16
Geriatric Psychiatry: Life Stress, Sociology, and Psychiatry

SECTION 17
Mental Health Issues in Women and Indian Minorities

SECTION 18
Culture, Spirituality, Anthropology and Psychiatry

SECTION 19
Community Psychiatry and Psychiatric Nursing

SECTION 20
Special Area of Interest

SECTION 21
Forensic Psychiatry and Mental Health Legislation

SECTION 22
Ethics and History of Psychiatry

CHAPTER 43

Child and Adolescent Psychiatric Disorders

NK Singh, Neena Bohra, Raju Sedhain, JN Vyas, Pramodh Bhardhwaj, NK Bohra, PB Behere, A Das, AP Behere, Dilip R Patel, Laura Murray, A Mulmule, SS Nathawat, Malavika Kapur, Jayati Simlai, Joyita Sinha, Christoday RJ Khess, Manju Mehta, Rajesh Sagar, RK Solanki, Varun S Mehta, N Parvez

43.1 EXAMINATION IN CHILD PSYCHIATRY

NK Singh

The child psychiatry assessment is similar in many ways to diagnostic in other medical disciplines in as much as it is constituted by the following main parts: the history of presenting problems; past history; family history; examination; specialized tests and consultations; and formulation (Table 1). There are, however, significant modifications which merit attention. It is important for the assessor to be adequately trained in interviewing skills which are necessary to elicit, understand and treat childhood mental, emotional and behavioral problems. This would help in clarifying the reason(s) for the referral of the child/family and in obtaining adequate factual data. It would be imperative for the examiner to establish a sense trust and confidence in the child and the family so that such information is reliably obtained. The elicitation of emotional responses and attitudes to past and current events and the observation of the behavior of the child and of the family during the interview session are greatly assisted if there is a feeling of trust and faith in the assessment process.

Table 1: An outline of a child psychiatric history

Age, sex, informants History of present illness including presenting complaints	Duration and course of illness Chronological development of problems Description along with descriptive quotes, wherever relevant Precipitating factors Treatment taken up to now
Relevant past history of medical or psychiatric problems Family history	Genograms Family dynamics History of similar problems
Development/personal history	Pregnancy and delivery history Temperamental characteristics Developmental milestones Reactions to separations, functions Schooling experiences

Clinicians vary in their practice in arranging the first interview session, with some preferring to see the whole family together whilst others may suggest talking the history from the parents (mainly the mother) in one or two sessions before seeing the child individually. It is useful for trainees to accustom themselves to the various approaches and to maintain flexibility. Often, assessing an order child or an adolescent on his/her own before talking to the family may strategically very important in order to obtain the trust of the adolescent and to maintain future engagement. Skills in interviewing families are useful for proper understanding of childhood psychiatric disorders. Nothing the following points may be of value:

- After introducing yourself, ask individual family members to introduce themselves.
- Children should be shown the available toys.
- The purpose of the interview should be outlined.
- Check factual details (e.g. age, sex, schools, ect.) from individual members of the family.
- Open-ended questions and questions which seek clarification of stated problems are useful, as are questions conveying empathy (It seems this really upset you; could you tell me something more about it?).

HISTORY OF PRESENT ILLNESS/ PRESENTING COMPLAINTS

Winning the co-operation and trust of both the parents and the children is an important aim of the initial interview. The child and the family need to feel sufficiently at ease before active elicitation of presenting complaints manifest and latent should be started. The areas which need to be covered include:

- Presenting problems which bring the family for consultation.
- Onset, duration, course, severity, frequency, modifying factors, situational variation (e.g. school versus home) and effect of the problems on the family.
- Interests, strengths and recreation activities.
- Assessment of general health (appetite, sleep, elimination, somatic complaints, etc.) relationships with family and friends, mood, activity and attention span, school performance.
- Any other problems which have not been previously mentioned.
- Steps taken by the individual or by the family to solve the problem(s) up to now.

FAMILY HISTORY

The assessment of the family serves many important functions, including finding out the role the family may have in the evolution of the problem (genetic or environmental) and also as a means of determining the level of support the child can potentially obtain from the family as part of the overall management plan. The areas which are usually required to be covered include:

- Family history of the same, or a similar, condition.
- Specific enquires to elicit history which could suggest the presence of depression or suicide; hyperactivity; learning disability; trouble with the law; bed-wetting; any other psychiatric problems; temperamental or constitutional traits; any significant medical problems.
- *Parents*: Age, occupations.
- *Siblings*: Age, problems.
- Detailed elicitation of each parent's personal history, including family of origin; their significant childhood experiences.
- Parent's marital history.
- Family structure and home circumstances.
- Quality of parenting; level of communication and problem-solving capacities.
- *Family relationships*: Acceptance, warmth, hostility, rejection or criticism, sibling's relationships.
- Parental views about the course of the problem(s) and their attempted solutions, including possible hindrances to obtaining such solutions.
- The family in the wider socio-cultural context.

DEVELOPMENT/PERSONAL HISTORY

A good child psychiatric assessment is incomplete without a detailed developmental history. It should start from an assessment of prenatal and parental factors, including the emotional circumstances and physical status surrounding the pregnancy, birth difficulties, prematurity, and the presence of other medical and congenital abnormalities. The subsequent development sequence should be carefully elicited, for it has the potential to provide valuable clues about the child's temperament and early formative experiences, and should include the following points:

- *Early mother-child relationship:* Early feeding and sleeping patterns; postpartum depression; mother's emotional view of the baby.
- *Constitutional-temperamental characteristics:* Activity level; easy or difficult baby; restlessness; crankiness.
- *Early developmental milestones:* The emphasis should be on descriptions and qualitative feelings surrounding the achievement of the milestones (neck-holding, sitting, crawling, walking, speaking); toilet training.
- History of separations from the primary caregiver(s) for more than a few days.
- *Behavioral and emotional difficulties:* Temper tantrums; phobias; nightmares; separation difficulties.
- The parenting styles of both parents (restrictive, permissive, authoritarian, etc.).
- Past illness and hospitalizations.
- Initiation into schooling; difficulties in early schooling; school performance.
- Peer relationships; play.
- Reaction to birth of sibling(s) (if applicable).

EXAMINATION OF THE CHILD

This is one of the most difficult part of the assessment process and occasionally somewhat daunting for the novice examiner. In very young children it may not be possible to conduct a formal mental status examination and observation of the child's behavior must always become an important part of the overall assessment (whether the child was verbal or nonverbal during the interview session). Points to be noted during 'observation' include:

- Appearance; grace of movement; nutritional status; right or left-handed; dress and hygiene; gross and fine motor co-ordination.
- Signs of neglect or injury.
- Activity level; span of attention; distractibility.
- Inhibition or disinhibition.
- *Attitude and feeling tone during the interview*: Shy, aggressive, oppositional, anxious to please, sad, miserable, etc.
- Choice and description of play.
- Tics, mannerisms, stereotypes and other involuntary movements.

- Eye contact with the examiner; spontaneous talk.
- Parents of interaction between child and parents; between other family members; reaction of child to separation; family communication.
- Any evidence suggesting the presence of delusions, hallucinations and thought disorder.

The physical examination of the child should form an extension of the description of observed behavior and includes a general medical assessment and a neurological screen. In the latter the following require to be assessed (it should be remembered that many of these are 'soft', non-logicalizing sign sand therefore their presence should be viewed as an indicator for further expert consultation):

- Straight line walking; gait and hoping on one foot.
- Presence of choreoathetoid movements.
- Copying patterns; drawing a man (observe grip and dexterity in drawing).
- Finger-thumb opposition; diadochokinesis (alternating pronation/supination); finger-nose pointing test.
- Standing on one foot (Denckla test); Romberg's test.
- Visual tracking movements; nystagmus.
- *Laterality:* School age children should make no mistakes in differentiating right from left; punching an imaginary bag or kicking an imaginary ball helps in including the dominant laterality.

Compared to the adult, mental status examination of the child is much less clear cut and does not lend itself to compartmentalization quit so easily. To be able to fill—in descriptively under the headings of a standard mental status examination, the examiner may require to make use of techniques other than simply talking: that is, play, drawing, games, etc. Broadly speaking, the mental status examination should cover information under the following heads:

- General appearance and behavior, including motor activity and overall demeanor, physical development in relation to age, unusual features, impulsivity.
- Consciousness.
- Orientation.
- Attention span and alertness; concentration; distractibility.
- *Affect:* Initial feeling tone; predominant mood; description of other emotional reactions to events during the interview session.
- Thought process and content, including phobias, worries and preoccupations, dreams and fantasies, wishes, delusions.
- Perceptual anomalies, including illusions, hallucinations, hearing, vision.
- Assessment of memory and intellectual functions.
- Responses to the interviewer; eye contact; interviewer's subjective response.
- *Language:* Articulation, speech, gesture and communication, expression.
- Awareness of problems; acceptance or denial; coping styles used up to now.

The individual assessment of the child needs to be arranged carefully. The establishment of trust and confidence in the examiner is of great importance, as has been pointed out earlier. The approach to the child should be informal and relaxed. After having noted the ease or difficulty with which the child was able to separate from his parent(s), he should be introduced to the toys, games and the drawing material in the room, including that he is quite welcome to play, draw or talk: "It's your choice". Generally speaking directly, through talking about dreams, three wishes', drawings, etc. The younger the child the more important it would be to utilize play, gauges and other indirect methods of elicitation of mental status material. It should be clear to the examiner that the purpose of play is to communicate with the child, so that the child is facilitated in expressing what he may find difficult to verbalize. It is also to observe the way find difficult to manages the impulses that arise within him. Comments and questions strategically asked during the play are likely to elicit valuable information for the assessor; it would be useful to point out that discussing the play events in the third person (rather than in the child's first person) is more likely to provide the necessary nonthreatening environment for the child to talk and develop themes in the play.

Drawings also are very useful in making an assessment of the child's neuropsychological developmental level, fantasies and feelings. The average child is able to draw symbolic representations by the time he is 5–6 years old. Observing the child while drawing may indicate about his self-esteem (for instance, one of the author's patients would draw, and almost always, in the initial assessment sessions, would crumple and throw away the drawing he had made, "because he had not drawn well"—despite the standard instruction from the examiner at the beginning of the child drew), as well as his motor co-ordination. After an initial open-ended invitation to draw, the child can be asked to draw specific scenes, including drawing a person, drawing his family, drawing the family doing something, the House – Tree – Person test or drawing a dream for a person sleeping (for which the initial drawing the clinician may do). The 'Squiggle game', is often useful for the clinician to make 'contact' with the child: the clinician draws an initial squiggle on a sheet of paper, and the child is then invited to make it into something. The clinician and the child take turns doing this and often a theme emerges from the series of squiggles thus drawn. Drawings may, in themselves, not be particularly revealing; rather, they often can provide openings for launching into discussions on related topics.

Psychological Assessment

In many situations, a psychological assessment carried out by a child psychologist may prove extremely valuable in the overall comprehensive assessment process. A long list of tests which can be used to assist the clinician in the list of tests which can be made. This includes tests for intelligence, development, personality, perceptuomotor functioning, educational can be obtained by the use of special questionnaires and/or rating scales.

Cognitive assessment or assessment of intellectual ability is conventionally assessed in the form of an intelligence quotient (IQ) which is defined as mental age/chronological age X 100, with the normal range being between 90 and 110 of late, however, the global precise value of the IQ is being less importance and most more emphasis is rightly being placed on the differential profile of strengths and weaknesses that emerges on testing on for example, the various subtests of the Wechsler Intelligence Scale for Children - Revised version (WISC - R). Malin (1968) has adapted the WISC - R for the Indian population. The WISC - R can be used for children of 6–15 years of age. For younger children (4 - 6 years old), the Wechsler Pre-School and Primary School Intelligence Scale (WPPSI) is recommended. Raven's Progressive Matrices, the Seguin Form Board, Bhatia's Battery of Performance Tests of Intelligence and the Hindi adaptation of the Stanford–Binet Scale are some of the other tests which can be used for cognitive assessment.

For children younger than 4 years of age, and particularly below 2 years, a number of instruments have been devised which assess the developmental status and which give a development quotient (DQ) which is defined as the tested developmental age/chronological age X 100. The Gesell Developmental Schedule is the best known of these. It has been adapted in India by Muralidharan (1970). The Vineland Social Maturity Scale and the Denver Developmental Screening Test are other scales which are used in the Indian setting.

The Wide Ranging Achievement Test (WRAT) and the Peabody Individual Achievement Test (PIAI) are popular tests for assessing academic achievement. The Bender Visual - Motor Gestalt Test is the best known among the tests for percetuo - motor abilities. The Thematic Apperception Test (TAT) for ages 8 years and above), the Children's Apperception Test (CAT) (for ages 3–7 years), the Rorschach Test and the Incomplete Sentence Tests are commonly used tests of personality for children.

It is important to recognize the advantages as well as the limitations of psychological tests. These are generally reliable in the hands of a competent psychologist, and the cognitive tests tend to have good validity in terms of school performance. The test results should always be interpreted in the overall context of assessment and caution needs to be exercised in conveying the information to parents, children or teachers. Fatigue, inadequate testing conditions and the use of inappropriate tests can influence the test results.

Finally, a word about information from other sources. It is a unique feature of assessment in child psychiatry that significant importance is attached to information obtained from school teachers, health workers or the family physician (if applicable). A common procedure adopted by this author is to sent out, through the parents (with their consent), a questionnaire to the school teacher which lists various problem behaviors and which the teacher is requested to fill in and send back. Valuable information can be obtained about children with attention deficit hyperactivity disorder by asking the parents and the teachers to feel out a questionnaire or rating scale, for example the Conners Teacher Rating Scale.

BIOLOGICAL INVESTIGATIONS

It is not very often that children referred for psychiatric assessment require biological investigation, but a significant number do and the investigations could include a wide variety of tests. The child psychiatrist would need to be familiar with various neuroimaging techniques, including the CT scan, magnetic resonance imaging, positron emission tomography, single photon emission computed tomography and magnetoencephalography. If the suspected diagnosis in a developmental disorder, then genetic and chromosomal assessments are going to be of value. A family medical history will give indications regarding the possibility of inherited disorders. Any detailed discussion of these investigations is beyond the scope of this chapter. The electroencephalogram (EEG) may have its main usefulness in diagnosing epilepsy. Other laboratory investigations, such as blood counts and biochemical psychiatry patient, unless there is a suspected physical disorder in association with the mental disorder.

FORMULATION

Having obtained the information from all the possible sources, the next task of the clinician is to put it all together as a 'formulation'. This involves summarizing the main features of the presentation, including predisposing, precipitating and perpetuating factors and forming a diagnosis with possible differential diagnoses. The process of formulating is vital to the assessment process because on it hinges the basic management plan. The prognosis and the short-term as well as long-term plans are discussed with a definite initial treatment plan being formulated. It is useful to plan a separate 'feedback' session with the family and usually the child is not included in the initial discussion with the parents, unless he is in the adolescent age group. The parents are invited to talk about their understanding of the emergent material and the therapist would do well to be sensitive to the feelings, including worries, that the family may have. Later, the child is included in the discussion and the clinician's understanding of the problem and the plan of management is conveyed to him also in age appropriate terms.

43.2 GENERAL PRINCIPLES OF THE CLINICAL INTERVIEW

Neena Bohra

The assessment of a child emotional state or of family functioning requires specific skills some general principals regarding interviewing and easement are useful to consider efficient communication requires unbroken can promote efficiency privacy will increase the amount of information shared during an interview and is especially important when sensitive psychosocial issue are being discussed in situation in which privacy cannot be easily attained (an open ward), pediatrician must always be aware that a patient (or family) may not be comfortable enough to share relevant information. Equally important is the need to explicitly address issue of confidentiality with patients and parents before clinical assessment.

Setting aside adequate time for an interview is important. The 1st goal is to build rapport with both family and child developmentally appropriate overtures to the child often start this process. Examples include playing peek-a-boo with a toddler and commenting on sports with a child who wearing a baseball cap.[1]

After and overture with the child, it is useful to allow the accompanying caregiver an opportunity to present his or her concern with practice, it takes no longer to focus on the concern of the patient and/or parent than to "lead" the interview. Centering the dialogue on the patient or family agenda often results in fewer misunderstanding.

Adolescent often seek medical care to discuss a hidden agenda such hidden agendas may realer to psychosocial issues, which the patient may not discuss unless he or she perceives that the physician has provided an appropriate opportunity during the visit.

Using a family centered approach increases this opportunity a primary determinate of malpractice claims is poor physician patient (or physician -family) Communication; from the patients perspective, "not being heard" is the central communication problem.

Family-centered interviewing improves data–gathering and increases patient satisfaction. Which in turn, improves compliance?

Much interview data can also be gathered through careful attention to nonverbal cues scanning for nonverbal cues and commenting on them is part of effective interviewing an adolescent who is expressionless and adverts his or her eyes is obviously uncomfortable if the physician notes this and inquires gently about what might be bothering the patient with psychosocial issues that are not addressed may return repeatedly or seek care elsewhere.

An interview is a reciprocal interaction and the way that a physician provides information can influence medical outcomes.

Patients respond to both verbal and nonverbal cues. Language should be clear and trained interpreters should be used whenever there is a chance that a language difference will impair communication in either direction. Although it is often tempting to use a child as an interpreter, this practice is strongly discouraged because parents may not be able to express their concerns comfortably and children may edit the information that is transmitted. It is useful to check in with parent can demonstrate that the pediatrician values the interaction and the relationship with the patient tone of voice when detailing a medication regimen will increase the likelihood that the patient or parent will understand the information. Providing feedback to talk with the parent or patient can demonstrate that the pediatrician values the interaction and the relationship with the patient and family maintaining eye contact and using a positive tone of voice when detailing a medication will understand the information providing legibly written instruction, a clear explanation of why the intervention is being used and instruction for follow-up will further increase compliance.

Although most pediatrician do not have the time or training to perform an in-depth psychiatric interview[2] they spend much of their time addressing concerns about children behavior. Family rarity with and use of available screening instruments allows the practitioner to follow-up on impressions regarding psychosocial concerns by getting more in depth data.

Teacher reports can also be useful if there is concern that parental perception may differ from the child's experiences at school. These check lists do not provide diagnoses but can help to determine what interventions or referral might be most appropriate. Even children who do not seem to have a specific disorder, but who are experiencing distress in context of parental discord or peer relationships, may require extra support or even referral for counseling.

TOPICS FOR ALL AGES

Emotional and behavior well-being should be assessed at every well child visit, beginning with the 1st visit even prenatal appointments can be useful in understanding a family expectation coping strategies, and level of streets. Setting basic ground rules for when and how to call for help is reassuring to parents.

As the child develops, anticipatory guidance about common stress point for parent resource is highly valued by most parents.

Using family centered interviewing does not mean that the pediatrician should eliminate an agenda for a given visit. The pediatrician should screen for maternal depression, a diseases that significant affects young children emotional development and medical outcomes. The development effects of maternal depression can be seen in the 1st week of life,when infants and in time with insecure physiologic responsiveness and changes in electrocephalographic activation maternal depression in associated with poor maternal responsiveness to the infant and in the optimal position to screen for obstetrician until 6 week postpartum.

Postpartum screening about mood and functioning can be done by using the US public health 2-question screen "have you had little interest or pleasure in doing things?"

It is important to remember that "baby blues" last only 10 days; mood symptoms that persistent beyond 10 days should be further evaluated. It is useful to have copies of formal screening measures such as the Edinburgh postnatal depression scale or the lack depression inventory in the office to assist with deciding which caregivers need referral for treatment. The majority of depressed parents will readily fill out a screening questionnaire, and most are relive red to be able to discuss their difficulties. The pediatrician who recognizes parental depression[3] and completes a referral may significantly improve the developmental course of me affected child.

Family violence is another common problem that is associated with the developmental consequences for children.

These are no simple demographic indicators of families at greatest risk for domestic violence: partner violence cuts across socioeconomics groups.

Many practitioners feel anxious inquiring about family violence but a quarry about family discourse easily leads to pertinent follow-up questions.

When the pediatrician hears about physical fighting in the home, he or she should ask about the current situation and assess family safety directly, including the child physical and emotional safety. Parents affected by partner violence should be given information about domestic violence resource in the community especially local shelters.

Women living in violent relationships rarely move out the 1st time a professional raises the issue; this delay, however should not be interpreter as noncompliance. Close follow-up with families after discussions of violence is critical, and that of their family. It is imperative that screening for child maltreatment, commonly associated with family violence, be undertaken any time a caregiver reports family violence.

There is much evidence that children are adversely affected by ongoing family violence. However, there is no clear clinical profile of an affected child. Common symptoms associated with family violence include aggression, behavioral deregulation, school failure and anxiety and mood symptoms.[4] Structured checklists, such as the child behavior checklist, are useful in screening for highly symptomatic children; obtaining data from >1 source (parent, teacher) is important. An assessment of children behavioral functioning should 1st considers the Child's[1] developmental stage.[4] The pediatrician who keenly observes the parent-child interaction and deftly interviews children will identify those with psychosocial problems. When coupled with appropriate intervention is associated with improved developmental outcomes.

USING A DEVELOPMENTAL APPROACH TO INTERVIEWING CHILDREN, INFANCY AND TODDLERHOOD[1-11]

Infants and toddlers have tremendous capacity for forming memories, although they do not have language available to describe them. This means that the frequent office or clinic visits before 3 years of age can collectively provide a "positive memory bank" for an individual child, which can then become the building blocks for a positive and meaningful physician relationship with the child and his other family. children at this stage of development are learning through sensory experiences. A soft tone of voice and gentle handing of the infant are important means of helping the infant develop a sense of trust and comfort with the practitioners. The practitioners who actively engages, even briefly, with young children will create these positive relationship building blacks furthermore, paying this kind of direct attention to the young child is almost always comforting to parents; infants and young children are highly adept at sensing parental anxiety.

Toward the end of the 1st years of life, the child begins to show focused attachment behavior forward his primary caregiver. By 10 months of age, the caregiver for emotional support when distressed. If by 18 months, the distressed child displays uncertainty in accessing support from the primary caregiver, the pediatrician should be concerned about the quality of the parent child attachment. The watchful practitioner can assess the developing attachment relationship because the typical health supervision visit is enough of a stressor for the toddler to yield important information about how he or she seeks comfort from the caregiver. The infant toddler social and emotional development, the checklist for Autisms in toddlers is also useful for children who make limited verbal and nonverbal social contact with their caregivers.

Preschool children: The verbal and cognitive capacities of preschoolers mean that they may anticipate physician visits with some anxiety. At this age, children commonly interpret medical procedures, such as needle sticks, as punishments for being bad.

The use of stickers and other small gifts may help to counteract this natural way of thinking and enrich the relationship with the preschool patient.

The preschool visit should also be used to address issues of emotional health and well-being. Although most children with mild behavior difficulties do not have significant psychiatric disorders, 1 in 10 preschoolers has a clinically significant emotional or behavior disorder, including attention-deficit/hyperactivity disorder (ADHD). Depression and anxiety disorder. Using a color-coded sticker in the chart when the parent notes behavioral sleep or eating difficulties allows the physician to inquire at a return visit if a suggested behavioral intervention was effective.

When basic intervention such as teaching the time out technique, do not seem effective, it is important to explore the symptoms further reassess the diagnosis and reconsider the plan, possibly including a mental health retrial. Reports of expulsions or suspensions in child-care or preschool settings should not be dismissed. Early aggression (even before age 3 years) is quite stable over time and is predicative of an evolving mental health problem.

Family-based interventions are effective. Although the longer the pattern of aggression and defiance persists the more difficult it is to treat another notable symptom is anerobia, which is of irritability. Anerobia is the most specific predictor of clinical significant depression in preschoolers whereas excessive crying is the most sensitive predictor. Persistent anxiety symptoms, such as fear of especially when the child anxiety impairs the family functioning (associated with parents missing work or the children's missing school).

School-aged children: As children reach school age, it is important to ask (in developmentally appropriate language) about their interests directly at the outset of any interaction. It can be helpful to document specific interests or activities in the patients chart to allow for follow-up queries at subsequent visits.

School-aged children look up to medical providers and the pedantries will strengthen the physician-patient relationship. This effort will be rewarded in the teen years, when the typical suspicion of adult authority is moderated by the teens sense of the provider as interested and caring.

A complete heath maintenance visit includes a review of the child emotional functioning. In the school-aged child the most common psychiatric disorder are attention-deficit/hyperactivity disorder.

Asking children and their parents about school achievement peer relationships and family functioning. Attention problems learning disorders and sometimes anxiety disorders can be identified in a discussion of school problems can indicate development delays and/or social skill deficits. The increasing incidence of pervasive developmental disorders requires the pediatrician to be familiar with this diagnostic category. Family functioning can provide clues about parental discord, child emotional or behavioral difficulties parental mental health problems or the effect of family stressors, such as poverty, community violence or domestic violence during the clinical interview careful tracking of the child affect or facial expression of emotion will provide information about his or her internal inquiry directly about what makes them feel sad or anxious is important.

Although the hyperactive form of ADHD presents by the school-age velars, the inattentive type is under-recognized, especially in girls. Children who are reported to have school difficulties should be screened for ADHD using readily available checklists such as the Conner rating scale for ADHD. Parents who described irritability or opposition may be alerting the pediatrician to a mood disorder. The age at which children begin using illegal drugs has been decreasing over the last decade. In 2004, 21.5% of 8th graders reported a lifetime use of illicit substance (see it is therefore important to discuss substance use with children in the prepubertal years.

Adolescent: A key developmental milestone for adolescents is gaining autonomy from their parents or caretakers pediatricians can support this autonomy by structuring the patient interaction to include time spent with the patient alone without the parent. This practice affords the adolescents a sense of privacy and increases the chance of gaining insight into issues that would not be discussed in front of parents confidently and the limits therefore should be discussed with both the patient and the parent together, before the parent leaves the room. Not all practitioners ask parents to leave the room during health maintainers visits although adolescents value this time and such interaction enhance the quality of information obtained and care provided. Physically examination of adolescent should also be conducted without the parents present, unless the parents requires otherwise.

Although adolescent has been traditionally viewed as a period of storm and stress most adolescents do not experiences more stress at this developmental stage than at others. Risk-taking behavior (use of alcohol, tobacco, or drugs; sexual activity) is common among adolescent reports peer pressure to take risk. Adolescents and most adolescents report peer pressure to take risk. Adolescence is also a period when the incidence of several major mental illness increases dramatically.

Major depression, bipolar disorder panic disorder and schizophrenia are chronic conditions that frequently present during adolescent; early stabilization of these illness may improve long-term outcomes. Rates of depression in tens are equivalent to these in adults and suicide is the 3rd most common cause of death in adolescent. Adolescent is a stage during which consolidation of sexual orientation generally occurs and this process especially for many youth who self-identify as homosexual, is associated with considerable stress, elevated levels of risk-taking behavior social stressors, sexual identity and orientation, substance abuse and emotional adjustment is recommended to ensure that all topics are covered in the interview. A commonly used format for adolescent interviewing is the home, health, education, employment, activities, drugs depression, safety, sexually, (HEADDSS) screen. Using an adolescent report questioning and having a provider form that prompts the provider to ask about these topics enhances screening in the primary care setting. Positive reinforcement for healthy behaviors should always be included in the interaction. It mental illness is suspected, a psychiatric review of symptoms should be part of the clinical interview. As part of such an assignment, suicidal ideation should also be discussed. Inquiring about suicide does not promote suicidal ideation. Suicidal ideation can be described as active (reflecting a through to harm oneself) or passive (a desire to be dead without a plan) having referral resource and a plan of action can make asking the question easier for the clinical.

For the parent, caring for an adolescent can be challenging maintains open communication between parents and their teenage children promotes positive adjustment for the adolescent however, parents sometimes feel disconnected from their adolescent in part because peer influence becomes more and more important during adolescent, resulting in a degree of withdraw from the parents. The pediatrician can play the role of parenting coach effectively at this developmental stage by modeling behavior for asking to meet with the adolescent alone to talk about teen issues and suggesting that the parent routinely do the same.

When the basic intervention involving the parents the child and school personnel do not lead to improve functioning referral to a mental health professional is indicated. It is important that pediatricians avoid commenting that mental health referral is a last resort. The need for mental health consultation should be expressed in terms of the joint need of the family and the physician and the family in the management of the other health care needs of the child remains intact. To be most effect, referral should begin with a call to the mental health provider after written permission to exchange health information is obtained from the parent. Result from parent or teacher reported screening instrument discussed in this section might be helpful to the receiving clinician.

PSYCHIATRIC CONSULTATION

A psychiatric consultation may be a valuable part of the assessment of a child's symptoms (including physical symptoms) or family stress or discord. The physician should inform both the parent and the child what the psychiatric consultation is intended to asses. The child consent is helpful and is usually easily obtained when the reasons for the referral are explained and the parents. Standardized is available to both the physician and the parents. Standardized guidelines for psychiatric assessment of infants, children and adolescents have been published by the American academy of the child and adolescent psychiatry and free, printable "facts for families" sheets on various psychiatric symptoms are available on the web need for a psychiatric consulation or referral can be expressed in areas where in the term of the joint need of the family and the physician for help in areas where the psychiatrist has special expertise, with the understanding that the collaboration of the physician and the family in the management of the other health care needs of the child will remain intact.

43.3 DEVELOPMENTAL ASSESSMENT OF CHILDREN

Raju Sedhain, JN Vyas

Developmental assessment is the process of mapping a child's performance compared with children of similar age. The comparison group is obtained from a representative sample of the population that the child comes from. Several factors contribute to performance varying greatly between different population groups.[12] In a multicultural society it can be challenging to find appropriate benchmarks for these standards.

This article reviews the literature on the assessment of child development. It aims to highlight what normal developmental parameters are, when and how to assess a child, and when to refer for specialist assessment.

SOURCES AND SELECTION CRITERIA

We searched PubMed, the *Cochrane Database of Systematic Reviews*, and reference lists of relevant publications using the subject headings and key words "development", "developmental assessment", "developmental delay", "disability", "mental retardation", "developmental screening tools", "screening", and "diagnosis". We also reviewed guidelines from the American Academy of Pediatrics[13] and the UK Healthy Child Programme.[14]

We have extensive clinical experience in developmental paediatrics in the United Kingdom and United States, which we drew on to comment on the extensive and potentially confusing technology currently used for developmental assessment.

What is Child Development?

Development is the process by which each child evolves from helpless infancy to independent adulthood.

Growth and development of the brain and central nervous system is often termed psychomotor development and is usually divided into four main domains:

- Gross and fine motor skills
- Speech and language
- Social and personal and activities of daily living
- Performance and cognition.

Fetal brain development starts by the fourth week of gestation and progresses rapidly throughout intrauterine life and early childhood. Brain development—the target of developmental surveillance and screening—reflects neurological maturation. It consists of a complex process of cell growth, migration, connection, pruning, and myelination, and it persists through at least the second decade. This fundamental phenomenon, which determines brain development, is a preprogrammed process that occurs in all children.

What is Normal Development?

The pattern of development is remarkably constant, within fairly broad limits, but the rate at which goals are achieved varies from child to child. Skills are acquired sequentially, with one goal acquired after another. Later goals often depend on achievement of earlier goals within the same field—for example, children must learn to sit independently before they can stand and then walk.

Descriptions of normal development, linked to the ability to perform a particular task at a particular age, relate to the performance of the average child. The acquisition of a key performance skill, such as walking, is referred to as a milestone. For each skill, the normal age range for attainment of the milestone varies widely. A median age is the age at which half a population of children acquire a skill. A limit age is the age at which a skill should have been achieved and is two standard deviations from the mean. It is important to know which milestones are most consistent. Smiling socially by the age of 8 weeks is a consistent milestone, whereas crawling is not. Crawling occurs at a widely varying time point, and some children with normal development never learn to crawl.

Genetic factors may determine the fundamental developmental potential, but environmental factors have crucial influences on the profile achieved. Positive experiences during early childhood may enhance brain development, particularly in the area of linguistic and social skills.

Box 1: Environmental causes of damage to brain development

Antenatal

- Early maternal infections, such as rubella, toxoplasma, cytomegalovirus
- Late maternal infections, such as varicella, malaria, HIV
- Toxins—for example, alcohol, pesticides, radiation, smoking
- Drugs—for example, cytotoxics, antiepileptics

Postnatal

- Infections—for example, meningitis, encephalitis, cytomegalovirus
- Metabolic disorders, such as hypoglycemia, hyponatremia or hypernatremia, dehydration
- Toxins—for example, lead, mercury, arsenic, chlorinated organic compounds, solvents
- Trauma, especially head injury
- Severe understimulation, maltreatment, or domestic violence
- Malnutrition, especially deficiency of iron, folate, and vitamin D
- Maternal mental health disorders, most commonly depression

Unfortunately, however, the brain is also vulnerable to various insults, particularly in the early embryonic stages, but also in later life (Box 1). Studies on abandoned Romanian children provide good evidence of how an adverse environment affects brain growth. Children who were institutionalized have smaller brains than those who were adopted abroad or brought-up in a family environment, including foster care in Romania.[15] Other studies showed significant gains in cognitive and language skills after abandoned children are taken into care.[16,17]

What is Developmental Delay?

Many clinicians use the term "global developmental delay" to mean a significant delay in two or more of the four main developmental domains listed above. Significant delay is defined as performance two or more standard deviations below the mean on age appropriate standardized norm-referenced testing (usually a secondary care procedure). In the United Kingdom and the United States, the term global developmental delay is usually reserved for younger children (typically under 5 years of age). In the UK learning disability is usually applied to older children, when IQ testing is more valid and reliable (although formal testing of IQ is rarely performed in clinical practice and the child's assessment is based on functional abilities). In the US, the term developmental disability or mental retardation is used in the over 5 age group.

The term developmental impairment or disorder covers a heterogeneous group of conditions that start early in life and present with delay or an abnormal pattern of progression in one or more developmental domain. Children with autism spectrum disorder fall into this category. In this context, the use of the term developmental delay has been challenged because it conveys a message that the child may "catch up," which is often not true.[18] Nevertheless, it remains in common use because it is well understood by professionals and parents.

How Common are Developmental Problems?

Global developmental delay affects 1–3% of children. About 1% (95% confidence interval 90–141 per 10 000) of children have an autism spectrum disorder.[19]

Structured assessment of a child's development aims mainly to clarify the quantity and quality of the child's developmental status.[20] However, the procedure also offers several advantages in terms of health promotion (Box 2).[21]

Children develop at different rates, and it is important to distinguish those who are within the "normal" range from those who are following a pathological course. We now have good evidence that early identification and early intervention improve the outcomes of children with developmental impairments.[22,23]

A persuasive body of work, which reviewed evidence from neurosciences, developmental psychology, social sciences, epidemiology (including animal and human studies), longitudinal studies, case series, and case reports,[24-26] describes the importance of the early years in promoting healthy brain development. This literature builds on the scientific understanding of brain development and finds that environments that do not promote healthy development have a cumulative and ongoing negative impact on a range of social, economic, and learning outcomes over the life course. This body of work emphasizes that early interventions are an effective way to improve children's outcomes than later remediation.

Given the importance of the early years, early intervention is crucial. Early intervention seems to be even more important for children with developmental disabilities than for children more generally, because learning is cumulative, and barriers to healthy development early in life impede development at each subsequent stage.[27,28]

Obviously, identification of abnormality must be followed by further action. Children develop relentlessly, and if they are on a deviant path the course becomes more difficult to change as time goes by. Early child health promotion, which includes support for parenting and treatment, is an effective investment that may prevent the need for more intensive, costly, and often less effective intervention later on. A series of systematic reviews of strategies for improving child development in 13 relatively deprived countries, published in the *Lancet*, found good evidence that interventions at pre-school age are highly cost effective.[29] A linked editorial stated that "Neglect of young children most in need is an outrage—and a huge strategic mistake."[30]

Box 2: Benefits of developmental assessment

- Early diagnosis and intervention
- Early diagnosis of conditions with a genetic basis, such as Duchene muscular dystrophy and fragile X syndrome, facilitates genetic counseling for families
- Provides carers with reliable information before a developmental problem becomes obvious and gives them more time to adjust to the child's difficulty and make appropriate management plans for their family
- Carers are reassured and relieved of anxiety if assessment shows that the child is within the normal range
- Early assessments can be compared with later ones, allowing the practitioner to follow a child's individual developmental trajectory
- Provides an opportunity to encourage good parenting and developmental stimulation

How do Children Present with Developmental Problems?

Children with developmental problems may present in several ways:

- In countries with routine child health surveillance or developmental screening practices, concerns may be raised at scheduled contacts
- In children with identified risk factors (such as prematurity) who have undergone developmental surveillance, developmental problems may be detected early
- Parents may recognize a delay or be worried about a child's behavior or social skills and seek professional advice (either through their health visitor, public health nurse, or general practitioner)
- Professionals in a nursery or day care setting may recognize deviant patterns of development and highlight their concerns to the family, thus prompting referral
- Concerns may be detected opportunistically at health contacts for other reasons, such as childhood illnesses, if questions are asked about development.

Development can be assessed at several levels, depending on the circumstances. Screening is a process to identify children at increased risk of having developmental difficulties that uses relatively brief and simple techniques, according to well recognized criteria.[31] Screening tests are inherently imperfect assessments because they have to balance the risk of missing a child with delays (sensitivity) versus erroneously identifying children without true delays (specificity).[32] Repeating the test after an appropriate time interval, or conducting a secondary screening with a more accurate and specific test, may improve test accuracy. The inherent trade-off of sensitivity and specificity makes screening controversial—it is promoted universally in some countries,[13] whereas others have a selective policy.[33]

The practice of child health surveillance and screening has changed in the UK since the introduction of the Healthy child Program (HCP) which supersedes Health for all Children IV. In the UK, the HCP offers every child and family a program that includes developmental reviews to facilitate early detection of, and action to deal with, developmental delay.[14] The emphasis is on a review at 2.5 years. The HCP is based on a model of "progressive universalism"—in other words, standard services that are available to everyone (universal) and extra services available to those who need them or are at risk (progressively more services provided according to need). It is basically a child health promotion program that includes opportunities for developmental surveillance and screening or case finding. It is a flexible and nonprescriptive programme that can be adapted locally according to population needs. Primary care practitioners should opportunistically ask flexible questions about a child's development at every visit where possible, as part of comprehensive medical care (Box 3). Children identified as at risk (often by a health visitor) may be referred for further assessment in primary or secondary care. Currently, standardized developmental screening tools are not routinely used in primary care in the UK.

By contrast, in the US the American Academy of Pediatrics (AAP) and many American state Medicaid programs recommend the use of standardized developmental screening tools during each routine healthcare visit. The AAP guideline for health supervision, *Bright Futures*,[34] suggests the use of structured developmental screens from the age of 18 months. The 2009 Affordable Care Act requires health insurance plans to cover preventive care,[35] as described in *Bright Futures*. Despite these federal protocols, strategy and implementation vary greatly between individual states.

How to Assess a Child's Development

A good starting point is to believe parents and carers who are worried about their child.

Box 4 lists factors that can result in a deviant pattern of development. It is important that these are elicited through appropriate history and examination. Ask about prenatal, perinatal, and postnatal events, including maternal health during pregnancy. Ask about the child's acquisition of developmental milestones (Table 2). The personal child health record ("red book" in the UK) is often a valuable source of information because it contains details of pregnancy, mode of delivery, condition at birth, Apgar scores, birth weight, birth head circumference, and newborn hearing screen results.

Box 3: Suggested opportunistic screening questions[46]

- Do you have any concerns about the way your child is behaving, learning, or developing?
- Do you have any concerns about the way he or she moves or uses his or her arms or legs?
- Do you have any concerns about how your child talks and understands what you say?
- Does your child enjoy playing with toys? Describe what he or she does while playing
- Has your child ever stopped doing something he or she could previously do?
- Does your child get along with others?
- Do you have any concerns about how your child is learning to do things for himself or herself?

Box 4: Developmental variation

Normal patterns

- Late talking or walking (including bottom shuffling) may be familial
- Language development may seem delayed at first in children of bilingual families, but counting total words in both languages typically compensates for perceived delay. Receptive language precedes language expression
- Black and Indian infants are more likely than white ones to have advanced motor skills[12]

Correctable causes of slow development

- Undernutrition (failure to thrive)
- Iron deficiency anemia
- Social isolation of the family or maternal depression
- Hypothyroidism

A sensitive but thorough environmental, social, and family history is essential, particularly asking about consanguinity and a family history of developmental problems or learning difficulties, which may point to metabolic problems or recessive conditions.

Many parents make video recordings of their child on a camera or mobile telephone and these may be invaluable for illustrating the past and present developmental profile. Table 3 lists the main physical examination features pertinent to developmental assessment. Always consider difficulties of hearing and vision when there are concerns about development.

Much information can be gained by observing the child entering and moving around the clinic while playing with a few age appropriate toys, such as blocks, toy cars, pull-along toys, paper, and crayons. Observation of the child at home or nursery can also prove invaluable, as can reports from other carers, such as nursery workers or school teachers. For those interested in further reading about developmental assessment and examination, we recommend a comprehensive review of methods and interpretation by Sharma.[36]

In primary care, when time is limited, clinicians with pediatric experience should base their assessment on clinical judgment and knowledge of the broadly normal range of child development. Table 2 contains normal milestones and gives some indicators of when to worry and Box 5 contains some important red flags for significantly disordered development, which should prompt early referral to secondary care for diagnostic assessment.

In children presenting with mild developmental delay in the absence of any red flags, primary care practitioners may consider basic investigations such as full blood count, bone profile, thyroid function tests, and measurement of vitamin D and creatine kinase. Some causes of mild developmental delay such as iron deficiency anemia can be easily treated. However, to avoid multiple venepuncture, investigations should be

Table 2: Normal developmental milestones

Age	Skills				Red flags
	Gross motor	*Fine motor and vision*	*Hearing, speech, and language*	*Social, emotional, and behavioral*	
6 weeks	Head level with body in ventral suspension	Fixes and follows	Becomes still in response to sound	Smiles	Unresponsive to sound or visual stimuli
3 months	Holds head at 90° in ventral suspension	Holds an object placed in the hand	Turns to sound	Hand regard, laughs, and squeals	Lack of social response or vocalization
6 months	No head lag on pull to sit; sits with support; in prone position lifts up on forearms	Palmar grasp of objects; transfers objects hand to hand	Vocalizations	May finger feed self	Poor head control, floppiness, not reaching
9 months	Crawls; sits steadily when unsupported and pivots around	Pincer grasp; index finger approach; bangs two cubes together	2 syllable babble, nonspecific—consonant-vowel, such as "mama"	Waves bye plays pat-a-cake; indicates wants; stranger anxiety emerging	Can't sit unsupported; no babble
12 months	Pulls to stand; cruises; may stand alone briefly; may walk alone	Puts block in cup; casts about	One or two words; imitates adults' sounds	Imitates activities; object permanence (the understanding that objects still exist when they cannot be seen) established; stranger anxiety established; points to indicate wants	Not communicating by gestures, such as pointing; not weight bearing through legs
18 months	Walks well; runs	Builds tower of 2–4 cubes; hand preference emerges	6–12 words	Uses spoon; symbolic play—"talking" on telephone; domestic mimicry—"helps" in household chores like sweeping, wiping surfaces	Not walking; no symbolic play; no words
2 years	Kicks ball; climbs stairs two feet per step	Builds tower of 6–7 cubes; does circular scribbles	Joins 2–3 words; knows some body parts; identifies objects in pictures	Can remove some clothes	Not joining two words; cannot run
3 years	Stands briefly on one foot; climbs stairs one foot per step	Builds tower of 9 cubes; copies a circle	Talks in short sentences that a stranger can understand	Eats with fork and spoon; puts on clothing; may be toilet trained	Not communicating with words; cannot climb stairs

deferred in children with moderate or serious delay, or red flags, because they will require a battery of tests in secondary care.

What Tools are Available for Developmental Assessment in Primary Care?

Professionals who work with children learn to recognize deviant patterns of development, but screening questionnaires and developmental screening tools can improve accuracy.[37,38]

Examples of screening questionnaires include: the ages and stages questionnaire (ASQ),[39] the parents' evaluation of developmental status (PEDS),[40,41] and the modified checklist for autism in toddlers (M-CHAT).[42] These surveys can be self-administered and can be answered by parents in the waiting room or during the consultation itself. These tools can help focus the consultation and increase the confidence of primary care practitioners in their referral decisions.

Several short (10–20 minutes) standardized assessment tools can be used to complement clinical impressions in primary care. Examples include the Denver developmental screening test, which is completed by an observer and gives "pass or fail" results in the four major developmental fields,[43] and the schedule of growing skills II. This last test is based on the standardized Sheridan stycar sequences,[44] and it objectively assesses the child's developmental level in nine subfields of development.[45] Both give visual maps of a child's developmental skills with clear cut-off points to guide referral to secondary care (Table 4).

When should a Child be Referred for Specialist Assessment?

The presence of a red flag (Table 2 and Box 5) is a clear indication for referral to secondary care. Referral is also recommended if there are concerns about the extent of

Table 3: Key features of the developmental examination

Key features on examination	*Possible diagnosis*
• Head circumference measured and plotted on centile chart and interpreted in context of height and weight centiles; consider measurement of parental occipitofrontal head circumference	• Microcephaly or macrocephaly
• *Dysmorphic features:* Does the child look like other family members? Are there any unusual features?	• Genetic, metabolic, or syndromic conditions, such as fragile X syndrome
• *Skin abnormalities:* Café au lait patches, axillary freckling, neurofibromas, or hypopigmented patches (ash leaf macules)	• Suggestive of neurocutaneous syndromes, such as neurofibromatosis or tuberous sclerosis
• Observation of child's movements to look for signs of unsteadiness, weakness, or spasticity; check tone, power, and reflexes where possible	• Underlying neurological disorder
• Child's ability to sit up and to stand up from lying down supine and to clear the floor on jumping from a standing position	• Muscle weakness suggestive of a muscular dystrophy
• Observation of eye movements and examination of eyes looking for cataracts, nystagmus, or wobbly eye movements	• Disorder of vision; underlying neurological condition
• General examination of respiratory and cardiovascular systems	• Underlying systemic disease
• Abdominal examination for hepatomegaly	• Metabolic disorder

Box 5: Red flags

These indicators suggest that development is seriously disordered and that the child should be promptly referred to a developmental or community pediatrician[21]

Positive indicators (the presence of any of the following)

- Loss of developmental skills at any age
- Parental or professional concerns about vision, fixing, or following an object or a confirmed visual impairment at any age (simultaneous referral to pediatric ophthalmology)
- Hearing loss at any age (simultaneous referral for expert audiological or ear, nose, and throat assessment)
- Persistently low muscle tone or floppiness
- No speech by 18 months, especially if the child does not try to communicate by other means such as gestures (simultaneous referral for urgent hearing test)
- Asymmetry of movements or other features suggestive of cerebral palsy, such as increased muscle tone
- Persistent toe walking
- Complex disabilities
- Head circumference above the 99.6th centile or below 0.4th centile. Also, if circumference has crossed two centiles (up or down) on the appropriate chart or is disproportionate to parental head circumference
- An assessing clinician who is uncertain about any aspect of assessment but thinks that development may be disordered

Negative indicators (activities that the child cannot do)

- Sit unsupported by 12 months
- Walk by 18 months (boys) or 2 years (girls) (check creatine kinase urgently)
- Walk other than on tiptoes
- Run by 2.5 years
- Hold object placed in hand by 5 months (corrected for gestation)
- Reach for objects by 6 months (corrected for gestation)
- Point at objects to share interest with others by 2 years

developmental delay or the lack of response to primary care interventions, such as health visitor advice or speech and language therapy.

What happens when a Child is Referred to a Specialist?

Children with developmental concerns are most often seen by community pediatricians who work as part of a multidisciplinary team, often in child development centers. Members of the team may include a nursery nurse, preschool teacher, speech and language therapist, physiotherapist, occupational therapist, and psychologist. The child usually has an initial consultation to clarify the nature of the developmental difficulties.

Investigations (blood and urine tests, cranial imaging) may be arranged at this stage or later. The child may then undergo a multidisciplinary team assessment and intervention package of care over several weeks, after which a diagnosis will be reached, a report issued, and recommendations for ongoing support made.

Examples of developmental instruments used in secondary care that are more accurate, sophisticated, and time consuming (2–3 hours) than those used in primary care include the Griffiths mental development scales, Bayley scales of infant development, and the Wechsler preschool and primary scale of intelligence. Specific instruments are also available for the diagnosis of developmental disorders such as autism spectrum disorder. Standardized structured parental interviews, such as the developmental, dimensional, and diagnostic interview and autism diagnostic interview-revised, complement objective assessments of the child, such as the autism diagnostic observation schedule.

Table 4: Developmental screening questionnaires

Instrument	*Method*	*Age range*	*Outcome*	*Availability*	*Validation, sensitivity, specificity data*
Parents' evaluation of developmental status (PEDS)	A parent reported questionnaire used to identify general developmental delay in primary care; takes 5 minutes to complete, 2 minutes to score	0–8 years	High, moderate, or low risk for developmental or behavioral problems	(www.pedstest.com)	Validated in a large diverse standardization sample; sensitivity of 74–79% and specificity of 70–80% in ages 0–8 years for detection of developmental delays and behavioral problems[47]
Ages and stages questionnaire (ASQ)	A parent reported questionnaire of 30 developmental items used to identify general developmental delay in primary care; takes 10–15 minutes to complete	4–60 months	Cut-off point guides need for further assessment	(www.brookespublishing.com)	Validated in a large diverse standardization sample; specificity ranges from 81% (16 months) to 92% (36 months), and 86% overall; sensitivity averages 72%; published validation studies[48]
Modified checklist for autism in toddlers (M-CHAT)	A parent report of 23 items used to screen for autism in primary care population; takes 2 minutes to complete	16–30 months	Cut-off point for further assessment	Freely available online (www.firstsigns.org/downloads/m-chat.PDF)	Published validation study[42]
Schedule of growing skills	Professional scores items in 9 developmental fields; takes 10–15 minutes to complete	0–59 months	Graphic profile of developmental age compared with chronological age; guidelines to aid professional judgment of next action	(www.gl-assessment.co.uk)	Original data validation study showed specificity of 94–100% and sensitivity of 44–82% in different fields;[49] validation of revised schedule showed high reliability Cronbach[44]
Denver developmental screening test	Professional scores items in 4 developmental fields	2–71 months	Graphic display of developmental age with "pass/fail" score compared with "normal" centiles	(www.denverii.com)	Originally validated in Colorado, US; later statistical study showed specificity of 43% and sensitivity of 83%[43]

43.4 ANXIETY DISORDERS AND POST-TRAUMATIC STRESS DISORDER IN CHILDREN AND ADOLESCENT

JN Vyas, Pramodh Bhardhwaj

Anxiety disorders are one of the most prevalent categories of pediatric psychopathology.[50] There is a range of prevalence estimates based on the type of epidemiologic study that is completed. Short assessment intervals and single collection points result in the lowest prevalence estimates. Childhood prevalence studies of having any anxiety disorder show that 3-month estimates range from 2.2% to 8.6%[51,52] and 6-month estimates range from 5.5% to 17.7%.[53,54] In contrast, retrospective studies with older adolescents and adults that use a lifetime interval typically report higher prevalence estimates. Lifetime prevalence estimates range from 8.3% to 27%.[55] Because pediatric anxiety disorders are relatively

Table 5: DSM-IV-TR criteria differences for anxiety disorders in youth	
Anxiety disorder generalized anxiety disorder	*Differences in criteria for youth requires only one associated symptom*

- *Social phobia:* Children must have the ability to develop age appropriate friendships.
- Children must endorse anxiety with adults and peers.
- Anxiety may be shown through crying, tantrums, freezing, or shrinking from social situations.
- Children do not need to recognize that the fear is excessive or unreasonable.
- *Obsessive compulsive disorder:* Children do need to recognize that the obsessions and compulsions are excessive or unreasonable.
- *Posttraumatic stress disorder:* Response to the traumatic event may be expressed through agitated or disorganized behavior rather than extreme fear, helplessness, or horror.
- Traumatic event may be re-experienced through the use of repetitive play about the trauma.
- Children may have scary dreams without recognizable content that is related to the event.
- Children may re-enact trauma-specific details.

common, there is an increasing interest in understanding the research and clinical issues related to the presentation and treatment of these disorders.

Anxiety disorders are diagnosed throughout the life span. The Diagnostic and Statistical Manual of Mental Disorders, Fourth Edition, Text Revision (DSM-IV-TR)[56] criteria are similar for youth and adults; however, there are some notable differences that need to be considered when diagnosing anxiety disorders in children and adolescents. Table 5 provides a summary of the differences in diagnostic criteria for pediatric anxiety disorders.

SEPARATION ANXIETY DISORDER

Clinical Presentation

The key feature of separation anxiety disorder (SAD) is excessive anxiety about separation from primary attachment figures (e.g. parents, grandparents). Children with SAD fear that harm will come to themselves or their attachment figures when separated. Other symptoms include distress at the time of separation, somatic complaints.

When separation occurs or is anticipated, nightmares with themes of separation, shadowing parents in the home, and sleeping with family members.[56] Children with SAD commonly refuse to attend school and are reluctant to go other places without their parents. To be diagnosed with SAD, symptoms must be more intense than expected for the child's developmental level, be present for at least 4 weeks, have an onset before 18 years of age, and cause significant distress or impairment. A distinguishing feature of SAD is that the child's anxiety is alleviated when with parents, whereas in other anxiety disorders, the presence of an attachment figure has minimal effect on symptom presentation.[57]

The SAD is common in youth with a prevalence rate of 3–5%.[58,59] It is more likely to occur in children compared with adolescents. Onset is typically at 7–9 years of age.[58,60] Common comorbid diagnoses include generalized anxiety disorder (GAD), specific phobia, attention-deficit hyperactivity disorder (ADHD), and social phobia (SP).[61]

Course and Outcome

The SAD can be short-lived or chronic and persistent. Last and colleagues[62] followed children in an anxiety clinic prospectively for 3–4 years and found that SAD had the highest remission rate (95.7%) of all the anxiety disorders. In another prospective study, young children in a community sample were assessed at age 3 (n = 60) and 3.5 years later (n = 44) to evaluate the stability of SAD.[63] At baseline, the children were classified as having clinical, subclinical, or nonclinical levels of separation anxiety. Children who met full diagnostic criteria for SAD compared with those with subclinical or nonclinical status were more likely to have comorbid disorders and high levels of internalizing symptoms. In addition, parents of children with clinical SAD experienced high levels of internalizing symptoms and general distress. At follow-up, many children showed a decline a separation anxiety symptoms and moved in the direction of subclinical or nonclinical status. The investigators suggested family and parental characteristics (e.g. inconsistency in limited setting) predict lower likelihood of remission of SAD. Foley and colleagues[64] assessed the short-term outcome of SAD in a community sample of twins (ages 8–17). At an average follow-up period of 18 months, SAD had remitted in 80% of the children. Persistent SAD was predicted by oppositional defiant disorder, impairment because of ADHD, and maternal marital dissatisfaction. Children with persistent SAD were significantly more likely than children with remitted SAD to develop a new depressive disorder within 18 months.

The SAD is a risk factor for development of anxiety and depressive disorders in adulthood. A controversy exists in the literature as to whether SAD increases the vulnerability for several anxiety disorders or specifically for panic disorder. Data from the Oregon Adolescent Depression Project[58] were used to determine the risk that SAD confers for new disorders in adulthood. Teenagers were evaluated at age 16, including retrospective reports of childhood psychopathology. They were assessed twice during adolescence and twice as adults. Most teenagers with a history of SAD developed new disorders as adults. The major outcomes were panic disorder[65] In a 7-year follow-up study of children treated for an anxiety disorder, children with SAD compared with children with GAD or SP were more likely to have other anxiety disorders, but not specifically panic disorder.[65]

The association between SAD and future psychopathology does not indicate causality. While SAD may be causal for later psychiatric disorders, it is also possible that SAD and adult panic disorder and depression are caused by a common underlying vulnerability. "If the latter is true, then it may also be true that SAD is a marker for severity of the underlying vulnerability."[58]

GENERALIZED ANXIETY DISORDER

Clinical Presentation

Generalized anxiety disorder (GAD) is a relatively new diagnosis in children and adolescents. In the DSM-III-R[66] a diagnosis of GAD required a minimum age of 18 years. Instead, youth with excessive worry were diagnosed with over anxious disorder (OAD) was omitted from the DSM-IV[67] and the age restriction was removed from the GAD diagnostic criteria. DSM-IV-TR criteria for GAD are similar for youth when compared with adults, with one exception. The differentiating factor is that youth are only required to endorse one associated symptom (i.e. restlessness, fatigue, difficulty concentrating, irritability, muscle aches or tension, or sleep difficulties), and three are required for a diagnosis of GAD in adults (*see* Table 5). Common domains of worry in children with GAD include health of significant others, personal performance, family matters, and world issues.[68]

Because the number of associated symptoms differentiates DSM-IV-TR criteria for GAD in children and adults, this domain has been an area of interest. Research has consistently shown that youth diagnosed with GAD typically endorse more than one associated symotom.[68,69] Three studies[68,70,71] show that restlessness is the most common and muscle tension is the least common associated symptom endorsed by youth with GAD.

There are limited data on the prevalence of GAD in youth, as it was not diagnosed in children and adolescents until the DSM-IV. The prevalence rate of OAD in early adolescents was estimated at approximately 3%.[72,73] The prevalence rate of OAD in early adolescents was estimated at approximately 3%[72,73] The National Comorbidity Survey, which included individuals ranging in age from 15 to 54 years old, provided GAD prevalence rates from 1.6% current to 5.1% lifetime.[74]

DSM-5 Diagnostic Criteria for Generalized Anxiety Disorder 300.02 (F41.1)

- Excessive anxiety and worry (apprehensive expectation), occurring more days than not for at least 6 months, about a number of events or activities (such as work or school performance).
- The individual finds it difficult to control the worry.
- The anxiety and worry are associated with three (or more) of the following six symptoms (with at least some symptoms having been present for more days than not for the past 6 months):
  Note: Only one item is required in children.
  - Restlessness or feeling keyed up or on edge.
  - Being easily fatigued.
  - Difficulty concentrating or mind going blank.
  - Irritability.
  - Muscle tension.
  - Sleep disturbance (difficulty falling or staying asleep, or restless, unsatisfying sleep).
- The anxiety, worry, or physical symptoms cause clinically significant distress or impairment in social, occupational, or other important areas of functioning.
- The disturbance is not attributable to the physiological effects of a substance (e.g. a drug of abuse, a medication) or another medical condition (e.g. hyperthyroidism).
- The disturbance is not better explained by another mental disorder (e.g. anxiety or worry about having panic attacks in panic disorder, negative evaluation in social anxiety disorder [social phobia], contamination or other obsessions in obsessive-compulsive disorder, separation from attachment figures in separation anxiety disorder, reminders of traumatic events in post-traumatic stress disorder, gaining weight in anorexia nervosa, physical complaints in somatic symptom disorder, perceived appearance flaws in body dysmorphic disorder, having a serious illness in illness anxiety disorder, or the content of delusional beliefs in schizophrenia or delusional disorder).

Course and Outcome

The GAD has a bimodal age of onset with an early onset occurring during childhood and adolescence and a later onset during adulthood.[74] Childhood-onset GAD is usually associated with a greater degree of psychopathology and a chronic course with fluctuations in symptoms severity.[75,76] Children with GAD and a comorbid diagnosis of depression often have a poorer prognosis, greater symptom severity, and longer duration of symptoms when compared with children without comorbid depression.[77] Because of high comorbidity rates between GAD and depression, there is speculation as to whether these are two distinct disorder. Researchers have suggested that GAD may be a subsyndrome to major depressive disorder (MDD) because of "sequential comorbidity," in which GAD typically precedes MDD.[78] Other researchers theorize that the disorders have "cumulative comorbidity," "meaning that the disorders tend to occur during a lifetime but not in a simultaneous manner".[78] Moffitt and colleagues[78] completed a prospective study following 1,037 participants 3 years to 32 years of age. Results showed a strong cumulative comorbidity from 11 to 32 years of age. Forty-eight percent of participants with MDD had a history of an anxiety disorder and 72% of participants with anxiety had a history of MDD. Findings did not provide strong evidence for sequential comorbidity because GAD was diagnosed first in 42% of participants and MDD was diagnosed first in 32% of participants. These results show a strong relationship between GAD and MDD; however, more longitudinal studies are needed to better understand the association.

SOCIAL PHOBIA

Clinical Presentation

Before the DSM-IV, social phobia (SP) was not diagnosed in children and adolescents. Youth who endorsed anxiety and avoidance of engaging with unfamiliar people were commonly diagnosed with avoidant disorder of childhood or adolescence. This diagnosis was excluded from the DSM-IV; children and adolescents who fear social and performance situations are now diagnosed with SP.

Diagnostic criteria for SP in youth are similar to adult criteria, with a few minor clarifications that take into account developmental differences between adults and children (*see* Table 5). The primary characteristic of SP is the same across all ages. Individuals with SP experience fear regarding social and performance situations because of anxiety that they will act in an embarassing way. Children with SP often have poor social skills and have difficulty initiating and maintaining interpersonal relationships.[79,80] Beidel and colleagues[79] found that in a clinical sample of 50 children (7–13 years old) with SP, 75% reported having few or no friends and 50% were not involved extracurricular activities. SP also seems to have an impact on children's functioning in the classroom. Muris and Meesters[81] found that higher SP symptoms in a nonclinical sample of children (10–12 years old) were associated with poorer general classroom functioning, increased difficulty with peer relationships. And lower self-esteem. Bernstein and colleagues[80] examined classroom functioning in a nonclinical sample of children with SP (7–10 years old) based on teacher reports. Results showed that children that greater severity of SP symptoms had poorer social and leadership skills. In addition, there was an association between the severity of SP symptoms and school difficulties: as SP severity increased, attention and learning problems also increased.

The rate of lifetime SP in a community sample of adolescents was found to be 1.6%,[82] and substantially high rate 14.9% in a clinical sample of children.[60] Mean age of onset for social phobia in clinical samples ranges from 11 to 12 years of age[60,83] and the rate of SP increases with age.[82] Essau and colleagues[82] found that the most commonly feared situations in adolescents were performing in front of others, public speaking, and engaging in conversations. The most frequent anxiety endorsed by these adolescents was the fear that something would happen to cause them to be embarrassed.

Beidel and colleagues[79] found that 60% of children with SP met criteria for another Axis I disorder. Thirty-six percent of the comorbid disorders were other anxiety disorders. The most common comorbid disorders included the following: 10% of children had GAD, ADHD, or specific phobia; 8% had selective mutism; and 6% had an affective disorder.

DSM-5 Diagnostic Criteria for Social Anxiety Disorder (Social Phobia) 300.23 (F40.10)

- Marked fear or anxiety about one or more social situations in which the individual is exposed to possible scrutiny by others. Examples include social interactions (e.g. having a conversation, meeting unfamiliar people), being observed (e.g. eating or drinking), and performing in front of others (e.g. giving a speech).
  Note: In children, the anxiety must occur in peer settings and not just during interactions with adults.
- The individual fears that he or she will act in a way or show anxiety symptoms that will be negatively evaluated (i.e. will be humiliating or embarrassing; will lead to rejection or offend others).
- The social situations almost always provoke fear or anxiety.
  Note: In children, the fear or anxiety may be expressed by crying, tantrums, freezing, clinging, shrinking, or failing to speak in social situations.
- The social situations are avoided or endured with intense fear or anxiety.
- The fear or anxiety is out of proportion to the actual threat posed by the social situation and to the sociocultural context.
- The fear, anxiety, or avoidance is persistent, typically lasting for 6 months or more.
- The fear, anxiety, or avoidance causes clinically significant distress or impairment in social, occupational, or other important areas of functioning.
- The fear, anxiety, or avoidance is not attributable to the physiological effects of a substance (e.g. a drug of abuse, a medication) or another medical condition.
- The fear, anxiety, or avoidance is not better explained by the symptoms of another mental disorder, such as panic disorder, body dysmorphic disorder, or autism spectrum disorder.
- If another medical condition (e.g. Parkinson's disease, obesity, disfigurement from burns or injury) is present, the fear, anxiety, or avoidance is clearly unrelated or is excessive.
  Specify if:
  Performance only: If the fear is restricted to speaking or performing in public.

Course and Outcome

A prospective longitudinal study that followed adolescents until 34 years of age showed that a diagnosis of SP during adolescence significantly increases the individual's risk for later onset depression.[84] Approximately 50% of participants with SP met criteria for a depressive disorder during the follow-up period, which placed them at a twofold risk compared with individuals without a diagnosis of SP. Several factors and SP characteristics were found to be associated with an increased risk for subsequent depression. The contributing factors were parental anxiety or major depression, female gender, childhood behavioral inhibition, and having more than two other anxiety disorders. The contributing SP characteristics were increased level of impairment, persistence of symptoms, and greater degree of severity.

In addition to the high rate of depressive disorders found in individuals diagnosed with SP, there is also a high rate of co-morbidity of SP and substance use disorders.[85] Buckner and colleagues[86] found that adolescents who were diagnosed with SP were more likely to be diagnosed with alcohol dependence and cannabis dependence during a follow-up period that ended at 30 years of age when compared with a adolescents who did not have a diagnosis of SP. Furthermore, the data provide evidence that SP in adolescents seems to be a unique risk factor for the development of subsequent substance dependence disorders. Because of the high comorbidity rates of subsequent depressive and substance dependence disorders, SP places youth at risk for long-term problems across domains of education, social relationships, and employment.

OBSESSIVE-COMPULSIVE DISORDER

Clinical Presentation

DSM-IV-TR requires either obsessions or compulsions to meet criteria for OCD.[56] Obsessions are recurrent intrusive thoughts, images, or impulses that cause excessive anxiety or distress. Compulsions are repetitive behaviors or mental acts that the individual feels compelled to perform in response to an obsession. To be diagnosed with OCD, The individuals must experience excessive distress, engage in obsessions or compulsions for greater than 1 hour per day, or experience functional impairment related to the OCD. Young children do not necessarily recognize their obsessions and compulsions as senseless or excessive.

Finally DSM-5 has come up with OCD under obsessive-compulsive and related disorder. And some changes have been made on it.

DSM-5 Criteria for OCD (Obsessive-Compulsive Disorder) 300.3 (F42)

- Presence of obsessions, compulsions, or both: Obsessions are defined by (1) and (2):
  - Recurrent and persistent thoughts, urges, or images that are experienced, at some time during the disturbance, as intrusive and unwanted, and that in most individuals cause marked anxiety or distress.
  - The individual attempts to ignore or suppress such thoughts, urges, or images, or to neutralize them with some other thought or action (i.e. by performing a compulsion).

  Compulsions are defined by (1) and (2):
  - Repetitive behaviors (e.g. hand washing, ordering, checking) or mental acts (e.g. praying, counting, repeating words silently) that the individual feels driven to perform in response to an obsession or according to rules that must be applied rigidly.
  - The behaviors or mental acts are aimed at preventing or reducing anxiety or distress, or preventing some dreaded event or situation; however, these behaviors or mental acts are not connected in a realistic way with what they are designed to neutralize or prevent, or are clearly excessive.

  Note: Young children may not be able to articulate the aims of these behaviors or mental acts.
- The obsessions or compulsions are time-consuming (e.g. take more than 1 hour per day) or cause clinically significant distress or impairment in social, occupational, or other important areas of functioning.
- The obsessive-compulsive symptoms are not attributable to the physiological effects of a substance (e.g. a drug of abuse, a medication) or another medical condition.
- The disturbance is not better explained by the symptoms of another mental disorder (e.g. excessive worries, as in generalized anxiety disorder; preoccupation with appearance, as in body dysmorphic disorder; difficulty discarding or parting with possessions, as in hoarding disorder; hair pulling, as in trichotillomania [hair pulling disorder]; skin picking, as in excoriation [skin-picking] disorder; stereotypies, as in stereotypic movement disorder; ritualized eating behavior, as in eating disorders; preoccupation with substances or gambling, as in substance-related and addictive disorders; preoccupation with having an illness, as in illness anxiety disorder; sexual urges or fantasies, as in paraphilic disorders; impulses, as in disruptive, impulse-control, and conduct disorders; guilty ruminations, as in major depressive disorder; thought insertion or delusional preoccupations, as in schizophrenia spectrum and other psychotic disorders; or repetitive patterns of behavior, as in autism spectrum disorder).

  Specify if:

  With good or fair insight: The individual recognizes that obsessive-compulsive disorder beliefs are definitely or probably not true or that they may or may not be true.

  With poor insight: The individual thinks obsessive-compulsive disorder beliefs are probably true.

  With absent insight/delusional beliefs: The individual is completely convinced that obsessive-compulsive disorder beliefs are true.

Specify if:

Tic-related: The individual has a current or past history of a tic disorder.

Prevalence of OCD in children and adolescents ranges from 1% to 4%.[87,88] The male-to-female ratio is approximately 3:2 in youth and changes to a slight female predominance in adulthood.[89] Common comorbid conditions are tic disorders, other anxiety disorders, ADHD, pervasive developmental disorders, and depression.[90]

Almost all children and adolescents with OCD have both obsessions and compulsions. One study showed that 93% of children with OCD experience multiple obsessions and 100% engage in multiple compulsions.[91] In a series of 70 consesutive cases of early onset OCD, the most common obsessions were concern about dirt or germs, danger to self or family, and symmetry; the most common compulsions were excessive washing, repeating rituals, and checking behaviors.[92]

Children with OCD present with a variety of obsessions and compulsions. Stewart and colleagues[93] used a principal component analysis to identify factors from the Children's Yale-Brown-Obsessive-Compulsive Scale (CY-BOCS)[94] in a sample of 231 children and adolescents with OCD. The CY-BOCS is a semistructured interview that assesses severity of OCD symptoms and includes a checklist of the types of obsessions and compulsions experienced. Four factors were identified as strongly associated with the presentation of pediatric OCD and accounted for 60% of the symptom variance: preoccupation with contamination/cleaning/aggressive somatic, symmetry/ordering/repeating/checking, sexual/religious themes, and hoarding.[93] There is evidence that suggests a similar four-factor structure is applicable across the life-span.[94] A dimensional approach is useful in understanding the heterogeneity in OCD.[93]

Course and Outcome

There is bimodal pattern to age of onset in OCD, with one peak in childhood and a second in adulthood.[95] Age of onset for pediatric OCD is typically around 10 years, with a range from 7.5 to 12.5 years.[89] In youth, the mean age at identification is 2.5 years after onset of the disorder this delay may be in part due to the secretive nature of the symptoms in many children.

In a meta-analysis of 16 pediatric samples (n = 521 participants) followed for 1 to 15.6 years, with the average period to follow-up of 5.7 years, a substantial number of children with OCD achieved remission of symoptoms.[96] In the pooled sample, 59% of participants no longer met criteria for the OCD diagnosis and 40% did not show any evidence of residual OCD symptoms at follow-up. Predictors of persistence of OCD diagnosis included earlier age of onset, longer duration of illness at ascertainment, and a history of impatient hospitalization.[96]

Pediatric Autoimmune Neuropsychiatric Disorders Associated with Streptococcal Infections

A small subgroup of children with OCD or tics has been classified as having pediatric autoimmune neuropsychiatric disorders associated with streptococcal infections (PANDAS).[97] This subset of children experiences a sudden onset of OCD or motor tics in association with group A streptococcal infections (e.g. "strep throat"). Diagnostic criteria for PANDAS include: (1) presence of OCD or tics, (2) prepubertal onset, (3) abrupt onset or episodic course of symptom severity, (4) exacerbations associated with streptococcal infections, and (5) exacerbations associated with neurologic abnormalities (e.g. hyperactivity, choreiform movements).[97] There is an increased rate of comorbid neuropsychiatric symptoms in children with PANDAS, including separation anxiety, impulsivity, hyperactivity, enuresis, and deterioration in handwriting.[97,98]

Although streptococcal infections are believed to be involved in the etiologic pathway leading to OCD in children with PANDAS, the mechanism is still under investigation. Research suggests that circulating autoimmune antibodies that cross-react with neuronal structures (particularly the basal ganglia) may play a key role in the pathogenesis of PANDAS.[99]

Case Examples

Rabindra is an 11-year-old boy presenting with a two-year history of intrusive, obsessive thoughts and compulsive, ritualistic behaviors. The obsessions began at around 9 years of age with concern about contamination of food. Rabindra would not eat anything that a family member had touched. Before preparing food, Rabindra required that his mother put on a clean outfit and thoroughly wash her hands. If he observed his mother touch the kitchen countertop or cough or sneeze during meal preparation, he demanded that she change clothes and wash her hands again. If she did not comply, Rabindra would not eat the food she prepared.

One of Rabindra's prominent intrusive thoughts was that meat was not thoroughly cooked. He asked his mother multiple times whether she had cooked the meat long enough. He worried that he or a family member might contract mad cow disease and die if the meat was not completely cooked. He refused to eat at restaurants because of his concerns about contamination and whether meat was completely cooked. He did not eat the hot lunch at school and brought his own lunch instead. Rabindra washed his hands multiple times during the day, using large amounts of soap and spending up to 30 minutes washing at a time. If he was interrupted, he restarted the compulsion that consisted of washing each hand an even number of times.

POST-TRAUMATIC STRESS DISORDER

Clinical Presentation

Clinical presentation of posttraumatic stress disorder (PTSD) in older children and adolescents in similar to that in adults. Older children and adolescents have a better understanding of the traumatic experiences and the long-term consequences than children.[100] Additionally, they have the cognitive abilities to describe symptoms of re-experiencing, avoidance, numbing, and dissociation. Carrion and colleagues[101] assessed the frequency and intensity of PTSD symptoms in children ranging from 7 to 14 years of age. The most frequent symptoms included: 83% engaged in avoidance of thoughts, feelings, and conversations associated with the trauma; 70% had distressing recollections and the inability to recall important aspects of the traumatic event; and 64% reported problems concentrating. Children rated irritability and anger, distressing dreams, and detachment from others as the most intense symptoms.

Clinical presentation of PTSD in young children tends to be markedly different than that in older children, adolescents, and adults. Young children are less likely to demonstrate emotional numbing and avoidance, which is likely because of the complicated cognitive introspection that is required.[100] Young children are more likely to exhibit overt aggression, destructive behavior, and repetitive play about the traumatic event. Because of these developmental differences in clinical presentation, it is less likely that young children will meet DSM-IV-TR criteria for PTSD.

DSM-5 Diagnostic Criteria for PTSD 309.81 (F43.10)

Posttraumatic Stress Disorder

Note: The following criteria apply to adults, adolescents, and children older than 6 years. For children 6 years and younger, see corresponding criteria below.

- Exposure to actual or threatened death, serious injury, or sexual violence in one (or more) of the following ways:
  - Directly experiencing the traumatic event(s).
  - Witnessing, in person, the event(s) as it occurred to others.
  - Learning that the traumatic event(s) occurred to a close family member or close friend. In cases of actual or threatened death of a family member or friend, the event(s) must have been violent or accidental.
  - Experiencing repeated or extreme exposure to aversive details of the traumatic event(s) (e.g. first responders collecting human remains; police officers repeatedly exposed to details of child abuse).

  Note: Criterion A4 does not apply to exposure through electronic media, television, movies, or pictures, unless this exposure is work related.
- Presence of one (or more) of the following intrusion symptoms associated with the traumatic event(s), beginning after the traumatic event(s) occurred:
  - Recurrent, involuntary, and intrusive distressing memories of the traumatic event(s).

  Note: In children older than 6 years, repetitive play may occur in which themes or aspects of the traumatic event(s) are expressed.
  - Recurrent distressing dreams in which the content and/or affect of the dream are related to the traumatic event(s).

  Note: In children, there may be frightening dreams without recognizable content.
  - Dissociative reactions (e.g. flashbacks) in which the individual feels or acts as if the traumatic event(s) were recurring. (Such reactions may occur on a continuum, with the most extreme expression being a complete loss of awareness of present surroundings.)

  Note: In children, trauma-specific reenactment may occur in play.
  - Intense or prolonged psychological distress at exposure to internal or external cues that symbolize or resemble an aspect of the traumatic event(s).
  - Marked physiological reactions to internal or external cues that symbolize or resemble an aspect of the traumatic event(s).
- Persistent avoidance of stimuli associated with the traumatic event(s), beginning after the traumatic event(s) occurred, as evidenced by one or both of the following:
  - Avoidance of or efforts to avoid distressing memories, thoughts, or feelings about or closely associated with the traumatic event(s).
  - Avoidance of or efforts to avoid external reminders (people, places, conversations, activities, objects, situations) that Posttraumatic Stress Disorder 145 arouse distressing memories, thoughts, or feelings about or closely associated with the traumatic event(s).
- Negative alterations in cognitions and mood associated with the traumatic event(s), beginning or worsening after the traumatic event(s) occurred, as evidenced by two (or more) of the following:
  - Inability to remember an important aspect of the traumatic event(s) (typically due to dissociative amnesia and not to other factors such as head injury, alcohol, or drugs).
  - Persistent and exaggerated negative beliefs or expectations about oneself, others, or the world (e.g. "I am bad," "No one can be trusted," "The world is completely dangerous," "My whole nervous system is permanently ruined").
  - Persistent, distorted cognitions about the cause or consequences of the traumatic event(s) that lead the individual to blame himself/herself or others.

  - Persistent negative emotional state (e.g. fear, horror, anger, guilt, or shame).
  - Markedly diminished interest or participation in significant activities.
  - Feelings of detachment or estrangement from others.
  - Persistent inability to experience positive emotions (e.g. inability to experience happiness, satisfaction, or loving feelings).
- Marked alterations in arousal and reactivity associated with the traumatic event(s), beginning or worsening after the traumatic event(s) occurred, as evidenced by two (or more) of the following:
  - Irritable behavior and angry outbursts (with little or no provocation) typically expressed as verbal or physical aggression toward people or objects.
  - Reckless or self-destructive behavior.
  - Hypervigilance.
  - Exaggerated startle response.
  - Problems with concentration.
  - Sleep disturbance (e.g. difficulty falling or staying asleep or restless sleep).
- Duration of the disturbance (Criteria B, C, D, and E) is more than 1 month.
- The disturbance causes clinically significant distress or impairment in social, occupational, or other important areas of functioning.
- The disturbance is not attributable to the physiological effects of a substance (e.g. medication, alcohol) or another medical condition.

  Specify whether:

  With dissociative symptoms: The individual's symptoms meet the criteria for posttraumatic stress disorder, and in addition, in response to the stressor, the individual experiences persistent or recurrent symptoms of either of the following:
  - *Depersonalization:* Persistent or recurrent experiences of feeling detached from, and as if one were an outside observer of, one's mental processes or body (e.g. feeling as though one were in a dream; feeling a sense of unreality of self or body or of time moving slowly).
  - *Derealization:* Persistent or recurrent experiences of unreality of surroundings (e.g. the world around the individual is experienced as unreal, dreamlike, distant, or distorted).

  Note: To use this subtype, the dissociative symptoms must not be attributable to the physiological effects of a substance (e.g. blackouts, behavior during alcohol intoxication) or another medical condition (e.g. complex partial seizures).

  Specify if:

  With delayed expression: If the full diagnostic criteria are not met until at least 6 months after the event (although the onset and expression of some symptoms may be immediate).

Posttraumatic Stress Disorder for Children 6 Years and Younger

- In children 6 years and younger, exposure to actual or threatened death, serious injury, or sexual violence in one (or more) of the following ways:
  - Directly experiencing the traumatic event(s).
  - Witnessing, in person, the event(s) as it occurred to others, especially primary caregivers.

  Note: Witnessing does not include events that are witnessed only in electronic media, television, movies, or pictures.

  Posttraumatic Stress Disorder 147
  - Learning that the traumatic event(s) occurred to a parent or caregiving figure.
- Presence of one (or more) of the following intrusion symptoms associated with the traumatic event(s), beginning after the traumatic event(s) occurred:
  - Recurrent, involuntary, and intrusive distressing memories of the traumatic event(s).

  Note: Spontaneous and intrusive memories may not necessarily appear distressing and may be expressed as play reenactment.
  - Recurrent distressing dreams in which the content and/or affect of the dream are related to the traumatic event(s).

  Note: It may not be possible to ascertain that the frightening content is related to the traumatic event.
  - Dissociative reactions (e.g. flashbacks) in which the child feels or acts as if the traumatic event(s) were recurring. (Such reactions may occur on a continuum, with the most extreme expression being a complete loss of awareness of present surroundings.) Such trauma-specific reenactment may occur in play.
  - Intense or prolonged psychological distress at exposure to internal or external cues that symbolize or resemble an aspect of the traumatic event(s).
  - Marked physiological reactions to reminders of the traumatic event(s).
- One (or more) of the following symptoms, representing either persistent avoidance of stimuli associated with the traumatic event(s) or negative alterations in cognitions and mood associated with the traumatic event(s), must be present, beginning after the event(s) or worsening after the event(s):

  Persistent avoidance of stimuli
  - Avoidance of or efforts to avoid activities, places, or physical reminders that arouse recollections of the traumatic event(s).
  - Avoidance of or efforts to avoid people, conversations, or interpersonal situations that arouse recollections of the traumatic event(s).

Negative alterations in cognitions
- Substantially increased frequency of negative emotional states (e.g. fear, guilt, sadness, shame, confusion).
- Markedly diminished interest or participation in significant activities, including constriction of play.
- Socially withdrawn behavior.
- Persistent reduction in expression of positive emotions.

- Alterations in arousal and reactivity associated with the traumatic event(s), beginning or worsening after the traumatic event(s) occurred, as evidenced by two (or more) of the following:
  - Irritable behavior and angry outbursts (with little or no provocation) typically expressed as verbal or physical aggression toward people or objects (including extreme temper tantrums).
  - Hypervigilance.
  - Exaggerated startle response.
  - Problems with concentration.
  - Sleep disturbance (e.g. difficulty falling or staying asleep or restless sleep).
- The duration of the disturbance is more than 1 month.
- The disturbance causes clinically significant distress or impairment in relationships with parents, siblings, peers, or other caregivers or with school behavior.
- The disturbance is not attributable to the physiological effects of a substance (e.g. medication or alcohol) or another medical condition.

  Specify whether:

  With dissociative symptoms: The individual's symptoms meet the criteria for posttraumatic stress disorder, and the individual experiences persistent or recurrent symptoms of either of the following:
  - *Depersonalization:* Persistent or recurrent experiences of feeling detached from, and as if one were an outside observer of, one's mental processes or body (e.g. feeling as though one were in a dream; feeling a sense of unreality of self or body or of time moving slowly).
  - *Derealization:* Persistent or recurrent experiences of unreality of surroundings (e.g. the world around the individual is experienced as unreal, dreamlike, distant, or distorted).

  Note: To use this subtype, the dissociative symptoms must not be attributable to the physiological effects of a substance (e.g. blackouts) or another medical condition (e.g. complex partial seizures).

  Specify if:

  With delayed expression: If the full diagnostic criteria are not met until at least 6 months after the event (although the onset and expression of some symptoms may be immediate.

Alternative criteria that are more developmentally appropriate to diagnose PTSD in infants and younger children have been proposed and are being evaluated.[102,103] Many of the adult PTSD symptoms depend on higher-level cognitive functions (i.e. memory, abstract thinking, emotional processing, language).[104] The criteria being investigated for younger children are less dependent on verbalizations and rely more on behavioral observations. The alternative criteria do not require young children to demonstrate an intense fear response during the traumatic even. The re-experiencing criteria emphasize posttraumatic play and play reenactment of the traumatic event. Young children are not required to exhibit avoidance behaviors related to the traumatic event or belief regarding a shortened future and recall of the event is not assessed. Instead it is proposed that young children demonstrate a numbing of responsiveness through constructed play, socially withdrawn behavior, and restricted range of affect. Young children need to show increased arousal similar to DSM-IV-TR criteria. The proposed criteria include an additional domain, which is related to the development of new fear and aggression (i.e. separation anxiety, fear of toileting alone, fear of the dark). The duration of the symptoms is still at least 1 month; however, the symptoms do not need to cause significant distress or impairment. These proposed criteria are not part of the DSM-IV-TR at this time.

Prevalence of pediatric PTSD was studied in the Great Smoky Mountains Study (GSMS), which is a longitudinal community study of childhood psychopathology that included 1,420 youths ranging in age from 9 to 16 years. At 16 years of age, 67.8% of participants reported exposure to at least one traumatic event and the trauma occurred more often during adolescence, as compared with childhood.[105] Of the participants exposed to trauma, 40.4% met criteria for a psychiatric disorder, compared with 25.5% of participants who were not exposed to trauma. Only 0.5% and painful recall were endorsed. Subclinical PTSD (i.e. one symptom of painful recall, hyperarousal, and avoidance) was present 2.2% of the youth and painful recall was present in 9.1% of the youth.

The occurrence of PTSD in a community sample of older adolescents is shown to be higher than reported in the GSMS that included younger children. From a sample of 384 adolescents with an average age of 17.9 years, 43% reported experiencing a traumatic event.[106] Of these participants, 14.5% met full DSM-III-R criteria for PTSD (i.e. 6.3% of total sample). The median age of onset of PTSD was 16 years. The rate of trauma did not significantly differ between males and females; however, females were six times more likely to meet criteria for PTSD. Adolescents diagnosed with PTSD were seven times more likely to develop another psychiatric disorder (most commonly major depression or substance dependence) compared with adolescents with no trauma exposure and four times more likely compared with other adolescents who experienced trauma but did not meet criteria for PTSD.

Course and Outcome

Risk factors associated with the development of PTSD in youth are based on factors before the trauma, related to the trauma, and following the trauma. Parental psychopathology and family conflict significantly increase the risk of youth experiencing a traumatic even.[107] Other risk factors related to the youth's life events, parental poverty, history of childhood maltreatment, poor family functioning, family history of psychiatric disorders, introversion or extreme behavioral inhibition, female gender, younger age, poor health, and history of psychiatric disorder.[108,109]

Risk factors for PTSD associated with the traumatic experience include the degree of trauma exposure and the parent's and child's subjective sense of danger.[110] Witnessing a threat to a primary caregiver during infancy, childhood, and adolescence is related to an increase in total number of PTSD symptoms.[111] Lack of social support, continued negative life events, parental reactions, and lack of post-trauma intervention are risk factors associated with poor outcome after the trauma.[110]

SUMMARY

Anxiety disorders are commonly diagnosed in children and adolescents. Prevalence rates range from 2% to 27% depending on the length of the assessment interval. Therefore, it is important to identify and treat pediatric anxiety disorder to reduce the long-term consequences. Although anxiety disorders often have similar clinical presentations in youth and adults. It is critical to understand the differences that may occur across the lifespan.

43.5 EATING DISORDER: ANOREXIA

Neena Bohra, NK Bohra

INTRODUCTION

Background

Anorexia nervosa is an eating disorder characterized by a weight loss of at least 15% of expected body weight,[112] a devastating fear of weight gain, relentless dietary habits preventing weight gain, and a disturbance in the way in which body weight and shape are experienced. It has potentially life-threatening physiologic effects as well as enduring psychological disturbance.

Although anorexia nervosa is often heralded by a desire to lose an insignificant amount of weight through dieting, once the weight loss is in progress, immunological and hormonal factors that may play a role in the malignant spiral down and maintenance of anorexia nervosa include leptins (involved with signally satiety) as well as alpha melanocyte stimulating hormone.[113]

According to the Diagnostic and Statistical Manual for Mental Disorders, Fourth Edition (DSM-IV), anorexia nervosa is defined as "the refusal to maintain body weight about 85% of predicted, an intense fear of gaining weight, undue influence of body shape or weight on self-image, and missing at least 3 consecutive menstrual periods."[114] An increase in morbidity and mortality is present in anorexia nervosa compared with other psychiatric disorders.

DSM-5 Diagnostic Criteria for Anorexia Nervosa

- Restriction of energy intake relative to requirements, leading to a significantly low body weight in the context of age, sex, developmental trajectory, and physical health. *Significantly low weight* is defined as a weight that is less than minimally normal or, for children and adolescents, less than that minimally expected.
- Intense fear of gaining weight or of becoming fat, or persistent behavior that interferes with weight gain, even though at a significantly low weight.
- Disturbance in the way in which one's body weight or shape is experienced, undue influence of body weight or shape on self-evaluation, or persistent lack of recognition of the seriousness of the current low body weight.

Coding note: The ICD-9-CM code for anorexia nervosa is 307.1, which is assigned regardless of the subtype. The ICD-10-CM code depends on the subtype (*See* below).

Specify whether:
(F50.01) Restricting type: During the last 3 months, the individual has not engaged in recurrent episodes of binge eating or purging behavior (i.e. self-induced vomiting or the misuse of laxatives, diuretics, or enemas). This subtype describes presentations in which weight loss is accomplished

primarily through dieting, fasting, and/or excessive exercise.

(F50.02) Binge-eating/purging type: During the last 3 months, the individual has engaged in recurrent episodes of binge eating or purging behavior (i.e. self-induced vomiting or the misuse of laxatives, diuretics, or enemas).

Specify if:

In partial remission: After full criteria for anorexia nervosa were previously met, Criterion A (low body weight) has not been met for a sustained period, but either Criterion B (intense fear of gaining weight or becoming fat or behavior that interferes with weight gain) or Criterion C (disturbances in self-perception of weight and shape) is still met.

In full remission: After full criteria for anorexia nervosa were previously met, none of the criteria have been met for a sustained period of time.

Specify current severity: The minimum level of severity is based, for adults, on current body mass index (BMI) (*See below*) or, for children and adolescents, on BMI percentile. The ranges below are derived from World Health Organization categories for thinness in adults; for children and adolescents, corresponding BMI percentiles should be used. The level of severity may be increased to reflect clinical symptoms, the degree of functional disability, and the need for supervision.

Mild: BMI >17 kg/m^2

Moderate: BMI 16–16.99 kg/m^2

Severe: BMI 15–15.99 kg/m^2

Extreme: BMI <15 kg/m^2

Pathophysiology

Anorexia nervosa is a disease that affects all organ systems. The principal systems affected are the cardiovascular and the endocrine systems. However, complications from other systems, including the GI, renal, reproductive, neurologic, orofacial, dermatologic and hematologic, are noted as well.

Frequency

United States

The prevalence of anorexia nervosa is 1%, with a bimodal pattern of onset, occurring in people aged 14 and 18 years. A point prevalence study performed in Rochester, Minnesota showed a prevalence of 145 and 113 cases per 100,000 people in 1988 and 1991, respectively. The disease is more common in industrialized countries where food is abundant and an emphasis is placed on a slender body shape and an overall thin appearance.

Although more common in women, with a female-to-male ratio of 10:1, approximately 10% of cases involve men. Gay and bisexual males are more likely to have an eating disorder than heterosexual males but they are more likely to have bulimia than anorexia.[115]

Anorexia nervosa is found mainly in the white (>95%) adolescent (>75%) populations of the middle and upper socioeconomic classes, although it can be observed in either sex and in people of any race, age, or social stratum.[116]

No influences have been found with respect to the month or season of birth.[117]

A 7% increased incidence in first-degree relatives may be related to an area on chromosome 1p at the DF1153721 locus.[118]

According to Mehler in 1997, certain groups are especially at risk, including dancers, long-distance runners, skaters, models, actors, wrestlers, gymnasts, flight attendants, college sorority members, and others for whom thinness is emphasized and overly rewarded.[119]

International

As mentioned above, anorexia nervosa is observed mostly in industrialized countries. However, a study performed in suburban London reported a prevalence of only 20.2 cases per 100,000 people, a much smaller figure than that observed in the United States.[120]

Mortality/Morbidity

Prognosis is guarded, and poor outcome is associated with longer duration of illness, late onset of illness, and more severe weight loss. Morbidity rates range from 10–20%; only 50% of patients completely recover. Of the remaining 50%, 20% remain emaciated, and 25% are thin.[121] The remaining 10% become overweight or die of starvation.

The following are prognostic factors and how they affect anorexia nervosa:

- Onset of anorexia nervosa before adulthood carries a more favorable outcome. However, onset at an age younger than 11 years is a poor prognostic factor.
- Although the degree of weight loss at the clinically noted onset of the involvement of the patient's organic systems is not predictive of outcome, a high weight loss at presentation predicts a poor outcome.
- Both a short duration of involvement of the patient's organic systems before admission and a short inpatient treatment period are associated with a favorable outcome.
- A good relationship between the parent and child tends towards a more favorable outcome. Bryant-Waugh et al. found a poor prognosis for patients from one-parent families, from families in which parents had been married before, and from families in which several generations lived together.[122]

Race

As mentioned earlier, no discrimination in race with respect to anorexia nervosa is observed, although the disease is observed more often in white adolescents than in black adolescents.

Sex

A predominance of anorexia nervosa in females is observed. Studies have reported a 10:1 female-to-male ratio. Treatment plans remain the same for both sexes.

Age

Although it is more frequently observed in the adolescent age group, anorexia nervosa has no age restrictions and can be observed in the young child and adult as well. Onset in both of the latter groups carries a poor prognosis.

CLINICAL EXAMINATIONS

History

Obtain patient history with the goal of developing a treatment plan and not with the thought of merely ruling out an eating disorder. With medical assessment, focus on the medical complications of altered nutrition. Seek a careful history detailing weight changes, dietary patterns, and excessive exercise. Determine weight and height.

A review of systems may reveal many positive responses. The following are symptoms commonly observed in patients with anorexia nervosa:

- Physical health concerns
- Mental health concerns
- Amenorrhea
- Concentration concerns
- Cold hands or feet
- Decision-making concerns
- Constipation
- Irritability
- Dry skin or hair loss
- Depression[123]
- Headaches
- Social withdrawal
- Fainting or dizziness
- Obsessiveness (food)
- Lethargy.

Physical Examination

Focus the physical examination on the changes commonly observed in anorexia nervosa. Vital sign changes include hypotension, bradycardia, and hypothermia. Other changes include dry skin, hypercarotenemia, lanugo body hair, acrocyanosis, atrophy of the breasts, and swelling of the parotid and submandibular glands. ECG reveals a prolonged cardiac output (QT) interval,[124] and echocardiography (ECHO) reveals a decreased ventricular mass and mitral valve prolapse. GI signs include intestinal dilation from constipation and diminished intestinal motility.

Mental Health Assessment

When performing a mental health assessment, focus on making a diagnosis, identifying concurrent emotional-behavioral illnesses, evaluating for the risk of suicide,[125,126] and exploring the psychosocial context of the symptoms.

The following are characteristic signs of inadequate energy (caloric) intake observed in patients with anorexia nervosa that are due to starvation-induced changes:

- Positive
  - Hypothermia
  - Acrocyanosis
  - Resting bradycardia (resting heart rate often 40–49 beats per minute)
  - Hypotension
  - Orthostatic lowered blood pressure or pulse
  - Loss of muscle mass
  - Low blood glucose (impaired insulin clearance)
  - Low parathyroid hormone levels
  - Elevated liver function
  - Low WBC count
- Negative
  - Normal fundi or visual fields
  - No organomegaly
  - No lymphadenopathy.

Causes

Anorexia nervosa is a complex condition based on various biologic, psychologic, and social issues. As such, referring to anorexia nervosa as a developmental condition rather than a mental condition is preferable. Therefore, commenting about predisposing, precipitating, and perpetuating factors is more useful than commenting about actual causes.

- Predisposing factors include the following factors that make a patient more vulnerable to developing an eating disorder:
  - Female sex
  - Family history of eating disorders[127]
  - Perfectionistic personality
  - Difficulty communicating negative emotions
  - Difficulty resolving conflict
  - Low self-esteem
- Precipitating factors relate most often to developmental tasks that cause intense intrapsychic conflict and unconscious feelings of anxiety related to developing into a mature sexual person; these factors interact with physiological and biological factors:

- In individuals aged 10–14 years, these factors are related to sexual development and menarche, which is associated with a spurt in weight gain. Societal influences intensify the fear of becoming 'fat'. This feeling is often intensified by a peer group that comments in a rejecting fashion. These individuals often diet and receive peer acceptance for weight loss; this emotional reinforcement combined with the physiological response of the body to the sudden loss of weight (when >5 lb) intensifies the likelihood of continued weight loss. Sudden weight loss with loss of fat causes a decrease in body temperature, which physiologically causes a subjective feeling of chills; this discomfort is relieved by increased physical activity, which causes further weight loss. The continuous downward spiraling of weight loss then causes secondary amenorrhea and loss of secondary sexual characteristics, which further worsens weight loss.
- In individuals aged 15–16 years, precipitating factors stem from independence and autonomy struggles. Ambivalence about growing up is present, and an abnormal transition from dependence to interdependence rather than independence occurs.
- In individuals aged 17–18 years, identity conflicts are more common. These patients do not make healthy transitions from leaving home to going to college or getting married.

- Perpetuating factors maintain the eating disorder:
  - Biologic issues refer to the signs and symptoms of starvation and to the aspects involved in refeeding the malnourished patient.
  - Psychologic issues encompass the coping strategies engendered by the eating disorders. According to Kreipe et al. in 2000, the treating clinician may threaten the homeostatic balance that has been achieved within the family system secondary to dealing with the patient with anorexia; negative emotions, such as anger and denial, may be directed at the clinician.[128]

DIFFERENTIAL DIAGNOSES

Achalasia
Celiac sprue
Chronic mesenteric ischemia
Clostridial cholecystitis
Clostridium difficile colitis
Constipation
Crohn disease
Cytomegalovirus colitis
Cytomegalovirus esophagitis
Esophageal motility disorders
Esophageal spasm
Esophageal stricture
Hyperthyroidism
Hypothyroidism
Irritable bowel syndrome
Malabsorption
Panhypopituitarism
Protein-losing enteropathy
Ulcerative colitis

Other Problems to be Considered

- Inflammatory bowel disease
- Cancer
- Chronic undiagnosed organic disease (infectious, congenital, or metabolic)
- Osteoporosis
- Osteopenia
- Myeloma
- Cardiac valvular disease
- Pellagra
- Occult infection (if heart rate is normal or elevated)
- Sheehan syndrome
- Cataracts
- Pediatric autoimmune neuropsychiatric disorders associated with streptococcal infection (PANDAS)[129]
- Rash (due to low zinc).[130]

WORK-UP

Laboratory Studies

Because an eating disorder is a clinical diagnosis, no specific diagnostic tests are available. However, perform the following laboratory tests to evaluate the patient:

- Obtain a CBC count with erythrocyte sedimentation rate (ESR).
- Perform urinalysis.
- Obtain blood chemistries analysis.
- Hyponatremia reflects excess water intake or the inappropriate secretion of antidiuretic hormone (ADH).
- Hypoglycemia is observed secondary to lack of glucose precursors in the diet or low glycogen stores.
- Renal function is generally normal except in the case of dehydration when the BUN level may be elevated.
- A hypokalemic hypochloremic metabolic alkalosis is observed with vomiting, and acidosis is observed in cases of laxative abuse.
- Protein and albumin are surprisingly normal because, although the amount of food intake is restricted, it usually contains high-quality proteins.
- Liver function test results are minimally elevated, but levels encountered in patients with active hepatitis are not observed.
- Dramatic elevations in cholesterol are observed in cases of starvation. This elevation may be secondary to (1) decrease in triiodothyronine (T3) levels, (2) low cholesterol binding globulin, and (3) leakage of intrahepatic cholesterol.
- Leukopenia, secondary to increased margination, and thrombocytopenia are observed. The leukopenia is not a sign that the patient is at an increased risk for infection.
- Hemoglobin levels are typically normal, although elevations are observed in states of dehydration. If anemia

is observed, it is not due to menstrual blood loss because these patients are usually amenorrheic. In such cases, further investigation is warranted.
- The ESR is normal. Elevations should prompt a search for an organic etiology as noted above.

Other Tests

- Cardiovascular complications account for most of the morbidity and mortality associated with this condition.
- An ECG is helpful in evaluating for a prolonged QT interval. ECG findings may include low voltage, prolonged QTc, and nonspecific T-wave changes.[124] In patients taking drugs with a prolonged QT, potential harmful dysrhythmias are possible.

Staging

Anorexia nervosa can be divided into an early or mild stage and an established stage.[128,131]

- Early or mild stage is defined by the following:
  - Mildly distorted body image
  - Weight 90% or less of average weight for height
  - No symptoms or signs of excessive weight loss
  - Use of potentially harmful weight-control methods or a strong drive to lose weight
- Established or moderate stage features include the following:
  - Definitely distorted body image that has not diminished with weight loss
  - Weight goal less than 85% of average weight for height associated with a refusal to gain weight
  - Symptoms or signs of excessive weight loss associated with a denial that any problems is present
  - Unhealthy means to lose weight, such as eating fewer than 1000 calories per day, purging, or excessive exercise.

TREATMENT

Medical Care

The medical modality is geared toward correcting and preventing the complications of anorexia nervosa.

- Monitoring of weight, vital signs, and serum electrolyte levels is important.
- Weight gain is a primary goal of treatment. Weight gain should not be excessive because rapid refeeding can lead to excessive bloating, edema, and, rarely, congestive heart failure (CHF).
- Outpatient treatment should only be done with very close monitoring, such as weekly weight measurement wearing only a gown.
- Family therapy should only be performed conjointly if the level of expressed emotion is not excessive;[132] simultaneous sessions can be more productive because if patients feel intense negative emotions from their families they are more likely to be noncompliant with treatment.
- Tube feeding often must be initiated on an inpatient basis when the patient's weight is less than or at 85% of expected weight because outpatient refeeding can be too uncomfortable and the weight gain can be too rapid for the patient to tolerate, sabotaging treatment.
- Prolongation of the QT interval is a contraindication for the use of tricyclic antidepressants because a prolonged QT may increase the risk of ventricular tachycardia and death.
- No treatment is needed for the euthyroid sick syndrome.
- Estrogen has no established effect on bone density in patients with anorexia nervosa, and vitamin supplementation with calcium should be started.
- Those at risk medically or psychiatrically require inpatient treatment. Indications for inpatient treatment include the following:
  - Low weight (≤85% of expected weight) or rapid weight loss
  - Lack of any weight gain
  - Significant edema
  - Severe electrolyte imbalance (life-threatening risks created by sodium and potassium derangements)
  - Temperature less than 36°C
  - Pulse less than 45 beats per minute
  - Altered mental status or other signs of severe malnutrition
  - Cardiac disturbances or other acute medical disorders
  - Psychosis or a high-risk of suicide
  - Symptoms refractory to outpatient treatment
- Individuals with anorexia nervosa may respond best to family therapy. Psychodynamic psychotherapy in combination with behavioral strategies is indispensable. Psychopharmacologic therapy is generally not helpful, although fluoxetine may stabilize recovery in patients who have already attained 85% of their weight.

Consultations

The approach to the treatment of individuals with anorexia nervosa is multidisciplinary. Consultations with specialists in adolescent medicine, nutrition, psychiatry or behavioral-developmental pediatrics, and psychology may be required.

Various psychological therapies have proven helpful in treating patients with anorexia nervosa, including the following:[133-135]

- Individual therapy (insight-oriented)
- Cognitive analytic therapy
- Cognitive behavior therapy
- Interpersonal therapy

- Motivational enhancement therapy
- Dynamically informed therapies
- Group therapy
- Family therapy
- Conjoint therapy
- Separated family therapy
- Multifamily groups
- Relatives and caregiver support groups.

Tube refeeding does not impair efficacy of any psychological therapies.[136]

Diet

Nutrition is an important part of the treatment for the individual with anorexia nervosa. A nutritionist or dietitian should be an integral part of the treatment plan because the well-recognized refeeding syndrome can occur during the early stages of refeeding the patient with anorexia. This syndrome encompasses cardiovascular collapse; starvation-induced hypophosphatemia; and dangerous fluctuations in potassium, sodium, and magnesium levels.

- According to Becker et al. in 1999, for adequate weight gain, the patient or family requires some "education on nutrition, adjustment of caloric and nutritional intake, and limitations on exercise and other modifications of behavior. Enteral or parenteral nutrition is reserved for patients with severe undernutrition that has been refractory to treatment by these methods."[137]
- In the moderate stage of anorexia nervosa, in addition to the above recommendations, providing structure to daily activities is necessary. This includes eating 3 meals a day. Also, parents should ensure that healthy food is available, but the patient should assume all responsibility for eating.
- In 1997, Mehler et al. proposed the following strategies to avoid the refeeding syndrome to avoid pitfalls during the refeeding period:[119]
  - Identify patients at risk
  - Measure serum electrolyte levels and correct abnormalities before refeeding
  - Obtain serum chemistry values every 3 days for the first 7 days and then weekly during the rest of refeeding
  - Attempt to increase daily caloric intake slowly by 200–300 kcal every 3–5 days until sustained weight gain of 1–2 pounds per week is achieved
  - Monitor the patient carefully for development of tachycardia[138] or edema
- Monitor for pellagra and administer niacin supplementation if needed.[139]

Activity

Limited physical activity (e.g. sports, exercise classes) is recommended. By limiting activity, energy expenditure is limited, thus assuring a balanced weight. Limitation of activity may also motivate the patient to maintain healthy eating habits in order to ensure a rapid return to favorite activities. Note that the disadvantage of curtailing activity is the removal of the patient's coping mechanism to deal with stress.

- Anorexia nervosa is based on caloric restriction and increased caloric expenditure that leads to excess exercise to control weight. Previous studies have described the use of exercise programs for hospitalized inpatients in which exercise was exchanged for weight gain and compliance. However, no guidelines were set forth in terms of type, intensity, and duration of exercise.
- A study by Thein et al. (2000) looked at a standard program designed for outpatient use, graduated in type of exercise, duration, and level of activity.[140] Without structure, patients could be exercising in potentially harmful ways and at very high intensities. This study showed that both the exercise and the control groups increased in body mass index (BMI) and body fat percentage. However, quality of life was increased in the exercise group, whereas the control group showed a decrease in all aspects of quality-of-life measures, although the difference was not statistically significant.

Medication

The use of medication for individuals with anorexia nervosa is limited to the treatment of medical complications. To treat osteopenia and to prevent further bone loss, dietary calcium (1000–1500 mg/day) and vitamin D (400 IU) are recommended. Estrogen replacement in the form of oral contraceptives has also been recommended for the treatment of osteopenia, although the benefits and minimal effective dose have not been established.

In anorexia nervosa, bone density is compromised, which can lead to an increase in fractures and early osteoporosis. The intake of calcium and other macronutrients that normally strengthen bone decreases because of poor nutrition. Studies of dehydroepiandrosterone (DHEA) using 50 mg, 100 mg, and 200 mg have reported a decrease in bone resorption, an increase in bone formation markers, and a possible association with resumption of menses (53%).[141]

The antiosteolytic and anabolic effects of DHEA have been noted to be secondary to the androgenic effects on bone mass and not secondary to the estrogenic effects, as was previously thought. Potential adverse effects include mild acne; decreases in cholesterol, high-density lipoprotein (HDL) and sex hormone binding globulin (SHBG) levels; insulin resistance, and hirsutism.

Limitations of the study by Gordon et al. included the small size, a question of compliance, and the self-reporting of activity levels and nutritional intake; no response relationship between the doses of 50 mg, 100 mg, or 200 mg was clear.[141]

Pharmacotherapy is generally not effective. In patients with anorexia nervosa who have already attained 85% of their expected weight, fluoxetine has been used to stabilize recovery. Zinc and cyproheptadine have not been useful.

Antidepressive and neuroleptic agents, although not reported to be effective, have a limited use in patients who have mood changes associated with anorexia nervosa. Their use is limited in patients with inadequate nutrition.

Selective serotonin reuptake inhibitors (SSRIs) are greatly preferred over the other classes of antidepressants.[142] Because the adverse effect profile of SSRIs is less prominent, improved compliance is promoted. SSRIs do not have the cardiac arrhythmia risk associated with tricyclic antidepressants. Arrhythmia risk is especially pertinent in overdose, and suicide risk must always be considered in the treatment of a child or adolescent with a mood disorder.

Physicians are advised to be aware of the following information and use appropriate caution when considering treatment with SSRIs in the pediatric population:

- Recently the UK Medicines and Healthcare Products Regulatory Agency (MHRA) issued an advisory that most SSRIs are not suitable for use by persons younger than 18 years for treatment of "depressive illness." After review, this agency decided that the risks to pediatric patients outweigh the benefits of treatment with SSRIs, except fluoxetine (Prozac), which appears to have a positive risk-benefit ratio in the treatment of depressive illness in patients younger than 18 years.
- Recently the US Food and Drug Administration (FDA) issued a public health advisory regarding reports of suicidality in pediatric patients being treated with antidepressant medications for major depressive disorder. This advisory reported suicidality (both ideation and attempts) in clinical trials of various antidepressant drugs in pediatric patients. The FDA has asked that additional studies be performed because suicidality occurred in both treated and untreated patients with major depression and thus could not be definitively linked to drug treatment.
- However, a recent study of more than 65,000 children and adults treated for depression between 1992 and 2002 by the Group Health Cooperative in Seattle found that suicide risk declines, not rises, with the use of antidepressants.[143] This is the largest study to date to address this issue.
- Currently, evidence does not support an increased risk of suicide in patients with obsessive-compulsive disorder (OCD) and other anxiety disorders who are treated with SSRIs.

Part of the pathophysiology of anorexia nervosa is a delay in gastric emptying, which can perpetuate the disorder by limiting the quantity of food that can be eaten. A study of cisapride (Propulsid) to improve gastric emptying did not show enhancement, but the patients did report a greater improvement in subjective symptoms during a meal.[144] However, in 2000, cisapride use in patients with anorexia nervosa or bulimia was advised against because of serious cardiac events associated with the drug (i.e. serious arrhythmias associated with prolonged QTc) and the risk of cardiovascular-related events in patients with eating disorders.

Follow-up

Further Inpatient Care

- Inpatient management should be approached in such a way as not to seem like punishment to the patient in order to preserve self-esteem and to prevent suicidality and hopelessness.
- The goals of inpatient therapy should be fully discussed with the family and the patient.
- The discussion elements should include development of a healthy meal plan, addressing underlying conflicts (low self-esteem, planning new coping strategies), and enhancing communication skills.
- Randomized controlled trials show that cognitive behavior therapy is very effective, especially in the setting of tube feeding.[145]
- In a study by McIntosh et al. that compared 3 psychotherapies, interpersonal psychotherapy and family therapy were also reported to be effective when the expressed emotion was not negative.[146]
  - Some patients who received nonspecific management appeared to have as good or better an outcome as those who received the other therapies
  - Interpersonal psychotherapy was the least effective
  - Cognitive behavior therapy outcomes were not as effective because of the large amount of psychoeducational material, large skills acquisition, and "the inability to generate alternatives to fixed cognition stemming from the cognitive rigidity of anorexia nervosa patients"[146]
  - Nonspecific management may be more successful because the therapy is provided by experienced clinicians, is practiced according to a detailed treatment manual, and institutes psychoeducation with a strong focus on normalizing eating with approaches such as smart food selection and quantities needed to gain weight. The rest of the sessions were based on issues presented by the patient. Key features of this type of therapy may include the nonspecific factor of empathy and therapeutic alliance. Because this is the first time this nonspecific management was studied, a replication of this study may be necessary
- Family involvement is a vital part of the process in the treatment of anorexia nervosa. Family group psychotherapy has been shown to be more cost-effective than family therapy and equally useful (weight gain measurements).[147]
- Robin et al. studied the effect of family relations on behavioral family systems therapy (BFST) versus ego-oriented individual therapy (EOIT) as treatment

modalities for adolescents with anorexia nervosa.[148] Although the difference was not statistically disparate, the results demonstrated a greater improvement in BMI in the BFST group. In addition, in this group, the mothers showed a decrease in negative communication and an increase in positive communication, whereas the mothers in the other group did not.

- Indications for hospital admission include the following:
  - Physiologic decompensation
    - Temperature less than 36°C
    - Pulse less than 45 beats per minute
    - Orthostatic differential greater than 30/min
    - Altered mental status, fainting, or other signs of significant malnutrition
    - Rapid or excessive weight loss that cannot be curtailed as an outpatient
  - Complications of weight control habits
    - Inability to break the cycle of disordered eating as outpatient
    - Inability to initiate effective outpatient psychotherapy.[128]

Further Outpatient Care

- Patients with anorexia nervosa may respond best to family therapy. Psychodynamic psychotherapy in combination with behavioral strategies is indispensable. Remember that anorexia nervosa is associated with suicide.
- For patients with the mild stage of anorexia nervosa, reevaluate in 1–2 months to check that the weight is not decreasing, that health is maintained, and that the patients have not developed bad eating habits. Surveillance is required to ensure that the patient has not progressed to the moderate stage.

Complications

- Most complications are secondary effects from starvation. Complications of anorexia nervosa include the following:
  - Orofacial—Dental caries
  - Cardiovascular[149]
    - Hypotension
    - Prolonged QT
    - Arrhythmias
    - Cardiomyopathy
  - GI
    - Delayed gastric emptying
    - Decreased intestinal mobility
    - Constipation
  - Endocrine and metabolic
    - Hypokalemia
    - Hyponatremia
    - Hypoglycemia
    - Hypothermia
    - Euthyroid sick syndrome
    - Hypercortisolism
    - Amenorrhea
    - Delay in puberty
    - Arrested growth
    - Osteoporosis
  - Renal—Renal calculi
  - Reproductive
    - Infertility
    - Low birth weight infant
  - Integumentary
    - Dry skin and hair
    - Hair loss
    - Lanugo body hair
  - Neurologic
    - Peripheral neuropathy
    - Ventricular enlargement
  - Hematologic
    - Anemia
    - Leukopenia
    - Thrombocytopenia
- Cardiac complications are the most common cause of death; the mortality rate is about 10%.
  - Cardiac effects include profound bradycardia, hypotension, decreased size of cardiac silhouette, and decreased left ventricular mass associated with abnormal systolic function. Patients with anorexia report fatigue and have an attenuated blood pressure response to exercise and reduction in maximal work capacity. An increased incidence of mitral valve prolapse without significant mitral regurgitation is also observed. Low potassium-dependent QT prolongation increases risk of ventricular arrhythmia[150]
  - Vital signs reflect hypotension with systolic pressures as low as 70 mm Hg and sinus bradycardia with heart rates as low as 30–40 beats per minute. These changes are a response to a decrease in basal metabolic rate. The mechanism may be due to an autonomic imbalance in heart rate regulation with increases in vagal activity and a reduction in sympathetic activity. These changes are physiologic cardiovascular responses, and treatment is unnecessary unless negative clinical sequelae are present. If ECG is performed, evidence of sinus bradycardia, ST-segment elevation, T-wave flattening, low voltage, and rightward QRS axis is apparent. All the aforementioned changes are clinically insignificant. The frequency of rhythm disturbances is most concerning, especially QT interval prolongation that may be an indication for those at risk for cardiac arrhythmias and sudden death

  - Cardiac decompensation is greatest during the initial 2 weeks of refeeding when the myocardium cannot withstand the stress of an increased metabolic demand. If the daily weight gain is 0.2–0.4 kg, then complications are limited
- Foremost in the gamut of endocrinologic complications is amenorrhea, which is actually part of the diagnostic criteria of anorexia nervosa.
  - Amenorrhea results from disorders in the hypothalamic-pituitary-ovarian axis in which levels of follicle-stimulating hormone (FSH) and luteinizing hormone (LH) are low despite low levels of estrogen. Reversion to the prepubertal state occurs; the LH response to gonadotropin-releasing hormone (GnRH) is blunted. This blunted response is insufficient to maintain menstrual integrity, and amenorrhea results
  - Weight loss and emotional instability play a role in amenorrhea, although persistence of amenorrhea has been observed in some patients despite a return to baseline weight
  - Amenorrhea persists in 5–44% of patients in whom weight gain has been documented. The explanation for this wide range has not been elucidated.
- Other changes related to endocrine function include a reduction in fertility, multiple small follicles in the ovaries, and decreased uterine volume and atrophy.
- Thyroid function is also affected, with laboratory data revealing a decrease in T3, thyroxine (T4), and an increase in reverse T3. These changes are characteristic of the euthyroid sick syndrome. Similar to the cardiac changes, these represent an adaptive mechanism and hormonal replacement is not necessary.
- An associated impaired release in vasopressin consistent with diabetes insipidus is present. This defect is of the neurogenic type; concentration of urine is observed after administering vasopressin. This affects 40% of those with anorexia nervosa and is reversible with weight gain.
- Osteopenia is a serious complication. Both cortical and trabecular bone are affected, and osteopenia persists despite estrogen therapy. Low levels of progesterone (accelerates remodeling) formation and decreased insulin-like growth factor-1 (IGF-1) levels, which stimulate type 1 collagen biosynthesis, contribute to bone loss. No established treatment is available; however, 1000–1500 mg/day of dietary calcium and 400 IU of vitamin D is recommended to prevent further bone loss and to maximize peak bone mass. Although exercise and hormonal replacement therapy have some benefit in perimenopausal women, exercise may be deleterious in patients with anorexia nervosa who have amenorrhea, and hormonal replacement may induce premature closure of bone epiphysis. Treatment with bisphosphonates is not indicated in adolescents.[151]
- Patients with anorexia nervosa have fewer GI complications than those with bulimia. Constipation is common. In addition, they still have prolonged GI transit, alterations in antral motility, and gastric atrophy. Prokinetic agents may accelerate gastric emptying, and the relief from gastric bloating can accelerate resumption of normal eating habits.
- Cerebral atrophy and loss of brain volume may be observed. Generalized muscle weakness is the most common neurologic symptom.
- Patients with anorexia nervosa typically have dry scaly skin, brittle hair and nails, and increased lanugo-type body hair.
- An increase in BUN levels, which reflects a level of dehydration and decreased glomerular filtration rate (GFR), is present. Electrolyte imbalances are secondary to vomiting, and potassium is most often affected. Other abnormalities include disturbances of calcium, magnesium, and phosphorus.

Prognosis

- As described in mortality/morbidity, outcome depends on various prognostic factors, including age at onset, weight loss at presentation, duration of symptoms, duration of inpatient care, and state of family relationships.
- Metacognition plays a role in predicting adverse outcomes or suicide, as does alexithymia.[152]
- The mortality rate in anorexia nervosa is 10–20%. Overall, 50% of patients recover completely. Another 20% remain emaciated, 25% are thin, and 5–10% remain overweight or die of starvation.[121]
- Joint family therapy is not as effective as separated family therapy when levels of maternal criticism are raised.[134]

MISCELLANEOUS

Medicolegal Pitfalls

- Maintain safety is important; therefore, hospitalization should not be shunned because anorexia nervosa is a complex chronic disorder associated with high comorbidity and significant mortality and complications.[153] It is difficult to treat due to the shame, denial, and lack of insight concomitant with the disorder.
- Restoring normal eating patterns is crucial because otherwise the restoration of health cannot occur.[154]

Special Concerns

A history of previous attempts, physical pain, drug use, and laxative use may correlate with a higher likelihood of suicide attempts.[125,126,155]

43.6 AUTISM SPECTRUM DISORDER

PB Behere, A Das, AP Behere

INTRODUCTION

The *pervasive developmental disorders* (PDDs) comprise a group of neuropsychiatric disorders characterized by specific delays and deviance in social, communicative, and cognitive development, with an onset typically in the first years of life. It is commonly associated with intellectual disability; they have distinctive features of behavioral and developmental disabilities which differentiate them from other developmental disorders.

According to DSM IV-TR Pervasive Developmental Disorders are characterized by severe and pervasive impairment in several areas of development like social interaction, communication skills and by presence of stereotypic behavior. This group of disorders include the Autistic Disorders, Rett's Disorder, Childhood Disintegrative Disorder, Asperger's Disorder and Pervasive Developmental Disorder Not Otherwise Specified.[156]

However the newly designed DSM-5 has made drastic changes in this group of disorders. The DSM-5 has removed the term Pervasive Developmental Disorder and has renamed it as Autism Spectrum Disorder. This spectrum group encompasses all types of Autism, Aspergers Disorder, Childhood Disintegrative disorder and the Pervasive Developmental Disorder Not Otherwise Specified.[157] Rett's Disorder has been eliminated from the current DSM-5 spectrum group.

This chapter will mainly deal with the spectrum group of disorders.

HISTORY

Leo Kanner (1943) first described a syndrome of "autistic disturbances". He described 11 children who presented between the ages of 2 and 8 years and who shared unique and previously patterns of behavior including social remoteness, stereotypy and echolalia. Autism was described as childhood onset schizophrenia in DSM I. The term Pervasive Developmental Disorders (PDDs) was first used in DSM III to describe disorders involved in the development of social skills and language, such as attention, perception, reality testing and motor movement. This also included, the term Infantile Autism as well as Childhood Onset Pervasive Developmental Disorder (with onset after age 30 months). In DSM-III, autism was also clearly differentiated from childhood schizophrenia and other psychoses for the first time. In 1944, Asperger described the clinical picture of four children with normal IQ who were socially odd, and inappropriate behavior, had good grammar and extensive vocabularies, poor non-verbal communication, circumscribed interests and poor motor coordination. Asperger syndrome was first included as a diagnostic category in DSM-IV (American Psychiatric Association, 2000) and ICD-10 (World Health Organization, 1996). Heller proposed the term *dementia infantilis* to account for children who develop normally for some period before profound developmental regression. His concept, also known as *disintegrative disorder,* is now included in the DSM-IV.[158,159]

AUTISM

Autism is also known as *early infantile autism, childhood autism or Kanner's autism.* It was coined by Leo Kanner in 1943.[160]

Epidemiology: The prevalence of autism is 5 cases per 10,000 individuals. The rate ranges from 2 to 20 cases per 10,000 individuals.[156] First epidemiological studies of autism reported the population prevalence at around 4 per 10,000.[161] Recent studies say that there is a prevalence of 13–30 per 10,000 for autism.[162] Autistic disorder is four times more prevalent in males than females.[163] Some studies find the ratio of male to females as 2.5:1.[164]

Course: The onset of autistic disorder is usually prior to 3 years. Manifestation of the disorder in infancy is difficult to define than those seen after 2 years of age. Mostly prior to 2 years the manifestations are subtle. They are identified by their parents as showing abnormalities or delays in the second year of life.[165]

Etiology: Autism is a neurodevelopmental disorder characterized by impaired communication and social interaction and repetitive behaviors. Several lines of evidence indicate that genetic, environmental, and immunological factors may play a role in its pathogenesis.[166] Genetic and familial factors are involved in causation of autism.[167] Families with multiple cases have been described. Concordance in monozygotic twins is reported to be as high as 70–90%. Concordance rates for autism in dizygotic twins appear no higher than among singleton siblings. Families with autistic children may contain members with 'autistic traits' such as social isolation or tendency toward repetitive behavior.[168] Autism occurs in a number of genetic conditions, among them Fragile X syndrome, Down syndrome, Cohen syndrome, Angel man syndrome and Rett syndrome. Main genes implicated to the causation of autism are 7q, 15q and 2q and 16 p.[169] Toxic exposure to heavy metals during first trimester of pregnancy can cause neurodevelopment harm leading to autism. These can be caused by lead, mercury, DDT, organophosphates, ethyl alcohol, manganese, PCB.[169] Thalidomide poisoning,[170] valproic acid[171] and misoprostol have also been found to have caused autism.[172] The TORCH group of infection particularly rubella has been implicated in the causative factor for autism. Studies have found that MMR vaccination may also lead to some cases of autism.[173] Studies of immunological function reveal a wide range of abnormalities, including decreased cellular immune capacity, decreased plasma complement component C4b, and increased humoral immune and autoantibody responses.[174] Children with autism show evidence of marked disruption in relationships between cortical–subcortical and cortical–cortical gray matter volumes. With repeated or extensive testing, EEG abnormalities are found in about 50% of individuals with autism. Event-related evoked potentials and magneto electroencephalography provides information about temporal and spatial aspects of brain functioning in autism. Studies using these methods show that individuals with autism have slowed face processing, decreased sensitivity to whether a face is upright or inverted, less effect to repeated presentation of a face, abnormal brain response to eye-gaze detection, abnormal hemispheric lateralization and different localization of processing within the cortex.[175] Increased serotonin and altered GABA and glutamate have been found in studies conducted in patients of autism. Recent studies suggest increased neurodegeneration, loss of neuronal cells, and increased production of oxidative stress elements.

Clinical Features

Symptoms of autism spectrum disorder (ASD) vary from one child to the next, but in general, they fall into three areas:

1. Social impairment
2. Communication difficulties
3. Repetitive and stereotyped behaviors.

Children with ASD do not follow typical patterns when developing social and communication skills. Parents are usually the first to notice unusual behaviors in their child. Often, certain behaviors become more noticeable when comparing children of the same age.

In some cases, babies with ASD may seem different very early in their development. Individuals become focused on certain objects, there is loss of eye contact, and they fail to engage in typical engaging play and babbling with their parents. Other children may develop normally until the second or even third year of life, but then start to lose interest in others and become silent, withdrawn, or indifferent to social signals. Loss or reversal of normal development is called regression and occurs in some children with ASD.

Social Impairment

Most children with autism have trouble engaging in everyday social interactions. Children with ASD may:

- Make little eye contact
- Tend to look and listen less to people in their environment or fail to respond to other people
- Do not readily seek to share their enjoyment of toys or activities by pointing or showing things to others
- Respond unusually when others show anger, distress, or affection
- Aloofness and failure to develop friendships
- Seeking people's company but lacking ability to engage in two-way social interactions
- Stilted, one-sided or repetitive social interactions
- Being socially passive while tolerating social approaches.
- Awkward, avoidant or indifferent eye contact
- Inability to understand social rules, e.g. make socially embarrassing comments unintentionally
- Impaired understanding of other people's motivations, perspectives or feelings
- Markedly impaired use of nonverbal behaviors to regulate social interaction, e.g. gestures
- Lack of spontaneously seeking to share enjoyment with others.

There is wide variation in social symptoms; there may be a total lack of awareness of another person. In the first year of life, some children with autism do not lift up their arms or change posture in anticipation of being held. Some children often make only in brief glances, but the eye contact is usually not directed for attention to objects or events. Other children make inappropriate eye contact, by turning someone else's head to gaze into their eyes, or tend to stare at other people's faces. Some children make indiscriminate and inappropriate approaches to strangers (e.g. may cling to a stranger).

Communication Impairment

According to normal developmental milestones, by the first birthday, typical toddlers can say one or two words, turn when they hear their name, and point when they want a toy. They make facial gestures and answers by nodding. It is estimated that only about half of children with autism develop functional speech. If a child with autism does begin to speak, their babbling is decreased. On the other hand, some children with autism are even loquacious; however, their speech tends to be repetitious and focused on preoccupations rather than continuing the speech in a goal directed manner. People with autistic disorder commonly use stereotyped speech including immediate and delayed echolalia, pronoun reversal, and neologisms. Speech usage is idiosyncratic, may consist of concrete and poorly constructed grammar may lack social meaning, and often lacks in inference and imagination. The speech is mostly monotonous and there is lack of prosody.

For children with ASD, reaching such milestones may not be so straightforward. For example, some children with autism may:

- Fail or be slow to respond to their name or other verbal attempts to gain their attention
- Fail or be slow to develop gestures, such as pointing and showing things to others
- Coo and babble in the first year of life, but then stop doing so
- Develop language at a delayed pace
- Learn to communicate using pictures or their own sign language
- Speak only in single words or repeat certain phrases over and over, seeming unable to combine words into meaningful sentences
- Repeat words or phrases that they hear, a condition called echolalia
- Use words that seem odd, out of place, or have a special meaning known only to those familiar with the child's way of communicating
- A delay in or lack of development of speech without any compensatory forms of communication, e.g. gesture or mime
- Significant difficulty in initiating and sustaining a conversation (in those with speech)
- Stereotyped or idiosyncratic use of language.

Restricted or Repetitive Interests and Activities

- Interests that is excessively narrow, intense or unusual
- Adherence to rigid routines
- Intolerance of change
- Stereotyped and repetitive motor mannerisms, e.g. hand flapping
- Persistent preoccupation with parts of objects.

There is presence of motor mannerisms such as hand-flapping, rocking, flipping objects or lining up toys in a fixed fashion. Some display sensory abnormalities. They are mostly preoccupied with rotator objects. These repetitive and sensory abnormalities can be a source of pleasure or self stimulation, which differentiates these behaviors from those seen in obsessive-compulsive disorder.

DSM IV Criteria for Autism

- Total of six (or more) items from (1), (2), and (3), with at least two from (1), and one each from (2) and (3).
  (1) ***Qualitative impairment in social interaction, as manifested by at least two of the following:***
    - Marked impairments in the use of multiple nonverbal behaviors such as eye-to-eye gaze, facial expression, body posture, and gestures to regulate social interaction
    - Failure to develop peer relationships appropriate to developmental level.
    - A lack of spontaneous seeking to share enjoyment, interests, or achievements with other people, (e.g. by a lack of showing, bringing, or pointing out objects of interest to other people)
    - Lack of social or emotional reciprocity (note: in the description, it gives the following as examples: not actively participating in simple social play or games, preferring solitary activities, or involving others in activities only as tools or "mechanical" aids)

  (2) ***Qualitative impairments in communication as manifested by at least one of the following:***
    - Delay in, or total lack of, the development of spoken language (not accompanied by an attempt to compensate through alternative modes of communication such as gesture or mime)
    - In individuals with adequate speech, marked impairment in the ability to initiate or sustain a conversation with others
    - Stereotyped and repetitive use of language or idiosyncratic language
    - Lack of varied, spontaneous make-believe play or social imitative play appropriate to developmental level

  (3) ***Restricted repetitive and stereotyped patterns of behavior, interests and activities, as manifested by at least two of the following:***
    - Encompassing preoccupation with one or more stereotyped and restricted patterns of interest that is abnormal either in intensity or focus
    - Apparently inflexible adherence to specific, non-functional routines or rituals
    - Stereotyped and repetitive motor mannerisms (e.g. hand or finger flapping or twisting, or complex whole-body movements)
    - Persistent preoccupation with parts of objects
- Delays or abnormal functioning in at least one of the following areas, with onset prior to age 3 years:
  - Social interaction
  - Language as used in social communication
  - Symbolic or imaginative play
- The disturbance is not better accounted for by Rett's Disorder or Childhood Disintegrative Disorder.

ASPERGER'S DISORDER

Asperger syndrome is defined by the presence of social impairment and repetitive behaviors and restricted interests, as in autism. However, in contrast to autism, there is no overall delay in language development. Normal or near-normal IQ is also the rule. The lack of clear language deviance usually leads to later clinical recognition than with other ASD, which is presumably a result of the normal or near-normal adaptive behavior early in life. The language in Asperger disorder is clearly not typical or normal. Individuals usually have poorly modulated speech, poor nonverbal pragmatic or communication skills, and intense preoccupations with circumscribed topics. They often have both fine and gross motor deficits, including clumsy and uncoordinated movements and odd postures. They usually are preoccupied with unusual topics.

The definitive data regarding the prevalence of Asperger's disorder is lacking.[156] However, some studies report a prevalence rate of 3 per 10,000 for Asperger disorder.[162] Males have greater ratio than females.

Clinical Features

- Normal or borderline intellectual ability
- Clumsiness
- Concrete, pedantic speech
- Lack of common sense
- Normal or even precocious speech development
- Better verbal than nonverbal skills on psychological assessments
- Intolerance of change
- Anxiety
- Stereotypic repetitive motor movements and mannerisms
- Persistent preoccupation with a part of object
- Curiosity to surrounding environment
- Aspergers child have executive dysfunction and non-verbal learning disorder.

DSM IV TR Criteria for Asperger's Disorder

- Qualitative impairment in social interaction, as manifested by at least two of the following:
  - Marked impairment in the use of multiple non-verbal behaviors such as eye-to-eye gaze, facial expression, body postures and gestures to regulate social interaction
  - Failures to develop peer relationships appropriate to developmental level
  - A lack of spontaneous seeking to share enjoyment, interests or achievements with other people (e.g. by a lack of showing, bringing or pointing out objects of interest to other people)
  - Lack of social or emotional reciprocity
- Restrictive repetitive and stereotyped patterns of behavior, interests and activities, as manifested by at least one of the following:
  - Encompassing preoccupation with one or more stereotyped and restricted patterns of interest that is abnormal either in intensity or focus
  - Apparently inflexible adherence to specific, non functional routines or rituals
  - Stereotyped and repetitive motor mannerisms (e.g. hand or finger flapping or twisting, or complex whole-body movements)
  - Persistent preoccupation with parts of objects.
- The disturbance causes clinically significant impairment in social, occupational or other important areas of functioning.
- There is no clinically significant general delay in language (e.g. single words used by the age of 2 years, communicative phrases used by the age of 3 years).
- There is no clinically significant delay in cognitive development or in the development of age appropriate self-help skills, adaptive behavior (other than in social interaction), and curiosity about the environment in childhood.
- Criteria are not met for another specific Pervasive Developmental Disorder or Schizophrenia.

CHILDHOOD DISINTEGRATIVE DISORDER (HELLER DISORDER)

It is a very rare disorder. Its prevalence rate 0.2 per 10,000.[176] The disorder manifests after an apparently normal development for the first 2 years of life. Receptive and expressive language functions are lost. Sometimes there is gross loss of attained toilet training leading to urine and fecal incontinence.[177] There is gross social disengagement. Individuals develop hand and finger stereotypes and simple rituals similar to those seen in autism. The deterioration continues for several months before reaching a plateau that is often difficult to distinguish from autism. In some cases, the deterioration progresses and motor dysfunction, epileptic attacks and neurological deficits.[178] Cerebral lipoidosis or leukodystrophy are thought to be causative factors, while in most cases a cause cannot be established. It remains quite unknown whether it constitutes an atypical variant of ASD or some meaningfully different syndrome.

Children with childhood disintegrative disorder tend to lose abilities that would normally allow them to take care of themselves. Some children with this disorder experience regression that occurs over a period of time and then becomes stable. Those individuals who have focal neurological findings and seizures have poorer outcomes. Many of children with this disorder deteriorate to a severe level of intellectual disability with a few retaining selected abilities in specific areas. Differential diagnosis of childhood disintegrative disorder requires obtaining a particularly thorough developmental history, history of course of illness, and neurological evaluation to rule out disorders including acquired epileptic aphasia.

This disorder is also known as *dementia infantilis or disintegrative psychosis*. The age of onset in most cases is between 3 and 4 years and may be insidious or abrupt. Initially there may be increased activity, irritability and anxiety then progressing into loss of speech and skills.

DSM IV TR Criteria for Childhood Disintegrative Disorder

- Apparently normal development for at least the first 2 years after birth as manifested by the presence of age-appropriate verbal and nonverbal communication, social relationships, play, and adaptive behavior.
- Clinically significant loss of previously acquired skills (before age 10 years) in at least two of the following areas:
  - Expressive or receptive language
  - Social skills or adaptive behavior
  - Bowel or bladder control
  - Play
  - Motor skills
- Abnormalities of functioning in at least two of the following areas:
  - Qualitative impairment in social interaction (for example, impairment in nonverbal behaviors, failure to develop peer relationships, lack of social or emotional reciprocity)
  - Qualitative impairments in communication (for example, delay or lack of spoken language, inability to initiate or sustain a conversation, stereotyped and repetitive use of language, lack of varied make-believe play)
  - Restricted, repetitive, and stereotyped patterns of behavior, interests, and activities, including motor stereotypes and mannerisms.
- The disturbance is not better accounted for by another specific Pervasive Developmental Disorder or by Schizophrenia.

ATYPICAL AUTISM OR PERVASIVE DEVELOPMENTAL DISORDER

This category should be used when there is a severe and pervasive impairment in the development of reciprocal social interaction, associated with impairment in either verbal or nonverbal communication skills or with the presence of stereotyped behavior, interests, and activities, but the criteria are not met for a specific Pervasive Developmental Disorder, Schizophrenia, Schizotypal Personality Disorder, or Avoidant Personality Disorder. For example, this category includes "atypical autism"— presentations that do not meet the criteria for Autistic Disorder because of late age at onset, atypical symptomatology, or sub-threshold symptomatology, or all of these. The atypicality may lie in the symptom pattern, its severity or age of first manifestation.

RETT SYNDROME

Rett syndrome is a progressive developmental disorder that affects 1 in 10,000–15,000 girls.[179] Rett's disorder is the only pervasive developmental disorder with a known genetic cause. Rett syndrome is an X-linked gene disorder. There is mutation in encoding methyl-CpG-binding protein 2. It is characterized by a relatively normal general and psychomotor development through the first 6–18 months of life. It is then followed by stagnation of developmental acquisitions and a rapid deterioration of behavior and mental status, resulting in apparently autistic-like features within less than 18 months. There is loss of purposeful use of the hands. Acquisition of normal grasp function is lost. There is presence of jerky ataxia of the trunk and limbs with unsteady gait and acquired microcephaly are some of the features. Spasticity more on the lower limbs may be present. Rett's disorder may be associated with epilepsy. The acquired microcephaly (after a normal head circumference at birth), associated with the loss of purposive hand movement and often a midline "handwashing" stereotypy is classical of Retts. There are no specific treatments currently available, although recent animal studies suggest that, potentially, the neural degeneration might ultimately prove to be reversible. At times, the manifestations can be similar to autistic disorder in that there is frequently impairment in language and social development along with presence of stereotyped motor movements. In particular, there is loss of acquired language, restricted interest in social contact or interactions, and the start of hand wringing, clapping or tapping in the midline of the body. Hyperventilation is mostly present. The child with Rett disorder actually may improve in social capabilities as time passes while progressively deteriorating in cognitive and motor function.

The DSM-5 has eliminated Rett's disorder from the autism spectrum disorder.

DSM-5: AUTISM SPECTRUM

One of the most important changes in the fifth edition of the Diagnostic and Statistical Manual of Mental Disorders (DSM-5) is to autism spectrum disorder (ASD). The revised diagnosis represents a new, more accurate, and medically and scientifically useful way of diagnosing individuals with autism-related disorders. In DSM-IV, patients could be diagnosed with four separate disorders: autistic disorder, Asperger's disorder, childhood disintegrative disorder, or pervasive developmental disorder not otherwise specified. Researchers found that these separate diagnoses many overlapping were found. The DSM-5 criteria's have features of all the above disorders. The Neurodevelopmental Work Group, led by Susan Swedo, MD, senior investigator at the

National Institute of Mental Health, recommended the DSM-5 criteria for ASD to be a better reflection of the state of knowledge about autism. The Work Group believes in a spectrum which will improve the diagnosis of ASD without limiting the sensitivity of the criteria, or substantially changing the number of children being diagnosed.[180]

People with ASD tend to have communication deficits, such as responding inappropriately in conversations, misreading nonverbal interactions, or having difficulty building friendships appropriate to their age. Again, the symptoms of people with ASD will fluctuate, with some individuals showing mild symptoms and others having much more severe symptoms. This spectrum will allow clinicians to account for the variations in symptoms and behaviors from person to person.[180]

Under the DSM-5 criteria, individuals with ASD must show symptoms from early childhood. The criteria in DSM-5 allow diagnosis to be made even for minor symptoms. It is an important change from DSM-IV criteria, which was geared toward identifying school-aged children with autism-related disorders, but not as useful in diagnosing younger children.

Some significant changes are:

- Eliminates pervasive developmental disorder and its subcategories.
- Rett syndrome, a genetic disorder, is not included in DSM-5, although girls with Rett syndrome often have ASD symptoms and may be diagnosed with ASD if they meet the criteria.
- Omits is to specify whether the ASD occurs "with or without accompanying language impairment."
- Changes the age of onset from "prior to age 3 years" in DSM-IV to symptoms present "in the early developmental period.

DSM-5 GUIDELINES

A. Persistent deficits in social communication and social interaction across contexts, not accounted for by general developmental delays, and manifest by 3 of 3 symptoms

A1. Deficits in social emotional reciprocity; ranging from abnormal social approach and failure of normal back and forth conversation through reduced sharing of interests, emotions, and affect and response to total lack of initiation of social interaction.

1. Abnormal social approach
   - Unusual social initiations (e.g. intrusive touching; licking of others)
   - Use of others as tools
2. Failure of normal back and forth conversation
   - Poor pragmatic/social use of language (e.g. does not clarify if not understood; does not provide background information)
   - Failure to respond when name called or when spoken directly to
   - Does not initiate conversation
   - One sided conversations/monologues/ tangential speech
3. Reduced sharing of interests
   - Does not share
   - Lack of showing, bringing, or pointing out objects of interest to other people
   - Impairments in joint attention (both initiating and responding)
4. Reduced sharing of emotions/affect
   - Lack of responsive social smile (note: the focus here is on the response to another person's smile; other aspects of emotional expression should be considered under A2).
   - Failure to share enjoyment, excitement, or achievements with others
   - Failure to respond to praise
   - Does not show pleasure in social interactions
   - Failure to offer comfort to others
   - Indifference/aversion to physical contact and affection
5. Lack of initiation of social interaction
   - Only initiates to get help; limited social initiations
6. Poor social imitation
   - Failure to engage in simple social games

A2. Deficits in nonverbal communicative behaviors used for social interaction; ranging from poorly integrated—verbal and nonverbal communication, through abnormalities in eye contact and body-language, or deficits in understanding and use of nonverbal communication, to total lack of facial expression or gestures.

- Impairments in social use of eye contact
- Impairment in the use and understanding of body postures (e.g. facing away from a listener)
- Impairment in the use and understanding of gestures (e.g. pointing, waving, nodding/shaking head)
- Abnormal volume, pitch, intonation, rate, rhythm, stress, prosody or volume in speech
- Abnormalities in use and understanding of affect (*Note:* Responsive social smile should be considered under A1, while affect that is inappropriate for the context should be considered under A3)
  - Impairment in the use of facial expressions (may be limited or exaggerated)
  - Lack of warm, joyful expressions directed at others
  - Limited communication of own affect (inability to convey a range of emotions via words, expressions, tone of voice, gestures)
  - Inability to recognize or interpret other's nonverbal expressions

- Lack of coordinated verbal and nonverbal communication (e.g. inability to coordinate eye contact or body language with words)
- Lack of coordinated nonverbal communication (e.g. inability to coordinate eye contact with gestures)

A3. Deficits in developing and maintaining relationships, appropriate to developmental level (beyond those with caregivers); ranging from difficulties adjusting behavior to suit different social contexts through difficulties in sharing imaginative play and in making friends to an apparent absence of interest in people.

1. Deficits in developing and maintaining relationships, appropriate to developmental level
   - Lack of "theory of mind"; inability to take another person's perspective (CA ≥4 years)
2. Difficulties adjusting behavior to suit social contexts
   - Does not notice another person's lack of interest in an activity
   - Lack of response to contextual cues (e.g. social cues from others indicating a change in behavior is implicitly requested)
   - Inappropriate expressions of emotion (laughing or smiling out of context) (*Note:* Other abnormalities in the use and understanding of emotion should be considered under A2)
   - Unaware of social conventions/appropriate social behavior; asks socially inappropriate questions or makes socially inappropriate statements
   - Does not notice another's distress or disinterest
   - Does not recognize when not welcome in a play or conversational setting
   - Limited recognition of social emotions (does not notice when he or she is being teased; does not notice how his or her behavior impacts others emotionally)
3. Difficulties in sharing imaginative play (*Note:* solitary imaginative play/role playing is NOT captured here)
4. Difficulties in making friends
   - Does not try to establish friendships
   - Does not have preferred friends
   - Lack of cooperative play (over 24 months developmental age); parallel play only
   - Unaware of being teased or ridiculed by other children
   - Does not play in groups of children
   - Does not play with children his/her age or developmental level (only older/younger)
   - Has an interest in friendship but lacks understanding of the conventions of social interaction (e.g. extremely directive or rigid; overly passive)
   - Does not respond to the social approaches of other children
5. Absence of interest in others
   - Lack of interest in peers
   - Withdrawn; aloof; in own world
   - Does not try to attract the attention of others
   - Limited interest in others;
   - Unaware or oblivious to children or adults
   - Limited interaction with others
   - Prefers solitary activities

B. Restricted, repetitive patterns of behavior, interests, or activities as manifested by at least 2 of 4 symptoms

1. Stereotyped or repetitive speech
   - Pedantic speech or unusually formal language (child speaks like an adult or "little professor")
   - Echolalia (immediate or delayed); may include repetition of words, phrases, or more extensive songs or dialog
   - "Jargon" or gibberish (mature jargoning after developmental age of 24 months)
   - Use of "rote" language
   - Idiosyncratic or metaphorical language (language that has meaning only to those familiar with the individual's communication style); neologisms
   - Pronoun reversal (for example, "You" for "I"; not just mixing up gender pronouns)
   - Refers to self by own name (does not use "I")
   - Perservative language (*Note: For perseveration on a specific topic, consider B3*)
2. Stereotyped or repetitive motor movements
   - Repetitive hand movements (e.g. clapping, finger flicking, flapping, twisting)
   - Stereotyped or complex whole body movements (e.g. foot to foot rocking, dipping, and swaying; spinning)
   - Abnormalities of posture (e.g. toe walking; full body posturing)
   - Intense body tensing
   - Unusual facial grimacing
   - Excessive teeth grinding
   - Repetitively puts hands over ears (*Note:* If response to sounds, consider B4)
   - Perseverative or repetitive action/play/behavior (*Note:* If 2 or more components, then it is a routine and should be considered under B2)
   - Repetitive picking (unless clear tactile sensory component, then consider B4)
3. Stereotyped or repetitive use of objects
   - Nonfunctional play with objects (waving sticks; dropping items)

- Lines up toys or objects
- Repetitively opens and closes doors
- Repetitively turns lights on and off

B2. Excessive adherence to routines, ritualized patterns of verbal or nonverbal behavior, or excessive resistance to change; (such as motoric rituals, insistence on same route or food, repetitive questioning or extreme distress at small changes).

1. Adherence to routine
   - *Routines:* Specific, unusual multiple-step sequences of behavior
   - Insistence on rigidly following specific routines (*note:* Exclude bedtime routines unless components or level of adherence is atypical)
   - Unusual routines
2. Ritualized patterns of verbal and nonverbal behavior
   - Repetitive questioning about a particular topic (distinguish from saying the same word or phrase over and over, which goes under B1)
   - Verbal rituals - has to say one or more things in a specific way or requires others to say things or answer questions in a specific way
   - Compulsions (e.g. insistence on turning in a circle three times before entering a room) (*Note:* Repetitive use of objects, including lining up toys, should be considered under B1).
3. Excessive resistance to change
   - Difficulty with transitions (should be out of the range of what is typical for children of that developmental level)
   - Overreaction to trivial changes (moving items at the dinner table or driving an alternate route)
4. Rigid thinking
   - Inability to understand humor
   - Inability to understand nonliteral aspects of speech such as irony or implied meaning
   - Excessively rigid, inflexible, or rule-bound in behavior or thought

B3. Highly restricted, fixated interests that are abnormal in intensity or focus; (such as strong attachment to or preoccupation with unusual objects, excessively circumscribed or perseverative interests.

- Preoccupations; obsessions
- Interests that are abnormal in intensity
- Narrow range of interests
- Focused on the same few objects, topics or activities
- Preoccupation with numbers, letters, symbols
- Being overly perfectionist
- Interests that are abnormal in focus
- Excessive focus on nonrelevant or nonfunctional parts of objects
- Preoccupations (e.g. color; time tables; historical events; etc.)
- Attachment to unusual inanimate object (e.g. piece of string or rubber band)
- Having to carry around or hold specific or unusual objects (not common attachment objects such as blankets, stuffed animals, etc.)
- Unusual fears (e.g. afraid of people wearing earrings)

B4. Hyper- or hyporeactivity to sensory input or unusual interest in sensory aspects of environment; (such as apparent indifference to pain/heat/cold, adverse response to specific sounds or textures, excessive smelling or touching of objects, fascination with lights or spinning objects).

1. High tolerance for pain
2. Poking own eyes
3. Preoccupation with texture or touch (includes attraction/aversion to texture)
   - Tactile defensiveness; does not like to be touched by certain objects or textures
   - Significant aversion to having hair or toenails cut, or teeth brushed
4. Unusual visual exploration/activity
   - Close visual inspection of objects or self for no clear purpose (for example, holding things at unusual angels) (no vision impairment)
   - Looks at objects, people out of corner of eye
   - Unusual squinting of eyes
   - Extreme interest or fascination with watching movement of other things (e.g. the spinning wheels of toys, the opening and closing of doors, electric fan or other rapidly revolving object)
5. In all domains of sensory stimuli (sound, smell, taste, vestibular, visual), consider:
   - Odd responses to sensory input (e.g. becoming extremely distressed by the atypical sound)
   - Atypical and/or persistent focus on sensory input
6. Unusual sensory exploration with objects (sound, smell, taste, vestibular)
   - Licking or sniffing objects (*Note:* As part of a ritual, consider B2; licking or sniffing people consider A1)

C. Symptoms must be present in early childhood (but may not become fully manifest until social demands exceed limited capacities)

D. Symptoms together limit and impair everyday functioning.

Level of severity: Table 6 shows level of severity.

OTHER CONDITIONS ASSOCIATED WITH AUTISM SPECTRUM

Sensory Problems

Many children with autism spectrum disorder (ASD) either over react or under react to certain sights, sounds, smells, textures, and tastes. Many dislike or show discomfort from a light touch or the feel of clothes on their skin. Some experience irritability from certain sounds, like of a machine, a ringing

Table 6: Levels of severity

Severity level	*Social communication*	*Restrictive movements*
Level 3 Requiring very substantial support	Severe deficits in verbal and nonverbal social communication skills cause severe impairments in functioning; very limited initiation of social interactions and minimal response to social overtures from others	Preoccupations, fixated rituals and/or repetitive behaviors markedly interfere with functioning in all spheres. Marked distress when rituals or routines are interrupted; very difficult to redirect from fixated interest or returns to it quickly
Level 2 Requiring substantial support	Marked deficits in verbal and nonverbal social communication skills; social impairments apparent even with supports in place; limited initiation of social interactions and reduced or abnormal response to social overtures from others	RRBs and/or preoccupations or fixated interests appear frequently enough to be obvious to the casual observer and interfere with functioning in a variety of contexts. Distress or frustration is apparent when RRB's are interrupted; difficult to redirect from fixated interest
Level 1 Requiring support	Without supports in place, deficits in social communication cause noticeable impairments. Has difficulty initiating social interactions and demonstrates clear examples of atypical or unsuccessful responses to social overtures of others. May appear to have decreased interest in social interactions	Rituals and repetitive behaviors (RRB's) cause significant interference with functioning in one or more contexts. Resists attempts by others to interrupt RRB's or to be redirected from fixated interest

telephone, or a sudden storm; sometimes they will cover their ears and scream. At times there may be no reaction to intense cold or pain.

Sleep Problems

Children with ASD tend to have problems falling asleep or staying asleep, or have other sleep problems. These problems make it harder for them to pay attention, reduce their ability to function, and lead to poor behavior. In addition, parents of children with ASD and sleep problems tend to report greater family stress and poorer overall health among themselves.[181]

Intellectual Disability

Many children with ASD have some degree of intellectual disability. When tested, some areas of ability may be normal, while others—especially cognitive (thinking) and language abilities—may be relatively weak. For example, a child with ASD may do well on tasks related to sight (such as putting a puzzle together) but may not do as well on language-based problem-solving tasks. Children with a form of ASD like Asperger syndrome often have average or above-average language skills and do not show delays in cognitive ability or speech.

The rate of coexisting severe to profound intellectual impairment is about 40%, mild to moderate cognitive impairments are found in 30% and normal intellectual functioning in another 30%.[158]

Seizures

One in four children with ASD has seizures, often starting either in early childhood or during the teen years.[182]

Fragile X Syndrome

Fragile X syndrome is a genetic disorder and is the most common form of inherited intellectual disability causing symptoms similar to ASD. The name refers to one part of the X chromosome that has a defective piece that appears pinched and fragile when viewed with a microscope. Fragile X syndrome results from a change, called a mutation, on a single gene. This mutation, in effect, turns off the gene. Some people may have only a small mutation and not show any symptoms, while others have a larger mutation and more severe symptoms.

Tuberous Sclerosis

Tuberous sclerosis is a rare genetic disorder that causes noncancerous tumors to grow in the brain and other vital organs. Tuberous sclerosis occurs in 1 to 4% of people with ASD.[183] A genetic mutation causes the disorder, which has also been linked to mental retardation, epilepsy, and many other physical and mental health problems. There is no cure for tuberous sclerosis, but many symptoms can be treated.

Gastrointestinal Problems

Some parents of children with ASD report that their child has frequent gastrointestinal (GI) or digestion problems, including stomach pain, diarrhea, constipation, acid reflux, vomiting, or bloating. Food allergies may also cause problems for children with ASD.

Co-occurring Mental Disorders

Children with ASD can also develop mental disorders such as anxiety disorders, attention deficit hyperactivity disorder

(ADHD), or depression. Research shows that people with ASD are at higher risk for some mental disorders than people without ASD.[184] Managing these co-occurring conditions with medications or behavioral therapy, which teaches children how to control their behavior, can reduce symptoms that appear to worsen a child's ASD symptoms.

Problematic Behavior

Perhaps the greatest challenge to those who interact with individuals across the autism spectrum is the presence of challenging behaviors. The individual may exhibit ritualistic or compulsive mannerisms, self-stimulatory behavior, refusal, withdrawal, self-injury/abuse, property destruction, or physical aggression.

Difficulties with Executive Function

There is persistent difficulty in organizing tasks. They perform one activity at one time. Multitasking is not possible. Executive functions also include deficits in the area of making transitions and organizing oneself.

Difficulties with "Theory of Mind"

Individuals on the autism spectrum have difficulty with theory of mind. In other words, they have difficulty inferring other people's mental states (e.g. thoughts, beliefs, desires, and intentions).

DIFFERENTIAL DIAGNOSIS OF AUTISM SPECTRUM DISORDER

- Developmental language disorder
- Mental retardation
- Acquired epileptic aphasia (Landau–Kleffner syndrome)
- Fragile X syndrome
- Chromosome 15 q11-13 duplication
- Schizophrenia
- Selective mutism
- Psychosocial deprivation
- Hearing impairment
- Visual impairment
- Traumatic brain injury.
- Metabolic disorders (inborn errors of metabolism, e.g. phenylketonuria)
- Emotional neglect.

MANAGEMENT

The management includes assessment, diagnosis, early intervention, treatment, counseling, skill training, vocational training, parent guidance and training. It is a multi-dimensional approach involving psychiatrists, pediatrician, psychologists, counselors, social workers, speech therapist, and audiologists.

Assessment includes:

- *History taking sources:* Parents, teachers, other caregivers, anyone with regular meaningful contact
- Developmental history
- Past medical history
- Family history
- Examination
- Direct observation of child's social, communication, and imaginative skills
- Psychological testing (nonverbal and verbal intellectual testing)
- Speech and language evaluation
- Tests of adaptive functioning
- Vocational assessment
- Physical examination including particular attention to the neurological examination, dysmorphology examination, and examination of the skin (preferably with a Wood's lamp to rule out hypopigmented macules of tuberous sclerosis)
- Audiological testing
- Laboratory testing
- Quantitative urinary amino acids
- EEG if suspicion of history of possible seizures
- Chromosomal analysis
- MRI if findings in history or examination
- Other laboratory testing based on findings from history and physical examination (e.g. organic acids, thyroid function tests, etc.).

Scales used for assessment

sometimes the doctor will ask parents questions about the child's symptoms to screen for ASD. Other screening instruments combine information from parents with the doctor's own observations of the child. Examples of screening instruments for toddlers and preschoolers include:

- Checklist of Autism in Toddlers (CHAT)
- Modified Checklist for Autism in Toddlers (M-CHAT)
- Screening Tool for Autism in Two-Year-Olds (STAT)
- Social Communication Questionnaire (SCQ)
- Communication and Symbolic Behavior Scales (CSBS). To screen for mild ASD or Asperger syndrome in older children, the doctor may rely on different screening instruments, such as:
- Autism Spectrum Screening Questionnaire (ASSQ)
- Australian Scale for Asperger's Syndrome (ASAS)
- Childhood Asperger Syndrome Test (CAST).
- Childhood Autism Rating Scale—strong evidence base, combines questioning of parents and targeted observation (CARS)
- Autism Diagnostic Observation Scale (ADOS); semi-structured interview that requires training to administer;

- Gilliam Autism Rating Scale (GARS-2); and
- Gilliam Asperger's Disorder Scale (GADS).

Cognitive and adaptive behavior evaluations as indicated below:
Cognitive evaluations include:
- The Differential Ability Scales (DAS),
- Stanford-Binet Intelligence Scales, Fifth Edition (SB5),
- Wechsler Intelligence Scale for Children-Fourth Edition (WISC-IV), and Wechsler Preschool and Primary Scale of Intelligence-Third Edition (WPPSI-III).

Adaptive behavior evaluations include:
- Scales of Independent Behavior-Revised (SIB-R) and
- Vineland Adaptive Behavior Scales (VABS).

Comprehensive speech/language/communication evaluations are obtained if language delays are present. Sensorimotor evaluations occur if motor development, sensory processing deficits, or mannerisms/stereotypes appear to be interfering with functioning.

Early Intervention

Studies has shown that intensive behavioral modification during early years can significantly improve cognitive and language skills in young children with ASD.[185] Early identification enables avoidance of unnecessary medical treatment and stress for parents. It provides for early guidance and genetic counseling and starting early interventions.[186] It is thought to be the best line of management.
These include:
- Starting as soon as a child has been diagnosed with ASD
- Providing focused and challenging learning activities at the proper developmental level for the child for at least 25 hours per week and 12 months per year
- Having small classes to allow each child to have one-on-one time with the therapist or teacher and small group learning activities
- Having special training for parents and family
- Encouraging activities that include typically developing children, as long as such activities help meet a specific learning goal
- Measuring and recording each child's progress and adjusting the intervention program as needed
- Providing a high degree of structure, routine, and visual cues, such as posted activity schedules and clearly defined boundaries, to reduce distractions
- Guiding the child in adapting learned skills to new situations and settings and maintaining learned skills.

It is claimed that effective early interventions include the following important components:[187]
- Provision at the earliest possible age
- High intensity, with the suggestion of a threshold of at least 20 hours per week spent one-to-one with the child
- Strongly based on parent involvement, training and support
- Various modules and training schemes to stimulate social and communicative functioning of the child in a developmentally oriented way
- Systematic instruction with individual goals, based on applied-behavioral analysis (ABA) and stepwise approach.
- Investment in attempts to generalize acquired skills to other settings of daily life.

Treatment

The main aims of the treatment of ASD are:[188]
- As much as possible to facilitate and stimulate the normal development of cognition, language and socialization
- To decrease autism-bound maladaptive behaviors such as rigidity, stereotypy, and inflexibility;
- To reduce or even eliminate nonspecific maladaptive behaviors such as hyperactivity, irritability and impulsivity.
- To alleviate stress and burden for the family.

The treatment of individuals with ASD should be multimodal, with a combination of family counseling, structured and special educational techniques, individual behavior modification, home training, and placement in special schools or day-care centers.

Medication treatment has not been shown to influence the core symptoms of ASD, but may be considered when troublesome target and comorbid symptoms such as aggression, temper tantrums, irritability, hyperactivity, self-injurious behavior, rigidity, anxiety and sleeping problems do not respond to behavioral interventions or seriously interfere with the application of these interventions.

Counseling for Parents and Family Support

Parents play a crucial role in management. They are first-line managers. Doctors need to prepare and educate parents and families on long-term treatment efforts. Parents should be informed about treatment options, including the need for family counseling or therapy. It is very important to inform parents about the diagnosis and implications for the future of the child. Parents may have difficulty in accepting the diagnosis. Once a family has a child with ASD, the risk of recurrence of ASD in subsequent children rises to 3–7%. Therefore, parents need appropriate counseling on genetic issues. During the different stages of development, the child and parents have different needs. For example, placement in a school that provides a specialized education can be enough for the first year, but when behavior management problems occur, more intensive counseling, behavioral therapy and/or medication may be an option. In some countries, patients and their families are organized into National Autistic Societies which hold information evenings where parents can meet each other and where 'nonprofessional' support is given. Most parents benefit from training courses aimed at skills building and reduction of problematic behavior. In adolescence, attention should be paid to sexuality issues that may be relevant to ASD—such as masturbation, inappropriate touching, privacy issues and public exposure.

Education

Adequate education is essential and necessary; studies have indicated that children who complete some form of education have a better outcome.[189] It is necessary for the teacher to be informed about the nature of autism and the child's needs. An autistic child at school needs extra individual attention, a very structured approach and special education programs, such as the Treatment and Education of Autistic and related Communication-handicapped Children program (TEACCH).[190] Parents play a great role again and they are made aware of their childs needs and requirements. It is a highly structured approach for autistic children at school. Based on principles from cognitive–behavioral theory, a system is developed with stepwise visualization of the actions needed to fulfill a task. Through this system, the life-environment can be structured, and parents can act as co-therapists and continue with the principles of TEACCH at home.

Vocational Training

Social support is again necessary. Stigma can be reduced by vocational training. Individuals can be trained so that they can take care of themselves to some extent. As a result, many individuals with autism require some form of community support. Projects have been established that involve autistic people living with more or less intensive supervision by a professional. Specialist-supported employment services have been designed for high-ability adults with autism.

Skills Training and Behavioral Therapy

Depending on clinical needs, a number of specific treatment modalities may be helpful. In cases of clumsiness or delays in motor development, there is an indication for sensorimotor training. Language and communication skills can be facilitated by means of language training. Occupational therapy and play therapy may be of use in some cases. For high-functioning autistic children, individual therapy can be an option. Social skills training programs, delivered on an individual or on a group basis.

Behavioral training based on classic and operant conditioning should be practized. There is a clear indication for specific behavioral interventions in cases of severely interfering and maladaptive behaviors such as stereotypes, self-injury and negativism. Reinforcement training, time out and token economy should be followed.

Pharmacotherapy

Antipsychotic medications are more commonly used to treat serious mental illnesses such as schizophrenia. These medicines may help reduce aggression and other serious behavioral problems in children, including children with ASD. They may also help reduce repetitive behaviors, hyperactivity, and attention problems. Risperidone has given best results in autistic children.[191]

Antidepressant medications, such as fluoxetine or sertraline, are usually prescribed to treat depression and anxiety but are sometimes prescribed to reduce repetitive behaviors. Some antidepressants may also help control aggression and anxiety in children with ASD.[192] Various studies reports that fluoxetine is useful in controlling repetitive behavior.[193]

Stimulant medications, such as methylphenidate (Ritalin), are safe and effective in treating people with attention deficit hyperactivity disorder (ADHD). Methylphenidate has been shown to effectively treat hyperactivity in children with ASD as well.[194]

Mood stabilizers such as lithium and valproic acid have been used to treat affective instability, impulsivity and aggression in individuals with ASD.[195] Antiepileptic are useful in cases of comorbid seizure disorders.

The alpha 2-adrenergic receptor agonist clonidine reduced irritability as well as hyperactivity and impulsivity in two double-blind, placebo-controlled trials.[196]

Pyridoxine, the water-soluble essential vitamin B_6, has been used extensively as a pharmacological treatment in autistic disorder. Many newer therapies like naltrexone therapy, music therapy, dietary supplements, hyperbaric oxygen, carnitine, vitamin C are being increasingly used to treat ASD.[197] Studies have been going on to treat ASD through stem cell therapy.[198]

AUTISM IN INDIA

Baltiwalla first described autism in India and described it as children showing schizophrenic symptoms,[199] but real clinical research and focus in autism in India started in late 1980's and early 1990's.[200] Daley found that Indian parents' initial symptom recognition in children who were eventually diagnosed with ASD was at a range of 6 to 10 months later than families in the West.[201]

Studies in India reports varying rates of prevalence of autism and ASD in India. Study made by Narayanan in late 1970 reports male to female ratio of 1.33:1.[202] Study reported by Srinath et al. in 1998 reports 30 cases of autism over a period of three years having male to female ratio of 7.5: 1, most of them developing symptoms by 30 months.[203] Malhotra and

Gupta reported 12 cases of CDD from 1989 to 1999 with a ratio of 5:1 for male to female. It was consistent with other studies. The only difference this study reports is the rapid onset of CDD in India than in other countries.[204] Comorbid mental retardation is common in India as reported by studies.

Autism was legally recognized by the government of India in 1999 as a disorder. Legal recognition has enabled such children to derive the benefits under Persons with Disability Act, i.e. equal opportunity, protection of rights, and prevention of discrimination (Persons with Disabilities Act, 1995). National Trust for the Welfare of Persons with Autism, Cerebral Palsy, Mental Retardation and Multiple Disabilities' (Act 44 of 1999) was set-up for well-being of individuals with autism. This organization strengthens facilities, provide support to disabled, deal with their problems and strive for their equal rights in society.[205]

Helplines in India for Autism

- Action for Autism (AFA)
- Academy for Severe Handicaps and Autism (ASHA)
- Autism Society of India (ASI)
- Society for Autistics in India (SAI)

SUMMARY

Autistic disorder and other pervasive developmental disorders are complex, early-onset disorders that usually lead to moderate-to-severe disability in domains of social, communicative, and flexible behavior. A more thorough understanding of these conditions and their treatment has developed over the past two decades. A coordinated, multidisciplinary approach to treatment that focuses on development of adaptive, social, and communicative functioning yields the best results.

RECOGNITION, REFERRAL, DIAGNOSIS, AND MANAGEMENT OF ADULTS WITH AUTISM: SUMMARY OF NICE GUIDANCE

Autism is a lifelong condition characterized by difficulties in social interaction and communication and by rigid or repetitive behaviors; it affects about 1.1% of adults.[206] Although some people's autism is diagnosed in childhood, for every three known cases, there are two individuals without a diagnosis who might need assessment, support, and interventions for autism at some point in their lives.[207] Four out of five adults with autism find that obtaining a diagnosis in adulthood is difficult or not possible,[208] and many who have all the core symptoms do not receive a formal diagnosis.[209] Particular problems arise in identifying high functioning autism (Asperger's syndrome), which may not be recognized until adulthood[210] or may be misdiagnosed as depression, personality disorder, or a psychotic illness. Inadequate identification and assessment of adults with autism not only leads to inadequate care but can also result in inadequate recognition and treatment of coexisting mental and physical health problems. Whereas care for children and young people is relatively well coordinated,[211] this is often not the case for adults. Falling between and being passed around services is a particular problem for adults with autism who have an IQ over 70 and do not have severe and enduring mental illness, as they may be excluded from both learning disabilities and mental health services.[208] Social and economic exclusion affects a large proportion of adults with autism. Unemployment or underemployment is a considerable problem for adults with autism, including the 44% of those who do not have a learning disability,[212] with almost 90% of this group unemployed.[213]

This chapter summarizes the most recent recommendations from the National Institute for Health and Clinical Excellence (NICE) on autism in adults.[214,215]

RECOMMENDATIONS

National Institute for Health and Clinical Excellence (NICE) recommendations are based on systematic reviews of best available evidence and explicit consideration of cost effectiveness. When minimal evidence is available, recommendations are based on the Guideline Development Group's experience and opinion of what constitutes good practice. Evidence levels for the recommendations are given in italic in square brackets.

General Principles

All staff working with adults with autism should have an understanding of:

- The nature, development, and course of autism
- The impact on personal, social, educational, and occupational functioning
- The impact of the social and physical environment.

Assessment for Autism

Consider assessment for possible autism when a person has:

- One or more of the following:
  - Persistent difficulties in social interaction
  - Persistent difficulties in social communication
  - Stereotypic (rigid and repetitive) behaviors, resistance to change or restricted interests and
- One or more of the following:
  - Problems in obtaining or sustaining employment or education
  - Difficulties in initiating or sustaining social relationships
  - Previous or current contact with mental health or learning disability services

- A history of a neurodevelopmental condition (including learning disabilities and attention-deficit/hyperactivity disorder) or mental disorder.

For adults with possible autism who do not have a moderate or severe learning disability, consider using the Autism Spectrum Quotient, 10 items (the AQ-10) (Table 7).[216] (If a person has reading difficulties, read out the AQ-10). If a person scores above 6 on the AQ-10, or clinical judgment suggests autism (taking into account any history provided by an informant), offer a comprehensive assessment for autism.

During a comprehensive assessment, inquire about and assess the following:

- Core autism signs and symptoms (difficulties in social interaction and communication and the presence of stereotypic behavior, resistance to change or restricted interests) that were present in childhood and have continued into adulthood
- Early developmental history, where possible
- Behavioral problems
- Functioning at home, in education, or in employment
- Past and current physical and mental disorders (for example, schizophrenia, depression, or other mood disorders; and anxiety disorders—in particular, social anxiety disorder and obsessive compulsive disorder)
- Other neurodevelopmental conditions
- Neurological disorders (for example, epilepsy)
- Communication difficulties (for example, speech and language problems, and selective mutism)
- Hypersensory and/or hyposensory sensitivities and attention to detail.

Carry out direct observation of core autism signs and symptoms especially in social situations.

Autism Spectrum Quotient—10 items (AQ-10): A quick referral guide for adults with suspected autism who do not have a learning disability.

Assessment of Challenging Behavior

When assessing challenging behavior, do a functional analysis (see "Interventions for challenging behavior" below), including identifying and evaluating any factors that may trigger or maintain the behavior, such as:

- Physical disorders
- The social environment (including relationships with family members, partners, carers, and friends)
- The physical environment, including sensory factors
- Coexisting mental disorders (including depression, anxiety disorders, and psychosis)
- Communication problems
- Changes to routines or personal circumstances.

Interventions for Autism

For adults with autism without a learning disability or with a mild learning disability, who are having difficulty obtaining or maintaining employment, consider an individual supported employment program.

An individual supported employment program should typically include:

Table 7: Autism spectrum quotient—10 items (AQ-10)

Please tick one option per question only	*Definitely agree*	*Slightly agree*	*Slightly disagree*	*Definitely disagree*
1. I often notice small sounds when others do not				
2. I usually concentration more on the whole picture, rather than the small details				
3. I find it easy to do more than one thing at once				
4. If there is an interruption, I can switch back to what I was doing very quickly				
5. I find it easy to "read between the lines" when someone is talking to me				
6. I know how to tell if someone listening to me is getting bored				
7. When I'm reading a story I find it difficult to work out the characters' intentions				
8. I like to collect information about categories of things (e.g. types of car, bird, train, plant, etc.)				
9. I find it easy to work out what someone is thinking or feeling just by looking at their face				
10. I find it difficult to work out people's intentions				

Scoring: Only 1 point can be scored for each question. Score 1 point for Definitely or Slightly Agree on each of items 1, 7, 8 and 10. Score 1 point for Definitely or Slightly Disagree on each of items 2, 3, 4, 5, 6 and 9. If the individual scores more than 6 out of 10, consider referring them for a specialist diagnostic assessment.

This test is recommended in *Autism: Recognition, Referral, Diagnosis and Management of Adults on the Autims Spectrum* (NICE clinical guideline 142). www.nice.org.uk/CG142

Key reference: Allison et al.[216]

- Help with writing CVs and job applications and preparing for interviews
- Training for the identified work role and work related behaviors
- Carefully matching the person with autism with the job
- Advice to employers about making reasonable adjustments to the workplace
- Continuing support for the person after they start work
- Support for the employer before and after the person starts work, including autism awareness training.

For the management of core symptoms of autism in adults, do not use anticonvulsants, chelation, drugs specifically designed to improve cognitive functioning (for example, cholinesterase inhibitors), oxytocin, secretin, drugs for testosterone regulation, hyperbaric oxygen therapy, antipsychotic medication, or antidepressant medication.

Interventions for Challenging Behavior

When deciding on the nature and content of a psychosocial intervention for challenging behavior, use a functional analysis. The functional analysis should facilitate the targeting of interventions by:

- Providing information, from a range of environments, on factors that seem to trigger the challenging behavior; and on the consequences of the behavior (that is, the reinforcement received as a result of their behavior)
- Identifying trends in the occurrence of challenging behavior, factors that may be evoking that behavior, and the needs that the person is trying to meet by behaving in that manner.

Psychosocial interventions for challenging behavior should include:

- Clearly identified target behavior(s)
- A focus on outcomes that are linked to quality-of-life
- Assessment and modification of environmental factors that may contribute to initiating or maintaining the behavior
- A clearly defined intervention strategy
- A clear schedule of reinforcement, and capacity to offer reinforcement promptly and contingently on demonstration of the desired behavior
- A specified timescale to meet intervention goals (to promote modification of intervention strategies that do not lead to change within a specified time)
- A systematic measure of the target behavior(s) taken before and after the intervention to ascertain whether the agreed outcomes are being met.

Consider antipsychotic medication in conjunction with a psychosocial intervention for challenging behavior when there has been no or limited response to psychosocial or other interventions (such as environmental adaptations). Antipsychotic medication should be prescribed by a specialist and quality-of-life outcomes monitored carefully. Review the effects of the medication after three to four weeks, and discontinue it if there is no indication of a clinically important response at six weeks.

Support for Families and Carers

Offer families, partners, and carers of adults with autism an assessment of their own needs, including personal, social, and emotional support; support in their caring role, including respite care and emergency plans; advice on and support in obtaining practical support; planning of future care for the person with autism.

Offer information, advice, training, and support to families, partners, and carers if they need help with the personal, social, or emotional care of the person with autism; or if they are involved in supporting the delivery of an intervention (in collaboration with professionals).

Overcoming Barriers

Primary and secondary care professionals currently have a limited knowledge of autism and its various presentations,[217] and this lack will need specific attention if the recommendations in this guideline are to be of real benefit. Two areas are of particular concern: initial identification in primary care, and autism symptoms being masked by comorbid conditions in secondary care.[218] Training in the identification and assessment of autism should be more prominent in the undergraduate and postgraduate education of health and social care professionals.

People with autism, particularly those who are more disabled by it, often fall through the gaps between medical and social care, especially if they do not present with a mental health disorder or learning disability. This presents challenges in developing integrated health and social care services that engage people with autism. Access to treatment for adults with autism is also limited and extends beyond mental healthcare to physical healthcare. The establishment of local autism strategy groups (which should be responsible for developing and managing local care pathways) and of associated multiprofessional teams should help to resolve this problem of access to treatment, but care is needed to ensure that adults with autism have access to the full range of healthcare services. However, it is the families of adults with autism who provide much of the care and support.[219] The guideline highlights that they too should receive specific support as without their involvement many interventions will be of limited benefit.

43.7 CHILD SUBSTANCE ABUSE

Dilip R Patel, Laura Murray

Increasing use and abuse of drugs, alcohol, and tobacco products by children and, adolescents is a significant threat to their physical as well as mental health. Substance abuse disorders are characterized by the following (Diagnostic and Statistical Manual of Disorders; International Classification of Diseases):

- Development of tolerance to the substance
- Withdrawal symptoms upon cessation of use
- Spending large amounts of time related to obtaining and using the substance
- Talking larger amounts for longer periods of time than intended
- A persistent desire or unsuccessful efforts to cut down or control substance use
- Impaired social, occupational, of recreational activities reduced due to substance-related behavior
- Continued substance abuse despite knowledge of persistent physical or psychological problems caused or exacerbated by the substance.

Certain behavior patterns are seen in most adolescents with drug abuse is characterized by impulsive drug-seeking behavior, with paroxysmal breaks in use and almost certain relapses; a common feature of all drug abusers (Frances and Miller, 1998; Comerica, Chewable, 2000). Many respects the behavior of drug abusers prior to the concept of drug abuse resembles that of juvenile delinquent; a number of minor socially disapproved acts, much as getting into fights, truancy, getting drunk at a young age, and smoking early (Comercial, Schwebel, 2000; Alderman,1997; Heischober, Hofmann, 1997). Tobacco-chewing was 29%. Many of the subjects were as young as 10 years of age (George et al. 1994; Patel, Greydanus, 1999). Malhotra et al. (1990) surveyed 500 students from Class XII at four public schools to find out their knowledge, perception about drug use, and reasons for starting drug use. They found that television and movies were the most important sources of information about drugs and tobacco use, only 12% thought smoking and alcohol were harmful, and peer influence was a major factor for alcohol and tobacco use. The authors further observed that improved education on drugs, showing television programs about dangers of drug abuse, and better family communication were useful to reduce drug use. Study suggested that parental communication about drug abuse was inadequate and that the students wanted more information (Mslhotra et al. 1990).

PREVALENCE IN UNITED STATES

In the United States, several, systemic national surveys monitor the epidemiology of tobacco use, alcohol use, and abuse of other illicit substances. Data form one such survey, Monitoring the Future Study by National Institute on Drug Abuse and University of Michigan's Institute for Social Research are presented in Table 8. In the United States, cigarette smoking, alcohol use, and marijuana use are the most common. In 2000, 54% of high-school students used an illicit drug by the time they entered 12th grade. Tobacco and alcohol are the first drug of abuse, and those who use either tobacco of alcohol were 65 times more likely to use marijuana; those who used marijuana were 104 times more likely to use cocaine compared to those who did not (Belcher, Shinitzky, 1998). Adolescents' perceptions of the harmfulness of drugs was found to be a key predictor of in their use of drugs. Retrospective data indicate that many 6th grade students had used inhalants, or tobacco. About 33% of marijuana smokers had started suing the drug in their 6th grade.

RISK FACTORS AND THEORIES OF ETIOLOGY

The etiology of substance use disorders (SUDs) in adolescents can be discussed in terms of predisposing or risk factors

Table 8: Monitoring the future study: Lifetime prevalence of substance abuse among high-school students in the United States, 2000

	8th grade	*10th grade*	*12th grade*
Any illicit drug	26.8%	45.6%	54.0%
Alcohol	51.7	71.4	80.3
Cigarettes	40.5	55.1	62.5
Smokeless tobacco	12.8	19.1	23.1
Marijuana	20.3	40.3	48.8
Inhalants	17.9	16.6	14.2
Hallucinogens	4.6	8.9	13.0
Lysergic acid	3.9	7.6	11.1
Diethylamide	4.5	6.9	8.6
Cocaine	3.0	3.5	2.5
Anabolic steroids	4.3	7.3	11.0
Methylenedioxy-methenamine (MDMA)			

(Table 9), and different theoretical constructs (patton, 1995; Fuller, Cavanaugh, 1995; Heyman, Adger, 1997; Heischober, Hofmann, 1997; Lipman, et al, 1998). No single factor or theory can fully explain the development of SUDs in adolescents. Belcher and Shinitzky (1998) note that behavioral, emotional, as well as environmental factors contribute to pediatric SUDs. Studies also indicate that the risk of SUDs increases as the number of risk factors increase (Patton, 1995).

One theory of the origin suggests that there stages that eventually lead to SUDs. Central to this theory is the idea that SUDs tend to begin past particular developmental stages, and seem to follow a sequential pattern of in evolvement in legal and illegal drugs. This pattern is described as the use of at least one class of drugs that licit for adults preceding another.

For example, alcohol or cigarettes precede the use of marijuana, and marijuana precedes the experiment with alcohol or cigarette; few try other illicit drugs without prior use of marijuana (Kandel, 1997; Kandel and Faust, 1995).

Researchers following adolescents with different drug using patterns over a 5- to 6-month interval identified four following stages; (1) beer or wine, (2) cigarettes or hard liquor, (3) marijuana, and (4) other illicit drugs.

Table 9: Risk and protective factors for substance abuse

Risk factors
- Low self-esteem
- Poor interpersonal relations with friends and parents
- Poor bonding with parents, family and community
- Low religious beliefs
- Poor coping and communication skills
- Inability to accept discipline
- Unwillingness to accept consequence of actions
- Difficulty delaying gratification
- Low academic achievement
- Learning disabilities, conduct disorders, attention deficit hyperactivity disorders
- Aggressive and impulsive behaviors
- Use of alcohol or tobacco at an early age
- Drug abuse by parents
- Drug abuse by friends

Protective factors
- Nurturing home environment
- Good communication within family
- Supportive and intact family
- Appropriate adult supervision
- Positive self-esteem
- Assertiveness
- Social competence
- Academic success
- Good school environment
- Good general health
- High intelligence
- Positive adult role models
- Peer group with positive personal attributes
- Religious involvement
- A personal sense of morality

There is large body of literature suggesting that cigarette smoking is often the gateway to more serious drug abuse (Kandel and Yamaguchi, 1993; Kandel, Marguiles, 1998). Milberger, Biederman, Faraone, and Chu (1997). Found that the onset of cigarette preceded or occurred simultaneously with onset of drug abuse.

This pattern seems to span across cultures, as it has also been observed in other countries such as France and Israel and Kandel, 1981). MacDonald has presented a model of drug seeking behavior and proposed that it occurs in a impressive manner from weekend use with friends to every use and dependence (Table 10) (MacDonald, 1984). Manual use of tobacco and alcohol products is the target for any pervasive strategy.

Some individuals may have a certain genetic predisposition toward alcoholism or other SUDs. Convergent evidence from twin, adoption, and biological response studies suggest that genetic factor may play a role in the etiology of alcoholism (Bohman, Sigardsson, and Cloninger, 1981; Cloninger, Bohman, and Sigvardsson, 1981). Heritability was estimated in one study at 0.31 in males and 0.22 in females (Pickens et al. 1991). Genetic association of the D2 dopamine receptor to alcoholism was first hypothesized based on the fact that the genetic variation in dopamine function could affect vulnerability towards abuse of reinforcing substances, et al. (1990) showed a strong association of the A1 allele of the D2 dopamine receptor gene and alcoholism.

Familial Characteristics

Another precursor may include certain familial characteristics. For example, among high-risk individuals, adverse interactions with the familial environment can orient the child toward enhanced risk for a negative outcome.

Three different types of parental characteristics have been suggested to predict initiation of substance use: parental substance use/abuse behaviors, parental attitude toward substances, and parent-child interactions (Kaminer and Bukstein, 1998).

Studies suggest that exposing a child to a caretaker's substance abuse behavior. Such as the nonfulfillments of parental responsibility, affect the child by providing negative models and by reinforcing similar behavior (Kaminer and Bukestin).

Other familiar characteristic often found among those with SUD include high stress, poor and inconsistent family management skills, increased separation, divorce, death, prison terms, and decreased family activities. Parent in substance-abusing homes also have fewer friend, and are less involved in recreational, social, religious, and cultural activities (Kumpfer and Demarsh, 1986).

Peer Influences

Peer relationship also have a significant effect on the initiation, development, and maintenance of substance abuse. Most

Table 10: Mac Donald's stages of substance abuse

Stage	*1. Learning the mood swing*	*2. Seeking the mood swing*	*3. Preoccupation with the mood swing*	*4. Using drugs to feel normal*
Mood alteration	Euphoria Normal	Euphoria Normal Some pain	Euphoria Normal	Euphoria Normal Definite pain marked pain
Feelings	Feels good; few consequences	Excitement; early guilt	Euphoric highs doubts; including severe shame and guilt; depression; suicidal thoughts	Chronic guilt; shame, remorse, depression
Drugs	Tobacco Marijuana Alcohol	All the above plus inhalants, hashish, depressants, methamphetamine, prescription drugs	All listed plus psilocybin, PCP, LSD, cocaine	Whatever is available
Sources	Peers	Buying	Selling	Anyway possible
Behavior	Little detectable change; moderate after-the-fact lying	Dropping extracurricular activities and hobbies; mixed friends (straight and drug user); dress changing; erratic school performance and truancy; unpredictable mood and attitude swings; manipulative behavior	"Cool" appearance; straight friends dropped; family fights (verbal or physical); stealing (police incidents) pathological lying; school failure; truancy, expulsion, jobs lost	Physical deterioration (weight loss, chronic cough); sever mental deterioration (memory loss and flashbacks); paranoia, volcanic anger, school dropout frequent overdosing
Frequency	Progress to weekend use	Weekend use progressing to four to five times per week some solo use	Daily; frequent solo use	All day everyday

Abbreviations: PCP = phencyclidine; LSD = lysergic acid diethylamide

substance use occurs due to social influences and can be attributed to the adolescent's immediate subculture and lifestyle (Kaminer and Bukestein, 1998).

The most consistent and reproducible finding in substance abuses research is the strong relationship between an individual's substance use behavior of his/her friends (Jessor and Jessor, 1977).

This may result from socialization or from a process of interpersonal in which adolescents with similar values and behaviors seek each other out as friends (Kandel, 1978). However, research suggests that substance abuse is more strongly tied to a developmental process involving bio-behavioral factors (Glantz and Pickens, 1992) syndrome of problem behavior (Jessor and Jessor, 1997) or general deviance (Newcomb, 1995).

Values and Beliefs

Individual and family values and beliefs are known to have an effect on the development of SUDs. Substance abuse is negatively correlated with conventional behaviors and beliefs, such as religious attendance, good school performance, and beliefs in the generalized expectations, norms, and values of society (Jessor, 1987). Substance abuse is positively correlated with risk-talking behavior, sensation-seeking behavior, early sexual activity, higher value of independence, and greater involvement in delinquent behavior (Jessor, 1987).

Psychiatric Comorbidity

Despite evidence in the areas of genetics, neurobiological mechanisms, and psychosocial precursors, many experts in the field point to psychiatric comorbidity as one of the primary reasons that a SUD may develop in any given individual. The presence of one or more comorbid psychiatric disorders is often noted in a adolescents with SUDs (Bukstein, Glancy, Kaminer, 1992; Riggs, Baker, Mikulich, Young, and Crowley, 1995). Psychiatric disorders in childhood, characterized by disruptive behavior disorders as well as mood of anxiety disorders, suggest an increased risk for the development of SUDs in many adolescents (Loeber, 1988; Christie et al. 1988; Buckstein, Brent, and constituent criteria such as aggression usually precede and accompany adolescent SUDs (Huizinga and Elliot, 1981; Loeber, 1988; Milin et al. 1991).

Sociocultural Factors

Asian-Americans adolescents, whose parents emigrated from India to United States face many unique risk factors. Some investigators surmise that intergenerational conflict may contribute to alcohol, tobacco, and other drug use among these youth (Bhattacharya, 1998). Bhattacharya (1998) examined family role and responsibility, socioeconomic factors, influence of gender specific roles, and cultural adaptation among these families in the United States.

The Euro-American culture is individual-oriented, while the Asian culture is family centered. In Asian families, oftentimes parental expectations for academic achievement during adolescence. Some Asian-Indian families in the United States may face socioeconomic difficulties and find it difficult to assimilate culturally. Like other cultures, drug and alcohol use by youth is considered morally wrong in to discuss drug use with parents and also to seek professional help. Among other factors contributing not only to substance abuse but also to other health risk behaviors among these adolescents in the United States (Bhattacharya, 1998).

RESILIENCY AND PROTECTIVE FACTORS

There are a number of children and adolescents who in spite of being at an increased risk for developing substance use disorders do not go on to develop such disorders. This has prompted a number of investigators to look at protective or resiliency factors. Some of these factors are listed in Table 9 (Belcher, Shinitzky, 1998; Comercil Schwebel, 2000; Heischober, Hofmann, 1997; Patton, 1995; Patel, Greydanus, 1999).

Table 11: General symptoms and signs of potential drug abuse

Behavioral and school work
• Mood swings, depressed mood, withdrawal
• Panic reaction, acute psychosis, paranoia
• Poor hygiene
• Lying, stealing, and runway behaviors
• Preferences for dress, music, movies identifying with drug culture
• Drug paraphernalia
• Conflicts with parents and authorities
• Poor insight and judgment
• Frequent absence from school
• Conflicts with teachers
• Poor school performance
Physical symptoms and signs
• Loss of appetite and weight loss
• Sleep disturbances
• Fatigue, malaise
• Frequent upper respiratory infections
• Nasal irritation, red eyes
• Chronic cough, wheezing, chest pain
• Hoarse voice
• High blood pressure
• Unexplained injuries
• Needle track, scratch marks, tattoos
• Severe acne, testicular atrophy
• Frequent blank stares
• Impaired short-term memory

Adapted from: Patel DR, Greydanus DE. Substance abuse; a pediatric concern. Indian Journal of Pediatrics. 1999; 66:557

ASSESSMENT

A complete history and physical examination are the cornerstones of substance abuse assessment. These can be aided by more focused interviews and use of standardized tests for further psychological evaluation.

The majority of children and adolescents who abuse drugs are unlikely to present with any specific signs or symptoms. A useful approach to identify substance abuse in the adolescent is to routinely perform brief psychosocial screening assessment at all regular visits and be vigilant for nonspecific symptoms and signs of substance abuse (Table 11) (Greydanus, 1996; Patton, 1995; Fuller and Cavanaugh, 1995; Heyman and Adger, 1997). History remains the most important, and often the only, diagnostic tool in cases of substance abuse as physical signs are none to minimal in the majority of cases, except in acute intoxications. History should be obtained from the patient and the parents separately in a confidential manner.

Golden ring et al. (1988) proposed a screening tool to assess psychosocial issues known by the acronym HEADSS (Home, Education/Employment, Activities, version applicable to substance abuse problems has been proposed by the State University of New York Health Science Center, Syracuse, USA (Fuller and Cavanaugh, 1995), known by the acronym HEAD FIRST

Home: Separation, Support, "Space to grow";
Education: Expectations, study habits, achievement;
Abuse: Emotional, verbal, physical, sexual;
Drugs: Tobacco, alcohol, marijuana, others;
Friends: Confidant, peer pressure, interaction;
Image: Self-esteem, looks, appearance;
Recreation: Exercise, relaxation, TV, video games
Sexuality: Changes, feelings, experience, identity;
Threats: Harm to self or others, running away.

Another example of an office screening tool is the RAFFT questionnaire used to identify adolescents who are at serious health risks from their drug use (Liepman, 1998; Robertson et al. 1998).

The RAFF questions for substance abuse are:

- Do you drink or take drugs to RELAX, feel better about yourself, or fit in?
- Do you ever drink or take or take drugs while you are ALONE?
- Do any of your closest FRIENDS drink or use drugs ?
- Does a close FAMILY member have a problem with alcohol or drugs?
- Have you ever gotten into TROUBLE from drinking or talking drugs?

Other more detailed screening instruments for adolescent substance use have been recommended by the United States, Adolescent Drinking Index (ADI), Adolescent Drug Involvement Scale (ADIS), Drug and Alcohol Problem (DAP)

Quick Screen, Personal Experience Screening Instrument for Teenagers (POSIT), Rutgers Alcohol Problem Index (RAPI), and Teen Addiction Severity Index (T-ASI) (further details can be accessed at website http://text.nlm.nih.gov).

The routine screening lest of urine (Table 12) to detect drugs of abuse is neither useful nor recommended in all cases as a diagnostic tool. The detection of drugs in the urine is influenced by many factors including route of administration, dose, individual differences in pharmacokinetics and metabolism, and liver or renal disease. Drug testing may be used as a monitoring tool during substance abuse treatment.

SPECIFIC SUBSTANCES OF ABUSE

There are numerous drugs of abuse, the most common being marijuana (cannabis), alcohol, and tobacco. Brief comments on common drugs of abuse are made in the following sections; more details about individual drugs of abuse and other relevant information can be obtained from the United States National Institutes on Drug Abuse at its website, and other standard references (American Psychiatric Association, 2000; Comerci, Schwebel, 2000; Heischober, Hofmann, 1997; Schwartz, Alderman, 1997; Schwartz, 1998).

Alcohol

In India, locally brewed alcohol, such as arrack which contains 40–50% alcohol, is widely consumed especially in coastal and rural areas (George et al. 1994). Another product, containing alcohol, called toddy, is fermented sap from palm trees. The effects of acute alcohol intoxication and health hazards associated with chronic use have been well documented in medical literature.

Marijuana

Marijuana is derived from the Cannabis sativa plant. Hashish or ganja is high-potency resin derived from the flowering tops of the plant; bhang is derived from the leaves and charas from resinous liquid of the plant. Bhang is traditionally consumed during various religious festivities. Chronic use leads to deterioration of learned behaviors. Marijuana use also causes chronic bronchitis and exacerbation of asthma and changes similar to tobacco smoking. It raises heart rate and blood pressure.

Table 12: Detection of drugs in urine

Drug	*Detection time*
Amphetamines	<48 hours
Barbiturates	Short-acting: 1 day Long-acting: 2–3 weeks
Cocaine metabolites	Acute use: 2–4 days
chronic use	2 weeks
Ethanol	2–14 hours
Opiates	Up to 2 days
Cannabinoids	Moderate use: 5 days Chronic use: 10:20 days
Methaqualone	2 weeks
Phencyclidine	Acute use: 1 week Chronic use: 3 weeks

Tobacco and Pan

Smoking and chewing (smoking less) tobacco are common in adolescents. Bidi it is made by wrapping less than 0.5 g of coarse tobacco dust in a dry tambourine (Diasporas melanoxyon) leaf (Sanharanarayana et al. 1998). It is relatively cheap, and readily available and smoked by children and adolescents particularly in rural communities (Krishnamurthy et al. 1997 Patel, Greydanus, 1999). Tobacco mixed with pan masala is commonly consumed by a large number of adolescents (Murlidhr, Upmanyu, 1996).

Areca nut and tobacco are known to be carcinogenic (Polasa et al. 1993; Babu et al. 1996; Bagwe et al. 1990).

The incidence of oral cancers is very high among those nut is also associated with development of oral submucous fibrosis among teenagers and adults (Babu, Sesikeran, Bhat, 1996).

It is also known to be genotoxic and clastogenic (Polasa et al. 1994; Babu et al. 1996; Bagwe et al. 1990). The carcinogenic effects are increased with concomitant use of alcohol (Ramchnrani, et al, 1998; Patel et al. 1994; Babau et al. 1996; Bagwe et al. 1990).

Pan consists of Piper betel leaves, areca catechu nuts, catechu from acacia catechu and slaked lime. Chewing pan is widely popular in India since ancient times. A pan is prepared by smearing the betel leaf with lime and catechu; and pieces of areca nut (or "Supari") and spices such as cardamom and cloves, are added (Ramchandani et al. 1998; Maher et al. 1994). Pan masala chewing has gained wide popularity among children and adolescents (Halarnkar, 1997).

Pan masala is dried complex mixture of areca nut, catechu, lime, cardamom, and unspecified flavoring argents with or without tobacco Halarnkar,1996; Trivedi et al. 1996). Pan masala or gutka is available in attractively packaged bags and is aggressively marketed (Halarnkar, 1997).

Heroin and Other Opioids

Keemam contains opioids, tobacco, and other unidentified substances. It is chewed as a paste taken with betel leaves and lime and is often mixed with pan masala. The paste is kept in mouth and slowly sucked. Keemam is addictive and leads to dependence and its discontinuation is manifested by withdrawal symptoms. Heroin is highly addictive and associated with serious health problems both physical and psychological (Schwartz, 1998). Intravenous use can lead to hepatitis and human immunodeficiency virus infections. Acute overdose has been associated with cardiorespiratory arrested of alternating wake fullness and drowsiness, eventually leading to central nervous system depression. Chronic use has been associated with a number of complications including venous thrombophlebitis, endocarditis, abscesses, cellulites, hepatitis, and pneumonia. Repeated use results in tolerance and addiction.

On cessation of use the user develops withdrawal syndrome characterized by drug craving, anxiety, irritability, insomnia, diarrhea, vomiting, cold flashes and kicking movements. Sudden withdrawal in a chronic user may be fatal.

Cocaine

Cocaine is a highly addictive drug. Smoking, injecting, sniffing or snorting are the main routes of administration of cocaine. Cocaine is a powerful central nervous system stimulant. It blocks the reabsorption of dopamine in the central nervous system. Various signs and symptoms associated with cocaine use include hypertension, hyperthermia, tachycardia, dilated pupils and peripheral vasoconstriction. The cocaine high is characterized by euphoria, hyperstimulation, decreased sense of fatigue and can last from 5 to 30 minutes depending upon route of administration and rapidity of absorption of cocaine. The abuser eventually develops tolerance and needs higher does to achieve the 'high'. Sudden death can occur even with first use of cocaine. Cocaine use can cause seizures and cardiorespiratory arrest and health. Chronic use is associated with paranoid behavior. Chronic snorting can result in ulceration and perforation of the nasal mucosa and septum.

Amphetamines

Amphetamines is a highly addictive central nervous system stimulant. Methamphetamine is a related drug with much higher potency with similar effects. Amphetamines can be taken orally, inhaled nasally, smoked, or injected. The rapidity and duration of effects vary depending on the route of administration.

Amphetamines cause increased wakefulness, insomnia, anorexia, tachypnea, euphoria, hyperthermia, irritability, confusion, tremors, seizures, hypertension, tachycardia, and paranoid reactions. Death can result from acute cardiac arrest.

Hallucinogens

Lysergic acid diethylamide (LSD) is a typical hallucinogenic drug. LSD is usually ingested in the form of tablets, capsules or liquid, often impregnated on blotting paper. The physical and psychological effects of LSD ingestion are unpredictable and depend upon the dose, user's mood and the context in which the drug is taken. Within half hour of ingestion there is emotional liability, delusions, visual hallucinations, distortion of time and space, distortions of sense (hearing colors and seeing sounds), rapid mood swings and often associated panic.

The feeling of euphoria is referred by the user as a 'trip' and adverse reactions as a 'bad trip'. Such trip can last use to 12 hours. An adverse experience is characterized by feeling of fear, loss of control, fear of death, and terrifying thoughts. Many users experience flashbacks often suddenly anywhere from within few days to a year after using LSD. Chronic use can lead to psychosis and depression.

Phencyclidine

Phencyclidine (PCP) can be snorted, smoked or eaten. It is a white crystalline powder that is soluble in an alcohol and water. Acute intoxication is manifested by in violent and often suicidal behaviors. Lowed by shallow respiration, profuse sweating, in-coordination, and generalized numbness. PCP use by adolescents can adversely affect their growth and cognitive abilities.

High dose of PCP lead to hypotension, bradycardia, bradypnea, vomiting, nystagmus, dizziness and drooling. Some may develop seizures and go into coma dental trauma. Prominent psychological signs associated coherent speech, and a sense of dissociation of one's self from the surrounding memory, depression, impaired speech, and weight loss.

Inhalants

Inhalants are easily available as household and industrial products. The different kinds of inhalants cause effects similar to general anesthesia.

There is initial stimulation, followed by loss of inhibition and eventually loss of consciousness with repeated inhalations.

The effects can last from several minutes to several hours depending upon use. Use of highly concentrated inhalants can result in cardiac arrest and health. Death can also consequences including hearing loss, peripheral damage. Serious liver and kidney damage can occur with repeated use of inhalants.

TREATMENT APPROACHES

Few adolescents present with acute intoxication to emergency departments. They need acute medical management on an emergent basis. The details of treatment of an acutely intoxicated patient can be found in standard medical and emergency texts and is beyond the scope of this chapter.

More often most drugs use adolescents present with nonspecific signs and symptoms resulting from chronic use and need comprehensive psychiatric treatment. There are various levels and modalities of treatment depending upon the severity if the problem (Buckstein, 1997; Center for Substance Abuse Treatment, 1999; Kranzler, et al. 1999; Liepman, 1998; Schwartz, Alderman, 1997).

Outpatient treatment program typically involves about 1 to 2 hour's meeting for 3 times a week; intensity of treatment can vary from 9 to 20 hours per week. Partial hospitalization or day treatment program is the most intensive outpatient treatment and consists of about 20 hours per week in a well-structured daily program working with the therapist 8 hours per day.

Some adolescents may need long-term residential (therapeutic communities) or inpatient treatment lasting anywhere from 6 months to up to 24 months. Inpatient programs are also used for detoxification treatments and following acute intoxication lasting from few days to several weeks. All these treatment programs incorporate various treatment modalities tailored to individual patient's needs.

The treatment of adolescent drug abuse should include the entire family. Behavioral approaches utilized in drug abuse treatment of adolescents include social skills development, family therapy and individual psychotherapy. Many adolescents have comorbid mental health conditions that need specific treatment in addition to treating substance abuse.

43.8 CHILD SEXUAL ABUSE: CURRENT SCENARIO IN INDIA

PB Behere, A Mulmule, AP Behere

INTRODUCTION

It is easy to understand the difficulties of children who suffered from malnutrition or starvation, plenty of nutritious food along with care can recover them so they can go on to lead normal lives. However, if malnutrition is severe can sometimes lead to long lasting effects on their growth and suffer physical impairments for the rest of their lives. Likewise children who suffer from abuse which if in the form of sexual abuse the damage is more likely to be permanent and the children to suffer emotional impairments for the rest of their lives. Sexual abuse is a traumatic life event with widespread negative psychological and sociological effects on victims of any gender.

Sexual abuse is highly organized and obviously secretive crime. Earlier it was believed that there were no child sexual abuses in India.[220] Gradually it was realized that many cases of sexual abuse are unreported or covered or protected in family itself and does not come out due to family pride.[221] With the time awareness increased and cases are surfacing out. Generally the victim is the only witness for the abuse thus it highly difficult to get evidence for the crime but if the support system and registering intermediary are well trained it becomes easy to obtain history. Women in our society have been psychologically conditioned to believe in what society has defined as their own promiscuity.[222]

DEFINITION

According to Child Sexual Abuse (CSA) bill 2012 'A person is said to commit "penetrative sexual assault" if he penetrates his penis, to any extent, into the vagina, mouth, urethra or anus of a child or makes the child to do so with him or any other person; or he inserts, to any extent, any object or a part of the body, not being the penis, into the vagina, the urethra or anus of the child or makes the child to do so with him or any other person; or he manipulates any part of the body of the child so as to cause penetration into the vagina, urethra, anus or any part of body of the child or makes the child to do so with him or any other person; or he applies his mouth to the penis, vagina, anus, urethra of the child or makes the child to do so to such person or any other person.'[223]

MAGNITUDE OF PROBLEM

Worldwide

This is a great issue currently discussed all over the world. WHO's estimation of 2002 states that 150 million girls and 73 million boys less than 18 years experienced forced sexual intercourse or other forms of sexual violence. While estimates from 2000 suggest that, 1.8 million children were forced into prostitution and pornography and 1.2 million were victims of trafficking.[224] Those cultures which promote objectification about women's behavior thus making them inferior than men had higher prevalence of sexual abuse. Highest prevalence rate of child sexual abuse in the world geographically was found in Africa (34.4%), USA and Asia had prevalence rates about 10.1% and 23.9% respectively while Europe showed the lowest prevalence rate (9.2%).[225]

India

A total of 33,098 cases of sexual crime against children were reported in country in 2011 as compared to 26,694 in 2010 that is the increase by 24%. Number of cases under procuration of minor girls increased from 679 to 862 in 2011, increase by 27% over 2010. A total of 7,112 cases of child rape were reported in country during 2011 as compared to 5484 in 2010, increase by 29.7%. State wise sexual abuse is highest in Madhya Pradesh highest (1,262) followed by Uttar Pradesh (1,088) and Maharashtra (818). These states account for 44.5% of total child rape cases reported in country.[226]

In India prevalence is less or there is a possibility that many of the cases are not reported or under reported. Sexual abuse is faced by nearly 53% of children; among them 52.94% were boys and 47.06% girls. In 50% of cases the abuser was in trusted relationship with the child. The significant finding was that contrary to the general perception, the overall percentage of boys was much higher than that of girls. Across the country, every second child was being subjected to other forms of sexual abuse and every fifth child was facing severe forms of sexual abuse.[227]

Rape occurs in India every twenty minutes. In 2011, more than 24 thousand cases were reported, i.e. about 70 a day. In Delhi new figures released by the Delhi Police reveals that a woman is raped every 18 hours or molested every 14 hours. The conviction rate is extremely low (26%) in India. There are 80,000 pending rape cases in India. The conviction rate is much higher in North India as compared to Maharashtra.[227]

Law and Changing Trends

Indian Panel Code Laws

Definition of rape and its punishment are discussed under IPC 375 and IPC 376 respectively.[220] Punishment for rape varies from capital punishment to seven years or life imprinsonment.[221] Intercourse by a man with his wife during separation is discussed under 376A of IPC and punishment varies from two years imprisonment with or without fine.[222] Intercourse by superintendent of jail, remand home, etc. is discussed under Section 376C of Indian Penal Code punishment and is liable for punishment for five years or fine.[223] Intercourse by any member of the management or staff of a hospital with any woman in that hospital is discussed under Section 376D. Here the punishment varies from imprisonment of five years or fine.[228]

Drawbacks of Indian Panel Code Laws

The ordinary criminal laws are totally inadequate to protect the women, who are victims of sexual abuse. Explanation to section 375 does not treat force sexual intercourse by a husband against the wife (above 15 years) as an offence. Section 376A also has the same reasoning. The Indian Panel Code needs to be reviewed. The existing definition of rape and molestation should be suitably amended to adequately address the various types of sexual assault. In fact, sexual assault on women should be made a specific offence requiring stringent punishment. There is no provision to deal with psychological trauma of the women. There are several cases pending in the court as the trial goes on for years. In several cases the girls have become adults by the time the final judgment comes through. The investigation of trial of sexual offences have to be made time bound. There is a need for special provision relating to medical examination of victim in the criminal procedure code. The mental health of victim needs to be attended to, as the trauma has to be reduced.[229]

JS Verma Committee Recommendations

The committee suggested ways to make rape laws stronger in country, and has submitted its report recently (23 Jan 2013). It is a 630 page report to government, suggesting amendment of criminal law to provide for higher punishment to rapists, including those belonging to police and public servant:

- Every complaint of rape must be registered by the police and civil society.
- It suggests that the punishment for rape should be rigorous imprisonment from seven years to life.
- Voyeurism, acid attacks is punished by imprisonment up to seven years in jail.
- Protocols for examination of rape victims for sexual abuse have been suggested.
- Special procedures for protecting persons with disabilities from rape and requisite procedures.
- It suggests various measures for complete reformation of political and judicial system is equally responsible for it.
- Thus, there is as urgent need to review the continuance of armed Forces Special Powers Act (AFSPA) and also recommends posting special commissioners for women's safety in conflicting areas.[230]

Antirape Bill

The bill was approved by Union Cabinet on 12th March 2013. The salient points suggested:

- The Bill provides stringent punishment for rapists and repeat offenders; it also includes offences like stalking, voyeurism, disrobing and acid attacks.
- The age of consent for sex has been increased to 18 years.
- This Bill replaces the existing antirape Ordinance, provides capital punishment for rapist if the act causes death for victim or leaves her in a permanent vegetative state. Repeat offenders may also get death penalty under the new law.
- Bill keeps rape as a gender-specific crime where only a male can be punished for committing such offence.
- The first offence will be bailable—a second offence will become nonbailable.
- The Bill prescribed a punishment ranging from 10 years to life imprisonment if someone is involved in trafficking a minor and a jail term of 14 years that may be extended

to life term if the offender is involved in trafficking more than one minor.

- For acid attack that caused harm to the victim, the offender will get a jail term of minimum 10 years, which can be extended to life term.[231]

Etiopathogenesis

Biologically it is noted that childhood abuse and maltreatment can shrink important parts of the brain. Reduced brain volume in parts of the hippocampus and subiculum could help to explain why childhood problems often lead to later psychiatric disorders, such as depression, drug addiction, schizophrenia and other mental health problems. This link could help us find better ways to treat survivors of childhood abuse. The child sexual abuse is such a traumatic event that it never disappears in adulthood.

Child Sexual Abuse Accommodation Syndrome (CSAAS)

This term has been recommended in view of why disclosure in case of child sexual abuse so difficult and at times retracted. Thus after a child under goes sexual abuse the following events occur; the child is warned to keep the sexual abuse a secret. In the initial period child feels trapped and helpless. Child's feelings of helplessness and fear of no one will believe the disclosure of abuse lead to accommodative behavior. On the contrary if the child does disclose, failure of family or professionals to protect child adequately and to support him, augment the child's distress and may lead to retraction of the disclosure.[232]

Imaging Findings

It was seen that EEG of the affected people had left hemispherical disturbances. EEG abnormalities were suggestive that victims are likely to have more self-destructive behavior and aggression. Observation on MRI suggests there is less activation of medial prefrontal cortex and anterior cingulated cortex suggesting poor arousal in children. In addition to this there is arrested development of left hemisphere along with poor integration with in left and right hemispheres.

Impact of Various Factors on Child Sexual Abuse

The consequences and after effects of child sexual abuse vary considerably depending on various factors such as the age, severity, frequency, duration of abuse. The relationship which a victim shares with the perpetrator, their type of abuse faced, whether any intervention was done for care and further rehabilitation of child, etc.

Positive Risk Factors

Female sex is one of the important and most crucial factor, followed by single child, adopted, step child, mentally or physically handicapped, in foster care, single parent or broken homes, poverty, social isolation, parents with mental illness, substance use history, some legal issues related to family.[233]

Clinical Presentation

Signs and Symptoms

Following are general changes noted when children is suffering from some form of sexual abuse: they had excess fearfulness, insomnia, amnesia, day dreaming, enuresis, encopresis, change in behavior in form of increased irritability, frequent anger outbursts especially towards male members of family, at times abusive, withdrawn, low self-esteem, suicidal, self mutilative behaviors, night mares, deterioration in school performance, decreased play.

Presentation of Victims of Child Sexual Abuse

Risk of mental illness in victims is twice than that of nonabused children. Child suffering from sexual abuse can have varied presentations ranging from dysthymia, recurrent depressive disorder, post-traumatic stress disorder, adjustment disorder, dissociative states, somatoform disorder, at times and eating disorders and can have disorders of sexual dysfunctions, personality disorders in future.

It is seen from several studies that women who faced child sexual abuse in their childhood are likely to suffer from depression or are suicide attempters twice than those not sexually abused. Rate of obesity in women were found to be higher in those victims of child sexual abuse.[234] Adverse Childhood Experiences (ACE) study in the United States, a study indicated that adults exposed to four or more adverse experiences in childhood were 12 times more likely to have attempted suicide than those who had no adverse experiences in childhood.[235]

Findings from the Australian component of the International Violence against Women Survey (IVAWS) had findings of 72% of women who experienced sexual abuse as a child are also likely to face violence in adulthood, in comparison to 43% of women who did not experience childhood abuse.[236]

Assessment and Evaluation of Case of Child Sexual Abuse

Consent and Confidentiality

Consent must be obtained not only for physical examination but also for interviewing it. Generally victim if older than 18 years can give consent or in most of the cases the primary care giver of the child. However, consent can be problematic, especially when the perpetrator is immediate family member or vested interest of some official authority is involved in case. In such issues the child protection authorities may need to be called into help for child's rights for the purpose of facilitating the medical evaluation.

Interview Techniques

To interview victims of CSA the interview should occur in a location the child perceives as a "safe place"(whichever it may be). They must be approached with extreme sensitivity and care irrespective of their age, gender. Team of experts present during the child interview may eliminate the need for multiple interviews generally a law person, consultant and social worker should be considered. Star the topic with neutral environment. Recognize yourself with child as some who is there to help him. Some record should be gathered about information during the interview; this may be a videotape, an audiotape, or notes. Each of these methods of data gathering has its strengths and weaknesses. It is usually optimal to interview the child before interviewing the parents. The rationale is that, in most cases, the child's statements and behavior are the primary means for determining whether sexual abuse occurred. Single detailed interview will suffice if done properly. To start with ask the child the reason for the interview. Tell child to describe what has happened with him in his verbatim. Try to interview in open questions rather than leading ones.

Sexual Abuse Recognition and Nondisclosure Inventory (SARDANI)

It is a questionnaire used in classrooms for survey to disclose the frequency of undisclosed sexual abuse among adolescents. The age group chosen is generally between 12 years and 15 years. Several studies were conducted using this scale had significant results.[237]

Guidelines for Forensic Medical Examination and its Reports in Sexual Abuse Cases

Government of Maharashtra has implemented new guidelines on 10th May 2013 for examination of rape victims. It was observed in a report studied by Dr Indrajit Khandekar that most of the questions enquired to rape victim were nonrelevant and posed major problems in delivering justice. He has framed some questions which should be considered while writing a forensic report in sexual abuse cases:

- Whether there is any evidence of sexual act and whether that was recent and forcible.
- What are types of injuries on the rape survivor's body, their numbers and location on the body.
- Whether any foreign body like hairs and blood/semen stains are found on her body.
- Describe her clothes and whether they are torn or containing blood/semen stains.
- Whether samples of her nail clippings, blood and vaginal swabs are collected for DNA test.[238]

These will overcome some of the loop holes such as the "finger test" which was done to report whether the victim is habitual to sexual intercourse; at the same time it will prevent the victim to undergo repeated humiliating examinations. The report is also valid in case the victim turns hostile.

Thus child sexual abuse is a multidimensional problem having legal, social and psychological implications. Hence, a team work is needed to asses and approach the problem. Detail assessment should be done by multidisciplinary team which includes:

- *Social worker:* For victim in community who did not confront.
- *Child and welfare committee officer:* For victim's support.
- *Police officer/Forensic Medical Expert:* Safety of other girls in community.
- *NGO's:* Helps in rehabilitation of victim.
- *Medical professionals:* Medical checkups.
- *Psychologist/Psychiatrist:* Counseling the victim.

Guidelines for the Media in Addressing the Issue of Child Sexual Abuse

- Media should bring the issue of child sexual abuse into public knowledge and debate but the issue is presented as a serious violation of rights, not only as an offence against children.
- Avoid showing crime methodology, sensationalization and undue prominence to the perpetrator.
- Besides drawing attention to the problem, media also needs to enlighten the public as what can be done to prevent such incidents and what needs and must be done if such an incident has taken place, including providing information on legal or other remedies, rights of the child.
- In all reporting, the media should aim for principle of best interest of the child in respect to convention on the rights of the child.[239]

Treatment

Treatment can be divided based on the physical findings and laboratory results into medical line of management such as treating acute genital infections, skin lesions, hemorrhages, pregnancy in case of adolescent abuse. In case of mental illness the treatment depends on symptom profile, family history, of mental illness, premorbid personality. Counseling, psycho education regarding anxiety management and behavior therapy sessions can also be provided if required. In some cases psychotropic medications and hospitalization can also be provided.

Prevention and Awareness

Early identification of a perpetrator can be made if certain points are considered:

- An adult shows undue attention towards a child
- Insists on touching, hugging, kissing, tickling or holding child even when child does not want
- Is overly interested in child's sexuality (talks about his growing body)
- Constantly maneuvers to get time alone or insists for such
- He tries to find time mostly with child rather than some one of his age
- They purchases expensive gifts for children or give money for no reason
- Frequently intrudes a child's privacy, (walks in on the child in bathroom)
- Allow children to consistently get away with undisciplined behavior.

Awareness About Parents and School Teachers

Teach child to trust their feelings and that it is ok to say no when somebody they know and care about them, does something they do not like, set and respect family boundaries, speak up when inappropriate behavior is seen or reported, talk about sexual abuse and teach proper names of body parts to children, educate children about difference between safe and unsafe touch, children also need to understand that people they know are capable of hurting them, encourage, affirm and acknowledge a child's opinions and feelings-giving them a sense of self-esteem and confidence, involve your child in setting up safety plan that is easy to remember, make a list for yourself and child-whom to call for advice, information, help. School children and teachers should be taught about these above points.

43.9 PHYSICAL ABUSE AND NEGLECT OF CHILDREN

JN Vyas, SS Nathawat

INTRODUCTION

Child maltreatment includes physical abuse and neglect, and happens in all countries and cultures. Child maltreatment usually results from interactions between several risk factors (such as parental depression, stress, and social isolation). Physicians can incorporate methods to screen for risk factors into their usual appointments with the family. Detection of physical abuse is dependent on the doctor's ability to recognize suspicious injuries, such as bruising, bite marks, burns, bone fractures, or trauma to the head or abdomen. Neglect is the most common form of child maltreatment in the western culture. It can be caused by insufficient parental knowledge; intentional negligence is rare. Suspected cases of child abuse should be well documented and reported to the appropriate public agency which should assess the situation and help to protect the child.

DEFINITIONS OF MALTREATMENT

The abuse and neglect (or maltreatment) of children is a worldwide problem, although its manifestations and extent vary. It is far more prevalent than is generally recognized. Child maltreatment has short-term and long-term physical, psychological, and social consequences. Professionals concerned about children's health and safety have an important part to play to address this problem; many physicians see their main responsibilities as identification and reporting of child maltreatment, although they could also have a role in prevention, treatment, and advocacy.

Physical abuse by parents or caregivers includes beatings, shaking, scalding, and biting. Although some forms of corporal punishment are widely accepted, many people think of any injury beyond immediate redness as abuse. However, harm might not be immediately evident, thus concerns about potential harm justify consideration as possible maltreatment.

Child neglect is omission of care, such as health care, education, supervision, protection from environmental hazards, meeting physical needs (e.g. clothing or food), and emotional support, resulting in actual or potential harm. Alternatively, neglect from a child's perspective is not adequately meeting a child's basic needs, regardless of the reasons. Several factors can contribute to neglect, such as parental depression, a child's disability, family violence, or an absence of community resources. Full comprehension of the problems underpinning neglect helps interventions to be tailored to the specific needs of the child and family.

PREVALENCE OF CHILD MALTREATMENT

Measurement of child maltreatment is inherently difficult, since it is rarely seen directly by people outside the immediate family, and is often unreported. However, data show that child abuse and neglect are not rare. Child maltreatment happens in all countries and in families of all racial and religious groups.

Different laws and child welfare systems, however, preclude comparisons across countries. Physicians and others can be reluctant to become involved. Thus, cases reported to child welfare agencies probably represent the tip of the iceberg.

Risk Factors

Child maltreatment seldom results from one cause; rather, many risk factors usually interact. Factors such as child's disability or a parent with depression predispose children to maltreatment. Within a family, intimate partner violence increases children's risk of abuse. In communities, factors such as dangerous neighborhoods or poor recreational facilities increase risk. Societal factors, such as poverty and associated burdens contribute substantially to risk of maltreatment. However, children in all social classes can be maltreated, and physicians need to guard against biases toward low-income families.

Protective Factors

By contrast, some resources buffer the effect of risk factors and protect children from maltreatment. Clinical experience suggests that protective factors include parental recognition of problems seeking help, a supportive grandparent, and accessible mental-health care. Child maltreatment generally results from a complex interplay between risk and protective factors. For example, a single mother with a colicky baby who has recently lost her job is at risk of maltreating the child, but presence of a loving grandmother might prevent abuse or neglect. Full understanding of factors contributing to maltreatment, and of a family's strengths, is key to effective intervention.

Prevention

Generally, medical responses to child maltreatment happen after maltreatment has taken place; prevention is preferable. Physicians can help in several ways. A continuing relationship with a family offers opportunities to develop trust and knowledge of their circumstances. Astute observation of parent-child interactions can reveal useful information. For example, does the relationship seem warm and comfortable or tense and hostile?

Parent education about medical disorders helps to ensure implementation of treatment; barriers to treatment should be addressed. Simple strategies such as writing down the treatment plan can help. Additionally, parenting advice might help with child rearing, thus diminishing the risk of maltreatment. Hospital-based programs for parents of newborn babies educating about infant crying and risks of shaking seem to prevent abusive head trauma.

Screening for risk factors and tackling known problems (often via referral to social or mental-health services) can strengthen families and reduce maltreatment. This role for the physician fits well with a broad view of health, and a professional mandate to help to ensure children's health and safety. Check-ups (preventive care) offer opportunities to screen for psychosocial disorders. The review of systems is standard in such visits. Its traditional focus on organ systems can be expanded to subjects such as feelings about the child, the parent's own functioning, possible depression, substance abuse, intimate partner violence, disciplinary approaches, and stressors and supports.

One approach is to systematically ask parents to complete a brief questionnaire about psychosocial issues while they are in the consulting room. This request should be phrased constructively with an empathic tone, and build on longstanding concern for children's safety. By starting a dialogue with topics familiar to physicians and parents, such as the presence of smoke detectors, the physician might be able to steer the conversation towards sensitive topics, such as drug use. Any concerns raised by such screens need at least brief assessment and initial management. This management could include a referral for further assessment and treatment. Frequent surgery visits can be scheduled for support and counseling, and to monitor the situation.

Physicians can advocate for promising interventions in the community. In some studies, programs that arrange home visits by nurses improved parental and family functioning and diminished the risk of child maltreatment, although evidence for their effectiveness has been mixed. Efforts and resources to help to ensure adequate nutrition and health care, and to address important risk factors such as parental depression or substance abuse are needed to strengthen families and enhance the health, development, and safety of children.

Assessment and Diagnosis

Detection of physical abuse is dependent on the clinician's ability to recognize suspicious injuries, do a careful and complete physical examination with the judicious use of ancillary tests, and to consider whether the history reasonably explains the physical findings. Absence of explanation for the injury, changing explanations, or one that is inconsistent with the child's developmental capabilities raises concern about abuse, as does delay in seeking medical care. A detailed medical history should include previous trauma, admissions to hospital, chronic illness, and adherence to treatment. A family history of easy bruising or fractures is important to elicit. Questions about substance or alcohol abuse, mental illness, intimate partner violence, discipline practices, stressors, or previous involvement of child protection services can be difficult to ask, but provide valuable insight into a family's functioning. Careful documentation, ideally with photographs, is necessary. An interdisciplinary approach is the best way to assess all possible risk factors; many hospitals have developed interdisciplinary teams for this purpose.

Bruises are the most common manifestation of physical abuse. Maguire and colleagues reviewed what patterns of bruising are diagnostic or suggestive of abuse. They identified differences between bruises that were not inflicted (accidental bruising) and those due to abuse. The frequency, number, and location of some bruises are linked to motor development. Bruises in infants younger than 9 months and who have not started walking should lead the physician to consider abuse or illness as likely causes. Accidental bruises are characteristically anterior and over bony prominences, such as shins and forehead, usually due to falls. Well-padded areas are unlikely to be bruised in the course of most childhood activities. Thus, bruises of buttocks, cheeks, and thighs suggest abuse. Some sites seldom get bruised in the course of children's activities (i.e. neck, ear, and genitalia). If an implement was used, bruises can carry an imprint.

Many factors affect the color of a bruise, including the depth of the injury, location, force of impact, vascularity of tissues, time since injury, skin color, and ambient lighting. Physicians might be asked to estimate the age of a bruise to identify possible perpetrators, to corroborate explanations for injuries, or to confirm that injuries happened at different times. However, to precisely date bruises is difficult.

Occasionally an underlying medical explanation for bruises exists—for example, idiopathic thrombocytopenic purpura, leukemia, coagulation disorders, or connective tissue disorders such as Ehlers-Danlos syndrome or osteogenesis imperfecta. Clues to suggest such a disorder should lie in the child's history and examination. Henoch Schonlein purpura, the most common vasculitis in young children, could be confused with abusive injury. Physicians should realize that the presence of a medical disorder does not preclude abuse.

Cultural practices need to be considered in the differential diagnosis. Cao Gio, commonly known as "coining," is a southeast Asian dermabrasion therapy and causes linear petechiae. Birthmarks and Mongolian spots can be confused with bruises. These marks are not tender and do not rapidly change color or size.

Bite marks have a characteristic pattern of one or two opposing arches with multiple bruises. They can be inflicted by an adult, another child, an animal, or by the patient. Bites by animals vary, but they usually have narrower arches than human bites, and are often deep. Self-inflicted bites are limited to accessible areas, especially the hands. Adult bites generally have more than an inch between the canines, and often cause the most prominent bruises. Many bites by another child suggest inadequate supervision and neglect. Distinction between adult and child bites is often difficult, and consultation with a forensic dentist can be helpful to identify the source of the bite. Photographs with a size standard are essential, and swabbing with sterile water or saline might recover genetic markers in saliva.

Childhood burns are frequently due to abuse. Many other burns happen because of inadequate supervision or neglect. The pattern or distribution of the burn can reveal the probable mechanism. Immersion burns, when a child is forcibly held in hot water, have clear delineation between the burned and the healthy skin, uniform depth, and might look like a sock or glove. There are often no splash marks since the extremity is held in the hot water. Symmetrical burns are especially suspicious, as are burns of the buttocks and perineum. Burns from hot objects such as curling irons, radiators, steam irons, metal grids, hot knives, and cigarettes have shapes that mirror those of the object. There are some unusual causes of abusive burns such as hair dryers, microwave ovens, and stun guns.

Neglect frequently contributes to childhood burns. Children, left at home alone, can be burned in house fires. A parent who has taken illegal drugs could cause a fire and be unable to protect a child. Children might pull hot liquids on to themselves while they are exploring their environment. Because spilt liquids cool quickly, such a burn is usually most severe and broad around the point of contact. Children might insert objects into an electrical outlet, usually resulting in no external burn, unless the child touched the electrical source. Burns from electric water heaters sometimes happen.

Several circumstances mimic abusive burns, such as brushing against a hot radiator, car seat burns, enuresis blanket marks, impetigo, and folk remedies such as moxibustion. Impetigo can resemble cigarette burns, but cigarette burns are usually 7–10 mm across; impetigo has lesions of varying size. Accidental cigarette burns are usually oval and superficial.

Establishing whether a burn was inflicted is dependent on the history, burn pattern, and the child's capabilities. A delay in seeking health care could be because the burn initially seemed minor, before blistering or becoming infected. Outside agencies should be consulted to corroborate the history and investigate the scene (e.g. testing the water temperature). Severe burns can lead to lifelong scarring and serious psychosocial sequelae. Prevention is key, such as setting hot water cylinders under 125°C.

Bone fractures are the second most common presentation of physical abuse after soft tissue injuries. No one lesion is absolutely a characteristic of abuse; however, some strongly suggest abuse. Although fractures in a child aged less than 1 year are highly suspicious of abuse, spiral or oblique fractures of the lower limb have been described in infants playing in static activity centers, and hairline fractures can take place in the tibia of newly walking toddlers.

The classic metaphyseal lesion (bucket handle fracture) usually suggests abuse, although it has been identified in children treated for equinovarus deformity and after a difficult delivery or cesarean section. Rib fractures are unusual in accidental trauma, even in motor vehicle crashes and falls from heights of more than 1.8 m. Rib fractures in children without mineral deficiencies are very rare after cardiopulmonary resuscitation. Chest physiotherapy rarely results in rib fractures. Rib fractures are unusual in healthy full-term infants as birth injuries, and usually occur in large babies (weighing more than 3300 g) and in difficult deliveries. Skull fractures happen in only 1–3% of children after falls from heights of less than 1.8 m and are usually linear, narrow, and uncomplicated.

Many or complex fractures of both sides of the skull and depressed or growing fractures (leptomeningeal cysts) are typical of abuse. Skull fractures with intracranial injury in infants are usually due to abuse, although simple skull fractures could have a thin adjacent subdural hematoma. Subperiosteal new bone could suggest trauma, but also occurs in several disorders. Physiological periosteal reaction is normally seen in children aged between 6 weeks and 6 months, and is generally symmetrical (Panel 1).

The differential diagnosis of fractures due to abuse includes noninflicted injury, trauma during delivery, osteogenesis imperfecta, rickets, copper deficiency, Caffey's disease, congenital syphilis, osteopenia of infancy, osteomyelitis, and normal variant. Osteogenesis imperfecta is usually a clinical diagnosis, but skin biopsy for collagen analysis might be needed if examination is not definitive. If any question about the correct diagnosis remains, the child should be placed in a protected environment while awaiting test results. Temporary brittle bone disease remains unproven and is not accepted as an explanation for fractures by most child abuse experts.

The American Academy of Pediatrics recommends a mandatory skeletal survey in all cases of suspected physical abuse in children aged under 2 years. Follow-up skeletal surveys 10 or more days later can help to detect occult fractures that might not have been apparent on first images. Similarly, a bone scan might detect occult fractures early on. Dating of fractures is an inexact science and clinicians should bear this in mind when offering time frames of injuries to investigating agencies or courts. However, radiologists can clearly differentiate recent fractures from old ones. Such differentiation remains invaluable in identification of children who have been subjected to repeated abuse, or whose injuries are shown to be inconsistent with given explanations.

Panel 1 Types of fracture by specificity for diagnosis of abuse[61]

High
- Classic metaphyseal lesion
- Rib (especially posterior)
- Scapula
- Spinous process
- Sternum

Moderate
- Several fractures, especially if bilateral
- Fractures of different ages
- Epiphyseal separations
- Vertebral body fractures
- Digital fractures
- Complex skull fractures

Low
- Subperiosteal new bone formation
- Clavicular fractures
- Long-bone shaft fractures
- Simple skull fractures

Abusive head injuries result from mechanisms including shaking, direct impact, penetration, and asphyxiation or hypoxia, alone or in combination. Hence, the term abusive head trauma is recommended. Although abusive head trauma is usually seen in infants, it is also seen in older children and adults. Results of studies strongly accord with the contention that adults do shake infants, and that shaking alone can cause widespread brain injury.

Abusive head trauma can result from frustration associated with a baby's crying or irritability. The adult usually holds the infant by the chest so they face each other, compressing the chest while violently shaking the infant to and fro. In some instances, the infant's head is also slammed against a hard surface. The exact force needed to cause shaking injuries is difficult to quantify. However, the American Academy of Pediatrics stated that such shaking is so violent that individuals observing it would recognize it as dangerous and likely to kill the child.

The characteristic findings of abusive head trauma, include subdural hemorrhage, retinal hemorrhages, and brain injury, particularly diffuse axonal injury, but these might not all be present. External signs of head trauma such as swelling, bruises, and skull fractures are sometimes present. Signs of trauma elsewhere, such as bruises, and rib or long bone fractures might be present. Signs and symptoms of abusive head trauma vary from none to mild and nonspecific, and to severe and life-threatening. Poor feeding, emesis, lethargy, and changes in neurological status (including limpness, irritability, seizures, and coma) and respiratory changes (including apnoea) have been reported. Consequently, the diagnosis of abusive head trauma could be missed and physicians need to be mindful of subtle manifestations. Publications about this subject generally suggest that severe abusive head trauma almost always results in the rapid onset of clinically significant signs or symptoms. shows the differential diagnosis of subdural hemorrhages (Panel 2). A detailed medical history, laboratory tests, and imaging will exclude many of the rare or obvious disorders.

Eye examination by an ophthalmologist with indirect ophthalmoscopy and dilated pupils (using eye drops unless pupils are fixed and dilated because of neurological state) is essential to properly assess the retina. Retinal hemorrhage is seen in about 85% of abusive head trauma cases, and can be unilateral or bilateral. The detailed characteristics

Panel 2 Differential diagnosis of subdural hemorrhage in infants and children

- Accidental or abusive trauma
- Birth trauma
- Congenital malformations (e.g. arteriovenous malformation)
- Coagulopathies (e.g. vitamin K deficiency in newborn babies, disseminated intravascular coagulation, hemophilia)
- Infection (e.g. septicemia, meningitis, and necrotizing encephalitis)
- Metabolic disorders (e.g. glutaric aciduria type 1, osteogenesis imperfecta)
- Tumor
- Vasculitis (e.g. Kawasaki disease)

of retinal hemorrhage are important for elucidation of the cause. Multiple retinal hemorrhages that extend to the peripheral retinal edge, and that affect several layers of the retina strongly suggest abusive head trauma. Traumatic retinoschisis can take place, with or without perimacular retinal folds. Such folds are usually confirmation of abusive head trauma from shaking, although a case report described crush injury of the head as a potential alternative mechanism. However, other studies of crush injury have not accorded with this finding.

Retinal hemorrhages are reported occasionally in patients with noninflicted head injury. Less common causes of such hemorrhage include meningitis, Henoch-Schönlein purpura and other vasculitides, glutaric aciduria, thrombocytopenia, and profound anemia. However, in such situations the hemorrhages are few and confined to the posterior pole. Substantial retinal hemorrhages are not caused by cardiopulmonary resuscitation. These bleeds are seen in 40% of newborn babies after vaginal delivery, but superficial retinal hemorrhages at birth resolve in less than 2 weeks and deeper intraretinal hemorrhages resolve within 6 weeks.

The CT remains the initial imaging modality for the child with possible abusive head trauma. It is better suited for detecting cerebral edema and subarachnoid hemorrhage than is MRI. MRI is a useful adjunct to CT, although it might not be possible in unstable patients, and is less sensitive in detection of subarachnoid blood and skull fractures than is CT. MRI can detect intraparenchymal lesions such as shearing injury and subdural hematomas better than CT, and therefore should be considered several days after initial CT scans. Caution should be exercised in dating of subdural hematomas with either CT or MRI.

Abdominal trauma accounts for substantial morbidity and mortality in abused children. Young children are especially vulnerable because they have large abdomens and lax abdominal musculature. Hollow organs can be ruptured by a blow or kick, and solid organs such as the pancreas can be injured, especially over the spine. Bleeding could result from trauma to an organ or from shearing of the vascular supply. Children can present with cardiovascular failure, often after a delay in care or diagnosis. Bilious vomiting in a young child without fever or peritoneal irritation suggests a duodenal hematoma, often due to abuse. Indeed, any of the abdominal organs can be injured as a result of abuse.

The manifestations of abdominal trauma are often subtle, even with severe injuries. Bruising of the abdominal wall is unusual. Damage can evolve slowly; there can be delayed perforation days after the injury, or bowel strictures, or a pancreatic pseudocyst weeks or months later. Timing of an abdominal injury is especially difficult.

Subtle presentations call for suspicion of abdominal trauma if other evidence of physical abuse is present. Physicians should screen urine and stool samples for blood, and check liver and pancreatic enzymes. A screening abdominal ultrasound should also be considered, although CT is preferable for detection of trauma to solid organs. Possible accidental mechanisms of injury, such as trauma in a bicycle handlebar injury should be considered. But, caution is needed in acceptance of unlikely explanations. Huntmer and colleagues noted no evidence that a fall down stairs led to small bowel perforation. Minor falls are also an unlikely explanation.

Neglect is the most prevalent form of child maltreatment in the USA, with potentially severe and long-lasting sequelae. Neglect has several manifestations that physicians might encounter. Initial questions a physician should consider are: Is this neglect? Have the circumstances harmed the child, or jeopardized the child's health or safety (Panel 3). For example, adherence to a treatment plan might be less than ideal, without clearly impairing a child's health. Inadequacies in the care children receive naturally fall along a continuum, so a range of responses should be tailored to the individual situation. Legal or public agency guidelines could discourage physicians from labeling many circumstances as neglect. They can still intervene to help to ensure that children's needs are adequately met.

There are usually many interacting factors that contribute to neglect. This situation demands a comprehensive assessment of possible underpinning problems—with child, parent, family, and community.

The system of health care should also be examined. Are there barriers to health care? Does a difficult or antagonistic

Panel 3 Manifestations of possible health-related neglect

- Nonadherence to treatment, jeopardizing the child's health
- Delay or failure in obtaining health care—medical, mental, or dental
- Nonorganic failure to thrive or severe obesity that is not being addressed
- Recurring injuries or ingestions suggesting inadequate supervision
- Drug-exposed newborn babies and children
- Exposure to environmental hazards—in and out of the home
- Poor hygiene or sanitation
- Inadequate attention to children's emotional and cognitive needs

relationship exist between the physician and the parent or the child, or both? For example, poor adherence to treatment for asthma could be due to the parent not understanding the treatment plan; the physician might not have communicated the plan clearly. Care is needed to avoid the assumption that the parent is responsible. For example, a complicated medical course does not mean poor adherence to treatment. In addition to probing for risk factors, strengths and resources (protective factors) should also be assessed; these are often crucial for effective intervention. A parent's interest to keep a child out of hospital, for example, can motivate adherence to treatment.

Physicians can notice other forms of neglect. For example, a child might have inadequate clothing or the family could be homeless—situations that can affect children's health. Children might not be enrolled in school. A child could have learning difficulties and the school's response inadequate. A broad view of health and interest in children's health and development includes attention to their environment. Neglect is a disparate problem that needs varied responses to address each case.

OUTCOMES

Child maltreatment has short and long-term medical, mental health, and social sequelae. Children in hospital who have been abused or neglected have more severe injuries, longer hospital stays, worse medical outcomes, higher hospital charges, and are more likely to die during the stay in hospital than other children admitted to hospital. Children with abusive head trauma have a worse short-term outcome than those with head trauma that was not inflicted. The above descriptions of different injuries due to abuse suggest their sizeable morbidity and mortality. Physically abused children are at risk of developing behavioral and functional difficulties, including conduct disorders, aggressive behaviors, decreased cognitive functioning, and poor academic achievement. Neglect is similarly associated with many potential problems.

In adulthood, maltreatment is associated with an increased risk for several health risk behaviors and physical and mental health disorders. Maltreated children are at risk of becoming abusive parents. Preliminary research has shown persistent neurobiological effects of abuse on the developing brain, which could account for some of these sequelae. Some children seem to be resilient and might not manifest sequelae of maltreatment, perhaps because of protective factors or interventions. The benefits of intervention have been seen in even the most severely neglected children, such as those from Romanian orphanages, who were adopted. Early intervention brings the greatest benefit.

REPORTING AND DOCUMENTATION

Many countries have laws mandating physicians and others to refer suspicions of child abuse or neglect to designated public agencies. The referrer does not need to be certain that maltreatment has taken place. The amount of suspicion that meets the threshold for reporting might be a judgment call. Consultation with an interdisciplinary team that is expert in child maltreatment, a pediatric expert, or the public agency, can help to make this decision. Reporting of child maltreatment is not easy. But ensuring the child's safety is the priority, and reporting could be life-saving.

Parental inadequacy or culpability is at least implicit, perhaps evoking anger. Physicians should inform families directly of their concerns and their report in a supportive manner. The referral can be explained as an effort to clarify the situation and provide help, or as a professional (and legal) responsibility. To explain what the ensuing process will probably entail is useful. Ideally, physicians should work cooperatively with the public agency to help ensure children's and families' needs are met.

Clear and comprehensive documentation is especially important because of the possible legal ramifications. Key statements or quotes should be copied verbatim, including the question that prompted the investigation. Physicians often avoid documenting awkward information, such as a parent's hostility toward a child or showing signs of drug abuse. However, such information can be important and should be objectively documented. Good documentation helps to ensure that crucial information is shared and contributes to appropriate interventions.

TREATMENT AND ADVOCACY

The interventions needed depend on the specific issues contributing to a child's maltreatment, and their sequelae, but there are some general principles that can be helpful. Physicians must know the local laws, regulations, and programs for child maltreatment. They are responsible for addressing medical problems, and for recognizing and reporting suspected maltreatment. Although they help to ensure children's safety, decisions about out-of-home placement are the responsibility of the public agencies. Substitute care is sometimes needed, at least temporarily. A comprehensive assessment of the child, the parents, and the family is key to guide appropriate interventions.

Neglect should initially be approached with unintrusive interventions. For example, if an infant's poor growth is due to an error in mixing formula milk, education of the parents and home visits by a nurse should be tried. By contrast, severe failure to thrive needs hospital admission, and in some circumstances (e.g. a mother with psychotic illness), out-of-home placement might be needed. If initial efforts fail, reporting to the public agency is necessary. Physicians should then try to remain involved, and offer families support and guidance. Physicians should also make a referral when other professional intervention is needed (e.g. treatment for substance abuse). The importance of addressing families' needs should not be overlooked. Access to nutrition programs or help with housing, for example, can be urgent. The problems that led to child maltreatment might need long-term support and monitoring, rather than quick fixes.

Advocacy on behalf of children and families can be to individuals, families, communities, and the society. Explaining to a parent that a hyperactive toddler is normal, albeit challenging, and offer alternatives to corporal punishment, illustrates advocacy on behalf of the child. Encouraging a depressed mother to accept treatment is also advocacy. Physician's efforts to strengthen families such as, encouraging father's involvement in childcare, are forms of advocacy. In the community, physician can be influential advocates for resource for children and families by, for example, supporting parenting programs. Working with colleagues in child protection, mental health, education, and law enforcement, physicians can help to address child maltreatment. Finally, in society, physicians can advocate for governmental policies and programs that support children and families. Physician advocacy fits well with a vision of improved child health in the 21st century.

WHEN TO SUSPECT CHILD MALTREATMENT: SUMMARY OF NICE GUIDANCE

Child maltreatment includes neglect; physical, sexual, and emotional abuse; and fabricated or induced illness. It may present in various ways to different healthcare professionals, who have a "duty . . . to be proactive in safeguarding children" but often find it difficult to act on what they find.

Child maltreatment has short and long-term harmful effects on a child's health and well-being; emotional, interpersonal development; and behavior; and in extreme circumstances it may lead to death. Children may present with both physical and psychological symptoms and signs that constitute alerting features of one or more types of maltreatment, which may also be observed as part of the interaction between the parent or carers and the child. The effects of maltreatment may continue throughout adulthood and include physical disability or disfigurement as well as the profound psychological consequences of anxiety, depression, substance misuse, and self-destructive or antisocial behaviors, which may lead to difficulties in forming or sustaining close relationships, sustaining employment, and parenting capacity.

Child maltreatment is under-recognized and inconsistently reported to children's social care by healthcare professionals in England and Wales. The recent death of Baby Peter is yet another reminder of the consequences of missing the alerting features of child maltreatment. The recently published guidance from the National Institute for Health and Clinical Excellence (NICE) aims to raise the awareness of healthcare professionals to the alerting features of child maltreatment. It also aims to support healthcare professionals who are not specialists in child protection in identifying children who may be being maltreated and who require further multiagency assessment to confirm or exclude child abuse or neglect. The scope of this guidance does not cover family and social risk factors, which may in themselves be alerting features. The guidance should not be used as a definitive diagnostic tool to prove or disprove maltreatment. This chapter summarizes key points in the NICE guidance.

KEY POINTS

NICE recommendations are based on systematic reviews of best available evidence. When minimal evidence is available, recommendations are based on the Guideline Development Group's experience and opinion of what constitutes good practice. For this guidance, the Guideline Development Group used a formal Delphi consensus process when the group did not reach a congruent opinion.

Alerting Features

The guideline recommendations refer to "alerting features" in the following categories.

Physical Features

Physical features include any serious or unusual injury with an absent or unsuitable explanation, and particularly in the following categories: abrasions, bites, bruises, burns, cold injuries, cuts, lacerations, ligature marks, petechiae, scalds, scars, and strangulation marks. They also include various sites of internal injury including fractures, spinal and intracranial injuries (including subdural hemorrhage), intra-abdominal and intrathoracic injuries, eye injuries (including retinal hemorrhage), and oral injuries. The recommendations describe specific attributes of these injuries and of the child that should lead the healthcare professional to consider or suspect child maltreatment; in so doing, the recommendations draw attention to the age and developmental stage of the child and the suitability of the explanation given by the parents or carers.

Clinical Presentations

Clinical presentations include:

- Unusual patterns of use of medical services and attendance at medical services;
- Discrepant clinical picture (including fabricated or induced illness);
- poor school attendance attributed to ill health; as well as

- Some particular indicators of ill health (apparent life threatening event; hypernatremia; ingestion of substances including poisoning; nasal bleeding; and near drowning).

Neglect

Neglect includes abandonment and several aspects of failure of provision and failure of supervision. Many of these features must be persistent for a healthcare professional to consider or suspect neglect. Aspects of neglect through failure of provision may include a child who persistently presents as dirty or smelly, with unsuitable clothing, severe infestations, with untreated tooth decay (when NHS treatment is available); whose home conditions are unhygienic or unsafe; or who receives inadequate provision of food or medication. Other aspects of neglect through failure of provision may include lack of adherence to necessary medical advice and persistent failure to engage with relevant child health promotion programs, such as immunization, health and development reviews, and screening. Failure of supervision may be indicated by injuries—for example, a burn, sunburn, an ingestion of a harmful substance, or an animal bite.

The Child's Emotional, Behavioral, and Interpersonal Functioning

This section includes a child's particular behaviors, emotional states, patterns of interpersonal functioning, and other aspects of the child's functioning. These behaviors comprise a wide range of features including aggression; fearfulness; dissociation; low self-esteem; indiscriminate contact or affection seeking; self harm; running away from home; body rocking; aspects of eating and feeding; and soiling and wetting behavior. Patterns of potential concern include age inappropriate behavior; marked change in emotional or behavioral state; and repeated, extreme, or sustained emotional responses by a child that are out of proportion to a situation and are not expected for his or her age and developmental stage.

Interactions Between Parent and Child

Several aspects of interactions between a child and the parent or carer may be harmful, especially when persistent. They include emotional unavailability and unresponsiveness from the parent or carer; hostility towards and rejection and scapegoating of a child; interactions and expectations that are inappropriate for the age of the child, including inappropriate threats or methods of disciplining; exposure to domestic abuse; using the child to fulfill the parent's or carer's needs (for example, involving the child in marital disputes); and failing to promote the child's socialization by isolation or lack of stimulation or education, or by involving the child in unlawful activities.

Terminology

The terms "consider" and "suspect" have been used in the guidance to indicate the level of concern with respect to the various alerting features. These two terms reflect the action(s) to be taken by the healthcare professional when encountering the particular alerting feature. The associated actions are intended to direct healthcare professionals to resources or ways of thinking that will enable them to overcome barriers to recognizing maltreatment. "Consider" means that maltreatment is one possible explanation for the alerting feature or is included in the differential diagnosis.

The actions will lead the healthcare professional to exclude maltreatment, to continue to keep the case under consideration, or to move to a stage of heightened concern where they suspect maltreatment.

"Suspect" means a serious level of concern about the possibility of maltreatment but is not proof of it. This may trigger a child protection investigation, which may indicate the need for starting child protection procedures and/or offering supportive services to the family or may lead to alternative explanations for the reported concerns being identified.

The guidance takes account of alternative causes of the alerting features, both in the recommendations and the processes associated with considering and suspecting child maltreatment.

Overcoming Barriers

Child maltreatment is a sensitive and emotive subject. Healthcare professionals face many obstacles to recognizing and responding to possible maltreatment. This guidance aims to empower and help them to overcome these obstacles, to encourage the appropriate course of action to protect the child or young person from further harm, and to reduce both delay in timely action and the high cost of abuse and neglect to individuals and to society. Support, supervision, education and training of 'front line staff' will be essential if this guidance is to be implemented successfully. Improving the quality of recognition should result in the right child being referred to specialist services for further assessment and protection from further maltreatment.

43.10 CONDUCT DISORDERS IN CHILDREN

JN Vyas

INTRODUCTION

The term conduct disorder refers to a persistent pattern of antisocial behavior in which the individual repeatedly breaks social rules and carries out aggressive acts that upset other people. It is the most common psychiatric disorder of childhood across the world, and the most common reason for referent to child and adolescent mental health services in western countries. Antisocial behavior has the highest continuity into adulthood of all measured human traits except intelligence. A high proportion of children and adolescents with conduct disorder grow up to be antisocial adults with impoverished and destructive lifestyles; a significant minority will develop antisocial personality disorder (psychopath). The disorder in adolescence is becoming more frequent in western countries and places a large personal and economic burden on individuals and society.

RELATION TO OTHER DISORDERS

Conduct disorder is one of the two disruptive disorders of childhood (also known s externalizing disorders); the other is the hyperkinetic syndrome (ICD-10), also known as attention-deficit hyperactivity disorder (DSM-IV). Conduct disorder and the hyperkinetic syndrome are distinct disorders but they often co-occur.

Juvenile delinquency is a legal term referring to an act by a young person who has been convicted of an offence, which would be deemed a crime if committed by an adult. Many but not all, recurrent juvenile offenders have conduct disorder. In this chapter the term conduct disorder is used as defined by ICD-10 diagnostic criteria; the term conduct problems will be used for less severe antisocial behavior.

Changes Made in DSM-5 Diagnostic Criteria for Conduct Disorder

The fifth edition of the *Diagnostic and Statistical Manual of Mental Disorders* (DSM-5) adds a descriptive features specifier to the diagnosis of conduct disorder for individuals who meet the full criteria for the disorder and who also present with limited prosocial emotions, such as limited empathy and guilt. The addition of the specifier will help specialize care and spur additional treatment and causal research.

Using the Specifier

Conduct disorder is characterized by behavior that violates either the rights of others or major societal norms. These symptoms must be present for at least three months with one symptom having been present in the past six months. To be diagnosed with conduct disorder, the symptoms must cause significant impairment in social, academic or occupational functioning. The disorder is typically diagnosed prior to adulthood.

In DSM-5, the criteria for conduct disorder are largely unchanged from DSM-IV, but the limited prosocial specifier is new to DSM-5. The specifier applies to those individuals with a more serious pattern of behavior characterized by a callous and unemotional interpersonal style across multiple settings and relationships. The specifier goes beyond the presence of negative behavior and reflects an individual's typical patterns in emotional and interpersonal functioning. People with conduct disorder who show this specifier display limited empathy and little concern for the feelings, wishes, and well-being of others.

Specializing Care and Spurring Research

Individuals with conduct disorder who meet criteria for the specifier have a relatively more severe form of the disorder and a different treatment response. Thus, the specifier will allow clinicians to more accurately identify and diagnosis individuals who need more intensive and individualized treatment. The specifier attempts to avoid stigmatizing language and focuses on a limited display of prosocial emotions such as empathy and guilt. The specifier will also encourage treatment research to refine what does and does not work for this group of individuals. In addition to treatment, the specifier will impact the research on persons with conduct disorder by designating groups of patients with more similar causal factors.

DSM-5 Diagnostic Criteria for Conduct Disorder

- A repetitive and persistent pattern of behavior in which the basic rights of others or major age-appropriate societal norms or rules are violated, as manifested by the presence of at least three of the following 15 criteria in the past 12 months from any of the categories below, with at least one criterion present in the past 6 months:

Aggression to people and animals:
- Often bullies, threatens or intimidates others.
- Often initiates physical fights.
- Has used a weapon that can cause serious physical harm to others (e.g. a bat, brick, broken bottle, knife, and gun).
- Has been physically cruel to people.
- Has been physically cruel to animals.
- Has stolen while confronting a victim (e.g. mugging, purse snatching, extortion, armed robbery).
- Has forced someone into sexual activity.

Destruction of property:
- Has deliberately engaged in fire setting with the intension of causing serious damage.
- Has deliberately destroyed others property (other than by fire setting).

Deceitfulness or theft:
- Has broken into someone else's house, building or car.
- Often lies to obtain goods or favors or to avoid obligations (i.e. "Cons" others)
- Has stolen items of non trivial value without confronting a victim (e.g. shoplifting, but without breaking and entering : forgery)

Serious violations of rules:
- Often stays out at night despite parental prohibitions, beginning before age 13 years.
- Has run away from home overnight at least twice while living in the parental or parental surrogate home, or once without returning for a lengthy period.
- Is often truant from school, beginning before age 13 years.

- The disturbance in behavior causes clinically significant impairment in social, academic, or occupational functioning.
- If the individual is age 18 years or older, criteria are not met for antisocial personality disorder.

Specify whether:

312.81(F91.1) Childhood-onset type: Individuals show at least one symptom characteristic of conduct disorder prior to age 10 years.

312.82 (F91.2) Adolescent-onset types: Individuals show no symptom characteristic of conduct disorder prior to age 10 years.

312.89(F91.9) Unspecified onset: Criteria for a diagnosis of conduct disorder are met, but there is not enough information available to determine whether the onset of the first symptom was before or after age 10 years.

Specify if:

With limited prosocial emotions: To qualify for this specifier, an individual must have displayed at least two of the following characteristics persistently over at least 12 months and in multiple relationships and settings. These characteristics reflect the individual's typical pattern of interpersonal and emotional functioning over this period and not just occasional occurrences in some situations. Thus, to assess the criteria for the specifier, multiple information sources are necessary. In addition to the individual's self-report, it is necessary to consider reports by others who have known the individual for extended periods of time (e.g. parents, teachers, co-workers, extended family members, peers).

Lack of remorse of guilt: Does not feel bad or guilty when he or she does something wrong (exclude remorse when expressed only when caught and/or facing punishment). The individual shows a general lack of concern about the negative consequences of his or her actions. For example, the individual is not remorseful after hurting someone or does not care about the consequences of breaking rules.

Callous-lack of empathy: Disregards and is unconcerned about feelings of others. The individual is described as cold and uncaring. The person appears more concerned about the effects of his or her actions on himself or herself rather than their effects on others, even when the result in substantial harm to others.

Unconcerned about performance: Does not show concern about poor/problematic performance at school, at work, or in other important activities. The individual does not put forth the effort necessary to perform well, even when expectations are clear, and typically blames others for his or her poor performance.

Shallow or deficient affect: Does not express feelings or show emotions to others, except in ways that seem shallow, insincere, or superficial (e.g. actions contradict the emotion displayed; can turn emotions "on" or "off" quickly) or when emotions expressions are used for gain (e.g. emotions displayed to manipulate or intimidate others).

Specify current severity:

Mild: Few if any conduct problems in excess of those required to make the diagnosis are present, and conduct problems cause relatively minor harm to others (e.g. lying, truancy, staying out after dark without permission, other rule breaking).

Moderate: The number of conduct problems and the effect on others are intermediate between those specified in "mild" and those in "severe" (e.g. stealing without confronting a victim, vandalism).

Severe: Many conduct problems excess of those required to make the diagnosis are present, or conduct problems cause considerable harm to others (e.g. forced sex, physical cruelty, use of a weapon, stealing while confronting a victim, breaking and entering).

SOCIAL PROBLEM OR MEDICAL DIAGNOSIS

Infringement of the rights of other people is a requirement for the diagnosis of conduct disorder. Since the manifestations include a failure to obey social rules despite an apparently intact mental state and social capacities, many have been the disorder as principally socially determined. Therefore, they believe that the responsibility for its cause and elimination lies with people who can influence the socialization process, such as parents, school teachers, social service departments, and politicians. There is some debate within child and adolescent psychiatry as to whether doctors and mental health professionals should be involved in any but the most complex causes. Some have argued that the involvement of medical personal carries the risk of their becoming agents of social control through the misapplication of diagnostic labels, which may lead to abuses of the kind seen in some totalitarian regimes.

However, advances in the last decade have shown there are substantial genetic and biological contributions to conduct disorder, and in some cases the symptoms may be responsive to medication. Work in the last 25 years mainly from the field of child and adolescent mental health has clarified many of the mechanisms contributing to the development and persistence of antisocial behavior, and has led to the development of effective treatment. As yet, these are not being widely used with the children and adolescents who need them. Therefore, psychiatrists need to be able to contribute to the planning and delivery of an appropriate service.

Clinical Features

Aggressive and defiant behaviors is an important part of normal child and adolescent which means ensures physical and social survival. Indeed, parents may express concern if a child is too acquiescent and unassertive. The level of aggressive and defiant behavior varies considerably amongst children, and it is probably most usefully seen as a continuously amongst children, and it is probably most usefully seen as a continuously distributed trail. Empirical studies do not suggest a level at which symptoms become qualitatively different, nor is there a single cut-off point at which they become impairing for the child or a clear problem for others. There is no hump towards the end of the distribution curve of severity to suggest a categorically distinct group who might, on these grounds, warrant a diagnosis of conduct disorder.

Picking a particular level of antisocial behavior to call conduct disorder' is therefore necessarily arbitrary. For all children, the expression of any particular behavior also varies according to the child's age; for example, physical hitting is at a maximum at around 2 years of age but delines to a low level over the next few years. Therefore, any judgment about the significance of the level of antisocial behavior has to be made in the context of the child's age. Before deciding that the behavior is abnormal or a significant problem, a number of other clinical features have to be considered.

- *Level:* Severity and frequency of antisocial acts, compared with children of the same age and gender.
- *Pattern and setting:* The variety of antisocial acts, and the setting in which they are carried out.
- *Persistence:* Duration over time.
- *Impact:* Distress and social impairment of the child: disruption and damage caused to others.

Change in Clinical Features with Age

The type of behavior seen will depend on the age and gender of the individual.

Younger Children, say from 3 to 7 years age, usually present with general defiance of adults' wishes, disobedience of instructions, angry outbursts with temper tantrums, physical aggression to people especially siblings and peers, destruction of property, arguing, blaming others for things that have gone wrong, and a tendency to annoy and provoke others.

In middle childhood, say from the ages of 8 to 11, the above features are often present. However, as the child grows older, stronger, including swearing, lying about what they have been doing, stealing others belongings outside the home, persistent breaking of rules, physical fights, bullying other children, cruelty to animals, and setting fires.

In adolescence, say from 12 to 17, more antisocial behaviors are often added: cruelty and hurting other people, assault, robbery using force, vandalism, breaking and entering houses, stealing from cars, driving and taking away cars without permission, running away from cars, driving and taking away cars without permission, running away from home, truanting from school, and the extensive use of narcotic drugs.

Gender Difference

Severe antisocial behavior is less common in girls, but it also has a different form. Girls are less likely to be physically aggressive and engage in criminal behavior. These include spitefulness, emotional bullying (such as excluding children from groups, spreading rumors so others are rejected by their peers), frequent unprotected sex leading to sexually transmitted diseases, drugs abuse, running away from home, and truancy from school. Compared with boys, fewer girls show the early onset pattern and more have an onset in adolescence.

Pattern and Setting

No single behavior carries special significance. The outlook is determined by the frequency and intensity of antisocial behaviors, the variety of types, the number of settings in which they occur, and their persistence. The main settings where antisocial behavior in children and adolescents is manifested are home, school, and in public. For general populations of children, agreement about the presence of antisocial behavior at home and at school is low—the correlation between parent and teacher ratings on the same measures is only 0.2 to 0.3. There are many children who are perceived to be mild to moderately antisocial at home but well behaved at school. However, for more severe antisocial behavior, their antimanifestations occur both at home and at school. The antisocial behaviors occur in public place, more commonly in adolescent that often leads to police involvement.

Persistence

Many children go through phases of becoming more defiant and argumentative for a few weeks of months. Sometimes this may be a reaction to a change in circumstances such as setting into a new school, adjusting to a new step parent or losing a friend or losing a friend or loved one. Only when difficult behavior has been present for say 6 months or more is it likely to indicate substantial problems.

Impact

At home the child is often subject to high levels of criticism and hotilty, and sometimes made a scapegoat for a catalog of family misfortunes. Frequent punishments and physical abuse are not uncommon. The whole family atmosphere is often soured and siblings are also affected. Maternal depression is often present, and families who are unable to cope may, as a last resort, give up the child to be measures to attempt to control the child and protect the other pupils, including sending the child out of the class, sometimes culminating in permanent exclusion from the school. This may lead to reduced opportunity to learn subjects on the curriculum and poor examination results. The child typically has few if any friends, as other children cannot tolerate his aggressive behavior. This often leads to exlusion from many group activities, games, and trips, also restricting the child's quality of life and experiences. On leaving school the lack of social skills, low level of qualifications, and presence of a police record make it harder to gain employment.

The experience of rejection and failure at home, at school, and with peers usually leads to a negative self-image and low self-esteem, but is not usually described by the young persons as actively distressing. In later adolescence intimate sexual relationships tend to be made with other young people who are also antisocial, and are frequently disruptive and violent.

Classification

The ICD-10 classification has a category for conduct disorders, (F91). According to the ICD-10 Clinical Descriptions and Guidelines, example of the behaviors on which the diagnosis is based include the following: excessive levels of fighting or bullying; cruelty to animals or other people; severe destructiveness to property; firesetting; stealing; repeated lying; truancy from school and running away from home; unusually frequent and severe temper tantrums; defiant provocative behavior; and persistent severe disobedience. Any one of these categories, if marked, is sufficient for the diagnosis, but isolated dissocial acts are not.

An enduring pattern of behavior should be present, but no timeframe is given and there is no impairment or impact criterion stated.

The ICD-10 Diagnostic Criteria for Research differ, requiring symptoms to have been present for at least 6 months, and the introductory rubric indicates that impact upon others (in terms of violation of their basic rights), but not impairment of the child, can contribute to the diagnosis. The research criteria take a menu-driven approach, whereby a cetain number of symptoms have to be present. It lists 15 behaviors to consider for the diagnosis of conduct disordes, which usually, but not exlusively, apply to older children and teenagers. They can be grouped into four classes.

1. Aggression to people and animals:
    - Frequently initiates physical fights (this does not include fights with siblings)
    - Has used a weapon that can cause serious physical harm to others (e.g. bat, brick, broken bottle, knife, gun)
    - Often stays out after dark despite parenting prohibition (beginning before 13 years of age)
    - Exhibits physical cruelty to other people (e.g. ties up, cuts or burns a victim)
    - Exhibits physical cruelty to animals.
2. Destruction of property:
    - Deliberately destroys the property of others (other than by fire-setting)
    - Deliberately sets fires with a risk or intention causing serious damage
3. Deceitfulness or theft:
    - Often lies or breaks promises to obtain goods or favors or to avoid obligations
    - Steals objects of nontrivial values without confronting the vitctim, either within the home or outside (e.g. shoplifting, burglary, forgery).
4. Serious violations of rules:
    - Is frequenctly truant from school, beginning before 13 years of age
    - Has run away from the parental or parental surrogate home at least twice or has run away once for more than a single night (this does not include leaving to avoid physical or sexual abuse)
    - Commits a crime involving confrontation with the victim (including purse-snatching, extortion, mugging)
    - Forces another person into sexual activity

- Frequently bullies others (e.g. deliberate infliction of path or hurt, including persistent intimidation, tormenting, or molestation)
- Breaks into someone else's house, building, or car.

To make a diagnosis, three symptoms from this list have to be present, one for at least 6 months. There is no impairment criterion. There are three subtypes: **conduct disorder confined to the family context** (F91.0) **unsocialized conduct disorder** (F91.1), where the young person has no friends and is rejected by peers, and **socialized conduct disorder** (**socialized conduct disorder** (F91.2), where peer relationships are normal. It is recommended that the age of onset be specified, with childhood onset type manifesting before age 10, and adolescent-onset type after, severity should categorized as mild, moderate, or severe according to the number of symptoms or impart on others (e.g. causing severe physical injury, vandalism, theft).

For younger children, say up to 9- or 10 years old, there is a list of eight symptoms for the subtype known as oppositional—defiant disorder (F9.3):

- Has unusually frequent or severe temper tantrums for his or her developmental level;
- Often argues with adults;
- Often actively refuses adult's requests or defies rules;
- Often, apparently deliberately, does things that annoy other people;
- Often blames others for his or her own mistakes or misbehavior;
- Is often 'touchy' or easily annoyed by others;
- Is often angry or resentful;
- Is often spiteful or vindictive.

To make a diagnosis of the oppositional-defiant type of conduct disorder, four symptoms from either this list or the 'main' conduct disorder 15-symptoms list have to be present, but no more than two from the later. Unlike the 'main' variant, there is an impairment criterion: the symptoms must be "maladaptive and inconsistent with the developmental level."

Where there are sufficient symptoms of a comorbid disorder to meet diagnostic criteria, the ICD-10 system discourages the application of a second diagnosis, and instead offers a single combined category. There are two major kinds; mixed disorder of conduct and emotions, of which depressive conduct disorder (F92.0) is the best researched, and hyperkinetic conduct disorder (F90.1). There is modest evidence to suggest these combined condition may differ somewhat from their constituent elements.

The DSM-IV system follows the ICD-10 research criteria very closely and does not have separate clinical guidelines. The same 15 behaviors are given for the diagnosis of conduct disorder 312.8, with almost identical wording. As for ICD-10, there symptoms need to be present for diagnosis. Severity, and childhood or adolescent onset are specification in the same way. However, unlike ICD-10, there is no division into socialized/unsocialized, or family-context-only types, and there is a requirement for the behavior to cause a clinically significant impairment is in social, academic, or social functioning. Comorbidity in DSM-IV is handled by giving as many separate diagnoses as necessary, rather than by single combined categories.

In DSM-IV, oppositional defend disorder is classification as a separate disorder on its own, and not as a subtype of conduct disorder. Diagnosis requires four symptoms from a list of eight behavior, which are the same as for ICD-10; but unlike ICD-10, all four have to be from the oppositional list, and many come from the main conduct disorder list. It is doubtful whether oppositional-defiant disorder differs substantially from conduct disorder in older children in any associated characteristics, and the value of designating it as a separate disorder is arguable. In this chapter, the term conduct disorder will henceforth be used as it is in ICD-10, to refer to all variants; oppositional-defiant disorder is included in this as a specific subtype.

Differential Diagnosis

Making a diagnosis of conduct disorder is usually is straight forward since parent readily volunteer the symptoms, although it is essential to obtain an independent report from school so as to overlook behavior in that context. Sometimes the diagnosis may be inappropriate since antisocial behavior may arise as part of other disorders such as autism or main, or not be severe enough to warrant a diagnosis. More commonly the diagnosis is correct but comorbid condition are missed. The differential diagnosis may include the following:

- **Hyperkinetic syndrome/attention-deficit hyperactivity disorder:** These are the names given by ICD-10 and DSM-IV respectively to very similar condition. For convenience the term hyperactivity will be used here. The condition is characterized by impulsivity, inattention, and motor overactivity. Any of these three sets of symptoms can be misconstrued as antisocial, particularly impulsivity which is also present in conduct disorder. However, none of the symptoms of conduct disorder are a part of hyperactivity so excluding conduct disorder should not be difficult. However, a frequent error should not be made to miss comorbid hyperactivity when conduct disorder is definitely present.
- **Adjustment reaction to an external stressor:** This can be diagnosed when onset occurs soon after exposure to an identifiable psychosocial stressor such as divorce, bereavement, trauma, abuse, or adoption. The onset should within 1 month for ICD-10, and 3 months for DSM-IV, and symptoms should not persist for more than 6 month after the cessation of the stress or its squeal
- **Mood disorder:** Depression can present with irritability and oppositional symptoms, but unlike typical conduct

disorder mood is usually clearly low and there are vegetable features; also more severe conduct problem are absent. Early manic-depressive disorder can be harder to distinguish, as there is often considerable defiance and irritability combined with disregard for rules, and behavior which violates the right of other. Sometime the mania only becomes obvious years later, but in retrospect was clearly driving the antisocial conduct. The greater risk, however, is to miss depressive symptoms in young people with definite conduct disorder. Low self-esteem is the norm in conduct disorder, as is a lack of friend or constructive pastimes. Therefore it is easy to overlook more pronounced depressive symptoms, particularly as they are usually not complained of by the young person. Systematic surveys reveal that around a third of children with conduct disorder have depressive or other emotional symptoms server enough to warrant a diagnosis.

- **Autistic spectrum disorders:** These are often accompanied by marked tantrums or destructiveness, which may be the reason for seeking a referral. Enquiring about other symptoms of autistic spectrum disorders should symptoms of autistic spectrum disorders should reveal their presence.
- **Dissocial/antisocial personality disorder:** In ICD-10 it is suggested that a person should be 17 years of age or older before dissocial personality is considered. Since at age 18 most diagnoses specific to childhood and adolescence no longer apply, in practice there is seldom difficulty. In DSM-IV conduct disorder can be diagnosed at over 18 years of age and so there is potential overlap. A difference in emphasis is the severity and pervasiveness of the symptoms of those with personality disorder, where by all individual's relationships are affected by the behavior pattern, and the individual's beliefs about his antisocial behavior are characterized by callousness and lack of remorse.
- **Subcultural deviance:** Some youths are antisocial and commit crimes but are not particularly aggressive or defiant. They are well adjusted within a deviant peer culture that approves of recreational drug use, shoplifting, etc. In some localities a third or more teenage males fit this description and would meet ICD-10 diagnostic guidelines for socialized conduct disorder.

Multiaxial Assessment

ICD-10 recommends that multiaxial assessment be carried out for children and adolescents, while DSM-IV suggests it for all ages. In both systems Axis 1 is used for psychiatric disorders which have been discussed above. The last three axes in both system cover general medical conditions, psychosocial problems, and level of social funcology. In the middle are two axes in ICD-10, which covers perosanlity disorders and general mental retardation.

It is essential to assess both specific and general mental retardation in individuals with conduct problems. Fully a third of children with conduct disorder also have specific reading retardation, defined as having a reading level of two standard deviations below that predicted by the person's IQ. While this may in part be due to a lack of adequate schooling, there is good evidence that the cognitive deficits often precede the behavioral problems. General mental retardation is often missed in children with conduct disorder unless IQ testing is carried out. The rate of conduct disorder rises several-fold as IQ falls below 50.

EPIDEMIOLOGY

Prevalence According to Age

Preschool Children

The prevalence of serious oppositional behavior in preschool children has been found to be between 4 and 9%.

Adolescents: The rate of oppositional disorder has been rated as being as high as 15% and that of sever conduct disorders between 6 and 12%.

Early onset versus adolescent-onset patterns: There are major differences between early adolescent onset. Those with an early onset display defiant and aggressive behavior before the age of 8, but is typically begins around 3 years of age. They grow older. However, not all young children with this early-onset pattern of problems progress to more severe difficulties later in childhood. Only about half of these child's symptoms persist; the remaining child symptoms improve subsequently. Compared with the adolescent-onset group, the early-onset children already at 3 years of age show a more difficult temperament (restlessness, inattention, negativity, irritability, etc.). At school age this group have cognitive, language, and motor deficits, reading difficulties, adverse family contexts, and poor parenting. By the age of 18 they have fewer friends and feel socially alienated, victimized, and are callous and suspicious. They continue behaving antisocially as adults. Some have called this group early onset-lifetime persistent.

Adolescent onset: About three times more common are the adolescent-onset group who have not shown significant antisocial behavior earlier in their lives, antisocially, so some call them an adolescence-limited group. The overall rate of arrests and convictions is somewhat lower than the childhood onset. Their behavior tends to be less aggressive and violent, less impulsive, they have fewer cognitive and neuropsychological deficits, tend to come from less dysfunctional family environments, and tend to have more adaptive social qualities. Crucially, among the adolescent-onset group, only a small group of individuals (less) than 10% of the total commence persistent antisocial activity in adulthood.

Sex difference: Conduct disorder is more common in boys at all ages, but the ratio of boys to girls depends on the type. In adolescence the ratio narrows to around 2:1. However, for DSM-IV conduct disorder, which includes several violent offences, the ratio is up to 10:01. Definitions that include abuse of drugs and precocious sexual activity show a greater proportion of girls.

Social class: Conduct disorder is three to four more common in children who are in socioeconomically deprived families with low income, or who receive state benefits or selfare, or who live in a poor neighborhood. Each of these indices overlap considerably, and each is a marker or many of the etiological factors discussed below.

Geographical location: Rates found in surveys carried out on Western countries such as the United Kingdom, the United States, France, New Zealand, and Canada have found very similar rates when comparable methods have been used.

Surveys in other locations such as Hong Kong and South America have found lower prevalence. Within countries, many, but not all, studies have found increased rates in urban compared with rural locations.

Etiology

Genes and environment: Conduct disorder cluster in families. Until the 1980s most twin studies of antisocial behavior showed a high concordance for monozygotic pairs at around 70–80%, suggesting a major share familial influence, a moderate unique environmental contribution for the individual, and only a limited genetic component.

Family Environment

Parent-child Environment

Fine-grained analysis by Patterson has shown that the moment-to-moment responses of parents towards children have a powerful effect on their behavior. In families with a conduct-disordered child, the children are likely to be ignored when they are behaving reasonably, but criticized and shouted at when they are misbehaving. The consequence is that to gain attention, they have to behave badly. What is perhaps surprising is that for these children who receive very little positive attention, they are prepared to elicit often unpleasant and Frankl hostile reactions from their parents rather than be ignored. By contrast, children who receive a reasonable amount of positive attention within the family tend to avoid behaving in a way that elicits negastates that children will behave in whatever way necessary to gain reasonable amount of attention.

Most emphasis in social learning theory has been on the harmful effect of negative behavior. However, other research has made it clear that the presence of positive parental behavior is equally the time by their parents, who do not respond to their overtures to join in activities, or praise them when they are behaving well. Not only does this make quiet prosocial activity less likely, but also no models are provided for the child to learn social skills such as turn-taking, negotiating skills, etc.

Parenting Practices

Conduct disorder is strongly associated with harsh erratic discipline, hostility directed at the child, lack of warmth, and poor supervision. However, up and inter vention studies show that these factors have a causal role in initiating and maintaining the child's disorder and are not just reaction to the child's behavior. The association of conduct disorder with large family size, and with broken homes (divorce, single parenthood, adoption), seem chiefly to be mediated by parenting practices and the previous characteristics of the individuals, rather than by the impact of a large family or broken home in themselves.

Psychiatric Disorder in Parents

Depression features commonly in mothers; alcoholism, drug abuse, and psychoses are not infrequent in parents of children with severe conduct disorder. These disorders exert their effects in childhood through the quality of interaction and parenting practices, and by affecting the inherited characteristics, of the child. There is no specialties child psychiatric disorder which is more common, but conduct problems are more frequent as are emotional disorders. Children of depressed mothers may have impaired cognitive and social development.

Criminality of the Father

As an environmental influence, this is important and may be mediated through parent-child interactions and parenting practices as described above, plus an antisocial set of values and living in a deprived neighborhood. It also represents an increased genetic risk.

Physical and Sexual Abuse

Physical and sexual abuse can lead to the emergence of conduct problems in girls or boys who were previously free of such problems. Kessler et al. found that physical aggression from the father was associated with a more than doubling of the rates of conduct disorder and Mebride-change found sexual and physical abuse associated with a wide range of poor outcomes. The difficulty in ascertaining their effect arises, as they are usually associated with multiple other risk factors such as poor parenting and rejection, in addition to a genetic predisposition. Widom, however, found that early childhood victimization only raised later criminality by 50 percent.

Obstetric Complications

Obstetric complications have no or only an extremely weak influence on antisocial behavior; Raine has suggested they contribute to violent behavior, but the evidence is unconvincing. There is more evidence that prenatal in utero exposure to alcohol and cocaine can impair brain development and lead to impulsivity and lower IQ, and hence antisocial behavior.

Environment Beyond the Family

School organization has been shown to affect the rates of antisocial behavior independently of home background. Poorly organized unfriendly schools with low staff morale, high staff turnover, and poor contact with parents have higher rates of conduct disorder even when catchment area characteristics have been allowed for.

Peer Influences

Conduct disorder is more likely in children who associate with friends who have an antisocial attitude, value aggression, and commit destructive and rule-breaking acts. Associating with deviant peers increases conduct problems independently of the individual's level of aggression. In adolescence, quite a lot of antisocial behavior is carried out with peers, sometimes in gangs. Together, conduct-disordered youths encourage and approve talk about antisocial activities and tend not to on delinquent acts. If children are rejected by their peers, the chance of later conduct problems is increased. This seems to apply particularly to early-onset conduct disorder. Treatments that put antisocial youths together in groups often increase the level of antisocial behavior.

Alcohol and Drugs

Many of the risk factors that lead to alcohol and drug abuse are similar to those for antisocial behavior. However, the relationship is more than just a passive overlap. Antisocial behavior increases the chances of substance abuse, and vice versa. Longitudinal surveys show that antisocial behavior in childhood and adolescence increases the risk of later alcohol- and drug-related problems, which peak in the twenties. ('Problems' refers to regular use of hard drugs or heavy drinking, with psychosocial impairment or medical complications as a result. This differs from the occasional or 'recreational' use of marijuana or hallucinogens, which is far more widespread, or alcohol use without crime as it causes disinhibition and is associated with a range of disorderly and violent offences. With alcohol, heavy drinking increase the chance of crime as it causes disinhibition and is associated with a range of disorderly and violent offences. With drugs, there is an increase in theft drugs may use violent methods to protect their business.

Neighborhood

Conduct problems are associated with overcrowding, poor housing, and poor neighborhood. How much these factors are causal or simply markers for other family or socioeconomic variables is unclear. Multivariate analyses suggest that when factors such as poor parenting and maternal depression are accounted from, neighborhood and poverty effects are not large. However, it is plausible that stressful living conditions with few amenities from children and many other demands on parents impair their ability to bring up their children constructively and responsively. Also areas where there are closet relationships between neighbors with high perceived social cohesion by residents and informal social controls have less antisocial behavior. Moving out of a deprived area reduces the rates of antisocial behavior.

Child Characteristics

Temperament and Personality

Infants with temperaments classified as difficult at 3 years of age are more likely to be referred for aggressive problems later on. The dimensions involved are behavioral impulsivity (lack of restraint), short attention span, and motor restlessness. Although not occurring at a clinical level, these are precisely the constituents of the hyperkinetic syndromes, together with the trait of negative emotionality (irritability, anger, and bad moods) they have a clear modest effect in predicting later antisocial behavior of the early-onset type. Social anxiety on the other hand is protective.

Thinking Style

Significant cognitive attributional bias has been shown in aggressive children and youths. They are more likely to perceive neutral acts by others as hostile, and are more, likely to believe conflicts can be satisfactorily resolved by aggression. As the individual becomes more disliked and rejected by his peers, the opportunity of or seeing things this way increases. By the late teenage years these youths can have a highly suspicious attitude, and be quick to perceive disrespect from others and sometimes react explosively. Social skills are lacking. Emotional processes in antisocial children have been little studied, although self-esteem, is often low and ecoexistent misery common. Youths with conduct disorder have been shown to plan their lives less than controls, so that they are more driven by events than in control of them.

IQ

Early-onset lifetime-persistent children have IQs between 8 and 10 points below controls. The relationship with antisocial behavior weakens after allowing for social class but is still present, although it only accounts for a few percent of the variance. It is not just the effect of missing schooling, since it is present before children go to school. Much of the association can be accounted for by the association with hyperactivity. It seems likely that low IQ alone does not confer much increased risk of antisocial behavior, but in the presence of adverse parenting and other risks, it has an interactive effect.

Physiological Characteristics

Physique has little influence on antisocial propensity. The relationship between testosterone (and other androgens) and antisocial behavior is complex. Levels vary with age, type of antisocial behavior, and social rejection, so that no straightforward conclusion can be drawn; certainly to date no obvious relationship has been shown between higher levels and more aggression.

However, autonomic arousal has shown a consistent, albeit modest, association with persistent antisocial behavior in young people. Their pulse rates are lower, their skin conductance is less, as is their rate of adresnaline and cortisol excretion. Some have postulated that this leads to less anxiety when taking risk. With wider picture of decreased central nervous system inhibition. With all these psysiological substrates and mechanism, the direction of effect is unlikely to be only biology-driven behavior, equally, confrontational situations, social dominance, peer rejection, and self-esteem do influence physiological parameters.

Course and Prognosis

Of those with early-onset conduct disorder (before 8 years of age about half persist with serious problems into adulthood. Of those with adolescent onset, the great majority (over 85 percent) desist in their antisocial behavior by their early twenties.

Many of the factors, children who do well despite adverse risk factors have been studied. However, these so-called 'resilient' children have been shown to have lower levels of risk factors, for example, a boy with supportive concerned parents. Protective factors are mostly the opposite end of the spectrum of the same risk factor; thus good parenting and high IQ are protective. Nonetheless there are factors associated with resilience independent of know adverse influences. These include a good relationship with at least one adult, who does not necessarily have to be the parent, a sense of pride and self-esteem, and skills or competencies.

Table 13: Factors predicting poor outcome

Onset: Early onset of severe problems (before age 8 years)
Phenomenology: Antisocial acts which are severe, frequent, and varied
Comorbidity: Hyperactivity and attention problems
Intelligence: Lower IQ
Family history: Parental criminality Parental alcoholism
Parentin: Harsh inconsistent parenting with high criticism, low warmth, low involvement, and low supervision
Wider environment: Low-income family in poor neighborhood with ineffective schools.

Table 14: Adult outcome

Antisocial behavior: More violent and nonviolent crimes (e.g. mugging, grievous bodily harm, theft, car crime, fraud)
Psychiatric problems: Increased rates of antisocial personality, alcohol and drug abuse, anxiety, depression and somatic complaints, episodes of self-harm and completed suicide, time in psychiatric hospitals
Education and training: Poorer examination results, more truancy and early school leaving, fever vocational qualifications
Work: More unemployment, low involvement with relatives, neighbors, clubs, and organizations
Social network: Few if any significant friends, low involvement with relative, neighbors, clubs and organizations
Intimate relationships: Increased rate of short-lived violent cohabiting relationships; partners often also antisocial
Children: Increased rates of child abuse, conduct problems in offspring, children taken into care
Health: More medical problems, earlier death

Adult Outcome

Studies of groups of children with early-onset conduct disorder indicate a wide range of problems not only confined to antisocial acts, as shown in Table 13.

What is clear is that not only are there substantially increased rates of antisocial acts, but that the general psychosocial functioning of children with conduct disorder when grown up is strikingly poor. For most of the characteristics shown in Table 14, the increase compared with controls in at least double for community cases who were never referred, an three to four times to referred children.

Pathways

The path from childhood conduct disorder to poor adult outcome is neither inevitable nor linear.

Different sets of influences impinge as the individual grows up and shape the life-course. Many of these can accentuate problems. Thus a toddler with an irritable temperament and short attention span, and where he can only get his way by behaving antisocially and grasping of what he needs. At school he may fall in with a deviant crowd of peers, where violence and other antisocial acts are talked-up and give him a sense of esteem. His generally poor academic ability and difficult behavior in class may lead him to truant increasingly, which in turn makes him fall further behind in education. He may then leave school with no qualifications and fail to find a job, and resort to drugs. To fund his drug habit he may resort to crime and, once convicted, find it even harder to get a job. From this example, it can be seen that adverse experiences do not only arise passively and independently of the young person's behavior; rather, the behavior predisposes them to end up in risky and damaging environments. Consequently, the number of adverse life events experienced is greatly increased. The path from early heperactivity into later conduct disorder is also net inevitable. In the presence of a warm supportive family atmosphere it is far less likely than if the parents are highly critical and hostile.

Other influences can, however, steer the individual away from an antisocial path. Examples are being separated from a deviant peer group, marrying a nondeviant partner, moving away from a poor neigborhood and military service which imparts skills (but not harsh boot camps).

TREATMENT

Evidence

Proven treatments include those which singly or in combination address:

- Parenting skills
- Child interpersonal skills
- Difficulties at school
- Peer group influences
- Medication for coexistent hyperactivity.

Parenting Skills

Parent management training aims to improve parenting skills. There are scores of randomized controlled trials showing that it is effective from children up to about 10 years old. They address the poarenting practices identified in research as contributing to conduct problems. A more detailed account is given in Scott. Typically, they include five elements.

1. **Promoting play and a positive relationship:** In order to cut into the cycle of deviant behavior and recriminations, it is important to instill some positive experiences for both sides and begin to mend the relationship. Teaching parents the techniques of how to play in a constructive and non-hostile way with their children helps them recognize the child's needs and to respond sensitively. The children in turn begin to like and respect their parents more, and become more secure in the relationship.
2. **Praise and rewards for sociable behavior:** Parents are helped to reformulate difficult behavior. For example, instead of shouting at the child not to run, they would praise him whenever he walks quietly; then he will do it more often. Though hundreds of such prosaic daily interactions, child behavior when it happens, with the result that it becomes less frequent.
3. **Clear rules and clear commands:** Rules need to be explicit and constant; commands need to be firm and brief. Thus shouting at a child to stop being naughty does not tell him what he should do, whereas telling him to play quietly, for example, gives a clear instruction which makes compliance easier.
4. **Consistent and calm consequences for unwanted behavior:** Disobedience and aggression need to be responded to firmly and calmly by, for example, putting the child in a room for a few minutes. This method of 'time out from positive reinforcement' sounds simple, but requires considerable skill to administer effectively. More minor annoying behaviors such as whining and shouting often repond to being ignored, but again parents often find this hard to achieve in practice.
5. **Reorganizing the child's day to prevent trouble:** There are often trouble spots in the day which will respond to fairly simple measures, such as putting siblings in different rooms to prevent fights on getting home from school, banning television in the morning until the child is dressed, and so on.

Treatment scan be given individually to the parent and child, which enables live feedback in light of the parent's progress and the child's response. Alternatively, group treatments with parents alone have been shown to be equally effective.

Trials show that parent management training is effective in reducing child antisocial behavior in the short-term, with moderate to large effect sizes of 0.5–0.8 standard deviations, and there is little loss of effect at 1 – or 3 year follow-up. parenting skills' interventions are successful use with delinquent boys.

Family Function

Functional family therapy, multisystemic therapy, and treatment foster care aim to change a range of difficulties that impede the effective functioning of teenagers with conduct disorder. Functional family therapy addresses family processes which need to be present, such as improving communication between parent and young person, reducing imterparental inconsistency, tightening up on supervision and monitoring, and negotiating rules and the sanctions to be applied for breaking them. Functional family therapy has been shown to reduce reoffending rates by around 50%. Other varieties of family therapy have not been subjected to controlled trials for young people with conduct disorder or delinquency, so cannot be evaluated for their efficacy.

In multisystemic therapy the young person's and family's needs are assessed in their own context at home and in their relationships with other systems such as school and peers. Following the assessment, proven methods of intervention are used to address difficulties and promote strengths. Multisystemic therapy differs from most types of family therapy, such as the Milan or systemic approach as usually practiced, in a number or ways.

- Treatment is delivered in the situation where the young person lives, for instance at home.
- The therapist has a low caseload (four to six families) and the team is available 24 hours a day.
- The therapist is responsible for ensuring appointments are kept and for making change happen—families cannot be blamed for failing to attend or 'not being ready' to change.
- Regular written feedback on progress towards goals from multiple sources in gathered by the therapist and acted upon.
- There is a manual for following the therapeutic approach and adherence is checked weekly by the supervisor.

Several randomized controlled trial attest to effectiveness, with reoffending rates typically cut by half and time spent in psychiatric inpatient care further reduced.

Treatment foster care is another way of improving the quality of encouragement and supervision that teenagers with conduct disorder receive. The young person lives with a foster family specially trained in effective techniques; sometimes it is ordered as an alternative to jail. Outcome studies show useful reductions in reoffending rates.

Child Interpersonal Skills

Most of programs to improve child interpersonal skills drive from cognitive-behavior therapy—there of the most effective are self-instructional training, the Anger Coping Program, and proself-instructional training, and promoting alternative thinking strategies (PATHS). These and other programs have in common training the young person to:

- Slow down impulsive response to challenging situations by stopping and thinking;
- Recognize his or her own level of physiological arousal, and his or her own emotional state;
- Recognize and define problems;
- Develop several alternative responses;
- Choose the best alternative based on anticipation of consequence;
- Reinforce his- or herself for use of this approach. Over the longer term they aim to increase positive social behavior by teaching the young person to:
  - Learn skills to make and sustain friendship;
  - Develop social interaction skills such as turn-taking and sharing;
  - Express viewpoints in appropriate ways and listen to others.

Typically, given alone, treatment gains with interpersonal skills training are good within the treatment setting, but they only generalize slightly to 'real life' situations such as the school playground. However, when they are part of a more comprehensive program, which has those outside the young person reinforcing the approach, they add to outcome gains.

Difficulties at School

These can be divided into learning problems to deal with specific learning probles such as specific reading retardation, for instance the reading recovery program. However, few of the programs have been specifically evaluated for their ability to improve outcome in children with conduct disorder although trials are in progress. Preschool education programs for high-risk populations have been shown to reduce arrest rates and improve employment in adulthood.

There are several schemes for improving classroom behavior, varying from those that stress improved communication such as 'circle time', and those that work on behavioral principles such as the good theme schemes have been shown to improve classroom behavior, and some specifically target children with conduct disorder.

Peer Group Influence

A few interventions have aimed to reduce the bad influence of deviant peers. However, a number have attempted this through group work with other conduct-disordered youths, but outcome studies showed a worsening of antisocial behavior. Current treatments therefore either see youths individually and try to steer them away from deviant peers, or work in small groups (say three to five youths) where the therapist can control the content of sessions. Some interventions for conduct disorder in group with well-functioning youth has led to favorable outcomes.

Medication of Coexistent Hyperactivity

Where there is comorbid hyperactivity in addition to conduct disorder several studies attest to a large reduction (effect size, 0.8 standard deviations or great) in both overt and covert antisocial behavior, both at home and at school. However, the impact on long-term outcome is unstudied.

Management

Engagement of the family is particularly important for this group of children and families as drop-out from treatment is high, at around 30–40%. Practical measures such as assisting with transport, providing childcare, holding sessions in the evening or at other times to suit the family will all help.

Many of the parents of children with conduct disorder may themselves have difficulty with authority/and officialdom and be very sensitive to criticism. Therefore, the approach is more likely to succeed if is respectful of their point of view, does not offer overly prescriptive solutions, and does not directly criticize parenting style. Practical homework tasks increase changes, as do problem-solving telephone calls from the therapist between sessions.

Parenting interventions may need to go beyond skill development to address more distal factors that prevent change. For example, drug or alcohol abuser in either parent, maternal depression, and a violent relationship with the partner are all common. Assistance in claiming welfare and benefits and help with financial planning may reduce stress from debts.

A multimodal approach is likely to result in large changers. Therefore involving the school in treatment by visiting and offering strategies for managing the child in class is usually helpful, as is advocating from extra tuition where necessary. If the school seems unable to cope despite extra resources, consideration should be given to moving the child to a different school that specializes in the management of behavioral difficulties. Avoiding antisocial peers and building self-esteem may be helped by encouraging the child to attend after-school clubs and holiday activities.

Where parents are not coping or a damaging abusive relationship is detected, it may be necessary to liaise with the social services department to arrange respite for the parents or a spell of foster care. It is important during this time to work with the family to increase their skills to the family. Where there is permanent break-down, long-term fostering or adoption may be recommended.

Opportunities for Prevention

Conduct disorder should offer good opportunities for prevention since:

- It can be detected early reasonably well;
- Early intervention is more effective than late intervention;
- There are a number of effective interventions.

In the United States a number of comprehensive interventions based on up-to-date empirical findings are being carried out. Perhaps the best known is Families and Schools Together. Here the most antisocial 10% of 5–6-year-old in schools in disadvantaged areas were selected, as judged by teacher and parent reports. They were then offered intervention, which was given for a whole year in the first instance and comprised the following:

- Weekly parent training, in groups with videotapes;
- An interpersonal sills' training program for the whole class;
- Academic tutoring twice a week;
- Home visits from the parent trainer;
- A paring program with sociable peers from the class.

RECOGNITION, INTERVENTION, AND MANAGEMENT OF ANTISOCIAL BEHAVIOR AND CONDUCT DISORDERS IN CHILDREN AND YOUNG PEOPLE: SUMMARY OF NICE GUIDANCE

Antisocial behavior and conduct disorders (including oppositional defiant disorder and conduct disorder) are the most common mental and behavioral problems in children and young people globally, with the frequency increasing in Western countries. In the United Kingdom 5% of mental and behavioral problems in children and young people (≤ 18 years) meet criteria for a conduct disorder, as do almost 40% of looked-after children, children who have been abused, and those on child protection or safeguarding registers. Conduct disorders are strongly associated with poor performance at school, social isolation, substance misuse, and involvement with the criminal justice system. A large proportion of children and young people with a conduct disorder will go on to be antisocial adults with impoverished and destructive lifestyles, especially if the conduct problems develop early, and a large minority will be diagnosed with antisocial personality disorder. Antisocial behavior and conduct disorders often coexist with other mental health problems, place a heavy personal and economic burden on individuals and society, and involve a wide range of health, social care, educational, and criminal justice services.

This chapter summarizes the most recent recommendations from the National Institute for Health and Clinical Excellence (NICE) on recognizing and managing antisocial behavior and conduct disorders in children and young people. The guideline was developed jointly with the Social Care Institute for Excellence (SCIE).

RECOMMENDATIONS

The NICE recommendations are based on systematic reviews of the best available evidence and explicit consideration of cost effectiveness. When minimal evidence is available, recommendations are based on the Guideline Development Group's experience and opinion of what constitutes good practice. Evidence levels for the recommendations are given in italic in square brackets.

Working Safely and Effectively

Health and social care professionals working with children and young people who present with behavior suggestive of a conduct disorder, or who have a conduct disorder, should be trained and competent to work with children and young people of all levels of learning ability, cognitive capacity, emotional maturity, and development.

Selective Prevention

Offer classroom based emotional learning and problem solving programs for children typically aged 3–7 years in schools where classes have a high proportion of children identified to be at risk of developing oppositional defiant disorder or conduct disorder resulting from any of the following factors:
- Low socioeconomic status
- Low school achievement
- Child abuse or parental conflict
- Separated or divorced parents
- Parental mental health or substance misuse problems
- Parental contact with the criminal justice system.

Provide these programs in a positive atmosphere and ensure the interventions are designed to:
- Increase children's awareness of their own and others' emotions
- Teach self-control of arousal and behavior
- Promote a positive self-concept and good peer relations
- Develop children's problem solving skills.

Typically the programs should consist of up to 30 classroom based sessions over the course of one school year.

Initial Assessment of Children and Young People with a Possible Conduct Disorder

Undertake an initial assessment for a suspected conduct disorder if parents or carers, healthcare or social care professionals, school or college, or peer group raise concerns about persistent antisocial behavior. [*Based on the experience and opinion of the GDG*]

Consider using the strengths and difficulties questionnaire (completed by a parent, carer, or teacher) and assess for the following complicating factors:
- A coexisting mental health problem (for example, depression, post-traumatic stress disorder)
- A neurodevelopmental condition (in particular, attention-deficit/hyperactivity disorder and autism)
- A learning disability or difficulty
- Substance misuse.

If there are complicating factors, refer the child or young person to specialist child and adolescent mental health services for a comprehensive assessment.

If there are no complicating factors, consider direct referral for an intervention.

Comprehensive Assessment

Standard components of this should include asking about and assessing:
- Core conduct disorders symptoms, including:
  - Patterns of negativistic, hostile, or defiant behavior in children aged under 11 years
  - Aggression to people and animals, destruction of property, deceitfulness or theft, and serious violations of rules in children aged over 11 years
- Current functioning at home, school, or college and with peers
- Parenting quality
- History of any past or current mental or physical health problems.

Assess for:
- The risks faced by the child or young person. If needed, develop a risk management plan for self-neglect, exploitation by others, self-harm or harm to others
- The presence or risk of physical, sexual, and emotional abuse in line with local protocols for the assessment and management of these problems.

Conduct a comprehensive assessment of parents or carers, covering:
- Positive and negative aspects of parenting—in particular, any use of coercive discipline
- The parent-child relationship
- Positive and negative adult relationships in the family, including domestic violence
- Parental wellbeing, encompassing mental health, substance misuse (including whether alcohol or drugs were used during pregnancy), and criminal behavior.

Parent Training Programs

Offer a group parent training program to the parents of those aged 3–11 years who have or are at high risk of oppositional defiant disorder or conduct disorder or are in contact with the criminal justice system because of antisocial behavior.

In these programs, involve both parents if possible and if in the best interests of the child or young person; and ensure that the programs:
- Typically have 10–12 parents in a group
- Are based on a social learning model, using modeling, rehearsal, and feedback to improve parenting skills
- Typically consist of 10–16 meetings, each lasting 90–120 minutes
- Adhere to the developer's manual (which should have been positively evaluated in a randomized controlled trial) and use all of the necessary materials to ensure consistent implementation of the program.

Foster Carer/Guardian Training Programs

Offer a group foster carer/guardian training program to foster carers and guardians of those aged 3–11 years who have or are at high risk of oppositional defiant disorder or conduct disorder or are in contact with the criminal justice system because of antisocial behavior.

In these programs, involve both of the foster carers or guardians if possible and if in the best interests of the child or young person; and ensure that the programs:

- Modify the intervention to take account of the care setting in which the child is living
- Typically have 8–12 foster carers or guardians in a group
- Are based on a social learning model using modeling, rehearsal, and feedback to improve parenting skills
- Typically consist of 12–16 meetings, each lasting 90–120 minutes.

Adhere to the developer's manual (which should have been positively evaluated in a randomised controlled trial) and use all of the necessary materials to ensure consistent implementation of the program.

Child Focused Programs

Offer group social and cognitive problem solving programs to those aged between 9 and 14 years at high risk of or with oppositional defiant disorder or conduct disorder or if they are in contact with the criminal justice system because of antisocial behavior.

Adapt these group programs to the children's or young people's developmental level and ensure that they:

- Are based on a cognitive behavioral problem solving model
- Use modeling, rehearsal, and feedback to improve skills
- Typically consist of 10–18 weekly meetings, each lasting two hours
- Adhere to the developer's manual (which should have been positively evaluated in a randomized controlled trial) and use all of the necessary materials to ensure consistent implementation of the program.

Multimodal Interventions

Offer multimodal interventions (for example, multisystemic therapy, in which a designated professional provides intensive support to the young person and their family in the home, school, and community, with the aim of reducing their antisocial behavior) to those aged 11–17 years for the treatment of conduct disorder.

In multimodal interventions, involve the child or young person and their parents and carers, and ensure that the interventions:

- Have an explicit and supportive focus on the family
- Are based on a social learning model with interventions provided at individual, family, school, criminal justice, and community levels
- Are provided by specially trained case managers
- Typically consist of 3–4 meetings a week for 3–5 months
- Adhere to the developer's manual (which should have been positively evaluated in a randomized controlled trial) and use all of the necessary materials to ensure consistent implementation of the program.

Improving Access to Services

Provide information about the services and interventions in the local care pathway, including the:

- Range and nature of the interventions provided
- Settings in which services are delivered
- Processes by which a child or young person moves through the pathway
- Means by which progress and outcomes are assessed
- Delivery of care in related health and social care services.

43.11 DEVELOPMENTAL CHILD PSYCHOPATHOLOGY

Malavika Kapur

In recent times, the discipline of child psychology has understandably merged into that of developmental psychology which is the study of normal development of physical, mental and social functions from conception to death. As against this, the study of child psychopathology continues to remain cross-sectional and that too simply as a downward extrapolation of psychopathology of adults.[240] It would make more sense if child psychopathology acquires a developmental perspective, since the study of pathology juxtaposed with that of normal developmental processes will offer clues to management which mere diagnosis is unable to provide. This is being attempted in the newly emerging area of developmental psychopathology. The task is far from complete, since there are considerable gaps in the information available. Also the classical diagnostic model will have to be revised radically before the normal development and corresponding pathology could be brought in line with each other. This task is rendered more formidable as viewed in the Indian context. There are very few Indian studies available and the western data cannot be directly applied to the Indian population, as child rearing variables are unique to each culture.

PORTRAITS OF CHILDHOOD: A HISTORICAL PERSPECTIVE

In the medieval times, childhood was not regarded as a psychologically distinct period. Children were merely viewed as underdeveloped adults at the fringes of society. In the 17th and 18th century philosophies, children were seen to have unique psychological, educational and physical needs. In the middle of the 19th century, a new approach to understanding of childhood emerged. Abstract speculations about child's nature being 'tabula rasa' (blank slate) were replaced by empirical efforts to record and study the behavior of the young. Charles Darwin did much to generate interest in the study of the development process, while Stanely Hall focused on children in different age groups. Alfred Binet made an attempt to distinguish intellectual development in normal and sub-normal children. Sigmund Freud startled the world with the suggestion that experiences of childhood account for the unusual behaviors of adulthood. By 1920, developmental psychology had come into public eye as the bearer of all practical solutions. John Watson's propagation of behaviorism as the force shaping the child's behavior took deep roots in the traditions of psychology. Several long-term and short-term studies on children were set in centers like Yale and Berkeley in the USA.

In India, the earliest document to record child development was Ayurveda.[241] It considered feeding practices as the central factor in the formation of personality. Breast feeding was seen as essential for the child's physical and mental health. The emotional state of the mother while feeding was also emphasized. Use of amulets, practice of certain feeding and bathing rituals were described in detail, both for healthy and sick infants. Physical and mental disturbances were attributed to planetary constellations or *'grahas.'* The use of toys to stimulate cognitive functions such as memory, intelligence and language were recommended.

In the contemporary Indian thinking, several workers have highlighted the special aspects of child rearing practices in India. Khatri[242] points out that traditional child rearing practices are persuasive in making the child dependent and submissive. He also argues that a female child is particularly vulnerable to mental health problems because of her early experiences. Ramanujam[243] suggests that in India, child rearing practices differ depending on the religious, ethnic and caste status of the family. He describes mother-child relationship as generally intimate and involved, but determined by adult considerations and values. There is a sudden increase in what is expected of a child when he is old enough to take minimum responsibility. Emotional needs of the child are considered secondary and the child often may be precocious due to environmental demands. In social relationships and modes of communication, the child becomes highly sensitive to those around. Ramanujam,[243] along with other workers such as Nandi,[244] Hoch,[245] Kakar[246] and Roland,[248] has noted that the separation and individuation of the self does not take place in the Indian children. This seems to promote prolonged infancy[246] and foster dependency.

Bassa[247] points out that in Indian families, child-rearing practices are characterized by overprotection, multiple caretaking, lack of firm and consistent limit-setting, precocious toilet training, and lack of control over anger and aggression. The mother, though emotionally and physically gratifying, is not empathically tuned to the individualized needs of the child.[245,248] It is interesting to note that from the days of Ayurveda to the present day, studies have focused a great deal on child rearing practices rather than on the nature of the child.

With regard to recent research in the area of developmental processes, Anandalakshmy[249] points out that the trend is by and large 'a theoretical' one and the variables studied are test-related and not theory-related. She emphasizes the need for culturally appropriate longitudinal studies, using observations of young children in natural setting as well as in controlled conditions.

After examining the period of childhood in the earlier times, now we shall look at a few theoretical models.

BASIC PRINCIPLES IN DEVELOPMENT

Developmental processes are not controlled by completely different and independent factors, such as nature versus nurture, continuity versus discontinuity in development, maturation versus learning, as seen in traditional approaches to biology and psychology. Principles of development are same for all the developing systems, be it an organ or an organism, i.e. they differentiate. This means that they progress from a relatively homogeneous state to a relatively heterogenous state. Though this is a well-known fact in the field of embryology, its relevance to psychology has not been explicitly stated.

The two descriptive principles, which account for biological as well as psychological development in humans and animals, are differentiation and hierarchical organization. As development proceeds, virtually in all organisms, behavior becomes more versatile and differentiated in all aspects. The growth occurs in a hierarchical fashion and optimal development occurs at certain *critical sensitive periods*. Apart from biological endowment and maturation, learning also plays an important role. Learning could be simple or complex, or through observation. Simple learning could be passive by habituation, or it could be an active effort from the child in terms of the reinforcements offered by self or environment.

It has been noted that in the early developmental stages of undifferentiated state, the potential for adaptation is limitless, while with differentiation certain amount of flexibility is lost.

THEORIES OF DEVELOPMENTAL PROCESSES

The models developed by various thinkers in the western context have dealt with aspects of development in a segmental fashion; justifiably so, as it is too vast an area to be comprehensively understood. Integration of the different theoretical models and disparate research findings is essential.

In the following section, some of the most influential theories, which highlight the developmental context with special focus on childhood, are briefly described.

Theories of Cognitive Development

One of the most influential theories of cognitive development is that of Jean Piaget.[250] According to Piaget, cognitive adaptation consists of two basic processes, 'assimilation' and 'accommodation', which the child uses in coping with the environment. *Assimilation* involves an organism incorporating, into its existing mental framework, new elements from the environment, while *accommodation* involves a modification of mental structure to fit new perceptions of the environment. For example, a four month old baby, when presented with a rattle, may grasp it in a way he has learnt earlier in a clumsy fashion (*assimilation*). Later, he does it more skillfully by accommodating his visual acuity, putting proper distance between himself and the rattle, and grasping it with specific movements (*accommodation*).

The four major stages described by Piaget are:

1. *Sensorimotor stage*: Birth to two years.
2. *Preoperational stage*: Two to seven years.
3. *Concrete operational stage*: Seven to eleven years.
4. *Formal operational stage*: Eleven years and above.

Piaget based his model on observation of his own children and subsequently tested out his theory on other children in a Genevan school.

Sensorimotor Stage

In the sensorimotor stage, the infant changes from automatic reflexive sucking to oral manipulation of any available object, becoming more purposive as he becomes older. This he specifically uses only for feeding himself. The grasp reflex of the newborn gives way to gross as well as fine motor movements for successful picking up of a football or a marble. At the end of this stage, the child grasps that he can kick a toy and make it move. The child also understands that objects, which disappear, may also be found or may come back.

Preoperational Stage

This stage lasts from two years to seven years and is characterized by an 'egocentric' perspective and failure to solve 'conservation' problems. In the next stage, these are achieved easily and hence it forms a contrast to the preoperational stage. Conservation problem, for example, refers to the child's inability to understand that when the same amount of water is poured into a shallow bowl and a tall tumbler, both the glass containers have equal amounts of water. The child would assume that the tall tumbler has more water in it. The preoperational child can view objects from only one perspective, that is, if there is a doll facing the child and the child is asked how a person, who is behind the doll but in front of the child, sees the doll, the child would say that the person sees the front of the doll, as the child sees himself.

The child, in this stage, fails to hold more than one perspective or category in his mind. He would, for example, say that a kilogram of cotton is more than a kilogram of stone as he takes only the volume as the determining factor. The logic is precausal; any two events occurring together are seen as cause and effect. A preoperational child views events around him in a very different fashion. This, in turn, can effect his understanding at a cognitive and emotional level. He may say that when he goes in a car, trees and electric poles follow him. Death or sickness in a parent may be seen by the child as being caused by himself.

Operational Stage

In the consequent operational stage, which occurs between seven and eleven years of age, the child can effectively understand the problems of conservation and reversibility. Cause and effect are now understood in a logical fashion.

Formal Operational Stage

In the formal operational stage of adolescence, the logical operations can be performed at an abstract level. Problems, such as the 'pendulum problem' in physics, can be understood by the youngster.

The Piagetian model highlights the sequential progress, which occurs in a hierarchical fashion, and focuses on the finer details of the development of thought process, at concrete level of logical operations as well as at an abstract level, making use of language and symbols. This model has been criticized on multiple grounds, such as the various states being more flexible than being envisaged by Piaget, the difficulty level of tests determining the stage of development than vice-versa, cross-cultural relevance, effect of training, and so on. But, this model essentially focuses on the developmental process of cognitive functioning.

Theories of Language Development

Development of language in children is a complex process, which has two distinct aspects. One is that of acquisition of skills related to the mechanism of speech and the other is that of language development. Speech develops from crying and babbling in infancy, progressively acquiring the ability to pronounce syllables, vowels and consonants clearly (articulation), and finally to have fluency (to say words or sentences without stammering). Children vary in their ability to acquire speech; while some acquire it early by ten months, others may take up to five years to speak sentences. A child, who understands spoken language but does not speak, is likely to have a normal speech. Occasional stammering is normal in a toddler. Speech problems that persist beyond six years may be considered as pathological.

Development of language, on the other hand, is a very complex process, wherein the child learns a series of symbols, gestures, grammar, etc. From a vocabulary of ten words by one year, he acquires a vocabulary of about two thousand words by the time he is six years old.

Of the several theories of language development, the most influential ones are those of Chomsky[251] and Skinner.[252] Skinner's model views all languages and language behavior in terms of stimuli and reinforcement contingencies. Skinner's followers highlighted the contextual nature of use of language in childhood. The development process in the context of child were minimized while environmental contributions were seen as the determining factors. In contrast, Chomsky's model redirected the thinking into a new area of developmental neurolinguistics. He proposed an internalized set of rules of grammar which govern language. He called this as *generative grammar*. It consists of 'inner/deep' and 'surface' structures. The infant is born with a *language acquisition device* constituting of an inner structure with certain language universals. Subsequent refinement, in terms of the grammar affecting the surface structure, is influenced by environment.

While the Skinnerian model may explain the learning of language by adults, the Chomskian model focuses on the developmental processes. Wide individual differences in the communication skills, especially in vocabulary, sex differences favoring girls, socioeconomic status of parents, influence of acquisition of language, could be accommodated within the Chomskian framework adequately.

Theories of Psychological Development

These theories focus on the emotional and social development. The foremost among these are the psychoanalytical theories, Sigmund Freud's[253] psychoanalytical theory being the most influential. His theory is predominantly a psychosexual theory of development, consisting of the oral, anal and phallic stages of development. The development occurs from the infant, whose mental apparatus works on the pleasure principle dominated by the absence of the capacity to differentiate between the self and others, to an adult capacity for genital sexuality and adult balance of ego, superego and id. Anna Freud[254,255] proposed a phasic theory of psychosexual development integrated with a theory of aggressive drive. Her description of ego development, in relation to the deployment of ego defenses, is her special contribution. In addition, she proposed the notion of the developmental line beginning with the biological unit of mother-and-child and the last step of adolescent struggle being loosening of the infantile ties, with the libidinal ties being transferred to objects of opposite sex outside the family.

Melanie Klein[256] stressed that the unconscious fantasies created in infancy affect whole of the subsequent life. Margaret Mahler[257] focused on the symbiotic relationship between the infant and the mother, and divided it into autistic, symbiotic, and separation-individuation phases. Separation anxiety is thus a resultant of the infringement of the biological mother-infant tie. Erik Erikson[258] proposed a theory where each stage is seen as a developmental crisis, imposing certain tasks on the developing organism. In his model, psychoanalytical concepts of aggression and sexual drives are integrated with social and cultural factors. Infants pass through stages of trust versus mistrust in the first year, autonomy versus shame and doubt in the second year, stages of initiative versus guilt between the second and the third year, and industry versus inferiority between the fifth and the twelfth year. Finally, adolescence is characterized by identity versus identity-diffusion.

Emerging from the background of psychoanalytical theories, Harlow's[259] experimental studies with primates and the work of ethnologists focusing on the survival function of the mother and offspring relationship in the animal kingdom, John Bowlby[260] proposed a model interaction between the infant and the mother leading to healthy emotional development. He introduced the term 'attachment' to describe this 'bond' between the infant and the mother. Ainsworth[261] defines attachment as "an affectional tie, one person or animal forms between himself and another specific one, a tie that bonds them in space and endures over time." According to Bowlby,[259] attachment behavior is characterized by:

- Behavior that initiates interaction, such as greeting, touching, embracing, calling, reaching, smiling, etc.
- Behavioral response to the mother's interactional initiative,
- Behavioral responses aimed at avoiding separations by clinging, crying, etc.,
- Entering new situations in the presence of the mother and withdrawal or fear in her absence.

Development of attachment behavior, in majority of infants to a specific individual, occurs around 9 months of age. By the 18th month, they would have attachment to more than one figure. The age, at which specific attachments occur, appears to be related to the infant's early interaction with his mother, as well as the level of cognitive development.

Several short-term and long-term effects are noted, by several workers in case of an insecure attachment or an absence of attachment. 'Separation anxiety' and 'stranger anxiety' are the two widely recognized conditions. Several studies focus on the harmful effects which go beyond the childhood in the form of lack of an ability to form relationships in adulthood, for example, conditions such as borderline personality and depressive disorders.

However, the concept of attachment has been criticized on the grounds that it may not be truly predictive of the later difficulties and that it is an interactional process between the infant and the mother, which is not a biological bond. But, the importance of the quality of caretaking in early childhood as a critical factor has not been questioned.

CONSTRUCT OF TEMPERAMENT

It is apparent to the least sophisticated parent that infants vary in vigor, liability of mood and their reaction to tiredness, hunger, boredom and play. A small group of infants are born with strong bias that favors certain moods and styles of reaction. These biases are considered temperamental properties. Some of the easily observable ones are activity, fussiness, fearfulness, sensitivity and attentiveness. These seem to be related to the future adjustment. The most influential workers to explore the area of temperament are Alexander Thomas and Stella Chess.[262] Out of the nine dimensions studied, they suggested three groups of children: 'easy to handle', 'difficult to manage' and 'slow to warm up to other people'. These dimensions also reflect concerns of American parents. A study of the same temperamental variables in an Indian context[263] has yielded similar results.

Of all the temperamental variables that have been studied, activity, irritability and fearfulness, and shyness (as against boldness) are reported to be fairly persistent qualities. The child's personality is thus a product of the child's temperament and the adult's reaction to it. For example, a shy child may thrive with a warm and encouraging mother, while it may become withdrawn with a hostile one. Social development of the child is determined by the child's temperament and exposure to the peer-group in early childhood, particularly in the setting of cooperative play.

Role of the Environment

All the theories highlight the importance of environment, particularly the family in its various spheres. Thus, stress in the context of family has a major role to play in the normal or pathological development. The area of stress in children, though very important, has been paid scant attention.

States of stress follow as an aftermath of traumatic experiences, natural or man-made disasters, parental mismanagement or overwhelming environments. Child's response to overwhelming stress may be understood in terms of the models of self-induced pathology, individual differences in vulnerability, one's alertness to them as well as presence of social support. However, these models do not include a developmental viewpoint. The reactions of children to high degree of stress vary according to the age of the child, ranging from mild and transient to severe psychopathology in the background of overwhelming experience of anxiety. Research on competent and creative coping by resilient children is currently gaining importance.

The various theories focus on segmental aspects of emotional or social development; none of them look at all the facets of development. Development of prosocial behavior through infancy to adolescence, though an important aspect, is not accommodated in these theories. Nor do they highlight the contexts of familial sociocultural milieu in terms of their contribution to normal development, despite their assertion that environment is an important contributor. However, all the theories are unanimous in that the childhood is a critical period in normal development where development proceeds from a simple to a complex state, and wherein inherited potential and environment have equally important roles to play.

CHILD PSYCHOPATHOLOGY IN DEVELOPMENTAL CONTEXT

The area of developmental psychopathology is still in its infancy. The multiaxial classificatory system of DSM-IV[264] and the multiaxial classificatory system of Rutter et al.[265] go beyond mere diagnostic classifications to a certain extent, and acknowledge the contribution of developmental delays, psychosocial stressors and organic pathologies in production of child psychopathology. However, the key issues in developmental psychopathology, namely age and sex related trends, the impact of environmental factors at each specific age and sex, are not taken cognizance of. The contribution of the various developmental theories, discussed earlier, is mostly ignored as non-contributory to classification and management.

A classification that juxtaposes the stages of normal development with the categories of dysfunction will contribute to our understanding of developmental psychopathology. This would help in (1) identifying the types of psychopathological disorders that are associated with impairments or distortions in certain areas of functioning, (2) discovering the nature of deviation with respect to quality, timing or reversibility, (3) disentangling the direction of causality of these deficits in terms of psychopathology or normal developmental functioning or vice-versa, and (4) examining the transaction between development in two or more domains of functioning.[266]

Several workers have attempted to evolve such frameworks. One such early effort to outline a conceptual scheme in the context of some better known theories, is proposed by Anthony.[267] He juxtaposed age and stages of psychoaffective development with various types of psychopathologies hypothesized to be associated with these stages. Achenbach and Edelbrock[268] have studied different age and sex groups with reference to psychopathology. Such a scheme may be useful in conceptualizing developmental psychopathology, but there has been very little empirical research in this area.

Some of the critical issues in classification of childhood psychopathology from a developmental perspective are:

- Continuity between childhood and adult normality or psychopathology.

- Definition of normality and deviance with respect to age, developmental tasks and progression of development over time.
- Differences between sexes in various types of psychopathology.
- Child rearing practices unique to each culture.

Longitudinal study of the course of development has shown that altogether there is some temperamental predictability from one year to next and that there is also considerable change over a period of time.[269] Among the characteristics, which tend to be most stable, are specific attributes such as achievement motivation, dependency and passivity in females, serious aggressive acting-out and intellectual mastery.[269] There is little support to the notion of continuity of personality from very early stage; there is stronger support for relationship between early temperamental characteristics of irritability, irregularity of biological functions and emotional intensity, and later development of emotional and behavioral disorders. The longitudinal study of the course of various disorders is an important aspect in understanding child psychopathology.

Certain unique features of childhood disorders are age and sex trends. A particular behavior may be diagnosed as normal at one age and pathological at the other. Examples are: bed-wetting in an infant and in a ten year old; school refusal in early childhood as a manifestation of separation anxiety and in adolescence leading to dropping out of school. Similarly, there are important sex differences in manifestation and distribution of emotional and behavioral problems over the course of development. In general, boys have higher rates of behavior deviation than girls and the tendency to behavior disturbance declines with age.[271]

Given the fact that all children, at some-time or the other, manifest behaviors that are more or less abnormal, how does one decide that a disturbance should not be neglected? The quantitative dimensions in judging the seriousness are intensity, frequency, duration, number and combination of symptoms. Fire-setting or serious violence may be considered as serious even if it occurs infrequently, while occasional school refusal or bed-wetting does not warrant attention. Some problems, such as sleep or eating problems, or minor fears, disappear as the child grows. However, particularly if they cluster as a syndrome which covary, these ought to be considered as problems serious enough to warrant attention.

Pervasive Developmental Disorders

It has been observed that severe disorders may have their onset in infancy and early childhood, or later in late childhood around eight years and adolescence. The early forms are represented by mental retardation, infantile autism, and other pervasive developmental disorders, typical or otherwise. In the latter group, one comes across schizophrenia, manic depressive psychoses or acute psychotic reactions. In the former group, the development is pervasively impaired. In mental retardation, organic etiology is definitely implicated, while in infantile autism a large number of workers like Ritvo[271] subscribe to an organic etiology. In the early days, Kanner[272] suggested a psychosocial etiology. This has since been disputed by workers in USA and UK, who favor an organic etiology.

Several workers have documented the frequency with which psychiatric disorders involve problems in social relationships and deviant communications. Apart from infantile autism, there is a paucity of work in the area of social relationships. Attachment theory focused on the bond between the mother and the child in infancy as being secure or insecure, while Mahler[257] focused on the symbiotic relationship between mother and infant. Bowlby[260] observed adverse effects of institutionalization in infancy, leading to poor social relationships and academic performance.

The author's own clinical observation of children, who present with autistic features, of average intelligence and linguistic abilities exhibited certain interesting features. These children showed normal cognitive and language development in early infancy up to a point of time and subsequently developed autistic behavior in response to difficult family and environmental situations. Social isolation of the child as well as parents, pathological interactions between the parents and the child, and drastic changes in the physical environment had been contributory, preceding the onset of disturbances. The deviant communication and social withdrawal from those around, were typically present. However, there was a definite evidence of presence of normal bonding in these children. Improvement in the living style often heralded improvement in the clinical status. The history was noncontributory in terms of birth complications, illnesses or family history of psychotic illness. It can be speculated that psychological stressors, in the stage where bonding and sensorimotor development are achieved, may lead to autistic features in the child. In response to difficulty in separating from the mother and the operation of precausal logic, social withdrawal and autism can develop.

In the older children and adolescents, the psychotic conditions are phenomenologically and possibly etiologically similar to adult forms, with minor variations. These seem to occur in latency of phallic stages and in the stage of concrete or formal operations, where the level of functioning is similar to that of adults.

Even in cases where there is evidence of minimal or gross brain damage, psychosocial factors may have compounding effects. An epileptic child may develop serious conduct or learning problems because of unhealthy interactions with parents involving neglect, understimulation, over-concern or lack of discipline. A young epileptic child, who is overprotected and not allowed to learn anything or who is totally isolated with understimulation, may appear like a psychotic or mentally retarded child. Severity of psychopathology may be a function of compounding factors, such as age, family context and additional stressors in which the illness occurs.

Attention Deficit Hyperactivity Disorder

This refers to a specific syndrome characterized by inattention, impulsivity and hyperactivity. Hyperactivity, which is pervasive across all situations and is persistent over time, differs from other psychiatric conditions and has a stronger association with cognitive deficits. Its long-term prognosis is worse as compared to situation-specific hyperactivity. For example, a boy, the only child of his parents, who is very bright and has no past history suggestive of brain damage, can become extremely overactive and disruptive, if pampered and overprotected, not being allowed to play and run around because the parent fears that he may get hurt, or if the parents are very strict and punitive, not allowing the child to play. The child may be quiet at home and becomes extremely overactive and disruptive in school or at other people's houses. Such children have overactivity which is situation-specific. This cannot be considered as a disorder in the true sense of the term. They would respond very well to counseling of parents and to behavioral management. From a developmental perspective, overactivity to certain extent in a toddler is normal. When overactivity occurs in all situations and at all times, and the child is incapable of attending to even a most interesting task, watching a cartoon film or playing a game, it can be considered as pathological. In addition, overactivity as such, whether in a normal child or in a hyperkinetic child, tends to diminish as the child grows older and disappears or reduces a great deal by adolescence.

An Indian study,[273] conducted in five to ten year old children, reported that simple hyperkinetics have significant deficits in terms of attention, form perception, reaction time, intelligence and social maturity. While conduct disordered children were similar to normals, the hyperkinetic conduct disordered children were in between the simple hyperkinetic and conduct disordered in their performance on the same variables. From a developmental perspective, when the onset is in infancy/early childhood, the core syndrome is that of attention deficit along with overactivity. As this occurs in the sensorimotor stage, there is a setback in the cognitive development. As the child grows older into middle childhood, the attention deficit, impulsivity and overactivity are compounded by conduct disturbance due to parental mismanagement. As the child grows into the late childhood and adolescence, overactivity reduces considerably while the attention deficit persists, leading to specific learning disabilities and school problems related to inattention. However, apart from conduct disturbance due to parental mismanagement, emotional and social development of these children appears to run a normal course, except when associated with aggressiveness.

In the Indian context, overactivity in preschoolers is not considered as a disturbance and is, in fact regarded as a predictor of high intelligence by the parents. This perhaps is true in a child without attention deficit, wherein hyperactivity is situational and is associated with conduct disturbances, while pervasive hyperactivity with poor attention span has associated cognitive deficits which are likely to retard the child's intellectual development.

Disturbances of Conduct and Emotion

Disorders of emotion and conduct, or internalizing and externalizing disorders, as described by Achenbach,[240] are a spectrum of disorders unique to childhood. *Internalizing disorders* consist of depression, withdrawal, anxiety, obsessions, somatic complaints and schizoid features. Children with these problems suffer themselves more than others do in their environment. *Externalizing disorders* reflect conflicts with the environment, as in conduct disorders. Conduct disorder is unquestionably the most researched upon area in child psychiatry and social psychology. The two kinds described are unsocialized and socialized conduct disorders. The former is characterized by lying, stealing, truancy, aggressive and antisocial behavior; while in the latter group, the youngster belongs to a peer group which indulges in similar antisocial activity. The socialized type has a better prognosis. The classic longitudinal study of Robins[274] points out that not all conduct disordered children grow up to be antisocial adults.

In spite of the lack of theoretical resolution, substantial progress has been made towards conventional integration of ideas of conduct disturbances. Both social learning and social control have provided important developments in the field. However, there have been etiological theories emphasizing biological, genetic, sociological and psychological variables.

Aggressive behavior is seen more frequently in males than females, though all children display physical aggression in the form of hitting, kicking, biting, taking objects away from other children and verbally abusing others. These behaviors are largely learnt by observing other models, such as parents, peers or others in the environment, who engage in aggressive behavior. The learning of aggressive behavior might also result from direct experience whereby the child is reinforced for responding in an aggressive manner when frustrated or provoked. For example, the mother may yield to child's demand of money or objects because he hits her, although she does not think he should be given what he asks for. There are instances of children aged seven or eight years actually terrorizing the whole household of grown-ups into submission. Sometimes, the child may not be given what he wants, though it is a just demand, unless he resorts to aggression. Once acquired, either vicariously or directly, aggressive behaviors are said to be maintained through contingent reinforcements.

Emotional disturbances refer to conditions which refer to abnormal development of emotions such as anxiety, fearfulness or depression. Emotional disturbance is a category exclusive to childhood problems, while emotional disorders consist of neuroses in childhood such as hysteria, anxiety, phobia and obsessive compulsive neurosis.[275]

Developmentally, studies have shown that most young children go through the phases of fearing objects that involve no objective threats. These, as a rule, become less frequent as the child grows older. Some fears are regarded as a normal part of development, like fear of noises, falling, strange objects. A fear, which persists beyond two years, may be considered as pathological. Fear of strangers is typical and is related to the development of normal attachment and separation anxiety. Other fears, similar to phobias in adults, also may present in older children. School refusal in the beginning of school career is usually linked with separation anxiety, while in an adolescent it may be linked with more serious psychopathology.

Sex differences in anxiety and fearfulness are not apparent in very young children. Specific fears and phobias are more common in girls, from school age onwards.

Majority of studies in India have focused on conduct disorders and delinquency of early and late adolescence. A study comparing normal children, children with disturbance of conduct, children with disturbance of emotion, and children with mixed disturbances of conduct and emotion in eight to twelve year olds, highlighted that conduct disorder was associated with lower intelligence, high aggression, difficult temperamental characteristics and more pre-, peri- and post-natal difficulties. On the other hand, children with emotional and mixed disturbances are almost like normal children in these variables. In all the three groups, in comparison with normals, there was more of marital disharmony in parents. These parents were rejecting in attitude and had deviant patterns of communication, along with an inconsistent pattern of discipline with their children. Though school adjustment was normal, sibling rivalry was present in all the three groups. Emotionally disturbed children, in addition, had poor interaction with peers and neighbors.

Neurotic conditions do occur in childhood, with some minor variations. Although allegedly on the wane in the western world, hysteria in children deserves a special mention as it is reported as widely prevalent in clinics in the Indian setting. Hysteria in children is phenomenologically similar to that in adults. In a sample of 70 children, between the age of eight and twelve years, Uma[276] found them to have well-adjusted personality prior to the onset. There were significantly large number of stressors, which were home- or school-related. Ninan and Kapur,[277] in a group of early adolescents, in addition to other stressors, also found evidence of sexual conflicts which could very well be age-related.

Hysteria, in children, seems to occur at the various developmental stress points, always within the context of families where verbalizing of conflicts is a taboo. For example, functional paralysis of lower limbs, in a child of four years, may occur due to loss of status following birth of a sibling. Problems of coping with school work in an average or dull child of ambitious parents, facing a punitive teacher in a new school, loss of face in front of the peer group in adolescents, are all stressors often encountered in the Indian context. Primary and secondary gains and modeling seem to be crucial variables which lend themselves to dynamically oriented as well as learning theory approaches to the understanding of the etiology of hysteria.

When one looks at the disorders of emotion and conduct, hysteria and somatization disorders, one is struck by the impact stress has at each stage of development in children. In infancy, it is the relationship with the family, while in the middle and late childhood, it is the relationship with peers and situations in schools which contribute significantly to the child's distress. In addition, often the boundaries between disorders may be fluid and symptoms belonging to different syndromes may occur simultaneously. What is essential is the understanding that the symptom represents the child's distress in an adverse environment at that point of time.

Scholastic Problems

Scholastic problems refer to school-related problems which are unrelated to low intelligence or sensory-motor handicaps. These could be related to faulty educational system, emotional or conduct disturbance, specific learning disabilities or a maturational lag, apart from environmental stressors related to poverty, illness or problems in the family. Scholastic backwardness of recent onset in an older child is likely to be due to emotional or conduct problems.

In India, one of the major problems presented in schools by teachers and in the clinics by parents is scholastic backwardness. Thirty nine percent of the normal and 44% of the disturbed 12–16 year olds are reported to have scholastic backwardness.[278] Scholastic backwardness of longer duration, beginning from early school years, may be related to low intelligence, specific learning problems, or attention deficit disorders.[279] Later onset appears to suggest factors related to emotional or conduct problems, or stressors in the environment. In a study by John,[280] of children between eight and twelve years, scholastic backwardness was found mostly in boys with average intelligence and social competence. Most of the children had problems with perceptuo-motor functions, along with specific difficulties in relation to reading, writing and arithmatic. Some had emotional problems secondary to scholastic problems.

Transient Developmental Disorders

There are yet some disturbances which are age-related and are described as developmental disturbances by Marilyn Erickson.[281] These are disturbances of sleeping, eating, elimination (enuresis, encopresis) and sexuality in adolescence. These problems are outcomes of interaction of biological endowments and family environment. These do not particularly signify pathology unless they assume pathological proportions. Sleeping and feeding problems are fairly common in preschoolers. These problems become disorders mainly through faulty upbringing. Interestingly, psychoanalytic concepts too have focused on oral, anal, phallic and oedipal phases, highlighting the importance of feeding, elimination and sexuality in the context of family, leading to pathology.

Natural sleep rhythms vary in children and mother's own poor sleep may induce the child to keep irregular hours. Feeding problems, faddiness, failure to thrive, and poor or bizarre eating habits appear to be related to maternal anxiety and overindulgence, and even at times to neglect by the mother. Bed-wetting and encopresis, which are normal in infancy, would generally lead to normal toileting habits by preschool years. However, children vary a good deal in developing bladder control, depending on physiological readiness and familiar tendency to delay. This may be considered as primary enuresis while those in whom bed-wetting occurs after bladder control has been gained earlier, is called as secondary enuresis.

Enuresis and encopresis, in the absence of organic pathology, appear to be related to severe emotional disturbance. A case of a five year old girl abandoned in an orphanage, or a twelve year old conduct disordered boy with lot of hostile feelings against the parents, are some examples of encopresis as expression of distress or hostility.

Developmental disorder in children is a term which is used in an ambiguous fashion. Pervasive developmental disorders represent disorders which are severely handicapping, chronic and pervasive while specific developmental disorders refer to chronic yet segmental disabilities which are not so severe in their impact on child's day-to-day life. Developmental disorders of sleeping, eating, elimination and sexuality are transient in nature and occur in particular stages of development like infancy or adolescence and are compounded by disruptive environmental factors.

In conclusion, the above description of psychopathological disorders barely touches upon the developmental context and only points towards that direction. Much work needs to be done with reference to each disorder, at different ages and in different psychological, social and cultural contexts as suggested by the theories as well as empirical findings. Developmental psychopathology aims at a new perspective which is in its nascent stage.[282]

Acknowledgment: The author gratefully acknowledges the help given by her husband Prof. RL Kapur, National Institute of Advanced Studies, Bengaluru.

43.12 MENTAL RETARDATION/INTELLECTUAL DISABILITY

Jayati Simlai, Joyita Sinha, Christoday RJ Khess

Mental retardation (MR) or intellectual disability (ID) is a descriptive term for subaverage intelligence and impaired adaptive functioning arising in the developmental period (< 18 y). MR/ID and other neurodevelopmental disabilities are seen often in a general pediatric practice.

Terminology for MR/ID has been particularly challenging as the term mentally retarded carries significant social and emotional stigma. The American Association for Intellectual and Developmental Disability (AAIDD) has been particularly influential in terminology changes such that most professionals working in the field now refer to mental retardation as intellectual disability. The DSM-5 has also adopted the new terminology.[283]

Developmental delay is often used inappropriately as synonymous with MR/ID. Developmental delay is an overly inclusive term and should generally be used for infants and young children (< 5 y) in which the diagnosis is unclear, such as those too young for formal testing.[283]

Approximately 10% of children have some learning impairment, while as many as 3% manifest some degree of MR/ID. The population prevalence of these combined disorders of learning rivals that of the common childhood disorder asthma.

MR/ID originates during the developmental period (i.e. conception through age 18 years) and results in significantly subaverage general intellectual function with concurrent deficits in functional life skills. The diagnosis of MR/ID requires an intelligence deficit of at least 2 standard deviations (SDs) below the mean IQ. This generally translates into an intelligence quotient (IQ) score of 70–75, given a population mean of 100. Equivalent deficits in at least 2 areas of functional life skills or adaptive skills also must be present to meet the diagnostic criteria for MR/ID. Adaptive skills encompass functional life skills within the domains of communication, self-care, home living, social and interpersonal skills, use of community resources, self-direction, functional academic skills, work, leisure, health, and safety.

The DSM-5 is widely changed the definition of MR/ID, relying less on specific IQ levels.[284] IQ scores can vary based on age, instrument, and practitioner. Furthermore, testing prior to school age does not correlate well with future performance. IQ scores can be measured using assessment instruments, such as the Stanford-Binet, Wechsler Adult Intelligence Scale (WAIS), or Wechsler Intelligence Scale for Children (WISC-IV). Nonverbal children can be tested with the Leiter International Performance Scale (Leiter-R).

The second component of diagnosis, adaptive skills, is usually measured with a self-reported or parent/caregiver-reported inventory, such as the Vineland Adaptive Behavior Scales, Second Edition (VABS-II). The DSM-5 diagnosis requires adaptive measurements of less than 2 SDs as compared to the population mean, with standard scores of 70 or less, in at least 2 of the following domains:[284]

- Conceptual skills (communication, language, time, money, academic)
- Social skills (interpersonal skills, social responsibility, recreation, friendships)
- Practical skills (daily living skills, work, travel)

MR/ID also can be categorized as syndromic, if associated with dysmorphic features, or nonsyndromic, if not associated with dysmorphisms or malformations. The understanding of specific MR/ID syndromes is expanding with recent molecular genetic advances. More than 800 recognized syndromes listed in the Online Mendelian Inheritance in Man (OMIM) database are associated with MR/ID, reflecting clinical diagnostic advances in the field. The most common associated chromosomal abnormality is trisomy 21, or Down syndrome. The most common X-linked abnormality associated with MR/ID is fragile X syndrome. However, for most cases of MR/ID, no specific genetic abnormalities are found.

Some forms of MR/ID are due to nongenetic factors and may be identifiable by their associated dysmorphisms and clinical presentation. Examples include prenatal exposure to teratogens (e.g. anticonvulsants, warfarin, alcohol) or prenatal thyroid dysfunction. Prenatal and postnatal exposure to lead and the associated decrement in IQ may increase an individual's chance of functioning in the MR/ID range. In DSM-5 new Intellectual Disability is used. The diagnostic criteria are given as follows.

DSM-5 DIAGNOSTIC CRITERIA FOR INTELLECTUAL DISABILITY (INTELLECTUAL DEVELOPMENTAL DISORDER)

Intellectual disability (intellectual developmental disorder) is a disorder with onset during the developmental period that includes both intellectual and adaptive functioning deficits in conceptual, social, and practical domains. The following three criteria must be met:

1. Deficits in intellectual functions, such as reasoning, problem solving, planning, abstract thinking, judgment, academic learning, and learning from experience, confirmed by both clinical assessment and individualized, standardized intelligence testing.
2. Deficits in adaptive functioning that result in failure to meet developmental and sociocultural standards for personal independence and social responsibility. Without ongoing support, the adaptive deficits limit functioning in one or more activities of daily life, such as communication, social participation, and independent living, across multiple environments, such as home, school, work, and community.
3. Onset of intellectual and adaptive deficits during the developmental period.

Note: The diagnostic term intellectual disability is the equivalent term for the ICD-11 diagnosis of intellectual developmental disorders.

Although the term intellectual disability is used throughout this manual, both terms are used in the title to clarify relationships with other classification systems. Moreover, a federal statute in the United States (Public Law 111-256, Rosa's Law) replaces the term mental retardation with intellectual disability, and research journals use the term intellectual disability. Thus, intellectual disability is the term in common use by medical, educational, and other professions and by the lay public and advocacy groups.

Specify current severity:

- 317 (F70) Mild
- 318.0 (F71) Moderate
- 318.1 (F72) Severe
- 318.2 (F73) Profound.

PATHOPHYSIOLOGY

MR/ID is the end result of many disorders of CNS function. Most individuals with significant intellectual impairment have no discernible structural abnormalities of the brain. CNS malformations, a visual correlate of the disorders, are diagnosed in 10–15% of cases; dysfunction is localized primarily to the cortical structures, including the hippocampus and the medial temporal cortex. The most common malformations consist of neural tube defects, hydranencephaly, and microcephaly. Less commonly, CNS malformations include disorders of migration (the lissencephalies) and agenesis of the corpus callosum.

Multiple congenital anomaly syndromes with malformations confined to non-neurologic organ systems may be present in 5% of all patients with MR/ID. Between 3% and 7% of cases may be associated with a wide array of inborn errors of metabolism complicated by multiorgan system disease. Alcohol exposure *in utero* may account for as many as 8% of those with mild MR/ID.

Most individuals with mild MR/ID and other learning disorders do not have other neurologic complications, CNS malformations, or dysmorphisms. They are more likely, however, to be born into families of low socioeconomic status, low IQ, and little education. The etiologic contribution of poverty to their poor cognitive function remains unclear. Clearly, however, poor cognitive functioning and MR are correlated positively with a life of poverty.

EPIDEMIOLOGY

Frequency

United States

The frequency of MR/ID of all degrees ranges from 1 to 3% of the population. The statistical definition of subaverage intelligence (2 SDs below the mean) would indicate a predicted prevalence of 2.5%.

International

A study with excellent ascertainment conducted in Aberdeen, Scotland, yielded a prevalence of 1 in 300 for severe MR and 1 in 77 for mild MR. Among those with severe MR were more boys than girls (male-to-female ratio 1.2:1), and among those with IQ >70, in the mild range of deficiency, boys exceeded girls by a ratio of 2.2:1.[285]

Although prevalence rates vary from country to country, the variance in prevalence may be attributed to ascertainment bias, the standardization methods employed from study to study, and a generalized upward drift in IQ scores over time. Even so, the greatest variance in statistics of prevalence is most likely to fall within the category of mild MR, a group for which the ascertainment bias is large.

MORTALITY/MORBIDITY

MR/ID itself is not necessarily associated with an increased premature death rate. However, individuals with severe to profound MR/ID experience a decreased life expectancy related to the underlying etiology or additional complicating neurologic disorders, such as epilepsy. Neurologic dysfunction resulting in immobility, significant oral motor incoordination, dysphagia, and aspiration confers a greater risk of premature death than MR/ID itself. When significant neurologic dysfunction is associated with other organ system anomalies, an individual's life expectancy is shortened further.

Respiratory disease is the most prevalent cause of death among individuals with profound MR/ID. In particular, respiratory infections were the leading cause of death among a Finnish cohort of children with MR/ID.[286] For those affected by mild MR/ID, life expectancy does not differ from that of the general population.

Comorbid psychiatric conditions are diagnosed more frequently in those with intellectual disabilities than in the general population. Even so, psychiatric disorders probably are underappreciated in this population.

Attention deficit/hyperactivity disorder (ADHD) is diagnosed in 8–15% of children and 17–52% of adults with MR. Self-injurious behaviors require treatment in 3–15%, particularly in the severe range of MR/ID. Major depression, bipolar disorders, anxiety disorders, and other mood disorders are the most common psychiatric diagnoses in adults with MR/ID. Obsessive-compulsive disorder, conduct disorder, tic disorders, and other stereotypic behaviors are also diagnosed more commonly in those with MR/ID. Schizophrenia may have a prevalence of 3% in individuals with MR/ID, compared to 0.8% in the general population.

In the 1970 Isle of Wight study, as many as 30% of children with MR/ID exhibited an emotional or behavioral disorder, compared to 6% of children in the general population. MR compounded by epilepsy conferred a 56% risk of comorbid psychiatric disease in this study.[287] Occult visual and auditory deficits occur in 50% of those with MR/ID, particularly when refractive errors are considered. The rates of transmittable diseases, including sexually transmitted diseases (STDs), hepatitis B, and *Helicobacter pylori* infection, are increased significantly among individuals with MR/ID. One in 5 individuals with MR/ID also has cerebral palsy (CP). As many as 20% of individuals with MR/ID have seizures. GI complications with MR/ID include feeding dysfunction, excess drooling, reflux esophagitis, and constipation. GU complications with MR/ID include urinary incontinence and poor menstrual hygiene.

A profound social morbidity affects individuals with MR/ID and their families. This morbidity can be measured in lost wages, dependence on social services, impaired long-term relationships, and emotional suffering.

Race

Consistent racial differences in prevalence of MR/ID and associated mortality rates are not known to exist.

SEX

The gender ratios for mortality and morbidity do not differ from the gender ratio noted in the severe/profound ranges of intellectual disability (i.e. male-to-female ratio, 1.2:1).

AGE

MR/ID refers to intellectual impairment that develops prior to the age of 18 years. Certain syndromes associated with MR/ID, such as Down syndrome, are associated with shorter life expectancy than the general population. In a comparison of those with MR/ID with and without Down syndrome from the California Department of Developmental Services cohort, excess mortality in the Down syndrome group tended to decrease with advancing age up to 35–39 years but increased thereafter. The increase in death rate from age 40 years was steeper in patients with Down syndrome than in those without Down syndrome.[288]

PRESENTING SIGNS/SYMPTOMS

The presenting symptoms and signs of MR/ID typically include cognitive skills delays, language delay, and delays in adaptive skills. Developmental delays vary depending on the level of MR/ID and the etiology. For example, in mild nonsyndromic MR/ID, delays may not be notable until the preschool years, whereas with severe or profound MR associated with syndromes or extreme prematurity, for example, significant delays in milestones may be noted from birth.

Language delay: One of the first signs of MR/ID may be language delays, including expressive language (speech) and receptive language (understanding). Red flags include no mama/dada/babbling by 12 months, no 2-word phrases by age 2, and parents reporting they are concerned that the child may be deaf.

FINE MOTOR/ADAPTIVE DELAY

Significant delays in activities such as self-feeding, toileting, and dressing are typically reported in children with MR/ID. Prolonged, messy finger feeding and drooling are signs of oral-motor incoordination.

Cognitive delay: Children with MR/ID have difficulties with memory, problem-solving and logical reasoning. This may be expressed early on with preacademic difficulties or difficulty following directions (particularly multipart directions).

Social delays: Children with MR may display lack of interest in age-appropriate toys and delays in imaginative play and reciprocal play with age-matched peers. Rather than their chronological age, play reflects their developmental levels.

GROSS MOTOR

Delays in gross motor development infrequently accompany the cognitive, language, and fine motor/adaptive delays associated with MR/ID unless the underlying condition results in both MR/ID and cerebral palsy. Subtle delays in gross motor acquisition, or clumsiness, may be identified in the developmental assessment.

BEHAVIORAL DISTURBANCES

Even before an age at which psychopathology can be identified, infants and toddlers who go on to have MR/ID may be more likely to have difficult temperaments, hyperactivity, disordered sleep, and colic.

Associated behaviors may include aggression, self-injury, defiance, inattention, hyperactivity, sleep disturbances, and stereotypic behaviors.

NEUROLOGIC AND PHYSICAL ABNORMALITIES

Prevalence of MR is increased among children with seizure disorders, microcephaly, macrocephaly, history of intrauterine or postnatal growth retardation, prematurity, and congenital anomalies. In the process of addressing somatic problems, assessment of a child's cognitive abilities is often overlooked.

Diagnoses of MR/ID and autism frequently overlap. Approximately 50–75% of those with autism (autistic disorder) also have MR/ID.[289] Some literature has suggested diagnostic shifts from MR to autism for unknown reasons.[290]

FAMILY HISTORY

Guidelines from the American Academy of Pediatrics recommend that the evaluation of a child with MR/ID includes an extensive family history, with particular attention to family members with MR, developmental delays, consanguinity, psychiatric diagnoses, congenital malformations, miscarriages, stillbirths, and early childhood deaths. The clinician should construct a pedigree of 3 generations or more.[291]

DEVELOPMENTAL ASSESSMENT

The American Academy of Pediatrics recommends developmental screening for all children at regular intervals. Methods include several parental surveys, such as the Parents' Evaluation of Developmental Status (PEDS), Ages and Stages Questionnaires (ASQ) and Child Development Inventories (CDI). Other instruments require direct observation, such as the Bayley Infant Neurodevelopmental Screener, Battelle Developmental Inventory, Early Language Milestone Scale, and Brigance Screens.

Key behavioral observations should focus on the child's communicative intent, social skills, eye contact, compliance, attention span, impulsivity, and style of play. For the diagnoses of developmental delay and MR/ID, an expanded neurodevelopmental and psychological examination is required. Various tests can be administered to assess language comprehension, language expression, nonverbal cognitive abilities, fine motor and adaptive abilities, attention span, memory, gross motor skills, and adaptive behaviors. The most common psychological tests for children include the Bayley Scales of Infant Development-III, the Stanford-Binet Intelligence Scale, the Wechsler Intelligence Scale for Children-IV, the Wechsler Preschool and Primary Scale of

Intelligence-Revised, and the Vineland Adaptive Behavior Scales-II.

PHYSICAL EXAMINATION

Head circumference: Measurement of all growth parameters must include head circumference. Microcephaly correlates highly with cognitive deficits. Macrocephaly may indicate hydrocephalus and is associated with some inborn errors of metabolism and may also be seen early on in some children later diagnosed with autism.[292,293]

Height: Short stature may suggest a genetic disorder, fetal alcohol syndrome, or hypothyroidism. Tall stature may suggest fragile X syndrome (FraX), Soto syndrome, or other overgrowth syndrome associated with MR/ID.

Neurologic: This examination should include assessments of head growth (for micro/macrocephaly), muscle tone (for hypotonia or spasticity), strength and coordination, deep tendon reflexes, persistent primitive reflexes, ataxia, and other abnormal movements such as dystonia or athetosis.

Sensory: Vision and hearing should always be tested in suspected cases of MR/ID. Children with disabilities and MR/ID are more likely than other children to have visual impairment (refractive errors, strabismus, amblyopia, cataracts, abnormal retinal pigmentation, and cortical blindness) and hearing deficits, particularly among those with severe impairments.

Skin: Cutaneous findings of etiologic interest include hyperpigmented and hypopigmented macules, such as café-au-lait macules (associated with neurofibromatosis type 1), and ash-leaf spots (associated with tuberous sclerosis), fibromas, and irregular pigmentation patterns.

Extremities: Examine for dysmorphic features and organ system dysfunction indicative of syndromes. Although MR/ID with multiple congenital anomalies and major malformations accounts for only 5–10% of all cases, most of these affected individuals have 3–4 minor anomalies, especially involving the face and digits.

CAUSES

Prenatal Conditions (Genetic)

Trisomy 21 or Down Syndrome

This disorder accounts for 25–50% of persons with severe MR; Down syndrome occurs in approximately 1 per 600 to 800 live births.

In infancy, this disorder is recognized by specific facial features, including flat facial profile, brachycephaly, up-slanted and narrow palpebral fissures, and anomalous auricles.

Hypotonia, joint hyperextensibility, neonatal jaundice, simian crease, shortened digits, and excess skin on the back of the neck contribute to the clinical features.

Congenital heart disease is present in approximately 40%. GI malformations are present in 5%. Congenital cataracts are found in 3%, and as many as 35% require treatment for strabismus or refractive error. Infantile spasms may develop in 5%.

The IQ score ranges from 25 to 50. Generally, verbal-linguistic skills lag behind visual-spatial skills and social performance is usually above the mental age.

In trisomy 21, gene expression of chromosome 21 is increased in a dosage-dependent fashion that varies by tissue type. While some trisomic 21 genes are not expressed at elevated levels, many are. Of those significantly increased, several encode proteins critical for mitochondrial function and for neurogenesis.

Other chromosomal abnormalities (e.g. deletions, duplications, translocations) may be present in as many as 25% of individuals with severe MR.

The most commonly occurring abnormalities of this class, detectable at the 500 band level of chromosomal analysis, are 5p- (i.e. Cri du chat syndrome) and 4p- (i.e. Wolf-Hirschhorn syndrome).

Cryptic subtelomeric deletions are diagnosed with increasing frequency as fluorescently tagged molecular DNA probes allow detection of deletions below the microscopic resolution of a standard karyotype.

Cryptic subtelomeric rearrangements now account for 5–6% of cases of idiopathic mental retardation.

Chromosomal analysis is undergoing further refinement with the application of gene array hybridization techniques that may detect abnormalities in up to 20% of cases of idiopathic mental retardation.

Fragile X Syndrome

The population prevalence of this disorder is approximately 1 in 3500 males, giving prevalence within the MR population of about 1 in 76. For males with severe MR, the prevalence rises to about 1 in 13. Other studies have found in populations of those with mental retardation positive fragile X studies in 5.9% of males and 0.3% of females.[294] About 1 in 2000 females carries the fragile X (FraX) gene. Current studies suggest that FraX is the most prevalent form of inherited MR.

Males with the full FMR1 trinucleotide repeat expansion (i.e. the full mutation) usually function in the moderate to severe range of MR.[295] Other features include testicular enlargement in the postpubertal period and minor facial anomalies (e.g. large forehead, elongated face, protuberant auricles, prominent chin).

Females with the full FMR1 trinucleotide repeat expansion may have no symptoms, although some have mild learning disabilities or even mild to moderate MR.

Mitral valve prolapse and seizures may occur.

Up to 20% of FraX males meet criteria for autism; autistic like behaviors can be present in affected females as well.

Direct DNA analysis of the FMR-1 gene is the method of choice for diagnosing both affected individuals with the full trinucleotide repeat expansion (>200 repeats) and unaffected carriers with the premutation (60–200 repeats).

Contiguous Gene Deletion Syndromes

Although less common, some of these syndromes can be readily identified clinically. The following syndromes often can be confirmed by utilizing a fluorescence *in situ* hybridization (FISH) probe to the deleted region in question.

Prader-Willi Syndrome

The Prader-Willi syndrome (PWS) involves deletion at 15q11-q13 (deletion of the paternally derived region).

Classic clinical features include neonatal and infantile hypotonia, feeding problems or failure to thrive in infancy, excessive weight gain with hyperphagia beginning between ages 12 months and 6 years, food compulsions, hypogonadism, global developmental delay, almond-shaped eyes, thin upper lip, and down-turned corners of the mouth.

The candidate gene within the Prader-Willi gene region is SNRPN, which encodes a ribonucleoprotein involved in mRNA splicing. How SNRPN contributes to the hypothalamic dysfunction that defines many clinical features of PWS is unclear.

It is the first known human disorder of genomic imprinting, leading to revolutionary changes in the field of molecular genetics and the understanding of uniparental disomy.

Negative FISH results in PWS may be due to maternal uniparental disomy (UPD) of chromosome 15 (2 number 15 chromosomes from the mother) and can be confirmed with molecular studies.

Angelman Syndrome

The Angelman syndrome (AS) also involves deletion at 15q11-q13 (deletion of the maternal copy of the gene region).

MR, absent speech, microcephaly, seizures, puppet like ataxic movements, inappropriate laughter, and facial dysmorphisms characterize AS.

The candidate genes within the AS critical region include UBE3A, whose protein product is important in the post-translational modification of proteins by ubiquitination, and GABRA3, a subunit of the GABAa receptor.

Negative FISH results in AS may be due to paternal UPD of chromosome 15 (2 number 15 chromosomes from the father) and can be confirmed with molecular studies.

Point mutations occasionally are found in AS with negative results on FISH and UPD studies.

Smith-Magenis Syndrome

Smith-Magenis syndrome (SMS) involves deletion at 17p11.2.

MR, short stature, brachydactyly, minor skeletal and facial anomalies, sleep disturbance, self-injurious behaviors, and other organ system malformations characterize this contiguous gene deletion syndrome.[296]

Although as many as 100 genes may be deleted in SMS, the physical characteristics are subtle.

CATCH 22 Syndrome

The CATCH 22 syndrome, which comprises DiGeorge syndrome (DGS) and velocardiofacial syndrome (VCF), involves deletion at 22q11.

Infants with classic DGS are identified readily by aplasia or hypoplasia of the thymus, T cell lymphopenia, conotruncal cardiac defects, oral-motor dysfunction, and facial dysmorphisms (e.g. low-set malformed ears, small jaw, palatal defects, hypertelorism, antimongoloid palpebral slant).

Minor variants may meet clinical criteria for the VCF syndrome. With a prevalence of 1 in 4,000 people, it is the most common known microdeletion disorder.

The majority of individuals with CATCH 22 have learning disabilities or mild MR and comorbid psychiatric disorders including schizophrenia and mood disorders with psychosis.

Williams Syndrome

The Williams syndrome involves deletion at 7q11.[297]

Characteristic facial features are described as "elfin." In the majority, valvular stenosis, poor growth, hypotonia, late-onset contractures, dental anomalies, infantile colic, oral-motor discoordination, and hyperacusis (i.e. hypersensitivity to sound) are reported. Infantile hypercalcemia may be transient and is often subclinical.

Mild to moderate MR, relative preservation of language, and associated weakness in visual-spatial development are typical.

Elastin is the candidate gene presumed responsible for some of Williams syndrome features, including supravalvular aortic stenosis.

Wolf-Hirschhorn Syndrome

The Wolf-Hirschhorn syndrome, also known as 4p-syndrome, involves deletion at 4p16.3.

Severe growth retardation, microcephaly, "Greek helmet" facies and orofacial clefts, and other midline fusion defects characterize this syndrome.

The region of deletion is gene dense, and an undefined number of genes may contribute to this phenotype.

Langer-Giedion Syndrome

This syndrome, also known as trichorhinophalangeal syndrome type II, involves deletion at 8q24.1.

Learning disabilities and the presence of MR vary.

Facial dysmorphisms include microcephaly, large ears, bulbous nose, broad nasal bridge, elongated philtrum, and sparse scalp hair. Multiple nevi and skeletal anomalies may be present.

Miller-Dieker Syndrome

The Miller-Dieker syndrome (MDS) involves deletion at 17p13.3.

Infants present with severe neurologic impairment, seizures, and hypotonia secondary to lissencephaly. The smooth cerebral cortex with absent or decreased gyral formation results from abnormal neuronal migration.

The identified gene LIS1 may function as a G protein subunit in cellular signal transduction that is important in telencephalon development.

Many contiguous gene deletion syndromes for which a FISH probe is not available have been recognized in association with MR. A comprehensive survey is beyond the scope of this article.

Single Gene Mutation Syndromes

Tuberous sclerosis

Hypopigmented cutaneous macules (i.e. ash-leaf spots), calcified intracranial cortical tubers with or without heterotopias, seizures, retinal hamartomas, and renal angiomyolipomas characterize this hamartomatous condition.

MR may or may not be seen in affected individuals; the presence of seizures is the factor most associated with poor cognitive outcome. Autism is a rather common finding in children with tuberous sclerosis associated with MR.

This is an autosomal-dominant inherited condition with about half of affected individuals resulting from a new mutation. Two genes have been identified, one at 9q34 (TSC1) and the other at 16p13 (TSC2). A variety of deletions, rearrangements, and point mutations have been implicated in tuberous sclerosis.

Rubinstein-Taybi Syndrome

Broad terminal phalanges, beaked nose, down-slanting palpebral fissures, epicanthal folds, and microcephaly characterize this syndrome.

Behavioral aspects include variable degrees of impulsivity, distractibility, instability of mood, and stereotypies.[298]

This is an autosomal-dominant inherited condition, with the majority of cases representing new deletions or point mutations of the CREB-binding protein gene (16p13.3).

Coffin-Lowry Syndrome

This syndrome is characterized by hypertelorism, down-slanting palpebral fissures, frontal prominence, thickened lips and nasal septum, as well as dental and skeletal anomalies.

It is an X-linked condition, with females having mild manifestations. The syndrome results from mutations in the RSK2 gene, which encodes a CREB kinase (Xp22.2-p22.1).[299]

Rett Syndrome

Developmental stagnation then regression, progressive microcephaly, seizures, ataxia, and autistic like behaviors are seen in affected females.

This X-linked dominant condition with presumed lethality for affected males is caused by mutations in MeCP2, a transcriptional repressor (Xq28).[300]

Smith-Lemli-Opitz Syndrome

Malformations consistent with holoprosencephaly sequence, syndactyly of toes 2 and 3, micrognathia, cleft palate, and moderate to severe MR are seen.

This autosomal-recessive inherited condition results from increases in 7-dehydrocholesterol (7-DHC) due to mutations in the 7-DHC reductase gene (11q12-q13).

Treatment with an oral cholesterol "cocktail" has shown some promise in this syndrome.

Costello Syndrome

Characteristic clinical features include polyhydramnios, failure to thrive, cardiac anomalies, and tumor predisposition.

Mean IQ is in the mild MR range, but the spectrum extends from severe MR to average intelligence. Affected males are lower functioning than females and have significantly more behavioral problems.[301]

Mutation in HRAS is identified, resulting in a gain of function of the encoded protein and increased activation of the cellular signaling pathway Ras-MAPK.[302]

Many other single-gene disorders are associated with MR with additional phenotypic and behavioral features including such problems as microcephaly, seizures, or short stature, with or without dysmorphic facies.

Recent advances in genetic linkage analysis techniques in families with multiple affected members have revealed more than 50 candidate genes along the X chromosome. In some kindreds with a pattern of X-linked nonsyndromic mild MR (XLMR), linkage analysis has identified candidate genes that code for interleukin receptors, G protein signaling factors, transcription factors, and transcriptional repressors.

ENVIRONMENTAL CAUSES

Fetal Alcohol Syndrome and Fetal Alcohol Effect

Alcohol results in a wide range of teratogenic effects.[303] The most severely affected individuals meet criteria for fetal alcohol syndrome (FAS) by demonstrating short palpebral fissures, dental crowding, camptodactyly flattened philtrum, thin vermillion border, flattening of the maxillary area, microphthalmia, prenatal and postnatal growth deficiency, microcephaly, and developmental delay.

Fetal alcohol effect (FAE) can be diagnosed only in the context of (1) maternal history of alcohol use and (2) a child with developmental and behavioral abnormalities that also manifests growth deficiency or the characteristic facial dysmorphisms.

The prevalence of FAS may be as high as 1.9 in 1000 live births and is the leading cause of MR in the western world. The impact of the milder FAE remains unknown. The teratogenic effects of alcohol may be responsible for as many as 8% of cases of mild MR. Alcohol's deleterious effects on cortical plasticity contribute to cognitive impairment.

Congenital Hypothyroidism

Congenital hypothyroidism (known as cretinism in the past) is a neurologic syndrome that results from severe thyroid hormone deficiency during the fetal period. In the infant, the syndrome comprises deaf mutism, moderate to severe MR, spasticity, and strabismus.

Normal fetal brain development requires sufficient production of both maternal and fetal thyroid hormones. Normal glandular production of T4 and T3 requires sufficient dietary intake of iodine.

Iodine deficiency may affect an estimated 800 million people worldwide. It can result in endemic goiter, fetal wastage, milder degrees of developmental delay, and endemic congenital hypothyroidism.

Perinatal/postnatal conditions: These conditions are responsible for fewer than 10% of all MR cases.

Congenital Cytomegalovirus (CMV)

Congenital rubella—No longer an important etiology in countries with high vaccination rates.

Intraventricular hemorrhage related to extreme prematurity—An important cause only in societies with advanced neonatal care and survival of the premature.

Hypoxic-ischemic encephalopathy—Always results in combined CP/MR.

Traumatic brain injury—Shaken baby syndrome, closed head injury sustained in motor vehicle accidents.

Meningitis—Decreasing in importance as the incidence of *Haemophilus influenzae* type B decreases in vaccinated populations.

- Trichomoniasis during pregnancy[304]
- Neurodegenerative disorders
- Differential diagnoses
- Autism
- Borderline intellectual functioning
- Child abuse and neglect, post-traumatic stress disorder
- Childhood disintegration disorder
- Cognitive deficits
- Depression
- Learning disorder, mathematics
- Learning disorder, reading
- Learning disorder, written expression
- Pervasive developmental disorder
- Rett's syndrome
- Severe communication/language disorder.

LABORATORY STUDIES

The examiner must determine the nature and extent of the laboratory investigation following a history and physical examination. Recommendations have been made by both the American Academy of Pediatrics[305] and the American Academy of Neurology.[306]

Availability of genetic testing, and thus recommendations for work-up, are changing rapidly. Chromosomal microarray and new sequencing techniques have revolutionized genetic testing.[307]

Array-based comparative genetic hybridization (CGH) or "microarray" is increasingly used in the evaluation of MR/ID and should be considered in the work-up of all children with MR/ID either after or as first-line instead of high-resolution karyotype and fragile-X testing (see below). The yield may be as high as 20%; however, a high false-positive rate can also confound interpretation.[307-310]

High-resolution karyotype (at the 650 band level of resolution at least) should be completed in all children with MR/ID.[305] Chromosomal abnormalities (trisomy 21 and others) may account for as many as 50% of those affected by severe to profound MR/ID.

Fragile X testing (i.e. DNA analysis of the FraX promoter region) should be ordered in all children with MR/ID.[306] In the postpubertal period, the clinical manifestations of Fragile X syndrome are likely to be readily apparent, such that DNA analysis can be ordered with more selectivity in this population. Sex chromosome aneuploidy is seen in as many as 5% of children with mild MR/ID or learning disabilities.

FISH probes are ordered as clinically indicated, as follows:

- Prader-Willi/Angelman syndrome
- Smith-Magenis syndrome

- CATCH 22
- Williams syndrome
- Wolf-Hirschhorn syndrome
- Cri du chat syndrome
- Langer-Giedion (trichorhinophalangeal) syndrome
- Miller-Dieker syndrome

Given their low yield, metabolic labs are not routinely ordered unless clinically indicated or newborn metabolic screen was not done or results are not available.[306]

- Plasma amino acids (aminoacidopathies)
- Urinary organic acids (organic acidopathies)
- Urinary mucopolysaccharides and oligosaccharides (mucopolysaccharidoses)
- Plasma 7-DHC (Smith-Lemli-Opitz syndrome)
- Thyroid function tests
- Very long-chain fatty acids (peroxisomal disorders)
- Creatine kinase (in the assessment of profound central hypotonia versus myopathy)
- Consider lead testing in children with risk factors.

IMAGING STUDIES

Brain MRI

Brain imaging should be conducted in any child with global developmental delays or MR/ID. The yield will be higher in the setting of an abnormal neurologic examination (e.g. microcephaly, focal neurologic finding and/or facial dysmorphisms).[306]

Brain MRI is generally preferred over CT scan because the former has greater resolution and enhanced detection of abnormalities in the progression and timing of myelination, demyelination, and heterotopic gray matter.

Head CT scan: This is the preferred imaging study for calcifications that may be identified with TORCH infections (i.e. toxoplasmosis, other infections, rubella, CMV, herpes simplex), when tuberous sclerosis is suspected, or if craniosynostosis is a concern.

Skeletal films: These assist with the phenotypic description, syndrome characterization, and assessment of growth.

Other Tests

Detailed assessment by a licensed professional is necessary to confirm the diagnosis of MR/ID. Some of the most commonly used tests in children include the following:

- Bayley scales of infant development
- Normalized for ages 2–49 months
- Subtest scores for receptive and expressive language, gross motor, fine motor, cognitive/problem-solving ability, and sustained attention
- Stanford-Binet intelligence scale: Normalized for ages 2 years to 23 years, fifteen subtests for assessment of 4 key areas of cognitive proficiency: verbal reasoning, abstract/visual reasoning, quantitative memory, and short-term memory

Wechsler preschool and primary scale of intelligence-revised (WPPSI-R)

- Normalized for ages 3 years to 7.25 years
- Twelve subtests for assessment of verbal and nonverbal intelligence

Wechsler intelligence scale for children–IV (WISC-IV)

- For ages 6 years to 16 years, 11 months
- Verbal and nonverbal intelligence scores derived from 12 subtests

Vineland adaptive behavior scales-II

- For neonates to adults
- Measures ability to perform daily activities required for personal and social sufficiency; adaptive or functional behaviors rated by interviewing the patient or parent/caregiver
- Deficiencies in at least 2 areas of adaptive skills required to meet the MR/ID diagnostic criteria.

ELECTROPHYSIOLOGIC STUDIES

- Auditory evoked potentials in the context of audiologic assessment
- Visual evoked potentials in cases of profound delay and suspected cortical blindness
- EEG is not recommended as part of the routine work-up of MR/ID unless the history is suggestive of seizures or a specific epileptic syndrome.[306]

HISTOLOGIC FINDINGS

- Pathologic analysis of cortical tissue by the Golgi method in the 1970s suggested that in cases of profound, unclassified MR, dendritic spines were decreased and/or had immature morphology. These findings have been confirmed in cortical autopsy material from individuals with Down syndrome and FraX. Dendritic spine morphology is related directly to the intradendritic microtubular components and their organization.
- Microtubules in dendrites of cortical neurons often are fragmented or in disarray in cases of developmental failure. In contrast, in some neuronal storage diseases associated with impaired cognition, dendritic spines are sprouted exuberantly beyond the developmental period and in ectopic locations. A relationship is implied, then, between dendritic spine morphology and number and cognitive development in the human.

MEDICAL CARE

Early identification of children with developmental delays is necessary to begin receiving early intervention services for children from birth to 3 years of age and early childhood education services for children aged 3–5 years, which are known to improve outcomes.

The mainstay of treatment of MR/ID is developing a comprehensive management plan for the condition. The complex habilitation plan for the individual requires input from care providers from multiple disciplines, including special educators, language therapists, behavioral therapists, occupational therapists, and community services that provide social support and respite care for families affected by MR/ID.

Preventive care: Unfortunately, routine preventive care for children and adults with MR/ID is lacking. Adaptive equipment (e.g. for nonambulatory patients) and extra time (e.g. double time slots) may be required to accommodate such patients. In addition, family members or other support persons may be helpful. Written plans (such as the Massachusetts Department of Developmental Services Annual Health Screening Recommendations and Health Record) are helpful for interdisciplinary team communication.

Physical activity and obesity are major contributors to disease in MR/ID. Very few programs exist that target healthy lifestyles (nutrition/diet, exercise, self-care, stress reduction) in those with MR/ID. Annual counseling and referral on these issues to community agencies and programs is recommended.[311] Medications (e.g. antipsychotics) should be titrated to reduce the risk of obesity and metabolic issues.

PAIN

Manifestations of pain in people with severe to profound MR/ID include crying, screaming, grimacing, protective postures (e.g. arching, fetal position), rocking, and aggression. Parent/caregiver input is key to interpretation of these behaviors, though validated tools have been used as adjuncts (such as the pediatric pain profile).

Common causes of acute pain include dental caries/abscesses, GERD, constipation, UTI, spasticity (when MR/ID is associated with cerebral palsy), pressure sores, and fractures.

In addition, neuropathic pain due to dysautonomia or motor spasms may create chronic disturbances. Treatment should be prompt and include NSAIDs or acetaminophen for mild pain, tramadol or equivalent for moderate pain, and opioids for severe pain as indicated, and management of sources of pain. Some suggest use of gabapentin for neuropathic pain if no sources are identified and there is a history of surgery, symptoms suggesting visceral hyperalgesia (e.g. associated with feedings or bowel movements), or symptoms of autonomic dysfunction and spasticity.

Written, verbal and pictoral forms of communication as well as gestures and demonstrations are helpful for those with MR/ID to ensure mutual understanding and improve treatment adherence.

Sedation/anesthesia: Patients with MR/ID requiring anesthesia may have different reactions than the general population, such as paradoxical reactions to benzodiazepines, and care should be taken to use the lowest dose and titrate slowly.

Sexuality/abuse: A significantly higher proportion of children and adults with MR/ID have experienced some form of abuse, with some estimates of up to 70%, which contributes to mental health issues. This should be addressed at each medical visit and especially in the setting of changes in behaviors, such as increased aggression.

No treatments are available specifically for cognitive deficiency. Although the pharmacologic enhancement of cognition (e.g. use of donepezil in patients with Down syndrome[312] is an area of interest, research on such nootropic (i.e. knowledge-enhancing) compounds is limited. Such drugs have not become part of the routine or even experimental clinical management of this population.

OTHER CONCERNS

Individuals in the United States older than 18 years are no longer under the guardianship of their biological parents. No exceptions are made for children with MR/ID. Most of these individuals, particularly those in the range of mild MR, are capable of making appropriate legal and medical decisions when adequately and appropriately informed of the decision outcomes.

Physicians have the duty to ascertain whether patients with MR/ID have the capacity to consent for medical treatments. This may be challenging and outside information and supports (e.g. family, caregivers, social workers) may be required to confirm the patients' understanding of the risks, benefits and alternatives to the procedure.

Some individuals may not be capable of comprehending the implications of the medical or legal matter at hand. In such cases, the decision is best made by a member of the biological family. The family member may obtain guardianship status for power of attorney over these matters. If a family member is unavailable to serve as guardian, then a guardian ad litem can be assigned by the court for assistance in such legal and medical matters. If a patient with MR/ID does not have the capacity to consent, then the patient's assent should be sought if possible.

Subsequent to the long history of forced sterilization of girls/women with MR/ID, varied federal, state, and local laws regulate sterilization of individuals with MR/ID. The American College of Obstetrician/Gynecologists provides guidance on informed consent for sterilization procedures in patients with ID/MR.[313]

Complex decisions, particularly those involving end of life, are perhaps best handled with the assistance of the ethics committee of the involved medical institution.

Failure to identify a genetic cause of MR/ID with risks to other family members or risks to the patient for future medical complications is potential medical/legal pitfalls.

Perhaps 1 in 8 convicts on death row in the United States has MR/ID. Many persons cannot fully comprehend the Miranda Rights and other critical concepts necessary to maneuver through the criminal justice system.

CONSULTATIONS

- Developmental pediatrician or psychologist
- Geneticist and counselor
- Psychiatrist
- Dentist
- Podiatrist
- Special education/educational therapist
- Occupational, speech and/or physical therapist
- Behaviorist
- Pharmacist
- Durable medical equipment providers
- Social services agencies/social workers
- Diet
  Nutritional supplements are of no proven benefit.

ACTIVITY

Because obesity is more prevalent in those with MR/ID, regular physical activity should be included in the management plan.[314] Adaptive exercise programs for those with concomitant physical disabilities should be recommended as needed.[311]

MEDICATION SUMMARY

No specific pharmacologic treatment is available for cognitive impairment in the developing child or adult with MR/ID.[315] Medications, when prescribed, are targeted to specific comorbid psychiatric disease or behavioral disturbances.

Development of nootropic drugs that may alter cognitive processes positively has been of interest to researchers. Medications currently prescribed for dementia, such as acetylcholinesterase inhibitors, are not accepted treatments for MR/ID, and clinical trials have not been conducted in children. Phosphodiesterase inhibitors enhance cortical plasticity in an animal model of fetal alcohol syndrome.

Although vitamin and mineral therapies have gained popularity, their efficacy has not been established in clinical trials. A randomized controlled study of antioxidants and/or folinic acid for 18 months in 156 infants with Down syndrome found no evidence to support the use of these supplements in this population.[316]

CENTRAL NERVOUS SYSTEM STIMULANTS

The most common class of drugs prescribed in this population is the psychostimulants because of the diagnosis of attention deficit with or without hyperactivity disorder (ADHD/ADD) in 6–80%. Few studies are available on stimulants in people with MR/ID and, in many studies, those with MR/ID have been specifically excluded. Available studies indicate that benefits vary and significant adverse events, such as severe social withdrawal, increased crying, drowsiness, and irritability have been noted, especially at higher doses of methylphenidate (0.6 mg/kg).[317]

Methylphenidate Hydrochloride

- Stimulates cerebral cortex and subcortical structures.
- Dextroamphetamine sulfate and racemic amphetamine
- Increase amount of circulating dopamine and norepinephrine in cerebral cortex by blocking reuptake of norepinephrine or dopamine from synapse.

Alpha-adrenergic Agonists

These agents are used commonly to modulate hyperactivity, aggression, tics, and dyssomnias. None of these drugs has an FDA-approved indication for MR/ID.

Clonidine Hydrochloride

Agonist at presynaptic alpha2-adrenergic receptors within brain stem. Clonidine reduces norepinephrine release at these sites, reducing sympathetic outflow and enhancing parasympathetic outflow. May reduce aggression by increasing release of GABA in frontal cortex and other brain regions.

Guanfacine

Presynaptic alpha2-adrenergic receptor agonist that stimulates alpha2-adrenergic receptors in brain stem, activating an inhibitory neuron, which in turn decreases vasomotor tone and heart rate. Similar reduction in potentially negative impact on academic performance and cognitive function.

Neuroleptic Drugs (Antipsychotics)

The neuroleptic drugs are the most frequently prescribed agents for targeting behaviors such as aggression, self-injury, and hyperactivity in people with MR/ID. These indications are generally off-label for MR/ID and caution is advised. Increasingly, they are more likely to be reserved for the older child or adult in whom intensive behavioral intervention has failed. Likewise, the prevalence of comorbid psychiatric disorders in MR/ID increases with age. Neuroleptics interact with receptors for a variety of brain neurotransmitters, including dopamine, serotonin, acetylcholine, histamine, and norepinephrine. Their ability to antagonize dopamine receptors appears to correlate with the efficacy of these drugs and imparts their antipsychotic properties. Likewise, antidopaminergic activity evokes extrapyramidal symptoms. Rarely, neuroleptic malignant syndrome may occur.

Risperidone

Atypical antipsychotic with fewer adverse neurologic effects and less propensity for extrapyramidal movements (e.g. pseudoparkinsonism, akathisia, acute dystonias, tardive dyskinesia).

Aripiprazole

A newer atypical antipsychotic, aripiprazole is indicated in acute bipolar mania and schizophrenia.

FURTHER OUTPATIENT CARE

Children with MR/ID should be evaluated regularly by a neurologist or neurodevelopmental pediatrician with a special interest in the etiology and management of cognitive disorders. The physician should have adequate knowledge of the educational, social, and support services available in the community; assessing the appropriateness of the patient's individualized habilitation is important.

To maximize the individual's functional independence, the following areas should be addressed by the physician at least annually:

- Treatment of associated impairments
- Pharmacotherapy
- Behavior management
- Educational services
- Recreational needs
- Family counseling.

The annual visit requires routine preventive medicine and coordination of specialized services such as dental and gynecologic care under sedation. Supplemental vaccines, including the influenza and hepatitis B vaccines, are particularly prudent for those in residential placements. A careful behavioral history is important to identify newly emerging maladaptive behaviors that may be treated effectively with behavior management. Examples of health care guidelines for individuals with MR/ID include the Massachusetts Department of Mental Retardation checklist.[318] If patients have coexisting motor impairments, the physician should monitor for secondary orthopedic disease. Advanced knowledge in the pharmacologic management of spasticity and rigidity allows the clinician to refer the patient for botulinum toxin injections or baclofen pump insertion when appropriate. Arthroplasty for progressive hip dislocation and/or tendon releases for progressive contractures due to spasticity may be required.

The health maintenance schedule for individuals with Down syndrome is well recognized. The American Academy of Pediatrics and American Academy of Family Practice have provided practice guidelines on the preventive care of children and adults with Down syndrome.[319] Ongoing vision and audiologic evaluation, thyroid function tests, and screening for atlantoaxial instability and obstructive sleep apnea are some important components. The American Academy of Pediatrics has recently provided practice guidelines for the health maintenance of children with Prader-Willi syndrome.[320]

ROLE OF PSYCHIATRIST IN MENTAL RETARDATION

The psychiatrist has multiple roles to play in the field of mental retardation. Besides the usual role as a diagnostician, therapist and researcher, the psychiatrist is often called as a consultant to various special schools or institutions for the mentally retarded. The environment at such places is different from the hospital set-up, where the psychiatrist acts as the chief coordinator of the therapeutic team. At such places, he is usually assigned the role of a medication consultant rather than being involved in the global therapeutic or rehabilitation work, leading sometimes to an impersonal type of attitude. Such a phenomenon can also lead to a negative image of the speciality. Therefore, for proper professional services to be provided to the retarded patients, a broader and more active approach is needed.

43.13 SPECIFIC DEVELOPMENTAL DISORDERS

Manju Mehta, Rajesh Sagar

Specific developmental disorders are disorders in which there is delayed development in a specific area or areas, other aspects of development being largely or entirely unaffected. These areas refer to deficiencies in the development of skills in the academic, language, and motor domains. The term 'developmental' implies persistence of the disorder in spite of advancing chronological age.

More and more children each year are being identified as having problems which affects their ability to attend and/or learn. Over the years, it has been given different labels like dyslexia, perceptual handicap, neurological impairment, minimal brain dysfunction, congenital word blindness, developmental aphasia, congenital aphasia, and educational handicap. One of the common reasons for scholastic problems in school is specific developmental disorders (SDD). But until very recent time, it was often not diagnosed due to lack of awareness and paucity of assessment tools.

CLASSIFICATION IN DSM-IV AND ICD-10

In DSM-III-R, these disorders were grouped together in Axis II of the diagnostic system and known as *specific developmental disorders*, but in DSM-IV they are promoted to Axis I and reclassified under the diagnoses of *learning disorder, motor skills disorder* and *communication disorder*. Learning disorders are divided into four categories, i.e. reading disorder, mathematics disorder, disorder of written expression and learning disorder, not otherwise specified (NOS). The motor skill disorder includes a sole subtype, i.e. developmental coordination disorder. The communication disorders include expressive language disorder, receptive language disorder, phonological disorder (formerly, developmental articulation disorder), stuttering, and communication disorder (NOS).

ICD-10 contains four subgroups of specific developmental disorders:

1. *Specific disorders of speech and language*: It includes specific speech articulation disorder, expressive language disorder, receptive language disorder, acquired aphasia with epilepsy (Landau-Kleffner Syndrome), other developmental disorders of speech and language, and developmental disorders of speech and language (unspecified).
2. *Specific developmental disorders of scholastic skills*: It includes specific reading disorder, specific spelling disorder, specific disorder of arithmetical skills, mixed disorders of scholastic skills, other developmental disorders of scholastic skills and developmental disorders of scholastic skills (unspecified).
3. *Specific developmental disorder of motor function.*
4. *Mixed specific developmental disorders.*

Although these are the psychiatric diagnostic labels, specific developmental disorders are subsumed under various labels by other classification system to include learning disability, learning disorder, specific learning disability (SLD), language impairment and communication disorder.

PREVALENCE

Due to lack of studies in India, the true prevalence of these disorders is not known. In conducting such researches, the problems exist in its definition, diagnostic criteria, type of settings and research design. The prevalence data available from developed countries suggests the reasonable estimate between 5% and 10% of specific developmental disorders.

According to DSM-IV, in United States, the prevalence of reading disorder and mathematics disorder is estimated at 4% and 1% respectively, of school-age children. The prevalence of developmental coordination disorder is 6% for children in age range of 5–11 years. The prevalence of various language disorders are between 2% and 5% for children.

Most of these are several times more common in boys than in girls.

COMMON FEATURES OF SPECIFIC DEVELOPMENTAL DISORDERS

1. Individual does not learn despite average intellectual potential and adequate opportunities.
2. Significant discrepancy exists between intellectual potential or academic aptitude and performance. The discrepancy is significant enough to require specialized intervention.
3. It is not due to direct result of mental retardation, medical or neurological illness, environmental factors, sensory, cultural or instructional deprivation.
4. These disorders have their onset during infancy or childhood.
5. There is an impairment or delay in the development of functions that are strongly related to biological maturation of the central nervous system.
6. They have a steady course without remissions and relapses that are characteristic of many mental disorders.

CLINICAL PRESENTATIONS

Broadly, specific developmental disorders are classified under the main categories of language and speech disorders, scholastic skill disorders and motor skill disorder.

Language and Speech Disorder

These disorders constitute the disturbance in the normal patterns of language acquisition, that too from the early stages of development. In normal children, the language acquisition varies widely; thus it is difficult to differentiate between 'normal variation' and 'delay.' ICD-10 suggests a delay that is "sufficiently severe to fall outside the limits of 2 standard deviations may be considered as abnormal". Whereas DSM-IV states "scores substantially below those obtained from standardized measures of both nonverbal intellectual capacity and receptive language development" for expressive language disorder. ICD-10 further states four main criteria for these disorders: severity, course, pattern and associated problems. The last of these include scholastic deficits, problems with interpersonal relationships, self-esteem, behavior and emotions. More than one language disorders may coexist in the same individual.

Specific Speech Articulation Disorder

This disorder is also known as developmental articulation disorder, developmental phonological disorder, dyslalia and lalling. The main feature of this disorder is deficiency in the development of speech sounds or correct articulation at appropriate ages but with normal level of language skills. This leads to omissions, substitutions, misarticulations, distortions and inconsistencies.

Expressive Language Disorder

This disorder is also known as 'developmental dysphasia or aphasia, expressive type.' The essential feature of this disorder is deficiency in the development in use of expressive spoken language at appropriate ages, but language comprehension is within normal limits. This includes restricted vocabulary, overuse of small set of general words, limited or immature sentence structure, difficulties in selecting appropriate words, syntactical errors, misuse of grammar, lack of sentence fluency and sequencing.

Receptive Language Disorder

This disorder is also known as developmental aphasia or dysphasia, receptive type, developmental Wernicke's aphasia and word deafness. The main feature of this disorder is failure in the development of ability to understand or comprehend language at appropriate ages. This includes inability to follow simple, routine instructions, grammatical structures or more subtle aspects of language (tone of voice, gestures, etc.). In almost all cases, expressive language is also severely disturbed. This disorder has the highest rate of associated socioemotional behavior disturbance among all of the developmental language disorders.

DSM-5 Diagnostic Criteria for Language Disorder 315.39 (F80.9)

- Persistent difficulties in the acquisition and use of language across modalities (i.e. spoken, written, sign language, or other) due to deficits in comprehension or production that include the following:
  - Reduced vocabulary (word knowledge and use).
  - Limited sentence structure (ability to put words and word endings together to form sentences based on the rules of grammar and morphology).
  - Impairments in discourse (ability to use vocabulary and connect sentences to explain or describe a topic BR series of events or have a conversation).
- Language abilities are substantially and quantifiably below those expected for age, resulting in functional limitations in effective communication, social participation, academic achievement, or occupational performance, individually or in any combination.
- Onset of symptoms is in the early developmental period.
- The difficulties are not attributable to hearing or other sensory impairment, motor dysfunction, or another medical or neurological condition and are not better explained by intellectual disability (intellectual developmental disorder) or global developmental delay.

DSM-5 Diagnostic Criteria for Speech Sound Disorder 315.39 (F80.0)

- Persistent difficulty with speech sound production that interferes with speech intelligibility or prevents verbal communication of messages.
- The disturbance causes limitations in effective communication that interfere with social participation, academic achievement, or occupational performance, individually or in any combination.
- Onset of symptoms is in the early developmental period.
- The difficulties are not attributable to congenital or acquired conditions, such as cerebral palsy, cleft palate, deafness or hearing loss, traumatic brain injury, or other medical or neurological conditions.

Scholastic Skills Disorders

The main feature of these disorders is impairment in the development of normal patterns of skill acquisition than would be expected based on intellectual ability. According to ICD-10, one of the basic requirements, for the diagnosis of these disorders, is clinically significant degree of impairment in the specified scholastic skill. These may be assessed on the basis of (1) severity, as defined in scholastic terms (i.e. a degree that may be expected to occur in less than 3% of school children), (2) on developmental precursors (i.e. the scholastic difficulties were preceded by developmental delays or deviance), (3) on associated problems (i.e. inattention, over activity, emotional or conduct difficulties), (4) on pattern (i.e. the presence of qualitative abnormalities that are not usually part of normal development, and (5) on response (i.e. that scholastic difficulties do not rapidly and readily remit with increased help at home and/or at school).

Other specific developmental disorders may coexist with specified scholastic skill disorder. Moreover, it is not a single disorder; rather it is heterogeneous and multidimensional.

Specific Reading Disorder

The essential feature of this disorder is significant impairment in skill development related to reading. There may be difficulties in recognition, oral reading skills (omissions, substitutions, distortions, slow rate, false starts, long hesitations, reversals), comprehension skills (inability to recall, to draw conclusions and inferences, and to use general knowledge as background information), decoding and performance of tasks requiring reading.

This disorder is also referred to as backward reading, specific reading retardation, and developmental dyslexia.

This disorder is often preceded by history of developmental language disorder. There may be difficulties in auditory (deficits in sound categorization or discrimination) or visual processing (letter discrimination problems). There may also be associated neurodevelopmental motor soft signs or abnormal neurologic signs.

Specific Spelling (Writing) Disorder

The main facet of this disorder, according to ICD-10, is impairment in the development of spelling skills, either orally or in writing, in the absence of history of specific reading disorder. In DSM-IV, it is known as 'disorder of written expression,' which suggests impairment in expressive writing abilities.

Impairments in writing include handwriting, spelling, written syntax, written discourse, grammatical or punctuation errors, and poor paragraph organization. It is a disorder in which child cannot combine auditory or visual verbal information into motor action needed for writing. Other factors that influence writing are attention, language, memory, visuomotor, audio-verbal, visuoverbal and combined processing deficits.

This disorder is also known as developmental dysgraphia and is classified under five types. This include pure agraphia (writing problems without any other significant language problems), aphasic agraphia (language based problems that interfere with written language), agraphia with alexia (deficits in reading and writing in absence of aphasia), apraxic agraphia (deficits in formation of graphemes when writing spontaneously) and spatial agraphia (problems writing in horizontal line and poor use of spacing).

Specific Disorder of Arithmetical Skills

This disorder is characterized by specific impairment of mathematical skills. The deficits relate to basic skills such as addition, subtraction, multiplication and division, rather than the more complex ones as algebra, trigonometry, geometry and calculus. The difficulties are regarded in failure to understand its concept, mathematical terms or signs, numerical symbols, standard arithmetical manipulations, insertion of decimal points, multiplication tables and poor spatial organization of arithmetical calculations.

There may be associated 'soft' neurological signs and impaired visuospatial or visual-perceptual skills.

This disorder is also known as developmental dyscalculia and is classified under six types. These include verbal dyscalculia (naming difficulties), practognostic dyscalculia (difficulty in mathematically manipulating objects, pictured or real), lexical dyscalculia (difficulty in reading mathematical symbols), ideognostic dyscalculia (difficulty in understanding mathematical concept and performing calculation mentally), and operational dyscalculia (difficulty in performing computations).

Motor Skill Disorder

Different terms are given to this disorder, such as clumsy child syndrome, developmental coordination disorder and developmental dyspraxia. This disorder is characterized by serious impairment in motor coordination with respect to chronological age and intellectual ability. This disorder is often associated with problems in visuospatial tasks.

In this disorder, there may be delayed motor milestones. They experience difficulty in feeding, dressing, walking, running, writing, drawing, and copying. In daily activities, they tend to drop things, also they have difficulty in learning to tie shoe laces, to fasten and unfasten buttons, and in games. Scholastic difficulties may occur in some children.

DIFFERENTIATING SPECIFIC DEVELOPMENTAL DISORDERS WITH MENTAL RETARDATION

Due to poor performance in school, language problems, clumsiness in motor coordination and associated behavioral problems, especially attention deficit and conduct disorders, many such children are erroneously labeled as mentally retarded. To differentiate specific developmental disorder with mental retardation, following are some of the guidelines:

- Developmental milestones and social maturity are normal in SDD child, as compared to the mental retardation.
- The child neither achieves equally with his/her age nor in ability in one/more specific areas, when provided with learning experiences appropriate for the child's age and ability levels. Mentally retarded have overall deficits in all areas.
- A child has a severe discrepancy between achievements and intellectual ability in one/more areas.
- Mentally retarded have uniform below average scores on standard intelligence tests; specific developmental disorder children have a discrepancy of scores on different subtests, related to their specific problem.

ETIOLOGY

The causes of specific developmental disorders are regarded as multiple. There is a general underlying assumption to support the presence of cerebral dysfunction which may be of unknown origin. Researchers have found that a cerebral dysfunction can alter the neurologic processes that affect learning and behavior.

The causes may be classified under medical, structural brain differences, psychophysiological, biochemical, genetic, and information processing and neuropsychological factors.

Table 15: Medical causes of learning disorders

A. Prenatal
- Alcohol consumption
- Cigarette smoking
- Cocaine use
- Malnutrition
- RH factor incompatibility
- Maternal insufficiency
- Maternal kidney malfunction
- Fetal infections
- Exposure to toxins

B. Perinatal
- Prematurity
- Anoxia
- Prolonged labor
- Premature separation of the placenta
- Mechanically assisted delivery
- Low birth weight

C. Postnatal
- Accidental head injury
- Stroke
- High fever
- Dehydration
- Brain tumor
- Meningitis
- Encephalitis
- Hypoglycemia
- Hypothyroidism
- Otitis media
- Epilepsy

Medical

It may be divided into prenatal, perinatal and postnatal causes (Table 15).

Structural Brain Differences

These are identified through techniques, which include autopsy studies, and CT and MRI studies.

Autopsy Studies

Previously, reading disorder was proposed of having incomplete cerebral dominance, but of late it was found to have asymmetry of temporal lobes, that occurs during the development of lateralization which is abnormal in both structure and sequence. This hypothesis has been supported by autopsy studies, which show increased number of neurons in the subcortical white matter of people with reading disorder, as well as left-right hemispheric symmetry in the temporal plane, and focal cortical dysgenesis with fibromyelinic plaques. The abnormal symmetry is apparently due to excessive nerve cells in the right hemisphere, rather than lack of development of neurons in the left hemisphere. Cortical dysgenesis occurs mainly in left hemisphere along the Sylvian fissure, which is due to abnormal neuronal migration. Fibromyelinic plaques are believed to be due to changes in microcirculation.

CT and MRI Studies

These show structural differences. Subjects with reading disorder have asymmetry of the occipital widths and temporal lobe volumes; also there is reversal of the typical pattern of brain structure asymmetry. Moreover, the reduction of volume in left hemisphere suggests relative risk for the development of language based skills.

Psychophysiological Studies

EEG, or more recently QEEG and event-related potentials (ERPs), investigations, in few, have revealed abnormal brain electric activity in the left temporal and parietal regions and in the medial frontal area.

It appears that there are differences among subjects with specific developmental disorder, but yet no conclusive results have been made through EEG, ERPs, position emission tomography (PET scan) or regional cerebral blood flow studies.

Biochemical Changes

These include abnormal neurochemical transmissions and glandular disorders.

Neurotransmitters

Imbalances in the production of neurotransmitters (such as serotonin, dopamine, norepinephrine, acetylcholine) are suggested to cause difficulties in neural impulse transmission and, in consequence, learning and behavior problems. Moreover, the effectiveness of psychostimulant drugs to improve attention and learning, and to decrease hyperactivity, supports the existence of neurochemical imbalance in some individuals with learning disorders.

Glandular Disorders

These include thyroid deficiencies and hypothyroidism. These abnormalities in young age can cause permanent damage to the brain, affecting overall intelligence, language functioning and motor abilities.

Genetic Causes

There is substantial evidence to suggest that some of the specific developmental disorders are significantly influenced by genetics. In this regard, reading and language disorders have received the most attention. Support of the heritability is provided by findings that there is a higher rate of these disorders in biological relatives than what would be expected in general. Twin studies have provided further such evidence, with monozygotic twins showing higher concordance of reading disorders than dizygotic twins. Linkage analysis studies have suggested that the learning disorders in some families are linked to variations in chromosome 15 and a gene located in one section of chromosome 6. More over, it has been suggested that some sex chromosome anomalies are correlated with learning disorders. Both 47 XXX and 47 XXY karyotypes are correlated with language and motor skill delay. Fragile X syndrome is also found to be related to developmental language disorders. Learning and language disorders have also been associated with genetically transmitted syndrome, such as cleft palate, some lysosomal storage diseases, and some craniofacial syndromes.

Current studies support the view that reading disorder is familial, heritable and heterogeneous in its mode of transmission.

Information Processing and Neuropsychological Factors

Various studies have revealed that these disorders are caused by underlying intrinsic deficits in specific areas, such as memory, visual processing, auditory and language processing, attention and executive functions.

- Typically, memory is studied through information processing perspective. Information processing is broadly defined, the way input is transformed, reduced, elaborated, stored, retrieved and used. Most models of memory include the structural components of sensory (initial copy or information), short-term (limited capacity and storage by rehearsal), and long-term (permanent storage with unlimited capacity).
- Visual processes include visual perception, visual analysis, appreciation of relevant visual features, visual memory and visuospatial ability (left to right scanning).
- Auditory and language processing skills include speech perception, vocabulary skills, linguistic short-term memory, information about syntactic or semantic structure and phonetic awareness.
- Attention disorders are frequently associated, and deficits in attention process include selective attention (ability to maintain attention to target stimuli in the presence of distracters), sustained attention (vigilance or maintenance of attention for an extended period), or focus of attention.
- Executive functions are also known as metacognitive skills, which refer an individual to engage in self-monitoring and self-appraisal.

ASSOCIATED DISORDERS

Individuals with specific developmental disorders may have other psychiatric or medical disorders (including related neurological disorders). They might also have social problems.

Other Psychiatric and Medical Disorders

In most cases, psychological problems are secondary to the frustrations and frequent failures consequent to their disabilities. In others, there may be a reflection of a dysfunctional nervous system.

Studies have revealed about one third patients to have learning disorders in youth diagnosed to have conduct disorder or personality disorder (especially, the borderline type).

The classification based on 'faulty wiring' or dysfunction suggests:

- Learning disorder, when dysfunctional areas interfere with receiving, processing, and expressing information.
- Language disorder, when dysfunctional area results in difficulty in receiving and expressing language.
- Development coordination disorder (motor skill disorder), when dysfunctional areas result in difficulty with gross or fine motor activities.
- Attention deficit hyperactivity disorder (ADHD), when dysfunctional areas result in hyperactivity, distractibility or impulsivity.
- Tourette's disorder, when dysfunctional areas relate to certain modulating tasks; this may also result in obsessive-compulsive disorder.

Attention Deficit Hyperactivity Disorder

Attention deficit hyperactivity disorder (ADHD) in one of the most common associated disorders. It is estimated that up to 40% of children with learning disorder have symptoms of ADHD.

The higher risk of comorbid ADHD suggested either there is a subtype of learning disorder plus ADHD with a common cause, i.e. derived from the concept of minimal brain dysfunction, or that learning disorder leads to ADHD as a secondary symptom.

Chromosomal Abnormalities

These include Turner's syndrome, fragile X syndrome, and others.

Tourette's Disorder

Tourette's disorder is a complex disorder that is commonly associated with ADHD and learning disorder. It is estimated that approximately 50% of children with Tourette's disorder also have a learning disorder. Some studies have revealed that severity of the learning disorder in, children with Tourette's disorder, tends to decrease over time; thus it represents a marker for improvement.

There might also be associated obsessive compulsive disorder.

Social Problems

There is a considerable association of specific developmental disorder with social dysfunction. SDD may directly contribute to peer problems by interfering with success in doing activities required to interact with certain age groups. This includes visual perception and visual-motor problems interfering with ability to do quickly the eye-hand activities, such as catching, hitting or throwing a ball.

Many such children have difficulty learning social skills and being socially competent. These children do not pick up social cues, such as facial expression, tone of voice, or body language and adapt their behavior appropriately.

COURSE

Language and Speech Disorders

The prognosis of both expressive and receptive language disorders is variable and depends on severity of the disorder, time of its detection and subsequent intervention, it is likely to have experienced through childhood or adulthood. Among these language disorders, articulation disorder has the best prognosis because of its early identification. Overall, the course of these disorders is closely related to the demands of language put on the individual.

Individuals having these disorders are at increased risk for socioemotional behavioral and other psychiatric disturbances.

Scholastic Skills Disorders

These disorders are often recognized during the early elementary schooling, although the types of scholastic difficulty depend on the grade level such tasks require. The impairment in the skills may be dependent over time on severity of impairment or, conversely, as the child moves though school and academic tasks become increasingly challenging, then the impairment may interfere more and more. This supports the variable prognosis for these disorders.

The prognostic variables are level of impairment, early educational experiences, vocational demands, and the coexistence of any other disabilities, illness, socioemotional and psychiatric problems.

Motor Skill Disorders

The course of these disorders is variable. In some cases, these may continue through adolescence and adulthood.

ASSESSMENT OF SPECIFIC DEVELOPMENTAL DISORDERS

A detailed assessment is necessary to arrive at the diagnosis of specific developmental disorder. A comprehensive schedule for assessment should include:

- *Detailed history:* Medical, developmental, academic, social, school and family.
- *Physical examination:* General, vision and hearing, speech apparatus, primitive reflex and involuntary movements.
- *Medical investigations:* EEG/sleep-recording, CT scan/MRI, if necessary. In language disorders, also include audiometry and brain stem evoked response.
- *Psychiatric assessment:* To find out associated comorbid conditions (hyperactivity, conduct disorder, etc.)
- Nonverbal and verbal communication.
- *Educational:* Formal (psychoeducational test) and informal measures.
- *Neuropsychological tests:* Intelligence, adaptive behavior, personality adjustment, and attention, concentration, visuomotor coordination, and memory.

MANAGEMENT

The treatment of specific developmental disorders may be classified under pharmacological, educational, behavioral, cognitive-behavior, information processing and neuropsychological and other interventions.

Pharmacological Interventions

The use of medication for specific developmental disorders remains controversial. There is no specific treatment for such disorders, but it is often used to control associated comorbid conditions, like ADHD or depressive disorder. The primary class of medications used is psychostimulants, such as methylphenidate, dextroamphetamine and pemoline. The improvements are short-term in nature and in perceptual-cognitive tasks. The other psychotropic drugs include antianxiety agents, antidepressants, and neuroleptics or major tranquilizers. Currently gaining recognition is the use of megavitamins, mineral supplements and specific dietary regimens.

Overall, findings have been equivocal and inconclusive with regard to learning and behavioral improvements. Moreover, adverse effects on learning may result from medications. Hence, currently there is only minimal support for pharmacological interventions for specific developmental disorders, although medications may hold promise for comorbid disorders.

Educational Interventions

The efforts in this educational interventions involve remedial and compensatory approaches, and are used through a multisensory approach for building in all areas of strength, while compensating for any area of weakness. These efforts are provided through regular classroom placement (to avoid stigma), with and without consultation services (special methods of instruction and curricula provided to classroom teacher), itinerant services (provided in regular classroom setting through trained special education teacher), resource room services (efforts are undertaken in the particular area of weaknesses, while the rest of the time is spent in regular classroom), self-contained classroom (spend all or most of the day for academic instruction), and separate special school (with restrictive environment; thus rarely used).

Intervention strategies depend on the assumption made about the etiology of the disorder and the deficit targeted for treatment. Also taken into account are student and instructional variables. Student variables include various mental processes, strengths and weaknesses, method of learning and understanding, remembering, problems solving, integration of new material, and monitoring their own progress. The approach to deal such problems is called strategy instruction and focuses on teaching individuals techniques for acquiring information. Instructional variables include an understanding of curricular content (analyzing the sequence of skills needed to master a concept or procedure).

Behavior Interventions

The principles of behavioral theory have been implemented widely in educational settings, with a significant influence on instructional strategies in a child with SDD. The behavioral treatment have been characterized by two basic strategies: (a) Nonspecific, i.e. modification of incompatible behaviors, and (b) Specific, i.e. direct modifications of academic and language deficits. Specific behavioral procedures, further may be subdivided into: (a) consequence strategies, or (b) stimulus control strategies.

Consequence strategies refer to the presentation of a reinforcer or punisher contingent on an observe behavior. Error correction methods as a consequence, such as feedback, feedback and rehearsal and positive practice have also been demonstrated to promote academic progress. (b) Stimulus control strategies include modeling, stimulus fading, prompting and delayed prompting. In modeling, the correct responses are first modeled by the teacher for the students. Stimulus fading involves a technique by which difficult discriminations are taught by slowly moving from an easy discrimination to the more difficult target discrimination skill needed. For example, to teach discrimination between the letters N and M, the first letter might be presented initially as much larger than the second. As the individual consistently identifies the letters appropriately, the size of the letters is systematically changed until the child is able to discriminate the letters when presented in equal sizes. Prompting refers to the presentation of an additional cue or discriminate stimulus, to elicit a particular response in a particular manner. For example, showing a picture of "pen" when presenting the word 'pen.' Delayed prompting refers to simply delaying the presentation of the cue or prompt with goal of systematically fading out the need to have the prompt presented. Corrective reading program includes modeling, behavioral rehearsal, immediate corrective feedback and frequent delivery of reinforcement from the teacher.

Cognitive-behavioral Interventions

Cognitive-behavioral interventions are based on the principle that thoughts, cognition and environmental factors influence overt behavior. Further, there is an interaction between overt behavior and cognition or feelings. In children with learning disabilities, there is a deficiency in their ability to regulate, organize, and execute cognitive functions in an efficient manner. Hence, goals of cognitive-behavioral interventions are to teach self-control, and self-regulation. The techniques commonly employed are self-assessment, self-monitoring, self-recording and self-reinforcement. The problem solving or self-instructional strategies are often taken up for treatment. Instruction in specific learning strategies involves teaching to provide practice, and this involves a 10-step method for developing these strategies: (a) test to determine student's current learning habits, (b) describe the learning strategy, (c) model the strategy, (d) verbally rehearse the strategy, (e) practice on controlled materials, (f) feedback, (g) test, (h) practice in grade materials, (i) feedback, and (j) test.

Information Processing and Neuropsychological Interventions

This is based on the assumption of underlying deficits in how information is processed. These processing deficits are manifestations of dysfunction in specific brain regions. The processes are inferred from observed behavior or neuropsychological assessment, and are the target of remediation or compensation.

Other Interventions

These disorders interfere with communicating with peers or family, success in sports and daily activities. Lack of success in school leads to poor self-image and low self-esteem. These can cause social, emotional, behavioral and other psychiatric disturbances.

It is necessary to educate the individual and family about the nature and cause of the disorder. It often helps to emphasize that the child has a unique way of learning rather than a disordered mechanism. Family conflicts and parenting issues have to be dealt for better understanding; often family counseling helps. Some children may need specific individual, group or family therapy.

Speech therapy is often helpful in child with language and speech disorders.

43.14 SLEEP DISORDERS IN CHILDREN AND ADOLESCENTS

RK Solanki

A recent survey of 1125 adolescents aged 15–18 from France, Great Britain, Germany, and Italy found that about 20% were sleepy in the daytime, 25% had insomnia symptoms, and 4% met established criteria for an insomnia disorder.[321,322] Sleep-wake disorders are common and have an important impact on the quality of life of children, but if they are promptly recognized and treated the outcome is favorable. Alertness is the inherent ability of the brain to sustain attention and wakefulness with little or no external stimulation;[323] sleepiness results from impaired daytime alertness.

MECHANISMS OF SLEEP-WAKE REGULATION

Whether a person is awake or asleep at any given time depends on the net balance between the circadian drive, which facilitates wakefulness, and the homeostatic drive, which facilitates sleep.[324-326]

The suprachiasmatic nucleus of the hypothalamus is the circadian timekeeper (biological clock); it receives photic input from the retina and regulates the timing and length of sleep. The hypocretin (orexin) neurons located in the dorsolateral hypothalamus, and their projections to the ventral forebrain and brainstem, serve as the major wakefulness promoting system.

Serum levels of melatonin, a sleep inducing hormone produced by the pineal gland, rise just before sleep onset. Around adolescence, the timing of release of melatonin shifts to a later time at night, rendering teenagers incapable of falling asleep before about 10:30 pm.

RECOGNIZING CHILDHOOD DAYTIME SLEEPINESS

As a general rule in a school age child, habitually falling asleep while traveling in a car or train for less than 30 minutes or while reading or watching television, or regularly napping on return home from school in the afternoon should raise suspicion about pathological daytime sleepiness. Excessive caffeine intake might also be a clue. Box 6 shows important disorders leading to daytime sleepiness, and Box 7 lists the neurobehavioral consequences of childhood daytime sleepiness.

SUMMARY

Sleep-wake disorders of diverse etiology affect about a fifth of children and adolescents and can greatly impact on their quality of life.

Inadequate sleep hygiene, circadian rhythm disorders, obstructive sleep apnea, restless legs syndrome, psychiatric disorders, and narcolepsy are most common in this age group.

The most common causes of childhood obstructive sleep apnea are adenotonsillar hypertrophy, craniofacial anomalies, and neuromuscular disorders.

Daytime sleepiness resulting from these conditions may impair concentration, attention span, memory, and behavior.

Daytime sleepiness can be managed by adherence to fixed bedtimes and waking times, planned naps, and medications.

Box 6: Disorders leading to daytime sleepiness in childhood and adolescence

Insufficient night sleep and enhanced night-time arousal
- *Inadequate sleep hygiene:*
  - Physical exercise late at night
  - Caffeine misuse
  - Misuse of alcohol, cigarettes, and illicit substances

Primary central nervous system disorders
- Delayed sleep phase syndrome
- Idiopathic hypersomnia
- Periodic hypersomnia
- Narcolepsy—cataplexy, idiopathic
- Narcolepsy secondary to neoplasms, trauma, inflammatory processes involving the dorsolateral hypothalamus
- Restless legs syndrome

Sleep-related breathing disturbance
- Obstructive hypoventilation, primary or secondary to Down's syndrome, obesity, hypothyroidism, or myopathies like myotonic dystrophy

Drugs
- *Prescription:* Benzodiazepines, barbiturates, antiepileptic drugs
- *Nonprescription:* Diphenhydramine, chlorpheniramine, illicit substances

Psychiatric
- Depression

Box 7: Neurobehavioral consequences of daytime sleepiness in childhood

- Loss of inhibition of the prefrontal cortex, leading to mood swings, impulsivity, and impaired attention and concentration, and increased vulnerability to accidents
- The ability to convert short-term memory into long-term memory (consolidation process) is impaired
- Verbal fluency and complex, divergent, and creative thinking are diminished.

Use of stimulants like caffeine and nicotine is more likely.

CLINICAL ASSESSMENT OF SLEEP-WAKE FUNCTION IN CHILDHOOD

History Taking

Record the time of going to bed, sleep onset time, rituals and habits used for facilitating sleep, presence of habitual snoring, restless sleep, mouth breathing, confusional arousals, sleep walking, sleep terrors, nightmares, bed wetting, whether the patient wakes up tired in the morning, wakeup times on school days and on weekends, daytime naps, drugs used to enhance alertness or to facilitate sleep, whether the patient uses caffeine, nicotine, or other drugs, and how sleepiness impacts on school and social functioning.

Examination

Record height, weight, body mass index, craniofacial anomalies, tonsillar hypertrophy, enlarged tongue base, "adenoid facies," overt sleepiness, labile or depressed mood, inattentiveness.

Sleep Laboratory Tests

Actigraphy and sleep logs—actigraphy provides longitudinal information about times of sleep onset and wake onset for up to two weeks. It is useful in evaluating insomnia and circadian rhythm disorders.

Nocturnal polysomnography measures multiple physiological variables during sleep. It is indicated when evaluating sleep apnea and periodic limb movements in sleep, or narcolepsy.

Multiple sleep latency tests—four or five planned nap opportunities are provided in a dark, quiet environment. The test measures the speed of falling asleep during the daytime and whether the transition from wakefulness is into REM (rapid eye movement) sleep or non-REM sleep.

Inadequate Sleep Hygiene

Inadequate sleep hygiene is by far the most common pediatric sleep-wake problem encountered by general practitioners. To begin with, teenagers are unable to fall asleep before 10:30 or 11 pm owing to a physiological shift in the timing of release of melatonin, which usually induces sleep at around 8:30 pm in preadolescence.[327] Social pressures like after-school sports, evening jobs, television, internet use, mobile phones, and homework may delay bedtime on school nights to between 11 pm and midnight. Caffeine, nicotine, and illicit drugs may also interfere with timely sleep onset. To compound the issue, where school usually starts between 7:15 and 7:45 am students have to awaken by about 6:30 am—yet teens need 9–9.5 hours of sleep to maintain optimum alertness.[328,329] Most adolescents are thus chronically sleep deprived. Management consists primarily of counseling about sleep hygiene (Box 8).

Box 8: Sleep hygiene measures for teenagers

- Go to bed only when sleepy
- Avoid nicotine
- Avoid caffeine and heavy exercise within two hours of bedtime as they may delay sleep onset
- Schedule 30 minutes of "quiet time" before getting into bed—no telephone, radio, television, or computer use
- Do your worrying before you get into bed, rather than afterwards; write down your worries or your next day's "to do" list onto a note pad that is kept in the bedroom
- Avoid clock watching at night—it is unnecessary
- Keep lights low, or off, in the bedroom or toilet at night

Try to wake at or about the same time, seven days a week

RESTLESS LEGS SYNDROME

Restless legs syndrome is an autosomal dominant, sensorimotor disorder characterized by insomnia due to a peculiar "creepy or crawling" feeling in the arms and legs at night, accompanied by an urge to move the limbs.[330] It is exacerbated by keeping the limbs still and is transiently relieved by movement. It interferes with going to sleep and staying asleep and may be accompanied by daytime fatigue, inattentiveness, or frank sleepiness. Restless legs syndrome in childhood is perhaps synonymous with "growing pains."[331] In adults, the favorable response of restless legs syndrome to dopamine receptor agonists like pramipexole and ropinrole or to dopamine precursors like carbidopa-levodopa seems to implicate dopamine deficiency in the pathogenesis. Close to two-thirds of children with restless legs may have low levels of serum ferritin;[330] iron is a cofactor in the synthesis of dopamine. Restless legs syndrome and attention deficit disorder are associated: in a community based questionnaire survey of 866 children aged 2–13.9 years, Chervin et al. found an odds ratio for significant hyperactivity and restless legs of 1.9.[332] Besides dopamine agonists, oral iron, clonazepam, and gabapentin have also been used to treat restless legs syndrome, but there have been no head to head randomized controlled trials to determine which treatment is most effective.

DSM-5 Diagnostic Criteria for Restless Legs Syndrome 333.94 (G25.81)

- An urge to move the legs, usually accompanied by or in response to uncomfortable and unpleasant sensations in the legs, characterized by all of the following:
  - The urge to move the legs begins or worsens during periods of rest or inactivity.
  - The urge to move the legs is partially or totally relieved by movement.
  - The urge to move the legs is worse in the evening or at night than during the day, or occurs only in the evening or at night.
- The symptoms in Criterion A occur at least three times per week and have persisted for at least 3 months.

- The symptoms in Criterion A are accompanied by significant distress or impairment in social, occupational, educational, academic, behavioral, or other important areas of functioning.
- The symptoms in Criterion A are not attributable to another mental disorder or medical condition (e.g. arthritis, leg edema, peripheral ischemia, leg cramps) and are not better explained by a behavioral condition (e.g. positional discomfort, habitual foot tapping).
- The symptoms are not attributable to the physiological effects of a drug of abuse or medication (e.g. akathisia).

NARCOLEPSY

Narcolepsy is characterized by irresistible sleepiness, vivid dreams at sleep onset (hypnagogic hallucinations), momentary paralysis at sleep onset, fragmented night sleep, and abrupt muscle tone atonia triggered by emotions like laughter, fright, or surprise (cataplexy). The cataplectic muscle weakness and atonia last only a few minutes, involve chiefly the extensor muscles, and are associated with absence of muscle stretch reflexes but fully preserved consciousness. The symptoms of narcolepsy result from impaired key arousal mechanisms and the intrusion of REM sleep on to wakefulness. The incidence is highest in the second decade and gradually declines thereafter. About a third of people with narcolepsy have onset before age 15.[333] The pathogenesis and sleep laboratory diagnostic features are summarized in Box 9.

General measures for managing narcolepsy, and indeed all daytime sleepiness, are adherence to fixed bedtime and morning wake-up time, and taking one or two planned naps of about 30 minutes each day. Pharmacological treatment of narcolepsy is with modafinil (level I evidence) or with regular or extended release preparations of methylphenidate or dexamphetamine sulfate (dextroamphetamine; level II evidence Cataplexy is treated using clomimipramine, protriptyline, or sodium oxybate. Emotional and behavioral problems may require fluoxetine (level II evidence), sertraline, and supportive psychotherapy. Teenagers should not drive if they have uncontrolled sleepiness, and should avoid working in locations where they could endanger themselves or others. Given the autoimmune nature of narcolepsy cataplexy, intravenous immunoglobulin at the onset of symptoms may be a novel treatment that warrants further study.[334]

Box 9: Pathogenesis of narcolepsy-cataplexy

- Genetic predisposition (presence of the histocompatibility antigen DQB1*0602 in over 95% of patients, compared with a 25–30% prevalence of the antigen in the general population)
- Acquired stress (head injury, infectious mononucleosis, bereavement, etc.) in many cases
- Degeneration of the hypocretin secreting neurons of the dorsolateral hypothalamus, leading to low to absent hypocretin-1 in the cerebrospinal fluid
- Impaired alertness and fragmented sleep

PSYCHIATRIC DISORDERS

Obsessive compulsive disorder, anxiety, depression, and psychophysiological disturbances may lead to insomnia. Substance misuse and drugs like fluoxetine might also play a role.

DELAYED SLEEP PHASE SYNDROME

The delayed sleep phase syndrome typically starts in adolescence, mostly in boys. Patients are habitually unable to fall asleep before 2 or 3 am and prefer to wake in the late morning or early afternoon. They show normal sleep quantity and quality when allowed to sleep freely but are very sleepy when they have to conform to more conventional sleep-wake schedules. A higher likelihood of HLA DR1 and the occasional familial clustering of delayed sleep phase syndrome suggest a genetic predisposition. Delayed sleep phase syndrome has been linked to polymorphisms in the period gene.[335]

Intrusion of REM sleep on to wakefulness leads to cataplexy, hypnagogic hallucinations, and sleep paralysis.

The condition must, however, be differentiated from school avoidance seen in adolescents with delinquent and antisocial behavior, as these individuals can indeed fall asleep at an earlier hour at night in the controlled sleep laboratory setting. Maintaining sleep logs and wrist actigraphy for 1–2 weeks is helpful in establishing the diagnosis.

"Bright light" therapy helps advance the sleep onset time. It consists of providing 2700–10,000 lux of bright light via a light box for 20–30 minutes immediately after waking in the morning. The phototherapy leads to gradual phase advancement (shifting back) of the sleep onset time at night. Taking 0.5–1 mg melatonin about 5.5 hours before sleep onset also helps in sleep phase advancement. Stimulant drugs can help counter residual daytime sleepiness.

SLEEP-RELATED BREATHING DISTURBANCE

Sleep disordered breathing is a continuum from primary snoring (snoring without sleep complaints) to frank obstructive sleep apnea. Obstructive sleep apnea is characterized by partial upper airway obstruction in the face of preserved thoracic and abdominal respiratory effort. In the United States, it is prevalent in about 2–4% of children, with a higher incidence in those born prematurely or of African-American ethnic origin.[336] The clinical manifestations include habitual snoring, mouth breathing, restless sleep, bed wetting, daytime fatigue, mood swings, and inattentiveness. Adenotonsillar hypertrophy, neuromuscular disorders, and craniofacial abnormalities such as retrognathia, maxillary hypoplasia, and macroglossia are important predisposing factors. Multiple predisposing factors may coexist, as seen in Down's syndrome. Primary snoring has a prevalence of 3–16%; it has been characterized as benign, but lately it too has been linked to neuropsychological impairments.

The upper airway is vulnerable to closure in childhood obstructive sleep apnea—the mean critical pressure at which the upper airway collapses is higher in children with obstructive sleep apnea than with primary snoring.[337] The combination of obesity, obstructive sleep apnea, sleep related hypoventilation with resultant hypercarbia from paradoxical chest and abdominal movement or diminished chest wall excursion, and daytime sleepiness comprise the Pickwickian syndrome. Box 10 shows the consequences of obstructive sleep apnea.

Unfortunately history alone cannot distinguish obstructive sleep apnea from primary snoring, which underscores the need for testing in a sleep laboratory. Sleep questionnaires are only marginally better than history taking. Sampling nocturnal oxygen saturation from an oximeter clipped to a finger is a reasonable diagnostic screen. The presence in each hour of sleep of two or more desaturation events of 4% or more and an oxygen saturation nadir below 90% suggest obstructive sleep apnea.[338] In a prospective study of 110 children undergoing tonsillectomy or adenotonsillectomy, the sensitivity and specificity of oximetry in the diagnosing obstructive sleep apnea when compared with history and clinical findings were 0.52 and 0.68 respectively ($P < 0.05$).[339]

Box 10: Consequences of childhood obstructive sleep apnea

Central nervous system

Sleep fragmentation leads to frontal lobe dysfunction. Animal model studies suggest the developing brain is particularly vulnerable.

- Cortical microarousals resulting from increased respiratory effort
- REM sleep and stages III-IV of non-REM sleep are suppressed
- Inattentiveness, impaired executive function and learning, mood swings, and hyperactivity can result.

Cardiovascular system

Intermittent hypoxemia causes pulmonary vasoconstriction, which can lead to cor pulmonale. It may also trigger increased sympathetic neural activity, which, if sustained, may alter baro-receptor function.

- Pulmonary hypertension
- Cor pulmonale
- Systemic hypertension.

Respiratory system

Most children maintain normal daytime blood gases and experience hypercapnia intermittently during sleep disordered breathing; this typically resolves with treatment.

- ↑breathing effort
- ↓ventilation, ↓O_2 saturation
- Central chemoreceptor reset.

Metabolism

- Reduced release of pulsatile growth hormone and raised resting energy expenditure
- Failure to thrive

Abnormal results on overnight oximetry suggest obstructive sleep apnea, but a normal result do not exclude it.

Impaired Glucose Tolerance

Nocturnal polysomnography is the gold standard for diagnosing obstructive sleep apnea and should be considered when oximetry results are equivocal. Nocturnal polysomnography can measure respiratory events and changes in the electroencephalogram due to obstructive sleep apnea. It is an expensive procedure, and sleep laboratories with equipment and staff geared to the needs of infants and toddlers are not always easily accessible. Nocturnal polysomnography can be bypassed in patients with marked adenotonsillar hypertrophy with classic history of obstructive sleep apnea: adenotonsillectomy can be done if overnight oximetry is positive, thus conserving sleep laboratory resources for patients in whom the diagnosis is less obvious.

Adenotonsillectomy is the most common treatment for sleep related breathing disturbance. About 20% of patients continue to have symptoms even after surgery; they are likely to be those with underlying craniofacial anomalies, obesity, or neuromuscular or neurological disorders. A therapeutic trial of continuous positive airway pressure breathing is recommended in these patients as it stents the airway and maintains its patency.

A recent Cochrane review of adenotonsillectomy commented on the ongoing debate about the criteria needed to diagnose sleep related breathing disturbance in children.[340] There are several reasons for this diagnostic uncertainty. Outdated and relatively insensitive polysomnographic interfaces (like nasal thermocouples or thermistors used for measuring oronasal breathing instead of nasal pressure transducers; mercury filled strain gauges for recording thoracoabdominal effort instead of respiratory inductive plethysmography) impair the detection of sleep related breathing disturbances. A meta-analysis of 12 large studies in which clinical history and examination were correlated with polysomnogram-based diagnosis of obstructive sleep apnea concluded that the clinical history and examination do not accurately predict childhood obstructive sleep apnea.[341] But the meta-analysis was not sufficiently critical—one of the 12 studies had excluded patients with upper airway anomalies and abnormal facial morphology, three studies were retrospective, and three used questionnaire surveys. Prospective studies using reliable, state of the art technology are scarce.

PARASOMNIAS

Parasomnias are undesirable phenomena that intrude on sleep, generally without any daytime consequences. Non-REM sleep parasomnias typically occur in the transition from the deeper into the lighter stages of sleep, about 2–3 hours after initial onset. The child wakes up agitated and confused or walks while asleep, with no recollection of the event the following morning. Most resolve spontaneously over a matter of months. When non-REM parasomnias become problematic, an underlying disorder such as sleep disordered breathing or restless legs syndrome is triggering partial arousals. Low dose clonazepam (0.25–0.5 mg) at bedtime controls most parasomnias. Nightmares are a REM sleep parasomnia and are usually seen in the early morning hours, when REM sleep is more prevalent.

DSM-5[342] Diagnostic Criteria for Parasomnias

Nonrapid Eye Movement Sleep Arousal Disorder

- Recurrent episodes of incomplete awakening from sleep, usually occurring during the first third of the major sleep episode, accompanied by either one of the following:
  - *Sleep walking:* Repeated episodes of rising from bed during sleep and walking about. While sleep walking, the individual has a blank, starring face; is relatively unresponsive to the efforts of others to communicate with him/her, and can be awakened only with great difficulty.
  - *Sleep terrors:* Recurrent episodes of abrupt terror accuses from sleep, usually beginning with a panicky scream. There is intense fear and signs of autonomic arousal, such as mydriasis, tachycardia, rapid breathing, and sweating, during each episode. There is relative unresponsiveness to efforts of others to comfort the individual during the episodes.
- No or little (e.g. only a single visual scene) dream imagery is recalled.
- Amnesia for the episodes is present.
- The episodes cause clinically significant distress or impairment in social, occupational, or other important areas of functioning.
- The disturbance is not attributable to the physiological effects of a substance (e.g. a drug of abuse, a medication)
- Coexisting mental and medical disorders do not explain the episodes of sleep walking or sleep terrors.

Coding note: For ICD-9-CM, code 307.46 for all subtypes. For ICD-10-CM, code is based on subtype.

Specify whether:

307.46 (F51.3) sleepwalking type.

Specify if:

With sleep-related eating.

With sleep-related sexual behavior (sexsomnia).

307.46 (F51.5) sleep terror type.

Nightmare Disorder 307.47 (F51.5)

- Repeated occurrences of extended, extremely dysphoric, and well-remembered dreams that usually involve efforts to avoid threats to survival, security, or physical integrity and that generally occur during the second half of the major sleep episode.
- On awakening from the dysphoric dreams, the individual rapidly becomes oriented and alert.
- The sleep disturbance causes clinically significant distress or impairment in social, occupational, or other important areas of functioning.
- The nightmare symptoms are not attributable to the physiological effects of a substance (e.g. a drug of abuse, a medication).
- Coexisting mental and medical disorders do not adequately explain the predominant complaint of dysphoric dreams.

Specify if:

During sleep onset.

Specify if:

With associated nonsleep disorder, including substance use disorders.

With associated other medical condition.

With associated other sleep disorder.

Coding note: The code 307.47 (F51.5) applies to all three specifiers. Code also the relevant associated mental disorder, medical condition, or other sleep disorder immediately after the code for nightmare disorder in order to indicate the association.

Specify if:

- *Acute:* Duration of period of nightmares is 1 month or less.
- *Subacute:* Duration of period of nightmares is greater than 1 month but less than 6 months.
- *Persistent:* Duration of period of nightmare is 6 months or greater.

Specify current severity:

Severity can be rated by the frequency with which the nightmares occur.

- *Mild:* Less than one episode per week on average.
- *Moderate:* One or more episodes per week but less than nightly.
- *Severe:* Episodes nightly.

Rapid Eye Movement Sleep Behavior Disorder 327.42 (G47.52)

- Repeated episodes of arousal during sleep associated with vocalization and/or complex motor behaviors.
- These behaviors arise during rapid eye movement (REM) sleep and therefore usually occur more than 90 minutes after sleep onset, are more frequent during the later portions of the sleep period, and uncommonly occur during day time naps.

- Upon awakening from these episodes, the individual is completely awake, alert, and not confused or disoriented.
- Either of the following:
  - REM sleep without atonia on polysomnographic recording.
  - A history suggestive of REM sleep behaviors disorder and an established synucleinopathy diagnosis (e.g. Parkinson's disease, multiple system atrophy).
- The behaviors cause clinically significant distress or impairment in social, occupational, or other important areas of functioning (which may include injury to self or the bed partner).
- The disturbance is not attributable to the physiological effects of a substance (e.g. a drug of abuse, a medication) or another medical condition.
- Coexisting mental and medical disorders do not explain the episodes.

Restless Legs Syndrome 333.94 (G25.81)

- An urge to move the legs, usually accompanied by or in response to uncomfortable and unpleasant sensations in the legs, characterized by all of the following:
  - The urge to move the legs begins or worsens during periods of rest or inactivity.
  - The urge to move the legs is partially or totally relieved by movement.
  - The urge to move the legs is worse in the evening or at night than during the day, or occurs only in the evening or at night.
- The symptoms in Criterion A occur at least three times per week and have persisted for at least 3 months.
- The symptoms in Criterion A are accompanied by significant distress or impairment in social, occupational, educational, academic, behavioral, or other important areas of functioning.
- The symptoms in Criterion A are not attributable to another mental disorder or medical condition (e.g. arthritis, leg edema, peripheral ischemia, leg cramps) and are not better explained by a behavioral condition (e.g. positional discomfort, habitual foot tapping).

Box 11: When should a general practitioner refer a child to a sleep specialist?

- The child chronically feels unrefreshed on waking up in the morning
- The school age child finds it difficult to stay awake in the classroom
- The school age child habitually falls asleep in the classroom or while riding in a car or train for less than half an hour, or naps on returning home from school
- The child habitually snores
- The child has difficulty falling asleep or staying asleep through the night that lasts over a month

The child has unexplained night time behaviors that keep family members awake.

- The symptoms are not attributable to the physiological effects of a drug of abuse or medication (e.g. akathisia).

REFERRAL TO SLEEP SPECIALIST

When a sleep problem persists despite institution of practical sleep hygiene measures listed in Box 9 or when it begins to impact the child's mood, behavior, and learning, it is appropriate to consider a referral to a sleep specialist (Box 11).

WHAT IS ON THE HORIZON?

The increasing awareness and prompt treatment of pediatric sleep-wake disorders can enhance the quality of life of children and adolescents. One bottleneck is the limited access to pediatric sleep specialists and sleep diagnostic laboratories. The sleep-related education and training of pediatric postgraduates needs to be enhanced, uniform technical standards for pediatric nocturnal polysomnography need attention, and evidence based guidelines for diagnosis and treatment of specific disorders need development. Genetic aspects of circadian rhythm disorders, narcolepsy, restless legs syndrome, and sleep apnea syndromes are receiving further study, as are the link between sleep and behavior and the development of hypocretin analog for the treatment of narcolepsy.[343] This exciting young field seeks to integrate many basic science and clinical disciplines.

43.15 ATTENTION-DEFICIT HYPERACTIVITY DISORDER

JN Vyas

INTRODUCTION

Attention-deficit hyperactivity disorder (ADHD) is a disorder of inattention, impulsivity, and hyperactivity that affects 8-12% of children worldwide. Although the rate of ADHD falls with age, at least half of children with the disorder will have impairing symptoms in adulthood. Twin, adoption, and molecular genetic studies show ADHD to be highly heritable, and other findings have recorded obstetric complications and psychosocial adversity as predisposing risk factors. Converging evidence from animal and human studies implicates the dysregulation of frontal-subcortical-cerebellar catecholaminergic circuits in the pathophysiology of ADHD, and molecular imaging studies suggest that abnormalities of the dopamine transporter lead ot impaired neurotransmission. Studies during the past decade have shown the safely and effectiveness of new nonstimulant drugs and long-acting formulations of methylphenidate and amphetamine. Other investigations have also clarified the appropriate role of targeted psychosocial treatments in the context of ongoing pharmacotherapy.

In the 20th century, attention-deficit hyperactivity disorder (ADHD) [in the diagnostic guise of very minimal brain dysfunction and other related terms] emerged as the first psychiatric disorder to be diagnosed and treated in children, with studies of stimulant treatment since 1937 and regulatory approval of stimulant treatment for children beginning in the 1960s. But despite the long research history and robust findings, divergent opinions controversy, clinical uncertainty, and scientific debate. Fortunately, as we enter the 21st century, fierce opinion has been replaced by data from empirical studies of epidemiology, cause, pathophysiology, and treatment.

EPIDEMIOLOGY AND DIAGNOSIS

The ADHD affects 8–12% of children worldwide, and results in inattention, impulsivity, and hyperactivity. The controversy about how to diagnose ADHD is seen in the differences between US diagnostic criteria for the disorder, as defined by the Diagnostic and Statistical Manual of the American Psychiatric Association (4th edition; DSM-IV), and the European diagnostic criteria for hyperkinetic disorder (HKD), as defined by the International Classification of Diseases (10th edition; ICD-10). Both classifications include children displaying developmentally inappropriate levels of inattention, hyperactivity, and impulsivity that begin in childhood and cause impairment to school performance, intellectual functioning, social skills, driving, and occupational functioning. But HKD criteria are more restrictive (Table 16) than the DSM-IV diagnosis of ADHD because they need a greater degree of symptom expression. Unlike the ICD-10, DSM-IV allows for three symptom-based subtypes of ADHD: mainly inattentive, mainly hyperactive-impulsive, or both combined. Evidence for the validity and clinical use of these subtypes is mixed, and current work has not yet resolved the ongoing controversy about whether a purely inattentive disorder exists that could be causally different from either ADHD or HKD.

DSM-IV ADHD is more prevalent than ICD HKD, a finding which has sometimes been misinterpreted to mean that ADHD is more common in the USA than in countries using ICD criteria. That controversy was resolved by a review of 50 epidemiological studies, which reported the prevalence of DSM-defined ADHD to be similar worldwide (Panel 4). Epidemiological studies show that the prevalence of ADHD is over estimated if the diagnosis does not adequately incorporate functional impairment into the diagnosis. In a US study, Wolraich and colleagues reported the prevalence of the disorder to be 16.1% if based on symptoms alone and 6.8% if functional impairment was needed. Similar results were reported from Australian and Germany studies.

Table 16: Differences between US and European criteria of ADHD or HKD

DSM-IV-ADHD	*ICD-10 HKD*
Symptoms: Either or both of following	All of following:
At least six of nine inattentive symptoms	At least six of eight inattentive symptoms
At least six of nine	At least three of five hyperactive symptoms
Hyperactive or impulsive symptoms	
At least one of four impulsive symptoms	
Prevasiveness	
Some impairment from criteria are met for more than one setting	Symptoms is present in more than one setting.

Panel 4 Diagnosis and epidemiology of ADHD

Prevalence: 6–12% worldwide
Sex ratio: Common in men
Social class: Common in lower economic status
Ethnic origin: Under-identified and treated in minority groups.
Age: Prevalence falls with age.

Epidemiological studies have shown that the male sex, low socioeconomic status, and young age are associated with a raised prevalence of ADHD. The male-to-female sex ratio for the disorder is greater in clinical studies than in community studies, which indicates that female individuals with the disorder are less likely to be referred for services than male individuals. This difference in referral rates by sex is probably because of ADHD being less disruptive in women than in men, and the raised population prevalence in male individuals could be due to their increased exposure to environmental sources of cause, such as head injury.

Although both DSM-IV and ICD-10 provide well-structured, criterion-based diagnoses for ADHD and HKD, they have several weaknesses. The diagnostic items, although well-described, do not have developmentally sensitive definitions to help doctors differentiate ADHD symptoms from developmentally healthy levels of inattention, hyperactivity, and impulsivity. Clinicians often receive diagnostic data from multiple informants (e.g. parent and teacher; parent and teenage child; adult with ADHD and spouse), but the DSM-IV and ICD-10 provide no guidelines to integrate this information. The weaknesses of the diagnostic system have led to critics of ADHD describing the diagnosis as subjective and much less credible than objective laboratory tests used in other medical specialties. This criticism is at odds with developments in medical testing studies that emphasize that the quality of a diagnosis derives from its reliability and clinical use and not from the apparent objectivity of the method of diagnosis. As reviewed elsewhere, the diagnosis of ADHD is reliable, i.e. well trained raters agree on the presence or absence of the disorder.

The ADHD diagnosis can predict clinically meaningful outcomes. Much work from both clinical and epidemiological studies shows that the disease puts children at risk for comorbidity with other psychiatric and substance use disorders. Some studies suggest that ADHD can put adults at risk for personality disorders, and at all ages, ADHD is associated with functional impairments such as school dysfunction, peer problems, family conflict, poor occupational performance, injuries, antisocial behavior, traffic violations, and traffic accidents. Because ADHD typically starts in early childhood, clinicians can practice primary and secondary prevention by alerting parents to the potential adverse outcomes associated with the disorder and by routinely screening for these conditions so that, if they emerge, they can be treated at an early stage and, if warranted, the treatment can be adjusted. More importantly, clinical errors will arise if clinicians rountinely discount symptoms of comorbid disorders as associated features of ADHD. In such cases, clinicians expose patients to the adverse effects of the untreated disorder and those problems could be further compounded if the choice of ADHD treatment exacerbates the untreated disorder (e.g. stimulant treatment can worsen tics and mania).

For several decades, the idea that ADHD persisted into adulthood was met with doubt. But, as reviewed by Faraone and colleagues, follow-up studies of ADHD persisted into adulthood. There is clearly an age-dependant decline in symptoms, but even when symptoms are not prominent enough to prompt a diagnosis, they are frequently associated with clinically significant impairments. As a result, by age 30 to 40 years, most individuals who had ADHD in childhood will no longer meet the full threshold criteria for the disorder, but about half will show continued impairing symptoms that are consistent with the DSM-IV diagnosis in partial remission. Yet, despite the partial remission of symptoms in adulthood, prospective follow-up studies show that when children with ADHD reach adolescence and adulthood, they are at high risk for such impairments.

Temporal trends in the use of stimulant drugs for ADHD have raised questions about possible over-identification and over-treatment. Several studies have shown increases in the prescription of stimulant drugs in the USA, Israel, Canada, and Europe, particularly in very young children (e.g. less than 5 years old) in whom differentiation of developmentally healthy levels of symptoms can be difficult and in whom more research is needed. Although these studies show increased pharmacological treatment of ADHD, they present little evidence for systematic over-treatment.

Specify whether:
314.01 (F90.2) Combined presentation: If both Criterion A1 (inattention) and Criterion A2 (hyperactivity-impulsivity) are met for the past 6 months.

314.00 (F90.0) Predominantly inattentive presentation: If Criterion A1 (inattention) is met but Criterion A2 (hyperactivity-impulsivity) is not met for the past 6 months.

314.01 (F90.1) Predominantly hyperactive/impulsive presentation: If Criterion A2 (hyperactivity-impulsivity) is must and Criterion A1 (inattention) is not met for the past 6 months.

Specify if:
In partial remission: When full criteria were previously met, fewer than the full criteria have been met for the past 6 months, and the symptoms still result in impairment in social, academic, or occupational functioning.

Specify current severity:
- *Mild:* Few, if any, symptoms in excess of those required to make the diagnosis are present, and symptoms result in no more than minor impairments in social or occupational functioning.
- *Moderate:* Symptoms or functional impairment between "mild" and "severe" are present.
- *Severe:* Many symptoms in excess of those required to make the diagnosis, or several symptoms that are particularly severe, are present, or the symptoms result in marked impairment in social or occupational functioning.

DSM-5 Diagnostic Criteria for Attention-deficit/Hyperactivity Disorder

- A persistent pattern of inattention and/or hyperactivity-impulsivity that interferes with functioning or development, as characterized by (1) and/or (2):
  1. *Inattention:* Six (or more) of the following symptoms have persisted for at least 6 months to a degree that is inconsistent with developmental level and that negatively impacts directly on social and academic/occupational activities:

     Note: The symptoms are not solely a manifestation of oppositional behavior, defiance, hostility, or failure to understand neurodevelopmental disorders tasks or instructions. For older adolescents and adults (age 17 and older), at least five symptoms are required.
     - Often fails to give close attention to details or makes careless mistakes in schoolwork, at work, or during other activities (e.g. overlooks or misses details, work is inaccurate).

Contd...

Contd...

- Often has difficulty sustaining attention in tasks or play activities (e.g. has difficulty remaining focused during lectures, conversations, or lengthy reading).
- Often does not seem to listen when spoken to directly (e.g. mind seems elsewhere, even in the absence of any obvious distraction).
- Often does not follow through on instructions and fails to finish schoolwork, chores, or duties in the workplace (e.g. starts tasks but quickly loses focus and is easily sidetracked).
- Often has difficulty organizing tasks and activities (e.g. difficulty managing sequential tasks; difficulty keeping materials and belongings in order; messy, disorganized work; has poor time management; fails to meet deadlines).
- Often avoids, dislikes, or is reluctant to engage in tasks that require sustained mental effort (e.g. schoolwork or homework; for older adolescents and adults, preparing reports, completing forms, reviewing lengthy papers).
- Often loses things necessary for tasks or activities (e.g. school materials, pencils, books, tools, wallets, keys, paperwork, eyeglasses, mobile telephones).
- Is often easily distracted by extraneous stimuli (for older adolescents and adults, may include unrelated thoughts). Is often forgetful in daily activities? (e.g. doing chores, running errands; for older adolescents and adults, returning calls, paying bills, keeping appointments).

Hyperactivity and impulsivity: Six (or more) of the following symptoms have persisted for at least 6 months to a degree that is inconsistent with developmental level and that negatively impacts directly on social and academic/occupational activities:

Note: The symptoms are not solely a manifestation of oppositional behavior, defiance, hostility, or a failure to understand tasks or instructions. For older adolescents and adults (age 17 and older), at least five symptoms are required.

- Often fidgets with or taps hands or feet or squirms in seat.
- Often leaves seat in situations when remaining seated is expected (e.g. leaves his or her place in the classroom, in the office or other workplace, or in other situations that require remaining in place).
- Often runs about or climbs in situations where it is inappropriate. (Note: In adolescents or adults, may be limited to feeling restless.)
- Often unable to play or engage in leisure activities quietly.
- Is often "on the go," acting as if "driven by a motor" (e.g. is unable to be or uncomfortable being still for extended time, as in restaurants, meetings; may be experienced by others as being restless or difficult to keep up with).
- Often talks excessively.
- Often blurts out an answer before a question has been completed (e.g. completes people's sentences; cannot wait for turn in conversation).
- Often has difficulty waiting his or her turn (e.g. while waiting in line).

Contd...

Contd...

- Often interrupts or intrudes on others (e.g. butts into conversations, games, or activities; may start using other people's things without asking or receiving permission; for adolescents and adults, may intrude into or take over what others are doing).

2. Several inattentive or hyperactive-impulsive symptoms were present prior to age 12 years.
3. Several inattentive or hyperactive-impulsive symptoms are present in two or more settings (e.g. at home, school, or work; with friends or relatives; in other activities).
4. There is clear evidence that the symptoms interfere with, or reduce the quality of, social, academic, or occupational functioning.
5. The symptoms do not occur exclusively during the course of schizophrenia or another psychotic disorder and are not better explained by another mental disorder (e.g. mood disorder, anxiety disorder, dissociative disorder, personality disorder, substance intoxication or withdrawal).

CAUSE

Genetics of ADHD

Is ADHD merely the extreme of a healthy variation exacerbated by adverse environmental circumstances rather than a medical disorder with biological causes? For many decades, studies have shown that ADHD is transmitted in families. According to twin and adoption studies, genes have a substantial role in the familial transmission of ADHD.

Heritability data from twin studies of the disorder or quantitative measures of its symptoms for Australia, Sweden, the UK, and many sites in the USA. These data, which estimate the heritability of ADHD to be 0.76, show that genes are very important in initiating ADHD. Pointed out that the estimated heritability have not changed from 1973 to 2004, despite intervening changes in diagnostic systems. Adoption studies also implicate genetic causes. Adoptive relatives of children with ADHD are less likely than biological relatives to have the disorder or associated syndromes.

Molecular genetic studies are beginning to unravel the complex genetics of ADHD. Genome scans of individuals with ADHD have used the method of linkage analysis to screen the genome for regions that might include disease-related susceptibility genes. With the exception of chromosome 17p11, genomic regions implicated by these studies do not overlap. For ADHD, the absence of repeated results across studies so far suggests that genes with moderately large effects are unlikely to exist, and for this reason, further studies need to have increased power of available linkage data.

The dopamine D4 receptorns (DRD4) is prevalent in the frontal-subcortical networks that are implicated in the pathophysiology of ADHD. Most DRD4 studies have assayed a variant known as the exon III 7-repeat allele, which produces an *in vitro* blunted response to dopamine. When data from analyses of this variant were pooled, the association with ADHD was significant in both case-control (odds ration 1.45) and family studies (1.16). Studies of the dopamine 5 receptor (DRD5) have analyzed a repeated sequence near the transcription start site. A study that combined 14 independent family studies of this variant reported an association of the 148-bp allele with ADHD (odds ration 1.2). Stimulant drugs that are effective against ADHD block the dopamine transporter and imaging studies have shown reduced dopamine-transporter binding in adults with the disorder. When pooled, studies of an ten-repeat sequence in the 3' untranslated region of the dopamine transporter gene ($SLC6A_3$) in ADHD estimate an odds ratio of 1.13. Dopamine β-hydroxylase is the main enzyme responsible for the conversion of dopamine to norepinephrine. Pooled family-based studies of this gene jointly suggest a significant association between ADHD and the 5' Taq1 polymorphism (odds ration 1.33).

Two genes involved in serotonergic transmission have been implicated in ADHD. A functional variant of the serotonin transporter gene ($SLC6A_4$) has been examined in several studies, leading to a meta-analysis odds ratio of 1.31. Several studies of the serotonin 1B receptor gene (HTR1B) have also been positive, with a nonfunctional marker showing a pooled odds ratio of 1.44.

Synaptosomal-associated protein of 25 kDa (SNAP25) is a neuron-specific protein involved in synaptic-vesicle transport and release. Mice that do not have the SNAP25 gene reduces their hyperactivity. Several studies assessed the association between the gene and ADHD in people and a meta-analysis of these studies recorded an odds ration of 1.19.

By contrast with these positive findings (Table 17), studies of other genes have produced equivocal or negative results, which include catechol-O-methyltransferase (COMT); monoamine oxidase (MAO); the norepinephrine transporter SLC6A2; and the 2A, 2C, and 1C norepinephrine receptors.

ENVIRONMENTAL RISK FACTORS FOR ADHD

Biological Adversity

Although the idea that particular foods or food additives might cause ADHD received much attention in the media, systematic studies have shown that this theory is wrong. By contrast with the mostly negative studies of dietary factors, lead exposure has been implicated in the pathophysiology of the disorder, although most affected children do not show lead contamination and many children with high lead exposure do not become affected with the disorder.

Several studies indicate that pregnancy and delivery complications raise the risk for ADHD. Specific complications implicated include toxemia or eclampsia, poor maternal health, maternal age, fetal postmaturity, long duration of labor, fetal distress, and antepartum hemorrhage. Complications associated with ADHD frequently lead to hypoxia and tend to include chronic exposures to the fetus (such as toxemia) rather than acute, traumatic events (such as delivery complications). Notably, the basal ganglia, which are commonly implicated in ADHD, are also one of the most metabolically active structures in the brain, and are particularly sensitive to hypoxic insults, which had shown to cause ending effects on dopaminergic functioning in animals.

Many studies confirm that prematurity, as indexed by lower birth weight, is a risk factor for ADHD, with one study showing that such effects could not be accounted for by potential confounders such as prenatal exposure to alcohol and cigarettes, parental ADHD, social class, and comorbid disruptive behavioral disorders in parents and offspring. Prospective studies of infants show that fetal exposure to maternal alcohol use leads to behavioral, cognitive, and learning problems that could present as ADHD. And studies of children with the disorder show an increased likelihood having been exposed to alcohol as a fetus.

A chronic exposure that has been extensively studied is maternal smoking during pregnancy. With exposure of the fetus to nicotine, maternal smoking can damage the brain at critical points in the developmental process. Animal studies in pregnant mice and rats have shown a correlation between chronic exposure to nicotine and hyperactive offspring. Because nicotinic receptors modulate dopaminergic activity and dopaminergic dysregulation could cause ADHD, maternal smoking could theoretically be regarded as a risk factor for the disorder. Furthermore, a review of 24 studies recorded an increased risk for the disorder in children whose mothers smoked during pregnancy.

PSYCHOSOCIAL ADVERSITY

Rutter's studies at London revealed six risk factors in the family environment that correlated significantly with childhood mental disturbances: severe marital discord; low social class; large family size; paternal criminality; maternal mental disorder; and foster placement. The aggregate of such adverse factors impaired development, rather than the presence of any one factor. Biederman and colleagues identified a positive association between Rutter's index of adversity and ADHD, measures of ADHD-associated psychopathology, impaired cognition, and psychosocial dysfunction.

Other cross-sectional and longitudinal studies have identified variables such as marital distress, family dysfunction, and low social class as risk factors for psychopathology and dysfunction in children. For example, the Ontario Child Health Study showed that family dysfunction and low income predicted the persistence and onset of one or more psychiatric disorders over a 4-year follow-up. Other published work has indicated that low maternal education, low social class, and single parenthood are important adverse factors for ADHD. Biederman and coworkers showed that chronic conflict, reduced family cohesion, and exposure to parental psychopathology (especially maternal psychopathology) were more common in ADHD families compared with control families. The differences between children with or without ADHD were not accounted for by social class or by parental history of major psychopathology. Many studies have shown maternal depression as a risk factor for psychological maladjustment and psychiatric disorder in children, and some data have suggested that depressed moods could lead mothers to perceive their children as more deviant than would be warranted by the child's behavior.

PATHOPHYSIOLOGY

The idea that dysregulation of dopamine and norepinephrine circuits underlies ADHD was initially suggested by the action of drugs for the disorder, which increase the synaptic availability of these neurotransmitters, and by animals showing that lesions in dopamine pathways create animal models of ADHD, as shown in developing rats and monkeys. As one of the most compelling animal models of ADHD, the spontaneously hypertensive rat (SHR) shows dopamine release abnormalities in subcortical structures.

Because executive dysfunction is common, although far from universal in ADHD, it has driven much neuropsychological theory about the disorder. Executive functions, which are controlled by frontal subcortical circuits, include inhibition, working memory, set-shifting, planning and sustained attention. This pattern of dysfunction has led to much debate about what core neuropsychological deficit might cause both ADHD symptoms and neuropsychological impairments. Candidates for core deficits include failure of inhibitory control; dysregulation of brain systems mediating reward and response cost; and deficit in arousal, activation, and effortful control. Deficits in arousal and effort lead to state-dependant cognitive deficits and a view of ADHD that emphasizes problems in regulating cognitive functions rather than core deficits in any single function. But, because no single neuropsychological impairments of the disorder could be heterogeneous and this heterogeneity probably corresponds to causal heterogeneity.

The pattern of neuropsychological deficit in ADHD patients has been interpreted as being caused by dysregulation of frontal-subcortical circuits. That hypothesis has now been confirmed by structural and functional neuroimaging studies showing patients to have small volume reductions in these regions. But other findings suggest that aberrant frontal-subcortical circuitry is not sufficient enough to explain the pathophysiology of the disorder. One study has reported widespread, albeit small (e.g. 4%) volume reductions throughout the brain, another has shown widespread cortical abnormalities, and others have implicated structures such as cerebellum and corpus callosum, which are outside the frontal-subcortical circuits.

Functional neuroimaging studies have assessed the degree of brain activation associated with neuropsychological tasks of attention and disinhibition. Because tasks are constructed so that ADHD and control individuals do equally well, activation differences indicate group differences in the neural systems used to accomplish the tasks. These studies are consistent with the structural studies locating abnormalities of brain activation in patients with ADHD in fronto-subcortical cerebellar circuits.

In the subcortical structures associated with ADHD, the striatum has been of particular interest because it is rich in dopaminergic synapses, is vulnerable to the perinatal hypoxic complications implicated in the disorder, and if not intact, it produces hyperactivity and poor inhibitory control in animals. *In vivo* neuroimaging studies in people showed that methylphenidate, which is used to treat ADHD, exerts its effects by binding to dopamine transporters, most of which are located in the striatum, and, as reviewed above, genetic studies have implicated the dopamine transporter gene in ADHD pathophysiology.

TREATMENT

For 40 years, the main treatments for ADHD (Panel 5) have been the stimulant drugs, methylphenidate and amphetamine, which are believed to enhance neurotransmission of dopamine and norepinephrine. The stimulant pemoline is less commonly used because of its hepatotoxic effects. Nonstimulant treatment has also been used, but for many years reduced efficacy and occurrence of side-effects had restricted their use. The average effect size for stimulants (0.91 for immediate release and 0.95 for long-acting versions) is greater than the average effects for nonstimulants (0.62), although much variability exists within classes.

Two clinically important developments in ADHD treatment have been the use of long-acting stimulant formulations and the nonstimulant, atomoxetine. Because the immediate release stimulants were effective for 3–6 h, multiple doses were needed to maintain their effectiveness during the day.

As Table 17 shows, clinicians now have many choices of stimulant drugs that allow them to choose the best regimen based on patients' needs for coverage throughout the day. The long-acting stimulants show effectiveness and side-effects similar to that seen for the immediate-release drugs.

Despite many decades of clinical use, stimulant drugs have been controversial because of concerns that they might cause ticks, substance abuse, and delay growth. Although early reports showed stimulants to raise the risk for tics in patients with a personal or family history of tic disorders, work in the past decade has challenged that view. Although these

Panel 5 Drug treatment for ADHD

Methylphenidate	Amfetamine	Modafinil
Pemoline	Amitriptyline	Desipramine
Imipramine	Clomipramine	Nortriptyline
Phenelzine	Selegiline	Clonidine
Guanfacine	Atomoxetine	Bupropion

Table 17: Duration of action of stimulant drugs

Methylphenidate	
Ritalin, methylin, focalin	3 hours
Concerta	10–12 hours
Ritalin LA	8–9 hours
Amfetamine	
Dexedrine	3 hours
Addrerall	6 hours
Adderall XR	10–12 hours

new data are reassuring, more information is needed in large studies for extended periods, to show that nonstimulants be considered for patients at risk for tic disorders.

Because stimulant drugs are controlled substances with addictive potential, concerns had been raised about children with ADHD being prone to abuse and addiction when used for many years. Because long-term, placebo controlled trials are not ethical, this issue can only be addressed by longitudinal, naturalistic studies. Meta-analyses of such studies have shown that rather than causing subsequent substance use disorders, the pharmacotherapy of ADHD has a significant protective effect, reducing the risk for substance use disorder by 50%.

Stimulants routinely result in appetite and weight loss, and most studies show that children with ADHD rather than with the stunting of growth in children with the disorder. Overall height seems to be unaffected if treatment is discontinued in adolescence and several long-term studies suggest that deficits in expected height are reversible even with continued treatment for 2–3 years, although no attenuation was recorded over 2 years in one study. Clinicians should continue to monitor growth in children treated with stimulant drugs.

Tricyclic antidepressants had been the best established nonstimulant treatment, until their use was curtailed because of reports of sudden unexplained death in four ADHD children treated with desipramine, although the causal link between desipramine and these deaths remains uncertain. Anticholinergic side-effects have also restricted clinical use of these drugs. Similar to the tricyclics, atomoxetine blocks the norepinephrine transporter, which is believed to attenuate ADHD symptoms by increasing norepinephrine in the synapse. However, unlike tricyclics, this compound does not have anticholingergic side-effects and has a safe cardiovascular profile.

Bupropion has shown modest efficacy in ADHD treatment in open-label and controlled trials. However, these studies have been small. Despite this uncertainty, bupropion is clearly efficacious for controlling cigarette smoking, which is increased in ADHD patients, and some studies suggest bupropion could be especially helpful for patients with comorbid depression, bipolar disorder, or substance abuse. Although buporpion is well tolerated by most patients, in rare cases it induces seizures. Thus, the drug should not be given to patients with a history of seizure disorders.

Modafinil, which has been used to promote wakefulness of narcolepsy, has also shown some efficacy against ADHD, initially in an open-label study in children. In a double-blind, placebo-controlled study of 223 children with the disorder, one 300 mg dose of modafinil per day greatly improved disease symptoms that were rated by teachers, clinicians, and parents. Modafinil doses of 400 mg per day had much better results than placebo, but did not add great beneficial effect to doses of 300 mg per day. All modafinil dosing regimens were well tolerated. The most common adverse events were insomnia, abdominal pain, anorexia, cough, fever and rhinitis. Two smalls studies also suggest the drug could be effective against adult ADHD.

Two α2-adrenergic agonists, clonidine and guanfacine, are also used in the treatment of ADHD but because of scarce efficacy and side-effect data, they are not routinely prescribed. Connor and colleagues did a meta-analysis of 11 studies and concluded that clonidine was significantly but only moderately effective against ADHD. Some work suggests that clonidine could be useful as an adjunct to stimulant treatment when symptoms of hyperactivity, impulsivity, and aggression are not well controlled, or if tics or sleep difficulties are present. The scarce data for guanfacine suggests that it could be moderately efficacious against ADHD and might also alleviate tics in children with ADHD and tic disorders. The most common side-effects of α2-agonists are sedation, drowsiness, and depression.

Many psychosocial interventions are used for children with ADHD both alone and in combination with drug treatment. Behavioral modification, which uses reward and response cost to change behavior, has been useful against symptoms and associated features of ADHD, and cognitive behavior therapy has shown positive results in adults with the disorder. But what is the relative value of pharmacological and psychosocial interventions for children with ADHD? This issue was recently resolved by a multisite study comparing drug management, intensive behavioral treatment, combined drug and behavioral treatment, and standard community care. For most ADHD symptoms, combined treatment and drug management groups showed greater efficacy than behavioral treatment and community-care groups. This pattern of effect continued to the 2-year follow-up. These analyses suggest that for children with ADHD, drugs should be the first-line treatment for the disorder. Nonetheless, other data from the MTA study (Multimodel Treatment of ADHD) indicate that behavioral treatment can be valuable for some patients. For clinicians, these findings suggest that, after drug treatment is successfully titrated, assessments of residual disabilities should guide subsequent decisions regarding psychosocial interventions.

CONCLUSION

The ADHD has emerged from the 20th century with a large amount of scientific work investigating its validity and clarifying clinical controversies. The disorder is highly prevalent worldwide, is associated with substatial life impairments, and frequently persists into adulthood. Hypotheses about the cause of ADHD have evolved from simple one cause theories to the view that it is a complex, multifactorial disorder caused by the confluence of many different types of risk factors (i.e. genetic, biological, environmental, psychosocial), with every type having a small effect on the increasing vulnerability to the disorder through their additive and interactive effects. If an individual's cumulative vulnerability exceeds a threshold, he or she will manifest the signs and symptoms of ADHD. This multifactorial view of ADHD is consistent with the recorded heterogeneity in its pathophysiology and clinical expression.

Although brain-imaging studies have documented both structural and functional pathological changes in frontal-subcortical-cerebellar circuits, imaging methods cannot be used as diagnostic methods. The same approach is true of the genetic variants associated with ADHD. These neurobiological data provide insights into cause and pathophysiology, but more work is needed before they can be considered diagnostically useful.

43.16 DIAGNOSTIC ISSUES IN CHILDHOOD BIPOLAR DISORDER

JN Vyas

In his early descriptions, Kraepelin observed that manic depression, although commonly presenting after puberty, can and does occur in children and adolescents.[344] Yet, despite this early insight, the field of psychiatry largely discounted the existence of bipolar disorder (BD) in children and viewed adolescent—onset BD as uncommon until recently.[345] Evidence demonstrating that a significant number of adults with BD report symptom onset before age 19 has led an explosion in the recognition of childhood BD over the past decade.[344] Children and adolescents including preschoolers, are being diagnosed with BD in rapidly increasing numbers.[344,346,347] The criteria for mania are being adjusted in children and adolescents to accommodate various presentations of emotional dysregulation into the paradigm of BD. For example, children with nonspecific symptoms of aggression, irritability, recklessness, and mood liability are being diagnosed with BD.[344] It has yet to be seen whether these presentations will develop in adulthood into what we have traditionally considered to be BD. This blurring of the diagnostic lines has led to significant controversy in the field of child and adolescent psychiatry. Currently there is little agreement on issues, such as the validity of the cardinal symptoms of elated mood and grandiosity, the role of irritability, whether mood episodes are episodic or continuous, the considerable overlap in symptoms with other childhood psychiatric disorders, and the validity of subthreshold presentations.[348] This Chapter introduces current thinking about this controversial diagnosis through two case examples.

IRRITABILITY AND AGGRESSION IN BIPOLAR DISORDER

Irritability is a nonspecific symptom common to a myriad of childhood psychiatric disorders. It is included in the DSM – IV criteria for such diverse diagnoses as disruptive behavior disorders, major depressive disorder, generalized anxiety disorder, and post-traumatic stress disorder.[349] Irritability is also commonly present in numerous additional psychiatric syndromes in children, including ADHD[348,351,352] and autism. Being present in nearly all manic youth to some degree, it is highly sensitive but has very low specificity in the detection of manic youth.[348]

Some researchers believe that chronic severe irritability in youth, accompanied by aggression and volatility, is the predominant mood state in children with BD, with elated or expansive mood playing a secondary role.[348] This controversial stance is countered by others who point out cross-sectional studies have consistently found a high prevalence of elated or expansive mood in samples of youth with BD.[348] These differences may be a result of researchers using different inclusion criteria. Overall, because of its lack of diagnostic specificity, irritability appears to be inadequate in making a diagnosis of mania in youth.[352]

EPISODIC VERSUS CONTINUOUS SYMPTOMS

The issue of whether BD must necessarily involve an episodic course has been addressed in both the child and adult literature. The classic thinking that adults with BD have complete interepisode recovery is now being called into question. Children presenting with mixed episodes have been described as often experiencing chronic symptoms that represent their baseline.[352-354] Geller has described a group of children with BD who present with chronic, continuous rapid-cycling, with long duration of episodes and with low rates of interepisode remission.[344] Some groups of researchers describe children suffering from chronic, manic symptoms, with mean durations of episodes up to 3 to 4 years, while others describe children with mixed states combined with complex cycling patterns between depression and mania. still others report chronic mixed states lasting for years, with rapid cycling between mania and depression as frequently as several times per day.[348] This cycling of mood multiple times within the course of a day, or greater than 365 episodes per year, has been defined as "ultradian" cycling and has been found to be present in 77% of one sample of children with BD.[344,350,355] Ultradian cycling is commonly referred to as "mood swings" or "mood lability."[344,350,356] "Ultrarapid" cycling is defined as a 5 to 364 episodes in a year and was found in 10% of a sample of children diagnosed with BD.[344,351,356] The general consensus is that BD in youth is more chronic and refractory to treatment than BD in adulthood, with many youth presenting with chronic problems regulating their mood, emotions, and behavior in response to stress and conflict.[344] However, some researchers argue that an episodic course is a key feature of BD that should be present to make the diagnosis, and that the diagnosis should not be made if mood episodes are not clearly demarcated.[348] While there are some researchers who believe that BD in children and adolescents can follow a chronic, continuous course, an episodic course continues to be a reasonable requirement for a conservative approach and increases the probability of making an accurate BD diagnosis.[348]

HALLMARK SYMPTOMS

Hallmark symptoms are symptoms that must be present for a diagnosis to have validity. The primary example of hallmark symptoms is the requirement that either depressed mood or anhedonia be present to meet DSM-IV criteria for a major depressive episode.[349] The DSM-IV does not currently include a similar hallmark symptom paradigm for diagnosing a manic episode. As such, an individual can have an irritable mood and no grandiosity and still meet full DSM-IV criteria for mania.

For example, a child who presents with a week-long history of irritability, distractibility, excessive talkativeness, increased goal-directed activity, and excessive risk-taking is considered to be in a manic episode by DSM-IV criteria.[349] This approach may be too loose and could lead to the misdiagnosis of some children with BD, who may in fact be suffering from other psychiatric disorders, such as severe ADHD.

Geller, in her NIMH study on BD in children and adolescence, refined her criteria for mania by requiring either elated/euphoric mood or grandiosity to be included in her cohort.[356] In other words, a child who presents with irritability as a primary mood state would have evidence of grandiosity to be diagnosed with BD. As in any area of child psychiatry, it is imperative to consider the child's developmental stage when evaluating a child with suspected BD using this approach. Normal childhood boasting, imaginary play portraying powerful figures, overactivity, and youthful indiscretions should not be considered as evidence of BD. In addition, the context in which the symptoms occur needs to be considered, as normally developing children may exhibit many of the same symptoms to varying degrees in certain situations or environment.[348] In general, to be included in marking a diagnosis of BD, a symptom should be pervasive and impairing. Although compelling, more studies are needed to solidity the use of grandiosity and elated/euphoric mood as hallmark symptoms of BD.[348,351,356]

Marked sleep disturbance has also been posited as a hallmark symptom of BD.[344] Frequently present in adult samples of mania, marked sleep disturbance appears to be less common in children, present in less than 50% of cases.[344] Hyperactivity, irritability, and dangerous play are more generic symptoms that are less likely to differentiate BD from other childhood psychiatric disorders.[344]

BD AND ADHD

The differentiation between BD and ADHD in children can be challenging. There is strong overlap between the disorders, with studies estimating that up to 80% of children with BD also have ADHD.[348] The reasons for this strong relationship are not entirely clear, although they may be related to similar risk factors, with ADHD representing an early presentation of BD in some children, early misdiagnosis of BD as ADHD or misdiagnosing BD in a child who has severe ADHD. Geller, in a widely cited study, found that symptoms of grandiosity, elated mood, hypersexuality (in the absence any history of sexual abuse or exposure to sexual activity), flight of ideas, and decreased need for sleep differentiated children with BD from children with ADHD alone.[355,357] She found irritability to be common in both cohorts, lending further support to the notion that irritability has low specificity in the diagnosis of BD.[13,14]

A child with ADHD should be suspected of having BD if symptoms begin after age 10 or appear abruptly in an otherwise healthy child.[358] Other factors that increase the likelihood of BD in a child diagnosed with ADHD include ADHD symptoms that come and go with changes in mood, severe mood swings, temper tantrums or rages, hallucinations or delusions, a strong family history of BD, or a lack of symptom response to stimulants in a child who previously responded positively to them.[358]

DIFFERENTIAL DIAGNOSIS

In addition to the above diagnostic considerations, a broader differential diagnosis of Jack's presenting symptoms must be considered. Jack's nonspecific presentation of chronic irritability and mood reactivity in the context of a history of abuse is fairly common in some clinical samples and can represent numerous different childhood psychiatric disorders. A savvy practitioner will probe much deeper into the history of Jack's symptoms to make this differentiation, including following Jack longitudinally and using collateral sources. ADHD, as discussed above, is an important consideration, as are other mood disorders, disruptive behavior disorders, pervasive developmental disorders, schizophrenia, substance abuse, post-traumatic stress disorder, a developing borderline personality disorder, and symptoms secondary to a medication or drug of abuse or a general medical condition.[348,350] Finally, developmentally appropriate symptoms and normal variations in mood need to be included on the differential.[348] Practitioners are advised to use caution in attributing symptoms to mania unless there is a clear temporal association with elevated, expansive or irritable mood.[348]

A particularly important consideration in the diagnosis of BD in children is the presence of other mood disorder. BD is thought to be on a continuum with other mood disorders based on severity, pervasiveness, and presence or absence of mania. Adjustment disorder with depressed mood is characterized as a response to a clear stressor that is mild and time limited.[359] The continuum advances through minor depression classified as depression not otherwise specified (NOS), dysthymia, and major depression with increasing degrees of severity.[359] The presence of mania is what defines BD. To a clinician, determining where a child fits on this continuum can be much more difficult than this straightforward description implies. However, the differentiation between unipolar depression and BD is of paramount importance, as the treatment is quite different. Children with unipolar depression misdiagnosed with BD are not only exposed to the significant side effect profiles associated with mood stabilizing medication, but their symptoms may not improve without treatment aimed specifically at unipolar depression. On the other hand, any child who presents with a unipolar depression should be carefully assessed for any history of mania, given the risk of antidepressant-induced mania and the increased risk of having a BD, particularly if the depression episode is characterized by rapid-onset, psychomotor retardation, or psychotic features.[344] Other factors that increase the risk of BD in a child presenting with depression include a positive family history of affective disorder, especially BD, and a history of antidepressant-induced manic symptoms.[344]

COMORBIDITY

In addition to considering the differential diagnosis, practitioners must also be cognizant of the role of comorbidity in childhood-onset BD. Comorbidity in children with BD has been found to be extremely high, up to 98% in some samples.[360] ADHD is the disorder most commonly found comorbid with BD, as discussed above. Anxiety disorders are also frequently comorbid, with some estimates ranging from 30% to 70%.[348] There is considerable overlap with behavioral disorders, such as conduct disorder, and rates of substance dependence are high and increase with age.[348]

EPIDEMIOLOGY

Although the prevalence of BD in youth has yet to be adequately established, the disorder is thought to have a lifetime prevalence of approximately 0.4% to 1.6%.[359,361] A recent large survey estimated that 2% of the population has BD-I or BD-II, and another 2.4% has subsyndromal symptoms.[362] Adults with BD report high rates of symptoms beginning before age 20, with some retrospective studies as high as 60%.[348] BD in adulthood occurs equally in males and females, although early-onset cases have been found to be predominantly male, particularly if symptoms begin before age 13.[344] When using a broader definition of BD in youth, estimates of prevalence have been as high as 1%.[363] Given that the lifetime prevalence of BD has been estimated to be 0.4% to 1.6%, a 1% prevalence in children would seen on the high side. This apparent discrepancy could be caused by a number of factors, including a shift downward in the age of onset, an increased ability to recognize the illness earlier, adult prevalence rates being underestimated, or the prevalence of the disorder increasing significantly.[344] It is also possible that given the controversies in the field, BD in children is being misdiagnosed and therefore over-diagnosed.

There is ample evidence from epidemiological studies that the rates of children and adolescents diagnosed with BD are increasing. For example, Blader and Carlson[346] found and almost sixfold increase in population-adjusted rates of hospital discharges of children with a primary diagnosis of BD from 1996 to 2004. Adolescent discharges increased fourfold.[346] While adult rates also increased significantly during this time period, the rates were far more modest, with a rise of 56%.[346] Because the characterization of BD in youth is still in its infancy, reliable incidence and prevalence numbers are not available. The disorder will need to be defined more specifically and the criteria universally agreed upon before this can happen.

In comparison with adults with BD, in which a depressed mood state predominates, children with BD have been found to have predominant mood states of mania or hypomania.[352] Prepubertal-onset mania may be more common in boys than girls.[364] In a recent study looking at sex differences in youth with BD, boys were found to present more commonly with a manic while girls presented more commonly with depressed mood.[365] Older children also presented with higher levels of manic mood than younger children, who presented more commonly with depressed mood.[365] Mixed states are also very common in children and adolescents.

TREATMENT

The treatment of BD in children should be comprehensive and include pharmacotherapy in addition to psychotherapeutic interventions.[344] Family and behavioral issues may be considerable and should be actively addressed.[366] The goal of psychotherapeutic interventions is to ameliorate symptoms, educate the child and family about BD, promote treatment adherence, reduce morbidity, and promote healthy growth and development.[344]

Most evidence for the efficacy of available psychopharmacologic treatments is extrapolated from adult studies and this is likely appropriate for the more classic presentation or narrow phenotype of BD in children.[344] However, there is limited evidence for the efficacy of mood-stabilizing medication in the broad-phenotype definition of BD in children. Hence, mood-stabilizing medication should be used cautiously and conservatively in this population. Pharmacotherapy with traditional mood stabilizers or atypical antipsychotics is considered the primary treatment of childhood BD.[344]

PROGNOSIS

Numerous studies have found the long-term prognosis of BD in adolescents to be similar to that of adults, with a few indicating worse outcomes.[344] Overall, the course of early-onset BD appears to be more chronic and refractory to treatment.[344] Of youth presenting with BD, 70%–100% eventually recover from their episode but up to 80% will experience at least one recurrence in the following 2–5 years.[348] For each year of illness the chances of recovery, defined as minimal or no symptoms for at least 8 consecutive weeks, have been estimated to decrease by 10%.[367] Early age of onset, long duration, low socioeconomic status, episodes of mixed symptom or rapid cycling, psychosis, subsyndromal symptoms, comorbid disorders, exposure to negative life events, and family psychopathology are all factors that have been linked to poor outcomes.[348,367] Low socioeconomic class, exposure to negative life events, and high expressed emotion or low maternal warmth have all been linked to poor outcomes, specifically in children and adolescents.[348,356]

In addition, some studies have linked rapid cycling, mixed episodes, comorbid disorders, and family conflicts with a worse prognosis.[350] Early onset of BD before age 12 has been associated with poor outcomes, including comorbid conduct disorder, anxiety disorders, and substance dependence, as well as suicidal behaviors, attempts, and completion.[351]

Youth diagnosed with BD–NOS (akin to the broad spectrum phenotype) as opposed to BD-I or BD-II (akin to the narrow spectrum phenotype) took longer to recover, and their symptoms recurred sooner, perhaps related to a more chronic, subsyndromal course that may be more resistant to the treatments used.[350] In addition, adolescents with persistent and abnormal elevated, expansive, or irritable mood who did not meet full DSM–IV criteria for mania did not go on to meet diagnostic criteria for BD by their early 20s, but did have higher rates of depression and other psychiatric disorders.[368] Overall, the course of BD in children and adults in marked by recurrence, significant impacts on functioning, decrease quality of life, and suicide.[369]

SUMMARY

Despite the lack of a consensus on the broad phenotype definition of BD in childhood, the consensus for the narrow-spectrum definition is quite strong.[350,370] Although mania in youth has not yet been conclusively shown to progress to classic adult BP, Geller's recent article demonstrating that a significant proportion of children diagnosed with BD using a narrow-spectrum definition do progress is compelling. In this study 44.4% of adult subjects with BD diagnosed in childhood had an episode of mania in adulthood.[356] This rate is 13 to 44 times higher than population prevalences, supporting the contention that using a careful diagnostic process, one can accurately identify cases of BD in childhood.[356] However, the surge in children being diagnosed with BD raises many questions and it is still not clear what the broad phenotype of BD actually represents. Children who fit the narrow-spectrum definition of BD should be treated as such, and clinicians can feel comfortable that the current state of the science supports the use of mood-stabilizing medication in this population. However, children fitting in to the broad phenotype should be treated more conservatively.

43.17 VERY EARLY INTERVENTION IN PSYCHOTIC DISORDERS

JN Vyas

It is well accepted that most serious psychiatric conditions begin in adolescence and are characterized by initial symptoms that predate the full manifestation of illness. This early period often consists of nonspecific symptoms, making accurate detection difficult. In fact, classification as "prodromal" is only possible retrospectively, after a patient has developed positive psychotic symptoms. To monitor these patients prospectively, we must identify and follow patients who are at risk for psychosis, understanding that this group may also include false positives who do not go on to develop psychotic illness. Improving detection of at-risk individuals gives us an opportunity to intervene earlier in the course of the disorder, creating a window of opportunity to improve outcome and decrease overall burden of illness.

The term "prodrome" indicates a period before the full manifestation of a psychotic illness, during which patients first experience changes in their emotions, cognition, or behavior that, although not meeting the threshold for the full disorder, indicate a deviation from the normal level of functioning. Much of the early research into prodromal symptoms is anecdotal, involving retrospective reports from first-break schizophrenia patients. Typical prodromal symptoms, in decreasing order of frequency, include: decreased concentration and attention, decreased motivation, depressed mood, sleep disturbance, anxiety, social withdrawal, suspiciousness, deterioration in role functioning, and irritability. These retrospective reports indicate that although some patients experience few or no prodromal symptoms and transition directly into full psychotic illness, others describe prodromal states lasting up to 20 years. The prodrome is operationally defined as the period bridging the transition between the nonaffected state and he psychotic phase of illness.

Comblatt and colleagues described two phases of the prodromal period: the early and late prodromal phases. The early prodromal phase typically occurs years before the onset of psychosis and consists of nonspecific symptoms, such as reduced concentration and motivation, irritability and depressed mood, anxiety, sleep disturbance, social withdrawal, suspiciousness, and impaired functioning. The late prodromal phase is believed to occur in the year before development of psychosis and is made up of symptoms that are closer to those experienced in the psychotic spectrum, but are considered subthreshold because they either occur transiently or are attenuated transient symptoms last at the most several days before subsiding spontaneously. Attenuated symptoms are those psychotic symptoms that the patient reports with less than full conviction. The patient questions the experience and expresses doubt as to the possibility of such symptoms and beliefs, magical thinking, thought disturbances, perceptual disturbances, ideas of references, changes in thought and speech patterns, and atypical behavior and appearance. This progression has been referred to as the march of symptoms from the nonspecific and negative to more specific, positive psychotic symptoms.

Retrospective data are limited in several ways, including recall bias and cognitive and emotional factors in the reporting patient and family members. To obtain a truly accurate picture of this critical period of time before full expression of psychosis it is necessary to prospectively follow subjects who have not yet developed psychosis. This monitoring requires the development of an approach that allows us to identify individuals who are at substantial risk for developing psychotic illness who can then be followed prospectively. The term "at-risk mental state" (ARMS) has been used to describe such populations who demonstrate clinical risk factors for subsequent psychosis. Ultra high risk (UHR), clinical high risk, and ARMS are terms that are used interchangeably to describe these individuals, who are also functionally impaired and generally help-seeking. A detailed discussion of these clinical risk factors follows.

Phenomenological research of these risk factors done in Germany has expanded on work by Gerd Huber, who described the symptoms that predate psychotic illness as basic because he believed that these symptoms were the basis or starting point for schizophrenia. Previously, behavioral observation of symptoms was emphasized. Huber, however, stressed the importance of a patient's subjective report of symptoms, proposing that patients were better reporters of early, more subtle changes in their cognitive, emotional, or physical status. These basic symptoms included subjective complaints of impaired energy, cognitive functioning, emotional functioning, motor functioning, bodily sensation, external perception, autonomic functioning, and tolerance to normal stress. Huber also discussed the progression of symptoms from the nonspecific, which he called level 1 symptoms, to the more specific, or level 2 symptoms. In addition, he talked about put post syndromes, which are clusters symptoms of behaviors that resemble prodromes, but occur before the prodrome and resolve spontaneously without immediately progressing to psychosis. Subsequent studies have shown that the presence of certain basic symptoms is in fact predictive of psychosis. Huber acknowledged that these symptoms serve as potential harbingers of other mental disorders also.

Over time, studies have shifted from examination of retrospective data of prodromal symptoms to prospective studies of at risk patients. This shift has led to a worldwide increased focus on identification and characterization of individuals who are vulnerable to the development of psychosis. Consistent with this, research has increasingly focused on enhancing the accuracy of risk prediction to optimize the risk/benefit ratio of clinical interventions and on development of interventions aimed at reducing the impact of emerging psychotic illness.

At the PACE Clinic (Personal Assessment and Crisis Evaluation) in Melbourne, three distinct high-risk groups have been identified and followed prospectively to assess the rate of conversion to psychosis, the effectiveness of clinical interventions, and exploration of potential biological markers. Subjects in these studies met inclusion criteria for at least one of the following groups:

- Attenuated Psychotic Symptoms Group, who experienced subthreshold, attenuated forms of positive psychotic symptoms during the past year;
- Brief Limited Intermittent Psychotic Symptoms Group (BLIPS), who have experienced episodes of frank psychotic symptoms that have not lasted longer than a week and have spontaneously abated; or
- Trait and State Risk Factor Group, who have a first-degree relative who has a psychotic illness or the identified client has a schizotypal personality disorder and they have

experienced a significant decrease in functioning during the previous year. Selection of these groups allowed the researches the ability to focus on a group of individuals at higher risk for developing psychosis than the general population. By combining trait (genetic risk) and state (functional decline) risk factors, they have in essence in on individuals who are at higher risk for developing psychosis, thus enhancing the predictive power for psychosis conversion.

As mentioned previously, the symptoms predating development of psychosis are often nonspecific and include inattention, irritability, and anxiety. In addition, the prodromal period often occurs in childhood and adolescence, when such symptoms may be seen in various psychiatric disorders. One method for improved detection of vulnerable individuals is to screen for attenuated or brief psychotic experiences in children who present with any behavioral changes or functional decline. In a prospective study of UHR individuals, Yung and colleagues found that clinical symptoms that were highly predictive of later development of included: lower global assessment of functioning (GAF) at baseline, longer duration of prodromal symptoms, presence of low- grade psychotic symptoms, depression, and disorganization. Presence of at least four of these symptoms yielded accurate detection of individuals at high risk for development of psychosis.

Retrospective studies of first-break schizophrenic patients have consistently shown that mood and anxiety symptoms are some of the earliest seen in the prodromal period. Early symptoms have included depression, irritability, guilt, anhedonia, mood swings, suicidal ideation, anxiety, decreased motivation, fatigue, decreased concentration, restlessness, and appetite and sleep distrurbance. Prospective studies have also shown early presentation of mood and anxiety symptoms in the UHR populations. Meyer and colleagues reported on their group of 24 adolescents who met criteria for one of the three UHR groups for a larger, prospective study. In this group of UHR teenagers, 50% received a diagnosis of major depression at baseline and 40% received a diagnosis of anxiety disorder, including (in decreasing order of frequency) anxiety disorder NOS, social phobia, generalized anxiety disorder, panic disorder, specific phobia, obsessive-compulsive disorder, and posttraumatic stress disorder. Svirskis and colleagues also found that their subjects who met criteria for one of the three UHR groups had a high number of lifetime mood, anxiety, or somatization disorder diagnoses. Among these UHR subjects, researchers found that the odds ratio for receiving a lifetime mood disorder diagnosis was 3.28 compared with asymptomatic subjects and 6.34 for receiving an anxiety or somatization diagnosis. What becomes difficult to ascertain is whether these mood anxiety symptoms represent comorbid conditions or are symptoms heralding a psychotic disorder. With further longitudinal studies, we can learn if those UHR patients who have mood and anxiety symptoms are more likely to develop an affective psychosis versus a nonaffective psychosis. It has been shown that recognition and treatment of depression in UHR patients is also important for the treatment of psychotic symptoms. In a study of nonpsychotic individuals experiencing "psychotic like experiences," 40% were determined to have depression at baseline. Of those who had depression, 67.5% remitted by 6-month follow-up and those who had remitted also reported a decrease in psychotic like experiences.

In their review of the prodromal psychosis, Yung and McGorry illustrated the path of events that can occur with patients experiencing prodromal symptoms of psychosis (Fig. 1). This path is a hypothetical course for patients, with the y-axis representing the severity of symptoms and x-axis the time scale. The first arrow indicates the point when the patient first notices some change in him of herself. These changes are not yet noticeable to family and friends, however. These changes may be vague and nonspecific, but are not psychotic. The second arrow indicates when these nonpsychotic but notable symptoms are also observed by family and friends, who may pick up on mood or behavioral changes. The third arrow indicates when the patient first notices psychotic symptoms in him or herself, which are not yet noticeable to others. The fourth arrow indicates when family and friends first notice psychotic symptoms in the patient and fifth arrow indicates the point of first psychiatric intervention.

The first attempts to improve clinical outcome focused on reducing the time between the fourth and fifth arrows, that is, to reduce the time that an individual experiences psychotic symptoms before receiving care. One meta-analysis looking at the relationship between duration of untreated psychosis (DUP) and outcome revealed that shorter DUP was associated with greater response to antipsychotic treatment, whereas another meta-analysis revealed that patients who had a longer DUP were more likely to have depression and anxiety at baseline and at 6- and 12-month follow-up and were more likely to experience more positive and negative symptoms and to have poorer overall functioning at 6- and 12-month follow-up.

The Norewegian TIPS study looked at the initiation of an early detection (ED) program to reduce duration of untreated psychosis. Patients in this ED area were compared with those from a parallel area that did not have such an intervention and both areas were indistinguishable in sociodemographic and treatment service variables. The ED-area patients were detected earlier in their illness than the control group (5-week median duration of illness for the ED area, as compared with 16 weeks for control group). At baseline, the patients from the ED area were in better clinical condition and had fewer negative symptoms and less risk for suicide. Both groups received the same treatment, but the ED-area group demonstrated fewer negative symptoms at 1-and 2-year follow-up and improved mood and cognitive scores.

These early intervention strategies, which are focused on initiating treatment with newly psychotic patients as quickly as possible to improve clinical outcome, are considered secondary prevention. To be considered primary prevention, the intervention should occur before the first presentation of psychosis, with hopes to prevent, delay, or reduce the onset of full illness. As we discussed previously, the prepsychotic symptoms are often nonspecific, so to improve efficacy of such interventions, groups have closed in on populations who had multiple risk factors and therefore were more likely to develop psychosis. Researchers have been intervening with these UHR groups, while monitoring the conversions to full psychotic illness. Going back to the hypothetical symptom courses in Figure 1, these groups are attempting to improve overall outcome by addressing the left-hand side of the symptom curve; by giving more services to patients at the first or second arrow, they hope to reduce the height of the overall curve.

The first step in this process is accurate identification of the target population. The Structured interview for Prodromal Syndromes (SIPS) is a structured diagnostic interview, somewhat analogous to the Structured Clinical Interview for DSM–IV (SCID), and is used to identify patients in the three UHR groups. The interview is made up of various components, including the Scale of Prodromal Symptoms (SOPS), the Schizotypal Personality Disorder Checklist, a family history questionnaire, and a GAF scale. The SIPS has established predictive validity, and groups can attain excellent interrater brief training.

After identifying patients as UHR, groups like the PACE clinic offer various intensive services, including case management, supportive counseling, and antidepressant medication, if needed. Intervening before presentation of illness raises concern of treatment being provided to false positives, meaning patients who would never have gone on to develop psychosis. Researchers have been mindful of this concern, only offering antipsychotic medications when the patient is clearly experiencing psychotic symptoms. Sensitivity is required when talking to the patients and families about their potential risk for psychosis, understanding the anxiety and stigma that such discussions can bring.

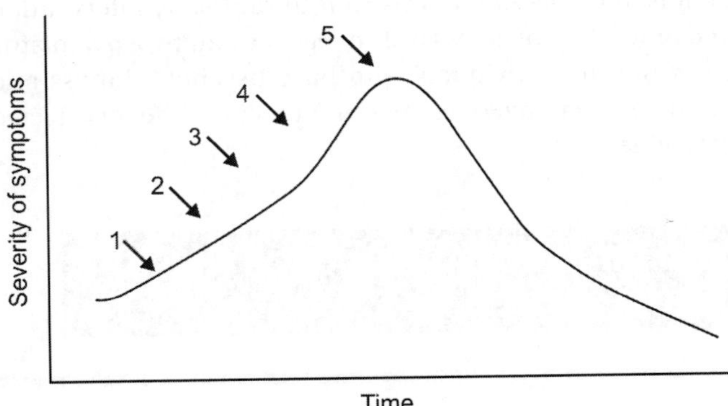

Fig. 1: Development of psychosis over time, with arrows indicating points of change noted by the patient or informants. *Arrow Points:* 1 = patient first notices some change in self, 2 = family or friends first notice some change in patient, 3 = patient first notices psychotic symptoms in self, 4 = family or friends first notice psychotic symptoms in patient, 5 = first psychiatric intervention. (From Yung AR, McGorry PD. The prodromal phase of first-episode psychosis: past and current conceptualizations.
Source: Schizophr Bull 1996; 22(2): 353-70 with permission.)

The rate of conversion from UHR to psychosis in these groups has ranged from 30% to 50%, which is much greater than the rates of first-episode psychosis in the general population or the short-term rates of symptom development in individuals at high genetic risk (e.g. siblings) in whom the life time risk is about 10%. This higher conversion rate indicates that the groups studied have been accurately identified as having increased vulnerability for psychosis. In some follow-up studies researchers have noted a reduction in the rate of conversion to psychosis over the years, which they acknowledge could be because of a dilution effect from enrolling patients who were false positives. The increased emphasis on early detection and attention to individuals who have nonspecific symptoms may be resulting in the selection of individuals who would never have gone on to develop psychosis. Instead of developing psychosis, these false-positive individuals could have resolution of symptoms or could go on to develop nonpsychotic disorders. The decreased conversion rate could also be attributable to patients becoming false false-positives, meaning that their trajectory was toward psychotic illness, but they were prevented from psychosis conversion by the interventions provided. At this point, it not possible to accurately distinguish between these possibilities.

TREATMENT/MANAGEMENT

The treatment goals in the UHR population are two fold: to treat the patient's current symptoms as the presenting disease and to improve immediate functioning, along with treating the current symptoms as risk markers for future disease. This process means monitoring the patient for worsening illness while using available interventions to minimize symptoms and improve patient's functioning. Groups working with the UHR population have attempted to engage patients in various psychosocial interventions using a recovery model of treatment. These interventions include case management; individual therapy, including psychoeducation and cognitive-behavioral therapy (CBT); multifamily support groups; and supported education and employment.

Studies have shown that CBT in UHR patients has resulted in decreased positive symptoms of psychosis and reduced likelihood of being prescribed an antipsychotic. There was evidence that those treated with CBT demonstrated decreased progression to psychosis compared with controls when baseline cognitive factors were controlled.

Treatment trials with medications are limited. An open study with aripiprazole in UHR subjects demonstrated improvements in prodromal symptoms without significant adverse events. A trial comparing needs-focused intervention (NFI) to NFI plus amisulpride revealed improved functioning with the combined group. There is also evidence to suggest that treatment with antidepressants can improve the outcome in these patients. A double-blind, placebo-controlled trial of olanzapine failed to show a significant effect of the drug. The low power of this study could have affected the outcome; the subjects in the placebo group had 2.5 times the rate of conversion to psychosis as the medication group.

Prospective studies following UHR patients and controls have shown that the UHR patients who later become psychotic demonstrated declines in visual memory and attentional set-shifting before becoming psychotic. Similarly, prospective MRI studies have shown a decrease in baseline thickness of anterior cingulated cortex (ACC) gray matter in UHR individuals who later become psychotic as compared with healthy controls and UHR subjects who did not become psychotic compared with UHR individuals who do not. Fornito and colleagues also demonstrate reduced ACC gray matter in UHR subjects who did not become psychotic. In this study, baseline ACC differences between the two high-risk groups predicted time to psychosis onset, with every 1 mm decrease in ACC thickness being associated with 20% increase in risk for psychosis. Waltergang and colleagues found that UHR subjects who later become psychotic had baseline thickening of the anterior genu of the callosum that was predictive of an individual's risk for conversion to psychosis. When baseline and repeat MRIs were done in UHR subjects, reductions in the gray matter volume of the hippocampus were seen after subjects developed psychosis.

FUTURE DIRECTIONS

The limited data regarding treatment of UHR patients underscores the need for further research in this populations and the importance of referring these patients to specialists. The Robert Wood Johnson Foundation launched a national program, the Early Detection and Intervention for the Prevention of Psychosis Program (EDIPPP), based on previous work done at the Portland Identification and Early Referral (PIER) program is Portland, Maine. This group, based at the Maine Medical Center, has used extensive community outreach and support to identify youth at risk for psychosis. The patients in the active treatment group were provided evidence - based psychosocial support and psychoeducation, and multifamily support group and medication treatment when needed. Patients at lower risk for psychosis were put into a comparison group that met with a case manager for monitoring, support, and referrals for additional treatment as needed but did not receive intensive services. The success of this program has been seen in the lower-than-expected rate of psychosis in the intensive services group at 1-year follow-up. Fourteen percent of the at-risk patients who enrolled in PIER experienced a full psychotic episode, which is lower than expected based on the conversion rates mentioned earlier (personal - communication).

Research in this UHR population presents an avenue of hope for patients and families struggling to cope with the debilitating effects of schizophrenia. As clinicians, we must be vigilant for individuals who present with the aforementioned risk factors and then carefully screen for unusual thought content, suspiciousness, grandiosity, perceptual disturbances, or disorganized communication. By referring these patients to specialty clinics that provide increased support and services, there is the potential that we can change the trajectory of their illness. Further research and funding is required to increase availability of such services and to reduce the time it takes patients to access care once ill. It is anticipated that this shift toward early intervention and prevention of illness will change the nature of psychiatric treatment in individuals who have psychotic illness and improve functional outcomes and quality of life for affected individuals.

43.18 COGNITIVE-BEHAVIORAL THERAPY AND DIALECTICAL BEHAVIOR THERAPY IN CHILDREN AND ADOLESCENTS

JN Vyas

Psychotherapy with children and adolescent present a set of challenges for the therapist that is qualitatively different from the challenges of psychotherapy with adults. Children and adolescents are not "little adults" and thus require a developmental approach to psychotherapy and modification of the treatment. Cognitive behavioral therapy (CBT) and modification behavior therapy (DBT) are two types of psychotherapy used in the treatment of children and adolescents. CBT is a psychotherapeutic model that posits that individuals with, for example mood and anxiety disorders, have cognitive distortions and behavioral deficits that can be targeted for change in therapy resulting in improvements in emotional, cognitive and behavioral functioning.[371] DBT is a principle-based psychotherapy developed by Linehan that blends standard cognitive-behavioral therapy with Eastern philosophy and meditation practices and shares elements with psychodynamic, client-centered, gestalt, paradoxical, and strategic approaches.[372] However, DBT is not uses with children and CBT with children is a subspecialty practice, so this chapter will focus on the developmental approach to the use of these treatments with adolescents as may be applicable to the practice of a general psychiatrist.

RESEARCH ON COGNITIVE BEHAVIORAL THERAPY AND ANXIETY IN ADOLESCENCE

Anxiety disorders are among the most command psychiatric disorder in children and adolescents.[373] However, the evidence base for treatment of anxiety in youths is relatively limited.[374] Initial studies of CBT for anxiety showed positive results.[375,326] More recently there have been several randomized controlled trials (RCTs) that have examined CBT in various formats including individual child,[375-377] family focused,[376-378] and group.[379] A number of these studies have demonstrated a significant effect of CBT compared with controls and alternate treatments.[380]

Recent systematic reviews of CBT for the treatment of anxiety disorders in youth appear to demonstrate benefit of CBT in comparison with waiting list or no-treatment controls. Cartwright and colleagues.[381] performed a meta-analyses of several studies that compared CBT with waiting list and found there to be a significant remission rate of diagnosed anxiety disorders in the CBT group compared with control. In addition, a more recent meta-analysis by James and colleagues[374] found similar results showing that just over half of subjects respond to CBT compared with a natural response rate of one-third.

Although CBT for anxiety disorders appears to be effective when compared with wait list and attention controls, two trials that compared CBT with educational support found no greater benefit to CBT.[382,383] Muris and colleagues[384] compared CBT with emotional disclosure and no treatment controls and found CBT to be superior to emotional disclosure; however, neither was significantly more effective than no treatment.

In a comparison of CBT literature, CBT for symptoms of anxiety appears to yield greater effect sizes than those for depression across studies. Chu and Harrison[380] conducted a comprehensive review of RCTs that tested CBT for anxiety and depression. Their findings suggest that CBT for anxious youth consistently yields moderate to large effects across variables in comparison with CBT for depression, which shows consistent but small effects. CBT appeared to produce comparatively greater behavioral and coping changes in anxiety samples, which support the possibility that different processes may mediate CBT for anxious and depressed youth.

The CBT and anxiety literature for children and adolescent has generally considered anxiety disorder such as social anxiety disorder, generalized anxiety disorder, and overanxious disorder as a single group.[374] However, these have been several studies that have examined other anxiety disorder such as post-traumatic stress disorder (PTSD) and obsessive compulsive disorder (OCD) specifically. To date, there are no rigorous RCT in children and adolescents with either phobias or panic disorder.

Although CBT is a well-documented intervention for adults with OCD, its effectiveness has not been extensively studied in youth populations. A recent comprehensive RCT[385] by the pediatric OCD treatment study team (POTS) comparing CBT and sertraline found the combination of treatments to be slightly more effective than CBT alone. Sertraline alone was proven to be significantly superior to placebo; however, the effect size of CBT alone was large than sertraline alone. This led the authors to the conclusion that children and adolescents with OCD plus a selective serotonin reuptake inhibitor (SSRI). Further RCTs and reviews have found similar results suggesting that CBT appears to be a promising treatment for OCD in children and adolescents.[386,387] Similarly, studies examining abuse-related PTSD in children and adolescents found trauma-focused CBT to be effective in not only reducing PTSD-related symptoms but also in reducing parallel depression and abuse-related shame when compared with child-centered therapy.[388,389]

In general, the reviewed studies have shown benefit for CBT in the treatment of anxiety disorders; however, there have been several methodological shortfalls identified.[390] The most significant of which appears to be difficulties in the process of randomization as well as limited active control comparison groups. In addition, study samples generally included children and adolescents with mild to moderate symptoms of anxiety mostly recruited from community and outpatient populations and did not include severe cases. Therefore, additional studies would be useful to further clarify the efficacy and effectiveness of CBT in treating child and adolescent anxiety disorders.

IMPLEMENTATION OF COGNITIVE BEHAVIORAL THERAPY FOR ANXIETY DISORDERS IN ADOLESCENTS

Anxiety disorders are associated with significant impairment in peer relationships, and family and school functioning. There is also an association with suicidal behaviors and comorbid psychiatric disorder such as depression and substance abuse.[374,381] CBT for adolescents is an empirically supported treatment, as described earlier. In this discussion, differences between CBT for adults and adolescents with anxiety disorder will be highlighted.

CBT for adolescents with anxiety can be conducted individually or in group. The most commonly used treatment manual was developed by Kendally and is called the "Coping Cat Program."[391] The program typically involves 16 to 20 sessions, which begin with skills training followed by exposure exercises. An acronym used in this program is FEAT (Feeling frightened, Expecting bad to happen, actions/attitudes that will help, review and, reward). The adolescent is taught to recognize anxious feelings and bodily sensations, identify and challenge cognitive distortions, develop a coping plan, and, finally, evaluate coping response and reward themselves appropriately.

These are some important developmental differences that may influence the manner in which CBT is performed in teenages.[391] First, their ability to recognize and process emotions is still developing, along with their ability to think in an abstract way. Using role-playing, stories and metaphors may be helpful in demonstrating some of the abstract CBT concepts given these developmental limitation. Adolescent also tend to be focused on the present and may have a difficult time envisioning how working on current difficulties will improved their future, especially when doing challenging exposure exercises. In the context of these considerations there are three distinct aspects of using CBT with adolescents will be discussed in more detail: alliance, role of parents, and homework/compliance.

Creating and alliance with adolescents is a different endeavor than with adults for a few reasons. First, adolescents are not usually the ones to initiate treatment. Parents or other outside influences are usually the ones to initiators of treatment. Adolescents are also at a stage in their development in which they are struggling with autonomy ad individuation. This may make it challenging to connect with and adult therapist, who may be seen as another authority figure in their life. Thus, collaboration in therapy is emphasized (consistent with the collaborative empiricism inherent in CBT) in addition to highlighting to confidentiality to improve the likelihood of creating a successful alliance. Furthermore, it has been found that active participation by teen and using his or her suggestions in session has been associated with positive treatment out comes.[392] Being too forceful in pushing a teen to talk about anxiety when he or she is not ready to has been shown to negatively affect the treatment alliance.[392]

Parents/caregivers have an influential role in the lives of most teens; therefore, they also have in important role in CBT. The literature is mixed with regard to outcome studies involving parents because it depends on the item of interest being measured.[378,393] Given that genetics and environmental modeling of anxiety have been well studied, involving parents may be valuable. They may help with the learning of coping skills, be "coaches" in exposure exercise, and help develop a behavioral rewards system to motivate the teen to work on anxiety and to remove any reinforcement of the teen's anxious behavior. In addition, parents may be valuable cotherapists who continue facilitating treatment gains when CBT is terminated.[378,393]

Homework is a key component of CBT. It well known that teens do not generally love homework, so it is challenging to design homework assignments that they will think worth their while. CBT homework creates opportunities to practice skill to build mastery and enhance capabilities. It also allows the therapist to assess whether the teen understands the material, as most will be reluctant to confess, if they are having trouble. To increase the likelihood that homework is completed, it is vital to begin with easily achievable assignments that have successful outcomes. In addition, having a reward system that is meaningful to the team is imperative.[394] The first step in dealing with noncompliance is to determine the reason, which may range from forgetting and avoidance, to the assignment being too difficult. The next step is to work on the homework together in session and strategize various ways for the homework to get done. It is important to keep in mind that although completing homework is essential, the teen should not be made to feel guilty or inadequate as the probability of homework being completed will drastically decrease.

The above principals can be applied to generalized anxiety disorder, social anxiety disorder, and to some extent, specific phobia. In working with teens with panic disorder many of the same techniques may be used. However, one important caveat is that there are usually more somatic symptoms in panic disorder with adolescents.[391] These may take the form of the classic cardiopulmonary symptoms, gastrointestinal symptoms, or neuromuscular symptoms such as trembling, numbness, and tingling. Therefore, it is essential to target these symptoms in CBT by doing relaxation exercises, cognitive restructuring, panic induction, and exposure therapy.[395]

Using CBT in the treatment of OCD and PTSD is more specialized than treating the above-mentioned disorders. There are a lot of similarities in treating adults and teens, including the importance of exposure with response prevention, but some of the developmental considerations mentioned earlier will come into play. Specifically, with OCD it is vital to recognize, relabel, and externalize intrusive thoughts as OCD, and develop strategies to cope with anxiety other than with compulsive behaviors. It is helpful to come up with a separate name for the OCD so that the teen can develop skills to conquer or manage the disorder so that in is not experienced as a part of the teen's identity.[387,396] CBT for PTSD in adolescents is similar to adults, with a few adaptations. It is important to take into account parental reactions and their coping strategies. Modifying both the adolescents and parents unhelpful trauma-related appraisals is vital.[397] with younger teens, using projective drawing and telling stories that reference the trauma my provide an opportunity to begin talking about the trauma.[398]

RESEARCH ON COGNITIVE BEHAVIORAL THERAPY AND DEPRESSION IN ADOLESCENCE

The CBT is the most studied nonpharmacologic intervention for the treatment of depression in youth.[371] Initial meta-analyses conducted throughout the late 1990s may have overestimated the effect sizes for CBT on measures of depression,[371] as recent meta-analyses have shown more modest effects. However, CBT for youth depression continues to be a promising intervention and appropriate treatment choice.

Initial studies found that CBT reliably outperformed wait list control and attention placebo conditions[399] and early meta-analyses found CBT outcomes to yield medium to large effect sizes.[400] In addition, Brent and colleagues[401] compared CBT to family therapy and a supportive therapy control and found that significantly more adolescents who received CBT than supportive therapy no longer met criteria for major depression, their data favored CBT over family and supportive therapy in reducing remising rates. Similarly, Wood and colleagues[402] found a brief CBT program to be superior to relaxation therapy alone, across multiple indices. Meta-analyses that pooled findings across early clinical trials documented consistent significant effect sizes for CBT.[399,400,403]

More recent investigations have brought into question the relative strength of CBT for the treatment of youth depression, the success of antidepressant medications in comparative clinical trials as well as the decreased effect sizes found in recent meta-analyses suggests that treatment effects may be more modest in clinical settings than previously thought. The publication of the Treatment for Adolescent Depression study (TDS) in 2004[404] showed outcomes for CBT that were less encouraging. However there was evidence that CBT may be beneficial in buffering youth against negative life stressors and suicidal thinking.[1] This led to the recommendation that the combination of fluoxetine and CBT for adolescent depression is the best treatment option and that CBT should be readily available as part of a comprehensive treatment strategy.[404] In contrast to the TADS study, a randomized controlled trial done by Goodyear and colleagues[405] looked at the effects of fluoxetine treatment alone and in combination with CBT in a population of moderately to severely depressed adolescents receiving routine clinical care and found that there was no evidence to support the combination treatment over fluoxetine alone. In addition, Weisz and colleagues[406] recently published the most comprehensive meta-analysis for CBT and depression in youth to date and found that the overall effects of psychotherapy treatment including CBT do not surpass and may actually lag significantly behind treatments for other youth conditions.

Although CBT for the treatment of adolescent depression appears to have a more modest effect in the valid treatment population than initially thought the effect has been shown to be significantly greater than zero across studies.[407] All things considered the results indicate that CBT for youth depression is a reasonable treatment option and should be available as part of a comprehensive treatment plan for depressed adolescents.

IMPLEMENTATION OF COGNITIVE BEHAVIORAL THERAPY FOR DEPRESSIVE DISORDERS IN ADOLESCENTS

As has been previously described, there are significant differences in the application of CBT for adolescents as compared with adults. The developmental considerations and the strategies for modifying the treatment approach described above for the use of CBT with anxiety disorders largely apply to the use of CBT with depression.

As described by Weersing and Brent[371] a review of the research on CBT for adolescents finds that there are four commonly studied models. The coping with depression for adolescents model (CWD-A) is the most studied,[408] whereas the Pittsburgh cognitive therapy model,[409] the brief cognitive therapy model used in the United kingdom,[402,409,410] and the TADS model[411] are also commonly found in the literature. CWD-A is a group therapy course that includes psychoeducation, pleasant activity scheduling, social skills training, and cognitive restructuring. In the Pittsburgh cognitive therapy model, the treatment was individual therapy driven by cognitive case conceptualization, with no preset exercises or homework and the content focused largely on cognitive restructuring, behavioral activation, and problem-solving skills. In the TADS model, the treatment was individual therapy with both required and optional family sessions. It blended elements of CWD-A the Pittsburgh cognitive therapy manual, and the investigators own expertise. Finally, in the brief cognitive therapy model, common CBT techniques were used but the interventions were low dose.[391] All of these models are based on fundamental CBT principles found in CBT models for adults. However, what is common to all of these models for adolescents is consideration of the developmental factors described above in the discussion of CBT for anxiety disorders. Consideration of these factors leads to modifications of the application of CBT appropriate to the stage of development of the patient.[412]

In the CBT models described above there are modifications for use with adolescents.[413] However, working with a 13-year-old and working with a 17-year-old can be quite different. Furthermore, chronological age does not determine capability and thus the developmental capacity of each adolescent must be determined in an ongoing manner. Many of the models described above use techniques to enhance learning and engagement in the therapy. For example, the use of cartoon strips to assist in the identification of negative cognitions.[414] However, the use of such a technique must be appropriately developmentally targeted, as some late adolescents will find such a technique irritating and in fact damaging to the alliance. In addition, each CBT model puts varying degrees of emphasis on cognitive versus behavioral components of treatment. In adolescents, assessment of the capacity of the adolescent to use cognitive constructs given their still-developing cognitive and abstraction capabilities is critical. Some adolescents will require greater emphasis on the behavioral strategies because of an inability to use the cognitive procedures.

Like CBT for anxiety disorders, CBT for depression models also recognize the role of family in the life of the adolescent. Most models either directly include or allow for family involvement in the treatment. Unfortunately, in studies conducted thus far, including families in the treatment has not been shown to add to the treatment gains that occur with CBT alone.[408,415]

As described above, CBT is often used in conjunction with antidepressant medication as part of a comprehensive treatment plan for a moderately to severely depressed adolescent.

RESEARCH ON DIALECTICAL BEHAVIOR THERAPY WITH SUICIDAL ADOLESCENT

Dialectical behavior therapy (DBT) is an empirically supported treatment[416,417] developed by Linehan[418] for adult women with borderline personality disorder who have chronic suicidal and nonsuicidal self-injurious behavior. To date, there are no published RCTs of dialectical behavior therapy for adolescent. However, there are two promising controlled studies of DBT modified for suicidal adolescent that have been published.[419,420] In the Rathus and Miller study,[419] 111 adolescent outpatients referred to an adolescent depression and suicide program received either 12 weeks of DBT or treatment as usual. It is not a randomized trial and adolescent with more severe symptomatology were referred for DBT. DBT was shown to reduce inpatient psychiatric days and treatment dropouts as compared with treatment as usual. Notably, there were no suicide attempts in the DBT group during the study. In Katz and collages[420] study, 62 adolescent inpatients received 2 weeks of either DBT or treatment as usual. DBT as compared with treatment as usual was found to reduce behavioral incidents during the hospitalization. There was also a 100% retention rate in the DBT program. In the 1-year follow-up, both treatments were found to reduce depression and suicidal ideation. Given the promising data generated by these studies, an RCT of 16 weeks of DBT for suicidal adolescent outpatients as compared with treatments as usual is currently under way in Norway.

IMPLEMENTATION OF DIALECTICAL BEHAVIOR THERAPY FOR SUICIDAL ADOLESCENTS

As mentioned above, DBT has been modified for use with adolescent. Miller and colleagues[372] have described the modifications for suicidal; adolescent outpatients in detail and Katz and Cox[421] have described the modifications for acute-care inpatients. In DBT, the treatment is always provides by a treatment team and not by an individual in isolation. The following discussion will provide a brief description of the differences between adult and adolescent DBT models.

Shorter Duration

Standard adult DBT is of 1-year duration. Although this duration of treatment may be used with adolescents, many programs have modified the duration of treatment. In their text, Miller and colleagues[372] describe a 16-week DBT program. The rationale for the shortening of treatment includes that adolescents may find it difficult to commit to 1 year of treatment. Service demands may also factor into the decision making on duration of treatment and currently there are no data in adolescents as to what is appropriate treatment duration. In many programs that do offer shorter length of treatment, the opportunity to either repeat the cycle or treatment or to "graduate" into a "graduate group" is available.

Multifamily Skills Training

In DBT for suicidal adolescents, modification have been made to the delivery of skills training groups. Given that adolescents reside with caregiver who play a significant role in their emotional experience, the caregivers, participate in the skills training groups. The principle is that the caregivers will require skills to effectively assist the adolescent in becoming skillful. The caregivers participate fully in the group in that they are there to learn the same skills as the adolescents and do the homework. The involvement of caregiver in the groups allows the skills trainer to observe the interactions between caregiver and adolescent and provide *in vivo* skills coaching. In stander DBT, individual therapists take phone calls from their patients to provide *in vivo* coaching on the use of skills during a crisis. In DBT for suicidal adolescents, this is also true but in addition the sills trainers take crisis calls from caregivers participating in the skill groups to provide the caregivers with *in vivo* coaching on applying the skills to their parenting.

Modification of the Wording of the Skills Manual

There is not currently a skills training manual for DBT for suicidal adolescents. Thus, the manual for skills training and the associated handouts are taken from the adult manual development by Linehan[422] Many program have modified the wording of the handouts to make them more "adolescent friendly"[372] However, there are no data on the use of any modifications to the skills manual.

Walking the Middle Path

In standard BT, there are four skills trading modules; core mindfulness, distress tolerance, emotion regulation, and interpersonal effectiveness. In the course of their work with adolescents, Miller and colleagues[372] found that the adolescent and his or her family had signification deficits that went beyond those that were addressed by the four existing modules in standard DBT. Miller and colleagues[372] identified a set of behavioral patterns that exist in the family constellations of suicidal adolescents and that parents, patients, and even therapists vacillate and become polarized along the three dimensions. Parents and therapists can become polarized along the dimension of excessive leniency versus authoritarian control, fostering dependence versus forcing autonomy and pathological normative behaviors versus normalizing pathological behaviors. The identification of these patterns led Miller and colleagues[372] to develop a fifth skills module for adolescents called "walking the middle path" to provide the skills necessary for adolescents and their caregivers to change these behavioral patterns. In this skills module the adolescent and his or her caregiver are taught basic behavioral principles, validation strategies, and how to think and act dialectically.

As Needed Family Sessions

Finally, in addition to including the caregiver in the skills—training group as described above, it is recognized that the adolescent is still residing in an environment that will be establishing contingencies for his or her behavior. As such, it is often necessary to meet with the adolescent and his or her family/caregiver for as-needed family therapy sessions.

In DBT for suicidal adolescents, the therapist uses a variety of strategies to help the adolescent understand his or her emotional experiences while at the same time working to get the adolescent to commit to change. The therapist uses behavioral chain analysis to elicit an understanding of the events of the day and allow for determination of what strategies might have been used to change the course of the events and allow for a more adaptive outcome.

RESEARCH ON COGNITIVE BEHAVIORAL THERAPY FOR SOMATOFORM AND EATING DISORDERS

Few studies have been conducted on the subject of CBT and somatoform illness in children and adolescents. Pain complaints, including recurrent abdominal pain in particular, are a common presentation in school-aged children and adolescents. However, there has been discrepancy as to effective management techniques.[423] Several recent studies have suggested the effectiveness of CBT intervention in reducing chronic pain syndromes in youth. Research by Sanders and colleagues[424] has shown that cognitive-behavioral intervention for recurrent abdominal pain was more effective than wait list intervention. In addition, CBT helped with reduction of pain symptoms more quickly, thoroughly, and for longer periods of time when compared with standard medical care.[425] Further RCTs by Duarte and colleagues[426] and Robins and colleagues[423] compared cognitive-behavioral family intervention with standard medical care to a control group that included patients receiving standard medical care alone. Both studies found a reduction in the amount of abdominal pain and the frequency of pain crises in the groups receiving cognitive-behavioral family therapy. Robins and colleagues reported reduction in both child and parent reported pain and somatisation. Sanders and colleagues reported the positive effects to be maintained at 6- and 12-month follow-up.[424] Duarte and colleagues[426] found that the CBT intervention was better for predicting and terminating pain episodes but not for dampening crises once started. Limitations of these studies included small sample sizes and selection bias in randomization. In addition, the CBT techniques used in treatment were not standardized across studies. Nonetheless, the results appear promising and suggest that combined medical and behavioral health intervention is effective in reducing perceived pain and somatisation in children and adolescent. Related empiric studies examining CBT for other commonly occurring pediatric pain disorders, including recurrent pediatric headache, have also yielded positive results demonstrating significant reductions in pain with CBT treatments.[427,428]

Similarly, few studies have focused on the area of CBT treatment for childhood and adolescent eating disorders. Finally-based models have proven to be effective in the treatment of adolescents with anorexia nervosa and bulimia nervosa;[429] however CBT remains largely unstudied as a treatment option in youth populations. CBT is the treatment of choice for adults with bulimia nervosa[429] and therefore may prove to be a useful intervention for bulimia in adolescents. A recent RCT by Schimdt and colleagues[430] compared the efficacy of family therapy and CBT guided self-care in adolescents with bulimia nervosa or eating disorder not otherwise specified. The findings suggest that CBT-guided self-care resulted in earlier reduction in binge eating than family therapy and that CBT had an advantage in terms of outcome and acceptability. Further research is required to further delineate the effectiveness and benefit of CBT for the treatment of eating disorders in children and adolescents.

SUMMARY

Although the benefits of CBT for anxiety and depressive disorders may not be as effective as once believed, it is nevertheless still an effective treatment and important part of the therapeutic armamentarium. To use CBT with adolescents, the therapist must factor in developmental considerations and use treatment models designed with these considerations mind. The effectiveness of DBT for suicidal adolescents remains unknown despite promising preliminary studies. However, there is no well-established, empirically supported treatment for suicidal adolescents and thus DBT has been widely implemented around the world. DBT for suicidal adolescents also is a modification of the adult approach factoring in developmental considerations. For the general psychiatrist who is treating adolescents, these treatments can have great utility in achieving desired outcomes but require familiarity with the principles described in this Chapter.

43.19 RECOGNITION AND MANAGEMENT OF PSYCHOSIS AND SCHIZOPHRENIA IN CHILDREN AND ADOLESCENTS

JN Vyas

Psychosis, including schizophrenia, comprises a major group of psychiatric disorders characterized by hallucinations and/or delusions (psychotic symptoms) that alter perception, thoughts, affect, and behavior, and which can considerably impair a child or young person's development, relationships, and physical health. Schizophrenia is estimated to affect 1.6 to 1.9 per 100 000 in the child population,[431,432] with prevalence increasing rapidly from age 14.[433] Psychosis and schizophrenia in children (age 12 years and under) and young people (up to age 17 years) are leading causes of disability[434] and are more severe and have worse prognosis than if onset is in adulthood, owing to disruption to social and cognitive development. Young people with schizophrenia tend to have a shorter life expectancy than the general population, largely because of suicide, injury, or cardiovascular disease,[435] the last partly from antipsychotic medication. Children and young people with transient or attenuated psychotic symptoms are at increased risk of developing psychosis or schizophrenia,[436] and delayed treatment can impair longer term outcomes,[437] making early recognition and intervention crucial.

This Chapter summarizes the most recent recommendations from the National Institute for Health and Clinical Excellence (NICE) guideline on psychosis and schizophrenia in children and young people.[438]

RECOMMENDATIONS

The NICE recommendations are based on systematic reviews of the best available evidence and explicit consideration of cost effectiveness. When minimal evidence is available, recommendations are based on the Guideline Development Group's experience and opinion of what constitutes good practice. Evidence levels for the recommendations are given in italic in square brackets.

GENERAL PRINCIPLES OF CARE

Health and social care professionals working with children and young people with psychosis or schizophrenia should be trained and competent to work with children and young people with mental health problems of all levels of learning ability, cognitive capacity, emotional maturity, and development. [*Based on the experience and opinion of the Guideline Development Group (GDG)*]

REFERRAL FROM PRIMARY CARE FOR POSSIBLE PSYCHOSIS

When a child or young person experiences transient or attenuated psychotic symptoms (such as possible or fleeting hallucinations or delusions) or other experiences suggestive of possible psychosis, refer for assessment without delay to a specialist mental health service such as child and adolescent mental health services or an early intervention in psychosis service (14 years or over). [*Based on the experience and opinion of the GDG*]

TREATMENT OPTIONS FOR SYMPTOMS NOT SUFFICIENT FOR DIAGNOSIS OF PSYCHOSIS OR SCHIZOPHRENIA

When transient or attenuated psychotic symptoms or other mental state changes associated with distress, sustained impairment in functioning, or help seeking behavior by the child or young person (or their parent or carer) are not sufficient for a diagnosis of psychosis or schizophrenia:[439,440]

- Consider individual cognitive behavioral therapy with or without family intervention, and
- Offer treatments recommended in NICE guidance for those with any of the anxiety disorders,[441,442] depression,[443] emerging personality disorder,[444,445] or substance misuse.[446-450]

[*Based on moderate to low quality evidence from randomised controlled trials in children and young people and on the experience and opinion of the GDG*]

Do not offer antipsychotic medication:

- For psychotic symptoms or mental state changes that are not sufficient for a diagnosis of psychosis or schizophrenia, or

- With the aim of decreasing the risk of psychosis.

[*Based on very low quality evidence from randomised controlled trials and an economic model in children and young people*]

REFERRAL FROM PRIMARY CARE FOR FIRST EPISODE PSYCHOSIS

Urgently refer all those with a first presentation of sustained psychotic symptoms (lasting four weeks or more) to a specialist mental health service, either to child and adolescent mental health services (age ≤17 years) or to an early intervention in psychosis service (≥14 years). Both services should include among their staff a consultant psychiatrist with training in child and adolescent mental health. [*Based on the experience and opinion of the GDG*]

ASSESSMENT OF FIRST EPISODE

Ensure that those with first episode psychosis receive a comprehensive multidisciplinary assessment, examining the following domains:

- Psychiatric (mental health problems, risk of harm to self or others, alcohol consumption, and history of prescribed and non-prescribed drugs)
- Medical, including medical history and full physical examination to identify physical illness (including organic brain disorders) and prescribed drug treatments that may result in psychosis
- Psychological and psychosocial (including social networks, relationships, and history of trauma)
- Developmental (social, cognitive, and motor development and skills, including coexisting neurodevelopmental conditions)
- Physical health and wellbeing (including weight and height, and information about smoking, diet, exercise, and sexual health)
- Social (accommodation; culture and ethnicity; leisure activities and recreation; and carer responsibilities—for example, of parents or siblings)
- Educational and occupational (attendance at school or college, educational attainment, employment, and functional activity)
- Economic (family's economic status).

[*Based on the experience and opinion of the GDG*]

TREATMENT OPTIONS FOR FIRST EPISODE PSYCHOSIS

Offer oral antipsychotic medication in conjunction with psychological interventions (family intervention with individual cognitive behavioral therapy). [*Based on high quality evidence from randomised controlled trials conducted in adults and an economic model using adult data from NICE's adult schizophrenia guideline*[451] *and on the experience and opinion of the GDG*]

If the child or young person and their parents or carers wish to try psychological interventions (family intervention with individual cognitive behavioral therapy) alone (without antipsychotic medication), advise that psychological interventions are more effective when delivered in conjunction with antipsychotic medication. If the child or young person and their parents or carers still wish to try psychological interventions alone, then offer family intervention with individual cognitive behavioral therapy. Agree a time limit (one month or less) for reviewing treatment options, including introducing antipsychotic medication. Continue to regularly monitor symptoms, level of distress, impairment, and level of functioning, including educational engagement and achievement (*Based on high quality evidence from randomised controlled trials conducted in adults and an economic model using adult data from NICE's adult schizophrenia guideline*[451] *and on the experience and opinion of the GDG*).

CHOICE OF ANTIPSYCHOTIC MEDICATION

This choice should be made by the parents or carers of younger children, or jointly with the young person and their parents or carers, and healthcare professionals. Provide age appropriate information and discuss the likely benefits and possible side effects of each drug, including:

- Metabolic (including weight gain and diabetes)
- Extrapyramidal (including akathisia, dyskinesia, and dystonia)
- Cardiovascular (including prolonging the QT interval)
- Hormonal (including increasing plasma prolactin)
- Other (including unpleasant subjective experiences).

[*Based on low to very low quality evidence from randomised controlled trials and observational studies conducted in children and young people; on high quality evidence from randomised controlled trials conducted in adults from NICE's adult schizophrenia guideline,*[451] *and on the experience and opinion of the GDG*].

HOW TO USE ORAL ANTIPSYCHOTIC MEDICATION?

Before starting antipsychotic medication, undertake and record the following baseline investigations:

- Weight and height (both plotted on a growth chart)
- Waist and hip circumference
- Pulse and blood pressure
- Fasting blood glucose, glycated hemoglobin (HbA_{1c}), blood lipid profile, and prolactin levels
- Assessment of any movement disorders

- Assessment of nutritional status, diet, and level of physical activity.

[Based on low to very low quality evidence from randomised controlled trials and observational studies conducted in children and young people; on high quality evidence from randomised controlled trials conducted in adults from NICE's adult schizophrenia guideline,[451] *and on the experience and opinion of the GDG]*.

Monitor and record the following regularly and systematically throughout treatment, but especially during titration:

- Efficacy, including changes in symptoms and behavior
- Side effects of treatment, taking into account overlap between certain side effects and clinical features of schizophrenia (for example, the overlap between akathisia and agitation or anxiety)
- The emergence of movement disorders
- Weight, weekly for the first six weeks, then at 12 weeks, and then every six months (plotted on a growth chart)
- Height every six months (plotted on a growth chart)
- Waist and hip circumference every six months (plotted on a centile chart)
- Pulse and blood pressure (plotted on a centile chart) at 12 weeks and then every six months
- Fasting blood glucose, HbA_{1c}, blood lipids, and prolactin levels at 12 weeks and then every six months
- Adherence
- Physical health.

The secondary care team should maintain responsibility for monitoring physical health and the effects of antipsychotic medication for at least the first 12 months or until the condition has stabilized. Thereafter, the responsibility for this monitoring may be transferred to primary care under shared care arrangements *[Based on the experience and opinion of the GDG, which was informed by low to very low quality evidence from randomised controlled trials and observational studies conducted in children and young people and on high quality evidence from randomised controlled trials conducted in adults from NICE's adult schizophrenia guideline*[451]*]*.

HOW TO DELIVER PSYCHOLOGICAL INTERVENTIONS?

When delivering psychological interventions take into account the child or young person's developmental level, emotional maturity, and cognitive capacity, including any learning disabilities, sight or hearing problems, or delays in language development (*Based on the experience and opinion of the GDG*).

Family intervention should:

- Include the child or young person, if practical
- Be carried out for between three months and one year
- Include at least 10 planned sessions
- Take account of the whole family's preference for either single-family intervention or multifamily group intervention
- Take account of the relationship between the parent or carer and the child or young person
- Have a specific supportive, educational, or treatment function and include negotiated problem solving or crisis management work.

[Based on the experience and opinion of the GDG, which was informed by high quality evidence from randomised controlled trials conducted in adults from NICE's adult schizophrenia guideline[451]*]*.

Cognitive behavioral therapy should be delivered on a one to one basis over at least 16 planned sessions (although longer may be needed) and should:

- Follow a treatment manual (adapting the approach to suit the age and developmental level of the child or young person) so that:
- They can establish links between their thoughts, feelings, or actions and their current or past symptoms, and/or functioning
- The re-evaluation of their perceptions, beliefs, or reasoning relates to the target symptoms
- Also include at least one of the following components:
- Normalizing, leading to understanding and acceptability of their experience
- Monitoring their own thoughts, feelings, or behaviors with respect to their symptoms or recurrence of symptoms
- Promoting alternative ways of coping with the target symptom
- Reducing distress
- Improving functioning.

[Based on the experience and opinion of the GDG, which was informed by high quality evidence from randomised controlled trials conducted in adults from NICE's adult schizophrenia guideline[451]*]*.

TREATMENT OF SUBSEQUENT ACUTE EXACERBATION OR RECURRENCE OF PSYCHOSIS OR SCHIZOPHRENIA

Offer oral antipsychotic medication in conjunction with psychological interventions (family intervention with individual cognitive behavioral therapy). *[Based on high quality evidence from randomised controlled trials conducted with adults and an economic model using adult data and on the experience and opinion of the GDG]*.

Offer family intervention to all families of children and young people with psychosis or schizophrenia, particularly for preventing and reducing relapse. Start this either during the acute phase or later, including in inpatient settings *[Based on high quality evidence from randomised controlled trials conducted in adults from NICE's adult schizophrenia guideline*[451] *and on the experience and opinions of the GDG]*.

HOSPITAL CARE

Before referral for hospital care, think about the impact on the child or young person and their parents, carers, and other family members, especially when the inpatient unit is a long way from where they live. Consider alternative care in the community wherever possible. If hospital admission is unavoidable, provide support for parents or carers when the child or young person is admitted. [*Based on the experience and opinions of the GDG, which were informed by the discussions of the topic group*].

PHYSICAL HEALTHCARE

General practitioners and other primary healthcare professionals should monitor the physical health of children and young people with psychosis or schizophrenia at least once a year, bearing in mind that people with schizophrenia are at higher risk of cardiovascular disease than the general population [*Based on the experience and opinions of the GDG*].

EDUCATION, EMPLOYMENT, AND OCCUPATIONAL ACTIVITIES

For children and young people of compulsory school age, liaise with their school and education authority, subject to consent, to ensure that ongoing education is provided [*Based on the experience and opinions of the GDG*].

OVERCOMING BARRIERS

Assessment and diagnosis of psychosis and schizophrenia in children and young people can be challenging because it has to take into account developmental factors and potential differential diagnoses and comorbid conditions, which differ from those in adults. The NICE guideline aims to reduce delayed recognition and increase accurate diagnosis and early uptake of evidence based treatments by supporting rapid referral of children and young people with suspected psychosis from primary care to a consultant psychiatrist with training in child and adolescent mental health (through either child and adolescent mental health services (CAMHS) or an early intervention in psychosis service). Ideally, trained staff in CAMHS should be embedded in the early intervention in psychosis service and take the lead for assessment and management of young people aged 14 and 17 years. The guideline advises that young people who enter early intervention in psychosis services at age 14 should receive follow-up from this service beyond the usual three year period to facilitate a smooth transition to adult mental health services.[452-455]

43.20 CHILD AND ADOLESCENT PSYCHOPATHOLOGY UPDATES

JN Vyas

Understanding pediatric psychopharmacology is often an important part of the practice of a general psychiatrist. A substantial number of children and adolescents are affected by a major psychiatric illness.[456,457] For many of these youths, medication management may be an important treatment option.[457] In addition, access to child and adolescent psychiatrists may be limited because child and adolescent psychiatry is an underserved medical subspecialty.[458] Considering that many pediatricians and family practitioners may feel treating these ill children is outside of their scope of practice, many of them are brought to general psychiatrist for treatment.[458]

There are some key issues for a general psychiatrist to consider before he or she begins prescribing psychotropic medications to children and adolescents. The most important is that agents that are effective in adults may not be effective in youths.[457] Similarly, medications that are well tolerated in adults may be associated with accentuated or additional risks when prescribed to young people. Thus, simply translating the practice of adult psychiatry to the pediatric population is not advisable.[457]

Historically, there has been a paucity of methodologically stringent data about the psychopharmacologic treatment of neuropsychiatric disorders in the pediatric population (with attention deficit hyperactivity disorder being a significant exception).[459] Fortunately, there has recently been a significant increase in research dedicated to the medication therapy of the pediatric population.[459] This Chapter is an effort to summarize those recent advances and bring the general psychiatrist up to date on the evidence-based psychopharmacologic treatment of children and adolescents.

ATTENTION DEFICIT HYPERACTIVITY DISORDER

Attention deficit hyperactivity disorder (ADHD) in one of the common and well-studied neuropsychiatric disorders in children and adolescents. It affects approximately 5% of children in the United States.[460] The gold standard of psychopharmacology for ADHD management has historically been psystimulants.[459] Stimulant treatment of ADHD has been studied for more than 70 years, longer even than antibiotics.[459]

Currently, stimulants can be conceptualized as falling into two fundamental groups: methylphenidate-based and amphetamine-based medications. In numerous randomized controlled trials, both classes of treatments have been shown to be generally well tolerated and superior to placebo, with a consistently large effect size.[461] No major differences in efficacy and tolerability have been found between methylphenidate- and amphetamine-based medications in the multiple studies comparing the two.[461] established that preferentially identifies responders to methylphenidate-versus amphetamine-based stimulants.

Originally, marketed stimulants were immediate-release formulations that required multiple daily dosing, often during the school day, a result of the stimulant's short half-lives. In order to address the shortcoming associated with the need for frequent dosing, long-acting formulations were developed. The benchmark stimulants used to treat ADHD, methylphenidate and dextroamphetamine, have been available in long-acting preparations since the 1918s. Ritalin SR and Dexedrine Spansules were the earliest long-acting formulations of methylphenidate and amphetamine, respectively. Although there were data that these early preparations were superior to placebo, clinical practice and further research found that these early long-acting formulations had significant variability in terms of both efficacy and duration of action.[462,463] Overall, they did not appear to offer substantial improvements over the original, immediate-release formulations.[462-464]

Because the first-generation formulations did not effectively achieve once-daily dosing, newer once-daily formulations of both methylphenidate and dextro-amphetamine were developed. Several oral versions of long-acting methylphenidate have been available for almost a decade (Concerta, Metadate, Ritalin LA) as have amphetamine-based treatments (Dexedrine ER and Adderall XR). In multiple, randomized controlled trials, these long acting formulations have been found to be therapeutically superior to placebo and generally well tolerated.[459-461] Differences between the medications remain primary related to duration and onset of action.[459-461]

Aside from the preparations described above, a transdermal formulation of methylphenidate has recently been developed: the methylphenidate-transdermal system (Daytrana). Methylphenidate transdermal consists of a mixture of methylphenidate contained in a polymer-based adhesive.[465] The medication diffuses out of the patch into the skin continuously over the recommended 9-hour wear time.[465] In a double-blind, placebo-controlled trial, the methylphenidate-transdermal system was well length of time the patch is worn can be adjusted to less than the standard 9-hour wear time in order to fit the schedule and demands of the individual child.[466]

Recent data suggest that there may be a difference in the onset and duration of action of d, l-methylphenidate versus d-methylphenidate.[467,468] One study reported that dexmethylphenidate may have a faster onset of action than d, I-methylphenidate.[12,13] However, conflicting reports exist as to the duration of action of the two formulations: one study has found d, I-methylphenidate to have a longer duration of action while another found that dexmethyphenidate lasted longer.[467,468] In short, despite potential differences in onset and duration of action, the two preparations appear to provide overall comparable symptom relief and tolerability.[467,468]

In addition to methylphenidate, as noted above, several long-acting formulations of amphetamine-based medications exit. Lisdexamfetamine (Vyvanse) has most recently entered the market. Lisdexamfetamine is a compound consisting of a pro-drug of dextroamphetamine.[461,469] This inactive formulation is metabolized into the active drug after ingestion and allows for once-daily dosing. Several placebo-controlled studies have found it be effective and safe in children.[461,469] No studies currently exist that compare the efficacy of Lisdexamfetamine with other long-acting formulations of amphetamine treatments.[461]

Stimulant in children and adolescents has raised questions regarding adverse cardiac events, in the past.[458,460] The rate of adverse cardiac events, including sudden death, in children treated with stimulant medication does not currently appear to exceed that of the general pediatric population.[458,460] At present, several guidelines do not recommend routine cardiac evaluation prior to stimulant treatment. A careful history for significant cardiac disease or symptoms and family history, looking particularly for sudden cardiac death, is recommended.[458,460] Consultation with a cardiologist for children with pre-existing cardiac disease or a concerning history is also recommended if considering stimulant treatment.[458,460]

Aside from stimulant treatment, there is one other Food and Drug Administration (FDA)-approved treatment for ADHD: a norepinephrine reuptake inhibitor, atomoxetine (Strattera). This has been shown to be generally safe and effective for the treatment of children, adolescents, and adults with ADHD.[461] Because of the larger effect size of stimulants when compared to atomoxetine, several treatment guidelines recommend atomoxetine as a second-line agent for the general ADHD population for those children who cannot tolerate stimulant treatment, whether because of underlying medical conditions, anxiety disorders, tic disorders, substance abuse problems, or intolerable side effects, these guidelines recommended atomoxetine as a first-line agent.[461]

Finally, α-adrenoceptor agonists, such as clonidine and guanfacine, have been prescribed off-label as alternatives or adjuvants to stimulant treatment. α-adrenoceptor agonists evidence for the treatment of tics.[470-472] However, there are also data to suggest/agonists may be generally safe and effective in treating ADHD and ADHD comorbid with tics.[473,474] In addition, some clinicians have used α-adrenoceptor agonists for sleep induction in children, although there is limited evidence to support this practice.[475]

Similar to stimulant treatment, previous formulations of α-agonists have required multiple daily dosing for the treatment of ADHD. In order to improve the utility of these medications, new long-acting formulations of both guanfacine and clonidine are being developed. Furthest along in development is a long-acting formulation of guanfacine, a selective α-2-agonist. Guanfacine ER (Intuniv) was studied in a randomized, placebo-controlled trial and found to be both safe and superior to placebo in children ages 6–17.[474] It has received an FDA-approvable letter for use in ADHD treatment.[476] In addition, a sustained-release formulation of clonidine (Clonicel) is being studied as part of the drug-development process.[477]

DISRUPTIVE BEHAVIOR DISORDERS

Disruptive behavior disorders (DBD), including oppositional defiant disorder and conduct disorder, are common diagnoses psychiatrists encounter when treating youth.[478,479] Aggression and aggressive behaviors are symptoms frequently targeted with pharmacotherapy.[478,479] When evaluating these children, characterizing the type of aggression they are displaying can be helpful in order to inform treatment decisions. Aggression in DBDs can be thought of as falling somewhere on a continuum between predatory aggression and impulsive/affect aggression.[480,481] predatory aggression involves planning and control while impulsive/affective aggression is characterized by reactivity, lack of planning, and minimal control.[480,481] This second, impulsive type of aggression in the type of aggression that appears to respond most robustly to pharmacotherapy.[480,481]

Recent data suggest that treating the impulsive/affective type of aggression associated with DBDs may reduce the many negative long-term consequences of DBDs.[481,482] It should be emphasized, however, that psychosocial interventions, such as family- and school-based interventions, as well as psychotherapy are recommended in many treatment guidelines as first-line interventions for DBDs.[482,483] Nevertheless, as part of a comprehensive treatment strategy/pharmacologic interventions are often considered and employed for affective/impulsive aggression, particularly when psychosocial interventions have been unsuccessful.[482,483]

When evaluating and treating a child with aggression as a potential target symptom for pharmacotherapy, it is recommended that a clinical first perform a meticulous assessment and diagnosis. Aggression is a nonspecific group of behaviors that may occur both in normal development and as understand and treat the underlying diagnosis that is resulting in the aggressive behaviors.[480,482] that is, aggression stemming from a primary mood disorder would be treated differently than one stemming from an anxiety disorder.[482] It is important to note that the treatment studies discussed below describe the treatment of youths with disruptive behavior disorders alone or comorbid with ADHD, generally free from other comorbid axis disorders.

In targeting this impulsive aggression associated with DBDs, clinicians have prescribed mood stabilizers, typical antipsychotics, and atypical antipsychotics off-label.[482] However, to date, there are no FDA-approved treatments for children and adolescents with DBDs.[476]

Historically, the typical antipsychotics and mood stabilizers were the mainstays of treatment for aggression in youth stemming from DBDs.[484,485] Haloperidol, in several studies, was found to be effective in reducing aggression in youth, particularly in those with irritability.[486] However, these studies found that the pediatric population appears to be significantly more vulnerable to extrapyramidal side effects of typical antipsychotics than the adult population.[487] Consequently, this side-effect profile appears to have significantly limited typical antipsychotics clinical utility in treating DBD-associated aggression in children and adolescents.

Among mood stabilizers, lithium and divalproic acid formulations (DVPX) have the most extensive literature supporting the treatment of DBDs in youth.[481,482,486,487] Both lithium and DVPX have been found to be more effective than placebo in treating aggressive symptoms in youth with DBDs.[481,482,486,487] However, the need for therapeutic drug monitoring and their side-effect profiles may limit their clinical use in youth with DBDs.[481,487]

The atypical antipsychotics appear to have become the most commonly prescribed medications in this patient population.[482,484] Risperidone, quetiapine, olazapine, and aripiprazole all have been studied in DBDs.[483] Among the atypical antipsychotics, risperidone has the most robust data supporting its use in children and adolescents.[488,489] Studies have found that risperidone may be beneficial both in the short-term and long-term treatment of aggressive behaviors associated with DBDs.[488,489]

There are less data on the use of other atypical antipsychotics in the treatment of DBDs in youths.[483] However, olanzapine, quetiapine, and aripiprazole have been studied in this population.[483] Olanzapine has been reported to effectively treat aggressive symptoms in youth with the combination of DBD and low IQ in retrospective and open-label trials.[490,491] However, side effects especially eight gain, were noted as significant problems for the study participants.[492,493] Similar to olanzapine, research on quetiapine in DBDs has shown some promise.[483] Several open-label studies have found that quetiapine is beneficial in DBDs and relatively well tolerated.[484-496] Aripiprazole, in one open label trial, has shown evidence of both safety and efficacy in treating children and adolescents with DBDs and aggressive symptoms.[497]

In summary, treating aggression associated with DBDs first involves careful evaluation and diagnosis to rule out other causes of the aggressive behavior. For impulsive/affective aggression stemming from DBDs and targeted with pharmacotherapy, typical antipsychotics, mood stabilizers, and atypical antipsychotics have been used. Side effects have limited the use of typical antipsychotics and mood stabilizers and it appears atypical antipsychotics, risperidone, in particular, have become a mainstay of treatment supported by evidenced-based data.

MAJOR DEPRESSIVE DISORDER

A key example of the pitfalls associated with extrapolating adult therapeutic data to children and adolescents is evident when one considers the pharmacologic treatment of major depressive disorder (MDD). Research into psychopharmacologic interventions for youth with MDD has identified significant differences in both efficacy and safety of antidepressants as compared to adults.[498]

Historically, tricyclic antidepressants (TCAs) have been a mainstay in the treatment of adult MDD. In spite of the development of selective serotonin reuptake inhibitors (SSRIs), they continue to have a role in the treatment of adult depression.[499] Pior to the 1980s, TCAs were also a primary treatment of pediatric depression.[500] However, once outcomes with tricyclics were studied in the pediatric population, no significant difference between TCAs and placebo was found.[500] There have been multiple negative randomized, controlled trials of TCAs in pediatric depression.[500-502] In addition, concerns regarding a narrow therapeutic index, anticholinergic side effects, ECG changes, and sudden death have raised in children and adolescents treated with TCAs.[503] Consequently, TCAs are not generally recommended as treatment for youth with MDD.[498]

Over the last 10 years, there has been a significant increase in the number of randomized, controlled trials related to the pharmacologic treatment of pediatric depression.[457] Currently, the only FDA-approved antidepressant for youth suffering from MDD is fluoxetine.[498] Several randomized, controlled trials have found fluxetine to be significantly more effective than placebo in treating depression in the pediatric population.[504,505] In addition to being effective for the acue treatment of MDD, a recent study found that fluxetine was effective in delaying the onset of relapse of depression in children and adolescents.[506]

Although this chapter focuses primary on psychopharmacologic treatment of children and adolescents, psychotherapeutic treatment is worth mentioning here regarding the treatment of pediatric MDD. There is methodologically stringent literature regarding the combination of medication and psychotherapy in this patient population. The treatment for adolescents with depression study was a multicenter, randomized clinical trial designed to study fluxetine alone, cognitive behavior therapy (CBT) alone, the combination of the two, and placebo in the treatment of adolescent depression.[507-509] This National Institute of Mental Health (NIMH)-funded study found that fluxetine was superior to both placebo and CBT, but that the combination of CBT and fluxetine was superior to the medication treatment alone.[508] In addition, it was found that the addition of CBT to fluxetine offered some protection against the emergence of suicidal events.[508]

Beyond the acute treatment of pediatric depression, there is very limited evidence regarding the treatment of refractory depression in youth. An NIMH-funded study, the treatment of SSRI-resistant depression in adolescents trial examined four different interventions in adolescents whose depression did not respond to treatment by an SSRI. They compared switching this group to another SSRI, venlafaxine, SSRI plus CBT, or venlafaxine plus CBT.[510] At the end of 12 weeks, they found no difference in clinical response between the venlafaxine group and the SSRI group. The addition of CBT did make a significant difference, however. The investigators found that adding CBT to either an SSRI or venlafaxine in this group was significantly better, in clinical response, than switching the medication alone.[510]

In addition to significant differences in efficacy between children and adults, there are important safety issues that are particular to the treatment of children and adolescents with MDD. In the forefront of the concerns has been the report of an associated increase in suicidal events in children and adolescents treated with SSRIs. In 2003, the FDA began looking into the effects of antidepressants on spontaneously reported suicidality (suicidal adverse events, suicidal ideation, and suicidal attempts).[511] The FDA evaluated the results of 24 randomized, controlled trials involving the treatment of youth with antidepressants and found a small but statistically significant increase in the occurrence of "suicidal adverse events" when compared to placebo. However, no completed suicides were reported throughout the students.[512] A second meta-analysis found a similar small increase in the relative risk for self-reported suicidality.[498] A black-box warning was placed on all antidepressants in 2004, regarding the risk of suicide in children and adolescents.[511] Overall, these studies have found an approximately 2% increase in the risk of suicidal ideation in youth who were treated with antidepressants versus those who were not.[498]

In addition, as stated above, the combination of CBT with medication appears to both add benefit and reduce the risk of suicidality in adolescents.[508] Treating moderate-to-severe depression in adolescents with both medication and CBT may, therefore, help to achieve the most rapid response with the smallest amount of risk.[508]

In addition to the concern regarding suicidality, treating children and adolescents with antidepressants raise concerns regarding the risk of pediatric bipolar disorder for several reasons. A child treated with an antidepressant because of a presentation consistent with MDD may develop manic or hypomanic symptoms after ignition of treatment.[513,514] This may be because of a latent bipolar disorder that was not evident on initial presentation.[514,515] Additionally, subclinical hypomanic symptoms may have been present prior to the presentation of MDD that were no elicited by the clinician.[514,515] Finally, a child may present with irritability and insomnia that is treated presumptively a MDD, but in fact represents a mixed episode. Treating such children with antidepressants risks producing more rapid cycling or worsening of manic and mixed symptoms.[515] Consequently, it is recommended that clinicians monitor children and adolescents beginning antidepressant treatment for the emergence of manic or hypomanic symptoms.[498] In addition, a meticulous clinical history with attention to the possibility of past manic or hypomanic symptoms and an examination of the family history for a history of bipolar disorder is recommended.[515]

BIPOLAR DISORDER

Pediatric bipolar disorder is a chronic and disabling condition.[515] Controversy has surrounded what constitutes the spectrum of pediatric bipolar disorder.[514-516]

Historically, there has been a dearth of research with methodologic rigor on the treatment of bipolar disorder in children and adolescents.[515,516] However, in recent years there has been a significant increase in the data available for treatment of these youth.[515,516] These studies of bipolar disorder primarily focus on youth in manic or mixed states.[515,516] Consequently, little is know still about the management of pediatric bipolar depression, the maintenance treatment of pediatric bipolar disorder, and the pharmacotherapy of major depression in youth with family histories of bipolar disorder.[515,516] At this point, there are three medication treatments approved by the FDA for the psychopharmacologic management of pediatric bipolar disorder: lithium for children aged 12 and up, and aripiprazole and risperidone for youth aged 10 to 17 in manic or mixed states.[515,516]

Lithium was one of the first medications used for the treatment of bipolar disorder in adults and remains an important mood stabilizer in that population.[491-520] In children and adolescents, there are prospective studies, several open label trials, and one randomized controlled trial supporting its use in pediatric bipolar dlsorder.[518-520] Many of these studies have lacked methodologic rigor and FDA approval of lithium in youth appears to be based primarily on data from adult studies.[518-520] More definitive research on lithium in children is currently being conducted with National Institute of Child Health and Human Development support. However, until more definitive data become available, it appears that lithium may be a relatively safe and effective treatment for adolescents in acute manic or mixed states.[518-520]

In addition to lithium, medications originally used to treat epilepsy, the anticonvulsants, have been used to treat bipolar disorder in both children and adults.[521] Divalproic acid-based preparations, carbamazepine, topiramate, and oxcarbazepine are the best studied of the anticonvulsants in the treatment of bipolar disorder.[515,516] Early research on DVPX consisted of open label trials and generally reported DVPX as effective in reducing mixed and manic symptoms in adolescents.[515,516] However, two recent randomized, controlled trials have provided contradictory results.[522,523] One three-site, National institutes of Health (NIH)-sponsored study found DVPX superior to placebo in treating manic symptoms in youth.[522] However, a larger, industry-supported, multisite study found no difference between DVPX and placebo.[523] Differences in study design and implementation may account for the discrepant results and more data on valproate's efficacy in comparison with placebo are still needed. Several studies have found that divalproate had efficacy equal to lithium in the acute treatment of pediatric bipolar disorder.[524,525]

Carbamazepine outcome data in youth is restricted to case reports. Currently, no controlled data are available to confirm or refute its use in children and adolescents.[516,526] Placebo-controlled data supporting its use in adults, however, may warrant further methodologically rigorous investigations into its use in the pediatric population.[527] Oxcarbazepine was studied in one randomized, controlled trial in youth with bipolar disorder.[528] This study found no statistically significant difference in efficacy between oxcarbazepine and placebo.[528]

In recent years, much of the research on pediatric bipolar disorder has focused on the atypical antipsychotics. As stated previously, risperidone and aripiprazole have FDA approval for the treatment of mixed and manic states in youth aged 10–17.[529] Risperidone, olanzapine, quetiapine, aripiprazole, and ziprasidone have all been studied in placebo-controlled clinical trials involving young people with bipolar disorder.[530-535] To date, all have been positive studies, that is, they have found that 'these atypical antipsychotics are more effective in the acute treatment of manic or mixed states in children than placebo.[530-535]

Most studies have been three-arm studies; they have looked at placebo, a supposed minimal-effective dose of the medication, and a higher dose.[530-535] In these three-arm studies, results indicate that both active-treatment arms were therapeutically superior to placebo and found no difference in treatment efficacy between the two doses of medication.[530-534] Although the higher doses showed no additional benefit, they did show an increase in side effects.[530-534]

In summary, three medication treatments are currently approved by the FDA for the treatment of youth in manic and mixed states: lithium for children ages 12 and up, and aripiprazole and risperidone for youths aged 10–17. Although the data are somewhat limited, lithium appears generally safe and effective in youth in manic or mixed states. In addition, since their advent, much of the research has focused on the atypical antipsychotics and, to date, all placebo-controlled trials have found the atypical antipsychotics more effective in treating manic or mixed states than placebo, The presumed minimally effective doses that have been studied in these trials have been found to be gas 'therapeutically effective as the higher dosages and with lower side effects.

ANXIETY DISORDERS

Anxiety symptoms and anxiety disorders are a common occurrence in childhood, with a diagnosable anxiety disorder occurring in 10%–20% of children.[536,537] Among medications, SSRIs have the most evidence supporting their use in youth with anxiety,although several medication groups have been studied.[536,537] Although the psychopharmacologic treatment of children and adolescents is the focus of this Chapter, psychotherapeutic treatment deserves a special mention, especially in the treatment of anxiety disorders.[536,537] In children with anxiety disorders, CBT has substantial evidence supporting its use and is often recommended in combination with medication therapy.[536,537]

In order to understand the research surrounding the pharmacologic treatment of pediatric anxiety disorders, it is helpful to think of them as falling in four basic categories: (1) broad anxiety disorders, which include generalized anxiety disorder, social phobia, traumatic stress disorder (PTSD); and (4) panic disorder.

Research concerning the pharmacologic treatment of the board anxiety disorders has primarily focused on the use of SSRIs.[536,543] Sertraline, fluoxetine, paroxetine, paroxetine and adolescents.[536-543] In addiction to these SSRIs, venlafaxine also has several recent randomized, controlled trials that indicate it may be more effective than placebo in reducing anxiety symptoms in youth with generalized anxiety disorder and social aphobia.[544-554] However, there are currently no FDA-approved medications for the treatment of these disorders in children and adolescents.

As stated above, in addition to medications, cognitive behavior therapy is often recommended in the treatment of these disorders.[536,537] However, there are limited data comparing the relative benefits of CBT and medications in this population[536,537] The NIMH is currently supporting a study (Child Adolescent Anxiety Multimodal Treatment Study) that is designed to compare sertraline treatment alone, CBT alone, and their combination in comparison with placebo in the treatment of social phobia and generalized anxiety disorder.[546]

In contrast to the broad anxiety disorders, there are several FDA-approved medications for the treatment of OCD in youth. To date, sertraline has FDA approval in children ages 6 and up, fluoxetine ages 7 and older, fluvoxamine ages 8 and up, and clomipramine for youth aged 10 and older. As with the broad anxiety disorders, SSRIs have the most robust research supporting their use in this population.[547-550] Sertraline, fluoxetine, fluvoxamine, and paroxetine all have positive randomized trials supporting their therapeutic superiority to placebo.[547-550]

Again; in contrast to the broad anxiety disorders there is evidence comparing CBT with medication management in OCD. In the Pediatric OCD Treatment Study, CBT alone, sertraline alone, and CBT plus sertraline were compared with placebo in youth aged 7–17 with OCD.[551] Data suggest that the combination of CBT plus sertraline was the most effective treatment and that both CBT alone and sertraline alone were more effective than placebo.[551] In addition, the results indicated that CBT alone was more effective treatment than sertraline alone in treating children with OCD.[551] In early-onset OCD, denned as OCD beginning before puberty, it has been found that family-based CBT is effective in reducing both obsessions and compulsions in preadolescent patients.[552]

The pharmacologic treatment of pediatric posttraumatic stress disorder has very limited evidence, and there are no medications currently approved by the FDA for this indication.[553] There are several case studies on both in patients and out-patients with PTSD reporting a reduction in anxiety symptoms with the use of clonidine.[555-557] In addition, quetiapine has been reportedly used with success in youth with PTSD in detention centers.[558] One controlled study exists that suggested propranolol was effective in reducing the symptoms of PTSD in the study population.[559]

In pediatric panic disorder, no controlled data exist regarding its pharmacologic treatment.[560] A pilot study of SSRI treatment in a small number of children indicated efficacy in reducing panic symptoms, but suggested the need for a benzodiazepine during treatment initiation.[561]

In summary, anxiety disorders are common disabling conditions affecting youth, but there is limited evidence regarding the pharmacotherapeutic interventions used to treat them. The broad anxiety disorders have evidence supporting the use of SSRIs, to reduce symptoms in children and adolescents. Similarly, SSRI management of OCD has significant data behind it. In contrast there is limited research on the psychopharmacologic management of pediatric PTSD and panic disorder. Multiple medication classes have been clinically used in this population, including SSRIs, α-agonists, and atypical antipsychotics although there are no FDA-approved medications anxiety disorders in youth.

AUTISM AND PERVASIVE DEVELOPMENTAL DISORDERS

Autism is the prototypic pervasive developmental disorder. It is characterized by dysfunction in socialization, language, and repetitive behaviors.[562,563] In addition to these core features, patients diagnosed with this disorder often struggle with other behaviors that impair their ability to function in daily life.[562,563] These include symptoms of inattention, hyperactivity, mood instability, and aggression.[562,563] As part of a comprehensive treatment plan, including school support, occupational and physical therapy, and social skills training, pharmacotherapy may be utilized to help youth manage the symptoms described above.[563]

One of the core features of autism is the presence of repetitive, stereotyped behaviors and compulsions. As in patients with OCD, several antidepressants have data supporting their use in reducing compulsions in autistic youth.[564] Fluoxetine has placebo-controlled data that indicate it may be more effective than placebo in reducing stereotyped behavior in autism, and may be generally well tolerated.[565,566] Citalopram, escitalopram, and sertraline all have open-trial data that indicate possible benefit in reducing compulsive behavior in these children.[567-570] Although benefit is suggested for these SSRIs, several studies found a significant occurrence of what some others have termed, "behavioral-activating side effects" with SSRl treatment In autistic youth, including aggression, agitation, and hyperactivity.[564-570] Aside from SSRIs, clomipramine, a tricyclic antidepressant, has been studied in this population.[571,572] Although clomipramine showed superior clinical efficacy to placebo, significant side effects were experienced by many of the patients, including urinary retention, worsening behavior, and sedation.[571,572]

Patients with autism often suffer from symptoms of inattention and hyperactivity. As with patients diagnosed with ADHD psychostimulants are the most well stunted medications for ADHD symptoms associated with autism.[573-575] A recent double blind, placebo-controlled crossover study was conducted investigating methylphenidate in youth with pervasive developmental disorders.[575] Methylphenidate was superior to placebo in reducing inattention and hyperactivity symptoms in this population, but at a significantly lower response rate than in typically developing children with ADHD.[575] In addition children in this study appeared to have a relatively high incidence of adverse events.[575] Amphetamine-based stimulants have very limited data in youth with autism, with the most recent data from the 1970s.[576-578] These data suggest poor tolerability for amphetamines in children with autistic spectrum disorders.[576-578] However, definitive studies with current methodologies are not yet available, except few.[579-582]

Aggression and self-injurious behaviors can be disabling for children with autism and have been the focus of many types of pharmacotherapy.[562] Currently, risperidone is the only FDA-approved medication to treat the irritability sometimes associated with pervasive developmental disorders.[562,583-585] Risperidone has several placebo-controlled trials that indicate it is efficacious in reducing aggression, tantrums, and self-injurious behaviors in the short- and long-term, and is generally well tolerated.[583-585] Quetiapine has also been studied, but has been found to have more modest benefit and more problematic side effects than risperidone in this population.[586,587] In addition, although olanzapine has been reported to have moderate efficacy in reducing aggressive symptoms, weight gain has been significantly problematic in the study populations.[588-590] Ziprasidone and aripiprazole have very limited data in this patient group.[591-595]

In addition to atypical antipsychotics, mood stabilizers have been used clinically to treat irritability and aggression in children with autism.[562,596,597] One placebo-controlled trial showed significant benefit of divalproex sodium in reducing aggressiveness and mood lability.[598]

Finally, to the core dysfunction of autism, impairment in social functioning, effective or FDA-approved pharmacotherapeutic interventions have not been identified at this point.[597,598] D-cycloserine, a glutamate agonist, which has shown limited success in the negative symptoms of schizophrenia, has been studied with mixed results in children with autism.[597,598] In addition, tetrahydrobiopterin, a compound involved in catecholamine synthesis, was found to have modest benefit in socialization in a small study of children with autism.[598]

In summary, many pharmacologic interventions have been used clinically for behavior dysfunctions related to pervasive developmental disorders. Unfortunately, treatment with respect to the core social dysfunction remains elusive. Medication treatment of associated behaviors involves identifying specific behaviors and targeting with medication appropriately. However, it should be noted that patients suffering from pervasive developmental disorders often display therapeutic and adverse reactions that differ significantly from those in the general pediatric population. As existing research is somewhat limited in this area, further methodologically stringent clinical trials are needed.

PSYCHOTIC DISORDERS

Early-onset schizophrenia and schizoaffective disorder are severe and chronic diseases.[599-601] Up to 33% of individuals with schizophrenia report having symptom onset before the age of 18.[599-601] Those patients who do have psychotic symptoms in their youth often have a less favorable prognosis than those with adult-onset psychotic disorders.[599-601] Effective treatment, therefore, is important, in this severely ill population. Since their advent, atypical antipsychotics appear to be, clinically, the most commonly used medications for pediatric psychotic disorders. However, recent research has suggested that first-generation antipsychotics may be equally effective acutely.[599,602] Definitive data and recommendations on which specific antipsychotic should be considered first line in children and adolescents with schizophrenia and schizoaffective disorder are not available. Currently, FDA-approved treatments include aripiprazole and risperidone for the treatment of adolescents aged 13–17 with schizophrenia.

Early studies on pediatric psychotic disorders focused on the first-generation antipsychotics, including haloperidol, thiothixene, thioridazine, and loxapine.[603-605] Haloperidol and Ioxapine have both been studied in comparison to placebo in adolescents and both were reported to be therapeutically superior to placebo.[603,604] However, both loxapine and haloperidol were associated with substantial rates of extrapyramidal symptoms (EPS) and sedation in comparison to placebo.[603,604] Thiothixene and thioridazine were compared in a similar study population and were found to reduce psychotic symptoms, but were associated with dose limiting sedation.[605]

Because of concerns' regarding the side effects of typical antipsychotics in juveniles, particularly EPS, the atypical antipsychotics have become much more commonly prescribed. Risperidone, olanzapine, and aripiprazole have been studied in comparison with placebo in the acute treatment of early-onset schizophrenia.[606-614] In addition, clozapine, in spite of its side-effect profile, has evidence to support its use in the treatment of refractory schizophrenia in youth.[615-618]

Risperidone was studied in a three-arm, placebo-controlled trial. The data suggest that both active treatments (1 mg/day-3 mg/day and 4 mg/day-6 mg/day) were superior to placebo in reducing psychotic symptoms. However, the higher dose treatment group had significantly greater extrapyramidal side effects than the lower dose group, with a similar degree of symptom reduction.[613] Olanzapine was studied in a blinded, 6-week, placebo-controlled, flexible dosing study in adolescents.[614] Treatment with olanzapine resulted in significantly greater reduction in symptoms than placebo. However, considerable weight gain (average of 4.3 kg), in addition to sedation and liver enzyme elevation, were noted with olanzapine treatment.[614] Recent data were published of a three-arm, placebo-controlled trial of aripiprazole in adolescents with schizophrenia.[612] In this study, both doses of aripiprazole (10 or 30 mg/day) were statistically superior to placebo in reducing psychotic symptoms, with no significant difference between the treatment arms. Significantly more EPS was noted in the aripiprazole-treatment groups with mild degrees of weight gain in comparison to placebo.[612]

With respect to treatment-resistant schizophrenia, clozapine remains the treatment of choice for adults.[615-618] The data in children are less robust, but consistently indicate that clozapine is superior to other typical and atypical antipsychotics for youths who have failed treatment with at least two previous antipsychotics.[615-618] Several open trials indicate clozapine is effective in reducing psychotic symptoms in youth with treatment-refractory schizophrenia.[615] in addition, clozapine has been compared to both haloperidol and high-dose olanzapine in double-blind comparison studies for treatment-resistant early-onset schizophrenia.[616-618] Clozapine was shown to be therapeutically superior in both studies. However, side effects, including seizures and neutropenia, remain a concern for patients treated with ciozapine.[615-618]

SUMMARY

There has been a significant increase in the number of methodologically rigorous studies concerning the psychopharmacologic treatment of children and adolescents in recent years. This has allowed clinicians to make better informed and more evidenced-based decisions when evaluating and treating youth. Although the research has increased in volume and rigor of late, further research is still needed. Studies evaluating the long-term safety of medication treatment in children and adolescents remain limited. In addition, data on head-to-head comparisons of medications are necessary. Comparisons of medication, psychotherapy, and the combination have begun, but further investigations are warranted. Finally, research into predictors of response and tolerability may aid in determining the optimal medication choices for particular patients. In conclusion, the consideration of pharmacologic treatment continues to be important for many children and adolescents with psychiatric illness.

43.21 PATERNAL PSYCHIATRIC DISORDERS AND CHILDREN'S PSYCHOSOCIAL DEVELOPMENT

JN Vyas

INTRODUCTION

Research evidence indicates that psychiatric disorders of parents are associated with an increased risk of psychological and developmental problems in their children. For example, parental depression has been associated with an increased risk of emotional and behavioral problems in children, and delay in cognitive development and infant growth.[619-621] The prevalence of psychiatric disorders affecting adults of parenting age is high and increasing worldwide.

Much research has focused on maternal psychiatric disorders. This is especially the case when research has examined the early years of children's lives[622]—a time of enormous cognitive and emotional development.[621,623] Several reasons exist for this focus on mothers. In many societies, women are the primary care givers for children, and thus have a greater role than men in their children's early development and socialization (however, the role of men is sometimes under emphasised).[624] Furthermore, several influential theories of child development—including psychodynamic theories and, recently, attachment theories[625]—emphazise the key role of mothers. Practical reasons could also exist for research to focus on mothers, because they might be more readily available than fathers and more willing to participate in research.[626]

Despite the dearth of research on paternal psychiatric disorders and, consequently, their effect on child development, they should be seriously considered.[627-629] Fathers' roles vary widely between different social and cultural groups, and substantial variability also exists both within any society and over time. For example, in intact families in the USA, fathers are now more overtly involved in child care than they were previously, although the absence of nonresidential fathers from their children's lives has increased.[622,627] On the whole, however, in most countries and cultures, fathers have an active role in child care; moreover, fathers seem to have more influence on their children's development than previously thought.[630-635] Therefore, the potential effects of psychiatric disorders on their ability to care for, and nurture, their children are important.

In most societies, parenting roles of mothers and fathers differ.[636] Men also have a different distribution of psychiatric disorders from that of women (e.g. they have higher rates of alcoholism and lower rates of depression); psychiatric disorders labeled identically may affect men and women differently. Overall, these factors suggest that paternal psychiatric disorders could differ greatly from maternal disorders in their effect on children; some research supports this hypothesis.[637,638]

Our aim was to review research publications on paternal psychiatric disorders, and children's health and psychosocial development. The effect of physical disorders is beyond the scope of this article, but reviews are available.[639] We first describe the research that has examined the associations between paternal disorders and child problems, focusing on paternal depression because it has been more thoroughly studied than other conditions. We then consider some mechanisms by which risk is transmitted from fathers to children (causal pathways), and whether some factors (effect modifiers) might exist that place some groups of children at high risk. Finally, we draw conclusions on clinical practice, service provision, and future research directions.

PATERNAL PSYCHIATRIC DISORDERS

Men differ from women in their distribution of psychiatric disorders. Here, we consider depression, anxiety, alcohol and substance abuse, bipolar disorder, and schizophrenia. These disorders are the most common, and most serious, mental illnesses affecting men; they all affect adults of parenting age; for most, peak onset is between 18 and 35 years of age.

Depression

Depression is the most comprehensively studied psychiatric disorder in terms of its effects on parents and, consequently, on their children. It has also the most substantial effect on health and wellbeing worldwide.[640] Most attention has been paid to maternal depression[621] (e.g. a recent search with PubMed yielded 2480 and 496 articles on depressive disorder in mothers and fathers, respectively), and especially postnatal depression. Environmental factors, such as the quality of parental care, can have a large effect on the development of infants.[641,642] Several longitudinal studies have shown increased rates of difficulties in infants and children after exposure to maternal postnatal depression, including high rates of emotional and behavioral problems,[643,644] delayed cognitive development,[645,646] and increased risk of depression and anxiety disorders in adolescence.[647]

Depression affects about 3–6% of men, which is about half of its prevalence in women.[648,649] Depression is characterized by persistent low mood, and loss of interest and energy. Other symptoms include irritability, anger, sleep problems, and poor concentration. Paternal depression during the postnatal period (measured at 8 weeks after birth) has been associated with an increased chance of subsequent behavioral and emotional problems in children.[638,650] Later in childhood, children of depressed fathers remain at increased risk. Meta-analysis studies[637,651] suggest effect sizes for internalizing (or emotional) and externalizing (or behavioral) problems of $d = 0{\cdot}24$ and $d = 0{\cdot}19$, respectively. These are small effect sizes, but are similar to those seen in studies on maternal depression.[644] Adolescent offspring of depressed fathers have an increased risk of various psychological problems including depression[652-654] and suicidal behavior.[651,655,656]

How do child disturbances differ, depending on whether a mother or a father is affected by depression? Adult offspring of mothers with depression have higher rates of depression than offspring of fathers with depression.[657] However, earlier in children's development the picture is mixed,[658] with a meta-analysis suggesting that, for behavioral problems, the effects of depression of either parent are equivalent, but for emotional problems maternal depression carries a greater risk than paternal depression.[637,638]

Anxiety Disorders

Anxiety disorders, including social anxiety, generalised anxiety, and post-traumatic stress disorder, are common in adults of parenting age (e.g. 2% of men are affected by generalized anxiety disorder).[659] Children whose parents have anxiety disorders have a two-fold increased risk of developing anxiety disorders.[660] Children of mothers with social phobia have reduced social responsiveness, suggesting that specific transmission might have a role in certain anxiety disorders.[661] Fathers might have an even greater influence than mothers in the development of children's social anxiety, because of the father's role in the socialization of children.[626] However, direct research evidence is lacking. In one study,[662] fathers with social anxiety disorder were less encouraging of their children's autonomy in a discussion task than fathers without the disorder—a difference not seen in mothers who participated alone. Additionally, fathers of children with social anxiety disorder have a higher risk of the same disorder.[663]

Post-traumatic stress disorder in fathers was associated with children developing the same disorder after an earthquake, whereas maternal post-traumatic stress disorder was not.[664]

Substance Abuse

The potential effect of paternal substance abuse (including alcohol) has been investigated more than that of mothers. This difference is partly because substance abuse is more common in men than in women. Rates vary widely worldwide, with 12-month rates ranging from 4% to 14% for alcohol abuse and from 1% to 5% for substance abuse.[659] Children of alcoholic parents are at increased risk for behavioral and emotional problems.[665,666] Longitudinal studies[666,667] have shown consistent associations between paternal alcoholism and an increased risk of conduct disorder, and substance abuse and dependence in children, with a possible higher risk in the sons than in the daughters of affected fathers. Paternal alcoholism is also associated with an increased risk of mood disorders and depressive symptoms in adolescents,[668] and increased academic underachievement, low self-esteem, and relational difficulties.[669,670] Scarce research exists directly comparing the effect of paternal versus maternal alcohol abuse, although paternal disorder seems to be more related to behavioral problems in offspring than maternal disorder, and maternal disorder more related to emotional problems.[670] Although most research has focused on adolescent and older children of alcoholic parents, some evidence suggests that infants and preschool-age children might also be at risk.[671-673]

There are important, and often overlooked, differences between parental substance abuse and alcohol abuse that might lead to different effects on children. Hogan[674] argued that families in which parents use illicit drugs—especially opiates and cocaine—are more likely to live in poverty than families of alcohol users. Furthermore, because opiates and cocaine are illegal drugs, secrecy might exist around their use, which could create isolation, decreased social support, public advocacy, and treatment for drug abusers and their families. Substantial variability exists in different countries, or even between settings within a single country. Empirical studies[675,676] showed that children from families in which fathers abused drugs, including cocaine or opiates, had more emotional and behavioral symptoms, and higher rates of psychiatric disorders, than those from families with fathers who abused alcohol, or no substances.

Bipolar Disorder and Schizophrenia

Although some research indicates that offspring of parents with schizophrenia or bipolar disorder are at increased risk of developing psychiatric disorders, research specifically investigating fathers has been limited. Adolescents whose parents have bipolar disorder are up to ten times more likely than adolescents with mentally healthy parents to develop bipolar disorder, and 3 to 4 times more likely to develop other psychiatric illnesses.[677,678] Similarly, children whose parents have diagnoses of schizophrenia are at increased risk of developing schizophrenia when they reach adulthood.[679] Only a few small studies have addressed risks for other psychiatric disorders in this group of children.[680,681] For both bipolar disorder and schizophrenia, whether having a father with the disorder poses any additional or different risks compared with having a mother with the disorder, is not clear.

MECHANISMS OF RISK TRANSMISSION

Understanding the mechanisms of risk transmission is crucially important to enable effective targeting of efforts at prevention and treatment. The potential mechanisms of risk can be broadly divided into three groups: genetic, environmental, and gene—environment interplay (Flow chart 1). Developed and adapted with permission from Goodman and Gotlib.[621]

Flow chart 1: Proposed mechanisms of risk transmission from fathers to children

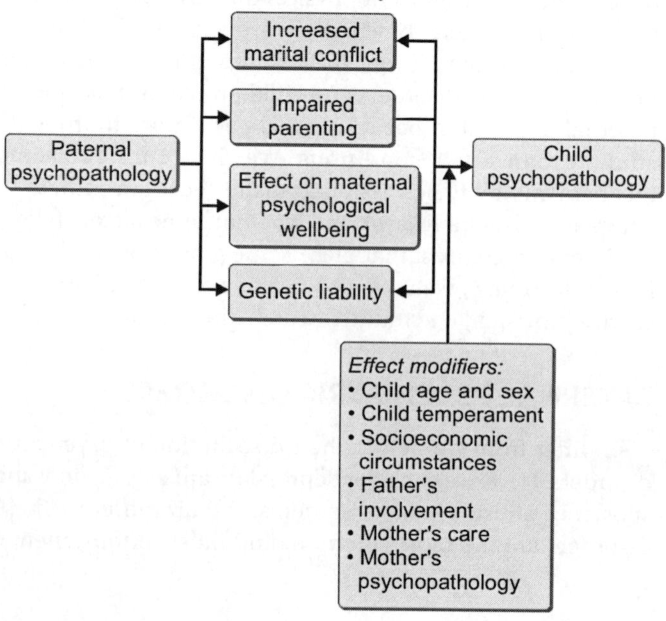

Genetic Mechanisms

The genetic contribution to psychiatric disorders is variable, being high in bipolar disorder and autism, and low in anxiety disorders;[682] genetic factors are important in most, if not all, psychiatric disorders. However, only a few, rare single-gene psychiatric disorders exist: genetic influence is more commonly the result of many genes, each having small effects.[683]

Environmental Mechanisms

Psychiatric disorders can affect the setting in which a child develops. Parental disorders can affect the choices a family makes about, for example, where to live, how much to engage with neighbors and the extended family, and what kind of activities to undertake. In this way, choices and opportunities for child development can be limited.

Psychiatric disorders can affect a father's performance at work and, if chronic and severe, can result in time off work, loss of income, and unemployment. The consequent socioeconomic hardship can then result in an increased risk that the child will develop a psychiatric disorder.[684]

Paternal disorders, like maternal disorders, can compromise the parents' ability to care directly for their offspring and the way in which they interact with their children, and adversely affect the parents' relationship. Parental disorders, such as depression, are associated with an increased risk of marital conflict and unhappiness, exposure to which, in turn, is associated with an increased risk of childhood behavioral problems.[685]

Psychiatric disorders can affect a father's involvement with his children in several ways. Some studies have shown that fathers with depression spend less time with their children than fathers without depression,[686,687] and that the quality of time spent with their children is less positive, with fewer activities such as reading, singing, and hugging, and higher rates of conflict.[688-690] Limited evidence exists on the involvement of fathers with their children during infancy. One study showed that paternal depression did not have any effect on the way fathers interacted with their infants,[691] by contrast with findings for maternal depression. This might be the result of the small size of the study (20 participants in each group); however, depression could affect the interaction of mothers and fathers with their infants differently, with fathers better able to maintain active engagement when depressed than mothers. However, depressed fathers could hold more negative views of their infants than do nondepressed fathers.[692] Most research on father—child relationships has been done in only a few countries, most notably the USA,[635,636] and thus might not be generalizable to other settings.

Depression in men is associated with impaired marital interactions. Depressed men make greater use of angry expressions and less positive expression in the interaction with their partner than do nondepressed men.[693] Couples show less positive behavior after positive remarks when the husband is depressed.[694] Marital conflict mediates the associations between some parental psychiatric disorders and child adjustment.[685,695] Indeed, conflict is a better predictor of poor child outcomes than is maternal depression.[696] Less evidence exists in this regard for depression affecting fathers than for that affecting mothers,[697,698] and marital conflict might affect children through different pathways in the context of paternal depression.

Gene: Environmental Interactions

The interactions between genetic and environmental factors have been increasingly studied in recent years, as initial findings in population studies suggested that some risk factors (such as exposure to life events) seem to only affect those with particular genetic endowments (gene—environmental interaction).[699] Although research on paternal psychiatric disorders is limited, children whose fathers have mental illness seem to be at increased risk of psychiatric illness, through both genetic endowment (an increased likelihood of a child carrying risk genes for depression if their father has a psychiatric disorder) and the influence of paternal psychopathological illnesses on the environment (e.g. through an increased risk of exposure to adverse life events if a father has a severe psychiatric disorder). In the case of antisocial behavior of fathers, such a double-risk effect seems to exist.[632] Paternal psychiatric disorders are also likely to influence children through gene—environment correlation (where genetic risk might influence the choice of specific types of environments), and epigenetic effects (where environmental exposures might influence the subsequent expression of specific genes).[682]

GROUPS AT RISK

The relation between paternal psychiatric disorders and an increased risk of adverse child outcomes is not linear. Several key effect modifiers exist, including characteristics of the child, such as sex, age, and temperament; and other contextual factors, such as socioeconomic status. These elements lead some children to be more vulnerable to the effects of paternal psychiatric disorders, and others to be more resilient.

Child Sex and Age

Boys seem to be more vulnerable than girls to the effects of their fathers' depression, especially early during development.[638] This finding has some similarities with data for maternal postnatal depression, although results are mixed,[645,646] whether these sex differences persist in adolescence is not clear. Similarly, sons of alcoholic fathers are at risk of developing conduct disorder, delinquency, and substance abuse,[667,700] but little is known about daughters of alcoholic fathers. One potential contributing factor might be the fact that fathers might spend more time with their sons than with their daughters: Lamb and Lewis[628] suggest that this is because they can identify better with a child of the same sex, or because of a belief that their knowledge and skills are more suited to raising a son than raising a daughter. Research from the USA suggests that fathers tend to be more involved with older children than with newborn babies.[628] As children age, fathers participate more with their children in social activities and homework and reading, and less in personal care and play.[701] This differential exposure might lead to an increased risk for sons of fathers with psychiatric disorders, compared with that for daughters.

Child Temperament

Children have individual characteristics that predispose them to be more or less affected by exposure to difficulties, such as paternal psychiatric disorders.[702-704] These characteristics—which can be persistent—are referred to as temperament features, and have been described as "vulnerability/resilience traits, which in adversity can activate processes which contribute to psychopathology or protect against it".[705] Studies showed associations between difficult temperament (children who were, for example, difficult to get settled, cried persistently, or found it difficult to adjust to small changes in routine or place) and depression and anxiety in both childhood and adult populations.[706-708] Children's temperament traits can influence or exacerbate paternal responses to them, and the interaction between difficult temperament and paternal disorder might lead to negative outcomes for the child. Children of alcohol-dependent fathers show temperamental difficulties,[709] which in turn might have a negative effect on parental behavior. For example, fathers with alcohol dependency tend to drink more alcohol after interacting with a difficult child if they think they will interact with the child again soon.[710,711] This finding does not imply that children cause alcoholism in their fathers, but suggests that a father's behavior can be influenced by difficult child behavior.

Paternal Income and Education

Studies in the general population have shown that prevalence of depression increases with poverty and socioeconomic disadvantage.[712] Socioeconomic disadvantage is also associated with increased rates of child psychiatric problems:[713] thus, some of the associations between parental psychiatric disorders and child disorders can be explained by confounding socioeconomic factors. Few studies[650] have controlled for these factors. Some studies of maternal depression[645,714,715] have shown that children of depressed mothers are at increased risk only if they also face socioeconomic adversity, suggesting that the stock of resilience is overcome by multiple adversities.[716] Similar research in fathers has yet to be undertaken, but could have important implications for the targeting of interventions to prevent psychiatric disorders in the offspring of parents with such difficulties.

Father Absence

Increasing interest exists in the adjustment of children whose fathers live in separate households. Several key factors, including economic support, quality of child—father relationship, and quality of parenting, are consistently related to child's adjustment.[717] However, there is limited research on paternal psychiatric disorders, with findings restricted to fathers with antisocial behavior. Research suggests that the presence of an antisocial father is associated with worse behavioral outcomes for children than if the antisocial father is absent.[632] Because of the extreme risks associated with antisocial parents, findings might well differ for other psychiatric disorders, but such research is lacking.

Clinical and Research Implications

How can clinicians use these findings? First, it is important to be aware of the possibility that some fathers might suffer from serious psychiatric disorders. This fact is often overlooked. For example, women are actively screened for postnatal depression in many countries; however, the possibility that men might also be depressed during this time has, until recently, been almost entirely ignored.[718] Findings that children could be at increased risk of behavioral problems when their fathers are depressed in the postnatal period,[650,719] as well as when their mothers are,[644] indicate an opportunity for potential intervention.

Second, questions about the effects of psychiatric disorders on men's functioning, including their role and relationships within the family, are likely to help a clinician to understand the family situation. Although one should not assume that children are at increased risk of emotional and behavioral problems simply because of a father's ill health, it is nonetheless wise to do a thorough assessment of those areas of child and family functioning that are most likely to be affected by paternal psychiatric disorders.[720]

Third, in most cases, another parent exists. The mistake that has often been made when assessing mothers—that of viewing the affected individual in isolation—should not be repeated in the case of fathers. The risk of psychiatric disorders co-existing in partners is increased and, even if a partner is not ill, the paternal disorder is likely to have had substantial effects on family life that might need to be addressed. However, in most cases, the other parent is an important source of support for both the father and the children, and this support should be mobilized.

Finally, the provision of good quality care and treatment to men with psychiatric disorders is key. Evidence is beginning to accumulate that the successful treatment of psychiatric disorders in parents can lead to improved outcomes for their children,[681,721] although this is not always the case.[722] In addition to the parental disorder, other aspects are potential targets for intervention. These include the interactions that fathers have with both their children and their partners.[685] Further work is needed to improve our understanding of these mechanisms.

Four areas of research might be important in this respect, both scientifically and clinically. Studies should be undertaken on fathers to assess the relation between their psychiatric disorders and their children's development; research in this area has already increased in recent years.[622,629,723] Such research can be challenging, since men are less likely to participate than women.[626,650] However, it is possible to redirect research towards fathers, with appropriate flexibility of approach.

CONCLUSION

Psychiatric disorders commonly affect adults of parenting age. Exposure to parental psychiatric disorders is associated with an increased risk of emotional, behavioral, and cognitive problems in children. Most research has been undertaken in the context of maternal psychiatric disorders. Although fathers—similarly to mothers—have mainly a positive influence in their children' lives,[631,634] recent findings have suggested that paternal psychiatric disorders can be associated with increased risk of adverse child outcomes, independent from maternal psychiatric wellbeing.[724-726] In some children, the patterns of risk associated with paternal disorders are different from those associated with maternal disorders, with boys potentially at increased risk. Additional focus on the mental health of fathers is likely not only to benefit them, but to create an opportunity to help improve the lives of their children.

43.22 DEPRESSION IN ADOLESCENCE

Neena Bohra, NK Bohra, Varun S Mehta, Christoday RJ Khess

INTRODUCTION

Unipolar depression is a universal health problem among adolescents globally, with a 1 year prevalence rate of 4–5% by mid-late adolescence. Suicide is the one of the foremost reasons of death within this age group with greater than 50% suicide victims reporting depression at the time of death. Social and educational impairments increased substance misuse, obesity are some of the consequences of untreated depression.

Depression is identified by an array of specific symptoms in the commonly used classificatory systems, i.e. ICD-10 (International Classification of Diseases-10) and DSM-5 (Diagnostic and Statistical Manual of Mental Disorders-5). The diagnostic features are identical in adolescents and adults in both the classificatory systems except that DSM-5 has a provision for irritable as supposed to depressed mood for adolescents. But depression in adolescents is not commonly identified due to its fluctuating nature, presence of irritability and mood reactivity or when presented with unexplained somatic complaints, eating disorders, school refusal, and decline in academic performance.

Depression in adolescents can also be seen as a juvenile form of corresponding disorder in adults due to its high recurrence in later stages of life. However, depression is likely seen in prepubertal children and has a distinct presentation than in adolescents and adults.

ICD-10 Criteria for major depressive disorder

Core symptoms (at least two must be present)

- Depressed mood present for most of the day and almost every day
- Loss of interest or pleasure in activities
- Decreased energy or increased susceptibility to fatigue

Associated symptoms

- Loss of confidence or self-esteem
- Unreasonable feelings of self-reproach or excessive inappropriate guilt
- Recurrent thoughts of death or suicide, or any suicidal behavior
- Diminished ability to think or concentrate
- Change in psychomotor activity, agitation, or retardation
- Sleep disturbance
- Change in appetite with corresponding change in weight

At least four of the above symptoms must be present for 2 weeks to diagnose a mild depressive episode, six to diagnose a moderate depressive episode, or eight for a severe depressive episode.

EPIDEMIOLOGY

Studies done in children have found the prevalence of depression below 1%. This difference increases considerably through the adolescent period. The cumulative probability of depression increases from 5% in early pubescence to 20% in late pubescence. The population prevalence, however, varies in different countries due to the methodological differences. Higher rates of adolescent depression has been reported in low-middle income countries, which could be because of large number of population in young age, but there is no conclusive evidence. The increase in recognition of the disorder in adolescents could have been contributory to increasing prevalence but the difference in the assessment methods and different taxonomies used in various studies makes it difficult to assess the changes in prevalence of depression over a period of time.

However, the most common reason for the increasing prevalence in adolescence are the biological and social changes observed by an increase in social understanding and awareness, alterations in the circuitry responsible for reward and danger coupled with high levels of stress, primarily in girls.

Epidemiological studies have found a significantly higher prevalence of depression in females after puberty (2:1) which is independent of the methods used for assessment, differences in help-seeking behavior or reporting of symptoms. This sex difference is linked to the hormonal changes in females during the pubertal period. However, it is unlikely that hormonal changes alone could be contributing to depression, but could be responsible for the sensitization of the brain following stress. Animal studies have found that estrogen sensitizes the prefrontal cortex to harmful effects of stress. However, the sex differences seem to blur in cases with neurodevelopmental or medical disorders who are diagnosed with depression.

CLINICAL OUTCOMES OF DEPRESSION IN ADOLESCENTS

It has been seen that 60–90% of adolescents suffering from depression remit within a year. However, 50–70% of them have recurrent depressive episodes within a span of 5 years. The onset of depression in adolescence is an outrider for suicide, anxiety disorders, bipolar disorders, substance use disorders, unemployment, and physical health problems. Consequently, their outcome in adults appears grimmer with only a scarce number of individuals attaining complete symptomatic as well as functional recovery with a substantial fraction having residual symptoms or impairment.

CAUSE AND PATHOGENESIS

Depression is a heterogeneous entity with multifactorial causation. The distal risk factor for inheritance interacts with early life adversities with temperament and personality attributes acting as mediators that predispose an individual to depression. The attributes akin to negative or decreased positive emotionality, behavioral inhibition and neuroticism contribute to depression. The interaction between the distal risk factors, proximal risk factors has also been shown to increase the sensitivity to the stressors by initiating changes in the neuroendocrine system which sows the seed for depression.

Familial and Genetic Risk

Scions of parents with depression have been found to have a three to four fold higher risk of depression in comparison to healthy parents for which genetic and nongenetic determinants are responsible. Fetal exposure during the prenatal and postnatal period in mothers suffering from depression constitutes an important risk factor in animals, but studies involving humans are not conclusive. However, maternal depressive symptoms continuing after the birth of child or psychosocial adversities have a bearing on the child as endowed by longitudinal studies, studies of children not genetically related to their mothers and maternal depression treatment trials. The impact of paternal mental health on depression is also being investigated and results are awaited.

Twin studies have shown that the heritability of depression loads up from zero to low in childhood to 30–50% in late adolescence. This modest rise in heritability is kindred to the adult population.

Anxiety and depression have been seen to share the same genetic susceptibility in family and twin studies but depression has been found to antecede anxiety in adolescence. Disruptive behavior disorders also share genetic susceptibility with depression. Some have suggested that adolescent onset depression symbolizes a strong genetic subform of depression, but this claim has not been substantiated.

Even though the genes responsible for depression were identified in some studies, they have not been replicated by others. This is contrary to other disorders like schizophrenia and bipolar disorder. The rationale could be that genes liable for depression function in a complex manner that we yet do not understand or we do not have the appropriate research design to detect it.

Psychosocial Risk Factors

Depression has also been linked to some environmental attributes like presence of stressful life events (e.g. personal injury, bereavement) and chronic adversity (e.g. abuse, family disharmony, bullying, poverty physical illness). However, such vulnerability can be a causative factor only in the ubiety of strong genetic risk. The stressful life events serve as predisposing factors in first episode of depression, female gender, adolescents with multiple traumatic events. Negative family relationships, peer victimization by bullying and maltreatment are the banal stressors for depression. Further, some of these children who are exposed to traumatic events (e.g. war, torture, orphanhood), suffering from HIV infection go on to develop long-term psychiatric disorders in the presence of family history or continuing trauma.

Gene-environment Interplay

The gene-environment interaction increases the risk of depression along with inherited factors by increasing the sensitivity to adversity and exposure to risky environment. Female gender has been specifically assailable to this interaction.

A variant of serotonin transporter gene (5-HTTLPR) has been shown to increase the risk for depression in the presence of environmental adversities, the findings being more sinewy for adolescent girls than boys. This variant has also been privy to increased activation of amygdala in response to fearful faces in healthy individuals. Though a recent meta-analysis fizzled to provide evidence for the 5-HTTLPR gene x environment interaction, it was sideswiped by other researchers who found proof for the presence of such an interaction especially in presence of maltreatment or medical illness.

Brain and Neuroendocrine Mechanisms

The inherited risk factors and psychosocial stressors mould the neural circuits and endocrine system at the helm for depression. Animal studies have shown that the adolescent brain is more susceptible to the genetic and environmental influences and have pinpointed those specific brain regions which are very much the same found to be altered in humans.

The circuits responsible for danger and learning of rewards have been found to be involved in depression among adolescents and adults.

The circuit that connects the amygdala to the hippocampus and prefrontal cortex (PFC) is highly activated in depression which can also be seen in healthy children, at risk children with behavioral inhibition and those with familial and genetic susceptibility for depression. This circuit is also linked to the HPA and so alterations in the HPA during stressful situations leads to changes in the cortisol levels and serotonin activity. The circuit interlacing the striatum with the PFC and the ventral dopamine-based systems has also been at fault. Reduced activity in this circuit has been inscribed in patients with depression.

Both these circuits continue to mature through adolescence with marked sex differences. Both the inherited and stress-related perturbations are liable for the disruption.

RESILIENCE

There are children who do not develop depression in the presence for familial predisposition and adverse events. The factors that shield them are high intelligence, good quality of interpersonal relationships, strong coping mechanisms and thinking styles. Thus, children who share warmth, acceptance, low hostility and low parental control with their parents are safeguarded even in the presence of risk factors. Also, the effects of child maltreatment and maternal depression are nullified in the presence of quality peer support.

However, the factors that increase the endurance to depression vary across different groups of children within the context of distinct risk factors.

Detection and Diagnosis

Depression lies on a continuum. Subsyndromal depression has been seen in adolescents not fulfilling the diagnostic criteria which is associated with impairment in functioning and poses a risk for a full blown episode. Low-risk intervention strategies and lifestyle changes should be promoted in such adolescents to forestall a depressive episode. Further to identify such individuals WHO has officiated various screening instruments which can be used in different settings. The Patient Health Questionnaire (PHQ-2) is a laconic tool that has been widely used to screen in primary care for depression in all age groups. The Strength and Difficulties Questionnaire (SDQ) is an appended tool to identify Attention Deficit Hyperactive Disorder (ADHD) and disruptive behavior. The Short Mood and Feelings Questionnaire and Children's Depression Inventory are auxiliary tools that solely target depression and change in symptom severity. The functioning of adolescent at home as well as school should be looked into for decrepitude in academic achievement, peer and family relationships. The risk for suicide should always be adjudged.

For the diagnosis of depression in adolescents, the information should be gathered from multiple informants to improve the reliability and validity. Standardized diagnostic interviews can also be used that aid in assessment.

Differential Diagnoses and Comorbidities

Dysthymia and adjustment disorder are the probable disorders that present with depressive symptoms. A stressor is known to precipitate adjustment disorder which does not last beyond 6 months after the removal of stressor. Dysthymia is a motif of chronic depression that is present throughout the day for at least one year in children and adolescents. Depression may overlay dysthymia in some of them. The presence of bipolar disorder should be ruled out in adolescents diagnosed with depression which is less common than unipolar depression in this age group (prevalence being < 0.1–1%). Though both disorders can predate or accompany depression or its symptoms, bipolar disorder can be singularized by unveiling of elated or irritable mood or enhanced energy of episodic nature. Chronic nonepisodic irritability has been defined as a major feature of severe mood dysregulation syndrome which is contrived to be a stark predictor of imminent depression.

At best a single comorbidity is seen in two-thirds of adolescents diagnosed with depression whereas 10–15% harbors two or more comorbidities. Anxiety is 12 times more probable, disruptive behavior is 4–11 times more probable; substance-use related disorders are 3–6 times more probable in adolescents with depression. Thus, 20% adolescents might satisfy criteria for generalized anxiety disorder, with lifetime rates of 50–70%.

Comorbidity is common in adolescents with greater severity of depression, which herald's poorer long-term prognosis and makes the treatment much more difficult. In case of comorbidities, both depression and comorbid psychiatric illness should be treated independently. In case of comorbid medical illness with depression, it might be difficult to find the primary cause as the relationship can be bidirectional, due to which both deserve equal attention.

TREATMENT

There are some aspects of treatment in adolescents which are different from adults. The most important of them being that the choice of treatment in adolescents which varies in different countries due the excessive concern regarding antidepressant use in children less than 18 years. Further, the long-term efficacy of medications and psychological interventions has not been consistently established.

Among the psychological interventions, cognitive behavior therapy (CBT) and interpersonal therapy (IPT) has been found to be effective in children. CBT has been found to be moderately effective in two separate meta-analysis with another study pointing towards its beneficial role when added to antidepressants in treatment resistant depression. To conclude, CBT has been found to be effective in milder forms of depression but its effectiveness in moderate-severe depression in adolescents is yet to be established. Though effectiveness of IPT has been found in some RCTs, more studies are needed to establish its role in adolescent depression.

With respect to pharmacotherapy, fluoxetine and escitalopram are the only two selective serotonin reuptake inhibitors found to be impressive, even though of modest impact. Fluoxetine can cause agitation in some patients and carries a risk of hypomania. Even though the use of SSRIs has an increased risk of suicide in adolescents younger than 25 years, a large meta-analysis has proved its use to be of greater benefit than the risk of suicide with the understanding that untreated depression might lead to suicide.

The combination of pharmacotherapy and psychotherapy has found conflicting results with the adolescent depression, antidepressants, and psychotherapy (ADAPT) trial not finding any change in outcome with the addition of CBT to fluoxetine whereas the Treatment for Adolescents with Depression Study (TADS) reporting improvement after combining fluoxetine to CBT for 12 weeks.

The delivery of appropriate health care to adolescents suffering with depression is a major concern in India and many other developing countries due to scarcity of resources. However, it has been seen that CBT delivered in primary care settings and school settings has been effective in mild or subthreshold depression. A report by WHO has highlighted the importance of treating adolescent depression among the mental health disorders in low to middle-income countries which was also supported by a study on adolescent survivors of war in northern Uganda in which IPT performed by local workers of the community resulted in significant improvement of depression in girls.

PREVENTION

A targeted and indicated approach rather than universal program has been found to be effective in the prevention of depression. The high-risk groups which require targeted strategy are offspring of parents with depression, adolescents with sub-threshold symptoms and adolescents with previous depressive episode. Group CBT has been found to be effective in reducing the incidence of depression but with limited benefit in adolescents whose parent has active symptoms of depression highlighting the importance of treatment of maternal depression. School-based CBT-oriented prevention has also found a place when addressed to adolescents with symptoms of depression. Other strategies such as positive thinking and conflict resolution have been beneficialthough parenting programs for adolescent depression have not been consistently effective.

43.23 SELF-HARM AND SUICIDE IN ADOLESCENTS

JN Vyas, N Parvez, Christoday RJ Khess

INTRODUCTION

Of lately, the major public health concerns in adolescents are self-harm and suicide. Self-harm in adolescents is more common and also largely concealed from health care services compared to suicide. Considering its dreadful outcome, suicide prevention strategies in adolescent age group should be of national importance. This chapter includes discussion on self-harm and suicide in the adolescent age group in terms of epidemiology; developmental and behavioral factors; outcomes; and treatment and prevention.

Adolescence can be defined in several ways, although there is no fixed agreement over any of the definitions. One of the ways is to define adolescence based on chronological age. Various studies use different ages as upper limits, which usually range from 18 to 25 years.

SELF-HARM

Self-harm includes deliberately harming oneself by poisoning or injury irrespective of the motives and intentions.[727,728] It includes both suicidal and nonsuicidal injury. The term is preferred instead of its separation into suicidal and non-suicidal variety because, intent is a dimensional phenomenon and there might be a difference in view between the patients and clinicians' view. Self-harm also remains a focus in national clinical guidelines.[727]

Epidemiology

Although data across countries vary considerably, community-based studies show that self-harm is seen in about 10% of adolescents. Some of the studies have suggested that suicidal intent may have been the reason behind their self-harm.[729-735] Data from the community suggests that self-harm is more common in females.[729-731,734] Although self-harm is common in adolescents, only about one in eight cases come to utilize health care services with rates being higher in females than male adolescents.[728,735] Also, the cases of self-harm in relation to overdose are the ones more likely to seek medical attention.[730,731]

Self-harm is more commonly seen beyond the age of 12 years onwards, especially in females. The male-to-female ratio between the ages 12 and 15 years is as high as one to five or six. It is very difficult to estimate the occurrence of self-harm in children younger than 12 years due to lack of data in general. The difference in frequency of self-harm between males and females tends to decrease in the late teen years as the behavior becomes increasingly common in males but levels off in females.[728,736] Higher rates of self-harm are seen in the lower socioeconomic groups.[737] Data from clinical services reveal a substantial increase in the number of cases of self-harm in the adolescent age group, especially from the late 1960s onwards. In 1990s, a trend towards an increased frequency was seen in female adolescents in the United Kingdom.[728] Although the exact cause for this increase is not known, the major contributing factors includes increased availability of drugs, medications, stress.

There are several modes of self-injury such as cutting self, self-battery and jumping from heights. According to community-based Child and Adolescent Self-harm in Europe (CASE) Study, the most common method adopted by adolescents is self-cutting while data from hospitals reveal self-poisoning as the most common method.[728,730,731,735] In few countries such as the UK, compounds containing paracetamol is frequently used for self-poisoning.[728]

A school survey in Australia and USA conducted using pubertal age as an assessment measure in adolescents aged 12 to 15 years reported that the onset of self-harm is related to the phase of puberty (mainly completed or late puberty) and not the chronological age, especially in females and for self-cutting behaviors. Other factors such as depression, substance use, and beginning of sexual activity independently contribute to the self-harm risk.[738] A neurodevelopmental vulnerability during this time puts the individual at an increased risk to affective disorders and behaviors that are risk taking, which explains the relationship between self-harm and affective symptoms in puberty.[739] Also, there might be an increased vulnerability to negative social cues such as criticism during adolescence.[740,741]

What are the reasons for self-harm? Community statistics suggest that the intent behind self-poisoning is more commonly suicide while self-cutting is more often to punish self or relieve tension. Those brought to hospital often admit the self-harm act to suicidal intent, escape from unbearable painful situations or a way adopted to show others their sorrow.[742-745] However, the clinical staff more often do not view self-harm behavior as being suicidal.[745] Although adolescents report suicidal intent, it is difficult to understand the extent of their true wish to die and their need to temporarily escape from an unbearable distressing situation.[744] Hence, we need to have a better understanding of the intentions behind self-harm or suicidal act.

The risk of recurrence of self-harm is also high in adolescence. A survey by CASE study reported that the risk of recurrence is more than double after an act of self-harm in the previous year (53% in male and 55% in female adolescents).[730] In a hospital survey conducted on a large number of adolescents in the UK, the risk of recurrence was 15% in the subsequent year.[728] This is clearly an underestimate when compared to the data from community. The risk of recurrence is more commonly seen in self-cutting compared to self-poisoning.[746] Common predictors of recurrence include depressive symptoms, sexual abuse, past history of self-harm, worries about sexual orientation.[747,748]

Etiology of Self-harm

Various genetic, psychological and social factors together contribute to self-harm in adolescents. Biological factors that predispose include serotonin imbalance, personality factors such as impulsivity and perfectionism, and cognitive susceptibilities such as reduced problem-solving skills. Psychiatric disorders such as depression and negative life events increase the risk of self-harm.[749,750]

Furthermore, factors such as impulsivity and exposure to self-harm by others increase the likelihood of conversion of self-harm or suicidal thoughts into actual suicidal.[732,751]

Poor parenting, parental divorce and family hardships are also associated with self-harm in children.[747,752,753] The independent contribution of these factors is emphasized by case-control studies.[754] Abuse (physical or sexual) is also an important factor associated with adolescent self-harm.[730,748]

Self-harm is also associated with negative life events.[741,755] The occurrence of self-harm is reported to be more in those experiencing stressful life events than in those who have self-destructive thoughts. Certainly difficulties in interpersonal relationships during adolescence (including difficulty in friendships, arguments with authority, loneliness, and interpersonal isolation) independently predict suicide attempts in late adolescence as well as in early adulthood.[753] Reports from school-based studies, both cross-sectional and prospective, suggest that an association exists between adolescent self-harm and bullying.[729,731,748] How bullying contributes to an increased risk of self-harm is not clearly understood. Also, research is needed to understand the effects of different modes of bullying on psychiatric health of an individual.

Being exposed to self-harm and suicide in others also increases the risk of self-harm in oneself,[729,731,748] most likely by providing a behavioral model especially in those who are vulnerable.[751] Self-harm can also be a reaction to common stressful events than just being a modeling type response.[756] Social transmission is another important mode that is associated with self-harm, especially in females.[746]

In either sex, self-harm also appears to have an association with the sexuality of an individual, especially sexual preference.[748] A study to find the relationship between self-harm and sexual preferences revealed that in comparison to the lesbian, gay, and bisexual (LGB) group, heterosexual individuals were six times less likely to have shown suicidal behavior.[757] Results from a systematic review also concluded that in comparison to heterosexual individuals, LGB individuals were four times more likely to have a history of attempted suicide.[758] Increased prevalence of mood and substance use disorders, victimization, bullying, and social stress and lower protective factors are suggested as possible mechanisms explaining the high occurrence of self-harm in the LGB group.[757-759]

Other factors known to predict suicidality are feelings of loss, being trapped and perceiving oneself as a burden.[760,761] Difficulties with social problem-solving is also associated with adolescent self-harm, although it is unclear to what degree this factor is associated with depression.[762] Need for perfection and self-criticism are also associated with adolescent self-harm.[741,744,763] A particular dimension of perfectionism, the belief that others have very high expectations of them, needs particular consideration because it can decrease ones level of tolerance to stressful life events and result in suffering.[741] Other factors associated with adolescent self-harm are low self-esteem,[748] social isolation,[765] impulsivity,[751] hopelessness[744] and poor parent-child attachment.[764] Impulsivity is suggested to be the common factor related to both child abuse and suicidality.[765] Also, being hopeful acts as a positive protective factor against self-harm, especially in girls.[748]

The presence of psychiatric disorders in young people who show self-harm behaviors appears to be very similar to that seen in the adults. Data from general hospitals suggests that psychiatric disorders are seen in 48%[766] to 87%[767] of those who harm self. Psychiatric disorders commonly associated with self-harm include depressive disorders, anxiety disorders, substance-related disorders, attention deficit hyperactivity disorder (ADHD) and conduct disorder. It is suggested that ADHD increases the severity of comorbid conduct disorder and depression, thereby increasing the risk of suicide in male adolescents.[768]

Personality disorders although not diagnosed prior to 18 years of age, are strongly related to self-harm and suicide. An early diagnosis of personality disorders can be justified in the presence of clear-cut pervasive and persistent symptoms. Follow-up studies of individuals diagnosed with emotionally unstable personality disorders prior to 18 years of age have reported increased self-harm behavior suggesting that early diagnosis of personality disorders is associated with self-harm behavior in adolescents.[769]

Substance abuse is a major risk factor for adolescent self-harm behavior. Data from community have reported that binge pattern of alcohol drinking is strongly associated with suicide attempts even in the absence of depressive symptoms.[770] This association is more pronounced in those aged less than 14 years. Though the pattern of substance use in those who show self-harm behavior is not clear, data from community suggests that there is a general increase in occurrence of self-harm across all groups of substances.[731] A study revealed that at least 14% adolescents give a history of substance abuse at the time of seeking medical attention, also such a history was more commonly seen in males.[728] Overall, it is seen that there is an increased occurrence of both suicidality and substance use during adolescence and impulsivity seems to be a risk factor connecting both.

Smoking appears to be associated with adolescent self-harm with hospital data suggesting that adolescents who smoked had four times increased risk of suicide than nonsmokers,[771] and also showed increased frequency of nonsuicidal self-injurious behaviors.[772] Even the data from community suggests a similar finding.[771] It is speculated that the association between smoking and self-harm is probably due to underlying depression, as both are ways of dealing with emotional problems or might even show a susceptibility to risk-taking behaviors. However, further research is required to reveal the contribution of lifestyle (e.g. smoking, drinking) as a risk factor for self-harm behavior. Important risk factors for self-harm and suicide during adolescent period are given in Table 18.

Outcome after Self-harm

Often adolescence self-harm behavior appears to stop by early adulthood, although it tends to persist in girls.[733]

Table 18: Risk factors associated with adolescent self-harm and suicide

Sociodemographic • Lower education status* • Sex (for self-harm females>males and for suicide males>females)—most countries* • Poor socioeconomic status* • Lesbian, gay, bisexual, or transgender sexual orientation
Individual negative line events and family adversity • Parental separation or divorce* • Parental psychiatric disorder* • History of physical or sexual abuse* • Adverse childhood experiences* • Parental death* • Family history of suicide* • Marital or family discord • Bullying • Interpersonal difficulties*
Psychiatric and psychological factors • Psychiatric disorders* (depression, anxiety, attention deficit hyperactivity disorder) • Drug and alcohol misuse* • Impulsivity • Low self-esteem • Poor social problem-solving • Perfectionism • Hopelessness*

All are risk factors for self-harm and *risk factors for suicide

Adolescent self-harm may be associated with an increased risk for affective disorders.[773] Even if self-harm occurs without any suicidal intent, there is a risk of future acts with suicidal intent.[774]

Prospective data indicates that whenever an act of self-harm results in seeking medical help, there is a future ten-times increased risk for adolescent suicide,[775] especially in those above 15 years old.[776,777] Similarly, data from retrospective studies shows that in people with death by suicide during late adolescent and early adulthood, there is a frequent history of self-harm behaviors,[778] particularly in males and those who previously received psychiatric care.

SUICIDE

Epidemiology

Adolescent suicides are often under reported by the authorities responsible for death verdicts. This probably occurs due to many of the possible suicides being classified as either accidental or undetermined.[779] The under-reporting of suicides is protective to the families from associated stigma. So, it is suggested that in the younger population, the rates of suicide must be very carefully compared. Also, national statistics are only normally available for comparison in individuals aged 10 to 24 years. Worldwide, suicide is the second leading cause of death in this age group, and the third leading cause of death in adolescent males. Also, in adolescent females aged 15–19 years, the leading cause of death appears to be suicide.[780]

Although, suicide is infrequent below 15 years of age (1–2 deaths per 100000 boys aged 5–14 years), the rates increase through adolescence (19.2 deaths per 100000 male adolescents aged 15–24 years) and into adulthood (286 deaths per 100000 men aged 25–34 years).[781] Each year, there are about 164000 self-inflicted deaths worldwide in those younger than 25 years.[780] Worldwide, the risk of completed suicide is 2.6 times greater in males when compared to females in the age group 15–19 years.[782] In some Asian countries, the suicidal rates are reported are greater in females across the age group 15–24 years.[783]

The frequency of suicide in youth varies worldwide with a higher prevalence reported in Russia, Japan, Hungary, Finland, Ukraine and Lithuania and lower prevalence in USA, Hong Kong, UK and Australia. Over the decades there has been a change in the suicide rates, with higher rates from the 1960s through to the 1980s and then a fall after 1990, particularly in males across 15–24 years age.[784]

Etiology of Suicide

The risk factors associated with both suicide and self-harm in adolescents are similar. Research on risk factors for suicide should emphasize not only on family history and psychiatric disorders but also on other risk factors. Risk factors such as family history of suicide, parental divorce, death of a parent, lower education status, and social isolation are more specific to suicide in adolescents (Flow chart 2).

Suicidal behavior tends to frequently run in families. Studies in twins suggest a higher concordance rate in monozygotic twins in comparison to dizygotic twins. Suicide in a monozygotic twin increased the risk in the other twin (by four times) even after other factors such as substance use, mood disorder and trauma were controlled.[785] The risk of suicide is four times higher in first-degree relatives of those individuals who have committed suicide. Suicidality in a family probably depends on the transmission of aggression.[786] This is consistent with the finding that serotonergic system is important to both suicidality and aggressive behaviors.[787]

Poor interpersonal relationships especially in the family seem to add to the transmission of suicidality. Family discord appears to be the most common cause of completed suicide.[788] Impulsivity raises the risk of suicidality and can also affect parents' capacity to offer an ideal environment.[789]

As suggested by psychological autopsy studies, the frequency of psychiatric disorders in adolescents is similar in cases suicide and self-harm, the most common being mood disorders.[790] In adolescent males, suicidal behavior appears to be related to psychopathology in even at the age

Flow chat 2: Risk factors associated with adolescent self-harm and suicide

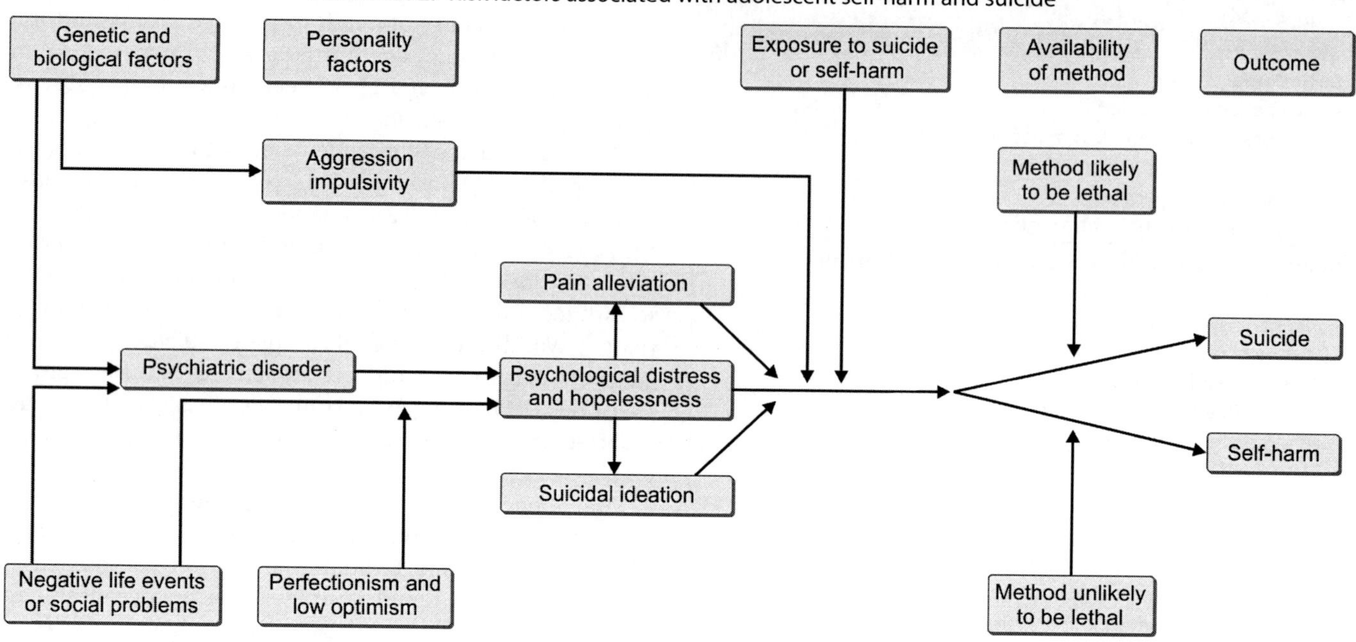

of 8 years age.[791] In the case of suicide in young people with substance use disorders, the frequency varies.[792] Personality disorders are reported in about 25% suicides, with a further 25% suicides showing relation to personality traits.[792] In some countries, suicides show a poor relation with psychiatric disorders, as the ease of access to means like pesticides and a lack of proper emergency services lead to high fatalities.[783]

In children below 14 years, psychosocial stressors especially problems in interpersonal relationship, are frequent precipitants for suicidal behaviors. When suicide in youth was studied using life chart method, atleast three groups were noted: those with chronic life and behavioral problems (Poor performance at school, relationship difficulties, childhood sexual abuse, violence, personality-related issues, low self-confidence); those with major psychiatric disorders; and those in whom it occurred as a response to life events.[778]

Mass media seems to have its own contribution in suicide and self-harm behaviors among adolescent especially, when the coverage is intense and includes the details of the methods employed.[793] As a result, guidelines have been established for a reporting of suicidal behaviors to decrease any unfavorable effect. The impact of media on self-harm and suicide is huge, as adolescents appear to be more vulnerable to the effect of media in general and the newer ones such as the social media in particular.[794] A bigger challenge would be in ensuring that the newer media provide support for the susceptible young people rather than encouraging self-destructive behaviors. Research in the area of online support groups and crisis helplines suggests that these can contribute to prevention of suicide and self-harm behaviors.

Prevention Measures for Self-harm and Suicide

The strategies for prevention of self-harm and suicide can either be population-based (using educational interventions) or aimed at high-risk groups such as those with history of self-harm or abuse (Table 19).

It is essential that the measures aimed at prevention of self-harm and suicide in adolescents should consider the characteristics associated with adolescent suicide and self-harm, such as address concerns about sexual orientation and bullying, target social transmission of self-harm and suicide, promote self-esteem and promote help-seeking behavior. School-based strategies for prevention of self-harm and suicide are evolving such as screening of high-risk groups, skills training, and gate keeper training.[795] Although there are reports suggesting that screening programmes can identify at-risk groups not recognized by school professionals,[796] they significantly burden mental health providers by giving false positives.[797] As the risk for suicide fluctuates with time, a one time screen will most likely yield false negatives. Also research suggests that the risk of suicidality in adolescent does not increase with mere questioning about suicidal ideation.[798]

Gatekeeper training includes training of adults and peers to effectively recognize warning signs for suicide. Such training can improve the knowledge and attitudes about suicide, promote help seeking, and reduce self-harm in the short-term.[799] Evidence also suggests that ensuring such training in a routine manner increases the knowledge about suicide in the gatekeepers and also increases capacity of community.[800] Another strategy at schools showing encouraging results in decreasing suicidal ideation is psychological skills training,[801]

Table 19: Strategies to prevent adolescent self-harm and suicide

Population measures • School-based programs (e.g. psychological skills training) • Gatekeeper training (e.g. teachers) • Restriction of access to means • Improved media reporting and depiction of suicidal behavior • Promoting help-seeking behavior • Public awareness campaigns • Helplines • Internet sources for help • Reduction of stigma related to psychiatric disorders
Measures for at-risk groups • Psychosocial interventions (e.g. adolescents with depression, sexual abuse, self-harm, etc.) • Screening high-risk population (e.g. young offenders) • Pharmacotherapeutic interventions

although some undesirable effects have also been reported.[802] Whole school approaches encourage help-seeking by positively altering the code and culture of a school without directly affecting suicide rates.[795] Further research is required into more school-based approaches.

An important approach to prevent adolescent suicide is by restricting the access to means. In areas with a high occurrence of suicide by using firearms, the risk of can be significantly reduced by controlling the availability and their safer storage.[803] Similarly, in rural areas with a high prevalence of suicide by consuming pesticides, safer storage will considerably decrease the risk.[804] Also, risk can be reduced by merely reducing the packet size of drugs frequently used by young people for poisoning.[805]

Psychosocial Interventions

The crisis related with adolescent self-harm can quickly respond to initial supportive psychotherapy. Specific interventions will be indicated especially in the presence of chronic and severe problems and when more harmful modes are encountered. Research related to psychosocial interventions is limited compared to the occurrence of self-harm in adolescents. It suggests poor response to family-problem-solving therapy,[806] motivational interviewing[807,808] and brief psychotherapy.[809] However, the studies lacked the power to satisfactorily test the effect of experimental treatment on repetition of self-harm. Although initially group therapy for recurrent self-harm showed some promise in reducing recurrence,[810] subsequent trials failed to reproduce the result.[811,812]

Overall, information on treatment recommendations for adolescent self-harm is minimal. After the encouraging results of dialectical behavior therapy in adults with emotionally unstable personality disorder, there is a lot of interest in its use in adolescent self-harm.[813] Results from randomized controlled trials are still awaited. Compared with psychiatric hospitalization, encouraging results are seen for multisystemic family-based therapy for suicidal individuals aged 10–47 years.

Most of the adolescents do not seek help. Studies have suggested that stigma, concerns about confidentiality and fear of receiving a psychiatric diagnosis were reported as barriers to seeking help, especially in females.[731] It is recommended that help-seeking be more acceptable with a notion that its very normal for anybody to have problems.[815] Culture also plays an important role not only in seeking help,[816] but also in the development of culture-specific interventions.

Pharmacotherapy

As newer antidepressants were prescribed, there were concerns about increased suicide risk in children and adolescents, which led to warnings being released by regulatory agencies. However, later it was seen that the benefits may outweigh the emergent suicidal risk.[817] Although, initially the early phases of treatment were suggested to be of highest risk, later no significant difference was noticed between the first and the subsequent months of antidepressant use. In fact it was seen that, the suicidal risk was maximum in the month prior to initiating antidepressant medications.[818] However, the warnings issued by the regulatory authorities had a marked effect on prescribing patterns.[819] Although the increase in suicidality with antidepressant use was initially reported in the USA and Netherlands, later this finding could not be replicated.[820]

There are no drug trials for adolescents with self-harm. Some indirect information is provided by trials for depression where antidepressant medications are compared with

Table 20: Challenges in prevention of adolescent self-harm and suicide

Understanding • Assessment of suicide risk • Subtyping of self-harm with individualized management • Factors associated with reduction of self-harm • Suicide or self-harm clusters • Impact of new media
Intervention • Development of new treatment options • Development of strategies to decrease stigma, promote help-seeking and enhance optimal utilization of health services • Improvement of access to psychiatric services • Better management of vulnerable groups from child or adolescent through adult services
Prevention • Protection against the deleterious effect of global challenges on mental health • Promoting newer media towards positive mental health and reduce its undesirable effects • Policies to promote restriction of access to means • Integration of policies on suicide and self-harm with other risk factors (e.g. substance abuse)

psychological interventions. The Multicenter Treatment of Adolescent Depression Study, showed that there was a significant decrease in suicidal ideation in the group receiving cognitive behavior therapy (CBT) in comparison to the group without CBT.[821] In two other trials, where CBT was compared with antidepressant medications, however, there was no difference in outcomes.[822,823]

CONCLUSION

Self-harm and suicide are important health issues in the adolescent population worldwide. However, there are several obstacles to their prevention and management (Table 20). Further research is required in the identification of subtypes of self-harm and suicide. An improved knowledge about risk factors associated with various levels of self-harm such ideation vs lethal attempts. In the light of diverse motives behind self-harm and suicide, a clear understanding of the meaning of the act is essential in better clinical management of it.

Only little progress has been made in the area of prevention and there is scarcity of evidence for effective treatment interventions. It will also be important to develop newer interventions (pharmacological and psychosocial) to decrease self-harm and suicide. The improvement in psychiatric health care services in terms of quality and accessibility is crucial. A continuity of care should be provided as the vulnerable individuals move from adolescence to adulthood. Another effective strategy is reducing the accessibility to means of committing suicide such as access to firearm and pesticides. Furthermore, the stigma associated with mental health should be tackled and timely help seeking should be encouraged. The inclusion of self-harm and suicide prevention in the national guidelines is also a welcome step forward.

43.24 PSYCHOTROPIC DRUGS IN CHILDREN AND ADOLESCENTS

PB Behere, A Das, AP Behere

INTRODUCTION

Child psychopharmacology is a relatively new field.[824] Over the past decades there have been a rise in number of psychiatric and neurobehavioral disorders in children and with it increase in number of children for psychiatric consultation.[825,826] There has been increasing use of psychotropic in children and adolescent. However, studies report that although there has been a surge in use of medications to treat childhood psychiatric disorders many a times these disorders are over diagnosed and over treated, there have been inadequate response, poor compliance, treatment have been stopped due to adverse drug reactions. Since this is comparatively a newer area there have been paucity of research in this field of childhood psychopharmacology.[824,827,828] Many of the drugs used are not yet approved by the FDA and they are used as off label drugs.[828] However, pharmacological treatment has become a potent force in controlling the psychiatric symptoms in children and it is now being increasingly used. This in a way manages the early onset illness, improves quality of life, reduces burden in caregivers and may help to alleviate the growing chance of adult psychiatric illness.[829] Psychiatrists must have foresight into potential side effects, family responses to similar psychotropic medications, the nature and intensity of the patient's illness, and most importantly psychosocial concerns. Intolerable side effects, poor efficacy, and ultimate perhaps a negative view towards medication that may have proved helpful. Lack of efficacy and ADEs are frequently cited as reasons for noncompliance in pediatric psychopharmacology.[830]

Utmost care is to be taken when prescribing psychiatric medications to children. Long-term side effects on the maturing and developing children may be potentially harmful. The essential consideration in using medications is being clear what the diagnosis and target symptoms that are focused for treatment, knowing the risks and benefits. While this is important for all of medicine, it is even truer in the treatment of children, whose bodies and nervous systems are not yet fully developed. Pharmacotherapy should not replace psychosocial and educational interventions.

DIFFERENCES OF ADULT AND CHILDHOOD PSYCHOPHARMACOLOGY

There is a definite difference of both pharmacokinetics and drug sensitivity pharmacodynamics properties in both children and adults. These differences occur throughout various stages of childhood and account.

Phelps et al.[831] laid emphasis on major issues to be implemented by clinician in treating children. This may give direction in making medication decisions, evaluating treatment effectiveness, and maintaining family involvement in the change process. These issues include assessing emotional and behavioral problems that may be appropriate for pharmacotherapy; identifying intervention goals; selecting empirically supported psychological interventions to accompany pharmacotherapy; and assessing therapy, readiness for change.

A number of factors other than age separate the practice of psychopharmacology with children from that with adults.

Physiological Factors

The rates at which medications are absorbed, distributed in the body, and metabolized by children differ markedly from adults.[832] When considering additional medications, the practitioner must take care to consider any adverse medication interactions that may occur from poly pharmacy (the use of more than one psychotropic simultaneously), an increasingly common practice in pediatric mental health. A number of physiologic and metabolic processes differ qualitatively as well as quantitatively when compared to adults. For example, different metabolic pathways predominate in the biotransformation of drugs. Children and adolescents may require larger doses of psychoactive medication per unit of body weight than adults to attain similar blood levels and therapeutic efficacy psychiatrist must pay attention to these physiological factors.[833]

Psychological Factors

Children may not be able to accurately describe their felling and symptoms. So for accurate diagnosis and proper prescription doctors must take information from all sources like parents, siblings, caregivers and teachers.[833]

Adherence to Treatment

For proper adherence to treatment both caregivers and parents should be give adequate psychoeducation about the illness, the importance of medication and the need for continuation of treatment. Parents as well as the child should be made aware of the side effects also. Children and adolescents do not always respond to treatment with psychotropic drugs in a similar way compared to adults. Also what is safe for adults might not be the case in children.[833]

THERAPEUTIC CONSIDERATIONS

Initially an assessment of the child's psychopathology should be made. This should be followed by a through physical examination to find out comorbid physical conditions. Stress should be made to rule out predisposition to side effects. The parents and caregivers should be made aware of the treatment side effects about giving the child a proper environment. They should be made aware of the precautions they should be following. The risk benefit ratio should be bargained and explained to the parents as well. Baseline scores and scale should be applied before starting treatment. Scales should be applied from time to time during periodic evaluation. Side effects should be managed. A physician should not rush into the treatment. All the above physiological and psychological factors should be remembered.

As the golden rule states ***start low and go slow.***

Diagnostic Process of Biological Therapy[834]

- Conduct a comprehensive psychiatric evaluation of the child or adolescent, including information from multiple sources, assessment of the family, and family history of psychiatric and medical disorders.
- Provide careful diagnostic and psychiatric symptom review with the patient and caregivers.
- Ensure a physical examination.
- Collect baseline laboratory and physical assessment data where warranted. Consider baseline rating scales of target symptoms.
- Determine indicated nonpharmacologic interventions for the diagnosed disorder.
- Consider the risks and benefits of pharmacotherapy.
- Consider the risks and benefits of specific medications relevant to the disorder.
- Conduct a formal consent procedure with the parent and youth. Give handouts on medications, where appropriate.

Principles to be Followed

American Academy of Child and Adolescent Psychiatry (AACAP) follows certain principles in the treatment of childhood psychiatric illnesses[835]

- Before initiating pharmacotherapy, a psychiatric evaluation is completed.
- Before initiating pharmacotherapy, a medical history is obtained, and a medical evaluation is considered when appropriate.
- The prescriber is advised to communicate with other professionals involved with the child to obtain collateral history and set the stage for monitoring outcomes and side effects during the medication trial.
- The prescriber develops a psychosocial and psychopharmacological treatment plan based on the best available evidence.
- The prescriber develops a plan to monitor the patient, short and long-term.
- Prescribers should be cautious when implementing a treatment plan that cannot be appropriately monitored.
- The prescriber provides feedback about the diagnosis and educates the patient and family regarding the child's disorder and the treatment and monitoring plan.
- Complete and document the assent of the child and consent of the parents before initiating medication treatment and at important points during treatment.
- The assent and consent discussion focuses on the risks and benefits of the proposed and alternative treatments.

- Implement medication trials using an adequate dose and for an adequate duration of treatment.
- The prescriber reassesses the patient if the child does not respond to the initial medication trial as expected.
- The prescriber needs a clear rationale for using medication combinations.
- Discontinuing medication in children requires a specific plan.

The AACAP stresses that this approach is absolutely necessary for safe, effective and proactive treatment and should help decrease the stigma from participating in psychiatric care. These recommended practices are implemented in an effort to eliminate demoralization experienced by patients and families receiving substandard treatment, "dropping out" of care or not seeking necessary treatment in the future.[835]

INDICATIONS AND CLASS OF PSYCHOTROPIC MEDICATION

Bipolar Disorder and Mood Stabilizers

Traditional mood stabilizers (i.e. lithium and antiepileptic) have greater benefits in children and adolescents than adults where study findings support greater benefits (i.e. reduction in mania) with second generation antipsychotics (SGAs). However, SGAs caused more weight gain and somnolence than mood stabilizers in youth than adults and SGAs caused greater weight gain in youth than adults. Also, the efficacy of combination therapy of two mood stabilizers compared with one antipsychotic agent at the present time is not known. Currently, the FDA has indicated risperidone, quetiapine and aripiprazole for use in children aged 10 or older and olanzapine for children aged 13 and older with bipolar disorder (i.e. mania and mixed mania); approved lithium for adolescents aged 12 and older; olanzapine for adolescents aged 13 and older; and aripiprazole and lithium as treatments to prevent the recurrence of bipolar symptoms in children and adolescents. There is currently insufficient evidence on treatment of bipolar depression in children and adolescents.[836,837] Few studies have documented use of lithium in bipolar disorders in pediatric populations. Lithium therapy has received widespread clinical use. There are in fact several controlled trials suggesting that lithium can be effective in the management of symptoms associated with bipolar disorder in adolescents.[838] Campbell and colleagues[839] have demonstrated the efficacy of lithium in treating aggressive behavior and conduct disorder; according to their findings, some children showed marked improvement. Anticonvulsants which were used in seizure have been found to be beneficial in controlling mania and aggression in children.[840]

The FDA has given approval for use of this class of drugs in seizures and in mania.

Depression and Antidepressant

The antidepressants may be divided into several classes, including the tricyclics, the selective serotonin reuptake inhibitors (SSRIs), monoamine oxidase inhibitors, and the atypical antidepressants. There has been a growing use of this class of drug to subside the features of depression like low mood, anhedonia, lack of sleep, decreased appetite. Tricyclics have not been found to be quite efficacious. There have been incidences of sudden deaths. So this class of drug have not been proposed for use in childhood depression.[841] Among SSRI sertraline escitalopram and fluoxetine have been found to be favorable while fluvoxamine has been proposed for use in OCD.[842] Bupropion have been found to reduce symptoms of ADHD.[843] The AACAP indicated that depressed patients treated with selective serotonin re-uptake inhibitors (SSRIs) have a relatively good response rate. The Treatment for Adolescents with Depression Study (TADS) compared treatments for moderate to severely depressed youth and found that 70% of those who received fluoxetine combined with weekly cognitive-behavioral therapy (CBT) had better responses.[844] Another important trial, the Treatment of Resistant Depression in Adolescent (TORDIA) study demonstrated that for adolescents with depression who do not response to an initial SSRI (i.e. fluoxetine, citalopram or paroxetine), a switch to another antidepressant (i.e. another SSRI or the selective serotonin and norepinephrine reuptake inhibitor (SNRI) venlafaxine combined with CBT should be considered for a better clinical response.[844]

Attention Deficit/Hyperactivity Disorder and Stimulants

Pharmacotherapy remains the primary treatment. Many studies have reports the effectiveness of stimulants. This class is mostly used to treat ADHD mostly the symptoms of inattention, impulsivity and hyperactivity. There use has been steadily rising.[840] Methylphenidate (Ritalin and others), a commonly used stimulant medication, has been demonstrated to exert significant positive effects on measures of attention and academic efficiency for children with ADHD.[845] They also reduce aggression in children of ADHD.[846] The amphetamines and methylphenidate are stimulant drugs that remain first-line treatments for ADHD with strong demonstrated efficacy in treating the core symptoms. Dextroamphetamine is approved by FDA for use in 3 years and above, while methylphenidate is used above 6 to 7 years of age. The nonstimulant SNRI drug, atomoxetine, was approved by the FDA to treat ADHD. It is the first non-stimulant to be approved by FDA for use in ADHD. Currently the alpha agonist like clonidine is also being increasingly used as a combination to treat symptoms of ADHD.

Schizophrenia and Antipsychotics

The atypical antipsychotics mostly form the bulk of treatment of schizophrenia in children. The atypical antipsychotics have replaced the traditional antipsychotics because of their favorable side effect profile. They have also been found to be favorable in treating the negative symptoms. Open label trials have reported the effectiveness of olanzapine, risperidone and quetiapine. The FDA approved several SGA agents for use in children and adolescents (aged 13–17) with schizophrenia after a wave of new placebo-controlled clinical trials were conducted and demonstrated efficacy in this population. Haloperidol was once the mainstay of treatment but because of the side effect profile it has been replaced by SGA. Clozapine has been approved as a last resort to treat childhood schizophrenia. Risperidone has been found to be the most efficacious drug in childhood psychosis, behavioral problem associated with mental retardation and pervasive developmental delay.[847-849]

Autism

Autistic disorders have been associated with impulsivity, inattention ritualistic behavior and temper outburst. In 2006, the FDA have approved the use of risperidone for use in the behavioral problems. Risperidone has been found to be the most efficacious drug in childhood psychosis, behavioral problem associated with mental retardation and pervasive developmental delay.[847-849] Other drugs useful are olanzapine and aripiprazole. As in ADHD clonidine have also been used in autism for control of aggression and irritability. Repetitive behavior, rigidity, obsessive-compulsive symptoms are being treated with SSRI like fluoxetine, fluvoxamine, citalopram, escitalopram.[850] Beta-blockers and mood stabilizers are also increasingly used to control behavioral problems. Stimulants also are helpful to reduce hyperactivity and inattention in children. Studies have reported improvement in children with autism.

Obsessive Compulsive Disorder

The AACAP Workgroup recommends cognitive-behavioral therapy (CBT) as the first-line of treatment for mild to moderate cases of OCD. The AACAP specifies that for youth with moderate to severe OCD, medication is indicated in addition to CBT. At the present time, there are four medications that have FDA approval for use in OCD in children and adolescents: the tricyclic antidepressant, clomipramine, for children aged 10 and over, and the SSRIs: sertraline (6 and older), fluoxetine (7 and older) and fluvoxamine (8 and older). Clomipramine was found to be more effective than SSRI. Also it was found in studies that when clomipramine was combined with CBT it gave a better outcome. However, SSRI are more commonly used because of a favorable side effect profile.[851,852]

Generalized Anxiety Disorder (GAD)/Separation Anxiety Disorder (SAD)/Specific Phobia

Although the non-OCD disorders (i.e. GAD, SAD, and Specific Phobias) are more prevalent than OCD in childhood, clinical studies on efficacy of treatments are far more limited. SSRI again are the mainstay of treatment. Clonazepam has been found to be effective in separation anxiety.[853] Combination CBT has also been found to be effective.

Disruptive Behavioral Disorders/Aggression and Conduct Disorder

Maladaptive aggression has been defined as a nonspecific, serious symptom accompanying many childhood disorders—i.e. oppositional defiant disorder (ODD), conduct disorder, ADHD and bipolar disorder. These problems have serious implications in socio-occupational functioning. Treatment of Maladaptive Aggression in Youth (T-MAY), sponsored by Rutgers Centre for Education and Research on Mental Health Therapeutics (CERT), provides recommendations for a standardized approach in dealing with maladaptive aggression seen in outpatient settings. CERT Guidelines indicate antipsychotics are the most studied class of drugs and have demonstrated the largest efficacy for disruptive/aggressive conditions, particularly risperidone versus placebo.[854] Lithium and carbamazepine have been effective in controlling the problematic behaviors. When associated with ADHD studies report stimulants are faster acting. However, combination of mood stabilizers and antipsychotics remain the best treatment option.

Tourette's Disorder

Haloperidol and pimozide have been the gold standard treatment for tourette's disorder. Recent studies have found clonidine to be equally effective.[834]

Enuresis

Behavioral modification remains the first-line of treatment in most cases. However, in pharmacological treatment desmopressin and imipramine have been found to be effective.

Mental Retardation

No specific pharmacological treatment is currently available for mental retardation. Specific behavioral techniques, parental skill training and counseling remains the mainstay of treatment. Comorbid disorders like seizures, behavioral problem, and psychosis are treated with specific medicines described as above.[834]

PSYCHOTROPIC DRUG FOR CHILDREN AND ADOLESCENTS (TABLES 21 TO 26)[855]

Table 21: Combination

Drug name	FDA approval/Indication	Pediatric dose	Warning
Fluoxetine and Olanzapine in combination	18 and older N/A	Pediatric dosing is currently unavailable or not applicable for this drug	Usage Black Box warning for fluoxetine/olanzapine combination formula increased the risk of suicidal thinking and behaviors in children and adolescents Possibly unsafe during lactation

Table 22: Antipsychotics

Drug name	FDA approval/Indication	Pediatric dose	Warning
Aripiprazole* (SGA)	10 and older for bipolar disorder, manic, or mixed episodes; 13–17 for schizophrenia and bipolar; 6–17 for irritability associated with autistic disorder	2–10 mg/kg/day	*Black Box warning for aripiprazole:* Not approved for depression in under age 18. Increased risk of suicidal thinking and behavior
Chlorpromazine† (FGA)	18 and older	0.25 mg/kg tid	May alter cardiac conduction; sedation; Neuroleptic Malignant syndrome; weight gain. Use caution with renal disease, seizure disorder
Clozapine* (SGA)	18 and older children	150–300 mg/day in children Adolescents: 200-600 mg/day	Agranulocytosis; seizures; myocarditis; other adverse cardiovascular and respiratory effects (*Note:* Clozapine is considered a treatment of last resort in children in whom trials of both FGA and SGA agents have failed
Haloperidol† (FGA)	3 and older	0.15–0.5 mg/kg/day	*Other precautions for haloperidol:* May cause sedation, orthostatic hypotension, photosensitivity, constipation, dry mouth, prolactin elevation
Olanzapine* (SGA)	18 and older; ages 13–17 as second line treatment for manic or mixed episodes of bipolar disorder and schizophrenia 18 and older	2.5–5 mg	Diabetes mellitus/weight gain/akathisia/dyslipidemia
Pimozide† (FGA)	12 and older ≤12 years	0.2 mg/kg/day > 12 years: 1–10 mg/day	*Other precautions for pimozide:* Dyskinesias, dry mouth, constipation, prolactin elevation, prolonged QTc interval. Possibly unsafe during lactation. Avoid abrupt withdrawal
Quetiapine*(SGA)	13 and older for schizophrenia; 18 and older for bipolar; 10–17 for treatment of manic and mixed episodes of bipolar disorder	100–300 mg	Diabetes mellitus/Weight gain/akathisia/dyslipidemia
Risperidone* (SGA)	13 and older for schizophrenia; 10 and older for bipolar mania and mixed episodes; 5 to 16 for irritability associated with autism	Usually 1–2 mg/day; other recommended doses: 3 mg/day—children; 6 mg/day—adolescents	
Thioridazine† (FGA)	2 and older	3 mg/kg/day	*Black Box warning for thioridazine:* Dose-related prolongation of QTc interval may cause torsade de pointes-type arrhythmias and sudden death. Use restricted to schizophrenia resistant to standard antipsychotic drugs

Contd...

Contd...

Drug name	*FDA approval/Indication*	*Pediatric dose*	*Warning*
Trifluoperazine[†] (FGA)	18 and older	0.5–10 mg/day	CNS collapse, CNS depression, blood dyscrasias, bone marrow depression, hepatic impairment. Safety in lactation is unknown
Ziprasidone* (SGA)	18 and older children	10 mg/day initial dose, maximum dose not established; 160 mg/day–adolescents	*Black Box warning for ziprasidone:* Not approved for depression in under age 18. Increased risk of suicidal thinking and behavior. Other precautions for ziprasidone: Prolonged QTc interval

**Precautions which apply to all atypical or second generation antipsychotics (SGA):* Neuroleptic Malignant Syndrome/Tardive Dyskinesia/ Hyperglycemia/Diabetes Mellitus/Weight Gain/Akathisia/Dyslipidemia

[†]*Precautions which apply to all typical or first generation antipsychotics (FGA):* Extrapyramidal symptoms/tardive dyskinesia

Table 23: Antidepressants

Drug name	*FDA approval/Indication*	*Pediatric dose*	*Warning*
Amitriptyline (Tricyclic [TCA])	18 and older 9–12 years	1–3 mg/kg/day >12 years: 50–100 mg/day	*Precautions for amitriptyline and other TCAs:* General caution for use in patients < 25 years; those with bipolar disorder or comorbid schizophrenia or cardiovascular diagnosis. Avoid abrupt withdrawal. Do not take if an MAOI was used within the past 14 days. EEG to be done prior to starting of this drug
Bupropion	18 and older	1–7 mg/kg/day	Anorexia and risk of seizures
Clomipramine (TCA)	10 and older (for OCD only)	Used for OCD >10 years: Max: 3 mg/ kg/day up to 100 mg/day in first 2 weeks; up to 200 mg/day	
Doxepin (TCA)	12 and older	N/A	Unsafe in lactation. Significant adverse effects to infant/breast milk production—contraindicated or requires cessation of breastfeeding
Scitalopram (SSRI)	18 and older; 12–17 (for major depressive disorder)	12–17 years: Max: 20 mg/day Taper dose gradually	*Black Box warning for escitalopram:* As noted above plus notes not to be used in children under 12 years of age
Fluoxetine (SSRI)	8 and older; 18 and older (for premenstrual dysphoric disorder)	5–30 mg/day	*Black Box warning for ziprasidone:* Not approved for depression in under age 18. Increased risk of suicidal thinking and behavior
Fluvoxamine (SSRI)	8 and older (for OCD only)	*Children:* 200 mg/ day *Adolescents:* 300 mg/day	
Imipramine (TCA)	6 and older (for bedwetting)	1–5 mg/kg/day; 150–250 ng/mL	
Sertraline (SSRI)	6 and older (for OCD only)	200 mg/day	
Paroxetine (SSRI)	18 and older children	*Adolescents:* 10–20 mg/day	*Note:* FDA changed classification of paroxetine from category C to D for scientific evidence of positive teratogenic effects. Paroxetine should be avoided in pregnancy if possible

Table 24: Mood stabilizing and anticonvulsant medications

Drug name	*FDA approval/Indication*	*Pediatric dose*	*Warning*
Carbamazepine	any age (for seizures)	10–50 mg/kg/day 8–12 mcg/mL (serum level)	*Black Box warning for carbamazepine:* Stevens-Johnson syndrome (particularly among Asians), aplastic anemia, agranulocytosis. *Other warnings/precautions:* Neutropenia, hyponatremia, induces metabolism of itself and some other drugs, decreased efficacy of oral contraceptives, teratogenicity, MAOI use within 14 days
Divalproex Sodium (Valproic acid)	2 and older	15–60 mg/kg/day 50–100 mcg/mL (serum level)	*Black Box warning for divalproex sodium:* Hepatotoxicity, teratogenicity, pancreatitis. urea cycle disorders, multiorgan hypersensitivity reaction, thrombocytopenia, polycystic ovaries
Lamotrigine	18 and older	15–5.0 mg/kg/day (25–200 mg/day)	Serious rashes including Stevens-Johnson syndrome and aseptic meningitis. *Other warnings/precautions:* Acute-multiorgan failure, withdrawal seizures, blood dyscrasias, hypersensitivity, suicidal ideation
Lithium Carbonate/ Citrate	12 and older	300–2,400 mg/day 0.5–1.2 mEq/L (serum level)	Toxicity above therapeutic serum levels. *Other warnings/precautions:* Renal function impairment, polyuria, tremor, diarrhea, nausea, hypothyroid, teratogenic effects. Special risk patients include those with significant renal or cardiovascular disease, severe debilitation, dehydration, sodium depletion
Oxcarbazepine	4 and older	5–30 mg/kg/day (150–1,200 mg/day)	*Warnings/precautions for oxcarbazepine:* Hyponatremia, suicidal ideation

Table 25: ADHD medications

Drug name	*FDA approval/Indication*	*Pediatric dose*	*Warning*
Amphetamine/ Amphetamine	6 and older (XR)	40 mg/day max 30 mg/day max	Abuse potential. Risk of sudden death and serious cardiovascular events. May cause hypertension, psychiatric adverse events and possible growth suppression
Atomoxetine	6 and older	*Children:* 0.5 mg/kg/day *Adolescents:* 40 mg/day	May cause serious cardiovascular events including sudden death, particularly in those with pre-existing structural cardiac abnormalities or serious heart problems; increase in blood pressure and heart rate; adverse psychiatric events and liver injury
Dexmethylphenidate/ Dexmethylphenidate	6 and older	20 mg/day maximum 30 mg/day maximum	
Clonidine: Immediate Release (IR)/Clonidine Extended Release (ER)	*IR:* not approved for children *ER:* 6–17 years old	Up to 0.4 mg/day	
Methylphenidate/ Methylphenidate ER and ER Suspension	6 and older	60 mg/day maximum	

Table 26: Psychotropic drugs: Side effects and teratogenic risk

Drug name	*Side effect*	*Teratogenic risk*	*Category*
Antipsychotic medications	• Akathisia and dystonic reactions are seen in children treated with SGAs but risk of tardive dyskinesia is small compared to FGAs • Weight gain is a significant problem with SGAs. *Other side effects:* Constipation, dry mouth, dizziness • Sedation/cognitive blunting may occur with FGAs and SGAs adolescent males at much greater risk for dystonic reactions than adults • Significant drop in neutrophils and increased risk of seizures with clozapine (should be used as treatment of last resort)	*FGAs:* Rare anomalies, fetal jaundice, fetal anticholinergic effects at birth *SGAs:* Gestational diabetes, large birthweight	*FGA:* C *SGA:* BC

Contd...

Contd...

Drug name	*Side effect*	*Teratogenic risk*	*Category*
Antidepressant medications	*TCAs:* Slowing of cardiac conduction Cardiac long QT syndrome may be mechanism be responsible for sudden death in children. *Other effects:* Dry mouth, urinary retention, sedation, constipation, weight gain and hypotension	*TCAs:* Fetal tachycardia, fetal withdrawal, fetal anticholinergic effects, urinary retention, bowel obstruction	D-amitriptyline, Imipramine, Nortriptyline C (other TCAs)
	MAOIs: Daytime sleepiness, dizziness, light headedness, low blood pressure, difficulty urinating, dry mouth, altered sense of taste, nervousness, muscle aches, insomnia and weight gain	*MAOIs:* Rare fetal malformations: rarely used in pregnancy due to hypertension	C
	SSRI side effects: Insomnia, sedation, appetite changes (up or down), nausea, dry mouth, headache, sexual dysfunction, Treatment emergent akathisia from SSRIs may be more evident in pediatric depression associated with bipolar disorder and greater suicide risk	*SSRIs:* Perinatal and cardiovascular complications, spontaneous abortions. Potential premature delivery and neonatal persistent pulmonary hypertension (PPHN)	C Paroxetine is D
	SNRIs: Nausea, insomnia, sedation, sexual dysfunction, sweating, hypertension and discontinuation syndrome	Potential premature delivery. Clinical outcome data sparse compared to SSRIs or TCAs	C
	Bupropion: Common side effects: headache, agitation, restless insomnia, weight loss, anorexia, sweating, tremor and hypertension	*Bupropion:* Risks unknown, but not recommended over SSRIs in pregnancy	C
Mood stabilizing and anticonvulsant medications	*Lithium common reactions:* Tremor, polyuria, polydipsia, weight gain, diarrhea, vomiting, drowsiness, cognitive impairment, muscle weakness, impaired coordination, anorexia, nausea, blurred vision, xerostomia, fatigue, alopecia, reversible leukocytosis , acne and edema	Lithium: Associated with increase in birth defects including cardiac anomalies (esp. Ebstein's anomaly) and behavioral effects.	D
	Valproate: Children younger than 2 years are at greatest risk for hepatotoxicity. *Common reactions:* headache, nausea/vomiting, loss of muscle strength, somnolence, thrombocytopenia, dyspepsia, dizziness, diarrhea, abdominal pain, tremor	*Valproate:* Neural tube defects lower IQ measures	D
	Carbamazepine: May cause dizziness, drowsiness, unsteadiness, impaired coordination, nausea/vomiting, blurred vision, nystagmus, rash, confusion	Neural tube defects, minor anomalies	D
	Lamotrigine: Children are at greater risk for rash than adults. May cause nausea, vomiting, dizziness, vertigo, visual disturbance, somnolence, ataxy, pruritus/rash, headache, pharyngitis, rhinitis, diarrhea, fever, loss of muscle strength	Unknown but there appears to be a high rate of cleft lip and palate	**C**
	Gabapentin: May cause dizziness, somnolence, ataxia, fatigue, peripheral edema, nystagmus, nausea, and vomiting, viral infection		C
	Pregabalin: Dizziness, somnolence, xerostomia, peripheral edema, blurred vision, weight gain, abnormal thinking, impaired coordination		C

CONCLUSION

With the increasing use of psychotropic in childhood psychiatric illness has helped to reduce the burden of illness. However, polypharmacy and off label drugs should be avoided. The increasing drug trials and research going on in the field of childhood psychopharmacology has brought about new guidelines and measures to prescribe drugs. However, the challenge of ensuring that children and adolescents receive evidence based mental health treatment requires a multi-disciplinary approach where children and families access and accept treatment, providers gain the necessary skills/knowledge and organizations and funding policies align to support them.

REFERENCES

General Principles of the Clinical Interview

1. Briggs-Gowan MJ, Carter AS, Irwin JR, et al. Brief infant-toddler social and emotional assessment: screening for social-emotional problems and delays in competence: J Padiatr Psychol. 2004;29:143-55.
2. Carlat DJ. The psychiatric review of symptoms: A screening tool for family physicians. AM Fame Physician. 1998;58:1617-24.
3. Ellington KD, Briggs-Gowan MJ, Carter AS, et al. Parent identification of early emerging child behavior problems: predicators of sharing parental concern with health providers. Arch Pediatr Adolescent Mec. 2004;158:766-72.
4. Kim-cohen J, Moffit TE, Taylor A, et al. Maternal depression and children antisocial behavior. Arch Gen Psychiatry. 2005;62:173-81.
5. McLennan JD, Kotelchuck M, Cho H: Prevalence, persistence, and correlates of depressive symptoms in a national sample of mothers of toddlers. J Am Acad Child Adolesc Psychiatry. 2001;40:1316-23.
6. Ozer Em, Adams SH, Lusting JL, et al. Increasing the screening and counseling of adolescent for risky healthy behaviors: A primary care interpenetration predicators. 2005;115:960-8.
7. Smith RC, Marshall-Dorsey AA, Osborn GG, et al. Evidence based guidelines for teaching patient-centered interviewing patient. Educ Couns. 2000;39:27.
8. Stein MT, Coleman WL, Epstein RM. "We have tried everything and nothing works": family-centered predicators and clinical problem-solving. J Dev Behav Pediatric. 2001;22:s55-s60.
9. Virshup BB, Oppenberg AA, Coleman MM. Strategic risk management: reducing malpractice claims through more effective patient-doctor communication. Am J Med Qual. 1999:14:153-9.
10. Weissman MM, Pilowski DJ, Wikramaratne PJ, et al. Remissions in maternal depression and child psychopathlogy. J Am A. 2006;295:1389-98.
11. Zukerman B, Parker S, Kaplan-sanoff M, et al. Healthy steps: a case study of innovation in pediatric practice. Pediatrics. 2004;114:820-6.

Developmental Assessment of Children

12. Kelly Y, Sacker A, Schoon I, Nazroo J. Ethnic differences in achievement of developmental milestones by 9 months of age: The Millennium Cohort Study. Dev Med Child Neurol. 2006;48:824-30.
13. American Academy of Pediatrics, Council on Children with Disabilities, Section on Developmental and Behavioral Pediatrics. Identifying infants and young children with developmental disorder in the medical home: an algorithm for developmental surveillance and screening. Pediatrics. 2006;118:405-20.
14. Department of Health. The Healthy Child Programme. 2009. www.dh.gov.uk/en/Publicationsandstatistics/Publications/PublicationsPolicyAndGuidance/DH_107563.
15. Sheridan MA, Fox NA, Zeanah CH, McLaughlin K, Nelson CA. Variation in neural development as a result of exposure to institutionalization early in childhood. Proc Natl Acad Sci USA. 2012;109:12927-32.
16. Windsor J, Wing CA, Koga SF, Fox NA, Benigno JP, Carroll PJ, et al. Effect of foster care on young children's language learning. Child Dev. 2011:82:1040-6.
17. Nelson CA, Zeanah CH, Fox NA, Marshall PJ, Smyke AT, Guthrie D. Cognitive recovery in socially deprived young children: the Bucharest Early Intervention Project. Science. 2007;318:1937-40.
18. Williams AN, Essex C. Developmental delay or failure to arrive? Dev Med Child Neurol. 2004;46:502.
19. Baird G, Simonoff E, Pickles A, Chandler S, Loucas T, Meldrum D, Charman T. Prevalence of disorders of the autism spectrum in a population cohort of children in South Thames: the special needs and autism project (SNAP). Lancet. 2006;368:210-5.
20. Blanchard LT, Gurka MJ, Blackman JA. Emotional, developmental, and behavioural health of American children and their families: a report from the 2003 national survey of children's health. Paediatrics. 2006;117:e1202-12.
21. Horridge KA. Assessment and investigation of the child with disordered development. Arch Dis Child Educ Pract. Ed2011;96:9-20.
22. Guralnik M. The effectiveness of early intervention. Paul H Brookes; 1997.
23. Gomby DS, Larner MB, Stevenson CS, Lewit EM, Behrman RE. Long-term outcomes of early childhood programs: analysis and recommendations. Future Child. 1995;5:6-24.
24. Shonkoff J, Phillips D (Eds). From neurons to neighborhoods: the science of early childhood development. National Academies Press; 2000.
25. Perry B. Childhood experience and the expression of genetic potential: what childhood neglect tells us about nature and nurture. Brain Mind. 2002;3:79-100.
26. McCain M, Mustard F. Reversing the real brain drain. Early years study final report, Ontario Children's Secretariat Toronto. Academy Press; 1999.
27. Heckman J, Masterov D. The productivity argument for investing in young children. Rev Agricult Econ. 2007;29:446-93.
28. KPMG. Reviewing the evidence on the effectiveness of early childhood intervention. Report to Department of Families, Housing, Community Services and Indigenous Affairs, Australia. 2011. www.fahcsia.gov.au/sites/default/files/documents/ 05_2012/childhood_int_effectiveness_report_0.pdf.
29. Engle PL, Fernald LC, Alderman H, Behrman J, O'Gara C, Yousafzai A, et al. Strategies for reducing inequalities and improving developmental outcomes for young children in low-income and middle-income countries. Lancet. 2011;378:1339-53.

30. Lake A. Early childhood development—global action is overdue. Lancet. 2011;378:1277.
31. Wilson JMG, Jungner G. Principles and practice of screening for disease. WHO Bull. 1968;22:473.
32. Cochrane AL, Holland WW. Validation of screening procedures. Br Med Bull. 1971;27:3-8.
33. Köhler L, Rigby M. Indicators of children's development: considerations when constructing a set of national child health indicators for the European Union. Child Care Health Dev. 2003;29:551-8.
34. Hagan JF, Shaw JS, Duncan PM (Eds). Bright futures: guidelines for health supervision of infants, children, and adolescents. 3rd edition. American Academy of Pediatrics, 2008. http://brightfutures.aap.org/pdfs/guidelines_pdf/1-bf-introduction.pdf.
35. HR 3962. To provide affordable, quality health care for all Americans and reduce the growth in health care spending, and for other purposes. 2009. http://housedocs.house.gov/rules/health/111_ahcaa.pdf.
36. Sharma A. Developmental examination: birth to 5 years. Arch Dis Child Educ Pract Ed. 2011;96:162-75.
37. Bax M, Whitmore K. The medical examination of children on entry to school. The results and use of neurodevelopmental assessment. Dev Med Child Neurol. 1987;29:40-55.
38. Voight RG, Llorente AM, Jensen CL, Fraley JK, Barbaresr WJ, Heird WC. Comparison of the validity of direct pediatric developmental evaluation versus developmental screening by parental report. Clin Pediatr. 2007:46:523-9.
39. Klamer A, Lando A, Pinborg A, Greisen G. Ages and stages questionnaire used to measure cognitive deficit in children born extremely preterm. Acta Paediatr. 2005;94:1327-9.
40. Glascoe FP. Parents' concerns about children's development: prescreening technique or screening test? Pediatrics. 1997;99: 522-8.
41. Glascoe FP. Evidence-based approach to developmental and behavioral surveillance using parents' concerns. Child Care Health Dev. 2000,26:137-49.
42. Robins D, Fein D, Barton M, Green J. The modified checklist for autism in toddlers: an initial study investigating the early detection of autism and pervasive developmental disorders. J Autism Dev Disord. 2001;31:131-4.
43. Glascoe FP, Byrne KE, Ashford LG, Johnson KL, Chang B, Strickland B. Accuracy of the Denver II in developmental screening. Pediatrics. 1992;89:1221-5.
44. Sheridan M, Sharma A, Cockerill H. From birth to five years: children's developmental progress. Routledge; 2007.
45. Bellman M, Lingam S, Aukett A. Schedule of growing skills II. NFER-Nelson; 1997.
46. Glascoe FP. A method for deciding how to respond to parents' concerns about development and behavior. Ambul Child Health. 1999;5:197-208.
47. Glascoe FP, Byrne KE. The accuracy of developmental screening tests. J Early Interv. 1993;17:368-78.
48. Squires J, Bricker D, Potter L. Revision of a parent-completed developmental screening tool: ages and stages questionnaire. J Pediatr Psychol. 1996;22:313-28.
49. Bellman MH, Rawson NS, Wadsworth J, Ross EM, Cameron S, Miller DL. A developmental test based on the Stycar sequences used in the National Childhood Encephalopathy Study. Child Care Health Dev. 1985;11:309.

Anxiety Disorders and Post-traumatic Stress Disorder in Children and Adolescent

50. Costello EJ, Egger HL, Angold A. The developmental epidemiology of anxiety disorders: phenomenology, prevalence, and comorbidity. Child Adolesc Psychiatr Clin N Am. 2005;14(4):631–48vii.
51. Costello EJ, Angold A, Burns BJ, et al. The great smoky mountains study of youth. Goals, design, methods, and the prevalence of DSM-III-R disorders. Arch Gen Psychiatry. 1996;53(12):1129-36.
52. Simonoff E, Pickles A, Meyer JM, et al. The Virginia twin study of adolescent behavioral development. Influences of age, sex, and impairment on rates of disorder. Arch Gen Psychiatry. 1997;54(9):801-8.
53. Beals J, Piasecki J, Nelson S, et al. Psychiatric disorder among American Indian adolescents: prevalence in northern plains youth. J Am Acad Child Adolesc Psychiatry. 1997;36(9):1252-9.
54. Costello EJ, Angold A, Keeler GP. Adolescent outcomes of childhood disorders: the consequences of severity and impairment. J Am Acad Child Adolesc Psychiatry. 1999;38(2):121-8.
55. Lewinsohn PM, Gotlib IH, Lewinsohn M, et al. Gender differences in anxiety disorders and anxiety symptoms in adolescents. J Abnorm Psychol. 1998;107(1):109-17.
56. American Psychiatric Association. Diagnostic and statistical manual of mental disorders, 4th edition, text revision. Washington, DC: American Psychiatric Association; 2000.
57. Suveg C, Aschenbrand SG, Kendall PC. Separation anxiety disorder, panic disorder, and school refusal. Child Adolesc Psychiatr Clin N Am. 2005;14(4):773-95.
58. Lewinsohn PM, Holm-Denoma JM, Small JW, et al. Separation anxiety disorder in childhood as a risk factor for future mental illness. J Am Acad Child Adolesc Psychiatry. 2008;47(5): 548-55.
59. Shear K, Jin R, Ruscio AM, et al. Prevalence and correlates of estimated DSM-IV child and adult separation anxiety disorder in the National comorbidity survey replication. Am J Psychiatry. 2006;163(6):1074-83.
60. Last CG, Perrin S, Hersen M, et al. DSM-III-R anxiety disorders in children: sociodemographic and clinical characteristics. J Am Acad Child Adolesc Psychiatry. 1992;31(6):1070-6.
61. Verduin TL, Kendall PC. Differential occurrence of comorbidity within childhood anxiety disorders. J Clin Child Adolesc Psychol. 2003;32(2):290-5.

62. Last CG, Perrin S, Hersen M, et al. A prospective study of childhood anxiety disorders. J Am Acad Child Adolesc Psychiatry. 1996;35:1502-10.
63. Kearney CA, Sims KE, Pursell CR, et al. Separation anxiety disorder in young children: a longitudinal and family analysis. J Clin Child Adolesc Psychol. 2003;32(4):593-8.
64. Foley DL, Pickles A, Maes HM, et al. Course and short-term outcomes of separation anxiety disorder in a community sample of twins. J Am Acad Child Adolesc Psychiatry. 2004;43(9):1107–14.
65. Aschenbrand SG, Kendall PC, Webb A, et al. Is childhood separation anxiety disorder a predictor of adult panic disorder and agoraphobia? A seven-year longitudinal study. J Am Acad Child Adolesc Psychiatry. 2003;42(12):1478-85.
66. American Psychiatric Association. Diagnostic and statistical manual of mental disorders, 3rd edition. Washington, DC: American Psychiatric Association; 1987.
67. American Psychiatric Association. Diagnostic and statistical manual of mental disorders, 4th edition. Washington, DC: American Psychiatric Association; 1994.
68. Layne AE, Bernat DH, Victor AM, et al. Generalized anxiety disorder in a nonclinical sample of children: symptom presentation and predictors of impairment. J Anxiety Disord. 2008;10.1016/j.janxdis.2008.08.003in press.
69. Masi G, Millepiedi S, Mucci M, et al. Generalized anxiety disorder in referred children and adolescents. J Am Acad Child Adolesc Psychiatry. 2004;43(6):752-60.
70. Kendall PC, Pimentel SS. On the physiological symptom constellation in youth with generalized anxiety disorder (GAD). J Anxiety Disord. 2003;17(2):211-21.
71. Tracey SA, Chorpita BF, Douban J, et al. Empirical evaluation of DSM-IV generalized anxiety disorder criteria in children and adolescents. J Clin Child Psychol. 1997;26(4):404-14.
72. Anderson JC, Williams S, McGee R, et al. DSM-III disorders in preadolescent children. Prevalence in a large sample from the general population. Arch Gen Psychiatry. 1987;44(1):69-6.
73. Bowen RC, Offord DR, Boyle MH. The prevalence of overanxious disorder and separation anxiety disorder: results from the Ontario child health study. J Am Acad Child Adolesc Psychiatry. 1990;29(5):753-8.
74. Wittchen HU, Zhao S, Kessler RC, et al. DSM-III-R generalized anxiety disorder in the national comorbidity survey. Arch Gen Psychiatry. 1994;51(5):355-64.
75. Bell-Dolan DJ, Last CG, Strauss CC. Symptoms of anxiety disorders in normal children. J Am Acad Child Adolesc Psychiatry. 1990;29(5):759-65.
76. Hoehn-Saric R, Hazlett RL, McLeod DR. Generalized anxiety disorder with early and late onset of anxiety symptoms. Compr Psychiatry. 1993;34(5):291-8.
77. Masi G, Mucci M, Favilla L, et al. Symptomatology and comorbidity of generalized anxiety disorder in children and adolescents. Compr Psychiatry. 1999;40(3):210-5.
78. Moffitt TE, Harrington H, Caspi A, et al. Depression and generalized anxiety disorder: cumulative and sequential comorbidity in a birth cohort followed prospectively to age 32 years. Arch Gen Psychiatry. 2007;64(6):651-60.
79. Beidel DC, Turner SM, Morris TL. Psychopathology of childhood social phobia. J Am Acad Child Adolesc Psychiatry. 1999;38(6):643-50.
80. Bernstein GA, Bernat DH, Davis AA, et al. Symptom presentation and classroom functioning in a nonclinical sample of children with social phobia. Depress Anxiety. 2008;25(9):752-60.
81. Muris P, Meesters C. Symptoms of anxiety disorders and teacher-reported school functioning of normal children. Psychol Rep. 2002;91(2):588-90.
82. Essau CA, Conradt J, Petermann F. Frequency and comorbidity of social phobia and social fears in adolescents. Behav Res Ther. 1999;37(9):831-43.
83. Strauss CC, Last CG. Social and simple phobias in children. J Anxiety Disord. 1993;7:141-52.
84. Beesdo K, Bittner A, Pine DS, et al. Incidence of social anxiety disorder and the consistent risk for secondary depression in the first three decades of life. Arch Gen Psychiatry. 2007;64(8):903-12.
85. Grant BF, Hasin DS, Blanco C, et al. The epidemiology of social anxiety disorder in the United States: results from the national epidemiologic survey on alcohol and related conditions. J Clin Psychiatry. 2005;66(11):1351-61.
86. Buckner JD, Schmidt NB, Lang AR, et al. Specificity of social anxiety disorder as a risk factor for alcohol and cannabis dependence. J Psychiatr Res. 2008;42(3):230-9.
87. Rapoport JL, Inoff-Germain G, Weissman MM, et al. Childhood obsessive-compulsive disorder in the NIMH MECA study: parent versus child identification of cases. Methods for the epidemiology of child and adolescent mental disorders. J Anxiety Disord. 2000;14(6):535-48.
88. Valleni-Basile LA, Garrison CZ, Jackson KL, et al. Frequency of obsessive-compulsive disorder in a community sample of young adolescents. J Am Acad Child Adolesc Psychiatry. 1994;33(6):782-91.
89. Geller D, Biederman J, Jones J, et al. Is juvenile obsessive-compulsive disorder a developmental subtype of the disorder? A review of the pediatric literature. J Am Acad Child Adolesc Psychiatry. 1998;37(4):420-7.
90. Geller DA. Obsessive-compulsive and spectrum disorders in children and adolescents. Psychiatr Clin North Am. 2006;29(2):353-70.
91. Geller DA, Biederman J, Faraone S, et al. Developmental aspects of obsessive compulsive disorder: findings in children, adolescents, and adults. J Nerv Ment Dis. 2001;189(7): 471-7.
92. Swedo SE, Rapoport JL, Leonard H, et al. Obsessive-compulsive disorder in children and adolescents. Clinical phenomenology of 70 consecutive cases. Arch Gen Psychiatry. 1989;46(4):335-41.
93. Stewart SE, Rosario MC, Brown TA, et al. Principal components analysis of obsessive-compulsive disorder symptoms in children and adolescents. Biol Psychiatry. 2007;61(3):285-91.

94. Scahill L, Riddle MA, McSwiggin-Hardin M, et al. Children's Yale-Brown obsessive compulsive scale: reliability and validity. J Am Acad Child Adolesc Psychiatry. 1997;36(6):844-52.
95. Stewart SE, Rosario MC, Baer L, et al. Four-factor structure of obsessive-compulsive disorder symptoms in children, adolescents, and adults. J Am Acad Child Adolesc Psychiatry. 2008;47(7):763-72.
96. Stewart SE, Geller DA, Jenike M, et al. Long-term outcome of pediatric obsessive-compulsive disorder: a meta-analysis and qualitative review of the literature. Acta Psychiatr Scand. 2004;110(1):4-13.
97. Swedo SE, Leonard HL, Garvey M, et al. Pediatric autoimmune neuropsychiatric disorders associated with streptococcal infections: clinical description of the first 50 cases. Am J Psychiatry. 1998;155(2):264-71.
98. Murphy ML, Pichichero ME. Prospective identification and treatment of children with pediatric autoimmune neuropsychiatric disorder associated with group A streptococcal infection (PANDAS). Arch Pediatr Adolesc Med. 2002;156(4):356-61.
99. Dale RC, Heyman I, Giovannoni G, et al. Incidence of anti-brain antibodies in children with obsessive-compulsive disorder. Br J Psychiatry. 2005;187:314-19.
100. Dyregrov A, Yule W. A review of PTSD in children. Child Adolesc Psychiatry Ment Health. 2006;11:176-84.
101. Carrion VG, Weems CF, Ray R, et al. Toward an empirical definition of pediatric PTSD: the phenomenology of PTSD symptoms in youth. J Am Acad Child Adolesc Psychiatry. 2002;41(2):166-73.
102. Scheeringa MS, Peebles CD, Cook CA, et al. Toward establishing procedural, criterion, and discriminant validity for PTSD in early childhood. J Am Acad Child Adolesc Psychiatry. 2001;40(1):52-60.
103. Scheeringa MS, Zeanah CH, Myers L, et al. New findings on alternative criteria for PTSD in preschool children. J Am Acad Child Adolesc Psychiatry. 2003;42(5):561-70.
104. Scheeringa MS, Zeanah CH, Drell MJ, et al. Two approaches to the diagnosis of posttraumatic stress disorder in infancy and early childhood. J Am Acad Child Adolesc Psychiatry. 1995;34(2):191-200.
105. Copeland WE, Keeler G, Angold A, et al. Traumatic events and posttraumatic stress in childhood. Arch Gen Psychiatry. 2007;64(5):577-84.
106. Giaconia RM, Reinherz HZ, Silverman AB, et al. Traumas and post-traumatic stress disorder in a community population of older adolescents. J Am Acad Child Adolesc Psychiatry. 1995;34(10):1369-80.
107. Costello EJ, Erkanli A, Fairbank JA, et al. The prevalence of potentially traumatic events in childhood and adolescence. J Trauma Stress. 2002;15(2):99-112.
108. Davidson JRT, Foa EB. Post-traumatic stress disorder: DSM-IV and beyond. Washington, DC: American Psychiatric Press; 1993.
109. Lonigan CJ, Phillips BM, Richey JA. Post-traumatic stress disorder in children: diagnosis, assessment, and associated features. Child Adolesc Psychiatr Clin N Am. 2003;12(2):171-94.
110. Pynoos RS, Nader K. Mental health disturbances in children exposed to disaster: prevention intervention strategies. In: Goldston SE, Yager J, Heinicke CM, et al. (Eds). Preventing Mental Health Disturbances in Childhood. 1st edition. Washington, DC: American Psychiatric Press; 1990.pp. 211-33.
111. Scheeringa MS, Wright MJ, Hunt JP, et al. Factors affecting the diagnosis and prediction of PTSD symptomatology in children and adolescents. Am J Psychiatry. 2006;163(4):644–51.

Eating Disorder: Anorexia

112. Slupik RI. Managing adolescents with eating disorders. Int J Fertil Womens Med. 1999;44(3):125-30. [Medline].
113. Fetissov SO, Harro J, Jaanisk M, et al. Autoantibodies against neuropeptides are associated with psychological traits in eating disorders. Proc Natl Acad Sci USA. 2005;102(41):14865-70. [Medline].
114. APA. Diagnostic and Statistical Manual of Mental Disorders, 4th edition. Washington, DC: APA; 1994.
115. Feldman MB, Meyer IH. Childhood abuse and eating disorders in gay and bisexual men. Int J Eat Disord. 2007;40(5):418-23. [Medline].
116. National Institute of Mental Health. National Comorbidity Survey (NCS) and National Comorbidity Survey Replication (NCS-R). Collaborative Psychiatric Epidemiology Surveys. Available at http://www.icpsr.umich.edu/CPES/. Accessed October 30, 2007.
117. Button E, Aldridge S. Season of birth and eating disorders: patterns across diagnoses in a specialized eating disorders service. Int J Eat Disord. 2007;40(5):468-71. [Medline].
118. Grice DE, Halmi KA, Fichter MM, et al. Evidence for a susceptibility gene for anorexia nervosa on chromosome 1. Am J Hum Genet. 2002;70(3):787-92. [Medline].
119. Mehler PS, Gray MC, Schulte M. Medical complications of anorexia nervosa. J Womens Health. 1997;6(5):533-41. [Medline].
120. Rooney B, McClelland L, Crisp AH, Sedgwick PM. The incidence and prevalence of anorexia nervosa in three suburban health districts in south west London, U.K. Int J Eat Disord. 1995;18(4):299-307. [Medline].
121. Speranza M, Loas G, Wallier J, Corcos M. Predictive value of alexithymia in patients with eating disorders: A 3-year prospective study. J Psychosom Res. 2007;63(4):365-71. [Medline].
122. Bryant-Waugh R, Knibbs J, Fosson A, Kaminski Z, Lask B. Long term follow up of patients with early onset anorexia nervosa. Arch Dis Child. 1988;63(1):5-9. [Medline].
123. Jordan J, Joyce PR, Carter FA, et al. Specific and nonspecific comorbidity in anorexia nervosa. Int J Eat Disord. 2008;41(1):47-56. [Medline].

124. Lesinskiene S, Barkus A, Ranceva N, Dembinskas A. A meta-analysis of heart rate and QT interval alteration in anorexia nervosa. World J Biol Psychiatry; 2007.pp.1-6. [Medline].
125. Franko DL, Keel PK, Dorer DJ, Blais MA, Delinsky SS, Eddy KT. What predicts suicide attempts in women with eating disorders?. Psychol Med. 2004;34(5):843-53. [Medline].
126. Holm-Denoma JM, Witte TK, Gordon KH, et al. Deaths by suicide among individuals with anorexia as arbiters between competing explanations of the anorexia-suicide link. J Affect Disord. 2008;107(1-3):231-6. [Medline].
127. Lilenfeld LR, Kaye WH, Greeno CG, et al. A controlled family study of anorexia nervosa and bulimia nervosa: psychiatric disorders in first-degree relatives and effects of proband comorbidity. Arch Gen Psychiatry. 1998;55(7):603-10. [Medline].
128. Kreipe RE, Birndorf SA. Eating disorders in adolescents and young adults. Med Clin North Am. 2000;84(4):1027-49, viii-ix. [Medline].
129. Puxley F, Midtsund M, Iosif A, Lask B. PANDAS anorexia nervosa—endangered, extinct or nonexistent? Int J Eat Disord. 2008;41(1):15-21. [Medline].
130. Roberts CM, Martin-Clavijo A, Winston AP, Dharmagunawardena B, Gach JE. Malnutrition and a rash: think zinc. Clin Exp Dermatol. 2007;32(6):654-7. [Medline].
131. Nicholls D, Viner R. Eating disorders and weight problems. BMJ. 2005;330(7497):950-3. [Medline].
132. Kyriacou O, Treasure J, Schmidt U. Expressed emotion in eating disorders assessed via self-report: an examination of factors associated with expressed emotion in carers of people with anorexia nervosa in comparison to control families. Int J Eat Disord. 2008;41(1):37-46. [Medline].
133. Morris J, Twaddle S. Anorexia nervosa. BMJ. 2007;334(7599):894-8. [Medline].
134. Eisler I, Simic M, Russell GF, Dare C. A randomised controlled treatment trial of two forms of family therapy in adolescent anorexia nervosa: a five-year follow-up. J Child Psychol Psychiatry. 2007;48(6):552-60. [Medline].
135. Rosenblum J, Forman S. Evidence-based treatment of eating disorders. Curr Opin Pediatr. 2002;14(4):379-83. [Medline].
136. Rigaud D, Brondel L, Poupard AT, Talonneau I, Brun JM. A randomized trial on the efficacy of a 2-month tube feeding regimen in anorexia nervosa: A 1-year follow-up study. Clin Nutr. 2007;26(4):421-9. [Medline].
137. Becker AE, Grinspoon SK, Klibanski A, Herzog DB. Eating disorders. N Engl J Med. 1999;340(14):1092-8. [Medline].
138. Krantz MJ, Mehler PS. Resting tachycardia, a warning sign in anorexia nervosa: case report. BMC Cardiovasc Disord. 2004;4:10. [Medline].
139. Jagielska G, Tomaszewicz-Libudzic EC, Brzozowska A. Pellagra: a rare complication of anorexia nervosa. Eur Child Adolesc Psychiatry. 2007;16(7):417-20. [Medline].
140. Thien V, Thomas A, Markin D, Birmingham CL. Pilot study of a graded exercise program for the treatment of anorexia nervosa. Int J Eat Disord. 2000;28(1):101-6. [Medline].
141. Gordon CM, Grace E, Emans SJ, et al. Changes in bone turnover markers and menstrual function after short-term oral DHEA in young women with anorexia nervosa. J Bone Miner Res. 1999;14(1):136-45. [Medline].
142. Ramoz N, Versini A, Gorwood P. Eating disorders: an overview of treatment responses and the potential impact of vulnerability genes and endophenotypes. Expert Opin Pharmacother. 2007;8(13):2029-44. [Medline].
143. Simon GE, Savarino J, Operskalski B, Wang PS. Suicide risk during antidepressant treatment. Am J Psychiatry. 2006;163(1):41-7. [Medline]. [Full Text].
144. Szmukler GI, Young GP, Miller G, Lichtenstein M, Binns DS. A controlled trial of cisapride in anorexia nervosa. Int J Eat Disord. 1995;17(4):347-57. [Medline].
145. Bergh C, Brodin U, Lindberg G, Sodersten P. Randomized controlled trial of a treatment for anorexia and bulimia nervosa. Proc Natl Acad Sci USA. 2002;99(14):9486-91. [Medline].
146. McIntosh VV, Jordan J, Carter FA, et al. Three psychotherapies for anorexia nervosa: a randomized, controlled trial. Am J Psychiatry. 2005;162(4):741-7. [Medline].
147. Geist R, Heinmaa M, Stephens D, et al. Comparison of family therapy and family group psychoeducation in adolescents with anorexia nervosa. Can J Psychiatry. 2000;45(2):173-8. [Medline].
148. Robin AL, Siegel PT, Moye A. Family versus individual therapy for anorexia: impact on family conflict. Int J Eat Disord. 1995;17(4):313-22. [Medline].
149. Matzkin V, Slobodianik N, Pallaro A, Bello M, Geissler C. Risk factors for cardiovascular disease in patients with anorexia nervosa. Int J Psychiatr Nurs Res. 2007;13(1):1531-45. [Medline].
150. Facchini M, Sala L, Malfatto G, Bragato R, Redaelli G, Invitti C. Low-K+ dependent QT prolongation and risk for ventricular arrhythmia in anorexia nervosa. Int J Cardiol. 2006;106(2):170-6. [Medline].
151. Golden NH. Eating disorders in adolescence: what is the role of hormone replacement therapy?. Curr Opin Obstet Gynecol. 2007;19(5):434-9. [Medline].
152. Woolrich RA, Cooper MJ, Turner HM. Metacognition in patients with anorexia nervosa, dieting and non-dieting women: a preliminary study. Eur Eat Disord Rev; 2007. [Medline].
153. Gowers SG. Management of eating disorders in children and adolescents. Arch Dis Child. 2008;93(4):331-4. [Medline].
154. Muscari M. Effective management of adolescents with anorexia and bulimia. J Psychosoc Nurs Ment Health Serv. 2002;40(2):22-31. [Medline].
155. Witte TK, Merrill KA, Stellrecht NE, Bernert RA, Hollar DL, Schatschneider C. "Impulsive" youth suicide attempters are not necessarily all that impulsive. J Affect Disord; 2007. [Medline].

Autism Spectrum Disorder

156. American Psychiatric Association. Diagnostic and Statistical Manual of Mental Disorders, 4th edition, text revision. DSM IV TR. 1994:69-84.

157. American Psychiatric Association. Diagnostic and Statistical Manual of Mental Disorders, 5th edition. DSM 5. 2013:50-59.
158. Rutter M. Treatment of autism. Journal of Child Psychology and Psychiatry. 2008;26:759-97.
159. Wiley Clinical Child Psychiatry, 2nd edition, 371-89.
160. Kanner L. Autistic Disturbances of Affective contact. Nervous child. 1943;2:431-8.
161. Lotter V. Epidemiology of autistic conditions in young children. Social Psychiatry. 1966;1:124-37.
162. Baird G, Simonoff E, Pickles A, Chandler S, Loucas T, Meldrum D, et al. Prevalence of disorders of the autism spectrum in a population cohort of children in South Thames: The Special Needs and Autism Project (SNAP). Lancet. 2006;368:210-5.
163. Fombonne E. The epidemiology of autism: A review. Psychological Med. 1999;29:769-86.
164. Treffet DA. Epidemiology of infantile autism. Archive of general Psychiatry. 1970;22:431-8.
165. Zwaigenbaum L, Bryson S, Rogers T, Roberts W, Brian J, Szatmari P. Behavioural manifestations of autism in the first year of life. International Journal of Developmental Neuroscience. 2006;23:143-52.
166. Kidd PM. Autism, an extreme challenge to integrative medicine. Part 1: The knowledge base. Alternative Medicine Review. 2002;7:292-16.
167. Bailey A, Le Couteur A, Gottesman I, et al. Autism as a strongly genetic disorder: evidence from a British twin study. Psychological Med. 1995;25:63-77.
168. Murphy M, Bolton PF, Pickles A, et al. Personality traits of the relatives of autistic probands. Psychological Med. 2000;30:1411-24.
169. Philip J. Landrigan. What causes autism? Exploring the environmental contribution. Current Opinion in Paediatrics. 2010;22:219-22.
170. Rodier PM. Converging evidence for brain stem injury in autism. Dev Psychopathological. 2002;14:537-57.
171. Moore SJ, Turnpenny P, Quinn A, et al. A clinical study of 57 children with foetal anticonvulsant syndromes. J Med Genet. 2000;37:489-97.
172. Bandim JM, Ventura LO, Miller MT, et al. Autism and Mobius sequence: an exploratory study of children in north-eastern Brazil. Arq Neuropsiquiatr. 2003;61(2A):181-5.
173. Chess S. Autism in children with congenital rubella. J Autism Child Schizophrenic. 1971;1:33-47.
174. Hornig M, Lipkin, WI. Infectious and immune factors in the pathogenesis of neurodevelopmental disorders: Epidemiology, hypotheses, and animal models. Mental Retardation and Developmental Disabilities Research Reviews. 2001;7: 200-10.
175. Grice SJ, Halit H, Farroni T, Baron-Cohen S, Bolton P and Johnson, MH Neural correlates of eye-gaze detection in young children with autism. Cortex. 2005;41:342-53.
176. Fombonne E. Epidemiological trends in rates of autism. Molecular Psychiatry. 2002;7:S4-S6.
177. Volkmar FR, Rutter M. Childhood disintegrative disorder: Results of the DSM-IV autism field trial. Journal of the American Academy of Child and Adolescent Psychiatry. 1995;34:1092-5.
178. Corbett J, Harris R, Taylor E, Trible M. Progressive integrative psychosis of childhood. Journal of Child Psychology and Psychiatry. 1977;18:211-9.
179. Kozinetz CA, Skender ML, MacNaughton N, Almes MJ, Schultz RJ, Percy AK, et al. Epidemiology of Rett syndrome: A population-based registry. Paediatrics. 1993;91:445-50.
180. American Psychiatric Association. Pocket book to DSM-5. 2013: 12-28.
181. Krakowiak P, Goodlin-Jones B, Hertz-Picciotto I, Croen LA, Hansen RL. Sleep problems in children with autism spectrum disorders, developmental delays, and typical development: a population-based study. Journal of Sleep Research. 2008;17(2):197-206.
182. Volkmar FR. "Medical Problems, Treatments, and Professionals." in Powers MD (Ed.) Children with Autism: A Parent's Guide, 2nd edition, Bethesda: Woodbine House, 2000.
183. Smalley SL. Autism and tuberous sclerosis. Journal of Autism and Developmental Disorders. 1998;28(5):407-14.
184. Leyfer OT, Folstein SE, Bacalman S, Davis NO, Dinh E, Morgan J, Tager-Flusberg H, Lainhart JE. Comorbid psychiatric disorders in children with autism: interview development and rates of disorders. Journal of Autism and Developmental Disorders. 2006;36(7):849-61.
185. Reichow B, Wolery M. Comprehensive synthesis of early intensive behavioral interventions for young children with autism based on the UCLA young autism project model. Journal of Autism and Developmental Disorders. 2009;39(1):23-41.
186. Charman T, Baird G. Practitioner review: Diagnosis of autism spectrum disorder in 2- and 3-year-old children. Journal of Child Psychology and Psychiatry and Allied Disciplines. 2002;43:289-305.
187. Kabot S, Masi W, Segal M. Advances in the diagnosis and treatment of autism spectrum disorders. Professional Psychology. 2003;34:26-33.
188. Rutter M. The treatment of autistic children. Journal of Child Psychology and Psychiatry. 1985;26:193-214.
189. Van der Gaag RJ. Multiplex developmental disorder: An exploration of borderlines on the autistic spectrum. Utrecht: Unpublished thesis, Utrecht University, 1993.
190. Mesibov G, Shea V, Schopler E. The TEACCH approach to autism spectrum disorders. New York: Plenum Press, 2004.
191. McCracken JT, McGough J, Shah B, Cronin P, Hong D, Aman MG, et al. Risperidone in children with autism and serious behavioral problems. New England Journal of Medicine. 2002;5:314-21.
192. Myers SM, Johnson CP. Management of children with autism spectrum disorders. Pediatrics. 2007;120(5):1162-82.
193. DeLong GR, Teague LA, McSwain KM. Effects of fluoxetine treatment in young children with idiopathic autism. Developmental Medicine and Child Neurology. 1998;40:551-62.

194. Research Units on Pediatric Psychopharmacology Autism Network. Randomized, controlled, crossover trial of methylphenidate in pervasive developmental disorders with hyperactivity. Archives of General Psychiatry. 2005;62(11): 1266-74.
195. Hollander E, Dolgoff-Kaspar R, Cartwright C, Rawitt R and Novotny S. An open trial of divalproex sodium in autism spectrum disorders. Journal of Clinical Psychiatry. 2001;62:530-4.
196. Fankhauser MP, Karumanchi VC, German ML, Yates A, Karumanchi SD: A double-blind, placebo-controlled study of the efficacy of transdermal clonidine in autism. J Clin Psychiatry. 1992;53:77-82.
197. Daniel A. Rossignol. Novel and emerging treatments for autism spectrum disorders: A systematic review. Annals of Clinical Psychiatry. 2009;21(4):213-36.
198. Dario Siniscalco. Stem Cell Research: An Opportunity for Autism Spectrum Disorders Treatment. Autism - Open Access. Siniscalco, Autism. 2012;2:2.
199. Batliwalla BM. A case study of a child showing schizophrenic behaviour. Indian Journal of Psychiatry. 1959;3:251-4.
200. Krishnamurthy V. A clinical experience of autism in India. Journal of Developmental and Behavioural Paediatrics. 2008;29(4):331-3.
201. Daley T, Sigman M. Diagnostic conceptualization of autism among Indian psychiatrists, psychologists, and paediatricians. Journal of Autism and Developmental Disorders. 2002;32(1):13-23.
202. Narayanan HS. A report of clinical observations and management in 7 cases of childhood autism. Indian Journal of Psychiatry. 1978;20:93-7.
203. Srinath S, Chowdhury J, Bhide AV, Narayanan HS and Shivaprakash. Descriptive study of infantile autism Nimhans Journal. 1989;7(1):77-81.
204. Malhotra S, Gupta N. Childhood disintegrative disorder - reexamination of the current concept. European Child and Adolescent Psychiatry. 2002;11:108-14.
205. Malhotra S, Vikas A. Pervasive Developmental Disorders: Indian Scene. JIACAM. 2008;1(3):1-11.
206. Brugha T, Cooper SA, McManus S, Purdon S, Smith J, Scott FJ, et al. Estimating the prevalence of autism spectrum conditions in adults: extending the 2007 Adult Psychiatric Morbidity Survey. NHS, Health and Social Care Information Centre, 2012.
207. Baron-Cohen S, Scott FJ, Allison C, Williams J, Bolton P, Matthews FE, et al. Autism spectrum prevalence: a school-based UK population study. Br J Psychiatry. 2009;194:500-9.
208. Taylor I, Marrable T. Access to social care for adults with autistic spectrum conditions. Social Care Institute for Excellence, University of Sussex, 2011.
209. Brugha ST, McManus S, Bankart J, Scott F, Purdon S, Smith J, et al. Epidemiology of autism spectrum disorders in adults in the community in England. Arch Gen Psychiatry. 2011;65:459-65.
210. Attwood T. Asperger's syndrome. Jessica Kingsley, 1997.
211. National Institute for Health and Clinical Excellence. Autism: recognition, referral and diagnosis of children and young people on the autism spectrum. (Clinical guideline 128) 2011. http://guidance.nice.org.uk/CG128.
212. Baird G, Simonoff E, Pickles A, Chandler S, Loucas T, Meldrum D, et al. Prevalence of disorders of the autism spectrum in a population cohort of children in South Thames: the Special Needs and Autism Project (SNAP). Lancet. 2006;368:210-5.
213. Barnard J, Harvey V, Potter D, Prior A. Ignored or ineligible? The reality for adults with autism spectrum disorders. National Autistic Society, 2001.
214. National Institute for Health and Clinical Excellence. Autism: recognition, referral, diagnosis and management of adults on the autism spectrum. (Clinical guideline 142) 2012. http://guidance.nice.org.uk/CG142.
215. National Institute for Health and Clinical Excellence. Service user experience in adult mental health: improving the experience of care for people using adult NHS mental health services. (Clinical guideline 136) 2011. http://guidance.nice.org.uk/CG136.
216. Allison C, Auyeung B, Baron-Cohen S. Towards brief "red flags" for autism screening: the short Autism Spectrum Quotient and the Short Quantitative Checklist for Autism in Toddlers in 1,000 cases and 3,000 controls. J Am Acad Child Adolesc Psychiatry. 2012;51:202-12.
217. Punshon C, Skirrow P, Murphy, G. The "not guilty verdict": psychological reactions to a diagnosis of Asperger syndrome in adulthood. Autism. 2009;13:265-83.
218. Nylander L, Gillberg C. Screening for autism spectrum disorders in adult psychiatric out-patients: a preliminary report. Acta Psychiatr Scand. 2001;103:428-34.
219. Esbensen AJ, Greenberg JS, Seltzer MM, Aman MG. A longitudinal investigation of psychotropic and non-psychotropic medication use among adolescents and adults with autism spectrum disorders. J Autism Dev Disord. 2009;39:1339-49.

Child Sexual Abuse: Current Scenario in India

220. Behere PB, Mulmule A. Sexual abuse in eight year old girl: Where do we stand legally? Ind J of Psycho Med. 2011;35(2): 30-2.
221. Behere PB, Mulmule A. Sexual abuse in children: Where are we heading? The Journal of Mahatma Gandhi Institute of Medical Sciences. 2008;18(1):6-11.
222. Behere PB, Mulmule A. Guest Editorial, Sexual abuse in women and Anti Rape bill: Lesson to learn from success and failure. The Health Agenda. 2013;1(2):27-30.
223. The protection of children from sexual offence bill, 2012. As passed by the Rajya Sabha on 10th May, 2012 (Last accessed 2012 Dec 20).

224. United Nations Study on violence against children. Available from: www.Unicef.org/violencestudy/reports.html. (Last accessed 2012 Dec 25).
225. Prevalence of child Sexual Abuse in Community and student samples: A Meta-Analysis. Available from: www.journalistsresource.org/studies. (Last accessed 2012 Dec 20).
226. National Crime Record Bureau 2011. Available from: ncrb.nic.in/chapter 6:crime against children, page 91, 95(89-98). (Last accessed 2012 Dec 30).
227. "Study on Child Abuse: India 2007" (PDF). Published by the Government of India, (Ministry of Women and Child Development). Available from: http://wcd.nic.in/childabuse.pdf. (Last accessed 2012 Dec 25).
228. Law against Rape, Punishment of Rape. Available from: www.businesswonder.com/Articles/(Last accessed 2013 March 13).
229. Available from: Childlineindia.org.in/cifgoals.htm. (Last accessed 2012 October 10).
230. Justice JS Verma Committee Report on Amendments to Criminal Law 23 Jan 2013. Available from: Http://ibnlive.in.com/news/full-text-justice-js-verma-committe-report-on-amendments-to-criminal-law/317383-53.html. (Last accessed 2013 January 26).
231. Anti Rape Bill. The Times of India. Available from: http://articles.timesofindia.indiatimes.com/(Last accessed 2013 March 22).
232. Roland et al. "The child sexual abuse accommodation syndrome". Child Abuse Negl. 2007;7(2):177-93.
233. Child Sexual Abuse—WHO, Available from www.who.int/violence_injury_prevention/.../en/guidelines_chap7 (last accessed 2013 October 5).
234. Rohde P, Ichikawa L, Simon G, Ludman E, Linde J, Jeffrey R, et al. Associations of child sexual and physical abuse with obesity and depression in middle-aged women. Child Abuse and Neglect. 2002;32:878-87.
235. Chapman D, Whitfield C, Felitti V, Dube S, Edwards V, Anda, R. Adverse childhood experiences and the risk of depressive disorders in adulthood. J Affect Dis. 82, 217-25.
236. Mouzos J, Makkai T. Women's experiences of male violence. Findings from the Australian component of the International Violence Against Women Survey (IVAWS). Canberra: Australian Institute of Crimonology. Available from: <http://www.aic.gov.au/documents/(Last accessed 17: 2014 Jan 30).
237. Faulkner N. Sexual abuse bibliography and references. Available from: http://www.prevent abuse now.com/. (Last accessed on 2013 May 10).
238. Ganjapure V. State formulates new guidelines for cops probing rape cases. Times of India. September 15, 2013. Available from: http://articles.timesofindia.indiatimes.com/(Last accessed on 2013 October 7).
239. Guidelines for the media in addressing the issue of child sexual abuse. Available from: nhrc.nic.in/Documents/Guidelines-forthemedia.pdf. (Last accessed on 2013 January 18).

Developmental Child Psychopathology

240. Achenbach TM. Research in Developmental Psychology: Concepts, Strategies and Methods. New York: Free Press; 1978.
241. Bhattacharya NL. Prasuthitantram, Streerogaa and Koumar Bhrutyam. Trans. Mysore: Government Ayurvedic and Unani College; 1956.
242. Khatri AA. Personality and mental health of Indians (Hindus) in the context of their changing family organization. In: Anthony EJ, Koupemik C (Eds). The Child in His Family. New York: Wiley; 1970, Vol. 1.
243. Ramanujam BK. Studies of changes in BM Institute of Mental Health. In: Roland CA (Ed). Psychoanalytic perspective of personality development in India. Samiksha. 1976;31(3):47-68.
244. Nandi A. Woman vs. womanliness in India: An essay in social and political psychology. In: Roland CA (Ed). Psychoanalytic perspective on personality in India. Samiksha. 1976;31(3):47-68.
245. Hoch EM. Research on cultural patterns and psychological development. ICMR Task Force Report on Psychological Problems of Children. New Delhi: ICMR; 1980.
246. Kalkar S. The Inner World: A Psychonalytic Study of Childhood and Society in India. New York: Oxford University Press; 1978.
247. Bassa DM. From the traditional to the modern: Some observations on changes in Indian parental and child rearing with special reference to identity formation. In: Anthony EJ, Koupemik C (Eds). The Child in His Family. New York: John Wiley; 1978, Vol. 1.
248. Roland CA. Psychoanalytic perspective on personality development in India. Samiksha. 1976;31(3):47-68.
249. Anandalakshmy S. Development processes. In: Pareek U (Ed). A Survey of Research in Psychology. 1971-76. Part II. Indian Council of Social Science Research. Bombay: Popular Prakashan; 1980.
250. Piaget J. The Child's Conception of the World. New York: Harcourt, Brace & World; 1929.
251. Chomksy N. Syntactic Structure. Hague: Mouton; 1957.
252. Skinner BF. Verbal Behaviour. New York: Appleton Century Crofts; 1957.
253. Freud S. The Ego and the Id. In: Standard Edition. London: Hogarth Press; 1923, Vol. 19.
254. Freud A. The concept of developmental lines. Psychonalytic Study of the Child. 1963;18:245-66.
255. Freud A. Normality and Pathology in Childhood. New York: International Universities Press; 1965.
256. Klein M. Contributions to Psychoanalysis; 1921-1945. London: Hogarth Press; 1948.
257. Mahler MS. On Human Symbiosis and the Vicissitudes of Individuation. New York: International University Press; 1968.
258. Erikson EH. Childhood and Society. New York: Norton; 1950.
259. Harlow H. Nature of love. Am Psychologist. 1958;13:673-85.
260. Bowlby J. Attachment and Loss. New York: Basic Books; 1980;Vol. 3.

261. Ainsworth MDS. The development of infant-mother attachment. In: Caldwell BM, Ricciuti HN (Eds). Review of Child Development and Research. Chicago: University of Chicago Press; 1973;3:1-94.
262. Thomas A, Chess S. Temperament and Development. New York: Brunner/Mazel; 1977.
263. Malhotra S, Malhotra A, Randhawa A. A child's temperament: Factorial validity. Indian J Clin Psy; 1983.pp.79-84.
264. American Psychiatric Association. Diagnostic and Statistical Manual of Mental Disorders, 4th edition, Washington DC: American Psychiatric Association; 1994.
265. Rutter M, Shaffer D, Shepherd M. A multiaxial classification of child psychiatric disorders. Geneva: WHO; 1975.
266. Garber J. Classification of childhood psychopathology: A development perspective. Child Develop; 1984;55:30-48.
267. Anthony EJ. The behaviour disorder of childhood. In: Mussen PH (Ed). Carmichael's Manual of Child Psychology. New York: John Wiley; 1970.
268. Achenbach TM, Edelbrock CS. The classification of child psychopathology: A review and analysis of empirical efforts. Psychol Bull; 1978;85:1275-301.
269. Kagan J, Moss HA. Birth to maturity: A study in psychological development. New York: John Wiley; 1962.
270. Lapouse R, Monk MA. An epidemiologic study of behaviour characteristics in children. Am J Publ Health; 1958;48: 1134-14.
271. Ritvo ER. Autism from adjective to noun. In: Ritvo ER (Ed). Autism: Diagnosis, Current Research and Management. New York: Spectrum; 1976.
272. Kanner L. Child Psychiatry, 4th edition, Springfield: Thomas; 1972 (Republished 1979).
273. Ommen A. A study of hyperkinetic syndrome of childhood. Unpublished doctoral thesis, Bangalore University; 1989.
274. Robins L. Deviant Children Grow Up. Baltimore: Williams and Wilkins; 1966.
275. Rutter M, Garmezy N. Developmental psychopathology. In: Handbook of Child Psychology. New York: John Wiley; 1983.
276. Uma H. Study of hysteria. Unpublished doctoral thesis. Bangalore University; 1988.
277. Ninan TP, Kapur M. A study of hysteria in early adolescence. NIMHANS J; 1989;7:43-7.
278. Rozario J. An epidemiological survey of prevalence and pattern of disturbances of school-going early adolescents. Unpublished M. Phil. dissertation, Bangalore University; 1988.
279. John A, Kapur M. Scholastic backwardness in a child guidance clinic population. NIMHANS J; 1986;4:55-9.
280. John A. A study of scholastic backwardness in a Child Guidance Clinic. Unpublished doctoral thesis, Bangalore University; 1988.
281. Erickson MT. Child Psychopathology. New York: Prentice Hall; 1978.
282. Rutter H (Ed). Scientific Foundations of Developmental Psychiatry. London: Heinemann Medical; 2006.

Mental Retardation/Intellectual Disability

283. Schroeder S, Gerry M, Gertz G, Velasquez F. Final Project Report: Usage of the Term "Mental Retardation:" Language, Image and Public Education. Social Security Administration; 2002.
284. American Psychiatric Association. APA DSM-5 Development: Proposed Revision: Mental Retardation. American Psychiatric Association DSM-5 Development. Available at http://www.dsm5.org/ProposedRevisions/Pages/proposedrevision.aspx?rid=384. Accessed; 2010.
285. Birch HG, Richardson SA, Baird D, Horobin G, Illsley R. Mental Subnormality in the Community: A Clinical and Epidemiologic Study. Baltimore: Williams & Wilkins; 1970.
286. Patja K, Mölsä P, Iivanainen M. Cause-specific mortality of people with intellectual disability in a population-based, 35-year follow-up study. J Intellect Disabil Res. 2001;45:30-40. [Medline].
287. Rutter M, Graham P. Epidemiology of psychiatric disorder. In: Rutter M, Tizard J, Whitemore P (Eds). Education, Health and Behavior. London, England: Longman Group; 1970.pp.178-201.
288. Strauss D, Eyman RK. Mortality of people with mental retardation in California with and without Down syndrome, 1986-1991. Am J Ment Retard. 1996;100(6):643-53. [Medline].
289. American Psychiatric Association. Diagnostic and Statistical Manual of Mental Disorders. 4th edition, Text Revision. Washington DC: American Psychiatric Association; 2000.
290. Shattuck PT. The contribution of diagnostic substitution to the growing administrative prevalence of autism in US special education. Pediatrics. 2006;117(4):1028-37. [Medline].
291. Moeschler JB, Shevell M. Clinical genetic evaluation of the child with mental retardation or developmental delays. Pediatrics. 2006;117(6):2304-16. [Medline].
292. Courchesne E, Carper R, Akshoomoff N. Evidence of brain overgrowth in the first year of life in autism. JAMA. 2003;290(3):337-44. [Medline].
293. Dawson G, Munson J, Webb SJ, Nalty T, Abbott R, Toth K. Rate of head growth decelerates and symptoms worsen in the second year of life in autism. Biol Psychiatry. 2007;61(4):458-64. [Medline].
294. Kenneth Lyons Jones. Smith's Recognizable Patterns of Human Malformations. Elsevier Saunders; 2006.pp.160-1.
295. Kaufmann WE, Abrams MT, Chen W. Genotype, molecular phenotype, and cognitive phenotype: correlations in fragile X syndrome. Am J Med Genet. 1999;83(4):286-95. [Medline].
296. Greenberg F, Lewis RA, Potocki L. Multi-disciplinary clinical study of Smith-Magenis syndrome (deletion 17p11.2). Am J Med Genet. 1996;62(3):247-54. [Medline].
297. Tassabehji M, Metcalfe K, Fergusson WD. LIM-kinase deleted in Williams syndrome [letter]. Nat Genet. 1996;13(3):272-3. [Medline].
298. Verhoeven WM, Tuinier S, Kuijpers HJ, Egger JI, Brunner HG. Psychiatric Profile in Rubinstein-Taybi Syndrome. A Review and Case Report. Psychopathology. 2009;43(1):63-8. [Medline].

299. Marques Pereira P, Schneider A, Pannetier S, Heron D, Hanauer A. Coffin-Lowry syndrome. Eur J Hum Genet; 2009. [Medline].
300. Amir RE, Van den Veyver IB, Wan M. Rett syndrome is caused by mutations in X-linked MECP2, encoding methyl-CpG-binding protein 2. Nat Genet. 1999;23(2):185-8. [Medline].
301. Axelrad ME, Schwartz DD, Fehlis JE, Hopkins E, Stabley DL, Sol-Church K, et al. Longitudinal course of cognitive, adaptive, and behavioral characteristics in Costello syndrome. Am J Med Genet A. 2009;149A(12):2666-72. [Medline].
302. Gripp KW, Lin AE, Stabley DL. HRAS mutation analysis in Costello syndrome: genotype and phenotype correlation. Am J Med Genet A. 2006;140(1):1-7. [Medline].
303. Autti-Ramo I, Fagerlund A, Ervalahti N. Fetal alcohol spectrum disorders in Finland: Clinical delineation of 77 older children and adolescents. Am J Med Genet A. 2006;140(2):137-43. [Medline].
304. Mann JR, McDermott S, Barnes TL, Hardin J, Bao H, Zhou L. Trichomoniasis in pregnancy and mental retardation in children. Ann Epidemiol. 2009;19(12):891-9. [Medline].
305. Moeschler JB, Shevell M. Clinical genetic evaluation of the child with mental retardation or developmental delays. Pediatrics. 2006;117(6):2304-16. [Medline].
306. Shevell M, Ashwal S, Donley D, Flint J, Gingold M, Hirtz D. Practice parameter: evaluation of the child with global developmental delay: report of the Quality Standards Subcommittee of the American Academy of Neurology and The Practice Committee of the Child Neurology Society. Neurology. 2003;60(3):367-80. [Medline].
307. Mefford HC, Batshaw ML, Hoffman EP. Genomics, intellectual disability, and autism. N Engl J Med. 2012;366(8):733-43. [Medline].
308. Liang JS, Shimojima K, Yamamoto T. Application of array-based comparative genome hybridization in children with developmental delay or mental retardation. Pediatr Neonatol. 2008;49(6):213-7. [Medline].
309. Sagoo GS, Butterworth AS, Sanderson S, Shaw-Smith C, Higgins JP, Burton H. Array CGH in patients with learning disability (mental retardation) and congenital anomalies: updated systematic review and meta-analysis of 19 studies and 13,926 subjects. Genet Med. 2009;11(3):139-46. [Medline].
310. Michelson DJ, Shevell MI, Sherr EH, Moeschler JB, Gropman AL, Ashwal S. Evidence report: Genetic and metabolic testing on children with global developmental delay: report of the Quality Standards Subcommittee of the American Academy of Neurology and the Practice Committee of the Child Neurology Society. Neurology. 2011;77(17):1629-35. [Medline].
311. Bazzano AT, Zeldin AS, Diab IR, Garro NM, Allevato NA, Lehrer D. The Healthy Lifestyle Change Program: a pilot of a community-based health promotion intervention for adults with developmental disabilities. Am J Prev Med. 2009;37(6 Suppl 1):S201-8. [Medline].
312. Kishnani PS, Sommer BR, Handen BL, Seltzer B, Capone GT, Spiridigliozzi GA, et al. The efficacy, safety, and tolerability of donepezil for the treatment of young adults with Down syndrome. Am J Med Genet A. 2009;149A(8):1641-54. [Medline].
313. ACOG Committee Opinion. Number 371. July 2007. Sterilization of women, including those with mental disabilities. Obstet Gynecol. 2007;110(1):217-20. [Medline].
314. Bartlo P, Klein PJ. Physical activity benefits and needs in adults with intellectual disabilities: systematic review of the literature. Am J Intellect Dev Disabil. 2011;116(3):220-32. [Medline].
315. Rueda JR, Ballesteros J, Tejada MI. Systematic review of pharmacological treatments in fragile X syndrome. BMC Neurol. 2009;9:53. [Medline].
316. Ellis JM, Tan HK, Gilbert RE, Muller DP, Henley W, Moy R, et al. Supplementation with antioxidants and folinic acid for children with Down's syndrome: randomised controlled trial. BMJ. 2008;336(7644):594-7. [Medline].
317. Wigal T, Greenhill L, Chuang S, McGough J, Vitiello B, Skrobala A. Safety and tolerability of methylphenidate in preschool children with ADHD. J Am Acad Child Adolesc Psychiatry. 2006;45(11):1294-303. [Medline].
318. Massachusetts Department of Developmental Services. Massachusetts Department of Developmental Services Annual Health Screening Recommendations. Available at http://www.mass.gov/Eeohhs2/docs/dmr/health_screening_checklist.pdf. Accessed; 2010.
319. Bull MJ. Health supervision for children with Down syndrome. Pediatrics. 2011;128(2):393-406. [Medline].
320. [Guideline] McCandless SE, Committee on Genetics. Clinical report—health supervision for children with Prader-Willi syndrome. Pediatrics. 2011;127(1):195-204. [Medline].

Sleep Disorders in Children and Adolescents

321. Ohayon MM, Roberts RE, Zulley J, Smirne S, Priest RG. Prevalence and patterns of problematic sleep among older adolescents. J Am Acad Child Adolesc Psychiatry. 2000;39:1549-56.[CrossRef][ISI][Medline]
322. American Psychiatric Association. Diagnostic and Statistical Manual of Mental Disorders, 4th edition, Washington, DC: American Psychiatric Association; 1994.
323. Millman RP. Excessive sleepiness in adolescents and young adults: causes, consequences, and treatment strategies. Pediatrics. 2005;115:1774-86.[Abstract/Free Full Text]
324. Hamada T, LeSauter J, Venuti JM, Silver R. Expression of Period genes: rhythmic and nonrhythmic compartments of the suprachiasmatic nucleus pacemaker. J Neurosci. 2001;21:7742-50.[Abstract/Free Full Text]
325. Sakurai T, Amemiya A, Ishii M, Matsuzaki I, Chemelli RM, Tanaka H, et al. Orexins and orexin receptors: a family of hypothalamic neuropeptides and G protein-coupled receptors that regulate feeding behaviour. Cell. 1998;92:573-85.[CrossRef][ISI][Medline]
326. Saper CB, Chou TC, Scammell TE. The sleep switch: hypothalamic control of sleep and wakefulness. Trends Neurosci. 2001;24:726-31.[CrossRef][ISI][Medline]

327. Carskadon MA, Wolfson AR, Acebo C, Tzischinsky O, Tzischinsky O, Seifer R. Adolescent sleep patterns, circadian timing, and sleepiness at a transition to early school days. Sleep. 1998;21:871-81.[ISI][Medline]
328. Carskadon MA. The second decade. In: Sleeping and waking disorders. Indications and techniques. Menlo Park: Addison-Wesley; 1982.pp.1-16.
329. Wolfson AR. Bridging the gap between research and practice: What will adolescent's sleep-wake patterns look like in the 21st century? In: Carskadon MA, (Ed). Adolescent sleep patterns. Biological, social and psychological influences. Cambridge: Cambridge University Press; 2002.p.200.
330. Kotagal S, Silber MH. Childhood onset restless legs syndrome. Ann Neurol. 2004;56:803-7.[CrossRef][ISI][Medline]
331. Walters AS. Is there a subpopulation of children with growing pains who really have restless legs syndrome? A review of the literature. Sleep Med. 2002;3:93-8.[CrossRef][Medline]
332. Chervin RD, Archbold KH, Dillon JE, Pituch KJ, Panahi P, Dahl RE. Association between symptoms of inattention, hyperactivity, restless legs, and periodic leg movements. Sleep. 2002;25:213-8.[ISI][Medline]
333. Challamel MJ, Mazzola ME, Nevsimalova S, Cannard C, Louis J, Revol M. Narcolepsy in children. Sleep. 1994;17(Suppl):17-20.
334. Dauvilliers Y, Carlander B, Rivier F, Touchon J, Tafti M. Successful management of cataplexy with intravenous immunoglobulins at narcolepsy onset. Ann Neurol. 2004;56: 905-8.[CrossRef][ISI][Medline]
335. Archer SN, Robilliard DL, Skene DJ, Smits M, Williams A, Arendt J, et al. A length polymorphism in the circadian clock gene Per3 is linked to delayed sleep phase syndrome and extreme diurnal preference. Sleep. 2003;26:413-5.[ISI][Medline]
336. Rosen CL, Larkin EK, Kirchner HL, Emancipator JL, Bivins SF, Surovec SA, et al. Prevalence and risk factors for sleep-disordered breathing in 8- to 11-year-old children: association with race and prematurity. J Pediatr. 2003;142:383-9.[CrossRef][ISI][Medline]
337. Marcus CL, Hamer A, Loughlin GM. Natural history of primary snoring in children. Ped Pulmonol. 1998;26:6-11.&link_type=DOI" >[CrossRef][ISI]
338. Marcus CL, McColley SA, Carroll JL, Loughlin GM, Smith PL, Schwartz AR. Upper airway collapsibility in children with obstructive sleep apnea syndrome. J Applied Physiol. 1994;77:918-24.[Abstract/Free Full Text]
339. Vavrina J. Computer assisted pulse oximetry for detecting children with obstructive sleep apnea syndrome. Int J Pediatric Otorhinolaryngol. 1995;33:239-48.[CrossRef][ISI]
340. Lim J, McKean M. Adenotonsillectomy for obstructive sleep apnoea in children. Cochrane Database Syst Rev. 2005;4:CD003136.
341. Brietzke SE, Katz ES, Roberson DW. Can history and physical examination reliably diagnose pedi-atric obstructive sleep apnea/hyponea syndrome? A systematic review of the literature. Otolaryngol Head Neck Surg. 2004;131:827-32.[CrossRef][ISI][Medline]
342. American Psychiatric Association. Desk Reference to the Diagnostic Criteria from DSM-5. Washington DC; 2013.
343. Mignot E, Taheri S, Nishino S. Sleeping with the hypothalamus: emerging therapeutic targets for sleep disorders. Nature Neurosci. 2002;5:1071-5.[CrossRef][ISI][Medline]

Diagnostic Issues in Childhood Bipolar Disorder

344. McClellan J, Kowatch R, Finding R, et al. Practice parameter for the assessment and treatment of children and adolescents with bipolar disorder. J Am Acad Child Adolesc Psychiatry. 2007;46(1):107-25.
345. Carison GA. Early onset bipolar disorder: clinical and research considerations. J Clin Child Adolesc Psychol. 2005;34(2):333-43.
346. Blader JC, Carlson GA. Increased rates of bipolar disorder diagnoses among U.S. child, adolescent, and adult inpatients. 1996-2004. Biol Psychiatry. 2007;62(2):107-14.
347. Wilens TE, Biederman J, Forkmer P, et al. Patients of comorbidity and dysfunction in clinically referred preschool and school-age children won bipolar disorder. J Childf Adolesc Psychopharmacol. 2003;13(4):495-505.
348. Birmaher B, Axelson D, Pavuluri M. Bipolar disorder. In: Martin A, Volkmar FR, editors. Lewis, Child and adolescent psychiatry: a comprehensive textbook, 4th edition. Baltimore: Lippincott Williams and Wilkims. 2007.pp.513-28.
349. American Psychiatric Association. Diagnostic and statistical manual of mental disorders, 4th edition, Text Revision (DSM-IV-TR). Washington (DC): American Psychiatric Association. 2000.
350. Pvaluri MN, Birmaher B, Naylor M. Pediatric disorder: a review of the past 10 years. J Am Acad Child Adolesc Psychiatry. 2005;44(9):864-71.
351. Demeter CA. Twonsend LD, Wilson M, et al. Current research in child and adolescent bipolar disorder. Dialogues Clin Neurosci. 2008;10(2):215-28.
352. Biederman J, Faraone SV, Wozniak J, et al. Further evidence of unique developmental phenotypic correlates of pediatric bipolar disorder: findings from a large sample of clinically referred preadolescents children assessed over the last 7 years. J Affect Disord. 2004;82:S45-58.
353. Biederman J, Mick E, Faraone SV, et al. A prospective follow-up study of pediatric bipolar disorder in boys with attention-deficit/hyperactivity disorder. J Affect Disord. 2004;82:S17-23.
354. Wozniak J, Biederman, J Kiely K, et al. Mania-like symptoms suggestive of childhood - onset bipolar disorder in clinically referred children. J Am Child Adolesc Psychiatry. 1995;34(7):867-76.
355. Geller B, Zimerman B, Williams M, et al. Prepubertal and young adolescent bipolar phenotype by gender, puberty and comorbid attention deficit hyperactivity disorder. J Child Adolesc Psychopharmacol. 2000;10(3):157-64.
356. Geller B Tillman R, Bolhofner K, et al. Child bipolar I disorder: prospective continuity with adult bipolar I disorder; characteristics of second and third episodes; predictors

of 8-year outcome. Arch Gen Psychiatry. 2008;65(10): 1125-33.
357. Geller B, Warner K, Williams M, et al. Prepubertal and young adolescent bipolarity versus ADHD: assessment and validity using the WASH - U - KSADS, CBCL and TRF. J Affect Disord. 1998;51(2):93-100.
358. Birmaher B. New Hope for Children and Adolescents with BP Disorder. New York: Three Rivers Press, a division of Random House, Inc. 2004.
359. Brent DA, Weersing VR. Chapter 5. 4. 1: Depressive disorders. In: Martin A, Volkmar FR, editors. Lewis Child and Adolescent Psychiatry: a comprehensive textbook, 4th edition. Baltimore: Lippincott Williams and Wilkins. 2007.pp.503-13.
360. Tillman R, Geller B, Bolhofner K, et al. Ages of onset and rates of syndromal and subsyndromal comorbid DSM-IV diagnoses in a prepubertal and early adolescent bipolar disorder phenotype. J Am Acad Child Adolesc Psychiatry. 2003;42(12):1486-93.
361. Weller EB, Weller RA, Danielyan AK, et al. Mood disorders in adolescents. In: Wiener JM, Dulcan MK (Eds). The American Psychiatric Publishing Textbook of Child and Adolescent Psychiatry, 3rd edition. Arlington (VA): American Psychiatric Publishing, Inc; 2004.pp.437-81.
362. Merikangas KR, Akiskal HS, Angst J, et al. Lifetime and 12-month prevalence of bipolar disorder spectrum disorder in the national comorbidity survey replication. Arch Gen Psychiatry. 2007;64(5):543-52.
363. Geller B, Luby J. Child and adolescent bipolar disorder: a review of the past 10 years. J Am Acad Child Adolesc Psychiatry. 1997;36(9):1168-76.
364. Weller EB, Weller RA, Danielyan AK, et al. Mood disorders in prepubertal children. In: Wiener JM, Dulcan MK (Eds). The American Psychiatric Publishing Textbook of Child and Adolescent Psychiatry, 3rd edition. Arlington (VA): American Psychiatric Publishing, Inc; 2004.pp.411-35.
365. Duax JM, Youngstrom EA, Calabrese JR, et al. Sex differences in pediatric bipolar disorder. J Clin Psychiatry. 2007;68(10):1565-73.
366. Belardinelli C, Hatch JP, Olvera RL, et al. Family environment patterns in families with bipolar children. J Affect Disord. 2008;107(1-3):299-305.
367. Birmaher B, Axelson D, Strober M, et al. Clinical course of children and adolescents with bipolar spectrum disorders. Arch Gen Psychiatry. 2006;63(2):175-83.
368. Lewinsohn PM, Rohde P, Seeley JR, et al. Treatment of adolescent depression: frequency of services and impact on functioning in young adulthood. Depress Anxiety. 1998;7(1):47-52.
369. Miklowitz DJ, Chang KD. Prevention of bipolar disorder in at-risk children: theoretical assumptions and empirical foundations. Dev Psychopathol. 2008;20(3):881-97.
370. Masi G, Perugi G, Millepiedi S, et al. Clinical implications of DSM-IV subtyping of bipolar disorders in referred children and adolescents. J Am Acad Child Adolesc Psychiatry. 2007;46(10):1299-306.

Cognitive-Behavioral Therapy and Dialectical Behavior Therapy in Children and Adolescents

371. Weersing R, Brent D. Cognitive behavioral therapy for depression in youth. Child Adolesc Psychiatr Clin N Am. 2006;15:939-57
372. Miller AL, Rathus JH, Linehan MM. Dialectical behavior therapy with suicidal adolescents. New York: Guilford Press; 2007.
373. Costello E, Egger H, Angold A. Prevalence and comorbidity. Child Adolesc Psychiatr Clin N Am. 2005;14:631-48.
374. James A, Soler A, Weatherall R. Cognitive behavioral therapy for anxiety disorders in children and adolescents. Cochrane Database Syst Rev. 2005;19(4):CD004690.
375. Kendall P, Flannery-Schroeder E, Panichelli-Mindel S, et al. Treating anxiety disorders in youth: a second randomized clinical trial. J Consult Clin Psychol. 1997;65:366-80.
376. Barret P, Dadds M, Rapee R. Family treatment of childhood anxiety: a controlled trial. J Consult Clin Psychol. 1996;64:333-42.
377. Kendall P. Treating anxiety disorders in youth: results of a randomized clinical trial. J Consult Clin Psychol. 1994;62:100-10.
378. Wood J, Piacentini J, Southam-Gerow M, et al. Family cognitive behavioral therapy for child and anxiety disorders. J Am Acad Child Adolesc Psychiatry. 2006;45:314-21.
379. Flannery-Schroeder E, Kendall P. Group and individual cognitive-behavioral treatments for youth with anxiety disorders: a randomized clinical trial. Cognit Ther Res. 2000;24: 251-78.
380. Chu B, Harrison T. Disorder-specific effects of CBT for anxious and depressed youth: a meta-analysis of candidate mediators of change. Clin Child Fam Psychol Rev. 2007;10:352-72.
381. Cartwright-Huttons S, Roberts C, Chitsabesan P, et al. Systematic review of the efficacy of cognitive-behaviour therapies for childhood and adolescent anxiety disorders. Br J Clin Psychol. 2004;43:421-36.
382. Last C, Hansen C, Franco N. Cognitive-behavioral treatment of school phobia. J Am Acad Child Adolesc Psychiatry. 1998;37:404-11.
383. Silverman W, Kurtines W, Ginsburg G, et al. Contingency management, self control, and education support in the treatment of childhood phobic disorders: a randomized clinical trial. J Consult Clin Psychol. 1999;67:675-87.
384. Muris P, Meesters C, Gobel M. Cognitive coping versus emotional disclosure in the treatment of anxious children: a pilot-study. Cogn Behav Ther. 2002;31:59-67.
385. The Pediatric OCD Treatment Study (POTS) Team. Cognitive-behavior therapy, sertraline, and their combination for children and adolescents with obsessive-compulsive disorder: the pediatric OCD treatment study (POTS) randomized controlled trial. JAMA. 2004;292(16):1969-76.
386. O'Kearney R, Anstey K, von Sanden C. Behavioral and cognitive behavioral therapy for obsessive compulsive disorder in children and adolescents. [review] Cochrane Database Syst Rev. 2006;18(4):CD004856.

387. Watson H, Rees C. Meta-analysis of randomized, controlled treatment trials for pediatric obsessive-compulsive disorder. J Child Psychol Psychiatry. 2008;49(5):489-98.
388. Cohen J, Deblinger E, Mannarino A, et al. A multi-site, randomized controlled trial for children with abuse-related PTSD symptoms. J Am Acad Child Adolesc Psychiatry. 2004;43(4):393-402
389. Deblinger E, Mannarino A, Cohen J, et al. A follow-up study of a multisite, randomized, controlled trial for children with sexual abuse-related PTSD symptoms. J Am Acad Child Adolesc Psychiatry. 2006;45(12):1474-84.
390. Brookman RR, Sood AA. Disorders of mood and anxiety in adolescents. Adolesc Med. 2006;17:79-95.
391. Roblek T, Piacentini J. Cognitive-behavior therapy for childhood anxiety disorders. Child Adolesc Psychiatr Clin N Am. 2005;14:863-76.
392. Creed TA, Kendall PC. Therapist alliance-building behavior within a cognitive-behavioral treatment for anxiety in youth. J Consult Clin Psychol. 2005;73(3):498-505.
393. Barmish AJ, Kendall PC. Should parents be co-clients in cognitive-behavioral therapy for anxious youth? J Clin Child Adolesc Psychol. 2005;34(3):569-81.
394. Hudson JL, Kendall PC. Showing you can do it: homework in therapy for children and adolescents with anxiety disorders. J Clin Psychol. 2002;58(5):525-34.
395. Hannesdottir DK, Ollendick TH. The role of emotion regulation in the treatment of child anxiety disorders. Clin Child Fam Psychol Rev. 2007;10:275-93.
396. Piacentini J, Langley AK. Cognitive-behavioral therapy for children who have obsessive-compulsive disorder. J Clin Psychol. 2004;60(11):1181-94.
397. Smith P, Yule W, Perrin S, et al. Cognitive-behavioral therapy for PTSD in children and adolescents: a preliminary randomized controlled trial. J Am Acad Child Adolesc Psychiatry. 2007;46(8):1051-61.
398. Shooshtary MH, Panaghi L, Moghadam JA. Outcome of cognitive behavioral therapy in adolescents after natural disaster. J Adolesc Health. 2008;42:466-72.
399. Lewinsohn P, Clarke G. Psychosocial treatments for adolescent depression. Clin Psychol Rev. 1999;19:329-42.
400. Reinecke M, Ryan N, Dubois D. Cognitive-behavioral therapy of depression and depressive symptoms during adolescence: a review and meta-analysis. J Am Acad Child Adolesc Psychiatry. 1998;37:26-34.
401. Brent D, Holder D, Kolko D, et al. A clinical psychotherapy trial for adolescent depression comparing cognitive, family, and supportive treatments. Arch Gen Psychiatry. 1997;54:877-85.
402. Wood A, Harrington R, Moore A. Controlled trial of a brief cognitive-behavioral intervention in adolescent patients with depressive disorders. J Child Psychol Psychiatry. 1996;37:737-46.
403. Michael K, Crowley S. How effective are treatments for child and adolescent depression? A meta-analytic review. Clin Psychol Rev. 2002;22:247-69.
404. Treatment for Adolescents with Depression Study Team (TADS). Fluoxetine, cognitive-behavioral therapy, and their combination for adolescents with depression: treatment for adolescents with depression study (TADS) randomized controlled trial. JAMA. 2004;292(7):807-20.
405. Goodyer I, Dubicka B, Wilkinson P, et al. Selective serotonin reuptake inhibitors and routine specialist care with and without cognitive behavioral therapy in adolescents with major depression: randomized controlled trial. BMJ. 2007;335(7611):142.
406. Weisz J, McCarty C, Valeri S. Effects of psychotherapy for depression in children and adolescents: a meta-analysis. Psychol Bull. 2006;132(1):132-49.
407. Klein J, Jacobs R, Reinecke M. Cognitive-behavioral therapy for adolescent depression: a meta-analytic investigation of changes in effect-size estimates. J Am Acad Child Adolesc Psychiatry. 2007;46(11):1403-13.
408. Lewinsohn PM, Clarke GN, Hops H, et al. Cognitive-behavioral treatment for depressed adolescents. Behav Ther. 1990;21:385-401.
409. Vostanis P, Feehan C, Grattan E, et al. A randomized controlled outpatient trial of cognitive-behavioral treatment for children and adolescents with depression: 9-month follow-up. J Affect Disord. 1996;40:105-16.
410. Kerfoot M, Harrington R, Harrington V, et al. A step too far? Randomized trial of cognitive-behavior therapy delivered by social workers to depressed adolescents. Eur Child Adolesc Psychiatry. 2004;13(2):92-9.
411. Rohde P, Feeny NC, Robins M. Characteristics and components of the TADS CBT approach. Cogn Behav Pract. 2005;12: 186-97.
412. American Psychiatric Association. Diagnostic and statistical manual, 4th edition. Washington (DC): American Psychiatric Association; 1994.
413. Shirk SR, Gudmundsen G, Kaplinski HC, et al. Alliance and outcome in cognitive-behavioral therapy for adolescent depression. J Clin Child Adolesc Psychol. 2008;37(3):631-9.
414. Clarke GN, Hornbrook M, Lynch F, et al. A randomized trial of a group cognitive intervention for preventing depression in adolescent offspring of depressed parents. Arch Gen Psychiatry. 2001;85:1127-34.
415. Clarke GN, Rohde P, Lewinsohn PM, et al. Cognitive-behavioral treatment of adolescent depression: efficacy of acute group treatment and booster sessions. J Am Acad Child Adolesc Psychiatry. 1999;38:272-79.
416. Linehan MM, Comtois KA, Murray AM, et al. Two year randomized trial and follow-up of dialectical behavior therapy vs. therapy by experts for suicidal behaviors and borderline personality disorder. Arch Gen Psychiatry. 2006;63: 757-66.
417. Verheul R, van den Bosch LM, Koeter MW, et al. Dialectical behavior therapy for women with borderline personality disorder: 12 month randomized clinical trial in the Netherlands. Br J Psychiatry. 2003;182:135-40.

418. Linehan MM. Cognitive-behavioral treatment of borderline personality disorder. New York: Guilford Press; 1993.
419. Rathus JH, Miller AL. Dialectical behavior therapy adapted for suicidal adolescents. Suicide Life Threat Behav. 2002;32: 146-57.
420. Katz LY, Gunasekara S, Cox BJ, et al. Feasibility of dialectical behavior therapy for parasuicidal adolescent inpatients. J Am Acad Child Adolesc Psychiatry. 2004;43:276-82.
421. Katz LY, Cox BJ. Dialectical behavior therapy for suicidal adolescent inpatients: a case study. Clin Case Stud. 2002;1:81-92.
422. Linehan MM. Skills training manual for treating borderline personality disorder. New York: Guilford Press; 1993.
423. Robins P, Smith S, Glutting J, et al. A randomized-controlled trial of a cognitive-behavioral family intervention for pediatric recurrent abdominal pain. J Pediatr Psychol. 2005;30(5):397-408.
424. Sanders M, Rebgetz M, Morrison M, et al. Cognitive-behavioral treatment of recurrent nonspecific abdominal pain in children: an analysis of generalization, maintenance and side effects. J Consult Clin Psychol. 1989;57:294-300.
425. Sanders M, Shepherd R, Cleghorn G, et al. The treatment of recurrent abdominal pain in children: a controlled comparison of cognitive-behavioral family intervention and standard pediatric care. J Consult Clin Psychol. 1994;62:306-14
426. Duarte M, Penna F, Andrade E, et al. Treatment of nonorganic recurrent abdominal pain: cognitive-behavioral family intervention. J Pediatr Gastroenterol Nutr. 2006;43:59-64.
427. Holden E, Deichmann M, Levy J. Empirically supported treatments in pediatric psychology: recurrent pediatric headache. J Pediatr Psychol. 1999;24:91-109.
428. Beames L, Sanders M, Bor W. The role of parent training in the cognitive behavioral treatment of children's headaches. Behav Psychother. 1989;20:167-80.
429. National Collaborating Centre for Mental Health. Eating disorders: core interventions in the treatment and management of anorexia nervosa, bulimia nervosa, and related eating disorders. London: National Institute for Clinical Excellence; 2004.
430. Schmidt U, Lee S, Beecham J, et al. A randomized controlled trial of family therapy and cognitive behavior therapy guided self-care for adolescents with bulimia nervosa and related disorders. Am J Psychiatry. 2007;164:591-98.

Recognition and Management of Psychosis and Schizophrenia in Children and Adolescents

431. Burd L, Kerbeshian J. A North Dakota prevalence study of schizophrenia presenting in childhood. J Am Acad Child Adolesc Psychiatry. 1987;26:347-50.
432. Gillberg C. Epidemiology of early onset schizophrenia. In: Remschmidt H (Ed). Schizophrenia in children and adolescents. Cambridge University Press; 2001.pp.43-59.
433. Thomsen PH. Schizophrenia with childhood and adolescent onset—a nationwide register-based study. Acta Psychiatr Scand. 1996;94:187-93.
434. World Health Organization. Division of Epidemiological Surveillance, Health Situation, and Trend Assessment. Global estimates for health situation assessment and projections 1990. World Health Organization; 1990.
435. Brown S, Kim M, Mitchell C, Inskip H. Twenty-five year mortality of a community cohort with schizophrenia. Br J Psychiatry. 2010;196:116-21.
436. Ruhrmann S, Schultze-Lutter F, Salokangas RKR, Heinimaa M, Linszen D, Dingemans P, et al. Prediction of psychosis in adolescents and young adults at high risk: results from the Prospective European Prediction of Psychosis Study. Arch Gen Psychiatry. 2010;67:241-51.
437. NHS Confederation. Early intervention in psychosis services. Briefing2011(219). www.iris-initiative.org.uk/silo/files/nhs-confederation-briefing-on-early-intervention-in-psychosis.pdf.
438. National Institute for Health and Clinical Excellence. Psychosis and schizophrenia in children and young people: recognition and management. (Clinical guideline 155.) 2013. http://guidance.nice.org.uk/CG155.
439. American Psychiatric Association. Diagnostic and statistical manual of mental disorders, fourth edition. (DSM-IV). American Psychiatric Association; 1994.
440. World Health Organization. The ICD-10 Classification of Mental and Behavioural Disorders: Clinical Descriptions and Diagnostic Guidelines. World Health Organization; 1992.
441. National Institute for Health and Clinical Excellence. Post-traumatic stress disorder (PTSD): the management of PTSD in adults and children in primary and secondary care. (Clinical guideline 26.) 2005. http://guidance.nice.org.uk/CG26.
442. National Institute for Health and Clinical Excellence. Obsessive-compulsive disorder: core interventions in the treatment of obsessive-compulsive disorder and body dysmorphic disorder (Clinical guideline 31.) 2005. http://guidance.nice.org.uk/CG31.
443. National Institute for Health and Clinical Excellence. Depression in children and young people: identification and management in primary, community and secondary care. (Clinical guideline 28.) 2005. http://guidance.nice.org.uk/CG28.
444. National Institute for Health and Clinical Excellence. Borderline personality disorder: treatment and management. (Clinical guideline 78.) 2009. http://guidance.nice.org.uk/CG78.
445. National Institute for Health and Clinical Excellence. Antisocial personality disorder: treatment, management and prevention. (Clinical guideline 77.) 2009. http://guidance.nice.org.uk/CG77.
446. National Institute for Health and Clinical Excellence. Alcohol-use disorders: diagnosis, assessment and management of

harmful drinking and alcohol dependence. (Clinical guideline 115.) 2011. http://guidance.nice.org.uk/CG115.

447. National Institute for Health and Clinical Excellence. Alcohol-use disorders: preventing the development of hazardous and harmful drinking. (Public health guidance 24.) 2010. http://guidance.nice.org.uk/PH24.
448. National Institute for Health and Clinical Excellence. Alcohol-use disorders: diagnosis and clinical management of alcohol-related physical complications. (Clinical guideline 100.) 2010. http://guidance.nice.org.uk/CG100.
449. National Institute for Health and Clinical Excellence. Drug misuse: psychosocial interventions. (Clinical guideline 51.) 2007. http://guidance.nice.org.uk/CG51.
450. National Institute for Health and Clinical Excellence. Drug misuse: opioid detoxification. (Clinical guideline 52.) 2009. http://guidance.nice.org.uk/CG52.
451. National Institute for Health and Clinical Excellence. Schizophrenia: core interventions in the treatment and management of schizophrenia in adults in primary and secondary care. (Clinical guideline 82.) 2009. http://guidance.nice.org.uk/CG82.
452. Pinfold V, Smith J, Shiers D. Audit of early intervention in psychosis service development in England 2005. Psychiatric Bulletin. 2007;31:7-10.
453. Borneo A. Your choice: results from the your treatment, your choice survey 2008— final report. 2008. www.rethink.org/how_we_can_help/our_campaigns/nice_schizophrenia_g.html.
454. Prescribing Observatory for Mental Health. Topic 10b Re-audit report: prescribing antipsychotics for children and adolescents. CCGI119 (data on file). London: Royal College of Psychiatrists, 2012.
455. De Hert M, Dobbelaere M, Sheridan EM, Cohen D, Correll CU. Metabolic and endocrine adverse effects of second-generation antipsychotics in children and adolescents: a systematic review of randomized, placebo controlled trials and guidelines for clinical practice. European Psychiatry. 2011;26:144-58.

Child and Adolescent Psychopathology Update

456. Kessler RC, Wang PS. The descriptive epidemiology of commonly occurring mental disorders in the United States. Annu Rev Public Health. 2008;29:115-29.
457. Vitiello B. Research in child and adolescent psychopharmacology: recent accomplishments and new challenges. Psychopharmacology. 2007;191:5-13.
458. Hoagwood K, Kelleher K, Feil M, et al. Treatment services for children with ADHD: a national perspective. J Am Acad Child Adolesc Psychiatry. 2000;39(2):198-206.
459. McClellan JM, Werry JS. Evidence-based treatments in child and adolescent psychiatry: an inventory. J Am Acad Child Adolesc Psychiatry. 2003;42(12):1388-400.
460. Pliska S, AACAP Work Group on Quality Issues. Practice parameter for the assessment and treatment of children and adolescents with attention-deficit/hyperactivity disorder. J. Am Acad Child Adolesc Psychiatry. 2007;46(7):894-921.
461. Findling R. Evolution of the treatment of attention-deficit/hyper-activity disorder in children: a review. Clin Ther. 2008;30(5): 942-57.
462. Swanson J, Wigal S, Wigal T, et al. A comparison of once-daily extended-release methylphenidate formulations in children with attention-deficit/hyperactivity disorder in the laboratory school (The COMACS study). Pediatrics. 2004;113(3): 206-16.
463. Pelham W, Sturges J, Hoza J, et al. Sustained release and standard methylphenidate effects on cognitive and social behavior in children with attention deficit disorder. Pediatrics. 1987;80(4):491-501.
464. Brown G, Ebert M, Mikkelse E, et al. Behavior and motor activity response in hyperactive children and plasma amphetamine levels following a sustained release preparation. J Am Acad Child Psychiatry. 1980;19:225-39.
465. Findling R, Bukstein O, Melmed R, et al. A randomized, double-blind, placebo-controlled, parallel-group study of methylphenidate transdermal system in pediatric patients with attention-deficit/hyperactivity disorder. J Clin Psychiatry. 2008;69:149-59.
466. Wilens T, Boellner S, Lopez F, et al. Varying the wear time of the methylphenidate transdermal system in children with attention-deficit/hyperactivity disorder. J Am Acad Child Adolesc Psychiatry. 2008;47(6):700-8.
467. Wigal S, Swanson J, Fiefel D, et al. A double-blind, placebo-controlled trial of dexmethylphenidate hydrochloride and d,l-threo-methylphenidate hydrochloride in children with attention-deficit/hyperactivity disorder. J Am Acad Child Adolesc Psychiatry. 2004;43(11):1406-14.
468. Muniz R, Brams M, Mao A, et al. Efficacy and safety of extended-release dexmethylphenidate compared with d,l-methylphenidate and placebo in the treatment of children with attention-deficit/hyperactivity disorder: a 12-hour laboratory classroom study. J Child Adolesc Psychopharmacol. 2008;15(3):248-56.
469. Biederman J, Boellner S, Childress A, et al. Lisdexamfetamine dimesylate and mixed amphetamine salts extended-release in children with ADHD: a double-blind, placebo-controlled, crossover analog classroom study. Biol Psychiatry. 2007;62:970-76.
470. Du Y, Li F, Vance A, et al. Randomized double-blind multicentre placebo-controlled clinical trial of the clonidine adhesive patch for the treatment of tic disorders. Aust N Z J Psychiatry. 2008;42(9):807-13.
471. Gaffney G, Perry P, Lund B, et al. Risperidone versus clonidine in the treatment of children and adolescents with Tourette's syndrome. J. Am Acad Child Adolesc Psychiatry. 2002;41(3):330-6.
472. Cummings D, Singer H, Krieger M, et al. Neuropsychiatric effects of guanfacine in children with mild Tourette syndrome: a pilot study. Clin Neuropharmacol. 2002;25(6):325-32.

473. Kurlan R, Goetz C, McDermott M, et al. Treatment of ADHD in children with tics: a randomized controlled trial. Neurology. 2002;58:527-36.
474. Biederman J, Melmed R, Patel A, et al. A randomized, double-blind, placebo-controlled study of guanfacine extended release in children and adolescents with attention-deficit/hyperactivity disorder. Pediatrics. 2008;121(1):73-84.
475. Carskadon M, Cavall A, Rosekind M, et al. Sleepiness and nap sleep following a morning dose of clonidine. Sleep.1989;12(4):338-44.
476. *Available at: www.fda.gov.*
477. *Available at: www.addrenex.com/lead_product.html.*
478. Bambauer K, Connor D. Characteristics of aggression in clinically referred children. CNS Spectr. 2005;10(9):709-18.
479. Nock M, Kaxdin A, Hiripi E, et al. Prevalence, subtypes, and correlates of DSM-IV conduct disorder in the National Comorbidity Survey replication. Psychol Med. 2006;36(5):699-710.
480. Findling R. Atypical antipsychotic treatment of disruptive behavior disorders in children and adolescents. J Clin Psychiatry. 2008;69(Suppl 4):9-14.
481. Pappadopulos E, MacIntyre J, Crismon M, et al. Treatment recommendations for the use of antipsychotics for aggressive youth. J Am Acad Child Adolesc Psychiatry. 2003;42(2):103-66.
482. Steiner H, Remsin L. Practice parameter for the assessment and treatment of children and adolescents with oppositional defiant disorder. J Am Acad Child Adolesc Psychiatry. 2007;46(1):126-41.
483. Findling R, Steiner H, Weller E, et al. Use of antipsychotics in children and adolescents. J Clin Psychiatry. 2005;66(Suppl 7):29-40.
484. Campbell M, Rapoport J, Simpson G, et al. Antipsychotics in children and adolescents. J Am Acad Child Adolesc Psychiatry.1999;38(5):537-45.
485. Ruths S, Steiner H. Psychopharmacologic treatment of aggression in children and adolescents. Pediatr Ann. 2004;33(5):319-27.
486. Campbell M, Small A, Green W, et al. Behavioral efficacy of haloperidol and lithium carbonate. A comparison in hospitalized aggressive children with conduct disorder. Arch Gen Psychiatry. 1984;41(7):650-6.
487. Malone R, Delaney M, Luebbert J, et al. A double-blind placebo-controlled study of lithium in hospitalized aggressive children and adolescents with conduct disorder. Arch Gen Psychiatry. 2000;57:649-54.
488. Reyes M, Buitelaar J, Toren P, et al. A randomized, double-blind, placebo-controlled study of risperidone maintenance treatment in children and adolescents with disruptive behavior disorders. Am J Psychiatry. 2006;163(3):402-10.
489. Turgay A, Binder C, Snyder R, et al. Long-term safety and efficacy of risperidone for the treatment of disruptive behavior disorders in children with subaverage IQs. Pediatrics. 2002;110(3):1-12.
490. Connor D, Fletcher K, Wood J, et al. Neuroleptic-related dyskinesias in children and adolescents. J Clin Psychiatry. 2001;62(12):967-74.
491. Biederman J, Mick E, Faraone S, et al. Risperidone for the treatment of affective symptoms in children with disruptive behavior disorder: a Post hoc analysis of data from a 6-week, multicenter, randomized, double-blind, parallel-arm study. Clin Therap. 2006;28(5):794-800.
492. Handen B, Hardan A. Open-label, prospective trial of olanzapine in adolescents with subaverage intelligence and disruptive behavior disorders. J Am Acad Child Adolesc Psychiatry. 2006;45(8):928-35.
493. Masi G, Milone A, Canepa G, et al. Olanzapine treatment in adolescents with severe conduct disorder. Eur Psychiatry. 2006;21:51-7.
494. Kronenberger W, Giauque A, Lafata D, et al. Quetiapine addition in methylphenidate treatment-resistant adolescents with comorbid attention-deficit/hyperactivity disorder, conduct/oppositional-defiant disorder, and aggression: a prospective, open-label study. J Child Adolesc. 2002;8(3):172-88.
495. Findling R, Reed M, O'Riordan M, et al. A 26-week open-label study of quetiapine in children with conduct disorder. J Child and Adolesc Psychopharmacol. 2007;17(1):1-9.
496. Findling R, Reed M, O'Riordan M, et al. Effectiveness, safety, and pharmacokinetics of quetiapine in aggressive children with conduct disorder. J Am Acad Child Adolesc Psychiatry. 2006;45(7):792-800.
497. Findling R, Blumer J, Kauffmann R, et al. Pharmacokinetic effects of aripiprazole in children and adolescents with conduct disorder. Presented at the XXIVth Collegium Internationale Neuro-Psychopharmacologicum Congress; 2004.
498. Birmaher B, Brent D, et al. Practice parameter for the assessment and treatment of children and adolescents with depressive disorders. J Am Acad Child Adolesc Psychiatry. 2007;46(11):1503-26.
499. Thase M, Nelson J, Papakostas G, et al. Augmentation strategies in the treatment of major depressive disorder. CNS Spectr. 2007;12(12 Suppl 22):3-5.
500. Geller B, Reisling D, Leonard H, et al. Critical review of tricyclic antidepressant use in children and adolescents. J Am Acad Child Adolesc Psychiatry. 1999;38(5):513-6.
501. Geller B, Cooper T, Graham D, et al. Pharmacokinetically designed double-blind placebo-controlled study of nortriptyline in 6- to 12-year-olds with major depressive disorder. J Am Acad Child Adolesc Psychiatry. 1992;31(1):34-44.
502. Birmaher B, Waterman S, Ryan N, et al. Randomized, controlled trial of amitriptyline versus placebo for adolescents with "treatment-resistant" major depression. J Am Acad Child Adolesc Psychiatry. 1998;37(5):527-35.
503. Wilens T, Biederman J, Baldessarini R, et al. Cardiovascular effects of therapeutic doses of tricyclic antidepressants in children and adolescents. J Am Acad Child Adolesc Psychiatry. 1996;35(11):1491-501.

504. Emslie G, Heiligenstein J, Wagner K, et al. Fluoxetine for acute treatment of depression in children and adolescents: a placebo-controlled, randomized clinical trial. J Am Acad Child Adolesc Psychiatry. 2002;41(10):1205-15.
505. Emslie G, Rush A, Weinberg W, et al. A double-blind, randomized, placebo-controlled trial of fluoxetine in children and adolescents with depression. Arch Gen Psychiatry. 1997;54(11):1031-7.
506. Emslie G, Heiligenstein J, Hoog S, et al. Fluoxetine treatment for prevention of relapse of depression in children and adolescents: a double-blind, placebo-controlled study. J Am Acad Child Adolesc Psychiatry. 2004;43(11):1397-405.
507. March J, Silva S, Vitiello B, et al. The treatment study for adolescents with depression study (TADS): methods and message at 12 weeks. J Am Acad Child Adolesc Psychiatry. 2006;45(12):1393-403.
508. March J, Silva S, Petrycki S, et al. Fluoxetine, cognitive-behavioral therapy, and their combination for adolescents with depression: treatment for adolescents with depression study (TADS) randomized controlled trial. JAMA. 2004;292(7):807-20.
509. March J, Silva S, Petrycki S, et al. The treatment for adolescents with depression study (TADS). Arch Gen Psychiatry. 2007; 64(10):1132-44.
510. Brent D, Emslie G, Clarke G, et al. Switching to another SSRI or to venlafaxine with or without cognitive behavioral therapy for adolescents with SSRI-resistant depression: the TORDIA randomized controlled trial. JAMA. 2008;299(23):901-13.
511. Libby A, Brent D, Morrato E, et al. Decline in treatment of pediatric depression after FDA advisory on risk of suicidality with SSRIs. Am J Psychiatry. 2007;164(6):884-91.
512. Brent D. Antidepressants and pediatric depression—the risk of doing nothing. N Engl J Med. 2004;351(16):1598-601.
513. Cheung A, Zuckerbrot R, Jensen P, et al. Guidelines for adolescent depression in primary care (GLAD-PC): II. Treatment and ongoing management. Pediatrics. 2007;120(5):1313-26.
514. McClellan J, Kowatch R, Findling R, et al. Practice parameter for the assessment and treatment of children and adolescents with bipolar disorder. J Am Acad Child Adolesc Psychiatry. 2007;46(1):107-25.
515. Findling R, Gracious B, McNamara N, et al. Rapid, continuous cycling and psychiatric co-morbidity in pediatric bipolar 1 disorder. Bipolar Disord. 2001;3:202-10.
516. Smarty S, Findling R. Psychopharmacology of pediatric bipolar disorder: a review. Psychopharmacology. 2007;191:39-54.
517. Findling R, Frazier J, Kafantaris V, et al. The collaborative lithium trials (CoLT): specific aims, methods, and implementation. Child Adolesc Psychiatry Ment Health. 2008;2(21):129-38.
518. Kafantaris V, Coletti D, Dicker R, et al. Lithium treatment of acute mania in adolescents: a placebo-controlled discontinuation study. J Am Acad Child Adolesc Psychiatry. 2004;43(8):984-93.
519. Kafantaris V, Coletti D, Dicker R, et al. Lithium treatment of acute mania in adolescents: a large open trial. J Am Acad Child Adolesc Psychiatry. 2003;42(9):1038-45.
520. Patel N, DelBello M, Bryan H, et al. Open-label lithium for the treatment of adolescents with bipolar depression. J Am Acad Child Adolesc Psychiatry. 2006;45(3):289-97.
521. Available at: http://bpca.nichd.nih.gov/clinical/studies/index.cfm.
522. Kowatch R, Findling, R, Schefer R, et al. Pediatric bipolar collaborative mood stabilizer trial.
523. Wagner K, Redden L, Kowatch R, et al. Safety and efficacy of Divalproex ER in youth with mania. AACAP; 2007.
524. Findling R, McNamara N, Youngstrom E, et al. Double-blind 18-month trial of lithium versus divalproex maintenance treatment in pediatric bipolar disorder. J Am Acad Child Adolesc Psychiatry. 2005;44(5):409-17.
525. Ginsberg L. Carbamazepine extended-release capsules: a retrospective review of its use in children and adolescents.Ann Clin Psychiatry. 2006;18(1):3-7.
526. Weisler R, Kalali A, Ketter T, et al. A multicenter, randomized, double-blind, placebo-controlled trial of extended-release carbamazepine capsules as monotherapy for bipolar disorder patients with manic or mixed episodes. J Clin Psychiatry. 2004;65:478-84.
527. Vieta E, Cruz N, Garcia J, et al. A double-blind, randomized, placebo-controlled prophylaxis trial of oxcarbazepine as adjunctive treatment to lithium in the long-term treatment of bipolar I and II disorder. Int J Neuropsychopharmacology. 2008;11(4):445-52.
528. Wagner K, Kowatch R, Emslie G, et al. A double-blind, randomized, placebo-controlled trial of oxcarbazepine in the treatment of bipolar disorder in children and adolescents. Am J Psychiatry. 2006;163(7):1179-86.
529. Delbello M, Findling R, Kushner S, et al. A pilot controlled trial of topiramate for mania in children and adolescents with bipolar disorder. J Am Acad Child Adolesc Psychiatry. 2005;44(6):539-47.
530. Wagner K, Nyilas M, Johnson B, et al. Long-term efficacy of aripiprazole in children (10-17 years old) with mania. AACAP; 2007.
531. Correll C, Auran C, Johsnon B, et al. Safety and tolerability of aripiprazole in children (10-17) with mania. AACAP; 2007.
532. DelBello M, Findling R, Earley W, et al. Efficacy of quetiapie in children and adolescents with bipolar mania: a 3-week, double-blind, randomized, placebo-controlled trial; 2006.
533. Pandina G, DelBello M, Kushner S, et al. Risperidone for the treatment of acute mania in bipolar youth. AACAP; 2007.
534. DelBello M, Findling R, Wang P, et al. Efficacy and safety of ziprasidone in pediatric bipolar disorder. APA Annual Meeting; 2008.
535. Tohen M, Kryzhanovskaya L, Carlson G, et al. Olanzapine versus placebo in the treatment of adolescents with bipolar mania. Am J Psychiatry. 2007;164(10):1547-56.
536. Williams T, Miller B. Pharmacologic management of anxiety disorders in children and adolescents. Curr Opin Pediatr. 2003;15:483-90.

537. Connoly S, Bernstein G, Work Group on Quality Issues. Practice parameter for the assessment and treatment of children and adolescents with anxiety disorders. J Am Acad Child Adolesc Psychiatry. 2007;46(2):267-83.
538. Birmaher B, Axelson D, Monk K, et al. Fluoxetine for the treatment of childhood anxiety disorders. J Am Acad Child Adolesc Psychiatry. 2003;42(4):415-23.
539. Clark D, Birmaher B, Axelson D, et al. Fluoxetine for the treatment of childhood anxiety disorders: open-label, long-term extension to a controlled trial. J Am Acad Child Adolesc Psychiatry. 2005;44(12):1263-70.
540. Cheer S, Figgit D. Spotlight on fluvoxamine in anxiety disorders in children and adolescents. Paediatr Drugs. 2001;3(10):763-781.
541. Research Unit on Pediatric Psychopharmacology Anxiety Study Group (RUPP). Fluvoxamine for the treatment of anxiety disorders in children and adolescents. N Engl J Med. 2001;344(17):1279-85.
542. Rynn M, Siqueland L, Rickels K, et al. Placebo-controlled trial of sertraline in the treatment of children with generalized anxiety disorder. Am J Psychiatry. 2001;158(12):2008-14.
543. Wagner K, Berard R, Stein M, et al. A multicenter, randomized, double-blind, placebo-controlled trial of paroxetine in children and adolescents with social anxiety disorder. Arch Gen Psychiatry. 2004;61:1153-62.
544. March J, Entusah R, Rynn M, et al. A randomized controlled trial of venlafaxine ER versus placebo in pediatric social anxiety disorder. Biol Psychiatry. 2007;62:1149-54.
545. Rynn M, Riddle M, Yeung P, et al. Efficacy and safety of extended-release venlafaxine in the treatment of generalized anxiety disorder in children and adolescents: two placebo-controlled trials. Am J Psychiatry. 2007;164:290-300.
546. *ClinicalTrials.gov.*
547. Riddle M, Reeve E, Yaryura-Tobias J, et al. Fluvoxamine for children and adolescents with obsessive-compulsive disorder: a randomized, controlled, multicenter trial. J Am Acad Child Adolesc Psychiatry. 2001;40(2):222-9.
548. Geller D, Wagner K, Emslie G, et al. Paroxetine treatment in children and adolescents with obsessive-compulsive disorder: a randomized, multicenter, double-blind, placebo-controlled trial. J Am Acad Child Adolesc Psychiatry. 2004;43(11): 1387-96.
549. Cook E, Wagner K, March J, et al. Long-term sertraline treatment of children and adolescents with obsessive-compulsive disorder. J Am Acad Child Adolesc Psychiatry. 2001;40(10):1175-81.
550. March J, Biederman J, Wolkow R, et al. Sertraline in children and adolescents with obsessive-compulsive disorder: a multicenter randomized controlled trial. JAMA. 1998;280(20):1752-6.
551. March J, Foa E, Gammon P, et al. Cognitive-behavior therapy, sertraline, and their combination for children and adolescents with obsessive-compulsive disorder; the pediatric OCD treatment study (POTS) randomized controlled trial. JAMA.2004;292(16):1969-76.
552. Freeman J, Garcia A, Fucci C, et al. Family-based treatment of early-onset obsessive-compulsive disorder. J Child Adolesc Psychopharmacol. 2003;13(Suppl 1):571-80.
553. Perrin S, Smith P, Yule W, et al. Practitioner review: the assessment and treatment of post-traumatic stress disorder in children and adolescents. J Child Psychol Psychiatry. 2000;41(3):277-89.
554. Seedat S, Stein D, Ziervogel C, et al. Comparison of response to a selective serotonin reuptake inhibitor in children, adolescents, and adults with posttraumatic stress disorder. J Child Adolesc Psychopharm. 2002;12(1):37-46.
555. Porter D, Bell D. The use of clonidine in post-traumatic stress disorder. J Natl Med Assoc. 1999;91(8):475-7.
556. Harmon R, Riggs P. Clonidine for posttraumatic stress disorder in preschool children. J Am Acad Child Adolesc Psychiatry.1996;35(9):1247-1249.
557. Lustig S, Botelho C, Lynch L, et al. Implementing a randomized clinical trial on a pediatric psychiatric inpatient unit at a children's hospital: the case of clonidine for post-traumatic stress. Gen Hosp Psychiatry. 2002;24:422-9.
558. Stathis S, Martin G, McKenna J, et al. A preliminary case series on the use of quetiapine for posttraumatic stress disorder in juveniles within a youth detention center. J Clin Psychopharmacol. 2005;25(6):539-44.
559. Famular R, Kinscherff R, Fenton T, et al. Propanolol treatment for childhood posttraumatic stress disorder, acute type. A pilot study. Am J Dis Child. 1988;142(11):1244-7.
560. Diler R. Panic disorder in children and adolescents. Yonsei Med J. 2003;44(1):174-9.
561. Renaud J, Birmaher B, Wassick S, et al. Use of selective serotonin reuptake inhibitors for the treatment of childhood panic disorder: a pilot study. J Child Adolesc Psychopharm. 1999;9(2):73-83.
562. Leskovec T, Rowles B, Findling R, et al. Pharmacological treatment options for autism spectrum disorders in children and adolescents. Harv Rev Psychiatry. 2008;16(2):97-112.
563. Aman M. Treatment planning for patients with autism spectrum disorders. J Clin Psychiatry. 2005;66(Suppl 10):38-45.
564. McDougle C, Kresch L, Posey D, et al. Repetitive thoughts and behaviors in pervasive developmental disorders: treatment with serotonin reuptake inhibitors. J Autism Dev Disord. 2000;30(5):427-35.
565. Cook E, Rowlett R, Jaselskis C, et al. Fluoxetine treatment of children and adults with autistic disorder and mental retardation. J Am Acad Child Adolesc Psychiatry. 1992;31(4):739-45.
566. Hollander E, Phillips A, Chaplin W, et al. A placebo controlled crossover trial of liquid fluoxetine on repetitive behaviors in childhood and adolescent autism. Neuropsychopharm. 2005;30:582-9.
567. Steingard R, Zimnitzky B, DeMaso D, et al. Sertraline treatment of transition-associated anxiety and agitation in children with autistic disorder. J Child Adolesc Psychopharm Springfielder. 1997;7(1):9-15.

568. Hellings J, Kelley L, Gabrielli W, et al. Sertraline response in adults with mental retardation and autistic disorder. J Clin Psychiatry. 1996;57(8):333-6.
569. Owley T, Walton L, Sat J, et al. An open-label trial of escitalopram in pervasive developmental disorders. J Am Acad Child Adolesc Psychiatry. 2005;44(4):343-8.
570. Namerow L, Thomas P, Bostic J, et al. Use of citalopram in pervasive developmental disorders. J Dev Behav Pediatr.2003; 24(2):104-8.
571. Reminton G, Sloman L, Konstantareas M, et al. Clomipramine versus haloperidol in the treatment of autistic disorder: a double-blind, placebo-controlled, crossover study. J Clin Psychopharm. 2001;21(4):440-4.
572. Sanches L, Campbell M, Small A, et al. A pilot study of clomipramine in young autistic children. J Am Acad Child Adolesc Psychiatry. 1996;35(4):537-44.
573. DiMartino A, Melis G, Ciancehetti C, et al. Methylphenidate for pervasive developmental disorders: safety and efficacy of acute single dose test and ongoing therapy: an open-pilot study. J Child Adolesc Psychopharm. 2004;14(2):207-18.
574. Handen B, Johnson C, Lubetsky M, et al. Efficacy of methylphenidate among children with autism and symptoms of attention-deficit hyperactivity disorder. J Autism Dev Disord. 2000;30(3):245-55.
575. Research Units on Pediatric Psychopharmacology (RUPP). Randomized, Controlled, Crossover Trial of Methylphenidate in Pervasive Developmental Disorders with Hyperactivity.
576. Volkmar F, Cohen D, Hoshino Y, et al. Phenomenology and classification of the childhood psychoses. Psychol Med. 1988;18(1):191-201.
577. Campbell M, Fish B, David R, et al. Response to tri-iodothyronine and dextroamphetamine: a study of preschool schizophrenic children. J Autism Child Schizophr. 1972;2(4): 343-58.
578. Campbell M, Small A, Collins P, et al. Levodopa and levoamphetamine: a crossover study in young schizophrenic children. Curr Ther Res Clin Exp. 1976;19(1):70-86.
579. Fankhauser M, Karumanchi V, German M, et al. A double-blind, placebo-controlled study of the efficacy of transdermal clonidine in children. J Clin Psychiatry. 1992;53(3):77-82.
580. Jaselskis C, Cook E, Fletcher K, et al. Clonidine treatment of hyperactive and impulsive children with autistic disorder. J Clin Psychopharmacol. 1992;12(5):322-7.
581. Posey D, Puntney J, Sasher T, et al. Guanfacine treatment of hyperactivity and inattention in pervasive developmental disorders: a retrospective analysis of 80 cases. J Child Adolesc Psychopharm. 2004;14(2):233-41.
582. Scahill L, Aman M, McDougle C, et al. A prospective open trial of guanfacine in children with pervasive developmental disorders. J Child Adolesc Psychopharm. 2006;16(5):589-98.
583. Research Units on Pediatric Psychopharmacology Autism Network (RUPP). Risperidone treatment of autistic disorder: longer-term benefits and blinded discontinuation after 6 months. Am J Psychiatry. 2005;162(7):1361-9.
584. McDougle C, Scahill L, Aman M, et al. Risperidone for the core symptom domains of autism: results from the study by the autism network of the research units on pediatric psychopharmacology. Am J Psychiatry. 2005;162(6):1142-8.
585. Aman M, Arnold E, McDougle C, et al. Acute and long-term safety and tolerability of risperidone in children with autism. J Child Adolesc Psychopharm. 2005;15(6):869-84.
586. Findling R, McNamara N, Gracious B, et al. Quetiapine in nine youths with autistic disorder. J Child Adolesc Psychopharm. 2004;14(2):287-94.
587. Martin A, Koenig K, Scahill L, et al. Open-label quetiapine in the treatment of children and adolescents with autistic disorder. J Child Adolesc Psychopharm. 1999;9(2):99-107.
588. Hollander E, Wasserman S, Swanson E, et al. A double-blind placebo-controlled pilot study of olanzapine in childhood/ adolescent pervasive developmental disorder. J Child Adolesc Psychopharm. 2006;16(5):541-8.
589. Kemner C, Willemsen S, deJonge M, et al. Open-label study of olanzapine in children with pervasive developmental disorder. J Clin Psychopharm. 2002;22(5):455-60.
590. Malone R, Cater J, Sheikh R, et al. Olanzapine versus haloperidol in children with autistic disorder: an open pilot study. J Am Acad Child Adolesc Psychiatry. 2001;40(8):887-94.
591. Duggal H. Ziprasidone for maladaptive behavior and attention-deficit/hyperactivity disorder symptoms in autistic disorder. J Child Adolesc Psychopharm. 2007;17(2):261-3.
592. Cohen S, Fitzgerald B, Khan S, et al. The effect of a switch to ziprasidone in an adult population with autistic disorder: chart review of naturalistic, open-label treatment. J Clin Psychiatry. 2004;65:110-3.
593. McDougle C, Kem D, Posey D, et al. Case series: use of ziprasidone for maladaptive symptoms in youths with autism. J Am Acad Child Adolesc Psychiatry. 2002;41(8):921-7.
594. Valicenti M, Demb H. Clinical effects and adverse reactions of off-label use of aripiprazole in children and adolescents with developmental disabilities. J Child Adolesc Psychopharm. 2006;16(5):549-60.
595. Shastri M, Alla L, Sabaratnam M, et al. Aripiprazole use in individuals with intellectual disability and psychotic or behavioral disorders: a case series. J Psychopharm. 2006;20(6):863-7.
596. Hardan A, Jou R, Handen B, et al. A retrospective assessment of topiramate in children and adolescents with pervasive developmental disorders. J Child and Adolesc Psychopharm. 2004;14(3):426-32.
597. Posey D, Kern D, Swiezy N, et al. A pilot study of D-cycloserine in subjects with autistic disorder. Am J Psychiatry. 2004;161(11):2115-7.
598. Danfors T, von Knorring A, Hartvig P, et al. Tetrahydrobiopterin in the treatment of children with autistic disorder. J Clin Psychopharm. 2005;25(5):485-9.
599. Kumra S, Oberstar J, Sikich L, et al. Efficacy and tolerability of second-generation antipsychotics in children and adolescents with schizophrenia. Schizophrenia Bulletin. 2008;34(1):60-71.

600. Correll C. Assessing and maximizing the safety and tolerability of antipsychotics used in the treatment of children and adolescents. J Clin Psychiatry. 2008;69(Suppl 4):26-36.
601. Thomas L, Woods S. The schizophrenia prodrome: a developmentally informed review and update for psychopharmacologic treatment. Child Adolesc Psychiatr Clin N Am. 2006;15:109-33.
602. Sikich L, Frazier J, McLellan J , et al. Double-blind comparison of first- and second-generation antipsychotics in early-onset schizophrenia and schizoaffective disorder: findings from the treatment of early-onset schizophrenia spectrum disorders (TEOSS) study. Am J Psychiatry. 2008; AiA:1-13.
603. Spencer E, Kafantaris V, Padron-Gayol M, et al. Haloperidol in schizophrenic children: early findings from a study in progress. Psychopharmacol Bull. 1992;28(2):183-6.
604. Pool D, Bloom W, Mielki D, et al. A controlled evaluation of loxitane in seventy-five adolescent schizophrenic patients. Curr Ther Res Clin Exp. 1976;19(1):99-104.
605. Realmuto G, Erickson W, Yellin A, et al. Clinical comparison of thiothixene and thioridazine in schizophrenic adolescents. Am J Psychiatry. 1984;141(3):440-2.
606. Bishop J, Pavuluri M. Review of risperidone for the treatment of pediatric and adolescent bipolar disorder and schizophrenia. Neuropsychiatr Dis Treat. 2008;4(1):55-68.
607. Armenteros J, Whitaker A, Welikson M, et al. Risperidone in adolescents with schizophrenia: an open pilot study. Am J Acad Child Adolesc Psychiatry. 1997;36(5):694-700.
608. Mozes T, Ebert T, Michal S, et al. An open-label comparison of olanzapine versus risperidone in the treatment of childhood-onset schizophrenia. J Child Adolesc Psychopharmacol. 2006;16(4):393-403.
609. Zalsman G, Carmon E, Martin A, et al. Effectiveness, safety, and tolerability of risperidone in adolescents with schizophrenia: an open-label study. J Child Adolesc Psychopharmacol. 2003;13(3):319-27.
610. Gothelf D, Apter A, Reidman J, et al. Olanzapine, risperidone, and haloperidol in the treatment of adolescent patients with schizophrenia. J Neural Transm. 2003;110(5):545-60.
611. van Bruggen J, Tijseen J, Dingemans P, et al. Symptom response and side-effects of olanzapine and risperidone in young adults with recent onset schizophrenia. Int Clin Psychopharmacol. 2003;18(6):341-6.
612. Findling R, Robb A, Nyilas M, et al. A multiple-center, randomized, double-blind, placebo-controlled study of oral aripiprazole for treatment of adolescents with schizophrenia. Am J Psychiatry. 2008;2:1-10.
613. Kushner S, Unis A, Copenhaver M, et al. Acute and continuous efficacy and safety of risperidone in adolescents with schizophrenia. AACAP; 2007.
614. Kryzhanovskaya L, Schulz C, McDougle C, et al. Efficacy and safety of olanzapine in adolescents with schizophrenia: results from a double-blind, placebo-controlled trial. 44th College of Neuropsychopharmacology; 2010.
615. Kranzler H, Kester H, Gerbino-Rosen G, et al. Treatment-refractory schizophrenia in children and adolescents: an update on clozapine and other pharmacologic inter-ventions. Child Adolesc Psychiatr Clin N Am. 2006;15:135-59.
616. Kumra S, Kranzler H, Gerbino-Rosen G, et al. Clozapine and "high-dose" olanzapine in refractory early-onset schizophrenia: a 12-week randomized and double blind comparison. Biol Psychiatry. 2008;63(5):524-9.
617. Kumra S, Frazier J, Jacobsen L, et al. Childhood onset schizophrenia. A double-blind clozapine-haloperidol comparison.Arch Gen Psychiatry. 1996;53(12):1090-7.
618. Shaw P, Sporn A, Gogtay N, et al. Childhood Onset Schizophrenia: a double-blind clozapine-olanzapine comparison. Arch Gen Psychiatry. 2006;63:721-30.

Paternal Psychiatric Disorders and Children's Psychosocial Development

619. Downey G, Coyne JC. Children of depressed parents: an integrative review. Psychol Bull. 1990;108:50-76.
620. Murray L, Cooper P. Intergenerational transmission of affective and cognitive processes associated with depression: infancy and the preschool years. In: Goodyer I (Ed). Unipolar depression: a lifespan perspective. Oxford: Oxford University Press, 2003.
621. Goodman S, Gotlib I. Risk for psychopathology in the children of depressed mothers: a developmental model for understanding mechanisms of transmission. Psychol Rev. 1999;106:458-90.
622. Cassano M, Adrian M, Veits G, Zeman J. The inclusion of fathers in the empirical investigation of child psychopathology: an update. J Clin Child Adolesc Psychol. 2006;35(4):583-9.
623. Gale CR, O'Callaghan FJ, Godfrey KM, Law CM, Martyn CN. Critical periods of brain growth and cognitive function in children. Brain. 2004;127:321-9.
624. Montgomery CM, Hosegood V, Busza J, Timaeus IM. Men's involvement in the South African family: engendering change in the AIDS era. Soc Sci Med. 2006;62:2411-9.
625. Bowlby J. Attachment and Loss: Attachment. London: Pimlico, 1997.
626. Bogels S, Phares V. Fathers' role in the etiology, prevention and treatment of child anxiety: a review and new model. Clin Psychol Rev. 2008;28:539-58.
627. Cabrera NJ, Tamis-LeMonda CS, Bradley RH, Hofferth S, Lamb ME. Fatherhood in the twenty-first century. Child Dev. 2000;71:127-36.
628. Lamb ME, Lewis C. The development and significance of father—child relationships in two-parent families. In: Lamb ME (Ed). The role of the father in child development. New Jersey: Wiley and Sons; 2004.
629. Phares V, Fields S, Kamboukos D, Lopez E. Still looking for Poppa. Am Psychol. 2005;60:735-6.
630. Flouri E. Fathering and adolescents' psychological adjustment: the role of fathers' involvement, residence and biology status. Child Care Health Dev. 2008;34:152-61.

631. Flouri E, Buchanan A. Early father's and mother's involvement and child's later educational outcomes. Br J Educ Psychol. 2004;74:141-53.
632. Jaffee SR, Moffitt TE, Caspi A, Taylor A. Life with (or without) father: the benefits of living with two biological parents depend on the father's antisocial behavior. Child Dev. 2003;74:109-26.
633. Lewis C, Lamb ME. Fatherhood: connecting the strands of diversity across time and space. Joseph Rowntree Foundation; 2006.
634. Sarkadi A, Kristiansson R, Oberklaid F, Bremberg S. Fathers' involvement and children's developmental outcomes: a systematic review of longitudinal studies. Acta Paediatr. 2008;97:153-8.
635. Lamb ME. The role of the father in child development. New Jersey: Wiley and Sons; 2004.
636. Engle PL, Breaux C. Fathers' involvement with children: perspectives from developing countries. In: Thomas NG (Ed). Social policy report. Ann Arbor: Society for Research in Child Development; 1998.
637. Connell AM, Goodman SH. The association between psychopathology in fathers versus mothers and children's internalizing and externalizing behavior problems: a meta-analysis. Psychol Bull. 2002;128:746-73.
638. Ramchandani P, Stein A, Evans J, O'Connor TG. Paternal depression in the postnatal period and child development: a prospective population study. Lancet. 2005;365:2201-2205.
639. Stein A, Ramchandani P, Murray L. Impact of parental illness or mental disorder. In: Michael Rutter DB, Daniel Pine, Stephen Scott, Jim Stevenson, Eric Taylor, Anita Thapar (Eds). Rutter's child and adolescent psychiatry. Oxford: Blackwells; 2008.
640. Murray CJ, Lopez AD. Alternative projections of mortality and disability by cause 1990-2020: global burden of disease study. Lancet. 1997;349:1498-504.
641. Gluckman PD, Hanson MA, Spencer HG, Bateson P. Environmental influences during development and their later consequences for health and disease: implications for the interpretation of empirical studies. Proc Biol Sci. 2005;272:671-7.
642. Bateson P, Barker D, Clutton-Brock T, et al. Developmental plasticity and human health. Nature. 2004;430:419-21.
643. Sinclair D, Murray L. Effects of postnatal depression on children's adjustment to school. Teacher's reports. Br J Psychiatry. 1998;172:58-63.
644. Beck CT. The effects of postpartum depression on child development: a meta-analysis. Arch Psychiatr Nurs. 1998;12: 12-20.
645. Hay DF, Pawlby S, Sharp D, Asten P, Mills A, Kumar R. Intellectual problems shown by 11-year-old children whose mothers had postnatal depression. J Child Psychol Psychiatry. 2001;42:871-89.
646. Murray L, Kempton C, Woolgar M, Hooper R. Depressed mothers' speech to their infants and its relation to infant gender and cognitive development. J Child Psychol Psychiatry. 1993;34:1083-101.
647. Halligan SL, Murray L, Martins C, Cooper PJ. Maternal depression and psychiatric outcomes in adolescent offspring: a 13-year longitudinal study. J Affect Disord. 2007;97:145-54.
648. Blazer DG, Kessler RC, McGonagle KA, Swartz MS. The prevalence and distribution of major depression in a national community sample: the National Comorbidity Survey. Am J Psychiatry. 1994;151:979-86.
649. Wilhelm K, Mitchell P, Slade T, Brownhill S, Andrews G. Prevalence and correlates of DSM-IV major depression in an Australian national survey. J Affect Disord. 2003;75:155-62.
650. Ramchandani PG, Stein A, O'Conner TG, Heron J, Murray L, Evans J. Depression in men in the postnatal period and later child psychopathology: a population cohort study. J Am Acad Child Adolesc Psychiatry. 2008;47:390-8.
651. Kane P, Garber J. The relations among depression in fathers, children's psychopathology, and father—child conflict: a meta-analysis. Clin Psychol Rev. 2004;24:339-60.
652. Beardslee WR, Gladstone TR, Wright EJ, Cooper AB. A family-based approach to the prevention of depressive symptoms in children at risk: evidence of parental and child change. Pediatrics. 2003;112:e119-e131.
653. Beardslee WR, Versage EM, Gladstone TR. Children of affectively ill parents: a review of the past 10 years. J Am Acad Child Adolesc Psychiatry. 1998;37:1134-41.
654. Klein DN, Lewinsohn PM, Rohde P, Seeley JR, Olino TM. Psychopathology in the adolescent and young adult offspring of a community sample of mothers and fathers with major depression. Psychol Med. 2005;35:353-65.
655. Lewinsohn PM, Olino TM, Klein DN. Psychosocial impairment in offspring of depressed parents. Psychol Med. 2005;35:1493-503.
656. Renk K, Oliveros A, Roddenberry A, et al. The relationship between maternal and paternal psychological symptoms and ratings of adolescent functioning. J Adolesc. 2007;30:467-85.
657. Currier D, Mann MJ, Oquendo MA, Galfalvy H, Mann JJ. Sex differences in the familial transmission of mood disorders. J Affect Disord. 2006;95:51-60.
658. Dierker LC, Merikangas KR, Szatmari P. Influence of parental concordance for psychiatric disorders on psychopathology in offspring. J Am Acad Child Adolesc Psychiatry. 1999;38:280-8.
659. Jenkins R, Lewis G, Bebbington P, et al. The National Psychiatric Morbidity surveys of Great Britain—initial findings from the Household Survey. Int Rev Psychiatry. 2003;15:29-42.
660. Merikangas KR, Dierker LC, Szatmari P. Psychopathology among offspring of parents with substance abuse and/or anxiety disorders: a high-risk study. J Child Psychol Psychiatry 1998;39:711-20.
661. Murray L, Cooper P, Creswell C, Schofield E, Sack C. The effects of maternal social phobia on mother-infant interactions and infant social responsiveness. J Child Psychol Psychiatry. 2007;48:45-52.
662. Bogels SM, Bamelis L, Van der Bruggen C. Parental rearing as a function of parent's own, partner's, and child anxiety status: fathers make the difference. Cognition Emotion. 2008;22:522-38.

663. Cooper PJ, Fearn V, Willetts L, Seabrook H, Parkinson M. Affective disorder in the parents of a clinic sample of children with anxiety disorders. J Affect Disord. 2006;93:205-12.
664. Kilic EZ, Ozguven HD, Sayil I. The psychological effects of parental mental health on children experiencing disaster: the experience of Bolu earthquake in Turkey. Fam Process. 2003;42:485-95.
665. Christensen HB, Bilenberg N. Behavioural and emotional problems in children of alcoholic mothers and fathers. Eur Child Adolesc Psychiatry. 2000;9:219-26.
666. Malone SM, Iacono WG, McGue M. Drinks of the father: father's maximum number of drinks consumed predicts externalizing disorders, substance use, and substance use disorders in preadolescent and adolescent offspring. Alcohol Clin Exp Res. 2002;26:1823-32.
667. Loukas A, Fitzgerald HE, Zucker RA, von Eye A. Parental alcoholism and co-occurring antisocial behavior: prospective relationships to externalizing behavior problems in their young sons. J Abnorm Child Psychol. 2001;29:91-106.
668. Chen YY, Weitzman ER. Depressive symptoms, DSM-IV alcohol abuse and their comorbidity among children of problem drinkers in a national survey: effects of parent and child gender and parent recovery status. J Stud Alcohol. 2005;66:66-73.
669. Harter SL. Psychosocial adjustment of adult children of alcoholics: a review of the recent empirical literature. Clin Psychol Rev. 2000;20:311-37.
670. Steinhausen HC, Göbel D, Nestler V. Psychopathology in the offspring of alcoholic parents. J Am Acad Child Adolesc Psychiatry. 1984;23:465-71.
671. Eiden R Das, Leonard KE, Morrisey S. Paternal alcoholism and toddler noncompliance. Alcohol Clin Exp Res. 2001;25: 1621-33.
672. Eiden RD, Edwards EP, Leonard KE. Mother—infant and father—infant attachment among alcoholic families. Dev Psychopathol. 2002;14:253-78.
673. Jaeger E, Hahn NB, Weinraub M. Attachment in adult daughters of alcoholic fathers. Addiction. 2000;95:267-76.
674. Hogan D. Annotation: the psychological development and welfare of children of opiate and cocaine users. Review and research needs. J Child Psychol Psychiatry. 1998;39: 609-19.
675. Fals-Stewart W, Kelley ML, Fincham FD, Golden J, Logsdon T. Emotional and behavioral problems of children living with drug-abusing fathers: comparisons with children living with alcohol-abusing and non-substance-abusing fathers. J Fam Psychol. 2004;18:319-30.
676. Kelley ML, Fals-Stewart W. Psychiatric disorders of children living with drug-abusing, alcohol-abusing, and non-substance-abusing fathers. J Am Acad Child Adolesc Psychiatry. 2004;43:621-8.
677. Hillegers MH, Reichart CG, Wals M, Verhulst FC, Ormel J, Nolen WA. Five-year prospective outcome of psychopathology in the adolescent offspring of bipolar parents. Bipolar Disord. 2005;7:344-50.
678. Henin A, Biederman J, Mick E, et al. Psychopathology in the offspring of parents with bipolar disorder: a controlled study. Biol Psychiatry. 2005;58:554-61.
679. Gottesman II, Shields J. A critical review of recent adoption, twin, and family studies of schizophrenia: behavioral genetics perspectives. Schizophr Bull. 1976;2:360-401.
680. Gross HE, Shaw DS, Moilanen KL. Reciprocal associations between boys' externalizing problems and mothers' depressive symptoms. J Abnorm Child Psychol. 2008;36:693-709.
681. Pilowsky DJ, Wickramaratne P, Talati A, et al. Children of depressed mothers 1 year after the initiation of maternal treatment: findings from the STAR*D-Child Study. Am J Psychiatry. 2008;165:1136-47.
682. Gordon JA, Hen R. Genetic approaches to the study of anxiety. Ann Rev Neurosci. 2004;27:193-222.
683. Rutter M, Moffitt TE, Caspi A. Gene—environment interplay and psychopathology: multiple varieties but real effects. J Child Psychol Psychiatry. 2006;47:226-61.
684. Solantaus T, Leinonen J, Punamaki RL. Children's mental health in times of economic recession: replication and extension of the family economic stress model in Finland. Dev Psychol. 2004;40:412-29.
685. Cummings EM, Keller PS, Davies PT. Towards a family process model of maternal and paternal depressive symptoms: exploring multiple relations with child and family functioning. J Child Psychol Psychiatry. 2005;46:479-89.
686. Bronte-Tinkew J, Moore K, Matthews G, Carrano J. Symptoms of major depression in a sample of fathers of infants. J Fam Issues. 2007;28:61-99.
687. Ballard C, Davies R. Postnatal depression in fathers. Int Rev Psychiatry. 1996;8:54-72.
688. Paulson JF, Dauber S, Leiferman JA. Individual and combined effects of postpartum depression in mothers and fathers on parenting behavior. Pediatrics. 2006;118:659-68.
689. Larson R, Pleck J. Hidden feelings: emotionality in boys and men. In: Bernstein D (Ed). Gender and motivation. Lincoln: University of Nebraska Press, 1999:25-74.
690. Lyons-Ruth K, Wolfe R, Lyubchik A, Steingard R. Depressive symptoms in parents of children under age 3: sociodemographic predictors, current correlates, and associated parenting behaviours. In: Halfon N, McLearn K, Schuster M (Eds). Child rearing in America. Challenges facing parents with young children. Cambridge: Cambridge University Press; 2002.
691. Field T, Hossain Z, Malphurs J. "Depressed" fathers' interactions with their infants. Infant Mental Health J. 1999;20:322-32.
692. Hart S, Field T, Stern M, Jones N. Depressed fathers stereotyping of infants labeled 'depressed'. Infant Mental Health J. 1997;18:436-45.
693. Du Rocher Schudlich T, Papp LM, Cummings EM. Relations of husbands and wives dysphoria to marital conflict resolution strategies. J Fam Psychol. 2004;18:171-83.
694. Johnson SL, Jacob T. Sequential interactions in the marital communication of depressed men and women. J Consult Clin Psychol. 2000;68:4-12.

695. Hammen C, Brennan PA, Shih JH. Family discord and stress predictors of depression and other disorders in adolescent children of depressed and nondepressed women. J Am Acad Child Adolesc Psychiatry. 2004;43:994-1002.
696. Murray L, Sinclair D, Cooper P, Ducournau P, Turner P, Stein A. The socioemotional development of 5-year-old children of postnatally depressed mothers. J Child Psychol Psychiatry. 1999;40:1259-71.
697. Low SM, Stocker C. Family functioning and children's adjustment: associations among parents' depressed mood, marital hostility, parent—child hostility, and children's adjustment. J Fam Psychol. 2005;19:394-403.
698. Leinonen JA, Solantaus TS, Punamaki RL. Parental mental health and children's adjustment: the quality of marital interaction and parenting as mediating factors. J Child Psychol Psychiatry. 2003;44:227-41.
699. Caspi A, Sugden K, Moffitt TE, et al. Influence of life stress on depression: moderation by a polymorphism in the 5-HTT gene.Science. 2003;301:386-9.
700. Loukas A, Zucker RA, Fitzgerald HE, Krull JL. Developmental trajectories of disruptive behavior problems among sons of alcoholics: effects of parent psychopathology, family conflict, and child undercontrol. J Abnorm Psychol. 2003;112:119-31.
701. Yeung WJ, Sandberg J, Davis-Kean P, Hofferth S. Children's time-use with fathers in intact families. J Marriage Fam. 2001;63:136-54.
702. Belsky J, Hsieh KH, Crnic K. Mothering, fathering, and infant negativity as antecedents of boys' externalizing problems and inhibition at age 3 years: differential susceptibility to rearing experience? Dev Psychopathol. 1998;10:301-19.
703. Bakermans-Kranenburg MJ, van Ijzendoorn MH. Genetic vulnerability or differential susceptibility in child development: the case of attachment. J Child Psychol Psychiatry. 2007;48: 1160-73.
704. van Zeijl J, Mesman J, Stolk MN, et al. Differential susceptibility to discipline: the moderating effect of child temperament on the association between maternal discipline and early childhood externalizing problems. J Fam Psychol. 2007;21:626-36.
705. Shiner R, Caspi A. Personality differences in childhood and adolescence: measurement, development, and consequences. J Child Psychol Psychiatry. 2003;44:2-32.
706. Goodyer IM, Ashby L, Altham PM, Vize C, Cooper PJ. Temperament and major depression in 11 to 16 year olds. J Child Psychol Psychiatry. 1993;34:1409-23.
707. Kelvin RG, Goodyer IM, Altham PM. Temperament and psychopathology amongst siblings of probands with depressive and anxiety disorders. J Child Psychol Psychiatry. 1996;37:543-50.
708. Masi G, Mucci M, Favilla L, Brovedani P, Millepiedi S, Perugi G. Temperament in adolescents with anxiety and depressive disorders and in their families. Child Psychiatry Hum Dev. 2003;33:245-59.
709. Eiden RD, Edwards EP, Leonard KE. Predictors of effortful control among children of alcoholic and nonalcoholic fathers. J Stud Alcohol. 2004;65:309-19.
710. Lang AR, Pelham WE, Johnston C, Gelernter S. Levels of adult alcohol consumption induced by interactions with child confederates exhibiting normal versus externalizing behaviors. J Abnorm Psychol. 1989;98:294-9.
711. Pelham WE, Lang AR. Can your children drive you to drink? Stress and parenting in adults interacting with children with ADHD. Alcohol Res Health. 1999;23:292-8.
712. Mojtabai R, Olfson M. Major depression in community-dwelling middle-aged and older adults: prevalence and 2- and 4-year follow-up symptoms. Psychol Med. 2004;34:623-34.
713. Meltzer H, Gatward R, Goodman R, Ford T. Mental health of children and adolescents in Great Britain. London: The Stationary Office; 2000.
714. Murray L, Hipwell A, Hooper R, Stein A, Cooper P. The cognitive development of 5-year-old children of postnatally depressed mothers. J Child Psychol Psychiatry. 1996;37:927-35.
715. Sohr-Preston SL, Scaramella LV. Implications of timing of maternal depressive symptoms for early cognitive and language development. Clin Child Fam Psychol Rev. 2006;9: 65-83.
716. Rutter M. Environmentally mediated risks for psychopathology: research strategies and findings. J Am Acad Child Adolesc Psychiatry. 2005;44:3-18.
717. Dunn J. Annotation: children's relationships with their nonresident fathers. J Child Psychol Psychiatry. 2004;45: 659-71.
718. Goodman JH. Paternal postpartum depression, its relationship to maternal postpartum depression, and implications for family health. J Adv Nurs. 2004;45:26-35.
719. Carro M, Grant K, Gotlib I, Compas B. Postpartum depression and child development: an investigation of mothers and fathers as sources of risk and resilience. Develop Psychopathol. 1993;5:567-79.
720. Rutter M. Psychiatric disorder in parents as a risk factor for children. In: Shaffer D, Phillips I, Enger NB (Eds). Prevention of mental disorder, alcohol and other drug use in children and adolescents. Rockville: Office for Substance Abuse, USDHHS; 1989.pp.157-89.
721. Sonuga-Barke EJ, Daley D, Thompson M. Does maternal ADHD reduce the effectiveness of parent training for preschool children's ADHD? J Am Acad Child Adolesc Psychiatry. 2002;41:696-702.
722. Forman DR, O'Hara MW, Stuart S, Gorman LL, Larsen KE, Coy KC. Effective treatment for postpartum depression is not sufficient to improve the developing mother—child relationship. Dev Psychopathol. 2007;19:585-602.
723. Phares V, Duhig M, Watkins M. Family context: fathers and other supports. In: Goodman SHG, IH (Eds). Children of depressed parents: mechanisms of risk and implications for treatment. Washington DC: APA; 2002.pp.203-25.
724. Velderman MK, Bakermans-Kranenburg MJ, Juffer F, van IJzendoorn MH. Effects of attachment-based interventions on maternal sensitivity and infant attachment: differential susceptibility of highly reactive infants. J Fam Psychol. 2006; 20:266-74.

725. Stein A, Woolley H, Senior R, et al. Treating disturbances in the relationship between mothers with bulimic eating disorders and their infants: a randomized controlled trial of video feedback. Am J Psychiatry. 2006;163:899-906.
726. Federman DD. The biology of human sex differences. N Engl J Med. 2006;354:1507-14.

Self-harm and Suicide in Adolescents

727. National Collaborating Centre for Mental Health. Self-harm: longer term management. NICE clinical guideline 133. London: National Institute for Clinical Excellence; 2011.
728. Hawton K, Hall S, Simkin S, Bale L, Bond A, Codd S, et al. Deliberate self-harm in adolescents: a study of characteristics and trends in Oxford, 1990-2000. J Child Psychol Psychiatry. 2003;44:1191-8.
729. De Leo D, Heller TS. Who are the kids who self-harm? An Australian self-report school survey. Med J Aust. 2004;181:140-4.
730. Madge N, Hewitt A, Hawton K, de Wilde EJ, Corcoran P, Fekete S, et al. Deliberate self-harm within an international community sample of young people: comparative findings from the Child and Adolescent Self-harm in Europe (CASE) Study. J Child Psychol Psychiatry. 2008;49:667-77.
731. Hawton K, Rodham K, Evans E, Weatherall R. Deliberate self-harm in adolescents: self-report survey in schools in England. BMJ. 2002;325:1207-11.
732. Hargus E, Hawton K, Rodham K. Distinguishing between subgroups of adolescents who self-harm. Suicide LW Threat Behav. 2009;39:518-37.
733. Moran P, Coffey C, Romaniuk H, Olsson C, Borschmann R, Carlin JB, et al. The natural history of self-harm from adolescence to young adulthood: a population-based cohort study. Lancet. 2012;379:236-43.
734. Centers for Disease Control and Prevention. Youth risk behavior surveillance-United States. 2009, MMWR Surveill Summ. 2010;59:1-142.
735. Olfson M, Gameroff MJ, Marcus SC, Greenberg T, Shaffer D. Emergency treatment of young people following deliberate self-harm. Arch Gen Psychiatry. 2005;61:1122-8.
736. Boeninger DK, Masyn KE, Feldman BJ, Conger RD. Sex differences in developmental trends of suicide ideation, plans, and attempts among European American adolescents. Suicide Life Threat Behav. 2010;40:451-64.
737. Burrows S, Laflamme L. Socioeconomic disparities and attempted suicide: state of knowledge and implications for research and prevention. Int J by Contr Saf Promot. 2010;17:23-40.
738. Patton GC, Hemphill SA, Beyers JM, Bond L, Toumbourou JW, McMorris BJ, et al. Pubertal stage and deliberate self-harm in adolescents. J Am Acad Child Adolesc Psychiatry. 2007;46:508-14.
739. Blakemore Sl. The social brain in adolescence. Nat Rev Neurosci. 2008;9:267-77.
740. Sebastian C, Viding E, Williams KD, Blakemore SJ. Social brain development and the affective consequences of ostracism in adolescence. Brain Cogn. 2010;72:134-45.
741. O'Connor RC, Rasmussen S, Hawton K. Predicting depression, anxiety and self-harm in adolescents: the role of perfectionism and acute life stress. Behav Res Ther. 2010;48:52-9.
742. Rodham K, Hawton K, Evans E. Reasons for deliberate self-harm: comparison of self-poisoners and self-cutters in a community sample of adolescents. J Am Acad Child Adolesc Psychiatry. 2004;43:80-7.
743. Hawton K. How patients and psychiatrists account for overdoses. In: Shepherd E, Watson K (Eds). Personal meanings. Chichester: Wiley; 1982.
744. Boergers J, Spirito A, Donaldson D. Reasons for adolescent suicide attempts: associations with psychological functioning. J Am Acad Child Adolesc Psychiatry. 1998;37:1287-93.
745. Hawton K, Cole D, O'Grady J, Osborn M. Motivational aspects of deliberate self-poisoning in adolescents. Br J Psychiatry. 1982;141:286-91.
746. Hawton K, Harriss L, Rodham K. How adolescents who cut themselves differ from those who take overdoses. Eur Child Adolesc Psychiatry. 2010;19:513-23.
747. O'Connor RC, Rasmussen S, Miles J, Hawton K. Self-harm in adolescents: self-report survey in schools in Scotland. Br J Psychiatry. 2009;194:68-72.
748. O'Connor RC, Rasmussen S, Hawton K. Predicting deliberate self-harm in adolescents: a six month prospective study Suicide Life Threat Behav. 2009;39:364-75.
749. Evans E, Hawton K, Rodham K. Factors associated with suicidal phenomena in adolescents: a systematic review of population-based studies. Clin Psychol Rev. 2004;24:957-79.
750. Klonsky ED. The functions of deliberate self-injury: a review of the evidence. Clin Psychol Rev. 2007;27:226-39.
751. O'Connor RC, Rasmussen S, Hawton K. Distinguishing adolescents who think about self-harm from those who engage in self-harm. Br J Psychiatry. 2012;200:330-5.
752. Fergusson DM, Lynskey MT. Childhood circumstances, adolescent adjustment, and suicide attempts in a New Zealand birth cohort. J Am Acad Child Adolesc Psychiatry. 1995;34:612-22.
753. Johnson JG, Cohen P, Gould MS, Kasen S, Brown J, Brook JS. Childhood adversities, interpersonal difficulties, and risk for suicide attempts during late adolescence and early adulthood. Arch Gen Psychiatry. 2002;59:741-9.
754. Beautrais AL, Joyce PR, Mulder RT. Risk factors for serious suicide attempts among youths aged 13 through 24 years. J AM Acad Child Adolesc Psychiatry. 1996;35:1174-82.
755. Madge N, Hawton K, McMahon EM, Corcoran P, De Leo D, de Wilde EJ, et al. Psychological characteristics, stressful life events and deliberate self-harm: findings from the Child & Adolescent Self-harm in Europe (CASE) Study. Eur Child Adolesc Psychiatry. 2011;20:499-508.
756. Joiner TE Jr. Contagion of suicidal symptoms as a function of assortative relating and shared relationship stress in college roommates. J Adolesc. 2003;26:495-504.
757. Fergusson DM, Horwood LJ, Beautrais Al. Is sexual orientation related to mental health problems and sexuality in young people? Arch Gen Psychiatry. 1999;56:876-80.

758. King M, Semlyen J, See Tai S, Killaspy H, Osborn D, Popelyuk D, et al. A systematic review of mental disorder, suicide, and deliberate self-harm in lesbian, gay and bisexual people. BMC Psychiatry. 2008;8:70.
759. Eisenberg ME, Resnick MD. Suicidality among gay lesbian and bisexual youth: the role of protective factors. J Adolesc Health. 2006;39:662-8.
760. O'Connor RC. Towards an integrated motivational-volitional model of suicidal behaviour. In: O'Connor RC, Platt S, Gordon J (Eds). International Handbook of Suicide Prevention: Wiley-Blackwell; 2011.
761. Van Orden KA, Wine TK, Cukrowicz KC, Braithwaite SR, Selby EA, Joiner TE Jr. The interpersonal theory of suicide. Psychol Rev. 2010;117:575-600.
762. Speckens AEM, Hawton K. Social problem-solving in adolescents with suicidal behaviour: a systematic review Suicide Life Threat Behav. 2005;35:365-87.
763. O'Connor RC. The relations between perfectionism and suicidality: a systematic review. Suicide Life Threat Behav. 2007;37:698-714.
764. Fergusson DM, Woodward LJ, Horwood LJ. Risk factors and life processes associated with the onset of suicidal behaviour during adolescence and early adulthood. Psychol Med. 2000;30:23-39.
765. Braquehais MD, Oquendo MA, Baca-Garcia E, Sher L. Is impulsivity a link between childhood abuse and suicide? Compr Psychiatry. 2010;51:121-9.
766. Al Ansari AM, Hamadeh RR, Matar AM, Marhoon H, Buzaboon BY, Raees AG. Risk factors associated with overdose among Bahraini youth. Suicide Life Threat Behav. 2001;31:197-206.
767. Manor I, Gutnik I, Ben-Dor DH, Apter A, Sever J, Tyano S, et al. Possible association between attention deficit hyperactivity disorder and attempted suicide in adolescents-a pilot study. Eur Psychiatry. 2010;25:146-50.
768. James A, Lai FH, Dahl C. Attention deficit hyperactivity disorder and suicide: a review of possible associations. Acta Psychiatr Scand. 2004;110:408-15.
769. Nock MK, Joiner TE Jr, Gordon KH, Lloyd-Richardson E, Prinstein MJ. Non-suicidal self-injury among adolescents: diagnostic correlates and relation to suicide attempts. Psychiatry Res. 2006;144:65-72.
770. Aseltine RH Jr, Schilling EA, James A, Glanovsky JL, Jacobs D. Age variability in the association between heavy episodic drinking and adolescent suicide attempts: findings from a large-scale, school-based screening program. J Am Acad Child Adolesc Psychiatry. 2009;48:262-70.
771. Bronisch T, Hofler M, Lieb R. Smoking predicts suicidality: Findings from a prospective community study. J Affect Disord. 2008;108:135-45.
772. Makikyro TH, Hakko HH, Timonen MJ, Lappalainen JA, Ilomäki RS, Marttunen MJ, et al. Smoking and suicidality among adolescent psychiatric patients. J Adolesc Health. 2004;34:250-3.
773. Fergusson DM, Harwood LJ, Ridder EM, Beautrais AL. Suicidal behaviour in adolescence and subsequent mental health outcomes in young adulthood. Psychol Med. 2005;35: 983-93.
774. Wilkinson P, Kelvin R, Roberts C, Dubicka B, Goodyer I. Clinical and psychosocial predictors of suicide attempts and nonsuicidal self-injury in the Adolescent Depression Antidepressants and Psychotherapy Trial (ADAPT). Am J Psychiatry. 2011;168:495-501.
775. Hamm K, Harriss L. Deliberated self-harm in young people; characteristics and subsequent mortality in a 20-year cohort of patients presenting to hospital. J Clin Psychiatry. 2007;68:1574-83.
776. Hawton K, Harriss L. Deliberate self-harm by under 15-year olds: characteristics, trends and outcome. J Child Psychol Psychiatry. 2008;49:441-8.
777. Hawton K, Bergen H, Kapur N, Cooper J, Steeg S, Ness J, et al. Repetition of self-harm and suicide following self-harm in children and adolescents. J Child Psychol Psychiatry. 2012;53:1212-9.
778. Fortune S, Stewart A. Yadav V, Hawton K. Suicide in adolescents: using life charts to understand the suicidal process. J Affect Disord. 2007;100:199-210.
779. Gosney H, Hawton K. Inquest verdicts: youth suicides lost. Psych Bull. 2007;31:203-5.
780. Patton GC, Coffey C, Sawyer SM, Viner RM, Haller DM, Bose K, et al. Global patterns of mortality in young people: a systematic analysis of population health data. Lancet. 2009;374:881-92.
781. Bertolote JM, Fleischmann A. Suicide and psychiatric diagnosis: a worldwide perspective. World Psychiatry. 2002;1:181-5.
782. Wasserman D, Cheng Q, Jiang GX. Global suicide rates among young people aged 15-19. World Psychiatry. 2005;4:114-20.
783. Li XY, Phillips MR, Zhang YP, Xu D, Yang GH. Risk factors for suicide in China's youth: a case-control study. Psychol Med. 2008;38:397-406.
784. Varnik A, Kolves K, Allik J, Arensman E, Aromaa E, van Audenhove C, et al. Gender issues in suicide rates, trends and methods among youths aged 15-24 in 15 European countries. J Affect Disord. 2009;113:216-26.
785. Roy A, Segal NL. Sarchiapone M. Attempted suicide among living co-twins of twin suicide victims. Am J Psychiatry. 1995;152:1075-6.
786. Brent D, Bridge I, Johnson B, Connolly J. Suicidal behaviour runs in families. A controlled family study of adolescent suicide victims. Arch Gen Psychiatry. 1996;53:1145-9.
787. Mann JJ. Neurobiology of suicidal behaviour. Nat Rev Neurosci. 2003;4:819-28.
788. Brent DA, Baugher M, Bridge J, Chen T, Chiappetta L. Age and sex-related risk factors for adolescent suicide. J Am Acad Child Adolesc Psychiatry. 1999;38:1497-505.
789. Brent DA, Mann JJ. Familial pathways to suicidal behavior-Understanding and preventing suicide among adolescents. N Engl J Med. 2006;355:2719-21.

790. Marttunen MJ, Aro HM, Henriksson MM, Lonnqvist JK. Psychosocial stressors more common in adolescent suicides with alcohol abuse compared with depressive adolescent suicides. J Am Acad Child Adolesc Psychiatry. 1994;33:490-7.
791. Sourander A, Klomek AB, Niemela S, Haavisto A, Gyllenberg D, Helenius H, et al. Childhood predictors of completed and severe suicide attempts: findings from the Finnish 1981 Birth Cohort Study. Arch Gen Psychiatry. 2009;66:398-406.
792. Houston K, Hawton K, Shepperd R. Suicide in young people aged 15-24: a psychological autopsy study. J Affect Disord. 2001;63:159-70.
793. Pirkis J, Nordemtoft M. Media influences on suicide and attempted suicide. In: O'Connor RC, Platt S, Gordon J (Eds). International Handbook of Suicide Prevention: Wiley-Blackwell; 2011.
794. Collings SC, Fortune S, Currey N, Hawton K, Wang J, Slim B. Media influences on suicidal behaviour: an interview study of young people in New Zealand. Auckland: National Centre of Mental Health Research, Information and Development; 2011.
795. Lake AM, Gould MS. School-based strategies for youth suicide prevention. In: O'Connor RC, Platt S, Gordon J (Eds). International Handbook of Suicide Prevention: Wiley-Blackwell; 2011.
796. Scott MA, Wilcox HC, Schonfeld IS, Davies M, Hicks RC, Turner JB, et al. School-based screening to identify at-risk students not already known to school professionals: the Columbia Suicide screen. Am J Public Health. 2009;99:334-9.
797. Gould MS, Marrocco FA, Hoagwood K, Kleinman M, Amakawa L, Altschuler E. Service use by at-risk youths after school-based suicide screening. J Am Acad Child Adolesc Psychiatry. 2009;48:1193-201.
798. Gould MS, Marrocco FA, Kleinman M, Thomas JG, Mostkoff K, Cote J, et al. Evaluating iatrogenic risk of youth suicide screening programs: a randomized controlled trial. JAMA. 2005;293:1635-43.
799. Aseltine RH Jr, James A, Schilling EA, Glanovsky J. Evaluating the SOS suicide prevention program: a replication and extension. BMC Public Health. 2007;7:161.
800. Platt S, Mclean J, McCollam A, et al. Evaluation of the first phase of choose life: the national strategy and action plan to prevent suicide in Scotland. Edinburgh: The Scottish Executive; 2006.
801. Thompson EA, Eggert LL, Randell BP, Pike KC. Evaluation of indicated suicide risk prevention approaches for potential high school dropouts. Am J Public Health. 2001;91:742-52.
802. Cho H, Hallfors DD, Sanchez V. Evaluation of a high school peer group intervention for at-risk youth. J Abnorm Child Psychol. 2005;33:363-74.
803. Brent D, Bridge J. Firearms availability and suicide: evidence, interventions and future directions. Am Behav Sci. 2003;46:1192-210.
804. Pearson M, Konradsen F, Gunnell D, Dawson AH, Pieris R, Weerasinghe M, et al. A community-based cluster randomised trial of safe storage to reduce pesticide self-poisoning in rural Sri Lanka: study protocol. BMC Public Health. 2011;11:879.
805. Hawton K, Simkin S, Desks J, Cooper J, Johnston A, Waters K, et al. UK legislation on analgesic packs: before and after study of long term effect on poisonings. BMJ. 2004;329:1076.
806. Harrington R. Kerfoot M, Dyer E, McNiven F, Gill J, Harrington V, Woodham A, et al. Randomized trial of a home-based family intervention for children who have deliberately poisoned themselves. J Am Acad Child Adolesc Psychiatry. 1998;37:512-8.
807. Cotgrove A, Zirinsky L, Black D, Weston D. Secondary prevention of attempted suicide in adolescence. J Adolesc. 1995;18:569-77.
808. Spirits A. Group treatment plus usual care decreased the risk of deliberate self harm in adolescents who repeatedly harm themselves. Evid Based Ment Health. 2002;5:55.
809. Donaldson D, Spirito A, Esposito-Smythers C. Treatment for adolescents following a suicide attempt: results of a pilot trial. J Am Acad Child Adolesc Psychiatry. 2005;44:113-20.
810. Wood A, Trainor G, Rothwell J, Moore A, Harrington R. Randomized trial of group therapy for repeated deliberate self-harm in adolescents. J Am Acad Child Adolesc Psychiatry. 2001;40:1246-53.
811. Hazell PL, Martin G, McGill K, Kay T, Wood A, Trainor G et al. Group therapy for repeated deliberate self-harm in adolescents: failure of replication of a randomized trial. J Am Acad Child Adolesc Psychiatry. 2009;48:662-70.
812. Green JM, Wood AJ, Kerfoot MJ, Trainor G, Roberts C, Rothwell J et al. Group therapy for adolescents with repeated self-harm: randomised controlled trial with economic evaluation. BMJ. 2011;342:682.
813. James AC, Taylor A, Winmill L, Alfoadari K. A preliminary community study of dialectical behaviour therapy (DBT) with adolescent females demonstrating persistent deliberate self-harm (DSH). Child Adolesc Mental Health. 2008;13:148-52.
814. Huey SJ Jr, Henggeler SW, Rowland MD, Halliday-Boykins CA, Cunningham PB, Pickrel SG, et al. Multisystemic therapy effects on attempted suicide by youths presenting psychiatric emergencies. J Am Acad Child Adolesc Psychiatry. 2004;43:183-90.
815. Fortune S, Sinclair J, Hawton K. Help-seeking before and after episodes of self-harm: a descriptive study in school pupils in England. BMC Public Health. 2008;8:369.
816. Cauce AM, Domenech-Rodriguez M, Paradise M, Cochran BN, Shea JM, Srebnik D, et al. Cultural and contextual influences in mental health help seeking: a focus on ethnic minority youth. J Consult Clin Psychol. 2002;70:44-55.
817. Bridge JA, Iyengar S, Salary CB, Barbe RP, Birmaher B, Pincus HA, et al. Clinical response and risk for reported suicidal ideation and suicide attempts in pediatric antidepressant treatment: a meta-analysis of randomized controlled trials. JAMA. 2007;297:1683-96.

818. Simon GE, Savarino J, Operskalski B, Wang PS. Suicide risk during antidepressant treatment. Am J Psychiatry. 2006;163:41-7.
819. Gibbons RD, Brown CH, Hur K, Marcus SM, Bhaumik DK, Erkens JA, et al. Early evidence on the effects of regulators' suicidality warnings on SSRI prescriptions and suicide in children and adolescents. Am J Psychiatry. 2007;164:1356-63.
820. Wheeler BW, Gunnell D, Metcalfe C, Stephens P, Martin RM. The population impact on incidence of suicide and non-fatal self-harm of regulatory action against the use of selective serotonin reuptake inhibitors in under 18s in the United Kingdom: ecological study. BMJ. 2008;335:542-5.
821. March J, Silva S, Petrycki S, Curry J, Well K, Fairbank J, et al. Treatment for Adolescents With Depression Study Team. Fluoxetine, cognitive-behavioral therapy and their combination for adolescents with depression: Treatment for Adolescents With Depression Study (TADS) randomized controlled trial. JAMA. 2004;292:807-20.
822. Melvin GA, Tenge BJ, King NJ, Heyne D, Gordon MS, Klimkeit E. A comparison of cognitive-behavioral therapy, sertraline, and their combination for adolescent depression. J Am Acad Child Adolesc Psychiatry. 2006;45:1151-61.
823. Goodyer I, Dubicka B, Wilkinson P, Kelvin R, Roberts C, Byford S, et al. Selective serotonin reuptake inhibitors (SSRIs) and routine specialist care with and without cognitive behaviour therapy in adolescents with major depression: randomised controlled trial. BMJ. 2007;335:142.

Psychotropic Drugs in Children and Adolescents

824. Sharma I. Child Psychopharmacology—Gaps in Knowledge. Jiacam. 1999;3:1-4.
825. Kessler RC, Wang PS. The descriptive epidemiology of commonly occurring mental disorders in the United States. Annu Rev Public Health. 2008;29:115-29.
826. McVoy M, Findling R. Child and Adolescent Psychopharmacology Update. Psychiatr Clin North Am. 2009;32(1):111-33.
827. Bourgeois FT, Mandl KD, Valim C, Shannon MW. Pediatric adverse drug events in the outpatient setting: An 11-year national analysis. Pediatrics. 2009;124(4):e744-e750.
828. Pediatric Psychopharmacology. Steven Domon, MD September, 2010.
829. Arango C, Parellada M, Moreno DM. Clinical effectiveness of new generation antipsychotics in adolescent patients. Eur Neuropsychopharmacol. 2004;14:471–9.
830. Safety and Efficacy Pharmacogenomics in Pediatric Psychopharmacology Christopher A. Wall, MD, Catherine Oldenkamp, MMSII, and Cosima Swintak, MD. Clinical Focus Primary Psychiatry. 2010;17(5):53-8.
831. Phelps L, Brown RT, Power T. Pediatric psychopharmacology: Combining medical and psychosocial intervention. Washington, DC: American Psychological Association, 2001.
832. Werry JS, Aman MG. Anxiolytics, sedatives, and miscellaneous drugs. In: J Werry and M Aman (Eds), Practitioner's guide to psychoactive drugs for children and adolescents; 2nd edition. New York: Plenum; 1999.pp.433-69.
833. Findling RL. Paediatric psychopharmacology: closing the gap between science and practice. Expert Opin Pharmacother, 2001;2:523-5.
834. Dorothy S. Child and adolescent psychiatry. Practical guideline; 2008.
835. Walkup J and the Work Group on Quality Issues: Bernet W, Bukstein O, Walter H, Arnold V, Benson RS, Beitchman J, Chrisman A, Farchione TR, Hamilton J, Keable H, Kinlan J, McClellan J, Schoettle U, Shaw J, Siegel M, Stock S. Practice Parameter on the Use of Psychotropic Medication in Children and Adolescents. J Am Acad Child Adolesc Psychiatry. 2009;48:9.
836. Correll CU, Sheridan EM, DelBello MP. Antipsychoticand mood stabilizer efficacy and tolerability in pediatricand adult patients with bipolar I mania: a comparative analysis of acute, randomized, placebo-controlled trials. Bipolar disorder. 2010;12:116-41.
837. American Academy of Child and Adolescent Psychiatry. 26 Appropriate Use of Psychotropic Drugs in Children and Adolescents—Magellan Health Services Bipolar Disorder Parents' Medication Guide for Bipolar Disorder in Children and Adolescents. Accessed websiteon September 25, 2012 http://www.aacap.org/galleries/default-file/aacap_bipolar_medication_guide.pdf.
838. Geller B, Cooper JB, Sun K, Zimmerman B, Frazier J, Williams M, Heath J. Double-blind and placebo controlled study of lithium for adolescent bipolar disorders with secondary substance dependency. Journal of the American Academy of Child and Adolescent Psychiatry. 1998;37:171-8.
839. Campbell M, Kafantaris V, Cueva JE. An update on the useof lithium carbonate in aggressive children and adolescents with conduct disorders. Psychopharmacology Bulletin, 1995;31:93-102.
840. Phelps L, Brown RT, Power T. Pediatric psychopharmacology: Combining medical and psychosocial intervention. Washington, DC: American Psychological Association; 2001.
841. Werry JS, Aman MG. Anxiolytics, sedatives, and miscellaneous drugs. In: J Werry, M Aman (Eds). Practitioner's guide to psychoactive drugs for children and adolescents. New York: Plenum; 1999.pp.433-69.
842. Alderman J, Wolkow R, Chung M, Johnston HF. Sertraline treatment of children and adolescents with obsessive-compulsive disorder or depression: Pharmacokinetics, tolerability and efficacy. Journal of American Academy of Child and Adolescent Psychiatry. 1998;37:386-94.
843. Barrickman L, Perry PJ, Allen AJ, Kuperman S, Arndt SV, Hermann KJ, Schumacher E. Bupropion versus methylphenidate in the treatment of attention deficit disorder. Journal of the Academy of Child and Adolescent Psychiatry. 1995;34:649–57.
844. Correll CU, Dratochvil CJ, March JS. Developments in Pediatric Psychopharmacology: Focus on Stimulants, Antidepressants, and Antipsychotics. J Clin Psychiatry; 2011.pp.72:5.

845. DuPaul GJ, Barkley RA, Conner DF. Stimulants. In: RA Barkley (Ed). Attention deficit hyperactivity disorder: A handbook for diagnosis and treatment. New York: Guilford Press; 1998. pp.510–51.
846. Hinshaw SP. Stimulant medication and the treatment of aggression in children with attention deficits. Journal of Clinical Psychology. 1991;17:393-407.
847. Armenteros JL, Whitaker AH, Welikson M, Stedge DJ, Gorman J. Risperidone in adolescents with schizophrenia: An open pilot study. Journal of the American Academy of Child and Adolescent Psychiatry. 1997;36:694-700.
848. Zuddas A, Pintor M, Cianchetti C. Risperidone for negative symptoms [Letter]. Journal of the American Academy of Child and Adolescent Psychiatry. 1996;35:838-9.
849. Perry R, Petaki C, Munoz-Silva DM, Armenteros J, Silva RR. Risperidone in children and adolescents with pervasive developmental disorder: Pilot trial and follow-up. Journal of Child and Adolescent Psychopharmacology. 1997;7:167-79.
850. Meyers SM, Plauche Johnson C. The Council on Children with Disabilities. Management of Children With Autism Spectrum Disorders. Pediatrics, Reaffirmed September 2010. 2007;120(5):1162-82.
851. Kodish I, Rockhill C, Varley C. Pharmacotherapy for anxiety disorders in children and adolescents. Dialogues Clin Neurosci. 2011;13:439-52.
852. Connelly SD, Bernstein GA. The Work Group on Quality Issues: Bernet W, Bukstein O, Arnold V, Beitchman J, Benson S, Kinlan J, McClellan J, Schoettle U, Shaw J, Stock S, Walter H. Practice Parameter for the Assessment and Treatment of Children and Adolescents With Anxiety Disorders. J Am Acad Child Adolesc Psychiatry. 2007;46:2.
853. Graae F, Milner J, Rizzotto L, Klein RG. Clonazepam in childhood anxiety disorders. Journal of the American Academy of Child and Adolescent Psychiatry. 1994;33:372-6.
854. Steiner H, Lemsing L. The Work Group on Quality Issues: Arnold V, Beitchman J, Benson S, Bernet W, Bukstein O, Kinlan J, Rue D, Shaw J, Schoettle U, Stock S, Walter H. Practice Parameter for the Assessment and Treatment of Children and Adolescents With Oppositional Defiant Disorders. J Am Acad Child Adolesc Psychiatry. 2007;46:1.
855. Magellan Health Services, Inc. Appropriate Use of Psychotropic Drugs in Children and Adolescents: A Clinical Monograph. Important Issues and Evidence-Based Treatments; 2007. pp.14-21.

FURTHER READING

Examination in Child Psychiatry

1. Adams PL, Fras I. Beginning Child Psychiatry. New York: Brunner/Mazel; 1998.
2. Anastasi A. Psychological Testing. 6th edition. New York: Macmillan; 1988.
3. Bhatia CM. Performance Tests of Intelligence Under Indian Conditions. Bombay: Oxford University Press; 1955.
4. Buck JN. The H-T-P technique: A qualitative scoring manual. J Clin Psychol. 1998;4:317.
5. Conners CK, Barkley RA. Rating scales and checkists for child psychopharmalogy. Psychopharmacol Bull. 1985;21:809.
6. Denckla MB. Revised neurological examination for subtle signs. Psychopharmacol Bull. 1985;21:773.
7. Haley J. Conducting the first interview. In: Haley J (Ed). Problem Solving Therapy. New York: Harper Colophon Books; 1978.
8. King RA. Practise parameters for the psychiatric assessment of children and adolescents. J Am Acad Child Adoles Psychiatry. 1995;34:1386.
9. Kulshreshtha SK. Manual of Stanford Binet Intelligence scale – Hindi adaptation of Third Revision. Form L-M. Allahabad: Manas Sewa Sansthan Prakashan; 1971.
10. Lewis M. Psychiatric assessment of infants, children, and adolescents. In: Lewis M (Ed). Child and Adolescent Psychiatry: A Comprehensive Textbook. Baltimore: Willians & Wilkins; 1991.
11. Malin AJ. Manual for Malin's Intelligence Scale for Indian Children. Nagpur: Child Guidance Centre; 1968.
12. Muralidharan R. Adaptive Development of Indian Children. VII Report. Delhi: NCERT; 1970.
13. Shapiro T. The psychodynamic formulation in child and adolescent psychiatry. J Am Acad Child Adoles Psychiatry. 1989;28:675.
14. Simmons JE. Psychiatric Examination of Children. 4th edition. Philadelphia: Lea & Febiger; 1987.
15. Winnicott DW. Therapeutic Consultations in Child Psychiatry. New York: Basic Books; 2001.

Eating Disorder: Anorexia

16. American Psychiatric Association. Desk Reference to the Diagnostic Criteria from DSM-5. Washington DC; 2013.
17. Morgan JF, Reid F, Lacey JH. The SCOFF questionnaire: assessment of a new screening tool for eating disorders. BMJ. 1999;319(7223):1467-8. [Medline].
18. Steiner H, Lock J. Anorexia nervosa and bulimia nervosa in children and adolescents: a review of the past 10 years. J Am Acad Child Adolesc Psychiatry. 1998;37(4):352-9. [Medline].
19. Steinhausen HC. Outcome of anorexia nervosa in the younger patient. J Child Psychol Psychiatry. 1997;38(3):271-6. [Medline].
20. Tan JO, Hope T, Stewart A, Fitzpatrick R. Control and compulsory treatment in anorexia nervosa: the views of patients and parents. Int J Law Psychiatry. 2003;26(6):627-45. [Medline].
21. Tchanturia K, Davies H, Campbell IC. Cognitive remediation therapy for patients with anorexia nervosa: preliminary findings. Ann Gen Psychiatry. 2007;6:14. [Medline].
22. Wade TD, Gillespie N, Martin NG. A comparison of early family life events amongst monozygotic twin women with lifetime anorexia nervosa, bulimia nervosa, or major depression. Int J Eat Disord. 2007;40(8):679-686. [Medline].
23. Ward L, Tricco A, Phuong P, Cranney A, Barrowman N, Gaboury I. Bisphosphonate therapy for children and adolescents

with secondary osteoporosis. Cochrane Database Syst Rev. 2007;(4):CD005324. [Medline].

24. Wildes JE, Marcus MD, Gaskill JA, Ringham R. Depressive and manic-hypomanic spectrum psychopathology in patients with anorexia nervosa. Compr Psychiatry. 2007;48(5):413-8. [Medline].

Child Substance Abuse

25. Alder I, Kandel DB. Cross-cultural perspectives on development stages in adolescent drug use. Journal Study of Alcohol. 1998;42:701-15.
26. American Psychiatric Association (2000). Diagnostic and Satirical Manual of Disorders (4th edition) Washington, DC, USA; Author.
27. Babu S, Sesikeran B, Bhat RV. Oral fibrosis among teenagers chewing tobacco, areca nut, and pan masala. Lancet. 1996;348:692.
28. Bagwe AN, Bangu UK, Gokhale, SV, Bhisey RA. Evaluation of the mutagenicity of 'pan masala', a chewing substance widely used in India. Mutation Research. 1990;241:349.
29. Banerjee DK. Editorial: Drugs and society. Journal of the Indian Medical Association. 1990;88(10):271.
30. Belcher HME, Shinitzky HE. Substance abuse in children; prediction, protection, and prevention. Archives Pediatric Adolescent Med. 1998;152:952.
31. Bhattacharaya G. Drug use among Asian-Indian adolescents: identifying protective/risk factors. Adolescence. 1998;33(129):169.
32. Blum D, Noble EP, Sheridan PJ, Montgomery A, Jagadeeswaran P, Nogami H, Briggs AH, Chon JB. Allelic association of human dopamine D2 receptor gene in alcoholism. JAMA. 1990;263:2055-60.
33. Bohaman M, Sigvardssonm S, Cloninger CR. Maternal inheritance of alcohol abuse Cross-fostering analysis of adopted women. Archives of General Psychiatry. 1981;38(9):965-9.
34. Buckstein OG. Practice parameters for the assessment and treatment of children and adolescents with substance use disorders. Journal of American Academy of Child and Adolescent Psychiatry. 1997;36(10 Suppl);1404-565.
35. Bukstein OG, Brent DA, Kaminar Y. Comorbidity of substance abuse and other psychiatric disorders in adolescents. American Journal of Psychiatry. 1989;146:1131-41.
36. Bukstein OG, Glancy LJ, Kaminer Y. Patterns of affective comorbidity on a clinical population of dually-diagnosed adolescent substance abusers. Journal of American Academy of Child and Adolescent Psychiatry. 1992;31:1041-5.
37. Center for Substance Abuse Treatment. Screening and assessing adolescents for substance abuse disorders. Treatment improvement protocols. United States Department of Health and Human Services, Washington, DC, USA, 1999.
38. Charles M, Masihi EJ, Siddiqui HY, et al. Culture, drug abuse and some reflections on the family. Bulletin on Narcotics. 1994; XLXI (1)67.
39. Christie KA, Bruke JD, Regier DA, Rae DS, Boyd JH, Locke BZ. Epidemiologic evidence for early onset of mental disorders and higher risk of drug abuse than young adults. American Journal of Psychiatry. 1988;145,971-5.
40. Cloninger CR, Bohman M, Sigvardsson S. Inheritance of alcohol abuse: Cross-fostering analysis of adopted men. Archives of General Psychiatry. 1981;38:861-8.
41. Comerci GD, Schwebel R. Substance abuse: an overview. Adolescent Medicine. 2000;11;79-101.
42. Frances RJ, Miller SI (Eds) (1998). Clinical Text-book of addictive Disorders, 2nd edition. New York: The Guilford Press.
43. Fuller PG, Cavanaugh RM. Basic assessment and screening for substance abuse in the pediatrician's office. Pediatric Clinics of North America. 1995;42:295.
44. Gavarasana S, Gorty P, Allam A. Illiteracy, ignorance, and willingness to quit smoking among villagers in India. Jpn. Journal Cancer Research. 1995;83:340.
45. George A, Varghese C, Sankaranarayanan R, Krishnan Nair M. Use of tobacco and alcoholic beverages by children and teenagers in low-income coastal community in South India. Journal of Cancer Education. 1994;9:111.
46. Glantz M, Pickens P. Vulnerability to drug, abuse, Washington DC: American Psychological Association. 1992;8(5):99-112.
47. Goldenring JM, Cohen E. Getting into adolescent heads. Contemporary Pediatrics. 1988;5:75.
48. Gupta PC. Survey of sociodemographic characteristics of tobacco use among 99, 598 individuals in Bombay, India using hand help computers. Tobacco Control. 1997;5:114.
49. Halarnkar S. Pan masala: a new way to die. India Today. 1997;8:44.
50. Heischober BS, Hofmann AD. Substance abuse. In: Hofmann AD, Greydanus DE (Eds). Adolescent Medicine, 3rd edition, Stamford, CT USA, Appleton and Lange; 1997. p.703.
51. Huizinga D, Elliot DS. A Nation Youth Study of drug use and delinquency in a national sample of youth. An assessment of casual of casual order. CO Behavioral Research Institute. Boulder. 1981.
52. World Health Organization. Internation Classification of Diseases (ICD 9) Clinical Modification. Los Angeles, CA, USA. 1988.
53. Jessor R. Problem-behaviour theory, psychological development and adolescent problem drinking. British Journal of Addiction. 1998;82:331-42.
54. Jessor R, Jessor SL. Problem behaviour and psychosocial development: A longitudinal study of youth. New York: Academic Press. 1997.
55. Kaminer Y, Buckstein O. Adolescent substance abuse. In: Frances RJ, Miller SI, et al, (Eds). Clinical Textbook of Addictive Disorders, 2nd edition. New York, USA: The Guilford Press. 1998; pp.346-73.
56. Kandel DB. Stages in adolescent involvement in drug use. Science. 1975;190:912-4.
57. Kandel DB. Longitudinal research on drug use: Empirical finding and methodological issues. New York; Hemisphere-Wiley. 1978.

58. Kandel DB. Epidemiological trends and implications for understanding the nature of addiction. In: Addictive States, O'Brien CP, Jaffe JH, (Eds). New York: Raven Press; 1992. pp. 23-40.
59. Kandel DB, Faust R. Sequence and stages in patterns of adolescent drug use. Archives of General Psychiatry. 1975;32:923-32.
60. Kandel DB, Kessler RC, Margulies RZ. Use: A developmental analysis. Journal of Youth and Adolescence. 1978;7:13-40.
61. Kandel DB, Yamaguchi K. From beer to crack: Development in drugs. American Journal of Public Health. 1993;83:351-855.
62. Kessler RC, McGonagle KA, Zhao S, et al. Lifetime and 12 months prevalence of DSM HIR psychiatric disorders in the United States. Archives of General Psychiatry. 1994;51:8-19.
63. Kranzer HR, Amin H, Modesto-Lowe V, Oncken. Psychiatric Clinics of North America. 1999;22:402-23.
64. Krishanamurthy S, Ramaswamy R, Trivedi U, Zacharish V. Tobacco use in rural Indian children. Indian Pediatrics. 1997;34;923.
65. Kumpfer KL, Demarsh J. Future issues and promising directions in the prevention of substance abuse among youth. Journal of Children in Contemporary Society. 1986;18:49-91.
66. Kushwala KP, Shing YD, Rathi AK, et al. Prevalence and abuse of psychoactive substances in children and adolescents. Indian Journal of Pediatrics. 1992;59:261.
67. Liepman MR, Keller DM, Botelho RJ, et al. Under sting and substance abuse by adolescents. Primary Care Clinics in Office Practice. 1998;25(1):132.
68. Loeber R. Natural histories of conduct problem, delinquency and associated substance use. In: Lahel BB, Kazdin AE (Eds). Advances in Clinical Child psychology. 1998;11:73-124.
69. Maher R, Lee AJ, Warnkulasuriya KAAS, Johnson R. Role of areca nut in the causation of oral substance related fibrosis: A case-control study in Pakistan. JO Pathol Med. 1994; 23:65.
70. Malhotra S, Kumar H, Anega S, et al. Substance abuse; Knowledge and perception in adolescents. Indian Pediatrics. 1990;27:488.
71. McDonald DI. Drugs, drinking, and adolescents. Chileago, USA, Year Book Medical Publishers, 1984.
72. Milberger S, Biederman J, Faraone SV, Wilens and Chu. Am J Addict. 1997;6:318-29.
73. Milin R, Halikas JA, Melter JE, et al. Psychopathology among substance abusing juvenile offenders. Journal of the American Academy of Child and Adolescent Psychiatry. 1991;30:569-74.
74. Murlidher V, Upmanyu G. Tobacco chewing, oral fibrosis, and anesthetic risk. Lancer. 1996;347:18.
75. Narayan KMV, Chadha SL, Hanson SL, et al. Prevalence and pattern of smoking in Delhi; cross sectional study. Bri International Med Journal. 1996;312:704-6.
76. Newcomb MD. Identifying high-risk youth: Prevalence and patterns of adolescent drug abuse. In: Rahdert E, Czechowicz D (Eds). Adolescent drug abuse: Clinical assessment and therapeutic interventions. National Institute on Drug Abuse. 1995:7-38.
77. Patel RK, Trivedi AH, Jaju R, et al. Ethanol potentiates the carcinogenicity of pan masala-an in vitro experience. Carcinogenesis. 1994;15(9):2017.
78. Patel DR, Gredanus DE. Substance abuse. Indian Journal of Pediatrics. 1999;66(4);557-67.
79. Patton LH. Adolescent substance abuse; risk factors and protective factors. Pediatric Clinics of North America. 1995;42:283.
80. Pickens RW, Svikis DS, McGue M, et al. Heterogeneity in the inheritance of alcoholism: A study of male and female twins. Archives of General Psychiatry. 1991;48(1):19-28.
81. Polasa K, Babu S, Shenolikar IS. Dose-dependent genotoxic effects of pan masala and areca nut in Salmonella typhimurium assay. Fed Chem Toxic. 1993;31:439.
82. Ramchandani AG, D'Souza AV, Borgess AM, Bhisey Ra. Evaluation of carcinogenic/co-carcinogenic activity of common chewing product, pan masala, in mouse skin, stomach and esophagus. Int Journal of Cancer. 1998;75:225.
83. Riggs SR, Alario A. Adolesscnet substance abuse. In: Goldestein MG, Lewis DC (Eds). Curriculum for Primary Care Physician Training Providence. Rohode Island, USA, Brown University. 2004.
84. Riggs PD, Baker S, Mikulich SK. Young, delinquent. Journal of American Academy of Child and Adolescent Psychiatry. 2003;34:764-71.
85. Robertson JA, Pant MA. Alcohol, sex and HIV infection. Drug Alcohol Depend. 1988;22:75.
86. Sankaranarayanan R, Duffy SW, Day Ne, et al. Case-control investigation of cancer of the oral. The floor of the mouth in southern India. Int Journal of Cancer. 1997;44:617.
87. Schwartz B, Alderman EM. Substance of a pediatrics in Review. 1997;18(6): 204.
88. Schwartz RH. Adolescent heroine use; a re-pediatrics. 1998;102(6);1461-6.
89. Sarma HK. (1996) Sociocultural perspective of substance abuse in India. Substance Use and Misusem. 1996;31(11):168-9.
90. Venkataraman S, Mukhopadhya A, Muliyil J. Trends of smoking among medical students. Indian Journal of Medical Research. 2002;104:316.
91. Trivedi AH, Balar DB, Shah PM, et al. Can genic and genotoxic effects of the tobacco substitute pan masala: Present status and likely future impact on the Indian population. Cancer Treatment Reviews. 1996;22:345.
92. Windle, M. Alcohol use and abuse. Alcohol Research World. 1991;15:5-10.

Physical Abuse and Neglect of Children

93. Ablin DS. Osteogenesis imperfecta: a review. Can Assoc Radiol J. 1998;49:110-23.
94. American Academy of Pediatrics Section on Radiology. Diagnostic imaging of child abuse. Pediatrics. 2000;105:1345-8.
95. American Academy of Pediatrics Section on Radiology. Shaken baby syndrome: rotational cranial injuries-technical report. Pediatrics. 2001;108:206-10.

96. Andronicus M, Oates RK, Peat J, Spalding S, Martin H. Non-accidental burns in children. Burns. 1998;24:552-8.
97. Angel C, Shu T, French D, Orihuela E, Lukefahr J, Herndon DN. Genital and perineal burns in children: 10 years of experience at a major burn center. J Pediatr Surg. 2002;37:99-103.
98. Asnes RS. Buttock bruises—Mongolian spot. Pediatrics. 1984;74:321.
99. Banaszkiewicz PA, Scotland TR, Myerscough EJ. Fractures in children younger than age 1 year: importance of collaboration with child protection services. J Pediatr Orthop. 2002;22:740-4.
100. Barlow KM, Thomson E, Johnson D, Minns RA. Late neurologic and cognitive sequelae of inflicted traumatic brain injury in infancy. Pediatrics. 2005;116:e174-e185.
101. Barnes PM, Norton CM, Dunstan FD, Kemp AM, Yates DW, Sibert JR. Abdominal injury due to child abuse. Lancet. 2005;366:234-5.
102. Baron JH. Corporal punishment of children in England and the United States: current issues. Mt Sinai J Med. 2005;72:45-6.
103. Barr RG, Trent RB, Cross J. Age-related incidence curve of hospitalized Shaken Baby Syndrome cases: convergent evidence for crying as a trigger to shaking. Child Abuse Negl. 2006;30:7-16.
104. Barsness KA, Cha ES, Bensard DD, et al. The positive predictive value of rib fractures as an indicator of nonaccidental trauma in children. J Trauma. 2003;54:1107-10.
105. Betz P, Liebhardt E. Rib fractures in children—resuscitation or child abuse?. Int J Legal Med. 1994;106:215-8.
106. Bifulco A, Bernazzani O, Moran PM, Jacobs C. The childhood experience of care and abuse questionnaire (CECA.Q): validation in a community series. Br J Clin Psychol. 2005;44:563-81.
107. Blakemore LC, Loder RT, Hensinger RN. Role of intentional abuse in children 1 to 5 years old with isolated femoral shaft fractures. J Pediatr Orthop. 1996;16:585-8.
108. Brahams D. Child abuse and the doctor's duty of care. Lancet. 1987;2:51.
109. Brooke OG, Lucas A. Metabolic bone disease in preterm infants. Arch Dis Child. 1985;60:682-5.
110. Brown D, Fisher E. Femur fractures in infants and young children. Am J Public Health. 2004;94:558-60.
111. Bulloch B, Schubert CJ, Brophy PD, Johnson N, Reed MH, Shapiro RA. Cause and clinical characteristics of rib fractures in infants. Pediatrics. 2000;105:E48.
112. Bullock K. Child abuse: the physician's role in alleviating a growing problem. Am Fam Physician. 2000;61:2977-78-80, 2985.
113. Bush CM, Jones JS, Cohle SD, Johnson H. Pediatric injuries from cardiopulmonary resuscitation. Ann Emerg Med. 1996;28:40-4.
114. Carpenter RF. The prevalence and distribution of bruising in babies. Arch Dis Child. 1999;80:363-6.
115. Carrigan TD, Walker E, Barnes S. Domestic violence: the shaken adult syndrome. J Accid Emerg Med. 2000;17:138-9.
116. Carty HM. Fractures caused by child abuse. J Bone Joint Surg Br. 1993;75:849-57.
117. Chalumeau M, Foix-l'Helias L, Scheinmann P, Zuani P, Gendrel D, Ducou-le-Pointe H. Rib fractures after chest physiotherapy for bronchiolitis or pneumonia in infants. Pediatr Radiol. 2002;32:644-7.
118. Chapman S, Hall CM. Non-accidental injury or brittle bones. Pediatr Radiol. 1997;27:106-10.
119. Chester DL, Jose RM, Aldlyami E, King H, Moiemen NS. Non-accidental burns in children—are we neglecting neglect?. Burns. 2006;32:222-8.
120. Chuang SS, Yang JY, Tsai FC. Electric water heaters: a new hazard for pediatric burns. Burns. 2003;29:589-91.
121. Coant PN, Kornberg AE, Brody AS, Edwards-Holmes K. Markers for occult liver injury in cases of physical abuse in children. Pediatrics. 1992;89:274-8.
122. Coffey C, Haley K, Hayes J, Groner JI. The risk of child abuse in infants and toddlers with lower extremity injuries. J Pediatr Surg. 2005;40:120-3.
123. Cumming WA. Neonatal skeletal fractures. Birth trauma or child abuse?. J Can Assoc Radiol. 1979;30:30-3.
124. Dahlenburg SL, Bishop NJ, Lucas A. Are preterm infants at risk for subsequent fractures?. Arch Dis Child. 1989;64:1384-5.
125. Davis RE. Cultural health care or child abuse? The Southeast Asian practice of cao gio. J Am Acad Nurse Pract. 2000;12: 89-95.
126. del Ciampo LA, Ricco RG, De Almeida CA, Mucillo G. Incidence of childhood accidents determined in a study based on home surveys. Ann Trop Paediatr. 2001;21:239-43.
127. Dias MS, Smith K, DeGuehery K, Mazur P, Li V, Shaffer ML. Preventing abusive head trauma among infants and young children: a hospital-based, parent education program. Pediatrics. 2005;115:e470-e477.
128. Drago DA. Kitchen scalds and thermal burns in children five years and younger. Pediatrics. 2005;115:10-6.
129. Dube SR, Felitti VJ, Dong M, Giles WH, Anda RF. The impact of adverse childhood experiences on health problems: evidence from four birth cohorts dating back to 1900. Prev Med. 2003;37:268-77.
130. Dubowitz H, Black M, Starr R, Zuravin S. A conceptual definition of child neglect. Crim Justice Behav. 1993;20:8-26.
131. Dubowitz H, Black M. Child neglect In: Reece RM, Ludwig S (Eds). Child Abuse: Medical Diagnosis and Management. Philadelphia PA: Lea & Febiger; 2001.pp.339-62.
132. Dubowitz H, Bross DC. The pediatrician's documentation of child maltreatment. Am J Dis Child. 1992;146:596-99.
133. Dubowitz H, Bross DC. The pediatrician›s documentation of child maltreatment. Am J Dis Child. 1992;146:596-9.
134. Dubowitz H, Giardino A, Gustavson E. Child neglect: guidance for pediatricians. Pediatr Rev. 2000;21:111-6.
135. Dubowitz H, Giardino A, Gustavson E. Child neglect: guidance for pediatricians. Pediatr Rev. 2000;21:111-6.
136. Dubowitz H, Guterman N. Prevention of Physical Abuse and Child Neglect In: Giardino A, Alexander R (Eds). Child Maltreatment: A clinical guide and reference. St Louis, MO: GW Medical; 2005.

137. Dubowitz H. Child neglect: the long-term medical management. The treatment of child abuse. Baltimore, MD: The Johns Hopkins University Press; 2000.
138. Dubowitz H. Preventing child neglect and physical abuse: a role for pediatricians. Pediatr Rev. 2002;23:191-6.
139. Dubowitz H. Preventing child neglect and physical abuse: a role for pediatricians. Pediatr Rev. 2002;23:191-206.
140. Dubowitz H. Preventing child neglect and physical abuse: a role for pediatricians. Pediatr Rev. 2002;23:191-6.
141. Dubowitz H. The neglect of childrens health care In: , Dubowitz H (Ed). Neglected children: research, practice and policy. Thousand Oaks, CA: Sage Publications; 1999.
142. Dubowitz H. What is Child Neglect? In: Dubowitz H, DePanfilis D (Eds). The Handbook for Child Protection. Thousand Oaks, CA: Sage; 2000.
143. Duhaime AC, Christian CW, Rorke LB, Zimmerman RA. Nonaccidental head injury in infants—the "shaken-baby syndrome". N Engl J Med. 1998;338:1822-9.
144. Durrant JE, Ensom Coalition on Physical Punishment of Children and Youth (2004). Joint statement on physical punishment of children and youth. Ottawa, Canada: Coalition on Physical Punishment of Children and Youth; 2004.
145. Edwards VJ, Holden GW, Felitti VJ, Anda RF. Relationship between multiple forms of childhood maltreatment and adult mental health in community respondents: results from the adverse childhood experiences study. Am J Psychiatry. 2003;160:1453-60.
146. Erdmann TC, Feldman KW, Rivara FP, Heimbach DM, Wall HA. Tap water burn prevention: the effect of legislation. Pediatrics. 1991;88:572-7.
147. Ewing-Cobbs L, Kramer L, Prasad M, et al. Neuroimaging, physical, and developmental findings after inflicted and noninflicted traumatic brain injury in young children. Pediatrics. 1998;102:300-7.
148. Feldman KW, Brewer DK. Child abuse, cardiopulmonary resuscitation, and rib fractures. Pediatrics. 1984;73:339-42.
149. Feldman KW, Schaller RT, Feldman JA, McMillon M. Tap water scald burns in children. Pediatrics. 1978;62:1-7.
150. Feldman KW. Pseudoabusive burns in Asian refugees. Am J Dis Child. 1984;138:768-9.
151. Flaherty EG, Sege R. Barriers to physician identification and reporting of child abuse. Pediatr Ann. 2005;34:349-56.
152. Forjuoh SN. Pattern of intentional burns to children in Ghana. Child Abuse Negl. 1995;19:837-41.
153. Frechette A, Rimsza ME. Stun gun injury: a new presentation of the battered child syndrome. Pediatrics. 1992;89:898-901.
154. Freitag R, Lazoritz S, Kini N. Psychosocial aspects of child abuse for primary care pediatricians. Pediatr Clin North Am. 1998;45:391-402.
155. Garcia VF, Gotschall CS, Eichelberger MR, Bowman LM. Rib fractures in children: a marker of severe trauma. J Trauma. 1990;30:695-700.
156. Geddes JF, Hackshaw AK, Vowles GH, Nickols CD, Whitwell HL. Neuropathology of inflicted head injury in children. I. Patterns of brain damage. Brain. 2001;124:1290-8.
157. Geddes JF, Tasker RC, Hackshaw AK, et al. Dural haemorrhage in non-traumatic infant deaths: does it explain the bleeding in 'shaken baby syndrome'? Neuropathol Appl Neurobiol. 2003;29:14-22.
158. Geddes JF, Vowles GH, Hackshaw AK, Nickols CD, Scott IS, Whitwell HL. Neuropathology of inflicted head injury in children. II. Microscopic brain injury in infants. Brain. 2001;124:1299-306.
159. Glaser D. Child abuse and neglect and the brain—a review. J Child Psychol Psychiatry. 2000;41:97-116.
160. Gnanaraj L, Gilliland MG, Yahya RR, et al. Ocular manifestations of crush head injury in children. Eye. 2007;21:5-10.
161. Grant P, Mata MB, Tidwell M. Femur fracture in infants: a possible accidental etiology. Pediatrics. 2001;108:1009-11.
162. Grayev AM, Boal DK, Wallach DM, Segal LS. Metaphyseal fractures mimicking abuse during treatment for clubfoot. Pediatr Radiol. 2001;31:559-63.
163. Gunn VL, Hickson GB, Cooper WO. Factors affecting pediatricians' reporting of suspected child maltreatment. Ambul Pediatr. 2005;5:96-101.
164. Gushurst CA. Child abuse: behavioral aspects and other associated problems. Pediatr Clin North Am. 2003;50: 919-38.
165. Hartmann RW Jr. Radiological case of the month. Rib fractures produced by birth trauma. Arch Pediatr Adolesc Med. 1997;151: 947-8.
166. Hazen AL, Connelly CD, Kelleher KJ, Barth RP, Landsverk JA. Female caregivers' experiences with intimate partner violence and behavior problems in children investigated as victims of maltreatment. Pediatrics. 2006;117:99-109.
167. Hennes HM, Smith DS, Schneider K, Hegenbarth MA, Duma MA, Jona JZ. Elevated liver transaminase levels in children with blunt abdominal trauma: a predictor of liver injury. Pediatrics. 1990;86:87-90.
168. Hildyard KL, Wolfe DA. Child neglect: developmental issues and outcomes. Child Abuse Negl. 2002;26:679-95.
169. Hobbs CJ, Wynne JM. Fractures in infancy: are the bones brittle? Curr Paediatr. 1996;6:183-8.
170. Hobbs CJ. ABC of child abuse. Fractures. BMJ. 1989;298:1015-8.
171. Hobbs CJ. Skull fracture and the diagnosis of abuse. Arch Dis Child. 1984;59:246-52.
172. Hoekelman RA. Child Health Supervision In: Hoekelman N, Friedman SB, Nelson NM, Seidel HM, Weitzman SL (Eds). Primary pediatric care. St Louis, MO: Mosby; 1997.
173. Holter JC, Friedman SB. Etiology and management of severely burned children. Psychosocial considerations. Am J Dis Child. 1969;118:680-6.
174. Huntimer CM, Muret-Wagstaff S, Leland NL. Can falls on stairs result in small intestine perforations?. Pediatrics. 2000;106:301-5.
175. Hymel K, Bandak F, Partington M, Winston K. Abusive head trauma? A biomechanics-based approach. Child Maltreatment. 1998;3:116-28.
176. Irazuzta JE, McJunkin JE, Danadian K, Arnold F, Zhang J. Outcome and cost of child abuse. Child Abuse Negl. 1997;21:751-7.

177. Jellinek MS, Murphy JM, Bishop S, Poitrast F, Quinn D. Protecting severely abused and neglected children. An unkept promise. N Engl J Med. 1990;323:1628-30.
178. Jenny C, Hymel KP, Ritzen A, Reinert SE, Hay TC. Analysis of missed cases of abusive head trauma. JAMA. 1999;281:621-6.
179. Jenny C. In: Cutaneous manifestations of child abuse. Child abuse: medical diagnosis and management. Philadelphia PA: Lippincott Williams, and Wilkins; 2001.pp.23-6.
180. Jenny C. Modes of presentation of inflicted childhood neurotrauma In: Reece RM, Nicholson CE (Eds). Inflicted childhood neurotrauma. American Academy of Pediatrics. 2003:49-64.
181. Joseph PR, Rosenfeld W. Clavicular fractures in neonates. Am J Dis Child. 1990;144:165-7.
182. Kaufman J, Zigler E. Do abused children become abusive parents?. Am J Orthopsychiatry. 1987;57:186-92.
183. Keenan HT, Runyan DK, Marshall SW, Nocera MA, Merten DF. A population-based comparison of clinical and outcome characteristics of young children with serious inflicted and non-inflicted traumatic brain injury. Pediatrics. 2004;114:633-9.
184. Kendall-Tackett K, Lyon T, Taliaferro G, Little L. Why child maltreatment researchers should include children's disability status in their maltreatment studies. Child Abuse Negl. 2005;29:147-51.
185. King J, Diefendorf D, Apthorp J, Negrete VF, Carlson M. Analysis of 429 fractures in 189 battered children. J Pediatr Orthop. 1988;8:585-9.
186. King WJ, MacKay M, Sirnick A, et al. Shaken baby syndrome in Canada: clinical characteristics and outcomes of hospital cases. CMAJ. 2003;168:155-9.
187. Kleinman PK, Marks SC Jr, Nimkin K, Rayder SM, Kessler SC. Rib fractures in 31 abused infants: postmortem radiologic-histopathologic study. Radiology. 1996;200:807-10.
188. Kleinman PK, Nimkin K, Spevak MR, et al. Follow-up skeletal surveys in suspected child abuse. Am J Roentgenol. 1996;167:893-6.
189. Kleinman PK. Diagnostic Imaging of Child. St Louis, MO: Mosby; 1998.
190. Kolko DJ. Characteristics of child victims of physical violence: research findings and clinical implications. J Interpers Viol. 1992;7:244-76.
191. Korbin JE. Neighborhood and community connectedness in child maltreatment research. Child Abuse Negl. 2003;27: 137-40.
192. Labbe J, Caouette G. Recent skin injuries in normal children. Pediatrics. 2001;108:271-6.
193. Lane WG, Rubin DM, Monteith R, Christian CW. Racial differences in the evaluation of pediatric fractures for physical abuse. JAMA. 2002;288:1603-9.
194. Lantz PE, Sinal SH, Stanton CA, Weaver RG Jr. Perimacular retinal folds from childhood head trauma. BMJ. 2004;328:754-6.
195. Leventhal JM, Thomas SA, Rosenfield NS, Markowitz RI. Fractures in young children. Distinguishing child abuse from unintentional injuries. Am J Dis Child. 1993;147:87-92.
196. Levin AV. Retinal hemorrhages and child abuse In: David TJ (Ed). Recent Advances in Paediatrics. London: Churchill Livingstone; 2000. pp.151-219.
197. Loder RT, Bookout C. Fracture patterns in battered children. J Orthop Trauma. 1991;5:428-33.
198. Ludwig S. Visceral manifestations of child abuse. In: Reece RM, Ludwig S (Eds). Child abuse: medical diagnosis and management. Philadelphia PA: Lippincott, Williams, and Wilkens; 2001.pp.157-76.
199. Lynch A. Child abuse in the school-age population. J Sch Health. 1975;45:141-8.
200. Lysack JT, Soboleski D. Classic metaphyseal lesion following external cephalic version and cesarean section. Pediatr Radiol. 2003;33:06.
201. MacMillan HL, Thomas BH, Jamieson E, et al. Effectiveness of home visitation by public-health nurses in prevention of the recurrence of child physical abuse and neglect: a randomised controlled trial. Lancet. 2005;365:1786-93.
202. Maguire S, Mann M, John N, et al. Does cardiopulmonary resuscitation cause rib fractures in children? A systematic review. Child Abuse Negl. 2006;30:739-51.
203. Maguire S, Mann MK, Sibert J, Kemp A. Are there patterns of bruising in childhood which are diagnostic or suggestive of abuse? A systematic review. Arch Dis Child. 2005;90:182-6.
204. Maguire S, Mann MK, Sibert J, Kemp A. Can you age bruises accurately in children? A systematic review. Arch Dis Child. 2005;90:187-9.
205. Mandelstam SA, Cook D, Fitzgerald M, Ditchfield MR. Complementary use of radiological skeletal survey and bone scintigraphy in detection of bony injuries in suspected child abuse. Arch Dis Child. 2003;88:387-90.
206. McMahon P, Grossman W, Gaffney M, Stanitski C. Soft-tissue injury as an indication of child abuse. J Bone Joint Surg Am. 1995;77:1179-83.
207. Mellick LB, Milker L, Egsieker E. Childhood accidental spiral tibial (CAST) fractures. Pediatr Emerg Care. 1999;15:307-9.
208. Mendelson KL. Critical review of 'temporary brittle bone disease'. Pediatr Radiol. 2005;35:1036-40.
209. Merten DF, Carpenter BL. Radiologic imaging of inflicted injury in the child abuse syndrome. Pediatr Clin North Am. 1990;37:815-37.
210. Merten DF, Radkowski MA, Leonidas JC. The abused child: a radiological reappraisal. Radiology. 1983;146:377-81.
211. Minns RA. Shaken baby syndrome: theoretical and evidential controversies. J R Coll Physicians Edinb. 2005;35:5-15.
212. Molina JA. Understanding the biopsychosocial model. Int J Psychiatry Med. 1983;13:29-36.
213. Morris AA, Hoffmann GF, Naughten ER, Monavari AA, Collins JE, Leonard JV. Glutaric aciduria and suspected child abuse. Arch Dis Child. 1999;80:404-5.
214. Morris S, Cassidy N, Stephens M, McCormack D, McManus F. Birth-associated femoral fractures: incidence and outcome. J Pediatr Orthop. 2002;22:27-30.

215. Naidoo S. A profile of the oro-facial injuries in child physical abuse at a children's hospital. Child Abuse Negl. 2000;24:521-34.
216. Olds DL, Eckenrode J, Henderson CR, Kitzman H, Powers J, Cole R, et al. Long-term effects of home visitation on maternal life course and child abuse and neglect. Fifteen-year follow-up of a randomized trial. JAMA. 1997;278:637-43.
217. Panel on Research on Child Abuse and Neglect. Commission on Behavioral and Social Sciences and Education National Research Council: Understanding child abuse and neglect. Washington, DC: National Academy Press; 1993.
218. Paulson JA. Pediatric advocacy. Pediatr Clin North Am. 2001;48:1307-18.
219. Perez CM, Widom CS. Childhood victimization and long-term intellectual and academic outcomes. Child Abuse Negl. 1994;18: 617-33.
220. Pierce MC, Bertocci GE, Janosky JE, et al. Femur fractures resulting from stair falls among children: an injury plausibility model. Pediatrics. 2005;115:1712-22.
221. Pounder DJ. Shaken adult syndrome. Am J Forensic Med Pathol. 1997;18:321-4.
222. Prange MT, Myers BS. Pathobiology and biomechanics of inflicted childhood neurotrauma. Inflicted childhood neurotrauma. American Academy of Pediatrics. 2003;237-44.
223. Prosser I, Maguire S, Harrison SK, Mann M, Sibert JR, Kemp AM. How old is this fracture? Radiologic dating of fractures in children: a systematic review. Am J Roentgenol. 2005;184:1282-6.
224. Reece RM, Ludwig S. Child abuse: medical diagnosis and management. Baltimore MD: Lippincott, Williams, and Wilkins; 2001.
225. Reece RM, Nicholson CE. Inflicted childhood neurotrauma. American Academy of Pediatrics; 2003.
226. Reece RM, Sege R. Childhood head injuries: accidental or inflicted?. Arch Pediatr Adolesc Med. 2000;154:11-5.
227. Renz BM, Sherman R. Abusive scald burns in infants and children: a prospective study. Am Surg. 1993;59:329-34.
228. Renz BM, Sherman R. Child abuse by scalding. J Med Assoc Ga. 1992;81:574-8.
229. Rizzolo PJ, Coleman PR. Neonatal rib fracture: birth trauma or child abuse?. J Fam Pract. 1989;29:561-3.
230. Roche KJ, Genieser NB, Berger DK, Ambrosino MM. Traumatic abdominal pseudoaneurysm secondary to child abuse. Pediatr Radiol. 1995;25(Suppl 1):S247-S248.
231. Rorke LB. Neuropathology of inflicted childhood neurotrauma In: Reece RM, Nicholson CE (Eds). Inflicted childhood neurotrauma (Concensus Development Conference). American Academy of Pediatrics; 2003.
232. Rutter M, O' Connor TG. Are there biological programming effects for psychological development? Findings from a study of Romanian adoptees. Dev Psychol. 2004;40:81-94.
233. Salehi-Had H, Brandt JD, Rosas AJ, Rogers KK. Findings in older children with abusive head injury: does shaken-child syndrome exist?. Pediatrics. 2006;117:e1039-e1044.
234. Satcher D, Kaczorowski J, Topa D. The expanding role of the pediatrician in improving child health in the 21st century. Pediatrics. 2005;115(suppl 4):1124-8.
235. Schuck AM, Widom CS. Understanding the role of neighborhood context in the long-term criminal consequences of child maltreatment. Am J Community Psychol. 2005;36: 207-22.
236. Schwend RM, Werth C, Johnston A. Femur shaft fractures in toddlers and young children: rarely from child abuse. J Pediatr Orthop. 2000;20:475-81.
237. Sedlack AJ, Broadhurst DD. Third national incidence study of child abuse and neglect: final report. Washington, DC: US Department of Health and Human Services; 1996.
238. Sewell RD, Steinberg MA. Chest compressions in an infant with osteogenesis imperfecta type II: No new rib fractures. Pediatrics. 2000;106:E71.
239. Sirotnak AP, Grigsby T, Krugman RD. Physical abuse of children. Pediatr Rev. 2004;25:264-77.
240. Sirotnak AP, Grigsby T, Krugman RD. Physical abuse of children. Pediatr Rev. 2004;25:264-77.
241. Skellern CY, Wood DO, Murphy A, Crawford M. Non-accidental fractures in infants: risk of further abuse. J Paediatr Child Health. 2000;36:590-2.
242. Smith SM, Hanson R. 134 battered children: a medical and psychological study. BMJ. 1974;3:666-70.
243. Socolar RR, Raines B, Chen-Mok M, Runyan DK, Green C, Paterno S. Intervention to improve physician documentation and knowledge of child sexual abuse: a randomized, controlled trial. Pediatrics. 1998;101:817-24.
244. Spevak MR, Kleinman PK, Belanger PL, Primack C, Richmond JM. Cardiopulmonary resuscitation and rib fractures in infants. A postmortem radiologic-pathologic study. JAMA. 1994;272:617-8.
245. Spivack BS, Margulies SS. Pathobiology and biomechanics of inflicted childhood neurotrauma In: Reece RM, Nicholson CE (Eds). Inflicted childhood neurotrauma. American Academy of Pediatrics. 2003:221-35.
246. Sponseller P. Pediatric musculoskeletal trauma. Curr Opin Orthop. 2000;11:461-7.
247. Sugar NF, Taylor JA, Feldman KW. Bruises in infants and toddlers: those who don't cruise rarely bruise. Puget Sound Pediatric Research Network. Arch Pediatr Adolesc Med. 1999;153:399-403.
248. Supreme Court of Judicature UK. Approved Judgment Neutral citation number: EWCA Crim. 1980, 2005 July 21; (Case nos: 200403277, 200406902, 200302848). (accessed May 24, 2007).
249. Surrell JA, Alexander RC, Cohle SD, Lovell FR Jr, Wehrenberg RA. Effects of microwave radiation on living tissues. J Trauma. 1987;27:935-9.
250. Svedin CG, Wadsby M, Sydsjo G. Mental health, behaviour problems and incidence of child abuse at the age of 16 years. A prospective longitudinal study of children born at psychosocial risk. Eur Child Adolesc Psychiatry. 2005;14:386-96.

251. Tenenbein M, Reed MH, Black GB. The toddler's fracture revisited. Am J Emerg Med. 1990;8:208-11.
252. Thomas PS. Rib fractures in infancy. Ann Radiol (Paris). 1977;20:115-22.
253. Thomas SA, Rosenfield NS, Leventhal JM, Markowitz RI. Long-bone fractures in young children: distinguishing accidental injuries from child abuse. Pediatrics. 1991;88:471-6.
254. US Department of Health and Human Services. Administration on Children Youth and Families. Child Maltreatment 2004. Washington, DC: US Government Printing Office; 2006.
255. van der Kolk BA. The neurobiology of childhood trauma and abuse. Child Adolesc Psychiatr Clin N Am. 2003;12: 293-317.
256. Wardinsky TD. Genetic and congenital defect conditions that mimic child abuse. J Fam Pract. 1995;41:377-83.
257. Waterston T, Rudolf M. Exploring the scope for advocacy by paediatricians. Arch Dis Child. 2000;82:428.
258. Waterston T. A general paediatrician's practice in children's rights. Arch Dis Child. 2005;90:178-81.
259. Wheeler DM, Hobbs CJ. Mistakes in diagnosing non-accidental injury: 10 years' experience. BMJ. 1988;296:1233-6.
260. Whitby EH, Griffiths PD, Rutter S, et al. Frequency and natural history of subdural haemorrhages in babies and relation to obstetric factors. Lancet. 2004;363:846-51.
261. Whittaker DK, Aitken M, Burfitt E, Sibert JR. Assessing bite marks in children: Working with a forensic dentist. Am Child Health. 1997;3:225-9.
262. Wilson SL, Kuebli JE, Hughes HM. Patterns of maternal behavior among neglectful families: implications for research and intervention. Child Abuse Negl. 2005;29:985-1001.
263. Worlock P, Stower M, Barbor P. Patterns of fractures in accidental and non-accidental injury in children: a comparative study. BMJ. 1986;293:100-2.
264. Wu SS, Ma CX, Carter RL, et al. Risk factors for infant maltreatment: a population-based study. Child Abuse Negl. 2004;28:1253-64.
265. Zimmerman S, Makoroff K, Care M, Thomas A, Shapiro R. Utility of follow-up skeletal surveys in suspected child physical abuse evaluations. Child Abuse Negl. 2005;29:1075-83.
266. Department for Children, Schools and Families. DCSF: referrals, assessments and children and young people who are the subject of a Child Protection Plan, England—year ending 31 Mar 2008 (additional tables including England summary tables and local authority tables). 2008. www.dcsf.gov.uk/rsgateway/DB/SFR/s000811/additional_tables.xls.
267. Data Unit Wales. Dataunitwales Dissemination Tool. 2009. http://dissemination.dataunitwales.gov.uk/webview/index.jsp.
268. Department of Health. National Service Framework for children, young people, and maternity services—core standards. London: DH; 2004.
269. Glaser D. Emotional abuse and neglect (psychological maltreatment): a conceptual framework. Child Abuse and Neglect. 2002;26:697-714.
270. Gilbert R, Kemp A, Thoburn J, Sidebotham P, Radford L, Glaser D, et al. Recognising and responding to child maltreatment. Lancet. 2009;373:167-80.
271. Wise J. Systemic failings in NHS contributed to death of Baby P. BMJ. 2009;338:b1967.
272. National Institute for Health and Clinical Excellence. When to suspect child maltreatment. 2009. (Clinical guideline 89.) www.nice.org.uk/CG89.
273. HM Government. Working together to safeguard children. London: Stationery Office; 2006.
274. National Society for the Prevention of Cruelty to Children. Child protection register statistics. 2009. www.nspcc.org.uk/Inform/resourcesforprofessionals/Statistics/ChildProtectionRegisterStatistics/england_wdf49858.pdf.
275. Gilbert R, Spatz Widom C, Browne K, Fergusson D, Webb E, Janson S. Burden and consequences of child maltreatment in high-income countries. Lancet. 2009;373:68-81.
276. MacMillan HL, Wathen CN, Barlow J, Fergusson DM, Leventhal JM, Taussig HN. Interventions to prevent child maltreatment and associated impairment. Lancet. 2009;373:250-66.
277. Welsh Assembly Government. National Service Framework for Children, Young People and Maternity Services in Wales. 2005. www.wales.nhs.uk/sites3/home.cfm?OrgID=441
278. Office of the United Nations High Commissioner for Human Rights. Convention on the Rights of the Child. 1990. www.unhchr.ch/html/menu3/b/k2crc.htm
279. National Institute for Health and Clinical Excellence. The guidelines manual. London: NICE; 2007.

Conduct Disorders in Children

280. Alexander IF, Holtzworth-Munrose A, Jameson PR. The Process and outcome of marital and family therapy research: review and Evaluation. In: Bergin AE, Gaarfied S (Eds). Handbook of Psychotherapy and Behavior Change. 1994.pp.595-630. Wiley, New York.
281. American Psychiatric Association. Desk Reference to the Diagnostic Criteria from DSM-5. Washington DC; 2013
282. American Psychiatric Association. Diagnostic and statistical manual of mental disorders, 4th edition. American Psychiatric Association, Washingtone, DC; 1994.
283. Anderson J, Williams S, McGee R, Silva P. DSM-III disorder in preadolescent children. Arch Gen Psychia. 1987;44:69-76.
284. Bank L, Marlowe JH, Reid JB, Patterson GR, Weinrott MR. A comparative evaluation of parent-training interventions for Families of chronic delinquents. Journal of Abnormal Child Psychology. 1991;19:15-33.
285. Bierman K, Grenberg M. Social skill training in the etiological theory through epidemiologically based preventive intervention trials. In: Mc Cord J, Tremblay R (Eds). Preventing antisocial behavior: interventions from birth to adolescence. Thouadn Oaks, CA. 1996.pp.162-95.
286. Bonman MI. Predisposition to criminality: Swedish adoption Studies in retrospect. In: Bock G, Goode J (Eds). Genetics of

criminal and antisocial behavior. Ciba Foundation symposium 194. Weley, Chichester; 1996. pp.99-114.

287. Caspi A, Lynam D, Moffitt T, Silva PS. Unraveling girls' Delinquency: biological, dispostional, and contextual contributions to adolescent misbehavior. Developmental Psychopathology. 2003;29:19-30.
288. Champion I. Psychology and Psychiatry, 1997;38:161-78. Up of London school children. Psychological Medicine; 25:161-78.
289. Cohen P, Cohen J, Kasesn S, et al. An epidemiological study of disorders in late childhood and adolescence I. Age and gender specific prevalence. J Child Psych Psychia. 1993;34: 851-68.
290. Coie J, Dodge K. Aggression and antisocial behavior. In: Damon W, Eisenbergg N (Eds). Handbook of child psychology: social, emotional and personality Development, Wiley, New York; Vol. 3. 1997.pp.779-862.
291. Conduct problems prevention Research Group. A developmental and clinical model for prevention of conduct disorder. Development and Psychopathology. 1992;4:509-27.
292. Dilalla LF, Gottesman I. Heterogeneity of causes of Delinquency and criminality: lifespan perspectives. Development and Psychopathology. 2004;1:339-49.
293. Dishion T, Andrews D. Preventing escalation in problem behaviors with high-risk young adolescents: immediate and 1-year outcomes. Journal of Consulting and Clinical Psychology. 1995;63:538-48.
294. Dishion T, Patterson G. The timing and severity of antisocial behavior: three hypotheses within an ecological framework. In: Stoff D, Breiling J, Maser J (Eds). Handbook of anstisocial behavior. Wiley, New York; 1997.pp.206-18.
295. Dodge K, Schwartz D. Social information processing Mechanisms I aggressive behavior. In: Stoff D, Breiling J, Maser J (Eds). Handbook of Antisocial Behavior. Wiley, New York; 1997.pp.171-80.
296. Durlak J. School-based prevention programs for children and adolescents. Sage, Thousand Oaks, CA; 1995.
297. Farrington D. The Twelfth lack Tizard Memorial Lecture: the development of offending and antisocial behavior from childhood: key findings from the Cambridge study in Delinquent Development. Journal of Child Psychology and Psychiatry. 1995;36:929-64.
298. Farrington DP. Early developmental prevention of juvenile Delinquency. Criminal Behaviour and Mental Health. 1994;4: 209-27.
299. Feldman R. The St Louis experiment: effective treatment of antisocial youths in prosocial peer groups. In: McCord J, Tremblay R (Eds). Preventing antisocial behavior: interventions from birth to adolescence. Guilford Press, New York; 1992. pp.233-52.
300. Gardner FME. Positive interaction between mothers and conduct-problem children: is there trainning for harmony as well as fighting. Journal of Abnormal Child psychology. 1987;15:283-93.
301. Goodman R, Meltzer H, Bailey V. The strengths and difficulties questionnaire: a pilot study on the validity of the self-report version. European Child and Adolescent Psychiatry. 1998;7:125-30.
302. Goodman R, Scott S. Comparing the strengths and difficulties questionnaires and the child behavior checklist: is small Beautiful? J Abnor Child Psycho. 1999;27:17-25.
303. Goodman R. Child and adolescent mental health services: Reasoned advice to commissioners' and providers. Maudsley discussion Paper No. 4. Institute of Psychiatry, London; 1997.
304. Gray J. The psychology of fear and stress. Cambridge University Press; 1987.
305. Henggeler SW. Multisystemic therapy: an overview of clinical Procedures, outcomes and policy implications. Child psychology and psychiatry Review. 1999;4:2-10.
306. Kazdi A. Conduct disorder. Behavioral approaches to Children. Journal of Child Psychology and Psychiatry. 1999;38: 161-78.
307. Kellam S, Rebok G. Building developmental and etiological theory through epidemiologically based preventive intervention trials. In: McCord J, Tremblay R (Eds). Preventing antisocial behavior: interventions from birth to adolescence. Gullfonl Press, New York; 1992.pp.162-95.
308. Kendall P, Braswell L. Cognitive, behavioral therapy for impulsive children. Guilford Press, New York; 1996.
309. Kesler R, Davis C, Kendler K. Childhood adversity and Adult psychiatric disorder in the US National Comorbidity Survey. Psychological Medicine. 1997;27:1101-9.
310. Lahey B, Loeber R. Framework for a developmental model of oppositional deviant disorder and conduct disorder. In: Herbet C. Quay. Routh D (Ed). Disruptive Behaviour Disorders in Childhood: essoys in honor of Plenum press, New York.; 1994. pp.139-80.
311. Lochamn J, Wells K. Social-cognitive intervention with aggressive children: prevention effects and contextual implementation intervention trials. In: Peters R, McMahon R (Eds). Preventing childhood disorders, Substance abuse and delinquency. Sage, Thousand Oaks, CA; 1996. PP, III-43.
312. Mayes L, Bornstein M. The development of children Exposed to cocaine. In development psychopathology: perspectives on J. Weisz); Cambridge University Press. 1997.pp.166-88.
313. Moffit T, Caspi AP, et al. Whole blood serotonin and family background relate to male violence. In: Raine A, Brennan P, Farrington D, Mednick S (Eds). Biological buses of violence. Plenum press, New York; 1997.pp.231-50.
314. Moffitt T, Caspi A, Dicckson N, Silva P, Standton W. Childhood -onset versus adolescent-onset antisocial conduct problems in males: natural history from ages 3 to 18 years. Development and Psychopathology. 1996;8:399-424.
315. Offord D, Boyle M, Racine Y. The epidemiology of antisocial behavior. In: Pepler D, Rubin K (Eds). The development and treatment of childhood ageression. Erlbaum, Hillsdale, NJ; 1991. pp.31-4.
316. Osborn S. Temperament and behavior disorders in children, New York University Press; 1980.
317. Patterson GR. Corcive family process. Gastalia, Eugene; 1982. pp.88-96.

318. Pelham W. Pharmacotherapy for children with attention-deficit hyperactivity disorder. School Psychology Review. 2003;22:199-227.
319. Raine A. Antisocial behavior and psychopathology: a biosocial Perspective and a prefrontal dysfunction hypothesis. In: Stoff D, Brelling, Maser J (Eds). Handbook of Antisocial behavior. Wiley, New York; 1997.pp.289-304.
320. Richman N, Stevenson J, Grahaum P. Preschool to school: Behavioral study: Academic Pres, London; 1982.
321. Robins L, Regier D (Eds). Heterogeneity of causes four Delinquency and criminality. Lifespan perspectives. Development and psychopathology. 2005;1:339-49.
322. Robins L. Deviant Children grown up, Williams and Wilkins, Baltimore, MD; 1966.
323. Rutter MP, Ousten J, Smith A. Fifteen thousand hours: secondary schools and their effects on Children. Harvard University press, Cambridge, MA. 1977; pp.15-24.
324. Rutter M, Quinton D. Parental Psychiatric disorder: effects on children. Psychological Medical. 1984;14:209-27.
325. Rutter M, Cox A, Tupling M, Berge M, Yule W. Attainment and adjustment in two geographical areas. Bri J Phy. 1975;126:493-509.
326. Rutter M, Giller H, Hagell A. Antisocial behavior by young People Cambridge University Press, 1998.
327. Rutter M, Tizard J, Whitmore K (Eds). Education, health and behavior. Longmans, London; 2003.
328. Sampson R, Raudenbush S, Earls F. Neighborhoods and Violent crime: a multilevel study of collective efficary. Science. 1997;277:918-24.
329. Scott S. Conduct disorder. In: Howlin P (Ed). Behaviroural approaches to Problems in childhood. Cambridge University Press; 1999.pp.1-27.
330. Scott S. Mental retardation. In: Rutter M, Taylor E, Hersov L (Eds). Child and adolescent psychiatry: Modern approaches, 3rd edition, Black Well Science, Oxford; 1994.pp. 616-46.
331. Shaffer D, Boyle M, et al. The NIMH Diagnostic Interview schedule for children version 2.3 (DISC 2.3): description, acceptability, prevalence rates, and performance in the MEGA study. J Am Acad Child and Adoles Psychia. 1996;35:865-78.
332. Silberg J, Meyer J, Pickeles A, et al. Heterogeneity among Juvenile antisocial behaviours. Findings from the Virginia Twin Study of Adloes CDI Behviroal De; 1996.
333. Stattin H, Romeljo A, Stenbacka M. Personal resources Underachievement in childhood and adolescence: causal relationships and underlying mechanisms. Psychologicla Bulletin. 1997;111:127-55.
334. Stattin H, Romelsjo A, Stendbacka M. Personal resources As modifiers of the risk for future criminality and analysis of protective factors in relation to 18 year old boys. British Jouruaal of Criminology. 1997;37:198-222.
335. Stressguth A. Fetal alcohol syndrome in older patients. Alcoholk. 1993;2:209-12.
336. Thomas A, Lynam D, Moffitt T, Silva P. Temperament and behavior disorders in children. New York University Press; 1968.
337. Tremblay Bothte, RE. Physical aggression, social dominance and testosterone levels at pubirty: A developmental perspective. In: Raine A, Breman P, Farringtom D, Mednick S (Eds). Biological Bases of Violence. 2006.
338. Trickett A, McBride-Chang C. The development impact of different forms of child abuse and neglect. Development Review. 1995;15:311-37.
339. Venables P. Pscholphysiology and crime: theory and data. In: Moffitt T, Mednick S (Eds). Biological contributions to crime causation. Nijhoff, Dordrecht; 1988.pp.3-13.
340. Webster Stratton C, Hollinsworth T, Kaolpacoff M. The Long-term effectiveness and clinical significance of three cost-effective training programs for families wit conduct-problem children. Journal of Consulting and Clinical Psychology; 1989.
341. Webster-Stratton C. Randomized trial of two parent-training Programs for families with conduct disordered children. Journal of Consulting and Clinical Psychology. 1984;52:666-78.
342. Widom C. Child abuse, neglect and witnessing violence. In: Stoff D, Breling J, Maser J (Eds). Handbook of antisocial behavior. Wiley, New York; 1997.pp.159-70.
343. World Health Organization. The ICD-10 classification of mental and behavioral disorders—diagnostic criteria for research. WHO, Geneva; 1992.
344. World Health Organization. The ICD-10 classification of mental and behavioral disorders—diagnostic criteria for research. WHO, Geneva; 1993.
345. Collishaw S, Maughan B, Goodman R, Pickles A. Time trends in adolescent mental health. J Child Psychol Psychiatry. 2004;45:1350-62.
346. Green H, McGinnity A, Meltzer H, Ford T, Goodman R. Mental health of children and young people in Great Britain, 2004: summary report. Office for National Statistics; 2005.
347. Fergusson DM, Horwood LJ, Ridder EM. Show me a child at seven: consequences of conduct problems in childhood for psychosocial functioning in adulthood. J Child Psychol Psychiatry. 2005;46:837-49.
348. Moffitt T. Life-course-persistent versus adolescence-limited antisocial behaviour: a 10-year research review and a research agenda. In: Cicchetti D, Cohen DJ (Eds). Developmental psychopathology. Volume 3: risk, disorder, and adaptation. Wiley; 2006.pp.570-98.
349. National Collaborating Centre for Mental Health. Antisocial personality disorder: treatment, management and prevention. British Psychological Society, Royal College of Psychiatrists; 2010.
350. Scott S, Knapp M, Henderson J, Maughan B. Financial cost of social exclusion: follow up study of antisocial children into adulthood. BMJ. 2001;323:191.
351. National Institute for Health and Clinical Excellence. Antisocial behaviour and conduct disorders in children and young people: recognition, intervention and management. (Clinical guideline 158.) 2013. http://guidance.nice.org.uk/CG158.
352. Goodman R, Meltzer H, Bailey V. The strengths and difficulties questionnaire: a pilot study on the validity of the self-report version. Eur Child Adolesc Psychiatry. 1998;7:125-30.

353. National Institute for Health and Clinical Excellence. Common mental health disorders: identification and pathways to care. (Clinical guideline 123.) 2011. http://guidance.nice.org.uk/CG123.
354. Barber AJ, Tischler VA, Healy E. Consumer satisfaction and child behaviour problems in child and adolescent mental health services. J Child Health Care. 2006;10:9-21.
355. National Collaborating Centre for Mental Health. Antisocial behaviour and conduct disorders in children and young people: recognition, intervention and management. British Psychological Society, Royal College of Psychiatrists [forthcoming].
356. Vostanis P, Meltzer H, Goodman R, Ford T. Service utilisation by children with conduct disorders—findings from the GB National Study. Eur Child Adolesc Psychiatry. 2003;12:231-8.
357. Scott S. Conduct disorders in children. BMJ. 2007;334:646-7.

Developmental Child Psychopathology

358. Brown RA. First Language: The Early Stages. Cambridge: Harvard University Press; 1973.
359. Cicchetti D. Editorial. Developmental psychopathology: Some thoughts on its evolution. Development and Psychopathology. 1989;1:1-4.
360. Gelfand DM, Peterson L. Child Development and Psychopathology. New Delhi: Sage; 1985.
361. Inhelder B, Piaget J. The Growth of Logical Thinking from Childhood to Adolescence. Boston: Little, Brown; 1958.
362. Kagan J. The Nature of the Child. New York: Basic; 1984.
363. Kashani JH, Orvaschel H, Rosenberg TK, Reid JC. Psychopathology in a community sample of children and adolescents: A developmental perspective. J Am Acad Child Adolesc Psychiatry. 1989;28:701-06.
364. Nannis E, Cowan P (Eds). Developmental Psychopathology and Its Treatment. San Francisco: Jassey Bass; 1988.
365. Papalia DE, Olds SW. Human Development, 3rd edition, New York: McGraw-Hill; 1986.
366. Rutter M, Tuma H, Lann IS (Eds). Assessment and Diagnosis in Child Psychopathology. New York: Guilford Press; 1988.
367. Stevenson JE (Ed). Recent Research in Development Psychopathology. Oxford: Pergamon; 1985.

Mental Retardation/Intellectual Disability

368. Ahn KJ, Jeong HK, Choi HS. DYRK1A BAC transgenic mice show altered synaptic plasticity with learning and memory defects. Neurobiol Dis; 2006. [Medline].
369. Capute AJ, Accardo PJ. Developmental Disabilities in Infancy and Childhood. Vol 1 and 2. Baltimore: Paul H Brookes. 1996: 1-619 and 1-521.
370. Developmental surveillance and screening of infants and young children. Pediatrics. 2001;108(1):192-6. [Medline].
371. Doheny KF, McDermid HE, Harum K. Cryptic terminal rearrangement of chromosome 22q13.32 detected by FISH in two unrelated patients. J Med Genet. 1997;34(8):640-4. [Medline].
372. Flint J, Wilkie AO, Buckle VJ. The detection of subtelomeric chromosomal rearrangements in idiopathic mental retardation. Nat Genet. 1995;9(2):132-40. [Medline].
373. Kirchhoff M, Gerdes T, Brunebjerg S. Investigation of patients with mental retardation and dysmorphic features using comparative genomic hybridization and subtelomeric multiplex ligation dependent probe amplification. Am J Med Genet A. 2005;139(3):231-3. [Medline].
374. Mao R, Wang X, Spitznagel EL. Primary and secondary transcriptional effects in the developing human Down syndrome brain and heart. Genome Biol. 2005;6(13):R107. [Medline].
375. Maulik PK, Mascarenhas MN, Mathers CD, Dua T, Saxena S. Prevalence of intellectual disability: a meta-analysis of population-based studies. Res Dev Disabil. 2011;32(2):419-36. [Medline].
376. Medina AE, Krahe TE, Ramoa AS. Restoration of neuronal plasticity by a phosphodiesterase type 1 inhibitor in a model of fetal alcohol exposure. J Neurosci. 2006;26(3):1057-60. [Medline].
377. Miyake N, Shimokawa O, Harada N. BAC array CGH reveals genomic aberrations in idiopathic mental retardation. Am J Med Genet A. 2006;140(3):205-11. [Medline].
378. Reiss S, Aman MG. Psychotropic Medications and Developmental Disabilities: The International Consensus Handbook. The Ohio State University Nisonger Center; 1998. pp.1-355.
379. Richardson SA, Koller H. Twenty-Two years. Cambridge, MA: Harvard University Press; 1996.pp.1-328.
380. Rubin IL, Crocker AC. Medical care for children and adults with developmental disabilities, 2nd edition. Baltimore, MD: Paul H Brookes Publishing Co, Inc; 2006.
381. Volkmar FR, Lewis M. Mental Retardation: Child and Adolescent Psychiatric Clinics of North America. Philadelphia: WB Saunders Company; 1996.769-993.

Specific Developmental Disorders

382. Ackerman P, Dykman R, Oglesby D. Sex and group differences in reading and attention disordered children with and without hyperkinesis. J Learn Disab. 1983;16:407-15.
383. Aman MG, Rojahn J. Pharmacological intervention. In: Singh NN, Beale IL (Eds). Current Perspectives in Learning Disabilities: Nature, Theory and Treatment. New York: Springer-Verlag; 1992.pp.478-525.
384. American Psychiatric Association. Desk Reference to the Diagnostic Criteria from DSM-5. Washington DC; 2013
385. Badian N. Prediction of good and poor reading before kindergarten entry: A nine-year follow-up. J Learn Disab. 2008;21:98-103.
386. Badian N. The prediction of good and poor reading before kindergarten entry: A four-year follow-up. J Spec Educ. 2006;16:309-18.

387. Bauer R. Memory processes in children with learning disabilities: evidence for deficient rehearsal. J Exp Child Psychol. 1979;24:415-30.
388. Beitchman JH, Nair R, Clegg MA, et al. Prevalence of psychiatric disorders in children with speech and language disorders. J Am Acad Child Psychiatry. 1986;25:528-35.
389. Bender B, Fry E, Penigton B, et al. Speech and language development in 41 children with sex chromosome anomalies. Pediatrics. 1983;71:262-7.
390. Bender B, Puck M, Salenblatt J, et al. Cognitive development of children with sex chromosome abnormalities. In: Smith SD (Ed). Genetics and Learning Disabilities. San Diego CA: College-Hill; 1986. pp.175-201.
391. Bigler E. Acquired cerebral trauma: Epidemiology, neuropsychological assessment and academic/educational deficits. J Learn Disab. 1987;20:516-7.
392. Bishop DVM, Edmundson A. Is otitis media a major cause of specific language disorders? Br J Dis Commun. 1986;21:321-38.
393. Blalock J. Persistent auditory language deficits in adults with learning disabilities. J Learn Disab. 1982;15:604-9.
394. Brandt I, et al. Brain growth, malnutrition and clinical consequences. J Perinat Med. 1980;9:324-37.
395. Burd L, Kaufman D, Kerbeshian J. Tourette syndrome and learning disabilities. J Learn Disab. 1992;25:598-604.
396. Colletti L. Relationship between pregnancy and birth complications and the later development of learning disabilities. J Learn Disab. 1979;12:659-63.
397. Cornine D, Silbert J, Kameenvi E. Direction Instruction Reading, Columbus, Ohio: Merrill; 1990.
398. DeFries J, Decker S. Genetic aspects of reading disability a family study. In: Malatesha R, Aaron P (Eds). Reading Disorders: Varieties and Treatments. New York: Academic Press; 1982.
399. DeFries J, Gillis J. Etiology of reading deficits in learning disabilities: quantitative genetic analysis. In: Pbrzut J, Hynd G (Eds). Neuropsychological Foundations of Learning Disabilities. San Diego: Academic Press; 1991.
400. Di Lollo V, Hanson D, McIntyre J. Initial stages of visual information processing in dyslexia. J Exp Psychol Human Percept Perform. 1983;9:923-35.
401. Duane D. Biological formations of learning disabilites. In: Obrzut J, Hynd G (Eds). Neuropsychological Foundations of Learning Disabilities. San Diego: Academic Press; 1991.
402. Elbert J. Short-term memory encoding and memory search in the word recognition of learning-disabled children. J Learn Disab. 1984;17:342-5.
403. Ellis E, et al. An instructional model for teaching learning strategies. Focus Except Child. 1991;23:1-23.
404. Engelmann S, Johnson G, Hanner S, et al. Corrective Reading Program. Chicago: Science Research Associates; 1978.
405. Finucci J, Gottfredson L, Childs BA. Follow-up study of dyslexic boys. Ann Dyslexia. 1985;35:117-36.
406. Finucci JM, Childs B. Are there really more dyslexic boys than girls? In: Ansara A, Geshwind N, Galaburda A, et al (Eds). Sex Differences in Dyslexia. Towson, MD: Orton Dyslexia Society; 1981.pp.1-9.
407. Gaddes W, Edgell E. Learning disabilities and brain function: A Neuropsychological Approach. New York: Springer-Verlag; 1985.
408. Gadiw K. Psychopharmacological assessment and intervention. In: Swanson HL (Ed). Handbook on the Assessment of Learning Disabilities. Austn, TX: Pro-ed; 1991.pp.351-72.
409. Galaburda AM, Kemper TL. Cytoarchitectonic abnormalities in developmental dyslexia: A case study. Ann Neurol. 1979;6:94-100.
410. Galaburda AM, Sherman GF, Rosen GD, et al. Developmental dyslexia: Four consecutive patients with cortical anomalies. Ann Neurol. 1985;18:222-3.
411. Grunau R, Low M. Cognitive and task-related EEG correlates of arithmetic performance in adolescents. J Clin Exp Neuropsychol. 1987;9:563-74.
412. Hagerman RJ, Sobesky WE. Psychopathology in fragile X syndrome. Am J Orthopsychiatry. 1989;59:142-52.
413. Hagin R, Kugler J. School problems associated with Tourette's syndrome. In: Cohen D, Brunn R, Leckman J (Eds). Tourette's syndrome and Tic Disorders: Clinical Understanding and Treatment. New York: Wiley; 1988.
414. Hagin RA, Beecher R, Pagano G, et al. Effects of Tourette syndrome on learning. In: Friendhoff AJ, Chase TN (Eds). Gilles de la Tourette Syndrome. New York: Reven Press; 1982.
415. Hallihan D, Reeve R. Selective attention and distractibility. In: Keogh B (Ed). Advances in Special Education. Vol 1, Greenwich, Conn: JAI Press; 1980.
416. Harris A, Sipay E. How to Increase Reading Ability: A Guide to Developmental and Remedial Methods. New York: Longman. 1990.
417. Harris E. The contribution of twin research to the study of etiology of reading disability. In: Smith S (Ed). Genetics and Learning Disabilities. San Diego: College Hill Press; 1986.
418. Haslam R, et al. Cerebral asymmetry in developmental dyslexia. Arch Neurol. 1981;38:679-704.
419. Healy J, Aram D. Hyperlexia and dyslexia: a family study. Ann Dyslexia. 1986;36:237-52.
420. Heller K, Holtzman W, Messick S. Placing Children in Special Education: A Strategy for Equity. Washington DC: National Academy Press; 1982.
421. Hetzel B, Hay I. Thyroid function, iodine nutrition and fetal brain development. Clin Endocrinol. 1979;11:445-60.
422. Hier D, et al. Developmental dyslexia: Evidence for a subgroup with a reversal of cerebral asymmetry. Arch Neurol. 1978;35:90-2.
423. Houselander J, et al. Infants born to narcotic addicted mothers. Psychol Bull. 1982;2:453-68.
424. Hunt RD, Cohen DJ. Psychiatric aspects of learning difficulties. Pediatr Clin N Am. 1984;31:471-97.
425. Hynd G. Neurological aspects of dyslexia: Comments on the balance model. J Learn Disab. 1992;25:110-3.

426. Johnson D, Myklebust H. Learning Disabilities: Educational Principles and Practices. New York: Grune and Stratton; 1967.
427. Kemper M, et al. Cognitive profiles and the spectrum of clinical manifestations in heterozygous fragile X females. Am J Med Genet. 1986;23:139-56.
428. Lyon G, et al. Neuropsychology and learning disabilities. In: Wong B (Ed). Learning About Learning Disabilities. San Diego: Academic Press; 1991.
429. Lyytinen H, Lorys-Vernon A. Neurodevelopmental changes in ERP components associated with automatic attention (MMN). J Clin Exp Neuropsychol. 1988;11:28.
430. Madison L, George C, Moeschler J. Functioning in the fragile X syndrome: A study of intellectual memory and communication skills. J Ment Defic. 1986;3:129-48.
431. McKinney J, Feagans L. Adaptive classroom behaviour of learning disabled students. J Learn Disab. 1983;16:360-7.
432. Meichenbaum D, Genest M. Cognitive behaviour modification: An integration of cognitive and behavioural methods. In: Kanfer FH, Goldstein AP (Eds). Helping People Change, 2nd edition, Elmsford NY: Plenum; 1980.pp.390-422.
433. Moray N. Attention selective processes in vision and hearing. London: Hutchinson; 1969.
434. Obrzut JE, Boliek CA. Neuropsychological assessment of childhood learning disorders. In: Swanson HL (Ed). Handbook on the Assessment of Learning Disabilities. Austin, TX: Pro-ed; 1991.pp.121-45.
435. Pennington B, Smith SD. Genetic influences on learning disabilities and speech and language disorder. Child Development. 1983;54:369-87.
436. Richards G, et al. Sustained and selective attention in children with learning disabilities. J Learn Disab. 1990;23:129-36.
437. Roberts R, et al. CT asymmetries in developmentally dyslexic adults. Dev Neuropsychol. 1988;43:231-7.
438. Rosenberger P, Hier D. Cerebral asymmetry and verbal intellectual deficits. Ann Neurol. 1980;8:300-4.
439. Rovert J. The psychoeducational characteristics of children with Turner syndrome. J Learn Disab. 1993;26:333-41.
440. Rumsey J, et al. Magnetic resonance imaging of brain anatomy in severe developmental dyslexia. Arch Neurol. 1986; 43: 1045-6.
441. Rumsey J, et al. MRI evaluation of the size and symmetry of the planum temporal in adolescent with developmental dyslexia. Brain Lang. 1990;39:289-301.
442. Rutter N. Prevalence and types of dyslexia. In: Benton A, Pearl D (Eds). Dyslexia: An Appraisal of Current Knowledge. New York: Oxford Press; 1978.
443. Segalowitz S, Brown D. Mild head injury as a source of developmental disabilities. J Learn Disab. 1991;24:551-9.
444. Shprintzen RJ, Goldberg RB. Multiple anomaly syndromes and learning disabilities. In: Smith SD (Ed). Genetics and Learning Disabilities. San Diego CA: College-Hill; 1986.pp.153-74.
445. Silver LB. Psychological interventions and therapies for children and adolescents with learning disabilities. Child Adolesc Psychiatr Clin N Am. 1993;2:323-37.
446. Silver LB. The relationship between learning disabilities, hyper-activity, distractibility and behavioural problem. J Am Acad Child Psychiatry. 1981;20:385-97.
447. Silver LB. The secondary emotional, social and family problems found with children and adolescents with learning disabilities. Child Adoles Psychiatr Clin N Am. 1993;2:295-308.
448. Singh NN, Deitz DE, Singh J. Behavioral approaches. In: Singh NN, Beale IE (Eds). Current Perspectives in Learning Disabilities: Nature, Theory, and Treatment. New York: Springer-Verlag; 1992.pp.375-414.
449. Spreen O. Prognosis of learning disability. J Consult Clin Psychol. 1988;56:836-42.
450. Stevenson J, et al. A twin study of genetic influences on reading and spelling ability and disability. J Child Psychol Psychiatry. 1987;28:229-47.
451. Swanson H. Relations among metamemory, rehearsal activity and word recall in learning disabled and nondisabled readers. J EducPsychol. 1983;53:186-94.
452. Swanson H. Semantic and visual memory codes in learning disabled readers. J Exp Child Psychol. 1984;37:124-40.
453. Taylor HG. Neuropsychological testing: Relevance for assessing children's learning disabilities. J Consult Clin Psychol. 1988;56:795-800.
454. Towbin A. Organic causes of minimal brain dysfunction: Perinatal origin of minimal cerebral lesions. JAMA. 1971;217: 1207-9.
455. Vaughn S, Hogan A. Social competence and learning disabilities a prospective study. In: Swanson H, Keogh B (Eds). Learning Disabilities: Theoretical and Research Issues. Hillsdale: Eribaum; 1990.
456. Willis WG, Hooper SR, Stone BH. Neuropsychological theories of learning disabilities. In: Singh NN, Beale IE (Eds). Current Perspectives in Learning Disabilities: Nature, Theory, and Treatment. New York: Springer-Verlag; 1992.pp.201-45.
457. Willows D. Visual processes and learning disabilities. In: Wong B (Ed). Learning About Learning Disabilities. San Diego: Academic Press; 1991.
458. Wright-Strawderman C, Watson B. The prevalence of depressive symptoms in children with learning disabilities. J Learn Disab. 1991;25:258-64.
459. Zeigler P, Holden L. Family therapy for learning disabled and attention-deficit disordered children. Am J Orthopsychiatry. 1988;58:196-210.

Attention-Deficit Hyperactivity Disorder

460. Abikoff H, Hechtma L, Klein RG, et al. Social functioning in children with ADHD treated with long-term methylphenidate and multimodal psychosocial treatment. J Am Acad Child Adolesc Psychiatry. 2004;43:820-9.
461. Adler LA, Chua HC. Management of ADHD in adults. J Clin Psychiatry. 2002;63(Supp 12):29-35.
462. Alexander GE, deLong MR, Strick PL. Parallel organization of functionally segregated circuits linking basal ganglia and cortex. Ann Rev Neurosci. 1986;9:357-81.

463. American Psychiatric Association. Desk Reference to the Diagnostic Criteria from DSM-5. Washington DC; 2013.
464. Angold A, Erkanli A, Egger HL, Costello EJ. Stimulant treatment for children: a community perspective. J Am Acad Child Adolesc Psychiatry. 2000;39:975-84.
465. Arcos-Burgos M, Castellanos FX, Pineda D, et al. Attention deficit/hyperactivity disorder in a population isolate: linkage to lociat 4q13.2, Sq33.3, 11q22, and 17p11. Am J Hum Genet. 2004;75:998-1014.
466. Autti-Ramo I. Twelve-year follow-up of children exposed to alcohol in utero. Dev Med Child Neurology. 2000;42:406-11.
467. Bakker SC, van der Meulen EM, Buitelaar JK, et al. A whole-genome scan in 164 Dutch sib pairs with attention-deficit/ hyperactivity disorder: suggestive evidence for linkage on chromosomes 7p and 15q. Am J Hum Genet. 2003;72:1251-60.
468. Barkely R. behavioral inhibition, sustained attention, and executive functions: constructing a unifying theory of ADHD. Psychol Bull. 1997;121:65-94.
469. Barkley RA, Edwards G, Laneri M, Fletcher K, Metevia L. Executive function, temporal discounting, and sense of time in adolescents with attention deficit hyperactivity disorder (ADHD) and oppositional defiant disorder (ODD). J Abnorm Child Psychol. 2001;29:541-56.
470. Barkley RA. Attention deficit hyperactivity disorder: a handbook for diagnosis and treatment. New York: Gulford; 1998.
471. Barkley RA. International consensus statement on ADHD. Clin Child Fam Psycho Rev. 2002;5:89-111.
472. Barkley. ADHD and the nature of self-control. New York: Guilford; 1997.
473. Battstra L, Hadders-Algra M, Neeleman J. Effect of antenatal exposure to maternal smoking on behavioural problems and academic achievement in childhood: prospective evidence from a Dutch birth cohort. Early Hum Dev. 2003;75:21-33.
474. Biderman J, Swanson J, Boellner SW, Lopez FA. Modafinil as therapy for ADHD in children: a 4-week, double-blind, placebo controlled study. In: ECNP, eds. Presented at the 17th annual Stockholm, Sweden. 2004;S364.
475. Biederman J, Faraone SV, Lapey K. Comorbidity of diagnosis in attention deficit hyperactivity disorder (ADHD). Child Adolesc Psychiatr Clin North Am. 1992;1:335-60.
476. Biederman J, Faraone SV, Monouteaux MC. Differential effect of environmental adversity by gender: Rutter's index of adversity in a sample of boys and girls with and without ADHD. Am J Psychiatry. 2002;159: 556-62.
477. Biederman J, Faraone SV, Monuteaux M, et al. Gender effects of attention deficit hyperactivity disorder in adults, revisited. Biol psychiatry. 2004;55:692-700.
478. Biederman J, Faraone SV. The Massachusetts General Hospital studies of gender influences on attention-deficit/hyperactivity disorder in youth and relatives. Psychiatr Clin North Am. 2004;27:225-32.
479. Biederman J, Lopez FA, Boellner SW, Chandler MC. A randomized, double-blind, placebo-controlled, parallel-group study of SLI381 (Adderall XR) in children with attention deficit hyperactivity disorder. Pediatrics. 2002;110:258-66.
480. Biederman J, Milberger S, Faraone SV, et al. Family-environmental risk factors for attention deficit hyperactivity disorde4r: a test of Rutter's indicators of adversity. Arch Gen Psychiatry. 1995;52:464-70.
481. Biederman J, Milberger Sv, Faraone S, et al. Impact of adversity on functioning and comorbidity in children with attention-deficit hyperactivity disorder. J Am Acad Child Adolesc Psychiatry. 1995;34:1495-503.
482. Biederman J, Monuteaux M, Seidman I, et al. Impact of executive function deficits and ADHD on academic outcomes in children J Consult Clin Psychol. 2004;72:757-66.
483. Biederman J, Quinn D, Weiss M, et al. Efficacy and safety of Ritalin L, a new, once-daily, extended-release dosage form of methylphenidate hydrochloride, in children with ADHD. Pediatric Drugs. 2003;5:833-41.
484. Biederman J, Thisted R, Greenhill L, Ryan N. Estimation of the association between desipramine and the risk for sudden death in 5 to 14-year-old children. J Clin Psychiatry. 1995;56:87-93.
485. Bird H, Gould M, Staghezza-Jaramillo B. The comorbidity of ADHD in a community sample of children aged 6 through 16 years. J Child Fam tud. 1994;3:365-78.
486. Boksa P, El-Khodor BF, Birth insult interacts with stress at adulthood to alter dopaminergic function in animal models: possible implications for schizophrenia and other disorders. Neurosci Biobehav Rev. 2003;27:91-101.
487. Botting N, Powls A, Cooke RW, Marlow N. Attention deficit hyperactivity disorders and other psychiatric outcomes in very low birthweight children at 12 years. J Child Psychol psychiatry. 1997;38:931-41.
488. Boyd TA, Ernhart CB, Greene TH, Sokol RJ, martier S, Prenatal alcohol exposure and sustained attention in the preschool years. Neurotoxicol Teratol. 1991;13:49-55.
489. Brown RT, Coles CD, Smith IE, et al. Effects of prenatal alcohol exposure at school age. II. Attention and behavior. Neurotoxicol Teratol. 1991;13:49-55.
490. Brownell MD, Yogendran MS, Attention-deficit hyperactivity disorder in Manitoba children: medical diagnosis and psychostimulant treatment rates. Can J Psychiatry. 2001;46:264-72.
491. Bussing R, Zima B, Perwien A, belin T, Widawski M. Children in special education programs: attention deficity hyperactivity disorder, use of services, and unmet needs. Am J Pub health. 1998;88:880-86.
492. Castellanos FX, Lee PP, Sharp W, et al. Developmental trajectories of brain volume abnormalities in children and adolescents with attention-deficit/hyperactivity disorder. JAMA. 2002;288:1740-8.
493. Castellanos FX, Tannock R. Neuroscience of attention-deficit/ hyperactivity disorder; the search for endophenotypes. Nat Rev Neurosci. 2002;3:617-28.
494. Cheon KA, Ryu YH, Kim YK, Namkoon g K, Kim CH, Lee JD. Dopamine transporter density in the basal ganglia assessed

with [1231] IPT SPET in children with attention deficit hyperactivity disorder. Eur J Nucl Med Mol Imag. 2003;30: 306-11.

495. Conners CK. Food additives and hyperactive children. New York: Plenum; 1980.
496. Connor DF, Fletcher KE, Swanson JM. A meta-analysis of clonidine for symptoms of attention-deficit hyperactivity disorder. J Am Acad Child Adolesc Psychaitry. 1999;38:1551-9.
497. Cox DJ, Humphrey JW, merkel RL, Penberthy JK, Kovatchev B. Controlled release methylphenidate improves attention during on road driving by adolescents with attention deficit/ hyperactivity disorder. J Am Board Fam Pract. 2004;17:235-9.
498. Crhsbie J, Schachar R, Deficient inhibition as a marker for familial ADHD. Am J Psychiatry. 2001;158:1884-90.
499. Daviss WB, Bentivoglio P, Racusin R, Brown KM, Bostic JQ, Wiley L. Bupropion sustained release in adolescents with comorbid attention-defict/hyperactivity disorder and depression. J Am Acad Child Adolesc Psychiatry. 2001;40:307-14.
500. Depfner M, Rothenberger A, Sonuga-Barke E. Areas for future investment in the field of ADHD: preschoolers and clinical networks. Eur Child Adolesc Psychiatry. 2004;13 (Suppl 1):1130-5.
501. Dilsaver SC, Henderson-Fuller S, Akiskal HS. Occult mood disorder in 104 consecutively presenting children referred for the treatment of attention-deficit/hyperactivity disorder in a community mental health clinic. J Clin Psychiatry. 2003;64:1170-6.
502. DiScala C, Lescohier I, Bathel M, M, Li G. Injuries to children with attention deficit hyperactivity disorder. Pediatrics. 1998;102:1415-21.
503. Dougherty DD, Bonab AA, Spencer TJ, Rauch SL, Madras BK, fischman AJ. Dopamine transporter density in patients with attention deficit hyperactivity disorder. Lancer. 1999;354: 2132-3.
504. Dowson JH, McLean A, bazanis E, et al. Impaired spatial working memory in adults with attention-deficit/hyperactivity disorder: comparisons with performance in adults with borderline personality disorder and in control subjects. Acta Psychiatr Scan. 2004;110:45-54.
505. Doyle AE, Faraone SV, seidman LJ, et al. Are endophenotypes based on measure sof executive functions useful for molecular genetic studies of ADHD? J Child Psychol psychiatri (in press).
506. Doyle R. The history of adult attention-deficit/hyperactivity disorder. Psychiatr Clin North Am. 2004;27:203-14.
507. Dresel S, Krause J, Krause KH, et al. Attention deficit hyperactivity disorder: binding of [99mTcJ TRODAT-1 to the dopamine transporter before and after methylphenidate treatment. Eur J Nucl Med. 2000;27:1518-24.
508. Durston S, Tottenham NT, Thomas KM, et al. Differential patterns of striatal activation in young children with and without ADHD. Biol Psychiatry. 2003;53:871-8.
509. Essau CA, Groen G, Conradt J, Turbanisch U, Petermann F, [Frequency, comorbidity and psychosocial correlates of attention deficit/hyperactivity disorder. Results of a Bermen adolescent study]. Fortschr Neurol Psychiatr. 1999;67:296-305.
510. Faraone S, Biederman J, Friedman D. Validity of DSM-IV subtypes of attention-deficit/hyperactivity disorder: a family study perspective. J Am Acad Child Adolesc Psychiatry. 2000;9:300-7.
511. Faraone S, Biederman J, Mick E. The age dependent decline of attention-deficit/hyperactivity disorder: a meta-analysis of follow-up studies. Psychol Med (in press).
512. Faraone SV, Biderman J, Zimmerman BA. Correspondence of parent and teacher reports in medication trials. Eur J Child Adolesc Psychiatry. 2005;14:20-7.
513. Faraone SV, Biederman J, Mick E, et al. Family study of girls with attention deficit hyperactivity disorder. Am J Psychiatry. 2000;157:1077-83.
514. Faraone SV, Biederman J, Monuteaux M, Spencer T. Long-term effects of extended release mixed amphetamine salts treatment of ADHD on growth. J Child Adolesc Psychopharmacol. 2005;15:191-202.
515. Faraone SV, Biederman J. Neurobiology of attention deficit hyperactivity disorder. In: Charney Ds, Nestler EJ (Eds). Neurobiology of mental illness, 2nd edition, New York, NY: Oxford University Press; 2004.
516. Faraone SV, Biederman J. Neurobiology of attention-deficit hyperactivity disorder. Biol Psychiatry. 1998;44:951-8.
517. Faraone SV, Doyle AE. The nature and heritability of attention deficit/hyperactivity disorder. Child Adolesc Psychiatr Clin North Am. 2001;10:299-316, viii-ix.
518. Faraone SV, Perlis RH, Doyle AE, et al. Molecular genetics of attention deficit/hyperactivity disorder. Biol Psychiatry. 2005;57:1313-23.
519. Faraone SV, Wilens T. Does stimulant treatment lead to substance use disorders? J Clin Psychiatry. 2003;64 (Suppl 11):9-13.
520. Faraone SV. Genetics of adult attention deficit hyperactivity disorder. In: Spencer T (Ed). Psychiatric Clinics of North America. Philadelphia. PA: Sauders Press; 2004.pp.303-21.
521. Faraone SV. Understanding the effect size of ADHD medications: implications for clinical care. Medscape Psychiatry ment Health. 2003;8(2).
522. Faroone SV, Sergeant J, Gillberg C, Biederman J. The worldwide prevalence of ADHD: is it an American condition? World Psychiatry. 2003;2:104-13.
523. Fischer M, barkley RA, Smallish L, Fletcher K. Young adult follow-up of hyperactive children: self-reported psychiatric disorders, comorbidity, and the role of childhood conduct problems and teen CD. J Abnorm Child Psychol. 2002;30:463-75.
524. Fogleman Y, Vinker S, Guy N, Kahan E. Prevalence of and change in the prescription of methylphenidate in Israel over a 2-year period. CNS Drugs. 2003;17:915-19.
525. Fung YK, Lau YS. Effects of prenatal nicotine exposure on rat striatal dopaminergic and nocitinic systems. Pharmacol Biochem Behav. 1989;33:1-6.
526. Gadow K, Sverd J, Sprafkin J, Nolan E, Ezor S. Efficacy of methylphenidate for attention-deficit hyperactivity disorder in children with tic disorder. Arch Gen psychiatry. 1995;52:444-55.

527. Gelfand DM, Teti DM, The effects of maternal depression on children. Clin Psychol Rev. 1990;10:329-53.
528. Geurts HM, Verte S, Oosterlaan J, Roeyers H, Sergeant JA. How specific are executive functioning deficits in attention deficit hyperactivity disorder and autism? J Child Psycho Psychiatr. 2004;45:836-54.
529. Graetz BW, Sawyer MG, Hazell PL, Arney F, baghurst P. Validity of DSM-IVADHD subtypes in a nationality representative sample of Australian children and adolescents. J Am Acad Child Adolesc Psychiatry. 2001;40:1410-7.
530. Greene RW, Biederman J, Faraone SV, et al. Social impairment in girls with ADHD: patterns, gender comparisons, and correlates. J Am Acad Child Adolesc Psychiatry. 2001;40:704-10.
531. Greenhill LL, Finding RL, Swanson JM. A double-blind, placebo-controlled, study of modified-release methylphenidate in children with attention-deficit/hyperacitivty disorder. Pediatrics. 2002;109:E39.
532. Guevara J, Lozano P, Wickizer T, Mell L, Gephart H. Utilization and cost of health care services for children with attention-deficit/hyperactivity disorder. Pediatrics. 2001;108:71-8.
533. Hack M, Youngstrom EA, Cartar L, et al. Behavioral outcomes and evidence of psychopathology among very low birth weight infants at age 20 years. Pediatrics. 2004;114:932-40.
534. Hawi Z, Lowe N, Kirley A, et al. Linkage disqulilibrium mapping at DATI, DRD5 and DBH narrows the search for ADHD suspectibility alleles at these loci. Mol Psychiatry. 2003;8:299-308.
535. He Y, Yang X, Xu F. Application of Conners Rating Scales in the study of lead exposure and behavioral effects in children. Zhonghua Yu Fang Yi Xue Za Zhi. 2000;34:290-3.
536. Hurt R, Schs D, Glover E, et al. A comparison of sustained-release bupropion and placebo for smoking cessation. N Engl J Med. 1997;337:1195-202.
537. Indredavik MS, Vik T, Heyerdahl S, Kulseng S, Fayers P, Brubakk AM, Psychiatric symptoms and disorders in adolescents with low birth weight. Arch Dis Child Fetal Neonatal Ed. 2004;89:F445-50.
538. Jensen PS, Hinshaw SP, Kraemer HC, et al. ADHD comorbidity findings from the MTA study: comparing comorbid subgroups. J Am Acad Child Adolesc Psychiatry. 2001;40:147-58.
539. Johansen E, Aase H, Meyer a, Sagvolden T. Attention-deficit/hyperactivity disorder (ADHD) behaviour explained by dysfunctioning reinforcement and extinction processes. Behav brain Res. 2002;130:37-45.
540. Johnston J, Lineberry, CG, Ascher, JA, et al. A 102 center prospective study of seizure in associated with bupropion. J Clin Psychiatry. 1991;52:450-6.
541. Kadesjo B, Gillberg C. The comorbidity of ADHD in the general population of Swedish school age children. J Child Psychol psychiatry. 2001;42:487-92.
542. Katz LJ, Goldstein G, Geckle M. Neuropsychological and personality differences between men and women with ADHD. J Attent Disord. 1998;2:239-47.
543. Klein Rg, Landa B, Mattes JA, Klein DF. Methylphenidate and growth in hyperactive children: a controlled withdrawal study. Arch Gen Psychiatry. 1988;45:1127-30.
544. Krause K, Dresel SH, Krause J, Kung HF, Tatsch K. Increased striatal dopamine transporter in adult patients with attention deficit hyperactivity disorder: effects of methylphenidate as measured by single photon emission computed tomography. Neurosci Lett. 2000;285:107-10.
545. Krause KH, Dresel SH, Krause J, Kung HF, Tatsch K, Ackenheil M, Stimulant like action of nicotine on striatal dopamine transporter in the brain of adults with attention deficit hyperactivity disorder. Int J Neuropsychoparmacol. 2002;5:111-3.
546. Lahey BB, Loeber R, Burke J, Rathouz PJ, Mc Burnett K. Waxing and waning in concert: dynamic comorbidity of conduct disorder with other disruptive and emotional problems over 7 years among clinic-referred boys. J Abnorm Psychol. 2002;111:556-67.
547. Lisska MC, Rivkees SA. Daily methylphenidate use slows the growth of children: a community based study. J Pediatr Endocrinol Metab. 2003;16:711-8.
548. Lou H. Etiology and pathogensis of attention-deficit hyperactivity disorder (ADHD); significance of prematurity and perinatal hypoxic-haemodynamic encephalopathy. Acta Paediatr. 1996;85:1266-71.
549. Lowe N, Kirley A, Hawi Z, et al. Joint analysis of DRD5 marker concludes association with ADHD confined to the predominantly inattentive and combined subtypes. Am J Hum Genet. 2004;74:348-56.
550. Lowe TL, Cohen DJ, Detlor J. Stimulant medications precipitate Tourette's syndrome. JAMA. 1982;247:1168-9.
551. Markussen-Linnet K, Dalsgaard S, Obel C, et al. Maternal lifestyle factors in pregnancy risk fo attention deficit hyperactivity disorder and associated behaviors: review of the current evidence. Am J Psychiatry. 2003;160:1028-40.
552. Michelson D, Adler L, Spencer T, et al. Atomoxetine in adults with ADHD: two randomized, placebo-controlled studies. Biol Psychiatry. 2003;53:112-20.
553. Michelson D, Allen AJ, Busner J, et al. Once-daily atomoxetine treatment for children and adolescents with attention deficit hyperactivity disorder: a randomized placebo-controlled study. Am J Psychiatry. 2002;159:1896-901.
554. Mick E, Biderman J, Prince J, Fischer MJ, Faraone SV. Impact of low birth weight on attention-deficit/hyperactivity disorder. J Dev Behav Pediatrics. 2004;114:932-40.
555. Mick E, Biederman J, Faraone SV, Sayer J, Klinman S. Case control study of attention-deficit/hyperactivity disorder and maternal smoking, alcohol use, and drug use during pregnancy. J Am Acad Child Adolesc Psychiatry. 2002;41:378-85.
556. Miller AR, Lalonde CE, McGrall KM, Armstrong RW, Prescription of methylphenidate to children and youth, 1990-1996. CMAJ. 2001;165:1489-94.

557. Miyake A, Friedman NP, Emerson MJ, Witzki AH, Howerter A, Wager TD. The unity and diversity of executive functions and their contributions to complex "Frontal Lobe" tasks: a latent variable analysis. Cognit Psycho. 2000;41:49-100.
558. Modestin J, Matutat B, Wurmle O. Antecedents of opioid dependence and personality disorder: attention-deficit/ hyperactivity disorder and conduct disorder. Eur Arch Psychiatry Clin Neurosci. 2001;251:42-7.
559. MTA Cooperative group. A 14-month randomized clinical trial of treatment strategies for attention deficit/hyperactivity disorder. Multi-modal treatment study of children with ADHD. Arch Gen psychiatry. 1999;56:1073-86.
560. MTA Cooperative Group. National Insititute of Mental Health Multimodel Treatment Study of ADHD follow-up: changes in effectiveness and growth after the end of treatment. Pediatrics. 2004;113:762-9.
561. MTA Cooperative Group. National Institute of Mental health Multimodel Treatment Study of ADHD follow-up: 24 month outcomes of treatment strategies for attention-deficit/ hyperactivity disorder. Pediatrics. 2004;113:754-61.
562. Murphy KR, Barkley RA, Bush T. Young adults with attention deficit hyperactivity disorder: subtype differences in comorbidity, educational, and clinical history. J Nerv ment Dis. 2002;190:147-57.
563. Nigg JT, Blaskey L, Stawicki J, Sachek J. Evaluating endophenotype model of ADHD neuropsychological deficit: results for parents and siblings of children with DSM-IV ADHD combined and inattentive subtypes. J Abnorm Psychol. 2004;113:614-15.
564. Nigg JT, Goldsmith HH, Sachek J. Temperament and attention deficit hyperactivity disor der: the development of a multiple pathway model. J Clin Child Adolesc Psychol. 2004;33: 42-53.
565. Nochols PL, Chen TC. Minimal brain dysfunction: a prospective study. Hillsdale, NJ, USA: Lawrence Erlbaum Associates; 1981.
566. Offord DR, Boyle MH, Racine YA, et al. Outcome, prognosis and risk in a longitudinal follow-up study. J Am Acad Child Adolesc Psychiatry. 1992;31:916-23.
567. Ogdie M, Macphie J, Minassian S, et al. A genome wide scan for attention-deficit/hyperactivity disorder in an extended sample: suggestive linkage on 17p11. Am J Hum Genet. 2003;72:1251-60.
568. Olfson M, Gameroff MJ, Marcus SC, Jensen PS. National trends in the treatment of attention deficit hyperactivity disorder. Am J Psychiatry. 2003;160:1071-7.
569. Palfrey JS, Levine MD, Walker DK, Sullivan M. The emergence of attention deficits in early childhood: a prospective study. J Dev Behav Pediatr. 1985;6:339-48.
570. Polution A, Powell CT. Slowing of growth in height and weight on stimulants: a characteristic pattern. J Paediatr Child Health. 2003;39:180-5.
571. Pomerleau O, Downey K, Stelson F, Pomerleau C, Cigarette smoking in adult patients diagnosed with ADHD. J Subst Abuse. 1996;7:373-8.
572. Raber J, mehta PP, Kreifeldt M, et al. Colobama hyperactive mutant mice exhibit 4 regional and transmitter-specific deficits in neurotransmission. J Neurochemistry. 1997;68:176-86.
573. Rapport MD, Moffitt C. Attention deficit/hyperactivity disorder and methylphenidate. A review of height/weight, cardiovascular, and somatic complaint side effects. Clin Psychol Rev. 2002;22:1107-31.
574. Rasmussen ER, Neuman RJ, Heath AC, Levy F, hay DA, Todd RD. Familial clustering of latent class and DSM-IV defined attention deficit/hyper-activity disorder (ADHD) subtypes. J Chind Psychol Psychiatr. 2004;45:589-98.
575. Rasmussen P, Gillberg C. Natural outcome of ADHD with developmental coordination disorder at age 22 years: a controlled, longitudinal, community-based study. J Am Acad Child Adolesc Psychiatry. 2000;39:1424-31.
576. Reid R, Hakendorf P, Prosser B. Use of psychostimulant medication for ADHD in South Australia. J Am Acad Child Adolesc Psychiatry. 2002;41:906-13.
577. Richardson GA, Day NL. Detrimental effects of prenatal cocaine exposure; illusion or reality? J Am Acad Child Adolesc Psychiatry. 1994;33:28-34.
578. Richters JE. Depressed mothers as informants about their children: a critical review of the evidence for distortion. Psychol Bull. 1992;112:485-99.
579. Riggs P, Leons S, Mikulich S, Pottle L. An open trial of bupropion for ADHD in adolescents with substance use disorder and conduct disorder. J Am Acad Child Adolesc Psychiatry. 1998;37:1271-8.
580. Roobins TW, James M, Own AM, et al. A study of performance on tests from the CANTAB battery sensitive to frontal lobe dysfunction in a large sample of normal volunteers; implications for theories of executive functioning and cognitive aging. J Int neuropsychol Soc. 1998;4:474-90.
581. Rugino TA, Copley TC. Effects of modafinil in children with attention-deficit/hyperactivity disorder: an open-label study. J Am Acad Child Adolesc Psychiatry. 2001;40:230-45.
582. Russel VA. The nucleus accumbens motor-limbic interface of the spontaneously hypertensive rat as studied in vitro by the superfusion slice technique. Neurosci Biobehav Rev. 2000;24:133-6.
583. Rutter M, cox A, Tupling C, Berger M, Yule W. Attainment and adjustment in two geographical areas: vol1. The prevalence of psychiatric disorders. Br J Psychiatry. 1975;126:493-509.
584. Safren SA, Otto MW, Sprich S, Winett CL, Wilens TE, Biederman J. Cognitive-behavioural therapy for ADHD in medication-treated adults with continued symptoms. Behav Res Ther. 2005;43:831-42.
585. Sagvolden T. Behavioral validation of the spontaneously hypertensive rat (SHR) as an animal model of attention-deficity/hyperactivity disorder (AD/HD). Neurosci Biobehav Rev. 2000;24:31-9.
586. Saigal S, Pinelli J, Hoult L, Kim MM, Boyle M, Psychopathology and social competencies of adolescents who were extremely low birth weight. Pediatrics. 2003;111:969-75.

587. Satterfield JH, Cantwell DP, Schell A, Blacschke T. Growth hyperactive children treated with methylphendate. Arch Gen Psychiatry. 1979;36:212-7.
588. Scahill L, Chappell PB, Kim YS, et al. A placebo-controlled study of guanfacine in the treatment of children with tic disorders and attention deficit hyperactivity disorder. Am J Psychiatry. 2001;158:1067-74.
589. Scahill L, Schwab-Stone M. Epidemiology of ADHD in school age children. Child Adolesc Psychiatr Clin N Am. 2000;9: 541-55.
590. Schmidt-Troschke SO, Ostermann T, Melcher D, Schuster R, Erben CM, Mathiessen PF. (The use of methylphenidate in children: analysis of prescription usage based in routine data of the statutory health insurance bodies concerning drug prescriptions). Gesundheitswesen. 2004;66:387-92.
591. Schneider JS, Sun ZQ, roeltgen DP. Effects of dopamine agonists on delayed response performance in chronic low-dose MPTP-treated monkeys. Pharmacol Biochem Behav. 1994;48:235-40.
592. Seidman JK, Valera E, Bush G. Brain function and structure in adults with attention-deficit hyperactivity disorder. In: Spencer T (Ed). Psychiatric clinics of North America. Philadelphia, PA: Saunders Press; 2004. pp.323-47.
593. Seidman L, Doyle A, Fried R, Valera E, Crum K, Matthews L. Neuropsychological function in adults with attention-deficity/ hyperactivity disorder. In: Spencer T (Ed). Adult ADHD, psychiatric clinics of North America: Elsevier Scinece; 2004. pp.261-82.
594. Sergeant J. EUNETHYDIS-searching for valid aetiological candidates of attention-deficit hyperactivity disorder or hyperkinetic disorder. Eur Child Adolesc Psychiatr. 2004;13 (Suppl 1):143-9.
595. Sergeant J. The cognitive-energetic model: an empirical approach to attention-deficit hyperactivity disorder. Neurosci Biobehav Rev. 2000;24:7-12.
596. Serveant JA, Guerts H, Huijbregts S, Schetes a, Oosterlaan J. The top and bottom of ADHD: a neuropsychological perspective. Neurosci Biobehav Rev. 2003;27:583-92.
597. Shywitz SE, Cohen DJ, Shaywitz BA. The biochemical basis fo minimal brain dysfunction. J Pediatr. 1978;92:179-87.
598. Sonuga-Barke EJ, Dalen L, Daley D, Remington B. Are planning, working memory, and inhibiton associated with individual difference sin preschool ADHD symptoms? Dev Neuropsychol. 2002;21:255-72.
599. Sonuga-Barke EJ. Casual models of Attention-deficit/ hyperactivity disorder: from common simple deficits to multiple developmental pathways. Biol Psychiatry. 2005;57:1231-8.
600. Sonuga-Barke EJ. The dual pathway model of AD/HD: an elaboration of neuro-developmental characteristics. Neurosci Biobhav Rev. 2003;27:593-604.
601. Sowell ER, Thompson PM, Welcome SE, henkenius AL, Toga AW, Peterson BS. Cortical abnormalities in children and adolescents with attention-deficit hyperactivity disorder. Lancet. 2003;362:1699-707.
602. Spencer T, Biderman J, Wilens T, Growth deficits in children with attention deficit hyperactivity disorder. Pediatrics. 1998;102:501-6.
603. Spencer T, Biederman J, coffey B, Geller D, Wilens T, Faraone S. The 4-year course of tic disorders in boys with attention-deficit/ hyperactivity disorder. Arch Gen Psychiatry. 1999;56:842-7.
604. Spencer T, Biederman J, Wilens T. Pharmacotherapy of attention dificit hyperactivity disorder. Child Adolesc Psychiatr Clin North Am. 2000;9:77-97.
605. Spencer T, Biederman J, Wilens T. Stimulant treatment of adult attention-deficit/hyperactivity disorder. Psychiatr Clin North Am. 2004;27:361-72.
606. Spirich S, Biderman J, Crawford MH, Mundy E, Faraone SV. Adoptive and biological families of children and adolescents with ADHD. J Am Acad Child Adolesc Psychiatry. 2000;39:1432-37.
607. State Rc, Frye MA, Altshuler LL, et al. Chart review of the impact of attention-deficit/hyperactivity disorder comorbidity on response to lithium or divalproex sodium in adolescent mania. J Clin Psychiatry. 2004;65:1057-63.
608. Stein B, Orlando M. ADHD treatment in a behavioral health care carve-out: medications, providers, and service utilization. J Behav Health Serv. Res. 2001;28:30-41.
609. Steinhausen HC, Drechsler R, Foldenyi M, Imhaf K, Brandeis D. Clinical course of attention deficit/hyperactivity disorder from childhood toward early adolescence. J Am Acad Child Adolesc Psychiatry. 2004;42:1085-92.
610. Stevens J, Harman JS, Kellenher KH. Ethnic and regional differences in primary care visits for attention-deficit hyperactivity disorder. J Dev Behav Pediatr. 2004;25:318-25.
611. Swanson JM, Sergeant JA, Taylor E, Sonuga-Barke EJS, Jensen PS, Cantwell DP, Attention-deficit hyperactivity disorder and hyperkinetic disorder. Lancet. 1998;351:429-33.
612. Sztmari P, Offord DR, Boyle MH, Ontario Child Health study: Prevalence of attention deficit disorder with hyperactivity. J Child Psychol psychiatry 1989;30:219-30.
613. Taylor E. Similarities and differences in DSM-IV and ICD-10 diagnostic criteria. Child Adolesc Psychiatr Clin North Am. 1994;3:209-26.
614. Taylor FB, Russo J, Efficacy of modafinil compared to dextroamphetamine for the treatment of attention deficit hyperactivity disorder in adults. J Child Adolesc Psychopharmacol. 2000;10:311-20.
615. Thapar A, Fowler T, Rice F, et al. Maternal smoking during pregnancy and attention deficit hyperactivity disorder symptoms in offspring. Am J Psychiatry. 2003;160:1985-89.
616. Todd RD, Joyner CA, Ji TH, Sun L, Reich W, Neuman RJ. Family factors and sampling approach differentially influence attention deficit/hyperactivity disorder subtypes. Mol Psychiatry. 2004;9:260-3.
617. Tourette Syndrome Study Group. Treatment of ADHD in children with tics: a randomized controlled trial. Neurology. 2002;58:527-36.

618. Tripp G, Ryan J, Peace K. Neuropsychological functioning in children with DSM-IV combined type attentiond eficit hyperactivity disorder. Aus NZ J Psychiatry. 2002;36:771-9.
619. Turner DC, Clark L, Dowson J, Robbins TW, Sahakian BJ. Modafinil improves cognition and response inhibition in adult attention-deficit/hyperactivity disorder. Biol Psychiatry. 2004;55:1031-40.
620. Van De Kamp J, Collins A. Prenatal nocitine alters nicotinic receptor development in the mouse brain. Pharmacol Biochem Behav. 1994;47:889-900.
621. van Dyck CH, Quinlan DM, Cretella LM, et al. Unaltered dopamine transporter availability in adult attention deficit hyperactivity disorder. Am J Psychiatry. 2002;159:309-12.
622. Vles JS, Feron FJ, Hendriksen JG, Jolles J, van Kroonenburgh MJ, Weber WE, Methylphenidate down-regulates the dopamine receptor and transporter system in children with attention deficit hyperkinetic disorder (ADHD). Neuropediatrics 2003;34:77-80.
623. Volkow ND, Swanston JM. Variables that affect the clinical use and abuse of methylphenidate in the treatment of ADHD. Am J Psychiatry. 2003;160:1909-18.
624. Volkow ND, Wang GJ, Fowler JS, et al. Dopamine transporter occupancies in the human brain induced by therapeutic doses of oral methylphenidate. Am J Psychiatry. 1998;155:1325-31.
625. Wells KC, Epstein JN, Hinshaw SP, et al. Parenting and family stress treatment outcomes in attention deficit hyperactivity disorder (ADHD): an empirical analysis in the MTA study. J Abnorm Child Psychol. 2000;28:543-53.
626. Westgard JO, Darcy T. The truth about quality: medical usefulness and analytical reliability of laboratory tests. Clin Chim Acta. 2004;346:3-11.
627. Wigal S, Swanson JM, Feifel D, et al. A double, placebo-controlled trial of dexmethylphenidate hydrochloride and d1-threomethylphenidate hydrochloride in children with attention-deficit/hyperactivity disorder. J Am Acad Child Adolesc Psychiatry. 2004;43:1406-14.
628. Wilcutt EG, brodsky K, Chhabildas N, et al. The neuropsychology of attention deficit hyperactivity disorder: validity of the executive function hypothesis. In: Gozal D, Molfese D (Eds). Attention deficit hyperactivity disorder from genes to patients. Totowa, NJ: Humana Press; 2005.
629. Wilcutt EG, Pennington BF, Chhabildas NA, Friedman MC, Alexander J. Psychiatric comorbidity associated with DSM-IV ADHD in a nonreferred sample of twins. J Am Acad Child Adolesc Psychiatry. 1999;38:1355-62.
630. Wilens T, Faraone SV, Biederman J, Gunawardene S. Does stimulant therapy of attention deficit hyperactivity disorder beget later substance abuse? Pediatrics. 2003;111:179-85.
631. Wilens T, Haight BR, Horrigan JP, et al. Bupropion XL in adults with ADHD: a randomized, placebo-controlled study. Biol Psychiatry. 2005;57:793-801.
632. Wilens T, Prince J, Spencer T, et al. An open trial of bupropion for the treatment of adults with attention deficit hyperactivity disorder and bipolar disorder. Biol Psychiatry. 2003;54:9-16.
633. Wilens TE, Spencer TJ, Biederman J, et al. A controlled clinical trial of bupropion for attention deficit hyperactivity disorder in adults. Am J Psychiatry. 2001;158;282-88.
634. Wilens TE, Spencer TJ. Combining methylphenidate and clonidine: a clinically sound medication. Option J Am J Child Adolesc Psychiatry. 1999;38:614-9.
635. Wilson MC. Coloboma mouse mutant as an animal model of hyperkinesis and attention deficit hyperactivity disorder. Neurosci Biobehav Rev. 2000;24:51-7.
636. Wolraich M, greenhill LL, Pelham W, et al. Randomized controlled trial of oros methylphenidate once a day in children with attention-deficit/hyperactivity disorder. Pediatrics. 2001;108:883-92.
637. Wolraich M, Wilson D, White W. The effect of sugar on behavior or cognition in children. JAMA. 1995;274:1617-21.
638. Wolraich ML, Hannah JN, Baugaertel A, Feurer ID, Examination of DSM-IV criteria for attention deficit/hyperactivity disorder in a country-wide sample. J Dev Behav Pediatr. 1998;19: 162-8.
639. Zito JM, Safer DJ, dosReis S, Gardner JF, Boles M, Lynch F. Trends in the prescribing of psychotropic medications to preschoolers. JAMA. 2000;283:1025-30.

Very Early Intervention in Psychotic Disorders

640. American Psychiatric Association. DSM-IV: diagnostic and statistical manual of mental disorders. 4th edition. Washington, DC: APA. 1994.
641. Andreasen NC, Endicott J, Spitzer RL, et al. The family history method using diagnostic criteria: reliability and validity. Arch Gen Psychiatry. 1977;34:1229-35.
642. Andreasson S, Allebeck P, Engstrom A, et al. Cannabis and schizophrenia. A longitudinal study of Swedish conscripts. Lancet. 1987;2:1483-6.
643. Arseneault L, Cannon M, Poulton R, et al. Cannabis use in adolescence and risk for adult psychosis: longitudinal prospective study. Br Med J. 2002;325:1212-3.
644. Beiser M, Erickson D, Fleming JAE, et al. Establishing the onset of psychotic illness. Am J Psychiatry. 1993;150:1349-54.
645. Bell RQ. Multiple-risk cohorts and segmenting risk as solutions to the problem of false positives in risk for the major psychoses. Psychiatry. 1992;55:370-81.
646. Bertelsen M, Jeppesen P, Petersen L, et al. Five – year follow-up of a randomized multicenter trial of intensive early intervention vs standard treatment for patients with a first episode of psychotic illness. Arch Gen Psychiatry. 2008;65(7):762-71.
647. Borgwardt SJ, Riecher – Rossler A, Dazzan P, et al. Regional gray matter volume abnormalities in the at risk mental state. Boil Psychiatry. 2007;61:1148-56.
648. Cameron ED. Early schizophrenia. Am J Psychiatry. 1938; 95:567-78.
649. Cannon TD, Cadenhead K, Cornblatt B, et al. Prediction of psychosis in youth at high clinical risk. Arch Gen Psychiatry. 2008;65(1):28-37.

650. Caspi A, Moffitt TE, cannon M, et al. Moderation of the effect of adolescent - onset cannabis use on adult psychosis by a functional polymorphism in the catechol-O-methyltransferase gene: longitudinal evidence of a gene x environment interaction. Biol Psychiatry. 2005;57:1117-27.
651. Conrad K, editor. Die beginnende schizophrenia. Stuttgart, Germany: Georg Thieme Verlag; 1958.
652. Corblatt BA, Lencz T, Obuchowski M, et al. The schizophrenia prodrome: treatment and high-risk perspectives. Schizophr Res. 2002;54:177-86.
653. Cornblatt BA, Lencz T, Smith CW, et al. The schizophrenia prodrome revisited: a neurodevelopmental perspective. Schizophr Bull. 2003;29:633-51.
654. Cornblatt BA. Lencz T, Smith CW, et al. Can antidepressants be used to treat the schizophrenia prodrom? Results of a prospective, naturalistic treatment study of adolescents. J Clin Psychiatry. 2007;68:546-57.
655. Craig TKJ, Garety P, Power P, et al. The Lambeth early onset (LEO) team: randomized controlled trial of the effectiveness of specialized care for early psychosis. Br Med J. 2004;329(7474):1067.
656. Culberg J, Mattsson M, Levander S, et al. Treatment costs and clinical outcome for first episode schizophrenia patients: a 3 - year follow-up of the Swedish "parachute project" and two comparison groups. Acta Psychiatr Scand. 2006;114(4): 274-81.
657. Fergusson DM, Horwood JL, Swain - Campbell NR. Cannabis dependence and psychotic symptoms in young people. Psychol Med. 2003;33:15-21.
658. Fornito A, Yung AR, Wood SJ, et al. Anatomic abnormalities of the anterior cingulated cortex before psychosis onset: an MRI study of ultra-high-risk individuals. Boil Psychiatry. 2008;64(9):758-65.
659. French P, Shryane N, Bentall RP, et al. Effects of cognitive therapy on the longitudinal development of psychotic experiences in people at high risk of developing psychosis. Br J Psychiatry. 2007;191:s82-7.
660. Gross G. The onset of schizophrenia. Schizophr Res. 1997;28:187-98.
661. Hall R. Global assessment of functioning: a modified scale. Psychosomatics. 1995;36:267-75.
662. Hawkins KA, Quinlan D, Miller TJ, et al. Factorial structure of the scale of prodromal symptoms. Schizophr Res. 2004;68(2-3):339-47.
663. Henquet C, Krabbendam L, Spauwen J, et al. Prospective cohort study of cannabis use, predisposition for psychosis, and psychotic symptoms in young people. BMJ. 2005;330:11-6.
664. Klosterkotter J, Ebel H, Schultze-Lutter F, et al. Diagnostic Validity of basic symptoms. Eur Arch Psychiatry Clin Neurosci. 1996;246:147-54.
665. Klosterkotter J, Hellmich M, Steinmeyer EM, et al. Diagnosing schizophrenia in the initial prodromal phase. Arch Gen Psychiatry. 2001;58:158-64.
666. Koehler K, Sauer H. Huber's basic symptoms: another approach to negative psychopathology in schizophrenia. Compr Psychiatry. 1984;25(2):174-82.
667. Larsen TK, Melle I, Auestad B, et al. Early detection of first - episode psychosis: the effect on 1-year outcome. Schizophr Bull. 2006;32(4):758-64.
668. Larsen TK. The transition from premorbid period to psychosis: how can it be described? Acta Psychiatr Scand. 2002;106: s10-1.
669. Marshall M, Lewis S, Lockwood A, et al. Association between duration of untreated psychosis and outcome in cohorts of first-episode patients. Arch Gen Psychiatry. 2005;62:975-83.
670. Mason O, Startup M, Halpin S, et al. State and trait predictors of transition to first episode psychosis among individuals with at risk mental states. Schizophr Res. 2004;71:227-37.
671. McGlashan TH, Miller TJ, Woods SW, et al. A scale for the assessment of prodromal symptoms and states. In: Miller TJ, Mednick SA, McGlashan TH, et al (Eds). Early intervention in psychotic disorders. Dordrecht, The Netherlands: Kluwer Academic Publishers. 2001.pp.135-49.
672. McGlashan TH, Zipursky RB, perkins D, et al. Randomized, double-blind trail of olanzapine versus placebo in patients prodromally symptomatic for psychosis. Am J Psychiatry. 2006;163:790-9.
673. McGorry PD, Singh BS. Schizophrenia: risk and possibility. In: Raphael B, Burrows GD (Eds). Handbook of Studies on Preventive Psychiatry. Amsterdam: Elsevier. 1995. pp.491-514.
674. Meares A. The diagnosis of prepsychotic schizophrenia. Lancet. 1959;1:55-8.
675. Mele I, Larsen TK, Haahr U, et al. Reducing the duration of untreated first-episode psychosis: effect on clinical presentation. Arch Gen Psychiatry. 2004;61:143-50.
676. Melle I, Johannesen JO, Friis S, et al. Early detection of the first episode of schizophrenia and suicidal behavior. Am J Psychiatry. 2006;163(5):800-4.
677. Melle I, Larsen TK, Haahr U, et al. Prevention of negative symptom psychopathologies in first-episode schizophrenia. Arch Gen Psychiatry. 2008;65(6):634-40.
678. Meyer SK, Bearden CE, Lux SR, et al. The psychosis prodrome in adolescent patients viewed through the lens of DSM - IV. J Child Adolesc Psychopharmacol. 2005;15(3): 434-51.
679. Meyer-Lindenberg A, Nichols T, Callicott JH, et al. Impact of complex genetic variation in COMT on human brain function. Mol Psychiatry. 2006;11:867-77.
680. Mihalopoulos C, McGorry PD, Carter RC. Is phase - specific, community-oriented treatment of early psychosis an economically viable method of improving outcome? Acta Psychiatr Scand. 1999;100(1):47-55.
681. Miller TJ, McGlashan TH, Rosen JL, et al. Prodromal assessment with the structured interview for prodromal syndromes and the scale of prodromal symptoms: predictive validity, interrater reliability, and training to reliability. Schizophr Bull. 2003;29(4):703-15.
682. Miller TJ, McGlashan TH, Woods SW, et al. Symptom assessment in schizophrenic prodromal states. Psychiatr Q. 1999;70:273-87.

683. Miller TJ. McGlashan TH, Rosen JL, et al. Prospective diagnosis of the initial prodromes: preliminary evidence of interrater reliability and predictive validity. Am J Psychiatry. 2002;159:863-5.
684. Moore THM, Zammit S, Lingford-Hughes A, et al. Cannabis use and risk of psychotic or affective mental health outcomes: a systematic review. Lancet. 2007;370:319-28.
685. Morrison AP, French P, Parker S, et al. Three - year follow-up of a randomized controlled trial of cognitive therapy for the prevention of psychosis in people at ultra - high risk. Schizophr Bull. 2007;33(3):682-7.
686. Pantelis C, Velakoulis D, McGorry PD, et al. Neuroanatomical abnormalities before and after onset of psychosis: a cross - sectional and longitudinal MRI comparison. Lancet. 2003;361:281-8.
687. Perkins DO, Gu H, Boteva K, et al. Relationship between duration of Untreated psychosis and outcome in first-episode schizophrenia: a critical review and meta-analysis. Am J Psychiatry. 2005;162(10):1785-804.
688. Petersen L, Nordentoft M, Jeppesen P, et al. Improving 1 - year outcome in first - episode psychosis. Br J Psychiatry. 2005;187(48):s98-103.
689. Phillips LJ, Yung AR, Yuen HP, et al. Prediction and prevention of transition to psychosis in young people at incipient risk for schizophrenia. Am J Med Genet. 2002;114:929-37.
690. Ruhrmann S, Bechdolf A, Kuhn K - U, et al. Acute effects of treatment for prodromal symptoms for people putatively in a late initial prodromal state of psychosis. Br J Psychiatry. 2007;191:s88-95.
691. Sullivan HS. The onset of schizophrenia. Am J Psychiatry. 1927;6:105-34.
692. Svirskis T, Korkelia J, Heinimaa M, et al. Axis - I disorders and vulnerability to psychosis. Schizophr Res. 2005;75:439-46.
693. Thorup A, Petersen L, Jeppesen P, et al. Integrated treatment ameliorates negative symptoms in first episode psychosis - results from the Danish OPUS trial. Schizophr Res. 2005;79-105.
694. Van Os J, Bak M, Hanssen M, et al. Cannabis use and psychosis: a longitudinal population - based study. Am J Epidemiol. 2002;156:319-27.
695. Varsamis J, Adamson JD. Early schizophrenia. Can Psychiatr Assoc J. 1971;16:487-97.
696. Veen ND, Selten JP, Van der Tweel I, et al. Cannabis use and age at onset of schizophrenia. Am J Psychiatry. 2004;161:501-6.
697. Waterfang M, Yung AR, Wood AG, et al. Corpus callosum shape alterations in individuals prior to the onset of psychosis. Schizophr Res. 2008;103(1-3):1-10.
698. Wood SJ, Brewer WJ, Koutsouradis P, et al. Cognitive decline following psychosis onset. Br J Psychiatry. 2007;191:s52-7.
699. Woods SW, Tally EM. Walsh BC, et al. Aripiprazole in the treatment of the psychosis prodrome. Br J Psychiatry. 2007;191:s96-101.
700. Yung AR, Buckby JA, Cosgrave EM, et al. Association between psychotic experiences and depression in a clinical sample over 6 months. Schizophr Res. 2007;91:246-53.
701. Yung AR, McGorry PD, Francey SM, et al. PACE: a specialized service for young people at risk of psychotic disorders. Med J Aust. 2007;187(7):s43-6.
702. Yung AR, McGorry PD. The prodromal phase of first-episode psychosis: past and current conceptualizations. Schizophr Bull. 1996;22(2):353-70.
703. Yung AR, Phillips LJ, Yuen HP, et al. Psychosis prediction: 12-month follow up of a high-risk (prodromal) group. Schizophr Res. 2003;60:21-32.
704. Yung AR, Phillips LJ, Yuen HP, et al. Risk factors for psychosis in an ultra high-risk group: psychopathology and clinical features. Schizophr Res. 2004;67:131-42.
705. Yung AR, Yuen HP, Berger G, et al. Declining transition rate in ultra high risk (prodromal) services: dilution or reduction of risk. Schizophr Bull. 2007;33(3):673-81.
706. Zammit S, ALlebeck P, Engstrom A, et al. Self reported cannabis use as a risk factor for schizophrenia in Swedish conscripts of 1969: historical cohort study. Br Med J. 2002;325:1199-203.

Depression in Adolescence

707. American Psychiatric Association. Diagnostic and statistical manual of mental disorders. Washington DC: American Psychiatric Association; 1994.
708. Angold A, Costello EJ, Erkanli A, Worthman CM. Pubertal changes in hormone levels and depression in girls. Psychol Med. 1999;29:1043-53.
709. Angold A, Costello EJ, Erkanli A. Comorbidity. J Child Psychol Psychiatry. 1999;40:57-87.
710. Angold A, Costello EJ. Depressive comorbidity in children and adolescents: empirical, theoretical, and methodological issues. Am J Psychiatry. 1993;150:1779-91.
711. Angold A, Costello EJ. Puberty and depression. Child Adolesc Psychiatr Clin N Am. 2006;15:919-37.
712. Asarnow JR, Jaycox LH, Duan N, et al. Effectiveness of a quality improvement intervention for adolescent depression in primary care clinics: a randomized controlled trial. JAMA. 2005;293:311-9.
713. Bardone AM, Moffitt TE, Caspi A, Dickson N, Stanton WR, Silva PA. Adult physical health outcomes of adolescent girls with conduct disorder, depression, and anxiety. J Am Acad Child Adolesc Psychiatry. 1998;37:594-601.
714. Birmaher B, Williamson DE, Dahl RE, et al. Clinical presentation and course of depression in youth: does onset in childhood differ from onset in adolescence? J Am Acad Child Adolesc Psychiatry. 2004;43:63-70.
715. Blakemore SJ. The social brain in adolescence. Nat Rev Neurosci. 2008;9:267-77.
716. Bolton P, Bass J, Betancourt T, et al. Interventions for depression symptoms among adolescent survivors of war and displacement in northern Uganda: a randomized controlled trial. JAMA. 2007;298:519-27.
717. Borner I, Braunstein JW, St Victor R, Pollack J. Evaluation of a 2-question screening tool for detecting depression

in adolescents in primary care. Clin Pediatr (Phila). 2010;49:947-53.

718. Brennan PA, Le Brocque R, Hammen C. Maternal depression, parent-child relationships, and resilient outcomes in adolescence. J Am Acad Child Adolesc Psychiatry. 2003;42:1469-77.
719. Brent D, Emslie G, Clarke G, et al. Switching to another SSRI or to venlafaxine with or without cognitive behavioral therapy for adolescents with SSRI-resistant depression: the TORDIA randomized controlled trial. JAMA. 2008;299:901-13.
720. Bridge JA, Yengar S, Salary CB, et al. Clinical response and risk for reported suicidal ideation and suicide attempts in pediatric antidepressant treatment: a meta-analysis of randomized controlled trials. JAMA. 2007;63:332-9.
721. Brody AL, Saxena S, Silverman DH, et al. Brain metabolic changes in major depressive disorder from pre- to post-treatment with paroxetine. Psychiatry Res. 1999;91:127-39.
722. Brotman MA, Schmajuk M, Rich BA, et al. Prevalence, clinical correlates, and longitudinal course of severe mood dysregulation in children. Biol Psychiatry. 2006;60:991-7.
723. Calear AL, Christensen H. Systematic review of school-based prevention and early intervention programs for depression. J Adolesc. 2010;33:429-38.
724. Casey BJ, Jones RM, Levita L, et al. The storm and stress of adolescence: insights from human imaging and mouse genetics. Dev Psychobiol. 2010;52:225-35.
725. Caspi A, Sugden K, Moffitt TE, et al. Influence of life stress on depression: moderation by a polymorphism in the 5-HTT gene. Science. 2003;301:386-9.
726. Clauss JA, Cowan RL, Blackford JU. Expectation and temperament moderate amygdala and dorsal anterior cingulate cortex responses to fear faces. Cogn Affect Behav Neurosci. 2011;11:13-21.
727. Cluver L, Gardner F, Operario D. Psychological distress amongst AIDS-orphaned children in urban South Africa. J Child Psychol Psychiatry. 2007;48:755-63.
728. Cole J, Ball HA, Martin NC, Scourfield J, McGuffin P. Genetic overlap between measures of hyperactivity/inattention and mood in children and adolescents. J Am Acad Child Adolesc Psychiatry. 2009;48:1094-101.
729. Collishaw S, Pickles A, Messer J, Rutter M, Shearer C, Maughan B. Resilience to adult psychopathology following childhood maltreatment: evidence from a community sample. Child Abuse Negl. 2007;31:211-29.
730. Collishaw S. Trends in adolescent depression: a review of the evidence. In: Yule W (Ed). Depression in childhood and adolescence: the way forward. London: Association of Child and Adolescent Mental Health; 2009. pp. 7-18.
731. Conradi HJ, Ormel J, de Jonge P. Presence of individual (residual) symptoms during depressive episodes and periods of remission: a 3-year prospective study. Psychol Med. 2010;8:1-10.
732. Costello EJ, Angold A, Burns BJ, Erkanli A, Stangl DK, Tweed DL. The Great Smoky Mountains Study of Youth. Functional impairment and serious emotional disturbance. Arch Gen Psychiatry. 1996;53:1137-43.
733. Costello EJ, Egger H, Angold A. 10-year research update review: The epidemiology of child and adolescent psychiatric disorders: I. Methods and public health burden. J Am Acad Child Adolesc Psychiatry. 2005;44:972-86.
734. Costello EJ, Erkanli A, Angold A. Is there an epidemic of child or adolescent depression? J Child Psychol Psychiatry. 2006;47:1263-71.
735. Costello EJ, Foley DL, Angold A. 10-year research update review: the epidemiology of child and adolescent psychiatric disorders: II. Developmental epidemiology. J Am Acad Child Adolesc Psychiatry. 2006;45:8-25.
736. Cyranowski JM, Frank E, Young E, Shear K. Adolescent onset of the gender difference in lifetime rates of major depression. Arch Gen Psychiatry. 2000;57:21-7.
737. Daviss WB, Birmaher B, Melhem NA, Axelson DA, Michaels SM, Brent DA. Criterion validity of the mood and feelings questionnaire for depressive episodes in clinic and non-clinic subjects. J Child Psychol Psychiatry. 2006;47:927-34.
738. Dunn V, Goodyer IA. Longitudinal investigation into childhood- and adolescence- onset depression: psychiatric outcome in early adulthood. Br J Psychiatry. 2006;188:216-22.
739. Eaves L, Silberg J, Erkanli A. Resolving multiple epigenetic pathways to adolescent depression. J Child Psychol Psychiatry. 2003;44:1006-14.
740. Emslie GJ, Ventura D, Korotzer A, Tourkodimitris S. Escitalopram in the treatment of adolescent depression: a randomized placebo-controlled multisite trial. J Am Acad Child Adolesc Psychiatry. 2009;48:721-9.
741. Engle PL, Black MM, Behrman JR, et al. The International Child Development Steering Group. Strategies to avoid the loss of developmental potential in more than 200 million children in the developing world. Lancet. 2007;369:229-42.
742. Evans DL, Charney DS, Lewis L, et al. Mood disorders in the medically ill: scientific review and recommendations. Biol Psychiatry. 2005;58:175-89.
743. Fava GA, Ruini C, Belaise C. The concept of recovery in major depression. Psychol Med. 2007;37:307-17.
744. Feder A, Nestler EJ, Charney DS. Psychobiology and molecular genetics of resilience. Nat Rev Neurosci. 2009;10:446-57.
745. Fleitlich-Bilyk B, Goodman R. Prevalence of child and adolescent psychiatric disorders in southeast Brazil. J Am Acad Child Adolesc Psychiatry. 2004;43:727-34.
746. Fletcher JM. Adolescent depression and educational attainment: results using sibling fixed effects. Health Econ. 2008;17:1215-35.
747. Forbes EE, Dahl RE. Neural systems of positive affect: relevance to understanding child and adolescent depression? Dev Psychopathol. 2005;17:827-50.
748. Forbes EE, Hariri AR, Martin SL, et al. Altered striatal activation predicting real-world positive affect in adolescent major depressive disorder. Am J Psychiatry. 2009;166:64-73.

749. Ford T, Goodman R, Meltzer H. The British child and adolescent mental health survey 1999: the prevalence of DSM-IV disorders. J Am Acad Child Adolesc Psychiatry. 2003;42:1203-11.
750. Foster CE, Webster MC, Weissman MM, et al. Remission of maternal depression: relations to family functioning and youth internalizing and externalizing symptoms. J Clin Child Adolesc Psychol. 2008;37:714-24.
751. Fox CL, Butler I. Evaluating the effectiveness of a school-based counselling service in the UK. Br J Guidance Counselling. 2009;37:95-106.
752. Garber J, Clarke GN, Weersing VR, et al. Prevention of depression in at-risk adolescents: a randomized controlled trial. JAMA. 2009;301:2215-24.
753. Goodman R, Ford T, Richards H, et al. The development and well-being assessment: description and initial validation of an integrated assessment of child and adolescent psychopathology. J Child Psychol Psychiatry. 2000;41:645-55.
754. Goodman R. The strengths and difficulties questionnaire: a research note. J Child Psychol Psychiatry. 1997;38:581-6.
755. Goodman SH, Gotlib IH. Risk for psychopathology in the children of depressed mothers: a developmental model for understanding mechanisms of transmission. Psychol Rev. 1999;106:458-90.
756. Goodyer I, Dubicka B, Wilkinson P, et al. Selective serotonin reuptake inhibitors (SSRIs) and routine specialist care with and without cognitive behaviour therapy in adolescents with major depression: randomised controlled trial. BMJ. 2007;335:142.
757. Goodyer I, Wright C, Altham P. The friendships and recent life events of anxious and depressed school-aged children. Br J Psychiatry. 1990;156:689-98.
758. Goodyer IM, Dubicka B, Wilkinson P, et al. A randomised controlled trial of cognitive behaviour therapy in adolescents with major depression treated by selective serotonin reuptake inhibitors. The ADAPT trial. Health Technol Assess. 2008;12:iii–iv. ix–60.
759. Goodyer IM, Herbert J, Altham PM, Pearson J, Secher SM, Shiers HM. Adrenal secretion during major depression in 8- to 16-year-olds, I. Altered diurnal rhythms in salivary cortisol and dehydroepiandrosterone (DHEA) at presentation. Psychol Med. 1996;26:245-56.
760. Goodyer IM, Herbert J, Tamplin A, Altham PME. Recent life events, cortisol, dehydroepiandrosterone and the onset of major depression in high-risk adolescents. Br J Psychiatry. 2000;177:499-504.
761. Gotlib IH, Hamilton JP, Cooney RE, Singh MK, Henry ML, Joormann J. Neural processing of reward and loss in girls at risk for major depression. Arch Gen Psychiatry. 2010;67: 380-7.
762. Green H, McGinnity A, Meltzer H, Ford T, Goodman, R. Mental health of children and young people in Great Britain, 2004. Basingstoke, UK: Palgrave Macmillan; 2005.
763. Guyer AE, McClure-Tone EB, Shiffrin ND, Pine DS, Nelson EE. Probing the neural correlates of anticipated peer evaluation in adolescence. Child Dev. 2009;80:1000-15.
764. Hammen C, Brennan PA. Severity, chronicity, and timing of maternal depression and risk for adolescent off spring diagnoses in a community sample. Arch Gen Psychiatry. 2003;60:253-8.
765. Hankin BL, Abramson LY, Moffitt TE, Silva PA, McGee R, Angell KE. Development of depression from preadolescence to young adulthood: emerging gender differences in a 10-year longitudinal study. J Abnorm Psychol. 1998;107:128-40.
766. Hariri AR, Drabant EM, Munoz KE, et al. A susceptibility gene for affective disorders and the response of the human amygdala. Arch Gen Psychiatry. 2005;62:146-52.
767. Hariri AR, Mattay VS, Tessitore A, et al. Serotonin transporter genetic variation and the response of the human amygdala. Science. 2002;297:400-3.
768. Harrington R. Adolescent depression: same or different? Arch Gen Psychiatry. 2001;58:21-2.
769. Hasler G, Pine DS, Kleinbaum DG, et al. Depressive symptoms during childhood and adult obesity: the Zurich cohort study. Mol Psychiatry. 2005;10:842-50.
770. Hawker DS, Boulton MJ. Twenty years' research on peer victimization and psychosocial maladjustment: a meta-analytic review of cross-sectional studies. J Child Psychol Psychiatry. 2000;41:441-55.
771. Hawton K, van Heeringen K. Suicide. Lancet. 2009;373:1372-81.
772. Hay DF, Pawlby S, Waters CS, Sharp D. Antepartum and postpartum exposure to maternal depression: different effects on different adolescent outcomes. J Child Psychol Psychiatry. 2008;49:1079-88.
773. Hetrick S, Merry S, McKenzie J, Sindahl P, Proctor M. Selective serotonin reuptake inhibitors (SSRIs) for depressive disorders in children and adolescents. Cochrane Database Syst Rev. 2007;3:CD004851.
774. Hollis C. Schizophrenia and allied disorders. In: Rutter M, Bishop D, Pine D, et al. (Eds). Rutter's child and adolescent psychiatry. 5. Oxford: Blackwell; 2008. pp. 737-58.
775. Hyde JS, Mezulis AH, Abramson LY. The ABCs of depression: Integrating affective, biological, and cognitive models to explain the emergence of the gender difference in depression. Psychol Rev. 2008;115:291-313.
776. Institute of Medicine. Preventing mental, emotional and behavioral disorders among young people: progress and possibilities. Washington DC: National Academies Press; 2009.
777. Jones L. Responding to the needs of children in crisis. Int Rev Psychiatry. 2008;20:291-303.
778. Karg K, Burmeister M, Shedden K, Sen S. The serotonin transporter promoter variant (5-HTTLPR), stress, and depression meta-analysis revisited: evidence of genetic moderation. Arch Gen Psychiatry. 2011;68:444-54.
779. Keenan-Miller D, Hammen CL, Brennan PA. Health outcomes related to early adolescent depression. J Adolesc Health. 2007;41:256-62.
780. Kendler KS, Gardner CO, Lichtenstein P. A developmental twin study of symptoms of anxiety and depression: evidence for genetic innovation and attenuation. Psychol Med. 2008;38:1567-75.

781. Kessler RC, Avenevoli S, Ries Merikangas K. Mood disorders in children and adolescents: an epidemiologic perspective. Biol Psychiatry. 2001;49:1002-14.
782. Khaw KT, Wareham N, Luben R, et al. Glycosylated haemoglobin, diabetes and mortality in men in Norfolk cohort of European prospective investigation of cancer and nutrition (EPIC-Norfolk). BMJ. 2001;322:15-8.
783. Kim-Cohen J, Caspi A, Moffitt TE, Harrington H, Milne BJ, Poulton R. Prior juvenile diagnoses in adults with mental disorder: developmental follow-back of a prospective-longitudinal cohort. Arch Gen Psychiatry. 2003;60:709-17.
784. Klein JB, Jacobs RH, Reinecke MA. Cognitive-behavioral therapy for adolescent depression: a meta-analytic investigation of changes in effect-size estimates. J Am Acad Child Adolesc Psychiatry. 2007;46:1403-13.
785. Kovacs M. The children's depression, inventory (CDI). Psychopharmacol Bull. 1985;21:995-8.
786. Kroenke K, Spitzer RL, Williams JB. The Patient Health Questionnaire-2: validity of a two-item depression screener. Med Care. 2003;41:1284-92.
787. Lau JY, Eley TC. Disentangling gene-environment correlations and interactions on adolescent depressive symptoms. J Child Psychol Psychiatry. 2008;49:142-50.
788. Leaf PJ, Alegria M, Cohen P, et al. Mental health service use in the community and schools: results from the four-community MECA Study. Methods for the epidemiology of child and adolescent mental disorders study. J Am Acad Child Adolesc Psychiatry. 1996;35:889-97.
789. Lewinsohn PM, Allen NB, Seeley JR, Gotlib IH. First onset versus recurrence of depression: differential processes of psychosocial risk. J Abnorm Psychol. 1999;108:483-9.
790. Lewinsohn PM, Klein DN, Seeley JR. Bipolar disorders in a community sample of older adolescents: prevalence, phenomenology, comorbidity, and course. J Am Acad Child Adoles Psychiatry. 1995;34:454-63.
791. Lewinsuhn PM, Pettit JW, Joivan TE, Seeley IR. The Symptomology of depressive disorder in adolescents and young adults. AmJ med Psychol. 2003;112:44-52.
792. Lewinsohn PM, Rohde P, Klein DN, Seeley JR. Natural course of adolescent major depressive disorder: I. Continuity into young adulthood. J Am Acad Child Adolesc Psychiatry. 1999;38:56-63.
793. Lewinsohn PM, Rohde P, Seeley JR, Klein DN, Gotlib IH. Natural course of adolescent major depressive disorder in a community sample: predictors of recurrence in young adults. Am J Psychiatry. 2000;157:1584-91.
794. Lewinsohn PM, Rohde P, Seeley JR. Major depressive disorder in older adolescents: prevalence, risk factors and clinical implications. Clin Psychol Rev. 1988;18:765-94.
795. Lopez A, Mathers C, Ezzati M, Jamison D, Murray C. Global burden of disease and risk factors. Washington: Oxford University Press and the World Bank; 2006.
796. Lopez-Duran NL, Kovacs M, George CJ. Hypothalamic-pituitary-adrenal axis dysregulation in depressed children and adolescents: a meta-analysis. Psychoneuroendocrinology. 2009;34:1272-83.
797. Ma J, Lee KV, Stafford RS. Depression treatment during outpatient visits by US children and adolescents. J Adolesc Health. 2005;37:434-42.
798. March J, Silva S, Petrycki S, et al. Treatment for Adolescents with Depression Study (TADS) team. Fluoxetine, cognitive-behavioral therapy, and their combination for adolescents with depression: Treatment for Adolescents with Depression Study (TADS) randomized controlled trial. JAMA. 2004;292: 807-20.
799. Milne BJ, Caspi A, Harrington H, Poulton R, Rutter M, Moffitt TE. Predictive value of family history on severity of illness: the case for depression, anxiety, alcohol dependence, and drug dependence. Arch Gen Psychiatry. 2009;66:738-47.
800. Moffitt TE, Caspi A, Taylor A, et al. How common are common mental disorders? Evidence that lifetime prevalence rates are doubled by prospective versus retrospective ascertainment. Psychol Med. 2010;40:899-909.
801. Mufson L, Dorta KP, Wickramaratne P, et al. A randomized effectiveness trial of interpersonal psychotherapy for depressed adolescents. Arch Gen Psychiatry. 2004;61:577-84.
802. Mufson L, Weissman MM, Moreau D, Garfinkel R. Efficacy of interpersonal psychotherapy for depressed adolescents. Arch Gen Psychiatry. 1999;56:573-9.
803. Nelson EE, Leibenluft E, McClure EB, Pine DS. The social re-orientation of adolescence: a neuroscience perspective on the process and its relation to psychopathology. Psychol Med. 2005;35:163-74.
804. Pargas RC, Brennan PA, Hammen C, Le Brocque R. Resilience to maternal depression in young adulthood. Dev Psychol. 2010;46:805-14.
805. Parker G, Brotchie H. Gender differences in depression. Int Rev Psychiatry. 2010;22:429-36.
806. Patel V, Araya R, Chatterjee S, et al. Treatment and prevention of mental disorders in low-income and middle-income countries. Lancet. 2007;370:991-1005.
807. Patel V, Fisher AJ, Hetrick S, McGorry P. Mental health of young people: a global public-health challenge. Lancet. 2007;369:1302-13.
808. Patel V, Fisher AJ, Hetrick S, McGorry P. Mental health of young people: a global public-health challenge. Lancet. 2007;369:1302-13.
809. Patton GC, Viner R. Pubertal transitions in health. Lancet. 2007;369:1130-9.
810. Pine DS, Cohen P, Johnson JG, Brook JS. Adolescent life events as predictors of adult depression. J Affect Disord. 2002;68:49-57.
811. Pine DS, Ernst M, Leibenluft E. Imaging-genetics applications in child psychiatry. J Am Acad Child Adolesc Psychiatry. 2010;49:772-82.
812. Pine DS. Developmental psychobiology and response to threats: relevance to trauma in children and adolescents. Biol Psychiatry. 2003;53:796-808.

813. Ramchandani P, Psychogiou L. Paternal psychiatric disorders and children's psychosocial development. Lancet. 2009;374:646-53.
814. Restifo K, Bögels S. Family processes in the development of youth depression: translating the evidence to treatment. Clin Psychol Rev. 2009;29:294-316.
815. Rice F, Harold G, Thapar A. The genetic aetiology of childhood depression: a review. J Child Psychol Psychiatry. 2002;43: 65-79.
816. Rice F, Harold GT, Boivin J, van den Bree M, Hay DF, Thapar A. The links between prenatal stress and off spring development and psychopathology: disentangling environmental and inherited influences. Psychol Med. 2010;40:335-45.
817. Richardson LP, Rockhill C, Russo JE, et al. Evaluation of the PHQ-2 as a brief screen for detecting major depression among adolescents. Pediatrics. 2010;125:e1097-103.
818. Risch N, Herrell R, Lehner T, et al. Interaction between the serotonin transporter gene (5-HTTLPR), stressful life events, and risk of depression: a meta-analysis. JAMA. 2009;301:2462-71.
819. Rosselló J, Bernal G. The efficacy of cognitive-behavioral and interpersonal treatments for depression in Puerto Rican Adolescents. J Consult Clin Psychol. 1999;67:734-45.
820. Rowe R, Rijsdijk FV, Maughan B, Eley TC, Hosang GM, Eley TC. Heterogeneity in antisocial behaviours and comorbidity with depressed mood: a behavioural genetic approach. J Child Psychol Psychiatry. 2008;49:526-34.
821. Rueter MA, Scaramella L, Wallace LE, Conger RD. First onset of depressive or anxiety disorders predicted by the longitudinal course of internalizing symptoms and parent-adolescent disagreements. Arch Gen Psychiatry. 1999;56:726-32.
822. Rutter M, Thapar A, Pickles A. Gene-environment interactions. Biologically valid pathway or artifact? Arch Gen Psychiatry. 2009;66:1287-9.
823. Saxena S, Maulik PK, Sharan P, Levav I, Saraceno B. Brief report – mental health research on low- and middle-income countries in indexed journals: a preliminary assessment. J Ment Health Policy Econ. 2004;7:127-31.
824. Shansky RM, Glavis-Bloom C, Lerman D, et al. Estrogen mediates sex differences in stress-induced prefrontal cortex dysfunction. Mol Psychiatry. 2004;9:531-8.
825. Sharan P, Gallo C, Gureje O, et al. World Health Organization-Global Forum for Health Research—Mental Health Research Mapping Project Group. Mental health research priorities in low- and middle-income countries of Africa, Asia, Latin America and the Caribbean. Br J Psychiatry. 2009;195: 354-63.
826. Shi J, Potash JB, Knowles JA, et al. Genome-wide association study of recurrent early-onset major depressive disorder. Mol Psychiatry. 2011;16:193-201.
827. Shyn SI, Shi J, Kraft JB, et al. Novel loci for major depression identified by genome-wide association study of sequenced treatment alternatives to relieve depression and meta-analysis of three studies. Mol Psychiatry. 2011;16:202-15.
828. Silberg J, Pickles A, Rutter M, et al. The influence of genetic factors and life stress on depression among adolescent girls. Arch Gen Psychiatry. 1999;56:225-32.
829. Silberg J, Rutter M, Neale M, Eaves L. Genetic moderation of environmental risk for depression and anxiety in adolescent girls. Br J Psychiatry. 2001;179:116-21.
830. Silk JS, Vanderbilt-Adriance E, Shaw DS, et al. Resilience among children and adolescents at risk for depression: mediation and moderation across social and neurobiological contexts. Dev Psychopathol. 2007;19:841-65.
831. Soares CN, Zitek B. Reproductive hormone sensitivity and risk for depression across the female life cycle: a continuum of vulnerability? J Psychiatry Neurosci. 2008;33:331-43.
832. Steinberg L, Dahl R, Keating D, Kupfer D, Masten A, Pine D. The study of developmental psychopathology in adolescence: integrating affective neuroscience with the study of context. In: Cicchetti D, Cohen D (Eds). Handbook of Developmental psychopathology. Vol. 2. New York: Wiley; 2006. pp. 710-41.
833. Stice E, Shaw H, Bohon C, Marti CN, Rohde P. A meta-analytic review of depression prevention programs for children and adolescents: factors that predict magnitude of intervention effects. Consult Clin Psychol. 2009;77:486-503.
834. Thapar A, Collishaw S, Potter R, Thapar AK. Managing and preventing depression in adolescents. BMJ. 2010;340:c209.
835. Thapar A, McGuffin P. A twin study of depressive symptoms in childhood. Br J Psychiatry. 1994;165:259-65.
836. Thapar A, Rice F. Twin studies in pediatric depression. Child Adolesc Psychiatr Clin North Am. 2006;15:869-81.
837. Todd RD, Neuman R, Geller B, Fox LW, Hickok J. Genetic studies of affective disorders: should we be starting with childhood onset probands? J Am Acad Child Adolesc Psychiatry. 1993;32:1164-71.
838. Tully EC, Iacono WG, McGue M. An adoption study of parental depression as an environmental liability for adolescent depression and childhood disruptive disorders. Am J Psychiatry. 2008;165:1148-54.
839. Uher R, McGuffin P. The moderation by the serotonin transporter gene of environmental adversity in the etiology of depression: 2009 update. Mol Psychiatry. 2010;15:18-22.
840. van Noorden MS, Giltay EJ, den Hollander-Gijsman ME, van der Wee NJ, van Veen T, Zitman FG. Gender differences in clinical characteristics in a naturalistic sample of depressive outpatients: the Leiden routine outcome monitoring study. J Affect Disord. 2010;125:116-23.
841. Verhulst FC, Ven der Ende V. Using rating scales in a clinical context. In: Rutter M, Bishop D, Pine D, et al. (Eds). Rutter's child and adolescent psychiatry. 5. Oxford: Blackwell; 2008. pp. 289-98.
842. Weissman MM, Pilowsky DJ, Wickramaratne PJ, et al. STAR*D-Child Team. Remissions in maternal depression and child psychopathology: a STAR*D-child report. JAMA. 2006;295:1389-98.
843. Weisz JR, McCarty CA, Valeri SM. Effects of psychotherapy for depression in children and adolescents: a meta-analysis. Psychol Bull. 2006;132:132-49.

844. WHO. mhGAP intervention guide for mental, neurological and substance use disorders in nonspecialized health settings: mental health Gap Action Programme (mhGAP). Geneva: World Health Organisation; 2010.
845. Windfuhr K, While D, Hunt I, et al. National confidential inquiry into suicide and homicide by people with mental illness. Suicide in juveniles and adolescents in the United Kingdom. J Child Psychol Psychiatry. 2008;49:1155-65.
846. Young JF, Mufson L, Davies M. Impact of comorbid anxiety in an effectiveness study of interpersonal psychotherapy for depressed adolescents. J Am Acad Child Adolesc Psychiatry. 2006;45:904-12.
847. Zuckerbrot RA, Cheung AH, Jensen PS, Stein RE, Laraque D. GLAD-PC Steering Group. Guidelines for adolescent depression in primary care (GLAD-PC): I. Identification, assessment, and initial management. Pediatrics. 2007;120:e1299-312.

CHAPTER 44

Basic Sciences

Sheela Jain, Uma Joshi, Aparna Garg, Sunila Chadda, AP Dadhich, LN Gupta, Pramodh Bhardhwaj, VS Randhawa, Geeta Mehta, GN Saxena

44.1 NEUROANATOMY

Sheela Jain

The human nervous system is the most complex, widely investigated and yet poorly understood physical system known to mankind. The organism has an ability to interact continually with a fluctuating environment without any loss of structural integrity. Basic to the interpretation of any behavior of man, from the simple knee jerk to the creation of a poem or splitting of the atom, lies the knowledge of the form and function of the nervous system. There is no guarantee of course that an understanding of anatomy and physiology will allow one to turn out a work of art or an invention. For that matter, such knowledge does not assure complete understanding of even less abstract functions.

ORGANIZATION

Nervous tissue is a special excitable tissue which is composed of (a) receptors cells, specialized to react to stimuli, (b) synapses, (c) neurons for the conduction of stimuli, and (d) effectors for responses.

Receptor Cells

These are present within the epithelial layers clothing the body's surfaces, with in the walls of blood vessels and solid and hollow viscera, and in muscles, tendons and ligaments. Plasma membrane of these cells is specialized to respond selectively to changes in the internal or external environment of the body.

Synapses (Synaptic Contacts)

These are the places where excitable cells (receptors, neurons, effectors) communicate with each other. There are two main types of synapses in the body: (1) electrical synapses identical with nerves; (2) chemical synapses characterized by release of neurotransmitter substances by one cell which alter the permeability of another cell for certain ions and thus alter their electric state (Fig. 1).

Neurons

These are the excitable cells and are specialized for reception, integration, transformation and transmission of coded information. In vertebrates, the neurons consist of a cell body, or soma, a specialized cytoplasm with a diploid nucleus and an excitable membrane. From the soma, one or more branching cytoplasmic processes enclosed in excitable membrane project and are called neurites. Depending upon the number of processes, the neurons are classified as pseudounipolar, unipolar, bipolar and multipolar neurons. Majority of the neurons in the human brain are considered to be multipolar. The neurites conducting toward soma are the dendrites. The axon, a single process that arises from a specialized portion of the cell body (the axon hillock), conveys information to other neurons.

In addition to neurons, the brain also contains several types of glial cells, which play several important roles in the nervous system. The oligodendrocytes and Schwann cells, found in the central and peripheral nervous system respectively, are concerned with the myelination. The myelin sheath facilitates the conduction of action potentials along the axons. Astrocytes serve a number of functions, including

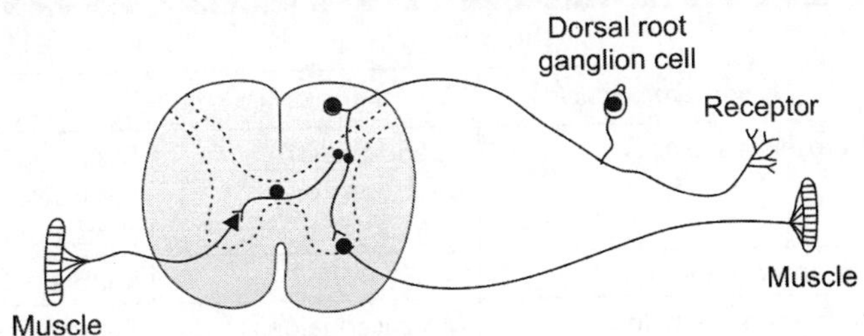

Fig. 1: Synaptic contact

participation in the formation of the blood-brain barrier, removal of neurotransmitters from the synaptic cleft, etc. The microglia are actually derived from macrophages and function as scavengers, eliminating the debris resulting from neuronal death and injury.

EMBRYOLOGY

During early differentiation, a thickened plate of ectoderm, neural plate, develops along the mid dorsal line of the embryo and is transformed by invagination into a neural tube. The neural tube detaches from the overlying ectoderm and thickens to develop into the spinal cord and brain. The rostral end of the neural tube, which ultimately forms the brain, differentiates into three primary brain vesicles (Table 1): (1) The prosencephalon or forebrain, which lies closest to the rostrum; (2) the mesencephalon or midbrain, which lies behind the prosencephalon; and (3) the rhombencephalon or hindbrain, which lies most caudally (Fig. 2).

Spinal Cord

The spinal cord averages 16" to 18" (40–45 cm) in length. It is nearly oval in cross-section, with the longer diameter in the transverse plane. The diameter is not uniform throughout its length. There are cervical and lumbar enlargements to accommodate the nerve supply to the upper and lower extremities. Caudal to the lumbar enlargement, the cord diminishes rapidly, having a cone shaped termination, called the conus medullaris, from the apex of which extends the filum terminale, which descends to be attached to the coccyx.

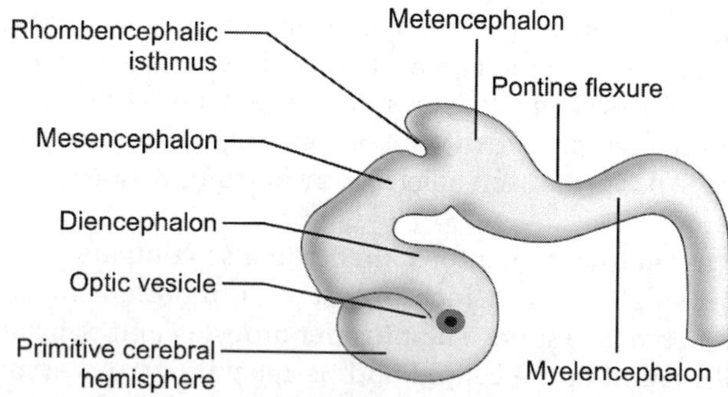

Fig. 2: Brain vesicles

The cord is divided into areas by several longitudinal grooves. A midline, ventral median fissure and a dorsal median septum, divide the cord into symmetrical halves. Each half of the cord is divided into columns called funiculi, by ventral-lateral, dorsal-lateral and dorsal-intermediate sulci. The cord is considered to be a segmental structure, since it gives rise to 31 pairs of nerves.

The spinal cord is enclosed in three membranes or meninges; these are, from without inwards, the dura, arachnoid and pia maters, which are separated from each other by subdural and subarachnoid spaces; the former being merely a potential space, the later being occupied by the cerebrospinal fluid (CSF).

Internal Structure

The cord is composed of two fundamentally different materials. The more peripheral part appears glistening white because of the fatty myelin sheaths covering the longitudinally running fibers contained in the areas. This region is called the white matter and is arranged as anterior, lateral and posterior funiculi; specific ascending and descending tracts run in each funiculus (Fig. 3). The ratio of white matter to gray matter varies from level to level in the cord, the actual amount of white matter being greatest in the cervical region.

Internal to the white matter lies an H-shaped mass of gray matter which appears less white, since it contains fine, non-myelinated fibers, together with all the neuronal cell bodies of the spinal cord. The gray matter, such as the white, extends through the length of the cord as columns. The posterior gray column consists of three parts, namely apex, caput and cervix. At the apex, the gray matter is of different consistency and is known as substantia gelatinosa. Just lateral to the cervix of the posterior column is an area of mixed white and gray. This is the reticular substance of the cord. The anterior columns are shorter and broader than the posterior, directed toward but not approaching the ventral lateral sulcus. The central canal exists throughout the spinal cord and also extends into the caudal half of the medulla oblongata, opening out above this into fourth ventricle. In the caudal part of the conus medullaris, it expands into a fusiform terminal ventricle. During life, it contains CSF and is lined by a columnar, ciliated epithelium, the ependyma.

Table 1: Fate of different parts of the neural tube and its cavities

Neural tube		*Adult brain component*	*Cavity*
Primary brain vesicle	*Secondary brain vesicle*		
Prosencephalon	Telencephalon Diencephalon	Right and left cerebral hemispheres, corpus striatum, thalamus, hypothalamus and associated parts, optic stalk, pars-nervosa of pituitary gland	Lateral ventricles
Mesencephalon	—	Midbrain	Cerebral aqueduct
Rhombencephalon	Metencephalon Myelencephalon	Pons and cerebellum Medulla oblongata, spinal cord	IV ventricle central canal

The various important tracts of spinal cord are depicted in Table 2.

THE PERIPHERAL NERVOUS SYSTEM

The peripheral nervous system comprises the *afferent*, or *centripetal*, fibers which connect the sensory end organs to the central nervous system, and the *efferent*, or *centrifugal*, fibers which connect the central nervous system to the affector apparatus. It includes the twelve pairs of cranial nerves, which arise from the spinal cord. The sympathetic trunks, with their various ganglia, also belong to this system.

THE CEREBROSPINAL NERVES

Spinal Nerves

The spinal nerves consist of numerous nerve fibers collected into bundles, which are enclosed in connective tissue sheaths. A small bundle of fibers is called fasciculus. Each fasciculus is surrounded by a connective tissue sheath, named the perineurium. Individual nerve fibers are ensheathed within the fasciculus by delicate connective tissue called the endoneurium. Fasciculi of large nerves are held together and invested by connective tissue, known as epineurium.

Out of 31 pairs of spinal nerves, there are 8 cervical, 12 thoracic, 5 lumbar, 5 sacral and 1 coccygeal. They emerge through the intervertebral foramina. Each nerve is connected with the spinal cord by ventral and dorsal roots, the latter being characterized by the presence of a spinal ganglion. Immediately beyond the spinal ganglia, the ventral and dorsal nerve roots unite to form the spinal nerve, which emerges through the intervertebral foramen, gives off recurrent meningeal branches, and then divides into a dorsal and a ventral branch, and then divides into a dorsal and a ventral ramus. At, or immediately distal to, its origin, the ventral ramus of each spinal nerve is joined by a gray ramus communicans

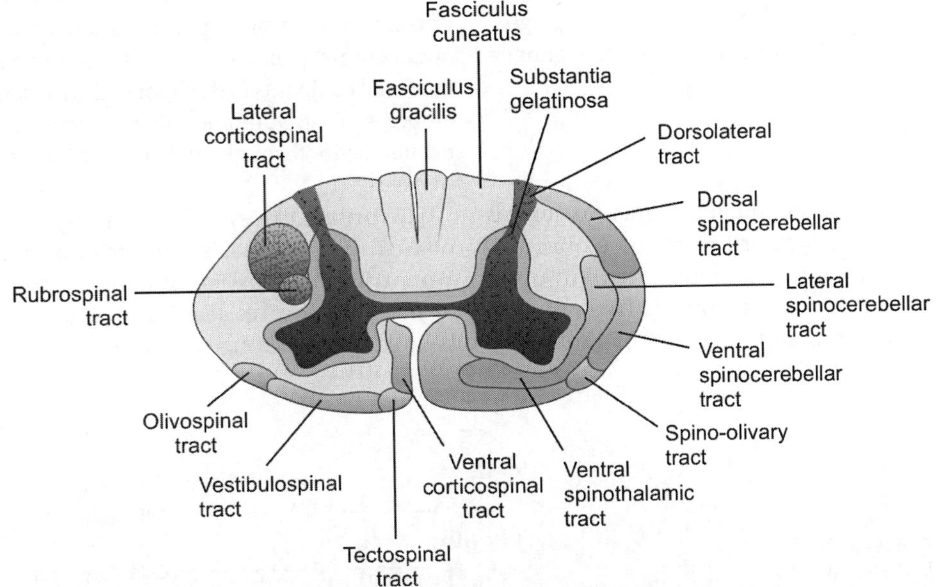

Fig. 3: Internal structure of neural tube

Table 2: Important tracts of spinal cord

Anterior column	*Lateral column*	*Posterior column*
Ascending tracts		
Ventral spinothalamic (light touch)	Dorsal and ventral spinocerebellar (reflex proprioception); lateralspinothalamic (pain and temperature); spinotectal (reflex visual); spino-olivary (reflex proprioception)	Fasciculus gracilis and fasciculus cuneatus (vibration, passive motion, joint, and two point discrimination)
Descending tracts		
Ventricle corticospinal (voluntary motion)	Lateral corticospinal (voluntary motion)	Fasciculus interfascicularis and septo-marginal
Vestibulospinal (balance reflex)	Rubrospinal (muscle tone and synergy)	Fasciculus (association and integration)
Tectospinal (audiovisual reflex) Reticulospinal (muscle tone)	Olivospinal (reflex)	

from the corresponding ganglion of the sympathetic trunk, while the ventral rami of thoracic and first and second lumbar nerves each contribute a white ramus communicans joining the corresponding sympathetic ganglion.

Cranial Nerves

The cranial nerves are customarily described as comprising of 12 pairs, which are referred to by numbers. Nerve I (olfactory) and II (optic) are not true nerves but fiber tracts of brain. Except for a part of nerve XI (accessory), which is derived from the upper cervical segments of the spinal cord, the caudal ten pairs emerge from the brainstem, in which lie their nuclei of origin.

The superficial origin of a cranial nerve is that area of the brain where the nerve appears or attaches (Fig. 4). Those cranial nerves, which have motor function, take their origin from collection of cells deep within the brainstem (motor nuclei), which are analogous to the anterior horn cells of the spinal cord. The sensory cranial nerves originate from collections of cells outside the brainstem, usually in ganglia, which may be considered analogous to the dorsal root ganglia of the cranial nerve.

Cranial Nerve I (Olfactory)

This term commonly refers to the olfactory tract on ventral portion of the frontal lobe, which arises from the olfactory bulb and continues posteriorly to end just lateral to optic chiasma, where it penetrates the cerebrum. This nerve is concerned with the olfaction, and disorders of smell may be caused by the lesions of nasal cavity, fracture of anterior cranial fossa, tumors of pituitary region and meningitis, etc.

Cranial Nerve II (Optic)

It contains nerve fibers arising from the inner layers of the retina, which proceed posteriorly, some crossing to opposite side, via the optic chiasma, to enter cranial cavity through optic foramen. Lesions of visual apparatus may manifest as retrobulbar neuritis, optic neuritis, papilledema and optic atrophy, leading to various visual defects.

Cranial Nerves III, IV and VI (Oculomotor, Trochlear, Abducens)

These are motor fiber going to muscles of eye, including levator palpebrae superioris. The motor nuclei of oculomotor and trochlear nerves lie in the mesencephalon, at the level of superior and inferior colliculi, respectively. The former emerges ventral to the crus cerebri, whereas later emerges dorsally through the superior medullary velum. Nucleus of the abducens nerve is situated in the substance of the pons, deep to the facial colliculus in the floor of the rhomboid fossa. The nerve emerges at the pontomedullary junction. The nerves enter the orbital cavity through superior orbital fissure and supply the muscles.

Disorders like syphilis, meningitis, encephalitis, cavernous sinus thrombosis, tumors of orbit and brain, cerebral hemorrhage, aneurysm of internal carotid artery, etc. may involve these nerves, leading to squint, diplopia, tilting of the head, nystagmus, ptosis, dizziness, etc.

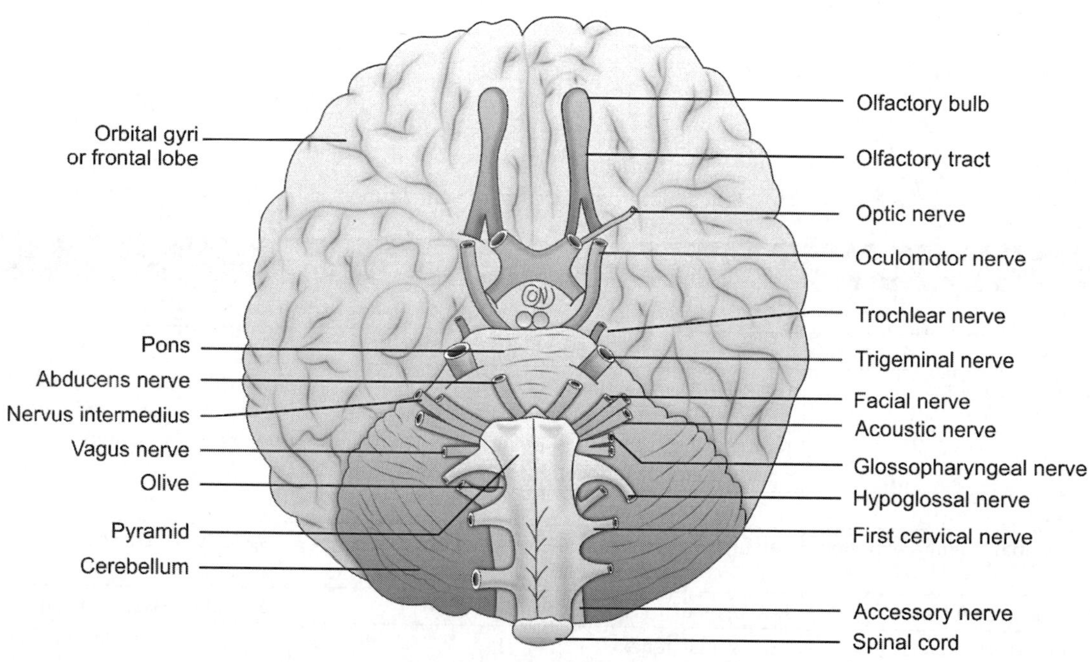

Fig. 4: Cranial nerves

Cranial Nerve V (Trigeminal)

It contains a large sensory root and a smaller motor root. The sensory or main portion arises from the cells in the large Gasserian ganglion, and penetrates the middle cerebellar peduncle to enter the pons. The peripheral fibers form (1) ophthalmic, (2) maxillary, and (3) mandibular divisions, which supply the skin of face, eye, teeth, paranasal sinuses and nasal cavity, etc. The motor fibers supply muscles of mastication.

Disorders like neuralgia, neuritis, tuberculosis, pontine diseases, cavernous sinus thrombosis, etc. may affect functioning of the nerve.

Cranial Nerve VI (Facial)

It is a mixed nerve. The motor fibers arise from the nucleus in substance of pons and supply muscles of face, including stapedius. The secretomotor activity of submandibular and sublingual glands is controlled by the superior salivatory nucleus. The nervus intermedius forms its sensory component and carries sensation of taste from anterior two-thirds of tongue.

Bell's palsy may be caused by chilling of face, middle ear infection, meningitis, tumors and fractures of skull, etc.

Cranial Nerve VIII (Acoustic)

It consists of two separate parts: cochlear (for hearing) and vestibular (for equilibrium).

Disorders like otitis media, infections and degenerative diseases, brain tumors, affect the functioning of VIII nerve. Sea sickness due to continuous movement of endolymph is characterized by vertigo, disturbance in equilibrium, nausea and vomiting.

Cranial Nerve IX (Glossopharyngeal)

It leaves the skull via the jugular foramen. Motor fibers arise from nucleus ambiguus, and pass to stylopharyngeus muscle. Parasympathetic fibers from the inferior salivatory nucleus pass via the Jacobson's nerve and supply the parotid gland. The sensory fibers arise from unipolar cells in petrous and jugular ganglia. Centrally, they terminate in the nucleus of tractus solitarius, while peripherally they supply general sensation to the pharynx, soft palate, tongue, auditory tube, tympanic cavity, and carotid body and carotid sinus.

Cranial Nerve X (Vagus)

The nerve contains afferent fibers, which originate in cells in jugular and nodose ganglia, and pass through the jugular foramen, to enter the medulla just behind the glossopharyngeal nerve. Motor fibers leave the medulla to join the sensory part of the nerve. Motor fibers supply muscles of pharynx, soft palate and larynx. Parasympathetic fibers control the activity of thoracic and abdominal viscera. The sensory fibers carry sensations from pharynx, larynx, thoracic and abdominal viscera.

Lesions of vagus nerve cause hoarseness of voice, cardiac arrhythmias, laryngeal paralysis, aphonia, dyspnea, etc.

Cranial Nerve XI (Accessory)

Two separate branches of the XI cranial nerve leave the skull together through the jugular foramen. The cranial fibers arise from the nucleus ambiguus and supply the intrinsic muscles of larynx, joining the vagus outside the skull. The spinal fibers arise from the upper five or six cervical cord segments, and supply part of the trapezius and sternocleidomastoid muscles.

Cranial Nerve XII (Hypoglossal)

This nerve is purely motor in distribution. The fibers arise from the hypoglossal nucleus in the substance of the medulla and supply the lingual musculature.

THE CEREBELLUM (LITTLE BRAIN)

The cerebellum, located in the posterior fossa of the skull behind the pons and medulla, is separated from the overlying cerebrum by an expansion of dura mater, the tentorium cerebelli. The surface of cerebellum contains many sulci and furrows, giving it a laminated appearance, which is accentuated by several deep fissures that divide the cerebellum into several lobes (Fig. 5). The cerebellum is composed of a small unpaired median portion, the vermis, and two large lateral masses, called the cerebellar hemispheres. The flocculonodular lobe includes the nodules of posterior vermis and flocculi, and is referred to as archicerebellum. The posterior part is considered as neopallium and paleopallium.

The white matter of the cerebellum contains three pairs of major projection bundles, the cerebellar peduncles. The superior cerebellar peduncle connects the cerebellum with mesencephalon and contains dentatorubral fibers, ventral spinocerebellar tract and uncinate fasciculus.

The middle cerebellar peduncle (brachium pontis) is the largest of the cerebellar peduncles. Fibers arise from the nucleus pontis. The inferior cerebellar peduncle (restiform body) arises from the upper lateral part of the medulla, ascends laterally and enters in the cerebellum. It carries dorsal spinocerebellar tract, external arcuate fibers, and fibers connecting olivary complex, reticular nuclei, vestibular nuclei and trigeminal nucleus with cerebellum.

CEREBELLAR FUNCTIONS AND DYSFUNCTIONS

The cerebellum is mainly a reflex center and exerts ipsilateral influence. In essence, the cerebellum receives an informational input from the cutaneous receptors,

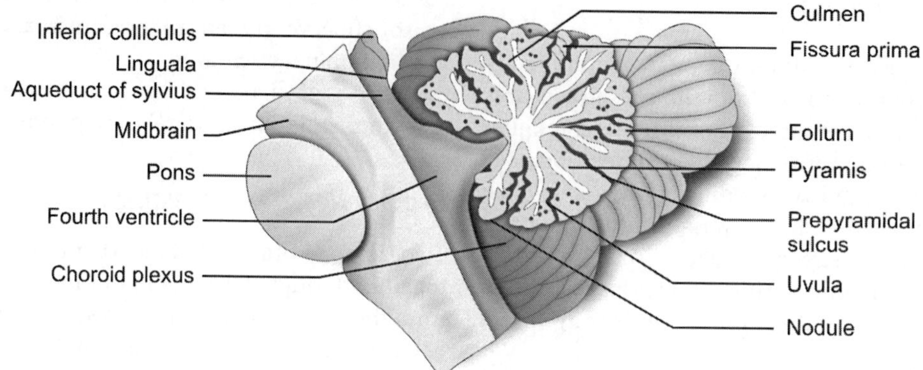

Fig. 5: Cerebellum

proprioceptors, eyes, ears, brainstem, reticular formation and cerebral cortex, which is integrated and then discharged to the motor controlling centers of the cerebrum and brainstem. Its normal functioning is necessary for smooth, coordinated, and effective locomotor responses to occur.

Functions

1. Maintenance of equilibrium (flocculonodular lobe).
2. Coordination of muscular activity, especially that of the extremities (neocerebellum).
3. Maintenance of muscle tone (neocerebellum).
4. Influence upon the extrinsic muscles of eye through cerebellovestibular connections.
5. Speech coordination.

Dysfunctions

Extensive injuries to cerebellum do not cause loss of sensory perception. Tumors of flocculonodular lobe, which occur not infrequently in children, cause disturbances of equilibrium. Disequilibrium in man is manifested by a tendency to fall backwards or laterally when standing, and by an unsteady staggering gait; it may be accompanied by sensation of spinning, nausea, etc. Paleocerebellar syndrome due to compression of anterior lobe of the cerebellum, or invasion of pineal body or other supratentorial tumors, is characterized by the exaggeration of the extensor tone of the limbs. Ataxia and dysmetria manifest in the presence of lesions of the neocerebellum. Increased tremors are indications of damage to the cerebellar nuclei. Hypotonia is also one of the manifestations of neocerebellar lesions. Cerebellar nystagmus presents as an inability to fix at an object with the eyes, resulting in repetitive conjugate drift of the visual axes away from the object, followed by a rapid return.

THE BRAINSTEM AND RETICULAR FORMATION

Brainstem is an important functional part of the nervous system. All its constituent parts (pons, medulla oblongata and midbrain) have a well-developed reticular formation. The reticular system functions by the connections of these parts of neural axis. The term reticular formation is applied to the network of gray and white matters in the medulla and in the tegmental areas of pons and midbrain.

General Characteristics

1. Reticular nuclei are deeply placed and have diffuse connections.
2. The conducting paths are polysynaptic.
3. They have ascending and descending components, and
4. They consist of somatic and visceral components.

Functional Associations of Reticular Formation

The reticular formation receives convergent information channels from all the principal parts of nervous system and in turn, it projects directly or indirectly back to all these regions, modulating their activities through complex and ill-understood mechanisms that involve synaptic neurotransmission, and local neuroparacrine as well as neuroendocrine effects.

Somatomotor and Sensory Control

Reticular formation forms a part of the complex of subregions of the nervous system, exerting controlling influences on activity pattern of skeletal muscles, ranging from relatively simple reflex loops, coarse to fine postural readjustments and positioning, to complicated patterns associated with intergroup and interpersonal communication and emotional expressions.

All the subregions of the nervous system, involved in the processing of somatosensory information, are subject to influences from reticular formation. Thus, the spinal and brainstem terminals of primary afferent fibers, their nuclear destinations and attendant interneurons, and the dendrites and somata of neurons projecting long axons to supraspinal centers, are all subject to reticular control.

Visceromotor Control

Cardiovascular readjustments and the activity of non-striated muscle and many glandular cells in the thoracoabdominal viscera are, of course, in most cases under the control of postganglionic autonomic neurons. Their preganglionic neuronal soma and dendrites are, either directly or through intermediary of local interneurons, partially controlled by reticulobulbar and descending reticulospinal fibers. Forebrain control of autonomic activities involves areas of orbitofrontal, cingulate, entorhinal cortices, the major limbic structures, medial and anterior groups of dorsal thalamic nuclei, and hypothalamic nuclei with destinations in reticular formation.

Neuroendocrine Control

Through the complex of ascending bundles accompanying the central and dorsal tegmental fasciculi, cholinergic and all varieties of monoaminergic fibers pass in side channels to reach and terminate in most, if not all, hypothalamic nuclei. Either directly, through the intermediary or other hypothalamic nuclei, or via the dopaminergic infundibular cells, the reticular neurons are one source of modification of the synthesis.

Biological Rhythms

A time base is imposed on all living systems by the intrinsic turnover rates of biological macromolecules, including the genetic apparatus of the cell, annual seasonal variations and daily environmental fluctuations.

States of Awareness

Awareness of environment and self is maintained by the reticular system. In man, lesions of brainstem may produce disturbances, ranging from fleeting unconsciousness to hypersomnia.

Sleep, Arousal and Perception

Two principal forms of sleep are recognized: deep or slow wave sleep (SWS) and rapid eye movements (REM) sleep. Arousal and awakening is accompanied in intact animals by a rapid, low amplitude, desynchronized waveform. An ascending activating reticular system, with a widespread bilateral radiation to most regions of the neocortex and limbic system, and desynchronization is necessary for wakefulness, attention and effective perception.

DIENCEPHALON

The diencephalon is almost completely hidden when the hemispheres are in place. Several parts are described, namely epithalamus, subthalamus, metathalamus, thalamus and hypothalamus.

Epithalamus

The epithalamus consists of the pineal body (epiphysis), habenular trigone, stria medullaris and habenular commissure. The epithalamus is continuous caudally with the pretectum of the mesencephalon.

Subthalamus

This is a transition zone between thalamus and tegmental portion of the mesencephalon. Both the red nucleus and the substantia nigra of the mesencephalon, protrude into the caudal portion of the subthalamus. Lateral to it, is the region where the internal capsule joins the cerebral peduncle. The hypothalamus lies medially and rostrally.

Metathalamus

Metathalamus is constituted by the medial and lateral geniculate bodies. Medial geniculate body is located dorsal to the lateral limit of the basis pedunculi, at the level of superior colliculus. It receives auditory impulses from the inferior colliculus nucleus, by way of brachium and projects upon the auditory cortex, on the superior aspect of the temporal lobe of the cerebrum, through the sublentiform fibers of the internal capsule.

The lateral geniculate body lies lateral and slightly more rostral. Dorsolaterally, it adjoins the lateral parts of the pulvinar. It serves as a thalamic relay between the retina and the visual area of the cerebral cortex. Optic tracts terminate in the lateral geniculate bodies and in the geniculocalcarine tract, arising from them. Various retinal areas have specific representation in the lateral geniculate body and there is a point-to-point relationship between it and the visual cortex.

Thalamus

External Morphology

This is the largest portion of the diencephalon and consists of two ovoid masses of gray matter. It is bounded ventrally by the hypothalamic sulcus; its caudal limit is at the level of posterior commissure and cerebral aqueduct; its rostral limit is at the interventricular foramen; and dorsally it is related to the stria medullaris and the roof of the third ventricle.

The lateral surface is intimately applied to the posterior limb of the internal capsule. The dorsal surface is free and slightly convex. The posterior part of thalamus overlaps the rostral mesencephalon. The stria and vena terminalis lie in a groove, which separates the lateral edge of the dorsal surface from the caudate nucleus. Medially, the dorsal surface is separated from the medial surface by the tenia thalami, the edge of the ependymal roof of the third ventricle. The caudal expanded part forms the pulvinar. The ventral surface adjoins the subthalamus; caudally it is continuous with the tegmental region of the mesencephalon, through which most ascending fibers enter the thalamus.

Internal Morphology

The thalamus is divided into a number of nuclear groups. The dorsal surface of thalamus has a thin covering of fibers, called the stratum zonale. Along the lateral surface is the external medullary lamina. Along the medial surface, beneath the ependymal lining of the third ventricle, is a homogeneous zone of gray substance called, the central gray. The stratum zonale sends fibers ventrally into the substance of the thalamus, following the internal medullary lamina. Rostrally, in the region of the anterior tubercle, the internal lamina splits, partially separating the anterior thalamus from the medial and lateral.

Thalamic Nuclei and Connections

The medial portion of the thalamus consists of dorsomedial and anterior nuclei. The dorsomedial group consists of the dorsomedial, submedial and habenulopeduncular tract nuclei. The lateral portion is divided into a dorsal and ventral tier of nuclei. The dorsal portion of the lateral nucleus consists of dorsolateral, posterolateral and pulvinar nuclei, from front to back. The ventral portion of the lateral thalamic mass consists of the anterior ventral, lateral ventral and posterior ventral nuclei (Fig. 6). In addition, there are two other scattered sets of nuclei, namely nuclei of the midline, and nuclei scattered in the internal medullary lamina.

Posteromedial ventral nucleus receives afferents from the trigeminothalamic tract. The efferents pass through the posterior limb of the internal capsule to areas 1, 2, and 3 of the postcentral gyrus. The posterolateral ventral nucleus receives ventral spinothalamic tracts and medial lemniscus. The efferents pass through the posterior limb of the internal capsule to areas 1, 2 and 3 of the postcentral gyrus. Afferents for the anterior ventral nucleus arise from the globuspallidus, via the fasciculus lenticularis and thalamic fasciculus. The efferent pass through the internal capsule to the frontal cortex. The lateral ventral nucleus receives afferents, chiefly from dentatothalamic fibers from the cerebellum. The efferents travel through the posterior limb of the internal capsule to motor area and to the premotor cortex, area 6. The anterior nucleus receives fibers of the mamilothalamic tract. The efferents have a wide distribution to areas 32, 23, 24 and 29. Dorsomedial and submedial nuclei receive afferents from prefrontal cortex, hypothalamus, the midline, lateral and ventral posterior thalamic nuclei, putamen and pretectal region. The efferents are also widely distributed to the hypothalamus, pretectal zone, anterior nucleus of the thalamus, striatum and the frontal lobe cortex.

Lateral dorsal and lateral posterior nuclei form the more rostral part of the dorsal tier of the lateral thalamic mass. Their afferents come from the other thalamic nuclei. The efferents are all thought to end in the parietal lobe, except the post-central gyrus. The nuclei of the midline receive terminals and many collaterals from the spinothalamic tracts, the trigeminothalamic tracts and the medial lemniscus. The efferents are distributed to the hypothalamus, basal ganglia, and medial and lateral thalamic areas.

Hypothalamus

The hypothalamus is the highest integration center for the autonomic nervous system. This region lies ventral to the hypothalamic sulcus. It consists of several parts, including the lamina terminalis, tubercinereum and mamillary bodies. The medial portion of the hypothalamus, is predominantly cellular, containing many nuclear groups. Among the most definite of these groups are the preoptic, supraoptic, paraventricular, ventromedial, dorsomedial and mamillary nuclei (Fig. 7). The lateral portion of hypothalamus contains scattered nerve cells and many longitudinally running myelinated fibers. The hypothalamus may also be subdivided transversely into a supraoptic area overlying the chiasma, a tubercle or central portion (containing the median eminence and the infundibulum), and the posterior mamillary region containing the mamillary bodies.

Afferent Connections

The afferent fibers originate from the cerebral cortex, basal ganglia and thalamus. Corticohypothalamic fibers arise from the frontal and parietal areas. Other fibers, originating in the olfactory centers, course to the hypothalamus by way of medial forebrain bundle, striaterminalis and fornix. Pallidohypothalamic tract ends in the ventromedial group of hypothalamic nuclei. Some fibers also reach the hypothalamus through ansa lenticularis.

The extralemniscal afferent system through the medial part of the brainstem reticular formation also appears to be the afferent connections to the hypothalamus.

Efferent Pathways

- Medial and lateral bundles of the descending fibers together constitute the medial forebrain bundle. Medial fibers descend close to the wall of the III ventricle and form the dorsal longitudinal fasciculus, which lies lateral to the cerebral aqueduct in the mid-brain. Lateral fibers descend through the lateral hypothalamic area and reach the midbrain by passing dorsolateral to the mammillary body.
- Mamillothalamic tract originates in the mammillary nuclei and ends in the anterior part of the thalamus, which further projects mainly to areas 23 and 24 of the cingulate gyrus. Electrical stimulation of area 24 elicits autonomic responses, which include changes in blood pressure, heart rate and respiration.
- Mamilotegmental tract enters in the tegmentum of the midbrain and through its connections with the cells of

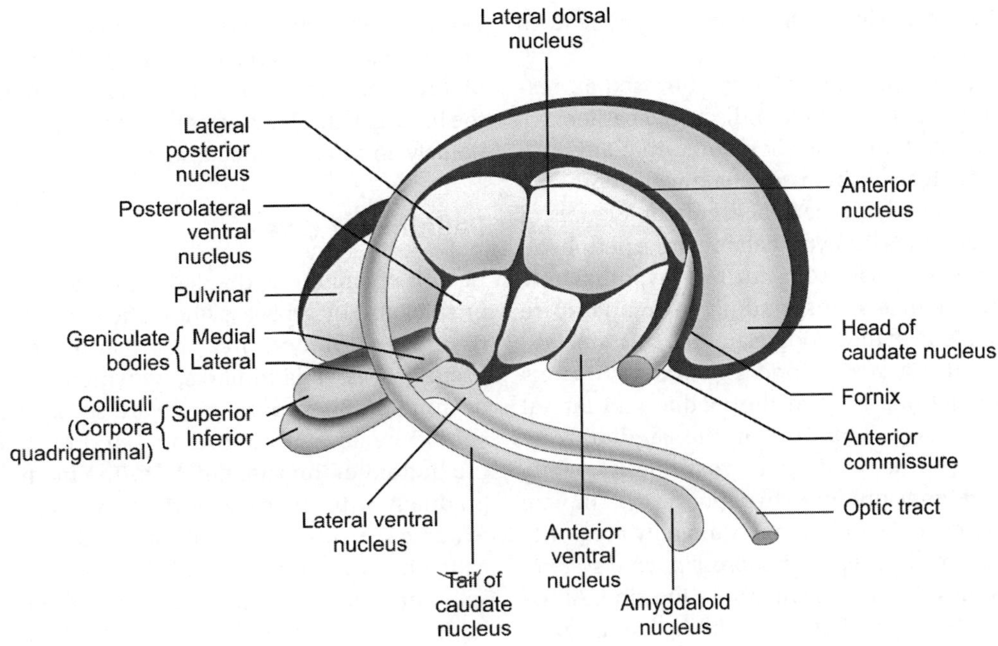

Fig. 6: Thalamus

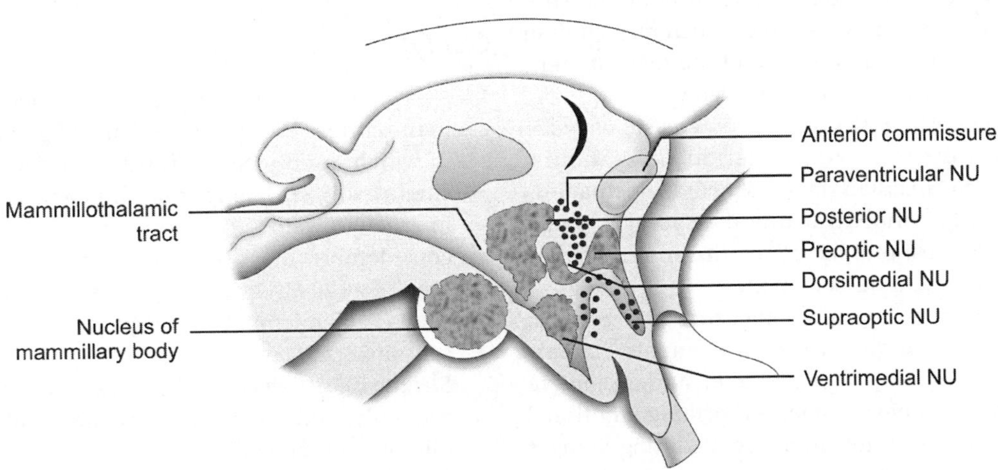

Fig. 7: Hypothalamus

origin of reticulospinal and other descending pathways. It provides a direct projection pathway from the hippocampus and hypothalamus to lower centers.

- Hypothalamo-hypophyseal tract; fibers of this tract originate in the supraoptic nucleus, course downwards through the median eminence and infundibulum, and are distributed to all parts of the neurohypophysis. Fibers from paraventricular nucleus and tuber cinereum also reach the neurohypophysis.

Hypothalamic Functions

Hypothalamus can be quoted as the 'head ganglion' of the autonomic nervous system, as it has important centers controlling it. The parasympathetic centers are situated in anterior and tuberal parts, while the sympathetic centers are situated posteriorly. These centers are under the inhibitory influence of frontal cortex, particularly the region above and around the rostrum of the corpus callosum. When this inhibitory influence is abolished, the animal exhibits 'sham rage' or the outbursts of rage. The other functions of hypothalamus are discussed below.

- Endocrine control is by influencing the activity of anterior pituitary, which releases the inhibitory factors. Some of these affect the target organ directly or through a second endocrine organ.
- Neurosecretion of oxytocin and vasopressin (ADH) is directly into the blood in the infundibulum and

hypophysial posterior lobe. Disturbances may lead to diabetes insipidus.

- The general autonomic effects on cardiovascular, respiratory and alimentary systems, as discussed earlier.
- Temperature regulation: In all homeothermic animals, production and loss of heat are balanced, with the hypothalamus providing a central regulator. Signals of body temperature reach the hypothalamus from peripheral thermodetectors and also from intrinsic hypothalamic themodetector neurons, responding to temperature changes in the blood of the hypothalamic circulation.
- Regulation of the intake of food and water: Regions with opposing actions exist in the medial and lateral hypothalamic zones. Ablation of the medial zone promotes hyperphagia, leading to gross obesity, while ablation of lateral zone promotes hypophagia or complete aphagia. Water balance and hemal osmolality are partly controlled by an osmoreceptor vasopressin renal system, which determines the rate of water loss in urine. Allied to this is a 'thirst' or 'drinking center' in the lateral zone, regulating water intake.
- *Sexual behavior and reproduction:* Through the hypophysial control of gonadotropin production, the hypothalamus controls aspects of reproduction, including gametogenesis, cyclic variations, and the development and maintenance of secondary sexual features.
- *Biological clocks:* Many tissues and organs show cyclic variations in function, with a period of 24 hours. Examples of such circadian rhythms include fluctuations in temperature, concentration of several plasma constituents, the eosinophilic count, the adrenocortical secretory activity and renal secretion.
- Emotions, fear, rage, aversion, pleasure and reward: Emotional states contain two main elements, namely subjective feeling or affective tone, and objective physical accompaniments, together forming emotional expression. For the full integration of both during changes in the internal and external environment and other cerebral activities, the essential structures are an intact hypothalamus, limbic system and prefrontal cortex.

Inflammations, vascular disturbances and neoplasms, in or about the hypothalamus, have led to many aberrant activities. Sometimes, these take the form of impaired memory, or of maniacal outbursts with excitement and destructiveness. Sudden and unreasonable seizures of crying and laughing may also occur. Anxiety states or periods of apathy may be seen. Loss of inhibitions, with indecent behavior, is not uncommon.

CEREBRUM: THE HIGHEST CENTER

The cerebrum occupies the greater part of the cranial cavity and covers the brainstem and cerebellum. It is divided into two lateral hemispheres by the sagittal fissure, into which dips a double fold of dura mater, the falx cerebri. The cerebral hemisphere consists of three parts: the pallium or cortex, the rhinencephalon, and the basal ganglia. Each cerebral hemisphere has three surfaces, namely dorsolateral, medial and basal.

Pallium or Cortex

Each hemisphere is divided into lobes by distinct fissures or sulci and by arbitrary lines. The central sulcus, the lateral fissure, the preoccipital notch, and the parieto-occipital fissure serve as landmarks, by which the frontal, parietal, occipital and temporal lobes are set apart. To these lobes should be added the insula (island of Reil), which lies at the bottom of the lateral fissure. The medial surface merges gradually with the basal surface. Among the most obvious features seen on the medial aspect of the brain is the corpus callosum, which consists of the rostrum, genu, body and splenium. The basal surface consists of the territory lying in a horizontal plane rostral to the temporal poles.

Cerebral Organization

Cell Types

1. *Pyramidal cells:* These are the most characteristic cells found in the cortex. They have the shape of pyramids, the apices of which are directed toward the brain substance. The single axon, springing from the base of cell, is directed internally toward the white matter. The size of the cell varies considerably. They are classified as small (10–12 microns), medium (20–30 microns), large (45–50 microns), and giant (>100 microns). These giant cells are the pyramidal cells of Betz.
2. *Stellate cells (Granule cells):* These are small polygonal or triangular cells, with a dark nucleus and measure 4 to 8 microns at their widest point.
3. *Fusiform cells (Spindle cells):* In these cells, the long axis of the spindle shaped cell is perpendicular to the surface. A dendrite is attached to each end of the cell.
4. *Horizontal cells (of Cajal):* These are small spindle shaped cells, with their axons extending horizontally.
5. *Ascending axon cells (of Martinotti):* These cells are small and polygonal in shape, with short dendrites.

Intracortical Fibers

These may be classified according to their direction as either radial or tangential. Radial fibers, run vertically, in fine bundles, toward the brain surface and include the axons of various cells of the cerebral cortex. Tangential fibers run horizontally parallel to the surface, and are often found in distinct bundle.

Layers

The six basic cortical layers, starting with the most external are:

1. *Molecular or plexiform layer (I):* It contains few cells; those present being the small stellate and horizontal types, and a fairly dense layer of tangential fibers.
2. *Outer granular layer (II):* It is made up of many closely packed, small pyramidal cells. Terminating with in this layer, are some axons from the deeper Martinotti's cells.
3. *Outer pyramidal layer (III):* It is made up of pyramidal cells, among which are scattered stellate and Martinotti's cells. A band of horizontal fibers, the bands of Kaes-Bechterew, may also be seen in the outer portion of this layer.
4. *Inner granular layer (IV):* The majority of cells are of small stellate variety. The entire layer contains a large number of horizontal fibers, the so called external band of Baillarger.
5. *Inner pyramidal layer (V):* It is composed chiefly of medium and large pyramidal cells. All axons of these cells enter the white substance.
6. *Fusiform layer (VI):* The predominant cells are fusiform cells. The axons of these cells enter the white substance.

Types of Cortex

There is considerably variation in thickness and cellular development in the cortical layers. In addition, there are differences in the total thickness of the cortex, the number of afferent and efferent fibers, and in the number, distinctness and position of horizontal bands. The regions with a readily identifiable six layered appearance are known as homotypical cortex, and are found in association of regions of the frontal, temporal and parietal lobes.

In contrast, some regions do not retain a six layered appearance, and are referred as the heterotypical cortex, which includes primary motor cortex (lacking a defined layer IV), and primary sensory regions (exhibiting an expanded layer IV) (Fig. 8).

Fibers of the Cortex

Afferent Fibers (Corticopetal)

In any area of the cortex, two types of afferent fibers are recognized; specific and non-specific. Specific fibers arise

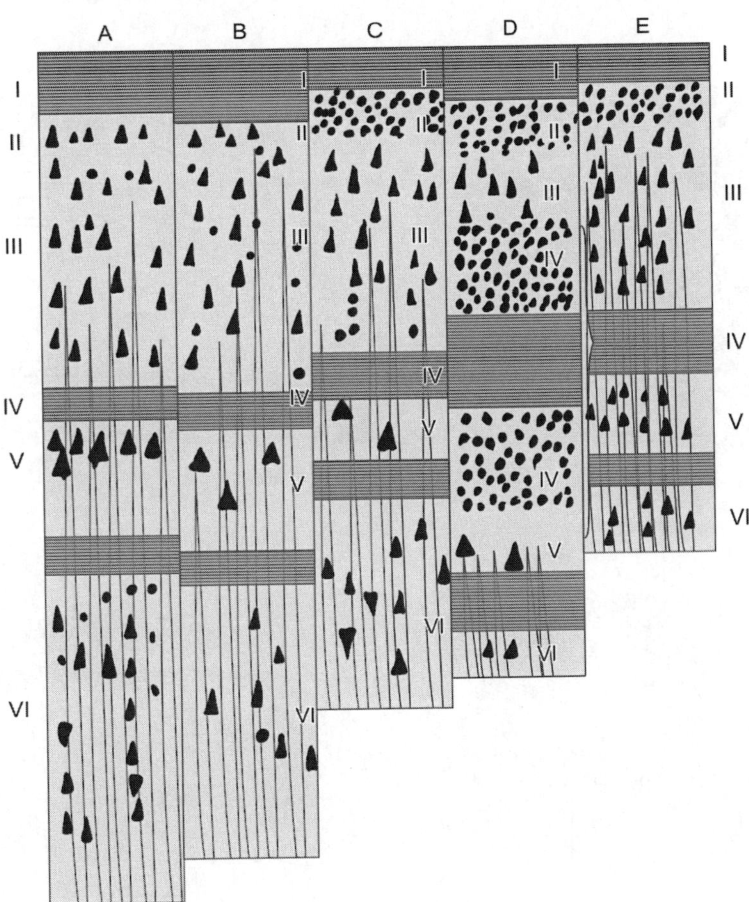

Fig. 8: Types of cortex

in nuclei outside the hemisphere and belong chiefly to the somesthetic, optic and auditory systems. They terminate in the primary sensory areas. Nonspecific fibers are the thalamocortical radiations arising in the elaborative or associational thalamic nuclei. They end in cortical areas adjacent to the primary sensory cortex.

Association Fibers

These fibers arise in one cortical area to terminate in the cortical areas of the same side. The distribution is mainly in areas 4 and 6, and the fibers terminate chiefly in layer IV and possibly in area III.

Commissural Fibers

These neurons arise in the cortex of one hemisphere, cross the midline, and are distributed to similar cortical areas of the opposite hemisphere. There are three major pathways, two of these, the anterior and hippocampal, interconnect parts of the archipallium. The third, the corpus callosum, by far the largest, unites the two neopallial hemispheres.

Efferent (Corticofugal) Fibers

These are of three sorts:

1. Projection fibers are the axons of pyramidal cells lying mainly in layer V. Among the fibers belonging to this group are corticothalamic, corticospinal, corticobulbar, corticorubral, corticostriate and corticopontine.
2. Association fibers arise chiefly from the small or medium sized pyramidal cells, particularly from the layer II and III, and to a lesser degree from layer V.
3. Commissural fibers are mainly from small and medium sized pyramidal cells.

Cortical Areas

Over the last 70–80 years, several investigators have mapped the cortex, according to variations in structural characteristics. The most widely used is the mapping of Korbinian Brodmann (Figs 9A and B), who divided the cortex of each hemisphere in to 44 areas. Using various sorts of electrical stimuli applied directly to the cortex, some of the cortical areas have been further subdivided and are demonstrated on the maps of Foerster (Figs 10A andB).

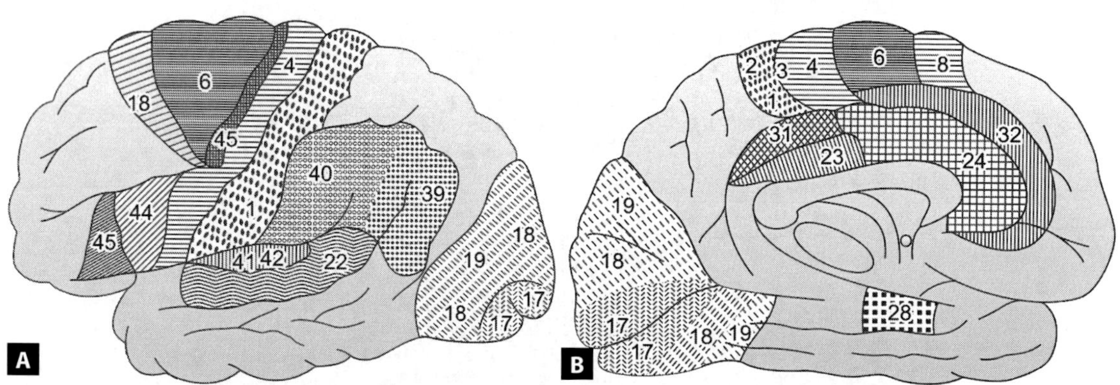

Figs 9A and B: Cortical areas I

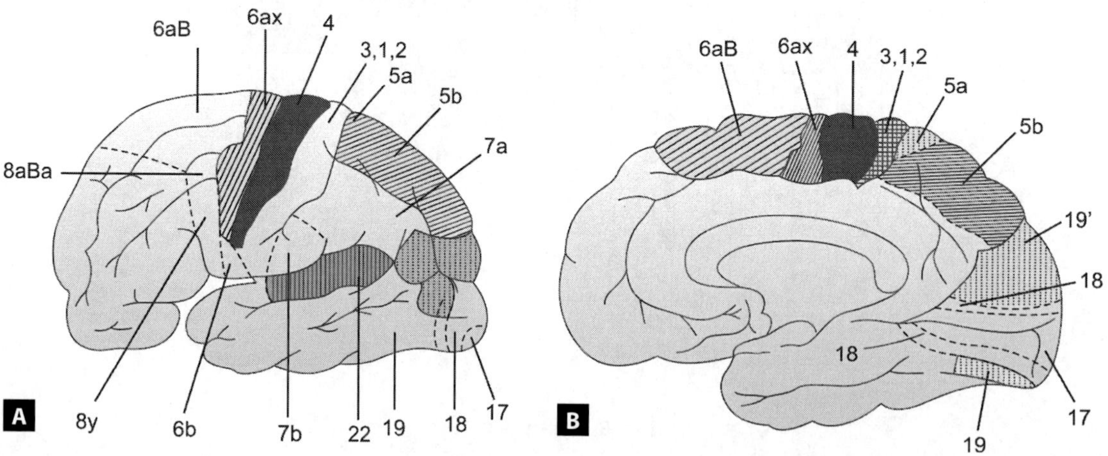

Figs 10A and B: Cortical areas II

Primary Sensory Areas and their Perception

1. *Somesthetic:* This is the region of the postcentralgyrus, including its medial extension into the paracentral lobule. It receives fibers from the posteromedial and posterolateral ventral nuclei via various thalamic radiations. Each small part of the body has a point for point representation of the cortex. The secondary cortex for this system has been described as lying around the inferior end of the central fissure, area 43, and a part of the rostral area 40.
2. *Visual:* This zone is located chiefly on the medial side of the hemisphere, in the walls of the calcarine fissure and includes portions of cuneus and lingual gyri. The entire area is indicated on the map as area 17. The visual perception are indicated as area 18 and 19.
3. *Auditory:* This region lies on the upper surface of the superior temporal gyrus, most of it facing the Sylvian fissure. The area is designated on map as areas 41 and 42. Area 22 is designated as perceptive area, and is interconnected with areas 41 and 42.
4. *Olfactory:* The primary cortical receptive zones seem to be prepyriform and periamygdaloid regions, the latter including the semilunar and ambient gyri. The chief associative region seems to be entorhinal area, mapped as area 28 and perirhinal area, the area 35.

Manifestations of Cortical Lesions

1. *Paralysis*: The term is used to denote loss or impairment of motor units. Flaccid paralysis is characterized by atonia, areflexia and, later, atrophies. Spastic paralysis is characterized by increased tone (hypertonia) and increased deep tendon reflexes (hyper-reflexia). The lesion is purely within the pyramidal or extrapyramidal system.
2. *Apraxia, or the loss of ability to perform purposeful movements:* It is associated with lesions of the dominant cerebral hemisphere, frequently involving the supramarginal gyms.
3. *Agnosia, or the loss of ability to recognize the important sensory stimuli:* Astereognosis is the inability to recognize the form and nature of objects by touch. The visual agnosia is the inability to recognize that which is seen. The lesion is usually located in the association area of that system.
4. *Aphasia* may be defined as the loss of power of expression by speech or writing. Receptive aphasia (alexia) or word blindness is usually due to the lesion affecting area 18 and 19. Expressive aphasia, or simply called as motor aphasia, is associated with the lesion of Broca's speech area 44.
5. *Ageusia* is loss of ability to taste. A central lesion is undoubtedly located in the parietal opercular region.
6. *Anosmia* is characterized by loss of smell. There is involvement of olfactory tracts, semilunar or ambient gyri.

PYRAMIDAL SYSTEM AND MUSCULAR ACTIVITY

The muscular activity is controlled from two levels of the central nervous system: (1) by neurons arising from the brainstem and cord (lower motor neurons), or final common path, and (2) by upper motor neurons, arising from the motor cortex of the cerebrum and descending through long projection pathways to synapse with the lower motor neurons.

Parts and Connections

The cells of origin, the giant pyramidal cells (of Betz) lie in the pyramidal, or motor cortex, which lies in the anterior lip of the central sulcus. It extends onto the lateral surface of the precentralgyrus superiorly, where it occupies more than half the precentral gyrus, covering the rostral portion of the paracentral lobule.

Pathways

From the giant pyramidal cells of area 4, efferent fibers descend by way of the corticospinal and corticobulbar pathways, to reach the ventral columns of the cord and the cranial motor nuclei, respectively. However, these tracts may contain fibers originating from smaller cells in area 4 as well as area 6. The corticospinal fibers, then pass through corona radiata, into the posterior limb of the internal capsule. At the rostral border of the midbrain, they join other descending cortical fibers in the formation of the cerebral peduncle (crus cerebri). The fibers then enter the rostral end of the pons and descend through its basilar part, into the pyramid of the medulla. In the caudal part of the medulla, about 80–90% fibers cross the median plane and descend as lateral corticospinal tracts; the remaining fibers descend uncrossed as ventral corticospinal tracts.

Clinical Manifestations and Pathology

In cases of lesions involving the pyramidal system, certain findings are commonly encountered: (1) all the cortical types of conditioned reflex are eliminated, the loss being most apparent in the hands and in the speech apparatus; (2) since the motor nerves (lower motor neurons) are intact, there is no degeneration of muscle, although some diminution of muscular size occurs owing to disuse. Since the pyramidal fibers are mainly excitatory, a lesion affecting only the true pyramidal cells or fibers would lead to the flaccid type of paralysis.

Specific pathologic changes occur due to injuries involving the motor cortex directly or damage to the spinal cord. Changes also occur due to the vascular accidents.

1. *Hemiplegia cruciata* is due to lesions involving the lateral aspect of the pyramidal decussation. There is paralysis of homolateral arm and contralateral leg.

2. *Hemiplegia alternata:* This is a symptom complex, in which there is an altered function of cranial nerves of the same side and altered function of one of the long pathways connected with the opposite side.
3. *Tetraplegia* usually occurs due to the lesion in the pyramidal region of the medulla. However, death usually occurs rapidly, owing to involvement of the respiratory or cardiac centers.
4. *Jacksonian epilepsy* occurs due to an irritative lesion at some point, on or near the motor cortex.

EXTRAPYRAMIDAL SYSTEM

In the broadest sense, the extrapyramidal system includes all parts of the central nervous system concerned with motor activity, except most of the cortical area 4 and the fibers which descend from it. For a time, among the lower animal forms, the reticular formation and, later the midbrain tegmental nuclei were sufficient for all motor activity. With the evolution of the fish, a nuclear mass, called the paleostriatum, appears corresponding to globus pallidus of higher forms. In reptiles and birds, the neostriatum develops, corresponding to the caudateputamen complex of man.

Generally, the extrapyramidal system is thought to provide a background motor pattern. In other words, this system sets up approximate positions of the body parts through the adjustment of large muscle groups, while the more refined, precise and specific activities of individual muscles are added by the pyramidal system.

Parts and Connections

Extrapyramidal Cortex

The extrapyramidal system represents an ancient motor mechanism, which has secondarily become dominated by cortical influence. The various extrapyramidal areas indicated on the cortical map are 2, 4, 43, 6, 8, 9, 19 and 24. The various components are:

1. *Corpus striatum:* It is explained along with basal nuclei.
2. *Substantia nigra:* This nuclear mass forms a zone between the midbrain tegmentum and basis pedunculi. At the level of subthalamus, it is almost continuous with pallidum. It extends as far caudally as the pons.

   Afferents: Striatonigral, pallidonigral and subthalamonigral fibers terminate at all levels of substantial nigra. In addition, corticonigral fibers synapse in the reticular portion of the cephalic end of the substantianigra.

   Efferents: Most of the efferents arise from the compact portion and end in the deep tegmental nucleus. There may be ascending fibers back to the striatum and pallium as well.
3. *Subthalamus:* This region, lying between the thalamus and hypothalamus, extends from the red nucleus to the internal capsule. In includes nuclear masses of zonaincerta, subthalamic nucleus and prerubral nucleus.

   Afferents for subthalamic nucleus arise in the corpus striatum, globuspallidus and cerebral cortex. Zonaincerta receives afferents mainly from the globuspallidus.

   Efferents pass to the tegmental reticular formation.
4. *Red nucleus:* It is a large, prominent cell mass, extending from the subthalamus through the tegmentum of mesencephalon to the caudal level of the superior colliculus. The nucleus has a 'capsule', made up of fibers entering or leaving its center.

   Afferents: Most of the afferent impulses are relayed from the prerubral field. Another large afferent contribution comes by way of the brachium conjunctivum from the dentate nucleus of the cerebellum.

   Efferents are widely distributed. Some enter the medial longitudinal bundle and relay in nuclei of cranial nerves III, IV and VI, and some, but not many, enter the rubrospinal tract. Many of the fibers first relay in reticular formation and then pass to the reticulobulbar and reticulospinal tracts.

Evaluation of the Extrapyramidal Circuit

The extrapyramidal system is mainly the regulator of large muscle masses of the trunk girdle and proximal parts of the limbs, while the pyramidal mechanism controls the muscles of the distal portions of the extremities.

Facilitation of movements occurs when certain portions of the cerebrum are stimulated in the absence of area 4 or its projections. These are areas 1, 2, 3, 5, 6a, 6b, 7, 8, 19, and 22. Suppression of the movement occurs usually due to the activity of medial reticular nuclei of the medulla. Thus, the normal muscular activity depends upon a balance between facilitation and suppression. If anything upsets this balance, the results are expressed in abnormalities of motor function. In practice, three general types of abnormality are seen: loss of certain movements; involuntary movements; and aberrations in states of muscle tone, i.e. hypotonia, spasticity or rigidity.

Abnormalities of Motor Function

The disorder of *tone* most frequently encountered is one of increase. Sometimes, the degree of hypertonia is so great that volitional and emotional movements are almost completely suppressed. In spasticity, the increase in tone is observed for the most part in the antigravity muscles, and may be the consequence of an interference with area 4s or its projection to the bulbar inhibitory center. When there is widespread pathologic change over much of the frontal lobe, or to a large segment of subcortical extrapyramidal centers, increased tone is seen in practically all muscle groups. The condition of generalized hypertonia is called rigidity.

In plastic rigidity, the hypertonia is constant, whereas in cogwheel rigidity, resistance to passive stretch is not smooth but is discontinuous.

Involuntary movements include tremors, choreiform movements, athetosis, hemiballism and dystonia. Tremors can be of various sorts. The postural (or alternating) tremors consist of the alternating contraction of opposing muscle groups-flexors and extensors, adductors and abductors—as seen in 'pill-rolling' tremors. Action (or intention) tremors always appear during voluntary acts, increasing in severity near the end of the action. Choreiform movements are rapid, dancing and jerky movements, while athetosis is a slow pattern of movement rather than an isolated act. It may occur, either at rest or in the course of voluntary action. Dystonic movements are slow, writhing and involuntary, with bizarre, grotesque tortions and twistings of the shoulders and pelvic girdles, as well as of the trunk. Hemiballism is characterized by involuntary movements of the entire limb. Rolling, wave-like patterns seem to flow down the arm from time-to-time.

Basal Ganglia and Corpus Striatum

The basal ganglia are a series of subcortical nuclear masses of gray matter, grouped together on the basis of their interconnections. The nuclei play an important role in dyskinesias. The various structures included under the general term, basal nuclei, are caudate nucleus, lentiform nucleus, amygdaloid complex and claustrum. The caudate nucleus and lentiform nucleus are commonly grouped together as the corpus striatum. The lentiform nucleus is divided into an internal globuspallidus and an external putamen, which are structurally distinct. The putamen resembles the caudate nucleus in its structure, and together, they constitute the neostriatum (or striatum). The neostriatum is well vascularized and highly cellular; the cells are small, multipolar cells.

The caudate nucleus is an arcuate mass, having a massive head lying in the floor of anterior cornu of the lateral ventricle, comparatively narrow body, projecting into the central part of the lateral ventricle, and a tail. The tail lies in the roof of the inferior cornu of the lateral ventricle and merges with the amygdaloid body.

The lentiform nucleus is shaped like a biconvex lens. Cut in section, it is seen to consist of two portions; a larger lateral part, which is darker incolor, is termed the putamen, while the smaller, medial portion is of a lighter tint, and is termed the globuspallidus. The lentiform nucleus is buried completely in the substance of the hemisphere.

Internal Organization

With the help of Golgi technique and electron microscopy, some general features have emerged. Striatal dendrites bear spines and axodendritic synapses, both related to spines and smooth interspine dendritic surfaces, and axosomatic synapses. Both asymmetrical (type I) and symmetrical (type II) synapses are present. Lesions in the cerebral cortex, thalamus or midbrain result in degeneration of asymmetrical synapses, which are presumably excitatory, in relation to both dendrites and to the cell somata.

Efferent Connections

The efferent fibers have their origin in the lentiform nucleus. Only few fibers originate in the putamen; a relatively large number of fibers come from the external division of the globuspallidus and a greatest number originate from the cells in its internal division.

1. *Fasciculus lenticularis:* The fasciculus courses medially from its origin in the globuspallidus, pierces the internal capsule and terminates in the interstitial and posterior commissural nuclei, the red nucleus, and some of the tegmental nuclei of mesencephalon.
2. *Pallidohypothalamic tract:* The tract initially follows fasciculus lenticularis, but later on leaves the fasciculus and terminates in the ventromedial hypothalamic nucleus.
3. *Pallidothalamic fibers:* These fibers constitute the thalamic fasciculus and are distributed to the lateral ventral nucleus of the thalamus.
4. *Ansalenticularis:* Fibers originate from all divisions of the lentiform nucleus and may also contain fibers from temporal and visual cortices. The fiber loop forward around the anterior border of the internal capsule and are traced into the hypothalamus and red nucleus. The fasciculus subthalamis comes from both divisions of globus pallidus; a few of its fibers originate in the putamen. After piercing the internal capsule, the fasciculus enters the lateral part of the subthalamic nucleus. Pallidonigral fibers are closely associated with the fasciculus subthalamicus and end in the substantia nigra.

Functions

The functions of the basal ganglia are somewhat complex. The pallidum may elaborate the simple motor and postural mechanisms of the brainstem into complex autonomic motor behavior. It is probably the center for gestures expression and reactive movements. The striatum elaborates and smoothes out the coarser motor integrations of the pallidum. Both are subordinate to the functions of the extrapyramidal cortex, which exerts a controlling influence over them. The subthalamic nucleus, red nucleus and substantial nigra probably have synergistic action, and are important in the integration of stereotyped behavior and the control of complex muscular movement. The basal ganglia not only elaborate and integrate voluntary motor behavior and make it smooth and effective, but the motor skills learned by the cortex can probably be relegated to these structures when they become automatic. The extrapyramidal system acts as a channel, in addition to the pyramidal system, through which volitional impulses are able to reach the pyramidal motor neurons in the brainstem and spinal cord. It is these habitual movements of daily life that are most impaired in diseases of this portion of the motor system.

Clinical Manifestations and Lesions

Paralysis agitans (Parkinson's disease): There is extensive degeneration of the globus pallidus and substantial nigra. The putamen and caudate nuclei are involved to a lesser degree, although the exact etiology is not known. There occurs rigidity of both plastic and cogwheel type. The trunk may assume a fixed posture. Postural tremors are more marked in the distal extremities.

Encephalitis: While Parkinsonism usually occurs later in life, encephalitis may lead to the appearance of these signs at any age. The most severe damage is in the globuspallidus and the reticular portion of the substantial nigra. There are tremors with associated trunk flexion.

Wilson's disease (Hepatolenticular disease): This is a rare, familial disease, usually fatal, occurring in young people. Cavitation and progressive degeneration of the putamen is the pathology. The disease is characterized by tremors, rigidity, muscle weakness, progressive dementia and emaciation.

Sydenham's chorea: This is a disease of children or adolescents. Petechial lesions in striatum and cortex have been described. There are quick, involuntary, asymmetrical, purposeless movements, increased by emotional stimuli.

Huntington's chorea: This is a disease of adults, due to degeneration in both the cortex and the basal ganglia. It is a hereditary disease, characterized by moderate to severe choreiform movements, coupled with progressive mental deterioration.

LIMBIC SYSTEM AND RHINENCEPHALON

During development, the superolateral aspects of the diencephalon gradually merge with the central areas of inferomedial surfaces of the hemispheres. Bordering the whole area of fusion on each side, a series of structures develop in the hemisphere wall, as the limbic lobe. Many structures of the limbic lobe are phylogenetically old, with an arched form, topographically interposed between the diencephalon and the cerebral neopallium. The various compartments of limbic system include:

1. *Olfactory nerves, bulb and tract (with the nervous terminalis, and the transient accessory olfactory bulb and vomeronasal nerve):* Olfactory nerves are the central processes of the olfactory cells in the nasal mucosa, which enter into the inferior surface of the olfactory bulb. The olfactory bulb and tract develop as a hollow diverticulum from the floor of the primitive cerebral hemisphere. The olfactory tract, near the anterior perforated substance, divides into medial and lateral olfactory striae, which merge with the paraterminal gyrus and the pyriform lobe.
2. *Anterior perforated substance:* An important land-mark on the cerebral base, it is continuous medially with the paraterminal gyrus. Laterally, it continue into prepyriform cortex and periamygdaloid area. Superiorly, it is continuous with corpus striatum. It gives passage to the central branches of anterior cerebral and middle cerebral arteries.
3. The pyriform lobe, including lateral olfactory gyrus, periamygdaloid area, uncus hippocampi and the entorhinal area (area 28).
4. *The amygdala (amygdaloid nuclear complex) is a series of neuronal masses, dorsomedial in the temporal pole. It is divided into two main groups:* The corticomedial and basilateral nuclei.
5. *Septal areas, including septum pellucidum and septum verum:* The main afferent connections to the septal nuclei are from the amygdaloid complex, the anterior perforated substance, the hippocampus via fornix, the midbrain reticular formation and hypothalamic nuclei. The efferent fibers are distributed to hippocampal formation via fornix, various hypothalamic nuclei and midbrain reticular formation, and to the habenular nuclei via the striamedullaris.
6. *The hippocampal formation, including:* (a) Pre-hippocampal rudiment, indusiumgriseum and longitudinal striae, and (b) gyrus fasciolaris, Ammon's horn, dentate gyrus, subiculum and related regions.
7. *The fornix and its various ramifications and divisions:* Fornix is the sole efferent system from the hippocampus. These fibers traverse the alveus and converge to form fimbria. The fimbria then continue as crus of the fornix. The two crura are interconnected as the commissure of the fornix. Anteriorly, the crura meet to form the body of the fornix.

   Thus, by different fornical fascicle, hippocampus efferents pass to septum pellucidum, cingulate gyrus, thalamic and hypothalamic nuclei, mamillary bodies and reticular formation of the midbrain.
8. *Striaterminalis:* Efferents from amygdaloid nuclear complex.
9. Striamedullaris thalami separate from the column of fornix, and reaches the habenular nucleus of same and opposite sides.
10. Cingulate and parahippocampal nuclei.

Functions

The limbic system in involved in higher integration of visceral, olfactory and somatic informations, and patterns of long- and short-term homeostatic responses. These include seeking and capturing prey, courtship, mating, rearing of young, subjective and expressive elements of emotional responses, balance between aggressive and communal behavior, and the formation of memory.

THE VENTRICLES OF THE BRAIN

The ventricular system of the brain includes two lateral ventricles, the third ventricle, the cerebral aqueduct and the fourth ventricle. The lateral ventricles communicate with the third ventricle through the interventricular foramen. The cerebral aqueduct connects the third ventricle with the fourth. The fourth ventricle communicates with the subarachnoid space, through the median foramen of Magendie and the lateral paired foramina of Luschka. The ventricular system is lined by a layer of ependymal cells. The ependymal roof of the third ventricle is covered by a layer of pia mater, known as the telachoroidea. The telachoroidea of the third ventricle is continuous with the pia mater lining the cerebral fissure. Vascular folds from the tela choroidea invaginate into the ventricle and form its choroid plexus. The ependymal membrane of the plexus is invaginated ahead of the vascular folds.

Cerebrospinal Fluid

The cerebrospinal fluid (CSF) is produced chiefly by filtration from the blood, through the semipermeable membranes of the choroid plexuses. Most of the fluid is formed in the lateral ventricles, and passes from there through the interventricular foramina to the third ventricles. Some contribution is made by the choroid plexus of the third ventricle, and the fluid then passes through the cerebral aqueduct into the fourth ventricle, where fluid is again added by the choroid plexus of that ventricle. From the fourth ventricle, the cerebrospinal fluid passes in to the subarachnoid cisterns around the medulla and central canal of the spinal cord.

BLOOD SUPPLY OF CENTRAL NERVOUS SYSTEM

Brain

The brain derives its arterial supply from the internal carotid and vertebral arteries. The internal carotid enters the cranial cavity through the carotid canal in the petrosa of the temporal bone. The vertebral artery, after coursing upwards through the successive transverse foramina of the upper six cervical vertebrae, enters the cranial cavity through the foramen magnum. The internal carotid courses through the cavernous sinus, where it gives off small branches to the semilunar ganglion, hypophysiscerebri and hypothalamus. It turns upwards at the anterior limit of the cavernous sinus, gives off ophthalmic, posterior communicating and anterior choroidal branches, and then divides into anterior and middle cerebral arteries.

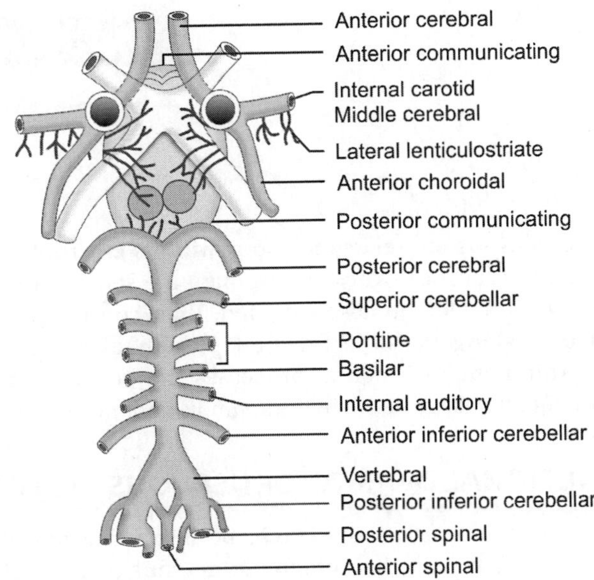

Fig. 11: Blood supply to brain

The intracranial portion of the vertebral artery extends forwards from the foramen magnum to the lower border of the pons, where it unites with its fellow to form the basilar artery. The basilar artery extends from the lower to the upper border of the pons, lying in its median sulcus, and terminates by dividing into right and left posterior cerebral arteries. The circle of Willis, at the base of the brain, is the principal arterial anastomotic trunk of the brain. Blood reaches to it via the vertebral and internal carotid arteries (Fig. 11).

The venous drainage from the brain is chiefly into the dural sinuses, the vascular channels lying with in the tough structure of the dura. The dural sinuses contain no valves and, for the most part, are triangular in shape.

Spinal Cord

Arterial supply of the spinal cord comes from the anterior and posterior spinal arteries, and from the spinal branches of the vertebral, intercostal, lumbar and sacral arteries.

The venous drainage of the spinal cord begins with the intramedullary veins, which emerge from it and empty into ventral and dorsal venous channels. These channels drain into the vertebral and segmental veins.

44.2 NEUROPHYSIOLOGY

Uma Joshi, Aparna Garg

The nervous system relates the body with its environment through the sensory structures. In man, the sensory input is not only mingled but also recorded. Thus, consciousness evolves making possible finer adaptation of behavior. The prominence of mental processes may obscure the fundamental linkage between the stimulus and the response.

FUNCTIONAL DIVISION OF NERVOUS SYSTEM

Functionally, the nervous system can be divided into somatic nervous system and the autonomic nervous system. The somatic nervous system is under the control of our will. It is concerned with the regulation and coordination of voluntary activities such as locomotion, speech, writing, etc. On the other hand, the autonomic nervous system is not under the control of our will. It consists of sympathetic nervous system, parasympathetic nervous system and ganglia. It regulates functions like the heart action, movements of the viscera, contraction of blood vessels and secretion of glands (Fig. 12).

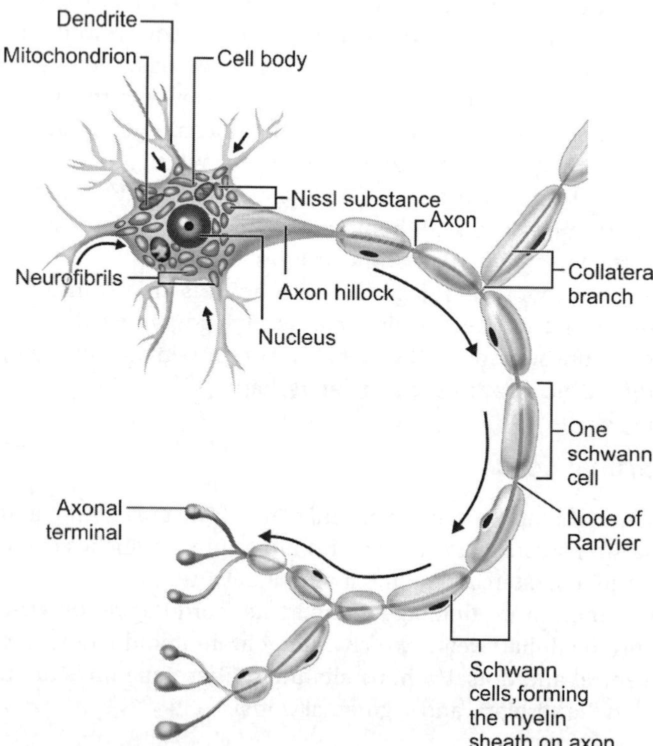

Fig. 12: Functional division of nervous system

Nerve Cell, Synapses and Transmission of Impulses

The basic structural unit of the nervous system is the nerve cell. A nerve cell, along with its axon and other processes, is referred to as a neuron. Nerve cells massed together form the gray matter, while axons or nerve fibers massed together form the white matter.

A nerve cell has processes of two varieties:

1. Axon
2. Dendrites.

Each cell has one axon and may have more than one dendrite. An axon tends to be straight and long, while dendrites branch like trees. An axon carries nerve impulse away from the nerve cell body, while a dendrite carries nerve impulse toward the cell body.

The nerve fibers are covered with a sheath of fatty matter, which is responsible for the difference in color between the gray and white matter. The sheath is called as myelin sheath. It provides insulation, protection, nutrition and helps in the conduction of impulses. The nerve fibers are arranged in bundles called fasciculi. Many fasciculi are enclosed by a layer called epineurium to form a nerve trunk.

CLASSIFICATION OF THE NERVE FIBERS

Nerve trunks can either be motor or sensory or can be of a mixed variety. Motor (or efferent) nerve trunks carry impulses from spinal cord and brain to the periphery and thus constitute the motor pathway. Sensory (or afferent) nerve trunks carry impulses from the periphery to the brain or spinal cord constituting the sensory pathway. Mixed nerve trunks carry impulses both way and link up the different nerve centers in the brain and spinal cord (Tables 3 and 4).

A nerve path for the passage of a nerve impulse is formed by a series of neurons placed one after another. The junctional region, where one nerve ends and the other begins, is called a synapse (Fig. 13). It is the basic functional unit of the CNS.

Functions of the Synapse

- Relay of nerve impulses.
- Dispersion of nerve impulses in all directions.
- Decides which impulses are to be allowed to pass and which ones are to be blocked.

Table 3: Erlanger's and Gasser's classification

Fiber type	*Function*	*Fiber diameter (μm)*	*Conduction velocity (m/s)*	*Spike duration*	*Absolute refractory period (ms)*
A					
A	Proprioception; somatic motor	12–20	70–120	0.4–0.5	0.4–1
B	Touch, pressure, motor	5–12	30–70		
Γ	Motor to muscle spindles	3–6	15–30		
δ	Pain, cold, touch	2–5	12–30		
B	Preganglionic autonomic	< 3	3–15	1.2	1.2
C					
Dorsal root	Pain, temperature, some mechanoreception, reflex responses	0.4–1.2	0.5–2	2	2
Sympathetic	Postganglionic sympathetics	0.3–1.3	0.7–2.3	2	2

Table 4: Based on physioclinical aspect

	Most susceptible	*Intermediate*	*Least susceptible*
Hypoxia	B	A	C
Pressure	A	B	C
Local anesthetics	C	A	B

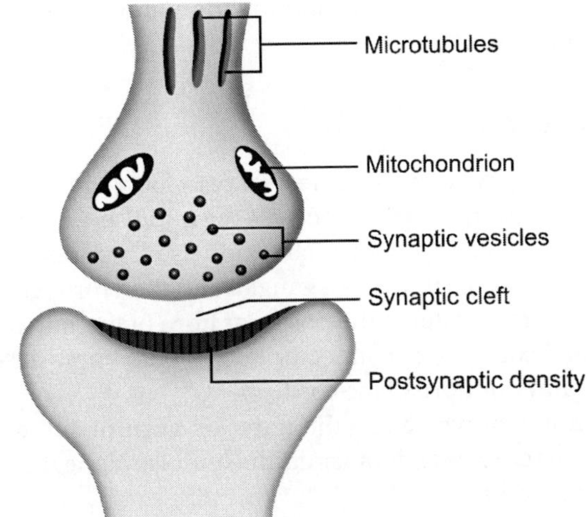

Fig. 13: Schematic representation of synapse

- Amplifies an incoming impulse, if needed, so that one impulse may elicit many outgoing impulses.
- Decreases the number of transmuted impulses, if needed.

The transmission of impulses is achieved by the following methods:

- Stimulus causes an axon to develop action potential.
- Action potential is propagated down the axon and reaches the presynaptic membrane.
- Now a chemical transmitter is released by the synaptic vesicles.
- The chemical transmitter comes out of synaptic membrane, crosses the synaptic cleft and gets attached to the receptor on postsynaptic membrane.
- The receptor chemical transmitter complex develops a local potential called the synaptic potential. This synaptic potential may be excitatory postsynaptic potential (EPSP) or inhibitory postsynaptic potential (IPSP).
- When EPSP is sufficiently strong enough, an action potential develops which is propagated down,

Central or Cerebrospinal Nervous System

The cerebrospinal system regulates the voluntary activities of the body. Motor impulses originate in the cerebrum and pass along the efferent nerve trunks to the various muscles.

Spinal Cord

The spinal cord is a conductor of impulses between the brain and the periphery.

- From periphery via spinal cord to the brain (afferent path).
- From brain via spinal cord to the periphery (efferent path).

The spinal cord also used in the reflex action. It begins at the medulla oblongata and ends in between the first and second lumbar vertebrae, where it tapers as the conus medullary. It is about 45 cm long and is divided in front by a deep anterior fissure and at the back by a narrow one. Spinal cord has two enlargements, the cervical and lumbar from which emerge the verve plexuses, to supply the upper and the lower limb. The nerve plexuses that emerge from the thoracic region form the intercostal nerves.

To the spinal cord are attached 31 pairs of spinal nerves. Each spinal nerve is attached to the spinal cord by two roots, the anterior and the posterior root. Efferent impulses originating in the brain pass down to the spinal cord and go along the anterior root of spinal nerves and reach the various muscles.

Afferent impulses reach the spinal cord through the posterior roots of the spinal nerves and then reach the brain.

Transverse section of the spinal cord reveals gray matter inside, surrounded by the white matter on the outside. The gray matter consists of two semilunar segments and is joined by a narrow strip of gray matter called the isthmus. In the center of isthmus, there is a canal called the central canal which contains cerebrospinal fluid. The gray matter is composed mainly of nerve cells and is supported by neuroglia cells and fibers.

The nerve cell in the spinal cord is arranged in groups. The anterior and posterior portions of each semilunar segment of gray matter are called as the anterior horn and posterior horn, respectively. Similarly, the lateral portion of each semilunar segment in the thoracic and upper lumbar region is called the lateral horn.

The white matter of spinal cord consists of myelinated nerve fibers which are held in position by connective tissue and by neuroglia cells and fibers. The white matter of the spinal cord can be divided in to a number of tracts. A tract is a bundle of fibers carrying one kind of impulse. There are two types of tracts that pass through the spinal cord. The descending tracts that originate in the cerebrum and pass down through the spinal cord to the organs, and the ascending tracts that start from the organs and pass through the spinal cord to the cerebrum. The descending tracts can be divided into pyramidal and extrapyramidal tracts (Fig. 14).

Pyramidal Tracts

The pyramidal tract is the longest tract, reaching up to the last segment of the spinal cord. Pyramidal tracts originate from Betz cells in precentral gyrus and cell in the parietal cortex of the cerebrum. They converge through corona radiata and reach the internal capsule. They give fibers to thalamus, pass to mid brain and give fibers to lentiform nucleus, pons and upper part of medulla, red nucleus, caudate nucleus, tegmental nucleus, motor cranial nerve nuclei and substantia nigra.

In the lower part of medulla, most fibers cross over to the opposite side to form the crossed pyramidal tract, while 15% remain on course to from the direct pyramidal tract. Fibers reach the anterior horn cells of spinal cord, and fresh fibers arise from the anterior horn cells of spinal cord and go to supply the muscles through anterior roots of the spinal cord.

The pyramidal tracts transmit the motor impulses to the voluntary muscles and also inhibit the muscles and spinal reflexes. Pyramidal system is responsible for nonpostural, fine, isolated, modifiable movement of small muscles at distal joints of limbs which form the basis for skills. Damage to the cells of crossed pyramidal tract may result in paralysis of various muscles of opposite side, increased muscle tone (rigidity and spasticity of paralysed muscles), and loss of superficial reflexes.

Damage to the cells of direct pyramidal tract results in paralysis of the muscles of the same side, flaccidity of the paralysed muscles, loss of reflexes and atrophy of the innervated muscles.

Extrapyramidal Tracts

It includes all descending tracts and nuclei other than the pyramidal tract.

It can be divided into two main types.

1. Extrapyramidal cortical projection fibers (including corticostriate fibers).
2. Descending pathways from suprasegmental nuclei to the anterior horn cells.

The extrapyramidal system contains both inhibitory as well as facilitatory fibers. It is a short-descending pathway that relays in various nuclei lying between cortex and spinal cord.

Functions

- It forms an alternative pathway for volitional impulses.
- It maintains tone, postural adjustment and equilibrium.
- It performs complex automatic associated movements:
- It exerts a tonic inhibitory control on lower centers.
- It forms a postural background against which fine voluntary movements are executed.
- It is responsible for accommodation and movements of external ocular muscles.

Reflex Action

The following structures are necessary to form a reflex arc:

- A sensory organ which receives the impulse, i.e. skin.
- A sensory nerve fiber which conducts this impulse to the cells in the posterior root ganglia and then through fibers to the gray matter in the posterior horn of the spinal cord.
- Spinal cord where connector nerves pass impulses on to the anterior horn of the cord.
- A motor nerve cell in the anterior horn of spinal cord which receives and transmits the impulse along the motor nerve fibers.
- A motor organ (e.g. muscle) which when stimulated by the motor nerve impulse, performs the action.

Reflex Arc

Sensory organ (receptor) → Sensory nerve (afferent limb) → Posterior root ganglion → Posterior horn cells (afferent cell) → Motor cells in anterior horn of spinal cord (efferent cell) → Motor nerve (efferent limb) → motor organ, i.e. muscle (effector).

Ascending Tracts or Sensory Tracts

Ascending tracts originate in neuromuscular spindle in muscles, tendon organ of Golgi in tendons, bones, joints,

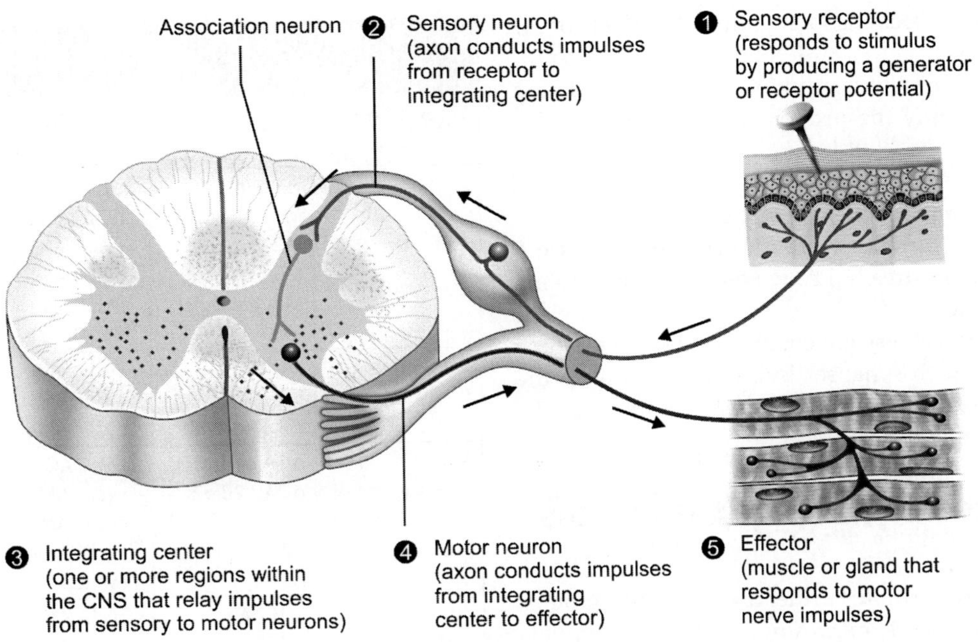

Fig. 14: Physiology of spinal cord

subcutaneous tissue, etc. They then pass through the spinal cord upwards into medulla and mid brain. Here, decussation of tracts takes place similar to the decussation seen with the descending tracts. From medulla, some of the tracts also pass on to cerebellum. From cerebellum, the tracts ascend upwards to the midbrain and then finally end in the sensory area of the cerebral cortex.

They are concerned with:

- Proprioception, passive movement, tone, position of limb in space.
- Pressure and touch.
- Perception, localization of sensation, tactile discrimination, special functions like writing, vibration sense and stereognosis (i.e. identification of objects coming in contact without seeing).
- Carry sensation of pain, temperature, itching and tickling; pleasant and unpleasant sensations.

Meninges

The brain and spinal cord are covered by the meninges which function to protect, carry blood and minimize effect of blow or concussion by secreting the cerebrospinal fluid (CSF).

The CSF is a clear alkaline fluid which acts as a buffer, protecting the brain and spinal cord, and conveying nourishment to the tissues of the CNS.

There are several interconnected cavities within the brain which form the ventricular system. These cavities contain the CSF. There are two lateral ventricles which lie one in each of the cerebral hemispheres and are connected to the third ventricle which lies between the thalamus, which in turn is connected to the fourth ventricle, lying between cerebellum and pons and medulla, by a narrow channel called as cerebral aqueduct.

The fourth ventricle has openings on its roof, which allow the CSF to pass into the subarachnoid space and in to the central canal of the spinal cord. As the subarachnoid space covers the entire brain and spinal cord, the CSF is able to reach all over the brain and cord until it is returned to the venous circulation by the arachnoid granulations in the superior sagittal sinus.

Thus, the delicate nervous tissue of the brain and spinal cord lies between the external layer of CSF in the subarachnoid space and the internal layer of the fluid in the ventricles of the brain and central canal of the spinal cord.

Neurotransmitter

Definition: Neurotransmitter are the chemical substances which are responsible for transmission of an impulse through a synapse.

Criteria for a neurotransmitter

- It should be synthesized by presynaptic neurons, and stored in the vesicles, which are present in the axon terminal.
- It should be released on stimulation of nerve.
- It travels a very small distance between presynaptic and postsynaptic membrane.
- It is associated with an enzyme for its inactivation.

- When applied extrisically should mimic the effects of the nerve stimulation.
- The drugs which modify the response to nerve stimulation should also modify the proposed action in a similar manner.

Neurotransmitters can also be of the subtypes such as:

- *Neuromediators:* These are synthesized in the neurons and poured into blood stream through terminals resembling synapses in structure.
- *Neuromodulators:* These are chemical substances which are associated with synapses but do not influence the effects of transmitters or of neuromediators, e.g. VIP, substance P (Table 5).

Table 5: Mechanism of action of the neurotransmitters by its receptors

Transmitter	*Receptor*	*Second messenger / MOA*	*Net channel effect*
Acetylcholine	Nicotinic M1 M2(cardiac) M3 M4(glandular) M5	...... ↑IP3, DAG ↓cyclic AMP ↓cyclic AMP ↑IP3, DAG ↑IP3, DAG	↑ Na , other small ions ↑ Ca ↑K
Dopamine	D1,D5 D2 D3, D4	↑cyclic AMP ↓cyclic AMP ↓cyclic AMP	↑K, ↓Ca
NE	α 1A,α1B,α1D α 2A,α2B,α2C β1 β2 β3	↑IP3, DAG ↓cyclic AMP ↑cyclic AMP ↑cyclic AMP ↑cyclic AMP	↓K ↑K, ↓Ca
5HT	5HT 1A 5HT1B 5HT1D 5HT 2A 5HT 2C 5HT3 5HT4	↓cyclic AMP ↓cyclic AMP ↓cyclic AMP ↑IP3, DAG ↑IP3, DAG .... ↑cyclic AMP	↑K ↓K ↓K ↑Na
Adenosine	A1 A2	↓cyclic AMP ↑cyclic AMP	
Glutamate	Metabotropic 2 Ionotropic AMPA, Kainate NMDA	....	↑Na ↑ Na, Ca
GABA	GABAA GABAB	.... ↑IP3, DAG	↑Cl ↑K, ↓Ca

CLASSIFICATION OF NEUROTRANSMITTERS

Broadly classified as:

a. *Biochemical classification:* Further divide into two groups:
   1. *Small molecule neurotransmitters:* These act rapidly and cause acute response. These are synthesized and packed into synaptic vesicles in the axon terminal
      a. Acetylcholine
      b. Biogenic amines
         - Catecholamines
         - Serotonin
         - Histamine
      c. Amino acid neurotransmitter
         - Gamma butyric acid (GABA)
         - Glycine
         - Glutamic acid or glutamate
         - Aspartic acid or aspartate
   2. *Neuropeptide transmitters:* Slow acting and have prolonged effect
      - Neuroactive peptides
      - Pituitary peptides
      - Peptides acting on gut and brain
      - Neuropeptides from other tissues

b. Physiological classification
   1. Excitatory neurotransmitters
   2. Inhibitory transmitters.

Brainstem

The brainstem is composed of midbrain, pons and medulla oblongata.

Reticular Formation

A very important component of the brainstem is the reticular formation. It constitutes one of the important regulatory mechanisms within the CNS. It is a diffuse, ill-defined mass of nerve cells and fibers situated at the central portion of the brainstem. It extends downwards into the spinal cord and upwards into the thalamus and subthalamus. The reticular system has both afferent and efferent connections. It receives afferent pathways bearing information to the brain from the environment, both direct afferent fibers as well as collaterals from the main afferent pathway to the cerebellum and thalamus (i.e. optic, olfactory, auditory, gustatory, spinal and trigeminal pathways). It receives afferent fibers from cerebellum, thalamus and cerebellum, basal ganglia, thalamus and cerebral cortex.

It sends efferent fibers to all parts of the cerebral cortex and both facilitatory and inhibitory fibers to the spinal cord. The reticular system is concerned with alerting and maintaining attention, production of sleep, initiation and maintenance of wakefulness, controlling the receptibility of stretch receptor in skeletal muscles, control of muscular activity and regulation of receptibility of peripheral sensory end organs. It also controls the threshold of central sensory pathways, regulates emotional expression and temperature regulation. The reticular system also contains centers for heart, center for regulation of blood pressure and for respiration. The reticular system also influences the endocrine system. It has a regulatory influence on conditioning and learning process, and on emotional and sexual behavior.

Both somatic as well as behavioral functions are connected in the reticular formation which explains that change in one can affect the functioning of other, e.g. change in emotional condition affecting the activity of heart and respiration. Worries and problems make it difficult to focus attention on prescribed task or sleep.

Medulla Oblongata

It is the upward continuation of the spinal cord and is continued above with the lower border of the pons. The medulla lies in the posterior cranial fossa. The medulla contains the nuclei for IX, X, XI and Xll cranial nerves. It also contains a mass of gray matter, the olivary body. The main feature of the medulla is that decussation of both the descending motor pathways and the sensory pathways occur here. It also contains the vital centers which control respiration and cardiovascular system. The medulla is an important center for reflex activity. Numerous reflex centers, like reflex center for closure of eyelids, vasomotor center, respiratory center, sweat secreting center, cardioinhibitory and acceleratory centers, cough center, center for sneezing, etc. lie here. The medulla is, therefore, indispensable for life.

Pons

The pons forms the middle portion of the brainstem. The pons contains a collection of gray matter called as nuclei pontis and Dieters· nucleus. The nuclei pontis receive fibers from the lobes of cerebral cortex and cerebellum. There are many fibers running transversally through the pons which link the two lobes of cerebellum and the cerebellum to the cerebral cortex. The pons forms the crossing place of these fibers which pass from one cerebral hemisphere to the cerebellum of opposite side. The Dieters' nucleus maintains the muscle tone and regulates posture. The pons function in conducting impulses as it contains the same ascending and descending pathways as the midbrain.

Midbrain

The midbrain forms the upper part of brainstem, through which runs the cerebral aqueduct, which connects the 3rd and 4th ventricles of cerebrum.

The midbrain consists of a pair of cerebral peduncles. Each peduncle is divided into two parts by a mass of pigmented gray matter, called the substantia nigra. The dorsal part is called the tegmentum and the ventral part, the basis pedunculi. The peduncles contain both cerebrospinal and cerebellar fibers. Sensory impulses pass upwards through tegmentum of midbrain while motor impulses pass downwards through the basis pedunculus.

Present in the tegmentum is an oval mass of gray matter called the red nuclei. The red nucleus is the center of righting reflexes and, along with Dieters nucleus in the pons, regulates muscle tone.

Cerebellum

The cerebellum is the largest part of hindbrain. lt occupies the posterior cranial fossa and is roofed over by the tentorium cerebelli, a fold of dura mater which separates it from the occipital lobes of cerebrum. The cerebellum is separated from the pons and medulla by the cavity of the 4th ventricle.

It consists of a central part, known as the vermis of cerebellum and is divided into the right and left hemispheres by a deep cleft into which dips another fold of the dura mater called falx cerebelli.

The surface of the cerebellum is ridged rather than folded into convolutions, the fissures between ridges being very much closer together than the sulci of the cerebral cortex.

The gray matter lies on the outside and the white matter on the inside. ln the white matter are present important masses of gray matter, such as the dentate nucleus and other nuclei. The gray matter of cerebellum contains large flask shaped cells, the Purkinje cells. Purkinje cells are connected to the red nucleus in the midbrain, to the Dieters' nucleus in the pons, and to the frontal lobe of the cerebrum through thalamus. The pathway cerebellum-thalamus-cerebral cortex pons cerebellum' is a means by which these cerebellum and cerebrum mutually influence one another's activities. It is by this pathway that the cerebellar hemispheres control voluntary movements.

The white matter of cerebellum contains both afferent and efferent fibers. Its principal connections are with the lobes of the cerebral hemispheres of the opposite side and with the brainstem. It also receives fibers from the spinal cord and is connected with the reflex centers of sight in the root of midbrain. It is also connected to the thalamus and with the auditory nerve.

The cerebellum controls bodily posture, equilibrium and volitional movements. It plays an important role in muscular coordination and maintenance of balance. It regulates the posture of eyeballs, head, trunk and limbs. The cerebellum forms a reflex center for the final control of posture. The cerebral cortex controls the movements of the opposite side of the body, the cerebellar hemispheres control the muscle tone and posture on their own side.

Damage to cerebellum may result in the following features:

- *Atonia:* loss of muscle tone.
- *Asthenia:* Weakness of the muscle.

- *Asynergia:* Lack of cooperation between agonist (flexor), antagonist (extensor), and synergist muscles.
- *Adiadochokinesia:* Inability to perform the act of alternate pronation and supination quickly. The movement are slow and irregular.
- *Dysmetria:* Force of muscular contraction is not well suited for the movements which the muscle is going to perform.
- *Decomposition:* The action, which can be performed in one movement is split up in to several movements.
- *Cerebellar ataxia:* In coordination of muscular contraction.
- *Nystagmus:* Jerky movements which occur when the eyeball moves from one side to other.

Cerebrum

The cerebrum occupies the front and upper portion of the cranial cavity, termed respectively the anterior and middle cranial fossa. It consists of two large hemispheres of gray matter and white matter. The outer layer of gray matter is termed the cortex. The two hemispheres are united at their bases by a mass of white matter, called the corpus callosum. Below the corpus callosum lie islands of gray matter, called the basal ganglia. The two hemispheres are separated, except at the corpus callosum.

The cerebral cortex is arranged in convolutions, with depressions in between the convolutions. These depressions are called sulci. The fissures and sulci divide the cerebral hemispheres into numerous lobes. The deepest sulci form the longitudinal and lateral fissures. The lobes of the cerebral hemispheres correspond in position to the bones beneath which they lie.

Each hemisphere is made up of gray matter on the outside and white matter on the inside. The gray matter is composed of neuronal cell bodies, while the white matter is composed of the axonal tracts.

Types of Nerve Fibers

The projection fibers serve to connect the cortex with the underlying part of CNS. These efferent projections are:

- Pyramidal fibers, which originate in the Betz cells in motor area of the cortex and pass through the internal capsule.
- Corticopontine fibers, which originate in the cortex and pass through the internal capsule and end in the nuclei pontis of pons.
- Corticostriate fibers, which originate from the frontal lobe, pass through the internal capsule and end in thalamus.

The afferent projection fibers are:

- Thalamocortical fibers, which originate from thalamus, pass through the internal capsule and end in the post-central gyrus, which is the tactile area of somoesthetic area.
- Optic radiations, which originate from lateral geniculate body, pass through the internal capsule and end in the occipital lobe.
- Auditory radiations, which originate from the medial geniculate body, pass through the internal capsule and end in temporal lobe.

The association fibers connect the different parts of the cortex of the same hemispheres.

The commissural fibers pass through the corpus callosum and connect the gray matter of the two hemispheres.

The cerebral cortex is thickest at the precentral gyrus and at the anterior part of the temporal lobe. It is thinnest in the frontal and occipital lobes. It consists of six layers. The most important layers are the outer pyramidal layer, the granular layer and the fusiform cell layer.

The outer pyramidal layer is concerned with intelligence and intellectual activities. The granular layer is concerned with reception and appreciation of sensory impulses. The fusiform layer fulfills instinctive activities, which arise from natural instincts such as feeding, excretion, and reproduction.

The cerebrum can be differentiated into different areas, depending on the function, e.g. association areas, motor area, and sensory area.

Motor Area: lt is that portion of the frontal lobe, anterior to the central sulcus, which on stimulation gives rise to motor response. This portion is known as precentral motor cortex. In this area, the whole body is represented upside down. The movements of the lowest part of the body are controlled by the area situated in the upper most part of the motor area. Stimulation of the motor area produces movements of a certain muscle or group of muscles of the opposite side of the body. The precentral motor cortex is divided into four areas, viz. 4, 8, 4S and 6.

Area 4 is the pure motor cortex and here the giant pyramidal cells or Betz cells are present. Pyramidal fibers arising here, pass through the anterior part of the posterior limb of the internal capsule and terminate in the anterior horn cells of the spinal cord.

Ares 8 is situated in the frontal gyrus and is involved in movements of the head and eye. Broca's area is also situated in the frontal lobe. It controls the movement of the muscles of tongue, lips and larynx.

Area 4S, called the suppressor band, is in front of area 4 and is involved in the control of tone of various muscles of the body, It is a part of reticulospinal tract, which is a part of extrapyramidal system.

Area 6, which is also called the premotor area, controls rhythmic cordinate movements of tongue, lips, larynx, pharynx and mandible which are necessary for chewing, swallowing, licking, grunting, etc. Area 6 forms a part of the extrapyramidal system.

Sensory Area: The sensory area of cerebral cortex includes postcentral gyrus, which receives impulses of light touch and pain.

The lingual gyrus in the occipital lobe is the visuosensory are receiving impulses of vision. The audiosensory impulses are received by areas in the temporal lobe. The impulses of taste are received in the postcentral gyrus. The smell area is located at the uncinate and hippocampal gyri.

Association Areas: These areas are located in the frontal lobe and the junction of parental, occipital and temporal lobe, and are connected to thalamus and hypothalamus by afferent and efferent fibers.

Stimulation of the frontal association are produces all the effects of the activity of the autonomic system. The impulses pass to the hypothalamus which controls all autonomic activities. The frontal association area is the seat of memory, intelligence, moral sense and social sense of an individual.

Limbic System

The term limbic system is applied to that part of the brain that consists of a rim of cortical tissue around the hilus and a group of associated deep structures such as the amygdala the hippocampus and the septal nuclei. It is mainly concerned with emotional expression and genesis of emotions. A small part of the limbic system is concerned with smell.

The afferent and efferent connections of limbic system form a closed circuit, called as Papez circuit.

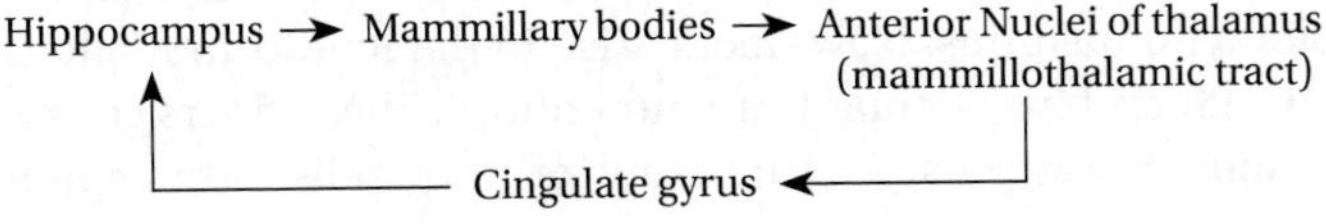

It has few connections with the neocortex, i.e. neocortical activity modifies the emotional behavior and vice versa. However, emotion cannot be turned on and off at will.

Another characteristic of the limbic system is the prolonged after-discharge following stimulation. This may explain in part the fact that emotional responses are generally prolonged than the stimuli that initiate them.

Functions

- The limbic system is concerned with autonomic responses in addition to role in olfaction. Along with hypothalamus, it is also concerned with sexual behavior, emotions of rage and fear and motivation.
- The autonomic responses produced are the changes in blood pressure and respiration.
- The stimulation of amygdala produces activities related with feeding (licking, chewing, etc.). Lesions produce moderate hyperphagia with indiscriminate ingestion of all kinds of food, also called as omniphagia.

Sexual Behavior

Mating is a basic but complex phenomenon, in which many parts of the nervous system are involved. The behavioral components, accompanying a series of spinal reflexes in the act (i.e. urge), and the coordinate sequence of events are regulated in the limbic system.

The basic responses are innate, so are present in all mammals, but learning plays a role in the mating behaviors. In humans, the sexual functions have become extensively encephalized and conditioned by social and psychic factors.

Relation with Endocrine Function

In primates, removal of gonads decreases sexual activity but hormonal administration revives the activity. Even the administration of hormone of opposite sex produces the sexual activity of same sex. Why that occurs is not yet clear.

In human female the removal of ovaries or menopause does not decrease libido, probably due to encephalization of sexual functions. Though the administration of hormones does increase the sexual activity.

In animals, lesions of limbic system in pyriform cortex or amygdala cause a marked intensification of sexual activity. Maternal behavior is depressed by the lesions of the cingulate gyrus.

Fear and rage are closely related emotions and mainly affected by limbic system. The external manifestations of fear, the avoidance reaction and rage (attack reaction), can be produced by the stimulation of hypothalamus.

Normally a balance is maintained between rage and its opposite, i.e. placidity. This balance can be disturbed by the lesion of amygdala and causes a state of abnormal placidity, and this state can be changed to a state of rage by destroying the ventromedian nucleus of hypothalamus.

It can be said that limbic system is the visceral brain for the higher control of autonomic activity, particularly that associated with emotions (like fear, grief, etc.).

Thalamus

Thalamus is a mass of gray matter which lies on the either side of the third ventricle. It is intimately interconnected with the cortex of frontal lobe and all sensory impulses after relaying in thalamus pass forward to cortex.

Functions

- By virtue of its connections with prefrontal cortex and hypothalamus, it is a reflex center concerned with emotional exteriorization.
- Prefrontal lobes are linked up with thalamus and hypothalamus by so many fibers passing in both directions that they together constitute an integrated nervous complex for higher intellectual activities, personality imotional affects and social behaviors,
- Thalamus is a part of the closed circuit (cortex-thalamus cortex), probably important in seizure generlization,
- Lession of thalamus results in ataxia, slowness of movement, and diminished muscle tone to the opposite side of the body.
- The thalamus relays skin, muscle and taste afferents to the postcentral cortex.
- The thalamus is an organ for sensation and the cerebral cortex is an organ for perception.
- Because of its to and fro connections with corpus striatum, lesion of the thalamus produces spontaneous movements (choreoathetosis).
- Thalamus is a relay station for visual and auditory impulses.

Hypothalamus

It is situated underneath the thalamus and forms a part of the wall and floor of the third ventricle. It has a blood supply six times richer than the cortex. It is concerned with integrated control of autonomic nervous system.

Functions

- It controls the secretion of posterior pituitary (ADH and oxytocin).
- It controls the secretion of anterior pituitary (ACTH, TSH, gonadotropins); hence is involved in the maintenance of the reproductive cycle of females.
- It controls the activity of autonomic nervous system (ANS). The stimulation of hypothalamus results in rise of blood pressure, secretion of adrenaline, quickening of the heart rate, cardiac slowing, and increased gastric and duodenal secretions (may result in gastric ulcer).
- It is the main center for regulation of temperature. Hypothalamus can modify muscular activity, sweat secretion, cutaneous circulation and pulmonary circulation.
- It is concerned with sleep. Mammillary body, located in the hypothalamus, is the center for sleep.
- Hypothalamus constitutes a part of the extrapyramidal facilitatory pathway. Lesions in the hypothalamus produce poverty of movement (which is a characteristic sign of Parkinson's disease).
- Along with thalamus, it is an important center for controlling emotional exteriorization.
- Along with limbic cortex and thalamus, it controls higher intellectual activities such as personality, emotional affects and social behaviors.
- Lesion in the hypothalamus can cause disturbance in carbohydrate and fat metabolism, and in sexual function.
- It is a site for hunger and satiety, and hence is implicated in obesity.
- Hypothalamus is a biological clock; it maintains the circadian rhythm.
- It also controls the gastric acid secretion.

Corpus Striatum

The corpus striatum consists of gray matter situated at the base of each hemisphere, in close relation to the internal capsule. It contains several nuclei called the basal ganglia. The anterior limb of internal capsule divides the striatum into two parts; the gray matter lying medially is the caudate nucleus and the gray matter lying external to internal capsule is the lentiform nucleus.

The lentiform nucleus is subdivided into two parts: the outer one is called the putamen and the inner one is called globus pallidus.

Caudate nucleus receives inhibitory fibers from the cerebral cortex. New fibers start here, which go to the thalamus. This circuit is involved in muscle tone. Stimulation decreases muscle tone and muscular contractions.

Fibers arising from the premotor area of the cerebral cortex are relayed to the globus pallidus and putamen, and go to hypothalamus. New fibers arise in the lentiform nucleus, which end in reticular formation nuclei. These fibers convey excitatory impulses to the anterior horn cells of the spinal cord.

Putamen and caudate nucleus receive afferents form thalamus and motor areas of cerebral cortex, and from brainstem. Efferents from these nuclei constitute nigrostriatal pathway and from globus pallidus efferent go to thalamus, subthalamic body, red nucleus and reticular formation, and substantia nigra.

The examples of lesions here include Parkinson's disease, encephalitis lethargica, and progressive lenticular degeneration.

The characteristic features of such lesions are:

- Striatal rigidity, due to increased tone (interruption of inhibitory pathway).
- Muscular weakness, due to interruption of the facilitatory pathways; the muscles get easily fatigued as a result of slight exhaustion.
- Involuntary muscular tremors of arms, hands or fingers due to some abnormal pattern of activity in reticulospinal pathways.
- Loss of facial emotional expression.

Internal Capsule

It is formed by fibers of great motor and sensory pathways, which link the cerebral cortex with the brainstem and spinal cord. In this part, the nerve fibers are closely packed together as they pass between the islands of gray matter. Thrombosis of the artery supplying the internal capsule may lead to hemiplegia (paralysis of muscles of opposite side) or hemianesthesia (loss of sensation on the opposite side).

The Autonomic Nervous System

The autonomic nervous system (ANS) is dependent on the central nervous system, with which it is connected by afferent and efferent nerves.

The ANS deals mainly with involuntary or automatic control of viscera. So, it is also called as the involuntary or visceral or vegetative nervous system, subdivided into two parts:

1. Sympathetic system, and
2. Parasympathetic system.

Sympathetic System

It lies in front of the vertebral column, and is associated and connected to the spinal cord by nerve fibers consisting of:

- 3 pairs of cervical ganglia.
- 3 pairs of thoracic ganglia.
- 4 pairs of lumbar ganglia.
- 4 pairs of sacral ganglia.
- The ganglia which reach the front of coccyx.
- Sympathetic plexuses
  - Cardiac plexus to heart and lungs.
  - Celiac plexus to organs of abdominal cavity.
  - Mesenteric plexus to organs of the pelvis.

The sympathetic nervous system is a double chain of ganglionated cords, extending from the base of skull and ending up in pelvis. These ganglia are intimately connected with CNS through spinal cord, by means of communicating branches which pass outwards from the cord to ganglia and inwards from ganglia to cord.

Table 6: Example of autonomic functions

Organ	*Action increased by*	*Action decreased by*
Heart	Sympathetic increase the table and force	Vagus decreases the rate and force
Bronchi	Vagus constricts	Sympathetics dilate
Stomach	Vagus constricts	Sympathetics dilate
Bladder	Sacral autonomic nerves contract	Sympathetics relax
Pupils	2nd cranial autonomic contract	Sympathetics dilate

Functions of Sympathetic System

- Supplies innervation to muscles of heart, involuntary muscles of all blood vessels and muscles of visceral organs, such as stomach, pancreas and intestine.
- Supplies motor secretory fibers to the sweat glands, and motor fibers to the involuntary muscles of the skin.
- Maintains tone of all muscles, including the tone of voluntary muscles.

Parasympathetic System

It consists of cranial autonomic nerves and sacral autonomic nerves.

Cranial Autonomic Nerve Fibers

- 3rd cranial nerve (oculomotor) reaches iris, and pupil of eye.
- 7th cranial nerve (facial) reaches face.
- 9th cranial nerve (glossopharyngeal) reaches the salivary glands.
- 10th cranial nerve (vagus) has wide distribution; it supplies many glands and organs such as, heart, airway, and upper part of CIT.

Sacral Autonomic Nerve Fibers

They pass out from the sacral region of spinal cord and form the nerves to pelvic viscera and together with sympathetic nerves form the plexuses which supply colon, rectum and bladder.

Majority of the organs have a dual supply of both sympathetic and parasympathetic nerves each acting in antagonism to the other. In other words, the activity of the organs being stimulated by one set of nerves is retarded or inhibited by the other set of nerves (Table 6).

44.3 NEUROPATHOLOGY

Sunila Chadda

INTRODUCTION

This chapter describe the neuropathological findings in a spectrum of psychiatric conditions, including the dementias. Neuropathology constitutes that branch of the clinical neuroscience which has traditionally achieved diagnoses of brain diseases by means of macroscopic and microscopic examination of the brain. It is currently a rapidly expanding discipline in which neuropathologists are beginning to implement molecular pathological methods in routine diagnosis, as well as maintaining active participation in research. There developments are providing new insights into the etiology and pathogenesis of many brain diseases, particularly the dementias. Despite this evidence of progress, some of the major psychoses continue to present a major challenge to neuropathology in that it has so far proved impossible to identify a cellular basis of disease.

It may be difficult to achieve a precise clinicopathological correlation for an individual patient with psychiatric symptoms, for a variety of reasons. First, although most dementing illnesses are associated with characteristic pathological lesions in the brain, a minority of demented patients may show very little in the brain, a minority of demented patients may show very little in the way of specific pathology. It is also puzzling to note that other individuals who have retained normal cognitive function until the end of life are found at postmortem examination to display remarkably advanced pathology of a type usually associated with dementia. Added to this are the complexities which emerged as a consequence of the frequent occurrence of mixed pathology in older patients. Several different diseases of the brain may apparently coexist in a single individual, and current thinking is forcing a reappraisal of the comorbidity of neurodegenerative conditions. Rather than merely coincidental coexistence, it is now held that some mixed pathology may represent synergy between particular neurodegenerative diseases.

It is undoubtedly true that there have been considerable advances in the neuropathological definition both of well-defined conditions such as Alzheimer's disease and of newer entities identified among the movement disorders. This progress in neuropathology could not have happened in isolation. Developments in cell- and tissue based methods in histopathology have occurred alongside major advances in neuroimaging, neurochemistry, neuropharmacology and molecular genetics as well as insights gained from the study of transgenic animals. There combined approaches have certainly highlighted certain disorders which appear to be the conventional distinctions between diagnostic categories in the psychiatric disease spectrum. They also point to the possibilities of new approaches to the assessment and classification of diseases of the brain. The lessons of history suggest the present dogma will surely change in the light of expanding knowledge. This applies to neuropathology particularly in those challenging areas of psychiatry in which neuropathology has had so little to offer. This chapter describes which may be detected in patients with psychiatric diseases.

RELATIONSHIP OF NEUROPATHOLOGY WITH PSYCHIATRY AND OTHER ALLIED DISCIPLINES

In examining the nature of these relationships, it is pertinent to ask what has been the contribution of neuropathology to the understanding of psychiatric disease up to the present time and which challenges remain outstanding at the outset of the 21st century. The potential division between these two disciplines is embodied in the view that neuropathology focuses on diseases of the brain while psychiatry is concerned with diseases of the mind. This notion has been explored recently by Lishman (1995), who came to the conclusion that neuropathology does indeed have much to offer in the field of psychiatry. The connection is both historic and contemporary. Neuropathology is based firmly in the traditions of classic neuroanatomy and saw the first clear delineation of some of those disorders which present with dementia, including general paralysis of the insane which was still common at that time. However, it was not until the start of the 20th century that neuropathology began to contribute significantly to the understanding of brain diseases. Alzheimer first described in the 1920s the neuropathology of the dementing illness now known by his name. Parkinsons's disease and Creutzfeldt-Jakob disease (CJD) were examined and characterized in the first half of the 20th century. However, other major disorders such as dementia with Lewy bodies (DLB) were recognized only quite recently.

As more and more brain diseases were subjected to microscopic secutiny by neuropathologists, this kind of analysis came to be seen as a standard of diagnosis against which others had to be measured. Inevitably neuropathology has fallen short of this high expectation in some significant areas of psychiatry but has had most to offer in the field of organic brain diseases, where there has been considerable and accelerating progress in the last two decades. Specialized techniques have been developed which are able to identity and localize specific proteins and DNA sequences within tissues and cells, thus generating a much more detailed view of brain pathology than that obtained through more traditional staining methods. A multidisciplinary approach has ensured that on the one hand molecular genetics has informal recent neuropathology searches while on the other the identification of novel pathological features has sometimes prompted the discovery research. A genuine explosion of knowledge has resulted which points the way to appropriate treatment strategies, particularly in the field of dementias.

DEVELOPMENT AND AGING OF THE BRAIN-PRESYMPTOMATIC PATHOLOGY

Development

The brain and spinal cord are formed in the embryo largely from cells derived from the progenitor neuroectoderm of the neural tube. Neuroectodermal cells give rise to neurons, astrocytes and oligodendroglia. The process of orderly cell division, migration, differentiation and outgrowth of processes is orchestrated by a variety of growth factors, notably platelet-derived growth factor A & B, transforming growth factor alpha and insulin-like growth factor. Bone-marrow-derived microglias invade the neural tube during early fetal life, and blood vessels grow into the developing nervous system from the surrounding mesoderm. Vascularization of the developing nervous system provides the opportunity for hormones and other blood-borne proteins to modulate differentiation. Many cells fail to completer the maturation process successfully, and are removed by a process of programmed cell and functions, characterized by their location, connections and transmitters. Astrocytes and oligodendroglia are also sophisticated cells which turn over slowly in normal circumstances. The process of development of the CNS continues in postnatal life, and only in late adolescence or early adult life can brain development be considered complete. There are some aspects of development which are directly relevant to the state of the central nervous system (CNS) in later life and particularly in relation to neurodegenerative disease. Among these are the putative roles of growth factors in ongoing neurotrophic support for aging nerve cells and the possibility that the recently recognized stem cells still present in the adult brain may retain full differentiation capacity. The implications of these findings for repair and regeneration in the mature brain are far clear but will become so with future research.

Aging Changes

Neurodegenerative disease which target particular subsets of nerve cells within the brain and spinal cord are devastating in their effect precisely because fully differentiated neurons are post-mitotic cells which, according to current thinking, are not replaced when lost. However, aging of the individual and of the brain does not invariably result shrinkage or atrophy with increasing age. Although this has been attributed in the past to neuronal loss, a more likely basis is now thought to be white matter shrinkage. Neuronal counts appear to be generally well preserved in the cortex in simple aging, although neuronal loss does occur in the substantia nigra of the brainstem. However, more subtle changes of neuronal atrophy and reduced functional integrity, combined with a loss in plasticity, may contribute significantly to declining brain function.

Most aged brains display changes in the vascular system which includes atheroma of the major vessels and small vessel hyalinization. These vascular abnormalities are frequently associated with small and large infarcts, which contribute to cognitive impairment in old age. However, minor degrees of vascular pathology in the brain should probably be considered as part of normal aging. Neuronal changes associated with aging include increasing accumulation of lipofuscin and ubiquitin. The expression of lipofuscin, a lysosomal associated pigment, is associated with cellular aging for reasons which are unclear. While it may partly reflect the metabolic waste disposal systems of long-lived cells, the fact that lipofuscin may appear during childhood in certain neuronal groups such as the olivary nucleus of the brainstem suggests that the causes many be more complex. Never cells and their processes also accumulate a protein known as ubiquitin during aging. As its name suggests, ubiquitin is a protein expressed in many cell types but which is not normally detectable in any significant amount in individual cells. Ubiquitin expression is certainly increased in normal aging but this process is accentuated in a number of neurodegenerative disease, particularly in the form of ubiquitin positive inclusions which may be intranuclear or intracytoplasmic. Astrocytes also show aging changes and upregulate their expression of glial fibrillary acidic protein (GFAP). Corpora amylacea are round amorphous basophilic bodies consisting largely of glycoprotein, which accumulate within the processes of astrocytes, particularly at the interface of brain tissue with the pia mater and ependyma, and around blood vessels. Microglial cells also display increasing activation in older subjects.

The concept has been advanced that aging changes may represent a step toward symptomatic neurodegenerative disease because they code the so-called brain reserve, coupled with the motion that diseases become clinically evident when there is a decline below a certain critical functional threshold. It is likely that a number of different insults might combine to accelerate this process toward the emergence of symptoms. The likely contribution of genetic factors to age-related phenotypic expression of disease is well illustrated by the observation that in Huntington's disease the greater the deviation from normal in the Huntington gene the earlier the diseases become apparent in the affected individual.

More generally, mRNA transcription is likely to become less reliable with aging such that proteins are generated which are less amenable to normal degradation and turnover.

Careful analysis suggests that most of the amyloid plaques seen in such individual are diffuse and made up of non-fibrillary amyloid. There considerable debate as to whether the presence of small number of neuritic plaques or of Lewy bodies is merely a feature of aging or whether these lesions are always pathological. Weight of opinion has now swung toward considering that these lesions do represent a presymptomatic phase of one or other of the common neurodegenerative diseases.

Although the brain atrophy somewhat with increasing age, the onset of specific pathology is not an inevitable consequence of aging. There are some individuals who remain cognitively intact and who display no neurodegenerative pathology even in extreme old age. As presently understood, these individuals are genetically well endowed to resist the onslaught of neurodegenerative diseases and have escaped, or have endured successfully, those environmental triggers which also predispose promote healthy brain aging could make a substantial contribution to the well-being of old age.

ANATOMY AND PATHOLOGY OF THE DEMENTIAS

Definition and Prevalence of Dementia

The many definitions of dementia have in common the motion that affected suffer deterioration of higher intellectual function while consciousness is preserved, and that the condition is relentlessly progressive. The deterioration encompass a number of cognitive deficits including memory impairment and impaired executive functioning and may be allied with specific problems such as aphasia, apraxia and agnosia. The dementing illnesses are largely conditions of later life occurring in middle and old age. In large surveys based both in hospital and in the community, the prevalence of dementia rises from between 5% and 10% of the population age 65 years and over to nearer 30% of those who have reached the age of 85 years and over. Given that individuals with dementia often survive for up to 10 years, the burden on families and on society is clearly very large. The encouraging fact is that a much larger proportion of elderly people remain relatively cognitively intact and are able to lead an independent life so far as their mental faculties are concerned.

The causes of dementia are many and include not just the common neurodegenerative diseases such as Alzheimer's disease (AD), but also infections, neoplasms, metabolic and other derangements of the CNS . Conversely, not all neurodegenerative diseases are necessarily accompanied by cognitive impairment. For instance may individuals with Parkinson's disease or motor neuron disease remain intellectually intact.

REGIONAL BRAIN INVOLVEMENT IN THE DEMENTING ILLNESS

No part of the brain is entirely exempt from involvement in one or other of the dementias, reflecting the range of causes and of the attendant signs and symptoms. Given the extent of gray matter which is involved in cognitive functions, and the white matter tracts which connect the different centers, it is hardly surprising that many different pathological conditions in the brain interfere with cognitive function. Inspection of the intact brain clearly identifies the involvement of the frontal and temporal lobes in certain diseases, while in others the occipital and parietal lobes may also appear atrophic, leading to a globally shrunken brain. The neuroanatomical features of the brain are considered elsewhere in this volume but in the present context, it is useful to confirm that while the major dementing illnesses result from pathology in the neocortex, in others the most obvious pathology is within the basal ganglia or thalami or even in the brainstem (Box 1). It is not surprising that in basal ganglionic diseases, dementia is frequently accompanied by movement disorders reflecting

Box 1: Main causes of dementia, cognitive decline and personality change

Neurodegenerative
- AD (15% Familial)
- DLB
- Pick's
- CBD
- PSP

Genetic
- Huntington's disease
- Familia AD
- Familial prion diseases

Developmental

Trauma
- Head injury, particularly repetitive (e.g. boxing)

Vascular
- Multi-infarct dementia and stroke
- Chronic subdural hematoma
- Binswanger's disease
- Amyloid angiopathy

Infective
- HIV/AIDS
- Prion diseases, including, CID (15% also genetic)
- Progressive multifocal leukoencephalopathy (JC virus)

Metabolic
- Alcohol abuse
- Drug misuse
- Hepatic encephalopathy

Neoplastic
- Frontal lobe tumors benign or malignant

Abbreviations: AD, Alzheimer's disease; CBD corticobasal degeneration; CJD, Creutzfeldt-Jakob disease; DLB, dementia with Lewy bodies; HIV/AIDS, human immunodeficiency virus/acquired immune deficiency syndrome; PSP, progressive supranuclear palsy.

the functional implications of damage to deep gray matter. Bilateral pathology in any component of the limbic system, including the hippocampus, temporal and entorhinal cortex, dentate gyrus, fimbria, mamillary bodies, thalamus, amygdale and the cingulated cortex, will lead to significant cognitive impairment. Even of the cerebellum, which may show significant pathology in many of the prion disease, has been implicated in cognitive function.

DIAGNOSIS OF DEMENTIA AND UNDERLYING PROTEINOPATHIES

Careful review of the clinical and family history, with the help of someone close to the patient if cognitive impairment is pronounced, usually leads to a likely diagnosis when the results of a full physical examination are taken into account. Neuroimaging may pinpoint focal lesions such as tumors, subdural hematomas and infarcts, as well as providing information on less specific but no less significant conditions such as brain atrophy. Atrophy is reflected in ventricular enlargement and sulcal widening, or diffuse white matter shrinkage. History of the progression of cognitive impairment will reveal whether this has been a steady or stepwise decline. Other significant factors in the history include the occupation and level of education, previous head injury, alcohol or drug intake, and infections of the CNS, while general examination may reveal a likely predisposing factor for, or symptom of, neurodegeneration. These signs would include vascular disease and high blood pressure, liver disease and the disease progresses and may remain so until the postmortem examination. More than one pathology may be present in the brain, giving rise to a potentially confusing clinical picture. The pathological diagnosis of dementias has evolved considerably in recent years. Comprehensive sampling of the brain, with exploratory immunocytochemistry as well as routine staining, is required to establish the diagnosis. Neuropathologists have come to realize that what for them may be a single diagnosis with a particular range of microscopic abnormalities may present with a wide diagnosis extremely difficult in life. A good example of this is the condition known as corticobasal degeneration.

It is now clear that many of the major neurodegenerative diseases actually represent disorders of protein metabolism in which the neurodegeneration is associated with the accumulation of insoluble deposits of protein within and between cells. Significantly advanced the understanding of neurodegenerative disorders, and is not merely of theoretical interest but also has implications for therapy. The major proteins to be deposited in the brain in this context are β amyloid (βA4), phosphorylated tau, α synuclein and prion protein. Because ubiquitin binds to proteins scheduled for degradation, many insoluble deposits are also ubiquitinated, Immunocytochemistry using antibodies specific for each of these accumulating proteins is a standard method for protein identification and localization in cells and tissues and is now indispensable in the neuropathological categorization of disease. Disorders in which an abnormal prtein is deposited are known as proteinopathies and include the amyloidopathies, tauopathies, synucleinopathies and prion disorders Table 1). Not all of these disorders result in cognitive impairment, depending on which neuronal systems are maximally affected.

Beta-Amyloidopathies

βA4 is derived from a normal transmembrane protein, β amyloid precursor protein (APP), coded from the corresponding gene on chromosome 21. The normal processing of APP involves cleavage by an α secretase which releases that portion of APP which is external to the cell in a secreted form of APP. The β amyloidogenic fragment of APP straddles the cleavage site at which α secretase operates. By definition therefore, the cleavage of APP produced by α secretase prevents the formation of an intact β amyloid fragment. In contrast, two further enzymes know as β and γ secretase target respectively expressed in neurons. The amyloidogenic fragment of APP gives rise to Aβ1-40 or Aβ1-42, depending on the β amyloid deposits seen in AD and are preferentially formed within the Golgi apparatus during intracellular tracking of the APP molecule. The β amyloidopathies include not only AD but also the associated vascular disorder of amyloid angiopathy.

Tauopathies

Hyperphosphorylated tau protein is another important insoluble protein deposited not only in AD but also in a wider spectrum of neurodegenerative diseases now defined as tauopathies. Most disease in this group display only tau positive inclusions, but AD is unusual in showing both tau and βA4 amyloid positive inclusions and deposits, thus qualifying as both a tauopathy and an amyloidopathy. Tau protein is one of the cytoplasmic microtubule associated proteins which neuronal cytoplasm. Consequently, tau is intimately concerned with the function of axonal transport and stabilization of neuronal shape and structure, and is found in axons throughout the nervous system. Other functions, including signal transduction, tau are known to exist, normally derived by alternative splicing from a gene on chromosome 17 and their distribution around the brain. The normal tau subtypes are further characterized by the presence of absence of inserts in the N-terminal and a repeat within the C-terminal. Phosphorylation of these normal tau isoform is a key step associated with neurodegeneration. Hyperphosphorylation of all isoforms is characteristic of AD, but in other tauopathies the reasons for tau aggregation are less well understood. Abnormally accumulating tau may be detected in neuritis, neuritic plaques, and in neurofibrillary tangles. In some diseases it is found also in glial cells. The different phosphorylated tau proteins are easily distinguished by Western blots, and the six isoforms found in AD form characteristic triplets. These aggregate into paired helical filaments which form the basis of neurofibrillary tangles (NFTs). Other tauopathies, including pick's disease, display a phosphorylated tau doublet of 60 and 64 kDa on Western blots, whereas corticobasal degeneration (CBD) and progressive supranuclear palsy (PSP) are both characterized by a doublet of 64 and 68 kDa. The differing tau molecular sequences form the background to the abnormal phosphorylation pattern seen in the different conditions included here. They also give rise to slightly different aggregated paired helical filaments which paired helical filaments are straight in PSP but are twisted is CBD.

Synucleinopathies

Alpha synuclein is a presynaptic protein encoded by a gene on chromosome 4 and maximally expressed in the gray matter. The role of α synuclein is normally associated with transfer of neurotransmitter vesicles to synapse, but its contribution to the generation of disease is poorly understood as yet. Certainly, α synuclein accumulates in the form of neuronal inclusions known as Lewy bodies which are found in Parkinson's disease and DLB. Lewy bodies are probably not in more likely than the classic inclusions to be harmful to neurons. Apart from Lewy body diseases, those disorders which form variants of multiple system atrophy display widespread α synuclein inclusions, particularly in glial cells (Dickson et al. 1999). Diseases which display α synuclein positive inclusion bodies have been designated the synucleinopathies.

DISORDERS MANIFESTING AS DEMENTIA

Alzheimer's Disease

This condition is characterized by a dementia of insidious onset and slow progression ultimately leading to death 10 years or more after the onset of the disorder. Although usually found in elderly individuals and of late onset, the characteristic neuropathological features of this condition were first described by Alzheimer in a woman in her fifties. Subjects who develop AD generally display a period of memory impairment preceding the onset of unambiguous dementia. AD is the most frequent cause of dementia, although its prevalence is variable, the estimates being sometimes confounded by methodological problems. Best estimates of the prevalence of AD are up to 10% of the population over 65 years, which clearly represents the vast majority of those affected by dementia individuals show AD pathology, either with other brain pathology or in isolation. Approximately 10% of cases of AD are familial. While AD is said to be uncommon in African and Asian population this may be more to do with decreased life expectancy in less affluent societies than with genuine ethnic differences in prevalence .

In AD the brain shows generalized atrophy with compensatory dilatation of the ventricular system. Atrophy is most pronounced in the frontal and temporal lobes. Microscopic evidence of pathology may be maximal in the medial temporal lobes but certainly involve the neocortex in other lobes of the brain, including the neocortex in other lobes of the brain, including the occipital lobes (although those display less overt atrophy). At the microscopic level, the lesions of AD characteristically comprise amyloid plaques, neurofibrillary tangles (NFTs), neuronal and synaptic loss, astrocytosis and microgliosis. These lesions are found at greatest density in a characteristic distribution involving the medial hippocampus, including the entrohinal cortex, the amygdala, and the neocortex of the occipital, frontal and temporal lobes. Amyloid depostis and NFTs may also be conspicuous in the basal ganglia, thalamic and even in the sustantia nigra, although the amyloid deposits in this location are of a more diffuse form than the complex neuritic plaques found in the neocortex in AD. Define plaques are made up of non-fibrillary amyloid whereas neuritic plaques contain a high proportion of amyloid fibrils. While conventional straining with hematoxylin cession be strongly suggestive of the presence of AD lesions special stains are required to demonstrate the full burden amyloid deposits and NFTs. Traditionally, a silver stain has generally been assessed on the basis Bielschowsky staining. Alternative silver methods include Gallyas and Bodian strains. Thioflavine staining is useful since the reagent fluoresces at the site of amyloid deposition, as congo red. Latterly, immunocytochemical techniques have been used for the specific demonstration of amyloid deposits (antibody to βA4 amylodi) and of NFTs (antibody to phosphorylated tau).

Amyloid plaques are extracellular accumulations of insoluble fibrillary and non-fribrillary material composed of βA4 amyloid. These microscopic deposits are of several different types. Neuritic plaques are composed of amyloid aggregates, often with a compact amyloid core, which are intersperse with, and surrounded by, expanded and damaged neuritic processes with associated astrocytic and microglial reactions. Diffuse plaques consist only of amorphous deposits of non-fibrillary amyloid lacking the neuritic and glial elements. Blood vessels within the gray matter and in the subarachnoid space may also accumulate βA4 within their walls, particularly if the burden of amyloid plaques is high in the neocortex. Occasionally only the dense amyliod core persists, and this lesion has been classically only the dense amyloid core persists, and this lesion has been classified as a burnt out plaque. It is generally supposed that amyloid deposits evolve from the diffuse to the neuritic form with advancing disease.

All amyloid plaques are visualized by immunocyto-chemical techniques which employ antibodies to βA4, and the AB42-43 molecular form of amyloid is particularly prevalent in plaques. Although β amyloid is predominant, other molecules also accumulate in plaques, including APP, alpha-1 antichymotrypsin, apolipoprotein E (ApoE). Complement and ubiquitin, as well as molecules associated with neuritis, including tau protein, neurofilaments, synaptophysin and neurotransmitters. Amyloid promotes the deposition of ubiquitin. Neuritic plaques are more characteristically found in the neocortex than in subcortical gray matter in AD, but those seen in the basal ganglia are generally diffuse. Vascular amyloid deposition is largely restricted to the cortex and subarachnoid space, sparing the white matter, and is present in the majority of cases of AD but may also occur in individuals who lack the other pathology of AD. This isolated pathology of blood vessels constitutes the condition known as cerebral amyloid angiopathy, which is associated with an increased risk of cerebral hemorrhage. The myeloid which is laid down in vessels is AB1-40.

Nerofibrillary tangles are intraneuronal aggregations of paired helical filaments largely composed of insoluble tau protein. Failure of normal tau to bind to microtubules may lead to hyperphosphorylation, and this in turn is associated with the development of paired helical filaments made up of protein strands of between 10 nm and 20 nm in diameter displaying regular constrictions which contribute to the twisted appearance of the helical strands. Unlike amyloid plaques, NFTs are often laminar in distribution in the neocortex. In AD, NFTs probably appear first in the CAL sector of the cornu ammonis, subiculum and entorhinal cortex of the medial temporal lobe. The amygdale is also involved. As AD progresses, NFTs involve more and more of the temporal cortex. The insular cortex and the cingulate gyri display NFTs in the large neurons of layer two as well as in deeper cortical layers in the worst affected areas. Glutamatergic neurons appear to be more vulnerable to NFTs than those using γ aminobutyric acid (GABA) or calbindin. NFTs may also be found in neurons within the basal ganglia, thalami and substantia nigra in advanced AD. Well-formed NFTs are visible with conventional staining and are generally flame shaped in the cytoplasm of pyramidal neurons in the cortex, whereas those in the midline structures, including the brainstem, are less angular in form. NFTs are rather basophilic on conventional H&E staining.

The presence of NFTs within neuronal cytoplasm indicates a profound derangement of neuronal function. Many affected neurons die and disappear in advanced stages of diseases, leaving the insoluble tangle as the only visible residue of the neuron it occupied previously. These ghost tangles may be very numerous in the hippocampus. NFTs and neuritic plaques are both highlighted by tau immunocytochemistry . Individual tau positive neuritic threads become increasingly prominent in late stages of AD. NFTs are not specific for AD, being found in aged non-demand subjects as well as in other neurodegenerative disease detailed below. However, if NFTs are present predominantly in the neocortex, and are accompanied by a heavy burden of β amyloid plaques, these lesions together are, a sufficient neuropathological substrate to substantiate a clinical diagnosis of AD. There is considerable evidence to suggest that number of amyloid plaques. Rare dementias are characterized by present of NFTs virtually in isolation in a form of tangel predominant dementia. Dementia pugilistica associated with a history of boxing, displays a preponderance of NFTs, although diffuse plaques and evidence of cerebrovascular disease may be present.

Neuronal loss is a prominent feature in late-state AD, and the neocortex frequently shows astrocytosis and many activated microglia, particularly in association with amyloid plaques. The mode of neuronal death is unclear, Beta amyloid is known from in-vitro experiments to be neurotoxic. Neuronal apoptosis has been implicated in AD following the demonstration of caspase 3 activation in response to the presence of amyloid both in vitro and in animal models. Caspase 3 activation is an important stage the apoptotic pathway and marks an irreversible commitment to the process of cell death. However, its demonstration in human AD cortex has not been well validated, and the contribution of apoptotic neuronal death to the atrophy seen in AD remains to be determined. Neuronal dysfunction and synaptic loss are more likely to be the key events underlying cognitive decline, and actual neuronal death may well be a late event. Understanding the pathogenesis of this process, particularly the initial trigger events, is vital for devising effective treatment strategies.

Hirano bodies are brightly eosinophilic rod-shaped neuronal inclusions composed of actin together with other proteins. They are seen best in the hippocampus along with granulovacuolar degeneration which may represent lysosomal accumulations degeneration which may represent lysosomal accumulations within neuronal cytoplasm. The clinical significance of these two microscopic features is not clear. Their distribution is considerably more limited than that of NFTs and amyloid deposits, and it is the latter two lesions which are used to grade the severity of the pathology in AD.

The loss of cholinergic neurons in AD, particularly in the temporal cortex, is confirmed by a measurable decline in acetylcholine in the cortex and by the clinical response, at least in some patients, to anticholinesterase agents given therapeutically. Cholinergic neurons are also lost in the nucleus of Meyner in the basal forebrain. Adrenergic neurons within the locus coeruleus in the brainstem are also likely to be depleted in AD.

The pathological diagnosis of AD depends on crucial assessment of a variety of brain sections for the presence of NFTs and amyloid plaques. The fact that these may be present in small numbers in non-demented aged subjects can cause diagnostic difficulty. Various histological staging schemes have been devised to address this problem and to ensure greater uniformity. The first of these was devised by Khachaturian (1985), based on a quantitative assessment of amyloid plaques in the brain. From 1988, the Consortium to Establish a Registry for Alzheimer's Disease CERAD) sought to refine thought to be suffering from AD, and 8 non-cemented controls, CERAD assessed the number of neuritic plaques based on the examination of five areas of the cortex, namely the middle frontal gyrus, the superior and middle temporal gyri, the inferior pariental lobule, the hippocampus and the entorhinal cortex, as well as the midbrain, including the substantia nigra. The CERAD criteria are listed in Box 2. The Bielschowsky silver stain was chosen for the comparative study since this method displayed neuritic plaques particularly well. Antibodies to β amyloid were also used but, this immunocytochemical technique decorated both diffuse and neuritic plaques, there was some difficulty in distinguishing between the two. While the clinical significance of the two types of assess neurotic plaques, which were coded as spares, moderate or frequent. When the age of the patient and the clinical history of dementia were taken into account, the investigators were able to stratify the diagnosis for an individual patient as definite, probable or possible AD based on the neuropathological findings.

Pathogenesis

The causes of AD are not known, although a number of risk factors have been recognized which are of help in understanding he pathogenesis. Among the factors linked to an increased risk of developing AD are older age, certain genetic factors such as ApoE ε4, a history of head injury, and a poorer level of education. There is some evidence of gender imbalance in the women generally survive longer with AD than do men, and hormone replacement therapy is emerging as potentially shown in patients of long-term anti-inflammatory treatment, in whom the risk of developing AD appears to be halved. This protective effect of anti-inflammation in the genesis of AD. Microglial activation and pro-inflammatory cytokine production are both characteristic of AD. Certain alleles of the interleukin 1 (1L-1) polymorphism, particularly 1L/1A/2, appear to be linked to an increased risk of sporadic AD.

Subject Down syndrome show precocious development of AD-type pathology and tend to develop widespread amyloid deposits by their fourth decade , which has been attributed to triple gene dose effect for APP, since this gene is found on chromosome 21. For reasons that are less clear, subjects with Down syndrome also have a tendency for premature development of NFTs. Apart from trisomy 21, mutations in the APP gene are associated with some familial cases of AD. Other genes which have been linked to early-onset familial AD are presenilin 1 (on chromosome 14) and presenilin 2 (on chromosome 1). Mutations are not present in the more common sporadic cases but these are influenced by the different alleles of the ApoE polymorphism (on chromosome 19). The ApoE ε4 alleles of the ApoE polymorphism (on chromosome 19). The ApoE ε4 allele is associated with an increased risk of late-onset AD, being over represented in cohorts of AD patients (Saunders 2000), whereas the most common allele, ε3, and the least common, ε2, do not show this association. In fact ApoE ε2 may be protective in regard to vulnerability to AD. It seems likely that possession of ApoE ε4 hastens the onset or AD in individuals who are susceptible for other reasons. However, ApoE ε4 is not necessarily predictive for AD, in that some individuals reach advanced old age while remaining cognitively intact despite having an ε4/4 genotype. The function of ApoE in the brain is not completely understood, although there is clearly some interaction with APP. Individuals possessing one or more ApoE ε4 alleles are more likely than those without to form amyloid deposits, and this has been well shown following head injury. Head injury is a known risk for AD, and the mechanism may be linked to deposition of β amyloid following APP upregulation, particularly in individuals with ApoE ε4 genotype. In contrast to AD, investigation of subjects with amyloid angiopathy appears to show overrepresentation of ApoE ε4 genotype. In contrast to AD, investigation of subjects with amyliod angiopathy appears to show overrepresentation ApoE ε2. A link between ApoE genotype and propensity for developing amyloid plaques is supported by studies of NFT-rich dementia occurring in very elderly subjects. Affected individuals have very few amyloid deposits and show a correspondingly low prevalence of ApoE ε4 allele.

Other pathogenetic mechanisms which have been implicated in AD include oxidative damage and withdrawal of neurotrophic factors, but the evidence for these mechanisms is not yet well substantiated. Cerebral hypoperfusion associated with vascular disease has been proposes as a common pathogenetic mechanism for AD.

Box 2: Consortium to Establish a Registry for Alzheimer's Disease (CERAD) criteria for diagnosis of Alzheimer's disease

- Brain weight
- Distribution of atrophy
- State of vessels
- Lacunar and large infarcts
- Pallor of substantia nigra
- Assessment of amyloid plaque density (various cortical areas including hippocampus, entorhinal cortex and Lewy bodies

DEMENTIA WITH LEWY BODIES

Patients with DLB display a fluctuating cortical dementia, usually but not always with some features of parkinsonism, which tends to be accompanied by hallucinations. This condition may be confused in life with multi-infarct dementia and indeed may coexist with it. Autopsy studies have established the presence of cortical Lewy body pathology in up to 25% of elderly demented patients with or without coexisting AD pathology. The causes of both Parkinson's disease and DLB remain elusive.

Lewy bodies are intracytoplasmic inclusions which were first identified in substantia nigra neurons in Parkinson's disease but are also present in other neuronal collections within the bainstem. However, approximately 10% of Parkinson's disease patients also develop increasing cognitive impairment amounting to dementia. When such patients come to autopsy a wider search in the cortex reveals the presence of neuronal cytoplasmic inclusions which are similar to, although not as obvious as, those in substantia nigra neurons, and these rounded inclusions are known as cortical Lewy bodies. Cortical Lewy bodies distend the cytoplasm and distort the nucleus, resulting in neuronal degeneration, but individual neurons are not markedly swollen. A major contribution to the understanding of Parkinson's disease was made with the discovery that these inclusions are largely composed of α synuclein, a presynaptic protein normally expressed in neurons. Cortical Lewy bodies are generally found in the deeper cortical layers of the temporal and cingulated gyri of the temporal and frontal lobes, often with associated spongiform change. Lewy bodies may be found in the amygdala and less commonly in the particle and occipital cortex. Lewy bodies also stain positively with ubiquitin since this protein is involved in the degradation of α synuclein and of parkin, another protein contributing to the pathogenesis of familial Parkinson's disease.

Small numbers of cortical Lewy bodies are frequently found in association with Parkinson's disease but appear to be subclinical. The dementing illness known as dementia with Lewy bodies is associated with large numbers of cortical Lewy bodies. There is an intriguing association with AD. The coexistence of AD and DLB has suggested to some that DLB is no more than one form of AD. Alternatively the two conditions may even be synergistic and each may promote the progression of the other. The exact nature of the relationship between the two pathologies remains to be elucidated.

VASCULAR DEMENTIAS

Individuals with evidence of vascular disease may display a stepwise deterioration of cognitive function in old age which in the absence of other neurodegenerative disease constitutes a vascular dementia.

Dementia associated with cerebrovascular disease is not generally associated with deposition of abnormal protein, with the exception of amyloid angiopathy. In terms of prevalence of the condition, vascular dementia is similar in importance to AD and DLB. Evidence of white-matter pathology associated with small-vessel disease is common and has been reported in up to half of all patients with AD. The exact prevalence of vascular dementia is difficult to determine. A recent study revealed cerebrovascular pathology in 78% of 209 community-based autopsies in 85-year-old individuals. The presence of cerebrovascular disease significantly enhanced the likelihood of dementia occurring in patients with early Alzheimer pathology. The notion that AD may be primarily a vascular disorder has also been advanced. In practice, some degree of vascular disease is frequently found together with the pathology of these two primary neurodegenerative diseases.

Changes in larger cerebral vessels is common in aging, leading to luminal narrowing and erosion of their smooth lining, with a consequent increased tendency for mural or occlusive thrombosis. Another common change is hyalinization of the walls of smaller vessels, which renders them inelastic. These vascular conditions separately or together may significantly compromise the blood supply to the brain occlusion of a major vessel supplying the brain tissue. Sometimes this sudden clinical event is followed by the appearance of overt dementia. It is supposed that the dementia represents the cumulative result of the immediately preceding brain injury and previous episodes of minor brain damage. In some individuals diagnosed with multi-infract dementia there may be no recollected episode of clinical stroke. Any condition which gives rise to multiple emboli to the brain, e.g. atrial fibrillation, may contribute to the onset of significant cognitive impairment. Vascular disease leads to significant loss of the white mater due to perivascular degeneration of tissue amounting to small lacunar infarcts. This is thought to be a sufficient substrate for dementia even in the absence of AD pathology, although there are as yet no agreed criteria for quantifying the extent and severity of vascular abnormality in the CNS.

Binswager's disease is a form of vascular brain damage which is not well understood. It appears to involve greater myelin loss in the cortical white matter than may be accounted for simply as a result of microinfarction, but some do regard it as an extensive form of lacunar infarction. Both lacunar infarcts and Binswager's disease are associated with hypertension and result in loss of white matter with compensatory dilatation of the ventricular system.

RARER DEMENTIAS

In this category are included a number of neurodegenerative conditions which have been characterized much more recently and are less common than AD. Most of these conditions are associated with the deposition of abnormal tau protein. Although tau inclusions are found most commonly in AD is also characterized by heavy deposits of β-amyloid as described previously. In the group of disorders considered in this section, tau inclusions are prominent in the absence of amyloid deposition. The disorders include Pick's disease, progressive supranuclear palsy (PSI), corticorbasal degeneration (CBD) and frontotemporal dementia with Parkinsonism associated with chromosome 17 (FTDP-17).

PSP has been known in the past as the Steele Richardson-Olszewski syndrome. Although each of these condition may display characteristic and distinctive pathological appearances there is in proactive a spectrum of pathology and clinical symtomatology spanning the tau-associated neurodegenerative disease (tauopathies), which may make exact diagnosis difficult.

Recent, developments in genetic analysis and characterization of the tau subtype which is expressed in the individual brain have proved to be of the most importance in clarifying the nature of the neurodegenerative condition in an individual patient. The different tau-associated neurodegenerative conditions may be distinguished on Western blots. Pick's disease is characterized by bands of 60 and 64 kDa phosphorylated tau, whereas PSP and CBD display bands of 64 and 68 kDa. In contrast, the phosphorylated tau of AD has a characteristic triple pattern of 60, 64 and 68 kDa.

Pick's disease was first described more than a hundred years ago, preceding the description of AD, and characterized by frontal lobe signs in the context of progressive dementia. This disorder may have come to attention relatively early in the study old dementias because its onset is at a somewhat younger age, usually in early middle life, and because of the characteristic extreme degree of brain atrophy. Most cases are sporadic and display a very striking frontal and temporal lobar atrophy which contrast markedly with the apparent macroscopic preservation of the remaining cortical structures. On closer examination the cerebral hemispheres may be asymmetric, with the atrophy affecting one side more than the other and with variable involvement of the basal ganglia leading to atrophy in these structures. The pathology of Pick's disease is characterized by the presence of swollen cortical neurons containing round inclusions or pick bodies. The presence of Pick bodies is frequently associated with spongiform change in the cortex and astrocytosis. These inclusions stain positively with the temporal lobe both in the granule and in the pyramidal cell as well as neurons of basal ganglia and periaqueductal gray matter. Neuronal loss may be found in the substantia nigra. Occasional tau-positive inclusions are also noted in glial cells in Pick's disease.

A familial form of Pick's inclusions but which has been described which also displays typical Pick inclusions but which has intriguing links to FTDP-17. Both disease show marked frontal and temporal lobar atrophy and are familial, but the microscopic pathology in FTDP-17 is of intraneuronal NFTs rather than Pick bodies. FTDP-17 commonly displays asymmetrical atrophy of the frontal lobe with corresponding loss of frontal lobe function, language deficits and Parkinsonism. Mutations of the tau gene have been detected in association with this condition, and the resulting tau deposits are widely distributed through the brain. Although this familial form of frontotemporal dementia is rare, it is of great interest in helping to elucidate the role of phosphorylated tau in neurodegenerative conditions. Mulated tau has an impaired ability to interact normally with microtubules, and NFTs are found in neurons while tau-positive inclusions are found in cells.

Progressive supranuclear palsy (PSP) presents as a movement disorder with cognitive impairment together with some rigidity and poverty of movement but without tremor, supranuclear gaze palsy is usually present. Although lobar atrophy is not seen macroscopically, there may be visible degeneration of the globus pallidus, periaqueductal gray matter, substantia nigra and lower brainstem nuclei, where neuronal loss and gliosis are also detected. The tau positive NFTs in the stem tend to be spherical or non-angulated, and are known as globose tangel. Tau-positive inclusions are characteristically prominent in glial cells, whose process takes on a tufted appearance. Microscopic involvement of the neocortex usually underlies the observed cognitive impairment. The tau of PSP displays a 64 and 68 kDa doulet on Westerm blot, and mutations of the tau gene are not generally detected. Coexistent pathology including that of AD and Parkinson's disease, as well as infarcts, may be present more often than expected.

Coticobasal degeneration (CBD) is primarily a pathological diagnosis which may underlie a range of symptomatology which includes cognitive impairment and movement disorder resistant to levodopa. Asymmetric cortical atrophy is generally present, and there may be white-matter and basal ganglionic degeneration as well as brainstem involvement. The substantia nigra is usually pale. The characteristic microscopic feature is the presence of very swollen or ballooned neurons with granular tau-positive inclusions in neurons and in neuritic threads. These are so abundant as to impart a brownish hue to the white matter naked-eye inspection. The Western blot pattern for tau protein is similar to that in PSP in that a 64 and 68 kDa doublet is seen. The condition may be sporadic or familial.

A familial dementia has been described in association with myoclonus and with mutations in the gene encoding the neuronal protein neuroserpin. The underlying neuropathology includes neuronal inclusions which stain positively with antineuroserpin pathy.

Acquired dementias are seen in some patients who are addicted to alcohol, and these include Korsakoff's psychosis. Apart from in the mammillary bodies and hypothalamus and which are preventable by thiamine, there is evidence for more widespread cortical atrophy and white matter loss in some alcoholics are an important component of the limbic system and are reduced in size in AD as well as in Wernicke's encephalopathy. The reasons for differences between alcoholics in cortical and white mater vulnerability, such that some become cognitively impaired while to involve genetic factors. Astrocytes in the basal ganglia and brainstem gray matter may display characteristically enlarged, pale and irregular nuclei, the change being know as Alzheimer II astrocytosis and associated with encephalopathy.

PRION DISEASE

Since the first description of Creutzfeldt-Jakob disease (CID) in the 1920s, this group of disorders has attracted attention to a degree which appears disproportionate to their prevalence of approximately 1 case per million of the population worldwide. The preoccupation with prion disorders is justified in that these dementing disorders may be both transmitted and inherited, although up to 90% are in fact sporadic with no evidence for either factor being the cause. The clinical features of sporadic CID characteristically include rapidly progressive dementia, myoclonus and periodic spike sin the electroencephalogram, in patients almost always over 50 years. However, the clinical diagnosis of CID is frequently suspected in individuals who subsequently prove to have AD, DLB, Pick's disease, paraneoplastic, syndrome or almost any other elementing condition.

Prion disorders are classified (Box 3) according to whether they are sporadic, dominantly inherited or acquired, and similar diseases are encountered in animals, notably scrape in sheep. Most prion diseases are characterized by the presence of immunocytochemically demonstrable prion protein which accumulates as an insoluble amyloid product within brain tissue. Resulting cell loss and astrocytosis may be profound and give rise to spongiform degeneration within the gray matter. The disease associated prion protein (PrP^{sc}) is derived from the normal form prp^{s}) by a post-translational conformational change. Prp^{s} is a cell surface protein encoded by a gene on chromosome 20 and expressed at high level in neurons but whose function is not yet understood. The fact that these diseases are also transmissible has been appreciated in scientific circles for many decades. Brain tissue from individual suffering from prion disorders is capable of transmitting the disease if injected into, or ingested by, a secondary host of the some or other susceptible species. Investigation of this phenomenon has rule out the presence of any conventional micro-organism, and the transmissible.

Cerebral cortex from a patient with sporadic Creutzfeldt-Jakob disease, displaying spongiform change throughout the layers of the cortex. Hematoxylin and eosin, original magnification x25 agent appear to be largely, if not entirely, made up of prion protein.

Prion disorders, and particularly CID, came to widespread public attention with the appearance of variant CID (vCID) in the wake of the UK epidemic of bovine spongiform encephalopathy. The total number of vCID cases has remained less than originally feared (Brown et al 2001). Affected individuals have generally become symptomatic at a younger age than patients with the sporadic form and have presented with a vague history of psychiatric and emotional disturbance prior to deterioration into a state of akinetic mutism. The reasons for the differences in clinical presentation between sporadic CID and vCID are not entirely clear, although the slower progression and the psychiatric presentation in the latter may reflect the more consistent involvement of basal ganglionic structures and the different form of the prion agent involved.

Box 3: Classification of prion diseases

Sporadic
- Creutzfeldt-Jakob disease (CID)
- Sporadic a fatal insomnia

Inherited
- Familia CID
- Gerstmann-Straussler-Scheinker syndrome
- Fatal familial insomnia

Acquired
- Kuru
- Iatrogenic (growth hormone and dural/corneal transplants)
- Variant CID

While the pattern of spongiform pathology and prion distribution is variable in sporadic CID, the histological appearances of vCID are uniformly predictable and consist of widespread florid prion plaques in the cortex. The cerebellum shows a particularly heavy load of prion protein. Reliable laboratory methods to detect PrP^{sc} in tissues include immunocytochemistry, histoblots and Western blots. These are useful in distinguishing CID from other dementias which may be associated with cortical spongiform change, including DLB and motor neuron disease with dementia. There is no reliable clinical test for detecting vCID in the early stage, when mild personality changes may be reported, and it remains a matter of urgency to develop such diagnostic tools. Increased signal in the thalamic pulvinar on magnetic resonance imaging is now used as one of the criteria of vCID, but this is not always present early in the disease and is not a feature of sporadic CID. Brain biopsy may be useful in confirming vCID, which predictably involves all of the cerebral cortex, in contrast to sporadic CID, in which the focal nature of the cortical changes renders biopsy unreliable. Biopsy may also exclude a treatable cause of dementia. However, surgical instruments have to be destroyed after the biopsy procedure because of the danger of transmitting infection. Detection of the 14-3-3 protein in cerebrospinal fluid is helpful but is not specific. Tonsillar tissue and gut-associated lymphoid tissue probably contain detectable prion protein before the onset of symptoms, but biopsy of these tissues is not a practicable option in all young people with new onset of psychiatric symptoms. Development of a suitable clinical test would have the advantages. While there is no evidence in sporadic CID that the agent is present in the blood, remains a possibility surgical instruments represent the chief concerns for the transmission of human prion disease during healthcare. As yet are no effective treatments for these conditions.

Mutations in the PrP gene, best known at codons 102, 178 and 210, are important factors in inherited prion, disease, but to mutation is present in sporadic CID or vCID. The natural valine/methionine polymorphism at codon 129 influences the phenotype of the disease as well as having an apparent effect on vulnerability. All patients with vCID have been methionine homozygotes up to the present time, and homozygous codon 129 is overrepresented among patients with sporadic CID.

HIV/AIDS

Soon after the onset of the AIDS epidemic, it became apparent that cognitive impairment often amounting to dementia was prominent complication of HIV/AIDS. The combination of a dementing illness with motor problems was designated the AIDS dementia complex (ADC) in the early 1980S. The pathological substrate for this was partially characterized in 1985 when giant cells were identified as the pathognomonic feature of HIV-related infection of the brain (HIV encephalitis. However, the advancing immune suppression which characterizes HIV/AIDS also predisposed to a variety of opportunistic infections and CNS lymphoma. Before the advent of effective combinations chemotherapy which can halt the decline into advanced immuosuppression. HIV encephalitis was present in up to 40% of subjects with AIDS and frequently accompanied by opportunistic conditions in the brain. Some of these, particularly cytomegalovirus encephalitis, progressive multifocal leukoencephalopathy and CNS lymphoma, could give rise to cognitive impairment in their own right.

The exact relationship between HIV encephalitis and dementia remains poorly understood despite considerable research. The two conditions may be discordant but, of HIV encephalitis and a high viral burden within brain tissue. HIV targets microglial cells and macrophages within the CNS through CD4 and chemokine cell surface receptors. Infected microglia probably give rise to giant cell. There is no general agreement that neurons, oligodendrocytes or endothelia evidence that astrocytes are restrictedly infected. Considerable neuronal loss is found in AIDS dementia, with evidence of synaptic, dendritic and axonal damage in HIV encephalitis, all leading to brain atrophy. Since neurons are not thought to be a direct target for HIV infection, neurotoxicity in HIV encephalitis may result from viral proteins **(gp120 and tat),** glutamate, free radicals or nitric oxide, but the favoured theory to proinflammatory cytokines **(TNF**α **and 1L -1**β**)** released by activated microglial cells and macrophages. Deprivation of neurotrophic factors and toxic molecules leaking across a deficient blood-brain barrier have also been implicated.

Combined antiretroviral therapy including protease inhibitors is effective in ameliorating or preventing HIV-associated dementia (HAD). However, it is clear that subtle neuropsychological impairment may still occur in treated subjects. Whether this relates to lingering inflammation within the brain is not known at present.

HUNTINGTON'S DISEASE

This autosomal-dominant condition was first described by George Huntington at the end of the 19th century. The initial presentation is usually with abnormal choreiform movements, which are followed by dementia. However, younger patients may first present with poverty of movement and rigidity, or an early disturbance of neuropsychological functions. The hyperkinetic form has been linked to maternal transmission. The disease cause atrophy and much more marked atrophy of the basal ganglia. Neuronal loss is detectable in the cerebral cortex but is maximal in the caudate nucleus and putamen, where microglia activation and severe astrocytosis are also found. The loss of GABA-containing spiny neurons in the caudated and putamen, which project to the lateral globus pallidus, results in decreased inhibitory control of the thalamic nuclei (Via subthalamic nuclei, medical globus pallidus and substantia nigra reticularis), which in turn increase their glutamatergic output to the cerebral cortex, leading to choreiform movements.

Following the identification of the Huntington gene of the short arm of chromosome 4, the inherited abnormality has been traced to a variable expansion in a trinucleotide triplet sequence, this expansion leading to accumulation of polyglutamine within the brain. Longer repeats are linked to earlier onset of the disease. The way in which this genetic abnormality is translated into brain specific cellular pathology is unknown despite intensive study and the development of transgenic mouse models. While it is clear that abnormal hunting gives rise to ubiquitin-positive intranuclear inclusions, the presence of these inclusions is not clearly linked to numerous inclusions, whereas they are sparse in the badly affected basal ganglia. It is also unclear why the systemic expression of hunting does not lead to disruption of cellular function in other tissues.

PATHOLOGY OF PSYCHOSES

Schizophrenia

Although there may be diagnostic overlap between schizophrenia and bipolar disorder, the diagnostic criteria are sufficiently distinctive at the two ends of the spectrum to allow for separate investigation of the epidemiology, causation and neuropathology of these disorders. Each of these disorders has a prevalence of about 1% of the population.

The pathological basis of schizophrenia has been singularly difficult to study. The disease has its onset in young adult life and affected individuals are likely to have had symptoms, and been treated with appropriate drug therapy, for a number of years. Neuroimaging studies have clearly identified ventricular dilatation present not only prior to the onset of treatment, but which may also antedate the onset of symptoms. The ventricular dilatation is accompanied by cortical diminution, particularly in the medial temporal lobe. Early stage of the disease correlates with decreased brain weight.

The identification of families with several affected individuals points to like genetic factors(s) predisposing to the condition and has allowed detection of at-risk individuals in the preclinical state. Although the responsible genetic factors are only now becoming clearer, this has not prevented longitudinal clinical and neuroimaging studies of risk of family members, which have established the presymptomatic characteristics. Some neuroimaging work also reveals that the two hemispheres are usually less asymmetrical than usual. This curious finding appears to represent a loss of the asymmetry which normally exists between cerebral hemispheres and which first appears during fetal life and suggests a very early onset for the structural abnormality which underlies the later appearance of schizopohrenia. Pathology studies have been supportive of a fetal origin. Neuronal arborization abnormalities rather than reduced neuronal number may underlie the cortical changes. The dorsal thalamus is also smaller than normal. Cortical cytoarchitectural abnormalities have been reported, but further studies are needed to substantiate these. Whether the primary defect is of genetic origin or the result of in-utero environmental influences remains controversial. Recent findings suggest that further neuroimaging abnormalities may be added to the earlier changes as the disorder progresses but this has yet to be replicated.

Bipolar Disorders

Ventricular dilatation with accompanying sulcal widening is also present in individuals presenting with mood disorder. Studies of untreated patients with bipolar disorder suggest reduced levels of serotonin metabolites in the raphe nuclei and the limbic system, implicating the serotonergic system in the pathogenesis, although results have been contradictory . Abnormalities in the size of the amygdale have been reported on neuroimaging. Identification of susceptibility genes for bipolar disorder which were different from those implicated in schizophrenia would support the view that these are independent entities. Bornavirus is reportedly detected more commonly in brain tissue of patients with major depression than in control healthy populations, but these findings may represent technical artifacts and await confirmation. There have been very few neuropathological studies of this male predominant psychiatric condition which usually presents in childhood. The ventricles do not appear to be enlarged in this condition and the brain has been various reported as normal or as enlarged, while there may also be focal atrophy in the parietal lobe and in the cerebellum. The number of brains examined precludes a reliable view of the neuropathological basis of such tissue from patients with disorders such as these which arise in childhood is obviously problematic.

CURRENT DEVELOPMENTS IN NEUROPATHOLOGY

Correlation with Neuroimaging

Although sophisticated neuroimaging is an almost routine part of the investigation of cognitive decline in current times, it is important to remember that none of these benefits were available just over two decades age. Before that time, accurate estimation of ventricular size or brain tissue volume was rarely possible in life. The clinical benefits of computerized tomography (CT), magnetic resonance imaging (MRI) and functional imaging have been enormous, and their potential in further research is by no means exhausted. It is salutary to note, however, that while MRI can instantly differentiate an ischaemic from a haemorrhage stroke the images still contain elements which have not yet yield to neuropathological correlation. These include the hyperintense white-matter foci seem on T2-weighted images in a wide variety of brain disorders.

Neuroimaging both serves and challenges the discipline of neuropathology. While imaging may confirm the global and lobar atrophy which is an expected element of many neurodegenerative conditions, it may also generate conditions-specific results which are consistently present and which require investigation. One example of this is the high signal seen on MRI in that part of the posterior part of the thalamus known as the pulvinar, in cases of vCID. Although this sign is now recognized as part of the diagnostic criteria, the exact pathological substrate remains to be determined; however, astrogliosis is a characteristic feature. The neuroimaging abnormalities in Schizophrenia and bipolar disorders are also evolving. A loss of the normal asymmetry between cerebral hemispheres, particularly in the temporal lobes, is now well known in Schizophrenia. An interesting recent development in AD research is the discovery that ApoE variants influence not only the hippocampal volume but also the degree of asymmetry, according to the different alleles. Functional imaging also provides insights into the pathogenesis of brain disorders. Using cell- and receptor-specific ligands, it is possible to highlight particular brain cell subsets. This approach has revealed that activated microglia appear early in the AD disease process and may not be a merely reactive phenomenon.

There are of course limitations to the diagnostic capabilities of neuroimaging. For instance, although ventricular dilatation and reduced periventricular white-matter signal intensity have been attributed by HIV encephalitis, these appearances are actually noninfections or lymphoma.

MOLECULAR DIAGNOSTICS

Psychiatric disease are occasionally the result of a single gene exerting an effect in isolation, and studies of families with many affected members have identified multations which direct attenuation to a likely role for particular gene-protein combinations in the causation of disease. Examples include APP and presenilin mutations in familial early-onset AD. Much more frequently, genes of small effect increase or decrease only slightly the genes of small effect increase or decrease only slightly their vulnerability of an individual to a particular disorder. The best known example of this phenomenon is the ε4 allele of the ApoE gene while there has been huge progress and a significant number of important gene discoveries in respect of AD, it is now clearer than even that sporadic AD results from the interaction of number of different genes which certainly include APP, presenilin-1 and presenilin-2 and ApoE ε4. Others for which there is mounting evidence include interlenrin-1 (1L-1α) and α1 macroglobution. A number of different mutations have been described in the presenilin-1 gene on chromosome 14. Presenilin-2 was subsequently located to chromosome 1, and mutations in this gene are a less common cause of autosomal-dominant AD. Research in the molecular biology of AD suggests that the preseniling may equate with γ secretase, which generates amyloid peptide from APP. Very rarely, mutations in the plaques are largely composed of AB42. With respect to the more common late-onset AD, individuals who are destined to develop the disease at an earlier age than those with non-ApoE γ secretase, which generates amyloid peptide from APP. Very rarely, mutation in the APP gen give rise to familial AD. In each of these cases the plaques are largely composed of AB42. With respect to the more common late-onset AD, individual who are prone to develop AD and who possess ApoE ε4 alleles appear to develop the disease at an earlier age than those with non-Apo-E4 genotypes. Well over half the population. Conversely not all individuals with an ApoE ε4/4 genotype develop AD, which suggests that other gene(s), as yet undiscovered, may be as important for disease susceptibility.

Beta amyloid appears to be central to the pathogenesis of AD. It is now know that the amyloidogenic peptide AB is produced under normal circumstances and is present in serum and CSF but is normally catabolized by an endopeptidase, inhibition of which accelerates AB4 deposition. The normal processing and degradation of proteins is the focus of much current research, with emphasis on extracellular protease and intracellular proteaes and aggresomal pathways. It is certainly possible that abnormal protein accumulation is the result of poor degradation as much as overproduction. Molecular neuropathology has made great strides in the field of tau metabolism, and tau immunocytochemistry has widended the focus in neurodegenerative disease beyond neuronal pathology. Tau-positive glial inclusions should not be regarded purely as an adjuvant to the pathological subclassfication of the tauopathies, and the contribution of glial pathology urgent further investigation.

CHARACTERIZATION OF ANIMAL MODELS

For some disease that affects the human nervous system, a naturally occurring animal model has long been known. Scrapple in sheep is a well-known of affected humans. Animals have also neuropathology to that of affected humans. Animals have also been used in transmissibility and pathogenesis studies in prion diseases and other infective diseases caused by retroviruses resembling HIV. However, it is the development of transgenic animals which has made the most significant contribution to the understanding of CNS disease processes. For instance, ubiquiting-positive nuclear inclusions were first identified in transgenic model of Huntington's disease which lead to their discovery in human diseases and the identification of related trinucleotide repeat disorders. Transgenic animal models have been used to elucidate not only the role of genetic mutations in AD and the metabolic relationships of β-amyloid and tau protein but also to investigate the therapeutic possibilities. Immunization of human APP transgenic mice with human AB peptide has been shown to reduction in behavioral impairment. Remarkably, antibodies to amyloid peptide administered peripherally to transgenetic mice can enter the brain and also induce clearance of β amyloid. Current and future research is likely to solve the remaining uncertainties regarding the exact relationship between β amyloid and tau pathology in AD.

CONCLUSION

The last two decades have seen major advances in the neuropathology of psychiatric disease, particularly the dementing illnesses. Neuropathology encompasses both a diagnostic and a research role, which is responsive to progress in other disciplines or itself provides the lead. Careful clinicopathological correlation will continue to be a cornerstone of further development in the endeavor to understand while on the one hand a single neuropathological entity such as the pathological lesions of corticobasal degeneration may have diverse clinical symptoms. Studies of this kind will help to elucidate the proximate cause of cognitive decline in patients who have pathology in their brains.

New approaches are challenging long-held concepts of particular pathologenetic pathways. The recognition that AD is less common in individuals who have been treated long-term with anti-inflammatory drugs raises the possibility that inflammation is a key pathogenetic factor, possibly through activation of microglia and perivascular macrophages, with consequent upregulation of cytokine release within the brain. This cascade is remarkably reminiscent of HIV-associated dementia. Similarly, reclassification of AD as a vascular dementia may be an unexpected development but in questioning current thinking, may open fresh lines of inquiry. Other long-held concepts being challenged include the dogma that neurodegeneration is extremely limited in adult life. The discovery of stem cells hold out the hope for regeneration of functional neuronal circuits possibly by transplantation but also by recruitment from and endogenous source. Before that can occur, the effects of deleterious genes and of environmental insults on the CNS stem cell population will further. Differentiation and functional transformation of already committed cells might also be a future goal. Closet to realization should be the proper understanding of disease processes which still present gaps in knowledge, e.g. the accumulation and intracellular processing in Huntington's disease. On a wider front, if it became clear that the presence of one pathology such as AD influenced or accelerated the development of another neurodegenerative condition, for instance DLB, this would be significant information in the quest for effective strategies to prevent or halt the progression of neurodegenerative diseases. Symptomatology may be further complicated by comorbid systemic disease affecting the brain, such as thyrotoxicosis, underlining the requirement to assets the whole patient.

Comparison between different neurodegenerative disorders may also yield insights. It is instructive to compare prion diseases with amyloidopathies such as AD, although transmissibility of β amyloid, unlike prions, has not been confirmed. Both disorders are commonly sporadic but are familial in 10–15% of cases; both are amyloidopathies, although the amyloid is made up of prion protein in the one and βA4 in the other, and both are associated with microglial inflammation. In each case surface precursor protein whose function is not yet understood. The difference appears to be that APP gives rise to βA4 far more readily than the corresponding change from a normal cell surface precursor protein whose function is not yet understood. The difference appears to be that APP gives rise to βA4 far more readily than the corresponding change from PrP^{sc}. However, both events probably occur within the endosome system after internalisation if the relevant cell surface molecule.

Developing classifications of dementia will legitimately be based on disorders of protein metabolism at least in part because of implications for therapy carefully planned. Pathological investigation of transgenic animals and of many human brain diseases, which remain largely speculative at present, is important. Understanding the steps in the pathway offers a real opportunity for devising new therapies which may ameliorate symptoms to prevent further deterioration. Prevention would allow healthy brain aging to be achieved. This may be seen as a goal which is relevant only to societies which are sufficiently affluent to be trouble by the disease of old age. In fact the burden of psychiatric disease is very heavy worldwide, and comparative studies are needed particularly with respect to ethnic and environmental influences which are likely to have an important influence.

44.4 NEUROPHARMACOLOGY

AP Dadhich

BRAIN ANATOMY

Impulses in neurons are transmitted by liberation of specific chemical substances, known as *neurotransmitters*. They are classified in to three types:

1. Monoamines, such as
   i. Catecholamines: Norepinephrine and epinephrine
   ii. Serotonin
   iii. Histamine
   iv. Acetylcholine
2. Neuropeptides, such as
   i. Thyrotropin releasing hormone (TRH)
   ii. Somatostatin
   iii. Neurotensin
   iv. Neuromedin N
   v. Corticotropin releasing factor (CRF)
   vi. Opioid peptides: enkephalins and endorphins
3. Amino acids, such as
   i. L-glutamate
   ii. L-aspartate
   iii. Gamma aminobutyric acid (GABA)
   iv. Glycine.

Brain consists of billions of neurons, which are integrated for performing various functions, such as cognition, affect and conation.

Neurotransmitter liberated from one neuron acts on the specific structure of the adjacent neuron (known as receptor) to elicit the action. The junction of two neurons is a synapse, with the space in between known as synaptic cleft. However, some other chemical substances are liberated from non-synaptic sites, which can change the effect by increasing or decreasing the responses of the neurotransmitters, and are known as *neuromodulators* (such as prostaglandins, interleukins, some neuropeptides and amino acids). There are certain agents which act as second messengers in mediating inter- and intracellular events, and are known as *neuromediators* (such as cyclic AMP and cyclic GMP).[1] Many times, a neuron liberates a chemical substance in the blood which acts in a hormonal manner to act on some distant neuronal receptor; it is known as *neurohormone*. Most of the peptides are included in this category.

To know the neurotransmission, it is essential to know the various parts of the brain responsible for processing the different information, their retention and their expressions. Brain is a complex organ, with different parts to perform different activities.

Cerebral Cortex

The two cerebral hemispheres are the largest parts of the brain, known as cortex. They are anatomically divided into frontal, temporal, parietal and occipital lobes, which are responsible for performing different functions, including somatosensory, visual, auditory and motor. The cerebral cortex has an uniform laminar appearance with in a local region. There are columnar sets of approximately 100 vertically connected neurons to form an elemental processing module. The specialized functions of cortical region are performed by the interplay by the module of connections among other regions of the cortex (cortico-cortical systems) and non-cortical areas (subcortical systems), linked to larger information processing.[2] These columnar bundles of neurons are interconnected and form the cortical areas termed as *association areas*. These areas receive information from primary cortical sensory regions, to produce higher cortical functions such as thoughts, memory, judgement and consciousness. They also have a role in conducting supervisory control over the autonomic nervous system, including cardiovascular and gastrointestinal activities, and integrate the somatic and vegetative functions.[3]

Limbic System

It consists of hippocampus, amygdaloid complex, septum, olfactory nuclei, basal ganglia and nuclei of diencephalon arranged at the subcortical border of the brain. They mainly perform the motivational and emotional functions. The parts of limbic system, such as the basal ganglia, neostriatum (caudate nucleus, putamen, globuspallidus and lentiform nucleus) form the essential part of the extrapyramidal motor system. Any damage to this system affects the involuntary movements of the body and produces extrapyramidal symptoms, including tremors and rigidity. Hippocampus is an essential part of the brain, responsible for formation of recent memory. Bilateral damage to this part produces marked recent memory disturbance.[4]

Diencephalon

It consists of the thalamus, situated in the center of the brain (under the cortex and the basal ganglia) and above the hypothalamus. The neurons of the thalamus are arranged into clusters or nuclei. These nuclei act as a relay between the incoming sensory pathway and the cortex. It has regulatory control on visceral functions, aphagia, adipsia and general sensory responses.

Hypothalamus

The hypothalamus is the main integrating part for the autonomic nervous system of the body. It also regulates the important functions of the body, such as regulation of the body temperature, water balance, intermediatory metabolism, blood pressure, sexual functions, circadian cycles of various physiological functions such as pituitary adrenocorticotrophic secretions, sleep and emotional reactions. These functions are mediated by individual hypothalamic nuclei and their interconnections.[5]

Midbrain and Brainstem

The mesencephalon, pons and medulla oblongata connect the cerebral cortex and thalamus-hypothalamus upwards and spinal cord downwards. This bridge consists of various important nuclei of cranial nerves and various incoming and outgoing tracts. This also contains reticular activating system, responsible for integration of the various sensory and motor activities of the body at periphery. Most of the neurons in these areas contain monoamines. This region is responsible for the central integration of reflex activity such as swallowing, vomiting, cardiovascular and respiratory system, and visceral afferent sensory information. Regulation of sleep, wakefulness, arousal and coordination of eye movements is performed by the reticular activating system. The neurons in these areas are more diffuse and non-specific.[6,7]

Cerebellum

It is situated at the posterior aspect of the pons, behind the cerebral hemispheres. It is a bilobular structure containing multiple folds projecting in to specific deep cerebellar nuclei to form motor cortex by way of the thalamus and the brainstem nuclei responsible for the vestibular functions (such as body position and posture). It is also responsible for maintaining the tone of antigravity musculature, providing continuous feedback during volitional movements of the trunk and extremities, and the visceral functions such as heart rate, and regulation of blood flow during change in posture.[2]

Spinal Cord

It runs from the caudal end of the medulla oblongata to the sacrum; it lies in the spinal canal of the vertebral column. It contains mass of nerve cells and tracts. The sensory informations from skin, muscles, joints and viscera are controlled locally in motor neurons and the primary sensory relay cells receive signals from higher levels. It contains various ascending and descending tracts with intersegmental connections. Sensory information flows in to the dorsal cord and motor impulses pass in the ventral portion. Preganglionic neurons lie in the intermediolateral column.

VARIOUS RECEPTORS: THEIR DISTRIBUTION AND FUNCTIONS IN CENTRAL NERVOUS SYSTEM

Cholinergic System

Cholinergic receptors are of two types: nicotinic and muscarinic. They are widely distributed in the CNS. Their main sites are in basal ganglia, forebrain, septohippocampal projection, striatum, nucleus accumbens and spinal motor neurons. Nicotinic receptors are present on the autonomic ganglia, widely distributed in CNS and in spinal cord. The muscarinic receptors are subdivided into M_1, M_2 and M_3 types. M_2 receptors are autoregulators. Cholinergic receptors are important in dementia, amnesia, Parkinson's disease, Huntington's chorea, convulsions and arousal. The neurotransmitter involved in cholinergic system is acetylcholine, synthesized by acetylation of choline in the neuronal cells, in the presence of the acetyl co-enzyme A catalyzing the reaction by choline acetyltransferase (CAT). Acetylcholine is stored in the vesicles in the neuronal cell and released in the synaptic cleft on neuronal stimulation and the ionic calcium also plays an important role in the release of the neurotransmitter. This transmitter reacts with the cholinergic receptor present on the surface of the adjoining neurons. After activating the receptor, it is hydrolyzed by cholinesterases and breaks down in to choline and acetic acid. This choline reappears in the synaptic cleft and is reutilized. Cholinergic neurons have a sodium-dependent uptake process for choline, which is the rate-limiting step controlling acetylcholine synthesis. The velocity of the transport process is dynamically regulated on the basis of the activity of the cholinergic neurons. Thus, the increased acetylcholine will stimulate the reuptake of choline and mechanisms of synthesis of acetylcholine. It reacts with the cholinergic receptor, which consists of proteins and has an high affinity to react with the cholinergic transmitter or cholinergic drugs to elicit the pharmacological action. Binding of the neurotransmitter with the receptor triggers a number of events affecting the neuronal activity.

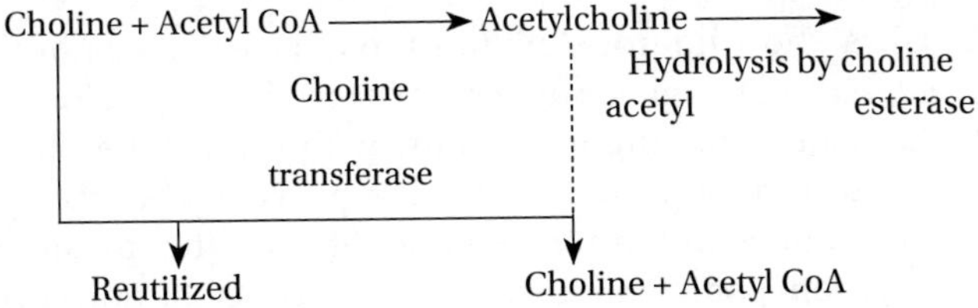

Adrenergic System

The main neurotransmitters are norepinephrine and epinephrine. Norepinephrine is synthesized in the neuronal cell, adrenal medulla and sympathetic nerve terminals from L-tyrosine, by the action of tyrosine hydroxylase and the action is catalyzed by ionic calcium to form levodopa, which undergoes decarboxylation to form dopamine and the action is catalyzed by pyridoxine phosphate. Further, dopamine is converted into norepinephrine by the action of dopamine β hydroxylase and the action is catalyzed by ionic calcium ascorbate and oxygen, which is stored in the neuronal cells and released on each stimulation to act on the adrenergic receptors present on the surface of the adjoining neuronal membrane and other cells. It is quickly oxidized by monoamine oxidase present intracellularly and catechol-O-methyl-transferase in plasma and converted in to 3-methoxy-4-hydroxy-mandelic acid and the inactive compound is excreted in urine.[1] The adrenergic receptors are of two types: alpha and beta, which are subdivided into α_1 situated postsynaptically and excitatory in nature. While α_2 are presynaptic autoregulatory and inhibitory in nature. Beta receptors are also of three types: β_1, β_2 and β_3, distributed on different structures and are usually inhibitory in nature. The effects of various adrenergic drugs and adrenergic nerve stimulation effects are mediated through these adrenergic receptors. They are mainly distributed selectively in pons, medulla oblongata, locus coeruleus, projections to cortex, hypothalamus, hippocampus and spinal cord (see Fig. 15). These receptors are responsible for control of emotions, mood, arousal, blood pressure, insomnia and hypertension.

Norepinephrine acts on the alpha receptors while epinephrine is agonistic for alpha and beta receptors. In central nervous system, there is a predominance of norepinephrine but epinephrine is also available, which is mainly synthesized in adrenal medulla.

On α_1 receptor, phenylephrine has a specific agonistic activity and prazosin has a specific antagonistic activity. Their effects are mediated through G-protein induced IP and DAG increased intracellular calcium.[8,9]

Clonidine is a selective agonist for α_2 receptor while yohimbine is selective antagonist for it. α_1 receptors are mostly post-synaptic excitatory in nature. The stimulation of presynaptic α_2 receptors leads to decreased release of norepinephrine from the nerve terminals. In CNS, there is more predominance of α_2 receptors. The effects of α_2 receptors are mediated by G-protein induced inhibition of adenyl cyclase, leading to decreased synthesis of cAMP. All three subtypes of beta receptors, i.e. β_1, β_2 and β_3, are present in central nervous system but their concentration varies at different sites. All the three types mediate their actions by stimulation of adenylcyclase enzyme, leading to increased secretion of cAMP. The β_3 adrenergic receptor has recently been found and is supposed to be present in adipose tissue and is responsible for lipolysis by adrenaline. Non-shivering pyrexia in rodents is also induced by activation of β_3 receptors.[10] β_1 receptors are mainly distributed on neurons. The specific agonist is dobutamine, while atenolol and metoprolol are the specific antagonists.

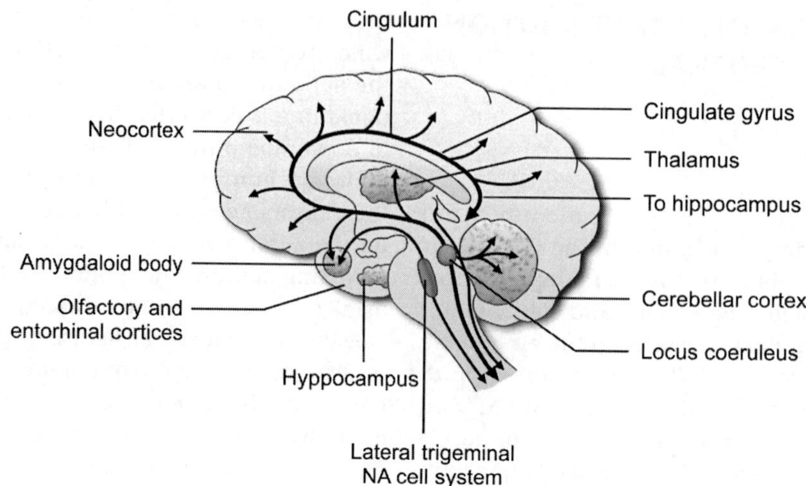

Fig. 15: Noradrenergic pathways in brain

The distribution of β_2 adrenergic receptors is on glial cells and vascular elements. Their specific agonist is terbutaline and the specific antagonists are butoxamine and ICI 118551.

The β_3 receptors are supposed to be existing on the lipid materials of the cell walls or the neuronal membrane, and adrenaline acts as an agonist while propranolol acts as an antagonist.

Norepinephrine is the main adrenergic neurotransmitter which acts on α_1 receptors of the neocortex and thalamus, which are prazosin sensitive depolarization and the response is mediated due to decrease in K^+ conductance.[11] A vasoactive polypeptide from intestine also stimulates α_1 receptor through cAMP synthesis in neocortical region.[12] α_1 receptor stimulation also take place by activation of phospholipase C, leading to release of IP_3 and DAG (inositol trisphosphate and diacylglycerol).

Alpha-2 receptors, distributed on adrenergic neurons, mediate their response by hyperpolarization on entry of K^+ conductance internally. The K^+ conductance is also regulated by other transmitters. α_2 receptors, along with the dopaminergic D_2 receptors are inhibiting the activity of adenylcyclase enzyme and reduce the synthesis of cyclic AMP. But in CNS, the effects of α_2 receptor are through receptor operated K^+ channel activation and suppression of the Ca^{++} channels, which can be mediated by pertussis toxin sensitive G-proteins of the α_2 receptors. Therefore, on the basis of ligands binding, the α_2 receptors are subdivided into three types. α_{2A}, α_{2B} and α_{2C}, but they all have the same signalling.[13]

Recently, the epinephrine containing neurons have been recognized by the discovery of the enzymatic assays. Epinephrine containing neurons have been observed in medullary reticular formation, which have connections with few pontine and diencephalic nuclei and course up to paraventricular nucleus of the dorsal midline thalamus. Their functions are not known so far.[14-16]

Dopaminergic System

Dopamine was supposed to be a precursor of nor-epinephrine previously. But now, it is recognized as a separate neurotransmitter having its own system. It is synthesized from levophenylalanine, an essential amino acid, by the action of hydroxylase enzyme in the liver and converted into L-tyrosine, which is taken up by adrenergic neurons. It undergoes hydroxylation by tyrosine hydroxylase and is converted into levodopa, which is converted into dopamine after decarboxylation by dopa decarboxylase. Dopamine is taken up by the synaptic vesicles and there it is converted into nor-epinephrine. More than 50% of the catecholamine is in the form of dopamine in the central nervous system. Distribution of dopaminergic areas is different from the areas of norepinephrine. Large quantity of dopamine is found in the basal ganglia, especially in the caudate nucleus, accumbens nucleus, olfactory tubercle, central nucleus of the amygdala, median eminence and some part of the cortex (see Fig. 16).

Dopaminergic neurons are morphologically classified into three types.

1. Ultra short neurons, within the amacrine cells of the retina and periglomerular cells of the olfactory bulb.
2. Intermediate length neurons, within the tuberobasal ventral hypothalamus that innervate the median eminence and intermediate lobe of the pituitary, incertohypothalamic neurons that connect the dorsal and posterior hypothalamus with the lateral septal nuclei, and small series of neurons within the perimeter of the dorsal motor nucleus of the vagus, nucleus of the solitary tract and the periaqueductal gray matter.
3. Long projection of the dopaminergic neurons between the dopamine containing nuclei in the substantia nigra, ventral tegmentum and their targets in the striatum, in the

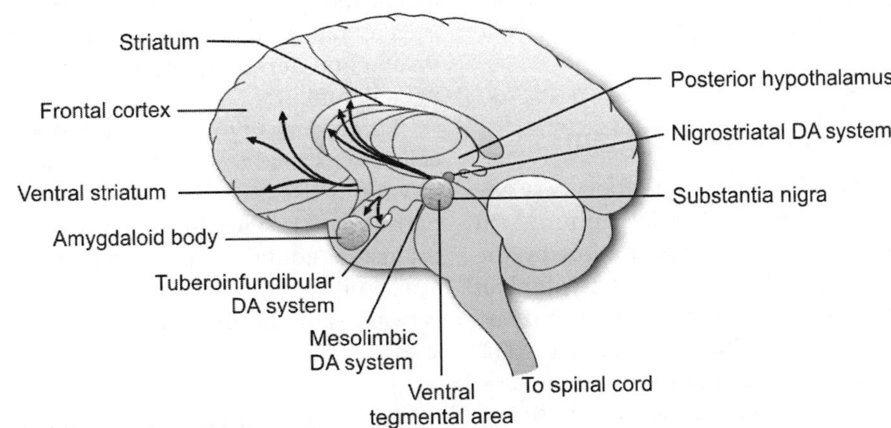

Fig. 16: Dopaminergic pathways in central nervous system

limbic zones of cerebral cortex and other major systems of the limbic system, except the hippocampus.[17] The actions of dopamine are mediated through its receptors and sub-receptors.

According to the pharmacological and biochemical basis, the dopaminergic receptors are divided into two subtypes D_1 and D_2. These receptors have different ligands having affinity to bind these receptors. Their agonists and antagonists are also of different nature. Drugs like benzazepines and SCH 23390 have a high affinity for D_1 receptors, while drugs like benzamides (as sulpiride, raclopride) and butyrophenones (as spiroperidol) have specific agonistic activity for D_2 receptors. On the basis of their nucleotide differences and genetic encoding, 5 subtypes have been found, which are subtypes of D_1 and D_2 receptors. D_1 receptor has a subtype D_5 receptor, described by Dearry et al[18] and Sunahara et al,[19] D_2 receptor has two isoforms, according to the length of the receptor. D_2 short receptor, denoted by D_2S, was described by Bunzow et al in 1988[20] and D_2 long receptor, denoted by D_2L, was described by Dal Toso et al, 1989.[21] The presence of D_3 and D_4 receptors was also described by Sokoloff et al in 1990[22] and Vantol et al in 1991,[23] respectively.

The D_1 and D_5 receptors mediate their responses through the activation of adenyl cyclase enzyme, while the D_2 receptors mediate their effects by inhibiting adenyl cyclase activity, and few other mechanisms associated are the suppression of Ca^{++} current with stimulation of K^+ conductance. The mechanisms involved in D_3 and D_4 receptors activities are not known so far.

The D_2 receptors are involved in the causation of schizophrenia and Parkinson's disease. There is direct correlation between the dose and affinity of the neuroleptics for D_2 receptors and inhibition of their responses by D_2 antagonists. Most of the antipsychotic drugs, when administered for longer time, cause extrapyramidal side effects including parkinsonian-like movement disorder and tardive dyskinesia. But, there are certain atypical antipsychotic drugs, which do not produce such effects. Both typical and atypical drugs bind to D_2, D_3 and D_4 receptors in nanogram quantity. D_3 receptor is present in mRNA in the nucleus accumbens and olfactory tubercle, and D_4 receptors have a high affinity for neuroleptics, like clozapine, which do not produce extrapyramidal reactions. Thus, the antagonism of D_3 and D_4 receptor has antipsychotic effects, while the Parkinsonian-like effects occurs due to D_2 dopaminergic stimulation and their increased activity in striatum nucleus.

Distribution of D_1 receptors is postsynaptically on intracerebral vascular beds in the CNS while the D_2 receptors are distributed in the basal ganglia, limbic cortex, hypothalamus and vomiting center. Thus, the dopaminergic pathway is spread out especially in the mesolimbic system, nigrostriatal system, and pituitary glands. The role of D_1 receptors is vasodilatation in these areas, while the D_2 receptors are presynaptic in nature and are concerned with emotional behavioral effects, psychotic effects, control of movements, neuroendocrine regulation and regulation of anterior pituitary hormones, prolactin release, and stimulation of CTZ (emesis). D_1 receptors stimulate G_s-proteins of adenylcyclase stimulation and increase production of cAMP. D_2 receptors mediate their effects by stimulation of G_i proteins of the substrate, leading to inhibition of adenylcyclase and decreased cyclic AMP production.

Selective agonist of D_1 receptors is SKF38393 and antagonist is SCH 23370. Non-selective agonists are dopamine and apomorphine, and the non-selective antagonists of D_1 receptor are phenothiazines and thioxanthines.

Selective agonists for D_2 receptor are lisuride and quinpirole, and antagonists with selectivity are sulpiride, metoclopramide and domperidone. Non-selective agonists for D_2 receptor are dopamine, apomorphine, bromocriptine, and non-selective D_2 antagonists are phenothiazines and thioxanthines.

Serotonin (5-hydroxytryptamine) System

Serotonin is an important neurotransmitter in CNS. It is synthesized from dietary essential amino acid levotryptophan, which undergoes hydroxylation by the enzyme tryptophan hydroxylase into 5-hydroxytryptophan (5-HTP). Then, it undergoes decarboxylation by the enzyme 5-HTP decarboxylase, to form 5-hydroxytryptamine (5-HT). After synthesis, it is stored in the mast cells and other tissues, and is liberated to act on the receptors on each impulse and then inactivated rapidly by monoamine oxidase and aldehyde dehydrogenase, by hydroxylation, and converted into an inactive metabolite, 5-hydroxyindole acetic acid (5-HIAA) excreted in urine.

5-HT 5-HTP is selectively distributed in brain at various sites, such as pons, midbrain, medulla oblongata, midline raphe nuclei, projections to cortex limbic system, hypothalamus and spinal cord (see Fig. 17). It is acting through the different receptors at different sites.

5-HT present in serum, called serotonin, and present in gut, called as enteramine, are synonymous terms for 5-HT. These tryptaminegic neurons are widely distributed in CNS, mainly in the nine nuclei lying adjacent to the midline (raphe) regions of pons and upper part of the brainstem. Serotonergic fibers from rostral raphe nuclei innervate forebrain, while the caudal raphe nuclei send fibers to brainstem and spinal cord. Median raphe nucleus has major contributions to the limbic system and dorsal raphe has its role in cortical regions and neostriatum.[14]

Large quantity of 5-HT is found in enterochromaffin cells of GIT, and taken up by the platelets and transported to various tissues. But, 5-HT cannot cross the blood brain barrier, so it is synthesized in the brain. The raphe nuclei of brainstem contains the serotonergic cells and neurons. It is also present in the pineal glands and hypothalamus, and is responsible for the release of various hormones of these sites.

Different Receptors Play Different Role in CNS

Serotonergic receptors are mainly divided in fourteen types, including their subtypes, at different places in the CNS. These subtypes have different ligands binding, couple to different intracellular signalling, and exhibit specific distributions in the CNS, and they are responsible for different behavioral effects. 5-HT_1 and 5-HT_2 are G-protein linked receptors, with seven transmembrane spanning domain motif while 5-HT_3 is ion-operated channel receptor, similar to the nicotinic receptor of acetylcholine a sub-unit.

Actually, 5-HT receptors are seven in number, i.e. 5-HT_1 to 5-HT_7 receptors. The 5-HT_1 receptor is further divided in to six subtypes such as 5-HT_{1A}, 5-HT_{1B}, 5-HT_{1C}, 5-HT_{1D}, 5-HT_{1E} and 5-HT_{1F}. All of these have different ligands and different sites, but have similar action to inhibit adenyl cyclase activity

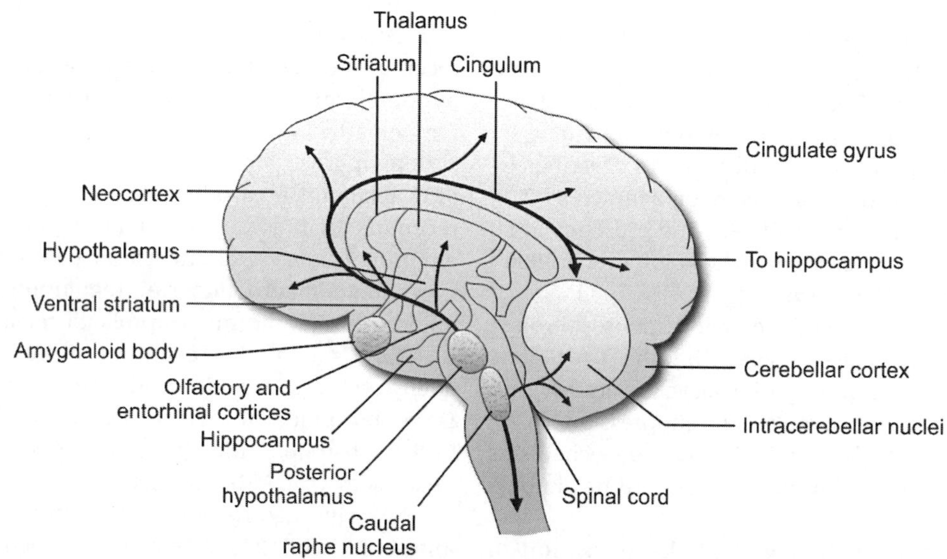

Fig. 17: Serotonergic system in brain

Serotonergic system is spread in CNS. The raphe nucleus has continuous collection of cell groups close to the midline throughout the brainstem. But for proper understanding they have been subdivided into rostral and caudal group. The raphe nuclei project to large number of structures extending from forebrain to occipital region. The caudal nucleus spreads fibers to cerebellum, posterior part of brain and spinal cord.

or to regulate the K^+ and Ca^{++} channels. 5-HT_1 receptor is an autoregulatory receptor in CNS and acts by inhibiting the cAMP and decreases or inhibits the release of 5-HT and other neurotransmitters.

5-HT_{1A} receptors are present on 5-HT neurons of the dorsal raphe nucleus and are responsible for temperature regulation.[15] They are also found in the hippocampus and amygdala nucleus and they are associated with anxiety and mood. Activation of 5-HT_{1A} receptor leads to opening of inward K^+ conductance and hyperpolarization leads to inhibition of neurons. The 5-HT_{1A} receptor can be activated by the drugs like buspirone and ipsapirone, which are used for the treatment of anxiety and panic episodes.[16] 5-HT_{1D} receptor is activated by the drug sumatriptan, used for the treatment of migraine.

In contrast to 5-HT_1 receptor, the 5-HT_2 receptor is activated by Phospholipase C, based on ligand binding through mRNA. 5-HT_2 receptors are abundant at post-synaptic sites in CNS and they are excitatory in nature and responsible for various behavioral responses. They act through IP_3 activation.

The 5-HT_2 receptors are subdivided in to 5-HT_{2A}, 5-HT_{2B}, and 5-HT_{2C} subtypes. 5-HT_{2A} receptors are abundant in number at forebrain, especially in the neocortex and olfactory tubercles, and some nuclei of brainstem. Two 5-HT mechanisms are involved in facial motor neurons excitability: (1) slow closure of resting K^+ conductance, leading to increasing membrane resistance, and (2) opening of the voltage sensitive K^+ conductance by hyperpolarization, as is done by ritanserin. In cerebral cortex, 5-HT_{2A} receptor agonists produce neuronal inhibition but not 5-HT itself. Ritanserin blocks the GABA mediated inhibitory interneuronal response at pyramidal neurons. The 5-HT_{2C} receptors are similar in structure and functions to 5-HT_{2A} receptors and distributed abundantly in the choroid plexus. They are supposed to be responsible for synthesis and regulation of CSF production.

5-HT_3 receptor type was first described in the peripheral autonomic neurons system, but later on detected in brain also. 5-HT_3 receptors are heterogenic in nature and are widely distributed in brain and periphery. They are responsible for behavioral anxiety, sleep, maintaining of body temperature, feeding, and pain perceptions.These receptors are present in the area postrema and nucleus tractussolitarious, which become desensitized by chronic exposure to 5-HT. The 5-HT_3 receptors lead to increase in Na^+ and K^+currents. 5-HT_3 receptors are associated with behavioral effects, like emesis, which are blocked by drugs, like ondansetron (controls drug-induced emesis).

5-HT_4 receptors are located on the nerve terminals of cholinergic and motor neurons. They are stimulatory in nature and act through the cAMP production. 5-HT_3 receptors are present in high concentration in area postrema of brain while they are in low concentration in forebrain. These receptors are transmitter-operated ionic channels, while the other 5-HT receptors are G-protein operated in nature. Sexual behavior and coordination of autonomic activities is also mediated by serotonin. It also has an important role in parkinsonism.

5-HT agonist, i.e. serotonin, can be increased by the following ways by the various drugs.

1. *5-HT uptake inhibitor:* Fluoxetine (a potent blocker) and trazodone (weak blocker)
2. *Increasing the release of 5-HT:* Fenfluramine and amphetamine.
3. *5-HT receptor different agonists:*
   - 5-HT_1 agonist are buspirone, sumatriptan, eltoprazine, ipsapirone
   - 5-HT_2 agonists are LSD and a methyl 5-HT
   - 5-HT_3 agonist is a methyl 5-HT
   - 5-HT_4 agonists are metoclopramide, cisapride, zacopride and renzapride.

   Specific antagonists of 5-HT receptors are as under:
   - 5-HT_1 antagonists are spiperone, methiothepine and quipazine
   - 5-HT_2 antagonists are cyproheptadine, mianserin, metergoline, quipazine, ritanserin
   - 5-HT_3 blockers are ondansetron, granisetron, tropisetrone (also metoclopramide and cisapride in high doses).
   - 5-HT_4 receptor is blocked by tropisetrone.
   - Drug like reserpine deplete the storage sites of 5-HT and inhibit the response of 5-HT.
   - Many antipsychotic drugs, like phenothiazines and butyrophenones, also have selective anti-5-HT actions.

LSD and other hallucinogenic agents interact with 5-HT, especially by the blockade of the 5-HT_2 receptors. It is also observed that LSD and 5-HT are both potent inhibitors of the firing of raphe neurons mediated by 5-HT. LSD and other hallucinogens are powerful excitatory agents on facial motoneurones that receive innervation from the raphe.[2] LSD has an inhibitory response on raphe neurons but the effect can be observed on the destruction of these neurons and the effect can be potentiated by administration of 5-HT precursors, like 5-HTP. So, the mechanisms of hallucinogenic drugs are still unexplainable.

Histaminergic System

Previously, histamine was supposed to be an autacoid in the peripheral system but it was observed that many antihistaminics had sedative and other effects, due to their effects on central nervous system. Recently, it has been observed that histamine is also an important neuro-transmitter in CNS. It is synthesized from levohistidine, an essential dietary amino acid, by decarboxylation by histidine decarboxylase enzyme, in the presence of pyridoxine (Vitamin B_6) as a co-factor.

The histamine is then stored in tissues, especially in the mast cells. If it is not in bound form or stored, it is rapidly inactivated by methylation, by histamine N-methyl-transferase to form N-methyl-histamine; it is further oxidized by monoamine oxidase (B type) in CNS and converted in to N-acetyl-histamine, which is excreted in urine. Three different types of histaminergic receptors have been observed in CNS, i.e. H_1, H_2 and H_3. The action of histamine is mediated on these receptors in a different manner.

On H_1 receptors, its actions are mediated by activation of phosphatidylinositol cycle, which increases the intracellular Ca^{++} concentration, while on H_2 receptors, the actions are mediated by activation of adenylcyclase system responsible for the synthesis of cAMP. The mechanism of H_3 receptor mediated actions is not known so far. Histamine is stored in mast cells or basophils, and is found with heparin complex in the cytoplasm of the neuronal cells.[1]

Most of the histamine containing neurons are distributed in the ventral posterior hypothalamus, which gives long ascending and descending tracts to the entire CNS. It has a characteristic pattern of other aminergic systems.[2] H_1receptors are located on glial cells, neurons and vessels. H_2 receptors are linked to activation of adenyl cyclase in concert with H_1 receptors. H_3 receptors have greatest sensitivity and selectivity to histamine located in basal ganglia and olfactory regions at presynaptic sites. On the basis of histaminic antagonists, this system is associated with regulation of arousal, maintenance of body temperature and vascular dynamics. Like other amines, histamine does not have its release and reuptake processes or any provoking actions.[24]

Amino Acid System

Many amino acids are present in the CNS. They are classified in two groups, such as the dicarboxylic amino acids (e.g. glutamate and aspartate having excitatory effects in CNS) and the monocarboxylic amino acids (e.g. GABA, Glycine, β alanine and taurine having inhibitory responses in CNS).[25,26] These amino acids have their selective antagonists, their receptors and subtypes.

Gamma amino butyric acid (GABA) is an important inhibitory amino acid in the brain. GABA mimicked effect stimulates the inhibitory nerves and these effects are blocked by picrotoxin antagonist. GABA is the only inhibitory amino acid found exclusively in crustacean inhibitory nerves. Release of GABA depends upon the frequency of the nerve stimulation and it increase the chloride (Cl^-) conductance of the affected cells.[27] GABA has an inhibitory response at interneuronal sites in the brain, while it mediates spinal cord. GABAergic inhibitory synapses have been observed between cerebellar Purkinje neurons and their targets in Deiter's nucleus. They are also present between small interneurones and major cells of cerebellar cortex, olfactory bulb, cuneate nucleus, hippocampus and lateral septal nucleus, and between the vestibular nucleus and the trochlear motoneurones. GABA also has an inhibitory response in cerebral cortex and between caudate nucleus and substantia nigra.

GABA is synthesized by an amino acid glutamic acid, by decarboxylase enzyme, and its effect is terminated by reuptake or by transamination of transaminase enzyme. Drugs, like bicuculline and picrotoxin, that block the GABAergic receptors, are selective antagonists of GABA. Drugs, like muscimol, mimic the GABAergic response and other drugs, like 2–4-diamino-butyrate, nipecotic acid and guvacine, inhibit the reuptake of GABA. Amino oxyacetic acid alters the turnover of GABA. GABA mediates its action through its subtypes, denoted by $GABA_A$ and $GABA_B$. The $GABA_A$ type receptors are post-synaptic and coupled with the chloride channels, mediating their role by increasing the chloride (Cl^-) conductance. The $GABA_B$ type receptors are pre-synaptic and mediate their response through second messengers. $GABA_A$ receptor proteins are well known because they are abundant in quantity and associated with various neuronal circuits.

GABA receptors are responsible for mediating actions of benzodiazepines and barbiturates. Recently, Franks and Lieb (1994)[28] reported the interactions between $GABA_A$ receptor and steroid anesthetic agents, volatile anesthetic agents and alcohol. On the basis of CDNA patterns, $GABA_A$ receptor appears to have about 15 subunits. $GABA_A$ receptors are associated with the nicotinic cholinergic receptor, having pentameric protein, in which the subunit assembles together around a central ion pore. There are multiple subtypes of $GABA_A$ receptors in the brain, which mediate different pharmacological actions. Thus, there are functional and anatomical differences among the subunits of $GABA_A$ receptors. There are α_1, β and γ are the main types of the subunits of $GABA_A$.

Glycine System

Glycine is also an inhibitory amino acid, acting through the specific receptors in the brain. The glycine receptors are distributed in the brainstem and spinal cord. These glycine receptors also have different subunits. Glycine receptors are present on the Ranshaw cells, which are blocked by strychnine. The association of glycine receptors with the GABA receptors is not known so far.

Glutamate and Aspartate Systems

Glutamate and aspartate are the stimulatory (excitatory) amino acids, widely distributed in all parts of the brain. There are different subtypes of excitatory receptors on the neurons. Glutamate receptors are inotropic channel operated receptors and metabotropic G-protein receptors. Metabotropic receptors are GTP proteins, while ionic-channel operated receptors are Na^+ or Ca^{++} operated paths, as described by Hollmann and Heinemann (1994).[29] Metabotropic receptors consist of a single seven transmembrane spanning protein, while the ligand gated channels are multi-subunit complexes.

Ionic operated channels are two types of subunits, on the basis of different agonists. These receptors are α-amino-3 hydroxy-5-methyl-4-isoxazole propionic acid (AMPA) and N-methyl-D-aspartate (NMDA) receptors. Different antagonists of these receptors act on different sites. Various open channel blockers, like phencyclidine (angel dust), act at glycine binding sites, while ifenprodil acts as a crossed channel blocker. The activity of NMDA receptor is pH dependent; it is also modulated by endogenous ligands, neurosteroids, arachidonic acid, redox reagents and polyamines (like spermine), and zinc. Blockade of NMDA receptors by these agents can be of competitive or non-competitive type. On genetic basis and different arrangements of amino acid patterns, the subtypes of NMDA receptor are AMPA and kainate receptors. Both are fast depolarizing receptors, present on glutamatergic synapses in the brain and spinal cord. The RNA pattern of AMPA and kainate receptors differs from each other. AMPA and kainate receptors are located along with NMDA receptors on various glutamatergic synapses. The NMDA receptors remains activated for longer time; that is from hours to days, called as long term potentiation. This activation can be observed in hippocampus area, as described by Bliss and Collingridge (1993).[30]

NMDA receptors are blocked by Mg^{++}, which inhibits the generation of action potential of the receptors. Long term potentiation of NMDA receptor is an important phenomenon for maintaining the learning and memory behavior. Inhibition of NMDA receptors can induce long term depression (LTD).[31] In few minutes, exposure of neurons to glutamate may lead to death of the neuronal cells and the same effect can be observed due to excessive stimulation of NMDA receptor by influx of Ca^{++} into the neurons. Ischemia and hypoglycemia of the brain also produce similar effects and death of the neuronal cells. Because both inhibit the reuptake of glutamate in the synapses, this leads to excessive stimulation of NMDA receptors. NMDA receptors are also involved in induction of epileptic seizure and NMDA increases the susceptibility to seizure activity. NMDA receptor antagonists are found to be anticonvulsants. Thus, glutamate receptors are involved in expression of various CNS activities and their disturbances are responsible in causation of neurological disorders and, even in schizophrenia and epilepsy.

Peptide System

Various peptides have been discovered which regulate one or another function of the neuronal cells. Few peptides, which were supposed to have limited actions on GIT or endocrine glands, are also found acting on CNS. These peptides are acting alone or along with other neurotransmitters. Thus, some neurons may have more than two possible transmitters.[32] These peptides independently regulate the neuronal functions at various sites of the CNS.

Central Nervous System Peptides

According to the sequence of amino acids, the families of peptides are ancestral or concurrent. The ancestral peptide is like substance P or the vasotocin family, in which species variation are in existence. The concurrent peptides are like endorphins and glucagon secretion family.

These peptides are different from other proteins in the length of the amino acid chain. There can be only more than two amino acids chain (like carnosine and anserine) or more than 40 amino acids (such as CRF—corticotropin releasing factor, or GRF—growth hormone releasing factor). But, most of the peptides have more than 90 amino acids. The important peptides present in brain are:

- TRH (thyrotropin releasing hormone)
- SRIF-28 (somatostatin)
- Neurotensin
- Neuromedin N
- CRF (corticotropin releasing factor).

Certain peptide resembles the peptides secreted from other parts of the body, such as intestine, pancreas, etc. These neuropeptides participate as chemical mediators in pathways, such as diverse behavior, thermoregulation, food and water consumption, sex, sleep, locomotion, memory, learning, reaction to pain, and stress responses. They are also responsible for the control of endocrinal functions. Most of the peptides can cross the blood-brain barrier to produce their effects. Their degradation is in the form of amino acids which also have biological activity. These peptides are found in brain as well as in peripheral organs, such as GIT, pancreas and adrenal glands. Some CNS peptides, like neurotensin and somatostatin, have dual role in brain and gut. These peptide receptors are found on glial cells. They are also localized in neurons that releases the transmitter or other neuropeptide or both. Neurotensin is found in neurons having dopamine synthetic enzyme in ventral tegmental area and arcuate nucleus of the hypothalamus. Reserpine inhibits the release of both dopamine and neurotensin in frontal cortex. Frontal cortex also contains cholecystokinins. Thus, there can be release of 3 to 6 peptides from a single neuron. TRH can be released with substance P on the median raphe nucleus and spinal cord. CRF can be released along with vasopressin, oxytocin and neurotensin in neurons of paraventricular nucleus of the hypothalamus. Somato-statin is released along with GABA at thalamic neurons.

The biosynthesis of the these peptides occurs by the transcription of mRNA sequence from DNA on the appropriate genes. Cyclic AMP also plays its role in activation of protein kinases A and C and casein kinase II for synthesis of the neuropeptides and regulation of their activity. They are degraded into small fragments by various peptidases. These enzymes are found bound to post- or pre-synaptic neural membranes or cytoplasm of the neurons, and extracellular fluids like CSF in the CNS. They often have a metal ion among their subunit responsible for cleavage of the target peptide.

Three major systems of endorphin peptides, named (a) pro-opiomelanocortin (b) pro-enkephalin and (c) pro-dynorphine, have been described by Bloom in 1988. Various peptides of glucagon family, such as glucagon vasoactive intestinal polypeptide (VIP), are secreted in duodenal mucosa, and related peptides are neuropeptides acting through their specific receptors in CNS. The main effects of the peptides are to increase the blood glucose. The existence of substance P receptors have been observed in CNS. Hypothalamic peptides are responsible to produce oxytocin, vasopressin, pro-opio-melanocortin, gonadotropin releasing hormone and growth hormone releasing hormone. Some more peptides such as somatostatin, cholecystokinin, encephalin and thyrotropin releasing hormone also have a role in CNS. Each peptide has its messenger roles at the cellular level. Synthesis of these peptides is performed in rough endoplasmic reticulum through mRNA. Different peptides act on the different receptors but there are no specific synthetic agonists or antagonists available so far. Only in the case of endorphin receptor, one plant alkaloid morphine and it derivatives, have been detected to have agonistic activity. Some non-peptide antagonists of neurotensin, such as cholecystokinin, have been developed recently, which have an important role in therapeutics.

Miscellaneous Neurotransmitters

Purines Transmitters

Three main anabolites of purine, adenosine monophosphate, adenosine triphosphate and adenosine it self act as neurotransmitter through P_1 and P_2 receptor.

P_1 receptors are G-proteins coupled receptors, divided into four subtypes, namely A_1–A_4. A_1 and A_2 receptors have adenosine as agonist while xanthine acts as their antagonist. A_1 receptor is responsible for inhibition of adenyl cyclase enzyme and activation of phospholipase C through stimulation of K^+ current regulation channel, while A_2 receptor activates the adenylcyclase activity. The P_2 receptors are activated by ATP and other triphosphates, and regulate the ionic gated channels. They are also subdivided into two subtypes, P_{2s} and P_{2y} which consist of coupling of G proteins. These receptors are distributed in various areas of the brain. Adenosine acts presynaptically throughout the cortex and hippocampus region, and inhibits the release of amino acid and amino acid transmitters. These responses are associated for maintaining the various effects, such as supracellular functions such as anxiety, stroke and epilepsy as described by Williams (1994).[33] Endogenous adenosine has been reported to inhibit mesopontine cholinergic neurons, through activation of K^+ channel conductance. This effect can be reversed by antagonists like caffeine and theophylline. These neurons are responsible for mediating the arousal response.

Diffusible Mediators

Certain potent agents act as mediators in physiological and pharmacological conditions. Biological membrane of the neuronal cells is rich in phospholipid materials, containing arachidonic acid. It undergoes phospholipid hydrolysis by phospholipase A_2, C and D. Phospholipases are activated by various factors, through a variety of receptors. The arachidonic acid undergoes two enzymatic pathways and produces various important regulators of physiological functions. Arachidonic acid under the effect of cyclooxygenase reaction forms prostaglandins and thromboxans, while lipoxygenases reactions lead to formation of leukotrienes, catabolites of eicosanoids and cytochrome P450. These arachidonic acid metabolites are diffusively distributed in whole of the brain and act as neuromodulators at various sites in CNS for long term potentiation and other forms of plasticity.[34]

Nitric Oxide

Previously, nitric oxide was supposed to be an important agent for regulating vascular tone and mediator of inflammation. But, after discovery of nitric oxide syntheses in brain, it was found to be an important mediator in CNS. Four types of this biosynthetic enzyme have been detected in brain. These are present on neurons, capillary endothelial cells, macrophages and on inducible enzymes. Their potent activator is nitroprusside and inhibitors are methylarginine and nitroarginine. Nitric oxide syntheses are responsible for the various activities in brain, such as long term potentiation, guanylyl cyclase activation, neurotransmitter release and reuptake, and enhancement of glutamate (NMDA) mediated neuro-toxicity. Nitric oxide binds on specific active sites of the target enzyme and regulates the activity of the enzyme such as regulation of guanylyl cyclase in neurons. Carbon monoxide also plays its role in binding of nitric oxide with the active site of the enzyme.

Cytokines

These are different polypeptides, embryological in origin, secreted widely by the cell body. These peptides act as regulators of various functions and effects on the target enzymes or cells, to perform synergistic, additive or opposite action. They are mainly effective on immune system macrophages and activation of T lymphocytes. These polypeptides are macrophage derived cytokinins, interleukin α, IL-1B, IL-16 and tumor necrosis factors α (TNFα). These have important roles in nervous system inflammation, such as in dementia after infection, recovery from traumatic injury, etc. Cytokinins have role in neurons and glial cells, and they interact with the growth hormones. Various studies have shown that neuronal or glial cells release growth enhancing and growth retarding factors under some pathophysiological conditions neurons, and astrocytes may liberate cytokines, which act as neuromodulators.

Neuropeptide Y

Recently, a new peptide has been found in the brain which consists of 36 amino acids. It has various roles in CNS and performs various homeostatic functions. Three subtypes of receptors for this peptide are distributed in different areas of the brain responsible for conducting various actions. These are Y_1, Y_2 and Y_3 neuropeptide receptors described by Munglani et al (1996).[35] Y_1 subtype receptors present on various sites and their functions are as given in Table 7.

Table 7: Neuropeptide Y receptor subtypes

No.	*Site*	*Action*
Y_1 Receptor Subtype		
1.	Dorsal roots ganglia and spinal cord	Analgesia
2.	Sympathetic nerve terminals	Hyperalgesia
3.	Vascular smooth muscle	Hypertension
4.	Amygdala	Anxiolytic/Sedation
5.	Hypothalamus	Ingestive behavior
Y_2 Receptor Subtype		
1.	Hypothalamus	Anorexia
2.	Rostral hippocampus	Enhanced memory
3.	Intestinal mucosa	Decreased secretions
Y_3 Receptor Subtype		
1.	Nucleus tractus solitarius	Reduction in vasomotor tone
2.	Adrenal medulla	Inhibits release of catecholamines

On dorsal root ganglia, spinal cord and on sympathetic nerve terminals, Y_2 receptors behave like Y_1 receptors and some actions are performed by Y_2 receptors.

Neuropeptide Y (NPY), when administered externally intrathecally, produces analgesia which is unaffected by opioid or α_2 receptor antagonists. This effect is mediated by Y_1 and Y_2 cortical receptors activation. Peripheral effect of NYP is enhancement of pain perception, in conjunction with noradrenaline. NPY stimulates food intake behavior and the effect is reversed by the drugs, such as anorexigenic agents, associated with lowering of NPY level in hypothalamus. NPY has anxiolytic effect with sedation. There is enhancement of memory by this peptide and it reverses the scopolamine-induced amnesia through activation of Y_2 receptors. Systemic administration of NPY causes vasoconstriction and rise of BP, while central administration leads to bradycardia, decreased cardiac output and fall of BP. So far, NPY_1 receptor antagonist, BRC-672, has been synthesized which can block this receptor.

DRUGS AND NEUROTRANSMITTERS

According to the action of drugs, they may be divided into two categories, like CNS depressants and CNS stimulants. General anesthetics (gases and volatile liquids), alcohol, hypnotics and sedatives, anxiolytic, narcotic analgesics, all are CNS depressants. They depress the excitable neurons in the CNS at different levels. These drugs decrease the amount of release of transmitters during nerve impulses, leading to depression of post-synaptic responses and ionic movements. Certain drugs have specific effects on some specific areas of the brain responsible for behavioral effects and some of these drugs may produce dependence.

Drug like pentylenetetrazol is a powerful stimulant while the drug methylxanthine is a weak stimulant of CNS. These stimulants mediate their effect, either by blocking the inhibitory response of the transmitter, or by direct neuronal excitation which increases the release of transmitter, leading to post-synaptic excitation and its prolongation. There are certain drugs which can modify the CNS functions. They are excitatory at one site and inhibitory at the other site. There are some drugs which are neither excitatory nor inhibitory in CNS. Such drugs are anticonvulsants, antiparkinsonian drugs, opioids and non-opioid analgesics, appetite suppressants, antiemetics, antimanics, tranquilizers and antipsychotic agents. These drugs act either directly or by alteration in the level of neurotransmitters.

44.5 PSYCHONEUROIMMUNOLOGY

LN Gupta, Pramodh Bhardhwaj

The term *psychoneuroimmunology* refers to the study of effects of psychological status on immune function. Since the psychological status of a person influences the function of immunocompetent cells through central nervous system and endocrine activity, and the immune cells can, in turn, influence neural functions and endocrine activity, the other terms like *neuroendocrinoimmunology* and *neuroimmunomodulation* have been applied to this phenomena.

The concept of 'resistance' to disease is as ancient as is the notion that such resistance could be modified experimentally. For example 'Ayurveda', the ancient Indian Medicine, contains concepts of natural and acquired immunity and approaches treatment by restoration of a balance of life forces and by an integrated relationship to environment. In the same line, the British authority Day, while describing the pathological process of tuberculosis, goes on to say that unhappiness is the cause of lowered body resistance. Elaborating on the multifactorial approach to disease, Salk speculates that illness may concern genetic, behavioral, social and immune relationship. Subsequent studies on diseases, where the resistance is considered as immunologic in nature (such as infectious diseases, cancer and autoimmune disease), documented the role of personality factors, stress and particularly failure of psychological defenses in onset and course of these illnesses. These studies clearly suggest that noxious emotions are immunosuppressive.

THE IMMUNE SYSTEM

The immunogenic response constitutes the principal means of man's defense against foreign substances. A substance must ordinarily be recognized as foreign in order to elicit an immune response. The major lymphoid organs are classified into either primary (central) or secondary (peripheral) lymphoid organs.

Primary lymphoid organs such as thymus, bone marrow and fetal liver are the major sites of lymphopoiesis. Here, lymphocytes differentiate from lymphoid stem cells, proliferate and mature into functional cells. In mammals, T-cells mature in the thymus, B cells in fetal liver and bone marrow. In primary lymphoid organs, the lymphocytes acquire their repertoire of specific antigen receptors in order to cope with antigenic challenges the individual receives during the life. The cells are selected for tolerance of self-antigens and are capable of recognizing only non-self antigens. Immunogens are drained into lymphoid organs, from where they are taken by macrophages. Macrophages catabolize most of the immunogen but retain a few molecules in partially degraded or completely undegraded state for presentation to lymphocytes for immune recognition. Macrophages handle the immunogen non-specifically.

In secondary or peripheral lymphoid organs such as spleen, lymph nodes, and mucosa-associated tissue, two kinds of lymphocytes (T and B) are present. The peripheral lymphoid tissue provides the environment in which lymphocytes can interact with each other and with antigens. It also disseminates the immune response. These functions are performed by phagocytes, macrophages, antigen presenting cells (APC's) and mature T and B cells in peripheral lymphoid organs.

Out of the two types of lymphocytes (T and B), B cells are derived from bone marrow stem cells in mammals and are characterized by large number of immunoglobulin molecules on their surface membrane. The immunoglobulins on the surface of B lymphocytes interact with antigen, a process which initiates antibody formation. The T lymphocytes are derived from thymus and do not have demonstrable immunoglobulin molecules on their surface membrane. Thus, the presence or absence of surface membrane immunoglobulins on lymphocytes serves to differentiate whether the cells are B or T in kind. The T lymphocytes also specifically react with antigen and are involved in cell-mediated immune reactions, and also serve a helper function in antibody formation. The consequence of immune response is termed immunity, when beneficial to the host, and hypersensitivity or allergy, when detrimental.

As a measure of immune response, the most commonly used measure is the T and B cell proliferation response to mitogens (plant derivatives which cause cells, particularly lymphocytes, to undergo cell division). Other measures of immune response include measures of antibody titer, number of antibody producing plaque-forming cells, NK cells (lymphocytes having no conventional surface antigen receptors) activity, the cytotoxic activity of cytotoxic-T lymphocytes, or absolute number and percentage of different immune cells (including B cells, T-cells or T-cell subsets) (see Table 8).

The immune system parallels the nervous system in many ways in its evolution and function. For instance, both systems have learning and memory functions based on cell-to-cell communication and they share many mediators, receptors and antigens. Both systems need an internal communication network which can control and interact with other organs.

Table 8: Cellular components of immune system

Cell type	*Immunogenic function*	*Soluble mediators*	*Comments*
Th lymphocytes	Augmentation of immunologic	IL2 reaction	IL2 promotes and maintains the growth of T lymphocytes
Ts/Tc lymphocytes	Suppression of immunologic reaction/mediate cell killing	IFN-Y	IFN-Y activates cytotoxic cells and macrophages, increases the expression of antigens of the major histocompatibility complex and inhibits viral infections
NK cells	Killing of virus-infected and tumor cells	IFN alpha	IFN alpha is inhibitory for viral replications, enhances NK cells activity, elevates expression of antigens of major histocompatibility complex
B lymphocytes	Production of antibody	Ig, IFN alpha	—
Macrophages	Phagocytosis and killing of infectious agents, antigen processing and presentation	IL1, IFN alpha	IL1 classically induces IL2 and drives thymocyte proliferation

Source: Adapted from Blalock (1989)[2]

The nervous system is directly connected to most other organs via nerves and also uses hypothalamic-pituitary-adrenal axis to send signals to the periphery. But in contrast, the immune system is composed mainly of free, mobile cells. Cell-to-cell interactions are intermittent and mostly concerned with internal communication. This communication with other organs is mostly cytokine-mediated.

Cytokines are a group of molecules secreted mostly by activated lymphocytes (then also called lymphokines) or other immune cells and involved in signalling between cells of immune system. Cytokines are effective in very low concentrations. This is due to their mode of action which involves binding to high affinity receptors on the cell surface, which transmits cytokine signals to the nucleus. Cytokines are hormone-like peptides or glycopeptides. They work in parallel with other signals arising from direct cell-to-cell contact, thus providing a communication network involved in every function of immune response. The term lymphokines originally referred to mediators released from lymphocytes. The immune system shares with nervous system an ability to signal via the hypothalamic-pituitary-adrenal axis through several cytokines, such as IL1, IL6 and TNF (tumor necrosis factor) which have direct effect on the hypothalamus or pituitary (Table 9).

Table 9: Neuro-endocrine effects of lymphokines and monokines

Lymphokine/Monokine	*Effects*
Interleukin-1 (IL1) (acts on hypothalamus and pituitary)	Causes fever Results in slow wave sleep Causes CRH release Causes ACTH and endorphin release Elevates glucocorticoid levels Stimulates GH and PRL (in humans) Inhibits TSH release (in rats) Stimulates somatostatin secretion Inhibits TRH synthesis Stimulates AVP release Stimulates IL-6 production
Interleukin-2 (IL2) (acts on pituitary) Interleukin-6 (IL6) (present in folliculo-stellate pituitary cells)	Stimulates release of ACTH, glucocorticoids PRL and GH Stimulates synthesis of TNF and IL1 Stimulates release of ACTH, glucocorticoids, GH and PRL
TNF	Inhibits GH release (directly) Stimulates ACTH adrenocortical secretion Inhibits TSH, T4 and T3 secretion Inhibits thyroid response to TSH Increases PRL release
IFN alpha and/or beta (acts on adrenal gland)	Induction of adrenal steroidogenesis Increases lodine uptake by thyroid cells Excites neurons Suppresses morphine withdrawalsymptoms Causes catalepsy, analgesia
Thymosin-alpha-1	Elevates ACTH and glucocorticoid (acts on nervous system) levels

Source: Adapted from Blalock (1989)[2]

NEUROIMMUNOMODULATION

Neural influences can modulate the immune response. Origin of this field may reside in classical conditioning (animal experiments of Pavlov), when it was shown that similar to many other physiological processes, immune reactions could be conditioned and conditioning induces immunosuppression. Subsequently, Jancovic and Isacovic (1973) showed that electrical stimulation of hypothalamus enhanced the *Arthus reaction*, a measure of immediate hypersensitivity. They also pointed out that lesions of anterior hypothalamus had effect on cellular immunity. Subsequent lesioning studies included not only anterior hypothalamus but other regions of hypothalamus and limbic system, such as hippocampus, the amygdala and mammillary bodies. The overall findings of these studies were that lesions in the anterior hypothalamus are immunosuppressive and this immunosuppression is not due to increased levels of corticosteroids but rather to increased suppressor activity of macrophages.

Similar lesioning studies were then conducted before and after hypophysectomy, which revealed that removal of pituitary gland abrogated many of the inhibitory effects of hippocampus and amygdala lesioning. Thus, many of the immunological alterations that are induced by central nervous system lesioning are mediated through the pituitary gland or other endocrine components. These changes in systemic immune function after manipulations of the central nervous system suggest that immune functions can be regulated by the brain. Another finding suggesting that brain and immune functions are related is that men and boys with dyslexia and left handedness have a higher incidence of autoimmune disease than other men and boys.

Subsequent clinical studies have clearly shown that stressful conditions may lead to a suppression of immune functions as response of lymphocytes to mitogens in vitro, or the ability to recover from infections. However, it is much more difficult to make direct connections at cellular level or molecular level that explain these observations. Broadly, there are two main routes by which events occurring in central nervous system could modulate immune function. Most lymphoid tissue receives direct sympathetic innervation, both to the blood vessels passing through the tissues and directly to the lymphocytes themselves. Thus, neural regulation of immune function is likely through sympathetic nervous system by the release of catecholamines at autonomic nerve endings and from adrenal medulla. Secondly, nervous system directly or indirectly controls the output of various hormones, in particular corticosteroids, growth hormone, thyroxine and adrenaline.

The role of sympathetic innervation to bone marrow has been postulated to help in regulation of production of hematopoietic stem cells and lymphocytes, as well as in migration of immature cells to thymus and their distribution within the thymus. Moreover, activation of sympathetic nervous system causes leukocytosis, lymphopenia and inhibition of natural killer cell activities. The thymus also secretes several immunoregulatory peptides and secretion of some of them is regulated directly by autonomic nerves or indirectly by pituitary hormones.

The hypothalamic-pituitary adrenal axis (HPA) is a model neuroendocrine system linking changes in central nervous system of alteration in target gland functions. Generally, the higher centers of brain maintain a tonic inhibition of HPA function. Certain conditions like environmental signals, sleep rhythms, physical and emotional stress alter this control, resulting in disinhibition and HPA overactivity. The signal is propagated first by release of corticotropin releasing factor (CRF) from the hypothalamus, which stimulates the synthesis and release of anterior pituitary hormone, adrenocorticotropin (ACTH), from its precursor, pro-opiomelanocortin (POMC), finally leading to increase in synthesis and release of adrenal cortical hormones, corticosterone and/or cortisol. CRF, ACTH and cortisol are all elevated in response to a variety of physical and emotional stress, and serve as prime factors in the maintenance of homeostasis and in the development of adaptive response.

Autoradiographic evidence indicates that the principal neuroanatomical site of action for the central effects of pituitary adrenal hormones lies within the limbic midbrain circuit and the ascending reticular activating system. The neurochemical mechanisms involved in the mediation of HPA effects on mood and mentation are complex in as much as stimulatory cholinergic and serotonergic system. In addition, gamma-amino-butyric acid (GABA)-ergic, opioid and the peptide systems influence HPA effects on mood and mentation. Vasopressin is also released during stress and stimulates ACTH release. Con-current with release of ACTH is the release of endogenous opiate beta-endorphin, also a part of POMC, cortisol and beta-endorphin feedback at the hypothalamic-pituitary level.

The hypothalamus contains mu, kappa and delta opioid receptors and injection of opioids directly into hypothalamus can stimulate HPA axis. Opioid receptors are present in the pituitary although their density in the anterior pituitary is rather low. Currently, the effects of opioids on the HPA axis are thought to be mediated by stimulating the release of CRF from the hypothalamus or by altering neurotransmitters that can alter hypothalamic releasing factors and/or release inhibitory factors. Data indicates that both mu and kappa receptors, but not delta opioid receptors, are involved in opioid-induced stimulation of CRF release from hypothalamus. Studies clearly suggest involvement of endogenous opioid system in the control of HPA axis.

Hippocampus and amygdala have independent effects on paraventricular nucleus (PVN) of hypothalamus. Central nucleus of amygdala is implicated in the stimulated HPA activity by stressors. The central nucleus of amygdala has a direct projection to the PVN, in which neuron cell bodies containing CRF, vasopressin and oxytocin are found, which triggers release of pituitary ACTH. The central nucleus of amygdala also has a projection to the bed nucleus of striaterminalis. Moreover, type II receptors are found in neurons of central nucleus of amygdala, which contains CRF, met-enkephalin, neurotensin and somatostatin. It is not yet clear if glucocorticoids regulate expression of any of these peptides in these neurons. Hippocampus has a generally inhibitory role in the control of HPA activity. The hippocampus, via the corticohypothalamic tract from the ventral subiculum, has both direct projections to the PVN and bed nucleus of striaterminalis, which sends projections to PVN that influence HPA activity.

The role of pituitary gonadal function in modulation of immune response has been suspected because of sex differences, in the prevalence of all autoimmune diseases. Estradiol potentiates mitogen induced B cell stimulation in men. Lymphocyte functions vary during the menstrual cycle. The greatest reduction in T lymphocytes is in the first half of the cycle. Other pituitary hormones can bind to specific receptors on lymphocytes. Usually all hormones, including many neurohormones or neurally mediated hormones which are known to be affected by stress, are stimulatory or inhibitory to various measures of immune function (Table 10). Melatonin, the pineal gland neurohormone, has been reported to stimulate immune function through opioidergic mechanisms.

Opioid peptides are considered responsible in some way for the effect on NK cell activity and tumor growth. Studies on peripheral blood cells from normal volunteers have shown that beta-endorphin and met-enkephalin enhances NK cell activity. Met-enkephalin has also been reported to alter activity of T lymphocytes from lymphoma patients, in vitro. There are evidences for the presence of opioid receptors on monocytes, neutrophils, lymphocytes and mast cells. Nevertheless, the indirect action via the HPA axis cannot be excluded. Finally, it may be mentioned that there are structural similarities between human leukocyte interferon (LIFN), corticotropin and endorphins. Therefore, there seems

Table 10: Immuno-regulatory effects of several hormones and neuropeptides

Hormone/ Neuropeptide	*Suppression of/ Inhibition of*	*Augmentation of/ Stimulation of*	*Other effects*
ACTH	Ig1 and IFN-γ synthesis IFN-γ mediated macrophage activation	B cell proliferation	–
Glucocorticoids	Lymphokine synthesis and effects	–	–
Estrogens	–	Number of lymphocyte functions	–
GH	–	Generation of T-cells	–
PRL	–	Thymulin secretion Lymphocyte proliferation	–
TSG	Tc and NK cell activity	Ig synthesis	–
hCG	T cell proliferation Mixed lymphocyte reaction		Generation of Ts cells
Alpha Endorphin	Ig synthesis and secretion	–	–
	Antigen specific helper T-cells		
Beta Endorphin	–	Ig and IFN-γ synthesis proliferation	Modulation of T-cell
		Generation of Tc cells NK cell activity	Chemotactic for monocytes and neutrophils
Leu or Met-enkephalin	Ig synthesis	IFN-γ synthesis NK cell activity	Chemotactic for monocytes
Substance-P	–	T-cell proliferation Macrophage phagocytosis	Degranulation of mast cells and basophils
AVP and oxytocin	–		Replacement of IL2 requirement for IFN-γ synthesis
Somatostatin	Histamine and leukotriene D4 release from basophil T-cell production	–	–
VIP	Mitogen stimulated T-cells through cAMP link Release of lymphocytes from popliteal nodes Migration of T lymphocytes into mesentric nodes	–	–
Alpha MSH	IL1 stimulated fever Monocytes secretion of IL2 Fibroblast production of prostaglandins Neutrophil migration	–	–

Abbreviations: Ig, immunoglobulin; IFN-γ, interferon γ; NK cells, natural killer T-cells; Ts cells, T suppressor cells; Tc cells, cytotoxic T-cells.
Source: Adapted from Blalock (1989)[2]

to be a very close relation between immune component and opioid peptide system.

The most important hormonal factors influencing the immune reactions are the glucocorticoids that inhibit most aspects of immune response, including the proliferation of lymphocytes, production of immunoglobulins, cytokines, etc. This inhibitory reaction occurs within the range of values induced by stress or inflammation. Since the pituitary adrenal functions are almost completely controlled by the brain, the system is an excellent example of neuroimmunomodulation. Physiological effects of other neural controlled anterior pituitary hormones on the immune response are more subtle (Table 10). GH deficient mice show thymic atrophy, involution of lymphatic tissue, and T-cell impairment, abnormalities that are reversible by GH treatment. Presence of GH receptors on lymphocytes support the view that these cells are GH regulated.

Prolactin (PRL) can also stimulate immune function. Human T and B lymphocytes bear PRL receptors and antibodies to PRL inhibit lymphocyte proliferation. Cyclosporine, an immunesuppressant drug, blocks the lymphocyte stimulating effect of PRL. Lymphocyte PRL dependency may be a manifestation not only of a response to pituitary-derived PRL but also of a response of an autocrine or paracrine system because lymphocytes can also synthesize and secrete PRL.

NEUROREGULATORS AND RECEPTORS COMMON TO IMMUNOCOMPETENT AND NEUROENDOCRINE CELLS

Immunocompetent cells contain a remarkable range of peptides, hormones and receptors, classically associated with neuronal tissue or endocrine cells (Table 11). The immune system of gut is innervated by sympathetic and parasympathetic nerves, one group of which contains vasoactive intestinal peptide (VIP). Vasoactive intestinal peptide secreted by nerves in the Payer's patches can modulate immune function by regulating the traffic of immunocompetent cells through the small bowel. Lymphocytes contain pro-opiomelanocortin (POMC) mRNA which codes for corticotropin, endorphin and alpha-melanocyte stimulating hormone. Lymphocytes also have receptors for these peptides, glucocorticoids and corticotropin releasing hormone (CRH). Lymphocyte secreted pituitary hormone is reportedly regulated by same factors that regulate pituitary. For example, ACTH secretion by lymphocytes is suppressed by glucocorticoids and is stimulated by CRF; TSH immunoreactivity of lymphocytes is suppressed by thyroid hormone; and lymphocyte GH is stimulated by GH-releasing hormone (GHRH) and is suppressed by somatostatin (Table 11).

NEUROENDOCRINE EFFECTS OF THE CYTOKINES

There are clear evidences that lymphokines act on brain. Activated immunocompetent cells (such as monocytes, lymphocytes and macrophages) can permeate the blood-brain barrier and take-up residence in the brain, where they secrete cytokines and other inflammatory mediators. Moreover a number of cytokines first discovered in immunocompetent cells are synthesized by glia. These include interleukin 1,2,4 and 6, and tumor necrosis factor (TNF-α). The co-localization of interleukin-1 receptor antagonist and interleukin-1 in the hippocampus, hypothalamus and other brain areas forms an intrinsic paracrine regulatory system. There are other binding sites on the cells of immune system, like neurotensin, substance P, GH, VIP, and insulin (Table 12).

The presence of common receptors and ligands on neuroendocrine system and immune system cells appears to

Table 11: Neuroendocrine peptides produced by the immune system

Peptide	*Cell/Tissue source*	*Comments*
ACTH	Lymphocytes and	Stimulated by CRH, macrophages, inhibited by glucocorticoids
GH	Lymphocytes	Stimulated by GHRH, inhibited by somatostatin
TSH	T-cells	Stimulated by TRH inhibited by thyroid hormones
PRL	Lymphocytes	–
hCG	T-cells	–
Enkephalins	Th cells	–
VIP	Mononuclear leukocytes, mast cells and polymorphonuclear leukocytes	–
AVP	Thymus	–
Oxytocin	Thymus	–
Neurophysin	Thymus	–

Source: Adapted from Blalock (1989)[2]

Table 12: Neuroendocrine peptide receptors in the immune system

Receptor	*Cellular/Tissue source*	*Comments*
ACTH	Murine spleen lymphocytes	ACTH receptors on human peripheral adrenal and lymphoid cells seems to be identical gene products
Beta-endorphin (non-opiate)	Lymphoblastoid cells	Binding not affected by opiate agonists and antagonists. Binding not through classical NH2 end of peptide but through COOH terminal of peptide
Encephalins (opiates)	Murine spleen	–
VIP	Lymphocytes	Coupled to adenylate cyclase system
GH	Lymphocytes	–
Substance-P	Lymphoblastoid cells	–
Insulin	Lymphocytes	–
Source: Adapted from Blalock (1989)[2]		

point out a biochemical basis for bidirectional communication between these two systems. These two systems contain and use the same set of signal molecules in the form of hormones, lymphokines and monokines for inter and intra-system communication and regulation. Moreover, they harbor the same set of receptors for the shared ligands. Thus, indicating biochemical integration of neuroendocrine and immune system. It seems obvious that a greater understanding of molecular aspects of neuroendocrine-immune interactions will have an impact on the immunological manifestations of stress and bereavement in humans. Now, we can hope to have an objective method of assessment of stress-related physical and psychological disorders through correlation of aberrant leukocyte receptor numbers and functions, and much more in the newly developed field, psychoneuroimmunology in terms of therapy and prophylaxis.

ROLE OF EMOTIONAL FACTORS IN PHYSICAL ILLNESS

Psychological health has been correlated with speed of recovery from infections. Prolonged convalescence from brucellosis and from influenza has been correlated with depression. Acute necrotizing gingivitis, in which the normal bacterial flora of mouth becomes invasive, is well known to be associated with acute stress. Personality and stress factors have been related to contact dermatitis. Suppressed weeping has been tied to attacks of urticaria. Emotions and personality factors have been linked to the onset and course of autoimmune diseases; these conditions are associated with physiological states of relative immune deficiency. There is a lack of suppresser T-cell function. Rheumatoid arthritis patients are described as quite introverted, reliable, conscientious, restricted in the expression of emotions (especially anger), conforming, self-sacrificing, sensitive to criticism, distant, overactive and busy, pseudo-independent to deny dependency, stubborn, rigid, and controlling. The onset of disease often follows either a period of psychological stress or interruption of ability to maintain previous patterns of defense and adaptation. Similar psychological findings have been reported in patients with other probably autoimmune diseases such as multiple sclerosis, systemic lupus erythematosus, Graves' disease, and ulcerative colitis. Rapidity of progression of disease, degree of incapacitation, and lack of response to treatment can be correlated with failure of psychological defense and concomitant anxiety, depression, and alienation.

Personality factors have been tied to the presence and the rapidity of dissemination of cancer in a large number of studies; rapid progression of cancer being associated with unsuccessful psychological defenses and psychic distress. Four consistent factors are found in reports of personality studies on some patients with cancer: the patient's loss of an important relationship prior to the development of tumor, the cancer patient's inability to express hostile feelings and emotion, the cancer patient's unresolved tension concerning a parent figure, and sexual disturbances. In summary, stress, failure of psychological defenses, and concomitant psychological distress are amply documented in a variety of clinical diseases that are associated with hypofunction and dysfunction of the immune system, suggesting that noxious affect (emotion) can be immunosuppressive.

IMMUNOLOGICAL ABNORMALITIES IN MENTAL ILLNESS

Immunoglobulins

Contradictory findings have been obtained in a considerable number of studies, regarding the presence and clinical correlation of abnormalities in immunoglobulins in psychiatric patients. Higher levels of IgM in withdrawn schizophrenia (and the lowest in paranoid patients) have been reported. A study reported significantly elevated IgG levels in acutely schizophrenic patients, and a drop in the level with increased phenothiazine dosage. Cerebrospinal fluid (CSF) immunoglobulins may have more clinical significance than serum levels. Research findings about immunoglobulin levels in mental illness are inconsistent, possibly reflecting clinical or treatment differences among patients.

Autoantibodies

An increased incidence of a variety of autoantibodies has been reported in conjunction with schizophrenia, including rheumatoid factor, antinuclear factor and antithymic antibodies. Heath has claimed the presence of specific antibrain antibody (taraxein) in schizophrenia. Although evidence, that auto-immunity plays a role in schizophrenia, is unconvincing, it seems clear that an increased incidence of nonspecific autoimmune reactions occur in conjunction with schizophrenic illness. However, evidences for altered immunological responsivity in schizophrenia are not convincing.

Revised antibrain antibody hypothesis proposed that schizophrenia may be caused by antibodies to neurotransmitter receptors, in whole or in part. For example, antidopamine receptor antibodies could act either as dopamine agonist or antagonist. In other investigations, self-directed cell-mediated immune responses to brain immunogens have also been found in schizophrenia patients. In a group of more than one thousand neuropsychiatric patients with dementia, mental retardation, cerebral atrophy, ethanol-induced brain deterioration and schizophrenia, about 90% of every patient group showed a cell-mediated immunity response to brain S-100 protein. High levels of antibodies to various viruses, such as herpes simplex virus and cytomegalovirus, in the CSF and in the serum of some schizophrenic patients has been reported in support of a viral hypothesis of etiology of schizophrenia. However, the evidences are at the best suggestive only. So far, there is no clear-cut evidence for a genetic marker for schizophrenia, although there are some reports of an association between the HLA-A9 immunogen and paranoid schizophrenia. The reports of relationship of grain consumption with onset of schizophrenia are largely inconsistent.

Large percentages of depressed patients show suppressed response on cellular immunity which subsides as depression is successfully treated. Psycho-active drugs also alter various parameters of immune cell numbers and functions. Lithium treatment has been found to enhance the immune activity. The immunoenhancing effects of lithium may be due to decreased suppressor T-cell activity. Chlorpromazine may cause transient decrease in leukocyte number in addition to decrease percentage and number of T-lymphocytes, decreased antibody production, decreased immunogen clearance from blood, formation of antinuclear antibodies, inhibited lymphocyte response to T- and B-cell mitogens, and 20–30% decrease in DTH response. Many other antipsychotic drugs (such as haloperidol, trifluoperazine and fluphena-zine) have been reported to suppress one or more parameters of immune response. Abnormal immunological reactivity might also be reflected in morphological abnormalities of lymphocytes. Some workers report deficient response to T-cell mitogens by lymphocytes from schizophrenic patients. In depression, studies shows that T- and B-cell responses were reduced in bereavement which was significantly reduced only in bereaved subjects with high scores on the depression scale.

Some studies report immunological abnormalities in other disorders like alcoholism, Alzheimer's disease, autism, cerebral dystrophy, criminal behavior, dementia, mental retardation, parkinsonism, etc. However, whether the reported abnormalities are the cause or consequence of the disorder remains unanswered. Only future research in this area may clarify the issue.

44.6 NEUROVIROLOGY

VS Randhawa, Geeta Mehta

Viral infections of the nervous system have been recognized by physicians for many centuries, though their cause was not understood. In 1884, Pasteur discovered the virus which caused rabies. The agent of poliomyelitis was demonstrated to be a virus.[36] Although many clinical syndromes were suspected to be of viral etiology, the technology was not available to isolate the agent and demonstrate its infectivity. It was particularly difficult to make viruses conform to Koch's postulates, the accepted criteria by which an agent was deemed to be responsible for a specific infection.

By 1941, herpes simplex was confirmed as a cause of encephalitis and, since then, many other viruses have been isolated from cases of meningitis and encephalitis.[37] The past few decades have seen enormous strides in our understanding of the infective nature of the so called 'slow virus' infections, and the more recent realization that they are caused by a novel form of infectious pathogen.

The past 12 years have seen the recognition of the pathogenic nature of retroviruses, which cause the acquired immune deficiency syndrome (AIDS) and HTLV-I associated myelopathy or tropical spastic paraplegia.[38] Every year newer techniques of immunology, molecular biology, and genetic engineering widen the range of tests available for diagnosis and refine their sensitivity and specificity, so that now it is possible to determine the presence of virus or viral constituents within body fluids and tissues in a matter of few hours.[39] What may not be so certain is whether the material demonstrated is the cause of clinical syndrome under investigation and the pathogenic mechanism by which it produces the disease manifestations.

Currently, neuropathogenic role has been attributed to at least 300 different viruses (over half of which are arthropode borne).[40,41] These infectious agents can produce neurological diseases such as meningitis, encephalitis, persistent CNS infections, and can cause a variety of neurobehavioral and neuropsychiatric disturbances (including amnesia, aphasia, depression, mania, psychosis, hallucinations and dementia). HIV type I virus has become a major cause of neuropsychological and neuropsychiatric morbidity.

Neurovirology is a quasi-separate discipline which spans the divide between many different specialities, including clinical virology, internal medicine, medical physics, neurophysiology, neuropathology, neuroradiology and the neurosciences. The special susceptibility of central nervous system cells to an extraordinary array of taxonomically disparate viruses had encouraged the development of this science.[5]

Classifying neuroviruses is important as it helps us to focus on specific aspects of the infectious agents and enhances our understanding of the subject in a better fashion. According to one classification, 'conventional' viruses have a well-defined protein structure and a genome which contains nucleic acid. Most of the neuroviruses come in this category. On the other hand, 'unconventional' agents refers to those infectious particles in which the protein structure has not been fully elucidated and a nucleic acid genome has not been demonstrated. Such 'unconventional' agents are thought to be responsible for kindred encephalopathies (e.g. Kuru, Creutzfeldt-Jacob disease, Gerstmann-Straussler syndrome).[40]

In another classification, the major neuroviruses are classified on the basis of chemical and physical properties. They are divided into groups (called families) based on size, shape, structure, and nucleic acid of the genomes (named with suffix viridae) (Table 13).[43] The simplest virion consists of protein shell or capsid which surrounds the nucleic acid core, or nucleocapsid. These are known as 'naked virions'. More complex viruses may be surrounded by a lipid layer, the envelope, which is derived from the membrane of an infected cell as the nucleocapsid buds from it. Such viruses are termed 'enveloped' viruses.

Viruses may also be classified on the basis of biological properties. To illustrate this, the Herpesviridae family has been classified accordingly (Table 14).

The neuroviruses may also be classified on the basis of portal of entry of entry in man (Table 15). The importance of this lies in studying the epidemiology of diseases and in initiating control measures, for instance in various arthopode-borne encephalitis.

PATHOGENESIS

The following are the steps involved in pathogenesis:

- Entry of virus to susceptible cell, multiplication and spread (Tables 15 and 16).[40]
- Host immune response.[44]
- Effect of virus on cell function.
- Viral clearance.

Pathogenesis of viral infections depends on the type of interactions between viral and host factors. A minimum amount of the viral inoculum is necessary to induce infection and this varies with the virulence of the organism and the robustness of the host defense mechanisms.[38] Some strains of

Table 13: Classification of major neuroviruses into families based on chemical and physical properties

Nucleic acid core	*Capsid symmetry*	*Virion*	*Viral size (nm*)*	*No. of genes (Approx)*	*Viral family*	*Viruses*
DNA	Icosahedral	Naked	70–90	30	Adenoviridae	Adenovirus
		Enveloped	100	160	Herpesviridae	Cytomegalovirus
	Complex	Complex coats	42	4	Hepadnaviridae	
RNA	Icosahedral	Naked	20–30	4–6	Picornaviridae	Polio
		Enveloped	50–70	10	Togaviridae	Rubella
		Naked	60–80	10–12	Reoviridae	
	Unknown	Enveloped	45–50	10	Flaviviridae	Japanese encephalitis
		Enveloped	50–300	10	Arenaviridae	
		Enveloped	100	4	Retroviridae	HIV
	Helical	Enveloped	90–100	3	Bunyaviridae	
		Enveloped	150–300	10	Paramyxoviridae	Measles
		Enveloped	75–180	5	Rhabdoviridae	Rabies

* nm–nanometer

Table 14: Classification based on biological properties of one of the important viral families, namely herpesviridae

Subfamily	*Growth cycle*	*Cytopathology*	*Latent infection*	*Official name*	*Common name*
Alpha herpes viruses	Short	Cytolytic	Neurons	Human herpes virus 1 Human herpes virus 2 Human herpes virus 3	Herpes simplex virus-type-I Herpes simplex virus-type 2 Varicella zoster virus
Beta herpes viruses	Long	Cytomegalic	Glands, Kidney	Human herpes virus 5	Cytomegalic virus
		Lymphotropic	Lymphnode	Human herpes virus 6 Human herpes virus 7	Human B cell lymphotropic virus RK virus
Gamma herpes viruses	Variable	Lymphoproliferative	Lymphoid tissue	Human herpes virus 4	Epstein-Barr virus

Table 15: Classification of neuroviruses based on portal of entry

Specific viruses	*Portal of entry*
Herpes simplex Varicella zoster Measles Mumps Adenoviruses Coxsackie (some) Echoviruses (some) Lymphocytic choriomeningitis Rubella	Respiratory tract
Polio Coxsackie Echo 'Kuru'	Gastrointestinal tract
Rabies HIV Arboviruses	Skin and Blood
Creutzfeldt-Jakob	Unknown

the same virus are more virulent than others. Once infection has become established, some viruses (such as rabies) cause mortality in almost 100% of cases, whereas others (such as rubella) carry a very low mortality and morbidity. Whether infection with a virus results in clinical disease depends on many factors, not all of which are understood.

Some viruses undoubtedly exhibit tropism for specific CNS cells. Neurotropism involves a complex chain of events which cascade and culminate in an exogenous virus, coercing the cells of nervous system to accept their sovereign role as an obligate intracellular parasite. An early and essential event is the recognition by the neurovirus, through the chemical configuration of its surface of specific receptors on the membrane of the cell of the nervous system. The impact of neurotropism on pathology is clear, inter alia it determines whether the virus causes a meningitis, an encephalitis or a myelitis or cerebellar crippling, whether it causes disturbances of personality and cognizance or frank mental disorder, whether conduction defects dominate the clinical picture, or whether the neurons are irrevocably lost. Neurotropism is arguably one of the most important of the attributes of the many viruses responsible for neurological affection but it does not explain everything.[40]

Host Immune Response

The first line of defense against viral invasion is the blood-brain barrier, which also keeps the CNS relatively isolated from the systemic immune system. Tight junctions connect CNS capillary endothelial cells, choroid plexus, epithelial cells and arachnoid cells, and, under normal conditions, these inhibit the passage of proteins and cells from the blood into the brain parenchyma and CSF. These tight junctions are not present between ventricular ependymal cells, so that here the flow of substances between CSF and extracellular spaces of the brain occurs more freely.[45]

Normally, the CNS has a relatively small population of immune cells. Lymphatic drainage within the brain has not been clearly demonstrated and the brain has no areas of lymphocyte concentration, such as in lymph nodes or reticuloendothelial system as we normally define them. Low levels of immunoglobulins are found in normal cerebrospinal fluid (CSF), but these immunoglobulins are derived solely from the blood. The few cells, that are able to enter through the blood-brain barrier under normal conditions, are primarily monocytes and lymphocytes. Plasma cells are not normally found in the CNS and the polymorphonuclear leukocytes found in the CSF are considered abnormal.

Normally, an immune response against virus sets within a few days after primary infection or almost immediately in an immunized host. But in the central nervous system which has been described as an 'immunologically privileged site', the picture may be different.[45-47] Immune responses in the CNS during infection are recruited from the systemic circulation in a relative selective and specific fashion.[44] Cell entry is immunologically specific and does not simply mirror the proportions of cell phenotypes of blood and differs from those that are found normally and those that follow non-specific rupture in the blood brain barrier, such as occurs after a traumatic injury (for example, a stab wound). During

Table 16: Paths followed by neuroviruses after gaining entry into host

Hemic path (Usual path)	Primary multiplication at site of entry	Pass along lymphatics to local lymph nodes	Multiplication in local lymph nodes
			Enter bloodstream causing primary viremia (short lasting)
			Viruses spread along blood to 'central foci' (liver, spleen or other organs with cell specifications)
	Reach specific target areas in nervous system	Cross blood-brain barrier	Extensive multiplication in 'central foci'; viruses re-enter bloodstream causing secondary viremia
– Neuronal path (rabies and herpes simplex encephalitis): Viruses gain access to CNS by ascending the axons of peripheral and cranial nerves. – Olfactory path: Firm evidence to prove the existence of this path is wanting.			

the viral infections, the blood brain barrier becomes 'leaky' and increased protein transudation occurs. Co-incident with the protein transudation is the increase in mononuclear cells entering the perivascular areas of brain parenchyma, meninges, subependymal areas and CSF. Natural killer cells, neutrophils, macrophages and T-cells constitute the initial mononuclear infiltrate, with B cells arriving relatively late. In addition to chemotactic factors that are released by activated inflammatory cells, the entry of cells into the CNS is also facilitated by activation of endothelial cells and expression of molecules on their cell surface that make them 'sticky' and allow circulating mononuclear cells to adhere to the vessel wall before entering. In addition, T-cells, when activated, also appear to express adhesion molecules on their cell surface.

Once a virus has infected cells in the brain and significant number of viral particles is replicated, then macrophages, T-cells and NK cells may be activated. Expression of viral proteins on the infected cell surface, along with class I molecules, may enable recognition of the viral infection by cytotoxic T-cells. In the CNS, microglia, astrocytes and vascular endothelial cells are candidates for antigen presenting cells. The activated macrophages contribute to the release of interleukin-l (IL-l) and can also release a number of other factors and cytokines that can enhance the inflammatory response.[49] Again, the inflammatory response is further enhanced by the cytokines released by activated T-helper cells, the proportion of cytotoxic or helper T-cells as well as other type of inflammatory cells entering the CNS vary with the type of viral infection.

In addition, inflammatory cell type that predominates in the brain parenchyma may not necessarily predominate in the meninges of CSF. Later, usually after the first week, a significant number of plasma cells are present within the CNS and are found elevated in the CSF as manifested by distorted CSF/serum ratios of immunoglobulin and the development of oligoclonal bands. As a result of local synthesis of antibody, the concentration of virus specific antibody increases. IgG is most commonly elevated, but lgM and IgA can be found as well.

Antibody acts as the principal immunodefense for some diseases (entero and arbovirus infections), while in others (HSV, CMV), cell mediated immunity (CMI) plays an important role. Antibody, which attaches to circulating virus particles, is effective in preventing infectivity of the virus, if it has neutralizing capabilities. Antibody can neutralize virus by several methods. It may prevent viral attachment to the cell membrane. It may prevent penetration of the virus after it has attached to the cell and then may enhance the ability of the cell to degrade the virus within a pinocytic vacuole. Antibody bound virus may result in complement activation and viral lysis. Virus that is bound by antibody may also be more easily phagocytosed by macrophages.[43]

Cell mediated antiviral actions are primarily against virus-infected cells. After antibody attachment to viral antigents on the host cell surface, antibody - dependent cellular cytotoxicity can occur via NK cells, macrophages or polymorphonuclear cells. Cell-mediated antiviral actions also include the elaboration of cytokines that enhance the immune response and, in the case of interferon (IFN), inhibit viral replication. Activation of immune system during viral infection can be a double-edged sword. In some viral infections, the immune response is responsible for more tissue damage than the virus itself. Other viruses are associated within increased frequency of autoimmune phenomena, resulting in tissue damage secondary to an overactive immune system.[43]

The integrity of host defense responses and the ability to mount an appropriate cellular and humoral response are critical. The range of viruses which may become pathogenic when the immune response is impaired, such as following cytotoxic chemotherapy for malignancy, immune suppression after organ transplantation or due to human immunodeficiency virus (HIV) infection, is increasing.[38]

Effect of Virus on Cell Functions

Viruses exhibit cell and organ specificity, indicating existence of surface receptors for virus on target cells *(cell tropism)*. The outcome of interaction of virus and host cell may be:

- *Cell transformation*: Virus infects the cells and its nucleic acid get integrated in the host cell DNA, leading to cell transformation. The virus is not generally produced from the infected cell.
- *Abortive infection*: Certain viruses are able to infect cells but do not replicate within them, this is called abortive infection. In it, there is either loss of some essential function in the cell due to mutation or production of interfering substances.
- *Cytolytic/cytocytic growth*: This results in cytopathic effect on host cell in the form of inclusion bodies and cell necrosis.
- *Noncytocidal productive growth*: This may result in persistent infections which may remain latent, inapparent (sub-clinical) or may progress to chronic infection.[43]

Virus Clearance

Virus is normally cleared within the first 1–2 weeks. Most inflammatory cells leave CNS relatively rapidly after virus clearance. The blood-brain barrier function usually normalizes within a week or two, as reflected by the normalization of the CSF albumin concentration,[48] CSF pleocytosis, cytokine pattern and the perivascular inflammatory response. Usually, the CSF antibody levels begin to return to normal within a few weeks but, in certain virus infections, antibody may persist for years. Plasma cells have been found to persist for months in the brain. Inflammatory cells may pass into the circulation or enter the cervical lymph nodes. The path way to cervical lymph nodes has not been elucidated.[45] In chronic viral infection of the CNS, inflammatory cells may persist in the brain parenchyma and CSF and levels of immunoglobulin may remain elevated. CD8+ T-cells can remain chronically elevated in the CSF during human immunodeficiency virus (HIV) infection, cytomegalovirus encephalitis and subacute sclerosing panencephalitis.

PATHOLOGY

Benign aseptic meningitis: Viral meningitis is much more common than bacterial meningitis but, as implied by its name, it carries a favorable prognosis. It is a relatively mild condition, yet there are exceptions and severe, sometimes fatal cases, are recognized. Because most patients with viral meningitis recover, postmortem studies are limited and there is a serious lack of information about the pathogenesis and pathology of the syndrome.[40,50]

Acute encephalitis: The term 'acute encephalitis' is entirely non-specific and is used clinically to describe many different syndromes with a catalogue of common features, all somewhat reminiscent of cerebral tumors or abscesses. They include acute or subacute onset, headache, fever, altered level of consciousness (ranging progressively from drowsiness and confusion to coma), meningeal irritation, disturbances of affect and speech, seizures, nystagmus, hemianopia and palsies.

Inflammation of brain or cord tissue is the hallmark of most acute virus encephalopathies. But, it is an entirely non-specific marker and merely signals an immune response without any regard to the nature of the stimulus. Edema is probably the first step of a developing inflammatory catastrophe. The edema is likely to increase with time and is destined to become a determinant factor within the unyielding confines of the cranium; the brain cannot expand to accommodate the water it accumulates as part of the inflammatory response. For example, pressure marks on the surface of fixed brain postmortem, particularly on the base and around the stem, is a characteristic feature of herpes encephalitis; fatal herniation of the uncus and of the cerebellar tonsils are dire consequences of the problem in vivo.

The cellular response in the patient CSF is invariable and usually monophasic, but it may be biphasic or even triphasic. The predominant infiltrating cells are always lymphocytes. A biphasic nature is particularly characteristic in infections with enteroviruses; a brief but quite intense polymorph response precedes the definitive lymphocytic infiltration. The triphasic nature is observed only in the severest cases, such as in acute necrotizing encephalitis. It is a result of tissue necrosis, which in turn stimulates a deployment of scavenging cells and polymorphs.

Acute Gray Matter Encephalitis and Myelitis

In the neurotropic 'non-enveloped RNA' viruses, causing this pathology, are enteroviruses. Among the enveloped viruses are herpes viruses and lenti viruses (HIV-1 and 2).

The histological appearance of neuronal death is that of neuronophagia. Neurons are set in gray matter and neuronophagia is a composite term used to describe the appearance of a CNS nodule, comprising one or more dead neurons surrounded by clusters of reactive microglial cells, astrocytes and lymphocytes. The dead neuron loses its ability to stain and within a few days is removed. This is one of the most significant aspects of virus infection of the CNS, an aspect that distinguishes the pathology of neuroinfection from virus infection of other organs. Neurons do not divide and consequently cannot be replaced after a cytolytic virus infection. Hence, the loss of neuronal tissue is irreversible; even though in all probability the lytic infection will be overcome and eliminated by host defense mechanism (with or without the help of antiviral therapy), damage to the nervous system and the resultant neurological crippling are certain to be permanent, even if subclinical. Loss of motor neurons in the spinal cord leads to lower motor neuron paralysis and death of motor cell in the respiratory center signal the onset of bulbar paralysis. The disappearance of neurons in the dominant temporal lobe can cause loss of speech and the dense amnesia, sometimes seen after recovery from herpetic encephalitis, is manifestation of neuronophagia in the limbic system.

The bedside physician, with skills to unravel the clinical enigmas of neurological disease, may some times exaggerate the importance of neurological foci and single structure involvement. Functional areas of the CNS are really all in fairly close anatomical proximity to each other. By contrast, viruses have a specific propensity to spread from cell to continuous cell, and they can move using both antegrade and retrograde axoplasmic flow relatively long distances via the cytoplasm of single nerve fiber. Secondary pathological processes (such as inflammation, glial cell loss, edema, vascular obstruction and rarefaction necrosis) are certainly not likely to respect the natural boundaries between one CNS structure and its neighbor. Lesions in one anatomical site are certain to exert a pathological influence on kindred areas in the CNS.

Acute White Matter Encephalitis and Myelitis

Acute disseminated leucoencephalomyelitis (ADE) (postviral encephalomyelitis; acute hemorrhagic leucoencephalitis; cerebellar ataxis; post-vaccinial encephalitis; transverse myelitis; ascending myelitis; acute paraplegic syndrome) represents a complex of syndromes.[5] The white matter of the CNS is white because it is predominantly myelin and consists mostly of myelinated nerve fibers. In ADE, the critical lesion is dissolution of myelin. The demyelination is characteristically patchy and centerd around the perivenous and perivenular spaces. In most cases, the myelinoclasis is complemented by brisk inflammatory response. Macroscopically, the brain (or cord) is swollen through edema; often there is herniation. Meningitis is usual and there are signs of perfusion failure, small hemorrhages and even necrosis. There is no firm information to explain the pathogenesis of ADE. Basically, there are three 'immunological' and a handful of other theories, but none is entirely satisfactory. One of the favourite hypothesis relates ADE to experimental allergic encephalitis (EAE) (or autoimmune).

ADE has five clinical phases. The first corresponds to the natural incubation period of the provoking infection which may be rubeola (measles), chickenpox, rubella, mumps, influenza or any other infection. Then follows the prodromal fever. The third phase corresponds to lysis of fever, fading of the rash (if any) and convalescence. It is at this point that disturbance in CNS occurs. Phase four begins 2–20 days following onset of prodromal illness. Typically, there is recrudescence of fever and suddenly the patient has rapid-onset encephalitis, cerebellar ataxia, myelitis or optic neuritis. Phase five of ADE corresponds to convalescence, remyelination and recovery, with or without permanent damage to the CNS.

DISEASES AND SYNDROMES

Acute Viral Diseases

These diseases result directly from viral invasion, i.e. the causative virus crosses the blood-brain barrier and is then present in the affected CNS tissue, fluid or both; for instance, most cases of acute viral meningitis and essentially all cases of acute encephalitis.

Herpes Simplex Encephalitis

It is an important condition because of many reasons:

- It has a complex pathology which can be used as a model to *illustrate many important neuropathogenic mechanisms.*
- It has been under scrutiny for well over half a century and occurs all over the world.
- It is the only viral encephalopathy at present amenable to specific antiviral chemotherapy.
- It may represent only the tip of an iceberg in that its prevalence measures only disease and might not measure the true incidence of HSV infections of the CNS. Many cases of HSE are never diagnosed because they are mild and do not demand investigation.

Herpes encephalitis is primarily a disease of gray matter, but such can be its intensity that extension to meninges and to white matter is inevitable. The target cells are primarily neurons, but oligodendrocytes, other glial cells and even ependymal cells are not necessarily exempt. Temporal-limbic structures are usually affected. Pathologically, there is acute necrotizing encephalitis with neuronal loss and perivascular lymphocytic infiltrates; intranuclear inclusion bodies in the neurons and the glia are characteristic. There is debate about whether HSE is the result of a current primary infection with an instantly acquired exogenous strain of HSV or whether it is the result of reactivation of latent virus or both mechanisms. It is worth postulating that there might be latent infection with HSV of at least a few brain cells in almost every adult beyond the age of 30 years. This can be the cause of a gray matter disease of cataclysmic proportions and of rapid evolution.

The presentation of HSE is protean. The onset of disease is often insidious, though it may be violent. A variety of behavioral changes may herald the onset of this disorder. Personality changes, some quite violent, may feature prominently. The acute syndrome is characterized by cognitive changes, focal neurological signs, seizures and eventual coma. Amnesia and some forms of aphasia may also be seen.

The diagnosis of HSE is a complex matter. Many diseases masquerade as HSE, some of which are treatable. Victims mostly present as neurological emergencies and intensive care can have decisive effect on the outcome. HSE cannot in any circumstance be diagnosed by antibody tests on serum alone.

The diagnoses can be reached by one of the four approaches. One is the direct identification of HSV by culture or by immunodetection in brain biopsy. The examination of the brain tissue is the 'gold standard'. Currently, it is the only approach that will yield a firm diagnosis (sensitivity 80–85%; specificity 100%) and in time to influence patient management. By immunofluorescence, a positive result can be obtained within 2–3 hours of biopsy. However from a clinical viewpoint, there are severe practical and ethical constraints in brain biopsy, though it is often essential to the differential diagnosis of clinically similar conditions.

Second is the demonstration of synthesis of HSV antibody within the CNS. Only when it can be shown, that the bulk of HSV antibody in CSF is not a transudate, can a safe diagnosis be made. A simple way to know this is to calculate the Klapper antibody index:

$$\frac{\text{CSF HSV antibody titer: serum HSV antibody liter}}{\text{CSF albumin concentration: Serum albumin concentration}}$$

In health, the index is less than 1.5 and in HSE, it lies above 1.9.

The third approach is histological demonstration of typical intranuclear eosinophilic inclusions (or, by electron microscopy, typical virions) in brain tissue and a significant specific immune response. The fourth approach, which is a recent development, is the use of the highly sensitive polymerase chain reaction (PCR) to identify viral DNA in the CSF.

Acute Parainfectious Neurological Syndromes

Here, the implicated virus does not cross into the CNS and is not present in the affected neural material. These forms develop 1–4 weeks after the onset of a variety of viral infections (see Table 17). These syndromes are believed mainly autoimmune in nature or show antibody and/or cell-mediated immune reactivity to neuroantigen.[41] An implication of this classification is that antiviral chemotherapy has little role in the management of these syndromes.

Congenital Defects

Viral invasion of the CNS in the fetus produces severe encephalitides with extensive inflammatory and necrotic lesions, as well as a variety of neural malformations and functional deficits (see Table 18) that are frequently accompanied by a number of teratogenic effects. The type and severity of these conditions depend on the etiologic agent as well as on the gestational development at the time of infection. The introduction of the rubella vaccination has considerably decreased the frequency of these congenital infections, at least in developed countries, but a limited number of cases of these devastating afflictions persist.

Subacute and Chronic Diseases

Recently, a number of well defined subacute and chronic neurological disorders have been recognized to be caused by persistent infections with conventional and unconventional viruses (Table 19). These disorders include both 'degenerative' noninflammatory diseases and demyelinating inflammatory diseases. These conditions are generally rare, but some are opportunistic diseases and develop preferentially in immunocompromised subjects; their number appears likely to increase in asssociation with the increasing number of immunocompromised individuals. An augmented incidence of Papovavirus-induced progressive multifocal leucoencephalopathy has already been noted as a consequence of the HIV pandemic.

Table 17: Parainfectious neurological syndromes and the viruses involved

Syndromes	*Triggering viruses*
Postinfectious encephalomyelitis	Measles, rubella, influenza and others
Guillain-Barre syndrome (Acute immune-mediated polyneuropathy)	VZV, mumps, CMV, HIV, and others
Reye's syndrome	VZV, influenza
von Economo's disease (Encephalitis lethargica)	Influenza

Table 18: Major neurological malformations and deficits associated with viral infections of the fetus

Diseases involved	*Viruses*
Microcephaly; hydrocephalus; limb hypoplasia; microgyria; cerebral calcifications; visual, auditory, motor and mental deficits	CMV, rubella HIV, HSV, others

Table 19: Subacute and chronic neuropathies caused by viruses

Disease	*Virus*
Subacute sclerosing panencephalitis Chronic progressive panencephalitis Progressive congenital encephalomyelitis Congenital cytomegalic inclusion disease AIDS-dementia complex and peripheral neuropathies	Measles Rubella Rubella CMV HIV
Spongiform encephalopathies	Unconventional viruses
Recurrent meningitis	Echo
Subacute encephalitis	Measles
Progressive multifocal leukoencephalopathy	JC polyomavirus
Persistent meningitis	

Subacute Sclerosing Panencephalitis (SSPE)

It is a rare condition associated with a persistent CNS infection with measles virus, but the nature and role of this persistence are mysterious. The encephalopathy occurs in children and in young adults, years after a natural, uncomplicated episodes of measles. After many years, the subacute disease declares itself with the insidious onset of behavioral, personality, intellectual and motor disabilities.

Laboratory analyses reveal elevated measles antibody titers. Cerebrospinal fluid reveals elevated protein with immunoglobulin G accounting for up to 60% of protein concentration and high measles antibody titers. The EEG is a key diagnostic tool, showing high amplitude bilateral and stereotyped complexes that repeat very 4–5 seconds. CT studies reveal enlarged ventricles and cortical, cerebellar and brainstem atrophy. PET scans show early subcortical hypermetabolism, followed by global cortical and hypometabolism.[42] Autopsy studies show gray and white matter microscopic abnormalities consisting of lymphocytic and plasma cell infiltrates.

Progressive Rubella Panencephalitis (PRPE)

It is more rate than SSPE. There are no clues about the pathogenesis of this very curious and exceptionally *rare* disease.[40] In clinical presentation, PRPE is not unlike SSPE, but there are differences such as the extended time course of the disease (10–15 years) and optic atrophy.

Progressive Multifocal Leukoencephalopathy (PML)

It is a rare disease caused by JC, a human polyomavirus occurring in occasional patients with some form of lymphoma, including Hodgkin's disease, more frequently in AIDS and rarely in sarcoidosis. The critical lesion appears to be in white matter where JC virus infects and destroys oligodendrocytes; in turn, this leads to foci of demyelination. Virus possibly also infects astrocytes, which assume strange multinucleated forms suggestive of a glioma. Patients typically present with an abrupt onset and focal neurological and neuropsychological signs, dependent on the site of lesions. Aphasia, hemineglect or visual field abnormalities, striking visuospatial disturbance and apraxia, are examples of specific neuropsychological syndromes that can be seen in the condition. The disease progresses rapidly with death occurring in 2–4 months in most cases. No unique diagnostic findings are seen in analyses of serum, blood, urine and the CSF; brain biopsy is the only means of making a certain diagnosis. Neuroimaging studies are helpful; multifocal areas of high signal intensity are typically seen in the white matter. CT findings also reveal non-enhancing lucent areas in the white matter. PET and SPECT studies may likewise reveal multifocal areas of reduced metabolic activity and blood flow respectively.[42] Some patients may show temporary improvement when treated with cytarabine, but in most cases the disease is irreversible, and it is invariably rapidly progressive.

Spongiform Encephalopathies/Unconventional Slow Viral Diseases

These are Creutzfeldt-Jakob disease, Kuru and Gerstmann-Straussler syndrome. These are characterized by long incubation period (on the order of 1/3rd of the host's life span), a clinical and pathological picture that is limited to the central nervous system (CNS), and invariably progressive, degenerative, and fatal course.[51-53]

The mystique of these diseases is a consequence of the unusual nature of the etiological agents.[54,55]

It is expected that an understanding of the nature of these agents will reveal new mechanisms of CNS disease and dysfunction, and will open up new areas of biology and molecular biology. The spongiform encephalopathies and Alzheimer's disease share several similarities: onset in middle to late years, primary pathology limited to the CNS, amyloid deposition in the brain, and sporadic and familial patterns of occurrence.[56] So, it is expected that an understanding of the spongiform encephalopathies may well assist in understanding basic mechanisms operating in Alzheimer's disease and other degenerative CNS disease of unknown etiology.

Persistent Meningitis

It is seen in subjects with inability to deploy specific immunoglobulins of adequate quality or quantity to eliminate an infection with enteroviruses (usually echoviruses). An curious eponymous condition, called Mollaret's meningitis, has been reported from time-to-time. This is recognized from recurrent episodes of neck stiffness, headache, lymphocytic CSF pleocytosis and fever. Each recurrence is by itself indistinguishable from single attack of benign aseptic meningitis, but in the latter condition the infection is rapidly eliminated.

Idiopathic (Viral) Neurological and Psychiatric Disorders

There are a number of neuropsychiatric disorders in which intensive research is being pursued with regard to the role of viruses and virus related genetic elements and some role of these have been found in these disorders (Table 20). Correlation between the presence of virus, viral genome or antibody titers are not very useful in determining causal relations for many reasons.[57] Firstly, most viruses are ubiquitous; it is estimated that 81% of adults over 35 years old have antibody to cytomegalovirus and that 40-50% of adults have antibody to the cold sore virus, herpes simplex type I (HSV-I).[58] It is likely that only a susceptible subject of infected persons would respond to virus in an unusual way that might cause mental illness. Secondly, exposure to and, thus infection by, a virus is determined in part by behavior.

Table 20: Some neurological and psychiatric disorders for which a viral origin has been suggested

- Demyelinating
  - Multiple sclerosis and its variants
  - Tropical spastic paraparesis (HTLV-I ?)
  - Behchet's disease
  - Other chronic myelopathies
- Degenerative
  - Amyotrophic lateral sclerosis
  - Parkinson's disease
  - Alzheimer's disease
- Psychiatric
  - Schizophrenia
- Vascular
  - Arteriosclerosis
  - Angitis
- Proliferative
  - Meningioma
  - Glioma
  - Other Tumors
- Others
  - Myalgic encephalomyelitis (or postviral fatigue syndrome)

Because of this, a high prevalence of infection amongst a target group may mean that the disorder they suffer from led them to expose themselves to the virus, not the virus caused the disorder, e.g., there is a high incidence of HSV-I antibody among the institutionalized retarded.[59] Rather than attributing mental retardation to HSV-I, we must recognize that level of contact and hygiene among the retarded might lead to spread of many common viruses. Thirdly, because viruses tend to be transmitted to family members, it is often not easy to differentiate genetic from viral etiology. Fourth, viruses are often not easy to detect; some do not provoke an immune response and therefore cannot be detected by antibody measures. In addition, incomplete or defective virus particles, which cannot be detected by culture methods, can cause disease. Finally, because developmental effects may not manifest for years after the original infection, it is difficult to connect mild infections with later sequele. Thus, it is not only difficult to prove that a virus causes illness, it is difficult to rule out viral causality because 'absence of proof is not proof of absence'.

Multiple Sclerosis (MS), Amyotrophic Sclerosis and Motor Neuron Disease

These remain as syndromes in which viral infections may be implicated.[60-62] For the present, there are no credible candidates. The list of agents isolated from patients with MS include HSV, para-influenza virus and CMV, among many others. Early serological tests suggested an association between MS and Human T-lymphotropic virus (HTLV). Recent surveys have confirmed the role of HTLV in the tropical manifestation of lateral column myopathy, but not in the nontropical forms nor in MS. Amyotrophic sclerosis bears some clinical similarity to poliomyelitis, and a small epidemic of this degenerative disease was recently observed in Guam.

Tropical spastic paraparesis may or may not be a particular epidemiological form of multiple sclerosis, but one characteristic feature has recently emerged. The syndrome occurs in the Caribbean, the Seychelles and West Africa, and more than half of those afflicted have serological evidence of exposure to human T lymphotropic virus type I (HTLV-1). In the same environment, fewer than 1 in 20 controls have demonstrable antibody.

Schizophrenia

It is a clinical syndrome without known cause. Despite numerous studies suggesting an association with genetic, toxic-metabolite, endocrine, viral-immunological and other biological factors, the etiology of schizophrenia is not known.[63,64] From time-to-time, there are claims of virus isolation from brain or lumbar fluid from patients with schizophrenia. None of the candidate viruses resisted critical study and theories about a single viral etiology for this disease remain entirely unproven. It may be that different viruses produce similar pathology.

Different case reports of patients presenting psychiatric symptoms during viral infections with herpes simplex encephalitis, varicella zoster encephalitis or subacute sclerosing panencephalitis have led to the suggestion that viral infections might play a role in the pathogenesis of schizophrenia. An increased incidence of schizophrenia, in children of mothers infected by an influenza epidemic in England in 1957 during pregnancy, point to a viral pathogenesis as well.[65] Epidemiological data have shown an increased number of manifestations of schizophrenia in winter born people.[64] Moreover, there are numerous studies, detecting raised titers of antibodies against certain viruses (Herpes simplex, measles, cytomegalovirus, varicella, bornavirus) in schizophrenic patients as compared to controls, and/or increased CSF/serum ratio of viral antibodies indicating a local synthesis of antibodies in the brain or CSF.[66,67]

Results of many psychoneuroimmunological studies indicate that about 20–50% of the schizophrenic patients show immune alterations. Many studies have reported elevated T helper lymphocytes ($CD4^+$) and/or elevated $CD4^+/CD8^+$ ratios.[68-70] These, along with reduced IL-2 levels (Interleukin-2) and increased number of IL-2 receptors, point to an activation of the immune system in schizophrenic patients.[71,72]

The viral and autoimmune hypothesis of schizophrenia may be thought of in relation to the role of viruses in molecular mimicry.[73-75] Viruses induce cells to change their identity, probably via expressing new or different members surface antigen; thus, they are not recognized as 'self', but as 'non-self', and therefore are attacked by their own immune cells. The close relationship of clinical features of schizophrenia and signs of immune activation as well may indicate that the immune activation represents only an epiphenomenon of schizophrenia.

In further studies, these results may be taken into account and schizophrenia patients may be subtyped by biological, especially immunological screening methods, into those with and without immune alterations to elicit more valid and compatible results.[75]

Myalgic Encephalomyelitis

Postviral fatigue syndrome, Royal free disease, Epidemic neuromyasthenia, Akureyi disease, Iceland disease, and Myalgic encephalomyelitis (ME), might or might not all refer to a single disease. Clinical experience suggests that there are probably three more or less distinct syndromes.[40] Onem perhaps best described as 'postviral neurasthenia', occurs during the months following an episode usually labelled 'glandular fever'. It resembles normal convalescence but is excessively protracted. The neurasthenia usually persists for no more than 6 months but, sometimes, it continues for up to 3 years.

The second syndrome has been reported to occur in sizeable epidemics, often in residential communities. Those affected complain of sudden onset of headache and muscle pain. There may be some myoclonus, some upper motor neuron-like paralysis and signs of brain stem involvement (nystagmus, vertigo, etc.). The disease last some 3 to 6 months, after which most patients recover, but in some individuals symptoms persist and the syndrome merges into the third category described next.

The third syndrome has earned the name, ME, for reasons which are not at all clear. The condition is best described as 'endemic', patients (more often women than men) frequently link the onset of symptoms with a viral illness, but the triggering episode (mild sore throat, fever, etc.) is considerably more vague than the clinical glandular fever preceding the true postviral neurasthenia (see above), and the incapacity that follows is rarely self-limiting.

Patients do not 'snap out' of the problem, but muscle fatigue after the slightest effort, myalgia and self-pitying depression may continue for as long as 20 years or even more.

Viral causes for all three syndromes have long been postulated, but no hypothesis has yet survived critical examination. Epstein-Barr virus (EBV) remains the favourite, if unlikely, nominee for the first of the three illnesses. No virus has so far emerged as likely candidate responsible for the epidemics, such as those at the Royal Free Hospital in London (over 300 cases) or 20 years earlier in Los Angeles (200 cases); for this reason, cynics have repeatedly offered a diagnosis of mass hysteria. Yet, this completely fails to address some of the quite clear-cut CNS signs witnessed by critical observers and one is left to conclude that something organic, and possibly viral, must be going on. Many experienced and wise practitioners are utterly convinced about the reality of ME as a disturbing cause of morbidity and a serious health problem.[5]

VIROLOGY LABORATORY TECHNIQUES

Virology laboratory tests, available to diagnose neuroviral agents, can be grouped into three categories (Table 21).[76,77]

Techniques in Directly Identifying Viruses/Viral Specific Structures/Antigen/Nucleic Acid

The indications are:

- When patient is presenting in the initial period of disease (also called *window period*).
- When rapid diagnosis has to be established in few hours.
- Immunodeficient cases, where serologic response is deficient.
- For diagnosis of new disease agents.

Electron Microscopy

It gives the best possibility for unearthing new viruses. However, the technique has low sensitivity and the specimen

Table 21: Categories of virology laboratory tests available to diagnose neuroviral agents

A	Techniques in directly identifying	Viruses	– Electron microscopy – Immune electron microscopy
		Viral specific structures	– e.g. Inclusion bodies in corneal smear of rabies cases
		Antigen	– ELISA/ Immunofluorescent techniques
		Nucleic acid	– Southern blot/Dot blot – In situ hybridization – Polymerase chain reaction (PCR)
B	Virus culture/ Isolation	Animal	– e.g. Intracerebral inoculation into suckling mice done for coxsackie viruses
		Embryonated egg inoculation	– e.g. Chorioallantoic membrane used for herpes viruses
		Cell culture	– e.g. Human embryonic kidney, a primary cell line used routinely
C	Measurement of antibodies	Different Techniques available	– ELISA, Latex agglutination, virus neutralization, immunofluorescence and others

should have 10^3-10^6 particles/mL, depending on the size of virus and nature of specimen for detection to occur.

Immune Electron Microscopy

It is an improvement over the above technique in which specific antibodies are used to concentrate the viruses in the specimen.

Dot Blot Hybridization And In Situ Hybridization

Both techniques are based on the fact that single stranded nucleic acid will reanneal in a characteristic way with complementary strands and if the latter are tagged, the detection is possible. In situ hybridization is used for probing directly viral nucleic acid in thin sections of tissue.

Polymerase Chain Reaction

It is a new and exquisitely sensitive technique to allow up to a million-fold amplification of DNA fragments. This enables it to pick a single viral genome in specimens containing thousands of cells. Recently, this technique was used to search CMV and other herpesviruses in brain tissue from schizophrenic patients.[39]

Virus Culture/Isolation

The indications are:

- It detects unexpected and totally new agents in certain clinical situations.
- It is a gold standard against which newer methods are compared and evaluated.
- It confirms serologic tests.

Virus culture has not been greatly successful in the diagnosis of CNS infections, largely due to difficulty of obtaining specimens of neural tissue. It may be possible to culture virus from other sources but this is seldom fruitful.

The brain, cord and retina are remote organs, anatomically and perceptually. Thus, their sampling for virological investigation poses problems and surrogate tests are often accepted for want of a better alternative. Cerebrospinal fluid is often fairly easily available. However, many patients with CNS viral infections suffer from cerebral edema and raised intracranial pressure, and there is a real risk of brain stem herniation and lumbar puncture can provoke the catastrophe. Thus, the aggressive neurovirologist has reason to temper his enthusiasm.

Viruses have varying range of host cell specificity; for this reason, it is important to inoculate specimens into several different types of cells when attempting isolation. In routine practice, it is usual to inoculate specimens into cultures of primary monkey and human kidney and of human embryo fibroblasts. These should cover most of the important human pathogens usually encountered.

The major drawback with virus isolation has always been the length of time required to grow and identify a virus, besides the difficulty in obtaining the right specimen at the right time and getting it to the laboratory quickly. Cytomegalovirus (CMV) can take 2 weeks or longer for isolation.

Measurement of Antibodies (Serologic)

The indications are:

- Conditions where good serologic tests are available.
- Testing for immunity.
- Testing effectiveness of viral vaccines.
- For epidemiologic purposes, especially to find past infection.

The criteria used for diagnosis by serology are:

- Two serum specimens are usually required: an 'acute' specimen (taken before day 7 of illness) and a 'convalescent' specimen (taken at least 1–2 weeks after the acute specimen). An increase of at least four-fold in the titer of antibody against a specific virus is indicative of infection with that virus.
- Specific IgM class antibodies in single specimen can be diagnostic. However, one should remember that the serological responses are delayed and a positive antibody index is not reliably obtained until after 10–15 days of neurological illness.
- Result of single sample containing antibodies (even IgG) can be important when these are against a truly exotic virus.
- Single sample can also be important in determining susceptibility of individual to risks, e.g. susceptibility to CMV of a proposed recipient of an organ transplant. Many assays are available to detect antibodies but it is beyond the scope of this chapter to go into their details.

Choosing A Test

Choosing the type of test(s) will depend on the type and stage of infection (Tables 22 and 23). Culture/isolation of viruses from CSF is problematical as a discriminatory test; specificity is very good but sensitivity is sadly lacking. As alternatives to virus culture, viruses in lumbar puncture fluid can be sought with an ever-increasing armamentarium of tests, including immunoflu-orescence, antigen detection and electron microscopy This is the virologist's dilemma; either he relies on tests of mediocre sensitivity and achieves nothing better than virus culture from CSF, or he recruits the exquisite sensitivity of the newer technologies; but sooner or later, he loses his bearings and his reputation. On the horizon, there may be promise of more sensitive tests on CSF, but in practical terms there is nothing at present available to improve on the relatively poor performance of virus culture.[5] It is hard to escape the conclusion that neurovirological diagnosis has

Table 22: Laboratory aids in neuroviral diagnoses

Viral antigen Or virus isolation	*Viral antibody*	*Neutralizing (NI) antibody*	*Antibody of IgM class*	*Interpretation of infection*
–	–	–	–	None
+	–/+	–	–	Early
+	+	+	+	Current
–	+	+	+	Recent
–	–/+	+	–	Old
-/+	+	+	+	Persistent

Table 23: Specimens and diagnostic tests of some important neuroviral agents

Virus	*Specimen*	*Culture/Isolation/Serology*
Rabies	Saliva, brain biopsy	Suckling mice, direct IF (Immunofluorescence) is preferable because of speed of diagnosis
Herpesvirus	Brain biopsy	Cell culture (HEL, HEp-2), Cytopathogenic effect (CPE) usually visible in 24–72 hours. Direct IF is rapid
Epstein-Barr (EB)	Blood, nasopharyngeal swab	Lymphoid cell culture, culture of EB virus not performed routinely
Varicella-zoster	Vesicle fluid	Cell culture (HEK), CPE usually visible in 4 days–2 weeks virus
Measles (rubella)	Nasopharyngeal swab, blood	Cell culture (PMK, HEK), CPE usually visible in 2–3 weeks
HIV	Blood, particularly leukocytes	Cell culture, antibody by ELISA and Western blot, routinely done
Dengue	Serum, CSF	Suckling mice, cell culture (vero)

not yet reached its apogee. Perhaps the future lies in imaging technology.

FUTURE DIRECTIONS

Animal model studies have clearly shown that the nervous system is a target for persistence by a wide spectrum of viruses and that neurotropic viruse can cause significant behavioral changes, without producing obvious histopathological alterations.[78] These findings have aroused suspicions (and hopes) that other and more widespread unexplained neurological and psychiatric disorders of man may be of similar etiologies. Because the suspicion of a viral etiology for 'idiopathic' nervous system disorders is of utmost importance, this area of research is currently one of great excitement. However, the difficulties encountered in this work are many and progress is inevitably slow. Frustration in this area is exemplified by the fact that, over the years, some 20 different viruses have been suggested as possible etiologic agents of multiple sclerosis. In schizophrenia, HIV has been added to the long list of viruses against which raised antibody titers have been detected in patients.[79,80] Thus, today it is impossible to predict whether and to what extent current suspects will be corroborated.

44.7 BRAIN IMAGING IN PSYCHIATRY

GN Saxena

INTRODUCTION

The development of non-invasive techniques for assessing brain structure, function, and chemistry has progressed rapidly since the innovation of computed tomography (CT) in the early 1970s though the current generation of imaging methods. A number of neuroimaging modalities are now commonly used in both clinical situations and for research. Contemporary neuroimaging modalities can be roughly divided into either structural modalities or functional modalities. Structure modalities include CT scan and magnetic resonance imaging (MRI). Functional modalities include position emission tomography (PET), single-photon emission computed tomography (SPECT), functional magnetic resonance imaging (FMRI), and magnetic resonance spectroscopy (MRS). All of these neuroimaging modalities will be discussed in this chapter. Although the focus of the chapter is the use of these neuroimaging modalities in clinical psychiatry, application for research will also be briefly addressed.

In general, neuroimaging techniques are used to aid in the differential diagnosis of neuropsychiatric conditions, usually to rule out a medical cause for altered mental status. Although there is great potential for future use of neuroimaging techniques to definitively diagnose psychiatric illness, currently not a single psychiatric illness can be definitively diagnosed with these tools. When a clinician is contemplating using the various currently available neuroimaging modalities, a number of factors must be considered, including the indications, risks, cost advantages, and limitations. This chapter reviews these factors and provides general guidelines for the use of neuroimaging in psychiatric practice.

STRUCTURE IMAGING MODALITIES

Computed Tomography

Technology

Standard X-ray imaging has been used as a medical diagnostic tool for over a century. X-rays are differentially attenuated, depending on the material through which they pass (higher attenuation in dense material such as bone and lower attenuation in less dense material such as air and fluid). All radiological procedures use different detection systems to quantitate attenuation. Standard X-rays procedures involve X-ray generators producing X-ray that pass in a unidirectional manner through tissue and then impact on X-ray sensitive film. Computed tomography (CT), developed in the1970s, is simply the use of standard X-rays with newer technology for acquisition and image reconstruction (Gibby and Zimmeerman 2007). CT scanners utilize multiple X-ray generators and detectors (scintillation crystals) arranged in a ring-like fashion. The body part of interest is placed inside this ring and X-ray pass through the tissue in a multidirectional manner. Instead of using X-ray sensitive film, the detectors send information regarding attenuation to a computer. In addition, the body part of interest is imaged in a slab—wise or slice-wise manner (thus the term "tomography") as it progresses through the CT scanner. After data acquisition, powerful computers are required to integrate and process the large volume of data that results from a CT scan in order to produce a completed CT image. In addition to standard CT imaging, newer methods of using CT continue to develop. For example, spiral CT uses a rapid acquisition sequence to assess perfusion and may be used in a number of clinical situations including when a pulmonary embolus is suspected. In CT angiography, contrast is utilized to assess the integrity of vasculature throughout the body. However, neither of these more recent innovations have great utility is psychiatric populations at this time.

CT with Contrast

As is the case for many standard X-ray procedures, the use of contrast agents with CT can increase the likelihood of identifying a lesion that may otherwise be missed or provide additional information about the lesion (Osborn 1994). Radio-opaque contrast material introduced intravenously allows visualization of lesions that compromise the integrity of the blood-brain barrier e.g. carebrovascular accident (CVA), tumor, inflammation because the contrast leaks from the intravascular space. Contrast media which enhance the visibility of pathology by CT are typically iodine-based and may be either ionic or nonionic. Ionic contrast is far less expensive than nonionic contrast, but is associated with a greater risk of side effects (Gibby and Zimmerman 1992). For example, idiosyncratic reactions occur in approximately 5% of cases where ionic contrast is used and includes hypotension, nausea, flushing, urticaria, and sometimes frank anaphylaxis. Risk factors for these idiosyncratic reactions to ionic contrast include age of less than 1 year or greater than 60 years, and a history of asthma, allergies, cerebrovascular disease, or prior contrast reactions (Shehadi 1982). In addition, chemotoxic reactions to ionic contrast can occur in the brain and the kidney. Chemotoxicity may present as impaired renal function or even renal failure, with the main risk factor being pre-existing renal insufficiency (Hayman et al, 1980). In the brain, chemotoxic reactions manifest as seizures. Such reactions occur in approximately 1 in every 10,000 cases but may develop in 1 to 10% of cases in which gross disruption of the blood-brain barrier is present (Witten et al, 1973). Nonionic contrast is less likely to cause idiosyncratic or chemotoxic reactions, but the cost remains several fold more than that of ionic contrast (White and Halden 1986).

Advantages and Limitations

- CT offers excellent spatial resolution (<1 mm) and is effective at distinguishing tissue with markedly different X-ray attenuation properties (e.g. bone versus soft tissue versus fluid versus gas).
- CT is useful for the detection of acute bleeding (less than 24 to 72 hours old) but less helpful in subacute bleeding (more than 72 hours old) and in severely anaemic patients (hemoglobin below 10 g/dL) (Osborn 1994). In addition, CT is an excellent modality for imaging bone. CT is the imaging modality of choice for acute trauma or when an acute bleed or ischemia is suspected.
- CT is not helpful in visualizing subtle white-matter lesions due to CTs poor ability to distinguish between the X-ray attenuation properties of different soft tissue densities.

- CT uses ionizing radiation and thus is strongly contraindicated in pregnancy. Woman of childbearing potential should undergo a pregnancy screen prior to having a CT scan.
- Patient anxiety is usually less during a CT scan than during an MRI because the scanning environment is more open, there is less noise associated with the procedure, and scanning time is relatively brief (~ 10 minutes for the brain).
- CT is best for patients with metallic implants (e.g. foreign bodies, some aneurysm clips, pacemarkers, etc.) as MRI is contraindicated in this patient population.

Magnetic Resonance Imaging

Technology

Magnetic resonance imaging (MRI) does not use X-ray but instead exploits the magnetic properties of hydrogen atoms in water molecules to construct a representation of tissue (Horowitz 1992). An MRI scanner is comprised of coil (or antenna) detectors arranged in a ring-like fashion. Initially, during an MRI scanning session, radiofrequency irradiation is produced by the scanner and directed at the body tissue. Next, the radiofrequency irradiation source is turned off. This results in relaxation of the hydrogen atom nuclei. As the hydrogen atom nuclei relax, they give off energy that is detected by MRI scanner coils. It is this signal that is measured by MRI scanner. Different components of the relaxation process exist and occur at different rates (called T1 and T2) in different tissues. Specific imaging parameters (T1-weighted versus T2-weighted) are selected according to the clinical circumstances.

T1-weighted images are typically used for optimal visualization of normal anatomy. T1-weighted images depict gray matter as dark and white matter as light. T2-weighted images (also referred to as proton density images) are typically used to detect areas of pathology. In T2-weighted images, blood appears dark (useful for detecting hemorrhagic) because of the paramagnetic properties of detecting regions with increased water appears light (useful for detecting regions with regions with increased water content such as tumors or edema).

Recent innovations in MRI technology include MR angiography, which utilizes contrast to assess the integrity of the vasculature. Magnetic resonance angiography has little utility in psychiatric populations at this time. Diffusion-weighted MRI is a newer MRI technique that detects the tiny random movements of water molecules (diffusion) in tissue (Albers 1998). This technique allows a map of the average apartment diffusion coefficient (ADC) to be calculated. Shortly after the onset of an ischemic stroke, the ADC of brain tissue is significantly reduced because of cytotoxic edema. Over several days, the rapid initial drop in ADC is followed by are turn to "pseudonormal" values at approximately 1 week, and by elevation above normal values subsequently. Diffusion-weighted MRI is remarkably sensitive in detecting and localizing acute regions of ischemia for chronic infarcts. Because of these properties, imaging modality of choice for situations where acute ischemia is suspected.

MRI with Contrast

Gadolinium is used as the contrast medium for MRI studies because of its paramagnetic properties (Bradley et al. 1993). Like CT contrast, it is introduced intravascularly. Once injected, gadolinium alters the local magnetic environment (i.e. tissue relaxation times). The use of MRI contrast highlights vascular structures and aids in the detection of pathology in areas where blood vessel walls or the blood-brain barrier is compromised. Gadolinium causes fewer and less severe side effects than does CT contrast, with only one reported death in over 5 million dosings.

Advantages and Limitations

- MRI provides excellent spatial resolution and superior soft-tissue contrast in comparison to CT (i.e. more useful for the visualization of white matter and white matter lesions). Also, while CT images are always axial images, MRI data can be resliced in any plane.
- MRI is superior for surveying the ***posterior fossa*** and brain stem.
- Fresh blood from acute bleed (< 48–72 hours) is not easily distinguished from gray matter. However, diffusion-weighted MRI may soon change this. Subacute bleeding (> 48–72 hours) or chronic hematomas are identified with MRI.
- MRI does not use ionizing radiation, and so it is preferable to CT in pregnancy, but still is relatively contraindicated.
- MRI is contraindicated in patients with metallic implants for the following reasons:
  - Metal can cause artifacts in MR images.
  - Mental can shift position or absorb heat within the magnetic field, causing burn injuries.
  - Mechanical devices such as pacemakers can malfunction within the magnetic field.
- As many as 10% of patients undergoing MRI scanning experience significant anxiety during the imaging session. This is likely due to a number of factors. MRI scanners are much deeper (often several feet deep) than CT scanners; patients generally perceive the MRI scanner as more tunnel-like and may experience claustrophobia. Pretreatment of potentially anxious patients with benzodiazepines or other sedatives/hypnotics before undergoing MRI may be helpful in these situations. Also, the noise associated with the procedure is much louder than with CT. lastly, the scanning time required more for MRI versus ~10 minutes for a CT of the brain).

CT versus MRI

- CT is the modality of choice for patients with acute bleeds or acute trauma, though diffusion-weighted MRI may soon become the modality of choice for assessing suspected acute brain ischemic events.
- MRI is superior to CT for the differentiation of white from gray matter and the identification of white from gray matter lesions.
- MRI is superior to CT for the detection of posterior fossa and brain stem pathology.
- CT is recommended if MRI is contraindicated (i.e. paramagnetic protheses; inability to tolerate scanner time, noise, or confinement).
- MRI is recommended if radiation exposure is contra-indicated (i.e. young children or women of childbearing potential).

INDICATIONS FOR USE OF STRUCTURAL IMAGING MODALITIES IN PSYCHIATRIC POPULATIONS

CT Scan

There have been numerous studies, dating back to 1978, assessing the utility of CT imaging in psychiatric populations. Across these studies, which represent a diverse population totaling 1,346 patients, 29.5% of patients exhibited diffuse cortical atrophy while 12% of patients exhibited focal abnormalities (Renshaw and Rauch 1999). The likelihood of detecting an abnormal finding increased with age, with an abnormal neurological examination, with an altered mental status, and with a history of head trauma or alcohol abuse. Based loosely on some of these findings, some investigators have proposed guidelines for the use of CT scanning in psychiatric populations with suggested indications, including confusion or dementia, presence of focal neurological signs, history of head trauma or seizures, new-onset psychosis, movement disorder, anorexia nervosa, prolonged catatonia, and new-onset major affective disorder or personality change after age 50 years (Weinberger 1984, Emsley et al, 1986).

MRI

When MRI became available in the 1980s, changes in the neuroimaging literature reflected a shift away from CT and toward these of MRI in psychiatric populations. To our knowledge, the largest study of the use of MRI in psychiatric populations was conducted at McLean Hospital over a 5-year period and included all 6200 patients who received an MRI during that time (Rauch and Renshaw 1995). Because finding and abnormality following structural neuroimaging is of questionable value if it does not alter the treatment or outcome, this study focused on treatable findings. The study found that 99 patients (1.6%) had unexpected and potentially treatable findings including hemorrhage, tempolar lope cysts, tumors, vascular malformations, and hydrocephalus. Most importantly, multiple sclerosis in the general population. (Lyoo et al 1996). For those psychiatric patients with newly diagnosed multiple sclerosis in this study, the largest subgroup had been diagnosed with refractory affective illness.

A number of studies have found an increased incidence of white matter lesions, more easily detected with MRI than CT, in psychiatric populations. When subsequent studies also revealed that as 30% of healthy control subjects over age 60 years have white matter abnormalities of no apartment clinical significance, researchers began to question the relevance of white matter lesions in psychiatric illness. More recently, however, strong evidence has been presented which suggests that subcortical and white matter lesions are more prevalent in patients with late life onset depression and psychosis (Becker et al 1995).

General Guidelines for Structure Neuroimaging

On the basis of existing data, the suggested criteria for appropriate structure brain imaging:

- Patients with acute changes in mental status (including changes in effect, behavior, or personality) plus at least one of three additional criteria:
  - Age greater than 50 years
  - Abnormal neurological exam (especially focal abnormalities)
  - History of significant head trauma (i.e. with extended loss of consciousness, neurological sequelae, or temporally related to mental status change in question).
- New onset psychosis.
  - New onset delirium or dementia of unknown cause.
  - Possibly for treatment refractory patents.

Possibly prior to an initial course of electroconvulsive therapy (may be helpful in identifying lesions that may lead to an adverse outcome such as aneurysm, tumors, arterovenous malformations, hydrocephalus, and basal ganglia infarction).

It is estimated that adherence to the criteria listed above should yield positive findings in 10 to 45% of cases. However, only 1 to 5% will produce findings that lead to specific medical intervention. Lastly, if structural neuroimaging is indicated, one should use MRI until the problem is an acute trauma or an acute bleed is suspected.

FUNCTIONAL: IMAGING MODALITIES

Positron Emission Tomography

Technology

Positron emission tomography (PET) uses positron-emitting isotopes to quantitate various measures of brain function (e.g. cerebral blood flow, cerebral glucose metabolism, neuroreceptor characterization, etc.) (Cherry and Phelps 1996). As the name indicates, these unstable isotopes emit positrons which then soon collide with the electrons of surrounding atoms. The annihilation event that occurs after a positron-collides with an electron produces gamma ray radiation. These gamma rays are what PET scanners detect.

A PET scanner consists of a ring of scintillation detectors designed to detect gamma rays. Opposing detectors in the ring are coupled from a coincidence circuit. Following a positron/electron annihilation event, the resulting gamma rays project from one another at 180°. When events are detected by opposing detectors, an annihilation event is presumed to have occurred at some point along the imaginary line connecting the opposing detectors. Lines of response, which localize the annihilation event in tissue, are produced from these coincidence events. Powerful computers are requires to sum all of the coincidence events, localize them in tissue, and then create cross-sectional images (tomographs).

Advantages and Limitations

- PET is the gold standard of functional neuroimaging modalities.
- Only PET can measure cerebral glucose metabolism.
- A larger number of radioligands, especially those used for neuroreceptor characterization, are available for PET.
- PET offers excellent spatial resolution (~ 4 mm).
- PET is very expensive and requires relatively rapid access to a cyclotron, which produces the positron-emitting radionuclides. Most PET centers have a cyclotron on the premises. However, because of the high cost of obtaining and maintaining a functional cyclotron some centers do not have a cyclotron on the premises. 18 F has a longer half-life (110 minutes) than other radionuclides such as 11C (20 minutes), 13N (10 minutes), and 15O (2 minutes), so 18FDG may be prepared using a cyclotron at one site and then transported to other sites as long as they are within hours (generally ~1-half-lives) of the site of synthesis.

Single Photon Emission Computed Tomography

Technology

A single photon emission computed tomography (SPECT) is most commonly used to construct images of regional cerebral blood flow, although it may be used for neuroreceptor characterization as well. As is the case with PET, SPECT detects gamma rays produced by unstable isotope component of radioligands. However, the gamma rays that SPET is designed to detect result from photon emission rather than the positron/electron annihilation events that PET is designed to detect. Gamma rays that result from photon emission behave differently from the gamma rays produced by positron/electron annihilation in that they do not project 180° from one another. Rather gamma rays resulting from photon emission project through the imaging field in a more random fashion. Thus, SPECT is unable to use coincidence circuits like those used in PET to localize the source of the annihilation event. This is the primary reason that SPET cameras have slightly poorer spatial resolution than PET cameras.

SPECT cameras are comprised of a ring of collimators and radiation detectors that are designed to detect gamma rays. SPECT collimators that are typically lead blocks containing thousands of very small holes. The collimators are placed between the subject and the radiation detectors. The holes in the collimator are long and narrow so that only photons of an essentially parallel trajectory are able to pass through and reach the detector.

Advantages and Limitations

- SPECT is more affordable than PET and does not require a cyclotron for production of nuclides.
- Currently, SPECT provides inferior spatial resolution (~6–8 mm) compared with PET.
- Typically, SPECT spatial resolution worsens as one attempts to image deeper brain structures, although this is becoming less of an issue with the introduction of newer generation SPECT cameras.

PET versus SPECT

- PET provides superior spatial resolution, especially for deeper brain structures.
- PET offers a broader array of radioligands for use in receptor studies and is the only modality that allows for the measurement of metabolism.
- SPECT is less expensive than PET and is more widely available.

INDICATIONS FOR USE OF FUNCTIONAL IMAGING MODALITIES IN PSYCHIATRIC POPULATIONS

Although functional neuroimaging modalities include PET, SPECT, and functional MRI, in clinical situations only PET and SPECT are used at this time. These modalities are now commonly used as aids for diagnosis and monitoring treatment in cardiology and oncology (including brain tumors). Also, the used of ligands for the diagnosis and assessment of basal ganglia diseases such as Parkinson's disease. Still, most applications of functional neuroimaging in psychiatry occur in the field of research. However, a clinical role for functional neuroimaging in dementia and seizures is evolving and showing promise.

Dementia

As characteristic functional neuroimaging profiles emerge for various forms of dementia, the role of PET and SPECT in the evaluation of dementia is expanding. For example, Alzheimer's disease is associated with characteristic hypoperfusion in bilateral temporoparietal regions.

Some studies have indicated that functional neuroimaging can offer better than 90% sensitivity and specificity in distinguishing Alzheimer's disease from other kinds of dementia (Silverman et al. 2001, Bonte et al. 2001). Currently, most forms of dementia are irreversible and specific diagnoses may not affect the treatment. Also, an adequate clinical examination is often all that is required to reach a diagnosis of dementia. However, since the introduction of cholinesterase inhibitors for treatment of dementia early diagnosis of Alzheimer's disease may have greater import than in the past. Some PET studies of healthy older subjects with normal cognitive function who are homozygous for the apolipoprotein E epsilon 4 allele (a gene associated with the development of Alzheimer's disease) reveal that these subjects have temporoparietal hypoperfusion before the onset of disease (Small et al. 1995, Reiman et al. 1996). Initiation of treatment, with cholinesterase inhibitors or other drugs being developed, in these individual prior to the onset of symptoms of dementia may prove to be of great value.

Seizures

Some seizers, especially complex partial seizers, are not always detected by electroencephalogram (EEG). EEG measures cortical surface electrical activity but is less efficacious if the seizure focus is deeper in the brain. PET and SPECT images typically demonstrate ictal hypermetabolism and interictal hypometabolism (Krausz et al. 1996, Theodore and Gaillard 2000). This allows for the detection of seizure foci during the predominant interictal period. To evaluate a possible seizure disorder, functional neuroimaging is usually performed in conjuction with EEG. PET is also useful for more precise localization of seizure foci in a patient with a known seizure disorder, if neurosurgical intervention is indicated.

PSYCHIATRIC NEUROIMAGING RESEARCH

The neuroimaging modalities that have been described in this chapter also have tremendous research potential. For example, specific structural MRI acquisition parameters result in morphometric quality structural images that may be used to precisely calculate the volumes of brain structures in individuals. Restings-stage PET and SPECT studies as described earlier may be used to compare regional cerebral blood flow or regional cerebral glucose metabolism between groups of subjects with psychiatric illness and healthy subjects.

FUNCTIONAL BRAIN IMAGING RESEARCH

fMRI

Expanding upon the basic principles underlying standard structural MRI used in clinical situations, functional magnetic resonance imaging (fMRI) allows investigators to assess brain function. Using either a standard or preferably, a high-speed MR scanner with specific image-acquisition parameters, indices of cerebral blood flow and blood volume can be measured. While structural MRI studies rely on excitation and relaxation of hydrogen atoms in water, fMRI takes advantage of the paramagnetic properties of hemoglobin to measure blood flow and volume.

fMRI has distinct advantages when compared to PET and SPECT, and these include:

- FMRI does not expose subjects to radiation and its relative safety has been documented.
- The spatial resolution of fMRI is at least equal to if not superior to that of PET.
- The temporal resolution of fMRI is vastly superior to that of PET or SPECT.

The major disadvantage of fMRI when compared to PET or SPECT is that no satisfactory techniques for receptor neuroiamging have yet been developed for fMRI.

IN VIVO NEUROCHEMICAL RESEARCH

PET and SPECT

A large number of radioligands used for neuroreceptor characterization are available for both PET and SPECT studies. Generally, each of these radioligands bind to a specific neuroreceptor, allowing PET or SPECT to quantity the spatial distribution of the receptor of interest. Radioligands are available for characterizing dopamine receptors (including D1, D2, and reuptake sites), serotonin receptors (including 5-HT1A, 5-HT2, and reuptake sites), benzodiazepine receptors, opoid receptors, and many other receptor systems. These receptor neuroimaging techniques can be used in a number of research paradigms, including comparing populations with and without psychiatric illness, to elucidate the pathophysiology of the psychiatric illness. It can perhaps aid in diagnosis as well as for determining pharmacodynamics and pharmacokinetics of available therapeutics and investigational compounds. Lastly, recent work has focused on using PET to study neuronal function at a level deeper than the surface receptors. Premlinary studies show promise for using PET to image second messenger systems and even gene expression (MacLaren et al. 2000).

MAGNETIC RESONANCE SPECTROSCOPY

Magnetic resonance spectroscopy (MRS) uses specific acquisition parameters and standard MR scanner just as fMRI does, although MRS measures the levels of various chemicals in the brain (Henry et al. 2001). The technique is very similar to that of nuclear magnetic resonance used in analytic chemistry. A number of MRS-visible nuclei can be assessed in vivo including phosphorus (31p) and hydrogen (1h). Phosphorous MR spectra provide quantitative data regarding phospholipids metabolites and markers of high energy phosphate metabolism. Proton (1H) MR spectra provide measures of N-acetyl aspartate (NAA, a cell marker specific for neurons) as well as some compounds that may be involved in cell membrane formation and second messenger systems. In addition, MRS is able to measure concentrations of some drugs in the brain including lithium (Renshaw and Wicklund 1988) and some fluorinated compared to other functional neuroimging modalities, MRS has less spatial resolution (from 1 to 150 cubic centimeters depending upon the spectra being generated) due tiits low sensitivity. It is, nonetheless, a valuable research tool. Currently, there is no clinical utility for MRS, though monitoring levels of drugs in the brain may be a future application.

SUMMARY

Neuroimaging technology has evolved considerably during the last few decades. Currently available neuroimaging modalities have increasing clinical utility in psychiatric populations. Although there are still substantial limitations on the amount of information that neuroimaging provides in the clinical setting, the continued evolution of neuroimaging technology offers great promise in the future.

REFERENCES

Neuropharmacology

1. Das PK, Bhatacharya SK, Sen P. Pharmacology. 1st edition. New Delhi: BI Churchill Livingstone; 1996. p. 212.
2. Bloom FF. Neurotransmission and the CNS. In: Hardman JG, Limbird JG, Molinoff PB, Ruddon RW (Eds). Goodman and Gilman's The Pharmacological Basis of Therapeutics. IX edition. New York: Mcgraw-Hill; 1996. p. 267.
3. Tononi G, Sporns O, Edelman GM. Re-entry and the problem of integrating multiple cortical areas stimulation of dynamic integration in the visual system. Cerbral Cortex. 1992;2: 310-35.
4. Zola-Morgan S, Squire LR. Neuroanatomy of memory. Ann Rev Neurosci. 1963;16:547-63.
5. Swanson LW. Organization of mammalian neuroendocrine system. In: Bloom FE (Ed). Handbook of Physiology. Bethesda, MD: American Physiological Society. 1986;Vol.IV(I). pp. 317-64.
6. Foote SL, Aston Jones GS. Pharmacology and physiology of central noradrenergic systems. In: Bloom FE, Kupfer DJ (Eds). Psychopharmacology: The Fourth Generation of Progress. New York: Raveen Press; 1994. pp. 335-45.
7. Mesulam MM. Structure and function of cholinergic pathways in the cerebral cortex, limblic system, basal ganglia and thalamus of the human brain. In: Bloom FE, Kupfer DJ (Eds). Psycho-pharmacology: The Fourth Generation of Progress. New York: Raveen Press; 1994. pp. 135-46.
8. Baraban JM, Coyle JT. Monoamine neurotransmitter in neural sciences. In: Bloom FE, Kupfer DJ (Eds). Psychopharmacology: The Fourth Generation of Progress. New York: Raveen Press, 1994.
9. Haranath PSRK, Sharif. Synopsis of Pharmacology with MCQs. 1st edition. Hyderabad: Kala Jyoti; 1995, Chap. II. pp. 3-9.
10. Emorine L, Blin N, Strosberg AD. The human b_3 adrenoceptor: The search for a physiological function. Trends PharmacolSci. 1994;15: 3-7.
11. Wang Z, McCormick DA. Control of firing mode of corticotectal and corticopontine layer V burst generating neurons by norepinephrine, acetylcholine and IS 3RACPD. J Neurosci. 1993;13:2199-216.
12. Magistretti PJ, Pellerin L, Martin JL. Brain energy metabolism: An integrated cellular prospective. In: Bloom FE, Kupfer DJ (Eds). Psycho-pharmacology: The Fourth Generation of Progress. New York: Raveen Press; 1994. pp. 657-70.
13. Bylund DB. Subtypes of $\alpha1$ and $\alpha2$ adrenergic receptors. FASEB J. 1993;6:832-9.
14. Dahlstrom A, Fuxe K. Evidence of the existence of monoamine containing neurons in the CNS. I. Demonstration of monoamines in the cell bodies of brainstem neurones. Acta Physiol Scand. 1964;232(Suppl. 62):1-55.
15. Gudelsky GA, Koeing JI, Meltzer HY. Thermoregulatory response to serotonin (5-HT) receptor stimulation in rat. Neuropharmacol. 1986;25:1307-13.
16. Aghajanian GK. Electrophysiology of serotonin receptor subtypes and signal transduction pathways. In: Bloom FE, Kupfer DJ (Eds). Psycho-pharmacology: The Fourth Generation of Progress. New York: Raveen Press; 1994. pp. 451-60.
17. Bjorklund A, Lindvall O. Catecholaminergic brainstem regulatory system. In: Bloom FE (Ed). Handbook of Physiology. Bethesda, MD: American Physiological Society; 1986;Vol.IV (I). pp.155-236.
18. Dearry A, Gingrich JA, Falardean P, et al. Molecular cloning and expression of the gene for a human D_1 dopaminergic receptor. Nature. 1990;347:72-6.
19. Sunahara RK, Guan HC, O'Dowd BF, et al. Cloning of the gene for a human D_5 receptor with higher affinity for dopamine than D_1. Nature. 1991;350:614-9.
20. Bunzow JR, Vontol HHM, Grandy DK, et al. Cloning and expression of a rate D_2 dopaminergic receptor CDNA. Nature. 1988;336:783-7.
21. Dal Toso R, Sommer B, Ewert M, et al. The dopamine D_2 receptor: Two molecular fors generated by alternative splicing EMBO J. 1989;8:4025-34.
22. Sokoloff P, Giros B, Martres MP, et al. Molecular cloning and characterization of a novel dopamine receptor D_3 as a target for neuroleptics. Nature. 1990;347:146-51.

23. Van Tol HHM, Bunzow JR, Guan HC, et al. Cloning of the gene for a human dopamine D_4 receptor with high affinity for the antipsychotic clozapine. Nature. 1991;350:610-4.
24. Schwartz JC, Arrang JM, Garbarg M, et al. Histamine. In: Bloom FE, Kupfer DJ (Eds). Psychopharmacology: The Fourth Generation of Progress. New York: Raveen Press; 1994. pp. 397-405.
25. Cotman CW, Kahle JS, Miller S, et al. Excitatory amino acid neurotransmission. In: Bloom FE, Kupfer DJ (Eds). Psychopharmacology: The Fourth Generation of Progress. New York: Raveen Press; 1994. pp. 75-85.
26. Kelly JS, Berat PM. Amino acid receptors in CNS. II. GABA in supraspinal regions. Inversen, et al. Handbook of Psychopharmacology. New York: Plenum Press. 1975;Vol. 4 (I). pp. 129-209.
27. Otsuka M. Gamma amino butyric acid and some other transmitter candidates in the nervous system: Pharmacology and the future of man. Proceedings of the Fifth International Congress of Pharmacology; 1973. pp. 186-201.
28. Franks NP, Lieb WR. Molecular and cellular mechanisms of general anaesthesia. Nature. 1994;367:607-14.
29. Hollmann M, Heinemann S. Cloned glutamate receptors. Ann Rev Neurosci. 1994;17:31-108.
30. Bliss TVP, Collingridge GL. A synaptic model of memory: Long term potentiation in the hippocampus. Nature. 1993;361: 31-9.
31. Mulekey RM, Malenka RC. Mechanisms underlying induction of homosynaptic long term depression in area CAI of the hippocampus. Neuron. 1992;9:967-75.
32. Hokfelt T, Fuxe K, Goldstein M, Johanson O. Immunohistochemical evidence for the existence of adrenaline neurons in the rat brain. Brain Res. 1994;66:235-51.
33. Williams M. Purinoceptors in CNS function target for therapeutic intervention. In: Bloom FE, Kupfer DJ (Eds). Psychopharmacology: The Fourth Generation of Progress. New York: Raveen Press; 1994. pp. 643-55.
34. Piomelli D. Arachidonic acid. In: Bloom FE, Kupfer DJ (Eds). Psychopharmacology: The Fourth Generation of Progress. New York: Raveen Press; 1994. pp. 397-405.
35. Munglani R, Hudspith MJ, Hunt SP. The therapeutic potential of neuropeptide Y. Drugs. 1996;52:371-89.

Neurovirology

36. Ackenheil M, Muller N. The Immune system and schizophrenia. In: Leonard BE, Miller K (Eds). Stress, the Immune System and Psychiatry. John Wiley & Sons; 1995. pp. 137-64.
37. Alexander RC, Spector SA, Casanova M, et al. Search for cytomegalovirus in the postmortem brains of schizophrenia patients using the polymerase chain reaction. Arch Gen Psychiatry. 1992;49:47-53.
38. Anderson M. Virus Infections of the Nervous system. In: Walton J (Ed). Brain's Diseases of the Nervous System. Oxford University Press; 1994. pp. 317-50.
39. Besedovsky H, Sorkin E. Network of immuno-neuroendocrine interactions. ClinExpImmunol. 1997;27:1-12.
40. Breard J, Costa O, Kardon C. Organization and functional relevance of neuroimmune networks. In: Leonard BE, Miller K (Eds). Stress, the Immune system and Psychiatry. John Wiley & Sons; 1995. pp. 17-46.
41. Colinge J. New Diagnostic Tests for prion diseases. N Engl J Med. 1996:335:963-5.
42. Corey L, Spear PG. Medical Progress. Infections with herpes simplex viruses. Part One. N Engl J Med. 1986;314:686-91.
43. Crnic LS. Behavioral Consequences of Virus Infection. In: Ader R, Fetten DL, Cohen N (Eds). Psychoneuroimmunology. Academic Press; 1991. pp. 749-69.
44. Cutler RWP, Watters GV, Hammerstad JP. The origin and turnover of cerebrospinal fluid albumin and gamma globulin in man. J Neurol Sci. 1969;10:259-68.
45. Dantzer R, Kelley KW. An integrated view of relationship between nervous and immune systems. Life Sci. 1989;44: 1995-2008.
46. De Armond SJ, Pruisner SB. Prion Diseases. In: Bloom FE, Kupfer DJ (Eds). Psychopharmacology: The Fourth Generation of Progress. Raven Press; 1995. pp. 1521-30.
47. Delisi LE, Goodman S, Neckers LM, et al. An analysis of lymphocyte subpopulations in schizophrenic patients.Biol Psychiatry. 1982;17:1003-9.
48. Ganguli R, Brar JS, Chengappa KNR, et al. Autoimmunity in schizophrenia : A review of recent findings. Ann Med. 1993;25: 489-96.
49. Ganquii R, Rabin BS. Increased serum interleukin 2 receptor concentration in schizophrenic and brain damaged subjects. Arch Gen Psychiatry. 1989;46:292.
50. Gorp WGV, Cumings JL. Neuropsychiatric aspects of infectious disorders. In: Kaplan HI, Saddock BJ (Eds). Comprehensive Textbook of Psychiatry. 6th edition. Baltimore: Williams & Wilkins; 1995. pp. 235-41.
51. Gottleib-Stematsky T, Zonis J, Aralazoroff A, et al. Antibodies to Epstein-Barr virus, herpes-simplex type I, cytomegalovirus and measles virus in psychiatric patients. Arch Virol. 1981;67: 333-9.
52. Hamilton RL, Wiley CA. Neurology of viral infections of the nervous system. In: Davis RL, Robertson DM (Eds). Textbook of Neuropathology. Baltimore: Williams & Wilkins; 1997. pp. 927-1062.
53. Hsich G, Kenney K, Gibbs CJ, et al. The 14-3-3 brain protein in cerebrospinal fluid as a marker for transmissible spongiform encephalopathies. N Engl J Med. 1996;335:924-30.
54. Karanth S, McCann SM. Anterior pituitary hormone control by interleukin 2. Proc Nat Acad Sci. 1991;88:2961-5.
55. King DJ, Scooper SJ. Viruses, Immunity and Mental Disorder. Br J Psychiatry. 1989;154:1-7.
56. Kristen K, Norrby E. Persistence of RNA viruses in the Central nervous system. Ann Rev Microbiol. 1986;40:159-84.
57. Laboratory diagnosis of viral diseases. In: White DO, Fenner F (Eds). Medical Virology. Academic Press; 1996. pp. 325-61.

58. Landsteiner K, Popper E. Ubertragung der Poliomyelitis acuta auf Affen. Z ImmunExpTher. 1909; 2:377.
59. Leland DS, French MLV. Virus isolation and identification. In: Lennette EW, Halonen P, Murphy FA (Eds). Laboratory Diagnosis of Infectious Diseases Principles and Practice. Vol II. Springer-Verlag; 1988. pp. 39-59.
60. Longson M. Virus infections of the central nervous system. In: Collier LH, Timbury MC (Eds). Topley and Wilson's Principles of Bacteriology: Virology and Immunity. Vol 4; 1990. pp. 452-78.
61. Masscrini C, Vita A, Basile R, et al. Lymphocyte subsets in schizophrenic disorders: Relationship with clinical, neuromorphological and treatment variables. Schizophr Res. 1990; 3:266-75.
62. Merill JE. Macroglia: neural cells responsive to cytokines and growth factors. Immunol Today. 1987;8:146-50.
63. O' Callaghan E, Sham P, Takei N, et al. Schizophrenia after prenatal exposure to 1957 alpha 2 influenza epidemic. Lancet. 1991; i: 1248-50.
64. Pruisner SB. Prions. In: Fields BN, Knipe DM, Howley PM (Eds). Fundamental Virology. Lippincott-Raven; 1996. pp. 1245-94.
65. Rabin BS, Ganguly R, Cunnick JE, et al. The central nervous system- immune system relationship. Clin Lab Med. 1988;8: 253-68.
66. Rabins PV, McMahon FJ. Neuropsychiatric aspects of multiple sclerosis and other demyelinating disorders. In: Kaplan HI, Saddock BJ (Eds). Comprehensive Textbook of Psychiatry. 6th edition. Baltimore: Wiliams& Wilkins; 1995. pp. 231-4.
67. Ravi V, Rakib A, Gangadhar DN, et al. IgM antibodies to eight common neurotropic viruses in the serum samples of schizophrenic patients, and controls from South India. J Neurovirol. 1996;2:213.
68. Reid AH, Martin KW, Ballinger BR, et al. The possible relationship of herpes simplex virus infection to cause retardation as severe mental handicap. Psychol Med. 1980;10:555-7.
69. Rowland PL. Motor neuron diseases and amyotrophic lateral sclerosis. Trends Neurosci. 1984;7:110-2.
70. Smith MG, Lennette EH, Reames HR. Isolation of the virus of Herpes Simplex and the demonstration of intranuclear inclusions in a case of acute encephalitis. Am J Path. 1941; 17:55-68.
71. Specter S, Bendinelli M, Friedman H. Virus and neuropsychiatric disorders: Facts and suppositions. In: Specter S, Bendinelli M, Friedman H (Eds). Neuropathogenic Viruses and Immunity. Plenum Press; 1992. pp. 1-12.
72. Torrey EF, Peterson MR, Brannon WL, et al. Immunoglobulins and viral antibodies in Psychiatric patients. Br J Psychiatry. 1978;132: 342-8.
73. Torrey EF, Torrey BB, Peterson MR. Seasonality of Schizophrenic births in the United States. Arch Gen Psychiatry. 1997;34: 1065-70.
74. Tyor WR, Johnson RT. Immune responses and the central nervous system. In: Specter S, Bendinelli M, Friedman H (Eds). Neuropathogenic Viruses and Immunity. Plenum Press; 1992. pp.15-37.
75. Villemain F, Chatenoud L, Galinowski A, et al. Aberrant T-Cell mediated immunity in untreated schizophrenia patients: Deficient Interleukin-2 production. Am J Psychiatry. 1989;146: 609-16.
76. Weinberger DR. The pathogenesis of schizophrenia: A neurodevelopmental theory. In: Nasarallah HA, Weinberger DR (Eds). Handbook of Schizophrenia. Vol. l. The Neurology of Schizophrenia. Elsiever Science; 1986. pp. 397-406.
77. Whitley R. Diagnosis and treatment of herpes simplex encephalitis. Ann Rev Med. 1981;32:335-40.
78. Wisniewski HM, Bruie ME, Fraser H. Infectious etiology of neuritic (senile) plaques in mice. Science. 1975;190:1108-9.
79. Wyatt RJ, Kirch DG, Egan MF. Schizophrenia: Neurochemical and Immunological studies. In: Kaplan HI, Saddock BJ (Eds). Comprehensive Textbook of Psychiatry. 6th edition. Baltimore: Williams & Wilkins; 1995. pp. 927-42.
80. Yolken RH. Summary of Meeting. J Neurovirol. 1996;2:196-7.

FURTHER READING

Neuroanatomy

1. Barson AJ. The vertebral level of termination of spinal cord during normal and abnormal development. J Anat. 1970;106: 489-97.
2. Brodal A. The reticular formation of the brainstem: Anatomical aspects and functional correlation. Edinburgh: Olivier and Boyd. 1957.
3. Calne DB. Parkinsonism. London: Arnold. 1970.
4. Carpenter MB, Peter P. Nigrostriatal and nigrothalamic fibers in the rhesus monkey. J Comp Neurol. 1972;144:93-116.
5. Carpenter MB, Sutin J. Human Neuroanatomy. VIII Edition. Baltimore: Williams and Wilkins, 1983.
6. Cowell TPS, Cowan WM. A study of thalamostriate relations in the monkey. Brain. 1956;79:364-90.
7. Housue EL, Pansky B. A Functional Approach to Neuroanatomy. 1960.
8. Ingram WR. Nuclear organization and chief connections of the primate hypothalamus. Res Publs Ass Res NervMent Dis. 1940; 20:195-244.
9. Kaplan HA. Arteries of the brain: Anatomic study. Acta Radiol. 1956;46:364-470.
10. Nauta WJH, Mehles WR. Projection of the lentiform nucleus in the monkey. Brain Res. 1966;I:3-42.
11. Ramon-Moliner E, Nauta WJH. The isodendritic core of the brainstem. J Comp Neurol. 1966;126:311-35.
12. Scheibel ME, Scheibel AB. Structural organization of nonspecific thalamic nuclei and their projection toward cortex. Brain Res. 1967;6:60-94.
13. Snider RS. Functional alterations of cerebral sensory areas by the cerebellum. Prog Brain Res. 1967;25:322-3.
14. Snider RS. Recent contributions to the anatomy and physiology of the cerebellum. Arch Neurol Psychiatr Chicago. 1950;64:196-219.

15. Webster KE. Structure and function of the basal ganglia: A non-clinical view. Proc Roy Soc Med. 1975;68:203-10.
16. Williams PL, Warwick R, Dyson M, et al. Gray's Anatomy. 1989.

Neurophysiology

17. Angleton JP. The Amygdala: Neurobiological Aspects of Emotion, Memory, and Mental Dysfunction. New York Wiley, 1992.
18. Filley CM. Neurobehavioral Anatomy, Niwot: University Press of Colorado, 1995.
19. Gazzaniga M. The Cognitive Neurosciences. Cambridge: MIT Press, 1995.
20. Kandel ER, Schwartz JH, Jessell TM. Principles of Neural Science. 3rd edition. New York Elsevier. 1991.
21. Khurana I. Textbook of Medical Physiology. Elsevier India. 2005.
22. Review of Medical Physiology by William F Ganong 22nd ed. McGraw-Hill. 2005.

Neuropathology

23. Aarsland D, Laake K, Larsen JP, et al. Donepezil for cognitive impairment in Parkinson's disease: A randomised controlled study. J Neurol Neurosurg Psychiatry. 2002;72(6):708-12.
24. Aarsland D, Perry R, Larsen JP, et al. Neuroleptic sensitivity in Parkinson's disease and Parkinsonian dementias. J Clin Psychiatry. 2005;66(5):633-7.
25. Alladi S, Mekala S, Chadalawada SK, et al. Subtypes of Dementia: A Study from a memory clinic in India. Dement Geriatr Cogn Disord. 2011;32(1):32-8
26. American Psychiatric Association (APA). Diagnostic and Statistical Manual of Mental Disorders, 4th edition. Text revision (DSM IV-TR). Washington, DC: American Psychiatric Association; 2000.
27. American Psychiatric Association (APA). Diagnostic and Statistical Manual of Mental Disorders, 5th edition. Text revision (DSM-5). Washington, DC: American Psychiatric Association; 2012.
28. Antinori A, Arendt G, Becker JT, et al. Updated research nosology for HIV-associated neurocognitive disorders. Neurology. 2007;69(18):1789-99.
29. Ballard C, Morris C, Kalaria R, et al. The k variant of the butyrylcholinesterase gene is associated with reduced phosphorylation of tau in dementia patients. Dement Geriatr Cogn Disord. 2005;19(5-6):357-60.
30. Bird T, Knopman D, Vanswieten J, et al. Epidemiology and genetics of frontotemporal dementia/Pick's disease. Annals of Neurology. 2003;54(suppl.5): S29-S31.
31. Bonanni L, Thomas A, Tiraboschi P, et al. EEG comparisons in early Alzheimer's disease, dementia with Lewy bodies and Parkinson's disease with dementia patients with a 2-year follow-up. Brain. 2008;131(pt 3):690-705.
32. Bowen DM, Procter AW, Mann DM, et al. Imbalance of a serotonergic system in Frontotemporal dementia: Implication for pharmacotherapy. Psychopharmacology (Berl). 2008; 196(4):603-10.
33. Braak H, Braak E. Pathoanatomy of Parkinson's disease. J Neurol. 2000;247 (Suppl2): II3-I10.
34. Braak H, Del Tredici K, Rub U, et al. Staging of brain pathology related to sporadic Parkinson's disease. Neurobiol Aging. 2003;24(2):197-211.
35. Burn D, Emre M, McKeith I, et al. Effects of rivastigmine in patients with and without visual hallucinations in dementia associated with Parkinson's disease. Mov Disord. 2006;21(11):1899-907.
36. Burns A, Folstein S, Brandt J, et al. Clinical assessment of irritability, aggression, and apathy in Huntington and Alzheimer disease. J Nerv Ment Dis. 1990;178(1):20-6.
37. Burton EJ, McKeith IG, Burn DJ, et al. Brain atrophy rates in Parkinson's disease with and without dementia using serial magnetic resonance imaging. Mov Disord. 2005;20(12): 1571-6.
38. Burton EJ, McKeith IG, Burn DJ, et al. Cerebralatrophy in Parkinson's disease with and without dementia: A comparison with Alzheimer's disease, dementia with Lewy bodies and controls. Brain. 2004;127(4):791-800.
39. Caine ED, Hunt RD, Weingartner H, et al. Huntington's dementia. Clinical and neuropsychological features. Arch Gen Psychiatry. 1978;35(3):377-84.
40. Centers for Disease Control and Prevention.1998 guidelines for treatment of sexually transmitted diseases. Morbid Mortal Weekly Rep. 1998;47:28-49.
41. Cysique LA, Brew BJ. Prevalence of non-confounded HIV-associated neurocognitive impairment in the context of plasma HIV RNA suppression. J Neurovirol. 2011;17(2):176-83.
42. Dalby MA. Effect of tetrabenazine in extrapyramidal movement disorders. Br Med J. 1969;2(5654):422-3.
43. Darshan S, Krewski D, Karyakina N, et al. Preventive risk management strategies for bovine spongiform encephalopathy and variant Creutzfeldt-Jakob disease in India. Int J Risk Assessment and Management. 2010;14(3-4):239-53.
44. David A. Lishman's organic psychiatry: A textbook of neuropsychiatry. John Wiley; 2009.
45. de Lau LM, Breteler MM. Epidemiology of Parkinson's disease. Lancet Neurol. 2006;5(6):525-35.
46. Delacourte A, Evers C. Familial CJD.Available from: http://www.alzheimer-europe.org/Dementia/Other-forms-of-dementia/Infectious-Diseases/Human-Prion-Diseases/Familial-CJD?#fragment-1.
47. Dewhurst K. The neurosyphilitic psychoses today: A survey of 91 cases. Br J Psychiatry. 1969;115:31-8.
48. Dichgans M, Herzog J, Gasser T. NOTCH3 mutation involving three cysteine residues in a family with typical CADASIL. Neurology. 2001;57(9):1714-7.
49. Dickson DW, Davies P, Mayeux R, et al. Diffuse Lewy body disease. Neuropathological and biochemical studies of six patients. Acta Neuropathol. 1987;75(1):8-15.
50. Dickson DW, Feany MB, Yen SH, et al. Cytoskeletal pathology in non- Alzheimer degenerative dementia: New lesions in diffuse Lewy body disease, Pick's disease, and corticobasal degeneration. J Neural Transm Suppl. 1996;47:31-46.

51. Dickson DW, Schmidt ML, Lee VM, et al. Immunoreactivity profile of hippocampal CA2/3 neurites in diffuse Lewy body disease. Acta Neuropathol. 1994;87(3):269-76.
52. Dickson DW. Neuropathology of Pick's disease. Neurology. 2001;56: S16-20.
53. Emre M, Cummings JL, Lane RM. Rivastigmine in dementia associated with Parkinson's disease and Alzheimer's disease: Similarities and differences. J Alzheimers Dis. 2007;11(4):509-19.
54. Finkenstaedt M, Szudra A, ZerrI, et al. MR imaging of Creutzfeldt-Jakob disease. Radiology. 1996;199:793-8.
55. Firbank MJ, Colloby SJ, Burn DJ, et al. Regional cerebral blood flow in Parkinson's disease with and without dementia. Neuroimage. 2003;20(2):1309-19.
56. Folstein SE, Jensen B, Leigh RJ, et al. The measurement of abnormal movement: Methods developed for Huntington's disease. Neurobehav Toxicol Teratol. 1983;5(6):605-9.
57. Forette F, SeuxML, Staessen JA, et al. The prevention of dementia with antihypertensive treatment: New evidence from the systolic hypertension in Europe (Syst-Eur) study. Arch Intern Med. 2002;162(18):2046-52.
58. Fröshaug H, Ytrehus A. A study of general paresis with special reference to the reasons for the admission of these patients to hospital. Acta Psychiatr Neurol Scand. 1956;31(1):35-60.
59. Gadgil NM, Chaudhari CS, Gohil SD, et al. Creutzfeldt-Jacob disease: An autopsy case report in tertiary care hospital. Indian J Pathol Microbiol. 2012;55(1):97-9.
60. Goldman JS, Farmer JM, Wood EM, et al. Comparison of family histories in FTLD subtypes and related tauopathies. Neurology. 2005;65(11):1817-9.
61. Gorno-Tempini ML, Dornkers NF, Rankin KP, et al. Cognition and anatomy in three variants of primary progressive aphasia. Ann Neurol. 2004;55(3):335-46.
62. Gregory CA, Serra-Mestres J, Hodges JR. Early diagnosis of the frontal variant of Frontotemporal dementia: How sensitive are standard neuroimaging and Neuropsychologic tests? Neuropsychiatry Neuropsychol Behav Neurol. 1999;12(2):128-35.
63. Hansen L, Salmon D, Galasko D, et al. The Lewy body variant of Alzheimer's disease: A clinical and pathologic entity. Neurology. 1990;40(1):1-8.
64. Harding AJ, Lakay B, Halliday GM. Selective hippocampal neuron loss in dementia with Lewy bodies. Ann Neurol 2002;51(1):125-8.
65. Harding AJ, Stimson E, Henderson JM, et al. Clinical correlates of selective pathology in the amygdala of patients with Parkinson's disease. Brain. 2002;125(Pt 11):2431-45.
66. Harper PS.The epidemiology of Huntington's disease. Hum Genet. 1992;89:365-76.
67. Harvey RJ, Skelton-Robinson M, Rossor MN.The prevalence and causes of dementia in people under the age of 65 years. J Neurol Neurosurg Psychiatry. 2003;74(9):1206-9.
68. Hassan I. Consultation-liaison psychiatry and prevention of severeneuroleptic sensitivity reactions in dementia with Lewy bodies. Australas Psychiatr. 2011;19(6):536-7.
69. Hebb C. CNS at the cellular level: Identity of transmitter agents. Annu Rev Physiol. 1970;32:165-92.
70. Hely MA, Reid WG, Adena MA, et al. The Sydney multicenter study of Parkinson's disease: The inevitability of dementia at 20 years. Mov Disord. 2008;23(6):837-44.
71. Huang Y, Halliday G. Can we clinically diagnose dementia with Lewy bodies yet? Translational Neurodegeneration. 2013;2(4):1-9.
72. Ibarretxe-Bilbao N, Ramirez-Ruiz B, Tolosa E, et al. Hippocampal head atrophy predominance in Parkinson's disease with hallucinations and with dementia. J Neurol. 2008;255(9):1324-31.
73. Ikeda M, Brown J, Holland AJ, et al. Changes in appetite, food preference, and eating habits in frontotemporal dementia and Alzheimer's disease. J Neurol Neurosurg Psychiatry. 2002;73(4):371-6.
74. Iudicello JE, Woods SP, Weber E, et al. Cognitive mechanisms of switching in HIV-associated category fluency deficits. J Clin Exp Neuropsychol. 2008;30(7):797-804.
75. Jarabek BR, Yasuda RP, Wolfe BB. Regulation of proteins affecting NMDA receptor-induced excitotoxicity in a Huntington's mouse model. Brain. 2004;127:505-16.
76. Joutel A, Vahedi K, Corpechor C, et al. Strong clustering and stereotyped nature of mutations in CADASIL patients. Lancet. 1997;350(9090):1511-5.
77. Junque C, Ramirez-Ruiz B, Tolosa E, et al. Amygdalar and hippocampal MRI volumetric reductions in Parkinson's disease with dementia. Mov Disord. 2005;20(5):540-4.
78. Kemp PM, Clyde K, Holmes C. Impact of 123I-FP-CIT (DaTSCAN) SPECT on the diagnosis and management of patients with dementia with Lewy bodies: A retrospective study. Nucl Med Commun. 2011;32(4):298-302.
79. Kertesz A, McMonagle P, Blair M, et al. The evolution and pathology of frontotemporal dementia. Brain. 2005;128: 1996-2005.
80. Klein JC, Eggers C, Kalbe E, et al. Neurotransmitter changes in dementia with Lewy bodies and Parkinson disease dementia in vivo. Neurology. 2010;74(11):885-92.
81. Knopman DS, Petersen RC, Edland SD, et al. The incidence of frontotemporal lobar degeneration in Rochester, Minnesota, 1990 through 1994. Neurology. 2004;62(3):506-8.
82. Kosaka K, Yoshimura M, Ikeda K, et al. Diffuse type of Lewy body disease: Progressive dementia with abundant cortical Lewy bodies and senile changes of varying degree--a new disease? Clin Neuropathol. 1984;3(5):185-92.
83. Kosaka K. Diffuse Lewy body disease in Japan. J Neurol. 1990;237:197-204.
84. Kothari K, Goyal S. Clinical profile of AIDS. J Assoc Physicians India. 2001;49:435-8.
85. Levy G, Tang MX, Louis ED, et al. The association of incident dementia with mortality in PD. Neurology. 2002;59:1708-13.
86. Li JY, Plomann M, Brundin P. Huntington's diseases a synaptopathy? Trends Mol Med. 2003;9(10):414-20.
87. Lippa CF, Smith TW, Perry E. Dementia with Lewy bodies: Choline acetyltransferase parallels nucleus basalis pathology. J Neural Transm. 1999;106(5-6):525-35.

88. Lippa CF, Smith TW, Swearer JM. Alzheimer's disease and Lewy body disease: A comparative clinicopathological study. Ann Neurol. 1994;35:81-88.
89. Litvan I, Bhatia KP, Burn DJ, et al. Movement Disorders Society Scientific Issues Committee report: SIC Task Force appraisal of clinical diagnostic criteria for Parkinsoni an disorders. Mov Disord. 2003;18(5):467-86.
90. Litvinenko IV, Odinak MM, Mogil'naya VI, et al. Use of memantine (Akatinol) for the correction of cognitive impairments in Parkinson's disease complicated by dementia. Neurosci Behav Physiol. 2010;40(2):149-55.
91. Loizou LA, Kendall BE, Marshall J. Subcortical arteriosclerotic encephalopathy: A clinical and radiological investigation. J Neurol Neurosurg Psychiatry. 1981:44(4):294-304.
92. Lucetti C, Logi C, Del Dotto P, et al. Levodopa response in dementia with Lewy bodies: A 1-year follow-up study. Parkinsonism Relat Disord. 2010;16(8):522-6.
93. Martin EM, Nixon H, Pitrak DL, et al. Characteristics of prospective memory deficits in HIV-seropositive substance-dependent individuals: Preliminary observations. J Clin Exp Neuropsychol. 2007;29(5):496-504.
94. Marttila RJ, Rinne UK. Dementia in Parkinson's disease. Acta Neurol Scand. 1976;54(5):431-41.
95. McArthur JC, Brew BJ, Nath A. Neurological complications of HIV infection. Lancet Neurol. 2005;4(9):543-55.
96. McCabe P, Sheard C, Code C. Pragmatic skills in people with HIV/AIDS. Disabil Rehabil. 2007;29(16):1251-60.
97. McGuinness B, Todd S, Passmore P, et al. Blood pressure lowering inpatients without prior cerebrovascular disease for prevention of cognitive impairment and dementia. Cochrane Database Syst Rev. 2009;(4):CD004034.
98. McKeith I, O'Brien J, Walker Z, et al. Sensitivity and specificity of dopamine transporter imaging with 123I-FP-CIT SPECT in dementia with Lewy bodies: A phase III, multi center study. Lancet Neurol. 2007;6(4):305-13.
99. McKeith I. Dementia with Lewy bodies and Parkinson's disease with dementia: Where two worlds collide. Pract Neurol. 2007;7(6):374-82.
100. McMurtray AM, Chen AK, Shapira JS, et al. Variations in regional SPECT Hypoperfusion and clinical features in frontotemporal dementia. Neurology. 2006;66(4):517-22.
101. Mehndiratta MM, Bajaj BK, Gupta M, et al. Creutzfeldt-Jakob disease: Report of 10 cases from North India. Neurol India. 2001;49(4):338-41.
102. Mendez MF, Chen AK, Shapira JS, et al. Acquired sociopathy and frontotemporal dementia. Dement Geriatr Cogn Disord. 2005;20(2-3):99-104.
103. Mendez MF, Shapira JS, Miller BL. Stereotypical movements and frontotemporal dementia. Mov Disord. 2005;20(6): 742-5.
104. Mercy L, Hodges JR, Dawson K, et al. Incidence of early-onset dementias in Cambridgeshire, United Kingdom. Neurology. 2008;71(19):1496-9.
105. Merrilees J. A model for management of behavioral symptoms in frontotemporal lobar degeneration. Alzheimer Dis Assoc Disord. 2007;21(4): S64-S69.
106. Middleton L, Kirkland S, Rockwood K. Prevention of CIND by physical activity: Different impact on VCI-ND compared with MCI. J Neurol Sci. 2008;269(1):80-84.
107. Miller BL, Darby A, Benson DF, et al. Aggressive, socially disruptive and antisocial behaviour associated with frontotemporal dementia. Br J Psychiatry. 1997;170:150-4.
108. Miller BL, Seeley WW, Mychack P, et al. Neuroanatomy of the self: Evidence from patients with frontotemporal dementia. Neurology. 2001;57(5):817-21.
109. Mollenhauer B, Förstl H, Deuschl G, et al. Lewy body and parkinsonian dementia: common, but often misdiagnosed conditions. Dtsch Ärztebl Int. 2010;107(39):684.
110. Molloy S, McKeith IG, O'Brien JT, et al. The role of levodopa in the management of dementia with Lewy bodies. J Neurol Neurosurg Psychiatry. 2005;76(9):1200-3.
111. Moretti R, Torre P, Vilotti C, et al. Rivastigmine and Parkinson dementia complex. Expert Opin Pharmacother. 2007;8(6):817-29.
112. Moroney JT. Meta-analysis of the Hachinski Ischaemic Score in pathologically verified dementias. Neurology. 1997;49:1096-1105.
113. Murgod UA, Saleem Q, Anand A, et al. A clinical study of patients with genetically confirmed Huntington's disease from India. J Neurol Sci. 2001;190(1):73-8.
114. Nagano-Saito A, Washimi Y, Arahata Y, et al. Visual hallucination in Parkinson's disease with FDG PET. Mov Disord. 2004;19(7):801-6.
115. Nath A, Schiess N, Venkatesan A, et al. Evolution of HIV dementia with HIV infection. Int Rev Psychiatry. 2008;20(1):25-31.
116. Neary D, Snowden JS, Gustafson L, et al. Frontotemporal lobar degeneration: A consensus on clinical diagnostic criteria. Neurology. 1998;51(6):1546-54.
117. Neumann J, Bras J, Deas E, et al. Glucocerebrosidase mutations in clinical and pathologically proven Parkinson's disease. Brain. 2009;132(7):1783-94.
118. Paulsen JS, Hoth KF, Nehl C, et al. Critical periods of suicide risk in Huntington's disease. Am J Psychiatry. 2005;162(4): 725-31.
119. Peters F, Perani D, Herholz K, et al. Orbitofrontal dysfunction related to both apathyanddisinhibition in frontotemporal dementia. Dementia Geriatric Cogn Disord. 2006;21:373-9.
120. Polnikorn N, Witoonpanich R, Vorachit M, et al. Penicillin concentrations in cerebrospinal fluid after different treatment regimens for syphilis. Br J Vener Dis. 1980;56(6):363-7.
121. Pringsheim T, Wiltshire K, Day L, et al. The incidence and prevalence of Huntington's disease: A systematic review and meta-analysis. Movement Disorders. 2012;27(9):1083-91.
122. Rana AQ, Yousuf MS, Naz S, et al. Prevalence and relation of dementia to various factors in Parkinson`s disease. Psychiatry Clin Neurosci. 2012;66(1):64-68.

123. Rankin KP, Baldwin E, Pace-Savitsky C, et al. Self-awareness and personality change in dementia. J Neurol Neurosurg Psychiatry. 2005;76(5):632-9.
124. Ratnavalli E, Brayne C, Dawson K, et al. The prevalence of Frontotemporal dementia. Neurology. 2002;58(11):1615-21.
125. Reddy HP, Willams M, Tagle DA. Recent advances in understanding the pathogenesis of Huntington's disease. Trends Neurosci. 1999;22(6):248-54.
126. Reger M, Welsh R, Razani J, et al. A meta-analysis of the neuropsychological sequelae of HIV infection. J Int Neuropsychol Soc. 2002;8(3):410-24.
127. Reiner A, Albin RL, Anderson KD.Differential loss of striatal projection neurons in Huntington's disease. Proc Natl Acad Sci USA. 1988;85(15):5733-7.
128. Riedel D, Ghate M, Nene M, et al. Screening for human immunodeficiency virus (HIV).dementia in an HIV clade C–infected population in India. J Neuro Virology. 2006;12(1): 34-38.
129. Román GC. Senile dementia of the Binswanger type: A vascular form of dementia in the elderly. JAMA. 1987;258(13):1782-8.
130. Ruberg M, Villageois A, Bonnet AM, et al. Acetyl cholinesterase and butyrylcholinesterase in frontal cortex and cerebrospinal fluid of demented and non-demented patients with Parkinson's disease. Brain Res. 1986;362(1):83-91.
131. Sanchez-Castaneda C, Rene R, Ramirez-Ruiz B, et al. Frontal and associative visual areas related to visual hallucinations in dementia with Lewy bodies and Parkinson's disease with dementia. Mov Disord. 2010;25(5):615-22.
132. Satoh K, Muramoto T, Tanaka T, et al. Association of an 11-12 kDa protease-resistant prion protein fragment with subtypes of dura graft-associated Creutzfeldt-Jakob disease and other prion diseases. J Gen Virol. 2003;84(Pt 10):2885-93.
133. Schoch PE, Wolters EC. Penicillin concentrations in serum and CSF during high-dose intravenous treatment for neurosyphilis. Neurology. 1987;37(7):1214-6.
134. Schroter A, Zerr I, Henkel K, et al. Magnetic resonance imaging in the clinical diagnosis of Creutzfeldt-Jakob disease. Arch Neurology. 2000;57(12):1751-7.
135. Seelaar H, Kamphorst W, Rosso SM, et al. Distinct genetic forms of frontotemporal dementia. Neurology. 2008;71(16): 1220-6.
136. Shah K, Qureshi SU, Johnson M, et al. Does use of anti hypertensive drugs affect the incidence or progression of dementia? A systematic review. Am J Geriatr Pharmacother. 2009;7(5):250-61.
137. Shankar NP, Atanu B, Sandip P, et al. Clinical profile of young-onset dementia: A study from Eastern India. Neurology Asia. 2007;13(2):103-8.
138. ShoulsonI, Odoroff C, Oakes D, et al. A controlled trial of baclofen as protective therapy in early Huntington's disease. Ann Neurol. 1989;25(3):252-9.
139. Sinforiani E, BanchieriL, Zucchella C, et al. Cognitive rehabilitation in Parkinson's disease. Arch Gerontol Geriatr Suppl. 2004;(9):387-91.
140. Snowden JS, Neary D, Mann DMA. Fronto-temporal lobar degeneration: Frontotemporal dementia, progressive aphasia, semantic dementia. New York: Churchill Livingstone, 1996.
141. Solbrig MV, Healy JF, Jay CA. Infections of the nervous System. In: Bradley WG, Daroff RB, Gerald MF, Marsden CD (Eds). The Neurological Disorders. 3rd edition. Boston: Butterworth-Heinemann; 2000. pp.1317-51.
142. Swanberg MM. Memantine for behavioral disturbances in frontotemporal dementia: A case series. Alzheimer Dis Assoc Disord. 2007;21(2):164-6.
143. Tiraboschi P, Salmon DP, Hansen LA, et al. What best differentiates Lewy body from Alzheimer's disease in earlystage dementia? Brain. 2006;129(pt 3):729-35.
144. Tournier-Lasserve E, Joutel A, Melki J, et al. Cerebral autosomal dominant arteriopathy with subcortical infarcts and leukoencephalopathy maps to chromosome 19q12. Nat Genet. 1993;3(3):256-9.
145. Troyer AK. Normative data for clustering and switching on verbal fluency tasks. J Clin Exp Neuropsychol. 2000;22(3): 370-8.
146. Uchiyama M, Nishio Y, Yokoi K, et al. Pareidolias: Complex visual illusions in dementia with Lewy bodies. Brain. 2012;135(8):2458-69.
147. Van Deerlin VM, Sleiman PM, Martinez-Lage M, et al. Common variants at 7p21 are associated with frontotemporal lobar degeneration with TDP-43 inclusions. Nat Genet. 2010;42(3):234-9.
148. Vonsattel JP, Meyers RH, Stevens TJ, et al. Neuropathological classification of Huntington's disease. J Neuropathol Exp Neurol. 1985;44(6):559-77.
149. Watt DC, Seller A. A clinicogenetic study of psychiatric disorder in Huntington's chorea. Psychol Med. 1993;23 (Suppl):1-46.
150. Will RG, Ironside JW, Zeidler M, et al. A new variant of Creutzfeldt-Jakob disease in the UK. Lancet. 1996;347(9006): 921-5.
151. Woods SP, Moore DJ, Weber E, et al. Cognitive neuropsychology of HIV-associated neurocognitive disorders. Neuropsychol Rev. 2009;19(2):152-68.
152. Woolley JD, Gorno-Tempini ML, Seelev WW, et al. Binge eating is associated with right orbitofrontal-insular-striatal atrophy in frontotemporal dementia. Neurology. 2007;69(14):1424-33.
153. World Health Organization and Alzheimer's disease International. Dementia: A Public Health Priority. Geneva, WHO Press, 2012.
154. Yadav S, Bentley P, Srivastava P, et al. The first Indian-origin family with genetically proven cerebral autosomal dominant arteriopathy with subcortical infarcts and leukoencephalopathy (CADASIL). J Stroke Cerebrovasc Dis. 2013;22(1):28-31.
155. Yamamoto R, Iseki E, Murayama N, et al. Correlation in Lewy pathology between the claustrum and visual areas in brains of dementia with Lewy bodies. Neurosci Lett. 2007;415(3):219-24.
156. Yip AG, Brayne C, Matthews FE. Risk factors for incident dementia in England and Wales: The Medical Research Council Cognitive Function and Ageing Study. A population-based nested case-control study. Age Ageing. 2006;35(2): 154-0160.

157. Zaccai J, McCracken C, Brayne C. A systematic review of prevalence and incidence studies of dementia with Lewy bodies. Age Ageing. 2005;34(6):561-6.
158. Zamboni G, Huey ED, Krueger F, et al. Apathy and disinhibition in frontotemporal dementia: Insights into their neural correlates. Neurology. 2008;71(10):736-42.

Psychoneuroimmunology

159. Ader R, Felten DL, Cohen N. Psychoneuroimmunology. 2nd edition. San Diego, California: Academic Press, 1991.
160. Blalock JE. A molecular basis for bidirectional communication between immune and neuroendocrine system. Physiol Rev. 1989;69:1-32.
161. Blalock JE. Psychoimmunoendocrinology. 2nd edition. Basel, Switzerland: Karger, 1992.
162. Chrousos G, Gold P. The concepts of stress and stress system disorders: Overview of Physical and behavioralhomeostatis, JAMA. 1992;267:1244-52.
163. Cooke A. Regulation of immune response. In: Evan R, Jonathan B, David M (Eds). Immunology. Mosby Year Book, 1993.
164. Felten DL, Cohen N, Ader R, et al. Central neural circuits involved in neural-immune interactions. In: Ader R, Felten DL, Cohen N (Eds). Psychoneuroimmunology. 2nd edition. San Diego: Academic Press, 1991, 3-25.
165. Irwin M, Hauger RL, Jones L, et al. Sympathetic nervous system mediates central corticotropin releasing factor induced suppression of natural killer cytotoxicity, J PharmacolExpTher. 1990;255:101-7.
166. Jankovic BD, Isacovic K. Neuroendocrine correlates of immune response. Int Arch Allergy Appl Immunol. 1973;45: 360-84.
167. Kelley KW, Arkins S, Li YM. Growth harmones, prolactin and insulin like growth factors: New jobs for old players. Brain Behav Immun. 1992;6:317-26.
168. Martin JB, Barchas JD. Neuropeptides in Neurologic and Psychiatric Disease. ARNMD Vol. 64, New York: Raven Press, 1986.
169. McEwen BS. Adrenal steroids, the hippocampus, and the amygdala: Relationship to anxiety and depression. Medicographia. 1994;16:60-3.
170. Payan DG, MacGills JP, Goetzl EJ. Neuroimmunology.Adv Immunol. 1986;39:299-323.
171. Pechnick RN. Effects of opioids on the hypothalamo-pituitary-adrenal axis.Ann Rev Pharmacol Toxicol. 1993;33:353-82.
172. Reichlin S. Neuroendocrine immune interactions. N Eng J Med. 1993;329:1246-53.
173. Roszman TL, Jackson JC, Cross RJ, et al. Neuroanatomic and neurotransmitter influences on immune function. J Immunol. 1985;135:769-72.
174. Solomon GF, Amkrant AA. Psychoneuroendocrinological effects on the immune response. Ann Rev Microbiol. 1981;35: 155-84.

Brain Imaging in Psychiatry

175. Adinoff B, Devous M. Scientifically unfounded claims in diagnosing and treating patients. Am J Psychiatry. 2010;167(5):598.
176. Albers GW. Diffusion-weighted MRI for evaluation of acute stroke. Neurology. 1998;51(Suppl 3),S47-S49.
177. Amen Clinics. 18 ways SPECT can help you. http://www.amenclinics.com/clinics/patients/18-ways-spect-can-help-you/. Accessed May 23, 2013.
178. Amen Clinics. How brain SPECT imaging can help with ADHD/ADD. http://www.amenclinics.net/conditions/ADHD/. Accessed May 23, 2012.
179. Amen Clinics. How brain SPECT imaging can help with anxiety and depression. http://www.amenclinics.net/conditions/Anxiety_Issues/. Accessed May 23, 2012.
180. Beker T, Rezt W, Hofmann E, et al. Some methological issue in neuroadiogical research in psychiatry. J Neur Transm. 1995;99: 7-54.
181. Belliveanu JW, Kennedy D, McKinstry RC, et al. Functional mapping of the human visual cortex by magnetic resonance imaging. Science. 1991;254:716-9.
182. Berman K, Meyer-Lindenberg A. Functional brain imaging studies in schizophrenia. In: Charney D, Nestler E (Eds). Neurobiology of Mental Illness. New York: Oxford University Press; 2004.pp.311-23.
183. Bonte FJ, Weiner MF, Bigio EH, et al. SpECT imaging in dementias. J Nucl Med. 2001;42:1131-2.
184. Bradley WG, Yuh WTC, Bydder GM. Use of MR imaging contrast agents in the brain. J Magn Reson Imag. 1993;3:199-218.
185. Bray S, Chang C, Hoeft F. Applications of multivariate pattern classification analyses in developmental neuroimaging of healthy and clinical populations. Front Hum Neurosci. 2009;3:32.
186. Brotman MA, Rich BA, Guyer AE, et al. Amygdala activation during emotion processing of neutral faces in children with severe mood dysregulation versus ADHD or bipolar disorder. Am J Psychiatry. 2010;167(1):61-9.
187. Burton R. Brain scam. Salon. May 12, 2008. http://www.salon.com/2008/05/12/daniel_amen/. Accessed May 23, 2013.
188. Calhoun VD, Maciejewski PK, Pearlson GD, Kiehl KA. Temporal lobe and "default" hemodynamic brain modes discriminate between schizophrenia and bipolar disorder. Hum Brain Mapp. 2008;29(11):1265-75.
189. Cherry SR, Phelps ME. Imaging brain function with positron emission tomography. In: Toga AW, Mazziotta JC (Eds). Brain Mapping: The Methods, Academic Press, San Diego; 1996. pp. 191-222.
190. deCharms RC. Applications of real-time fMRI. Nat Rev Neurosci. 2008;9(9):720-9.
191. Derubeis RJ, Siegle GJ, Hollon SD. Cognitive therapy versus medication for depression: treatment outcomes and neural mechanisms. Nat Rev Neurosci. 2008;9(10):788-96.

192. Dougherty DD, Rauch SL. Psychiatric Neuroimaging Research: Contemporary Strategies. American Psychiatric Publishing, Washington DC, 2001.
193. Emsley RA, Stander D, Bell PSH, et al. Computed tomography in psychiatric patients. S Afr Med J. 1986;70:212-4.
194. Etkin A, Wager TD. Functional neuroimaging of anxiety: a meta-analysis of emotional processing in PTSD, social anxiety disorder, and specific phobia. Am J Psychiatry. 2007;164(10): 1476-88.
195. Evans KC, Dougherty DD, Pollack MH, Rauch SL. Using neuroimaging to predict treatment response in mood and anxiety disorders. Ann Clin Psychiatry. 2006;18(1):33-42.
196. Flaherty LT, Arroyo W, Chatoor I, et al. Brain imaging and child and adolescent psychiatry with special emphasis on SPECT. Arlington, VA: American Psychiatric Association, Council on Children, Adolescents and Their Families; 2005.
197. Gibby WA, Zimmerman RA. A-ray computed tomography. In: Mazziotta JC, Gilman S (Eds). Clinical Brain Imaging: Principles and Applications, FA Davis, Philadelphia; 1992. pp. 2-38.
198. Gillihan SJ, Parens E. Should we expect "neural signatures" for DSM diagnoses? J Clin Psychiatry. 2011;72(10):1383-9.
199. Gonzalez RG, Fischman AJ, Guimaraes AR, et al. Functional MR in the evalution of dementia: Correlation of abnormal dynamic cerebral blood volume measurements with changes in cerebral metabolism on positron emission tomography with fluorodeoxyglucose. Am J Neororadiol. 1995;16: 1763-70.
200. Gotlib IH, Hamilton JP. Neuroimaging and depression: current status and unresolved issues. Curr Dir Psychol Sci. 2008;17:159-63.
201. Hamani C, Mayberg H, Snyder B, Giacobbe P, Kennedy S, Lozano AM. Deep brain stimulation of the subcallosal cingulate gyrus for depression: anatomical location of active contacts in clinical responders and a suggested guideline for targeting. J Neurosurg. 2009;111(6):1209-15.
202. Hartshone MF. Single photon emission computed tomography. In: Orrison WW Jr, Lewine JD, Sanders JA, et al. (Eds). Functional Brain Imaging. Mosby, New York, 1995
203. Hayman LA, Evans RA, Fahr LM, et al. Renal consequences of rapid high dose contrast. Am J Radiol. 1980:134:553-5.
204. Haynes JD, Rees G. Decoding mental states from brain activity in humans. Nature Rev Neurosci. 2006;7(7):523-34.
205. Herny ME, Frederick BB, Moore CM, et al. Magnetic resoilur spectroscopy in psychiatric illness. In: Dougherty DD, Rauch SL (Eds). Psychiatric Neuroimaging Research: Contemporary Strategies, American Psychiatric publishing, Washington DC; 2001.pp.291-334.
206. Horowitz AL. MRI physics for Radiologists: A Visual Aproach Springer-Verlag, New York, 1992.
207. Hyman SE. The diagnosis of mental disorders: the problem of reification. Ann Rev Clin Psychol. 2010;27(6);155-79.
208. Ingvar DH, Lassen NA. Quantitative determination of relionl cerebral blood flow in man. Lancet. 1961;2:806-7.
209. Insel T, Cuthbert B, Garvey M, et al. Research domain criteria (RDoC): toward a new classification framework for research on mental disorders. Am J Psychiatry. 2010;167(7):748-51.
210. Jonnson KA, Renshaw PF, Becker JA, et al. Comparison of functional MRI and SPECT in Alzheimer's disease. Neurology. 1995;45(Suppl), S874.
211. Keener MT, Phillips ML. Neuroimaging in bipolar disorder: a critical review of current findings. Curr Psychiatry Rep. 2007;9(6):512-20.
212. Kido DK, Sheline YI. Neuroimaging for neuropsychiatry. In: Fogel BS, Schiffer RB (Eds). Neuropsychiatry, Lippincott, Williams & Wilkins, Baltimore, MD. 1996.
213. Kim HF, Schulz PE, Wilde EA, Yudofsky SC. Laboratory testing and imaging studies in psychiatry. In: Hales RE, Yudofsky SC, Gabbard GO (Eds). The American Psychiatric Publishing Textbook of Psychiatry. 5th edn. Arlington, VA: American Psychiatric Publishing; 2008.pp.19-72.
214. Krausz Y, Bonne O, Marciano R, et al. Brain SPECT imaging of neuropsychiatry disorders. Eur J Radiol. 1996;21:183-7.
215. Leonard JP, Nowotnik DP, Neieinck RD. Technetium-99m-d 1-HM-PAO: A new radiopharmaceutical for imaging religion brain perfusion using SPECT: A comparison with iodile-123 HIPDM. J Nucl Med. 1986;27:1819-23.
216. Leuchter AF. Healing the Hardware of the Soul: Enhance Your Brain To Improve Your Work, Love, and Spiritual Life, by Daniel Amen (book review). Am J Psychiatry. 2009;166(5):625. *http://ajp.psychiatryonline.org/data/Journals/AJP/3890/09aj0625.PDF. Accessed May 23, 2012.*
217. Lyoo IK, Seol HY, Byun HS, et al. Unsuspected multiple sclerosis in patients with psychiatric disorders: A magnetic resonance imaging study. J Neuropsychiatr Clin Neurosci. 1996;8:54-9.
218. MacLaren DC, Toyokuni T, Cherry SR, et al. PET imaging of trangene expression. Boil Psychiatr. 2000;48:337-48.
219. Mayberg HS, Lozano A, Voon V, et al. Deep brain stimulation for treatment-resistant depression. Neuron. 2005;45(5): 651-60.
220. McIntosh AM, Owens DC, Moorhead WJ, et al. Longitudinal volume reductions in people at high genetic risk of schizophrenia as they develop psychosis. Biol Psychiatry. 2011;69(10): 953-8.
221. National Institute of Mental Health. Research domain criteria (RDoC). *http://www.nimh.nih.gov/research-funding/rdoc. Accessed May 23, 2012.*
222. Orison WW Jr, Sanders JA. Clinical brain imaging: Computerized axial tomography and magnetic resonance imaging. In: Orrison WW Jr, Lewine JD, Sanders JA, et al. (Eds). Functional Brain Imaging, Mosby, New York. 1995.
223. Osborn AG. Diagnostic Neuroradiology. Mosby Year Book, St. Louis, 1994.
224. Rauch SL, Renshaw PF. Clinical neuroimaging and psychiatry. Harv Rev Psychiatr. 1995;2:297-312.
225. Reiman EM, Caselli RJ, Yun LS, et al. Preclinical evidence of Alzheimer's disease in persons homozygous for the epsilon 4 allele for apolipoprotein E. New Engl J Med. 1996;334:752-8.

226. Reivich M, Kuhl D, Wolf A, et al. Measurement of local cerebral glucose metabolism in man with 18F-2-deoxy -d-glucose. Acta Neurol Scand. 1997;56(Suppl 64)190-1.
227. Renshaw PF, Wicklund S. In vivo measurement of lithium in humans by nuclear magnetic resonance spectroscopy. Boil therapeutic administration. An J Psychitr. 1988;23:465-75.
228. Renshaw PF, Guimaraes AR, Fava M, et al. Accumulation of fluxetine and norfluoxetine in human brain during therapeutic administration. Am J Psychiatr. 1992;149:1592-994.
229. Renshaw PF, Rauch SL. Neuroimaging in clinical psychiatry. In: Nicholi AM Jr. (Ed). The Harvard Guide to Psychiatry, 3rd ed., Belknap Press, Cambridge, MA, 1999. pp. 84-97.
230. Renshaw PF, Wicklund S. In vivo measurement of lithium in humans by nuclear magnetic resonance spectroscopy. Boil therapeutic administration. An J Psychitr. 1988;23:465-75.
231. Schwartz JM, Baxter LR Jr, Mazziotta JC, Gerner RH, Phelps ME. The differential diagnosis of depression: Relevance of positron emission tomography studies of cerebral glucose metabolism to the bipolar-unipolar dichotomy. JAMA. 1987;258(10):1368-74.
232. Shehadi WH. Contrast media adverse reactions: Occurrence, recurrerce, and distribution patterns. Radiology. 1982;143:11-7.
233. Silverman DH, Small GW, Chang CY, et al. Positron emission tomography in evaluation of dementia: Regional brain metabolism and long-term outcome. J Am Med Assoc. 2001; 286:2120-7.
234. Small GW, Mazziotta JC, Collins MT, et al. Apolipoprotein E type 4 allele and cerebral glucose metabolism in relatives at risk for familial Alzheimer's disease. J Am Med Assoc. 1995;273: 942-7.
235. Theodore WH, Gaillard WD. Positron emission tomography in neocortical epilepsies. Adv Neuro. 2000;84:435-46.
236. Wahlund K, Kristiansson M. Aggression, psychopathy and brain imaging: review and future recommendations. Int J Law Psychiatry. 2009;32(4):267.
237. Weinberger DR. Brain disease and psychiatric illness: When should a psychiatrist order a CAT scan? Am J Psychiatr. 1984; 141:1521-7.
238. White RI, Halden WJ. Liquid gold: Low-osmolality contrast media. Radiology. 1986;159:559-60.
239. Within DM, Hirsch RD, Hartman GW. Acute reactions to urographic contrast medium: Incidence, clinical characteristics, and relationship to history of hypersensitivity states. Am J Radiol. 1973;119:832-40.

CHAPTER 45

Psychological and Social Culture Sciences

CR Mukundan, Jyoti Ahuja, Radha Prabhu, PSDV Prasadarao, V Kumaraiah, SK Verma, A Puri, RC Chowdhary, Hemant Vyas, AP Dadhich, Mridula Vyas, Sai Krishna Tikka, Christoday RJ Khess, SC Bhargav, Umesh S, SS Nathawat, Vijaya Nathawat

45.1 NEUROPSYCHOLOGY

CR Mukundan, Jyoti Ahuja, Radha Prabhu

William Osler, first used the term *neuropsychology* in the beginning of the twentieth century to represent a study that combined the neurologists' and physiological psychologists' common interest in brain function.[1] Lashley[2] gave wide publicity for the then newly coined term in his book, *'The Neuropsychology of Lashley'*. Currently, neuropsychology is defined as "the study of the relation between brain function and behavior". Although, the study draws information from many disciplines, e.g. anatomy, biology, ethology, pharmacology, physiological psychology, and philosophy- the central focus is on the development of a science of human behavior based on the function of the human brain. Neuropsychology deals with the study of the mechanisms which are responsible for human thinking, learning and emotion, how do these mechanisms operate, and what are the effects of changes in brain states upon human behavior? The main theme of neuropsychological investigation is that, to understand human behavior, we need to understand the human brain.

Since earliest times, humans have tried to examine internal mechanisms that control human behavior. Mental processes have been variously located in the soul, the heart (Empedocles, ca. 495–435 BC) and in the brain (Alcmaeon, 500 BC). Plato (427–347 BC) believed in the soul, of which the brain constituted the rational part. Aristotle (384-322 BC) believed that the heart was the source of mental processes while the brain functioned as a radiator to cool the blood. Physicians such as Hippocrates (460-370 BC), however, argued strongly for the brain hypothesis, no doubt influenced by their clinical experience.

It is now recognized that simply knowing that the brain controls behavior is not sufficient. Formulation of a complete hypothesis requires knowledge of how it controls behavior. This has given rise to the issue of localization of functions; the notion that specific areas of the brain control specific behaviors. Modern thinking about the mind began with Descartes[3] (1596–1650) who believed in a unitary mind, which is the reasoning or rational entity. He believed that since the mind was indivisible, theories of subdivided brain function could not be correct. Modern neuroscientists debated this and dismissed the mind simply as a term to represent the activities of the brain. The argument for the localization function began with the phrenological theories of Gall and Spurzheim, who evolved the 'science' of phrenology: the study of the relation between the skull's surface features and a person's faculties.[4] Their elaborate theory evoked widespread ridicule and fell into disrepute, especially owing to the work of Flourens, who developed the technique of lesioning the brains of animals in order to examine the changes in the behavior. He concluded that there is no localization of function in the cerebrum, advocating Descartes' idea of a holistic, indivisible mind. Lashley similarly came to doubt that psychological functions could be successfully localized.

Subsequently, the concept of localization again began to gain momentum owing to the extensive work on language localization. Bouillard (1825) presented evidence from his clinical studies that speech functions are localized in the frontal lobes, possibly within the left hemisphere. In 1836, Dax presented a series of clinical case reports demonstrating that disorders of speech were constantly associated with lesions of the left hemisphere. Broca,[5] in 1863, described a syndrome consisting of inability to speak despite the presence of intact vocal mechanisms and normal comprehension, associated with lesions of a specific area in the left frontal lobe. This syndrome subsequently came to be known as 'Broca's aphasia', and the area he described, as 'Broca's area'. Thus, he synthesized the theory of localization of function and neuroanatomy, and further elaborated the concept of cerebral dominance of language in the left hemisphere. However, Wernicke[6] (1874) dissented with the localizationist view and proposed that there is more than one language area in the brain. He corroborated this by describing a syndrome known as 'Wernicke's aphasia' resulting from damage to the left temporal gyrus. Patients suffering from this disorder could speak fluently, but their speech was confused and made little sense; and they were unable to understand or repeat what was said to them despite normal hearing abilities.

The debate on localization continued throughout the 19th century. However, *neuropsychology* received recognition as a distinct discipline only after the World War II, aided by the developments in the fields on neurosurgery, psychometry, and technology. The basic assumption in *neuropsychology* is that every neural tissue in the brain has a specific function. Thus, a lesion in any part of the brain would result in changes in cognitive processing and affective responses of the individual. Several cognitive functions, such as learning and memory, are complex and are associated with different areas of the brain. A focal lesion can, therefore, produce not only focal functional deficits, but also interrupt a functional network engaged in complex psychological functions. Impairment of function can be measured using appropriate tests and associations between site of lesion and impairment can thus be established. It is necessary to remember, however, that while a one-to-one relationship has been established between the motor and sensory cortex and motor and sensory function, this is not a rule for the rest of the brain.

Neuropsychology is divided into two main areas: clinical and experimental neuropsychology. *Clinical neuropsychology* deals with patients who have structural lesions of the brain, and employs a variety of specialized testing procedures to examine the functional changes associated with damage to specific areas of the brain. Emphasis is on behavioral assessment methods, which would reflect changes in psychological functions owing to brain damage or lesion. The information thus gathered helps in practical clinical work, such as aiding diagnosis of brain lesions and rehabilitating brain-injured patients; and for scientific investigation of brain-behavior relationships. In contrast, in experimental neuropsychology, both normal subjects with intact brains and patients with brain lesions are studied. Varieties of laboratory techniques are employed to study higher functions and their structural correlation. Event related potential and EEG studies, used to investigate cognitive processes, are examples of such techniques.

GENERAL PRINCIPLES OF NEUROPSYCHOLOGY

Principles of Cerebral Asymmetry

Dax and Broca discovered, over a century ago, that damage to the left hemisphere alone results in speech and language impairments. Their conclusion, that the left hemisphere plays a special role in language, not shared by the right hemisphere, is widely accepted today. In 1874, Hughlings-Jackson proposed that the right hemisphere might have some special perceptual function to complement the language function of the left hemisphere. This proposition has now gained widespread acceptance, owing to systematic work on hemisphere specialization in the 1960s by researchers, who carried out extensive neuropsychological investigations of neurosurgical patients with focal lesions. In 1957, Scoville and Milner[7] demonstrated severe anterograde memory impairment in a patient who had medial temporal lobe resection, which was found to persist over 35 years of follow-up. This revolutionized the study of memory. Milner,[8,9] in a number of subsequent studies, demonstrated impaired verbal learning abilities in persons with left temporal lobe lesions, and impaired visual perception and visual learning among patients with right temporal lobe lesions. The linking of verbal and nonverbal memory deficits, with the left and right hippocampi respectively, remains the cornerstone of all current research on the neuropsychology of memory. It is largely due to these efforts that it is now accepted that there is a functional lateralization within the cortex, with the left and the right hemispheres each performing their own specialized functions.

The functions of the left hemisphere include processing verbal material and spoken sounds, verbal learning and memory, language and speech, sequential processing, refined movement and auditory reception. The right hemisphere is involved in visual spatial processing, processing of non-verbal material such as geometric and tonal patterns, visual learning and memory, emotion, nonverbal memory and processing of music and melody. The core function of the right hemisphere is the ability to carry out parallel processing, whether the material is nonverbal or verbal. Similarly, the core function of the left hemisphere is the ability to process information serially, whether the material is verbal or non-verbal. Therefore, mode of information processing is considered the main principle of cerebral lateralization. Laterality can be affected by environmental and cultural factors, besides genetic factors such as gender and handedness. For example, non-European languages, such as Chinese or Japanese, may have more right hemisphere involvement, since there is more prosody in them. Similarly, cerebral organization of left-handers and females appears to have less functional asymmetry than that of right-handers and males.

Principle of Cerebral Localization

Another way of looking at the functions of the cortex is in terms of specific areas or lobes specialized for specific functions. We have already discussed the role of understanding localization of functions within the brain, in relation to the early developments in neuropsychology. The cerebral cortex is structurally divided into four lobes: frontal, parietal, occipital, and temporal lobes. This division has also helped to delineate the functional differences amongst the lobes on the left and right sides. Although we can attribute different functions to each of the lobes, it is necessary to consider the basic fact that higher functions are complex and need participation of different areas of the brain. Therefore, localization of a specific function generally signifies the specific role an area of the brain has in its total performance. It is necessary to understand that it is not always possible to assign discrete packets of cognitive activity to different pieces of cortical tissue. Human behavior is extremely complex and this complexity of processes requires continual interaction of different area. Also, there are multiple solutions to different problems and different regions may play greater or lesser roles in particular aspects of processing, depending on the strategies used. However in general, the functions mediated by each of these lobes are as enumerated in Table 1.

Table 1: Functions and impairments associated with the frontal, parietal, temporal and occipital lobes

Area	*Function*	*Impairments associated with damage*
Frontal	Execution of motor movement Initiation, planning, programming, sequencing and organization of movement Programming of motor speech Ideation Abstraction and concept formation Initiation and planning of action Judgment Memory Intellectual functions Emotions	Disturbances of motor function Poor movement programming Broca's aphasia Loss of divergent thinking Poor strategy formation Reduced spontaneity Impulsivity Impaired associative learning Impaired temporal memory Impaired anticipatory functions Poor delayed response/working memory Loss of inhibition/impaired social behavior Altered sexual behavior
Parietal	Tactile localization and discrimination Fine touch, sensation Proprioception Kinesthesia Stereognosis *Gnosis:* Recognition of received tactile, visual or auditory input *Praxis:* Storage of program or visuokinesthetic motor engrams necessary for motor sequences *Body schema:* Postural model of body, body parts and their relation to the environment *Language:* Comprehension of words, interpretation of tone, loudness and timing of words	Disorders of tactile function Visual or tactile agnosia Apraxias Constructional apraxia Disorders of language (such as alexia and agraphia) Acalculia Contralateral neglect Disorders of visuospatial functions and spatial ability Body schema disturbances Right-left confusion
Temporal	Auditory reception Language comprehension Sound modulation Perception of music Memory Learning of higher order visual tasks and auditory patterns Emotion Motivation Personality	Disturbances of auditory sensation and perception Disturbances of language comprehension Disorders of visual perception Poor long-term memory Impaired organization and categorization of material Poor contextual use Changes in personality, affect and sexual activities
Occipital	Visual reception Synthesis and integration of visual information Perception of visuospatial relationships Formation of visual memory traces Prepositional construction in language comprehension and speech Formation of visuokinesthetic motor engrams	Impaired visual reception Disturbances of selection of visual input Impaired visuospatial organization

NEUROPSYCHOLOGICAL ASSESSMENT

After World War II, a number of neuropsychological laboratories were established in Europe and North America. These have been principally responsible for the development of neuropsychological assessment as a tool in clinical neurology and psychiatry. Neuropsychological assessment has several goals in a clinical setting. The primary goals of neuropsychological assessment are:

- To diagnose the presence of cortical damage or dysfunction, and localize it where possible.
- To provide an accurate and unbiased estimate of an individual's functionally cognitive capacity.
- To monitor course and outcome of treatment, and provide information about the potential for resuming previous lifestyle.
- To facilitate patient care and rehabilitation. Serial assessments can provide significant information about the rate of recovery and help in planning treatment strategies.
- Behavioral assessments are highly sensitive indices of change and can often detect changes even before structural changes are evident.
- It has an important role in neurosurgery; the information gathered from neuropsychological testing is important in deciding neurosurgical strategies. Assessment before and after surgery helps to evaluate the changes in functioning as a result of the surgery.
- Cognitive profile and cognitive deterioration in functional psychoses can be most adequately assessed using neuropsychological tests.

Administration of behavioral tests and their interpretation can use either a psychometric or an ideometric approach. The *psychometric approach* relies on rigid assessment procedures for measuring behavior and psychological functions, and uses norms for comparing individual performance and interpretation of data. This mode of assessment is most suitable when one wants to know the potentialities and functional efficacy of an individual in comparison with his or her peer group. The *ideometric approach*, on the other hand, is more flexible, and takes into account individual factors during assessment and interpretation. In clinical practice, the emphasis is on detecting deficits in behavior and cognitive functions, as they have diagnostic implications. A syndrome profile and analysis provide not only important diagnostic clues but also help in differential diagnosis. A profile of impaired functions serve as guideline for monitoring the progress/recovery from disease as well as for formulating rehabilitative strategies for the patient. Though a totally mutually exclusive one-to-one relationship has not been established with respected to specific functions and structures of the brain, there exists a stronger relationship between deficits and lesions in the brain. Because of this reason, the latter approach is found most suitable for clinical applications.

The steps involved in neuropsychological assessment are:

- Clinical or diagnostic review of history of present illness.
- Detailed interview of patient and significant others to elicit details of onset, course, degree and nature of cognitive and personality changes; and profile of premorbid functions.
- *Selection and administration of appropriate neuropsychological tests:* Most neuropsychological assessments begin or end with some general measures of intelligence, which are invaluable in providing a base level of cognitive functioning. The Wechsler Adult Intelligence Test is one intelligence test used for this purpose. However, a comprehensive neuropsychological assessment requires a series of different tests. Hence, researchers have developed neuropsychological batteries, administered routinely as a group. A useful neuropsychological battery should satisfy certain important criteria such as high degree of validity, thoroughness, ease of administration and scoring, cost and time efficiency, adaptability and flexibility. Validity refers to the sensitivity of a test to elicit a deficit known to be associated with a certain lesion in the brain.

There are essentially two kinds of test batteries: formal batteries of tests, which are commercially available, and informal batteries, assembled for use with particular populations of patients. Some of the most widely used formal batteries are:

Halstead-Reitan Battery

This battery is composed of a series of tests devised by Halstead[10] in the late 1940s. The battery originally comprised of seven tests selected for their ability to discriminate between patients with frontal lobe lesions and other patient groups and normal controls. The current version of the battery consists of about 10 basic subtests. These include: Wechsler Intelligence Scale, Category Test, Critical Flicker-Fusion Test, Tactile Performance Test, Rhythm Test, Speech-Sounds Perception Test, the Finger-Oscillation Test and the Time-Sense Test. Other auxiliary tests sometimes included in the battery are the Trail Making Test and the Aphasia Screening Test. Although widely used, this battery has been criticized for a variety of reasons. The tests are not theoretically based; their neuroanatomical significance has not been adequately established, memory functions are poorly assessed, and the battery is not comprehensive (there are no measures of somatosensory, praxic and gnostic functions).

Luria's Neuropsychological Investigation[11,12]

Generally considered the most comprehensive battery available, it also has a number of other advantages. This battery has a basis on sound theoretical principles, the neuroanatomical significance of deficits is established, and it is thorough, inexpensive, and flexible. Luria has not proposed any formal test battery. His findings are based on original observations and examinations of patients (mainly war victims) with lesions of the brain. Luria is considered the founder of modern clinical neuropsychology because of the extensive clinical data he gathered and documented. His account of behavioral and functional deficits relates to large and extensive lesions, which were not then investigated by any currently known methods. This is a handicap for the present user, especially if the lesion is relatively small, as the classical deficits described by Luria may be absent in such cases. Some of his most significant contributions are: (a) understanding of functional interactions between different areas of the brain, (b) formulation of different functional systems with networking of different areas, (c) extensive understanding of the functions and role of the frontal lobes and frontal cortex in regulation of behavior, and (d) understanding the principles of lateralization based on successive and simultaneous processing.

Luria[11] spoke of 11 major higher cortical functions in man, and devised test procedures for comprehensive evaluation of each of these functions. These functions include:

- *Motor function:* Subdivided into three areas, motor functions of the hands, oral praxis, and speech regulation of the motor act.
- *Rhythmic function:* Subdivided into perception/motoric reproduction of pitch relationships and of complex rhythmic structures.
- *Tactile function:* Composed of simple cutaneous and deep tactile sensation and complex higher-order tactile functions called stereognostic ability.
- *Visual function:* Composed of visual perception, spatial orientation, and intellectual operations in space.
- *Receptive speech function:* Subdivided into phonemic hearing, word comprehension, simple sentence comprehension, and complex sentence comprehension.
- *Expressive speech function:* Subdivided into articulation, nominative functions, narrative speech and grammatical expressions.
- *Writing function:* It has two basic components, phonetic analysis of verbal material and the motor aspect of writing.
- *Reading function:* It includes reading individual letters, simple words and complex words.
- *Arithmetic function:* Composed of two basic abilities, namely arithmetic operation and comprehension of number structures.
- *Memory function:* It has three important aspects, namely learning, retention and retrieval, and logical memorization.
- *Intellectual function:* It includes aspects such as preliminary synthesis, concept formation and problem solving skills, which are provided by assessment of general neuropsychological competence and estimate of IQ.

Luria-Nebraska Neuropsychological Battery

This battery is the result of an attempt by Golden[13] to standardize the Luria test procedures. Although Golden and his colleagues have made widespread claims of the diagnostic efficiency of this instrument, the battery has not yet received the same degree of acceptance.

Although formal batteries are easy to obtain, many neuropsychologists believe that readymade batteries are not as good as informal batteries designed for use with specific populations.[14] Such a battery will comprise of various items, such as focal tests of sensory-motor functions, tests of attentional processes, regulation of motor actions, perception, verbal and visual integration, language functions, learning, memory, thinking, emotions and personality.

NEUROPSYCHOLOGICAL REHABILITATION

Brain injury leads to a variety of neuropsychological deficits in various cognitive and emotional areas, such as attention, memory, regulatory functions, language and speech functions, and personality. Neuropsychological rehabilitation aims at helping the patient overcome these deficits and helping to improve the patient's functioning, as far as possible, to premorbid levels. Rehabilitation is an active process, in which services are provided to the disabled person in order to reduce impairment, to facilitate optimum acquisition of skills, and to overcome the disability.[15] The primary task in neuropsychological rehabilitation is to understand the nature of the disabilities that follow CNS injury, in order to facilitate optimum social and occupational adaptation. An understanding of pathological states provides insight into patterns of impairment, and prognosis for recurrence or recovery of function.

Various mechanisms have been proposed for recovery of function after injury, but a substantial portion of recovery is thought to involve reorganization of remaining undamaged tissue, or reorganization of tissue around the area of lesion. The concept of brain plasticity is the base of rehabilitation. Some researchers believe that the brain has an unlimited potential for recovery and reorganization after injury. Several neural mechanisms have been suggested as being important in mediating recovery, such as regeneration and re-establishment of connection between neurones, sprouting of new nerve fibers, denervation supersensitivity and disinhibition of potential compensatory zones. The evidence indicates that there are always residual and permanent deficits after brain damage. Extensive recovery after brain damage is an exception rather than a rule.

Although, there is little data on long-term recovery, evidence seems to suggest that:

- Recovery is likely in complex behaviors that comprise many components through processes that are referred to as behavioral compensation.
- Recovery is more pronounced after incomplete lesions.
- Recovery is unlikely for specific functions controlled by localized brain areas, if the entire area is removed.

Rehabilitation methods commonly used include retraining, (a) in basic functions such as attention, short-term memory, and information processing, (b) in functional skills, such as activities of daily living and professional skills, and (c) in problem solving skills, which teach the patient to approach problems of daily life in a planned manner.

A rehabilitation program must take into account various individual factors that may influence learning and recovery. These include medical problems, physical handicaps, motivational factors, environmental problems and activity patterns. The rehabilitation system must be prepared to deal with each of these areas of difficulty. An important practical aspect to consider in conducting a remediation program is the emotional state of the patient. One emotional factor, which can interfere with the success of the program, is denial of the problem by the patient. A remediator must develop strategies to overcome denial and create awareness of the problem by demonstrating the existence of the problem to the patient. There are patients, who are acutely and overwhelmingly aware of their inability to perform and this may become associated with depression and feelings of failure. It is important to maintain motivation in the face of depression. Rewards, praise and immediate feedback can be helpful in such cases. Prognosis is primarily a function of the motivational status in the patient. If amotivation itself is a result of brain lesion, the chances of recovery and adjustment are poor. Extensive frontal lobe lesions and subcortical lesions often produce severe amotivation and apathy in a patient. There are no easy and short methods to encounter absence of motivation. Patients with severe memory deficits are also poor candidates for successful rehabilitation. However, it may be improper to decide in advance, if a patient is unlikely to benefit from retraining programs and reject such cases. Only repeated and sustained efforts can confirm with certainty that a patient is unlikely to benefit from active retraining programs. In the prevailing psychosocial situation in India, it is essential to organize family support for such patients for their maintenance and daily upkeep.

It is a common finding that a patient undergoing a retraining program shows a greater general improvement, than specific cognitive facilitation, in the initial stages. Many of the head trauma patients will have insight into their own handicap, especially in comparison with their premorbid level of efficiency and personal acumen. The loss of skills and abilities throw them into states of incompatibility and uncertainty. These patients react in a highly positive manner to the initial beneficial effects of therapeutic contact and retraining, with a sense of enhanced cognitive confidence and spurt in motivation. It is a extremely important that the initial enthusiasm is reinforced and maintained in cautious way by the therapist, as true cognitive enhancement and functional recovery may follow only at a slower pace.

NEUROPSYCHOLOGICAL DEFICITS IN FUNCTIONAL AND NEUROPSYCHIATRIC DISORDERS

The central nervous system, more specifically the brain, is now believed to be implicated in most of the functional disorders, such as schizophrenia, depression, mania, obsessive, compulsive disorders (OCDs), psychopathy, and childhood disorders such as learning disability. There are also a number of neuropsychiatric conditions, such as alcohol dependence and neurological conditions with profound psychiatric symptomatology such as dementia, which are characterized by neuropsychological deficits. Some of these are reviewed here.

Schizophrenia

Since several decades, neuropsychological deficits in functions such as attention and information processing, learning and memory, language, conceptual and executive functions have been identified to be associated with schizophrenia. Researchers have put forth several hypotheses to explain impaired brain functioning in schizophrenia patients. These include the theories of dissociation of attention, inability to sustain attention, and filtering deficits. The information processing model suggests that schizophrenia patient has a defective 'filtering mechanism', which decides which stimuli a person should respond to and which he should ignore. This leads to an information overload. Abstraction deficits, commonly found in these patients, are considered secondary to the primary attention deficit.

Researchers attempted to organize previous findings into a model in the 1980s. Ciompi[16] explained cognitive deficits in terms of a vicious circle of different components of personal, social and physiological components. The vicious circle is a positive feedback, in which elements in a loop exacerbate one another, resulting in a continuous worsening of deficits. Gjerde[17] elaborated this model and suggested that social perceptions and interactions, commonly found severely impaired in schizophrenia, arise since the cognitive deficits prevent adequate acquisition of interpersonal coping skills. This leads to a heightened arousal, which limits intellectual capacities. Frith[18] emphasized the role of willed intention for motor actions. While the intention to perform an act may not be defective in schizophrenia, decision-making regarding what action would be appropriate seems to be impaired. Decades of research in schizophrenia demonstrate that a generalized neuropsychological deficit is a characteristic feature of schizophrenia. Initial studies of the neuropsychological aspects of schizophrenia focused on whether a profile of deficits could be drawn which would differentiate this illness from organic conditions. However, the current understanding is that schizophrenia is fundamentally a disease of the brain and neuropsychological deficits are but a part of the illness. Deficits have been found associated with symptom type and severity. Assessment of these deficits helps to clear the clinical picture by appropriate treatment strategies and plan rehabilitation programs.

Early studies done in this area focused on diagnostic issues, i.e. whether a neuropsychological profile can differentiate between schizophrenia, neurological and psychiatric conditions.[19,20] While a comprehensive and definite profile of deficits has not been established, several consistent findings have emerged. An extensive body of research brought forth the question of whether schizophrenia is a lateralized disorder, particularly of left temporal and frontal regions, or of interhemispheric communications affecting these regions. Another view is that it is a bilateral frontal disorder. A review of the literature on laterality and schizophrenia shows that when hemispheric functional activation favored the right hemisphere, patients were characterized as chronic, process, nonparanoid and had premorbidly poor functioning.[21,22] When activation favored the left hemisphere, patients were termed acute, reactive and paranoid.[22]

Current findings clearly demonstrate that global deficits are seen consistently on standard neuropsychological batteries, such as the Halstead-Reitan battery. Saykin et al[23] found that patients with schizophrenia performed at least one standard deviation below normal controls on all neuropsychological tests. Researchers are now debating whether this generalized dysfunction is a reflection of major impairment in core aspects of functioning, such as attention, memory and problem solving. Attention deficits have been studied extensively in schizophrenia as a central function in perception, recall of information and planning of motor acts. Impairments in selective and sustained attention have been reported.[24] Recent studies use sensitive tests, such as the continuous performance test and backward masking procedures.[25] Studies show that performance on the tests is influenced by test condition of distraction.

Memory impairments have also been consistently reported. Patients with schizophrenia have difficulty in acquisition of both verbal and visual material. This was considered to suggest a bilateral involvement, though recent Positron emission tomography[26-28] studies have shown that acquisition is essentially a left frontal function. Tests, such as Wechsler's Memory Scale (WMS) and Wechsler's Adult Intelligences Scale (WAIS) have been widely used, and the performances on these tests suggest that a majority of the sample exhibits memory deficits. The influence of attention on the tests of intelligence and memory was studied by Gold et al.[29] They concluded that memory impairments were observed across paradigms differing in the extent of their attention demands, suggesting that both attention and memory deficits were present in schizophrenic patients in a relatively independent manner. They further suggested that memory impairments in schizophrenia involves several aspects and includes deficits in encoding, retrieval and recognition. Another major function found to be uniformly impaired is abstraction. Tests such as Proverb tests, Tactual performance test, Category test and the Wisconsin card sorting tests have been used to demonstrate difficulties in abstract reasoning and problem solving.[29]

The profile of deficits implies that there is dysfunction in several interconnected brain regions. There is strong evidence of frontal lobe impairment and researchers have now found that the deficits in this condition are similar to that in frontal lobe lesions.[30] This explains difficulties in problem solving, set shifting and volitional difficulties. The memory deficits, however, indicate the role of the medial temporal lobe and other subcortical structures.[23] Tamlyn et al,[31] however, suggest that the pattern of memory impairment demonstrated by schizophrenia patients is similar to that seen in classic amnesic syndromes.

The conclusive evidence of several studies is that there is definite impairment of neuropsychological functioning in schizophrenia. These impairments are now seen as a symptom of the illness and understanding these deficits plays a major role in the management of this illness.

Mood Disorders

Neuropsychological deficits have been clearly identified in mood disorders, particularly in depression. Initial studies concentrated on whether a neuropsychological profile could be used to aid diagnosis, i.e. to differentiate mood disorders from other psychotic conditions (such as schizophrenia) and organic conditions (such as dementia). However, no clear neuropsychological diagnostic markers of mood disorders have been established. In addition, it is difficult to identify a single framework or theory of the nature and underlying process of neuropsychological functioning.

Early studies focused on comparing the performance of patients of mood disorders with other psychotic conditions, such as schizophrenia. These researchers found that depressives had more difficulty in tasks involving the non-dominant hemisphere.[19,20] Reitan's modification of Halstead-Neiman Aphasia screening test and WAIS showed that mood disordered patients made most of their errors on items requiring functioning of the nondominant parietal area and to lesser degree, the frontal area.[32] While some researchers found mild dominant hemispheric deficits, most studies clearly indicated that there is predominant right hemisphere dysfunction in affective patients. Their performance on tasks involving the dominant temporal and parietal areas was similar to that of normal subjects.

Although patients with mood disorders show deficits in area such as abstract reasoning, perceptual discrimination and verbal fluency, the most common subjective complaint is of memory deficits. Initial research on memory in mood disorders highlighted deficits in all aspects of memory, such as registration, learning and retention.[33] Later, researchers such as Weingarter et al.[34] reported that depressed patients used weak or incomplete encoding strategies to organize and transform events. Watts et al.[35] found that while depressed patients are able to use imagery as a memory aid, they definitely have difficulty in organizing components of information, and this reflects an impairment of encoding. These deficits were initially thought to be related to attention and motivational deficits often seen in depressive disorders.

However, recent studies have clearly established that the finding of impaired memory functioning in major depression is not simply attributable to reductions in motivation.[36] Current research attempts a detailed fractionalization of different aspects of memory. With respect to short-term memory, Squire and Zouzounis[37] state that the subjective complaint of poor concentration and short-term memory is what distinguishes depressive from amnesics. However, on tests such as Digit Span, depressive do not show any impairment.[38] In contrast to short-term memory, majority of studies shows evidence of impaired recall and recognition for both verbal and visuospatial material.[39] Impairment has also been noted in semantic memory as seen by Calev et al.,[40] who conclude that depressives had a specific deficit in retrieving information meaningfully organized in their semantic memory. However, implicit memory seems to be preserved, as most researchers found that depressive performed poorly only on explicit tasks.[41] Mini-Mental State Examination, Verbal Fluency test, Rivermead Behavioral Memory test, Digit Span test, Digit Symbol Substitution test, Wordstem Completion test, Silly Sentences test and the National Adult Reading test have been used in to assess memory in patients with mood disorders.[42] A recent study by Elliot et al[43] reports impair-ments in tests of recognition memory, working memory and planning in patients with unipolar depression. They hypothesized that these impairments may be a result of perceived failure on one task influencing performance on other tasks suggesting a catastrophic response to failure.

Most research in this area has focused on unipolar depression. Very few studies give us a comprehensive picture of the nature of neuropsychological deficits in bipolar affective disorders. The distinction between unipolar and bipolar categories is likely to be of importance, as the two conditions may produce different kind of deficits. However, assessment of patients with mania is difficult with standard neuropsychological procedures; though these patients show deficits, which sometimes persist in the euthymic state. Among patients with mania, learning is often accompanied by intrusions from idiosyncratic word associations. Several studies have shown that the degree of neuropsychological deficits is proportional to the severity of manic symptoms.[44] It is reversible when the patient improves and may normalize in remission, although the deficits in older bipolar patients can persist beyond the disappearance of affective signs.

Studies have also attempted to compare neuropsychological profiles between unipolar and bipolar depression to see whether deficits are different in mania and depression, and between depression of the unipolar and bipolar type. However, manic patients have proved to be difficult to access with standard psychological procedures. One study[45] reports the presence of learning impairments accompanied by intrusions from idiosyncratic word associations formed by the patients. These were also found to be at a much higher degree than observed in other studies of psychotic depression and schizophrenia. Comparisons between cognitive performance in the unipolar and bipolar depressed states are often confounded by the severity of depression and related factors that are difficult to control.

Researchers have consistently found affective disorder patients to have performance deficits on neuropsychological measures. Most of the studies have been carried out in depressive patients. Depending on the measures used, 'affectives' have typically performed better than schizophrenics. Most deficits for affectives appear on tasks that reportedly measure primarily right or non-dominant hemisphere functioning. Specific neuropsychological tests have focused mainly on memory, and depressives have been found to have deficits in the stages of encoding, effortful cognitive processing and executive functions.

Obsessive-compulsive Disorders

Although the precise etiology of obsessive-compulsive disorders (OCD) is still unknown, data gathered in recent years has led to a gradual shift from psychological to biological explanations for the disorder. Altered neurological functioning is now recognized as an important etiological factor in OCD. Some of the factors, pointing to an organic etiology in OCDs are the high concordance rates of this disorder in monozygotic twins, positive response to neurosurgery, and its association with neurological disorders, like temporal lobe epilepsy and postencephaliticparkinsonism.

The primary task of any theory of OCD is to explain why innocuous stimuli, like dirty hands, can evoke the extreme concern that these patients display, and why repeated performance of compulsive acts fail to relieve this concern. In trying to explain these facts, research has consistently tried to examine structures most involved in emotional regulation and response feedback, i.e. the frontal lobes, basal ganglia, and the interconnections of these structures with the limbic system. Investigation of lobe dysfunction in OCD is intuitively appealing for a variety of reasons. The frontal lobes play an important role in programming, regulating, and verifying ongoing motor activity, modulating goal-directed behavior, and have intimate connections with the sensory, motor, and limbic systems. Behavioral disruptions associated with frontal lobe dysfunction include failure to adapt to changing environmental conditions, which can lead to stereotyped, perseverative and nonadaptive behaviors, very similar to the stereotyped and repetitive thoughts and actions seen in OCD. Similarly, the basal ganglia, which has rich interconnections with the entire cortex and limbic structures, is involved in regulating motor movement and sensory information. It has suggested that basal ganglia structures function as a gating station for information, and are important in filtering irrelevant from relevant stimuli. Disruption of the basal ganglia system is thus hypothesized to leave the individual unable to disregard irrelevant stimuli, resulting in inappropriate response patterns such as compulsive orderliness, checking and washing.

A variety of neuroimaging studies have also documented frontal lobe or basal ganglia dysfunction among at least a subset of OCD patients.[46] Apart from abnormal frontal or basal ganglia functioning, attention has also been placed on overactive neural labelling of stimuli as dangerous, causing the individual to be overaroused. Some neuroanatomic theories[47] have hypothesized that there may be a functional disconnection between sensory systems and response output systems. Thus, feedback about the adequacy of a completed act cannot reach the motor or emotional systems, leading to high arousal and persistent/compulsive behavior.

The neuropsychological perspective has great value in aiding an understanding of this disorder. It's value lies in its ability to identify brain regions most involved in the disorder, regardless of whether this involvement is primary or secondary to the disorder. Identification of normal and abnormal processes involved in the disorder can help identify risk factors for OCD and delineate clinical areas for consideration. Further, neuropsychological assessment can help in: (a) providing data to further support the neuroanatomic hypothesis of frontal/basal ganglia involvement; (b) identification of cognitive strengths, weaknesses, and alterations in information processing associated with the disorder. Regardless of whether they are primary or secondary to the disorder, identification of these deficits and strengths may suggest additional areas for clinical intervention, as they may serve to maintain obsessive-compulsive patterns.

Some limitations of neuropsychological data, however, need to be kept in mind:

- Neuropsychological tests do not differentiate between frontal lobe and basal ganglia dysfunction.
- If the structural dysfunction is not marked enough to disrupt cognitive tasks, neuropsychological tests of frontal functions may not show deficits or dysfunction.
- Cognitive deficits may be secondary to the disorder, rather than representing a cause or maintaining influence, which must be kept in mind while interpreting data.

A review of the neuropsychological studies of OCD shows two groups of findings. One group of studies have tended to support hypotheses of frontal lobe or caudate dysfunction, whereas other studies have failed to find deficits on frontal functions, but have instead documented visuospatial and memory deficits as prominent.

Findings of Frontal Dysfunction

Flor-Henry et al.[48] found that OCD patients showed lower performance on attentional, language, nonverbal auditory perception, psychomotor performance, spatial learning, and abstraction tasks as compared to a group of normal controls. They interpreted these results as indicative of frontal, particularly left frontal lobe, dysfunction and hypothesized that obsessions were a result of inhibition of verbal motor programs. Insel, et al.[49] were, however, unable to replicate these results. Their results agreed with those of Flor-Henry et al., only for the tactile performance test (TPT). While poor performance on the TPT can indicate difficulties in spatial organization or memory, the lack of specificity of this test makes it difficult to interpret in terms of brain function. Khanna et al.[50] reported in a single case study, that they found evidence of frontal lobe dysfunction in a patient who developed OCD 3 years following head injury. Direct evidence of apparent frontal dysfunction was obtained by Behar et al.,[51] who evaluated 17 adolescents and matched controls. Differences obtained in tests sensitive to frontal dysfunction were significant. They also found deficits in the ability to organize an approach and process an adequate amount of information at one time, which is a function of the frontal lobes.

More recently, Malloy[52] obtained measures of general intelligence, memory attention and frontal lobe function, and found abnormal scores only on the Wisconsin Card Sorting Test (WCST). This, however, was seen only in subset of OCD patients, judged as 'increasingly psychotic, lower functioning, having poorer prognosis and lower intelligence'. Of particular note, was the absence of deficits obtained on other neuropsychological tests sensitive to frontal lobe dysfunction, viz. the Luria Nebraska test and Verbal Fluency test. Head et al,[53] in testing the ability to shift set in OCD patients, replicated the above findings. All the above studies were in agreement in finding no significant deficits on memory tasks.

Findings of Memory and Visuospatial Deficits

Zielinski et al.[54] and Boone et al.[55] examined OCD patients and matched controls on tests sensitive to frontal lobe, as well as verbal and nonverbal memory deficits. Both studies found decreased performance on tests of visuospatial memory, but adequate performance of tests of frontal lobe abilities (including the WCST), and attention and verbal memory. Otto et al.[56,57] replicated these results. Boone et al. found pronounced visuospatial deficits for patients with OCD, who had a family history of the disorder. Similar deficits are also found among patients with Tourette's syndrome. The above studies have consistently shown that OCD patients have normal frontal, attentional and intellectual abilities, but impaired visuospatial abilities. Recent research has tried to examine the reasons for these two different sets of findings. It now appears that comorbid depression may be an important factor accounting for this difference. Review of data suggests that studies with patients having comorbid depression, or a more severe form of the illness, documented prominent frontal lobe deficits. Visuospatial/memory deficits appear more prominent in samples with no comorbid depression and purer samples of OCD.

To summarize findings from the neuropsychological tests in OCD, no clear consensus is yet available. However, current literature stresses the need for subtyping OCD, at least by the presence of depression or schizotypal features. These findings also direct increasing interest on tasks involving cognitive shifts and visuospatial memory. The limited findings of performance deficits on tasks involving trial and error learning and shifting task set are consistent with neuroanatomic theories emphasising frontal lobe and basal ganglia dysfunction. Particularly, these findings are consistent with theories emphasising that OCD involves a disruption in response feedback. The urge to repeat compulsive acts could thus be a result of difficulty in attending to feedback about and confirming the adequacy of behaviors already performed. For example, compulsive checking may result from a loss of task set, leading to chronic doubt and repetitive need to check and confirm the absence of potential danger.

Memory deficits represent another cognitive dysfunction that may inhibit the ability to confirm the accuracy of an obsessive concern or the adequacy of a compulsive act. Memory reconstructions of past events/acts often help to decrease anxiety associated with obsessions of harm or negligence. Likewise, the confirmation of a compulsive act (e.g. 'did I turn off the stove?') relies on memory. Disruptions on the clarity of memory for these acts may feel a need to repeat a compulsive act. Visual memory is used more frequently in the review of personal acts. It is significant that OCD patients have consistently shown visuospatial memory deficits. Some studies indicating poor or immature approach to complex copying tasks suggest that a poor perceptual strategy may contribute to memory difficulties.

Theories focusing on the role of neuropsychological dysfunction in the cause and maintenance of OCD are especially compelling in cases of OCD symptoms emerging following head injury or specific brain pathophysiology. Whereas neurological abnormalities may contribute to the emergence of OCD in select cases, it is nonetheless crucial to ask whether the abnormalities are necessary for the development of the disorder. Controlled neuropsychological research focusing on frontal and memory disturbances, with stringent methodology and design, is necessary to clarify many of these issues.

Alcohol Dependance

Recent studies on alcohol dependance have found significant cognitive impairment, ranging from poor performance on neuropsychological tests to cortical atrophy and dementia. Several variables have been studied as predictors of impairment. These include family history of alcohol dependence, number of years of drinking, age of the subject, amount of alcohol consumed and presence of classic symptoms of alcohol dependence. Various hypotheses have been proposed to account for the deficits.

The 'premature aging' hypothesis[58] states that the type of damage inflicted on the brain by alcohol is essentially that of accelerated senescence. Studies reveal[59,60] that the pattern of deficits displayed by normal elderly bears a striking resemblance to the 'selective' deficits of alcohol dependent individuals. On the other hand, the 'global impairment' theory[61] observes that prolonged exposure to alcohol induces uniform impairment of cognitive functions. However, current studies[62,63] indicate that alcohol does produce selective damage to specific functional areas of the brain.

Several researchers emphasise that alcohol dependant individuals show a selective impairment of right hemispheric functions and that alcohol somehow selectively damages the right, more than the left, cerebral hemisphere. This is supported by the performance of these subjects on verbal and nonverbal (performance) tests. More specifically, the 'frontal deficit' hypothesis posits the primary locus of damage in alcoholics to the frontal lobes, with impairment in other functional areas being attributable to insufficient or abnormal integration from the frontal cortex. Numerous investigators have consistently found alcohol dependant individuals to be impaired on tests of functions considered localized in the frontal lobes. A study by Corville[64] also suggests that there may be an etiologic deficit, which may actually precede the development of alcoholism and may contribute to precipitating the disorder. Frontal lobe dysfunction in volitional control and problem solving skills may predispose an individual to alcohol abuse. Retrospective and high-risk studies have supported this theory. Another hypothesis suggests a deficit in sensitivity to internal cues, such as internal scanning, may act as a precursor to chronic alcoholics.

Researchers have also examined the possibility of left hemisphere deficits in alcoholics.[65] This hypothesis suggests that there is primary disruption of cerebral functioning at subcortical levels in alcoholics. Short-term, as well as chronic changes, in subcortical structures and in pathways of neural transmission projecting to the cortex may account for some of the dysfunctions observed in higher associative and integrative processes. Research done in this area suggests a clear but diffuse pattern of deficits in alcoholics, based on controlled and longitudinal studies. Consistent impairments have been found in a variety of cognitive processes. These include spatial and visuoperceptual analysis, location learning, memory and problem solving abilities. Verbal abilities have been relatively spared within the alcoholic syndrome. Intelligence quotient is usually found to be within normal limits, especially when the tests are loaded highly on verbal items.

General intellectual function in alcoholics has also been explored. The WAIS has been extensively used to study cognitive functions in this group and studies show that subjects performed poorly on block design. Deficient performance was also seen in digit symbol, visuoperceptive analysis and location learning. Though verbal IQ was distinctively better than performance IQ, arithmetic may be severely impaired. In addition, adaptive behaviors, such as problem solving and abstraction, are most likely to be affected by chronic alcoholism. Several studies[66-68] document the poor performance of alcoholics on Trail Making Test, Halstead Category test, and the Wisconsin Card Sorting test. Ron[65] states that "the ability to solve problems, to perform complex psychomotor tasks and to manipulate abstract concepts appears to be particularly affected".

The effects of chronic alcohol abuse falls into two major categories: the Korsakoff amnesic syndrome and other non-amnesic psychological deficits.

Wernicke-Korsakoff Syndrome

The salient features of this condition, as described by Wernicke in 1881, were ataxia, ocular symptoms, and mental confusion. The main features are: (a) profound difficulty or total inability in acquiring new verbal and nonverbal information, (b) retrograde amnesia, (c) preservation of immediate memory, learned behavior such as speech, language, gestures, and activities of daily living, (d) presence of confabulation (a falsification of memory occurring in clear consciousness in association with an organically derived dementia), and (e) lack of initiative and spontaneity, and blunting of affect.

The neuropsychological deficits associated with this condition, include poor performance in tests that involve new learning such as verbal passages, visual reproduction and paired associate learning. Other features include poor orientation and mental control. Apart from the Wernicke-Korsakoff syndrome, chronic alcohol abuse leads to widespread cerebral changes. Some of the neuropsychological deficits in chronic alcohol abuse are discussed below. One test, extensively used with chronic alcoholics, is the WAIS. Golden et al.[69] have reviewed studies done with WAIS and summarized the findings. Overall, alcoholics produced near normal scores on verbal tests, except in the arithmetic subtest. However, on the performance subtest, most researchers have found that alcoholics performed more poorly on block design, digit symbol and object assembly, indicating deficient paired associate learning, visuoperceptive analysis and location learning. On the Halstead-Reitan battery, alcoholics show deficits in the category test, tactual performance test, finger oscillation test and the trail making test. Alcoholics also seem to have limited ability to process spatial and temporal information. Tests that measure adaptive behavior (such as problem solving, abstraction and other 'higher order' processes) show consistent deficits in chronic patients. Several researchers report poor performance on abstraction tests. Memory and learning have also been found to be impaired, as seen on tests such as Benton Visual Retention Test (BVRT) and the Wechsler Memory Scale (WMS).

Overall, neuropsychological profiles of chronic alcohol intaker show a clear and rather diffuse pattern of deficits. Impairment is evident in functions such as memory, spatial and visuoperceptual analysis, location learning and problem solving abilities. Verbal abilities seem to be relatively preserved. These findings have also been validated by physiologic data, such as electroencephalograph and evoked potential studies.

NEUROPSYCHOLOGY OF AGING AND DEMENTIA

Researchers have held widely differing views on the relationship between normal aging and dementia. One view holds that following a peak period during early adulthood, intellectual abilities enter into a steady decline; thus, cognitive decline is seen as an intrinsic part of normal aging.[70] A contrary view, which is gaining increasing support, is that there is no decline in intellectual function with advancing age, except in elderly individuals who acquire diseases of the central nervous system.[71] Current knowledge regarding the effects of age on the structure and function of the human brain has been steadily increasing. It is now accepted that while aging is accompanied by decline in psychomotor skills and motor output, intellectual decline is not a necessary component of normal aging. There is no decline in verbal abilities and abstract thinking, and an individual can maintain a high level of participation in decision-making. True intellectual decline starts when degenerative processes begin in the brain. These degenerative processes of the brain, which affect a large proportion of affected individuals (although they can occur at any age), are known as dementia.

Syndromes of Dementia

The dementia is a pathological process (not part of the normal aging process) in the brain that results in the progressive loss of cognitive functions, including memory, learning, attention and judgment. This includes decline in planning and decision-making abilities, and affective changes, such as emotional withdrawal and lack of interest. Volitional inadequacies often result in loss of initiative and goal-directed behavior. Most prominent is the progressive deterioration of memory, especially recent memory. In time, the dementing process erodes all aspects of thought, felling, and behavior, eventually resulting in death. An estimated 5% of the population, over the age of 65 years in the United States, is thought to be severely demented, while another 10% is thought to be mildly to moderately demented.[72] Dementia can result from a variety of causes, such as neuronal changes in the brain, vascular insufficiency, multiple infarcts, and metabolic and hormonal imbalances. Although some forms of dementia are treatable, most are not.

Neuropsychology of dementia essentially refers to a study of the various components that constitute dementia and their evaluation. The objectives of neuropsychological evaluation are: (1) to determine whether the patient has dementia, (2) to assess the magnitude of the illness, and (3) to assess the assets and liabilities of the affected person for purposes of rehabilitation. Prior to neuropsychological testing, it is necessary to conduct a thorough evaluation of the patient's condition and the course of the illness. This includes:

- An interview with a collateral or significant other, to elicit information about premorbid functioning and onset, course and nature of cognitive loss and behavioral changes in the patient.
- Recording of history/clinical course of the dementing illness (including impairments in memory, orientation, judgement, planning, personality, affect, language, behavior patterns, and other symptomatology).
- Mental status examination of the patient.

Neuropsychological procedures are an important part of the evaluation of a patient with dementia, primarily to provide objective verification of impaired cognition and support the clinical diagnosis of dementia. In addition, these procedures are useful as outcome measures of pharmacological and surgical interventions, and for deciding rehabilitation strategies and priorities. A neuropsychological evaluation gives information about the presence and severity of cognitive deficits, and helps decide whether the presenting complaints are due to cognitive dysfunction or to a nonorganic condition. In an organic condition, test performance will provide evidence consistent with the presenting complaints. It is often difficult to distinguish depression from dementia, and neuropsychological testing can be helpful in this discrimination. In a pseudodementing condition, real and consistent deficits would not be seen on neuropsychological test performance. Depression is usually characterized by variable performance, and the patient will make fewer errors given the benefits of time. Sad mood and anhedonia are often indicators that distinguish depression from the mild apathy and withdrawal seen in dementia.

Frontal neuropsychological evaluation in this condition must cover the following areas:

- *Attentional processes:* These can be evaluated by observation as well as formal testing. Arousal and distractibility are assessed by behavioral observation. Tests such as Digit span, Visual scanning and Serial subtraction are also useful for assessing attention.
- *Comprehension and language functions:* These are assessed by asking questions, which the patient must understand and respond appropriately. Speech output and evidence of difficulties with expressive speech must be examined.
- *Psychomotor functions:* These are assessed using tests of opticspatial coordination, tests of motor alternation and kinetic melody.
- *Learning and memory functions:* These include evaluation of episodic and semantic memory, memory in day-to-day life, sensory memory, working memory, immediate recall, delayed recall, verbal and visual memory.
- *Visuospatial and integrative functions:* Both perceptual and executive functions may be impaired, and this area therefore requires careful assessment.
- Presence of focal deficits in various sensorimotor functions.

Dementia in Alzheimer's Disease

This is one of the most common forms of dementia. Neuropsychological studies of patients diagnosed with AD have generally shown a distinct pattern of cognitive dysfunction. Three types of neuropsychological dysfunction are commonly seen in these patients: (i) memory impairments, (ii) language and naming deficits, and (iii) visuospatial dysfunction. Impaired memory is usually the first noticeable symptom, followed by increasing problems with language. Symptoms of aphasia become more pronounced, following which memory problems increase severely and remote memory is also disturbed. The final stage is characterized by severe and global cognitive impairments in all intellectual abilities.

Neuropsychological investigations in AD have focused on the nature and course of memory, language, and visuospatial deficits. Memory dysfunction is a hallmark of AD, and detailed assessment of verbal/visual memory, immediate recall, and delayed recall are important for diagnostic evaluation. Progressive language impairments and executive motor problems are other cognitive dysfunctions that increase as the illness progresses. General strategy of assessment in dementia usually involves an assessment of general intellectual functions (e.g. using WAIS, Progressive Matrices, and other tests of intelligence), attention, memory, language and fluency, problem solving and executive functions, and praxis and constructional ability. In addition, affective and personality changes, such as lack of initiative, apathy, lack of concern, impulsivity or aggressiveness, are also often associated with this condition and must be carefully evaluated.

Subcortical Dementia

Dementia of subcortical origin is differentiated from dementia due to lesions involving the cerebral cortex. In subcortical dementia, the primary structures involved are thalamus, basal ganglia and brainstem structures. Cortical dementia produces prominent impairment of higher mental functions such as memory, language, visuospatial skills and praxis. In contrast, subcortical dementia present with prominent impairment in the areas of mood, drive, attention and arousal; evidenced by affective disorders, apathy, mental inertia, forgetfulness, and poor problem solving strategies. Subcortical dementia also present with prominent neuropsychiatric conditions, which may precede or occur concomitantly with the intellectual decline.

Rehabilitation of Patients with Dementia

Rehabilitation in dementia is now an important aspect of health care policy in developed countries, and a variety of psychosocial agencies have been set-up to provide structured services to persons afflicted with this condition. In India, however, the onus of responsibility of care usually lies on the family of the affected person. This makes effective rehabilitation complex, and family counseling is a vital function of the treating agency. In dealing with the family, it is important for the counselor to remember that family members are not trained caregivers, and that they also need help in dealing with their own emotional distress about the condition of the patient. An effective rehabilitation program must take into account the following factors:

- *Psychoeducation about the disease:* It is necessary to explain the nature of the disease and the kind of symptoms and changes it has brought on. It is also essential, however difficult it may be, to explain that the disease is progressive and the patient will not recover. It is necessary to consider the effect the patient's illness may be having on the spouse. Intensive counselling may be necessary to help the spouse understand the nature of the illness and to learn to live with it.
- *Providing a conducive environment:* A normal home environment may not be an ideal one for a dementing patient, as the input of a multitude of environmental stimuli may be too much for the patient to handle. However, the family must be advised to continue their normal lifestyle and activities, as far as possible. Some degree of isolation of the patient with the household may be the best solution. The family should try to limit/reduce the quantity of information and stimuli the patient has to handle or process.
- *Orientation of the patient:* Family members can help patient cope with early stages of forgetfulness, by readily providing cues and information. Other interventions may be required as patient becomes disoriented to time, place, and person. Reality Orientation Therapy[73] is a structured technique that helps facilitate orientation. The essence of the technique is to reinforce a less complex real world to the patient, to which he can orient more adequately. Many subsequent studies have found the technique effective (see Miller[74] for review).
- *Communicating with the patient:* It is essential to use simple forms and levels of communication with the patient. Only one piece of information should be given to the person at a time, rather than several pieces of information, which he may not be able to process. Encouraging the patient to make visual associations with verbal material may also be helpful.
- *Dealing with emotional responses of the patient:* Often, patients may display anxiety and depression in the early stages, or lack of emotional responsivity as the disease progresses. Family members should deal with the patient firmly but gently, with a view to help him calm down. Shouting at the patient or trying to convince him of his mistake will only be disturbing and depressing to him, and will be counterproductive. A mature and supportive approach would be most useful in helping him deal with his conflicts.

CHILD NEUROPSYCHOLOGY

Recent years have witnessed the emergence of child neuropsychology, as a distinct subspeciality within clinical neuropsychology. Clinical observations and research reports strongly suggest that brain impairment is at least a contributing factor in many of the functional and behavioral disorders seen in children and adolescents with psychopathology. There is strong evidence that brain dysfunction in childhood is associated with increased risk for psychiatric disorder in children with documented brain damage[75] and in children with soft neurological signs. Conversely, there is a relatively high rate of neurological dysfunction among children with psychiatric disorders, even when cases of known brain damage are excluded.[76] This may often remain undetected in routine neurological examination.[77] Accurate detection in this population often requires the use of more comprehensive procedures than are commonly employed.

Various factors are responsible for this increased interest and activity in child neuropsychology. A significant percentage of children suffer from learning disabilities and other developmental handicaps of neurodevelopmental origin. This has accentuated an important role for neuropsychological assessment, which can help both in the identification of problems and in devising appropriate educational plans. In addition, advances in medical care have brought about a dramatic increase in the number of children who survive conditions that can have a potentially adverse impact on the developing brain. This has created a greater need for the careful assessment of the extent, pattern, and developmental significance of possible neuropsychological sequele in these survivors of serious childhood illness.[78]

There is now a growing realization of the important differences in brain-behavior relationships between children and adults. Children differ from adults in types of brain insult commonly experienced, the behavioral effects manifested, pattern of recovery of functions after injury, and the modifying effects of ongoing developmental change. An appropriate assessment of brain-behavior relationship in children, therefore, cannot be based simply on scaled-down versions of assessment methods used with adults. Various neuropsychological batteries have been developed specifically for use with children. Reitan and his colleagues developed two versions of the Halstead-Reitan Neuropsychological Battery for children: the Reitan-Indiana Neuropsychological Test Battery for Children (ages 5–8 years) and the Halstead Neuropsychological Test Battery for Children (ages 9–14 years). Both versions have been found to discriminate effectively between normal children and those with brain damage. The Luria-Nebraska Neuropsychological Battery-Children's Revision is another battery developed for use with children. This was developed by Golden[13] for children ranging from 8 to 12 years of age.

A number of recent studies have begun to examine whether there are any distinguishing neuropsychological features associated with specific forms of child psychopathology, such as autism, attention deficit disorder, and learning disability.

Learning Disabilities

The study of learning disabilities has been one of the most extensive areas of investigation in child neuropsychology. Central nervous system dysfunction is now believed to have primary etiological significance in this disorder. Neuropsychological assessment can be of great value, both in identification of specific dysfunction in particular learning dimensions and in the formulation and evaluation of specific educational plans.

Neuropsychological theories of learning disabilities have used a cybernetic model of learning, based on the steps that occur during learning; the 'input-integration-memory-output' model.[79] Learning disability can occur due to impaired ability to carry out any of these steps. Input disabilities refer to perceptual disabilities, e.g. visual or auditory perceptual disabilities, which can impair learning. Integration disabilities refer to impairments in the ability to understand what is perceived; inability to sequence and contextualize from concepts, and organize information. Memory disabilities are often observed in children with learning disabilities, who show marked deficits in short-term memory. Output disabilities refer to difficulty in retrieving information from the brain. In addition, persons with learning disability often have trouble coordinating gross and fine motor movements. Each individual will have his own individual profile of disabilities, with there being no stereotyped profile. Assessment of the disability profile can have great value in understanding the etiology of the condition, as well as in devising appropriate remediational and educational programs for each patient.

Autism

This is currently an area of great interest and activity, and cognitive factors are currently believed to play a vital role in the etiology of this condition. Three major theories of autism proposed in the recent years are: (i) theory of mind deficits,[80] (ii) executive function deficits,[81] and (iii) theory of weak central coherence.[82] The theory of mind deficits proposes that autistic individuals lack the ability to 'mentalize', i.e. to attribute independent mental states to self and others in order to predict and explain action. This theory of impaired understanding of mental states is now well replicated, though the findings have not been universal. A number of questions remain unanswered, e.g. some researchers point out that language/memory dysfunction, lack of motivation, or artefacts of task structure could influence the results of these studies. Recent studies speak of autism as being associated with executive function deficits, i.e. difficulties in high-level planning and control of behavior. Executive function refers to the ability to maintain an appropriate problem-solving set for attainment of some future goal, including planning, impulse control, maintaining set, organized search, and flexibility of thought and action. The third cognitive model of autism suggests that autistic children have an unusually weak drive for central coherence. Frith and Happe[82] propose that autists lack the ability to interpret stimuli in a global way, or construct meaning from complex and diverse information. Thus, they tend to process information piecemeal, rather than in context. This theory also explains splinter/savant skills seen in some individuals with autism. This is a promising field of investigation, and further examination of these theories is essential to gain a clearer understanding of the neuropsychology of autism.

Attention-deficit Hyperactivity Disorder

Neuropsychological investigations have found several types of deficits in children with this disorder. These include:

- *Attention deficits:* Children with attention-deficit hyperactivity disorder (ADHD) have been found to perform poorly on tasks involving sustained attention or vigilance. These tasks involve three aspects: maintenance of attention over time; extent to which attention is self-directed and organized; and the amount of effort that is invested. Selective attention, which refers to the ability to focus on critical target stimuli while ignoring irrelevant stimuli, has also been found impaired. These children are highly distractible, and are usually unable to ignore irrelevant stimuli.

- *Inhibitory control deficits, leading to impulsivity and disinhibition:* This refers to behavior that arises from lessened control on response inhibition. Deficits in inhibitory control have been shown in children with ADHD.
- *Arousal differences:* Evidence from studies examining the impact of stimuli on autonomous and central functioning point consistently to an 'under-reactivity' to environmental stimulation. Thus, there is considerable evidence to state that defective attention, inhibition, and arousal and reinforcement processes have both immediate and long-term impact on the behavior and cognitive functioning of hyperactive children.

Neuropsychologists are now attempting to examine the presence and nature of cognitive deficits in the entire spectrum of child psychiatric conditions. This research has so far yielded promising results, and has been valuable both in increasing understanding of childhood disorders, as well in rehabilitation and management. Neuropsychological rehabilitation has been found to be effective in a number of the above conditions, such as ADHD, and cognitive retraining is been recognized as an important adjunct to other forms of treatment (pharmacological and psychological) in child mental health.

Problems and Issues in Child Neuropsychology

As already mentioned, there are a number of important differences in brain-behavior relationships between children and adults, and there are a number of complications which arise in the neuropsychological assessment of children.[83-87] Some of the important factors that often obscure the assessment of brain-behavior relationships in children include:

- *Nonspecific effects of brain damage*: Effects of brain damage become more specific as functional organization of the cerebral hemispheres becomes more established (around 5–7 years of age). Thus, effects of brain damage tend to be less specific in children, and decrements in general intelligence are usually the chief manifestation of early childhood brain injury.[83] There is therefore, considerable overlap or redundancy between standard measures of intelligence and test batteries used for assessing neuropsychological functioning in children.
- *Developmental changes:* It is essential to use a developmental approach in child assessment. Tests and measures, that are appropriate for the age range of the children being assessed and which are sensitive to the child's increasing competence over time, should be used.
- Absence of a baseline of premorbid functioning in cases of early brain damage.
- Blurred distinction between neurodevelopmental anomalies and normal variation in rate and pattern of acquisition of function.[88]
- Absence of a standard nosology for classifying childhood neurodevelopmental disorders.
- Extent to which deficits can sometimes be 'silent' until later developmental periods.
- Difficulty in specifying a precise time of onset for various forms of brain pathology.

In addition, there are a number of practical difficulties in assessing a brain-impaired child, such as: (i) problems in maintaining behavioral compliance and attention for long periods, (ii) inability of younger children to provide a reliable subjective report of deficits, which makes it necessary to rely on parents and teacher's reports, and (iii) problems in assessing children with special handicapping conditions, such as sensory loss, motor impairments, and physical disabilities.[89]

Rehabilitation

Although child neuropsychologists are relative newcomers to the field of pediatric rehabilitation, they are now entering the area in increasing numbers. They possess a unique combination of skills and knowledge in various areas, including neurocognitive functions, child development and psychopathology, and behavioral treatment and psychotherapy. Thus, their roles include not only assessment and treatment consultation, but also the actual delivery of treatment services. It is now being increasingly recognized that neuropsychological assessment is invaluable for formulating treatment plans, monitoring treatment progress, and adjusting the child's rehabilitation programs as needed.[90,91] Greater systematic research into the link between neuropsychological assessment and treatment is a vital need in child neuropsychology today.

45.2 THEORIES OF LEARNING

PSDV Prasadarao, V Kumaraiah

The behaviors of an organism can be classified as either inherited or acquired. Those behaviors which an organism is not endowed with by its biological heritage are said to be acquired or learned. Learning is the process of being modified, more or less permanently, by what happens in the environment around the organism, by what we do, or by what we observe. What we learn is to make relatively simple responses to the immediate aspects of our environment. This also involves the modification of inborn responses and is often referred to as conditioned response learning. Almost all activities of life are influenced by learning and it is basic to many functions of life. It plays an important role even in such complex aspects of human behavior as personality, social relations, and acquisition of various mental disorders. All organisms have the capacity to profit from the experience, hence they acquire the behaviors needed for effective functioning in the environment; such ability is generally termed as *learning* which is a central process in all behaviors of every organism.

The topic of learning has long been one of major interests to psychologists and various definitions of learning have been suggested. One most accepted definition is: "learning is any relatively permanent change in behavior (or behavior potential) produced by experience".[92] This definition restricts use of the term learning only to relatively lasting changes in behavior. Temporary alterations such as those due to drugs or illness are not included. Moreover, it refers to changes in *behavior potential*as well as to changes in overt behavior as changes in the potential for new behaviors can occur even in the absence of such behaviors. Since the potential for such behavior would now exist, whereas it did not exist before, learning may be said to have occurred. Learning is used only for changes in behavior stemming from experience. Changes deriving from such factors as fatigue, physical growth or recovery from physical injury are not viewed as instances of learning. This definition, however, does not mention of 'improvements' in behavior as learning can yield undesirable as well as desirable outcomes.[93]

Heredity sets the limits of our capacity to learn. A supportive environment allows an individual to mature and be ready to learn and the experience provides the exposure and stimulation, while training and practice determine what is learned. A wide range of behaviors such as skills, knowledge, attitudes, opinions, ideals and values are learned.[93]

What we learn is acquired mostly through conditioning, which is said to be dependent on the association between various stimuli and responses. While learning affects behavior, it is generally viewed as taking three major forms, namely, classical conditioning, operant conditioning and social learning. Classical conditioning occurs under conditions in which one stimulus is followed by another stimulus. As a result of such pairing, the first stimulus often gains the ability to evoke reactions which, initially, could be produced only by the second. Operant conditioning is based upon the fact that our actions often produce positive or negative effects. Thus, we tend to behave in ways which yield outcomes we find pleasant or which help us to avoid or escape from outcomes we find unpleasant. According to the social learning perspective, the individual acquires new behaviors through exposure to the actions of others and by modeling them. Most of our behaviors are, presumably, learned through classical conditioning. Many of the abnormal behaviors such as phobias are acquired through conditioning.[94]

CLASSICAL CONDITIONING

Pavlov, while conducting experiments on digestive processes, serendipitously noted that the dogs salivate when they caught sight of the pan in which their food was served or when they saw the person who served the food. This phenomenon was termed as *psychic secretion*. Following this observation, he inferred that through repeated pairing with food, these stimuli had become conditioned signals for the delivery of food due to their repeated pairing with food; these dogs learned that when these specific stimuli were present, food would soon follow and hence they would respond to these stimuli similar to how they spontaneously respond to food. Subsequently, Pavlov started working on the conditioning process. While studying the process of *classical conditioning*, thus termed later, Pavlov inserted a rubber tube into the salivary glands of dogs through a surgical procedure. These dogs were placed in an apparatus which could restrain the movements of the dogs and which would help record the amount of saliva secreted during the process of conditioning. Initially, a neutral stimulus (e.g. a bell) which had previously been shown to have no noticeable effect upon the dog's rate of salivation was presented for a brief period of time. A second stimulus, known to exert a strong effect upon salivation (e.g. meat powder) was then quickly delivered. The bell (the neutral stimulus) was termed the conditioned stimulus (CS) as at first it did not cause the dogs to salivate. The meat powder was termed the unconditioned stimulus (UCS) as it produced salivation the first time it was presented, without any prior conditioning. Each pairing of these two stimuli served into as a conditioned trial, and such trials were presented repeatedly. Since the response (salivation) to the bell occurred only after repeated pairing (i.e. conditioning) it was termed conditioned response (CR). Since response to the meat powder occurred without any conditioning in a spontaneous fashion, it was named unconditioned response (UCR). In this experiment, conditioning is said to have occurred if the CS (bell) presentation, following pairings of the CS-UCS, results in the elicitation of a conditioned response (salivation), which usually resembles the UCR. Pavlov's[95] work with the conditioning of salivation of dogs paved the way to later understanding, development and explanations of the classical conditioning paradigm.[96]

Basic Principles of Classical Conditioning

Acquisition

The number of times the conditioned and unconditioned stimuli are paired and presented, influences the degree of conditioning. The more the number of such pairings, the greater is the ability of the CS to evoke a CR. The strength of conditioning first increases rapidly and then levels off as the number of CS-UCS pairings increase. The strength of conditioning is measured by the magnitude, latency and probability of occurrence of the conditioned response. Moreover, the time interval between the presentation of the CS and UCS plays an important role. For example, when the interval between these stimuli was about 0.5 seconds, the conditioning is said to be stronger. However, such interval varies depending on the nature of the conditioned response in question. For motor responses, such as eye blinks or the withdrawal of limbs, the ideal time interval is found to be 0.5 seconds. For autonomic nervous system (e.g. salivation and changes in heart rate) responses, longer intervals would also lead to conditioning.[97,98]

Stimulus Generalization

Once conditioning has taken place for a given conditioned stimulus, the organism tends to respond in the similar fashion to other stimuli resembling the already conditioned CS. Such process is known as stimulus generalization. By this process of conditioning, our past experience and learning would generalize to new stimuli and events. The process of generalization, thus, serves a useful function in our everyday life.[93]

Discrimination

When one of two similar stimuli is followed by a UCS while the other is not, the tendency to respond to the first stimulus is strengthened, while tendency to respond to the second is weakened. This is known as discrimination. Discrimination involves two processes: initially the individual learns to pay attention to the appropriate stimulus dimensions and later the conditioned responses are attached to the CS.[93]

Extinction and Spontaneous Recovery

When a CS is presented repeatedly without it being followed by a UCS, the ability of the CS to elicit CRs decreases. If the CS is presented again at a later time, its ability to evoke CRs reappears. This phenomenon is called as spontaneous recovery.[93]

Cognitive Processes in Classical Conditioning

Initially, the classical conditioning has been understood to have occurred entirely due to the principle of contiguity, as the learning occurs at the central nervous system level due to the pairing of two stimuli.

However subsequently, a cognitive interpretation of classical conditioning has gained support with less emphasis on the contiguity model. According to the cognitive perspective, what is learned in classical conditioning is an expectancy that the UCS will follow the CS. When a CS is repeatedly paired with the UCS, the CS becomes a 'signal' to the subject that the UCS is coming, and the subject responds accordingly. Research has shown the importance of the predictability of the UCS-CS occurrence rather than its frequency.[99,100]

The role of cognitive perspective in classical conditioning has been explained by "blocking" experiments, in which subjects are exposed to repeated pairings of a light and an electric shock until the light becomes a CS. A second stimulus (e.g. sound) is then added so that both the light and the noise occur together prior to the shock. In such an experimental condition, the second stimulus (i.e. sound) should become a conditioned stimulus since it is consistently paired with the shock. However, it does not happen in the experimental condition; when the sound is later presented alone, it does not elicit a conditioned response. The sound is considered "blocked" from becoming a CS due to the previous conditioning to the light.[101] In the cognitive perspective, it is explained that since the light already predicts the occurrence of the shock, the new stimulus (the sound) is irrelevant because it provides no new information. Since the new stimulus does not add to the subject's ability to predict the shock, it fails to become a conditioned stimulus.[102]

Rescorla-Wagner Model of Classical Conditioning

Attempts have been made to explain learning theories that are either distinctly 'molecular' or 'molar'. Rescorla-Wagner model of learning,[103] a molecular learning approach, has received attention.

This model attempts to account for Pavlovian conditioning with more than one CS as it was noticed that it is not possible to present a single CS during the process of conditioning. For example, if a tone is presented as a CS, that tone is heard against a background of certain other stimuli such as ambient noise, illumination, smells, tastes, etc. constituting the background. When such background remains constant between conditioning trials, it can be considered as a single stimulus. Thus, the standard Pavlovian classical conditioning procedure can be viewed as an alternative between: (1) the background alone during the intertrial intervals (without the UCS); and (2) the background plus the CS during the trials (with the UCS).

The Rescorla-Wagner model follows two assumptions:

1. The strength of conditioned stimulus gained during a specific conditioning trial is proportionate to the difference between the strength of conditioning prior to the trial and the asymptotic strength of conditioning. Unreinforced trials are considered like conditioning trials except that the asymptote is zero.
2. The strength of conditioning of a basic compound stimulus (i.e. more than one CS) is the sum of the strengths of the individual components; hence on a reinforced trial with a compound stimulus, both the conditioned stimuli contribute to the pretrial level of conditioning. This determines the amount gained on a trial depending on the unconditioned stimulus.[103]

The Rescorla-Wagner model explains the phenomenon of 'blocking'. When the compound has background plus a single CS, if an UCS is first presented during the intertrial interval without the presentation of any conditioned stimulus, the conditioning associated with the background will block further conditioning to any CS superimposed upon it. The Rescorla-Wagner model has certain significant clinical implications.[103]

OPERANT CONDITIONING

We learn to engage in behaviors which produce positive outcome. We also learn a complex action that helps us to obtain such positive outcomes as money, status and success, which are termed positive reinforcers as they tend to strengthen our responses which precede them. We always tend to engage in behaviors which help us to avoid or escape from unpleasant outcomes or stimuli. Such undesirable events are termed negative reinforcers, and their effect upon behavior is that they strengthen responses which lead to their termination or removal. In operant conditioning (also termed as instrumental conditioning), the reinforcer is contingent upon the occurrence of the response and thus follows the response in time. Thus, conditioning is based on the fact that behavior often produces consequences. As a result of such contingencies, we acquire responses which yield desirable outcomes (positive reinforcers) or which help us to avoid or escape from undesirable behaviors (negative reinforcers). Reinforcement is a procedure in which a response produces a stimulus change and as a result becomes more probable. A positive reinforcement is any stimulus or event which when present increases or maintains the strength of a response. A negative reinforcement is any stimulus or event which when terminated or removed increases or maintains the strength of a response.[104] Skinner in his conceptualization focused on the observable consequences of behavior.

Thorndike's theory of behavior—*the law of effect*—has formed the basis for the origins of operant conditioning which was later developed by Skinner. According to the law of effect, if a response is followed by "satisfying" consequences, it will be strengthened and if followed by an unpleasant or negative state of affairs, it will be weakened. Following the work of Thorndike[105] and Skinner,[106] learned responses have been developed by procedures using operant conditioning. The major feature characterizing the operant conditioning is that the organism assumes an active role in the learning process, unlike the classical conditioning in which the organism plays a passive role. The experimenter manipulates the experimental situation in such a way that the organism cannot obtain reward or cannot escape from punishment of some kind until and unless it makes a particular response. When reward is made contingent on the prior occurrence of a particular response, such method is called as instrumental or operant conditioning. In this process, the organism plays an instrumental role in producing rewards for itself or in escaping from or avoiding some unpleasant situation or punishment by operating on the environment. In essence, a contingent relationship is established between the occurrence of a potential response and the presentation or nonpresentation of a reinforcer during the process of operant conditioning. The nature of the conditioned stimulus, the response, and the reinforcement are the independent variables in operant conditioning; similar to the classical conditioning paradigm, their relationship and the timing are critical factors in operant conditioning.[93,107]

Basic Procedures of Operant Conditioning

There are three basic aspects involved in the operant conditioning experiment: (1) the experimental plan uses procedures involving reward or punishment and such operations of reward or punishment are termed reinforcement, (2) the experimental plan leads an organism to either produce or withhold some specified response, (3) a discriminative cue- a stimulus that tells the organism in effect, when reinforcement can be obtained and when it cannot be obtained—will be used in some experimental plans; the discriminative cue sets the appropriate occasion for the behavior that leads to reinforcement. In such experiments, where discriminative cue is used, the response will not be reinforced if it occurs when the discriminative cue is absent, or vice versa.[94]

According to the operant conditioning, the analysis of behavior involves the assessment of relationships between three basic aspects, namely antecedents (a) or the stimulus conditions, behaviors (b) that the organism engages in, and consequences (c) that follow and either strengthen or weaken the behaviors that produce them. The relationships existing among these elements are called contingencies. Such contingencies are expressed in such a way that if antecedent stimuli (a) are present and behavior (b) is emitted, then consequences (c) will occur.

Antecedents which signal the likely occurrence of specific behavioral consequences in a given situation are known as discriminative stimuli. Such discriminative stimuli guide the behaviors of organisms so that the individual could involve in appropriate behaviors and which would always lead to positive consequences.[94]

Hulse, Deese and Egeth[108] described eight experimental paradigms using the operant conditioning. The following four paradigms involve active production of a response by the organism in conjunction with reinforcement operations of reward or punishment. These include (a) reward training; (b) discrimination training; (c) escape training; and (d) avoidance training.

- *Reward training:* In a typical instrumental conditioning, a hungry rat is placed in a Skinner box which is fixed with a lever connected to an automatic recording devise and a magazine of pellets of food. When the lever is pressed, the magazine automatically delivers a pellet of food into the box. The hungry rat when placed in this box, explores and when accidentally presses the lever, it would lead to the delivery of food pellet. If the rat presses the lever once again, it would learn that pressing lever would lead to appearance of food. Following such experience, the rat would start pressing the lever repeatedly in order to obtain food in the Skinner Box. In reward training, essentially, the organism performs a critical response or set of responses and achieves the reward. Though the organism receives a reward after making a particular response, such response which precedes the reward need not be physically related to the actual delivery of the reward. What is essential in the instrumental conditioning is that the reward must follow the response in a systematic relationship.
- *Discrimination training:* In the Skinner box, a discriminative cue—white light—is fixed; the light is turned on when the rat is placed in the box and reward training is initiated. Following the reward training, the light is turned off and the food magazine is disconnected from the lever so that lever pressing would no longer lead to appearance of food. Subsequently, the light is turned on and the food magazine is reconnected to the lever and now the lever pressing would lead to the appearance of food. Such trials are alternated wherein 'light-on' in the box leading to appearance of food and 'light-off' with no food. Eventually, after a number of periods in which the light is turned on and off and reinforcement is delivered or withheld, accordingly the animal learns that lever pressing during the 'light-on' condition would lead to appearance of food whereas lever pressing during 'light-off' condition would not lead to such reinforcement. In this experiment, the discriminative cue (i.e. light) sets the occasion for lever pressing and the animal learns when to press and when not to, in order to receive the reinforcement.
- *Escape training:* In this experiment, a dog is placed in one of a two-compartment box, and these two compartments are separated by a sliding door. Both the compartments are fixed with floor made of stainless steel bars so that electricity can be passed into each of the compartments separately by turning on the electricity into the box in order to produce shock in the animal. When the current is 'on' in one compartment, it is off in the other. The door is arranged in such a way that the dog can jump from the first compartment into the second when electricity is passed in the former compartment. During the process of the experiment, the door drops and electricity is passed into the first compartment. The shock continues until the dog jumps over the hurdle and reaches the second compartment in which the shock is not present. In the 'safe' compartment, the dog can rest until the experimenter again drops the door and turns on the shock in the second compartment. The dog must then jump the hurdle once again, moving back to the previous compartment. The process of shock in one compartment followed by escape to the 'safe' compartment continues for several trials leading to the learning in the dog to jump into the safe compartment when shock is presented in the previous compartment so that it can escape the shock. Thus, in escape training, the noxious stimulus is presented before the critical response occurs and the critical response increases in its rate of appearance or probability.
- *Avoidance training:* In this experiment, the apparatus used for the escape training is modified and a light is added in both the compartments. The dog is initially placed in the first compartment with the light 'turned-off'. Now the light is 'turned-on' in the first compartment (a discriminative cue) and 10 seconds later shock is provided into this compartment. The dog can avoid the shock by jumping into the 'safe' compartment during the 10-second interval period between the onset of the discriminative cue and the onset of the shock. Here, the discriminative cue sets the occasion for the dog's response. When the dog jumps into the safe compartment, it can rest. Similar trial is conducted in the second compartment. In this paradigm also, initially, the discriminative cue has no effect on the behavior of the dog. However, after a few trials during which the latency of the response to the shock may decrease considerably and the dog learns to respond to the discriminative cue and jumps to the second compartment before the shock comes on. Thus,

unlike the other approaches, in the avoidance training, the critical response prevents the noxious stimulus from appearing.

The following procedures require active withholding or omission of a response on the part of an organism in order to obtain reward or avoid punishment. These paradigms include: (a) punishment training, (b) omission training, (c) discriminated punishment, and (d) discriminated omission training.

- *Punishment training*: In this experiment, initially a lever pressing response is established using the reward training in the animal. Following this, the contingency is changed so that now the lever pressing leads to electric shock rather than appearance of food pellets. In such a situation, the animal must learn to inhibit or withhold the lever-pressing response in order to avoid the shock. Since the animal becomes passive and would not emit a response in such a punishment situation, in order to avoid the unpleasant consequence, this process is called as passive avoidance learning. Thus, in punishment training, the noxious stimulus occurs after the critical response and such critical response decreases in its rate or probability.
- *Omission training*: This paradigm follows an experimental situation in which initially the simple reward training is used; following the establishment of reward training in the animal, then the contingencies are changed so that: (1) lever pressing no longer leads to appearance of food pellet, but (2) not pressing the lever is reinforced. This is executed by dropping a food pellet into the food cup at the end of each 5-second interval period when the animal does not press the lever. This experimental situation leads the organism to learn to withhold or omit the response in order to get the reinforcement.
- *Discriminated punishment, and D. discriminated omission training*: In these procedures, a discriminative cue is added that sets the occasion for reinforcement during the process of punishment training or omission training. In a typical situation, a light is used as a discriminative cue, and the contingencies are arranged such that onset of light sets the occasion for omitting lever pressing in order to obtain rewards or to avoid punishment. When the discriminative cue is absent, i.e. when the light is off, simple reward training is introduced again into such a paradigm.

These experimental paradigms have wide range of applications, e.g. parents learn that rewards given when children withhold some kind of unwanted behavior can sometimes prevent the recurrence of the unwanted behavior. Such principle is found to be effective when it is combined with punishment for the unwanted behavior. Discriminative cues in everyday life are used in terms of verbal commands; those set the occasion for the omission of a specific response in question. Discriminated punishment training is used by warning the children that unless a specific maladaptive response is omitted, punishment will ensue; consequently they learn to omit such unwanted responses in the presence of a specific discriminative cue, but might indulge in such behaviors when the same discriminative cue is absent.[108]

Cognitive interpretation of operant conditioning: The cognitive perspective of operant conditioning assumes that mere response consequences do not automatically strengthen or weaken a specific behavior; they provide the information about the behavior-environment relations—the likely consequences of specific behaviors under certain conditions; past reinforcement and negative consequences motivate the organism through anticipation of future outcome. According to the cognitive perspective, the behaviors of an organism are largely governed by the expectation of resultant outcome.[109] In the operant conditioning paradigm, the response consequences involve two aspects, namely, (a) they *inform* and (b) they *motivate* the organism. Thus, the cognitive basis of operant conditioning is an expectancy that certain behaviors lead to specific outcomes under specific conditions,[110] and such information is stored in the central nervous system which influences the feelings and actions through cognitions. The awareness—contingency between a specific behavior and its consequences—also plays a significant role. It is also said that the best predictor of an individual's behavior is the 'perceived' contingency rather than the 'actual' contingency.

According to the cognitive interpretation of operant conditioning, the individual tends to perform a response if aware of the contingency between that behavior and its consequences and if he is motivated for or against the consequences. Thus, the cognitive paradigm focuses on the role of awareness. In operant conditioning, awareness involves knowing the relationships between responses and their probable consequences.

MOWRER'S TWO-FACTOR THEORY OF LEARNING

Mowrer's theory was developed in three stages: stage one dealt with the discover of anxiety reduction as a reinforcing agent; stage two with the dual nature of learning; and the stage three with the revised two factor theory of learning. Since the 1950s, Mowrer[111,112] has extended his two-factor theory to applications in the area of mental health.[113]

Anxiety Reduction as a Reinforcing Agent

Mowrer, in 1939, introduced that anxiety reduction serves as a reinforcing agent; anxiety motivates human beings and its reduction reinforces behavior, resulting in a sense of relief. Mowrer, assuming that all reactions are learned, emphasized that fear motivates and reinforces the human behavior. Painful stimuli, arising from organic need or injury, produce a defense reaction. The stimulus-response sequence involved, preceded by neutral stimuli that have been associated by contiguity, acquires the capacity of eliciting a fear or anxiety reaction.[113]

Dual Nature of Learning

In 1947, Mowrer extended his theory and proposed that two basic learning processes, namely, (1) conditioning by association (solution learning), and (2) problem-solving (sign learning) are important. Learning by contiguity, which involves the autonomic nervous system, is considered as sign learning, whereas in solution learning, the problems are solved those are drive-reducing and pleasure producing. In 1953, Mowrer's dual nature of learning was termed as 'two-factor theory', which acquired more vocabulary and was discussed in relation to the human nervous system. According to the new approach, the solution learning involves the central nervous system and the skeletal musculature resulting in certain voluntary, instrumental response patterns which are called as 'acts' or 'habits'. Whereas the sign learning involves the autonomic nervous system and visceral-vascular tissue resulting in such involuntary reactions as 'attitudes', 'feelings', or 'meanings'. The former exemplifies the law of effect as formulated by Thorndike and elaborated by Hull, and the latter exemplifies associative learning or conditioning as defined by Pavlov.[113]

According to Hull, by the 'solution learning' the individual learns ways to reduce drives and looks for solutions to resolve drive needs (such as hunger, thirst, and sex). By the sign learning, the individual looks for signs of danger, such as indications leading to one's fears and aversions.[114]

Mowrer revised his two-factor theory in 1956, in which he distinguished between sign learning as fear conditioning and solution learning as habit formation. According to him, the individual learns to involve in behaviors that would reduce fear. To Hull, learning is governed by 'drive reduction' (hunger, thirst, and sexual satisfaction), and the fear conditioning is controlled by 'drive induction'. The solution learning results when drive is reduced and is mediated by the central nervous system and skeletal muscles and voluntary behavioral responses. Whereas the sign learning results when a neutral stimulus is paired with drive reduction and is mediated by the autonomic nervous system. This involves glands and smooth muscles and involves the emotional responses.[113]

In 1960s, Mowrer reformulated the two-factor theory, in which he considered all learning as conditioning or sign learning, solution learning being merely a derivative or 'special instance' of conditioning. The drive of fear is incremental, learning occurring with its reduction; and the drive of sex is decremental, learning occurring with its alleviation. Whereas incremental reinforcement is characterized by punishment, decremental reinforcement is rewarding. Accordingly, Mowrer used the term 'incremental' to reinforcement involved in punishment (drive induction) and thus likely to produce active or passive avoidance behavior, and used the term 'decremental' to the reinforcement which reward (drive reduction) provides.[115]

Stampfl and Levis,[116-118] based on Mowrer's two-factor theory, proposed such therapeutic techniques as 'implosion' and 'flooding' to deal with conditioned emotional responses. Stampfl and Levis hypothesized that psychopathology, occurring due to past experiences with punishment and pain, leads to strong emotional reactions to initially nonpunishing stimuli (classical conditioning). This is followed by the conditioned stimuli which motivate for developing responses leading to escape or avoidance of the source of the conditioned aversive stimulation (instrumental conditioning). They also emphasized the role of past conditioning experiences which may tend to function as conditioned emotional stimuli. Accordingly, Stampfl and Levis believed that extinction of the conditioned emotional responses occurs when the total conditioned stimulus complex is presented without the presentation of the unconditioned stimulus, thus supporting the need to utilize implosion and flooding as therapeutic methods in dealing with such conditioned emotional responses as phobias.

HULL'S DRIVE REDUCTION THEORY

Hull's scientific approach has been variously termed as 'mathematico-deductive', 'logico-deductive', 'hypothetico-deductive' and 'logico-empirical'. Hull synthesized the principles of classical conditioning and trial and error learning under one unitary concept of reinforcement, namely, drive reduction. Hull believed that there is a connection between a stimulus and a response, and that the 'neurological substrata' plays a role in the formation of such connections between stimulus and response.[119] According to Hull, whenever a response process is closely contiguous to a stimulus process, and this association occurs near in time to the reduction of a drive, the association is strengthened. Reinforcement is defined in terms of drive reduction. Drive, in turn, is defined in terms of physiological 'needs' of the organism.

Hull proposed that learning occurs when a response is reinforced and when it reduces a drive. According to him, "whenever an effector activity (R) is closely associated with rapid diminution in the motivational stimulus (SB or SG), there will result an increment (A) to a tendency for that stimulus to evoke that response".[120] Learning occurs with reinforcement as behaviors that are rewarded tend to be repeated. Hull's main principle, the postulate of reinforcement and learning, is responsible for the behavior. The strengthening of a stimulus-response connection is contingent upon the reinforcement's quantitative properties, wherein the larger the reward, the more effective it is. If a response is not rewarded, it will not produce learning. Thus, larger rewards and which are more immediate in time following a behavior are more effective in bringing about learning. Drive reduction is reinforcing and it increases the habit strength which is said to be basic to any learning. Learning is negatively accelerated and gradual, because the habit strength follows the 'law of diminishing return'.[120]

Hull focused on the overt and observable behavior (acts) rather than on the minute physiological elements (such as muscular contractions). However, he did not reject the role of such cognitive aspects of behavior as purpose, ideas, intelligence, insight, values and knowledge which are implied in the behavior itself, assuming that they are the properties of molar behavior.[120]

Habit Strength

Habit strength ($_SH_R$) is a learned association between a stimulus and a response; *'H'* stands for habit, *'S'* represents the stimulus trace and *'R'* the resulting action of behavioral response. 'H' denotes the magnitude of a change in the state of the conduction structure of the nervous system whereby the propagation of the neural impulse; *'S'* is routed into the efferent fibers leading to the organs which execute the reaction, *'R'*.[121] Thus, habit is an S-R connection, a relatively permanent connection established due to the effect of reinforcement A habit generalizes to similar stimuli. Habit is considered as "a combination of (1) the stimulus event; and (2) a relatively permanent condition or organization left by the reinforcement within the nervous system.[122] In order to establish a habit, both reinforcement and contiguity are essential. According to Hull's law of habit formation, "if reinforcements follow each other at evenly distributed intervals, everything else constant, the resulting habit will increase in strength as a positive function of the number of trials".[120]

Hull[114,122] emphasized that if occurrence of receptor activity (a stimulus) and effector activity (a response) in a temporal contiguity leads to the diminution of a need (drive reduction), it results in an increase in the tendency of occurence of such afferent impulse to evoke that reaction subsequently. Such increment in successive reinforcements would lead to habit strength ($_SH_R$). Drives interact with habit strength to produce performance ($D \times {_SH_R}$). Hull also assumed that every response results in an increment of reactive inhibition (I_R), irrespective of whether it is reinforced or not, and this acts as a negative drive and with increase in IR (reactive inhibition) the strength of the response preceding it becomes weakened. For example, since I_R (fatigue) is a drive, the reduction of this state is reinforcing and therefore is capable of strengthening any response that precedes it in contiguity. Moreover, since I_R leads to cessation of activity, a resting response is conditioned to the CS. This process is known as 'conditioned inhibition' ($_SI_R$), And the sum inhibition results from a combination of both I_R and $_SI_R$. Hence, behavior equals $D \times ({_SH_R} - I_R + {_SI_R})$. With the removal of the UCS (reinforcement), inhibition exceeds the strength of excitation leading to extinction.

Hull also emphasized on the concept of secondary reinforcement and secondary drive. "When a neutral stimulus (one that does not act either as a drive or as a reinforcer) is paired with a sudden reduction in a drive stimulus, the neutral stimulus tends to acquire reinforcing properties".[119] Thus, it becomes a secondary reinforcer.

Hull's hypothetico-deductive system has been challenged on two points: (1) the parameters used by Hull were basically the products of animal studies, and (2) the drive reduction cannot be the basic process in all learning.[123]

SOCIAL LEARNING THEORY

Various limitations have been explained while applying the classical and operant animal learning models to the human behavior, due to the alleged narrowness in the application of the laboratory experimental data to such specific clinical areas as psychopathology and psychotherapy. The human capacity for language and thinking is said to provide ability to bypass simple conditioning processes. These verbal and social skills also enable the individual to benefit from the learning experiences of the significant others even when he is not formally present in the learning situation. The individual benefits from learning experiences from other individuals within the immediate environment while acquiring verbal and social skills.

Moreover, acquisition of certain complex intellectual, social and moral behaviors, cannot be explained in mere simplistic approaches utilizing the S-R learning paradigms. Such approaches have been criticized as they cannot adequately explain certain aspects of human life, such as acquisition of novel responses, language and social development, the role of language and thinking in behavior control. Moreover, the experimental data in laboratory studies as well as natural environment studies indicate that even the animals are active, curious, and explore the environment for new stimulation and, accordingly show variations in responses to the environment. This also has lead to the assumption that learning is an active process which has multiple and complex environmental influences. Moreover, findings from various experiments illustrate that organisms observe the events in the immediate environment and attempt to imitate the same under similar situations, though the extent of observational learning varies across species. Thus, the conditioning principles have been criticized saying that they are overly simplistic and mechanistic, too restricted in relying on animal laboratory paradigms, and too narrow in the behaviors.

Consequently, attempts have been made to broaden behavioral learning principles by extending to 'characteristically human' aspects of individuals and their social environment.[124,125] Such approaches have been variously termed as 'social learning', 'vicarious learning', 'imitation', 'observational learning' and 'modeling'. The usage of these terms has been with no clear distinction among them. Social learning perspective determines the content of a person's repertoire and is determined by his previous experience and personal characteristics.

The social learning theory (SLT), basically developed by Bandura, rejects the exclusive role of such specific internal motivational forces as needs, drives and impulses of an individual in the process of learning. The SLT also rejects the explanations of behaviors solely based on the conditioning paradigm, claiming that it exclusively deals with the external causal factors. Consequently, the SLT propounds the interactional approach, wherein a causal two-way interaction between the internal (i.e. personal dispositions) and the external (i.e. situational determinants) factors determine the behavior of an individual, with an emphasis on the cognitive mediational-personal factors.[126] Moreover, according to this approach, the behaviors and aspects have mutual interaction among themselves. SLT assumes that (a) the organisms respond to novel stimuli in their environment and engage in behaviors that procure changes in environmental stimulation; and (b) behavior of a peer model is imitated by the observer when placed under similar conditions. The SLT also acknowledges biological factors as predisposing conditions that modulate learning and behavior. Reciprocal determinism, the thesis that the individuals are active agents in determining their own goals, is central to the SLT model. The SLT perspective, further emphasizes a multidimensional interaction between biological, environmental and other organismic variables (cognitive, emotional and psychophysiological).

According to Bandura, "man is neither an internally impelled system nor a passive reactor to external stimulation. Rather, psychological functioning involves a reciprocal interaction between behavior and its controlling environment. The type of behavior that a person exhibits partly determines his environmental contingencies which, in turn, influence his behavior".[127]

The upsurge, according to Kanfer and Phillips,[124] in the development of social learning model is due to: (1) the dissatisfaction with therapeutic applications of the conditioning models, (2) incorporates more complex social phenomena within the explanatory systems of learning theories in competition with other models, (3) the recognition that uniquely human capacities require special consideration, and (4) the confluence of streams of interest in related phenomena within social, developmental, clinical and learning psychology.

EYSENCK'S THEORY OF INCUBATION

Eysenck[128-130] laid emphasis on his concept of 'neurotic paradox' (i.e. repeatedly engaging in behaviors that are maladaptive, self-defeating, and frequently punished by the society). Eysenck,[128] modifying the law of extinction, stressed that when the conditioned stimulus alone is presented without it being followed by unconditioned stimulus, it may either lead to extinction or enhancement of the conditioned response. Such enhancement of the conditioned response is termed as incubation of the anxiety/fear response. To Eysenck, the conditioned stimuli which do not produce drives tend to lead to extinction, whereas the conditioned stimuli that produce drives (e.g. fear/anxiety, sexual responses) lead to enhancement (incubation).

According to Eysenck, the maladaptive fear responses can be innate, or acquired through learning. He attempted to explain why some phobias are more prevalent among individuals than certain others, by challenging the theory of equipotentiality and emphasizing the role of 'preparedness' of Seligman[131] which states that certain conditioned stimuli are biologically prepared to be conditioned more readily with anxiety responses than others. Such innate phenomenon sensitizes the individual to certain stimuli and facilitates the maladaptive conditioning of fear responses to such stimuli.[129]

The anxiety response is generally acquired through classical conditioning, which may occur due to traumatic or subtraumatic, or due to single-trial learning, or repeated presentation of the CS-UCS in contiguity. Conditioned responses, when not reinforced (i.e. during CS-only presentation) may extinguish. However, in certain conditions, presentation of 'CS-only' produces incubation (enhancement of the conditioned response) which leads to the development and maintenance of neurotic responses. Incubation tends to occur with those conditioned stimuli which acquire drive properties during the process of conditioning. Such drive properties of the conditioned stimulus make the conditioned response functionally equivalent to the unconditioned response, thus providing reinforcement for the CS-only presentation. Thus, a positive feedback cycle sets in, which produces conditioned response enhancement instead of extinction. Conditions such as *short* CS-only presentation, *strong* unconditioned stimulus, and certain personality characteristics (high neuroticism and introversion) of an individual tend to facilitate the incubation of fear responses during the CS-only presentation. Due to the process of incubation, the conditioned responses exceed the unconditioned responses in strength and the neurotic responses increase slowly over a period of time with occasional exposure to CS-only. Thus, Eysenck's theoretical explanations have significant implications for understanding the neurotic behaviors.[129]

CLINICAL APPLICATIONS

The study of learning plays a significant role in clinical psychology and in understanding human personality. Moreover, the learning theories help us in understanding the origin of various mental disorders and formulate effective intervention strategies, accordingly. The theoretical contributions of various theorists such as Pavlov, Hull,

Guthrie, Mowrer and Tolman shed light on the development and treatment of psychopathology. Theories explaining acquisition, response maintenance, and generalization of various clinical disorders paved way for objective and appropriate explanations of these disorders. Accordingly, the modern behavior therapy has derived its therapeutic procedures from learning theories, specifically the classical, instrumental and social learning theories.

The classical conditioning has formed the basis for many complex human behaviors. It helps us to understand how we learn emotional responses that underlie our attitudes and social behaviors. Though some theoretical constructs are criticized for the "lack of direct experimental support, Pavlov's concepts of excitation and inhibition have been incorporated into various modern theories.[103,122,132-134]

Pavlov explained the psychopathology by extending his theoretical models. According to Pavlov, extreme cortical irradiation of the inhibitory process leads to sleep, whereas extreme excitation leads to active behavior. When there is a clash between the excitatory and inhibitory processes and the intense stimulation, it leads to psychopathology resulting in symptoms such as hysteria, neurasthenia, depression, mania, and catatonia.[96]

The research findings suggest that classical conditioning processes play an important role in the development of some psychosomatic disorders, in which physical symptoms are caused by psychological factors. In asthma patients, the asthmatic attacks occur in the presence of specific stimuli such as dust and certain emotional stimuli (conditioned stimuli) which can be explained by the process of classical conditioning, as evidenced by the fact that such asthmatic attacks could be induced by presenting the conditioned stimuli.[135]

Application of classical conditioning principles in the area of mental health started when Watson and Rayner[136] demonstrated the acquisition of phobic reaction in a child called *'Little Albert'*. Jones[137] first used classical conditioning principles to eliminate fear in a child called *'Peter'*.

Inspired by Pavlovian theory, Salter[138,139] developed 'conditioned-reflex therapy' assuming that a neurotic individual suffers from an excess of inhibition which blocks his normal output of excitation. Therapy, therefore, is designed to encourage the patient to express feelings directly. Wolpe's[140] 'assertive' response approach represents a similar conceptualization and technique.

According to Wolpe, anxiety could be neutralized if "a response antagonistic to anxiety can be made to occur in the presence of the anxiety-evoking stimuli so that it is accompanied by the complete or partial suppression of the anxiety response".[140] This theoretical principle, *reciprocal inhibition,* has lead to the development of specific techniques such as systematic desensitization, which has been effectively used in the management of phobias.

The classical conditioning paradigm explains the initiation, maintenance and relapse of drug abuse. According to this approach, stimuli repeatedly present during drug taking can modulate the behavioral and pharmacological effects of drugs. Such stimuli generate drug-like behavioral and physiological effects which is termed as 'drug-mimicking'. Moreover, the drug-associated stimuli can produce effects opposite to those produced by the drugs themselves, which is termed as 'drug-mirroring'.[141]

Classical conditioning model also explains such phenomena as tolerance and craving in alcohol dependence. According to this model, the individual uses available situational cues to predict the onset of drug action and reacts by generating an anticipatory counter response that dampens the drug's action.[142] According to Ludwig and Wikler,[143] presence of exteroceptive (e.g. physical setting or drinking companions) or interoceptive (e.g. emotional states) stimuli (cues) associated with heavy drinking/withdrawal elicits craving, thereby predisposing the individual to take alcohol. Thus, consumption further intensifies the craving and leads to loss of control. This model assumes that craving occurs due to: (1) the presence of conditioned stimuli that elicit the internal state, and (2) the convergence of certain situational factors that determine how the internal state is labeled. When these are active, the individual takes the first drink, leading to increased craving and finally going to loss of control drinking. The classical conditioning model has been adopted in the treatment of alcohol dependence. Classical conditioning procedures are also effective in treatment of substance abuse. Such approaches have included counterconditioning (aversion therapy) and extinction procedures. Various aversive conditioning procedures based on this paradigm have been in use in the intervention of alcohol dependence.

Aversion therapy, based on classical conditioning, played a significant role in behavior therapy, which was applied to specific clinical disorders such as addictive behaviors and sexual deviance. The goal of aversion therapy is to eliminate or decrease an undesirable response by repeatedly pairing it with an aversive event (e.g. physical discomfort produced by electric shock).[94]

Operant conditioning contributed significantly to the therapy utilizing learning principles. Essentially, operant conditioning explains the acquisition of new behaviors, and modifying the maladaptive response patterns by systematic application of rewards and punishment. Though earlier researchers have contributed to the theoretical formulations, Skinner's theoretical contributions played a significant role in formulating a system of assessment and a distinct clinical research method in the area of behavior therapy. Operant conditioning has made a substantial impact in certain areas, specifically, child psychology, learning disabilities and rehabilitation of institutionalized psychiatric patients.[144]

Humans learn many complex behaviors through shaping, which is based on the operant conditioning paradigm. In shaping, in order to teach complex new behaviors, reinforcement for successive approximations is used. For example, shaping is involved in learning a language and in developing educational skills.

Extinction (gradual disappearance of a learned response) of operant behaviors occurs when a particular response is not reinforced. This principle accounts for many changes in human behavior. When previously reinforced behaviors are no longer reinforced, the organisms tend to abandon them and replace them with responses which have a potential to be reinforced.

The operant conditioning model has been used to explain the acquisition, maintenance and modification of problem drinking. According to this model, problem drinking is developed through selective reinforcement of incipient components of behavior. When the behavior is established, the intermittent occurrence of reinforcement enhances the resiliency of the behavior. Modification of drinking behavior requires removal of positive reinforcers (i.e. extinction) and/or application of punishment. A variety of positive (i.e. money, tokens, social interaction) and negative (e.g. electric shock, social isolation) reinforcers have been in use within the operant paradigm (e.g. punishment, escape, token economy and contingency contracting) to modify drinking behavior.[145]

Many behaviors have immediate positive consequences and later negative consequences. Responses such as smoking, drinking, drug use and criminal acts can be explained in an operant paradigm since these behaviors have immediate positive effects, though they may have negative consequences at a later time. It is difficult to deal with such behaviors as the immediate positive reinforcement for such behaviors overrides the negative consequences that may occur subsequently.

Mowrer's two factor theory explains the acquisition and maintenance of anxiety. This theory involves two key assumptions: (a) anxiety is an acquired drive in the classical conditioning paradigm in which a neutral stimulus (CS) is paired with an UCS, and (b) this anxiety motivates instrumental or avoidance behavior which, in turn, is reinforced by the reduction of the underlying anxiety drive.[94]

Bandura[127] described behavior modification within the social learning perspective. Bandura's[127] social learning theory explains the human functioning of both deviant and pro-social behaviors which are assumed to be acquired and maintained on the basis of three distinct processes: (a) certain behaviors are primarily under the control of external stimulus events and follow classical conditioning paradigm, (b) some behaviors are under the influence of external reinforcement, the main focus of operant conditioning paradigm, and (c) some behaviors are influenced by cognitive-mediational processes, which are said to be the most influential system of control. According to the social learning perspective, such cognitive mediational processes as vicarious learning, symbolic activities and self-control mechanisms play a significant role in the response patterns.

Bandura's work on the principle of vicarious learning was a significant contribution to the field of behavior therapy, which emphasized on the learning through observation with a view of experience which lacks any internal processing of incoming information.[144]

SLT assumes central role to self-efficacy mechanism in explaining how thoughts affect actions and how behavior patterns are selected by the individual.[146] The SLT model suggests that individual's beliefs about alcohol and their ability to cope with the demands of everyday life are crucial determinants of how psychologically dependent on alcohol the individual becomes, cultural norms, role models, and learned expectations influence the drinking behavior and play a central role in determining drinking patterns. The cognitive activities such as anticipation, expectancy, memory about history of use and modeling play the primary role as determinants of behavior. The situational determinants of drinking behavior (e.g. modeling effects, reactivity to alcohol cues) are modulated by these cognitions. Thus, the underlying psychological principle of an SLT model of alcohol use differs from a biological perspective.[125]

Bandura[127] also explained the determinants of sexual deviance using the social learning perspective. According to him, parents model deviant patterns of sexuality, and such behaviors are maintained through direct and vicarious reinforcement. Moreover, such sexual activities may become self-reinforcing due to the tension-reducing characteristic of such activities, along with immediate sexual gratification.[147]

Thus, the basic theoretical paradigms—classical, operant and social learning, a few among many—play a significant role in understanding various disorders in the area of mental health. Accordingly, despite certain controversies, the learning theories provide insights into understanding the disorders and formulating intervention strategies utilizing specific theoretical paradigms. Such approaches have been proved to be effective in mental health.

ACKNOWLEDGMENTS

The authors gratefully acknowledge the comments of Dr H Mishra, Additional Professor, Department of Clinical Psychology, NIMHANS, for his valuable comments on a previous draft of this chapter.

45.3 MEASUREMENT IN PSYCHIATRY

SK Verma, A Puri

MEASUREMENT

Everything that exists, exists in some quantity and can be and must be measured. It is measurement which makes a science exact, objective, reliable, replicable and valid. Psychiatry is no exception to this. Measurement refers to assigning of numerals, according to some principle. One may consider a person having a particular trait, like anxiety or depression, or not having it. This refers to categorization of persons in terms of mutually exclusive classes.

These classes can be assigned values of 0 or 1 (not having/having). This is the crudest form of measurement, called as *nominal scale.* But the either and or type of existence of such characteristics is not always possible, and in fact much finer shades usually exist and their measurement should be possible. Case study method, phenomenological studies, epidemiological studies, field surveys, classification of psychiatric disorders, etc. may be included here, where the differentiation between one disorder and another is based on such a nominal scale of categorization. However, when it includes severity of illness or rating of degree of improvement, one goes to a higher level of measurement.

The next higher or finer type of measurement is when some degree is added, such as: nil/mild/moderate/severe/profound—or always absent/sometimes present/often present/very often/always present—or very small/small/large/very large, etc. Thus, people can be arranged in some order-ascending or descending, with regard to a trait/characteristic/symptom, e.g. intelligence. 'A' may be more intelligent than 'B', 'B' may be more intelligent then 'C', and so on. They, then, can be assigned numerals in that order; the most intelligent having the highest score followed by others, till the lowest intelligent who gets the lowest possible value. Such a scale is called an *ordinal scale.*

Further fineness can be added, when the intervals between any two consecutive numbers are equal, e.g. difference between scores of 1 and 2 is same as the difference between 2 and 3 or between 3 and 4, etc. This is called an *interval scale.*

Most of the scales presently used in Psychiatry have this much accuracy or refinement, i.e. either they show some definite order (ascending or descending) or they have in addition to it, equal difference between any two consecutive values. The limitation of all such scales lies in the fact that it is very difficult to have an absolute zero point in such measurements. For example, it cannot be defined at the present moment what is zero intelligence or, zero anxiety, or zero depression, etc. in an absolute sense. This kind of measurement is possible in physics where one knows the zero value, e.g. weight, length, etc. Such a scale is called a *ratio scale,* e.g. where it is possible to say with accuracy that 50 is double of 25 and half of 100. However, even with this limitation, much can be achieved and has been achieved in the field of Psychiatry.

AREAS OF MEASUREMENT IN PSYCHIATRY

The field of Psychiatry has been fast expanding. But measurement or measuring instruments have not been able to keep pace with it, particularly the finer type of measurements mentioned above. There is some arbitrariness in defining the boundaries of these areas. However, an attempt is made here to show the work done and to classify it to the extent possible, with particular emphasis on work done in India. For the sake of convenience and simplicity, the work done is classified as follows:

- Definition and classification of mental disorders.
- Interview schedules.
- Measurement of cognitive functions.
- Measurement of personality variables.
- Miscellaneous scales.

Needless to say, some of the instruments mentioned could have been grouped differently, depending upon the emphasis given to the use to which they are put. Some of the more common and useful/promising instruments are briefly described.

Definition and Classification of Mental Disorders

Attempts have been made from time to time to define and classify mental disorders, but as yet no universally acceptable and satisfying definition and/or universally acceptable classification have been found. Following the leads of the so called 'antipsychiatry' movement in the west, some persons in India have started to doubt the very existence of the mental disorders. However, mental disorders are continued to be diagnosed, treated and researched in the psychiatric and general hospitals by the mental health professionals. Alternate models are being suggested and tried to a limited extent.

Mental disorders are mostly ill-understood and underestimated problems, particularly in our country, where they are often considered as physical diseases.[148] The new Mental Health Act of 1987 defines mentally ill person as a person who is in the need of treatment by the reason of any mental disorder, other than mental retardation.[149] The term mental disorder, referring to a clinically significant and identifiable behavioral or psychological syndrome or pattern that occurs in an individual, has clinical usefulness for making treatment and management decisions; has wide acceptability among clinicians and researchers; has usefulness for educating people including health-professionals, family members and others; and finally adequately reflects current knowledge about the existence of specific disorders. Development of increasingly reliable, valid and clinically useful classification system is an ongoing process.[150] A majority of hospitals/clinics in India are still using either the ICD-9,[151] or DSM-IIIR[152] with minor modifications here and there, although, after extensive field testing across the word, ICD-10[153] and DSM-IV[154] and now recently DSM-5 have come and already have been started at a few psychiatric clinics. Dissatisfaction with ICD-9 was prevalent because of its conceptual heterogeneity and a tendency to give concessions to various disparate schools of thought, while DSM-IIIR had a complicated structure posing numerous problems for the general mental health services of the developing world, which often work under tremendous constraints of personnel and resources. Even DSM-5 which recently came-up is criticized by various eminent psychiatrists of the world and did not address the above mentioned issues.

It was felt that some consideration needed to be given to the socioeconomic status, as in many developing countries poverty, and sociocultural deprivation result in special mental health problems.[155] The need for multiaxial classification, with additional assessment of severity of illness, has been suggested by many workers. The classification needs to be simple, practical, bias-free, manageable and acceptable to the population, if it has to stay and be used. There is also a long felt need to develop a parallel but simple, management oriented classification that can be easily taught, learnt and effectively used by less trained, nonmedical paraprofessionals working in the community. Some work in this direction has been done at a number of centers in India, e.g. Chandigarh, Bengaluru, Delhi, Lucknow and Ranchi.

Dissatisfaction with the existing system has led to a search for alternate models and terminology. Some psychiatrists and psychologists have sought refuge in the ancient Indian medical system. For example, Prof. KC Dube at Agra[156,157] has attempted to describe the nosology and the therapy of mental illness in Ayurveda, comparing it with the ICD-8. Dr. HG Singh,[158-161] at Gurukul Kangri University, Hardwar, has been persistently writing on the types of mental illness, personality types and psychotherapy as described in Ayurveda and Yogic systems, as well as giving their equivalents from modern psychiatry and psychology. Similarly, the Ayurvedic Research Unit and Department of Clinical Psychology at NIMHANS, Bangalore have also brought out a number of theoretical articles on the subject,[162,163] and related symptoms/syndromes like suicide, dhat syndrome, near death experiences, etc.[164-170]

However, little systematic, empirical work with these suggested models has been done and these individual, feeble, half-hearted attempts at evolving a more satisfactory, alternative, Indian classificatory system have not been popular in clinical practice also.

Interview Schedules

The most common form of psychiatric evaluation is done through direct face-to-face contact with subjects or patients. There may or may not be a fixed schedule for the type of questions asked and a fixed way of conducting this interview. Depending upon the relative structuring (fixedness) of this procedure, these interviews are called as unstructured (complete freedom), semi-structured (some are fixed, while others are open ended questions and variable questions) or highly structured (fixed questions with a standardized way and sequence of questions). There are a number of unstructured, unstandardized schedules used in psychiatry in majority of clinics in India. However, some of the more structured interview schedules have been standardized for specific purposes only and are used in various psychiatric researches, particularly when dealing with groups. For such schedules, carefully collected reliability and validity data are also available. Some of these schedules are sometimes used for individual case studies also and thus used for limited purpose only. A number of standardized western psychiatric interview schedules have been translated/adapted for use in Indian situations also. These relatively structured and well standardized interview schedules include the following:

- Present State Examination (PSE)[171,172]
- Indian Psychiatric Survey Schedule (IPSS)[173]
- Health Staff Interview (HSI)[174]
- Key Informant Interview Schedule[175]
- Childhood Psychopathology Measurement Schedule (CPMS)[176]
- Structured Interview Schedule for DSM-III (SCID)[177]
- Schedule for Affective Disorders and Schizophrenia (SADS)[178]
- Renard Diagnostic Interview[179]
- Clinical Interview Schedule[180,181]
- Diagnostic Interview Schedule[182]
- Clinical Global Impression Scale[183]
- Smart et al. Modified Youth Survey Drug Use Questionnaire[184]
- Explanatory Model Interview for Catalogue (EMIC)[185]
- Developmental Psychopathology Check List (DPCL)[186]
- Primary Care Psychiatric Questionnaire (PPQ)[187]
- The Schedule for the Assessment of Psychiatric Disability (SAPD)[188]

Whereas, some of these standardized interview schedules are for general psychiatric examination of patients and for general screening purposes, others are for specific research studies only. Then, there are standardized ways of collecting basic sociodemographic data which are needed for comparison of results from different studies. Unless the data are grouped in a common way, sometimes cross-cultural comparisons are just not possible. Several attempts to adopt common methodologies are, therefore, made for collecting data in a specific desirable way. For this purpose, Indian Council of Medical Research and World Health Organization have contributed in a big way, bringing together researchers from different areas to sit together, discuss and evolve common methodologies for this purpose, and to use them for multi-centric studies, e.g. Self-Reporting Questionnaire; Reporting Questionnaire for Children; Schedule for Standardized Assessment of Patients with Depressive Disorders; Home Risk Cards; Subjective Well-Being Scale; Quality of Community Life Scale, etc.

Several writers have described certain desirable features that should be considered while using or evaluating structured interview. These are as follows:

- The source of information should be specified in order to reduce unreliability of information variance resulting from various sources of information.[189]
- Structured interviews should define terms so that clinicians are consistent in their use of the terms.[190]
- Guidelines for determining the presence or absence of specific signs & symptoms should be given.[189]
- Structured interviews should prompt clinicians to gather information to determine whether the criteria for a particular diagnosis are present, by specifying what questions should be asked. This can be viewed as increasing the construct validity of the diagnosis.[191]
- Structured interviews should collect information in a format so that diagnosis can be made in a logical fashion and the same data will always yield the same diagnosis. This can be facilitated by the use of computer programs.[189]
- The structured interviews should give information about the possible pitfalls in coming to the right conclusions in a specific situation(s) or with a specific population.
- The structured interview should include questions or prompts in the local language, using simple, unambiguous and day-to-day language (not using difficult, vague words).
- The structured interview schedule should be brief, reliable, valid, simple and attractive for psychiatrists, who are hard-pressed for time and should be flexible enough to change with the gain in knowledge about the diagnostic system, categorical or dimensional, etc.

There have been many criticisms of the structured interview schedules. They have been described as highly subjective, unreliable, cumbersome,[192,193] disruptive to development of a therapeutic alliance with the patient, lengthy, time consuming,[190] etc. However, they have a distinct advantage of substantially increasing thereliability of diagnosis, of reducing the errors arising from differences in interviewer techniques of questioning, interviewer expectations and differences in definition of terms.[191]

Helzer[193] has shown that it is possible to have structured interview schedules with a proper balance, to make them attractive to a non-researcher, practising psychiatrists also. These interview procedures have ushered in a 'comeback' of the interview, particularly of the stand taken by some psychiatrists and psychologists that there is little point in administering elaborate and often lengthy tests when one can just as well as use the criterion measure itself, i.e. the psychiatric interview, rather than the test.

The unstructured and in-depth interviews should also be not lost sight of in this, as they also have an important role to play, both as an exploratory, hypothesis producing, item constructing technique, as well as dynamic and therapeutic methods in dealing with psychiatric disorders. However, these by definition also, are rather too flexible to be standardized in the usual manner, although broad guidelines can be given, as in psychoanalytic interviews, marital counseling, student counseling, etc. A detailed discussion, however, is beyond the scope of the present chapter.

Measurement of Cognitive Functions

There are four main reasons for measurement of cognitive functions in psychiatry:

1. This is necessary for the assessment of cognitive deficit, which helps in the psychiatric diagnosis and determining the type and degree of the organic damage.
2. It helps in making the rehabilitation plans by pointing out the areas of intact cognitive functions, which are the assets for such purposes—and areas that are in need of cognitive retraining as well as the identification of the starting point for such retraining.
3. It also helps in evaluation and comparisons of various therapies for psychiatric patients.
4. It helps in assessing improvement over time in individual cases, with or without treatment, as well as the rate of improvement.

In the case of children, measurement of cognitive functions serves an additional purpose, i.e. the assessment of the development of mental abilities in children, whether it is slow, delayed or within normal range. Early detection of developmental delays can help in taking timely remedial steps and reversing this process, failing which an irreversible or permanent damage may take place, resulting in mental retardation. In many cases, it is preventible, hence the need and importance of measurement of cognitive functions in children, is paramount.

Cognitive means knowing about ourselves and about the world around us. It is mainly through our sense organs and nervous system, and includes attention, concentration, perception, memory, intelligence, learning, judgement and thought processes. There are a number of psychological tests measuring these functions in adults. Some of these are well known and well standardized, reliable and valid measures of cognitive functions.

A psychological test is a standardized way of comparing the behavior of two or more individuals at any given time, or of the same individual at different periods of time. Standard is that in terms of which we measure other things. Most of the tests are simple, easy and quick standard measures which can be learned readily. However, there are some that need careful prolonged training under competent supervision, only after which they can be administered in a reliable way. The organic test batteries are examples of such tests.

A list of some of the tests of cognitive functions is given below, with suitable examples wherever considered necessary.

Tests of Attention and Concentration

The capacity to arouse and sustain attention varies with individuals and with time. In some of the psychiatric illnesses, attention becomes poor and/or fluctuates; hence a good and reliable measure of attention and concentration is considered desirable for any test battery. There are a number of psychological measures for this purpose and they include digit span test of concentration, Eysenck's digit test of concentration, color cancellation test, and addition and substraction test, digit symbol substitution test, letter cancellation test, Knox cube imitation test, etc.[194] These are very easy, brief and simple measures, and norms are available for most of them. These tests are also included in most of the test batteries.

Tests for Physical Mental Alertness or Retardation

Individuals differ with regard to psychomotor alertness or retardation. In some psychiatric disorders, one expects some degree of psychomotor retardation, e.g. in depression. Tests like minnesota block reversal tests, pencil tapping test, reaction time, response time, total time and productivity per unit of time, etc. give some indication about it. Gross retardation becomes visible even to naked eye; it is only the milder form of retardation and its degree that requires some finer measurements with the help of psychological tests.

Intelligence Tests

Assessment of intelligence or abilities is required in psychiatric disorders for mainly two reasons: for the diagnosis of mental retardation, which in spite of its limitations, is still mainly based on IQ. Assessment in children,and for differential loss of intellectual functions. The latter helps in:

- Diagnosis of organic brain disorder
- Localization and lateralization or organic brain disorder
- Rehabilitation of patients by assessment of intact functions and of impaired functions
- Assessment of improvement in different functions with time or treatment.

A large number of intelligence tests have been developed and standardized for different age groups and for different abilities and aptitudes. Some of the well-known and well-standardized popular tests of intelligence are given here.

Intelligence Tests for Children

For children below five years, especially for those below two years, there exist development schedules, which describe developmental milestones that are achieved at particular ages and give DA (developmental age) and DQ (developmental quotient) of the child.

$$DQ = \frac{\text{DA (developmental age)}}{\text{CA (chronological age)}} \times 100$$

The ratio of DA to CA is multiplied by 100 to remove decimal points and negative signs, in case of low intelligence, which are at times confusing to most people. It is expected that under normal conditions, DQ would correlate well with later IQ.

$$IQ = \frac{\text{MA (mental age)}}{\text{CA (chronological age)}} \times 100$$

But unfortunately, it is not always necessary in case of children[195] who may have different levels of sensory stimulation at different age levels, may have organic damage or specific organic disorders, resulting in differential developmental delays or loss of functions. Some of the scales measure social age (SA) and social quotient (SQ), e.g. Vineland Social Maturity Scale, so called because of the greater emphasis placed on the social milestones. Similarly, some scales give different quotients for different functions, e.g. Gessell's Developmental Schedule gives five types of quotients, one overall DQ, and four specific quotients, viz. Motor, Adaptive, Language and Personal-Social. Nancy Bayley Scale gives two quotients-Motor and Mental, though the basic principle is the same. These scales, re-standardized in the Indian conditions, include the following:

- Vineland Social Maturity Scale, Nagpur adaptation by Malin[196]
- Gessell's Developmental Schedule, Indian adaptation[197]
- Nancy Baley Scales, adapted at Baroda[198]
- Developmental Screening Test[199]
- Cattell's Infant Intelligence Scale, Indian adaptation,[200] etc.

For little older children, some of the popular tests in use in India are:

- Gessell's Drawing Test[201]
- Seguin Form Board Test[202,203]
- Draw-a-Man Test[204]
- Bhatia's Battery of Performance Tests of Intelligence[205]

- Malin's Intelligence Scale for Indian Children (MISIC)[206]
- Indian adaptation of Stanford-Binet Test[207]
- Bureau of Psychology, UP, Allahabad's Group Verbal Tests of Intelligence
- Proteus Maze Test[208]
- Raven's Colored Progressive Matrices[209]
- Raven's Standard Progressive Matrices[210]
- Cattell's Culture Fair Tests of Intelligence
- Jalota's Group Verbal Intelligence Test[211]
- Differential Aptitude Test Battery, etc.

Many of these tests have been adapted in different Indian languages also.

Intelligence Tests for Adults

Some of the intelligence tests mentioned earlier are for adults also, e.g.

- Bhatia's Battery of Performance Tests of Intelligence[212]
- Stanford-Binet Test[207]
- Proteus Maze Test[208]
- Standard Progressive Matrices,[210] etc.

In addition, there are some tests which are for adults only, e.g.

- Wechsler Adult Intelligence Performance Scale (WAPIS), Indian adaptation[213]
- Hindi WAIS-R Verbal Scale[214,215]
- Advanced Progressive Matrices,[216] etc.

For elderly subjects (above 50 years of age), some of the above tests are used as such, while others use different norms. For examples, Raven's Colored Progressive Matrics has separate norms for elderly, although this test was mainly to be used for children. This is because of deterioration of intellectual functions that occurs with normal aging process. Another test for older subjects is the Set Test[217] wherein they are required to name cities, colors, animals and fruits, etc. Elderly persons have been reported to be poorer performers, as compared to younger adults. For WAIS-R Verbal Tests and for Bhatia's Battery of Performance Tests of Intelligence, modification in scoring and norms for different age, sex and education groups have been developed.

Mental age and age scales have definite disadvantages, like mental growth reaching matured level (plateau), the concept of IQ as a ratio between MA and CA no longer holds good for adults. So, most adult tests nowadays use what is called as 'Deviation IQ' in place of classical IQ, which depends upon the transformed scores with mean for particular age group taken at 100 and obtained standard deviation fixed at 15 to 16. This method has the added advantage of comparability of age groups having different standard deviations, e.g. a person at say 1 standard deviation above the mean will always be 115 IQ for any age group. It also makes constancy of IQs possible with age.

Intelligence tests have been classified in many different ways, e.g. global assessment vs. assessment of different abilities, individual vs. group intelligence tests; verbal vs. nonverbal performance or non-verbal non-performance tests; timed vs. powered tests, etc. It is not possible to describe them at length here. However, some of the important issues and features with regard to the assessment of intelligence are mentioned here. Education is one of the important variables affecting intelligence test scores in India, as educational facilities and opportunities are not easily and equally available to all, because of many non-cognitive factors like poverty, family responsibility, distance from schools and other socioeconomic factors. Recently, some attention to these factors has been given in India, in terms of providing separate norms for different age, sex and educational groups.[212,214,215,218-221]

Some of the tests had been developed a long-time back and these old norms need revision. Work in this direction has already begun, e.g. Draw-a-Man Test,[204] and Bhatia's Battery of Performance Tests of Intelligence.[212] Work with other test batteries has also been started, e.g. Raven's Standard Progressive Matrices, Seguin Form Board Test, Raven's Colored Progressive Matrices, Malin's Intelligence Scale for Indian Children, at some centers in India.

There has been some criticism of the global concept of intelligence and it is suggested that at least verbal and performance abilities should be measured separately. With Wechsler's Intelligence Scales (for children and adults), factorial studies have revealed these as the two strongest components. As and when required, other more specific tests may also be used.

There are many problems encountered in the measurement of intelligence, such as poor test-retest reliabilities at lower age groups (e.g. with developmental schedules),[195] the value of time, spirit of competition, the concept of working for a score etc., particularly in the case of mental retardation[222] and in the area of manutrition.[223]

Tests of Memory

Many neurotic patients complain about impaired memory or forgetfulness, while some, mainly organic patients, are definitely found to be so on standardized and comprehensive memory scales, like Wechsler's Memory Scale,[224] Boston Memory Scale,[225] PGI Memory Scale,[226,227] etc. Out of these, PGI Memory Scale has been specially constructed and standardized for Indian Population, with separate norms for specific and education groups, and is in our national language Hindi. Interestingly, on this test, the profiles of normals and neurotics were found to resemble, while they were found to be different from those of organic and psychotic (mainly schizophrenic) groups. However, organic and schizophrenic groups did not differ from each other significantly. The ten areas of memory included both verbal and non-verbal areas, like memory for recent, remote and immediate events, capacity for forming new associations, verbal and nonverbal memory, mental control (balance), recognition and visual retention.

Besides the above mentioned batteries of memory tests, there exist other memory scales also, which form part of many tests of intelligence or organic test batteries. Such single memory tests include Digit Span Test, Memory for Letters, for Words and for Sentences, Comprehension Tests (stories), etc.

Tests of Perceptual-motor Functions

Most of the patients of organic brain syndrome have been shown to have impaired perceptual-motor functions on standardized tests. For this purpose, a number of tests have been used in India, e.g. Bender Visual-Motor Gestalt Test,[228-230] Nahor and Benson Scale,[231] Hooper's Visual Organization Test,[232,233] Benton Visual Retention Test,[234] etc. All these are primarily western instruments; some work in this area has been done in India, but so far, no new tests seem to have been constructed to suit Indian conditions or special norms prepared for them, with the lone exception of a Smell Matching Test.[235]

Organic Test Batteries

While a number of highly specialized, time consuming, complex test batteries like Luria-Nebraska Test Battery and Halstead-Reitan Neuropsychological Test Battery are available, and some unpublished work is going on to adapt them to Indian conditions at Ranchi and Delhi, work with Indian Test Batteries is also available from Bengaluru, Chandigarh, Delhi and Ranchi centers mainly.[236-241] However, published manual is available only for PGI Battery of Brain Dysfunction (PGI BBD),[241] with detailed instructions for administration, scoring and interpretation, thus enabling other researchers to use it in different studies on epileptics, head trauma, alcoholics, and other cases. PGI BBD include five subtests, viz. PGI Memory scale, WAIS Verbal scale, Bhatia's short revised scale, Bender-Gestalt scale, and Nahor and Benson Scale, and gives a profile on nineteen variables derived from them, as well as a total dysfunction rating score. This is an important area and requires much more concerted efforts by many researchers in order to bear any worthwhile results.

Tests for Abstraction, Judgment, though Disorder and other Related Concepts

Capacity for abstract thinking has been reported to be impaired in certain groups of psychiatric disorders. This leads to concrete thinking in some and may be attributed to faulty filtering mechanism, overinclusion or over-generalization in others. Similarities and Proverbs have been used to measure thought disorders.[242] A Grid Test of Schizophrenic Thought Disorder, when used with Indian subjects, failed to differentiate them.[243] Other tests like Sentence Completion Tests, Finding Absurdities in Pictures, Story Completion Tests, Word Association Tests, Thematic Apperception Test, Children Apperception Test, etc. can also be used to reflect thought disorders. A Linguistic Competence Test Battery[244] has been developed to measure language ability which, it is claimed, is not impaired in schizophrenics; rather linguistic competence determines manifest symptomatology and type of schizophrenia and neurosis.[245] Balodhi[246] has suggested analysis of logical structure of a sentence, as a test for the assessment of thought disorder.

However, these tests have been found to be related to educational levels of the subjects; thereby justifying the use of education-wise norms. For example, on Proverbs and Similarities Tests, it has been found that whereas schizophrenic patients show poor performance when compared to education matched controls. Illiterate/low-literate normal showed even poorer scores as compared to literate schizophrenics.[242] The acceptance rate of the Grid Test for schizophrenic thought disorder was found to be poor in our population.[243] Many subjects, with low education and low test sophistication level, show great resistance and hesitation when asked to rate unknown persons, particularly on negative criteria like cruel, mean, selfish, etc. Besides, other groups of psychiatric patients (like manics) have also been found to score low on this test, suggesting thereby that this is not a specific deficit limited to schizophrenia alone.

Measurement of Personality Variables

This is an area where maximum work seem to be have been done in India and abroad, as reflected in the various year books and handbooks of measuring instruments,[246-248] as well as in different review articles.[249-255] Unfortunately, most of it is still of a repetitive nature or consists of translation of existing questionnaire and rating scales, standardized in the West, without giving due attention to the 'IOC' ('in our culture') aspect.

The instruments in this area are too numerous to be included here, but can be broadly grouped into:

- Personality questionnaires/inventories/rating scales/checklists/criteria for making a diagnosis/interview schedules, etc.
- Projective techniques

It is possible to list only some of the important ones, particularly the ones frequently used/reported and/or standardized in India, with local norms and/or those well adapted/translated.

Personality, as broadly and operationally defined, would include all those characteristics that help predicting what a given person would do in a given situation, under a given mood; but here it is, for convenience sake, defined in a limited sense to include only noncognitive factors, as we have already dealt with cognitive factors and their measurements in the earlier section.

Questionnaires/Rating Scales

Some of the personality questionnaires and rating scales, that have been constructed specially for Indian clinic population, include: PGI Health Questionnaires N-1[256] and N-2,[257] PGI Locus of Control Scale,[258] PGI Achievement Value Index,[259] Subjective Well Being Scale,[260] PGI Well Being Measure,[261] PGI Quality of Life Scale,[262] SPD Scale,[263] Yoga Attitude Scale,[264] Role Stress Questionnaire,[265] Sinha's Anxiety Scale,[266] Dysfunction Analysis Questionnaire,[267] Psychiatric Disability Scale,[268] Amritsar Depressive Inventory,[269] Presumptive Stressful Life Events Scale,[270] Adjustment Inventory for Older People,[271] Jodhpur Multiphasic Personality Inventory (Forms I, II, III for Psychoneurotic, Psychotic and Psychosomatic Disorders,[272] Rajas and Tamas Inventory,[273] P-Questionnaire,[274] Sexuality Scale,[275] Suicidal Intent Questionnaire,[276] CIP Ward Behavior Objective Rating Scale,[277] Murthy's Multiphasic Personality Questionnaire,[278] Thakur Death Anxiety Scale,[279] Learned Helplessness Scale,[280] *Aapaka Vyaktitwa: Ek Naidanik Janch*,[281] Authoritarian Traits Inventory,[282] Command Hospital Questionnaire (to study belief in '*karma*'),[283] Reddy's Alienation Scale,[184] Mishra's Sexual Impotence Rating Scale,[284] Neeliyara's Motivation Scale,[285] Premenstrual Assessment Forms,[286] and Anger Assessment Checklists (for adolescents and parents),[287] etc.

Other psychological tests, that are translations, adaptations or modifications of the well-known personality tests standardized elsewhere, include: Hindi PEN Inventory,[288] Cornell Medical Index Health Questionnaire,[289] Personality Trait Inventory,[290] Spielberger's State-Trait Anxiety Inventory,[291] Illness Behavior Questionnaire,[292] Marital Adjustment Questionnaire,[293] Beck's Inventory for Measuring Depression,[294] Baron's Ego Strength Scale,[295] Rathus Assertiveness Schedule,[296] Junior Eysenck Personality Inventory,[297] Cattell's Anxiety Scale,[298] Neuroticism Scale Questionnaire,[299] Taylor's Manifest Anxiety Scale,[300] Sarason's Anxiety Scales for Children (GASC and TASC),[301] Bells's Adjustment Inventory,[302] Self-esteem Inventory,[303] Self Rating Questionnaire,[304] Dependence Proneness Scale,[305] Bortner Rating Scale,[306] Tripathi Personal Preference Schedule,[307] Middlesex Hospital Questionnaire,[308] Minnesota Personality Inventory,[309] Goldberg's General Health Questionnaire,[310] Sexual Knowledge and Attitude Scale,[311] Leyton Obsessional Inventory,[312] Toronto Alexithymia Scale,[313] Miller's Hope Scale,[314] Moos Menstrual Distress Questionnaire,[315] Bellak et al's Ego Function Assessment (Modified) Scale,[316] David's Insight and Treatment Outcome Questionnaire,[317-319] Vaugham's Questionnaire of Copying Styles in Schizophrenia,[320] Zuckerman et al. Sensation Seeking Scale,[321] Nielsen and Eaton's Senior Medical Student's Attitude Toward Psychiatry Questionnaire,[322] McKenna et al. Quality of Life Scale,[323] and Bond's Defense Style Questionnaire,[324] etc.

In addition, there have been a number of symptom rating scales and checklists frequently used and only very broadly confined to the limits of personality tests-depending upon the way one defines personality. These includes: Scale of the Assessment of Negative Symptoms,[325] Scale for the Assessment of Positive Symptoms,[326] Hamilton's Rating Scale for Depression,[327,328] Lader and Wing's Symptom Rating Scale,[329] Zigmond and Snaith's Hospital Anxiety and Depression Scale,[330] Levin et al. Neurobehavioral Rating Scale,[331] Simpson-Angus Extra-pyramidal Side Effect Scale,[332] Simpson Tardive Dyskinesia Rating Scale,[333] Schooler and Kane Criteria for Tardive Dyskinesia,[334] Kanner et al. Hassles and Uplifts Scale,[335] Caplan et al. Social Support Scale,[335] Schwartz et al. Cognitive Somatic Anxiety Questionnaire,[336] Bernstein and Putnam's Questionnaire of Experiences of Dissociation,[337] Hyperactive Behavior Checklist,[338,339] Abbreviated Conner's Teacher's Rating Scale,[338,339] Observer Rating Scale,[338,339] Child Behavior Questionnaire,[338,339] and Cognitive Failure Scale of Broadbent et al,[340] etc.

Many of the above tests have been translated in one or more Indian languages at different places. While some of the scales are being used in India in original form as well as in adapted/translated terms, depending upon the educational level of the subjects and their language. Others have not been translated/adapted and are being used with educated samples only.

There are many difficulties in translating/adapting a foreign test to Indian situations and languages because of the cultural differences.[341] The majority of the clinic population in India is rural, illiterate/low-literate and unsophisticated in the use of these tests. They require simple tests which are easy to comprehend and the medical model of presentation in terms of symptoms or complaints is found to be more acceptable to them. The difficulty levels of some of the tests/adaptations are found to be very high,[342] and many tests are poorly standardized and/or have high social desirability response biases.[343]

Unfortunately, there is little agreement among workers about the exact number of personality factors and/or of these constructs. Test constructors have come out with a large number of tests measuring overlapping dimensions or traits, and some of the tests measuring the same dimensions corelate very poorly among themselves, e.g. Anxiety scales, Extraversion scales, Type A personality tests, etc. There are very few measures of personality disorders and of personality dynamics, and whatever are there, are not well-standardized, leaving a lot to be desired.

Despite all this, the literature in this area is fast growing and there is increasing awareness and concern about the quality of personality measurements through these questionnaires and relating scales.

Projective Techniques

Whereas most of these questionnaires and rating scales are subject to motivational distortions, and other response biases, projective techniques are relatively free form them, though they suffer from some other limitations. Views violently differ with regard to even the employment of projective techniques in clinical settings. There are some psychologists who would not like others to use them without intensive and prolonged training with large number of subjects. On the other hand, there are others, who not only do not want to have anything to do with them themselves, but also want to throw away these instruments as invalid and useless ones. Truth however, seems to lie somewhere in between these two warring positions, for projective techniques have shown definite advantages over other tools and can be gainfully employed to provide additional, useful and reliable/valid information about the patients. But obviously, they are not answers for everything and cannot be blamed for all the ills or limitations of psychometric approach to human behavior. Judiciously used, they can have a useful role to play in personality assessment.

In case of projective techniques, the stimulus material is relatively unstructured and vague. It can be interpreted differently by different persons. These techniques differ from one another with regard to the degree of vagueness or structure. There are some tests, which are relatively more structured than others, e.g Rorschach Inkblot Test is more unstructured than Thematic Apperception Test or Children Apperception Test. The aim of all these tests is relatively disguised, i.e. one is never sure how his responses would be interpreted or evaluated, with the result that possible effects of motivational distortion are considerably reduced, if not eliminated altogether. However, in some cases, this may also lead to increased anxiety, and this is one of the reasons for the recommendation that projective tests should not be the first test to be used with anxious subjects. Some of the tests can be described as completion tests, e.g. Sentence Completion Test, Story Completion Test, Picture Completion Test, Make a Picture Story Test, etc. Others may be described as interpretation tests like Rorschach, TAT, CAT, etc. Still others are some which can be grouped as construction techniques, e.g. Draw A Person Test, Draw A Hut Test, Play, Draw A Penis Test, etc. In fact, there are a variety of overlapping ways to classify projective techniques.

As opposed to other psychometric tests, projective techniques aim more at the description of personality, rather than attempt at actually measuring it. They are relatively less objective and less amenable to reliability and validity exercises. Scoring and interpretations are complex; administering them more of an art to be mastered, a skill to be developed. All these are generally true for some of the techniques like Rorschach, but there are also different approaches to it, like Objective Rorschach, Multiple Response Rorschach, besides various objective indexes (e.g. Elizur's Hostility Scores, Pitrowsky's Signs of Organicity, Prognostic Rorschach Index, Homosexuality Index, etc.). It is because of these variations that projective tests are frequently described as more of 'techniques' rather than specific tests. However, one can argue both ways. There are a number of reliability and validity studies reported with them. By far, the commonest tests used in India psychiatric researches include Rorschach Ink Blot Test with Indian norms,[344-346] Holtzman Inkblot Techniques,[347,348] Thematic Apperception Test-Indian Adaptation,[349] Children Apperception Test—Indian Adaptation,[350] Sentence Completion Test (a number of scales in India are available), Draw A Person Test (requires only paper and pencil; Interpretations are based on the work of Karen Machover, with Indian workers providing some additional validating research),[357] Rosenzweig Picture Frustration Study (Indian adaptation of both child and adult forms), Malhotra and Wig's Vignetts,[352] and Murthy's Pictures for Attitudinal Research.[353] Others include Kahn Test of Symbol Arrangement,[354] Dosanjh D Test,[355] Word Association Tests, Three Wishes Test, etc.

Out of these, the maximum work has been done with Rorschach Test, for which norms are available with varied populations including normals,[356] army personnel,[357] epileptics,[358] neurotics,[359] impotence cases,[360] schizophrenics,[361-363] depressives, etc. The Rorschach test consists of ten standard inkblots, five of them noncolored, i.e. black, white and gray colors (cards I, IV, V, VI, VII) and five colored ones, with two cards having red color (II, III) and three being multicolored ones (VIII, IX, X). Scoring depends upon location (whole, major and minor details, unusual detail area, space, etc.), determinants (form, color, movements, shading, vista, etc.) and contents (human, animal, anatomy, object, nature, plant, sex, etc.), mainly. This test is rated as one of the most frequent five tests used in India for psychodiagnostics. Pershad and Dubey[364] have shown that Rorschach indices should not be interpreted in absolute terms, rather they depend upon the number of responses per protocol. Some researchers prefer Holtzman Inkblot Technique (HIT) because of this and for its greater objectivity in scoring.[347]

One of the main uses of Rorschach has been in detecting early schizophrenic (or preschizophrenic) patients, and for differential diagnosis, but it has been used for other purposes as well, e.g.

- *Detecting organicity*: The validity of Pitrowsky's signs of organicity has not been substantiated by Indian researches, though it is sometimes reported to be helpful in selected cases.
- *Measuring hostility*: Elizur's hostility scoring procedure has been used in a number of studies in India and has met with moderate success.
- *Screening psychopathology*: Sometimes used for selection of candidates for various jobs. Although, as such no research data is available for this purpose, it is reported to be successful in keeping out those who are later likely

to develop psychiatric disorders or were suffering from it already.

- Studying *personality patterns* of different groups of subjects, e.g. doctors, engineers, hysterics, psychopaths, drug addicts, alcoholics, prisoners, criminals, etc.
- Selecting candidates with greater degree of originality, creativity, *ego strength*, leadership quality, etc.
- Indicating *prognosis* in individual cases suffering from psychiatric disorders.
- Evaluating *treatment outcomes.*
- Assessing *degree of improvement*, if any, in individual cases.

Perusal of literature points to dissatisfaction with relatively uneconomic, time consuming, traditional procedures of evaluation in most of the projective tests, with increasing demands for the briefer techniques. While not replacing the more intensive projective methods, they offer important, at times dramatic, insights to time-harassed clinicians. These briefer, more objective modifications in the case of Rorschach include Multiple Choice Rorschach, P. O'Reilly's Objective Rorschach, Rorschach Inetrview, Process Anaysis, Objective Counseling, etc.[365] A recent extensive review of Rorschach studies[346] shows that it faces an uncertain future and possible eclipse.

There are a number of scoring methods available (Rorschach's, Rapaport's, Beck's, Klopfer's, Kumar's, Prabhu's, Asthana's, etc.) also for computing different indexes based on specific signs. On the one hand, some psychologists prefer 'global' descriptive approach which depends upon the relative expertise of the tester; on the other hand, some prefer a more limited and a more objective 'sign' approach. Both these approaches have their advantages and limitations.

Recently, a new inkblot series, the somatic inkblot series (SIS), has come up. Developed by an American Psychiatrist, Wilfred A. Cassell, SIS continues Rorschach's conceptualization that individuals project their own unique mental imagery into ambiguous and semiambiguous visual stimuli.[366-369] SIS has five forms (cards, booklets and videotapes). It provides multidisciplinary enhancement, not available when Rorschach was developing the inkblot techniques. The test is found to be reliable and valid in India.[370-376] Recently, a new association (Somatic Inkblot Society) has come out with a research journal, SIS Journal of Projective Psychology and Mental Health (1994), the first of its kind in India.

Murray's thematic apperception test (TAT) has over a dozen methods of scoring, made on thirty pictures and one blank card (20 for each age and sex group, e.g. boy/gird/man/woman, or any combination of these), including that of Murray himself, in terms of *needs, presses* and *outcome.* The method by Vorhous is the one which has gained wider acceptance among various workers, but other methods are also in use, like the one developed by Bureau of Psychology, UP, Allahabad. The clinician, when pressed for time, may also use an overall global impression for limited use, e.g. in assessing the personality of patients in therapy or in evaluating the outcome, comparing it with earlier studies. TAT has been adapted and abridged at Allahabad (Bureau of Psychology, UP) and by Uma Choudhary at Calcutta. The TAT manuals published by Bureau of Psychology, Allahabad and by Uma Choudhary, try to adopt an eclectic approach, and both have changed the original pictures to suit Indian conditions while keeping their need values intact. The number of cards has been reduced to ten for each age and sex group.

Miscellaneous Scales

Some of the psychiatric instruments do not fall in clear-cut categories. They are, for convenience sake, put in this group of miscellaneous scales. Some of these may have been put in more than one category also, depending upon the way one looks upon them or, upon the use to which they can and have been put. These include a number of scales to measure socioeconomic status,[377-383] rating of symptoms and of improvements,[384] tools to study family interaction,[385,386] parental attitude scales,[387,388] social support scales,[389,390] perceived burden scales,[391] attitude toward mental illness and related issues,[392-395] family jointedness scale,[396] patient's satisfaction in a general hospital,[397] family typology scale,[398] behavior rating scale for mentally handicapped,[399] a modified version of KAS behavior inventory,[400] repertory grid technique,[401] symptom checklist for hyperactive children,[402] etc.

Other Related Issues

One of the most important problems facing psychiatric research is the lack of sophistication in the use of statistical designs and measurement techniques in the published work. A number of studies relate to this problem, both in India and abroad. The number of articles pointing out this, and the figures they quote about the percentage of articles with such deficiencies or errors (70–100%), are indeed staggering, both for medical and psychiatric research.[403-407]

Many of these deficiencies are because of carelessness and therefore are easily avoidable. Also, more attention needs to be given to the training of psychiatric residents, with regard to statistics and research methodology. Another related issue in the published work is the lack of awareness about the possible sources of errors and biases in the data collection. Even if the basic experimental design and statistical treatment of the data are excellent or flawless, if the basic data is not reliable or not collected as planned, any amount of later treatment can not rid it of these biases. This is often the case when different studies, trying to replicate the original one, are not able to confirm the earlier findings. They, then, add to the prevailing confusion, with misleading, invalid and contradictory results and conclusions.

Then, there is also the question of ethical consideration in such researches. In most of the research institutes, lately, ethical committees have been formed and ethical clearance is one of the essential requirements of any research project, even before it is considered for financial support by such national bodies as the Indian Council of Medical Research, Indian Council of Social Science Research, or even by foreign financial sources, like the WHO. Still, all research projects may not have been financed, and in such self-financed researches also, it is the awareness of ethical issues, which has to be given it due share by the researchers, e.g. the question of confidentiality, informed consent, benefit to the subject/patient by the research, invasion of patient's privacy, imposition of one's own value system on the patient, among many others.

SUMMARY AND SUGGESTIONS

The above review of measurements in psychiatry points out clearly the following conclusions:

- A lot of effort is being made in this area of measurement in psychiatry and the attempts have met with some, though limited, success. There are a number of tools to measure many cognitive, noncognitive, personality, diagnostic, and outcome related measures.
- There are a variety of objective measurement tools available in most areas, including interview schedules, questionnaires, rating scales, projective techniques, etc. for measuring many areas of human behavior in which psychiatrists might be interested. They need to be critically examined, modified and updated from time-to-time and cross-validated in different cultures and subcultures before use.
- The quality of these instruments is improving with increasing attention being paid to objectivity, reliability, validity, cross-validity, local norms, cut-off points, difficulty levels and various confounding variables, like tendency to give socially, desirable responses, 'yeah saying' and 'nay saying', tendency to choose middle responses or extreme responses, halo effect in rating scales, and many other response tendencies that may bias the test results. This is a continuous process and needs to be continually addressed.
- Increasing attention is also being given to the cross-cultural variables in measurement, like the culturally appropriate items and questions, understood even by the unsophisticated, rural subjects with the lowest educational levels, who form the bulk of our clinic population in India today. Sophistication levels of the instruments have to be kept at culturally acceptable and appropriate forms, neither at a level too high and complex, not at too low and crude a level. At the same time, attempts are afoot to understand both the similarities and differences among different cultures on a number of variables at diagnostic, therapeutic and intervention levels, and also to measure them in definite quantitative terms.
- In spite of all this, however, in many areas we still find the measurement tools developed in the West, being used with utter disregard for the IOC (in our culture), mentioning sometimes even apologetically, about the lack of availability of well-standardized tools in our country, for our population. Partly, this is also because of the lack of expertise in sufficient numbers, with the lame excuse that too few have to look after too many and, therefore, hardly find sufficient time for such researches that are needed for it. Partly, this may also be because of lack of understanding of need for local norms and, to some extent, our lack of knowledge of the work already done, most of which remains unpublished or is published in some remote journals in India or abroad. There is a need to share knowledge and experience with other co-workers in India. The phrase, 'no work seems to have been reported in this area from India', is often found in Indian research and found, more often than not, to be untrue. This has often resulted in wasteful, avoidable efforts, which have gone into the duplication of the similar work at different places. For example, some of the research tools have been translated in Hindi at many different places, often without being aware of the existence of such work at other centers.
- The reasons for our lagging behind the other developed countries are many and include the lack of trained manpower and financial resources. There are markedly fewer trained psychiatrists and clinical psychologists in India, as compared to those in the developed countries. Financial resources in this area are meagre. We are still dominated by older generation of academicians at many places, majority of whom had little training in, and unfortunately also seem to have little faith in, the more sophisticated statistical and research methodological techniques. Rather, there is a mistrust among them, most probably a fear, of the numbers, and the unmistakable resistance to systematically analyze their vast experience, which they would still like to quote, as and when they please, in qualitative and descriptive terms only.
- Fortunately, the situation is gradually but definitely changing, with the need and importance of culturally appropriate psychometric tools acceptable, suitable, reliable, and valid for our (majority of whom are rural, uneducated or poorly educated, and unsophisticated about these tools) being recognized by such national bodies as ICMR, ICSSR, NCERT, Indian Psychiatric Society, Indian Psychological Association, Indian Association of Clinical Psychologists, and by the international bodies like World Health Organization, and by individual crusaders among the professionals. It is in the interest of Psychiatry in India that it should remain so and gain momentum in the years to come.

45.4 EPIDEMIOLOGY AND RESEARCH METHODS

RC Chowdhary, Hemant Vyas

INTRODUCTION

Epidemiology can be defined as 'the study of the distribution and determinants of health-related states or events in specified populations' (Last 1995) or simply as examinations of the frequency and associations of disease. It includes the study of causes, in terms of etiological or risk factor but does not include the study of pathophysiological mechanisms, which is the province of biomedical research. These two approaches, however, are obviously complementary, and the fundamental methods used are the same. Both 'psychiatric epidemiologists' and 'biological psychiatrists' pay close attention to case identification, control selection, accurate measurement and minimizing bias in executing and interpreting research studies. Both can choose from a variety of research methods to study a particular issue, constrained by what is practicable.

Research—as simply 'the organized quest for new knowledge' (Last 1995)—has a long history, whereas epidemiology is generally regarded as having begun (in 1849) with John Snow's famous localization of an outbreak of cholera in London to a particular water pump. The methods that both employ have, however, been considerably developed since that time, particularly over the last 50 years or so, and continue to be refined. It is, only comparatively recently that the case report and case series have been superseded by controlled studies of the causes and treatments of disease (Hennekens & Buring 1987). Much of contemporary medicine remains on comparatively shaky scientific foundations, and it is only through carefully conducted further study that we will be able to further improve on what we can currently offer our patients. Laboratory-based basic science ('blue skies research') and population-based epidemiology aim to deliver a greater understanding of the causes of disease, with the prospect of earlier detection, better treatment and even prevention. Therapeutic and health services research seeks to refine currently available treatments, optimize their delivery to those most likely to benefit, and be able to test any new therapies as and when they arise. Progress may seem frustratingly slow, but that is inevitable if the science is to be rigorously conducted and evaluated.

Epidemiology and research methods also underpin clinical practice in other ways. Several components of public health necessarily use such principles in determining disease prevalence and needs assessment for planning services, implementing and evaluating disease screening and assessing the population impact of causative factors with a view to prevention. The application of epidemiological and statistical principles to everyday clinical decisions used to be described as clinical epidemiology (Sackett et al. 1991) and has, over the past 10 years or so, led to the development and implementation of evidence-based medicine.

ETHICAL CONSIDERATIONS

The ethics of clinical research rest upon and are little different from the ethics of clinical practice. The fundamental principles of least harm, confidentiality and informed consent, which are the cornerstones of good clinical practice, are the same (Wing 1981). Clinicians and medical researchers both confront these issues daily. The principal difference between the two is that research does not aim to directly benefit an individual, although it may do so, whereas clinical practice does have this aim but may not. Even this distinction is muddied when one considers innovative clinical practice and audit.

Above all, do no harm: Most research does not lead to any harm to those involved. Indeed, there is some evidence that patient outcomes are better if treated within the disciplined context of a clinical trail than in routine clinical practice. Some procedures are physically or 'mentally' invasive, but usually lead only to transient discomfort and distress. This is also true of pharmacological evaluation studies. If a comparatively new product is being tested, then some insurance or indemnity agreement may be necessary for potentially serious adverse effects. Provided any risks are minimized and frankly acknowledged, so that truly informed consent is possible, these types of study do not pose any particular ethical issues.

There have, however, been extensive recent discussions about whether placebo-controlled trials are ethical in serious diseases, the recommendation in the fifth revision of the Declaration of Helsinki (Vastag 2000) that they should no longer be conducted. This is a complex issue, as place placebo-controlled trials provide their own check of internal validity—and trials comparing new and old drugs need to be much larger than these if they are to have enough power to show true equivalence rather than just no difference. It may not be ethically acceptable to compare any new antipsychotic or antidepressant drug against placebo, given that the evidence for the efficacy of the standard treatments is generally regarded as overwhelming, but it is definitely unethical to conduct research that cannot deliver a reliable answer. Many medical trials get round this problem by comparing a new treatment plus standard care versus standard treatment. At the very least, researchers clearly need to pay close attention to what kind of treatment participants are offered at the termination of a trial, particularly if they have been treated with placebo.

Maintain confidentiality: Research data are technically part of a person's medical record and are, therefore, confidential. Scientific data should generally be stored anonymously and in a locked facility. Issues of confidentiality rarely give rise to problems during research projects—it should be communicated to the patient's own doctor, and usually to the patient, as it is in the latter's best interests to do so.

Obtain informed consent: Particular attention needs to be paid to the process of enrolling participants in any study. Potential subjects should be able to give 'fully informed consent' in that they fully appreciate the purpose and nature of the study, as well as the potential risks and benefits to them. This is an unarguable principle but easier said than done. Even people of above average IQ have difficulty understanding some scientific concepts (e.g. randomization), cannot be expected to grasp subtle academic points, and can only be meaningfully informed about and retain the principal risks involved (cf. consent to clinical treatments). The information given obviously has to be selective, but there is no guidance on how. It is cleared, however, that there is a potential for conflict interest if patient's clinicians are seeking to enroll them in their own studies—if so, an independent clinician should be involved in seeking consent.

There may be particular issues about obtaining valid informed consent in people with psychiatric disorders and learning disabilities, but these are often overstated in a potentially prejudicial way (Roberts et al. 2002). Patients who are detained (or imprisoned) are rarely included in, and often specifically excluded from, most research and clinical trials in particular. They may well still be capable of consenting to a study and are arguable worse served by a dearth or complete absence of relevant treatment information. Some recent reports, highlighted in a number of American and European newspapers, have suggested that even relatively stable psychotic patients may fail one or more of a number of criteria that establish whether somebody is able to give informed consent. Some work indicates that this problem is related more to cognitive impairment than psychotic symptoms, and can be overcome by spending more time with potential subjects (Carpenter et al. 2000).

Ethical issues arise during the planning, conduct and analysis stages of any investigation. A worthwhile study needs to address a genuinely unresolved question with robust methods that are likely to provide a useful answer. It is therefore desirable to conduct a systematic review of the available evidence before at new study, both to check the question has not already been answered and to inform design. Studies which are poorly designed or likely to be inconclusive are unethical, as they expose patients to unnecessary and potentially dangerous interventions. If there is a sound rationale for doing a particular study, a research protocol needs to be submitted along with answers to standard questions to local Ethical Committees.

Ethical Committee practices vary, however, from region to region and country to country. This has given rise to the unsatisfactory situation where an ethical application for a multicenter trial may be approved in one region, but rejected in another (Savulescu et al. 1996). Research participants should not be paid for doing research, but they are entitled to receive compensation for, e.g. travel and subsistence expenses. It need hardly be said that fraudulent analysis or presentation of the results of a study are unethical, as they are at best misleading and could actually endanger lives. Fraud is rare, however; sloppy research and conclusions not supported by the data are much more common.

ARCHITECTURE OF CLINICAL RESEARCH

There are essential three classes of clinical research study (Feinstein 1985):

- *Descriptive observational studies:* These usually describe the characteristics of a clinical population without a control group, and are, therefore, suitable only for hypothesis generation rather than testing. Examples include case reports and series, audit, qualitative studies and surveys.
- *Analytical observational studies:* These generally compare two subject groups, cases and controls, and are suitable for hypothesis testing. Ideally, the study and control groups are similar in all but the characteristic of main interest, i.e. demographically similar, but with and without disease (in case-control studies) or having been subject to a particular exposure or not (in cohort studies).
- *Experimental studies:* These can be used to directly infer causation or to assess the effect of treatment, as something is given or done to an experimental group but not to a control group (of patients). Controlled trials have similar strengths as experimental studies in laboratory settings, but efforts to minimize bias and measurement error are usually greater in trials, and random treatment allocation is rare in lab work.

These distinctions are not absolute. Some audits and surveys include control groups, while some cohort studies (e.g. of the prognosis of a disease) do not. Similarly, some so called 'clinical trials' are not experimental and are merely uncontrolled case series.

There is also another types of research that does not fit easily into this scheme—so-called *secondary research*—that is, systematic reviews and meta analyses of the existing literature. These can generate the most reliable results of all and are increasingly used to inform the development of clinical guidelines.

DESCRIPTIVE STUDIES

Case Reports and Case Series

There are simple descriptions of clinical observations, sometimes with results of investigations, in one or a small group of patients. The patients tend to be opportunistically identified from a single location, subject to all kinds of selection biases and hence unrepresentative. Any unusual constellation of features may be coincidental in the absence of a control group. For example, it was quit common 10 years or so ago to see reports of two or more 'specific' delusional syndromes in a particular patient when the patient may simply have had an unusual case of schizophrenia. Case studies are susceptible to misdiagnosis, bias and measurement error. This makes them unreliable (and often unrepeatable).

However, case reports and series should generally be regarded as means of only identifying priorities or hypotheses for further and more comprehensive study (Box 1). Clinical experience is essentially a series of extended case series, in which one is most likely to remember the most dramatic successes and failures (recall bias).

Clinical Audit

Audit, as the 'examination of the extent to which a condition, process or performance conforms to predetermined standards or criteria' (Last 1995), is not strictly speaking a research method, but is included here as it typically uses research methods and arguably should be conducted routinely by every medical practitioner. The key distinguishing features include the measurement of clinical performance against a standard, some attempt to improve this performance and then a re-audit, to 'close the audit cycle', to assess any improvement. In a sense, if patients are studied before and after some initiative, they could be regarded as their own controls but 'historical controls' are notoriously prone to bias as there are so many influences on medical services, patients' well-being and outcomes over time. The same concerns are pertinent in so-called 'mirror image' studies of the effects of treatments in what are essentially uncontrolled trials.

Box 1: Characteristics, strengths and limitations of case reports and series	
Describe the clinical features or outcome in one or more patients	
Strengths	
•	Arise from clinical practice
•	Quick and easy
•	May have important general implications
Limitations	
•	Apparent associations may be due to coincidence
•	Nonsystematic retrospective studies
•	Unreliable results: Misdiagnosis, measurement error, bias and confounding (see further)

Almost any aspect of clinical care can be audited, which can be conveniently classified as:

- *Service structure,* e.g. personnel, equipment;
- *A process of care,* e.g. note-keeping, investigation use and utility, treatments;
- *Clinical outcomes,* e.g. morbidity, mortality.

Clinical outcomes are arguably the most important, as they measure local clinical effectiveness, but can be difficult to define and measure. Outcomes are rarely systematically recorded in hospital records.

Audit has some potential to improve local services, but the evidence for its impact on clinical care is very limited and its effects are modest (O'Brien et al. 2002a, b). Guyatt (1996) have helpfully summarized the optimal, if somewhat stringent, criteria for assssing the quality of a clinical audit report (Box 2). In the absence of any really good pragmatic guides to (psychiatric) audit, critical appraisal criteria can usefully highlight the chief issues to be considered in designing an audit project.

These criteria are however far from exhaustive. Other important issues to consider include the completeness of case ascertainment and data collection, and any bias in assessing case records/data extraction. Training, experience and support are required in audit study design, particularly for quality control of data collection and management, as with all research. It is therefore concerning that clinicians who might otherwise be hesitant to conduct observational research will attempt clinical audit without any methodological expertise or assistance.

Box 2: Critical appraisal of a clinical audit	
I.	*Are the criteria (standards) valid?*
•	Was an explicit and sensible process used to identify, select, and combine evidence for the criteria?
•	What is the quality of the evidence used in framing the criteria?
•	Was an explicit and sensible process used to consider the relative values of different outcomes?
•	Are the judgments of the experts who established the criteria was weak, have the criteria been prospectively evaluated and shown to improve patient outcomes?
II.	*Were the criteria applied appropriately?*
•	Did the process of applying the criteria meet scientific standards (e.g. auditors blind to practitioner or institution identity, admixture of index cases as accuracy checks, random or consecutive sampling, and adequate sample size)?
•	What is the impact of uncertainty associated with evidence and values on the criteria-based of process of care?
III.	*Can you use the criteria in your own practice setting?*
•	Have the criteria been field-tested for feasibility of use in diverse settings?
•	Are the criteria up-to-date?

Qualitative Studies

Most medical research is quantitative, in that variables are 'objectively' measured in numerical terms and summarized or analyzed statistically. Qualitative research of peoples' experiences, feelings, values and other types of opinion are seen as increasingly important. Complex issues and behaviors may not be easily amenable to quantitative approaches and may be better explored qualitatively. Qualitative studies may thus complement and even inform quantitative approaches by, e.g. generating ideas and hypotheses for further testing and assisting in questionnaire development where relevant variables are not obviously apparent. They are often useful adjuncts to clinical trials, to identify why people might wish to participate or not, establish the feasibility of the trial and thus reduce difficulties in recruitment and follow-up.

Qualitative studies are not necessarily subjective or unscientific. Data are usually gathered with semistructured interviews, in focus groups and/or through observation. Objectivity can be ensured by recording these observations, on audio or video-tape, and obtaining independent ratings by multiple passing through the recordings, and/or with a variety of increasingly sophisticated software programs. Direct quotations, addressing a clearly formulated initial question a clear account of the researchers' perspectives and the explicit consideration of various explanations of the data all serve to improve the validity of a qualitative study. Each of the main approaches to data collection have their own advantages and disadvantages: individual interviews elicit specific opinions but may not generalize; a focus group can establish a group norm, but minority views may be obscured; and direct observation of behavior (rather than just attitudes) in natural settings may give the strongest results, but may lose individual detail. The best methods depend upon the phenomenon under investigation, but as a general rule, it is desirable to collect data from more than one source. In addition, recent studies are increasingly adopting 'purposive sampling', to derive representative samples with desirable demographic characteristics. The essential features, strengths and limitations of qualitative studies are summarized in Box 3.

There are, in addition, two qualitative approaches that habitually use quantitative techniques, particularly questionnaires, to deliver consensus in controversial areas, such as therapeutic approaches to particular disorders. The two most commonly used are the so-called *Delphi or Delphic process* and the *nominal group (or expert panel) technique*. Both approaches require the initial definition of a problem and the selection of 'experts'. Questionnaires elicit responses to a range of therapeutic options, which participants rate anonymously; that process continues or 'iterates', with participants receiving feedback on how their response compares with that of the group, and the opportunity to change their initial response, until consensus is achieved.

Box 3: Essential features, strengths and limitations of qualitative studies	
Collect data on opinions, to generate ideas and hypotheses (i.e. inductive rather than deductive reasoning)	
Strengths	
•	Offers insight when research is not well-established or conventional theories seem inadequate
•	Have validity, provided they are well-conducted
•	Can inform and improve quantitative research
Limitations	
•	Prone to researchers' bias in the collection and analysis of data
•	Without direct observation, attitudes do not necessarily equate to behavior
•	May lack reliability, particularly if only one rater analyses responses

There are slight differences in how the experts are selected, the questionnaires constructed and results fed back to participants; see Jones & Hunter (1995) for further details. These techniques have not been widely used, in psychiatry or medicine, but have already been used to assist in the development of clinical guidelines for the use of psychological therapies in the UK and the management of bipolar disorder in the USA. In all such uses, consensus-delivering techniques are complementary to, but should not replace, the systematic review of the literature arid grading of recommendations desirable for valid clinical guidelines.

Surveys

Survey is an ambiguous word, being merely 'the systematic collection of information' (Last 1995). Indeed, one sees at least three different uses of the word in the medical literature. It is relatively common to see the term 'questionnaire survey', particularly in accounts of often hastily cobbled together questions being set out in the hope of eliciting opinions about medical training or practice, usually obtaining low, uninformative response rates. These are, in fact, simply poor qualitative studies or case series. The term survey is more accurately applied to *two-phase epidemiological surveys* (screening questionnaire then interview) to determine the prevalence of a disease and other types of cross-sectional study. These should not be confused with surveillance studies, e.g. the active or passive monitoring of adverse drug effects in phase IV 'clinical trials'. The key feature of *cross-sectional studies* is that they simultaneously ascertain the presence of absence of disease and the presence or absence of an exposure, at one particular point in time. They are, therefore, studies of prevalence or frequency and sometimes called so, and cannot reliably distinguish between cause and effect.

These studies need to pay particular attention to potential biases in population sampling. In an attempt to ensure that the population studied is representative, surveys tend to take a random sample from, e.g. census data, the electoral roll or even a telephone directory. All of these are probably better than attempting to accost people in the street, but will, of course, miss those who move frequently, do not pay their 'community charge' or do not have a telephone—and psychiatric patients are probably over-represented in each category. Patients will be difficult to contact at home if they are currently hospitalized or in prison. Making false associations through 'sampling bias' is known as *Berkson's fallacy (or bias).*

Close attention must equally be paid to how potential participants are approached. In large studies, such as two-phase epidemiological surveys of rare illnesses, it is standard to send out postal questionnaires because interviewing everybody would be too costly. Edwards et al (2002) systematically reviewed randomized controlled trials to compare methods of maximizing response rates to postal questionnaires; they found that response was approximately doubled when questionnaires were sent out by recorded delivery, were short, and were designed to be of interest to participants and when monetary incentives were offered. Response rates were also increased by such factors as personalizing questionnaires and letters, using stamped returned envelopes, contacting participants before sending questionnaires, follow-up contact, providing non-responders with a second questionnaire and even using colored ink. Questionnaires including sensitive questions were less likely to be returned. It is a general rule of clinical interviewing and questionnaire design that questions should be unambiguous and two questions should not be combined in one. Consideration of these issues is crucial to obtaining a response rate, in the region of 80–90%, which allows confidence in the results. Telephone or personal contact for a relatively brief interview may be more successful, particularly in a psychiatric population, as those affected with psychiatric disorders are known to be less likely to respond to questionnaires. A particular type of cross-sectional survey, the ecological or correlational study, avoids the potential problems of response bias by examining pre-existing data on exposures and outcomes in populations rather than individual. Usually routinely collected data on disease rates is compared with data on the general level of exposure between particular geographical regions.

In summary, descriptive observational research is comparatively quick and easy, and useful to develop new hypotheses, but cannot reliably test hypotheses or discern causal relationships. The main features of the individual types of study are summarized in Table 2. Those interested in further information are referred to excellent introductory (Hennekens & Buring 1987) or detailed (Feinstein 1985) epidemiology textbooks, a serried of recent articles in the Lancet (Grimes & Schulz 2002) or Lawrie et al. (2000).

ANALYTICAL STUDIES

Case-control Studies

In a case-control study, individuals with a particular condition or disease (the cases) are selected and compared with individuals without the condition or disease (the controls). The case-control comparison is the frequency of previous exposures or attributes potentially relevant to the development of the condition or disease under study. In essence, therefore, disease status is determined before exposure status. The development and increasing use of case-control studies, such that they are now the most common type of study published in medical journals, has largely followed their initial use in cancer epidemiology. Their relatively simple approach can identify important effects. They are particularly suitable in rare diseases or those that take a long time to develop, as in mist psychiatric disorders. Many potential exposures can be investigated simultaneously (Box 4).

Case-control studies also have to deal with various types of 'information bias' as the exposure is being assessed retrospectively. In particular, if subjects are asked whether or not they have been exposed, 'recall bias' commonly arises because those affected 'search after meaning' in seeking an

Table 2: Summary features of descriptive observational studies

Type of study	*Essential features*	*Advantages*	*Disadvantages*
Case report	Observations in a single case	Cheap and easy way of generating hypotheses	Liable to coincidence, error, bias and confounding
Case series	Disease characteristics in a number of cases	May be the best information on very rare diseases	No comparison group, so cannot test hypotheses
Audit	Examines service provision and outcome	Gives information on service delivery	Unreliable estimate of effectiveness
Qualitative study	Elicits opinion	Can illuminate complex issues	May be unreliable
Cross-sectional study	Measures rates of disease	Identifies patterns of disease	Cannot distinguish cause and effect
Ecological study	Measures associations of disease	Can use prerecorded data	Describes populations rather than individuals

Box 4: Case-control studies	
Compare cases and controls on the relative frequencies of one or more exposure	
Strengths	
•	Relatively quick and inexpensive
•	Suitable for rare diseases
•	Can evaluate distant and multiple exposures
Limitations	
•	Unsuitable for rare exposures
•	Susceptible, in particular, to selection bias
•	Susceptible to recall bias and reverse causality

explanation for their illness. This can apply equally to relatives or carers. Perhaps the best example of this in the psychiatric literature comes from studies of the association between life events and depression, where depressed mood may also influence the recall of particular events. For this reason, life events researchers now focus on so called 'independent events' such as bereavement, and especially those that can be verified as preceding the outcome, to avoid the possibility of 'reverse causality'. Similar difficulties can affect researchers, with 'observer bias' resulting from researchers not being blind to, or being able to guess, disease status and searching more rigorously for exposures in the cases. Some of these problems can be reduced, but not avoided entirely, by using pre-recorded exposure information.

One of the common methods to deal with selection bias is to match cases and controls on one or more important characteristics, e.g. sex. This has the advantage of improving the power of the study, but runs the risk of seriously limiting the number of suitable subjects, over matching and reducing associations, and makes it impossible to examine the effects of the matched variables statistically. It is usually better, therefore, to measure any potential confounder and to correct for it statistically unless the effect of a confounder is particularly large and can only be quantified with difficulty. Either approach, however, requires that the investigators know what the confounders are or might be.

For these reasons, exposures are, in general, more reliably related to particular diseases in prospective cohort studies. Shulz & Grimes (2002a) have, however, recently suggested five guidelines for investigators planning (or appraising) case-control studies:

- Explicitly define case diagnosis and eligibility criteria.
- Select controls from the same population as cases, independent of the exposure of interest.
- Train data gatherers to elicit exposure in a similar manner from cases and controls, e.g. using memory aids to facilitate and balance recall in both.
- Blind the data gatherers to case or control status (or at least to the main hypothesis of the study).
- Address confounding factors, either in the design stage or during analysis.

Cohort Studies

Cohort studies first classify subjects according to whether or not they have been exposed to a suspected risk factor, or have a particular attribute, and then follow the exposed and nonexposed for a period of time (often years) to compare the frequency of an outcome such as disease. Prospective follow-up obviously needs to be sufficiently long and complete that enough subjects develop the condition of interest, without losing too much information from dropouts, to be able reliably to compare disease rates. The principal advantage of cohort studies is, therefore, that there is rarely any debate about whether or not the exposure predated the onset of disease, and this can be measured without any bias in relation to disease status. For this reason, it can be argued that poorly understood diseases should first be evaluated in cohort studies, and once potential confounders have been reliably identified, case-control studies can then proceed more economically (although the reverse is usually the case). Cohort studies also have the ability to study multiple possible outcomes of a single exposure. They are, however, expensive and time-consuming, usually include relatively few cases and are unsuitable for studying rare diseases (unless the outcome is very common amongst those exposed, i.e. the attributable risk percentage is high).

Cohort studies are mainly liable to two types of bias. First, participants who drop out of the study or move away and become uncountable are likely to differ from those that do not, often because they have developed the condition or disease of interest. As a general rule, follow-up rates of less than 80% are liable to deliver unreliable results. Second, the assignment of disease or outcome status can be subject to 'observer bias' unless such outcomes are rigorously defined and outcome assessors are blind to exposure status. In psychiatric studies, this demands at least a structured psychiatric interview. Cohort studies are less liable to the other main sources of bias because of the prospective collection of data (Box 5).

EXPERIMENTAL STUDIES

It should already be apparent that, even in a medical sense, experimental studies are not synonymous with clinical trials. A clinical trial is any kind of study designed to establish the effects of a particular therapeutic intervention. This includes uncontrolled trials and phases I (development) and phase IV (surveillance) studies in evaluating new treatments. The randomized control trial (RCT) is the gold standard of medical experimentation, but there are an increasing number of variants (Table 3).

Table 3: Summary of the features of clinical trials

Type of study	*Essential features*	*Advantages*	*Disadvantages*
Uncontrolled 'trials'	All subjects are given one treatment	Cheap and easy	No controls
Controlled trials	Two treatments are compared	Relatively straightforward	No randomization
Randomized control trials	Random allocation of treatment	Randomization reduces selection bias and confounding	Expensive and time-consuming
Cluster trials	Groups of individuals are randomized	Can assess the efficacy of certain health services	Often difficult to find enough clusters to give adequate power
Crossover trial	Subjects are their own controls	Can study treatment of rare, chronic disorders	Historical controls; order effects; carryover effects
N-of-1 trial	A single subject	Can establish effectiveness in an individual patient	As above, only applicable to certain types of chronic diseases

Box 5: Summary of the essential features of cohort studies

Typically, those exposed or not are identified and then followed-up to compare frequency of subsequent disease

Strengths

- Ideal for rare exposures
- Can examine many outcomes of a single exposure
- Generally less liable to bias than other observational studies, particularly recall bias and reverse causality

Limitations

- Can be expensive and lengthy
- Usually unsuitable for rare diseases
- Losses to follow-up can affect validity

General Issues

What is the Aim of the Study?

Clearly, the question has to be clinically relevant (i.e. the answer would help clinicians and their patients to make therapeutic decisions), ethically acceptable, and not have been satisfactorily answered already (e.g. in a systematic review or meta-analysis).

Which Patients are to be Studied?

A 'pure' highly selected group in an 'explanatory' trial may generate findings of little representative ness or generalizability. Broad inclusion criteria and minimal exclusions will serve to avoid the 'disappearing patient phenomenon', particularly when one allows for those who refuse to participate. For example, many psychiatric trials exclude patients with co morbid substance abuse, thus excluding about half of all potential participants, with the result that the study results may be inapplicable in approximately half of all patients that psychiatrists see and will probably overestimate the benefits of the new treatment (given that co-morbid patients are notoriously reluctant to comply with medical interventions). Excluding those under the age of 16 to 18 years or over the age of 60 to 65 years means that child, adolescent and old-age psychiatrists are often obliged to prescribe drugs with little information from clinical trials and may actually have to prescribe a drug 'off licence'. Excluding involuntarily-detained patients has the effect that psychiatrists treating the most severely ill patients are often doing so in the absence of any reliable evidence.

Which Interventions and how?

In a drug trial, one needs to consider the dose, type, formulation and route of administration of the medication. If comparing a new and a standard treatment, one can easily make the new drug look better (e.g. less toxic) by choosing a high dose of standard drug as the comparator (Geddes et al 2000). How the optimum dose of a drug is achieved and the dosing schedules require careful consideration. An important choice has to be made between allowing only fixed doses and allowing clinicians in the trial to tailor the dose to a particular patient. Fixed-dose trials generally give results that are easier to interpret, but they are obviously different from how a drug is used in clinical practice, and many patients will receive nonoptimal doses. Flexible dosing is more clinically representative, but difficult if not impossible to achieve without unbinding the responsible clinicians. One must also decide what, if any, other drugs are permissible for participating patients. For example, antipsychotic trials usually permit the concomitant prescription of one or more anticholinergic drugs and 'rescue' medication for behavioral disturbance.

How Long?

Many trials in psychiatry are short, lasting 6 weeks or less. This is simply because they are easier to do. Long trials are complex, expensive and liable to suffer from large numbers of people dropping out of the trial for various reasons. Clinical trials, particularly if we advise our patients to stay on a drug for a year or more, but trials which suffer from more than a 20% dropout over the duration of the study deliver results of dubious representative ness and reliability.

Is Blinding Possible?

Controlled trials may be open (if the doctors and patients both know what treatment is given), single-blind (if the patient is not told what treatment he is getting), or triple-blind (if, in addition, the outcome assessors do not know what treatment a patient has received). The purpose of single-, double- and triple-blinding is to improve the reliability of trial findings, by reducing observer bias. Single- and double-blinding also reduce placebo effects. Blinding is, however, rarely entirely complete. Patients and doctors can quite often guess whether that patient has received an active treatment according to whether they have responded or not and whether they have side effects. Single- and double-blinding are also difficult, if not impossible, in psychotherapy trials. Even in comparative drug trials, particular side-effects can suggest that a specific drug has been administered: e.g. trials of the tricycle antidepressants have commonly included anticholinergic compounds in the placebo, and trials which use this approach generally find less advantage of tricycles over placebo than those which have not (Moncrieff et al. 1998). Having independent outcome assessors can go some way to mitigating these problem, but suggestive information can still be given away by the patients or picked up by the observers. A useful method to quantify the success or otherwise of blinding in a trial is to simply ask patients, clinicians and/or outcome raters what treatment they think a particular patient has received—if blinding has been successful, they should score no better than chance (Even et al. 2000). However, blinding is not as important (nor the same) as allocation concealment.

Which Outcomes should be Measured and how?

Clinical outcomes can be measured either categorically or continuously. Dichotomous categorical outcomes are probably the most clinically meaningful, as the doctor and patient can choose a particular treatment accordingly. 'Dead or alive' is the standard and least subject to bias outcome, but these events are too rare for practical use in psychiatric studies. Typical alternatives are 'readmitted or not', 'recovered or not', or 'relapsed or not', but it can be difficult to measure these. In may psychiatric trials, recovery or relapse have been determined from somewhat arbitrary cutoff points on symptom severity or behavioral scales.

Controlled Trials

Uncontrolled trials are a means of establishing whether a treatment works at all and what sort of adverse effects are prominent, but an unreliable one. The absence of a control group means that some, or even all, of these apparent effects could be attributable to many different causes (the types of patient, severity of disease, a true treatment effect, placebo effect, etc.). If any treatment is given or taken with enough enthusiasm some people will benefit.

Controlled trials are obviously necessary if a particular treatment is to be evaluated against placebo or against a pre-existing treatment, but even controlled studies tend to overestimate therapeutic benefits. For example, there were numerous reports of apparent benefits from renal dialysis in schizophrenia until a series of randomized control trials found no beneficial effects (Carpenter et al. 1983). The main potential problem with controlled trials is that patients getting the new treatment tend to be selected (consciously or not) to have a slightly less severe illness and/or better prognosis, so that the beneficial effects of the new drug or procedure are typically overestimated by 30% (Schulz et al. 1995, Juni et al. 2001).

Randomized Control Trials

Randomization has two main purposes. First and for most, it evenly distributes both the known and, more importantly, the unknown confounders (e.g. age, sex, prognostic factors) of the therapeutic effect in the two treatment groups. Secondly, it avoids the potential selection biases described above—this, however, depends on allocation concealment. To be properly randomized, a trial should use a randomization schedule that is not predictable or known. For example, if patient treatment is allocated by, dates of birth, days of admission to hospital, etc. it is possible for investigators to subvert the treatment allocation process by finding reasons to include or exclude particular patients.

Random numbers should therefore be generated to assign particular treatment (although tossing a coin is acceptable), the assignment should be sealed in opaque envelopes, kept in a locked cabinet and only opened by someone (preferably indifferent to the trial result) when a suitable patient has consented to participate. This may sound extreme, but Chalmers et al. (1983) have shown that approximately 58% of published studies without randomization find a significant treatment effect, and 24% with randomization that allowed 'easy cheating' found a significant effect, whereas a significant effect was found in only 9% of studies in which subverting randomization was judged to be difficult. Randomization is not bona fide without allocation concealment. This is reflected in some 'trial quality scores', which award marks for randomization but subtract them if the allocation is not convincingly concealed. It should be noted that phase II ('dose-ranging') and phase III ('comparative') trials, as part of drug development, may or may not be randomized.

People, even doctors, can cheat with sealed envelopes, however. Envelopes can also get lost or destroyed, thereby subverting the allocation sequence. Ideally, therefore, a 'central randomization method' should be used. Once a patient has consented to participate, an investigator contacts a separate center (by telephone, fax or computer), the patient's baseline data are entered, and then a computer algorithm allocates the next treatment and the operator informs the investigator. This has the advantage that everyone involved knows who is in the trial immediately and baseline data collection is complete. It is more costly than using sealed envelopes, but touch-tone phone systems and the internet have made central randomization more generally applicable and affordable. Indeed, computer can operate the system 24 hours a day for global multicenter trials. A computer can also implement stratification or minimization to ensure that prognostic factors are balance between the treatment arms.

Various methods of randomization are sometimes used to ensure that trial groups are balanced in terms of number and/or patient characteristics.

- *Blocked randomization* simply randomizes patients in groups (of four, six, etc.) to ensure that numbers are equal in the two groups.
- *Stratified randomization* allocates patients on the basis of prognostic variables to ensure that these are evenly distributed, but requires an additional schedule for each stratum.
- An alternative is *minimization (or adaptive) randomization* in which each patients is allocated to a particular group by minimizing any differences in important variables as each particular patient is entered into the trial (Pocock 1983).

The problem with all these procedures is that they can under some circumstances, if poorly designed or implemented, increase the chances of unblinding the allocation (Schulz & Grimes 2002b). They are, however, essential in small trials. In large trials of say more than 500 patients, properly conducted simple randomization will usually, but not always, generate sufficiently even groups by chance alone.

Cluster Trials

One other important variant of randomization is to randomize subjects in groups of clusters rather than as individuals. These so called 'cluster trials' are most commonly used in evaluating more global aspects of health services than one particular treatment or where allocation of individual subjects is not practicable (Gilbody & Whitty 2002). For example, educating general practitioners about the detection and treatment of depression is ideally suited to cluster randomization, as general practitioners tend to work in group practices and it would be difficult in practice to educate one partner without that being communicated to another. The main disadvantage of cluster randomization is that the unit of randomisation should be the unit of analysis, so that large numbers of clusters are required to give the trial adequate power.

Explanatory versus Pragmatic Trials

The randomized control trial has given clinical therapeutics a sound scientific base but measures treatment efficacy rather than clinical effectiveness (i.e. whether a treatment works rather than whether it works in clinical practice). Randomization generally increases the scientific quality of 'internal validity' of a trial, but can lead to problems with 'external validity' if patients who are included differ systematically from all potential participants. This is a type of selection bias which can limit the representatives of the population being studied and the generalizability of the results. Pragmatic trials typically have less restrictive inclusion criteria and can therefore have greater generalizability. However, patients who are able to give informed consent and willing to be randomized may be just as likely, or even more so, to participate in an explanatory trial.

The distinction between explanatory and pragmatic trials is also not as clear as when the terms were introduced in 1967 (McMahon 2002). At that time, trials tend to exclude patients who violated the study protocol by, e.g. not complying with their treatment. The pragmatic approach was to include all violators, as they had been part of the therapeutic programme (see 'intention to treat' analysis below), but this has now become standard. These days, an 'explanatory' trial is typically a small trial, with highly selective entry criteria, which focus on one specific issue and often uses intermediate or surrogate outcome measures. A 'pragmatic' trial is usually larger, with broad entry criteria, in which the interventions can feasibly be provided in routine health care and the outcome is a major clinical event (Hotopf et al., 1999). Both types of trial are desirable, as they address different information needs. There is a common tendency to regard pragmatic trials as 'good' and explanatory trials as unrepresentive, but treatment control is usually more careful in explanatory studies and no-one would argue that this is undesirable. Neither trial type will be truly representative, because only those prepared to be randomized will be included.

Crossover Trials

These are trials in which all participants receive two or more interventions, one after the other, with the two groups receiving a different treatment first (Louis et al., 1984). Patients may randomize to receive a particular intervention first or second. Crossover trials are a real option in relatively rare diseases when the numbers of available participants may not permit a randomized parallel-group controlled trial. It is, however, probably preferable to attempt to conduct multicenter parallel-group trials in such instances. A second potential advantage of crossover trials in more apparent than real. If one of the treatment options is placebo, then a crossover trial gets round potential ethical concerns about not giving people effective treatment that may be required.

There is, however, no reason, particularly in short-term trials, why all patients allocated to placebo cannot be offered active treatment after the cessation of the trial, and if there is a genuine need to test a new treatment against placebo then it cannot be unethical to conduct such a trial.

There are, however, several disadvantages of crossover trials. These amounts to the difficulties in ensuring that the trial is long enough to ensure therapeutic effects are manifest in reasonable number of participants, but short enough to avoid contaminating the results with natural fluctuation in a chronic disease. There are very few conditions in which disease activity is constant over time. There is also the problem of effects from one treatment carrying over into the second time period and the potential for drug interment, but this introduces new difficulties with sudden cessation of potentially effective treatments and in ensuring the washout period is long enough to be effective, but short enough to be ethical. The one type of crossover trial which is probably underutilized is the N-of-l trial in which a particular patient is given two treatments blind. This has some potential in individual patients in individual patients in which it is simply not known which treatment they should receive but obviously requires a consenting patient and co-operation from the hospital pharmacy (Guyatt et al. 1986).

Need for Large-scale Trials in Psychiatry

Most of the first 2000 controlled trials in patients with schizophrenia included less than 60 participants (Thornley & Adams 1998). This sample size could only detect very large treatment effects. Trials comparing two active agents ('comparative studies') require much larger groups (as the difference in effects is generally much smaller). The main reason for larger trials is that very large effects are rare in medicine. Large trials are needed chiefly to avoid missing a modest but clinically worthwhile benefit simply because the trial is underpowered. They also reduce random error and produce a more precise estimate of the treatment effect. The logical extension of this argument is to the so called 'mega trial', in which thousands of patients are randomized to particular treatments (Peto et al., 1993, Warlow 2002). This gives the best opportunity of reliably identifying moderate treatment effects. Such trials can benefit from computerized randomization (which allows enrolment 24 hours a day worldwide), minimizing data requirements and using simple objective outcome measures, but still require tremendous organization. There is, however, no doubt the psychiatrists, like many medical specialists, are over-reliant on the pharmaceutical industry to evaluate new products and are years behind our colleagues in cardiology and neurology in carrying out large independent trials. Trials in psychiatry can be said to have particular problems, but large randomized 'sample trials have been conducted in comparably difficult' patients, whit epilepsy and traumatic brain injury.

SPECIFIC STATISTICAL ISSUES

Multiple Hypothesis Testing in Trials

A power calculation is necessary before any trial to determine how many participants will be required to detect a specific finding at a given level of statistical significance. One therefore needs a defined primary outcome measure and a means of estimating how many participants may develop it (for a dichotomous outcome) or the likely mean change in a continuous measure and some idea of its likely variance (in standard deviation units). There is, however, a drive to considering several outcomes, including those from the patient's point of view. These might include measures of adverse effect frequency, levels of functioning, or quality-of-life measures, as 'surrogate outcome measures'. Multiple outcome measures may be thought of as giving better coverage of therapeutic response, but increase the chances of finding statistically significant differences by chance alone.

Intention-to-treat Analysis

Generally speaking, using a continuous measure (e.g. a symptom severity score) gives more statistical power than using a dichotomous or categorical one, but less relevance. The latter has particular advantages when it comes to dealing with the results in participants who have dropped out of the trial before its completion. All trials should conduct intention-to-treat analyzes of the results in all participants randomized to one treatment of another, regardless of whether they completed the trial-to include treatment failures and avoid overestimating the benefits of treatment (McMahon 2002).

Checking Randomization

It is also briefly worth mentioning one statistical test that should not be conducted in clinical trials (or indeed most other studies). It make little sense to statistically compare descriptive variables in two or more treatment groups 'to test the success of randomization'. Not only is it inappropriate to conduct statistical tests for which there is no hypothesis, but if randomization is truly random, then every now and then some descriptive variables will differ between allocated groups. Note, however, that it is necessary to check that the randomization process has not been subverted, and important to detect and describe baseline imbalances. An imbalance in a major prognostic factor between the treatment and control groups may not reach 'statistical significance' but may still be enough to materially influence the outcome in the two groups and hence lead the trial to over-or underestimate the treatment effect. Thus, baseline statistical comparisons are overused, but tests of interactions between potential moderators and mediators of therapeutic effects are underused (Pocock et al. 2002).

Systematic Reviews and Meta-analysis

Any one study-no matter how large or well conducted—needs independent replication. If, as is often the case, study results vary, systematic reviews and meta-analysis can help deliver consensus. These are examples or 'secondary research' in that they synthesize the available relevant evidence in a given research area. They are generally seen as increasingly important because, provided they are done well, they provide the single most reliable piece of evidence on a particular topic. Systematic reviews identify and cite studies in a pre-specified and reliable way; while meta-analysis provide an overall numerical effect across several studies. Although a systematic review has some value without an accompanying meta-analysis, the main advantage of a meta-analysis is that it is more precise and less biased than the estimate of effect from any one study. However, if the review has been flawed and collects only a biased selection of studies, this will yield a biased summary estimate of the true effect. Done properly, systematic reviews are important for two main reasons. First, as alluded to above, any individual study, no matter how rigorously conducted, analyzed and interpreted, can only be an estimate of the true underlying effect and needs to be independently replicated, but subsequent studies often apparently disagree with the original for a wide variety of reasons. Second, the amount of literature in many areas is now so vast that doctors need access to high-quality review articles which reliably and conveniently provides an up-to-date summary. In addition, systematic reviews and meta-analyzes are a crucial first step for planning future research and providing the evidence-base for valid clinical guidelines.

Systematic reviews have the following key components:	
•	The formulation of a specific question
•	Prespecification of the types of article to be included and excluded
•	Pre-specification of the outcome(s) of interest and important potential confounders or effect modifiers, and of any planned subgroup comparison
•	Use of several search strategies to identify articles from a number of sources (chiefly computerized databases), supplemented by searching through the references of included studies and preferably by contacting researches for any published or unpublished studies of which they are aware; this is sometimes augmented by a hand search of key journals and/or by searching the 'gray literature' in, e.g. textbooks, theses, etc, and other unpublished studies
•	Identifying the relevant articles and extracting the relevant data.

Properly conducted systematic reviews are, therefore, time-consuming, protocol-driven studies in their own right. The key feature is that such a review be repeatable, i.e. given your methods other researchers, would identify the same articles and draw the same conclusions. Reliability is augmented if two or more researchers independently examine the (electronic) searches to identify papers for possible inclusion and search through such papers for data to be extracted. Oxman & Guyatt (1988) helpfully devised eight questions for assessing the quality of research reviews (Box 6). The Department of Health (2001) psychotherapy guidelines, e.g. included only reviews that met at least six of these eight criteria.

The desirability of contacting other researchers for any unpublished studies is that 'publication bias' is a large threat to the validity of a systematic review. *Publication bias* is the tendency for researchers to be more likely to write up, and (especially leading) journals to publish, positive than negative studies it is possible that summary estimate will be biased-although this can be checked statistically (Gilbody & Song 2000). Publication bias is more likely if one searches only one database (e.g. Mediline is biased toward North American studies, whilst BID and Psychlit are more biased toward European studies). This is also the case if one extracts only English language articles ('language bias') as there are empirical examples of European' researchers reporting negative results in their native language and positive results in English (although the reverse has also been described).

Meta-analyzes mathematically combine the results of different studies to give one summary estimate of a given effect. Different studies may find apparently incompatible results for several reasons, including inadequate power, measurement error and different liabilities to bias and confounding. Simple 'vote-counting' summary techniques, comparing the number of positive studies to the number of 'negative' studies, are unreliable as they do not include an assessment of study size or quality and themselves have low power. Large studies tend generally to be of higher quality quality and provide more precise estimates of any given effect than smaller studies and should have relatively greater influence on a summary effect.

The choice of techniques to perform and interpret meta-analysis is wide, and anyone undertaking a meta-analysis should have expert statistical advice and support. Under some circumstances, if there is substantial heterogeneity between studies, which cannot be explained, it may not be appropriate

Box 6: Guidelines for assessing research reviews	
•	Were the questions and methods clearly stated?
•	Were comprehensive search methods used to locate relevant studies?
•	Was explicit methods used to determine which articles to include in the review?
•	Was the validity of the primary studies assessed?
•	Was the assessment of the primary studies reproducible and free from bias?
•	Was variation in the findings of the relevant studies analysed?
•	Were the findings of the primary studies combined appropriately?
•	Were the reviewers' conclusion supported by the data cited?

to generate an overall estimate of effect at all. In other cases, e.g. where the review combines a number of studies with poor methodology (e.g. trials with poor allocation concealment) and yields an apparent benefit of 20–30%, seemingly clinically worthwhile effects and merely be due to bias. In other works, the treatment may have no effect and the apparent effect could simply be due to poor methodology.

While no one can seriously challenge the desirability of systematic reviews, there remain many critics of meta-analysis. Meta-analysis certainly has its limitations, but not all of the most frequent criticisms are justified.

More pertinent criticisms of meta-analysis include that they are unreliable if they include few outcome events and if there were only a small number of small studies. Importantly, since meta-analysis was devised to deal with the results form randomized control trials, there are still no way of satisfactorily combining the results of randomized and nonrandomized clinical trials, and the liabilities to bias in observational research require great caution in interpreting a meta-analysis of observational studies. A particular problem occasionally arises where a meta-analysis disagrees with the results form a large RCT or when two or more meta-analyzes of the same issue find opposing results. Nonetheless, the advantages of meta-analysis generally outweigh the problems. Two recent articles have proposed standardized methods of reporting the results of observational and experimental meta-analyzes (Moher et al., 1999, Stroup et al., 2000) which are complementary to similar articles on the reporting of individual randomized control trials and serve as excellent introductions for potential reviewers. Particularly interested readers are referred to an excellent book (Egger et al. 2001) that discusses all the foregoing in far greater detail.

CAUSAL INFERENCE

Factors to Consider as Possible Explanations for Research Findings

Any association found in medical research could theoretically be attributable to one or more of the following explanations; chance, reverse causality, bias and/or confounding.

Chance

Chance or 'random error', and the related issues of study power and statistical significance are important factors to be considered. Suffice to say here that if a study is insufficiently powered, whether the result is positive or 'negative', chance remains a likely explanation. Further, studies which do not find a statistically significant association are, in fact, neutral rather than negative studies unless they have been specifically powered to be able to show 'non-equivalence', and this generally requires several hundreds of subjects in each group. In other words, a lack of evidence of an effect is not the same as evidence of a lack of effect.

Reverse Causality

Reverse causality simply refers to the situation where a disease causes the apparent exposure rather than vice versa. This is particularly likely in case-control and descriptive studies. For example, the original descriptions of an association between schizophrenia and low social class have subsequently been attributed to social downward drift after the onset of the disorder (although there are now suggestions that living in a city or overcrowding many have an etiological role). Similarly, non-independent life events can often follow depression rather than precede it.

Bias

Bias can be defined as 'any process at any stage of inference which tends to produce results or conclusions that differ systematically from the truth' (Sackett 1979). There are numerous subtypes of bias that can arise at any stage of research, and Sackett mentions 35, but there are two broad categories: selection (or recruitment) bias and information (measurement or observation) bias. These can be usefully subdivided according to whether they a primarily introduced by researchers or subjects themselves (Box 7).

Selection Bias Stems from an absence of comparability between the groups being studied. This tends to arise either because researchers recruit form an unrepresentative population of subjects, e.g. hospital inpatients (*Sampling bias).* The only way to avoid this is to randomly sample form population registers, but such attempts can always fail because of non-representative participation by subjects (*response bias*). Random samples are those in which every individual in a population has an equal chance of being included or excluded in a study, but nonresponse is far from random. As a rule, people are more likely to participate in research if they perceive a likely benefit for themselves or people like them, but the determinants of research participation have been poorly studies. These issues are particularly important in case-control studies as they do not have the advantage that surveys and cohort studies do of being able to identify a representative sample of controls from among large numbers of noncases. Randomized control trials use the same patients as potential subjects and controls prior to randomization. At least in such cases, it is possible to compare those who are identified and participate with those who do not in terms of possibly important confounders.

Box 7: The main types of bias in medical research	
Selection bias	
•	*Sampling:* Non-representative identification/recruitment of subjects.
•	*Response:* Unrepresentative participation by subjects
Information bias	
•	*Interviewer:* Differential data recording in subject groups by researchers.
•	*Recall:* Historical data is selectively filtered by subjects

Important subtypes of sampling bias include:

- Admission (Berkson) bias—where hospitalization rates differ for particular exposure/disease groups such that the relationship between exposure and disease is distorted in hospitalized patients;
- Referral filter bias—when patient referrals from primary to secondary care increase the concentration of rare exposures and sever diseases;
- Diagnostic purity bias—where the exclusion of comorbidity results in a nonrepresentative sample;
- Membership bias—where group affiliation is used to identify subjects, e.g. members of a patients' organizaiton, hospital staff controls;
- Historical control bias—where secular changes in disease definition, exposures, treatments, etc. render such controls incomparable;
- Ascertainment bias—where two groups of subjects are recruited in different way and differ because of this.

Important subtypes of response bias include:

- Non-respondent bias—as non-respondents are often those who are most ill—and the reverse situation of volunteer bias;
- Unacceptable disease bias;
- Missing data bias—e.g. on sensitive questions about sexuality, etc.

Information (measurement or observation) bias arises through the systematic misclassification of disease or exposure, or both, by researchers and the instruments they use of subjects themselves. If people know they are being observed, they tend to normalize their behavior and minimize any perceived deviation from the norm ('attention bias'). Examples of this include the so-called 'Hawthorne effect'. Similar principles may at least partly underlie the often remarkably beneficial effects of simply asking patients, e.g. with eating disorders, to monitor certain aspects of behavior.

Interviewer bias arises when researchers are not blind to exposure or disease status and tend to alter their approach, unconsciously or not. If the exposure is measured after disease, 'exposure suspicion bias' can influence both the intensity and the outcome of a search for exposures in affected subjects. Conversely, 'diagnostic suspicion bias' can arise if researchers strive harder to detect observers, researchers and patients, tend to make observations the concur with their expectations ('expectation bias').

Recall bias is the equivalent of interviewer bias, but introduced by subjects rather than researchers. Subjects generally tend to alter their response in the direction they perceive is desired by the investigator ('obsequiousness bias'). Patients and their relatives are likely to 'search after meaning' for possible exposures to explain their disease (also called 'rumination bias'). A good psychiatric example is the maternal recall of obstetric complications in their schizophrenic children—although this can potentially be cross-cheeked with obstetric records. Conversely, if subjects know they have been exposed, they may be more likely to report symptoms of a disease.

Confounding

Confounding arises when the effects of two processes are not separated. It can be defined as 'the distortion of the apparent effect of an exposure brought about by the association with other factors that can influence the outcome' (last 1995). Put another way, confounding mixes the effects between an exposure and a disease and a third factor associated with both. This can lead to a false association (positive confounding) or obscure a true association (negative confounding). A confounder is therefore an independent risk or protective factor for a disease that varies systematically with another exposure. Further, a confounder is in a triangular relationship with the other variables, rather than on the causal pathway. For example, there is increasing evidence that being born and raised in cities is a risk factor of schizophrenia. The social drift of previous generations of people with schizophrenia could, however, account for this association, i.e. genetic liability to schizophrenia and urban drift could positively confound the apparent association between urban upbringing and the disease. Age, sex and social class are common confounders. Confounders can however, only, exert effects if they differ between study groups, and confounding can, sometimes, be reduced in the design stage or measured and controlled.

Controlling Confounding

The common methods for reducing confounding are:

- Randomization (as in RCTs)
- Restriction
- Matching

Restriction is done by selecting only subjects who have a particular range of values of a potential confounder, e.g. social class *Matching,* on the other hand, at least in 'individual matching', selects case-control pairs with similar properties, e.g. age and sex. Rather confusingly, 'frequency matching' lies somewhere between restriction and individual matching, as the values of particular variables are 'balanced' overall between two groups. Matching reduces confounding and improves statistical power, but is not to be used lightly. Identifying potential subjects becomes more difficult; one cannot study a association between the disease and exposure on the matched variable (although this may be possible with balanced groups, and interactions with matched variables can be studied), and if one inadvertently matches on variables that are not confounders this will actually tend to reduce statistical power. In general, therefore, it is preferable to measure the potential confounder and control for it statistically. Matching is, however, preferable if it is difficult to accurately measure or classify confounders (e.g. genetic liability to depression).

Statistical control of confounding involves two methods. The first is a 'stratified analysis' where a potential confounder such as age is treated by separating subjects into age groupings, or 'strata'. Standardized mortality rates are an example of this. The second, although related approach, is to conduct multivariate analyzes using regression. As before, however, if it is difficult to measure a confounder accurately; attempted statistical control for it is likely to leave some 'residual confounding'. This is particular problem when so-called proxy measures are used, e.g. using paternal social class as an index of childhood environment. If, as is common, adjustment for confounding reduces the association, residual confounding should be considered. On the other hand, confounding can be overcontrolled if two variables are strongly related or if an apparent confounder actually lies on the causal pathway. This is a particular potential problem in psychiatric studies, as our knowledge of the mechanisms of most psychiatric disorders is rather limited. Statistical control for confounding should, therefore, always present both uncorrected and adjusted values of associations.

Language of Risk

A risk factor is 'an attribute or exposure that is associated with an increased probability of an outcome, such as disease' (Last 1995). The term is, however, rather loosely used and merits clarification and subdivision. Offord & Kraemer (2000) suggest that there are three different types of risk factor:

- A fixed marker—a risk factor that cannot be changed, e.g. sex;
- A variable marker—a risk factor that can be manipulated but, even so, does not change the risk of an outcome;
- A causal risk factor—which is both manipulable and changes the probability of an outcome.

For example, poverty is a risk factor for conduct disorder, but evidence thus far suggests that increasing income does not reduce the risk; whereas improving parenting practice does appear to reduce the incidence. This refinement of terms, which may seem rather abstract, has important implications. First, risk factors are not necessarily causal. Second, risk factors may differ in different populations and at different points in the history of disease. Greater attention to these definitions might well help to shed further light on the etiology and even pathogenesis of psychiatric disorder and is obviously required in considering the development of new therapeutic or preventative approaches. Etiological research and screening programs might best focus on fixed or variable (trait) markers, which pathophysiological and therapeutic studies should arguably focus on causal risk factors and state-related changes.

Criteria for Causality

Establishing causation in multifactorial disorders in clearly complex and difficult. Old models, such as Koch's postulates and causes being 'necessary and sufficient', are inadequate. Bradford Hill Proposed some criteria for deciding whether an exposure caused and outcome (Box 8). Of these, perhaps the most important is that of establishing a temporal sequence, in demonstrating that the cause precedes the outcome, and that of an increase in the risk as the degree of exposure increases (a dose-response relationship). The strength of the association, i.e. size of the odds ratio of relative risk is another important guide. Some authorities recommend that newly identified exposures or risk factors should only be taken seriously if the odds ratio is at least 3, at least until replication. Replication with different study designs and different methods is crucial. Finally, any observed association should have biological plausibility, based on what is known about pathophysiology.

DEVELOPING YOUR OWN RESEARCH IDEAS

Doing research is intellectually stimulating and rewarding, the best way of appreciating the strengths and limitations of different approaches, and can even generate valuable new knowledge. An enquiring mind, careful planning and a determination to finish are enough for many research projects. Personal and financial assistance are not essential for descriptive and case-control studies, or systematic reviews, although they do help. On the other hand, sizeable grants and research teams are generally required for cohort studies, most clinical trials and technological investigations.

- *Have an idea*: These may arise form clinical observations discussion with other staff or reading the journals. Published articles often discuss what further studies are required. Simply attempting to replicate a particular study with minor alterations to clarify on issue can

Box 8: Bradford Hill's criteria for causation	
•	Temporal sequence
•	Dose-response relationship
•	Strength of association
•	Consistency
•	Biological plausibility

be an important contribution. Turning the idea into a question may help focus the idea, by clarifying the aims and hypotheses, and suggest a research design. It can be helpful to think in terms of the 'four part clinical question' patient problem, exposure, outcome, and control subjects or interventions. Note that one aim and hypothesis is generally preferable, as it is more likely to be thoroughly address than when attempting to answer two or more.

- *Review the relevant literature*: Truly original ideas are very rare, getting up to speed with the available research is often the most time-consuming process in preparing a study, but is time well spent. It will identify what needs to be done, identify the strengths of weaknesses of particular research designs, what measures are potentially relevant, etc. If there is no recent good review article then you should write one or, preferably, do a systematic review. If you are thinking about a therapeutic question, look at the Cochrane Library. If you are prepared to do a systematic review, consider writing a Cochrane review, as you will get considerable methodological support and training to do it.
- *Consider the advantages and disadvantages of the various research designs*: You must realistically evaluate what you are able to do. What sort of patients and controls, and how many of them, do you have access to? It is wise to study the sorts of patients you are likely to see anyway in you clinical work. How much time will you have? If, e.g. you have one 4-hour session a week for research, and each subject's measures will take an hour, it will take you at least 6 months to recruit and assess 50 patients and 50 controls. Even this can only start once you have ethical approval (let alone grant funding) and have conducted a pilot study. Will you have any help? One assistant will halve the time required and will be able to ensure that any measures have 'inter-rater reliability' if that is required.
- *Write a research protocol*: At this stage it is worth consulting and experienced researcher and/or statistician if you have not already done so, statistical and methodological support is very important at all stages of study. Good research supervision will help to focus you idea, clarify the design and advise on sensible statistics. A protocol is essential for properly planning the study and will serve as a template for any ethical approval or grant applications you need to apply for.

A protocol starts with a title and *Introduction*. This should discuss the issue you are addressing, briefly summarized the main finding and limitations of previous studies, and describe the aims of your study. If you are attempting to answer a particular question, as is preferable, you should predict what you expect to fine and rephrase the prediction as a negative ('the null liypothesis'). You may find it helpful, in writing the introduction, to ask yourself why does this study need to be done, at this time and in this way?

The protocol should them describe the precise *methods* you mend to employ, particularly how you will identify and define subjects, the measurements you plan to make and the main statistical techniques you will use. Cases and controls should be as representative as possible of the entire populations form which they come. Controls are usually even more difficult to identify and recruit. Any psychiatric diagnoses must be verified, preferably by actually interviewing all the subjects—although this well take about an hour or more with most of the available structured psychiatric interviews.

Inclusion and exclusion criteria are usually based on diagnosis and demographics, such as age. Do not make inclusion criteria too restrictive or exclusion too numerous, as your study will lose representativeness and the ability to examine any differences with in you patient group, and may well suffer form the 'disappearing patient' phenomenon (sometimes called 'Lasagna's law'). Inclusions are best kept to the diagnosis of interest, and exclusions limited to important potentially confounding conditions such as for example, neurological disease.

You must then describe the *measurements* you plan to make measures should ideally be reliable, valid, objective and standard. Only directly relevant data should be collected, to minimize the amount of time it takes you and the subjects to complete the study. Using at least some of the measures in some of the previous studies will aid comparison and clarification. Basic demographics (age, sex, social class) can be obtained from simply, asking the subjects, although some descriptors (e.g. Intelligence) will require specific scales. Relevant disease parameters, such as duration, medication and number of admissions, can be easily and fairly reliably obtained from case notes. Symptom severity is generally worth measuring and may be the outcome of primary interest. These variables may modify any affects you discover, either in reality or as confounders. Important potential exposure and confounders need to be measured, as do outcomes. If you are interested in something for which there is no scale or questionnaire, it is probably better to devise one yourself than to forcefully adapt something else. Devised instruments should be focused, brief and clear. If you need a simple measure of severity, e.g. do not be afraid to ask subjects to mark a cross on a 10 cm line, as such visual analogue scales are often surprisingly useful.

You will also need to give some thought to how the data will be recorded, stored, checked and analyzed. This and indeed all other aspects of your study can and should be examined in pilot study.

- *Do a pilot study*: This may use up time and subjects, but is a crucial determinant of whether your aims, subject recruitment plans and methods are realistic. As important, a pilot study will give you the best available information for power calculation to determine exactly how many subjects you will need to examine in the study. Further, many grant-giving bodies and ethical committees now require evidence form pilot studies to ensure that ideas are feasible before giving monies or subjecting participants to projects that are unlikely to give clear-cut results.

- *Plan the statistical analysis*: Before you start collecting data. The test used will depend on the types and likely distribution of your data (i.e. parametric or non-parametric statistics), whether you are simply describing subjects or comparing them (i.e. descriptive or inferential statistics), the number of groups, and any planned analysis of potential confounders (e.g. by subgroups, analyzes of covariance, regression).
- *Write a patient information sheet and consent from*: Writing these will help you present your research idea in the sort of lay language that is required for ethical approval submissions (which always require information and consent sheets and often place the greatest emphasis on them) and may be required for some grant giving bodies.
- *Keep your data safe and backed up*: Store your protocol, correspondence, any patient records and collected data in a locked, fireproof filling cabinet. Make regular copies of backups of your data and store this separately from your computer, preferably in a fireproof safe. All too often, computers are stolen, or floods and fire danger research offices, and data from important studies are irretrievably lost. Unfortunately, most researchers do not start to make regular backups until they have suffered some kind of major data loss.
- *Write your paper*: A good protocol will provide you with the bulk of the introduction and methods sections of any papers you write to get your research published. The purpose of a paper is to communicate the essence of a research project so that it can be appraised in the context of others. An introduction should briefly summarize what is known and what needs to be in a particular areas. A detailed methods section should be written so as to allow your study to be exactly replicated (if any one so desires). The results section should only give important positive and negative findings. The discussion should consider the results, strengths and limitations, and implication of your findings in the context of other studies. While you are waiting for the research to be published, you could always try to answer the new questions it will inevitably raise.

COMMONLY USED PSYCHIATRIC INTERVIEWS AND RATING SCALES

It is not possible here to describe all the properties of all the available interviews and rating, scales used in psychiatric research, even if that were desirable. Rather, we shall describe the principal features of the main tools for general usage.

Structured Psychiatric Interviews

These are detailed, time-consuming and generally only recommended for use by trained personnel. However, they share the ability to improve the reliability of diagnosis of the major disorders, over standard clinical approaches, which is why they were first developed.

Present State Examination (Wing et al. 1974)

The present state examination (PSE) is a semistructured interview with probes for each symptom and a detailed list of signs to be evaluated. These are generally rated as absent, mild/possible and moderate/definite. It only covers the past 4 weeks, unless augmented by additional duration questions. There are 140 items in total, with particularly detailed coverage of different types of sensory distortion and delusion. This and the detailed appendix of how to score items are a great introduction to psychopathology for trainees. There is a computer program ('Catego') that can generate diagnoses for the major disorders but not for personality disorder, in children and adolescents, or the learning disabled.

Versions 7 and 8 were first used in two large international collaborations: the US, UK Diagnostic Project and the International Pilot Study of Schizophrenia. The current version, PSE-10, was slightly adapted to generate most DSM-IIIR and then DSM-IV diagnoses as well as ICD-10. It is the central component of the *Schedules of Clinical Assessment for Neuropsychiatry (SCAN),* which has become the standard instrument for clinical assessment worldwide (Wing et al., 1990) and is complementary to the US-derived instruments for community screening.

Schedule for Affective Disorders and Schizophrenia (Endicott & Spitzer 1978)

The schedule for affective disorders and schizophrenia (SADS) is entirely structured, with symptom rating criteria contained within the interview schedule. Symptom severity is assessed—on a 7-point scale where 3 or more is usually 'clinically significant'—for current episode, the previous week, the point of maximal severity and any previous episode. Not surprisingly, this can take up to 2 hours. There are now several versions available, including those for lifetime assessments, sensitivity to change and for children and adolescents. The SADS is not useful for organic disorders or anorexia, however. The same research group also developed a separate instrument, the Structured Clinical Interview for

DSM (SCID), with the advantage that it is suitable for both clinical and research use, but the disadvantage that it is rarely used for either.

Diagnostic Interview Schedule (Robins et al. 1981)

The diagnostic interview schedule (DIS) was specifically devised to be useful in all settings and for use by lay interviewers after 1–2 weeks training, so that prevalence of DSM-III disorders (except organic and mental retardation) could be determined. The resulting Epidemiological Catchment Area (ECS) study of more then 18000 urban residents if five US sites was extremely influential, although there are serious questions about the sensitivity of the tool (and particularly for schizophrenia). The DIS was revised to be suitable for DSM-IIIR but, rather embarrassingly, the subsequent National Co-morbidity Survey found rather different (usually higher) prevalence's (Narrow et al., 2002). Nonetheless, the DIS was then transformed, in line with ICD-10 and DSM-IV, into the *Composite International Diagnostic Interview (CIDI).*

The development of the CIDI has been sponsored by WHO (Robins et al., 1988), and is generally recommended for initial community screening to be followed by professional interviewing with the SCAN. Both are now available in several languages. These instruments are likely to become increasingly favored over others, but will of course need amendment when DSM-V appears.

Symptom Severity Rating Scales

The following are the most frequently used scales to assess symptoms, their severity and to monitor any change.

- *Brief Psychiatric Rating Scale* (BPRS; Overall & Gorham 1962): Originally composed of 16 general itmes (5 observational), rated 0-7, this was then revised to 18 (to include observations of excitement and disorientation), and some version include up to 25 items. The semi-structured interview schedule is brief (18 minutes) and delivers reliable ratings, but the instrument is better for psychosis than depression or anxiety.
- *Krawieeka or Manchester Scale* (Krawieeka et al. 1977): Devised of rating chronic psychosis, with four symptoms and four signs (later revised to separate flat and incongruous affect) scored 0-4. No interview sehedule is available, however.
- *Positive and Negative Symptoms Scale* (Kay et al. 1987): Measures general psychopathology (16 items), as well as positive and negative symptoms (7 items each) on a scale of 1–7 where 3 is mild. The PANSS takes longer than the BPRS but has been carefully validated against other instruments, especially for schizophrenia. Not to be confused with the Scale for the Assessment of Positive Symptoms (SAPS) and the equivalent for negative Symptoms (SANS; Andeasen 1982) is by far the best option if negative symptoms are the focus of the study. It has 30 items, scored 0–5, in five domains (affective flattening, alogia, avolitionapathy, anhedonia-asociality, and attentional impairment).
- *Hamilton Rating Scale for Depression* (HRSD; Hamilton 1960): The original 21 items are commonly reduced to 17 (excluding the comparatively rare depersonalization, paranoia and obsessionality items, and missing out diurnal variation as this was thought to be related to the subtype of illness rather than severity). It is clinician rated, taking all available information into account. Although it is by far the most commonly used scale for depression, it is commonly misused as a diagnostic instrument, is biased toward biological symptoms over subjective distress, and has an unstable factor structure, similar criticisms apply to the *Hamilton Rating Scale for Anxiety* (HRSA; Hamilton 1959) although this too has been extensively used for severity and change assessments.
- *Beck Depression Inventory* (BDI; Beck et al. 1961): Self-completed 21-item inventory, which is sensitive change, but biased to cognitive items.
- *Montgomery-Asberg Depression Rating Scale* (MADRS; Montgomery and Asberg 1979): Specifically designed as 10 items sensitive to change, it has good psychometric properties.
- *Hospital Anxiety and Depression Scale* (HADS; Zigmond and Snaith 1983): Specifically intended as a screening tool in medical patients, it contains seven items each on self-rated depression and anxiety (scored 0-3) and is valid and sensitive to change.
- *State-Trait Anxiety Inventory* (STAI; Spielberger et al. 1970): Two separate self-rated scales of 20 items each, which only take a few minutes to complete, and the state scale is sensitive to change.

The most widely used scale for obsessional symptoms is probably the Leyton Obsessional Inventory. There are few good scales for mania severity, which generally suffer from a difficulty capturing mixed states. Any of the various versions of the General Health Questionnaire (GHQ) are suitable for (postal) screening for psychiatric morbidity in the general population, although the follow-up interview is now rarely done with the Clinical Interview Schedule as was originally intended.

45.5 RESEARCH MEASUREMENT AND STATISTIC

AP Dadhich, Mridula Vyas, Sai Krishna Tikka, Christoday RJ Khess

INTRODUCTION

The term statistics literally means 'numerical data', and statistics as a discipline is the science of assembling and interpreting numerical data (Bland 2000). Some form of numerical analysis is useful in most research, and all doctors should be able to understand and interpret the findings presented in medical journals that inform their clinical practice.

Almost all statistics are based on the premise that study of a sample of people with a condition allows the inference of something more general about the population from which they came. To do this, studies need to be valid (i.e. well designed and conducted) and present clear results using the appropriate tests. Statistics is concerned not merely with the results of an experiment or study, but also with its design. Badly designed studies are unlikely to yield reliable results, no matter how sophisticated the statistical analysis may be.

RESEARCH MEASUREMENT

Types of Data

Data is conventionally classified as either discrete or continuous. Discrete data can only take a limited set of possible values (e.g. socioeconomic status, sex) whereas continuous data have a potentially infinite series of values (e.g. height, temperature). In practice, the accuracy of data measurement usually means that continuous parameters such as height are measured to the nearest unit and are actually discrete variables. This qualification is not usually very important, however. Discrete data can be further subdivided into four types according to their properties:

- Nominal or categorical
- Ordinal
- Interval
- Ratio.

Nominal or categorical data have values which are qualitatively different from one another but have no particular order (e.g. diagnosis). When there are only two possible values (e.g. gender), nominal data are sometimes are also referred to as dichotomous. Ordinal data have a logical order in their values, but the differences between each of the values are not necessarily equal and the measurement has no true zero point (e.g. social class I-V, ward observation level). Interval and ratio data have very similar properties; in both, the differences between values are equal (e.g. the differences between a value of 1 and 2 is the same as the differences between 33 and 34). Ratio data have the additional properties of having a true zero point (i.e. a complete absence of the quantity), though this distinction is rarely important. Distinguishing the various data types may seem like an irrelevant abstraction, but is essential in determining the correct method of data description and analysis. Discrete interval, discrete ratio and continuous data can be analyzed using a group of related techniques called Parametric statistics, subject to a limited number of additional considerations. Data which are nominal or ordinal are analyzed using nonparametric or distribution-free methods.

A further distinction in study data is made between variables that are dependent and those that are independent. Dependent variables are the characteristics we wish to investigate, whereas an independent variable refers to the data classification. For example, in a study where one compared the whole brain volume of patients with various psychiatric diagnoses, diagnosis would be the independent variable and brain volume the dependent variable.

Validity and Reliability of Measurement

- Validity is whether an instrument measures what it purports to measure.
- Reliability is whether repeated measurements of the same data give similar results.

There are several methods of determining the reliability and validity of a measure.

Validity

Validity of measurement can be assessed in many ways, but perhaps the simplest form of validity is when something 'looks right'. When a scale 'looks right' at brief inspection then it is said to have face validity. A related measure of validity is content validity. This refers to the individual items or content of scale. For example an anxiety scale containing many items about psychosis is likely to have poor content validity.

Types of validity	
•	Face validity
•	Content validity
•	Criterion validity
•	Construct validity
•	Internal consistency

With a new measurement technique there is often a gold standard against which it can be compared. If the new measurement gives consistently different result it cannot be valid. This form of validity is called criterion validity and should not be confused with reliability or repeatability, although the concepts are similar. If there is no clear gold standard then one has to compare the new measure with another measure of uncertain validity to see if it gives the results one could reasonably expect. For example, a scale measuring suicidal ideation might be found to predict deliberate self-harm. This property of having an appropriate relationship with other variables is known as construct validity. A final measure of the validity of a scale is whether the items on a scale are related to one another. This is known as internal consistency and can be measured using Cronbach's alpha (Bland and Altman, 2002).

Reliability

Researchers and clinicians often wish to obtain data from patients. Sometimes obtaining the information may be long and protracted (e.g. full clinical interview) or on other occasions it may entail the risk of harm to the patient (e.g. direct measurement of the CSF levels of drugs). In order to obtain the information more quickly, or with less risk to the patient, new methods may emerge whose levels of agreement with the old techniques needs to be assessed. Measurements using a given technique should also be repeatable from researcher to researcher. For example: during a 10 year cohort study of people with schizophrenia it would be unlikely for the same researchers to be present throughout the whole study. We therefore need to be satisfied that, given the same material, the researchers would have a high level of agreement on its measurement.This form of reliability is sometimes known as inter-rater reliability.

The quantification of reliability between different raters (inter-rater) or between different methods in general can be accomplished by a number of means depending on the data type. For categorical data (e.g. whether someone has schizophrenia or not) the reliability of the results are usually measured using the kappa (K) statistic. Kappa is calculated according to the following formula:

$$K = \frac{P_o - P_e}{1 - P_o}$$

Where Po is the proportion of observed agreement and Pe is the proportion of agreement expected by chance. Consider the example show in Table 4, where two observers interview 100 patients and decide whether they have schizophrenia or not. In 50 cases, Observer 1 and Observer 2 agree that the person has schizophrenia, and in 20 that they do not, out of a total sample of 100. Therefore the observed agreement (pn) is 0.7 or 70%. This is spuriously high, however, as the rates would agree by chance alone on a number of occasions. The expected chance agreement can be calculated as follows: for each cell where there observed agreement the row total is multiplied by the column total and divided by the total sample size. This comes to 60 × 70/100(42) and 40 × 30/100(12). Adding these together and dividing by the total sample size gives 56% expected agreement by chance alone.

Therefore:

$$K = \frac{(70/100) - (56/100)}{1-56/100} = 0.32$$

(A relatively unreliable result).

This method can be extended to situations where diagnoses or measurements are made in three or more ranked categories (e.g. no, borderline and definite diagnoses of mental illness), in which case kappa can be modified, or weighted, to account for partial agreement.

The reliability of interval, ratio or continuous measurements can be measured by a variety of other methods. The most misused method is to consider the association or correlation between the ratings of two or more observers using the Pearson or Spearman correlation coefficient. This approach is unsuitable because one investigator may consistently under-rate or over-rate compared with his colleague, and yet the degree of correlation between their scores could be very high. For example, one researcher may consistently over-rate the presence of positive symptoms compared with another at the same center, but because the over-rating is consistent, the correlations between scores may be perfect despite the fact that the raters never agree. A useful alternative to this approach is to use the intraclass correlation coefficient (ICC).

The ICC distinguishes the bias in the measurement from random variation of the instrument and produces a more accurate and representative value of reliability. I can also be adapted to situations where there are several observers and can be easily calculated from an analysis of variance (ANOVA) table (Streiner & Normal 1996).

No statistical text is however a substitute for clear graphical representation. The common error in representing agreement between two or more investigators is to plot the observations on a graph where the values given by each investigator are represented on each axis. This approach is similar to the method of correlation and can lead to misleading results. A more informative approach is to plot the difference between the investigators measurements against the mean of the

Table 4: Example showing the level of agreement and disagreement between two observers

		Observer		
		Present	*Absent*	*Total*
Observer 2	Present	50	10	60
	Absent	20	20	40
	Total	70	30	100

measurements. Plotting the difference against the average will demonstrate whether the difference between the two methods is generally very small or very large. A mean difference between the methods can be calculated and, in situations where the mean difference is not zero, whether or not one methods gives systematically higher or lowers scores than the other can be evaluated. Limits of agreement can be added around the average difference (as $d \pm 2s$) as a further refinement by calculating the mean difference (d) and its standard deviation (s). When these limits of agreement do not incorporate any clinically meaningful difference, the two methods may be used interchangeably (Bland & Altman 1986).

Reliability	
•	Can be between methods or raters (inter-rater) or within the same instrument or rater repeated on more than one occasion (intrarater, test-retest)
•	Can be graphically represented on a Bland-Altman plot
•	Should not be measured by the simple correlation of different investigators' scores

STATISTICS

Probability and Risk

Probability and risk are interchangeable terms and to quantify uncertainty or the chance of an observation (or event) occurring. Probability always takes a value between 0, indicating that an event cannot occur, and 1 where it is certainty. The probability of an event can be easily understood by referring to an unbiased six-sided dice. If we ask ourselves the probability of throwing a 6, almost intuitively we come up with the solution 1 in 6, or 0.167. Without realizing it, we are undertaking the following calculation:

Probability = number of events/number of possible events.

We know that each side of the dice is equally likely (if the dice is unbiased) and that there are six sides. Therefore the probability that any side will turn face up is 1 in 6. The probabilities of events in medicine are rarely quite as simple as this although the principles are the same. Consider a study of the probability of readmission following an acute episode of schizophrenia. In a study of 100 people over 1 year, let us say that 40 are readmitted. What is the probability of readmission over 1 year? From the above calculation we see that it is 40 (the number of events) divided by 100 (the number of possible events). Therefore the probability or risk of readmission is 0.4 or 40%.

There are alternative ways of stating the possibility that an event will occur. Those who are familiar with betting will recognize the term odds. This statistic is simply the ratio of events of interest to the nonevents. To take the example of the dice, the odds of throwing a 6 are 1 (the number of events) divided by (the number of nonevents) 5.

Where there is only one group of people and we wish to give an estimate of the chance with which an event with occur, the odds or probability will usually suffice. Odds and probability can be converted into one another using the following formulae:

$$\text{Odds} = \frac{P}{1 - P} \text{ (probability of an event/probability of nonevent)}$$

$$P = \frac{0}{(1 + 0)} \text{ (p, probability; 0, odds)}$$

In a clinical trial we generally compare the probability or odds of one or more outcomes in the two groups. If the treatment is efficacious, the probability of the adverse event (like relapse) will be less in the treated (or experimental group) than it is in the control group. These probabilities, or risk, are sometimes called the experimental event rate (EER) and control event rate (CER) respectively. The experimental event rate is defined as the probability of an event in the experimental group, and the control event rate is defined as the probability of an event in the control group. These terms are usually applied to undesirable events but are applicable to both undesirable and desirable events.

Consider, for example, a trial where patients are randomized to receive either haloperidol or placebo. One hundred people are treated in the haloperidol group and 100 are treated with placebo. Fifty people in the placebo group relapse over the course of the 6 week trial and 20 relapse in the haloperidol-treated group. We can represent the data in the form of a 2 × 2 (contingency) table, as shown in Table 5. The probability (or risk) of relapse in the haloperidol-treated group is 20/100 or 0.2. This is called the experimental event rate. Alternatively we could also say that the odds of relapse were 20/80 or 0.25.

The probability of relapse in the placebo-treated group is 50/100 or 0.5. This is called the control event rate. Alternatively, we could also say that the odds of relapse are 0.5/0.5 or 1.

These probability or odds can be combined to give a single measure of treatment effect. The simplest and most useful things to do are to divide probabilities or odds in the two groups, giving the relative risk and odds ratio respectively. Alternatively we could subtract the probabilities from each other giving an absolute risk or risk difference.

In the above example EER=0.2 and CER=0.5. Dividing these two risks we get 0.2/0.5 or 0.4 (40%). This is known as the relative risk (RR),

Table 5: Contingency table showing relapse in haloperidol and placebo-treated patients

	Relapse	*Nonrelapse*	*Total*
Haloperidol	20	80	100
Placebo	50	50	100

$$\text{Relative risk} = \frac{\text{EER}}{\text{CER}}$$

Alternatively one could also say that the risk of relapse is reduced by 60% in the experimental group relative to the control group. This is known as the relative risk reduction (RRR).

$$\text{RRR} = 1 - \text{RR, or RRR} = \frac{\text{CER} - \text{EER}}{\text{CER}}$$

Given the odds of relapse are 0.25 in the experimental group and 1 in the control group, their ratio (the odds ratio) is 0.25 divided by 1, or 0.25.

$$\text{Odds ratio} = \frac{\text{Odds of the event in the experimental group}}{\text{Odds of the event in the control group}}$$

Another way of summarizing the difference between groups is to subtract the individual estimates of the probability of outcomes from one another. It makes no mathematical sense to subtract and odds from another odds so we will concentrate on the probabilities or risks. In the example above, the risk of relapse (EER) in the experimental groups was 0.2 (or 20%) and the risk of relapse in the control group (CER) was 0.5. By subtracting these figures we can also say that the risk difference is 0.3 (30%). This is called the risk difference or absolute risk reduction (ARR).

Absolute risk reduction (ARR) = CER - EER.

Incidence and Prevalence

Epidemiology is the study of disease in populations. In many cases epidemiologists study populations by taking what they hope is a representative sample and inferring something about the population from which they were drawn. In order to this, two numerical concepts must be introduced: incidence and prevalence. Incidence is the number of new cases arising in a given population in a defined time period. For instance, schizophrenia has an incidence of 2–3 cases per 10,000 populations per year. Incidence is in fact an event rate, and the experimental and control event rates mentioned above are also incidence rates. Prevalence is the number of people within a population who have the disease of interest at any given time. The prevalence of schizophrenia is sometimes quoted as 0.5 per 100 (0.5%), meaning that at any time point, 5 in 1000 people fulfill diagnostic criteria for schizophrenia. Prevalence can be measured at a single point in time (point prevalence) or over a given time period (e.g. 1 month prevalence). Incidence and prevalence are related to each other though chronicity. When a disease is chronic, prevalence will be high relative to incidence. When a disease is acute and short lived, the incidence may be high, but because few cases persist, prevalence will remain low.

Using data on incidence epidemiologists can investigate candidate risk factors. For example, when two populations exist, one of which is exposed to an agent (e.g. sheep dip) while the other is not, incidence of a disease (e.g. depression) can be measured in both groups. If the incidence of depression is greater in the exposed groups, this suggests that sheep dip may cause depression. It would be unusual for the results of an epidemiological study to be as simple as this. Frequently two populations may differ on a number of other variables which may be associated with both the disease and exposure, in which case the study is said to be confounded. Quite often, the measurement of the disease frequency itself may be biased by a number of factors. Subjects to these considerations, the ratio of the incidence in the exposed group to the incidence in the unexposed group is also referred to as the relative risk. Similarly, the subtraction of one risk from the other is referred to as the absolute risk (or risk difference) and has similar properties to the absolute risk reduction mentioned earlier.

The size of a relative risk or odds ratio is not however the only determinant of the importance of a putative risk factor or the incidence or prevalence of a disease. Analogously to the EER of 0.02/0.2 example above, a rare risk factor with a relative risk of 10 will be less important at a population level than a common risk factor with a relative risk of 2. The concept of population attributable risk quantifies this relationship where, if an attributable risk is 10%, then removing that risk factor from the general population could avoid 10% of cases.

DESCRIPTIVE STATISTICS

It is difficult to make sense of a particular dataset without summarizing its main characteristics in a meaningful way. In particular we often wish to know of what constitutes a typical value and the spread or distribution of other values around that number. There are several numerical and graphical methods of summarizing datasets.

Measures of Central Tendency or Location

The average (or measure of central tendency or location) is a general term for the typical value from a distribution and can be measured in a number of ways. First of all, let us consider that we have measured the height of 10 people in the street and we have obtained the following values (cm):

100, 120, 98, 132, 80, 140, 160, 138, 122, 108

Mean

The mean is simply the sum of all the values divided by the number of values. In our example this equals:

(100+120+98+132+80+140+160+138+122+100)/10 = 119 cm

Algebraically

$$\text{Mean } (\bar{X}) = \frac{\Sigma x}{n}$$

(Where ∑x is used to denote the sum of all observations, and n is the total frequency or number of values).

Median

The median, or middle value, can be calculated by ranking the numbers from smallest to largest and talking the middle one. If there is an even number of values, the median is calculated by taking the arithmetic mean of the two middle values.

80,98,100,100,120,122,132,138,140,160

the median is 121.

Mode

The mode is the easiest measure of central tendency to calculate as it is simply the most common value. As all of the numbers in our dataset occur once, with the exception of 100 which occurs twice, the mode is 100.

The relative benefits of the mean, median and mode are not apparent until one considers different datasets and the effect of extreme values on each estimate. For example, if socioeconomic status were measured in 100 individuals on an ordinal scale of 1 to 6, the mean social class would be somewhat meaningless, as the differences between each point are not equal. The median would give a much more meaningful estimate of central tendency. The mean also gives a poor estimate of central tendency when there is skew in a distribution (i.e. when there are a disproportionately large amount of either small values or large values). In situations where the distribution is symmetrical (e.g. Normal distribution, distribution), the mean, median and mode all take the same value and are equally good measures of central tendency. In skewed data, however, these statistics diverge.

Measures of Dispersion

As well as describing the central location of a dataset, a statement of the data spread or dispersion is also helpful. There are several ways of doing this, and the best method often depends on type of data and its distribution. The simplest method of describing dispersion is simply to give the range of values from smallest to largest. This measure is called the range and can be usefully represented on a 'box and whisker plot'. Another method, less influenced by extreme values, is to rank the distribution from smallest to largest value and divided the distribution into equal parts called quantiles. The most commonly used methods divide the distribution up in to 4 quarters using 3 quartiles, or into 100 parts using 99 percentiles. By stating the difference from the first quartile (Q1) to the third quartile (Q3) we obtain the interquartile range (Q3-Q1) or IQR. Occasionally this range is further divided by 2 to obtain the semi-interquartile range. It is worth noting also that the second quartile and 50th percentile will always be equal to the median. This method is more robust to skewness but lacks the many useful mathematical properties of other methods.

A more popular method of determining spread is to measure how much each value differs from the mean and divide it by the number of values in the distribution. If we were to sum all of the differences we would however arrive at a value of 0 for every data set. Therefore the sign (+or –) of each deviation is ignored. Each deviation is then added together for every value and then divided by the number of observations. This gives the mean deviation. Another method of overcoming the problem of differences summing to 0 is to square each deviation from the mean first. This value is always positive and is sometimes referred to the sum of squares. This figure is then divided by the total number of values minus 1 to give the mean square about the mean. This measure has the more familiar name of the variance. Algebraically,

$$\text{Variance} = \frac{\Sigma\,(x - \bar{x})}{n - 1}$$

The standard deviation (SD) is simply the square root of this value. The reason for dividing the squared deviations by n–1 rather than n is that, given that you know the mean, the number of independent ways a data set can vary is always one less than the number of values. To illustrate, if a distribution of numbers had only one value, any measure of dispersion would be meaningless. Where a distribution has two values, it is possible to calculate how much each one varies around the mean, but dividing by n (2) would give a very misleadingly small estimate of the population variance from which the sample was drawn. n -1 is sometimes called the degrees of freedom. When a distribution is skewed, the variance or standard deviation may mislead, as they are based on the deviations around the mean. When the mean is a poor estimate of central tendency, the variance and standard deviation will also be poor estimates of dispersion. Table 6 summarizes descriptive statistics appropriate for various types of data.

INFERENTIAL STATISTICS

Introduction

In the previous section we considered the various ways in which data may be described. In many circumstances, however, one wishes to know whether two or more groups of measurement are different, or to be more precise, whether

Table 6: Descriptive statistics for various types of data

	Nominal	*Ordinal (i.e. ranked)*	*Interval or ratio*
Central tendency	Proportion	Median	Mean
Dispersion (speed)	NA	Interquartile range	Variance or SD

Table 7: Hypothesis testing and statistics power

	Population	
Sample study finding	*There is a difference*	*No difference*
There is a difference (reject H0)	Correct (true positive)	Incorrect (false positive) type error P = α
There is no difference (accept H0)	Incorrect (false negative) Insufficient power Type II error P = $(1 - \beta)$	Correct (true negative)

the difference is likely to be true or likely to have arisen by chance.

Conventionally, when we conduct a statistical test we are testing the statement, or null hypothesis (Ho), that there is no difference between two or more groups. When we conduct a test for no association (correlation or regression analysis) we test for no association. Any P-value from a statistical test is simply the probability that the difference or association between variables is due to chance (i.e. a false positive). The arbitrary threshold for statistical be set significance is $p = 0.05$ (5/100 or 1 in 20), although the threshold can be set at any value, sometimes called alpha. When a statistical test is significant at $p \leq 0.05$, we reject the null hypothesis that there is no difference or association. If one finds no association or difference, then the null hypothesis cannot be rejected and there is no association or difference between two or more variables (true negative). Alternatively, we may find no difference when our study is not large enough or measurement is too imprecise. This often happens when the spread of values is very large, or when the effect one is trying to detect is very small. The probability that a study will not find a differences should one exist (false negative, or type II error) is sometimes called beta. $1-\beta$ is the probability that we will find a significant difference should one exist and is sometimes referred to as the power of a study. The above concepts are demonstrated in Table 7.

The power of a study should always be considered in advance to ensure that a study is going to be large enough to reliably address a given research question. Underpowered studies are both unethical and a waste of effort. In order to calculate the power of a study and the number of people required to reject the null hypothesis, we need to set the level of statistical significance we required (usually $p = 0.05$) and the likely size of the treatment effect. If one requires a very high level of statistical signification (e.g. $p< 0.01$) one needs to recruit a far greater number of participants. Similarly, if comparatively small effects are envisaged, a much larger number of participants will be required than if the effect is very large.

There are a number of methods for calculating the standardized difference. When there are two groups of patients and the mean value and standard deviations in each group are known, then the standardized difference is given by:

$$\text{Standardized difference} = \frac{\bar{x}_1 - \bar{x}_2}{\text{Pooled standard deviation}}$$

The means and standard deviations for each group will not be known with total accuracy (else there would usually be no point in doing the study), but they can often be estimated from existing data. Cohen's d, Hedge's g and Glasses Δ are related measures of standardized difference (or effect size) and are sometimes quoted in meta-analysis.

One-tailed and Two-tailed Tests of Significance

In the above examples we have referred to the probability of rejecting the null hypothesis being alpha or p-value. In rejecting the null hypothesis, one is usually inferring that two or more groups are unequal in terms of a depended variable (by dependent variable we mean the variable that is being compared between the groups), but that the difference might lie in either direction (e.g. group A>B or vice versa). Whichever group is bigger than the other is likely to be of some interest. For example, in a trial of olanzapine versus risperidone, we would be interested to know whether olanzapine was better than risperidone, but we would be equally interested in the reverse. Occasionally, researchers have preconceptions about the direction of the difference and only test for a significant difference in one direction. Therefore, the null hypothesis becomes Ho: 'olanzapine is not better than risperidone' instead of Ho: 'there is no difference'. In order to test whether there is a significant difference in one direction only, a one-tailed test (so called because only one tail of the distributions or differences is examined) is performed. If the investigator wishes to test for a difference in either direction, a two-tailed test will be conducted. However, one-tailed tests are almost never appropriate, as we are usually interested in a difference in either direction. The effect of using a one-tailed test is to increase the chance of finding a significant result, and this can lead to spurious positive findings (type I error) (Bland & Altman 1994).

Multiple Significance Testing

Many published studies describe several significance tests which may generate conflicting results that are difficult to interpret. Part of this difficulty arises because, if many statistical tests are conducted, around one in twenty will show a significant result by chance alone. In an attempt to correct for the chance finding of a positive result, multiple significance tests are sometimes 'corrected'. The Bonferroni adjustment is perhaps the most commonly used of many methods for correcting significance tests.

False positive results occur (by definition) with a frequency of around 5% when the significance level is set to $p = 0.05$. When we conduct one significance test and find it to be significant, we are in fact saying that 'the probability of finding this result, or one that is more extreme, is less than one in twenty if the null hypothesis is true'. Therefore, if two independent tests are conducted simultaneously and the null hypothesis is true, the chance that one of them will be significant is 1 - (the probability that they are both non-significant) = $1-(0.95)^2$ or 0.1 (approximately). The probability of a false positive increases with each independent test and approximates to the following relationship:

The probability that one or more significance tests will be positive when the null hypothesis is true	=	Significance level (α) (usually 0.05) × Number of individual significance tests

There are a number of approaches to this problem. The most conservative approach is the Bonferroni method which corrects for multiple significance testing by setting a higher threshold for statistical significance. The result of the correction is that the significance level for each individual test ($p_{corrected}$) when multiplied by the number of individual tests will be 0.05. By rearranging the above formula, we can see that if we conduct an independent test and we want an overall significance level of 0.05, then the significance of individual findings will need to be (approximately):

$$P_{corrected} = \frac{0.05}{\text{Number of significance tests}}$$

Therefore, if we test two hypothesis, then the level of statistical significance require for each comparison will be approximately 0.025 or 2.5%.

Confidence Intervals

P-values tell the investigator how likely it is that the difference found in a study is due to chance. Studies often quote very small p-values in the hope that this demonstrates the certainty of their result. However, the p-value takes no account of the precision of the estimate and the likely range of plausible values that the value might take. For example, a treatment might to be better than placebo at improving scores on the Hamilton Depression Rating Scale and be significant at p=0.01 but have a wide range of possible effect sizes, some of which may not be clinically significant.

Confidence intervals are the range of plausible values that a variable may take in the 'real world' or population as a whole. For example, if a clinical trial showed that chlorpromazine was more effective than placebo for preventing relapse with a relative risk of 2.3 (with a 95% confidence interval of 1.2 to 3.5). We could be 95% certain that the true treatment effect lay between 1.2 and 3.5. The result is also statistically significant; as the confidence interval does not overlap 1 (the point of no effect or equal risk) though the range of possible risk ratios stretches from 3.5 (potentially very clinically important) to 1.2 (somewhat less clinically impressive). The result could also be said to be somewhat imprecise. By increasing the number of people in the study we could obtain a more precise estimate of the treatment effect. Alternatively we could combine several studies together in a meta-analysis producing a summary measure of treatment effect with an proved precision (and hence narrower confidence interval).

Statistical Distributions

Many variables in medicine follow a known distribution. For example, height and IQ follow an approximately normal distribution which is more or less symmetrical around a central mean. In a normal distribution it is also possible to say that 95% of possible values lie from the mean minus 1.96 x the standard deviation to the mean plus 1.96 x the standard deviation. Normally distributed variables also enable us to perform parametric statistical tests which have greater power than their nonparametric equivalents. Even if raw data in one study are not normally distributed, the sample means in several studies generally are (this is sometimes called the central limit theorem).

Parametric and Nonparametric Statistics

When we complete a study, we usually want to do one of two things:

- Test the hypothesis that some measurement is different between two or more groups of people;
- Test the hypothesis that there is a relationship between two or more variables.

In order to test these hypotheses we have to re-frame each question as a null hypothesis (Ho: there is no difference or association), decide which p-value would lead us to reject this hypothesis and then conduct the appropriate statistical test. The correct choice of statistical test will depend on certain parametric assumptions:

- Continuous data or at least interval discrete data;
- Each unit of data collection should be independent of any other;
- Data should be normally distributed;
- The variance of each group should be approximately equal.

Where data meet these criteria we can use relatively powerful parametric statistical tests which use all of the data values, but where these criteria are not met we may need to use nonparametric statistics (distribution free tests) which require the conversion of raw values into ranks before analysis (Siegel 1988).

Parametric statistics are relatively robust to minor departures from a normal distribution, contrary to the common misperception that normally is the greatest underlying requirement. Where data are not normally distributed, it is often possible to transform them to normal distribution by taking the log or squaring each value.

TESTING FOR DIFFERENCES

Chi-squared (χ^2) Test

The χ^2 test is one of the most important statistical tests. It is one of the most commonly quoted tests in published papers, and other more complicated analyses can be derived from it. The χ^2 test is a nonparametric test which is most commonly used to test whether the proportion of people with or without a certain characteristic differs between two or more independent groups. For example, the proportion of people improving on a certain drug, or the numbers of people of male gender in healthy controls compared with patients with schizophrenia. When conducting a χ^2 analysis, it can be helpful to represent the data in the form of a 2 × 2 table. Consider the data, shown in Table 8, from a study comparing the sexes of people with schizophrenia and healthy controls. The proportions of male subjects in both groups differ slightly; the null hypothesis is that 'there is no difference in the proportion in the population from which this sample was drawn.' In order to test the hypothesis we need to calculate the expected table values if there were no true difference between the groups. In order to do this, we multiply the row total by the column total for each cell and divide it by the total sample size, although in this case it seems perhaps intuitive that the expected values will each be 30. Once we have the observed and expected values from each cell, we can calculate the value of χ^2 using the formula:

χ^2 test	
•	Is distribution free
•	Compares expected with observed frequencies
•	Should be modified when cell values are small
•	The value of χ^2 and the degrees of freedom should always be stated

$$\chi^2 = \Sigma = \frac{(O - E)^2}{E} = 1.2\ (\rho = 0.27)$$

Because the probability of falsely rejecting the null hypothesis is 0.27, we cannot assume a difference in the population from which the sample was drawn. In practice χ^2, and the resulting ρ-value, are almost always calculated by computer.

Table 8: Example of subject group by gender

	Male	*Female*	*Total*
Schizophrenia	27	33	60
Healthy controls	33	27	60
Total	60	60	120

t-test

The *t*-test is one of the most common statistics quoted in medical research. There are two common uses of the *t* distribution. The two sample *t*-test is used to examine differences in the means between two populations, provided there are independent samples from each, when the data are continuous or at least interval and approximately normally distributed with equal variances. Data from the same group measured on two separate occasions or from two different groups, where each individual member of one group is matched on key characteristics with an individual member of the other group, should be analyzed by considering differences in scores between occasions, or between members of each pair, In such cases the paired *t*-test is applicable. You can also use a one-sample *t*-test to compare a sample mean with a known population mean; for example, you could compare the mean age of patients with dementia with the mean age of all elderly patients in a general hospital.

t-test	
•	Is a parametric statistical test
•	Compares the mean values of two independent groups
•	Is relatively robust to departures from parametric assumptions
•	The value of t and the degrees of freedom should always be stated

$$t = \frac{\text{Observed difference in means}}{\text{Standard error of the observed difference}}$$

with $n_1 + n_2 - 2$ degrees of freedom (where $n_1 + n_2$ is the total number of people in both samples combined). This tests the null hypothesis that there is no difference in the means of the two populations from which the samples were drawn. *t* becomes larger (and is more likely to be significant) as the difference in means increases, or when the standard error decreases (e.g. when the sample size increases). The significance of *t* can be obtained from tables, although it is usually calculated within the various statistical packages available.

Mann-Whitney U-test

The Mann-Whitney U-test is used when the aim is to show a difference between two groups in the value of an ordinal, interval or ratio variable. It is the nonparametric version of the *t*-test, which latter should be used for interval, ratio or continuous data unless there are large departures from the parametric assumptions. The process of calculating the test statistic is very simple. It is worth noting that the test can detect differences in the spread as well as the location (median) of two variables, even when the medians are very similar (Hart 2001). Therefore, when presenting the results of Mann-Whitney tests, the median of each group should be presented along with a description of the skewness of each sample (e.g. a box plot). The Mann-Whitney test also assumes that the two groups are independent. Where the measurements are paired (i.e. are two measurements from the same individual), the Wilcoxon matched pairs test should be used instead.

Analysis of Variance

All of the previous tests have concerned two groups of observations. When there are three or more groups, one rests the null hypothesis that there is no difference in the group means by examining the variances.

Consider the data, shown in Table 9 from three groups of 4 patients. There are several sources of variation in this sample.

Mann-Whitney U-test	
•	Is distribution free
•	Is based on ranked values
•	Is used to compare the medians of two independent groups
•	The value of U and the degrees of freedom should always be stated

First, there is the total variation of the whole sample. To calculate this value one calculates the sample variance, ignoring the group to which each measurement belongs. This is sometimes called the total mean squares (MS_{total}) or total variance. Second, there is the variation of the group means about a grand mean of all observations. This is sometimes called the between-groups variance ($MS_{between}$) or sometimes MS_{treat}. Finally, there is the variation between the group measurements and their individual group means. This is sometimes called the within-groups mean square or residual mean squares ($MS_{residual}$) or within-groups variance. The relationship between these sources of variation is:

Table 9: Ages of three groups of 4 patients			
	Ages	*Mean*	*Variance*
Depressed	47,52,58,66	55.75	66.9
Bipolar	25,28,32,45	32.5	77.7
Schizophrenic	18,27,28,32	28.75	71.6
Mean of whole sample = 39, variance = 214.5			

$$SS_{total} = SS_{between} + SS_{residual} \ (MS = \frac{SS}{df})$$

If each of the groups is drawn from the same population with equal population means, the between-groups variance will be comparable to the within-groups variation ($MS_{residual}$). Alternatively, if the three groups have different population means, the between-groups variation will be large compared with the within-groups variance. In order to test which one of these situations is more likely, we use the test statistic F:

$$F = \frac{\text{Variation between samples}}{\text{Variation within samples}} = \frac{(MS_{between})}{(MS_{residual})}$$

In the example above, the total variance is calculated from the whole sample (as if they were not in groups). The between groups sum of squares is the sum of squared deviations between the group means and the overall mean multiplied by the number of observations in each group. The residual sum of squares is calculated usually by subtraction.

Most statistical packages when performing an analysis of variance (ANOVA) will produce an output similar to that shown in Table 10. The sum of squares is just the sum of the squared difference between each value and its corresponding mean. By dividing by the degrees of freedom, we can calculate the within groups ($MS_{residual}$), between groups ($MS_{between}$) and total variance.

In the above example, F=11.9, which is significant, being less than 0.05. We can therefore reject the null hypothesis that there is no difference between the groups.

ANOVA can also be extended to the analysis of data which can be classified a number of ways. For example, in an observational study measuring memory performance score, patients may be classified by diagnosis, sex and treatment. If one wished to compare memory score by diagnosis, a one-way ANOVA (as above) could be conducted. However, if gender and treatment also affected memory score, the difference might not be due solely to the effect of diagnosis alone. To avoid this potential pitfall, a factorial ANOVA can include any number of the factors in a single experiment. The resulting analysis could give the effect of each factor independently, but can also provide information about interactions between factors. For example, a factorial ANOVA could detect that memory scores may be impaired in males with schizophrenia but not females, whereas a one-way ANOVA might fail to detect any differences.

Table 10: Analysis of variance table					
	Sum of squares	*Degrees of freedom*	*Mean square*	*F*	*Sig.*
Between groups	1711.500	2	855.75	11.9	0.003
Within groups	648.500	9	72.1		
Total	2360.000	11	214.5		

ANOVA	
•	Is a parametric statistical test
•	Tests the null hypothesis that the mean values of three or more independent groups are equal
•	The test statistic F is the ratio of the between-groups to within-groups variance
•	The value of F and the two degrees of freedom should always be stated
•	ANOVA has a nonparametric equivalent called the Kruskal-Wallis test (one-independent grouping only)

TESTING FOR ASSOCIATION

Testing for an association between two variables is a common analysis in medical statistics and one that it sometimes misused (Table 11). Often such analysis are undertaken in the hope that one variable causes a change in another, but the direction of effect cannot be inferred solely from the results of the analysis (i.e. association is not causation).

Correlation

Consider the sample data, given in Table 12, from patients in an inpatient ward in whom performance IQ and duration of psychosis in months were measured. If we plot a graph of these values, we can see that they appear to be related to one another (Fig. 1).

In order to show a relationship we need to test the null hypothesis that there is no association between the two variables. If the parametric assumptions are met, we can calculate Pearson's product-moment correlation coefficient. If the assumptions are not met, we can use Spearman's rank correlation coefficient, which is the corresponding distribution-free test. We will calculate both for the same data set.

Pearson's correlation coefficient (r) can take any value from -1 to +1. A correlation coefficient of 1 would indicate perfect positive correlation (both values rise together) where as a correlation coefficient of -1 indicates perfect negative correlation. A correlation coefficient of 0 suggests that there is no relationship between two variables. Pearson's correlation coefficient is calculated using the method of least squares which tries to minimize the differences between each data point and a line of best fit. For the dataset shown above, the correlation coefficient is –0.69 and the significance of the result is p=0.026. This show that duration of psychosis and performance IQ have a moderate to strong negative relationship with each other and that the relationship is significant at p< 0.05. In other words, as the duration of psychosis goes up, the performance IQ goes down, and the null hypothesis (that the correlation coefficient is zero and there is no relationship) can be rejected.

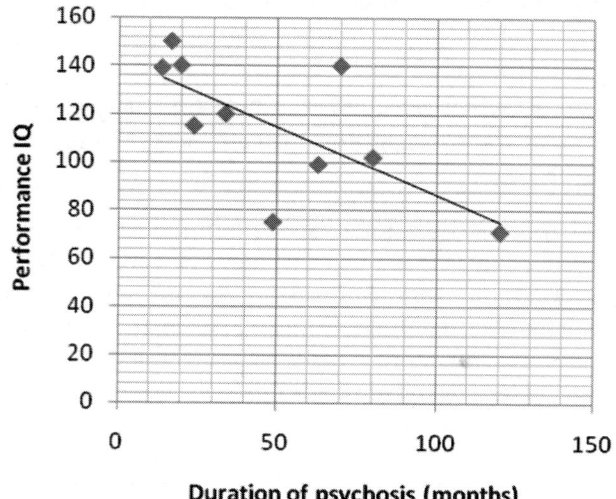

Fig. 1: Scatter plot of performance IQ against duration of psychosis, with line of best fit shown

Table 11: Summary of tests for differences

Two groups	*Categorical*	*Ordinal (ranked)*	*Interval or continuous*
Unpaired	Chi-squared test	Mann-Whitney U-test	Independent t-test
Paired	McNemar test	Willcoxon matched pairs	Paired t-test
Three or more groups Unordered and unpaired	Chi-squared test	Kruskal-Wallis test	Analysis of variance (ANOVA)
Paired	Cochrane Q test	Friedman test	Repeated measures (ANOVA)
Reference from Altman (1991) or Swinscow and Campbell (1996)			

Table 12: Sample data on duration of psychosis and performance IQ

Duration of psychosis (months)	20	14	17	24	49	120	80	63	34	70
Performance IQ	140	139	150	115	75	71	102	99	120	140

Pearson's correlation coefficient	
•	Is a parametric statistical test
•	Measures the observed association between two variables
•	Its significance or confidence interval should always be stated
•	Is derived using the method of least squares

Spearman's rank correlation coefficient (p) can be calculated using the same dataset and is not dependent on a normal distribution of values. The value will lie between -1 and +1 and its interpretation is similar to that of Pearson's coefficient. In this case Spearman's correlation coefficient is –0.64, p= 0.044. The result is still significant, although slightly less so than before. This is results the fact that distribution-free tests tend to have less power to detect associations or differences than parametric tests and yield more conservative estimates if data is normally distributed. Spearman's coefficient however tends to exaggerate the association between variables when there are many tied values, in which case other measures may be more appropriate.

The simple correlation example shown above can be extended to the situation where there is a third variable. In our example, this might be age or premorbid IQ. It is possible to calculate a partial correlation coefficient to take account of this confounder. Table 13 summaries statistical test for association.

Spearman's correlation coefficient	
•	Is a distribution-free test
•	Converts raw values to ranks before measuring their association
•	Tends to inflate the strength of the association when there are many tied values, in which case other tests may be more appropriate

Regression Analysis

Regression analysis is the study of relationships between two or more variables and is usually conducted for the following reasons:

- When we want to know whether any relationship between two or more variables actually exists;
- When we are interested in understanding the relationship between two or more variables;
- When we want to predict a variable given the value of others.

Table 13: Statistical tests for association

Data	*Test*
Categorical data	Kappa
Ranked data	Spearman's rank correlation coefficient
Continuous or interval data	Pearson's correlation coefficient

In its simplest form regression analysis is very similar to correlation; in fact the underlying mathematical models are virtually identical. Regression analysis can however be used where there are many explanatory variables and where various data types are used together. The general regression model is:

$$Y = a + bX_1 + cX_2 + \ldots\ldots + \text{error}$$

Where a is a constant, X_1, X_2, etc. are the predictor variables, and the error term is the difference between the observed and predicted values of r. A practical example of the above equation using the performance IQ data might take the following form:

$$\text{IQ} = 149 - 0.57 \text{ X duration of psychosis}$$

The error term is omitted here and is assumed to have a mean of 0. The distances between each data point and the line of best fit summarizing their relationship are called the residuals. These are the differences between the observed and predicted values and are a measure of the unexplained variation. The model can be extended to more complicated examples, e.g. brain volume using the variables diagnosis, height and IQ. The equation might take the following form:

$$\text{Total brain volume} = 10 \text{ x diagnosis} + 0.03 \text{ x height} + \text{IQ} / 20$$

Diagnosis is a categorical variable, and therefore it makes no sense to allocate a number to each diagnostic category as there is no order in the categories. Therefore, we have to include a number of a "dummy variables" each one indicating the presence or absence of a diagnosis. The example above would be a suitable model when only one diagnosis is considered, as the variable diagnosis will only have to take values of 1 or 0.

Most statistical packages have a variety of methods for doing this. The most common methods are called forward entry, backward entry and stepwise. Forward entry is a method of regression analysis whereby the predictor variable most significantly associated with the dependent variable is included in the model first, and if other predictor variables are also significantly associated with the dependent variable, they are entered into the model. Backward entry regression enters all of the terms into the regression equation first and removes successive terms if they do not predict the dependent variable. Stepwise regression is a combination of forward and backward entry methods.

The Table 14 in the regression analysis was titled ANOVA as regression and ANOVA use virtually identical underlying models. For instance, one could conduct a regression

Table 14: Analysis of variance table for a regression analysis in SPSS

ANOVA					
Model	*Sum of Squares*	*Df*	*Mean square*	*F*	*Sig.*
1 Regression	6098.446	2	3049.223	22.744	0.001
Residual	938.454	7	134.065		
Total	7036.900	9			

analysis where IQ was the dependent variable and duration of psychosis was the predictor. If we had done that we would have arrived at the same answer as an ANOVA.

Linear regression	
•	Is a parametric statistical test
•	Tests the null hypothesis that there is no relationship between a predictor variable and a dependent variable
•	Uses the test statistic F to test for the significance of the regression model used
•	Can incorporate interaction terms
•	The value of F, the degrees of freedom, and R^2 should be stated
•	Can often be helpfully combined with the use of graphs or other descriptive statistics

SURVIVAL ANALYSIS

Survival analysis, as its name implies, was originally related to the drawing of inferences from numerical data on length of life. However, the methods of survival analysis may be applied to the amount of time elapsing before any particular event, such as relapse, in the history of an individual. The quantity which is the subject of a survival analysis is the 'time to outcome', or survival time, of the individuals under study (Altman & Bland 2002). The survival time is the difference between two times or dates. The terminal event in psychiatric applications will not usually be death of subject, but some other kind of event.

Perhaps the most important thing to appreciate about survival analysis is that by the end of any study the event will probably not have occurred in all patients. We will not know when or even whether they experience the event, only that they have not yet done so by the end of the study. Patients may also be lost to follow-up during the course of a study or may experiences an event which is not the event of interest but means that their data is in effect 'censored'. An example of this might be the death of a patient from a lung tumor during the course of an antipsychotic trial to prevent relapse in schizophrenia. In survival analysis, it is assumed that those patients lost to follow-up have the same prognosis as those remaining in the study.

Significance Tests Applied to Survival Analysis

The purpose of undertaking a survival analysis and plotting a Kaplan-Meier curve is usually to demonstrate that the time to some event is greater in one group than in another. In such cases it is usual to perform a significance test to rest the null hypothesis that the survival times are equal. The most common method of comparing two or more survival functions is the *log rank test.* This test is distribution-free and effectively yields a value which can be checked against statistical tables in order to give the significance level of the result. The log rank test assumes that survival times are at least ordinal and that the risk of one group relative to another does not change with time. This 'relative risk' is sometimes called the hazard function or ratio and the assumption that it is constant is called the *proportional hazards assumption.* The terms relative risk and hazard ratio, though they may be similar for specific time points, are not terms which should be used synonymously (Parmar & Machin 1995).

More complex methods of analyzing survival data may be very useful, especially when two groups differ in the presence of one or more prognostic factor. Ideally, their effects should be corrected for in a type of multiple regressions. The most common regression model applied to survival analysis is called *Cox's proportional hazards.*

MULTIVARIATE STATISTICS

Multivariate statistics refers to analyses in which there are multiple (more than one) dependant variables. This situation often arises in medicine when more than one outcome measurement is made (e.g. PANSS, BPRS, etc.) or sometimes when the same measurement is repeated on more than one occasion. A common mistake in the analysis of such data is to perform a series of one-way ANOVAs for each dependent variable separately. The problem with that approach is that every one-way ANOVA increase the chances of at least one type I error (false positive). In addition, the dependent variables are often correlated with one another, and including each variable in the same analysis can provide the researcher with more information (e.g. interactions between variables) than if several analyses are conducted separately. To overcome these problems, a series of multivariate techniques have been devised (Norman & Streiner 1999).

Survival analysis	
•	Is useful when the outcome is time to an event
•	Assumes that dropouts have the same prognosis as those remaining in the study
•	A Kaplan-Meier curve illustrates survival data
•	Methods of data analysis include the log rank test and Cox's proportional hazards

Multivariate Analysis of Variance

In order to compare two or more group means we would conventionally conduct a one-way ANOVA. In more complicated situations, where are several *independent* variables, a factorial ANOVA would be the appropriate technique. If one wishes to compare means between several groups while controlling for a confounder (e.g. when measuring current IQ in people with various diagnoses, one might with to control for premorbid IQ) the appropriate model is called an *analysis of covariance or ANCOVA.* Finally, when there are two or more dependent variables the amended ANOVA model is called a multivariate analysis of variance or MANOVA which can also be adapted to control for confounding variables (MANCOVA). The general mathematical model used in all of these approaches is very similar and often referred to as the general linear model (GLM).

Factor Analysis (Flow chart 1)

Another method of dealing with large datasets is the technique of factor analysis. Factor analysis is a method of data reduction in which many variables are collapsed into a smaller number of different variables called factors. The variables can be reduced in this way when two or more variables are highly correlated and can effectively be replaced by a single factor without the loss of much information. Factors are effectively condensed statements of relationships between a set of variables and are sometimes referred to as latent traits or variables and also as hypothetical constructs.

Multivariate ANOVA	
•	Is a parametric statistical technique
•	Is based on the general linear model
•	Is a relatively computer intensive technique
•	A common test statistic is Hotelling's T^2, although others exist

One of the best known uses of factor analysis was in the field of intellectual ability. Spearman observed that the performances of people on a wide variety of tests of intellectual ability were highly correlated. Spearman, among others, thought that the reason for this finding was that performance on tests of intellectual ability could be explained by a single trait we now know as IQ. Evidence from factor analysis, and from other research, suggests this human abilities can indeed be explained partly by such a single factor. Research in the field of personality variation has also shown that human personality can be thought of as having five latent dimensions using the technique of factor analysis.

Taking a hypothetical example, if we measured the following list of variables on every admission to a hospital we might obtain the factors shown in figure above. This suggests that any patient's observed behavior may be explained by three latent traits (arbitrarily) called hostility, mania and depression. It is worth noting that the names of the factors are descriptive and not derived scientifically.

Factor analysis, as outlined above can be used for data reduction or data exploration. A further technique has evolved called confirmatory factor analysis (CFA) or structural equation modeling which can be used to test hypotheses about underlying factor structure (Kline 1994).

Flow chart 1: Factor analysis of patient's admission data

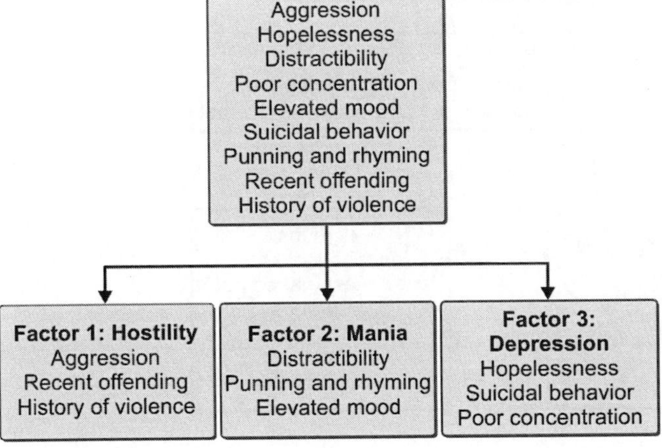

Cluster Analysis (Fig. 2)

Cluster analysis is the name given to a set of techniques which ask whether people can be grouped into categories on the basis of their similarities or differences. It began when biologists began to classify plants on the basis of their various phyla and species and wanted to derive a less subjective technique. It has been applied to diagnostic classification in a similar way. To take a theoretical example, conventional categories of functional psychotic illness (depression, bipolar disorder and schizophrenia) are thought by many to be somewhat unsatisfactory concepts. They do not predict outcome particularly well and seem to share many risk factors. A researcher might attempt to collect data from people with psychosis and empirically derive their own categories using cluster analysis. The mathematical details are too complicated to explain here, but basically

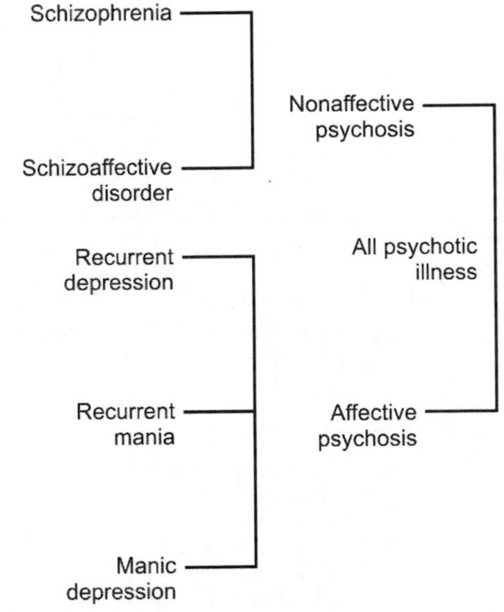

Fig. 2: Dendrogram of hypothetical cluster analysis of psychotic patients

the researcher should first decide whether he wishes to use a hierarchical or partitioning method. Hierarchical methods involve the measurement of various variables on each subject. These variables are then compared between subjects and the clusters are derived in such a way as to minimize the differences (*'Euclidian distance')* between members within a category and to maximize the differences between people belonging to different categories. Each categories represented with a dendrogram. Partitioning techniques assume each category is unique from all the others and are less commonly used.

Factor analysis	
•	May be obtained by several methods
•	Can be used to simplify large data sets
•	Produces latent variables or hypothetical constructs
•	Rotations may be oblique or orthogonal

META-ANALYSIS

A meta-analysis is the weighted average of the results from two or more studies. A meta-analysis is often conducted alongside a systematic review, but the terms are not synonymous. A meta-analysis of several studies may be misleading without a systematic review, since nonsystematic reviews are more prone to bias, particularly in selectively citing studies which support a particular point of view. A meta-analysis of such studies will then provide a spuriously precise estimate of any overall effect failing to take into account other studies. Publication bias is also a threat to the validity of a meta-analysis, even when there has been a previous systematic review. Publication bias is the tendency for small, usually negative studies to remain unpublished. Finally, for studies to be meaningfully combined, the results must be broadly similar from study to study. When study results vary more than one would expect by chance, the results are said to demonstrate statistical heterogeneity. The finding of heterogeneity should prompt investigators to search for an explanation. Causes include differences in the characteristics of study participants and differences in methodology (Flow chart 2).

Common multivariate techniques in psychiatry	
•	Multivariate analysis of variance
•	Factor analysis
•	Cluster analysis

There are in fact a range of meta-analytic methods from which to choose. The choice of method will depend upon the measure of effect used in the individual studies and the presence or absence of heterogeneity. If the results of individual studies do not show heterogeneity, fixed-effects analyses should be used. These assume that there is a single underlying effect and that each individual study is an unbiased estimator of that effect. When heterogeneity is present, random-effects analyses should be used. These do not assume a single underlying treatment effect which is generally less precise than the corresponding fixed-effects analysis since the heterogeneity is also incorporated into the confidence interval of the overall effect estimate.

Fixed-effects Analysis

Fixed-effects meta-analysis is a two-step process. The first step is to calculate a common unit of treatment effect, usually an odds ratio or relative risk of an event or a difference in

Flow chart 2: Data representation

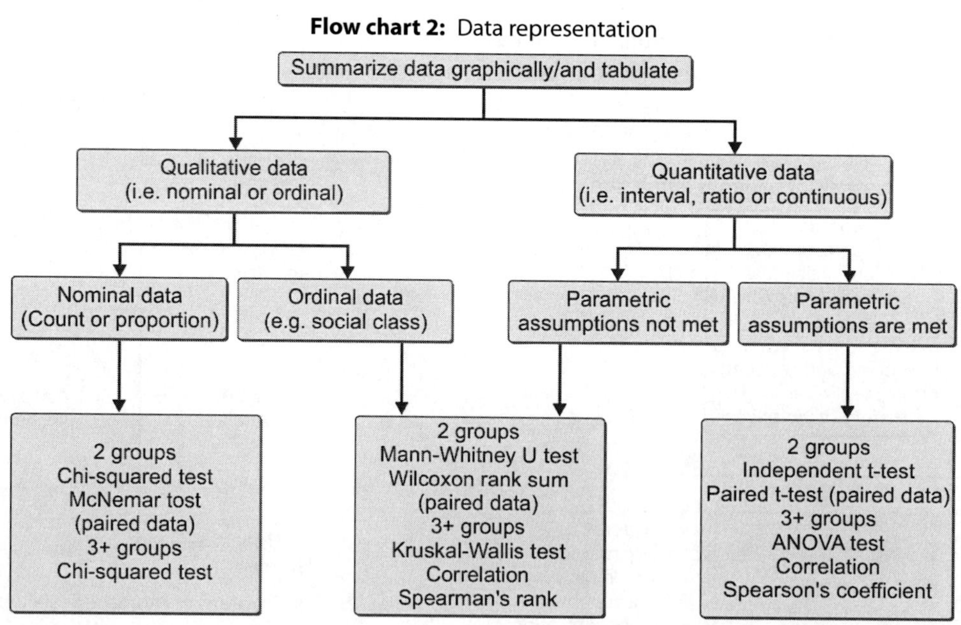

two means for continuous data, for each individual studies. The second stage is to calculate a summary statistic which is a weighted average of the results from individual studies. The weights used are usually the inverse of the variance (the square of the standard error) from the individual studies. Larger studies, which provide a more precise estimate of overall treatment effect, and have a relatively small variance, are given more weight than smaller trials with larger variances. This method can be expressed algebraically:

$$\theta_{IV} = \frac{\Sigma w_i \theta_i}{\Sigma w_i}$$

Where θ_{IV} is the pooled result using fixed-effects (inverse variance) analysis, θ_i is the result of individual studies, and w_i, is the weight given to individual studies.

$$W_i = \frac{1}{SE(\theta_i)^2}$$

Where SE (θ_i) is the standard error of the results of individual studies. The heterogeneity statistic Q is calculated as:

$$Q = \Sigma w_i (\theta_i - 0_{iv})^2$$

Random-effects Models

Random-effects analysis sometimes referred to as DerSimonian and Laird random-effects models (DerSimonian & Laird 1986), do not assume one underlying treatment effect. The effect sizes from individual studies are assumed to be normally distributed with variance τ^2. The individual weights (w_i) for each included study are then:

$$W_i = \frac{1}{SE(\theta_i)^2 + r^2}$$

Where SE (θ_i) is the standard error of the results of individual studies. And the pooled overall effect is:

$$\theta_{DL} = \frac{\Sigma w_i \theta_i}{\Sigma w_i}$$

Where θ_{DL} is the pooled result using random-effect (DL=DeLaird) analysis, θ_i is result of individual studies, and w_i is the weight given to individual studies.

As heterogeneity (and therefore τ^2) increase, the study weights given to individual studies will become more similar, and relatively more weight will be given to smaller studies compared with fixed-effects models. Random-effects models are more conservative than fixed-effects models, giving wider confidence intervals around the overall summary estimate.

Measuring Publication Bias

In order to assess whether the sample of studies you have obtained is likely to be biased because of selective publication or identification, a number of graphical and numerical methods are available. The simplest method of all is to construct a funnel plot. Essentially a funnel plot is a plot of the study effect size against its precession. The effect size is usually measured as a mean difference or standardized difference, for continuous data, or a relative risk or odds ratio for dichotomous or event-like data. Relative risks and odds ratios are usually plotted on a log scale so that effect sizes favoring an effect are plotted an equal distance away from the line of no effect as those showing an equal effect, but in the opposite direction.

Concerning meta-analysis	
•	Fixed-effects analysis-assume no or low heterogeneity and a single underlying effect
•	Fixed-effects analysis-usually weight the results by the reciprocal of their variance
•	Random-effects analyses-allow for heterogeneity, to give an average treatment effect across studies
•	Random-effects analysis-incorporate heterogeneity as well as study variance into the weights given to individual studies
•	Publication bias may be suggested by funnel plot asymmetry

Qualitative Data Analysis

The aim of most medical research is top quantity differences or relationships between one or more group people according to an exposure or experimental factor. However, sometimes researchers wish to interpret or explain something and may use qualitative rather than quantitative research methods in order to accomplish this. Qualitative research methods have been developed in order to provide reproducible and reliable methods of addressing questions usually about the beliefs or attitudes of group of people.

Good qualitative research has several features. Firstly the perspective of the researcher must be considered in some detail. Secondly, the results should be confirmed using two or more methodologies (triangulation) and the theoretical framework to the study should be described. Numerous papers on the subject of qualitative research have been published by the BMJ and are available by searching bmj.com using the search terms 'qualitative research'.

45.6 GENETICS IN RELATION TO PSYCHIATRY

SC Bhargav, Umesh S, Christoday RJ Khess

INTRODUCTION

The completed full sequence of the human genome has recently been announced, an astonishing achievement coming only two years after the publication of the draft sequence in 2001. We are now in the postgenomic age, and it is important to keep pace with the rapid advances in genetics as applied to psychiatry. The number of human genes has turned out to be surprisingly small at around 30000, and the molecular diversity of created proteins is greatly increased by a variety of processing mechanisms beyond DNA transcription. The principal aim of genetics is to relate genotype to phenotype, and in the last ten years over 1200 genes that cause human illness have been identified. There are also complex general and tissue-specific regulatory mechanisms that control gene expression, and important inherited (epigenetic) control factors that are not directly coded by DNA. Our genetic inheritance influences almost all disease to a greater or lesser extent, and this is particularly true of psychiatric disorders. Some of the best-established findings in psychiatry related to the role of genetic factors in determining the risk of developing a disorder.

Genetic Code and Mechanisms of its Transmission

Inheritances can be interpreted in several ways. Culture is transmitted from one generation to the next through the experience of a social environment that persists and changes more slowly than the generational period. Information can be passed on over generations though stable media—books, photographs, recordings, and other such artifacts. The inheritance of genetic factors is mediated by the generational passage of deoxyribosenucleic acid (DNA). DNA consists of four nucleotide bases, adenine (A), thymine (T), cytosine (C), guanine (G), arranged in two anti-parallel strands where phosphate bonds link individual bases and the strands bind through hydrogen bonds in according to the base pairing rule—A with T, C with G- which is the basis of the copying mechanism that ensures DNA fidelity during replication. This vertical flow of information dictates the development and maintenance of the human form.

Structure of the Chromosome

Long linear molecules of DNA exist in the cell nucleus in association with a variety of histones and other chromosome-associated proteins; the whole complex (called chromatin) forms a discrete structure, the chromosome. Chromatin is packed at several levels: the DNA duplex wraps around a protein complex (nucleosome) in a bead-on-string fashion, the beads coil into a 30-nm chromatin fiber, which in turn is formed into twisted loops that radiate from a protein scaffold (Fig. 3).

During cell division, further compaction occurs, rendering the chromosome visible under light microscopy. The structure shows differential staining patterns with certain chemicals, producing the classical banded appearance at metaphase. This has an underlying functional basis, with light staining areas (using Giemsa dye) being gene-rich and dark bands gene-poor. The phase of the cell cycle during which DNA replicates also differs between bands.

In humans, chromosomes exist as 22 matched autosomes and one heteromorphic pair of sex chromosomes. The autosomal pairs are numerically labeled depending on their size (1 being the largest); sex chromosomes are labeled as XX (females) and XY (males). Thus a normal complement in a woman can be described as 46, XX, the digit indicating total chromosome number or diploid count, the letters the sex chromosome status. Human chromosomes have an obvious macrostructure during certain stages of cell division. A primary constriction, the centromere, divides the chromosome into two arms: a short (termed 'p') and a long ('q'). The centromere contains a particular type of repeated DNA motif (alpha-satellite), hypoacetylated histones and centromere-specific proteins, some of which may have motor functions to drive chromosomes along microtubules during cell division. At the end of human chromosomes are other specialized structures called telomeres where a repeated sequence (TTAGGG) caps the free chromosome end, acting as a halt to replication. Telomeres are replicated themselves by a separate enzymatic mechanism involving telomerase. During any cell division there is loss of telomeric DNA which telomerase serves to correct in undifferentiated cells. In differentiated cells, however, telomerase is not expressed, and shortening of telomeres occurs with aging, leading eventually to cellular malfunction.

Formation of Gametes: Meiotic Division

The germ cells (ova and sperm) differ from other (somatic) cells in that they only contain one chromosome from each original pair (haploid count). This is the end product of meiotic division, a reduction mechanism that involves recombination and random chromosome assortment. It is a two-stage process. The first division involves chromosome doubling (during the prophase stage in which the chromosomes also condense and the nuclear membrane dissolves), each chromosome being linked at the centromere to its new partner. Each part of this doublet is now termed a sister chromatid, and the doublets to each chromosome of the pair appose each other so that the highly important process of recombination can occur. DNA segments (over 300bp in length) are exchanged between the chromatids of homologous chromosomes, a process (synapsis) that involves the formation of bridges (seen as chiasmata under the light microscope) in a synaptonemal complex. Specific proteins (including human Rad51) can bind to a single strand of the DNA duplex and recognize a complementary strand in the DNA of the other homologous chromosome. In an energy-dependant step a heteroduplex junction is formed, with breakage, crossover and reunion of DNA between the homologues. Rearranged DNA is important in maintaining diversity within the genome, and hence its adaptability to differing and changing environments. Recombination can also act to repair DNA, preserving its fidelity; the template-scanning functions allow correction of damage caused by external (alkylating substances, radiation) and internal (reactive oxygen species) agents and errors due to the replication process itself.

Each paired sister chromatid unit has a specific protein containing disk (kinetochore) at their fused centromere region which interacts and binds with a microtubule-based apparatus that radiates from two anchoring structures (poles) spaced apart within the cell. Though the addition or subtraction of molecular subunits to microtubules the spindle apparatus can 'pull' or 'push' chromosomes within the cell, either bringing them to the equator of the spindle (congression) as a prerequisite for recombination or separating them to opposite poles (segregation) prior to the formation of daughter cells. The kinetochores are orientated towards one pole or the other, and after recombination the individual members of the homologous chromosome pair are drawn towards the poles. Such segregation is a random event introducing a mixture of paternal and maternal derived chromosomes into the germ line, adding another element of adaptive variation into the transmitted genome. Meiosis-I is completed, after the formation of two clusters of segregated chromosomes, by the disappearance of the spindle apparatus, the formation of new nuclear membranes, and finally by the ingression of the cell membrane in a closing purse string fashion to separate into two daughter cells. The second meiotic division (Meiosis-II) does not involve DNA duplication—it is a reduction division, so that each gamete contains only half the original chromosomal material. The sister chromatids that were fused at the centromere during Meiosis-I are split and pulled (random orientation with respect to the poles ensuring random selection) to two new poles by the spindle apparatus of Meiosis-II. Four gametes are thus produced from each original cell, each containing only 23 chromosomes (normally either 23, X or 23, Y). The above description is simplified, and a large number of complex interactions occur involving molecular motors, checkpoint systems that control progress from one phase to the next, the spindle apparatus and kinetochores. In fact a significant proportion of all proteins produced by a cell are involved in the (seemingly simpler) process of somatic mitosis where there is neither recombination nor reduction division (Scholey et al. 2003).

In the male germ line all four gametes are retained as sperm; however, in the formation of ova only one of the four gametes survives as an ovum, the others form polar bodies.

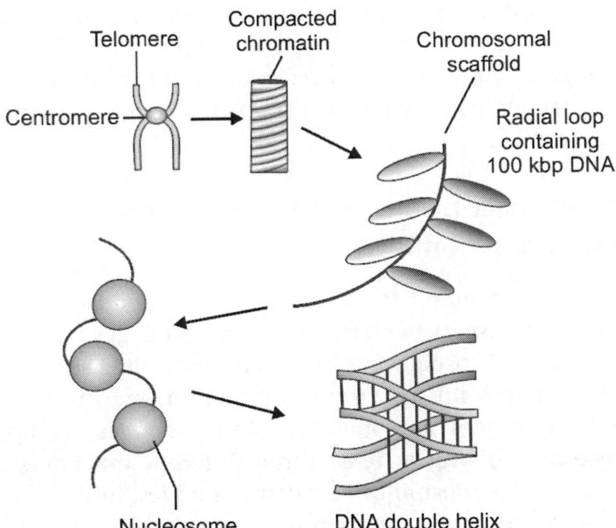

Fig. 3: The various levels of DNA compaction at metaphase: from the level of the whole chromosome (upper left), to the duplex DNA helix itself (lower right)

Gene

This is the basic unit of genetic information that lies within each chromosomal DNA sequence. Originally the term 'gene' was used in an abstract sense to explain why some traits seemed to be inherited. In fact the relationship between genes and proteins (Beadle's 1930s concept of 'one gene, one enzyme') was conceived well before the structure of DNA was known. The gene is now taken to mean a stretch of DNA that contains the information (genetic code, read as triplets of nucleotides) necessary to direct amino acids into the correct sequence order during protein assembly in the cytoplasm (using ribonucleic acid, RNA, intermediates), or to direct the formation of RNA molecules that are end-products in themselves. The products of so called RNA genes have structural, enzymatic or regulatory functions. Information in DNA is copied into messenger RNA (mRNA), which in turn acts as a template for polypeptide assembly through

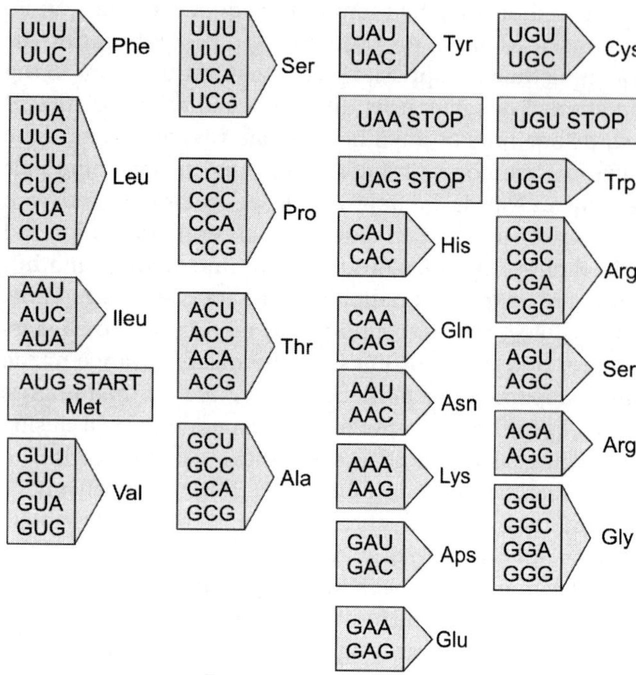

Fig. 4: The genetic code in mRNA, left hand side of columns indicates the coding triplets. Columns are arranged by order of the second nucleotide in each 'triplet (U [uracil], C, A or G). The amino acid coded for is given on the right using the standard chemical abbreviations. Note the start (methionine) and stop codons. The code can easily be referred 'back' to DNA or 'forward' for tRNA triplets

interaction with transfer RNAs (tRNAs) that are conjugated to specific amino acids. The emphasis is on functionality—a gene is that segment of the chromosome that directs the formation of a functional product. Many sequences within the genome bear great similarity to active genes but are either completely untranscribed, or their mRNAs are untranslated. Such pseudo genes produce no functional product. Within the gene the basic unit of information is the codon—a triplet of three nucleotide bases whose presence in a sequence will lead to a specific amino acid insertion into a protein. The genetic code maps DNA codons to amino acids, and the code has a degree of redundancy (degeneracy), with several different codons linked to individual amino acids (a triplet can be taken from four nucleotides in 64 different ways, but there are only 20 different amino acids). Some codons do not code for amino acids, but dictate operational events during protein formation such as initiation and termination of polypeptide chain assembly (start and stop codons; start codons also code for methionine the initial amino acid in any polypeptide (Fig. 4).

Transcription: DNA to mRNA

To describe transcription in relation to DNA sequence a nomenclature based on the sugar chemistry of DNA has developed. The fifth carbon of deoxyribose (the 5′-carbon; pronounced 'five prime') is bound to a phosphate moiety, the third to a hydroxyl group. Diphosphate bonds are formed between the 3' and 5' of the first sugar leaving the first 5' free (the '5'-end') and the last 3' of the DNA free (the 3'-end). This gives a direction to the DNA sequence. Thus transcription of DNA into RNA begins at the 5'-end of DNA and proceeds in the 3'-direction. Normally a sequence of bases exists on either side of the ORF that is transcribed into mRNA but not translated into protein (untranslated regions; UTRs). RNA, normally single stranded, differs from DNA in its sugar backbone (ribose instead of deoxyribose) and the replacement of thymine with uracil bases. During transcription the duplex DNA is partly unwound to allow access to the key enzyme DNA-dependant RNA polymerase (RNA pol) (There are three forms of RNApol in eukaryotes: RNApol I, which creates ribosomal or rRNA; RNApol II which creates messenger of mRNA; and RNApol III, which creates transport or tRNA). The initial event is binding of an initiation protein to a nontranscribed promoter sequence (normally containing a TATA nucleotide motif or box) near the 3'-end of the ORF. A complex of proteins that includes transcription factors (co-activators) and activator proteins that link to more distant enhancer elements in the DNA sequence itself help closely regulate transcriptional activity and also position RNApol correctly at the start of the ORF. Abnormalities in these regulatory proteins or the DNA motifs in the promoter and enhancer elements that they bind have been increasingly recognized as pathogenic in addition to direct alterations within gene sequence itself. In some cases the altered enhancer sequence (that up-regulates transcription) can be hundreds of kbp distant from the gene under regulation. Figure below summarizes the gene unit and its regulatory elements. Not shown on this diagram are silencer motifs that act to down-regulate transcription by binding specific proteins (repressors). Taken together this complex set of interacting proteins serves to position and stabilize RNApol at the transcription start site and to offer many targets for cellular line-tuning of transcriptional activity (Fig. 5).

Post-transcriptional Modification and Regulation of mRNA

All DNA within an ORF is initially transcribed into mRNA (primary transcript), but the sequence that codes for amino acids (exon) is usually interrupted by noncoding sequences (introns) that must be removed to form mature mRNA before translation into protein. RNA processing is a complex process involving at least three different mechanisms. A 7-methylguanosine cap structure is added to the 5'-end of mRNA during transcription and immediately after transcription a polyadenylate tail (a sequence of repeated adenine nucleotides) is added at the 3'-end. These are essential to mRNA stability, protecting it from enzyme (exonuclease) attack as well as facilitating export from the nucleus and efficient translation. Introns are spliced out in the spliceosome, an assemblage of proteins and small nuclear ribonucleoproteins (snRNP) that recognize terminal intronic sequences (largely conserved dinucleotides). The exons are often spliced together in different ways depending on up- and down-regulating protein and tissue-specific signals. In this way the mammalian genome vastly increases its repertoire of protein types above the relatively limited number of human genes available. Neurons have a specific splicing regulatory system, dysfunction in which can lead to several disorders. Chromosome 17 linked frontotemporal dementia and Parkinsonism is associated with mutations in the tau gene, leading to aberrant function of tau in microtubule assembly. Eleven exons are normally spliced into six different protein isoforms. Exon 10 has a number of repeated microtubule binding domains, and various mutations are associated with increased spliced-in copies of this exon leading to neurodegenerative disease. In spinal muscular atrophy there are mutations or small deletions at the exon splice sites, and the abnormal protein (called survival of motor neuron protein, SMN) may lead to a deficit in snRNP recycling essential to spliceosome function. Other neurological disorders (e.g. spinocerebellar ataxia 8 and amyotrophic lateral sclerosis) may also involve splicing dysfunction. NOVA proteins are a class of neuron-specific splice regulators that are produced from genes on chromosomes other than those harboring the genes they act on (and are termed *trans*-acting, as opposed

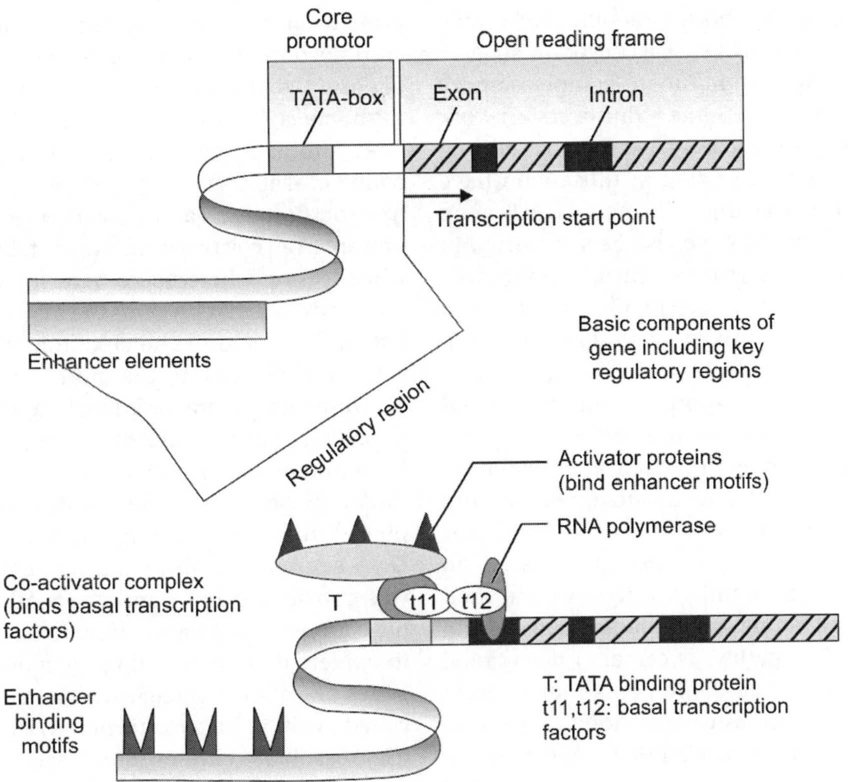

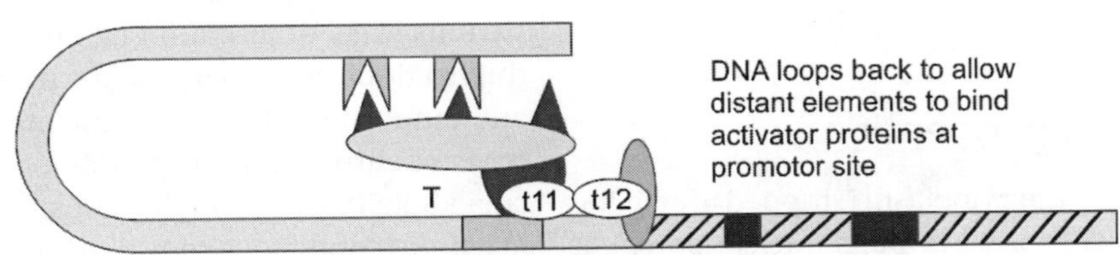

Fig. 5: The basic elements of eukaryotic gene structure and regulation

to *cis*-acting elements from elsewhere on the same DNA duplex as the gene). High levels of NOVA2, for example, seem restricted to cerebral cortex, hippocampus and dorsal spinal cord. They have KH-binding domains (cf. the similar domain in fragile-X linked mental retardation protein) of a type implicated in splicing activity. NOVA1 is a similar splice regulator restricted to CNS regions controlling movement, and disruption leads to loss of inhibitory control of motor neurons (paraneoplastic opsoclonus myoclonus ataxia) (Dredge et al. 2001).

mRNA is also modified by the process of RNA editing, which changes its coding function by converting cytosine residues to uracil, and adenine to inosine, using a series of specific editing enzymes (termed ADAR, APOBECI and ACF) (Keegan et al. 2001). In mammals most of the ADAR-edited transcripts are expressed in the CNS, increasing again the amount of CNS protein diversity. Inosine-modified RNAs may act to target specific types of mRNA such as the brain-specific small nucleolar RNAs (snoRNAs) that are complementary to mRNA for the $5HT_{2c}$ receptor. Some (controversial) work suggests that $5HT_{2c}$ receptor mRNAs have reduced editing in schizophrenia or increased editing in those who have committed suicide. Editing changes in the GLUR-B gene (prefrontal cortex and striatum) have also been reported in Alzheimer's and Huntington's disease and in schizophrenia.

Finally, altering their decay rate regulates the levels of mRNAs. mRNAs are differentially stable and, although most mRNAs have a fixed half-life, there are a large number in which the levels change in response to environmental stimuli. Decay usually begins with shortening of the 3'-poly-A tail. An initial trimming in the nucleus is followed by a substantial deadenylation after movement of the processed mRNA into the cytoplasm via pores in the nuclear membrane. This is followed by rapid cleavage of the 5'-cap by a variety of factors. Decay of mRNA is tightly controlled by *cis*-acting elements, including some motifs in the 3' - and 5'-UTRs of genes. Signaling pathways can alter decay rate. Interleukin-2 mRNA has 3' and 5' elements that interact with extracellular stimuli such as calcium ionophores and phorbol esters. Aberrant stop codons in mRNA, that generate signals to stop synthesi prematurely, are also recognized and eliminated by rapid decay, helping maintain the fidelity of the RNA. This effect can help minimize the damage caused by premature stop codon abnormalities seen in many patients with disease such as Duchenne muscular dystrophy (Wilusz et al. 2001).

Translation: mRNA to Polypeptide

Once mRNA has moved to the cytoplasm (stripped of splicing proteins and actively transported through nuclear pores), it associates with ribosomes in the final steps towards protein synthesis. Again the process is complex. Cytoplasmic translational factors must bind the mRNA to allow it to interact with the ribosome. In some cases inhibiting factors will prevent its translation (e.g. ferritin mRNA is usually inhibited by aconitase which binds with the initial 30 bp, forming a loop that cannot link to ribosomes; only in the presence of cellular iron which binds aconitase is this inhibition removed). Normally a large multiprotein initiation complex forms that positions the mRNA correctly in the ribosomal groove. Amino acids are shuttled to the ribosomal complex attached to tRNA molecules by genetic code-reading activating enzymes. Each tRNA molecule has one anticodon complementary to the codons on the template strand of duplex DNA and carries the amino acid dictated by the genetic code.

Genome Outside Genes

Chromatin is the term used to describe the nucleic-acid-protein complex that gives structure as well as function to the chromosome. As cells leave mitosis or meiosis, large stretches of chromatin become de-condensed and dispersed through the nucleus; Genes are embedded within this 'true' chromatin or euchromatin. Other areas do not de-condense but remain compact at all stages of the cell cycle. This in general is termed heterochromatin (and classified as constitutive when it is present in all cell types and stage of differentiation; facultative when it is only heterochromatic in certain cells, such as the Barr body which represents the inactivated X-chromosome in females). Constitutive heterochromatin predominates around the centromeres and telomeres of the chromosome. The centromeres are bracketed by long stretches of large repeats of several hundred nucleotides length (satellite DNA), which form into dense heterochromatic coding regions (C-bands). This replicates at a different time of the cell cycle (late S phase) from euchromatin, and has large blocks of repeated DNA sequences. Although, historically, heterochromatin was considered inert, more recently it has been shown to have a host of regulatory functions, especially those related to epigenetic programming. In general it contains very few genes but has the capacity to silence genes (a phenomenon called position-effect variegation) that are positioned within it by reason of a chromosomal rearrangement.

Gene Mutations

At the simplest level, mutation can be taken to mean an alteration from normal in the DNA sequence of chromosomes. Various sizes of mutation can be delineated, ranging from duplications and deletions of whole chromosomes (trisomy and monosomy) through segmental changes involving short parts of chromosomes (partial monosomy and trisomy), to small deletions and duplications that only affect a few genes at a time (contiguous gene syndromes).

From the discussion of the genetic code it is clear that the ORF must be read correctly by the polymerase enzyme for the correct amino acids to be assembled into polypeptide.

Any change in the sequence of base pairs of DNA within the ORF can lead to errors in reading, and such mutations usually involve one or a few bases (point mutations). If mutations occur in the germ line they can be transmitted, and some will arise during the natural process of recombination. Others are caused by errors in the systems that preserve DNA fidelity or by external mutagenic agents (radiation, chemicals). Outside the ORF, mutation gives rise to the great variety of noncoding polymorphisms that are used as tools to study patterns of inheritance and co-segregation. Within the ORF, however, the results can alter transcription. Most changes involve the substitution of one base for another, and 50% of substitutions lead to *missense mutations* where a triplet coding for one amino acid is altered to one that codes for a different amino acid. Depending on the position of the amino acid within the polypeptide and the type of amino acid substituted, this can result in increased or decreased protein activity through to complete loss of function. *Nonsense mutations* (30%) arise when the substitution changes the codon to a stop signal; these are often pathological and usually lead to a decreased level or complete absence of any mRNA formed. The mechanism for silencing the production of the abbreviated mRNA is unclear. The exon position of the nonsense mutation is also important; those in the terminal exons have been sometimes found to have less effect. *Nonsense mutations* may also produce 'exon skipping' where the exon containing the stop codon is completely bypassed during transcription and an aberrant mRNA is formed. *Silent mutations* are those without phenotype consequence. The redundancy built into the genetic code means that substitution may lead to an alternative triplet for the same amino acid (synonymous mutation). Insertions and deletions of bases, however, can lead to drastic consequences due to frame shift mutations. Here the entire downstream sequence of the reading frame is disrupted, resulting in a very aberrant mRNA. The disruption is maximal when the deletion or insertion is not a multiple of three (which leads to a resumption of correct frame reading after the mutation has been transcribed).

Mutations can also cause differences in the way mRNA is spliced together. *Splice-junction mutations* as a source of human disorder are not rare (near 10% of all mutations). Failure of splicing may occur or mutations may lead to *de novo* splice site formation in aberrant positions. The cell may attempt compensation for loss of a splice site by splicing at a second illegitimate site (cryptic splice site), or by exon skipping (as in spinal muscular atrophy). Mutation in 5' and 3' UTRs can also be pathogenic. 5' disruption can lead to disturbance of translational efficiency (as in Charcot-Marie-Tooth syndrome), and 3' disruption to changed mRNA stability (Mendell & Dietz 2001). Finally, mutations in remote gene promoter and regulatory elements are increasingly recognized.

Patterns of Inheritance

Complementary genes on both the paternally and maternally derived autosomes in a cell are normally both transcribed (biallelic expression), and a gene mutation on the chromosome derived from one parent usually leads to a reduction (haploinsufficiency), not absence, of a gene product. The level of product may be sufficient for normal cell function, with no phenotypic consequences unless the complementary gene is also mutated. This situation would present as a classical recessive inheritance pattern. At the other extreme, when silencing or down-regulation of one gene of a pair is functionally uncompensated by the other, the resulting illness would show a dominant pattern.

Mendel studied such phenotype patterns in plant breeding experiments, and suggested that quantal genetic factors were being inherited. Disorder due to the inheritance of a single mutated gene (monogenic disorders) are often said to be Mendelian. Recessive conditions rely on mutations in both genes of the pair—the affected person is usually homozygous for the same mutation. If the gene mutations in the paternally and maternally derived chromosomes differ, the offspring is said to be a compound heterozygote. The chances of inheriting rare gene mutations from both parents is increased if they are themselves closely related, and an increased rate of consanguinity is often found in recessive disorder. With more common recessive disorder such as cystic fibrosis (1:2500 live births) the frequency of mutations in the population is high. Either new mutation is frequent, or heterozygous carriage, confers some reproductive advantage. If both parents carry one copy of the mutant gene then, on average, one in four of their children will be affected. No cases may occur in previous generations, the disease being apparent only in the children-'horizontal' inheritance.

Dominant disorders are more common than recessive (7:1000 live births as opposed to 2-3: 1000) and more likely to be associated with late-onset conditions. Fully dominant conditions result in a phenotype whether the person is heterozygous or homozygous for the mutant genes. Affected individuals are found in every generation ('vertical' inheritance), and around half of any sibship is affected. Fully dominant disorder are rare, and usually the clinical outcome is variable—especially in heterozygotes because of reduced penetrance, measured as proportion of people heterozygous for the mutation who show any phenotypic feature.

Mutations in genes on the sex chromosomes form a third Mendelian group. Males can only pass on their Y chromosome to their sons, so that there will be no male-to-male vertical inheritance in X-linked conditions, but affected males are more common in X-linked pedigrees. The mothers of affected males will be carriers of the gene mutation, and either be unaffected (X-linked recessive) or affected (X-linked dominant).

Sometimes one gene may interact with another gene on the same or a different chromosome to influence the expression of a phenotype—a situation termed epistasis. In psychiatry an interesting example of this is shown by the effect on the risk of dementia of interactions between variations in the gene for apolipoprotein E, variations in the gene for amyloid protein, and variations at a separate gene locus on chromosome 10 (Lendon & Craddock 2001). Mutations in completely different genes may cause the same clinical picture (locus heterogeneity). Early - onset Alzheimer's disease provides an example, with mutations known in genes for presenilin I (Chromosome 14), presenilin II (Chromosome 1) and amyloid precursor protein (chromosome 21). Conversely some disease may result from different pathogenic mutations within one single gene (allelic heterogeneity). Over 600 different mutation (mainly missense) resulting in cystic fibrosis are known in the cystic fibrosis transmembrane conductance regulator gene (CFTR).

Nonmendelian Inheritance

Quantitative Trait Loci

When the genetic contribution to a disorder is shared by several (oligogenic) or many (polygenic) genes the clinical phenotype is the result of the additive or interactive contributions at each locus. Variation in any single gene associated with a trait is neither necessary nor sufficient on its own to account for the phenotype, and the expression of the phenotype is best described under a liability/threshold model. Many aspects of psychopathology and descriptions of personality can be viewed as quantitative variables where clinical or pathological states represent extremes of a normal continuum of genetic and environmental variation found in the general population. This contrasts with the categorical approach we apply when classifying someone as being depressed or not, using standard criteria. Common conditions and attributes such as hypertensions, obesity, cognitive abilities and personality dimensions are understood as quantitative traits, and it is likely that this mode will best explain some aspects of common psychiatric conditions such as depression, anxiety and personality disorders. Quantitative trait loci (QTL) are genes that contribute to the variance of a continuous trait, as distinct from single gene mutations that may have a major effect on risk of disease.

Dynamic Mutations

Most inherited disorders do not fall neatly into Mendel's classes. Partial penetrance is the most common difference, but there are many others. Anticipation is said to occur when a disease has an earlier age-at-onset and increased severity in succeeding generations; it was originally proposed by Mott in 1910, who examined psychiatric illness in parent-offspring pairs. Since then it has been frequently described in psychiatric illness, especially bipolar disorder (Blackwood & Muirs 2001). One possible cause is a dynamic mutation involving transgenerational expansion of repeat sequences that alter nearby gene expression dependent on their size. The classical dynamic mutation is the (noncoding) triplet repeat expansion associated with fragile X syndrome. Over 20 neurological and developmental conditions are now known to be associated with expanded repeats of nucleotide triplets, but not all involve transgenerational repeat expansion. Those repeats that exist in the ORF of genes (coding dynamic mutations) often have CAG as the repeated triplet base, which then codes for a polyglutamine tract within the protein (Sugar & Rubinsztein 2003). This is the case in Huntington's disease, where the gene on the short arm of chromosome 4 has over 35 CAG triplets within the first exon, and the size of the repeat is related to age-at-onset of the disorder, explaining up to 60% of the variance. The aberrant protein (huntingtin) contains a polyglutamine sequence that alters its function (a gain of function effect). It may interact with nuclear transcription factors and similar proteins to disrupt the expression of other genes. It also forms abnormal complexes with cytoplasmic and nuclear proteins that may be toxic and play a role in neurodegeneration. In fact all eight known CAG expansion diseases have a clinical picture involving neurodegeneration (and all are also typically late-onset). The noncoding repeat in fragile-X syndrome, is at the 5' untranslated end of exon 1, and leads to methylation-driven gene silencing. Other noncoding repeats are known. The myotonic dystrophy type I repeat (CTG) is located at the 3 UTR of the gene, and the pathology is thought to arise from accumulation of abnormal mRNA in the nucleus that then interferes with splicing and other functions. Myotonic dystrophy type 2 is associated with a tetranucleotide repeat (CCTG) in a completely different gene (ZNF9 on chromosome 3), again untranslated but this time in the first exon. The strikingly similar clinical picture may result from similar patterns of mRNA accumulation leading to general effects on function of the cell nucleus (Ranum & Day 2002). Apart from the neurodegenerative conditions and disorders that are associated with learning disability such as myotonic dystrophy and fragile X syndrome, no convincing evidence has yet emerged for the involvement of repeat expansions in any form in general psychiatric illness.

Epigenetics, Imprinting and Parent-of-origin Effects

Epigenetic mechanisms are those events occurring during development that lead to stable changes in the ability of cell to transcribe DNA. These alterations are heritable from parent to child without involving direct mutations in the DNA itself. There are at least three interacting routes by which such controls on expression are effected: chromatin remodeling, histone alteration and DNA methylation. The latter two may act sequentially to establish the stable state represented by the former. Thus DNA methylation may be the signal for histone modification that may then act to recruit other chromatin modeling proteins, which rearrange chromatin into a stable unexpressed state. DNA methylation occurs mainly at CpG sequences and follows a developmental route that differs between male and female genomes. Its main function seems to be as a signal that recruits cellular factors leading to the transcriptional silencing of associated coding regions of DNA. Originally it may have developed as a repressor of unwanted transcription of the widespread transposable elements that occur in mammalian genome, as well as to differentially regulate developmental gene expression. In the zygote the genome inherited from the father is actively stripped of methylation within hours of fertilization, whereas methylation of the genome inherited from the mother passively decreases in later cleavage divisions. This demethylation seems to be an essential 'slate-cleaning' process removing most (but importantly not all) of the inherited parental chromosomal DNA methylation patterns. An extensive *de novo* remethylation follows, that then decreases in a tissue-specific fashion, releasing coding regions from their inactive states to produce the necessary proteins for cellular proliferation and differentiation. After methylation, erasure differences between the developmental routes in male and female embryos lead to sexually dimorphic methylation patterns in somatic cells. In germ cells, however, further reprogramming is needed to remove those methylation pattern that escaped the first general round of demethylation. This is followed by sex-specific re-methylation, completed in developing sperm at a very early stage (premitotic) but much later in ova (pre-meiotic stage). Thus methylation is one way in which the cell can 'mark' or 'imprint' its DNA in a sex-specific pattern.

It has been pointed out that DNA methylation is a system of 'cellular memory' that senses that a silent state is to be stabilized and invokes the mechanisms required for this (Jaenisch & Bird 2003). However, the actual primary marks that set this in play are still unclear. Both in somatic and germ cells the establishment of the correct methylation pattern is very important, and several disorders can result from its disruption. Some chromosomal regions that escape the first round of embryonic demethylation end up with differential imprinting between loci inherited from mother or father. In such cases monoallelic gene expression is the normal outcome. Such genes usually come in clusters, and there is often a local DNA region that acts as a specific imprint control center, as in the Prader-Willi/Angelman region.

Disruption of this specific imprinting pattern by deletions, uniparental disomy (both chromosomes of a pair originating from only one parent) or imprinting center mutations can result in these syndromes. Other genes that are normally differentially imprinted include several important fetal growth factors (such as the insulin related series). Disruption of epigenetic mechanisms may have a consequences for cognitive development (Reik and Walter 2001). More generally, such mechanisms (epimutations) may underlie many non-Mendelian features of psychiatric disorders: discordance in monozygotic twins, age-at-onset effects, sex-specific expression as well as parent-of-origin effects. In fact there is an abundance of parent-of-origin effects described for psychiatric disorder, including bipolar disorder and schizophrenia.

Mitochondrial (Cytoplasmic) Inheritance

The mitochondria contain DNA that resides outside the nucleus and thus does not segregate in meiosis. In man the mitochondrial DNA (mtDNA) is small (around 16.5 kb), has been entirely sequenced and contains genes particularly involve with oxidative phosphorylation. Since sperm have no mitochondria, inheritance is purely maternal. However, most cell have several copies of this genome, and mutations have been associated with a variety of human neurodegenerative diseases, including a form of deafness. The mutation may only occur in some of the copies, and the expression of the conditions can be very variable.

POPULATION GENETICS

Family, Adoption and Twin Studies

Any disease with a significant genetic causation will tend to aggregate in families, and comparison of rates of illness in relatives with the general population rate will provide a measure of the strength and nature of the genetic contribution. Clustering of disease in families may be entirely the result of shared environment, for example when infections are related to poor living conditions, or shared genetic inheritance as in the case of Huntington's disease where all affected individuals in a family have inherited a mutated huntingtin gene. However, most psychiatric condition are influenced by a mixture of genetic and environmental factors, and to dissect the relative contributions of nature and nurture on family members the two main strategies available are twin and adoption studies.

In general the association between a genetic risk factor and a disease in a population can be expressed as relative risk (RR) defined as the ratio of the incidence of disease in an 'exposed' group and 'unexposed' groups and measured by studying the illness in population cohorts. To study aggregation of disease within families, it is useful to compare the relative risk of illness in specific groups of relatives with the general population risk. Data is often most easily obtained from siblings, and the relative risk (or risk ratio) for relatives (λr) or specifically for siblings (λs) is frequently used to evaluate the strength and significance of familial aggregation of a disease. λs is defined as the recurrence risk to siblings compared with the risk of the disorder in the general population. A high value of λs reflects a strong genetic effect : for example, in a single gene disorder with dominant inheritance such as Huntington's disease, λs is about 5000; and in cystic fibrosis, a recessive disorder, λs is around 500. Few psychiatric illnesses show such clear-cut familial aggregation. For schizophrenia λs is about 10, and in complex disorders λs greater than 2 is generally taken to indicate a significant genetic component. Caution is needed when evaluating λ because the value depends on the population prevalence of the disease and in general a strong genetic effect in a common disease will generate a smaller λ than the same effect in a rare disease.

Analysis of Segregation

If a disease, measured as a discrete trait is found to be heritable, it is often useful to know whether or not the disease follows Mendelian rules, or if more complex modes of inheritance need be considered. The laws of Mendelian inheritance allow precise predictions of the expected number of affected and unaffected offspring of affected parents, measured as segregation ratios. These ratios also allow prediction of the population frequencies of a disease, and the statistical methods of segregation analysis applied to data on the observed frequencies of a disease in families and the general population lead to predictions of whether the disease is caused by one or more loci.

Family and population data have been extensively studied to elucidate mode of genetic transmission of schizophrenia. A highly influential book (Gottesman 1991) reviewing the results of several family studies in schizophrenia conclude that the risk of developing schizophrenia in relatives of probands with the disorder is significantly increased in all classes of relatives. In summary the life-time risk of developing schizophrenia and related illness was around 1% in the general population, 10% among first-degree relatives, dropping to about 3% in second-degree relatives. Offspring both of whose parents had schizophrenia had a 40–50% chance of becoming ill. A review of several more recent studies using strict diagnostic criteria (kindler 2000) found rather similar rates of schizophrenia in these classes of relative, confirming that schizophrenia is a familial disease.

Segregation of illness in families is not consistent with a model of schizophrenia as a simple homogeneous condition cause entirely by a defect in a single major gene or even two or three genes. The mode of inheritance remains unclear, perhaps because schizophrenia is a heterogeneous group of conditions. Genetic findings to date suggest that several, perhaps many, genes are implicated and both Mendelian and non-Mendelian modes of inheritance are possible in different subgroups of the disorder. A multifactorial threshold model gave the best fit to observed family data (McGue & Gottesman 1989). However, in the absence of reliable biological markers, at-risk relatives who carry the genetic risk without developing symptoms cannot be reliably identified, so segregation studies in families based only on clinically defined cases may provide an incomplete picture. There is evidence from linkages studies to suggest that in some families the illness can be attributed to the effect of a single locus, though such families may be uncommon (Blackwood et al. 2001).

Family and population studies in bipolar disorder using strict diagnostic criteria have confirmed an increased risk of bipolar disorder in relatives of bipolar probands, with and estimated relative risk in first-degree relatives of 5–10% (Craddock & Jones 1999). Similar studies of unipolar depression have reported relative risk of 1.5–3 for first-degree relatives, variation in results being due to differences in diagnostic criteria and varied estimates of the population prevalence of depression. Affective disorders are probably a heterogeneous group of conditions, and subgroups such as depression with onset early in adult life may show increased familiarity. Because unipolar depression is common in general population, heritability can be measured from large community based twin registers, and estimates of heritability are in region 30–40% (Sullivan et al. 2000). A further observation from the Virginia twin register was an almost complete correlation between generalize anxiety disorder and major depression, indicating that the same genetic factors contribute to depression and anxiety (Kendler et al. 1992).

The mode of inheritance of mood disorders is not well understood, and it is probable that a variety of genetic, epigenetic and environmental factors contribute to the risk of illness. Some studies of the segregation of the disorder in families support a model in which single genes of relatively large effect cause illness in some families and different genes will be responsible for illness in different families (major genes with locus heterogeneity) (Rice et al. 1987, Blackwood et al. 1996). There is also evidence that in many cases of the disorder, segregation is incompatible with a single major locus and illness may develop as the result of additive or interacting gene variants, each one alone being neither sufficient nor necessary for illness to develop (polygenic model) (Craddock et al. 1997). Further complexity arises when we consider that other genetic and epigenetic effects may be important in some but not all families. Genomic imprinting mediated by DNA methylation was proposed as an explanation of an apparent parent-of origin effect in linkage studies on chromosome 18p in bipolar disorder. Mitochondrial inheritance is another possible explanation of maternal inheritance in a subgroup of families. However, the mitochondrial hypothesis was not supported when the whole mitochondrial genome was sequenced in nine bipolar probands from families showing exclusively maternal transmission (McMahon et al. 2000).

Adoption Studies

Adoption studies are one of the most powerful ways to disentangle genetic from environmental influences on a disease. There are three main designs of adoption studies, and the choice of design will depend on the available methods of ascertainment.

- *Parent as proband*: One of the first studies of the adopted offspring of mother diagnosed with schizophrenia was carried out in Oregon, where 47 individuals, adopted shortly after birth when their mother were receiving institutional care, were traced in adulthood (Heston 1966). Rates of illness among these adoptees were compared with those in 50 adopted offspring of mothers without psychiatric illness. The striking finding of the Oregon adoption study was a significant increase in schizophrenia in the adoptees whose mothers were schizophrenic: 5/47 compared with 0/50 in the control group. Similar findings have come from a much larger, more recent Finnish study of adopted offspring of mothers with schizophrenia (Tienari et al. 2000).
- *Adoptee as proband*: In this approach, adopted children who become ill are ascertained and rates of illness are compared in their biological and their adoptive families. Studies carried out in Demark, where national registers facilitate the tracing of adopted children, showed that 20% of 118 biological relatives and only 6% of 224 adoptive relatives had a diagnosis of schizophrenia. This difference between adoptive and biological relatives was significant (Kety et al. 1994). To remove any doubts about the reliability of earlier diagnostic methods, Kendler et al. (1994) re-analyzed the data from the Danish study, applying strict DSM-III criteria and confirmed a diagnosis of schizophrenia in 8% of first-degree relatives of schizophrenic adoptees, contrasting with only 1% among relatives of control adoptees with no history of schizophrenia.
- *Cross-fostering design*: This compares the rate of illness in two groups of adoptees: one group has ill parents and after adoption has been raised by well parents, the second group has well biological parents but has been brought up in a family where a parent has become ill. Children adopted shortly after birth will still have experienced the pre-and perinatal environment provided by their biological mother and after adoption may suffer greater stress by virtue of being an adoptee. These potential limitations of adoption studies were addressed by the cross-fostering design. The possibility of strong shared environmental influences *in utero* was addressed by Kety (1976), who studied the rate of illness in a group of paternal half siblings of schizophrenic adoptees and demonstrated an increased incidence of schizophrenia in paternal half siblings that could not be attributed to pre- and perinatal effects. Also children adopted into a home where an adoptive parent becomes ill do not have an increased risk of illness.

Adoption studies in bipolar disorder have similarly confirmed increased rates of affective disorder in biological compared with adoptive relative of adoptees.

Twin Studies

Monozygotic (MZ) or identical twins result from a single fertilized ovum and therefore share all genes, whereas dizygotic (DZ) or fraternal twins are the result of the implantation of two separate fertilized ova and generally share about 50% of genes and are no more alike than other siblings. Since, in general, twins share a very similar cultural, family and educational environment, a comparison of MZ and DZ twins allows an estimate of genetic as well as environmental contributions to their phenotype. Concordance rate measures the similarity of phenotype between twins. If both members of a pair of twins develop a disease they are said to be concordant for that condition. For a fully genetic disease showing a dominant pattern of inheritance, concordance will be 100% in MZ twins and around 50% in DZ twins. In the case of a recessive disorder, DZ concordance will be about 25% when a disease is entirely due to environmental causes we expect to find no difference in concordance rates in MZ and DZ twin pairs. Most psychiatric disorders are likely to be a result of both genetic and nongenetic factors, and concordance rates in MZ twins may be quite small, but a significant genetic contribution will be indicated by the comparison of MZ and DZ rates. The simplest way to measure this is pairwise concordance defined as the number of pairs of twins where both are affected divided by the total number of pairs studied. More commonly the proband wise concordance is quoted, and this is the number of affected co-twins with an affected proband divided by the total number of co-twins in the study. The mode of ascertainment of the sample of twins used in the study is very important and, unless an entire population has been systematically screened, probandwise concordance will be different from pairwise concordance because some twins will be counted twice if they have been independently ascertained for probandwise analysis.

In a classic twin study of schizophrenia, Gottesman & Shields (1972) found in their sample 11 concordant and 11 discordant pairs of MZ twins and 3 concordant and 30 discordant DZ pairs of twins. This gives pairwise concordance rate of 11/22 = 50% for MZ and 3/33 = 10% for DZ twins. In the same sample, proband concordance was calculated to be 58% for MZ twins and 12% for DZ twins. The difference between the two methods of analysis arose because in 4/11 pairs of concordant MZ twins both of the twins were ascertained independently, so in effect counted twice, to calculate pairwise concordance. Similarly 1/3 pairs of concordant DZ twins were ascertained independently. This illustrates the importance of ascertainment in twin studies. Both analyses yielded significant differences between MZ and DZ concordance, proving a genetic effect. Early reports have been substantially supported by several more recent twin studies where probandwise concordance for MZ twins ranged between 40% and 65% compared with a range of 0% to 30% in DZ twin pairs (Cardno & Gottesman 2000). An important study fo the offspring of MZ twins discordant for schizophrenia found that the children of unaffected co-twins inherited the same increased risk of schizophrenia as their cousins who were offspring of the affected twin (Kringlen & Cramer 1989). This suggests that the interpretation of 'environmental' risk in twin studies requires explanation because environment may include epigenetic risk factors that influence the expression of a gene in an individual but do not involve changes in the genome. Twin studies in schizophrenia report a concordance rate for MZ twins of around 50%, but it would be wrong to conclude that half of the variation in phenotype can be attributed to peri- or postnatal causes; the risk attributed to 'environment' includes nontransmitted biochemical effects on genes, for example the random variation that occurs in DNA methylation, a process that may alter gene expression but is not heritable.

In bipolar disorder twin studies yield essentially similar findings as in schizophrenia. MZ concordance rates of 40% to 60% are significantly greater than DZ concordance rates, and the risk of bipolar illness in the offspring of MZ twins discordant for the disorder was the same among offspring of the affected and unaffected co-twins (Jones et al. 2002).

Mapping and Finding Genes

When family, adoption twin studies have identified a substantial genetic contribution to a disease, different strategies can be followed for identifying genes. A 'functional' approach requires the selection of candidate genes to be directly examined for mutations.

The selection of candidate genes is usually based on knowledge of the biology or pharmacology of the disease; but because, for most psychiatric conditions, we have no clear understanding of the underlying neurobiology, the range of possible candidates could include most of the 10000 or more genes expressed in the brain. A 'positional' strategy aims to identify the approximate chromosomal location of genes using the methods of linkage analysis in families, association studies in populations, or mapping of cytogenetic anomalies in individuals. Regions of the genome thus identified are further examined by association studies, and candidates are selected from the genes known to reside within the region of linkage. A positional approach has been successful in identifying genes responsible for many single-gene disorders—including cystic fibrosis, Huntington's disease, muscular dystrophy and some familial cases of Alzheimer's disease—and does not rely on prior knowledge of the biology of the disease permitting the discovery of previously unknown genes.

Linkage Analysis

Linkage studies look for the co-segregation of polymorphic DNA markers with disease in families. Studies on single large pedigrees, on many small two-generation families or on large numbers of pairs of affected siblings are widely adopted strategies.

The basis of linkage analysis is the recombination that takes places between pairs of homologous chromosomes during meiosis. On average, recombination takes place at two places on each chromosome during every meiosis, and the recombination fraction is the probability that a recombination event will occur between two markers or between a marker and a disease locus. Recombination fraction is a useful measure because over short distances it is a measure of the physical distance between two markers on a chromosome. When two genes are physically far apart on a chromosome they will usually become separated by recombination during meiosis and will assort independently of each other just as if they were on separate chromosomes (Mendel's Law of Independent Assortment). In general, the closer a polymorphic marker is to a disease locus, the more likely it is that the two will remain together from one generation to the next, because the chance of a recombination taking place between them is proportional to the physical distance that separates them. If two points are separated by a million base pairs of DNA (megabase Mb) then recombination will occur between them roughly once in every 100 meiosis, which is 100 generations, and the statistical unit to describe this rate of recombination is termed the centimogan (cM). The effect of recombination is analogous to cutting a pack of cards. The chance that two card will be separated by the cut is proportional to how far apart they are in the pack and two consecutive cards are the least likely to be separated by repeated cutting. Genes far apart on the same chromosome co-segregate randomly and have a 50:50 chance of remaining on the same chromosome following meiosis. In a family linkage study the recombination fraction (θ) will therefore lie between 0 (indicating that a polymorphic marker is a physical part of the gene responsible for the disease so the marker and the gene never become separated) and 0.5 (completely independent assortment of marker and gene). For analysis of linkage the recombination fraction between a marker and disease locus can be measured directly in a family or group of families simply by counting the number of recombinant individuals, divided by the total number of offspring. In large families, calculation of linkage is complex and the recombination fraction is estimated by the method of maximum likelihood and calculated using 'linkage' computer programs (OTT 1999). The conventional statistical method to test for linkage is to calculate the LOD (Log of the odds) score from the recombination fraction. It is conventionally accepted that a LOD score of 3 (odds in favor of linkage of 1000:1) is considered proof of linkage and conversely a LOD score of – 2 (odds against linkage of 100:1) is accepted as exclusion.

Linkage analysis is an important tool for the analysis of genetic loci, exploiting the immense amount of sequence variation found across the human genome. Typically a genome wide screen for linkage in a group of families multiply affected by a disease will employ several hundred microsatellite markers or several thousand SNPs chosen to be evenly space at intervals of less than 10 cM across all chromosomes. Regions of interest may be further examined with a denser series of markers. Many independent linkage studies, including whole genome scan in large collections of multiply affected families or affected pairs of siblings, have been reported in schizophrenia and manic depressive illness with some encouraging convergence of results (Reley & McGuffin 2000, Baron 2002).

Some genes of apparently larger effect have been detected in studies of extended families, although these may be relatively rare causes of illness in the general population. Large numbers of affected pairs of siblings are easier to recruit than large pedigrees, and if very large cohorts are studied the approach is suited to the detection of genes of small effects predicted under a polygenic model. However, if substantial locus heterogeneity is present, this approach requires unrealistically large samples. A large number of linkage projects using both strategies have been completed in the past two decades, and evidence for linkage, supported by more than one study, has emerged in several chromosomal regions. In a single family, carriers of a reciprocal translocation t (1:11)(q42.2;q21) which was stably inherited in a large Scottish pedigree were shown to have very high rates of major psychiatric illness when compared with noncarriers. The strongest evidence for linkage (LOD score of 7.1) was found with a phenotype that included both schizophrenia and affective psychosis, and linkage was also found at this region in families from the finish population (Blackwood et al. 2001, Ekelund et al. 2000). Candidate genes for schizophrenia, Disrupted in Schizophrenia I (DISC1) and Disrupted in Schizophrenia 2 (DISC2) were detected by closing the translocation breakpoint (Millar et al. 2000). Chromosome 22q11 is another region where a chromosomal abnormality has initially focused the search for genes. A small interstitial deletion at this location causes the velocardiofacial syndrome (VCFS), and patients with the disorder have characteristic congenital abnormalities in addition to carrying a substantially increased risk of psychosis. The deletion encompasses several candidate genes—including genes coding catechol-O-methyltransferase (COMT) and the G-protein-coupled receptor kinase 3 (GRK3), for which there is some evidence for association in schizophrenia and bipolar disorder. Linkage to a region on chromosome 6p was identified in Irish families, and evidence has been recently presented that a candidate gene in that region, Dysbindin, is associated with schizophrenia (Straub et al. 2002). On Chromosome 8p several groups have reported linkage, and the gene Neuregulin-1 (NRGI) shows association with schizophrenia in the Icelandic and Scottish populations (Stefansson et al. 2002, 2003). Other regions identified by linkage in families with schizophrenia include 13q, 6q, 2p, 5q, 6q, 10p and 13q. The focus is now to identify genes at these regions of interest and to study the expression patterns and biological functions of candidate genes in the regions.

Association Studies

Linkage analysis is performed on families with more than one affected relative whereas association studies compare the frequency of alleles of a DNA marker in population of patients and healthy controls. In the search for genes these two approaches are entirely complementary. The idea of association is simpler and is well known through the long-established association between HLA subtypes and some common disease, including diabetes, rheumatoid arthritis and ankylosing spondylitis. When one allele of a DNA polymorphism, for example a SNP or a microsatellite marker, is found more commonly in a disease population than controls the marker and disease are said to be associated or in 'linkage disequilibrium'. This could occur because the polymorphic marker itself is a variant that directly influences the phenotype. One example is the association of late-onset Alzheimer's disease with ApoE4. The frequency of ApoE4 is about 0.4 in individuals with Alzheimer's disease compared with 0.15 in controls. This QTL increases the liability to develop dementia but is neither sufficient nor necessary to cause illness. Linkage disequilibrium may also occur between a disease and a polymorphic marker situated very close to the disease-related gene but not involved in causing the disease phenotype. When the market and the disease gene are physically close on the genome they are less likely to become separated by recombination over many generation.

The ideal setting for an association study would thus be a completely isolated island population where the disease had been introduced many generations previously by a single founder and all the people with the disease being studied were descended from that person. In practice, association studies are successfully carried out, for example in European populations, provided cases and controls are carefully matched for age and ethnic origin. Linkage disequilibrium typically extends over very short distances of a few hundred kilobases, giving much higher resolution for mapping genes than be achieved by linkage strategies.

Candidate Genes

Genes coding proteins related to neurotransmitter function, including dopamine, noradrenaline, serotonin, GABA and glutamate neurotransmission, have been extensively investigated in schizophrenia and bipolar disorder by association studies and directly formulations by sequencing. Evidence that variants in neurotransmitter-related gene have a substantial causative role in schizophrenia remain unconfirmed, but studies on the gene on chromosome 22 coding for the enzyme COMT, which show significant association with schizophrenia, provide and illustration of the difficulties of establishing a link between a candidate gene and a complex disorder such as schizophrenia. The gene coding COMT is a strong candidate for a role in schizophrenia because of its biological function and its chromosomal location. COMT is one of the enzymes that degrades catecholamines, and the gene that codes it is located within the small region on chromosome 22 deleted in patients with velocardiofacial syndrome, a condition that carries and increased risk of schizophrenia. Numerous linkage and association studies around this region had produced conflicting results but very strong association was detected by Shifman et al. (2002). In this study the important factors contributing to the detection of association were the large sample size (4800 controls and over 700 patients), a homogeneous study population and the use of several polymorphic markers in the association study (12 SNPs across the gene were genotyped), allowing analysis of association with individual markers and also with haplotypes made up of groups of these markers. The evidence from this study suggests that variants of the COMT gene are risk factors in schizophrenia.

Monoamine oxidase (MAO), another key enzyme in amine metabolism, has shown association with bipolar disorder in some studies, but the effects are small and not replicated. Specific serotonin reuptake inhibitors (SSRIs) are mainstay of pharmacotherapy in the treatment of depression, and it is logical that their substrate, the human Serotonin Reuptake Transporter (h SERT), and its gene on the long arm of chromosome 17 have been the focus of intensive study. A polymorphism (a variable number tandem repeat or VNTR) affects the function of the gene, and there is evidence that the 12-repeat allele modestly increases the susceptibility to bipolar disorder in Caucasian populations. The primary function of aminergic neurotransmitters is to interact with a postsynaptic receptor to achieve their signaling actions. These membrance-bound receptor proteins are key candidates for dysfunction in psychiatric illness. The serotonergic receptor system has been examined both at the sequence level and by association analysis for seven of the 5HT receptor types, with very mixed results—with both positive and negative findings in abundance (Potash & Depaulo 2000).

Dopaminergic receptors have been more extensively studied in patients with schizophrenia than with bipolar disorder, and here again the results have been mixed. An example is DRD5 the gene encoding the type 5 dopamine receptor, which is found especially in the limbic and frontal cortex in human brain. This is strongly associated with schizophrenia but not bipolar disorder (Muir et al. 2001) and yet lies within a region of linkage to bipolar disorder on chromosome 4. The confusing results that emerge from association studies of neurotransmitter systems may arise because studies are too small to detect genes that are components of polygenic system.

Cytogenetic Studies

Cloning disrupted genes from rare chromosomal rearrangements has been a very fruitful approach for a wide variety of inherited neurological conditions because—in contrast to linkage and association studies, where the results, even if positive, define broad areas at the molecular level—abnormalities of chromosomes can precisely pinpoint the position of disrupted genes (Evans et al. 2001). Example of the success of this approach are:

- The discovery of the novel genes DISC1 and DISC2 at the breakpoint of a translocation on chromosome 1 in a family with schizophrenia;
- The analysis of candidate genes including COMT, PRODH2 and the G-protein-coupled receptor kinase 3 (GRK3) in the region on chromosome 22 deleted in the velocardiofacial syndrome.

A small pedigree was described with a t (9;11) (p24; q23) translocation co-segregating with affective disorders. Five relatives who carried the translocation had bipolar disorder and one had early-onset recurrent major depression. A mannosyltransferase gene was shown to be disrupted by the chromosome 11 break point (Baysal et al. 2002) and labeled DIBDI (Disrupted in Bipolar Disorder 1) a 15-exon brain-expressed gene that is possibly involved in protein N-glycosylation. This is one of the first novel genes decribed thought to have a role in bipolar disorder.

45.7 FUNDAMENTAL OF PSYCHOLOGY

SS Nathawat, Vijaya Nathawat

INTRODUCTION

The case can be made that of all the disciplines that are essential for the study of psychiatry, knowledge of psychology is the most important. However, until recently, psychology (or behavioral science) has represented a very small component of the general medical curriculum. Most psychiatrists on commencing higher training have therefore, had relatively little exposure to psychology, yet have elected to specialize in the medical discipline whose essence is the study and treatment of abnormal experience and behavior. Such individuals will enter higher training with a good background in anatomy, physiology and pharmacology yet may have relatively little knowledge and understanding of the scientific basis of perception, emotion, congnition and personality.

What is 'psychology'? The definition depends on the view of psychology to which you subscribe. The behavioral approach, which we will consider later in detail, has traditionally defined psychology as the 'study of behavior' because behavior is observable and measurable. In contrast, cognitive psychologists have offered definitions of psychology along the lines of 'the science of mental life'. It may be possible of course to incorporate all of these elements and offer and integrated definition such as the science of behavior and mental life.

Traditional View of Science

The traditional view of 'science emphasizes a number of basic principles which have proven of great value in the history and development of science. In fact, 19th-century scientists thought that all the major problems of science had been answered by the development of grand theories such as Newton's mechanics, thermodynamics and Darwin's theory of evolution, and that only the details were left to be filled in. The basic principles on which these developments were considered to depend are as follows.

Observation and Fact

In medicine of course observation of signs plays a crucial role in diagnosis; the collation of such signs and other symptoms is then used to provide descriptive classification systems such as that used in the American Diagnostic and Statistical Manual (DSM-IV) and the World Health Organization's International Classification of Disease system (currently ICD-10).

Description and Classification

To return to the medicopsychiatric classification systems such as DSM-IV and ICD-10, these systems of diagnosis and classification are not theoretically based systems, but, instead, are systems agreed by committees who change their minds every few years. In fact, it is more accurate to state that the systems contain a mishmash of theories, as powerful individuals on the committees horse-trade their favorite diagnoses with each other. Hardly the way to do science! Until psychiatry therefore has a theoretically based and empirically supported diagnostic and classification system, it will remain at the level of mere descriptive science.

Theory and Hypothesis

Theories group together facts and description in a way that provides an overall working model relevant to the domain in question. A good theory, as the philosopher Karl Popper stated, is both useful and falsifiable; i.e. a good theory should generate hypotheses which may be novel and surprising and which can be tested in manmade or 'natural' experiments. One of the classic examples is that of Einstein's theory of relativity, which predicted that light would bend in a gravitational field, a prediction that was dramatically upheld when the light from a distant source was shown to bend as it passed the sun.

Experiment

Hypotheses derived from scientific theories may be tested in manmade and natural experiments in order to decide whether or not the experimental outcome is that predicted by the hypothesis. Experiments have to be carefully designed in order for us to be sure that the variable that the experimenter manipulates (the independent variable) is truly the one that leads to differences in the variable that is measured (the dependent variable). If the experimental outcome is due to some other confounding variable rather than the one that is manipulated, then the experiment is invalid.

Behaviorism

Behaviorism was a reaction against the 'introspectionist' approach to psychology, where armchair psychologists sat and recorded their own mental processes. The American

Psychologist J B Watson was the leading figure of the behavioral approach to psychology. Watson argued that the study of the mind was a scientific irrelevance because the mind is unobservable, and indeed he subsequently focused primarily on the environment. He argued that only behavior is observable and therefore that a science of psychology must be a science of behavior. Behaviorists drew on the work of the Russian physiologist Ivan Pavlov. Pavlov was awarded the Nobel Prize for his work on the physiology of digestion. In the course of subsequent work on salivation in the dog, he noticed that the dogs began to salivate on seeing the attendant who normally fed them. Pavlov made those observations the basis for his subsequent study of the conditioned reflex (or 'conditional reflex' in Pavlov's own terms). His most famous studies were of bell-ringing and salivation in dogs.

Two other significant figures in behavioral psychology were Edward Thorndike and B F Skinner. Thorndike became famous for his study of how cats learned to escape form puzzle boxes; over a number of trials the cats were found through trial-and-error learning to escape more quickly from the boxes. Thorndike's so-called law of effect stated that responses were either more likely or less likely to occur according to the consequences that they produced. B F Skinner continued Thorndike's study of learning based on the consequences of behavior. Many behaviorists accepted that thoughts and feelings had a causal role to play in our behavior, but because they were unobservable were not within the domaion of science. In contrast to these 'methodological behaviorists', Skinner espoused a so-called 'radical behaviorist' philosophy which stated that, although such private events existed, they played no causal role in behavior but were merely by products of internal physiological processes. Skinnner stated that the true determinants of behavior were the environment and the organism's genetics and learning history, which were both represented neurophysiologically.

Classical Conditioning

This type of learning was originally identified by Pavlov, and hence is also known as Pavlovian Conditioning. The basic paradigm is shown in Figure 6. The figure shows that an unconditioned stimulus (UCS) such as food leads to an unconditioned response (UCR) such as salivation. The pairing of an initially neutral stimulus such as a bell with the UCS eventually leads the bell to become a conditioned stimulus (CS) for the conditioned response (CR) of salivation. Pavlov demonstrated that conditioning occurs optimally if the CS occurs just prior to the UCS, that conditioning will generalize to other stimuli that are similar to the original CS, and that the CR will gradually extinguish over a number of trials if the CS is presented on its own without the UCS.

One of the main applications of classical conditioning to adult psychological disorders has been through an analysis of 'conditioned emotional responses'. The idea is

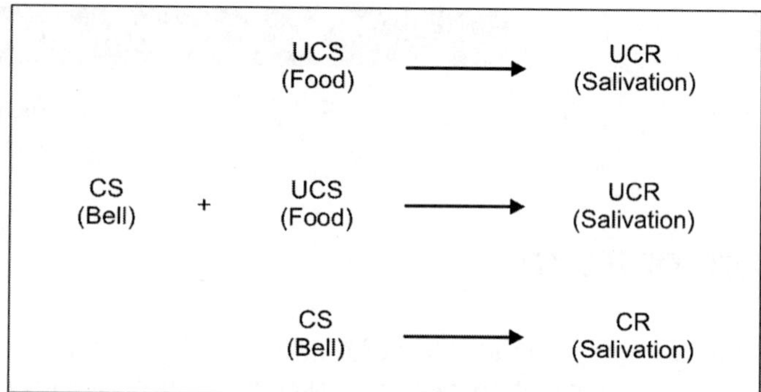

Fig. 6: An outline of classical (pavlovian) conditioning
Abbreviations: (U)C, (un) conditioned; S, stimulus; R, response

that the pairing of been through an analysis of 'conditioned emotional responses'. The idea is that the pairing of a neutral stimulus with an aversive or traumatic UCS which produces and unpleasant emotional response will lead the neutral stimulus to produce conditioned emotional response. A famous early demonstration of this sequence was carried out by Watson and Rayner (1920) with a 1-year-old child named little Albert. The child was happily playing with a white rat (the CS) when a loud noise (the UCS) behind him produced a startle reaction and considerable distress (the UCR). After a few such pairings of the white rat and the noise, the white rat eventually produced an unpleasant emotional reaction (the CR) or its own. This reaction generalized to other similar objects such as white rabbits (and even to Santa's beard !). This type of conditioning has been incorporated into learning models for the development of clinical phobias, for example a child traumatized by being bitten or frightened by a dog may develop a phobia of dogs.

Operant Conditioning

Both Skinner and Thorndike emphasized that classical conditioning was one type of learning that applied in the main to more reflex-like or autonomic nervous system behavior. In contrast, they argued that voluntary behavior is dependent on its consequences for whether or not it is likely to be repeated. More formally, Skinner stated that operant (or 'instrumental') conditioning is based on the three-term contingency of discriminative stimulus, response, and outcome. A discriminative stimulus indicates whether or not a particular continency applies; e.g. a green light might indicate that any pressing of a lever in a Skinner box would lead to a food reward. The outcome can be positive (e.g. food) and therefore the likelihood of the response increases – that is, it is positively reinforcing – or it can be punitive (e.g. electric shock) in which case the response is punished and is less likely to occur again under those stimulus conditions.

Other key concepts in operant conditioning are negative reinforceiment, schedules of reinforcement, and shaping. In contrast to the punishment procedure described above in which a response is less likely to occur because the outcome is unpleasant, in negative reinforcement the response is more likely to occur because it switches off an aversive stimulus such as shock or loud noise. For example, a rat that learns to avoid a section of its cage because it has received mild foot shock in the past has learned via negative reinforcement : moving away terminated the aversive experience. The term 'schedule of reinforcement' refers to the fact that in many situations not every response is reinforce; e.g. people are typically rewarded with money for their work once a week or once a month (a fixed-internval schedule), though some individuals on piecework are rewarded for the amount that they produce (normally a 'fixed-ratio' schedule). One of the properties of these partial rather than continuous reinforcement schedules is that the behavior is more resistant to extinction: thus, if reinforcement is no longer presented, an individual who has been rewarded for every response will normally stop responding sooner than someone who has received partial reinforcement. The term 'shaping' refers to the technique where by the organism is initially rewarded for responses that only vaguely resemble the desired response, but gradually the reinforce response approximates closer the desired response. For example, a performing dog in a circus is unlikely to pirouette three times and then roll over straight away, but through shaping by successive approximations to the desired behaviors, the dog could be trained to do so. A clinical example of the use of shaping procedures is in skill acquisition training for individuals with learning disabilities.

Escape and avoidance are two further important type of operant conditioning. In escape learning, the organism receives an aversive stimulus such as an electric shock, which a particular response such as pressing a lever will remove. In avoidance learning, an initial discriminative stimulus signals that if the appropriate response does not occur, then the aversive stimulus will be presented. One well-known variant on escape/avoidance learning is Seligman's (1975) 'learned helplessness'. In learned helplessness task, the organism initially receives noncontingent punishment, i.e. the aversive stimulus is received whatever response the animal makes. The contingency is then changed such that a response would lead to escape from the aversive stimulus, but the typical finding is that the animal remains helpless and does not find the escape response. Seligman propose that learned helplessness could provide a model for the acquisition and maintenance of depression in humans.

Behavior Therapy

A classic demonstration of behvior therapy was carried out by Mary Cover Jones (1924). Following in the Little Albert tradition, she successfully treated a young boy's fear of rabbits by having him eat in the presence of a rabbit, while gradually bringing the rabbit closer to him over a number of occasions. The basic idea of the encouragement of a response such as eating which is incompatible with fear was further elaborated by Joseph Wolpe (1958). Wolpe first taught phobic adults a muscle relaxation technique, which they then used whilst imagining increasingly fearful stimuli—a technique that Wolpe called systematic desensitization. Although sometimes still use, behavior therapists now generally prefer to use actual exposure to the feared object or situation when this is possible rather than just working in imagination (e.g. Marks 1987). This technique is termed graded exposure, the phobic individual gradually works through a hierarchy towards the feared stimulus. For example, a dog phobic may work through a hierarchy from a photograph of a puppy, photograph of a larger dog, video of a puppy, video of a larger dog, puppy through a one way mirror, etc. The phobic individual and therapist work as a team in a collaborative relationship, and the patient only moves on to the next stage of the hierarchy when he feels ready to do so. Exposure-based treatments have proved particularly effective in the treatment of anxiety disorders.

Two-factor Learning Theory

One of the classic theories on which behavior therapy was based was Mowrer's (1939) two-factor theory of the acquisition and maintenance of fear. Mowrer proposed that both classical and operant conditioning were involved. The first step was that an originally neutral stimulus acquired fearful properties by being paried with a frightening or painful event, i.e. through a classical conditioning procedure (e.g. as in the case of Little Albert). The second step is that through a process of operant conditioning, the individual learns to reduce the fear by avoidance of the relevant object or situation, and hence avoidance behavior is reinforced. Much of the focus of behavioral interventions in anxiety and obsessional disorders has therefore included exposure to the feared object or situation, a procedure that is repeated until the fear response reduces substantially. However, it is now well recognized that not all fears are acquired in accordance with the two factor theory (Rachman1990) and that not all so-called fears or phobias are based on anxiety but that some are based on disgust reactions (Power & Dalgeish 1997) . Most people with a fear of flying have never actually flown, so their fear could not have been acquired by classical conditioning in the situation itself. Conversely, not everybody who has experienced a traumatic event while flying (e.g. a hijack) develops a phobia. Instead, the observationof someone else (e.g. a parent) being fearful about an object or situation (known as 'vicarious' or 'observational' learning) is also a common source of fears and phobias.

Psychoanalysis

Psychoanalytic theory has been important historically in information views concering personality, consciousness and psychological interventions. However, psychoanalysis, the treatment developed by Sigmund Freud based on psychoanalytic theory, lost popularity largely because of criticisms regarding its efficacy (Eysenck 1969). Furthermore, many critics have suggested that psychoanalysis is not scientific, as it is not open to refutation by experimentation. More recently psychoanalytic theory has undergone somewhat of a renaissance. Two main factors have contributed to this renewed interest. First, there has been a huge amount of attention devoted to the phenomenon of 'recovered memories' in adult survivors of child sexual abuse (Conway 1997, Davies and Dalgleish 2002). Findings such as this have forced research attention to the issue of whether or not it is possible to have no memory of an experience for many years, only for it to resurface in later life. Recent studies with in the domain of cognitive psychology have shown that repression can be induced in the laboratory (Conway 2001). Findings such as this have forced a re-examination of basic psychoanalytic concepts. Secondly, recent advances in our understanding of how unconscious processes can influence over behavior (e.g. studies of 'blind-sight' patients, studies of the effects of subliminal perpetual priming, and the study of explicit versus implicit memory system) have made some of Freud's proposals on the role of the unconscious appear more plausible and, critically, empirically testable.

Unconscious

Freud did not simply see the unconscious as an inactive storehouse of past memories, but rather as a system of wishes, fantasies, impulses and memories that actively influenced our thought, actions, symptoms, dreams, mistakes, accidents and emotions. He proposed that the unconscious was derived from innate drives of which we could never become directly conscious, and repressed material which was typically of an unpleasant personal nature. One of the key points, Freud proposed about the unconscious was that it defied time and logic and was not constrained by reality. For example, painful memories could be recalled from many years past as if they were happening now and had lost none of their emotional impact (This phenomenon is observed in descriptions of the re-experincing of traumatic memories in post-traumatic stress disorder). In a similar manner, opposite and contradictory thoughts and impulses can be held in the unconscious; the same person can be both loved and hated at the same time.

Psychic Energy

Freud believed that the mind was fuelled by psychic energy very much in the way that physical energy is needed to fuel a physical machine. This energy, or ' libido' as it was called, he initially considerd to be derived from the life-preserving drives, 'Eros'. Freud added a second set of life-destroying drives, 'Thanatos', which typically manifested themselves as aggression towards the self or toward others.

The comparison that Freud made between psychic energy and physical energy led to him adopting the so-called 'principle of constancy'; namely, that by analolgy with the laws of themodynamiccs, psychic energy can never be created nor destroyed, but can only be changed from one form to another. For example, if sexual energy is blocked from being expressed through the normal channels, then it has to be expressed in other forms. In milder cases these forms could be disguised in dreams, in symptoms such as headaches, or in excessive intellectual activity, and so on. However, in more extreme cases Freud suggested that severe psychological disorders including anxiety, depression and obsessional disorders resulted from the blocking of sexual energy.

Repression

Freud used the term 'repression' in various ways in his writings in order to refer to either the conscious or the unconscious avoidance of painful or unwanted information—in particular, information about the self or the self in relation to significant others. Freud used repression as a general term therefore to refer to almost an defence mechanism. However, his daughter, Anna Freud, in 1937 provided a systematic list that, along with repression (in the specific sense of an unconscious avoidance of an unacceptable impulse or idea), include a number of other defence mechanisms such as reaction formation, sublimation and projection. Recently, Anderson and Green (2001) provided an elegant demonstration of experimentally induced memory repression in the laboratory. They showed that if a memory that is associated with something familiar is actively avoided every time that familiar object is seen, then the memory becomes repressed and the avoided time is later difficult to remember.

Developmental Stages

Freud proposed that the child passes through a series of developmental stages labeled the oral, anal, phallic, latency and genital phases. The main sources of pleasure in the oral, and phallic stage are the mouth, the anus and the genitals, respectively. One of the additional proposals is that fixation can occur at different stages of development which can either be apparent as personality traits, or revealed at times of stress. Typical oral characteristics are talkativenses, gred, gullibility and generosity, whereas typical anal characteristics include obstinacy, orderliness and miserliness.

Transference and Countertransference

Freud's early collaborator, Josef Breuer, found that one of his hysterical patients, Anna O, developed very strong feelings towards him in the course of his treatment of her, Breuer was unable to cope with the strength to her feelings and terminated her treatment. The feelings that the patient has for the therapist are called transference. Originally, therefore, transference was seen as a nuisance that impeded the therapeutic process, but Freud later recongnized the therpetutic potential of transference. He believed that transference was a re-enactment in the relationship with the therapist of earlier significant relationships and provided an opportunity to examine their nature via the exploration of fantasies and feelings in the transference relationship. In fact, the exploration of transference is considered to be the key therapeutic tool in psychoanalytic work, because it provides insight into past and present relationships and allows the working through of related conflicts and problems. The intimate situation in which the therapist and patient are placed and the fact that the psychoanalyst sits behind the patient are methods which encourage transference. The technique of free association, whereby the patient is meant to say whatever comes into his or her mind, also allows the patient to dwell on fantasies about the therapist which the more directive therapies such as behavior therapy and cognitive therapy would typically steer the patient away from.

The fact that patient have strong reactions to their therapists does not preclude the fact that threrapists may have strong reactions, both positive and negative, to their patients. Such reactions are called countertransference and again can either be seen as nuisance phenomena that have no relevance to the treatment process or can be used in the course of therapy as a source of important information about the therapeutic relationship.

Cognitive Psychology

The general area of cognitive psychology is a broad one that overlaps with other disciplines such as linguistics, philosophy, artificial intelligence and anthropology, and indeed a new discipline of 'cognitive science' has emerged from this overlap. There is as yet no one grand theory in cognitive psychology, but, instead, there is a general agreement that, whatever form they might take, internal mental states play important causal roles in the generation of action (Bolton & Hill 1996). Beyond this, there is agreement that the system must process information from a range of sensory inputs, that this information needs to be transformed in various ways so that, e.g. meaningless sequences of sounds can be interpreted meaningfully, and that there must be an overall system that co-ordinaties these multiple functions. Most of this information processing occurs outside of awareness, and we only become aware of the extent to which it is automatic when we put our foot on the 'break' while sitting in the passenger seat, or drive home to the flat that we used to live in rather than the one that we've just move to.

Perception and Attention

The German physicist and physiologist Hermann von Helmholtz is considered to be the father of the science of perception. Long before Freud had developed his ideas on the dynamic unconscious, Helmboltz, in the 1860s, had argued that perception must be based on 'unconscious inferences' (Power 1997). For example, when we look at an object at different distances it looks the same size, even though the physical size of the object on the retina is very different (so-called'object constancy'); the same object can be looked at from different angles yet appears to preserve its shape (so-called' shape constancy'); and an object can be viewed under different lighting conditions and appear the same color (so-called 'color constancy'). Although the unconscious perceptual processes which give rise to these constancies have clear advantages, the fact that processing necessarily distorts the incoming information can under other circumstances lead to disadvantages which, at one extreme can produce mildly amusing perceptual illusions, and at the other extreme can lead the individual to perceive life-threatening danger where there is none.

One of the central questions in the perception and attention literature has been the extent to which sensory information is analyzed prior to conscious awareness, Broadbent (1958) argued that this input is analyzed at the superficial physical level and that only input that reaches awarness is analyzed for its meaning. Subsequent work on attention, however has suggested that the sensory input can be analyzed for meaning without the individual having to be aware of the input; in the so-called 'cocktail party phenomenon' and individual can be attending to one conversation, but suddenly become aware of his or her name being spoken in another conversation. This phenomenon demonstrates that the unattended information must have been analyzed for meaning for the switch of attention to happen.

Memory

One of the questions that cognitive psychology has addressed is the form that internal representation of the world takes. Do we remember visual scenes as if they were video-recorded sequences ? Or conversations as if they were tape-recorded? Given the arguments that couples have about who said what to whom and when, it might seem unlikely that memory is in any way veridical in the manner of tape and video-records. The question then is to what extent is memory a reconstruction, one part truth to nine parts fiction? This question has bedeviled recent debates about the possibility of repressed truamatic memories versus the possibility of false memories in cases of sexual abuse (Davies & Dalgleish 2002).

In his classic book on cognitive psychology, Ulric Neisser (1967) took an extreme constructivist view that the process of remembering is like the palacontologist who, on the basis of a couple of small bone, constructs a whole dinosaur. More recently, Neisser has stepped back from this extreme view in the recognition that memory can sometimes be surprisingly accurate. We must recognise too that in the development of childhood vulnerability for later adult disorders, the child may be given conflicting information, i.e. difficult to intergrate in memory; e.g. a mother may repeatedly insist to the child that she love him above all else, though her action may clearly contradict her statements. There is no reason, of course, why there could not be more than one memory (or group of memories) of a particular event or person; a number of current views of memory would be consistent with such a possibility. In such cases, some of the aims of therapy may be to help the adult identify such discrepancies, to work through the consequent emotions, and to reintegrate the memories into a more realistic overall representation of the person or the event (Power & Dalgleish 1997).

A further question that cognitive psychologist ask about memory is what the basic psychological units are. To this question there have been numbers answers and few if any condusions. One of the types of internal representation that has played a significant role, from the work of Bartlett early in the 20th century onwards, is the schema. Piaget also use the term 'Schema' in his studies of child development, and Beck in his account of cognitive therapy. Although there is considerable variation in the use of the term (Power & Champion 1986), schemata refer to unitary representations of regularly encountered objects, events and situations, and activation of one part of a schema leads automatically to activation of all other parts.

Reasoning

An assumption made by many philosophers and psychologists is that people use formal logical rules in reasoning. Perhaps the clearest account of such a system was provided by Jean Piaget in his studies of child development. However, there is now a considerable body of research that demonstrates the limits of the adult capacity for reasoning, though the debate still continues over whether errors are the result of performance limitations (e.g. working memory being limited in processing capacity) or whether there is no such thing as 'mental logic'.

Three main types of reasoning task are deduction, induction, and probability judgment. Deduction is the drawing of a conclusion from a set of premises; induction is the drawing of a general rule on the basis of one or a limited number of instances; and probability judgements involve a statement about the likelihood of an event occurring. As an example of deductive reasoning, for the premises:

If I pass exams I'll study medicine at university.

If I fail my exams I'll go into politics and become prime minister.

I've passed my exams.

The valid and perhaps fortunate conclusion is that I will study medicine at university. As an example of problems that can arise with inductive reasoning, Wason and Johnson-Iaird (Johnson-Iaird 1988) presented subjects with the series of digits '2 4 6' and asked them to discover the underlying rule through the production of additional examples. Most subjects set about confirming the possible the rule 'even numbers increasing by two' by generating large numbers of positive instance of the rule, instead of attempting to disconfirm the ruel by generating negative instances such as '7 8 9'. Had they done so, they would have eventually discovered that the rule was 'any three increasing numbers'. This confirmatory bias is one of the many biases that are evident from studies of reasoning. Other bases have been examined in an elegant series of studies by Kahneman and Tversky (Kahnemaan et al. 1982). For example, the availability bias lead subjects to say that more words begin with the letter 'R' than have 'R' in the third letter, because it is easier to generate words beginning with 'R'. In a similar manner to the influence of biases introduced by schemata in memory, these reasoning biases can be quite benign in their effects and even on occasion lead us to be blissfully ignorant of our faults. However, under othe circumstances the same biases can lead depressed individuals to conclude that they are insignificant and that life is not worth living, or paranoid individuals to conclude that their neighbors really are against them.

Cognitive Therapy

Unlike psychoanalysis and behaviorism, where theory and therapy are very closely connected, cognitive therapy and cognitive psychology have developed almost independently of each other. Thus, it would be feasible to derive a cognitive-based therapy from current cognitive science that constrasted with current cognitive therapy on most points; or more optimistically, it may be possible to bring cognitive therapy closer to cognitive science (Power 2001).

The theory has been developed by Beck (1976) and is based on the idea that dysfunctional schemata arise in childhood typically in problematic parental relationships. These schemata normally remain dormant until later in life when a negative life event or stress occurs which activates them. For example, if the schemata focus on the need to feel love by everybody and the first serious raltionship goes wrong, the individual is vulnerable to becoming depressed. As a consequence of these activated schemata, the individual become overwhelmed with negative automatic thoughts such as 'I am unlovable', 'Nobody has ever relly loved me', and so on, thoughts which lead the individual into a stage of depression.

The therapy has 4 main components:

1. *Education:* The depressed or anxious individual may have little information about depression of anxiety, or may have mistaken information such as a belief that a panic attack

is the same as a heart attack. One of the useful features of congnitive therapy is the fact that individuals are provided with information about the condition they are experiencing and about the procedures used in cognitive therapy.

2. *Goal-setting and graded activities:* Many depressed individuals withdraw from their normal activities, and the resultant inactivity may help to maintain the state of depression (e.g. reduce opportunity to experience reward). One of the key strategies of both congnitive therapy and behavior therapy is the identification of what these activates might be, and then setting activities or homework to be carried out between clinical sessions. The activities typically begin with easier ones and then gradually build up to more difficult ones in order to lessen the chance of failure early on in therapy.
3. *The identification of negative automatic thoughts:* A key step in cognitive therapy is helping the individual to identify the negative automatic thoughts that are intimately connected with feelings of depression and anxiety. These may be identified in the clinical sessions themselves—e.g. by asking the individual to role-play a difficult encounter—or they can be identified as homework by asking the individual to keep a diary of such thoughts in the situations in which they arise. Once identified, the individual is then encouraged to test their validity, to question them, and to check for the evidence for and against them.
4. *Challenging dysfunctional schemata*: The identification and challenging of negative automatic thoughts leads into the final phase of cognitive therapy, which is challenging the dysfunctional schemata that underlie the negative thoughts. In depression, these core beliefs typically center on the need to be loved or the need to do well at all costs. The depressed individual tends to take a one-sided view of past achievements in love and work and may feel hopless about the possibility of any future success; although some of these views may well be realistic, the problem for the therapist is to disentangle genuine failures from the imagined ones, so that individuals can take a more balanced view of themselves and their future.

Personality

Personality is the term used to describe consistency in peoples behavior, for one time to the next and from one situation to another. This is based on a fundamental assumption that certain behaviors characterize a person in a wide variety of situations. Critically, this view involves the belief that knowledge of an individual's personality will allow the prediction of how a given person will behave, even in situations in which the individual has never been observed before. Examples of the use of this predictive approach includes personality assessment used in officer selection in the second World War, and in selecting individuals for particular occupations, e.g. the sales force.

Nomothetic Versus Idiographic Approaches

It has been traditional to categories personality models into nomothetic or idiographic approaches. The nomothetic approach encompasses theories that portray personality in terms of shared attributes, i.e. there are a limited number of variables on which people differ. Within the nomothetic approach there are two main categories: type or trait approaches. Type theories are categorical in nature, i.e. are noncontinuous. An example of the type approach with in psychiatry is the use of diagnostic categories for specific personality disorders: you either have an antisocial personality disorder or you do not. The trait approach also advocates that there are a limited number of personality variables on which people differ; however, the critical difference is the notion that these variables are continuous in nature (akin to individual variation in height and weight). An example of the trait approach is Eysenck's three dimensions of personality: neuroticism, extraversion and psychoticism (Eysenck & Eysenck 1975). Theorists who favor the idiographic approach argue that the nomothetic type/trait method loses the individuality of the person. For example, two people could have the same scores on each of Eysenck's three dimensions of personality, but the viewed by others as quite different people. The idiographic approach considers each individual as unique. Psychodynamic and social learning, theories are examples of nomothetic approaches.

Measuring Personality

If personality is to be assessed, then one needs a measuring instrument that is both valid and reliable. The type of instrument that is developed clearly depends on the underlying theoretical model favored.

Projective personality tests were developed from an idiographic, psychodynamic perspective, in particular that deeper layers of an individual's personality contain repressed wishes, impulses and desires that are not always accessible by conscious self-report. The essence of projective techniques is that they can bypass the individual's defence mechanisms by presenting stimuli which are ambiguous or unstructured. The examinee then has to impose some structure on the stimuli, and in doing so, reveals his own wishes, desires, impulses, etc. The two most widely used instruments are the Rorschach inkblots and the thematic apperception test (TAT). The Rorschach inkblots were developed by a Swiss Psychiatrist, Hermann Rorschach in 1921. The stimuli consist of 10 symmetrical ink blots, some colured, some black and white. Examinees are asked to report what they 'see' in the ambiguous ink blot. The examinees' responses are thought to reflect their deep personality structure. By way of example, focusing on the small details of the ink blots can suggest compulsive rigidity. The TAT was developed by Morgan and Murray (1935) and consists to 30 pictures of various scence; the examinee is asked to tell a story about each picture. As with the Rorschach, the product is thought to reflect the examinee's motives, conflicts, etc.

Attempts to evaluate the validity of the projective techniques have produced disappointing results. Several studies have compared projective test scores from psychiatric groups and healthy individuals, and have shown little if any difference between groups in pattern of responding. Defenders of projective techniques argue that such studies are irrelevant, that the projective techniques are a means of facilitating communication between clinical and examinee, and that when used as part of a comprehensive clinician and evaluation, they help to provide a richer understanding of the person. Projective techniques are not widely used by clinical psychologists in the UK, largely because of concerns over reliability and validity.

Dimensions of Personality

From a nomothetic perspective, if one believes that individuals can be described on a limited number of personality traits, how many traits are require? Allport and Odbert (1936) identified 18,000 words referring to personality traits in the unabridged English dictionary. It is clear that many of these words have similar meaning, and many attempts have been made to try to identify the core number of traits that are required in order to provide a full economic description of an individual's personality.

Cattell (1957) used the technique of factor analysis to reduce trait name to 16 personality factors, express as dimensions, e.g. tense verus relaxed, outgoing versus reserve. Cattell's factors can be measured using his 16-PF self-report questionnaire (Cattell et al. 1970). Further workers have proposed that a smaller number of dimensions can be used, and that each individual's personality can be described in terms of relative location on each of these dimensions.

The 'Big Five'

More recently, a number of investigators have conducted extensive factor-analytic studies and proposed that five dimensions are required in order to accurately describe and individual's personality structure (Norman 1963, Costa & MeCrae 1992a) (Table 15). It is proposed that the richness of each individual's personality can be described in terms of relative placement on each of these five major dimensions of personality. Many studies using many different methods and questionnaires, conducted across different cultures, have generally found these same basic dimensions of personality. There has been a growing consensus that these 5 dimensions provide an economic method for describing a wide variety of individual differences. The 'Big Five' dimensions of personality can be measured using questionnaires such as the NEO Personality Inventory (Costa & McCrae 1992b).

Table 15: The 'Big Five' personality dimensions

Factor name	*Scale dimensions*
Extroversion	Talkative/silent Adventurous/cautious Sociable/reclusive
Agreeableness	Goodnature/irritable Not jealous/jealous Cooperative/negativistic
Conscientiousness	Fussy, tidy/careless Responsible/undependable Scrupulous/unscrupulous
Neuroticism	Poised/nervous, tense Calm/anxious Composed/excitable
Openness to	Artistically sensitive/artistically insensitive
Experience	Intellectual/unreflective, narrow Imaginative/simple, direct

Situational Approach

Personality, by definition, is thought to be at stable phenomenon across situations and time. However, critics argue that refining instruments in order to perfect prediction of how individuals behave is a fruitless exercise as there is no such thing as stability in how people behave, i.e. people behave differently according to the situation in which they find themselves. Mischel (1968) is the most famous proponent of this viewpoint. He argued that studies which measured the behavior of individuals across situations reported correlations which were not particularly impressive (e.g. r = 0.3). Mischel proposed that this is because human behavior is largely determined by the characteristics of the situation itself rather than by stable characteristics of the person. A compromise position is that behavior is determined by the interaction, between the individual's personality traits and a particular situation. More recent research using more refined constructs of personality (such as the 'Big Five' has found impressive stability over time, e.g. 10-year stability for extraversion 0.7–0.8 and for neuroticism 0.6–0.78 (Costa & McCrae 1977).

Emotion

Emotion lies at the very heartland of psychiatry. Many psychiatric disorders are characterized by abnormalities of emotional state, e.g. sadness in depressive disorders, fear in anxiety disorders, disgust in obsessive-compulsive disorder and some eating disorders. However, for many years emotional experience was considered to be out with 'the domain of respectable scientific enquiry in psychology, as emotions were not overt, quantifiable behaviors. However, with the development of cognitive psychology, there have been significant advance in our understanding of the perception and experience of emotional states, and cognition, emotion and behavior interact.

How Many Emotions are there?

As with personality traits, there have been disagreements as to the number of core emotions. The work of Paul Ekman has proved hugely influential in showing, that six basic facial expressions are apparently universally recognized across cultures: happiness, sadness, anger, surprise, disgust and fear (Ekman 1980). However, some authors have argued against trating 'surprise' as a basic emotion. Therefore, a number of authors now propose that there are five basic emotions. (Oatly & Johnson – Laird 1987, Power & Dalgleish 1997). Facial expressions of human emotion are clearly key communication signals. Recent studies have shown that certain clinical disorders are characterized by a recognition deficit for specific emotions, e.g. people with Huntington's disease and people suffering from obsessive-compulsive disorder show severe deficits in recognizing facial expressions of disgust, whereas people with lesions restricted to the amygdala are especially impaired in recognizing facial expressions of fear (Cader et al. 2001).

Theories of Emotion

An influential early theory of emotion, the James-Lange theory, stated that physiological responses are central and precede the experience of emotion. William James (1884) stated that 'common sense says .... we meet a bear are frightened and run .... the hypothesis to be defended here is that the order of the sequence is incorrect ...... the more rational statement is we feel afraid because we tremble'. James thus focused on the experience of emotion as a consequence of perception of body state. A contrasting model of emotional experience was proposed by Walter Cannon (1927). He manipulated peripheral feedback in animals and noted that surgical isolation of the viscera did not impair emotional behavior and that artificial induction of visceral changes did not appear to produce emotional behavior. Cannon also pointed out that, in general, sympathetic reactions to arousing stimuli are too slow to account for the speed of subjective emotional reactions. Cannon proposed that emotional stimuli produced two paralled effects in the brain: one that produced emotional experience and one which produced the somatic changes that readied the organism to respond ('fight or flight'). Thus, in this model, physiological changes were viewed as a consequence, not the cause, of emotional experience.

PSYCHOBIOLOGY

Psychobiology is the branch of psychology that concerns itself with the interface between biological processes and behavior. The range of topics under this umbrella term is huge, including the study of nerve transmission, behavioral genetics, hormones and behaviors, psychopharmacology, biological bases of memory and learning and neuropsychology.

A basic psychobiological tenet is that psychological disorders can result from pathogenic physical processes of external or internal origin. External pathogens include invasive agents such as harmful organisms and toxins which, when introduced into the body, can cause disease and temporary or permanent physical damage. Physical trauma may also cause temporary or permanent damage to the organism, e.g. closed head injury leading to changes in cognition, affect and personality. A number of psychiatric conditions are clearly the result of pathogenic physical processes of external or internal origin. For example, in multi-infarct dementia, a series of small strokes lead to the increased death of brain matter and consequent general intellectual and personality impairments in the sufferer. External agents include psychoactive drugs taken either deliberately or accidentally which can clearly lead to a wide range of psychological problems, e.g. drug induced psychosis. However, it is critical to note that, psychobiology posits bidirectionality, i.e. that while biology can clearly affect behavior, it is equally the case that environment and experience can significantly impact upon biology (Rosenweig & Bennert 1972).

Diathesis–Stress Models

It is clear that there is considerable individual variation in the development of psychiatric disorder. For example, following extreme stress or trauma, some individuals may develop conditions such as PTSD, whereas others who have experienced exactly the same stress or do not. How is this explained? The diathesis–stress model posits that a pre-existing vulnerability (Diathesis) renders an individual more susceptible to particular diseases. Diathesis-stress models have been proposed for a number of psychiatric conditions, including psychosomatic disorders such as gastric ulcer, myocardial infarctions and eczema, and conditions such as schizophrenia and certain types of severe depression. In these disorders, the interaction between a vulnerability and some form of physical or psychosocial stress forms the central part of the model.

Diathesis–stress models are now common place, not only in the biomedical approach, but in a range of psychological and social models also, though the diathesis or vulnerability factor is expressed at a psychological (e.g. sensitivity to the experience of loss) or social level (e.g. a lack of social support from other individuals) rather than at a physical level. A good illustration of this is the work of Brown and Harris (1978) in relation to social factors and risk of depression. They proposed that certain vulnerability factors (lack of a confiding relationship, loss of mother before age 11, 3+children aged < 15-year-old at home, unemployed status) rendered women particularly at risk of depression in the face of certain severe provoking factor (life events) such as deaths, illness/accidents to significant others, job or residence change, etc.

Genes and Behavior

The relative contribution of genetic versus environmental factors to various psychological attributes (e.g. intelligence) has been vigorously debated for may years. Twin studies have been used extensively to try to inform the debate. The typical study compares the intelligence quotient (IQ) of monozygotic (MZ, identical) twins reared together with dizygotic (DZ, non-identical twins) reared together. Generally the correlation between the IQs of the MZ tiwns is significantly higher than that of the DZ twin. However, the greater similarity in IQ may not be simply attributable to genetic factor; MZ twins may have more similar environments than DZ twins. MZ twins clearly look alike (and sometimes are dressed alike), and this may encourage others to treat them more similarly than nonidentical twins. Importantly, significant adults (parents and teachers) may develop the same expectations for MZ twins. Thus there may be strong environmental pressures that contribute towards the similarity in the measured intelligence of MZ twins. In order to try and tease apart the relative contribution of genetic from environmental factors, several studies have capitalizes on occasions where MZ twins have been reared apart (e.g. given up for adoption soon after birth). In one study MZ twins who were reared apart during their formative years showed strong similarities in IQ: about 70% of the variance in IQ was found to be associated with genetic variation, not substantially less than that observed in MZ twins reached together (Bouchard et al. 1990). Evidence such as this indicates that identical genotypes lead to highly similar IQs even when the identical twins grow up in different environments. Critics of such studies argue, however, that the allocation of environments to adopted twins is not truly random, and that twins often are raised in similar types of environments, and that the case for the relative genetic contribution towards IQ has been overstated. With recent developments in the 'new genetics' and mapping of the human genome, a plethora of studies have emerged which aim to identify the relative genetic contribution to a number of psychiatric disorders.

Motivation

Pressure of space prevents a detailed review of the psychobiology of motivation; however, two topics which have particular relevance for psychiatry will be briefly presented: threat and reward.

Threat: Human evolution required the development of an effective series of mechanisms to quickly perceive and respond to threatening stimuli. Cannon (1927) proposed that the perception of threat triggers intense sympathetic arousal which mobilize the individual for 'fight or flight'. Psysiological changes which occur include heart accelearation, inhibition of intestinal peristalsis, pupillary dilatation and the opening of respiratory passages. It has become increasingly clear that the limbic system, in particular the amygdala, plays an important role in the perception and appraisal of threat. LeDoux (1996) has proposed that two paralled neural pathways are activated when a potentially threatening stimulus is encountered: the 'low road' and the 'high road'. The stimulus is first processed in the sensory region of the thalamus, and a 'glimpse' of information about the stimulus is shuttled down a short, quick and dirty route to the amygdala. This triggers the amygdala to start to respond to the possible danger/threat. A slower route involves more detailed processing of the stimuli by the cortex. If this cortical analysis confirms that genuine threat exist, additional signals for action are passed down to the amygdale. However, if the analysis indicates that the stimulus is not a threat, then the 'fight or flight' response is terminated. The amygdala is thus seen as playing a central role in the perception of threat. Recent neuroimaging studies have confirmed that the amygldala is activated in threatening situations, e.g. when patients with post-traumatic stress disorder are exposed to trauma reminders (Liberzon et al. 1999). The amygdale also appear to play a critical role in memory formation for emotional experience (Cahill et al.l 1995).

Reward: In a pioneering experiment, Olds and Milner (1954) cronically implanted electrodes in various brain regions of rats. They discovered that the rats would learn to press a lever if rewarded with a brief burst of electrical stimulation in certain regions of the hypothalamus and limble system. The rewarding efect of this electrical stimulation was remarkable. The rats pressed the level at rates as high as five thousand times per hour. They pressed for 15–20 hours until they fell asleep exhausted, and , on awakening, immediately restarted lever pressing. When forced to choose between food and self-stimulation, hungry rats often opted for self-stimulation. One interpretation of these findings was that the brain stimulation mimicked the natural reward system. Self-stimulation was most effective when applied to the medial forebrain bundle, which connects the ventral tegmental area with the nucleus accumbens. This pathway utilizes dopamine as a neurotransmitter, and it has been established that dopamine plays a crucial role in the physiology of reward. This has clear relevance for psychiatry in that the dopaminergic system is thought to be impicated in the pathophysiology of a variety of psychiatric disorders (e.g. schizophrenia), and dopaminergic agonists and antagonists are widely used treatments in psychiatry (Anhedonia, e.g. may reflect a dysfunction of an endogenous reward system).

Developmental Psychology

In this brief section, the main piagetian development stages will be outlined and criticized in light of more recent evidence. Then two specific developmental topics of particular relevance for psychiatry will be discussed: attachment ands theory of mind.

Piagetian Theory

Developmental psychology has been hugely influenced by the work of the Swiss psychologist Jean Piaget. Piaget proposed that the mental life of the child is qualitatively different from that of the adult. He believed that children were active contributors to their own learning. By acting on the environment a child constructs internal structures, and it is these structures and not the environment, that controls the way a child thinks. He proposed that all children go through a fix series of developmental stages; sensorimotor; concrete operational (including preopeartional and formal operational).

Sensorimotor stage: This stage extends from birth to roughly 18 months. Initially, the infant utilizes reflex responses such as sucking and grasping, before gaining more motor control and progressing to intiating his own behavior. In the first few months of life, in the mind of the infant, and object only exists as long as it is actively perceived, e.g. a toy dropped out of sight no longer exists. However, at around 12 months the object becomes permanent and the child will look for it (e.g. if it is hidden under a blanket). Active experimentation with objects then commences, e.g. pressing a toy to make it squeak.

Concrete operational state: This stage is thought to extend from about 2 to12 years of age. Piaget proposed that this stage marks the transition between the literalness of perception and the ability for abstract thinking that characterizes the next developmental stage. Between 18 months and 7 years a child is in the preoperational period. During this period, the child begins to represent actions with symbols, which is illustrated by their rapid progress in acquiring language. Similarly, at about 2 years of age children begin to engage in symbolic play, e.g. a chair being ridden as a horse. During this period the child is egocentric, e.g. the child can only describe things from his own perspective. At around age 7 years, the child begins to see the perspective of other people and also master the principle of conservation. Between 7 years and 12 years, the child enters the full concrete operational stage. For example, in demonstrating the principle of number conservation, an experimenter lays out a row of six red and a row of six blue counter side by side on a table, and asks the child 'are there more red counters or blue counters on the table?'; most children will say that threre are the same number of red and blue counters. Next the researcher perform a transformation, e.g. pushing the red counter closer to each other to destroy the one-to-one alignment with the blue counters (the row of red counters is now shorter than the blue row). The child is now asked the same question as previously. Children younger than 7 years of age typically respond 'There are more blue counters' those over 7 typically reply 'There are the same number of each'. Piaget interpreted this kind of finding as illustrative of the younger child's inability to reason logically, because of lack of understanding of general principles such that the number of objects in a set is independent of their spatial layout. By 7 years, the child is able to solve problems related to concrete events but has difficult with abstract thought.

Formal operational stage: This last developmental stage is though to extend from 12 years onwards. During this phase, the child begins to apply concrete operations to hypothetical situations, thus showing abstract thought. The adolescent develops the ability to form hypothese to explain unfamiliar phenomena. During this development stage the individual can think logically and can do so with respect o abstract objects, and is a considered to have reached cognitive maturity.

Criticisms of Piagetian Theory

Many developmental psychologists would agree with several of Piaget's general claims, e.g. that cognitive development is influnced by an interaction between biological and environmental factors, that children play an active role in acquiring knowledge and making sense of their world, and that children's thinking is sometimes qualitatively different from adults. However, some researcher, notably Margaret Donaldson, have challenged some of Piaget's views. Donaldson (1978) argued that Piaget underestimated (a) young children's logical competence and conceptual understanding (b) the influences of contextual factors on children's performance, and (c) the extent to which children's performance depends on their familiarity with the specific contents of the particular task. By way of illustration, the conservation of number task describe above was repeated by Donaldson (1978), however, on this occasion, the transformation (pushing the row of red counters closer together) instead of being carried out by an adult experimenter was carried out by 'naughtly teddy who like to mess up games'. With this modification, many more 4–6-year-old responded correctely that there were still equivalent numbers of red and blue counters. Donaldson (1978) argued that in Piaget's original version of that task the deliberate nature of the transformation misleads the children into inferring that the action is relevant to the question which immediately follows it, and the child misinterprets the question as referring to length. Donaldson proposed that the young child actively attempts to make sense of the total situation by attending not only to what is said, but also to how it is said, and that the child also makes inferences about other people's intentions. Donaldson argued that young children are capable of logical reasoning, but they are more likely to be able to demonstrate this in circumstances where the task make sense to the child.

Further work also suggests that babies are born with a predisposition to look at human faces. Johnson and Morton (1991) showed that newborns preferentially look longer at a schematic face compared with a scrambled face or a blank pattern. Studies such as these suggest that infants are far more congnitively competent than Piaget initially proposed.

Attachment

A safe, secure and loving bond between parent and child is clearly an important foundation for optimal development. We largely learn how to be parents by our own experience as children and by observing others. What type of mothers do motherless mothers make? Harlow and colleagues in Wisconsin conducted a widely cited experiment using rhesus monkey.

Subsequent research with human infants has largely supported the view that neglect can lead to significant problems in the later life of the neglected child. Bowlby (1973) has been a strong advocate of the view that disturbance of a child's initial attachment to the mother will leave the child less secure in late life. Follow-up studies of children reared in inadequate institutional care have shown that many developed significant social impairments, e.g. constantly craving attention or, in contrast, showing marked apathy towards others (Provence & Lipton 1962). While early environment is clearly critical in term of learning and socialization, animal studies also indicate that quality of the early environment directly influence brain development. Rosenzweig and Bennett (1972) studied rats who were either rared in bare surroundings or in a cage that was environmentally enriched (running wheels, apparatus to climb on, etc.) after 80 days in the enriched environment, rats had developed 23% more neural interconnections than control rats raise in bare conditions. Evidence such as this indicates that the developing brain is markedly influenced by environmental stimulation.

Theory of Mind

As started above, Piaget propsed that in the concrete operational stage of development, children are initially egocentric and only at about 7 years can they appreciate the difference between another person's point of view and their own. More recetly, 'theory of mind' studies have suggested that children can take the perspective of another person at about 4 years of age. A theory of mind is the ability to appreciate that minds contain mental states, e.g. beliefs, desires, intentions, and to use this knowledge to predict another person's actions. Theory of mind is commonly assessed using test which evaluate a child's understanding of false beliefs. Recently, theory of mind deficits have been implicated in psychological models which attempt to explain disorders such as autism and schizophrenia.

REFERENCES

Neuropsychology

1. Osler W. Specialism in the general hospital. Bull John Hopkins Hosp. 1913;24:167-71.
2. Lashley KS. Brain Mechanisms and Intelligence. Chicago: University of Chicago Press, 1929.
3. Descartes R. Triate de l'homme. Paris: Angot, 1664.
4. Mann L. On the Trail of Process. New York: Grune and Stratton, 1979.
5. Broca P. Sur le siege de la faculte du langagearticule. Bull SocAnthropol 1885;6:377-396. cf. Kolb.
6. Wernicke C. Der aphasischesymptomekomplex. Breslau, Poland: Cohn and Weiger, 1874.
7. Scoville WB, Milner B. Loss of memory after bilateral hippocampal lesions. J Neurol Neurosurg Psychiatry. 1957;20:11-21.
8. Milner B. Interhemispheric differences in the localization of psychological processes in man. Br Med Bull. 1971;27:272-303.
9. Milner B. Effects of different brain lesions on card sorting. Arch Neurol. 1963;9:90-103.
10. Halstead WC. Brain and Intelligence. Chicago: University of Chicago, 1947.
11. Luria AR. Higher Cortical Functions in Man. New York: Basic Books, 1966.
12. Luria AR. Higher Cortical Functions in Man. New York: Basic Books, 1981.
13. Golden CJ. The Luria-Nebraska Children's Battery: Theory and form. In: Hind G, Obrzut J (Eds). Neuropsychological Assessment and the School-aged Child. New York: Grune and Stratton, 1981.
14. Kolb B, Whishaw IQ. Fundamentals of Human Neuropsychology. New York: WH Freeman, 1990.
15. Diller L, Gordon WA. Rehabilitation and Clinical Neuropsychology. In: Filskov SB, Boll TJ (Eds). Handbook of Clinical Neuropsychology. New York: John Wiley, 1981.
16. Ciompi L. Affectologic: Uber die Strukker der Psyche und ihre Entwicklung. Stuttgart: Klett-Cotta, 1982.
17. Gjerde PF. Attentional capacity dysfunction and arousal in schizophrenia. Psychol Bull. 1983;93:339-41.
18. Frith CD, Done DJ. Towards a neuropsychology of schizophrenia. Br J Psychiatry. 1988;153:437-51.

19. Taylor MA, Greenshop B, Abrams R. Lateralized neuropsychological dysfunction in affective disorder and schizophrenia. Am J Psychiatry. 1979;136:1031-4.
20. Weckowitz TE, Tam CI, Mason J, et al. Speed in test performance in depressed patients. J Abnor Psychol. 1978;87:578-82.
21. Bilder RM, Mukherjee S, Rieder RO. Symptomatic and neuropsychological components of defect states. Schizophr Bull. 1985;11:409-20.
22. Liddle PF. Schizophrenia syndromes, cognitive performance and neuropsychological dysfunction. Psychol Med. 1987;17: 49-63.
23. Saykin AJ, Gur RC, Gur RE, et al. Neuropsychological function in schizophrenia: Selective impairment in memory and learning. Arch Gen Psychiatry. 1991;48:618-24.
24. Gold JM, Harvey PD. Cognitive deficits in schizophrenia. Psychiatr Clin N Am. 1993;16:295-312.
25. Braff DL, Sacuzzo DP. The effects of antipsychotic medication on speed of information processing in schizophrenia. Am J Psychiatry. 1982;139:1127-32.
26. Cabeza R, Grady CL, Nyberg L, et al. Age related differences in neural activity during memory encoding and retrieval: A positron emission tomography study. J Neurosci. 1997;17: 391-400.
27. Fletcher PC, Frith CD, Grasby PM, et al. Brain systems for encoding and retrieval of auditory-verbal memory. Brain. 1995;118:401-16.
28. Shallice T, Fletcher P, Frith CD, et al. Brain regions associated with acquisition and retrieval of verbal episodic memory. Nature. 1994;368:633-5.
29. Gold JM, Randolph C, Carpenter CJ. Forms of memory failutre in schizophrenia. J Abnor Psychol. 1992;101:487-501.
30. Goldberg TE, Weinberger DE, Pliskin NH, et al. Recall memory deficit in schizophrenia: A possible manifestation of prefrontal dysfunction. Schizophr Res. 1989;2:251-8.
31. Tamlyn D, McKenna PJ, Mortimer AM, et al. Memory impairment in schizophrenia: Its extent, affiliations and neurospychological character. Psychol Med. 1992;22:101-15.
32. Flor-Henry P, Yeudall LT. Neuropsychological investigation of schizophrenia and manic-depressive psychosis. In: Gruzelier J, Flor-Henry P (Eds). Hemisphere Asymmetries of Function and Psychopathology. New York: Grune and Stratton, 1983.
33. Stenberg DE, Jarvik ME. Memory functions in depression. Am J Psychiatry. 1976;33:219-24.
34. Weingarten H, Cohen RM, Murphy DL. Cognitive processes in Depression. Arch Gen Psychiatry. 1981;38:42-7.
35. Watts FM, Dalgleish T, Bourke P, et al. Memory deficit in clinical depression: Processing resources and structure of materials. Psychol Med. 1990;20:345-9.
36. Robbins TW, Joyce EM, Sahakian BJ. Neuropsychology and imagine. In: Handbook of Affective Disorders, 2nd edition. Edinburgh: Churchill Livingstone, 1992. cf. Ref. 42.
37. Squire L, Zouzounis JA. Self ratings of memory dysfunction: Different findings in depression and amnesia. J Clin Exper Neuropsychol. 1988;10:727-38.
38. Austin MP, Ross M, Murray C, et al. Cognitive function in major depression. J Affect Dis. 1992;25:21-30.
39. Brand AN, Jolles J, Gispen-de Wied C. Recall and recognition memory deficits in depression. J Affecte Dis. 1992;25:77-86.
40. Calev A, Nigal D, Chazan S. Retrieval from semantic memory using meaningful and meaningless constructs by depressed, stable bipolar and manic patients. Br J Clin Psychol. 1989;28:67-73.
41. Bazin N, Perruchet P, De Bonis M, et al. The dissociation of explicit and implicit memory in depressed patients. Psychol Med. 1994;24:239-45.
42. Iisley JE, Moffoot APR, O'Carroll RE. An analysis of memory dysfunction in major depression. J Affect Dis. 1995;35:1-10.
43. Elliot R, Sahakian BJ, McKay AP, et al. Neuropsychological impairments in unipolar depression: The influence of perceived failure on subsequent performance. Psychol Med. 1996;26:975-90.
44. Henry GH, Weingarten H, Murphy DL. Idiosyncratic patterns of learning and word association during mania. Am J Psychiatry. 1971;128:56-66.
45. Crowin J, Perelow E, Fieve R, et al. Memory deficit in depression. J Affect Dis. 1990;21:173-83.
46. Baxter LR, Schwartz JM, Mazziotta JC. Cerebral glucose metabolism rates in nondepressed patients with obsessive compulsive disorder. Am J Psychiatry. 1988;145:1560-63.
47. Insel TR. Toward a neuroanatomy of obsessive-compulsive disorder. Arch Gen Psychiatry. 1992;49:739-44.
48. Flor-Henry P, Yeudall LT, Koles ZJ, et al. Neuropsychological and power-spectral EEG investigations of the obsessive-compulsive syndrome. Biol Psychiatry. 1979;14:119-30.
49. Insel TR, Donnelly EF, Lalakea ML, et al. Neurological and neuropsychological studies of patients with obsessive compulsive disorder. Biol Psychiatry. 1983;18:741-51.
50. Khanna S, Narayanan HS, Sharma SD, et al. Post-traumatic OCD: A single-case report. Indian J Psychiatry. 1985;27:337-40.
51. Behar D, Rapoport JL, Berg CJ, et al. Computerized tomography and neuropsychological test measures in adolescents with obsessive compulsive disorder. Am J Psychiatry. 1984;141:363-9.
52. Malloy P. Frontal lobe dysfunction in obsessive compulsive disorder. In: Perecmen E (Ed). The Frontal Lobes Revisited. IRBN Press, 1987.
53. Head D, Bolton D, Hymas N. Deficit in cognitive shifting ability in patients with obsessive compulsive disorder. Biol Psychiatry. 1989;25:929-37.
54. Zielinski CM, Taylor MA, Juzwin KR. Neuropsychological deficits in obsessive compulsive disorder. Neuropsychiatr Neuropsychol Behav Neurol. 1991;4:110-26.
55. Boone KB, Ananth J, Philpott L. Neuropsychological characteristics of nondepressed adults with obsessive compulsive disorder. Neuropsychiatr Neuropsychol Behav Neurol. 1991;4:96-109.
56,57. Otto MW, Baer J, Jenicke MA. Neuropsychological aspects of obsessive compulsive disorder: Frontal lobe and memory functions. cf. Otto MW. Normal and abnormal information processing. Psychiatr Clin N Am. 1992;15:825-48.

58. Fitzhugh LC, Fitzhugh KB, Reitan RM. Adaptive abilities and intellectual functioning in hospitalized alcoholics: Further considerations. Quart J Stud Alcohol. 1965;21:414-23.
59. Goldstein G, Shelley CH. Field dependence and cognitive, perceptual and motor skills in alcoholics: A factor analytic study. Quart J Stud Alcohol. 1971;32:29-40.
60. Ryan C, Butters N. Learning and memory impairment in young and old alcoholics: Evidence for the premature aging hypothesis. Alcoholism: Clin Exper Res. 1980;4:288-93.
61. Bowden SC. Brain impairment in social drinkers? No cause for concern. Alcoholism. 1987;11:407-10.
62. Bolter JF, Hannon R. Cerebral damage associated with alcoholism: A re-examination. Psychol Rec. 1980;30:165-79.
63. Gordon SM, Kennedy BP, McPeake JD. Neuropsychologically impaired alcoholics assessment, treatment considerations and rehabilitation. J Subs Abuse Treat. 1988;5:99-104.
64. Corville CB. Effects of Alcohol on the Nervous System of Man. Los Angeles: San Lucas Press, 1995.
65. Ron MA. Brain damage in chronic alcoholism: A neuropathological, neuroradiological and psychological review. Psychol Med. 1977;7:103-12.
66. Molloy MP. A neuropsychological investigation of the memory disorder found in chronic alcoholism.Unpublished Masters Thesis, University of Melboume. cf. Walsh KW. Ed. Understanding Brain Damage. New York: Churchill Livingstone, 1976.
67. Parker ES, Noble EP. Alcohol consumption and cognitive functioning in social drinkers. J Stud Alcohol. 1977;38:1240-46.
68. Loberg T. Alcohol misuse and neuropsychological deficits in man. J Stud Alcohol. 1980;41:119-28.
69. Golden CJ, Moses JA, Coffman JA, et al. Clinical Neuropsychology. London: Grune and Stratton, 1983.
70. Wechsler D. Measurement of Adult Intelligence. Baltimore: Williams and Wilkins, 1944.
71. Goldstein G. Normal ageing and the concept of dementia. In: Golden CK, Vicente PJ (Ed). Foundations of Clinical Neuropsychology. New York: Plenum Press, 1983.
72. National Institute of Health. The Dementias: Hope Through Research. Bethesda: NIH Publications (No. 81-2252), 1981.
73. Folsom JC. Reality orientation for elderly mental patients. J Geriatr Psychiatry. 1968;1:291-307.
74. Miller E. Psychological strategies in the treatment and management of dementias. In: Copeland, JRM, Abou-Saleh MT, Blazer DG (Eds). Principles and Practice of Geriatric Psychiatry, New York: John Wiley and Sons, 1994.
75. Rutter M, Graham P, Yule W. A Neuropsychiatric Study in Childhood. Clinics in Developmental Medicine Nos. 35-36. London: Spatics International Medical Publications/ Heinermann Medical Books, 1970.
76. Tramontana MG, Sherrets SD, Golden CJ. Brain dysfunction in youngsters with psychiatric disorders: Application of Selz-Reitan rules for neuropsychological diagnosis. ClinNeuropsychol. 1980;2:118-23.
77. Rutter M. Brain damage syndromes in childhood: Concepts and findings. J Child Psychol Psychiatry. 1977;18:1-21.
78. Tramontana MG, Hooper SR. Assessment Issues in Child Neuropsychology. New York: Plenum Press, 1988.
79. Silver LB. Developmental learning disorder. In: Lewis M (Ed). Child and Adolescent Psychiatry. Baltimore: Williams and Wilkins, 1991.
80. Baron-Cohen S, Leslie AM, Frith U. Does the autistic child have a 'theory of mind'? Cognition. 1985;21:37-46.
81. Ozonoff S, Pennington B, Rogers S. Executive function deficits in high-functioning autistic children: Relationship to 'theory of mind.' J Child Psychol Psychiatry. 1991;32:1081-6.
82. Frith U, Happe F. Autism: Beyond the 'theory of mind.' Cognition. 1994;50:115-32.
83. Murphy FC, Sahakian BJ. Neuropsychology of bipolar disorder. British Journal of Psychiatry. 2001;178:S120-27.
84. Morrison G. O' Carroll RE, McCreadie RG. The long term course of cognitive impairment in schizophrenia. Trends in cognitive science. 2004;7:234-54.
85. Halligan PW, David AS. Cognitive neuropsychiatry: towards a scientific psychopathology. Nature Neuroscience. 2001; 2:209-15.
86. Simonoff E, Pickles A, Charman T, Chandler S, Loucas T, Baird G. Psychiatric disorders in children with autism spectrum disorders; prevalence, comorbidity, and associated factors in a population-derived sample. J Am Acad Child Adolec Psychiatry. 2008;47:921-9.
87. Hartley SL, Sikora DM, McCoy R. Prevalence and risk factors of maladaptive behaviour in young children with autistic disorder. J Intellect Disabil Res. 2008;52:819-29.
88. Rogers SJ, Hepbum S, Wehner E. Parent reports of sensory symptoms in toddlers with autism and those with other developmental disorders. J Autism Dev Disord. 2003;33:631-42.
89. Rapin I, Tuchman R. Autism: definition, Neurobiology, screening, diagnosis. Pediatr Clin North Am. 2008;55: 1129-46.
90. Serveant JA, Guerts H, Huijbregts S, Schetes A, Oosterlaan J. The top and bottom of ADHD: a neuropsychological perspective. Neurosci Biobehav Rev. 2003;27:583-92.
91. Barkley RA, Edwards G, Laneri M, Fletcher K, Metevia L. Executive function, temporal discounting, and sense of time in adolescents with attention deficit hyperactivity disorder (ADHD) and oppositional defiant disorder (ODD). J Abnorm Child Psychol. 2001;29:541-56.

Theories of Learning

92. Tarpy RM, Mayor RE. Foundations of Learning and Memory. Glenview: Scott, Foresman, 1978.
93. Baron RA, Byrne D, Kantowitz BH. Psychology: Understanding Behavior. 2nd edition. NewYork: Holt, Rinehartand Winston, 1980.
94. Wilson GT, Cleary KD. Principles of Behavior Therapy. Englewood Cliffs, New Jersey: Prentice-Hall, 1980.

95. Pavlov IP. Conditioned Reflex. Transl. Antrep GV. London: Oxford, 1927.
96. Turkkan JS. Classical conditioning: The new hegemony. Behav Brain Sci. 1989;12:1989.
97. Garcia J, McGowan BK, Green KF. Biological constraints on conditioning. In: Black AH, Prokasy WF (Eds). Classical Conditioning: Current Research and Theory. New York: Appleton, 1972.
98. Andrews EA, Braveman NS. The combined effects of dosage level and interstimulus interval on the formation of one-trial poison-based aversions in rats. Animal Learning and Behavior. 1975;3:287-9.
99. Rescorla RA. Probability of shock in the presence and absence of CS in fear conditioning. J Compar Physiol Psychol. 1968;66: 1-5.
100. Bolles RC. Reinforcement, expectancy, and learning. Psychol Rev. 1972;79:394-409.
101. Kamin LJ. Predictability, surprise, attention, and conditioning. In: Campbell BA, Church RM (Eds). Punishment and Aversive Behavior. New York: Appleton, 1969.
102. Rachlin H, Logue AW. Learning. In: Hersen M, Kazdin AE, Bellack AS (Eds). The Clinical Psychology Handbook. New York: Pergemon Press, 1983.
103. Rescoria RA, Wagner AR. A theory of Pavlovian conditioning: Variations in the effectiveness of reinforcement and non-reinforcement. In: Black AH, Prokasy WF (Eds). Classical Conditioning: Current Research and Theory. New York: Appleton, 1972.
104. Wittig AF. Psychology of Learning. New York: McGraw-Hill, 1981.
105. Thorndike ES. Animal Intelligence. New York: Macmillan, 1911.
106. Skinner BF. The Behavior of Organisms: An Experimental Analysis. New York: Appleton-Century, 1938.
107. Smith RE, Sarason IG, Sarason BR. Psychology: The Frontiers of Behavior. New York: Harper & Row, 1982.
108. Hulse SH, Deese J, Egeth H. The Psychology of Learning, 4th edition. Tokyo: McGraw-Hill Kogakucha, 1975.
109. Bandura A. Self-efficacy: Toward a unifying theory of behavioral change. Psychol Rev. 1977;84:191.
110. Bolles RC. Learning theory. 2nd edition. New York: Holt, Rinehart and Winston, 1979.
111. Mowrer OH. Psychotherapy theory and research. New York: Ronald, 1953.
112. Mowrer OH. Abnormal reactions or actions? (An auto-biographical answer). Dubuque, Iowa: Brown, 1966.
113. Sahakian WS. Introduction to the Psychology of Learning. Chicago: Rand McNally College Publishing Company, 1976.
114. Hull CL. A Behavior System: An Introduction to Behavior Therapy Concerning the Individual Organism. New Haven: Yale University Press, 1952a.
115. Mowrer OH. Learning Theory and Symbolic Processes. New York: Wiley, 1960.
116. Stampfl TG, Levis DJ. The essentials of implosive therapy: A learning-theory-based psychodynamic behavioral therapy. J AbnorPsychol. 1967;72:496-503.
117. Stampfl TG, Levis DJ. Learning theory: An aid to dynamic therapeutic practice. In: Eron LD, Callahan R (Eds). Relationship of Theory to Practice in Psychotherapy. Chicago: Aldine, 1969.
118. Stampfl TG, Levis DJ. Implosive therapy: A behavioral therapy. In: Spence JT, Carson RC, Thibaut JW (Eds). Behavioral Approaches to Therapy. Morristown: General Learning Press, 1976.
119. Hill WF. Learning: A Survey of Psychological Interpretations. London: Methenn& Co., 1963.
120. Hull CL. A Behavior System: In Introduction to Behavior Therapy Concerning the Individual Organism. New Haven: Yale University Press, 1952b.
121. Hull CL. Conditioning: Outline of a systematic theory of learning. In: Henry NB (Ed). The Psychology of Learning. Forty-First Yearbook of the National Society for the Study of Education. Part II. Chicago: University of Chicago Press, 1942.
122. Hull CL. Principles of Behavior. New York: Appleton-Century-Crofts, 1943.
123. Mishra H. Therapeutic Procedures of Behavior Modification. Unpublished PhD Thesis. Bangalore: Bangalore University, 1974.
124. Kanfer FH, Phillips JS. Learning Foundations of Behavior Therapy. New York: John Wiley & Sons, 1970.
125. Abrams DB, Niaura RS. Social Learning theory. In: Blane HT, Leonard KE (Eds). Psychological Theories of Drinking and Alcoholism. New York: The Guilford Press, 1987.
126. Bandura A. Social Learning Theory. Englewood Cliffs: Prentice Hall, 1977.
127. Bandura A. Principles of Behavior Modification. New York: Holt, Rinehart and Winston, 1969.
128. Eysenck HJ. A theory of the incubation of anxiety fear responses. Behav Res Ther. 1968;6:309-22.
129. Eysenck HJ. The learning theory model of neurosis: A new approach. Behav Res Ther. 1976;14:251-68.
130. Eysenck HJ. The conditioning model of neurosis. Behav Brain Sci. 1979;2:155-66.
131. Seligman MEP. Phobias and preparedness. Behav Ther. 1971;2: 307-20.
132. Arnsel A. The role of frustrative nonreward in noncontinuous reward situations. Psychol Bull. 1958;55:102-19.
133. Rescoria RA. Pavlovian conditioned inhibition. Psychol Bull. 1969;72:77-94.
134. Rescoria RA, Lo Lordo VM. Inhibition of avoidance behavior. J Compar Physiol Psychol. 1965;59:406-12.
135. Dekker E, Groen J. Reproducible psychogenic attacks of asthma. J Psychosom Res. 1973;17:359-63.
136. Watson JB, Rayner R. Conditioned emotional reactions. J Exper Psychol. 1920;3:1-14.
137. Jones MC. The elimination of children's fears. J Exper Psychol. 1924;1:383-90.

138. Salter A. Conditioned Reflex Therapy. New York: Farrar, Straus, 1949.
139. Salter A. The theory and practice of conditioned reflex therapy. In: Wolpe J, Salter A, Reynas LJ (Eds). The Conditioning Therapies. New York: Holt, Rinehart and Winston, 1965.
140. Wolpe J. Psychotherapy By Reciprocal Inhibition. Stanford: Stanford University Press, 1958.
141. Siegel S. Drug-anticipatory responses in animals. In: White L, Tursky B, Schwartz GE (Eds). Placebo: Theory, Research and Mechanisms. New York: Guilford Press, 1985.
142. Siegel S. Tolerance to the hyperthermic effect of morphine in the rat is a learned response. J Compar Physiol Psychol. 1978;92:1137-49.
143. Ludwig AM, Wikler A. "Craving" and relapse to drink. QJ Stud Alcohol. 1974;35:108-30.
144. Newell R. Developments in behavior therapy. In: Dryden W. Developments in Psychotherapy: Historical Perspectives. London: Sage, 1996.
145. George WH. Marlatt GA. Alcoholism: The evolution of behavioral perspective. In: Galanter M (Ed). Recent Developments in Alcoholism. Vol. I. New York: Plenum Press, 1983.
146. Bandura A. Self-efficacy mechanism in human agency. Am Psychol. 1982;37:122-47.
147. O'Leary KD, Wilson GT. Behavior Therapy. Englewood Cliffs: Prentice-Hall, 1976.

Measurement in Psychiatry

148. Dube KC. Cultural factors in the treatment of schizophrenia. Indian J Psychiatry. 1978;20:132-6.
149. The Mental Health Act 1987 (No. 14 of 1987). Published in the Gazette of India, Extraordinary, Pt II Sec I dated 22nd May 1987.
150. Wig NN, Saxena S. Recent development in psychiatric diagnosis and classification. Continuing Medical Education Program. Indian Psychiatric Society. 1982;1:53-62.
151. World Health Organisation. International Classification of Diseases. Chapter V. 9th Rev. Geneva: WHO, 1978.
152. American Psychiatric Association. Diagnostic and Statistical Manual of Mental Disorders, 3rd edition. Washington DC: APA, 1987.
153. World Health Organisation. ICD-10. Classification of Mental and Behavioral Disorders (Clinical Descriptions and Diagnostic Guidelines). Geneva: WHO, 1992.
154. American Psychiatric Association. Diagnostic and Statistical Manual, 4th edition. Washington DC: APA, 1994.
155. Kastrup M, Wig NN. Transcultural perspective in the multiaxial classification. Indian J Soc Psychiatry. 1986;2:289-300.
156. Dube KC, Dube S, Kumar A. Psychiatric syndromes in Ayurveda with description of epilepsy and alcoholism. In: Kiev A, VenkobaRao A (Eds). Readings in Transcultural Psychiatry. Madras: Higginbothams, 1982. pp. 1-10.
157. Dube KC. Nosology and therapy of mental illness in Ayurveda. Compar Med. 1979;2:87-92.
158. Singh HG. Atharva Vedic approach towards insanity (unmada). Vedic Path. 1976;41:71-5.
159. Singh HG. Apasmar (epilepsy): An Atharva-Vedic description and care. Vedic Path. 1977;42:34-7.
160. Singh HG. Personality typology of Yoga. Vedic Path. 1980;43:23-31.
161. Singh HG. Psychopathology and Atharva Veda. Vedic Path. 1983;45:38-45.
162. Ramu MG, Venkataram BS, Jankiramaiah N. Manovikaras with special reference to udvega (anxiety) and vishada (depression). NIMHANS J. 1988;6:41-6.
163. Mahal AS, Chaturvedi DS, Ramu MG, et al. A clinical study of unmada (unmadalakshanasamuchayaadhyana). Indian J Psychiatry. 1977;19:19-26.
164. Shamsundar C. Psychiatric symptoms and cause-effects in Indian mythology. NIMHANS J. 1991;9:87-90.
165. Balodhi JP. Holistic approach in psychiatry: Indian view. NIMHANS J. 1991;9:101-4.
166. Balodhi JP. Indian mythological views on suicide. NIMHANS J. 1992;10:101-5.
167. Pasricha S. Near death experiences in South India: A systematic survey in Channapatna. NIMHANS J. 1922;10:111-8.
168. Raguram R, Jadhav S, Weiss M. Historical perspectives on dhat syndrome. NIMHANS J. 1994;10:117-24.
169. Chaturvedi SK, Chandra PS, Issac MK, et al. Is there a female dhat syndrome? NIMHANS J. 1993;11:89-93.
170. Wing JK, Cooper JE, Sartorious N. The measurement and classification of psychiatric symptoms. Cambridge: Cambridge University Press, 1974.
171. Wig NN, Menon DK, Murthy RS. Hindi version of Present State Examination: Problems of translation and application in Indian setting. Indian J Psychiatry. 1982;24:309-27.
172. Kapur RL, Kapur M, Carstairs GM. Indian Psychiatric Survey Schedule (IPSS). Soc Psychiatry. 1974;9:71-6.
173. Murthy RS, Wig NN. Community Psychiatry in India: Organization, service and training. In: Kiev A, Venkoba Rao A (Eds). Readings in Transcultural Psychiatry. Madras: Higginbothams, 1982. pp. 85-99.
174. Wig NN, Suleiman MA, Routledge R, et al. Community reaction to mental disorders: A key informant study in three developing countries. Acta Psychiatr Scand. 1980;61:111-7.
175. Malhotra S, Varma VK, Verma SK. Temperament as determinant of phenomenology of childhood psychiatric disorders. Indian J Psychiatry. 1986;28:263-76.
176. Spitzer RL, Williams JBW. Instruction manual for the structured clinical interview for DSM-III (SCI-D). New York: New York State Psychiatric Institute, 1983.
177. Spitzer RL, Endicott J. Schedule for Affective Disorders and Schizophrenia. Technical Report. New York: New York State Psychiatric Institute, 1977.
178. Helzer J, Robina L, Croughan J, et al. Renard Diagnostic Interview. Arch Gen Psychiatry. 1981;38:383-98.
179. Godlberg DP, Cooper B, Eastwood MR, et al. A standardized psychiatric interview for use in community surveys. Br J Prevent Soc Med. 1980;24:18-23.

180. Sen B. Psychiatric phenomena in primary health care: Their extent and measure. Indian J Psychiatry. 1987;29:33-40.
181. Robins SL, Helzer J, Croughan NA, et al. National Institute of Mental Health Diagnostic Interview Schedule. Arch Gen Psychiatry. 1981;38:381-9.
182. Guy W. Clinical Global Impressions. In: Guy W, et al. ECDEU Assessment Manual for Psychopharmacology. Rockville: NIMH, 1976. pp. 217-22.
183. Basu D, Varma VK, Malhotra S. Alienation and psychoactive substance use. Indian J Soc Psychiatry. 1992;8:24-34.
184. Channabasavanna SM, Raguram R, Weiss MG, et al. Enthonography of psychiatric illness: A pilot study. NIMHANS J. 1993; 11:1-10.
185. Kapur M, Barnabas I, Reddy MV, et al. Development of a checklist for assessment of childhood psychopathology in the Indian setting. Indian J Clin Psychology. 1994;21:40-52.
186. Srivasan TN, Suresh TR. Non-specific symptoms and screening of nonpsychotic morbidity in primary care. Indian J Psychiatry. 1990;32:770-82.
187. Thara R, Rajkumar S, Valecha V. Schedule for the Assessment of Psychiatric Disability: A modification of DAS-II. Indian J Psychiatry. 1988;30:47-53.
188. Spitzer RL, Williams JBW. Quoted In: Goldstein G, Hersen M. Eds. Handbook of Psychological Assessment. Pergamon Press, USA, 1984.
189. Spizer DG, Ehler JG. Structured psychiatric interviews for adults. In: Goldstein G, Hersen M (Eds). Handbook of Psychological Assessment. Pergamon Press, USA, 1984. pp. 291-304.
190. Kendell. Quoted In: Goldstein G, Hersen M (Eds). Handbook of Psychological Assessment.Pergamon Press, USA, 1984.
191. Burgoyne. Quoted In: Goldstein G, Hersen M (Eds). Handbook of Psychological Assessment.Pergamon Press, USA, 1984.
192. Helzer. Quoted In: Goldstein G, Hersen M (Eds). Handbook of Psychological Assessment. Pergamon Press, USA, 1984.
193. Catell RB. Guide to Mental Testing. University of London Press, 1948.
194. Bhakoo ON, Kaur S, Narang A, et al. A longitudinal study of variations in developmental quotients (DQs) in the first 30 months of life. Indian J ClinPsychol. 1977;4:59-68.
195. Malin AJ. Nagpur adaptation of Vineland Social Maturity Scale. Lucknow: Indian Psychological Corporation, 1972.
196. Murlidharan R. Indian adaptation of Gessell's Developmental Schedules. Delhi: NCERT, 1968.
197. Phatak P. Motor and mental development of Indian babies from 1 month to 30 months. Indian Ped. 1969;6:18-22.
198. BharathRaj J. Manual of Developmental Screening Test (DST). Mysore: All Indian Institute of Speech and Hearing, 1983.
199. Koshy V, Sharma SD. Standardization of the Cattell's Infant Intelligence Scales in India. Indian J Psychiatry. 1984;26: 327-30.
200. Verma SK, Pershad D, Kaushal P. Gessell drawing tests as a measure of intelligence in the mentally retarded children. Indian J Ment Retard. 1972;5:64-8.
201. Bharath Raj J. AIISH norms on Seguin Form Board with Indian Children. Mysore: All India Institute of Speech and Hearing, 1971.
202. Pershad D, Verma SK, Randhawa A. Preliminary report on a performance test of intelligence on 4-8 years old children. Indian J Clin Psychology. 1979;6:125-30.
203. Phatak P. Revision and extention of Phatak Draw-a-Man Scale for Indian children of age group 2.5 to 16.5 years. Psychol Stud. 1984;29:34-46.
204. Bhatia CM. Performance Tests of Intelligence. Bombay: Oxford University Press, 1955.
205. Malin AJ. Malin's Intelligence Scale for Indian children. Indian J Ment Retard. 1977;4:15-25.
206. Kulshreshtha SK. Stanford-Binet Intelligence Scale: Hindi adaptation of third revision. 1960. L-M form. Allahabad: Manas Sewa Sansthan Parkashan, 1971.
207. Porteus SD. Poteus Maze Test: Fifty year's application. California: Pacific Books, 1965.
208. Raven JC. Colored Progressive Matrices. London: Lewis, 1962.
209. Raven JC. Standard Progressive Matrices. London: Lewis, 1958.
210. Jalota S. Manual of Directions for the Group General Mental Ability Test (GMAT) in Hindi. Delhi: Psychocentre, 1973.
211. Verma SK, Pershad D, Malhotra A, et al. The revised Bhatia's Short Battery of Performance Tests of Intelligence for Adults (A Handbook). Agra: National Psychological Corporation, 1988.
212. Ramalingaswarmy P. Measure of Intelligence Among Adult Indians. New Delhi: NCERT, 1975.
213. Verma SK, Pershad D, et al. Hindi WAIS-R Verbal Scale. Unpublished Final Report of an ICMR Project. New Delhi,1983.
214. Verma SK, Pershad D, Gupta LN, et al. Standardization of Hindi WAIS-R Verbal Short Scale. Bull PGI. 1984;18:70-9.
215. Bhogle S, Jaiprakash I. Normative data on Advanced Progressive Matrices for Indian University Students. Indian J Clin Psychol. 1994;21:53-7.
216. Isaacs B, Akhtar J. The Set Test: A rapid test of mental functions in old people. Age and Ageing. 1972;18:70-9.
217. Verma SK, Pershad D, Shukla TR, et al. Standardization of Hindi WAIS-R Verbal. In: Pershad D, Verma SK (Eds). The Concept and Assessment of Intelligence (Indian Perspective). Agra: National Psychological Corporation, 1988. pp. 90-120.
218. Pershad D, Verma SK. The Concept and Assessment of Intelligence (Indian Perspective). Agra: National Psychological Corporation, 1988.
219. Ramalingaswamy P. The use of Block-Design Test among literate low-economic group of people: A comparative study on North Indian and South Indian Population. Indian J Psychol. 1965;41:27-32.
220. Bhakoo ON, Gupta AN, Chopra JA, et al. A prospective study of neonatal neurological examination including electroencephalographs in high risk babies and its co-relation with subsequent neurological and mental development. ICMR Enquiry Final Report, 1976.
221. Verma SK. Intelligence assessment in the mentalyretardates: Some experiences. Indian J Ment Retard. 1971;4:10-4.

222. Wig NN, Mehta S, Verma SK. Methodological shortcomings of previous studies on malnutrition and mental development. Asian J Psychol Educ. 1981;8:25-36.
223. Wechsler D, Stone CP. Manual. Wechsler Memory Scale. New York: Psychological Corporation, 1945.
224. Pershad D, Verma SK. Evaluation of Boston Memory Scale. Indian J ClinPsychol. 1975;2:51-6.
225. Pershad D. Construction and Standardization of Clinical Tests of Memory in Hindi. Agra: National Psychological Corporation, 1977.
226. Pershad D, Wig NN. A battery of simple tests of memory for use in India. Neurol India. 1976;24:86-93.
227. Verma SK, Wig NN, Shah DK. Validation of Bender Gaestalt Test in Indian psychiatric patients. Indian J Applied Psychol. 1972;9:65-7.
228. Bender L. A visual motor gestalt test and its clinical use. New York: American Orthopsychiatric Association, 1938.
229. Bhargave M, Sandhu R. Guidelines for Bender Visual Motor Gestalt Test. Lucknow: Ankur Psychological Agency, 1987.
230. Pershad D, Verma SK. Cross-validation of a screening test for organic brain disease. Neurol India. 1976;26:107-10.
231. Hooper HE. Manual-Hooper Visual Organisation Test. Los Angeles: Western Psychological Services, 1966.
232. Pershad D, Verma SK. Clinical utility of Hooper's Visual Organisation Test (VOT): A preliminary investigation. Indian J Clin Psychol. 1980;7:67-70.
233. Shukla TR, Jha J, Mishra MN. The diagnostic usefulness of Benton Revised Visual Retention Test of Brain Damage. Psychol Stud. 1971;16:35-41.
234. Abraham A, Mathai KV. The effect of right temporal lobe legions on matching of smells. Neuropsychologia. 1983;21:277-81.
235. Kapur M. Measurement of organic brain dysfunction. Indian J Clin Psychol. 1978;5:1-9.
236. Kapur M. A short screening battery of tests to detect organic brain dysfunction. J Clin Psychol. 1978;34:104-11.
237. Mukundan CR, Reddy GNN, Hegde AS, et al. Neuropsychological and clinical recovery in patients with head trauma. NIMHANS J. 1987;5:23-31.
238. Pershad D, Verma SK, Malhotra S, et al. Utility of psychological tests in the diagnosis of brain dysfunction cases. Indian J Applied Psychol. 1984;21:25-32.
239. Pershad D, Verma SK, Malhotra S, et al. Screening of organic brain dysfunction. Indian J Psychiatry. 1984;26:349-55.
240. Pershad D, Verma SK. Handbook of PGI Battery of Brain Dysfunction (PGI-BBD). Agra: National Psychological Corporation, 1990.
241. Varma VK, Suri A, Kaushal P. Abstract thinking in schizophrenia. Indian J Psychiatry. 1973;15:123-30.
242. Verma SK, Pershad D, Menon DK. A preliminary investigation with a grid test of schizophrenic thought disorder. Indian J Clin Psychol. 1978;5:33-6.
243. Varma VK, Aggarwal RK, Das K, et al. Linguistic competence and psychopathology: Construction of a test of linguistic competence. Indian J Psychiatry. 1985;25:183-91.
244. Varma VK, Das K, Jiloha RC. Correlation of linguistic competence with psychopathology. Indian J Psychiatry. 1985;27:193-9.
245. Balodhi JP. Logical structure of a sentence as a tool for the assessment of thought disorder (Ancient Indian View). Indian J Psychiatry. 1986;28:253-7.
246. Pestonjee DM. Second Handbook of Psychological and Social Instruments. Delhi: Concept, 1988.
247. Pareek U, Rao TV. Handbook of Psychological and Social Instruments. Baroda: Samasthi, 1974.
248. Long L, Mehta PH. The First Mental Measurement Hand-book for India. Delhi: NCERT, 1966.
249. Wig NN, Pershad D, Verma SK. The use of psychometric tools in Indian psychiatric research. Indian J Clin Psychol. 1974;1:8-14.
250. Wig NN, Verma SK, Pershad D. Development of psychological tests in India: An overview of current situation. Indian J Clin Psychol. 1983;10:429-37.
251. Verma SK, Pershad D. Psychometric assessment in India: An overview of literature in the last decade with particular emphasis on cultural and methodological problems. In: Kulshreshtha SP, Rahinwal DN (Eds). Recent Advance in Educational and Psychological Testing in India. Dehradun: Jugal Kishore, 1984. pp. 1-25.
252. Verma SK. Development of psychological tools: 10 years experience. J Rajasthan Psychiatr Soc. 1978;1:43-56.
253. Verma SK. A note on psychological tests: Are they essential? Indian J Clin Psychol. 1077;4:193-7.
254. Verma SK. Psychodiagnostics: An evaluation. Psychol Stud. 1993;38:101-13.
255. Venkatesh S, Verma SK, Siddiqui RS. Neuropsychological assessment in organic brain pathology: An overview. Psychol Stud. 1993;38:125-34.
256. Verma SK, Wig NN, Pershad D. Manual for PGI Health Questionnaire. N-1. Agra: National Psychological Corporation, 1985.
257. Verma SK. Construction and standardization of PGI Health Questionnaire. N-2. Agra: Psychological Research Cell, 1978.
258. Menon DK, Wig NN, Verma SK. Manual for PGI Locus of Control Scale. Varanasi: Rupa Psychological Centre, 1988.
259. Menon DK, Wig NN, Verma SK. Manual for PGI Achievement Value Index. Varanasi: Rupa Psychological Centre, 1988.
260. Nagpal R, Sell H. Subjective Wellbeing. SEARO, Health Papers. New Delhi: WHO, 1985.
261. Verma SK, Verma A. General Wellbeing Measure. Lucknow: Ankur Psychological Agency, 1989.
262. Modgil AC, Verma SK, Kaur K. PGI Quality of Life Scale (Revised form). Indian J Clin Psychol. 1986;13:175-84.
263. Pasricha S, Wig NN, Verma SK. SPD Scale: Preliminary data. Indian J Clin Psychol. 1975;2:95-6.
264. Grover P, Verma SK, Pershad D, et al. Manual for PGI Yoga Attitude Scale. Varanasi: Rupa Psychological Centre, 1988.
265. Pareek U. Role Stress Scale Manual. Ahmedabad: Navin Publications, 1983.

266. Sinha D. Sinha Anxiety Scale. Varanasi: Rupa Psychological Centre, 1968.
267. Pershad D, Verma SK, Malhotra A, et al. Measure of Dysfunction and Dysfunction Analysis Questionnaire (DAQ). Agra National Psychological Corporation, 1984.
268. Murthy RS, Anuradha D, Pershad D, et al. Psychiatric Disability Scale: Preliminary report. Indian J Clin Psychol. 1975;2:183-7.
269. Singh G, Verma HC, Verma RS, et al. A new depressive inventory (Amritsar Depressive Inventory). Indian J Psychiatry. 1974;16: 183-8.
270. Singh G, Kaur D, Kaur H. Presumptive Stressful Life Events Scale (PSLES): A new stressful life events scale for use in India. Indian J Psychiatry. 1984;26:107-14.
271. Ramamurthy PV. An Adjustment Inventory for older people. J Psychol Res. 1969;13:162-5.
272. Joshi MC, Malik AK. Jodhpur Multiphasic Personality Inventory (JMPI). (Forms I, II, III for Psychoneurotic, Psychotic and Psychosomatic disorders). Varanasi: Rupa Psychological Centre, 1983.
273. Lakshmibai AJ, Murthy HN, Nagalakshmi SV. Rajas and Tamas in psychological disturbances. Indian J Clin Psychol. 1975;2: 135-8.
274. Arora M, Varma VK. A psychoticism scale in Hindi. I. Construction and initial tryouts. Indian J Psychiatry. 1980;22: 225-9.
275. Kumar P. Development and standardization of sexuality scale. J Person Clin Stud. 1988;4:108-10.
276. Gupta SC, Anand R, Trivedi JK. Development of a suicide intent questionnaire. Indian J Psychiatry. 1983;25:57-62.
277. Kaur N, Nizamic A, Shulka TR. Construction of a ward behavior observation rating scale for psychiatric patients. J Person Clin Stud. 1987;3:166-70.
278. Barnabas I, Nagalakshmi SV. Clinical utility of Multiphasic Questionnaire. NIMHANS J. 1993;11:39-42.
279. Thakur GP, Thakur M. Thakur Death Anxiety Scale. Varanasi: Rupa Psychological Centre, 1984.
280. Dhar U, Kohli S, Dhar S. Manual for Learned Helplessness Scale. Bhiwani: Haryana Council of Psychological Research, 1987.
281. Mishra VD, Gupta KM. Manual for AapkaVyaktitva: EkNaidanikJanch (Your Personality: A Clinical Investigation). Varanasi: BundiMahal, 1975.
282. Varma VK, Akhtar S, Kaushal P, et al. Measurement of Authoritarian traits in India. Indian J Psychiatry. 1973;15:156-65.
283. Saldanha D, Goel DS, Rathee SP, et al. Personality profiles of coronary cases. Indian J Psychiatry. 1973;15:156-65.
284. Shrivastava S, Kumaraiah V, Mishra H. Behavioral intervention in the management of male sexual dysfunction. NIMHANS J. 1993;11:149-53.
285. Neeliyara T, Nagalkshmi SV. Motivation for change in alcohol dependent individuals NIMHANS J. 1993;11:155-9.
286. Chandra PS, Chaturvedi SK, Gururaj G. Identification and assessment of premenstrual symptoms and syndrome in women: An epidemiological approach to the investigation. NIMHANS J. 1994;12;1-8.
287. Karpe S, Kumaraiah V, Mishra H, et al. Behavioral intervention of anger outbursts in adolescents. NIMHANSJ. 1994;12: 163-7.
288. Menon DK, Verma SK. Manual for Hindi PEN Inventory. Varanasi: Rupa Psychological Centre, 1988.
289. Wig NN, Pershad D, Verma SK. Abridged manual of CMI Health Questionnaire (Hindi). Agra: National Psychological Corporation, 1983.
290. Sen NN. Personality Trait Inventory. Delhi: Psychological Foundation, NCERT, 1966.
291. Spielberger CD, Sharma S, Singh M. Development of Hindi edition of the State-Trait Anxiety Inventory. Indian J Psychol. 1973;48:11-20.
292. Bhat VK, Gauba S. A marital adjustment questionnaire in Hindi. Indian J Clin Psychol. 1978;5:29-32.
293. Anjmany S, Nandi DN. Adaptation of Beck, et al. An inventory for measuring depression. Indian J Psychiatry. 1973;15: 386-91.
294. Hasan SQ. A study towards adaptation of Baron's Ego Strength Scale. Indian J Psychol. 1970;45:349-52.
295. Gupta BS. Adaptation of a Hindi Version of the Junior Eysneck Personalty Inventory. Br J Soc Clin Psychol. 1971;10: 189-90.
296. Kapur SD. Hindi version of Cattell's Self Analysis Form on IPAT Anxiety Scale Questionnaire. New Delhi: Psychocentre, 1970.
297. Kapoor K. Hindi version of The Neuroticiam Scale Questionnaire (NSQ). Indian J Psychol. 1965;49:93-8.
298. Krishnan B. Adaptation of Taylor's Manifest Anxiety Scale. Mysore: Mysore University, 1966.
299. Nijhwan HK. Anxiety in School Children. New York: Halstead, 1972.
300. Mohsin SM, Shamshad M. Bell's Adjustment Inventory: Hindi adaption. Patna: Psycho-Scientific Works, 1970.
301. Prasad MS, Thakur GP. Development of an inventory to measure self-esteem. ISPT J Res. 1977;1:33-5.
302. Harding TW, Dearange MV, Baltazar J. Mental dirorders in primary health care: A study of their frequency and diagnosis in four developing countries. Psychol Med. 1980;10: 231-41.
303. Sinha JBP. A test of dependence proneness. J Psychol Res. 1968;12:66-70.
304. Raju GG, Krishnaswamy S, Verghese A. Usefulness of Bortner Rating Scale in the measurement of Type A behavior pattern. Indian J Psychiatry. 1987;29:373-6.
305. Tripathi RR. Tripathi Personal Preference Schedule: Manual. Varanasi: Raghuvir Sharan, 1973.
306. Srivastava ON, Bhat VK. The Middlesex Hospital Questionnaire (MHQ): Standardization of Hindi version. Indian J Psychiatry. 1974;16:283-6.
307. Singh B. Development of some MMPI scales in Indian conditions. Indian Psychol Rev. 1967;3:151-3.

308. Gautam S, Nijhawan M, Kamal P. Standardization of Hindi version of Goldberg's General Health Questionnaire. Indian J Psychiatry. 1987;29:63-6.
309. Singh RA, Malhotra S, Avasthi A, et al. Sexual knowledge and atitude of medical and non-medical students. Indian J Soc Psychiatry. 1987;3:126-36.
310. Agarwal AK, Goel PK, Gupta SC. Application of the Leyton Obsessional Inventory in an Indian population. Indian J ClinPsychol. 1987;14:72-6.
311. Sriram TG, Chaturvedi SK, Gopinath PS, et al. Assessment of Alexithymia: Psychometric properties of Toronto Alexithymia Scale (TAS): A preliminary report. Indian J Psychiatry. 1985;29: 133-8.
312. Sharma S, Jindal SK, Bahera D, et al. Hindi adaptation of an instrument to measure hope: Some preliminary observations. Indian J Soc Psychiatry. 1992;8:57-66.
313. Jatana A, Verma A, Verma SK. A study of menstrual distress before, during and after menstrual phases. Mind. 1991;17: 10-2.
314. Basu J. Applicability of the ego function assessment scale as a guided interview schedule on schizophrenics, neurotics and normals: A preliminary report. Psychol Stud. 1993;38:119-24.
315. Kulhara P, Chakrabarti S, Basu D. Insight and psychosis I. An empirical study. Indian J Soc Psychiatry. 1992;8:40-4.
316. Kulhara P, Basu D, Chakarbarti S. Insight and psychosis II. A pilot study comparing schizophrenia and affective disorder. Indian J Soc Psychiatry. 1992;8:45-8.
317. Akhtar S, Jagwat T. Restrained psychiatric outpatients: Necessity, justification on violation of human rights. Indian J Psychiatry. 1993;35:115-8.
318. Raghuram R. An exploratory study of coping styles in schizophrenic patients. Indian J Psychiatry. 1993;35:22-6.
319. Basu D, Varma VK, Malhotra S, et al. Sensation Seeking Scale: Indian adaptation. Indian J Psychiatry. 1993;35:155-8.
320. Alexander PJ, Kumaraswamy N. Senior medical students' attitude towards psychiatry: Relationship with carreer interest. Indian J Psychiatry. 1993;35:221-4.
321. Mohanty A, Das BS, Mukundan CR, et al. Cognitive outcome and quality of life after aneurysmal subarchnoid haemorrhage. Part II. Quality of life. NIMHANS J. 1993;11:119-24.
322. Arya DK, Avasthi AA, Verma SK, et al. Defense styles in post-graduates form different medical specialities. Indian J Soc Psychiatry. 1992;8:48-51.
323. Andreasen NC. Scale for Assessment of Negative Symptoms. Iowa: University of Iowa, 1982.
324. Andreasen NC. Scale for Assessment of Positive Symptoms. Iowa: University of Iowa, 1984.
325. Hamilton M. A rating scale for depression. J Neurol Neurosurg Psychiatry. 1960;23:56-62.
326. Hamilton M. Development of a rating scale for primary depressive illness. Br J Soc Clin Psychol. 1967;6:278-96.
327. Abraham A, Kamaraiah V. Electromyograph feedback: Treatment outcome in anxiety neurosis. Indian J Psychiatry. 1994;36:70-3.
328. Chaturvedi SK, Chandra PS, Channabasavanna SM, et al. Detection of anxiety and depression in cancer patients. NIMHANS J. 1994;12:141-4.
329. Misra S, Rao SL. Divided attention in head injury. NIMHANS J. 1994;12:157-62.
330. Simpson A. Extrapyramidal side effect scale. Acts Psychiatr Scand. 1970;212(Suppl.):9-12.
331. Datta S, Subhalakshmi TP, Jayaseelan L, et al. Risk factors for tardive dyskinesia. Indian J Psychiatry. 1994;36:22-4.
332. Schooler NR, Kane JM. Research diagnosis of tardive dyskinesia. Arch Gen Psychiatry. 1982;39:486-7.
333. Dubey SN. A study of life stress and social support of drug addicts. Indian J Clin Psychol. 1993;20:21-4.
334. Sargunaraj D, Kumaraiah V. The reliability and translation of STAI, CASQ, EPI and I-E Scale. J Person Clin Stud.1991;7:99-101.
335. Katoch V, Jhingan HP, Saxena S. Level of anxiety and dissociation in patients with conversion and dissociative disorders. Indian J Psychiatry. 1994;36:67-9.
336. Sethia P, Sinha SP. Selective attentional deficits among pervasively and situationally hyperactive children. J Commun Guid Res. 1993;10:137-44.
337. Sharma A, Sethia P, Sinha P. Behavior problems of hyperactive children. Indian J ClinPsychol. 1994;21:6-10.
338. Verma SK, Dubey BL, Khan HA. The cognitive failure scale (CFS) in Hindi: Some initial experiences. J Clin Psychiatry. 1982;6:205-10.
339. Verma SK. Measurement of positive mental health: Some theoretical and practical considerations. Indian J Clin Psychol. 1988;15:6-11.
340. Verma SK. The difficulty levels of some personality tests in Hindi. Indian J Clin Psychol. 1974;1:15-8.
341. Verma SK, Menon DK, Malhotra A. Response tendencies in a questionnaire without questions. Indian J Clin Psychol. 1980;7:151-5.
342. Rorschach H. Psychodiagnostik. Bern: Emst Bircher, 1921.
343. Dubey BL. A pragmatic view of Rorschach Inkblot Technique. Agra: National Psychological Corporation, 1982.
344. Prabhu GG. Herman Rorschach: A centenary tribute. NIMHANS J. 1984;2:77-92.
345. Shukla TR. Psychodiagnostic efficacy of Holtzman inkblot technique under Indian conditions: A normative study. Indian J Clin Psychol. 1976;3:189-98.
346. Holtzman WH. Holtzman Inkblot Technique: Administration and Scoring Guide. New York: Psychological Corporation, 1958.
347. Choudhary U. Indian adaptation of Thematic Apperception Test. Calcutta: Bookland, 1967.
348. Choudhary U. Children Apperception Test. Delhi: Mansayan, 1961.
349. Solanki PPS, SenMazumdar DP. A study of emotional indicators on Draw-a-Person Test with normal and emotionally disturbed female children of lower socio-economic group. Indian J Clin Psychol. 1975;2:13-7.
350. Malhotra HK, Wig NN. Vignettes for attitudinal research in psychiatry. Indian J Psychiatry. 1975;17:195-201.

351. Murthy RS. Features of Mental Disorders. Department of Psychiatry. NIMHANS. Bangalore, 1986.
352. Pramanik KB, SenMazumdar DP. Use of Kahn Test of Symbol Arrangement (KTSA) for assessment of developmental lag and utilization of cognitive ability in emotionally disturbed (ED) children. Indian J Clin Psychol. 1977;4:81-4.
353. Dosanjh NL, Gulati R. Dosanjh (D) Test. Indian J Clin Psychol. 1981;10:439-44.
354. Prabhu GG. The Rorschach technique with normal adult Indians. Indian Psychol Rev. 1967;3:97-106.
355. Dubey BL. Rorschach indices of psychiatric patients in army. Indian J Clin Psychol. 1977;6:175-9.
356. Vagrecha YS, SenMazumdar DP. Relevance of Pitrowski's signs in relation to intellectual deficit in organic (epileptic) and normal subjects. Indian J Clin Psychol. 1974;1:64-6.
357. Akhtar S, Pershad D, Verma SK. A Rorschach study of obsessional neurosis. Indian J Clin Psychol. 1975;2:139-43.
358. Dubey BL. Rorschach analysis of impotence cases and their response to psychotherapy. Indian J Clin Psychol. 1977;4: 145-9.
359. Sandhu JS. Rorschach responses in schizophrenia. Indian J Clin Psychol. 1978;5:145-53.
360. Bagadia VN, Anand S, Saraf K, et al. Analysis of Rorschach Test of 250 cases of schizophrenia. Indian J Psychiatry. 1971;13: 248-52.
361. Kumar P. The Rorschach test in schizophrenia and normal groups. Indian J Psychol. 1963;38:121-4.
362. Pershad D, Dubey BL. A proposed statistical design for Rorschach indices. Indian J Clin Psychol. 1977;4:191-2.
363. Verma SK. A cross-validation of an objective Rorschach. DM&SP Dissertation. CIP, Ranchi, 1966.
364. Cassell WA. Body symbolism and the Somatic Inkblot Series. Alaska: Aurora Pub. Co., 1980.
365. Cassell WA. SIS-II Manual. Alaska: Aurora Pub. Co., 1990.
366. Cassell WA. SIS-I Video.SIS Centre. Alaska: Anchorage, 1992.
367. Cassell WA. The Somatic Inkblot Series: Continuing Rorachach's conceptualization. SIS J Proj Psychol Ment Health. 1994;1:3-14.
368. Cassell WA, Dubey BL, Pershad D. SIS Video: Practiotioner's Manual. Alaska: SIS Centre, 1994.
369. Dubey BL, Cassell WA. Some experiences with Somatic Inkblot Series. Br J Proj Psychol. 1993;38:19-47.
370. Dubey BL, Cassell WA. Somatic Inkblot Technique: Evaluation and current status. Mind. 1993;19:22-31.
371. Pershad D, Dubey BL. Reliability and validity of Somatic Inkblot Series in India. SIS J Proj Psychol Ment Health. 1994;1:33-8.
372. Rathee SP, Goel DS, Chawla Ml, et al.A study of Somatic Inkblot Series-I in coronary cases. SIS J Proj Psychol Ment Health. 1994; 1:51-64.
373. Saldanha D, Goel DS, Rathee SP, et al. Personality profiles of coronary cases. Indian J Psychiatry. 1993;35:197-9.
374. Verma SK, Pershad D, Nehru R. Cross-validation of SIS-II in psychiatric population. SIS J Proj Psychol Ment Health. 1994;1:15-8.
375. Kuppuswami B. Socio-economic Status Scale (Urban). Delhi: Mansayan, 1962.
376. Trivedi G, Pareek U. Socio-economic Status Scale (Rural). Delhi: Mansayan, 1964.
377. Gupta SC, Sethi BB. Development of a socio-eonomic scale for urban population. Indian J Psychiatry. 1979;23:371-9.
378. Indian Council of Medical Research. New Delhi. Socio-economic Status Scale. Unpublished manuscript, 1966.
379. Khanna BC, Verma SK. Socio-economic status and its measurement: Some experiments with Kuppuswami's scale. Indian J Clin Psychol. 1976;3:59-62.
380. Verma SK, Khanna BC. Socio-economic status and its measurement: A critical evaluation. Indian J Clin Psychol. 1976;3:63-72.
381. Kulshreshtha SP. Socio-economic Status Scale (SESS) for Rural and Urban. Dehradun: Institute for Studies in Psychological testing, 1980.
382. Wig NN, Gupt AN, Khatri R, et al. A prospective study of psychiatric and menstrual disturbances following tubal ligation. Indian J Med Res. 1977;66:581-90.
383. Shetty G, Mahal AS. A tool to study family interaction. Indian J Psychiatry. 1977;19:67-70.
384. Henderson S, Duncan Jones P, McAulcy M, et al. The patient primary group. Br J Psychiatry. 1978;132:74.
385. Saxena U. Indian Adaptation of Parental Attitude Research Instrument (PARI). M-Form. Indian Psychol Rev. 1976;13:1-7.
386. Bhatti RS, Channabasvanna SM, Prabhu LR. A tool to study the attitude of parents towards the management of mentally retarded children. Child Psychiatry Quart. 1985;18:1-9.
387. Aneshensel CS, Stone JD. Stress and depression: A test of the buffering model of social support. Arch Gen Psychiatry. 1982; 39:1392.
388. Eaton WW. Life events, social supports and psychiatric symptoms: A reanalysis of the New Heaven data. J Health Soc Behav. 1978;19:230.
389. Pai S, Kapur RL. The burden on the family of a psychiatric patient: Development of an interview schedule. Br J Psychiatry. 1981;138:332-3.
390. Srinivasa Murthy R, Aurora M. Attitude changes in medical post-graduates following short term training in psychiatry. Indian J Clin Psychol. 1976;3:165-9.
391. Srinivasa Murthy R. Rural community sttitudes to mental disorders. Indian J Clin Psychol. 1977;4:141-4.
392. Verghese A, Beig A. Public attitude towards mental illness: Vellore study. Indian J Psychiatry. 1974;16:8-14.
393. Sethi BB, Chaturvedi PK, Saxena NK, et al. A comparative study of attitudes of key relatives towards schizophrenic patients and patients of disturbed family. Indian J Psychiatry. 1982;24: 126-9.
394. Khatri AA. Manual of the Scale to Measure Jointedness of Families in India. Ahemdabad: BM institute, 1970.
395. Timmappaya A, Pareek U, Chattopadhyay S, et al. Measuring satisfaction in a general hospital. Indian J Soc Work. 1971;32: 295-304.

396. Bhatti RS, Channabasvanna SM, Prabhu LR, et al. A Manual of Family Typology Scale. Bangalore: NIMHANS, 1985.
397. Kushlick A, Blunden R, Cox G. A method for rating behavior characteristics for use in large scale surveys of mental handicap. Psychol Med. 1973;3:466.
398. Kapur RL, Chandrasekhar CR, Kapur M, et al. Social dysfunctioning as a measure of serverty of psychiatric illness. Indian J Psychiatry. 1981;23:27-32.
399. Sachdev PS, Chawla HM, SubhaRao G, et al. A repertory grid comparison of endogenous and neurotic depression. Indian J Psychiatry. 1983;25:46-51.
400. Chawla PL, Shasthri G, Sundaram KR, et al. A study of pervalence and pattern of hyperactive syndrome in primary school children. Indian J Psychiatry. 1981;23:313-22.
401. Rao NSN, Seth AK, Murthy NS, et al. Some statistical deficiencies in medical research journals in India. Indian J Med Res. 1977; 66:696-703.
402. Gore SM, Jones IG, Ryther EC. Misuse of statistical methods: Critical assessment of articles of BMJ from January to March, 1976. Br Med J. 1977;1:85-8.
403. Verma SK. A critical analysis of research in clinical psychology in India. Bombay Psychologist. 1982;4:75-82.
404. Verma SK. Uses and misuses of statistics in Indian psychiatric research: Observation based on papers published in Indian Journal of Psychiatry. In: Srivastav RN, Verma BL, Shukla GD (Eds). Principles and Practice of Statistics in Medical Research Publications. Bombay: Himalaya Pub. House, 1985. pp. 88-93.
405. Verma BL, Shukla GD, Srivastav RN. Current status of statistics in medical research publications. In: Srivastav RN, Verma BL, Shukla GD (Eds). Principles and Practice of Statistics in Medical Research Publications. Bombay: Himalaya Pub. House, 1985. pp. 56-70.
406. Verma SK. Data Analysis. In: Rajkumar S, Thara R, Nagaswami V (Eds). The Natural History of Schizophrenia. Madras: SCARF Publications, 1989. pp. 173-8.
407. American Psychiatric Association. Desk Reference to the Diagnostic Criteria from DSM-5. Washington DC, 2013.

FURTHER READING

Neuropsychology

1. Bruce D. On the origin of the term 'neuropsychology'. Neuropsychologia. 1985;23:813-4.
2. Reitan RM. Manual of administering and scoring the Reitan-Indiana neuropsychological battery for children (aged 5 through 8). University of Indiana Medical Center, 1964.
3. Umholm B, Ottosson J. Memory functions in endogenous depression. Arch Gen Psychiatry. 1961;5:101-7.
4. Walsh KW. Understanding Brain Damage. New York: Churchill Livingstone, 1991.
5. Hort J, O'Brien JT, Gainotti G, et al. EFNS guidelines for the diagnosis and management of Alzheimer's disease. Eur J Neurol. 2010;17:1236-48.
6. Fuh JL, Wang SJ, Cummings JL. Neuropsychiatric profiles in patients with Alzheimer's disease and vascular dementia. J Neurol Neurosurg Psychiatry. 2005;76(10):1337-41.
7. National initiative for Autism. The National Autism Plan for Children. Screening and assessment, 2003. *http://www.nas.org.uk/nas/isp/pooly.jsp?d-368&a=2178 (accessed July 18, 2011).*
8. Honda H, Shimizu Y, Nitto Y, et al. Extraction and refinement strategy for detection of autism in 18-months-old: a guarantee of higher sensitivity and specificity in the process of mass screening. J Child Psychol Psychiatry. 2009;50:972-81.
9. Wong V, Hul LH, Lee WC, et al. A modified screening tool for autism (checklist for autism in toddlers [CHAT-23] for Chinese children, Pediatrics. 2004;114:166-76.
10. Ozonoff S, Goodlin-Jones BL, Solomon M. Evidence-based assessment of autism spectrum disorders in children and adolescents. J Clin Child Adolesc Psychol. 2005;34:523-40.
11. Pennsylvania Department of Public Welfare, Pennsylvania autism assessment and diagnosis expert workgourp; supporting quality diagnostic practices for persons whit suspected autism spectrum Resources/Documents/Pdf/Publication/PA-ASD-Diagnosis Expert Workgourp.pdf (accessed June 15,2009).
12. Charman T, Baird G. Practitioner Review: diagnosis of autism spectrum disorder in 2-and -3 year-old children. J Child Psychol Psychiatry. 2002;43:289-305.
13. Sagvolden T. Behavioral validation of the spontaneously bypertensive rat (SHR) as an animal model of attention-deficity/hyperactivity disorder (AD/HD). Neurosci Biobehav Rev. 2000;24:31-9.
14. Russel VA. The nucleus accumbens motor-limbic interface of the spontaneously hypertensive rat as studied in vitro by the superfusion slice technique. Neurosci Biobehav Rev. 2000;24: 133-6.
15. Doyle AE, Faraone SV, Seidman LJ, et al. Are endophenotypes based on measure sof executive functions useful for molecular genetic studies of ADHD? J Child Psychol Psychiatri (in press).
16. Sonuga-Barke EJ, Dalen L, Daley D, Remington B. Are planning, working memory, and inhibiton associated with individual difference sin preschool ADHD symptoms? Dev Neuropsychol. 2002;21:255-72.
17. Tripp G, Ryan J, Peace K. Neuropsychological functioning in children with DSM-IV combined type attentiond eficit hyperactivity disorder. Aus NZ J Psychiatry. 2002;36: 771-9.
18. Wilcutt EG, brodsky K, Chhabildas N, et al. The neuropsychology of attention deficit hyperactivity disorder: validity of the executive function hypothesis. In: Gozal D, Molfese D (Eds). Attention deficit hyperactivity disorder from genes to patients. Totowa, NJ: Humana Press, 2005.
19. Seidman L, Doyle A, Fried R, Valera E, Crum K, Matthews L. Neuropsychological function in adults with attention-deficity/hyperactivity disorder. In: Spencer T (Ed). Adult ADHD, psychiatric clinics of North America: Elsevier Scinece, 2004; 261-82.

20. Geurts HM, Verte S, Oosterlaan J, Roeyers H, Sergeant JA. How specific are executive functioning deficits in attention deficit hyperactivity disorder and autism? J Child Psycho Psychiatr. 2004;45:836-54.
21. Dowson JH, McLean A, Bazanis E, et al. Impaired spatial working memory in adults with attention-deficit/hypeactivity disorder: comparisons with performance in adults with borderline personality disorder and in control subjects. Acta Psychiatr Scan. 2004;110:45-54.
22. Roobins TW, James M, Own AM, et al. A study of performance on tests from the CANTAB battery sensitive to frontal lobe dysfunction in a large sample of normal volunteers; implications for theories of executive functioning and cognitive aging. J Int Neuropsychol Soc. 1998;4:474-90.
23. Miyake A, Friedman NP, Emerson MJ, Witzki AH, Howerter A, Wager TD. The unity and diversity of executive functions and their contributions to complex "Frontal Lobe" tasks: a latent variable analysis. Cognit Psycho. 2000;41: 49-100.

Measurement in Psychiatry

24. Anderson HH, Anderson GL. Introduction to Projective Techniques. New York: Prentice Hall, 1951.
25. Banko JJ, Carpenter WT. On the methods and theory of reliability. J Nerv Ment Dis. 1976;163:307-17.
26. Faustman WO, Moses JA, Caemansky JG. Limitations of the mini mental state examination in predicting neuropsychological func-tioning in psychiatric sample. Acta Psychiatr Scand. 1990;81:126-31.
27. Kaplan HI, Sadock BJ, Grebb JA. Synopsis of Psychiatry (Behavioral Science, Clinical Psychiatry), 8th edition. New Delhi: BI Waverly, 1998.
28. Lewis G, Pelosi AJ. The case-control study in psychiatry. Br J Psychiatry. 1990;157:197-207.
29. Robins LN, Barrett JE. The Validity of Psychiatric Diagnosis. New York: Raven Press, 1989.
30. Taube CA, Mechanic D, Hohmann AA. The Future of Mental Health Services Research. Maryland: NMH, 1987.
31. Taylor MA, Abrams R, Faber R, Almy G. Cognitive tasks in the mental status examination. J Nerv Ment Dis. 1980;168:167-70.
32. Wetzler S, Katz MM. Contemporary Approaches to Psychological Assessment. Monograph No. 1. New York: Brunner/Mazel, 1989.
33. Whitworth RH, Larson CM. Differential diagnosis and staging of Alzheimer's disease with an aphasia battery. Neuropsychiatr Neuropsychol Behav Neurol. 1988;1:255-65.

Genetics in Relation to Psychiatry

34. Antonarakis SE, Krawezak M, Cooper DN. The nature and mechanisms of huma gene mutation. In: Service CR, et al (Eds). The metabolic & molecular bases of inherited disease. McGraw-Hill, New York; 2001.pp.343-77.
35. Baron M. Manic-depression genes and the new millennium: poised for discovery. Molecular Psychiatry. 2002;7:342-58.
36. Blackwood D, Muir W. Molecular geneties and the epidemiology of affective disorder. Annals of Medicine. 2001;33:242-7.
37. Blackwood DH, Fordyce A, Walker MT, et al. Schizophrenia and affective disorders—cosegregation with a translocation at chromosome 1q42 that directly disrupts brain—expressed genes:clinical and p300 findings in a family, American Journal of Huma Genetics. 2001;69:428-33.
38. Botstein D, Risch N. Discovering genotypes underlying huma Phenotypes: past successes for mendelian disease, future approaches for complex disease, Nature Genetics. 2003;33 (supp):228-37.
39. Cardno AG, Gottesman H. Twin studies of schizophrenia: from bow-and-arrow concordances to star wars Mx and functional genomics. American Journal of Medical Genetics. 2000;97:12-7.
40. Craddock N, Jones I. Genetics of bipolar disorder. Journal of Medical Genetics. 1999;36:585-94.
41. Cradock N, Van Eerdewegh P, Reich T. Single major locus models for bipolar disorder are implausible. American Journal of Medical Genetics 1997;74:18-20.
42. Dredge BK, Poydoride AD, Darnell RB. The splice of life: alternative splicing and neurological disease. Nature Reviews Neuroscience. 2001;2:43-50.
43. Ekeludnd J, Lachtermann D, Hovatta 1, et al. Genome wide scan for schizophrenia in the Finihish population: evidence for a locus on Chromosome 7q22. Human Molecular Genetic. 2000;9:1049-57.
44. Evans KL, Muir WJ, Blackwood DH, Porteous DJ. Nuts and bolts of psychiatric geneties: building on the human genome project. Trends in Genetic. 2001;17:35-40.
45. Fishre SE, Francckes C, Marlow AJ, et al. Independent genome-wide scan identity a chromosome 18 quantitative trait locus influencing dyslexia. Nature Genetics. 2002;17:35-40.
46. Friedgberg EC. DNA damage and rapair. Nature. 2003;421: 436-40.
47. Gottesman H, Shiedl J. Schizophrenia and genetics a twin study advantage point. Academic Press, New York Gratacos M, Nadan M, Martin Santos R et al 2001 A polymorphic Genomic deplication on human chromosome 15 is a susceptility gene locus, on 13q-33, Hatro for panic and provide disorders. Cell 106 :267-379 gene locus, on 13q33, are associated with bipolar disorder to two independent pedigree series. American Journal of Human (Genetides). 1972;72:1131-1, 1, 245-54.
48. Gottesman H. Schizophrenia genesis: the origins of madness. Freema, New York; 1991.
49. Heston LL. Psychiatric disorders in foster home reared children of schizophrenic mothers. British Journal of Psychiatry. 1966;112:819-25.
50. Jaensih R, Bird A. Epigenetic regulation of gene expression. How the genome integrates intrinsic and environmmental signals. Nature Genetics. 2003;33(suppl):245-54.
51. Jenuwein T, Allis CD. Translating the histone code. Science. 2001;293:1074-80.

52. Jones I, Kent L, Craddock N. Genetics of affective disorders. In: McGuffin P, Owen MJ, Gottesman 11 (Eds). Psychatric genetics & genomics. Oxford University Press. Oxford; 2002.pp.211-45.
53. Keegan LP, Gallo A, O'Connell MA. The many roles of an RNA editor, Nature Reviews Genetics. 2001;2:869-78.
54. Kendler KS, Gruenberg AM, Kinney DK. Independent diagnoses of adoptees and relatives as defined by DSM-III in the provincial and national samples of the Danish Adoption Study of Schizophrenia. Archives of General Psychiatry. 1994;51:456-68.
55. Kendler KS, Neale MC, Kessler RC, et al. Major depression and generalized anxiety disorder. Same genes, (partly) different environments? Archives of General Psychiatry. 1992;49:716-22.
56. Kendler KS. Schizophrenia genetics. In: Sadock BJ, Sadock VA (Eds) Kaplan and Sadock's comprehensive textbook of psychiatry, 7th edition. Lippincott, Williams & Wilkins. Philadelphia; 2000.pp.1147-59.
57. Kety SS, Wender PH, Jacobsen B, et al. Mental illness in the biological and adoptive relatives of schizophrenic adoptees. Replication of the Copenhagen Study in the rest of Denmark. Archives of General Psychiatry. 1994;51:442-55.
58. Kety SS. Studies designed to disentangle genetic and environmental variables in schizophrenia: some epidemological questions and answers. American Journal of Psychiatry. 1976;133:1134-7.
59. Kringlen F, Cramer G. Offspring of monozygotic twins discordant for schizophrenia. Archives of General Psychiatry. 1989;46:873-7.
60. Lendon C, Craddock N. Susceptibility gene(s) for Alzheimer's disease on chromosome 10. Trends in Neurosciences. 2001;24: 557-9.
61. Maison C, Batlly D, Peters AH, et al. Higher order structure in pericentric heterochromatin involves a distinct pattern of histone modification and an RNA component. Nature Genetics. 2002;30:329-34.
62. McGue M, Gottesman H. A single dominant gene still cannot account for the transmission of schizophrenia. Archives of General Psychiatry. 1989;46:478-80.
63. McGuffin P, Owen MJ, Gottesman H. Psychiatric genetics and genomics. Oxford University Press, Oxford; 2002.
64. McMahon FJ, Chen YS, Patel S, et al. Mitochondrial DNA sequence diversity in bipolar affective disorder. American Journal of Psychiatry. 2002;157:1058-64.
65. Mendell JT, Dietz HC. When the message goes away: disease-producing mutations that influence mRNA content and performance. Cell. 2001;107:411-4.
66. Millar JK, Wilson-Annan JC, Christic S, et al. Disruption of two novel genes by a translocation co-segregating with schizophrenia. Human Molecular Genetics. 2000;22:1415-23.
67. Muir WJ, Thomson ML, McKeon P, et al. Markers close to the dopamine D5 receptor gene (DRD5) show significant association with schizophrenia but not bipolar disorder. American Journal of Medical Genetics. 2001;105:152-8.
68. Ott J. Analysis of human genetic linkage. Johns Hopkins University Press, Baltimore; 1999.
69. Park ET, Kazazian HH Jr. Mobile elements and the human genome. Nature Reviews Genetics. 2000;1:134-44.
70. Potash JB, DePanlo JR Jr. Searching high and low; a review of the genetics of bipolar disorder. Bipolar Disorders. 2000;2: 8-26.
71. Ranom IP, Day JW. Dominantly inherited, non coding microsatellite expansion disorders. Gurrent Opinion in Geneties & Development. 2002;12:266-71.
72. Reik W, Walter J. Genomic imprinting: parental influence on the genome. Nature Reviews Genetics. 2001;2:21-32.
73. Rice J, Reich T, Andreasen NC, et al. The familial transmission of bipolar illness. Archives of General Psychiatry. 1987;44: 441-7.
74. Riley BP, McGuffin P. Linkage and associated studies of schizophrenia. American Journal of Medical Genetics. 2000;97: 23-44.
75. Scholey JM, Brust-Mascher I, Mogilner A. Cell division. Nature. 2003;422:746-52.
76. Shifihan S, Bronstein M, Sternfeld M, et al. A highly significant association between a COMT haplotype and schizophrenia. American Journal of Human Genetics. 2002;71: 1296-1302.
77. Stankiewiez P, Lupski JR. Genome architecture, rearrangements and genomic disorders. Trends in Genetics. 2002;18:74-82.
78. Stefansson H, Sarginson J, Kong A, et al. Association of neuregulin I with sehizophrenia confirmed in a Seottish population. American Journal of Human Genetics. 2003;72: 83-7.
79. Stefansson H, Sigurdsson E, Steinthorsdottir V, et al. Neuregulin 1 and susceptibility to schizophrenia. American Journal of Human Genetics. 2002;71:877-92.
80. Straub RE, Jiang Y, MacLean CJ, et al. Genetic variation in the 6p22.3 gene DTNBPI, the human ortholog of the mouse dysbindin gene, is associated with schizophrenia. American Jounal of Human Genetics. 2002;71:337-48.
81. Sugars KL, Rubinsztein DC. Transcriptional abnormalities in Huntington disease. Trends in Genetics. 2003;19:233-8.
82. Sullivan PF, Neale MC, Kendler KS. Genetic epidemiology of major depression: review and meta-analysis. American Journal of Psychiatry. 2000;157:1552-62.
83. Tienari P, Wynne JC, Moring J, et al. Finnish adoptive family study: sample selection and adoptee DSM-III-R diagnoses. Acta Psychiatrica Scandinavica. 2000;101: 433-43.
84. Wilusz CJ, Wormington M, Peltz SW. The cap-to-tail guide to mRNA turnover. Nature Reviews Molecular Cell Biology. 2001;2:237-46.

SUGGESTED READING

Epidemiology and Research Methods

1. Al-Shahi R, Warlow C. Using patient identifiable data for observational research and audit. British Medical Journal. 2000;321:1031-2.

2. Andreasen NC. Negative symptoms in schizophrenia: definition and reliability. Archives of General Psychiatry. 1932;39:784-8.
3. Assmann SF, Pocoek SJ, Enos LE, Kasten LE. Subgroup analysis and other (mis)uses of beseline data in clinical trials. Lancet. 2000;355:1064-9.
4. Barker S, Lavender T, Morant N. Client and family narratives on schizophrenia. Journal of Mental Health. 2001;10:199-212.
5. Beck AT, Ward CH, Mendelson M, et al. An inventory for measuring depression. Archives of General Psychiatry. 1961;4:561-71.
6. Bedi N, Chilvers C, Churchill R, et al. Assessing effectiveness of treatment of depression in primary care: partially randomized preference trial. British Journal of Psychiatry. 2000;177:312-8.
7. Carpenter WT Jr, Sadler JH, Light PD, et al. The therapeutic efficacy of hemodialysis in schizophrenia. New England Journal of Medicine. 1983;308:669-75.
8. Carpenter WT Jr. Gold JM, Lahti AC, et al. Decisional capacity for informed consent in schizophrenia research. Archives of General Psychiatry. 2000;57:533-8.
9. Chalmers TC, Celano P, Sacks HS, Smith H Jr. Bias in treatment assignment in controlled clinical trials. New England Journal of Medicine. 1983;309:1358-61.
10. Charlwood P, Mason A, Goldacre M, et al. Health outcome indicators: Several mental illness. Report of a working group to the Department of Health. National Centre of Health Outcomes Development, Oxford. 1999.
11. CSBS. Schizophrenia. Clinical Standards Board for Scotland, Edinburgn. 2001.
12. Department of Health. Treatment choice in psychological therapies and counseling. Evidence based clinical practical guideline. Department of Health, London. 2001.
13. Dowrick C, Dunn G, Ayuso-Mateos JL, et al. Problem solving treatment and group psychoeducation of depression: multicentre randomized controlled trial. Outcomes of Depression International Network (ODIN) Group. British Medical Journal. 2000;321:1450-54.
14. Duffen R, Lelliott P. Auditing electroconvulsive therapy: The thin cycle. British Journal of Psychiatry. 1998;172: 401-5.
15. Edwards P, Roberts L, Clarke M, et al. Inceasing response rates to postal questionnaires: systematic review. British Medical Journal. 2002;324:1183.
16. Egger M, Smith GD, Aluman DG. Systematic reviews in health care. Meta-analysis in context. BMJ Books, London. 2001.
17. Endicott J, Spitzer RL. A diagnostic interview schedule for affective disorders and schizophrenia. Archives of General Psychiatry. 1978;35:837-44.
18. Even C, Siobud-Dorocant E, Dardennes RM. Critical approach to antidepressant trials. Blindness protection is necessary, feasible and measurable. British Journal of Psychiatry. 1999;174:93-4.
19. Feinstein AR. The architecture of clinical research. Saunders, Philadelphia. 1985.
20. Geddes J, Freemantle N, Harrison P, Bebbington P. Atypical antipsychotics in the treatment of schizophrenia: systematic overview and meta-regression analysis. British Medical Journal. 2000;321:1371-8.
21. Gilbody S, Whitty P. Improving the delivery and organization of mental health services: beyond the conventional randomized controlled trial, British Journal of Psychiatry. 2002;180:13-8.
22. Gilbody SM, House AO, Sheldon TA. Outcomes research in mental health. British Journal of Psychiatry. 2002;181:8-16.
23. Gilbody SM, Song F. Publication bias and the integrity of psychiatry research. Psychological Medicine. 2000;30:253-8.
24. Grimes DA, Schulz KF. Descriptive studies: what they can and can not do. Lancet. 2002;359:145-9.
25. Guyati G, Sacket D, Taylor D W, et al. Determining optimal therapy-randomized tirals in individual patients. New England Joural of Medicine. 1986;314:889-92.
26. Hamilton M. A rating scale for depression. Journal of Neurology Neurosurgery & Psychiatry. 1960;23:56-62.
27. Hamilton M. The assessment of anxiety states by rating. British Journal of Medicine. 1959;314:889-92.
28. Hennekens CH, Buring JE. Epidemiology in medicine. Little Brown, Boston. 1987.
29. Hotopf M, Churchill R, Lewis G. Pragmatic randomized controlled trials in psychiatry. British Journal of Psychiatry. 1999;175:217-23.
30. Jones J, Hunter D. Consensus methods for medical and health services research. British Medical Journal. 1995;311:378-80.
31. Juni P, Altman DG, Egger M. Systematic reviews in health care: Assessing the quality of controlled clinical trials. British Medical Journal. 2001;323:42-6.
32. Kmemer HC, Stice E, Kazdin A, et al. How do risk factors work together? Mediators, moderators and independent, overlapping, and proxy risk factors. American Journal of Psychiatry. 2001;158:848-56.
33. Krawieeka M, Gold Berg D, Vaughan M. A standardized psychiatric assessment scale for rating chronic psychotic patients. Acta Psychiatrica Scandinavica. 1977;55:299-308.
34. Last JM. A dictionary of epidemiology. Oxford University Press, Oxford. 1995.
35. Lawric SM. Clinical trial methodology: In: Reid I, Anderoson I (Eds) The fundamentals of psychopharmacology: the definitive guide, Martin Dunitz, London. 2002.
36. Lawrie SM, McIntosh AM, Rao S. Critical appraisal for psychiatry Churchill Livingstone, Edinburgh. 2000.
37. Lewis G, Pelosi AJ. The case-control study in psychiatry. British Journal of Psychiatry. 1990;157:197-207.
38. Louis TA, Lavori PW, Bailar JC 3rd, Polansky M. Crossover and self-controlled designs in clinical research. New England journal of medicine. 1984;310:24-31.
39. Marslxdl M, Lockwood A, Bradley C, et al. Unpublished rating scales: a major source of bias in randomized controlled trials

of treatments for schizophrenia. British Journal of Psychiatry. 2000;176:249-52.
40. McMahon AD. Study control, violators, inclusion criteria and defining explanatory and pragmatic trials. Statistical Medicine. 2002;21:1365-76.
41. Moher D, Cook DJ, Eastwood S, et al. Improving the quality of reports of meta-analyses of randomized controlled trials: the QUOROM statement. Lancet. 1999;354:1896-1900.
42. Monerieff J, Wessely S, Hardy R. Meta-analysis of trials comparing antidepressants with active placebos. British Journal of Psychiatry. 1998;172:227-31: discussion 232-4.
43. Montgomery SA, Asberg M. A new depression scale designed to be sensitive to change. British Journal of Psychiatry. 1979;134:382-9.
44. Narrow WE, Race DS, Robins LN, Regier DA. Revised prevalence estimates of mental disorders in the United States: using a clinical significance criterion to reconcile 2 surveys' estimates. Archives of General Psychiatry. 2002;59:115-23.
45. Naylor CD, Guyatt GH. Users guides to the medical literature. XI: How to use an article about a clinical utilization review. Evidence-Based Medicine Working Group Journal of the American Medical Association. 1996;275:1435-9.
46. O'Brien T, Oxman AD, Davis DA, et al. Audit and feedback: effects on professional practice and health care outcomes (Cochrane review). In: The Cochrane Library, Issue 3. Update Software, Oxford. 2002a.
47. O'Brien T, Oxman AD, Davis DA, et al. Audit and feedback versus alternative strategies: effects on professional practice and health care outcomes (Cochrane review). In: The Cochrane Library, Issue 3. Update software, Oxford. 200b.
48. Offord DR, Kraemer HC. Risk factors and prevention. Evidence Based Mental Health. 2000;70:70-71.
49. Overall JE, Gorham DR. The Brief Psychiatric Rating Scale. Psychological Reports. 1962;10:799-812.
50. Oxman AD, Guyatt GH. Guidelines for reading literature reviews Canadian Medical Association Journal. 1988;138:697-703.
51. Peto R, Collins R, Gray R. Large-scale randomized evidence: large, simple trials and overviews of trials. Annals of the New York Academy of Sciences. 1993;703:314-40.
52. Pocock SJ, Assmann SE, Enos LE, Kasten LE. Subgroup analysis, covariate adjustment and baseline comparison in clinical trial reporting: current practice and problems. Statistical Medicine. 2002;21:2917-30.
53. Pocock SJ. Clinical trials: a practical approach. John Wiley, Chichester. 1983.
54. Roberts LW, Warner TD, Brody JI, et al. Patient and psychiatrist ratings of hypothetical schizophrenia research protocols: assessment of harm potential and factors influcening participation decisions. American Journal of Psychiatry. 2002;159:573-84.
55. Robins LN, Helzer JE, Croughan J, Rateliff KS. National Institute of Mental Health Diagnostic Interview Schedule: its history, characteristics, and validity. Archives of General Psychiatry. 1981;38:381-9.
56. Robins LN, Wing J, Wittehen HU, et al. The Composite International Diagnostic Interview: an epidemiologic instrument suitable for use in conjunction with different diagnostic systems and in different cultures. Archives of General Psychiatry. 1988;45:1069-77.
57. Sackett DL, Haynes RB, Guyatt GH, Tugwel P. Clinical epidemiology: a basic science for clinical medicine. Little, Brown, Boston. 1991.
58. Sackett DL, Straus SE, Richardson WS, et al. Evidence-based medicine: how to practice and teach EBM. Churchill Livinstone, Edinburgh. 2000.
59. Sackett DL. Bias in analytic research. Journal of Chronic Diseases. 1979;32:51-63.
60. Savulescu J, Chalmers I, Blunt J. Arc research ethics committees behaving unethically? Some suggestions for improving performance and accountability. British Medical Journal. 1996;313:1390-93.
61. Schulz KF, Chalmers I, Hayes RJ, Altman DG. Empirical evidence of bias: dimensions of methodological quality associated with estimates of treatment effects in controlled trials Journal of the American Medical Association. 1995;273;408-12.
62. Schulz KF, Grimes DA. Case-control studies: research in reverse Lancet. 2002a;359:431-4.
63. Schulz KF, Grimes DA. Unequal group sizes in randomized trials: guarding against guessing. Lancet. 2002b;359:966-70.
64. Schulz KF, Grims DA. Case-control studies: research in reverse Lancet. 2002a;359:432-4.
65. Spielberger CD, Gorusch RL, Lushene R. STAI-Manual For the State-Trait Anxiety Inventory. Consulting Psychologists Press, Palo Alto. 1970.
66. Stroup DF, Berlin JA, Morton SC, et al. Meta-analysis of observational studies in epidemiology. Journal of the American Medical Association. 2000;283:2008-12.
67. Thornlcy B, Adams C. Content and quality of 2000 controlled trials in schizophrenia over 50 years. British Medical Journal. 1998;317:1181-4.
68. Vastag B. Helsinki discord? A controversial declaration. Journal of the American Medical Association. 2000;284: 2983-5.
69. Warlow C. Advanced issues in the design and conduct of randomized clinical trials: the bigger the better? Statistical Medicine. 2002;21:2797-805.
70. Wing J. Ethics and psychiatric research. In: Bloch S, Chodoff P (Eds) Psychiatric ethics. Oxford University Press, Oxford, 1981. pp.277-94.
71. Wing JK, babor T, Brugha T, et al SCAN. Schedules for Clinical Assessment in Neuropsychiatry. Archives of General Psychiatry. 1990;47:589-93.
72. Wing JK, Copper JE, Sartorius N. The measurement and classification of psychiatric symptoms: Cambridge University Press, Cambridge. 1974.
73. Zigmond AS, Snaith RP. The Hospital Anxiety and Depression Scale. Acta Psychiatric Scandinavia. 1983;67: 361-70.

Research Measurement and Statistic

74. Altman DG, Bland JM. Time to event (survival) data. British Medical Journal. 2002;317:468-9.
75. Altman DG. Practical statistics for medical research. CRC Press, Boca Raton, Florida. 1991.
76. Bland JM, Altman DG. Statistical methods for assessing agreement between two methods of clinical measurement. Lancet, 1986.pp.307-10.
77. Bland JM, Altman DG. Statistics notes: Cronbach's alpha. British Medical Journal. 1997;314:572.
78. Bland JM, Altman DG. Statistics notes: one and two sides tests of significance. British Medical Journal. 1994.pp.309-48.
79. Bland JM, Altman DG. Survival probabilities (the Kaplan-Meier method). British Medical Journal. 1998.
80. Bland JM, Altman DG. Validating scales and indexes. British Medical Journal. 2002;324:606-7.
81. Bland JM. An introduction to medical statistics. Oxford University Press, Oxford. 2000.
82. DerSimonian R, Laired N. Meta-analysis in clinical trials. Controlled Clinical Trials. 1986;7:177-88.
83. Egger M, Smith GD, Altman DG. Systematic reviews in health care: Meta-analysis in context. BMJ Books, London. 2001.
84. Gore SM, Altman DG. Statistics in practice. BMJ books, London Hand DJ, Taylor CC 1987 Multivariate analysis of variance and repeated measures. Chapman and Hall, London. 1982.
85. Hart A. Mann-Whitney test is not just a test of medians: differences in spread can be important. British Medical Journal. 2001;323:391-3.
86. Kline P. An easy guide to factor analysis. Rouledge, London. 1994.
87. Normal GR, Streiner DL. PDQ statistics. BC Decker, Hamilton, Ontario. 1999.
88. Parmar MKB, Machin D. Survival analysis: a practical approach. Wiley, Chichester. 1995.
89. Perneger TV. What's wrong with Bonferroni adjustments. British Medical Journal. 1998;316:1236-8.
90. Pocock SJ. Clinical trials: a practical approach. Wiley, Chichester, 1993.
91. Siegel S. Nonparametric statistics. McGraw-Hill, Singapore, 1998.
92. Styreiner DL, Norman GR. Health measurement scales: a pratical guide to their development and use. Oxford University press, Oxford. 1996.
93. Swinscow TDV, Campbell MJ. Statistics at square one. BMJ Publishing Group, London. 1996.

Fundamental of Psychology

94. Allport GW, Odbert HS. Trait names: a psychological study. Psychological Monographs 17 (Whole No. 211), 1936.
95. Anderson MC, Green C. Suppressing unwanted memories by executive control. Nature. 2001;410:366-9.
96. Back AT. Cognitive therapy and the emotional disorders. Meridian, New York, 1976.
97. Barker C, Pistrang N, Elliott R. Research methods in clinical psychology, 2nd edn. Wiley, Chichester, 2002.
98. Bolton D, Hill J. Mind, meaning and mental disorder: the nature of causal explanation in psychology and psychiatry. Oxford University Press, Oxford, 1996.
99. Bouchard TJ Jr, Lykken DT, McGue M, et al. Sources of human psychological differences; the Minnesota Study of Twins Reared Apart. Science. 1990;250(4978):223-8.
100. Bowlby J. Separation and loss. Basic Books, New York, 1973.
101. Broadbent DE. Perception and communication. Pregamon, Oxford, 1958.
102. Brown GW, Harris T. Social origins of depression. Tavistock, London, 1978.
103. Cahill I, Babinsky R, Markowitsch HJ, McGaugh JL. The amygdala and emotional memory. Nature. 1995;377: 295-6.
104. Calder AJ, Lawrence AD, Young AW. Neuropsychology of fear and loathing. Nature Reviews Neuroscience. 2001;2(5):352-63.
105. Cannon WB. The James-Lange theory of emotions: a critical examination and an alternative theory. Americal Journal of Psychology. 1927;39:106-24.
106. Cattell RB, Eber HW, Tatsuolca MM. Handbook for the sixteen personality Factor Questionnaire (16 PF). Institute for personality and Ability Testing, Illinois, 1970.
107. Cattell RB. Personality and motivation: Structure and measurement. Harcoart, Brace and World. New York, 1957.
108. Conway MA. Recovered memories and false memories. Oxford University Press, Oxford, 1997.
109. Conway MA. Repression revisited. Nature. 2001;410:319-20.
110. Costa PT, McCrae RR. Age differences in personality structure revisited; studies in validity, stability and change. Aging and Human Development. 1966;8:261-75.
111. Costa PT, McCrae RR. Four ways five factors are basic. Personality and Individual Differences 1992a;13:653-5.
112. Costa PT, McCrae RR. Revised NEO Personality Inventory (NEO PI-R) and NEO Five factor Inventory (NEO-FFI) Professional Mannual, Psychological Assessment Resources, Odessa, FI, 1992b.
113. Damasio AR. Descartes' error, Papermac/Macmillan, London, 1994.
114. Davies GM, Dalgleish T (Eds). Recovered memories: seeking the middle ground, Wiley, Chichester, 2002.
115. Donaldson M. Children's minds. Fontana, Glasgow, 1978.
116. Ekman P. The face of man: expressions of human emotions in a New Guinea village. Garland STPM, New York, 1980.
117. Eysenck HJ, Eysenck SBG. Hand book of the Eysenck Personality Questionnaire. Hodder & Stoughton: London, 1975.
118. Eysenck HJ. The effects of psychological therapy. Science House, New York, 1969.
119. Frend A. The ego and the mechanisms of defence. Twvistock, London, 1937.

120. Frith U. The neurocognitive basis of autism. Trends in Cognitive Sciences. 1997;1:73-7.
121. Gibson FJ, Walk RD. The "visual cliff". Scientific American. 1960;202:64-71.
122. Gleick I. Chaos: making a new science. Heinemann, London, 1988.
123. Harlow H, Harlow M. Learning to love. American Sciencist. 1966;54:244-72.
124. James W. What is an emotion? Mind. 1884;9:188-205.
125. Johnoson M, Morton J. Biology and cognitive development the case of face recognition. Blackwell, London, 1991.
126. Johnson Laird PN. The computer and the mind: an introduction to cognitive science, Fontana, London, 1988.
127. Jones MC. A laboratory study of fears: the case of peter. Pediatric Seminars. 1924;31:308-15.
128. Kahneman D, Slovic P, Tversky A. Judgement under uncertainty; heuristics and biases. Cambridge University Press, Cambridge, 1982.
129. Karni A, Meyer G, Jezzard P, et al. Functional MRI evidence for adult motor cortex plasticity during motor skill learning. Nature. 1995;377(6545):155-8.
130. LeDoux J. The emotional Brain. Simon & Schuster, New York Liberzon I, 1996.
131. Marks I. Fears, phobias and ritualsl. Oxford University Press, Oxford, 1987.
132. Mischel W. Personality and assessment. Wiley, New York, 1968.
133. Morgan CD, Murray HA. A method for investigating fantasies: the thematic apperception test. Archives of Neurological Psychiatry. 1935;34:289-306.
134. Mowrer OH. A stimulus response analysis of anxiety and its role a reinforcing agent. Psychological Review. 1939;46: 553-65.
135. Neisser U. Cognitive psychology. Appleton-Century-Crofts, New York, 1967.
136. Norman WT. Toward an adequate taxonomy of personality attributes: replicated factor structure in peer nomination personality ratings. Journal of Abnormal and Social Psychology. 1963;66:574-83.
137. Oatley K, Johnson Laired PN. Towards a cognitive theory of emotions. Cognition and Emotion. 1987;1:29-50.
138. Olds J, Milner P. Positive reinforcement produced by electrical stimulation of septal area and other regions of rat brain. Journal of Comparative Physiological Psychology. 1954;47: 419-27.
139. Power MJ, Champion IA. Cognitive approaches to depression: a theoretical critique. British Journal of Clinical Psychology. 1986;25:201-12.
140. Power MJ, Dalgleish T. Cognition & emotion; from order to disorder, Psychology Press, Hove, W Sussex, 1997.
141. Power MJ. Conscious and unconscious representations of meaning In: Power MJ, Brewin GR (Eds) The transformation of meaning in psychological therapiews. Wiley, Chichester, 1997.
142. Power MJ. Integrative therapy from a cognitive behavioural perspective. In: Holmes J, Bateman A (Eds). Integration in psychotherapy: models and methods, Oxford University Press, Oxford, 2001.
143. Prowence S, Lipton R. Infants in institutions, International Universities Press, New York, 1962.
144. Rachmari SJ. Fear and courage, 2nd edn. Frecman, New York, 1990.
145. Robertson IH, Murre JM. Rehabilitation of brain damage; brain plasticity and principles of guided recovery. Psychological Bulletin. 1999;125(5):544-75.
146. Rorschach H. Psychodiagnostic. Bircher, Bernc, 1921.
147. Rosenzweing M, Bennett E. Cerebral changes in rats exposed individually to an enriched environment. Journal of Comparative & Physiological Psychology. 1972;80: 304-13.
148. Schacter S, Singer J. Cognitive, social and physiological determinants of emotional state. Psychological Review. 1962; 769:379-99.
149. Seligman MEP. Helplessness. WH Freeman, San Francisco, 1975.
150. Seligman MEP. Phobias and preparedneess. Behaviour Therapy. 1971;2:207-20.
151. Semenoff B. Projective techniques, Wiley, London, 1976.
152. Taylor SF, Amdur R, et al. Brain activation in PTSD in response to trauma-related stimuli. Biological Psychiatry. 1999;45(7): 817-26.
153. Watson JB, Rayner R. Conditioned emotional reactions. Journal of Experimental Psychology. 1920;3:1-14.
154. Wolpe J. Psychotherapy by reciprocal inhibiton. Stanford University Press, Stanford, 1958.

CHAPTER 46

Pharmacological and Other Methods of Treatment

Niraj Ahuja, Shree Ram Ghimire, Avinash De Souza, Nilesh Shah, VN Vahiya, Anjali Chabbria, Dinesh Mohan Das, Neha Singh, Christoday RJ Khess, Jayati Simlai, BS Chavan, Priti Arun, Eesha Sharma, Urvakhsh Mehta, Jagadisha Thirthalli, BN Gangadhar, V Balasubramaniam, Sachchidanand Singh, Anushul Khichy, JN Vyas, G Prasad Rao, Bikramaditya Jaiswal, VS Chadda, RK Solanki, Anjanik Kr Ranjan, Neena Bohra, NK Bohra, BK Singh

46.1 ANTIPSYCHOTIC DRUGS

Niraj Ahuja, Shree Ram Ghimire

Antipsychotics are those psychotropic drugs, which are used for the treatment of psychoses and psychotic symptoms. These are also known as *major tranquilizers, neuroleptics, ataractics, anti-schizophrenic drugs* and *D_2-receptor blockers*, but the term *antipsychotic* appears to be the most appropriate.

Before the advent of antipsychotics, the treatment of psychiatric disorders (particularly psychotic disorders) had often been merely institutionalization, sometimes associated with the use of other treatment which now seems either ridiculous or fantastic or mostly both. The first report of successful treatment of psychoses came from India (Sen and Bose, 1931), using Rauwolfia serpentina extract (reserpine). Unfortunately, this report was ignored until 1954 when Nathan Kline confirmed this finding.

Phenothiazines were synthesized in 1883, while evolving alternative methods of synthesis of methylene blue. Charpentier (1949–1950) first synthesized chlorpromazine while developing a more potent antihistaminic than promethazine. In 1952, Jean Delay and Pierre Deniker brought about a revolution in psychopharmacology with the introduction of chlorpromazine. The admission patterns of the mental hospitals of that era show a sudden decrease in the number of inpatients, after treatment with chlorpromazine was instituted. Janssen later synthesized haloperidol, a butryophenone derivative, in Belgium in 1958. Later, he used pimozide for the treatment of schizophrenia in 1968. Clozapine was introduced in the US market in 1990 as a treatment for refractory schizophrenia, although it was synthesized as early as in 1959.

CLASSIFICATION AND PROPERTIES OF ANTIPSYCHOTICS

The available antipsychotic drugs are described in Table 1 discussed in detail below.

PHENOTHIAZINES

Aliphatics

Chlorpromazine (CPZ)

- *Half Life (hours):* 10–30 hours
- *Therapeutic Plasma Concentration:* 30 to 500 ng/mL
- *Dose Range:* 300–1500 mg/day (oral); 50–100 mg (parenteral; IM only)
- *Strengths Available:* 10 mg; 25 mg; 50 mg; 100 mg; 200 mg (oral); 25 mg/mL (parenteral).

Common Side Effects

Sedation (+++); hypotension (+++); EPS (+); anti-cholinergic side-effects (++); galactorrhea, amenorrhea, impaired ejaculation, tachycardia, cardiac arrhythmias, mydriasis, weight gain, jaundice, agranulocytosis, seizures.

Comments

- It is also indicated in the treatment of intractable hiccoughs, nausea and vomiting, eclampsia (earlier chlorpromazine, promethazine and pethidine were given

Table 1: Classification and properties of antipsychotics

Examples of drugs	*Examples of Trade Names**	*Oral dose range (mg/day)*	*Parenteral dose range (mg)*	*Equivalent dose (Equal to 100 mg of CPZ)*	*Common side effects****		
					Sedation	*Hypotension*	*EPS***
Phenothiazines							
Aliphatics							
• Chlorpromazine (CPZ)	Megatil	300–1500	50–100 IM only	100	+++	+++	+
• Triflupromazine	Siquil	100–400	30–60 IM	25–30	++	++	++
Piperidines							
• Thioridazine	Thioril	300–800	–	95–100	+++	++	+
Piperazines							
• Trifluoperazine	Espazine	15–60	1–5 IM	5	+	+	+++
• Prochlorperazine	Stemetil	45–150	40–80 IM	15	+	+	+++
• Fluphenazine hydrochloride	Anatensol	5–30	–	2	+	+	+++
• Fluphenazine decanoate	Prolinate	–	25–50 IM every 1–3 weeks	0.7 (for 25 mg IM every 2 wks)****	+	+	+++
• Thioproperazine	Majeptil	15–45	–	5	+	+	++++
Thioxanthenes							
Aliphatics							
• Chlorprothixene	(Taractan)	75–600	25–75 IM	50–75	+++	++	++
Piperazines							
• Thiothixene	(Navane)	6–60	2–6 IM	5	+	++	++
• Flupenthixol	Fluanxol	3–40	–	–	±	±	+
• Flupenthixol Depot	Fluanxol Depot	–	20–40 IM every 2–4 weeks	****	±	±	+
Butyrophenones							
• Haloperidol	Senorm	5–100	5–20 IM	2	+	+	+++
• Haloperidol decanoate	Senorm-LA	–	25–250 IM	****	+	+	+++
• Trifluperidol	Triperidol	0.5–8.0	2.5–5.0 IM	0.6	±	±	+++
Diphenylbutylpiperidines							
• Pimozide	Orap	4–20	–	2	+	+	++
• Penfluridol	Flumap	20–60 mg once every week	–	3.5 (Probably for 20 mg given	+	+	++
Indolic derivatives (Dihydroindolones)							
• Molindone	(Moban)	50–225	–	10	++	0	+
Dibenzoxazepines							
• Loxapine	Loxapac	25–100	–	10–20	+	+	++
Atypical antipsychotics							
Dibenzodiazepines							
• Clozapine	Sizopin	50–450	–	50	+	+	0
Substituted benzamides							
• Sulpiride	(Dolmatil)	400–1800	–	200	+	+	0
• Remoxipride	(Roxiam)	60–1200	–	–	+	+	0
Benzisoxazoles							
• Risperidone	Sizodon	2–10	–	–	±	+	±
Benzisothiazolyl							
• Ziprasidone	–	–	–	–	±	+	0

Contd...

Contd...

Examples of drugs	Examples of Trade Names*	Oral dose range (mg/day)	Parenteral dose range (mg)	Equivalent dose (Equal to 100 mg of CPZ)	Common side effects***		
					Sedation	Hypotension	EPS**
Arylpiperidylindole							
• Sertindole	(Serdolect)	12–24	–	–	±	+	±
Thienobenzodiazepine							
• Olanzepine	(Zyprexa)	5–20	–	–	+	++	0
Dibenzothiazepine							
• Quetiapine	(Seroquel)	300–750	–	–	+	+	±
Others							
Rauwolfia Alkaloids							
• Reserpine	Serpasil	–	–	–	++	++	+

* The trade names given in brackets indicate that the drug is not available in India as yet and the names mentioned are popular trade names in the US market.
** EPS means Extrapyramidal symptoms.
*** 0 = Absent; ± = Probable/very little; + = Mild; ++ = Moderate; +++ = Severe.
**** 40 mg of flupenthixol decanoate every 2 weeks = 25 mg of fluphenazine decanoate every 2 weeks = 100 mg of haloperidol decanoate every 4 weeks.

as *lytic cocktail*), heat stroke, tetanus, intractable pruritus, severe pain in malignancies, acute intermittent porphyria, mental retardation with behavior problems, and as pre-anesthetic medication.
- The lethal dose is 26 g.

Triflupromazine

- *Examples of Trade Names:* Siquil
- *Dose Range:* 100–1200 mg/day (oral); 30 to 60 mg IM (parenteral)
- *Strengths Available:* 10 mg; 25 mg (oral); 3 mg/mL; 10 mg/mL; 20 mg/mL (parenteral; IM only)
- *Equivalent Dose (Equal to 100 mg. of CPZ):* 25–30 mg

Common Side Effects

Sedation (++); hypotension (++); EPS(+++) (especially akathisia); anticholinergic side-effects (++), laryngospasm, respiratory depression, agranulocytosis, seizures.

Comments

- A good antiemetic.
- Sometimes used in obsessive compulsive disorder (in small doses) and alcoholic psychoses.

Other Aliphatic Phenothiazines

Levomepromazine or Methotrimeprazine (Levoprome; Nozinan):
- *Dose Range:* 50–400 mg/d (oral); 50 mg (IM/IV slowly)
- *Equivalent Dose (Equal to 100 mg of CPZ):* 66 mg

Comments

- It is effective in treatment refractory schizophrenia (probably has a profile similar to clozapine).
- It is also used in postherpetic neuralgia and trigeminal neuralgia (when given parenterally, the analgesic effect is comparable to that produced by morphine).
- There is no dependence potential.

Alimemazine or Trimeprazine (Theralene):
- *Dose Range:* 10–75 mg/day (oral)

Comments

- It has a marked antihistaminic action; sometimes used as an antiallergic in combination with other antihistaminics.
- It is less effective than CPZ; no longer used as an antipsychotic.

Promazine (Sparine):
- *Dose Range:* 40 to 1000 mg/day (oral); 200 mg IM, 50–150 mg IV (parenteral)

Comments

- It has been used in treatment of eclampsia (with or without pentobarbital), delirium tremens (DT), and heroin withdrawal syndrome.
- It is less effective than CPZ; not used frequently nowadays.

Prothipendyl (Tolnate):
- *Dose Range:* 240–1000 mg/day (oral); 80–240 mg IM/IV (parenteral).

Comments

- It is a weak antipsychotic, less effective than CPZ, and not used frequently nowadays.
- It has been used in agitation in elderly, mental retardation with aggression, tremor, oculogyric crises and torticollis.

Piperidines

Thioridazine

- *Half-life (Hours):* 26–36 hours
- *Dose Range:* 300–800 mg/day (oral); 1–4 mg/kg in children (oral); 25 mg IM (parenteral)
- *Strengths available:* 5 mg; 10 mg; 25 mg; 50 mg; 100 mg (oral)
- *Equivalent Dose (Equal to 100 mg of CPZ):* 95–100 mg

Common Side Effects

Sedation (+++); hypotension (++); EPS (+); retinopathy (resembling retinitis pigmentosa) if given in high doses (1600–4000 mg/day) for long periods of time. No eye changes reported in dose range of 600–800 mg/day. Also galactorrhea, amenorrhea, impaired ejaculation, tachycardia, cardiac arrhythmias, mydriasis, weight gain

Comments

- It should not be given in doses of more than 800 mg/day.
- It is not recommended in children below 2 years of age.

Mesoridazine

- *Dose Range:* 50–400 mg/day (oral); 25 mg IM (parenteral)
- *Equivalent Dose (Equal to 100 mg of CPZ):* 35–50 mg.

Common Side Effects

Sedation (+++); hypotension (++); EPS (+); anticholinergic side-effects (++); galactorrhea, amenorrhea, impaired ejaculation, tachycardia, cardiac arrhythmias, mydriasis, weight gain.

Comments

It is a metabolite of thioridazine.

Piperacetazine

- *Dose Range (mg/day):* 25–160 mg/day (oral)
- *Equivalent Dose (Equal to 100 mg of CPZ):* 10 mg

Common Side Effects

Sedation (+++); hypotension (++); EPS (++); anticholinergic side-effects (++).

Comments

It is not used frequently nowadays.

Propericiazine or Periciazine

- *Dose Range:* 75–150 mg/day (oral)
- *Equivalent Dose (Equal to 100 mg of CPZ):* Less effective than CPZ.

Common Side Effects

Sedation (+); hypotension (+); EPS (+); anticholinergic side-effects (++).

Comments

- It is a link between piperidines and piperazines, both structurally and clinically.
- It is not used frequently nowadays.
- It is also indicated in chronic pain (probable central analgesic effect) and impulse control disorders.

Sulforidazine

- *Dose Range:* 150–300 mg/day (oral)
- *Equivalent Dose (Equal to 100 mg of CPZ):* 50 mg.

Common Side Effects

Sedation (+++); hypotension (+); EPS (++); anticholinergic side-effects (++).

Comments

It is a metabolite of thioridazine.

Piperazines

Trifluoperazine

- *Dose Range:* 15–60 mg/day (oral) 1–5 mg IM or IV (Not more than 10 mg IM/IV in 24 hours) (parenteral)
- *Strengths Available:* 5 mg (oral); 1 mg/mL (parenteral)
- *Equivalent Dose (Equal to 100 mg of CPZ):* 5 mg.

Common Side Effects

Sedation (+); hypotension (+); EPS (+++); anticholinergic side-effects (±); galactorrhea, amenorrhea, impaired ejaculation, tachycardia, cardiac arrhythmias, mydriasis.

Comments

- It may be beneficial in severe, intractable anxiety in small doses (1–5 mg/day).
- It is not recommended below 3 years of age.

Prochlorperazine Maleate

- *Dose Range:* 45–250 mg/day (oral); 40–80 mg IM (parenteral)
- *Strengths Available:* 5 mg; 25 mg (oral); 12.5 mg/mL; 25 mg/mL (parenteral)
- *Equivalent Dose (Equal to 100 mg of CPZ):* 15 mg.

Common Side Effects
Sedation (+); hypotension (+); EPS (+++).

Comments
- It has a good antiemetic effect, especially in migraine, and drug and alcohol withdrawal syndromes.
- It is not used frequently nowadays.
- It is not recommended in children.

Thioproperazine Mesylate

- *Dose Range:* 15–45 mg/day (up to 90 mg/day) (oral); 7.5–15 mg IM/IV (parenteral)
- *Strengths Available (Oral):* 5 mg (oral); parenteral form not available in India
- *Equivalent Dose (Equal to 100 mg of CPZ):* 5 mg.

Common Side Effects
Sedation (+); hypotension (+); EPS (++++).

Comments
- It has a powerful antiemetic effect.
- It is a very potent neuroleptic, especially in treatment-refractory patients.
- It has been given as a '*chemical shock*', i.e. high doses given for a few days and then stopped.
- It should be used with caution in bronchial asthma.

Fluphenazine Hydrochloride

- *Examples of Trade Names:* Anatensol
- *Half Life (hours):* 72–96 hours
- *Therapeutic Plasma Concentration:* 0.13–2.8 ng/mL
- *Dose Range:* 5–30 mg/day (oral)
- *Strengths Available:* 1 mg (oral)
- *Equivalent Dose (Equal to 100 mg of CPZ):* 2 mg.

Common Side Effects
Sedation (+); hypotension (+); EPS (+++); anticholinergic side-effects (±).

Fluphenazine Decanoate (Depot Preparation)

- *Examples of Trade Names:* Prolinate; Fludecan; Anatensol decanoate
- *Half-life (Hours):* 7–9 days (single dose); 14.3 days (multiple doses)
- *Dose Range:* 12.5–50 mg IM every 1–3 weeks (parenteral)
- *Strengths Available:* 25 mg/mL (parenteral)
- *Equivalent Dose (Equal to 100 mg of CPZ):* 0.7 mg (for 25 mg IM given every 2 weeks).

Common Side Effects
Sedation (+); hypotension (+); EPS (+++).

Comments
- The enanthate form is also available (though not in India); decanoate form is longer lasting and produces less EPS.
- It is indicated in schizophrenia, particularly where drug compliance is a problem.

Other Piperazine Phenothiazines

Acetophenazine maleate (Tindal):
- *Dose Range:* 40–400 mg/day (oral)
- *Equivalent Dose (Equal to 100 mg of CPZ):* 16 to 25 mg.

Common Side Effects
Sedation (+); hypotension (++); EPS (+++).

Comments
- It is not used frequently nowadays.

Perphenazine (Trilafon; Fentazin):
- *Therapeutic Plasma Concentration:* 0.8–1.2 ng/mL
- *Dose Range:* 16–64 mg/day (oral); 5–10 mg IM (parenteral)
- *Equivalent Dose (Equal to 100 mg of CPZ):* 10 mg.

Common Side Effects
Sedation (+); hypotension (++); EPS (+++).

THIOXANTHENES

Aliphatics

Chlorprothixene

- *Dose Range:* 75 to 900 mg/day (oral); 25–75 mg IM (parenteral)
- *Equivalent Dose (Equal to 100 mg of CPZ):* 50 mg.

Common Side Effects
Sedation (++); hypotension (++); EPS (+).

Comments
- It is chemically related to CPZ.
- It has an antidepressant effect in small doses (50 mg/day).

Piperazines

Thiothixene

- *Examples of Trade Names:* Navane; Not available in India
- *Half-life (hours):* 36 hours
- *Therapeutic Plasma Concentration:* 2–57 ng/mL
- *Dose Range:* 6 to 60 mg/day (oral); 2–6 mg IM (parenteral)
- *Strengths Available:* 1 mg; 2 mg; 5 mg; 10 mg; 20 mg (capsules); 5 mg/mL (liquid); 2 mg/mL (parenteral)
- *Equivalent Dose (Equal to 100 mg of CPZ):* 5 mg.

Common Side Effects

Sedation (+, sometimes insomnia); hypotension (++); EPS (++); lenticular opacities with prolonged use.

Comments

- It is the most potent thioxanthene; it is chemically related to thioproperazine.
- The lethal dose is 2.5–4.0 g.
- It is particularly useful in negative symptoms of schizophrenia.

Flupenthixol

- *Examples of Trade Names:* Fluanxol
- *Dose Range:* 3–18 mg/d (oral); Maximum dose 40 mg/d
- *Strengths Available:* 0.5 mg; 1 mg; 3 mg (oral)
- *Equivalent Dose (Equal to 100 mg. of CPZ):* 1 mg

Common Side Effects

Sedation (±, activating); hypotension (±); EPS (+); galactorrhea, amenorrhea, loss of libido, weight gain.

Comments

- It has a stimulating, and probably antidepressant and mood-stabilizing, effect in small doses. Large doses have an antipsychotic effect.
- It has no active metabolites.
- The possible mechanism of action is by D_2 receptor blockade, central anti-adrenergic effect, peripheral anti-serotonergic and anticholinergic effect.
- It should be used with caution in excited or agitated patients because of activating effect.
- It is not indicated below 12 years of age.
- It is particularly useful in negative symptoms of schizophrenia.

Flupenthixol Decanoate (Depot Preparation)

- *Examples of Trade Names:* Fluanxol depot
- *Dose Range:* 20–40 mg (Maximum dose = 100 mg) deep IM every 2–4 weeks (parenteral)
- *Strengths Available:* 20 mg/mL; 40 mg/2 mL; dissolved in low-viscosity vegetable oil (parenteral)
- *Equivalent Dose (Equal to 100 mg of CPZ):* 40 mg of flupenthixol decanoate every 2 weeks = 25 mg of fluphenazine decanoate every 2 weeks.

Common Side Effects

Sedation (+); hypotension (±); EPS (++); galactorrhea, amenorrhea, loss of libido, weight gain.

Comments

- It is chemically related to fluphenazine decanoate; the cis-isomer is a thousand times more potent than the trans-isomer. It has no active metabolites.
- It is probably better than fluphenazine decanoate in schizophrenia with depressive symptoms.
- It has no prophylactic effect in bipolar disorder.
- It should be used with caution in excited or agitated patients because of the activating effect.
- It is indicated in schizophrenia, particularly where drug compliance is a problem.
- It is not indicated below 12 years of age.

Clopenthixol

- *Examples of Trade Names:* (Sordinol)
- *Dose Range (mg/day):* 10 to 180 mg/d (oral); Parenteral depot preparation available.

Common Side Effects

Sedation (++); hypotension (+); EPS (++); decreased libido.

Comments

- It is chemically related to perphenazine.
- It has a rapid onset of onset.
- It is sometimes used in the management of hypersexuality.

BUTYROPHENONES

Haloperidol

- *Examples of Trade Names:* Serenace; Senorm; Depidol; Relinase; Halopidol; Halidol; Trancodol; Larenase; Normadol; Halorid; Seradol
- *Half-life (hours):* 24 hours
- *Therapeutic Plasma Concentration:* 5 to 20 ng/mL
- *Dose Range:* 5 to 100 mg/d (oral); 5–20 mg IM/IV (Parenteral)
- *Strengths Available:* 0.25 mg; 1.5 mg; 2 mg; 2.5 mg; 5 mg; 10 mg; 20 mg (tablets); 2 mg/mL; 10 mg/mL (liquid); 5 mg/mL (parenteral)
- *Equivalent Dose (Equal to 100 mg of CPZ):* 2 mg.

Common Side Effects

Sedation (+); hypotension (+); EPS (+++); insomnia, organic catatonic syndrome, neurotoxicity (with lithium), galactorrhea, amenorrhea, impotence, sudden death.

Comments

- Several studies have shown that lower doses (about 10 mg) are as effective or more effective than higher doses.
- Should be used with caution with lithium.
- Apart from its use in psychoses, it is also indicated in Tourette's syndrome (and other tic disorders), infantile autism (pervasive developmental disorders), delirium (e.g. delirium tremens), Huntington's chorea, and Sydenham's chorea.

Haloperidol Decanoate

- *Examples of Trade Names:* Senorm-LA; Depidol-LA
- *Half Life (hours):* 21 days
- *Dose Range:* 25 to 250 mg every 2–4 weeks (parenteral)
- *Strengths Available:* 50 mg/mL (parenteral); 100 mg/mL (100 mg/mL dose not yet available in India)
- *Equivalent Dose:* 100 mg/every 4 weeks is equal to about 5 mg/day of haloperidol.

Common Side Effects

Sedation (+); hypotension (+); EPS (+++); insomnia, organic catatonic syndrome, neurotoxicity (with lithium), galactorrhea, amenorrhea, impotence, sudden death.

Comments

It is indicated in schizophrenia (particularly chronic schizophrenia, catatonic schizophrenia, and acute schizophrenia), where drug compliance is a problem.

Trifluperidol

- *Examples of Trade Names:* Triperidol
- *Dose Range:* 0.5–8.0 mg/d (oral); 2.5–5.0 mg IM/IV (parenteral)
- *Strengths Available:* 0.5 mg (oral); 2.5 mg/mL (parenteral)
- *Equivalent Dose (Equal to 100 mg of CPZ):* 0.6.

Common Side Effects

Sedation (±; can cause insomnia); hypotension (±); EPS (+++; especially akathisia ++++).

Comments

- It has a rapid onset of action.
- It is not recommended below 5 years of age.

Droperidol

- *Dose Range:* 5 to 20 mg (oral); 5–10 mg IM; 5–15 mg IV (parenteral)
- *Strengths Available:* 10 mg tablets; 1 mg/mL liquid (oral); 12.5 mg/mL; 5 mg/mL (parenteral)
- *Equivalent Dose (Equal to 100 mg of CPZ):* 10.

Common Side Effects

Sedation (+); hypotension (+); EPS (++); chills, shivering.

Comments

- It has a rapid onset and is a brief acting drug; it is used in anesthesia.
- It is also used as an antiemetic.

Benperidol

- *Examples of Trade Names:* (Frenactyl, Anquil)
- *Dose Range:* 0.25 to 1.5 mg/day (oral; maximum dose 5mg/d); 0.5 to 2.0 mg IM/IV (parenteral).

Common Side Effects

Sedation (+); hypotension (±); EPS (+++, 350 times more than CPZ and 8 times more than haloperidol).

Comments

- It is a very potent neuroleptic.
- It is sometimes used for '*temporary and reversible neuroleptic castration*' for hypersexuality/antisocial sexual behavior.

Melperone/Methylperone

- *Dose Range:* 100–600 mg/day (oral)
- *Equivalent Dose (Equal to 100 mg of CPZ):* Less effective than CPZ.

Common Side Effects

Sedation (+); hypotension (+); EPS (+).

Comments

- It is a butyrophenone with atypical properties.
- It has an anxiolytic effect in small doses.
- It is probably more effective in treatment refractory schizophrenia.

Methylperidol

- *Dose Range:* 15–60 mg/day (oral)
- *Equivalent Dose (Equal to 100 mg of CPZ):* Less effective than CPZ.

Common Side Effects

Sedation (+); hypotension (±); EPS (++).

Fluspirilene (Depot Preparation)

Dose Range: 3–12 mg IM once every week (parenteral).

Common Side Effects

Sedation (±, Activating); hypotension (+); EPS (+).

Comments

It has a rapid onset of action (as unlike in other depot preparations, no hydroxylation is needed).

Fluanison

- *Dose Range:* 2.0–6.25 mg/day (oral; Liquid)
- *Equivalent Dose (Equal to 100 mg of CPZ):* Less effective than CPZ.

Common Side Effects
Sedation (+); hypotension (+); EPS (++); 'dullness'.

Comments
- It has a rapid onset of action.
- It also has a short duration of action, therefore is not suitable for maintenance treatment.

Floropipamide

- *Dose Range:* 120–360 mg/day (oral)
- *Equivalent Dose (Equal to 100 mg of CPZ):* Less effective than CPZ.

Common Side Effects
Sedation (+); hypotension (±); EPS (±, probably lowest EPS in butyrophenones).

Comments
It was claimed to possess 'delayed hypnogenic effect', i.e. no immediate sedation but allowing normal nocturnal sleep to occur.

DIPHENYLBUTYLPIPERIDINES

Pimozide

- *Examples of Trade Names:* Orap; Pimodac; Neurap; Mozep; Larap; Monozide
- *Half-life (hours):* 55 hours
- *Dose Range:* 4–20 mg/day (oral)
- *Strengths Available:* 2 mg; 4 mg; 10 mg (oral)
- *Equivalent Dose (Equal to 100 mg of CPZ):* 1 mg.

Common Side Effects
Sedation (+); hypotension (+); EPS (+++); cardiac arrhythmias, prolonged QT interval, sudden death.

Comments
- It has a long duration of action.
- It is the most specific D_2 (dopamine) blocker.
- It ia indicated in schizophrenia (particularly indicated in treatment of negative symptoms of schizophrenia, in small doses), delusional disorders (monosymptomatic hypochondriacal psychosis), and Tourette's syndrome.
- Regular EKG should be done while on regular pimozide treatment. Presence of cardiac arrhythmias is a contraindication for the use of pimozide.
- It is not recommended under the age of 12 years.

Penfluridol

- *Examples of Trade Names:* Flumap; Semap; Penflur
- *Half-life (hours):* 65–70 hours
- *Dose Range:* 20–60 mg given once every week (oral)
- *Strengths Available:* 20 mg (oral)
- *Equivalent Dose (Equal to 100 mg of CPZ):* 3.5 mg (Probably for 20 mg given every week).

Common Side Effects
Sedation (+); hypotension (+); EPS (++).

Comments
- It has a long duration of action.
- It was earlier withdrawn from the world market due to its effect on pancreas.
- It is indicated in schizophrenia (particularly chronic schizophrenia, catatonic schizophrenia, and acute schizophrenia), where drug compliance is a problem.

INDOLIC DERIVATIVES (DIHYDROINDOLONES)

Molindone Hydrochloride

- *Half-life (hours):* 10–20 hours
- *Dose Range:* 50–225 mg/day (oral)
- *Equivalent Dose (Equal to 100 mg of CPZ):* 10 mg.

Common Side Effects
Sedation (+, probably activating); hypotension (0); EPS (+); EKG changes common.

Comments
- It does not cause any weight gain; may cause weight reduction.
- The chemical structure is similar to hallucinogenic tryptamine derivatives, like bufotenin and psilocybin.
- Although it has both antipsychotic and antidepressant activities in animal studies, it is only an antipsychotic in clinical setting.

Oxypertine

- *Dose Range:* 60–300 mg/day (oral)
- *Strengths Available:* 10 mg; 40 mg (oral);

Common Side Effects
Sedation (+ in high doses; activating in small doses); hypotension (0); EPS (+); nausea, vomiting, dizziness.

Comments
- The chemical structure is similar to 5-HT, LSD, and reserpine.

- It is indicated in schizophrenia, particularly in the treatment of negative symptoms of schizophrenia and schizophrenia with associated depression.
- It is not recommended in children.

DIBENZOXAZEPINES

Loxapine Succinate

- *Examples of Trade Names:* Loxapac
- *Half-life (hours):* 5–19 hours
- *Dose Range:* 25–100 mg/day (oral) (Maximum dose = 250 mg/day); 12.5–50 mg IM (parenteral)
- *Strengths Available:* 10 mg; 25 mg (capsules); 25 mg/mL (liquid concentrate); parenteral form not available in India
- *Equivalent Dose (Equal to 100 mg of CPZ):* 10–20 mg.

Common Side Effects

Sedation (++); hypotension (+); EPS (++); anticholinergic side-effects (+); seizures.

Comments

- It has a rapid onset of action.
- It is not recommended in children.

DIBENZODIAZEPINES

Clozapine

- *Examples of Trade Names:* Sizopin, Lozapin, Leponex; Skizoril
- *Half-Life (hours):* 4–12 hours
- *Therapeutic Plasma Concentration:* > 350 ng/mL
- *Dose Range:* 100–450 mg/day (oral); Begin with 12.5 mg twice daily; Maximum dose 900 mg/day
- *Strengths Available:* 25 mg; 100 mg (oral); 50 mg/2 mL; parenteral form not available in India
- *Equivalent Dose (Equal to 100 mg of CPZ):* 50 mg.

Common Side Effects

Sedation (++); orthostatic hypotension (+); EPS (±; virtually no dystonia, rigidity, parkinsonism, akinesia, rabbit syndrome, TD or NMS); agranulocytosis (0.8% of patients; 50% cases occur in first 12 weeks and 75% in first 6 months of treatment); seizures (1–5% ; more likely at higher doses; EEG abnormalities in > 50% patients on clozapine); hypersalivation, hyperthermia, weight gain, tachycardia, cataplexy.

Contraindications:

- History of agranulocytosis or seizures
- Nonpsychotic depression
- Blood dyscrasias
- Impaired liver function
- Coma or co-administration with other CNS depressants
- Co-administration of drugs with a risk of agranulocytosis (e.g. carbamazepine, captopril, sulfonamides, co-trimoxazole, propylthiouracil)
- Known hypersensitivity to drug

Comments

- It is an atypical antipsychotic, effective against both positive and negative symptoms of schizophrenia.
- It produces less EPS (less tremor and akathisia, no dystonia or rigidity) and has a very low incidence of tardive dyskinesia and neuroleptic malignant syndrome.
- Originally developed in 1958, it was withdrawn from several countries around 1975 due to fatal agranulocytosis (most cases occurred in Finland). It was re-introduced recently (1990), due to good response shown in some (about 30–60%) of the treatment-resistant or treatment-intolerant chronic schizophrenics.
- It is currently indicated in treatment-refractory chronic schizophrenics, although also effective in acute schizophrenia and treatment-resistant mania.
- It is available under a management system which ensures weekly/bi-weekly WBC counts (in first 18 weeks; 1/month thereafter) for early detection of agranulocytosis.
- It has a probable beneficial effect in TD.
- It improves water intoxication syndrome (causing hyponatremia) in schizophrenia.
- It has no effect on prolactin; thus has no sexual or reproductive side effects.
- The possible mechanism of action is potent serotonergic ($5\text{-}HT_{1C}$ and $5\text{-}HT_2$), $alpha_1$-adrenergic, histaminic (H_1), and muscarinic activity. It produces preferential blockade of D_1 and D_4 receptors as compared to D_2 receptor (also acts preferentially in mesolimbic and amygdaloid than in nigrostriatal pathways).
- The lethal dose is 2.5–4.0 g.
- It is not recommended below 16 years of age.

SUBSTITUTED BENZAMIDES/ ORTHOPRAMIDES

Sulpiride

- *Dose Range:* 400–1800 mg/day (oral)
- *Strengths Available:* 200 mg (oral)
- *Equivalent Dose (Equal to 100 mg of CPZ):* 200

Common Side Effects

Sedation (±; Insomnia can occur); hypotension (+); EPS (±); galactorrhea, hyperprolactinemia, amenorrhea.

Comments

- It is chemically related to metoclopropamide.
- It has a rapid onset of action.
- It is a broad spectrum antipsychotic, indicated in psychosis, especially schizophrenia. It is effective in treatment of both

negative and positive symptoms of schizophrenia. It is probably also effective in psychotic depression.
- It is not recommended below 14 years of age.

Remoxipride

- *Half-life (Hours):* 3–7 hours
- *Dose range:* 60–1200 mg/day (oral).

Common Side Effects
Sedation (+; can cause insomnia); hypotension (+); EPS (0).

Comments
- The drug has been withdrawn from the world market by the manufacturers due to several cases of aplastic anemia.
- It is highly selective for D_{2b} receptors (a subtype, a short form, of D_2 receptors).

Raclopride

- *Dose Range:* Up to 8 mg/day (oral).

Tiapride

Dose Range: 300 to 1200 mg/day (oral).

Amisulpride

- *Dose range:* 400 to 1200 mg/day (oral)
- *Strengths available:* 50 mg; 200 mg (oral).

Common Side Effects
Insomnia can occur, with anxiety and agitation; hypotension (+); EPS (±); galactorrhea, hyperprolactinemia, amenorrhea, less weight gain.

Comments
- It is a broad spectrum antipsychotic.
- It should not be used in patients with prolactin-dependent tumors, e.g. pituitary gland prolactinemias, breast cancer.

RAUWOLFIA ALKALOIDS

Reserpine

- *Examples of Trade Names:* Serpasil
- *Half-life (hours):* 33 hours
- *Dose range:* 0.5 to 50 mg/day (oral)
- *Strengths available:* 0.25 mg; 1.0 mg (oral); 2.5 mg/mL (parenteral)
- *Equivalent Dose (Equal to 100 mg of CPZ):* 2 mg.

Common Side Effects
Sedation (++); hypotension (++); EPS (+); drug induced depression; can become severe, with suicidal ideation.

Contraindications:
- Parkinsonism
- History of depression
- Blood dyscrasias
- Impaired liver function
- Coma
- Coadministration of other CNS depressants, monoamine oxidase inhibitors, digitalis, quinidine, or antihypertensives
- Peptic ulcer disease
- Ulcerative colitis.

Comments
- It is an alkaloid derivative of *Rauwolfia serpentina.*
- It is not used as an antipsychotic nowadays.

PYROLISOQUINOLINES

Piquindone

Dose Range: Up to 120 mg/day (oral)

Comments
- It has a rapid onset of action.
- It is beneficial for negative symptoms.

BENZOQUINOLIZINES

Benzquinamide

Dose Range: up to 200 mg/day (oral).

Common Side Effects
Sedation (++); hypotension (++); EPS (+).

Comments
- The actions are similar to those of reserpine, though duration of action is shorter (24–30 hours), onset of action is faster, and it is less potent.
- It depletes monoamines presynaptically; this effect is blocked by pretreatment with monoamine oxidase inhibitors (MAOIs).
- It is used as an antiemetic. It has a doubtful efficacy as antipsychotic.

Tetrabenazine

- *Examples of Trade Names:* Revocon
- *Dose Range:* 35 to 300 mg/d (oral); 50 mg IM (parenteral).

Common Side Effects
Sedation (+); hypotension (+); EPS (±).

Comments
- The actions are similar to those of reserpine, though duration of action is shorter (24–30 hours), onset of action is faster, and it is less potent.

- It depletes monoamines presynaptically; this effect is blocked by pretreatment with monoamine oxidase inhibitors (MAOIs).
- It is used sometimes in the treatment of TD, and Tourette's syndrome. It is used in animal studies in place of reserpine.

BENZISOXAZOLE DERIVATIVES

Risperidone

- *Examples of Trade Names:* Sizodon; Respidon; Risdone; Risperdal; Rispid; Rozidal, Rispond
- *Half-life (hours):* 2.8 hours (Risperidone); 20.5 hours (9-hydroxy-risperidone); 24 hours (average half life for the active moiety)
- *Dose range:* 2–10 mg/d (oral; maximum 16 mg/d); given in twice daily doses
- *Strengths available:* 1 mg; 2 mg; 3 mg; 4 mg (oral; tablets); 1 mg/mL (liquid).

Common Side Effects

Sedation (± ; can also cause insomnia); hypotension (+); EPS (±; more on higher doses, i.e. > 6 mg/day); less TD and NMS; weight gain (dose related), agitation, headache, prolongation of QT interval (in some patients), rhinitis.

Comments

- It is an atypical antipsychotic, first in a class of SDAs (serotonin-dopamine antagonists). It is also the first benzisoxazole derivative.
- It has greater affinity for 5-HT_2 receptors than for D_2 receptors. It also has a high affinity for α_1 and α_2 adrenergic receptors, and H_1 histamine receptors. It is devoid of anticholinergic activity.
- Its major metabolite, 9-hydroxy-risperidone, has potent antipsychotic efficacy.
- It is indicated in schizophrenia and is effective in the treatment of both positive and negative symptoms; it also alleviates affective symptoms associated with schizophrenia.
- It is not recommended below 15 years of age.

BENZISOTHIAZOLELS

Ziprasidone

Common Side Effects

Sedation (± ; can also cause insomnia); hypotension (+); EPS (±); less TD and NMS.

Comments

- It is an atypical antipsychotic.
- It has a high affinity for 5-HT_{2C} and 5-HT_{1C} receptors, D_2 receptors, and a_1 adrenergic receptors.
- It is indicated in schizophrenia, effective in treatment of both positive and negative symptoms. It also alleviates affective symptoms associated with schizophrenia.
- It is not recommended below 15 years of age.

ARYLPIPERIDYLINDOLES

Sertindole

- *Dose Range:* 12 to 24 mg/d (oral); given in once daily dose
- *Strengths Available:* 4 mg; 12 mg; 16 mg; 20 mg (oral).

Common Side Effects

Sedation (±); hypotension (+); EPS (±); less TD and NMS; weight gain, dry mouth, nasal congestion, dizziness, decreased ejaculatory volume, prolongation of QT interval (in some patients).

Comments

- It is an atypical antipsychotic.
- It has a high affinity for 5-HT_{2c} and 5-HT_{2A} receptors, D_2 receptors, and a_1 adrenergic receptors.
- It is effective in treatment of both positive and negative symptoms of schizophrenia. It is not indicated in management of acute schizophrenia.
- It is not recommended with concomitant use of potassium non-sparing diuretics, ketoconazole and quinidine.

THIENOBENZODIAZEPINES

Olanzapine

- *Examples of Trade Names:* Olan, Olimelt
- *Dose Range:* 5–20 mg/d (oral); given in once daily dose
- *Strengths Available:* 5 mg; 7.5 mg; 10 mg (oral).

Common Side Effects

Sedation (+); hypotension (+); EPS (±); weight gain, dizziness, dry mouth, constipation.

Comments

- It is an atypical antipsychotic.
- It has a high affinity for 5-HT_{2A}, 5-HT_{2C} and 5-HT_3 receptors, D_1, D_2 and D_4 receptors, M_1 muscarinic, and H_1 histamine receptors.
- It is indicated in schizophrenia, effective in treatment of both positive and negative symptoms.
- It is not recommended below 18 years of age.

DIBENZOTHIAZEPINES

Quetiapine Fumarate

- *Dose Range:* 300–450 mg/day (oral; maximum 750 mg/d); given in twice daily doses
- *Strengths Available (Oral):* 25 mg; 100 mg; 200 mg

Common Side Effects*

Sedation (+); hypotension (+); EPS (±); dizziness, constipation, dry mouth, cataracts (in animal experimentation in dogs; so 6 monthly ophthalmological check-up is advocated while on quetiapine).

Comments

- It is an atypical antipsychotic.
- It has a greater affinity for 5-HT_2 receptors, a_1 and a_2 adrenergic receptors, and D_1 receptors.
- Ii is indicated in schizophrenia, effective in treatment of both positive and negative symptoms. It also alleviates affective symptoms associated with schizophrenia.

LONG-ACTING ANTIPSYCHOTIC PREPARATIONS

A large number of psychotic patients are uncooperative and have poor drug compliance. So, it may be at times difficult to ensure proper administration of antipsychotics, particularly on an outpatient basis. Since discontinuation of antipsychotic medication often leads to a relapse, long-acting preparations of antipsychotics are valuable in treatment. They may be given in a depot form intramuscularly or administered orally. Recent studies have shown that the use of long-acting depot preparations is not associated with increase in any of the negative treatment outcomes (like EPS, TD, NMS).

There are about 20 different preparations available (the first 5 are currently available in India), but the most often used ones are:

- Fluphenazine decanoate (25–50 mg IM, every 2–3 weeks)
- Haloperidol decanoate (50–250 mg IM, every 4 weeks)
- Flupenthixol decanoate (20–40 mg IM, every 2–3 weeks)
- Penfluridol (20–40 mg, oral every 1 week)
- Pimozide (8–40 mg oral, every 24 hours)
- Pipothiazine undecylenate and palmitate (50–200 mg, every 2–4 weeks)
- Fluspirilene (3–12 mg IM, once every week)
- Perphenazine enanthate (100 mg IM, every 2–3 weeks)
- Bromperidol decanoate (40–300 mg, every 4 weeks)
- Clopenthixol decanoate (50–600 mg, every 1–4 weeks)
- Zuclopenthixol decanoate (50–400 mg, every 1–4 weeks).

ATYPICAL ANTIPSYCHOTICS

A search for an antipsychotic drug that acts only on limbic system but has no effect on extrapyramidal system has led to the development of a heterogeneous group of drugs, collectively known as '*atypical antipsychotics*'. These drugs are effective antipsychotics without producing extrapyramidal side effects (i.e. *antipsychotics without being neuroleptics*) and do not cause elevation of serum prolactin levels. These are characterized by a selective limbic dopamine blockade, D_4 receptor blockade, or a combination of potent 5-HT_2 and weak D_2 antagonism. 5-HT_2 antagonism increases dopamine turnover in striatal areas and reduces the chances of EPS. Such a drug will be less likely to have the serious side effects, like tardive dyskinesia and neuroleptic malignant syndrome, and will be much safer. Recent research has indicated that several mechanisms may underlie 'atypicality'.

Atypical antipsychotics are characterized by the following biochemical and clinical atypicalities.

- They do not produce catalepsy in rats (a predictor of EPS) at doses that block conditioned avoidance response (a predictor of antipsychotic activity).
- They do not produce akinesia in humans.
- They do not elevate the prolactin levels in humans (so, no effect on tubero-infundibular pathway).
- They have a considerably lower potential for causing EPS, including TD (so, no effect on nigro-striatal pathway). Hence, they are antipsychotics that are truly not neuroleptics.

Clozapine is one such drug, but it causes significant agranulocytosis and seizures. Risperidone is currently being used extensively as a model drug of this nature. The atypical antipsychotics (most of which are still under development) can be tentatively classified as under.

Selective Dopamine Receptor Blockers

These include sulpiride (D_2), remoxipride (D_2), raclopride (D_2), amisupride (D_2), tiapride (D_2), nafedodride ($D_{3/4}$), SCH39166 (D_1), SCH23390 (D_5), and NNC010687 (D_1).

Partial D_2 Receptor Agonists (Autoreceptor Agonists)

These include terguride, preclamol, roxindole, and talipexole.

Nondopaminergic Antipsychotics

These include ritanserin (5-HT_2 antagonist), ondansetron (5-HT_3 antagonist), raclopride (5-HT_3 antagonist), milacemide (glutamate agonist), rimcazole (glutamate agonist), bretazenil (benzodiazepine receptor partial agonist), remoxipride (sigma receptor antagonist), and tiospirone (sigma receptor antagonist).

*(0 = Absent; ± = Probable/Very Little; + = Mild; ++ = Moderate; +++ = Severe).

Drugs Acting Via Dopaminergic as well as Via Other Receptor

These include risperidone ($5\text{-}HT_2 + D_2$ antagonist), melperone ($5\text{-}HT_2 + D_2$ antagonist), olanzapine ($5\text{-}HT_2 + D_2$ antagonist), ziprasidone ($5\text{-}HT_2 + D_2$ antagonist), zotepine ($5\text{-}HT_2 + D_2$ antagonist), sertindole ($5\text{-}HT_2 + D_2 + a_1$ antagonist), amperozide ($5\text{-}HT_2 + D_2 + a_1$ antagonist), clozapine ($5\text{-}HT_2 + D_1 + D_2 + a_1$ antagonist), and savoxepine ($5\text{-}HT_2 + D_1 + D_2 + a_1$ antagonist).

INDICATIONS

Although used earlier (historically) as urinary antiseptics and antihelminthics (use was stopped due to toxicity), the current *indications* for the use of antipsychotics include:

Organic Psychiatric Disorders

- Delirium (in small doses; e.g. *haloperidol*)
- Dementia (for psychotic features and agitation)
- Delirium tremens (and psychoses occurring in drug and alcohol withdrawal states; e.g. *haloperidol*)
- Drug-induced psychosis (e.g. *haloperidol* in amphetamine-induced psychosis)
- Other organic psychoses (e.g. organic hallucinosis, organic delusional disorder, secondary mania)

Non-organic Psychotic Disorders

- Schizophrenia
- Schizo-affective disorder
- Acute psychoses
- Mania (with or without lithium)
- Major depression (for psychotic features, and agitation; along with antidepressants)
- Delusional disorder, including monosymptomatic hypochondriacal psychosis (e.g. *pimozide*).

Child Psychiatric Disorders

- Attention deficit disorder with hyperactivity (in low doses, when stimulant medication is either not available or is contraindicated; e.g. *thioridazine*)
- Infantile autism and other pervasive developmental disorders (e.g. *haloperidol*)
- Conduct disorders in children, presenting with aggression (rarely used)
- Enuresis (sometimes used; e.g. *thioridazine* in low doses)

Neurotic and Other Psychiatric Disorders

- Severe, intractable, and disabling anxiety (occasionally, in low doses, e.g. *thioridazine*)
- Intractable obsessive compulsive disorder (e.g. low doses of *haloperidol*)
- Anorexia nervosa (e.g. *chlorpromazine*)
- Premature ejaculation (retarded ejaculation as a side effect of *thioridazine* is sometimes used).

Medical Disorders

- Huntington's chorea (e.g. *haloperidol*)
- Intractable hiccoughs (e.g. *chlorpromazine* used rarely in low doses)
- Nausea and vomiting (rarely, in low doses)
- Neuroleptanesthesia (*droperidol* with fentanyl, a meperidine-like drug)
- Tic disorders, e.g. Gilles de la Tourette syndrome (e.g. *haloperidol*)
- Ecclampsia (*chlorpromazine*, promethazine and pethidine are given as *lytic cocktail*)
- Heat stroke (e.g. *chlorpromazine*)
- Tetanus (e.g. *chlorpromazine* for muscle spasms and rigidity)
- Intractable pruritus (rarely used)
- Severe pain in malignancies (e.g. *chlorpromazine*)
- Preanesthetic medication (e.g. *chlorpromazine,* rarely used).

PHARMACOKINETICS

The orally administered antipsychotics are absorbed erratically and variably from the gastrointestinal tract, with uneven blood levels. Intramuscular and intravenous administration provide much more reliable blood levels. On an average, the oral liquid dose produces a peak level at 1½ hours, while the intramuscular dose peaks at 30 minutes.

The antipsychotics are highly lipophilic and highly protein-bound. They easily enter areas with good blood supply like brain, lung, kidneys and fetus, and accumulate there. They are not dialyzable.

The half-lives of all antipsychotics are long and theoretically a single dose administration per day is enough to produce sustained therapeutic blood levels. However in practice, divided doses are given initially to avoid side effects. Later, an attempt is made to give the whole dose or a major part of total daily dose at night. Steady state plasma levels are usually reached in 5–10 days. Once the drug is withdrawn, it may remain in body for many days to many months.

The main metabolic pathway is through liver (hepatic microsomal enzymes). Oxidation and conjugation are the most important methods of metabolism. Many of the metabolites, e.g. mesoridazine (for thioridazine) and reduced haloperidol (for haloperidol), are also active. Chlorpromazine has more than 150 metabolites, some of which are active. The excretion of the metabolites is through kidneys and liver (enterohepatic circulation).

Most of the antipsychotics tend to have a *therapeutic window*. If the blood level is below this 'window', the drug is ineffective. If the blood level is higher than the upper limit of the 'window', there is toxicity or the drug is again ineffective.

GENERAL GUIDELINES AND DOSAGE

- Take *informed consent* from the patient and/or close relative(s) before starting antipsychotics.
- Select therapeutic goals (*target symptoms*) at the beginning of treatment to monitor improvement.
- Discover patient's *drug attitude*, try to ensure cooperation, and warn about possible side effects (patient and family *education*).
- Use *low doses*, particularly of low potency drugs (like chlorpromazine and thioridazine). PET studies show that the maximal D_2 receptor occupancy (70–90%), needed for antipsychotic efficacy, occurs at modest doses. Use high doses or *megadoses* only as a last resort.
- Use high potency drugs (like haloperidol), if *higher doses* are needed. The BNF (British National Formulary) has specified 'advisory maximum daily doses' of antipsychotics for routine clinical use. Any dosage above the specified maximum dose is considered a high dose. Some examples of high doses specified by BNF include chlorpromazine (1000 mg), pimozide (20 mg), clozapine (900 mg), haloperidol (100 mg), thioridazine (800 mg), trifluoperazine (none) and loxapine (250 mg), among many others.
- When using parenterally, combine *benzodiazepines* with high potency antipsychotics to ensure the use of lower doses of antipsychotics (e.g. haloperidol with diazepam).
- If no improvement is seen after 2–4 weeks of reaching the maximum dose of the drug, then slowly taper the drug and give *another antipsychotic* from a different class.
- Antipsychotics in any dosage are best avoided in *non-psychotic children*.
- *Side effects* are more common in elderly and in presence of organic mental disorders. Therefore, use smaller doses in these populations.
- Avoid *low potency drugs* (and use low doses of high potency drugs) in the presence of cardiac illness, closed angle glaucoma or BHP, in elderly, and in delirium.
- Avoid *high potency drugs* in patients with history of EPS and parkinsonism.
- A patient's *previous drug response history* concerning a particular antipsychotic is likely to be a reliable guide for selecting the antipsychotic during the current episode.
- Suicidal patients should not be given thioridazine, loxa-pine and pimozide, as they are cardiotoxic in over-dosage.
- If patient is to be put on any *long-acting depot antipsychotic* for maintenance therapy, it is logical to start the patient first on the oral form of the same antipsychotic.
- The *minimum effective* CPZ equivalent dose in schizophrenia appears to be 400 mg/d. However, the dose needs to be individualized for each patient.
- Antipsychotic treatment can often be started in *outpatient* department. However, *inpatient* treatment may be indicated in patients who are noncompliant to treatment, are treatment resistant or intolerant, are homicidal or suicidal, present with co-morbid medical disorders, are unmanageable at home, or have unclear diagnosis.
- Abrupt discontinuation of antipsychotics can lead to an *antipsychotic withdrawal syndrome* (characterized by agitation, insomnia, nausea, vomiting, diarrhea, malaise, rhinorrhea and diaphoresis) within 2 weeks of stoppage. Therefore, a slow tapering of dose is preferable when antipsychotics are to be discontinued.
- *Co-morbid depression* (with schizophrenia) may need to be treated with antidepressants or ECT. Some antipsychotics (like thioridazine, chlorpromazine and flupenthixol) also have an antidepressant effect while others (e.g. fluphenazine, and pimozide) may exacerbate depression.
- Routine use of *antiparkinsonian agents* is not justified as not all patients are affected and TD may be unmasked or worsened by them. However, in patients with prior history of severe EPS, young men (more prone to dystonia), and patients in whom EPS might impair compliance (particular in the outpatient setting), the need of these agents may be assessed in a case-to-case basis.
- Prescription of *more than one antipsychotic* at the same time is usually not a good treatment policy.
- *Drug holidays* as well as *intermittent targeted therapy* are not recommended.
- Do not use antipsychotics in *non-psychotic individuals* (e.g. severe anxiety) unless there are compelling reasons to do so. Also, do not use antipsychotics to control *uncooperative or excited patients* before a diagnosis is made.
- Some of the following factors may adversely influence *drug compliance*:
  - Poor patient (and family) education regarding the drug.
  - Nonavailability (or lack of easy availability) of drug, or costly medication (lack of financial resources).
  - Excessively complex drug regimen.
  - Poor patient-therapist relationship.
  - Early onset of side-effects, with or without late onset of beneficial effects.
  - Rapid onset of beneficial effects and lack of awareness of need to continue maintenance medication.
  - Perceived stigma of having a mental disorder and being on medication
  - Presence of paranoid ideation, absent insight, denial, anxiety or fear, passive-aggression, or co-morbid substance use disorders.

SIDE EFFECTS

The antipsychotics are safe drugs, with a high therapeutic index and wide margin of safety in dosages. Adult patients have survived even after 10,000 mg of chlorpromazine given in one day.

In spite of this safety, a wide range of side effects does occur with the use of antipsychotics even in the therapeutic doses.

The side effects are listed in Table 2, with their mechanisms of causation and management.

CONTRAINDICATIONS AND CAUTIONS

Some of the contraindications and cautions of antipsychotic use are listed here.

- Parkinsonism
- Glaucoma (use phenothiazines with caution)
- Blood dyscrasias or bone marrow depression
- Severe hepatic or cardiac disease
- Coma or coadministration of other CNS depressants
- History of neuroleptic malignant syndrome or tardive dyskinesia

Table 2: Side effects of antipsychotics

Side effect	*Probable cause*	*Maximum with (For example)*	*Minimum with (For example)*	*Management*
		Autonomic side effects		
• Dry mouth	Muscarinic cholinergic blockade	Chlorpromazine	Haloperidol	Usually none; tolerance develops; occasionally pilocarpine 2%.
• Constipation	Muscarinic cholinergic blockade	Chlorpromazine	Haloperidol	Usually none; tolerance develops; bulk (or other) laxatives.
• Cycloplegia	Muscarinic cholinergic blockade	Chlorpromazine	Haloperidol	Usually none; tolerance develops; sometimes pilocarpine 2%.
• Mydriasis	Muscarinic cholinergic blockade	Thioridazine (Chlorpromazine causes miosis)	Haloperidol	Usually none; tolerance develops; sometimes pilocarpine 2%.
• Urinary retention	Muscarinic cholinergic blockade	Chlorpromazine	Haloperidol	Usually none, if only hesitancy occurs; tolerance develops. Rule out BHP. Bethanethol or Catheterization for retention.
• Central anticholinergic syndrome (delirium)	Muscarinic cholinergic blockade	Chlorpromazine	Haloperidol	Physostigmine (neostigmine does not enter CNS). Diazepam, sometimes. General supportive care.
• Orthostatic (postural) hypotension	α_1 adrenergic blockade	Chlorpromazine	Haloperidol	Usually none; tolerance develops. Change in posture slowly. When severe, use plasma expanders, raise legs, other supportive measures, and change drug.
• Impotence	α_1 adrenergic blockade	Chlorpromazine	Haloperidol	Decrease dose. If severe, change the medication.
• Impaired ejaculation	α_1 adrenergic blockade	Thioridazine	Haloperidol	Decrease dose. If severe, change the medication.
		Extrapyramidal side effects (EPSE)		
• Parkinsonian syndrome (especially tremor)	Dopaminergic (D_2) receptor blockade in striatal areas	Haloperidol	Clozapine	Antiparkinsonian anticholinergics, benzodiazepines, also change of medication or reduction of dose
• Akathisia	—do—	Haloperidol	Clozapine	—do— (also β-blockers for akathisia)
• Acute dystonia	—do—	Haloperidol	Clozapine	—do—; Rule out hypocalcemia
• 'Rabbit' syndrome (peri-oral tremor)	—do—	Haloperidol	Clozapine	—do—

Contd...

Contd...

Side effect	*Probable cause*	*Maximum with (For example)*	*Minimum with (For example)*	*Management*
• Tardive dyskinesia (late onset orofacial dyskinesia)	Dopaminergic (D_2) receptor supersensitivity	Not known (probably equal with all other antipsychotics)	Clozapine	Treatment unsatisfactory, though several drugs are available. Prevention is best
• Neuroleptic malignant syndrome (Hyperpyrexia, EPS, high CPK, catatonic symptoms, and autonomic dysfunction)	Not known	Probably haloperidol	Not known (less with clozapine)	Bromocriptine, dantrolene, baclofen. General supportive care; occasionally ECT.
Other central nervous system effects				
• Seizures	Decreased seizure threshold	Chlorpromazine (High doses)	Trifluoperazine	Decrease dose. Change to a safer antipsychotic
• Sedation	α adrenergic blockade	Chlorpromazine (High doses)	Haloperidol	This side-effect may be beneficial. Otherwise decrease dose, change drug. Give single dose only at night.
• Depression or	Decreased catecholamine Pseudo-depression	Not known levels in brain	Not known	Decrease dose. Change drug. Occasionally antidepressants or ECT.
Metabolic and endocrine side effects				
• Weight gain	Not known	Almost all antipsychotics	Molindone Exercise.	Change drug. Dietary control.
• Galactorrhea	Increased prolactin released with/ without amenorrhea	Haloperidol due to dopaminergic blockade in hypothalamus	Thioridazine; Atypical antipsychotics	None. Change drug.
Allergic side effects				
• Cholestatic jaundice	Hypersensitivity reaction	Chlorpromazine	Haloperidol	Change drug; benign course. Supportive care.
• Agranulocytosis (very rare)	Hypersensitivity reaction	Clozapine	Haloperidol	Stop drug immediately; treat infection; isolation; general supportive care. Figastrim may be useful.
Cardiac side effects				
• EKG changes	Anticholinergic effect	Chlorpromazine	Haloperidol	None. Change drug, if severe.
• Sudden death (very rare)	Probably ventricular	Not known fibrillation	Not known	None.
Ocular side effects				
• Granular deposits in cornea and lens	Not known (probably photosensitivity)	Chlorpromazine (High doses for long duration)	Haloperidol	Change drug.
• Pigmentary retinopathy resembling retinitis pigmentosa	Not known	Thioridazine only (Dose-related)	All other antipsychotics	Never give more than 800 mg/day of thioridazine. Prevention only.
Dermatological side effects				
• Contact dermatitis	Allergic	Chlorpromazine	All other treatment. (By handling)	Avoid handling. Symptomatic treatment antipsychotics
• Photosensitivity reaction	Not known (probably photosensitivity)	Chlorpromazine (High doses)	All other antipsychotics	Avoid excessive exposure to sunlight. Use sunscreen.
• Blue-gray metallic	Not known (probably discoloration photosensitivity)	Chlorpromazine (High doses for long duraion)	All other antipsychotics	Change drug.

- Severe hypertension or hypotension (use phenothiazines with caution)
- Severe brain damage
- Pregnancy and lactation (use with caution)
- Seizures (use with caution)
- Pheochromocytoma.
- Benign hypertrophy of prostate (use antipsychotics with anticholinergic activity with caution, e.g. thioridazine, chlorpromazine).

ANTIPSYCHOTICS—EQUIVALENT DOSES

Antipsychotic drugs vary greatly in potency (not the same as efficacy) and this is usually expressed as differences in 'neuroleptic' or 'chlorpromazine' 'equivalents'. Some of the estimates relating to neuroleptic equivalents are based on early dopamine binding studies and some largely on clinical experience or even inspired guesswork. BNF maximum doses for antipsychotic drugs bear little relationship to their 'neuroleptic equivalents'. Table 3 gives some approximate equivalent doses for conventional drugs. Values given should be seen as a rough guide when transferring from one conventional drug to another. An early review of progress is essential.

It is inappropriate to convert SGA doses into 'equivalents' since the dose-response relationship is usually well-defined for these drugs. Dosage guidelines are discussed under each individual drug. Those readers eager to find chlorpromazine equivalents for the newer drugs are directed to the only published paper listing such data.

Table 3: Equivalent doses of antipsychotics as per Maudsley Guidelines 2012

Drug	*Equivalent dose (consensus)*	*Range of values in literature*
Chlorpromazine	100 mg/day	–
Fluphenazine	2 mg/day	2–5 mg/day
Trifluoperazine	5 mg/day	2.5–5 mg/day
Flupentixol	3 mg/day	2–3 mg/day
Zuclopenthixol	25 mg/day	25–60 mg/day
Haloperidol	3 mg/day	1.5–5 mg/day
Sulpiride	200 mg/day	200–270 mg/day
Pimozide	2 mg/day	2 mg/day
Loxapine	10 mg/day	10–25 mg/day
Fluphenazine depot	5 mg/week	1–12.5 mg/week
Pipotiazine depot	10 mg/week	10–12.5 mg/week
Flupentixol depot	10 mg/week	10–20 mg/week
Zuclopenthixol depot	100 mg/week	40–100 mg/week
Haloperidol depot	15 mg/week	5–25 mg/week

NICE GUIDELINES: ANTIPSYCHOTICS – GENERAL PRINCIPLES OF PRESCRIBING

- The lowest possible dose should be used. For each patient, the dose should be titrated to the lowest known to be effective (see section on minimum effective doses); dose increases should then take place only after 2 weeks of assessment during which the patient is clearly showing poor or no response. With depot medication, plasma levels rise for 6–12 weeks after initiation, even without a change in dose. Dose increases during this time are therefore inappropriate.
- F or the large majority of patients, the use of a single antipsychotic (with or without additional mood-stabilizer or sedatives) is recommended (see section on antipsychotic polypharmacy). Apart from exceptional circumstances (e.g. clozapine augmentation) antipsychotic polypharmacy should be avoided because of the risks associated with QT prolongation and sudden cardiac death.
- Combinations of antipsychotics should only be used where response to a single antipsychotic (including clozapine) has been clearly demonstrated to be inadequate. In such cases, the effect of the combination against target symptoms and the side effects should be carefully evaluated and documented. Where there is no clear benefit, treatment should revert to single antipsychotic therapy.
- In general, antipsychotics should not be used as 'PRN' sedatives. Short courses of benzodiazepines or general sedatives (e.g. promethazine) are recommended.
- Responses to antipsychotic drug treatment should be assessed by recognized rating scales and be documented in patients' records.
- Those receiving antipsychotics should undergo close monitoring of physical health (including blood pressure, pulse, ECG, plasma glucose and plasma liquids).

46.2 ATYPICAL ANTIPSYCHOTICS

Avinash De Souza, Nilesh Shah

INTRODUCTION

The atypical antipsychotics—clozapine, risperidone, olanzapine, quetiapine, and ziprasidone—have important implications for the long term pharmacotherapy of schizophrenia. All antipsychotics have actions at dopamine-2 receptors, but the atypical agents behave differently than the conventional antipsychotics at those receptors. In addition, the atypical antipsychotics block serotonin-2 receptors. These differences in receptor-binding profiles provide the basis for 2 theories that explain why the 2 classes of antipsychotics are similar in efficacy but different in side effect profile, especially in their propensity to cause motor side effects such as extrapyramidal symptoms and tardive dyskinesia. These antipsychotics have been grouped into a new therapeutic class often referred to as *atypical*. Grouping these new agents together, despite some dissimilarities, helps to distinguish them as a class from most of the older conventional antipsychotics, which are clearly less tolerable and possibly less effective for negative symptoms.

Clinical characteristics, such as propensity for or lack of motor side effects such as extrapyramidal side effects (EPS) and tardive dyskinesia, can separate the atypical agents from the conventional drugs. Underlying the different clinical profiles are differences in receptor binding, especially at dopamine-2 (D2) and serotonin-2A (5-HT2A) receptors. While these drugs are bound to a receptor, that receptor is blocked from the naturally occurring substance, in this case, dopamine or serotonin. The improved tolerability of atypical antipsychotics is linked to reduced D2 receptor blockade in parts of the brain where side effects are mediated. This reduced blockade, in turn, may be linked to antagonism of 5-HT2A receptors, a drug's ability to quickly dissociate from D2 receptors, or both.

MECHANISMS OF ACTION OF ATYPICAL ANTIPSYCHOTICS

All antipsychotics have actions at D2 receptors in the brain. One way to distinguish the atypical antipsychotics from the conventional agents is that they block 5-HT2A receptors as well as D2 receptors and have fewer motor side effects such as EPS than the conventional antipsychotics have at standard doses. One atypical antipsychotic (quetiapine) has no more EPS than placebo. Additionally, at least 2 antipsychotics (olanzapine and risperidone) have shown greater efficacy than a conventional antipsychotic for negative symptoms, and 3 (olanzapine, ziprasidone, and quetiapine) do not raise prolactin levels like the conventional drugs do. Ziprasidone is associated with less weight gain compared with conventional and other atypical antipsychotics. Atypical antipsychotics have antipsychotic actions with much reduced or no motor side effects like EPS and tardive dyskinesia. Theoretically, this effect could be the result of blockade of 5-HT2A receptors in addition to D2 receptors.

The presence of serotonin in some dopamine pathways, such as the nigrostriatal pathway, inhibits the release of dopamine, whereas in the mesolimbic dopamine pathway, serotonin has little or no effect. In other words, when 5-HT2A receptors are blocked, dopamine is released in the nigrostriatal dopamine pathway but is not released in the mesolimbic dopamine pathway. In the nigrostriatal pathway, this reaction may reverse some of the D2 blockade by atypical antipsychotics through a process called disinhibition. When serotonin receptors are blocked in this pathway, dopamine levels increase. The naturally occurring dopamine is then "disinhibited" and fills D2 receptors, preventing blockade by the antipsychotic agent. With less D2 blockade in nigrostriatal pathways, motor side effects are reduced. However, disinhibition in the nigrostriatal pathway does not affect the blockade of D2 binding in the mesolimbic dopamine pathway, since few 5-HT2A receptors are in the mesolimbic dopamine pathway; thus antipsychotic actions are preserved. According to this hypothesis, antipsychotics are atypical when their 5-HT2A antagonism superimposed on their D2 antagonism reduces their D2 binding enough to reverse motor side effects but not enough to reverse antipsychotic effects.

How many, if any, of the atypical properties are due to serotonin antagonism remains open to debate. There are at least 16 receptors where 1 or more of the new drugs interact. In addition, no 2 atypical agents have an identical receptor-binding profile, providing a possible explanation for some of the differences clinicians observe from one drug to another and from one patient to another. These ancillary pharmacologic properties, in addition to 5-HT2 and D2 antagonism, include binding to D1, D3, and D4 receptors; to 5-HT1A, 5-HT2C, 5-HT3, 5-HT6, and 5-HT7 receptors; to α1-adrenergic, α2-adrenergic, histamine H1, and muscarinic cholinergic receptors; and to serotonin and norepinephrine reuptake pumps. Many of the old antipsychotics bind to α1-adrenergic, muscarinic, and histaminic receptors in addition to D2 receptors; however, a few traditional antipsychotics also bind to the 5-HT2A receptor just like the new antipsychotics. These include loxapine, chlorpromazine, and thioridazine.

Another hypothesis of atypicality is that, although all antipsychotics have actions at D2 receptors, the dopamine blockade with atypical agents lasts only long enough to cause an antipsychotic action but not long enough to cause the side effects associated with conventional agents. Theoretically, it takes only a quick blockade of the D2 receptor to cause an antipsychotic action, but a longer-lasting action to cause motor side effects such as EPS. Thus, if the antipsychotic has "hit-and-run" actions, also called rapid dissociation, it dissociates from D2 receptors after antipsychotic actions are established but before motor side effects are induced. According to this hypothesis, lack of motor side effects comes from low D2 binding due to rapid dissociation, not reversal by 5-HT2A antagonism. Support for the hit-and-run hypothesis of atypical antipsychotic action is based in part on evidence from positron emission tomography scans of patients taking antipsychotics, which shows that when D2 binding in the striatum is high, even in the presence of high 5-HT2A binding in the cortex, motor side effects still occur.

Also, rapid dissociation from the D2 receptor *in vitro* is a good predictor of low potential for motor side effects. Since rapid dissociation occurs more readily when the drug has low potency, low-potency agents (i.e. those requiring higher milligram doses such as clozapine and quetiapine) have faster dissociation from the D2 receptor than high potency agents (i.e. those requiring lower milligram doses such as risperidone), with intermediate-potency agents such as olanzapine in the middle. This hierarchy roughly correlates with the tendencies of these drugs to cause motor side effects within the group of atypical antipsychotics and also sets all of them apart from the conventional antipsychotics. This difference between low- and high-potency atypical antipsychotics also points to the need for careful dosing, especially with the high-potency agents, to maximize antipsychotic action but minimize side effects such as movement disorders. One of the consequences of fast dissociation is that the drug is gone from the receptor until the next dose. Natural dopamine can then bathe the receptor for a while before the next dose of the drug. It is possible that a bit of real dopamine in the nigrostriatal dopamine system is all that is needed to prevent motor side effects. If enough natural dopamine is available in the nigrostriatal pathway to minimize these side effects but not enough is available in the mesolimbic dopamine system to reactivate psychosis between doses, the drug will have atypical antipsychotic clinical properties.

Either 5-HT2A antagonism or fast dissociation from D2 receptors may define the atypicality of an antipsychotic. To have little or no motor symptoms from an antipsychotic, it is clear that D2 receptor binding in the striatum must be less than that caused by conventional antipsychotics. Pure 5-HT2A antagonism by itself does not result in robust antipsychotic actions. However, 5-HT2A antagonism can reduce D2 antagonism and thereby reduce motor symptoms without reversing antipsychotic actions. If, however, this 5-HT2A antagonism is overwhelmed by too much D2 antagonism, it cannot result in such atypical antipsychotic actions. Another route to reducing D2 receptor binding appears to be a shorter binding time, also known as rapidly dissociating from the D2 receptor. Many of the agents with atypical antipsychotic clinical properties "hit" the D2 receptor hard enough to cause antipsychotic effects and then "run" before they cause motor side effects like EPS. Although these agents are classified as antipsychotics, the nomenclature should not intimidate clinicians interested in using these agents. Instead, one can demystify them by calling them serotonin-dopamine antagonists, or, by seeing the similarities with antiparkinsonian agents, dopamine modulators. Hopefully, with a basic understanding of the mechanism of action of these agents, clinicians in both psychiatry and primary care will be able to recognize their benefits and manage their side effects more effectively.

ATYPICAL ANTIPSYCHOTICS

Clozapine, the prototype of atypical antipsychotics, was introduced for clinical use in a small number of countries in the early 1970s. However, shortly after introduction there were fatalities reported, subsequently attributed to a risk, albeit low (<1%), for clozapine to cause agranulocytosis. This led to a severe curtailment in its use, and it was not until the 1980s that the drug was reintroduced in North America, this time with the requirement of mandatory blood monitoring on a regular basis. Because of this history, clozapine use has been restricted to those individuals who have failed to respond to alternative antipsychotics. An important contribution of clozapine was its ability to dissociate antipsychotic action from EPS action—a feature that encouraged researchers to exploit this dissociation in other drugs. In North America, the reintroduction of clozapine was followed by other antipsychotics that fit the atypical profile: risperidone, olanzapine, and more recently, quetiapine. Sertindole was submitted to the US Food and Drug Administration (FDA) for approval but was subsequently withdrawn owing to cardiac conduction issues, specifically prolongation of the QTc interval. Ziprasidone is another atypical antipsychotic that has undergone extensive phase III testing and has recently been approved by the FDA, with some extended testing to assure its safety with regard to QTc prolongation. In parts of Europe and Asia, two other atypical antipsychotics have been approved for use, amisulpride and zotepine.

SIDE EFFECTS OF ATYPICAL ANTIPSYCHOTICS

Efforts to develop newer antipsychotics have been driven by two goals: improved efficacy and a more benign side effect profile. Since their introduction into clinical use, antipsychotics have been associated with a number of troublesome side effects that have, in turn, been linked to compliance problems. The first agents available, e.g. chlorpromazine, were discovered serendipitously. Since they acted on several aminergic and cholinergic receptors, they commonly gave rise to a variety of side effects such as dry mouth, urinary and bowel motility disturbances, sedation, and cardiovascular complications. With the recognition that they seemed to effect their antipsychotic response through D2 blockade, efforts shifted to the development of selective D2 antagonists, e.g. haloperidol, and these antipsychotics were identified as high-potency conventional antipsychotics. Unfortunately, this increased potency at the D2 receptor came at the cost of an increased risk of EPS, the side effects that came to characterize this class of typical antipsychotics. Paradoxically, the atypical antipsychotics have returned us to a class of compounds that are more heterogeneous in their receptor profile. As a result, although we have made significant gains in relegating EPS and prolactin side effects to the background, new side effects, related to the promiscuous receptor profile of the atypicals, are now emerging.

A review of all side effects is beyond the scope of this chapter. The focus here is confined to those side effects linked to D2 blockade (EPS and hyperpolactinemia), as well as weight gain and impaired glucose tolerance, which have been identified as the most problematic adverse effects with the current group of atypical antipsychotics.

Antipsychotic-induced EPS have been associated with the drugs' D2 blockade at the level of the nigrostriatal pathway. A major advantage of atypical antipsychotics is their relative freedom from this group of side effects. Once again, though, it must be pointed out that the comparative doses for the conventional antipsychotics in many of the initial clinical trials were inappropriately high. In addition, atypical antipsychotics are not equal along this dimension. Risperidone's risk is dose-related, as is olanzapine's, although the latter seems to carry a comparatively lower risk of overt EPS, perhaps related to its inherent antimuscarinic activity. Clozapine and quetiapine carry a very low risk of EPS. This has been attributed to their very fast dissociation from the D2 receptor, which results in lower D2 occupancy across time. Tardive dyskinesia (TD) occurs in approximately 25% of individuals exposed to ongoing use of typical antipsychotics, a figure that is even higher in certain subgroups, e.g. the geriatric population. With their decreased risk of acute EPS, it has been postulated that the atypical antipsychotics may carry a diminished risk of TD, since sustained EPS have been identified as a risk factor for TD. A diminished risk of TD has been established for clozapine, the atypical that has been available longest, and the early data for other atypicals seem promising in this respect. At least some of the newer antipsychotics have been shown to have antidyskinetic properties in individuals who have existing TD owing to previous antipsychotic exposure.

All typical antipsychotics have been linked to a risk of elevated prolactin, associated with D2 blockade of the tuberoinfundibular pathway. As a class, the atypical drugs are free of sustained prolactin elevation, although one of them, risperidone, still has a relatively high incidence of this side effect. The precise reason for this is not clear; however, a higher peripheral level of risperidone plus 9-hydroxyrisperidone in the plasma (as related to the brain) may be responsible, since the prolactin-elevating effects of antipsychotics are exerted outside the blood-brain barrier, whereas their antipsychotic efficacy arises from their central effects. The more immediate consequences of hyperprolactinemia, e.g. galactorrhea and amenorrhea, cannot be overlooked in the clinical setting. In addition, there is growing concern regarding potential long-term consequences; although not well understood, these may include osteoporosis, altered immune function, and risk for certain types of cancer.

Weight gain has always been an issue with antipsychotics, but as a side effect it has historically been overshadowed by the risk of EPS. Atypical antipsychotics, as a class, carry a much lower risk of EPS but a much greater risk of weight gain. Olanzapine and clozapine seem particularly problematic in this respect. It has been suggested that ziprasidone may be largely free of this side effect, but this drug has not seen widespread clinical use. The mechanisms underlying this drug-induced weight gain are not entirely clear; both the serotonin 5-HT2C and the histamine H1-blocking activity of these drugs have been implicated. The degree of weight gain can be substantial, e.g. as much as 30 pounds or more, a problem made more serious by other features of the population who must receive ongoing antipsychotic therapy. Patients with schizophrenia tend to have poor levels of nutrition, a 70% prevalence of smoking, and little or no preventative health care, so the cardiovascular risks associated with weight gain take on even greater importance. Another issue coming to the fore is the potential impact of atypical antipsychotics on glucose tolerance. A growing number of reports indicate new-onset diabetes in individuals being treated with atypical antipsychotics, and evidence gathered to date has indicated that risk of diabetes mellitus and/or impaired glucose tolerance may be at least twice as common in individuals on atypicals than in patients on typical agents. Again, drugs such as clozapine and olanzapine seem to be the worst offenders. In fact, a recent study suggests that the overall incidence of diabetes in patients taking clozapine may rise to an astronomical 37% in 5 years of follow up—a consequence at least as troubling as the TD problems associated with the typical antipsychotics. Early data suggest that risperidone may be less problematic along these dimensions; data on quetiapine and ziprasidone are lacking.

Yet another related problem is increased levels of lipids, specifically triglycerides. The underlying mechanisms are not clear, but the overall impairment of glucose tolerance seems to be consistent with insulin resistance. These changes could simply be secondary to weight gain, but the precise relationship is not clear, and there is the possibility that these glucose/lipid abnormalities are independent. The second possibility is particularly worrisome because weight gain, glucose intolerance, and lipid abnormalities are all independent risk factors for cardiovascular mortality. Regardless of etiology, regular weight monitoring and glucose/lipid profile assessments are now advocated for patients receiving atypical antipsychotics.

CONCLUSION

Although it is widely agreed that schizophrenia is a heterogeneous disorder with multiple dimensions, we still treat it with a single drug that includes a cocktail of receptor blockades. A more sophisticated pharmacological approach would be to define the different dimensions, develop targeted treatments for each, and combine these drugs in a flexible manner to address a patient's individual requirements along the different dimensions. Until such a time is reached, we hope that the intelligent use of atypical antipsychotics, with particular attention to weight gain and impaired glucose tolerance, combined with active and focused psychosocial rehabilitation, shall be our ally.

46.3 ANTIDEPRESSANTS

VN Vahiya, Anjali Chabbria, Dinesh Mohan Das

Depression, as a disease entity, consists of varying presentations which cover a wide spectrum. It could be a feeling of sadness at some real loss, pervasive disappointment or a major psychiatric disorder that appears spontaneously without any psychosocial triggers. Up till about five decades ago, the popular concept, that depression was a response to stresses and strains of life, resulted in different kinds of psychotherapy as the preferred treatment modality. A relatively recent emergence of knowledge concerning neurotransmitters, neuroreceptors and neuroamines has led to a search for specific biological abnormalities associated with mood and thought disturbances. This has now resulted in the use of antidepressant medications as the treatment of choice for almost every case of depression. Loss of sleep, appetite or libido, loss of weight and other biological symptoms of depression are amongst the indicators for prescription of antidepressant medication. Suicidal thoughts or preoccupation, which often occur in depression, may be treated with antidepressant medication. However, other biological therapies, especially ECT, should be considered in patients where suicide is assessed to be a likely occurrence.

Proponents of evidence-based medicine have gathered data to justify the use of antidepressant medicine in spite of occurrence of treatment emergent symptoms, as benefits far outweigh drug-related adverse effects. The role of psychotherapy, behavior therapy, meditation and other non-drug therapies as an adjunct of antidepressive medicine is favorably reported in the contemporary literature.

HISTORY

A search for effective antipsychotic drugs led to accidental discovery of imipramine, the first specific antidepressant drug. Kuhn observed the calming and antidepressant effects of imipramine.

This observation subsequently led to the discovery of a series of tricyclic and heterocyclic antidepressant drugs. In the preimipramine era, amphetamines and other psychostimulants were administered for their mood elevating effects amongst depressed patients. These were nonspecific drugs with a high-risk of dependence. Iproniazid and antituberculous drugs had also been noted to have exhibited mood elevating actions. MAO inhibiting properties of iproniazid led to the use of MAO inhibitors (MAOIs) in the treatment of depression.

The earlier tricyclic antidepressant drugs, often referred to as the first generation compounds, had four major pitfalls, namely:

1. Slow onset of action (4–6 weeks)
2. Anticholinergic properties (dryness of mouth, constipation, blurring of vision)
3. Cardiotoxicity (conduction defects and sudden cardiac deaths)
4. Lethality in overdose.

A series of so-called newer compounds have been synthesized with the aim of circumventing these pitfalls. It is pertinent to note that the first generation antidepressant compounds continue to be substantially the most potent antidepressant drugs. The newer compounds, which are equiefficacious, have less side effects and in some instances, less effective than the first generation antidepressants (Table 4).

BIOLOGICAL BASIS OF ANTIDEPRESSANT DRUG THERAPY

The benzyl ring forms the core of antidepressant drugs. Depending upon the number of benzyl rings in their chemical

Table 4: Years of development of the various pharmacological classes of antidepressants

1957–1970	TCAs (tricyclic antidepressants)
1970–1980	NARIs (noradrenaline epinephrine reuptake inhibitors)
1980–1990	SSRIs (selective serotonin reuptake inhibitors)
1990–2000	RIMAs (reversible inhibitors of monoamine oxidase)
	SNRIs (serotonin and noradrenaline reuptake inhibitors)
	NaSSAs (noradrenergic and specific serotonergic antidepressants

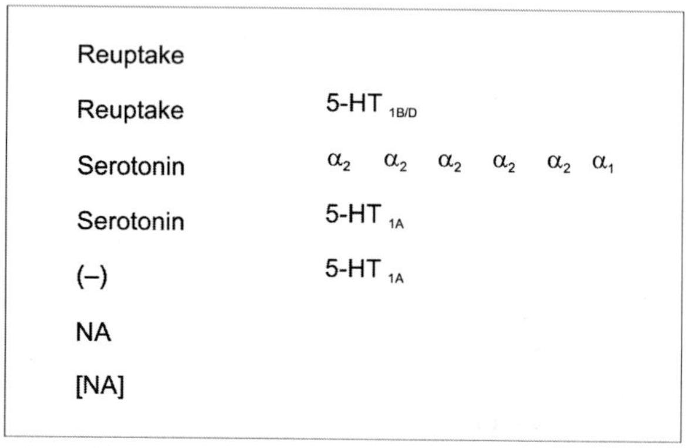

Reuptake

Reuptake $5\text{-HT}_{1B/D}$

Serotonin α_2 α_2 α_2 α_2 α_2 α_1

Serotonin 5-HT_{1A}

(–) 5-HT_{1A}

NA

[NA]

Fig. 1 Schematic representation of the modulation of serotonergic and noradrenergic neurotransmission in the hippocampus by presynaptic receptors located on serotonergic nerve terminals

structure, antidepressants are classified as tricyclic and heterocyclic compounds. The heterocyclic compounds can be further grouped as monocyclic, bicyclic and tetracyclic compounds. The largest number of antidepressant drugs belong to the tricyclic group (Fig. 1).

The cyclic compounds block the reuptake of serotonin and norepinephrine in the nerve synapse. This increases the availability of these biogenic amines at the receptor sites in the brain and other tissues. The differential potency of various antidepressant drugs on either serotonin or norepinephrine, along with their action on other amines and neurotransmitters (like acetylcholine and dopamine), account for the differential efficacy and different side effect profiles of individual drugs.

CLASSIFICATION

Depending upon the specificity of blocking the different receptor sites, the antidepressant drugs currently available can be grouped as;

- *Cyclic compounds (Table 5):*
- *Specific serotonin reuptake inhibitors (SSRIs):*
  - Fluoxetine (e.g. Fludac)
  - Paroxetine (not currently available in India)
  - Fluvoxamine (not currently available in India)
  - Sertraline (e.g. Zosert)
  - Citalopram
- *Norepinephrine serotonin reuptake inhibitors (NSRIs):*
  - Venlafaxine (e.g. Effexor; not currently available in India)
- *Norepinephrine serotonin reuptake enhancer (NSREs):*
  - Tianeptine (Stablon)
- *Norepinephrine serotonergic antidepressant drug (NSADs):*
  - Mirtazapine (Remeron; not currently available in India)
- *Dopaminergic antidepressant drugs:*
  - Amineptine (Survector)
- *Monoamine oxidase inhibitors:*
  - Phenelzine
  - Tranylcypromine
- *Atypical antidepressants:*
  - Bupropion
  - Nefazodone
  - Trazodone
- *Reversible inhibitors of MAO-A (RIMAs):*
  - Brofaromine
  - Moclobemide

DESCRIPTION OF SOME COMMONLY USED ANTIDEPRESSANTS

Tricyclic Antidepressants (Table 5)

Examples are imipramine (e.g. depsonil), amitriptyline (e.g. tryptomer), dothiepin (e.g. prothiaden), doxepin (e.g. spectra), nortriptyline (e.g. sensival).

Pharmacokinetics

Absorption

Tricyclic antidepressants (TCAs) are fairly well absorbed after oral administration. Administered initially in divided doses, the long half life permits a gradual transition towards a single dose given at bedtime. This is done safely up to 150 mg of imipramine. However, higher doses produce strong anticholinergic effects, like slowing of gastric motility resulting in slowing or erratic absorption of other drugs taken concomitantly.

Distribution

Once absorbed, the lipophilic compounds are widely distributed. They have a strong protein binding.

Plasma level range of 100–250 ng/mL correlates with antidepressant activity of imipramine (Nortriptyline 50–150 ng/mL; desipramine 100–250 ng/mL).

Metabolism

Oxidation occurs by hepatic microsomal enzymes. Most tricyclics are completely eliminated within 7–10 days.

Table 5: Tricyclic antidepressants

Antidepressant	*Usual dose*	*Extreme dose*	*Dosage*	*Amine effect*	*Sedation*	*Anti-cholinergic*	*Hypo-tension*	*Cardiac effects*	*Seizures*	*Weight gain*
Tertiary amine tricyclic										
Amitriptyline	100–200	25–300	O and I	NE, 5HT	+++	+++	+++	+++	++	++
Clomipramine	100–200	25–250	O	NE, 5-HT	++	+++	++	+++	+++	++
Doxepin	100–200	25–300	O	NE, 5-HT	+++	++	+++	++	++	++
Imipramine	100–200	25–300	O and I	NE, 5-HT	++	++	++	+++	++	++
Tri-imipramine	75–200	25–300	O	NE, 5-HT	+++	+++	++	+++	++	++
Secondary amine tricyclic										
Amoxapine	200–300	50–600	O	NE, DA	+	+	++	++	++	+
Desipramine	100–200	25–300	O	NE	0/+	+	+	++	+	+
Maprotiline	100–150	25–225	O	NE	++	++	++	++	+++	+
Nortriptyline	75–150	25–250	O	NE	+	+	+	++	+	+
Protriptyline	15–40	10–60	O	NE	0/+	++	++	+++	++	+

5HT blockage: Weight gain
Anti-cholinergic: Dry mouth, constipation, urinary retention, blurred vision, cognitive impairment, worsened TD
H_1 blockade: Sedation, cognitive impairment
Noradrenergic reuptake blockade: Postural hypotension
5HT reuptake inhibition: Nausea, diarrhea, and reduced appetite

An exceptionally long acting tricyclic antidepressant is protriptyline.

Adverse Effects

Allergic
Rash (rare); somewhat more frequent with maprotiline.

Anticholinergic
Blurred vision (common); narrow angle glaucoma may worsen; dry mouth (common); constipation (common); urinary retention (occasional), especially in elderly male patients with prostate problems; sweating - increased or decreased (infrequent); sinus tachycardia (common); speech blockage, mental clouding (occasional), confusion, delirium (rare).

Cardiovascular
Postural hypotension, dizziness (occasional); hypertension (rare); sinus tachycardia (common anticholinergic effect); premature atrial or ventricular beats (infrequent); antiarrhythmic effect, myocardial depression (additive with antiarrhythmic drugs); pedal edema (occasional)—may worsen congestive heart failure; EKG - ST segment depression, T-wave flattened or inverted, QRS prolongation.

Gastrointestinal
Constipation (common anticholinergic effect); nausea, vomiting, heart burn (infrequent).

Neurological
Central anticholinergic effects as above (vary considerably with different drugs); drowsiness (varies considerably with different drugs); muscle tremors, twitches, jitteriness (occasional); extrapyramidal symptoms (rare); paresthesias, fatigue, weakness, ataxia (infrequent); seizures—with overdose or in patients with known seizure disorder; hallucinations, delusions, activation of schizophrenia or mania (in bipolar disorder).

Sexual Dysfunction
Impotence and delayed or painful ejaculation in men; delayed orgasm in women; decreased libido and anorgasmia; increased central serotonergic function responsible for sexual side effects, does not appear to affect sexual dysfunction with Trazodone.

Specific Serotonin Reuptake Inhibitors

Examples are fluoxetine (e.g. fludac), fluvoxamine, paroxetine, sertraline (e.g. zosert), citalopram. Fluoxetine and sertraline are the only brands available in India at present.

Pharmacokinetics

Absorption
Fluoxetine is well absorbed from gastrointestinal tract (GIT). Food has little effect in slowing absorption, so can be given with or without food. Peak plasma levels are attained within 6–8 hours.

Distribution
Fluoxetine is 95% protein bound; widely distributed and found in breast milk.

Elimination
Fluoxetine is demethylated in liver to norfluoxetine. Half-life of fluoxetine is 2–3 days and of norfluoxetine is 7–9 days. Steady state is reached after 4 weeks. As a result of long half-life, increase in dosage does not always result in immediate increase in the pharmacological action.

Effects on Specific Organs and Systems

Cardiovascular
No major changes in BP, small drops (3 mm Hg) reported in cardiac-healthy depressed patients. No major EKG changes.

Respiratory System and Skin
Shortness of breath and fibrotic changes; skin rashes common (3–4%). The drug must be discontinued in the event of any allergic phenomenon.

Gastrointestinal
Nausea in a dose dependent fashion, due to increase in central peripheral serotonin level. Anorexia and diarrhea are also reported. Weight loss of up to three pounds is reported with this drug.

Blood
Hyponatremia reported in elderly patients and alcoholic patients in withdrawal state.

Neurological
Anxiety, insomnia and sedation.

Precautions and Adverse Effects

Neurological
Headache, insomnia, drowsiness, anxiety, nervousness, akathisia like reaction and tremors, seizures (0.2%), hypomanic reaction (more than 1%). Rarely, movement disorders may be seen.

Gastrointestinal
Nausea, diarrhea, anorexia, dyspepsia.

Skin
Rashes 3–4%, develop in patients on SSRIs.

Pulmonary System
Allergic reaction, like fibrosis and dyspnea may be seen.

Sexual Dysfunction
Decreased or delayed orgasms, delayed ejaculation, impotence in 4% of all patients have been reported.

Miscellaneous
Hypoglycemia specially in diabetic patients may be seen. Overdosages are less dangerous, overdose of up to 3000 mg/day without long-term consequences have been reported.

Augmentation of Response

Drugs used for augmentation of response include trazodone, stimulants, and buspirone.

Dosage

The therapeutic dose is 20–80 mg/day. It is advisable to start at 20 mg a day; if tolerated, continue for four weeks and watch for the response.

Depressed usually respond to 20–40 mg a day. If not, the drug can be increased to 80 mg/day. Obsessive-compulsive disorder (OCD) patients may need higher doses.

Venlafaxine

It is not currently available in India.

Chemistry

It is a phenylethylamine, structurally different from the existing antidepressants.

Pharmacokinetics

Venlafaxine is absorbed from the GIT and has a half-life of five hours. It should be administered in twice or thrice daily dosage. It is metabolized by cytochrome P450-2D6.

The metabolite is O-desmethyl-venlafaxine, whose activity is similar to the parent compound and has a half-life of 11 hours.

Pharmacodynamics

It is a nonsedative reuptake inhibitor of serotonin, norepinephrine and dopamine.

Adverse Effects and Precautions

Common adverse effects include nausea, somnolence, dry mouth, dizziness, constipation, nervousness, asthma, sweating, anorexia, blurred vision, abnormal ejaculation, impotence, increase in BP, particularly in patients treated with more than 300 mg daily.

Drug Interactions

Since it causes weak inhibition of cytochrome P450-2D6, co-administration of drugs like cimetidine should be done carefully; no interaction with lithium, diazepam or ethanol has been reported.

Trazodone

Structure

Trazodone is a triazolopyridine derivative and is structurally unrelated to other antidepressants. In fact, the triazolo ring resembles alprazolam.

Pharmacokinetics

Given orally, it is well absorbed; food significantly increase its absorption up to 20% and lengthens the time to peak plasma concentration (one hour fasting and two hour nonfasting). Drug intake with food decreases the peak level of plasma concentration and hence the side effects.

The half life is 5–9 hours; the steady state level is reached in less than four days. Metabolism of trazodone is by hepatic hydroxylation and oxidation.

Pharmacodynamics

Trazodone is a weak serotonin reuptake blocker. This action is of little significance. It blocks the postsynaptic $5HT_2$ receptors. Blockade at this site causes stimulation of other receptors of 5HT. The agonist action at $5HT_{1C}$ is postulated to have some behavioral consequences. The short-term use of trazodone has an adrenergic blocking action. The alpha receptor blockade causes dry mouth, orthostatic hypotension, priapism, down regulation of receptor; H_1 and muscarinic receptor blockade is negligible.

Clinically, the drug is effective in mild to moderate depression with anxiety and insomnia. In the geriatric population, the drug is useful, as it has low anticholinergic side effect, less orthostatic hypotension compared to tricyclic antidepressants (TCAs). Dizziness is a common side effect in the elderly.

Effects on Specific Organ Systems

Though treatment is relatively safe for cardiovascular system, orthostatic hypotension may develop shortly after ingesting the drug and resolve in 4–6 hours. It is preferably to be avoided in arrhythmias.

Contraindications

Contraindications include seizure disorder, current or previous diagnosis of anorexia nervosa and/or bulimia, history of head trauma, CNS tumor or other organic brain diseases.

Caution

Caution needs to be observed in the presence of EEG abnormalities, recent withdrawal from benzodiazepines and/or alcohol, psychotropic agents that reduce seizure threshold, lithium, and known history of substance abuse.

Dosage and Administration

The drug is available in 50 and 100 mg tablets; starting dose range is 200–225 mg/day. If no improvement after a week, raise to 450 mg/day. Increase in dose should not exceed 100 mg/day in a three day period; single dose should not exceed 150 mg.

Monoamine Oxidase Inhibitors

They are used less commonly due to dietary precaution to prevent hypertensive crisis. The commonly used monoamine oxidase inhibitors (MAOIs) include phenelzine, isocarboxazid, tranylcypromine, non-specific inhibitors of MAO_A (clorgyline; useful for rapid cycling bipolar disorder) and MAO_B (selegiline; used in parkinsonism).

Pharmacokinetics

These are well observed after oral administration. The hydrazine MAOIs are metabolized by acetylation.

Pharmacodynamics

Monoamine oxidase (MAO) concentration is highest in liver, GIT, CNS and sympathetic nervous system. MAO_A in GIT is responsible for metabolism of dietary tyramine. Inhibition of MAO_A by MAOIs leads to hypertensive crisis, due to increased tyramine in circulation.

MAO_A decreases metabolism of norepinephrine, serotonin and phenylethylamine. Both MAO_A and MAO_B decrease dopamine metabolism.

In addition to inhibition of MAO, MAOIs have additional neurochemical effects, like inhibition of catecholamine and serotonin reuptake.

Specific Effects

These include decreased sleep, insomnia, daytime drowsiness, significantly decreased amounts of rapid eye movement (REM) sleep, hypotension due to vascular effects (centrally and peripherally), and hepatotoxicity.

Indications

Monoamine oxidase inhibitors (MAOIs) are effective in panic disorder with agoraphobia, PTSD, eating disorders, social phobia and pain disorder. In atypical depression, MAOIs are preferred.

Precautions and Adverse Effects

These include orthostatic hypotension, weight gain, edema, sexual dysfunction, and insomnia; myoclonus, muscle pains, and paresthesias (secondary to pyridoxine deficiency); less cardiotoxic and less epileptogenic; contraindicated in pregnancy; tyramine containing foods (e.g. cheese) induce hypertensive crisis; SSRIs and MAOIs combination avoided due to risk of serotonin syndrome.

Dosage

- *Phenelzine:* 15 mg/day; increased to 45 mg/day in first week and 90 mg/day by fourth week.
- *Tranylcypromine and isocarboxazid:* Test dose of 10 mg; 30 mg/day by first week.

When switching over from MAOIs to TCAs or SSRIs, a gap of two weeks should be given for enzymes to be resynthesized.

RIMAs (Reversible Inhibitors of MAO_A)

The dietary restrictions and hypertensive crisis associated with MAOIs led to the decline of their use in 1970s.

The discovery, that MAO exists in two forms, led to the development of more selective inhibitors of the enzyme. MAO_A inhibitors, moclobemide and brofaromine are all reversible inhibitors of MAO.

Novel RIMAs do not interact with dietary tyramine. However, caution must be used in combination with venlafaxine and SSRIs to prevent 'serotonin syndrome'. Caution is also needed when they are used with over-the-counter agents, such as cimetidine or nasal decongestants.

Most of the clinical data of RIMAs is on moclobemide. Moclobemide 300–600 mg/day was comparable with fluoxetine 20–40 mg/day in its efficacy. Patients on moclobemide, however, complained of sleep problems due to its activating effects.

RIMAs may also be effective in social phobias and panic disorders.

Mirtazapine

It is a new antidepressant with a mode of action that differs from currently used agents and is best referred to as noradrenergic and specific serotonin antidepressant (NaSSA).

It is well absorbed from GIT. Peak plasma levels are reached in two hours. The drug is demethylated and oxidated followed by conjugation. The demethylated metabolite is also active. Eighty-five percent of the drug is eliminated in urine and 15% in feces.

Half-life

Half-life of mirtazapine is 20–40 hours; so once daily dosage is sufficient.

Dosage

The starting dose is 15 mg/day for four days; increased to 30 mg/day for ten days; if effective, continue at 30 mg/day. If there is not sufficient improvement, the dose can be increased to 45 mg/day.

Tolerability and Safety

It has little or no effect on heart rate, BP or body temperature. There are no anticholinergic, serotonergic and adrenergic side effects. It has less sexual dysfunction and low seizure inducing properties.

ANTIDEPRESSANTS USED IN SPECIFIC CLINICAL CONDITIONS

- *Cardiac problems:*
  - *Angina:* Mianserin, SSRIs
  - *Arrhythmias:* Best avoided
  - *Cardiac failure:* No important effect
  - *Hypertension:* Nortriptyline, mianserin, SSRIs
  - *Myocardial infarction:* Avoid all antidepressants for first two months; if absolutely indicative, use SSRIs ormianserin
- *Epilepsy:*
  - *Low-risk:* Doxepin, MAOI, moclobemide, SSRIs
  - *Moderate risk:* Mianserin, nefazodone, trazodone, TCAs, venlafaxine
  - *High-risk:* Amoxapine, maprotiline
- *Diabetes:*
  - Tricyclic are safe, unless the diabetes is brittle.
  - May cause hypoglycemia during fluoxetine treatment.
  - Fluoxetine side effects (like tremor, nausea, sweating and anxiety) can mimic the symptoms of hypoglycemia.
- *Breastfeeding:*
  - Preferably all antidepressants should be avoided.
  - If absolutely indicated, low dose TCAs (amitriptyline, nortriptyline, desipramine), or fluoxetine
- *Old age:*
  - *Lower risk:* Desipramine, mirtazapine, lofepramine, moclobemide, nortriptyline, SSRIs, trazodone, tryptophan, venlafaxine
- *Pregnancy*: All drugs to be avoided preferably.
- *Renal disease:*
  - *Low-risk:* TCAs (nortriptyline, amitriptyline, imipramine), moclobemide, mianserin
  - *Moderate risk:* MAOIs, SSRIs, trazodone, venlafaxine, mirtazapine, nefazodone
- *Liver disease:*
  - *Low-risk:* Mianserin, paroxetine
  - *Moderate risk:* SSRIs, mirtazapine, moclobemide, nefazodone, trazodone, TCAs venlafaxine
  - *High-risk:* Lofepramine, MAOIs
- *Sexual dysfunction*: Nefazodone, moclobemide.

Common Drug Interactions

Drugs	TCAs	SSRIs	MAOIs
Lithium	Well used, rarely-myoclonus, seizure and neurotoxicity	Two cases of toxicity	No interaction
Carbamazepine (CBZ)	Plasma level of TCAs decreased by 40-50%	Increases CBZ level by 25%	CBZ structurally related to TCAs, so interaction postulated
Neuroleptics haloperidol	Increased level of TCAs 2–3 times; (Imipramine, desipramine, nortriptyline) Phenothiazine and TCA used concurrently, serum level of both rises, increased anticholinergic effects	Clozapine levels increase six fold. With pimozide, increased side effects	-
OC pills	Akathisia, decreased tricyclic effectiveness, increased toxicity	-	
Alcohol	Increased sedation, decreased threshold inhibits alcohol dehydrogenase	No effects	Potential effects
Benzodiazepines	Enhanced sedation	Increases level of benzodiazepines.	-

CHOOSING AN ANTIDEPRESSANT

When to start? Which drug? How much? How long? When to stop? One is faced with these questions, especially while dealing with recurrent and chronic depressions.

Treatment strategies that provide long-term, prophylactic efficacy are now recommended.

Frank et al categorized outcomes of treatment according to five R's, i.e. Response, Remission, Relapse, Recovery, and Recurrence (Fig. 2). The relationships between these outcomes and the three phase of treatment (acute, continuation and maintenance therapy) is reviewed.

The first positive step towards *recovery* is a significant *response* to treatment. Continuation pharmacotherapy then begins, the goals of which are prevention of *relapse* and *remission*. *Remission* is defined as a return to the patient's premorbid or well-self, even if only for a few weeks.

A patient, who achieves a stable remission for at least 4–6 months, is assumed to have recovered from the index depressive episode. A *relapse* is defined by a return of depressive symptoms at a syndromal level at any point in time, between the initial response and the end of continuation therapy.

Maintenance pharmacotherapy is recommended to follow continuation therapy for most patients with a history of recurrent episodes of depression (history of frequent/multiple prior episodes of depression, a seasonal pattern of mood disturbance, and a family history of affective disorder).

Maintenance pharmacotherapy is provided with the same antidepressant agent(s) used during the acute and continuation therapy.

More recurrence occurs in the ultra-low dosage group. How long should the antidepressant be given? Probably as long as the benefits outweigh the costs.

ANTIDEPRESSANTS: SUMMARY OF NICE GUIDELINE

Effectiveness

The *severity* of depression at which antidepressants show consistent benefits over placebo is poorly defined. In general, the more severe the symptoms, the greater the benefit. Antidepressants are normally recommended as first-line treatment in patients whose depression is of at least moderate

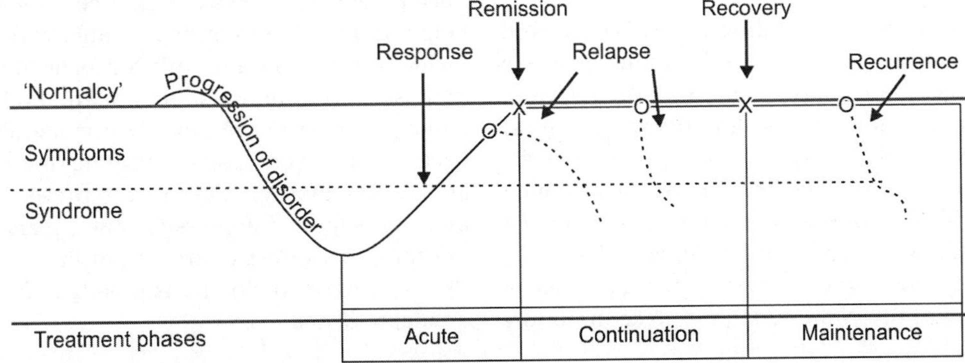

Fig. 2: A diagram of five possible outcomes (response, remission, relapse, recovery, and recurrence) during the three phases of treatment of depression (acute, continuation, and maintenance)

severity. Of this patient group, approximately 20% will recover with no treatment at all, 30% will respond to placebo and 50% will respond to antidepressant drug treatment. This gives a number needed to treat (NNT) of 3 for antidepressant over true no-treatment control and an NNT of 5 for antidepressant over placebo. Note though that response in clinical trials is generally defined as a 50% reduction in depression rating scale scores, a somewhat arbitrary dichotomy, and that change measured using continuous scales tends to show a relatively small mean difference between active treatment and placebo.

In patients with subsyndromal depression it is difficult to separate the response rate to antidepressants from that to placebo; antidepressant treatment is not indicated unless the patient has a history of severe depression (where less severe symptoms may indicate the onset of another episode), or if symptoms persist. Patients with dysthymia (symptom *duration* of at least 2 years) benefit from antidepressant treatment; the minimum duration of symptoms associated with benefit is unknown. In other patients, the side effects associated with antidepressant treatment may outweigh any small benefit seen.

Onset of Action

It is widely held that antidepressants do not exert their effects for 2–4 weeks. This is a myth. All antidepressants show a pattern of response where the rate of improvement is highest during weeks 1–2 and lowest during weeks 4–6. Statistical separation from placebo is seen at 2–4 weeks in single trials (hence the idea of a lag effect) but after only 1–2 weeks in (statistically more powerful) meta-analyses. Thus, where large numbers of patients are treated and detailed rating scales are used an antidepressant effect is evident at 1 week. In practice using simple observations, an antidepressant effect in an individual is often seen by 2 weeks. It follows that in individuals where no antidepressant effect is evident after 2 weeks' treatment, a change in dose or drug may be indicated.

Choice of Antidepressant and Relative Side Effects

Selective serotonin re-uptake inhibitors (SSRIs) are well tolerated compared with the older tricyclic antidepressants (TCAs) and monoamine oxidase inhibitors (MAOIs), and are generally recommended as first-line pharmacological treatment for depression. There is no evidence of any clinically meaningful difference in efficacy between SSRIs, although sideeffect profiles differ. For example, paroxetine has been associated with more weight gain and a higher incidence of sexual dysfunction, and sertraline with a higher incidence of diarrhea than other SSRIs. Newer dual re-uptake inhibitors such as venlafaxine and duloxetine tend to be tolerated less well than SSRIs but better than TCAs. With all drugs there is marked interindividual variation in tolerability which is not easily predicted by knowledge of a drug's likely adverse effects. A flexible approach is usually required to find the right drug for a particular patient.

As well as headache and GI symptoms, SSRIs as a class are associated with a range of other side effects including sexual dysfunction, hyponatremia and GI bleeds. TCAs have a number of adverse cardiovascular effects (hypotension, tachycardia and QTc prolongation), and are particularly toxic in overdose. MAOIs have the potential to interact with tyramine-containing foods to cause hypertensive crisis. All antidepressant drugs can cause discontinuation symptoms with short half-life drugs being most problematic in this respect.

Drug Interactions

Some SSRIs are potent inhibitors of individual or multiple hepatic cytochrome P450 (CYP) pathways and the magnitude of these effects is dose-related. A number of clinically significant drug interactions can, therefore, be predicted. For example fluvoxamine is a potent inhibitor of CYP1A2 which can result in increased theophylline serum levels, and fluoxetine is a potent inhibitor of CYP2D6 which can result in increased seizure risk with clozapine.

Antidepressants can also cause pharmacodynamic interactions. For example, the cardiotoxicity of TCAs may be exacerbated by drugs such as diuretics that can cause electrolyte disturbances.

Potential pharmacokinetic and pharmacodynamic interactions between antidepressants have to be considered when switching from one antidepressant to another.

Suicidality

Antidepressant treatment has been associated with an increased risk of suicidal thoughts and acts, particularly in adolescents and young adults leading to the recommendation that patients should be warned of this potential adverse effect during the early weeks of treatment and know how to seek help if required. All antidepressants have been implicated, including those that are marketed for an indication other than depression (e.g. atomoxetine). It should be noted that; (1) although the relative risk may be elevated above placebo rates in some patient groups, the absolute risk remains very small, and; (2) the most effective way to prevent suicidal thoughts and acts is to treat depression, and (3) antidepressant drugs are the most effective treatment currently available. For the most part, suicidality is greatly reduced by the use of antidepressants.

Duration of Treatment

Antidepressants relieve the symptoms of depression but do not treat the underlying cause. They should, therefore, be taken for 6–9 months after recovery from a single episode (to cover the assumed duration of most single untreated episodes). In those patients who have had multiple episodes, there is evidence of benefit from maintenance treatment for at least 2 years; no upper duration of treatment has been identified. There are few data on which to base recommendations about the duration of treatment of augmentation regimens.

Next Step Treatments

Approximately a third of patients do not respond to the first antidepressant that is prescribed. Options in this group include dose escalation, switching to a different drug and a number of augmentation strategies. The lessons from STAR*D are that a small proportion of nonresponders will respond with each treatment change, but that effect sizes are modest and there is no clear difference in effectiveness between strategies.

Use of Antidepressants in Anxiety Spectrum Disorders

Antidepressants are first-line treatments in a number of anxiety spectrum disorders.

CONCLUSION

More and more treatment modalities will be available with advances in neurophysiological mechanisms of psychiatric illness. Antidepressants in development are being defined from various classes, with different mechanisms of action; serotonergic agents presently dominate the field.

All the new antidepressants so far discovered have failed to surpass the plateau of efficacy of the classical antidepressants (TCAs and MAOIs). The new antidepressants generally have an improved side effects profile. The search for an antidepressant drug which has a rapid onset of action, greater efficacy and is cost-effective, as compared to less expensive antidepressants still continues.

46.4 NEWER ANTIDEPRESSANTS FOR THE TREATMENT OF DEPRESSION IN ADULTS

Neha Singh, Christoday RJ Khess, Jayati Simlai

Antidepressants are prescribed mainly for people with depression, although some are also used for anxiety disorders and other conditions, including chronic pain and enuresis. They are one of the most commonly prescribed medications (more than 43 million prescriptions were written for them between April 2010 and March 2011 in England and more than this in USA and other countries).[1]

Antidepressants were developed in the 1950s, and their mechanism of action is thought to be by increasing the levels of extracellular synaptic neurotransmitters such as serotonin, noradrenaline, and dopamine; they also have other effects, including increasing hippocampal neurogenesis. The original antidepressants were known as tricyclics because of their chemical structure. Since the 1980s, a new generation of antidepressants has been developed and marketed based on their mode of action. The nomenclature for referring to these newer drugs is confusing as they can be classified by several criteria, including the target molecule and the number of neurotransmitter sites involved.[2] Box 1 lists antidepressants grouped according to the current nomenclature used by the World Health Organization.[1-6]

This article focuses on selective serotonin reuptake inhibitors (SSRIs) and other newer antidepressants [using the World Health Organization's nomenclature (Box 1)] and their use in adults presenting with depressive disorders. We have excluded nonreversible monoamine oxidase inhibitors such as phenelzine as recent guidelines recommend these should usually be prescribed only by specialist mental health professionals and cautiously.[3] Our article does not cover the use of antidepressants in children and adolescents or depression in bipolar disorder.

The use of antidepressants is increasing worldwide—for example, in the United Kingdom, antidepressant prescribing doubled between 1993 and 2005; this has been explained by small changes in the proportion of patients receiving longer treatment.[6] However, evidence also exists of overuse: in one study about a quarter of those taking antidepressants had never had a depressive disorder.[7]

Patient health questionnaire (PHQ-9)

Question 1

Over the past two weeks how often have you been bothered by any of the following problems?	*Score*			
	Not at all	*Several days*	*More than half the days*	*Nearly every-day*
• Little interest or pleasure in doing things	0	1	2	3

Contd...

Contd...

• Feeling down, depressed, or hopeless	0	1	2	3
• Trouble falling/staying asleep, sleeping too much	0	1	2	3
• Feeling tired or having little energy	0	1	2	3
• Poor appetite or overeating	0	1	2	3
• Feeling bad about yourself or that you are a failure or have let yourself or family down	0	1	2	3
• Trouble concentrating on things, such as reading the newspaper or watching television	0	1	2	3
• Moving or speaking so slowly that other people could have noticed. Or the opposite: being so fidgety or restless that you have been moving around more than usual	0	1	2	3
• Thoughts that you would be better off dead or of hurting yourself in some way	0	1	2	3
Add the individual scores together to get a total score. Of those patients who score 10 or more in primary care, most (7.6% of all patients in primary care) will have a score 10–14, which indicates either subthreshold depression or moderate depression;[10,11] a smaller proportion (3.4% of all patients in primary care) will have a score of 15–19, indicating moderate to severe depression; and the smallest proportion (2% of all patients in primary care) will have a score of ≥20)				
Question 2				
If you indicated any problems, how difficult have these problems made it for you to do your work, take care of things at home, or get along with people?				
Not difficult at all	Very difficult			
Somewhat difficult	Extremely difficult			

Box 1: World Health Organization's current nomenclature for antidepressants, with examples of current drugs

- *Nonselective monoamine reuptake inhibitors:*
  - *Tricyclic antidepressants:* Imipramine, amitriptyline (Limbival)*, clomipramine, lofepramine, amoxapine
  - *Noradrenaline reuptake inhibitors:* Desipramine, nortriptyline, maprotiline
- *Selective serotonin reuptake inhibitors:*
  - Fluoxetine (Fludawn)*, fluvoxamine (Voxamin), zimelidine, paroxetine (Panex-CR), sertraline, citalopram, escitalopram (S-celepra)
- *Monoamine oxidase inhibitors (nonselective):*
  - Phenelzine, tranylcypromine, isocarboxazid
- *Monoamine oxidase A inhibitors:*
  - Moclobemide, toloxatone
- *Other antidepressants:*
  - *Serotonin noradrenaline reuptake inhibitors:* Venlafaxine (Venfax-PR), duloxetine
  - *Noradrenaline dopamine reuptake inhibitors:* Nomifensine, bupropion
  - *Noradrenaline and selective serotonin antagonists:* Mirtazapine (Mirazep)
  - *Serotonin antagonist and reuptake inhibitor:* Trazodone
  - *Melatonin receptor agonist with 5-HT2C receptor antagonist properties:* Agomelatine
  - *Serotonin partial agonist:* Gepirone

Note: *Listed in the WHO's list of essential medicines for use in depressive disorders

WHAT ARE THE INDICATIONS FOR ANTIDEPRESSANT USE IN DEPRESSION?

The guideline from the National Institute for Health and Clinical Excellence (NICE) on managing depression recommends that doctors be alert for depression in patients with a history of depression or who have a chronic health problem with functional impairment.[3] Consider asking patients two screening questions for depression: "during the last month have you often been bothered by feeling down, depressed, or hopeless?" and "during the past month have you often been bothered by having little interest or pleasure in doing things"?[8] An answer of "yes" to one of these indicates possible depression. A "no" answer to both questions virtually rules out depression. A further assessment with a depression inventory such as the patient health questionnaire (PHQ-9)[9] or the hospital anxiety and depression scale (HADS)[12] is helpful for measuring the severity of the depression and for monitoring changes in response to treatment. This strategy is similar to measuring blood pressure when treating hypertension and is part of successful programs to manage depression in primary care.[13] The initial assessment of a depressed patient includes the items listed in Table 6.

The NICE guideline, which is based on systematic reviews of the evidence and explicit consideration of cost effectiveness, recommends that antidepressants should not be used for persistent, subthreshold symptoms or mild depression as the risk to benefit ratio is poor unless the patient has a history of moderate to severe depression or persisting low level symptoms, or other interventions have not worked.[3] For people with moderate to severe depression NICE recommends antidepressants initially, as well as high intensity psychological interventions, combined treatments, collaborative care, consideration of referral, and further interventions.[14]

Table 6: Assessment of a patient with suspected depression

History item	*Reason for item*
Previous episodes	Depression is a recurrent disorder and it is important to know which treatments (drug and nondrug) have worked in the past and to consider long-term antidepressant treatment to prevent relapse
Suicidality and suicide history	Taking a history will guide whether to use medication, which medication to use, and how closely to monitor
Severity and duration	Severity can be measured by symptom inventories—e.g. the patient health questionnaire, the hospital anxiety and depression scale, the Beck depression inventory, and the Center for Epidemiological Studies depression scale. The more severe and enduring the episode, the more likely the initial need for antidepressant medication
Evidence of psychosis	Patient may need antipsychotic medication in addition to antidepressants and advice from secondary care
Bipolarity	Evidence of past manic or hypomanic episodes would warrant advice from secondary care
Comorbid health conditions and other medication	To improve the accuracy of diagnosis in people with chronic physical problems consider asking about feelings of worthlessness, poor concentration, and thoughts of death
	Consider the role of medication in causing depression—e.g. steroids or interferon
	Be aware of the potential for drug interactions with antidepressants
Use of complementary therapies	In one US survey about half of depressed women had tried alternative therapies for depression.[14] Asking about complementary therapies is an opportunity for clinician and patient to collaborate in a management plan and to check for potential interactions
Adherence	Patients are likely to stop and start medication without clinician advice
Functional and social assessment	The assessment of social support, social networks, and social functioning is important in establishing the impact of the disorder and planning treatment. If the patient is not coping at home or work, increase the intensity of the treatment

Table 7: Effectiveness using individual patient data based on six studies (718 outpatients) of paroxetine or imipramine versus placebo.[18] Values are scores except where stated otherwise

Severity (NICE criteria)	*Hamilton depression rating scale-17*	*PHQ-9*	*HADS-D*	*BDI-II*	*Number needed to treat compared with placebo over six to eight weeks*
Severe	≥23	≥20	≥15	≥29	4
Moderate	19–22	10–19	11–14	20–28	11
Mild	14–18	6–9	8–10	14–19	16

Abbreviations: PHQ-9, the patient health questionnaire (9 item); HADS-D, the hospital anxiety and depression scale (German version); BDI-II, Beck depression inventory II.

The ranges are indicative only, and there is some evidence that they are not exactly equivalent.[19] Treatment decisions also need to consider other factors, such as patient preference, duration of depression, and impact on function.

HOW WELL DO THE NEWER ANTIDEPRESSANTS WORK?

How well the newer antidepressants work has become a controversial topic owing to concern about publication bias. A meta-analysis of 35 randomized controlled trials sourced from the Food and Drug Administration (which included unpublished data) found that antidepressants were clearly effective only in patients with severe levels of depression (Hamilton depression rating scale scores of ≥28).[15] However, this meta-analysis has been criticized for its statistical methods, and commentators have asserted that patients included in the trials were unlikely to be severely depressed and that the long-term effects of antidepressants on preventing relapse were ignored.[16] A reasonable quality recalculation of the data from the original meta-analysis found that antidepressants had some effect regardless of the severity of the depression, although the authors of this paper declared significant competing interests.[17]

It is difficult to assess efficacy by comparing depression inventory scores as these scales focus on symptoms rather than function and are treated as ratio scales when in fact they are ordinal. It may be more helpful to consider the numbers needed to treat for significant improvement (rather than changes in rating scale scores) when comparing antidepressants with placebo using individual patient data in a meta-analysis (Table 7).[18] Table 7 shows that for those with severe depression four people need to be treated with an antidepressant over two months for one extraperson to get better compared with taking a placebo over the same period. This reinforces the need to add in psychological therapies or to try more than one antidepressant for patients with severe depression. For people with mild to moderate depression, the initial choice of drug or nondrug treatment should be guided by patient preference and availability of resources.[19]

The NICE guideline suggests that all newer antidepressants are equally effective. However, there is some debate about this. A meta-analysis of 117 head to head randomized controlled trials of 12 new generation antidepressants that included almost 26,000 patients showed a slightly better response rate with four of them: escitalopram, mirtazapine, sertraline, and venlafaxine.[20] The meta-analysis included patients from primary and secondary care and the differences were assessed at only eight weeks. Escitalopram and sertraline showed better acceptability (on the basis of overall withdrawal rates), which, if cost and patient history of drug response were not an issue, would make them potential first line SSRIs. However, a larger, updated meta-analysis of 234 studies failed to find any differences in efficacy among "second generation" antidepressants.[21] A recent systematic review of reboxetine concluded that it was an ineffective and potentially harmful antidepressant.[22] Individual patients show large differences in response to antidepressants, and there is currently no reliable way to predict who will respond to which treatment.

HOW SAFE ARE THE NEWER ANTIDEPRESSANTS?

The safety concerns for antidepressants range from adverse effects that make patients feel unwell or prone to stopping medication through to an increase in suicidal thoughts to death either from completed suicide or cardiac arrhythmias. Most adverse events are mild, although one in six patients treated with second generation antidepressants discontinue treatments in randomized controlled trials because of intolerable adverse effects.[23] However, as these data come from a meta-analysis of randomized controlled trials, the experience of adverse effects and withdrawal may be different in everyday patients.

Table 8 shows the common adverse effects and suggested management options. A systematic review of harms from second generation antidepressants found that sexual dysfunction was commonly reported, with between half and two-thirds of patients experiencing some sexual dysfunction.[23] The highest incidence of sexual dysfunction was with citalopram, paroxetine, and venlafaxine; mirtazapine had the lowest rate. Sexual dysfunction is likely to be under-reported in the clinical trials as they rely on spontaneous reporting.[24] Nausea, vomiting, diarrhea, dry mouth, sweating, headache, dizziness, and weight gain are other commonly reported adverse effects with SSRIs. Venlafaxine seems more likely than SSRIs to be associated with nausea and vomiting; sertraline has higher rates of diarrhea; mirtazapine and paroxetine cause more weight gain than other SSRIs.

In patients aged over 65 years a cohort study of more than 60,000 patients in UK primary care with a new diagnosis of depression found that SSRIs increased the risk of falls (hazard ratio 1.66, 95% confidence interval 1.58–1.73) and that citalopram, escitalopram, and fluoxetine were associated with hyponatremia (hazard ratio 1.52, 1.33–1.75).[25] Trazodone, mirtazapine, and venlafaxine were associated with an increase in all-cause mortality. Most adverse effects occurred in the first month after starting the antidepressants.

Box 2 outlines the main concerns about interactions and contraindications for different drug classes.

HOW COST EFFECTIVE ARE THE NEWER ANTIDEPRESSANTS?

A trial of SSRIs and supportive psychotherapy versus supportive therapy alone in the treatment of mild to moderate depression in UK general practice found that adding SSRIs to supportive therapy was cost effective, with mean costs of £90 (€108; $140) per point improvement in the Hamilton depression rating scale and £14854 per quality adjusted life year gained.[31] The NICE guideline found that there was weak evidence that escitalopram was more cost effective than three other antidepressants. It also reported a weak trend showing that SSRIs may be more cost effective than tricyclic antidepressants.[3]

How do the Newer Antidepressants Compare with Older Pharmacological Treatments for Depression?

The second generation antidepressants seem to be as effective as the tricyclics and monoamine oxidase inhibitors. The major differences are in the frequency and type of adverse effects, ease of dosing, and lethality in overdose. A Cochrane review of antidepressants versus placebo for treating depression in primary care found that the number needed to harm (NNH for withdrawal owing to adverse effects over six to eight weeks) ranged from 4–30 (median 17) for tricyclic antidepressants and from 20–90 (median 23) for SSRIs.[32] For tricyclics, the most common side effects are related to their anticholinergic action and include dry mouth, constipation, and urinary retention. A major consideration in prescribing antidepressants is the risk of their being taken in overdose and the consequences of such an act. Tricyclic antidepressants are associated with a higher case fatality ratio (the ratio of the number of deaths caused by self-poisoning to nonfatal self-poisoning episodes for a particular drug), with case fatality ratios of 13.8 compared with 2.5 for venlafaxine, 1.9 for mirtazapine, and 0.5 for SSRIs.[33]

Table 8: Adverse effects and suggested management

Adverse effect	*Comment*	*Management*
Dizziness	Occurs in about one in 10 people who take second generation antidepressants and is more common with venlafaxine and less common with sertraline or fluoxetine	Check blood pressure standing and lying; symptoms may improve over time; decrease dose or change treatment. Ensure adequate fluid intake
Sedation	More common with trazodone but can occur with all second generation antidepressants	Sedation may be desirable; it may improve over time. Change time of dosing and treatment
Dry mouth	Probably dose related	Tolerance may develop; change treatment; suggest sugarless gum or saliva substitutes
Sexual dysfunction	Common but often not asked about	Consider reducing dose, waiting for the effects to improve, switching to a different antidepressant (some evidence exists for lower rates of sexual dysfunction with mirtazapine, moclobemide, duloxetine and bupropion), or consider sildenafil
Insomnia	Common problem but hard to distinguish from insomnia caused by depression	Change time of dosing (earlier or later may help), pay attention to sleep hygiene, try a different antidepressant, or possibly try short course of benzodiazepine, zopiclone, or low dose trazadone
Suicidal thoughts	Antidepressants may paradoxically increase suicidal thoughts in those aged under 30	Review often (within a week of starting antidepressants and continue until no longer clinically needed). No evidence exists that asking about suicide makes people more likely to harm themselves. Prescribe small amounts of medication. Prescribe antidepressants that are less lethal in overdose (such as SSRIs). Venlafaxine has a greater risk of death from overdose than other newer antidepressants, although the greatest risk is with the tricyclics (except for lofepramine)[3]
Anxiety	Often occurs when starting SSRIs	Consider using a benzodiazepine for no longer than two weeks
Hyponatremia	Particularly a problem in the elderly and more common with SSRIs	Check sodium before and after starting treatment, and consider changing to mirtazapine if it becomes problematic
Serotonin syndrome	Characterized by changes in mental state (e.g. confusion or agitation), autonomic instability (e.g. high temperature, shivering, sweating, changes in blood pressure), and neuromuscular hyperactivity (e.g. clonus or hyper-reflexia). Seen particularly with SSRIs and other drugs that effect serotonin	Stop the antidepressant. Use supportive measures such as hydration, management of hyperthermia, and benzodiazepines. Consider cyproheptadine or chlorpromazine in severe cases
Discontinuation syndrome	More common with SSRIs that have a short half-life (e.g. paroxetine or venlafaxine)	Decrease dose over four weeks. Warn the patient

Abbreviation: SSRIs, selective serotonin reuptake inhibitors

In general, the newer antidepressants can be started at their therapeutic dose and given once a day whereas the older antidepressants need to be started at a low dose and gradually increased to their therapeutic levels, sometimes splitting the dose over the day.

How are the Newer Antidepressants Taken and Monitored?

Which Antidepressant to Use First?

The NICE guidelines on depression recommend an SSRI as the first choice of antidepressant.[3] Measurement of change in symptoms should be monitored with depression rating scales.

How soon they will Work and what to do if They Do not Work?

The usual advice is that antidepressants should start working after one to two weeks, although a meta-analysis of placebo controlled trials of SSRIs found that the therapeutic response is greatest in the first week.[34] The advice on when to see the patient after the first visit differs by guideline and varies from one to two weeks, more often if there are suicidal thoughts at the baseline assessment. The guidelines also differ on when to change management if the patient is not showing signs of improvement. Canadian guidelines suggest that if there is less than a 20% reduction in scores at six weeks then a change in treatment (such as an increase in dose) should be

Box 2: Precautions when prescribing for depression

- *Interactions with SSRIs*
  - *Tramadol or oxycodone:* In older people interactions between antidepressants (usually SSRIs) and tramadol or oxycodone form about a third of reported drug interactions.[26] This interaction can result in a serotonin syndrome at any age.
  - *ST John's Wort:* This induces liver CYP450 enzymes so may decrease levels of SSRIs; also, using St John's wort with SSRIs may precipitate a serotonin syndrome.
  - *Tricyclic antidepressants:* SSRIs may prevent the metabolism of tricyclics through the CYP450 enzyme system, resulting in toxic levels of the tricyclic.
- *Hepatic disease:* Hepatic disease increases the half-life of antidepressants, so a decrease in the usual dose is needed.
- *Pregnancy and breastfeeding:* If psychotherapies are unavailable or ineffective in depressed women who are pregnant, balance the risks of any potential damage to the fetus from antidepressants with the benefits of antidepressant treatment. A recent systematic review found that 10 of the 12 small studies showed little evidence of effect on the neurodevelopmental outcome of infants exposed to antidepressants.[27] NICE states that in pregnancy amitriptyline, imipramine, nortriptyline, and fluoxetine have lower risks than other antidepressants and that imipramine, nortriptyline, and sertraline are present in breast milk at relatively low levels.[28]
- *Heart disease:* About one in five people with coronary heart disease have major depression, which is associated with a worse prognosis. In patients with heart disease, tricyclic antidepressants are best avoided because of their risk of causing arrhythmias and postural hypotension; SSRIs should be tried first, with baseline electrocardiography.[29] Concerns have been expressed about venlafaxine, as in high doses it can exacerbate hypertension.
- *Bleeding:* Selective serotonin reuptake inhibitors and serotonin noradrenaline reuptake inhibitors are associated with an increased risk of gastrointestinal bleeding as they reduce platelet aggregation (although the absolute increase risk is low, the number needed to harm is 411 people prescribed an SSRI for a year).[30] Patients at increased risk include those with peptic or liver disease and those receiving anticoagulant, antiplatelet, or nonsteroidal anti-inflammatory drugs. Proton-pump inhibitors may reduce the risk of gastrointestinal bleeds from SSRIs.

considered.[24] The NICE guidance recommends that if there is no improvement after three to four weeks the treatment should change.[3] The Macarthur Foundation on Depression in Primary Care suggests that a five point drop in the PHQ-9 score from baseline is a sign of adequate treatment and a two to four point drop warrants an increase in medication dose.[11] For those with insomnia, agitation, or anxiety (other than those with chronic anxiety) the NICE guidelines advise treatment with a benzodiazepine for no longer than two weeks to avoid dependence.[3]

If a patient shows no response to the initial antidepressant, the first steps are to check adherence, increase the frequency of appointments, consider the addition of psychotherapy, increase the dose of antidepressant, and consider changing to another antidepressant. The evidence for the effectiveness of an increase in dose or a switch to another antidepressant is not strong. If choosing to change medications, consider a different SSRI and then an antidepressant of a different pharmacological class. After this step, other strategies are best considered after consultation with specialist services and may include augmentation with other drugs (such as lithium, triiodothyronine or second generation antipsychotics) or combination antidepressant treatment.[35] For all these strategies, the effect size is modest and the number of side effects is significantly increased.

Switching Antidepressants

Switching from SSRIs to tricyclics generally means reducing the dose of the SSRI and slowly increasing the dose of the tricyclic from low doses. Fluoxetine, because of its longer half-life, should be stopped four to seven days before starting the tricyclic at a low dose. Monoamine oxidase inhibitors should generally be stopped for two weeks before starting other antidepressants. When switching from a tricyclic to an SSRI the dose of the tricyclic should be halved and the SSRI added before further reducing the dose of the tricyclic. It is wise to consult local prescribing guidelines, seek specialist advice, and read the specific product details of the antidepressant before switching antidepressants.

Stopping Antidepressants

There is no evidence that antidepressants cause psychological dependence, are "addictive," or that people develop tolerance to their actions. However, about a third of patients report discontinuation symptoms when stopping antidepressants, with the greatest risk occurring with paroxetine, venlafaxine, and amitriptyline. The symptoms include affective, gastrointestinal, neuromotor, vasomotor, neurosensory, and other neurological symptoms, which usually occur within five days of stopping treatment. They are best managed by avoiding abrupt withdrawal so that the dose is reduced over four weeks and by reassuring the patient that the symptoms usually disappear after a few days. If the symptoms are severe then the original antidepressant may need to be reintroduced and the dose tapered more gradually.

46.5 MOOD STABILIZING DRUGS

Avinash De Souza

INTRODUCTION

Simply defined, mood stabilizers are medicines used in treating mood disorders such as bipolar disorder and depression. Bipolar disorder is characterized by mood swings in which the individual cycles between mania and depression. The symptoms fluctuate from euphoria and limitless energy in the manic phase to the depths of depression with little energy, guilt, sadness, decreased concentration, lack of appetite, and sleep disturbance. Because of the wide range of symptoms, from mania to depression, bipolar disorder is often called manic depression. Mood stabilizers are used to treat acute mania, hypomania (a mild form of mania), mixed episodes (when mania and depression coexist in an episode), and depression. Following the acute episode, mood stabilizers are used in maintenance therapy to prevent the cyclical relapse of abnormal mood elevations and depressions.

MOOD STABILIZERS

The goals of maintenance treatment with a mood stabilizer are to:

- Reduce residual symptoms
- Prevent manic or depressive relapse
- Reduce the frequency of cycling into the next manic or depressive episode
- Improve functioning
- Reduce the risk of suicide.

LITHIUM

Lithium was one of the first mood stabilizers used in the treatment of bipolar disorder. Lithium is a simple ion not unlike sodium found in table salt (sodium chloride). Lithium comes in two forms—lithium carbonate and lithium citrate. Lithium carbonate is available in immediate—and controlled—release capsules and tablets. Lithium also comes in a liquid preparation in the form of lithium citrate. Over several decades of clinical experience, lithium has been shown to be effective not only in treating mania but also in preventing relapse of mania and depression in bipolar disorder. Lithium was the most important mood stabilizer for many years, but another mood stabilizer—Depakote (divalproex)—has since surpassed lithium for the treatment of bipolar disorder. The reason is that lithium has many troublesome side effects, including nausea, diarrhea, weight gain, and mental sluggishness, and there is a risk of lithium toxicity when the amount of lithium, as measured by serum levels, exceeds its narrow therapeutic range. Monitoring of lithium blood levels is very important to prevent lithium toxicity.

ANTICONVULSANTS AS MOOD STABILIZERS

The introduction of anticonvulsants to the treatment of mood disorders emerged as one of the most significant advances in modern psychiatry. Carbamazepine has been used for more than two decades to treat bipolar disorder without an approved indication for this purpose from the US Food and Drug Administration (FDA). (Divalproex and Lamotrigine) are the only two anticonvulsants approved by the FDA for treatment of seizure and bipolar disorders; the other anticonvulsants are indicated primarily for treatment of epilepsy. The use of a medication for its approved indication is called labeled use. In clinical practice, however, physicians often prescribe medications for unlabeled ("off-label") uses when published clinical studies, case reports, or their own clinical experiences support the efficacy and safety of those treatments. Based on a number of clinical studies, some medications with antiepileptic properties are also effective for treating bipolar disorder, despite the lack of an FDA-approved indication for this purpose. Some may wonder why an anticonvulsant that is effective for controlling seizures also works for bipolar disorder. How is this paradox explained? The application of anticonvulsants in psychiatry was due in part to serendipity. With certain types of epilepsy, individuals sometimes manifest psychiatric symptoms, including hallucinations, agitation, and changes in mood. When such patients were treated with phenytoin, an anticonvulsant, their seizures, as well as their psychiatric symptoms, were stabilized. These observations spurred clinical investigations of other anticonvulsants, including carbamazepine and valproic acid (and valproate), to determine if they also offered benefits in treating mood disorders. It is not totally clear why some anticonvulsants are effective for seizures and bipolar disorder. The anticonvulsants, which have very complex effects on the central nervous system, may be effective by controlling "kindling" in the areas of the brain from which the psychiatric disorder emanates. Kindling is a phenomenon that occurs when repeated subthreshold stimulation is applied to certain regions of the brain and sensitizes them, setting off a cascade of events leading to seizures or manic behavior. By decreasing electrical conduction or neurotransmitter activity in unstable brain cells, anticonvulsants are effective in controlling seizures and bipolar illness.

SECOND-GENERATION ANTIPSYCHOTICS AS MOOD STABILIZERS

Antipsychotics are frequently prescribed in combination with a mood stabilizer, such as lithium, to treat acute mania. An antipsychotic is helpful for rapidly reducing mania, especially during the interval of time until the mood stabilizer, which has a slower onset of action, takes effect. Generally, the psychiatrist would discontinue the antipsychotic after mania abates, maintaining mood stabilization with the mood stabilizer alone. This was the conventional practice when only the older, first-generation antipsychotics were available. The long-term use of conventional antipsychotics was not advisable then because the older agents were associated with significant risks of tardive dyskinesia (disabling, late-onset movement disorders) and extrapyramidal symptoms, which are side effects that affect coordination and movement. Moreover, the conventional agents can exacerbate depressive symptoms in some patients. This strategy—that is, the long-term use of an antipsychotic to treat bipolar disorder—changed when the newer, second-generation antipsychotics became available. These antipsychotics have significantly reduced the risk of tardive dyskinesia and extrapyramidal symptoms and have fewer of the bothersome side effects commonly seen with the conventional agents. Furthermore, they appear to have a wider spectrum of therapeutic activity than the conventional agents. They can do more than just reduce mania; they appear to have mood stabilizing properties and can prevent relapse when used in maintenance therapy. Olanzapine, for example, is currently the only second-generation antipsychotic approved by the FDA for acute mania and maintenance therapy for relapse prevention in bipolar illness. The others are also effective anti-manic agents, but it is not clear whether they also possess mood-stabilizing properties for long-term maintenance therapy. However, some preliminary data show that other second-generation antipsychotics may be effective mood stabilizers as well.

BENEFITS OF MOOD STABILIZERS

Mood stabilizers can help relieve or reduce the symptoms of the illness and also the impact it may have on daily life. They can reduce the need for admission to hospital or shorten the length of stay and help you be able to work and live independently. Mood stabilizers can be used to treat high or low mood as well as reducing the number of times you are ill or the severity of your illness. It may take time to notice the benefits of the medication so it may be worth comparing your highs and lows before you started the medication with how you are while taking the medicine. Lithium has been shown to reduce the risk of suicide in bipolar disorder. Mood stabilizers are generally needed over a long period and you should discuss with your doctor if you intend to stop them as they should be stopped slowly to prevent you becoming ill. It is important that these medications are taken regularly for them to provide their full benefit. Mood stabilizers usually have to be taken for at least 2–5 years.

WHAT EXACTLY IS A MOOD STABILIZER?

Two decades ago, there was 1 drug in the mood stabilizer category: lithium carbonate. Carbamazepine was used in refractory cases and in a small number of specialty clinics. Valproate was entering the scene as a novel and effective mood stabilizer. Since then, it seems that every new anticonvulsant is evaluated for its mood-stabilizing properties. More recently, the atypical antipsychotic drugs have emerged as promising treatments for bipolar disorder, and the evidence supporting their efficacy rivals that of anticonvulsant medications. Other agents, such as calcium-channel blockers, have also been evaluated but have shown little evidence of mood-stabilizing properties. Guidelines for the treatment of bipolar disorder now focus on lithium, a selected number of anticonvulsants and an increasing number of atypical antipsychotic drugs as the principal agents. How does the finding that seemingly disparate classes of medication have a common domain of efficacy shape our definition of what constitutes a "mood stabilizer" and our understanding of their mechanisms of action?

There has been substantial debate about the definition of a mood stabilizer. In general, these definitions are based on antimanic, antidepressant and prophylactic properties to varying degrees, and they usually require 2 of the 3 effects. If we apply such a definition to the agents listed here, more differences than similarities emerge. Lithium remains the gold standard, but patient selection is probably the most important variable in ensuring its effectiveness, because patients with a classic course of illness, family history and good interepisode functioning show the best response. Nonetheless, most patients, regardless of their subtype of illness and clinical features, are exposed at some point in their treatment to lithium. It may indeed become more widely prescribed because of its antisuicide effects, including its ability to prevent suicide in patients who do not have a complete response to the drug. Although valproate remains a widely prescribed agent, it seems to be of limited value in bipolar depression, particularly as monotherapy. Carbamazepine remains an often-underused treatment option that may have a broad range of efficacy. Lamotrigine is the only newer anticonvulsant that is supported by unequivocal evidence as a treatment for bipolar disorder but with its effects, for the most part, limited to the depressed phase and perhaps rapid cycling in patients with type II bipolar disorder. Gabapentin and topiramate were found to be ineffective in bipolar disorder in randomized clinical trials. Atypical antipsychotics as a class have been shown to be effective antimanic agents and their prophylactic and antidepressant effects continue to be studied, with particularly good evidence for olanzapine from randomized clinical trials and for clozapine, at least from open-label studies. The diversity of the agents and the differences in their clinical profiles make it hard to generalize across the agents and determine what distinguishes them as mood stabilizers. Does this call into question our somewhat ambiguous definition of a mood stabilizer?

It may be that overlapping mechanisms of action underlie the mood-stabilizing properties of the agents described here. There has been much progress over the past decade in elucidating the mechanism of action of mood-stabilizing drugs, in particular, lithium and valproate. It is interesting that these 2 drugs share many common targets. Both have wide effects on signal transduction pathways within the cell, and both regulate the expression of a number of important target genes such as BCL-2 and GRP78, which are important in preventing cell death and toxicity. More recently, cellular biology has shown that both lithium and valproate have robust neuroprotective effects after a variety of insults both in cultured cells and in intact animal models. The overlap of targets between these 2 diverse agents is remarkable and, in my view, quite unexpected. Carbamazepine shares some, but not all, these effects, whereas lamotrigine has not been studied widely enough for one to draw many conclusions. Even less is known about the atypical antipsychotics, although several laboratories have published data on the neuroprotective effects of these latter agents, which have some broad similarities to those of both lithium and valproate.

If regulation of signal transduction and its downstream effects is the way in which mood stabilizers work, we are left with a very incomplete picture, particularly for the atypical antipsychotics in contrast with the rather impressive data on their clinical effects. Where do we go next? From a clinical point of view, it seems likely that with more time the picture will become more complex and that specific patient variables in this heterogeneous disorder may be predictive in choosing the right agent for a specific patient. Furthermore, defining a drug as a mood stabilizer may be less relevant than the clinical profile of a specific agent. For instance, certain agents may be more helpful for the depressive part of the illness, namely, lamotrigine, and others for mania, namely, valproate. Such distinctions may be more definitive than assigning drugs to the broader category of mood stabilizers. At a mechanistic level, the shared targets of lithium and valproate remain very intriguing. A concerted effort should be made to understand whether these targets are shared by other agents, such as lamotrigine and atypical antipsychotics. It is also possible that the biologic targets of these agents may show similar variation based on their clinical differences.

INDIVIDUAL DRUG

Lithium

Lithium is effective in the acute treatment of manic and depressive episodes and in the prevention of recurrent manic and depressive episodes. In addition, lithium has been reported to decrease the mood instability that plagues many patients between episodes.

Pharmacokinetics and Drug-Drug Interactions

Lithium is available in tablets or capsules as carbonate salt or as lithium citrate in syrup form. A 300 mg tablet of lithium carbonate contains 8 mEq or mmol of lithium; 5 cc of the citrate syrup also contains 8 meq of lithium. Lithium is readily absorbed after oral administration; no parenteral forms are available. Standard preparations lead to peak serum levels in 1.5–2 hours; slow release forms lead to peak serum levels in 4–4.5 hours. Lithium is excreted almost entirely by the kidneys, with a half-life between 14 and 30 hours (Normally the lithium clearance is about one-fourth of the creatinine clearance). The rate of lithium clearance is faster in younger persons and decreases in association with diminished glomerular function and age.

Therapeutic and toxic effects of lithium are correlated with serum levels, which are correlated, to a lesser extent, with oral dose. Therefore, safe and effective administration of lithium requires that serum levels be monitored. The relatively long half-life of lithium means that steady state levels after a dosage change will not occur for 5–7 days. Trough levels are typically reported, and these are traditionally sampled 12 hours after the last dose. If this procedure is not followed, the results are likely to be unreliable and misleading. The availability of a slow release form and the practice of switching from a multiple dose regimen to a once daily regimen may confuse the interpretation of serum levels. In general, a patient whose lithium regimen changes from twice a day to once a day can expect a 10–26% increase in 12-hour lithium levels.

Lithium is distributed in total body water, is not protein bound, and is not metabolized. Changes in hydration will affect lithium levels, with episodes of dehydration leading to higher levels. Lithium excretion, and therefore serum levels, can be affected by changes in renal function. Decreases in glomerular filtration rates, either due to age or disease, will decrease lithium clearance. In addition, sodium deficiency (secondary to diet, medication, or other causes) will increase lithium reabsorption and increase lithium levels. Thiazide diuretics increase lithium levels by 30–50%. Furosemide appears to have no direct effect on lithium levels, although lithium levels should be monitored in any patient beginning treatment with a diuretic because of potential changes in total body fluid. Many types of medications have been reported to increase lithium levels, including some nonsteroidal anti-inflammatory agents and angiotensin converting enzyme inhibiting antihypertensive agents. Although there have been reports of enhanced neurotoxicity, including the development of neuroleptic malignant syndrome, when lithium was administered in conjunction with a neuroleptic (especially haloperidol), most investigators have found that these medications can be safely combined at standard doses, and are, in fact, used together quite commonly without severe adverse effects.

Side Effects and Toxicity

Up to 75% of patients treated with lithium experience some side effects. These side effects vary in clinical significance; most are either minor or can be reduced or eliminated by lowering the lithium dose or changing the dosage schedule. For example, Schou has reported a 30% reduction in side effects among patients treated with an average lithium level of 0.68 meq/liter compared to those with an average level of 0.85 meq/liter. Side effects, that appear to be related to peak serum levels (e.g. tremor that peaks within 1–2 hours of a dose), may be reduced or eliminated by using a slow release preparation or changing to a single bedtime dose.

Dose-related Side Effects

These include polyuria, polydipsia, weight gain, cognitive problems (e.g. dulling, impaired memory, poor concentration, confusion, mental slowness), tremor, sedation or lethargy, impaired coordination, gastrointestinal distress (e.g. nausea, vomiting, dyspepsia, diarrhea), hair loss, benign leukocytosis, acne, and edema. Side effects persisting despite dosage adjustment may be managed with other mediations (e.g. b-blockers for tremor; diuretics for polyuria, polydipsia or edema; topical antibiotics or retinoic acid for acne). Gastrointestinal disturbances can be managed by administering lithium with meals or switching lithium preparations (especially to lithium citrate).

Lithium may cause benign ECG changes associated with repolarization. Less commonly, cardiac conduction abnormalities have been associated with lithium treatment. Anecdotal reports have linked lithium with other ECG changes, including the exacerbation of existing arrhythmias and, less commonly, the development of new arrhythmias.

The most common renal effect of lithium is impaired concentrating capacity due to reduced renal response to ADH, manifested as polyuria and/or polydipsia. Although the polyuria associated with early lithium treatment may resolve, persistent polyuria (ranging from mild and well tolerated to severe nephrogenic diabetes insipidus) may occur. Polyuria can frequently be managed by changing to a once daily bedtime dose. If the polyuria persists, management includes ensuring that fluid intake is adequate and that the lithium dose is as low as possible. Some clinicians have found that decreasing the total daily protein intake, in conjunction with a nutritional assessment, is helpful. If these measures do not ameliorate the problem, then concurrent administration of a thiazide diuretic (e.g. hydrochlorothiazide at a dose of 50 mg/day) may be helpful. The dosage of lithium will usually need to be decreased (typically by 50%) to account for the increased reabsorption induced by thiazides. In addition, potassium levels will need to be monitored, and potassium sparing diuretics are reported to be effective in treating lithium induced polyuria and do not cause potassium depletion. Amiloride may be started at 5 mg twice a day and may be increased to 10 mg twice a day, as needed.

Hypothyroidism occurs in 5–35% of patients treated with lithium, is more frequent in women, tends to appear after 6 to 18 months of lithium treatment, and may be associated with rapid cycling. Lithium induced hypothyroidism is generally reversible when lithium is discontinued. However, lithium induced hypothyroidism is not a contraindication to continuing lithium treatment. When lithium is continued, the associated hypothyroidism is easily treated by administration of levothyroxine. In addition to the classic signs and symptoms of hypothyroidism, patients with bipolar disorder are at risk of developing depression and/or rapid cycling as a consequence of suboptimal thyroid functioning. If these symptoms occur in the presence of laboratory evidence of suboptimal thyroid functioning, then thyroid supplementation and/or discontinuation of lithium should be considered.

Idiosyncratic Side Effects

A small number of case reports describe exacerbation or first occurrence of psoriasis associated with lithium treatment. Some of these patients improved with appropriate dermatological treatment and/or when the lithium dose was lowered. In some cases, however, lithium seemed to block the treatment and the condition cleared only after lithium was discontinued. In addition, occasionally patients experience severe pustular acne that does not respond well to standard dermatological treatments and only resolves once the lithium has been discontinued (This is in contrast to the more common mild to moderate acne that can occur with lithium treatment and that is usually responsive to standard treatments.

Much concern has been raised about whether long-term lithium exposure may cause irreversible kidney damage. Approximately 10–20% of patients receiving long-term lithium treatment (more than 10 years) display morphological kidney changes—usually interstitial fibrosis, tubular atrophy, and sometimes, glomerular sclerosis. These changes may be associated with impairment of water reabsorption, but not with reduction in glomerular filtration rate or development of renal insufficiency. Although irreversible renal failure due to lithium has not been unequivocally established, there are two case reports of probable lithium induced renal insufficiency. Additionally, several studies show that a small percentage of patients treated with lithium may develop rising serum creatinine concentrations after 10 years or more of treatment.

Toxicity and Overdose

Toxic effects of lithium become more likely as the serum level rises. Most patients will experience some toxic effects with levels above 1.5 mEq/liter; levels above 2.0 mEq/liter are commonly associated with life-threatening side effects. For many patients, the therapeutic range within which beneficial effects outweigh toxic effects is quite narrow, so that small changes in serum level may lead to clinically significant alterations in the beneficial and harmful effects of lithium. Elderly patients may experience toxic effects at lower levels and have a correspondingly narrower therapeutic window.

Signs and symptoms of early intoxication (with levels above 1.5 mEq/liter) include marked tremor, nausea and diarrhea, blurred vision, vertigo, confusion, and increased deep tendon reflexes. With level above 2.5 mEq/liter, patients may experience more severe neurological complications and eventually experience seizures, coma, cardiac dysrhythmia, and permanent neurological impairment. The magnitude of the serum level and the duration of exposure to a high level of lithium are both correlated with risk of adverse effects. Therefore, rapid steps to reduce the serum level are essential. In addition, during treatment for severe intoxication, patients may experience '*secondary peaks*', during which the serum level rises after a period of relative decline; the clinician must therefore, continue to monitor serum levels during treatment for severe intoxication. The patient with lithium intoxication should be treated with supportive care (e.g. maintenance of fluid and electrolyte balance), and steps should be taken to prevent further absorption of the medication (e.g. induction of emesis in the alert patient, gastric lavage).

Hemodialysis is the only reliable method of rapidly removing excess lithium from the body and is more effective than peritoneal dialysis for this purpose. Criteria for use of hemodialysis in lithium intoxication are not firmly established, and the decision to dialyze must take into account both the patient's clinical status and the serum lithium level. While most authorities agree that dialysis should be used in instances when clinical signs of intoxication are severe, it is not clear that a clinically tolerated high lithium level is by itself an indication for dialysis.

Implementing Lithium Treatment

Prior to beginning lithium treatment, the patient's general medical history should be reviewed, with special reference to those systems that might affect, or be affected by, lithium therapy (i.e. renal, thyroid, and cardiac functioning). In addition, pregnancy or the presence of a dermatological disorder must be ascertained.

In general, laboratory measures and other diagnostic tests are recommended based on knowledge of pathophysiology and anticipated clinical decision, rather than on evidence from experimental studies that indicate their clinical utility. The decision to recommend a test is based on the probability of detecting a finding that would alter treatment and the expected benefit of the resulting alteration in treatment. Recommended tests fall into three categories: baseline measures that are used to facilitate the later interpretation of laboratory tests (e.g. ECG, CBC); tests of determine whether different or additional treatments are needed (e.g. pregnancy, thyroid stimulating hormone level); and tests to determine whether the standard dosage regimen of lithium needs to be altered (e.g. creatinine level).

Valproate

Valproate has been studied alone and in combination with other mood stabilizers in all phases of bipolar disorder.

Pharmacokinetics and Drug–Drug Interactions

Valproate is commercially available in the United States in a wide variety of preparations: valproate (available in capsules and syrup), divalproex sodium (an enteric-coated, stable coordination compound containing equal proportions of valproic acid and sodium valproate), and divalproex sodium sprinkle capsules (containing coated particles of divalproex sodium that can be ingested intact or pulled apart and sprinkled on food). There are only minor differences in the pharmacokinetic properties of these different preparations, and valproate is the common compound in plasma. Valproate, in both capsules and syrup, is rapidly absorbed after ingestion; peak serum concentrations are reached within 2 hours. Peak serum concentrations of divalproex sodium are attained within 3 to 8 hours. The plasma half-life of both valproate and divalproex sodium ranges from 6–16 hours.

The relationship between valproate serum concentrations and mood stabilizing effects is not fully defined. The range considered therapeutic for epilepsy is 50–100 μg/mL. A recent study of the use of valproate in patients with acute mania found that the beneficial effects increased markedly with levels above 45 μg/mL and certain adverse effects increased markedly with levels above 125 μg/mL.

Because valproate is extensively metabolized by the liver and is highly protein bound, interactions may occur with other metabolized or protein bound drugs. In addition, valproate weakly inhibits drug oxidation, so serum concentrations of drugs that undergo oxidative metabolism (e.g. phenobarbital, phenytoin, and tricyclics) can be increased when co-administered with valproate. Conversely, valproate serum concentrations can be decreased by coadministration of microsomal enzyme inducing drugs (e.g. carbamazepine) or increased by drugs that inhibit metabolism (e.g. fluoxetine). Also, serum valproate free fraction concentrations can be increased and valproate toxicity precipitated by coadministration of other highly protein bound drugs (e.g. aspirin), which can displace valproate from its protein binding sites.

Side Effects and Toxicity

Minor side effects of valproate, such as sedation or gastrointestinal distress, are common initially and typically resolve with continued treatment or dosage adjustment. In addition, the medication has a wide therapeutic window. Inadvertent overdose in uncommon, and purposeful overdose is less likely to be lethal than with lithium. However, the medication can rarely cause life-threatening reactions, and patients must be relied upon to report the often quite subtle symptoms of these reactions promptly.

Dose-related Side Effects

Common dose-related side effects of valproate include gastrointestinal distress (e.g. anorexia, nausea, dyspepsia, vomiting, diarrhea), benign hepatic transaminase elevations, tremor, and sedation. Patients with past or current hepatic disease may be at increased risk for hepatotoxicity. Mild, asymptomatic leukopenia and thrombocytopenia (reversible upon drug discontinuation) occur less frequently.

Other side effects often bothersome to the patient include hair loss (usually transient), increased appetite, and weight gain.

Persistent gastrointestinal distress associated with valproate can be alleviated by dosage reduction, change of preparation (use of the divalproex sodium formulation rather than valproic acid), or by administration of a histamine-2-antagonist (e.g. famotidine or cimetidine). Tremor can be managed with dosage reduction or co-administration of β-blockers. If mild, asymptomatic thrombocytopenia occurs, a decrease in valproate dosage will usually restore the platelet count to normal. Similarly, cases of mild, asymptomatic leukopenia (total WBC count above 3000 and polymorphonuclear leukocyte count above 1500) is usually reversible upon dosage reduction or discontinuation.

Idiosyncratic Side Effects

One recent uncontrolled report indicated that 80% of women receiving long-term valproate treatment for epilepsy before the age of 20 had polycystic ovaries or hyperandrogenism. The implications of this for women who take valproate for bipolar disorder (both for acute and perhaps maintenance treatment) need to be assessed. Rare, idiosyncratic, but potentially fatal adverse events include irreversible hepatic failure, pancreatitis, and agranulocytosis. Patients taking valproate need to be instructed to contact their psychiatrist immediately if they develop symptoms of these conditions.

Toxicity and Overdose

Valproate has a wide therapeutic window, and unintentional overdose is, therefore, uncommon. Signs of overdose include somnolence, heart block, and eventually coma. Deaths have been reported. Overdose can be treated with hemodialysis and/or naloxone.

Implementing Valproate Treatment

Before initiating valproate treatment, a general medical history should be taken, with special attention to hepatic, hematological, and bleeding abnormalities. Ideally, liver function and hematological measures should be obtained at baseline prior to drug administration to evaluate general medical health.

Valproate may be initiated in low, divided doses to minimize gastrointestinal and neurologic toxicity. Dosage should generally be started at 250 mg three times a day, with the dose increased every few days as side effects allow. The dose is then titrated upward by 250–500 mg/day every several days according to response and side effects, generally to a serum concentration between 50 and 100 μg/mL (with a maximum adult daily dose of 60 mg/kg per day). Patients with acute mania may tolerate larger initial doses of up to 20 mg/kg per day (valproate loading) and more rapid dosage increments than elderly patients and patients who are hypomanic, euthymic, or depressed. Once the patient is stable, valproate dosage regimens can be simplified to enhance convenience and compliance.

Asymptomatic hepatic enzyme elevations, leukopenia, and thrombocytopenia do not reliably predict life-threatening hepatic or bone marrow failure. In conjunction with careful monitoring of clinical status, educating patients about the signs and symptoms of hepatic and hematological dysfunction and instructing them to report these symptoms if they occur is essential. Some investigators believe that routine monitoring of hematological and hepatic function in otherwise healthy patients with epilepsy receiving long-term valproate treatment is not necessary. Nevertheless, most psychiatrists perform clinical assessments, including tests of hematological and hepatic function, at a minimum of every 6 months for stable patients who are taking valproate. Patients who cannot reliably report signs or symptoms of toxicity need to be monitored more frequently.

Carbamazepine

Carbamazepine has been studied alone and in combination with other mood stabilizers in the treatment of all phases of bipolar disorder.

Pharmacokinetics and Drug–Drug Interactions

Carbamazepine is available in a wide variety of preparations, including solutions, suspensions, syrups, and newly developed chewable and slow release formulations. All of these preparations appear to have similar bioavailability.

Peak plasma carbamazepine concentrations are generally obtained between 4 and 8 hours after ingestion, but peaks as late as 26 hours have been reported. The elimination half-life of carbamazepine ranges from 18 to 55 hours. With maintenance treatment, carbamazepine induces its own metabolism and its half-life may be decreased to 5–26 hours.

Because carbamazepine also induces the metabolism of other drugs metabolized by the liver and is highly protein bound, it can have clinically important interactions with other drugs stemming from changes in protein binding and hepatic metabolism. Carbamazepine decreases the plasma levels of many medications metabolized by the liver, including neuroleptics, benzodiazepines (except clonazepam), tricyclic antidepressants, anticonvulsants, sex steroids and hormonal contraceptives, and thyroid hormones.

Conversely, carbamazepine serum concentrations can be increased by drugs that inhibit carbamazepine metabolism, including erythromycin, calcium channel blockers (diltiazem and verapamil, but not nifedipine or nimodipine), and serotonin reuptake inhibitors.

Side Effects and Toxicity

Up to 50% of patients receiving carbamazepine experience side effects and the drug is associated with potentially serious adverse reactions.

Dose-related Side Effects

The most common side effects of carbamazepine include neurological symptoms, such as diplopia, blurred vision, fatigue, nausea, and ataxia. These effects are usually dose related, transient, and often reversible with dosage reduction. Elderly patients, however, may be more sensitive to the side effects.

Less frequent side effects include skin rashes, mild leukopenia, mild thrombocytopenia, hyponatremia, and (less commonly) hyposmolality, and mild liver enzyme elevations (occurring in 5–15% of patients). Mild asymptomatic leukopenia is not related to serious idiopathic dyscrasia and usually resolves with dosage reduction or spontaneously with continuation of carbamazepine treatment. In the event of asymptomatic leukopenia, thrombocytopenia, or elevated liver enzymes, the carbamazepine dosage can be reduced and, with severe ranges, the drug is discontinued.

Hyponatremia may be related to water retention due to carbamazepine's antidiuretic effect. Hyponatremia occurs in 6–31% of patients, is rare in children but probably more common in the elderly, occasionally develops many months after the initiation of carbamazepine treatment, and sometimes necessitates carbamazepine discontinuation. In addition, carbamazepine may decrease total and free thyroxin levels and increase free cortisol levels, but these effects are rarely clinically significant.

Idiosyncratic Side Effects

Rare, idiosyncratic, but serious and potentially fatal side effects of carbamazepine include agranulocytosis, aplastic anemia, hepatic failure, exfoliative dermatitis (e.g. Steven-Johnson Syndrome), and pancreatitis. Although these side effects usually occur within the first 3 to 6 months of carbamazepine treatment, in some cases they occur after more extended periods of treatment. Routine blood monitoring does not reliably predict blood dyscrasias, hepatic failure, or exfoliative dermatitis. Thus, in addition to careful monitoring of clinical status, it is essential to educate patients about the signs and symptoms of hepatic, hematological, or dermatological reactions and instruct them to report symptoms if they occur.

Other rare side effects include systemic hypersensitivity reactions, cardiac conduction disturbances, psychiatric symptoms (including sporadic cases of mania and psychosis), and, very rarely, renal effects (including renal failure, oliguria, hematuria, and proteinuria).

Toxicity and Overdose

Carbamazepine may be fatal in overdose (deaths have been reported with ingestion of more than 6 g). Signs of impending carbamazepine toxicity include dizziness, ataxia, sedation, and diplopia. Acute intoxication can result in hyperirritability, stupor, or coma. The most common symptoms of carbamazepine overdose are nystagmus, ophthalmoplegia, cerebellar and extrapyramidal signs, impairment of consciousness, convulsions, and respiratory dysfunction. Cardiac symptoms may include tachycardia, arrhythmia, conduction disturbances, and hypotension. Gastrointestinal and anticholinergic symptoms may also occur. Management of carbamazepine intoxication includes symptomatic treatment, gastric lavage, and hemoperfusion.

46.6 SEDATIVE HYPNOTIC AND ANXIOLYTIC DRUGS

BS Chavan, Priti Arun

The primary use of drugs, classified as sedative, hypnotic and anxiolytic is to produce calmness and sleep. All central nervous system depressants have some antianxiety effects. A sedative drug reduces daytime activity and calms the recipient; an anxiolytic drug reduces pathological anxiety; and a hypnotic drug produces drowsiness and facilitates the onset and maintenance of sleep. In addition to inducing sleep and reducing pathological anxiety, the various sedative and hypnotics are used as antiepileptic agents, muscle relaxants, antipanic agents, in the treatment of alcohol withdrawal states and as anesthetic agents.

The first agent used as sedative and hypnotic was bromide (1853). Other sedative-hypnotic drugs used before 1900 were chloral hydrate, paraldehyde, urethan and sulfonal. Barbital was introduced in 1903 and phenobar-bital in 1912. Barbiturates were most commonly used sedative-hypnotics till 1961 when chlordiazepoxide was introduced. Since then, many benzodiazepines have been synthesized and marketed.

Benzodiazepines, variously referred to as antianxiety agents, anxiolytics and minor tranquillizers, are prescribed more often and preferred over barbiturates and other drugs because:

- Benzodiazepines have a higher therapeutic index. Doses as high as 50 times of therapeutic dose do not endanger life
- Benzodiazepines do not affect other bodily systems. However, an intravenous injection of diazepam (or lorazepam) might lower the blood pressure
- Benzodiazepines have lower abuse liability as compared to barbiturates
- Benzodiazepines also have antiepileptic properties and are thus preferred in the management of alcohol withdrawal state
- Benzodiazepines do not alter disposition of other drugs by microsomal enzyme induction
- A specific benzodiazepine antagonist (flumazenil)[2] has now been synthesized and used in benzodiazepine overdose poisoning.

BENZODIAZEPINES

Benzodiazepines are the most commonly prescribed group of anxiolytics and sedatives. Benzodiazepines were primarily introduced as anxiolytics and hypnotics. The recent indications for their use include panic disorder, phobia, epilepsy, bipolar disorder, muscle spasms and as anesthetic agents.

Classification

The basic chemical structure of benzodiazepines consists of a benzene ring, fused to the seven sided diazepine ring containing two nitrogens at position 1 and 4 (Fig. 3). Most of the benzodiazepines have another benzene ring attached to the carbon at position 5 on the diazepine ring.

Benzodiazepines can be classified according to substitution at the diazepine ring.

- *2-keto-benzodiazepine:* Keto group is attached to carbon atom at position 2. For example, chlordiazepoxide, diazepam, flurazepam and chlorazepate.
- *3-hydroxy-benzodiazepine*: Hydroxy group is attached to carbon atom at position 3. For example, oxazepam, lorazepam and temazepam.
- *Triazolo-benzodiazepines:* Triazolo ring is attached to nitrogen atom at position 1 and carbon atom at position 2. For example, alprazolam, triazolam.
- *Nitro-benzodiazepines:* Nitrogen atom is attached at position 7 of benzene ring. For example, clonazepam.
- *Imidazo-benzodiazepines:* Imidazo ring is fused to nitrogen at position 1 and carbon at position 2. For example, midazolam.

Pharmacokinetics

- *Absorption:* Benzodiazepines are commonly given orally and are absorbed from small intestine as the benzodiazepines are weak bases and are relatively less ionized in the alkaline environment of small intestine. The rate of oral absorption depends on many factors, including lipophilicity. The absorption of diazepam, lorazepam and alprazolam is rapid. Oxazepam is absorbed at a slower rate than other benzodiazepines. Absorption after

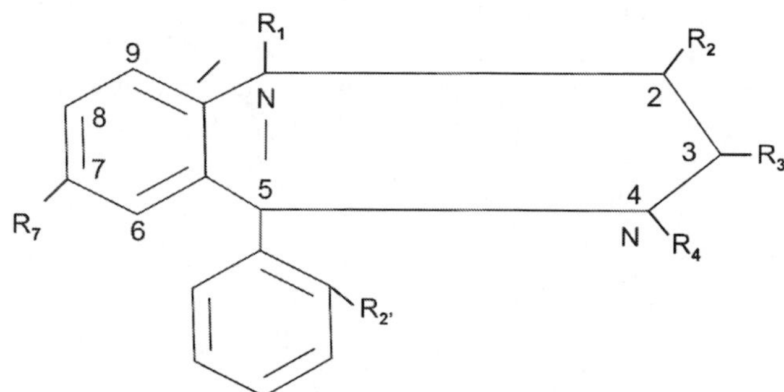

Fig. 3: General structure of benzodiazepines

intramuscular route is unreliable. However, lorazepam has rapid and reliable absorption after intramuscular route.

- *Distribution:* Lipid solubility of benzodiazepines determines the rate at which they enter the central nervous system. For example, diazepam and triazolam are more lipid soluble than chlordiazepoxide and lorazepam, and thus have a rapid onset of action. Most of the benzodiazepine agents are able to cross the placental barriers and thus can reach the fetus during pregnancy. Benzodiazepines also have high protein binding property which varies from 60%–95%.
- *Biotransformation:* Redistribution of benzodiazepines from brain to other tissues is an important means of terminating their actions. However, metabolic transformation to more water soluble metabolites is necessary for clearance of these drugs from the body. Metabolism takes place in liver by dealkylation (Phase 1) and conjugation (Phase 2) reactions. Metabolites of some of the benzodiazepines are pharmacologically active and have a much longer half-life than the parent compound. Water soluble metabolites of benzodiazepines are excreted via kidney (Flow chart 1).

Chlordiazepoxide, diazepam, clorazepate and flurazepam have plasma half-life of 30 to more than 100 hours, because of their active metabolites (desmethyl diazepam) which is slowly metabolized. The plasma half-life can be as high as 200 hours in persons who are genetically slow metabolizers. Patients with hepatic disease, as well as elderly persons, are at risk of toxic effects of benzodiazepines after repeated doses. Oxazepam and lorazepam have short half lives of 10 to 30 hours, because they are directly metabolized by glucuronidation. Triazolam has the shortest half-life of 2–3 hours. The half-life of lorazepam varies from 10–15 hours.

Flow chart 1: Metabolism of benzodiazepines

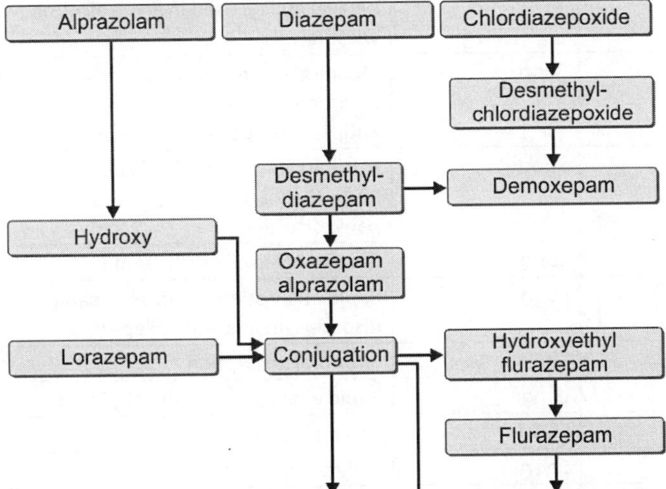

Pharmacodynamics

Benzodiazepines bind to a specific receptor (benzodiazepine receptor) which is closely associated with gamma-amino-butyric acid (GABA) binding sites. GABA is a major inhibitory enzyme in the brain. Benzodiazepine binding increases influx of chloride ions into the cell and thereby causes hyperpolarization.

Pharmacological Actions

Central Nervous System

Benzodiazepines selectively act on polysynaptic neuronal pathways throughout the central nervous system (CNS). The effects on the midbrain reticular formation are most important, as this part of brain is involved in the maintenance of wakefulness. Mesencephalic reticular formation is very sensitive to the effects of benzodiazepines. Benzodiazepines are not truly GABA-mimetic because they are inactive when GABA is depleted. The simulation of the effects of GABA by benzodiazepines may be due to an action of the drug to antagonize a protein that inhibits the binding of GABA to its receptors.

Seizures, elicited by repetitive stimulation of the amygdala, are prevented by both diazepam and phenobarbital. Benzodiazepines prevent the spread of seizure rather than suppress the action on the cerebellum. Benzodiazepines decrease the firing rate of Purkinje cells.

The mechanism of the paradoxical excitement, that is occasionally caused by benzodiazepines, is not known. Benzodiazepines are known to affect the brain turnover of various neurotransmitters. Benzodiazepines decrease the turnover of norepinephrine. The turnover of dopamine is increased at some sites and decreased at other sites. In addition, 5-HT turnover is also decreased.

Respiration

The therapeutic doses of various sedatives and hypnotics in normal individuals do not have any effect on respiration. However, sedatives-hypnotics, even at therapeutics doses can produce significant respiratory depression in patients with obstructive pulmonary diseases. Effects on respiration are dose related and the cause of death in overdose poisoning is often depression of medullary respiratory center.

Cardiovascular System

Hypnotics and sedatives in therapeutic doses do not have significant effects on cardiovascular system. Anesthetic doses of diazepam may moderately decrease left ventricular stroke volume and cardiac output, leading to decrease in systolic pressure and reflex increase in systemic peripheral resistance and heart rate. At toxic doses, myocardial contractibility and vascular tone may be depressed by central and peripheral effects, leading to circulatory collapse.

Gastrointestinal Tract

There is no experimental evidence that benzodiazepines have significant direct effects on the gastrointestinal tract.

NICE Guideline

Drugs used as hypnotics	*dose (mg/day)*
Lormetazepam	0.5–1.5
Oxazepam	15–30
Nitrazepam	5–10
Temazepam	10–20
Zaleplon	10
Zopiclone	3.75–7.5
Zolpidem	5–10
Melatonin	2
Promethazine (not licensed)	25–50

Clinical Uses

Anxiety

In psychiatry outpatient department, anxiety is the most common symptom. Anxiety is also commonly associated with adjustment disorders, depression, obsessive compulsive disorder, and many other psychiatric as well as medical illnesses. The most common use of benzodiazepines in psychiatry is in the treatment of anxiety. Benzodiazepines are effective both in anxiety neurosis as well as anxiety symptoms associated with other psychiatric and medical illnesses. However, most of the patients, in addition to antianxiety drugs, need counseling or psychotherapy.

All the benzodiazepines are equally effective. The choice of a particular benzodiazepine is made on the basis of its pharmacokinetic properties. A long-acting benzodiazepine may be preferred for persistent and sustained anxiety, while a short acting benzodiazepine is ideal for situational and short lasting anxiety. Short acting benzodiazepines are also preferred for insomnia when day time drowsiness is not desired. Table 9 shows pharmacokinetic properties of some of the commonly used benzodiazepines.

Guidelines for prescribing antianxiety drugs:

- Benzodiazepines should be prescribed in lowest effective doses, for shortest duration.
- Abuse liability of benzodiazepines should be kept in mind. Short acting benzodiazepines have higher abuse liability.
- Patients with history of alcohol and drug abuse are more likely to abuse benzodiazepines.
- Benzodiazepines should not be mixed with alcohol, opiates and antihistaminic drugs.

Table 9: Pharmacokinetic properties of selected benzodiazepines

Drug	*Adult dose (Range)/day*	*Strengths available*	*Average elimination half life (Hours)*	*Short/Long acting*	*Comments*
Diazepam	5–60	2, 5, 10 mg (tablets) 5 mg per mL (injection)	100 (50–100)	Long	Rapid absorption. Used in acute alcohol withdrawal. Poor intramuscular bioavailability
Chlordiaze-poxide	15–100	5, 10, 25 mg (tablets)	100	Long	Medium rate of absorption. Poor in bioavailability. Used in acute alcohol withdrawal
Alprazolam	0.5–6	0.25, 0.5, 1 mg (tablets)	12	Short	Medium absorption. Has antidepressant and antipanic property
Lorazepam	2–6	1, 2 mg (tablets)	15	Short	Medium absorption. Rapid absorption from IM sites. Used in anxiety and panic disorder
Nitrazepam	10–50	5, 10 mg (tablets)	30	Long	Commonly used as a hypnotic
Clonazepam	0.5–10	0.5, 1, 2 mg (tablets)	34	Long	Rapid absorption. Effective in panic disorders, mania and epilepsy
Oxazepam	30–120	15, 30 mg (tablets)	8	Short	Slow oral absorption
Flurazepam	15–30	15 mg (tablets)	100	Long	Rapid absorption. Used as hypnotic
Triazolam*	0.125–0.25	0.125, 0.25 mg (tablets)	2	Short	Rapid absorption
Midazolam*	1.0–5.0	1 mg/mL; 5 mg/mL	2.5	Short	Only parenteral preparation available

* Not available in India

- Organic cause of anxiety (e.g. thyroid dysfunction, caffeinism, medication) should be ruled out.
- Length of therapy should be decided in the beginning and need for longer therapy should be frequently reassessed.
- When drug is to be discontinued, drug should be slowly tapered off.
- Benzodiazepines should be prescribed under strict medical monitoring in patients of obstructive pulmonary disease and in those with hypersensitivity to benzodiazepines.

Insomnia

The main aim in the treatment of insomnia is to induce sleep as quickly as possible, maintenance of sleep, and patient should awake refreshed in the morning (no drowsiness). All the benzodiazepines in adequate doses will produce hypnotic effect. However, the choice of a benzodiazepine as a hypnotic depends upon its pharmacokinetic properties. Nitrazepam, flurazepam and triazolam are preferred as hypnotics.

Most benzodiazepines decrease sleep latency and diminish the number of awakenings as well as increase the awakening threshold. The time spent in stage 2 (non-REM) sleep is increased by all benzodiazepines. Benzodiazepines decrease time spent in slow wave sleep (stage 3 and 4). All benzodiazepines also increase the REM latency.

Epilepsy and Seizures

Most of the central nervous system depressants have some property of suppressing the seizure activity. Clonazepam and diazepam are commonly used in the treatment of epilepsy. Intravenous diazepam is still the drug of choice in the treatment of status epilepticus.

Muscle Relaxation

Benzodiazepines are known to depress polysynaptic reflexes and may even depress transmission at neuromuscular junction at higher doses. Benzodiazepines have shown improvement in decerebrate rigidity in cats and spasticity in patients of cerebral palsy. Diazepam is commonly used for muscular relaxation in joint disease and muscle spasms.

Alcohol Withdrawal State

Long-acting benzodiazepines are the drugs of choice in the treatment of alcohol withdrawal state. These are preferred over barbiturates and other sedatives because of their anticonvulsant property, high therapeutic margin, low abuse potential and cross-tolerance with alcohol.

Panic Disorders

Alprazolam and clonazepam are commonly used in the treatment of panic disorders as well as phobic disorders.

Bipolar Disorder

Clonazepam is effective in the management of acute mania and also as an adjunct to lithium therapy, because antipsychotic drugs have more side effects and social stigma. Clonazepam is also used in the prophylaxis of bipolar disorder in combination with lithium.

Other Indications

Benzodiazepines are very effective in the treatment of drug induced akathisia. Benzodiazepines have also been used in the treatment of nausea or vomiting caused by chemotherapy. Sedative-hypnotics have also been used as an adjunct to anesthesia.

Drug Interactions

Cimetidine, disulfiram, isoniazid and estrogens increase the metabolism of benzodiazepines. Plasma levels of phenytoin and digoxin may be increased by benzodiazepines. Benzodiazepines will have additive CNS depression, when combined with alcohol, opiates and antihistamines.

Adverse Effects

- The *most common undesirable effects* are drowsiness, excessive sedation, impaired motor coordination, confusion and memory loss. These effects are more pronounced in first 7–10 days and gradually tolerance develops to most of these side effects. Thus, the patient is advised not to drive and operate machinery in the first few days. The less common side effects are dizziness, ataxia, blurred vision, nausea or vomiting, and epigastric distress. Anterograde amnesia has also been reported with the use of benzodiazepines. More serious side effects (overdose and CNS depression) develop when benzodiazepines are combined with other CNS depressants. Benzodiazepines can produce respiratory depression in patients of pulmonary obstructive disease. There is some evidence that benzodiazepines are teratogenic and their use during pregnancy is not advised. Benzodiazepines are also excreted in milk.
- *Hypersensitivity*: Allergic reaction to benzodiazepines are rare. Occasionally, generalized itching, rashes, and swelling of eyelids and lips may develop.
- *Idiosyncrasy*: Benzodiazepines may cause paradoxical effects, e.g. excitement, hostility and antisocial acts. The exact mechanism is not known. Alteration in dose (increase or decrease) may eliminate these effects. Rarely, chlorpromazine may be required.
- *Tolerance and dependence:* Benzodiazepines are generally known to have low abuse liability, as compared to barbiturates and many other CNS depressants. When benzodiazepines are used in low doses for a short period,

there may not be any evidence of tolerance, dependence or withdrawal (Table 10). Dependence on benzodiazepines will depend upon:

- Length of time benzodiazepines have been used,
- Daily dose the patient has been taking,
- Half-life of the benzodiazepine, and
- Rate at which drug is tapered off.

Abrupt discontinuation of a benzodiazepine, particularly of a short acting benzodiazepine, will result in severe withdrawal, if the drug has been used for long periods in high doses. Appearance of withdrawal may be delayed up to 2–3 days in short-acting benzodiazepines and 10–14 days in case of long-acting benzodiazepines.

The common withdrawal symptoms consist of anxiety, irritability, insomnia, fatigue, headache, tremors, muscle twitching, and sweating. Severe withdrawal symptoms may include nausea, loss of appetite, paranoia, depression, convulsions, depersonalization and derealization. On many occasions, distinction between relapse/re-emergence of anxiety symptoms on sudden withdrawal and specific benzodiazepine withdrawal state is difficult. The symptoms listed above in severe category suggest a specific withdrawal state. The occurrence of dependence will be minimized by cautious prescription of benzodiazepines in lowest effective dose for shortest period and need of longer prescription should be frequently reassessed.

BENZODIAZEPINE ANTAGONIST

Flumazenil is a competitive antagonist at the benzodiazepine receptors. It may also have some agonist actions. Because of a short-half live (t½, 1 hour), it has to be given in repeated intravenous doses (0.2–0.5 mg) in benzodiazepine overdose. The response is very quick and patient may become alert in 5 minutes. In addition to the management of benzodiazepine overdose, it may also be useful in the diagnosis of benzodiazepine overdose. Sedation and respiratory depression due to nonbenzodiazepines are not reversed with flumazenil.

Table 10: Common withdrawal symptoms of benzodiazepines

- Mild
  - Anxiety
  - Insomnia
  - Headache
  - Irritability
  - Weakness
- Moderate
  - Muscle twitching
  - Tremors
  - Sweating
  - Difficulty in concentration
- Severe
  - Loss of appetite
  - Nausea
  - Depression
  - Withdrawal seizures
  - Paranoia
  - Depersonalization
  - Derealization

BUSPIRONE

Buspirone relieves anxiety without sedation. Unlike benzodiazepines, it lacks hypnotic, anticonvulsant, and muscle relaxant properties. Its mechanism of action is not known. Buspirone has binding affinity for $5HT_1$, $5HT_2$ and D_2 receptor binding sites. It does not bind to the GABA chloride receptor complex and, thus, does not reverse benzodiazepine withdrawal state.

The absorption of buspirone after oral administration is nearly 100%, but it undergoes extensive first pass metabolism which limits its bioavailability to about 3%. The half-life of buspirone varies from 2 to 11 hours.

The most common side effects associated with buspirone include dizziness, nausea, headache, nervousness, light headedness, dry mouth, and diarrhea. Buspirone has little effect on respiratory system, the heart, blood pressure, platelets, smooth muscle, or the autonomic nervous system.

Buspirone is indicated for the treatment of generalized anxiety disorder. It has also been tried in performance anxiety, social phobia, and major depressive disorder with mixed results. It has been found useful for augmentation of serotonin-specific reuptake inhibitors (SSRIs) used in the treatment of obsessive compulsive disorder. It has also been tried in cocaine, phencyclidine, tobacco, and alcohol withdrawal with mixed results.

CHLORAL HYDRATE

It is the oldest synthetic drug used as a hypnotic. Chloral hydrate is a liquid, irritant to buccal and gastric mucosa, and has a horrible, burning taste. It is metabolized in liver and is converted to an active metabolite (trichloroethanol) by alcohol dehydrogenase enzyme. Trichloroethanol is conjugated to glucuronic acid and is extracted in urine. After the discovery of benzodiazepines, chloral hydrate is no more used as a hypnotic.

BARBITURATES

Because of higher abuse potential, low therapeutic range and serious interaction with other drugs, barbiturates are not used nowadays as hypnotic and antianxiety agents. However, barbiturates are still used for the treatment of seizure disorders and general anesthesia. Benzodiazepines have replaced the barbiturates as hypnotics, sedatives and antianxiety agents.

ANTIDEPRESSANTS

Tricyclic antidepressants, such as doxepin and amitriptyline, produce considerable sedation and are used in the management of anxiety symptoms associated with depression. However, because of anticholinergic and other side effects, antidepressants are rarely used in the treatment of anxiety symptoms.

BETA-ADRENERGIC BLOCKING AGENTS

Beta-adrenergic blocking antagonist, such as propranolol, have been widely used in the treatment of anxiety symptoms. Beta blockers are more effective when somatic symptoms of anxiety are more predominant, such as sweating, palpitation, tremors and tachycardia.

ZOPICLONE

Zopiclone is from a new class of anxiosedative agents, the cyclopyrrolones, which are structurally unrelated to benzodiazepines. Cyclopyrrolones also act on the GABA receptors but at a site distinct from that of the benzodiazepines.

It has a short duration of action as well as shorter onset. Zopiclone has a potent hypnotic effect. After oral administration, zopiclone is absorbed rapidly with peak plasma concentration occurring in about 60 minutes. Bioavailability is about 80% and the elimination half-life is 3.5–6.5 hours.

The usual dose of zopiclone is 7.5 mg at night-time. The dose may be reduced to half in elderly patients and in patients with severe hepatic failure.

The side effects include bitter taste, dry mouth, drowsiness, nausea and headache. It does not have any interaction with ranitidine and care should be exercised when used concurrently with tri-imipramine and alcohol.

NICE Guidelines for prescribing hypnotics:

- Use the lowest effective dose
- Use intermittent dosing (alternate nights or less) where possible
- Prescribe for short-term use (no more than 4 weeks) in the majority of cases
- Discontinue slowly
- Be alert for rebound insomnia/withdrawal symptoms
- Advise patients of the interaction with alcohol and other sedating drugs
- Avoid the use of hypnotics in patients with respiratory disease or severe hepatic impairment and in addiction-prone individuals

46.7 ELECTROCONVULSIVE THERAPY

Eesha Sharma, Urvakhsh Mehta, Jagadisha Thirthalli, BN Gangadhar

Electroconvulsive therapy (ECT) is a treatment modality for psychiatric disorders, wherein passing an electric current through the scalp, under medical supervision, produces a seizure. It is used in the treatment of a wide range of psychiatric disorders particularly when other treatments are unlikely to produce effect quickly, have failed or are not well tolerated.

HISTORY OF ELECTROCONVULSIVE THERAPY

Owing perhaps to a supposition that epileptic seizures and schizophrenia were antagonistic to each other, a number of methods of inducing seizures were being sporadically used since the 16th century to cure different types of psychiatric disorders.

In 1938, Italian neurologist Ugo Cerletti and his colleague Lucio Bini, after several trials of electrically inducing seizures in animals, applied the same to a patient with delusions. The patient improved after 11 treatment sessions without significant side effects. This was a huge improvement over the very unpleasant effects of camphor and metrazol that were used earlier. Max Fink and others later conducted rigorous scientific research on ECT, including randomized controlled trials. This was followed by refinements in ECT practice, including the use of muscle relaxants to prevent fractures from violent convulsions, replacement of sine-wave stimulus with pulsed, square-wave stimulus and the use of unilateral ECT to reduce cognitive deficits. With the advent of psychotropic medications, there was a decline in the use of ECT. Negative coverage on ECT in media also contributed to this decline.

In 1985, the National Institute of Mental Health and the National Institutes of Health of the USA conducted a consensus-developing conference on ECT. The consensus stated that there is a definite therapeutic role for ECT in certain conditions, even though it may be a controversial treatment with significant cognitive side effects. Professional bodies of several countries, including USA, UK, Austria, Canada, Australia, Denmark, Netherlands, Germany, and India have offered professional guidelines for the practice of ECT, covering various issues like consent, unilateral ECTs, delivery protocol, education and training, and the role of ECT in current practice. These developments in the last 2–3 decades have renewed practice and acceptability of ECT.

ELECTRICAL ASPECTS

Electrical stimulation generates a seizure, the essential therapeutic ingredient in ECT. The electric stimulation comprises of a predecided amount of electricity passing over a prefixed duration of time. The scalp and skull offer some impedance to the passage of electricity. The stimulation parameters have to be arranged to overcome the impedance and deliver enough charge to produce a seizure. An understanding of the electrical aspects of ECT is essential to maximize benefit and minimize adverse effects.

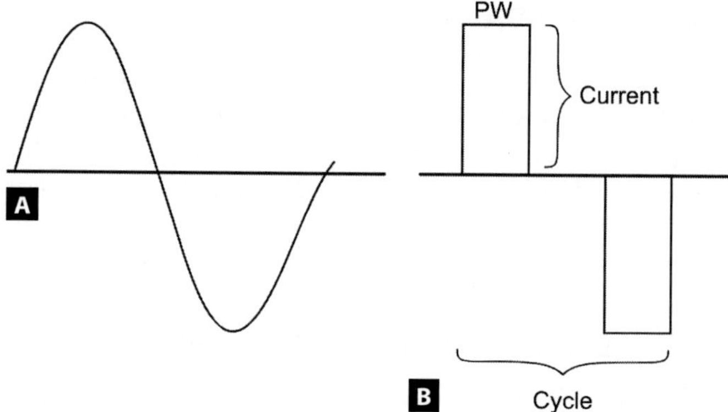

Figs 4A and B: Shapes of waveforms of stimulus. (A) Sine wave (B) Pulse wave. PW, pulse-width in milliseconds; current in Amperes; a pair of pulses in the opposite directions make a cycle

Impedance

This is the resistance to flow of current. Impedance is determined by the quality of electrode contact with the patient's skin. It is reduced with the use of conducting gel on the electrodes, the shape of the electrodes, making sure the site of contact is clean and holding electrodes firmly at the site during administration of stimulus. Convex electrodes are used for bitemporal ECT, and concave for bifrontal so as to maximize surface area of contact to facilitate current passage. Impedance also results from varying electrical properties of the skin, hair, skull, blood vessels, meninges, brain and cerebrospinal fluid. Some ECT machines are able to determine the amount of dynamic resistance and adjust the voltage accordingly, while other machines assume preset estimates of resistance. Most contemporary ECT machines deliver a constant current—they dynamically adjust the voltage to ensure prefixed amperage.

Waveform (Figs 4A and B)

Initial ECT machines delivered sine-wave stimulus. The slow rising and trailing edges of the sine wave unnecessarily stimulated the brain tissue with subthreshold stimuli and through the postdepolarization refractory period respectively. This reduced efficiency of the stimulus and also increased adverse effects. The sine wave was hence modified to eliminate the rising and trailing edges, to retain only the peaks as brief pulses, 1–2 millisecond wide. Further, intermittent stimulation using pulses is more efficient, as it allows the neuronal tissue to recover from the refractory period. Thus, compared to a constant-voltage sine wave, a constant-current brief pulse stimulus is more efficient; the latter needs less than a third of the stimulus dose of the former, when given to a patient with same impedance (Table 11).

Brief pulse ECT produces lesser:
- Postictal disorientation
- Postictal EEG suppression
- Amnesic effects on standard memory tests than sine wave ECT.

Characteristics of the Brief Pulse

- *Amplitude*: This is the height of the pulse wave and gives the amount of current flowing. It is measured in milli ampere (mA) or ampere (A). This is prefixed in a constant current type of ECT machine. It should be kept between 0.5 and 1A (optimal value 0.8A).

Table 11: Comparison of waveforms

Parameter[2]	*Current*	*Voltage*	*Frequency*[3]	*Width*[4]	*Duration*[5]	*Impedance*	*Energy*[6]	*Charge*[1,6]
Brief pulse	**0.8 A**	160 V	**100 pps**	**1 ms**	**1 s**	200 Ohm	12.8 J	80 mC
Sine wave	0.6 A	**120 V**	50 Hz	—	**0.5 s**	200 Ohm	36 J	300 mC

1. At conventional threshold settings, sine: pulse = 3:1
2. Parameters which can be chosen by the operator are in **bold** face
3. Frequency = Number of cycles/second; PPS = Pulses per second
4. Width: Relevant only to pulse stimuli
5. Stimulus duration: Total period for which the stimulus train is applied
6. Unit of energy is Joule (J) and of charge, Millicolomb (mC). Latter is preferred for indicating the stimulus dose.

- *Polarity*: Unipolar pulses are all in one direction while bimodal pulses are delivered in both positive and negative phases. Most devices give bimodal pulses.
- *Pulse width*: This is the duration, in milliseconds (ms) of each pulse. In brief square wave pulses the width may vary between 0.5 and 1.5 ms. Pulse width tells us the duration for which neurons are stimulated by a single pulse. Wider pulses may be inefficient because the chronaxie of the mammalian neurons is in the range of 0.1–0.2 ms. 'Ultra-brief' pulses, now being increasingly researched, are of the order of ≤0.5 ms, and may be more efficient (i.e. use less charge) at seizure elicitation. In depression, use of ultra-brief pulse ECT is likely to cause less adverse cognitive effects without seriously compromising efficacy. It is not explored in other disorders.
- *Pulse frequency*: This is the number of pulses, or the number of pulse pairs in bipolar ECT stimulus delivered in a second and is also measured in Hertz (Hz). It should be reflective of the refractory period of the neurons, as higher pulse frequencies may lead to stimulation of neurons during their refractory period. Indeed, stimulus at 50 pulses per second has been shown to be more efficient (i.e. seizure is elicited at a lower stimulus intensity) than that at 200 pulses per second. However, for stimulation of deeper structures and while using ultra brief pulses, higher frequencies may be needed to aid stimulation by temporal summation.
- *Stimulus duration*: Stimulus duration, measured in seconds(s), is the total length of stimulation. It is usually kept between 0.2 and 4s. It has been demonstrated that increasing the duration of stimulation by varying pulse frequency/pulse width decreases the threshold for stimulation.

Electrode placement: Four types of electrode placement have been used.

1. *Bitemporal*: The electrodes are placed bilaterally about 2.5 cm above the midpoint of an imaginary line joining the outer canthus of eye to the external auditory meatus.
2. *Bifrontal*: The electrodes are placed 5 cm superior to the outer angle of the orbits.
3. *Unilateral*: For right-handed patients, one electrode is placed in the right temporal position and the second electrode is placed just to the right of the vertex, the highest point on the skull. Efficacy of treatment does not vary with which side ECT is administered; however, cognitive side effects may be more with the dominant hemisphere.
4. *Left anterior right temporal (LART)*: One electrode is placed in the right temporal position. The second electrode is placed on the left side, 5 cm anteriorly to the bitemporal position.

The main purpose of variations in electrode placement is to strike a balance between therapeutic efficacy and cognitive adverse effects. Factors important here are—distance between electrodes and the brain region directly beneath the electrodes. In bitemporal placement, the electrodes are placed furthest apart. The larger the brain area between electrodes, the greater is the number of seizure foci generated, and, to stimulate all of these, a higher dose of stimulation is required. Bitemporal stimulation produces the most well generalized seizure activity in the brain, but at the cost of highest amount of cognitive side effects. In contrast, unilateral placement has less brain area between the electrodes. Lower charge is required for stimulation, however, for a well-generalized seizure the dose has to be kept much higher than the threshold. Similar sites in the two cerebral hemispheres have complementary roles in higher mental functions. Areas directly below the stimulating electrode have the largest current density and likely to suffer maximum adverse effects. Understandably, stimulating identical areas on the two sides would result in greater cognitive side effects. Unilateral or LART placements reduce this risk. Overall, unilateral placement is cognitively safer but may be slightly less efficacious than bitemporal placement; bifrontal ECT may have the best balance of efficacy and adverse effect.

Stimulus Used for Treatment

Seizure threshold stimulus is defined as the lowest stimulus (in millicoulombs) at which an adequate seizure is produced. Though the induction of seizure is necessary for clinical response, it is not in itself sufficient. Elegant studies have demonstrated therapeutic inferiority of ECT using charge at threshold level, more so with unilateral application. Hence, suprathreshold stimulus is used. Both efficacy and side effects are related to the degree by which stimulus exceeds seizure threshold rather than the absolute magnitude of the stimulus. Hence, a well-balanced decision should be taken regarding the degree by which the stimulus should exceed threshold-level. Generally, stimulus used is 1.5–2 times higher in bilateral ECT and 4–6 times higher in unilateral ECT.

Determination of the seizure threshold can be done by the following methods:

- *Dose titration method*: Increasing doses of electrical stimulus are given till the patient gets an adequate seizure. From the next session suprathreshold doses are used. Empirical dose titration is the most favored method currently. Threshold is known to increase with number of sessions in the ECT course. Therefore, if ECTs are to be continued beyond two weeks, threshold should be re-estimated and dose adjusted accordingly.
- *Formula-based method*: Threshold is estimated here by taking into account various influencing factors like age, sex, concurrent drugs, etc (e.g. three times the age in years = threshold).
- *Fixed dose method*: Here all patients are given a same pre-fixed dose. This method is outdated, as a majority of the

patients would be receiving a dose much higher than is required.

The total stimulus given is calculated by the following formula: Charge (mC) = Current (mA) × Stimulus duration (s) × Frequency (pulse per second) × Pulse width (ms). For example for a current of 0.8 A, pulse width of 1 ms, pulse frequency of 100 and a train length of 1.5 ms, the charge provided will be 120 mC. The determined dose of stimulus may be administered by altering any of these variables. It may be useful to note that a dose of 120 mC is approximately equivalent to the electricity used in lighting a 40 watt bulb for less than a second's duration.

Frequency of Treatment

Electroconvulsive therapies are usually administered twice or thrice weekly, during acute treatment. The efficacy does not vary greatly between the two regimens. Speed of improvement is greater with thrice weekly ECTs but this comes with a higher likelihood of cognitive side effects. The total number of ECTs that are to be given for adequate treatment is not fixed. The patient has to be evaluated after each session for response. If a patient with depression has not shown any response after six sessions, ECT may be abandoned. If definite but only partial response is noted, continuing ECT for 12 sessions may be tried.

Continuation and Maintenance ECT (C-ECT and M-ECT)

The ECT is generally used to achieve remission in acute illness. Subsequently, without adequate pharmacological prophylaxis, relapse rates may be very high. For some patients pharmacological interventions fail to prevent relapse. Continuation ECT may be used when—the index episode has responded well to ECT, early relapse occurs despite adequate pharmacotherapy or drugs are not well tolerated, and psychosocial and medical factors are conducive to continuing ECT. By definition, C-ECT is used to prevent relapse of index illness episode. It is used over first 6 months after remission. M-ECT is used to prevent further episodes or recurrences of illness. It is continued beyond 6 months. The frequency may be variable in both. No consensus recommendations exist for these regimens; however, clinical data suggests reduced relapse rates in schizophrenia, bipolar illness and major depression. Evidence regarding cognitive deficits is lacking and hence careful monitoring of the same is recommended.

Focal Electrically Administered Seizure Therapy

Focal electrically administered seizure therapy (FEAST) is a novel and different ECT procedure. This incorporates modifications in three aspects of stimulation, (1) the directionality or mode of current, (2) polarity of electrodes and (3) electrode placement. It has been held that generalization of seizure is vital in the therapeutic efficacy of ECT. However, anodal stimulation of the prefrontal cortex with cathodal inhibition of the surrounding cortex, in depression produced therapeutic effects. In conventional bilateral ECT with bidirectional pulses, the two electrodes alternatively act as anode and cathode. Unidirectional pulses are more efficacious at seizure generation, in that the thresholds are much lower, and allow use of unipolar electrodes. Also, cognitive side effects are understandably lesser with a restricted area of stimulation.

Magnetic Seizure Therapy

Transcranial magnetic stimulation (TMS) induces an electric current within the brain by an electrically generated magnetic field outside it. The TMS used at convulsive parameters can produce seizures. This is now being used in a novel technique called magnetic seizure therapy or magnetic seizure therapy (MST). Similar to ECT, a short general anesthesia is used during seizure induction. MST is capable of focally stimulating the brain rather than the widespread stimulation in ECT. Preliminary data show that it may have antidepressant efficacy with lesser cognitive side effects.

MECHANISM OF ACTION

von Meduna had postulated that ECT affects the chemical composition of the brain and the changes resulting thereof are therapeutic. Several studies have tried to study what really is the therapeutic change effected by ECT. It seems that repetitive stimulation leads to longstanding changes that are more relevant to the effects of ECT rather than the transient effects of a single stimulation. ECT has a wide spectrum of action. It has been used in depression, mania, psychosis, catatonia, suicidality, epilepsy, and neurological disorders, etc. Notably, it helps in depression and mania, two seemingly opposite conditions. These observations suggest that complex processes are at play.

Psychological Theories

These were among the earliest theories to explain the mechanism of action of ECT and reflect the then prevailing models of mental illness. They have now been discarded, and currently hold only academic and historical interest, as they cannot be verified. *Psychoanalytic theories* propounded 'fear' of ECT, 'regression' to a stage of infancy, and 'punishment' for bad behavior. The efficacy of modified ECT and of real over sham ECT is evidence against these theories. One of the non-psychoanalytic theories spoke of 'brain damage' caused by ECT, however no evidence of brain damage has been seen on autopsy specimens or neuroimaging. The other theory talked about ECT induced 'amnesia' making the patient 'forget' his illness-related behaviors. Modifications in ECT technique that reduce cognitive side effects do not affect its therapeutic efficacy.

Neurophysiological Theories

Neurophysiological changes observed with ECT reflect an increase in inhibitory neurotransmission and neuropeptides. Markers of this inhibitory process, that terminates seizures, correlate with efficacy of ECT. The occurrence of generalized and repeated seizures has been long held as the therapeutic ingredient of ECT. In support of this, isolated or sub-convulsive stimuli show weaker or no therapeutic effect. An extended activation of corticosubcortical circuits is needed for efficacious ECT. ECT also has an anticonvulsant action. Over a course of ECTs seizure threshold increases and seizure duration decreases, the former being associated with therapeutic benefit. On the EEG, slow wave activity increases. There is a marked increase seen in the interictal EEGs during a course of ECT. This change persists for weeks after ECT completion. It may reflect the inhibition of cortical pyramidal cells by GABAergic interneurons or a summation of long duration after-hyperpolarization in the deep cortical pyramidal cells. Therapeutic effects are more with greater postictal suppression, i.e. slow-wave activity that has an earlier onset, is of higher amplitude and low frequency.

ECT reduces cerebral blood flow and glucose metabolism. This change, seen more in the anterior frontal regions in the immediate postictal period, lasts from weeks to months and is associated with superior clinical outcome. Diminished functional activity in specific brain regions may be a key neurophysiological change underlying therapeutic effect of ECT. The prefrontal cortex, with its critical role in integration of cognition and emotion, is one such area. ECT also increases the permeability of the blood-brain barrier. This may theoretically facilitate entry into the brain, of coadministered psychotropic drugs, thus increasing their efficacy.

Neurochemical and Neuroendocrine Theories

Depression and other psychiatric disorders have altered serotonergic, norepinephrinergic or dopaminergic neurotransmission in key brain regions. Such changes may be due to pathology at the neurotransmitter, receptor, or signal transduction levels. A downregulation of postsynaptic β-1 and noradrenergic autoreceptors (α2), upregulation and sensitization of postsynaptic 5-HT_1A serotonergic receptors, a downregulation of dopaminergic autoreceptors and upregulation of postsynaptic dopamine receptors is seen following a course of ECT. These may be responsible for the antidepressant and anti-Parkinsonian (via increase in dopaminergic transmission) action of ECT. To account for the delayed therapeutic effects of ECT, intracellular changes have been studied. It is seen that ECT leads to an increase in calcium influx and stimulation of protein synthesis via C-fos protooncogene.

Neuroendocrine dysfunction, predominantly in the hypophysiopituitary-adrenal (HPA) axis, is associated with depression. ECT induces a widespread endocrine release including prolactin, corticotropin, cortisol, thyroid-stimulating hormone (TSH), arginine vasopressin (AVP), neuropeptide Y (NPY), β-endorphin and growth hormone. However, most of these endocrine changes are reflective of general responses to any kind of stress and are nonspecific.

Neuroanatomic Theories

The neuroanatomic theories center around two main processes—neurogenesis and synaptic plasticity. Stress, both psychological and environmental, can cause neuroanatomical changes in sensitive brain areas, like the hippocampus. Depressed individuals have been shown to have lower hippocampal volumes compared to healthy controls. This has been attributed to the degenerative and antiproliferative effects of hormones like cortisol that are released under stress. Hypercortisolemia is reversed with ECT. Studies in rats and nonhuman primates have shown increased, rather restored, hippocampal volumes following ECT. Brain derived neurotrophic factor (BDNF) is an important neuropeptide that aids survival and growth of neurons and synapses, via tyrosine kinase-B and MPA-kinase pathways. Increase in BDNF levels is seen in a sustained and dose-dependent manner following ECT. As for synaptic plasticity, repeated electrical stimulation of a circuit can produce lasting therapeutic changes by long-term potentiation (LTP).

ADVERSE EFFECTS AND COMPLICATIONS OF ECT

Common Adverse Effects

Headache, muscular ache, body ache, drowsiness, nausea, vomiting, weakness, and anorexia are transient and benign side effects of ECT. They are easily managed with symptomatic treatment.

Missed or Inadequate Seizure

A well-modified seizure occurs as a faint tonic phase followed by clonic activity of skeletal muscles, accompanied by a typical seizure pattern on EEG. Absence of these changes and the presence of only focal seizures is termed as a *missed seizure*. Previously, minimum duration of typical seizures was prescribed. However, duration of seizure has been observed to be unrelated to clinical outcome. Hence, observation of well-generalized tonic phase followed by clonic phase of seizure should be considered to be adequate seizures. A missed seizure may happen due to a number of reasons—insufficient stimulus intensity, high dynamic impedance (male gender, older age), premature stimulus termination, concurrent medication (benzodiazepines, antiepileptic drugs), hypercarbia, high dose of anesthetic agent, dehydration, and later ECT sessions. Restimulation with a higher stimulus may be done after a gap of 20 seconds, as neurons may be in refractory period due to the previous stimulation. Preoxygenation with 100% oxygen is seen to lower seizure threshold and is used in cases of inadequate or missed seizures. EEG monitoring can reveal the occurrence of a seizure when motor seizure is not seen. Proconvulsant drugs, such as etophylline, can be given before anesthesia in selected cases, where ECG and EEG monitoring are possible. Reviewing concurrent medication, correcting dehydration and electrolyte imbalance, using a lower dose of anesthetic agent, giving twice weekly ECT instead of thrice weekly ECT and use of stimulus with lower pulse-frequency are other measures that can be taken, depending on the likely cause.

Prolonged Seizure and Tardive Seizure

A prolonged seizure is one that goes on for longer than 90 seconds of motor seizure or 120 seconds of EEG seizure. Nonconvulsive status epilepticus can go unrecognized without EEG monitoring. A tardive seizure is a late return of seizure activity during the recovery period after ECT. Risk factors for these are—younger age, female gender, earlier treatment sessions, concurrent medication (e.g. lithium, theophylline), neurological disorder and electrolyte imbalance. The principles of management are to maintain oxygenation throughout, to monitor EEG activity when available, and to abort the seizure with anesthetic agent or benzodiazepines.

Prolonged Apnea

Pseudocholinesterase, or butyrylcholinesterase, is a nonspecific cholinesterase enzyme that hydrolyzes many different choline esters, significant among which are succinylcholine, heroin, and cocaine. With normal plasma levels of this enzyme, almost 90 to 95% of the succinylcholine administered during ECT anesthesia is hydrolyzed, and only 5–10% reaches the neuromuscular junction. Skeletal muscle function recovers within 5 minutes after a single bolus of succinylcholine. In individuals with pseudocholinesterase deficiency, larger amounts of succinylcholine reach the neuromuscular junction leading to prolonged depolarization and flaccid paralysis of the muscles. This results in prolonged apnea and the patient requires 30–60 minutes of assisted ventilation, till the drug is washed off. For such patients, atracurium is a better choice for muscle relaxation, as it does not require pseudocholinesterase for metabolism and is eliminated via Hoffman elimination pathway. Pseudocholinesterase deficiency, an inherited condition, is common among the Hindu Arya Vysya community and it exists as an autosomal recessive trait in Persian Jews. Recent organophosphorous poisoning also increases the likelihood of prolonged apnea. Pseudocholinesterase enzyme activity can be assessed using the Acholest Test Paper. However, routine use of this test is neither practical nor reliable.

ECT Emergent Mania or Organic Euphoria

Like during treatment with antidepressants, some patients who are undergoing ECT for depression or mixed affective state may develop hypomanic or manic symptoms. These may worsen with continued ECT. Typical features of mania like mood elevation, increased psychomotor activity, distractibility, and reduced need for sleep are seen in clear sensorium. The latter distinguishes this from delirium with euphoria that has in addition disorientation, confusion and memory deficits. There are no standard guidelines for management of ECT emergent mania. Some practitioners stop ECT and wait and watch. Manic symptoms may resolve spontaneously. If they do not resolve or depressive symptoms relapse, restarting ECT may be considered. Some practitioners stop ECT and add on a mood stabilizer.

Transient Neurological Phenomenon

Dyspraxia, lateralized inattention and dysphasia can occur rarely, as complications of ECT. They are transient and resolve within a couple of weeks of stopping ECT.

Prolonged Postictal Confusion

All patients undergoing ECT develop a variable period of disorientation with impaired attention, memory and praxis. This develops immediately after the seizure, and usually resolves spontaneously within an hour. Some patients may develop prolonged confusion after ECT, often mimicking an acute organic psychosis. It is characterized by disorientation, memory deficits, restlessness, agitation, aggression, hallucinations, etc. Bilateral ECT, sine waveform, frequent sessions, older age group, concurrent psychotropic drugs, pre-existing cognitive impairment and neurological disorders are risk factors. Using parenteral antipsychotics and benzodiazepines helps to control the crisis. Further, stopping or spacing out sessions, using unilateral ECT, and reviewing concurrent medication is needed.

Cognitive Adverse Effects

The ECT-induced cognitive impairment is the most controversial and most common argument by opponents to the practice of ECT. Cognitive adverse effects are not associated with therapeutic response; rather they may interfere with the assessment of clinical response in a given patient. This may result in premature termination of ECT, leading to early relapse, or prolonged administration of ECT, leading to increased risks. Much research in the last two decades has looked at the nature of these impairments, variables that affect the degree of impairment, and neurobiological mechanisms underlying them. Memory is the most commonly affected cognitive domain. Both retrograde and anterograde amnesia are seen with ECT. Memory for events a few minutes before ECT administration is commonly lost. There is impaired recall of the temporal sequence of events. Usually, these cognitive deficits do not interfere with activities of daily living. After termination of ECT, the retrograde amnesia shrinks and disappears over weeks to months. Chronic retrograde amnesia seen in occasional patients may not be solely attributable to ECT. Personality, persisting symptoms and other nonspecific factors should be considered.

A recent meta-analysis of 84 studies, with nearly 3000 subjects, examined the degree, pattern and progression of cognitive impairment produced by ECT. Cognitive impairments occurring in the subacute period (up to 3 days after ECT course), in the short-term (4–15 days) and in the long-term were reported. Medium-large deficits in episodic memory and executive functioning occurred during the subacute period. Episodic memory deficits were more for verbal than visual memory, for delayed recall than immediate recall, and for unstructured information (word lists) than organized contextualized information (short story). In executive functioning, set shifting and planning showed greater impairments than processing speed, spatial problem solving and global cognition [(as estimated on mini mental status examination (MMSE)]. No deficits were seen in attention, working memory, intellectual ability, abstract reasoning and creative ability. In the short-term follow-up, deficits were seen mainly in verbal paired associates delayed recall. No persisting cognitive deficits were seen after 15 days. Persisting deficits (some even up to 6 months) seen in multiple cognitive domains reported in some studies, might be due to persisting cognitive impairment in depression rather than ECT-induced cognitive deficits. For some patients, subjective complaints of retrograde amnesia may persist even without objective impairment.

Electrode placement (bilateral more than unilateral), stimulus waveform (sine wave more than brief and ultrabrief pulse), frequency of ECT sessions, total number of ECT sessions and stimulus dosage are important moderators of cognitive adverse effects. The anesthetic technique, type and dose of anesthetic drug used and preoxygenation, concomitant medication (including lithium at higher end of therapeutic range) and pharmacological and neuropsychological mitigation approaches, may also have an important bearing. Older age does not seem to play an important role.

A detailed discussion of neurobiological mechanisms is out of the scope of this chapter. Hypertensive surge during ECT and seizures may cause cerebral edema and increased protein diffusion across the blood-brain barrier. This is turn can disturb neuronal functioning and predispose to cognitive impairment. Hypercortisolemia induced by seizures has the potential to disrupt dendritic spines and cause shrinkage of the hippocampus leading to memory deficits. Increase in glutamatergic activity during seizure may contribute to neuronal loss via excitotoxicity.

Cardiovascular Effects of ECT

During ECT, there is initial parasympathetic outflow followed by sympathetic outflow. Immediately after stimulation there is bradycardia and even asystole in some cases. This is followed by tachycardia, increase in blood pressure (up to 200 mm Hg systolic) and in some cases, dysrhythmias. The latter changes are secondary to massive catecholamine release triggered by electrical stimulation as well as the seizure generated. In a young, healthy person these changes may be clinically nonsignificant. However, one must be mindful of such changes in a patient with compromised cardiac functioning. The oxygen demand on the myocardium, which is related to the rate-pressure product (i.e. systolic pressure X heart rate), may increase considerably (by up to 8 times) and may lead to cardiac insufficiency. The massive arterial hypertension seen has the potential to cause intracerebral hemorrhage. Following cessation of seizure, there is reduction in blood pressure and heart rate, towards normal in about 10–15 minutes. This reduction may take more than an hour and parallels the reduction in circulating catecholamines. Hemodynamic responses are lesser with unilateral than bilateral ECT.

Cerebrovascular Effects of ECT

There is marked increase in cerebral blood flow during ECT, with the maximum blood flow velocity in the middle cerebral artery increasing up to two times more than pretreatment. Oxygen demand and consumption increase. This may not be adequately compensated for by the increase in cerebral blood flow, thus leading to a delivery-demand mismatch. The raised systemic blood pressure may hinder autoregulation of cerebral pressure, leading to elevated intracranial tension. Aneurysmal rupture may be a complication of raised intracranial tension, making cerebral aneurysms a relative contraindication to ECT.

PROCEDURE

ECT Unit

An ECT unit is an essential part of every inpatient psychiatry set up. It comprises of three contiguous rooms, the capacity and size of which is determined by the number of patients likely to be receiving ECT.

- *Waiting room*: This is a room where patients wait before ECT. It should have an informal and relaxing environment.
- *Treatment room*: This is the room where all the equipment for ECT and routine and emergency care of patients is kept. All electrical equipment should be properly grounded. Patients are assisted onto a trolley and prepared for treatment in this room. It should be visually shielded and soundproofed from the waiting room. It should be large enough to allow for unrestricted movement of the staff.
- *Recovery room*: It should be easily accessible from the treatment room. It should be large enough to accommodate all the recovering patients. Time for recovery may vary from 5 to 30 minutes. Before the first patient is shifted out of the recovery room, 3–4 more patients would have received ECT and have come into the recovery room. The patient should have regained orientation and should be able to walk without support. The recovery room should be equipped with a pulse oximeter for monitoring each unconscious patient, a blood pressure monitor, an oxygen source, suction equipment and emergency drugs and equipment.

Staff

Medical staff includes a qualified psychiatrist with training in ECT administration, an anesthetist, and assistants as may be deemed necessary. Nursing staff includes one trained nurse with managerial responsibility, who is the overall in-charge of the ECT services. Total number of nurses would again depend on the number of patients undergoing ECT. One nurse should accompany every patient during all stages of treatment. Nurses should be trained in basic emergency interventions, like cardiopulmonary resuscitation. Trained attendees are required to assist during all stages of treatment.

Equipment

The ECT machine should be constant current, square-wave pulse, with a wide output range, and preferably with EEG monitoring. A back up arrangement should be available, in case of malfunction.

- Electrodes and conducting gel
- Trolley with a firm base, cot sides and tilt facility should be available for each patient. The patient will lie on this from the start of treatment till recovery.
- Anesthesia machine
- Anesthetic drugs should be available as per protocol being followed in the unit
- Oxygen supply
- Suction apparatus
- *Monitoring equipment:* Logbook that contains clinical details of all patients undergoing ECT. A blood glucose testing kit, stopwatch for measuring seizure duration, sphygmomanometer, electrocardiograph, pulse oximeter
- *Miscellaneous items:* Disposable gloves, mouth gags, airways, syringes, needles, intravenous cannulae, sticking tape, scissors, swabs, skin cleansers, facility for appropriate disposal of used items
- *Emergency equipment:* Cardiac defibrillator, laryngoscope, laryngeal masks, endotracheal tubes and associated connectors, intravenous infusion sets, fluids, stethoscope, thermometer, ice packs, and an emergency drug box, the contents of which will have been agreed by local protocol.

Consent

A written informed consent is mandatory before ECT is used for a given patient. Consent may be given by the patient, where the patient is able to comprehend the procedures and implications, or by a relative. Usually, consent is taken for a course of ECT sessions. A maximum number of stipulated sessions should thus be told to the patient. At some centers, consent is renewed before each session. Patient has a right to refuse treatment at any point during the treatment, even after consenting initially. The treating psychiatrist should preferably obtain consent. The patient should be given adequate information about indication for ECT, alternative treatment options, risks and benefits of treatments, and right to refuse treatment. Active discussion should be encouraged during this process. Administration of ECT to involuntarily admitted patients and those incapable of providing informed consent is subject to regulation or limitation.

Preparation

The purpose of pre-ECT evaluation is:

- To rule out medical conditions, especially cardiovascular and intracranial, that may relatively contraindicate ECT or pose anesthetic risk
- To identify factors that may contribute to adverse effects from ECT
- To get details of past ECT, if any, the indication for it, efficacy and adverse effects
- To review concurrent medication that may interfere with seizure generation, anesthesia or contribute to adverse effects

The indication for ECT should be clearly ascertained. A detailed medical and psychiatric history, detailed physical examination and mental status examination are mandatory in all patients. A fundus examination should be done to look for any evidence of raised intracranial tension. Other specific features to look for are loose teeth, adequacy of mouth opening and handedness (determined by hand, leg and eye preference). Partial dentures/loose teeth must be removed before the procedure. Investigations required prior to ECT vary as per local protocol. Hemoglobin estimation, liver and renal function tests, blood sugar, and serum electrolytes and ECG are usually done. Specific investigations may be needed depending on the medical status of the patient. Anxious patients may be given a nonbenzodiazepine sedative on the night prior to ECT administration. Patients should be advised to keep the scalp oil-free. The patient should be on empty stomach for at least 6 hours prior to ECT administration, to minimize the risk of aspiration. Fluids should be restricted from at least 2 hours prior to ECT. Bladder should be emptied. An intravenous line should be secured and maintained till the patient has recovered from anesthesia without any complications following the procedure. Some practitioners give atropine (0.6 mg) thirty minutes before the procedure. This helps to dry secretions and protect the heart against vagal inhibition. However, a waiting patient with dry mouth may drink water. Therefore, more commonly, atropine is given on the table. Some centres prefer to omit atropine.

Concomitant Medication Use with ECT

It is common practice to use ECT once a patient does not respond, or responds inadequately to pharmacotherapy alone. In this scenario an important question posed for the clinician is whether to continue the medication along with ECT or stop them. Interaction between ECT and medication may be manifold:

- Medication may interfere with seizure generation
- Medication may have interaction with the anesthetic drugs
- Medication may increase cardiovascular risk
- Medication may increase cognitive side effects
- Discontinuation of medication may lead to relapse once ECT has been terminated.

There are no clear recommendations in this area. The following points may be noted.

- Antidepressants can be continued during ECT. They may not play an adjuvant role, however, they may help prevent relapse following ECT. No significant increase in cognitive side effects is seen with their use. Patients on SSRIs may have prolonged seizures, especially with fluoxetine that has a long half-life. MAOIs, especially the irreversible ones, should be used with caution because of possible cardiovascular instability.
- Antipsychotics can be safely continued. They, too, may help prevent relapse following ECT.
- Lithium is proconvulsant and has been reported to increase cognitive side effects with ECT. Lithium increases the neuromuscular blockade induced by succinylcholine and predisposes the patient to excessive and severe confusion and delirium when serum lithium level is in the upper level of therapeutic range. Continuation during ECT should be based on a cost-benefit analysis.
- Antiepileptic drugs (AEDs) being used for psychiatric illnesses may pose obvious problems in seizure generation. Higher doses of stimulation required would increase cognitive side effects. AEDs being used for seizure disorder may help prevent prolonged seizures. Carbamazepine may prolong action of succinylcholine.
- Benzodiazepines can interfere with seizure generation. They may also decrease duration of observed seizure. Ideally they should be discontinued before ECT. If they must be used, e.g. in anxious patients or those who are dependent on them, short-acting benzodiazepines may be preferred. Another approach is to use flumazenil, a short-acting benzodiazepine receptor antagonist, just before ECT. It is not seen to affect seizure duration or ECT efficacy.
- Stimulant medication can cause prolonged seizures, besides having cardiovascular effects in the form of dysrhythmias and elevation of blood pressure.
- Protective medication for comorbid medical illnesses should be continued during ECT. These include anti-hypertensives, antianginals, antidysrhythmics, bronchodilators and antacid or antireflux therapy. These can be given up to 2 hours before ECT with small sips of water. Antidiabetic medication should be withheld until after recovery, lest it complicate hypoglycemia during seizure. Patients with glaucoma may need change in muscle relaxant used. Patients on long-term steroids may need supplementary doses.

Anesthesia

Modification of ECT came from the understanding that the therapeutic ingredient in ECT is the central seizure and not the peripheral convulsion. It implies use of intravenous anesthesia, neuromuscular blockade, with mechanical ventilation, and electrical stimulation to generate a therapeutic seizure, in that order. It reduces risk of fracture and cardiovascular morbidity posed by unmodified ECT. ECT has now become a 'low risk' medical treatment, with a risk of death or serious injury as rarely as 1 in 50000, which is even lesser than the risk during childbirth. The goals of modified ECT are:

- To overcome musculoskeletal risk by decreasing convulsive motor activity
- To attain complete loss of consciousness without completely suppressing cerebral seizure
- To prevent hypoxia
- To manage adverse effects of electrical stimulation and seizure

The electrical stimulus used in ECT seldom lasts longer than 8 seconds, and the seizure activity usually lasts 30–60 seconds. The duration of anesthesia required is about 3–5 minutes, just enough to cover the period of muscle relaxation, electrical stimulus and resultant seizure. This is achieved with the use of short acting intravenous agents like methohexital, thiopental sodium, or propofol. The main purpose of anesthesia is to avoid perception by the patient of muscle paralysis especially in the event of a partial or missed seizure. Complete skeletal muscle paralysis, along with paralysis of respiratory muscles, can invoke panic and fear in the patient. A generalized seizure itself produces the desired amnesia. Intubation is usually not required unless there is increased risk of aspiration, as with history of gastroesophageal reflux disease or morbid obesity.

The ideal anesthetic for ECT should have the following characteristics:

- Smooth and rapid induction
- Minimal or no antagonistic effects on seizure
- Short duration activity with rapid recovery
- Hemodynamic stability
- Attenuation of the physiological effects of ECT
- No injection pain

A detailed description of all the available anesthetic agents is beyond the scope of this chapter. Methohexital is the first choice anesthetic agent for ECT, and all other agents are compared to this for efficacy. It does not have significant effects on seizure and hemodynamic status. Thiopental sodium (most commonly used in India, at 2–4 mg/kg) may shorten seizure duration, when compared to methohexital. It may also increase frequency of sinus bradycardia and ventricular extrasystole, both of which in turn may impair intracranial hemodynamics. Propofol is a safe anesthetic agent with minimal side effects. When used in doses above 1mg/Kg it may, however, lower seizure duration. Due to its safe cardiac profile, it is the drug of choice in elderly patients. Etomidate has the potential to prolong seizures and may have utility where maximal stimulus fails to produce a convulsion. It has a safe cardiac profile, however, emetic side effects and confusional state may be greater in the postictal state, delaying recovery. Ketamine has the potential to increase pulse and blood pressure and consequently increase intracranial tension. It has limited utility for ECT anesthesia. Volatile anesthetics are more time consuming, have no advantage when compared to the intravenous agents and are currently not in use for modified ECT. Dose of the anesthetic agent is initially calculated by body weight. In subsequent sessions it may be modified depending on the effects on seizure generation and response to ECT.

Neuromuscular blockade during ECT is done with the aim to reduce risk of trauma and severe muscular pain following ECT. It should also suppress abdominal muscle contraction to avoid aspiration of stomach contents. Succinylcholine is the drug of choice, in a dose of 0.5 to 1 mg/Kg. For complete muscle relaxation, as for patients with orthopaedic complications, cachexia or osteoporosis, doses up to 1 to 2 mg/Kg are needed. Electrical stimulus should be given only after fasciculations due to succinylcholine have completely subsided. Direct stimulation may produce tetanic contraction of the masseter muscle. This is not necessarily indicative of inadequate muscle relaxation. It may however pose dental risks and bite blocks should be used. Succinylcholine is avoided if there is possibility of malignant hyperthermia, neuroleptic malignant syndrome, history of recent organophosphorous poisoning, pseudocholinesterase deficiency, history of bradyarrhythmias and sensitivity to potassium releasing effects of succinylcholine. The latter may happen in paraplegia, burn injuries, and congenital muscle disease. Use of a non-depolarising muscle relaxant like mivacurium is preferred where potassium release can be a problem, while atracurium is favored for pseudocholinesterase deficiency. Atracurium has a long duration of action and reversal with atropine and edrophonium may be required. Mechanical ventilation with 100% oxygen should be done till return of spontaneous and regular respiration.

Use of atropine or glycopyrronium, anticholinergic drugs, is to prevent prolonged bradycardia after electrical stimulation. There is increased risk of bradycardia with concomitant use of β-blockers and calcium channel antagonists, and with strong likelihood of subconvulsive responses.

ECT Administration

The patient lies supine on the trolley. The clothing is loosened. Oxygen (100%) is given through a face mask. The anesthetic agent is injected, followed by muscle relaxant, using a separate syringe, intravenously. During anesthesia, oxygenation is maintained by intermittent positive pressure ventilation (IPPV). A bite block is inserted prior to stimulation, to protect the tongue and dentition. The chin of the patient is held up to keep the jaw tight against the 'bite block.' Disposable bite blocks (tightly rolled and taped 4-inch swabs) are preferred to reusable bite blocks to reduce risk of transmitting infection. The electrical stimulus is delivered by the psychiatrist at the chosen electrode placement site. The electrodes should be held firmly at the site. Forceps type of electrodes are not recommended. Seizure duration is recorded from the onset of first tonic activity to the last clonic activity. Pulse, BP and other vital parameters must be monitored before and after the procedure. ECG monitoring is considered mandatory; this has distinct merits, especially in the elderly. Pulse oximetry helps to determine adequate ventilation and oxygenation. Following cessation of seizure, IPPV is continued till spontaneous regular breathing resumes. Excessive secretions in oropharynx should be cleared by suction. The patient is put in a left lateral position and is then shifted to the recovery room. The patient should remain under observation till he/she is steadily ambulant and oriented.

Seizure Monitoring

It is imperative that the seizure is monitored and its occurrence confirmed. Seizure in unmodified ECT is a dramatic behavioral event. Special care, however, is required to monitor seizure during modified ECTs. The typical grand mal seizure on an EEG comprises of widespread high frequency spike waves (polyspike activity), followed by slower 3 cycles/sec or 3 Hz spike and wave complexes. The ictal EEG has the following sequential components, occurring immediately after the stimulus:

- *Phase 1:* 1–3 sec; High frequency, nonspecific, low amplitude waves.
- *Phase 2:* 10–20 sec; hypersynchronous polyspikes, 10 Hz, recruiting rhythm

- *Phase 3:* 20–40 sec; rhythmic spike and wave complexes of 3.0–3.5 Hz.

This is followed by a phase of relative or complete suppression of electrical activity (postictal suppression). A grand mal motor seizure comprises of initial tonic contraction of muscles, followed by a longer clonic phase of rhythmic alternating contraction and relaxation of muscles of the limbs on both sides of the body. Often there may be a 'latent period' before seizure initiation after the end of the electrical stimulus.

Several factors that may produce a dissociation between a generalized cerebral seizure and visible convulsive activity. The anesthetic agent and muscle relaxant produce unconsciousness and muscle relaxation, respectively. In addition, a patient may be on medication like antiepileptic drugs. All of these will reduce convulsive activity. A motor seizure is shorter than EEG seizure; only 70% the length of the cerebral seizure. It was earlier held that an adequate seizure was one with ≥ 15 sec of motor or ≥ 25 sec of cerebral seizure activity. It was thought that seizures lasting shorter than this duration may actually be a result of focal seizure activity. Similarly, occurrence of facial seizures alone reflects focal activity and is inadequate. It has been seen in multiple studies that the length of seizure does not correlate with clinical efficacy. An adequate seizure is one that is well generalized, the duration of the seizure having lesser importance. Notably, elderly patients have clinical benefit even with short duration seizures.

Methods of monitoring seizure are the following:

- *Timing of convulsion*: The time from the end of electrical stimulation to the end of generalized (i.e. bilateral and clonic) convulsive activity is recorded. Any persisting clonic activity in one of the limbs is recorded separately. This is a simple, inexpensive method. It ensures that the treating psychiatrist confirms the induction of a tonic-clonic convulsion. It is useful where EEG monitoring is unavailable. The disadvantages are that seizure activity may be confused with muscle contraction during stimulation; it is heavily influenced by muscle relaxant and may be abolished by the same; it underestimates cerebral seizure activity.
- *Cuff technique*: A blood pressure cuff is tied on one of the upper or lower limbs. The pressure is elevated to above the level of anticipated systolic rise during seizure activity, after administration of the anesthetic agent but before the muscle relaxant is given (in the opposite limb). The purpose is to prevent muscle relaxant from reaching vein of the opposite cuffed limb, such that after electrical stimulation nearly unmodified convulsive activity can be seen in that limb. Fasciculations occurring in other parts of the body do not occur in the cuffed limb. The ECT stimulus is applied and the time noted. At the start of the tonic phase of seizure in this limb, the cuff is released. The last clonus on the cuffed limb denotes the seizure termination. This method is inexpensive and is valuable when total paralysis is desirable and also when EEG monitoring is unavailable. However, this too has limitations. Cuff pressure needs continual maintenance. It may be left inflated after ECT increasing risk of trauma in frail patients and risk of clotting in patients with sickle-cell disease. The cuff-method underestimates cerebral seizure activity.
- *EEG monitoring*: This is the most direct available means of measuring seizure activity. It has particular utility in the occurrence of brief convulsions, in scenarios where complete paralysis is desired and in the detection of focal and prolonged seizures. However, it requires training, and the cost of equipment and treatment goes up. Recent recommendations state that at least a two channel EEG recording is desirable. On single channel recording, it is hard to distinguish artifacts from true seizures at times and focal from generalized seizures. Prefrontal-mastoid positioning of EEG electrodes is used—one electrode placed in the middle of the eyebrow on the forehead and the other over the ipsilateral mastoid. Recent Royal College of Psychiatrists recommendations have mandated the use of EEG during all ECT sessions.

STATUS AND PRACTICE OF UNMODIFIED ECT

Unmodified ECT is given without the administration of a muscle relaxant. Although most organizations proscribe unmodified ECT, it is being practiced in the following exceptional situations:

- Lack of adequate anesthesiological support in several centers
- Patients who urgently require ECT, and there is no time to ascertain fitness for anesthesia
- In situations where anesthesia cannot be administered, e.g. with inaccessible veins
- Contraindications for anesthesia or muscle relaxants (e.g. cardiorespiratory disorders)

Reluctance towards use of unmodified ECT is because of its unwanted physiological effects. The vigorous motor convulsion poses significant risk of musculoskeletal complications like compression fracture, joint dislocation, muscle or ligament injury, backache, and broken teeth. Blood pressure surge can lead to hemorrhage. Pretreatment anxiety is high. The patient is usually fully aware of the elements of ECT procedure and may recall them later. Physical restraints applied and experience of subconvulsive stimuli may be disturbing. Emergence from postictal confusion is prolonged. Conceptually and visually unmodified ECT is unesthetic.

The World Psychiatric Association states that where unmodified ECT is mandatory, a case-by-case decision should be made, taking into consideration clinical factors, evidence of efficacy, informed consent and available alternative treatments. Clinicians could also consider a facility that has the required resources for modified ECT. The patient may be shifted to such a center instead of accepting unmodified ECT as the only course. The only official guidelines on the use of unmodified ECT have been given in a joint statement of the Indian Association of Private Psychiatry, Indian Psychiatric Society and Indian Association of Biological Psychiatry.

The Indian guidelines state that use of unmodified ECT should not be considered a recommended routine practice. A case-by-case selection has to be made, considering the 'strong indication' for ECT, nonavailability of modified ECT, and that benefits of a suboptimal technique clearly outweigh the risks. Bilateral electrode placement should be preferred in unmodified ECT to minimize chances of slow or nonresponse. If available, 100% oxygen by mask should be given starting before electrical stimulus and extending to the onset of regular breathing after the end of seizure. The electrical dose used in unmodified ECT should be the lowest stimulus at which an adequate seizure is produced. This lowers musculoskeletal side effects, postictal confusion, and cognitive impairment. After each session, benefit and side effects of ECT should be assessed and decision about continuing ECTs reviewed. Recommendations are also made in these guidelines to regarding minimization of musculoskeletal risks, comorbid medical illnesses, dental examination, informed consent, and use of restraints.

Benzodiazepine modified ECT: It is another option where facilities for modified ECT are unavailable. Diazepam, preferred for its superior muscle relaxant action, is administered in a dose of 10 mg intravenously 1–3 minutes before the procedure or 10–15 mg orally 1–2 hours prior to the procedure. Somnolence is induced leading to reduced awareness and anxiety of ECT. Musculoskeletal side effects are reduced, as is postictal restlessness and confusion. Use of benzodiazepines is not seen to significantly raise seizure threshold.

INDICATIONS

Depression

Most ECT trials have focused on depression. Evidence from multiple trials that use a doubled-blind randomized sham controlled, placebo-controlled or other antidepressant medication controlled study designs have demonstrated a significant superiority of ECT in short-term treatment of depression. The effect sizes for the superiority of ECT have been in the range of 0.8–0.9, which are considered large. These studies demonstrate that ECT has an incontrovertible role in depression.

The presence of vegetative (endogenous/melancholic) symptoms predict a good response. The other predictors are good response to previous ECTs, shorter duration of illness, good premorbid adjustment, and absence of anxiety as well as hypochondriacal symptoms. The neurobiological predictors of response are cortisol nonsuppression (dexamethasone suppression test), short REM latency and normal P300 evoked potential amplitude. ECT appears to be equally effective for both bipolar and unipolar depression.

ECT is commonly used as a second line of treatment, when drugs have failed or are not tolerated. Even when ECT fails to produce sufficient antidepressant effect, subsequent course of antidepressant drugs yield better response. ECT is used selectively as the first line treatment in severe depressive illness with one or more of the following features:

- Catatonic stupor
- Psychotic symptoms
- Suicidal risk
- Pregnancy and lactation
- Co-existing medical conditions, where antidepressant drugs are contraindicated.

Mania

In randomized controlled trials in mania, ECT was found to be superior to sham ECT, lithium, or the combination of lithium and haloperidol. Another double-blind randomized clinical trial demonstrated equal efficacy of ECT alone compared to ECT with sodium valproate in treatment of acute mania. Unilateral ECT is less potent than bilateral ECT. No empirical research is available to support more frequent ECTs in acute mania. In lithium unresponsive acute mania, no comparative evaluation of ECT with other alternatives (e.g. carbamazepine, sodium valproate) is available. ECT given during acute mania has no demonstrable effect on the long-term course of bipolar disorder. Bifrontal electrode placement appears to have a faster response, with comparable or fewer cognitive side effects.

Schizophrenia and Other Psychoses

The therapeutic effects of ECT were first documented in schizophrenia. When used alone, acute therapeutic effects are inferior to adequate doses of neuroleptics. Concurrent ECT can accelerate or augment the response to acute neuroleptic therapy and may be used in selected patients who have a limited response to drug therapy alone and when both a rapid global improvement and a faster reduction in symptomatology are desired. This has been noted as the post common indication of ECT in schizophrenia. The most common accompanying symptoms of schizophrenia for which ECT is prescribed are catatonia, aggression and suicidal behaviors, in that order. ECTs, however, do not seem to confer advantage over continued neuroleptic therapy when introduced in mid-course of the latter. In neuroleptic refractory positive symptom schizophrenia, ECT was found effective only in open trials. The efficacy of ECTs with negative symptoms is uncertain. The long-term effect of ECT on the course of illness is unknown. The only study which examined this has evidence to suggest that patients who received ECT had better outcome at five years than those who did not. No studies have compared newer antipsychotics with ECTs. As in patients with mania, bifrontal ECT in schizophrenia also has superior clinical and cognitive outcomes than bitemporal ECT. Patients with catatonic schizophrenia respond faster to ECT than patients with noncatatonic schizophrenia.

The Royal College of Psychiatrists has limited the use of ECTs to the following:

- Schizophrenia, with predominant depressive symptoms.
- Schizophrenia, with inability to tolerate 500 mg or less of chlorpromazine equivalents or poor response to the same.
- Specific subgroups, such as acute catatonic states, acute drug-induced psychosis, schizophreniform disorders, acute paranoid syndrome, schizo-affective disorders.

Other Neuropsychiatric Disorders

ECTs have been found to be useful in the following conditions in some open trials, though firm evidence is still lacking.

- Neuroleptic malignant syndrome
- Obsessive compulsive disorder
- Parkinson's disease
- Fugue/twilight states in epilepsy
- Panhypopituitarism, hypothyroidism, mild glucose intolerance
- Other organic psychosyndromes, i.e. delirium.

CONTRAINDICATIONS

The ECT administration in medically compromised and elderly subjects requires careful consideration of the contraindications. Fortunately, technical advances in recent years have rendered the old time contraindications into relative contraindications. There are very few absolute contraindications excepting raised intracranial tension. However, there are certain special circumstances when administration of ECT demands more skill and care. Some refer to these as 'relative contraindications'; increased risk of ECT in such patients should be weighed against the expected therapeutic benefits from ECT. The risk of the patient's psychiatric illness and the side effects of antidepressant medications must be weighed against the risk associated with ECT and anesthesia. If ECT is indicated, and particularly when alternative treatments are more risky and/or less efficient, efforts must be made to overcome these relative contraindications. These include recent cerebrovascular accident, cardiovascular conduction defects, high-risk pregnancy, and aortic and cerebral aneurysms and phaeochromocytoma. These are discussed (more appropriately) as ECT in 'special populations' below. The emphasis is on cardiovascular effects of ECT, complications to be anticipated, and the special precautions to be followed in psychiatric patients who have a coexisting medical illness.

ECT IN SPECIAL POPULATIONS

Children and Adolescents

The indications for electroconvulsive therapy in children and adolescents are similar to those in adults, like severe prepubertal depression, mania and other psychiatric disorders when more conservative treatments have been unsuccessful. Review of existing literature indicates that ECT could be safe and effective for these indications. Mood disorders and catatonia have better response rates than psychotic disorders. Preliminary studies on cognitive outcomes after ECT in this group suggest no differences when compared to psychiatric controls. Prolonged seizures should be anicipated. The presence of mental retardation is not a contraindication. Even though it is not a first line of treatment for psychiatric disorders in childhood or adolescence, ECT is often under-utilized in children and adolescents. A systematic selection of children with appropriate indications and a dedicated post-ECT evaluation of symptoms and cognitive functions would yield optimal results.

Geriatric Population

Old age is not a contraindication in an otherwise healthy individual. In fact, several studies predict a better response in old age. The additional risk involved because of physical problems does not appear to be greater than continuing depression and side effects of antidepressants. Duration of postictal confusion increases with age. Special consideration must be given to the baseline cognitive abilities and comorbid medical disorders of an elderly patient prior to treatment with ECT. Threshold of stimulus required to elicit a seizure is high in elderly. Prolonged postictal confusion should be anticipated. Cognitive side effects occur with a frequency similar to that in younger individuals. Using unilateral ECTs can minimize these side effects.

Pregnancy

The ECT has been administered in all trimesters of pregnancy without untoward effects. General anesthetic agents, anticholinergics and muscle relaxants used in ECT are not reported to have teratogenic effects. Prolonged apnea due to pseudocholinesterase deficiency and risk of pulmonary aspiration (especially in 2nd and 3rd trimesters) due to prolonged gastric emptying in pregnancy should be pre-empted. Special measures and modifications of ECT procedures are required to minimize the risk of complications in pregnant patients undergoing ECT. These include, liaison with obstetrician to assess risk of abortion or preterm delivery, adequate oxygenation and muscle relaxation, and mildly left lateral positioning compared to supine position to reduce pressure on great vessels. Fetal monitoring during ECT should be reserved for high-risk pregnancies.

The Medically Ill

The cardiovascular effects of ECT contribute to significant morbidity. It is hence necessary to review this aspect with emphasis. Given this effect on the cardiac function (see above) during the seizure, changes (albeit benign) are expected in the rhythm. These are best demonstrated if EKG monitoring is practiced during ECT. Vagal arrhythmias include those of atrial, junctional or nodal origin, as well as sinus bradycardia, sinus arrest, atrial premature contractions, paroxysmal atrial tachycardia, atrial flutter, atrial fibrillation, first-, second-, or third-degree atrioventricular block, and premature ventricular contractions during the sinus bradycardia. Rarely though, the other abnormalities (not so benign) occur. They are noted during the sinus tachycardia and include bigeminy, trigeminy, ventricular tachycardia and ventricular fibrillation. Other transient EKG changes (both ischemic and nonischemic) are recorded even in normal subjects but more often in cardiac patients. These are peaked 'T' waves, inverted 'T' waves and S-T segment depression. Thiopentone produces more EKG abnormalities than methohexital. EKG abnormalities are rarely present beyond the acute postictal phase.

Anticholinergic (atropine or glycopyrrolate) premedication, used by most practitioners for modified ECT, contributes to larger RPP. In patients with normodynamic cardiac function, atropine premedication as a routine may not be indicated. Nonconvulsive stimulus produces only the vagal effect, leading to bradycardia and has the potential to prolong the asystole. The use of atropine may be limited to the ECT session, in which threshold is estimated by titration method. Although it is generally believed that nonconvulsive stimuli are not associated with any CNS morbidity, the cardiac risks should be seriously considered. The sympathoadrenal outflow associated with the convulsive response counteracts the vagal cardiac inhibition and a nonconvulsive stimulus, hence, fails to overcome the vagal inhibition.

The tricyclic drugs, although by themselves affect cardiac rate and rhythm, do not increase CVS risk during ECT. Likewise, lithium can contribute to increased CNS morbidity with ECT and prolong suxamethonium effect, but poses no extra risk to CVS morbidity in the absence of other electrolyte disturbances. Benzodiazepines, by virtue of increasing seizure threshold and hence causing subconvulsions, may contribute indirectly to CVS risks.

Pre-ECT Medical Evaluation of High-risk CVS Patient

The ECT evaluations should be titrated to each patient with the knowledge of pre-existing CVS disease. A detailed physical examination should include careful evaluation of cardiac function. Stress test is preferred over coronary angiogram, as the former evaluates the functional integrity of the heart. Echocardiography is increasingly used to assess myocardial function, akinetic segments and size of the individual chambers. Consultation with a cardiologist should be obtained in all patients who have had known ischemic attacks, valvular disease (operated or otherwise), and in patients with congestive cardiac failure. Routine metabolic investigations (such as serum digitalis levels, prothrombin time, arterial blood gas levels) may be required. Medical evaluation is best repeated at intervals, even during the course of ECTs, rather than merely declaring the patient's fitness at the start of the ECT course. Detecting early evidence of compromised cardiac function effectively prevents morbidity related to ECT.

Individual Cardiac Disorders

Systemic hypertension due to pheochromocytoma calls for the treatment of the latter, prior to ECT. Control of hypertension should be achieved using indirect antiadrenergic drugs (e.g. clonidine) or calcium channel blockers (e.g. nifedepine) or angiotensin converting enzyme inhibitors (e.g. enalapril). Beta-blockers, like propranolol or esmolol, are indicated in patients with myocardial ischemia with hypertension, although prolonged bradycardia may occur. In hypertensives, ECT may cause larger elevations of ictal and postictal hypertensive responses; an occasional patient may need intravenous antihypertensives. Sublingual nifedepine (5–10 mg) before ECT has been found to be effective in controlling ictal and postictal hypertension. Rarely, nitroglycerine infusion (0.01%) may be necessary to maintain blood pressure (around 140–150 mm Hg) in patients with myocardial ischemia.

Dysrhythmias detected before ECT should be corrected. Digitalis is helpful in atrial fibrillation. Blood levels of the drug should be within therapeutic range to prevent the risk of sinoatrial arrest. The conversion of atrial fibrillation to sinus rhythm can dislodge thrombi. ECT has been known to facilitate this conversion, thus increasing the risk of embolism. Anticoagulation therapy before ECT may help prevent the risk of embolism in such patients. Transesophageal echocardiogram may be performed to check for atrial clots. Nevertheless, atrial fibrillation is the most common dysrhythmia in patients receiving ECT. Other dysrhythmias are rare, often benign and self-limiting. A number of medications are available to control the more complicated ones. The discussion about these is beyond the scope of this chapter.

Cardiac pacemakers are of three types: fixed rate, synchronous (triggered by P/R waves) and demand (inhibited by P/R waves). Modified ECT is safe in patients with cardiac pacemakers. Electrical stimulus applied across scalp during ECT does not usually interfere with the pacemaker, unless poor grounding exists in the electromedical equipment used, such as ECT and EEG machine. ECT with a pacemaker results in fewer cases of arrhythmias than without pacemakers as heart rate is controlled by pacemaker. However, hypertensive episode may still occur. Pre-ECT X-ray should confirm intact insulation around pacemakers wires. A cardiologist's opinion should be sought for a routine check of pacemaker funcion and decision on the optimal mode of the pacemaker for safe pacing. The patient should be sufficiently paralyzed with muscle relaxants. The demand pacemakers, which are more commonly used, can be inhibited by the discharges from muscle potentials during succinylcholine depolarization and during the clonic phase of the seizure, if the paralysis is inadequate. A ring magnet should, therefore, be available to convert the demand mode to fixed rate mode, if severe bradycardia occurs.

Congestive cardiac failure poses a special challenge as these patients are more sensitive to increases in myocardial oxygen demand and can potentially progress to frank decompensation. It should be adequately controlled using digitalis, diuretics and vasodilators, including on the morning of each ECT session. The hypertensive response during the seizure may at times precipitate failure and pulmonary edema. Therefore, the ictal hypertensive response should be well controlled. The dose of barbiturates for anesthesia should be carefully titrated, as these are myocardial depressants.

In *recent myocardial infarction (<3 months),* the merits of ECT should be more carefully assessed against those of risks associated with ECT. The complications of myocardial infarction should be controlled before ECT with appropriate medications or revascularization procedures. Well compensated old myocardial infarction (>6 months) is no contraindication for ECT. Nevertheless a comprehensive cardiac assessment is necessary as discussed already.

Other Medical Disorders

Vascular malformation in systemic as well as cerebral circulatory systems, poses risks during ECT. The cerebral autoregulatory mechanism responds to the increase in peripheral blood pressure by increasing intracranial pressure. Aneurysms should be repaired, otherwise they may rupture and bleed during the hypertensive responses to ECT. Drugs such as hydralazine, propranolol or nitroprusside have been advised to contain dramatic elevations of blood pressure in patient with multiple cerebral aneurysms.

Cerebrovascular accidents can lead to severe affective states necessitating use of ECT; more so because these patients may be intolerant to antidepressants. No additional risk is anticipated if ECT is used 3 moths after a stroke; although even one month-poststroke patients have received ECT uneventfully. While the above points are applicable to thromboembolic strokes, more care and monitoring of blood pressure is required for patients with hemorrhagic strokes.

ECT should be withheld when there is evidence for *raised intracranial pressure* (ICP). Use of dexamethasone should be considered in other patients with intracranial space occupying lesion, but without raised ICP, to prevent elevations of ICP during ECT.

Stimulus electrodes should be placed away from the *craniotomy* site, preferably equidistant from the skull defect, to avoid abnormally high charge densities.

Epileptic patients may develop severe psychiatric disorders, necessitating use of ECT. Antiepileptic drugs can prevent induction of seizures, although seizure can be obtained using a large stimulus dose. Yet some patients may not obtain a seizure at all. There are no standard guidelines to overcome this problem. Discontinuing the antiepileptics abruptly may result in status epilepticus during ECT. Closely monitoring the plasma levels of the antiepileptic drugs and maintaining them at the lower end of the therapeutic range may be useful. It is important to anticipate and be prepared to manage the possibility of prolonged seizure or even status epilepticus.

Dementia of degenerative type itself poses no additional risks for ECT. Major depression and severe agitation occurring in these patients can be successfully and safely treated with ECT.

In patients with *ventriculoperitoneal shunts,* the patency of the shunt should be confirmed before referring them for ECT.

There are no consistent reports of the effect of ECT on blood sugar levels in patients with *diabetes mellitus*. Both hypoglycemic and hyperglycemic attacks have been reported. Since the patient is fasting before ECT, it is often recommended to skip the oral hypoglycemic medications and short-acting insulin on the morning of the ECT. The dose of long-acting insulin should be halved.

Thyroid dysfunction can be a primary or subclinical pathology in certain depressive states. In the former case, the CVS effects of the endocrinopathy should be properly evaluated and if abnormal, should be brought under control. Beta-blockers help to overcome the risks from thyroid storm in patients with hyperthyroidism during the seizure.

The ECT in patients with *dyselectrolytemia* should be considered after treating the underlying cause and correcting the electrolyte imbalance. Hyperkalemia may be worsened with succinylcholine. Hypokalemia is associated with prolonged apnea. Hypernatremia may cause increase in seizure threshold and hyponatremia may contribute to prolonged seizures.

In patients with *asthma* or *chronic obstructive pulmonary disorders*, pretreatment with bronchodilators, systemic anticholinergic agents and preoxygenation are suggested to reduce rates of exacerbations. Theophylline may be avoided because of its risk of causing prolonged seizures or even statusepilepticus.

Anecdotal reports are aplenty illustrating the safe use of ECT in several medical conditions coexisting with the psychiatric disorders needing ECT. However, a general rule is to anticipate occult or apparent medical morbidity in the elderly patient going for ECT. All elderly patients (preferably even those 45 years or older) should undergo a careful and detailed physical examination, supplemented with appropriate laboratory tests. It is further recommended that in selected patients repeat medical evaluations should be conducted during the course of ECT and preferably at least once a week.

46.8 PSYCHOSURGERY

V Balasubramaniam, Sachchidanand Singh, Christoday RJ Khess, Jayati Simlai

The term *psychosurgery* includes many procedures. While there is not much ambiguity as to whether a particular procedure can be grouped under psychosurgery, it is difficult to give a comprehensive definition of psychosurgery. According to the National Commission for the Protection of the Human Subjects of Biomedical and Behavioral Research, "psychosurgery means brain surgery on (1) normal brain tissue of an individual, who does not suffer from any physical disease, for the purpose of changing or controlling the behavior or emotions of such individual, or (2) diseased brain tissue of the individual, if the sole object of the performance, is to control, change, or affect any behavioral or emotional disturbance of such individual".[36] Subsequently, the word 'primary' was substituted for the word 'sole'. Psychosurgery has been defined by this author as "referring to those procedures aimed at giving relief in disorders of thought, feeling or behavior (i.e. psychiatric disorders), by operations aimed at eliminating anatomically or functionally, certain areas in the brain".[37] Various other definitions are available and are more or less equivalent in their ambit.

There are some reservations regarding the use of the term psychosurgery. Part of this reluctance arises from the fact that at some time in history (and even now in some quarters) psychosurgery was considered to be empirical, unphysiological and irrational, and capable of inflicting more damage than giving benefit to the patient. So, the term *functional surgery* was proposed to circumvent this. But, this term encompasses the management of conditions other than psychiatric disorders. Some have preferred the term *psychiatric surgery* but there seems to be no special advantage; hence the term psychosurgery will be used here, because it is well known and it is still accepted, though not universally.

HISTORY OF PSYCHOSURGERY

The history of psychosurgery is closely linked with the history of neurosurgery. This need occasion no surprise as the various psychosurgical procedures are but exquisite examples of the precision that neurosurgery can offer. Arguing from the neatly circumscribed perforations in the excavated skulls, it has being held by some that psychosurgery must have had an early start and that these skulls are evidences of the handiwork of the pioneers. This is unlikely, because from the early days of human evolution, it was the heart that was held in esteem and considered as seat of emotions, as contemporary expressions like 'heartfelt' testify. The brain was considered, at best as another organ. Moreover, the so-called mental disorders were thought to arise from black magic or due to visitations from evil spirits (views that are still prevalent). So, it is unlikely that these procedures were done for psychiatric disorders; they could have been performed for relief of headaches due to brain tumors.

Anyway, specific record of 'forays' in psychiatric surgery can only be seen in the nineteenth century. According to Valenstein, Burkhardt in 1891 resected parts of cerebral cortex to treat psychiatric disorders.[38] The same author states that later Puusepp disconnected the frontal and parietal lobes in some psychiatric conditions.[38] These procedures were attended with some success in the hands of the innovators. Then, Freud entered the field and psychosurgery was pushed to the background. There were other reasons also. Psychosurgery, to be really successful, depended on refined neurosurgical techniques; and neurosurgery was just being developed into a superspeciality by pioneers like Harvey Cushing, Walter E Dandy and others.

PSYCHOSURGERY IN INDIA

In India, psychosurgery antedated the introduction of neurosurgery by some years. The earliest report was published by Govindaswamy in 1944.[39] In this report, thirteen out of twenty five cases improved. Ten years later, Nambiar reported on the results of 'free hand' leukotomy;[40] 89% of his cases did well.

With the establishment of neurosurgical centers, neurosurgeons began tackling psychiatric problems too.

REVIVAL OF PSYCHOSURGERY

The rebirth of psychosurgery can be said to be have begun in a correct way in the year 1936, when John Fulton and Jacobsen reported on the ameliorating effects of frontal lobe ablations on chimpanzees.[41] According to Lima, these and Bickener's observation of a patient of Dandy, in whom large portions of the frontal lobes had been removed, prompted the performance of frontal lobe ablative procedures on the humans by the combined efforts of EgazMoniz and Lima.[42] Then came a deluge and a large number of patients had been tackled. All these were only leukotomy or its modifications. There were many other procedures which came under the term psychosurgery. The history of these procedures is detailed in the sections dealing with the specific operations to maintain continuity.

All these procedures were done, either by open craniotomy or through a burr hole. Bony landmarks were used as guidelines.

In 1948, stereotaxic surgery was done on human patients and reported by Spiegel and Wycis.[43] These techniques were quickly adopted for psychosurgery, as the advantages were many. The most important is that stereotaxic techniques gave a precision unobtainable by other methods. Bilateral, multiple and repeat procedures could be done easily and with safety. It can be said that the resurrection of psychosurgery is mainly due to the availability of stereotaxic methods.

For a meaningful application of the various psychosurgical procedures in different psychiatric disorders, it is necessary to have a model of the brain and its functioning and the various disease processes.

This should not be taken to mean that the functions and pathology of mental illnesses have been correctly elucidated. But, without a model, the deployment of a particular procedure for a specific illness may be difficult and may border on empiricism and born out of personal preferences. The appropriate procedure may not be done because one does not have a model, and so the results would not be good. For example, leukotomy would not work for a retarded patient with aggressive behavior.

The personality of an individual, the various thought processes and the decision to act in response to stimuli (either introceptive or extroceptive) depend on the frontal lobes, particularly that part of the brain lying rostral to the motor strip (The term frontal lobe actually includes all the area in front of the central sulcus). From the frontal lobe, thoughts arise and are reinforced by inputs from the cingulate region, the area responsible for affect and drive. This is what Papez calls as the 'stream of thought'.[44] The frontal lobes depend for their work on the influences from the thalamus (the median nucleus and nuclei of internal medially lamina) and the hypothalamus. These thought processes are modified by memory records from the hippocampus and ultimately reach the action centers, namely the amygdala and other areas[45] (Flow chart 2).

This is at best a rough model and may not conform to all the theories regarding mind and the various mental activities.

A discussion of psychosurgery can be done from the point of view of the various disorders or the different operations.

Flow chart 2: Behavioral brain

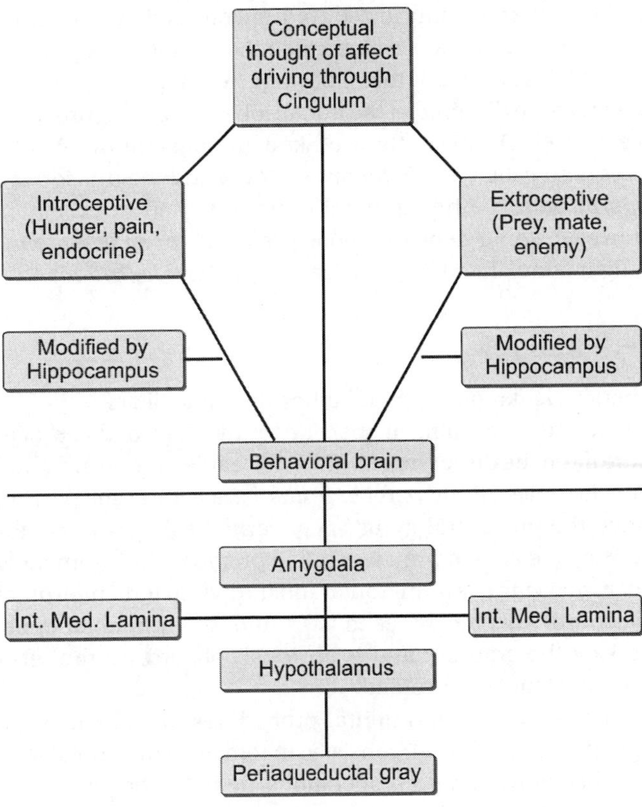

Here, the approach followed will be from the various procedures. Since, the very first and most employed procedure was leukotomy, many tend to equate (not quite correctly) psychosurgery with only leukotomy. Many procedures come under psychosurgery. They are:

- Frontal lobe operations
  - Leukotomy
  - Cingulomotomy
- Thalamic operations
- Callosal operations
- Operations of sedative neurosurgery.

There are a few more procedures done exclusively for very limited (or controversial) indications. One such example is the operations for homosexuality. These procedures will not be discussed here.

LEUKOTOMY

History

As has been indicated, it was the experimental work of Fulton and others that led to lobotomy being performed by Moniz and Lima. It must be said that earlier Moniz and Lima were thinking about some such sort of procedure and in this connection Fulton uprightly remarked "we should not forget that he (Moniz) had considered surgical interference long before learning of our (Fulton and Jacobsen's) results.[46] While Moniz and Lima introduced leukotomy, it was the work of Freeman and Watts which made the operation popular in USA.[12] Some even felt that it became 'too popular'. Since the object was to disconnect the frontal lobes, various approaches were used. Of these, the well known ones are the frontal ones, also called as *orbital undercutting* and the *transorbital approaches.*[47,48] The temporal route was used by Freeman. However, some neurosurgeons preferred '*open leukotomy*'. Knight popularized the practice of *stereotaxic leukotomy.*[49]

Terminology

Literally, leukotomy means cutting the white fibers.

Before proceeding further, the terminology of this procedure has to be discussed. As indicated earlier, the term frontal lobe includes all the parts in front of the central sulcus. But, since the precentral gyrus is concerned solely with motor activity, the area in front was called premotor. This somehow got mixed with the term frontal and the hybrid term prefrontal was born. This term means in front of the frontal lobe, i.e. outside the cranium and is obviously absurd. So the term prefrontal must be avoided.

The earlier experimental procedures, on which these operations were based, consisted in removing the frontal lobe by lobectomy. But, such operations are not to be performed for psychiatric conditions today.

Lobotomy means merely cutting into the frontal lobe and this was the kind of operation done in the earlier days by Freeman and Watts, and others. In these procedures, the frontal lobes are disconnected from the other structures, either partially or totally.

Leukotomy means cutting of the white fibers and perhaps describes the procedure most accurately, as the aim of the operation is only to cut the white fibers. This is the best term to describe the operative procedure.

Anatomical and Physiological Basis

The frontal lobe connects to the medial nucleus of the thalamus and also to the hypothalamic nuclei. In addition, fibres run into the cingulate gyrus. This inferior orbital cortex of the frontal lobe is different from the rest of the frontal lobe structurally (in being less agranular) and functionally (in being more like the limbic system). This connects to the temporal lobe through the uncinate fasciculus and also indirectly to the amygdaloid nucleus (through the temporopolar bundle).

All these connections are two way connections. The original procedure of Moniz was a massive disconnection. From experimental observations and from studies on postmortem material, it is now clear that best results are obtained only by division of the frontothalamic and frontohypothalamic connections. These fibers are best caught at the bottle neck just below the head of the caudate nucleus. It can be said that the aim of the various approaches is only to reach these fibers. The operation is described by many terms, e.g. modified leucotomy, subcaudate leukotomy or basofrontal tractomy. When cut here, the undesirable sequele are minimal. As to how they are approached and how they are divided, depends on the preference and convenience of the individual surgeons. The plethora of names employed to describe these operations testifies to the various different approaches and techniques (Fig. 5).

Modus Operandi of the Procedures

How does leukotomy work? The thalamus acts as an integrating station (like the synthesizer in an orchestra) for the sensory, motor and affective impulses. These are then passed on to the frontal lobe for appropriate action. In this, the medial nucleus of the thalamus has an important part of play. This nucleus connects to the frontal agranular cortex (excluding the inferior orbital cortex). The process of thinking is ultimately the function of the frontal lobe and the responses to the various stimuli (endogenous or exogenous, or even those that arise de novo) all originate from the frontal lobe. The appropriate action depends on this 'thought process' in the frontal lobe. Whether this means that the mind is in the frontal lobe cannot be discussed here. The 'command' from the frontal lobes arises after modification by ethical considerations (which again depend on or arise from the frontal lobes). When this frontal lobe control is missing, as when under the influence of alcohol, an antisocial unethical behavior results. In schizophrenia, there is a fundamental disorder of the process of thinking and the behavior of the patient is a consequence of this disordered thinking, i.e. wrong thinking and 'appropriate action'. This is at best a simplistic model. In leukotomy, these disordered thoughts are prevented from reaching the thalamus and hypothalamus.

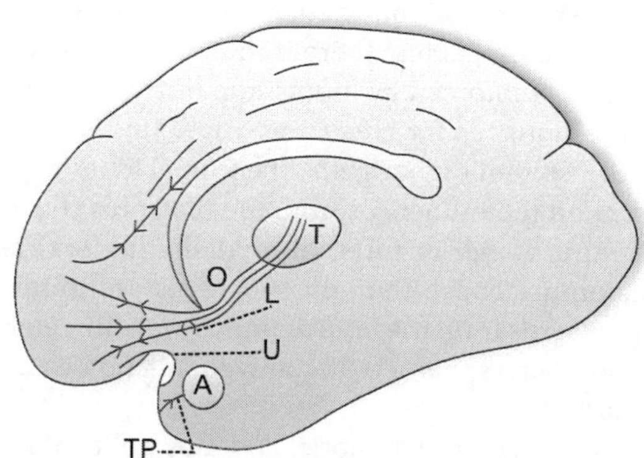

Fig. 5: Frontal lobe connections. For sake of clarity, only single lines have been drawn. Site of leukotomy is indicated

Indications

Leukotomy is indicated in schizophrenia, manic depressive psychosis, depressive psychosis and schizoaffective disorders. In the hands of most workers, paranoid and simple schizophrenia do best. In the hands of Freeman, hebephrenic and catatonics have done well.[50] Patients with suicidal tendencies respond well to this procedure.

Timing of the Operations

One of the most vexing questions is the timing of the operation in psychiatric illness. What is discussed here with regard to leukotomy applies with equal force to the other procedures. It had been found that patients taken up for surgery, decades after having been in an institution, did not do well. As Freeman says, lobotomy should not be considered as a 'final heroic remedy'.[11] On the other hand, surgery certainly is not to be offered soon after the diagnosis is made. The usual escape out of this is to state that operations are advised after 'reasonable' period of trial with drugs and other measure. The problem comes in the expression 'reasonable' and also how much of drugs and what drugs. There is no use in delaying surgery because a drug is likely to be discovered in near future or a drug is being marketed elsewhere and is not available to the patient. Naturally, these conditions and limitations will vary. But, it can be said that 3–4 years of trial with available drugs and methods should be the main indication to think of surgery.

Techniques

The fibers can be divided by:

- Craniotomy
- Through a burr hole
- By stereotactic method.

Craniotomy

A bicoronal osteoplastic craniotomy is performed. By approaching though the frontal poles, the fibers are divided at the subcaudate level. This point is about 6 cm from the frontal tip. The cut starts about 10 mm from the medial surface and is 10 mm long. The division is done by suction. Hemostasis is achieved by directly controlling the bleeding points.

Burr Hole

The same area can be reached through a burr hole and the division performed by a small retractor. Here the bleeding, if any, is controlled by temporary packing.

Stereotactic Method

The same disconnection can be achieved by destroying the fibers by radiofrequency current, by radioactive seeds, or by injection of chemicals.

Complications and Sequelae

In open operations and when done through burr hole, there are chances of bleeding. This can be controlled under vision or by temporary packing when burr holes are employed.

Sometimes, seizures can follow leukotomy. Seizures can occur after any procedure that cuts into the brain and so cannot be considered as detracting from the value of a particular procedure. There are no other significant complications or sequele.

Nearly all psychosurgical procedures have to be bilateral (for exceptions, see under amygdalotomy). Both sides can be done at the same sitting.

Objections against Leukotomy

Soon after the introduction of leukotomy, as usually happens, enthusiasm for a new procedure overtook balanced judgment. Many cases were done by many surgeons. The outcome in some operations was far from laudable. Some of the patients were rendered absolutely 'wooden', which made the relatives of the patients wonder whether they have exchanged one problem for another. In addition, complications like hemorrhage and occurrence of seizures were held up to discredit the procedures.

The operations done earlier were extensive. Now that it is known which fibers are to be divided, the sequele are minimal. Further the earlier cuts were taken too far laterally and this resulted in interruption of the uncinate fasciculus, leading to woodenness.

Hemorrhage can be properly tackled nowadays. Seizures can be controlled by anticonvulsants, as they are after any cerebral operation.

Results

The results of leukotomy are good if proper care is taken in the selection of the patients. There are many reports available on this. According to Freeman, out of 455 cases operated by various methods, 45% of frontal lobotomy and 65% of transorbital leukotomy did well.[50] Knight[51] reported 70% success and Hirose 66%.[52] In the series of Kalyanaraman and Ramamurthi, out of 11 cases of leukotomy for various conditions, there were 4 cases of schizophrenia, of whom 3 did well.[53] In the author's series of 34 cases, 76% did well.[54]

THALAMOTOMY

Since the major connections of the frontal lobe are to the median nucleus of the thalamus, in an attempt to get the best of both bargains, operations were directed at this nucleus to get the maximum effect of a leukotomy with minimal side-effects. This procedure can only be done by stereotaxic technique. The results are fairly good for chronic painful conditions, but not so for schizophrenia. Further, there is today no need for this operation, as even the leukotomy is only a restricted one.

OPERATIONS ON THE CINGULUM

It is said that operations on the cingulum were suggested by John Fulton as a sort of restricted frontal leukotomy. But nowa-days, they are not performed for schizophrenia. They are employed in certain neurotic states and drug dependence.

History

Perhaps the work of Fulton and the paper of Papez prompted operations on the cingulate gyrus. Scoville reported surgery directed by the cingulate gyrus.[55] According to the same author, Whity, and later Le Beau and Pecker, described their experience with open cingulectomy. With the introduction of stereotaxic techniques, Foltz and later Ballantine performed stereotaxic cingulomotomy.[56,57]

In India, from the beginning, cingulomotomy was done by stereotaxic techniques. The first report was in 1973.[58] Later, cingulomotomy for pain was reported by Ray.[59] Subsequently, a few additional reports have appeared.

Terminology

While the earlier operations were cingulectomy (i.e. excision of cingulate gyrus), the stereotaxic procedure consisted in disconnecting the bundle of white fibers (the cingulum) and so, cingulomotomy is the proper term.

Anatomical and Physiological Basis

The cingulate gyrus, along with the medial part of the frontal lobe, is concerned with affect and drive. Motivation also arises from this area. Connections are seen between this region and the frontal lobe. In addition, there is a distinct band of white fibres streaming through the gyrus. This is the cingulum bundle. The cingulum bundle is a part of the Papez circuit.

This circuit, which was described by James W Papez, was a notable one, as for the first time a structural basis for emotional feeling was given. It is a closed loop, wherein fibers from the hippocampus stream out as the fornix, which ends in the hypothalamic nuclei (particularly in the mamillary bodies); from here, they go as the mamillo-thalamic bundle (bundle of Vicq d' Azyr) to the anterior thalamic nucleus, which connects to the cingulum. The cingulum joins the hippocampus, thus closing the loop (Fig. 6).

Modus Operandi

Affect, motivation and drive, all are governed by the influences from the cingulate region and the area around it. Affect or emotional feeling is a part of one's behavior occurring proximal to emotional expression. The temporal continuum of emotional feeling is mood. Drive and motivation are necessary for goal directed behavior. The termination of such an act is also due to the same factors. Suppose the drive is pathological, then one continues the act in spite of the goal having been achieved or even if the goal is not there. This is particularly so for 'small' acts. The result is the patient goes on doing the same thing repeatedly all the time knowing that this is purposeless. This is unlike in a schizophrenic, who has a psychosis and is unaware of the disordered thinking or the action resulting from this. The patient with obsessive compulsive disorder, however, can not help repeating the action. This is seen well in patients who (at least in the early stages of their problem) often invent excuses as to why they are doing the act. The same thing is seen in some types of drug dependent individuals. Their usual (and genuine) refrain is "doctor I want to get rid of this habit but I cannot help it". In all these types of patients, the drive does not 'turn itself off' and so continues to be there, and the patient has to keep on doing the same act, however much he is unwilling to do so.

In addition, there is another factor at work in drug dependent individual. In some patients, the effects of the withdrawal symptoms are so strong that they run back to the drugs. Most of the withdrawal symptoms are sympathomimetic in nature and are probably initiated through hypothalamo-cingulate connections. These hypothalamic connections join at the level of the foramen of Munro and so

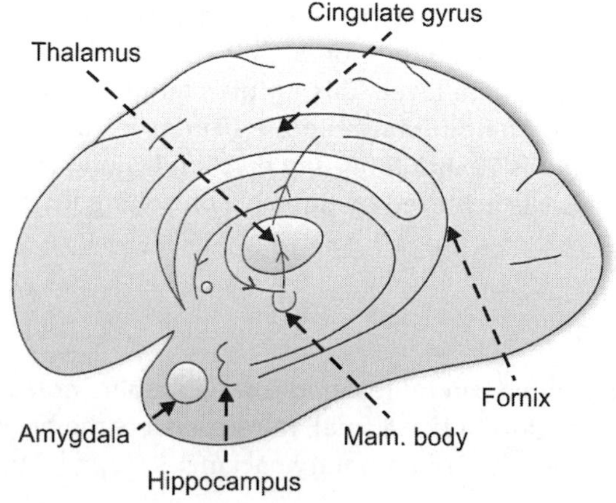

Fig. 6: Papez circuit

can be easily disconnected by placing the stereotaxic lesions at this level.

This is at best a simplistic description of the modus operandi of the procedure.

Indications

The most common indications are obsessive compulsive disorders and mood disorders. It has also been performed for alleviation of pain in chronic painful states. It was found that when a patient with a chronic painful state had cingulomotomy, not only did the pain disappear but also simultaneously any dependence on drugs (acquired as a result of repeated administration) was also abolished. A few case of drug dependence were treated by cingulomotomy by some. But in our series, cingulomotomy was done mostly for the management of dependence. The indications are also listed below:

- Schizophrenia
- Schizoaffective states
- Anxiety disorders (severe)
- Certain painful conditions
- Obsessive compulsive disorder
- Drug dependence.

Of these, schizophrenia and schizoaffective disorder are not clear cut indications, as the procedure has only limited value. Painful conditions fall outside the realm of psychosurgery.

Cingulomotomy has been found to be very useful in obsessive compulsive disorder and drug dependence.

A word of caution has to be given in the selection of drug dependent individuals. Firstly, there must be a genuine desire on the part of the patient to give up the drug. Secondly, the factors which led to the dependence must be analyzed and tackled before offering surgery. In this connection, the author classifies 'addicts' into those that are basically 'psychopathic', have 'ego' problems, and have taken to addiction as an outlet. In such patients, merely correcting the dependence would not help. This is where a preliminary therapy by psychiatrists becomes invaluable. In the second group are those who have become dependent by chance. The classical example is a person who has a chronic painful problem and takes pethidine or some such drug, and very soon becomes an addict. It is likely that there may be a basic psychopathic state in some of these. But, it is not correct to say that all drug dependent persons are basically psychopathic to start with. In many of these, the psychopathic state is the result of repeated administration of drug. It must be mentioned that experimentally, even animals can be made addicts. Recent research into endorphins has raised the possibility that in many, there is an underlying defect in the endorphin metabolism and thus dependence can be termed a metabolic disease.[60]

Timing of Operation

The two problems, obsessive compulsive disorder and drug dependence, can often be well treated by psychiatric therapy. But, surgery must be advised if after a reasonable trial of these measures the patient does not recover.

Techniques

Since open cingulectomy is no longer performed, only *stereotaxic cingulomotomy* will be described. This consists in making a lesion (one on each side) in the cingulum bundle. The operation can be done bilaterally at one sitting. The actual placement of the lesion (i.e. target) varies with individual surgeon's preferences. They are all indicated in (Fig. 7). This author places the lesion in the cingulum in line with the foramen of Munro, as it has been shown that all the fibers can be 'caught' here. The lesions can be made by any method. The author uses injection of an oil-wax mixture.

Complications and Sequelae

Injury to the neighboring arteries, the pericallosal or the callosomarginal, has to be borne in mind.

Objections

The questions often asked are, what type of deficits can one expect from cingulomotomy. These have to be balanced against the quality of life these patients had before the surgery. It is obvious that a severe deficit cannot be accepted in exchange for getting rid of the obsession or drug dependence. It has been the uniform experience of all workers that whatever deficit occurs, balances against the good quality of life after surgery.

However, there were no significant sequele in the 160 patients operated by Ballantine.[57] According to Gachs, though

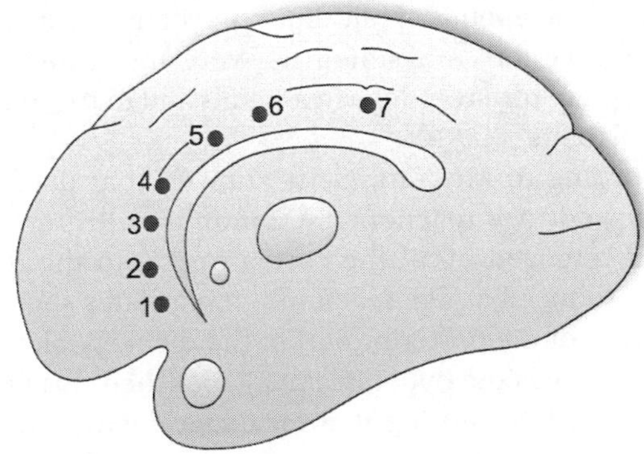

Fig. 7: Various targets for cingulomotomy. The Author's target is indicated by number 5

there was temporary inertia and urinary incontinence, "on the contrary the patient's efficiency was always improved".[61] Again, there was no significant fall in intelligence in the series of Laitenen and Vilkki.[62]

Results

In the author's series of 119 patients with drug dependence, 80% were cured. This was reported in 1986.[61] Out of one batch of 50 patients in the author's series, 13 were randomly selected and subjected to intensive psychological assessment both pre- and postoperatively. All could not be tested, because of the practical difficulties. The details of the assessment have already been reported. The conclusion was, "it is evident that stereotaxic cingulomotomy does not produce any type of neurological or psychological deficit in an appreciable number of cases. Only in two cases, there has been a slight fall in practical reasoning. Highly significant improvement was seen in immediate and recent memory after operation ($p < 0.01$). In general, there is no deficit attributable to the operation *per se*".[63,64] In a recent series of the authors, out of 26 patients, 76% improved.[65]

SEDATIVE NEUROSURGERY

The term sedative neurosurgery was introduced by Sano of Tokyo to cover those procedures, designed to quieten a patient.[66] Sedative neurosurgery has been embroiled in controversy, both among the specialists and the lay public because of:

- The fear of misuse against convicts and minorities
- The bogey of creating a monster by poorly performed procedures, and
- By comparison with what was thought to be similar behavior among animals

  All these will be discussed later in the chapter.

History

Though the therapeutic applications of sedative neurosurgery came in very late, physiologists were interested in the mechanism of rage reactions in animals and in the measures to control them.

According to McLean, Geltz showed that decorticate dogs showed rage reactions.[67] Cannon and Britton observed that removed of all the cortex rostral to the diencephalon produced a rage reaction.[68] It was later shown that destruction of the posterior part of the diencephalon (what is now known as the hypothalamus) abolished this rage.[67] It must be noted that during all these times, the hypothalamus was not recognized as an entity. Parenthetically, it may be mentioned that (in inverse proportion to its importance) even now it has no distinct name of its own, except as being described as something below the thalamus. Subsequently, many ablative and stimulation experiments were done involving the hypothalamus and the periaqueductal grey.

Interestingly, the role of the hypothalamic nuclei and the periaqueductal grey was investigated much earlier than that of the amygdala.

As indicated earlier, Papez described the circuit, where he hypothesized an ensemble of structures subserving emotional feeling.[44] There was one notable omission and this was the amygdala. This structure, ironically, holds the key to emotional behavior.

Part of the reason for the slow rate of accumulation of knowledge of the behavioral system was due to the fact that this system was closely linked with olfaction, which was in any way diminishing in importance in human beings.

One other reason was the bogey raised by the experiments of Brown Schafer (later repeated by Kluver and Bucy), which reported a set of sequelae following bilateral temporal lobectomy in monkey.[69,70] It was feared that any interference similar to their ablations in human beings might produce the same Kluver-Bucy syndrome.

All these notwithstanding, two important landmark papers followed one another, in 1963, by Narabhayashi on amygdalotomy and, in 1966, on hypothalamotomy by Sano (both from Tokyo).[66,71] Still, there was reluctance to accept these procedures. A few centers, however, did perform either of the two operations.

In Madras, both these operations were performed, depending on the indications. Many papers were published on this from 1967.[72-76]In no other center had this been done. The advantage was that the benefits of the two procedure could be compared.

Terminology

The two procedures, which have been used, are amygdalotomy (which means cutting into the amygdala) and hypothalamotomy. Strictly, the latter operation must be correctly termed PVM hypothalamotomy (discussed below). Amygdalectomy was once done by the transventricular route for epilepsy.

Anatomical and Physiological Basis

Emotional reactions consist of emotional feeling (which is subjective) and emotional expression (which is objective). Some call only the latter as emotional behavior. Emotional behavior can be of any kind, but here aggressive behavior will be discussed, as this is the one that needs treatment.

Aggressive behavior is closely linked with olfaction. The full details of this can be obtained from current literature. Here, only a brief outline is given. Broca described a set of structures around the brain stem and because of a fancied resemblance to a ring, it was called the *limbic system* (or *limbic brain*). But, the actual number of structures to be included is not definitely established. The term is still retained because of its prolonged usage. An alternative term, the *behavioral brain* has put been put forward.[45] Among the structures this limbic system includes, two are relevant to our discussion. They are the amygdaloid nucleus and the hypothalamus.

The amygdaloid nucleus is situated in front of the apex of the temporal horn. It lies mostly superomedial to the temporal horn. The amygdaloid nucleus has two main divisions; one, which is olfactory in function, and another, which is concerned with behavior. The nucleus receives afferents from many areas including olfactory fibers. The efferents run mainly in two streams: (1) a phylogenetically older one called, striaterminalis and (2) a recently acquired tract called the ventral amygdalohypothalamic tract. Through both these tracts, the amygdaloid nucleus makes connections with the hypothalamus.

The hypothalamus has many nuclei, of which the posteroventral nucleus is of interest in behavioral mechanisms. It connects to the amygdala and to the periaqueductal grey. Developmentally, this nucleus corresponds to the pernifornical nucleus of the canines. When stimulated in these, it produces a rage reaction.

Modus Operandi

To understand the mechanism of relief by these procedures, a study of aggression in animals, vis a vis aggression in humans, has to be made.

Aggression in animals, other than humans, is of two types: (a) predatory, and (b) nonpredatory. In *predatory aggression*, the animal has to kill the prey in front and, so in such combats, the lethal weapons (claws, etc.) are used and the prey is killed. Most often, the prey belongs to a species not the same as the attacker. In *nonpredatory aggression*, on the other hand, fights are usually between members of the same species and often arise from rivalry for mates or territorial infringements. None of the contenders die (except by accident) and this is because the lethal weapons are not employed.

The decision to employ lethal weapon or not is borne out of recognition of the animal in front. This is mostly by olfactory cues. It is here that the amygdaloid nucleus plays an important part, as it receives olfactory inputs on one side and also connects to the hypothalamus, the executive centre in charge of an attack. This is supported by laboratory studies, wherein stimulation of hypothalamic nuclei causes rage reaction whereas stimulation of amygdala causes only modification of hypothalamically induced rage.

The amygdaloid nucleus and the hypothalamic nuclei, together with other areas like the thalamic nuclei, etc. form the behavioral brain. There is even an hierarchical type of organization to be observed here.[45]

In the two types of aggression in nonhuman animals, different emotional feelings precede the emotional behavior (viz the attack). In predatory aggression, it is one satisfying hunger, i.e. the victim is prospective food. There is no feeling of hatred or anger. In nonpredatory aggression, there is the desire to protect one's property and here there is no desire to kill. One of the contenders will have to retreat. There is no fight to death, since there is no 'ego problem'. There is a teleological explanation too for this. If animals indulging in nonpredatory aggression kill each other, then it will be the end of the species, and the laws of Nature will not allow this. Such combats have necessarily got to be only 'sham', a mere 'sabre-rattling'.

With this background, if we study the psychopathic aggression in humans, it will be noted that the patient who attacks the person in front, may do so without provocation and the victim often is a total stranger. Nor is there any rancour. This is somewhat similar to predatory aggression, though not identical.

Apart from these two types of aggression, there is another type of aggression peculiar to humans. This has no parallel in the rest of the animal kingdom. Actually, there is not even a suitable name for this; though some prefer the term *agonistic aggression*. Here, the killing is not for purposes of eating. This arises from a different mechanism. It is best called *social aggression*.[77]

It was necessary to elaborate on the nature of aggression, mainly to stress that only one type of human aggression, viz *'psychopathic aggression'*, will respond to sedative neurosurgery. The rage reaction that is seen in brain damaged individuals, in postepileptic behavioral disorders and as part of the spectrum of temporal lobe epilepsy, all belong to the group of psychopathic aggression. These will respond to surgery directed at the various structures of the behavioral brain, viz amygdala, hypothalamic nuclei and the periaqueductal grey. But, best results are obtained only in procedures directed at the first two. Non-psychopathic aggression, arising as it does from a different set of mechanisms, will not respond to sedative neurosurgery. Fears or even hopes that this type of surgery will help to 'cure' criminals and other groups are based on wrong analysis of the mechanisms. Similarly, there is no way of 'increasing' the aggressive behavior by incorrect sedative neurosurgery. The absence of a sense of social etiquette, etc. and the resultant violent behavior following leukotomy, are very different from this.

Indications

The indications for both amygdalotomy and hypothalamotomy are the same. Many behavioral disorders usually do not respond to conventional drug therapy. Most drugs act for sometime but ultimately they are effectless. These behavioral disorders range from mere hyperkinesis, wherein the child is restless and wanders listlessly, to extremely severe form of assaultive behavior. These may follow a variety of causes; some of the commoner ones are (a) prolonged uncontrolled epileptic seizures, (b) retarded cerebral development of varied causes, or (c) part of a severe paranoid schizophrenia.

The relation of seizures to the behavior may vary from case to case. The behavioral disorders may coexist with seizures; or may follow a long history of seizures. Rarely, they may alternate with seizures.

Patients with hemispherical damage may exhibit behavioral disorders along with seizures and hemiplegia.

All these patients benefit by these procedures.

Timing

The types of behavioral disorders, which need sedative neurosurgery, vary in intensity. As things stand today, there is no drug which is uniformly successful in controlling these disorders. Such being the case, the timing of the operation will depend more on factors, other than merely medical. In most instances, the surgery is done to quieten the patient and also to make life bearable for the relatives. And many of the parents would opt for surgery quite early. It is easy to appreciate their stand, if one remembers that living with an aggressive and retarded child (or worse adult) day in and day out is nightmarish. In our experience, the prime indication is the end of tolerance of the parent(s).

Techniques

The two operations of sedative neurosurgery, amygdalotomy and hypothalamotomy are best done by stereotaxic technique. But, amygdalotomy can be done by open technique also.

Stereotaxic Amygdalotomy

The target is the center of the amygdaloid nucleus. This lies 4 mm in front of the apex of the temporal horn. The major part of the nucleus is superomedial to the temporal horn tip. The amygdaloid lesions can be made by any preferred method. The author has used oil wax injection, diathermy coagulation and mechanical destruction by loop. Both sides have to be done. Narabhayashi stages the procedure one side at one time.[71] But, the author does both sides at one sitting.[72]

In certain cases of infantile hemiplegia, there is a gross atrophy of one hemisphere and the patient has aggressive behavior. Only in such cases, unilateral amygdalotomy directed at the damaged side is sufficient.[78]

Amygdalectomy by Open Method

Excision of the amygdaloid nucleus can be done by open technique. After a temporal craniotomy, the temporal lobe is exposed. The temporal horn is opened into and, through this, the amygdaloid nucleus is removed by suction.[79] This procedure is ideally suited for temporal lobe epilepsy with unilateral focus. For behavior disorders, both sides will have to be done, either successively or at one sitting. The author has employed both methods in few cases. Recently, a trans-sylvian route has also been advocated.[80]

Complications and sequelae: Anosmia does not occur after the procedure, as the amygdala is not primarily concerned with olfaction. Memory loss cannot occur, unless the surgical procedure involves the hippocampus mistakenly.

In the overall series of 330 cases reported by the author, three developed suicidal tendencies after the operation. In one, this was corrected by modified leukotomy. Two patients, who had aggressive behavior and suicidal tendency before surgery, did not improve as far as the suicidal tendency was concerned, and one of them committed suicide.

One of the greatest deterrents to the employment of amygdalotomy has been the bogey of KluverBucy syndrome following surgery. This has arisen out of the experiments conducted by Brown and Schafer, and Kluver and Bucy. This has been indicated earlier. It can be asserted categorically that KluverBucy syndrome has not occurred after bilateral amygdalotomy. On the other hand, one of the author's cases, who had KluverBucy syndrome, improved after amygdalotomy.

Hypothalamotomy

Hypothalamotomy is also done by stereotaxic techniques. Like amygdalotomy, it has to be done on both sides. But, it is always done one side at a time, with a minimum of one week interval between the two sides.

The target is the posteroventral medial nucleus of the hypothalamus. This nucleus belongs to the sympathomimetic portion of the hypothalamus. It is identified by stimulation performed during operation and the area showing the maximum of sympathomimetic effects is chosen for elimination. This is best done by thermal or radiofrequency coagulation.

Complications: Diabetes insipidus may occur temporarily, after the procedure. Sometimes, hemorrhagic pulmonary edema has occurred following hypothalamotomy.

Objections: A retarded, but aggressive patient, after sedative neurosurgery will still be retarded but quiet. Often the mistake the surgeon may commit is not to make the relatives realise the limitations. Sometimes, the quiet attitude of the patient is mistaken for woodenness, and this has been held up against the surgery.

Amygdalotomy or Hypothalamotomy?

Either of the two operations can be performed with equal success. But as indicated already, most surgeons perform only one of the procedures, to the pointed exclusion of the other and the results with either procedure are parallel. But, both the operations have been preformed in Madras and this has provided a opportunity to compare the two procedures.[81,82]

We feel that amygdalotomy can be done first and, if it does not work, hypothalamotomy can be done. It has also been shown that hypothalamotomy done after amygdalotomy need be only on one side.

Results

Results of Amygdalotomy

There are no established methods of assessing behavioral disorders, which may range from hyperkinesis to severe assaultive behavior. Most surgeons depend on their own individual methods of assessment. While this makes comparison difficult, still it can be seen easily that the overall results are definitely good. The author's method of assessment of psychosurgery patients is given below:

- Where there is no need of any drug. Patient is able to mingle easily with others
- Very much docile and given to occasional outbursts only
- Manageable when given drugs, though not leading a useful life
- Transient improvement, but relapsed
- No change
- Died.

In a recent series of Narabayashi, 88% had moderate to dramatic improvement, while 12% had slight improvement.[83] Ramachandrananalyzed a group of 46 cases (operated by the author), who were taken up from mental hospital. All these had bilateral amygdalotomy for postepileptic behavior disorder, schizophrenic aggression and other types. Aggressive was reduced in 58% of cases.[84] In the author's series of 330 cases, 78% had good results.

Results of Hypothalamotomy

The same grading, as for amygdalotomy, has been employed by the author. In a series of 78 cases of the author, 72.9% had good results.[64] Sano had 95% good results.[85]

MULTIPLE OPERATIONS

Some patients, who have complex problems, may need multiple operations. These can be done after suitable interval between each procedure. Thus, an aggressive patient with an obsessive impulse to break all things made of glass (one of author's patients) needed amygdalotomy and cingulomotomy.

AN APPRAISAL OF PSYCHOSURGERY

In today's context, an appraisal of psychosurgery becomes obligatory if anyone has to recommend or perform it.

Psychosurgery is the most discussed of all procedures in surgery. In addition, much opprobrium has been placed upon it by scientists and nonscientists. Psychiatry deals with diseases of the 'mind'. To many, even psychiatric disorders are not akin to other disorders of the brain. So, they feel that psychosurgery, which has to deal with mental disorders, must be equally uncertain in scope and performance. Such arguments are not based on proper studies of psychiatric disorders. Without getting involved with the complex problem of what mind is, it can be said that psychiatric disorders do arise from the brain. The inability to identify the pathology is due to limitations of the present day diagnostic methods. Of late, the structural origin of psychiatric problems are beginning to gain acceptance, thanks to advances in molecular physiology and other subjects. Recent work has implicated D_2 receptor mechanisms in schizophrenia; or again this disease may also arise from faults in the glutamatergic system.[86,87] These indicate that, like any other human malady, psychiatric disorders too many have structural basis. So, psychosurgical procedures are not mere shots in the dark.

WHY IS THERE SO MUCH UPROAR ABOUT PSYCHOSURGERY?

Psychosurgery is often discussed, and points for and against are given out, not only by scientists involved in it but also by others like the general public, science fiction writers, the media, etc. It must be accepted that since psychosurgery deals with human beings, everyone has a right to take part in the discussion and so nontechnical persons can participate. But, including them very early in the debate will only lead to chaos.

Pseudoreligious objections have been raised against psychosurgery, by claiming that it destroys the soul or cuts away the conscience. Psychiatric disorders are accepted to be disorders of the mind and have nothing to do with the soul. Nor does the 'soul' reside in the brain and the objection is pointless.

It has been said that psychosurgery leaves the patient wooden and like a vegetable. The bad results of psychosurgery are only due to bad techniques. They are not the outcome of the procedures themselves but are due to wrong placement of lesions or an extensive lesion. We saw an example of this under leukotomy, wherein a too lateral a cut would involve the uncinate fasciculus and leave the patient wooden.

Many feel that psychosurgical procedures are empirical. This is perhaps the most unjustified criticism. Most psychosurgical procedures have followed years of experimental work on animals.[88] For example, leukotomy evolved out of experiments conducted by John Fulton, and also clinical observations on a patient, in whom a penetrating injury had disconnected the frontal lobe. Yet strangely, leukotomy is the one procedure most criticized. Perhaps it is so, because it is well known. In a similar way, the description of Papez circuit paved the way for behavioral amelioration by surgery. One has only got to read the original paper of Papez to know the meticulous experimental and clinical observations, on which the paper is based.

The hypothalamus was a common target for many experimental neurophysiologists interested in behavioral mechanisms. The neurophysiological work done on amygdala has been equally striking, as the number of papers testify.

And yet the common refrain is that psychosurgical procedures are not based on laboratory data. Can anything be more unfair? Arguing in the same line, in how many surgical procedures involving other regions can such backup by physiologists is available.

But, one thing must be admitted. These experimental procedures were on nonhuman animals. They were, however, backed by astute clinical observations on human beings, who had suffered neurological deficits due to diseases or injury.

The one unanswerable objection would be that there were no animal models of the disease process. But, psychiatric disorders cannot have animal models because of the different nature of the human psyche.

Another fear about psychosurgery is that they would be employed on murderers and persons convicted of criminal assaults, etc. This fear is groundless. As would be evidenced from the discussion earlier, the type of aggression, wherein the persons attacks (or kills) belongs to what is called social aggression. This is of a different type. In these acts, the person, who is committing them, is aware of the implications and so, tries to hide as happens in a murder; or the person has been so much 'brainwashed' that he, temporarily or permanently, justifies his act. This happens in hired assassins. It is also exemplified by military aggressions or religious wars, wherein the frontal lobe inhibition is suppressed by propaganda. These are very different from psychopathic aggression and will not respond to sedative neurosurgery.

The dangers of making an individual more violent by surgery, either deliberately or by accident during the procedure, have been held up to discredit sedative neurosurgery. Deliberate production of an aggressive individual, by surgery directed at the amygdala, is not possible.[89] Making an ablation, as what Cannon did, might produce 'sham rage' but not a motivated, well-directed aggressive behavior. Frontal lobe disconnection might produce aggressive behavior because it removes the usually available inhibitory role played by the frontal lobes. But, this can happen in persons who take alcohol or certain hallucinogenic drugs. Surely in these cases, the fault is not in the procedure but rests with the person who performs it.

Error, during sedative surgery, cannot make the patient more aggressive. This operation is as much prone to go wrong as any other surgical attempt and so this should necessitate more care during performance rather than an outright condemnation of the very procedure.

Psychosurgical procedures are like any other procedure in surgery. They need care in planning, skill in performance and a thorough awareness of the merits and drawbacks of the operation. They are not to be performed by the 'casual operator'; they should not be considered as 'minor' procedures. This was one of the gravest mistakes of the earlier era. The specialist neurosurgeon, preoccupied as he was with more challenging brain tumors and other problems connected with the brain, was not too keen in doing procedure like leukotomy (except for a few) and so any one who wanted to do, went and did a leukotomy. This is not to decry the pioneering attempts of the trail blazers but to stress that psychosurgical procedures do need as much care as removal of a brain tumor.

Psychosurgical procedure should be performed, only after adequate trial with the nonoperative method; and even after this, there must be a constant interaction between the neurosurgeon, who performs the operation, and the psychiatrist, who was handling the patient earlier. Even more than this, after the operation the psychiatrist has to be available for proper rehabilitation. Performing a leukotomy and setting the patient back in society straightway can produce many problems and a slow re-acclimatization is needed. If all these conditions are observed, psychosurgery will regain a respectable status and will not be considered as somewhere in between witchcraft and black magic.

TECHNIQUES OF STEREOTAXIC SURGERY

A brief description of stereotaxic surgery is given, as most of the psychosurgical procedures are performed this way.

In stereotaxic surgery, the area to be disconnected or eliminated is called the *target*. This is localized by using three parameters, as we are dealing with a three dimensional structure. The *parameters* (called *coordinates*) are calculated with reference to specific points of reference, like the anterior commissure. To visualize these reference points, one many have to do contrast studies with air, or pantaopaque. Where MRI can be done, this can be dispensed with.

Under local analgesia or general anesthesia, the stereotaxic frame is fixed and the reference points visualized. The coordinates for the target are calculated. The electrode is then advanced to the target.

For leukotomy or cingulomotomy, once the electrode is in place, elimination is done by any suitable method.

The most common method is to use radiofrequency generator and make the lesions. Diathermy current has also been used. Injection of a mixture containing pantaopaque, almond oil and beeswax is also employed. Destruction by radioactive seeds is equally good.

For amygdalotomy, verification of electrode placement is done by depth EEG, elicitation of evoked potentials and stimulation.

For hypothalamotomy, the selection of the target depends on stimulation effects. Where possible, postoperative radiograph or MRI can be done.

Guidelines for the Clinical Use of Psychosurgery

Neurosurgical procedures for psychiatric disease are reserved for patients who are refractory to pharmacologic, psychotherapeutic, or electroconvulsive therapies. The patient's psychiatrist is the only individual who may recommend a surgical procedure, and must provide detailed documentation regarding the course of therapy, and the reasons for discontinuation of therapy. It is the responsibility of the psychiatrist to follow the recovery of the patient postoperatively. The family of the patient must also express interest in the surgery, as well as support for the recovery process. It is important to determine that the interests of the family are directed to the best outcome for the patient.

The severity of the psychiatric disease takes precedence over the chronicity of the disorder, although refractory cases have usually failed treatment for five years. Quantitative data is usually obtained, including the Yale-Brown Obsessive Compulsive Scale, the Beck Depression Inventory, and the global assessment of function. Each institution typically has its own criteria for psychosurgical procedures. The Cingulotomy Committee at the Massachusetts General Hospital, for example, is a multidisciplinary board of neurosurgeons, psychiatrists, and neurologists, who all must clinically evaluate the patient. Electroencephalogram, magnetic resonance imaging, electrocardiogram, neuropsychological testing, and laboratory testing are all required in addition to an extensive review of the medical record. All involved family members and committee members must give consent for the surgery.

Future Directions

Functional neurosurgery, somatic therapies, and beyond the future of psychosurgery, like its past, is linked to the developments of neurosurgery, neurology, psychiatry, and cognitive neuroscience. As pharmacologic treatments become more efficacious, there will be less need for neurosurgical intervention, but refractory cases will be more challenging. Greater understanding of the neurobiology of emotion through basic research or cognitive neurology will result in more rational and more precise techniques.

Advanced neuroimaging techniques will also contribute to the translation of investigative findings to human intervention. Furthermore, other interventions in the clinical neurosciences for conditions such as epilepsy, Parkinson's, or chronic pain will find greater application in the neuropsychiatric arena. Again, it is important to recognize psychosurgery as one of many interventions historically referred to as somatic therapies. Somatic, or physical treatment for psychiatric disease is best exemplified by psychosurgery and electroconvulsive therapy, formerly known as shock therapy.

Another method of nonsurgically modulating electrical activity in the brain is transcranial magnetic stimulation (TMS). A coil is placed against the scalp, and a pulse of radiofrequency electric current is passed through it, creating a magnetic field that results in depolarization of the superficial cortex.[90] The neural response is dependent on the site, number, and intensity of the applications. TMS has been employed as a neurophysiologic tool for the investigation of cortical excitability, but has also been shown to induce changes in neurochemistry that are similar to those found with antidepressants or electroconvulsive therapy.[90] Reports and metastudies have been ambiguous, but repeated TMS applications to the area adjacent to the left prefrontal cortex are being explored for antidepressant activity. The most prominent adverse effect of repeated TMS is the precipitation of seizures, thought to result from increased cortical excitability.[90]

One of the promising future directions of psychosurgery is the combination of surgical and electrical approaches. While electroconvulsive therapy delivers a nonspecific electrical surge to the brain, and TMS causes disruption or excitation of more focal areas, there are more circumscribed uses of electrical manipulation that are currently employed. The use of implantable electrodes for focal modulation of the vagus nerve and the basal ganglia are promising treatments for epilepsy and Parkinson's disease and may have relevance for neuropsychiatric disorders.[91-100] The vagus nerve relays information that can function in an autonomic feedback loop, and also delivers signals to the forebrain via the parabrachial nucleus and locus ceruleus, both of which have important connections to crucial limbic system structures such as the amygdala.[101-113] Vagal nerve stimulation acts via an electrode attached to the nerve in the neck, coupled to a pulse generator implanted in the chest wall. It is currently being used for treatment-refractory epilepsy patients, with encouraging and sustainable results.[114] It has also been explored as a treatment for refractory depression, and in a multicenter trial of 30 patients has led to a sustainable reduction in depressive symptoms in 12 patients.[101,104] Vagal nerve stimulation has been shown to increase serotonergic and noradrenergic transmission in the brain, and has also been posited to improve limbic system blood flow. Adverse effects in the postoperative period include pain, cough, vocal cord paralysis, hoarseness, and nausea. Asystole has been reported to occur transiently in a small amount of patients, but there were no persistent effects. Dyspnea and voice alteration have also been associated with stimulation. In general, though, the procedure has been tolerated well in epilepsy patients, and may hold promise in the neuropsychiatric population.

Deep brain stimulation (DBS) is a technique used to modulate basal ganglia and thalamic function in order to attenuate the symptoms of Parkinson's disease.[105-109] Chronic electrical stimulation of basal ganglia structures such as the globus pallidus internus and subthalamic nucleus are achieved by an implantable electrode coupled to a pulse generator, and has been found to ameliorate bradykinesia, tremor, rigidity, as well as postural and gait abnormalities.[86] Stimulation of the ventral intermediate nucleus of the thalamus has been shown to attenuate tremor. DBS has been shown to be highly efficacious, especially in younger Parkinson's patients. Adverse effects of DBS result from the surgical procedure itself, most notably intracerebral hemorrhage. More common effects are perioperative or stimulation-related confusion.[90]

The technique of chronically stimulating focal brain structures may hold promise as an alternative to ablative neurosurgery for psychiatric disorders. In patients with coexisting Parkinson's and OCD, the subthalamic electrodes and the use of DBS was found to ameliorate compulsive symptoms in addition to the motor abnormalities.[91] It has also been widely recognized that stimulation of the subthalamic nucleus can also result in an improvement of mood. Interestingly, bilateral stimulation of the subthalamic nucleus in patients with Parkinson's has been reported to induce laughter as well as acute depression. Stimulation of other brain sites have also been shown to affect psychiatric symptoms. DBS of the internal globus pallidus has been shown to decrease symptoms of anxiety in Parkinson's patients independently of motor symptoms.[110] Thalamic stimulation has been suggested to attenuate the tics associated with Tourette's. Bilateral stimulation of the anterior limbs of the internal capsule has been shown to be beneficial in attenuating the effects of OCD, and suggests DBS as an alternative to ablative capsulotomy.[104] As the functional neuroanatomy underlying OCD, depression, and other psychiatric disease continues to be elucidated, DBS may become more frequently employed.[111]

Again, it is important to note that the stimulation ultimately results in an inhibition of neural activity, and thus is the functional equivalent of lesioning. The prominent difference, of course, is that the functional lesion is controllable and reversible. Furthermore, whereas it has not proven possible in the past to do controlled studies with destructive lesions, it may prove feasible with these inhibitory stimulators. The stimulator can be implanted and activated at various time points in certain patients. In this manner, an ethically appropriate study could finally answer whether such surgery is efficacious.[112] Furthermore, such stimulators could be implanted at more than one target site and relative efficacy of various targets could be tested. Such studies would be a major advance in the field. Most of the psychosurgical procedures described in this review have been destructive rather than constructive, and, indeed, lesioning in one form or another has been the mainstay of neurosurgical treatment of psychiatric disease.

The advances in neurobiology over the last decade have created the future possibility for constructive psychosurgery—an intervention that augments or stimulates neural function for therapeutic benefit rather than ablating it. The stereotactic delivery of genetic or cellular material with specific functions to specific brain areas holds the promise of augmenting rather than inhibiting neural function.[113] As the complex genetic factors of psychiatric disorders are elucidated, specific gene replacement strategies in focal areas may become viable therapeutic modalities. The expression of gene products in the brain by modified herpes, adeno- or adenoassociated viruses is already being explored for brain tumors and other neurologic dysfunctions such as epilepsy, and can conceivably play a role in psychiatric disease. Another future direction of neurosurgical intervention will be the delivery of cellular products such as stem cells to degenerated or malfunctioning brain regions. Stem cell research is currently in an explosive phase, and is beset with its own complex ethical questions. The introduction of modified neural stem cells as a therapeutic modality has already had experimental success in other neurologic disorders,[114] and may hold potential for psychiatric disease.

46.9 PSYCHOPHARMACOLOGICAL DRUGS

Jayati Simlai, Anushul Khichy, JN Vyas

INTRODUCTION

Psychotropic drugs are widely used in medical practice so that most clinicians are likely to have under their care a number of patient receiving treatment with psychoactive medication (Table 12). Practitioners, therefore, need to have an understanding of the uses and side effect of psychotropic drugs, particularly of the way in which such medication can interact with drugs used to treat other medical disorders.

The majority of psychotropic drugs are prescribed for the treatment of depressive and anxiety disorders. The reflects the frequency of these conditions in both primary care and general hospital settings; accordingly, drugs treatment for anxiety and depression will often be instituted both by general parishioners and hospital clinicians. Similarly, while the principal use of antipsychotic drugs in the treatment of schizophrenia, such agents are also frequently used in general hospitals in the management of organic psychoses.

Table 12: Classification of clinical psychotropic drugs

Name	*Examples of classes*	*Indications*
Antipsychotic	Phenothiazines Butyrophenones Substituted benzamides	Acute treatment of schizophrenia and mania, prophylaxis of schizophrenia
Antidepressant	Tricyclic antidepressants Monoamine oxidase inhibitors Selective serotonin-reuptake inhibitors	Major depression (acute treatment and prophylaxis), anxiety disorders, obsessive-compulsive disorder (S-HT-uptake blockers)
Mood stabilizer	Lithium (Lithium-SR) Carbamazepine Valproate (Valprid-CR)	Acute treatment of mania, prophylaxis of recurrent mood disorder
Anxiolytic	Benzodiazepines Azapirones (buspirone)	Generalized anxiety disorder
Hypnotic	Benzodiazepines Cyclopyrrolones (zopiclone) Imidazopyridines (zolpidem)	Insomnia

Finally, while treatment with mood-stabilizing drugs, such as lithium, will generally be initiated by psychiatrists, patients receiving long-term therapy may well require treatment for coexisting medical disorders, because of which a knowledge of the effects of lithium on different body systems and its liability to produce adverse drug interactions will be required.

DRUG OVERDOSE

The effects of deliberate or accidental overdose of psychotropic drugs will also involve physicians. Related to this is the general point that when prescribing psychotropic drugs, particularly for depressed patients, the risk of overdose should always be considered. If such a risk is present the practitioner should:

- Ensure that medication is dispensed small amounts
- Consider asking a close relative to supervise the medication
- Use a relatively nontoxic, if possible.

Pharmacokinetic Factors

Most psychotropic drugs are highly lipophilic and well absorbed from the gastrointestinal tract. They are metabolized by the layer to water-soluble derivatives which are eliminated by the layer to water-soluble derivatives which are eliminated by the kidney hence their half-life will be prolonged in patients with hepatica renal impairment must be considered. For example, selective cartooning reuptake inhibitors are potent inhibitor of hepatic cytochrome P-450 enzymes and can thereby increase plasma levels of co-administered drugs such as warfare.

Withdrawal of Psychotropic Medication

Psychotropic and many other classes of drugs produce neuro-adaptive changes during their repeated administration. Readjustment has to occur when drug treatment is stopped, and this may appear clinically as a withdrawal or abstinence syndrome. Characteristic abstinence syndromes have been described for the antidepressants and anxiolytics, while the sudden discontinuation of lithium can provoke a 'rebound' mania; hence it is prudent to withdraw psychotropic drugs slowly whenever possible. It is clearly also important to be label to distinguish withdrawal syndromes from relapse of the disorder being treated.

Compliance and Concordance with Treatment

In psychotropic drug prescribing, compliance is an even greater problem than in general therapeutics. Psychoactive drugs frequently have unpleasant side effects. Psychoactive drugs frequently have unpleasant side effects and, whiled side effects are experienced early in treatment, several days may elapse before a therapeutic response is evident. In addition, patients may not see the need for treatment or believe that it can help them. Careful explanation accompanied by written instructions is taken.

It is increasingly recognized that the successful and safe use of medication requires a collaborative relationships between patient and doctor. The team 'concordance' may, therefore, be preferred to 'compliance', which carries the implicit assumption that the patient's job is to obey instructions. It is, therefore, important to acquire an understanding of the patient's attitude to his or her illness as well its treatment. For example, discussion that helps patients to weigh the advantages and disadvantages of drug treatment ('compliance therapy') has been shown to benefit those with schizophrenia.

Antidepressant Drugs

All currently employed antidepressant drugs, through one mechanism or another, increase the activity of serotoninergic (5-hydroxytryptamine, 5-HT) and/or noradrenergic neuronergic activity in the CNS. The pharmacological actions of both noradrenaline (norepinephrine) and 5-HT in the synapse are terminated by specific reuptake pumps that draw these neurotransmitter back into the presynaptic never ending. Most antidepressant potentiate the action of 5-HT and noradrenaline by blocking this reuptake process.

Tricyclic Antidepressants

Pharmacology

Tricyclic antidepressant inhibit the neuronal uptake of nor adrenaline (nor epinephrine) and 5-HT. They have numerous other pharmacological properties, but these are though to contribute to their adverse effect profile rather than their therapeutic activity. However, some of these adverse effects, for example, sedation, can prove beneficial in certain circumstances.

Principal Drugs

These are amitriptyline, clomipramine, desmethylimipramine, doxepin, imipramine, lofepramine, and nortriptyline.

Indications and Use

Tricyclic antidepressant are still the most widely prescribed drug treatment for the management of depressive illness, but their use, particularly in less severe depressive states, is waning in favors of newer compound that are severe depressive states, is waning in favors of newer compounds that re better tolerated. However, none of the newer antidepressants is more efficacious than the tricycles and their therapeutic activity in severely ill patients is not as well established. For this reason, unless there are specific contraindications, tricyclic antidepressants should be preferred in depressed inpatients or in those with marked melancholic features.

Depressed patients with prominent sleep disturbance and anxiety should be treated with a sedating antidepressant such as amitriptyline; for other patients, less sedating compounds such as lofepramine or nortriptyline can used. To obtain tolerance to side effects, it is usual to begin treatment at a low dose, for example 25–50 mg of amitriptyline at night, and to increase the amount over about 2–3 weeks to the usual therapeutic dose, which ranges between 75 and 20 mg daily for amitriptyline and imipramine. Tricyclic antidepressants have long half-lives and a single daily dose taken at night is unsuitably appropriate. Patients should be warned about side effects because this help to ensure compliance in the early stages of treatment. They should also be advised that a clear therapeutic response may not appear for up of 2–4 weeks.

It treatment is successful, it is usual to continue the antidepressant for 4 to 6 months at the original dose if tolerance allows (so called 'continuation therapy'). This reduces the risk of early relapse by about half. Some patients have to continue up to 5 years or even lifelong with antidepressant drugs. This should be considered in those who have had more than two episodes of depression in the previous 5 years, particularly if the episodes have been severe in terms of symptomatology and impact on work and social functioning.

Side Effects

As well as inhibiting the uptake of noradrenaline (norepinephrine) and 5-HT, tricyclic antidepressants possess antagonist properties at a variety of neurotransmitter receptors, including Muscarine cholinergic receptors, α_4-adrenoceptors, and H_1-histamine receptors. These receptors' antagonist effects account for most of the adverse effect profile of these agents, particularly their anticholinergic properties (Table 13). Tricyclics also possess membrane-stabilizing effects that underline their most serious side effect of cardiotoxicity, which can be particularly problematic in tricyclic overdose, where ingestion of less than 1 g can sometimes prove fatal. Lofepramine, however, is relatively safe in overdose. Tricycles should be used with caution in patients with cardiovascular disease. They also lower the seizure threshold and can thereby aggravate pre-existing epilepsy or sometimes cause seizures *de novo*.

Drug Interactions

Tricyclic antidepressants antagonize the hypothesize effect of α_2-adrenoceptor agonists such as condone, but can be safely combined with trioxides and angiotensin-converting enzyme (ACE) inhibitors. The ability of tricycles to block noradrenaline (norepinephrine) reuptake can lead to hypertension with systemically administered noradrenaline and adrenaline (epinephrine). Tricycles should not be used in conjunction with antiarrhythmic drugs, particularly amiodarone. Plasma levels of tricycles can be increased by numerous other drugs including cimetidine, sodium valproate, calcium-channel blockers, and selective serologic-reuptake inhibitors (SSRIs).

Table 13: Some adverse effects of tricyclic antidepressants

Pharmacological action	*Adverse effects*
Muscarinic-receptor blockade (anticholinergic)	Dry mouth, tachycardia, blurred vision, glaucoma, constipation, urinary retention, sexual dysfunction, cognitive impairment
α_1-Adrenoceptor blockade	Drowsiness postural hypertension. Sexual dysfunction, cognitive impairment
Histamine H_1-receptor blockade	Drowsiness, weight gain
Membrane-stabilizing properties	Cardiac conduction defects, cardiac arrhythmias, epileptic seizures
Other	Rash, edemas, leukopenia, elevated liver enzymes

Newer Antidepressants

Principal Drugs

These can be classified as follows:
- *Selective 5-HT reuptake inhibitors (SSRIs):* Catalpa, fluoxetine, fluvoxamine, pirouetting, restrainers
- Selective noradrenaline (norepinephrine)-reuptake inhibitors; reboxetine
- Selective noradrenaline and serotonin-reuptake inhibitors; venlafaxine
- *Monoamine-receptor antagonists:* Mirtazapine, nefazodone, and trazodone.

Pharmacology

The actions of SSRIs are essentially confined to inhibition of 5-HT reuptake. Their use is associated with a sustained increase in brain 5-HT neurotransmission. By contrast, reboxetine inhibits only the reuptake of noradrenaline (norepinephrine). Venlafaxine (Venfax-PR) is a potent blocker of 5-HT reuptake and at higher doses blocks the reuptake of noradrenaline as well. Nefazodone and trazodone have weak 5-HT_2 receptors, and trazodone is a potent α_3-adrenoceptor antagonist at 5-HT_2 receptors, and trazodone is a potent α_3-adrenoceptor antagonist at 5-HT_2 receptors antagonist, but in addition blocks inhibitory presynaptic α_2-adrenoceptors, resulting in an increased release of noradrenaline.

All these compound lack the cardiotoxicity and the anticholinergic effects of conventional tricyclic antidepressants. They are therefore safer in depressed subjects they have equal efficacy to tricycles by, as noted above, it is not clear it this extends to the most severely ill patients.

Indications for Use

The newer antidepressants should be used to treat patients in whom the use of tricyclic antidepressants is contraindicated because of their anticholinergic and cardiotoxic effects. In addition, some patients in whom the use of tricyclic antidepressants is causes fewer side effects. The lack of sedation associated with SSRIs, reboxetine, venlafaxine, and nefazodone can be beneficial in outpatients striving to carry out their usual activities. Unlike tricyclic antidepressants, appropriate in patients in whom weight gain would weight gain would be undesirable. Finally, in patients where the risk of overdose cannot be minimized, the newer drugs may be minimized the newer drugs may be preferred because of their lower acute toxicity.

Side Effect

The main adverse effects of the newer antidepressants are shown in Table 14. The major distinction between compounds is whether or not they are sedating. The sedating antidepressants have the advantage of improving sleep at an early stage but may impair cognitive function, while the reverse is true at an early stage but may impair cognitive function, while the reverse is true for SSRIs, venlafaxine, and reboxetine. Like tricyclic antidepressant, the newer compounds appear to lower seizures threshold to some extent, though this effect may be less with trazodone and SSRIs. SSRIs may increase the risk of upper gastrointestinal bleeding, particularly if given conjunction with nonsteroidal anti-inflammatory drugs (NSAIDs).

Drug Interactions

SSRIs with the exception of citalopram slow the metabolism of numerous other drugs including warfarin, theophylline, anticonvulsants, antipsychotics, and tricyclic antidepressants. Dangerous interactions, characterized by 5-HT neurotoxicity have been reported between SSRIs, Venlafaxine (Venfax-PR), and monoamine oxidase inhibitors (MAOIs). At least 5 weeks should, therefore, elapse between stopping fluoxetine and prescribing a monoamine oxidase inhibitor. SSRIs may also

Table 14: New antidepressants

Drug	*Mechanism*	*Adverse effects*
SSRIs	5-HT-reuptake blockade	Nausea, insomnia, headache, anxiety, rash, sweating, sexual dysfunction, low sodium state, extrapyramidal movement disorders (rare), seizure (rare)
Venlafaxine (Venfax-PR)	5-HT-and noradrenaline (norepinephrine)-reuptake blockade	Nausea, headache, insomnia, sweating, anxiety, hypertension (high doses), sexual dysfunction
Reboxetine	Noradrenaline-reuptake blockade	Dry mouth, sweating, constipation, insomnia
Trazodone	5-HT_2-receptor antagonism α_1-Adrenoceptor blockade	Sedation, dizziness, nausea, postural hypotension, priapism (rare), cardiac arrhythmias (rare)
Nefazodone	5-HT_2-receptor antagonist	Headache, fatigue, dizziness, dry mouth, nausea, somnolence
Mirtazapine (Mirazep)	5-HT_2 / α_2-receptor agonist	Sedation, weight gain, abnormal liver function tests, reversible agranulocytosis (rare)

produce 5-HT toxicity in combination with lithium. Trazodone and mirtazapine (Mirazep) may increase the sedative effects of other centrally acting drugs. Nefazodone can raise plasma levels of terfenadine, causing a risk. Reboxetine should not be given with other agents that might potentiate noradrenaline (norepinephrine) function (such as MAOIs) or increase blood pressure (such as ergot derivatives).

Monoamine Oxidase Inhibitors

Pharmacology

Monoamine oxidase inhibitors (MAOIs) block the enzyme monoamine oxidase, which deaminates the neurotransmitters, 5-HT, noradrenaline (norepinephrine), and dopamine. Monoamine oxidase exists in two forms, known as type A (which deaminates noradrenaline and 5-HT) and type B (which preferentially deaminates dopamine and tyramine). Conventional MAOIs irreversibly deactivate both type A and type B monoamine oxidase. This has two main consequences of importance for MAOI use:

1. There is a potential for serious food and drug interaction; and
2. The consequent drugs and food restrictions need to be continued for 2 weeks after cessation.

Recently a new MAOI, moclobemide, has been introduced. This differs from conventional MAOIs in that its inhibition of monoamine oxidase only. This leads to an increase in brain noradrenaline and 5-HT level, other amines such as tyramine are little affected. These factors make moclobemide much less likely than the older monoamine oxidase inhibitors to produce adverse food and drug interactions, giving it a significant safety in the treatment of moderately depressed outpatients. Studies have not thus far demonstrated its efficacy in the patients groups for whom conventional MAOI treatment is currently reserved.

Principal Drugs

These are isocarboxazid, phenelzine, tranylcypromine, and moclobemide.

Indications and Use

Conventional MAOIs are rarely used as a first choice of antidepressant, except where a patient is known to have responded to them in the past. They are usually reserved for subject who have failed to respond to tricyclic antidepressants, newer antidepressant, or electro convulsive therapy. Where a very useful antidepressant effect can often by achieved.

Phenelzine and tranylcypromine are the two most commonly prescribed MAOIs. The usual therapeutic dose for phenelzine is between 30 and 90 mg daily. As with tricyclic antidepressants, patients should be informed about side effect and advised that a therapeutic response from monoamine oxidase inhibitor may not be apparent for 3 to 4 weeks. Once a response is obtained, it is usually necessary to continue treatment for several months.

Side Effects

Monoamine oxidase inhibitors may cause the following side effects:

- *Central nervous system:* Dizziness, muscular twitching, insomnia, confusion, mania
- *Cardiovascular:* Tachycardia, postural hypotension, hypertensions
- *Other:* Dry mouth, blurred vision, impotence, peripheral edema, hepatocellular damage, leukopenia.

Food and Drug Interaction

The major hazard of conventional MAOI treatment is through interaction with indirect sympathomimetics, that is, agents that release noradrenalin from nerve endings. The usual source of the interaction is tramline in certain foodstuffs, especially cheese and meat extracts. Tyramine is usually metabolized by monoamine oxidase in the gut wall and liver, but in patients taking MAOIs large amounts may enter the systemic circulation, resulting in hypertension and even cerebrovascular accidents. Similar adverse effects have been cerebrovascular accidents. Similar adverse effects have been reported when sympathomimetic drugs, such as amphetamines or ephedrine, are administered to patients taking monoamine oxidase inhibitors. Ephedrine or its derivatives are frequently present in cold cures; patients must therefore be warned against self-medication without seeking advice.

Hypertensive episodes resulting from the interaction of sympathomimetic drugs and monoamine oxidize inhibitors are best treated with an α_2-adrenoceptor antagonist. If one is unavailable, intramuscularly chlorpromazine is an alternative.

MAOIs also produce important interactions with other commonly used drugs, including opiates, insulin, and oral hypoglycemic agents. Except in special circumstances, combination with tricyclic antidepressants is best avoided. Combination with tricyclic antidepressants is best cause a 5-HT neurotoxicity syndrome and is contraindicated.

From the foregoing it will be apparent that conventional monoamine oxides inhibitors should only be prescribed to patients capable of adhering to the necessary dietary restrictions. Written instructions listing prohibited foods should be provided. No additional medication should be given until the possibility of an adhering to the necessary dietary restrictions. Written instructions listing prohibited foods should be provided. No additional medication should be given until the possibility of an adverse drug interaction has been escaladed.

Moclobemide

Moclobemide is well tolerated, although insomnia and nausea may occur. Unlike conventional monoamine oxides inhibitors, moclobemide does not cause significant interaction with tyramine, and adverse drug interactions also seem to be less likely. However, caution is recommended when prescribing with opiate, and combined use with SSRI and sympathomimetic agents should avoided. Because of the reversible nature of moclobemide's interaction with monoamine oxidase and its short half-life (about 3 hour), monoamine oxidase activity is restored within a days of stopping treatment.

MOOD-STABILIZING DRUGS

Lithium (Lithium-SR)

Pharmacology

Lithium salts have inhibitory effects on receptor-transudation system, particularly second messengers such as cyclic-AMP and phosphoinositol. Lithium also produces marked increase in some aspects of brain 5-HT function.

Indications and Use

The main uses of lithium are:

- Prophylaxis recurrent affective disorders, especially mania depressive illness
- Acute treatment of mania
- Augmentation of antidepressant medication in patients with resistant depression.

The excretion of lithium from the body is critically dependent on the kidney. Since there is little margin between the therapeutic plasma level of lithium (0.5–0.8 mmol/L) and those causing toxicity (>1.2 mmol/L), the introduction of lithium therapy should be preceded by clinical and laboratory assessment of renal function. Renal function tests should include urine analysis and estimations of plasma ketone and electrolyte levels, with measurement of creatinine levels if there is any suspicion of impaired renal function.

Patients should initially be treated with 200 to 400 mg daily or lithium carbonate, usually as a single dose at night. Slow-release preparations of lithium are available, but their pharmacokinetic *in vivo* are very similar to those of the standard preparation. Dosage should be adjusted every 5 to 7 days on the basis of plasma lithium exterminations obtained approximately 12 hour after the last dose. For prophylaxis of recurrent mood disorders, plasma levels of 0.5–0.5 mmol/L usually satisfactory; but some patients-particularly those with an acute manic episode—may require levels (0.8–1.0 mmol/L). Most patients achieve adequate plasma levels with lithium carbonate dosages of between 600 and 1200 mg daily, and following this their lithium requirement is generally stable.

In the sense of clinical indication it is usually sufficient to check lithium levels monthly. Lithium can also cause hypothyroidism, so thyroid function test should be performed prior to treatment and at 6-monthly intervals thereafter. If necessary, lithium can be combined with thyroxin replacement therapy. Sudden withdrawal of lithium in bipolar patients can cause an acute rebound mania and should be avoided if at all possible.

Side Effects

Many patients suffer from a fine tremor and nausea; diarrhea may occur especially at the start of treatment (Table 15). Some degree of thirst and polyuria is common, and few patients develop nephrogenic diabetes insipidus, caused by lithium probably through the effect of ADH on the renal tubule. Most patients taking lithium have a demonstrable impairment of tubular concentrating ability, although this is rarely of clinical significance. Glomerular function is not usually affected by lithium, but glomerular damage and interstitial fibrosis have been reported following lithium toxicity. There are reports that long-term renal impairment. However, this risk is low provided the plasma concentrations of lithium are kept within the therapeutic range and episodes of toxicity are avoided.

Up to 80% of the lithium filtered by the renal glomeruli is reabsorbed by the proximal tubule. Conditions such as diarrhoea and excessive sweating, which induce renal sodium retention, also in increased lithium reabsorption by the kidney and elevated plasma lithium levels.

Table 15: Some adverse effects and interactions of lithium

Central nervous system	Drowsiness, lethargy, headache, memory impairment, fine tremor
Cardiovascular system	Conduction defects (rare)
Gastrointestinal system	Nausea, vomiting, diarrhea
Genitourinary system	Polydipsia, polyuria, nephrogenic diabetes insipidus
Endocrine system	Hypothyroidism (T4↓TSH↑) hyperglycemia, hyperparathyroidism
Other	Leukocytosis, skin rash, weight gain
Drug interaction (lithium level)	Diuretics, NSAIDs, metronidazole, spectinomycin, ACE inhibitors
Signs of toxicity (plasma level: >1.2 mmol/L)	Nausea, vomiting, coarse tremor, drowsiness, dysarthria, seizures, coma, renal failure, cardiovascular collapse.

Abbreviations: T4, thyroxine; TSH, thyroid stimulating hormone; NSAIDs, non-steroidal anti-inflammatory drugs; ACE, angiotensin-converting enzyme

Drug Interactions

Thiazide diuretics, through their effects on sodium excretion, increase lithium reabsorption and can produce lithium toxicity unless the dose of lithium is reduced and plasma concentrations carefully monitored. It is said that loop and potassium-sparing diuretics are less likely to alter lithium clearance, but it is prudent to monitor lithium level carefully when using these drugs. Plasma lithium levels may also be increased by concomitant administration of NSAIDs, and a similar effect may be produced by metronidazole. Lithium levels may be increased by ACE inhibitors and lowered by theophylline. While the effects of lithium on cardiac conduction are usually considered benign, the effects of cardiac glycosides on conduction may be potentiated. Lithium can cause neurotoxicity (at normal plasma levels) with calcium-channel blockers and carbamazepine. Finally, lithium may increase the liability of antipsychotic drugs to cause extrapyramidal movement disorders.

Lithium Toxicity

Acute lithium toxicity usually appears at plasma levels above 1.2 mmol/L. Early sings are coarse tremor, drowsiness, and dysarthria. Higher plasma concentration (>2.0 mmol/L) can lead to seizures, coma, and death. Since lithium toxicity is potentially fatal, any suspicion of intoxication should lead to the immediate withdrawal of lithium treatment and close monitoring of serum lithium and plasma electrolyte and creatinine concentration. Severely ill patients with high serum lithium levels may require dialysis.

Carbamazepine

Pharmacology

Like certain other anticonvulsant drugs, carbamazepine blocks neuronal sodium channels. The relationships of this effect to its therapeutic action in affective disorder is uncertain. Similarly to lithium, carbamazepine facilitates some aspects of brain 5-HT neurotransmission.

Indications and Use

Carbamazepine is effective in the acute treatment of mania and in the prophylaxis of bipolar affective disorder. It is used in patients who have difficulty to lithium therapy, when it may be given in combinations with lithium.

The dose range of carbamazepine employed to treat patients with affective illness is similar to that used in the treatment of seizure. Initial treatment should be with 100 mg of carbamazepine twice daily, with the dose increased a according to tolerance over next 2– 2 weeks. The effective range in the treatment of bipolar disorders is generally between 600 and 1200 mg daily, although some patients require higher closes. Plasma level monitoring may be used to help avoid toxicity.

Side Effects

Dizziness, dreaminess, and nausea are common early in treatment, particularly with rapid dose titration, but tolerance to these effects usually develops. Persistent ataxia and diplopia may indicate plasma carbamazepine level in the toxic range. A moderate degree of leukopenia is often seen during carbamazepine treatment and agranulocytosis can occasionally develop, such that it is prudent to monitor the white cell count as well as the carbamazepine level during treatment. Skin rashes are also quite common. Other rarer adverse effects include hyponatremia and live cell damage. Circulating thyroid hormone level may be lowered by carbamazepine treatment, but thyroid-stimulating hormone (TSH) levels by carbamazepine in the normal range and clinical hypothyroidism is unusual. Carbamazepine can impair cardiac conduction and should be used with caution in patient with cardiovascular disease.

Drug Interactions

Carbamazepine increases the metabolism of a number of other drugs, including tricyclic antidepressant, haloperidol, oral contraceptive agents, wireman, and other anticonvulsants. A similar mechanism may underlie the decline in the plasma carbamazepine level sometimes seen during continued treatment. The carbamazepine level may be increased by erythromycin and by some calcium-channel blockers, such as digitized and verapamil. Reversible neurotoxicity has been reported when carbamazepine is combined with lithium.

Sodium Valproate (Valprid-CR)

Pharmacology

Valproate is a simple branch-chin fatty acid with a mode of action that is unclear, although there is some evidence that it can slow the breakdown of the inhibitory neurotransmitter Y-amino butyric, but whether it also underlies the psychotropic effects is unclear.

Indications and Use

Like carbamazepine, sodium valproate was first introduced as an anticonvulsant. Recent studies have shown that it is clearly effective in the management of acute mania: the drug is licensed for this purpose in the United State, but not in the United Kingdom. In the United States, vaporize is widely used in the longer term prophylaxis of bipolar disorders, but there is little evidence for this indication from randomized trials.

Valproate can be started at a dose of 400 to 600 mg daily, which may be increased once or twice weekly to between 1 and 2 g daily. Plasma levels of valproate do not correlate well with either its anticonvulsant or mood-stabilizing effects, but it has been suggested that efficacy in the treatment of mood disorders is usually apparent when plasma levels are above 50 µg/ml.

Side Effects

Common side effects of valproate include gastrointestinal disturbances, tremor, sedation, weight gain, and transient hair loss. Serious side effects are rare, but fatal hepatic toxicity has been reported, as has acute pancreatitis. Valproate may also thrombocytopenia and inhibit platelet aggregation, and increases in plasma ammonia have been reported.

Drug Interactions

Valproate potentiates the effects of central sedatives. It has been reported to increase the side effect of other anticonvulsants (without necessarily improving anticonvulsant control). IT may increase plasma levels of phenytoin and Tricyclic antidepressant.

ANTIPSYCHOTIC DRUGS

Conventional (Typical) and Atypical Agents

Pharmacology

Antipsychotic drugs, also known as major tranquilizers or narcoleptics, are a group of agents of varied structure that are used to treat schizophrenia and other psychoses. Conventional or typical ant psychotic agents have in common the ability to block dopamine receptors in the central nervous system, and it is likely that their antipsychotic effect is caused by blocked of dopamine D_2-receptors in mesolimbic and mesocortical brain regions.

Atypical antipsychotic drugs have been developed more recently. These have a varied pharmacology, but a much lower likelihood than conventional agents of producing extrapyramidal side effect at therapeutic doses. Some are highly selective dopamine D2-receptor antagonists with selectivity for mesolimbic dopamine receptors, for example sulpiride and amivity for mesolimbic dopamine receptors (for example, risperidone, olanzapine, and quetiapine have high affinities for the 5-HT_2 receptor that exceed their affinities for the D_2-receptor. Finally, clozapine is also a potent 5-HT receptor antagonist but a weak D2-receptor antagonist, which accounts for its particularly low-risk if include extrapyramidal movement disorders.

Principal Drugs

These are the:

- *Conventional (typical) antipsychotic drugs:* Chlorpromazine, haloperidol, flupenthixol, fluphenazine and trifluoperazine
- *Atypical antipsychotic drugs:* Amisulpride, olanzapine, quetiapine, risperidone, sulpiride.

Indications and Use

Antipsychotic drugs are sued mainly in the management of schizophrenia. They are also used to treat mania and are sometimes given to depressed patients who have psychotic symptoms or who are particularly agitated. Antipsychotic drugs are also used in the management of disturbed behavior arising from other cause (for example, confessional states), but their use as nonspecific: tranquilizing agents should (if possible) be limited to short-term use because of potentially serious side effects.

In the treatment of acute confessional states, haloperidol, in doses of 1.0–5.0 mg is often helpful. This can be administered either orally or parent rally, with the dose repeated after an hour if the patient remains disturbed. Cardiovascular and respiratory sideeffect are unlikely with this drugs, but acute destinies can occur and should be treated appropriately (Table 16). Antipsychotic drugs such as risperidone are used for the treatment of confused elderly patients. It is worth nothing that some groups of demented patients particularly those with Lewy body type dementia may suffer severe extrapyramidal effect from comparatively low doses of antipsychotic dugs.

The treatment of patient with schizophrenia or mania with antipsychotic drugs requires careful mentoring and persistence because the full therapeutic response may be delayed for some weeks. Furthermore, the dose of antipsychotic drugs required may vary considerably from patient to patient, and also within the same patient at different stages of the illness. Lower doses of conventional antipsychotic drugs are now employed for the treatment of these disorders, since an adequate blockage of dopamine D2-receptors can be obtained with oral doses of 5–10 mg of haloperidol daily or 200–400 mg of chlorpromazine. Higher doses of these agents can produce sedation and behavioral calming, but at the expense of movement disorders and decreased compliance subsequently.

If a patient has responded to an antipsychotic drug it is usual to continue the medication for a number of months into remission. Frequently it is necessary to administer medication on a long-term basis to prevent relapse, in which case the use of long-acting intramuscularly preparations will improve compliance. The deaconates of fluphenazine, flupenthixol, and haloperidol are most commonly used.

Atypical antipsychotic drugs should be used when patients experience extrapyramidal movement disorders on low doses of typical agents. In addition, clozapine can be effective in up to 50 per cent of patients with schizophrenia whose symptoms have not responded to typical antipsychotic drugs. It is effective in the treatment of both positive and negative symptoms of schizophrenia; the latter often showing a poor responses to typical agents. Whether the other atypical agents are effective in treatment-resistant patients is not yet fully clear. Clinical impression is that some patients can indeed show a useful response, but the frequency of a positive outcome may be less than with olanzapine.

Side Effects

Movement Disorder

Through their blockade of brain dopamine receptors, typical antipsychotic drugs produce a variety of extrapyramidal movement disorders that can mimic signs of basal ganglia disease (Table 16). Many patients exhibit symptoms of Parkinsonism very similar to those of the idiopathic disorders, although tremor is less prominent. A side effect that appears early in treatment is acute dystonia, which can present with abnormal postures of dramatic muscular spasms involving the face and limbs. Laryngeal spasm with respiratory distress can also occur. A history of recent antipsychotic drugs use can help avoid misdiagnoses (it is not unusual, for example, for such reactions to be viewed as 'hysterical'). Another movement disorder that patients and very distressing is Akathisia, which is a state of motor restlessness, often with agitation and dysphoria, distinguishing this reaction from symptoms arising from the underlying psychiatric disorders may not be easy.

All these movement disorder may be treated by a reduction in dosage of the antipsychotic drug or by the introduction of anticholinergic medication such as Benztropine. However, anticholinergic drugs should not be prescribed routinely with antipsychotic medication because of the risk of misuse of their euphoria effects.

Later in treatment, thrive duskiness may develop. This consists of involuntary repetitive movements, usually involving the tongue and lips, though other parts of the body may be involved. The condition may be associated with a super sensitivity of postsynaptic dopamine receptors in the Basel ganglia. Unfortunately, this disorder cannot be treated easily, and anticholinergic medication may make it worse. If possible, the antipsychotic drug should be stopped, but this decision is often difficult because of the risk of relapse of the psychiatric disorder.

Atypical antipsychotic drugs are much less likely to cause movement disorders. Risperidone, however, is a potent D2-receptor antagonist as well as a 5-HT_2- receptor antagonist and can produce some movement disorders at the upper end its dose range (above 4–6 mg daily). Whether atypical antipsychotic drugs are generally less likely to cause tardive dyskinesia is not yet clear. The risk does appear to be less with clozapine, olanzapine, and risperidone.

Neuroleptic Malignant Syndrome

A rare but potentially very serious reaction to antipsychotic drugs is the neuroleptic malignant syndrome (Table 16). The syndrome is characterized by fever, rigidity, and altered consciousness, together with tachycardia and labile blood pressure. Laboratory investigations usually reveal a leukocytosis together with markedly levels of creatinine phosphokinase. Antipsychotic drug treatment should be withdrawn immediately if the neuroleptic malignant syndrome is suspected. Management in an intensive care facility may be needed to deal with cardiovascular, respiratory, and renal complications, Treatment with a dopamine-receptor agonist,

Table 16: Extrapyramidal disorders and antipsychotic drugs

Disorder	*Description*	*Treatments employed*
Dystonic reaction	Involuntary muscle contraction, especially face and jaw, oculogyric crisis	Benztropine (1–2 mg IM or IV) Diazepam (10 mg IV)
Akathisia	Sense of subjective motor restlessness, continual pacing	Reduce dose of antipsychotic drug Benztropine (1–6 mg daily) Propranolol (40–120 mg daily) Diazepam (10–30 mg daily)
Parkinsonism	Rigidity, bradykinesia, tremor	Reduce dose of neuroleptic Benztropine (1–6 mg daily)
Tardive dyskinesia (late onset)	Choreoathetoid movements, especially tongue, lips, and jaw	Withdraw antipsychotic drug Vitamin E Atypical antipsychotic drug
Neuroleptic malignant syndrome (rare)	Fever, muscular rigidity, coma, death	Discontinue neuroleptic Intensive care support Bromocriptine Dantrolene

Table 17: Atypical antipsychotic

Drug	*EPS1*	*Prolactin*	*Weight gain*	*Adverse effects*
Amisulpride (Maxpride)	+	↑	+	Insomnia, agitation, nausea, constipation, Q-T prolongation (rare)
Sulpiride	+	↑	+	Insomnia, agitation, abnormal liver function tests
Clozapine	0	0	+++	Agranulocytosis—white cell monitoring mandatory, myocarditis and myopathy (rare), fatigue, drowsiness, dry mouth, sweating, tachycardia, postural hypotension, nausea, constipation, ileus, urinary retention
Olanzapine (Olan/Olan-MD)	+/0	0	+++	Somnolence, dizziness, edema, hypotension, dry mouth, constipation
Quetiapine (Q-win SR)	0	0	++	Somnolence, dizziness, postural hypotension, dry mouth, abnormal liver function tests, Q-T prolongation (transient)
Risperidone (Rispond)	+	↑	++	Insomnia, agitation, anxiety, headache, impaired concentration, nausea, abdominal pain

such as bromocriptine, and the antiplasticity agent dantrolene may be beneficial.

Other Side Effects of Antipsychotic Drugs

Antipsychotic drugs, especially chlorpromazine and thioridazine, can produce a variety of side effect due to blockade of mescaline receptors and α-adrenoceptors (Table 17). Other side effects include:

- *Endocrine:* Elevated prolactin levels, amenorrhea, and galactorrhea
- *Skin:* Rashes, pigmentation, and photosensitivity (especially phenothiazines)
- *Other:* Precipitation of seizures, hypothermia (especially chlorpromazine) cardiac arrhythmias (pimozide), weight gain cholestatic hepatitis, leukopoenia, and retinitis pigmentosa (thioridazine in doses >800 mg daily).

Drug Interactions

Antipsychotic drugs potentiate the effects of other central sedatives. They may delay the hepatic metabolism of tricyclic antidepressants and antiepileptic drugs, leading to increased plasma levels of these agents. The hypotensive properties of chlorpromazine and thioridazine may enhance the effects of antihypertensive drugs. Antipsychotic, drugs particularly pimozide and thioridazine, can increase the Q-T interval and should not be given with other drugs likely to potentiate this effect, such as antiarrhythmics, astemizole, terfenadine, cisapride and tricyclic antidepressants. There are also reports about clarithromycin and erythromycin. Clozapine should not be given with any agents likely to potentiate its depressant effects on the white cell count such as carbamazepine, cotrimoxazole, and penicillamine. SSRIs slow the hepatic metabolism and increase blood levels of several antipsychotic drugs, including haloperidol, risperidone, and olanzapine.

ANTIANXIETY AGENTS

Benzodiazepines

Pharmacology

Benzodiazepines enhance the action of the neurotransmitter γ-amino butyric acid (GABA) in the central nervous system by binding to a specific benzodiazepine receptor located in a complex with a GABA receptor and a chloride-ion channel. The pharmacological effects of benzodiazepine are attributed to the facilitation of GABA neurotransmission.

Principal Drugs

These are alprazolam, chlordiazepoxide, flurazepam, lorazepam, lormetazepam, nitrazepam, and diazepam.

Indication and Use

The prescription of benzodiazepines is now decreasing following concern about their liability to produce dependence. Alternative therapies are available for most anxiety-related disorders, and it is recommended that the duration be short. The major indication for the use of benzodiazepines is to help patients in a crisis, when generalized anxiety and insomnia are causing function impairment and reducing their ability to cope. Patients should be advised that the drug treatment will be of short duration to help them manage their immediate difficulties.

All benzodiazepines have hypnotic and anxiolytic properties. The major distinction of clinical importance is their length of action, Derivatives with relative lack of a hangover effects are preferred. Some benzodiazepines, for example diazepam, have long half-lives and are metabolized to active compounds. These may be used for the treatment of anxiety;

either in the form of regular dosing, or on the now preferred 'as required' basis with an agreed maximum daily dose.

Side Effects and Interactions

Benzodiazepines have a low acute toxicity. Their adverse effects are extensions of their clinical effects and include the following: drowsiness, psychomotor impairment, dizziness, ataxia, and paradoxical aggression (rare). Benzodiazepines potentiate the effects of other centrally acting sedatives, particularly alcohol. The effects of benzodiazepine are potentiated by cimetidine.

Patients who have taken clinical doses of a benzodiazepines for more than a few months may show a withdrawal syndrome when the medication is stopped. In many respects, this syndrome resembles an anxiety state, but perceptual disturbances and acute dysphoria may also occur. It is thus apparent that benzodiazepines can cause physical dependence, and, although the withdrawal syndrome is less severe than that seen following the cessation of barbiturates, patients frequently find it extremely difficult in stop their medication. A gradual reduction is usually best. Generally, withdrawal from a long-acting benzodiazepine is easier than from a short-acting preparation, and if patients taking short-acting benzodiazepine have difficulty withdrawing, then a switch to a long-acting preparation may be helpful.

Other Drugs that Increase Brain GABA Function

Zopiclone, Zolpidem, and Zaleplon

Zopiclone is a cyclopyrrolone derivative marketed for the treatment of insomnia. It binds to a site close to the benzodiazepine receptor and thereby facilitates brain GABA function. By contrast to the benzodiazepines, which reduce the amount of slow-wave (deep) sleep at night, zopiclone has little effect on sleep architecture and is relatively free from a daytime 'hangover' effect. It is claimed to be less likely than benzodiazepine hypnotics to produce tolerance and withdrawal effects, but cases have been reported. The most common adverse effects of zopiclone include bitter taste, nausea, dry mouth, irritability, and headache.

Zolpidem is an imidazopyridine derivative, which also binds to a site close to the benzodiazepine receptors. It has a very short duration of action and, like zopiclone, has little effect on sleep architecture or daytime performance. Its possible adverse effects include nausea, dizziness, headaches, and diarrhea. Zaleplon is a pyrazolopyrimidine derivative with pharmacological properties similar to zopiclone and zolpidem. However, its half-life is only about an hour which means that it can be used to re-induce sleep after nocturnal waking.

Clomethiazole

Clomethiazole also binds at the GABA-receptor complex, but its clinical effects resemble those of barbiturates rather more than those of the benzodiazepine. It can cause serious respiratory depression in overdose, particularly in dominant on with alcohol. Because of it short half-life (4–5 hours), clomethiazole is also used as a hypnotic in the elderly, where dependence has not been reported.

Drugs Altering Monoamine Function

Buspirone

Buspirone is a 5-HT 1A-receptor agonist structurally unrelated to benzodiazepines. It is effective in the treatment of generalized anxiety disorder (less so in patients previously exposed to benzodiazepine) buspirone does not cause significant sedation or cognitive impairment and appears unlikely to cause dependence. It does not have hypnotic properties. Side effects include nervousness, dizziness, and headache.

Other Drugs

Tricyclic antidepressants and SSRIs are effective in the management of patients with a range of anxiety disorders, including generalized anxiety. They are generally preferred to benzodiazepines for the treatment to agoraphobia with and without panic attacks. SSRIs are also effective in the treatment of obsessive-compulsive disorder and social phobia, but tricycles (with the exception of clomipramine) are not.

46.10 DRUG THERAPY OF SCHIZOPHRENIA

G Prasad Rao

Schizophrenia is a chronic, debilitating psychotic mental disorder that affects about 1% of people. A new generation of medications and recent developments in neuropathology, brain imaging, and molecular genetics have led to a greater understanding of the pathophysiology of schizophrenia and to improved treatment. Nonetheless, it remains an enigmatic illness that places a substantial burden on patients, their families, and society.

CLINICAL CHARACTERISTICS

Schizophrenia has varied and ominous symptoms that generally begin in late adolescence or early adulthood and usually continue throughout life. Most patients have a history of behavioral dysfunction primarily social and learning difficulties. Diagnostic features of schizophrenia include auditory hallucinations (generally voices that converse with or about the patient) and delusions (often the paranoid belief that external forces are conspiring against the patient). Patients may have some insight that the voices are internal thoughts and that the delusions cannot possibly be true, but these phenomena remain persistent and troubling. In addition to these overt psychotic, or "positive," symptoms, various deficits, or "negative" symptoms, occur, including an inability to pay attention, the loss of a sense of pleasure, the loss of will or drive, disorganization or impoverishment of thoughts and speech, flattening of affect, and social withdrawal (Table 18). Positive and negative symptoms vary in intensity over time; patients may have predominantly one type at any particular time. Cognitive dysfunction, including a decreased ability to focus attention and deficiencies in short-term verbal and nonverbal memory, is also a core feature of the illness, which predicts vocational and social disabilities for patients. Criminal behavior *per se* is not a concomitant of schizophrenia, but patients may commit violent acts in response to hallucinations or delusions or because of frustration in social interactions. The life-time prevalence of suicide is about 10% among patients with schizophrenia.

Table 18: Diagnostic features of schizophrenia (DSM-IV)

At least two of the following characteristic symptoms lasting at least one month:

- Delusions
- Hallucinations
- Disorganized speech
- Grossly disorganized or catatonic behavior
- Negative symptoms, such as affective flattening

(Only one characteristic symptom is required if delusions are bizarre or hallucinations consist of a voice keeping up a running commentary on the person's behavior or thoughts or two or more voices conversing with each other).

Dysfunction in work, interpersonal relationships, or self-care throughout most of the illness; a level of functioning markedly below the level the patient had achieved or might reasonably have been predicted to achieve before the onset of illness.

Any of the above symptoms lasting in full or attenuated form, at least six months.

Mood disorder not prominent after the onset of psychotic symtoms (if psychotic symptoms always occur during mood disturbance severe enough to meet the criteria for bipolar disorder or a manor depressive disorder, the diagnosis is schizoaffective disorder).

Illness not due to a medication or other medical conditions or substance abuse.

Illness not part of autism or another pervasive developmental disorder.

Pathophysiology

Schizophrenia is a uniquely human illness. Although none of us know to what extent our perception of the world is merely a construct of our own minds, persons with schizophrenia are confronted with this existential dilemma throughout most of their lives. Their struggle to decide if the voices or suspicions they experience are real is part of their inability to discern relevant information from their surroundings. Indeed, the hallucinations and delusions, which initially seem mysterious, can often be traced to misprocessed information. Persons with schizophrenia are hypervigilant, responding to external stimuli as well as to internal thoughts that most other persons can ignore. In addition to this deficit in sensory gating, patients have difficulty processing information in short-term memory to assess its significance. For example, a college student who is becoming psychotic may report that he hears strange people who are hiding in the walls, whispering about his appearance. This symptom demonstrates his inability to filter out the noise of the dormitory and his lack of the skills necessary to learn the identity of the other students around him—both of which heighten his insecurity about himself.

Schizophrenia and Dopamine

The conceptualization by biomedical researchers of schizophrenia as the manifestation of deficits in elementary brain processes was facilitated by observations of certain drug effects. Many drugs that cause psychoses resembling schizophrenia (e.g. stimulants) increase dopaminergic neurotransmission. All currently available antipsychotic drugs that alleviate symptoms of schizophrenia decrease dopaminergic neurotransmission. Decreased dopaminergic neurotransmission, in turn, diminishes the distractibility that characterizes patients with schizophrenia and improves their perceptual abilities. Patients treated with such drugs concomitantly experience a decrease in the intensity of their hallucinations and delusions, and the patients are therefore better able to manage their behavior.

The dopamine theory of schizophrenia has several flaws, however, first, blockade of dopaminergic neurotransmission does not fully alleviate symptoms of schizophrenia. Second, although positive symptoms of schizophrenia are diminished when dopaminergic neurotransmission is decreased by antipsychotic medications, levels of dopamine metabolites and receptors, when measured in patients before and after treatment, are still generally within the wide range of normal values. Third, the role of dopamine in the brain is more complex than that of acting as a simple switch for psychotic symptoms. During acute psychotic episodes, many persons with schizophrenia appear to have increased occupancy of receptors in the basal ganglia by dopamine, as measured by the displacement of radioactive ligands on single photon emission computed tomography. However, decreased dopaminergic activity in the cerebral cortex of the frontal lobe may also be one of the factors contributing to the cognitive impairment commonly found in persons with schizophrenia. Investigation of the pathophysiology of schizophrenia has, therefore, extended beyond dopamine, and researchers exploring the pharmacologic treatment of schizophrenia, while not abandoning dopamine as a target, have extended their field of inquiry to include other neurotransmitters.

Evidence of Multiple Types of Brain Dysfunction

No single lesion in the brain appears to be responsible for causing schizophrenia. Rather, multiple genetic and environmental factors contribute to disturbances in brain function and development that result in schizophrenia. Inhibitory interneurons are particularly affected, as shown by a quantifiable decrease in their number, diminished expression of the enzymes that synthesize the inhibitory neurotransmitter γ-aminobutyric acid (GABA), diminished expression of neuropeptides such as cholecystokinin and somatostatin that are released during neurotransmission, and decreased migration of neurons into the cortex from the underlying white matter. In addition to these specific changes in interneurons, there is a general loss of cortical neuropil, defined as the dendrites and axons that connect neurons, reflecting the failure of both pyramidal and inhibitory neurons to form synaptic connections. In some areas of the brain, the total number of neurons is diminished as well.

In a finding consistent with this neuropathology, magnetic resonance imaging (MRI) shows enlarged ventricles and diminished volume in several regions of the brain, including the hippocampus and the superior temporal cortex. Analysis with magnetic resonance spectroscopy suggests diminished neuronal content in both the hippocampus and the prefrontal cortex, as indicated by levels of the neuronal amino acid N-acetyl aspartate. Despite apparently diminished brain tissue, functional brain imaging by means of positron-emission tomography and functional MRI reveal hyperactivity in the hippocampus and dorsal lateral prefrontal cortex, perhaps consistent with the loss of inhibitory neuron function.

Genetic Findings in Schizophrenia

The diversity of neurobiologic findings in schizophrenia is mirrored by the multiplicity of genetic findings. Genetic epidemiologic findings, such as greater concordance with respect to schizophrenia among monozygotic twins than among dizygotic twins and a high incidence of illness among adopted children whose biologic mothers have schizophrenia, point to a significant heritable component that accounts for about 70% of the risk. However, schizophrenia does not appear to be monogenic, and there are a number of chromosomal loci for which linkage to the illness has been replicated. Single-nucleotide polymorphisms associated with schizophrenia, some of which have been shown to diminish neuronal functions, have been found in genes within these loci, including a G-protein regulator on chromosome 1, a protein on chromosome 6 associated with synaptic structure, a growth factor on chromosome 8 associated with synaptic growth, a response modulator on chromosome 13 that influences N-methyl-D-aspartate glutamate, a receptor on chromosome 15 for acetylcholine, and an enzyme on chromosome 22 that affects dopamine metabolism. The glutamatergic, cholinergic, and dopaminergic neuronal mechanisms affected by these genetic factors have been related to various aspects of cognitive dysfunction involving the inability to perceive and remember information.

In addition to the genetic factors, the environmental component of the pathogenesis of schizophrenia, accounting for the remaining 30% of the risk, includes perinatal and childhood brain injury and psychosocial stress over life events such as separation from the family.

Pathophysiology and Pharmacologic Treatment

An acute psychotic episode in a person with schizophrenia appears to reflect a convergence of pathologic processes that can include an increase in the neurotransmission of dopamine (perhaps in response to stress), one or more genetic factors that alter the neurotransmitter mechanisms regulating the activity of cortical neurons, and nongenetic factors that have caused a loss of neurons and their connections. The result is a brain that is hypersensitive to stimuli and unable to regulate its response through normal inhibitory mechanisms. The decrease in the number of neurons and interneuronal connections that store and process information further diminishes the ability of the brain to sort the incoming information into what is known and what is unknown. Persons with schizophrenia therefore experience the world as overwhelming and commonly form the delusion that an evil force is controlling them or the world around them, or both.

The pharmacologic approach to this manifestation of psychosis has centered on the neurotransmitters that control the response of neurons to stimuli. Neurons that store and process information, such as the pyramidal neurons found in the cerebral cortex, are regulated by many other neurons. Inhibitory interneurons, which regulate cortical neurons, are a primary source of such regulation. The interneurons monitor and inhibit pyramidal-neuron activity. The activity of both pyramidal and inhibitory neurons is

Table 19: Examples of antipsychotic drugs and doses

Medication	*Daily dose (mg)*
First generation antipsychotic agents	
Chlorpromazine (Thorazine)	150–1000
Perphenazine	8–64
Trifluoperazine	5–60
Thiothixene	5–60
Haloperidol	2–25
Second-generation antipsychotic agents	
Clozapine	100–900
Risperidone	2–10
Olanzapine	5–20
Quetiapine	75–750
Ziprasidone	40–160
Aripiprazole	15–30
Amisulpride	400–1200
Intramuscular dose (every 2–4 week)	
Depot preparations	
Fluphenazine decanoate	12.5–50
Haloperidol decanoate	50–200
Flupentixol decanoate	20–100
Risperidone microspheres	25–50

further modulated by dopaminergic neurons, as well as by serotonergic, cholinergic, and noradrenergic neurons, which send afferents into the cortex. The receptors for dopamine, serotonin, and acetylcholine provide additional targets for newer antipsychotic drugs (Table 19).

ANTIPSYCHOTIC TREATMENT

First-generation Antipsychotic Agents

The first antipsychotic, or neuroleptic, drug used to treat schizophrenia was chlorpromazine. Its antipsychotic effects were identified incidentally, when it was tested as an antihistamine in subjects who happened to have schizophrenia. Later research established that blockade of dopamine receptors is the therapeutic mechanism for the effectiveness of chlorpromazine in schizophrenia and prompted the development of increasingly potent dopamine antagonists. Drugs such as haloperidol are more than 100 times as potent as chlorpromazine as antipsychotic agents, but they also are more likely to have parkinsonian side effects caused by dopamine blockade in the basal ganglia. Furthermore, despite their increasing potency, newer drugs in this group of first-generation agents that block dopamine receptors are no more effective than chlorpromazine.

Efficacy

Initial administration of first-generation antipsychotic drugs such as haloperidol and chlorpromazine in a patient with schizophrenia results in an immediate blockade of dopamine D2-receptors and a partial antipsychotic effect. Further therapeutic effects develop over the course of six to eight weeks, a period of time that correlates with decreased release of dopamine from presynaptic terminals. About 20% of patients have complete remission of their symptoms. Most patients have some response but also have continuing symptoms. However, many severe, chronic symptoms associated with schizophrenia, such as catatonic withdrawal, that were observed before the era of commonly prescribed antipsychotic agents are rarely seen today, perhaps because of drug treatment. After an episode of psychosis, continued treatment with antipsychotic agents can significantly decrease the probability of relapse. Several reports of two-year studies showed that approximately 30% of patients have a relapse during treatment with first-generation antipsychotic drugs, as compared with 80% without treatment.

Side Effects

Antipsychotic effects occur because of the blockade of neurotransmission between the dopaminergic neurons of the ventral tegmental area and the neurons in the limbic and cortical forebrain that perform higher level information processing. However, the ventral tegmental neurons are members of an extensive family of neurons descended from a common embryologic ancestor that also use dopamine or related catecholamines, such as norepinephrine, as their neurotransmitter. The melanocytes, which synthesize melanin as a catecholamine polymer, are part of this family. The side effects of neuroleptic drugs encompass effects on the entire group of neurons of this lineage (Table 20).

The most obvious side effects are involuntary movement disorders arising from the extrapyramidal system, many of which mimic the effects of Parkinson's disease and reflect the blockade of dopaminergic transmission between the dopaminergic neurons of the substantia nigra and the dorsal neostriatum. Symptoms include dystonia, akathisia, bradykinesia, and tremor. Elderly patients may be at increased risk for hip fractures as a result of drug associated movement disorders. As with all patients who have involuntary movement disorders, patients with schizophrenia are distressed but generally have difficulty describing the problem. Hence, they may appear in physicians' offices with vague reports of their symptoms. Akathisia, a severe state of restlessness that is difficult to distinguish from agitation, is a major cause of non-compliance with the drug regimen. Treatment with propranolol (20–80 mg per day) is useful for controlling akathisia. Bradykinesia, decreased spontaneous movement and slowed voluntary movement, mimics the effects of

Table 20: Common side effects of first-generation and second-generation antipsychotic drugs

First-generation antipsychotics
• Movement disorders, such as dystonia, bradykinesia, tremor, akathisia, choreoathetosis • Anhedonia • Sedation • Moderate weight gain • Temperature dysregulation, poikilothermy: cold in cold environments, warm in warm environments • Hyperprolactinemia, with galactorrhea and amenorrhea in women and gynecomastia in men; decreased sexual function in both • Postural hypotension • Sunburn • Prolonged QT interval, risk of potentially fatal arrhythmia (with thioridazine)
Second-generation antipsychotics
• Moderate-to-severe weight gain (with olanzapine, clozapine) • Diabetes mellitus • Hypercholesterolemia • Sedation • Moderate movement disorder–hypotension • Hyperprolactinemia (with risperidone) • Seizures (with clozapine) • Nocturnal salivation (with clozapine) • Agranulocytosis (with clozapine) • Myocarditis (with clozapine) • Lens opacities (with clozapine)

depression. Treatment with anticholinergic, antiparkinsonian drugs, such as benztropine (2–6 mg per day in divided doses), is helpful. Tardive dyskinesia, a choreoathetotic movement disorder, develops in about 30% of patients, generally after several years of treatment. Orofacial movements such as grimacing are common manifestations. Tardive dyskinesia does not respond to anticholinergic agents; it resolves slowly after the withdrawal of first-generation drugs, but it may be irreversible.

Death caused by the administration of antipsychotic drugs is rare but can occur through several mechanisms. Temperature dysregulation can lead to a severe neuroleptic malignant syndrome, in which the patient's temperature exceeds 40°C (104°F) and brain death ensues. The occurrence of such an extreme outcome is related to both environmental heat and the presence of a Taq A polymorphism in the D2 dopamine-receptor genotype. Preventive measures include hydration and caution in the administration of anticholinergic agents in high-temperature environments, because the agents block perspiration. Neuroleptic malignant syndrome is treated by rapid cooling, and dantrolene can be administered to inhibit the release of calcium in muscle cells and thus attenuate the metabolic changes caused by the hyperthermia. Dopamine agonists, such as bromocriptine, can be administered to reverse the pathogenic dopamine blockade.

A prolonged QT interval is a side effect of several antipsychotic drugs, and the possibility of this abnormality limits the dose of thioridazine, in particular. To what extent a prolonged QT interval predisposes a patient to the potentially fatal torsade de pointes arrhythmia is unknown, but the incidence of sudden death among patients treated with antipsychotic drugs is 0.015% per year—about twice the rate reported in the normal healthy population.

Second-generation Antipsychotic Agents

A second generation of antipsychotic agents has been introduced into clinical practice over the past 15 years in an attempt to improve therapeutic effects and decrease the side effects associated with first generation dopamine blocking drugs. All second generation drugs share the D2-dopamine-receptor antagonism of first generation drugs, but second-generation drugs are less tightly bound to the D2-receptor, and D2 receptor antagonism is no longer the sole therapeutic mechanism. Hence, there are similarities in the general scope and time course of the effects of first- and second-generation drugs, but there are clinically important differences in both the therapeutic effects and the side effects.

Clozapine

Clozapine is the first atypical antipsychotic drug, so designated because it has antipsychotic effects without the adverse effects on movement of the first-generation drugs. In addition, clozapine has enhanced therapeutic efficacy, as compared with the first-generation drugs.Therefore, it was introduced into clinical practice in the United States despite a serious known adverse effect: an increased incidence of agranulocytosis. Patients taking clozapine must undergo frequent monitoring of the leukocyte count (weekly for the first six months and every two weeks thereafter, including the first four weeks after the patient has discontinued the drug). Since the incidence of agranulocytosis is 0.39% and the death rate among patients who take clozapine is 0.013%, dispensing by pharmacies must be linked to proof of monitoring to prevent patients from receiving the drug without adequate follow-up. Myocarditis has been reported in 0.032% of patients receiving clozapine, with a fatality rate of 0.012%. Although all antipsychotic drugs lower the threshold for seizure, this effect is more pronounced with clozapine. Nevertheless, for 30% of patients who do not have a response to other treatments, clozapine has substantially enhanced therapeutic effects that justify its use. Clozapine reduces suicidal behavior, although a decrease in the rate of death by suicide has not yet been fully established.

Clozapine has significant antagonist effects at D1, D2, and D4 dopamine receptors, as well as at norepinephrine and serotonin receptors. An unexpected effect is that patients who are smokers and who have a response to clozapine also decrease their cigarette smoking. It has been hypothesized that heavy smoking among persons with schizophrenia is an attempt at self-medication, and indeed, nicotine does briefly improve several aspects of brain function. Clozapine increases the synaptic release of acetylcholine, a fact that may account in part for its enhanced therapeutic effect, and concomitantly provides patients with an alternative to the use of nicotine, which is a cholinergic agonist.

Newer Second-generation Agents

The enhanced antipsychotic action of clozapine was initially thought to be due to its antagonism of both D2 dopaminergic and 5-hydroxy-tryptamine (5-HT) of type 2A (5-HT2A) serotonergic receptors. Drugs with a similar combined dopamine–serotonin antagonism, including risperidone, olanzapine, quetiapine, and ziprasidone are all effective antipsychotic agents. Like clozapine, these drugs have an efficacy that is equivalent to or exceeds the efficacy of first-generation antipsychotic agents, without many of the extrapyramidal effects of the first-generation drugs. These newer agents also entail a greatly reduced risk of tardive dyskinesia. Their increased efficacy with respect to negative schizophrenic symptoms is particularly noteworthy, and the rate of relapse is significantly less than that with the first-generation drugs. For example, in a one year, multisite trial, patients taking the second generation drug risperidone had a 25% rate of relapse, as compared with a rate of 40% for patients taking the first-generation drug haloperidol.

Other second-generation drugs have a different putative mechanism, involving refinements of action at dopamine receptors. Aripiprazole was characterized by mixed agonism and antagonism at dopamine receptors in preclinical studies, and investigators proposed that the drug enhanced low levels of dopaminergic transmission, thus improving cognition, but blocked higher levels of transmission that might cause psychosis. Aripiprazole also has effects at serotonergic receptors. Amisulpride is an antagonist at D2 and D3 dopamine receptors. Both aripiprazole and amisulpride have antipsychotic effects that are associated with a lower risk of movement disorder than that associated with first-generation agents.

Side Effects

Although only clozapine causes agranulocytosis in a substantial proportion of patients, many second-gene-ration drugs produce clinically significant weight gain—for example, 5.4 kg (11.9 lb) in a recent 14-week trial of olanzapine.

Weight gain of 20 kg (44 lb) or more can occur with longer term treatment. Diabetes mellitus has been increasingly reported in patients treated for more than five years with second generation antipsychotic agents, presumably in association with weight gain; there is also some evidence of the development of insulin resistance. In a few cases, life-threatening ketoacidosis has occurred. Cholesterol levels increase by 10% after 14 weeks of treatment with olanzapine. Ziprasidone and amisulpride at recommended doses cause less weight gain than do other antipsychotic drugs. Second-generation antipsychotic agents can sometimes induce obsessive compulsive symptoms, which may reflect antagonism of serotonergic neurotransmission.

Cognitive Improvement

The extent to which second generation antipsychotic agents improve cognition in patients with schizophrenia is controversial. First-generation antipsychotic agents have moderate effects on cognition, improving the patient's ability to pay attention to tasks. Studies comparing first-generation and second-generation drugs show that about 30 to 70% of patients receiving second-generation drugs have improvement on neuropsychological tests of cognitive function, particularly in assessments of attention and short-term memory. Improvement in these cognitive functions is seen in only 30% of patients receiving first generation drugs. The additional improvement in those receiving second-generation antipsychotic drugs, however, may not translate directly into an improved quality-of-life for all patients. Furthermore, whether the difference in improvement in cognitive functions reflects the differential effects of the two groups of drugs on dopamine or on other neurotransmitters such as serotonin or acetylcholine is unknown. Low doses of haloperidol (5 mg per day), a first-generation antipsychotic drug, have effects on neurocognition equivalent to those of the second-generation drug risperidone, suggesting a positive effect from the blockade of low level dopamine D2-receptors that was masked at the higher doses used for previous comparisons with second-generation agents.

Treatment Guidelines

The treatment of schizophrenia requires experience in performing a differential diagnosis of mental disorders and in assessing a patient's potential for suicide and violence. Optimal management includes psychological, social, and occupational therapies. Physicians who are not psychiatrists are often consulted in the first stages of illness, and many chronically ill patients receive maintenance pharmacotherapy from their family physicians.

Treatment of a First Psychotic Episode

Immediate treatment of a patient after a first psychotic episode improves his or her long-term outcome and does not obscure the later differential diagnosis. The usual presenting features are hallucinations or delusions, or both, generally accompanied by anxiety, behavioral withdrawal, angry outbursts, and suicidal thoughts. Most psychiatrists initially prescribe a second-generation antipsychotic (other than clozapine, because of the incidence of side effects), in divided doses. Less disturbed sleep patterns and decreased anger and anxiety should be observed within the first day or two of treatment, with gradual improvement in other symptoms in the first week and near-maximal effects in six to eight weeks. Lack of improvement in the first one to four weeks should prompt an increase in the dose, followed by a change to another drug, usually clozapine or another second-generation drug after an additional four to six weeks, if the response remains inadequate. As in all illnesses in which suicidal intent is a factor, the patient's risk of death paradoxically increases as other symptoms improve.

Maintenance Treatment

After the first episode has resolved, the patient should continue treatment for at least one year and then should be re-evaluated. A variety of psychotherapeutic approaches are particularly helpful and can support the patient's rehabilitative efforts and increase insight about the illness. Many clinicians engage patients in weight loss programs prospectively.

Indications for Clozapine

Clozapine is not a first-line drug, because of the possibility of agranulocytosis. The indication for treatment with clozapine is either the lack of an adequate response with other second-generation or first-generation antipsychotic agents or the patient's inability to tolerate side effects, such as akathisia, of other antipsychotic agents. In practice, both highly functional and highly dysfunctional patients are prescribed clozapine. Patients who are already highly functional sometimes have additional benefits, including a return to meaningful employment, that justify the increased risk of agranulocytosis, myocarditis, and seizures. Highly dysfunctional patients for example, patients who have persistent, troubling psychotic and behavioral symptoms, including suicidal intent, despite treatment with other antipsychotic drugs may respond to no other medication.

Role of First-generation Antipsychotic Agents

Many patients continue to receive first-generation antipsychotic agents, and most treatment algorithms for patients with schizophrenia suggest a trial with a drug from this group for patients who do not have a response to second-generation drugs. Patients receiving first-generation antipsychotic agents are monitored yearly for tardive dyskinesia. In most cases, tardive dyskinesia that is diagnosed early is reversed when the patient is switched to a second-generation drug. Tardive dyskinesia that involves involuntary tongue and chewing movements is more manageable if patients use good dental hygiene to retain their own teeth.

Antipsychotic drugs that are administered in a depot injection are associated with lower rates of relapse than medications that are administered orally, because of the greater likelihood that the patient will receive the medication. Haloperidol and fluphenazine are available in the form of depot injections in the United States, and flupenthixol and risperidone are available as depot preparations in Europe.

Choice of an Antipsychotic Drug

All antipsychotic drugs are effective for positive symptoms of acute psychosis. Second-generation drugs are preferred because of their greater effects on negative symptoms and cognitive function and because they are associated with a lower rate of relapse and a lower incidence of movement disorders. Consistent therapeutic differences among second-generation drugs, other than clozapine, have not been established; thus, the response of the individual patient must be used to guide selection.

First-generation antipsychotic agents administered as a depot injection, despite the risk of tardive dyskinesia, remain the optimal therapy for patients who have a relapse because of poor adherence to a regimen of oral medication. Similarly, choosing to administer a drug with potentially fatal side effects, such as agranulocytosis and myocarditis, in the case of clozapine, is an acceptable treatment decision when patients have not had a response to other drugs. Furthermore, clozapine may be associated with a decreased risk of suicide; if so, the increase in mortality from agranulocytosis and myocarditis might be compensated for by the decrease in mortality from suicide, and clozapine could rationally be prescribed more frequently. The possibility of weight gain may influence the choice among second-generation drugs. For the patient in whom diabetes develops, ziprasidone may be an alternative. However, although ziprasidone is as effective as the first-generation drug haloperidol, its efficacy relative to that of other second-generation drugs has yet to be evaluated.

Antipsychotic drugs are often not the sole therapy for schizophrenia. Depression is common and is frequently treated with antidepressants. Patients with schizoaffective symptoms who have periods of excitement and agitation that fulfill the criteria for mania are often treated with mood stabilizers such as lithium carbonate or valproic acid. Patients with anxiety and sleep disturbance can be treated with benzodiazepines.

Early Intervention

The lower likelihood of extrapyramidal side effects associated with the second-generation antipsychotic drugs has made intervention earlier in life more acceptable to young patients and their parents. A small number of the children with severe attention deficit disorder and the teenagers with conduct disorder who are seen in primary care pediatric clinics already have most of the symptoms that make up a diagnosis of schizophrenia or bipolar disorder.

Clinicians are often either reluctant to diagnose schizophrenia or unaware that it appears as early as six years of age. The presence of hallucinations and delusions is sometimes dismissed as childhood fantasy. However, affected children are deeply troubled and may be suicidal or even homicidal. They may have a good response to second-generation drugs, although weight gain can be particularly severe in this age group. In addition, many children present with only subclinical signs of schizophrenia, including unmanageable aggressive reactions, psychosocial difficulties, attention and learning disabilities, and odd behavior. Because these symptoms are also typical of attention deficit disorder, the children are frequently treated with stimulant drugs such as methylphenidate before overt symptoms of psychosis appear or are fully recognized. How stimulant treatment might contribute to the possibility of the later development of psychosis is unknown.

During adolescence and early adulthood, treatment with risperidone may delay the transition from the prodromal phase to the first episode of psychosis for at least six months. The clinical importance of this delay in the longer term has not yet been established. Delay of the onset of psychosis has historically been associated with an improved prognosis, but because psychosis does not ultimately develop in all children who have prodromal signs, the risk and benefit of such treatment are not clear.

The critical period for intervention may be quite early. Many of the genes that have been identified as candidates for contributing to schizophrenia are intimately involved with brain development, and deficits in brain development have been observed in the fetuses and newborn infants of women with schizophrenia. Additional developmental abnormalities may occur through an exaggeration of the neuronal cell death that normally occurs in adolescence. Interventions directed at problems during brain development have not yet been developed, but they may be a necessary part of the full treatment of schizophrenia.

46.11 DRUG TREATMENT OF ALZHEIMER'S DISEASE

Christoday RJ Khess, Bikramaditya Jaiswal, Jayati Simlai

Alzheimer's disease is a chronic neurodegenerative disorder characterized by memory impairment, prominent psychiatric symptoms and behavioral abnormalities which then leads to impairment in activities of daily living. It is estimated that Alzheimer's disease is currently affecting around 25 million people worldwide and this figure is rapidly increasing in both developed and developing countries.[115,116]

Among the treatment of Alzheimer's disease are both pharmacological and nonpharmacological interventions. Among the pharmacological agents are cholinesterase inhibitors, neuroprotective strategies and other agents to reduce behavioral disturbances. Another important component of treatment includes close association between family members and other caregivers responsible for the patient[117] and clinicians.

DIAGNOSIS

In the elderly most common form of dementia is Alzheimer's disease. The onset and progression of Alzheimer's disease follows a characteristic pattern, and a probable diagnosis can be made on the basis of clinical history. Alzheimer's disease is associated with specific neuropathological changes seen in the brain on histological examination and a definitive diagnosis can be made only at autopsy.

According to the DSM-IV-TR, Alzheimer's dementia is defined as the gradual onset and continuing cognitive decline involving memory impairment and one or more of aphasia, apraxia, agnosia, and disturbance in executive functioning. These impairments each cause significant impairment in social or occupational functioning and represent a significant decline from a previous level of functioning. The deficits must not be due to other central nervous system conditions or systemic conditions or the result of substances, must not occur exclusively during the course of a delirium, and must not be accounted for by another Axis I disorder. Diagnosis is further classified into subtypes as with or without behavioral disturbance and with early (before age 65) or late onset.[116] Specific criteria for Alzheimer's disease were defined by the NINCDS-ADRDA in 1984. These criteria are similar to the DSM-IV-TR criteria but also add features that support, are consistent with, or make the diagnosis uncertain or unlikely.[118]

The patients with Alzheimer's disease presents with gradual decline in short-term memory function,[119,120] language function[121] and visuospatial deficits.[122,123] In the later phase of illness other symptoms such as seizures, gait abnormality and motor and sensory abnormalities may appear.[118]

Along with memory impairment, there are also behavioral and functional impairment associated with Alzheimer's disease. The disease progress from disturbance in instrumental activities of daily living in earlier phase to loss of basic activities of daily living as the disease enters advanced phases.[124] Similarly behavioral disturbances such as apathy and mood changes may present from earlier stages and progress over the course of the illness.[117] In the middle and later stages psychosis and agitation appears.[125]

There are certain laboratory studies which can be done to identify reversible causes of dementia along with other coexisting illness commonly found in elderly. Among these commonly done tests are thyroid-function tests, serum electrolyte, vitamin B_{12} measurement, hematocrit value, blood urea nitrogen, liver function tests and blood glucose levels.[126]

Neuroimaging has an important role in diagnosis of Alzheimer's disease. CT scan or MRI should be done in every patient of dementia at least once during the course of their illness.[129] Other neuroimaging tests includes positron emission tomography (PET) or single photon emission CT which can also be done.[127,128]

TREATMENT

Antiamyloid Therapies

There are no currently available antiamyloid therapies. After an observation that immunization with Aβ causes reduction of signs of Alzheimer's disease in transgenic mice that has amyloid precursor protein mutation, a program was implemented to vaccinate humans.[129] The clinical trial was interrupted because of development of encephalitis in few of the patients.[130] Within the trial when postanalysis of a subgroup of patients was done at a single site, it was observed that those patients who generated Aβ antibodies had a reduction in disease progression.[128] Passive immunization represents an alternative and perhaps a safer vaccination strategy.[131]

β and γ secretases are the enzymes which acts on amyloid precursor protein to liberate toxic fragment of amino acid Aβ. Active study is being underway to study the role of inhibitors of these enzymes.[132] Cholesterol metabolism is intimately involved in the generation of Aβ, and based on this finding it is suggested that there may be a role of statins in reducing the accumulation of Aβ.[133] Other strategies such as reducing aggregation of Aβ or use of analogs of insulin degrading enzymes may be explored.[134]

Neuroprotective Approaches

There is a variety of mechanisms through which Aβ protein seems to exert its neurotoxic effects. These include glutamatergic excitotoxic signals, free radical oxidative injury, tau protein hyperphosphorylation, lipid peroxidation of cell membranes and inflammation. These mechanisms have been targeted by various neuroprotective strategies in a bid to reduce generation and accumulation of Aβ so as to prevent cell injury. There are animal data available but no human data which proves that these approaches are neuroprotective.

Antioxidants

Vitamin E is an antioxidant which has been shown to slow nerve damage and delay cell death in cell cultures. No benefit for cognition or function compared to baseline or change in rate of cognitive decline were found when vitamin E, selegiline, both drugs together was compared with placebo in a randomized, placebo-controlled trial.[135] However, patients on vitamin E, selegiline, or the combination of both exhibited delay by about 5–7 months in reaching endpoints of poor outcome (death, institutionalization, or significant functional decline).[136-138] Currently vitamin E is not recommended for treatment of Alzheimer's disease.

Memantine

Memantine is a noncompetitive NMDA receptor antagonist that has neuroprotective functions. Currently it has been approved for the treatment of moderate to severe Alzheimer's disease. Memantine is known to modulate glutamatergic excitatory signals or may have some effects on hippocampal neuronal function which may lead to symptomatic improvement.[139] Memantine has shown efficacy for both cognitive and functional improvement.[140] Dose range of Memantine is 10–20 mg per day. It is effective and well-tolerated when added to cholinesterase inhibitors.

Anti-inflammatory Agents

In the postmortem examination of patients with Alzheimer's disease there were microscopic evidence of inflammation in the brain.[141] Based on this observation there were number of clinical trials with NSAIDs (nonsteroidal anti-inflammatory drugs) or steroidal drugs. There was no benefit with prednisone,[142] diclofenac,[143] rofecoxib and naproxen[144] as compared to placebo. So, there is no evidence for the use of anti-inflammatory drugs in Alzheimer's disease.

Hormone Replacement Therapy

Epidemiological evidence suggested that hormone replacement therapy has benefit in improving cognitive functioning and delaying cognitive decline and was shown to be beneficial in the treatment of dementia in two controlled trials. But the results showed no benefit of estrogen over placebo on cognition in women with Alzheimer's disease.[145,146] Therefore, estrogen is not indicated in the treatment of dementia.

Cholinesterase Inhibitors

The first class of medications approved by FDA for the treatment of Alzheimer's disease was the cholinesterase inhibitors—tacrine, donepezil, rivastigmine, and galantamine. These agents are reversible inhibitors of the enzyme acetylcholinesterase, which degrades acetylcholine in the synaptic cleft, thereby increasing the availability of intrasynaptic acetylcholine.[147,148] Tacrine is now rarely used because of its hepatotoxic side effects.[149] Second-generation cholinesterase inhibitors have fewer side effects, and have more convenient dosage regimens because of their duration of action.

Starting dose of donepezil is 5 mg per day, which can be hiked after one month to 10 mg per day. The suggested dose range of galantamine is 16–32 mg per day given twice a day (e.g. 8 mg twice daily). The starting dose is 8 mg per day, and after a minimum of 4 weeks, the dose can be increased. Further dose increases should be based on tolerability, with a minimum time period of 4 weeks on the previous dose.[150] The suggested dosage range of Rivastigmine is 3–12 mg per day. Patients should be initiated with 1.5 mg twice a day and gradually increased (usually by every 2–4 weeks) until the maximum daily dose of 12 mg per day is reached or titrated to the patient's tolerability.

Use of cholinesterase inhibitors is shown to help patients with Alzheimer's disease to maintain their activities of daily living; they also tend to have less behavioral abnormalities.[150] Further studies are needed to find out whether cholinesterase inhibitors can be used in advanced stages of Alzheimer's disease as improvement is seen in only few studies.[151]

Side effects of cholinesterase inhibitors include diarrhea, nausea, insomnia, vomiting, muscle cramps, fatigue, anorexia, bradycardia and syncope. Side effects of these drugs can be reduced by slowly titrating the dose upwards.[150] The drug should be started at low doses and slowly hiked upwards depending on the tolerability. Gastrointestinal side effects could be minimized by giving drugs with meals.

Although there is no suggested optimal duration of treatment as most of the trials are for six months only, studies have shown that patients with Alzheimer's disease who continue treatment with cholinesterase inhibitors continue to have benefit for 2–3 years.[152]

All of these agents show similar efficacy, and there is insufficient evidence comparing these agents to each other. There are no data on whether or how to switch from one agent to another. Certain indications such as severe side effects, allergic reactions, family preference, and no response after six months of trial may warrant changing from one cholinesterase inhibitor to another.[150] There are no studies regarding concurrent use of two cholinesterase inhibitor together and so, this is not advisable. Though cholinesterase inhibitors is commonly given in combination with memantine.[153]

Other Treatments for Cognitive Deterioration

Ginkgo biloba has antioxidant properties and has been studied in the treatment of Alzheimer's disease. In some trials, small statistically significant effects have been found for *Ginkgo biloba* in comparison to placebo in patients with Alzheimer's disease.[154] A trial is currently under progress to see the effects of *Ginkgo biloba* in reducing the rate of development of Alzheimer's disease.

Management of Neuropsychiatric Symptoms and Behavioral Disturbances

About 80% of patients with Alzheimer's disease have comorbid neuropsychiatric symptoms as reported in most studies.[125] To avoid the risk of additional side effects and additional expenses psychological management should be tried before pharmacologic agents in case of comorbid behavioral abnormalities.[155] A number of nonpharmacologic interventions such as light exercise, relaxation, music, video or audio tapes of care givers, sensory stimulation can be tried.[147,155,156] While treating associated behavioral disturbances, it would be better to explore nonpharmacologic interventions because of their relatively benign nature.[147]

For the treatment of behavioral changes in patients with Alzheimer's disease there are few randomized, controlled trials using optimal psychopharmacologic agents. Recommendations are made on the basis of small trials. Atypical antipsychotics are preferred drugs for the treatment of associated psychosis or other behavioral disturbances. There are fewer side effects as compared to typical antipsychotic drugs such as extrapyramidal symptoms and other tardive movement disorders. Olanzapine and risperidone are mostly supported as an efficacious agent by double-blind, controlled trials in reducing psychosis patients with Alzheimer's disease.[157-160] There is clear superiority of neuroleptic agents over placebo for the treatment of dementia as shown by meta-analysis of neuroleptic agents. Mood stabilizers or antidepressants can be used alone or in combination with antipsychotic agents in cases of inadequate responses to the treatment of agitation.

Mood stabilizers such as Carbamazepine or Divalproex sodium can be used to reduce behavioral disturbances in patients with Alzheimer's disease.[161] Studies using Divalproex sodium for its effects on agitation have shown mixed results.[162,163]

Several clinical trials have been done to address the role of antidepressants for the treatment of depression in patients with Alzheimer's disease. The results are both in favor and against the use of antidepressants in similar number of studies using placebo as comparison. Both trials have used selective serotonin-reuptake inhibitors and tricyclic antidepressants. Studies having a rigorous study design and involving severely depressed patients tended to show positive effects. Because of their fewer side effects combined serotonin and noradrenergic-reuptake inhibitors are commonly used in elderly patient whereas tricyclic antidepressants which have anticholinergic side effects are used less often. Selective serotonin reuptake inhibitors are most frequently used by most clinicians when treating depression in patients with Alzheimer's disease.[164-166]

Health Maintenance and General Medical Treatment

With the progression of Alzheimer's disease, various conditions such as malnutrition, lung infections, pneumonia, bed sores and fractures develop that may lead to death.[167] So, these conditions should be appropriately managed. Health maintenance activities such as exercise, control of diabetes and hypertension, use of eye glasses and hearing aids as needed should be encouraged by clinicians in early stages of Alzheimer's disease.[168] In later phases of the disease, basic requirements such as skin care, nutrition, hydration, and safety should be addressed.

Alliance with Caregivers

An essential element for the treatment of patients with Alzheimer's is alliance between the clinician and the caregiver. It is the responsibility of the caregivers to supervise patients who live in the community and to frequently visit and provide assistance when the patient is institutionalized. Providing and administering medication, implementing psychological management, taking care of the general health and wellbeing of the patients are also some of the other responsibilities of caregivers. Caregivers must make decisions regarding advance directives, financial management, driving, removal of fire arms, and home safety among others.[169]

Caregiver burden associated with caring for loved ones with dementia is great. Caregiving is emotionally and physically demanding because the patient has less ability to communicate, eventually may not recognize the caregiver and frequently exhibits inappropriate and difficult behavior. Many times, caregivers consider their health as relatively poor as found in many studies.[170] Caregiving is emotionally and physical demanding as the patients becomes more dependent on the caregivers with the passage of time. Behavioral disturbances are a major source of caregiver burden and also increases risk for caregiver depression and anxiety and other somatic symptoms. Studies also show that compared to noncaregivers they engage in fewer preventive health activities.[170] Therefore, treatment of demented patients must also include addressing the needs of, and when appropriate treating the caregivers. Intervention for reducing caregiver burden includes psychoeducation about Alzheimer's disease and comprehensive support such as individual and family counseling and support groups. There is reduction in psychological distress by these interventions but they are not able to reduce caregiver's burden.[171,172]

CONCLUSION

A better understanding of the natural history of Alzheimer's disease has been achieved and appropriate trial designs and outcomes for the various stages of this condition have been developed. There is clear evidence of the benefits for the treatment of symptoms in mild to moderately severe AD using cholinesterase inhibitor and memantine. However, there is cautious optimism for successful disease modification using several agents currently being studied. Treatment guidelines must be constantly updated to take into account new evidence.

46.12 TREATMENT OF CHRONIC INSOMNIA

JN Vyas

CLINICAL PROBLEM

Insomnia is defined as difficulty with the initiation, maintenance, duration, or quality of sleep that results in the impairment of daytime functioning, despite adequate opportunity and circumstances for sleep.[173,174] (Difficulty with sleep maintenance implies waking after sleep has been initiated but before a desired wake time). Most research studies adopt an arbitrary definition of a delay of more than 30 minutes in sleep onset or a sleep efficiency (the ratio of time asleep to time in bed) of less than 85%.[173] However, in clinical practice, a patient's subjective judgment of sleep quality and quantity is a more important factor. Transient insomnia lasts less than one week, and short-term insomnia one to four weeks.

Chronic insomnia—insomnia lasting more than one month[175]—has a prevalence of 10-15%[174,176] and occurs more frequently in women, older adults, and patients with chronic medical and psychiatric disorders.[173] It may follow episodes of acute insomnia in patients who are predisposed to having the condition and may be perpetuated by behavioral and cognitive factors, such as worrying in bed and holding unreasonable expectations of sleep duration.[177] Consequences include fatigue, mood disturbances, problems with interpersonal relationships, occupational difficulties, and a reduced quality-of-life.

Taking a careful history from the patient and a bed partner, if present, usually allows accurate categorization of the causes of insomnia. Asking the patient to keep a diary documenting times of sleep for one to four weeks may be helpful. Polysomnography is rarely needed unless there is a strong suspicion of sleep-disordered breathing or periodic limb movement disorder or unless insomnia fails to respond to treatment.[178]

Insomnia can be classified as primary or secondary (Table 21).[175] The pathogenesis of primary insomnia is unknown, but available evidence suggests a state of hyperarousal. As compared with controls, patients with insomnia show increased global cerebral glucose metabolism on positron emission tomography when awake and asleep, increased beta activity and decreased theta and delta activity on electroencephalography during sleep, an increased 24-hour metabolic rate, and higher levels of secretion of adrenocorticotropic hormone and cortisol.[180]

Insomnia secondary to other causes is more common than primary insomnia (Table 21)[179] and must be excluded or treated before making a diagnosis of primary insomnia. If insomnia persists despite treatment of secondary causes, then therapy for primary insomnia should be instituted. Several causes of the disorder may be present in a single patient. Circadian-rhythm disorders, such as shift-work sleep disorder and delayed-sleep-phase syndrome (a delay in the sleep period of more than two hours relative to conventional times), and voluntary insufficient sleep syndrome should be considered in the differential diagnosis, but these are not considered forms of insomnia.

Table 21: Classification of adult insomnia*

Primary insomnia: • Idiopathic insomnia—Insomnia arising in infancy or childhood with a persistent, unremitting course • Psychophysiologic insomnia due to a maladaptive conditioned response in which the patient learns to associate the bed environment with heightened arousal rather than sleep; onset often associated with an event causing acute insomnia, with the sleep disturbance persisting despite resolution of the precipitating factor • Paradoxical insomnia (sleep-state misperception)—Insomnia characterized by a marked mismatch between the patient's description of sleep duration and objective polysomnographic findings
Secondary insomnia: • Adjustment insomnia—Insomnia associated with active psychosocial stressors • Inadequate sleep hygiene—Insomnia associated with lifestyle habits that impair sleep • Insomnia due to a psychiatric disorder—Insomnia due to an active psychiatric disorder, such as anxiety or depression • Insomnia due to a medical condition—Insomnia due to a condition such as the restless legs syndrome, chronic pain, nocturnal cough or dyspnea, or hot flashes • Insomnia due to a drug or substance—Insomnia due to consumption or discontinuation of medication, drugs of abuse, alcohol, or caffeine

* Modified from the classification of adult insomnia adopted by the International Classification of Sleep Disorder[179]

STRATEGIES AND EVIDENCE

Cognitive Behavioral Therapies

Cognitive behavioral therapies (Table 22) comprise a group of techniques that address the factors that help perpetuate

Table 22: Types of cognitive behavioral therapy

• *Stimulus-control therapy** – Go to bed only when sleepy – Use the bedroom only for sleeping and sex – Go to another room when unable to sleep in 15–20 minutes, read or engage in other quiet activities, and return to bed only when sleepy; repeat if necessary – Have a regular wake time regardless of the duration of sleep – Avoid daytime napping • *Sleep-restriction therapy*† – Reduce time in bed to estimated total sleep time (minimum, 5 hour) – Increase time in bed by 15 minutes every week when estimated sleep efficiency (ratio of time asleep to time in bed) is at least 90% • *Relaxation therapy*‡ – *Physical component:* Progressive muscle reaxation, biofeedback – *Mental component:* Imagery training, meditation, hyponosis • *Cognitive therapy*‡ – Education to alter faulty beliefs and attitudes about sleep, such as that a minimum of 8 hours of sleep a night is required for health • *Sleep-hygiene education*‡ – Correct extrinsic factors affecting sleep, such as environmental disruption (pets or snoring bed partner); bedroom temperature; fixation on the bedside clock; use of alcohol, nicotine, or caffeine; lack of exercise or exercise too close to bedtime

* Description are from Bootzin et al.[181]
† Description are from Spielman et al.[181]
‡ Description are from Hauri[181]

chronic insomnia, regardless of the cause. Stimulus-control therapy assumes that insomnia is a maladaptive response to factors such as bedtime and the bedroom environment (for example, regularly reading or watching television in bed rather than sleeping) and requires a learning process to reassociate the bed with sleep.[181] Sleep-restriction therapy is based on the premise that people with insomnia can learn to increase their sleep time by inducing temporary sleep deprivation through voluntarily reducing their time in bed.[182] Relaxation therapies are predicated on the hypothesis that insomnia is associated with hyperarousal.[183] The cognitive component of such therapies involves the education of the patient about sleep needs, the correction of unrealistic expectations, and a discussion of anxiety and catastrophic thinking, such as exaggerating to oneself the consequences of poor sleep. Sleep-hygiene education addresses extrinsic factors that can perpetuate insomnia, such as noise in the bedroom and the use of caffeine.[183]

Many randomized, controlled trials have demonstrated the efficacy of cognitive behavioral therapies in primary insomnia. Two large meta-analyses[176,184] concluded that, as compared with placebo, such therapies result in improvements in initial sleep-onset latency and total sleep time (by about 30 minutes for each measure, on average) and the number and the duration of awakenings. About 50% of patients show meaningful clinical improvement.[185]

Treatment generally combines several approaches. Although data support the efficacy of the various individual components of therapy with the possible exceptions of sleep-hygiene education and cognitive therapy alone,[173] combined therapies are more effective than individual techniques alone.[186] The mean reported duration of follow-up after completion of cognitive behavioral therapy is six months, with sustained benefits noted in most studies. Few studies of longer than one year have been performed.[173]

In most studies, cognitive behavioral therapy has been administered by psychologists, with an average of six sessions (totaling 5.8 hours) per patient.[173] Meta-analysis suggests that individual therapy is somewhat more effective than group therapy.[176] Trainees in the fields of psychology and psychiatry,[187] community health nurses,[185] and primary care counselors[188] have successfully administered this therapy during four to six sessions of 20–50 minutes each. Successful results have also been reported when therapy (consisting of 3–10 sessions) was delivered by primary care physicians who had received three hours of training from a psychologist experienced in treating insomnia.[189] A study of abbreviated cognitive behavioral therapy, administered by junior clinical psychologists in two sessions of 25 minutes in duration two weeks apart, showed significant benefit sustained for at least three months.[190] Self-help treatment by means of videotapes[191] or written material[192] has also proved beneficial.

Pharmacologic Therapies

Classes of prescription medications that are used for the treatment of insomnia include benzodiazepines, benzodiazepine-receptor agonists, and sedating antidepressants. Benzodiazepines that are approved by the Food and Drug Administration (FDA) for use in insomnia include drugs of long, intermediate, and short half-life, whereas approved benzodiazepine-receptor agonists include drugs of intermediate, short, or ultrashort half-life (Table 23). Benzodiazepines act through the benzodiazepine γ-aminobutyric-acid–receptor complex by affecting chloride flux. Benzodiazepine-receptor agonists bind to the same receptor complex but have different affinities for various receptor subclasses.

Nonprescription products that are marketed for the treatment of insomnia include sedating histamine-1–receptor antagonists (diphenhydramine and doxylamine) and melatonin, but the use of these drugs is not supported by rigorous data. Randomized, controlled trials of the histamine-1–receptor antagonists suggest that they improve sleep subjectively, but conclusions are limited by a small number of subjects, a short duration of drug administration, and a lack of objective measurements; morning sedation is a recognized side effect.[193] Studies of melatonin, which have involved small numbers of subjects treated for short periods with various doses and formulations, have demonstrated conflicting results.[194]

Many randomized trials have shown the efficacy of benzodiazepines and benzodiazepine-receptor agonists in relieving short-term insomnia, but no studies extend beyond six months of use. A meta-analysis of 22 studies of benzodiazepines or the benzodiazepine-receptor agonist zolpidem[195] demonstrated that these medications resulted in significant improvements in sleep latency, total sleep time, number of awakenings, and sleep quality. In a subgroup of nine studies that included relevant data, the average patient receiving medication fell asleep faster than 71% of controls, slept longer than 76%, woke less often than 74%, and reported better-quality sleep than 73%. Short-acting agents had the greatest effect on sleep latency, whereas agents with an intermediate or long duration had the greatest effect on total sleep time.

Another meta-analysis of benzodiazepine therapy (including short, intermediate, and long-acting agents) confirmed the beneficial effects of this class of drug on total sleep time but did not find a significant effect on sleep latency.[196] Studies of the benzodiazepine-receptor agonist zaleplon (Sonata) have shown a 50% reduction of sleep latency as compared with baseline but have had no significant effect on total sleep time—a result that is consistent with the very short half-life of the drug.[197,198] Zaleplon, administered 3.5 hours

Table 23: Medications for insomnia approved by the FDA

Medication	*Duration of action*	*Half-life (hr)*[†]	*Dose*	*Indications*	*Side effects*	*Contraindications or drug interactions*
*Benzodiazepines**						
Temazepam (Restoril)	Intermediate	8–15	7.5–30 mg	Mainly for sleep-maintenance insomnia[‡]	Drowsiness, dizziness incoordination	
Estazolam (ProSom)	Intermediate	10–24	0.5–2 mg	Mainly for sleep-maintenance insomnia[‡]	Drowsiness, dizziness, incoordination	
Triazolam (Halcion)	Short	2–5	0.125–0.25 mg insomnia [‡]	Mainly for sleep-onset	Amnesia, drowsiness, dizziness, incoordination	Drugs that induce CYP3A4 (including ketoconazole and nefazodone)
*Benzodiazepine-receptor agonists**						
Eszopiclone (Lunesta)	Intermediate	5–7	1–3 mg	Mainly for sleep-maintenance insomnia[§]	Unpleasant taste, dry mouth, dizziness drowsiness	Drugs that induce CYP3A4 (including ketoconazole and nefazodone)
Zolpidem (Ambien)	Short	3	5–10 mg	Mainly for sleep-onset insomnia[‡]	Drowsiness, dizziness, occasionally amnesia	Possibly drugs that induce CYP3A4[¶]
Zaleplon (Sonata)	Ultrashort	1	5–20 mg	For sleep-onset or sleep maintenance insomnia[‡‖]	Drowsiness	Possibly drugs that induce CYP3A4[¶]
Melatonin-receptor agonist						
Ramelteon (Rozerem)	Short	2–5	8 mg	Mainly for sleep-onset insomnia	Drowsiness, dizziness, increased prolactin levels	Drugs that induce CYP1A2 (especially fluvoxamine), hepatic failure, pregnancy

[*] All medications listed her bind to the γ-aminobutyric acid A receptor. All of the agents are contraindicated in pregnancy. They should not be combined with alcohol and should b used only with caution in patients taking other central nervous system depressants. Physicians should consider all factors carefully before prescribing these agents in patients with a history of substance abuse. Flurazepam and quazepam are also approved by the FDA for treatment of insomnia, and clonazepam is sometimes prescribed. However, Because of the long half-lives of these drugs, thy are generally not recommended. Lower does should always be used in the elderly, in debilitated patients, and in those with hepatic insufficiency.

[†] Half-life refers to the drug and its active metabolites

[‡] This drug was approved by the FDA for short-term management of insomnia (generally lasting 7–10 days).

[§] This drug was approved by the FDA for the treatment of insomnia.

[¶] This drug may need to have its does lowered.

[‖] For sleep-maintenance insomnia this drug is administered on waking during the night.

after lights out with 4 hours more sleep permitted, did not result in any daytime drowsiness or cognitive impairment.[199] A six-month study of eszopiclone, a benzodiazepine-receptor agonist with an intermediate half-life that was recently approved for use in the United States, showed a 50% reduction in sleep latency and 65% reduction in wake time after the onset of sleep as compared with baseline.[200] Studies with zolpidem have shown that intermittent use (three to five times a week) can also be effective in chronic insomnia, with sustained benefit on nights the drug is taken and sleep that is no worse than baseline on nights without medication.[201,202]

Withdrawal effects, especially rebound insomnia, are rare after the discontinuation of long-duration benzodiazepines and tend to be mild after the discontinuation of intermediate-acting benzodiazepines.[203-205] However, marked rebound insomnia has been reported after the discontinuation of triazolam, a shorter-acting drug,[206,207] usually lasting one to three nights.[207,208] In contrast, withdrawal studies of zolpidem have shown little or no rebound insomnia,[197,199,203,206,207,209] and no rebound insomnia was noted after withdrawal of zaleplon.[197,199] The rate of withdrawal of benzodiazepines should be individualized, depending on the half-life and dose of the drug, the duration of therapy, and whether the insomnia is acute or chronic.[208]

Several cases of anterograde amnesia, the day after the use of triazolam have been reported, but the prevalence of this side effect is unknown.[210] Whereas studies have shown variable deficits in memory following the use of benzodiazepines of varying half-lives,[211] clinically significant amnesia seems largely limited to the short-acting agents. Amnesia, including that associated with sleep-related eating, has been described with the use of zolpidem,[212,213] but far less frequently than with triazolam. The most prominent side effects of long-acting benzodiazepines are daytime sleepiness, dizziness, and incoordination.[205] These effects may also occur with intermediate-acting agents, but less frequently; they are rare with short-acting agents such as triazolam and generally occur only with high doses.[205] Side effects are more frequent in the elderly, and dose reductions are needed. The use of long-acting benzodiazepines has been associated with an increased risk of falls and hip fractures in older patients.[214]

A problem with most studies of these agents is their limited duration. The mean treatment duration of the 22 studies included in the meta-analysis noted above was 12 days (with a maximum of 35 days).[195] Short-term tolerance, measured by deterioration in sleep measures with time, has not been noted with the use of temazepam for 8 weeks, the use of zolpidem continuously for 4–5 weeks[197,203,206,209,215] or intermittently for 12 weeks,[202] or the use of zaleplon for 4 to 5 weeks.[197,199] The longest trial, involving six months of treatment with eszopiclone, showed a sustained beneficial effect without development of tolerance.[200]

Sedating antidepressants have been increasingly prescribed for chronic insomnia,[210] despite a paucity of data from randomized trials to support this practice. Small, randomized trials have demonstrated the efficacy of trazodone in treating insomnia in patients with depression.[217,218] A 14-day trial comparing trazodone, zolpidem, and placebo in patients with primary insomnia showed improvement in sleep latency and duration (as assessed by questionnaire) with trazodone as compared with placebo but less effect than with zolpidem.[219] A four-week study of the tricyclic antidepressant doxepin in the treatment of primary insomnia showed significant improvements in sleep latency (21% reduction from baseline), sleep efficiency (13% increase from baseline), and total sleep time (13% increase from baseline).[220] Side effects of tricyclic antidepressants include dry mouth, postural hypotension, drowsiness, cardiac arrhythmias, and weight gain, whereas trazodone can produce hypotension, constipation, and priapism. Mirtazapine, a tetracyclic antidepressant that has adrenergic and serotoninergic antagonist actions, reduces wake time after the onset of sleep, enhances sleep efficiency, and increases the duration of slow-wave sleep in normal subjects,[221] but data are lacking on its effects in primary insomnia.

Pharmacologic Therapy versus Cognitive Behavioral Therapy

Several randomized, controlled studies have compared cognitive behavioral therapy with pharmacologic therapy and with combined therapy. One study comparing the efficacy of triazolam with cognitive behavioral therapy showed a shorter sleep latency with triazolam at two weeks but equal latencies at four weeks.[222] Another study comparing the efficacy of zolpidem with cognitive behavioral therapy showed that the latter was superior throughout the study.[223] Follow-up at four to six weeks after the discontinuation of medication and the completion of cognitive behavioral therapy showed a sustained benefit only for the cognitive behavioral therapy groups in both studies. A meta-analysis comparing studies of cognitive behavioral therapy with those of hypnotics showed similar short-term outcomes during treatment, except that cognitive behavioral therapy resulted in a greater reduction in sleep latency.[224]

Several studies have compared a combination of cognitive behavioral and drug therapy with cognitive behavioral therapy alone.[215,223,225] All of these reports have shown that at 10 to 24 months of follow-up, improvements are maintained for cognitive behavioral therapy alone but not for combined therapy. The most likely explanation is that patients are less committed to learning and practicing cognitive behavioral therapy techniques if they can control insomnia with medications. In contrast, cognitive behavioral therapy that was instituted while attempting to taper doses of benzodiazepines for patients with long-standing chronic insomnia resulted in a higher percentage of patients who were drug-free, as compared with tapering alone.[226,227]

AREAS OF UNCERTAINTY

Cognitive behavioral therapy has been well established as effective in chronic primary insomnia, but its role in secondary insomnia, especially insomnia as a result of psychiatric disorders, has not been systematically tested. Further studies are needed to demonstrate whether primary care physicians can obtain successful results by teaching behavioral techniques in a small number of sessions compatible with the flow of a busy practice. For patients with chronic primary insomnia who do not benefit adequately from cognitive behavioral therapy, questions remain regarding the role of long-term drug therapy. Although studies of treatment with benzodiazepine-receptor agonists for as long as six months have demonstrated efficacy without evidence of tolerance, it is not known whether these results are sustained over longer periods. Melatonin-receptor agonists have shown benefit in randomized trials.[228,229] Ramelteon has just received FDA approval, but more published data and clinical experience with the drug will be needed to determine its role in insomnia management.

Guidelines from Professional Societies

In 1999, the American Academy of Sleep Medicine published evidence-based practice measures for the nonpharmacologic treatment of chronic insomnia.[230] Stimulus control therapy, progressive muscle relaxation, biofeedback, sleep-restriction therapy, and multicomponent cognitive behavioral therapy were recommended. Insufficient evidence was available to recommend sleep-hygiene education, imagery training, or cognitive therapy alone as single therapies. A preliminary report of a June, 2005 conference on insomnia that was sponsored by the National Institutes of Health notes that both cognitive behavioral therapy and benzodiazepine-receptor agonists are effective in treating insomnia but that the long-term effectiveness of the agonists requires further study.

SUMMARY AND RECOMMENDATIONS

Secondary causes of insomnia must be identified and addressed before a diagnosis of primary insomnia is made. Effective treatment is available for most patients with chronic primary insomnia, such as the patient described in the vignette. Both cognitive behavioral therapy and pharmacologic therapy with benzodiazepines or benzodiazepine-receptor agonists are effective in the short-term, but data beyond six months are lacking to support pharmacologic therapies. One should recommend first a course of cognitive behavioral therapy involving stimulus control, relaxation, sleep hygiene education, or other techniques discussed above. Primary care physicians may refer patients to sleep specialists or psychologists trained in this therapy but may alternatively choose to familiarize themselves with the techniques, given the prevalence of primary insomnia and some data to support that even a few short sessions of therapy delivered by primary physicians can produce significant benefits. Cognitive behavioral therapy should not generally be combined with the use of hypnotic agents, given data suggesting that such an approach reduces the long-term benefit of cognitive behavioral therapy.

Although long-term data are lacking, most sleep specialists recommend long-term use of pharmacologic therapy in a subgroup of patients with chronic primary insomnia who do not respond to cognitive behavioral therapy. Careful monitoring for efficacy, tolerance, and side effects is essential, especially in the elderly. For insomnia that is predominantly associated with the onset of sleep, off label use of zolpidem or zaleplon should be considered. For insomnia that is predominantly associated with maintenance of sleep, intermediate acting benzodiazepines such as temazepam can be tried, but these drugs may soon be supplanted by eszopiclone. Zaleplon can also be administered on waking in the latter part of the night. There is little role today for long-acting benzodiazepines in the management of insomnia, unless a coexisting anxiety disorder is present.

46.13.1 RECENT ADVANCES IN THE DIAGNOSIS AND MANAGEMENT OF MIGRAINE

VS Chadda

The World Health Organization considers that severe migraine can be as disabling as quadriplegia.[231] The disorder affects as many of 15% of adults in North America and Western Europe and world wide; and is probably one of the most common reasons for patients to see their doctors. Traditionally, headache is given little time in medical teaching, but headache science is advancing rapidly, fuelled by developments in treatment and neuroscience, and there is a sense of excitement perhaps unrivalled in neurology. Many recent advances have particular relevance to clinical practice in terms of both diagnosis and management.

HEADACHE CLASSIFICATION: IMPROVING AND SIMPLIFYING THE DIAGNOSIS OF MIGRAINE

The development and promulgation of the International Headache Society's diagnostic criteria in 1988 was an important milestone, giving clear guidance and having wide-spread acceptance. Migraine was defined by the component clinical parts of an attack so that the most important tool for the clinician was a good history (Box 3).[232] The second edition of the international classification of headache disorders (ICHD-II)[233] has seen fine tuning of the migraine classification and refining of important issues around frequent headache. Some issues merit highlighting.

Childhood Migraine

The classification of migraine has been modified for children by allowing headaches with fewer features. It seems clear that migraine is common in children, that the attacks are shorter than in adults, and that associated attack features, such as throbbing or unilateral pain or the presence of photophobia and phonophobia, are less common. Most adults who attend their general practitioner with disabling primary headache have migraine,[234] and in my experience migraine is also the most common basis for referral to a headache clinic in children.

Box 3: Simplified diagnostic criteria for migraine (from ICHD-II[233])

Repeated attacks of headache lasting 4–72 hours that have these features:

- Normal physical examination
- No other reasonable cause for the headache
- At least two of:
  - Unilateral pain
  - Throbbing pain
  - Aggravation of pain by movement
  - Moderate or severe intensity of pain
- At least one of:
  - Nausea or vomiting
  - Photophobia and phonophobia

In addition to straight forward migraine, further thought has been given to the childhood periodic syndromes—cyclical vomiting, abdominal migraine, and begin paroxysmal vertigo of childhood—which so often portend migraine in adolescence and adulthood. These syndromes need careful evaluation, although it seems clear that they have a strong association with migraine.

Chronic Daily Headache

Perhaps the most controversial issue in headache classification and management is how to deal with the problem of frequent, daily or near daily headache (Box 4). Some 5% of Western European populations have headache on at least 15 days a month for, on average, four or more hours a day. If one includes shorter lasting headaches, then chronic daily headache is simply a syndrome defined by frequency of headache.[235] It is not just tension-type headache, nor is it all just due to medication overuse. Chronic daily headache is often incorrectly equated with the concept of transformed migraine, a term now superseded by the definition of chronic migraine, which is a subset of chronic daily headache (Box 5). When a doctor gets a history of frequent headache they need to pursue its basis.

Box 4: Classification of chronic daily headache

Headache on ≥15 days a month that may be due to a range of underlying mechanisms and may be complicated by, or caused by, drug overuse

Primary headache

For >4 hours daily

- Chronic migraine—An IHCD-II[233] term for, in essence, migraine without aura for ≥15 days a month. Transformed migraine is a more useful term in clinical practice (box 5 has a current working definition)
- Chronic tension-type headache
- Hemicrania continua
- New daily persistent headache—An IHCD-II[233] term, but I find a more generic approach useful[236]

For <4 hours daily

- Chronic cluster headache—Patients may have >4 hours of headache a day, but the attacks themselves are generally <4 hours duration
- Chronic paroxysmal hemicrania
- Short lasting unilateral neuralgiform headache attacks with conjunctival injection and tearing (SUNCT)
- Hypnic headache

Secondary headache (list not exhaustive)

- Post-traumatic—Head injury, iatrogenic, post-infectious
- Inflammatory—Giant cell arteritis, sarcoidosis, Behçet's syndrome
- Chronic infection of the central nervous system

Medication overuse headache

Box 5: Chronic migraine (modified criteria of the ICHD-II[233])

- Current or prior headache fulfills criteria for migraine without aura (see Box 3)
- Headache on ≥15 days a month
- At least 8 headache days a month for the previous 3 months fulfilling at least one of the following:
  - Criteria C and D for migraine without aura
  - Criteria C and D for migraine without aura with the exception of a single sub-criterion, and not meeting criteria for tension-type headache
  - Headache that the patient believes to be migraine and is relieved by a 5-$HT_{1B/1D}$ receptor agonist
- Not attributable to another disorder, including medication overuse headache

CORE ISSUES FOR GENERAL PRACTITIONERS

In clinical practice there seem to be two core issues for general practitioners: who has sinister or secondary headache, and how can migraine be differentiated from tension-type headache.

Secondary Headache

Although little new development has occurred in this area, some coverage is appropriate. In determining the likelihood of secondary headache, the most crucial clinical feature to elicit is the length of the history. Patients with a short history require prompt attention and may need quick investigation and management. Patients with a longer history generally require time and patience rather than speed. Certain features of the presentation demand attention:

- Pain of sudden onset
- Fever
- Marked change in pain character or timing
- Neck stiffness
- Pain associated with higher center complaints
- Pain associated with neurological disturbance, such as clumsiness or weakness
- Pain associated with local tenderness, such as of the temporal artery.

If a positive diagnosis that is benign cannot be made, patients with a headache that is of recent onset or with neurological signs require brain imaging with computed tomography or magnetic resonance imaging. Patients with a history of recurrent headache for a year or more that fulfills the criteria for migraine (Box 3), and with a normal physical examination, rarely show positive results on brain imaging (only about 1/1000 images). A brain tumor is rarely the cause of a headache, particularly so if it is isolated and long term.[237] Severity is a poor marker of secondary headache, with the most severe and disabling headaches being primary headaches.

Differentiating Migraine and Tension-type Headache

There are two key ways to differentiate migraine from tension-type headache. Firstly, migraine is in essence head pain with associated features whereas tension-type headache is featureless head pain. This small compromise of the International Headache Society criteria results in a pragmatic test that generally yields a useful clinical answer. Secondly, migraine has biological signatures that tension-type headache does not seem to, namely the inherited tendency to headache when confronted with particular triggers (Table 24). Determining whether a patient has a family history of headache, especially if it is migraine, and questioning about trigger factors help to differentiate migraine from tension-type headache. Details of a patient's susceptibility to triggers also provides important information about the patient's biology and offers a management strategy in terms of reducing headache by sensible behavioral change. Testing the reliability of this approach to distinguishing migraine from tension-type headache would be extremely useful but is complicated by there being no known biological marker

Table 24: Differentiating migraine from tension-type headache

Characteristics	*Migraine*	*Tension-type headache*
Pain features of acute attacks	Throbbing	Boring or squashing
	Worsening of pain with movement	No effect of head movement
Associated features	Nausea or vomiting	None
	Photophobia and phonophobia	
Triggering Factors	Altered sleep patterns (too Little or too Much)	Psychological stress
	Skipping meals	
	Overexertion	
	Change in stress Level (too much or relaxation)	
	Excess afferent Stimuli (such as Bright lights)	
	Weather change	
	Chemical (delayed Headache after Alcohol or glyceryl Trinitrate)	
	Menstruation	

against which to judge the outcome. In clinical practice, however, erring on the side of diagnosing migraine has few drawbacks and offers many options for management.

GENETICS OF MIGRAINE: EXPLAINING TO PATIENTS WHY THEY HAVE THE PROBLEM

It seems logical to suppose that all sufferers of primary headaches have a genetic predisposition that is in some way activated by physiological and other life events, such as poverty, although the only genetic associations yet identified are for migraine. Migraine genetics offer a useful tool in clinical practice for helping to explain to patients that they were born with a tendency to headache—by establishing that their parents also had headaches, or by pointing out that the triggers listed in Table 24 do not produce headache universally, the doctor can explain the cause. This is useful in allaying fear and setting the groundwork for improving the problem.

The first concrete example of inherited migraine was the identification of missense mutations in the Cav2.1 subunit of the gene for the P/Q type, voltage gated, calcium channel on chromosome 19 in families with familial hemiplegic migraine. Since then, other cases of familial hemiplegic migraine have been found to be caused by mutations in the ATP1A2 gene, which encodes the α_2 subunit of the Na^+/K^+ pump, and in the SCN1A gene for the neuronal voltage-gated sodium channel.

The overall message is of migraine as an ionopathy, a disorder based on abnormal ion channels whose strategic function and anatomical distribution in the brain determine the clinical phenotype. If genetics can explain why patients have headaches and what the biochemical disorder may be, then we can ask the question, "Where is the problem?" or, framed in the terms of classic neurology, "Where is the lesion?"

PATHOPHYSIOLOGY OF HEADACHE—WHERE IS THE LESION?

Classic neurology, as promulgated by Gowers, sought to provide anatomical answers to clinical questions. This approach has been successful, but the problems of primary headache will need a physiological approach. To some extent, human functional imaging starts to do this.

In the 1960s and 1970s migraine was considered a vascular phenomenon and is still often referred to incorrectly as a vascular headache. Wolff summarized in his classic book the referral patterns of structures that produced intracranial pain, taking a view that migraine aura was due to vasoconstriction and that the subsequent headache was due to a reactive vasodilatation. Olesen debunked this link. The spreading depression theory points out that the changes in blood flow follow metabolic demand—vasoneuronal coupling. Considering features of the attack that do not occur in all cases (such as nausea, photophobia, and phonophobia) or of the premonitory phase (such as yawning or diuresis), the vascular hypothesis seems unattractive.

The lesion should be considered a functional concept. What structure or network of structures would produce a syndrome whose core features are unilateral head pain and sensitivity to light, sound, smells, and head movement, as well as have the potential to alter brain blood flow, be influenced by sleep or changing sleep patterns, and alter broadly cortical function in terms of attention and concentration. Brainstem aminergic neurones, such as the noradrenergic neurones of the locus coeruleus, could potentially have these broad effects, so the hypothesis would predict functional imaging changes in the brainstem, indeed in the pons.

Functional Brain Imaging in Migraine

Positron emission tomography in acute migraine has shown activations in the rostral brainstem that persisted after successful treatment of the attack but are not present interictally.[238] These changes are not seen in experimentally induced ophthalmic division pain[239] or in other primary headaches, such as cluster headache[240] or paroxysmal hemicrania.[241] Indeed, we and others have consistently observed activation in the dorsolateral pons in both spontaneous and triggered episodic migraine.[242-245] Moreover, in chronic migraine, defined as migraine without aura that occurs on ≥15 days a month for more than six months,[233] the same area of the dorsolateral pons is activated,[246] suggesting that infrequent and frequent migraine are ends of a shared spectrum. Use of blood oxygen level dependent (BOLD) contrast functional magnetic resonance imaging holds the promise of studying single patients and determining the site of abnormal activation. Moreover, magnetic resonance angiography has shown that the blood flow changes seen in migraine[244] and cluster headache[240] are simply a result of ophthalmic division pain,[247,248] not a cause of the syndrome.

Functional neuroimaging has recently shown that the changes in the dorsolateral pons in migraine lateralize with the attack: studies of typical migraine triggered by glyceryl trinitrate have revealed left sided brain activation in patients with left sided attacks, right sided activation in patients with right sided attacks, and bilateral activation in patients with bilateral pain.[245] These data suggest that the dorsolateral pons is pivotal in the phenotypic expression of migraine. These changes in brain activation persisted after resolution of the pain with a triptan, were not present interictally, and were not seen in a control group who were scanned but in whom migraine did not develop. Moreover, the pontine change was not seen during the dull bilateral headache induced by glyceryl trinitrate in either controls or migraineurs.[245] The extent to which the changes observed form part of a unique response to brain dysfunction elsewhere, or are themselves the pivotal changes, remains to be determined.

The implication of the studies for clinicians is to be able to tell patients that we are confident that the disorder is one that is localized in the brain. It seems clear that migraine is not a disorder of blood vessels but one of brain function. To this end we can assure patients who feel odd during attacks, perhaps have trouble concentrating, or simply feel a little befuddled that this is normal, indeed expected of a brain disorder of this type. More importantly, these insights must lead to new directions for the development of much needed new preventive treatments.

MIGRAINE—WHAT NEW TREATMENTS CAN WE EXPECT?

Triptans, selective 5-$HT_{1B/1D}$ receptor agonists, were the main advance in migraine treatment during the latter part of the 20th century. Many migraine sufferers were liberated in a way that they had not previously known, clinical trial guidelines were refined and revised, and clinical studies were well organized and uniform. After sumatriptan, came zolmitriptan, naratriptan, rizatriptan, almotriptan, eletriptan, and frovatriptan; donitriptan has now finished preclinical development. Ergotamine, the mainstay of specific acute treatment for most of the 20th century after its initial description in the 19th, now has few indications in which it is the treatment of choice. It is clear what patients want—rapid, complete, and consistent pain relief— but not entirely established how they make preference decisions among the available treatments. What is established is that most patients do have preferences for individual triptans when asked. Box 6 sets out some situations in which the various triptans may be

Box 6: Clinical stratification of acute migraine treatment

Failed analgesics or NSAIDs

First tier-Sumatriptan 50 mg or 100 mg rizaptriptan 10 mg, almotriptan 12.5 mg, eletriptan 40 mg, zolmitriptan 2.5 mg (all tablets)

For slower effect or better tolerability-Naratriptan 2.5 mg, frovatriptan 2.5 mg (tablets)

Infrequent headache-Ergotamine 1–2 mg tablet, dihydroergotamine nasal spray 2 mg

Early nausea or difficulties taking tablets

- Sumatriptan* 20 mg nasal spray, zolmitriptan 5 mg nasal spray, rizatriptan 10 mg dissolvable wafer, zolmitriptan 2.5 mg disperisible

Headache recurrence

- Ergotamine 2 mg (perhaps most effective taken rectally, usually with caffeine), naratriptan 2.5 mg tablet, eletriptan 80 mg dispersible

Poor tolerance of acute treatments

- Naratriptan 2.5 mg, frovatriptan 2.5 mg (tablets)

Early vomiting

- *Sumatriptan 25 mg suppository, sumatriptan 6 mg subcutaneous injection

Menstrually related headache

- Prevention—Ergotamine tablet taken at night, estrogen patches
- Treatment—Triptans, dihydroergotamine nasal spray

Rapidly developing symptoms

* Sumatriptan 6 mg subcutaneous injection, dihydroergotamine 1 mg intramuscular injection

Table 25: Preventive treatments in migraine*

Agent	*Dose**	*Selected side effects*
Commonly used drugs		
Pizotifen	0.5–2 mg daily	Weight gain, drowsiness
β blocker (propranolol)	40–120 mg twice daily	Reduced energy, tiredness, postural symptoms, contraindicated in asthama
Tricyclics (amitriptyline, dothiepin , nortriptyline)	25–75 mg nightly	Drowsiness (some patients are very sensitive and may need only a total dose of 10 mg, though 1–1.5 mg/kg body weight is generally required for a response.
Anticonvulsants:		
Valproate	400–600 mg twice daily	Drowsiness, weight gain, tremor, hair loss, fetal abnormalities, hematological or liver abnormalities
Topiramate	25–100 mg twice	Paresthesiae, cognitive dysfunction, weight loss, renal stones, glaucoma
Gabapentin	900–3600 mg daily	Dizziness, sedation
Methysergide	1–4 mg daily	Drowsiness leg cramps, hair loss, retroperitoneal fibrosis (1 month drug holiday required every 6 months)
Flunarizine	5–10 mg daily	Drowsiness, weight gain, depression, parkinsonism
Metabolic enhancers		
Riboflavin	400 mg daily	
Coenzyme	100 mg thrice daily	
Non-pharmaceuticals		
Feverfew		
Butterbur		
Other preventives with controlled evidence for efficacy		
Lisinopril	10–20 mg daily	Cough
Candesartan	16 mg daily	
No convincing controlled evidence		
Verapamil		
Shown to have no effect by controlled trials		
Nimodipine		
Clonidine		
Fluoxetine		

helpful, based on the results of meta-analyses of large scale controlled trials[249-251] and clinical experience.

New Treatments and Unmet Needs

Three unmet needs come readily to mind—new preventive drugs, acute treatments without vascular effects, and new strategies for managing intractable migraine.

Preventive drugs—On average, two-thirds of patients will have a 50% reduction in headache frequency with most preventive drugs.[252] They can then choose between the potential for sleepiness, exercise intolerance, erectile impotence, nightmares, dry mouth, weight gain, tremor, hair loss, or fetal deformities as possible side effects. The fact that migraineurs are prepared to accept such side effects indicates the level of disability they experience. The recent positive results from clinical trials of topiramate show its utility in migraine.[253,254] Table 25 shows the range of options for prevention, none of which is ideal.

Nonvascular acute treatments are required for those patients who cannot take triptans and ergot derivatives. Publication of a clinical trial where BIBN4096BS, a potent calcitonin gene-related peptide (CGRP) antagonist, was effective in treating acute migraine,[255] simultaneously answers the question of whether nerves or blood vessels are of primary pathophysiological importance and provides the promise of a new treatment that is safe for patients with cardiovascular disorders. This advance was predicted by laboratory work more than a decade ago, and the translation of the basic experimental work to clinical practice illustrates the importance of basic neurobiology to advancing clinical practice. It is now clear that vasoconstriction is not necessary for aborting acute migraine, recently confirmed by the demonstration that sildenafil, a phosphodiesterase inhibitor, can induce migraine without changes in cerebral vessel diameter.

Treatment for intractable migraine—Patients with intractable migraine require a new way forward, this may at last be at hand. Controlled observations of occipital nerve stimulation in chronic migraine are extremely promising.[246] There is good evidence from animal studies of a clear interaction between trigeminal and cervical afferents in the trigeminocervical complex, and a controlled trial has been initiated to examine this approach.

The future for migraine sufferers seems bright as the combination of good clinical research, basic neuroscience, and clinical investigation is delivering both understanding and new treatments for this common and disabling disorder.

46.13.2 DIAGNOSIS AND MANAGEMENT OF HEADACHES IN YOUNG PEOPLE AND ADULTS: SUMMARY OF NICE GUIDANCE

JN Vyas

Headaches are a common problem that many clinicians in primary and secondary care find difficult to treat.[256,257] Once the serious causes of headache have been excluded (such as infection, tumor, bleeding, and arteritis), the major health and social burden of headaches can be attributed to primary headache disorders (cluster headache, migraine, and tension-type headache) and headache caused by the overuse of medications. Straightforward advice is needed for anyone working in the NHS on the diagnosis and treatment of these common disorders and the prevention of medication overuse headache.

This article summarizes the most recent recommendations from the National Institute for Health and Clinical Excellence (NICE) on the diagnosis and management of headaches in young people and adults.[258]

RECOMMENDATIONS

NICE recommendations are based on systematic reviews of the best available evidence and explicit consideration of cost effectiveness. When minimal evidence is available, recommendations are based on the Guideline Development Group's experience and opinion of what constitutes good practice. Evidence levels for the recommendations are given in the full version of this article on bm.com.

ASSESSMENT: INDICATIONS FOR CONSIDERING ADDITIONAL INVESTIGATION

- Evaluate people who present with headache and any of the following features, and consider the need for further investigations or referral (or both):[259]
  - Worsening headache with fever
  - Sudden onset headache that reaches maximum intensity within five minutes
  - New onset neurological deficit
  - New onset cognitive dysfunction
  - Change in personality
  - Impaired level of consciousness
  - Recent (typically within the past three months) head trauma
  - Headache triggered by cough, valsalva (trying to breathe out with nose and mouth blocked), or sneeze
  - Headache triggered by exercise
  - Orthostatic headache (headache that changes with posture)
  - Symptoms suggestive of giant cell arteritis
  - Symptoms and signs of acute narrow angle glaucoma
  - A substantial change in the characteristics of their headache.
- Consider further investigations or referral (or both) for people who present with new onset headache and any of the following:
  - Compromised immunity, caused, for example, by HIV or immunosuppressive drugs
  - Age under 20 years and a history of malignancy
  - A history of malignancy known to metastasize to the brain
  - Vomiting without other obvious cause.

DIAGNOSIS

- Diagnose primary headaches such as tension-type headache, migraine, or cluster headache according to the features in Table 26.
- Be alert to the possibility of medication overuse headache in people whose headache developed or worsened while they were taking the following drugs for three months or more:
  - Triptans, opioids, ergots, or combination analgesic drugs on 10 days a month or more, or

Table 26: Diagnosis of tension-type headache, migraine, and cluster headache[256-260]

Headache feature	*Tension-type headache*		*Migraine (with or without aura)*		*Cluster headache*	
Pain location*	Bilateral		Unilateral or bilateral		Unilateral (around the eye, above the eye, and along the side of the head or face)	
Pain quality	Pressing or tightening (non-pulsating)		Pulsating (throbbing or banging in young people aged 12–17 years)		Variable (can be sharp, boring, burning, throbbing, or tightening)	
Pain intensity	Mild or moderate		Moderate or severe		Severe or very severe	
Effect on activities	Not aggravated by routine activities of daily living		Aggravated by, or causes avoidance of, routine activities of daily living		Restlessness or agitation	
Other symptoms	None		Unusual sensitivity to light or sound (or both), or nausea or vomiting (or both). †Aura symptoms can occur with or without headache; they are fully reversible, develop over at least 5 minutes, and last for 5–60 minutes. Typical aura symptoms include visual symptoms such as flickering lights, spots or lines, or partial loss of vision (or a combination thereof); sensory symptoms such as numbness or pins and needles (or both); and speech disturbance		On the same side as the headache: red or watery eye (or both); nasal congestion or runny nose (or both); swollen eyelid; forehead and facial sweating; constricted pupil or drooping eyelid (or both)	
Duration of headache	30 minutes to continuous		4–72 hours in adults; 1–72 hours in people aged 12–17 years		15–180 minutes	
Frequency	<15 days a month	≥15 days a month for more than 3 months	<15 days a month	≥15 days a month for more than 3 months	1 every other day to 8 per day,‡ with continuous remission§ >1 month	1 every other day to 8 per day,‡ with continuous remission§ <1 month in a 12 months period
Diagnosis	Episodic tension-type headache	Chronic tension type headache¶	Episodic migraine (with or without aura)	Chronic migraine with or without aura)**	Episodic cluster headache	Chronic cluster headache

* Headache pain can be felt in the head, face, or neck.
† See full guideline for further information on the diagnosis of migraine with aura.
‡ The frequency of recurrent headaches during a cluster headache bout.
§ The pain-free period between cluster headache bouts.
¶ Chronic migraine and chronic tension-type headache commonly overlap; if the patient has any features of migraine, diagnose chronic migraine.
** The National Institute for Health and Clinical Excellence has developed technology appraisal guidance on botulinum toxin type A for the prevention of headaches in adults with chronic migraine.

– Paracetamol, aspirin, or a nonsteroidal anti-inflammatory drug (NSAID), either alone or in any combination, on 15 days a month or more.

MANAGEMENT

All Headaches

- Do not refer people diagnosed as having tension-type headache, migraine, cluster headache, or medication overuse headache for neuroimaging solely for reassurance.
- Include the following in discussions with the person with a headache disorder:
  - A positive diagnosis, including an explanation of the diagnosis and reassurance that other pathology has been excluded, and
  - The options for management, and
  - Recognition that headache is a valid medical disorder that can have a serious impact on the person and his or her family or carers.
- Explain the risk of medication overuse headache to people who are using acute treatments for their headache disorder.

Tension-type Headache

- Consider aspirin, paracetamol, or an NSAID for acute treatment, taking into account the person's preferences, comorbidities, and risks of adverse events.

Because of an association with Reye's syndrome, do not offer preparations containing aspirin to people aged under 16 years.

- Do not offer opioids for acute treatment.
- Consider a course of up to 10 sessions of acupuncture over five to eight weeks for the prophylactic treatment of chronic tension-type headache.

Migraine with or without Aura

- Offer combination therapy with an oral triptan and an NSAID, or an oral triptan and paracetamol, for acute treatment, taking into account the person's preferences, comorbidities, and risk of adverse events. For people aged 12–17 years consider a nasal triptan in preference to an oral triptan.
- For people in whom oral preparations (or nasal preparations in people aged 12–17 years) for acute treatment are ineffective or not tolerated:
  - Offer a nonoral preparation of metoclopramide or prochlorperazine, and
  - Consider adding a nonoral NSAID or triptan if these have not been tried.
- Offer topiramate or propranolol for prophylactic treatment according to the person's preference, comorbidities, and risk of adverse events. Advise women and girls of childbearing potential that topiramate is associated with a risk of fetal malformations and can impair the effectiveness of hormonal contraceptives. Ensure they are offered suitable contraception.
- If both topiramate and propranolol are unsuitable or ineffective, consider a course of up to 10 sessions of acupuncture over five to eight weeks or gabapentin (up to 1200 mg/day) according to the person's preference, comorbidities, and risk of adverse events.
- Advise people with migraine that riboflavin (400 mg once a day) can reduce the frequency and intensity of migraine in some people.

Combined Hormonal Contraceptive Use by Women and Girls with Migraine

- For those who have migraine with aura, do not routinely offer combined hormonal contraceptives for contraception.

Menstrual Migraine

- For women and girls with predictable menstrual related migraine that does not respond adequately to standard acute treatment, consider treatment with frovatriptan (2.5 mg twice a day) or zolmitriptan (2.5 mg twice or three times a day) on the days that migraine is expected.

Cluster Headache

- Offer oxygen and a subcutaneous or nasal triptan for acute treatment.
- When using oxygen for acute treatment:
  - Use 100% oxygen at a flow rate of at least 12 L per minute with a non-rebreathing mask and a reservoir bag, and
  - Arrange provision of home and ambulatory oxygen.
- When using a subcutaneous or nasal triptan, ensure the person is offered an adequate supply of triptans. This should be calculated according to the person's history of cluster bouts, taking into account the manufacturer's maximum daily dose.
- Consider verapamil for prophylactic treatment during a bout of cluster headache. If unfamiliar with its use for cluster headache, seek specialist advice before starting verapamil, including advice on electrocardiographic monitoring.

Primary Headaches during Pregnancy

- Offer pregnant women paracetamol for the acute treatment of migraine. Consider the use of a triptan or an NSAID after discussing the woman's need for treatment and the risks associated with the use of each drug during pregnancy.
- Seek specialist advice if prophylactic treatment for migraine is needed during pregnancy.
- Seek specialist advice if treatment for cluster headache is needed during pregnancy.

Medication Overuse Headache

- Explain to people with medication overuse headache that it is treated by withdrawing the drugs that are overused.
- Advise people to stop taking all overused acute headache drugs for at least one month and to stop abruptly rather than gradually.
- Advise people that headache symptoms will probably get worse in the short term before they improve and that there may be associated withdrawal symptoms. Provide them with close follow-up and support according to their needs.
- Consider prophylactic treatment for the underlying primary headache disorder in addition to withdrawal of overused drugs.

Overcoming Barriers

The use of combination therapy as the first choice treatment for migraine is innovative and should improve acute treatment. Compliance may, however, be better when people take one drug only, and the guideline provides this alternative. Alongside other considerations, patient preference should inform choice of acute migraine treatments. At the time of publication (September 2012), not all the recommended drugs had marketing authorisation in the United Kingdom for the indication specified or for young people. Prescribers should follow relevant professional guidance and take full responsibility for the decision when prescribing drugs that do not have marketing authorization. Because topiramate is recommended as first line agent for migraine prophylaxis, prescribers and patients will need to be aware of its safe use in women and girls of childbearing potential. Its enzyme inducing potential means that many hormonal contraceptives may be unreliable. Prescribers should consult authoritative guidance, such as the *British National Formulary* (*BNF*) or guidance from the Royal College of Obstetricians and Gynaecologists Faculty of Sexual and Reproductive Healthcare,[5] when advising on contraceptive use. In treating those with cluster headaches, general practitioners and oxygen supply companies should ensure that an urgent supply of oxygen is readily available. Challenges around medication overuse headaches include the need to recognize the risk factors, plus early preventive advice. Advice to stop taking drugs abruptly may not be welcome, especially as a definite diagnosis can be made only after the headaches resolve, which occurs in only half of those who succeed in stopping. No recommendation has been made for other therapist delivered interventions, such as manual therapy, exercise, cognitive behavioral therapy, or self management programs because of the absence of evidence. The guideline makes research recommendations in some of these areas.

46.14 ATYPICAL ANTIPSYCHOTICS FOR BIPOLAR DISORDER

JN Vyas

The term atypical antipsychotic is used to describe N. a group of medications that have efficacy in treating psychosis but have little or no propensity to cause extrapyramidal symptoms (EPS). Atypical antipsychotic agents have higher affinity to 5-HT2A receptors than to dopamine D2 receptors, and it has been argued that this unique property gives these medications a lower propensity towards EPS and increased efficacy against negative symptoms. Clozapine is the prototype of atypical antipsychotic agents. Although clozapine was used initially to treat psychosis as early as the 1970s, its use was rapidly abandoned because of deaths associated with agranulocytosis. The demonstration of the benefit of clozapine in treating refractory psychosis in the 1980s fuelled development of other atypical antipsychotic agents.

During the past decade, several atypical antipsychotic agents, including risperidone, olanzapine, quetiapine, ziprasidone, aripiprazole, and amisulpride, became available in various parts of the world. Case reports and open studies documenting the usefulness of atypical antipsychotic agents in bipolar disorder provided a much-needed impetus for the pharmaceutical industry to embark on comprehensive clinical trial development programs to examine the efficacy of atypical antipsychotic agents in various phases of bipolar disorder. Olanzapine was the first to be examined in double-blind, placebo-controlled and for prevention of mood episodes. Trials of risperidone, quetiapine, ziprasidone, and aripiprazole, examined the antimanic efficacy of the other atypical antipsychotic agents. To date only quetiapine has been examined for its antidepressant agents. To date only quetiapine has been examined for its antidepressant properties and aripiprazole for prophylaxis in double-blind, placebo-controlled studies. No double-blind trials to date have reported on the efficacy of clozapine or amisulpride in bipolar disorder.

The results of double-blind trials suggest that the atypical antipsychotic agents examined to date have antimanic, antidepressant, and prophylactic properties in bipolar disorder. Atypical antipsychotic agents reduce dopamine transmission through blockade of or partial agonism for dopamine D2 receptors: this action might explain their antimanic effect, because mania is reported to be associated with dopaminergic hyperactivity. More importantly, the ability of atypical antipsychotic agents to block or down-regulate 5-HT2A receptors may be associated with relief or prevention of depressive symptoms.

This article reviews the data from double-blind, controlled trials investigating the efficacy of atypical antipsychotic agents in acute mania, in acute bipolar depression, and in continuation and maintenance treatment of bipolar disorder.

ACUTE MANIA PLACEBO-CONTROLLED MONOTHERAPY STUDIES

Each of the five atypical antipsychotic agents currently available in North America (i.e. risperidone, olanzapine, quetiapine, ziprasidone, and aripiprazole) has been examined in at least two placebo-controlled double-blind trials for treatment of acute mania. All studies with the exception of ziprasidone studies used changes in the Young Mania Rating Scale (YMRS) (>14 on the MRS for ziprasidone studies). And all studies excluded patients with substance abuse. Manic patients with and without psychotic features were included in all studies; patients with mixed episodes and rapid cycling were included in some studies but not in others.

Because of the simarity of these trials, comparative data from these trials are reviewed using the following clinically meaningful efficacy measures: (1) changes in the primary efficacy measure, (2) onset of action, (3) resonse rates, (4) remission rates, (5) patient subgroups, and (6) induction of depression.

CHANGES IN THE PRIMARY EFFICACY MEASURE

Each of the 10 studies showed that the atypical antipsychotic agent was superior to placebo in treating acute manic symptoms as indicated by significantly greater reductions on the primary efficacy measure. In addition, a study that examined the efficacy of risperidone versus placebo versus haloperidol with a 3-week primary end-point also showed superiority of risperidone in comparison with placebo. The mean difference of reduction on primary efficacy measure between an atypical antipsychotic agent and placebo in these studies ranged from - 3.97 to - 12.4. The averages of the mean differences in the primary efficacy measure in the two studies for each of the atypiocal antipsychotic agents (or three studies for resperidone) were remarkably similar (-6.05 for olanzapine. -5.94 for quetiapine, -5.07 for aripiprazole, and -5.05 for ziprasidone), but risperidone had slightly larger reductions (-7.9). The greater average reduction for risperidone resulted mainly from a larger reduction in YMRS scores (-12.4) observed in the India study, which enrolled more severely ill manic patients than the other acute mania studies.

ONSET OF ACTION

Medications that work faster may lead to savings in significant health care costs by reducing hospitalization days. The earliest day at which a medication separates from a placebo might indicate how quickly a medication works in treating manic symptoms. The earlier studies that examined the efficacy of atypical antipsychotic agents used day 7 as the first postrandomization measurement day, but more recent studies have used day 2. The first olanzapine study did not show separation from placebo until week 3. The starting dosage of olanzapine in this study was only 10 mg. However, which is somewhat lower than the dose clinicians routinely use for treating acute mania. In the second olanzapine study, which used 15 mg as the starting dose, separation from placebo was shown on day 7, the first postrandomization measurement date. Risperidone studies used day 3 as the first measurement date. One study showed separation on that day; the other showed separation on day 7. The quetapine studies had very slow dose titration schedules (100 mg on day 1 increased by 100 mg day until day 4 and to 600 mg on day 5). This slow titration schedule may, to some extent, have accounted for the lack of separation from placebo until day 21 in the quetiapine studies. The combined analysis of two quetiapine monotherapy studies, however, revealed a separation from placebo on day 4. Both ziprasidone studies showed separation from placebo in changes in MRS scores on day 2, and aripiprazole studies showed separation on day 4.

RESPONSE RATES

Clinicians are more interested in the number of patients who respond to a given agent than in the mean reductions in YMRS scores for a group of patients. Therefore all clinical trials report rates, and the response is typically defined as a 50% or greater reduction on the primary efficacy measure score (YMRS or MRS) or "much or very much improvement" on the Clinical Global Impression-Improvement (CGI-I) Scale. The differences in response rates between an active agent and a placebo (placebo-corrected response rate) from each study for each agent should provide an estimate of true response to the medication.

The placebo-corrected response rates on YMRS ranged from 8% to 37%. The placebo-corrected response rates were similer in the monotherapy studies for olanzapine (24.4% and 21.9%), ziprasidone (15% and 16.8%), and aripiprazole (21% in both studies), but the differences in response rates were substantial between the three studies for risperidone (15%, 19%, and 37%) and for quetiapine (26% and 8%). The differences in the severity of mania in patients enrolled in the three risperidone studies may account for the differences in response rates, but the severity of mania was similar in the two quetiapine studies.

The mean placebo-corrected response rates (i.e. the average response rates from placebo-controlled trials for each agent) were in the range of 16%–23.3% for risperidone, 23.2% for olanzapine, 17% for quetiapine, 21% for aripiprazole, and 15.9% for ziprasidone). Overall, the results of these studies suggest that there is an incremental response rate of about 20%–25% with active medication overplacebo.

REMISSION RATES

Patients who meet criteria for response may still have significant manic symptoms, because response requires only a 50% reduction in rating scale scores. Remission should be the goat of therapy, but there is no consensus as to what constitutes remission. Furthermore, only the risperidone, olanzapine, and quetiapine studies reported remission rates; the aripiprazole and ziprasidone studies did not.

Remission rates will probably vary depending on the definition used. Olanzapine and quetiapine monotherapy studies used a score of 12 or lower on YMRS to define remission. Using this definition, remission rates were 20%

to 25% higher with olanzapine than with placebo at weeks 3 and 4, respectively, In the two studies comparing quetiapine with placebo, the remission rates for quetiapine were 4% and 24.5%, respectively, higher than placebo at week 12. The two risperidone studies using a more stringent definition of 8 or lower on the YMRS and 12 or lower on the Montgomery-Asberg Depression Rating Scale (MADRS) reported remission rates that were 11%–36%, respectively, higher than placebo at week 3.

PATIENT SUBGROUPS

The proportion of patients with mixed episodes varied, and only a few studies reported on the outcome for mixed patients separately. Both the placebo-controlled trials of olanzapine monotherapy included patients with mixed episodes, and both studies showed that the magnitude of change in YMRS scores in patients with mixed episodes was similar to that in patients with manic episodes. Both the quetiapine studies and two of the risperidone studies excluded mixed patients. The third risperidone study. Which included mixed, patients, reported similar reductions in YMRS scores in patients with mixed and manic episodes (–28.7 versus –22.5); however, only 6% of patients in this study had a mixed episode. In the trial with ziprasidone, patients in the manic and mixed subgroups had comparable improvements in MRS scale scores (–13.1 and –11.2). The aripiprazole study included significant number of mixed episode patients, but the results for these patients were not reported separately.

Most studies with risperidone and both quetiapine studies excluded patients with rapid cycling. The aripiprazole study included patients with rapid cycling, but results were not reported. Although both olanzapine in 45 patients with a rapid cycling course than with placebo (–13.9 versus –4.1 P = 0.01).

All the studies included patients with and without psychotic features. In general, the results suggested that the magnitude of improvement in YMRS scores was similar in patients with and without psychotic features and were significantly greater than the improvement seen with placebo.

INDUCTION OF DEPRESSIVE SYMPTOMS

Although conventional antipsychotic agents have been reported to induce depressive symptoms in manic patients, there is no evidence to suggest that atypical antipsychotic agents have the same liability. In one of the olanzapine studies that reported this outcome, the proportion of patients in the olanzapine group who experienced a clinically detectable worsening of depression was similar to that in the placebo group (11.1% versus 17.9%;P=0.42). Similarly, mean reductions in MADRS scores in the risperidone group were greater in one study, suggesting that risperidone also does not have a propensity to induce depression. Both quetiapine studies found greater mean reductions in MADRS scores in the quetiapine group than in the placebo group and that the incidence of treatment-emergent depression was similar in the quetiapine and the placebo groups. The aripiprazole and ziprasidone studies have not reported on this outcome measure.

DOUBLE BLIND ACTIVE COMPARATOR STUDIES FOR ACUTE MANIA

Studies that compared atypical antipsychotic monotherapy with conventional antipsychotic or lithium or divalproex monotherapy are summarized here.

With the exception of ziprasidone, all atypical antipsychotic agents currently available in North America have been compared with haloperidol monotherapy for treatment of acute mania. The olanzapine and aripiprazole studies had no placebo groups; the risperidone and quetiapine studies included placebo comparator groups. The primary endpoint for acute mania included placebo comparator groups. The primary endpoint for actue mania was at 6 weeks in the olanzapine study and at 3 weeks in the risperidone, quetiapine, and aripiprazole studies. None of the studies showed any significant differences in changes on the YMRS scores or in response rates between the atypical antipsychotic agent and haloperidol. In the general, the incidence of EPS was higher in the haloperidol. In general, the incidence of EPS was higher in the haloperidol group in all studies.

Olanzapine, risperidone, and quetiapine were also compared with lithium monotherapy. The results showed that each of these atypical antipsychotic agents is as effective as lithium monotherapy in treating acute mania. Olanzapine was compared with divalproex in two double-blind studies with conflicting results. In one trial of 248 patients, changes in YMRS total scores were significantly greater with olanzapine (-13.4) than with divalproex (-10.4P < 0.03). In a smaller trial (n=120), there was no significant difference between the two treatments.

The placebo-controlled trials of atypical antipsychotic agents show similar mean changes in YMRS scores and response rates, suggesting that there are no significant differences in the efficacy of the various atypical antipsychotic agents for treating acute mania. The best way to establish similarity or difference in efficacy, however, is to conduct a head-to-head comparator study, and only one such study has been conducted to date for acute mania. In this 3-week trial, olanzapine was compared with risperidone in the treatment of 329 patients with nonpsychotic acute mania. Results showed no differences in chages in YMRS scores or responder rates between the two groups. The mean improvement in MADRS score was significantly greater with olanzapine than with risperidone, but because the difference in score was only one point. The clinical significance of this finding remains unclear.

COMBINATION THERAPY STUDIES

The combination of an atypical antipsychotic agent and a mood stabilizer is commonly used in clinical practice, and studies suggest that up to 80% of patients receive combination therapy. Because of the wide-spread use of combination therapy, a number of recent studies compared the efficacy of an atypical antipsychotic agent (olanzapine in one study, risperidone in two studies, and quetiapine in three studies) plus in mood stabilizer with a mood stablizer pluse placebo for treating acute mania. The duration of these studies varied from 3 weeks to 6 weeks.

All six studies numerically greater reductions in the primary efficacy measure of YMRS or MRS scores, but only four studies showed statistical superiority of combination therapy over mood stabilizer monotherapy. In the failed risperidone study, when patients treated with carbamazepine (which reduced the plasma concentration of risperidone by 40%) were excluded, YMRS total scores at endpoint were significantly greater with risperidone than with placebo (mean difference, 5.4:P=0.04–7). This result suggests that carbamazepine induction of risperidone metabolism may have accounted for the failure of this study on the primary efficacy meausre. In the failed quetiapine study, the combination group had numerically greater reductions in YMRS scores, but the differences were not significant because of the excellent response to a mood stabilizer along in this study population. The combined analysis of the two quetiapine (14.1%, 22%–34%) plus mood stabilizer plus placebo, indicating that the combination treatment provides a clinically meaningful increase in response rates. In all studies, weight gain was more common with combination therapy than with mood stabilizer monotherapy. Somnolence and dry mouth were more common with olanzapine and quetiapine; EPSs were more common with risperidone in one study.

ACUTE BIPOLAR DEPRESSION

Although bipolar patients experience depressive symptoms three times more commonly than mania, only two studies examined the efficacy of atypical antipsychotic agents in the treatment of acute bipolar depression in double-blind, placebo-controlled trials.

OLANZAPINE (OLAN)

As with mania, olanzapine was the first atypical antipsychotic agent to be assessed for its efficacy in acute bipolar I depression. Eight hundred thirty-three patients were randomly assigned to olanzapine, 5–20 mg day (n = 370), placebo (n = 377), or olanzapine plus Huoxetine combination (OFC) (n = 86) for 8 weeks. Both olanzapine and OFC were significantly superior to placebo at all visits and at endpoint on the primary efficacy measure of reduction in depressive symptoms as measured by the MADRS. Further, OFC was superior to olanzapine from week 4 to week 8. Remission rates were 24.5% for the placebo group. 32.8% for the olanzapine group, and 48.8% for the OFC group. The incidence of manic switch was not different among the three groups (placebo 6.7%, olanzapine 5.7, and OFC 6.7%). The adverse-event profile was similar for the olanzapine and OFC groups, with weight gain, somnolence, increased appetite, dry mouth, and asthenia occurring more commonly than in the placebo group. Nausea and diarrhea were more common in OFC group than in the olanzapine group.

Patients with acute mania (n=731) were treated with open-label olanzapine, 5 to 20 mg daily. Patients who responded during a 6- to 12-week period and met criteria for randomization (n=136) for 52 weeks. Approximately one-third of patients had a mixed index episode, one-fifth had psychotic features during the index manic episode, and about half of the patients in each group had a history of rapid cycling.

A significantly greater number of patients in the olanzapine group completed the study (53 versus 13), and fewer patients in the olanzapine group discountinued the study for lack of efficacy (64 versus 78) compared with the placebo group. Time to relapse into a mood episode (based on hospitalization, symptomatic rating scale criteria, or Diagnostic and Statistical Manual IV syndromic criteria) was significantly longer in the olanzapine group than in the placebo group. Significantly fewer patients in the olanzapine group that in the placebo group (46.7% versus 80.1%) had a relapse into a mood episode. Relapse rates were significantly lower in the olanzapine group than in the placebo group for manic episodes (16.4% versus 41.2%) and for depressive episodes (34.7% versus 47.8%).

QUETIAPINE (Q-WIN SR)

In contrast to the olanzapine study, patients in the quetiapine study include both bipolar I (66.9%) and bipolar II (33.1%) depressed patients who were randomly assigned to treatment with quetiapine, 300 mg/day (n=172), quetiapine, 600 mg/day (n=170), or placebo (n=169) for 8 weeks. Patients in the quetiapine group were started on 50 mg/day and titrated upwards so that the target dose was reached by day 4 in the 300-mg group and by day 8 in the 600-mg group. Both quetiapine groups separated from the placebo group on the primary efficacy measure of change in MADRS scores from week 1 to week 8 including endpoint. Response rates were significantly greater for quetiapine groups (56% for 600 mg and 55% for 300 mg) than in the placebo group (31%). The incidence of treatment emergent mania was similar in the three groups (2.4%, 3.5%, and 4.1%, respectively). Treatment-emergent adverse events. Such as dry mouth, sedation, somnolence, and dizziness, were more common in both quetiapine groups than in the placebo group. But no differences in EPS or sexual adverse events were observed among the groups.

CONTINUATION AND MAINTENANCE THERAPY

In contrast to the extensive evidence for the efficacy of atypical antipsychotic agents in treating acute mania, the evidence for their efficacy in the continuation and maintenance treatment of bipolar disorder is limited, with the exception of olanzapine. No consensus exists as to what constitutes continuation or maintenance therapy for bipolar disorder.

PLACEBO-CONTROLLED MONOTHERAPY STUDIES

A 1-year study examined the efficacy of olanzapine, and a 6-month study assessed the efficacy of aripiprazole after an acute manic episode in the continuation/maintenance treatment of bipolar disorder. Quetiapine was examined only for continuation treatment of mania. No placebo-controlled, double-blind studies reported on the efficacy of risperidone, ziprasidone, or clozapine in continuation-/maintenance treatment.

ARIPOPRAZOLE

Patients with acute mania or mixed episode were treated with open-label aripiprazole, 15–30 mg/day, for 6-18 weeks, and those who met criteria for stabilization (i.e. a YMRS score of 10 or lower and a MADRS score of 13 or lower for four consecutive visits or 6 weeks) were randomly assigned to double-blind maintenance treatment with aripiprazole (n=78) or placebo (n83) for 26 weeks. Time to relapse of a mood episode defined as a discontinuation from study because of lack of efficacy, was significantly longer for the aripiprazole group than for the placebo group. Fewer patients in the aripiprazole group (24%) than in the placebo group (43%) had a relapse of a mood episode (P=0.013). A subanalysis showed that the difference between the two groups was significant for manic but not for depressive relapse. No significant differences were noted between the two groups in frequency of adverse events such as EPS, weight gain, or prolactin levels.

OLANZAPINE (OLAN) VERSUS DIVALPROEX SODIUM (DIVALPRID-OD)

Patients with acute mania (n=251) were randomly assigned to olanzapine, 5–20 mg day, or divalproex, 500–2500 mg/day for a 3 week acute phase and a 44-week maintenance phase. Overall, no episode, a manic episode, or a depressive episode were noted between the two groups. Although the median time to remission of mania was significantly shorter in the olanzapine group than in the divalproex group, the rates of remission into mania at 47 weeks using the last observation carried forward method were not significantly different between the two groups. Treatment emergent events such as weight gain, somnolence, dry mouth, increased appetite, and akathisia were more common in the olanzapine group. The incidence of nausea and nervousness was higher in the divalproex group.

DOUBLE-BLIND COMBINATION THERAPY STUDIES

Olanzapine is the only atypical antipsychotic agent that has been examined in combination with a mood stabilizer plus placebo in a double-blind trial. Patients who met criteria for remission within 6 weeks of olanzapine plus lithum or valproate treatment for an acute manic episode were randomly assigned to receive double-blind olanzapine, 5 to 20 mg day (n=46), or placebo (P=0.014). Time to discontinuation was longer in the combination group than in the monotherapy group (111 versus 82 days; P=0.049), but the time to syndromic relapse into a mood episode, manic episode, or a depressive episode was not different between the two groups. Of the patients who were asymptomatic at entry into the relapse prevention phase, the time to symptomatic relapse into a mood episode was significantly longer for those receiving combination therapy than for those treated with monotherapy (median time to relapse: 163 versus 42 days, respectively: P=0.023). There was no significant difference in the incidence of EPS in the two groups.

SUMMARY

Atypical antipsychotic agents have been widely investigated for their efficacy in acute mania. The data to date suggest that olanzapine, risperidone, quetiapine, aripiprazole, and ziprasidone are effective, with no significant differences in antimanic efficacy among these agents. These agents are effective as an alternative to lithium or divalproex as monotherapy or in combination with these mood stabilizers. The date concerning their utility in acute bipolar depression and maintenance treatment of bipolar disorder are limited. The studies to date suggest that olanzapine has modest acute antidepressant properties but probably has efficacy comparable to lithium and divalproex in preventing manic and depressive episodes. Quetiapine seems to have robust antidepressant properties, but these date need to be replicated in further trials before quetiapine can be recommended as a first line agent for acute bipolar depresssion. Aripiprazole has shown promise in preventing manic episodes in one 6-month study, but further studies with at least 1-year duration and larger sample sizes are needed before this agent can be recommended as a monotherapy for prophylaxis of bipolar disorder. It is currently unknown if risperidone, aripiprazole, and ziprasidone have any efficacy in treating acute bipolar disorder. Overall, the atypical antipsychotic agents as a group represent an effective and relatively safe addition to the armamentarium for the treatment of bipolar disorder.

46.15 ATYPICAL MOOD STABILIZERS: ATYPICAL ROLE FOR ATYPICAL ANTIPSYCHOTICS

JN Vyas

Bipolar disorder is a common and disabling illness that exacts an immeasurable toll on individuals, their families and society as a whole. Historically, it has been described as comprising episodes of mania and depression separate by periods of near normality. In recent years this nescient view that bipolar disorder comprises distinct phases with full functional recovery in between has been challenged, with increasing recognition of 'subtypes' such as bipolar I, II and III and the presence of mixed states of depression and mania that are often no-responsive to treatment. The poor detection, diagnosis and management of bipolar depression has often been blamed for the extensive morbidity associated with bipolar disorder. However, current research suggests that poor inter-episode functioning in perhaps more common that previously thought and that it may in fact be 'normal' such that there are not only state but also trait deficits as well.

Given the clinical complexity of bipolar disorder it is no surprise that managemnt is equally sophisticated. The acute phases often encessitate urgent and sometimes involuntary treatment. However, even emergency treatment has to be tempered against the risk if aggravating the illness. Hence, in order to achieve stability without compromising prognosis clinicians have broadened their pharmacologic armamentarium. In this regard the atypical antipsychotics have proven to be exceptionally 'atypical'. In practice, their use has extend beyond the bounds of their conventional ancestors. As a class they have established efficacy in the treatment of psychoses and are now increasingly positioned as 'anti-agitation' and 'anti-bipolar' agents. Beyond acute treatment they are increasingly used in maintenance with the aim of preventing relapse. One reason why this has occurred is that many of the usual treatments have documented efficacy but lack equivalent effectiveness in practice. Atypical antipsychotics both as adjunctive medication and as mono therapy have managed to bridge this gap and are now widely prescribed in patients with bipolar disorder.

MANIA

Atypical antipsychotics are used widely for the treatment of mania, however, the strength of evidence regarding efficacy varies considerably across agents. Several have been shown to be effective in randomized-controlled, clinical trials suggesting that in the treatment of acute mania there may be a 'class effect' for atypical antipsychotics.

OLANZAPINE

The most extensively studied atypical antipsychotic is olanzapine, the efficacy of which in the treatment of acute mania and prevention of manic relapse has been demonstrated by several clinical trials. Three and 4-week randomized placebo-controlled trials with more than 5 manic (or mixed) patients in each limb have been conducted using a double-blind, parallel group study design. In these two studies and drop of 50% or more in the total Young Mania Rating Scale (YMRS) score was reported for 48.5% and 64.8% of patients treated with olanzapine but only 24.2% and 42.9% of patients treated with placebo in the first and second study respectively. Furthermore post hoc analyses of pooled data showed that olanzapine was effective in the treatment of acute mania irrespective of patient characteristics, psychosis, and mixed or pure status.

A much larger 12-week, randomized double-blind, parallel group study, compared patients with bipolar mania on haloperidol (n = 234). Both were equally effective in achieving remission, however, patients became more rapidly depressed in the haloperido-treated group whereas olanzapine resulted in a significantly greater improvement in quality of his indices.

When compared with conventional mood stabilizers in the treatment of acute mania olanzapine has been shown to be as effective is lithium in a 4-week randomized, double-blind trial (olanzapine n = 15; lithium n = 15; and somewhat better than divalproex in a 3-week, randomized, double-blind study (olanzapine n = 125; divalproex n = 123). Adjunctively, olanzapine has been shown to be superior to monotherapy in a 6-week, double-blind trial in which patients with acute mania non-responsive to adequate lithium or valproate monotherapy were randomized to adjunctive olanzapine (n = 229) or placebo (n = 115). Hence clinically, olanzapine is used widely both as an adjunct or on its own in the treatment of acute maniaand perhaps even more so now that it can be administered intramuscularly.

ARIPIPRAZOLE

Three double-blind, placebo-controlled trials, each of 3 weeks duration, have assessed the efficacy of aripiprazole in the treatment of acute mania or mixed bipolar episodes. Keck et al. included 130 and 132 patients in the aripiprazole and placebo groups respectively, while the other studies comprised 137 patients on aripiprazole and 135 patients on placebo. All three studies used a > 50% reduction in YMRS score from baseline as a response rate endpoint, and all three found significantly greater reduction these scores from day 4 onwards in the aripiprazole-treated group.

In a longer 3-month comparator trial, acutely manic bipolar patients were randomized to treatment with haloperidol (n = 172) or aripiprazole (n = 175; 22). Less than a third of the patients (29.1%) on haloperidol and just over half the patients (50.9%) on aripiprazole responded to treatment and completed the 12-week trial. However, the apparent superiority of aripiprazole relative to haloperidol may largely be a function of tolerability as opposed to efficacy.

QUETIAPINE

Two 12-week, multicenter, double-blind clinical trials referred to as STAMP 1 and STAMP 2 of quetiapine monotherapy for the treatment of acute mania in bipolar I patients have been conducted. Pooled data from these two very similar trials that compared quetiapine (n = 209), lithium (n = 98), haloperidol (n = 99), and placebo (n = 198 showed that quetiapine was superior to placebo and equivalent to haloperidol or lithium as measured by reduction in YMRS scores. Furthermore, quetiapine has been shown to be effective as an adjunct to mood stabilizers lithium and divalproex in a 3-week, double-blind, parallel group study of manic bipolar patients randomized to placebo (n = 100) or quetiapine (n = 91) with significantly greater reduction YMRS scores for patients treated with quetiapine (–13.76) than for placebo (-9.93). This has been further corroborated in a recent 3-week, double-blind adjunctive study of manic patients randomized to placebo (n = 203) or quetiapine (n = 196). In this larger study a significant difference in YMRS scores, favoring quetiapine emerged at the end of the first week of treatment.

ZIPRASIDONE

In a double-blind placebo-controlled study of manic or mixed episode bipolar patients the reduction in MRS scores was greater in the ziprasidone mono-therapy group (n = 140) when compared with the smaller placebo group (n = 140) when compared with the smaller placebo group (n = 70) at the end of the 3-week trial. However, the difference between the groups was apparent from day 2 and at the end of the trial the reductions in scores were –7.8 and –12.4 for the placebo and ziprasidone groups, respectively. In an adjunctive trial of similar duration (3 weeks) lithium-treated manic bipolar patients were randomized to additional placebo (n = 103) or ziprasidone (n = 102). Significant improvement in the latter group on day 4 in the trial suggested faster onset of action with ziprasidone adjunctive therapy than with lithium alone, however, outcomes between the two groups were not significantly different at the end of the study.

RISPERIDONE

Risperidone monotheray has been shown to be effective for the treatment of mania in two double-blind trials. In the first study 125 patients were randomized to risperidone and 1345 to placebo and 56 and 42% of patients in each group completed the trial. Statistically significant differences in YMRS scores were achieved on day 3 and maintained to the 3-week endpoint. In the second study with slightly larger numbers of patients (146 and 144 in the risperidone and placebo groups respectively) an even greater improvement as measured by YMRS scores was noted, with a reduction of –23.2 = 13.5 for the risperidone group and –10.8 ± 13.5 for the placebo group.

When compared with lithium (n=15) and haloperidol (n=15) was shown to have equivalent efficacy. This is in keeping with findings from open-labeled studies that report its monotherapeutic efficacy in the treatment of mania. However, adverse events such as extrapyramedial side-effects suggest that the dosage in bipolar disorder may need to be lower than that used in schizophrenia.

Open-labeled combination studies of risperidone and mood stabilizers suggest that risperidone is effective in the treatment of mania, as do adjunctive trials. Indeed, two such double-blind studies of risperidone adjunctive treatement have been conducted over a period of 3 weeks for the treatment of acute mania. Yatham et al. randomized manic or mixed episode bipolr patients on lithium, divalproex or carbamazepine to risperidone (n = 75) or placebo (n = 75) and at the endpoint YMRS scores were reduced by 14.5- and 10.3-points in the antipsychotic and placebo groups, respectively. However, these reductions were not statistically significant. In the study by Sachs et al manic or mixed episode patients being treated with lithium or divalproex were randomized to adjunctive therapy with risperidone (n = 52), haloperidol (n = 53) or placebo (n = 51). Compared with the placebo-treated group the reductions in YMRS scores were significantly greater in the haloperidol- and risperidone-treated groups.

Clozapine, Surprisingly, there have been no documented double-blind clinical trials of clozapine in the treatment of bipolar disorder. One open-labeled 3-week trial of acutely manic bipolar patients that were randomized to clozapine (n = 15) and chlorpromazine (n = 12) as adjunctive treatment of lithium showed significant reductions in YMRS scores in the clozapine-treated patients when compared with the chlorpromazine-treated patients. However, this difference was only apparent at the 2-week time-point and disappeared at the 3-week time-point, suggesting perhaps a difference in speed of response rather than overall efficacy. However, a retrospective study involving 117 patients with acute mania that showed significant improvement in Clinical Global Impression scores (6.0 ± 1.0 to 4.3 ± 1.2, mean ± SD), and Global Assessment Functioning (GAF scores 37.8 ± 12.6 to 68.9 ± 14.7, mean ± SD), suggests that clozapine does have efficacy in this patient population.

AMISULPRIDE

There is no published data to date with respect to the use of amisulpride in the treatment of acute mania, however, a 3-month, multicenter, open-labeled trial, combining either valproate and amisulpride, or valproate and haloperidol, is in progress and the results of this study should be known in 2005.

Acute manic patients often present in an agitated state resulting sometimes in violent and aggressive behavior. Clinically many of the atypical antipsychotics are routinely used for the treatment of acute agitation and aggression, in particular olanzapine and ziprasidone that can be administered intramuscularly, however, there are few studies systematically examining the use of these agents in this context with the majority of data coming from studies in patients with schizophrenia.

In a double-blind placebo-controlled study comparing an atypical antipsychotic and a benzodiazepine, bipolar patients were randomized to intramuscular placebo (n = 51), olanzapine (n = 99) or lorazepam (n = 51) and assessed for a period of 24 h. Olanzapine was overall equivalent to lorazepam and superior to placebo. Similarly, in two randomized, fixed-dose, double-blind 24-h studies intramuscular ziprasidone has been shown to be effective for the control of psychotic-agitated patients with bipolar subtype schizoaffective disorder.

Summary

There is good double-blind placebo-controlled evidence to support the use of olanazapine, aripiprazole, quetiapine, risperidone, and ziprasidone in the treatment of acute mania. These agents are effective both as monotherapy and as adjuncts to mood stabilizers; however. The evidence for the use of clozapine and amisulpride is much less robust. To date, only open-labeled evidence exists with respect to clozapine and the use of amisulpride awaits further studies. Similarly, although in practive, atypical antipsychotics are widely used for the management of acute behavioral disturbance in patients with bipolar disorder the evidence supporting such use is minimal and the issue merits further research.

BIPOLAR DEPRESSION

Bipolar depression is the predominant mood state of patients with bipolar disorder and the phase of the illness that is associated with the greatest morbidity and risk of suicide.

Olanzapine

Akin to its use in acute mania, olanzapine has been trailed both as monotherapy and in combination, for the treatment of bipolar I disorder with a Montogomery-Asberg Depression Rating Scale (MADRS) score of 20 or more were randomized to olanzapine (n = 370), olanzapine/fluoxetine combination (n = 86) or placebo (n = 377). With respect to MADRS scores, both arms containing olanzapine were superior to placebo from weeks 1 to 8 with the olanzapine/fluxetime combination showing further superiority when compared with olanzapine alone from weeks 4 to 8. From baseline to endpoint a ≥50% improvement in MADRS score, was achieved by 56.1% of patients treated with the olanzapine/fluoxetine combination, 39.0% of patients treated with olanzapine alone and 30.4% of patient streated with placebo. A similar trend was observed with respect to overall remission trend was observed with respect to overall remission and time to response and time to remission with the olanzapine/fluoxitine combination bettering olanzapine alone, which in turn was better than placebo. Interestingly, treatment emergent mania did not significantly differ across the groups suggesting an independent antidepressant effect.

Quetiapine

The potential antidepressant use of quetiapine in the management of bipolar depression was noted in a 4-month, multicentered, open-labeled trial, in which patients with bipolar I disorder, among other diagnoses, were randomized to quetiapine (n = 554) or risperidone (n = 175) in combination to usual therapy. Positive results have also been posted in a small preliminary 8-week, open-label trial of adjunctive quetiapine therapy, in bipolar depressed patients with five of eight patients completing the trial and demonstrating reductions in 21-item Hamilton Depression Rating Scale (HAMD-21) scores. However, definitive data has emerged with the completion of the first double-blind trial of quetiapine in depressed bipolar I (n=358) or bipolar II (n=181). Patients treated with quetiapine, at either dose, demonstrated significantly greater improvement as measured by MADRS and HAMD scores from the very first week through to the study endpoint 8 weeks later. Overall MADRS scores improved by –16.7, –16.4 and –10.2 for the 300 mg/day and 600 mg day quetiapine groups and placebo, respectively. It is of interest to note that the effect size of the 600 mg daily dose of quetiapine was 0.75, compared with 0.31 for the olanzapine depression trial described above.

Risperidone

An antidepressant effect for risperidone is suggested by case series and one preliminary study. In the latter, an open-label trial conducted in 44 depressed bipolar II patients, risperidone was added to usual treatment and HAMD scores improved from the first week of the study, implicating risperidone in the prevention of depressive relapse recurrence in bipolar disorder.

Summary

The evidence of antidepressant efficacy for atypical antipsychotics in bipolar depression is for less substantive than that for the treatment for acute mania and a class effect cannot be argued. However, clinically in the treatment of both bipolar and major depression many of the atypical antipsychitics are routinely used to small doses in combination with antidepres-sants to augment their actions and sometimes exert an independent antidepressant effect. Clearly further research is necessary but it seems likely that some of the atypical antipsychotics will likely possess antidepressant properties.

TREATMENT RESISTANCE

Numerous clinical studies have demonstrated the efficacy of atypical antipsychotics in the treatment of manic mixed states and subgroup analyses suggest their utility in the prevention of manic relapse. However, randomized-controlled trials addressing specific cohorts of patients with mixed mania or depressive mixed states have yet to be conducted.

The same applies to rapid cycling, a well described phenomenon that has thus for been investigated little with respect to the role of atypical antipsychotics, even though clinically these agents are used widely in patients with this pattern of illness. Data from open-labeled studies or subanalyses of rapid-cycling patients in treatment studies, suggest that atypical antipsychotics, in particular quetiapine and olanzapine, may have a therapeutic role.

A major problem in managing patients with mixed states or rapid cycling mood episodes is that they often fail to respond to treatment. Indeed partial or complete non-response to mood stabilizers is a common and perplexing problem that eventually occurs in approximately a third of patients with bipolar disorder. This usually necessitates the use of adjunctive medications and in this context open-labeled, naturalistic and retrospective chart review studies suggest that atypical antipsychotics such as clozapine, risperidone, olanzapine, and quetiapine may have a therapeutic role. However, the benefit of such polypharmacy in terms of overall functional outcome is questionable.

MAINTENANCE

The efficacy of olanzapine as monotherapy and as adjunctive therapy with conventional mood stabilizers in the maintenance phase of bipolar disorder has been demonstrated in a number of longitudinal studies. In a long-term study, which compared olanzapine (n=125) with divalproex (n = 126) in the treatment of manic patients (YMRS score of ≥20), olanzapine was more effective with respect to symptomatic remission, however, there was no statistical difference between the two groups with respect to the time to symptomatic or syndromal recurrence of may affective episode. At the end of the 47-week study almost a quarter (23.6%) of olanzapine and a fifth (17.9%) of divalproex-treated patients had gained 7% of more of their baseline weight. In another randomized double-blind comparison study patients with bipolar I disorder were treated with either olanzapine (n = 217) or lithium (n = 214) over a period of 12 months. The study reported that the two agents were equally effective in preventing depression but that olanzapine was superior to lithium in preventing mania. Therefore not surprisingly, olanzapine (n = 225) has also been shown to be superior to placebo (n = 136) in preventing relapse into both mania (16.4% vs. 41.2%) and depression (34.7% vs. 47.8%) in another 12-month, double-blind randomized study in patients with bipolar I disorder. Similar data favoring mood stabilizer (lithium or valproate) combination with olanzapine (n = 51) over placebo (n = 48) has been found in an adjunctive study in which the median time to manic or depressive relapse was 163 days as opposed to 42 days.

In a double-blind relapse prevention trial, euthymic bipolar I patients were randomized to aripiprazole (n = 78) or placebo (n = 83) for 26 weeks. Manic relapse was significantly lower for aripiprazole- (5%) than for placebo-treated (19%) patients, and the difference for depressive relapse (aripiprazole 9%, placebo 11%) was not significant.

Adverse Effects of Atypical Antipsychotics

When first introduced the atypical antipsychotics were lauded for their lack of extrapyramidal side-effects and clearly in the management of chronic illnesses such as schizophrenia and bipolar disorder this is an important advance. However, apart from common and usually transient side-effects such as dry mouth and dizziness it has become increasingly apparent that individual agents are associated with a number of more serious adverse effects.

Olanzapine

Weight gain is evident from as early as 3 weeks of treatment with olanzapine and is a major safety concern, especially with long-term use. Amongst the atypical antipsychotics, the average weight gained is second only to clozapine ranging form approximately 3 kg over 3 weeks to 6 kg over 6 months. Olanzapine also increases the risk of hyperlipidemia, which is an independent risk factor for heart disease and is linked to type 2 diabetes mellitus. Despite this, patients comply with olanzapine more to than placebo and discontinuation because of adverse events is not significantly different to that with risperidone or valproate.

Risperidone

Risperidone, like other atypical antipsychotics, is associated with significant weight gain, but to a much lesser extent than olanzapine or clozapine. However, it is not associated with hyperlipidemia or dibetes and is the only atypical antipsychotic associated with a significant risk of sustained hyperprolactinemia and extrapyramidal side-effects.

Quetiapine

Quetiapine-associated weight gain equivalent to that seen with risperidone and like risperidone there is no significant association with type 2 diabetes or hypertriglyceridemia. However, unlike risperidone quetiapine is not associated with hyperprolactinemia or extrapyramidal side-effects.

Ziprasidone

It is not associated with weight gain and extrapyramidal, side-effects are no greater that those with placebo (S6). However significant safety concern is QTc interval prolongation and the potential risk of torsades be point. In practice, these conduction abnormalities are unlikely to be of significance except in patients with electrolyte abnormalities, alcoholism and pre-existing cardiac disease where additional caution a advisable.

Aripiprazole

Aripiprazole is a relatively new agent and thus far appear to be on path with placebo in terms of weight gain and extrapyramidal side effects. It also has no association with QTs proplogation or hyperprolactinemia but can cause prolonged somnolence.

Clozapine

Clozapine has the greate propensity toward weight gain and like olanzapine increases the risks of type 2 diabetes and hyperglyceridemia. It is the most pronematical of the atypical antipsychotics as it is also associated with a significant risk of agranulocytosis, of approximately 1% and causes a similar rate of seizures when titrated rapidly or administered in hugh doses. However, it incurs the lowes risk of extrapyramidal side effects and is thus reasonably vetolerated.

CONCLUSION

The atypical antipsychotics do appear to have a potential role in the treatment of bipolar disorder, especially its acute phases, and in particular mania. It would be erroneous to assume that this would extend to other phases of the illness or that atypical antipsychotics could be used long-term without concern. Clearly, these issues need to be explored further, however, it is likely that some of the atypical antipsychotics will prove to be effective in both depression and mania and may also have a role in maintenance therapy. Use of the term 'mood-stabilizer' to describe atypical antipsychotics is somewhat premature however, the evidence thus far, and that on the horizon, suggests that in the content of bipolar disorder pharmacotherapy, the long-term use of atypical antipsychotics may not remain 'atypical' for long.

46.16 VAGUS NERVE STIMULATION AND DEEP BRAIN STIMULATION

RK Solanki, JN Vyas

The authors are supported in part by research grants from the National Alliance for Research on Schizophenia and Depression and the Stanley Foundation, by a National Institute of Neurological Disorder and Stroke grant (R01-AG40956), by a National Institute of Mental Health grant (ZN), and by a grant from the Defence Advanced Research Projects Agency. The Brain Stimulation Laboratory also has received grant support from Cyberonics (vagus nerve stimulation (VNS) and Neotonus (transcranial magnetic stimulation) for clinical trials. Non of the authors has equity or financial conflicts. Drs George and Bohning hold a patent for interleaving transcranial magnetic stimulation with functional magnetic stimulation with functional magnetic resonance imaging (fMRI) as a neuroscience tool and an invention disclosure (with Drs Bohning and Nahas) to use fMRI to determine the optimum treatment settings for VNS. The authors would research advances with Burke Barrett, formerly of Cyberonics, and Dr Jake Zabara.

VAGUS NERVE STIMULATION

Two somatic treatment the brain routinely used as therapies in neurology offer promise as antidepressant treatments-in neurology offer promise as antidepressant treatments-vagus nerve stimulation (VNS) and deep brain stimulation (DBS). Recent studies in epilepsy patients, as well as those in primary depressed patients, suggest that VNS has significant antidepressant effects. In this chapter, we describe the VNS method, the clinical studies to date in depression, and potential antidepressant mechanisms of action interpreted in light of current theories concerning the antidepressant mechanisms of medications and electroconvulsive therapy

(ECT). Stimulation of cranial nerves can alter brain function. In fact, throughout the past century, researchers have investigated how stimulation of the cranial nerves, especially the vagus nerve, produces observable brain effects.

The vagus nerve is actually nerve is actually a cable of nerve fibers that regulates the body's autonomic functions, which are important in a variety of emotional tasks. Most students are familiar with the vagus nerve's efferent functions, when it serves as the messenger for signals from the brain to the viscera. Tradionally, the vagus nerve has been considered a parasympathetic efferent nerve (controlling and regulating autonomic functions such as heart rate and gastric tone). The afferent role of the vagus (fibers carrying signals originating in the periphery to the brain) has been underemphasized in the traditional literature. The vagus is actually a mixed nerve composed of about 80% afferent sensory fibers carrying information to the brain from the head, heck, thorax, and abdomen (Foley and DuBois 1937).

Researchers have convincingly documented extensive projections of the vagus nerve via its sensory afferent connections in the nucleus tractus solitarius to diverse brain regions (MacLean 1990). For example, as early as 1938, Bailey and Bremer found that VNS in the cat elicited synchronized electroencephalogram (EEG) activity in the orbital cortex. In 1949, MacLean and Pribram stimulated the vagus nerve and recorded EEG activity from the cortical surface of anesthetized monkeys. They found that VNS caused inconsistent slow waves to the generated from the lateral frontal cortex (Maclean 1990). Shortly after that, Dell and Olson (1951) studied the effects of VNS in awake cats with high cervical spinal lesions. They found that VNS evoked a slow-wave response in the anterior rhinal sulcus, as well as in the amygdala.

Reasoning from this body of literature, as well as evidence that deep breathing (e.g. Lamaze or yoga) can calm the brain (Sovik 2000), presumably through activation of vagus afferents, Zabara (1985a, 1985b, 1992) reported an anticonvulsant action of VNS on experimental seizures in dogs. Zabara hypothesized that VNS could prevent or control the motor and autonomic components of epilepsy. Penry and others then ushered in the modern clinical application of VNS in 1988 by using an implanted device to treat epilepsy in human patients (Penry and Dean 1990).

Although the route of entry into the brain is constrained, VNS offers the potential for modulating and modifying function in several important brain regions through transsynaptic connections. (For a detailed discussion of vagus circuitry, see George et al. 2000; Henry 2002; Ter Horst and Streetland 1994.) These brainstem and limbic anatomical connections can be shown in nonhuman animals and, with functional neuroimaging, in humans.

The oncogene c-fos is a general marker for cellular activity. In rats, c-fos studies showed increased activity in the amygdala, cingulated, locus coeruleus, and hypothalamus while the vagus was being stimulated (Naritoku et al, 1995). Furthermore, the signal into the brain from VNS can be amplified or reduced by modifying the activity in several of these key relay nuclei.

In an important study that established the potential for combining VNS with general or local pharmacology, Walker and colleagues (1999) outlined a possible role of the nucleus tractus solitatius in how VNS reduces seizures. By micro-injecting the nucleus tractus solitarius with either γ-aminobutyric acid (GABA) agonists or glutamate antagonists while seizing animals also were receiving VNS, they found that increased GABA or decreased glutamate in the nucleus tractus solitarius blocked seizures. Indirectly, these findings suggest that VNS may change nucleus tractus solitarius GABA and glutamate concentrations, with secondary changes in the function of specific limbic structures noted earlier (e.g. amygdala, cingulated, insula, and hippocampus).

In summary, incoming sensory (afferent) connections of the vagus nerve provide direct projections to many of the brain regions implicated in neuropsychiatric disorders. These connections provide a basis for understanding how VNS might be a portal to the brain stem and connected limbic and cortical regions. These pathways likely account for the neuropsychiatric effects of VNS, and they invite additional theoretical considerations for potential research and clinical applications. Functional imaging studies in humans have largely confirmed this important neuroanatomy of the vagus (Henry 2002; Henry et al. 1998, 1999).

Methods

The broad term vagus nerve stimulation generally refers to several different techniques used to stimulate the vagus nerve, including studies in animals in which the vagus was accessed through the abdomen and diaphragm. However, for virtually all him a studies, VNS refers to stimulation of the left cervical vagus nerve with a commercial device: the VNS Therapy System (Cyberonics, Houston, TX)(An important exception to this rule was the recent work that used a modified VNS Therapy System to stimulate both subdiaphragmatic vagus nerves for the treatment of obesity [Roslin and kurian 2001])

VNS has been commercially available for the treatment of resistant partial-onset seizures in Europe since 1994 and in the United States since 1997. More than 22,000 people with epilepsy worldwide have been treated with the VNS Therapy System. Typically, although not always, epilepsy patients considering VNS have had unsatisfactory seizure control despite treatment with multiple medications. In many ways, VNS resembles implanting a cardiac pacemaker. With VNS, the electrical stimulation is delivered through a pulse generator-an implantable, multiprogrammable, bipolar pulse generator (about the size of a pocket watch)—that is implanted in the left chest wall to deliver electrical signals to the left vagus nerve through a bipolar lead. Thus, VNS resembles in some ways DBS (Limousin et al. 1995, 1998), with the main differences being the location of the end wire (left cervical vagus nerve with VNS, deep brain nuclei with DBS); the need for breaching the skull, with consequent risks in DBS but not VNS; and the nature of the electrical pulse (intermittent and relatively low frequency stimulation [<100 Hz] with DBS). In VNS, the electrode is wrapped around the vagus nerve in the neck and is connected to the generator subcutaneously. The VNS implantation surgery is typically an outpatient procedure most commonly, but not exclusively, performed neurosurgeons.

A personal computer or handheld personal digital assistant (PDA) and an infrared wand control the VNS Therapy System is designed to shut off in the presence of a constant magnetic field. Each patient is given a small handheld magnet that, when held over the pulse generator, turns off stimulation. When the magnet is removed, normal programmed stimulation resumes. This allows patients to control and temporarily eliminate stimulation-related side effects during key behaviors such as public speaking (voice tremor) and heavy exercising (mild shortness of breath).

USE IN EPILEPSY

VNS has been most extensively studied as a treatment for epilepsy. Two double-blind studies (Ben-Menachem et al. 1994) have been conducted in patients with epilepsy, with a total of 313 treatment-resistent completers. In this difficult-to-treat group, the average decline acutely in seizure frequency was about 25–30% compared with baseline.

VNS, as now delivered, generally has not been shown to be a substitute for anticonvulsant medications. In some patients, the dosage levels or numbers of antiepileptic medications have been decreased with the addition of VNS. VNS is increasingly being used in children with epilepsy, in part because VNS does not have negative cognitive effects, which are common with other anticonvulsants (Heck et al. 2002; Helmers et al. 2001).

In patients with epilepsy, the long-term efficacy of VNS is either maintained or improved, while the frequency of adverse events generally decreases as patients accommodate to stimulation (Salinsky et al. 1996), Data from uncontrolled observation suggest that, contrary to a tolerance effect, improvement in seizure control is maintained or may increase over time to the anticonvulsant actions of VNS. The patient with the longest exposure to VNS has had the system operating for 13 years.

Several different programmable variables are involved in developing how to deliver VNS. (These are also an an issue with other forms of electrical brain stimulation-DBS and transcranial magnetic stimulation [TMS]). These "use parameters" include the pulse width of the electrical signal (130, 250, 500, 750, 1000 μs), the stimulation intensity (0.25–4.00 mA is clinically tolerated), the frequency of stimulation (1–145 Hz), the length or duration of uninterrupted stimulation (7–70 seconds), and the length of time between trains of stimuli (0.2 second to 180 minutes). I general, the initial epilepsy use parameter settings were derived from the animal studies in which acute anticonvulsant effects were found. The initial epilepsy studies compared efficacy in two groups, on the basis of different use parameters: a high-stimulation group (500-μs pulse width, 30 Hz, 30 seconds on, 5 minutes off) and a low-stimulation group (130-μs pulse width, 1 Hz, 30 seconds on, 90–180 minutes off). Most of the VNS epilepsy efficacy and safety data come from trials with use parameters similar to those used in the high-stimulation group in the initial epilepsy studies. Similarly, most of the data concerning VNS effects to other neuropsychiatric disorders (depression, anxiety) involve VNS at use parameters similar to those used in the high-stimulation group in the initial epilepsy studies. These use parameters are not likely the maximally effective choices for different diseases or even individuals. It is also unlikely that the same parameters work equally well in all conditions. Epilepsy physicians commonly switch nonresponding patients to use parameters different from their current settings. However, there has been no clear proof that changing settings improves efficacy. Further work to understand the translational neurobiology of these use parameter choices, and how they relate on clinical symptoms, is an important area for future growth of the field.

EFFECTS IN DEPRESSION

The increasing literature in psychiatry indicates that anticonvulsants medications (e.g. carbamazepine) or devices (e.g. ECT) have mood-stabilizing or antidepressant effects. In early 1998, several lines of evidence suggested that VNS might have antidepressant effects. (For a full discussion of this reasoning, see George et al. 2000.) In the initial decision to perform a clinical trial of VNS in depression, the knowledge of vagus connections in the brainstem, particularly the role of the locus coeruleus, was crucial. Additional supporting information came from 1) mood effects on VNS observed in patients with epilepsy (Elger et al. 2000), 2) evidence from positron emission tomographic (PET) imaging that VNS affects the function of important limbic structures, 3) the long history of anticonvulsant medications being useful in treating mood disorders (Ballenger and Post 1978), and 4) neurochemical studies in both animals and humans that reported that VNS alters concentrations of monoamines within the central nervous system (transmission of serotonin, norepinephrine [Krah] et al 1998, 2000, 2001], GABA, and glutamate) (Walker et al. 1999). The initial openlable VNS depression study involved four sites (Medical University of South Carolina, Charleston; Columbia-New York States Psychiatric Institute, New York; University of Texas Southwestern Medical Center-Dallas; Baylor-Houseton) and initially involved 30 subjects to clarify the effectisize and look for response predictors (Sackeim et al, 2001b). The study design involved selecting patients with treatment-resistant, chronic, or recurrent major depressive episode (MDE) (unipolar or non-rapid-cycling bipolar) and then adding no antidepressant medications. No stimulation was given for the first 2 weeks following implantation, creating a single-blind placebo phase and allowing for surgical recovery. All patients met eligibility criteria by failing at least two adequate treatment trials in the current MDE according to the Anti-depressant Treatment History Form (Prudic et al. 1996; Sackeim et al. 1990).

Of the 59 subjects who completed the study (1 patient improved during the recovery period before the device was turned on permanently and was not included), the response rates after 3 months of treatment were 30.5% for the primary 28-item Hamilton Rating Scale for Depression measure, 34.0% for the Montgomery-Asberg Rating Scale for Depression, and 37.3% for the Clinical Global Impression-Improvement Scale score (1 or 2). Interestingly and perhaps importantly, 2 patients developed hypomania. VNS was well tolerated in this group; side effects were similar to those encountered by epilepsy patients. The most common side effect was voice alteration or hoarseness, 60.0% (36/60), which was generally mild and related to the intensity of the output current. No adverse cognitive effects occurred (Sackeim et al. 2001a), sures after 8 weeks of therapy, likely because because their depression had lifted. Prior antidepressant treatment resistance correlated with a poor VNS response. For example, non of the 13 patients who had not responded adequately to more than seven research-defined adequate antidepressant trials in the current episode responded to VNS, whereas 39% of the remaining 46 patients did respond (P=0.0057).

This cohort has now been followed up regularly for more than 2 years. Changes in psychotropic medications and in VNS stimulus parameters were allowed during this long-term follow-up. Results seen at the end of the 10-week acute phase largely appear to have continued and even improved over 9 months of long-term maintenance VNS treatment (Marangell et al. 2002). According to the last observation carried forward, response rates were 30.5% (18/59) after 3 months, 42.4% (25/59) after 1 year, and 42.4% (25/59) after 2 years of VNS. Remission rates were 15.3% (9/59) at 3 months, 27.1% (16/59) at 1 year, and 22.0% (13/59) at 2 years. By 2 years, two deaths, unrelated to VNS, had occurred, and four patients had withdrawn for other reasons. At 24 months, 48/59 (81.4%) were still receiving active VNS therapy. These naturalistic open results suggest, but do not prve, that long-term beneficial effects are associated with VNS therapy for patients with chronic or recurrent treatment-resistant depression. Longer-term VNS therapy was generally well tolerated (Nahas et al., in press).

These encouraging initial open-label results led to market approval for VNS in the treatment of chronic or recurrent depression in Canada and served as the basis for a recent United multisite double-blind trial of VNS for chronic or recurrent, low to moderate treatment-resistent depression. In this trial, VNS failed to show a statistically significant difference in acute response from the sham group. The sham response was 10%, and the active response was 15% (-Rush et al., in press). There are several possible explanations for the differences between the 30% response rate in the double-blind study. Some placebo response was likely in the open study and the 15% active acute response was likely in the open study, likely because of the complex nature of the double-blind trial. However, a VNS antidepressant dose-response relation was not evident, although this does exist for epilepsy and was the basis for the initial double-blind epilepsy trials. Finally, an attempt at screening out highly treatment resistant individuals was no fully successful.

As in the initial open study, at the end of the acute phase, subjects continued to receive VNS therapy, the response rate in this cohort approached that seen in the open study (35%). The long-term outcome of a highly treatment-resistant group like this is unknown. To assess whether the presence of the VNS therapy influenced the long-term course, these D-02 data were compared with those of a control group with similar entry criteria that simply received treatment as usual (George et al., in press). The 205 depressed subjects who received VNS (D-02) were compared with 124 subjects who received treatment as usual (D-04) over the course of 1 year. The two groups had similar baseline demographic, psychiatric, and mood disorder treatment histories. VNS (D-02) subjects had a statistically significant greater improvement per month when compared with treatment-as-usual (D-04) subjects across 12 months of therapy (P=0.001), by repeated-measures linear regression on the Inventory of Depressive Symptomatology-Self-Rated (Rush et al. 1986). These results suggest that, when compared in a nonrandomized fashion with usual standard of care (D-04) for 1 year, VNS therapy (D-02) provides a statistically significant benefit for depression symptoms in a chronic or recurrent treatment-resistent depression population. The company is continuing to gather long-term data on these subjects and is organizing further studies. These results have been presented to the U.S. Food and Drug Administration (FDA) for potential approval of VNS as a therapy for treatment-resistant depression. Thus, no double-blind, prospective, randomized, controlled evidence exists for VNS as an antidepressant in patients with primary depression. However, open (Harden et al. 2000) and double-blind (Elger et al. 2000) studies showed that VNS has antidepressant effects in epilepsy patients with comorbid depression.

ACUTE CHANGES IN PAIN

Perception in Depressed Patients

Previous research suggested that VNS affects pain perception in epilepsy patients, with acute VNS decreasing pain thresholds (pronociceptive) (Ness et al. 2000) and chronic treatment increasing pain thresholds (antinociceptive)

(Kirchner et al. 2000). These studies did not address whether different VNS device parameter settings had varying effects on pain perception. Divergent studies, as discussed in more detail later, suggested that different device parameters are associated with unique fiber activation and different regional brain activation. Borckardt and colleagues at the Medical University of South Carolina thus examined the effects of different VNS device parameters on pain perception in depressed adults with a thermal pain paradigm (Borckardt et al. 2005). Pronociceptive effects (pain enhancing) were found for VNS output current, frequency, and interaction of current and frequency. The effects of VNS on pain perception were most pronounced during the first 3 seconds of the thermal pain procedures. Subjects' levels of depression did not predict VNS-induced changes in pain threshold. However, large individual differences were seen with the 4 specific device settings associated with the largest changes in pain threshold. Further work with VNS as a potential treatment for chronic pain appears warranted.

Clinical Summary and Conclusion

Although VNS is highly promising as a potential long-term treatment for recurrent mood disorders, no propective, randomized, double-blind data currently exist for use of VNS to treat primary depression. The double-blind data showing efficacy in treating depression within the context of epilepsy, and the long-term positive open results in treatment-resistant primary depression, suggest that VNS is an area with future promise. More research is needed.

Mechanisms of Action

What are the potential mechanisms by which VNS relieves symptoms of depression? A lack of consensus exists about the underlying pathophysiology of the depressions, and many different mechanisms of action are proposed for the currently effective and approved antidepressant treatments. Any potential VNS antidepressant mechanism of action must account for the known route of entry of VNS into the brain and also must be able to explain the relatively slow onset of antidepressant action of VNS, with continued improvement over long time frames such as 1 year. What might be happening at a neurobiological level, starting at the vagus nerve and entering the brain, over slow periods in the depressed patients who respond to VNS?

Neurotransmitters and Cerebrospinal Fluid

Both clinical and animal studies indicate that VNS likely results in changes in serotonin, norepinephrine, GABA, and glutamate, which are all neurotransmitters implicated in the pathogenesis of major depression. VNS in animals activates the locus coeruleus, the main source of central nervous system (CNS) norepinephrine-containing neuronal cell bodies (Krahl et al. 1998, 2000). In patients with epilepsy, VNS appears to increase 5-hydroxyindoleacetic acid-a metabolite of serotonin. Because many of the currently available thearapies are believed to work through changes in the same neurotransmitters (serotonin or norepineprine), VNS might be acting through mechanisms similar to antidepressant medications. It was thus surprising that a recent study of effects of VNS on cerebrospinal fluid (CSF) changes in depressed patients over time failed to confirm the finding of serotonin metabolite (Carpenter et al. 2004). The two studies differed in their study subjects (epilepsy and depression), VNS use parameters, and concomitant medications, which might explain the discrepancy. Further studies are needed, but enough data have accumulated to date to conclude that VNS acts on norepinephrine and serotonin systems and that this may be an important mechanism in explaining VNS antidepressant actions.

ANTIDEPRESSANT EFFECTS SECONDARY

To Anticonvulsant Action

A popular theory about ECT is that it invokes natural anticonvulsant cascades that then reregulate a system and improve depression. Several other anticonvulsant medications, including carbamazepine and lamotrigine, also have antidepressant effects, and the anticonvulsant effects of VNS are well established. VNS may improve depression by manipulating anticonvulsant systems in the brain. Recent work by Dean and colleagues (2002) in epilepsy patients with VNS implanted for 6–12 months showed the powerful and persistent anticonvulsant effects of VNS. These researchers used TMS to study the effects of acute VNS on motor threshold and the cortical silent period following a TMS pulse. Motor threshold and cortical silent period are TMS measures of cortical excitability. The most interesting finding was that in epilepsy patients who had been receiving VNS for more than 6 months, a significant decrease in motor cortex excitability occurred while VNS was on, compared with 30 minutes after VNS was turned effects. Further work is needed to understand the mechanisms by which VNS stops seizures and whether these are the same or similar mechanisms as those working to improve mood in depression.

Changing Regional Functional Anatomy

Structural and functional imaging studies over the past 20 years in emotion regulation and depression have drawn attention to a "functional neuroanatomy of depression." One of the current main concepts is that clinical depression arises through an imbalance in prefrontal-limbic circuits. Several imaging studies over the past 10 years have examined antidepressant treatments and how they cause changes in these circuits. Through the know projections of the vagus nerve, VNS could theoretically cause changes in these limbic and orbitofrontal regions. Functional imaging studies with VNS have now shown that VNS, repeatedly and over time, causes changes in these key brain regions (Bohning et al. 2001; Henry et al. 1998,1999; Lomarev et al. 2002; Mu et al. 2003).

Studies combining functional brain imaging with VNS offer the promise of elucidating the antidepressant mechanisms of action of VNS. Fast imaging methods such as functional magnetic resonance imaging (fMRI) can show the immediate effects of VNS, whereas slower imaging methods such as single-photon emlocion computed tomography (SPECT) and PET can show the longer-term changes associated with constant VNS over time as a therapy (Chae et al. 2003). We have recently succeeded in performing blood oxygen level-dependent fMRI studies in depressed patients implanted with VNS as part of the initial pilot clinical study and a more recent larger double-blind trial. An initial study and a more recent larger double-blind trial. An initial study that used the interleaved VNS/fMRI technique showed that VNS immediately activates many anterior para-limbic regions, including the orbitofrontal cortex, insula, and medial temporal lobe (Bohning et al. 2001). A follow-up study that used the same technique showed that VNS at 5 Hz had a smaller brain effect than did VNS at 20 Hz (Lomarev et al. 2002). Most recently, we have serially scanned 17 depressed patients in the D-02 study with the VNS/fMRI interleaved technique (Mu et al. 2003). Patients were scanned at the first moments when VNS was turned on and again 2 weeks later after a ramp-up phase, when the VNS intensity was intechnique after 10 weeks of VNS therapy. These imaging data are consistent with the notion that repeated daily VNS causes immediate cortical increases and limbic (cingulated and orbitofrontal) decreases and that, over time, these immediate effects change as the system changes its dynamic homeostasis.

This prefrontal-limbic neuronatomical theory of VNS antidepressant mechanisms of action accounts for the known projections and role of the vagus afferents, as well as the very slow and gradual time frame involved in resetting a dynamic system. As a corollary, the antidepressant effects of gamma-knife surgery and other surgical lesion treatments for depression also take 6 months to a year before reaching peak effect.

Perhaps the most important information for the entire field of VNS as theory is improved understanding of the different effects of use parameters on VNS brain effects. This information can be partially gathered in animal studies, although it is difficult to implant VNS in small animals, and they then are immobile for most of the day. Inter-leaving VNS with fMRI can help solve the riddles of how different VNS use parameters differentially affect the brain. Future work with this methodology holds promise for rapidly and efficiently refining the more than 500,000 different combinations of VNS pulse width, frequency, intensity, trainlength, and length of time turned off.

Stress Sensitization

Another important concept in depression pathogenesis is stress sensitization. This term applies to the phenomenon in which repeated mild stresses, over time, build up to a point at which an animal is sensitized to developing depression (Antelman 1988; Antelman et al. 1991; Kalivas et al. 1988; Post 1980; Post et al. 1986). Thus, a single stressful even would not produce depression, but repeated daily stresses will. Reasoning within this stress sensitization paradigm, one wonders whether VNS might be constantly and repeatedly diminishing the abnormal brain reaction to stress inherent in depression. Thus, theoretically, with each new stress that a depressed patient encounters, VNS might be blunting an otherwise amplified pathological reaction. Then the brain gradually is able to return to homeostasis without the pathological feedback from repeated stresses.

Patients taking selective serotonin reuptake inhibitors (SSRIs) commonly report that a stressful life event is no longer as stressful to them as it was before they were taking medications. Our group has similarly observed patients in VNS depression trials tolerate stressful events much better than they did before they were receiving VNS. Learning whether and to what degree VNS might "stress inoculate" or reduce anxiety and the pathological overreaction of a depressed individual to a stressful event is important. VNS may improve depression by gradually reducing the downstream effects of stressful life events, thus enabling corrective brain responses over time. This mechanism of action would account for the slow onset of antidepressant action, the continued improvement overtime, and the relatively low rates of relapse (because stressful events that precipitate relapse are less neurobiologically potent during VNS regulation). To gree VNS affects serum or urinary cortisol, thyroid function, or other hypothalamic-pituitary-adrenal axis measures, such as the dexamethasone suppression test. Further research is needed.

Overall Vagus Nerve Stimulation Summary

In summary, more work is needed to establish whether VNS is an effective antidepressant and, if so, to determine what mechanisms are responsible for causing these changes. From the relatively few studies to date, it appears that VNS could improve depression through several of the current antidepressant mechanism models. Strong data support the anticonvulsant properties of VNS, as well as the changes VNS causes in regional brain activity, both acutely and gradually may produce brain changes through mechanisms not shared by other medications or devices.

Deep Brain Stimulation

The most antomically discrete, and invasive, method of stimulating deep brain structures is called DBS (Ashby and Rothwell 2000; Bekhtereva et al. 1972; Kumar et al. 1998; Olanow et al. 2000) et al 2000; Tarsy 2001).

Use in Parkinson's Disease

In DBS, a thin electrode is inserted directly into the brain. Then different currents are applied at varying depths until the desired effects are achieved. High-frequency (>80 Hz) electrical stumulation of the middle thalamus or subthalamic nucleus has been found effective in PD (Damier 1998, Limousin et al. 1995, 1998). Stimulation can be performed at high frequencies (>50 Hz), which are thought to create a transient functional lesion and inhibit a brain region from normal participation in brain activity. Alternatively, low frequency stimulation may intermittently activate a region (Grill 1999; Grill and Mclntyre 2001).

Mood Effects

Although DBS has not been used to treat major depression, mood effects of the stimulation have been reported. In one patient with PD who had never had depression, the testing of the stimulation caused the acute onset of tearfulness, sadness, and despair. These symptoms remitted immediately when the surgeon moved the stimulator aware from the substantia nigra, directly below the subthalamic nucleus. Transient acute depression was evoked 5 seconds after 130-Hz DBS of the left substantia nigra and ceased 90 seconds after DBS was stopped. Others also have reported that unilateral or bilateral DBS of the subthalamic nucleus resulted in involuntary laughter, humor well-being that lasted for several minutes until the stimulation intensity was lowered or discontinued (Kumar et al. 1998). This emotional reaction was accompanied by improved parkinsonian symptoms.

Other studies during diagnostic DBS prior to neurosurgical ablations also have reported emotional reactions. Microstimulation of the nucleus ventralis caudalis (somatosensory) was accompanied by a strong affective component of visceral pain similar to that previously observed in the patient during a comorbid PD panic attack (Lenz et al. 1995). Weeping, anxiety, and depression were reported to be elicited during neurosurgery in unanesthetized PD patients with 32-Hz stimulation for several seconds of ventral arterionucleus, ventral lateral pars oralis, and other thalamic nuclei as well as pallidum septum and hyphthalamus (Schaltenbrand et al. 1973). Different emotional reactions occurred while stimulating nucleus ventralis laterlis with the floating electrode (Il'inskii 1970).

Bondarchuk and Smirnov (1969) summarized the effects of diagnostic and therapeutic DBS via long-term implanted electrodes in a large sample of patients with PD: positive emotional states occurred after stimulation of the centrum medianum area of the thalamus. Interestingly, high frequency (ablative) DBS and also stereotaxic destruction of the anterior thalamic nuclei resulted in relief from intractamus was one of the brain strucutures in which Health and colleagues recorded EEG correlates of pleasure during orgasm (Heath 1964; Heath and Guerrero-Figueroa 1968). Thus, recent and older case report data indicate that DBS has the potential for short-term alteration of mood. However, this are has not been systematically studied in a controlled setting, and only recently have investigators been able to use powerful concurrent functional neuroimaging to trace the circuits that are activated during stimulation.

DATA IN OBSESSIVE–COMPULSIVE DISORDER

Obsessive–compulsive disorder (OCD) is perhaps the major psychiatric disorder for which the most is know about regional brain pathology (Baster 1990). Briefly, many functional and structural imaging studies have implicated the orbitofrontal cortex and the caudate nucleus in OCD pathogenesis (Breiter et al. 1996; Rauch et al. 194). Additionally, treatment responses to medications and behavior therapy are modest at best for most OCD patients (Goodman 1999; McDougle et al. 1991). Over the past 20 years, neurosurgical ablation of the cingulated gyrus has continued to be offered as an option for treatment-resistent patients (Ballantine et al. 1987; Cosgrove and Rauch 1995; Kurlan et al. 1990; Spangler et al. 1996). This surgery likely interrupts fibers connecting the orbitofrontal cortex to the cingulated gyrps and other limbic regions. Reasoning from this literature, Nuttin and colleagues (1990; Spangler et al. 1996). This surgery likely interrupts fibers connecting the orbitofrontal cortex to the cingulated gyrus and other limbic regions. Reasoning from this literature, Nuttin and colleagues (1999) reported the first series of patients with OCD treated with DBS of the anterior limb of the internal capsule. These initial reports have been followed by continued positive reports (Greenberg et al. 2000, 2003; Nuttin et al. 2003). Double-blind studies are now under way.

Use in Depression

As discussed earlier, one of the more common, but likely incomplete, theories concerning DBS and the brain is that high-frequency DBS results in a functional ablation, or the switching off and inhibition of ongoing neuronal activity, although this theory needs more informed research (Grill 1999). Use of DBS of the subthalamic nucleus or globus pallidus is increasing in patients with PD whose symptoms have not responded to medications.

Major depression occurs in up to 40% of patients with PD (Cummings 1993; Tom and Cummings 1998). Mood changes with DBS treatment in patients with PD are now being studied.

Many neurologists and neurosurgeons have commented that there may be a post-DBS hypomania in the month following surgery. Thus, clinicians are interested in whether DBS might be used for treatment-resistant depression. Although the functional neuroanatomy of normal mood regulation in health and the pathological changes in major depression are becoming better understood knowledge in this are lags drastically behind the beuroanatomical knowledge of motor dysfunction in PD or the circuitry of OCD. A key recent concept is that mood is regulated through changes in activity in the anterior paralimbic circuit (amygdala, seprum, anterior cingulated cortex, anterior temporal poles, and orbitofrontal cortex) and that this system functions abnormally in major depression. Neurosurgical ablation of the anterior cingulate gyrus or the anterior limb of the internal capsule has been used for many years for treatment-resistant depression. Neurosurgical ablation of the anterior cingulated gyrus or the anterior limb of the internal capsule has been used for many years for treatment-resistant depression. Additionally, some researchers have indicated that the DBS-related improvements in patients with OCD are actually more mood related than pure OCD symptoms.

With these theories in mind, several researchers in the United States are beginning small series of DBS studies in patients with treatment-resistent depression. Extreme caution is needed in these studies, particularly given the checkered history with respect to brain surgery (frontal lobotomies) for psychiatric diseases in the early 1900s. It is important to proceed cautiously in patients who have failed almost all available treatments and to integrate knowledge gained from these pilot studies with information from brain imaging and animal models of depression.

In addition to the incomplete knowledge about where to place the DBS leads, this are alacks complete knowledge of the mechanisms of action of DBS and how these are affected by the different use parameters.

CONCLUSION

In summary VNS and DBS represent important new technologies that may rapidly develop into established treatments for depression. Both are approved and commonly used for other neuropsychiatric disorders. The initial pilot and later randomized studies of VNS for the treatment of depression are encouraging, but further studies are needed to provide prospective randomized, controlled data on efficacy. Few published data are available on the use of DBS for depression, although these reports from patients with PD and OCD hint that this may be an emerging treatment option in the years to come. Both of these treatments, along with TMS, represent a new class of brain treatments that build un knowledge of regional brain activity in disease pathogenesis. Much more information is needed, however, about the neurobiological basis of depression and the translational effects initiated by brain stimulation with VNS, DBS, or TMS.

46.17 COMPLEMENTARY MEDICINE IN PSYCHIATRY

Jayati Simlai, Anjanik Kr Ranjan, Neena Bohra, NK Bohra

Complementary medicines are either used as an alternative or in addition to conventional medicine (Zimmerman and Thompson, 2002). Their use by those with chronic disorders such as cancers, with their associated physical and psychological problems, is well documented (Eisenberg et al, 1993; Ernst and Cassileth, 1999). In psychiatric patients, estimates of their use range from 8 to 57%, with the most frequent use being in depression and anxiety. A population-based study from the USA found that 9% of respondents had anxiety attacks, 57% of whom used complementary medicines; 7% of respondents reported severe depression, with 54% of these using complementary medicines (Kessler et al, 2001). Another survey from the USA reported mental disorders in 14% of respondents, 21% of whom used complementary medicines (Unutzer et al, 2000). Usage was highest (32%) in respondents with panic disorder. In studies restricted to those with psychiatric disorders, usage ranged from 13 to 54% (Knaudt et al, 2001; Wang et al, 2001; Alderman and Kiepfer, 2003; Matthews et al, 2003). Complementary medicines are also used by those seen by liaison psychiatrists and a recent study of cancer patients showed that 25% took substances with psychoactive properties (Werneke et al, 2004a). Complementary medicines can be grouped into herbal remedies, food supplements, including vitamin preparations, and other organic and inorganic substances, including omega-3 fatty acids. Some people take food supplements and vitamin preparations in high doses, often outside the safety margins recommended by the food Standards Agency (Food Standards Agency, 2003). People with mental health problems may take complementary medicines to treat anxiety and depression or to counter side effects of conventional treatments, for example tardive dyskinesia and weight gain. Some seek a more holistic approach to treatment, others hope that complementary medicines have fewer or no side-effects, and many with chronic anxiety and depression understandably feel disillusioned by the apparent ineffectiveness of conventional treatment. The aim of this review is to acquaint psychiatrists with the complementary medicines routinely encountered in clinical practice, to review the evidence base for their purported effectiveness and to discuss potential adverse effects and interactions.

COGNITIVE ENHANCERS

Cognitive enhancers are either used in the treatment of dementia to enhance mental performance or to prevent cognitive decline in healthy people. This can be achieved by increasing choline availability in the brain, e.g. by inhibiting acetylcholinesterase. Alternative noncholinergic neuroprotective strategies have been postulated; these include antioxidants scavenging free radicals, thereby reducing neurotoxicity, and anticoagulants increasing cerebral blood flow (Spinella, 2001). Suggested herbal cognitive enhancers include ginkgo, ginseng, hydergine, which is an ergot (*Claviceps purpurea*) derivative, and solanaceous plants, including potatoes, tomatoes and aubergines (Table 27).

Although in some individuals with Alzheimer's disease ginkgo biloba has been reported to improve cognitive performance (Birks et al, 2002; Kanowski and Hoerr, 2003), another trial did not show any benefit in elderly people with Alzheimer's disease of vascular type or age-associated cognitive impairment (van Dongen et al, 2003). Whether the effect in those with Alzheimer's disease is equivalent to that of synthetic cholinesterase inhibitors is debatable (Itil et al, 1998; Wettstein, 2000; Schreiter Gasser and Gasser, 2001. Hydergine was reported to lead to significant improvement of cognitive impairment in dementia, but most studies were performed before standardized dementia criteria were agreed (Olin et al, 2001). The results for panax ginseng and vitamin E were inconclusive (Sano et al, 1997; Vogeler et al, 1999). Solanaceous plants may exercise strong cholinergic effects by inhibiting not only acetyl- but also butyrylcholinesterase. However, no clinical studies have been conducted to determine their effects on cognition. They may augment cocaine toxicity via the same mechanism (Krasowski et al, 1997).

ANXIOLYTICS AND SEDATIVES

Anxiolytics and sedatives essentially have the same underlying mechanisms of action. The stronger the agent the greater the sedative effect, leading to coma in extreme cases. Four mechanisms of action have been implicated (Spinella, 2001): (a) binding to gamma-aminobutyric acid (GABA) receptors leading to hyperpolarization of the cell membrane through increased influx of chlorine anions; (b) inhibition of excitatory amino acids, thereby also impairing the ability to form new memories; and (c) calcium channel blockade, decreasing the release of neurotransmitters into the synaptic cleft. Most complementary medicines prescribed for anxiolysis/sedation (e.g. kava-kava, valerian, passion flower and chamomile) are GABAergic, though for some such as hops the mechanism of action remains unknown. As expected, all remedies can lead to drowsiness when taken in high doses and can potentiate the effect of synthetic sedatives.

The most researched substance is kava-kava (*Piper methysticum*), which originated from Polynesia and was traditionally used for religious rituals (Chevallier, 1996). Kava has an anxiolytic effect that has been established in several RCTs (Pittler and Ernst, 2003). Kava has been associated with several cases of liver toxicity (Natural Medicines Database, 2004a), Which has led to its voluntary withdrawal from the UK market. Valerian (*Valeriana officinalis* or *Valeriana edulis*) is a sedative believed to have been known to Galen and Dioscorides, which has maintained its importance throughout the centuries (Spinella, 2001). In 1845, Coffin described it as 'an excellent sedative..... predisposing the mind to quietness and the body to sleep.' Valerian may have comparable efficacy to oxazepam (Dorn, 2000; Ziegler et al, 2002). However, a systematic review on the effectiveness of valerian in insomnia produced inconclusive results (Stevinson and Ernst, 2000).

Passion flower (*Passiflora incarnata*) contains chrysin, a partial agonist to benzodiazepine receptors. One study comparing passion with oxazepam found both to be equally effective (Alkhondazadeh et al, 2001a); more trials are need to confirm the effect. No data are available on chamomile and hops. Chamomile (*Chamaemelum nobile* or *Matricaria recutita*) contains apigenin which binds to benzodiazepine receptors (Viola et al, 1995). The mechanism of action for hops (*Humulus lupulus*) remains unclear. Bach flower remedies are a combination of 38 flowers and seem to have no effect (Ernst, 2002). Melatonin extracted from the pineal gland may improve sleep in those with delayed sleep phase disorder, but no benefit has been shown in the treatment of primary sleep disorder (MacMahon et al, 2005). It may also improve initial sleep quality in older adults with insomnia (Olde Rikkert and Rigaud, 2001), but its role as a treatment for insomnia in those with Alzheimer's disease remains disputed (Cardinali et al, 2002; Singer et al, 2003).

ANTIDEPRESSANTS AND AUGMENTATION THERAPY

All known synthetic antidepressants act via the enhancement of serotonergic and noradrenergic neurotransmission. Most complementary antidepressants are thought to work through the same pathways. The mechanism of action for selenium is not clear but does seem to be different. Its antioxidant qualities may reduce nerve cell damage (Benton, 2002), and it is also known to facilitate conversion from thyroxine (T4) to thyronine (T3); T3 substitution is one possible means of augmentation of antidepressants in conventional psychiatry. There are no clinical studies but

Table 27: Cognitive enhancers

Substance	*Postulated mechanism of action*	*Effectiveness*	*Side-effects*	*Potential drug interactions*
Ginkgo	Antioxidant: destroying free radicals implicated in cell damage (Oken et al, 1998; Tabet et al, 2000); ↑cerebral blood flow through platelet activation factor inhibition and nitric oxide pathways (Maclenan et al, 2002; Ahlemeyer and Krieglstein, 2003); cholinergic effects (Tang et al, 2002)	Possible improvement of cognitive function, activities of daily living and mood in those with Alzheimer's disease or other cognitive decline, but recent results inconsistent (Birks et al, 2002; Kanowski and Hoerr, 2003; van Dongen et al, 2003)	↑Bleeding time. Case reports of intracerebral hemorrhage (Matthews, 1998; Benjamin et al, 2001); possibly adverse effects on male and female fertility (Ondrizek et al, 1999)	Antithrombolytic agents (Medical Economics, 2000)
Panax ginseng	Interference with platelet aggregation and coagulation (Medical Economics, 2000); Neuroprotection through nicotinic activity (Lewis et al, 1999), antioxidant effects (Lee et al, 1998)	Improvement of mental arithmetic and abstraction; age-delaying properties unproven (Vogeler et al, 1999); one recent trial reporting marginal improvement in mini-mental state examination and improvement in memory tests (Tian et al, 2003)	Insomnia, mania, hyper-and hypotension, ↑vaginal bleeding (Medical Economics, 2000)	Insulin and oral hyperglycemics, anti-thrombolytic agents, MAOIs (phenelzine), loop diuretics (Medical Economics, 2000)
Hydergine (ergoloid)	↑Cholinergic activity (Le Poncin-Lafitte et al, 1985); reversal of age-related decline of choline acetyltransferase (Dravid, 1983) and muscarinic receptors (Amenta et al, 1989); modulation of all monoaminergic neuro- transmitter systems (Markstein, 1985)	Significant improvement in dementia patients; hydergine was more effective at higher doses and in younger patients (Olin et al, 2001)	Cholinergic and monoaminergic side-effects possible; risk of psychotic recurrence	Serotonergic antidepressants, cholinesterase inhibitors
Vitamin E	Antioxidant (Tabet et al, 2000)	Behavioral but no cognitive improvement with combination of vitamin E with selegiline; possibly delay of residential care using vitamin E (Sano et al, 1997)	High doses: ↑risk of bleeding due to antagonism of vitamin K-dependent clotting factors (Liede et al, 1998)	Anticoagulants including aspirin, clodipro-gel, warfarin (Corrigan, 1982; Liede et al, 1998) and herbal anticoagulants such as Ginkgo, garlic and ginseng; possible prevention of nitrate tolerance (Watanabe et al, 1997); possible ↑effect of slidenafil and related phosphodiesterase-5 inhibitors
Solanaceous plants	Inhibit acetylcholinesterase and Butyrylcholinesterase (Krasowski et al, 1997)	No study available	Cholinergic poisoning through dietary intake possible (Krasowski et al, 1997)	Prolonged action of pan-curonium, other myorelaxants and cocaine through, inhibition of butyrylcholinesterase (Krasowski et al, 1997)

low selenium levels have been associated with depression, anxiety and hostility (Hawkes and Hornbostel, 1996), and high dietary intake or supplementation has been associated with mood improvement. The apparent therapeutic effect may be dose-dependent (Bonton and Cook, 1991; Benton, 2002). Like lithium, there may be a narrow therapeutic index. A recent report by the Food Standard Agency (2003) reduced the recommended limits of safe daily intake. Trials may be most promising in those with a low baseline selenium level.

The most robust clinical data are available for St John's wort (Hypericum perforatum). These have been extensively reviewed in meta-analyses (Linde et al, 1996; Williams et al, 2000; Whiskey et al, 2001; Roder et al, 2004; Werneke et al, 2004b; Linde et al 2005) which have found a decrease in effect size over time when tested against placebo. The more recent meta-analyses mostly suggest that the effectiveness of St John's wort is limited to mild depression, and more homogeneous studies targeting patients with mild depression are required (Roder et al 2004; Werneke et al, 2004b; Linde et al, 2005).

However, four of these meta-analyses have demonstrated equivalence to standard antidepressants (Linde et al, 1996; Whiskey et al, 2001; Roder et al, 2004; Linde et al, 2005). One recent trial using high doses (up to 1800 mg) of St John's wort reported equivalence to paroxetine in those with moderate or severe depression (Szegedi et al, 2005). Hyperforin, which inhibits the reuptake of monoamines, is thought to be most likely active component (chatterjee et al, 1998; Miiller et al, 1998). Thus, the use of extracts with maximum hyperforin content should be examined more systematically (Werneke et al, 2004b).

Folate and S-adenosylmethionine are in the same biochemical pathway, with folate being required to synthesize methionine, the direct precursor of S-adenosylmethionine facilitates many methylation reactions required for the synthesis of many neurotransmitters (Bottiglieri et al, 2000; Morris et al, 2003). Thus, those with high levels of homocysteine may be more likely to become depressed, or possibly less likely to respond to antidepressant treatment. Interestingly, hypothyroidism can lead to an increase in homocysteine levels (Roberts and Ladenson, 2004) and this may contribute to the associated depression. In clinical studies, folate has been reported to be effective only when added to antidepressant therapy (Taylor et al, 2004).

Parental S-adenosylmethionine has been reported to be superior to placebo (Bressa, 1994), and equivalence to imipramine has been demonstrated in two RCTs (Delle Chiaie et al, 2002; Pancheri et al, 2002). The onset of action may be more rapid (Fava et al, 1995). Oral S-adenosylmethionine may require doses four times as high as the parenteral formulation (Delle Chiaie et al, 2002). Finally, omega-3 fatty acids are known to stabilize membranes and to facilitate monoaminergic, serotonergic and cholinergic neurotransmission (Haag, 2003) but their antidepressant effect has not been convincingly demonstrated in clinical studies (Marangell et al, 2003; Su et al, 2003). Omega-3 fatty acids are possibly effective when added to lithium in the treatment of bipolar affective disorder (Bowden, 2001).

ANTIPSYCHOTICS, AUGMENTATION AND TREATMENT OF TARDIVE DYSKINESIA

Only two complementary medicines have been suggested for the treatment of psychosis. Ravwolfia (Rauvolfia serpentina) extracts were traditionally used before synthetic antipsychotics became widely available, several alkaloid derivatives, including reserpine, being introduced in the 1950s (Malamud et al, 1957). Ravwolfia originates from India and was mentioned in Ayurvedic medicine around 700 BC (Chevallier, 1996). It blocks vesicular storage of monoamines, allowing them to be more easily degraded by monoamine oxidases in the cytoplasm. As a consequence, the amount of neurotransmitter available on depolarization of the cell membrane is reduced (Spinella, 2001), which may lead to a reduction in dopamine and the resolution of psychotic symptoms. However, serotonin and noradrenaline will also be less available, which explains why reserpine readily precipitates depression. An alternative strategy is the augmentation of antipsychotic treatment with omega-3 fatty acids, but the results of clinical trials remain inconclusive (Joy et al, 2003).

Attempts have been made to treat tardive dyskinesia with vitamin E. This treatment strategy relies on the assumption that tardive dyskinesia not only results from dopamine receptor supersensitivity but also related to the oxidative tissue damage of antipsychotic drugs (shamir et al, 2001; Lohr et al, 2003). Meta-analysis of ten small trials has indicated that vitamin E protects against deterioration of tardive dyskinesia (Soares and McGrath, 2001); one recent trial has reported improvement (Zhang et al, 2004). A far more powerful antioxidant than vitamin E is melatonin, which attenuates the dopaminergic activity in the striatum as well as the release of dopamine from the hypothalamus (Shamir et al, 2001; Lohr et al, 2003). However, as with omega-3 fatty acids, clinical trials have been inconclusive (Shamir et al, 2000, 2001), and larger trials are required to test its therapeutic effectiveness.

ANTIADDICTIVES

Although there are many addictive plants, few have been identified as having the potential to counter addiction. Such may be ibogaine, which is derived from the West-African shrub *Tabernanthe iboga*. It has hallucinogenic properties and is traditionally used in religious ceremonies and initiation rites, but has also been claimed to counter nicotine, cocaine and opitate addiction, via blocakade of dopamine release in the nucleus accumbens (and the dopamine response in general) in chronic cocaine and users (Maisonnuve and Glick, 2003). Ibogaine also binds to the cocaine site of the serotonin transporter (Stately et al, 1996), but its therapeutic value is limited as it is highly neurotoxic and can cause irreversible cerebellar damage (Maisonneuve and Glick, 2003); as a result, further clinical studies have been abandoned. A synthetic derivative 18-methoxycoronaridine has similar reported effects but no cerebellar toxicity or specific effects on the serotonin transporter (Maisonneuve and Glick, 2003). To date 18-methoxycoronaridine has only been tested in animal experiments where it has been shown to reduce cocaine, morphine and alcohol intake in rats (Rezvani et al, 1997; Glick et al, 2000).

Passion flower has also been used to ameliorate the effects of opiate, cannabis, benzodiazepine and nicotine addiction, but clinical data are limited (Dhawan et al, 2002a,b, 2003; Akhondzadeh et al, 2001b). Likewise, valerian has been tried in benzodiazepine withdrawal (Poyares et al, 2002) and St John's Wort has been used for the treatment of alcohol dependence (De Vry et al, 1999; Rezvani et al, 1999; Overstreeet et al, 2003b), but effectiveness has not been established. Kudzu, Japanese arrowroot (Pueraria lobata), has traditionally been used for the treatment of alcoholic hangover. The active ingredient, purerarin, counteracts the anxiogenic effects associated with alcohol withdrawal (Overstreet et al, 2003a). Kudzu also contains two potent, revesible inhibitors of human alcohol dehydrogenase isozymes (Keung, 1993), but an effects has only been demonstrated *in vitro* (Lin and Li, 1998). One small trial among those with chronic alcohol misuse has not shown any difference from placebo (Shebek and Rindone, 2000). Further trials are required to test genuine therapeutic potential, perhaps using more standardized formulations of the active ingredient.

DISCUSSION

This review demonstrates that the evidence base for the use of psychotropic complementary medicines is available for St John's Wort and Kava, both of which are used extensively in various cultures. However, trials of St John's Wort need improved definition of inclusion criteria (Werneke et al, 2004b), and Kava has been withdrawan due to concerns about hepatotoxicity. Further RCTs are required to assess other promising agents such as selenium and S-adenosylmethionine for the treatment of depression, ideally in individuals showing the corresponding deficiencies at baseline. This may lead to new therapeutic approaches for treatment-resistant depression. Valerian and passion flower should be tested as anxiolytics and sedatives; their potential value in the treatment of addiction also requires further clarification. The role of omega-3 fatty acids as an adjunct to antipsychotics and melatonin as a treatment or prophylactic agent for tardive dyskinesia remain ambiguous, both requiring trials with sound methodology.

This review outlined only a limited range of complementary medicines used for the treatment of common psychiatric problems. Clearly there are many more remedies that may be taken to improve general health or to counter the side-effects of conventional treatments. Clinicians need to be aware of and enquire about such forms of self-medication, since all remedies may interact with prescribed medication or have associated side-effects in their own right. For instance, patients may take phytoestrogens, such as black colosh (*Actaea racemosa*), wild yam (*Dioscorea composita*) or dong quai (*Angelica sinensis*) to counter sexual side-effects, and this might pose a problem in patients with oestrogen receptor-positive breast cancer (Werneke et al, 2004a). For the same reason, patients may also try evening primrose oil (*Oenothera biennis*), which could decrease the effect of sodium valproate (Miller, 1989). Kelp (*Laminaria digitata* or *Fucus vesiculosus*) may be taken to counter weight gain, but can contain substantial amounts of iodine and can interfere with treatment for thyroid function disorders. Iodine taken together with lithium may have additive hypothyroid effects (Natural Medicines Comprehensive Database, 2004b).

Given the complex pattern of potential interactions, clinicians should not be afraid to discuss complementary medicines with their patients. Although some patients may choose to use complementary medicines as alternatives to conventional treatment, many may decide to use them in addition to prescribed medications. Complementary medicines have-rightly or wrongly—a very positive 'natural' reputation among significant sections of the population, and therefore can be popular with those from a wide variety of cultural backgrounds. This may lead to higher acceptance and adherence compared with conventional drugs, making it important to be 'willing and prepared to work in partnership with patients' beliefs and preferences-provided their actions are safe' (Brugha et al, 2004). Also, she do not know whether the agreed use of complementary medicines could in itself improve insight and subsequently lead to greater adherence to conventional treatment regimens. This emphasizes the importance of further research on complementary medicines focusing on promising agents such as passion flower, valerian and S-adenosylmethionine, which appear to be obvious candidates for further RCTs. In addition, it might be important to consider patients' attitudes and preferences in future studies, possibly targeting those demanding complementary medicines.

Finally, clinicians need to be aware of side-effects associated with complementary medicines and any interactions with other treatments. They should be able to identify hazards, advising patients accordingly and avoiding uncritical encouragement of potentially harmful use. Ignorance in this area, given the independent usage of complementary medicines, may lead to criticism and possibly litigation (Cohen and Eisenberg, 2002). Equally, patients should be encouraged to disclose information about complementary medicines to healthcare professionals. These discussions need to be conducted sensitively in order to avoid alienating patients who may feel that they have not been taken seriously or have been criticized for using complementary medicines. Such discussions can be complex and may demand more time than is available in designed to meet this challenge, with consideration being given to specialist clinics providing regular updated advice to both clinicians and patients.

46.18 PHARMACOLOGICAL PREVENTION OF MIGRAINE

JN Vyas

People who have migraine experience intermittent attacks of unilateral, pulsating, and moderate to severe headache with associated nausea or photophobia and phonophobia (or all these symptoms). These attacks typically start before the age of 40, often in childhood or teenage years, and occur most commonly from the second to the fourth decade of life.[261] Attacks may be infrequent or frequent. Chronic migraine is diagnosed when attacks regularly occur on more than 15 days a month. Box 7 shows the International Headache Society's classification criteria for migraine without aura.

Recent population studies have shown the worldwide prevalence of migraine to be greater than 10%. The prevalence of migraine in the United States has been estimated at 18% for women, 6% for men, and 12% overall.[262,263] Migraine clearly affects women more than men, and its etiology also seems to have a hereditary component. The World Health Organization ranks migraine 19th on the list of diseases worldwide that cause disability. In spite of recent advances in treatment options for migraine, both acute and preventive, these treatments continue to be underused,[263,264] which leaves patients with unnecessary suffering and increases the burden on the healthcare system. We review the different types of preventive treatment and discuss how they should be used to treat migraine effectively.

SOURCES AND SELECTION CRITERIA

The content of this chapter is based in part on guidelines from the United States Headache Consortium, which use an evidence based medicine format but include data up to 1997 only.[265] We also included guidelines on the management of migraine from the European Federation of Neurological Societies.[266,267] In addition, we used Cochrane reviews as well as peer reviewed publications in headache and neurological journals obtained from Medline searches.

Box 7: International Headache Society's classification criteria for migraine without aura[261]

At least five attacks fulfilling criteria A-C
- A: Headache attacks lasting 4–72 hours (untreated or unsuccessfully treated)
- B: Headache has at least two of the following characteristics:
  - Unilateral location
  - Pulsating quality
  - Moderate or severe pain intensity
  - Aggravation by, or causes avoidance of, routine physical activity
- C: During headache at least one of the following occurs:
  - Nausea or vomiting
  - Photophobia and phonophobia
- D: Not attributed to another disorder

When to Consider Prevention for Migraine

Specific clinical guidelines on when it is clinically appropriate to start preventive treatment vary between different countries and organizations. A high frequency of migraine, inadequate responsiveness to drugs used to treat migraine acutely, and migraines that greatly interfere with activities of daily life are accepted criteria for starting preventive treatment.[265-267] Box 8 lists the European Federation of Neurological Societies and American Academy of Neurology guidelines for starting preventive treatment. It is important to consider coexisting medical conditions and psychological diagnoses when deciding on a preventive treatment. A single drug may effectively treat the coexisting condition and prevent migraines in some circumstances. The importance of the discussion between practitioner and patient about preventive drugs and the reasons for considering their use is often overlooked. Shared decision making, which ensures that the patient understands the reasons for starting preventive treatment and feels comfortable with the drug chosen, increases the likelihood of adherence to the preventive treatment plan. Because overuse of analgesics and other acute drugs may make preventive drugs less effective, the patient should also be instructed to limit their use.[268] Simple analgesics should ideally be used on fewer than 15 days a month and combination analgesics and other acute drugs be limited to 10 days a month.

What are the Goals of Preventive Treatment?

The goals of preventive treatment mirror the criteria for starting these drugs. The major targets of preventive treatment are reduced frequency and severity of migraine headaches, and it is helpful to communicate this to the patient.[265-267] An important point to stress early on is that migraine has no cure, and the goal is to manage and reduce the burden of the

Box 8: Criteria for starting preventive treatment[266,267]

- Quality of life, business duties, or school attendance is severely impaired
- Two or more attacks a month
- Migraine attacks do not respond to acute drug treatment
- Frequent, very long, or uncomfortable auras occur

disease. The patient's disability is reduced if these main goals are achieved. Other goals of preventive treatment include reduced use of acute drugs and fewer visits to the emergency room or doctor's surgery. Patients also need to understand that it may take time for a drug to become effective, most often two to three months at an adequate dose. Asking patients to keep a headache calendar or diary is an effective way to monitor progress.

What do the Treatments Prevent?

The pathogenesis of migraine is not completely understood. Studies of patients prescribed commonly used drugs for preventing migraine have shown that these drugs suppress cortical spreading depression. However the complex mechanisms of action of migraine preventive drugs are unclear.

What Drugs are Available for the Prevention of Migraine?

Although preventive options for migraine may be either pharmacological or non-pharmacological, we will discuss the pharmacological option only. Certain β-blockers, calcium channel blockers, tricyclic antidepressants, and antiepileptic drug are considered first line preventive treatments, and many other drugs are considered second and third line options.[265] Only five drugs are currently approved by the Food and Drug Administration (FDA) for prevention of episodic migraine. These are propranolol, timolol, valproate, topiramate, and methysergide. OnabotulinumtoxinA (Botox) is now FDA approved for the treatment of chronic migraine. European and US treatment recommendations have only a few minor differences (Table 28).[265,266] The evidence for the recommendations is derived from clinical trials where available.

Table 28: Drugs for the prevention of migraine

Drug	*Target dose*	*Common adverse drug reactions*	*Strength of evidence (US)*†	*Strength of evidence (Europe)*‡
β-blockers				
Propranolol	80–160 mg once daily	Hypotension	A	A
Metoprolol	25–100 mg once-twice daily	Hypotension	B	A
Atenolol	25–100mg once daily	Hypotension	B	NA
Calcium channel blockers				
Flunarizine	5–15 mg once daily	Weight gain, tardive dyskinesia	NA	A
Verapamil	80–120 mg once-three times daily	Bradycardia, hypotension	B	NA
Amlodipine	5–10 mg once daily	Edema	NA	NA
Other antihypertensives				
Lisinopril	20 mg once daily	Cough	NA	C
Candesartan	16 mg once daily		NA	C
Antidepressants				
Amitriptyline	25–75 mg once daily	Anticholinergic side effects	A	B
Nortriptyline	10–100 mg once daily	Anticholinergic side effects	C	NA
Fluoxetine	10–40 mg once daily		B	NA
Venlafaxine	75–150 mg twice daily	Drowsiness, urinary retention	NA	B
Anticonvulsants				
Valproate	250–500 mg twice daily	Weight gain, tremor, hair loss	A	A
Topiramate	50–100 mg twice daily	Nephrolithiasis, acute glaucoma	A	A
Gabapentin	300–1200 mg three times daily	Drowsiness, dizziness	B	C
Lamotrigine	50–300 mg once daily	Stevens-Johnson syndrome	NA	NA
Zonisamide	25–400 mg once daily	Nephrolithiasis, sulfonamide allergy	NA	NA
Supplements and herbs				
Riboflavin	200 mg twice daily		B	C
Coenzyme Q10	100 mg three times daily	Gastrointestinal upset	NA	C
Magnesium	400–600 mg once daily	Diarrhea	B	C
Others				
Methysergide	2 mg once daily	Retroperitoneal fibrosis	A	
OnabotulinumtoxinA	155 U		A	

QD = once daily; BID = twice daily; TID = three times daily.

†Taken from American Academy of Neurology practice parameter.

‡Taken from European Federation of Neurological Societies guidelines.

β Blockers

Propranolol and metoprolol have been evaluated in randomized placebo controlled trials for their efficacy in migraine prevention. A Cochrane review of available studies in 2004 concluded that propranolol is effective in preventing migraines in the short-term, with insufficient data to make a conclusion regarding long-term treatment.[269] Sustained release options offer the benefits of once daily dosing and improved compliance. β blockers are a good choice of preventive drug for patients with coexistent hypertension, but they should not be used for patients with asthma and must be used with caution in patients with depression.

Calcium Channel Blockers

Flunarazine—a calcium channel blocker not available in all countries—causes a mild reduction in the frequency of migraine attacks.[270] Calcium channel blockers that are more widely available, such as amlodipine and verapamil, are effective options for some patients. As with most other antihypertensive drugs, hypotension and pedal edema are side effects to watch out for, but otherwise these drugs are well tolerated.

Other Antihypertensive Drugs

Several drugs belonging to the angiotensin converting enzyme inhibitor class and the angiotensin receptor blocker class have been studied as potential treatments for preventing migraine, although because of a lack of definitive data for migraine prevention, these drugs are second or third tier options. A randomized, placebo controlled, crossover study showed that lisinopril, an angiotensin converting enzyme inhibitor, decreased both the number of days with migraine and headache severity by 20%.[271] One randomized controlled trial found that candesartan, an angiotensin receptor blocker, reduced the number of days of migraine a month by nearly five days compared with placebo.[272] Both these classes of drugs may be alternative choices for patients with or without hypertension who do not tolerate, or do not respond to, β-blockers or calcium channel blockers.

ANTIDEPRESSANTS

Amitriptyline, a tricyclic antidepressant, has been shown to be effective in preventing migraine in several randomized controlled trials and is considered a first line option in the US.[273] The dose of amitriptyline used to prevent migraine is lower than the recommended dose to treat depression, and benefits in migraine are independent of improvement in depression. The effective use of other tricyclics, such as protriptyline and nortriptyline, has been reported, but high level evidence to support their use is lacking. Patients may experience anticholinergic side effects such as dry mouth and constipation when taking tricyclic drugs. Selective serotonin reuptake inhibitors have proved to be no more effective than placebo for preventing migraine attacks.[274] The serotonin and noradrenaline reuptake inhibitor venlafaxine has been shown to be effective in prevention of migraine compared with placebo and selective serotonin reuptake inhibitors. One randomized controlled trial found that venlafaxine decreased the number of days with migraine compared with placebo.[275] Serotonin and noradrenaline reuptake inhibitors may be appropriate for patients with chronic pain from other conditions, such as fibromyalgia.

ANTIEPILEPTIC DRUGS

Several antiepileptic drugs have been shown to be effective in preventing migraine in randomized controlled trials, and valproate and topiramate are generally considered first line treatment choices since a Cochrane review in 2008 found them to be effective.[276-279] The same Cochrane review also concluded that the class as a whole is generally well tolerated and can help reduce the frequency of migraine attacks.[277] Valproate must be used with caution in women of childbearing age because of its association with neural tube defects in offspring. Warn patients about weight gain, hair loss, and tremor when prescribing valproate. Topiramate has been associated with weight loss.[278] A history of renal stones is a relative contraindication for using topiramate. Topiramate may be effective in treating chronic migraine and may be useful in patients whose headaches are complicated by overuse of acute drugs. The evidence that gabapentin is effective in preventing migraine is variable, and it is not considered a first line treatment choice. Gabapentin is helpful for patients with other pain conditions, but it has to be taken three times a day. Lamotrigine may be useful for patients who have migraine with aura.

SUPPLEMENTS AND HERBS

Several vitamins, minerals, and herbal remedies can be used to prevent migraine and may appeal to patients who wish to avoid taking daily prescription drugs. These treatments offer the benefits of few adverse drug reactions and drug interactions. Butterbur, or *Petasites hybridus*, is effective but warn patients to use only properly processed plant extracts because the leaves of the plant are potentially carcinogenic. Petasites decreases the frequency of migraine attack, and one study found a statistically significant decrease (≥50%) in the frequency of migraine.[279] Coenzyme Q10 can decrease the frequency of attacks, but it has little effect on the severity of migraine and does not reduce the use of acute drugs.[280] Magnesium oxide and riboflavin (vitamin B-2) have also been shown to reduce the frequency of attacks.[281,282] A negative Cochrane systematic review and meta-analysis of studies that examined the effectiveness of feverfew, derived from the *Tanacetum parthenium* plant, has limited its use.[283]

OTHER DRUGS

Methysergide, an ergot derivative, is an effective preventive option. Its use is limited to six month periods with recommended drug holidays because of the potential development of retroperitoneal, pleural, and cardiac valve fibrosis. Although it was approved by the FDA for prevention of migraine, methysergide is no longer available in the US. Its major metabolite, methylergonovine, is however used by some practitioners.

BOTULINUM TOXIN A

The use of botulinum toxin A has gained a great deal of attention in recent years. The results of trials to date have not proved clear efficacy over placebo in episodic migraine, and it is known to be ineffective for tension-type headache.[284] However, the FDA has approved botulinum toxin A for the treatment of patients with chronic migraine, and it is licensed in the United Kingdom for the same indication.[285] It is administered every three months as 155 units distributed over 31 injection sites, which include the forehead, temporalis muscles, suboccipital areas, upper posterior cervical musculature, and trapezius muscles.

COMBINATION TREATMENT

For patients who fail to respond to single preventive drugs, the use of more than one drug may prove effective—for example, a combination of propranolol and amitriptyline.

When should Preventive Treatment be Discontinued?

The frequency of follow-up visits is tailored to the patient's individual needs and response to treatment. Guidelines for discontinuing preventive drugs are arbitrary, and treatment decisions should be made on a case by case basis. For example, if coexisting conditions are being treated, the clinician might decide not to discontinue drugs. Drugs might need to be discontinued slowly in patients who react to quick changes in medication. Drugs are usually discontinued in patients who have shown no clear benefit after an adequate trial duration.

46.19 MANAGEMENT OF CHRONIC EPILEPSY

VS Chadda

Epilepsy can be defined pragmatically as the occurrence of at least two unprovoked epileptic seizures. It is the most common serious neurological condition in adults, directly affecting over 400,000 people in the United Kingdom and up to 60 million people worldwide.[286] Prevalence of epilepsy in developed countries is about 0.5%; however, the lifetime risk of a person having a nonfebrile epileptic seizure is much higher at 2 to 5%, implying, for most patients, remittance of the condition or premature death.

Risk of a second seizure occurring within two years of the first event is about 50%. Early treatment with antiepileptic drugs after the first seizure does not affect the long-term prognosis, with 75–80% achieving remission at five years, irrespective of whether treatment began after the first seizure or only after a recurrence.[287,288] Treatment is therefore typically reserved for people who have had at least two seizures; the risk of a third seizure in these patients is over 70%. A tailored approach to treatment should always be adopted, since there could be circumstances in which treatment after a first seizure is appropriate (for example, presence of a structural lesion on neuroimaging) or deferred (for example, in those with very infrequent seizures).

Most people with epilepsy eventually become free of seizures on antiepileptic drugs. Nevertheless, about 20–30% of patients continue to have seizures despite treatment.[289] By extrapolating this proportion to the UK, an estimated 100,000 people with epilepsy need continuing, hospital based medical treatment. Of this group, over 35,000 will have more than one seizure a month. Epilepsy carries an increased risk of morbidity and premature mortality with standardized mortality rates two to threefold higher than the general population.[290,291] This raised risk is partly due to the underlying cause of the epilepsy but is also a direct result of seizures, such as an increased risk of accidents (including drowning) and sudden unexpected death in epilepsy (a condition that affects at least 500 people with epilepsy in the UK annually). On this basis, seizure remission, wherever possible, is a major goal.

The implications of chronic epilepsy extend beyond continued seizures, and encompass cognitive difficulties, mood disturbance, and lifestyle issues, the effective treatment of which involves a coordinated response from both primary and secondary care.

The purpose of this review was to examine the literature on how to manage adults with chronic epilepsy.

WHO GETS EPILEPSY?

The incidence of epilepsy is increased in childhood, at least partly because of brain malformations, perinatal cerebral insults, and genetic disorders, and in later life, usually as a result of cerebrovascular disease. Nevertheless, seizures could start at any age and may follow a cerebral insult, such as head injury, intracranial infections, or tumours. The risk of developing epilepsy increases in the presence of learning disability or after a prolonged or lateralized febrile convulsion in childhood. Genetic factors contribute either directly (for example, in the autosomal dominantly inherited condition tuberous sclerosis) or in a more complex pattern of polygenic inheritance. Overall, genetic factors are thought to contribute to about 40% of people with epilepsy.

WHAT IS THE GOAL OF EPILEPSY TREATMENT?

In all people with epilepsy, the goal should be to achieve seizure freedom. Reducing a person's seizures by 50%, for example, from six seizures to three seizures a month might have a minimal effect on quality of life.[292] This is largely because of the restrictions to a person's lifestyle that remain until seizure freedom, such as the inability to drive, difficulties obtaining work, and maintaining a relationship. Nevertheless, antiepileptic drugs have both idiosyncratic and often more predictable chronic side effects, and seizure freedom should not be relentlessly pursued at the expense of quality of life; intrusive side effects also have a negative effect on quality of life.[292] Common side effects that lead to withdrawal of drug treatment include drowsiness, dizziness, lethargy, and cognitive slowing. These side effects are a particular concern for combination antiepileptic drug treatment.

HOW IS EPILEPSY MANAGED?

The diagnosis of epilepsy is clinical—that is, it is made on the basis of a description of the seizure by both a patient and a witness. It is mandatory to try to obtain a witness description, which is often more informative than the person's account of the event, which may be confounded by loss of awareness, confusion, and amnesia. Investigations such as a brain scan by magnetic resonance imaging or an electroencephalography recording should be used to corroborate clinical suspicion and not as screening tests, owing to the presence of both false positive and false negative information. Patients should be referred to a specialist for evaluation if a seizure is suspected, but drug treatment is typically started only after a second seizure. The choice of initial monotherapy has been guided by several important studies (including, most recently, SANAD)[293,294] and advice from the National Institute for Health and Clinical Excellence (NICE).[295] The antiepileptic drug strategy should be tailored to each patient's seizure type, epilepsy syndrome, cotreatment, comorbidity, lifestyle issues, and preferences (Box 9).

Specialists should adjust the dose of the selected drug to achieve optimal seizure control, making increments if seizures continue in the absence of side effects and, for some drugs

Box 9: Information needs

General epilepsy information
- Explanation of what the condition is
- Classification
- Investigations
- Syndrome
- Epidemiology
- Prognosis
- Genetics
- Sudden unexpected death in epilepsy

Antiepileptic drugs
- Choice of drug
- Efficacy
- Side effects
- Adherence
- Drug interactions
- Free prescriptions

Seizure triggers
- Lack of sleep
- Alcohol and recreational drugs
- Stress
- Photosensitivity

First aid
- General guidelines

Issues for women
- Contraception
- Preconception
- Pregnancy and breastfeeding
- Menopause

Lifestyle
- Driving regulations
- Employment
- Education
- Leisure
- Relationships
- Safety at home

Possible psychosocial consequences
- Perceived stigma
- Memory loss
- Depression
- Anxiety
- Maintain mental well-being
- Self-esteem
- Sexual difficulties
- Support organizations
- Address and telephone numbers

such as phenytoin, being guided by assays of serum drug concentrations. Zealous adherence to quoted therapeutic ranges of serum antiepileptic concentrations is, however, not appropriate. These data should always be secondary to the clinical picture of whether the person continues to have seizures or dose related side effects from antiepileptic drugs. Blood levels of antiepileptic drugs should also be monitored to detect nonadherence to the prescription, suspected toxicity, and in the management of specific clinical conditions such as status epilepticus, organ failure and pregnancy, in which serum levels may fall resulting in the re-emergence of seizures.

Treatment should be initiated and continuing therapy should be planned by the specialist. If management is straightforward, continuing drug treatment can be prescribed in primary care if local circumstances or licensing allow. The duration of each treatment trial before deciding on continuing or changing to an alternative drug depends on the occurrence of side effects and seizure frequency. For example, it will take longer to establish whether a drug has been effective in a patient with very infrequent seizures than in a patient with daily or weekly seizures.

WHAT AFFECTS SEIZURE CONTROL AND PROGNOSIS IN CHRONIC EPILEPSY?

Several factors influence prognosis, and specifically, the chance of patients becoming seizure-free. Perinatal neurological insult and learning disability are associated with an increased risk of developing chronic epilepsy. Only about 10% of people with an epileptic structural lesion on magnetic resonance imaging, such as hippocampal sclerosis, achieve seizure freedom with drug treatment alone. For some of these, epilepsy surgery offers the best chance of becoming seizure-free and improving quality of life.[296]

An important factor in the probability of subsequent remission is the frequency of seizures within the first six months after seizure onset; 95% of patients with two seizures in the first six months achieve a five year remission, compared with only 24% of those with more than ten seizures.[297] The probability of seizure remission decreases significantly with each successive treatment failure. About 50% of people become seizure-free with their first antiepileptic drug, whereas only 11% who discontinued the first appropriate drug owing to a lack of efficacy become seizure-free on a second drug, and only 4% become seizure-free on a third drug or beyond.[298] A recent series of studies has suggested, however, that this view is overly pessimistic. For example, in a review of the effect of 265 drug changes in 155 people with chronic epilepsy, 16% were rendered seizure-free after introduction of one drug, whereas a further 21% had a considerable reduction in seizure frequency. Overall, 28% of the cohort was rendered seizure-free by one or more changes to their drug treatment.[299]

WHAT ARE THE FACTORS TO CONSIDER IF SEIZURE CONTROL IS SUBOPTIMAL?

Is the Diagnosis Correct?

A patient's failure to respond to adequate trials of antiepileptic drugs should prompt specialists to review the diagnosis. One study showed that up to 20–30% of people attending tertiary referral centers with presumed chronic epilepsy did not in fact have the condition, with the most common differential diagnoses being dissociative seizures and neurocardiogenic or cardiac syncope.[300]

Is the Drug Treatment Appropriate?

Some antiepileptic drugs could exacerbate seizure disorders if used injudiciously. The most common examples are the use of carbamazepine, oxcarbazepine, phenytoin, pregabalin, and gabapentin in primary generalized epilepsy, all of which can exacerbate not only absences and myoclonic jerks but also convulsive seizures.[301] Therefore, a patient's seizure disorder must be classified accurately, although this is not possible in some instances and drugs with a broad spectrum of activity should be used.

NICE GUIDELINES ON ANTIEPILEPTIC DRUG TREATMENT[295]

What Other Medications and Illnesses Need to Be Considered?

Other nonepilepsy drugs may lower the seizure threshold, including antimalarial compounds (such as chloroquine, mefloquine), smoking cessation drugs (such as bupropion), antidepressants, and antipsychotics (such as amitriptyline and clozapine). Use of these drugs should be questioned if seizure control is suboptimal. Systemic illnesses, such as sepsis, renal or hepatic disease, or an endocrine disturbance, may cause treatment failure and should be investigated.

Is Adherence to Treatment Adequate?

If there are doubts about adherence to treatment, the patient and carer should be questioned sensitively about this. Serum concentrations of antiepileptic drugs can also be obtained. Inspecting the packaging and drugs themselves may rarely yield prescribing or dispensing errors. If adherence is a problem, consider using dossett boxes, prepackaged treatment packs, and reminder services (such as alarms or regular, timed text messages).

Has the Patient had a Good Trial with a Maximally Tolerated Dose of all Major Antiepileptic Drugs?

People with poorly controlled epilepsy are usually under the care of a specialist neurology team. If seizures continue despite a maximally tolerated dose of individual first line drugs, specialists should trial a combination of two first line drugs for that seizure type. The chance of dual therapy controlling seizures, if monotherapy has been unsuccessful, is 10–15%. If dual therapy does not help, the drug which seems to have the most effect and fewest side effects should be continued, and the second drug should be gradually replaced with an adjunctive drug. NICE guidelines may help in selecting an alternative, second line antiepileptic drug (Table 29).[295] The chance of a 50% reduction in seizures from the addition of a second line drug is 20–50%, with the chance of the patient becoming seizure-free less than 10%.

If the second-line drug is effective, consider withdrawing the initial drug. Prescription of an unhelpful second line drug should not be continued. If adjunctive treatment is ineffective or not tolerated, discuss this with the person, and possibly refer them to a tertiary epilepsy specialist. Current NICE guidelines recommend other antiepileptic drugs to consider at this point for focal epilepsy, such as lacosamide, eslicarbazepine acetate, pregabalin, zonisamide, retigabine, and tiagabine, as well as the older substances phenobarbitone and phenytoin.[295]

Over the past 20 years, the number of antiepileptic drugs available has increased markedly (see Figure 8 and Table 29). Similarities exist between drugs in terms of efficacy and indications, but there is a wide range of dosing strategies, pharmacokinetic and pharmacodynamic interactions, and side effect profiles. This complexity has led to a degree of "prescribing paralysis" among nonspecialists, and clinicians will often retreat to established and trusted drugs, rather than considering more contemporary and newly licensed drugs.

Which Drug should the Patient Try Next?

With a large number of drugs to choose from, how do specialists choose drugs rationally—that is, tailor the choice of treatment to an individual? Many placebo=controlled trials of adjunctive antiepileptic drugs have formed the bases on which individual drugs have been licensed. Establishing which drug is the most effective and well tolerated by comparing these trials is difficult because of different trial designs, patient selection, and outcome measures. Nevertheless, detailed analysis shows no clear statistical difference between the drugs in terms of efficacy and tolerability,[302,303] and therefore one drug cannot be stated as conclusively better than another.

Table 29: NICE guidelines on antiepileptic drug treatment[295]

Epileptic seizure type	*First line treatment*	*Adjunctive treatment*	*Other drugs to consider on referral to tertiary care*	*Do not consider (may worsen seizures)*
Generalised tonic-clonic	Carbamazepine, lamotrigine, oxcarbazepine,* sodium valproate	Clobazam, lamotrigine, levetiracetam, sodium valproate, topiramate	—	Carbamazepine, gabapentin, oxcarbazepine, phenytoin, pregabalin, tiagabine, vigabatrin
Tonic or atonic	Sodium valproate	Lamotrigine*	Rufinamide*, topiramate*	Carbamazepine, gabapentin, oxcarbazepine, pregabalin, tiagabine, vigabatrin
Absence	Ethosuximide, lamotrigine,* sodium valproate	Ethosuximide, lamotrigine,* sodium valproate	Clobazam, clonazepam, levetiracetam,* topiramate,* zonisamide*	Carbamazepine, gabapentin, oxcarbazepine, phenytoin, pregabalin, tiagabine, vigabatrin
Myoclonic	Levetiracetam,* sodium valproate, topiramate*	Levetiracetam, sodium valproate, topiramate*	Clobazam, clonazepam, piracetam, zonisamide*	Carbamazepine, gabapentin, oxcarbazepine, phenytoin, pregabalin, tiagabine, vigabatrin
Focal	Carbamazepine, lamotrigine, levetiracetam, oxcarbazepine, sodium valproate	Carbamazepine, clobazam, gabapentin, lamotrigine, levetiracetam, oxcarbazepine, sodium valproate, topiramate	Eslicarbazepine acetate, lacosamide, phenobarbital, phenytoin, pregabalin, retigabine, tiagabine, vigabatrin, zonisamide	—

*At the time of publication of NICE guidelines in January 2012, this drug did not have UK marketing authorization for this indication or population.

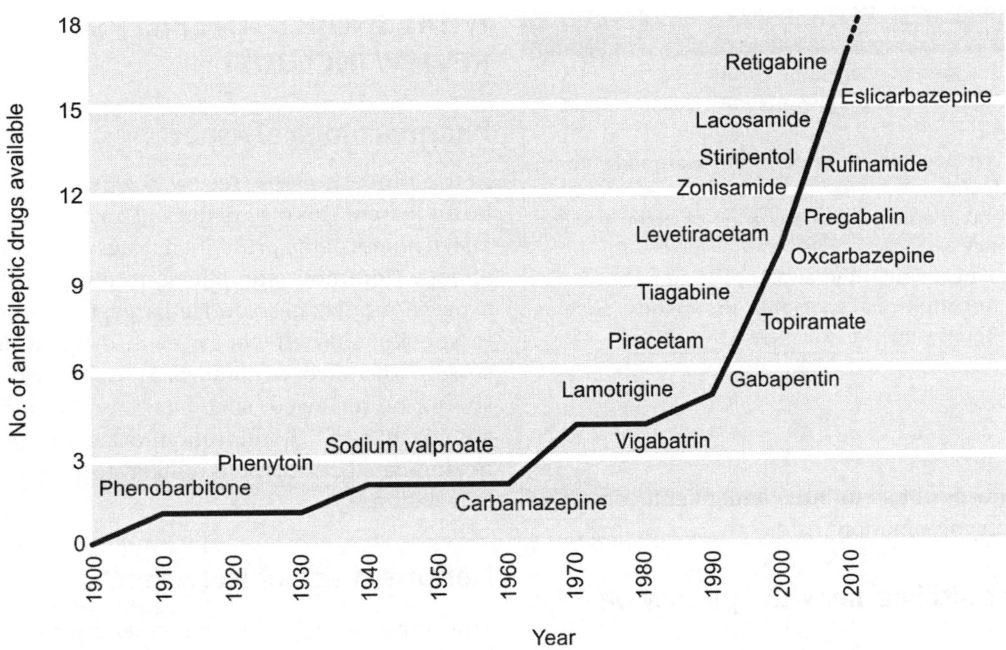

Fig. 8: Antiepileptic drugs available in the UK over the past 20 years, in addition to acetazolamide, clobazam, clonazepam, and ethosuximide

Head-to-head trials of adjunctive and combination treatments offer greater potential for establishing a drug hierarchy. Few such studies exist, and those that have been undertaken frequently evaluate outcome measures other than seizure frequency, such as mood changes and aggression.[304] These goals are laudable but do little to inform which drug or combination to recommend next for people with refractory epilepsy to improve seizure control.

In reality, the choice of the third or fourth antiepileptic drug or beyond is complex and involves looking at the evidence, clinical experience, and individual characteristics and concerns. For example, in people with comorbidities such as migraine, choosing a drug with adjunctive preventative properties for migraines may be beneficial (such as topiramate, sodium valproate, pregabalin, or gabapentin). In people with anxiety or depression, compounds that are also indicated for generalized anxiety disorder (such as pregabalin) or other drugs with mood stabilizing properties (such as valproate and lamotrigine) may be worth considering earlier than other substances. In people with an elevated body mass index, consider avoiding pregabalin, sodium valproate, and gabapentin, and consider instead topiramate and zonisamide, which are commonly associated with weight loss.

The presence of cotreatments, particularly those affected by enzyme inducing drugs, may influence the choice of drug. Oral anticoagulants may need an increased dose to maintain appropriate anticoagulation levels, and hormonal contraceptives are rendered less effective, even with a dose adjustment, in the presence of drugs such as carbamazepine, phenytoin, and higher dose topiramate. Other drugs with favorable pharmacokinetics, such as levetiracetam, may be better choices. Teratogenicity is a clear concern with all drugs, and particularly in combinations including sodium valproate.[305]

How can the Total Drug Load be Minimized?

It is important to reduce and discontinue antiepileptic drugs if their prescription has not aided seizure control and they are suspected of giving rise to adverse effects. Reduction of the number of antiepileptic drugs frequently results in patients feeling better and improved seizure control.[306] The rate at which these drugs should be withdrawn in this situation is controversial and should be planned and supervised by specialist services. Some drugs can be safely withdrawn fairly rapidly, but conventional withdrawal occurs over a period of weeks. This period is particularly important in the withdrawal of benzodiazepines and barbiturates, which could precipitate status epilepticus if withdrawn too rapidly.[307] Making only one drug change at a time is recommended, to determine cause and effect if there is any improvement or deterioration.

What about Epilepsy Surgery?

In focal epilepsy, if satisfactory seizure control cannot be achieved by antiepileptic drugs, consider an evaluation for epilepsy surgery. This treatment is especially indicated if a lesion with concordant clinical features has been detected on magnetic resonance imaging, but should be considered in patients with a focal onset epilepsy and ongoing seizures

Box 10: Triggers for referral to secondary care

- All patients with a suspected epileptic seizure
- All patients who continue to have epileptic seizures (that is, active epilepsy)
- Patients who have possible side effects, both acute and chronic, from drug treatment
- Patients with stable epilepsy but a change of circumstances, such as pregnancy
- Consideration of treatment withdrawal
- Patients needing additional specialist information, such as preconception counseling

despite optimal doses of two to three antiepileptic drugs (as monotherapy or in combination).

How Often should People with Epilepsy be Reviewed?

Current NICE guidelines recommend that all people with epilepsy should have a yearly structured review. In adults, this review may be undertaken by a general practitioner or specialist, depending on how well the epilepsy is controlled and the presence of specific lifestyle issues, such as consideration of pregnancy, driving regulations, or drug cessation (Box 10). At this review, people should have access to written and visual information, counseling services, timely and appropriate investigations, and tertiary services (Box 9). In particular, if seizures are not controlled or diagnosis is uncertain, patients should be referred to tertiary services for further assessment.[295]

WHAT SHOULD AN EPILEPSY REVIEW INCLUDE?

Pharmacological Aspects

At the annual epilepsy review, the person's treatment should be discussed. This discussion will include an evaluation of the effectiveness of the prescribed drugs and presence of adverse effects. Common side effects to almost all drugs include drowsiness, dizziness, and lethargy; these effects, in addition to specific side effects for each drug, should be actively sought. The effect of comorbidities and use of cotreatments should be reviewed, such as the oral contraceptive pill or anticoagulants.[308] Routine monitoring of antiepileptic drugs is not indicated because it is unlikely to alter drug management in isolation.

Nonpharmacological Aspects

The implications and consequences of chronic epilepsy should be considered, which often are more devastating than the seizures themselves. Patients should be given general safety advice about cooking with a microwave oven, safe bathing, and recreational activities. The driving regulations should be discussed if appropriate, and patients should be reminded that a one year period of seizure freedom is required before being eligible to drive. Issues regarding epilepsy, antiepileptic drugs, contraception, and pregnancy should be considered in women of childbearing age and further advice sought from a specialist if relevant. A discussion of reasonable expectations and limitations with regard to the prognosis and the prospects for independent living, leisure and social life, and employment is also important.

46.20 MANAGEMENT OF SEASONAL AFFECTIVE DISORDER

BK Singh

Low mood associated with a certain season (usually winter) is very common. For example, in the UK, up to 6% of adults have "recurrent major depressive episodes with seasonal pattern", commonly known as seasonal affective disorder (SAD).[309-311] People with SAD consult in primary care more often than age- and gender-matched control groups; patients also receive more prescriptions and are referred more often to secondary care.[312] Around 6–35% of patients require hospitalization for SAD at some point.[313] Here we discuss the management of adults with SAD, and in particular light therapy.

SEASONAL AFFECTIVE DISORDER

The SAD involves symptoms typical for depression (e.g. lowered mood, energy loss, fatigue) and also atypical symptoms (e.g., hypersomnia, increased appetite and eating, carbohydrate craving, weight gain).[309,310,314] Some specialists have questioned the value of considering "SAD" as a separate diagnostic category from nonseasonal depression;[315] and of note it is classified as a subset of recurrent major depressive or bipolar disorder rather than as a separate category by both the Diagnostic and Statistical Manual of Mental Disorders (DSM-IV; see Box 11) and the World Health Organization's International Statistical Classification of Diseases and Related Health Problems (ICD-10).[309,316]

WHAT CAUSES SAD?

Evidence suggests that SAD has a genetic element, with genes affecting serotonin metabolism (which has a seasonal pattern) being implicated in seasonal mood variations.[317,318] Melatonin, a hormone secreted by the pineal gland during darkness, has also been implicated in the etiology of SAD. It is important in the regulation of daily or 'circadian' rhythms (e.g. the sleep-wake cycle) and seasonal or 'circannual' rhythms (e.g. regulating reproduction in many mammals).[319] The time at which the plasma melatonin concentration rises occurs later in patients with than without SAD.[320] Nocturnal melatonin secretion can be suppressed by light (e.g. a light intensity of around 3000 lux suppresses melatonin secretion by around 70%; see Box 12 for examples of light intensities measured in lux).[321,322]

WHO GETS SAD?

The mean age of onset of SAD is around 27 years; it can occur in childhood, when rates among girls and boys are similar.[323,324] Women are up to four times more likely than men to be affected during the reproductive years.[317,325] In older adults, prevalence rates decline and the genders are equally likely to be affected.

Clinical Course

Episodes of SAD last around 4 months.[313,326] Around 60% of patients diagnosed with SAD continue to have a seasonal disturbance of mood and/or behavior in the long-term, while around 20% have complete remission within several years of first diagnosis.[317] Some patients have manic or hypomanic episodes in spring and summer.[327] SAD can markedly impair quality of life in winter, but this may return to normal in summer.[328,329]

Box 11: DSM-IV criteria for "with seasonal pattern" within recurrent major depressive disorder or major depressive episodes in bipolar disorder[309]

- Regular temporal relationship between the onset of major depressive episodes and a particular time of the year (e.g. fall [autumn] or winter)
- Full remissions (or a change from depression to mania or hypomania) at a characteristic time of year (e.g. spring)
- In the last two years, two major depressive episodes that demonstrate the seasonal relationship and no nonseasonal episodes
- Seasonal episodes substantially outnumber nonseasonal episodes that may have occurred over the individual's lifetime

Box 12: Examples of light intensities measured in lux[322,323]

Moonlight: 0.2 lux
Winter's day: 20 000 lux
Bright sunny summer's day: 100 000 lux

Box 13: Structured Interview Guide Hamilton depression rating Seasonal Affective Disorder (SIGH-SAD): an interview covering HAM-D21 plus Atypical Depression Supplement of 8 items giving HAM-D29[330-332]

- *Current SAD episode criteria*: Total SIGH-SAD 20 or more, including HAM-D21 10 or more and Atypical Depression Supplement 5 or more
- *Response*: A reduction of at least 50% from baseline
- *Remission*: Score falls to below 8[333]

Diagnosis

Various rating scales have been used to measure symptoms in SAD (e.g. the 21-item and 17-item versions of the Hamilton Depression Rating Scale [HAM-D21 and HAM-D17, respectively] and the six-item depression subscale [HAM-D6]).[326] The gold standard of diagnosis is a structured interview to determine whether patients fulfil DSM-IV criteria (see Box 13).[317]

CONVENTIONAL ANTIDEPRESSANTS

Acute Treatment of SAD

The suggestion that serotonin metabolism is disordered in SAD underlies the use of selective serotonin reuptake inhibitors (SSRIs) for acute treatment of patients with the condition; however, there have been few good-quality clinical trials of such intervention.[334]

One five-week randomized placebo-controlled trial, involving 68 adults with SAD, found a higher response rate with fluoxetine 20 mg daily (59% *v* 34% with placebo, $P < 0.05$).[335] A second, eight-week, placebo-controlled trial, involving 187 adults with SAD and a mean baseline HAM-D29 of around 36, found a greater change in mean HAM-D29 with sertraline 50 to 200 mg daily (-17.90 *v* -13.39 with placebo, difference 4.51, 95% CI 0.76–8.28).[331]

Fluoxetine and sertraline are licensed for major depressive episodes, although SAD is not specifically mentioned in the summaries of product characteristics (SPCs) for these drugs.[336,337]

Prevention of SAD Episodes

Given that SAD may recur, long-term and maintenance treatment may be needed.[338]

Pooled data from three randomized trials, involving a total of 1042 patients who started treatment before onset of SAD symptoms in autumn, suggested that compared with people on placebo, there was a lower recurrence rate among those on bupropion 150 to 300 mg daily (a noradrenaline and dopamine reuptake inhibitor not licensed in the UK for this indication, and not commonly used for SAD in UK practice; 16% *v* 28%; relative risk [RR] 0.56).[313,339] However, no P values were stated for this difference.

LIGHT THERAPY

Why Use Light Therapy?

No clear mechanism of action has been established for light therapy in SAD. One theory is that morning bright light counters disordered circadian rhythms in patients with SAD.[340,341] Other theories suggest that light may also have direct effects on some neurotransmitters (e.g. serotonin).[318]

What does Light Therapy Involve?

Light therapy involves daily scheduled exposure to fluorescent light boxes, dawn simulators (devices that slowly increase the room illumination over a period of around 90 minutes during sleep), or incandescent light visors (shaped like baseball caps with light sources shining from the brim down into the wearer's eyes). The "dose" of light is determined by the intensity and duration of exposure.[342]

ASSESSING LIGHT THERAPY

Methodological Difficulties

Several factors make designing trials of light therapy difficult. For example, the appropriate "minimum dose" of treatment is unclear, and it is hard to find a credible control condition since patients are not "blind" to therapy, and treatment expectations may contribute to a positive outcome.[342,343] The acceptable maximum dose for a low-light control is not known.

In addition, it is difficult to combine the results of light therapy trials in a meta-analysis due to differences between studies in terms of the doses of light used; the methods of delivery (e.g. light box, dawn simulation or visor); comparator treatments; and populations.[344]

Clinical Efficacy of Light Therapy

A systematic review of randomized controlled trials of bright light therapy (at least 3000 lux-hours daily) for SAD found eight studies involving a total of 360 patients with a maximum of 300 lux for controls, and lasting 7–42 days.[345] The effect sizes for a significant reduction in depression symptom severity with bright light were consistently positive across the studies. However, there was significant heterogeneity among the studies, indicating that they should probably not be combined statistically.

The same review also identified five randomized controlled trials (involving a total of 133 patients) assessing dawn simulation (increasing light exposure from 0 lux to around 200–300 lux, over 1.5–2.5 hours) with controls receiving less than 5 lux and/or less than 15 minutes of treatment; the effect size for a significant reduction in symptom severity was reported as moderate to large.[345]

In a meta-analysis of five randomized controlled trials of light visors, no difference between light intensities of 3500–7600 lux, 400–650 lux, and under 100 lux was found; however, the authors stated that the combined statistical power of the studies was insufficient to demonstrate a significant effect.[343]

A recent update of the National Institute for Health and Clinical Excellence (NICE) guideline on the management of depression in adults has reviewed the data on light therapy for depression with a seasonal pattern.[344] This review included 20 randomized controlled trials, comparing light therapy (ranging from 176–15 000 lux daily) with waiting list control management, "attentional" control (e.g. sham light box), or active treatment controls (e.g. cognitive behavioural therapy [CBT], fluoxetine). Compared with waiting-list control, bright light reduced depressive symptoms more (e.g. weighted mean difference [WMD] in SIGH-SAD score -10.4, 95% CI -15.99 – -4.81); however, bright light did not differ significantly from attentional control or active treatments. The review concluded that it was unclear whether the superior effectiveness of the light therapy compared with waiting list management was more than a placebo effect. Another possibility is that light therapy was as effective as fluoxetine or CBT. The NICE review also concluded that dawn simulation did not reduce symptoms more than attentional control.[345]

No published randomized controlled trials have assessed the combination of light therapy and antidepressants in SAD.[341]

Unwanted Effects of Light Therapy

Unwanted effects of light therapy include eye strain or visual disturbances (in 19–27% of patients), headache (13–21%), agitation (6–13%), nausea (7%), sweating (7%) and sedation (6–7%).[317] These effects are generally mild and subside with time or with reduction of the dose.[317] Hypomania can also occur.[317,332]

PRACTICALITIES OF LIGHT THERAPY

Regulations

Light therapy devices intended as treatment for disease, which do not achieve their principal intended action on the human body by pharmacological, immunological or metabolic means, come within the scope of the Medical Device Directive and should carry a CE mark.[346]

Stopping and Restarting Light Therapy

There are few data on stopping and restarting light therapy. Specialists suggest that patients on light therapy generally continue treatment until the time of their usual spontaneous remission; it can be stopped abruptly.[332] In rare cases where a patient experiences a relapse, treatment can be resumed for several weeks.

If light therapy is felt to be effective, it can be resumed in subsequent years before, or with the appearance of, the first symptoms (e.g. difficulty waking, daytime fatigue, carbohydrate craving) prior to the onset of depression.[347,348] However, this may be unnecessary, as patients do not always become depressed every winter.[349]

OTHER TREATMENTS

Cognitive Behavioral Therapy

Two randomized controlled trials of CBT in patients with SAD have been published.[350,351]

The first was a pilot study involving 23 patients who received group CBT tailored to SAD (1.5 hour sessions twice weekly, with four to six participants per group), light therapy (10 000 lux for 45 minutes in the morning and 45 minutes in the evening), or both, for six weeks.[350] SIGH-SAD scores improved from pre- to post-treatment with no significant difference between groups (only graphical information presented). At the 1 year follow-up, no patients treated with CBT (with or without light therapy) the previous winter met SIGH-SAD criteria for relapse, compared with 62.5% of patients who had received light therapy only (P = 0.005).

The second study, involving 61 patients with a mean pretreatment SIGH-SAD score of around 28.6, compared four strategies for SAD: CBT (1.5 hour sessions twice weekly, with four to eight participants per group, for six weeks); light therapy (10,000 lux for 45 minutes in the morning and 45 minutes in the evening for one week, then flexible dosing for five weeks); both of these treatments for six weeks; and waiting list control management (minimal contact monitoring for six weeks; then treatment with light therapy).[351] All three active-treatment groups had a significant fall in SIGH-SAD scores (post-treatment scores: CBT only 12.9; light only 12.7; CBT plus light 8.5) and scores in all these groups were lower than that in the waiting list control group (23.1; P < 0.05 for each active treatment).

Self-help and Complementary Treatments

An NHS direct patient leaflet on SAD recommends lifestyle changes to reduce symptoms, including exercise, a healthy diet and trying to get as much natural sunlight as possible.[347]

A systematic review of complementary and self-help treatments for depression identified one randomised controlled trial that assessed vitamin D therapy as treatment for SAD (involving only 15 patients but suggesting the treatment was more effective than light therapy); one that assessed vitamin B_{12} as treatment for SAD (involving 27 patients, which found no benefit); and one that assessed *Ginkgo biloba* for prevention of SAD relapse (involving 27 patients, which also found no benefit).[352]

One randomized trial, involving 27 patients with SAD, compared bright light (2500 lux between 2 pm and 4 pm daily), physical exercise (training on a stationary bicycle between 1 pm and 2 pm daily), and "no treatment" for one week.[353] The two active treatments reduced depressive symptoms (HAM-D21 fell by 64.5% with light and 68.5% with exercise, each P < 0.001 *v* baseline) while "no treatment" did not (change in score 4.9%, not significant).

Negative Ion Generators

The environmental concentration of negative air ions varies greatly (for example, it is higher in humid, vegetated environments and at the seashore, and lower in urban environments and heated or air conditioned interiors).[332] It is thought that sustained exposure to negative air ionization may elevate mood, although no definitive mechanism of action for this effect has been established.[333]

One double-blind randomized controlled trial involved only 25 patients with SAD, who received negative ions from an electronic device for 30 minutes shortly after rising (between 5.30 am and 8.30 am), for 20 days, at one of two doses.[354] More of those who received the higher density of ions achieved remission (58% with 2.7 × 106 ions/cm^3 *v* 15% with 104 ions/cm^3, P = 0.025).

What do Guidelines Say?

American Psychiatric Association guidelines published in 2000 suggest that the entire range of treatments for major depressive disorder may also be used to treat patients with SAD, either in combination with, or as an alternative to, light therapy.[355] As first-line treatment, the guidelines recommend light therapy as a time-limited trial, primarily in out-patients with clear seasonal patterns of symptoms. For patients with more severe depression, the guidelines recommend light therapy as a potential adjunct to psychopharmacologic intervention.

British Association for Psychopharmacology guidelines published in 2008 state that antidepressants are a first-line treatment for moderate and severe major depression in adults irrespective of depression type, and that CBT may be used in addition.[334] For SAD, the guidelines state that light therapy is a first-line acute treatment but that effective prophylaxis against relapse is then needed, including consideration of an antidepressant. The limited evidence available suggests that bupropion or CBT helps to prevent recurrence the following winter.

Canadian Network for Mood and Anxiety Treatments (CANMAT) guidelines published in October 2009 recommend "second-generation" antidepressants (e.g. SSRIs) or CBT first line for major depressive disorder, and medication plus CBT as second-line treatment.[356,357] For SAD, they recommend light therapy first-line.[341]

The final draft of the NICE guideline on depression in adults, updated for publication in October 2009, suggests that people with depression with a seasonal pattern should be treated according to the strategy offered in the guideline for major depressive disorder in general.[344] Recommendations include an antidepressant (normally an SSRI) or CBT for mild to moderate depression, or both for moderate or severe depression; and that CBT should be offered for relapse prevention. The draft guideline also states that although there are a large number of studies that address the efficacy of light therapy in people with seasonal depression, they are difficult to interpret due to methodological differences. It goes on to propose that patients with winter depression who wish to try light therapy in preference to antidepressant or psychological treatment should be advised that the evidence for the efficacy of such therapy is uncertain.

The various guidelines appear to have reached different conclusions about light therapy because they included different studies and analysed primary data or published meta-analyses.[358]

CONCLUSION

Seasonal affective disorder (SAD) describes a subtype of major depression which has a seasonal pattern (usually winter depression and remission or hypomania during spring and summer). It includes atypical symptoms such as hypersomnia, carbohydrate craving and weight gain. A common approach is to treat the condition as for non-seasonal depression, for example, using SSRI antidepressants and/or cognitive behavioral therapy (CBT).

Light therapy has been suggested for treating people with SAD. Trials of such therapy are complex as they need a plausible control arm, and methodological differences between published trials have made the results hard to interpret. In addition, reviews and guidelines of light therapy have included different trials and reached contradictory conclusions. Nevertheless, bright light therapy in the early morning, using a light box or dawn simulation, appears to be a reasonable first-line approach to relieve depressive symptoms, instead of, or as well as, drug therapy and/or CBT when the patient has mild or moderate symptoms; people with more severe symptoms should be treated with antidepressant drugs, with or without light therapy and/or CBT.

For prevention of subsequent episodes, there is limited evidence for a benefit of CBT or bupropion (an unlicensed indication in the UK)

46.21 CHOLINESTERASE INHIBITORS AND MEMANTINE FOR SYMPTOMATIC TREATMENT OF DEMENTIA

RK Solanki

WHAT ARE CHOLINESTERASE INHIBITORS AND MEMANTINE?

The most common types of dementia are Alzheimer's disease, vascular dementia, mixed dementia, dementia with Lewy bodies, and frontotemporal dementia. At present, four drugs are licensed in the UK for the management of Alzheimer's disease, the cholinesterase inhibitors (donepezil, rivastigmine, and galantamine) and memantine, a partial antagonist of N-Methyl-D-aspartate (NMDA) receptors (Table 30). The use of these drugs in other types of dementia has been investigated, with the most convincing evidence coming from studies of dementia with Lewy bodies and Parkinson's disease dementia. There is currently no evidence to support the use of cholinesterase inhibitors or memantine in frontotemporal dementia or mild cognitive impairment.

Cholinesterase inhibitors increase the availability of acetylcholine at the synaptic cleft by preventing its breakdown by the enzyme acetylcholinesterase. Galantamine also modulates nicotinic acetylcholine receptors, and rivastigmine inhibits butylcholinesterase, but the importance of these additional properties is unknown. Memantine is believed to act by reducing glutamate mediated excitotoxicity.

HOW WELL DO THEY WORK?

Cholinesterase Inhibitors in Mild-to-moderate Alzheimer's Disease

A 2008 systematic review and meta-analysis of placebo-controlled and comparative studies of donepezil, galantamine, and rivastigmine in Alzheimer's disease included 22 trials of

Table 30: Licensed indications for cholinesterase inhibitors and memantine in the UK

	Donepezil	*Rivastigmine*	*Galantamine*	*Memantine*
Mild Alzheimer's disease	Yes	Yes	Yes	No
Moderate Alzheimer's disease	Yes	Yes	Yes	Yes
Severe Alzheimer's disease:				
UK	No	No	No	Yes
US	Yes	No	No	Yes
Mild to moderate Parkinson's disease dementia	No	Yes	No	No
Vascular dementia	No	No	No	No
Mild cognitive impairment	No	No	No	No
Dementia with Lewy bodies	No	Yes	No	No
Frontotemporal dementia	No	No	No	No

good or fair quality. On a commonly used measure of cognition, the Alzheimer's disease assessment scale cognitive section (ADAS-cog), 14 studies showed that all three cholinesterase inhibitors showed a modest mean benefit of about 2.7 points (95% confidence interval 2.3–3.0) on the 70 point ADAS-cog compared with placebo after three to six months of treatment. Most studies reporting measures of function such as the Alzheimer's Disease Cooperative Study's activities of daily living inventory (ADCS/ADL), also significantly favored active treatment.[359] There is currently no evidence to support the use of one cholinesterase over another.

The clinical meaningfulness of the reported small changes on clinical scales is the subject of considerable controversy; one group suggests that a four point change over six months on the ADAS-cog scale is clinically important.[360] It has also been suggested that the apparent small mean improvements on clinical scales may be driven by a small percentage of patients deriving substantial benefit while the remainder do not benefit at all. Attempts to more accurately define characteristics of this group of potential responders are currently under way.

However, recent studies have considered response to treatment as "reduced worsening than expected if left untreated." A pooled data analysis from three randomized controlled trials using a definition of "clinical worsening" incorporating cognition, global outcome, and function reported that more placebo patients showed clinical worsening from baseline over the six month trial period compared with those taking donepezil (30% *v* 14%, giving a number needed to treat of six),[361] highlighting the possibility that apparent "nonresponders" are still able to derive benefit from treatment. Assessing multiple domains in this manner is, arguably, a more clinically meaningful outcome measure since it helps determine whether the patient's condition as a whole is deteriorating.

Cholinesterase Inhibitors in Severe Alzheimer's Disease

Donepezil is licensed in the US, but not the UK, for severe Alzheimer's disease. However, two separate randomized controlled trials in patients with severe Alzheimer's disease in community or nursing home settings found that donepezil significantly improved cognitive function and, in the nursing home study, preserved general function.[362,363] A more recent 2010 post hoc pooled analysis included three multinational randomized controlled trials of donepezil and reported significant benefits for patients with severe Alzheimer's disease on the severe impairment battery (SIB), a tool for assessing cognition in patients for whom floor effects (when everyone scores at the bottom of the scale) limit the use of the MMSE.[364] Similar findings have been published in a double blind, placebo-controlled study in 10 European countries for galantamine in severe Alzheimer's disease.[365] These data suggest that there are untreated patients with severe disease in the community and nursing home settings who could benefit from treatment. In the UK, however, use of cholinesterase inhibitors in severe disease remains outside current licence indications and guidance from the National Institute for Health and Clinical Excellence (NICE).

Current NICE guidance relating to cholinesterase inhibitors and memantine:[366,367]

- Donepezil, galantamine, and rivastigmine are recommended as options for management of mild-to-moderate Alzheimer's disease and for people with dementia with Lewy bodies who have noncognitive symptoms that cause significant distress to the individual
- Memantine is recommended as an option for severe Alzheimer's disease and for people with moderate Alzheimer's disease who are unable to take cholinesterase inhibitors

- Cholinesterase inhibitors and memantine are not recommended for use in patients with vascular dementia or mild cognitive impairment except as part of properly constructed clinical studies
- Treatment should be initiated by a specialist in the care of patients with dementia, and carers' views should be sought
- Treatment should continue only if thought to be having a worthwhile effect on cognitive, functional, or behavioral symptoms
- Patients continuing with treatment should be reviewed regularly either by a specialist or according to local shared care protocols
- Assessment of the severity of Alzheimer's disease should not rely purely on cognitive measures (such as the mini-mental state examination (MMSE).

MEMANTINE IN ALZHEIMER'S DISEASE

Contrary to a manufacturer sponsored analysis recommending memantine for mild Alzheimer's disease, a 2006 Cochrane review[369] and a 2011 independent meta-analysis[11] found no difference between memantine and placebo on any cognitive measure.

In moderate-to-severe Alzheimer's disease, for which memantine is licensed in the UK, a Cochrane review of data from three pooled randomized controlled trials supported a beneficial effect at six months on cognition (2.97 points on the 100 point severe impairment battery (95% confidence interval 1.68–4.26), P < 0.0001), activities of daily living, and behavior which was detectable clinically.[368]

The available randomized controlled trials examining the effect of adding memantine for patients whose Alzheimer's disease was already stabilized with cholinesterase inhibitors provide conflicting evidence.[369] In a study of 404 patients who had been stabilized for six months with donepezil, the addition of memantine for six months produced a statistically significant improvement over placebo on cognition, global measures, and activities of daily living.[370] In a subsequent study of patients with mild or moderate Alzheimer's disease stabilized with any cholinesterase inhibitor, addition of memantine was no better than placebo on various assessments.[371] More recently, the DOMINO study—a 12 month, double blind, randomized controlled trial of people with moderate to severe Alzheimer's disease already taking donepezil—reported no significant benefit of the combination of donepezil and memantine compared with donepezil alone in terms of cognitive or functional measures.[372]

LONG-TERM TREATMENT

It is difficult to draw firm conclusions about long-term treatment as most controlled treatment trials average six months. Generalizability of data from the longest running placebo-controlled trial published[373] was limited by the multiple washout design and high drop-out rate (70%) and was excluded from the Cochrane review. However, the DOMINO study reported that continuation of donepezil was associated with greater cognitive and functional benefit over 12 months compared with discontinuation (1.9 points (1.3–2.5), P < 0.001) on the standardized MMSE.[372]

VASCULAR DEMENTIA

A meta-analysis of eight large randomized controlled trials of antidementia drugs (three of donepezil, two of galantamine, one of rivastigmine, and two of memantine; trial duration 24–28 weeks; including both published and unpublished data) in patients with vascular dementia reported modest but significant cognitive effects in favor of cholinesterase inhibitors based on the ADAS-cog (or VaDAS-cog) measure in all trials, ranging from −1.10 (−2.15 to −0.05) points for rivastigmine to −2.17 (−2.98 to −1.35) points for donepezil, similar to that reported in trials in Alzheimer's disease.[374] However, there was no consistent benefit in terms of global measures or activities of daily living, and patients in the cholinesterase inhibitor (but not memantine) treatment arms had a significantly increased risk of adverse events compared with placebo groups.

Although current evidence has led to the approval of antidementia drugs for use in Alzheimer's disease but not in vascular dementia, many patients in clinical practice have both Alzheimer's disease and cerebrovascular pathology; several population based studies of autopsy results have identified the most common pathological substrate for dementia is combined Alzheimer's pathology and cerebrovascular disease.[375] Most industry sponsored trials of cholinesterase inhibitors have concentrated on rigid diagnoses of either Alzheimer's disease or vascular dementia to the exclusion of many "real life" patients who have overlapping pathology and multiple comorbidities. Subanalyses of patients with mixed dementia suggest that those with Alzheimer's disease plus cerebrovascular disease benefit from treatment with cholinesterase inhibitors: for example, a large randomized controlled trial of galantamine included 592 patients with mild to moderate vascular dementia or Alzheimer's disease plus cerebrovascular disease and reported improvements in cognitive and global functioning over six months in the latter group of a similar magnitude to that reported in the trials of Alzheimer's disease.[376] Clinicians should thus not be dissuaded from treating patients with Alzheimer's disease who also have vascular risk factors or pathology.

DEMENTIA WITH LEWY BODIES AND PARKINSON'S DISEASE DEMENTIA

Dementia with Lewy bodies and Parkinson's disease dementia are overlapping clinicopathological conditions existing within a spectrum of Lewy body disorders and are both associated with marked cholinergic deficits. A randomized controlled trial of rivastigmine in dementia with Lewy bodies included 120 participants with an MMSE score ≥10 and reported significant treatment benefits on measures of neuropsychiatric symptoms, but not on cognitive or global measures, over 20 weeks.[377] In a subsequent 24 week trial of 541 participants with mild to moderate Parkinson's disease dementia, the number needed to treat for significant improvement or avoidance of clinically significant worsening on global measures was seven.[378] Trials of memantine in patients with either Parkinson's disease dementia or dementia with Lewy bodies have reported similar results: one study of a combined group of patients with dementia with Lewy bodies or with Parkinson's disease dementia reported improvements in global outcomes (mean difference of 0.7 points on the Alzheimer's disease assessment scale clinicians' global impression of change (ADAS-CGIC), P = 0.03),[379] while a second study reported improved global outcomes in dementia with Lewy bodies but not Parkinson's disease dementia.[380]

At present, only rivastigmine is licensed for use in Parkinson's disease dementia, and neither cholinesterase inhibitors nor memantine are licensed for use in dementia with Lewy bodies. NICE guidance does not refer to dementia with Lewy bodies or Parkinson's disease dementia with respect to treatment of cognitive symptoms with cholinesterase inhibitors or memantine, but recommends use of cholinesterase inhibitors for treatment of noncognitive symptoms in dementia with Lewy bodies and suggests that the recommendations may be useful when considering treatments for Parkinson's disease dementia. The evidence suggests that it is appropriate to offer patients with dementia with Lewy bodies or with Parkinson's disease dementia a trial of a cholinesterase inhibitor. It is also worth noting that many patients with dementia with Lewy bodies or Parkinson's disease dementia also have noticeable Alzheimer's disease pathology,[381] and many patients in the clinical setting will have mixed pathology.

HOW SAFE ARE THEY?

Cholinesterase Inhibitors

The meta-analysis from the 2006 Cochrane review of cholinesterase inhibitors in Alzheimer's disease showed that patients in treatment arms were more likely than those in placebo arms to report a single adverse event (number need to harm of seven) and that donepezil was associated with fewer adverse events than the other cholinesterase inhibitors.[382] A meta-analysis of trials of cholinesterase inhibitors and memantine showed that cholinesterase inhibitors were associated with an increased risk of syncope (odds ratio 1.53 (95% confidence interval 1.02–2.30), number needed to harm = 143) but not falls.[383]

Memantine

Overall, memantine is associated with fewer and less serious side effects than the cholinesterase inhibitors. Meta-analysis shows similar rates of withdrawal due to adverse events in memantine and placebo arms.[368]

WHAT ARE THE PRECAUTIONS?

Cholinesterase Inhibitors

Most adverse effects of cholinesterase inhibitors arise from direct cholinergic effects or via increased vagal tone. Importantly, this necessitates caution in the presence of sick sinus syndrome and atrioventricular block. Caution is advised in patients with chronic obstructive pulmonary disease or asthma, urinary retention, and those with a history of peptic ulcer, although these are not absolute contraindications and many patients with these conditions can be successfully prescribed cholinesterase inhibitors. Depending on the nature and severity of the condition, it may be necessary to request relevant specialist advice, and memantine is an alternative option in many cases.

Table 31: Cholinesterase inhibitor and memantine preparations

	Tablet	*Capsule*	*Orodispersible tablet*	*Oral solution*	*Transdermal patch*
Donepezil	Yes 23 mg in US	—	Yes	—	—
Galantamine	Yes*	Yes	—	Yes*	—
Rivastigmine	—	Yes*	—	Yes*	Yes
Memantine†	Yes	—	—	Yes	—

*Twice daily dosing required; all other preparations are administered once daily
†Previously 10 mg twice daily, now 20 mg once daily

The most common adverse effects of the cholinesterase inhibitors are nausea, vomiting, diarrhea, abdominal pain, anorexia, and dizziness, and these can generally be reduced by dose titration. The rivastigmine transdermal patch is associated with reduced gastrointestinal adverse events compared with the capsule formulation.[384]

Although there are potential synergistic or additive interactions between cholinesterase inhibitors and other drugs that may slow heart rate, there is no indication to routinely stop digoxin or atenolol before a cholinesterase inhibitor can be prescribed. All cholinesterase inhibitors will interfere with the effects of anticholinergic drugs and may exaggerate the effects of muscle relaxants used during anesthesia.

A comprehensive review of the available data on cardiovascular adverse events concluded that serious events were rare and outlined a clinical protocol that included screening and monitoring using pulse rate in asymptomatic, nonbradycardic patients.[385]

Memantine

Other than hypersensitivity to the drug or its excipients, there are no absolute contraindications to memantine. Although caution is advised when there is a history of seizure, the effect of memantine on seizure activity has not been systematically evaluated, and animal studies suggest that it may have both pro-convulsant and anticonvulsant effects mediated via the NMDA receptor system.

The most common side effects of memantine are constipation, dizziness, headache, hypertension, and somnolence.

How are They Taken and Monitored?

Memantine and cholinesterase inhibitors are available in a variety of preparations (Table 31). Start these drugs at low doses and gradually titrate up to minimize the risk of adverse events. Individualize treatment plans according to comorbidities (see section on precautions). Patients taking cholinesterase inhibitors should have their pulse checked regularly, although there are no clear data on which to base the frequency of monitoring. One clinical protocol suggests that this should be monthly during dose titration and then six monthly.[385] There are no data to support routine use of electrocardiography before starting treatment.

REFERENCES

Newer Antidepressants for the Treatment of Depression in Adults

1. NHS Information Centre for Health and Social Care. www.ic.nhs.uk/services/prescribing-support-unit-psu/using-the-service/reports-publications-and-presentations/reports/national-prescribing-costs-and-items
2. Nutt D. Beyond psychoanaleptics—can we improve antidepressant drug nomenclature? J Psychopharmacol. 2009;23:343-5.
3. National Institute for Health and Clinical Excellence. The treatment and management of depression in adults (update). (Clinical guideline 90.) 2009. http://guidance.nice.org.uk/CG90.
4. Hetrick SE, McKenzie JE, Merry SN. The use of SSRIs in childhood and adolescents. Curr Opin Psychiatry. 2010;23(1): 53-7.
5. Reid S, Barbui C. Long term treatment of depression with selective serotonin reuptake inhibitors and newer antidepressants. BMJ. 2010;340:c1468.
6. Moore M, Yuen HM, Dunn N, Mulee MA, Maskell J, Kendrick T. Explaining the rise in antidepressant prescribing: a descriptive study using general practice research database. BMJ. 2009;339:b3999.
7. Pagura J, Katz LY, Mojtabai R, Druss BG, Cox B, Sareen J. Antidepressant use in the absence of common mental disorders in the general population. J Clin Psychiatry. 2011;72:494-501.
8. Arroll B, Khin N, Kerse N. Screening for depression in primary care with two verbally asked questions: cross sectional study. BMJ. 2003;327:1144-6.
9. Nease DE, Malouin JM. Depression screening: a practical strategy. J Fam Pract. 2003;52:118-26.
10. Arroll B, Goodyear-Smith F, Kerse N, Hwang M, Crengle S, Gunn J, et al. The prevalence of depression among Maori patients in Auckland general practice. J Primary Health Care. 2009;1(1):26-9.
11. Macarthur Foundation. www.depression-primarycare.org. 2009.
12. Bjelland I, Dahl AA, Haug TT, Neckelmann D. The validity of the hospital anxiety and depression scale. An updated literature review. J Psychosomatic Research. 2002;52(2):69-77.
13. Gilbody S, Bower P, Fletcher J, Richards D, Sutton AJ. Collaborative care for depression: a cumulative meta-analysis and review of longer-term outcomes. Arch Intern Med. 2006;166:2314-21.
14. Wu P, Fuller C, Liu X, Lee H-C, Fan B, Hoven CW, et al. Use of complementary and alternative medicine among women with depression: results of a national survey. Psychiatric Services. 2007;58:349-56.
15. Kirsch I, Deacon BJ, Huedo-Medina TB, Scoboria A, Moore TJ, Johnson BT. Initial severity and antidepressant benefits: a meta-analysis of data submitted to the Food and Drug Administration. PLoS Med. 2008;5(2):e45.
16. Horder J, Matthews P, Waldmann R. Placebo, Prozac and PLoS: significant lessons for psychopharmacology. J Psychopharmacol2010; http://jop.sagepub.com/content/25/10/1277.
17. Fountoulakis KN, Moller H-J. Efficacy of antidepressants: a re-analysis and re-interpretation of the Kirsch data. Int J Neuropsychopharmacol. 2011;14:405-12.
18. Fournier JC, DeRubeis RJ, Hollon SD, Dimidjian S, Amsterdam JD, Shelton RC, et al. Antidepressant drug effects and

depression severity: a patient-level meta-analysis. JAMA. 2010;303:47-53.

19. Cameron IM, Cardy A, Crawford JR, du Toit SW, Hay S, Lawton K, et al. Measuring depression severity in general practice: discriminatory performance of the PHQ-9, HADS-D and BDI-II. Br J Gen Pract. 2011;61(588):e419-26.
20. Cipriani A, Furukawa T, Salanti G, Geddes J, Higgins J, Churchill R, et al. Comparative efficacy and acceptability of 12 new-generation antidepressants: a multiple-treatments meta-analysis. Lancet. 2009;373:746-58.
21. Gartlehner G, Hansen RA, Morgan LC, Thaler K, Lux L, van Noord M, et al. Comparative benefits and harms of second generation antidepressants for treating major depressive disorder. Ann Intern Med. 2011;155:772-85.
22. Eyding D, Lelgemann M, Grouven U, Harter M, Kromp M, Kaiser T, et al. Reboxetine for acute treatment of major depression: systematic review and meta-analysis of published and unpublished placebo and selective serotonin reuptake inhibitor controlled trials. BMJ. 2010;341:c4737.
23. Gartlehner G, Thieda P, Hansen RA, Gaynes BN, Deveaugh-Geiss A, Krebs EE, et al. Comparative risk for harms of second-generation antidepressants: a systematic review and meta-analysis. Drug Safety. 2008;31:851-65.
24. Lam RW, Kennedy SH, Grigoriadis S, McIntyre RS, Milev R, Ramasubbu R, et al. Canadian Network for Mood and Anxiety Treatments (CANMAT) clinical guidelines for the management of major depressive disorder in adults, 3rd edition. Pharmacotherapy. J Affect Disord. 2009;117(Suppl 1):S26-43.
25. Coupland C, Dhiman P, Morriss R, Arthur A, Barton G, Hippisley-Cox J. Antidepressant use and risk of adverse outcomes in older people: population based cohort study. BMJ. 2011;343:d4551.
26. Mark TL, Joish VN, Hay JW, Sheehan DV, Johnston SS, Cao Z. Antidepressant use in geriatric populations: The burden of side effects and interactions and their impact on adherence and costs. Am J Geriatric Psychiatry. 2011;19:211-21.
27. Gentile S, Galbally M. Prenatal exposure to antidepressant medications and neurodevelopmental outcomes: a systematic review. J Affect Disord. 2011;128:1-9.
28. National Institute for Health and Clinical Excellence. Antenatal and postnatal mental health: clinical management and service guidance (Clinical guideline 45.) 2007. http://guidance.nice.org.uk/CG45.
29. Depression, antidepressants and heart disease. Drug Ther Bull. 2008;46(4):29-32.
30. Andrade C, Sandarsh S, Chethan KB, Nagesh KS. Serotonin reuptake inhibitor antidepressants and abnormal bleeding: a review for clinicians and a reconsideration of mechanisms. J Clin Psychiatry. 2010;71:1565-75.
31. Kendrick T, Chatwin J, Dowrick C, Tylee A, Morriss R, Peveler R, et al. Randomised controlled trial to determine the clinical effectiveness and cost-effectiveness of selective serotonin reuptake inhibitors plus supportive care, versus supportive care alone, for mild to moderate depression with somatic symptoms in primary care: the THREAD (THREshold for AntiDepressant response) study. Health Technol Assess. 2009; 13(22).
32. Arroll B, Elley CR, Fishman T, Goodyear-Smith FA, Kenealy T, Blashki G, et al. Antidepressants versus placebo for depression in primary care. Cochrane Database Syst Rev. 2009;3:CD007954.
33. Hawton K, Bergen H, Simkin S, Cooper J, Waters K, Gunnell D, et al. Toxicity of antidepressants: rates of suicide relative to prescribing and non-fatal overdose. Br J Psychiatry. 2010;196:354-8.
34. Taylor MJ, Freemantle N, Geddes JR, Bhagwagar Z. Early onset of selective serotonin reuptake inhibitor antidepressant action: systematic review and meta-analysis. Arch Gen Psychiatry. 2006;63:1217-23.
35. Connolly KR, Thase ME. If at first you don't succeed: a review of the evidence for antidepressant augmentation, combination and switching strategies. Drugs. 2011;71(1):43-64.

Psychosurgery

36. National Commission for the Protection of Human Education and Welfare. 1977, Part III, USA.
37. Balasubramaniam V. Psychosurgery in India and Abroad.Col. Pandalai Oration. Indian J Surgery. 1976;(Conference number): 271-4.
38. Valenstein ES. In: Valenstein ES (Ed). The Psychosurgery Debate. San Francisco: Freeman and Company, 1980.
39. Govindaswamy MV, Balakrishana Rao DN. Bilateral frontal leucotomy in Indian patients. Lancet. 1944;1:466-8.
40. Nambiar KC. Some Researchers and Thoughts. (Private Publication), 1954.
41. Fulton JF, Jacobsen F. The functions of the frontal lobes: A comparitive study in monkey, chimpanzee and man. II International Neurological Congress, London. 1935.pp.70-1.
42. Lima A. In: Paul C Bucy (Ed). Egas Moniz in Neurosurgical Giants: Feet of Clay and Iron. New York: Elsevier, 1985.
43. Spiegel EA, Wyeis HT. Pallidothalamotomy in Chorea. Arch Neurol Psychiatry. 1950;64:295-6.
44. Papez JW. A proposed mechanism of emotion. Arch Neurol Psychiatry. 1937;38:725-44.
45. Balasubramaniam V, Kanaka TS. Behavioural brain: A physiological concept. Proceedings of the Institute of Neurology, Madras. 1979;8:4-21.
46. Fulton JF. Functional Localisation in the Frontal Lobes and Cerebellum. London: Oxford University Press, 1949.
47. Freeman W, Watts JM. Psychosurgery in the Treatment of Mental Disorders and Intractable Pain. Springfield, Illinois: Charles C Thomas, 1950.
48. Scovile WB. Late results of orbital undercutting. Am J Psychiatry. 1960;117:525-532.
49. Knight GC. Stereotactic tracotomy in the surgical treatment of mental illness. J Neurol Neurosurg Psychiatry. 1965;28: 304-10.

50. Freeman W. Frontal lobotomy in early schizophrenia. In: Hitchcock E, Laitinen L, Vaernet K (Eds). Psychosurgery. Springfield, Illinois: Charles C Thomas, 1972.
51. Knight GC. Bifrontal stereotaxic tractomy in the substanti-ainnominata. In: Hitchcock E, Laitinen L, Vaernet K (Eds). Psychosurgery. Springfield, Illinois: Charles C Thomas, 1972.
52. Hirose S. The case selection of mental disorder for orbitovental medial undercutting. In: Hitchcock E, Laitinen L, Vaernet K (Eds). Psychosurgery. Springfield, Illinois: Charles C Thomas, 1972.
53. Kalyanaraman S, Ramamurthi B. Stereotaxic basofrontal tractotomy. Neurol India. 1973;21:113-8.
54. Balasubramaniam V. In Psychosurgery. Madras: Private Publication, 1989.
55. Scoville WB. Psychosurgery and other lesions of the brain affecting human behaviour. In: Hitchcock E, Laitinen L, Vaernet K (Eds). Psychosurgery. Springfield, Illinois: Charles C Thomas, 1972.
56. Foltz EL, White LE. Pain relief by frontal cingulumotomy. J Neurosurg. 1962;19: 89-100.
57. Ballantine Jr. HT, Cassidy WL, Flanagan NB, et al. Stereotaxic anterior cingulumotomy for neuropsychiatric illness and intractable pain. J Neurosurg. 1967;26:488-95.
58. Balasubramaniam V, Kanaka TS, Ramanujam PB. Stereotaxic cingulumotomy for drug addiction. Neurol India. 1973;21: 65-6.
59. Roy TK. Stereotactic cingulate lesions for intractable pain in malignant conditions: A report of five cases. Neurol India. 1983;31:55-8.
60. Dole VP, Nyswander ME. Heroin addiction: A metabolic disease. Arch Int Med. 1987;120:19-25.
61. Gaches J, Le Beau J, Choppy M. Psychosurgery in severe obsessive syndromes. In: Hitchcock E, Laitinen L, Vaernet K (Eds). Psychosurgery. Springfield, Illinois: Charles C Thomas, 1972.
62. Laitinen LV, Vikki J. Stereotaxic ventral anterior cingulumotomy in some psychological disorders. In: Hitchcock E, Laitinen L, Vaernet K (Eds). Psychosurgery. Springfield, Illinois: Charles C Thomas. 1972.
63. Viruthagirinathan BS, Balasubramanium V, Kanaka TS. Psychological appraisal in drug addiction. Neurol India. 1983; 31:37-40.
64. Balasubramanium V. Vistas in stereotaxic surgery. Neurol India. 1986;34:225-40.
65. Balasubramanium V, Chidambaram B. Stereotaxic cingulumotomy-Second look. Neurol India. 1990;38:559-62.
66. Sano K. Sedative stereoencephalotomy, fornicotomy, upper mesencephalic reticulotomy and posteromedial hypothalamotomy. In: Tokizane T, Schade JP (Eds). Progress in Brain Research: Correlative neurosciences. Part B. Clinical studies. Amsterdam: Elsevier. 1966.pp.350-72.
67. MacLean PD. The hypothalamus and emotional behaviour. In: Haymaker W, Anderson E, Nauta WJH (Eds). The Hypothalamus. Springfield, Illinois: Charles C Thomas, 1969.
68. Cannon WB, Britton SW. Studies on the conditions of activity in endocrine glands. XV. Pseudo-affective medulloadrenal secretion. Am J Physiol. 1925;72:283-90.
69. Brown S, Schafer EA. An investigation into the function of the occipital and temporal lobe of the monkey's brain. Trans Roy Phil Soc. 1988;1798:303.
70. Kluver H, Bucy PC. Preliminary analysis of functions of the temporal lobes in monkeys. Arch Neurol Psychiatry. 1939;42: 979-1000.
71. Narabayashi H, Nagao T, Saito Y, et al. Stereotaxic amygdalotomy in behavioural disorders. Arch Neurol. 1963;9:1-16.
72. Balasubramaniam V, Ramamurthi B, Jaganathan K, et al. Stereotaxic amygdalotomy. Neurol India. 1967;15:115-221.
73. Balasubramaniam V, Ramamurthi B. Stereotaxic amygdalotomy for behaviour disorders. Confinia Neurologica. 1970;32:367-72.
74. Balasubramaniam V, Kanaka TS, Ramanujam PB, et al. Stereotaxic Hypothalamotomy. Indian J Surg. 1971;33:227-30.
75. Balasubramanium V, Kanaka TS, Ramanujam PB, et al. Stereotaxic surgery for behaviour disorders. In: Hitchcock E, Laitinen L, Vaernet K (Eds). Psychosurgery. Springfield, Illinois: Charles C Thomas, 1972.
76. Balasubramanium V, Kanka TS, Ramanujam PB, et al. Stereotaxic hypothalamotomy. Confinia Neurologica. 1973;35: 138-43.
77. Balasubramanium V. In: Human Aggression. Private Publication, Madras, 1989.
78. Balasubramaniam V, Kanaka TS. Why hemispherectomy? ApplNeurophysiol. 1975;38:197-205.
79. Niemeyer P. Trasventricular amygdala hippocampectomy in temporal lobe epilepsy. In: Baldwin M, Baiky P (Eds). Temporal Lobe Epilepsy. Illinois: Charles C Thomas, 1968.
80. Yasargill MS, Wieser HC. Selective amygdalohippocampectomy at the University Hospital, Zurich. In: Engel Jr. J (Ed). Surgical Treatment of Epilepsy. New York: Raven Press. 1987.
81. Balsubramaniam V, Kanaka TS. Amygdalotomy and hypothalamotomy: A comparative study. Proceedings of the Institute of Neurology, Madras. 1973;3:67-74.
82. Balasubramaniam V, Kanaka TS. Amygdalotomy and hypothalamotomy. A comparative study. Confinia Neurologica. 1975;37: 195-201.
83. Narabayashi H. Stereotaxic amygdalatomy. In: Eleftherious BE. (Ed). Neurobiology of the Amygdala. New York: Plenum, 1972.
84. Ramachandran V, Balasubramaniam V, Kanaka TS. Follow up of patients treated with stereotaxic surgery. Indian J Psychiatry. 1974;16:295-300.
85. Levkowitz Y, Ng M. Transcranial magnetic stimulation and antidepressive drugs share similar cellular effects in rat hippocampus, Neuropsychopharmacology. 2001;24:608-16.
86. Limousin P, Krack P, Pollak P, Benazzouz A, Ardouin C, Hoffmann D, Benabid AL. Electrical stimulation of the subthalamic nucleus in advanced Parkinson's disease. N Engl J Med. 1998;339:1105-11.

87. Lindquist C, Kihlstrom L, Hellstrand E. Functional neurosurgery—a future for the gamma knife? Stereotact. Funct. Neurosurg. 1991;57:72-81.
88. MacLean PD. Psychosomatic disease and the bivisceral brain Q: recent developments bearing on the Papez theory of emotion, Psychosom. Med. 1949;11:338-53.
89. Mairet A. De la demence melancolique: contribution a l'etude de la periencephalite localisee, et a le'etude des localisations cerebrales d'ordre psychique, Paris & Masson, 1883.
90. Malhi GS, Sachdev P. Novel physical treatments for the management of neuropsychiatric disorders, J Psychosom Res. 2002;53:709-19.
91. Mallet L, Mesnage V, Houeto JL, Pelissolo A, Yelnik J, Behar C, Gargiulo M, Welter ML, Bonnet AM, Pillon B, Cornu P, Dormont D, Pidoux B, Allilaire JF, Agid Y. Compulsions, Parkinson's disease, and stimulation, Lancet. 2002;360:1302-4.
92. Mark VH, Ervin FR. Violence and the Brain, Harper & Row, New York, 1970.
93. Martuza RL, Chiocca EA, Jenike MA, Giriuna IE, Ballantine HT. Stereotactic radiofrequency thermal cingulotomy for obsessive compulsive disorder, J Neuropsychiatry Clin Neurosci. 1990;2:331-6.
94. Mayberg HS, Starkstein SE, Sadzot B, Preziosi T, Andrezejewski PL, Dannals RF, Wagner Jr HN, Robinson RG, Selective hypometabolism in the inferior frontal lobe in depressed patients with Parkinson's disease. Ann Neurol. 1990;28:57-64.
95. Mayberg HS, Starkstein SE, Peyser CE, Brandt J, Dannals RF, Folstein SE. Paralimbic frontal lobe hypometabolism in depression associated with Huntington's disease. Neurology. 1992;42:1791-7.
96. Milner B. Effects of different brain lesions on card sorting. Arch. Neurol. 1963;9:90-100.
97. Mindus P, Edman G, Andreewitch S. A prospective, long-term study of personality traits in patients with intractable obsessional illness treated by capsulotomy. Acta Psychiatr. Scand. 1999;99:40-50.
98. Moniz E. Essai d'un traitement chirugical de certaine psychoses, Bull. Acad. Med. 1936;115:385-93.
99. Moniz E. Prefrontal leucotomy in the treatment of mental disorders. Am J Psychiatry. 1937;93:1379-85.
100. Montoya A, Weiss AP, Price BH, Cassem EH, Dougherty DD, Nierenberg A, Rauch SL, Cosgrove GR. Magnetic resonance imaging-guided stereotactic limbic leukotomy for treatment of intractable psychiatric disease. Neurosurgery. 2002;50: 1043-9.
101. National Omission for the Protection of Human Subjects of Biomedical and Behavioral Research. Use of psychosurgery in practice and research: report and recommendations of National Commission for the Protection of Human Subjects of Biomedical and Behavioral Research. Fed Regist. 1977;42:26318-32.
102. New World. Future of psychosurgery in doubt. Nature. 1973; 224:128-9.
103. JM Nielsen, LL Jacobs. Bilateral lesions of the anterior cingulated gyri Bull Los Angel Neurol Soc. 1951;16:231-4.
104. Nuttin B, Cosyns P, Demeulemeester H, Gybels J, Meyerson B. Electrical stimulation in the anterior limbs of the internal capsules in patients with obsessive-compulsive disorder. Lancet. 1999;354:1526.
105. Nuttin B, Gybels J, Cosyns P, Gabriels L, Meyerson B, Andreewitch S, Rasmussen S, Greenberg B, Friehs G, Rezai AR, Montgomery E, Malone D, Fins JJ. Deep brain stimulation for psychiatric disorders, Neurosurg Clin N Am. 2003;14:xv–xvi.
106. Papez JW. A proposed mechanism of emotion. Arch Neurol Psychiatry. 1937;38:725-43.
107. Pascual-Leone A, Catala MD, Pascual AP. Lateralized effect of rapid-rate transcranial magnetic stimulation of the prefrontal cortex on mood. Neurology. 1996;46:499-502.
108. Penfield W, Evans J. The frontal lobe in man: a clinical study of maximal removals. Brain. 1935;58:115-33.
109. Price BH, Adams RD, Coyle JT. Neurology and psychiatry: closing the great divide. Neurology. 2000;54:8-14.
110. Price BH, Baral I, Cosgrove GR, Rauch SL, Nierenberg AA, Jenike MA, Cassem EH. Improvement in severe self-mutilation following limbic leucotomy: a series of 5 consecutive cases. J Clin Psychiatry. 2001;62:925-32.
111. Puusepp L. Alcune considerazioni sugli interventi chirugici nelle malattie mentali, G. Accad. Med. Torino. 1937;100:3-16.
112. Robinson D, Wu H, Munne LA, Ashtari M, Alvir JM, Lerner G, KoreenA,ColeK,BogertsB.Reducedcaudatevolumeinobsessive-compulsive disorder. Arch Gen Psychiatry. 1995;52: 393-8.
113. Rodgers JE. Psychosurgery: Damaging the Brain to Save the Mind, Harper-Collins, New York. 1992.
114. Rossi F, Cattaneo E. Opinion: neural stem cell therapy for neurologic diseases: dreams and reality. Nat Rev Neuroscience. 2002;3;401-9.

Drug Treatment of Alzheimer's Disease

115. Ferri CP, Prince M, Brayne C, et al. Global prevalence of dementia: a Delphi consensus study. Lancet. 2005;336:2112-7.
116 Diagnostic and statistical manual of mental disorders text revision, 4th edition. DSM-IV. Washington, DC: American Psychiatric Association; 2000.
117. Kawas CH. Early Alzheimer's disease. N Engl J Med. 2003;349:1056-63.
118. McKhann G, Drachman D, Folstein M, Katzman R, Price D, Stadlan EM. Clinical diagnosis of Alzheimer's disease: report of the NINCDS-ADRDA Work Group under the auspices of Department of Health and Human Services Task Force on Alzheimer's Disease. Neurology. 1984;34:939-44.
119. Greene JD, Baddeley AD, Hodges JR. Analysis of the episodic memory deficit in early Alzheimer's disease: evidence from the doors and people test. Neuropsychologia. 1996;34:537-51.
120. Pillon B, Deweer B, Agid Y, Dubois B. Explicit memory in Alzheimer's, Huntington's, and Parkinson's diseases. Arch Neurol. 1993;50:374-9.

121. Price BH, Gurvit H, Weintraub S, Geula C, Leimkuhler E, Me-sulam M. Neuropsychological patterns and language deficits in 20 consecutive cases of autopsy confirmed Alzheimer's disease. Arch Neurol. 1993;50:931-7.
122. Esteban-Santillan C, Praditsu-wan R, Ueda H, Geldmacher DS. Clock drawing test in very mild Alzheimer's disease. J Am Geriatr Soc. 1998;46:1266-9.
123. Kirk A, Kertesz A. On drawing impairment in Alzheimer's disease. Arch Neurol. 1991;48:73-7.
124. Galasko D, Bennett DA, Sano K, et al. An inventory to assess activities of daily living for clinical trials in Alzheimer's disease: the Alzheimer's Disease Cooperative Study. Alzheimer Dis Assoc Disord. 1997;11:S33-S39.
125. Mega MS, Cummings JL, Fiorello T, Gornbein J. The spectrum of behavioral changes in Alzheimer's disease. Neurology. 1996;46:130-5.
126. Knopman DS, DeKosky ST, Cummings JL, et al. Practice parameter: diagnosis of dementia (an evidence-based review): report of the Quality Standards Subcommittee of the American Academy of Neurology. Neurology. 2001;56:1143-53.
127. Silverman DH, Small GW, Chang CY, et al. Positron emission tomography in evaluation of dementia: regional brain metabolism and long-term outcome. JAMA. 2001; 286:2120-7.
128. Hock C, Konietzko U, Streffer JR, et al. Antibodies against beta-amyloid slow cognitive decline in Alzheimer's disease. Neuron. 2003;38:547-54.
129. Schenk D, Barbour R, Dunn W, et al. Immunization with amyloid-β attenuates Alzheimer's disease like pathology in the PDAPP mouse. Nature. 1999;400:173-9.
130. Orgogozo JM, Gilman S, Dartigues JF, et al. Subacute meningoencephalitis in a subset of patients with AD after A beta42 immunization. Neurology. 2014;61:46-54.
131. Wolfe MS. Therapeutic strategies for Alzheimer's disease. Nat Rev Drug Discov. 2002;1:859-66.
132. Seimers ER, Quinn JL, Kaye J, et al. Effect of LY450139, a functional g-secretase inhibitor on plasma and cerebrospinal fluid concentrations of Ab and cognitive functioning in patients with mild to moderate Alzheimer's disease. Am Acad Neurol 2004;101(Suppl):S17.
133. Petanceska SS, DeRosa S, Olm V, et al. Statin therapy for Alzheimer's disease: will it work? J Mol Neurosci. 2002; 19:155-61.
134. Windisch M, Hutter-Paier B, Rockenstein E, Hashimoto M, Mallory M, Masliah E. Development of a new treatment for Alzheimer's disease and Parkinson's disease using anti-aggregatory beta synuclein derived peptides. J Mol Neurosci. 2002;19:63-9.
135. Sano M, Ernesto C, Thomas RG, et al. A controlled trial of selegiline, alpha-tocopherol, or both as treatment for Alzheimer's disease. N Engl J Med. 1997;336:1216-22.
136. Engelhart MJ, Geerlings MI, Ruitenberg A, et al. Dietary intake of antioxidants and risk of Alzheimer disease. JAMA. 2012;287:3223-9.
137. Esposito E, Rotilio D, Di Matteo V, Di Giulio C, Cacchio M, Algeri S. A review of specific dietary antioxidants and the effects on biochemical mechanisms related to neurodegenerative processes. Neurobiol Aging. 2002;23:719-35.
138. Zandi PP, Anthony JC, Khachaturian AS, et al. Reduced risk of Alzheimer disease in users of antioxidant vitamin supplements: the Cache County Study. Arch Neurol. 2004;61:82-8.
139. Parsons CG, Danysz W, Quack G. Memantine is a clinically well tolerated N-methyl-D-aspartate (NMDA) receptor antagonist a review of preclinical data. Neuropharmacology. 1999;38:735-67.
140. Reisberg B, Doody R, Stöffler A, Schmitt F, Ferris S, Möbius HJ. Memantine in moderate to severe Alzheimer's disease. N Engl J Med. 2003;348:1333-41.
141. Finch CE, Longo V, Miyao A, et al. Inflammation in Alzheimer's disease. In: Chesselet MF (Ed). Molecular mechanisms of neurodegenerative diseases. Totowa NJ: Humana Press; 2001. pp. 87-110.
142. Aisen PS, Davis KL, Berg JD, et al. A randomized controlled trial of prednisone in Alzheimer's disease. Neurology. 2000;54:588-93.
143. Scharf S, Mander A, Ugoni A, Vajda F, Christophidis N. A double-blind, placebo-controlled trial of diclofenac/misoprostol in Alzheimer's disease. Neurology. 1999;53:197-201.
144. Aisen PS, Schafer KA, Grundman M, et al. Effects of rofecoxib or naproxen vs placebo on Alzheimer's disease progression: a randomized controlled trial. JAMA. 2003;289:2819-26.
145. Henderson VW, Paganini Hill A, Miller BL, et al. Estrogen for Alzheimer's disease in women: randomized, double-blind, placebo-controlled trial. Neurology. 2000;54:295-301.
146. Mulnard RA, Cotman CW, Ka was C, et al. Estrogen replacement therapy for treatment of mild to moderate Alzheimer disease: a randomized controlled trial. JAMA. 2000;283:1007-15.
147. Doody RS, Stevens JC, Beck C, et al. Practice parameter: management of dementia (an evidence-based review): report of the Quality Standards Subcommittee of the American Academy of Neurology. Neurology. 2001;56:1154-66.
148. Small GW, Rabins PV, Barry PP, et al. Diagnosis and treatment of Alzheimer's disease and related disorders: consensus statement of the American Association of Geriatric Psychiatry, the Alzheimer's Association, and the American Geriatrics Society. JAMA. 1997;278:1363-71.
149. Watkins PB, Zimmerman HJ, Knapp MJ, Gracon SI, Lewis KW. Hepatotoxic effects of tacrine administration in patients with Alzheimer's disease. JAMA. 1994;271:992-8.
150. Cummings JL. Use of cholinesterase inhibitors in clinical practice: evidence-based recommendations. Am J Geriatr Psychiatry. 2003;11:131-45.
151. Tariot PN, Cummings J, Katz IR, et al. A randomized, double-blind, placebo-controlled study of the efficacy and safety of donepezil in patients with Alzheimer's disease in the nursing home setting. J Am Geriatr Soc. 2001;49:1590-9.
152. Rogers SL, Doody RS, Pratt RD, Ieni JR. Long-term efficacy and safety of donepezil in the treatment of Alzheimer's disease:

final analysis of a US multicentre open label study. Eur Neuropsychopharmacol. 2000;10:195-203.

153. Tariot PN, Farlow MR, Gro-ssberg GT, Graham SM, McDonald S, Gergel I. Memantine treatment in patients with moderate to severe Alzheimer disease already receiving donepezil: a randomized controlled trial. JAMA. 2004;291:317-24.
154. Oken BS, Storzbach DM, Kaye JA. The efficacy of Ginkgo biloba on cognitive function in Alzheimer disease. Arch Neurol. 1998;55:1409-15.
155. Cohen-Mansfield J. Nonpharmacologic interventions for inappropriate behaviors in dementia: a review, summary, and critique. Am J Geriatr Psychiatry. 2001;9:361-81.
156. Cohen-Mansfield J, Werner P. Management of verbally disruptive behaviors in nursing home residents. J Gerontol A Biol Sci Med Sci. 1997;52:M369-M377.
157. Katz IR, Jeste DV, Mintzer JE, Clyde C, Napolitano J, Brecher M. Comparison of risperidone and placebo for psychosis and behavioral disturbances associated with dementia: a randomized, double-blind trial. J Clin Psychiatry. 1999;60:107-15.
158. De Deyn PP, Rabheru K, Rasmussen A, et al. A randomized trial of risperidone, placebo, and haloperidol for behavioral symptoms of dementia. Neurology. 1999;53:946-55.
159. Street JS, Clark WS, Gannon KS, et al. Olanzapine treatment of psychotic and behavioral symptoms in patients with Alzheimer's disease in nursing care facilities: a double-blind, randomized, placebo-controlled trial. Arch Gen Psychiatry. 2000;57:968-76.
160. Brodaty H, Ames D, Snowdon J, et al. A randomized placebo-controlled trial of risperidone for the treatment of aggression, agitation, and psychosis of dementia. J Clin Psychiatry. 2013;64:134-43.
161. Tariot PN, Erb R, Podgorski C, et al. Efficacy and tolerability of carbamazepine for agitation and aggression in dementia. Am J Psychiatry. 1998;155:54-61.
162. Porsteinsson AP, Tariot PN, Erb R, et al. Placebo-controlled study of divalproex sodium for agitation in dementia. Am J Geriatr Psychiatry. 2001;9:58-66.
163. Porsteinsson AP, Tariot PN, Erb R, Gaile S. An open trial of valproate for agitation in geriatric neuropsychiatric disorders. Am J Geriatr Psychiatry. 1997;5:344-51.
164. Lyketsos C, Sheppard JM, St-eele CD, et al. Randomized, placebo-controlled, double-blind clinical trial of sertraline in the treatment of depression complicating Alzheimer's disease: initial results from the Depression in Alzheimer's Disease study. Am J Psychiatry. 2000;157:1686-9.
165. Katona CL, Hunter BN, Bray J. A double-blind comparison of the efficacy and safety of paroxetine and imipramine in the treatment of depression with dementia. Int J Geriatr Psychiatry. 1998;13:100-8.
166. Taragano F, Lyketsos C, Mangone CA, Allegri RF, Comesanac Diaz E. A double-blind, randomized, fixed dose trial of fluoxetine vs. amitriptyline in the treatment of major depression complicating Alzheimer's disease. Psychosomatics. 1997;38:246-52.
167. Chandra V, Bharucha NE, Schoenberg BS. Conditions associated with Alzheimer's disease at death: case-control study. Neurology. 1986;36:209-11.
168. Magenheim MJ. Preventive health maintenance. In: Duthie EH Jr, Katz PR (Eds). Practice of geriatrics, 3rd edition. Philadelphia: WB Saunders. 1998:11-5-29.
169. Schulz R, O'Brien AT, Bookwala J, Fleissner K. Psychiatric and physical morbidity effects of dementia caregiving: prevalence, correlates, and causes. Gerontologist. 1995;35: 771-91.
170. Mittelman MS, Ferris SH, Shulman E, Steinberg G, Levin B. A family intervention to delay nursing home placement of patients with Alzheimer disease: a randomized controlled trial. JAMA. 1996;276:1725-31.
171. Brodaty H, Green A, Koschera A. Meta-analysis of psychosocial interventions for caregivers of people with dementia. J Am Geriatr Soc. 2003;51:657-64.
172. Brodaty H, Green A, Koschera A. Meta-analysis of psychosocial interventions for caregivers of people with dementia. J Am Geriatr Soc. 2013;51:657-64.

Treatment of Chronic Insomnia

173. Morin CM, Hauri PJ, Espie CA, Spielman AJ, Buysse DJ, Bootzin RR. Nonpharmacologic treatment of chronic insomnia: an American Academy of Sleep Medicine review. Sleep. 1999;22:1134-56.
174. Costa e Silva JA, Chase M, Sartorius M, Roth T. Special report from a symposium held by the World Health Organization and the World Federation of Sleep Research Societies: an overview of insomnias and related disorders—recognition, epidemiology, and rational management. Sleep. 1996;19:412-6.
175. The international classification of sleep disorders, revised: diagnostic and coding manual. Rochester, Minn.: American Sleep Disorders Association. 1997.
176. Morin CM, Culbert JP, Schwartz SM. Nonpharmacological interventions for insomnia: a meta-analysis of treatment efficacy. Am J Psychiatry. 1994;151:1172-80.
177. Spielman AJ, Caruso LS, Glovinsky PB. A behavioral perspective on insomnia treatment. Psychiatr Clin North Am. 1987;10:541-53.
178. Littner M, Hirshkowitz M, Kramer M, et al. Practice parameters for using polysomnography to evaluate insomnia: an update. Sleep. 2003;26:754-60.
179. The international classification of sleep disorders: diagnostic & coding manual, IC-DS-2, 2nd edition. Westchester, Ill.: American Academy of Sleep Medicine; 2005.
180. Perlis ML, Smith MT, Pigeon WR. Etiology and pathophysiology of insomnia. In: Kryger MH, Roth T, Dement WC (Eds). Principles and practice of sleep medicine, 4th edition. Philadelphia: Elsevier/Saunders; 2005.pp.714-25.
181. Bootzin RR, Epstein D, Wood JM. Stimulus control instructions. In: Hauri PJ (Ed). Case studies in insomnia. New York: Plenum Medical Book; 1991.pp.19-28.

182. Spielman AJ, Saskin P, Theorpy MJ. Treatment of chronic insomnia by restriction of time in bed. Sleep. 1987;10:45-56.
183. Hauri PJ. Sleep hygiene, relaxation therapy, and cognitive interventions. In: Hauri PJ (Ed). Case studies in insomnia. New York: Plenum Medical Book; 1991.pp.65-84.
184. Murtagh DRR, Greenwood KM. Identifying effective psychological treatments for insomnia: a meta-analysis. J Consult Clin Psychol. 1995;63:79-89.
185. Espie CA, Inglis SJ, Tessier S, Harvey L. The clinical effectiveness of cognitive behaviour therapy for chronic insomnia: implementation and evaluation of a sleep clinic in general medical practice. Behav Res Ther. 2001;39:45-60.
186. Edinger JD, Wohlgemuth WK, Radtke RA, Marsh GR, Quillian RE. Cognitive behavioral therapy for treatment of chronic primary insomnia: a randomized controlled trial. JAMA. 2001;285:1856-64.
187. Turner RM, Ascher LM. Therapist factor in the treatment of insomnia. Behav Res Ther. 1982;20:33-40.
188. Morgan K, Dixon S, Mather N, Thompson J, Tomeny M. Psychological treatment for insomnia in the management of long-term hypnotic drug use: a pragmatic randomised controlled trial. Br J Gen Pract. 2003;53:923-8.
189. Baillargeon L, Demers L, Ladouceur R. Stimulus control: non-pharmacologic treatment for insomnia. Can Fam Physician. 1998;44:73-9.
190. Edinger JD, Sampson WS. A primary care “friendly” cognitive behavioral insomnia therapy. Sleep. 2003;26:177-82.
191. Riedel BW, Lichstein KL, Dwyer WO. Sleep compression and sleep education for older insomnias: self help versus therapist guidance. Psychol Aging. 1995;10:54-63.
192. Mimeault V, Morin CM. Self-help treatment for insomnia: bibliotherapy with and without professional guidance. J Consult Clin Psychol. 1999;67:511-9.
193. Meoli AL, Rosen CL, Kristo D, et al. Oral nonprescription treatment for insomnia: an evaluation of products with limited evidence. J Clin Sleep Med. 2005;1:173-87.
194. Rogers NL, Dinges DF, Kennaway DJ, Dawson D. Potential action of melatonin in insomnia. Sleep. 2003;26:1058-9.
195. Nowell PD, Mazumdar S, Buysse DJ, Dew MA, Reynolds CF III, Kupfer DJ. Benzodiazepines and zolpidem for chronic insomnia: a meta-analysis of treatment efficacy. JAMA. 1997;278:2170-7.
196. Holbrook AM, Crowther R, Lotter A, Cheng C, King D. Meta-analysis of benzodiazepine use in the treatment of insomnia. CMAJ. 2000;162:225-33.
197. Elie R, Ruther E, Farr I, Elilien G, Salinas E. Sleep latency is shortened during 4 weeks of treatment with zaleplon, a novel nonbenzodiazepine hypnotic. J Clin Psychiatry. 1999;60:536- 44.
198. Walsh JK, Vogel GW, Scharf M, et al. A five week, polysomnographic assessment of zaleplon 10 mg for the treatment of primary insomnia. Sleep Med. 2000;1:41-9.
199. Walsh JK, Pollak CP, Scharf MB, Schweitzer PK, Vogel GW. Lack of residual sedation following middle-of-the-night zaleplon administration in sleep maintenance insomnia. Clin Neuropharmacol. 2000;23:17-21. [CrossRef][ISI][Medline]
200. Krystal AD, Walsh JK, Laska E, et al. Sustained efficacy of eszopiclone over 6 months of nightly treatment: results of a randomized, double-blind, placebo-controlled study of adults with chronic insomnia. Sleep. 2003;26:793-9.
201. Walsh JK, Roth T, Randazzo A, et al. Eight weeks of non-nightly use of zolpidem for primary insomnia. Sleep. 2000;23: 1087-96.
202. Perlis ML, McCall WV, Krystal AD, Walsh JK. Long-term, non-nightly administration of zolpidem in the treatment of patients with primary insomnia. J Clin Psychiatry. 2004;65:1128-37.
203. Voshaar RC, van Balkom AJ, Zitman FG. Zolpidem is not superior to temazepam with respect to rebound insomnia: a controlled study. Eur Neuropsychopharmacol. 2004;14:301-6.
204. Vogel GW, Morris D. The effects of estazolam on sleep, performance, and memory: a long-term sleep laboratory study of elderly insomniacs. J Clin Pharmacol. 1992;32:647-51.
205. Roth T, Roehrs TA. A review of the safety profiles of benzodiazepine hypnotics. J Clin Psychiatry 1991;52(Suppl): 38-41.
206. Monti JM, Attali P, Monti D, Zipfel A, de la Giclais B, Morselli PL. Zolpidem and rebound insomnia a double-blind, controlled polysomnographic study in chronic insomniac patients. Pharmacopsychiatry. 1994;27:166-75.
207. Soldatos CR, Dikeos DG, Whitehead A. Tolerance and rebound insomnia with rapidly eliminated hypnotics: a meta-analysis of sleep laboratory studies. Int Clin Psychopharmacol. 1999;14:287-303.
208. Greenblatt DJ, Harmatz JS, Zinny MA, Shader RI. Effect of gradual withdrawal on the rebound sleep disorder after discontinuation of triazolam. N Engl J Med. 1987;317:722-8.
209. Scharf MB, Roth T, Vogel GW, Walsh JK. A multicenter, placebo-controlled study evaluating zolpidem in the treatment of chronic insomnia. J Clin Psychiatry. 1994;55:192-9.
210. Rothschild AJ. Disinhibition, amnestic reactions, and other adverse reactions secondary to triazolam: a review of the literature. J Clin Psychiatry. 1992;53(Suppl):69-79.
211. Roth T, Hartse KM, Saab PG, Piccione PM, Kramer M. The effects of flurazepam, lorazepam, and triazolam on sleep and memory. Psychopharmacology (Berl). 1980;70:231-7. [CrossRef][ISI][-Medline]
212. Canaday BR. Amnesia possibly associated with zolpidem administration. Pharmacotherapy. 1996;16:687-9.
213. Morgenthaler TI, Silber MH. Amnestic sleep-related eating disorder associated with zolpidem. Sleep Med. 2002;3:323-7.
214. Mendelson WB. Clinical distinctions between long-acting and short-acting benzodiazepines. J Clin Psychiatry. 1992;53(Suppl):4-7.
215. Morin CM, Colecchi C, Stone J, Sood R, Brink D. Behavioral and pharmacological therapies for late-life insomnia: a randomized controlled trial. JAMA. 1999;281:991-9.
216. Walsh JK, Schweitzer PK. Ten-year trends in the pharmacological treatment of insomnia. Sleep. 1999;22:371-5.
217. Kaynak H, Kaynak D, Gozukirmizi E, Guilleminault C. The effects of trazodone on sleep in patients treated with stimulant antidepressants. Sleep Med. 2004;5:15-20.

218. Nierenberg AA, Adler LA, Peselow E, Zornberg G, Rosenthal M. Trazodone for antidepressant-associated insomnia. Am J Psychiatry. 1994;151:1069-72.
219. Walsh JK, Erman M, Erwin CW, et al. Subjective hypnotic efficacy of trazodone in DSM3-R primary insomnia. Hum Psychopharmacol. 1998;13:191-8.
220. Hajak G, Rodenbeck A, Voderholzer U, et al. Doxepin in the treatment of primary insomnia: a placebo-controlled, double-blind, polysomnographic study. J Clin Psychiatry. 2001;62:453-63.
221. Aslan S, Isik E, Cosar B. The effects of mirtazapine on sleep: a placebo controlled, double-blind study in young healthy volunteers. Sleep. 2002;25:677-9.
222. McClusky HY, Milby JB, Switzer PK, Williams V, Wooten V. Efficacy of behavioral versus triazolam treatment in persistent sleep-onset insomnia. Am J Psychiatry. 1991;148:121-6.
223. Jacobs GD, Pace-Schott EF, Stickgold R, Otto MW. Cognitive behavior therapy and pharmacotherapy for insomnia: a randomized controlled trial and direct comparison. Arch Intern Med. 2004;164:1888-96.
224. Smith MT, Perlis ML, Park A, et al. Comparative meta-analysis of pharmacotherapy and behavior therapy for persistent insomnia. Am J Psychiatry. 2002;159:5-11.
225. Hauri PJ. Can we mix behavioral therapy with hypnotics when treating insomniacs? Sleep. 1997;20:1111-8.
226. Baillargeon L, Landreville P, Verreault R, Beauchemin JP, Gregoire JP, Morin CM. Discontinuation of benzodiazepines among older insomniac adults treated with cognitive-behavioural therapy combined with gradual tapering: a randomized trial. CMAJ. 2003;169:1015-20.
227. Morin CM, Bastien C, Guay B, Radouco Thomas M, Leblanc J, Vallieres A. Randomized clinical trial of supervised tapering and cognitive behavior therapy to facilityate benzodiazepine discontinuation in older adults with chronic insomnia. Am J Psychiatry. 2004;161:332-42.
228. Zammit G, Roth T, Erman M, et al. Double-blind, placebo-controlled polysomnography and outpatient trial to evaluate the efficacy and safety of ramelteon in adult patients with chronic insomnia. Sleep. 2005;28:A228-A229.
229. Zemlan FP, Mulchahey JJ, Scharf MB, Mayleben DW, Rosenberg R, Lankford A. The efficacy and safety of the melatonin agonist betamethyl-6-chloromelatonin in primary insomnia: a randomized, placebo-controlled, crossover clinical trial. J Clin Psychiatry. 2005;66:384-90.
230. Chesson AL Jr, Anderson WM, Littner M, et al. Practice parameters for the nonpharmacologic treatment of chronic insomnia: an American Academy of Sleep Medicine report: Standards of Practice Committee of the American Academy of Sleep Medicine. Sleep. 1999;22:1128-33.

Recent Advances in the Diagnosis and Management of Migraine

231. Menken M, Munsat TL, Toole JF. The global burden of disease study—implications for neurology. Arch Neurol. 2000;57 418-20.
232. Goadsby PJ. Advances in headache management. In: Haskard D, (ed). Horizons in medicine. Vol 17. London: Royal College of Physicians, (in press).
233. Headache Classification Committee of the International Headache Society. The international classification of headache disorders (second edition). Cephalalgia. 2004;24(suppl 1): 1-160.
234. Tepper SJ, Dahlof CG, Dowson A, Newman L, Mansbach H, Jones M, et al. Prevalence and diagnosis of migraine in patients consulting their physician with a complaint of headache: data from the landmark study. Headache. 2004;44: 856-64.
235. Goadsby PJ, Dodick D, Silberstein SD. Chronic daily headache for clinicians. Hamilton, Canada: BC Decker. 2005.
236. Goadsby PJ, Boes C. New daily persistent headache. J Neurol Neurosurg Psychiatr 2002;72(suppl 2):ii6-9.
237. Goadsby PJ. To scan or not to scan in headache: that is the question. BMJ. 2004;329:469-70.
238. Weiller C, May A, Limmroth V, Juptner M, Kaube H, Schayck RV, et al. Brain stem activation in spontaneous human migraine attacks. Nature Med. 1995;1:658-60.
239. May A, Kaube H, Buechel C, Eichten C, Rijntjes M, Jueptner M, et al. Experimental cranial pain elicited by capsaicin: a PET-study. Pain 1998;74:61-6.
240. May A, Bahra A, Buchel C, Frackowiak RSJ, Goadsby PJ. Hypothalamic activation in cluster headache attacks. Lancet. 1998;352:275-8.
241. Matharu MS, Cohen AS, Frackowiak RSJ, Goadsby PJ. Posterior hypothalamic activation in paroxysmal hemicrania. Ann Neurol (in press).
242. Afridi S, Giffin NJ, Kaube H, Friston KJ, Ward NS, Frackowiak RSJ, et al. A PET study in spontaneous migraine. Arch Neurol. 2005;62:1270-5.
243. Denuelle M, Fabre N, Payoux P, Chollet F, Gereud G. Brainstem and hypothalamic activation in spontaneous migraine attacks. Cephalalgia. 2004;24:775-814.
244. Bahra A, Matharu MS, Buchel C, Frackowiak RSJ, Goadsby PJ. Brainstem activation specific to migraine headache. Lancet. 2001;357:1016-7.
245. Afridi S, Matharu MS, Lee L, Kaube H, Friston KJ, Frackowiak RSJ, et al. A PET study exploring the laterality of brain-stem activation in migraine using glyceryl trinitrate. Brain. 2005;128: 932-9.
246. Matharu MS, Bartsch T, Ward N, Frackowiak RSJ, Weiner RL, Goadsby PJ. Central neuromodulation in chronic migraine patients with suboccipital stimulators: a PET study. Brain. 2004;127:220-30.
247. May A, Buchel C, Turner R, Frackowiak RSJ, Goadsby PJ. Neurovascular dilatation of intracranial vessels in experimental headache. Cephalalgia. 1999;19:464-5.
248. May A, Buchel C, Turner R, Goadsby PJ. MR-angiography in facial and other pain: neurovascular mechanisms of trigeminal sensation. J Cereb Blood Flow Metab. 2001;21:1171-6.
249. Tfelt-Hansen P. Efficacy and adverse events of subcutaneous, oral, and intranasal sumatriptan used for migraine treatment: a systematic review based on number needed to treat. Cephalalgia. 1998;18:532-8.

250. Ferrari MD, Goadsby PJ, Roon KI, Lipton RB. Triptans (serotonin, 5-HT$_{1B/1D}$ agonists) in migraine: detailed results and methods of a meta-analysis of 53 trials. Cephalalgia. 2002;22: 633-58.
251. Tfelt Hansen P, De Vries P, Saxena PR. Triptans in migraine. A comparative review of pharmacology, pharmacokinetics and efficacy of triptans in migraine. Drugs. 2000;6:1259-87.
252. Silberstein SD, Goadsby PJ. Migraine: preventative treatment. Cephalalgia. 2002;22:491-512.
253. Brandes JL, Saper JR, Diamond M, Couch JR, Lewis DW, Schmitt J, et al. Topiramate for migraine prevention: a randomized controlled trial. JAMA. 2004;291:965-73.
254. Silberstein SD, Neto W, Schmitt J, Jacobs D. Topiramate in migraine prevention: results of a large controlled trial. Arch Neurol. 2004;61:490-5.
255. Olesen J, Diener HC, Husstedt IW, Goadsby PJ, Hall D, Meier U, et al. Calcitonin gene-related peptide (CGRP) receptor antagonist BIBN4096BS is effective in the treatment of migraine attacks. N Engl J Med. 2004;350:1104-10.

Diagnosis and Management of Headaches in Young People and Adults: Summary of NICE Guidance

256. Latinovic R, Gulliford M, Ridsdale L. Headache and migraine in primary care: consultation, prescription, and referral rates in a large population. J Neurol Neurosurg Psychiatry. 2006;77:385-7.
257. Weatherall MW. Acute neurology in a twenty-first century district general hospital. J R Coll Physicians Edinb. 2006;36:196-200.
258. National Institute for Health and Clinical Excellence. Headaches. Diagnosis and management of headaches in young people and adults. (Clinical Guideline 150.) 2012. http://guidance.nice.org.uk/CG150/Guidance.
259. Faculty of Sexual and Reproductive Healthcare Clinical Effectiveness Unit. Drug interactions with hormonal contraception. 2011. www.fsrh.org/pdfs/CEU guidancedruginteractionshormonal.pdf.
260. National Institute for Health and Clinical Excellence. Botulinum toxin type A for the prevention of headaches in adults with chronic migraine. (Technology appraisal guidance 260.) 2012. http://guidance.nice.org.uk/TA260.

Pharmacological Prevention of Migraine

261. Headache Classification Committee of the International Headache Society. The international classification of headache disorders. 2nd edition. Cephalalgia. 2004;24(suppl 1):1-160.
262. Silberstein SD, Lipton RB, Dodick DW. Wolff's headache and other head pain. 8th edition. Oxford University Press, 2008.
263. Stovner LJ, Hagen K, Jensen R, Katsarava Z, Lipton RB, Scher AI, et al. The global burden of headache: a documentation of headache prevalence and disability worldwide. Cephalalgia. 2007;27:193-210.
264. Lipton RB, Bigal M, Diamond M, Freitag F, Reed ML, Stewart WF, et al. Migraine prevalence, disease burden, and the need for preventive therapy. Neurology. 2007;68:343-9.
265. Silberstein SD. Practice parameter: evidence-based guidelines for migraine headache (an evidence-based review): report of the quality standards subcommittee of the American Academy of Neurology. Neurology. 2000;55:754-62.
266. Evers S, Afra J, Frese A, Goadsby PJ, Linde M, May A, et al. EFNS guideline on the drug treatment of migraine- revised report of an EFNS task force. Eur J Neurol. 2009;16:968-81.
267. Antonaci F, Dumitrache C, De Cillis I, Allena M. A review of current European guidelines for migraine. J Headache Pain. 2010;11:13-9.
268. Mathew N, Kurman R, Perez F. Drug induced refractory headache—clinical features and management. Headache. 1990;30:634-8.
269. Linde K, Rossnagel K. Propranolol for migraine prophylaxis. Cochrane Database Syst Rev. 2004;2:CD003225.
270. Reveix Herault L, Cardona A, Ospina E, Carrillo P. Effectiveness of flunazarine in the prophylaxis of migraine: a meta-analytical review of the literature. Revista de Neurol. 2003;36:907-12.
271. Schrader H, Stovner L, Helde G, Sand T, Bovim G. Prophylactic treatment of migraine with angiotensin converting enzyme inhibitor (lisinopril): randomized, placebo controlled, crossover study. BMJ. 2001;322:19.
272. Trovnik E, Stovner L, Helde G, Sand T, Bovim G. Prophylactic treatment of migraine with an angiotensin II receptor blocker: a randomized controlled trial. JAMA. 2003;289:65-9.
273. Couch JR, Hassanein RS. Amitriptyline in migraine prophylaxis. Arch Neurol. 1979;36:695-9.
274. Moja L, Cusi C, Sterzi R, Canepari C. Selective serotonin re-uptake inhibitors (SSRI) for preventing migraine and tension-type headaches. Cochrane Database Syst Rev. 2005;3:CD002919.
275. Ozyalcin S, Talu G, Kiziltan E, Yucel B, Ertas M, Disci R. The efficacy and safety of venlafaxine in the prophylaxis of migraine. Headache. 2005;45:144-52.
276. Jensen R, Brinck T, Olesen J. Sodium valproate has a prophylactic effect in migraine without aura: a triple-blind, placebo-controlled crossover study. Neurology. 1994;44:647-51.
277. Mulleners WM, Chronicle EP. Anticonvulsants in migraine prophylaxis: a Cochrane review. Cephalalgia. 2008;28:585-97.
278. Silberstein SD, Neto W, Schmitt J, Jacobs D. Topiramate in migraine prevention: results of a large controlled trial. Arch Neurol. 2004;61:490-5.
279. Lipton RB, Gobel H, Einhaupl, Wilks K, Mauskop A. Petasites hybridus root (butterbur) is an effective preventive treatment for migraine. Neurology. 2004;63:2240-4.
280. Sandor PS, Di Clemente L, Coppola G, Saenger U, Fumal A, Magis D, et al. Efficacy of coenzyme Q10 in migraine prophylaxis: a randomized controlled trial. Neurology. 2005;64:713-5.

281. Schoener J, Jacquy J, Lenaerts M. Effectiveness of high-dose riboflavin in migraine prophylaxis—a randomized controlled trial. Neurology. 1998;50:65-9.
282. Peikert A, Wilimzig C, Kohne-Volland R. Prophylaxis of migraine with oral magnesium: results from a prospective, multi-center, placebo-controlled and double-blind randomized study. Cephalalgia. 1996;16:257-63.
283. Pittler MH, Ernst E. Feverfew for preventing migraine. Cochrane Database Syst Rev. 2004;1:CD002286.
284. Evers S, Vollmer-Haase J, Schwaag S, Rahmann A, Husstedt IW, Frese A. Botulinum toxin A in the prophylactic treatment of migraine—a randomized double-blind, placebo-controlled study. Cephalalgia. 2004;24:838-43.
285. Diener HC, Dodick DW, Aurora SK, Turkel CC, DeGryse RE, Lipton RB, et al. Onabotulinumtoxin A for treatment of chronic migraine: results from the double-blind, randomized, placebo-controlled phase of the PREEMPT 2 trial. Cephalalgia. 2010;30:804-14.

Management of Chronic Epilepsy

286. Ngugi AK, Kariuki SM, Bottomley C, Kleinschmidt I, Sander JW, Newton CR. Incidence of epilepsy: a systematic review and meta-analysis. Neurology. 2011;77:1005-12.
287. Leone MA, Solari A, Beghi E. Treatment of the first tonic-clonic seizure does not affect long-term remission of epilepsy. Neurology. 2006;67:2227-9.
288. Marson A, Jacoby A, Johnson A, Kim L, Gamble C, Chadwick D. Immediate versus deferred antiepileptic drug treatment for early epilepsy and single seizures: a randomised controlled trial. Lancet. 2005;365:2007-13.
289. Annegers JF, Hauser WA, Elveback LR. Remission of seizures and relapse in patients with epilepsy. Epilepsia. 1979;20:729-37.
290. Cockerell OC, Johnson AL, Sander JW, Hart YM, Goodridge DM, Shorvon SD. Mortality from epilepsy: results from a prospective population-based study. Lancet. 1994;344:918-21.
291. Lhatoo SD, Johnson AL, Goodridge DM, MacDonald BK, Sander JW, Shorvon SD. Mortality in epilepsy in the first 11 to 14 years after diagnosis: multivariate analysis of a long-term, prospective, population-based cohort. Ann Neurol. 2001;49:336-44.
292. Gilliam F. Optimizing health outcomes in active epilepsy. Neurology. 2002;58(suppl 5):S9-20.
293. Marson AG, Al-Kharusi AM, Alwaidh M, Appleton R, Baker GA, Chadwick DW, et al. The SANAD study of effectiveness of valproate, lamotrigine, or topiramate for generalised and unclassifiable epilepsy: an unblinded randomised controlled trial. Lancet. 2007;369:1016-26.
294. Marson AG, Al-Kharusi AM, Alwaidh M, Appleton R, Baker GA, Chadwick DW, et al. The SANAD study of effectiveness of carbamazepine, gabapentin, lamotrigine, oxcarbazepine, or topiramate for treatment of partial epilepsy: an unblinded randomised controlled trial. Lancet. 2007;369:1000-15.
295. National Institute for Health and Clinical Excellence. Clinical guideline 137. NICE, 2012.
296. Wiebe S, Blume WT, Girvin JP, Eliasziw M. A randomized, controlled trial of surgery for temporal-lobe epilepsy. N Engl J Med. 2001;345:311-8.
297. MacDonald BK, Johnson AL, Goodridge DM, Cockerell OC, Sander JW, Shorvon SD. Factors predicting prognosis of epilepsy after presentation with seizures. Ann Neurol. 2000;48:833-41.
298. Kwan P, Brodie MJ. Early identification of refractory epilepsy. N Engl J Med. 2000;342:314-9.
299. Luciano AL, Shorvon SD. Results of treatment changes in patients with apparently drug-resistant chronic epilepsy. Ann Neurol. 2007;62:375-81.
300. Smith D, Defalla BA, Chadwick DW. The misdiagnosis of epilepsy and the management of refractory epilepsy in a specialist clinic. QJM. 1999;92:15-23.
301. Chaves J, Sander JW. Seizure aggravation in idiopathic generalized epilepsies. Epilepsia. 2005;46(suppl 9):133-9.
302. Marson AG, Kadir ZA, Hutton JL, Chadwick DW. The new antiepileptic drugs: a systematic review of their efficacy and tolerability. Epilepsia. 1997;38:859-80.
303. Marson AG, Hutton JL, Leach JP, Castillo S, Schmidt D, White S, et al. Levetiracetam, oxcarbazepine, remacemide and zonisamide for drug resistant localization-related epilepsy: a systematic review. Epilepsy Res. 2001;46:259-70.
304. Meador KJ, Loring DW, Hulihan JF, Kamin M, Karim R. Differential cognitive and behavioral effects of topiramate and valproate. Neurology. 2003;60:1483-8.
305. Meador KJ, Baker GA, Browning N, Clayton-Smith J, Combs-Cantrell DT, Cohen M, et al. Cognitive function at 3 years of age after fetal exposure to antiepileptic drugs. N Engl J Med. 2009;360:1597-605.
306. Albright P, Bruni J. Reduction of polypharmacy in epileptic patients. Arch Neurol. 1985;42:797-9.
307. Duncan JS, Shorvon SD, Trimble MR. Discontinuation of phenytoin, carbamazepine, and valproate in patients with active epilepsy. Epilepsia. 1990;31:324-33.
308. Hosking PG, Duncan JS, Sander JW. The epilepsy nurse specialist at a tertiary care hospital-improving the interface between primary and tertiary care. Seizure. 2002;11:494-9.

Management of Seasonal Affective Disorder

309. American Psychiatric Association. Diagnostic and Statistical Manual of Mental Disorders. 4th edition, text revision. American Psychiatric Association, 2000.
310. Michalak EE Wilkinson C, Dowrick C, Wilkinson G. Seasonal affective disorder: prevalence, detection and current treatment in North Wales. Br J Psychiatry. 2001;179:31-4.
311. Thompson C, Thompson S, Smith R. Prevalence of seasonal affective disorder in primary care; a comparison of the seasonal health questionnaire and the seasonal pattern assessment questionnaire. J Affect Disord. 2004;78:219-26.
312. Eagles JM, Howie FL, Cameron IM, Wileman SM, Andrew JE, Robertson C, et al. Use of health care services in seasonal affective disorder. Br J Psychiatry. 2002;180:449-54.

313. Modell JG, Rosenthal NE, Harriett AE, Krishen A, Asgharian A, Foster VJ, et al. Seasonal affective disorder and its prevention by anticipatory treatment with bupropion XL. Biol Psychiatry. 2005;58:658-67.
314. Rosenthal NE, Sack DA, Gillin JC, Lewy AJ, Goodwin FK, Davenport Y, et al. Seasonal affective disorder: a description of the syndrome and preliminary findings with light therapy. Arch Gen Psychiatry. 1984;41:72-80.
315. Hansen V, Skre I, Lund E. What is this thing called "SAD"? A critique of the concept of seasonal affective disorder. Epidemiol Psichiatr Soc. 2008;17:120-7.
316. World Health Organization. International statistical classification of diseases and related health problems 10th revision, version for 2007 (ICD-10). 2007. http://apps.who.int/classifications/apps/icd/icd10online.
317. Lam RW, Levitt AJ, (Eds). Canadian consensus guidelines for the treatment of seasonal affective disorder. 1999. http://ubcsad.bc-alter.net/CCG%20SAD%201999.pdf.
318. Sohn CH, Lam RW. Update on the biology of seasonal affective disorder. CNS Spectr. 2005;10:635-46.
319. European Medicines Agency. Assessment report for Circadin. 2007. www.emea.europa.eu/humandocs/PDFs/EPAR/circadin/H-695-en6.pdf.
320. Lewy AJ, Bauer VK, Cutler NL, Sack RL, Ahmed S, Thomas KH, et al. Morning vs evening light treatment of patients with winter depression. Arch Gen Psychiatry. 1998;55:890-6.
321. Macchi MM, Bruce JN. Human pineal physiology and functional significance of melatonin. Front Neuroendocrinol. 2004;25:177-95.
322. McIntyre IM, Norman TR, Burrows GD, Armstrong SM. Human melatonin suppression by light is intensity dependent. J Pineal Res. 1989;6:149-56.
323. Avery DH, Eder DN, Bolte MA, Hellekson CJ, Dunner DL, Vitiello MV, et al. Dawn simulation and bright light in the treatment of SAD: a controlled study. Biol Psychiatry. 2001;50:205-16.
324. Swedo SE, Pleeter JD, Richter DM, Hoffman CL, Allen AJ, Hamburger SD, et al. Rates of seasonal affective disorder in children and adolescents. Am J Psychiatry. 1995;152:1016-9.
325. Magnusson A, Stefansson JG. Prevalence of seasonal affective disorder in Iceland. Arch Gen Psychiatry. 1993;50:941-6.
326. Martiny K, Lunde M, Simonsen C, Clemmensen L, Poulsen DL, Solstad K, et al. Relapse prevention by citalopram in SAD patients responding to 1 week of light therapy. A placebo-controlled study. Acta Psychiatr Scand. 2004;109:230-4.
327. Magnusson A, Partonen T. The diagnosis, symptomatology, and epidemiology of seasonal affective disorder. CNS Spectr. 2005;10:625-34.
328. Michalak EE, Tam EM, Manjunath CV, Solomons K, Levitt AJ, Levitan R, et al. Generic and health-related quality of life in patients with seasonal and nonseasonal depression. Psychiatry Res. 2004;128:245-51.
329. Michalak EE, Murray G, Levitt AJ, Levitan RD, Enns MW, Morehouse R, et al. Quality of life as an outcome indicator in patients with seasonal affective disorder: results from the Can-SAD study. Psychol Med. 2007;37:727-36.
330. Williams JBW. A structured interview guide for the Hamilton Depression Rating Scale. Arch Gen Psychiatry. 1988;45:742-7.
331. Moscovitch A, Blashko CA, Eagles JM, Darcourt G, Thompson C, Kasper S, et al. A placebo-controlled study of sertraline in the treatment of outpatients with seasonal affective disorder. Psychopharmacology. 2004;171:390-7.
332. Terman M, Terman JS. Light therapy for seasonal and nonseasonal depression: efficacy, protocol, safety, and side effects. CNS Spectr. 2005;10:647-63.
333. Terman M, Terman JS, Ross DC. A controlled trial of timed bright light and negative air ionization for treatment of winter depression. Arch Gen Psychiatry. 1998;55:875-82.
334. Anderson IM, Ferrier IN, Baldwin RC, Cowen PJ, Howard L, Lewis G, et al. Evidence-based guidelines for treating depressive disorders with antidepressants: a revision of the 2000 British Association for Psychopharmacology guidelines. J Psychopharmacol. 2008;22:343-96.
335. Lam RW, Gorman CP, Michalon M, Steiner M, Levitt AJ, Corral MR, et al. Multicenter, placebo-controlled study of fluoxetine in seasonal affective disorder. Am J Psychiatry. 1995;152:1765-70.
336. Eli Lilly and Company Limited. Prozac 20 mg hard capsules, and 20 mg per 5 ml oral liquid. Summary of product characteristics, UK. Eli Lilly and Company Limited, 2009.
337. Wockhardt UK Ltd. Sertraline 50 mg and 100 mg film-coated tablets. Summary of product characteristics, UK. Wockhardt UK Ltd, 2009.
338. Westrin A, Lam RW. Long-term and preventative treatment for seasonal affective disorder. CNS Drugs. 2007;21:901-9.
339. Terman JS, Terman M, Lo ES, Cooper TB. Circadian time of morning light administration and therapeutic response in winter depression. Arch Gen Psychiatry. 2001;58:69-75.
340. GlaxoSmithKline UK. Zyban 150 mg prolonged release film-coated tablets. Summary of product characteristics. GlaxoSmithKline UK, 2009.
341. Ravindran AV, Lam RW, Filteau MJ, Lespérance F, Kennedy SH, Parikh SV, et al. Canadian Network for Mood and Anxiety Treatments (CANMAT) clinical guidelines for the management of major depressive disorder in adults. V. Complementary and alternative medicine treatments. J Affect Disord. 2009;117:S54-64.
342. Eastman CI. Is bright light therapy a placebo? In: Partonen T, Magnusson A (Eds). Seasonal affective disorder, practice and research. Oxford University Press, 2001.
343. Thompson C. Evidence-based treatment. In: Partonen T, Magnusson A (Eds). Seasonal affective disorder: practice and research. Oxford University Press, 2001.
344. National Institute for Health and Clinical Excellence. Depression in adults (update). 2009. www.nice.org.uk/nicemedia/pdf/DepressionUpdateFullGuideline.pdf.
345. Golden RN, Gaynes BN, Ekstrom RD, Hamer RM, Jacobsen FM, Suppes T, et al. The efficacy of light therapy in the treatment of mood disorders: a review and meta-analysis of the evidence. Am J Psychiatry. 2005;162:656-62.

346. EurLex. 31993L0042. Council directive 93/42/EEC of 14 June 1993 concerning medical devices. 1993. http://eur-lex.europa.eu/LexUriServ/LexUriServ.do?uri=CELEX:31993L0042:EN:HTML.
347. NHS Direct. Seasonal affective disorder. http://cks.library.nhs.uk/patient_information_leaflet/seasonal_affective_disorder.
348. Directgov. 2009. VAT relief on products and services for disabled people. www.direct.gov.uk/en/DisabledPeople/FinancialSupport/Taxreliefandreductions/DG_10028495.
349. National Light Hire. VAT exemption. 2009. www.sad-lighthire.co.uk/exemption.html.
350. Rohan KJ, Roecklein KA, Tierney Lindsey K, Johnson LG, Lippy RD, Lacy TJ, et al. A randomized controlled trial of cognitive-behavioral therapy, light therapy, and their combination for seasonal affective disorder. J Consult Clin Psychol. 2007;75:489-500.
351. Rohan KJ, Lindsey KT, Roecklein KA, Lacy TJ. Cognitive-behavioral therapy, light therapy, and their combination in treating seasonal affective disorder. J Affect Disord. 2004;80:273-83.
352. Jorm AF, Christensen H, Griffiths KM, Rodgers B. Effectiveness of complementary and self-help treatments for depression. MJA. 2002;176:S84-96.
353. Pinchasov BB, Shurgaja AM, Grischin OV, Putilov AA. Mood and energy regulation in seasonal and non-seasonal depression before and after midday treatment with physical exercise or bright light. Psychiatry Res. 2000;94:29-42.
354. Terman M, Terman JS. Treatment of seasonal affective disorder with a high-output negative ionizer. J Altern Complement Med. 1995;1: 87-92.
355. American Psychiatry Association. Practice guideline for the treatment of patients with major depressive disorder (revision). Am J Psychiatry. 2000;157(4 suppl):1-45.
356. Parikh SV, Segal ZV, Grigoriadis S, Ravindran AV, Kennedy SH, Lam RW, et al. Canadian Network for Mood and Anxiety Treatments (CANMAT) clinical guidelines for the management of major depressive disorder in adults. II. Psychotherapy alone or in combination with antidepressant medication. J Affect Disord. 2009;117:S15-25.
357. Lam RW, Kennedy SH, Grigoriadis S, McIntyre RS, Milev R, Ramasubbu R, et al. Canadian Network for Mood and Anxiety Treatments (CANMAT) clinical guidelines for the management of major depressive disorder in adults. III. Pharmacotherapy. J Affect Disord. 2009;117:S26-43.
358. Anderson IM, Haddad PM. CANMAT guidelines for depression: clear and user-friendly. J Affect Disord. 2009;117:S3-4.

Cholinesterase Inhibitors and Memantine for Symptomatic Treatment of Dementia

359. Hansen RA, Gartlehner G, Webb AP, Morgan LC, Moore CG, Jonas DE. Efficacy and safety of donepezil, galantamine, and rivastigmine for the treatment of Alzheimer's disease: a systematic review and meta-analysis. Clin Interv Aging. 2008;3:211-25.
360. Rockwood K, Fay S, Gorman M, Carver D, Graham JE. The clinical meaningfulness of ADAS-Cog changes in Alzheimer's disease patients treated with donepezil in an open-label trial. BMC Neurol. 2007;7:26.
361. Wilkinson D, Schindler R, Schwam E, Waldemar G, Jones RW, Gauthier S, et al. Effectiveness of donepezil in reducing clinical worsening in patients with mild-to-moderate Alzheimer's disease. Dement Geriatr Cogn Disord. 2009;28:244-51.
362. Winblad B, Kilander L, Eriksson S, Minthon L, Batsman S, Wetterholm AL et al. Donepezil in patients with severe Alzheimer's disease: double-blind, parallel-group, placebo-controlled study. Lancet. 2006;367:1057-65.
363. Black SE, Doody R, Li H, McRae T, Jambor KM, Xu Y, et al. Donepezil preserves cognition and global function in patients with severe Alzheimer disease. Neurology. 2007;69: 459-69.
364. Cummings J, Jones R, Wilkinson D, Lopez O, Gauthier S, Waldemar G, et al. Effect of donepezil on cognition in severe Alzheimer's disease: a pooled data analysis. J Alzheimers Dis. 2010;21:843-51.
365. Burns A, Bernabei R, Bullock R, Cruz Jentoft AJ, Frolich L, Hock C, et al. Safety and efficacy of galantamine (Reminyl) in severe Alzheimer's disease (the SERAD study): a randomised, placebo-controlled, double-blind trial. Lancet Neurol. 2009;8:39-47.
366. National Institute for Health and Clinical Excellence. Donepezil, galantamine, rivastigmine and memantine for the treatment of Alzheimer's disease. NICE technology appraisal guidance 217. NICE, 2011.
367. National Collaborating Centre for Mental Health. Dementia: A NICE–SCIE Guideline on supporting people with dementia and their carers in health and social care. National Clinical Practice Guideline Number 42. NICE, 2006 amended 2011.
368. McShane R, Areosa SA, Minakaran N. Memantine for dementia. Cochrane Database Syst Rev. 2006;(2):CD003154.
369. Schneider LS, Dagerman KS, Higgins JP, McShane R. Lack of evidence for the efficacy of memantine in mild Alzheimer disease. Arch Neurol. 2011;68:991-8.
370. Tariot PN, Farlow MR, Grossberg GT, Graham SM, McDonald S, Gergel I. Memantine treatment in patients with moderate to severe Alzheimer disease already receiving donepezil: a randomized controlled trial. JAMA. 2004;291:317-24.
371. Porsteinsson AP, Grossberg GT, Mintzer J, Olin JT. Memantine treatment in patients with mild to moderate Alzheimer's disease already receiving a cholinesterase inhibitor: a randomized, double-blind, placebo-controlled trial. Curr Alzheimer Res. 2008;5:83-9.
372. Howard R, McShane R, Lindesay J, Ritchie C, Baldwin A, Barber R, et al. Donepezil and memantine for moderate-to-severe Alzheimer's disease. N Engl J Med. 2012;366:11-21.
373. Courtney C, Farrell D, Gray R, Hills R, Lynch L, Sellwood E, et al. Long-term donepezil treatment in 565 patients with Alzheimer's disease (AD2000): randomised double-blind trial. Lancet. 2004;363:2105-15.

374. Kavirajan H, Schneider LS. Efficacy and adverse effects of cholinesterase inhibitors and memantine in vascular dementia: a meta-analysis of randomised controlled trials. Lancet Neurol. 2007;6:782-92
375. Schneider JA, Arvanitakis Z, Bang W, Bennett DA. Mixed brain pathologies account for most dementia cases in community-dwelling older persons. Neurology. 2007;69:2197-204.
376. Erkinjuntti T, Kurz A, Gauthier S, Bullock R, Lilienfeld S, Damaraju CV. Efficacy of galantamine in probable vascular dementia and Alzheimer's disease combined with cerebrovascular disease: a randomised trial. Lancet. 2002;359:1283-90.
377. McKeith I, del Ser T, Spano P, Emre M, Wesnes K, Anand R, et al. Efficacy of rivastigmine in dementia with Lewy bodies: a randomised, double-blind, placebo-controlled international study. Lancet. 2000;356:2031-6.
378. Emre M, Aarsland D, Albanese A, Byrne EJ, Deuschl G, De Deyn PP, et al. Rivastigmine for dementia associated with Parkinson's disease. N Engl J Med. 2004;351:2509-18.
379. Aarsland D, Ballard C, Walker Z, Bostrom F, Alves G, Kossakowski K, et al. Memantine in patients with Parkinson's disease dementia or dementia with Lewy bodies: a double-blind, placebo-controlled, multicentre trial. Lancet Neurol. 2009;8:613-8.
380. Emre M, Tsolaki M, Bonuccelli U, Destee A, Tolosa E, Kutzelnigg A, et al. Memantine for patients with Parkinson's disease dementia or dementia with Lewy bodies: a randomised, double-blind, placebo-controlled trial. Lancet Neurol. 2010;9:969-77.
381. Ballard C, Ziabreva I, Perry R, Larsen JP, O'Brien J, McKeith I, et al. Differences in neuropathologic characteristics across the Lewy body dementia spectrum. Neurology. 2006;67:1931-4.
382. Birks J. Cholinesterase inhibitors for Alzheimer's disease. Cochrane Database Syst Rev. 2006;(1):CD005593.
383. Kim DH, Brown RT, Ding EL, Kiel DP, Berry SD. Dementia medications and risk of falls, syncope, and related adverse events: meta-analysis of randomized controlled trials. J Am Geriatr Soc. 2011;59:1019-31.
384. Winblad B, Cummings J, Andreasen N, Grossberg G, Onofrj M, Sadowsky C, et al. A six-month double-blind, randomized, placebo-controlled study of a transdermal patch in Alzheimer's disease—rivastigmine patch versus capsule. Int J Geriatr Psychiatry. 2007;22:456-67.
385. Rowland JP, Rigby J, Harper AC, Rowland R. Cardiovascular monitoring with acetylcholinesterase inhibitors: a clinical protocol. Adv Psychiatric Treat. 2007;13:178-84.

FURTHER READING

Antipsychotic Drugs

1. Agarwal AK, Aga VM, Khalid A. Physical methods of treatment in schizophrenia: Indian perspective. In: Kulhara P, Avasthi A, Verma SK (Eds). Schizophrenia: The Indian Scene. Chandigarh: Searle; 1997. pp. 114-48.
2. American Psychiatric Association. Practice guidelines for the treatment of patients with schizophrenia. Am J Psychiatry. 1997;154 (Suppl.4):1-63.
3. Bhatara VS, Sharma JN, Gupta S, et al. Rauwolfia serpentina:The first herbal antipsychotic. Am J Psychiatry. 1997;154:894.
4. Bishara D, et al. Upcoming agents for the treatment of schizophrenia. Mechanism of action, efficacy and tolerability. Drugs. 2008;68:2269-96.
5. Casey DE, et al. Efficacy and safety of bifeprunox in patients with an acute exacerbation of schizophrenia: results from a randomized, double-blind, placebo-controlled, multicenter, dose-finding study. Psychopharmacology (Berl). 2008;200:317-31.
6. Citrome L, et al. Iloperidone for schizophrenia: a review of the efficacy and safety profile for this newly-commercialised second-generation antipsychotic. Int J Clin Pract 2009;In Press.
7. Citrome L. Olanzapine pamoate: a stick in time? Int J Clin Pract. 2009;63:140-50.
8. Cosi C, et al. Partial agonist properties of the antipsychotics SSR181507, aripiprazole and bifeprunox at dopamine D2 receptors: G protein activation andprol actin release. Eur J Pharmacol. 2006;535:135-44.
9. Cutler AJ, et al. Four-week, double-blind, placebo- and ziprasidone-controlled trial of iloperidone in patients with acute exacerbations of schizophrenia. J Clin Psychopharmacol. 2008;28:S20-S28.
10. Davis JM, Metalon L, Watanabe MD, et al. Depot antipsychotic drugs:Place in therapy. Drugs. 1994;47:741-73.
11. Glazer WM, Kane JM. Depot neuroleptic therapy:An under-utilized treatment option. J Clin Psychiatry. 1992;53:426-33.
12. Hirsch SR, Barnes TRE. Clinical use of high-dose neuroleptics. Br J Psychiatry. 1994;164:94-6.
13. Indanpaan-Heikkila J, Alhava E, Olkinuora M, et al. Agranulocytosis during treatment with clozapine. Eur J Clin Pharmacol. 1977;11:193-8.
14. Kane JM, et al. Long-term efficacy and safety of iloperidone: results from 3 clinical trials for the treatment of schizophrenia. J Clin Psychopharmacol. 2008;28:S29-S35.
15. Kane JM, Freeman HL. Towards more effective antipsychotic treatment. Br J Psychiatry. 1994;165 (Suppl. 25):22-31.
16. Kerwin RW. The new atypical antipsychotics. Br J Psychiatry. 1994;164:141-8.
17. Lauriello J, et al. An 8-week, double-blind, randomized, placebo-controlled study of olanzapine long-acting injection in acutely ill patients with schizophrenia. J Clin Psychiatry. 2008;69:790-9.
18. Lehman AF, Steinwachs DM, et al. Patterns of usual care for schizophrenia: Initial results from the Schizophrenia Patient Outcomes Research Teams (PORT) Client Survey. Schiz Bull. 1998:24:11-20.
19. McElvoy JP, Hogarty GE, Steingard S. Optimal dose of neuroleptic in acute schizophrenia. Arch Gen Psychiatry. 1991;48:739-45.
20. McKenna PJ, Bailey PE. The strange story of clozapine. Br J Psychiatry. 1993;162:32-7.

21. Potkin SG, et al. Efficacy and tolerability of asenapine in acute schizophrenia: a placebo- and risperidone-controlled trial. J Clin Psychiatry. 2007;68:1492-500.
22. Potkin SG, et al. Efficacy of iloperidone in the treatment of schizophrenia: initial phase 3 studies. J Clin Psychopharmacol. 2008;28:S4-11.
23. Ray WA, et al. Atypical antipsychotic drugs and the risk of sudden cardiac death. N Engl J Med. 2009;360:225-35.
24. Seeman P. An update of fast-off dopamine D2 atypical antipsychotics. Am J Psychiatry. 2005;162:1984-5.
25. Shahid M, et al. Asenapine: a novel psychopharmacologic agent with a unique human receptor signature. J Psychopharmacol. 2009;23:65-73.
26. Stone CK, Garver DL, Griffith J, et al. Further evidence of a dose-response threshold for haloperidol in psychosis. Am J Psychiatry. 1995;152:1210-2.
27. Tarazi FI, et al. Differential regional and dose-related effects of asenapine on dopamine receptor subtypes. Psychopharmacology (Berl). 2008;198:103-11.
28. Taylor DM. Olanzapine pamoate – blockbuster or damp squib? Int J Clin Pract. 2009;63:540-1.
29. Thompson C. The use of high-dose antipsychotic medication. Br J Psychiatry. 1994;164:448-58.
30. Weiden PJ, et al. Safety profile of iloperidone: a pooled analysis of 6-week acute-phase pivotal trials. J Clin Psychopharmacol. 2008;28:S12-S19.

Atypical Antipsychotics

31. Allison DB, Mentore JL, Heo M, et al. Antipsychotic-induced weight gain: a comprehensive research synthesis. Am J Psychiatry. 1999;156:1686-96.
32. Kapur S, Remington G. Serotonin dopamine interaction and its relevance to schizophrenia. Am J Psychiatry 1996;153:466-76.
33. Kelland MD, Freeman AS, Chiodo LA. Serotonergic afferent regulation of the basic physiology and pharmacological responsiveness of nigrostriatal dopamine neurons. J Pharmacol Exp Ther. 1990;253:803-11.
34. Leucht S, Pitschel-Walz G, Abraham D, Kissling W. Efficacy and extrapyramidal side-effects of the new antipsychotics olanzapine, quetiapine, risperidone, and sertindole compared to conventional antipsychotics and placebo. A meta-analysis of randomized controlled trials. Schizophr Res. 1999;35:51-68.
35. Remington G, Kapur S. Atypical antipsychotics: Are some more atypical than others? Psychopharmacology (Berl.). 2000;148:3-15.
36. Seeman P, Lee T, Chau-Wong M, Wong K. Antipsychotic drug doses and neuroleptic/dopamine receptors. Nature. 1976;61:717-9.
37. Seeman P. Dopamine receptor sequences. Therapeutic levels of neuroleptics occupy D2 receptors, clozapine occupies D4. Neuropsychopharmacology. 1998;7:261-84.
38. Waddington JL, Scully PJ, O'Callaghan E. The new antipsychotics, and their potential for early intervention in schizophrenia. Schizophr Res. 1997;28:207-22.

Antidepressants

39. Anderson IM, et al. Evidence-based guidelines for treating depressive disorders with antidepressants: a revision of the 2000 British Association for Psychopharmacology guidelines. J Psychopharmacol. 2008;22:343-96.
40. Baldassarini JR. Drugs and Treatment of Psychiatric Disorders: Depression and Mania. In: Hardman JG, Limbird JG, Molinoff PB, Ruddon RW (Eds). Goodman and Gilman's The Pharmacological Basis of Therapeutics, 9th edition. New York: Mcgraw-Hill, 1996.
41. Cookson J. Side effects of antidepressants. Br J Psychiatry. 1993;163 (Suppl 20):20-4.
42. Flanagan RJ. Fatal toxicity of drugs used in psychiatry. Hum Psychopharmacol. 2008;23 (Suppl) 1:43-51.
43. Frazer A. Antidepressants. J Clin Psychiatry. 1997;6:56.
44. Friedman RA, et al. Expanding the black box–depression, antidepressants, and the risk of suicide. N Engl J Med. 2007;356:2343-6.
45. Gartlehner G, et al. Comparative benefits and harms of second-generation antidepressants: background paper for the American College of Physicians. Ann Intern Med. 2008;149:734-50.
46. Kaplan HI, Sadock BJ, Grebb JA. Synopsis of Psychiartry, 7th edition. Baltimore: Williams and Wilkins; 1994.
47. Kaplan HI, Sadock BJ. Comprehensive Textbook of Psychiatry, 6th edition. Baltimore: Williams and Wilkins; 1995.
48. Kirsch I, et al. Initial severity and antidepressant benefits: a meta-analysis of data submitted to the Food and Drug Administration. PLoS Med. 2008;5:e45.
49. Leonard BE. Mechanism of action of antidepressants. CNS Drugs. 1996;4(Suppl 1):1-12.
50. Mulder RT, et al. Antidepressant treatment is associated with a reduction in suicidal ideation and suicide attempts. Acta Psychiatr Scand. 2008;118:116-22.
51. National Institute for Health and Clinical Excellence. Depression (amended) management of depression in primary and secondary care. 2007.http://www.nice.org.uk.
52. Papakostas GI, et al. A meta-analysis of early sustained response rates between antidepressants and placebo for the treatment of major depressive disorder. J Clin Psychopharmacol. 2006;26:56-60.
53. Rudorfer VM, Potter ZW. Antidepressants: A comparative review of clinical pharmacology and therapeutics of newer vs. older drugs. Drugs. 1989;37:713-38.
54. Sambunasis A, et al. Development of new antidepressants. J Clin Psychiatry. 1996;6:21.
55. Simon GE, et al. Suicide risk during antidepressant treatment. Am J Psychiatry. 2006;163:41-7.
56. Taylor MJ, et al. Early onset of selective serotonin reuptake inhibitor antidepressant action: systematic review and meta-analysis. Arch Gen Psychiatry. 2006;63:1217-23.
57. Thasse M. Maintenance treatment of recurrent affective disorder. Current Opinion in Psychiatry. 1993;6: 16-21.

58. Tondo L, et al. Suicidal status during antidepressant treatment in 789 Sardinian patients with major affective disorder. Acta Psychiatr Scand. 2008;118:106-15.

Mood Stabilizing Drugs

59. Aichhorn W, et al. Influence of age, gender, body weight and valproate comedication on quetiapine plasma concentrations. Int Clin Psychopharmacol. 2006;21:81-5.
60. American Psychiatric Association. Practice guideline for the treatment of patients with bipolar disorder (revision). Am J Psychiatry. 2002;159(Suppl 4):1-50.
61. Anon. Using lithium safely. Drug Ther Bull. 1999;37:22-4.
62. Baldessarini RJ, et al. Decreased risk of suicides and attempts during long-term lithium treatment: a meta-analytic review. Bipolar Disord. 2006;8:625-39.
63. Baldessarini RJ, et al. Effects of the rate of discontinuing lithium maintenance treatment in bipolar disorders. J Clin Psychiatry. 1996;57:441-8.
64. Bassilios N, et al. Monitoring of glomerular filtration rate in lithium-treated outpatients - an ambulatory laboratory database surveillance. Nephrol Dial Transplant. 2008;23:562-5.
65. Bauer MS, Mitchner L. What is a "mood stabilizer"? An evidence-based response. Am J Psychiatry. 2004;161(1):3-18.
66. Bergemann N, et al. Valproate lowers plasma concentration of olanzapine. J Clin Psychopharmacol. 2006;26:432-4.
67. Biel MG, et al. Continuation versus discontinuation of lithium in recurrent bipolar illness: a naturalistic study. Bipolar Disord. 2007;9:435-42.
68. Bowen RC, et al. Less frequent lithium administration and lower urine volume. Am J Psychiatry. 1991;148:189-92.
69. Cavanagh J, et al. Relapse into mania or depression following lithium discontinuation: a 7-year follow-up. Acta Psychiatr Scand. 2004;109:91-5.
70. Collins JC, et al. Divalproex, lithium and suicide among Medicaid patients with bipolar disorder. J Affect Disord. 2008;107:23-8.
71. Coyle JT, Duman RS. Finding the intracellular signaling pathways affected by mood disorder treatments. Neuron. 2003;38(2):157-60.
72. Falk WE, et al. Lithium prophylaxis of corticotropin-induced psychosis. JAMA. 1979;241:1011-2.
73. Fehr C, et al. Increase in serum clomipramine concentrations caused by valproate. J Clin Psychopharmacol. 2000;20:493-4.
74. Franks MA, et al. Bouncing back: is the bipolar rebound phenomenon peculiar to lithium? A retrospective naturalistic study. J Psychopharmacol. 2008;22:452-6.
75. Geddes JR, Burgess S, Hawton K, Jamison K, Goodwin GM. Long-term lithium therapy for bipolar disorder: systematic review and meta-analysis of randomized controlled trials. Am J Psychiatry. 2004;161(2):217-22.
76. Gitlin M. Lithium and the kidney: an updated review. Drug Saf. 1999;20:231-43.
77. Goodwin FK, et al. Suicide risk in bipolar disorder during treatment with lithium and divalproex. JAMA. 2003;290: 1467-73.
78. Goodwin GM. Recurrence of mania after lithium withdrawal. Implications for the use of lithium in the treatment of bipolar affective disorder. Br J Psychiatry. 1994;164:149-52.
79. Gunes A, et al. Inhibitory effect of valproic acid on cytochrome P450 2C9 activity in epilepsy patients. Basic Clin Pharmacol Toxicol. 2007;100:383-6.
80. Guzzetta F, et al. Lithium treatment reduces suicide risk in recurrent major depressive disorder. J Clin Psychiatry. 2007;68:380-3.
81. Harris EC, et al. Excess mortality of mental disorder. Br J Psychiatry. 1998;173:11-53.
82. James L, et al. Informing patients of the teratogenic potential of mood stabilising drugs; a case notes review of the practice of psychiatrists.J Psychopharmacol. 2007;21:815-9.
83. James L, et al. Mood stabilizers and teratogenicity - prescribing practice and awareness amongst practising psychiatrists. J Ment Health. 2009;18:137-43.
84. Johnston AM, et al. Lithium-associated clinical hypothyroidism. Prevalence and risk factors. Br J Psychiatry. 1999;175:336-9.
85. Livingstone C, et al. Lithium: a review of its metabolic adverse effects. J Psychopharmacol. 2006;20:347-55.
86. Meador KJ, et al. Cognitive function at 3 years of age after fetal exposure to antiepileptic drugs. N Engl J Med. 2009;360:1597-605.
87. Moncrieff J. Lithium: evidence reconsidered. Br J Psychiatry. 1997;171:113-9.
88. Moore CM, et al. Brain-to-serum lithium ratio and age: an in vivo magnetic resonance spectroscopy study. Am J Psychiatry. 2002;159:1240-2.
89. Morris RG, et al. Clinical study of lamotrigine and valproic acid in patients with epilepsy: using a drug interaction to advantage? Ther Drug Monit. 2000;22:656-60.
90. Morriss R, et al. Lithium and eGFR: a new routinely available tool for the prevention of chronic kidney disease. Br J Psychiatry. 2008;193:93-5.
91. Muller-Oerlinghausen B, Berghofer A, Ahrens B. The antisuicidal and mortality-reducing effect of lithium prophylaxis: consequences for guidelines in clinical psychiatry. Can J Psychiatry. 2003;48(7):433-9.
92. National Institute for Clinical Excellence. The clinical effectiveness and cost effectiveness of newer drugs for epilepsy in adults. Technology Appraisal 76. 2004. http://www.nice.org.uk.
93. Perlis RH, et al. Effect of abrupt change from standard to low serum levels of lithium: a reanalysis of double-blind lithium maintenance data. Am J Psychiatry. 2002;159:1155-9.
94. Sajatovic M, et al. Treatment adherence with lithium and anticonvulsant medications among patients with bipolar disorder. Psychiatr Serv. 2007;58:855-63.
95. Sandson NB, et al. An interaction between aspirin and valproate: the relevance of plasma protein displacement drug–drug interactions. Am J Psychiatry. 2006;163:1891-6.
96. Sanofi-Aventis. Summary of Product Characteristics. Depakote tablets. 2009. http://emc.medicines.org.uk.
97. Sanofi-Aventis. Summary of Product Characteristics. Epilim. 2009. http://emc.medicines.org.uk.

98. Severus WE, et al. What is the optimal serum lithium level in the long-term treatment of bipolar disorder – a review? Bipolar Disord. 2008;10:231-7.
99. Suppes T, Webb A, Paul B, Carmody T, Kraemer H, Rush AJ. Clinical outcome in a randomized 1-year trial of clozapine versus treatment as usual for patients with treatment-resistant illness and a history of mania. Am J Psychiatry. 1999;156(8):1164-9.
100. Tohen M, Ketter TA, Zarate CA, Suppes T, Frye M, Altshuler L, et al. Olanzapine versus divalproex sodium for the treatment of acute mania and maintenance of remission: a 47-week study. Am J Psychiatry. 2003;160(7):1263-71.
101. Tohen M, Vieta E, Calabrese J, Ketter TA, Sachs G, Bowden C, et al. Efficacy of olanzapine and olanzapine-fluoxetine combination in the treatment of bipolar I depression. Arch Gen Psychiatry. 2003;60(11):1079-88.
102. Tyrer SP. Lithium and treatment of aggressive behaviour. Eur Neuropsychopharmacol. 1994;4:234-6.
103. Wei Z, Mousseau DD, Richardson JS, Dyck LE, Li XM. Atypical antipsychotics attenuate neurotoxicity of beta-amyloid (25-35) by modulating Bax and Bcl-X(l/s) expression and localization. J Neurosci Res. 2003;74(6):942-7.
104. Yazici O, et al. Controlled lithium discontinuation in bipolar patients with good response to long-term lithium prophylaxis. J Affect Disord. 2004;80:269-71.

Sedative Hypnotic and Anxiolytic Drugs

105. Armour A, et al. A randomized, controlled prospective trial of zolpidem and haloperidol for use as sleeping agents in pediatric burn patients. J Burn Care Res. 2008;29:238-47.
106. Buscemi N, et al. Efficacy and safety of exogenous melatonin for secondary sleep disorders and sleep disorders accompanying sleep restriction:meta-analysis. BMJ. 2006;332:385-93.
107. Buscemi N, et al. The efficacy and safety of exogenous melatonin for primary sleep disorders. A meta-analysis. J Gen Intern Med. 2005;20:1151-8.
108. Costa E. (Symposium) The benzodiazepines: From molecular biology to clinical practice. New York: Raven Press; 1983.
109. Dailey JW. Sedative, hypnotic and anxiolytic agents. In: Craig CR, Stelzel RE (Eds). Modern Pharmacology. Boston: Little Brown; 1990. pp. 440-9.
110. Erman M, et al. An efficacy, safety, and dose-response study of Ramelteon in patients with chronic primary insomnia. Sleep Med. 2006;7:17-24.
111. Goldberg HL, Finnerty RJ. The comparative efficacy of buspirone and diazepam in the treatment of anxiety. Am J Psychiatry. 1979;136:1184.
112. Harvey SC. Hypnotics and sedatives. In: Gilman AG, Rall TW, Nies AS, Taylor P (Eds). The Pharmacological Basis of Therapeutics. New York: Pergamon Press; 1990. pp. 339-49.
113. Jacobs GD, et al. Cognitive behavior therapy and pharmacotherapy for insomnia: a randomized controlled trial and direct comparison. Arch Intern Med. 2004;164: 1888-96.
114. Kalpan HI, Sadock BJ. Pocket Handbook of Psychiatric Drug Treatment. New Delhi: BI Publication; 1993. pp. 52-64.
115. Krystal AD, et al. Long-term efficacy and safety of zolpidem extended-release 12.5 mg, administered 3 to 7 nights per week for 24 weeks, in patients with chronic primary insomnia: a 6-month, randomized, double-blind, placebo-controlled, parallel-group, multicenter study. Sleep. 2008;31:79-90.
116. Krystal AD, et al. Sustained efficacy of eszopiclone over 6 months of nightly treatment: results of a randomized, double-blind, placebo-controlled study in adults with chronic insomnia. Sleep. 2003;26:793-9.
117. Laurence DR, Bennet PN. Clinical Pharmacology. New York: Churchill Livingstone; 1992. pp. 264-9.
118. Medicines and Healthcare Products Regulatory Agency. Restrictions on the import of unlicensed Melatonin products following the grant of a marketing authorisation for Circadin® 2 mg tablets. 2008. http://www.mhra.gov.uk
119. Mini L, et al. Ramelteon 8 mg/d versus placebo in patients with chronic insomnia: post hoc analysis of a 5-week trial using 50% or greater reduction in latency to persistent sleep as a measure of treatment effect. Clin Ther. 2008;30:1316-23.
120. Morgan K, et al. Psychological treatment for insomnia in the regulation of long-term hypnotic drug use. Health Technol Assess 2004;8:11-68.
121. Morin CM, et al. Valerian-hops combination and diphenhydramine for treating insomnia: a randomized placebo-controlled clinical trial. Sleep. 2005;28:1465-71.
122. National Institute of Clinical Excellence. Insomnia-newer hypnotic drugs. Zaleplon, zolpidem and zopiclone for the management of insomnia. Technology Appraisal 77. http://www.nice.org.uk. 2004.
123. Polc P. Electrophysiology of benzodiazepine receptor ligands: Multiple mechanisms and sites of action. Progress Neurobiol. 1988;31:349-423.
124. Poyares D, et al. Chronic benzodiazepine usage and withdrawal in insomnia patients. J Psychiatr Res. 2004; 38:327-34.
125. Rao S, Sherbauink RW, Prasad K, et al. Cardiopulmonary effects of diazepam. Clin Pharmacol Ther. 1973;14:182-9.
126. Roth T, Roehrs TA. A review of the safety profiles of benzodiazepine hypnotics. J Clin Psychiatry. 1991;52 (Suppl 9):38.
127. Suhner A, et al. Impact of melatonin on driving performance. J Travel Med. 1998;5:7-13.
128. Tripathi KD. Essentials of Medical Pharmacology. New Delhi: Jaypee Brothers; 1992. pp. 333-42.
129. Uhde TW, Tancer MEW. Benzodiazepine receptor agonists and antagonsits. In: Kaplan HI, Sadock BJ (Eds). Comprehensive Text Book of Psychiatry. Baltimore: Williams & Wilkins; 1995. pp. 1957-60.

Electroconvulsive Therapy

130. American Psychiatric Association. The practice of electroconvulsive therapy: Recommendations for the treatment, training, and privileging: A Task Force Report of the American Psychiatric Association. Washington, DC. 2001.

131. Andrade C, Kurinji S, Sudha S, Chandra JS. Effects of pulse amplitude, pulse frequency, and stimulus duration on seizure threshold: a laboratory investigation. The Journal of ECT. 2002;18(3):144-8.
132. Andrade C, Shah N, Tharyan P, Reddy MS, Thirunavukarasu M, Kallivayalil RA, et al. Position statement and guidelines on unmodified electroconvulsive therapy. Indian Journal of psychiatry. 2012;54(2):119-33.
133. Andrade C. Dose calculation with brief-pulse ECT demystified. Indian Journal of Psychiatry. 2010;52(3):276-8.
134. Andrade C. Molecular mechanisms underlying electroconvulsive therapy-induced amnestic deficits: A decade of research. Indian Journal of Psychiatry. 2008;50(4):244-52.
135. Andrade C. Unilateral ECT and dosing. Indian Journal of Psychiatry. 2000;42(4):442-3.
136. Bolwig TG. How does electroconvulsive therapy work? Theories on its mechanism. Canadian Journal of Psychiatry Revue canadienne de psychiatrie. 2011;56(1):13-8.
137. Charlson F, Siskind D, Doi SA, McCallum E, Broome A, Lie DC. ECT efficacy and treatment course: a systematic review and meta-analysis of twice vs thrice weekly schedules. Journal of Affective Disorders. 2012;138(1-2):1-8.
138. Chung KF, Wong SJ. Stimulus dose titration for electroconvulsive therapy. Psychiatry and clinical neurosciences. 2001;55(2): 105-10.
139. Devanand DP, Dwork AJ, Hutchinson ER, Bolwig TG, Sackeim HA. Does ECT alter brain structure? The American Journal of Psychiatry. 1994;151(7):957-70.
140. Dierckx B, Heijnen WT, van den Broek WW, Birkenhager TK. Efficacy of electroconvulsive therapy in bipolar versus unipolar major depression: a meta-analysis. Bipolar Disorders. 2012;14(2):146-50.
141. Eitan R, Lerer B. Nonpharmacological, somatic treatments of depression: electroconvulsive therapy and novel brain stimulation modalities. Dialogues in Clinical Neuroscience. 2006;8(2):241-58.
142. el-Mallakh RS. Complications of concurrent lithium and electroconvulsive therapy: a review of clinical material and theoretical considerations. Biological Psychiatry. 1988;23(6):595-601.
143. Endler NS. The Origins of Electroconvulsive Therapy (ECT). Convulsive Therapy. 1988;4(1):5-23.
144. Gangadhar BN, Thirthalli J. Frequency of electroconvulsive therapy sessions in a course. The Journal of ECT. 2010;26(3): 181-5.
145. Gleiter CH, Nutt DJ. Chronic electroconvulsive shock and neurotransmitter receptors—an update. Life Sciences. 1989;44(15):985-1006.
146. Grover S, Mattoo SK, Gupta N. Theories on mechanism of action of electroconvulsive therapy. German Journal of Psychiatry. 2005;8(4):70-84.
147. Haskett RF, Loo C. Adjunctive psychotropic medications during electroconvulsive therapy in the treatment of depression, mania, and schizophrenia. The Journal of ECT. 2010;26(3):196-201.
148. Jahangard L, Haghighi M, Bigdelou G, Bajoghli H, Brand S. Comparing efficacy of ECT with and without concurrent sodium valproate therapy in manic patients. The Journal of ECT. 2012;28(2):118-23.
149. Kellner CH, Knapp R, Husain MM, Rasmussen K, Sampson S, Cullum M, et al. Bifrontal, bitemporal and right unilateral electrode placement in ECT: randomised trial. The British Journal of Psychiatry: The Journal of Mental Science. 2010;196(3):226-34.
150. Krystal AD, Weiner RD. ECT seizure therapeutic adequacy. Convulsive Therapy. 1994;10(2):153-64.
151. Loo CK, Katalinic N, Martin D, Schweitzer I. A review of ultrabrief pulse width electroconvulsive therapy. Therapeutic Advances in Chronic Disease. 2012;3(2):69-85.
152. Loo CK, Schweitzer I, Pratt C. Recent advances in optimizing electroconvulsive therapy. The Australian and New Zealand Journal of Psychiatry. 2006;40(8):632-8.
153. Naguib M, Koorn R. Interactions between psychotropics, anaesthetics and electroconvulsive therapy: implications for drug choice and patient management. CNS Drugs. 2002;16(4):229-47.
154. Payne NA, Prudic J. Electroconvulsive therapy: Part I. A perspective on the evolution and current practice of ECT. Journal of Psychiatric Practice. 2009;15(5):346-68.
155. Peterchev AV, Rosa MA, Deng ZD, Prudic J, Lisanby SH. Electroconvulsive therapy stimulus parameters: rethinking dosage. The Journal of ECT. 2010;26(3):159-74.
156. Petrides G, Tobias KG, Kellner CH, Rudorfer MV. Continuation and maintenance electroconvulsive therapy for mood disorders: review of the literature. Neuropsychobiology. 2011;64(3):129-40.
157. Pompili M, Lester D, Dominici G, Longo L, Marconi G, Forte A, et al. Indications for electroconvulsive treatment in schizophrenia: a systematic review. Schizophrenia Research. 2013;146(1-3):1-9.
158. Prudic J. Strategies to minimize cognitive side effects with ECT: aspects of ECT technique. The Journal of ECT. 2008;24(1):46-51.
159. Rabheru K. Maintenance electroconvulsive therapy (M-ECT) after acute response: examining the evidence for who, what, when, and how? The Journal of ECT. 2012;28(1):39-47.
160. Robertson C, Fergusson G. Electroconvulsive therapy machines. Adv Psychiatr Treat. 1996;2:24-31.
161. Royal College of Psychiatrists' Special Committee on ECT. The ECT Handbook: The third report of the Royal College of Psychiatrists' Special Committee on ECT. 2nd edition. Scott AIF. 2005.
162. Sackeim HA. Convulsant and anticonvulsant properties of electroconvulsive therapy: towards a focal form of brain stimulation. Clinical Neuroscience Research. 2004;4(1-2):39-57.
163. Sanchez Gonzalez R, Alcoverro O, Pagerols J, Rojo JE. Electrophysiological mechanisms of action of electroconvulsive therapy. Actas Espanolas de Psiquiatria. 2009;37(6):343-51.
164. Semkovska M, McLoughlin DM. Objective cognitive performance associated with electroconvulsive therapy for depression: a systematic review and meta-analysis. Biological Psychiatry. 2010;68(6):568-77.

165. Spellman T, Peterchev AV, Lisanby SH. Focal electrically administered seizure therapy: a novel form of ECT illustrates the roles of current directionality, polarity, and electrode configuration in seizure induction. Neuropsychopharmacology: official publication of the American College of Neuropsychopharmacology. 2009;34(8):2002-10.
166. Swartz CM, Nelson AI. Rational electroconvulsive therapy electrode placement. Psychiatry (Edgmont (Pa: Township)). 2005;2(7):37-43.
167. Swartz CM. 4 ECT electrode options: Which is the best for your patient? Current Psychiatry. 2006;5(3):114-5.
168. Swartz CM. ECT dosing by the benchmark method. German Journal of Psychiatry. 2002;5(1):1-4.
169. Tharyan P, Adams CE. Electroconvulsive therapy for schizophrenia. The Cochrane Database of Systematic Reviews. 2005(2):CD000076.
170. UK ECT Review Group. Efficacy and safety of electroconvulsive therapy in depressive disorders: a systematic review and meta-analysis. Lancet. 2003;361(9360):799-808.
171. Versiani M, Cheniaux E, Landeira-Fernandez J. Efficacy and safety of electroconvulsive therapy in the treatment of bipolar disorder: a systematic review. The Journal of ECT. 2011;27(2):153-64.
172. Wagner KJ, Mollenberg O, Rentrop M, Werner C, Kochs EF. Guide to anaesthetic selection for electroconvulsive therapy. CNS Drugs. 2005;19(9):745-58.

Psychopharmacological Drugs

173. Adli M, Berghofer A, Linden M, et al. Effectiveness and feasibility of a standardized stepwise drug treatment regimen algorithm for inpatients with depressive disorders: results of a 2-year observational algorithm study. J Clin Psychiatry. 2002;63:782-90.
174. American Psychiatric Association. Practice guideline for the treatment of patients with major depressive disorder (revision). Am J Psychiatry. 2000;157(Suppl):145. [Full Text]
175. Amsterdam JD, Maislin G, Potter L. Fluoxetine efficacy in treatment resistant depression. Prog Neuropsychopharmacol Biol Psychiatry. 1994;18:243-61.
176. Ananth J, Parameswaran S, Gunatilake S. Side effects of atypical antipsychotic drugs. Curr Pharm Des. 2004;10:2219-29.
177. Anderson IM. Selective serotonin reuptake inhibitors versus tricyclic antidepressants: a meta-analysis of efficacy and tolerability. J Affect Disord. 2000;58:1936.
178. Angst F, Stassen HH, Clayton PJ, Angst J. Mortality of patients with mood disorders: follow-up over 3438 years. J Affect Disord. 2002;68:167-81.
179. Ansorge MS, Zhou M, Lira A, Hen R, Gingrich JA. Earlylife blockade of the 5HT transporter alters emotional behavior in adult mice. Science. 2004;306:879-81.
180. Barbosa L, Berk M, Vorster M. A doubleblind, randomized, placebocontrolled trial of augmentation with lamotrigine or placebo in patients concomitantly treated with fluoxetine for resistant major depressive episodes. J Clin Psychiatry. 2003;64:403-7.
181. Bauer M, Dopfmer S. Lithium augmentation in treatment resistant depression: metaanalysis of placebocontrolled studies. J Clin Psychopharmacol. 1999;19:427-34.
182. Bauer M, Forsthoff A, Baethge C, et al. Lithium augmentation therapy in refractory depression update 2002. Eur Arch Psychiatry Clin Neurosci. 2003;253:132-9.
183. Belmaker RH. Bipolar disorder. N Engl J Med. 2004;351: 476-86.
184. Benkert O, Muller M, Szegedi A. An overview of the clinical efficacy of mirtazapine. Hum Psychopharmacol. 2002;17(Suppl 1):S23-S26.
185. Bennett AJ, Lesch KP, Heils A, et al. Early experience and serotonin transporter gene variation interact to influence primate CNS function. Mol Psychiatry. 2002;7:118-22.
186. Bertolino A, Frye M, Callicott JH, et al. Neuronal pathology in the hippocampal area of patients with bipolar disorder: a study with proton magnetic resonance spectroscopic imaging. Biol Psychiatry. 2003;53:906-13. [-CrossRef][ISI][Medline]
187. Bottlender R, Rudolf D, Strauss A, Moller HJ. Moodstabilisers reduce the risk of developing antidepressant induced maniform states in acute treatment of bipolar I depressed patients. J Affect Disord. 2001;63:79-83.
188. Bowden CL, Calabrese JR, McElroy SL, et al. A randomized, placebocontrolled 12-month trial of divalproex and lithium in treatment of outpatients with bipolar I disorder. Arch Gen Psychiatry. 2000;57:481-9.
189. Brannan SK, Mallinckrodt CH, Brown EB, Wohlreich MM, Watkin JG, Schatzberg AF. Duloxetine 60 mg once daily in the treatment of painful physical symptoms in patients with major depressive disorder. J Psychiatr Res. 2005;39:43-53.
190. Briley M. Clinical experience with dual action antidepressants in different chronic pain syndromes. Hum Psychopharmacol. 2004;19(Suppl 1):S21-S25. [CrossRef][ISI][Medline]
191. Caspi A, Sugden K, Moffitt TE, et al. Influence of life stress on depression: moderation by a polymorphism in the 5HTT gene. Science. 2003;301:386-9.
192. Ciechanowski PS, Katon WJ, Russo JE. Depression and diabetes: impact of depressive symptoms on adherence, function, and costs. Arch Intern Med. 2000;160:3278-85.
193. Cohen D. Atypical antipsychotics and new onset diabetes mellitus: an overview of the literature. Pharmacopsychiatry. 2004;37:1-11.
194. Coyne JC, Fechner Bates S, Schwenk TL. Prevalence, nature, and comorbidity of depressive disorders in primary care. Gen Hosp Psychiatry. 1994;16:267-76.
195. de Montigny C. Lithium addition in treatment-resistant depression. Int Clin Psychopharmacol. 1994;9(Suppl 2):31-5.
196. DeBattista C, Solvason HB, Poirier J, Kendrick E, Schatzberg AF. A prospective trial of bupropion SR augmentation of partial and nonresponders to serotonergic antidepressants. J Clin Psychopharmacol. 2003;23:27-30.
197. Dell'Osso B, et al. Switching from serotonin reuptake inhibitors to duloxetine in patients with resistant obsessive compulsive disorder: a case series. J Psychopharmacol. 2008;22:210-3.

198. Demyttenaere K, De Fruyt J, Stahl SM. The many faces of fatigue in major depressive disorder. Int J Neuropsychopharmacol. 2005;8:93-105.
199. DeRubeis RJ, Gelfand LA, Tang TZ, Simons AD. Medications versus cognitive behavior therapy for severely depressed outpatients: meta-analysis of four randomized comparisons. Am J Psychiatry. 1999;156:1007-13.
200. Detke MJ, Wiltse CG, Mallinckrodt CH, McNamara RK, Demitrack MA, Bitter I. Duloxetine in the acute and long-term treatment of major depressive disorder: a placebo and paroxetineb controlled trial. Eur Neuropsychopharmacol. 2004;14:457-70.
201. Diagnostic and statistical manual for mental disorders, 4th edition: DSMIV. Washington, D.C.: American Psychiatric Association; 1994.
202. Eriksson T. Anti-androgenic treatment of obsessive-compulsive disorder: an open-label clinical trial of the long-acting gonadotropin-releasing hormone analogue triptorelin. Int Clin Psychopharmacol. 2007;22:57-61.
203. Fava M, Papakostas GI, Petersen T, et al. Switching to bupropion in fluoxetine resistant major depressive disorder. Ann Clin Psychiatry. 2003;15:1722.
204. Feiger A, Kiev A, Shrivastava RK, Wisselink PG, Wilcox CS. Nefazodone versus sertraline in outpatients with major depression: focus on efficacy, tolerability, and effects on sexual function and satisfaction. J Clin Psychiatry. 1996;57(Suppl 2):53-62.
205. Feighner J, Targum SD, Bennett ME, et al. A doubleblind, placebocontrolled trial of nefazodone in the treatment of patients hospitalized for major depression. J Clin Psychiatry. 1998;59:246-53.
206. Fineberg NA, et al. Escitalopram prevents relapse of obsessive-compulsive disorder. Eur Neuropsychopharmacol. 2007;17:430-9.
207. Furukawa TA, Streiner DL, Young LT. Is antidepressant benzodiazepine combination therapy clinically more useful? A meta-analytic study. J Affect Disord. 2001;65:173-7.
208. Geddes JR, Carney SM, Davies C, et al. Relapse prevention with antidepressant drug treatment in depressive disorders: a systematic review. Lancet. 2003;361:653-61.
209. Geddes JR, Freemantle N, Mason J, Eccles MP, Boynton J. SSRIs versus other antidepressants for depressive disorder. Cochrane Database Syst Rev. 2000;2:CD001851CD001851.
210. Gibbons RD, Hur K, Bhaumik DK, Mann JJ. The relationship between antidepressant medication use and rate of suicide. Arch Gen Psychiatry. 2005;62:165-72.
211. Gijsman HJ, Geddes JR, Rendell JM, Nolen WA, Goodwin GM. Antidepressants for bipolar depression: a systematic review of randomized, controlled trials. Am J Psychiatry. 2004;161:1537-47. [Abstract/Full Text]
212. Goldman LS, Nielsen NH, Champion HC. Awareness, diagnosis, and treatment of depression. J Gen Intern Med. 1999;14:569-80.
213. Goldstein DJ, Lu Y, Detke MJ, Lee TC, Iyengar S. Duloxetine vs. placebo in patients with painful diabetic neuropathy. Pain. 2005;116:109-18.
214. Goldstein DJ, Lu Y, Detke MJ, Wiltse C, Mallinckrodt C, Demitrack MA. Duloxetine in the treatment of depression: a doubleblind placebocontrolled comparison with paroxetine. J Clin Psychopharmacol. 2004;24:389-99.
215. Goodwin FK, Jamison KR. Manic depressive illness. New York: Oxford University Press; 1990.
216. Greco T, Eckert G, Kroenke K. The outcome of physical symptoms with treatment of depression. J Gen Intern Med. 2004;19:813-8.
217. Guelfi JD, Ansseau M, Timmerman L, Korsgaard S. Mirtazapine versus venlafaxine in hospitalized severely depressed patients with melancholic features. J Clin Psychopharmacol. 2001;21:425-31.
218. Hariri AR, Drabant EM, Munoz KE, et al. A susceptibility gene for affective disorders and the response of the human amygdala. Arch Gen Psychiatry. 2005;62:146-52.
219. Hawley CJ, Pattinson HA, Quick SJ, et al. A protocol for the pharmacologic treatment of major depression: a field test of a potential prototype. J Affect Disord. 1998;47:87-96.
220. Hemmelgarn B, Suissa S, Huang A, Boivin JF, Pinard G. Benzodiazepine use and the risk of motor vehicle crash in the elderly. JAMA. 1997;278:27-31. [Abstract]
221. Henry C, Sorbara F, Lacoste J, Gindre C, Leboyer M. Antidepressant induced mania in bipolar patients: identification of risk factors. J Clin Psychiatry. 2001;62:249-55.
222. Hirschfeld RMA, Keller MB, Panico S, et al. The National Depressive and Manic Depressive Association consensus statement on the undertreatment of depression. JAMA. 1997;277:33
223. Jiang W, Krishnan RR, O'Connor CM. Depression and heart disease: evidence of a link, and its therapeutic implications. CNS Drugs. 2002;16:111-27.
224. Johnson J, Horwath E, Weissman MM. The validity of major depression with psychotic features based on a community study. Arch Gen Psychiatry. 1991;48:1075-81. [Abstract]
225. Jorge RE, Robinson RG, Arndt S, Starkstein S. Mortality and poststroke depression: a placebo-controlled trial of antidepressants. Am J Psychiatry. 2003;160:1823-9.
226. Judd LL, Akiskal HS, Maser JD, et al. A prospective 12 year study of subsyndromal and syndromal depressive symptoms in unipolar major depressive disorders. Arch Gen Psychiatry. 1998;55:694-700.
227. Judd LL, Paulus MJ, Schettler PJ, et al. Does incomplete recovery from first lifetime major depressive episode herald a chronic course of illness? Am J Psychiatry. 2000;157:1501-4.
228. Katona C. Managing depression and anxiety in the elderly patient. Eur Neuropsychopharmacol 2000;10(Suppl 4):S427-S432.
229. Keck PE Jr, Perlis RH, Otto MW, Carpenter D, Ross R, Docherty JP. Treatment of bipolar disorder 2004. Expert consensus

guideline series. Minneapolis: McGrawHill Healthcare Information; 2004.

230. Keck PE Jr. Bipolar depression: a new role for atypical antipsychotics? Bipolar Disord. 2005;7(Suppl 4):34-40.
231. Keller MB, Lavori PW, Rice J, Coryell W, Hirschfeld RM. The persistent risk of chronicity in recurrent episodes of nonbipolar major depressive disorder: a prospective followup. Am J Psychiatry. 1986;143:24-8.
232. Keller MB, Ryan ND, Strober M, et al. Efficacy of paroxetine in the treatment of adolescent major depression: a randomized, controlled trial. J Am Acad Child Adolesc Psychiatry. 2001;40:762-72.
233. Kendler KS, Davis CG, Kessler RC. The familial aggregation of common psychiatric and substance use disorders in the National Comorbidity Survey: a family history study. Br J Psychiatry. 1997;170:541-8.
234. Kennedy SH, Lam RW. Enhancing outcomes in the management of treatment resistant depresssion: a focus on atypical antipsychotics. Bipolar Disord. 2003;5(Suppl 2):36-47.
235. Kessler RC, McGonagle KA, Zhao S, et al. Lifetime and 12 month prevalence of DSM IIIR psychiatric disorders in the United States: results from the National Comorbidity Survey. Arch Gen Psychiatry. 1994;51:8-19.
236. Kroenke K, Spitzer RL, Williams JB, et al. Physical symptoms in primary care: predictors of psychiatric disorders and functional impairment. Arch Fam Med. 1994;3:774-9.
237. Kroenke K, West SL, Swindle R, et al. Similar effectiveness of paroxetine, fluoxetine, and sertraline in primary care: a randomized trial. JAMA. 2001;286:2947-55.
238. Krystal AD, et al. Long-term efficacy and safety of zolpidem extended-release 12.5 mg, administered 3 to 7 nights per week for 24 weeks, in patients with chronic primary insomnia: a 6-month, randomized, double-blind, placebocontrolled, parallel-group, multicenter study. Sleep. 2008;31:79-90.
239. LotufoNeto F, Trivedi M, Thase ME. Meta-analysis of the reversible inhibitors of monoamine oxidase type A moclobemide and brofaromine for the treatment of depression. Neuropsychopharmacology. 1999;20:226-47.
240. MacGillivray S, Arroll B, Hatcher S, et al. Efficacy and tolerability of selective serotonin reuptake inhibitors compared with tricyclic antidepressants in depression treated in primary care: systematic review and meta-analysis. BMJ. 2003;326:1014. [Medline]
241. Mann JJ, Currier D, Quiroz J, Manji HK. Neurobiology of severe mood and anxiety disorders. In: Siegel GJ, Albers RW, Brady S, Price D (Eds). Basic neurochemistry: molecular, cellular and medical aspects, 7th edition. San Diego, Calif.: Elsevier (in press).
242. Martin A, Young C, Leckman JF, Mukonoweshuro C, Rosenheck R, Leslie D. Age effects on antidepressant induced manic conversion. Arch Pediar Adolesc Med. 2004;158:77-380.
243. Masan PS. Atypical antipsychotics in the treatment of affective symptoms: a review. Ann Clin Psychiatry. 2004;16:3-13.
244. McEwen BS. Effects of adverse experiences for brain structure and function. Biol Psychiatry. 2000;48:721-31. [CrossRef][ISI][Medline]
245. Melfi CA, Chawla AJ, Croghan TW, Hanna MP, Kennedy S, Sredl K. The effects of adherence to antidepressant treatment guidelines on relapse and recurrence of depression. Arch Gen Psychiatry. 1998;55:1128-32.
246. Milak MS, Parsey RV, Keilp J, Oquendo MA, Malone KM, Mann JJ. Neuroanatomic correlates of psychopathologic components of major depressive disorder. Arch Gen Psychiatry. 2005;62:397-408.
247. Misri S, Burgmann A, Kostaras D. Are SSRIs safe for pregnant and breastfeeding women? Can Fam Physician. 2000;46:631-3.
248. Montejo AL, Llorca G, Izquierdo JA, RicoVillademoros F. Incidence of sexual dysfunction associated with antidepressant agents: a prospective multicenter study of 1022 outpatients. J Clin Psychiatry. 2001;62(Suppl 3):10-21.
249. Montgomery SA, Reimitz PE, Zivkov M. Mirtazapine versus amitriptyline in the long-term treatment of depression: a doubleblind placebocontrolled study. Int Clin Psychopharmacol. 1998;13:63-73.
250. Mueller TI, Leon AC, Keller MB, et al. Recurrence after recovery from major depressive disorder during 15 years of observational followup. Am J Psychiatry. 1999;156:1000-6.
251. Mulder RT, Watkins WG, Joyce PR, Luty SE. Age may affect response to antidepressants with serotonergic and noradrenergic actions. J Affect Disord. 2003;76:143-9. [CrossRef][ISI][Medline]
252. Narrow WE, Rae DS, Robins LN, Regier DA. Revised prevalence estimates of mental disorders in the United States: using a clinical significance criterion to reconcile 2 surveys' estimates. Arch Gen Psychiatry. 2002;59:11-51-3.
253. Nieuwstraten CE, Dolovich LR. Bupropion versus selective serotonin reuptake inhibitors for treatment of depression. Ann Pharmacother. 2001;35:1608-1613.
254. Nobler MS, Sackeim HA. Electroconvulsive therapy. In: Helmchen H, Henn F, Lauter H, Sartorius C (Eds). Contemporary psychiatry. Heidelberg, Germany: Springer; 2001. pp. 42-534.
255. Olfson M, Shaffer D, Marcus SC, Greenberg T. Relationship between antidepressant medication treatment and suicide in adolescents. Arch Gen Psychiatry. 2003;60:978-82.
256. Pampallona S, Bollini P, Tibaldi G, Kupelnick B, Munizza C. Combined pharmacotherapy and psychological treatment for depression: a systematic review. Arch Gen Psychiatry. 2004;61:714-9.
257. Parsey RV, Hastings RS, Oquendo MA, et al. [11C]McN5652 binding to the serotonin transporter in human brain: lower binding during a major depressive episode. Am J Psychiatry (in press).
258. Peet M. Induction of mania with selective serotonin reuptake inhibitors and tricyclic antidepressants. Br J Psychiatry 1994;164:549-50. [Abstract]
259. Peretti S, Judge R, Hindmarch I. Safety and tolerability considerations: tricyclic antidepressants vs. selective serotonin reuptake inhibitors. Acta Psychiatr Scand Suppl. 2000;403:1725. [Medline]

260. Practice guideline for the treatment of patients with bipolar disorder (revision). Am J Psychiatry. 2002;159(Suppl):150.
261. Prien RF, Kupfer DJ, Mansky PA, et al. Drug therapy in the prevention of recurrences in unipolar and bipolar affective disorders: report of the NIMH Collaborative Study Group comparing lithium carbonate, imipramine, and a lithium carbonateimipramine combination. Arch Gen Psychiatry. 1984;41:1096-104.
262. Prudic J, Olfson M, Marcus SC, Fuller RB, Sackeim HA. Effectiveness of electroconvulsive therapy in community settings. Biol Psychiatry. 2004;55:301-12. [CrossRef][ISI][Medline]
263. Quitkin FM, Stewart JW, McGrath PJ, et al. Columbia atypical depression: a subgroup of depressives with better response to MAOI than to tricyclic antidepressants or placebo. Br J Psychiatry Suppl. 1993;21:30-4.
264. Reynolds CF III, Frank E, Perel JM, et al. Nortriptyline and interpersonal psychotherapy as maintenance therapies for recurrent major depression: a randomized controlled trial in patients older than 59 years. JAMA. 1999;281:39-45.
265. Rothschild AJ, Williamson DJ, Tohen MF, et al. A doubleblind, randomized study of olanzapine and olanzapine/fluoxetine combination for major depression with psychotic features. J Clin Psychopharmacol. 2004;24:365-73.
266. Rowbotham MC, Goli V, Kunz NR, Lei D. Venlafaxine extended release in the treatment of painful diabetic neuropathy: a doubleblind, placebocontrolled study. Pain. 2004;110:697-706.
267. Ruck C, et al. Capsulotomy for obsessive-compulsive disorder: long-term follow-up of 25 patients. Arch Gen Psychiatry. 2008;65:914-21.
268. Rush AJ, Armitage R, Gillin JC, et al. Comparative effects of nefazodone and fluoxetine on sleep in outpatients with major depressive disorder. Biol Psychiatry. 1998;44:314.
269. Rush AJ, Kupfer DJ. Strategies and tactics in the treatment of depression. In: Gabbard GO (Ed). Treatment of psychiatric disorders, 3rd edtion. Washington DC: American Psychiatric Press. 2001.pp. 141-739.
270. Sachs GS, Lafer B, Stoll AL, et al. A doubleblind trial of bupropion versus desipramine for bipolar depression. J Clin Psychiatry. 1994;55:391-3.
271. Sackeim HA, Haskett RF, Mulsant BH, et al. Continuation pharmacotherapy in the prevention of relapse following electroconvulsive therapy: a randomized controlled trial. JAMA. 2001;285:1299-307.
272. Schatzberg AF, Haddad P, Kaplan EM, et al. Serotonin reuptake inhibitor discontinuation syndrome: a hypothetical definition. J Clin Psychiatry. 1997;58(Suppl 7):5-10.
273. Sheline YI, Gado MH, Kraemer HC. Untreated depression and hippocampal volume loss. Am J Psychiatry. 2003;160:1516-8.
274. Shelton RC, Tollefson GD, Tohen M, et al. A novel augmentation strategy for treating resistant major depression. Am J Psychiatry. 2001;158:131-4.
275. Simon GE, VonKorff M, Heiligenstein JH, et al. Initial antidepressant choice in primary care: effectiveness and cost of fluoxetine vs. tricyclic antidepressants. JAMA. 1996;275:1897-902. [Abstract]
276. Simon JS, Aguiar LM, Kunz NR, Lei D. Extended release venlafaxine in relapse prevention for patients with major depressive disorder. J Psychiatr Res. 2004;38:249-57.
277. Skapinakis P, et al. Antipsychotic augmentation of serotonergic antidepressants in treatment-resistant obsessive-compulsive disorder: a meta-analysis of the randomized controlled trials. Eur Neuropsychopharmacol. 2007;17:79-93.
278. Smith D, Dempster C, Glanville J, Freemantle N, Anderson I. Efficacy and tolerability of venlafaxine compared with selective serotonin reuptake inhibitors and other antidepressants: a meta-analysis. Br J Psychiatry. 2002;180:396-404. [Abstract/Full Text]
279. Soomro GM, et al. Selective serotonin re-uptake inhibitors (SSRIs) versus placebo for obsessive compulsive disorder (OCD). Cochrane Database Syst Rev. 2008;CD001765.
280. Spiker DG, Weiss JC, Dealy RS, et al. The pharmacological treatment of delusional depression. Am J Psychiatry. 1985;142:430-6.
281. Stahl SM, Entsuah R, Rudolph RL. Comparative efficacy between venlafaxine and SSRIs: a pooled analysis of patients with depression. Biol Psychiatry. 2002;52:1166-74. [CrossRef] [ISI]-[Medline]
282. Stahl SM. Placebocontrolled comparison of the selective serotonin reuptake inhibitors citalopram and sertraline. Biol Psychiatry. 2000;48:894-901.
283. Stark C, Hall D, O'Brien F, Smith H. Suicide after discharge from psychiatric hospitals in Scotland. BMJ. 1995;311:1368-9.
284. Storch EA, et al. Aripiprazole augmentation of incomplete treatment response in an adolescent male with obsessive-compulsive disorder. Depress Anxiety. 2008;25:172-4.
285. Suri R, Burt VK, Altshuler LL. Nefazodone for the treatment of postpartum depression. Arch Women Ment Health. 2005;8:55-6.
286. Swenson JR, O'Connor CM, Barton D, et al. Influence of depression and effect of treatment with sertraline on quality of life after hospitalization for acute coronary syndrome. Am J Cardiol. 2003;92:1271-6.
287. Taylor CB, Youngblood ME, Catellier D, et al. Effects of antidepressant medication on morbidity and mortality in depressed patients after myocardial infarction. Arch Gen Psychiatry. 2005;62:792-8. [Abstract/Full Text]
288. Taylor FB, Prather MR. The efficacy of nefazodone augmentation for treatment resistant depression with anxiety symptoms or anxiety disorder. Depress Anxiety. 2003;18:83-8.
289. Thase ME, Entsuah AR, Rudolph RL. Remission rates during treatment with venlafaxine or selective serotonin reuptake inhibitors. Br J Psychiatry. 2001;178:234-41. [Abstract/Full Text]
290. Thase ME, Mallinger AG, McKnight D, Himmelhoch JM. Treatment of imipramine resistant recurrent depression, 4th edition. A doubleblind crossover study of tranylcypromine for anergic bipolar depression. Am J Psychiatry. 1992;149:195-8.
291. Thase ME, Rush AJ. When at first you don't succeed: sequential strategies for antidepressant nonresponders. J Clin Psychiatry. 1997;58(Suppl 13):23-29.

292. The World Health Report 2002—reducing risks, promoting healthy life. Geneva: World Health Organization; 2002.
293. Thies Flechtner K, Muller Oerlinghausen B, Seibert W, Walther A, Greil W. Effect of prophylactic treatment on suicide risk in patients with major affective disorders: data from a randomized prospective trial. Pharmacopsychiatry. 1996;29:103-7.
294. Tohen M, Jacobs TG, Grundy SL, et al. Efficacy of olanzapine in acute bipolar mania: a doubleblind, placebocontrolled study. Arch Gen Psychiatry. 2000;57:841-9.
295. Tohen M, Vieta E, Calabrese J, et al. Efficacy of olanzapine and olanzapinefluoxetine combination in the treatment of bipolar I depression. Arch Gen Psychiatry. 2003;60:1079-88. [Erratum, Arch Gen Psychiatry. 2004;61:176.] [Abstract/Full -Text]
296. Treatment for Adolescents with Depression Study (TADS) Team. Fluoxetine, cognitive-behavioral therapy, and their combination for adolescents with depression: Treatment for Adolescents with Depression Study (TADS) randomized controlled trial. JAMA. 2004;292:807-20. [Abstract/Full Text]
297. Treatment of depression—newer pharmacotherapies. Evidence report/technology assessment no. 7. Washington DC: Agency for Health Care Policy and Research, 1999. (AHCPR publication no. 99E013.)
298. Trivedi MH, Rush AJ, Crismon ML, et al. Clinical results for patients with major depressive disorder in the Texas Medication Algorithm Project. Arch Gen Psychiatry. 2004;61:669-80.
299. UK ECT Review Group. Efficacy and safety of electroconvulsive therapy in depressive disorders: a systematic review and meta-analysis. Lancet. 2003;361:799-808.
300. Vinkers DJ, Gussekloo J, van der Mast RC, Zitman FG, Westendorp RG. Benzodiazepine use and risk of mortality in individuals aged 85 years or older. JAMA. 2003;290:2942-3.
301. Wecker L, James S, Copeland N, Pacheco MA. Transdermal selegiline: targeted effects on monoamine oxidases in the brain. Biol Psychiatry. 2003;54:1099-104.
302. Wisner KL, Gelenberg AJ, Leonard H, Zarin D, Frank E. Pharmacologic treatment of depression during pregnancy. JAMA. 1999;282:1264-9.
303. Yatham LN. Newer anticonvulsants in the treatment of bipolar disorder. J Clin Psychiatry. 2004;65(Suppl 10):2835.
304. Zisook S, Rush AJ, Albala A, et al. Factors that differentiate early vs. later onset of major depression disorder. Psychiatry Res. 2004;129:127-40.

Drug Therapy of Schizophrenia

305. Abi-Dargham A, Rodenhiser J, Printz D, et al. Increased baseline occupancy of D2-receptors by dopamine in schizophrenia. Proc Natl Acad Sci USA. 2000;97:8104-9.
306. Adler LE, Hoffer LD, Wiser A, Freedman R. Normalization of auditory physiology by cigarette smoking in schizophrenic patients. Am J Psychiatry. 1993;150:1856-61.
307. Aghajanian GK, Marek GJ. Serotonin model of schizophrenia: emerging role of glutamate mechanisms. Brain Res Brain Res Rev. 2000;31:302-12.
308. Akbarian S, Kim JJ, Potkin SG, Hetrick WP, Bunney WE Jr, Jones EG. Maldistribution of interstitial neurons in prefrontal white matter of the brains of schizophrenic patients. Arch Gen Psychiatry. 1996;53:425-36.
309. American Psychiatric Association. Practice guideline for the treatment of patients with schizophrenia. Am J Psychiatry. 1997;154(Suppl):1-63.
310. Benes FM, Kwok EW, Vincent SL, Todtenkopf MS. A reduction of nonpyramidal cells in sector CA2 of schizophrenics and manic depressives. Biol Psychiatry. 1998;44:88-97.
311. Berkeley G. A treatise concerning the principles of human knowledge. Dublin, Ireland: Jeremy Pepyat, 1710.
312. Biederman J, Lerner Y, Belmaker RH. Combination of lithium carbonate and haloperidol in schizoaffective disorder: a controlled study. Arch Gen Psychiatry. 1979;36:327-33.
313. Bilder RM, Goldman RS, Volavka J, et al. Neurocognitive effects of clozapine, olanzapine, risperidone, and haloperidol in patients with chronic schizophrenia or schizoaffective disorder. Am J Psychiatry. 2002;159:1018-28.
314. Bressan RA, Costa DC, Jones HM, Ell PJ, Pilowsky LS. Typical antipsychotic drugs–D(2) receptor occupancy and depressive symptoms in schizophrenia. Schizophr Res. 2002;56:31-6.
315. Buchanan RW, Breier A, Kirkpatrick B, Carpenter WT Jr. Positive and negative symptom response to clozapine in schizophrenic patients with and without the deficit syndrome. Am J Psychiatry. 1998;155:751-60.
316. Buchanan RW, Kreyenbuhl J, Zito JM, Lehman A. The schizophrenia PORT pharmacological treatment recommendations: conformance and implications for symptoms and functional outcome. Schizophr Bull. 2002; 28:63-73.
317. Carlsson A. Antipsychotic drugs, neurotransmitters, and schizophrenia. Am J Psychiatry. 1978;135:165-73.
318. Caroff SN, Mann SC. Neuroleptic malignant syndrome. Med Clin North Am. 1993;77:185-202.
319. Castner SA, Williams GV, Goldman-Rakic PS. Reversal of antipsychotic-induced working memory deficits by short-term dopamine D1-receptor stimulation. Science. 2000;287: 2020-2.
320. Cecil KM, Lenkinski RE, Gur RE, Gur RC. Proton magnetic resonance spectroscopy in the frontal and temporal lobes of neuroleptic naïve patients with schizophrenia. Neuropsychopharmacology. 1999;20:131-40.
321. Chowdari KV, Mrinics K, Semwal P, et al. Association and linkage analyses of RGS4 polymorphisms in schizophrenia. Hum Mol Genet. 2002;11:1373-80.
322. Chumakov I, Blumenfeld M, Guerassimenko O, et al. Genetic and physiological data implicating the new human gene G72 and the gene for D-amino acid oxidase in schizophrenia. Proc Natl Acad Sci USA. 2002;99:13675-80.
323. Conley RR, Tamminga CA, Kelly DL, Richardson CM. Treatment-resistant schizophrenic patients respond to clozapine after olanzapine non-response. Biol Psychiatry. 1999;46:73-7.

324. Cornblatt BA, Lencz T, Kane JM. Treatment of the schizophrenia prodrome: is it presently ethical? Schizophr Res. 2001;51: 31-8.
325. Cox B, Lee TF. Do central dopamine receptors have a physiological role in thermoregulation? Br J Pharmacol. 1977;61:83-6.
326. Cramer J, Rosenehck R, Xu W, Henderson W, Thomas J, Charney D. Detecting improvement in quality of life and symptomatology in schizoph-renia. Schizophr Bull. 2001;27:227-34.
327. Creese I, Burt DR, Snyder SH. Dopamine receptor binding predicts clinical and pharmacological potencies of antischizophrenic drugs. Science. 1976;192:481-3.
328. Csernansky JG, Mahmoud R, Brenner R. A comparison of risperidone and haloperidol for the prevention of relapse in patients with schizophrenia. N Engl J Med. 2002;346:16-22. [Erratum, N Engl J Med 2002;346:1424.]
329. Czobor P, Volavka J, Sheitman B, et al. Antipsychotic-induced weight gain and therapeutic response: a differential association. J Clin Psychopharmacol. 2002;22:244-51.
330. Daniel DG, Zimbroff DL, Potkin SG, Reeves KR, Harrigan EP, Lakshminarayanan M. Ziprasidone 80 mg/day and 160 mg/day in the acute exacerbation of schizophrenia and schizoaffective disorder: a 6-week placebo controlled trial. Neuropsychopharmacology. 1999;20:491-505.
331. de Haan L, Beuk N, Hoogenboom B, Dingemans P, Linszen D. Obsessive-compulsive symptoms during treatment with olanzapine and risperidone: a prospective study of 113 patients with recent-onset schizophrenia or related disorders. J Clin Psychiatry. 2002;63:104-7.
332. Diagnostic and statistical manual of mental disorders, 4th edition. DSM-IV. Washington, D.C.: American Psychiatric Association; 1994.
333. Egan MF, Goldberg TE, Kolachana BS, et al. Effect of COMT Val108/158 Met genotype on frontal lobe function and risk for schizophrenia. Proc Natl Acad Sci USA. 2001;98:6917-22.
334. Erlenmeyer-Kimling L. Early neurobehavioral deficits as phenotypic indicators of the schizophrenia genotype and predictors of later psychosis. Am J Med Genet. 2001;105:23-4.
335. Farde L, Hall H, Ehrin E, Sedvall G. Quantitative analysis of D2 dopamine receptor binding in the living human brain by PET. Science. 1986;231:258-61.
336. Frazier CJ, Buhler AV, Weiner JL, Dunwiddie TV. Synaptic potentials mediated via alpha-bungarotoxin-sensitive nicotinic acetylcholine receptors in rat hippocampal interneurons. J Neurosci. 1998;18:8228-35.
337. Freedman R, Silverman MM, Schwab PJ. Patients' awareness of extrapyramidal reactions to neuroleptic drugs: possible evidence for the role of catecholamines in perception. Psychiatry Res. 1979;1:31-8.
338. Gardos G, Casey DE, Cole JO, et al. Ten-year outcome of tardive dyskinesia. Am J Psychiatry. 1994;151:836-41.
339. Gearon JS, Kaltman SI, Brown C, Bellack AS. Traumatic life events and PTSD among women with substance use disorders and schizophrenia. Psychiatr Serv. 2003;54:523-8.
340. Gilmore JH, van Tol J, Kliewer MA, et al. Mild ventriculomegaly detected in utero with ultrasound: clinical associations and implications for schizophrenia. Schizophr Res. 1998;33: 133-40.
341. Glassman AH, Bigger JT Jr. Antipsychotic drugs: prolonged QTc interval, torsade de pointes, and sudden death. Am J Psychiatry. 2001;158:1774-82.
342. Goodman LS, Gilman A (Eds). The pharmacological basis of therapeutics: a textbook of pharmacology, toxicology, and therapeutics for physicians and medical students. 3rd edition. New York: Macmillan; 1965.pp.165-6.
343. Grace AA, Bunney BS. Induction of depolarization block in midbrain dopamine neurons by repeated administration of haloperidol: analysis using in vivo intracellular recording. J Pharmacol Exp Ther. 1986;238:1092-100.
344. Green MF, Marder SR, Glynn SM, et al. The neurocognitive effects of low dose haloperidol: a two year comparison with risperidone. Biol Psychiatry. 2002;51:972-8.
345. Green MF. What are the functional consequences of neurocognitive deficits in schizophrenia? Am J. Psychiatry. 1996;153:321-30.
346. Greene R. Circuit analysis of NMDAR hypofunction in the hippocampus, in vitro, and psychosis of schizophrenia. Hippocampus. 2001;11:569-77.
347. Hagg S, Spigset O, Bate A, Soderstrom TG. Myocarditis related to clozapine treatment. J Clin Psychopharmacol. 2001;21:382-8.
348. Hershman KM, Freedman R, Bickford PC. GABAb antagonists diminish the inhibitory gating of auditory response in the rat hippocampus. Neurosci Lett. 1995;190:133-6.
349. Herz MI, Marder SR. Schizophrenia: comprehensive treatment and management. Philadelphia: Lippincott Williams & Wilkins; 2002.
350. Hoek HW, Brown AS, Susser E. The Dutch famine and schizophrenia spectrum disorders. Soc Psychiatry Psychiatr Epidemiol. 1998;33:373-9.
351. Hogarty GE, Goldberg SC, Schooler NR, Ulrich RF. Drug and sociotherapy in the after care of schizophrenic patients, 2nd edition. Two-year relapse rates. Arch Gen Psychiatry. 1974;31:603-8.
352. Hogarty GE, Schooler NR, Ulrich R, Mussare F, Ferro P, Herron E. Fluphenazine and social therapy in the aftercare of schizophrenic patients: relapse analyses of a two-year controlled study of fluphenazine decanoate and fluphenazine hydrochloride. Arch Gen Psychiatry. 1979;36:1283-94.
353. Honigfeld G, Arellano F, Sethi J, Bianchini A, Schein J. Reducing clozapine related morbidity and mortality: 5 years of experience with the Clozaril National Registry. J Clin Psychiatry. 1998;59(Suppl 3):3-7.
354. Ichikawa J, Dai J, O'Laughlin IA, Fowler WL, Meltzer HY. Atypical, but not typical, antipsychotic drugs increase cortical acetylcholine release without an effect in the nucleus accumbens or striatum. Neuropsychopharmacology. 2002;26:325-39.
355. Jeste DV, Lohr JB. Hippocampal pathologic findings in schizophrenia: a morphometric study. Arch Gen Psychiatry. 1989;46:1019-24.

356. Johnson SW, Palmer MR, Freedman R. Effects of dopamine on spontaneous and evoked activity of caudate neurons. Neuropharmacology. 1983;22:843-51.
357. Jordan S, Koprivica V, Chen R, Tottori K, Kikuchi T, Altar CA. The antipsychotic aripiprazole is a potent, partial agonist at the human 5-HT1A receptor. Eur J Pharmacol. 2002;441:137-40.
358. Kane J, Honigfeld G, Singer J, Meltzer H. Clozapine for the treatment-resistant schizophrenic: a double-blind comparison with chlorpromazine. Arch Gen Psychiatry. 1988;45:789-96.
359. Kane JM, Carson WH, Saha AR, et al. Efficacy and safety of aripiprazole and haloperidol versus placebo in patients with schizophrenia and schizoaffective disorder. J Clin Psychiatry. 2002;63:763-71.
360. Kane JM, Davis JM, Schooler N, et al. A multidose study of haloperidol decanoate in the maintenance treatment of schizophrenia. Am J Psychiatry. 2002;159:554-60.
361. Kane JM, Marder SR, Schooler NR, et al. Clozapine and haloperidol in moderately refractory schizophrenia: a 6-month randomized and double-blind comparison. Arch Gen Psychiatry. 2001;58:965-72.
362. Kapur S, McClelland RA, VanderSpek SC, et al. Increasing D2 affinity results in the loss of clozapine's atypical antipsychotic action. Neuroreport. 2002;13:831-5.
363. Keefe RS, Silva SG, Perkins DO, Lieberman JA.The effects of atypical antipsychotic drugs on neurocognitive impairment in schizophrenia: a review and meta-analysis. Schizophr Bull. 1999;25:201-22.
364. Kramer MS, Gorkin R, Dijohnson C. Treatment of neuroleptic-induced akathisia with propranolol: a controlled replication study. Hillside J Clin Psychiatry. 1989;11:107-19
365. Kubicki M, Shenton ME, Salisbury DF, et al. Voxel based morphometric analysis of gray matter in first episode sc-hizophrenia. Neuroimage. 2002;17:1711-9.
366. Leonard S, Gault J, Hopkins J, et al. Association of promoter variants in the alpha7 nicotinic acetylcholine receptor subunit gene with an inhibitory deficit found in schizophrenia. Arch Gen Psychiatry. 2002;59:1085-96.
367. Leucht S, Pitschel-Walz G, Engel RR, Kissling W. Amisulpride, an unusual "atypical" antipsychotic: a meta-analysis of randomized controlled trials. Am J Psychiatry. 2002;159: 180-90.
368. Levinson DF, Umapathy C, Musthaq M. Treatment of schizoaffective disorder and schizophrenia with mood symptoms. Am J Psychiatry. 1999;156:1138-48.
369. Lindenmayer JP, Czobor P, Volavka J, et al. Changes in glucose and cholesterol levels in patients with schizophrenia treated with typical or atypical antipsychotics. Am J Psychiatry. 2003;160:290-6.
370. Madison DV, Nicoll RA. Norepinephrine decreases synaptic inhibition in the rat hippocampus. Brain Res. 1988;442: 131-8.
371. Marder SR, Essock SM, Miller AL, et al. The Mount Sinai conference on the pharmacotherapy of schizophrenia. Schizophr Bull. 2002;28:5-16.
372. Marder SR, Van Putten T, Mintz J, Lebell M, McKenzie J, May PR. Low and conventional dose maintenance therapy with fluphenazine decanoate: two-year outcome. Arch Gen Psychiatry. 1987;44:518-21.
373. McEvoy JP, Freudenreich O, Wilson WH. Smoking and therapeutic response to clozapine in patients with schizophrenia. Biol Psychiatry. 1999;46:125-9.
374. McGorry PD, Yung AR, Phillips LJ, et al. Randomized controlled trial of interventions designed to reduce the risk of progression to first episode psychosis in a clinical sample with subthreshold symptoms. Arch Gen Psychiatry. 2002;59:921-8.
375. McGuffin P, Riley B, Plomin R. Genomics and behavior: toward behavioral genomics. Science. 2001;291:1232-49.
376. Meltzer HY, Alphs L, Green AI, et al. Clozapine treatment for suicidality in schizophrenia: International Suicide Prevention Trial (InterSePT). Arch Gen Psychiatry. 2003;60:82-91.
377. Meltzer HY. Clinical studies on the mechanism of action of clozapine: the dopamine-serotonin hypothesis of schizophrenia. Psychopharmacology (Berl). 1989;99(Suppl: S18-S27.
378. Nordstrom A, Farde L, Halldin C. Time course of D2-dopamine receptor occupancy examined by PET after single oral dose of haloperidol. Psychopharmacology (Berl). 1992;106:433-8.
379. Park S, Holzman PS, Goldman-Rakic PS. Spatial working memory deficits in the relatives of schizophrenic patients. Arch Gen Psychiatry. 1995;52:821-8.
380. Pickar D, Labarca R, Doran AR, et al. Longitudinal measurement of plasma homovanillic acid levels in schizophrenic patients: correlation with psychosis and response to neuroleptic treatment. Arch Gen Psychiatry. 1986;43:669-76.
381. Pisani F, Oteri G, Costa C, Di Raimondo G, Di Perri R. Effects of psychotropic drugs on seizure threshold. Drug Saf. 2002;25:91-110.
382. Satanove A, McIntosh JS. Phototoxic reactions induced by high doses of chlorpromazine and thioridazine. JAMA. 1967;200:209-12.
383. Schaeffer JL, Ross RG. Childhood onset schizophrenia: premorbid and prodromal diagnostic and treatment histories. J Am Acad Child Adolesc Psychiatry. 2002;41:538-45.
384. Selemon LD, Rajkowska G, Goldman-Rakic PS. Abnormally high neuronal density in the schizophrenic cortex: a morphometric analysis of prefrontal area 9 and occipital area 17. Arch Gen Psychiatry. 1995;52:805-18.
385. Sernyak MJ, Desai R, Stolar M, Rosenheck R. Impact of clozapine on completed suicide. Am J Psychiatry. 2001;158: 931-7.
386. Sernyak MJ, Leslie DL, Alarcon RD, Losonczy MF, Rosenheck R. Association of diabetes mellitus with use of atypical neuroleptics in the treatment of schizophrenia. Am J Psychiatry. 2002;159:561-6.
387. Siris SG. Suicide and schizophrenia. J Psychopharmacol. 2001;15:127-35.
388. Small JG, Hirsch SR, Arvanitis LA, Miller BG, Link CG. Quetiapine in patients with schizophrenia: a high and low-dose

double-blind comparison with placebo. Arch Gen Psychiatry. 1997;54:549-57.

389. Smith S, Wheeler MJ, Murray R, O'Keane V. The effects of antipsychotic-induced hyperprolactinaemia on the hypothalamic-pituitary-gonadal axis. J Clin Psychopharmacol. 2002;22:109-14.
390. Spohn HE, Lacousiere RB, Thompson K, Coyne L. Phenothiazine effects on psychological and psychophysiological dysfunction in chronic schizophrenics. Arch Gen Psychiatry. 1977;34:633-44.
391. Stefansson H, Sigurdsson E, Seinthorsdottir V, et al. Neuregulin 1 and susceptibility to schizophrenia. Am J Hum Genet. 2002;71:877-92.
392. Straub RE, Jiang Y, MacLean CJ, et al. Genetic variation in the 6p22.3 gene DTNBP1, the human ortholog of the mouse dysbindin gene, is associated with schizophrenia. Am J Hum Genet. 2002;71:337-48.
393. Suzuki A, Kondo T, Otani K, et al. Association of the TaqI A polymorphism of the dopamine D(2) receptor gene with predisposition to neuroleptic malignant syndrome. Am J Psychiatry. 2001;158:1714-6.
394. Swanson JW, Holzer CE III, Ganju VK, Jono RT. Violence and psychiatric disorder in the community: evidence from the Epidemiologic Catchment Area surveys. Hosp Community Psychiatry. 1990;41:761-70.
395. Tamminga CA, Thaker GK, Buchanan R, et al. Limbic system abnormalities identified in schizophrenia using positron emission tomography with fluorodeoxyglucose and neocortical alterations with deficit syndrome. Arch Gen Psychiatry. 1992;49:522-30.
396. Thompson PM, Vidal C, Giedd JN, et al. Mapping adolescent brain change reveals dynamic wave of accelerated gray matter loss in very early-onset schizophrenia. Proc Natl Acad Sci USA. 2001;20:543-50.
397. Tran PV, Hamilton SH, Kuntz AJ, et al. Double-blind comparison of olanzapine versus risperidone in the treatment of schizophrenia and other psychotic disorders. J Clin Psychopharmacol. 1997;17:407-18.
398. Tsuang M. Schizophrenia: genes and environment. Biol Psychiatry. 2000;47:210-20.
399. Venables PH. Input dysfunction in schizophrenia. Prog Exp Personality Res. 1964;1:1-47.
400. Volavka J, Czobor P, Sheitman B, et al. Clozapine, olanzapine, risperidone, and haloperidol in the treatment of patients with chronic schizophrenia and schizoaffective disorder. Am J Psychiatry. 2002;159:255-62. [Erratum, Am J Psychiatry 2002;159:2132.]
401. Wolkowitz OM, Pickar D. Benzodiazepines in the treatment of schizophrenia: a review and reappraisal. Am J Psychiatry. 1991;148:714-26.
402. Woo TU, Whitehead RE, Melchitzky DS, Lewis DA. A subclass of prefrontal gamma-aminobutyric acid axon terminals are selectively altered in schizophrenia. Proc Natl Acad Sci USA. 1998;95:5341-6.
403. Wyatt RJ, Henter ID. The effects of early and sustained intervention on the long-term morbidity of schizophrenia. J Psychiatr Res. 1998;32:169-77

Complementary Medicine in Psychiatry

404. Ahlemeyer B, Krieglstein J. Neuroprotective effects of Ginkgo biloba extract Cellular and Molecular Life Sciences. 2003;60: 1779-2.
405. Akhondzadeh S, Kashani L, Mobaseri M. et al. Passion flower in the treatment of opiates withdrawal: a doble-blind randomized controlled trial. Journal of Clinical Pharmacy and Therapeutics. 2001b;26:369-73.
406. Akhondzadeh S, Naghavi HR, Vazirian, M. et al. Passion flower in the treatment of generalized anxiety: a pilot double-blind randomized controlled trial with oxazepam. Journal of Clinical Pharmacy and Therapeutics, 2001a;26:363-7.
407. Alderman CP, Kiepfer B. Complementary medicine use by psychiatry patients of an Australian hospital. Annals of Pharmacotherapy. 2003;37:1779-84.
408. Amenta F, Cavalloti C, Franch F, et al. 1989. Mascarinic cholinergic receptors in hippocampus of the aged rat: effect of long-term hydergine administration. Archives internationals de pharmocodyanamine et de Theropie297:225-34.
409. Benjamin J, Muir T, Briggs K, et al. A case of cerebral haemorrhage—can Ginkgo biloba be implicated? Postgraduate Medical Journal. 2001;77:112-3.
410. Benton D, Cook R. Selenium supplementation improves mood in a double-blind crossover trial. Biological Psychiatry. 1991; 29:1092-8.
411. Benton D. Selenium intake, mood and other aspects of psychological functioning. Nutrition and Neurosciences. 2002; 5:363-74.
412. Birks J, Grimley Evans J, Van Dongen M. 2002. Ginkgo biloba for cognitive impairment of dementia. Cochrane Library, Issue 2. Oxford: Update Software.
413. Boerner RJ, Sommer H, Berger W, et al. 2003. Kava-kava extract L1150 is as effective as opipramol and buspirone in generalized anxiety disorder an 8-week randomized, double-blind multi-centre clinical trial in 129 out-patients. Phytomedicine. 10:(suppl.), 38-49.
414. Bottiglieri T, Laundy M, Crelin R, et al. 2000. Homocysteine, folate, methylation, and Neurology. Neurosurgery and Psychiatry, 69:228-32.
415. Bowden CL. Novel treatments for bipolar disorder. Expert Opinion in Investigating Drugs, 2001;10:661-71.
416. Bressa GM. S-adenosyl-methionine (SAMe) as antidepressant: meta-analysis of clinical studies. Acta Neurologica Scandinavica. 1994;154(Suppl.):7-14.
417. Brown BG, Zhao XQ, Chait A, et al. Simvastatin and niacin, antioxidant vitamins, or the combination for the prevention of coronary disease. New England Journal of Medicine. 2001; 29:1583-92.

418. Brugha T, Rampes H, Jenkins R. Surely you take complmentary and alternative medicines? Psychiatric Bulletin. 2004;28: 36-9.
419. Cardinali DP, Gvozdenovich E, Kaplan MR, et al. A double blind-placebo controlled study on melatonin efficacy to reduce anxiolytic benzodiazepine use in the elderly. Neuroendocrinology Letters. 2002;23:55-60.
420. Carman JS, Post RM, Buswell R, et al. Negative effects of melatonin on depression. American Journal of Psychiatry. 1976; 133:1181-6.
421. Chatterjee SS, Nolder M, Koch E, et al. Antidepressant activity of Hypericum perforatum and hyperforin: the neglected possibility. Pharmacopsychiatry. 1998;31(suppl.):7-15.
422. Chevalier A. The Encyclopedia of Medicinal Plant. London: Dorling Kindersley, 1996.
423. Coffin AI. Botanic Guide to Health and Natural Pathology of Diseases. London: J Caudwell, 1845.
424. Cohen MH, Eisenberg DM. Potential physician malpractice liability associated with complementary and integrative medicinal therapies. Annals of Internal Medicine. 2002; 136:596-603.
425. Committee on safety of medicines and medicines control Agency. Reminder: St John's wort (Hypericum perfortum) interaction. Current Problems in Pharmacovigilance. 2000; 26:6-7.
426. Corrigan JJ Jr. The effect of vitamin E on warfarin-induced vitamin K deficiency. Annals of the New York Academy of Sciences. 1982;393:361-8.
427. Cott JM. In vitro receptor binding and enzyme inhibition by hypericum perforatum extract. Pharmacopsychiatry. 1997; 30(sppl.):108-12.
428. De Vry J, Maurel S, Schreiber R, et al. Comparison of Hypericum extract with imipramine and fluoxetine in animal model of depression and alcoholism. European Neuropsychopharmacology. 1999;9:61-8.
429. Delle Chiaie R, Pancheri P, Scapicchio P. Efficacy and tolerability of oral and intramuscular S-adenosyl-L-methionine 1,4-butanedisulfonate (SAMe) in the treatment of major depression: comparision with impiramine in 2 major multicenter studies. American Journal of Clinical Nutrition. 2002;76 (Suppl.):11725-65.
430. Dhawan K, Dhawan S, Chhabra S. Attenuation of benzodiazepine dependence in mice by a trisubstituted benzoflavone moiety of Passiflora incarnata Linneaus: a non-habit forming anxiolytic. Journal of Pharmacy and Pharmacological Science. 2003;6:215-22.
431. Dhawan K, Kumar S, Sharma A. Reversal of cannabinoids (delta9-THC) by the benzoflavone moiety from methanol extract of Passiflora incarnata Linnaeus in mice: a possible therapy for cannabinoid addiction. Journal of Pharmacy and Pharmacology. 2002a;54:875-81.
432. Diaper A, Hindmarch I. A double-blind, placebo-controlled investigation of the effect of two doses of a valerian preparation on the sleep, cognitive and psychomotor function of sleep-disturbed older adults. Phytotherapy Research. 2004;18:831-6.
433. Dinh LD, Simmen U, Bueter KB, et al. Interaction of various Piper methysticum cultivars with CNS receptors in vitro. Planta Medica. 2001;67:306-11.
434. Dorn M. Efficacy and tolerability of Baldrian versus oxazepam in non-organic and non-psychiatric insomniacs: a randomized, double blind, clinical comparative study Forschende Kamplementarmedizin und Klassische Naturheikunde. 2000; 7:79-84.
435. Dravid AR. Deficits in cholinergic enzymes and muscarinic receptors in the hippocampus and striatum of senescent rats: effect of chronic hydergine treatment. Archives internationals Pharmcodynaamie et de Therapie. 1983;264:195-202.
436. Eisenberg DM, Kessler RC, Foster C, et al. Uncoventional medicine in the United States. Prevalence, costs and pattern of use. New England Journal of Medicine. 1993;328:246-52.
437. Ernst E, Cassileth BR. How useful are unconventional cancer treatment? European Journal of Cancer. 1999;35:1608-13.
438. Ernst E. "Flower remedies" : a systematic review of the clinical evidence. Wiener Klinische Wochenschrift. 2002;30:963-6.
439. Fava M, Giannelli A, Rapisarda V, et al. Rapidity of onset of the antidepressant effect of parenteral S-adenosyl-L-methionine. psychiatry Research. 1995;56:295-7.
440. Fisher AA, Purecell P, Le Couteur DG. Toxicity of Passiflora incarnata L. Journal of Clinical Toxicology. 2000;38:63-6.
441. Food Standards Agency. Expert Group on vitamins and Minerals (2003) Safe Upper Levels for Vitamins and Minerals. http://www.foodstandards.gov.uk
442. Friedel HA, Goa KL, Benefield P. S-adenosyl-L-methionine. A review of its pharmacological properties and therapeutic potential in liver dysfunction and affective disorders in relation to its physiological role in cell metabolism. Drugs. 1989; 38:389-416.
443. Fugh-Berman A. Herb-drug interactions. Lancet. 2000; 355:134-8.
444. Glick SD, Maisonneuve IM, Dickinson HA. 18-MC reduces methamphetamine and nicotine self-administration in rats. Neuroreport, II. 2000;2013-5.
445. Hagg M. Essential fatty acids and the brain. Canadian Journal of Psychiatry. 2003;48:195-203.
446. Hamilton M. Development of a rating scale for primary depressive illness. British Journal of Social and Clinical Psychology. 1967;6:278-96.
447. Hawkes WC, Hornbostel L. Effects of dietary selenium on mood in healthy men living in a metabolic research unit. Biological Psychiatry. 1996;39:121-8.
448. Herxheimer A, Petrie KJ. Melatonin for the prevention and treatment of jet lag. Cochrane Library, issue 4. oxford : Update Software, 2003.
449. Houghton PJ. The scientific basis for the reputed activity of Valerian. Journal of Pharmacy and Pharmacology. 1999; 51:505-12.
450. Itil TM, Ahmed I, Kunitz A, et al. The pharmacological effects of Ginkgo biloba, a plant extract, on the brain of dementia patients in comparison with tacrine. Psychopharmacology Bulletin. 1998;34:391-7.

451. Jaroszewski JW, Olafsdottir ES, Wellendorph P, et al. Cyanohydrin glycosides of Passiflora: distribution pattern, a saturated cyclopentane derivative from P, guatemalensis, and formation of pseudocyanogenic alpha-hydroxyamides as isolation artifacts. Phytochemistry. 2002;59:501-11.
452. Joy CB, Mumby-Croft R, and Joy LA. 2003. Polyunsaturated fatty acid supplementation for schizophrenia. Cochrane Library, issue 4. oxford : Update software.
453. Jussofie A, Schmiz A, and Hiemke C. 1994. Kavapyrone enriched extract Piper methysticum as modulator of the GABA binding site in different regions of rat brain. Psychopharmacology. 116:469-74
454. Kanowski S, Hoerr T. Gingkgo biloba extract EGb 761 in dementia: intent-to-treat analyses of a 24-week, multi-center, double-blind, placebo-controlled, randomized trial. Pharmacopsychiatry. 2003;36:297-303.
455. Kessler RC, Soukup J, Davis RB, et al. The use of complementary and alternative therapies to treat anxiety and depression in the United States. American Journal of Psychiatry. 2001; 158:289-94.
456. Keung WM. Biochemical studies of a new class of alcohol dehydrogenase inhibitors from Radix puerariae. Alcoholism, Clinical and Experimental Research. 1993;17:1254-60.
457. Klepser TB, Klepser ME. Unsafe and potentially safe herbal therapies. American journal of Health-System Pharmacy. 1999; 56:125-38.
458. Knaudt PR, Connor KM, Weisler RH, et al. Alternative therapy use by psychiatric outpatients. Journal of Nervous and Mental Disease. 2001;187:692-5.
459. Krasowski MD, McGehee DS, Moss J. Natural inhibitors of cholinesterases: implications for adverse drug reactions. Canadian Journal of Anaesthesia. 1997;44:525-34.
460. Le Poncin-Lafitte M, Rapin JR, Duterte D, et al. Learning and cholinergic neurotransmission in old animals: the effect of Hydergine Pharmacology. 1985;16:(suppl.):57-63.
461. Lee BM, Lee SK, Klim HS. Inhibition of oxidative DNA damage, 8-OHdG, and carbonyl contents in smokers treated with antioxidants (vitamin E, vitamin C, beta-carotene and red ginseng). Cancer Letters. 1998;132:219-27.
462. Lehrl S. Clinical efficacy of kava extract WS 1490 in sleep disturbance associated with anxiety disorders. Results of a multicenter, randomized, placebo-controlled, double-blind clinical trial. Journal of Affective Disorders. 2004;78:101-10.
463. Lewis R, Wake G, Court G, et al. Non-ginsenoside nicotinic activity in ginseng species. Phytotherapy Research. 1999; 13:59-64.
464. Liede KE, Saxen LM, et al. Increased tendency towards gingival bleeding caused by joint effect of alpha-tocopherol supplementation and acetylsalicylic acid. Annals of Medicine. 1998;30:542-6.
465. Lin RC, Li TK. Effects of isoflavones on alcohol pharmacokinetics and alcohol-drinking behavior in rats: American Journal of Clinical Nutrition. 1998;68(suppl.):15125-55.
466. Linde K, Berner M, Egger M, et al. St John's wort for depression. Meta-analysis of randomized controlled trials. British Journal of Psychiatry. 2005;186:99-107.
467. Lohr JB, Kuczenski R, Niculescu AB. Oxidative mechanisms and tardive dyskinesia. CNS Drugs. 2003;17:47-62.
468. Maclennan KM, Darlington CL, Smith PF. The CNS effects of Ginkgo biloba extracts and ginkgolide B. Progress in Neurobiology. 2002;67:235-57.
469. Maclennan KMA, Broomfield NM, Espie CA. A systematic review of the effectiveness of oral melatonin for adults (18 to 65 years) with delayed sleep phase syndrome and adults (18 to 65 years) with primary insomnia. Current psychology Reviews. 2005;1:103-13.
470. Maisonneuve IM, Glick SD. Anti-addictive actions of an iboga alkaloid congener: a novel mechanism for a novel treatment. Pharmacology Biochemistry and behavior. 2003;75:607-618.
471. Malamud W, Barton WE, Fleming AM, et al. The evaluation of the effects of derivatives of Rauwolfia in the treatment of schizophrenia. American Journal of Psychiatry. 1957; 114:193-200.
472. Marangell LB, Martinez JM, Zboyan HA, et al. A double-blind, placebo-controlled study of the omega-3 fatty acids docosahexaenoic acid in the treatment of major depression. American Journal of Psychiatry. 2003;160:996-8.
473. Markstein R. Hydergine: interaction with the neurotransmitter systems in the central nervous system, journal of pharmacology. 1985;16(suppl.)-17.
474. Mash DC, Staley JK, Pablo JP, et al. Properties of ibogaine and its principal metabolite (12-hydroxy ibogamine) at the MK-801 binding site of the NMDA receptor complex. Neuroscience Letters. 1995;192:53-6.
475. Mathews JM, Etheridge AS, Black SR. Inhibition of human cytochrome P450 activities by kava extract and kavalactones. Drug Metabolism and Disposition. 2002;30:1153-7.
476. Matthews MK jr. Association of Ginkgo biloba with intracerebral hemorrhage. Neurology. 1998;50:1993-94.
477. Matthews SC, Camacho A, Lawson K, et al. Use of herbal medications among 200 psychiatric outpatients: prevalence, patterns of use, and potential dangers. General Hospital Psychiatry. 2003;25:24-6.
478. Medical Economics. PDR (Physicians' Desk Reference) for Herbal Medicines 2nd edition, Montavle, NJ: Medical Economics Company, 2000
479. Meseguer E, Taboada R, Sanchez V, et al. Life-threatening Parkinsonism induced by kava-kava. Movement Disorders. 2002;17:195-6.
480. Miller LG. Herbal medicinals: selected clinical considerations focusing on known or potential drug-herb interactions. Archives of Internal Medicine. 1989;158:2200-11.
481. Mischoulon D, Fava M. Role of S-adenosyl-L-methionine in the treatment of depression: a review of the evidence. American Journal of Clinical Nutrition. 2002;76(suppl.):11585-615.
482. Morris WE, Singer A, Wonnemann M, et al. Hyperforin represents the neurotransmitter reuptake inhibiting constituent of Hypericum extract. Pharmacopsychiatry. 1998; 31(suppl.):16-21.
483. Munoz-Hoyos A, Sanchez-Forte M, Molina-Carballo A, et al. Melatonin's role as an anticonvulsant and neuronal protector:

experimental and clinical evidence. Journal of Child Neurology. 1998;13:501-9.

484. Natural Medicines Comprehensive Database. http://naturaldatabase.com.Product search:kava. 1998
485. Natural Medicines Comprehensive Database. http://naturaldatabase.com.Product search:iodine. 2004b.
486. Natural Medicines Comprehensive Database. http://naturaldatabase.com.Product search:selenium. 2004c.
487. Natural Medicines Comprehensive Database. http://naturaldatabase.com.Product search:Folic acid. 2004d.
488. Natural Medicines Comprehensive Database. http://naturaldatabase.com.Product search: Indian snakeroot. 2004e
489. Natural Medicines Comprehensive Database. http://naturaldatabase.com.Product search:iboga. 2004f.
490. Natural Medicines Comprehensive Database. http://naturaldatabase.com.Product search:kudzu. 2004g.
491. Neary JT, Bu Y. Hyperforin inhibits uptake of serotonin and norepinephrine in astrocytes. Brain Research. 1999; 816:358-63.
492. Nemets B, Stahl Z, Belmaker RH. Addition of omega-3 fatty acid to maintenance medication treatment for recrurrent unipolar depressive disorder. American Journal of Psychiatry, 2002;159:477-9.
493. Oken BS, Storzbach DM, Kaye JA. The efficacy of Ginkgo biloba on cognitive function in Alzheimer disease. Archives of Neurology. 1998;55:1409-15.
494. Olde Rikkert MG, Rigaud AS. Melatonin in elderly patients with insomnia. A systematic review. Gerontology and Geniatrics, 2001;34:491-7.
495. Olin J, Schneider L, Novit A. et al. Hydergine for dementia. Cochrane Library, issue 4. Oxford: Update Software, 2001.
496. Ondrizek RR, Chan PJ, Patton WC, et al. Inhibition of human sperm motility by specific herbs used in alternative medicine. Journal of Assisted Reproduction and Genetics. 1999;16:87-91.
497. Overstreet DH, Keung WM, Rezvani AH, et al. Herbal remedies for alcoholism: promises and possible pitfalls. Alcoholism, Clinical and Experimental Research. 2003a;27:177-85.
498. Overstreet DH, Kralic JE, Morrow AL, et al. NPI-031G (Puerarin) reduces anxiogenetic effects of alcohol withdrawal or benzodiazepine inverse or 5-HT(2C) agonists. Pharmacology, Biochemistry and Behavior, 2003b;75:619-25.
499. Pancheri P, Scapichio P, and Chiale RD. A double-blind, randomized parallel-group, efficacy and safety study of intramuscular S-adenosyl-L-methionine 1,4-butanedisuphonate (SAMe) versus imipramine in patients with major depressive disorder. International Journal of Neuropsychopharmacology. 2002;5:287-94.
500. Perovic S, Miiller WE. Pharmacological profile of hypericin extract. Effect on serotonin reuptake by postsynaptic receptors. Arneimittelforschung. 1995;45:1145-8.
501. Pittler MH, Ernst E. Kava extract for treating anxiety. Cochrane Library, issue 4. Oxford: Update Software, 2003.
502. Poyares DR, Guilleminault C, Ohayon MM, et al. Can valerian improve the sleep of insomniacs after benzodiazepine withdrawal? Progress in Neuropsychopharmacology and Biological Psychiatry. 2002;26:539-45.
503. Rezvani AH, Overstreet DH, Perfumi M, et al. Plant derivatives in the treatment of alcohol dependency. Pharmacology, Biochemistry and Behavior. 2003;75:593-606.
504. Rezvani AH, Overstreet DH, Yang Y, et al. Attenuation of alcohol consumption by a novel nontoxic ibogaine analogue (B-methoxycoronaridine) in alcohol-preferring rats. Pharmacology, Biochemistry and Behavior. 1997;58:615-9.
505. Roberts CC, Ladenson PW. Hypothyroidism. Lancet. 2004; 363:793-803.
506. Roder C, Schaefer M, Leucht S. Meta-analysis of effectiveness and tolerability of treatment of mild to moderate depression with St. John's Wort. Fortschritte der Neurologie Psychiatrie. 2004;72:330-43.
507. Sano M, Ernesto C, Thomas RG, et al. A controlled trial of selegeine alpha-tocopherol or both as treatment for Alzheimer's disease. New England Journal of Medicine. 1997;336:1216-22.
508. Schelosky L, Raffauf C, Jendroska K. Kava and dopamine antagonism. Journal of Neurology, Neurosurgery and Psychiatry. 1995;58:639-40.
509. Schmitz M, Jackel M. Comparative study for assessing quality of life of patients with exogenous sleep disorders (temporary sleep onset and sleep interruption disorders) treated with a hops-valerian preparation and a benzodiazepine drug. Wiener Medizinische Wochenschrift. 1998;148:291-8.
510. Schreiter-Gasser U, Gasser T. A comparison of cholinesterase inhibitors and ginkgo extract in treatment of Alzheimer's dementia. Fortschritte der Medizin Originalien. 2001;119:135-6.
511. Shamir E, Barak Y, Plopskey L, et al. Is melatonin treatment effective for tardive dyskinesia? Journal of Clinical Psychiatry. 2000;61:556-8.
512. Sharmir E, Barak Y, Shalman I. Melatonin treatment for tardive dyskinesia: double-blind, placebo controlled, crossover study. Archives of Genetic Psychiatry. 2001;58:1049-52.
513. Shebek J, Rindone JP. A pilot study exploring the effect of Kudzu root on the drinking habits of patients with chronic alcoholism. Journal of Alternative and Complementary Medicine. 2000;6:45-8.
514. Sheppard SG. A preliminary investigation of ibogaine: case reports and recommendation for further study. Journal of Substance Abuse and Treatment. 1994;11:379-85.
515. Sher L. Role of thyroid hormones in the effects of selenium on mood, behavior, and cognitive function. Medical hypotheses. 2001;57:480-3.
516. Singer C, Tractenberg RE, Kaye J. et al. Alzheimer's Disease Cooperative Study. A multicenter, placebo-controlled trial of melatonin for sleep disturbance in Alzeheimer's disease. Sleep, 2003;26:893-901.
517. Soares KVS, McGrath JJ. Vitamin E for neuroleptic-induced tardive dyskinesia. Cochrane Library, issue 4. Oxford: Update software, 2001
518. Spinella M. Psychotherapeutic herbs, in the Psychopharmacology of Herbal Medicine, Cambridge, MA:MIT Press. 2001, p. 278.
519. Staley JK, Ouyang Q, Pablo J. Pharmacological screen for activities of 12-hydroxyibogamine: a primary metabolite of the indole alkaloid ibogaine. Psychopharmacology. 1996;127:10-8.

520. Stevinson C, Ernst E. Valerian for insomnia: a systematic review of randomized clinical trials. Sleep Medicine. 2000;1:91-9.
521. Stoll AL, Severus WE, Freeman MP, et al. Omega 3 fatty acids in bipolar disorder: a preliminary double-blind, placebo-controlled trial. Archives of General Psychiatry. 1999; 56:407-12.
522. Su KP, Huang SY, Chiu CC, et al. Omega-3 fatty acids in major depressive disorder. A preliminary double-blind, placebo-controlled trial. Europeon Neuropsychopharmacology. 2003; 13:267-71.
523. Szegedi A, Kohnen R, Dienel A, et al. Acute treatment of moderate to severe depression with hypericum extract WS5570 (St John's wort): randomized controlled double blind non-inferiority trial against paroxetine. BML. 2005;330:503-6.
524. Tabet N, Birks J, Grimley Evans J. Vitamin E for Alzheimer's disease. Cochrane Library, issue 4. Oxford. Update Software. 2000.
525. Tang F, Nag S, Shiu SY, et al. The effects of melatonin and Ginkgo biloba extract on memory loss and choline acetyltransferase activities in the brain of rats infused intracerebroventricularly with beta-amyloid. Life Sciences. 2002;71:2625-31.
526. Taylor MJ, Carney S, Geddes J, et al. Folate for depressive disorders. Cochrane Library, issue 1. Oxford: Update Software, 2004.
527. Teufel-Mayer R, Gieitz J. Effects of long term administration of Hypericum extracts on the affinity and density of the central serotonergic 5HTIA and 5HT2A receptors. Pharmacopsychiatry. 1999;30(suppl. 2):113-6.
528. Thiele B, Brink I, Ploch M. Modulation of cytokine expression by Hypericum extract. Journal of Genetic Psychiatry and Neurology. 1994;7(suppl. 1):560-2.
529. Tian JZ, Zhu AH, Zhong J. A follow-up study on a randomized, single-blind control of King's Brain pills in treatment of memory disorder in elderly people with MCI in a Beijing community Zhongguo Zhong Yaa Za Zhi. 2003;28:987-91.
530. Unutzer J, Klap R, Sturm R, et al. Mental disorders and the use of alternative medicines: results from a national survey: American Journal of Psychiatry. 2000;157:1851-7.
531. Van Dongen M, van Ressum E, Kessels A, et al. Ginkgo for elderly people with dementia and age-associated memory impairment: a randomized clinical trial. Clinical Epidemiology. 2003;56:367-76.
532. Viola H, Wasowski C, Levis de Stein M. Apigenin, a component of Matricaria recutita flowers, is a central benzodiazepine receptors-ligand with anxiolytic effects. Planta Medica. 1995;61:213-6.
533. Vogeier BK, Pittler MH, Ernst E. The efficacy of ginseng. Asystematic review of randomized controlled trials. Europeon Journal of Clinical Pharmacology. 1999;55:567-75.
534. Wang JL, Patten SB, Russel ML. Alternative medicines use by individuals with major depression. Canadian Journal of Psychiatry. 2001;46:528-33.
535. Watanabe H, Kakihana M, Ohtsuka S, et al. Randomized, double-blind, placebo-controlled study of supplemental vitamin E on attenuation of the development of nitrate tolerance. Circulation. 1997;96:2545-50.
536. Werneke U, Earl J, Seydel C, et al. Potential health risks of complementary alternative medicines in cancer patients. British Journal of Cancer. 2004a;90:408-13.
537. Werneke U, Horn O, Taylor D. How effective is St John's wort? The evidence revisited. Journal of Clinical Psychiatry. 2004b;65:611-7.
538. Werneke U. Alternative nutrition therapies in cancer—the evidence. Clinical Nutrition Update. 2003;8:6-8.
539. Wettstein A. Cholinesterase inhibitors and gingkgo extracts-are they comparable in the treatment of domentia? Comparison of published placebo-controlled efficacy studies of at least six months. Phytomedicine. 2000;6:393-401.
540. Whiskey E, Werneke U, Taylor D. A systematic review of Hypericum perforatum in depression. International Clinical Psychopharmacology. 2001;16:239-52.
541. Williams JW, Mulrow CD, Chiquette E. A systematic review of newer of pharmacotherapies for depression in adults. Annals of Internal Medicine. 2000;132:743-56.
542. Wolfman C, Viola H, Paladini A, et al. 1994. Possible anxiolytic effects of chrysin, a central benzodiazepine receptor ligand isolated from Passiflora coerulea. Pharmacology. Biochemistry and Behavior. 47:1-4.
543. Wolkowitz OM. Rational polypharmacy in schizophrenia. Annals of Clinical Psychiatry. 1993;5:79-90.
544. Zhang XY, Zhou DF, Cao LY, et al. The effect of vitamin E treatment on tardive dyskinesia and blood superoxide dismutase: a double-blind placebo-controlled trial. Clinical Psychopharmacology. 2004;24:83-6.
545. Ziegler G, Ploch M, Miettinen-Baumann A, Efficacy and tolerability of valerian extract LI 156 compared with oxazepam in the treatment of non-organic insomnia—a randomized, double-blind, comparative clinical study: European Journal of Medical Research. 2002;25:480-6.
546. Zimmerman RA, Thomspon LM Jr. Prevalence of complementary medicines in urologic practice. A review of recent studies with emphasis on use among prostate cancer patients. Urology Clinics of North Americal. 2002; 29:1-9.

BIBLIOGRAPHY

Atypical Antipsychotics for Bipolar Disorder

1. Alvir JMJ, Lieberman JA, Safferman AZ, et al. Cozapine-induced agranulocytosis-incidence and risk factors in the United States. N Engl J Med. 1993;329(3):162-7.
2. Baker R, Zarate C Jr, Brown E, et al. A three-week comparison of olanzapine versus risperidone in the treatment of bipolar mania: improvement in manic and depressive symptoms and treatment adherence [abstract15]. Presented at 156th American Psychiatric Association Annual Meeting. San Francisco, CA, 17-22, 2003.
3. Berk M, Ichim L, Brook S. Olanzapine compared to lithium in mania: a double-blind randomized controlled trial. Int Clin Psychopharmacol. 1999:14(6):339-43.

4. Bourin M, Auby P, Swanik S, et al. Aripiprazole vs. haloperidol for maintained treatment effect in acute mania. Eur Neuropsychopharmacol. 2003;13:S333.
5. Bowden CL, Grunze H, Mullen J, et al. A randomized double blind placebo controlled efficacy and safety study of quetiapine or lithium as monotherapy for mania in bipolar disorder. J Clin Psychiatry, in press.
6. Calabrese JR, Keck PE Jr, Macfadden W, et al. A randomized double blind placebo controlled trial of quetiapine in the treatment of bipolar I or II depression. Am J Psychiatry. 2004. in press.
7. Chengappa KNR, Baker RW, Shao LX, et al. Rates of resonse, euthymia and remission in tow placebo-controlled olanzapine trials for bipolar mania. Bipolar Disord. 2003;5(1)-5.
8. DelBello MP, Schwiers ML, Rosenberg HL, et al. A double-blind. Randomized, placebo-controlled study of quetiapine as adjunctive treatment for adolescent mania. J Am Acad Child Adolese Psychiatry. 2002;41(10):1216-23.
9. Esparon J, Kolloori J, Naylor GJ, et al. Comparison of the prophylactic action of flupenthixol with placebo in lithium treated manic-depressive patients. Br J Psychiatry. 1986;148:723-5.
10. Ghaemi SN, Sachs GS, Baldassano CF, et al. Acute treatment of bipolar disorder with adjunctive risperidone in outpatients. Can J Psychiatry. 1997;42(2):196-9.
11. Hadjakis WJ, Marcus R, Abou-Gharibia N, et al. Aripiprazole in acute mania: results from a second placebo-controlled study. Bipolar Disord. 2004;6:39-40.
12. Hirschfeld RMA, Keck PE, Kramer M, et al. Rapid antimanic effect of risperidone monotherapy: a 3-week multicenter, double-blind, placebo-controlled trial. Am J Psychiatry. 2004;161(6):1057-65.
13. Ichim L, Brook S. Olanzapine compared to lithium in mania: a double-blind randomized controlled trial. Inn Clin Psychopharmacol. 2001;12:213-23.
14. Jibson MD, Tandon R. New atypical antipsychotic medications. J Psychiat Res. 1998:32(3-4):215-28.
15. Jones M, Huizar K, Randomised, double-blind, controlled data on the treatment of mania with quetiapine. Eur Psychiatry. 2004;19:206S-7S.
16. Judd LL, Akiskal HS, Schettler PH, et al. The long-term natural history of the weekly symptomatic status of bipolar I disorder. Arch Gen Psychiatry. 2002;59-(6):530-7
17. Kane J, Honigfeld G, Singer J, et al. Clozapine for the treatment-resistent schizophrenic a double-blind comparison with chlorpromazine. Arch Gen Psychiatry. 1988;45(9):789-96.
18. Kane JM. Newer antipsychiotic drugs-a review of their pharmacology and therapeutic potential. Drugs. 1993:46(4):585-93.
19. Keck PE, Marcus R, Tourkodimitris S, et al. A placebo-controlled, double-blind study of the efficacy and safety of aripiprazole in patients with acute bipolar mania. Am J Psychiatry. 2003;160(9):1651-8.
20. Keck PE, McElroy SL, Strakowski SM, et al. Factors associated with maintenance antipsychotic treatment of patients with bipolar disorder. J Clin Psychiatry. 2001;62(12):975-80.
21. Keck PE, Versiani M, Potkin S, et al. Ziprasidone in the treatment of acute bipolar mania: a three-week, placebo-controlled, double-blind, randomized trial. AM J Psychiatry. 2003;160(4):741-8.
22. Khanna S, Vieta E, Lyons B, et al. Risperidone in the treatment of acute bipolar mania: a double-blind, placebo-controlled study of 290 patients, Eur Neuropsycho-pharmacol. 2003;13: S314-5.
23. Leysen D, Linders JTM, Ottenheijm HCJ. 5-HT2 antagonists: a concept for the treatment of schizophrenia. Curr Pharm Des. 1997;3(4):367-90.
24. Mclntyre R, Brecher M, Paulsson B. Quetiapine as monotherapy for bipolar mania: a double blind randomized parellel group placebo controlled trial. Eur Neuropsycho-pharmacol. 2004. in press.
25. Sachs G, Chengappa KNR, Suppes T, et al. Quetiapine with lithium or divalproex for the treatment of bipolar mania: a randomized, double-blind, placebo-controlled study. Bipolar Disord. 2004:6-(3):213-23.
26. Sanchez R, Marcus, Carson WH, et al. Aripiprazole in the maintenance treatment of bipolar disorder. Eur Psychiatry. 2004:19:-204S.
27. Schs GS, Gorssman F, Ghaemi SN, et al. Combination of a mood stabilizer with risperidone or haloperidol for treatment of acute mania: a double-blind. Placebo-controlled comparison of efficacy and safety. Am J Psychiatry. 2002;59(7): 1146-54.
28. Segal J, Berk M, Brook S. Risperidone compared with both lithium and haloperidol in mania: a double-blind ramdomized controlled trial. Clin Neuropharmacol. 1998:21-(3):176-80.
29. Segal S, Riesenberg RA, Ice K, et al. Ziprasidone in mania: a 21-day randomized, double-blind, placebo controlled trial. Eur Neuropschopharmacol. 2003;13:S345-6.
30. Smulevich A, Khanna S, Erdekens M, et al. Acute and continuation risperidone monotherapy in bipolar mania: a 3 week placebo controlled trial followed by a 9 week double-blind trial of risperidone and haloperidol. Eur Neuropsychopharmacol, in press.
31. Tarazi FI, Zhang KH, Baldessarini RJ. Long-term effects of olanzapine, risperidone, and quetiapine on serotonin IA, 2A and 2C receptors in rat forebrain regions. Psychopharmacolgy (Berl). 2002;161(3):-263-70.
32. Tohen M, Baker RW, Althuler LL, et al. Olanzapine versus divalproex in the treatment of acute mania. Am J Psychiatry. 2002;159(6):1011-7.
33. Tohen M, Bowden C, Calabrese J, et al. Olanzapine's efficacy of relapse prevention in bipolar disorder: a randomized double-blind placebo-controlled 12-month clinical trial. Bipolar Disord. 2004;6:26-7.
34. Tohen M, Chengappa KNR, Suppes T, et al. Efficacy of olanzapine in combination with valprorate or lithium in the treatment of mania in patients partially nonresponsive to valprorate or lithium monotherapy. Arch Gen Psychiatry. 2002;59(1):62-9.
35. Tohen M, Chengappa KNR, Suppes T, et al. Relapse prevention in bipolar I disorder: 18-month comparison of olanzapine

plus mood stabilizer vs mood stabilizer alone. Br J Psychiatry. 2007;2(1)4:184:337-45.
36. Tohen M, Goldberg JF, Arrillaga AMGP, et al. A 12-233k, double-blind comparison of olanzapine vs haloperidol in the treatment of acute mania. Arch Gen Psychiatry. 2003;60(12):1218-26.
37. Tohen M, Jacobs TG, Grundy SL, et al. Efficacy of olanzapine in acute bipolar mania: a double-blind, placebo-controlled study. The Olanzipine HGGW Study Group. Arch Gen Psychiatry. 2000;57(9):841-9.
38. Tohen M, Ketter Ta, Zarate CA, et al. Olanzapine versus divalproex sodium for the treatment of acute mania and maintenance of remission: a 47-week study. Am J Psychiatry. 2003;160(7):1263-71.
39. Tohen M, Sanger TM, McElroy SL, et al. Olanzapine versus placebo in the treatment of acute mania. Olanzapine versus placebo in the treatment of acute mania. Olanzapine HGEH Study Group. Am J Psychiatry. 1999:156(5):702-9.
40. Tohen M, Vieta E, Calabrese J, et al. Efficacy of olanzipine and olanzapine-duoxetine combination in the treatment of bipolar I depression. Arch Gen Psychiatry. 2003;60-(11);1079-88.
41. Tohen M, Zarate CA Jr. Antipsychotic agents and bipolar disorde. J Clin Psychiatry.1998;59(Suppl 1):38-48.
42. Tohen MF, Marneros A, Greil W, et al, Olanzapine versus lithium in replapse recurrence prevention in bipolar disorder: a randomized double blind controlled 12 month clinical trial. Am J Psychiatry. 2004. in press.
43. Yatham LN, Grossman F, Ghaemi SN, et al. Combination of a mood stabilizer with risperidone or placebo in the treatment of acute mania: international, double blind, randomized, controlled trial. Br J Psychiatry. 2003:in press.
44. Yatham LN, Liddle PF, Dennie J, et al. Decrease in brain serotonin 2 receptor binding in patients with major depression following desipramine treatment: a positron emission tomography study with fluorine-18-labeled setoperone. Arch Gen Psychiatry. 1999;56(8):705-11.
45. Yatham LN, Liddle PF, Shiah IS, et al. Effects of rapid tryptophan depletion on brain 5HT2 receptors: a PET study. Br J Psychiatry. 2001;178:448-53.
46. Yatham LN, Paulsson B, Mullen J, et al. Quetiapine versus placebo in combination with lithium or divalroex for the treatment of bipolar mania. J Clin Psychopharmacol. 2004;24(6):599-606.
47. Yatham LN. Brain imaging investigations of dopaminergic pathways in mood disorders. In: soares JC (Ed). Brain imaging in affective disorders. New York: Marcel Dekker. 2003.
48. Yatham L, Grossman F, Augustyns I, Vieta E. Ravindran A. Mood stabilizers plus risperidone or placebo in the treatment of mania. Int Clin psychopharmacol. 2003;18:227-35.
49. Zajecka JM, Weisler R, Sachs G, et al. A comparison of the efficacy, safety, and tolerability of divalproex sodium and olanzapine in the treatment of bipolar disorder. J Clin Psychaitry. 2002:63(12):148-55.
50. Zarate CA Jr. Antipsychotic drug side effect issues in bipolar manic patients. J Clin Psychiatry. 2000;60(Suppl8):52-61.

Atypical Mood Stabilizers: Atypical Role for Atypical Antipsychotics

51. Akiskal H, Pinto O, The evolving bipolar spectrum. Prototypes I, II, III, and IV. Psychiatr Clin North Am. 1999;22:517-34.
52. Allison D, Mentore J, Heo M, et al. Antipsychotic-induced weight gain: a comprehensive research synthesis Am J Psychiatry. 1999;156:1686-96.
53. Atkin K, Kendall F, Gould D, Freeman H, Lirerman J. O'sullivan D. Neutropenia and agranuloytosis. Patients receiving clozapine in the UK and Ireland Br J Psychiatry. 1996;169:483-8.
54. Baldessarini RJ, Hennel J, Wilson M, et al. Olanzapine versus placebo in acute mania: treatment responses in subgroups. J Clin Psychoparmacol. 2003;23:370-6.
55. Barbini B, Scherillo P, Bendetti F, Crespi G, Colombo C, Smeraldi E. Response to clozapine in acute mania is more rapid than that of chlorpromazine. Int Clin Psychopharmacol. 1997;12:109-12.
56. Berk M, Dodd S, Malhi G. Bipolar missed states: the diagnosis and clinical salience of bipolar mixed states. Aust N Z J Psychiatry. 2005;6:530-9.
57. Berk M, Ichim L, Brook S. Olanzapine compared to lithium in mania: a double-blind randomized controlled trial. Inn Clin Psychopharmacol. 1999;14:339-43.
58. Borin M, Auby P, Swanink R, et al. Aripiprazole versus haloperidol for maintained treatment effect in acute mania. Annual Meeting of the American Psychiatric Association, 17-22, 2003. San Francisco. USA, 2003.
59. Brecher M, Huizar K. Quetiapine monotherapy for acute mania associated with bipolar disorder (STAMP 1). Bipolar Disord. 2003;5(suppl 1):35-6.
60. Brecher M, Huizar K. Quetiapine vs. placebo for acute mania associated with bipolar disorder (STAMP 1). Bipolar Disord. 2003;5(suppl 1):35.
61. Calabrese J, Macfadden W, Mccoy R, Minkwitz M, Wilson E, Mullen J. Double-blind, placebo-controlled study of quetiapine in bipolar in bipolar depression. American Psychiatric Association 2004. annual Meeting-Abstracts on disk. 157th Annual Meeting of American Psychiatric Association, American Psychiatric Association , New York, NY, USA, 2004.
62. Ciapparelli A, Dell'osso L, Pini S, Chiavacci M, Fenzi M, Cassano G. Clozapine for treatment-refractory schizophrenia, schizoaffective disorder, and psychotic bipolar disorder: a 24-month naturalistic study. J Clin Psychiatry. 2000;61:329-34.
63. Daniel DG, Brook S, Warrington L, Loebel A, Murray S. IM ziprasidone in agitated psychotic patients with bipolar diagnoses. Arch Gen Psychiatry. 2002;59:530-7.
64. Degner D, Bleich S, Muller P, Hajak G, Adler L, Ruther E. Clozapine in the treatment of mania. J Neuro-psychiatry Clin Neurosci. 2000;12:283.
65. Delbello M, Schwiers M, Rosenberg H. Strakowski S. A double-blind, randomized, placebo-controlled study of quetiapine as adjunctive treatment for adolescent mania. J Am Acad Child Adolesc Psychiatry. 2002;41:1216-23.

66. Frye M, Ketter T, Leverich G, et al. The increasing use of polypharmaco-therapy for refractory mood disorders: 22 years of study. J Clin Psychiatry. 2000;61:9-15.
67. Fuller M, Shermock K, Secic M, Grogg A. Comparative study of the devemipment of diabetes mellitus in patients taking risperidone and olanzapine. Pharmacotherapy. 2003;23:1037-43.
68. Ghaemi S, Katzow J. The use of quetiapien for treatment-resistant bipolar disorder: a case series. Ann clin Psychiatry. 1999;11:137-40.
69. Gianfrancesco F, White R, Wang R, Nasrallah H. Antipsychotic-induced type 2 diabetes: evidence from a large health plan database. J Clin Psychopharmacol. 2003;23:328-35.
70. Goodnick P, Jerry J. Aripiprazole: profile on efficacy and safety. Expert Opin Pharmacother. 2002;3:1773-81.
71. Goodwin F, Jamison K. Manic-depressive illness. New York, USA: Oxford University Press, 1990.
72. Green A, Tohen M, Patel J, et al. Clozapine in the treatment of refractory psychotic mania. Am J Psychiatry. 2000;157:982-6.
73. Guille C, Sachs G, giiaemi S. A naturalistic comparison clozapine, risperidone, and olanzapine in the treatment of bipolar disorder. J Clin Psychiatry. 2000;61:638-42.
74. Hadiakis W, Marcus R, Abou-Gharbia N, et al. Aripiprazole in acute mania: results from a second placebo-controlled study. Bipolar Disord. 2004;-6(suppl 1)39-40.
75. Hirschfeld R, Keck PE, Karcher K, Kramer M, Grossman F. Rapid anti-manic effect of risperidone monotherapy: a three-week, multicenter, randomized, double-blind, placebo-controlled trial. American Psychiatric Association Annual Meeting. 17-22, 2003; San Francisco, CA, USA, 2003.
76. Iqbal M, Rahman A, Husain Z, Mahmud S, Ryan W, Feldman J. Clozapine: a clinical review of adverse effects and management Ann Clin Psychiatry. 2003;15:33-48.
77. Joines M, Huizar K. Quetiapine as monotherapy for mania associated with bipolar disorder. 43rd Annual NCDEU Conference. Boca Raton, FL. USA, 2003;158.
78. Jones M, Huizar K. Quetiapine monotherapy for acute mania associated with bipolar disorder (STAMP 1 and STAMP 2). Bipolar Disord. 2003;5(suppl 1):57.
79. Judo L, Akiskal H, Schettler P, et al. The long-term natural history of the weekly symptomatic status of bipolar I disorder. Arch Gen Psychiatry. 2002;59:530-7.
80. Keck P Jr, Marrcus R, Tourkodimitris S, et al. A placebo controlled, double-blind study of the efficacy and safety of aripiprazole in patients with acute bipolar mania. Am J Psychiatry. 2003;160:1651-8.
81. Keck P, Mcelroy S, Arnold L. Ziprasidone: a new atypical antipsychotic. Expert Opin Pharmacother. 2001;2:1033-42.
82. Keck P, Mcelroy S. Bipolar disorder, obesity, and pharmacotherapy-associated weight gain. J Clin Psychiatry. 2003;64:1426-35.
83. Keck PE Jr, Versiani M, Potkin S, West Sa, Giller E, Ice K. Ziprasidone in the treatment of acute bipolar mania: a three-week, placebo-controlled, double-blind, randomized trial. Am J Psychiatry. 2003;160:741-8.
84. Kelly D, Love R. Ziprasidone and the Qtc interval: pharmacokinetic and pharmacodynamic considerations. Psychopharmacol Bull. 2011;35:66-79.
85. ketter T, Wang P, Nowakowska C, marsh W. New medication treatment options for bipolar disorder. Acta Psychiatr Scand. 2004;110(suppl 422):18-33.
86. Khanna S, Vieta E, Lyons B. Grossman F, Kramer M. Risperidone monotherapy in mania: a double-blind randomized controlled trial. Clin Neuropharmacol. 1998;21:176-80.
87. Koro C, Fedder D, L Italian G, et al. An assessment of the independent effects of olanzapine and risperidone exposure on the risk of hyperlipidemia in schizophrenic patients. Arch Gen Psychiatry. 2002;59:1021-6.
88. Lindenmayer J, Czobor P, Volavka J, et al. Changes in glucose and cholesterol levels in patients with schizophrenia treated with typical or atypical antipsychotics. Am J Psychiatry. 2003;160:290-6.
89. Malhi G, Checkley S, Olanzapine in the treatment of psychiatric in the treatment of psychotic depression. Br J Psychiatry. 1999;174:460.
90. Malhi G, Ivanovski B, Szekeres V, Olley A. Bipolar disorder: it's all in your mind? The neuropsychological profile of a biological disorder. Can J Psychiatry. 2009;49:813-9.
91. Malhi G, Lagopoulos J, Owen a, Yatham L. Bipolaroids: functional imaging in bipolar disorder. Acta Psychiatr Scand. 2004;110(suppl. 422):46-54.
92. Malhi G. Mitchell P, Salim S. Bipolar depression: management options. CNS Drugs. 2003;17:9-25.
93. Malhi G. Weight gain: gained by waiting. Acta Psychiatr Scand. 2003;108:249-51.
94. Mcelroy S, Frye M, Denicoff K et al. Olanzapine in treatment-resistent bipolar disorder. J Affect Disord. 1998;49:119-22.
95. Mcintyre R, Mancini D, Basile V, Srinivasan J, Kennedy S. Antipsychotic-induced weight gain bipolar disorder and leptin. J Clin Psychopharmacol. 2003;23:323-7.
96. Mcquade RD, Sanchez R, Marcus R, et al. Aripiprazole for relapse prevention in bipolar disorder: a 26-week placebo controlled study. Int J Neuropsychopharmacol. 2004;7(suppl. 1):s161.
97. Mehan K, Zhang F, David S, et al. A double-blind, randomized comparison of the efficacy and safety of intramuscular injections of olanzapine, lorazepam, or placebo in treating acutely agitated patients diagnosed with bipolar mania. J Clin Psycho-pharmacol. 20031;21:389-97.
98. Meyer J. A rstrospective comparison of weight, lipid, and glucose changes between risperidone, and olanzapine treated impatients: metabolic outcomes after 1 year. J Clin Psychiatry. 2002;63:425-33.
99. Michell P, Malhi G, Ball J. Major advances in bipolar disorder. Med J Aust. 2004;181:207-10.
100. Milev RV, Abraham G, Voutsilakos F, Hoaken P. Open-label add-on quetiapine for bipolar depression: an eight-week trial. American Psychiatric Assiciation Annual Meeting, 1-6, 2004 New York, NY. USA, 2004.

101. Mitchell P, Malhi G. Bipolar depression – phenomenological over-view and clinical characteristics. Bipolar Disord. 2004;6:530-9.
102. Mitchell P, Malhi G. The expanding pharmacopoeia for bipolar disorder. Annu Rev Med. 2002;53:173-88.
103. Monkul S, Malhi G, Sores J. Anatomical abnormalities in bipolar disorder: do they exist and do they progress? Aust N Z J Psychiatry. 2011;39:222-6.
104. Mullen J, Jibson M. Switzer D. a comparison of the relative safety, efficacy, and tolerability of quetiapine and risperidone in outpatients with schizophrenia and other psychotic disorders: the quetiapine experience with safety and tolerability (QUEST) study. Clin Ther. 2001;23:1839-54.
105. Mullen J, Paulsson B. Quetiapine in combination with mood stabilizers for the treatment of acute mania associated with bipolar disorder. Bipolar Disord. 2003;5(suppl 1):70.
106. Narendran R, Young C, Valenti A, Pristach C, Pato M, Grace J, Olanza-pine therapy in treatment-resistent psychotic mood disorders: a long-term followup study. J Clin Psychiatry. 1999;11:137-40.
107. Nemeroff C. Safety of available agents used to treat bipolar disorder: focus on weight gain J Clin Psychiatry. 2003;64:532-9.
108. Osser D, Najarian D, Dufrense R. Olanzapine increases weight and serum triglyceride levels. J Clin Psychiatry. 1999;60: 767-70.
109. Pacia S, Devinsky O. Clozapine-related seizures: experience with 5,629 patients. Neurology. 1994;44:2247-9.
100. Parker G, Malhi G, Malhi G, Are atypical antipsychotic drugs also atypical antidepressants? Aust N Z J Psychiatry. 2001;35:631-8.
111. Sachs G, Chengappa K, Suppes T, et al. Quetiapine with lithium or divalproex for the treatment of bipolar mania: a randomized, double-blind, placebo-controlled study. Bipolar Disord. 2004;6:213-23.
112. Sachs G, guile C. Weight gain associated with use of psychotropic medications. J Clin Psychiatry. 1999;60 (suppl. 21):16-9.
113. Sachs G, Sanchez R, Marcus R, et al. Aripiprazine versus placebo in acute mania: results from a second study. 55th Meeting of the Institute of Psychiatric Service Boston MA, USA, 2008.
114. Sajatovic M, Brescan D, Perez D, et al. Quetiapine alone and added to a mood stabilizer for serious mood disorders. J Clin Psychiatry. 2001;62:728-32.
115. Sajatovic M, Mullen JA. Sweitzer DE. Efficacy of quetiapine and risperidone against depressive symptoms in outpatients with psychosis. J Clin Psychiatry. 2002;63:1156-63.
116. Sanger T, Grundy S, Gibson P, Namjoshi M, Greaney M, Tohen M. Long-term olanzapine therapy in the treatment of bipolar I disorder: an open-label continuation phase study. J Clin Psychiatry. 2001;62:273-81.
117. Sanger T, Tohen M, Vieta E, et al. Olanzapine in the acute treatment of bipolar I disorder with a history of rapid cycling. J Affect Disord. 2003;73(1-2):155-61.
118. Shi L, Namijoshi MA, Zhang, G et al. Olanzapine versus haloperidol in the treatment of acute mania clinical outcomes. Health-related quality of life and work status. Int Clin Psychopharmacol. 2002;17:227-37.
119. Suppes T, Webb A, Paul B, Carmody T, Kraemer H, Rush A. Clin-ical outcome in a randomized 1-year trial of clozapine versus treatment as usual for patients with treatment-resistant illness and a history of mania. Am J Psychiatry. 1999;156: 1164-9.
120. Tandon R. Safety and tolerability: how do newer generation 'atypical' antipsychotics compare? Psychiatr Q. 2002;73:297-311.
121. Tohel M, Goldberg JF, Gonzalez-Pinto Arrllaga AM et al. A 12-week, double-blind comparison of olanzapine vs haloperidol in the treatment of acute mania. Arch Gen Psychiatry. 2003;60:1218-26.
122. Tohen M, Baker R, Altshuler L, et al. Olanzapine versus divalproex in the treatment of acute mania. Am J Psychiatry. 2002;159:1011-7.
123. Tohen M, Bowden C, Calabrese J, et al. Olanzapine's efficacy for relapse prevention in bipolar disorder: a randomized double-blind, placebo-controlled 12-month clinical trial. Bipolar Disord. 2003;5(suppl 1):89.
124. Tohen M, Bowden CL, Calabrese JR, et al. Olanzapine's efficacy for relapse prevention in bipolar disorder: a randomized double-blind, placebo-controlled 12-month clinical trial. Bipolar Disord. 2003;5(suppl 1):89.
125. Tohen M, Chengappa K, Suppes T, et al. Efficacy of olanzapine in combination with valproate or lithium in the treatment of mania in patients partially nonresponsive to valproate or lithium monotherapy. Arch Gen Psychiatry. 2002;59: 62-9.
126. Tohen M, Chengappa K, Suppes, T et al. Relapse prevention in bipolar disorder: 18-month comparison of olanzapine plus mood stabilizer vs. mood stabilizer alone. Br J Psychiatry. 2004;184:337-45.
127. Tohen M, Jacobs T, Grundy S, et al. Efficacy of olanzapine in acute bipolar mania: a double-blind, placebo-controlled study. The olanzapine HGGW study group. Arch Gen Psychiatry. 2000;57:841-9.
128. Tohen M, Ketter TA, Zarate CA, et al. Olanzapine versus divalproex sodium for the treatment of acute mania and maintenance of remission a 47-week study. Am J Psychiatry. 2003;160:1263-71.
129. Tohen M, Marneros A, Bowden CL, et al. Olanzapine vs. lithium in relapse prevention in bipolar disorder: a randomized double-blind controlled 12-month clinical trial. Bipolar Disord. 2003;5(suppl 1):89.
130. Tohen M, Sanger T, Mcelroy S, et al. Olanzapine versus placebo in the treatment of acute mania. Olanzapine HGEH study group. Am J Psychiatry. 1999;156:702-709.
131. Tohen M, Vieta E, Calabrese J, et al. Efficacy of olanzapine and olanzapine-fluoxetine combination in the treatment of bipolar I depression. Arch Gen Psychiatry. 2003;60:1079-88.

132. Vieta E, Brugue E, Gccolea JM, et al. Acute and continuation risperidone monotherapy in mania. Hum psychopharmacol. 2004;19:41-5.
133. Vieta E, Colom F. Psychological Interventions in Bipolar Disorder: from wishful thinking to an evidence-based approach. Acta Psychiatr Scand. 2004;110(suppl. 422):34-38.
134. Vieta E, Gasto C, Colom F et al. Role of risperidone in bipolar II: an open 6-month study. J Affect Disord. 2001;67(1-3):213-9.
135. Vieta E, Gasto C, Colom F, Martinez A, Otero A, Vallero J. Treatment of refractory rapid cycling bipolar disorder with risperidone. J Clin Psychopharmacol. 1998;18:172-4.
136. Vieta E, Goikolea J, Corbella B, et al. Risperidone safety and efficacy in the treatment of bipolar and schizoaffective disorders: results from a 6-month, multicenter, open study. J Clin Psychiatry. 2001;62:818-25.
137. Vieta E, Herraiz M, Parramon G, Goecolea J, Fernandez A, Benabarre A. Risperidone in the treatment of mania: efficacy and safety results from a large, multicentre, open study in Spain. J Affect Disord. 2002;72:5-19.
138. Vieta E, Herrtz M, Parramin G, Goecolea J, Fernandez A, Benabarre A. Risperidone monotherapy in mania. Hum Psychopharmacol. 2004;19:41-5.
139. Vieta E, Parramon G, Padrell E, et al. Quetiapine in the treatment of rapid cycling bipolar disorder Bipolar Disord. 2002;4:335-440.
140. weisler R, Dunn J, English P. Adjunctive ziprasidone for bipolar maina: short and long-term data. Int J Neuropsychopharmacol. 2004;7(suppl 1):s327.
141. Yatham L, Binder C, Riccardelli R, Leeblnc J, Connolly M, Kusumakar V. Risperidone in acute and continuation treatment, of mania. Int Clin Psychopharmacol. 2003;18:227-35.
142. Yatham L, Grossman F, Augustyns I, Vieta E, Ravindran A. Mood stabilizers plus risperidone or placebo in the treatment of acute mania. International double-blind, randomized controlled trial. Br J Psychiatry. 2003;182:141-7.
143. Yatham L, Grossman F, Augustyns I, Vieta E. Ravindran A. Mood stabilizers plus risperidone or placebo in the treatment of mania. Int Clin psychopharmacol. 2003;18:227-35.
144. Yatham L. Acute and maintenance treatment of bipolar mania: the role of atypical antipsychotics. Bipolar Disord. 2003;5 (suppl 2):7-19.
145. Yatham LN, Mullen J. Quetiapine in combination with mood stabilizer for the treatment of acute mania associated with bipolar disorder. Int J Neuropsychopharmacol. 2004;7 (suppl 1):s330.

Vagus Nerve Stimulation and Deep Brain Stimulation

146. Antelman SM. Stresson-induced sensitization to subsequent stress: implications for the development and treatment of clinical disorders, in Sensitization in the Nervous System. Edited by Kalivas PW, Barnes CD. Caldwell, NJ, Telford Press, 1988.pp.227-54.
147. Antelman SM, Kocan D, Knopf S, et al. One brief exposure to a psychological stressor induces long-lasting, time-dependent sensitization of both the cataleptic and neurochemical responses to haloperidol. Life Sci. 1991;51:261-6.
148. Ashby P, Rothwell J. Neurophysiologic aspects of deep brain stimulation. Neurology 2000;55(12, supple 6):S17-S20.
149. Bailey P, Bremer F. A sensory cortical representation of the vagus nerve. J Neurophysiol. 1938;2:405-12.
150. Ballantine HT Jr, Bouckoms AJ, Thomas EK, et al. Treatment of psychiatric illness by stereotactic cingulatomy. Biol Psychiatry. 1987;22:807-19.
151. Ballenger JC, Post RM. Therapeutic effects of carbamazepine in affective illness: a preliminary report. Commun Psychopharmcol. 1978;2:159-75.
152. Baxter LR. Brain imaging as a tool in establishing a theory of brain pathology in obsessive compulsive disorder. J Clin Psychiatry. 1990;51(Suppl):22-5.
153. Bekhtereva NP, Bondarchuk AN, Smirnov VM, et al. Therapeutic electric stimulation of deep brain structures. Vopr Neirokhir. 1972;36:7-12.
154. Ben-Menachem E, Manon-Espaillat R, Risctanovic R, et al. Vagus nerve stimulation for treatment of partial seizures, 1: a controlled study of effect on seizures. First International Vagus Nerve Stimulation Stody Group. Epilepsia. 1994;35:616-26.
155. Bohning DE, Lomarev MP, Den-slow S, et al. Feasibility of vagus nerve stimulation-synchronized blood oxgenation level dependent function MRI. Invest Radiol. 2001;36:470-9.
156. Bondarchuk AN, Smirnov VM. Effects of electric stimulation on the thalamic median center in man. Fiziol Zh SSSR Im I M Sechenova. 1969;55:408-13.
157. Borckardt JJ, Kozel FA, Anderson B, et al. Vagus nerve stimulation affects perception in depressed adults. Pain Res Manag. 2005;10:9-15.
158. Breiter HC, Rauch SL, Kwong KK, et al. Functional magnetic resonance imaging of symptom provocation in obsessive-compulsive disorder. Arch Gen Psychiatry. 1996;53:595-606.
159. Carpenter LL, Moreno F, Kling MA, et al. Effects of vagus nerve stimulation cerebrospinal fluid monoamine metabolites, norepinephrine, and gamma aminobutyric acid concentrations in depressed patients. Biol Psychiatry. 2004;51:418-26.
160. Chae JH, Nahas Z, Lomarev M, et al. A review of functional neuroimaging studies of vagus nerve stimulation (VNS). J Psychiatr Res. 2003;37:443-55.
161. Cosgrove GR, Rauch SL. Psychosurgery. Neurosurg Clin N Am. 1995;6:167-76.
162. Cummings JL. The neuroanatomy of depression. J Clin Psychiatry. 1993;54(Suppl):14-20.
163. Damier P. The stimulation of deep cerebral structures in the treatment of Parkinson's disease. Eur Neuropsychopharmacol 1998;8:S89-S13,04.
164. Dean AC, Wu AT, et al. Motor cortex excitability in epilepsy patients treated with vagus nerve stimulation. American Epilepsy Society Meeting, 2002.
165. Dell P, Olson R. Secondary mesencephalic, diencephalic and amygdalian projections of vagal visceral affernces. C R Seances Soc Biol Fil. 1951;145:1088-91.

166. Elger G, Hoppe C, Falkai P, et al. Vagus nerve stimulation in associated with mood improvements in epilepsy patients. Epilepsy Res. 2000;42:203-10.
167. Foley JO, DuBois F. Quantiative studies of the vagus nerve in the cat, I: the ration of sensory and motor studies. J Comp Neurol. 1937;67:49-67.
168. George MS, Sackeim HA, Rush AJ, et al. Vagus nerve stimulation: a new tool for brain research and therapy. Biol Psychiatry. 2000; 47:287-95.
169. George MS, Rush AJ Sackeim H, et al. A one-year comparison of vagus nerve stimulation (VNS) with treatment as usual for treatment-resistant depression. Biol Psychiatry. (in press).
170. Goodman WK. Obsessive-compulsive disorder: diagnosis treatment. J Clin Psychiatry. 1999;60(suppl 18):27-32.
171. Greenberg BD, Murphy DL, Rasmussen SA. Neuroanatomically based approaches to obsessive-compulsive disorder: neurosurgery and transcranial magnetic stimulation. Psychiatr Clin North Am. 2000;23:671-86.
172. Greenberg BD, Price LH, Rauch SL, et al. Neurosurgery for intractable obsessive-compulsive disorder: critical issues. Neurosurg Clin N Am. 2003;14:199-212.
173. Grill WM Jr. Modeling the effects of electric fields on nerve fibers: influence of tissue electrical properties. IEEE Trans Biomed Eng. 1999;46:918-28.
174. Grill WM, McIntyre CC. Extracellular excitation of central neurons: implications for the mechanisms of deep brain stimulation. Thalamus Relat Syst. 2001;1:269-77.
175. Harden CL, Pulver MC, Ravdin LD, et al. A pilot study of mood in epilepsy patients treated with vagus nerve stimulation. Epilepsy Behav. 2000;1:93-99.
176. Heath RG. Pleasure response of human subjects to direct stimulation of the brain: physiologic and psychodynamic considerations, in The Role of Pleasure in Behavior. Edited by Heath RG. New York, Hoeber. 1964.pp.219-43.
177. Heath RG, Guerrero-Figueroa R. Stimulation of the human brain: spontaneous and evoked electroencephalographic responses. Acta Neurol Latinoam. 1968;14:116-24.
178. Heck CN, Helmers SL, DeGiorgio CM, et al. Vagus nerve stimulation therapy, epilepsy, and device parameters: scientific basis and recommendations for use. Neurology. 2002;59(suppl 4):S31-S37.
179. Helmers SL, Wheless JW, Frost M, et al. Vagus nerve stimulation therapy in pediatric patients with refractory epilepsy: retrospective study. J Child Neurol. 2001;16:843-8.
180. Henry TR. Therapeutic mechanisms of vagus nerve stimulation. Neurology. 2002;59(suppl 4):S15-S20.
181. Henry TR, Bakay RA, Votaw JR, et al. Brian blood flow alterations induced by therapeutic vagus nerve stimulation in partial epilepsy, I: acute effects at high and low levels of stimulation. Eplepsia. 1998;39:983-90.
182. Henry TR, Votaw JR, Pennell PB, et al. Acute blood flow changes and efficacy of vagus nerve stimulation in partial epilepsy. Neurology. 1999;52:1166-73.
183. Il'inskii IA. Emotional-affective re-actions evoked by electro-stimulation of the ventrolateral nucleus of the optic thalamus. Vopr Neirokhir. 1970;34:26-2.
184. Kalivas PW, Duffy P, Abhold R, et al. Sensitization of mesolimbic dopamine neurons by neuropeptides and stress, in Sensitization in the Nervous System. Edited by Kalivas PW, Barnes CD. Caldwell, NJ, Telford Press, 1988, pp. 119-43.
185. Kirchner A, Birklein F, Stefan H, et al. Left vagus nerve stimulation suppersses experimentally induced pain. Neurology. 2000;55:1167-71.
186. Krahl SE, Clark KB, Smith DC, et al. Locus coeruleus lesions suppress the seizure attenuating effects of vagus nerve stimulation. Epilepsia. 1998;39:709-14.
187. Krahl SE, Senanayake SS, Handforth A. Seizure suppression by systemic epinephrine is mediated by the vagus nerve. Epilepsy Res. 2000;38:171-5.
188. Krahl SE, Senanayake SS, Hand-forth A. Destruction of peripheral Cfibers does not alter subsequent vagus nerve stimulation-induced seizure suppression. Epilepsia. 2001; 42:586-9.
189. Kumar R, Lozano AM, Kim YJ, et al. Double-blind evaluation of subthalamic nucleus deep brain stimulation in advanced Parkinson's disease. Neurology. 1998;51:850-5.
190. Kurlan R, Kersun J, Ballantine HT Jr, et al. Neurosurgical treatment of severe obsessive-compulsive disorder associated with Tourette's syndrome. Mov Disord. 1990;5:152-5.
191. Lenz FA, Gracely RH, Romanoski AJ, et al. Stimulation in the human somatosensory thalamus can reproduce both the affective and sensory dimensions of previously experienced pain. Nat Med. 1995;1:910-913.
192. Limousin P, Pollak P, Benazzouz A, et al. Effect of parkinsonian signs and symptoms of bilateral subthalamic nucleus stimultion. Lancet. 1995:345(8942):91-95.
193. Lomarev M, Denslow S, Nahas Z, et al. Vagus nerve stimulation (VNS) synchronized BOLD fMRI suggests that VNS in depressed adults has frequency/dose dependent effects. J Psychiatr Res. 2002;36:219-227.
194. MacLean PD. The Triune Brain in Evolution: Role in Paleocerebral Functions. New Tork, Plenum, 1990.
195. Marangell LB, Rush AJ, George MS, et al. Vagus nerve stimulation (VNS) for major depressive episodes: longer-term outcome. Biol Psychiatry. 2002;51:280-7.
196. Mark VA, Barry H, McLardy T, et al. The destruction of both anterior thalamic nuclei in a patient with intractable agitated depression. J Nerv ment Dis. 1970;150:266-72.
197. McDougle CJ, Price LH, Goodman WK, et al. A controlled trial of lithium augmentation in fluvoxamine-refractory obsessive-compulsive disorder: lack of efficacy. J Clin Psychopharmacol. 1991;11:175-84.
198. Mu Q, Bohning DE, Nahas Z, et al. Acute VNS using different pulse widths produces varying brain effects. Biol Psychiatry. 2004;55:816-25.

199. Nahas Z, Marangell LB, et al. Two-year outcome of vagus nerve stimulation (VNS) therapy for major depressive episodes. J Clin Psychiatry (in press).
200. Naritoku DK, Terry WJ, Helfert RH, et al. Regional induction of Fos immunoreactivity in the brain by anticonvulsant stimulation of the vagus nerve. Epilepsy Res. 1995;22: 53-62.
201. Ness TJ, Fillingim RB, Randich A, et al. Low intensity vagal nerve stimulation lowers human thermal pain thresholds. Pain 2000;85:81-5.
202. Nuttin B, Cosyns P, Demeulemeester H, et al. Electrical stimulation in anterior limbs of internal capsules in patients with obsessive-compulsive disorder. Lancet. 1999; 354(9189):1526.
203. Nuttin BJ, Gabriels LA, Cosyns PR, et al. Long-term electrical capsular stimulation in patients with obsessive-compulsive disorder. Neurosurgery. 2003;52:1263-72.
204. Olanow CW, Brin MF, Obeso JA. The role of deep brain stimulation as a surgical treatment for Parkinson's disease. Neurology. 2000;55(12, Suppl 6):S60-S66.
205. Penry JK, Dean JC. Prevention of intractable partial seizures by inter-mittent vagal nerve stimulation humans: preliminary results. Epilepsy. 1990;31:S40-S43.
206. Post RM. Behavioral sensitization and kindling: implications for affective illness and its treatment with carbamazepine. Rivesta de Psichiatria. 1980;1:71-79.
207. Prudic J, Haskett RF, Mulsant B, et al. Resistance to antidepressant medications and short-term clinical response to ECT. Am J Psychiatry. 1996;153:985-92.
208. Rauch SL, Jenike MA, Alpert NM, et al. Regional cerebral blood flow measured during symptom provocation in obsessive-compulsive disorder using oxygen 15-labeled carbon dioxide and positron emission tomography. Arch Gen Psychiatry. 1994; 51:62-70.
209. Roslin M, Kurian M. The use of electrical stimulation of the vagus nerve to treat morbid obesity. Epilepsy Behav. 2001; 2:S11-S16.
210. Rush AJ, Giles DE, Schlesser MA, et al. The Inventory of Depressive Symptomatology (IDS): preliminary findings. Psychiatry Res. 1986;18:65-87.
211. Rush AJ, George MS, Sackeim HA, et al. Vagus nerve stimulation (VNS) for treatment-resistent depressions: a multi-center study. Biol Psychiatry. 2000;47:276-86.
212. Rush AJ, Marangell LB, George MS, et al. Vagus nerve stimulation (VNS) therapy for treatment-resistant depression: a randomized, controlled acute phase trial. Biol Psychiatry (in press).
213. Sackeim HA, Prudic J, Devanand DP, et al. The impact of medication resistance and continuation pharmacotherapy on relapse following response to electroconvulsive therapy in major depression. J Clin Psychopharmacl. 1990;10:96-104.
214. Sackeim HA, Keilp JG, Rush AJ, et al. The effects of vagus nerve stimulation on cognitive performance in patients with treatment-resistant depression. Neuropsychiatry Neuropsychol Behav Neurol. 2001;14:53-62.
215. Sackeim HA, Rush AJ, George MS, et al. Vagus nerve stimulation (VNS) for treatment-resistent depression: efficacy, side effects, and predictors of outcome. Neuropsychopharmacology. 2001b;25:713-728.
216. Salinsky MC, Uthman BM, Ristanovic RK, et al. Vagus nerve stimulation for the treatment of medically intractable seizures: results of a 1-year open-extension trial. Arch Neurol. 1996;53:1176-80.
217. Schaltenbrand G, Spuler H, Wahren W, et al. Vegetative and emotional reactions during electrical stimulation of deep structures of the brain during stereotactic procedures. Z Neurol. 1973;205:91-113.
218. Sovik R. The science of breathing-the yogic view. Prog Brain Res. 2000;122:491-505.
219. Spangler WJ, Cosgrove GR, ballantine HT Jr, et al. Magnetic resonance image-guided stereotactic cingulatomy for intractable psychiatric disease. Neurosurgery. 1996; 38:1071-6.
220. Tarsy D. Deep brain stimulation and movement disorders. Epilepsy Behav. 2001;2(suppl):S45-S54.
221. Ter Horst GJ, Streetland C. Ascending projections of the solitary tract nucleus in Nucleus of the Solitary Tract. Edited by Robin I, Barraco A. London, CRS Press, 1994.
222. Tom T, Cummings JL. Depression in Parkinson's disease: pharmacological characteristics and treatment. Drugs Aging. 1998;12:55-74.
223. Walker BR, Easton A, Gale K. Regulation of limbic motor seizures by GABA and glutamate transmission in nucleus tractus solitarius. Epilepsia. 1999;40:1051-7.
224. Zabara J. Peripheral control of hypersynchronous discharge in epilepsy. Electroencephalogr Clin Neurophysiol. 1985a; 61S:S162.
225. Zabara J. Time course of seizure control to brief, repetitive stimuli. Epilepsia. 1985b;26:518.
226. Zabara J. Inhibition of experimental seizures in canines by repetitive vagal stimulation. Epilepsia. 1992;33:1005-12.

CHAPTER 47 Psychotherapies

DN Nandi, AN Basu, JN Vyas, SS Nathawat, Ajit Avasthi, Hitesh Khurana, Sandeep Grover, Munish Aggarwal, AR Garg, Neena Bohra, NK Bohra, Sujata Malik, Ashok Singhal

47.1 PSYCHOANALYSIS

DN Nandi, AN Basu

WHAT IS PSYCHOANALYSIS?

Psychoanalysis denotes, firstly, a technique of treating mental disorders by psychological means; secondly, a procedure for the investigation into those human psychical processes which are not accessible otherwise; and thirdly, a psychological theory based upon the psychological data, obtained from the above-mentioned investigation, which has been accumulated under a scientific discipline. As this scientific discipline emphasizes, in a major way, the unconscious mental processes, it is sometimes described as '*depth psychology*'.[1]

Thus, psychoanalysis may be designated both as an art and a science as depicted in Flow chart 1.

Flow chart 1: Psychoanalysis

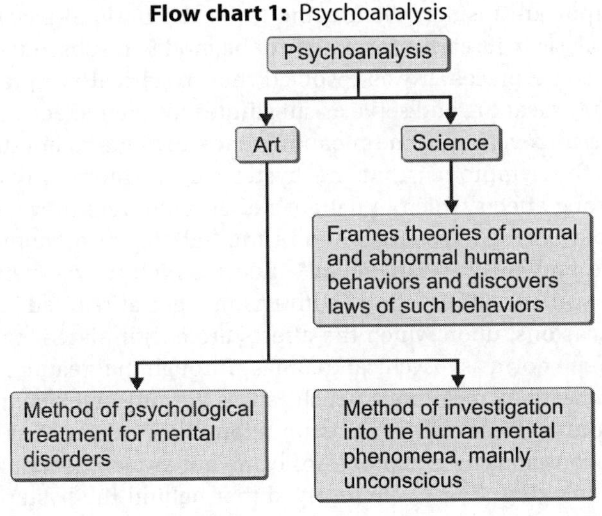

HISTORICAL OVERVIEW

Psychoanalysis may be said to be a product of twentieth century, as the world came to know of it with the publication of Sigmund Freud's (1856–1939) 'Interpretation of Dreams' in the year 1900. But, as is usual with every birth, it also had a long period of gestation.

Psychoanalysis originated in the keen perception and meticulous clinical observation of Freud, the renowned neurologist and physician of Vienna. Freud himself coined the term, '*psychoanalysis*'.

Thus, a new science developed in an effort to understand the nature of functional nervous diseases which baffled the physicians. The medical profession of the late nineteenth century was caught in a puzzle of the psychical factors involved in the enigmatic 'hysteria'. A decisive turn was taken in the eighties of the nineteenth century when Freud was studying and working in Vienna.

It is a remarkable fact in the history of psychoanalysis that the names of two patients of nervous disorder, Fraulein 'Anna O' and Elizabeth von R, are uttered with affection and respect along with its discoverer, Freud. Freud's two mentors, the Viennese physician Josef Breuer (1842–1925) and the Parisian physician JM Charcot (1835–1893) were also associated with the discovery of psychoanalysis.

Fraulein 'Anna O' was treated by Breuer in the year 1881-82 for her disturbed sight and speech, paralyzed limbs, and recoiling from food, after her father's death. From the state of normal behavior, she used to slip into the role of a recalcitrant child with alarming symptoms which later came to be categorized as symptoms of hysteria.

During the course of her treatment, Breuer found to his astonishment that one day, while the girl narrated the details of one of her severe episodes, the symptoms gradually disappeared. Breuer, then, supplemented his procedure by inducing hypnosis, and the results were startlingly successful. But, the improvement was unfortunately not permanent.

Freud was watching keenly this treatment affair, as he was made aware of the whole treatment story by Breuer himself in their frequent discussion over the matter. Anna O's case stimulated Freud's thinking and it came to be a turning point in his thought process regarding the mechanism of mental disorders. It came to his mind that hysterical symptoms must have some powerful psychogenic factors in their origin. Later, Freud, in 1895, formulated his idea in words: "hysterical symptoms originate through the energy of the mental process being withheld from conscious influence and being diverted into bodily innervation (conversion)."

In 1885, Freud had gone to Paris and had his famous encounter with Charcot. Freud tried to draw his attention to the 'talking cure' or 'chimney-sweeping', as 'Anna O' nicknamed the method by which she was relieved of her symptoms several times. In hypnosis, she would pour out her forgotten or 'strangulated' episodes along with their emotional contents and, thus would be spontaneously relieved of her traumatic past events. Charcot also demonstrated that in hypnosis, hysterical symptoms could be induced in persons. It indicated that hysteria could be removed by thought alone. In the whole treatment procedure, the cathartic effect came to be recognized as of great importance and significance.

After intensive training in the hypnotic method under Charcot, Freud returned to Vienna and began to use hypnosis in the treatment of nervous diseases in 1887. But, it appeared to him that by this method, though some patients were found to be cured temporarily, yet actually the symptoms were suppressed to a major extent. Moreover, by 1892, Freud realized that his ability to hypnotize was very limited. In that year, in treating Elizabeth von R, he abandoned hypnosis altogether, as she could not be hypnotized. This was the first case that Freud treated completely with waking suggestion.

There is no pinpoint date for the discovery of the technique of free association. It gradually developed during the years from 1892 to 1896, starting with the treatment of Elizabeth von R who reproached Freud, on one occasion, for interrupting her flow of thoughts by questioning her and applying pressure on her forehead and insisting upon her for her past memories.

Originally, Freud used to command the patient to talk about the origin of the symptoms during hypnosis. The patient, responding, produced a series of memories accompanied by intense affect. At the end of the session, the patient was asked to forget all the disturbing memories. Subsequently, Freud abandoned hypnosis, and adopted suggestion and pressure technique on the forehead during the patient's waking state.

On the whole, it may be said that Anna O's case initiated Freud to think of psychogenic factors of mental disorders. He realized that somatic changes could be brought about by mental influences. On the other hand, Elizabeth von R's case urged him to shift from the hypnotic method to the method of free association. The former is the basis of the theory, while the latter is the foundation of the technique of psychoanalysis. Historically, the 'Studies on Hysteria',[2] jointly written by Freud and Breuer, may be marked as the precursor of psychoanalytic thoughts. In 1893, Breuer and Freud published 'The Psychical Mechanism of Hysterical Phenomena' and, two years later, it was elaborated and incorporated into the 'Studies on Hysteria',[2] with the aforesaid joint paper as its opening chapter. Five case histories, a theoretical paper by Breuer, and a final chapter by Freud, are the other contents of the book. The book was not well received by the then medical circle. Breuer was so disturbed by some reviews that he lost confidence in his own theory. But Freud, undaunted, carried on being supported by Wilhelm Fliess, an ENT specialist, whose ability of bold speculation and framing of hypotheses had strongly attracted Freud.

Freud's gradual emphasis on sexual etiology of neurosis also refrained Breuer from further investigation. Freud[3] says in this context: "when I later began more and more resolutely to put forward the significance of sexuality in the etiology of neuroses, he was the first to show the reaction of distaste and repudiation which was later to become so familiar to me, but which at that time I had not yet learnt to recognize as my inevitable fate." Furthermore, the attachment of the patient towards the physician, with indications of sexual motivation, which Breuer must have discovered during the treatment of 'Anna O', scared him and ultimately refrained him from further venture into psychoanalysis. Breuer could not understand the universal nature of this patient-physician relationship in psychoanalytical setting. The patient-physician relationship was later recognized as the ultimate basis of psychoanalytic treatment and was designated as 'transference'.

Investigations of Breuer and Freud yielded several important results which came to be the basis of psychoanalysis in its earlier form, only to be modified subsequently in some places. It was resolved that hysterical symptoms carry meaning and serve as substitutes for mental acts; that the uncovering of the meaning leads to the amelioration of the symptoms; that the hysterical symptoms involve strong affects which in patient's earlier life were prevented from normal discharge; and in the 'talking cure' method, the previously 'strangulated' affects, which were diverted in somatic innervation (conversion), get abreacted. The occasions, upon which the affects are accumulated, came to be known as 'psychical traumas'. Through the treatment, a 'catharsis' comes about, which causes the cure of the patient. From all these results, an assumption of the existence of the unconscious mental processes came out as an essential line of thinking. It was also resolved that behind the hysterical symptoms exist the subject's experiences of affective life and the interaction of unconscious mental forces.

After Breuer had withdrawn from the treatment of hysterical patients by cathartic or abreaction method, Freud ushered in fresh developments in the realm of technique for the treatment of such patients. As has been mentioned earlier, free association method was introduced. In this method, the patient is asked to recline on a couch and relax. Then, he has to refrain from any conscious thinking but to watch his spontaneous or involuntary ideas that come up in his mind. They are to be communicated to the physician, even if they seem to be unpleasant, senseless or irrelevant. The patient should not hide any idea.

Although it was named free association, yet Freud recognized that it was not truly speaking 'free'. Because, the ideas that emerged were determined by the unconscious material. The material that came out was not the actual forgotten memories, which were seen to be produced in hypnosis, but was a real hint for those forgotten experiences. The physician was to, by obeying some rules, interpret and reconstruct the forgotten experiences. Thus, new development made the treatment method so different from the hypnotic and cathartic method, and under it the doctor-patient relationship brought about so many fresh results, that Freud gave it the name of '*psychoanalysis*' in 1896. Thus, he was provided with the technique for studying the meaning of dreams, slips of the tongue, forgetfulness, and other mistakes and errors. Psychoanalysis, over and above its role as a healing technique, was thus lifted to an interpretative art for human behavior, as well as a theory of human personality.

The decade of 1890s was very significant in the history of psychoanalysis. During this period, Freud himself suffered from an attack of psychoneurosis. He started his self-analysis in 1897, and it yielded new results out of his own psychical turmoil. The existence of infantile sexuality and incestuous desires were hinted at. The concept of 'Oedipus complex' began to take form. The importance of dream analysis in psychoanalysis was recognized. Full-fledged theories of unconscious motivation, mechanisms of repression, resistance, defense and transference, theory of anxiety and etiology of the neuroses, were evolved.

Next comes the period from 1900 to 1910, when Freud developed the instinct theories. He also chalked out the course of biological sexual development of the child. At this time, Freud's sexual theory came under attack by his two close collaborators, Adler followed by Jung. This, in spite of the fact that, Freud indicated the importance of factors other than sex in mental disorders.

In the years from 1910 to 1920, a complete psychoanalytic theory about the total human personality emerged: the structure of the personality being formed by the id, ego and superego. The concept of narcissism was made clear, and a new theory of instincts, with aggression as one of its two pillars, was envisaged.

After 1920 till the present day, psychoanalysis has been enriched with theoretical expansion by Freud himself and also by many of his coworkers. Some of his followers deviated from him in some respects and some have added new dimensions to his thoughts. Many of his metapsychological speculations have been supported and many of his hypotheses have been experimented and validated by many workers; again, many have been challenged also. But, whatever the deviations and shifts of emphasis are, it can be said without any doubt that the basic structure of psychoanalysis remains the same as was built by Freud. All the deviations and dimensions emanate from that basic structure. In that sense, psychoanalysis is Freudian and both the deviants and post-Freudians are Freudian.[2-7]

THEORETICAL CONSIDERATIONS OF THE STRUCTURE AND WORKING OF THE MENTAL APPARATUS

Our immediate acquaintance with the human mental apparatus occurs through our consciousness. We need not explain its validity and describe it. But, the question is whether the consciousness is equivalent to our whole mental life. By trekking the path of symptoms of mental illness, dreams, various kinds of slips or errors and human psychical development, we gather the knowledge of an area of our mental life which is called, unconscious. Here, a spontaneous hypothesis may crop up regarding the localization of conscious and unconscious mental life, because the idea (imaginary) underlying it is that our mental apparatus is extended in space and made up of some parts, the conscious and the unconscious being two of them. But, the assumption regarding the localization does not lead us far, as it does not help us in understanding the working of our mental apparatus.

In his earlier description of the mental apparatus, Freud[8] made a tripartite division of the human psyche; the conscious, the preconscious and the unconscious. The conscious, being the external territory, acts like the outer cortex of the mind. The preconscious and the unconscious are the internal territories, of which the unconscious lies in the innermost of the mental apparatus. The external territory of our mental life is very narrow, because it is the region of perception, and any perception is of momentary nature. The internal territory encompasses most of our mental life. The outermost layer of the mind is responsible for the conscious phenomena, whereas the materials of the preconscious area can be made conscious through easy efforts (memorization), but the unconscious region is not easily accessible. The main features of the unconscious, in the words of Freud,[8] are "exemption from mutual contradiction, primary process (mobility of cathexis), timelessness, and replacement by psychical reality".

This tripartite division of mind is called the topographical description of mental apparatus. But, Freud[9] in his later conceptual developments, due to some obvious difficulties in explaining the features of narcissistic disorders, along with self-esteem and self-love in megalomania where ego is found to be the object of its own love, replaced the topographical view by the structural-cum-functional view regarding the mental apparatus of which the id, the ego and the superego are the three pillars. Here, it must be kept in mind that this conceptual change does not invalidate the concept of the unconscious; rather, it makes the unconscious a dynamic one. This concept of the unconscious remained as one of the main cornerstones of psychoanalysis. The conscious and the unconscious (including the preconscious) are the attributes of the mental apparatus being expressed through the three dynamic agencies, namely id, ego and superego.

Id

The oldest agency, or the original state of the human mental apparatus, is named as id. A new born baby comes to this world with this original state of psychical apparatus. It is the repository of everything that is inherited. It is totally unconscious; therefore, it is the most inaccessible part of the human mind. Human instinctual needs find their psychical expression in it. Hence, it is "a chaos, a cauldron full of seething excitations". It is not a coherent organization. In it there is no value judgment, no reasoning and no sense of time. Therefore, it is full of contradictions. The opposites remain in it side by side. It has no direct link with the world of reality.

The id has its own world of perception. Its drives are instinctual and it has feelings of pleasure-unpleasure. The instinctual drives in it are compounded out of fusion in varying proportions of two primal forces: *Eros* (life or pleasure) and *Thanatos* (death). The only urge of these drives is satisfaction which generates pleasures. In the id, everything is positive, there is nothing negative. The core of human mental apparatus is formed by the id.

Ego

From the moment of birth of a baby, a portion of the id undergoes a special change or development under the influence of the external world, which may be ascribed as the cortical layer of the id. This development is manifested through the function of an agency, called the ego. The ego is principally determined by the individual's experience of the real world as presented to him. It is the agency which conducts the sense of perception and muscular action, i.e. it has control over motility. It is a coherent organization of mental processes which acts as an intermediary between the instinctual impulses (i.e. the id) and the external world (i.e. the reality). As it is the agency for perception and motility, it receives stimuli from and acts on the external world. Hence, it has at its command all sorts of perceptions and voluntary actions. Thereby, it acts as a protective shield, like the external cortical layer of an organism, against the unfavorable stimuli. It stores up experiences, avoids excessive stimuli, adapts itself to the situation, and by learning and activity brings change in the external world. It has the capacity to gain control, in a round-about way, over the demands of the instincts.

It strives to avoid tension (unpleasure), roused by the instincts (id-demands), by lowering that tension which means seeking for pleasure. In that way it serves the id. But, in that pursuit it has to recognize the world of reality. Therefore, it can be said that in its activity it is guided by the *reality principle.* Occasionally, the ego severs its connection with the conscious or external world and withdraws into sleep, and at that time exercises censorship on dreams and brings a change in its own organization, and consequently, into the other functions of the mind. The ego is invested with the energy from the id, because it is an emergent from the id. Therefore, to speak in a functional sense, though the ego operates in the conscious province of the mental life, the unconscious region is not out of its bounds. It is mostly conscious and partly unconscious. The relation between the id and the ego has been compared by Freud[9] to that of a rider and the horse, the man on the horseback being the ego who has to control the superior strength of id, the horse. In doing so, the ego transforms the will of the id as its own.

Superego

The long period of human childhood dependence upon parents leaves upon the mental apparatus the marks of its influence which is manifested in the ego. Thus, there is a change in the ego. Gradually, this trace of parental influence stands apart from the ego and acts as a special agency, the superego. This parental influence includes in it not only the marks of the actual parents but also of the family, race, nation, tradition of the past as well as of the present, and religion. In the superego is reflected also the individual's attitude towards his parents. As a matter of fact, the child's triangular relationship with his parents, what is known as the *Oedipus complex*, is involved in it. By way of identification, the parental images are introjected with all their love-hate ramifications. According to the nature of relationship of the child with its parents, a code of morality is built up in the superego which the ego has to obey as the child obeys his parents. If the ego fails to come to a compromise with the superego, the superego torments the ego with the sense of guilt along with its derivatives, giving rise to a disaster in the psychic life.

The process of the formation of the superego is mostly unconscious. Hence, this process of derivation brings it into close relation to the id. In that way, it reaches deep down into the id, and thereby it is further away from the consciousness than the ego is. So, it partakes in a major way the characteristics of the id. In describing the characters of the three agencies, Freud[9] says : "From the point of view of instinctual control of morality, it may be said of id that it is totally nonmoral, of the ego that it strives to be moral, and of the superego that it can be supermoral and then becomes as cruel as only the id can be". Thus, it is seen that the poor ego has three severe, and sometimes tyrannical, masters—the external world, the superego, and the id. For a healthy mental life, these three agencies must act in perfect harmony.

It may be noted here that the ego and superego of an individual do not remain the same all through his life. They undergo gradual change and development. At the outset, the ego is very feeble and the superego is not well established. Grossly speaking, it may be said that, at birth, a child is totally id. Through gradual development, due to experience, the ego and the superego become differentiated and begin to function as separate entities. First of all, the ego is body-ego and it feels itself omnipotent. For the full development of the ego, the child is required to pass through the experience of reality testing for a considerable period of his early life; and for that of the superego he has to undergo parental, interpersonal and cultural influence throughout the period of his childhood dependence. The influence of the family, tradition, race and nation percolate through the parental figures and education.

It may be mentioned here for clarification that the concept of ego was not the same all through during Freud's different phases of discovery. In his preliminary thought, around 1908–1910, he failed to see the unconscious role of the ego which became clear only afterwards on his observation of the facts of ego-drives (ego-instincts) and repression. Thereby, he could develop his structural theory.

Thus, on the whole, it is envisaged that all the three agencies are ingrained in the unconscious; the id being totally unconscious, the ego partly unconscious and partly conscious, and the superego having much of its being in the unconscious and its minor portion being conscious. All these three entities function in an intimate relationship for their being submerged in the unconscious; there is a mutual interchange of energy among them.[4, 9-11]

THEORY OF INSTINCTS

The instincts are the forces, the sources of which are the organs of the body. These forces act behind the tensions generated by the needs of the id. The instincts are the mental representations of the somatic demands or needs, which are manifested in the mental level as impulses or drives. As the needs are varied, the usual practice is to enlist innumerable number of apparently distinct instincts. But, Freud could trace back the roots of all those instincts to two basic instincts only.

In his earlier conceptual classifications, Freud[9] differentiated instincts in two broad divisions: *sexual instincts* and *ego instincts* (or the instincts of self-preservation). But, later he realized that the differentiation between the sexual and ego instincts is not tenable, because the self-preservative instincts are also of sexual nature; they can take the subject's own ego as their object of love. Further, it was explored that all these instincts can replace one another in respect of object and aim; one instinct can derive satisfaction from the other. This character is most clearly found in sublimation where both the object and the aim of an instinct are changed, and finds satisfaction in a new object and aim.

Finally, Freud[9,12] recognized two classes of instincts; life instincts or *eros*, and death (or destructive) instincts or *thanatos*. The former aims at unity and the latter works for disintegration. These two basic instincts operate against each other or they work in combination with each other. The interplay of these two makes creation what it is. Both of these classes of instincts are in operation from the beginning of creation. Though they are opposite in nature and work against each other, yet they can never remain in isolation. Sometimes, one fulfills the aim of the other.[1, 9-10]

DEVELOPMENT OF PSYCHOSEXUAL FUNCTION

The term 'sexual' in psychoanalysis denotes a wide range of activities over and above the genital performances. In psychoanalysis, 'sexual' and 'genital' are not synonymous. All 'genital' events are 'sexual', but all 'sexual' events are not 'genital'. Therefore, the following three points must be kept in mind, while considering the development of the sexual function:

1. Sexual life of an individual starts immediately after his birth.
2. The scope of 'sexual' is wider than that of 'genital'.
3. Sexual life consists of the activities of the different zones of the body which bring pleasure to the individual. These activities may or may not coincide with the functions of reproduction.[13]

Freud[1] introduced the term *'libido'* for the dynamic manifestation of the sexual instincts in human mental life, i.e. libido is made up of sexual instincts, the sources of which are the organs of the body, mainly erotogenic zones. Contributions to the libido come from all the functional processes of the body which bring pleasure. Thus, the libido or sexual instinct manifests through different zones of the body, but it follows a definite course of development. In a new born baby, the sexual functional processes of the body, which bring pleasure, take the form of a sort of constellation or come under an organization.

First of all, the child's oral zone plays the leading role in the formation of this organization. The new born child comes in contact with the external reality in connection with the experience of hunger and its satisfaction through the mouth. His first perception is connected with the oral incorporation; he has to judge whether an object is edible. Along with this oral perception is connected the attainment of pleasure, a pleasure gained through the satisfaction of the roused stimulation of the erogenous oral mucous membrane. This is evident in the thumb-sucking of the child.

The oral sexual phase is followed by the anal phase or anal organization of the development of the sexual function or of the libido development. During this period, the anal erogenous zone becomes the chief executive through the acts of defecation and holding back the fecal mass. The stimulation of the rectal mucosa is tied up with both discharge and retention. This phase is technically known as anal-sadistic, because cruel or aggressive drives, along with sexual drives, are fulfilled through it. This phase is also connected with the appearance of teeth and strengthening of the muscular apparatus.

Next comes the phallic phase, in which the genitals (penis in the case of a boy and clitoris in the case of a girl) attain importance in the life of the child, as the concentration of the sexual excitement appears there. The libido is organized around this and a sort of genital orgasm is attained at this period.

The manifestation of libido, or the development of sexual function, occurs one after another through these three organizations or phases and is completed within the fourth or fifth year of life of a child. But, this does not mean that one does not function when the other appears. Always they overlap with one another; in one phase the characteristics of another are present. The phases are so named according to the predominance of a particular erotogenic zone.

Here, one thing should be noted. The last phase has been named as phallic phase, not genital phase, in spite of the fact that the concentration of sexual excitement is around the genital organ. Freud[10] reserved the term 'genital phase' for the sexual organization which appears after puberty when the whole system matures for reproduction.

In the course of the sexual development, there occurs a very important event. Though the phases of development pass from one stage to another, yet some portion of a component sexual instinct may remain behind, attached to a previous zone in the course of the libido's forward march. This state of affairs gives rise to '*fixation*', which may impede the subsequent normal sexual development. This situation is very important for the onset of neuroses.

Infantile Sexuality

On the basis of analytic data from the adult patients, and subsequently by child observation, Freud was convinced of the appearance of sexuality in a child from the moment of his 'extrauterine' existence. Certainly, the aim of this infantile sexuality is not the 'union of the two sexes in the sexual act'. The infantile sexuality includes such activities as are forerunner of forepleasure in adult life, and which are also of perverse nature from the adult point of view. This sexuality may be autoerotic in nature as it takes the child's own body as the object. Every kind of excitation-muscular, affective, intellectual or even painful-in the child may become a source of sexual pleasure. Hence, psychoanalysis had to enlarge the concept of sexuality.

Through experience with his patients, Freud came to the conclusion, during the beginning years of his discovery, that sexual etiology played the most powerful role in many forms of neuroses, mainly in hysteria. The root of this sexual etiology was grounded in a patient's early childhood experience. Freud gathered from many patients that one of their parents had attempted or achieved their 'seduction' in their childhood. But, later, Freud came to the realization, on examination of facts and analysis of data, that these 'childhood seductions' had in fact never occurred, but were fantasies of the childhood. They were reversal of the desired role. It was actually a wish of the patient in his childhood to have a passive sex experience before puberty. Hence, the trauma of 'childhood seduction' was, in most of the cases, not an actuality but a fantasy. It was rooted in the infantile sexuality, though the parental behavior might have contributed to it.[10,13,14]

Oedipus Complex

Oedipus complex is the climax of infantile sexuality. In a straight way, it means a child's love for the parent of opposite sex and hate towards the parent of same sex.

The instinctual components of the libido find their satisfaction, first by being autoerotic, and then when they are diverted on to the external world, mother becomes the object. With the onset of the oral phase, mother's breast becomes the object of libidinal cathexis. Then, gradually, with the advance of age through different phases of libidinal development, mother (or mother substitute) as a whole person turns to be its object. Approximately between the age from two to five, there occurs a convergence of the sexual impulses with the libidinal or sexual energy, and consequently, the phallic phase rises to its height when a boy turns towards his mother as his libidinal or sexual object in a fresh way. This choice of an object leads him towards an attitude of rivalry and hostility towards the father. In the case of a girl, the picture emerges in quite the reverse way. That is, the father becomes her object of choice and the mother is her rival. This is the main content of the Oedipus complex. In every normal human being, the development and resolution of the Oedipus complex is of great importance in shaping his personality and erotic life. A normal individual learns gradually to master this complex, whereas a neurotic remains involved in it and produces symptoms.[1,4,10,13]

Biphasic Sexual Development

It is a biological peculiarity with the human species that the sexual development occurs in two installments. The libidinal development of a child comes to an end with the reaching to the phallic phase at about the age of five. Then there is a period of rest or silence, which is called the period of latency, and during which various types (e.g. ethical, social, etc.) of restraints are built up to act as defenses against affects related to the Oedipus complex. This latency period continues till the advent of puberty, when renewed intensity of sexual instinct comes forth and the Oedipus complex is revived in the unconscious with various modifications. The course it takes is determined by the early experiences of child's sexuality, i.e. his experience in libidinal development through different phases. This biphasic development of human sexuality contains, to a great extent, the determining factors of neurotic breakdown, if it does not pass through the stages properly.[4,10,13]

REPRESSION AND RESISTANCE

The concept of 'repression' was mooted in Freud's mind since his discussion with Breuer about the case of 'Anna O'. Breuer could elicit the following story from the girl during her hypnoid state:

"The girl had been nursing her father during his illness. One night, while she was on duty by his bedside and was waiting for the doctor to come, she fell in a slumber with an arm on the back of the chair. In her doze, she dreamt that a snake was coming out of the wall towards her father. She tried to reach the snake, but it seemed that her arm was the snake. On waking, she found that her arm was benumbed".

In the course of the treatment of this girl, Breuer discovered to his astonishment that after she had recalled the episode in hypnosis, the paralysis vanished. Thus, it was acknowledged that though the event remained cut off from the consciousness, yet it continued to exert influence upon her mind and found expression in symptoms. This was no ordinary forgetting, but had some dynamic forces or motives acting behind it. Hence, it was concluded that the episode was repressed. The impulses, that came into her mind, were not compatible with the ethical standard and integrity of her conscious mind or ego. The ego shut them off and obstructed their satisfaction. But, those impulses found their expression in symptoms. The symptoms were substitutive satisfaction of impulses.

In analysis, the existence of repression is evident from the act of resistance by the patient to the treatment. He opposes, unconsciously, the revelation of his unpleasant memories. As these are not ego-syntonic, the ego withdraws interest from them and pushes them back in the unconscious, so that they may not become conscious. Resistance is another side of repression. Like repression, it is also a dynamic force and is mostly unconscious. It is a conservative force which creates greatest difficulty in treatment and, consequently, to the cure of the patient.

Another very important source of resistance is the secondary gain from illness. As the neuroses are the expression of conflicts between the ego and the impulses, the symptoms are the product of a compromise formula between the two. Therefore, in spite of the sufferings from the symptoms, the patient also achieves satisfaction by their presence. Furthermore, due to the diseased condition, the patient can manipulate, to some extent, the environment to his favor. Thus, he draws some privileges from the persons around him. These secondary gains create a formidable resistance on the way of the repressed materials to come out.

The repression has another style of functioning. When a libidinal impulse is thwarted in its expression or satisfaction, that repressed drive may turn back to its earlier phase of development or earlier attitude towards its object. That is, the libido, instead of going forward, '*regresses*' to an earlier position. A major quantity of the libidinal energy may remain fixed in that position. This is a situation of morbidity.

Again, as the symptoms are substitutive impulse satisfaction, they also cannot escape ego's repressive act fully. Hence, the symptoms undergo modification and displacement—as the dream materials undergo—and, therefore, it becomes difficult to recognize them as impulse satisfaction. This is more true in the symptoms of hysteria than in obsessional neurosis, where the stronger emphasis is upon the function of the ego which erects an insurmountable dam against the onset of flash flood of instinctual drives.

Freud discovered that the act of repression starts from the early childhood period and that the children are more vulnerable to repression than the adults. The act of repression can go on unconsciously as the ego's root remains in the unconscious. Freud was of the opinion at the beginning that the repression must have a sexual bearing, but later he realized that aggression was another factor which contributes to repression.[2,4-6,10,13,15]

DEFENSE MECHANISMS

Resistance and defense are interrelated concepts. Resistance is that unconscious tendency in the patient's mind which opposes the total treatment procedure and, consequently, does not allow the reasonable ego to win over the diseased condition.

Defense refers to the unconscious mechanism or operations of the mental apparatus which make the resistance fruitful. These operations are carried by the ego. As the symptoms are the products of a compromise between impulses and reality, i.e. the symptoms are the compromise formation of the conflicts, the purpose of the resistance and defense is to defend the neurosis from exposure. The neurosis finds its satisfaction in the symptoms. So, its exposure or breaking of the symptoms entail pain on the ego. Hence, the ultimate purpose of resistance and defense is to avoid pain which arises due to a conflict between the impulses and the reality. Thus, it may be said that the defenses are of the ego and, are mostly aimed at the impulses.

Anna Freud[16] gave special importance to locating and analyzing the defense of the ego in therapeutic work. The important defense mechanisms which are found during the analytic work may be listed as follows: regression, repression, reaction formation, isolation, rationalization, projection-introjection-identification, turning against the self, reversal, conversion, and sublimation of instinctual aims.

Regression

In this mechanism, the normal behavior is replaced by activities in fantasy, the content of which always shows a return to the infantile mode of gratification. In it, the ego abandons the matured path of gratification and takes resort to pregenital or less objectionable (to the ego) attitude towards its object of gratification. Fixation, if any, in the course of sexual development helps the ego to determine its regressive path. For example, when an adult behaves like a child in his eating habits or otherwise finds pleasure in that, it may be said that he has regressed to the infantile mode of gratification. In analysis, it is found that the patient's free-association materials move back from the present situations to earlier experiences and remain fixed in the past, i.e. in the materials of early childhood experiences. This is known as regression.

Repression

It is the mechanism in which the ego excludes from the consciousness all the psychological contents which it cannot fit in harmoniously in its scope. This is the principal mechanism of the infantile ego, which is too weak to withstand, postpone and modify any impulse. The repressed impulses do not cease to exist by mere expulsion from the consciousness. They remain in the unconscious as dynamic forces, as they are backed by instincts. To deal with these pent-up or repressed impulses, the ego has to take further steps. They are:

1. Further reinforcements of repression, and
2. Finding out substitute channels for outlet of the impulses.

Suppose a child finds that, with the advent of his new baby-brother, his mother's love for him is divided. He feels jealousy and rivalry towards his little brother. Consequently, he becomes aggressive towards him, but he represses his aggression for fear of punishment or further loss of love. But, he may channelize his aggression through some other activity, for example, by breaking the little brother's toy.

Reaction Formation

The ego may take an acceptable attitude to keep at a distance, an ego-alien impulse. Thus, love may cover-up unconscious hate, shyness serve as a defense against exhibitionism, and so on. The conscious attitude is the polar opposite of the repressed ego-alien tendency. This is also known as *overcompensation*. In the previous example, the child may feel in his consciousness, an extraordinary concern for the welfare of the new born brother and behave accordingly. In this way, his unconscious hate and aggression for the little brother, is covered-up or over-compensated.

Isolation

In this defense, the ego-alien tendencies, which appear in consciousness, are separated from all other mental contents as if they do not belong to the ego. In this way, they are made innocuous. Isolation is mainly found in obsessive-compulsive neurotics. By rituals like touching, washing, etc. the ego separates the ego-alien tendency from itself. This is also called as the *restriction of the ego*. For example, a person, by repeatedly washing his hands, may isolate an unsocial sexual desire from himself or by frequent touching of a particular object, may restrict his ego from venturing into an unsocial desire.

Rationalization

It is a method to support an attitude with false reasons. The ego selects, from the coexisting motivations, only those which are acceptable to it. In doing so, it intellectualizes the tendency which it displays by suppressing the ego-alien ones. For example, the fox of the fable rationalizes its indifference towards grapes with the argument that grapes are sour, though the fox was greedy of the grapes.

Projection-introjection

Projection is the mechanism by which the ego attributes its own intolerable sexual and aggressive impulses to the outside person or agency. For example, a spinster, who has repressed her sex impulse, may develop the delusion that her male neighbors are trying to molest her sexually. That is, she projects her own desire for sex upon others.

In introjection, the reverse process is adopted when the ego incorporates or re-establishes the lost object in itself by way of identification. Sometimes, it becomes a part of the superego. When a female child plays with her doll, feeds the doll, bathes it and makes it go to sleep, she is only displaying her introjected mother in her behavior.

Turning against the Self

Sometimes the ego, instead of expressing hostility against the other person, represses the hostility but ventilates it against the own self in the form of self-criticism and self-accusation. Thus, hate towards others can be transformed into self-hatred. A child may suppress his hatred towards his parents and develop the idea that he himself is hateful.

Reversal

In this mechanism the ego, by way of fantasy, reverses the real situation and takes that to be otherwise. By this method, the external reality is denied and, thus, the external threat is averted. This is also called *denial in fantasy*. The fear of examination may be averted by a boy by imagining (with a belief) that there will be no examination due to political disturbance in the town.

Conversion

By this mechanism, the ego-alien tendencies are totally repressed and given expression on the physiological or somatic level. Hysterical paralysis, convulsions, etc. are products of this mechanism. For example, due to the repressed aggression, one's arms may be paralyzed, lest he kills his object of aggression.

Sublimation

This is the most normal defense. The unacceptable tendency is substituted or replaced by another one which is appropriate for relieving the original tendency and at the same time has a social value. Thus, sexual impulses are substituted by creative activities. In this category, a form of altruism may be included. Rejection by the lover may induce one to divert his energy into human welfare, or artistic and literary activities.

DREAM

Dream analysis lifted psychoanalysis from a therapeutic process to a full-fledged *depth psychology*. Dream is the phenomenon where unconscious is demonstrated. Actually speaking, Freudian hypotheses regarding human mental structure are proved and illustrated in dream analysis. In dream, the functions of the id, ego and superego, and the conflicts among them, are easily understandable. Knowledge gained through dream made it possible to understand the patterns of diseased as well as normal minds. It was also gathered that the dynamics of the formation of dreams and that of the symptoms are same. Dream and disease, both, are the outcome of the conflicts among the three: id, ego and superego. Whereas the dream is temporary, the disease continues. Moreover, as the dream is a way of fulfilling the unconscious wishes, it has an adaptive value; the tension due to unfulfilled desires are released in dream. Therefore, dream exerts a palliative influence upon the mind. Contrarily, the disease is painful, brings suffering to the mind and is maladaptive.

A dream is a phenomenon of normal mind. But, it is a state of mental derangement in the sleep condition with 'illusions' and 'hallucinations' as its main features. Therefore, the knowledge of dream is very illuminative; it shows that the mental mechanism, which is responsible for producing a pathological state, is also found to be present in the normal mind. Thus, the analysis of dream saved psychoanalysis from the blame or charge that it bases its understanding of the normal mind on pathological data. Furthermore, through the understanding of dream symbolism, it has been possible to decode the symbolism in human archaic thought, language, mythology and folklore. Thus, it is said that the interpretation of dreams is the '*royal road to the knowledge of the unconscious activities of the mind*'.[17]

The formation of dream can occur in two ways:

1. An unsocial or an unattainable impulse which, in our waking and real life situation is not practicable and hence is generally suppressed, finds its way during sleep to exert influence upon the ego, because the ego inhibition at that time is slackened; the ego in sleep withdraws itself from reality. The ego has an inherent tendency to turn away from the external reality; therefore it wishes to sleep. Thus, the suppressed material of the waking life finds a passage towards manifestation in dream.
2. Again, a repressed thought or desire may achieve reinforcement during sleep from the unconscious element, i.e. from the id impulses. That reinforcement may cause the repressed thought or desire to come out in dream by shattering down the resistance of the ego. Thus, a dream may be formed either by ego relaxation or by id pressure. However, the mechanism of dream in both cases is the same; it takes the forms of 'illusions' and 'hallucinations'.

The primary functions of dream are, on the one hand to protect sleep, and on the other, to fulfill the wish of the dreamer. As the dream is a compromise-structure, which arises from the conflicts among the agencies of the mental apparatus, it can fulfill the double function. In its function as a protector or guardian of sleep, dream strives to relieve tensions generated by the unattainable wishes which, if not removed, might prevent the person from sleeping. Suppose a doctor is required to get up early in the morning and reach the hospital in time to attend his duty. He goes to sleep with an anxiety for his duty and his sleep gets disturbed. But, he begins to see a dream that he is already in the hospital as a patient, who is not required to get up early in the morning. He sleeps on. Thus, by dreaming, his sleep has been protected.

In dream, the stimuli from instinctual impulses are lowered to some extent by altering their original stature and are, thus, made to conform with the ego (i.e. made ego-syntonic). In this way, the dream helps to sleep or fulfill the wish to sleep. Again, the dream allows the repressed instinctual impulses (i.e. id demands) to obtain a satisfaction in its compromise manifestation. This is also a fulfillment of wish. For example, a person has a hidden desire for sexual enjoyment with a forbidden object—suppose with his friend's wife. He dreams of having sexual intercourse with a lady whose name is the same as his friend's wife's, though the appearance of the lady in the dream is different from that of his friend's wife's. The lady in the dream stands for the person's desired object and accords him wish-fulfillment.

The dreams of children and a few dreams of adults, such as dreams of food or drink (hunger or thirst), are direct expressions of wishes arising from some organic needs. But, the great majority of dreams are disguised expressions of wishes or desires, repressed but operative and powerful in the unconscious. All dreams are, somehow or the other, wish-fulfillments. Dreaming is an indirect device for the gratification (in its compromise structure) of unfulfilled wishes, which have been repressed into the unconscious owing to the unsuitability of such wishes in waking life or in reality. Various wishes are always working in the human mind and seeking gratification. Some of them are conscious and the ego, which has formed a moral ideal, finds that a gratification of those wishes is incompatible with that ideal; consequently, it attempts to check or control them. Many of these wishes, which are sexual and aggressive in character, do not however come to consciousness at all. If these wishes were known to the ego, they could be condemned as immoral and unworthy of gratification in any form.

When a man is awake, his ego is in a position to exercise control over his ideas, thoughts, wishes and impulses. He can make a distinction between perception and mere idea, between truth and falsity, and can form a more or less coherent view of things and events presented to him in perception. But, when he is asleep, the control of the ego is relaxed and all sorts of combination of ideas make their appearance. The unconscious wishes, which are ordinarily kept in check, seek their gratification through these combinations of ideas presented in dream, which are taken to be real objects and events by the ego which has temporarily, in sleep, lost its critical faculty. Moreover, the original impulses get altered or distorted and become tolerable to the ego in dream; hence, there is a satisfaction of the wishes and, at the same time, sleep is not disturbed.

Dream Mechanism

The mechanism by which the original impulses (or events) are distorted in dreams, due to compromise formula, is known as '*dream-work*'. In sleep, the ego is not totally paralyzed. Its influence is found in the distortion imposed upon the unconscious material to be manifested in dream which would not be too unacceptable to the ego. Hence, at the face of constant resistance from the ego, the original unconscious materials are altered. Therefore, the *manifest content* of a dream should be distinguished from its *latent content*. The dream, as it actually presents itself while being dreamt or as it is remembered and narrated soon after by the dreamer when he arises from his sleep, is the manifest dream content. The unconscious impulses, most of which are of sexual and aggressive nature, constitute the latent dream content. The latent content is the material which we search for in the dream interpretation; it lies behind the manifest content and is the source of dream. Consequently, it may be said that the manifest content is the distorted or disguised version of the latent content.

The unconscious desire, which is always seeking to reach consciousness, is confronted by a repressive force of the ego. This activity of the ego has been personified as the '*censor*'. The rigid control, which the censor exercises over all thoughts and desires, and which determines whether a particular idea or desire is to be admitted into consciousness and, if admitted, in which form that would be done, is described as '*censorship*'. The censor takes an active share in compelling and producing the distortion of unconscious ideas and desires into the manifest content. Thoughts and desires, which cannot evade the censor while a man is awake, appear in consciousness while he falls asleep; but before they do so, they disguise themselves in different ways in order that they may appear to be acceptable to the ego. The disguise of the manifest content is effected so that the dream may escape the vigilance of censor and, so, enter consciousness.

The different processes, through which the different elements of the latent content of dream become disguised in the form of various objects of the manifest content, are known as 'dream mechanism' or 'dream-work.' There are four such mechanisms. They are:

1. Condensation
2. Displacement
3. Dramatization
4. Secondary elaboration.

These mechanisms are carried in cooperation with the censorship of the ego.

'*Condensation*' is that process by which the various elements in the latent dream thoughts are fused together in the manifest content of the dream. For example, a single figure in dream may be built up by a fusion of the different traits belonging to different persons. The hair of the person in a dream may represent a particular person and the dress may represent another, who are associated with the dreamer by way of various impulses and desires. Here, the different persons related to dreamer's reality life get fused in one figure in dream. The process of condensation in dream-work is invested with the activity of symbolization. '*Symbolization*' is a perfect method of condensation, as by it many qualities and features may be fused together in one thing and those may also be kept secret. In a symbol, the latent content of the dream is kept in disguise very easily. A symbol speaks of many things at a time.

'*Displacement*' is that process, by which the psychic importance is transferred to a given element in the manifest content from certain elements in the latent content, which seems to be quite unrelated to the former. Suppose, a woman sees a snake in her dream but does not get afraid of it, whereas in the next-sequence of the same dream she finds a small stick lying on her path and gets terribly horrified.

'*Dramatization*' is the mechanism, by which an idea in latent content is turned into an action. By this process, abstract ideas of the latent content are turned into concrete images in the manifest content of the dream. For example, the idea of the ownership of an object may be translated into an image in the dream that the dreamer is sitting on that object.

'*Secondary elaboration*' is the process of giving a coherent and sensible form to the different elements of the latent dream content. It gives the whole matter a form not unacceptable to the ego. In this task of dream-work, in different ways, the ego applies the mechanism of '*projection*' with the unconscious motive to distort the latent content. For example, one may see in dream that he is hated by a person, which is actually his hatred towards that person.

Thus, on the whole, it is understood that the most important purpose served by the dream-work is to disguise the latent dream content in such a way as to evade the censorship of the ego. The latent dream content always represents ungratified wishes which are mostly of obnoxious nature according to the ego's value scale.

Questions are raised that if dream is fulfillment of wishes as well as protector of sleep, how do the punishment dreams and anxiety dreams fit in that formula. The latent contents of these types of dreams undergo the least distortion. What purpose is served by that? A little reflection shows that the punishment-dreams also serve the purpose of wish-fulfillment, though not of the instinctual impulses, but of the mind's critical, censoring and punishing agency. Moreover, it must be kept in mind that dreams are the product of conflict and they are of compromise-structure. What causes anxiety to the ego may bring satisfaction to id.

Anxiety dreams are extreme cases where dreaming cannot protect sleep. That does not mean that these types of dreams do not fulfill their purpose. Such a dream alerts and, consequently, wakes the ego only when it finds that it alone would not be able to protect ego's wish to sleep. It cannot be said that a nightwatchman, whose business is to guard the sleeping town, fails in his duty if he raises the alarm, finding no other alternative and awakens the people to save them from the machinations of the dacoits. On the other hand, it may be said that the watchman has done his duty faithfully. In anxiety dreams, the manifest dream takes the role of a faithful watchman, as the dream content rouses the dreamer and saves him from further severe anxiety. With the break of sleep, the ego is saved.

Extreme anxiety dreams, such as dreams related to psychical trauma of early life, or dreams of shell shock in the battlefield or such others, take back the dreamer to his original situation of shock, and by repeating that situation in dream the ego tries to bear that shock by reconciling with that situation through repetition.[13,17]

PSYCHOANALYTIC METHOD

We have seen before that the fundamental method of psychoanalysis is free-association. But, free-association method had to be sharpened, by making it associated with other processes, before it could be used as a scientific method for psychoanalytic therapy and investigation.

Psychology (and naturally, psychoanalysis) is a field where the observer and the observed are human personalities. Mainly verbal communication is the way of conveying each other's motivation. But, there are so many impediments in the way that, unless they are overcome, no scientific investigation is possible.

First of all, there is no reason that, in ordinary circumstances, a person would disclose his mind to another person through verbal communication. Secondly, it is impossible for a person to give a full account of his thoughts and imaginations as he himself does not know all of them. Thirdly, because of individual differences, it becomes difficult for the observer to understand the mind of the observed. And lastly, every observer has some blind spots in his own personality, due to which he overlooks those in others. Here comes the contribution of psychoanalysis which, as a scientific method, overcomes all these obstacles.

To the physician comes the sick person; he wants help, to get rid of his maladies. Therefore, he will be more willing, unlike a healthy person, to put aside all his resistances against opening his mind to the analyst. So, in free-association his intimate thoughts will be reflected. Thus, the patient's desire to be cured is an effective guarantee for unreserved self-revelation, i.e. a portion of the patient's ego is ready to work with the therapist for its own cure. This portion of the ego may be called the '*reasonable ego*', as opposed to the '*pathological ego*' which resists the treatment. The 'reasonable ego' makes an alliance with the analyst for analytic work. This is called the '*working alliance*'. Moreover, after a considerable period of working through with the help of 'working alliance', a special type of emotional tie is developed between the patient and the analyst. This relationship is called as '*transference*'. It becomes the main tool in psychoanalytic treatment. Thus, free association, with all these phenomena, makes the psychoanalytic communication a success.

Again, the method of dream interpretation has to be taken in the psychoanalytic treatment method. According to Freud, the dream is the royal road to the unconscious mind.

The obstacles due to individual differences can be surmounted by prolonged study, frequent sittings and, above all, by empathy. Psychoanalysis has been able to understand the preverbal and primitive unconscious mental processes. Thereby, it is possible to understand the mind of another person, how much different it may be in sociocultural aspects from the therapist.

The obstacle of the analyst's own blind spot can be surmounted by a training in psychoanalysis. The analyst himself has to be thoroughly analyzed to cleanse him of all the blind spots of his own mental processes. As psychiatry deals with mental patients, it has to take note of the psychoanalytic methods. Without some training in psychoanalysis, psychiatry cannot venture successfully in the realm of psychical disorders, because psychiatry has to face all the obstacles psychoanalysis faces. Only intellectual knowledge, without the emotional and direct experience of the psychoanalytic situation, is not enough.[18]

Technique

Understanding of the dream phenomenon has led psychoanalysis to evolve its own particular and specialized technique for the treatment of the mental patients. The dream itself is a state of severe mental disorder, a psychosis with all its complicated network. But it is of short duration, and with the awakening, the ego again comes to its normal functioning. In sleep, the ego is detached from reality and suffers a setback under the influence of the internal world, the id and the superego forces; but with the break of sleep, the ego regains its reality connection and is able to overcome the internal pressures. Here is the clue from which we can derive the technique for a cure of the patient (i.e. the suffering ego of the patient).

The ego has to serve its three masters—the reality, the id and the superego, and at the same time, it has to keep in order its own organization and maintain its autonomy. But, when the pressure from its masters is too heavy to bear, its gives in and pathology starts. Then, the connection with the reality is disturbed.

The disorganized ego comes to the analyst for help. The analyst, who represents reality and at the same time an ally from outside, has to help the sick ego in its fight against its internal enemies. The position of the analyst is like the reality-world, which helps the ego in reality testing and in regaining reality sense, after it comes out of illusions and delusions during sleep state with the break of sleep. The analyst and the sick ego work together as a unit, to overcome the pressures of the id and the superego. The function of the analyst is to give back the sick ego its "mastery over the lost province of his mental life".[13] In this joint function, the sick ego must promise 'complete candor' and the analyst must lend his analyzing ego to the patient. This is the basis of the working alliance, which may be called the first step in technique.

Working Alliance

In this, alliance is reflected the patient's realistic and non-neurotic attitude towards the analyst. Due to this, the patient can undergo the strain of treatment and work with the analyst against his (patient's) own transference reactions. This is a form of patient-analyst relationship, quite different from transference relationship. Behind this lies the patient's purposeful desire, the desire to overcome his neurosis. According to Greenson,[5] "the reliable core of the working alliance is formed by the patient's motivation to overcome his illness, his sense of helplessness, his conscious and rational willingness to cooperate, and his ability to follow the instructions and insight of the analyst. The actual alliance is formed essentially between the patient's reasonable ego and the analyst's analyzing ego". In this relationship, the patient, due to identification with the analyst, is able to separate his reasonable ego from his experiencing ego. But, one must be cautious that too much reasonableness in analysis is a sign of *pseudoworking alliance*.

As analysis progresses, it happens usually that the patient fails to pour out his materials passively and obediently, and refuses to accept the realistic attitude pointed out by the analyst. A remarkable thing happens at this stage. The patient is no longer satisfied with the analyst in seeing him only as his adviser and healer. He sees in him something more. A new relationship, apart from the working alliance, develops in which the total psyche, unlike the working alliance, is involved. Freud[13] says in this regard, "on the contrary, the patient sees in him the return, the reincarnation of some important figure out of his childhood or past, and consequently transfers on to him feelings and reactions which undoubtedly applied to this prototype". This is known as '*transference*'.[5,10,13]

Transference

Transference is a form of relationship between the patient and the analyst. It is "a transference of feelings on to the person of the physician".[12] This relationship crops up as a universal phenomenon during the course of the psychoanalytic treatment. This phenomenon distinguishes psychoanalysis from any other form of psychotherapy. Transference is the pivotal point around which the theoretical and technical aspects of psychoanalysis evolve.

Like other psychoanalytic concepts, the concept of transference developed in a progressive way with the maturity of Freud's experience and thinking. He first mentioned it in his 'Psychotherapy of hysteria' in the book 'Studies on Hysteria'.[2] There, he describes it as the result of 'false connection', because old relationships or feelings are transferred by the patient on to the person of the physician through a false connection. "Feelings connected with past wishes (which have been excluded from consciousness) emerge and become experienced in the present as a consequence of the false connection".[19] At the outset, Freud[4] thought it to be an obstacle to the treatment, as this relationship gives rise to resistance. And, it would be impossible to carry on analysis unless this resistance is met. He was "greatly annoyed at this increase in psychological work".[2] But, he soon realized that the whole process of transference followed a law.

Freud[2] narrates his first experience with a patient regarding transference as follows: "in one of my patients, the origin of a particular hysterical symptom lay in wish, which she had many years earlier and had at once relegated to the unconscious, that the man she was talking to at the time might boldly take the initiative and give her a kiss. On one occasion, at the end of a session, a similar wish came up in her about me. She was horrified at it, spent a sleepless night, and at the next session, though she did not refuse to be treated, was quite useless for work."

In the narration of the Dora case,[14] the phenomenon of transference becomes more clear. There he says, "what are transferences? They are new editions or facsimiles of the impulses and fantasies which are aroused and made conscious during the progress of the analysis; but they have this peculiarity, which is characteristic for their species that they replace some earlier person by the person of the physician. To put it another way: a whole series of psychological experiences are revived, not as belonging to the past, but as applying to the person of the physician at the present moment." Gradually, Freud realized that "transference, which seems ordained to be the greatest obstacle to psychoanalysis, becomes its most powerfully, if its presence can be detected each time and explained to the patient.[14]

Greenson[5] defines transference as follows: "transference is the experiencing of feelings, desires, attitudes, fantasies, and defenses towards a person in the present which do not fit that person, but are a repetition of reactions originating in regard to significant persons of early childhood, unconsciously displaced onto figures in the present".

Transference may be of two types: positive, and negative. The feelings and other mental states which are of affectionate or erotic type are called positive; and those which are of hostile or aggressive type are named as negative. Both the types may arise in the patient during the course of analysis.

In psychoanalytic treatment, it is found that the patient's interest is focused on the analyst and the symptoms of the disease are replaced by different reactions towards the analyst that is, the patient diverts the emotional content of his disease towards the analyst. When this situation is achieved, it is called as *transference neurosis*; "it is a new edition of the old disease".[5]

The term 'transference neurosis' is used in another sense also. In hysteria, obsession and phobia, the patient makes his mental energy to flow down to the external world, unlike psychotic patients whose mental energy is withdrawn from the external world. Therefore, in this sense the malady of the former is designated as 'transference neurosis' and that of the latter is called '*narcissistic disorder*'.

Counter-transference

The concept of transference entails the concept of '*counter-transference*.' Like transference, counter-transference is also a manifestation of the doctor-patient relationship, occurring in psychoanalytic treatment situation. But, it differs from the former in that it is viewed from the doctor's total feelings towards his patient, arising as reactions of the patient's influence upon his (doctor's) unconscious. The 'counter' in counter-transference may thus indicate a reaction in the analyst which implies a parallel to the patient's transferences (as in 'counterpart') as well as reaction to them (as in 'counteract').[19] The counter-transference reactions may provoke blind-spots in the analyst and, consequently, in such situations he would overlook or sidetrack the patient's real difficulties. Hence, like transference reactions of the patient, if not properly handled, the counter-transference reactions of the therapist, if not properly controlled, may jeopardize analysis. Therefore, the analyst must always be aware of his own reactions and be on guard, and be able, on the strength of his analytical training and insight, to tackle this phenomenon. Analyst's ability in this regard will yield success in his analytical work. So like transference, this also can be regarded as a useful tool in the hands of the therapist. Moreover, "the observation of counter-transference reactions may also be of diagnostic importance".[19] In psychiatric practice, the physician must be aware of this phenomenon in his own mind, because this may lead him, if not properly understood, to wrong diagnosis and management.

The success of the psychoanalytic treatment depends upon the proper analysis of the patient's transference relationship. It has been pointed out before, that there develops a resistance in patient in looking towards his inner world and, consequently, towards the treatment as well. After the development of transference, the purpose of analysis is to do away with this resistance phenomenon. This is the period of '*working through*'.

Indications and Contraindications

Whether a patient is suitable for psychoanalytic treatment, it is necessary for the analyst, first of all, to ascertain that the patient is suffering from mental conflicts for a long time, the conflicts which arise within the structure of his own personality. Next important factor required for this treatment is the ability to develop transference on the part of the patient. For this reason neuroses, such as hysteria, obsession, neurotic depression, character disturbances, and psychosomatic illnesses, are most suitable fields for psychoanalytic treatment. The analyzability of perversions, impulse neuroses, addictions, delinquencies, and borderline cases, are questionable and should be determined by the special features of the individual cases.[5]

Psychoanalytic treatment is time-consuming, costly and painful (psychically). Therefore, only the patients, who are strongly motivated, will work wholeheartedly with the treatment. The patient's suffering due to symptoms will enable him to undertake the treatment. Moreover, acute and fresh cases always present a better indication for psychoanalysis than chronic and old ones. The absence of favorable indications for psychoanalytic treatment are its points of contraindications. Generally, aged persons are not suitable for psychoanalysis. Feeble-mindedness, severe physical illness and severe disturbances of speech are hindrances to this treatment lack of cooperation, on the part of the patient and his important family members, will never yield good result. Sometimes, many patients' life situations may oppose this treatment.

Narcissistically oriented and psychotic patients generally are not suitable for psychoanalysis, because they lack the capacity to develop transference reactions. Withdrawn type and emotionally uninvolved persons are also not suitable for psychoanalysis.[5]

Either for indications or for contraindications, one should not take these factors rigidly. The ultimate criterion for the suitability of a case for psychoanalytic treatment is its actual response in analytic situation. Therefore, *trial-analysis* for a brief period is the best method for selection for psychoanalysis.

DEVIANTS

Like any other scientific discovery, psychoanalysis did not remain confined under the sole authorship of its discoverer, Sigmund Freud. A constantly growing group of workers gathered around him. Some of them followed him and elaborated his findings, some discovered new vistas, and some also deviated from the fundamentals of its discoverer.

Among the deviants, Alfred Adler (1875–1961) and Carl Gustav Jung (1875–1961) were the main contenders.

Alfred Adler

Adler attacked Freud's libido theory and propounded the '*organ inferiority theory*'. According to this theory, a person tends to compensate in his psychic life his sense of organ inferiority, by the compensatory act he tries to attain superiority. In an extension of this theory, Adler further put forward that a child, because he is small, feels inferior. Thus, a universal feeling of inferiority is generated in human beings. This sense of inferiority gives rise to the tendency of dominating or the desire to become superior. Too much intensity in this tendency may generate neurosis in a person.

According to Adler, masculinity means striving for power. And, as the position of women is inferior in society, femininity is the symbol of inferiority. So, every man and woman strives to attain masculine power. This is technically known as '*masculine protest*'. In neurosis, the disease condition is sometimes used by the patient as a way to gain superiority or to dominate. Thus, one becomes neurotic in one's attempt to achieve the future goal of possessing power. Therefore, not the past experience, but the future imagination, makes one a neurotic. This is a point of departure from Freud, as Freud laid much emphasis on the past.

Adler disagreed with Freud also in respect of the importance of sex in neurosis. According to him, ego's craving for power is at the root of mental disorder. The neurotic lacks a proper balance between his individualistic urges and the social drives. His style of life is not in harmony with the community living, as he aims to attain superiority by avoiding the difficulties of the reality. Adler's school of thought is known as '*Individual Psychology*', because it emphasized the importance of individual differences in personality, which are rooted in the differences in the environment of early childhood.

Adler advocated short-term treatment and his technique was to attack the patient's difficulties. He gave more emphasis to the parent-child relationship in his treatment procedure. To him, dream was not merely the fulfillment of earlier wishes; it revealed patient's attitude towards his present problems. It was considered also as rehearsal of his future ambitions.

Adler's theory and practice are considered by the psychoanalysts as being hasty and superficial. It is not depth psychology. The treatment procedure is based on common sense truth of our daily life. But, in some cases it yields good results, especially in the case of children. Adler's conception of '*style of life*' is a valuable contribution to the psychology of personality.[3,6,20]

Carl Gustav Jung

Jung, along with Freud, was a collaborator in founding the International Psychoanalytical Society in 1911 and was its first president. But at the end of the first two years, he deviated considerably from Freud and displayed himself as an analytical psychologist instead of a psychoanalyst.

Jung was vastly experienced in dealing with psychotics, and he was also well versed in philosophy, myths, symbolism, literature and culture of different countries. All these made a great impact upon his contributions to psychoanalysis.

As we have seen, Freud laid great emphasis on the predisposing cause of neurosis, which he traced in the Oedipus complex of the small child. Jung, on the other hand, noted the '*exciting cause*' to be the source of neurosis. In spite of maladjusted early life, some adults carry on well if no problem of adult life blocks their way. When any problem or 'exciting cause' in adult life demands some extra psychic energy than an individual can muster, he is likely to fall a victim of mental breakdown. That is, when an individual fails to solve any problem of his present life, he regresses to his earlier mechanism in handling the situation.

Jung's main point of departure from Freud was his interpretation of the libido. He did not accept Freud's sexual theory of neurosis. Libido to Jung was much broader than merely having sexual character. In his scheme, libido stands for total psychical energy; it includes both Freud's libido and Adler's 'will for power'. Jung's libido finds its manifestation in growth, reproduction and all other kinds of activities. To a child, libido is a source of pleasure, not for its sexual character, but for its having an outlet in nutrition and growth. Child's interest in mother lies in the fact that she is the food-providing or the nourishing being. Therefore, the child's attachment to his mother, before the Oedipus complex period, is rooted in the urge to live, for self-preservation, and not in sex.

Thus, it is seen that sexual libido is only a part of Jung's scheme of the libido. He laid emphasis on the improper parent-child interaction in the genesis of neurosis. And consequently, the importance of mother came to fore in his theory of psychoanalysis. In his scheme, sex does not play any important role in human personality before puberty. Thus, there is lack of stress on biological aspects of the human being.

Though Freud saw Jung's ideas as betrayal to the fundamental concepts of psychoanalysis, which he built up by postulating the importance of sex or libido in framing the human personality, yet later his findings on "narcissism led him to combine libido and the other life instincts under the name of *Eros*, which is essentially the same as Jung's libido,......"[20] But, to overcome his theoretical difficulties, he postulated death instinct as the opposite tendency of Eros. This pair of opposites—Eros and Thanatos—makes what life and creation are.

Jung also framed pairs of opposites, of which the pair of *introversion* and *extroversion* is best known. The introvert has an inward and the extrovert an outward thrust, in the subjective and the objective worlds, respectively. Individuals differ according to the predominance of introversion and extroversion in them. In every individual, there are also male and female sides, side by side (*anima* and *animus*). In a well-rounded personality, all these aspects must be developed in a balanced form. The task of therapy is to make this development possible.

Jung envisaged another polarity too: The polarity of conscious and unconscious. According to him, there are two layers of the unconscious, the deeper among them is the *collective* or *racial unconscious*. It is the storehouse of our inheritance, coming down from our primitive ancestors. It is the storehouse of instincts or drives (id) gathered through countless generations. In collective unconscious reside the *archetypes*, which are the modes of primitive ways of thinking. The drives refer to the ways of acting and the archetypes signify the ways of thinking. The latter crop up in dreams, fantasies, delusions, and in myths and fairy tales. More superficially, between collective unconscious and conscious, lies the *personal unconscious* which is equivalent to Freud's preconscious and unconscious.

The analyst's participation, through his own free-association in connection with the patient's dreams, is a specialty of Jung's technique. He took analysis as a mutual process, in which both the patient and the analyst are to participate. He used dreams as indicators of disturbed mind, as well as of the unconscious way of looking to the future. He encouraged his patients to be immersed in their own cultural milieu in respect of mythology and to give free expression to them in free-association.[3,6,20]

POST-FREUDIANS

Actually, the expansion of psychoanalysis started during and after the First World War, when the cases of 'shell-shock' neurosis posed a great problem to the psychiatrists. Freud's concepts were applied in those cases and good results were obtained. With the advance of time the cleavage between Freud and the deviants lost its sharp edge. Rigid adherence to Freud was also abandoned even by his close associates, as through experience they could gain more knowledge about the human psyche and could explore new vistas of psychoanalysis. They differed from Freud in some respects, though their foundation was in Freudian thought. Second World War accelerated the progress of psychoanalysis more rapidly, because it made opportunities for psychoanalysis to be applied in new situations in the background of war.[21] In England, Anna Freud (1895–1982) and Melanie Klein (1882–1960) worked intensively with children, and in America, Erich Fromm (1900–1979), Karen Horney (1885–1952), Harry Stack Sullivan (1892–1949) and Erik Erikson (1902–1997) contributed in different ways to psychoanalysis.

Anna Freud

She introduced a new trend in psychoanalysis, by laying greater emphasis on the function of the ego or the conscious mind. Her book, 'The Ego and the Mechanism of Defense,'[16] brought a new era in psychoanalysis in respect of ego analysis, instead of id analysis. The analysis of the ego, thus, paved the way to the understanding of its defensive mechanism through which the pattern of transformation of the instincts was also realized. This new technique, and the resultant knowledge, enabled psychoanalysis to understand the structure of the personality. Anna Freud came to her conclusion through her work with children. But, on experiment, it was found that those were equally applicable to the adults.[21,22]

On the whole, though Anna Freud accepted orthodox Freudian theory, yet she attached more importance to the ego and its defenses. She attached equal importance to the environment of the child, especially to the parents' attitude towards the child, but never underestimated the significance of the unconscious and instinctual factors. According to her, superego starts to come into being during the fourth year of the child, and among the human drives, the sexual ones are of high importance.

Anna Freud was of the opinion that as young as a child of 3 years could be brought under analytical treatment. But, for younger children, free-association could not be applied. Hence, the child must be allowed to walk, talk, tell stories and play games, and all these activities must be utilized in treatment work. One has to be very cautious in interpretation in child analysis, because the child-ego is undeveloped. Moreover, transference in child cannot reach its required height. Intensive cooperation has to be sought from the parents during the treatment period.[16,21]

Melanie Klein

Her main contribution to psychoanalysis centers around child analysis and the origin of superego. Freud[10] hinted at the harshness of the child superego; Klein established this fact by her data obtained from child analysis. She threw more light on the function of death instinct. Karl Abraham (1877–1925), a brilliant co-worker of Freud, was engaged in dealing with psychotic patients. By using Freud's latest discovery on aggression (death instinct) in clinical work, he was able to uncover in more detail the earliest developmental stages of a child. But, unfortunately he lived a very short span of life.

Abraham's unfinished work was carried to an appreciable height by his able pupil, Klein. She applied Abraham's ideas in the analysis of children and, thereby she developed play-therapy, replacing the free-association method, as children could hardly give free-association. Instead of only talking, she encouraged the children under her treatment to play freely with toys provided to them.

Klein's new technique brought in the field of psychoanalysis a variety of new harvests. The child's unintegrated ego reacts to his mother's breast, which is the object (to the child) in the external world, sometimes gratifying and sometimes frustrating. To the child, mother becomes sometimes good and protective, and sometimes bad and persecutory. In this way, in the child's mind, the ideas of '*good object*' and '*bad object*' are introduced. And, since the child introjects and incorporates these ideas, by which his fantasies are also oriented, they are manifested in future in the form of a severe superego, more severe and ruthless than the real mother. The persecutory anxiety, which in turn if intense, may disintegrate the child's ego and usher in a depressive episode. Klein names this early stage as '*paranoid-schizoid position*'. Here, she gave more emphasis to the aggressive drives than any other.

Going through proper child rearing experiences, the child comes to realize gradually that good and bad are the two aspects of the same object, mother. Thus, comes his sense of reality.

Klein's work made it possible to realize that the Oedipus complex and the superego begin to take shape much earlier in the child than Freud thought of. Thus, child analysis, what was inaccessible to psychoanalysis, was made accessible by the work of Klein. She started analysis with a child as little as two years of age. She could trace the existence of sexual and aggressive fantasies, including Oedipal wishes, in the child from his first year of life. In therapeutic practice, she usually did not seek the cooperation of the parents, as that might distort the treatment situation.[21,23]

Karen Horney

Horney is one of the main exponents of that psychoanalytical school which is of the opinion that social factors play an important role in the genesis of neurosis. She challenged the biological foundation of psychoanalysis propounded by the orthodox Freudians. As a result, she proceeded to carry out analysis by leaving aside the instinct and sexual development theories. Horney took Freud as an antifeminist and started a crusade against him. She was influenced by Marxism during her practice as analyst in Berlin and that must have contributed to her social factor theory. According to her, the basis of sexual difference between man and woman lies not in biological factors, but in social factors. Her notion of personality is based on the idea that an individual functions in a social frame-work and interacts with the environment. Hence, neurosis is a product of the culture.

Horney's main theoretical contention was her concept of the self. She propounded the ideas of the '*actual self*', the '*real self*' and the '*idealized self*'. The self that experiences, is the 'actual self'; and the self that works as the guiding principle for healthy integration of human personality, is the 'real self'. The 'idealized self' is the glorified image, which encompasses all the aspects of personality and rises to an attitude of self-sufficiency. In the unconscious stratum, it is the source of '*neurotic claims*'. So, the goal of Horney's therapy is '*self-realization*'.[6,21]

Erich Fromm

Fromm was born in Germany and was influenced by Freud on the psychological side and by Marx on the sociological side, at the same time. His primary interest had always been in the problems of relationship between the individual and the society. He rather gave a Marxian bias to the Freudian psychology. When he shifted to the USA, his convictions were stimulated by his close associations with Horney and Sullivan. Fromm challenged Freud's biological orientation of instinct theory and developed his own theory of personality based on human learning and cultural training.

Fromm disagrees with Freud mainly on two points:

1. The basis of the neurotic problem is not the frustration in instinctual life, but it is a product of the failure in the specific type of relatedness of the individual with the society and the world, and
2. The relationship between man and society is constantly in a flux; it is not static.

According to him, man is born with fewer predetermined courses of behavior than animals. Therefore, man's nature, his emotions and his anxieties are the products of culture. Consequently, man is his own creation.

Fromm does not believe in main's innate traits. So to him, man is innately neither social nor antisocial. There is in man no innate *eros* or *thanatos*. It is the privilege of man that he possesses the most flexible nervous system, with which he can adapt enormously. This cultural orientation of human personality is the outstanding contribution of Fromm to psychoanalysis.[6,21]

Harry Stack Sullivan

He was an American psychiatrist, whose theories are the product of his clinical experiences. According to him, all human behaviors depend upon two factors:

1. Satisfaction of drives, and
2. Sense of security.

Drives come from man's innate biological needs and are met accordingly, e.g. food, sleep, sex, etc. The sense of security comes from cultural influence. Man's action, language, thoughts, and imaginations contribute to his sense of security, and all these are shaped by his culture. Man, as a child, is taught to do and think what his culture teaches under the threat of withdrawal of approval or punishment. Therefore, when there is a conflict between his satisfaction of drives and culture, he develops a feeling of badness and there is consequent insecurity and discomfort. Thus, man is the product of his culture. Any attempt to undo the influence of culture produces anxiety. Only a modification in the influence upon and reaction of the individual within the general framework of the culture can be brought. There lies the function of the therapist, who can induce self-esteem and self-confidence in the patient and, thus, avert the sense of insecurity. Sullivan views the therapeutic situation as a situation of interpersonal relationship. The position of the therapist in his scheme is that of a participant observer in the framework of interpersonal relationship. But, the therapist must take a detached role. The cure of the patient lies in the gradual realization (i.e. development of insight) by the patient of what is going on between himself and others, i.e. society.

Sullivan developed a theory of personality development according to his own ideas. In this development, he gave emphasis to interpersonal relationship. According to him, human personality develops through different stages of life, starting from infancy and traversing through childhood, juvenile era, preadolescence, adolescence, and ending and culminating in adulthood. To him, sex is an important factor for personality development in adolescence only. Sullivan developed his theory of personality purely on his clinical experience, with more emphasis on the cultural aspect than on the biological side of human life.

A few words may be noted here. One should not think that Horney, Fromm and Sullivan noticed first the impact of culture on human personality, and they and their followers are the only culturally-oriented psychoanalysts. If we notice the progressive development of Freud's thought, we find that the germ of the concept of cultural influence upon man made itself visible occasionally throughout his writings at different times, though in the first phase of his discovery it was not accorded such importance. With the publication of his 'Totem and Taboo',[24] his interest in cultural concept was manifested clearly; the ideas were further advanced in 'The Future of An Illusion',[25] 'Civilization and Its Discontents',[26] and in some other writings. Therefore, the origin of the cultural concept is also found in Freud's writings. The cultural group of psychoanalysts in America has only taken the thread from him and has been working with dexterity in this regard. It must be appreciated that their work has advanced psychoanalysis to a wider horizon.[6,21]

Erik Erikson

Erikson, in developing his theory of personality, concentrated on Freud's infantile sexuality; but in doing so, he gave emphasis to child's development beyond puberty. According to him, ego is the main tool of personality, by which it organizes everything. He showed eight stages of the ego, which roughly coincide with Freud's psychosexual stages. These stages are accompanied by psychological crises typical to them. They are depicted in Table 1:[27]

According to Erikson, the five physical modes of functioning of the erotogenic zones of the body, if malfunction, may cause abnormality in the personality development. These modes of functioning are: (1) passive incorporation, (2) active incorporation, (3) retention, (4) elimination, and (5) intrusion. In the course of development of a child, if proper trust cannot be invested in the mind of the child, it may cause

Table 1: Erikson's developmental stages

Developmental stages		*Accompanied by psychological crises*
1.	Oral-sensory (Infancy)	Basic trust versus mistrust
2.	Muscular-anal (Early childhood)	Autonomy versus shame, doubt
3.	Locomotor-genital (Play age)	Initiative versus guilt
4.	Latency (School age)	Identity versus inferiority
5.	Puberty and adolescence	Industry versus role confusion
6.	Young adulthood	Intimacy versus isolation
7.	Adulthood	Generative versus stagnation
8.	Maturity	Integrity versus despair

severe abnormality. From trust develops an identity (e.g. with parents, teachers, etc.) which is essential for mental health. A crisis in identity leads to the development of symptoms. Therefore, the trust of the patient upon the healer is the main foundation of Erikson's psychoanalysis.

ASSESSMENT

One of the functions of psychoanalysis is to treat mental disorders. Treatment of mental diseases is undoubtedly a noble work. Moreover, psychoanalysis stretches its helping hand to psychiatry in understanding mental diseases. There was a time when psychiatry was groping in dark, as it could not establish any cause-effect relationship among the phenomena of mental diseases and aspects of life. Symptoms of mental diseases appeared meaningless. In that respect, psychiatry was in no way in a better position than 'ghost-theory'. Psychoanalysis lifted psychiatry from its helplessness. With the advent of psychoanalysis, with its determinism in the field of mental disorders, everything there—the minutest experiences, behavior, imagination, thought, fantasy and action, i.e. all symptoms were given proper meaning and 'appropriate' place in the cause-effect chain. Thus, psychoanalysis showed psychiatry the light to follow, and by following which it could enter the dark, and till then unknown, region of the human mind. Thus, there was a revolution in psychiatry in understanding of the mental diseases scientifically.

The functions of psychoanalysis as a therapeutic method and as a helping agency to psychiatry are no mean contributions. But, the importance of psychoanalysis does not lie in these facts. There are so many methods of treating mental disorders which can cure many-a-case of psychic abnormality. Again, there are so many auxiliary arts and sciences which have become unavoidable to psychiatry. All these bring no distinction to psychoanalysis.

The real importance and significance of psychoanalysis rests with the fact that it did not remain confined within the sphere of abnormal mind or mental disorder, i.e. as a healing art. It stretched its investigations into the functioning of the normal human mind, developing itself as an independent science of human mind.

The progressive march of human civilization, from its primitive stage to the up-to-date form, is the handiwork of human mind. Psychoanalysis, under the genius of Freud, pervades all the stages and spheres of the man's long march along the road of civilization—primitive, ancient, medieval and modern, and socioeconomic, cultural, group and individual. Psychoanalysis explores the inner sources of all sorts of creative works—mythology, religion, law, ethics, classical literature, folklore, war and peace, social developments, arts, and sciences. In the field of education, it has influenced pedagogy enormously. It is known to all that after the First World War, Freud was invited by the League of Nations to contribute to the common pool of thoughts for international understanding and peace, on the behalf of psychoanalysis. Above all, psychoanalysis has shown in a new way the uniformity of human mind all over the world. Man's joy and sorrow, his love and hate, his fear and courage are similar everywhere; whether he is in icy Greenland or in tropical forests of Africa, or in primitive society of Andaman or in a modern city of Europe, matters little. Here lies the unity of man, in spite of all his apparent diversities. This is an exploration upon which man will have to work for centuries to come. In this way, psychoanalysis will be employed in the task for future human cultural development.

Some argue that the conclusions of psychoanalysis are not valid for all men as those were evolved by Freud on the basis of his findings in a typical atmosphere and society of Vienna. But, the results yielded from the subsequent application of psychoanalysis to a wider field have repudiated the above criticism. Moreover, the conclusions of psychoanalysis were obtained by deep dissection of human mind. When by dissection of the human body, an inner anatomy or mechanism of physiology was discovered, the question whether that dissected body was of a rich aristocrat or of a beggar, or that was of a farmer or of an intellectual, was never pertinent. Fundamentally, the physiological mechanism is same for every man under the law of uniformity of nature. Only the outer manifestations may differ. Similarly, in the realm of mental dissection, the questions of race, nation, religion, caste, creed and status are futile.

The validity of psychoanalysis as a therapeutic measure has been challenged by many. Among them, Eysenck[28] is the most vociferous. He rejects the efficacy of psychoanalysis altogether, on the basis of his research data. According to him, the percentage of cure among the patients without the use of psychoanalysis is very high; whereas those in whom psychoanalysis was used are found to be cured in a significantly lower percentage. But, the fallacy in his research process was pointed out by Rosenzweig;[29] Eysenck's conclusion was based on a wrong method of data selection. It is very difficult to assess the result of psychoanalysis properly, because there are no valid and dependable methods for the assessment of basic psychodynamic variables. Unlike Eysenck, Schijeilderup[30] has shown marked efficacy of psychoanalysis on personality of the patients under treatment.

All these facts show only that many more studies are needed in this regard. Furthermore, the question of validity is a relative one. In every science, say for example physics, a valid theory of today may be required to be changed tomorrow to accommodate new facts. That does not invalidate the science and it is no discredit to it. On the other hand, it proves its openness, which is an essential mark of a scientific method. It has never been said that psychoanalysis has been able to explain satisfactorily all the phenomena of human life. It is enough for a science that it attempts at explaining the immense number of facts with a minimum number of assumptions and, at the same time, raises new and appropriate questions, invites further application and explanation, and in this way it always remains open.

Thus, the achievement of psychoanalysis lies in its being a science (or a scientific method) which has yielded a bounteous harvest of knowledge in the realm of mind, and knowledge is power.[31-35] With this power of knowledge, it has brought within its purview every human being.

Besides psychoanalysis, due to its inherent nature, has not kept itself confined in the task of exploring human mental affairs only. It has developed a point of view for looking at human activities; it has built up a world-view, rather a philosophy of outlook. In that way it moulds human thought. Psychoanalysis is one of those four scientific thoughts—the other three being Darwin's theory of evolution, Marx's theory of dialectical materialism and Einstein's theory of relativity—of modern world, which have influenced the human thinking at its bottom; more truly, have revolutionized it.

A few words about the scope of psychoanalysis in India will not be irrelevant here. Psychoanalysis urges us to look inward. Only by knowing ourselves we can strengthen our ego, we can resolve our conflicts between the 'inner' and 'outer'. Psychoanalysis teaches us to sit in solitude and dive deep within and face our inner self. That is the golden way along which we can reach a harmonious state of mind. Similarly, India has to her credit the heritage and tradition of Yoga which asks us to sit in quietness and meditate. For thousands of years, Indian tradition has been 'looking within'. Therefore, Indian mind is the fertile field where psychoanalysis can reap the reward of the psychoanalysts' hard and sincere effort. Though the birth of psychoanalysis is in the West, yet it received the stiffest opposition from there because of the West's predominating external orientation, failing to realize the significance of 'looking inward.' Indian scene is just the reverse.

Let us conclude with the words of Radhakrishnan:[31] "the system of Yoga asks us to resort to quietness and meditation.... Even worship is a means to gain solitude...." "Freud's great contribution to mental therapy is in his view that much of the unhappiness in the world is traceable to unconscious conflict which can be overcome by realizing and resolving the conflict. When the personality is divided or distracted, there can be no effective work or happiness. There is the need for the single eye within, the closest correspondence between the secret thoughts and the overt desires. We cannot find out easily our secret impulses or deep desires. We cannot find ourselves, unless we use our leisure and solitude in contemplation. However, difficult it may be, it is still the appointed way."

47.2 PSYCHOTHERAPY

DN Nandi, AN Basu

Since antiquity, man has sought to develop methods or means which would take care of his problems. In that context, the treatment of priest, local healer or other primitive physician does not depend upon specific physiological effects but nonetheless leads to improvement. The process may be designated magico-religious and primitive but perhaps belongs to the general category of faith healing. How a condition is treated in any society depends upon the relevant concepts of causality. Primitive cultures recognize simple injuries and can identify some fractures; most have a concept of immobilization and even the setting of bones. On the other hand, primitive cultures vary widely in the degree to which they accept naturally occurring diseases. This applies in particular to psychiatric disorders, which Simmons explains primarily as due to prevalence of witchcraft.

TOWARDS DEFINING PSYCHOTHERAPY

It is difficult to arrive at an acceptable definition of psychotherapy. Dorlands' Illustrated Medical Dictionary defines it as "the treatment of emotional and mental problems". Somewhat more circumspect, Webster's and Noyes and Kolbdescribe psychotherapy as "the treatment of emotional and mental problems by psychological means". This definition, while more satisfying in some ways, tends to exclude the treatment of psychosomatic illnesses such as ulcerative colitis, peptic ulcer, asthma and so on. Perhaps the most acceptable definition is the one given by Wolberg, which is as follows:

"Psychotherapy is the treatment, by psychological means, of problems, of an emotional nature, in which a trained person deliberately establishes professional relationship with the patient, with the object of (1) removing, modifying or retarding existing symptoms, (2) mediating disturbed patterns of behavior, and (3) promoting positive personality growth and development".

The final use of psychotherapy has introduced a new dimension into the field of psychotherapy; a dimension that deals, on the one hand, with the problems of immaturity of so-called normal persons and, on the other, with characterologic difficulties associated with inhibited growth previously considered inaccessible to treatment.

HISTORICAL PERSPECTIVES

One attribute not emphasized in most definitions, but nonetheless crucial, is that the therapist's method has specific effects on the patients. The importance of nonspecific factors in treatment outcome was already recognized by Hippocrates and these were differentiated from specific treatment factors. Franz Mesmer was highly successful in treating a broad range of disorders, though he believed that his cures were the consequence of a specific therapeutic agent, which he called 'animal magnetism'. Two hundred years later, we know only too well that the empirical distinction between nonspecific faith-healing effects (which in psychopharmacology are conveniently subsumed under the concept of the placebo effect) and specific therapeutic effects is difficult to draw.

The importance of psychological factors and their effect on disease was recognized by Patanjali. Reassurance, support, and even counseling and meditation were seen as an ancillary part of medical treatment by physicians through ages. The study of hypnotic phenomena in the early nineteenth century came close to providing a specific method of treatment, and the increased recognition of functional disorders helped identify the maladies to which it could most appropriately be applied. It remained for Sigmund Freud to develop the rationale necessary to make psychological treatment a specific therapy. The influence of Freud's ideas was probably even greater outside the field of Medicine than within it; we are probably too close to fully appreciate their stature. It can be said that if Marx created 'Economic Man', Freud created 'Psychological Man'.

CHOICES OF TECHNIQUES

No psychotherapeutic method exists today that is applicable to all patients or germane to the operations of all therapists. The techniques by which transformations come about accord with the skill of the therapist who applies them and with the facility of the patient to accept and utilize preferred interventions. Since psychotherapy is a learning process, the techniques, to which a patient is exposed, will work best if they coordinate with his unique method of learning. Some persons learn best through cognitive operations, finding out the reasons that underlie their problems and acquiring an understanding of their self-defeating behavior and its origins. Such persons are attracted to insight-oriented methods of psychotherapy. Others learn by following suggestions of authoritative persons whom they respect. Some learn through action and doing, i.e. achieving positive reinforcements in their environment for adaptive behaviors; some learn through experiencing a corrective emotional experience with their therapist or with another human being who is used as a substitute therapist; others learn through example (modeling), which provides them with models of thinking and behavior. Some learn best when subjected to psychological shock, attack, or confrontation that challenges their habitual defences. These and additional kinds of learning usually act in combination within each individual. What is challenging for a therapist is discerning the form of learning that each patient can best utilize and then working to adopt techniques that are best suited for the particular patient's learning propensities. An important issue is to identify a way of detecting a patient's optimal modes of learning.

VARIETIES OF PSYCHOTHERAPY

The various psychotherapies may conveniently be divided into three main groups: supportive therapy, re-educative therapy and re-constructive therapy. Radical divergencies in technique of these therapies are more apparent than real, many distinctions vanishing as soon as romantic differences are resolved. To describe the countless permutations of therapy that exist today would be an impossible task, since all practitioners evolve a unique format influenced by their background and character structure. Besides, they become more diverse every year as an increasing number of professionals enter the psychotherapeutic field introducing their own unique technical modifications.

Supportive Psychotherapy

This is the most commonly practiced form of psychotherapy and is the generic name for a variety of procedures, whose characteristics depend a greater deal, as in all psychotherapy, upon the therapist's personal style. This attempt to offer a standardized description must be somewhat idealized. Supportive psychotherapy is required where basic ego structure is sound, having broken down under the impact of extraordinary severe strains that sap the vitality of the individual. An attempt is made to bring the patient to an emotional equilibrium as rapidly as possible, with amelioration of symptoms, so that the patient can function again at his normal level. There is no intent to change the personality. In many cases, this is all that is needed. Supportive measures, thus, may be utilized as the principal treatment or may be combined with other forms of psychotherapy or even pharmacotherapy.

Guidance

Guidance includes a number of procedures that provide active help in the form of fact-finding and interpretation, such as child guidance, employment/vocational guidance, educational guidance, health and social welfare. Many counseling and casework methods relate to this kind of care.

Guidance may be the only type of treatment to which some patients will respond. Desperately helpless in the grip of life situation, such individuals have neither the motivation nor the strength to work with a technique that requires self-direction. On the other hand, acceptance of advice may be tantamount to giving up their independent style of functioning. Hence, a judicious assessment has to be made regarding the feasibility of guidance in a particular patient.

Tension Control

More subdued than anxiety, of which it is undoubtedly a component, tension activates many disturbing physiological behavioral tendencies. Tolerance of the effects of tension varies from individual to individual. Since tension is so discomforting, it is little wonder that escape from it constitutes a chief preoccupation of human beings, who will eagerly utilize any device to get rid of it. It is often one of the earliest signs of emotional disturbance.

Massage has been used traditionally in India to provide relief from tension. Muscular relaxation exercises have been used for many years; the best known modern exercises are those of Jacobson, Rippan and Fletcher, Yates, and Neufeld. Meditation has a long history, especially with Hinduism, Buddhism (particularly Zen cult) and Raja Yoga. More recently, transcendental meditation has attracted a large group of people. Experimental studies have shown that these methods do alleviate tension, while lowering oxygen consumption, metabolic rate and cardiac output.

Biofeedback training is a recent entry into the arena of self-regulated tension control.

Some practitioners, utilizing tension control as a primary treatment method, employ a combination of techniques, for example, progressive relaxation, skin galvanometry, hypnosis and meditation.

Milieu Therapy (Environmental Adjustment Sociotherapy)

In milieu therapy, an attempt is made to identify and eliminate provocative environmental irritants, whether at the place of vocation, or at home, or elsewhere, to the extent possible. Therapeutic nursery schools, residential treatment centers, halfway houses, day-care centers, rehabilitation centers, nursing homes, and other institutions have attempted to apply principles of milieu therapy.

Very often, patients are so bound to an existing life situation, either because of a sense of loyalty or because of a feeling that they have no right to express their demands, that environmental distortions are tolerated as unalterable, about which they may be unaware. The therapist may have to interfere actively with environmental aspects before the patient shows a maximal response to therapy.

Externalization of interest: It may become necessary to encourage patients with anxiety, depression or excessive somatic concern, to resume activities that were once meaningful to them or help them to develop new diversion for leisure time.

Occupational Therapy

Occupational therapy (OT) is more than merely recreational and diversionary, and may be the sole means of entering into the inner world of the withdrawn and regressed patient. The occupational therapist has already become an important member of the psychiatric team.

The objectives of OT also include improvement in work, socialization and activities of daily living. Accordingly, prevocational guidance, work adjustment, self-care and other services are offered to the patients in various set-ups.

Creative Arts Therapies

The usefulness of art therapy, music therapy, drama therapy, dance movement therapy and other creative arts therapies is being increasingly recognized and utilized with individuals, their families and other groups in outpatient clinics, apart from their use in the mental hospital settings.

Other Methods

Other methods include reassurance, prestige suggestion, pressure and coercion, persuasion, confession and ventilation, which have stood the test of time. They seem to provide certain people with a mental crutch, especially when a psychological analysis is either difficult or impossible. Then perhaps, substitution of pursuance of philosophic precepts for destructive habit patterns is lesser of the two evils.

Re-educative Psychotherapy

In re-educative therapy, the aim is achievement of a more extensive process than is achieved in supportive therapy. It is, in fact, attempted to remodel the patient's attitude and behavior in line with more adaptive life integration. There is less emphasis on searching for causes than on promoting new and better forms of behaviors. It is the presumption that individuals, with help from a therapist, have within themselves the ability to reorganize their values and behavior patterns. Therefore, this therapy comes to be included under re-educative therapy. Other measures, which will be discussed here, include therapeutic counseling, directive psychotherapy, relationship therapy, attitude therapy, distributive analysis and synthesis, interview psychotherapy, somatic therapy and certain philosophical approaches.

Client-centered Therapy (Nondirective Psychotherapy)

Carl Rogers, and his approach, has been popular with the psychologists, although in recent years the impact of psychoanalytic concepts and behavior therapy has made a dent into his hold. Nevertheless, his concepts are still employed and many aspects are utilized in group work, play therapy, and religious, marital and industrial counseling.

Essentially, the therapy is based on the idea that a human being is possessed of innate goodness and actualizing tendencies, leading to a 'balanced', realistic behavior. The guiding principle of client centered therapy is oriented around the fact that the client (or patient) is the one responsible for his own destiny and he possesses the right of choice of the solution for his problems, irrespective of the choice of the therapist. Residual in each individual are resources for growth that need merely to be released to enable the person to achieve maturity.

The therapy consists of attentive listening to the client's communications for content and feeling, which are accepted in a tolerant, non-judgmental way, and are to act as a catalyst of growth, avoiding any attempt to impose any directions on the client.

Directive Approaches

Here, the therapist assumes an active role, identifying which of the basic problems of the patient is to be taken care of, the immediate and the long-term objectives, and sorting out an action-plan. The goals are, in fact, in the hands of the therapist, who makes an effort to dissect, tear down, rebuild and resynthesize the personality. The various methods include:

Rational emotive psychotherapy

Albert Ellis gave this name to cognitive therapy procedures that combine formulations from semantic, persuasive and directive therapies. Treatment tactics are organized around the hypothesis that aberrant emotions are controlled by the faulty thinking processes, such as illogical "self-talk and internalized sentences". Generally, a search will reveal the origin of illogical ideas in the attitudes of parents, teachers and peers, usually supported by the culture. The therapist brings this to the notice of the patient, revealing the irrational links, and teaches the patient how to rethink and reverbalize these in a "more logical, self-helping way".

Confrontation

Thorne employed a number of techniques under the title 'directive psychotherapy'. This method entailed confrontation of the patient with factual information in an effort to get the patient re-evaluate his own attitudes.

Programmed psychotherapy

Young suggested that the patient be given a series of significant problems and appropimate solutions to illuminate and revise existing assumptions.

Direct decision therapy

The patient is asked to state as clearly as possible the nature of his problems and the goals he wishes to achieve. The patient and therapist jointly re-examine past decisions that created the problems and the options now available. Once the patient has made a decision to change, the various methods available are then discussed.

Reality therapy

It is another directive method, organized around the central theme of 'identity as a core problem'. The patient is guided away from methods by which he avoids reality and is motivated towards success.

Casework Therapy

Social workers have traditionally employed guidance or counseling techniques based on interviewing, home visits or visits to the client's place of vocation, with the aim to help individuals find a solution to problems of social adjustment. This include three steps, namely, the case study, the plan and the working out of the plan with the client. The casework method has been enriched by knowledge from psychoanalysis, psychology, sociology and other behavioral sciences. Interpersonal and social problems are resolved, both to help the clients meet unfulfilled need and to adapt more adequately in their relationship with people and society.

Relationship Therapy and Attitude Therapy

The focus of the treatment is organized around the patient-therapist relationship. The relationship is the vehicle that both promotes change and serves as a target for an enquiry into the basic interpersonal patterns. In 'relationship therapy' (*attitude therapy*), the therapist provides a corrective emotional experience for the patient by absorbing the patient's neurotic behavior and not responding to it with expected anger or indignation.

Psychobiologic Therapy (Distributive Analysis and Synthesis, or Distributive Analysis)

Adolf Meyer, founder of the psychobiologic school, emphasized that in studying human behavior, it was necessary to take into account everything significant in the life history of the patient, including heredity, body build, temperament, developmental history, illness, traumatic experiences, and the interaction of the individual with parents, siblings and other important persons. Once a blueprint is obtained of the formative and presently operating influences in the patient's neurosis, the therapist strives to help the patient make constructive use of what has been discovered. Incidently, history taking in any psychiatric patient is based on this approach.

Crisis Intervention

A crisis may precipitate around any incident that overwhelms one's coping capacities. The stimulus itself bears little relationship to the intensity of the victim's reaction. Every individual is a potential candidate for a breakdown in the adaptive equilibrium, if the stress is sufficiently severe. The two important variables are, the 'meaning' of the calamity for the individual, and 'flexibility' of one's defenses, i.e. the prevailing ego strength.

The immediate response to a cataclysmic situation, such as the sudden death of a loved one, a violent accident, or an irretrievable shattering of security, is a dazed shock reaction. Almost immediate response is denial, accompanied by numbness and detachment. At the core of this cycle of denial and twisted repetitive remembering is, the mind's attempt to protect itself by repressing what had happened and to heal itself by reprocessing and working through the traumatic experience in order to reconcile it with the present reality situation.

These patients are receptive to minimal help with appreciable improvement. The goal is rapid emotional relief and not basic personality modification. Normally, six sessions therapy is sufficient, unless warranted more by the patient. The techniques include reassurance, confrontation with active interpretation of resistances, narcoanalysis, environmental manipulation, hypnotic probing, guidance and psychotropic medication and, if required, brief hospitalization. These are sort of turning points, for better or for worse. At times, however, maladaptive behavior is more apparent and may lead to suicide. Yet, where the patient possesses a motivation for change, crisis therapy may register a significant change and the patient may attain a level of functioning that is superior to that before the onset of crisis.

Biofeedback

Biofeedback is particularly acceptable to those who are fearful of the labels of psychotherapy and psychiatric illness. It has been shown that an individual may become aware of changes in bodily functions, of which one is ignorant by using electronic instruments. Changes in skin temperature, blood pressure, muscle tension and brain wave patterns can be known or displayed, and the subject gradually learns how to reproduce such feelings and states to secure desired physiological effects.

Biofeedback is being employed in migraine, hypertension, phobias, low backache, cerebral palsy, upper motor neurone hemiplegia, irritable bowel syndrome and several other neuropsychiatric conditions. A powerful placebo effect accompanies biofeedback instrumentation, but this does not entirely account for the benefits.

In the technique of biofeedback, a meditative state of deep relaxation is conducive to the establishment of voluntary control by allowing the individual to become aware of subliminal imagery, fantasies and sensations. A blood pressure apparatus and electrocardiographic machines are employed to control blood pressure and heart rate. There is some evidence that penile tumescence, the operation of sphincters, respiratory activities, optic and stomach functions may be mediated through special instruments in this way, helping impotence, fecal incontinence, excess gastric acidity, asthma and myopia. Work in these areas is still incomplete.

Philosophical and Religious Approaches

The basic aim of psychotherapy is to effectuate a change in value systems through an altered perception of one's inner self. Philosophical and religious approaches accomplish the same purpose through a different means with an effort to bring about peace of mind. Since psychological needs are diverse, no single religious or philosophical credo appeals to all persons. Thus, ungratified mothering will open the door to acceptance of a system that promises protection, love and pleasure from some goddess or 'God-mother' or 'Earth mother', if not immediately, then in the hereafter. It is interesting that in organizing values, modern humankind still exploits philosophical systems that parallel those developed hundreds or even thousands of years ago; for example, *Mahabharata*, *Ramayana*, *Koran* and *Bible*, apart from other writings, such as *Vedas* and *Brahmanas*, which continue to guide and be quoted.

Mysticism

The mystical striving is twofold; first, there is an attempt to achieve communion with the Absolute (the Highest, the One, God, *Brahma*, the Order of the Heaven, Being of beings) and second, a desire to grasp through introspection, the ultimate nature of reality. The Absolute, whatever the religion, establishes stability, methodical arrangement, and permanence in the universe. Since, it is impossible to approach it through the senses, the establishment of the Absolute is attempted by epistemological arguments, by mandates in sacred writings (presumably divinely inspired and enforced through religious discipline), and by mystical experiences.

A search for the Absolute has preoccupied philosophers and theologians throughout the ages. Its most prominent forms have been found in the Eastern systems, for example, the *Hindu* and *Buddhist* religions, which promote a different nature of reality and goal of absorption in mystical essences towards ecstatic enlightenment (*'moksha', 'nirvana'*), In all mystical systems, direct personal experience is approached through states of absorption, in which the individual becomes aware of oneness with the Absolute.

Historically, *Hinduism* preceded *Buddhism*. Essentially, it conceived of an absolute spirit, the *Brahma*, as the source and goal of all things. *Brahma*, *Vishnu* and *Shiva* respectively represent creation, preservation and destruction. There is a generally accepted doctrine of 'Karma', which makes humans accountable in the present life or in their reincarnation, because of transmigration of souls, for their good and bad actions.

Modern Hindu systems of philosophy are employed to help the distressed. Vahia conceives of three basic sources of conflict or disturbed peace of mind: too intense emotional attachment to external things, such as possessions, status and power, which inevitably produces destructive competitiveness; a delusion that humans with their finite mind can understand cosmic reality, which is actually beyond human comprehension; and in harmonious interaction with other people, presence of (a) excessive attachments, (b) too powerful emotions, yearnings, including love, (c) inordinate jealousy, or (d) unreasonable anger.

While these conflicts are universal, the special way in which they operate is unique for each individual. Three main categories of people exist, and the approach will differ in each. Firstly, there are those who operate on the basis of intellectual understanding; then there are second, who are swayed primarily by sentiments and emotion; while the third are insistent on a practical solution, without analyzing the problem or bothering about feelings.

Yoga

Yoga, a form of Hindu mysticism, had its origins in an idealistic monism, the *Vedanta* philosophy. The *Yoga* system advocates identification of the soul (*Atman*) with its final aim being union with the supreme being (*Pramatma*). This is brought about by the following eight steps:

1. Self-control (*Yama*), obtained by such devices as chastity, nonstealing, nonviolence, truthfulness, and avoidance of greed.
2. Religious observance (*Niyama*), through chanting of the Vedic hymns, austerity, purity and contentment.
3. Assumption of certain positions (*Asana*).
4. Regulation of the breath (*Pranayama*), with controlled rhythmic exhalation, inhalation, and temporary suspension of breathing.
5. Restraint of the senses (*Pratyahara*).
6. Steadying of the mind (*Dharana*), through fixation on some part of the body, such as the nose or navel.
7. Meditation (*Dhyana*), on the true object of knowledge, the supreme spirit, to the exclusion of other things in life.
8. Profound contemplation (*Samadhi*), with such complete absorption and detachment that there is insensitivity to heat and cold, pain and pleasure.

The Yogin, who arrives at the perfection of the last three stages (*Samyana*), achieves an ecstatic mystical state that stimulates the ability to have an awareness of the past and the future, and of what happened in the previous births. Proper application of the *Samyana* promises a complete release of the intellect from the self, purity and eternal liberation in the form of separation of matter from spirit (*Raja Yoga*). The ultimate goal is fusion with the absolute, during which the person experiences the higher wisdom and the most profound truth of being.

Buddhism

A young prince, *Gautama Sidhartha*, at the age of 29, during the sixth century BC, struck with the suffering of humankind, deserted his family to search for the true meaning of life. After years of wandering, one day under a fig tree (known later as the 'Bo Tree' or the 'tree of enlightenment'), he suddenly achieved a glimpse of truth. Among the teachings of *Buddha*, as he later came to be known, were the three basic concepts:

- The soul of a person, after death, goes on to reside in higher or lower animals, depending upon his deeds. *Nirvana*, a peaceful state of oblivion, is acquired, when the soul no longer has its individuality.
- Release from conscious existence is hastened by pursuing the eightfold path of righteousness of faith, intention, conduct, livelihood, effort, thinking and meditation.
- There is no supreme God.

Subsequently, the teachings of *Buddha* underwent revision. *Buddha*, himself, came to be considered as God.

Zen Buddhism

Among the *Buddhist* sects, *Zen Buddhism* is the most difficult to explain and has attracted many psychotherapists. *Satori* (enlightenment and awakening) experience is predicated on a suspension of the reasoning faculties. *Zen* is dedicated to the idea that one may solve all problems through intuition and enlightenment, rather than through logical abstraction. Essentially, it is an achievement of the extraordinary '*Satori experience*' ('oneness with *Buddha*'), which is devoid of emotion and intellectual content, through study with a Zen Master. The various methods employed are: meditation on a '*koan*', a riddle for which there is not set solution; solving paradoxes, such as 'what is the sound of one hand clapping'; random activities, such as flower arrangements, practising archery.

The solution to any of the problems is not through customary modes of problem-solving; somehow the student must work out a reply that will satisfy the Zen Master.

In the process of doing this, the student will have developed a unique mode of conceptualizing reality that dissociates him from habitual points of reference.

Cultist Movements

A growing number of movements have developed, that appeal usually to young people seeking to dissociate themselves from the cultural values and norms. The cults appeal to school dropouts, borderline cases or just unhappy people. The heads of such organizations are usually charismatic, intelligent and well read people.

- *Hare Krishna Movement*: In 1965, AC *Bhaktivedanta Phapupada* went to the United States to bring to the needy the benefit of his transcendental teachings, including *Bhakti Yoga*, which endorses restriction on diet, sex, intoxication, gambling and aggression. The *Hare Krishna* movement sponsors community-living, devoted to the worship of *Lord Krishna*, one of the incarnations of God *Vishnu*, 'to help man in distress'. The movement has received widespread publicity, especially in western countries.
- *Transcendental Meditation* (TM): Transcendental meditation (TM) has been publicized in the western countries since the 1960s, by *Maharishi Mahesh Yogi*, and has found favor with many young people of a generation which vigorously questioned the values of western societies. It was claimed that after regular periods of meditation for even a few months, the individual becomes more resilient to the stresses of life, works with increased efficiency and is less likely to be dependent on alcohol, drugs or tobacco. Later research purported to show that TM improves reaction time and intelligence, and helps in recovery from hypertension, asthma and a variety of other conditions. TM is accompanied by a number of physiological changes, like fall in oxygen consumption, metabolic rate, cardiac output, blood lactate, respiratory rate and pulse rate. However, these physiological changes may not be specific to TM, as they have been reported in other low arousal states.

  Maharishi Mahesh Yogi was able to establish an International University of Creative Intelligence in Meru in Switzerland (MICI) in the 1970s, and has recently announced in newspaper, a new unified field theory to explain the forces of nature and to bring perfection to every area of national life.
- *Brahma Kumaris Movement*: Brahma Kumaris World Spiritual University, founded in 1937 with headquarters at Mt. Abu (Rajasthan, India), was declared to be dedicated to spiritual, moral and intellectual upliftment of humanity. It is now affiliated to the Department of Public Information of the United Nations, as a non-government organization and is proclaimed to be independent of traditional politics and religions. Their main therapy is through *Raja Yoga*. The University, through 1750 *Raja Yoga Centres*, located over 35 countries of the world, offers courses which are stated to combine both knowledge and practice in areas of spiritual study, *Raja Yoga*, transformation of character, development of social harmony and humanitarian service.
- *Bhagwan Rajneesh*: The oldest of the eleven children of a Jain cloth merchant, Rajneesh Chandra Mohan was born in 1931. He experimented with meditation and at the age of 21, while studying philosophy at Jabalpur (India), he claimed he had achieved enlightenment.

  During his landmark years, he plunged deep into every religion and into the fountainheads of human thought, chewing at length both the western philosophers, from Plato to Marx, and the oriental school, from Zen to Tao to Hinduism. In an era of atheism and of existentialistic art and literature, Rajneesh, changing his name first to Zorba and then to Osho, came selling a hedonistic philosophy of 'here and now', a philosophy of pleasure, a philosophy of 'letting go'. He believed in the inspiring effects of divine influence testified by the fact that a human being has the potentiality for extraordinary response to the proper authoritative mandates. Faith cures are 'irrefutable'. Under favorable circumstances, the ravages of physical and psychological illness may be palliated. Some may even be permanently resolved.

Existentialism

Existentialism as a philosophy has attracted many a people in Europe and United States. It is more or less oriented around the writings of Soren Kierkegaard (1813–1855). Drawing from Kierkegaard's original conceptions, psychiatrists such as Karl Jaspers, Ludwig Binswanger, Viktor Frankl and Medard Boss adapted existentialist ideas within a framework of psychotherapy:

- The basis of existence is a sum of nothingness that vitalizes the self with meaningfulness.
- The self reaches its highest stature in its struggle with anxiety, guilt, and the ubiquitous threat of death.
- The self reaches its fullest development in the experience of love, which is indeed the keystone of existence.
- With the shattering of love, the self suffers from damage and returns to nothingness.
- 'Existential neurosis' is the inability to see meaning in life.
- 'Being in the world' and 'I am' convey self-acceptance, tolerance of limitations, ability to scale down ambitions, acknowledgement of prevailing creativity, self-realization, and self-determination shorn of neurotic cultural values and demands.

Logotherapy is a special existential approach, elaborated by Viktor Frankl, which includes two distinctive re-educative procedures: paradoxical intention and dereflection.

Existential approach proposes to fulfill the innate spiritual drive in man by exploring the 'meaning of human existence'. The 'will to meaning' is one of the deepest motivating forces of humanity. When human beings no longer question the meaning of their existence, they become ill, as this creates an 'existential vacuum'.

Western religious approaches

Religious healing, recorded in successes of Jesus, is legendary, "and great multitudes came unto him, having with them those that were lame, blind, dumb, maimed, and many others, and cast them down at Jesus' feet, and he healed them".

Reconstructive Psychotherapy

Reconstructive psychotherapy assumes that the past inimical experiences have retarded the normal psychosocial growth process and are now promoting in the individual immature strivings and emotions that come into conflict with reality on the one hands, and on the other with the person's own incorporated system of ideals and standards.

Reconstructive psychotherapy is distinguished from supportive and re-educative therapy by the degree and quality of insight mobilized. In supportive therapy, efforts at insight are minimal, while in re-educative therapy, they are more extensive but are at a conscious level. In Reconstructive therapy, the objective is to bring the individual to an awareness of crucial unconscious conflicts and their derivatives. The various methods used have drawn inspiration from psychoanalytic theories.

Classical Psychoanalysis

Sigmund Freud's formulations are more or less accepted as the basis for present day classical psychoanalysis. (For details see Chapter 58). The technique of free association, lying on couch, and passivity on the part of analyst are purely designed to encourage passive dependence and regression. It is generally accepted that psychoanalysis is useful only in persons who have reached a relatively mature state of personality development.

Because Freudian psychoanalysis is a transference analysis, all means of increasing the transference are employed. These include assumption by the therapist of an extremely passive role; analysis of dream material; maintenance of an intense contact with the patient during no less than four or five visits a week; and the 'basic rule' of verbalizing whatever comes to mind, however, fleeting, repulsive or seemingly inconsequential (this is known as 'free association'). Besides enhancing the evolution of transference, this helps in overcoming resistance and in dismantling psychological defense mechanisms. The therapist fights off all temptations towards 'small talk' or to react. The therapist interferes only when resistance to free association develops. Dream analysis is used constantly as an additional method of penetrating the unconsciousness. Unresolved infantile conflicts slowly emerge in the transference process and are managed by timely interpretations.

Since Oedipus complex is considered to be the nucleus of every neurosis, its analysis and resolution in transference constitutes a primary focus. If the Oedipus complex is not revealed, or its pathologic manifestations are not thoroughly analyzed and worked through, or forgotten memories of early childhood experiences are not restored, treatment is considered incomplete.

The therapist must also constantly guard against manifestations of the destructive counter-transference which, disguised and varied, are mobilized by the unresolved problems and pressing needs within the therapist. Common forms of counter-transference are subtle radiatic attacks on the patients, impulse to be pompous and omnipotent, or reject the patient. Because of counter-transference, a personal analysis (analysis of the therapist) is considered essential.

Kleinian Psychoanalysis

Melanie Klein developed a biological theory that has gained a great deal of prominence among English psychoanalysts and has a large following in South America, Spain and Switzerland. Kleinian principles are believed to be basic to a dynamic conception of child psychology. These can be summarized as follows:

- The Oedipus complex emerges during the first year of the life.
- The superego is organized soon after birth.
- In the initial contracts with reality, the child fuses emotional feelings in relation to objects (mother, breast, nipple, etc.) with the objects themselves. Thus, objects that inspire pleasure are 'good objects' and those that provoke pain are 'bad objects'.
- The infant does not have the knowledge "that loss, frustration, pain and discomfort are usually temporary and will be followed by relief".
- Any change in the tension-alleviating state, such as a less easy grasp of the nipple or diminution in the flow of milk, will suffice to change the pleasant stimulus into an unpleasant one. The child will then love and hate the breast and mother simultaneously on all or none basis.
- The infant conceives of coitus as an act of biting, with oral incorporation of the penis by the mother.
- Penis and vagina are regarded as dangerous; the penis equated with breast and vagina with a biting mouth.
- 'Envy' operates from the time of birth and is distinct from jealousy. Jealousy is based on love, it aims at possession, while envy is a two-person relationship. Greed aims at the possession of all the goodness that can be extracted from the object.
- The assault on the breast around the sixth month (when passive sucking is replaced by biting) enables the infant to react to anxiety with attack. This oral sadism is vital to personality development. At the time, a persecutory, 'paranoid-schizoid position' prevails. Later, the 'whole

object', consisting of 'good' or 'bad' breast or mother between 6 months and one year is introjected, leading to guilt, fear of loss and feelings of depression (the so called 'depressive position').

Neurotic defenses are evaluated around paranoid, schizoid or depressive personalities, described as *projective identification.*

Ego Analysis

Fairbrain, one of the earliest to emphasize the importance of the ego, developed object-relation theory. The main features of this theory are:

- Behavior is determined by forces other than instincts in the form of response sequences encompassed under 'ego'.
- The ego, as an entity, has an autonomy separate from both instinct and reality.
- A greater emphasis must be put on the effect of environment on health.
- Personality is more plastic and modifiable, even beyond the period of childhood, than is traditionally believed.

Neo-Freudian and Non-Freudian (Post-Freudian Psychoanalysis)

As a technique, classical (Freudian) psychoanalysis is applicable to a class of patients who are able to devote themselves to and tolerate the rigors of a long-term intensive exploratory process. Patients are thus afforded an opportunity to experience, to understand and to resolve in a dynamic, protected atmosphere conflicts of which they were previously unware. Deviation from this approach varies from minor divergences to major disagreements, especially with regard to cultural factors. This deviation from the classical psychoanalysis is exemplified by the following schools of psychotherapy.

Individual psychology (Alfred Adler)

Although Alfred Adler was one of the first to contribute to ego psychology, he is rarely given credit for this work. Also his work in child guidance, group therapy, family therapy, community psychiatry, and social therapy has not received the attention it deserved.

Around 1910, Adler broke with Freud over the importance of infantile sexuality and libido theory. According to him, social factors were important in the causation of mental disorders. He believed that each individual was unique and had an individual psychology. The basic helplessness of the human infant, magnified by the existing body or organ defect, creates a feeling of inferiority ('Organ inferiority') leading to 'will to power'. The constellation of impulses, attitudes and strivings, marshalled to overcome inferiority and to achieve power, are shaped into an elaborate 'lifestyle'. The outcome of this may be (a) successful compensation with good adjustment, or (b) over compensation with various kinds of faulty adjustments, or (c) 'fictive goals', such as retreat into illness as a means to power.

Adler rejected the concept of 'penis envy' and regarded women's 'masculine protest' as an objection to their subordinate economic and social roles.

Analytical psychology (Carl Jung)

Carl Jung acknowledged the existence of bodily libido and said that it issues from universal forces or 'life urge'. While observing that the symbolic productions of the neurotics and the psychotics bear a resemblance to those of primitive people, Jung speculated on the existence of 'collective unconscious', a hereditary portion of mind that contained the imprints of ancestral experience.

A study by Jung of associations, dreams, fantasies, etc. seemed to suggest the presence of the thought processes called 'archetypes'. He divided the psyche into a superficial part, the 'persona', which represented a social mask; a less superficial aspect, the 'ego', which was only to some extent conscious; and a deeply unconscious part, the 'collective unconscious', which contained archetypes. There had to be a balance between the conscious and the unconscious aspects, such as the balance between the masculine 'animus' element and the feminine 'anima' element.

Jung evolved a theory of personality character and divided people into two types: introverts and extroverts. He stated that analysis consisted of four stages, namely catharsis, explanation, education and transformation. He is also credited with the clinical application of the 'word association test'.

Therapeutic modifications of Sandor Ferenczi

Sandor Ferenczi, while remaining loyal to Freudian theories, introduced certain modifications of his own, e.g. he advised setting a time limit to analysis a means of accelerating the end of treatment.

Will therapy (Otto Rank)

Otto Rank laid emphasis on Freud's original idea that the process of birth, with separation of the child from mother, constitutes a trauma from which the child never recovers. 'Birth trauma' is of crucial importance in his therapy.

Some of the present day transactional approaches draw their tactics from Rank, while the client-centered therapy appears to be related to his philosophy of 'self-realization'. Also, the school of Casework appears to be oriented towards his concepts of 'helping process'.

Active psychoanalysis (Wilhelm Stekel)

Wilhelm Stekel related himself perceptively and rapidly to the immediate problems of his patients, applying himself forcefully to bring them to an awareness of their conflicts. His chief contribution was in elucidating the technique of 'dream interpretations' in particular, especially their symbolic significance. He stressed on what we now call as 'counter-transference'. He was also particularly interested in the sexual disorders.

Character analysis and organ therapy (Wilhelm Reich)
Wilhelm Reich was a psychoanalyst, who said that neurosis was due to a conflict between the repressed instinctual and the ego-repressing forces. He described the analysis of resistance, including character resistance, and insisted that this was necessary before the patient could accept and integrate the content of the unconscious.

Later, his new ideas made a reformation of his hypothesis necessary. Character or 'bio-energy' therapy resulted in liberation of emotions produced by the mobilization of 'organ therapy'. In 'organ therapy', the muscles of the patient's back, chest, jaw, abdomen and extremities are pressed firmly to elicit emotional reactions, and to liberate associations and memories. This therapy, later called by Reich as 'vegetotherapy', is now being practiced under the name of '*bio-energetics*'.

Dynamic-cultural school of psychoanalysis
The works of Wilhelm Reich, Eric Fromm and Anna Freud have made significant contributions to ego psychology. The sociologically oriented therapists term this as the 'dynamic-cultural' school. The distinctive features of this school are as follows:

There is a shift from biological to sociological events, from concern with the past to the patient's present day contacts, and from preoccupation with the fixation of libido to concentration on growth and maturation.

The 'school' accents character structure above all the other aspects of personality. Distorted character drives make for defects in the interpersonal relationships and oppose normal biological and social needs.

Eric Fromm believes that social forces encourage irrational mechanisms in a person's relationships with the group and promote the isolation of the person from others.

A primary need is for closeness with, and approval from, a significant individual.

Gestalt therapy ('Humanistic', 'Third force')
Drawing from the gestalt theory and employing concepts from psychoanalysis, a transactional form of therapy was evolved that proposed to bring fragmented elements of personality into a unified whole. According to this theory, ideally an object ('figure') and its field ('ground') should blend into a harmonious assemblage ('gestalt'). The therapy requires a search for repressed material, the mechanisms through which repression is maintained, as well as the specific needs for repression. To organize a mature figure-ground gestalt, it is essential that the individual restore to his total being, the dissociated aspect. Guidance in bringing these to awareness is indispensable.

One technique is to animate and hold conversations with parts of one's body. Sometimes, the 'empty chair' technique is used, the patient being urged to imagine a parental figure or any important figure settling in a nearly empty chair and then to talk to upbraid or question the visionary occupant, followed by changing the seats and acting the part of the person ('role reversal').

Transactional analysis
Eric Berne, a psychoanalyst, suggested that there are three different 'ego states' in all persons: the first, the child within the person; the second, the external parental agency (parent); and the third, the grown-up, mature, reasonable adult-self. Each of these aspects of the person perceives reality differently. The three states are constantly operating in response to the needs of the person and the kind of pastimes and games that he is indulging at the time.

During therapy, the three ego states, displayed in the relationship with the therapist, are interpreted to the patient. The function of the child and the parent within the patient, and the origin of these states in the life history are ventilated. Ultimately, the adult becomes stronger and displaces the child and parent.

Neo-Freudians
Harry Stack Sullivan, Karen Horney and Eric Fromm together formed, what came to be known as the Neo-Freudian School of Analysts. Although differing in details, they are united in the following conceptual beliefs.

The social and cultural, rather than biological, factors are basic to the understanding of human nature.

The instinct and libido theories are outdated. The Oedipus complex, the formation of superego and the alleged inferiority of women are cultural and non-universal traits, and although there may be a biological foundation for oral and anal stages, these can be greatly modified by cultural factors.

Emphasis is placed on 'interpersonal relationships' in the formation of character and in the production of anxiety and neurosis.

It is asserted that instead of character arising from sexual development, the sexual development is an index of character. In this view, it is not the sexual behavior that determines character but the character that determines sexual behavior.

Karen Horney

There are two traits that Horney believes are present in all neurotics.

- *Rigidity in reaction*: The neurotic brings to all human relationships, a tendency to act in a predetermined way, unlike a normal who is flexible.

- *Discrepancy between potentialities and accomplishments*: A neurosis, as defined by Horney, is "a psychic disturbance brought about by fears and defenses against these fears, and by attempts to find compromise solutions for conflicting tendencies".

Whereas Freud saw the Oedipus complex as the foundation of all neurosis, Horney explains neurosis in terms of 'basic anxiety', which is described as a feeling of being small, insignificant, helpless, endangered in a world that is out to cheat, attack, humiliate, betray and envy. Such feelings arise in childhood, especially in those who have never experienced 'the blissful certainty of being wanted'.

For such reasons, the potentially neurotic child has to repress his hostility and grows up feeling that the world is a frightening and dangerous place. In order to escape anxiety, the tends to develop neurotic personality traits, such as striving for affection.

Later, Horney came to the conclusion that all the traits concealed only three basic attitudes, namely, moving towards people, moving against people, and moving away from people. If it were possible to hold on to any one attitude, the individual might be able to get through life reasonably safely. The conflict among these three tendencies constitutes the core of any neurosis and is therefore described as the 'basic conflict'.

Eric Fromm

Fromm describes certain 'psychic mechanisms', analogous to the 'neurotic character traits' of Karen Horney, by which man tries to relate himself to the society. These can be summarized as follows:

- Assimilative process
  - Moral masochism; the need to be dependent and to rely on others in a weak and helpless manner, often disguised as 'love', 'devotion' or 'loyalty'.
  - Sadism; wish to make others dependent upon oneself and to make them suffer.
  - Destructiveness; attempts to eliminate any possible threat or basis of comparison.
  - Automaton conformity; attempts to wipe out, by conformity, the differences which exist between oneself and others.
  - Love; genuine love is a repression of productiveness and implies care, respect, responsibility and knowledge.
- Socialization processes
  - The receptive character; all things he wishes must come from an outside source, and this is passively accepted.
  - The exploitative character; he tries to satisfy his desires by force or cunning and is aggressive.
  - The hoarding character; he is mainly concerned with hoarding and saving, and is ordinarily punctual.
  - The marketing character; he exists to adopt one selfor' selling oneself' to others.
  - The productive character; a normal person who is capable of genuine love attachment to others.

Harry Stack Sullivan

In Sullivan's system, the individual is seen as seeking freedom from anxiety, achievement of security, and release from tension under all circumstances. The experience may be selectively ignored, dissociated, or its meaning willfully misunderstood. Interpersonal relations do not relate merely to what goes on between two or more real people. There may be 'fantastic personifications' or 'ideal figures', with whom the individual 'interacts', and by a process called as 'parataxic distortion', one may attribute to others traits taken from significant people in one's past. Therapy will attempt to remove such distortions.

According to Sullivan, at any time, a large area of mind remains unattended. Freudian unconsciousness is seen as 'selective inattention', Sullivan's picture of mind is rather like the state of affairs seen by the driver of a car on a dark night; characterized by the focus (Freudian conscious), the surrounding area (selective inattention corresponding to Freudian preconscious) and the total darkness behind the car (dissociation or Freudian unconscious).

Miscellaneous therapies

Innovative therapies came about largely as a revolt against the semantics and rigidness of the traditional therapies. It is beyond the scope of this chapter to describe all these therapies. Besides, new techniques are evolving every year. Currently, more than 250 kinds of psychotherapy are in use.

Emotive Release Therapy (Body Therapies)

Breuer and Freud, in the late 1800s, developed the cathartic method, which served as a precursor of psychoanalysis. The chief task was to induce the patient to give utterance to the traumatic event 'with an expression of affect'. These ideas still form a part of the philosophy behind abreactive, emotionally oriented, release therapies, such as scream therapy, narcotherapy, primal therapy and the like.

a. *Scream therapy*: Scream therapies have been developed to liberate the fundamental 'survival-based' feeling frozen within the individual by society. In a group setting, the emphasis is placed on screaming to express feelings, rather than to talk about them.

   There are basic screams of fear, pain, need, anger and pleasure. Confrontations, encounter methods, and marathons are utilized to loosen feelings.
b. *EST*: Founded in 1971, as 'Erhard Seminars Training (EST)', it is essentially organized around a two-week-end, experience designed to transform the participants' ability to 'clear up' disabling life situations. Honesty of revelation is stressed and much of the effectiveness is based on surprise or shock.

c. *Primal therapy*: When basic needs of a child are unmet, the pain caused is diverted by shutting off the need. Substitute gratifications ensure, usually symbolically, and become the mode of functioning of the 'unreal self'. Primal therapy constitutes a systematic assault on the unreal self 'which eventually produces a new quality of being, normality'. There can be no resolution until the 'primal pains' are re-experienced consciously.

Guided Imagery

Sigmund Freud earlier employed a technique which required the patients to imagine while he pressed their foreheads. He later abandoned this technique in favor of free association and interpretations of dreams.

Some therapists find that imagery plays important role in treatment of a number of disorders.

a. *Psychoimagination therapy*: This is an existentially based therapy, organized around how patients view themselves from the inside and how they believe other people view them.
b. *Psychosynthesis*: While relaxed on a couch, the patient is asked to visualize and relive the unpleasant situations, and to let the emotions come out as freely as possible.

Ericksonian Psychotherapy (Strategic Therapy)

Acting differently with each patient as counselor, analyst, referee, arbiter, mentor or accepting authority, MH Erickson (perhaps the most outstanding hypnotist in the United States) emphasizes the uniqueness of each individual who requires an original mode of approach. He considers himself and his words, intonations, manner of speaking and body movements as methods which could promote change.

Hypnosis

Hypnosis or hypnotherapy has gained an increasing acceptance among the medical professionals of late, and has been employed both as a therapeutic adjunct and as a research tool for the investigation of many complex aspects of human behavior.

Suggestion, which influences the individual profoundly in a positive way, is the rationale behind its use. Hypnosis is a particular state of mind, which is known to exist but is at present incompletely defined. Hypnosis is usually descried in terms of characteristics which are associated with it. It has been shown that hypnotic and post-hypnotic suggestions may produce the following effects:

- An increase in psychomotor speed and endurance, as well as a decrease in physical fatigue.
- An increase in the span and duration of attention.
- An increase in the speed of learning.
- An increase in the speed of association, mental alertness, concentration and general mental efficiency.
- An improvement in the application of abstract abilities in relation to actual usefulness.
- An improvement in the speed of ready comprehension.
- A heightened sense of enjoyment in performance.
- Obviously, there are new areas in which hypnosis can be extremely helpful. Hypnotic suggestions facilitate many a behavioral techniques, such as systematic desensitization, role-playing, behavior reversal, time projection, emotive imagery, anxiety relief, Ellis' rational emotive therapy, among others.

Group Psychotherapy

Definition and Related Considerations

Group psychotherapy encompasses a variety of forms and goals, which include relief from psychological symptoms, modification of social for family relationships, and a permanent change in attitudes or other aspects of the relatively stable organization of an individual's mental activity and behavior which comprise personality.

A group of individuals, who are appropriately called patients within the setting of a psychiatric service, meet regularly with one or more trained professionals to interact by verbal interchange and other communicative behavior. Groups for psychopathic individuals should be in the context of a specialist institution or service (e.g. therapeutic community). Other groups may comprise of couples with marital difficulty (marital therapy), or the relatives of patients, or several members of one family (family therapy). Additional varieties include '*marathon groups*' lasting for 6–48 hours, and peer self-help groups, such as Alcoholics Anonymous (AA) and Depressives Anonymous.

Therapeutic ingredients

As in individual psychotherapy, there are three main types of psychotherapy: supportive, re-educative and reconstructive. Some issues, such as the importance of the relationship between patient and therapist receive less attention, while others, such as the provision of new interpersonal situations from which the patients may learn, receive an extra dimension in the group setting. The methods include advice, explanation, instruction, suggestion and display of emotions, with the focus usually on the present and future, rather than on the past. In contrast, the approach derived from the psychoanalytic theory is directed towards an awareness and understanding of unconscious mental activity and uses the techniques of free association, overcoming resistance, dismantling defense mechanisms, and analysis of dreams, transference and counter-transference.

Group psychotherapy can also provide therapeutic events which are specific to this form of treatment. An atmosphere of trust, openness, concern, tolerance and support, with controlled negative feedback, has been termed as 'group cohesiveness' and may be therapeutic in itself.

Organizing group psychotherapy

- After a patient has been selected, he should be examined individually by the conductor.
- Patients should not meet socially outside the hospital.
- Any significant change in life situation must be reported to the group.
- It may be made clear that repeated disruptive behavior may lead to exclusion from the group.
- Severely psychotic, paranoid, and excessively narcissistic individuals should not be included in group therapy.

Various forms of groups

Various methods from open groups, with provision to include a new member at any stage, to closed groups exist. Usually a group consist of 10–12 members; less than 30 members constitute a 'small' group, while over 30 members form a 'large' group. The treatment usually lasts from 6 months to 18 months or more, with weekly or biweekly meetings lasting for 90 minutes.

Personality, a degree of self-awareness, knowledge and experience determine the efficacy of a group conductor. The conductor should open each group meeting formally and introduce new group members, if any. During the last 15 minutes of the session, he may decide to prompt previously silent members by asking them for their comments. The groups may include the conductor, other staff members, trainee conductors and the patients. The patients should comprise at least 60% of the group. The groups may be selected with regard to any criterion, such as homogeneity of presenting problems, religious inclinations, and like.

The patient attending a group may also receive individual psychotherapy, if required. On the other hand, a patient being treated by individual psychotherapy may also join a group.

Psychodrama

Moreno introduced a group therapy method in 1925, which is now used as sociodrama, axiodrama, role playing and analytic psychodrama. This has also been incorporated into modern gestalt, encounter and marathon therapy.

The technique, which is often followed, is that the 'star' (the patient) is groomed for the roles to play with representatives of important people in the patient's past and current life ('auxiliary egos'), whose needs for insight preferably fit in with the parts they assume. The director (therapist), who knowing the problems, decides which life situations from the patient's history are to be re-enacted, thus helping "to bring his personal and collective drama to life and to correct it".

In the hands of a skilled therapist, psychodrama is a valuable adjunct in helping patients work through resistances towards translating their insight into action.

CONTRAINDICATIONS FOR PSYCHOTHERAPY

- *Older age:* As a person becomes more and more rigid as he grows, flexibility being essential to modification, it implies that a young person is more likely to benefit from psychological intervention and, therefore, a patient should preferably be 40 years or younger, especially for psychodynamically-oriented psychotherapy.
- *Low intelligence:* Intelligence should be average at least, so that a meaningful relationship can be established.
- *Poor motivation:* Motivation is essential. The patient should be keen on the changes which he may have to imbibe in order to achieve the set goals.
- *Antisocial personality disorder:* Absence of relatedness to others is the single most negative predictor of psychotherapy response. The person with antisocial personality, however, may benefit from certain types of psychotherapy, such as group therapy with other antisocial personalities.

Meloy believed that sadistic cruelty to others, total absence of remorse, and lack of emotional attachment are the key distinguishing factors that lead to inability to engage in therapy.

Are Psychotherapies different for Children and Adolescents?

Psychotherapies can be adapted to the needs of children and adolescents, depending on the mental disorder. For example, the NIMH-funded Treatment of Adolescents with Depression Study (TADS) found that CBT, when combined with antidepressant medication, was the most effective treatment over the short term for teens with major depression. CBT by itself was also an effective treatment, especially over the long term. Studies have found that individual and group-based CBT are effective treatments for child and adolescent anxiety disorders. Other studies have found that IPT is an effective treatment for child and adolescent depression. Psychosocial treatments that involve a child's parents and family also have been shown to be effective, especially for disruptive disorders such as conduct disorder or oppositional defiant disorder. Some effective treatments are designed to reduce the child's problem behaviors and improve parent-child interactions. Focusing on behavioral parent management training, parents are taught the skills they need to encourage and reward positive behaviors in their children. Similar training helps parents manage their child's attention deficit/hyperactivity disorder (ADHD). This approach, which has been shown to be effective, can be combined with approaches directed at children to help them learn problem-solving, anger management and social interaction skills. Family-based therapy may also be used to treat adolescents with eating disorders. One type is called the Maudsley approach, named after the Maudsley Hospital in London, where the approach was developed. This type of outpatient family therapy is used to treat anorexia nervosa in adolescents. It considers the active participation of parents to be essential in the recovery of their teen. The Maudsley approach proceeds through three phases:

Weight restoration: Parents become fully responsible for ensuring that their teen eats. A therapist helps parents better understand their teen's disease. Parents learn how to avoid criticizing their teen, but they also learn to make sure that their teen eats.

Returning control over eating to the teen: Once the teen accepts the control parents have over his or her eating habits, parents may begin giving up that control. Parents are encouraged to help their teen take more control over eating againity.

When the teen has reached and maintained a healthy weight, the therapist helps him or her begin developing a healthy sense of identity and autonomy. Several studies have found the Maudsley approach to be successful in treating teens with anorexia.

ILL THERAPIST: THERAPISTS' REACTIONS TO PERSONAL ILLNESS AND ITS IMPACT ON PSYCHOTHERAPY

Sooner or later, most people get sick. If they are fortunate, the illness is brief and they recover. In other instances, the illness is long-term, recurrent, chronic or even terminal. Psychotherapists are no exception to this and are no less vulnerable to these exigencies than other human beings. Relatively little has been written until recently regarding the counter-transference aspects of the illness in the therapist. Available literature on the topic has noted such defenses as denial, omnipotent fantasies, and reaction formation against dependency and weakness. Illness has been seen as a problem for 'older' therapists, but of course, it may occur at any age.

Personal illness creates conscious and unconscious dilemmas for therapists, and the psychotherapy relationship may be strongly affected by the ways in which these dilemmas are managed. Illness or thinking about illness, can stimulate a variety of potential reactions for a therapist, including a challenge to one's defenses, shame and envy, and realistic worries about one's clinical decisions and over all therapeutic practice. Concerns for the ill therapist fall into two categories:

1. how much (if any) information about the therapist's illness to be given to a patient, and
2. how to work therapeutically with the patient's reactions.

While there are no clear guideline, the authors recommended a flexible common-sense approach, with the central focus always on the patient's reactions to information or changes in the therapy. According to the authors, it is the ethical responsibility of every therapist to be prepared ahead of time for illness or unavoidable absence and to see that his patients are provided for, in the event of such an emergency.

TEAMWORK

The WHO Expert Committee on Mental Health made an important statement in the first report that "the dynamic conception of psychiatry implies a progressive and integrated application of biological, psychological, social and anthropological science to the study of the etiology, pathology, and treatment of psychiatric disorders. The committee wishes to stress this view because it believes that any partial explanation of the facts of mental disorders, for example, in terms of individual psychopathology, neurophysiological concepts, or purely social causation will not lead to the most effective understanding of their causation, (and) will not lead to the most effective understanding of their causation, prevention and treatment".

The practice of such psychiatry demands teamwork. It is clear that the responsibility must be shared by all persons who are capable of assuming even a small part of it, regardless of their professions and occupations. The traditional team consists of psychiatrist, clinical psychologist, psychiatric nurse and psychiatric social worker, but changing conditions of practice since World War II have, however, to some extent altered this conception toward that of a constantly changing team membership.

There are areas where a given profession can contribute its unique skills and information, more than others at any given time. The team is regarded as a group of specialists or consultants, each playing a special role as well as having some sort of therapeutic functions. No small part of the overall difficulty we experience is a function of the fact that almost everything in some way or the other, affects human behavior. The quality and extent of the external and internal forces, with which we must be concerned, are constantly changing and not even their variance is constant.

Individuals may have medical problems, psychological problems, or social problems, but they are not problems in isolation; each one involves the others. In fact, the traditional team is still too limited and there is a scope for expansion. Thus, teachers may be utilized for reading and writing disabilities, speech therapists for stammering, and rehabilitation workers for special losses of functions. This applies not only to psychiatric clinics or mental hospitals, but also in the community, where general practitioners, family physicians, general social workers, priests or religious heads, or rehabilitation officers and others are all capable or taking a more active part in preventive mental health and patient care.

The draws attention to the fact that there are inevitably different shades of teamwork, ranging from the most intimate doctor-nurse partnership or even only therapists' participation, e.g. in psychiatric clinics where the function is primarily psychotherapy with adults, as in such cases the interference of another member in the treatment program may adversely influence the therapeutic relationship, right down to the 'team' composed of everybody who has any official dealing with the patient.

Functioning of the Team

Two important considerations have to be kept in mind; the selection of an appropriate team leader and the selection of individuals who will serve as his team-mates. It is usually essential to have a designated leader. This not only encourages well-balanced and coordinated therapy, but also allows for the full utilization of even personal quality and acquired skill which is available. The background training of the psychiatrist, and his affiliation with the discipline of Medicine, is presumed to put him in the best position for the assumption of responsibility of the total treatment of the patient, particularly in a hospital set-up. But the roles vary, for instance, in developing a proper program for extra-mural care, the role of traditional team may be minimal, and the skills of different nonpsychiatric health workers, teachers, magistrates, employers, religious leaders, and labor leaders may be more important. While the leader is the first member of the team selected, the choice of his team-mates is not less important. In the field of mental health, as in other fields, teams are often composed of highly trained professional persons who have achieved a high level of educational development with an accompanying need for status recognition. Such people often have difficulty in 'working under a chief' but they do find it possible to 'work with a leader'.

Abuse of Teamwork

The entry of professionals of varied disciplines into the mental health field is, nevertheless, not without its dangers, for there are always aggressive and over-enthusiastic participants, who do not recognize or accept their limitations of functions. Insisting that they are not 'helpers' or counselors, but 'psychotherapists', they may plunge recklessly into the psyche of the patient, in this way potentially harming the patient as well as endangering their own professional stature.

A number of nonmedical professionals, like clinical psychologists and social workers working in psychiatric clinics and child guidance centers and having gained considerable supervised psychotherapeutic experience, have sent themselves in private practice as adult and child psychotherapists. Some case workers have even sought to give up their identity with the social work field on the basis that they have established themselves in a new profession. Such persons, say the psychiatrists, constitute a potential public health menace, of which they themselves are completely unaware. There is no room for inter-professional jealousies, or tolerance for an individual who 'stands upon the prerogatives of his profession'. Teamwork, and teamwork upon a vast scale, is not only desirable but is demanded by the complexity and enormity of the problem.

PSYCHOTHERAPY AND MEDICATION

It is possible to widen the scope of psychoanalysis without destroying it. The approach uses both medication and psychoanalysis, or psychoanalytic psychotherapy, started as a combined approach at the Hackensack Medical Centre. A revolutionary idea just three decades ago, the concept of using medication along with psychotherapy in treating patients has even today not gained wide acceptance. But many psychiatrists, especially those trained in recent years, stress biological treatment and eschew psychoanalysis altogether, convinced that it is ineffective. It appears that biological treatment alone, or with psychotherapy, has come to stay.

47.3 PSYCHOLOGICAL THERAPIES

JN Vyas, SS Nathawat

INTRODUCTION

Psychotherapies are 'tanking' cures, symptom relief is provided via the medium of a personal relationship, within the context of professional service or contract. Psychotherapy is not new and has been practised in some form or other for thousands of years. Every culture has devised ways of providing support, guidance and consolation for individuals at times of great stress. Often this has occurred via religions agencies, but in Western, secular society, it is increasingly being regarded as the state's role to protect the 'souls' of its people. Hence, following major disasters, or the disappearance of a child, it is expected that counselors will automatically be supplied to comfort and help the stressed, shocked or bereaved. As Western cultures have become more technological and 'rational', psychological modes of healing have become more formalized and 'scientific'. Individuals have come to rely less on family and other social support systems, and much more upon formal organizations and health care.

All psychotherapies consist of two elements: Professional service and personal attachment. There is a formal contractual arrangement between therapist and client, with the delivery of specific psychological technology and expertise. This takes place in the context of personal relationship, in which a bond develops between the two (or more) individuals engaged in the process.

The contribution of psychological therapies to the treatment of people suffering from mental illness is being increasingly recognized. In 1996, the Department of Health produced a strategic review of policy in relation to psychotherapy service in England. The importance of delivering evidence-based psychotherapies, to those individuals most in need of treatment, has been emphasized in the National Service Framework for Mental Health (for highlighted the importance of treatment choice in relation to psychological treatments and counseling (Department of Health 2001).

Common Factors

Although, there are many different types of therapies and diverse approaches to the relief of psychological suffering, all psychotherapies have key common ingredients. These can be divided into three categories: support factors, learning factors and action factors (Lambert and Bergin 1994). Examples are listed in Box 1. The supportive factors include important aspects of therapy such as reassurance, and warmth and empathy from the therapist. Another supportive factor, the therapeutic alliance, has been found consistently to correlate positively with therapeutic outcome (Horvath and Luborsky 1993, Gaston et al. 1998, Martin et al. found to be particularly important (Horvath and Symonds 1991). The therapeutic has been conceptualized in a variety of different ways but includes the following:

- The ability of the patient to work purposefully in therapy
- The capacity of the patient and therapist to form a strong affective bond between them
- The therapist's skill at providing empathic understanding
- An agreement between the client and therapist about goals and tasks
- The ability of the therapist to identify and repair ruptures to the alliance.

Learning factors include giving advice, gaining insight, and the assimilation of problematic experiences. Action factors include modeling testing of solutions, and mastery.

Types of Psychotherapy

There are many different types of psychotherapy, but most can be grouped into four main categories: Cognitive-behavioral therapies, psychodynamic-relational therapies, experiential-expressive therapies; and systemic therapies (Box 2). Cognitive-behavioral therapies have a shared emphasis upon the identification of maladaptive practices or thoughts produced by faulty learning or reasoning, and the correction of such problems in the context of a collaborative relationship. Modern psychodynamic therapies which have been heavily influenced by interpersonal theory (Sullivan 1953) focus upon the correction of deeply ingrained and increase patterns of attachment, or problematic ways of relating to others.

Box 1: Common ingredients of psychological treatment

Support factors	*Learning factors*	*Action factors*
Release of tension	Advice	Facing fears
Trust	Feedback	Mastery
Reassurance	Insight	Working through
Structure	Exploratory rationale	Modeling
Warpathy Therapeutic alliance	Assimilation of problematic	Testing solutions
Acceptance	experiences	

Box 2: Different kinds of psychotherapy

Cognitive-behavioral therapies	*Psychodynamic-relational therapies*	*Experiential-expressive therapies*	*Systemic therapies*
Behavior therapy	Psychodynamic therapy	Client- centerd psychotherapy	Family
Personal construct theory		Gestalt therapy	Variously group therapies
Rational-emotive therapy		Counseling	Therapeutic
Dialectical behavioral therapy			Communities
Interpersonal therapy			
Cognitive-analytic therapy			
Psychodynamic-interpersonal therapy			

The patient-therapist relationship is recognized as a powerful medium through which problematic patterns of relating can be elucidated and modified, experiential-expressive therapies aim to restore well-being through the self-expression of distress. A supportive and safe framework is provided for the individual(s), within which to identify and find solutions to problems. Systemic therapies share a common approach in viewing an individual's behavior as the product of a system. Emphasis is placed upon changing or altering the system rather than the individual.

The distinction between different therapeutic approaches is becoming gradually more blurred, and there is greater integration between different therapeutic approaches. Some therapies such as interpersonal therapy (Klerman and Weissman 1993) share elements of both cognitive-behavioral and relational approaches. Cognitive analytic therapy (Ryle 1990) is another example of an integrative therapy which combines cognitive techniques within a framework of dynamic understanding. Psychonamic-interpersonal therapy (Hobson 1985) combines elements of dynamic therapy, relational and experiential-expressive approaches.

PSYCHODYNAMIC THERAPY

Psychodynamic therapies developed from the work of Freud in the late 19th and early 20th century. Early theory (i.e. pre-1950s) focused upon the salience of motivation forces or innate drives (e.g. sexual drive or libido) or which individuals are or partially unaware. Such drives resulted in unacceptable wishes or impulses which were kept out of conscious awareness, but resulted in the development of symptoms (either physical or emotional). Treatment was aimed at providing patients with awareness of (or insight into) these unacceptable wishes or conflicts, which could then be modified or resolved. Other key aspects of Freudian theories have been revised over the years. For example, in relation to development, other theories such as Erikson (1950) and Mahler have focused on more social and interpersonal aspects of development, and extended the developmental period to include late life.

In the 1950s, greater emphasis was placed on the role of attachment and on the important influence of early carer-infact/child relationship upon the stability and quality of relationships with significant others in adult life. This move, from a focus on the individual's internal conflicts, to an emphasis on the interactions he has with others, is represented by the development of object relations theory (Kernberg 1980). Writers such as Faireburn (1954) and Guntip (1969) suggested that the primary innate drive in humans is to form a strong bond with a good object (i.e. person). This process begins during (some may argue even before) infancy and is characterized by complex two-way interactions between carer and infant. A stable, supportive, reciprocal relationship between carer and infant is regarded as the essential cornerstone for both emotional and cognitive development. Gradual separation of child from carer, with the eventual development of independent functioning by the child, is seen as a key development process. Disruption to the carer-infant relationship can occur at any stage, but early disruption produces long-term maladaptive patterns of behavior in relation to others. Positive caring relationships are perceived as producing 'good objects' within people, whereas negative or abusive early relationships result in 'bad objects'. Objects are metaphors for the internalization of emotional experiences. A preponderance of good over bad objects results in the individual being able to tolerate uncertainty, trust others and engage in warm and meaningful reciprocal relationships. A preponderance of bad objects over good objects produces difficulties in being able to care for and trust others, or tolerate disappointment. Thus, relationships are brittle and stormy. Objects relations theory has much in common with the later ideas of schema-focused cognitive therapy, although initially the two approaches may seem very different.

Transference

Transference in its most basic form is the projection onto an individual of feelings and assumptions, which are derived from a previous important relationship (usually childhood). The feelings are experienced as real and there is no insight about their true derivation. A somewhat concrete, but real example of this involves a woman who was tortured and abused by her father when she was a child. He was a small man who wore round rimless glasses. As an adult, she regarded all men who wore such glasses as potential abusers. She described a hatred for her tutor at college, who she felt picked on her unfairly and humiliated her in class. This was not a view shared by her friends. It was only later on in therapy that she realized that, although her tutor did not wear glasses, he had certain facial characteristics which resembled those of her father. She realized that her perception of him had been clouded by her previous traumatic experiences.

Freud originally conceptualized transference as only occurring within psychotherapy, so that patients who had experienced such feelings as love, anger or a profound sense of gratitude towards their therapist may be expressing feelings which originated from relationships in early childhood, particularly with their parents. Freud broadened his view to accept that transference reactions occur throughout ordinary life and are part of most, if not all, relationships. The most common example of transference is 'falling in love'.

The psychodynamic therapy, transference is used as an important (if not the most important) tool to understand an individual's difficulties or problems with relationships. Such problems come alive in therapy, and are re-enacted between the therapist and client. Analysis and interpretation of the transference is one of the most powerful therapeutic agents in psychoanalytic psychotherapy.

The core conflictual relationship theme method (CCRT), developed by Loborsky (Luborsky and Crits-Christoph, 1990), can be used to objectively assess elements of the transference. Narratives from sessions of therapy are analysed according to three components: types of wishes, responses from other, and responses of the self. From this material, central relationship pattern, both adaptive and maladaptive, can be identified. The CCRT can be used to inform interpretations (see next subsection).

The term counter transference is used in a number of different ways by psychodynamic therapists. It most commonly refers to the therapist's emotional response to the client. The therapist's response will be made up of own 'transference' feelings, which have a basis in the therapist's own prior experiences, and the therapist's reaction to the client's transference towards him. If a therapist can distinguish these two elements of the counter trasference, he can gain valuable insight into the client's problems and ways relating to others.

Interpretations

Interpretations are one the main therapeutic tools used in dynamic therapies to aid conscious awareness of underlying conflicts or problem. They are attempts by the therapists to link conscious or and unconscious determinants by the therapist to link conscious and unconscious determinant of an experiences, feeing or symptom. An interpretation is not a dogmatic statement by the therapist, which is treated as being correct even if the patient disagrees with it. This, however, is how it is often portrayed. Interpretations are best understood as suggestions or tentative hypotheses which the patient is able to consider, and either agree with or reject.

There are a variety of measures which can be used to measure transference interpretations. Empirical research on the usefulness of interpretations has been reviewed by Pipar et al. (1993). Most studies of the effects of transference interference interpretations have been conducted on short-term therapies. Two aspects of transference interpretations have been studied: dosage (how many interpretations per session) and accuracy. The best outcome results are achieved from low frequency and high correspondence of transference interpretations (i.e. accuracy). For patients who score highly on objects relations transference interpretation variables can account for up to 40% of the outcome variance.

Object Relations

Quality of object relations refers to a person's lifelong pattern of relationships, identified on a dimension ranging from primitive to nature. A measure has been developed by Azim and colleagues (1991) which enables patient's level of object relations to be rated on a nine-point scale. The measure is interview based and requires two 1-hour sessions to complete. Lifelong patterns of relationships are explored in reference to criteria that characterize five levels of object relations: primitive, searching, controlling, triangular, and nature. The criteria refer to behavioral manifestations, regulation of affect, regulation of self-esteem, and historical antecedents. A tendency towards more mature object relations means the person enjoys equitable relationships characterized by love, tenderness and concern for objects of both sexes. There is a capacity to mourn and tolerate unobtainable relationships. A tendency towards primitive object relations means the person reacts to perceived separation or loss of object, or disapproval or rejection by the objects, with object intense anxiety and affect. There is inordinate dependence on the object who provides a sense of identity for the person.

Psychological Mindedness

Psychological mindedness is the ability to identify dynamic or intrapsychic components and to relate them to one's difficulties. An individual is considered to be psychologically minded if the person is willing to talk about intrapsychic and interpersonal problems, has the capacity and motivation for behavioral change, and is interested in what motivates other people' behavior.

McCallum and Piper (1997) have developed a procedure for assessing psychological mindedness assessment procedure (PMAP). The subject is asked to watch two brief video clips of simulated patient-therapist scenarios. After viewing videos, the person being assessed is asked for his general impressions of what is troubling the 'patient' on the tape. The person's responses are assessed by an individual assessor who grades the individual according to nine levels of psychological mindedness. They range from level 1, where a subject can recognize the patient's emotional state on the tape to level 9 where the subject is able to recognize that the 'patient' on the tape is behaving in a defensive way to protect herself from her true feelings.

Patients who score low on psychological mindedness are more likely to drop out of therapy. There is also a strong positive correlation between psychological mindedness and work in therapy. There is also some, but not conclusive, evidence that psychological mindedness is also associated with outcome.

Defense Mechanisms

Defense mechanisms are psychological strategies that are used to protect individuals from unbearable emotional distress. They protect individuals from unbearable emotional distress. They are universal phenomena which all of us use

Box 3: Common defense mechanisms
Mature
Sublimation—partial expression of unacceptable desires in modified way which makes them acceptable or even desirable
Suppression—partial prevention of unpleasant of feelings at times when their expression would be socially unacceptable, but ability to acknowledge feelings at other times
Anticipation—being able to anticipate and plan for distressing or difficult emotional events
Altruism—meeting one's own emotional needs by helping others
Humor—defusing difficult or conflictual situations by seeing funny side
Intermediate/neurotic
Displacement—transfer of negative feelings to a less threatening object
Repression—anxiety-provoking thoughts are prevented from being made conscious
Isolation—over-reliance upon self
Reaction formation—opposite reaction to hide underlying true feelings
Immature
Projection—internal anxiety are attributed to an outside cause
Schizoid fantasy—over-reliance upon fantasy to cope with life's disappointments
Passive aggression—transformation of angry or aggressive impulses into passive resistance or refusal to comply with realistic goals
Acting out—socially unacceptable behavior prompted by underlying aggressive impulses (behavior is usually self-injurious or directed at a key other person with whom the person is in conflict)
Hypochondriasis—unacceptable feelings are converted into concerns about illness
Dissociation—difficult feelings are split off from conscious awareness, and the individual becomes unconnected to reality (e.g. may develop fugue state or severe physical symptomatology)
Splitting—people are perceived as being either all good or all bad

at times to limit and constrict awareness so that threatening cues, either from the inner or outer environment, can be excluded. They appear to be invoked automatically and not under conscious control, and are psychological measures which allow stressful situations to be coped with by distorting reality (Box 3). In a fascinating study, Valliant et al. (1986) studied the defence mechanisms of 307 healthy middle-aged men followed up for 40 years and described the defence styles associated with coping and success. On the basis of this work the defense mechanisms measured in the study were grouped into hierarchical categories: mature, neurotic and immature defenses. Individuals who tended to use mature defences had a better long-term outcome (both physical and mental) than those who used immature defences.

A small number of empirical studies of defensive mechanisms in relation to psychiatric disorder provide a degree of support for the validity of some aspects of psychodynamic theory. There is evidence that persecutory delusions reflect a defensive attributional style which protects the individual against feelings of low self-esteem (Lyon et al. 1994). Panic disorder patients have a heightened use of reaction formation and undoing (Brusch et al. 1995). These findings are consistent with psychodynamic formulation of panic that proposes that negative effects are threatening to panic patients because they represent a threat to the relationship to a significant other on whom the individual feels dependent. Patients with dysthymia score highly on immature defense mechanisms (Bloch et al. 1993), and patients with a diagnosis of personality disorder use immature and primitive defensive mechanisms (Paris et al. 1996).

The activation of mature mechanisms often result in a positive response from others (e.g. individuals who use humor or altruism are generally seen as likeable), whereas immature mechanisms may provoke a negative and response from others. Thus, mature defenses are more adaptive and result in greater stability. Most individuals employ a repertoire of defense mechanisms, but when placed under stress of pressure, less mature defenses tend to be deployed.

An analysis of an individual's repertoire of defense mechanisms can be a useful indicator of how that person may behave during psychotherapy. However, a finer grading system of categories of defensive control processes, which integrates both psychodynamic and schema-focused cognitive theory, may also be useful in understanding maladaptive ways of coping with street and anxiety (Horowitz et al. 1997). The categories include:

- Shifting attention
- Juggling concepts about a topic
- Sliding meanings and values
- Premature disengaging from topics
- Blocking apt modes of representation
- Shifting time span
- Using poor ideational linkage strategies
- Engaging inappropriate arousal levels
- Shifting self-other roles
- Rigidly stabilizing compromise roles
- Altering valuation schemas (e.g. idealization or denigration of others).

Evidence Base

There are relatively few studies of psychodynamic therapies, in contrast with the large evidence base available for cognitive and behavioral interventions. In the last 15 years, there have been three systematic reviews. Svartberg and Stiles (1991) reviewed 19 studies and found a negative outcome. Crits-Christoph (1992) focused on short-term interventions and included 11 studies, with favorable results for dynamic therapies. A more recent review by Anderson and Lambert (1995) included 26 studies and provided conclusions more similar to that of Crits-Christoph. Further evaluation of psychodynamic therapies is urgently required.

BEHAVIORAL METHODS

In many early descriptions of behavioral approaches, emphasis was placed on the role of learning in the etiology, maintenance and treatment of psychiatrics problems. It was generally held that learning was a crucial concept in three main ways. First, some disorders were associated with a lack of learning, e.g. enuresis, or psychopathic behavior. Second, some disorders were associated with overlearning, e.g. obsessional rituals and phobias. Third, some disorders were associated with loss of previous learning, by neurological dysfunction, e.g. aphasia, or through insufficient or inappropriate reinforcement as in institutionalization. These nations provided the rationale for the application of learning theory to the amelioration of psychiatry problems. The links between behavioral approaches and learning theory have gradually become less direct, and methods of behavior change have been sought from winder experimental psychology and other areas.

Systematic Desensitization (SD) (General Exposure)

The original technique developed by Wolpe (1958) involved three stages:

1. Training the patient to relax (see next subsection).
2. Constructing with the patient a hierarchy of anxiety—arousing situations.
3. Presenting phobic items for the hierarchy in a graded way, while the patient inhibits the anxiety by relaxation.
4. In this way the patient, while never experiencing intolerable anxiety, proceeded from mildly frightening situations to previously terrifying ones.

Progress up the hierarchy can be made in imagination, in real life (*in vivo*) or by a combination of both, depending on such factors as the availability of the feared objects or situation and how easily the graded steps can be used. The balance of evidence suggests that *in vivo* SD is more effective, possibly because the treatment setting is more like the real-life situation, thus facilitating generalization.

When SD is being conducted in imagination, the length of the session is generally about 40 minutes, depending on how long it takes to get the patient relaxed; moving up steps in the hierarchy rarely extends beyond 30 minutes. The number of sessions required varies (anything from 10 to 100 being possible), depending on the complexity of the problem and on the number of hierarchies to be worked through, for it is seldom that a patient presents with a single well-defined phobia. Patients are expected to practice at home what they have learned in the clinical session.

The following illustrates a section of a typical hierarchy for a patient with a phobia of shopping:

1. Entering a quiet shop to purchase one article, e.g. a newspaper, with the exact purchase money in hand
2. Waiting behind one person, otherwise as (1)
3. Purchasing more than one article, as (1)
4. As (3), but having to wait for change
5. Asking to see an article before purchasing
6. As (4), but waiting in a queue of several people.

When SD is carried out *in vivo*, the patient is instructed how to relax and how and when to use relaxation in the clinic; but the actual desensitization is done in the real situation. Often this 'homework' can be done while the patient is accompanied by way of breaking down the hierarchy into smaller steps. SD is one of the most intensively investigated of all kinds of psychological therapy, with over one hundred studies looking simply at the relative importance of the various elements involved. There is little doubt its effectiveness, and it is extensively used as a treatment for phobic anxiety.

Relaxation

Behavior therapists are not the only practitioners of relaxation, as other therapists have used it extensively. Nevertheless, since Wolpe (1958) advocated Jacobson's (1938) technique it has earned a firm place in the behavioral armamentarium. Its role has also gradually extended. Formerly, when used alone, it was regarded as a control procedure lacking the essential conditioning element of SD; but gradually evidence accumulated showing that it was often at least as effective as the treatment with which it was compared: this was particularly striking when it was being used as a control procedure with which to compare biofeedback (see below). It has now earned a place in its own right as an effective treatment for anxiety management, headaches, chronic pain, hypertension and other problems. A useful review of relaxation procedures has been provided by Lichstein (1988).

Flooding (Rapid Exposure)

Flooding involves exposing patients to a phobic object in a nongrated manner with no attempt to reduce anxiety beforehand. As with SD, flooding can be conducted *in vivo* or in imagination. In the latter case it is often referred to as implosive therapy, and as such was originally put forward as a psychoanalytic technique, with some similarity to abreaction.

A recent application of imaginal flooding is to post-traumatic stress disorder (Cooper and Chum 1989).

Typically the patient is placed alone in a room with the phobic object, says a cat, and is required to stay there until the fear has diminished. It is argued that fear is maintained by the patient's avoidance of the phobic object or situation, and that if avoidance is not allowed the fear will diminish. The flooding session must be of long duration, normally an hour or more, to be effective. In general, the patient should stay in contact until there are clear indications of marked fear reduction; some reduction is normally seen after 15 minutes. Ending before this may represent avoidance and could exacerbate the problem. This brings out a resemblance to SD which may not be obvious at first sight. In the initial stages of flooding, the anxiety is very high but, due to emotional exhaustion or habituation, after a time it starts to decline so that each recurrence of the frightening stimulus, e.g. a movement of the cat towards the patient, no longer leads to increased anxiety and the stimulus-response link between the cat and the fear has weakened. Another likely reason for success is the subject's 'reality testing' of the situation, whereby he discovers that he is less afraid of the phobic object than he had expected to be.

Several studies have compared flooding with SD in the treatment of phobias. Most have shown that there are no major differences in outcome. Flooding seems to be more effective with obsessive—compulsive patients when combined with response prevention.

The decision whether to use flooding or not is by mutual agreement of patient and therapist. Most patients find it less frightening than they had imagined and it is usually much quicker acting than SD.

Flow chart 2 Cognitive processes

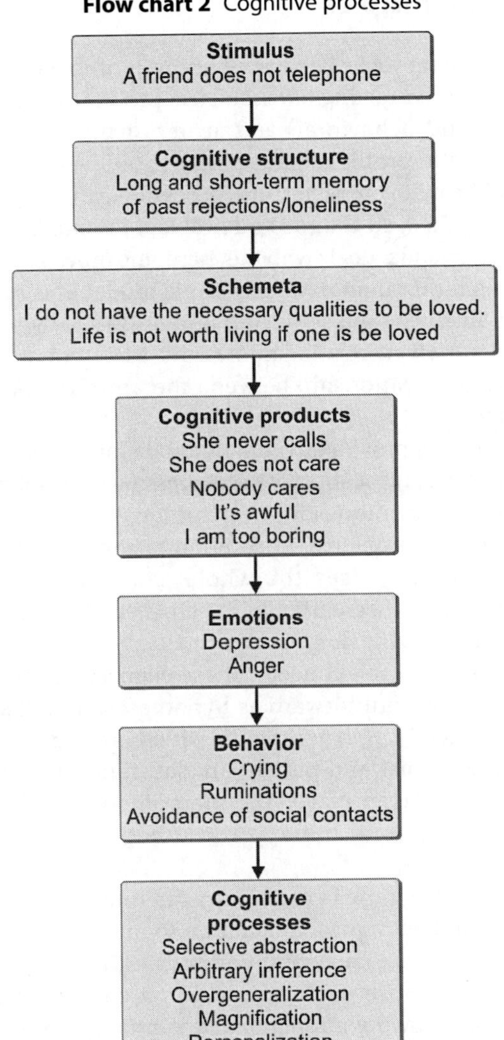

COGNITIVE THERAPY

Cognitive or cognitive–behavioral therapy refers to a method of therapy based on a theory of the emotional disorders (Ellis 1962, Beck 1967), a body of experimental and clinical studies (Blackburn 1988) and well-defined therapy techniques (Beck et al. 1997), Beck and Emery 1985, Hawton et al. 1989, Blackburn and Davidson 1990). Theoretically, the emphasis is on information processing; that is, individuals react, feel and behave according to how they process the information contained in their environment (Flow chart 2).

Cognitive approaches to treatment were first developed for the management of depressive illness and labelled as cognitive therapy (Beck 1964) or as rational-emotive therapy (RET) (Ellis 1962). The theoretical and experimental studies were criticized (e.g. sere Ledwigde 1978, Coync and Gottlib 1983), but a more general positive reaction has led to a mushrooming of basic research and of therapeutic applications to discovers other than depression. The general principles of cognitive therapy will be described, followed by its specific applications. The main characteristics of cognitive therapy are described in Box 4.

Box 4: How cognitive–behavioral therapy differs from other psychotherapies
• Open, explicit
• Structured, e.g. agenda
• Sets behavioral tasks
• Therapist more active
• Mainly uses here-and-now rather than past
• Does not use symbolism
• Uses specific cognitive techniques

General Principles

Cognitive therapy, like behavior therapy, is problem oriented. It is aimed at correcting psychological problems (emotional, cognitive and behavioral) and at improving coping skills (dealing with problem situations) to alleviate patient's distress. The main characteristics of cognitive therapy are that it is time limited, structured and problem oriented; it follows an explicit agenda, deals with the 'here-and-now', and adopts a learning rather than psychodynamic model. It is scientific method, involving the setting up and testing of hypotheses. Patients are given regular homework assignments, and a collaborative relationship between therapist and patient is developed.

Patients are provided with a rationale for understanding their problems, a vocabulary for expressing themselves, and a training in techniques for overcoming distressing affects and for solving problems. In addition to cognitive methods, cognitive therapy uses the whole gamut of behavioral techniques described earlier in the chapter. This is done not only to change behavior but also to change interpretations, expectations and self-concept. These changes are not taken for granted, but put forward as hypotheses, and discussed after the behavioral experiments, which are repeated until both the therapist and patient are satisfied that cognitive changes have taken place. The main differences between cognitive behavioral therapy and other therapies are in Box 5.

Cognitive therapy is more than the routine application of a series of techniques. In addition to mastering the basic therapeutic skills (Truax and Carkhuff 1967), the therapist must conceptualize each case within a cognitive therapy framework following a functional analysis which is similar to that described earlier in this chapter. The focus is on the cognitive factors which maintain emotional disturbance and maladaptive behavior. Blackburn and Davidson (1990) described the main areas of enquiry to reach a formulation in cognitive therapy. These are:

- *Definition of the problem*: What are the major complaints? Which particular functions are affected?
- *Objective factors*: What are the current stresses, main past traumatic events and current living situation?
- *Internal vulnerability factors*: What are the main attitudes and beliefs which the patient holds about himself and his world?
- *Mediational cognitive factors*: What are the typical automatic thoughts which are expressed and which processing errors do they contain?
- *Current themes*: The recurring theme, for example, failure, loss of control, loss of love, or low self-image, will indicate particular vulnerabilities and help the therapist to hypothesise about basic schemata.
- *Coping skills*: What are the typical methods of dealing with problems? In what are these helpful or unhelpful?
- *Emotions*: What are the predominant emotions and what situations trigger them?

Box 5: Elements of supportive psychotherapy	
•	The interview
•	Reassurance
•	Explanation
•	Guidance and suggestion
•	Ventilation

Specific Techniques

The techniques first described for the treatment of depression (Beck et al. 1979) are applicable, with some modifications and additions, to many different discovers (Hawton et al. 1989): for example, anxiety, obsessional—compulsive and eating discovers, somatic problems, sexual dysfunction and chronic psychiatric handicaps. Beck (1987) has described the cognitive dysfunctions which maintain depression. These are seen at three levels of thinking and cognitive therapy techniques are aimed at modifying each of these levels. An example is given in Flow chart 2.

The general aims of cognitive therapy are:

- To monitor negative automatic thoughts
- To recognize connections between cognitions, affect and behavior
- To examine evidence for and against distorted automatic thoughts
- To substitute more reality—oriented interpretations
- To learn to identify and alter dysfunctional schemata.

The automatic thoughts (so called because they are the habitual and reflexive commentaries that we make to ourselves and of which we are not necessarily fully conscious) are the basic data of cognitive therapist elicit and modify these thoughts, which maintain low or anxious or angry moods and dysfunctional behavior (e.g. inactivity, ruminating, checking, bingeing, avoiding, etc.). The patient can be helped to access these thoughts through direct questioning, inductive questioning (a series of questions which guide the patient to discover the related automatic thought), using moments of strong emotion, re-enacting situations in role plays, using mental imagery to recreate situations or using behavioral tasks to trigger the thoughts. The patient is asked to keep a diary (the 'daily record of dysfunctional thoughts'), using changes in emotions as cues to monitor thinking. These records are also used to practice challenging the automatic thoughts and substituting alternative interpretations which may lead to less distressing emotions. A variety of other techniques can also be used to modify automatic thoughts: for example, examing the evidence for and against, listing probabilities and collecting information which may invalidate the original interpretation. The basic principle in all these techniques is

Flow chart 3 Downward-arrow technique

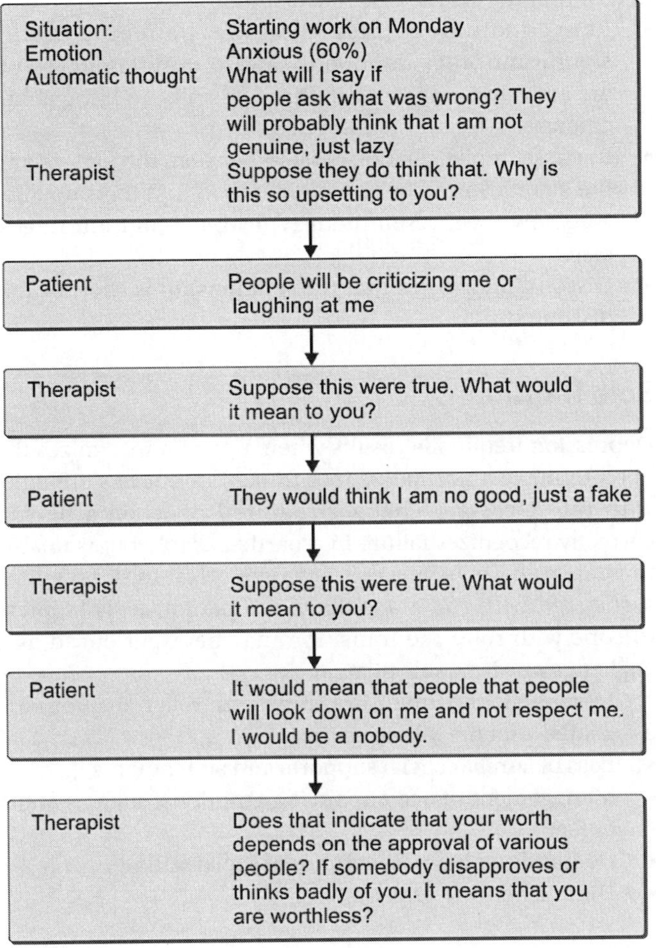

that the patient is thought to consider his thoughts not as facts but as interpretations which may be more or less fictional in terms of the feelings and the behavior that they trigger.

Identifying the basic schemata or beliefs lead the patient to process information in idiosyncratic ways typically occurs later on in therapy and is generally more difficulties and abstract than identifying automatic thoughts. It is also more difficult to modify the schemata, particularly in the personality discovers (Beck and Freeman 1990).

The schemata are inferred from the implicit or explicit rules which are exemplified in the automatic thoughts. The therapist and the patient, in collaboration, must look for common themes, for the 'shoulds' which are applied to the self and to others, and for the logical implications of automatic thoughts, by, for example, the 'downward arrow technique', of which an example (from Blackburn and Davidson 1990) is given in Flow chart 3.

As with the automatic thoughts, modifying the schemata is done through collaborative discussion and the use of behavioral tasks. Thus, the patient may be asked to weight up the advantages and disadvantages of holding the belief, to examine the evidence for and against the belief, to question the validity of to the personal contract, to consider the short-term and long-term utility of the personal rule, to disobey the rule in a behavioral assignment and test the consequences. The latter technique is similar to response prevention in behavior therapy.

Evidence Base

There are numerous studies of cognitive—behavioral therapy which support its efficacy for a wide variety of disorder, including depressive disorder, anxiety states, somatization and other neurotic conditions.

INTERPERSONAL PSYCHOTHERAPY

Interpersonal psychotherapy (IPT) is a structured, individual, time-limited (12–16 sessions) psychotherapy which has been shown to be effective in clinical trials of major depressive disorder and bulimia nervosa.

There are many different types of interpersonal psychotherapy, but IPT refers specifically to the model of treatment proposed by Klerman and Weissman (Klerman et al. 1984). It is of particular interest because it was devised by a biological psychiatrist and an epidemiologist.

The IPT is based on the work of Harry Stack-Sullivan (1953). Sullivan taught that psychiatry includes the scientific study of people and processes between people rather than focusing exclusively on the mind, society or the brain; hence the unit of clinical study is the patient's interpersonal relation at any one particular time.

The IPT has two foci: to reduce depressive symptoms and to deal with the social and interpersonal problems associated with the onset of the symptoms. The initial sessions are devoted to establishing the treatment contract, dealing with the depressive symptoms, and identifying the problem areas. During the initial session, both the depression and the interpersonal problems are accomplish six tasks:

1. Being dealing with the depression
2. Complete an interpersonal inventory and relate the depression to the interpersonal context
3. Identify the principal problem areas
4. Explain the rationale and intent of interpersonal therapy
5. Set a treatment contract with the patient
6. Explain the patient's expected role in the treatment.

Relating Depression to the Interpersonal Context

Once the review of the depression has been completed, the therapist should direct the patient's attention to the onset of symptoms and to the reason for seeking treatment what has going on in the patient's social and interpersonal life that is associated with the onset of symptoms? The review of key persons and issues often follows easily. If not, it is useful to being an inventory of current and past relationships to get a full picture of what the important current social interactions are in the patient's life.

The systematic review of current and past interpersonal relationships involves an exploration of the patient's important relationships with others' beginning with the present. This may be done during the session or the psychotherapist may ask the patient to write an autobiographical statement containing interpersonal information.

In this inventory, the following should be gathered about each personal who is important in the so on:

- Interactions with the patient, including frequency of contact, activity shares, and so on
- The expectations of each party in the relationship, including some assessment of whether these expectations were or are fulfilled
- A review of the satisfactory aspects of the relation, with specific, detailed examples of both kinds of interactions
- The ways the patient would like to change the relationship, whether through changing his or her own behavior or bringing about changes in the other person
- Although the inventory is constructed in the first two sessions, it may be added to less systematically as treatment progresses.

Problem Areas

It is important to define the problem areas because they can help the psychotherapist formulate a treatment strategy with the patient. Since IPT is short-term, it is usually concentrated on one or two of the four problem areas that depressed patients commonly encounter. The main problem areas are usually:

- Grief
- Interpersonal disputes with spouse, lover, children, or other family members, friends, or co-workers
- Role transitions—a new job, leaving one's family, going away to school, relocation in a new home or area, divorce, economic or other family changes
- Interpersonal deficits—loneliness and social isolation.

Diagnosis of Interpersonal Disputes

For the therapist to choose role disputes as the focus of IPT, the patient must give evidence of current overt conflicts with a significant other. Such disputes are usually revealed in the patient's initial complaints or in the course of the interpersonal inventory. In some IPT research, role disputes with the spouse have been the most common problem area. In practice, however recognition of important interpersonal disputes in the lives of depressed patients may be difficult.

In developing a treatment plan, that the therapist first determines the stage of the role dispute:

- Renegotiation implies that the patient and the significant other are openly aware of differences and are actively trying, even if unsuccessfully, to bring about changes.
- Impasse implies that discussion between the patient and the significant other has stopped and that the smouldering, low-level resentment typical; of 'cold marriages' exits.
- Dissolution implies that the relationship is irretrievably disrupted.

Role Transitions

Depression frequently results when a person recognizes the need to make a normative role transition but has difficulty with the necessary changes required or when a person correctly recognizes failure in a particular role but is unable to change the behavior or to change roles. In depressions associated with role transitions, the patient feels helpless to cope with role. The transition may be experienced as a challenge one is unable to meet.

In general, difficulties in coping with role transitions are associated with the following issues:

- Loss of familiar social supports and attachments
- Management of accompanying emotions, such as anger or fear
- Demands for a new repertoire of social skills
- Diminished self-esteem.

Training

Didactic seminar: In a 2–5 day seminar, an attempt is made to help therapists identify what they are already doing that is like IPT, what they are doing that is not IPT, and the special skills needed for the IPT approach. This takes the form of an exegesis of the written material with extensive clinical illustration using videotaped case material.

Supervised Casework

After the didactic seminar, therapists are assigned between two and four training cases each, on which they receive weekly super vision on a session-by-session basis. This is done on the telephone or in person after the supervisor has received the videotape of the session. Both trance and supervisor have videotape equipment and tapes available, so that they can watch specific segments as they discuss the session. The primary purpose of the supervision is boundary marking or helping the therapist learn which techniques are included and which are excluded in IPT. It is also helpful if the supervisor reviews the ratings made by the patient during the session as well as the observer ratings.

SUPPORTIVE PSYCHOTHERAPY

This form of psychotherapy is as variously defined as it is widely used. Block (1979) describes it as a form of psychological treatment given to patients with chronic and disabling psychiatric conditions 'for whom basic change is not seen as a realistic goal.' This definition emphasizes the notion of therapy as a prop or crutch and envisages the objectives of such an approach as the promotion of the patient's best possible psychological and social functioning, the bolstering of his self-esteem and self-confidence, the cultivation of his sense and contact with reality, the prevention of relapse, and, in certain instances, the transfer of the source of support from professional to family of friends.

However, other definitions of supportive psychotherapy stress its role in enabling individuals to cope with and overcome psychological difficulties presenting more acutely. For example, Royal College of General Practitioners' report (1981) on prevention of psychiatry disorders in general practice emphasized the importance of supportive intervention in enabling the individuals to negotiate 'psychosocial transitions'—particular life events and challenges which produce psychological reactions, symptoms and disorders commonly seen in patients presenting to general practitioners, health visitors and social workers. The objectives of such supportive psychotherapy include the minimising of the impact of the threatening event, the provision of protection and relief from responsibilities during the crisis or transition, the encouragement of the expression of emotions and talking through the difficulties, and support for the individual in his attempts to seek out new directions in life.

Supportive psychotherapy is also conceived of as the use of psychological means to build individuals up to point where they can devote themselves to more profound, time-consuming and complex psychotherapeutic interventions and as a temporary expedient to contain individuals who are actually ill and who are awaiting the therapeutic impact of other forms of psychiatric treatment, most notably pharmacological.

There is much more general agreement as to what constitutes the key elements of the supportive forms of psychotherapy. It is now recognized that an interview itself can exercise a psychotherapeutic effect—that the mere act of a doctor listening carefully to what the patient is saying, and enabling the patient to gives a full account of his situation and problems, can result in a significant improvement. This realization has led in turn to attempts to dissect out those characteristics of the interview which may exercise particularly beneficial effect. To date, the bulk of the effort has been directed at identifying interview techniques which facilities case detection but the implications for the facilitation of therapy seem clear. Among the interview techniques which appear important are the therapist's ability to note verbal and nonverbal cues, to ask questions in a sequence from open to closed, to avoid using too many direct questions and to emphasise the importance of understanding the here-and-now situation (Marks et al. 1993).

Reassurance provided by a therapist equipped to use the therapeutic relationship constructively, able to be both detached, and compassionate and skilled in listening and providing information simply and comprehensively, is one of the basic elements of the supportive form of psychotherapy. Reassurance can be used to good effect to relieve fears, boost self-confidence and promote hope. But it is not without its problems. To promote a patient's hopes unreasonably by providing false reassurance or to intervene prematurely before the patient has explained his situation fully, may be effective initially but eventually prove useless or worse. However, as Kessel (1979) has pointed out in a thoughtful essay on the subject, such a view at least partly reflects the perspective of the specialist psychotherapist concerned with the explorationing a patient from his responsibilities and of getting between a patient and his recognition of underlying causes can be avoided once it is recognized.

Explanation is likewise an important element in psychotherapeutic support. Whereas reconstructive forms of psychotherapy emphasise non-directiveness, a degree of therapeutic passivity and active therapeutic interventions limited to the provision of interprectation, the supportive forms encourage the explanations by the therapist of such diverse matters as the nature of the patients symptoms, the choice of treatment, and the likely outcome. Explaining to a patient quite why are common can itself be reassuring and therapeutically effective. The goal is not so much to increase self-understanding as to enhance the patient's ability to cope by clarifying the nature of the problem faced, the symptoms experienced and/or the treatment recommended.

Guidance and suggestion involve the provision of direct and indirect advice. In general, therapists are encouraged to refrain from advising patients, yet in supportive therapy teaching a patient how and when to ask for help is often a crucial component. Advice may be necessary with regard to particular problems, such as optional ways of relating to a particularly difficult relative or handling a job interview, or to general issue, such as making contact with members of the opposite sex. Occasionally, advised is ineffective, and persuasion, involving the therapist in a more direct, controlling role, is required. Suggestion involves the therapist using such techniques as the showing or withholding of approval in attempts to modify a patient's situation. Suggestion operates in all forms of psychotherapy, and it has even been postulated that the suitability of an individual for treatment is dependent on his potential openness to the suggestive influence (Strupp 1978). Variables which appear to regulate the forcefulness of suggestion include the significance of the therapist to the patient, the degree to which the patient is or can become dependent and the depth of the patient's anxiety or depression. Individuals whose coping strategies have been overwhelmed are believed to be particularly prone to cling with desperation to any potential helping resource and to respond dramatically to proffered advice, reassurance and guidance.

In recent years, the value of ventilation of feelings within the psychotherapeutic setting has received support, and interest has been stimulated in the old notion of catharsis by the rise of the so-called 'emotive release (body) therapies'. It does seem useful for patients to be able to express emotions such as anger, frustration and despair openly. Unfortunately, the amount and quality of emotional expression has rarely been assessed independently and related to outcome, so its value has received little direct experimental verification.

Supportive psychotherapy is widely used in psychiatric settings, in general practice and in settings in which patients with short-lived yet intense emotional crises are seen.

COUNSELING

There has been an enormous expansion of counseling services in primary care in the UK over the last twenty years. The most commonly practiced form is non-directive counseling. In this, the client is given opportunities to explore, discover and clarify ways of living more resourcefully. This occurs in the context of therapeutic relationship, within which the counselor uses a range of skills to facilitate the client's resolution of his problems. Counseling is based upon the general factors present in all kinds of psychotherapy (see Box 1). These include, developing a working relationship with the client, within a supportive frame-work; encouraging a frank and open discussion of the client's problems; adopting a non-judgmental attitude; the release of emotional distress and the facilitation of problem solution. Other forms of counseling, which involve specific tasks, are also used widely in the NHS setting. This can include information—giving (e.g. genetic counseling) or brief structured guidance (e.g. alcohol counseling).

The evidence base in support of counseling as an efficacious treatment is mixed. However, a recent, large, well-conducted study in primary care, has shown that there is no significant difference between counseling and cognitive therapy for the treatment of depression (Ward et al. 2001).

GROUP THERAPY

There are many different forms of group therapy. They all, however, share certain characteristics. In addition to factors common to all therapies, groups enable people to share experiences and interact with each other, in a safe setting. Individuals within the group give and receive help from the other members. Yalom (1970) summarized the factors of group psychotherapy which can have beneficial (curative) effects:

- Installation of hopes
- Universality
- Imparting of information
- Altruism
- Corrective recapitulation
- Development of socializing techniques
- Imitative behavioral
- Interpersonal learning
- Catharsis
- Group cohesiveness.

Groups can be divided into the educational or therapeutic, fixed or open, and short- or long-term. Educational groups are common in the heathcare setting, and are usually time-limited and very structured. They usually have a clear leader and a timetable. Members of the group are invited to comment on the information they have been given and to discuss it.

Therapeutic groups are either fixed or open. Fixed implies that the membership of the group is determined before its start and does not change. 'Open' means that the membership of the group gradually changes over times; as one person leaves, another may join.

Most of the individual forms of therapy discussed above can be delivered in a group format, including CBT and psychodynamic therapy. Although the effects of group work are difficult to evaluate, over seven hundred studies have reported outcomes for various forms of group psychotherapy (Fuhriman and Burlingame 1994). Several meta-analytic studies have been carried out, some showing no difference between group therapy and individual therapy (Robinson et al. 1990, Tillitski 1990) and some reporting an advantage for individual therapy over group (Dush et al. 1983; Hemmings and Gretter 1987). Given the diversity of different treatment approaches, lengths of treatment, and conditions for which group therapy has been provided, the results are difficult to interpret.

Most analytic groups are 'slow, open' groups, this means they run for a lengthy period of time (several years) over which older members of the group may leave, and new members join. The group leaders may also change. Most members stay in the group for at least 2 years. Group members agree (before entry) to have no other contact with each other, outside the group setting. They are known to each other only by their first names. Most groups consist of 6–8 members, plus one or two therapists, and may meet either once or twice weekly. One group session usually lasts 90 minutes.

Groups of this nature are powerful mediators of change. Individuals within the group are faced with a variety of different interpersonal experiences. They may have to cope with an old member leaving the group, assimilate new people into the group, cope with peer relationships and also relationships with authority, as symbolized by the group leader. In addition, they have to interact with the other group members on a personal basis.

Transference and counter transference issues may become evident and played out within the group. As people get to know each other within the group, a cohesiveness develops, and the group becomes more than a set of individuals. This transpersonal network of communication is sometimes referred to as the group matrix.

As group work of this nature is quite intensive and expensive, it is usually only offered in the healthcare sector to individuals who have chronic psychological problems and a pattern of interpersonal disturbance.

Psychodrama

Psychodrama is a form of group therapy that was developed by Moreno. It usually occurs in a closed group setting. Each member of the group has an opportunity to become the focus particular enactment. Other members of the group role play the person's family or friends. A particular problem will be re-enacted and discussed by the group, from which new understanding and solutions are generated. The enactments usually generate strong feeling in the person represented, but also resonate with other members of the group, who may share similar difficulties. Members can also swap roles, to help them appreciate the problem from a different perspective.

FAMILY THERAPY

Family therapy was developed in the 1950s. It involves working with the whole family or at least several family members. It is most widely practiced in child and adolescent psychiatry, but is also used in a variety of other setting, including the treatment of schizophrenia in adults (Kuipers et al. 1992) and the treatment of mental health problems in the elderly (Richaedson et al. 1994). There are many different forms of family therapy, but systemic family approaches are among the most commonly practiced forms. In systemic family therapy, the whole family is seen as a system, in which the behavior of one individual is understood as a reaction to other parts of the system. For example, the development of emotional symptoms in a child whose parents are experiencing marital difficulties, may be understood as a way of trying to keep the parents together. Alleviation of the symptoms will only occur if the fundamental problems with the system are addressed.

Another form of family therapy is attachment-based family therapy (ABFT) (Diamond and Siqueland 1995). The underlying assumption of ABFT is that poor attachment bonds, high conflict, harsh criticism, and low affective attunement can lead to physical or emotional neglect, abuse and abandonment. This kind of negative family environment inhibits children from developing the internal and interpersonal coping skills needed to buffer against the family, social and community stressors that can cause or exacerbate depression. An equally important assumption of ABFT is that attachment failures can be resolved, parents can become better caregivers, and adolescents can rebuild trust and communication with their parents.

Evidence Base

There is a paucity of well-designed randomized controlled trials of systems therapies with children and adolescents and those trials that do exist evaluate older therapies. Methodological limitations of existing research include the use of unrepresentative participants, small sample sizes and wide age ranges. There is a lack of credible no—treatment or alternative—treatment controls, tests of clinical as opposed to statistical significance, and conceptually relevant outcome measures that examine underlying interactional mechanisms. The term 'family therapy' encompasses a wide range of interventions and it is not always clear what treatment intervention has been delivered. Nevertheless, there is good evidence for the effectiveness of systemic family therapies in the treatment of conduct disorders, substance misuse and eating disorders, and some support for their use as second-line treatments in depression and chronic illness (Cottrell and Boston 2002). Family and parenting interventions for juvenile delinquents and their families may have beneficial effects on reducing time spent in institutions and their criminal activity (Woolfenden et al. 2002).

COUPLE THERAPY

Couple therapy involves the psychotherapeutic treatment of married or cohabiting partners. It is usually reserved for situations where there is clear marital or relationship conflict. Relatively little couple therapy is offered on the NHS, but it is widely available from nonstatutory agencies such as RELATE.

There have been relatively few evaluations of couple therapy, and many of the problems highlighted above in relation to the evaluation of family therapy are equally relevant to couple therapy.

EYE MOVEMENT DESENSITIZATION AND REPROCESSING (EMDR) AND OTHER ULTRA-BRIEF THERAPIES

The late 1980s and the 1990s saw the emergence of a cluster of very brief therapies, sometimes labeled 'power' therapies. These include 'the five-minute phobia cure', TFT (Thought Field Therapy) and EMDR. Only EMDR (eye movement desensitization and reprocessing) has an established evidence base (Foa et al. 2000). EMDR was developed by Shapiro (1995) as a technique for mitigating the impact of traumatic memories. It was subsequently developed into a more comprehensive treatment for PTSD. The technique involves cognitive behavioral and emotional aspects. The patient is asked to hold in the bodily sensations associated with that traumatic image. The clinician then moves his or her fingers back and forth approximately 25 cm in front of the patient's pace while the patient tracks the moving fingers with his eyes. After approximately 20 back and forth eye movements (saccades) the clinician stops and asks the patient to go of the memory, take a deep breath and provide feedback on any changes in the image, body sensations, emotions or thoughts about the self. This is repeated until the image beings to fade. The second stage is the installation of a positive cognition. The eye movements are the central stage in what is an eight-stage treatment process for which specific training and treatment manuals are available.

There is debate about whether the eye movements are necessary or sufficient for the treatment, and it seems likely that EMDR works because it is an accelerated form of behavior exposure and cognitive reprocessing.

For such a new treatment, the evidence base is remarkably strong, with 12 good randomized, controlled trials comparing EMDR with wait list or other brief treatments, and there are four dismantling studies for PTSD. EMDR appears to be as effective as cognitive therapy or drug treatment and somewhat more efficient. The evidence base is, however, limited by the multiple traumatic events.

The other ultra-brief therapy which has a robust evidence base is Richard Bryant's Four Session Cognitive Therapy for Acute Stress Disorder (Bryant et al. 1998). This has been shown in several trials to be a highly effective treatment in reducing the symptoms of acute stress disorder and somewhat more efficient. The evidence base is, however, limited by the fact that most studies have treated single rather than multiple traumatic events.

The second cluster of brief treatments are those grouped under the rubric of psychological debriefing, including such packages as critical instant stress debrifing (CISD). These are psychological interventions delivered shortly after a major traumatic event, either individually or in groups. They aim to reduce or prevent the development of subsequent psychological disorders, such as PTSD, major depressive disorders. The Cochrane Review (Rose et al. 2002) has clearly demonstrated that a single episode of psychological debriefing delivered in the days higher rates of subsequent PTSD in those who were debriefed compared with those who were not. Orner and Schnyder (2003) have recently comprehensively reviewed the whole area of 'early intervention after trauma.'

EFFICACY AND EFFECTIVENESS OF PSYCHOLOGICAL INTERVENTIONS

In any discussion of outcome, it is important to distinguish between efficacy and effectiveness. Efficacy refers to the performance of treatment in a (randomized) controlled trial, whereas effectiveness refers to its performance in a clinical setting. Randomized controlled trials of psychological treatment usually recruit highly selected patient populations, have strict exclusion criteria, and usually employ experienced or expert therapists to conduct the treatment, which is manual based and monitored closely. In clinical settings, patients have heterogeneous problems, therapy is not manual based, and is much less closely supervised or scrutinized than in a trial, and therapists have different degrees of expertise. It is perhaps not surprising that psychotherapies perform better in trial settings than in ordinary clinical settings (Weisz et al. 1995).

Psychotherapy researchers were one of the first group of investigators to adopt meta-analytic methods, within the field of psychiatry, to evaluate outcome. The first meta-analytic reviews of psychotherapy were published in the 1970s. At the time of writing this chapter, meta-analytic review have become the gold standard in terms of evaluating the efficacy of a particular treatment approach.

Although meta-analyses have many positive aspects, some caution is required regarding their use in relation to psychotherapy outcome. Most meta-analyses of psychotherapy combine different patient groups, different treatments, evaluate change over different periods of time, and employ different outcome measures. These difficulties should, however, diminish somewhat with the passage of time as more trials are published. It is only in relation to cognitive-behavioral treatments that there are sufficient studies at presents which meet the homogeneity that the meta-analytic method requires (for example, all studies using the same outcome measure in the same condition).

Major Depressive Disorder (MDD)

Many of the large reviews of the efficiency of psychotherapy in major depression are now quite old and do not include many studies using modern psychotherapy techniques. Nevertheless, three reviews have focused on the efficiency of psychotherapy contrasted with pharmacotherapy: the Quality Assurance Project (1983), Steinbruek et al. (1993) and Conte et al. (1986). The most influential of these, the Quality Assurance Project, showed an effect size for psychotherapy of 0.69, for tricyclic antidepressants of 0.55 and for monoamine oxidase inhibitors of 0.39. The Depression Guidelines Panel (1993) reported somewhat differently from most meta-analyses in that the effect size is not given but there is an expected response rate for each therapy. There are a relatively small number of studies on brief dynamic psychotherapy and only one on interpersonal psychotherapy in this review. Although cognitive therapy is undoubtedly efficacious in depression, whether it is more or less effective than other treatments is controversial (Wampold et al. 2002). Two key studies are also worthy of attention: Hollon et al. (1992), Elkin (1994).

Specific/Simple Phobia: Key Review

Emmelkamp (1994) reviews behavior treatments for specific phobias. Overall improvement rates appear to be achieved in approximately 75% of cases. The general conclusion is that exposure is more effective than systematic desensitization and that *in vivo* exposure is the most effective. Treatments for circumscribed specific phobias can be brief, being carried out in a single prolonged session of 2 hours or over two four sessions at weekly intervals. Key studies are Ost (1989), Liddell et al. (1994).

Generalized Anxiety Disorder

Durham and Allan's review (1993) is important because they reviewed studies that had used the Hamilton Anxiety Scale and the State Trait Anxiety Inventory as outcome measures. Their results show that CBT produces best results, but there are some important qualifications. The rates of improvement varied markedly from study to study, CBT was not always the best treatment, and outcome and rates of improvement were modest, though significantly better than placebo drugs or anti-anxiety medication. Not all studies had reasonable follow-up periods. Approximately, 55% of those who had received cognitive therapy were in the normal range on the two above measures at the end of treatment, and this compared with 22% who had received behavior therapy without cognitive intervention. Key studies are Power et al. (1990), Butler et al. (1991), Durham et al. (1994).

Panic Disorder

Gould et al. (1995) carried out a meta-analysis on 43 controlled studies for the treatment of panic disorder. Treatments included pharmacological treatment, cognitive-behavioral interventions, and combined pharmacological and CBT treatments. The long-term analysis favored CBT above either CBT combined with pharmacotherapy or pharmacotherapy alone. However, there was a paucity of trials in which CBT was directly compared with antidepressant medication. Key studies Marks et al. (1993), Clark et al. (1994), Gauld et al. (1995).

Social Phobia

There is one good meta-analysis of 10 trials of behavior and cognitive therapy (Chambless and Gillis 1993). There were significant effects both on the positive symptoms of social phobia and on the fears of negative evaluation that social phobics have. Given the chronicity of this disorder, follow-ups were relatively brief at 1–6 months. A key study is Heimberg et al. (1990).

Post-traumatic Stress Disorder

The most comprehensive review is that by Foa et al. (2000). They point out that most studies have either been on Vietnam veterans or female rape victims. Effective techniques appear to be anxiety management, stress inoculation, training and cognitive restructuring. The role of exposure-based treatments remains controversial. The evidence-base for psychodynamic psychotherapy is unclear largely because of the poor quality of the studies. Although not part of Foa's review it is perhaps worth emphasizing that as yet there is little evidence base for post-disaster counseling or post-disaster psychological debriefing. A recent review by Rose et al. (2002) found no evidence for any benefits of post-disaster debriefing.

Psychological Treatments in Primary Care

A systematic review by Churchill et al. (2001) has been conducted on the effectiveness and costeffectiveness of brief psychological treatments for depression in primary care. Low overall quality scores were recorded for many of the trials, and interpretation of the finding was limited by identification of probable bias in the funnel plots and heterogeneity and sensitively analyses. Patients receiving variants of CBT were significantly more likely to improve than those receiving treatment as usual. There was very little available information concerning a comparison of CBT with other psychological treatments.

Seven trials of counseling in primary care have been evaluated in a recent systematic review (Bower et al. 2002). Counseling produced significantly greater clinical effectiveness in comparison with usual care, and the levels of satisfaction with counseling were not sustained. Four trials reported that the total costs of counseling were similar to those for controls, so it may be underpowered. Further high-quality trials of all types of psychological treatment (both brief and long-term) are required.

CONCLUSION

There is growing evidence that psychological treatment is efficacious for a wide variety of psychiatric disorders. However, in comparison to the evidence base for pharmacological treatment, there are still relatively few randomized controlled trials which have investigated the efficacy of funding for psychotherapy research and the enormous resources available to the pharmaceutical industry for the development and evaluation of psychotropic treatment. The vast majority of randomized controlled trials of psychological treatment which have been published in the last 10 years involve evaluations of cognitive behavioral therapy (or its derivatives). There is therefore a sound and robust evidence base for its use in clinical settings. Other psychological treatment approaches have not been evaluated to the same extent, and there is a clear need for further evaluation of these interventions.

47.4 GROUP PSYCHOTHERAPY

Ajit Avasthi

INTRODUCTION

Differentiation into groups is an inevitable concomitant of man's living a social life. A social group grows out of and requires a situation which permits meaningful inter-stimulation and meaningful response between the individuals involved; common focusing of attention, common stimuli and/or interests, and the development of certain common drives, motivations or emotions. Reciprocal relationships, sense of unity, we-feeling, common interests, similar behavior and group norms are considered as essential characteristics of social group. These groups are ever changing according to situations and needs. Group setting is universal phenomenon in every society, from our family units, to the classroom; to the persons we surround ourselves with at work, at play, and at home. Because of powerful and unique therapeutic experience, the group setting is being used not only by mental health professionals but also by lay persons also. Interpersonal relationships play an important role in human psychological development, and have therapeutic implications. A number of specialized groups have been developed to function in a supportive and therapeutic mode in nonpsychiatric medical settings in addition to self-help groups and group interventions in psychiatric settings. In group-settings, patients are provided with varied array of interpersonal relationships that, with proper guidance, will permit them to identify, explore, and alter maladaptive interpersonal behavior. Group therapy is a widely practiced mode of psychotherapy that is applicable to a wide range of human problems and in a vast number of clinical settings, viz., inpatient, outpatient, community, half way homes etc. The advent of widespread managed care and population-based care systems have opened an era of group psychotherapy and its teaching because economic issues are important for this kind of care.

HISTORICAL BACKGROUND

Group psychotherapy began at the turn of the 20th century when Joseph Pratt, a Boston physician, identified the positive effects of assembling and teaching patients with tuberculosis in groups who were unable to afford sanatoria. Using regular group meetings, he emphasized on strict hygienic measures and optimistic attitude as a part of their management. The role of charismatic leadership and its dynamics was later reinforced by Freud and then applied by Redl in group-settings. During the First World War, psychologically informed clinicians had extensive experience of the treatment of traumatized soldiers which further led the progress of group psychotherapy. The role of Tavistock Clinic at London by Crichton-Miller and his colleagues is notable. In 1920s, the concept of group analysis was put forward by Trigant Burrow; this lead to a paradigm shift with a vision of the group as a whole. Burrow conceptualized humans as a social being and group as the natural focus of treatment. His aim was to make conscious both latent and repressed meanings through the here-and-now interaction within a group. In the United States, teachings of John Dewey about child centered education spilled over social work and by 1930s social work group had become well recognized as a social work method comparable with, though differing from case work. During the Second World War, advances in group psychology led to further progress in this field. In the postwar period, group psychotherapy moved from inspirational and didactic models to psychodynamic and analytic models. Group analytic tradition, initially based on ideas of Trigant Burrows, was further strengthened by Foulkes and his associates with series of publications and foundation of several associations. The "Tavistock" approach that originated from the work of Bion and his colleagues became popular, especially in staff training and consultancy.

Jacob Moreno introduced the concept of group psychodrama. Yalom's interpersonal approach was documented in his most influential book *"Theory and Practice of Group Psychotherapy"*. Moreno founded the American Society for Group Psychotherapy and Psychodrama in 1942. The Society was later named as the *International Association for Group Psychotherapy*, an umbrella organization for all approaches. All this led to upsurge in the systematic approach and reporting of group psychotherapy. Over the years group methods played an active part in the reconstruction of mental health services throughout Europe in the post-war phase. Subsequent years, especially the 70s saw a large number of empirical investigations of the 'new groups'. In the 80s, there was a shift of interest towards biological treatments. Nevertheless, substantial evidence regarding the efficacy of group treatments, and mounting pressures from third party payers to employ more cost effective treatments, renewed interest in group managements.

CLASSIFICATION OF GROUP THERAPIES

Using two basic indicators, i.e. specificity of goals and levels of leadership activity, group therapies can be broadly classified as:

- Goal-specific therapy with high level of leader activity as in structured groups in centers for alcohol and drug dependence.
- Goal-directed therapy with lower level of leader activity like problem-solving and psychoeducational groups for homogeneous populations (e.g. eating disorders or offenders).
- Nonspecific goals with high level of leader activity as in groups for psychodrama, music therapy, short-term dynamic and systems-centered groups.
- Nonspecific goals with low level of leader activity as in support groups, art psychotherapy and psychotherapy groups viz., interpersonal (Yalom and colleagues), Tavistock (Bion or group-as-a-whole) and group-analytic schools.

Group psychotherapy can also be divided based on the basic methods employed in the therapy into: activity, supportive, problem-solving, psychoeducational, and psychodynamic therapies. However, all the various types of group therapy rely on same fundamental procedures, i.e. the selection and grouping of members seeking help, who have regular meetings together with one or more trained therapist. *Activity group approach* has been used extensively in rehabilitation programs related with refugees, social work, and fostering and adoption programs in form of group activity like exercise or cooking. *Supportive group approach* aims to reduce the deleterious effects of social isolation, bring people out of social withdrawal states and provide opportunities for problem sharing. These groups are useful to serve patient populations with chronic mental and physical illnesses including mental retardation. *Problem-solving groups* resolve a defined and sometimes circumscribed problem, viz, Alcoholics Anonymous, Al-anon, Gamblers Anonymous, and groups for people with poor impulse control, eating disorders or smoking. In *psychoeducational groups* the participants are given the role of students rather than seen as sick, and are provided information through lectures, discussions, and suitable reading material. *Psychodynamic groups* aim to create personal change through nondirective free-associative therapy. In the psychodynamic group model structure describes the 'architecture' of interpersonal relations of group ascribed in terms of the setting and its boundaries, and in terms of bond between each individual, therapist and the group as a whole. Process deals with the fluid and dynamic fluctuations of emotion and experience. It includes the business of relating and communication, the changes of association, and intermember responses. The content of a group's exchange involves visible and audible events. Further 3 different models of psychodynamic therapy are described. The interpersonal group therapy model takes into account the intra-group interactions, including those between the leader and other members of group in totality and does not differentiate the leader from rest of the members. This group provides opportunity for change in maladaptive interpersonal beliefs and behaviors through feedback from others and experimentation with healthy behaviors. The Tavistock model looks at the interactions in the group in the form of two-body psychology between two parties, i.e. the leader and the rest of the group is used for personal exchange. The therapist plays a role in the analysis and interpretation of defenses against primitive anxieties. The Group analytic model tries to incorporate elements of above two models. It considers the leader as structurally different to other group members as in Tavistock model, but at the same time encourages the leader to work in the group with individuals as well as with the group as a whole like the interpersonal model. This three-body psychological approach proceeds through the dynamic interaction of each individual, the leader, and the group as a whole.

PRACTICAL FOUNDATIONS: NEED FOR GROUP PSYCHOTHERAPY

Earlier understanding of group therapy involved a passive assimilation of information delivered by an inspirational leader about group process. However, over the years the understanding has changes and it emphasizes on understanding the role of interaction and sharing with fellow sufferer as the main factor in group process. Simultaneously, "let's place them in a group" as a matter of convenience has been replaced by a more articulated rationale based on the unique merits of group process for the particular patients referred for treatment. With this change in the basic foundations, group psychotherapy became a very powerful method of treatment because of its expediency, cost-effectiveness and staff-efficiency, i.e. the need to respond to the large number of patients who seek symptomatic relief.

THEORETICAL FOUNDATIONS

Even though group process originated as a purely pragmatic approach towards large number of patients, psychoanalytic model exerts the primary thrust in the progression of group process and current understanding. Contemporary theories of group psychotherapy may be contrasted along a number of critical discussions. Parloff, for example, has differentiated theories in terms of the focus of therapist's interventions into Interpersonalists (Individual), Transactionalists (relationship within the group) and Integralists (group-as-a-whole). Interpersonalists generally seek to resolve intrapsychic conflicts and view the group as especially effective in facilitating the interpretations of resistance and transference phenomena.

Transactionalists are mainly interested in member to member relationship and portray the group as providing a unique opportunity for stimulating idiosyncratic modes of relating and responding to a wide range of individual styles. Integralists place primary emphasis on group-as-a whole process. Membership in a therapy group presumably evokes shared unconscious conflicts or motivations around issues of dependency and intimacy.

However, over the years there has been a fair amount of blending and joining of the best of each theory into a workable model. Further, few dynamic therapists worked without integrating individual, interpersonal, and group as a whole threads into their practices. By the 1990s, theoretical innovation and refinement had led to the emergence of other schools of thought in the group therapy like systems theory, self-psychology, existential psychiatry object relations and Lacania psychology, which tries to redefine group psychoanalysis and interpersonal therapy into a joined model which leads ways of understanding the phenomena that take place within the unfolding of psychotherapy groups.

DISTINGUISHING THE TYPES OF GROUPS

At this point it is necessary to make some preliminary distinctions among all these groups which, so far, have been described together, but which in fact differ considerably in their aims and in the methods used to realize these aims. Broadly the group situations could be divided into: group psychotherapy, group counseling, and group discussion. Similarly to individual psychotherapy, *group psychotherapy* tries to effect a significant change in the personality of each member of the group. As with individual psychotherapy, normal social rules are suspended, and each member of the group is expected to reveal his thoughts and feelings with complete freedom, on the understanding that the psychotherapist will be able to maintain the safety of the group and protect each member from any adverse consequences. On the other hand, *group counseling* has a more definite and directed aim. It is concerned with relieving particular problems and with modifying specific situations. To this end, it may be necessary to bring about changes in some attitudes and relationships, but fundamental changes in the structure of personality are not specifically sought. *Group discussions* are done with primary aim of education. The focus of the group work is not upon specific problems, but is upon topics that are presented for development and elucidation. The processes that take place in this group are used to develop and elucidate the topics, and thus they become an educational tool. In contrast to above types of group, in activity groups, the members come together in first instance to take part in some shared activity such as acting, painting etc, in which the leader attempts to make use of occasion provided and the group situation, to help members in other ways.

PRACTICAL ASPECTS OF GROUP PSYCHOTHERAPY

Selection and composition: Group composition remains the most important role of the therapist as it determines the outcome of group therapy. Selection criteria aim to optimize the 'fit' between the requirements and resources of the individual and those of the group. The general characteristics of the patients that determine their selection for group psychotherapy are:

- Motivation to change
- Ability to perform group activity
- Ability to explore problem areas compatible with group goals
- Interest to share problems of self and others
- Ability to sympathize or empathize with other's needs and problems.

Subjects are considered unfit for group therapy if they have the following characteristics:

- Incompatibility with group norms for acceptable behavior
- Intolerance to group setting
- Interpersonal problems with one or more members
- Tendency to assume deviant role, be it subdued, hostile or aggressive
- Patients in acute crisis or having major problems of self-disclosure.

If selection and composition of group are not given due importance, it can lead to high dropout rates and disruption of the therapy situation. Over the years objective measures have been developed to supplement the clinical judgement in selection process. The commonly described instruments for objective measures include Group Therapy Questionnaire and the Group Selection Questionnaire. Another empirical approach to selection emerges from the use of personality inventories such as the NEO-Five Factor Inventory.

Setting: Among the most important pragmatic decisions taken by the therapist is to choose an appropriate meeting place. A setting with privacy and freedom from distraction is essential. The group meeting place should be consistently available and of adequate size and having comfortable sitting arrangement. There is always a need of circular sitting arrangement so that all of the members are able to see each other. Some therapists advocate coffee and tea at meeting place in order to increase the sociability of the setting.

Optimal size: The optimal size for group psychotherapy range from five to nine members, determined by the most practical considerations. Group with fewer numbers will not generate enough interaction, while in group with higher number of members with more members it becomes difficult to examine and understand all of the interactions.

Time boundaries: This is a fundamental part of the therapy, which involves duration, punctual beginnings and endings and predictable frequency of its meetings and breaks. There is a clinical consensus that the optimal duration for group session should be between 60 and 120 minutes. Usually 20–30 minutes are required for the group to warm up, and at least 60 minutes are essential to discuss the major themes of a session. After 2 hours, most therapists find themselves fatigued and the group becomes tired and repetitious. The frequency of group meetings can vary from once a day (inpatient setting), to once a week (outpatient groups) and to once a month as in clinic medication-support group. A once weekly schedule is most commonly followed for outpatient groups and well suited for supportive or specialized groups.

Open vs closed groups: Some groups have a set number and composition of patients. If members leave, no new members are taken in and it is termed as a closed group. An open group is one in which there is more fluidity of membership, new members are taken on whenever old members leave.

Inpatient vs outpatient groups: Although the therapeutic factors that account for change in the small inpatient group are similar to those in the outpatient setting, there are qualitative differences. Relatively high turnover of patients in inpatient group and shorter stay complicates the process of cohesion and imbibing insight, in comparison to outpatient group. Advantage of inpatient group is extragroup interactions, as they live in the same surroundings.

Homogeneous and heterogeneous groups: Homogeneous groups can be utilized for those presenting with similar clinical pictures like phobias, anxiety, or depression. This kind of groups can also be used for those with a similar personality structure or life history, particularly those in socially extreme categories. Heterogeneous groups share one strong characteristic, like diagnosis such as eating disorders, or attribute of personality change like intelligence, with a diversity of presenting problems or social backgrounds.

STAGES IN GROUP FORMATION

Patients who are prepared by the therapist for a group experience tend to continue in treatment longer and report less initial anxiety than do those who are not so prepared. Hence, preparation consists of therapist's explanation before the first session, about the procedure in as much detail as possible and answering all the questions the patients have. Once the members are inducted, the group goes through a process of formation or development, which consists of four indistinct stages of development, i.e. rebeginning, subgrouping, work phase and termination. In the *re-beginning phase* the group's focus is on its external boundary and the common group concerns center on being in or out. In the *sub-grouping phase* the external boundary has usually stabilized and the group members turn their attention to participants within the group to find new alliances. In the *work phase* members start seeing others revealing themselves. The boundary between preconscious and conscious, denied and acknowledged, talked about and not talked out, becomes more obvious. There is surge in group cohesiveness and a marked drop in conflict. In *termination phase*, the group's best functioning members are preparing for discharge. Members concern themselves again with the external boundary. Discharge and aftercare plans are discussed and out-of-group life is a focus.

For the therapist, it is important to review the key points at the termination phase. A review and reinforcement of individual change which has occurred in the therapy should be done and the therapist should guide the departing client to a resolution of the relationships with the therapist and group members. Further the individual is prepared to face future life demands with the tools provided in the therapy.

THERAPEUTIC FACTORS IN GROUP PSYCHOTHERAPY

Researchers have identified a number of mechanisms of change in group therapy, that is, the curative or therapeutic factors. Yalom has derived an atheoretical, 11-factor inventory of the therapeutic mechanisms operating in group therapy, which includes:

- Instillation of hope
- Universality
- Imparting of information
- Altruism
- Development of socializing techniques
- Imitative behavior
- Catharsis
- Corrective recapitulation of the primary family group
- Existential factors
- Group cohesiveness
- Interpersonal learning.

There is a complex interdependency among the three therapeutic factors of cohesiveness, self-disclosure and feedback that promotes a working through process that is also apparent in interpersonal learning-output within the group and productive and enduring intrapsychic changes in object and self-representations. Of the above described therapeutic factors, the mechanism of cohesion is now being considered to be the most central to the therapy. It is considered to be a therapeutic mechanism in itself and also considered to facilitate the action of other therapeutic factors. There is growing consensus that cohesion is the best definition of the therapeutic relationship in group.

THERAPIST'S BASIC TASKS IN GROUP THERAPY

The therapist plays the important role in establishing and maintaining the group and resolving the problems faced in group setting. The therapist's activity is summarized below:

- Establishing a therapy group
  - Group selection and composition
  - Manage the setting (open vs closed group)
  - Deciding about time issues, i.e. frequency and length of sessions
  - Managing boundaries and membership issues
  - Selection of a cotherapist for the group
- Creating a therapy group
  - Formulation of appropriate goals
  - Selection of patients who can perform group task
  - Preparing patients for group therapy
- Constructing and maintaining a therapeutic environment
  - Allow and cultivate free-floating discussion
  - Location and resolution of common problems and focal conflicts of group
  - Use procedural aids as appropriate
- Analysis and interpretation
  - The therapist works as both therapist as well as group member.
  - Analysis of transference issues and provide metaphorical constructions for defenses and resistances
  - Interpretation and therapist use of counter-transference
  - Translate from the language of unconscious (individual or group) behavior to conscious behavior
- Leadership activity
  - Therapist provides holding, containment and reflection
  - Model a capacity for open direct communication
  - Maintain therapeutic neutrality
  - Provide linking communications
  - Clarification and confrontation with individuals
  - Bring background events to foreground or vice-versa
  - Attention to omissions, avoidance or denial
  - Maintain silence-lead from behind.

TECHNIQUES OF GROUP THERAPY

Although similar psychotherapeutic techniques are used by individual and group therapists, a number of interventions, are unique to group therapy, which include working in the here and now, use of transference and therapist transparency and use of various procedural aids.

Working in the 'here and now': In group therapy, interpersonal learning requires a leader, who is well versed in the techniques of working in 'here and now'. The focus consists of a rotating sequence of affect-evocation followed by affect- examination. For the first stage, i.e. the stage of emotional experience, the therapist needs a set of techniques that will plunge the group into the immediate interpersonal interactions. For the second stage, clarification and understanding of emotional experience, the therapist needs a set of techniques that will help the group transcend itself to examine and interpret its own experiences.

Use of transference and therapist transparency: True transference influences the nature of the group discourse. To work effectively with transference in the therapy group, therapist must help patients to recognize, understand and change their distorted attitudinal sets. Two major approaches or techniques facilitate transference resolution in therapy group. The first involves consensual validation by other group members of the patient's distorted views, while second approach makes use of increased therapist transparency.

Procedural aids: At times, therapeutic armamentarium of group leader can be expanded with procedural aids, i.e. the use of written summaries, videotaping, and structured exercises.

Modification of Basic Techniques for Specialized Clinical Settings

The therapist must learn to modify fundamental group therapy principles and techniques in order to work in some specialized clinical settings with following basic steps:

1. *Assessment of clinical setting:* The therapist must carefully determine the immutable clinical restraints surrounding the group, and take steps to change those factors that might hinder the group.
2. *Formulation of goals:* The therapist must formulate appropriate goals within the existing clinical restraints. Yalom described six achievable goals for the inpatient setting, which are engaging patients in the therapeutic process, teaching patients that talking helps, problem spotting, decreasing isolation, allowing patients to be helpful and alleviating hospital-related anxiety.
3. *Modification of traditional techniques:* The therapist must retain the basic principles of group therapy but alter techniques to adapt to the clinical setting and to fulfill the formulated goals. Four essential modifications are to adopt a radically shortened time frame, show direct support, emphasize the 'here- and- now' and provide structure.

ETHICAL ISSUES IN GROUP PSYCHOTHERAPY

Effective group work with minimal adverse outcomes requires ethical practice. The therapist must have knowledge base, technical skills and certain personality characters in order to attain ethical competence in group psychotherapy. Such competence entails knowing both the rules established by one's profession, federal, state, and local statutes, and the case law that guides practice. Beyond a mastery of rules and laws, decision-making about ethical issues requires the group psychotherapist's possession of additional tools.

- At times despite having adequate knowledge base and technical skills, the therapist may not be able to practice ethics unless he has certain personal qualities to utilize the resources well. Five virtues of the moral practitioner which the therapists must possess include compassion, discernment (cognitive ability to understand the workings of an ethical problem), trustworthiness, integrity and conscientiousness.
- Many guidelines are available for ethical practice of group psychotherapy. However, the primary resource for the therapist is the set of ethical principles that underlie professional ethical codes and that have been accepted within the helping professions since antiquity-beneficence, nonmaleficence, respect for autonomy, fidelity and justice.
- In the group therapy situation the same action often serves both as beneficence and nonmaleficence, and at times these principles can be at odds with one another. This occurs more often in group setting because multiple parties are being treated simultaneously and may be differentially affected by the same intervention or process. Obtaining an informed consent that comprehensively outlines potential benefits, risk, and methods employed in the group is one way that group therapists apply the principle of respect for autonomy. With adequate information, prospective members can make meaningful decisions about whether there is congruence between the goals of the group and their personal goals and whether the methods are ones which clients are willing to use. Interventions designed to ensure that members maintain one another's confidentiality are also in the service of the respect for autonomy principle. The emphasis on confidentiality also conforms to the principle of nonmaleficence as lapses in confidentiality can have serious negative impact on the concerned member's extra group life. The therapist need to maintain fidelity by he or she remaining loyal to the client and acting in accordance with the trust the client has placed in him or her. Further, fidelity requires that the therapist be governed by each group member's interests rather than his or her own interests. The principle of justice requires that the therapist be responsive to the special needs of different groups of people, particularly groups that have been subjected to oppression and discrimination.
- At time the ethical principles can be at odds with one another and thus creating ethical dilemmas. The therapist should have an ability to identify circumstances in which these principles may be in conflict with one another. Often, the first sign that an ethical dilemma has arisen is the therapist's subjective sense of unease. The therapist needs to determine the relative strength of the ethical principles in relation to the particular circumstance and find the means to accommodate them which is often known as balancing. By balancing ethical principles, the therapist can identify an ethically grounded course of action.
- The therapist must also possess a systematic decision-making process to resolve conflicts satisfactorily and develop an ethically defensible course of action. Haas and Malouf's system of decision making process is one that has achieved particular prominence. This system directs to proceed through two phases of resolving ethical dilemma. The first is the gathering of information and the second involves decision making process itself.
- However it is important to remember that various ethical guidelines tend to relate to the common rather than unusual situations that therapists encounter. They also tend to be generic and fail to capture the nuances of situations in which ethical problems can emerge. Although, they are generally useful in everyday practice, but this generality also limits their usefulness. These limitations require that group therapists have something else available to negotiate those challenges that emerge in everyday practice.

SELECTION OF GROUP PSYCHOTHERAPY: ACCORDING TO DISORDERS

Studies have shown that group approaches offers promise as an intervention when used as an adjunct to medications in dealing with patients suffering from various mental health problem and also for physical illnesses. Among the various models psychoeducational model and supportive models have been used more frequently for many disorders.

Schizophrenia and other psychotic disorders: Group therapy is useful to manage problems of social isolation, to develop social skills and coping resources and to learn about appropriate interactions in the group. Further the group interventions have also been used to manage antipsychotic induced side effects like weight gain. Schizophrenia patients perform best in supportive groups or group interventions based on cognitive behavioral principles that help them to manage their symptoms and formulate coping strategies for day-to-day problems.

Personality disorders: Working with patients of personality disorders creates difficult clinical problems due to several causes, i.e. inability to form a stable therapeutic alliance, mood fluctuations, poor impulse control, limited reflective ability and self-destructive gestures. Short-term group therapy based on cognitive, behavioral and psychodynamic approaches has shown promising results. Long-term therapies have been encouraging but have not been evaluated.

Anxiety disorders: Group psychotherapy, when combined with psychotropic drugs shows good results in patients with anxiety disorders. People with high degree of anxiety require a good, trusting relationship with therapist before they actually enter into therapy group. Homogeneous groups are advocated in patients with PTSD and to some extent in patients with social phobias. Patients with somatoform disorders get benefit from small, homogeneous and supportive group. In eating disorders, an educational approach, followed by encouragement of interpersonal learning and intrapsychic exploration, is recommended.

Mentally retarded people/pervasive developmental disorders: The needs for closeness, love, sharing and acceptance are as important to the mentally retarded population as to all other members of our social structure. If these needs are dealt with realistically and if their existence is accepted as a normal part of personality development, it becomes possible for retarded individuals to change those disruptive behaviors that alienate families and professionals. A responsive, active, limit-setting but accepting therapist provides the framework to assist the retarded clients in reducing hyperactive and impulsive behavior patterns and to improve realistic socialization responses. Group therapy may also be an important modality for better understanding and developing crucial social skills among the children diagnosed with a pervasive developmental disorder.

Dementia: Recent reports suggest that group methods may be useful for patients suffering from Alzheimer's disease as well as for their caretakers. Group therapy utilizing techniques derived from psychodrama (such as dance, rhythm, and songs) and from storytelling (focusing on general human themes related to different life stages) help improve quality of life of demented patients as they socialize with one another and remember and make associations to situations and events they experienced earlier in their lives. Psychoeducational group approach for caregivers of Alzheimer's patient is effective in decreasing the distress.

Trauma victims: Group work with trauma victims, viz., survivors of sexual abuse, war trauma and torture and other kinds of violence, is comparatively new field in group psychotherapy. These groups provide an environment in which victims can realize their own potential for self-healing.

Couple groups: This group-analytic approach, first described by Foulkes has been developed to resolve marital problems in marital groups. These groups serve for people in stable but troubled relationships in which there is some pernicious collusion.

Elderly people: This remains an area of relatively new therapeutic exploration. A number of groups have been found useful in helping the elderly persons to face their problems, improve their functioning, and feel happier about them. Psychodynamically oriented group therapy with older adults tries to address existential, system, diagnostic and cohort issues. Themes of physical health, disability, narcissism and shame have also been addressed.

Alcohol and drug dependent patients: Group psychotherapy adds a significant therapeutic dimension in management of this population through a variety of group strategies.

Medically ill: Group therapies have been used for those with acute conditions (renal dialysis and organ transplantation), chronic conditions (diabetes, irritable bowel syndrome, and rheumatic disease), and life-threatening conditions (metastatic cancers). For these conditions, usually the groups are homogeneous, short-term and psychoeducational in nature. These groups stress on the importance of compliance with treatment regimes and opportunities to share and explore affective consequences of the conditions.

GROUP PSYCHOTHERAPY: INDIAN TRADITION

In the words of Swami Vivekananda, the difference of the life style between Indian and American societies becomes crystal clear, *"In the West, they are trying to solve the problem of how much a man can possess, and we are trying in India to solve the problem of on how little a man can live".* India's religion and philosophy contains invaluable psychological material that makes the Indian psychologist's task much easier, provided they dare look beyond their British-American psychological orientation.

Vedas, Upanishads. Sankhya-yoga, Bhagavad-Gita and several other Hindu spiritual systems can create important place in the international strategies of Westem oriented psychologists. In *Bhagavad-Gita,* the therapist *Krishna* makes some important comments relating to group situations.

According to traditional Indian system, society is regarded as functional organization and conflict with social tradition causes alienation. Lack of understanding of others, as well as self, causes inability to make decisions. A mature person needs to be free from social distraction and yet at the same time he should be able to help others in the attainment of happiness. One should consider the effects of his actions on others.

Four basic steps of the 8-fold path of *Sankhya-Yoga* as prescribed by *Maharishi Patanjali:*
- Practice of truth, nonviolence, restrained sex and nonstealing
- Practice of keeping body clean, mind content, persistence, reading and faith in the God
- Practice of breathing exercise and physical postures
- Meditation.

The other components like theoretical advice, discussion, teaching and reply of individual queries do require greater theoretical and practical adjustments in the existing psychotherapeutic framework.

EFFICACY OF GROUP INTERVENTIONS

The empirical foundation for understanding group treatments has grown substantially since the earliest investigations of group process and outcome in the years immediately following World War II. Of course, the sophistication and methodological rigor of the research projects varies tremendously from simple questionnaires administered to a single treatment group, to highly complex multivariate approaches conducted with large numbers of patients in multiple group settings. Initial formal surveys of the outcome of group psychotherapy and T-group first appeared during the early 1960s. These initial reviews offered highly tentative conclusions regarding the efficacy of group interventions. However, the later literature in the field of group psychotherapy suggests that group treatments represent a powerful therapeutic intervention, with positive outcomes in alcoholism, anxiety disorders, bereavement, bulimia, depression, schizophrenia, and sexual abuse. Data from recent well-designed and well-controlled studies attest to the value and utility of groups as a primary form of psychiatric treatment.

Schizophrenia: Over the years many studies (some of which are shown in Table 2) have evaluated the efficacy of different types of group psychotherapy as an adjunctive treatment in the management of schizophrenia. Most of these studies have compared one type of group intervention with other type of group intervention or individual psychotherapy for various target symptoms. Most of these studies have shown that group interventions are effective as an adjunct for management of psychotic symptoms, increasing treatment adherence and compliance, decreasing relapse and rehospitalization and reducing the treatment emergent side effects like weight gain.

Bipolar disorders: As is seen in schizophrenia, group interventions have also been found to be useful as adjunctive measures for the management of bipolar disorders (some of the studies are shown in Table 3) for reducing the relapse rates, improving the interpersonal functioning and productivity, social adjustment and overall functioning.

Depression: In a review, Oei et al. (2008) reported that group cognitive behavior therapy was effective for a range of samples and diagnostic subgroups of depression and it compares well

Table 2: Group interventions for schizophrenia

Authors	*Target*	*Type of intervention and comparison group*	*Outcome*
Miller and Mason, 2001	Treatment adherence	Group intervention versus individual therapy	Group therapy intervention had better treatment adherence
Newton et al. 2005	Recent onset auditory hallucinations	Group CBT	Significant reductions in auditory hallucinations with group CBT compared to wait list during the treatment phase
Barrowclough et al. 2006	Persistent psychotic symptoms	Group CBT	No significant difference with usual measures in reducing hallucinations and delusions but had important benefits in reduction of feelings of hopelessness and self-esteem
Drury et al. (1996 a,b) and Drury (1999) RCT (N=40)	Positive psychotic symptoms, especially delusions	Group and individual CBT versus structured activity	CBT better than structured activity in symptoms reduction; symptoms also reduced at a faster rate
Wykes et al. 1999	Treatment resistant auditory hallucinations	Group intervention versus wait list control prior to therapy	Patients showed significant improvement over the treatment period in insight, experience of hallucinations, and number of coping hallucinations strategies which were maintained at follow-up; no changes during waiting period
Bechdolf et al. 2004 RCT (N=80)	Hospitalization, relapse and compliance rate, psychopathology	Group CBT versus group psychoeducation (PE)	Group CBT patients had decreased hospitalization and relapse rate; increased compliance rate; maintained psychopathological improvement at post term and follow-up

Contd...

Contd...

Authors	*Target*	*Type of intervention and comparison group*	*Outcome*
LI et al. 2005 (N=101; sample of Chinese people; RCT)	Knowledge about illness, symptoms and functioning	Group family education administered by nurses versus treatment as usual	Family education effective in improving knowledge, symptom scores and functioning
Chien et al. 2007 RCT	Families' burden of care and functioning; patients' functioning, symptoms, and rehospitalization rates	Family psychoeducation group program versus routine psychiatric outpatient care	Found to be beneficial on all outcome measures
Chien et al. 2004 RCT; N=32 families in each group	Patients' psychosocial functioning, use of mental health services, and rehospitalization	Mutual support multiple-family-group intervention compared with psycho-education intervention and standard care	Mutual support intervention was associated with greater improvements in patients' functioning and rehospitalization and stable use of mental health services compared with the other two
Newton et al. 2005 N=22 (using a waiting list control)	Persisting auditory hallucinations	Group CBT	Significant reductions in auditory hallucinations over total treatment phase, but not over waiting period
Penn et al. 2009 (65 participants with schizophrenia spectrum disorders and persistent hallucinations)	*Primary outcomes*: Auditory hallucinations, beliefs about voices Secondary outcomes: psychotic symptoms, self-esteem, social functioning, insight, depression, and hospitalization	Group CBT versus enhanced group supportive therapy	Outcomes improved through 12-month follow-up in both therapy groups, with enhanced ST having more specific impact on auditory hallucinations, and CBT impacting general psychotic symptoms
Alvarez-Jiménez et al. 2008 (Meta-analysis)	Antipsychotic-induced weight gain in patients with first episode or chronic schizophrenia	Adjunctive non-pharmacological interventions, either individual or group interventions, or CBT as well as nutritional counseling	Effective in reducing or attenuating antipsychotic-induced weight gain compared with treatment as usual; effects maintained over follow-up
Chien, 2008 (RCT; N= 68 Chinese families of schizophrenia sufferers in Hong Kong)	Patient and family functioning, duration of re-hospitalization	Family psychoeducation and mutual support group vs a routine care group	Greater improvements on patient and family functioning and shorter lengths of hospitalizations compared with the routine care group
Weber et al. 2006 (individuals with schizophrenia or schizoaffective disorder taking atypical antipsychotics)	Body weight, body mass index, waist–hip ratios, and fasting glucose levels	16 week cognitive behavioral group intervention	Group that received CBT lost more weight than treatment as usual group although the difference was not statistically significant
Kingsep et al. 2003 N=33 (individuals with schizophrenia and co-morbid social anxiety)	Anxiety, Psychopathology, Depression, QOL and Enjoyment and satisfaction	Cognitive behavioral group treatment (CBGT) versus waitlist control (WLC)	All outcome measures displayed statistical improvement in the intervention group compared with no change in the control group; treatment gains were maintained at follow-up
Pekkala et al. 2009 (Review; the Cochrane collaboration)	Compliance, relapse	All relevant RCTs (10 included) focusing on psychoeducation for schizophrenia and/or related serious mental illnesses involving individuals or groups	All studies of group education included family members; compliance with medication significantly improved in a single study using brief group intervention (at one year) but other studies produced equivocal or skewed data. Any kind of psychoeducational intervention significantly decreased relapse or readmission rates at nine to 18 months follow-up compared with standard care

Table 3: Group interventions for bipolar affective disorder

Retzer et al. 1991 (20 bipolar and 10 schizoaffective disorder patients)	Relapse rate, interactional style measure	Group psychoanalytic psychotherapy	Significant reduction in relapse rate at 3 years follow-up in both diagnostic groups
Cerbone et al. 1992 (43 bipolar patients)	Number of affective episodes, productivity, interpersonal functioning	Group psychoanalytic psychotherapy	Improvements on all measures
Hallensleben et al. 1994 (N=37)	Self-reported benefit	Group psychoanalytic psychotherapy	Most patients felt the benefit
Palmer et al. 1995 (4 bipolar out patients; single group repeated measures)	Internal States Scale (ISS), Social Adjustment Scale (SAS), Symptoms Checklist-90 (SCL-90)	Group CBT (17 weekly and 6 monthly sessions)	Improvement in mood and social adjustment
Kanas et al. 1998 (12 bipolar patients)	Attendance rate, coverage of intended topics	Group psychoanalytic psychotherapy	72% attendance, 81% topic coverage, greater cohesion, less avoidance and conflict
Patelis-Siotis et al. 2001 (open label study)	Functioning	Group CBT (14 weekly sessions) in addition to pharmacotherapy	Significant increase in psychosocial functioning as assessed by Global Assessment of Functioning scale and the Medical Outcomes Survey SF-36
Saksa et al. 2009 (review of CBT for early psychosis)		Group versus individual CBT	Findings suggest that group CBT may be a more effective modality

Table 4: Group interventions for children and adolescents

Kellner, 1999 (N=7 adolescents)	Anger and aggression	Group anger management program (included psychoeducation, anger discrimination training, writing down incidents of anger, and training in prosocial responses to anger	Significant improvement on both teacher and parents versions of the conduct subscale of the connors rating scale
Snyder et al. 1999 (N=50, adolescent psychiatric in patients)	Acquisition of anger management skills, and effective transfer and implementation of those skills in naturally occurring social interactions	Brief manual-based group therapy intervention (4 session) for anger management given over 2 weeks period	Effective for training adolescent psychiatric inpatients in methods of anger management
Clarke et al. 1999 (N=123 adolescents with major depression or dysthymia from a community sample)	Depression	Group CBT (adolescent only versus adolescent plus parents) versus waiting list control group	Higher depression recovery rate and greater reduction in self-reported depression with group CBT; no significant difference in outcomes for adolescent only and adolescent plus parent cohorts

with drug treatment and other forms of psychological therapy including individual cognitive behavior therapy and group therapy is more cost-effective in comparison to individual therapies or medications.

Anxiety disorders: Group interventions have also been evaluated in a range of anxiety disorders. Van Ingen et al. (2009) evaluated the efficacy of group cognitive behavior therapy for a group of patients with primary diagnosis of generalized anxiety disorder, panic disorder with agoraphobia, social phobia, specific phobia or obsessive compulsive disorder. Of the 31 participants, 17 treatment completers (defined by a minimum of 20 sessions in a flexibly bounded psychotherapy group) achieved significant reductions in anxiety related dysfunction.

Children and adolescents: Since maturational limitations make it difficult to utilize traditional forms of nondirective talk therapy for children and adolescents, therapeutic groups for children and adolescents typically employ expressive

Table 5: Group interventions for dual diagnosis patients

Aubrey et al. 2003 Quasi experiment; N = 56 outpatients with dual diagnosis	Substance use and mental health outcomes, QOL, functioning	Group therapy based on staged treatment (monthly sessions for 9 months) versus treatment as usual	Decreased alcohol consumption per client report but not clinician report; no differences in drug use outcomes or treatment progress; No group differences in mental health outcomes; Improvement in QOL; no differences in hospitalization, community functioning, or work outcomes
Bellack et al. 2006 Experiment; N = 175 outpatients with severe and persistent mental illness and cocaine, heroin, or marijuana dependence	Substance use outcomes, activities of daily living	Group behavioral treatment (motivational interviewing and contingency strategies) versus supportive group therapy for 6 months	Increased total and continuous abstinence; increased proportion of negative urine drug screens; no difference in days with drug problems or number of days drugs used; improved ability to complete activities of daily living
James et al. 2004 Experiment; N = 63 outpatients with nonorganic psychotic disorder and harmful substance use or dependence	Substance use and mental health outcomes; hospitalization rate	Integrated treatment (supportive group therapy and education, medication management) for 6 weeks versus one psychoeducational session with treatment as usual	Decreased alcohol, drug, marijuana and polysubstance use; decreased severity of dependence; decreased psychiatric symptoms; decreased medication use; decreased rate of hospitalization
Weiss et al. 2000 Quasi experiment; N = 45 outpatients with bipolar disorder and substance dependence	Abstinence, mental health outcomes, medication compliance, hospitalization	Integrated group therapy for 12–20 sessions versus no treatment	Decreased drug use; increased total and consecutive days of abstinence; no difference in days of use or alcohol use; no group differences in mental health outcomes; no group differences in medication compliance or hospitalizations
Weiss et al. 2007 Experimental; N = 62 with bipolar disorder and substance dependence	Abstinence rate, mental health outcomes, group attendance	Integrated group therapy versus group therapy focused on substance abuse (20 sessions)	Decreased alcohol use; decreased total substance use; improved abstinence; no group differences in mental health outcomes; improved group therapy attendance

media (e.g. symbolic play, art and crafts, video games, *yoga*) to facilitate emotional communication. Studies have shown that group interventions have useful for management of anger and aggression (see Table 4). Group cognitive behavior therapy has been found useful for management of depression in children and adolescents.

Dual diagnosis: Group interventions have also been evaluated for management of patients with dual diagnosis. Studies (Table 5) have shown that group interventions not only reduce the intake of substance but also lead to improved mental health outcome.

FUTURE DIRECTIONS AND CONCLUSION

Group psychotherapy is a widely practiced mode of treatment employed in a diverse range of settings with a proven degree of effectiveness. It makes use of a host of therapeutic factors that are unique to this type of therapy. Therapists must understand the particular mechanisms of change at work in varied kinds of groups and employ appropriate methods to facilitate them and to achieve the desired goals.

The current overview of group psychotherapy clearly documents the unique learning opportunities available in group treatments. Contrary to individual therapies, there is much less 'talking about' outside interpersonal difficulties and more 'living through' relationship issues within the context of treatment. The group psychotherapy situation is less contrived and therefore more likely to approximate the patient's day-to-day reality; that is, to stimulate the very conflicts that promoted the patient to seek treatment in the first place. The group modality also has the potential to evoke uniquely powerful process to effect changes in those maladaptive patterns. Sharing self-doubts, angry feelings, and blocks in the area of intimacy with a group of contemporaries is decidedly different from disclosing those same feelings to a therapist who does not reciprocate. Struggling with peers to understand common interpersonal dilemmas, while at the same time striving to construct facilitative group norms, represents a unique learning environment with characteristics not found in the one-to-one treatment setting. The correspondence of these interpersonal processes to outside relationship increases the probability that learning will generalize beyond the immediate context of treatment.

Group leaders make use of very specific techniques and interventions that include working in the here- and- now, therapist transparency, and the use of various procedural aids to suit any specialized setting.

Recently, the notion of evidence-based practice has gained further acceptance and momentum. The establishment of the American Group Psychotherapy Association (AGPA) task force has played a major role in this. In the Western world, evidence based practice has increasingly become a matter of public policy. Many would argue that the overall cost-efficiency and effectiveness of both outpatient and inpatient group psychotherapy have already been amply demonstrated. However, it is likely that in the near future individual clinicians will be asked to provide convincing evidence that the particular forms of group psychotherapy they practice actually work with their particular types of patients.

Group therapies which are specific, documentable and replicable are being favored now-a-days. There seems to be a trend towards electic group therapies which are characterized by technical integration. Attempts are now being made in educating group therapy practitioners. This is exemplified by provision of guidelines for teaching a basic course in group psychotherapy, highlighting issues involved in the ethical practice of group psychotherapies.

47.5 FAMILY AND MARITAL THERAPY

Ajit Avasthi, Hitesh Khurana, Sandeep Grover, Munish Aggarwal

INTRODUCTION

The family is a group of mutually interacting people, living together with the purpose of proper growth and development of its constituting members. With time, its structure and functions have undergone tremendous changes, yet it formed the basic unit of human civilization in all cultures.[36] The family fulfills the individual's need for food, shelter and protection against external dangers. It helps in achieving social affiliation and establishing affectional bonds. It provides the individual an opportunity for personal identity, shaping sexual behavior, social roles and responsibilities. Thus, family clearly helps in determining individual's role as husband-wife; mother-father or children, etc.[37] Family provides the individual a direction for establishing relationship with society. It can be imagined that without family, society would have been full of chaos.

The smallest group of mutually interacting individuals and doing the functions of a family is that of the marital or cohabiting partners. They may be drawn together for emotional reasons, empathic attraction,[37] similarities,[38] or complementarity.[39] Each partner unconsciously desires to fulfill its needs from this union; the psychic identity of marital couple also derives from this union, they interact and re-differentiate to start a new family.

FAMILY AND MENTAL DISORDER

Many times in psychiatry, the identified patient may be the product of pre-existing family psychopathology. The family members often relate to each other through interlocking neurotic roles that maintain a homeostasis at a maladaptive or pathological level. Family members consciously or unconsciously accommodate such roles and resist their resolution. Interacting in this way, a controlling or authoritarian parents may produce a rebellious or excessively compliant offspring; an over protected child may feel helpless or may become compulsively independent or defiant. A patient with delusions may induce delusion in the other through close interacting and interdependent roles. Two or more family members emotionally may be at war with the other, yet unconsciously in order to fulfill the needs they may scapegoat the children and avoid explicit discord. The mother may involve the child against the father, who drinks frequently, which ultimately increases relational distance between the children and father too.

Psychological interventions in the form of family therapy may help in all such situations including family violence that is becoming increasingly common.[40] Reduction in expressed emotions of family members has been shown to be effective in reducing rate of schizophrenia relapses.[41] Outcome of depressive illness has been better in couple therapeutic approach compared to individual therapy.[42] Thus, family therapeutic approaches have an established role in the relationship problems as well as in the DSM-IV axis I disorders.[42-49]

HISTORY OF FAMILY AND MARITAL THERAPY

Since very early in the development of psychiatry, the psychiatrist's and psychotherapist's focus of treatment has been resolution of the individual's symptoms. Freud too believed that neurotic symptoms of a person date back to unhealthy interactions with parents during childhood. However, he aimed to isolate the individual, adopt a role of substitute family member and developed a transference relationship to resolve symptoms. Even long after him, the therapist's primary focus remained on the individual symptoms. Consequently, the patient might improve in therapist's office but regress back in the family.

Family therapy is a specialized form of psychotherapy, where in the client are the family rather than individual and interactions within the unit is focus of therapy. Family therapy differs from family psychiatry. *Family therapy* refers to the treatment of cases where pathology primarily lies in the interaction between individuals and only secondarily in the one or more individuals. Modus operandi of family therapy is intricate and focuses on whys and the where's of interactions. In contrast, *family psychiatry* refers to treatment of families where pathology is primarily in one or more individuals and only secondarily in the family interaction. The term family therapy refers to a systematic method of psychotherapeutic intervention on the multiple interlocking emotional disturbances of a family group.[44] It is also defined as any psychotherapeutic method that explicitly focuses on altering the interaction between or among family members and seeks to improve functioning of family or its subsystems and/or functioning of the individual members of the family.[45]

Origin of the family therapy can be traced to the practice of Child Guidance Clinics at the turn of the century.[46] However, it was only in the latter half of the twentieth century when family therapy saw a steady growth and gained importance as method of treatment.[47,48] Ackerman[37] published the first book on family therapy in 1958. Later on, Howell[49] had been the primary advocate of the family therapists for at least twenty years. In the light of these facts, it is sufficient to say that impact of family therapy on the general adult psychiatry practice had been rather late and marginal.[50]

Family therapy found its way into the general practice through the studies searching for the identification of schizophrenogenic families. In 1950s, studies had primarily focused on mother-child symbiotic relationship in the causation of schizophrenia.[49] Bowen[51] held that genetic loading of emotional immaturities of grandparents and parents generate symptoms of schizophrenia in a vulnerable child. Wynne and coworkers[52] reported a pseudomutual and pseudohostile type of communication pattern in the families of schizophrenics, which blocked the psychic development of the individual. These authors concluded that members of such a family may develop schizophrenia when they resist change in interactional pattern on exposure to hostile and coercive external environment in adulthood or through shift or loss of family members. In the same way, skewed relationships, i.e. when one parent competes with the adult and establishes a special bond with the child, had also been found causally linked with the development of schizophrenia.[53] High level of expressed emotions has been consistently linked to the increased probability of relapse in schizophrenia.[41]

Family therapy came of age in seventies. At this time, family therapists began to address themselves to a wider range of disorders with lesser emphasis on patients with schizophrenia and their families. The Philadelphia Child Guidance Clinic under Salvador Minuchin's leadership became one of the world's premier Family Therapy Center, though it established itself completely in 1980's.[54] Mara Selvini Palazzoli played a major role in setting up institute of family study in Milan, Italy. She was one of the four psychoanalytically trained psychiatrists who became famous as Milan Group, the other three being Gianfranco Cecchin, Giuliana Prata and Luigi Bosco. They made an important observation on how families having members with schizophrenia defeated the attempts of the therapist to change their functioning. They proposed the term '*Families in schizophrenic transaction*.' Milan Group also developed techniques of circular interviewing, triadic and reflexive questioning and structuring of session. In late seventies, family therapists emphasized on the use of scientific and solution focused methods of treatment. They felt that telling families what to do and not to do does not always work, at times indirect and paradoxical methods may be needed.[45]

In eighties, many new methods like cognitive approach[55] and systemic family therapy of Luciana LA'bate were developed. In the same decade narrative approaches and technique of externalizing the problems also developed.[45] Thereafter, there has not been any significant new development. However, the role of family therapy as one among the therapeutic modalities became firmly established. The growth of family therapy had been rather theoretical. During this phase, a large number of papers were published regarding effectiveness of this therapy. Comparative studies on family therapy also helped establish it on firm footing. As a result, a new phase in practice incorporating concepts for different schools became popular among therapists. Currently, trends over the different parts of the world suggest that family therapy is becoming firmly established method of choice for couple problems. Secondly, it is proven to be effective for both relationship problems and Axis-I disorders. It has also generated new respect for diverse family forms.[44]

Marital and couple therapy also uses the same principles as of family therapy. In this context, it is difficult to trace the development of couple therapy independent of developments in family therapy. It can be viewed as special form of family therapy, where the presenting members are couple. The term couple therapy is preferable as the presenting members may be cohabiting partners or in homosexual or lesbian relationship. Marital therapy, when viewed as method of improving harmony between the married couple, existed in one or other form since the ancient times. Egyptian deities existed exclusively for the purpose of assuring a happy marital union in addition to a fertile one. Hebrews were known for prescribing certain ritualistic behaviors, which would ensure a happy married life. Instructions on the sexual techniques in the form of love manual were quite popular among the Indians and Arabians.[56] However, the conceptual framework of marital therapy and the practice of using couples in the clinics for interpersonal problems started in the late nineteenth century. In 1920s and 1930s, Pope Popenor conducted seminars on marital relations in United States. At about the same time, Havelock Ellis and Magnus Hirschfeld in Europe were attempting to study sexual dysfunctions in the context of marital relationships. The interest in sexual dysfunction of marital partners further developed in 1960s and 1970s following the studies by William Masters and Virginia Johnson, leading to newer therapeutic techniques and more crystallized results. Till 1960s, the marital partners were usually seen in the clinics individually.[56] It is only for the past 50 years that seeing couples jointly in marital clinics has increased.

GENERAL FACTORS GOVERNING THE FAMILY

A family works as a system in which different family members interact with each other for achieving mutually agreed goals. This interaction is determined by slowly evolved family rules which are allowed by the family members, mostly without being aware of those. In an adequately functioning family, these rules ensure the overall growth of its members and as a group.

The family becomes dysfunctional when these rules fail to accommodate (i) growth needs of its family member (ii) satisfactory achievement of joint outcome, and (iii) does not include means for using outside world to expand and change itself. Then one or more vulnerable family members may demonstrate a symptomatic behavior and present as the identified patients, demanding identification and correction of dysfunction.[49]

The family rules may be identified through the interpersonal interaction between various members that determine family structure, leadership patterns, role structures and role functioning, communication and family adaptive patterns.

Family Structure

The term family structure refers to the repetitive pattern of interaction (or transactions, as called by Minuchin) between various family members. Systemic family therapy outlines three basic subsystems in the family[47]

- *The spouse/couple sub-system*: It contains the relationship between couples, their functioning and roles.
- *The parental subsystems:* It contains the role of parents and their functioning.
- *The siblings subsystems:* It contains the children's relationship, their functioning and roles.

Minuchin[57] considered different members as subsystems, within the broad system of family. The family members interact among themselves according to certain rules, which determine the boundaries of subsystem. A family comprising of the above subsystems can function according to generic/hierarchical or idiosyncratic/irregular family rules. In family operating under generic/hierarchical rules parents are in the control of the situation, there is a good communication and family functions with mutually agreed rules and roles. Whereas, in a family operating under idiosyncratic/irregular rules the parents are not in control and children may be running the family.[47]

The pattern of transactions between any two members is determined by psychological rules called boundaries. It is a dynamic concept, i.e. consistency of boundaries and therefore subsystems may change. The boundaries are determined by various criteria such as age, sex, roles, cultural influences etc. Boundaries between various subsystems can be open, diffused or closed. *Open boundaries* allow the members of the subsystem to carry out their functions without any undue interference and have transactions with the other systems. They are ideal because they are firm yet flexible, permitting maximum adaptation to change. The *closed or rigid boundaries* prevent the members to have a meaningful transaction with other subsystems. It hinders support and limit adaptation in the family. On the other hand, with *diffused boundary,* the interpersonal differences between the members are few and they are extremely sensitive to each other's influences. As the result, with diffused boundaries the distinction of various subsystems is lost. The various sub-systems interfere with each other's working. At the time of change effective guidance cannot take place.[47] Enmeshment and disengagement in relationship also define type of boundaries. Enmeshed members behave as with diffused boundary between them. Whereas disengaged relatives who are emotionally isolated, have rigid boundaries.

With change in family's developmental needs, due to addition or loss of members or because of external stressors, the consistency of different subsystems may change through alignment. In this process, two or more family members may reshape their boundaries to alter the transaction pattern between them. Such type of alignment is called coalition if it works against a family member. Alliance, on the other hand, is a positive or emotionally neutral type of alignment. However, it has an aggressive potential against others. The concept of alignment also includes the phenomenon of triangulation and conflict detouring. In *triangulation,* the two members in a conflict do not work it out together but a third person is brought in who becomes the part of conflict process. In *conflict detouring,* the members in a conflict, pass the conflict to the third party and remain in stable relationship. When one or both parents and child are the parties in this phenomenon, it is also called *cross generation* alliance. If detouring results in scapegoating of the third party, it is called *detour attacking.* But if it results in identification of third party as sick or in need of concern by the detouring members it is called *supportive detouring.*[57]

Leadership Pattern

Leadership in the family context is the capacity to decide what should happen in and to the family. One or more persons in the family may be in a role as leader. Leadership in the family is important for the family in dealing with stressor, problem solving and maintaining homeostasis. It may be determined on the bases of age, sex, education and prevailing cultural patterns in the family, etc. In the matrilineal families, mother is assigned this role, whereas the same role in the patrilineal families is assigned to the father. In pathological families, the choice of leadership, its acceptability and functional adequacy is usually determined by the conflicts of the individual members.

In a particular family, mother may have a controlling and authoritative role because of the strong dependency needs of the husband or because of sickness such as alcoholism in the husband. Husband may dominate because of his own strong narcissistic needs or culturally dominant male aggressiveness and refusal to accept female roles. Such conflicts may produce ambivalent reactions in the other family members also. Leader may also have ambivalent feeling in its authoritative role. Under this situation, the leader may be a nominal leader, assigning executive duties to the other family member, who is generally next in hierarchy. In a seriously disturbed family, no clear leadership pattern may be apparent and its members may work autocratically. Decision-making process and its implementation depend upon the leadership pattern. Under a highly authoritative leadership, decision-making may have a dictatorship pattern whereas in more accommodating families it may have even a democratic way.

Leadership pattern is a longitudinal process depending on persons involved and nature of conflict. There may be changes in the leadership pattern at various times. In the absence or sickness of father, the mother may take over the role of a leader and similarly in absence of parents, one of the siblings may take over this responsibility.

Role Assignment

Roles are prescribed and are repetitive behaviors involving a set of reciprocal activities with other family members.[58] Each family member has a part to play, assigned to him by the family and its cultural heritage. The given role has a potential of emotional health or illness. The idea of *role* has been used to denote prescription, description and evaluation of one's action. The assigned role thus demands a specific and consistent behavior by family members.

Formal roles, the more general roles, depend on factors like age, sex, etc., and the person has no choice over selection of such role, such as the elder family members have a prominent role of nurturing the children, males and females have distinct sex roles such as mother-father, husband-wife, son-daughter, etc. Because of the unique characteristics of individuals determining those roles, such roles are also said to be allocated based on achievement.

Informal roles, on the other hand are not so stylized or patterned. These roles are the loosely patterned ways of behavior, which are usually learnt in childhood and adolescence and are acquired often unconsciously, and are therefore difficult to sort out through cognitive operations. The selection of such roles allows the persons a choice. Therefore, informal roles are allocated because of adoption, where the individual is free to adopt one, the other, or no role at all. Such as, a student may choose to study science or humanities or neither of these.

Fictive roles are the unreal or the imaginary roles taken either in a jest or play or because of defects in reality testing. Such roles are allocated based on assumption, which may change from time to time. Therefore, these roles are also called assumed roles. Any of the roles may be explicit or implicit. Explicit roles occur at the surface of interpersonal relationships, therefore can be easily identified and acknowledged. Implicit roles, on the other hand, are usually hidden from the awareness and are acknowledged with difficulty.

In a normal family, the individuals perform the roles as per sociocultural expectations and with an adequate degree of skill. Family members may adopt *complementary or reciprocal* roles, which fit well with each other's functioning and are generally adaptive in nature. Such as father may have a role to collect raw food material and mother may have complementary role of cooking and one or more children may adopt the role of serving. Symmetrical roles on the other hand denote two family members on equal footing.

In maladaptive situations, one or more family members may have conflicting roles. *Role conflict* refers to a situation where the particular member has difficulty in fulfilling the role obligations because of the incompatible expectations. Role conflict may be in the form of *role diffusion,* when more than one member performs the same role or in the form of *role ambiguity,* when there is no formal recognition of the role a particular member is performing.

The family members in conflict may induce each other to change their roles to meet each other's expectations through various manners such as praising, blaming or coaxing, etc. If these techniques are successful, these may produce sufficient complementarity, without correcting the ideational incongruence. In this way, through *role induction* the conflict instead of being solved is circumvented.[58]

In *role dislocation,* the family members attempt to avoid the conflict by shifting the role, which is the seat of conflict to some other one. This may occur through manners operating implicitly, thus difficult to detect. Role relocation during the course of therapy may take place through resolution of conflict and release of accompanying anxiety. Behaviorists find abnormal roles and leadership patterns due to maladaptive behavior getting rewarded. Along with the communication problems, the roles and the leadership pattern make a strong ground for behavior family therapist to work.

Roles in the family can be assessed by asking following questions[59]

- Who is the breadwinner in the family?
- Who forms the rules in the family?
- Who discusses the family problems?
- Who does the household chores?

Communication Pattern

Whenever two living organisms exist together, they would maintain a contact with each other, to meet their external and internal demands. To fulfill this requirement, communication serves a significant purpose. It facilitates specialization, maturation and differentiation of the individual. Communication is an organizing principle of nature that all biological and social organizations are characterized by the need and the ability to communicate. Depending on the level of sophistication, the individual may utilize verbal and/or nonverbal ways of communication. Interpersonal communication is characterized by the expressive acts of one or more persons followed by conscious or unconscious perception of these actions by other persons and a reply expressing that observation has been perceived. It is the awareness of being perceived that establishes the interpersonal relationships.

Human communication is a dynamic process, influenced by psychological, physiological, and external environmental factors. Depending on the influence of these factors, the pattern of communication may change, but it is impossible not to communicate. Even silence, lack of gestures and affective responses has messages concealed in them to be conveyed.

The pattern of communication can be studied through answering the following questions:

- What is the situation?
- Who are the participants in the situation?
- What is being communicated?
- What channel is being utilized?
- What change has this communication brought?

Communication is clear when the words spoken have an explicit meaning and are spoken to the person concerned. It is unclear when it is mediated by a third person, which reduces the clarity of the message by creating a 'noise' effect. Thus, the message conveyed would be different from the message received. This is called indirect communication. The double bind may be considered as an extreme form of unclear communication where the person addressed is conveyed two incompatible messages simultaneously in a situation out of which he cannot get out. Communication may be verbal when it occurs through written or spoken words, or nonverbal when it is through the means other than language, such as through gestures, appearance and other artifacts. Communication may be paradoxical when simultaneously the statement conveys a message just opposite of what is intended to be conveyed.

Adaptive Patterns

Adaptive patterns refer to the family functioning and management of problems in stressful situations. It involves the methods of conflict resolution and mobilization of social support to deal with stressors. Conflict may be resolved either through adapting an adequate problem solving strategy or through coping, which may be emotional and/or goal-directed. Social support refers to informal and formal relationships and groups through which individual receives moral, cognitive skills necessary to master stressful experiences.

GENERAL PRINCIPLES OF FAMILY THERAPY

The family serves as the intermediate link between the individual and the community. It provides individuals a milieu for their multidimensional development, improving interpersonal skills, ensuring the proper development of participating members, contributing and utilizing the community resources effectively. Thus, the ideal family therapy ensures a proper development of individual, improvement in interpersonal relationship for the individual's well being, and improvement in the family-community interaction. Therefore, while treating a family a high degree of flexibility may be required depending on the dimension of dysfunction. It may start as family therapy but later on individual or dyadic therapies may also be required and vice-versa. In the individual therapy, the therapist establishes a close relationship with the disturbed individual and helps him to resolve the adverse situation and reintegrate him in the family. Whereas in the dyadic therapy, the interaction between any two family members is the focus, the most common being the dyad of husband-wife, when the dyadic therapy takes form of the marital therapy. Thus, in the family therapy it is the whole family rather than a particular identified patient who is the target for effecting a positive change. In this way, the process of family therapy can be viewed as a group therapy process where the individuals having different kinds of problems learn to adjust through direct attention of the therapist through a group experience.

Despite differences in the methods, most of the family therapies find roots in the psychotherapeutic techniques for the individual patients. Technically the family therapy is an extension of individual psychotherapy techniques and puts the same kind of demands on the therapist as in the individual therapy but to a higher magnitude. The therapist may choose any technique for a family depending upon the school of his training or experience. The therapist must be well versed with the technique he selects. As in individual therapy, the therapist should be able to establish an empathic relationship with the different family members in order to identify and evaluate the existing tensions and enmity among various members. As the therapy progresses, he should be able to identify the conflicts, vulnerability of the individuals and their efforts to cope with the feeling of guilt-shame in order to compensate for their shortcomings. Difficulty in identification or conceptualizing these areas of vulnerabilities should be recognized as failure to establish empathy.

In the extreme form of empathic failure, the therapist may be involved in collusion with one or more family members and blame or confront a particular scapegoated member. Somewhat harder to recognize are the problems of subtle rejections, criticism, competing with any particular member or sexualizing the therapeutic process. Counter-transference in family therapy may obstruct the therapeutic process and requires its identification and resolution. Especially in marital therapy, it may exist as competing with the same sex spouse for the approval of the other. It may also be identified through therapist's arbitrariness in selecting what to respond to or ignore. These problems must be managed adequately or these may lead to non-cooperativeness or even treatment discontinuance by the one or more family members.

INDICATIONS AND CONTRAINDICATIONS FOR FAMILY THERAPY

As stated, the aims of the family therapeutic process can be summarized into achieving improvement in functioning and interpersonal relationships. Hence, there can be a wide variety of indications for the family therapy and there does not appear to be any absolute contraindication.

Indications[46,60-61]

- Problems in the relationship within the family (e.g. primary marital discord, existence of communication or generation gap).
- Interdependence of symptoms (e.g. the wife's depression being contingent on the husband's alcohol consumption and vice versa).
- Symptomatology in one individual reflecting a dysfunctional family background (e.g. emotional disorder, delinquency or violent behavior, abuse of a child).
- Development of stress/symptoms in other family members when one family member improves (e.g. development of depression in wife following husband's giving up drinking).
- Failure of individual therapy (may be because family conflicts have not been handled).
- Problems presented solely to produce some desirable change in the relationship even when there is no overt relationship problem.
- Separation difficulties.
- Family, which is severely disorganized, functioning badly in poor socioeconomic situations.
- Inadequate resources for individual treatment of more than one family member needing individual treatment.
- Child abuse and other forms of relationship abuse.
- Psychiatric illness requiring assessment for family therapy (if any of the above indication is met with): Neuroses (anxiety and depression), adjustment disorders, conduct and/or emotional disorder of the childhood, substance abuse (not dependence), sexual dysfunctions (other than sexual deviations).

Contraindications[46]

Family Factors

- Family in the process of breaking up
- Families characterized by deeply-ingrained psychopathology
- Families having major psychopathology unrelated to family interactions in more than one family member
- Families in which tense, dysfunctional equilibrium is present, attempt to change may lead to severe decompensation
- Presence of family sectors (e.g. extra-marital relations, homosexual tendencies) not accessible to therapy
- Family members staying apart
- Presence of situational constraints such as inability to afford cost, give up other activities to participate in the session, legal complication in the family
- Nonavailability of the key family member
- Unwillingness to accept the therapy
- Family presenting very late in the course of problem
- Severe medical illness
- Escalating physical harm.

Therapist Factors

- Lack of training/commitment/empathy
- Inflexibility
- Poor psychological mindedness, judgmental attitude, cultural biases
- Therapist having problems similar to the clients' problems
- Therapist in social relations with the family/family member.

FAMILY ASSESSMENT

Conducting an assessment interview requires not only clarity of thought and purpose on the part of therapist, but also requires tact, judgment, intuitive sensitivity and a degree of imagination. It demands a specific level of clinical skill to maintain a balance between disclosure and privacy, as insufficient disclosure precludes effective assessment while lack of privacy because of asking for over-elaborate details may induce in the patient, a sense of having been exposed and violated.[62] Therefore, assessment of family demands an initial training and supervision of the therapist's learning. Many models of family assessment have been developed by the therapists depending upon the theoretical school of their practice. These models are summarized in the Table 6. All these resemble one another closely.

McMaster Model[63] and Process Model[64]

McMaster model of functioning and process model of family functioning consider the six aspects of family functions. There is only slight difference between these two (Table 7).

Problem solving and task accomplishment: Both McMaster's and process model consider three types of tasks for the family: basic, developmental and crisis tasks. Basic task take the physiological needs of the family into consideration, e.g. provision of food, shelter, health care. The developmental tasks are the specific tasks required at different stages of life. These may vary from individual to individual. A well-functioning family is sensitive to the needs of individual and makes necessary adjustments to meet these needs. Crisis tasks are those for which family has to exercise their maximum skill and utilize resources. Such problems are often in case of death, migration, illness of family member, etc. Additionally, McMaster model also considers affective problems such as hostility or distrust between family members and communication about different problems to the concerned members. The effective families solve their problems more effectively as compared to the problem families.[55]

Roles: Problem solving always requires that family members do their roles effectively. McMaster model distinguishes between necessary and other roles performed by family members. It involves the various roles being assigned to the family members (allocation) and fulfillment of those roles by the family members (accountability).[55] The necessary roles include provision of material resources, nurturance, and life skill development. The other roles are those which are unique to a family member such as scapegoating or idealizing a family member. The effective families are able to maintain family function and fulfill their roles while the disturbed families do not have consistency in their role functioning and have poor accountability in family functioning.[55]

Table 7 shows comparison between McMaster and process model. The process model describes roles as either traditional or idiosyncratic. The traditional are same as the necessary roles describe by McMaster model. Idiosyncratic roles encompass other roles that often depict severe family pathology.

Control: This term is same as behavior control in McMaster model. It denotes the influence of family members on one another. It also includes leadership pattern. It refers to how family shapes the members' behavior in domains of

Table 6: Models for family assessment

•	McMaster model of family function
•	Process model of family functioning
•	Structural approach
•	Triaxial scheme
•	Circumplex model
•	Darlington family assessment system

Table 7: Comparison of McMaster and process model

Process model	*McMaster model*	*Assessment*
Problem solving	Task accomplishment	• Identify the task, exploring the alternative approaches, selecting the approach and taking action, monitoring results and making adjustment
Communication	Communication and affective expression	• Verbal or nonverbal, sufficient, direct topic of communication instrumental (about daily activities), emotional or neutral
Affective involvement	Affective involvement	• Degree and quality of involvement, whether because of real need or any other cause
Affective responses Affective involvement		• It concerns with the range and appropriateness of the family members' emotional interaction
Behavioral control	Control	• Who controls whom and how, leadership, control: rigid, flexible, etc.
Roles	Roles	• Traditional or necessary roles, idiosyncratic or other roles
---	Values and norms	• All social, moral religious concerns that are acceptable and not acceptable to family

dangerous situations, development of socialization skills, and satisfying/regulating biological needs and drives.[65]

Behavior control can be rigid, flexible, laissez-faire and chaotic. *Rigid control* is high on predictability but low on adaptability and constructiveness. It may work well in managing day-to-day activities but not when some change is required. This aspect may encourage punitive behavior leading to subversion, passive aggressive behavior, power struggle and displacement of anger. *Flexible control* is predicable, constructive and can adapt well to changing circumstances. Its supportive and educational influences help family members to participate and to identify with the ideals and rules of family. *Laissez-faire* means "anything goes." Inertia and indecisiveness are the rules for such control. This control may be fully predictable but low on constructiveness. Such control often creates insecurity, attention seeking among children. In the situations outside family where high standard of behavior is required, it often becomes difficult to adapt. *Chaotic* control *does* not have any fixed pattern and may have rigidity and indecision of *laissez-faire* style depending on whims of family member. Of all the type of controls, this is the most pathological.

Affective involvement: Affective involvement is the degree and quality of family members' concern for others. The following types of involvement are listed in both models:

- *Lack of involvement (uninvolved of the process model)*: Family members live like strangers. They are generally alienated.
- *Interest devoid of feelings*: In such cases, family members seem involved with one another due to sense of duty, need to control or curiosity.
- *Narcissistic involvement*: One family member is involved with others because of his feeling of self-importance rather than due to concern or caring for the persons.
- *Empathic involvement*: This is the real understanding of needs of those with whom the subject is involved.
- *Enmeshment*: The family members are over concerned, about each other. The responses to each other's needs are often exaggerated.

Affective response: It refers to how the family members emotionally interact with each other. Healthy families have appropriate ways of responding to each others' emotional needs and have full range of emotional interaction, whereas, unhealthy families use limited means of interacting with each other.[65]

Communication: This dimension is considered by all models of assessment. The McMaster model considers only verbal communication as it is easy to assess. A clear communication, whether verbal or non-verbal, is often desirable. Healthier families use clear and direct communication while unhealthy families use unclear and indirect means of communication.[30]

Values and norms: This aspect includes the sum total of all those moral, religious and social values, which are and are not acceptable to the family as a whole. However, McMaster model does not include it in the assessment but it is certainly of great value for therapist to know all these. These values and norms may include many minor issues, e.g. fixing bed time and meal time of family members to many complex issues such as drug use and discussing about sex among children.

Triaxial System of Assessment.[66]

As proposed by Tseng and McOermott[66] triaxial system divides the family dysfunction in three categories as shown in Table 8.

Circumplex Model[67-69]

This model is based on measurement of cohesiveness and adaptability/flexibility and communication of the family in different situations. Cohesion measures emotional bonding

Table 8: Triaxial system of family assessment

Axis I (Family development dysfunction)	*Axis II (Family subsystem dysfunction)*	*Axis III (Family group dysfunction)*
A. Developmental dysfunction • Difficulty in establishing satisfactory marital relationship • Childbearing family dysfunction • Childrearing family dysfunction • Maturing family dysfunction-problems of differentiation and separation • Contracting family dysfunction	**A. Spouse-system dysfunction** • Complimentary marital dysfunction-unequal marital relationship • Conflicting marital dysfunction-couples in conflict • Disengaged marital dysfunction-couples are emotionally uninvolved • Incompatible marital dysfunction	**A. Structural- functional dysfunction** • Under performing families • Over structured/rigid families • Emotionally overinvolved families • Emotionally detached families • Disorganized families
B. Developmental complications and variations • Family crisis associated with separation (divorce) • Single parent family • Remarriage with children already present • Chronic unstable family-Frequent moves, separations, etc.	**B. Parent child subsystem dysfunction** • Parent centered dysfunction • Child related dysfunction • Parent child interaction dysfunction • Parent child triangular dysfunction **C. Sibling subsystem dysfunction** • Sibling rivalry, etc.	**B. Social dysfunction** • Socially isolated families • Socially deviant families • Special theme families (commonly shared themes, mysteries, secrets, cultural beliefs, etc.)

Table 9: Family types as per circumplex model

Balanced functioning	*Mid-range functioning*	*Extreme*
• Flexibly separated • Flexibly connected • Structurally separated • Structurally connected	• Chaotically separated • Rigidly separated • Chaotically connected • Rigidly connected • Flexibly disengaged • Structurally disengaged • Flexibly enmeshed • Structurally enmeshed	• Chaotically disengaged • Chaotically enmeshed • Rigidly disengaged • Rigidly enmeshed

that family members have towards one another. It includes dimensions of emotional bonding, family involvement, marital relationship, parent–child relationships, internal boundaries and external boundaries. Adaptability here refers to how far family permits change (morphogenesis) and stability (morphostasis). It consists of dimensions of leadership, discipline, negotiation, roles and rules. Communication scale includes dimensions of listeners' skills, speakers' skills, self-disclosure, clarity, continuity and respect/regard.

Assessment of these three measures is usually done using self-reported scales, e.g. the family adaptability and cohesion evaluation scale (FACES). The original instrument is three item self report scales, which was later replaced by 33-item FACES II, and the 20-item FACES III and FACE IV scale. Using the assessment, families can be designated to one of the 16 subtypes as shown in Table 9.

Critics of this model often conclude that correspondence of the model and measurement devices is more frequently assumed. The balanced functioning families are not always better functional than those classified in extremes.[70]

The Darlington Family Assessment System[71]

This model differs from the other models as it not only considers family as a system but the individuals of the family as well. The assessment is done using a structured procedure: the Darlington Family Intervention Schedule and Darlington Family Rating Scale. Both have acceptable levels of reliability and validity but the evaluation of these tools in family studies is quite limited.[71]

After the initial assessment, the family problems should be summarized, preferably in the form of a formulation. Formulation serves as an intermediate link between the assessment and therapy.[72,73] The complaints may be formulated with a view to different therapeutic approaches. Such formulations have been shown to have some predictive value in the outcome of the treatment and should be discussed with the family in order to select the type of therapeutic approach needed. This step may be a difficult one, as it requires the therapist to strike a balance between his skills in the particular psychotherapies and level of the psychological mindedness of the participating individuals, their motivation, ego strength and ability to enter a sustained therapeutic relationship. Therapist for his own ease may discuss only those therapeutic approaches in which he feels comfortable as at present evidence is not sufficient to suggest if a particular approach is superior to the other.[62]

SCHOOLS OF FAMILY THERAPY

The therapists may differ in the method of dealing with the troubled family but the goals remain essentially the same. Their aim may be achieved by improving communication styles, accept one another's handicaps without scapegoating and developing strategies to avoid conflicts. The therapist may choose any of the following models to deal with the troubled family.

Psychodynamically Oriented Family Therapy

This approach for family therapy is based on the principles of psychodynamics and object relations.[62,73] Earlier therapists were mostly trained in individual psychoanalytical therapy. They viewed psychopathology of the family on the psychodynamic principles quite similar to the individual therapy. Hence, the existing family pathology was assumed to result from psychodynamic/developmental failures at various stages of family development. Bowen[51] considered the family as an individual in which different members are unable to become emotionally autonomous and hence behave like an 'undifferentiated ego mass.'

Ackerman,[37] another pioneer of this school and founder of Ackerman Institute of Family Therapy considered the family pathology to be the outcome of 'interlocking pathology' of the individual family members.

Different persons with their own psychopathology exist in the family in such an equilibrated state with each other that it does not ensure the proper functioning of family. It is therefore assumed that parental psychopathology which once gets established, exerts pressure in the vulnerable areas of the personality of individual.

Thus, the failed individuation, poor separation of self and non-self, projection and manipulation of the parents, replaces the orderly negotiation in resolving disagreement.[74,75] Each parent tries to recreate a new family depending on blocks in his personality development, thereby, creating a situation that repeats the incomplete aspects of one's personality. The process (because of its unconscious motives) remains largely unrecognized and thus, undermines the chance of parents successfully resolving what is seen as current interactional conflict.

The therapist helps the family members to recognize the incompatible defensive system. His primary aim is to provide the family members insight rather than motivating them to change. In comparison to other approaches, the therapist

Table 10: Psychoanalytic approach to family and marital therapy

Listening to unconscious: Provides material for construction of object relations of family. This step can be mastered through self-analysis, experience, peer review and supervision
Maintaining neutral position: Therapist has to hold a position of 'involved impartiality.' He has to make no preference regarding any of the family members; continuing with marriage or divorce
Creating psychological space: The therapist's ability to hold and tolerate anxiety provides the couple a transitional space where couple can portray and reflect current functioning, modify projective identification. The couple in turn also learns how to deal with current and future anxieties
Use of therapist self: The therapist's openness to learning and supervision, an understanding of own object relations in psychoanalysis. The use of self is useful as a diagnostic and therapeutic instrument
Negative capability: Capability of being in uncertainties, mysteries, doubts without any irritation reaching after facts and reasons
Transference and counter-transference: Transference gives rise to ideas, feelings, or behavior in the therapist, i.e. counter-transference Counter-transference must be analyzed as it can be a useful instrument to reach patient's unconscious
Interpretation of defenses and anxieties: Material gained through content of dreams, fantasies and interviews; formation of developmental hypothesis
Termination: When family has sufficient holding capacity and unconscious projective identifications have been recognized. Capacity to work together is restored. Relating intimately and sexually gratifying. The couple can envision its future development, can provide holding environment for its family

with psychodynamic orientation is more passive and makes fewer comments (Table 10). Due to the advancement of other systems, this model is becoming less popular among family therapists. Recently however, the emotionally focused therapy and approaches based on object relation theory have gained some acceptance.[74] No doubt, this model is the mother of many other systems of family therapy. The Milan school is one such classical example.

Structural Family Therapy

This approach of family therapy is purely based on the systems theory. Systems theory, as proposed by Von Bertalanffy[76] is a general theory of the organization of parts or subsystems into the whole. The system is a set of objects with relationship between the objects and between their attributes. Von Bertalanffy[76] identified open and closed systems. *Closed systems* are those, which do not interact with surrounding environment. Such systems tend to reach the equilibrium state through entropy, i.e. a tendency to reach the simplest possible state. *Open systems,* on the other hand, interact with the environment to varying degree, do not show entropy and tend to reach a steady state if the boundaries of the system and environment remain unchanged, through the property of *equifinality.* The subsystem is a component of the system. The family system is usually a part of larger suprasystem which can be the neighborhoods, community, etc.

The properties of a system which the family therapists have found useful in family therapy are as follows:

- Each family system and subsystem has emotional boundaries, which determine the interaction of various family members.
- Boundaries are semipermeable.
- Family system tends to reach a relative steady state by equifinality, i.e. the same end point may be reached despite differing starting points.
- Communication and feedback mechanisms between various parts are important in functioning of the family system.
- Behavior of individuals in a family is better understood based on circular causality, i.e. behavior of one individual affects the behavior of other and vice-versa.

Structural family therapy may also be called as boundary mending therapy as the therapist primarily focuses on correction of boundaries. The therapist views the individuals in their family context and sees the pathology occurring within the individual in the family context or at its interface. The structural model sees the homeostatically maintained family structure being regulated by repeated transactional patterns among and within its subsystems which are separated from each other in terms of boundaries and which regulate the flow of ideas, affect and event. The family therapist enters in alliance with the family to assess the boundary pattern and thereafter works on the boundaries to restrict them. He may achieve this by primarily focusing on current interactional pattern rather than the psychological antecedents of the individual behavior. The interactional patterns are directly handled to teach, redefine roles and rules; align them in coalition, thereby modifying the interpersonal boundaries to facilitate achieving autonomy for individual members within the family structure.

Strategic Family Therapy[77]

Classical strategic family therapists viewed the patient's symptoms as the representation of unsuccessful attempts to solve the existing problems that have become self-reinforcing.

Therefore, one unsuccessful attempt generates a series of problems according to the laws of circular causation. In the social context, the symptoms are viewed as the patient's attempts to break out of the impossible situations in which they are bound by the family, and the interpersonal functions they serve. Thus, the goal of the therapist is to use the complaints as an entry point and correct the sequence of dysfunctional behavior.

Strategic therapist uses the following four types of questions in any exploratory and interventive session.

Lineal questions: These are asked to orient the therapist to the client's situation and are based on lineal assumptions about the nature of mental phenomena. The intent behind these questions is predominantly investigative. The therapist behaves much like an investigator or detective trying to unravel a complex mystery. The basic questions are "Who did What," "Where" "When," and "Why?" Most interviews begin with at least some lineal questions. This is often necessary in order to "join" the family members through their typically lineal views of their problematic situation. With this mode of inquiry, the therapist tends to adopt a reductionistic stance in trying to determine the specific cause of the problem. Efforts are made to tease things apart so that the origin of the problem eventually becomes clearly delineated.

Circular questions: Circular questions tend to be characterized by a general curiosity about the connectedness of events that include the problem, rather than a specific need to know the precise origins of the problem. If the therapist has established cybernetic orientation toward mental process, and has developed skills in maintaining a conceptual posture of circular hypothesizing, these questions will come easily and freely. Two general types of circular questions, "difference questions" and "contextual question," have been associated with fundamental patterns of symmetry and complementarities. Several subtypes, including category difference questions, temporal difference questions, category-context questions, and behavioral effect questions, have been described.

Strategic questions: These are asked in order to influence the client or family in a specific manner, and are based on lineal assumptions about the nature of the therapeutic process. The intent behind these questions is predominantly corrective. It is assumed that instructive interaction is possible. The therapist behaves like a teacher, instructor, or judge, telling family members how they erred and how they ought to behave (albeit indirectly in the form of questions).

Reflexive questions: These are intended to influence the client or family in an indirect or general manner, and are based on circular assumptions about the nature of the process taking place in the therapeutic system. The intent behind these questions is predominantly facilitative. It is assumed that family members are autonomous individuals and cannot be instructed directly.

Thus, the therapist behaves more like a guide or coach encouraging family members to mobilize their own problem-solving resources. One major presupposition behind these questions is that the therapeutic system is co-evolutionary and what the therapist does is to trigger reflexive activity in the family's pre-existing belief systems. These questions are reflexive in that they are formulated to trigger family members to reflect upon the implications of their current perceptions and action and to consider new options.

The therapist endeavors to interact in a manner that opens space for the family to see new possibilities and to evolve more freely of their own accord. Even though reflexive questioning is also intended to influence a family in a therapeutic direction, it remains a more neutral mode of inquiry than strategic questioning because it is more respectful of the family's autonomy.

Well-developed skills in maintaining a conceptual posture of neutrality contribute to the probability that an influencing question will be reflexive rather than strategic. What is missing in all these questions is the emotional tone used in asking the questions. In the strategic therapy, the therapist devises the specific strategies to solve the family's problems. Clearly, depending on the strategy devised, there can be number of strategic therapies. According to Hayes[77] there are two major models of strategic therapy: the brief/communication model developed at Mental Research Institute and a blend of different strategic and structural models developed by Haley Madnes and Erickson.

All these therapies tend to bring second order change, i.e. changing the pattern of family interaction or structure which is more lasting than change in the symptomatic behavior without altering interactions. In this approach, the therapist takes a covert control on the family in therapeutic system. The distinction between systemic therapies of Milan Group[78] and strategic therapies is not well marked. To many authors it is just the difference in the level of systematization, the Milan Group being most systematized in their approach. In fact, all therapies can be called systemic as all view the family as system. Behavior therapy is least systematized type of therapy.

The strategic therapist may not share the goals with family members and prescribe behaviors to solve problems according to his hidden agenda. He may take help of *paradox and counter-paradox* situations, which are especially helpful in families resisting a change. The therapist may paradoxically prescribe a behavior that is to be eliminated. The family can defeat the prescribed behavior only by giving up the symptoms. Thus, this method requires an active involvement from the patient and family than the other two methods. Clearly, the classical strategic methods are indirect. Most of the therapists work on these methods when more explicit or direct methods fail to bring sufficient change.

Table 11: Strategic methods of family therapy	
Reframing	*Giving new meaning to a behavior either in the context or content*
Paradox	• Communicating or prescribing just the opposite of what is desired. Challenge represent a simple form of paradox
Rituals	• Prescribing or modifying family tradition, e.g. religious celebration, birth days, reunions, outings, even day task
Metaphors	• Use of some anecdotes, short stories, analogies encompassing the family situation to bring about change
Externalizing	• Redefining, objectifying or personifying the problem in a way to decrease conflict, undermining sense of failure
The Greek chorus	• The consultation/supervision group observing through one way mirror and sending a series of message in the therapy room, such as support messages, public opinion polls, disagreement with therapist, advice, creating surprise or confusion

Other indirect methods used by the strategic therapist are given in Table 11.

Experiential Family Therapy[44]

Though experiential therapists (Carl Whitaker, Waiter Kempler) subscribe to the views held by the therapists from other schools, they downplay the theory in what they do. They feel it is difficult to help the family without becoming involved in intense interaction with them. It is the existential encounter, which promotes change in the family. Thus, the experiential therapist may at time even be outrageous to the family. He is more active, interpretive and directive to the families.[79] Because of the difficult nature of intervention, the therapy did not gain much popularity. Only highly experienced therapists dare practice this method.

Behavioral Social Exchange Therapy

This method of family therapy is based on the principle of behavioral conditioning. It views family as an agency that encourages the adaptive behavior through reward in the way that ensures a long term reciprocation of desired behavior and reward in a situation where benefits outweigh the costs. Any maladaptive behavior in the normal functioning family is not given any reinforcement, thereby, helping it to become extinct. Behavior therapist sees the deviant behavior as an outcome of a number of interacting feedback processes. According to Whaler,[80] any behavior is the outcome of operation of larger cybernetic systems. He described *positive and negative reinforcer traps,* i.e. a maladaptive behavior gets a positive or negative reinforcement repeatedly. In case a person manifests behavioral symptoms, it can be the outcome of deficits in communication, rewarding the maladaptive behavior or the deficient reward system. The therapeutic aim is to help the family in deciding appropriate rewarding strategy, which can be achieved through deciding the observable behavioral goal and changing the contingencies for interpersonal behavior. Communication training with emphasis on clear and direct expression of positive feeling, ideas and plans is a good starting point. Thereafter, structured problem solving approach encourages the family members to list the problems and to think/generate various possible solutions. It also encourages them to discuss the advantages and disadvantages of each proposed solution and then to agree to choose the best feasible option. Later, it helps to formulate and implement a plan and to review the results of the interventions carried out.[81] Compared to other schools, the behavioral family therapists are more precise in defining the criteria, method and the outcome measures.

Vector Therapy[82,83]

The term vector has been derived from physics that is defined as a force of a known magnitude and direction of action. The vector therapy views the individual as being acted upon by emotional forces within the field of family, in the space of life. The individual's actions or responses can be assumed to be the sum total of emotional forces acting on him. The forces if evaluated to be positive can be utilized in the therapy or removed should they be negative. The purpose of vector therapy is to readjust the pattern of emotional forces in the life space to bring relief and benefit to the individuals and families within the life space. Instead of treating the individual, the vector therapy focuses on the impact of various emotional forces on each member.

In the life space, the forces can be within the individual (e.g. self-directed anger) or in the coalition care of a particular member by individuals or detouring partners. When it deals with the forces outside the family, indeed, this approach conceptualizes, working in family's supra-system. The vector therapy, therefore, involves prescription of:

- Change in magnitude of forces, e.g. to decrease aggression.
- Change in the direction of emotional force with no change in magnitude, e.g. father to direct anger at mother instead of child.
- Change in length of duration for which emotional force operates, e.g. father to work away from home.
- Change in the quality of emotional force, e.g. father to be affectionate to his child rather than being aggressive.

To affect these changes, the sources of emotional forces may have to be moved temporarily or permanently, e.g. father to work outside the home, etc. Thus, vector therapy may allow the family to break and result in new better working families from the fragments.[14] This concept is more a family psychiatry approach, which did not gain much acceptance.

Functional Family therapy[84]

Functional family therapy is family intervention program that focuses on children and teens. It mainly involves the children who are at-risk or already involved in juvenile delinquencies. It consists of three specific intervention phases which are sequential and interlinked viz. engagement and motivation, behavior change, and generalization. The interventions in each phase are organized coherently, which allows clinicians to maintain focus in contexts that often involve considerable family and individual disruption.

The assessment focuses on how the problem behaviors occur in the context of the family relationships. It also helps to identify the risk factors and the protective factors in the family. In addition it helps to identify what can be the possible targets of the intervention program. It consists of an average 8–12 sessions for mild cases and up to 30 hours of direct service (e.g. clinical sessions, telephone calls, and meetings involving community resources) for more difficult cases. Sessions are usually spread over a 3-month period.

Spirituality and Family Therapy

Spiritual domain stands alongside biological and psychological domains of health. Dynamics of prayer significantly influence the people's interaction. Prayer gives a feeling of an experience of relationship with deity. It de-escalates hostile emotions and reduces emotional reactivity, enhances relationship and partner orientation, facilitates empathy, encourages people to take responsibility for problem solving, and results in more positive marital interaction.[85] Prayers help the couples to relax, increased ability to think and improves the overall health of the couple.[85] Spirituality also gives a feeling that God or divine power is interested in humans and acts upon within their relationship to promote beneficial change.[86] Some authors even recommend educating and working with clergymen as part of family therapy process.[87]

MARITAL THERAPY

Marital therapy is a form of psychotherapy aimed to modify the psychological interaction between the married or cohabiting partners who are in conflict with one another along one or a variety of parameters which may be social, emotional, sexual, economic, parental, etc.

It can be better conceptualized as the special type of family therapy. All psychopathologies seen in a family can be present in marital couples also. Thus, marital therapy shares its thinking with all schools of family therapy. Family therapy methods are applicable to couples too; it is only being described separately here for certain minor differences. Marital therapy has a wider goal than of marital counseling. Marital counseling is usually problem focused and concentrates only on the conflict concerning the couple at the moment, whereas marital therapy puts a greater emphasis on restructuring the interactional pattern between the couple.[88]

Scope of Marital Therapy

Marriage tends to be universal in the human race. Most of the happily married couples would tend to be similar in characteristics of interaction but the unhappy marriages tend to be unhappy in their own way and may break. Marital separation, divorce and their after affects cause great stress on the psychological and physical functioning of both individuals. The trend for marital breakdown or divorce is on rise.

There has been global rise in divorce rates from 1960 to 1980 in United States, with current anticipated divorce rates as high as 50%.[89] With high rates of marital discords, there is increased incidence of adult psychopathology like depression, suicide,[90] and alcoholism. A discordant marriage may have a heavier impact than divorce on the children.[91,92] Different studies conclude that psychiatric and physical illness occurs more frequently in people with disrupted marriages.[93]

Moreover, the help-seeking by the patients living in stressful marriage is on the increase, therefore, creating a demand for marital help on the therapist. In a particular study, nearly 40% patients reported marital problems as one of the reasons of their help seeking.[94,95]

Marital Pathology

Maintaining marital satisfaction requires certain efforts and commitment from both partners. The marital partners may be 'alike' and 'different' in a variety of ways. Each partner needs affection, recreation, companionship, sex, approval and status.

Marriage may be one of the ways of overcoming the developmental blocks and handicaps by the neurotic people. A woman may marry to an alcoholic man in order to fulfill her narcissistic needs. Such marriages may mean cajoling, seduction and burden to either or both partners.

Paradoxically negative emotions, either giving or receiving, may keep marital couple together. Anxieties, hostility and abnormalities of coping of the neurotic may be transferred to the spouse, which may be complicated by reactive guilt, remorse or attempts at separation. Therefore, inviting an attack from the healthier or the sick partner may perpetuate the chain of indignation, anger and counter attack by the marital partner. They may blame each other for their shortcomings, mediocrities and even the symptoms.[96] The couple in marital conflict may remain in relationship even when it appears unsatisfactory. Both partners may feel fulfillment of fewer than the required needs, remain unwilling to part and blame the relationship for unhappiness.

Object relations theory has emerged as most applicable psychodynamic model of marital interactions.[97] As adults too, the individuals remain unconsciously attached to the conflicts with the early objects, which they may re-enact with the marital partner through repetition compulsion, which may be maintained through collusion and reciprocity. Faulty mutual projective identification, inadequate containment, introjective identification and identification of the marital partners with the aggressors in the early life may also lead to unhappiness in the partners.[98]

Sager[99] described three levels of conscious and unconscious marital contracts, non-fulfillment of which may lead to intense emotional reactions. The first is conscious and expressed in the form of if I give you X, you give me Y. The second is conscious but in which one partner assumes that I have done X, so I must get Y. The third is unconscious; expectation at this level may be irrational and contradictory. For example, 'A' may expect the distressed 'B' to please 'A' so that 'A' may extend help to 'B' because of the unconscious motives. It evokes an intense emotional reaction, which puzzles both the partners.

This form of contract leads to the most severe kind of marital discord.

Behavioral and Communication Pathology

A good communication is essential for any healthy relationship. Many behaviorists feel that the marital partners are generally dissatisfied because their communication is inadequate. Communicating one's feeling involves both verbal and nonverbal components. While communicating, it is important to be aware of what is said and how it is said. In marital relationships, it is often an exchange of personal messages that is almost never learnt. Virginia Satir[100] believes that all martial partners have emotional needs of one or other type, which they hope to have met in marriage. It is important that in communication other's emotional needs should be fulfilled.

A healthy communication between marital partners serves following functions:

- It defines a relationship as one partner becomes aware that message is coming from partner
- Cognitive processing of the message generates feelings and ideas about the partner and possible ways of responding
- Sending back own message with verbal and nonverbal component.

In a satisfactory relationship, reciprocity of communication is essential. It involves doing or saying the things that are pleasing to the other partner. Such interaction often called by many workers as *pleases*, gives strength and satisfaction to the marital bond. *Coercion* is another form of communication, which can maintain the relationship as pathological one. It involves making the partner feel unpleasant the way communication occurs between them. Paradoxically, the partner has a sense of satisfaction and the relationship continues. *Negative emotional responses* are another form of expressions/words/action, which are unpleasant. Such responses the partner may consider rewarding especially when there is paucity of pleasant interaction. Some response is better than none.

In a study by Yalcin and Karahan,[101] use of couple communication program consisting of 10 sessions, each lasting for one and half hour duration, resulted in better adjustment between the couple. As compared to a control group, the couple communication program resulted in significant difference after the conclusion of the program and after a follow-up period of three months.

Indications and Contraindications for Marital Therapy

Like for family therapy, there are relative contradictions for marital therapy as well. The reader must note that the indications for this therapy are conceptually quite similar to those of family therapy.

Indications (Modified from Medelson and Polonsky)[98]

- Presence of unresolved conflict and stress in the relationship
- One partner who has changed as the result of individual treatment and which has increased the stress in the relationship
- Gross distortions in the relationships, which disrupt the reality
- One partner having mental illness, staying in equilibrium with a healthy partner through collusive defense, which results in emergence of symptoms in the healthy partner when the sick one starts improving.
- During individual therapy when difficulty with the partner becomes the major focus
- When the marital therapy may augment the gains of individual therapy
- Likelihood of breaks in relationships due to transference and counter-transference
- Sexual dysfunction of psychological origin.

Contraindications for Marital Therapy (Modified from Medelson and Polonsky)[98]

- Unwillingness of partner to cooperate
- Inability to control hostility by one or both partners

- The other partner having active psychosis or being emotionally fragile
- When one partner begins to decompensate in the course of marital therapy
- When one partner is extremely paranoid, not able to tolerate the therapist's collaboration with the other partner
- Manipulative partner, trying to sabotage the therapy
- The individual's unwillingness to share the information with the partner, which may be required for therapeutic effect
- When the partner consciously resists the therapeutic change.

Assessment of the Couple

Most of the times couple presents for the therapy, with ambivalent feelings towards the marital problems. They may fear criticism from the therapist. They should be able to perceive that their presenting for therapy means their readiness to change and a willingness to stay together. Their present agony may be severe, but a good adjustment in the past should ensure the therapist that their pathology can be reversed. The therapist in the first few sessions would be able to see their attitude towards each other and himself that would provide a sufficient background for the therapist to decide the type of therapy that should be chosen. In case both the partners present together, it also provides opportunity to see the communication styles, which are usually morbid in the disturbed couple. In order to make an objective assessment of the marital difficulties, standardized tools may be used, e.g. Style of conflict inventory for personal relationships, influences tactics scales, etc.

Presentation of the Couple

- Factors leading to request for therapy
- Threat to integrity as seen by each partner
- Motivation of each partner for treatment and their expectations.

Individual Assessment

- Adaptive and defensive patterns
- Self-images, personal values and goals
- Family history, expectations of relationships in the family of origins, interpersonal relationship patterns, patterns of dealing with anger
- Past long-term relations, in comparison with present relations.

Couple Assessment

- Role of individual expectations, values, goals and conflicts in relationship
- Effect of each partner's adaptive patterns on the other
- Need for control by one partner on the other
- Mutual trust and ability to share
- Importance of individual and mutual dependency issues
- Communication pattern
- Affection, empathy and mutual support
- Sexual adjustment
- *Daily interactions*: Sharing, flexibility of roles, rivalry and competition, balance of power
- Areas of major conflict in relationship including development, intensity and means of resolving conflict.

Relationship with Family, Including Childhood Friends

Task of marital therapy

Whenever the marital partners present for therapy, it may mean the willingness of both partners to change and stay together. Thus, the therapist through the communication skills helps the partners to create a positive change in their development, makes them visualize their weaknesses and accept them. If at all, these goals are not accessible and separation is inevitable, the therapist should help the partners to separate with minimum remorse and guilt.

Technique of Marital Therapy

The process of marital therapy is multifaceted which finds its basis in almost all theoretical formulations of inducing a behavior change. The choice of technique usually depends on the therapist's experience. Marital therapy may be psychoanalytically oriented or may involve techniques of behavior and sex therapy. It may share its foundations with the family therapy and group therapy. Greene[102] described six types of classical marital therapies as shown in Table 12, based on method of interviewing.

Crisis counseling focuses on modifying the sociocultural forces on the situational basis. Classical psychotherapeutic approach may be utilized when the spouses have widely divergent goals. One partner may manifest a severe acting out behavior whereas the other may be completely unaware of it.

Table 12: Types of marital therapies

Classical marital therapies	*Combined marital therapies*
• Supportive marital therapy—crisis management • Intensive marital therapy • Classical psychoanalytical psychotherapy • Collaborative psychotherapy • Concurrent psychotherapy • Conjoint psychotherapy • Combined therapies	• Simple therapy • Conjoint family therapy • Combined collaborative therapy • Marital group therapy

In dealing with such problem, both partners are seen by the separate therapists who do not communicate with each other. They focus more on the individual problems, with marriage in background.

Collaborative approach involves separate therapists for both partners, however the therapists share the information with each other by regular scheduled meetings.[103] In *concurrent therapy,* both partners are seen by the same therapist individually. Therapist in this model tries to create insight into each individual's own behavior which affects the other partner adversely.[104] This therapy should be avoided when there is a personality disorder or severe paranoid reactions.

In the *conjoint marital therapy,*[105] both the partners see the therapist together. This particular technique is particularly more popular among the therapists because of it being economical and also brings out the marital dynamics more clearly. It also provides an opportunity to identify and resolve the conflicts at the earliest. Combined therapies may involve combination of two or more of these therapies.

Table 13: Factors affecting marital satisfaction according to object relation marital therapy

- Projective and introjective identification processes are not mutually gratifying
- Containment of the spouse's projection is not possible
- Un-arousing projective identification of the genital zone cannot be modified by sexual experience
- Aspects of the love object have to be split off and experienced in a less threatening situation, leading to triangulation involving a child, hobby, friend, parent or lover

Table 14: Goals of object relation marital therapy

- To recognize and provoke the couple's mutual projective and introjective identification
- To improve the couples' contextual holding capacity so that partner can fulfill each other's need for attachment, and autonomy and developmental progression
- To promote individuation of spouses and differentiation of needs including the need for individual therapy or psychoanalysis
- To return the family with confidence to the tasks of the current developmental stage in the couple's life cycle

SCHOOLS OF MARITAL THERAPY

Psychoanalytic Model

Object relation couple therapy: Object relation couple therapist primarily assumes that a marital relationship can be ungratifying if the couple does not have adequate projective identification, containment, and introjective identification fails.

The object relation marital therapist creates a therapeutic environment in which a couple's pattern of defenses can be displayed, recognized and understood; couple's capacity to distinguish each other's projections from aspects of self, containment and to take back the projections is improved. The therapist helps the couple to perceive each other free from self. The process is reinforced by the pleasure of becoming more loving and lovable towards the object.

However, goals of the object relation therapy are difficult to specify. Most of the object relation therapist opine that goal setting often restrict the progress of therapy. The broader reasons for conflicts and goals to achieve in object relation couple therapy are shown in Tables 13 and 14 respectively.

Emotionally focused couple therapy: Based on attachment theory[106] emotionally focused therapy posits that seeking and maintaining contact with few others is a primary motivating factor for establishing social relationships with others.[62] This is also an innate survival mechanism, which provides a secure base in stressful situations. Any disapproval or rejection of one partner's effort to seek attachment with other partner generates a spiral of negative interactions, which ultimately make relations unsatisfactory. The therapist works with the couple with a goal to recognize feelings and mechanisms triggered by individual's vulnerability and risk of rejection.[107] This therapy has been particularly found useful in couples having severe traumatic experiences.[108] Some workers rate this therapy superior in outcome, in comparison with other modes.[109]

Client-centered Model

This approach is based on the work of Carl Rogers.[110] It helps the couple to clarify their own thinking and feeling about the various issues. The therapist follows the lead to the patients and does not introduce material based on the preconceived scheme, other than the basic assumption that the client possesses the ability to improve.

Transactional Model

Relying on the theories of Eric Berne, the therapist examines the transactions between the spouses as they occur in the here and now. A determination is made as to whether the patient is acting as a parent, child or adult. The therapist provides the couple with active feedback about their interactions as they occur.[111]

Systems Theory Model

Derived from general systems theory, it views the marital unit as a system in equilibrium. Disequilibria are equivalent to discomfort and produce stress, which is felt by the partners. The role of the therapist is to monitor the emotional forces from moment to moment, as they unfold through the interactions of the couple. Therapy is geared to modify whatever tension states exist.

Behavioral Marital Therapy

As in family therapy, principles of behavior therapy also find their application in marital therapy. Stuart[112] suggested the effectiveness of mutual reinforcement strategy in making behavioral changes in the couples.

In marriage, the individuals adopt behaviors, which are most rewarding and least costly in terms of efforts. Each of the partners expects fairly equal sharing of rewards and costs. In problematic marriages, sharing is either unequal or has not reached the expected level which leads to vicious negative interactions. In behavioral exchange therapy, the couple designs the tasks with the help of therapist and carries out on give-and-get basis.

Tasks identified in the therapy must be positive, repeatable, specific, and realistic so that these may be reinforced by the other partner easily, e.g. partners may agree that wife would serve husband the morning tea, and in return, husband would be expected to dust the bed.

Behavioral exchange training can be usefully employed with the majority of couples with relationship problems. Some couples, whose recurrent communication problems lead to resentment and misunderstanding, can be helped through communication skill training. The therapist asks the couple to discuss a topic in his presence and identifies the faulty communication patterns which may be destructive criticism, generalizations, mind reading, bringing up the past, putting oneself in the right and partner in the wrong, using logical argument as a weapon, raising the voice, etc.
The therapist helps the couple in identifying these faults and encourages to replace each of these with ones listed below:

- Express one's own feeling instead of imputing feeling in the other partner
- Use specific examples and stick to the point
- Avoid mind reading
- Taking responsibility for own actions
- Avoid monologues
- Examine nonverbal communication

The therapist may give instructions or may use role modeling. Hometask[113] should also be prescribed and feedback can be given by the therapist based on video or audio recordings.

DIVORCE MEDIATION

Rate of marriages terminating in divorce is globally on rise. Nearly 50% of marriages in the west end in divorce.[54] Divorce mediation is a medical model to seek a comfortable divorce rather than go into cumbersome legal procedure. Divorce mediation therapist helps the couple in reducing anger and bitterness during and after the divorce process is over. Such mediation produces a high level of agreement and satisfaction with the decisions, decreased expenditure and reduced post divorce litigations.[114] Divorce mediation is more successful when the focus is on communication pattern and on problem solving pattern.[115-116]

Kressel et al.[117] identified four patterns of divorce namely, enmeshed, autistic, direct and disengaged on the bases of three intercorrelated factors like degree of ambivalence, frequency and openness of communication and level and overtness of conflict. They concluded divorce mediation was most successful in direct and disengaged group; postdivorce adjustment of these groups was also better than the other two groups. For the legal purpose, decision for divorce reached in the course of mediation must be confined by the court. Haynes[118] held the view that divorce mediation often requires expertise in negotiation and bargaining. The couple therapist should undergo some training to acquire these skills.

ROLE OF SEX THERAPY IN MARITAL THERAPY

Sex therapy and marital therapy may be considered different from each other as both require different type of training and skill for the therapist, yet both may be viewed as two different sides of the same coin. Many a times it is difficult to recognize the difference between the symptoms of marital dysfunction and sexual dysfunction. The couple primarily presenting for marital discord would also manifest sexual symptoms, which may relate to primary etiology through a link of circular causation. Similarly, the patient with sexual dysfunction may present with marital disturbance too. In either of the case, combined sex and marital therapy finds it application. Irrespective of the situation, whenever the couple presents with sexual dysfunction, a complete medical examination is always indicated.

The relationship of marital and sexual dysfunction seems to be a crucial factor in determining the initial focus of the therapy.

Based on temporal correlation between the types of dysfunctions, three categories of couples can be identified:[99]

1. Sexual dysfunction produces secondary marital discord. Sex therapy is generally the treatment of choice in this situation, especially when sexual dysfunction existed before the relationship problems between the spouses.
2. Marital discord in other areas impairs sexual functioning. For such couples conjoint therapy may be the treatment of choice. Sex therapy may be indicated if the couple's positive feelings outweigh their negative feelings.
3. Severe marital discord with basic hostility obstructs the possibility of good sexual functioning. Sex therapy is usually contraindicated. However, sensate focus technique with no genital gratification may be prescribed for helping the couple work through hostilities, poor

communication, fear of emotional closeness and difficulties in verbalizing desires. The procedure of taking turns giving and receiving pleasure may be prescribed. This procedure can be utilized as an evaluative test to determine several interactional and intrapsychic factors, thus helping the therapist to arrive at most urgent and fruitful priorities for therapeutic intervention.

Treatment of couple may be in conjoint or individual interviews. It should be ensured that couple understands physiology of normal sexual response. An educative approach of the therapist usually helps the couple to lower down unrealistic romantic demands and expectations. Whenever couple is beset with sexual dysfunction, a complete medical examination is always indicated.

There is nothing pathological about some difference in the level of sexual desires of partners. In case of gross deficits, chronic problems like depression, past-traumatic experience etc., must be ruled out. Emotions like anger, shame, and fear about performance also contribute to low levels of desires. Arousal and orgasmic dysfunction such as anorgasmia in females, premature ejaculation and erectile dysfunction in males are frequently reported. Once anatomical and physiological causes have been ruled out, stop-start and squeeze techniques advocated by Masters and Johnson may be prescribed.

Medications such as sildenafil, tadalafil, verdenafil may be prescribed in suitable cases. Paraphilias, if present, are usually reported first by the sexual partner or on encountering some legal complication. Behavioral techniques with motivation enhancement are usually helpful in such cases.

Effectiveness of Family Therapy Or Couple Therapy

Family therapy has been widely researched regarding its effectiveness. It has been found to be effective in relationship problems. In addition it has been found to be helpful in various psychiatric disorders.

Relationship Distress

In a systematic review of meta-analyses of couple therapy mostly consisting of behavioral or emotionally focused couples therapy, Shadish and Baldwin[119] found that the average treated couple fared better than 80% of couples in control groups. In a meta-analysis of twenty-three studies, Wood et al.[120] found that both these approaches are equally effective for mildly distressed couple, while emotionally focused couple therapy was more effective in moderately distressed couple. The results suggest that for distressed couples, emotionally focused couples therapy is currently the treatment of choice.

Snyder et al.[121] compared insight oriented marital therapy with behavioral therapy and found that 4 years after treatment, only 3% of cases in the former group were divorced compared to 38% in the latter.

Hypoactive Sexual Desire

Systemic reviews of therapies involving cognitive and behavioral measures showed that 50–70% of cases showed improvements in levels of desire following therapy, but in up to 50% of cases, improvement was not sustained at three-year follow-up, though improvement in sexual satisfaction continued.[122]

Female Sexual Pain Disorders

Couples-based cognitive behavioral sex therapy was found to be effective in a systematic review of outcome studies by Meston and Bradford[123] for reducing dyspareunia and vaginismus in women with vulvar vestibulitis syndrome.

Male Erectile Disorder

In a study by Banner and Anderson[124] in fifty-three cases of acquired erectile dysfunction, combination of cognitive behavior sex therapy and sildenafil was found to be effective in 48% of cases while sildenafil alone was effective only in 29% of cases.

Domestic Violence

In a narrative review of six studies by Stith and Rosen[125] couples therapy was found to be effective in reducing domestic violence. In addition studies suggest that multicouple therapy may be more effective than single-couple therapy.[126]

Juvenile Delinquency

Both randomized trials and nonrandomized trials have shown that functional family therapy significantly reduces recidivism for a wide range of juvenile offense patterns.[49] Moreover studies have shown that functional family therapy reduces the cost of treatment.[127] It also significantly reduces potential new offending for siblings of treated adolescents.[128]

Anxiety Disorders

In a review of 12 studies of couples-based treatment for panic disorder for agoraphobia, by Byrne et al.[129] it was found that partner assisted cognitive-behavioral exposure therapy was as effective as individual based cognitive-behavioral treatment.

In a review by Renshaw et al.[130] of five trials of systemic couple's therapy or family-based approaches to the treatment of OCD, it was shown that such approaches are atleast as effective as individually based cognitive behavior therapy for adults with OCD.

Mood Disorders

Depression: Systemic couples therapy, family therapy based on the McMaster model, emotionally focused couple's therapy; behavioral marital therapy, cognitive marital therapy, and conjoint interpersonal therapy have been found to be effective in narrative reviews of controlled trials of systemic intervention for depression.[131] These therapies were found to be effective alone or in combination with antidepressant medications.[131]

Bipolar disorder: In systematic reviews and meta-analyses, systemic therapy was found to significantly reduce relapse rates in people with bipolar disorder when included in multi-modal programs involving mood-stabilizing medication.[131]

Alcohol Abuse

In a systematic narrative review of 38 controlled studies of systematic interventions for the treatment of alcohol problems it was concluded that these approaches were effective in helping the families promote the family members with alcohol problem to continue in treatment and recover.[132]

Schizophrenia

Pfammatter et al.[133] in a review of meta-analysis concluded that as compared to medication alone, approaches which in addition to antipsychotic medications included psychoeducational family therapy had lower relapse and rehospitalization rates and improved medication adherence.

In a longitudinal prospective study by Bressi et al.[134] using the Milan school model of systemic family therapy, it was found that the relapse rate was 15% in the experimental group while it was 65% in the control group after one year, but no significant difference was found at 2 year follow-up.

Chronic Physical Illness

In a meta-analysis of seventy studies, Martire et al.[135] found that couple therapy was effective in alleviating depression in patients with chronic illnesses like cancer, heart disease, and dementia. Also systemic interventions for relatives of people with these illnesses and family therapy were found to be effective in alleviating caregiving burden, depression and anxiety.

FAMILY THERAPY IN INDIA

Family therapy in India is still in its evolutionary phase. History of Indian Psychiatry is marked with shortage of psychiatrists and psychiatric beds.[136] Faced with shortage of beds, Dr Vidya Sagar at Mental Hospital, Amritsar, resorted to keeping such patients in tents along with their family members. Patients were treated without being separated from the family. This outpatient tent approach with family orientation was basically a family psychiatry approach. This approach helped to educate the family members and participate in the treatment. In addition, it also reduced stigma associated with mental illness.

The success of tent approach stimulated the staff members at NIMHANS, Bangalore, to carry out similar experiments, which ultimately culminated in setting up family psychiatric center at NIMHANS in 1976. The center receives referrals from outside the institute too. The therapeutic approach identifies whole family as a sick unit and thus all family members participate in treatment. The therapist is doubly supervised by a supervisor and family psychiatry team for guidance, clarification. The family and patient are admitted to the ward for 2–3 weeks. Outdoor treatment may continue for 3–6 months. Therapist most of the times follows an eclectic approach. Till date, this is the only structured family therapy unit setup in India. It also offers training to the students/professionals associated with mental health promotion.[46] However, in general hospital psychiatry units (GHPU) patients are admitted with the family members, wherein they participate in the treatment of the patients and are provided education about the illness.

Psychosexual clinics exist in many of the teaching hospitals but no specific center for couple therapy has been established. One such clinic being run by the Department of Psychiatry at PGIMER, Chandigarh, since 1987 on a regular basis, has contributed some scientific data in this field.

Effectiveness of Family Intervention in India

Psychoeducational family programs have resulted in the prevention of relapse among patients with chronic schizophrenia[137] and led to an improvement in the attitude of the family members towards mentally ill people.[138]

Pai et al.[139,140] showed that the home intervention group had higher improvements in symptoms, better social functioning and reduced burden for carers as compared to the routine hospital care at six months follow-up. At the end of two years, the intervention group continued to have better clinical status and fewer hospital admissions. However, there was no significant difference in social functioning and caregiver burden. In a randomized control trial in caregivers of schizophrenia, structured psychoeducational intervention was shown to result in significantly better outcome than routine out-patient care in areas of psychopathology, disability, caregiver-support and caregiver satisfaction.[141]

ETHICS AND FAMILY THERAPY

Family and couple therapy generally works on the general ethics and other guidelines laid for psychotherapeutic relationships. The knowledge of ethics is of utmost importance. Without this, it is just like driving a car perfectly but on the wrong side, which is disastrous for both the driver and others on the road. Without ethical practice, family therapy is likely to manifest its adverse effects as with pharmacotherapy. It can result in disinterest of members in treatment, nonresolution of symptoms and in the extreme cases can result in litigations.

The ethics for the therapy may differ from culture to culture. However, there are some common guiding principles, e.g. Hippocratic principle-first do no harm to the patient. Following ethical principles that should be respected for any psychotherapeutic process:[45,142]

Autonomy: The therapist must respect autonomy of the individual in the family. Each individual in the family has right to freedom. Even if therapist disagrees with any individual, he/she must be respected if his/her opinion is not causing any harm to the individual or any other family member.

Fidelity: The therapist has to be faithful and loyal to his clients. It helps in establishing trustworthy meaningful relations.

Justice: This principle states that all people should be treated equally in the family unless there is a compelling reason, e.g. marital infidelity, child abuse, etc.

Informed consent: Informed consent is not just any ethical or legal obligation. It ensures the participation of all concerned and has the potential for enhancement of clinical work. It emphasizes the patient's role in making treatment decisions.[143]

The informed consent can be given only when the objectives, goals, duration, risks and complications have been properly discussed with the family members. It helps to ally the Client's anxiety as patient would be aware of the proceedings of the psychotherapy.[143]

It is particularly necessary to have consent when treatment outcome at any stage is likely to be hazardous or when no one mode of treatment is clearly superior to other. At times, the outcome may be quite unpredictable. All these situations are frequent in psychotherapy.

While taking the informed consent of the clients, consideration should be given to the cognitive level of the clients.[142] Moreover, informed consent should be an on going process, clients should be informed regularly about the changing treatment needs and any change in treatment plan should be informed to the client and informed consent to be taken for the same.[144]

If the therapist is a trainee, then she/he must inform the client regarding their status and must take help of their supervisors at regular intervals.[142]

Therapist values: The value is the enduring belief that specific modes of conduct or end state of existence are personally or socially preferable to others.[145] The therapist's own value system is often a hindrance in any form of psychotherapeutic relationship, especially when the therapist is a trainee. It may often lead to biases in assessment and setting up of deliberate/nondeliberate hidden agenda that can affect the family members adversely. Therapist values can be more interfering especially when spirituality and religiosity are being considered allies in therapy if used judicially/ethically.

Competence of therapist: Therapist should be aware of his/her competence, regarding his knowledge, training and experience in a particular type of psychotherapy. Also, therapist should be aware of his emotional state while dealing with the clients. If the therapist anticipates that his personal problems would interfere in carrying out therapy in an effective manner, they should refrain from initiating or continuing the therapy. Therapist should take the help of his/her colleagues as the need arises during the course of therapy, regarding his competence and personal/emotional problems that may interfere with the progress of therapy.[142]

Confidentiality: It is against the interest of patient to reveal what client has said in any form of therapy. In family therapy situations, there is more risk of sharing client's confidential information with other family members especially when individual or subsystems of the family are seen separately.

In the introductory intake session of therapy it is always recommended to set the limits of confidentiality with regard to what is to be revealed and what not. Before the therapy begins, all family members should agree with the policies for the treatment. There are situations when the information received during the conduct of therapy cannot be confidential.[142] The situations include a parent abusing the child or someone is harboring homicidal/suicidal ideas. Parents' sexual life need not be discussed/revealed to children. For the matters which are not clear it is advisable that therapist take help of seniors/colleagues before finalizing a contract.[142]

Most of the times breaches in confidentiality are due to overlapping and/or inappropriately diffuse boundaries in the therapist role as a professional and "family member". The danger of such breach is more often when the therapist treats a family who is a social contact of the therapist also. Hence, it is not advisable to the therapist to treat the family or a friend or anyone in his social relations.[146]

Communication medium: Role of communication media in family and marital therapy situations is very limited. It can be used at best to handle the individual problems, fixing and cancellation of session appointment. Use of telephone may be permissible. However, again it is the therapist's duty to decide that what has been revealed on phone should be discussed in session with other family members or not. Use of e-mail (and other internet devices) should not be recommended as these are likely to mishandled/revealed to third person at many points of transmission between therapist and patient and vice versa. Further, use of e-mail/internet devices does not ensure that information conveyed by patient or therapist has been conveyed to the other party instantaneously. It depends on individual variations in checking the message on this source.[147] In the institutional setting where someone else e.g. secretary/computer operator handles the messages to be conveyed to therapist—use of internet for communication should be sincerely discouraged.

Boundaries in psychotherapy: Boundaries in psychotherapy is an important issue and at times difficult to answer. At times nonsexual boundary crossings can help to strengthen the client-therapist relation. But at the same time it can cause immediate or long-term harm to the client or severe the therapist-patient alliance.[107] The various behaviors that are considered as boundary violation includes, seeking sexual favors, giving or accepting gifts, meetings outside the therapy situations, disclosure about own fantasies and dreams.[107]

Dual relationship: Dual relationship too poses ethical problems which are more likely to a rise in small groups and communities. Dual relationship is the one in which there are one or more distinct kind of relationships with the same person. For instance, a therapist who has a relationship with someone as an employer or neighbor. Such relationships can be affirming, assuring, enriching as well as exploitative. There is no acknowledgment whatsoever of any potential benefits of dual relationships. For the fear of exploitation in any form, most of the therapists and ethical bodies recommend avoidance of dual relationships. Some workers also feel that such concerns at times may be unduly exaggerated and likely to be counterproductive. The 2001 version of American Association of Marital and Family Therapy code of ethics strongly recommend avoidance of dual relationships with clients, students, supervisors, employees and with research participants.[148]

CONCLUSION

The theoretical models of family and marital therapy view the whole family and presenting couple as the patient. There is a gross over lap of the different schools of family and marital therapy. At times, family therapy and marital therapy may be indistinguishable. In this chapter, both are described separately for the purpose of clarity only, as some of the pathological features are described predominantly for family or couple separately in the different texts. Such sick unit can be treated as a whole through one or the other models of psychotherapy. As yet, there is little evidence of one method being better than the other. The therapist, after careful evaluation, may select one of the models of psychotherapy depending on his skill, motivation of members and their psychological mindedness. Depending on the need, the therapist may add the other techniques.

While treating a marital couple, the therapist may prescribe techniques of sex therapy too. Substantial body of research suggests family and couple therapy to be effective methods for ameliorating marital and family discord. A few studies comment about superiority of emotionally focused therapy and behavioral methods. Results of long-term outcome studies are still awaited. It is hoped that concern about negative impact of increasing number of nuclear families, family breakups, divorce and marital separation will continue to provide impetus for further research.

47.6 CURRENT STATUS AND FUTURE DIRECTION IN COUPLE THERAPY

JN Vyas, SS Nathawat

INTRODUCTION

The fundamental challenges of psychotherapy research whether evaluating individual, Couple, or family interventions are to identify effective treatments, understand their underlying mechanisms of change, and delineate aspects of the therapist, client, or context that influence their outcome. One examine the effectiveness of couple-based interventions for treating general relationship distress as well as coexisting emotional, behavioral, and physical health problems.

PREVALENCE AND IMPACT OF COUPLE DISTRESS

Couple therapy continues to gain in stature as a vital component of mental health services. There factors contribute to this growing recognition: (a) the prevalence of couple distress in both community and clinic samples; (b) the impact of couple distress on both the emotional and physical well-being of adult partners and their offspring; and (c) increased evidence of the effectiveness of couple therapy not only in treating couple distress and related relationship problems but also as a primary or adjunct treatment for a variety of individual emotional, behavioral, or physical health disorders.

Couple distress is prevalent in both community epidemiological studies and in research involving individual treatment samples. In the United States, the most salient indicator of couple distress remains a divorce rate of approximately 50% among married couples (Kreider and Fields 2002), with about half of these occurring within the first seven years of marriage. Independent of divorce, the research literature suggests that many, if not most, marriages experience periods of significant turmoil that place them at risk for dissolution or symptom development (e.g. depression or anxiety) in one or both partners at some point in their lives. In a recent national survey, the most frequently cited causes of acute emotional distress were relationship problems including divorce, separation, and other marital strains (Swindle et al. 2000). Other recent studies indicate that maritally discordant individuals are over-represented among individuals seeking mental health services, regardless of whether they report marital distress as their primary complaint (Lin et al. 1996). In a study of 800 employee assistance program (EAP) clients, 65% rated family problem as "considerable" or "extreme" (Shumway et al. 2004).

The linkage of relationship distress to disruption of individual emotional and physical well-being emphasizes the importance of improving and extending empirically based strategies for treating couple distress. Research indicates that couple distress covaries with individual emotional and behavioral disorders beyond general distress in other close relationships (Whisman et al. 2000). Moreover, couple distress-particularly negative communication-has direct adverse effects on cardiovascular, endocrine, immune, neurosensory, and other physiological systems that, in turn, contribute to physical health problems (Kiecolt-Glaser and Newton 2001). Nor are the effects of couple distress confined to the adult partners. Gottman (1999) cites evidence indicating that "Marital distress, conflict and disruption are associated with a wide range of deleterious effects on children, including depression, withdrawal, poor social competence, health problems, poor academic performance, a variety of conduct-related difficulties, and markedly decreased longevity" (p.4). In brief, couple distress has a markedly high prevalence: has a strong linkage to emotional, behavioral, and health problems in the adult partners and their offspring: and is among the most frequent primary or secondary concerns reported by individuals seeking assistance from mental health professionals.

EFFECTIVENESS OF COUPLE THERAPY IN TREATING RELATIONSHIP DISTRESS

How effective is couple therapy? Few reviews affirm that various versions of couple therapy produce moderate, statistically significant, and often clinically significant effects in reducing relationship distress.

Since Christensen and Heavy's (1999) review of couple therapy in the Annual Review of Psychology, several qualitative and quantitative (meta-analytic) reviews of couple therapy have appeared. Shadish and Baldwin (2003) reviewed six previous meta-analyses of studies comparing couple therapy versus no-treatment control groups, including four published reviews (Dunn and Schwebel 1995, Hahlweg and Markman 1988, Johnson et al. 1999, Shadish et al. 1993) and two unpublished reviews (Dutcher 1999, Wilson 1986). The samples of couple therapy studies included in each of these reviews ranged from {Johnson et al. (1999) review of emotion-focused couple therapy (EFCT)} to 163 {Shadish et al. (1993) review of couple and family therapy, of which 62 studies emphasizing couple therapy were reanalyzed by Wilson (1986)}. Mean effect sizes across these six meta-analyses ranged from approximately 0.50 (Wilson 1986) to 1.30 (Johnson et al. 1999). Based on their review of these studies, Shadish and Baldwin (2003) reported an overall mean effect size of 0.84 for couple therapy, indicating that the average person receiving treatment for couple distress was better off at termination than were 80% of individuals in the no-treatment control group.

Shadish and Baldwin (2003) also noted that mean effect size for couple therapy was generally comparable to or larger than that obtained by alternative interventions ranging from individual therapy to medical interventions. They found little evidence of differential effectiveness across different theoretical orientations to couple therapy, particularly once other covariates (e.g. reactivity of measures) were controlled. Noting the small number of couple therapy approaches listed by the American Psychological Association Division 12 Task Force (Chambless and Hollon 1998) as either well established EFCT and insight-oriented couple therapy (IOCT), Shadish and Baldwin (2003) argued that clinicians should also consider such as cognitive-behavioral, systemic, and eclectic approaches to couple therapy as viable approaches to treating general couple distress. They also noted that numerous studies of couple therapy (particularly those emphasizing behavioral treatments) raised unanswered questions regarding their clinical representative ness in that they failed to use clients referred through usual routes and experienced therapists in actual clinic settings. Finally, among those studies reporting data from follow-up at six months or longer, treatment effects tended to be reduced but still significant.

Findings from alternative viewpoints or more recent research provide complementary perspectives to conclusions reached by Shidish and Baldwin in their 2003 summary. One such addition involves a follow-up meta-analysis of 30 randomized experiments with distressed couple contrasting BCT with a no-treatment control (Shadish and Baldwin 2005). Their more recent analysis included 13 studies (7 published in journals and 6 unpublished dissertations) not includes the Shidish et al. (1993) review. Overall, these 30 Studies of BCT yielded a mean effect size of 0.59, which was smaller than the mean effect size of 0.84 for couple therapy pooled across theoretical approaches reported by Shadish and Baldwin (2003), and which indicated that the average individuals in the control condition. In accounting for the more recent, smaller effect size obtained for BCT was better off at the end of treatment than were 72% of individuals in the control condition. In accounting for the more recent, smaller effect size obtained for BCT, the authors noted the consequence of including no published dissertation with smaller sample sizes and small or negative effect size. They also reported that of the various components comprising behavior couple interventions (e.g. communication training, problem-solving training, contingency contracting, behavior exchange, desensitization, cognitive restructuring, and emotional expressiveness training), only communication and problem-solving training led to larger effects, whereas use of cognitive restructuring actually lead to smaller effects. Shadish and Baldwin (2005) found that the effects of BCT were unrelated to "dose" (defined by number and length of sessions), reactivity of the dependent variables considered (e.g. self-report measures of affect or cognition versus observation ratings of communication behavior), or clinical representativeness.

Other than BCT, the sole approach to couple therapy evaluated in multiple trials is EFCT, which combines an experiential, intrapsychic focus on inner emotional experience with an emphasis on cyclical, self-reinforcing interaction (Johnson et al. 1999). In four randomized trials, EFCT was superior to a waiting-list control condition in reduction relationship distress, yielding recovery rates of 70–73% and a weighted mean effect size of 1.31 (Johson 2002).

In addition to the two couple therapy approaches evaluated in multiple clinical trials, several approaches have demonstrated positive outcomes in treating couple distress in only one trial. Fist Snyder and Wills (1989) compared insight-oriented approaches to couple therapy with behavior approaches in a controlled clinical trial involving 79 distressed couples. The insight oriented condition emphasized the interpretation and resolution of confliction emotional processes related to development issues, collusive interactions, and maladaptive relationship patterns. At termination after approximately after approximately 20 sessions, couple in both treatment modalities showed statistically and clinically significant gains in relationship satisfaction compared with a wait-list conditions were 1.01 and 0.96, respectively; treatment gains were substantially maintained at six-month follow-up. However, at experienced divorce, in contrast to only 38% of couples in the behavior condition had experienced divorce, in contrast to only 3% of couples treated in the insight-oriented condition (Snyder et al. 1991).

More recently, findings have emerged for an integrative behavior approach to couple therapy (IBCT; Jacobson and Christensen 1996) that combines traditional behavior techniques for promotion change (specifically, communication and behavior-exchange skills training) with strategies aimed at fostering emotional acceptance. Interventions aimed at increasing acceptance include promoting tolerance and encouraging partners to appreciate differences and to use them to enhance their marriage. In the largest randomized clinical trial of couple therapy ever conducted, Christensen and colleagues (2004) compared the expanded IBCT with traditional BCT by assigning 134 distressed couple to the two conditions, stratified into moderately and severely distressed group. Couples in IBCT made steady improvements in satisfaction throughout the course of treatment. Whereas BCT couple improved more quick than IBCT couple early in treatment but then platitude later in treatment. Both treatment produced similar levels of clinically significant improvement by the end of treatment (71% of IBCT couples and 59% of BCT couples were reliably improved or recovered, based on self-reports of overall relationship satisfaction).

Although various specific approaches to couple therapy have now demonstrated effectives in reducing relationship distress in controlled trial, a substantial percentage of individuals fail to show significant improvement from these treatments and an even greater percent of individuals show deterioration in gains at follow-up. Specifically, previous research has shown that about one-third of couples fail to achieve significant gains from treatment, and in only half of treated couples do both partners show significant improvement in marital satisfaction at termination. Moreover, assessment at two years or longer after termination indicates significant deterioration among 30–60% of treated couples (Cookerly 1980, Jacobson et al. 1987, Snyder et al. 1991). Such finding have fostered two alternative lines of attack for treating couple distress: (a) distillation and emphasis of common factors hypothesized to contribute to beneficial effects across "singular" treatment approaches, and (b) pluralistic models incorporating multiple components of diverse treatment approaches.

Adopting the former strategy, Sprenkle and Blow (2004) argued that common mechanisms of change cutting across the diverse couple therapies account for the absence of significant differences in their overall effectiveness. They cited and three types or classes of common factors characterizing psychotherapy in general, and three factors specific to couple or family therapy. Common factors viewed as generics to psychotherapy include (a) client characteristics (e.g. learning style, perseverance, and compliance with instructions or assignments), (b) therapist characteristics (e.g. abilities to foster a therapeutic alliance and to match activity level to clients' expectations or preferences),

(c) characteristics of the therapeutic relationship (e.g. emotional connectedness and congruence between the therapist's and client's specific expectations or goals), (d) expectancy or placebo effects, and (e) nonspecific interventions promoting emotional experiencing, cognitive mastery, and behavioral regulation. Those common factors viewed by Sprenkle and Blow (2004) as specific to couple or family therapies include (a) emphasis on the interpersonal context in which specific problems occur, (b) inclusion of multiple members of the extended family system in direct treatment, and (c) fostering an expanded therapeutic alliance across partners or multiple members of the family as a whole. To date, there has been little research documenting specific treatment effects attributable to proposed common factors—and no efforts in designing couple treatment approaches explicitly intended to maximize the therapeutic impact of common factors (Sexton et al. 2004).

An alternative to the common factors approach involves efforts to incorporate active, specific treatment components for diverse approaches into multicomponent interventions in a systematic manner. Such approaches have variously been described as "integrative" (e.g. Gurman 1981, 2002) or "pluralistic" (Snyder 1999), and are distinguished from eclecticism by their systematic selection or synthesis within a conceptually coherent model. Gurman (2002) described a "depth-behavioral" integrative approach to couple therapy that emphasizes the critical interrelation of intrapsychic and interpersonal factors in couple interactions and defines the goal of couple therapy as the loosening and broadening of each spouse's implicit matrix of assumptions, expectations, and requirements of intimate interpersonal contact. This is accomplished through interpretation, cognitive restructuring, and creation of therapeutic tasks to promote each spouse's exposure to those aspects of him- or she and his or her partner that are blocked form awareness. Snyder (1999) proposed a hierarchical approach to couple therapy incorporating structural, behavioral, and cognitive techniques earlier in the therapeutic sequence and drawing on insight-oriented techniques termed "affective reconstruction" later in treatment primarily if relationship problems prove resistant to the earlier interventions. In affective reconstruction, previous relationships, their affective components, and strategies for emotional gratification and anxiety containment are reconstructed, with a focus on identifying for each partner recurring maladaptive patterns in their interpersonal conflicts and coping styles across relationships. In addition, interventions examine ways in which previous coping strategies vital to prior relationships represent distortions or inappropriate solutions for emotional intimacy and satisfaction in the current relationship. Neither the integrative depth-behavioral approach proposed by Gurman (2002) nor the pluralistic approach advocated by Snyder (1999) has been subjected to empirical evaluation, although both approaches build on couple treatment approaches previously supported in randomized clinical trails.

EFFECTIVENESS OF COUPLE THERAPY IN TREATING COMORBID DISORDERS

The co-occurrence between overall couple distress and specific relationship problems, as well as individual emotional or behavioral disorders, has been well established in the research literature over the past decade. Based on these findings, new couple-based treatments have emerged for treating distressed couples for whom one or both partners have coexisting emotional, behavioral or physical health problems (Snyder and Whisman 2003). Snyder and Whisman (2004a) examined the covariation between general relationship distress and problems in specific areas of the couple's relationship in a sample of 1020 community couples and 50 couples in therapy, based on partner's scores on the Marital Satisfaction Inventory–Revised (Snyder 1997). Results indicated that individuals reporting moderate or higher global relationship distress were five to six times more likely than nondistressed persons to report specific relationship problems in the areas of physical aggression, the sexual relationship, finances, and child rearing. Whisman (1999; Whisman and Uebelacker 2005) evaluated the association between marital distress and 12 months prevalence rates of 13 psychiatric disorders in 2538 married persons comprising the National Comorbidity Survey. Results indicated that martially distressed persons were two to three times more likely than were nondistressed persons to experience disorders involving mood, anxiety or substance abuse.

The co-occurrence between overall couple distress and specific individual or relationship problems has led to three couple-base treatment strategies for addressing these comorbid difficulties (Baucom et al. 1998). The first uses general couple therapy to reduce overall relationship distress based on the premise that martial conflict serves as a broad stressor that contributes to the development, exacerbation, or maintenance or specific individual or relationship problems. The second strategy involves developing disorder-specific couple interventions that focus on particular partner interactions presumed to directly influence either the co-occurring problems or their treatment. The third couple-based strategy involves partner-assisted intervention in which one partner serves as a "surrogate therapist" or coach in assisting the other partner with individual problems.

Couple-based Treatment of Specific Relationship Problems

Couple-based interventions have been well established as effective in treating two specific components of relationship functioning: difficulties in the sexual relationship and problems of physical aggression. Recent findings also suggest the effectiveness of couple therapy in treating couples dealing with issues of infidelity.

- *Sexual difficulties:* Epidemiological data indicate that 43% of women and 31% of men will experience sexual dysfunction during their lifetime (Laumann et al. (1999). A recent review of couple-based treatments for sexual dysfunctions (Regev et al. 2003) concluded that (a) sex therapy, primarily consisting of sensate focus, is comparable to communication therapy in primary and secondary an orgasmic women; (b) couples receiving couple therapy in addition to sex therapy demonstrate more pronounced and comprehensive treatment gains, including significantly more intense experiences of sex and sexual desire: and (c) sex therapy positively influences both sexual and marital problems, whereas general couple therapy appears to facilitate resolution of marital problems only. Baucom et al. (1998) identified several couple-based interventions with documented effectiveness in treating female sexual dysfunctions related to lifelong or situational orgasmic disorders, male partners participate with their female partner in techniques of sensate focus; toward the end of treatment, women are coached in sharing effective techniques of masturbation with their partners. Couple-based interventions also assist couples in discussing and resolving specific difficulties they experience in their sexual interactions. Findings have affirmed the efficacy of couple interventions in treating women with primary or secondary orgasmic disorders, with improvement rates ranging from 65% to 90%. Additional evidence supports combining general behaviorally oriented couple therapy with orgasm-consistency training in the treatment of women reporting hypoactive sexual desire (Hurlbert et al. 1993). Baucom et al. (1998) noted that few studies of couple-based interventions have targeted male sexual disorders despite evidence that sexual and marital problems are more closely linked in men than in women and despite reports of recent increases in male complaints of low sexual desire.
- *Physical aggression:* Mild to moderate physical aggression (e.g. pushing, grabbing, shoving, or slapping) occurs in more than half of couples seeking couple therapy (Holtzworth-Munroe et al. 2003). Among couple therapy samples, as much as 85% of partner aggression is reciprocal, with both partners engaging in primarily low levels of aggression. Moreover, psychological aggression (e.g. verbal abuse or threats of violence) predicts physical abuse a year later (Murphy and O'Leary 1989). Although most therapists agree that couple therapy is inappropriate for couples characterized by severe physical aggression (primarily violence by male partners resulting in female partners' injuries), couple-based interventions have been effective in treating mild to moderate levels of aggression. Such interventions emphasize anger management (e.g. recognition of anger, time-outs, and self-regulation techniques) and communication skills (e.g. emotional expressiveness and problem solving). In their review of randomized trials comparing conjoint treatment to gender-specific treatment, Holtzworth-Munroe et al. (2003) concluded that conjoint couple therapy that has a direct and specific focus on eliminating violence "may be as effective as the more widely utilized gender specific treatments". A more recent study compared the outcomes of a domestic violence focused treatment for 51 couples randomly assigned to either individual couple therapy, a multi-couple group treatment, or a no-treatment comparison group (Stith et al. 2004). Male partner rates of physical aggression at six-month follow-up were highest in the comparison group (66%) and lower in the multi-couple group (25%) than in the individual-couple therapy group (43%). Moreover both marital aggression and acceptance of physical aggression decreased significantly among participants in the multi-couple group therapy but not among participants in either the individual-couple therapy or no-treatment comparison conditions, a finding that suggests the multi-couple group format has an incremental impact in changing underlying attitudes toward relationship aggression.
- *Extramarital affairs:* Research suggests that on average, between 1.5% and 4% of married individuals will engage in extramarital sex in any given year (Allen et al. 2005), and approximately one in three men aged 60–69 and one in five women aged 40–49 report engaging in extramarital sex at some point in their lives (Wiederman 1997). Although couples report extramarital affairs as a leading cause of divorce and couple therapists describe infidelity as among the most difficult problems to treat (Whisman et al. 1997). Until recently there has been almost no empirical study of interventions for couples dealing with affairs. Atkins and colleagues (2005b) examined treatment outcomes for 19 couples reporting an affair by one of the partners participating in the randomized trial of IBCT versus BST by Christensen and colleagues (2004) reported findings from a replicated case study of an integrative approach designed specifically to assist couples recovering from an extramarital affair. The six-month intervention comprised three phases that targeted (a) coping with initial emotional and behavioral disruption of individual and relationship functioning following discovery or disclosure of the affair; (b) exploring individual, relationship, and outside contextual factors contributing to the initial onset or maintenance of the affair; and (c) reaching an informed decision about how to move on, either individually or as a couple. At termination, the majority of participants in the

study reported less emotional and marital distress, and individuals whose partner had participated in the affair reported greater forgiveness toward their partner.

Couple-based Treatment of Mental and Physical Health Problems

Research has documented the effectiveness of couple-based interventions for a broad range of emotional and behavioral dysfunctions, including alcohol and related health problems. Promising couple-based interventions have also recently emerged for a variety of other difficulties; interventions that have received at least preliminary empirical evidence of their effectiveness are described here.

- *Substance-use disorders alcohol-* and drug-use disorders comprise the most common psychiatric disorders in the general population, with lifetime prevalence rates of 23.5% and 11.9%, respectively (Kessler et al. 1994). BCT for alcoholism and drug abuse aims to alter couple and family interaction patterns to promote a family environment more conducive to abstinence and sobriety (e.g. by reducing the partner's recurring complaints about past drinking and promoting attention to positive aspects of current sober behavior), as well as to improve communication and positive activities (Fals-Stewart et al. 2003). BCT for alcohol and drug abuse typically involves 15–20 outpatient couple sessions over five to six months.

  Recently, Fals-Stewart and colleagues (2005a) examined the clinical efficacy and cost-effectiveness of a shortened version of BCT with 100 alcoholic male patients and their partners. In the shortened version, couples participated in only 6 rather than 12 conjoint sessions; alcoholic clients participated in an additional 12 weekly individual sessions. Results indicated that those assigned to the clients receiving standard BCT, thereby supporting the cost-effectiveness of this shortened intervention.

  - *Mood disorders:* Lifetime prevalence rates for major depressive episode and dysthymia are estimated at 17.1% and 6.4%, respectively (Kessler et al. 1994). Three clinical trials have shown that behavioral couple interventions for depression emphasizing behavior exchange, communication and problem-solving skills, and cognitive interventions (e.g. cognitive reframing and directing attention to positive change) are effective in relieving depression when provided to martially distressed couples with a depressed partner (Gupta et al. 2003). Furthermore, compared with individual-based therapies. BCT has the incremental benefit of improving overall relationship satisfaction. Clinical guidelines for providing BCT for depressed individuals are provided by Beach and Gupta (2003). Similarly, conjoint couple therapy incorporating components of interpersonal psychotherapy for depression aimed at helping depressed individuals better understand and negotiate their interpersonal relationships has been shown to be effective in treating depression (Foley et al. 1989). More recently, Leff et al. (2000) reported promising results for systemic couple therapy, using interventions designed to reduce problematic patterns of interacting, for depressed married individuals with a critical spouse. Finally, Dessaulles et al. (2003) compared 14 sessions of EFCT with pharmacotherapy in treating wives' major depression in 18 couples randomly assigned to treatment condition. Both interventions were equally effective in reducing depressive symptoms although there was some evidence that women receiving EFCT made greater improvement following termination than those receiving pharmacotherapy.
  - *Anxiety disorders:* Excessive anxiety is one of the most frequent mental health problems in the United States, with a lifetime prevalence rate of developing any anxiety disorder at 24.9% (Kessler et al. 1994). In their review of couple-based interventions for anxiety disorders, Baucom et al. (2003) noted that anxiety disorders may negatively impact couple functioning by disrupting interaction patterns, intention to the needs of the non-anxious partner. Baucom et al. (2003) described ways in which efficacious treatments for anxiety disorders (e.g. exposure and response prevention) cognitive restructuring and relaxation training can be incorporated into either (a) partner-assisted interventions using the partner to assist with exposure exercises and provide support or (b) couple-based interventions focusing on ways in which couple functioning maintains anxiety symptoms, as well as ways in which the anxiety influences couple functioning. In their review of specific couple-based interventions for various anxiety disorders, Baucom et al. (1998) concluded that partner-assisted exposure treatment of obsessive-compulsive disorder is at least as effective as treating the patient without such assistance; they also determined that exposure interventions for agoraphobia may show enhanced benefit from involving the partner even when there is no overt relationship distress, a conclusion affirmed in a recent review by Byrne et al. (2004).
  - *Pain and physical illness:* Over the past 15 years, psychosocial pain researchers have become increasingly interested in the role that partners play in how patients adjust to pain and in involving partners in psychosocial pain-management efforts (Keefe et al. 2006). For example, partners can encourage patients in acquiring more effective pain-control strategies, and can be discouraged themselves from criticizing appropriate coping skills. Enforcing the patient's rest,

or insisting that pain medication is the only way to manage pain. Moreover, couple-based interventions for chronic pain-and for physical illness more generally-can help partners to cope with their own emotional struggles with caretaking, promote more effective communication around pain and emotional distress, and facilitate couple processes for providing emotional and tangible support, dealing with conflict, and expressing affection and intimacy (Keefe et al. 2006).

Keefe and colleagues (1996) randomly assigned 88 patients with osteoarthritis knee pain to spouse-assisted coping skills training, a conventional coping skills training condition alone, or an arthritis education and partner-support control condition. Patients in the spouse-assisted coping skills training condition received training in a variety of cognitive and behavioral pain-coping skills (e.g. relaxation, imagery, distraction techniques, activity pacing, goal setting, and cognitive restructuring) and they and their partners received training in various couples skills (e.g. joint practice, communication skills, behavioral rehearsal, problem solving, and maintenance training). Patients in the partner-assisted coping skills training had the best outcomes across multiple criteria, whereas those in the arthritis education-social support control condition had the worst outcomes. Moreover, patients in the partner-assisted coping skills training who showed increases in marital adjustment were more likely to show lower levels of psychological disability, physical disability, and pain behavior at 12 months follow-up.

Couple-based interventions for patients dealing with cancer have resulted in similar findings. Specifically, Keefe and colleagues (2005) recently completed a study that tested the effects of a partner-guided pain management intervention for 78 patients with end of life cancer pain. The intervention delivered by a nurse, integrated information about cancer pain with training in three pain-coping skills and emphasized the role these skills could play in controlling patient and partner emotional responses and relational exchanges. Results indicated that patients receiving this intervention tended to report reduced levels of pain, and that their spouses improved in their sense of efficacy for helping the patient control pain and tended to report reduced levels of caregiver strain.

Finally, recent study examined the impact of an eight-session couple therapy for nine couples in which one partner was diagnosed with a terminal illness (Mohr et al. 2003). Conjoint sessions emphasized (a) helping patients and their partners to find meaning together through examining beliefs, goals, and values; (b) increasing intimacy, emotional support, and reciprocity; and (c) facilitating conversations about death and dying. Results indicated improvements in couples' relationship quality and significant decreases in patients' distress about dying and the frequency of partner's worry about their partner dying.

Emerging treatments for other disorders: Couple-based treatments continue to be developed at an increasing pace for a broad spectrum of individual emotional, behavioral and health-related difficulties. Although evidence for these treatments' effectiveness remains primarily anecdotal, several noteworthy exceptions exist; Monson et al. (2004) described recent findings form cognitive behavioral couple treatment of post-traumatic stress disorder (PTSD) in a pilot study of seven couples in which the husband was diagnosed with PTSD secondary to Vietnam combat experiences. The treatment emphasized three components involving psycho education about PTSD and relationship problems, communication skills training and interventions targeting cognitions contributing to the association between PTSD and relationship problems. Following the 15-session treatment, clinicians' and partner's ratings of the veterans' PTSD symptoms showed significant improvement, with effect sizes exceeding 1.00; the veterans' self-reported reductions in PTSD symptoms were not statistically significant (in part due to the small sample), but still yielded a moderate effect size of 0.64. Wives' own ratings of anxiety also improved with this couple-based intervention, and both partners reported improved social functioning in the household.

Finally, two couple-based treatments have been developed for couples in which one partner has been diagnosed with borderline personality disorder (BPD). The first (Fruzzetti and Iverson 2006) builds on dialectical behavior therapy (DBT) for individuals with BPD. In a sample of 22 couples participating in a six session couples group, decreases in invalidating behaviors (e.g. dismissive, minimizing, or rejecting statements) and increases in validating responses (e.g. acceptance and understanding) pre- to post-treatment predicted decreased levels of individual and relationship distress in a moderately distressed sample (Lillis and Fruzzetti 2004). More recently, Kirby and Baucom (2004) reported results of a couple-based group intervention combining elements of DBT with cognitive behavioral couple therapy (CNCT) for 10 couples in which one partner had been diagnosed with BPD and had already received individual DBT. Following 16 two-hour sessions (with five couples per group), the women partners showed less depression and related negative affect, increases in positive affect, and improved ability to regulate their own emotions; effect sizes ranged from 0.72 to 1.00.

PROCESSES OF CHANGE IN COUPLE THERAPY

How does couple therapy work? Although each of the empirically supported approaches to couple therapy posits specific processes or mechanisms of change, there has been little research explicitly indicating these proposed mechanisms as responsible for observed therapeutic effects. Three briefly describe three approaches to examining change processes in couple therapy. And then summarize the few available empirical findings related to change mechanisms in the context of theoretical formulations underlying the major approaches to couple therapy.

Methods of Investigating Change Processes

- *Regression analysis of mediation:* Probably the best-known and most widely used approach for examining change processes in therapy involves use of regression analysis, following procedures outlined by Baron and Kenny (1986), for establishing mediation effects. Using these guidelines, a proposed mediating variable (e.g. communication processes) is shown to account (either entirely or partially) for the relation between some predictor variable (e.g. treatment condition status) and some outcome variable (e.g. relationship satisfaction) when the following four conditions are met: (a) The predictor affects the criterion (e.g. treatment leads to increased relationship satisfaction); (b) the predictor affects the mediator (e.g. treatment leads to gains in communication skills); (c) the mediator affects the criterion (e.g. gains in communication skills lead to increased relationship satisfaction). Controlling for the predictor; and (d) the relation between the predictor and the criterion is reduced (partial mediation) or eliminated (complete mediation) after controlling for the relation between the mediator and the criterion. In moderated mediation (see Whisman and Snyder 1997), the mediating or change mechanisms are demonstrated to have a stronger effect for one group than for another (e.g. mediating effects of therapeutic alliance for couples receiving BCT versus EFCT, or effects of behavior-exchange skills training for younger couples relative to older ones).
- *Hierarchical linear modeling analysis of change process:* More recently, couple researchers (e.g. Doss et al. 2005) have examined the relation between proposed mechanisms of change and outcome variables through the use of hierarchical linear modeling (HLM; Raudenbush and Bryk 2001), also known as growth curve analysis. This approach to identifying change mechanisms involves two steps. First, multiple assessments of some criterion variable are used to estimate a trajectory, or growth curve, which allows investigators to describe the nature of change for a given criterion or outcome within a sample. In the second step of growth curve analysis, the parameters summarizing change of each person are treated as new dependent variables that are then predicted from other within or between-subject variables proposed as mechanisms of change.
- *Task analysis of change processes:* A third approach to investigating change processes involves task analysis of proximal outcomes that occur within or between sessions by focusing on specific therapeutic events (Heatherington et al. 2005, Rice and Greenberg 1984). Such task analysis involves disassembling the therapeutic process into smaller, measurable in-session units or events to capture the actual sequence of therapist-client interactions and then delineating the linkage of these events to proximal or "mini" outcomes that presumably build on each other and contribute to molar, more distal outcomes (e.g. relationship satisfaction at termination). For example, an investigator examining presumed mechanisms of change in EFCT might examine events delimited by therapist clarification of underlying primary attachment-related fears and the client's owing and expressing those fears in a "softened" manner, and the linkage of this sequence to the other partner's likelihood of shifting from antagonistic or defensive responses to empathic or nurturing ones.

Empirical Findings Regarding Change Processes

Previous reviews (e.g. Gottman 1998, Lebow 2000) have generally concurred in their conclusion that little empirical evidence exists regarding presumed mechanisms of change in couple therapy. Such conclusions rest in part from disappointing findings from mediation analyses adopting the traditional regression approach. For example, whereas BCT emphasizes the importance of improving communication skills as a means of reducing relationship distress-and although such skills do typically increase among couples receiving BCT several studies have failed to find an association between the magnitude of changes in communication behaviors and gains in relationship satisfaction. Similarly, although CBCT has been shown to produce positive change in targeted cognitions (e.g. expectancies and attributions), changes in these cognitions have not been linked to couples' gains in satisfaction following CBCT (see Whisman and Snyder 1997 for a summary of relevant studies).

However, recent findings drawing on HLM and task analysis offer encouragement regarding significant developments in identifying change mechanisms in couple therapy. For example, Doss et al. (2005) use hierarchical growth curve analysis to examine mechanisms of change in 134 couples randomly assigned to either traditional BCT or ICBT. Both therapies were effective in increasing emotional acceptance and improving communication behaviors across the course of therapy; however, these changes differed by treatment modality in a manner consistent with their respective presumed change mechanisms. Specifically, acceptance increased significantly more for couples in IBCT than for couples in BCT, whereas couples in BCT showed larger gains in positive communication. Moreover, examination of change separately in the first and second halves of therapy indicated that change in targeted behaviors was a powerful mechanism of change early in therapy, whereas in the second half of therapy, emotional acceptance was more strongly related to changes in relationship satisfaction.

Task analysis has been used successfully to examine change processes in both IBCT and EFCT. In a pilot study with 12 distressed couples randomly assigned to either IBCT or traditional BCT (Cordova et al. 1998), couples in IVCT showed relatively more constructive detachment (i.e. talking about problems without blaming or being compelled to solve them-both indicators of acceptance) over the course of therapy and more " soft expressions" of emotion in late sessions relative to earlier ones. Changes in husbands' and wives' constructive detachment from early to late sessions predicted couples' gains in relationship satisfaction.

The most compelling findings regarding specific change processes in couple therapy have emerged using a task-analysis approach to investigating change in EFCT. An early study by Johnson and Greenberg (1998) comparing partner exchanges in "best" sessions of three successfully treated couples versus those for three couples with poor outcome showed that high-change couples exhibited more frequent "softening" events in which a previously critical partner expressed vulnerability and asked for comfort and connection from his or her spouse. A second report regarding three task analytic studies of EFCT (Grenberg et al. 1993) showed that (a) couples receiving EFCT demonstrated more shifts from hostility to affiliative behaviors than did wait-list couples; (b) best sessions as identified by couples were characterized by more depth of experiencing and affiliative and autonomous statements than were sessions identified as poor' and (c) intimate, emotionally laden self-disclosure by one partner was more likely to lead to affiliative statements by the other partner than were other randomly selected responses. Finally, a recent task analysis of four EFCT sessions by Bradley and Furrow (2004) found that emotional experiencing and the disclosure of attachment-related affect and fears were the key client features of successful softening events; consistent with proposed mechanisms of change in EFCT, specific therapist interventions linked to softening events involved intensifying a couple's emotional experience and promoting intrapsychic awareness and interpersonal shifts in attachment-related interactions.

PREDICTORS OF COUPLE THERAPY OUTCOME

Methods of Identifying Predictors of Treatment Outcome

- *Identifying prognostic indicators from analyses of main effects:* In evaluating predictors of treatment outcome, investigators have made a distinction between prognostic indicators, which predict response to a particular treatment (or response across treatments, irrespective of specific approach), and prescriptive indicators, which predict response to one versus another treatment (Hollon and Najavits 1988). Identifying a prognostic indicator requires only evaluating the association between the predictor variable and some outcome measure. This can be done by regressing post-treatment outcome scores on the predictor, controlling for pretreatment scores on the outcome variable: similar analyses can be done with dichotomous outcomes (e.g. clinical significance outcomes) using logistic regression analyses. The overwhelming preponderance of research on predictors of response to couple therapy has emphasized the delineation of these more general prognostic indicators.
- *Identifying prescriptive indicators from analyses of interactions:* Evaluating whether some variable predicts outcome to one specific treatment versus another treatment-that is, identifying prescriptive indicators-requires testing for an interaction or moderator effect. Prescriptive indicators are examined using the aptitude-treatment interaction (ATI) paradigm (Coronbach and Snow 1977, Dance and Neufeld 1988). In using regression to identify prescriptive indicatoes, one tests for a significant treatment X predictor interaction indicating that the association between the predictor and treatment outcome varies as a function of the type of treatment (i.e. that type of treatment moderates the association between the predictor and outcome). Alternative approaches for identifying prescriptive indicators exist when using analysis of individual growth curves (Rogosa 1991).

Research design requirements for identifying prescriptive indicators are more rigorous than those for identifying more general prognostic indicators, particularly as these relate to adequate power for detecting effects (Whisman and McClelland 2005).

Empirical Findings Regarding Predictors of Couple Therapy Outcome

- *Prognostic indicators of treatment response:* Over the past several decades, a substantial body of research has identified general prognostic indicators of response to couple therapy including demographic, relationship, and individual characteristics. Most of these findings have been derived from controlled clinical trials of BCT and are reviewed in greater detail by Whisman et al. (2005); exception are noted where applicable.

Several studies have found that younger couples respond more favorably to BCT (Baucom 1984, Hahleweg et al. 1984, O'Leary and Turkewitz 1981), Whereas others have found no association between age and treatment outcome (Crowe 1978, Jacobson et al. 1986). In addition, Crowe (1978) found that less-educate couples had better response to BCT than those with higher education. A prediction study collapsing across behavioral and insight-oriented treatment conditions (Snyder et al. 1993) found that initial status of being unemployed or employed in a position of unskilled labor predicated poor treatment outcome four years after termination. In a controlled trial of IVCT versus traditional BCT, couples who were married longer showed greater treatment gains, regardless of condition (Atkins 2005a).

Results from various studies indicate that couples having the greatest difficulties in their relationship are less likely to benefit form treatment, with initial levels of relationship distress accounting for up to 46% of the variance in treatment outcome (Johnson 2002). Lack of commitment and behavioral steps taken toward (Beach and Broderick 1983, Hahlweg et al. 1984) but not in another (Jacobson et al. 1986). Hahlweg et al. (1984) found that BCT outcome was predicted by negative communication behavior. Snyder et al. (1993) found that poorer outcome to couple therapy was predicted by lower relationship quality, greater negative relationship affect and disengagement, and greater desired change in the relationship. By contrast, initial levels of relationship distress were not significantly related to treatment outcome in a study of EFCT (Johnson and Talitman 1997), although partners' therapeutic alliance accounted for 22% to the variance in response to treatment.

Greater interpersonal sensitivity and emotional expressiveness-as determined by measures of "femininity"– have been found to predict better outcome at termination (Baucom and Aiken 1984) and long-term follow-up (Snyder et al. 1993) but were not predictive in a third study (Jacobson et al. 1986). Couples in which partners exhibit a higher degree of traditionality (i.e. higher affiliation needs in the wife and higher independence needs in the husband) have been shown to have poorer response to BCT (Jacobson et al. 1986). Partner's higher levels of depressed affect have been linked to poorer outcome in one study (Snyder et al. 1993) but not in another (Jacobson et al. 1986).

PRESCRIPTIVE INDICATORS OF TREATMENT RESPONSE

In contrast to findings regarding general prognostic indicators of response to couple therapy, research identifying prescriptive indicators of couple treatment response has been rare. An early study by O'Leary and Turkewitz (1981) suggested that younger couples responded better to behavioral interventions emphasizing behavior-exchange skills, whereas older couples showed more favorable response to general communication skills training. More recently, research comparing IBCT with traditional BCT suggests that severely distressed couples may respond more favorably to BCT than to IBCT during the initial stages of treatment, although both treatments produce equivalent gains at outcome and preliminary findings indicate that IBCT may produce more enduring gains at extended follow-up (Atkins and Christensen 2004). Moreover, exploratory analyses from this clinical trial reported by Atkins et al. (2005a) suggested that sexually dissatisfied couples showed slower initial response but more consistent gains overall in IBCT versus BCT.

47.7 ENDURING EFFECTS FOR COGNITIVE BEHAVIOR THERAPY IN THE TREATMENT OF DEPRESSION AND ANXIETY

JN Vyas, AR Garg

Psychosocial interventions have long been touted as providing enduring change. Not only are they said to reduce existing distress or improve functioning, they are believed to do so in a manner that produces lasting change overtime. The question is whether this is true: Do psychosocial interventions truly produce enduring effects, and, if so, how do they compare with other major interventions like psychoactive medications?

Enduring effects can be of at least two kinds. Treatment effects reduce existing problems that would not have gone away on their own they can be said to be enduring to the extent that the problem does not come back. In such instances, all that is required to document that a treatment has an enduring effect is that the changes produced be stable overtime. If problems return at a lesser rate or intensity than would have been the case if the treatment had not been provided. Preventive effects reduce risk for future problems. Such effects may not be immediately apparent in terms of the outcomes of interest; rather, their beneficial effects may become apparent only over time. Nonetheless, to have an enduring effect, an intervention must set in motion causal processes that interrupt the sequence of events leading to the onset or return of the disorder. That means that even delayed effects must reflect on going causal processes that may be subject to detection.

If Psychosocial interventions do have enduring effects, how would they be detected? For an effect to be said to endure, its benefits must extend beyond the end of the period of intervention. When enduring effects are absolute (when symptoms do not return or expected onsets do not occur), then no comparison is required other than the lack of change from the end of treatment overtime. When enduring effects are probabilistic (when symptoms do return to some extent or onsets do occur for some), then gains must be maintained or deterioration forestalled relative to some type of comparison condition. With respect to treatment, evidence for enduring effects is most compelling when subsequent symptom return is reduced relative to some other equally efficacious intervention and the relative value of those effects is best established by comparison to the most efficacious continuing interventions.

Efficacious treatments can fall into at least three categories, depending on their mechanisms of action and the nature of the underlying disorder. Some may be purely palliative; that is, they suppress the expression of symptoms so long as they are applied but do nothing to address the processes that drive the underlying disorder. Other interventions may be curative in the sense that they eliminate or reverse the underlying process that would otherwise lead to be prophylactic. These interventions eliminate or offset processes that contribute to risk for future onsets. Both curative and prophylactic interventions can be said to have enduring effects, with the former keeping symptoms form coming back (relapse) and the latter preventing wholly new onsets (recurrence).

Existing intervention can be classified with respect to this typology. As effective as medications are for many psychiatric disorders, there is no evidence that they are anything more than palliative; that is, they suppress symptoms so long as they are taken, but often do little to alter the course of the underlying disorder or to reduce subsequent risk once their use is discontinued. The cognitive and behavioral interventions, on the other hand, actually may be curative and possibly even prophylactic; that is, there is evidence that they produce lasting change or even reduce future risk. To the extent that this is true, it means that patients need not stay in treatment forever or that disorders can actually be prevented and possibly never even expressed (Hollon et al. 1992b). Dynamic-interpersonal and humanistic-experiential interventions typically have not been tested in a way that would allow for the detection of enduring effects.

This article highlights the evidence for the statements above. The bulk of the evidence to date comes from the literature on depression and the anxiety disorders and involves the cognitive and behavior therapies (collectively referred to throughout the review as CBT). Typically, this takes the form of comparisons between patients treated to remission with CBT versus medication, then followed over time following treatment termination.

TREATMENT AND PREVENTION OF DEPRESSION

Depression is one of the most prevalent of the psychiatric disorders and a leading cause of disability worldwide. Although most patients remit from any given episode, symptoms often come back at some later time, and depression is now considered to be a largely recurrent disorder (when it is not chronic). Several different types of interventions have been shown to be efficacious in its treatment (see Hollon et al. 2002 for a review). Antidepressant medication (ADM) has been shown to be superior to placebo controls in literally thousands of trials and tends to suppress symptoms for as long as it is continued or maintained, but there is no evidence that it does anything to reduce underlying risk once its use is terminated. Both interpersonal psychotherapy (IPT) and CBT appear to be about as efficacious as ADM with respect to the reduction of acute distress: moreover, IPT appears to have a greater breadth of effect with respect to enhancing the quality of relationships, whereas CBT appears to be more enduring than ADM. More purely behavioral interventions have not been tested often, but have performed well in recent trials. Family-focused therapy shows promise in preventing relapse or recurrence in bipolar disorder, but has been little tested in unipolar depression. More traditional dynamic psychotherapy has fared poorly in direct comparisons with other interventions (although questions can be raised about the adequacy with which it has been implemented), and humanistic-experiential therapies have not been often tested.

Cognitive Therapy and the Prevention of Relapse

Among the various efficacious interventions, cognitive therapy (CT) has produced the most consistent evidence of enduring effects. In this variant of CBT, patients are trained to collect information in a systematic fashion to offset the influence of maladaptive information processing strategies and to conduct behavioral experiments to test the accuracy of their negative beliefs (Beck et al. 1979). Patients also are encouraged to examine the accuracy of their beliefs using a series of logical tools (cognitive restructuring), and a premium is placed on teaching the patient to do the therapy for him- or herself, in recognition of the chronic recurrent nature of depression. Preparation for termination is addressed from the beginning of therapy (Serving to justify the extensive use of homework) and explicit practice is provided in relapse prevention throughout.

Patients treated to remission in CT appear to be about half as likely to relapse following treatment termination as are patients treated to remission with medications. In recent studies patients with moderate to severe depression were found to be more likely to respond to 8 weeks of treatment with either CT or ADM than with pill-placebo (a demonstrable treatment effect); by 16 weeks, response rates to the two active interventions were virtually identical (just under 60%) (DeRubeis et al. 2005). At that point, patients who had responded to medications were randomly assigned to continuation ADM or withdrawn onto pill-placebo and followed over the ensuing year. Patients who responded to CT terminated treatment and were allowed no more than three booster session (not more than one per month) over that same interval.

Even when nonadherence was taken into account, prior CT did as well as continuation medication. This suggest that prior CT has an enduring effect that is at least as large in magnitude as keeping patients on medications, a purely palliative intervention that is the current standard of treatment for recurrent depression (Am Psychiatric Assoc. 2000).

This is one of the most robust findings with respect to enduring effects in the literature. In several earlier trials, patients treated to remission in cognitive therapy were only about half as likely to relapse as were patients treated to remission with medications alone following treatment termination (Blackburn et al. 1986, Kovacs et al. 1981, and Simons et al. 1986), and no more likely to relapse than were patients continued on medication (Evans et al. 1992). Only two studies have failed to find enduring effects for prior CT (Perlis et al. 2002, Shea et al. 1992); one involved the use of a medication (fluoxetine) with a particularly long half-life, and questions have been raised about the adequacy of the therapy provided in the other (Jacobson and Hollon 1996).

Although promising, these findings do not speak directly to the prevention of recurrence, defined as the onset of wholly new episodes (Frank et al. 1991). Depressed patients appear to be at elevated risk for symptoms return (relapse) for the first six to nine months following initial response to medications when it is likely that the underlying episode has yet to run its course (Hollon et al. 1990). No good pharmacotherapist would withdraw patients from medications so soon after initial response. And it has become standard practice to continue patients on medications for at least six months after initial remission. Clearly, the early withdrawal practiced in the studies just described was done for research purposes only and does not reflect standard clinical practice. Nonetheless, studies of this kind do established that CBT has an enduring effect that lasts beyond the end of treatment. Current medical practice is moving in the direction of maintaining patients with a history of recurrence (the vast majority of all depressed patients) on medication indefinitely (Am Psychiatric Assoc. 2000). In that context, it would be important to know if CBT's enduring effects extend to the prevention of recurrence.

There are reasons to think that the effects might prevent recurrence. In the Hollon et al. 2005 study, to continued follow patients who survived without relapse for another year (months 13–24 following the end of acute treatment). Patients who survived the full year of continuation treatment without relapse were withdrawn from medications at that time and compared to patients with a history of prior exposure to CT. Given that all of these patients had gone a full 12 months without relapse following initial remission, they were assumed to be fully recovered fro the treated episode and any subsequent return of symptoms was considered to represent the onset of a wholly new episode (recurrence). Only 5 of 20 recovered patients with a history of prior exposure to CT experienced a recurrence during that second year of naturalistic follow-up relative to 7 of 14 patients treated to recovery with medications alone. Taking attrition into account, the adjusted recurrence rates were 17.5% for prior CT versus 53.6% for prior continuation ADM, with a hazard ratio of 0.15 (meaning that prior CT reduced risk for recurrence relative to medication withdrawal by about 85%). Although larger studies are needed, these findings suggest that CT's enduring effect may extend that this is true, it would mean that CT is not only curative (by virtue of bringing the treated episode to an end), but also possibly prophylactic (in the sense of forestalling the onset of wholly new episodes).

Two studies found that CBT's enduring effect was robust whether it is provided alone or in combination with medications (Blackburn et al. 1986, Evans et al. 1992), but a third found that relapse rates were higher when CT was provided in combination with medication relative to CT alone or CT plus placebo (Simons et al. 1986). Moreover, the existing combinatorial trials were all conducted with the older tricyclic medications; it remains to be seen if newer medications with less problematic side effects and broader profiles of action will undermine CT's enduring effects.

There also are indications that CBT or related interventions may have enduring effects when provided after medications have been used to reduce acute distress, for example, Paykel and colleagues found that adding CT to medication treatment for partial responders not only helped resolve residual symptoms but also reduced risk for subsequent relapse after the end of the psychosocial treatment (Payke et al. 1999). Even more interestingly, Fava and colleagues found that adding an patients in continuation treatment reduced risk for recurrence following medication withdrawal (Fava et al. 1998). Finally, an innovative integration of acceptance and meditation called "mindfulness-based cognitive therapy" has been shown reduce risk for relapse and recurrence following treatment termination in patients first treated to remission with medications (Teasdale et al. 2000).

There are even indications that CBT may have a preventive effect when provided to children and adolescents at risk (Gillham et al. 2000). Clarke and colleagues have conducted a pair of studies in adolescents at risk by virtue of having a parent with a history of depression; in both trials, training in skills designed to facilitate affective regulation reduced risk for subsequent diagnosable disorder (Clarke nondepressed subjects selected on the basis of problematic cognitive style both in children (Jaycox et al. 1994) and college effects, since the benefits are obtained long after the intervention is over.

Other types of interventions simply have not been adequately tested. Dynamic psychotherapy has rarely been found to be efficacious with respect to acute treatment; although it is possible to have an enduring effect in the absence of any immediate effect; it is unlikely that such an effect would be detected. IPT has been shown to prevent relapse or recurrence when continued (Klerman et al. 1974) or maintained (Frank et al. 1990), but there is little evidence of any enduring effect once its use is terminated (Hollon et al. 2002). IPT was included in the National Institute of Mental Health Treatment of Depression Collaborative Research Program along with CT and medications, but medication treatment was extended for the first several moths of the post-treatment follow-up (Shea et al. 1992).

In a disorder such as depression, patients who experience a relapse or recurrence following medication withdrawal are likely to seek additional treatment; if symptom return is not monitored in an ongoing fashion, the outcome of interest will likely be missed because subsequent treatment will reduce the distress before the next assessment. Given that patients withdrawn from medications typically experience more symptom return, they are more likely to require additional treatment. Periodic assessments focused solely on current symptom levels typically fail to detect such differences because the effects of subsequent treatment tend to offset the very symptom return that led patients to get back on medications in the first place (Evans et al. 1992).

Mechanisms Underlying Enduring Change

How do cognitive and behavior therapies produce their enduring effects? Cognitive theory suggests that change in what people believe and the way they process information is the primary mechanism of change in CT (Beck 1991). Several studies have shown that thinking does change over the course of therapy; however, the kinds of "surface-level' automatic negative thoughts found in the stream of consciousness typically change as much in pharmacotherapy or other successful interventions as they do in CT (Imber et al. 1990, Simons et al. 1984). What does appear to change in a more specific fashion are the underlying beliefs and information-processing propensities often found in depression, such as core beliefs about the self or the way an individual explains the causes of negative life events. Such core beliefs and information-processing styles tend to lie dormant until activated by negative affect or external stress and serve as the stable cognitive predispositions in a larger diathesis-stress model of depression (Hollon et al. 1992b).

Enduring Effects in Behavior Therapy

Recent studies suggest that more purely behavioral interventions may also produce enduring effects. In a component analysis, Jacobson and colleagues found that the behavioral strategies use in the early stages of CT produced as much change as the complete treatment package when extended over the full course of therapy (Jacobson et al. 1996). Most critically for the current discussion, there was no evidence of differential risk for relapse following treatment termination (Gortner et al. 1998). This led to the articulation of a more fully realized contextual intervention between behaviors and outcomes and eschews attention to the content of cognitions (Jacobson et al. 2001, Martell et al. 2001). In a recent trial, BA was found to be as efficacious as ADM with respect to acute treatment (Dimidjian et al. 2005) and as enduring as CT with respect to the prevention of subsequent relapse and recurrence (KS Dobson, SD Hollon, S Dimidjian, KB Schmaling, RJ Kohlenberg, R Gallop, S Rizive, JK Gollan, DL Dunner, NS Jacobson, manuscript in preparation). Given that therapists pay little attention to thought content in BA (other than noting the role of rumination in maintaining behavioral avoidance), it is clear that direct efforts to beliefs and information-processing proclivities may not be required to produce enduring change. However, it remains possible that these largely behavioral strategies work through underlying cognitive mechanisms to produce their enduring effects (Bandura 1997).

Prevention of Bipolar Disorder

Patients with bipolar are at risk for episodes of mania or hypomania as well as depression. Genetic factors play greater role in bipolar disorder than in unipolar depression, and course is marked by frequent relapse and recurrence. Medication forms the core of treatment and most patients are maintained indefinitely on lithium or mood stabilizers to forestall symptom onset (especially mania), with antidepressants often added to deal with depressive symptoms (Am Psychiatric Assoc. 2002).

Psychosocial interventions typically are used in an adjunctive fashion and it has only been in recent years that empirical studies have demonstrated their value. Teaching patients to detect prodromal signs and seek prompt medical help has been shown to reduce the frequency of onset of full manic episodes (Perry et al. 1999), and interpersonal and social rhythm therapy has been found to reduce frequency of depressive relapse (Malkoff-Schawartz et al. 1998). Family focused treatment, designed to reduce stress and improve communication, has been found to reduce the frequency of mania and depression both during and after the end of treatment (Miklowitz et al. 2003). This represents one of the few instances in which enduring effects have been documented for any psychosocial intervention other than CBT.

Lam and colleagues found that adding CT to medication management over a six-month period reduced risk for subsequent relapse relative to medications alone for the rest of the year in bipolar patients not currently in episode (Lam et al. 2003) A subsequent follow-up found that this advantage was maintained over the next year and a half, but largely reflected differences that emerged during and shortly after treatment (Lam et al. 2005). Thus, although CT had a beneficial effect (in that patients did better during treatment when CT was added to medications), it is not clear that it had an enduring effect such that patients previously treated with CT were at any lower risk of relapse once its use was terminated than were patients receiving medication only a direct comparison of the conditional probabilities of relapse for each specific interval following the termination of the psychosocial treatment would have been of interest.

However, survival analyses based on time to first relapse are not the best way to detect enduring effects when differences emerge during treatment, since high-risk patients are more likely to be retained (and thus remain at risk) by the more efficacious treatment (Holon et al. 2002). Thus, it is possible that documented success of CT in preventing relapse during its initial application led to the differential retention of more high-risk patients going into the later months of the follow-up, thereby obscuring possible enduring effects. In this regard, it is of interest that patients previously treated with CT spent fewer months in episode during the extended follow-up than did patients treated with medication management alone, an index that would not be biased by differential retention. This suggests that CT with bipolar patients may have the same kind of enduring effect that has been found so often in unipolar depression.

PANIC AND THE ANXIETY DISORDERS

Is there evidence for enduring effects in other disorder? Such evidence does exist, especially with respect to panic and the anxiety disorder, although it is not as well documented as for depression and is largely limited to CBT (Hollon and Beck 2004). In this section, we review panic and the anxiety disorders.

Catastrophic Cognitions in Panic and Agoraphobia

As for depression, different theoretical models exists and each posits different interventions for panic disorder and agoraphobia. Biological models view panic as the consequence of the spontaneous discharge of neural centers deep in the brain stem or limbic system and treat the symptoms with medications (Lydiard et al. 1996). Behavioral models regards panic attacks to be a conditioned response to internal or external cues that need to be extinguished via exposure; agoraphobia is regarded as reinforced avoidance behavioral that needs to be suppressed through response (Barlow and Lehman 1996). Cognitive models emphasize the role of catastrophic misinterpretations of benign bodily sensations and encourage patients to test the accuracy of their beliefs via inducing the physiological sensations that they most fear (Back and Emery 1985, Clark 1986). Interventions based on all three models have been shown to be both specific and efficacious in the treatment of panic disorder (DeRubeis and Crits-Christoph 1998).

There are consistent indications that treatment effects achieved with the psychosocial interventions are more likely to endure following treatment termination than are those obtained with medications (Roth and Fonagy 2005). For example, sharp and colleagues (1996) found that patients treated with CBT (alone or in combination with medication) were more likely to maintain gains at a six-month post-treatment follow-up than were patients treated with fluvoxamine alone. Loerch and colleagues (1999) found that adding CBT enhanced response relative to either moclobemide or placebo alone and that those patients in the latter two conditions were far more likely to seek additional treatment across a naturalistic follow-up. In perhaps the best of the early trails, Clark and colleagues (1994) found CT superior to either imipramine (an older tricyclic ADM) pharmacotherapy or applied relaxation in a sample of patients with panic disorder (and each superior to a wait-list control); across a subsequent six-month follow-up, only 5% of the CT patients relapsed following treatment termination, compared with 40% of the patients withdrawn for medications. Moreover, as specified by theory, CT produced a reduction in catastrophic cognitions that was greater than that of either of the other two active treatments, and the frequency of such beliefs at the end of treatment predicated subsequent risk for relapse following treatment termination.

Barlow and colleagues (2000) also found an enduring effect for prior CBT, as well as a cautionary note with regard to its combination with medication. In a multisite study, patients with panic disorder (with or without mild agoraphobia) were randomly assigned to three months of weekly acute treatment followed by six months of monthly maintenance treatment with either CBT or imipramine, each alone and in combination, or pill-placebo, again alone and in combination with somewhat better still by the end of maintenance treatment. Imipramine produced higher quality response among treatment completers, but CBT was more enduring.

This pattern of findings suggests that if adding medication suppresses CBT's enduring effect, it does so through largely pharmacological mechanisms. For example, it is possible that the presence of active medication acts to retard learning, either by suppressing interoceptive cues ion a manner that slows the process of habituation (behavioral) or by reducing the opportunity for disconfirmation of catastrophic expectations (cognitive). That is, medication may operate through biological mechanisms that suppress the occurrence of panic for so long as it is taken, but that interfere with other learning-based mechanisms that would have produced more lasting change.

This is not first time that the addition of medications has undermined the enduring effect of a psychosocial intervention. In an earlier trial, Marks and colleagues combined either exposure of relaxation with alprazolam (a high-potency benzodiazepine) or placebo in a factorial design. Agoraphobic patients treated with the combination of exposure plus alprazolam showed a higher rate of relapse than did patients treated with the combination of exposure plus placebo (Marks et al. 1993). It would appear that medication is more likely to interfere with the enduring effects of CBT for panic and agoraphobia than has been the case to date in the treatment of depression.

The precise nature of the mechanisms involved remains unclear, but it is possible that they will vary as a function of the nature of the disorder and the specific medication. Disorders such as panic with rapid symptom onset may be more susceptible to interference effects than are disorders with greater temporal stability such as depression. At the same time, patients are particularly likely to attribute change to fast-acting medication such as alprazolam, and any medication that produces rapid and transitory change in affective states is particularly likely to induce state-dependent learning. Moreover, medications with short half-lives are particularly likely produce discontinuation effects, making them harder to withdraw and increasing the risk of relapse following termination. In fact, the sequential application of CBT has been used facilitate withdrawal from high-potency benzodiazepines such as alprazolam, which can provoke rebound panic attacks following discontinuation (Bruce et al. 1999, Otto et al. 1993). It remains to be seen whether such a sequential strategy will prove useful in helping patients withdraw from never antidepressants with short half-lives, such as venlafaxine or paroxetine, and whether those medications will interfere with CBTs enduring effect if provided in combination during active treatment.

There are few indications that either dynamic-electric or humanistic-experiential interventions are efficacious in the treatment of panic disorder, much less have enduring effects. More purely behavioral interventions tend to produce gains that endure (Arntz and Van den Hout 1996, Ost and Westling 1995), although enduring effects have not been clearly documented. Presence of agoraphobic avoidance predicts poorer overall response, and tests of enduring effects have been few (Bouchard et al. 1996). Nonetheless, it is clear that CBT has an enduring effect in the treatment of panic disorder. As in the treatment of depression, this effect is most evident in comparisons to drugs and represents one of the main advantages of CBT over medications.

Hypochondriasis and Concerns about Physical Illness

Patients with hypochondriasis believe they have a physical illness and take little comfort from medical reassurance. Although common in medical settings, the disorder has rarely been studied empirically and has long been thought to be impervious to treatment. Cognitive theory suggests that hypochondriasis is a consequence of an enduring tendency to misinterpret innocuous physical sensations as symptoms of a serious illness, much as in panic disorder, with the key difference being the perceived imminence of the medical catastrophe (Warwick and Salkovskis 1990). Patients in CT are encouraged to examine the evidence for their beliefs and to conduct behavioral experiments in which they induce symptoms by focusing attention on their body. Reassurance seeking and "body checking" are discouraged to reduce the operation of safety behaviors, and patients are encouraged to keep a daily record of negative thoughts and rational responses.

Recent studies suggest the efficacy of this approach. Warwick and colleagues (1996) found CT superior to a wait-list control after four months treatment, with gains essentially maintained at a three-month follow-up. Clark and colleagues (1998) found CT superior to a wait-list control on all measures and better than behavioral stress management on symptoms of hypochondriasis, with gains essentially maintained over a subsequent 12-month follow-up. Barsky and Ahern (2004) found that six sessions of CBT (similar but not identical to the approach described above) produced greater change in symptoms of hypochondriasis compared with usual medical care across a 12-month post-treatment follow-up.

Given that hypochondriasis has long been thought to be refractory to treatment, these findings are most promising; this is especially the case for indications that gains endure over time following treatment termination. Evidence for enduring effects would be even more compelling if prior CBT were to prove more stable over time than some alternative intervention stress management, no other treatment (including medications) has yet been found to be efficacious in the treatment of hypochondriasis.

Generalized Anxiety Disorder and the Primacy of Worry

In recent years, cognitive symptoms like pervasive apprehension and worry have come to be seen as the core symptoms of generalized anxiety disorder (GAD) (Brown et al. 1994). CBT involving the combination of relaxation training and cognitive restructuring has been found to be both efficacious and specific in a number of comparisons to other interventions and control conditions, and applied relaxation has shown promise in a smaller number of trial (DeRubeis and Crits-Christoph 1998). More purely behavioral interventions based on exposure are difficult to implement, since there is often no clear external referent to target. Medication treatment is often problematic; minor tranquilizers can induce dependence and tend to lose potency with prolonged use. And antidepressants do nothing to reduce future risk (Nathan and Gorman 1998). More traditional forms of psychotherapy have long been touted, but rarely tested.

Treatment gains for CBT are generally well maintained over time, both in adults (Borkovec and Rusico 2001) and in geriatric populations (Stanley et al. 2003). Differences favoring cognitive strategies sometimes have emerged following treatment termination relative to more purely behavioral interventions (Borkovec and Costello 1993), and Durham and colleagues (2003) recently reported that patients in CBT exhibited lower overall symptom severity and less interim treatment in 8–14 years following treatment terminations than did patients receiving either dynamic or pharmacological treatment.

Nonetheless, there is a general sense that more can be done with the treatment of GAD. For example, Borkovec and colleagues (2002) found that interpersonal difficulties remaining after treatment with CBT predicted poorer status across follow-up, and they called for the inclusion of strategies that targets these problems. Similarly, Fava and colleagues (2005) found that adding strategies designed to promote a sense of well-being enhanced the efficacy of CBT, with gains maintained across a one-year follow-up. Finally, Ladouceur and colleagues (1999) have dropped relaxation training entirely to focus on more purely cognitive targets such as intolerance of uncertainty and cognitive avoidance. A recent controlled trial found this more purely cognitive intervention superior to a delayed treatment control; 77% of all participants treated with CBT no longer met criteria for GAD following treatment (Ladouceur et al. 2000). In a subsequent trial, participants provided with group CBT did better than a waist-list control and continued to improve across a 24-month follow-up (Dugas et al. 2003) It remains to be seen how this approach will compare to more conventional renditions of CBT that incorporate more explicitly behavioral components, but treatments effects for each appear to be well maintained over time.

Interpersonal Anxiety and Social Phobia

Social phobia (also known as social anxiety disorder) tends to begin early in life and often follows a chronic course (Davidson et al. 1993). Social phobia involves an undue fear of evaluation by others and the accompanying desire to avoid situations in which scrutiny is anticipated. A number of pharmacological agents have been found to reduce distress, including the monoamine oxidase inhibitors and, more recently, the selective serotonin reuptake inhibitors (SSRIs) (Hidalgo et al. 2001). Behavioral approaches base on exposure to social situations (often supplemented with training in social skills) generally have been efficacious, although gains have not always been well maintained over time (DeRubeis and Crits-Christoph 1998). Cognitive approaches target beliefs regarding personal defects that could lead to ridicule or censure by others in social situations (Beck and Emery 1985), and a recent extension focuses on the elimination of safety behaviors that retard the disconfirmation of those beliefs (Well et al. 1995).

Although the effects produced by exposure alone have not always been stable over time, they do appear to be more enduring than are those produced by medications. Blomhoff and colleagues (2001) found that sertraline (an SSRI) was superior to exposure therapy in a primary-care sample, but that patients treated with the psychosocial intervention continued to improve across a subsequent year-long follow-up, whereas those treated with sertraline (alone or in combination) tended to deteriorate after treatment termination (Haug et al. 2003). Similarly, a naturalistic study of long-term treatment outcomes in social phobia found that concomitant use of benzodiazepines during active treatment was associate with greater risk of relapse in patients treated with exposure (Fava et al. 2001). These reports are reminiscent of the findings in panic and agoraphobia that adding medication may undermine the enduring effects of CBT (Barlow et al. 2000, Marks et al. 1993). There are also indications that the addition of cognitive restructuring facilitates the maintenance of gains produced by exposure to social situations (e.g. Butler et al. 1984, Heimberg et al. 1993).

Perhaps the best evidence for the enduring effects of CBT in social phobia comes form a two-site comparison to medications that did a particularly nice job of controlling for allegiance across sites and conditions (Heimberg et al. 1998). In that trial, patients with social phobia were randomly assigned to cognitive behavioral group therapy (CBGT) alone, phenelzine (a monoamine oxidase inhibitor) alone, pill-placebo, or educational-supportive group therapy. Both active treatments were superior to the two control conditions;

phenelzine produced somewhat faster response than did CBGT, but rates of response were comparable by the end of acute treatment (12 weeks). Responders to the two active treatments were provided with six months of additional maintenance treatment and then tracked across a subsequent six-months of additional maintenance treatment termination. The result shown in that, there was clear evidence for an enduring effect for the psychosocial intervention; none of the patients previously treated with CBGT relapsed following treatment termination versus 33% of the patients previously treated with phenelzine (100% versus 67% survival) (Liebowitz et al. 1999).

Clark and colleagues have suggested that patients with social phobia focus undue attention on their image of themselves in social situations and engage in safety behaviors (strategies designed to protect them from feared consequences) that make them appear less socially skilled and prevent them from learning that they can handle the feared encounters (Wells et al. 1995). Patients are videotaped engaging in various social situations, both with and without safety behaviors, and are then invited to watch both tapes and rate themselves on various characteristics. Patients typically find that they appear more relaxed and socially skilled when they drop their safety behaviors and that their internal images of themselves are more negative and self-derogatory than they actually appear. Moreover, patients show greater change in beliefs and greater reductions in anxiety when they drop their safety behaviors in exposure situations.

Clark and colleagues have argued that targeting self-focused attention and encouraging patients to drop their safety behaviors during exposure can facilitate their capacity to learn from experience and hasten their response to treatment. A recent comparison suggests that this newer individual approach may be superior to more conventional CBGT, which had been done in groups to take advantage of the opportunities afforded for exposure to social situations (Stangier et al. 2003). In another recent comparison, Clark and colleagues found that patients with social phobia who were treated with individual CBT in the manner described above showed greater reductions in measures of social phobia across 16 weeks of active treatment than did patients treated with either fluoxetine or placebo. Moreover the advantage observed for CBT relative to medication was essentially maintained across three months of booster treatment and was still evident at a 12-month follow-up following treatment termination (Clark et al. 2003). These findings, combined with those obtained by Liebowitz and colleagues (1999) with CBGT, suggest that CBT for social phobia has an enduring effect not found with medication.

Specific Phobias and the Perception of Danger

Specific phobias involve an intense fear of certain objects or situations and a corresponding desire to avoid being in their presence. Behavior therapy suggests that phobias are established via traumatic conditioning and maintained by avoidance behaviors that prevent their extinction (Mowrer 1948). Behavioral interventions such as systematic desensitization and exposure plus response prevention are clearly efficacious and represent the current standard of treatment (DeRubies and Crits-Christoph 1998). Gains typically are well maintained, although return of fear (spontaneous recovery) sometimes does occur, especially when contextual cues favor the retrieval of memories associated with fear acquisition rather than extinction (Bouton 1993). Being on a psychoactive substance during exposure appears to alter those cues (Mystkowski et al. 2003), and treatments has been shown to be more enduring when provided in the absence of medications (Marks et al. 1972).

Cognitive theory posits that individuals with specific phobias perceive greater danger or risk in the feared situation than do other people and suggests that such beliefs often are activated only in the presence of the feared object (Beck and Emery 1985). Ost and colleagues have had great success with single-session cures by adjusting the nature of the exposure to test the idiosyncratic beliefs expressed by patients as they approach the object of their fears (Hellstrom et al.1996, Hellstorm and Ost 1995, Ost et al. 1997). Other groups have obtained similar results (Thom et al. 2000, Thorpe and Salkovskis 1997). Whether this approach will enhance the stability of change relative to more purely behavioral interventions remains to be seen, but it does appear to facilitate the rapidly of change.

Obsessive-Compulsive Disorder and Personal Responsibility

Obsessive-compulsive disorder (OCD) is characterized by obsessive thoughts and images that evoke anxiety and compulsive behaviors or ritualistic mental acts that serve to reduce distress. OCD tends to be a chronic recurrent disorder. Naturalistic data suggest that full remission is rate and relapse is common after partial remission (Eison et al. 1999); nearly half of all patients will show a chronic course (Skoog and Skoog 1999). Comparison across studies indicates that patients with OCD show a low rate of placebo response than do patients with other types of anxiety disorders (Huppert et al. 2004).

Exposure plus response prevention (ERP) is both efficacious and specific in the treatment of OCD (DeRubies and Chits-Christoph 1998). Although it need not be the case, ERP for this disorder typically is presented as a test of the consequences of choosing not to act to undo the obsessions, making it a largely cognitive behavioral intervention. Pharmacotherapy with the serotonin reuptake inhibitor (SRI) clomipramine and the other selective SSRIs has also been shown quite substantial for both approaches, with up to two-thirds of all the patients showing clear improvement and about one-third of all patients showing full recovery. Nonetheless, symptoms tend to persist at moderate levels for most patients, and few controlled comparisons have tracked the maintenance of gains over extended periods.

Foa and Kozak (1996) reviewed studies that examined the long-term outcome of OCD patients had maintained response up to two-and-a-half years after treatment terminations. By way of contrast, the available double-blind discontinuation medication trials show a different picture (Romano et al. 2001); relapse rates often are high and typically exceed those for continuation medication (Koran et al. 2002, Pato et al. 1988, Ravizza et al. 1996). Hembree and colleagues (2003) conducted a naturalistic follow-up of patients treated with ERP, serotonergic medications, or their combination. Although difference were not evident across the whole sample, patients previously treated with ERP had less severe symptoms than did patients who were not among those not currently on medications.

Foa and colleagues (2005) provided the first direct comparison of ERP versus medications in the treatment of OCD in a study that afforded an opportunity to evaluate the stability of response following treatment termination. In that trial, adults patients with OCD of at least one-year duration were randomly assigned to ERP or clomipramine pharmacotherapy, each alone and in combination, or a pill-placebo control. Acute treatment lasted for 12 weeks and was quite intense; exposure sessions were conducted daily for the first three weeks and dosages levels were pushed aggressively (as appropriate) to a maximum of 250 mg/day. At the end of treatment, all three active treatments were superior to pill-placebo, ERP was superior to medications alone, and adding medication did little to enhance response to ERP. Response rates among all assigned were 62% for ERP, 70% for combined treatment, 42% for clomipramine alone, and 8% for placebo.

Treatment responders were than monitored over a subsequent 12-week period following the end of active treatment. ERP was discontinued and patients who responded to clomipramine (alone or in combination) were tapered off medications over a four-week period. Relapse was defined as a return to pretreatment levels of severity or a clinical state that warranted resumption of treatment.

As for depression (but unlike panic disorder), there was no indication that adding medications during acute treatment did anything to undermine the enduring effect of CBT; the rate of survival without relapse following ERP alone was 89% versus 87% for the combination.

The literature is mixed with respect to the relative benefits of ERP versus more purely cognitive approaches (Van Oppen et al. 1995, Mclean et al. 2001, Vogel et al. 2004). Salkovskis (1999) suggests that people who are prone to OCD have exaggerated beliefs about personal responsibility and argues that making that a focus of treatment during exposure can enhance response and contribute to the stability of gains. The only trial to date to explore that approach found good maintenance of gains over a six-month follow-up, but did not provide comparisons to either more conventional ERP or medication treatment (Freeston et al. 1997). More studies are clearly needed comparing such different versions of CBT (and each to medication maintenance), but results to date suggest that CBT for OCD has an enduring effect not found for medications.

Post-traumatic Stress Disorder

Post-traumatic stress disorder (PTSD) involves the occurrence of a distinctive set of symptoms in response to traumatic events; symptoms include increased arousal, persistent avoidance, flashbacks and intrusive recollections, affective constriction, and a sense of interpersonal detachment. The nature of the trauma can be diverse, including sexual and other assaults, motor vehicle and other accidents, and combat trauma, with the last the most refractory to treatment (Bradley et al. 2005). Not everyone who experiences trauma develops PTSD, but for those who do, it often becomes chronic. Simple debriefing strategies applied in an unselective fashion immediately after trauma may actually increase the risk for developing PTSD (Mayou et al. 2000), but preventive interventions applied in a more selective fashion to targeted populations appear to reduce subsequent risk (Bryant et al. 1998, Foa et al. 1995).

Although PTSD tends to be a chronic condition that does not remit spontaneously once it is established, treatment with several different types of interventions appears to lead to large initial gains that are often well maintained over time (Bradley et al. 2005). Prolonged exposure (flooding), stress-inoculation training (combining relaxation training and controlled breathing with some limited cognitive restructuring), and cognitive reprocessing of the trauma have all been shown to be efficacious in the treatment of PTSD. Some studies suggest that prolonged exposure may have a more sustained effect than does stress-inoculation training (Foa et al. 1991), and that adding stress-inoculation to prolonged exposure may underline the enduring effects of the latter (Foa et al. 1999), but those indications are neither robust across trials nor consistent across research groups (Marks et al. 1998, Resick et al. 2002, Tarrier et al. 1999). Eye-movement desensitization and reprocessing continues to be controversial; although typically superior to control conditions (Marcus et al. 1997; Wilson et al. 1995, 1979), there is little evidence of specific efficacy and it sometimes is outperformed by other active interventions (Devilly and Spence 1999, Ironson et al. 2002, Taylor et al. 2003). ADM (especially the SSRIs) has been shown to be efficacious and is less likely to induce dependence than are minor tranquilizers or alcohol, but does nothing to reduce risk once its use in discontinued (Ballenger et al. 2004).

Resick and colleagues developed an approach called cognitive processing therapy that targets specific maladaptive beliefs related to safety, trust, and self-esteem (Resick and Schnicke 1992). In this approach. Patients are encouraged to write detailed descriptions of the traumatic event and read them back to the therapist as a form of exposure, and the implications are then discussed. In a recent trial, cognitive processing therapy was found to be at least as efficacious and enduring as prolonged exposure and superior to a minimal treatment control; patients in the control condition showed comparable gains when provided subsequent active treatment (Resick et al. 2002).

Ehlers and Clark (2000) have argued that PTSD becomes persistent when individuals process trauma in a way that leads to a continued sense of current threat. As they describe, the paradox of PTSD form a cognitive perspective is that memories for prior events create a current state of anxiety, which usually implies a sense of impending threat. This sense of current threat is seen as a consequence of the combination of excessively negative appraisals of the implications of the prior trauma and disturbance of autobiographical memory characterized by poor elaboration and perceptual priming. This model differs from earlier cognitive formulations by specifying more fully the processes contributing to the maintenance of distress and addressing the idiosyncratic nature of the appraisals made by different individuals. As such, it represents an evolution in therapy that may well guide the development of the next generation of cognitive interventions.

In a recent trial, Ehlers and colleagues (2003) applied this approach to the treatment of a sample of motor vehicle accident survivors who met criteria for persistent PTSD. Potential participants were first asked to self-monitor symptoms for a three-week period, and those who fell below criteria for subsequent risk were excluded (about 12%). Those who did not recover with self-monitoring alone were then randomly assigned to treatment with this newly elaborated version of CT, a self-help booklet based on those same principles, or repeated assessments only. Treatment lasted for three months, with subsequent assessments at six and nine months following the start of treatment. Participants treated with CT were less likely to meet criteria for PTSD at the end of treatment than were participants provided with either self-help or assessment only (21% versus 79% and 72%, respectively). Although the sample as a whole continued to improve over time, CT retained its relative advantage over the other conditions; only 11% of the participants who received CT met criteria for PTSD at the nine-month follow-up relative to 61% of the self-help participants and 55% of the assessment-only controls.

These studies provide support for the notion that the effects of CBT endure in the treatment of PTSD. The absence of comparisons to efficacious medication treatments such as the SSRIs makes it hard to demonstrate this effect as persuasively as can be done for other disorders, but it is clear that the effects of treatment do not erode over time. Thus, the preponderance of evidence appears to suggest that CBT has an enduring effect in the treatment of PTSD.

CONCLUSION

Cognitive behavior therapy (CBT) appears to have an enduring effect in the treatment of depression and the anxiety disorders that reduces risk for subsequent symptom return. This enduring effect is most evident in comparison to medication treatment, which appears to be largely palliative in nature, and represents one of the major advantages for CBT. Clear documentation exists relative to medication treatment with respect to depression, panic, social phobia, and OCD. Despite the absence of comparisons to prior medication treatment, there is also evidence of stability of gains for several of the other anxiety disorders (tests for enduring effects are largely lacking in other disorders). There are indication that adding medications may undermine the enduring effects of CBT in some instances; such interference could be a consequence of either pharmacological or psychological mechanisms and may vary as a function of medication and disorder. With the exception of family-focused treatment for bipolar disorder, there are few indications that other psychosocial interventions have enduring effects, although this possibility has rarely been explored. The nature of the underlying mechanisms remains to be determined, but CBT appears to have an enduring effect in the treatment of depression and the anxiety disorders that may preclude the need for extended medication treatment.

47.8 BEHAVIORAL MEDICINE

JN Vyas, SS Nathawat

OVERVIEW

Founded in the 1970s, behavioral medicine is a relatively new subspecialty that emerged out of curious roots. Importantly, among these was the realization that many medical problems have their genesis, and perhaps cure, in behavioral actions. Perhaps one of the clearest examples of mainstreaming of behavioral medicine is the Healthy People 2010 initiative of the US Department of Health and Human Services (2000). This initiative is explicitly biobehavioral in perspective, formulating health as the interplay of behavior and biology interacting with the social and physical environment. The goals of this initiative are to increase both the quality and years of healthy life, and to eliminate the health disparities. The approach to achieving these goals recognize the importance of behavioral factors and focuses on leading health indicators that impact health and well-being (i.e. physical activity overweight and obesity, tobacco use, substances abuse, responsible sexual behavior, mental health, injury add violence, environmental quality, immunization and access to health care). This integrative approach to the determinants of health is central to behavioral B medicine.

The second founding attribute of behavioral medicine is a conviction that behavior is a crucial subject matter in its own right in medicine and that underlying motivations and personality structure, although interesting, may not be crucial in determining change in health. Thus, the focus on behavior alone reflects one pole in the familiar and doctrinaire struggles between psychodynamic and behaviorist intellectual tradition.

Perhaps a third characteristic of behavioral medicine is its opportunism we use this term advisedly and without any pejorative connotations. Psychosomatic medicine flourished as research discipline to study the physiological and psychological underpinnings of many diseases. As clinical subspecialty, it provided psychotherapy for patients ermined to have "psychosomatic illnesses" but focused particularly on a limited subset of illnesses (the so-called "holy seven"). General psychiatry and even consultation-liaison psychiatry left certain important clinical area uncovered. None of these movements in psychiatry was oriented toward improving patients' compliance or modifying their many risk enhancing behaviors. Similarly, psychiatry did not seem to offer special programs other than supportive psychotherapy for specialized groups of patients with diverse medical problems, such as chronic pain or anticipatory nausea associated with chemotherapy.

Despite the extraordinarily successful growth in consolation psychiatry, such services were oriented primarily toward inpatient setting. Little was being done in outpatient setting to address the intersection of psychiatry and medicine. Thus, a fourth characteristic of behavioral medicine is its in interdisciplinary focus on outpatient setting. As the economics of medicine have shifted from inpatient setting and specialty consolation to managed care, outpatient treatment, and health maintenance, new opportunities for the emerging field of behavioral medicine have arisen, and behavioral medicine concepts have become more integrated into mainstream care.

Finally, behavioral medicine straddles medicine, psychiatry, psychology, and public health. It tends to focus not just one the patient but also larger health policy matters such as social class, race and ethnicity, risk screening, and communication of medical information to diverse populations.

WHAT IS BEHAVIORAL MEDICINE?

Behavioral medicine is an interdisciplinary field concerned with the development and integration of behavioral and biomedical science, knowledge, and techniques relevant to health and illness and the applications of this knowledge and these techniques to prevention, diagnosis, treatment, and rehabilitation. Among these, five primary factors deserve further comment in characterizing the unique nature of behavioral medicine approaches to health care.

First, behavioral medicine is inherently and absolutely interdisciplinary. Traditional (Western) Medical Care divided problems and patients by disciplinary boundaries and encouraged independent treatment approaches. Contemporary care often characterized as multidisciplinary, is organized as a summation of component disciplines true interdisciplinary care involve an integration and melding of the component disciplinary approaches such that the original component distinctions are no longer important and a new complex approach is created that is more than the sum of its parts.

Second, behavioral medicine is staunchly entrenched in the scientific method and is founded in empirical data an emphasis of scientific research and empirical support for theories and intervention has been a hallmark of the field. The field has an always emphasized the development of knowledge at least as much as the application of knowledge and technology to care of patients. In this way, behavioral medicine is different from "alternative medicine" approaches, which are based on a fundamental mistrust of science and a disregard for scientific (Western) method.

A third characteristic of behavioral medicine is one of the clearest distinctions between it and conventional psychiatry and psychology emphasis is placed on a medical disorder rather than on a psychiatric or behavioral problem, the behavioral medicine specialist addresses foremost that which is held to be the principle problem of the patient a medical disease, while understanding that secondary psychiatric symptoms are common with health problems and must also be treated to ensure optimal health.

Fourth, behavioral medicine has a primary focus on the integration of behavioral and biomedical sciences to solve problems related to health and illness. Behavioral medicine assumes equally strong understanding of and familiarity with biomedical and behavioral sciences, it is the integration of these disciplines that truly distinguishes the field from other areas of medicine. With this approach behavioral medicine is applicable (potentially) at any point along the health-illness continuum.

Thus, a fifth characteristic of behavioral medicine is that it is not limited to particular activities (e.g. epidemiology assessment, intervention) or techniques (e.g. biofeedback, education, medication) behavioral medicine is a general approach to health care health service delivery, medical research and public health.

The behavioral medicine approach cuts across health care disciplines in an attempt to fully address the complex are of biopsychosocial factors in any particular disease presentation. With regard to discipline, the behavioral medicine practitioner could be a primary care physician, internal medicine specialist, psychiatrist, psychologist, or nurse, more likely, an interdisciplinary team of experts that represents all of these, and perhaps additional, disciplines.

History and Development of the Field

The recognition that behavioral factors influence health and illness date from Hippocrates, intellectual and clinical interest in behavioral factors in health and health care, however, has waxed and waned through the years. Four major factors came together in the late 1960s and early 1970s to renew such interest and motivate the establishment of behavioral medicine.

Morbidity and mortality patterns were changing, as were health care programs. Infectious disease, the primary killers of the previous generation, were treated and prevented with unparalleled success. Now the major health problems in terms of morbidity, mortality, and disability were chronic illnesses with undeniable lifestyle and behavioral correlates (e.g. heart disease, cancer, diabetes, chronic pain syndromes). These disorders did not appear to fit readily into the traditional infectious disease model, which had been so successful with the major illnesses of the past. Moreover, with improved health, demystification of medicine, and the knowledge that many chronic illnesses have predisposing lifestyle factors, patients became more interested in what they could do to influence their health (self-management). This recognition culminated with the US government publication of Healthy people, which articulated the major health goals for the millennium. The report indicated that the major health issues for the nation have behavioral and lifestyle components and called for prevention and intervention programs that address these issues.

Consultation-liaison psychiatry focused on delivery of pragmatic (Often crisis-based) care to medical surgical inpatients but offered relatively little in the way of preventive services, health promotion, or outpatient services. Psychoanalysis, became increasingly oriented toward research (both physiological and epidemiological) concerning mind-body or biopsychosocial relationships. Behavioral approaches had demonstrated success in several areas of mental health. In part because clear operational goals are implicit in any behavioral intervention, the data from such techniques were measurable and the efficacy was impressive. For the first time, data were available that demonstrated reliable change elicited by behavioral technologies, an interest developed at this time for broadening the application of behavioral technologies.

Developments in the area of psychophysiology combined with behavior theory to create biofeedback. The pioneering work of Neil Miller demonstrating operant control of autonomic responses in animals and humans had a profound influence in fostering the field's development. Biofeedback demonstrated possible mechanisms by which behavior change can affect physiological mechanisms of disease.

The concepts of stress and coping have been a major underpinning of the field of behavioral medicine, because these concepts have commonly been seen as linking the mind and the body. Whereas traditional psychiatry has been interested in stress as a cause or effect of many mental disorders, behavioral medicine has emphasized stress as discussed different under subheading.

PHYSICAL ACTIVITY

Mounting research provides ever more compelling evidence of the merits of an active life style. Exercise can have marked benefits on cardiovascular and respiratory fitness, body composition (i.e. body mass, fat content), muscle strength, endurance, and flexibility. In addition, physical activity is associated with (1) reduced risk for osteoporosis or bone loss in postmenopausal women using weight-bearing exercise, (2) increased strength from resistance weight training in geriatric populations, (3) psychological health and effective treatment of some emotional disorders (e.g. anxiety, depression and addictive behaviors), (4) prevention and treatment of obesity, (5) significant improvement in chronic pain conditions (arthritis and low back pain), (6) increased longevity, and (7) improvements in quality of life. Yet, only an estimated 15% of American adults regularly engage in moderate physical exercise, and 40% engage in no leisure physical activity at all.

The physiological mechanism linking health improvement with activity is unknown, but some suggestions include: (1) strengthening of the heart muscle, increasing its size, and improving its functioning; (2) increase of high density lipoprotenin cholesterol; (3) reduction of triglycerides; (4) decreased likelihood for development of hypertension and reduction of diastolic blood pressure; (5) reduction of blood glucose levels, increasing insulin receptors and the effectiveness of insulin; (6) promotion of skeletal muscle size and weight, increased burning of calories, and increased resting metabolic rate; and (7) reduction of the stickiness of fibrins that leads to blood clots.

Dietary Risk Factors

The influence of diet on health has changed considerably thought the years as common nutritional-deficiency diseases such as rickets and scurvy have become rare in the US. Although dietary habits still contribute significantly to ill health, the primary cause tends to no longer be a deficiency of nutrients, but rather an oversupply.

In the top 10 causes of death, dietary fats are associated with increased risk of coronary heart disease and cancer, stroke diabetes, and atherosclerosis (US Department of Health and Human Services 1991, 2000). In addition, increases in dietary fiber can mitigate important health problems, such as diabetes cardiovascular disease, and cancer; excessive sodium use increases the likelihood of hypertension for some individual; and supplemental calcium not only can decrease blood pressure but also helps maintain bone density.

Data on the ill effects of obesity suggest that increases in body mass index (weight kilograms divided the square of the height in meters) are strongly associated with increases in morbidity and mortality. Excess visceral adipose tissue is associated with metabolic disorders, such as diabetes, hypercholesterolemia, hypertriglyceridemia, and hypertension. Similar to the data showing health benefits from less exercise, data from newer studies suggest greater health benefit from small weight losses. A 10% loss of body weight, for instance, has been found to normalize blood pressures in obese hypertensive patients and to reduce blood glucose levels lipid and lipoprotein levels.

Smoking

Addiction to nicotine may be the most serious medical problem in the US. Tobacco use causes more deaths than alcohol, firearms, motor vehicles, and illegal drugs combined. On the basis of a review of the literature from 1977 to 1993, cigarette smoking was found to cause 30% of all cancer, 21% of deaths from bestir disease, and 19% of all a deaths combined (McGinnis and foege 1993). It is thought that 20% of low-weight births, 8% of preterm deliveries, and 5% of all prenatal deaths could be eliminating smoking during petulancy (US Department of Health and Human Services 1990). Furthermore, evidence accumulated in the last 10 jars implicates environmental to backs smoke as a risk skater for nonsmokers. Despite in tensile programs, low cessation rates have remained a perplexing problem, hence, structured in tureen duos of late have attempted to incorporate methods that individuals have used on their own to quit. These programs are aimed at targeting the specific "stage" of quitting in a bash the individual in operating.

Screening Behavior and Risk Appraisal

Screening and risk assessment are becoming increasingly colorant in clinical medicine, and behavioral medicine is focusing more on the complexity of the problems attendant with such assessment. Screening involves the systematic application of a test to invitee individuals at sufficient task of a specific disease to benefit from further investigation or direct preventive action, among people who have not sought medical action on account of symptoms. Risk appraisal involves providing people with risk information on which to base sisal and lifestyle decisions. Of course, screening has been with us for many years in forms such as chest X-rays and amniocentesis, while appraisal of risk such as cigarette looking are very familiar. However, two factors have led to recent growth in the area.

The first is the increased sophistication with which biological pathways related to disease are being identified, for example, cardiovascular risk assessment has advanced beyond the measurement of bold pressure and total. Hemostatic factors, and inflammatory makers in the risk profile. Similarly, There are many screening indications in cancer. Premalignant polyps (adenomas) are early markers for colorecta cancer prostate-specific for prostate cancer, and human papilloma virus seropositivity is marker for cervical cancer.

The second factor leading to increased focus on screening is the explosion of genetic sophistication, which has led to identification of genotypes for several common disorders such as breast cancer, colon cancer, and early onset Alzheimer's disease. This new knowledge has led to the development of genetic screening, aimed at identifying genetic susceptibility to disease in individuals or their offspring genetic counseling in which people are advised about disease risk usually on the basis of family history has also been expanding.

This growth of medical screening and risk appraisal raises important issues in behavioral medicine individuals who previously regarded themselves as healthy may be identified as being ill or at high-risk for illness. The World Health

Organization has argued that screening is only justified if there is evidence for an effective treatment, together with reason to believe that early treatment will result in better outcome. Unfortunately, screening tests are often developed more rapidly than treatments, so clinical conditions may be identified without any treatment or preventive action being available. Early identification can have undesirable consequences, such as the lowering of parental and school expectations in children, difficulties with employment and insurance in adults, and the need to make difficult decisions about preventive surgery which may have unpleasant side effects or uncertain benefits.

This is concern that medical and genetic screening may have adverse emotional effects. Some screening procedures involve a period of distress and uncertainty, even for individuals who prove to have negative results, because test findings may not be instantly available. Fortunately, while transient distress is common, few studies has as yet identified long-term adverse emotional effects of screening. Nevertheless, screening requires careful attention to the psychological experience of participants as well as to the psychological experience of participants as well as to clinical outcomes, and counseling programs may be required for emotionally vulnerable individuals. The need for counseling in conjunction with screening has been recognized for many years in relation to HIV and Huntington's disease, but now with the profuse-soon of screening indications, this knowledge is increasingly relevant to larger numbers of patients.

Screening is likely to become increasingly central to behavioral medicine over the next few years. Already screening clinics are being seen as valuable sites for health behavior change and preventive advice, since people attending them may be sensitive to general health issues and, therefore, responsive to advice. Genetic screening may also, therefore, responsive to advice. Genetic screening may also interact with health behavior change programs. For example, there is evidence that particular genetic polymorphisms may enhance motivation for smoking cessation. However, screening results can have complex effects on health behavior that are not yet well understood. Negative results may lead to a false sense of security, while positive results can be greeted with fatalism rather than providing an added impetus for taking preventive action.

PERSONALITY FACTORS

Personality factors have long been thought to predisposes an individual to illness. Probably the best known personality risk factor is the type a behavior pattern a term first coined in the 1950s and its association with coronary artery disease. The original definition described type a behavior as an action-emotion complex that individuals use to confront their environment and challenges. This hard-driving behavior pattern included aggression competitiveness impatience and specific behaviors such as muscle tension alertness rapid and emphatic vocal style accelerated pace of activities, emotional responses of affectability or covert hostility and above average anger. Early studies found approximately two times the frequency of coronary artery disease compared with that of nontype.

Stress, Coping, and Illness

The most common psychosocial variable associated with illness onset has to do with the ever elusive concept of stress, one of the most controversial and pervasive notions in health care today. Poor management of stress has been associated with an increased occurrence of heart disease, coronary artery disease, poor diabetes control chronic pain conditions, and significant distress.

Stressors have been associated with numerous pathological changes in biochemical and immunological activities. Research on the relationship of stress and the likelihood of becoming ill has clearly pointed out that nation for illness in ordinary human experiences, just as genetics alone does not cause mental illness. Characteristics of the stressor presumed to mediate its impact include its magnitude, duration, novelty, and predictability and the temporal sequence of events. Relevant person factors include biological vulnerabilities, response thresholds, age at exposure, personality style (e.g. self-efficacy, optimism, and sense of coherence). In addition, the person's appraisal of the stressful situations (i.e. the degree of threat, perceptions of control, previous experience, and what coping resources of options are available) has been found to be critical in determining psychological and physiological reactions to stress. Individuals who appraise situations as more threatening, important and uncontrollable report more physical symptoms and emotional distress. On the basis of the empirical evidence, coping skills training programs teach patients the importance of particular coping strategies in enhancing health.

POPULATION PERSPECTIVE

Sociodemographic Factors

The origins of behavioral medicine as a discipline lie in individual biobehavioral processes and the impact of emotions and behavior on health outcomes. Another major strand has been added to this interdisciplinary field via behavioral and psychosocial epidemiology. It has been known for centuries that the experiences of illness depends on the social environment as well as individual behavior and biology. People living in poverty, migrants, and ethnic minorities have suffered a greater disease burden and more premature mortality since records began. In the 19th and early 20th century, much of this excess was caused by material deprivation, under nutrition, unsanitary living conditions and exposure to infectious organisms. But despite the general much infectious disease in the 20th century, social inequalities in morbidity and mortality have persisted. There are socioeconomic gradients in many of the leading causes of depth, including coronary heart disease, stroke, respiratory disease and many cancers, chronic conditions such as arthritis and ulcers, and in suicide and mental illness. Behavioral medicines researchers have been very involved in tracing hose pathways in the hopes of influencing public policy. After all, the "etiology" of so much of the premature mortality is "behavioral" or "societal" in nature.

Modified from the work of professor sir Michael Marmot, schematically diagrams the putative path ways by which socioeconomic factors act. Note that these pathways involve some of the major themes of behavioral medicine, in particular health behavior and stress related psycho physiological mechanisms. Armor notes that social adult working and nonworking life, building on the substrate of early life and genetic factors. These chronic experiences determine patterns of health behavior and disturbances in stress related autonomic, neuroendocrine, and risk factor profiles that are prejudicial for health. For example, people in lover socioeconomic status categories (as defined by occupation, income, as did educational background) tend to have jobs over which they have little control; they have relatively little influence over decision-making, the pace of work, or how their works is carried out. Low job control in turn leads to heightened blood pressure and disturbances in the diurnal rhythm of the output of the hypothalamic pituitary–adrenocortical axis. Monotonous, uncontrollable work may also increase depressive symptoms and be associated with deleterious health habits such as lack of physical exercise. Thus, behavioral medicine operates within a population framework and touches on issues of culture and social organization as well as on individual health outcomes.

Behavioral Medicine Techniques: Clinical Applications

Although behavioral medicine shares many applications and techniques with traditional medical and behavioral approaches to health care, several aspects are unique and characteristic of the field. Five specific clinical activities have been synonymous with behavioral medicine across several areas of an application and clinical populations.

Biobehavioral Assessment

Biobehavioral assessment involves the coordinated and in-targeted evaluation of biomedical and behavioral factors in the health status and quality of life of the patient. Careful behavioral analysis is a hallmark of this approach with a detailed specification of the frequency, amplitude, duration, quality, and correlates of key health behaviors. Behavioral analysis emphasizes a systematic search for function (continged) relationships of the cues in the environment (discriminative stimuli), "signs, symptoms, or problems" (behavioral responses), and consequences of the behaviors (reinforcers). The frequent clincal observation that chronic pain patients in the presence of the floor nurse (discriminative stimuli), "signs, symptoms, or problems: (behavioral responses), and consequences of the behaviors (reinforcers). The frequent clinical observation that chronic pain patients in the presence of the floor nurse (discriminative stimulus) increase their rates and intensity of pain complaints and behavior (behavioral responses), resulting in greater likelihood of narcotics administration (positive reinforcement) exemplifies these contingent relationships. Direct observation of the patient's behavior in problem setting is preferred to self-reports of symptoms and analysis of internal (mental) "causes."

Behavior Management

Behavior management is the use of learning principles (particularly operant and classical conditioning to encourage and direct health behavior change. This approach emphasize a functional analysis and contingency management to assist patients in making desired behavior change to achieve health goals. A functional analysis is a case conceptualization. Similar to the case of the pain, patient with an escalating narcotic intake described before, that emphasizes empirical contingent (predictable) relationships between the person's behavior and the environment. Contingency management is the systematic manipulations of the probabilistic relationships (contingencies) between the terms of the functional analysis (i.e. discriminative stimuli, behavioral responses, and reinforcing stimuli). An example of this strategy is to schedule narcotics administrations at regular intervals (time contingent) rather than as needed (pain behavior contingent) which removes the contingency between pain behaviors and narcotic reinforcement, thereby decreasing (after perhaps an initial extinction burst) the probability (and strength) of the (behavioral response) pain complaints and behaviors. Again, these clinical techniques have been direct outgrowth of basic psychological laboratory research.

Cognitive-educational Approaches

Cognitive–educational approaches have been based primarily on the health belief model. The health belief model emphasizes the role of the individual's beliefs about health and the meaning of symptoms, including beliefs about the likely effects of behavior change on health outcomes and beliefs about the ability to make worthwhile behavior change. This model asserts that such beliefs and anticipated costs and benefits of health behaviors, whether accurate or not, are critical determinants of health choices that have direct effects on clinical outcomes. Clinical approaches from this perspective emphasize education and cognitive change as key factors for improving health. The social and education psychology literatures provide extensive information about variable (e.g. credibility, perceived similarity) that enhance persuasion and provide the empirical foundation for efforts toward cognitive change. These health education-based approaches have played a particularly significant role in community and public health interventions.

Treatment for Stress-related Illness

Stress responses are complex reaction patterns with physiological, cognitive, behavioral, and social components. As a result, prevention and treatment of stress-related illness have concentrated on several important dimensions. The characteristic approach of behavioral medicine is to help individuals be more competent in managing their behaviors and emotions in reaction to taxing aspects of their environment or their medical illness. Self-management and effective command of one's health and environment depend on possessing the necessary cognitive and behavioral skills and being able to employ those skills. Goals for treatment do not entail eliminating stress (or the medical problem) but aim toward helping the patient to learn the skills to function adequately despite stressful situations.

Individuals who rely more on active coping efforts to manage problems generally tend to adapt better to life stressors and experience. Active efforts to seek information and support and to problem solve have been related to better adjustment in a variety of populations, including medical patients with diverse disorders, family caregivers, and healthy adults. Furthermore, research has shown that persistent avoidance or passive coping, such as denying, fantasizing, minimizing, acceptation the situation and venting negative emotions, is maladaptive and an important risk factor associated with many medical illnesses as well as emotional distress.

One of the key areas of focus has been on arousal reducing techniques, such as biofeedback, relaxation training, diaphragmatic breathing, meditation, self-hypnosis, and the use of exercise to reduce or counter stress. The rationale for these stress management techniques assumes that an increased level of physiological arousal is manifested by a combination of increased muscle tension and increased sympathetic nervous system activity. In addition, specific training in reducing thoughts that increase arousal and learning more adaptive behaviors in response to a variety of stressful situations are emphasized in behavioral medicine's integrated multicomponent approach to managing stress-related illness.

Biofeedback

Biofeedback as a tool for the treatment of tension dates to the early 1970s and has been used to provide information on physiological changes that were once thought involuntary. With repeated training, patients can produce and detect physiological change to bring under control many aspects of autonomic arousal (e.g. blood pressure, heart rate, musculoskeletal tension, and peripheral vascular blood flow).

The effects of biofeedback are often produced by the person's attempts at relaxation or mental imagery. Treatment of a range of problems, such as anxiety, headaches temporomandibular joint difficulties, and a variety of chronic pain problems, has been useful with the techniques of biofeedback. However, for the most part, it is fair to say that biofeedback has not shown to be any more effective in reducing arousal and helping with these illnesses that the following stress management strategies:

Relaxation Training

The oldest arousal-reducing or stress management techniques for a variety of medical problems, especially cardiovascular reactivity, are the various forms of relaxation training: (1) progressive muscle relaxation, the systematic tensing and relaxing of major muscle groups: (2) autogenic training specific self-instruction to relax: (3) various forms of meditation, including the "relaxation response" and (4) diaphragmatic breathing. These nonhuman ecological treatments for stress-related disorders have been a major landmark in the field: a large body of evidence has accumulated showing diminished stress-related symptoms. The various techniques allow an individual a way of countering arousal in anticipation, moderation its intensity, inhibiting it, or assisting in recovery from stressful encounters.

Tension is associated with physiological changes that may or may not be noticeable (e.g. heart rate, blood pressure, and respiratory rates). Regular practice of progressive muscle relaxation teaches individuals to gradually relax skeletal muscles and quiet the autonomic nervous system. Individuals are taught to become more familiar with the effects of stress on musculoskeletal tension and to counter act these reactions by acquainting themselves with the sensations of both tight and relaxed musculature throughout the whole body. Tainting begins with the tensing and relaxing of multiple muscle groups, and individuals are eventually asked to achieve relaxation by merely recalling the sensations associated with the release of tension. Successful training aids the individual in greater awareness of muscle tension and its physiological and provides an ability to reduce arousal in an efficient manner. Emphasis is placed on transferring the relaxation efficient to real-life situations (also called applied relaxation)—the physician's office, work site, traffic jams, or everyday interactions with others.

Exercise

Whereas a formidable body of evidence has accumulated underscoring the long-term benefits of exercise, the specific stress-reducing effects have been more anecdotal than empirical. Evidence indicates that aerobic exercise tends to lower blood pressure across a wide variety of hypertensive individuals-from mildly to moderately hypertensive patients, in adolescent to geriatric populations, and even in those with advanced end-organ damage such as renal dialysis patients persons who are aerobically fit are better able to meet a physical demand with less sympathetic activation than their less fit counterparts. Individuals secrete less catecholamine, have reduced heart rates, and have lower peripheral vasoconstriction at the same exercise workload. Moreover, review of the literature suggest that exercise may be effective in reducing the risk for development of essential hypertension.

Cognitive Therapy

Another focus of stress management techniques has been on the specific thoughts that decrease arousal and reduce the effects of stress. The area that has shown the greatest promise has been cognitive therapy. To decrease persistent negative emotions and help patients adapt to events for which they have little or no control, individuals are taught cognitive strategies, such as restructuring irrational beliefs and replacing distorted, unrealistic, negative, or worry thoughts with rational, optimistic and "what and see" beliefs.

Aside from unusual catastrophic events (e.g. prison of war, rape victimization by terrorists), stress is often perception or an attribution by the patient. Moreover thoughts about a situation always precede arousal (whether the individuals is aware of the thought or not) therefore individuals are taught to identify events that increase emotional distress or arousal, analyze specific aspects of event that are upsetting, and learn whether they are over reacting or distorting events unnecessarily.

Pain Management: An Example of Adaptation and Progress in Behavioral Medicine

Pain management has been a significant emphasis of behavioral medicine since its curliest days. Pain control is also one of the areas of greatest success and documented and efficacy. The development of pain management approaches in behavioral medicine parallels to the development of the field in general and the historical, political, and socioeconomic factors of the times.

Phase I: Mental Control of Pain Sensations

Initial efforts to conceptualize chronic pain syndromes emphasized psychiatric concepts that influence pain reports (e.g. summarization, hypochondriasis, hysteria, secondary gain). Psychotherapeutic approaches were then employed to resolve conflicts and redirect attention. Most notable was the use of mental techniques like hypnosis to redirect attention and modify perception directly at a cognitive level. Considerable success was attained. Particularly with painful procedures, acute pain, and relatively circumscribed pain syndromes. Dissatisfaction grew out of inconsistency of results, lack of generalization to chronic pain, and in attention to dysfunction and disability.

Phase II: Biofeedback to Regulate Painful Processes

Biofeedback approaches offered an integrated psycho-physiological (Mind-body) approach to pain. Biofeedback developed out of the need to address disease process and dysfunction. Moreover, biofeedback was congruent with the basic notion of self-regulation that permeates the field and arose from successful laboratory research demonstrating reliable visceral leering phenomena. Biofeedback approaches enjoyed considerable success when disease processes were well understood although the mechanism of action is still under considerable debate. Dissatisfaction grew out of limited applications, lack of generalization, and limited attention to disability.

Phase III: Behavioral Rehabilitation to Restore Function

The marriage of operant psychology and rehabilitation medicine brought the next wave of influence on behavioral medicine pain management (1976). This approach indirectly addressed pain by directly modifying pain behaviors, functional capacities, and use of health care technologies. For example, patients were taught to gradually increase their exercise tolerance while staff and families systematically reinforced attempts at healthy functional behavior and did not reinforce "pain behaviors" (e.g. guarding, bracing, limping, grimacing, complaints of pain). Greater emphasis was placed on reducing impairment and disability associated with pain than on alleviation of the subjective experience of pain. For the first-time, rigorous outcome data were available supporting behavioral approaches to reducing pain, distress, and disability. Dissatisfaction grew out of limited acceptability to patients, lack of generalization, and limited attention to pain.

Phase IV: Comprehensive Integrated Biomedical and Behavioral Technologies

Before the 1980s, pain management approaches were primarily singular. Practitioners adopted one of the aforementioned approaches or gradually converted and retrained as the prevailing modes developed. Moreover, behavioral care was not well integrated with biomedical approaches. The 1980s, saw the development of the multidisciplinary pain center, providing a conscious attempt to integrate the preceding three behavioral approaches with each other and with biomedical technologies. Patients were typically treated in highly structured inpatient setting to control their environments and were exposed to mental techniques, biofeedback, operant conditioning. Cognitive therapy, physical rehabilitation, occupational therapy, vocational counseling, analgesic management, and innovative neurosurgical pain control technologies. With such comprehensive approaches it was difficult to determine which elements were primarily responsible for observed effects. Dissatisfaction grew out of limited access limited generalizability of finding and techniques and high cost of treatment.

Phase V: Health Services Delivery Accountability Models

The 1990s, brought a renewed emphasis on accountability clinical outcomes were weighed against cost of treatment in ever more sophisticated ways. Most multidisciplinary inpatient pain centers have closed or are in financial trouble at this time. The emphasis in care has centered on cost containment, and comprehensive inpatient programs have found it difficult to justify sufficient incremental benefits over more focused outpatient programs. Current research focuses on distilling the finding from comprehensive treatment package, determining essential treatment components evaluating patient treatment matching, and exploring more efferent delivery systems. Prevention of chronicity and disability managements have taken center stage in the new millennium.

CONCLUSION

In this chapter, we have tried to describe some of the historical and ideological underpinnings of behavioral medicine. The field has made impressive strides in a short-time by offering unique behavioral interventions in diverse medical settings.

Paradoxically, the interdisciplinary focus, which responsible for much of its progress, also entails some problems. Behavioral medicine programs are rarely found in their own "departments" and instead are typically housed in departments of psychiatry psychology or family medicine. In such settings the behavioral medicine practitioner or academic may be relatively isolated as a lone voice for the behavioral medicine perspective. More recently some free-standing departments and programs in behavioral medicine have been developed at several notable institutions such as Harvard and the University of California san Francisco and behavioral medicine has become a part of many medical school curricula professional societies such as the society of behavioral medicine. The American Psychosomatic Society provide academic and clinical leadership through their behavioral journals and annual conferences. It remains to be determined setting for long-term behavioral medicine programs.

47.9 PSYCHOANALYSIS, PSYCHOANALYTIC PSYCHOTHERAPY, AND SUPPORTIVE PSYCHOTHERAPY

Neena Bohra, NK Bohra

Psychotherapy was defined by Harry Stack Sullivan (1954) as primarily a verbal interchange between two individuals in which one of these individuals is designated an expert and the other is a help seeker. Munford et al. (1984) explored in their meta-analysis of the cost-offset effects outpatient mental health treatments, most of which were short-term. They found that outpatient psychotherapy care were less expensive and effective. Furthermore, these reductions occurred dominantly in the more expensive inpatient medical services.

PSYCHOANALYTICALLY-ORIENTED PSYCHOTHERAPIES

Primary to the psychodynamic (psychoanalytically oriented) treatments is the importance of the patient feeling engaged and involved in the work. Through the exploration of the patient's conflicts evidenced in symptoms, metaphors, and symbols, both defensive patterns and disturbances in present interpersonal relationship can be identified in the treatment setting as well as in the patient's life. The therapist's ability to hear what the patient has to say and to understand its meaning is central to all psychoanalytically-oriented treatments (Solnit 2000). This facet of treatment demands skill in neutral listening and the ability to identify with the patient's perspective and worldview while not losing one's own.

The therapist is always listening for the continuity present, but hidden, between sessions (Coleman 1968). The therapist operates on the hypothesis that each session is related to the previous one. The psychoanalyst and the psychodynamic psychotherapist listen to the patient's subjective experience of the world, interpersonal and internal conflicts, and cognitive defenses that result in the day-to-day changes in moods, thoughts, and behaviors (Moihl and McLaughlin 1997; Silberman and Certa 1997).

In the initial phase of treatment, the therapeutic alliance (i.e. the working alliance) is developed (Greenson 1965; Zetzel 1956). The therapeutic alliance is the reality-based relationship between the analyst (or the therapist) and the patient that forms the basis of working together in a cooperative manner (Sonnenberg et al. 1997). The therapeutic alliance is nurtured through the identification of the patient's initial anxieties about beginning treatment. Fostering the therapeutic alliance is a part of the therapist's establishment of the conditions under which the patient can favorably hear and deal with the interpretations that the therapist will give later in the treatment (Ponsi 2000).

Psychoanalysis

Psychoanalysis was development by Sigmund Freud beginning in the late nineteenth century. Originally, Freud used hypnosis to recover forgotten memories related to traumas of early childhood. Historically, the progressed from hypnosis to the 'Pressure technique' and finally to the modern approach of using free association. Perhaps Freud's most important and lasting discovery was the contribution of psychic reality to development and conflict formation. Freud found that it was the subjective experience of events in childhood—that is, the psychic reality of the events—rather than the presence or absence of the actual events, that affected development and conflict formation. This discovery led Freud to denitrify the role of the unconscious and unremembered experiences of childhood and to develop a mechanism, psychoanalysis, to discover and bring these memories into awareness.

The dangers of neglecting the actuality of traumatic events have been highlighted in recent years and must always be considered by the therapist. In the treatment of children, this is particularly important because of the need to intervene to protect the child. Often a neglect of the reality of trauma results if the therapist does not understand that the patient's recall is a mixture of both subjective factors and objective fact, neither of which can be ignored.

Freud identified dreams, slips of the tongue, and free association as important windows on the influence of childhood and the present conflicts of the patient. From the psychoanalytic view, and understanding of the conflicts experienced in childhood is important to gaining knowledge and changing present behavior (Brenner 1976). The conflicts of childhood are called the childhood neurosis.

Conflicts are patterns of feelings, thoughts, and behavior that were 'learned' (i.e. incorporated into brain function and patterning) during childhood. 'Neurotic' conflicts result in the patient's feelings of anxiety and depression; somatic symptoms; work, social, sexual inhibition; and maladaptive interpersonal relations. Typically, such conflicts are between libidinal (i.e. sexual/bodily) and aggressive wishes. Libidinal wishes can be thought of as longing for sexual and emotional gratification or more generally as positive feelings and affects (Kernbeg 2001). Aggressive whishes are destructive desires (or, as they are more often conceptualize, today; negative feelings and affects) that either are primary or result from frustration and deprivation.

The concept of sexual wishes is quite broad in psychoanalysis and is not limited to only genital feelings. Sexual wishes include wishes to be held and touched, to control, to eat, and many others. This concept of sexuality was another of Freud's major contributions; his discovery, and the subsequent confirmation through child observation, of the intimate relationship between children and their bodies. It is through their bodies that children come to know mother, father and the world. It is hard to overemphasize the radical change in thinking that resulted from beginning to think of the child as having thoughts, feeling, and fantasies and as not being a 'tabula rasa' or a 'small adult'.

The goal of psychoanalysis is the elucidation of the childhood neurosis (i.e. conflicts) as it presents in the transference neurosis. This is a major undertaking that requires a reasonably psychiatrically healthy individual who can sustain the treatment. Psychoanalysis is frequently criticized for being used to treat reasonably psychiatrically healthy people. In fact, however, this is the tradition of medicine. For example, one may ask who receives triple bypass surgery: the individual with a single left main descending artery occlusion or the individual who is having a myocardial infarction and in the end stage of congestive heart failure? Clearly, the answer is the former. This underscores the frequently forgotten point that medical treatments are given to patients rather than to diseases. All medical treatments, including psychoanalysis, make certain requirements of the patient. These requirements must be considered when the treatment is prescribed, psychoanalysis is very demanding of patients. It requires an individual who is able to access his or her fantasy life in an active, experiencing manner and is able to leave it behind at the end of a session (Table 15).

Psychoanalysis focuses on the recovery of childhood experiences as they appear in the relationship with the

Table 15: Psychoanalysis: goal, selection criteria, duration, techniques

Goal	Resolution of the childhood neurosis as it presents itself in the transference neurosis
Selection criteria	Experiences conflict that is primarily oedipal Experiences conflict as internal Is psychologically minded Is able to obtain symptom relief through Understanding Has supportive relationships available in both the present and the past
Duration	Four to five sessions per week; 3–6 years, average duration
Techniques	Free association Therapeutic alliance Neutrality Abstinence Defense analysis Interpretation of transference

analyst (Chessick 2000; Coltrera 1980; Freud 1912a/1958; Gill 1982; Greenson 1967). This recreation in the doctor-patient relationship of a conflicted relationship with a childhood figure is the transference neurosis. Frequently, the transference is paternal or maternal, but it need not be. Sibling, aunt, uncle, and grandparent transferences are all important parts of psychoanalytic work. The transference neurosis (in contrast to transference phenomena) is the sustained appearance of the transference over time. When the transference neurosis is present, the patient experiences the analyst in a similar manner as he or she once did the significant figure from the past. Frequently, this experience is accompanied by other elements of the past being experienced in the patient's life.

Transference is a ubiquitous phenomenon that is increasingly able to be studied empirically (Fried et al. 1992; Luborsky and Crits-Christoph 1990). Several empirical studies support the importance of addressing the transference for a successful outcome of psychodynamic treatment (Brodaty 1983; Donovan 1984: Frances and Sperry 1983; Luborsky and Crits-Chistoph 1990; Malan 1975, 1976, 1980; Marziali 1984; Marziali and Sullivan 1980). Transference is the result of our tendency to see the past in the present, to exclude new information, and to see what is familiar to us. This "looking for the familiar" results in our reacting and responding in ways that are characteristic of our relationships with significant figures from our past. The analyst's relative abstinence (i.e. avoiding gratiflying wishes) and neutrality (i.e. not encouraging one side or another of the patient's conflict-either the wishes or the defenses and prohibitions) help create a setting in which the transference can emerge and, more important, in which it can be observed and understood by the analyst and the patient. It is the contrast between the patient's experience of the analyst in the transference and his or her experience in the therapeutic alliance that facilitates. The recognition that the transference thoughts and feelings are self-generated.

Table 16: Transference and countertransference

Transference	Seeing the past in the present Seeing the familiar Excluding new information
Countertransference	
Concordant	Identifying with the patient's feelings (the therapist feels as though he/she were the patient)
Complementary	Reacting to the patient's feelings (the therapist feels as though he/she were the transference figure)

The transference is not a total distortion of the doctor-patient relationship. Rather, it is often an elaborations (without confirming information) of an observation the patient has made about the analyst or his or her office. Reality serves as the foundation on which the transference is constructed. The patient's understanding of the transference aids in the recall of the past and the recovery of lost feelings.

Counter transference is the analyst's transference response to the patient. At time, countertransference is also used to describe the analyst's specific neurotic responses to the patient's transference (Table 16). However, this is not clearly different from the first, more general, definition (Blum 1986; Sandler et al. 1973). Countertransference is also ubiquitous and it is not limited to the psychoanalytic setting. In fact, it can be an important part of any relationship, particularly the doctor-patient relationship; when present, it may be intense and enduring. Countertransference is increased by life stress and unresolved conflicts in the analyst. It can appear as either an identification with or a reaction to the patient's conscious and unconscious fantasies, feelings, and behaviors (Racker 1957). Through analysis of his or her own countertransference reactions, the analyst recognizes subtle aspects of the transference relationship and is better able to understand the patient's experience (Searles 1965). Skill in recognizing countertransference and transference is an important part of the psychiatrist's armamentarium in all treatment settings, particularly those involving consultation-liaison psychiatry, in which the doctor-patient or nurse-patient relationships can be the major reason a consultation was requested.

The design to the psychoanalytic treatment situation fosters the patient's observing capacity so that transference neurosis can be analyzed (Stone 1961). Transference is not unique to the psychoanalytic situation. It occurs throughout life in all areas and is a frequent 'accompaniment to hospitalization of any kind. Entering a hospital, having one's clothes removed, having one's name forgotten, being required to eat when told, and having to submit to medical procedures constitute a highly regressive experience that facilitates the appearance of transferences. The ability to recognize transference phenomena as they appear in all doctor-patient relationships is very important. Psychoanalysis is unique in its efforts to establish a setting in which the transference, when it appears, can be used as a vehicle for understanding.

Modern psychoanalysis continues to require frequent meetings of the analyst and analysand–usually, four to five sessions per week (Freud originally met with his patients six times per week). This frequency of sessions is continued, on the average, for 3–6 years. This intensity of meetings is necessary for the patient to develop sufficient trust to explore his or her inner fantasy life. In addition, given the number of events that occur daily in a life, the frequent meetings enable the patient to explore fantasies rather than only the reality-based perceptions of life events (Freud 1912b/1958). Individuals who are in crisis and who, therefore, are very concerned and focused on the real events. In their life are not good candidates to enter psychoanalysis. Psychoanalysis focuses on the patient's experience and fantasies of his or her life rather than on the real events. A crisis does not allow the patient the opportunity to explore fantasies. In general, the patient in psychoanalysis is encouraged to use the couch so that the patient's focus on fantasies rather than on reality will be further facilitated. In addition, the analyst usually sits out of view, allowing the patient better to elaborate his or her fantasies about the analyst.

Free association is a major element in the technique of psychoanalysis. Freud described free association through an analogy of a train ride (Freud 1913/1958). He suggested that if the analyst and analysand were riding together on a train and the analyst were blind, the analysand would not forget to describe the beautiful mountains or the ugly coal slags. This analogy is meant to convey the sense of the patient's reporting of all thoughts that come to mind without censorship and without dismissing them as too trivial. In point of fact, free association is difficult to attain, and much of the work of psychoanalysis is based on identifying those places where free association breaks down (i.e. the occurrence of a defense, clinically experienced by the analyst as resistance). When the patient is able to achieve the highest level of free association, the neurotic conflicts have been removed and termination is near.

Early in treatment, the analyst establishes a therapeutic alliance with the patient that allows for a reality-based consideration of the demand so the treatment and for a working collaboration between analyst and analysand toward the patient's understanding himself or herself (Grenson 1965) Meissner 1998; Zetzel 1956). The analyst focuses on analyzing the defenses the patient uses to minimize conflict and disturbing affects (Freud 1912/1958, 1913/1958 1914/1958). Defenses such as intellectualization, reaction formation, denial, repression, and to other neurotic cognitive mechanisms are identified and repeatedly interpreted to the patient. Though the analysis of defense, the working alliance strengthens and the patient's ability to observe internal fantasies increases. In addition, the patient's comfort with talking about his or her feelings with the analyst increases. In this way, the transference grows more available and can be analyzed.

The analysis of the patient's dreams is an important element of psychoanalytic treatment (Freud 1911/1958, Reiser 2001; Sharpe 1961; Ursano et al. 1998). Dreams, as well as slips of the tongue and symptoms, express the conflicts of the patient in 'metaphor', evidencing the out-of-awareness (i.e. unconscious) elements of the conflict. The building blocks of dreams are recent life events. Dreams express both a present and a childhood conflict in much the same way that a rebus expresses a story. The grammar of the dream process different from that of conscious thought. Rather than following logic and time sequence, dreams are constructed by condensation of multiple meanings and the use of symbols. There are no universal symbols. The symbols, perhaps better thought symbolic vehicles available to any given person, are from the 'dictionary' of meanings developed as part of the individual's life experience, both in childhood and in adulthood. Thus, dreams (and slips of the tongue and symptoms) are a means for the patient to understand the feelings and thoughts that influence his or her life, that are out of awareness, and that often are derived from childhood experiences, beliefs, and views of the interpersonal world and familial behavior (Weiss and Sampson 1986).

The primary goal of psychoanalysis is the establishment of transference relationship and the subsequent analysis of this relationship. It is this primary focus that distinguishes psychoanalysis from psychodynamic psychotherapy. The specific treatment effects of psychoanalysis grow from the experience and analysis of transference, reawakened affects, cognitions, and behaviors linked with significant individuals in the patient's past. In the context of the arousal associated with these figures and the simultaneous understanding the experience, behavioral change occurs (Loewald 1984).

The analyst uses a number of techniques in his or her intervention, including interpretation and clarification (Bibring 1954; Glove 1968; Sandler et al. 1973). Classically, an interpretation is the linking together of the patient's experience of an event in the present with the transference experience of the analyst and the childhood-significant figure. Rarely are interpretations actually given in one sentence in one session. More frequently, interpretations occur over a period during which the past, the present, and the transference experiences are linked together (Tables 17 and 18).

Medications are infrequently used in psychoanalysis, although some analysts are attempting to use psychoanalysis with medication in the treatment of persons, with affective disorders. Psychoanalysis is actually a highly supportive treatment for the individual who experiences frequent

Table 17: Defense mechanisms
Repression
Intellectualization
Reaction formation
Regression
Displacement
Sublimation
Reversal
Splitting
Denial
Projection
Inhibition
Projective identification
Asceticism
Omnipotence
Isolation of affect
Devaluing
Identification with the aggressor
Primitive idealization

Table 18: Principle of psychoanalytic technique	
Neutrality	The analyst maintains a neutral stance favoring neither the patient's wishes (i.e. id) nor the patient's condemnations of these wishes (i.e. superego)
Abstinence	The analyst does not gratify the patient's desire or expectation that the analyst act like the person from the past. Rathe, the analyst helps the patient see and understand this process

contact, quiet inquiry, and intellectual understanding as a supportive environment (De Jonghe et al. 1992; Wallerstein 1986, 1989). The supportive elements and their contribution to the treatment process have been less discussed in psychoanalysis than in other treatments. The need for medication may indicate the patient's need for medication may indicate the patient's need for medication may indicate the patients' need for greater support than can be provide in the psychoanalytic treatment.

The analyst operates under several guiding principles that facilitate the analysis of the transference. These principles include (1) neutrality, by which the analyst favors neither the patient's wishes (i.e. id) nor the condemnations of these wishes (i.e. superego), and (2) abstinence, where by the analyst does not provide gratification to the patient similar to that of the wished-for object (Freud 1915 [1914/1958)]. It is helpful is understanding the rule of abstinence to recognize a definition of transference used by joseph Sandler, Sandler et al. (1973) described transference as the role pressure placed on the analyst to conform to the behaviors of the significant individual from the past. Therefore, transference is experienced by the analyst as an expectation from the patient that the analyst will behave in a certain manner. Abstinence is the avoidance of becoming this figure in reality and gratifying these wishes or beliefs. The therapist's abstinence leads to his or her being somewhat silent but not withholding in order better to observe how the patient organizes his or her psychic world. This stance must be explained and the patient educated about the reason for this stance.

The assessment of a patient for psychoanalysis must include diagnostic considerations as well as an assessment of the patient's ability to make use of the psychoanalytic situation for behavioral change. These considerations include the patient's psychological mindedness; the availability of supports in his or her real environment to sustain the psychoanalysis, which can be felt as quite depriving; and the patient's ability to experience and simultaneously to observe highly charged affective states.

Because of the frequency of the sessions and the duration of the treatment, the cost of psychoanalysis can be prohibitive. Low-fee clinics frequently make available a substantial amount of treatment to some patients who could not otherwise afford it.

Psychoanalysis has been useful in the treatment of obsessional disorders, anxiety disorders, dysthymic disorders, and moderately sever personality disorders. Individuals with substantial preoedipal pathology, usually indicated by chaotic life settings and an inability to establish a supportive dyadic relationship, as is often seen in patients with narcissistic, borderline, schizoid, paranoid, and schizotypal personality disorders, are usually not thought to be candidates for traditional psychoanalysis. In the present climate of emphasis on cost-effectiveness, psychoanalysis is more frequently recommended after a course of brief psychotherapy has proved to be either ineffective or insufficient.

PSYCHOANALYTIC PSYCHOTHERAPY (TABLE 19)

Psychoanalytically-oriented psychotherapy also known as psychoanalytic psychotherapy, psychodynamic psychotherapy, and explorative psychotherapy is a psychotherapeuticprocedurethatrecognizesthedevelopment of transference and resistance in the psychotherapy setting (Brush 1974; Fromm-Reeichmann 1950). Both long-term and brief psychodynamic psychotherapy and long-term and brief psychodynamic psychotherapy are possible. In the past, the terms brief psychotherapy and long-term psychotherapy were frequently use synonymously with supportive psychotherapy and explorative psychotherapy, respectively. However, brief and long-term more accurately describe the duration rather than the technique, focus or goal

Table 19: Psychoanalytic psychotherapy

Goal	Defense and transference analysis with limited reconstruction of the past
Selection criteria	When a narrower focus and less comprehensive outcome is acceptable. The same selection criteria as in psychoanalysis are used, but they can include more seriously disturbed patients who can use understanding to resolve symptoms when supportive elements are available in the treatment
Duration	One to three sessions per week from 1–6 years on average
Techniques	Therapeutic alliance Face to face Free association Defense and transference interpretation More use of clarification, suggestion, and learning through experience than in psychoanalysis

of psychoanalytically-oriented psychotherapy (Budman and Gurman 1983; Errenra et al. 1967; Ursano and Dressler 1977). In addition, newer methods of delivering psychotherapy-including intermittent psychotherapy, which is provide in episodes over an extended period of time, and sequential brief psychotherapy, in which medication is continued after the termination of the psychotherapy—are becoming more common than classical long-term psychotherapy.

Brief psychotherapy, in particular, requires the therapist to confront his or her own ambitiousness and perfectionism as well as any exaggerated ideal of personality structure and function. The time limits of brief psychotherapy give the therapy its unique characteristic and distinguish it from long-term psychotherapy and psychoanalysis (Ursonaon and Drssler 1974). Steirlin (1968) identified two treatment factors that are important to understanding the effectiveness of psychotherapy: the "propitious moment" and the "shared past" Brief psychotherapy uses the propitious moment to create personality change, whereas long-term treatment uses the shared past that develops between therapist and patient. Both the propitious moment and the shared past carry psychotherapeutic advantages and disadvantages, emphasizing certain technical possibilities and limiting others.

Following World War II, the interest in psychoanalysis resulted in a rapid growth in the demand for psychotherapy. This growing demand considerably increased the resultant pressure on psychiatrists to develop briefer and less intense forms of psychotherapy than psychoanalysis. In addition, the community mental health movement, and more recently, the increasing cost of mental health care, have stimulated efforts to find briefer forms of psychotherapy (Milrod et al. 1997). At present, brief psychotherapy is an important part of the psychiatrist's armamentarium (Kay 1997).

Psychoanalytic psychotherapy is usually more focused than the extensive reworking of personality undertaken in psychoanalysis (Dewald 1978). In addition, psychoanalytic psychotherapy is oriented somewhat more to the here and now and there is less of an attempt to reconstruct the developmental origins of conflicts. Psychoanalytically-oriented psychotherapy may take as its entire goal the analysis of a set of defenses that are interfering with the patient's development. The accomplishment of this task may substantially open up the patient's life and development.

Psychoanalytic psychotherapy recognizes and interprets transference when it occurs. However, the entire treatment is not directed toward the establishment and analysis of the transference in the thorough manner of a psychoanalysis. Long-term psychodynamic psychotherapy includes more transference work than do the brief psychodynamic psychotherapies. Psychoanalytic psychotherapy also makes use of techniques that are not available in psychoanalysis. This allows for its application to a broader range of patients, including those with psychotic regressive potentials such as borderline personality disorder.

Usually, patients in long-term psychoanalytic psychotherapy are seen one, two or three times per week; twice per week is desirable in that this frequency allows for sufficient intensity for the transference to unfold and to be interpreted. Patient and therapist meet in face-to-face encounters and free association is encouraged. Psychoanalytic psychotherapy may extend from several months to several years, at times taking as long as psychoanalysis. The length of treatment is determined by the number of focal problem areas undertaken in the treatment. Medications can be used in psychoanalytic psychotherapy and provide another means of titrating the level of regression a patient may experience. The therapist uses interpretations and clarifications as in psychoanalysis. In addition, however, the therapist may use other interpretative techniques such as suggestion, practice of new behavior patterns and experiences, and confrontation (Bilbring 1954). Practice in this context (classically called manipulation) refers to learning from experience, such as pointing out that the therapist does not respond in the expected transferential manner. Confrontation is not 'Fighting' but rather pointing out to the patient when something is being denied or avoided.

The same patients who are treated in psychoanalysis can be treated in psychoanalytic psychotherapy. However, the focus of the treatment is much narrower and the expected outcome less comprehensive. At times, the supportive elements of a psychoanalytic psychotherapy can interfere with the patient's full experience of his or her conflicts, which can be more evident to the patient in a psychoanalysis. The psychosocial problems and internal conflicts of patients who could not be treated in psychoanalysis, such as those with major depression, schizophrenia, and borderline personality disorder, can be addressed in a long-term psychoanalytic psychotherapy. The long-term contributions of psychoanalytic psychotherapy to the treatment of major depression and schizophrenia, for which biological treatments have proved efficacious for some of the major symptoms, require further study. Patients with these diagnoses use psychotherapy to modify illness-onset conditions and facilitate readjustment, recovery, and integration into family and community. In long-term psychoanalytic psychotherapy, the regressive tendencies of such patients can be titrated with greater elements of support, the use of medication as needed, greater reality feedback through the face-to-face encounter with the therapist.

The opening phase of psychodynamic psychotherapy is often marked by activation of magical expectations of the patient and the belief that past pains will now be resolved. During the initial phase, the therapist may make few comments and usually accepts the positive transference of the patient. Important aspects of the current problems, the patient's characteristic defense mechanisms and coping styles, and the developmental roots of the central issue become clearer during this phase. In the middle phase of treatment, resistance is likely to appear, as well as the negative transference. The patient experiences the frustration that not all the wished-for changes are occurring. Defenses are identified and analyzed, and usually the transference is sufficiently evident to be worked with.

The patient must be educated about transference phenomena and develop sufficient observing ego to participate with the therapist in wondering about this aspect of his or her internal life. The transference is not suddenly interpreted to the patient, nor should one assume that the patient knows that it is expected or desirable to talk about feelings toward the therapist. It is the skills of the therapist that allows him or her to know when to introduce this topic to the patient and how to help the patient increasingly to explore this area of feelings and thoughts. In the end phase of treatment, termination and the patient's resistances to termination are prominent. Termination is based on having reached a series of life goals that allows the patient to continue on a normal developmental path, Ideal treatment goals are not the end point. Rather, the reestablishment of normal development and the removal of obstacle to the normal recovery processes are the goals of treatment. The patient's increased capacity to understand his or her conflicts and to analyze conflicts independently indicates that the end of treatment will occur shortly.

Interpersonal Psychotherapy (Table 20)

Interpersonal psychotherapy (IPT) is psychotherapy developed by Klerman and colleagues (Klerman et al. 1984a, Markowitz 1998; Rounsaville et al. 1985b). Whether conducted briefly or longer term, IPT focuses on current interpersonal problems in outpatient nonbipolar, nonpsychotic depressed individual. IPT has been the major psychotherapeutic modality used in combined psychotherapy and pharmacological treatment studies. This psychotherapy has also been used for the treatment of drug abuse. It did not, however, have a notable impact on outcome when patients were already participating in a well-run treatment program that included weekly group psychotherapy (Rounsaville et al. 1983, 1985a). IPT derives from the interpersonal school of psychiatry that originated with Adolf Mayer and Harry Stack Sullivan. The understanding of social supports and of attachment provides further theoretical underpinning for this form of psychotherapy. IPT focuses on reassurance, clarification of feeling states, improvement in interpersonal communication, testing of perception, and interpersonal skills rather than on personality reconstruction.

Table 20: Interpersonal psychotherapy

Goal	Improvement in current interpersonal skills
Selection	Outpatients, nonbipolar, nonpsychotic depression
Duration	Short-and long-term Usually once-weekly meeting
Techniques	Reassurance Clarification of feeling states Improvement of interpersonal communication Testing perceptions Development of interpersonal skills Medication

Interpersonal psychotherapy (IPT) has been primarily used in the treatment of depressed patients. (AF Frank et al. 1991; O 'Hara et al. 2000). In the opening phase of IPT, a detailed symptom history is taken, usually using a structured interview. The symptoms are reviewed with the patient, and the patient receives explicit information about the natural course of depression as a clinical condition. There is an emphasis on legitimizing the patient in the sick role. A second major task of this phase is the assessment of the patient's interpersonal problem areas. There is an attempt to identify one or more of four problem areas: grief reaction, interpersonal disputes, role transition, and interpersonal deficits. Each of these areas is thought to be related to depression.

The middle phase of treatment is directed toward resolving the problem area or areas. Clarifying positive and negative felling states, identifying past models for relationships, and guiding and encouraging the patient in examining and choosing alternative courses of action constitute the basic techniques of handling each problem area (Weissman and Markowitz 1994). The focus is kept on current dilemmas and not past interpersonal relationships. Interpersonal events, rather than intrapsychic or cognitive events, are the focus of IPT.

Much of IPT is based on psychodynamic theory (Markowitz et al. 1998). The therapist's attitude is one of exploration, similar to the attitude in other insight-oriented psychotherapies when applied in a medical model. Applying the dictum of working "from the surface to the depths" results in much of the resemblance of IPT to psychodynamic psychotherapy. However, Klerman and colleagues found it is useful to highlight the differences between these approaches to standardize a psychotherapeutic technique. Collaborative clinical trials have demonstrated the advantage of maintenance IPT in enhancing social functioning during recovery from depression and in reducing symptoms and improving functioning during the acute phase of a depressive episode. These effects require 6–8 months to become apparent. Depressed patients undergoing combined pharmacotherapy and IPT have the best outcomes (DiMascio et al. 1997; Weissman et al. 1981). IPT has also been effective in the treatment of postpartum depression, improving symptoms and social adjustment (O Hara et al. 2000).

Comparison of Psychodynamic, Interpersonal, and Cognitive Psychotherapies

Because interpersonal cognitive psychotherapies are related to the psychodynamic model, there is a high degree of overlap in the problem areas identified in any given patient in these treatments. The conceptualization of the problem, however, is different. In many ways it is complementary rather than mutually exclusive. The psychoanalytic, interpersonal, and cognitive psychotherapies share explorative and change-oriented goals. Cognitive psychotherapy focuses on the patient's thinking; IPT on the patient's interpersonal relations and social supports, and psychoanalytically-oriented treatments on the internal experience of the patient and its relationship to past experience. Cognitive and interpersonal psychotherapies are most frequently used to treat depression rather than to treat an entire range of psychopathology. No studies using well-defined psychodynamic psychotherapies and medication have been performed. In this area, IPT and cognitive psychotherapy have been more closely studied.

IPT, cognitive psychotherapy, and the traditional psychodynamic psychotherapies can be compared. All three modalities are complex methods of treatment that must be tailored to the individual and the therapist requires a considerable amount of time to acquire competency in administering these treatments (Beck et al. 1997).

The relationship between therapist and patient and the establishment of a therapeutic alliance are essential in IPT, cognitive psychotherapy, and the psychoanalytically-oriented treatments. Extensive exploration of the patient's thoughts and feelings, including those involving the therapist, is a major portion of the work. In addition, in all three, the therapist attempts to maintain an investigative, collaborative, and nonjudgmental stance.

In practice, cognitive is similar to the analysis of defense in the psychodynamic approaches. Understanding defenses focuses the patient and therapist on the hidden cognitive distortions that result in the patient's faulty perception of both the internal and the external world. In the dynamic model, defense mechanisms from conflict. The defenses, however, distort perception and cognition resulting in distortions that are similar to those that are the focus of cognitive psychotherapy. In cognitive psychotherapy, cognitions are seen as the causative agent of the patient's distress. Much of the work in identifying these cognitions and alerting the patient to them is similar to the understanding and interpretation of defense in the psychodynamic psychotherapies. The schemata underlying the faulty cognitions of cognitive psychotherapy are unconscious assumptions, which in the psychodynamic model are viewed as being derived from earlier experience. Both treatments share the importance of identifying these unconscious patterns of behavior and of making them know to patient. To the extent that a psychodynamic psychotherapy focuses on the here-and-now experience of the patient rather than on the here-and-now experience of the patient rather than on the reconstruction of past experience, its similarity to cognitive psychotherapy increases. Frequently, the understanding of a defensive pattern used by a patient to handle and ongoing conflict can be the end point of a well conducted psychodynamic psychotherapy. In such a case, the outcomes for cognitive and psychodynamic individual psychotherapy might be quite similar.

With regard to the degree of structure and directiveness, however, the two types of psychotherapy are different. In psychodynamic psychotherapy, the structure of the session is largely determined by the flow of the patient's thoughts and the interaction of these thoughts with the therapist interpretive comments. In contrast, cognitive psychotherapy sessions are structured by an agenda that serves to focus the patient's thought and activities. In psychodynamic psychotherapy, the role of the therapist is limited to that of an empathic interpreter and sharer of the patient's experiences, whereas in cognitive psychotherapy the therapist may direct, prescribe, enjoin, educate, train, or role-play as well. Furthermore, in cognitive psychotherapy more emphasis is placed on directly altering psychopathology rather than on facilitating its alleviation through insight and resolution of inferred underlying conflicts.

IPT is most closely related to the psychodynamic object relations perspective. Understanding internal objects rests on understanding the actual interpersonal relationships of the patient, including his or her relationship with the physician. Both interpersonal and psychodynamic psychotherapy share a focus on identifications and transference, which in IPT is defined as past models for relationships in addition, in IPT particular attention is paid to withdrawal and detachment, areas related to defenses in the psychodynamic model and to faulty cognitions in the cognitive mode. Interpersonal rather than intrapsychic or cognitive events are identified in IPT. This frequently means that the interpersonal psychotherapist's attention is directed toward the same area of disturbance as is the cognitive or psychodynamic psychotherapist's. However, the identified "problem—interpersonal deficits, faulty cognitions, or intrapsychic conflict—is different.

The difference in the interventions used by these psychotherapies are more striking than the differences in their goals or in problems they target for treatment (DeRubeis or et al. 1982). To what extent it is the differences in psychotherapeutic treatment, not the similarities, that produce behavioral change is not clear. Both cognitive and interpersonal psychotherapy use more directive and behavioral interventions than do psychodynamic approaches. IPT and cognitive psychotherapy make more use of teaching new behavioral skills. More than the cognitive and interpersonal treatments, the psychodynamic psychotherapies rely on the patient to activate and practice new behaviors without direction. The briefer psychotherapies (i.e. IPT, cognitive psychotherapy, and brief psychodynamic psychotherapy) lack the extended working-thought and application period of psychoanalysis and of intensive (i.e. long-term psychodynamic psychotherapy).

Table 21: Supportive psychotherapy

Goal	Support of reality testing Provision of ego support Maintenance or re-establishment of use level of functioning
Selection criteria	Very healthy individual faced with overwhelming crises patient with ego deficits
Duration	Days, months, or years–as needed
Techniques	Predictable availability of therapist Use of interpretation to strengthen defenses Maintenance of reality-based working relationship grounded in support, concern and problem solving Suggestion, reinforcement, advice, reality testing, cognitive restructuring, reassurance, limit setting, and environmental interventions Medication Psychodynamic life narrative

Supportive Psychotherapy

The term supportive is generally used to distinguish a type of psychotherapy that is less ambitious, less intensive, and less anxiety-provoking than those designated psychoanalytic, insight-oriented, exploratory, or expressive. Universally, supportive psychotherapy is ranked as the most important type of psychotherapy to learn during residency training (Langsley and Yager 1988), despite its centrally supportive therapy has traditionally been described only vaguely, as residual category of treatment for patients not suitable for other forms of therapy—a modality defined more by what it is not than by what it is. More recently, there has been a growing interest in supportive therapy as a worthy subject in its own, right, and increasing numbers of articles and books have been devoted to describing or studying it (Novalis et al. 1997; Pinsker 1997; Rockland 1989b; Werman 1984).

The concept of supportiveness tends to be defined from diverse, often conflicting theoretical, technical, or practical perspectives, and proposed differences between supportive and other psychoanalytically derived therapies do not necessarily hold true in practice. Twice-weekly psychotherapy, for example, has been labeled "supportive" by authors distinguishing it from psychoanalysis, but "psychoanalytic" by others comparing it with less intensive treatments (Holmes 1995). Techniques theoretically specific to supportive therapy may also be integral to psychoanalysis (De Jonghe et al. 1994; Wallerstein 1986). Outcomes in patients randomly assigned to "supportive" versus "expressive" therapies may be surprisingly similar (Hellerstein et al. 1998).

In current thought, supportiveness is seen as an essential element in all forms of psychotherapy, which differ in degree rather than presence of supportive techniques (Ornstein 1986; Rockland 1993). Supportive psychotherapy may best be viewed as one pole on a continuum of therapies with only relatives differences in goals, indications, theoretical bases, strategies, and techniques (Table 21).

Goals

The goals of psychoanalysis and psychoanalytic psychotherapy encompass so broad an array of intrapsychic, interpersonal, adaptive, behavioral, and symptomatic changes that they cannot be distinguished definitively from those of supportive psychotherapy. However, most authors emphasize amelioration of symptoms, maintenance or restoration of function, improved self-maintenance or restoration of function, improved adaptation to internal and external stresses as the distinctive goals of supportive therapy (Dewald 1994; Freyberger and Freyberger 1994; Holmes 1995; Kernberg 1999; Munich 1997). These stand in contrast to the goals of psychoanalysis and psychoanalytic therapy, which center on reversing underlying pathology and restructuring personality.

This dichotomy is clearest in cases where supportive therapy aims to maintain or restore function. It is uncertain whether long-term improvement in symptoms, self-esteem, or life-functioning can occur without concomitant changes. In ego structure—at least in the absence of a continuing relationship with the therapist an "auxiliary ego". Therefore, whereas separation of patient and therapist (resolution of the transference) is an implicit goal of psychoanalytic therapies, it is less important in supportive therapy, where decreased intensity rather than termination of treatment may be more appropriate in the long-term (Dewald 1994). When the patient in supportive therapy is able to sustain improvement

Table 22: Goals	
Supportive therapy	*Psychoanalytic therapy*
Maintenance of function	Reversal of pathology
Restoration of function	Restructuring of personality
Coping with pathology	Resolution of unconscious conflict
Alleviation	Understanding of symptoms

autonomously, the outcome becomes more similar to that sought by psychoanalytic therapies (Table 22).

Indications

Because there are relatively few data to support the assignment of patients to one or another therapy type personal predilection of the therapist often plays a prominent role in the prescription of supportive versus psychoanalytic psychotherapy. Most often, insight-oriented therapy automatically considered the treatment of first choice and supportive therapy is assigned to those patient who are not considered amenable to change. Some authors, however, have suggested that the two types of treatment should be considered on a more equal basis, because a briefer or less intense treatment may be in many patient's best interest as a treatment of first choice (Pinsker 1997; Rockland 1989b). Furthermore, research has recently demonstrated that supportive therapy, as defined by technique, may be used to attain the same goals as expressive or insight-oriented therapy (Hellerstien et al. 1998). Such considerations become especially relevant as economic pressures force clinicians to prescribe the most efficient among potentially effective treatments.

In common clinical practice, patients at both ends of the health-sickness continuum receive supportive psychotherapy. Those who are generally very psychiatrically healthy and well adapted but who have become impaired in response to stressful life circumstances and those which overwhelming stress or crises-particularly those which include traumas or disasters—may seek help and be a candidate for supportive psychotherapy. The relatively psychiatrically healthy candidate for supportive psychotherapy is a well-adapted individual with good social support and interpersonal relations, flexible defenses, and good reality testing who is experiencing an acute crisis, making use of social supports, not withdrawing, and anticipating resolution of crisis. Although functioning below his or her usual level, this patient remains hopeful about the future and makes use of resources available for problems solving, respite, and growth. This patient uses supportive psychotherapy to reconstitute more rapidly, to avoid errors in judgment by "thinking out loud", to relieve minor symptomatology, and to grow as an individual by learning about the world.

The more typical candidate for supportive psychotherapy has significant deficits in ego functioning the following:

- *Poor reality testing:* These patients show an inability to separate fact from fantasy and to recognize boundaries between self and others. They may become psychotic under stress of psychodynamic psychotherapy and develop psychotic transferences.
- *Poor impulse control:* Such patients need promptly to discharge affects through actions that are often destructive to themselves or others. They are not able to contain and examine feelings as is required by more explorative, insight-oriented psychotherapies.
- *Poor interpersonal relations:* Patients who are unable to form and maintain stable relationships that include reasonable levels of trust and intimacy are limited in their capacity to maintain therapeutic relationships that include reasonable levels for trust and intimacy are limited in their capacity to maintain therapeutic relationships as well, especially those that arouse powerful feelings.
- *Poor balance of affects:* This category includes patients who are overwhelmed by anger or anxiety and those who experience little or no affect of any sort.
- *Lack of ability to sublimate:* These patients are unable to channel energy into creative and socially useful activities, reflecting their low ability to master affects and impulses pleasurably.
- *Low capacity for introspection:* Because self-observation is a necessary step toward the attainment of insight, these patients do poorly in psychotherapies that require self-reflection and curiosity about themselves and their interpersonal relations.
- *Low verbal ability:* Most clinicians do not include high intelligence as a prerequisite for insight-oriented psychotherapy. However, patients for psychodynamic psychotherapies do need to be able to identify and communicate their thoughts and feelings intelligibly to the therapist and to derive relief from doing so.

A variety of other factors have been proposed as exclusion criteria for insight-oriented psychotherapy and as possible indications for supportive psychotherapy (Table 23). Motivation has been stressed by many authors. However, it has yet to be determined whether motivation for symptom change, for behavioral change, for a relationship with the therapist, or for insight (among others) is crucial in assigning patients to explorative/change-oriented versus supportive psychotherapy (Bloch 1979). Alexithymic patients are generally referred for supportive rather than insight psychotherapy. Such patients are characterized by an inability to find words to describe their emotions; they tend to describe-situational details and symptoms rather than feelings (Sifneos 1975). These patients are thought to be prone to psychosomatic illnesses and likely unsuited for insight-oriented psychotherapy (Sifneos 1972, 1972–1973, 1975). However, studies of patients with the traditional psychosomatic illness have found them to be quite variable

Table 23: Characteristics of candidates for supporting psychotherapy
Type I: Patient impaired by overwhelming crisis, trauma, or disaster and functioning below usual level in response to a crisis
Generally very psychiatrically healthy
Well adapted
Good social supports
Good interpersonal relations
Flexible defenses
Good reality testing
Hopeful about future
Uses resources
Type II: Patient has chronic ego deficits and impaired functioning
Impaired with impulse control
Difficult with impulse control
Limited ability to sublimate
Limited interpersonal relations
Frequently high levels of aggression
Limited ability to self-soothe/refuel
Low verbal ability and capacity for introspection

in their response to psychotherapy (Kellner 1975). Patients who are very passive and who lack the conviction that their own efforts are effective may be candidates for supportive rather than insight-oriented psychotherapy (Werman 1981). Some have suggested that a certain level of dependency may be necessary for patients to do well in supportive therapy, and that those with a high need for autonomy are poorly suited for this treatment (Freyberger and Freyberger 1994). Patients who derive substantial practical benefit from their illness, such as financial or emotional support (i.e. secondary gain), may also be appropriate candidates for supportive psychotherapy rather than an insight-oriented approach (Persson and Alstrom 1983). However, severe antisocial traits generally predict poor response to supportive therapy, as they do to insight-oriented therapy.

Ego strength and the ability to form relationship may be more important than diagnosis in the selection of patients for supportive psychotherapy (Warman 1994). Patient with lower ego strength and lower motivation for therapy have been found to be benefit more from supportive techniques than from those specific to exploratory therapy (Horowitz et al. 1984). More attention needs to be paid to which characteristics of the patient may best predict a good response to supportive psychotherapy as opposed to merely a poor response to psychoanalytic psychotherapies. Delineation of the personal qualities needed to benefit from supportive psychotherapy remains an important task for future research.

Theoretical Basis

Psychoanalytic theory is generally viewed as the basis for supportive therapy, although certain aspects are especially emphasized (Werman 1988). Theories of unconscious motivation and defense, internalized objects, and ego psychology inform supportive as well as psychoanalytic therapies (Holmes 1995; Kernberg 1999). However, practice of supportive therapy draw more heavily on the work of Kohut and the British Object Relations School than on Freudian metapsychology (Buckley 1994). Thus, the emphasis is less on conflict resolution, as achieved by analysis of transference, than on establishment of a positive and coherent sense of self, mediated by the relationship between patient and therapist.

From this theoretical perspective, the therapist provides a "holding environment" in which patients feel secure, understood, and valued and a relationship through which they can develop a more realistic, less negatively biased view of themselves and others (Winston et al. 1986). Therapeutic gain stems from the gradual internalization of aspects of the therapist and the therapeutic relationship, which replace internalized 'bad' objects (i.e. critical, punitive, rejecting) to form a stable core of positive identity. From the point of view of attachment theory, the patient forms as secure attachment to the therapist as a necessary precursor to developing increased autonomy.

Theoretical frameworks from outside psychoanalysis have been increasingly used to expand the techniques of supportive therapy. The theory of social constructionism has suggested a strategy of working with patients to derive positive meanings from adverse life experiences (Holmes 1995). Religiously based concepts of mindfulness and self-acceptance have provided the foundation for techniques to support self-destructive patients through change-oriented therapy (Shearin and Lineehan 1994). Cognitive and behavioral theories, with their emphasis on conscious thought, behavioral change, learning, and problem solving, inform many of the techniques of supportive therapy. In general, supportive therapy derives from a broader theoretical base than psychoanalytic theory alone (Table 24).

Strategies

The basic strategy of psychoanalytic therapy is to uncover and resolve unconscious conflicts underlying the difficulties that the patient brings to treatment. This implies understanding the genesis of such conflicts in early relationships and reworking the defensive structure that has evolved to manage them. By contrast the basic strategy of supportive therapy is to map out the patients major area of life difficulty and ameliorate them in whatever way possible rather than to discover causes (Kernberg 1999: Rosenthal et al. 1999).

Central to this strategy is helping the patient to strengthen adaptive defenses, diminish use of maladaptive defenses, and

Table 24: Theoretical emphasis

Supportive therapy	*Psychoanalytic therapy*
Self-psychology	Conflict theory
Ego psychology	Object relations theory
Behavioral psychology	Ego psychology
Cognitive psychology	

Table 25: Strategies

Supportive therapy	*Psychoanalytic therapy*
Fostering of positive transference	Analysis of transference
Containing the unconscious	Revealing the unconscious
Strengthening defenses	Loosening defenses
Regulation of affects	Mobilization of affects
Clarifying the present	Reconstructing the past
Minimizing regression	Facilitating "regression in the service of the ego"

improve the balance of impulse and defense—for example, by avoiding overwhelming stress, reducing excessively harsh self-criticism, or containing overly intense impulses (Dewald 1994; Holmes 1995; Kernberg 1999). This strategy entails a focus on the conscious thoughts and feelings of the patient rather than on the unconscious, and on strengthening rather than losing defenses. Similarly, the attempt is to minimize rather than foster regression, and to help the patient contain rather than mobilize affects.

As in psychoanalytic treatment, the relationship between patient and therapist forms the basis of supportive therapy. However, whereas in the former the relationship serves as a means for clarifying and correcting the patients projections and distortions (i.e. transference), in the latter it provides an object of identification and a source of security and reassurance (Dewald 1994; Pinsker 1994). In psychoanalytic therapy, the neutrality and abstinence of the therapist mobilize anxiety; in supportive therapy, the transparency and spontaneity of the therapist diminish it.

Improved self-esteem may be a goal of both psychoanalytic and supportive therapies, but the strategies for attaining that goal differ. In psychoanalytic treatment, self-esteem is enhanced by fostering the patient's understanding of the unconscious mental content that undermines it. In supportive therapy, self-esteem is enhanced by helping the patient to improve adaptive functioning and minimize emotional discomfort and by fostering the patient's introjection of the therapist's acceptance and positive regard (Table 25).

Techniques

Although supportive therapy is often dismissed as mere "hand holding" or "paid friendship," skillful practice of supportive psychotherapy may actually be more difficult than that of change-oriented psychotherapy because the patient may have less capacity to engage beneficial with a therapist (Wallace 1983). Understanding unconscious motivation, psychic conflict, the patient-therapist relationship, and the patient's use of defense mechanisms is essential to comprehending the patient's strengths and vulnerabilities. This knowledge is critical to providing support as well as insight (Bellak and Siegel 1983; Karen Horney Clinic Medical Board 1981; Rockland 1989a).

The basic stance of the therapist in supportive therapy is quite different from that of the therapist conducting psychoanalytic psychotherapy. Rather than being abstinent and neutral, the therapist is both active and reactive, more readily taking positions, answering questions, giving advice, reassuring, praising, and educating the patient. The therapeutic style tends to be more conversational than that in insight-oriented therapy and less one of silent listening (Pinsker 1994). By his or her activity, judicious sharing of personal factual information, planned use of verbal and nonverbal reinforcement, and willingness to intervene with practical help when necessary, the supportive therapist presents as more of a real person and less of a "blank screen" than the psychoanalytic therapist.

The structure of supportive therapy is less intensive and more flexible than that of psychoanalytic therapy (Stafford-Clark 1970). Typical frequency of meetings ranges from weekly to monthly, and sessions may be brief or full-length. More-frequent meeting may be appropriate in times of crisis, and unscheduled telephone calls may be viewed as central to the treatment rather than as deviations to be understood and interpreted.

A particular technical challenge in supportive treatment is the therapist's need to maintain spontaneity without acting impulsively or out of counter-transference. For example, the therapist must use reinforcement without becoming coercive, give advice or information without presenting as omnipotent (Nurnberg 1984), and respond flexibly to the patient's needs without becoming anxiously protective or overindulgent.

The therapist who is predictably available and safe (i.e. who accepts the patients and puts aside his or her own needs in the service of the treatment) assumes some of the holding functions of the good parent. In such a therapeutic situation, the patient is able to identify with and incorporate the well-functioning aspects of the therapist-such as the capacity for self-observation and the ability to tolerate ambivalence (Adle 1982; Pine 1976). Similary, permitting the patient to see himself or herself mirrored in the therapist as a part of an idealized parental figure over long period may stabilize new internal structure and behaviors. This approach is in contrast to psychoanalytically-oriented psychotherapy, in which such attitudes are generally interpreted rather than accepted.

Patients in supportive psychotherapy frequently develop intensely dependent and ambivalent relationships with the therapist. These relationships often paralleled the separation-individuation on process of normal child development

(Adler 1982). Patients may recapitulate with the therapist the alternating autonomy and approachement experienced with the parent. The therapist's respect for the patient's autonomy and need for "refueling" may be important in strengthening the patient's independence and facilitating return to health. The containment of affect is also an important supportive function (Adler 1982; Kernberg 1975, 1984). Patients in need of supportive psychotherapy typically fear the destructive power of their rage and envy. They may be helped to modulate their emotional reactions by the reliable presence of the therapist and a therapeutic relationship that remains unchanged in the face of emotional onslaughts.

The doctor-patient relationship in supportive psychotherapy does not require the patient to observe and report on his or her own feelings and behavior to the same extent as in the change-oriented, explorative psychotherapies. In addition, the therapist acts more as a guide and a mentor. There is unanimous agreement among writers on supportive psychotherapy that fostering a good working relationship with the patient is the first priority. Studies indicate that in the case of more severely ill patients, this may take many months, in contrast to work with psychiatrically healthier patients, in which the therapeutic alliance tends to develop early or not at all (Docherty 1989; AF Frank and Gunderson 1990).

Many of the active interventions of supportive psychotherapy are based on the principle of "substitutive psychotherapy" (Werman 1994), in which the psychotherapy substitutes for capacities that the patient lacks. This is sometimes stated as the therapist acting as an "auxiliary ego" for the patient. The deficient ego capacities for which substitution is needed may include basic elements of self-perception, such as attainment of a stable sense of self-over time and a clear recognition of boundaries between self and others. Techniques that may support the patient's deficient ego functions include suggestion, reinforcement, clarification, limit setting, environmental interventions, and concurrent use of medication (Dewald 1994; Rockland 1989b; Werman 1984).

Patients may be encouraged to discuss alternative behaviors, goals, and interpretations of events (Castel-nuovo-Tedesco 1986). The therapist tries to reinforce the most adaptive defenses of which the patient is capable while discouraging use of more primitive defenses. To do so effectively, the therapist must judge the capacities of the patient and the degree to which a primitive defense might be necessary for the patient's equilibrium. This judgment is particularly important when assessing the primitive defenses of patients with schizophrenia (Mc Glashan 1982) or limited self-mutilation in those with severe personality pathology (Holmes 1985).

Reassurance takes a variety of forms in supportive psychotherapy, including supporting an adaptive level of denial (such as that employed by a patient in coping with a terminal illness), the patient's experience of the therapist's empathic attitude, or the therapist's empathic attitude, or the therapist's reality testing of the patient's negatively biased evaluations (Werman 1984). Reassuring a patient is not easy (Pette 1982). Reassurance requires a clear understanding of what the patient fears. Overt expression of interest and concern may be reassuring to a patient who fears rejection but threatening to one who fears intrusion. In a similar vein, Rockland (1989a, 1989b) stressed the need to tailor interventions to fit the character traits and unconscious transference of the patient. Thus, the therapist may stress independence in the case of a patient who fears passivity or loss of control and may give advice and direction to a clinging, dependent patient. Intellectualize language may be more effective with obsessional patients and emotionally toned language with histrionic patients.

Communication of the therapist's knowledge of the patient and his or her circumstances is a pedagogical aspect of supportive psychotherapy (Werman 1981). The therapist uses simple, concrete language that has personal meaning of the patient. The therapist may discuss with the highly inhibited patient the advantages of being more assertive or spontaneous, or may point out to the patient with poorly developed social controls the dangers of impulsive behavior. In this manner, the therapist function as as auxiliary superego. In both the very constricted patient and the very impulsive patient, the therapist's recognition and accurate naming of the patient's affects may aid the patient in recognized and differentiating emotional stages, a necessary prerequisite to tolerating and modulating affect (Pine 1976).

Intellectualized interpretations may also be useful in discussing dreams in supportive psychotherapy (Werman 1978). In addition, these interpretations may foster and increased capacity for self-obsevation (Ermutlu 1977). A technique that has been used for the latter purpose consists of suggesting that pathological behavior is the product of a "sick part" of the patient that is distinct from the patient as a whole. This "induced dichotomy of personality" helps the patient recognize both pathological behaviors and the better-functioning aspects of himself or herself and fosters the patient's identification with the more mature, adoptive traits.

The suitability of an interpretation may depend more on the manner in which it is given than on its content (Pine 1986). In supportive psychotherapy, interpretations are phrased to relieve the patient of the pressure to make an immediate response. The therapist tries to communicate that although the interpretation may be painful, he or she will stick by the patient thought the patient's discomfort. Interpretations can best be made at times of low emotional intensity. The patient can also be given advance warning that a potentially painful comment is going to be made. Such techniques are directed toward sufficiently modulating the patient's emotional response so that the interpretation can be tolerated and processed.

Supportive psychotherapy with special patient populations may require special techniques. Rates and Rockland (1994) described supportive therapy with schizophrenic patients as occurring in three phases; stabilization, maintenance, and working through/termination. Although applying techniques common to most supportive therapies, they particularly stressed the need for a collaborative (versus an authoritarian) patient-therapist relationship, in which goal and parameters of treatment are negotiated bilaterally. Use of the therapeutic interaction as a means of reality testing is also especially important in work with schizophrenic patients.

With somatizing patients who may habitually express feelings through physical symptoms, the first step may be to get the patient talking about him—or herself, while supplying information and advice relevant to the problem (Freyberger and Freyberger 1994). As the therapeutic alliance develops, the patient is encouraged to express more feelings in recounting his or her life story to the therapist. This supportive phase of treatment may prepare some patients to understand emotional cause and effect in their lives and help them begin to appreciate the workings of unconscious process.

Supportive therapy with medically ill patients may entail providing the patient with a safe place to ventilate anger and grief over illness-related loss and disability (Freyberger and Freyberger 1994). A specific therapeutic tasks is to help the patient maintain optimism and a problem-solving approach and avoid becoming entirely preoccupied with illness. Assisting patients in modulating their expressions of anger and dependency may be crucial in maintaining their interpersonal support networks.

Efficacy

Relative few studies have assessed the efficacy of supportive therapy. Most data come from studies in which supportive psychotherapy was used as a control in testing the efficacy of other treatments (Conte and Plutchik 1986). In such studies, the procedures used in supportive psychotherapy tend to be poorly specified, and no attempts are made to correlate individual supportive techniques with outcome (Conte 1994). There are no studies in which supportive psychotherapy has been compared with no treatment or minimal treatment.

Despite its limitations, the research literature offers some evidence that supportive psychotherapy is an effective treatment. The Menninger Psychotherapy project assessed long-term (i.e. up to 10 years) explorative and supportive psychotherapy in a group of patients with mixed symptomatic and personality pathology (Wallerstein 1986). A major result of the study was that psychoanalytic therapy was less effective, and supportive therapy was more effective, then expected. In general, the techniques of supportive therapy produced improvement in functioning and ego strength comparable to those of expressive and insight-oriented techniques. This result is consistent with the idea that sophisticated support itself promotes structural change in some patients.

More recently, this result was conformed in a group of patients with, Axis II Cluster C disorders who were treated with either supportive or confrontational dynamic psychotherapy (Hellerstein et al. 1998). Outcomes were comparable in the two groups. At 6 months, the patients who received supportive therapy remained improved in interpersonal functioning, especially in increased assertiveness (Rosesenthal et al. 1999). The cases of supportive therapy patients who experienced good outcomes were characterized by highly positive therapeutic alliances throughout treatment, a finding that confirms the importance of the patient-therapist relationship in this type of treatment.

Studies of patients with anxiety disorders have also demonstrated the efficacy of supportive therapy. The effects of imipramine therapy plus behavior therapy have been compared with those of imipramine therapy plus supportive psychotherapy in a group of patients with agoraphobia, mixed phobia, or simple phobia (Kleina et al. 1983; Zitrin et al. 1978). The expected benefit of adding behavioral techniques to supporting psychotherapy was not found; patients in both groups fared equally well. Similar results were reported by Alstronm et al. (1984a, 1984b), who found that psychodynamically-oriented supportive psychotherapy was as effective as behavior therapy in the treatment of patients with agroaphobial and social phobia. These results may indicate that the active ingredient in both supportive psychotherapy and behavioral treatments is the encouragement of the patient to expose him—or herself to the feared situation (Klein et al. 1983). A study of supportive psychotherapy in combination with antidepressants has also shown the combined-treatment -group to do best (De Jonghe et al. 2001).

Research in the psychotherapy of schizophrenia has failed to demonstrate the benefit of explorative, expressive techniques (Gomes-Schwartz 1984). By contrast, the use of supportive techniques appears more promising (Hogarty et al. 1974; Munich 1997). May (1968) found the inpatients with nonchronic schizophrenia had somewhat better outcomes when treated with supportive psychotherapy and antipsychotic medication than when treated with medication alone. When these approaches were used singly, however, medication was more effective than psychotherapy. A later study compared medication plus explorative, insight-oriented psychotherapy with reality—adaptive supportive psychotherapy in patients with schizophrenia (Gunderson et al. 1984; Stanton et al. 1984). Patients receiving supportive therapy spent less time in the hospital and performed better in major life roles than did patients receiving insight therapy, a finding seemingly at variance with the lower intensity and cost of supportive treatment.

A large body of research exist indicating that supportive psychotherapy is an effective component of treatment for patients with a variety of medical illnesses. Karush et al. (1969) reported that ulcerative colitis patients with high dependency and low ego strength improved both somatically and emotionally after supportive psychotherapy, but not after insight-oriented treatment. The best results were found in cases in which the therapist was viewed as warm, understanding, and optimistic and a positive working relationship was formed. Forester et al. (1985) assessed the effects of supportive psychotherapy on patients undergoing radiation treatment. The psychotherapy, which consisted of educational clarification of emotional issues and ventilation of feelings, resulted in less emotional distress and fewer complaints of side effects in treated patients compared with those in the control group, who received no psychotherapy. Mumford et al. (1982) reviewed controlled studies of psychotherapy treatment of patients recovering from myocardial infarction and surgery and found positive effects on experience of pain, cooperation with treatment, incidence of complications, speed of recovery, and number of days in the hospital. The psychotherapies focused on educating the patients about their illnesses and treatments, but also included varying amounts of cognitive and behavioral techniques, ventilation, and reassurance in the context of a supportive relationship. Schindler et al. (1989) demonstrated that supportive therapy reduced medical complications, use of pain medication and length of hospital stay in patients undergoing coronary artery bypass surgery, studies of patients with gastrointestinal disease suggest that those who receive supportive therapy fare better and maintain their improvement compared with those receiving medical treatment alone (Conte 1994; Freyberger and Freyberger 1994). A dramatic study by Spiegel et al. (1989) showed that women with metastatic breast cancer who received supportive group therapy had less depression, anxiety, and pain and survived 19 months longer than control patients.

The evidence to date, although preliminary, suggest that supportive psychotherapy can be effective in both psychiatric and medical illnesses and may be more cost effective than more intense psychotherapies. More research is needed regarding the indications, contraindications, and techniques of supportive psychotherapy.

Education

The importance of individual psychotherapy to the practicing clinician make mandatory the inclusion of instruction on psychotherapy in psychiatric residency training. The skill learned in psychotherapy-both the ability to intervene and the ability to recognize transference, countertransference, and defense—are important in many other treatment modalities. The clinician skilled in recognizing these phenomenon is better able to perform a wide array of treatments, including medication management, family therapy, inpatient psychiatric treatment, and consultation-liaison.

The fundamental skills of establishing the therapeutic alliance, understanding the relationship of transference to anxiety and regression, and providing support are central to psychiatric care. Learning psychodynamic psychotherapy provides the opportunity to work with a specific treatment modality as well as to become skilled in a wide array of areas central to clinical care. Learning long-term psychodynamic psychotherapy is not the equivalent of learning the brief psychotherapies or supportive psychotherapy (Levenson and Strupp 1999; Vaughan et al. 2000), however, it may be true that the long-term psychotherapist is best prepared for using the briefer psychotherapy, in which there are fewer opportunities to make mistakes and to correct them. In this era of managed care, it is even more likely that the psychiatrist will be called on to supervise others conducting psychotherapy. For this reasons also, skills in psychotherapy are necessary.

Psychiatric residents must develop skills to apply all psychotherapeutic treatment modalities and to understand their indications and contraindications. Psychoanalysis, with its extended intensive training requirements, is essentially a subspecialty area and is now generally pursued postresidency. It offers the opportunity for specific patients to gain broad-based understanding in a generally supportive environment. Supportive psychotherapy, the mainstay of psychiatric treatment, is much more complicated than is often recognized. The understanding of which patient for which treatment at which time is as critical for the prescription of psychotherapy as it is for the prescription of psychopharmacological agents (Frances et al. 1984). Given the decrease in the number of psychoanalysts in medical school education, learning the indication for referral for psychoanalysis may be increasingly difficult for future psychiatrists.

The brief psychotherapies are best taught in conjunction with the discussion of the principles of long-term psychotherapy and in the context of learning psychodynamic formulations of pathology and the ways in which defenses, transferences, and counter-transferences appear in the psychotherapeutic dyad. The resident can then begin to learn the unique constraints and advantages that accrue within a brief period as well as the unique advantages of long-term psychotherapeutic work. The resident must also learn the advantages and disadvantages of intermittent psychotherapy and sequential psychotherapy with continued medication treatment. Though contrasting the psychotherapies, the trainee learns appropriate patient selection and technical procedures to accomplish psychotherapy. Such training requires both familiarity with the psychotherapy literature and supervise clinical experiences in the various psychotherapies. All physicians should be versed in brief supportive psychotherapy as a technique distinct from pure 'Counseling' and education.

The evaluation of the patient is an important part of initiating any psychotherapy. Seeing psychotherapy as a modality that must be prescribed in duration, focus, and intensity and with a plan similar to pharmacological treatment of a patient enhances the resident's sense of mastery, accomplishment, and competence in dealing psychotherapeutically with a broad range of patients (Luborsky and Auerbach 1985).

CONCLUSION

Individual psychoanalytically-oriented and supportive psychotherapies are an effective treatment for a wide range of symptoms and disorders. These treatment modalities require accurate diagnosis, treatment planning, and consistent application of principles and technique. Various types of psychotherapy are now well described. Further research is needed to identify which psychotherapy is most effective for which patient. The identification of specific type of change associated with different psychotherapies may aid this process.

The psychoanalytic treatment-psychoanalysis and psychoanalytic psychotherapy now span the range of approaches from brief to long-term and focal to broad based (Kernberg 1999). Interpersonal psychotherapy has primarily been used in research, both highlighted in this form of therapy is the importance of focusing on the social relationships as an aspect of understanding the psychoanalytic components of personality and mind-brain interaction. Interpersonal psychotherapy, cognitive psychotherapy, and supportive psychotherapy have more of an empirical research base than do the more specific psychoanalytic treatments. Research studies with more rigorous designs and conducted over longer periods are needed. Supportive psychotherapy, probably the most widely practiced of the psychotherapies, continues to be lacking in specific research. Better delineation of the specific technique in supportive psychotherapy will aid this development.

Clinicians require training in each of the psychotherapy modalities and in their application in stand-alone treatment plans and used intermittently or in combination of sequence with medication. Such training will enable them to better recognize the relationship of the psychotherapies to each other and the potential therapeutic benefits and costs associated with each.

47.10 INTERPERSONAL PSYCHOTHERAPY

JN Vyas

Interpersonal psychotherapy (IPT) is a time-limited, interpersonally focused, psychodynamically informed psychotherapy that has the goals of symptom relief and improving interpersonal functioning. IPT is concerned with the *'interpersonal context'*—the relational factors that predispose, precipitate and perpetuate the patient's distress. Within IPT interpersonal relationships are the focus of therapeutic attention as the means to bring about change, with the aim of helping patients to improve their interpersonal relationships or change their expectations about them. In addition, the treatment also aims to assist patients to improve their social support network so that they can better manage their current interpersonal distress (Stuart and Robertson, 2003).

HISTORY AND EVOLUTION OF INTERPERSONAL PSYCHOTHERAPY (IPT)

From the late 1970's American psychiatry turned its focus to evidence-based medicine, in particular the randomized control trial. The traditional clinical view was that most interventions seemed to work for depression. With the advent of antidepressant medications, and their apparent effectiveness in treating depression, it was necessary to compare these with the established psychological therapies. The timeframe for the therapy 'control' treatment was determined by the research design, rather than being drawn from any evidence base. As such, the traditional assumption that IPT was of 16 weeks duration was based upon academic considerations, not clinical ones. In order to standardize what seemed to comprise the elements of good psychotherapy, researchers led by Gerald Klerman devised a treatment that integrated what was thought to be the essence of medical psychotherapy and constructed a treatment program that would fit neatly within a treatment trial. Klerman and colleagues believed that, given depression invariably had an impact on communication and interpersonal interactions, as well as consequences for the patient's marriage, family, work and community activities, this was a worthy focus for psychotherapeutic intervention. The development of IPT therefore did not follow the conventional path of a theory leading to practice. However, several theories are considered influential in the development of IPT including the attachment theory of Bowlby and his successors, and communication theory (Stuart and Robertson, 2003). Whilst IPT made no assumptions about etiology of depression, the social risk factors for depression as identified by Brown and Harris (1978), Paykel, Weissman and Prusoff (1978), and Henderson (1988) also influenced the development of the approach. IPT first appeared as the control treatment for studies investigating the efficacy of antidepressant medications (Klerman, Weissman, Rounsaville and Chevron, 1984). Like many serendipitous findings in science, IPT was found to be of comparable efficacy to medication in these studies and earned itself a place alongside Aaron Beck's cognitive behavior therapy (CBT) as a credible candidate for investigation as an active treatment. For many years IPT remained little known outside academic circles in the USA and Europe, unlike CBT. In the late 1990's, there was an increased interest in IPT amongst clinicians. This culminated in the formation of the International Society for IPT (ISIPT) in 2000. Since that time, dissemination of IPT has increased momentum within some mental health circles. The recent inclusion of IPT in the focused psychological strategies for the Medicare funded Better Outcomes in Mental Health and Better Access to Mental Health programs has resulted in increased exposure for and interest in IPT across Australia. The structure of IPT. There are five distinct phases in the IPT approach; assessment, the initial sessions, middle sessions, termination sessions or conclusion of acute treatment, and maintenance sessions. In the assessment phase, the therapist completes a standard clinical interview and determines the suitability of IPT for the patient. If the patient is suitable the therapist proceeds through the initial sessions of IPT including socializing the patient to IPT, which is referred to as 'creating the IPT focus', completing an interpersonal inventory, developing an interpersonal formulation and contracting the patient to a specific number of sessions. In the middle sessions, the therapist and patient address the relevant problem areas (ideally one but can be more more) using key IPT techniques. During the termination phase, or what is often referred to as the conclusion of acute treatment phase, the therapist and patient review progress in the problem areas and plan for future problems.

Maintenance sessions can be conducted to prevent relapse or to work through any remaining problems, but only after a new contract is negotiated. The focus should remain on interpersonal issues and the short to midterm nature of IPT should be kept in mind. Each of these stages is now explained in more detail.

Initial Assessment for IPT Suitability

The 'assessment phase' of IPT determines whether the patient is a suitable candidate for IPT. Nonspecific issues are considered such as suitability for any psychological intervention, motivation for change, ego strength, adequacy on nonpsychological treatments, and so forth that the following characteristics can increase the likelihood that patients will benefit from IPT:

- A relatively secure attachment style
- The ability to relate a coherent narrative of their interpersonal network and specific interpersonal interactions; a specific interpersonal focus for distress
- A good social support system.

Perhaps the most critical judgment is whether the IPT intervention resonates with the patient's view of their psychological distress. The assessment phase ends with a treatment contract with the patient to proceed with a specific number of IPT sessions and to work on one or more specific interpersonal problems.

Initial Sessions

The initial sessions of IPT include a number of specific tasks. The primary goals are to develop an interpersonal formulation, which is a detailed hypothesis about why the patient is having interpersonal difficulties, and to gauge the patient's social support in general. The interpersonal formulation is a modification of Engel's Biopsychosocial model, integrating the four IPT problem areas. Intrinsic to this process is the development of an *interpersonal inventory* (IPI). The IPI functions as the main structural component of this process with a specific focus of the patient and therapist on:

- Current relationships
- The history of the patient's current problems as applied to that relationship
- Information that is relevant to the process of resolving the problem area, for example attachment style, communication style, and patterns of interaction
- Setting appropriate treatment goals. With the completion of the interpersonal inventory, an interpersonal focus is formulated using the four IPT problem areas.

Middle Sessions

In the middle sessions of IPT the therapist and patient address one or more of the four IPT problem areas using key IPT techniques. Whilst working on these issues the therapist is mindful of the patient's attachment style and communication style. In general, after identifying specific problems during the assessment and initial phases, the therapist gathers more information about the specific problem area(s). Both patient and therapist then work to develop solutions to the problem, such as improving the patient's communication skills or modifying his or her expectations about a dispute. A suitable solution is selected, and the patient attempts to implement it between sessions. In subsequent sessions the patient and therapist work to refine the solution(s) and implement these accordingly. The four problem areas and a number of key IPT techniques are outlined later.

Concluding Acute Treatment and Maintenance Treatment

Rather than using the traditional psychoanalytic model in which 'termination' is a severing of the therapeutic relationship, in IPT, the provision of acute treatment comes to an end as specified by the therapeutic contract. This does not necessarily signify the end of the therapeutic relationship. It is often agreed that the patient and therapist will have further therapeutic contacts via a new negotiated contract. The specific goals at the conclusion of treatment are to foster the patient's independent functioning and to enhance his or her sense of competence. Ideally, IPT teaches patients new communication skills, helps them to develop insight into how they communicate their needs, and helps them to establish more functional social support networks, all in the service of improving interpersonal functioning. The therapist should review the progress made in therapy, and give as much positive feedback to the patient as is genuinely possible. A review of the problems identified in the interpersonal inventory and progress in dealing with these, as well as reviewing associated symptomatic improvement should be conducted. A summary of the positive changes that the patient has made in improving his or her communication and in developing an improved social support network should also be undertaken. Credit for change should be ascribed primarily to the patient. Although the therapist has served as a 'coach,' the patient has done the difficult work and has implemented the changes discussed.

The IPT should be conceptualized as a two-phase treatment, in which a more intense acute phase of treatment focuses on resolution of immediate symptoms, and a subsequent maintenance phase follows with the goal of preventing relapse and maintaining productive interpersonal functioning. In addition to being supported by theory, research, and experience, this model also fits well with current clinical best practice. In clinical practice, IPT can be seen to follow a family practice or general practitioner model of care, in which short-term treatment for an acute problem or stressor is provided until the problem is resolved. Once resolved the therapeutic relationship is not terminated. As with a general practitioner, the therapist makes him or herself available to the patient should another crisis occur, at which time another time-limited course of treatment is undertaken. In the interim, the therapist may want, in the same fashion as the general practitioner, to provide periodic maintenance sessions.

The conclusion of acute treatment is a mutually negotiated and agreed ending of intense intervention. This includes a review of the patient's progress in resolving the interpersonal problems first identified in the interpersonal inventory, planning for future problems that may arise in the problem area, and anticipating the emergence of new interpersonal problems. The patient's responses to the end of acute treatment should be discussed in order to prevent the potential of symptom intensification, and to emphasize to the patient that the therapeutic relationship has been a successful experience for the patient. A new contract for maintenance sessions should be negotiated if indicated and if both parties are able to continue. When a patient's symptoms are recurrent or unresolved, maintenance sessions can be contracted, usually at a less frequent interval to monitor interpersonal problems and further develop interpersonal skills as required. This must be a structured and predetermined course of treatment, similar to how the initial phase of treatment was structured. The IPT problem areas within the four problem areas, interpersonal processes are made more understandable for the patient. The four IPT problem areas are:

- *Grief*
- *Interpersonal disputes* (role disputes)
- *Role transitions*
- *Interpersonal sensitivity* (Interpersonal deficits).

Psychosocial stressors from any of the problem areas can lead to psychological distress or psychiatric syndromes, in particular when combined with an attachment disruption in the context of a poor social support network.

Interpersonal Disputes

Interpersonal disputes (initially known as *role disputes*) should be selected as a problem area when overt or covert disputes are contributing to the patient's problems or illness. Disputes are often covert as patients fail to mention disputes that are too painful, or they think are unsolvable such as many disputes within families. As a consequence, these covert disputes may only become obvious during a thorough assessment. Examples of disputes according to Stuart and Robertson (2003) include the following:

- *Overtly hostile conflict*, e.g. domestic violence, verbal abuse
- *Betrayals*, e.g. infidelity, impropriety, conflicting loyalties within a family
- *Disappointment*, e.g. unmet expectations at work or school
- *Inhibited conflicts*, e.g. anger at a partner's illness or disability.

Attachment theory speculates that disruptions in an individual's intimate attachments, such as those caused by interpersonal disputes, make vulnerable individuals more likely to suffer psychological distress. (Stuart and Robertson, 2003). Most minor disagreements are usually resolved by individuals over time and do not constitute significant stressors in their lives. Interpersonal disputes are of clinical significance when their resolution is beyond the patient. Interpersonal disputes can present as acutely distressing, smoldering and persistent or as a relationship in dissolution. Ultimately, IPT intervenes in disputes by assisting the patient to revisit the process of resolving the dispute or helping the patient move towards an acceptable dissolution of the relationship.

In order for this process to occur, the therapist must understand the 'state of play' in the dispute. In IPT this is achieved by staging the dispute. Disputes are identified as one of three stages: *negotiation* where there are ongoing attempts by both parties to bring about change; *impasse* which implies that the attempts at resolving the dispute have stalled and communication efforts to resolve the dispute and associated affect are less likely to be occurring; and *dissolution* when the process is at such an advanced stage that the goal of interventions in IPT is to help the patient move on from the relationship, and undergo a role transition

(Stuart and Robertson, 2003). Intervention in interpersonal disputes in IPT involves enhancement of communication of attachment needs and problem solving styles, and modifying expectations on the part of the patient.

Role Transitions

Adaptation to change is at the core of adaptation to life. All interpersonal relations occur in a complex psychosocial setting and individuals experience these relationships consistently within that setting. Though some transitions, such as loss of health may be seen as wholly negative by the patient, most change involves elements that are perceived as good and bad. In IPT, role transitions are assumed to be a focus of treatment when the patient develops psychological distress in the context of change. Invariably, the change is experienced as a loss. Like interpersonal disputes, role transitions are varied in their nature. Examples according to Stuart and Robertson (2003: 184) include:

- *Situational role transitions*, e.g. job loss, promotion, graduation, migration
- *Relationship role transitions*, e.g. marriage, divorce, step-parenthood
- *Illness related role transition*, e.g. diagnosis of chronic illness, adaptation to pain or physical limitations
- *Post-event role transition*, e.g. post-traumatic symptoms, refugee status. Interventions in role transitions aspire to help the patient to:
  - Define the old role and new role in a balanced and realistic way that is more acceptable to the patient.
  - Accept the emotional component of the loss of the 'old role' and the perceived challenges of the 'new role'.
  - Develop and implement skills and attitudes that overcome the perceived challenges of the 'new role'.

Grief

At some stage in the life cycle we all experience grief and loss. This process can be complicated by a variety of factors that necessitate grief-oriented therapy to navigate a path toward completion of the process. Many authors have theorized about the intrapsychic processes that mediate an individual's progress through grief and loss, and many share a view that the human being who suffers loss progresses through a myriad of emotional responses including sadness, despair, anger, and anxiety, and ultimately progresses to initiate new interests and relationships to replace the relationship that has been lost (Stuart and Robertson, 2003). In IPT, grief is considered to be relevant as a complicated bereavement. The basic tasks of working with grief in IPT according to Stuart and Robertson (2003) are:

- Diagnosing grief as a problem area
- Clarification of the circumstances of the loss
- Linking the timing of the loss to the onset of symptoms
- Helping the patient accept painful affect associated with the loss
- Helping the patient communicate the loss to others
- Recreating the relationship with the deceased
- Helping the patient utilize existing social supports and develop new attachments.

Interpersonal Deficits/Sensitivity

The IPT problem area of interpersonal sensitivity relates to a difficulty in forming and maintaining relationships that often results in loneliness and social isolation. The consequent impoverished social support network leads to interpersonal problems, and often psychiatric problems such as depression due to attachment needs not being met. This is particularly likely if a social stressor occurs such as a transition or death. Attempts at improving one's social supports are often frustrated by poor communication and relationship skills. In the original descriptions of IPT, the term interpersonal 'deficits' was used (Klerman et al. 1984). Deficits can be seen as pejorative term and therefore the term 'sensitivity' has been suggested as an alternative by Stuart and Robertson (2003). Interpersonal sensitivity is manifested in many ways. This includes patients who report having few friends, and repeated relationship failures or conflict with others. Patient behavior during sessions is also a clinical marker of sensitivity including passivity and hostility toward the therapist. A difficulty in forming a relationship with the therapist may also indicate interpersonal sensitivity. Whilst the true nature of interpersonal sensitivity is a pervasive process ingrained in the patient, IPT seeks to intervene by helping the patient resolve a current interpersonal stressor. The scope of possible intervention in a structured and focal treatment in the process is most effective if it is limited to an acute or current problem. By nature, the patient with interpersonal sensitivity will have known no different in their life experience. On this basis, attempts to elaborate and alter a complex problem in such a focus may serve to further reinforce the patient's pervasive sense of failure in relationships. A focus on the manifestations of interpersonal sensitivity in a current interpersonal problem in the 'here-and-now', will enable the patient and therapist to crystallize the patient's interpersonal difficulties in an accessible and meaningful way.

The IPT helps reduce the patient's isolation and assist in their expansion of social repertoire via the following interventions according to Stuart and Robertson (2003: 216):

- Optimizing the patient's current relationship functioning
- Helping the patient establish new supportive relationships
- Resolving the patient's acute interpersonal stressor.

The process involves the therapist in a review of old relationships, current relationships and the relationship with the therapist to obtain a better understanding of relationship patterns that assist and impede the formation and maintenance of relationships.

The therapist aims to optimize the functioning of current relationships through assisting the client to reconnect with old relationships and form new relationships. The therapy relationship can serve as a modeling experience for the patient who proceeds through the stages of forming and maintaining a relationship, and then managing the evolution and termination of the relationship with the therapist. At a fundamental level this relationship acts as a secure base for the patient to form and maintain other relationships.

INTERPERSONAL PSYCHOTHERAPY (IPT) TECHNIQUES

The IPT therapists should be proficient in basic micro-counseling and psychotherapy skills. Additionally, there are a number of specific techniques that are central to the success of IPT, although not unique to IPT. This includes nondirective and directive exploration, clarification, encouragement of affect, communication analysis, role play, problem solving (or decision analysis), and the therapeutic relationship (Stuart and Robertson, 2003). Three key techniques are briefly outlined below.

The Therapeutic Relationship

In IPT the establishment of a productive therapeutic alliance is more important than any technique. A basic tenet of IPT is that all interventions should be therapeutic and should enhance the alliance. Of course, the IPT therapist needs to draw boundaries when necessary and to be active and directive as required, as it is a structured therapy. There is effectively a balance between activity and active listening (Weissman et al. 2007). Furthermore, the therapeutic relationship is not viewed in terms of transference in that difficulties within the therapeutic relationship are addressed in the here and now in terms of the clients' wider interpersonal network, rather than being about a past relationship. For example, if a client is angry about the therapist running late, the client is encouraged to express this in a way that enhances their existing interpersonal skills, and there is an exploration of how the anger and its expression may affect relationships within their wider interpersonal network.

The therapeutic relationship can be used in IPT as a means to gather information, and as a means of attending to the patient's attachment needs and helping them to experience a successful relationship. The therapist can use the relationship indirectly as a means to bring about therapeutic change, for example modeling different communication patterns. Most importantly, the therapeutic relationship provides the safe background against which change may occur.

Encouragement of Affect

This technique is used to help patients express, understand and manage affect (Weissman et al. 2007). According to Stuart and Robertson (2003, 125) there are several goals regarding the use of affect in IPT:

- To assist the patient to recognize his or her immediate affect
- To assist the patient to communicate his or her affect more effectively to others
- To facilitate the patient's recognition of affect that may have been suppressed, or that the patient may find painful to acknowledge.

Of particular importance is the therapist's attention to and facilitation of *'process affect'*—affect displayed during the conduct of therapy—as opposed to *'content affect'*—affect about past events or interactions outside of the therapeutic relationship (Stuart and Robertson, 2003). This can serve to increase the patient's awareness of feelings they may be unaware of such as anger or guilt. The therapist also encourages patients to express a range of feelings during sessions and explores with them how these feelings can be expressed safely outside of sessions to resolve disputes and enhance their interpersonal network.

Communication Analysis

Disordered communication is hypothesized to be a primary reason for interpersonal problems. In particular, the therapist is attuned to ambiguous and indirect verbal and nonverbal communication that could be changed to more direct, less ambiguous verbal communication (Weissman et al. 2007). Recent incidents and past incidents of note are explored in some detail to detect these difficulties and to explore alternate and more effective ways of communicating. The detail is required to offset what are often biased accounts by patients who typically put the blame on the other party, or in more self-deprecating patients who put excessive blame on themself. Sources of information also include in-session communication with the therapist and collateral information from other sources. Communication analysis often leads on to other techniques such as problem solving and role-play. In terms of change the therapist may also serve as a role model for communication. The overall goals of communication analysis according to Stuart and Robertson (2003) are:

- Identify communication patterns and responses elicited from others
- Identify the client's contribution to communication problems
- Motivate the client to communicate more effectively
- Learn new and more effective skills.

IPT Treatment Intervention

Following an initial assessment including a standard clinical interview, for instance, Brendan was diagnosed with a major depressive disorder, in partial remission. Various treatment options were considered and IPT was chosen primarily because of the evidence base for depression and the interpersonal context for his presenting problems, i.e. the difficulties with the supervisor, death of his mother, and impoverished social network. These are conceptualized within IPT as an interpersonal dispute, grief, and interpersonal sensitivity respectively. During the initial sessions an interpersonal inventory was completed including obtaining further information about key relationships with his parents, brother, best friends, and past friendships including girlfriends. The therapist was of the opinion that his attachment style was *'insecure avoidant'*. He was contracted for an initial set of 12 sessions with the initial seven sessions being weekly, and then tapered to fortnightly for the next three sessions and the last two sessions being monthly. A formulation regarding his symptoms and contributing factors was presented at the initial session that served to 'create the IPT focus.' He was informed that the sessions would address the three problem areas relevant for him, and the focus would not be on symptoms specifically or on major points of intervention in other therapies such as cognition or the unconscious. The role of patient and therapist were also discussed.

Therapy then progressed into the middle sessions where the three problem areas were addressed directly whilst the therapist was mindful of Brendan's insecure attachment style, and that he was quite introverted. The decision to address the dispute with his supervisor first was made collaboratively based on the immediacy of the dispute. The therapist also believed that Brendan would need time to feel comfortable with therapy and the therapeutic relationship before he could address the more emotive issue of the death of his mother. Each session began with a check in with the aim of linking his mood with interpersonal events. During the middle sessions the therapist elicited affect from Brendan as required, whilst also attending to the therapeutic relationship. A core goal of IPT is to generate solutions to the problem areas and, with this in mind, solutions were generated on how to address his supervisor's behavior. This involved assisting him to communicate his needs to the supervisor, but only once his expectations of the supervisor and the potential solutions were reviewed. The review indicated that his supervisor's behavior was not personal to Brendan. This was elicited via the technique of communication analysis. Nevertheless Brendan wanted to be more assertive with his supervisor. The therapist and Brendan brainstormed ways of doing this and practiced what to say and different scenarios using the technique of role-play. Once the dispute was addressed the therapy then progressed to the problem area of grief.

The link between the development of his depressive symptoms and the ill health and death of his mother was made explicit. He was asked to describe the sequence of events related to her illness and death. He was then encouraged to 'recreate' his relationship with his mother. The full spectrum of process affect was elicited, not just acceptable affect such as sadness. In particular, he expressed anger and guilt regarding her death, two emotions he had not acknowledged before. Therapy then proceeded to utilize new and existing social supports and develop new interests to improve his interpersonal functioning and life in general. This dovetailed well into the problem area of sensitivity. Brendan wanted to develop new confidantes and he therefore sought to develop a stronger relationship with a maternal aunt and a family friend. He also started socializing more with some of the quieter men from work and joined a weekly pool tournament at a local tavern. Whilst he was anxious and distant at first he was starting to relax more at these events. There were girls involved and he was also starting to talk to them more often. He felt confident that many of the girls had similar interests to him. He also 'made friends' with his best friend's girlfriend so he wasn't alienated from his best friend's life. Brendan acknowledged that he was unlikely to attempt these activities without the knowledge that he could count on the therapist for support and guidance. The therapist considered this to be analogous to the 'secure base' function of the patient therapist relationship.

Once the problem areas were addressed effectively, the therapy proceeded into the termination sessions. This included traditional termination interventions such as relapse prevention, as well as planning for future interpersonal issues that arose, and recognizing the interpersonal competencies that Brendan had established. The opportunity to discuss feelings about the termination of sessions was provided to prevent symptom intensification or other maladaptive forms of communicating concerns or discomfort with regard to termination. Brendan advised that he would miss the sessions as he enjoyed having someone to talk to openly, but he felt ready to put more emphasis on his new and developing relationships. He was advised that maintenance sessions were available should he relapse.

IPT Research

Although IPT was developed in the 1970s, it came to prominence in the *National Institute of Mental Health Treatment of Depression Collaborative Research Program* (Elkin et al. 1989). This was a multi-center study of over 250 depressed adults who were assigned randomly to one of four treatments: IPT, cognitive-behavioral therapy, imipramine, and placebo ('clinical management'). Amongst more severely depressed patients, IPT was comparable to imipramine on several outcome measures, and had a mean outcome better than placebo. Subsequent re-analysis of the data also concluded that IPT was superior to placebo, and superior to CBT for the severely depressed group. Two subsequent studies have reinforced the efficacy of IPT for major depression, although the most recent study has suggested that CBT was superior to IPT for severe depression (Luty et al. 2007). This study also suggested that patients with anxious and avoidant personalities perform better with CBT than IPT (Joyce et al. 2007). Since the NIMH study, IPT has been adapted for the treatment of a range of conditions and the evidence base has continued to develop. IPT has demonstrated efficacy for bulimia nervosa (Fairburn et al. 1991), group therapy application (Wilfley et al. 2002), as a maintenance treatment for depression in old age (Reynolds et al. 1999), and as a maintenance treatment for recurrent major depression (Frank 1991; Frank et al. 2007). Applications of IPT have also been developed for a range of other conditions and either have demonstrated effectiveness or are being studied currently. This includes depression in adolescence, dysthymic disorder, social anxiety disorder, and borderline personality disorder (Weissman et al. 2007).

The inclusion of IPT in the focused psychological strategies for the *Better Outcome* and *Better Access* programs funded by Medicare is an acknowledgment of the value of the evidence base. Suggestions for further research include the optimal dosage and duration of sessions, identifying the 'active components' of IPT, and exploring who would benefit most from IPT in terms of how the patient explains the cause of their symptoms.

Why IPT?

There are many reasons why psychotherapists should consider IPT as a therapy worth learning more about and adding to their clinical expertise. This includes the following:

- A well-documented evidence base as outlined above
- IPT's minimal use of jargon and manualized format allows the therapist with good basic psychotherapy skills and experience to quickly become competent
- The approach is modified easily for a range of conditions whilst still following the same evidence based format
- The approach is intuitively appealing for many therapists especially for presentations related to grief and relationship problems
- IPT is likely to be applicable to patients with a wide range of problems, as almost all illnesses involve interpersonal problems
- It is important that practitioners are familiar with a variety of empirically based treatments
- It is pure speculation as to why the uptake of IPT has been lower than other therapies such as CBT. Two possibilities include the following:
  - The dominant paradigm of psychology training programs and the self-help movement has been on internal cognition, in contrast to the emphasis of IPT on interpersonal functioning and affect. This has resulted in the potential complimentary nature of IPT with cognitive focused therapies being overlooked in favor of their competing differences, and at first glance IPT being viewed as 'counterintuitive'.
  - Consistent with the above point, despite the evidence base of IPT it has been taught rarely in university settings, thereby preventing the dissemination of the modality to a broader audience. This in turn has led to a dearth of trainers and supervisors that frustrates many practitioners' attempts to receive supervision or advanced training in IPT. This is especially the case in Australia. Further training in IPT training and accreditation standards in IPT have been a key concern for the International Society of IPT. Draft guidelines for level A to D certification were established but consensus was never reached. However, there is a general acknowledgment that an experienced psychotherapist can reach basic competency by completing an introductory workshop of 2–3 days duration, reading a manual, and then completing 2–3 supervised cases with an experienced IPT therapist including weekly supervision for the duration of the case with audiotaped or videotaped sessions. Becoming an IPT practitioner involves taking basic psychotherapy training and modifying it for use with a specific set of strategies and problem areas (Weissman et al. 2007). One study showed that selected, experienced psychotherapists can perform IPT competently at a high level after as little as one supervised case (Rounsaville et al. 1986). Competency should not be confused with specialization or being recognized as an expert or at trainer level. In Australia there are difficulties obtaining the relevant training and supervision because of the small number of experienced IPT practitioners.

CONCLUSION

IPT stands in contrast to other therapies through an emphasis on the effects of a person's external interpersonal environment upon their mental health. There are sufficient clinical trials to conclude that IPT is an efficacious time limited treatment for a range of conditions, in particular, depression and bulimia. The structured and manualized format of IPT makes it relatively easy to learn and apply. Further research is required for different treatment durations, to establish the active components, and to determine minimum training standards. Nevertheless the research to date highlights its bona fides and supports its place alongside CBT within the medicare funded focused psychological strategies.

47.11 BEHAVIOR THERAPY

JN Vyas

Behavior therapy developed as a scientific approach to human behavior change. The search for an understanding of the process of learning moved from the field of philosophy to the newly developing field of psychology late in the nineteenth century. Association theory had already been developed by the British school of philosophical empiricism, but it was Pavlov and his co-workers who demonstrated the basic principles of learning by contiguity and the way in which new connections could be acquired, generalized, and extinguished. In the United States, first Thorndike and then Skinner and his colleagues demonstrated how the environment alters behavior and introduced principles such as reinforcement, punishment, and stimulus control. In broad terms, Skinner postulated that the environmental consequences of behavior determined which actions would be strengthened and which would be weakened over time.

These developments were contemporary with the development of psychoanalytic theory and practice, and beginning in the 1950s numerous attempts were made to integrate the more recently developed learning theories and psychoanalytic theory. These attempts failed to gain acceptance from either psychoanalytic theorists or learning theorists, perhaps because they did not lead to new testable proposition. Thus, behavior therapy developed as an alternative way of understanding and treating disordered behavior, being sparked by the failure to demonstrate the efficacy of psychoanalysis. Among the basic principles underlying the conceptual basis for behavior therapy are the following:

- Both normal and abnormal behaviors are assumed to be learned and maintained in the same way; thus, procedures that alter normal behaviors will also be useful in altering deviant behavior. An example of this is positive reinforcement, which affects a wide range of behaviors across a variety of different species and which has proven useful in modifying many problem behaviors.
- The social environment plays a key role in the development and maintenance of both normal and abnormal behaviors. A consequence of this view is that the patient's environment may need to be altered to maintain newly acquired behaviors and prevent relapse.
- The major focus of treatment is on the behavior problem itself, and thus, specification of both the behaviors to be changed and the circumstances presently maintaining those behaviors is an important facet of assessment and treatments. Behaviors requiring treatment will usually be broken up into discrete components, each of which will be treated using individually tailored procedures depending on the behavior and its antecedents and consequences.
- Behavior therapy is based on a scientific approach to treatment. Treatment procedures must be well specified so that they can be replicated by others; this involves the development of detailed treatment manuals. Treatment procedures must be evaluated in controlled experiments and the active components of treatment separated from inactive components by additive clinical experimental designs.

Social-cognitive learning theory (Bandura 1986) has now become the most widely accepted theoretical underpinning of behavior therapy. This theory incorporates elements of both Pavlovian and Skinnerian theories but goes beyond these in postulating an interaction between environment, behavior, and cognitive processes. Not only does the environment affect the person, but the person can alter his or her personal environment, thus affecting future behavior. Reinforcement is viewed not as the automatic effect of reward but rather as a source of information about the potential effects of future behavior. Similarly, classical conditioning is no longer viewed as an automatic result of the occurrence of two stimuli occurring closely in time. Experimental work has demonstrated that prior experience and recognition of the relatedness of events are often crucial to this type of learning. Hence, cognitive processes are recognized as important modulators of behavior.

Basic research is beginning to unravel the biology of learning. It is now clear that learning leads to neurochemical changes in the central nervous system. Work with the simple organism *Aplysia,* a sea mollusk, has revealed that when this animal learns avoidance behavior, the chemical structure of cells in the nervous system is altered. When the avoidance behavior disappears—for example, through repeated exposure—the chemical changes are reversed (Kandel 1989). Hence, there is a reciprocal interaction between biological processes in the central nervous system and behavior changes resulting from environmental influences. Because psychotherapy involves learning new ways of behaving, and learning produces neurochemical changes, the behavior changes associated with therapy should be detectable by imaging methods. In a study of patients with obsessive-compulsive disorder (OCD), positron emission tomography was used to investigate changes in rates of glucose metabolism in the cerebrum before and after treatment with behavior therapy (Baxter et al. 1992). Rates of glucose metabolism in the right head of the caudate nucleus changed when the OCD was successfully treated but did not change in patients who did not respond to treatment. Moreover, these changes were similar to those produced by antidepressant treatment.

In addition to developments in theory and practice, behavior therapy has reached into new areas of endeavor. These include the development of behavioral pediatrics and behavioral medicine, which have in turn taken behavior therapy into preventive medicine. Another active area of research involves investigations of the interaction between behavior therapy and pharmacological treatments. Finally, the development of effective manualized therapies derived from perspectives other than behavior therapy not only allows comparisons of behavior therapy with these procedures but also allows the testing of differing hypotheses regarding the processes by which therapeutic behavior change occurs.

It should be recognized that behavior therapy is not a monolithic procedure; rather, it involves the application of a variety of well-specified therapeutic procedures that have been packaged to treat or prevent a variety of disorders. The large number of applications of behavior therapy to the wide variety of psychiatric problems and the extensive research literature preclude a comprehensive account in this chapter. Thus, the focus will be on applications in a few common disorders.

THERAPEUTIC PROCEDURES

In the following paragraphs, some therapeutic procedures commonly used in behavior therapy are detailed. Many of these procedures form one component of a more complex therapeutic package that has been designed for a particular psychiatric disorder and tested in controlled outcome studies. It should be recognized that certain procedures common to all therapies are employed in such therapeutic packages—including a therapeutic rationale and therapeutic instructions—and that a satisfactory therapeutic relationship is as essential to behavior therapy as it is to other psychotherapies.

Systematic Desensitization

Systematic desensitization, a procedure introduced by Wolpe (1958), is most often used in the treatment of phobias (see "Anxiety Disorders" section later in this chapter). After a thorough exploration of the patient's phobia, a hierarchy of feared situations along one dimension is created—for example, for a patient with height phobia, looking down from the second floor of a building to looking down from a skyscraper, with many gradual steps in between. The patient is then taught deep muscle relaxation (see "Relaxation Training" subsection below) and next visualizes the first item in the hierarchy for some 20 30 seconds, signaling if any anxiety has been aroused. When the visualization of the first scene has produced no anxiety on two repetitions, the therapist moves on to the next item in the hierarchy. Because there may be some recrudescence of anxiety between sessions, it is usually wise to drop back a couple of items and to proceed forward from there.

Some patients have difficulty visualizing feared scenes and may need coaching (e.g. to imagine colors and specific details of a particular scene). Systematic desensitization is little used today, having been largely superseded by the use of direct exposure to the feared situation, as will be described in the next subsection. The procedure is useful, however, in extremely fearful patients who will not venture into the feared situation, when it is used before exposure to the feared situation.

Exposure Therapy (Programmed Practice)

Exposure therapy, sometimes known as *programmed practice,* is one of the most investigated and frequently used therapies in the treatment of phobias, including agoraphobia. There are several variants of this therapeutic procedure, although all begin with the construction of a hierarchy of feared situations along a particular dimension. The simplest variant of exposure therapy is known as *exposure instructions.* The therapist helps the patient construct the first few steps in a hierarchy of the feared situation. For example, for the patient with agoraphobia who is housebound, this involves walking a few yards from the front door, then walking half a block, then walking a block, and so on. With the use of the hierarchy, a course is laid out along which the patient is instructed to walk alone. The instructions are to walk as far as possible until mild anxiety is evident. At least one session, lasting approximately 30 minutes, should be held each day. The patient repeats each walk until the anxiety has dissipated and then he or she begins to walk farther. A diary is kept for each trial. At the next session the diary is reviewed, progress is attended to and praised, and any stumbling blocks are discussed and a solution for them is found. Progress is usually slow at first, with occasional setbacks, but as the patient gains experience with the method, he or she is able to make faster progress and eventually can proceed on his or her own.

In *therapist-assisted exposure* the therapist accompanies the patient to the feared situation and provide direct coaching on facing it. In such cases the therapist may challenge the patient to experience maximal anxiety levels. In addition, the therapist may explore the thoughts of the patient during the exposure experience so that distorted cognitions can be directly challenged.

Group exposure therapy combines individualized exposure instructions and practice with group education concerning the phobia (usually panic disorder with agoraphobia) and with a discussion of the participants' experiences during exposure to the feared situation.

Such group sessions are usually 3 hours in duration, comprising a 30-minute educational session, an exposure session with individual practice, and a 45-minute debriefing session. Group sessions are often held daily for 10–14 days.

Flooding is a form of exposure therapy in which patients are exposed to the maximal phobic situation and kept in that situation until their fear dissipates. Although this form of treatment produces positive results more rapidly than does graduated exposure, it may be associated with much discomfort and therefore is rarely used today.

Cognitive Therapy

Although behavior therapy, as its name implies, tends to focus on the current behavior of the patient, from the earliest days of behavior therapy there was at least some focus on the specific cognitions accompanying a particular disorder. The importance of distorted cognitions has been particularly recognized in the treatment of the anxiety disorders, depression, and the eating disorders. The typical approach to cognitive therapy involves a thorough exploration of the thoughts and feelings preceding, during, and following a particular behavior (e.g. binge eating or purging). For patients who have difficulty recalling such thoughts, self-monitoring is often useful. Once the cognitions have been clearly identified, the reality of such thoughts is considered in detail. When the patient recognizes the unrealistic nature of the thoughts, such thinking can be challenged *in vivo* by the patient or behavioral experiments designed further to test the reality of such thinking can be devised.

The following case history is an example of the use of cognitive therapy: A philosophy student in her late 20s had a sudden panic attack while presenting a paper in her class. She then had several further attacks (apparently precipitated by thoughts of failure), lost her appetite, and began to lose weight. In addition, she began to avoid leaving home unless accompanied by her husband. She was evaluated within a month of the start of her symptoms. During the initial interview, it became clear that this ambitious young woman thought her life was out of control, that she was a failure, that she could not continue with her projected career as a philosopher, and that her life was essentially over. She was particularly afraid that her wealthy and successful husband would divorce her and find a more suitable companion. Because she was a philosopher and supposedly a logical individual, the therapist asked her to examine the reality of her beliefs. Within the first session she was able to see that her beliefs were unrealistic. She immediately began practicing leaving home alone, challenging her unrealistic thinking when it recurred. Within a few sessions she no longer felt anxious, was able to resume her studies, had no phobic limitation, and once more felt secure in her marriage. At 1-year follow-up she remained, by her assessment, symptom free.

It should be noted that cognitive procedures are usually combined with behavior change procedures, and that many behavior therapies are now referred to as *cognitive behavioral* therapies.

Reinforcement

Reinforcement consists of making an event contingent on the performance of a behavior that one wishes to change, *Positive reinforcement* is said to occur when the contingent application of the event strengthens the behavior. Positive reinforcers are usually viewed as pleasant (e.g. food, attention, praise, money). All therapists use verbal attention to reinforce particular themes during therapy sessions. Behavior therapists tend to use such reinforcement in a more precise manner, making attention or praise contingent on the occurrence of the behavior that is being strengthened. Although positive reinforcement is an aspect of all therapeutic encounters, it is most often used to strengthen prosocial behaviors in children with conduct disorder or in persons with schizophrenia.

Negative reinforcement refers to a process by which a particular behavior removes the reinforcing event, thus strengthening the behavior. The events used in a negative reinforcement paradigm are usually regarded as unpleasant. For example, in the treatment of anorexia nervosa the often-used threat of tube feeding serves as a negative reinforcer, because the patient can avoid the negative occurrence (i.e. NG tube feeding) by eating and gaining weight. In addition to using reinforcement within a therapeutic package of some kind, the psychiatrist must review patients' current behavior to identify reinforcers that might be maintaining the pathological behavior. It is also clear that staff attention to problem behaviors increases the frequency of such behaviors. Therefore, nursing and medical staff at all levels should be trained in the application of social reinforcement and extinction procedures. Research has shown that untrained nursing staff attend to problem behaviors more frequently than they attend to prosocial behaviors of patients. Such an approach causes an increase in the frequency of problem behaviors.

Extinction

Removal of positive reinforcement weakens behavior and may lead to its total disappearance. This procedure is known as *extinction.* From a clinical viewpoint, extinction can be used only in environments such as an inpatient unit or a classroom in which reinforcement can be controlled, although relatives of patients can be taught to use extinction in the home. The withdrawal of positive reinforcement may lead to an *extinction burst,* in which the unwanted behavior briefly increases in frequency or strength. If the procedure is being applied by relatives in the home setting, it is important to warn them that an increase in the problem behavior may occur at first, so that they do not abandon the attempt to control the behavior through extinction.

Punishment

The punishment paradigm consists of the application of an aversive stimulus contingent on the unwanted behavior, with the aim of rapidly bringing the behavior under control. Punishment is used infrequently in behavior therapy and only in situations in which the behavior in question threatens physical harm and in which more benign procedures such as positive reinforcement or extinction have failed. An example of the application of punishment is given in the subsection on ruminative vomiting, a life-threatening condition in infancy. The use of punishment, because it raises difficult ethical issues, is usually supervised by a committee that should include an informed layperson. In addition, if the use of punishment does not bring the unwanted behavior rapidly under control, the punishment paradigm should be reviewed for the accuracy of its use and/or stopped.

Aversion Therapy

Aversion therapy, which should not be confused with punishment, is based on the principle of classical conditioning and involves pairing an aversive stimulus with the unwanted behavior. An example of such a paradigm is the pairing of nausea (induced with emetine) with the drinking of alcohol in the treatment of alcoholism. It has been shown that such classical conditioning is more powerful if it involves the same physiological system as the one involved in the unwanted behavior. Thus, drinking is paired with nausea in the case of alcoholism because both involve the gastrointestinal system. One of the problems with aversive therapy is that exposure to the original stimulus (in this case, drinking alcohol) tends to weaken the classically conditioned response and lead to relapse. Therefore, in the original application of such conditioning, booster sessions were found to delay relapse. Nonetheless, the tendency toward relapse after aversion therapy has led to a decrease in enthusiasm for the use of aversion therapy in general.

Biofeedback

The principal aim of biofeedback procedures is to magnify a response that is not accessible to a patient and to provide feedback regarding changes in that response over time. For example, small muscle contractions are not usually discriminable by patients. Such responses can be amplified through the use of electronic monitoring, and a signal can be displayed, either visually or in the form of a continuous tone, that is proportional to the muscle contraction being measured. In this way, the patient can be informed about the degree of contraction and can potentially learn either to increase or to decrease the contractions, depending on the aim of therapy. Thus, in the case of nerve or muscle damage the aim would be to increase contractions in selected muscles, whereas in the case of tension headache the aim would be to reduce tension in the affected muscles. Biofeedback has many potential applications—for example, in fecal incontinence, through training of the anal sphincter; in hypertension, through displaying blood pressure values and allowing patients to discover methods to control their blood pressure; and in Raynaud's disease, through enhancing temperature control. Using small portable biofeedback units, patients can practice in their own homes, and thus learning can be transferred from the office to the patients' own environment.

Relaxation Training

Relaxation training is a relatively simple therapeutic technique that is useful in a variety of conditions (discussed later in this chapter) and often forms a component of a behavior therapy treatment package. Patients are first presented with a rationale. For example, a patient who has tension headaches would be told that muscles tense up as a result of anxiety and this can lead to pain; if the patient were to learn to relax his or her muscles, such pain could be lessened. Patients are then seated comfortably in a chair and are taught to tense and then relax each muscle group systematically. Soon they are able to induce relaxation fairly quickly simply by relaxing all their muscles. Patients are encouraged at the same time to visualize a pleasant, relaxing scene or to use a simple mantra to control distracting thoughts. Patients are given a tape recording of relaxation instructions and are encouraged to use the tape for some 20 minutes each day at home. After several treatment sessions with intervening home practice, patients are taught rapid relaxation techniques, in this procedure, patients are taught to scan their bodies intermittently for tense muscles and to bring on the relaxation response rapidly using the word *relax,* which they have previously paired with a deeply relaxed state. This procedure can then be used during the course their everyday lives.

Modeling

Modeling refers to a procedure in which a desired behavior is performed by a therapist with the aim of having his or her patient copy that performance. It may be necessary to break a complex behavior pattern into its component parts and model each segment of that behavior sequentially until the entire sequence can be performed by the patient. Reinforcement such as praise is used as the patient gradually masters the desired behavior. The patient is then encouraged to try out the behavior at home. Modeling has been used to treat children's phobias through encouragement to expose themselves to the feared situation; in social skills training in disorders such as schizophrenia; in marital counseling; and in training in better parenting skills.

Social Skills Training

Social skills training is used in the rehabilitation of patients with schizophrenia (discussed later in this chapter), in the treatment of social phobia, particularly when the phobia is combined with avoidant personality disorder; and in any patient in whom a particular social skills deficit is apparent. The first step is to analyze the social skills deficit in concrete behavioral terms—for example, avoiding eye contact, a slumped body posture that is not conducive to interpersonal communication, or speaking too softly. More appropriate behavior is then gradually developed by means of modeling and social reinforcement, together with opportunities for the patient to (practice the new behaviors e.g. in a group setting). The patient is next encouraged to practice the new behaviors in his or her own environment. Videotapes of the patient performing the desired behavior may also be employed so that the therapist can give detailed feedback on progress.

Anxiety Disorders

Panic Disorder With or Without Agoraphobia

Agoraphobia (and the simple phobias) has been a central focus of behavior therapy since Wolpe's description of systematic desensitization first appeared (Wolpe 1958). The work in this area is an excellent example of the continual refinement of therapeutic hypotheses and procedures based on the results of clinical trials. On the basis of his findings from animal experiments in which fear responses were induced and then treated (Wolpe formulated the hypothesis that if a response that inhibits anxiety occurs in an anxiety-provoking situation, then the anxiety response will be weakened—an example of the principle of *reciprocal inhibition*). In his animal experiments, Wolpe used food to inhibit fear while the animal was exposed to gradually intensifying fear-arousing situations. In humans, relaxation was used to inhibit anxiety; hence, in the clinical application of systematic desensitization, deep muscle relaxation is paired with the imagination of feared scenes presented in a graded hierarchy, beginning with those provoking the least fear and gradually progressing to more fear-arousing scenes. Research in the field was catalyzed by the development of an analog model of phobia, namely, snake fears (Lazovik and Lang, 1960). This model allowed for a more rapid delineation of the active and inactive components of systematic desensitization than would have been possible if research had been limited to clinical populations.

Findings from analog research challenged the theory on which systematic desensitization was based. Therapeutic instructions were found to be an essential component of desensitization, and removal of such instructions from the therapeutic package weakened the efficacy of treatment. This finding was not entirely surprising, given that therapeutic instructions have been found to be a major component of all psychotherapies. Such instructions comprise information concerning the therapeutic rationale, a description of the therapeutic procedures to be used, and, perhaps most important, an assessment of the outcome that might be expected from treatment. More surprising was the finding that pairing relaxation with feared scenes was not essential for successful outcome, nor was a gradual approach to the feared situation in imagination. This finding challenged the central notion of reciprocal inhibition. Ultimately, exposure to the feared situation itself was found to be the critical ingredient for successful treatment.

Many controlled clinical trials have demonstrated the effectiveness of graded exposure therapy in the treatment of agoraphobia (Taylor and Arnow 1988). Long-term studies have shown that improvement is well maintained for periods of up to 7 years (Fava et al. 1995). Involving a spouse (or friend) in the treatment process adds to the effectiveness of exposure therapy, probably because the patient's practice in the feared situation is better supported. The addition of couples training in communication skills enhances maintenance of the effects of exposure therapy. Such enhanced communication may allow the couple to adjust better to the agoraphobic individual's newfound freedom of movement, a change that may be stressful for some couples. Overall, exposure therapy is associated with dropout rates of approximately 10%, and more than 80% of patients demonstrate marked improvement. However, exposure therapy may be less effective in reducing panic attacks than in reducing or eliminating phobic behavior.

Behavior Therapy for Panic Disorder

Several studies suggest that the catastrophic interpretation of panic symptoms rather than the frequency of panic attacks is the critical element associated with the severity of agoraphobia. Catastrophic cognitions fall into three categories: (1) fear of illness, (2) fear of loss of control, and (3) fear of embarrassment while having a panic attack. It is hypothesized that persons susceptible to such cognitions misinterpret either mild symptoms of anxiety or other body changes (e.g. dizziness on standing up suddenly) in a catastrophic manner, leading to spiraling anxiety that culminates in a panic attack. It follows that therapy aimed at correcting such misinterpretations should lead to a reduction in panic. Such therapy consists, first, in identifying the type of cognitions experienced by the patient and, second, having the patient expose himself or herself to situations in which the catastrophic cognitions occur, essentially demonstrating to himself or herself that the feared consequences do not occur in reality (e.g. despite a fear of having a heart attack because of an accelerating heart rate, no heart attack occurs). In addition, some physical symptoms leading to the catastrophic thinking patterns can be induced in the therapy situation (e.g. in the case of dizziness, spinning the patient in a chair) and the reality of the frightening thoughts can thus be directly disconfirmed.

Controlled studies have demonstrated the effectiveness of this treatment in reducing panic attacks; between 50% and 90% of patients achieved remission of their symptoms in the various studies (e.g. Barlow et al. 1989; Clark et al. 1994; Craske et al. 1995). Follow-up studies reveal some relapse in symptoms of panic, although, for the most part, maintenance of treatment effects is good. In a study by Fava et al. (1995) in which panic disorder patients with agoraphobia received 12 sessions of behavioral therapy with *in vivo* exposure, 67% remained in remission for at least 7 years.

Combination Therapy

In general, it appears that the most effective treatment of agoraphobia with panic is a combination of pharmacological treatment and exposure therapy. For example, in a study comparing exposure therapy with and without treatment with fluvoxamine, the addition of medication was found to enhance the outcome of exposure therapy (de Beurs et al. 1995). For patients with agoraphobia who have not experienced panic attacks, exposure therapy alone should suffice. Behavior therapy may also be useful in the discontinuation of treatment with alprazolam, as demonstrated in a study comparing a slow tapering of medication with and without behavior therapy. Patients receiving the combined treatment were more successful in discontinuing alprazolam therapy and were significantly less anxious and depressed after medication discontinuation than those not receiving behavior therapy (Bruce et al. 1995).

Simple Phobia

Because medication appears to have little place in the treatment of simple phobia, the approach to this problem that is most often used is graded exposure therapy. Such treatment is usually fairly easy to arrange and involves the patient's gradually approaching the feared object or situation. Therapist-aided exposure may be used in which the therapist accompanies the patient into the phobic situation and directly arranges exposure trials, or the therapist may simply use instructions regarding the practice of exposure and request that the patient keep a record of such practice. This record is examined at subsequent treatment sessions, and solutions to problems encountered by the patient are worked out. Most patients with simple phobia respond rapidly to such treatment, and follow-up studies suggest that gains are well maintained.

Social Phobia

The number of studies of the treatment of social phobia, once a rather neglected area of research, is now increasing (Heimberg and Barlow 1991; Heimberg et al. 1993). Findings of controlled studies suggest that the behavioral treatment of choice is a combination of exposure therapy and cognitive restructuring. One study found that the addition of cognitive restructuring to exposure therapy prevented relapse. The principal area of focus for cognitive change is in eliciting the details of the social phobic patient's fears of negative evaluation by others and challenging the reality of these ideas. Exposure therapy in social phobia is more difficult to arrange than in the case of simple phobia or agoraphobia because social situations are less controllable by the patient than other phobic situations and may become more intense than expected. Moreover, many social interchanges are of short duration and therefore do not provide the more prolonged exposure characteristic of the therapy for other phobias. Hence, careful planning of exposure situations, ensuring sufficient number of opportunities for exposure, and providing support for failure experiences when the social situation is more intense than was planned are all important aspects of the treatment of social phobia.

Obsessive-Compulsive Disorder

There have been remarkable advances in the treatment of OCD with behavior therapy, although the results of treatment are not completely satisfactory. Deriving from basic work concerning the relationship between anxiety and avoidance behaviors such as compulsions, *response prevention* of compulsive rituals has become one of the cornerstones of behavior therapy in this condition (Stanley and Turner 1995). The thesis is that the compulsive behaviour does not allow for reality testing of the fear. Thus, patients' fear of contamination leading to illness and death is reinforced by the fact that they do not become sick or die as long as they engage in hand washing.

The main therapeutic procedure is to prevent the patient from engaging in compulsive acts such as hand washing after exposure to "contaminating" situations. This may be accomplished by means of a gradual approach on an outpatient basis in which the patient, perhaps aided by a relative, abstains from engaging in compulsive behavior after exposure to the feared situation. A hierarchical approach is taken, in which the patient begins with the easiest situation and gradually moves toward more difficult tasks. On an inpatient basis, a more intensive approach can be taken—for example, preventing the patient from engaging in hand washing for a period of several days while providing a supportive relationship. The efficacy of this approach was first demonstrated in controlled single-case studies and since then has been examined in a number of controlled clinical trials.

Although response prevention results in marked diminution in compulsive behavior, it does not usually eliminate the fear of contamination. Controlled studies have demonstrated that exposure to contaminating situations results in marked diminution in contamination fears but relatively little change in rituals (Steketee et al. 1982). The combination of the two treatments (exposure plus response prevention) is clearly superior to either one alone. Finally, it has been shown that the addition of desensitization in imagination—focusing on the imagined catastrophic consequences of contamination—results in superior maintenance of recovery. Thus, a three-part behavior therapy dealing with separate components of the disorder appears to be most effective: response prevention for rituals, exposure therapy for phobic anxiety, and imaginal desensitization for obsessive worry.

Relatively little is known about the efficacy of combinations of behavior therapy and pharmacological treatment. A review of the literature suggests that patients in medication studies drop out at higher rates and experience somewhat less positive results than do patients in studies involving behavior therapies. Kozak et al. (2000) studied patients with OCD who were treated with exposure plus response prevention (ERP) alone, clomipramine alone, or the combination. ERP monotherapy produced a response rate similar to that for the combination condition, and both of these conditions resulted in greater improvement than did the clomipramine-alone condition. Furthermore, at follow-up 3 months after the end of treatment, the ERP-alone and combination groups continued to experience greater improvement than did the clomipramine-alone group.

Mood Disorder

Major Depression

The effectiveness of a cognitive-behavioral approach to treating unipolar nonpsychotic depression has been studied extensively in controlled clinical trials. In this treatment, the contingencies maintaining the depressed mood, often conceptualized as a relative lack of environmental reinforcement, are examined. Among the therapeutic procedures used are (1) problem solving combined with the teaching of coping skills to enhance the reinforcement deficit and (2) an examination of self-defeating cognitions, followed by the psychiatrist's teaching the patient to recognize such thoughts, to challenge them, and to substitute more adaptive thinking. Because antidepressant therapy can be viewed as the standard treatment for major depression, much recent research has been aimed at clarifying the relative effectiveness of pharmacological therapy and cognitive-behavioral therapy (CBT) and the effectiveness of the combined treatments (Clarkin et al. 1996).

In one of the first studies to examine this issue systematically, Kovacs et al. (1981) found that both imipramine therapy and CBT produced improvement in depressive symptomatology in a 12-week treatment period and that CBT was marginally superior. At 1-year follow-up, both groups of patients maintained their improvement; however, there was a suggestion that those receiving CBT showed less relapse than those receiving imipramine. In the large-scale National Institute of Mental Health Treatment of Depression Collaborative Research Program (Elkin et al. 1989), CBT, interpersonal therapy (IPT), and antidepressant medication were compared in a multicenter trial. The results suggested that all three therapies were effective but that medication was more effective in cases of severe depression.

Other studies have found that of patients who respond to therapy, those receiving CBT in combination with a tricyclic antidepressant show less tendency to relapse than those receiving antidepressants alone (Simons et al. 1986). Given that patients receiving antidepressants tend to improve more quickly than those receiving CBT, the preferred treatment for major depression would seem to be a combination of CBT and an antidepressant.

Patients with chronic major depression often have serious and unremitting courses. Some studies have reported that responses to CBT are similar to those observed for other forms of psychotherapy or for antidepressant medication. A multicenter trial (Keller et al. 2000) evaluated 662 patients with chronic, nonpsychotic major depression who were randomly assigned to receive 12 weeks of treatment with antidepressant medication (nefazodone), a cognitive-behavioral approach specifically designed to treat chronic depression, or a combination of both treatments. The combination of CBT with nefazodone resulted in significantly greater response (73%) than did either CBT or nefazodone alone (both 48%). Thus, this study supports the clinical notion that a combination of psychotherapy with CBT plus medication may be very useful to patients with chronic depression.

Social skills training has also been used to treat major depression. Such training involves the teaching of more assertive behavior that would be expected to increase social interaction and strengthen environmental reinforcement. Controlled studies have shown that this approach is as effective as CBT. Indeed, one must conclude from a survey of the literature that behavior therapy, IPT, and time-limited focused psychotherapy are all equally effective in the treatment of major depression although superior maintenance has been demonstrates only in the case of CBT and IPT at this time. This raises the theoretical issue regarding what procedures might be shared by these different approaches to treatment and whether they affect depressed mood through the same or different psychological processes.

Other Depressive Disorders

The place of behavior therapy in more severe depression (e.g. cases meeting research criteria for endogenous depression) is less certain, due to a relative lack of controlled treatment studies in this area. Early work suggests, however, that CBT may be quite effective in both outpatient and inpatient populations and may be a useful alternative to treatment with medication. This modality may perhaps be helpful in patients who are not able to tolerate adequate dosage of antidepressant medication or as an adjunctive treatment combined with medication. CBT has also appeared to be useful in the treatment of dysthymia in initial uncontrolled studies.

Disorders of Eating

The three major disorders of eating are *anorexia nervosa, bulimia nervosa,* and *binge-eating disorder* (BED), the latter often associated with obesity. The development of behavior therapy differs significantly between these three disorders for different reasons. In the case of anorexia nervosa, the relative rarity of the disorder has militated against the conducting of controlled clinical trials, and very little is known about the comparative effectiveness of different approaches to treatment over the long-term. Bulimia nervosa, although common, markedly increased in prevalence toward the end of the 1970s, and clinical research is now in a state of relative maturity. BED has only recently attracted research attention, and therefore much less is known about the treatment of this disorder, although it would appear that treatments effective in bulimia nervosa are also effective in BED.

Anorexia Nervosa

The behavioral approach to the treatment of anorexia nervosa is aimed at the restoration of normal body weight, usually within an inpatient setting. It is widely agreed that weight restoration in the severely emaciated patient is the first objective of treatment. Next, there would be an attempt to deal with whatever problems appear to have precipitated and are maintaining the eating disorder. Crisp et al. (1991) viewed anorexia nervosa as an avoidance of maturation (a weight and shape phobia); thus, weight restoration is viewed as exposing the patient to problems that are being avoided through starvation (i.e. an exposure therapy).

Single-case controlled research, a useful approach when dealing with a relatively rare disorder, has revealed three procedures that promote increased caloric intake: reinforcement of weight gain in small increments, feedback of information regarding progress (usually accomplished by daily weight and caloric consumption feedback), and the serving of large meals even though the patient will at first leave most of the food untouched. These procedures are used in the context of a carefully negotiated therapeutic contract and a well-designed ward milieu (Agras 1987). Such programs lead to steady weight gain, and studies suggest that behavior therapy is more efficient than other treatment approaches, resulting in shorter hospital stays for equal amounts of weight gain. The only large-scale controlled study of an inpatient behavioral approach to weight restoration suggested that behavior therapy may be relatively more effective in the, less severe case of anorexia nervosa.

Research has also been directed toward evaluating outpatient treatments for anorexia nervosa. One study compared inpatient and outpatient care for anorexia nervosa in a randomized controlled trial (Crisp et al. 1991). Surprisingly, the results of outpatient care equaled those of inpatient care, in that weight gains in the patients receiving outpatient care were equivalent to those in the patients receiving inpatient care, and weight gains in the patients in these groups were superior to those in patients who received no treatment. This study requires replication by other investigators because of methodological problems, including a high rate of dropout from the study. Nonetheless, in an era in which the duration of hospitalization for the anorexic patient is becoming ever shorter, this study may point the way to the future of treatment of anorexia.

Bulimia Nervosa

The upsurge in the number of young women seeking treatment for bulimic symptoms in the late 1970s presented clinicians with a difficult problem because no effective treatment methods had been described for this condition. The work of Fairburn (1981), who first described a CBT for bulimia, has led to the appearance of a large number of controlled trials in the last decade. It is generally agreed that the social pressure for women to remain thin has increased during the past 15 years. This pressure leads a subgroup of young women to restrict their caloric intake markedly and to form rigid rules relating to food, leading to an increased probability of binge eating and eventually, because of threatened weight increase, to purging. It is also probable that the most susceptible young women are those who markedly restrict their food intake despite being genetically programmed for having a fuller figure. Research has shown that some bulimic individuals have a markedly increased energy efficiency, maintaining normal body weight in the absence of purging on a mean daily caloric intake of approximately 1,400 calories. They also tend to eat very little early in the day, which sets the scene for binge eating later in the day.

CBT is aimed at overcoming the dietary restriction and distorted thinking patterns that are believed to maintain bulimia nervosa. The basic components of CBT include self-disclosure to significant others, thus increasing social control over the secretive bulimic behaviors; gradual reintroduction of the consumption of three adequate meals each day; slow introduction of "feared" binge foods to the diet; challenge of distorted cognitions regarding food intake; and a relapse prevention program (Agras 1987; Fairburn 1981). Controlled studies have demonstrated that CBT is more effective in reducing binge eating and purging than are awaiting-list control condition; a pill placebo; psychoeducational treatment; nondirective psychotherapy combined with self-monitoring of eating behavior; stress management; and, in some studies, behavior therapy (i.e. a treatment omitting the procedures aimed at correcting distorted thinking patterns). In other studies, CBT and behavior therapy have been found to be equivalent in effectiveness in reducing binge eating and purging, although patients receiving CBT almost always have psychiatrically healthier attitudes toward weight and shape, attitudes that are specifically targeted by CBT. Overall, some 55% of patients with bulimia recover with the use of CBT, and the majority maintain their gains over follow-up periods of up to 5 years (Fairburn et al. 1993). A substantial proportion of those not fully recovering have a subclinical eating disorder at follow-up.

Combination Therapy

Because both CBT and antidepressant medication have been used in the treatment of bulimia nervosa, the relative effectiveness of these different approaches to treatment and their combination has been investigated. Studies have shown that CBT is superior to antidepressant medication in reducing binge eating and purging and that the combined treatment is no more effective than CBT alone. It appears, however, that the combined treatment more effectively reduces depression and emotionally induced eating, and there is tentative evidence that, as in depression, the combined treatment leads to better maintenance of improvement (Agras et al. 1992; Mitchell et al. 1990). More recently, Walsh et al. (1997) conducted a study in which two antidepressants, desipramine and fluoxetine, were used. These investigators substituted fluoxetine when desipramine was ineffective; such a model is more similar to that used by practitioners. Walsh and colleagues found that the sequential use of these medications was as effective as CBT and that there was a marginally improved effectiveness when medication was combined with CBT.

Other Approaches to Treatment

It has been shown that an adaptation of IPT—an approach that was first demonstrated to be effective in the treatment of depression—to eating disorders is as effective as CBT (Fairburn et al. 1991). This is an interesting finding, given that no attention was paid to eating disturbances in the interpersonal treatment. This suggests that IPT and CBT may work by different processes. There is much evidence that negative affect, frequently arising from interpersonal conflicts, triggers binge eating. It may be that IPT works by reducing negative affect, whereas CBT works by reducing dietary restraint.

Binge-Eating Disorder

The research in bulimia nervosa has resulted in the rediscovery of a subset of obese individuals who binge eat but do not purge. The proportion of overweight individuals who binge eat increases with increasing levels of adiposity, from 10% in mildly obese persons to more than 40% in severely obese persons. Moreover, it appears that these individuals are less successful in their weight loss attempts than are their nonbinge-eating counterparts. The similarity of this disorder to bulimia nervosa suggests that treatments effective in that condition should be effective in BED. Initial research has shown this hypothesis to be true: both CBT and IPT have been demonstrated to be equally effective in reducing binge eating in controlled studies (Agras et al. 1994; Wilfley et al. 1993). As is the case with bulimia nervosa, although antidepressant medication appears effective, adding therapy with such medication to CBT does not result in a significant additional reduction in binge eating. However, those receiving antidepressant treatment lose more weight than those not receiving medication.

The optimal approach for treating the obese binge eating patient is to begin treatment with CBT and follow this with weight loss treatment that does not demand overly restrictive dieting. Patients with BED who stop binge eating and who maintain abstinence also maintain their weight losses.

Psychotic Disorders

The behavioral approach to the treatment of psychotic disorders may be viewed as being adjunctive to pharmacological treatment and directed toward amelioration of specific problem behaviors or, more broadly, toward the social rehabilitation of the disturbed individual. These aims are accomplished using methods deriving from operant conditioning. Thus, precise definition of the problem behavior, combined with the use of reinforcement in various forms, is the core of the approach for patients with either disturbed behavior that does not improve with the use of medication or limitations in social and vocational skills secondary to the psychotic process.

Some of the first applications of behavior therapy were to severely disturbed individuals with chronic psychoses. The early successes of reinforcement therapy, demonstrated largely in single-case experiments, led to many applications in the mental hospital, in which a large number of problems, including aggressive and disruptive behavior, delusional behavior, depression, and apathy, were found susceptible to change (Kazdin 1977). Ayllon and Azrin (1965) demonstrated the effectiveness of using tokens with chronic psychotic patients, thus broadening the range of backup reinforcers that could be used to motivate individuals. One of the most sophisticated applications and testings of a token economy system was the experiment conducted by Paul and Lentz (1977) comparing a social-learning program with a more traditional milieu therapy program. This experiment had many noteworthy features, including the use of multiple outcome measures, continuous monitoring of staff behavior to ensure proper operation of programs, collection of long-term follow-up data, and computation of the cost-effectiveness of the two programs. Patients in both treatment programs showed progress, but those in the social-learning program showed significantly greater improvement across a range of prosocial behaviors, required less medication, and maintained their gains more successfully during the 18-month follow-up. Moreover, the social-learning program was the most cost-efficient of the two programs.

Whereas the token economy focused on generating skills useful to most patients, social skills training, delivered within complex and sophisticated rehabilitation programs and based on a detailed analysis of each patient's interpersonal deficits, now forms a more individualized approach to the patient with schizophrenia. Among the skills taught are maintaining eye contact, reacting more quickly to interpersonal communication, trying intonation, and reinforcing prosocial responses from others. Techniques such as modeling prosocial behaviors are often used. In addition, the patient and family members may be taught more effective conflict resolution through the use of role playing, video feedback and practice. A number of controlled studies have demonstrated that clinically meaningful changes in behavior occur as a result of social skills training, improvements of up to 70% in social functioning are made, and hospital stays are shortened.

In recognition of the fact that environmental stress is a factor affecting the outcome of treatment in schizophrenic patients, the effectiveness of a behavioral family-based treatment has been studied intensively (Falloon et al. 1985). The main focus of such treatment has been problem solving at the family level. When families are unable to use the problem-solving approach successfully, training in communication skills is added to the program. Specific behavior problems impeding the process of therapy are dealt with using appropriate behavior change techniques. Compared with patients undergoing individual treatment, those receiving behavioral family therapy showed a 10-fold decrease in the number of days spent in the hospital or in jail during follow-up. In addition, the number of days spent in residential facilities decreased 30-fold. Thus, we may conclude that behavioral family treatment is an effective adjunct to the treatment of chronic schizophrenia. Few exacerbations are observed with family behavioral approaches compared with individual approaches or routine care. In addition, family behavioral treatment resulted in lower levels of rejecting attitudes by family members and reduced levels of tension in the patients (Mueser et al. 2001) as compared with a supportive family therapy approach.

BEHAVIORAL MEDICINE

Behavior therapy has been applied to a number of medical disorders, including essential hypertension, hypercholesterolemia, and obesity; headache; sleep disturbance; gastrointestinal problems; and asthma. In addition, therapeutic procedures have been developed for problems common to many medical disorders such as compliance with medication taking and the response to stress.

Obesity

Behavioral treatment for mild to moderate obesity contains the following elements: (1) self-monitoring; (2) reinforcement of an increase in activity levels; (3) slowing of the eating rate; (4) narrowing of the stimuli associated with eating; (5) adherence to a low-fat, high-fiber, heart-healthy diet; and (6) use of reinforcement and self-reinforcement to attain short-term goals. This treatment package has been shown to be more effective than more traditional dietary approaches to weight control, psychotherapy, and even pharmacological treatment in a large number of controlled studies. The degree of weight loss achieved by the average patient is modest, usually averaging approximately 0.5 kg per week of treatment. Treatment programs of 16 weeks' duration result in a mean weight reduction of 8–10 kg. Weight loss is enhanced when reinforcement procedures, such as refund of a monetary deposit depending on weekly weight loss, are used. There is, however, marked variability in weight loss between individuals: some patients do not lose weight, whereas others lose more than 15 kg over the same period. The reasons for such variability are unclear, although there is evidence that poor adherence to the treatment regimen and particularly to self-monitoring is associated with a poorer outcome. In addition, biological factors—for example, adaptation of basal metabolic rate to dietary restriction—may vary between individuals. Finally, as discussed earlier in this chapter, the obese binge-eating patient appears to have more difficulty in losing weight than does the obese nonbinge-eating patient.

Group therapy is the most usual behavioral approach to the treatment of obesity and may have advantages over individual treatment in that a wide variety of problem situations and their solutions are presented in a group context. Maintenance of weight loss appears to depend on the continued practice of behaviors learned during treatment. The most crucial of these are adherence to a healthy diet and eating style and continued exercise. Patients who continue to practice these behaviors have been shown to maintain or even increase their initial weight losses up to 5 years after treatment. Those who do not continue such behaviors tend to regain all of the weight that they lost, and some regain even more weight.

Behavior therapy has also been used to enhance the maintenance of weight loss with a very-low-calorie diet (VLCD), a treatment regimen used in moderately to severely obese patients. YLCDs were initially associated with a series of deaths in obese patients undergoing such treatment. These deaths were caused by inadequate protein in the diet accompanied by potassium deficiency which in susceptible individuals led to ventricular fibrillation. Modern variants of the diet with adequate protein, minerals, and vitamins have proved safe when used with careful medical supervision. One controlled study demonstrated that weight regain after completion of a 12-week VLCD was less in a group of patients who were also receiving behavior therapy than in a group of patients who were not receiving this adjunctive treatment.

Clinical studies suggest that mean weight losses of 20 kg or more might be expected with this combination of treatments, as well as marked improvement in cardiovascular risk factors including blood pressure, serum cholesterol levels, and even sleep apnea.

Relapse Prevention and Longer-term Treatment

Longer-term follow-up studies have demonstrated difficulty with weight regain after acute weight loss (Brownell and Wadden 1986; Stunkard and Penick 1979). The theory of relapse proposed for the addictions but applicable to the treatment of obesity suggests that relapse (i.e. a return to previous behaviors) occurs when a patient who has insufficient ways to cope is confronted by a high-risk situation, problem, or emotional state. Precipitants to overeating often include negative affective states while alone or positive affective states in social situations. Cognitive-behavioral approaches have begun to address the relapse issue.

In a study addressing long-term treatment, Perri et al. (1988) treated a group of obese patients using behavioral techniques. Participants were then randomized to a no-treatment control group and to four other groups, each of which used a variety of behavioral approaches. All of the behavioral groups had continued therapist contact biweekly for an additional year. Problem situations were discussed and new strategies developed to help patients cope without resorting to eating at high-risk times. The participants in the no-treatment control group regained approximately one-half the weight they had lost during the year, whereas the participants in all of the behavioral groups maintained weight losses. In sum, continued therapist contact, longer treatment, and cognitive-behavioral approaches appear necessary for greater weight loss maintenance.

Combined Treatments

As is the case with other disorders, the question arises with regard to whether the effects of behavior therapy and medication might be synergistic. Several studies involving the combination of appetite-suppressant drugs, such as fenfluramine, and behavior therapy have been reported. The most impressive of these found an advantage in terms of weight loss for the group receiving fenfluramine at the end of treatment (Craighead et al. 1981). However, at 1-year follow-up this result was reversed, with those receiving medication regaining more weight than those receiving behavior therapy. The combined-treatment group lost less weight at this time than did those who were treated with behavior therapy alone. It may have been the case that patients receiving medication attributed their weight losses to the medication and thus did not practice the behavior changes needed to maintain the weight losses. The withdrawal of fenfluramine and dexfenfluramine from the market because of their linkage with cardiac valvular damage in a substantial number of cases has reduced the number of available appetite suppressant agents. Sibutramine has been approved for use in the treatment of obesity, and phentermine remains on the market because there is no evidence of a relationship between cardiac damage and the latter medication.

Wadden et al. (2007) found that the addition of a behavioral approach and a portion-controlled diet to pharmacological management of obesity significantly improved weight loss and patients' satisfaction with treatment outcome. At 12 months, obese patients had lost 4.1% of their initial body weight with sibutramine treatment alone, 10.8% when behavioral treatment was added to sibutramine, and 16.5% when behavioral treatment plus a meal-replacement approach using prepackaged food was added to sibutramine treatment.

Headache

The research literature on the treatment of both tension and migraine headache suggests that relaxation and bio-feedback procedures are equally effective. Relaxation training is simpler to apply and should thus be the preferred treatment. Both relaxation training and biofeedback are more effective in reducing the number and intensity of tension or migraine headaches than either no treatment or treatment with various types of placebos. One study, however, suggests that patients who do respond to relaxation training may benefit from bio-feedback. Follow-up studies show good maintenance for patients who improved with treatment; however, a fairly large percentage of individuals, perhaps 40%, are nonresponders. For the responder, studies have suggested that booster sessions may lead to lowered relapse rates. The mechanism of action of relaxation training and related procedures in the treatment of headache is uncertain, although it seems likely that lowering of sympathetic nervous system activity is the basis for the effect.

Primary Insomnia

Sleep disturbance uncomplicated by other psychiatric or physical disorders is a common problem in medical practice. Given the potential deleterious effects of long-term use of hypnotic agents, it should not be treated for longer than a few days with medication. Thus, the discovery and testing of nonpharmacological approaches to the treatment of sleep-onset insomnia are important.

Two behavior therapy approaches to sleep disturbance have been shown to be effective in controlled studies. Both of these approaches decrease the amount of time before sleep onset as measured by self-report and polysomnography. The first of these treatments, relaxation training, is based on the rationale that anxiety and other distractions preventing sleep onset can be controlled with such training. The second treatment, stimulus control, is based on the theory that sleep onset should be signaled by a narrow range of stimuli—that is, being in bed in a dark room and feeling drowsy—and that for many patients with sleep-onset disturbance the connection between these stimuli and sleep has broken down. Thus, stimulus control treatment consists of removing distractions such as books, television, and radio from the bedroom. In addition, patients are instructed to get up if they do not fall asleep within 10 minutes and are further instructed not to go back to bed until they are drowsy. It has been shown that this treatment is more effective than relaxation training (Lacks et al. 1983). The preferred treatment approach to uncomplicated sleep-onset disturbance should now be stimulus control training combined with discontinuance of hypnotic medication.

Stress Management

Relaxation training is useful in ameliorating many symptoms of stress, including anxiety, tension headache, and sleep disturbance. In addition, relaxation training appears to modify the Type-A behavior pattern, an independent risk factor for cardiovascular disease. Type A behavior, which may represent a maladaptive response to life stress, consists of aggressive striving, time urgency, irritability, and impatience. A long-term controlled study involving patients who had myocardial infarction demonstrated that it was possible to modify this pattern of behavior with an educational treatment regimen based on relaxation training and that reduction in Type A behavior was associated with fewer recurrent myocardial infarctions (Friedman et al. 1984).

Adherence to a Medical Regimen

A number of controlled studies have demonstrated that behavior change approaches can improve adherence to the medical regimen, particularly medication taking. Appointment keeping, one of the first steps in adherence, has been shown to improve with the use of simple reminder strategies (e.g. a telephone call or a reminder card). Controlled studies suggest that appointment keeping can be improved from levels of approximately 70% to levels of more than 90% with the use of these simple; strategies, thereby improving the cost-effectiveness of medical care (Gates and Colborn, 1976).

Compliance with medication taking has also been shown to be poor: approximately half of all patients take medication as prescribed, a further 20% take medication approximately 80% of the time, and the remainder take either no medication or very little medication. Behavior change strategies are aimed at several aspects of the problem (Agras 1989). First, the patient's expectations about the effectiveness of the proposed treatment are explored. If the patient does not expect the treatment to work, he or she will be unlikely to adhere to the prescribed regimen. For example, a negative experience of a relative or friend with the prescribed treatment may affect the expectations of a patient regarding outcome. Education regarding the short- and long-term benefits of the medical regimen is important in helping to promote a positive expectation regarding treatment. Second, the complexity of the regimen should be examined, because it has been shown that the more complex the regimen, the poorer the compliance. This includes an examination of all the medications that the patient is currently taking and an attempt to fit the new medication into the current regimen. Third, it has been demonstrated that patients quickly forget instructions given by their physicians; this underlines the need for written instructions. Fourth, it appears important to tie medication taking to other regularly scheduled behaviors (e.g. mealtimes, bedtime) and to have the pills stored in such a way that they are easily accessible at such times. Finally, the early handling of side effects to medication appears critical in maintaining adequate adherence. Patients with preexisting symptoms similar to the side effects of a medication appear particularly likely to prematurely discontinue taking medication. Identification of such symptoms before beginning medication is therefore important.

Cancer

One important role of behavior therapy in the treatment of patients with cancer is the reduction of anxiety and nausea associated with cancer chemotherapy, an example of classical conditioning. Relaxation training can be used for patients who do not respond to modern antiemetic agents. Controlled studies demonstrate that such treatment is effective in reducing anxiety, nausea, and vomiting. Unfortunately, little is known about the comparative effects of medication and relaxation training in reducing nausea and vomiting or whether these two treatment modalities augment each other. A second role of behavior therapy is to enhance coping with cancer. In a randomized controlled study involving patients in whom malignant melanoma had been newly diagnosed, Fawzy et al. (1993) used a structured 6-week group intervention with components including health education, stress management, coping skills, and supportive group psychotherapy. There were several interesting findings. First, the group receiving the intervention used significantly more active-coping methods than did the control (usual care) group. Second, the active-treatment group experienced notable immunological changes. Third, at 6-year follow-up there was a strong trend for recurrence to be lower, and survival to be longer, in the active-treatment group. These results are similar to those of Spiegel et al. (1989), who employed a 1-year program of supportive expressive group psychotherapy in women with breast cancer. After 1 year of treatment, the group receiving active treatment showed markedly less anxiety and pain than did the control group. In addition, at 10-year follow-up, length of survival time was superior for the group receiving the active treatment. Because the two treatments differed from one another, it is possible that some common mechanism was responsible for the observed results.

Disorders of Childhood

Behavior therapy for children's disorders has been based on the use of operant conditioning, particularly the application of reinforcement procedures. This model emphasizes that behavior is a function of its consequences. Maladaptive behaviors are hypothesized to be learned as a result of complex reinforcement and punishment schedules in specific social environments. By analyzing the contingencies surrounding a behavior, one may change it by altering those contingencies. More recently, therapeutic procedures found to be useful in adults (e.g. in the treatment of anxiety disorder, depression, and OCD) have been successfully applied to children. Selected areas in the treatment of children's disorders are reviewed in the following subsections.

Autism

Autism, a pervasive developmental disorder, is no longer considered to be psychogenic in origin and is now viewed as a central nervous system disorder (Cohen and Shaywitz, 1982). Lovaas et al. (1971, 1979) made an important contribution to our understanding of autism by identifying the perceptual problem of *stimulus over-selectivity*. When a variety of stimuli are presented to autistic children, as is the case in almost every social contact, only one portion is attended to, and there is a lack of response to the complex stimulus and its meaning. In one study, normal children were able to respond to each component (auditory, visual, and tactile) of a complex cue, while the autistic child responded selectively to only one cue and not the others. Thus, the autistic child's response to situations often appears bizarre. No evidence of sensory deficits is found. When simple cues are presented to autistic children, behavioral responding is more consistent. When well-defined cues are used, along with immediate and tangible reinforcers, desired behaviors can gradually be shaped. Behavioral excesses (e.g. tantrums, aggression, self-stimulatory behaviors) may be either punished (using, for example, time-out from reinforcement, in which a child might be put in a room alone for a few minutes contingent on disruptive behavior) or, if mild, ignored with the aim of weakening them (an example of the removal of reinforcement, i.e. extinction), therapists and parents can be trained to teach autistic children in this way, and environments can be designed to reinforce desired behaviors systematically. Lovaas (1977) also developed methods to teach language skills to autistic children. Such children are able to learn but require very specific programming. Verbal skills are taught progressively, first with the use of reinforcement for attending to the teacher, then by the use of imitation, then by labeling objects, followed by stating simple sentences. Autistic children are able to improve their language skills substantially with this method; however, improvement is correlated with IQ, and maintenance depends on continued reinforcement. Increasing language skills can also initiate socialization in children with severe language deficiencies.

In a controlled study, Lovaas (1977) provided intensive treatment to young autistic children and their parents. Parents, along with children, applied a home-based program using operant procedures over a 2-year period. The children received reinforcement for learning, communication, and social behaviors. After the trial, 47% of the children in the intervention group had been placed in regular first-grade classroom (and IQ levels had markedly increased compared with pretreatment levels), whereas none from the no-treatment control group were able to be placed in such a classroom setting. These results suggest that such early, intensive, and comprehensive treatment may be very useful in autism. Improvements in language and social functioning have also been supported in other studies using intensive behavioral programming, as summarized by Rogers (1998).

Combination Treatment

In a controlled study, Campbell et al. (1978) investigated the use of haloperidol or placebo versus contingent or non-contingent reinforcement in a language training program for hospitalized autistic children. Medication reduced stereotypical and withdrawn behavior in older, not younger, children, whereas contingency management improved ward behaviors and compliance and imitation in the language training program. The group receiving haloperidol and contingent reinforcement showed the greatest improvement.

Conduct Disorder

Parents often seek help for their children's behavior problems, including aggressiveness, destructiveness, oppositional behavior, temper tantrums, and other negative behaviors (e.g. whining, screaming, threatening). Numerous studies have described a high rate of what Patterson (1976) described as *coercive interactions* in families of these children. Parents of these children respond with coercive behaviors when attempting to control their children's misbehavior. Patterson described a negative reinforcement model in which the coercive behavior of the parent may be reinforced by the reduction of the aversive behavior of the child. Unfortunately, the parent also models punitive behaviors to the child, who is then trained to behave similarly. In addition, parents may, without intending to, positively reinforce the deviant behaviors, either by attending to them or by fulfilling a demand accompanied by the deviant behavior (Wahler

1976). Often a parent will spend considerable effort and time with a child in attempting to abort a temper tantrum, and this approach may in fact reinforce the behavior.

To address such problems, the primary research effort has been in training parents to use social learning techniques to shape more adaptive and prosocial behaviors in their children. Such programs (Patterson 1976) have taught parents to monitor both prosocial and deviant behaviors, develop positive reinforcement systems (e.g. contingent point systems for obtaining rewards), use extinction (i.e. ignoring) for minor misbehaviors, and use punishment (e.g. time-out) for serious infractions. Christophersen et al. (1972) examined the use of a home reinforcement system (i.e. token economy) with observations by parents and reliability checks by the experimenters. The token economy is a systematic use of contingent reinforcement using tokens (often points or stars) earned by the child for prosocial behaviors and later used to purchase privileges or desired items. This approach led to a marked reduction in deviant behaviors and increase in prosocial behaviors.

Christophersen et al. (1976) also compared the parent training and home token economy system with conventional outpatient treatment for children with conduct disorder. Parents using the token economy reported a 67% reduction in deviant behavior, whereas those using traditional treatment reported only a 34% reduction. Similar systems have been designed and have been found useful in the classroom, psychiatric inpatient programs, and residential treatment programs for children with behavioral disturbances.

There are, however; limits to the efficacy of such programs. It has been shown, for example, that marital discord is associated with conduct disorder in children. In such cases, improvement is unlikely until the marital discord has been addressed. Other complicating parental factors may include depression, substance abuse, or other psychopathology that will require therapeutic attention for the child to improve using behavioral techniques.

Kazdin and colleagues (Kazdin et al. 1987) reviewed in great detail the behavioral treatments for conduct and oppositional disorders and suggested that the more severe the conduct disorder, the more guarded the outcome. They studied the combined effects of parent management training (using behavioral techniques described earlier in the chapter) and a cognitive behavioral problem-solving skills training approach for the children, the latter approach aimed at improving maladaptive thinking patterns. Such patterns seen in aggressive children, they noted, include the lack of problem solving skills and the tendency to believe that others are antagonistic toward them. Those children receiving the combined treatment exhibited less aggressive behavior at home and in school, along with greater overall prosocial behaviors, than did the contact-control group, both following treatment and at 1-year follow-up. Further controlled work is much needed so that more powerful therapies for this important disorder can be developed.

Kazdin (1987) and others advocated earlier treatment for children and their families, that is, treatment before the children became heavily involved in antisocial behaviors and involved in the juvenile justice system. Such research should focus on early intervention to minimize the severity of the conduct disorder and the frequency of antisocial behaviors.

One study (Dumas and Wahler 1985) evaluated mother-child dyads participating in a parent-training program for children with conduct disorder. Mothers who had a low level of community contact (i.e. insular mothers) used more aversive control toward their children than did mothers with a higher level of community contacts. Children of the insular mothers were more aggressive than those of noninsular mothers in general, and in particular when responding to negative maternal behavior. Increasing contacts with friends and social supports in the community may help reduce negative interpersonal interactions.

A number of studies now report that behavioral techniques and parent management training for the treatment of childhood conduct problems can produce significant improvement in child behavior (reviewed by Kazdin 1998). Maintenance of these gains has been found in follow-ups of 1–3 years; one program has even reported maintenance of gains for 10–14 years (Long et al. 1994).

Attention-deficit/Hyperactivity Disorder

Attention-deficit/hyperactivity disorder (ADHD) and associated learning disabilities may occur in more than 5% of children in the United States. Hyperactive children demonstrate excessive motor activity, distractibility, and impulsivity, which cause adjustment difficulties both at home and in school. These children often have difficulty when concentration is required for task completion. Behavioral studies using contingent reinforcement of desired behaviors in this population demonstrated that when teachers differentially attended to and reinforced appropriate classroom behavior, deviant behavior was reduced (Becker et al. 1967). Children who were rewarded for increasing academic work through use of free time or through participation in preferred classroom activities made considerable academic gains that were well maintained. Maintenance in school-related gains has been enhanced by the addition of parental reinforcement (Ayllon et al. 1975). When children brought home a good-behavior letter, one indicating cooperation and a reduced level of deviant behavior, they could select home-based rewards (e.g. praise, more allowance money); failure to bring home the letter resulted in an earlier bedtime or withholding of allowance.

Ayllon et al. (1975) evaluated academic performance in children who had been taking methylphenidate and who continued to do poorly academically. When methylphenidate therapy was discontinued, their hyperactivity increased. A token program was instituted whereby first work in math and then work in both math and reading were reinforced. Not only did academic performance improve, but the hyperactivity decreased. The behaviors incompatible with learning were reduced if the child was successful academically. A number of studies have begun to evaluate whether interactive effects exist when both behavioral and pharmacological interventions are used. Controlled studies suggest that medication reduces hyperactive behaviors but does little for either the learning deficits or the impulsive and aggressive behaviors associated with this disorder (Gadow 1985). Thus, a combination of behavior therapy and medication is most commonly used in the treatment of ADHD.

Combination Treatment

Pelham et al. (1993) compared an intensive behavioral intervention with pharmacological treatment (methylphenidate) for children with ADHD. Although both the behavioral and the pharmacological interventions resulted in significant improvements in hyperactive and impulsive behaviors, the effect sizes were greater with the pharmacological treatment. A major clinical trial, the Multimodal Treatment Study of Children with ADHD (1999), examined whether intensive behavioral treatment, when combined with pharmacological treatment, provided added benefits. The subjects who received the combination of behavior therapy plus medication did not differ in measures of hyperactivity from those receiving medication alone. However, those receiving behavior therapy plus medication showed greater improvements than did the medication-alone group in a number of areas—oppositional and aggressive symptoms, social skills, parent-child relations, and achievement in reading—compared with those children who received only the behavioral intervention without medication or the community intervention. These findings suggest that the combination of behavioral and pharmacological treatment may be useful to maximize treatment response in children with ADHD.

Ruminative Vomiting

Ruminative vomiting is seen in infants and in mentally retarded individuals of all ages. Milk, or food in the case of the older child, is regurgitated and spat out. Because in—infancy this condition is often life threatening, the principal approach to treatment has been within a punishment paradigm. Punishment is much less useful as a therapeutic procedure than positive reinforcement, because there are unwanted side effects such as aggressive behavior and there is always the possibility of inflicting physical harm. For the most part, punishment is used only in situations in which the behavior to be changed threatens injury to the patient and only when procedures using positive reinforcement have been found not to lead to improvement. In institutions where punishment processes are frequently used, it is essential that an oversight committee be appointed to monitor the use of punishment.

Infants with ruminative vomiting regurgitate their food mouthful by mouthful, which leads to malnutrition and dehydration and thus poses a threat to life. One approach to treatment is to use the principle of punishment, whereby an unpleasant event is made contingent on each episode of regurgitation. In one controlled study, a drop of lemon juice on the tongue was used as the unpleasant event. During baseline measurement, before treatment was begun, the infant ruminated between 40% and 70% of the time the infant was awake (Sajwaj et al. 1974). Once lemon juice was presented contingent on spitting up food, the rate of ruminative vomiting decreased steadily. Punishment was then briefly removed, and rumination quickly returned to original baseline levels, confirming the effectiveness of lemon juice as a punishing event. Reintroduction of punishment led to disappearance of the behavior and a return to normal weight, with no relapse at 1-year follow-up. Similar procedures have been used successfully in mentally retarded ruminating individuals.

Childhood Depression

Behavioral treatment of childhood depression has been added on the demonstrably successful treatment of adult depression using either social skills training or a more comprehensive CBT package. The treatment package used with depressed children is similar to that used with adults and is aimed at decreasing depressive thinking, enhancing social skills, and increasing pleasant activities. Several controlled single-case studies have shown the effectiveness of either the whole cognitive-behavioral package or an element of the package (e.g. social skills training). However, many of these studies focused their assessment of improvement on the specific skills taught, rather than on depression. In one controlled study, it was found that some 50% of adolescents no longer met criteria for depression after treatment, whereas little change was observed in the waiting-list control group. There was continued improvement over a 2-year follow-up: fewer than 10% met criteria for depression at 1 year, and fewer than 20% met criteria at 2 years. This finding suggests that although not everyone improves, the effects of treatment are long lasting. Interestingly, adding therapy for the parents of these children produced no added benefits. Other studies suggest that younger children respond equally well to treatment, but, as with adults, there tends to be no difference between different types of active treatment.

In a randomized controlled trial of adolescents with major depression, Brent et al. (1997) found that CBT resulted in a higher rate of remission (65% achieved absence of depression) compared with individual supportive therapy (39%) or systemic family therapy (38%). The rate of remission was also greater with CBT compared with the other treatments.

Behavioral Pediatrics

As in the case of adults, behavioral approaches have been used increasingly in pediatric populations with medical problems. Chronic diseases in childhood often require complex behavior changes for optimal treatment. Such is the case, for example, for the child with insulin-dependent diabetes mellitus who must comply with medications, diet, and exercise. Epstein et al. (1981) developed an educational intervention aimed at increasing knowledge and skills, using instruction, feedback concerning performance, and reinforcement. The content included insulin dosage, diet, exercise, self-administration of insulin, and the signs and symptoms of hypoglycemia. Parents participated, encouraging child adherence. Substantial improvements were made: urine samples were negative for glucose in 27% of cases during treatment, 39% after treatment, and 45% at 2-month follow-up. Reinforcement systems have also been used to help children adhere to the demands of hemodialysis (Magrab and Papadopoulou, 1977). Children were encouraged to adhere to diet and were rewarded with prizes for improvements in weight and in potassium and blood urea nitrogen levels. Similar reinforcement approaches have been helpful in larger populations, such as for the encouragement of attendance at dental facilities by low-income families (Reiss et al. 1976).

Modeling has proved useful in reducing children's fears before medical procedures. Melamed and Siegel (1975), in a randomized, controlled study, studied children who were about to have surgery. One group of children in the study viewed a film about a child coping with hospitalization and medical procedures, whereas the control group saw a film on another topic. Directly after this film, the experimental group demonstrated more physiological arousal. However, before surgery and a month later, both self-report of fear and physiological arousal were notably less in the experimental group. Fewer children in the experimental group required pain medication after surgery or complained of side effects, and more returned to eating solid foods sooner. This procedure is an excellent example of the use of modeling to aid in adaptive coping with a stressful life event.

47.12 COGNITIVE THERAPY: CURRENT STATUS AND FUTURE DIRECTIONS

JN Vyas, SS Nathawat

OVERVIEW

From its inception more than 45 years ago,[149-151] cognitive therapy has been theory driven. Specifically, Beck's objectives for deriving and evaluating this system of psychotherapy involved an overall plan to construct a comprehensive theory of psychopathology that maps clearly onto the treatment approach, to investigate scientific support for the theory, and to test the efficacy of therapeutic interventions.[151,152] Cognitive theory and therapy were first developed for depression[149-151] and later systematically applied to suicide prevention,[153] anxiety disorders,[154] personality disorders,[155] substance abuse,[156] and most recently, schizophrenia.[157,158]

Cognitive therapy (CT), often discussed under the generic label cognitive behavior therapy (CBT), is now widely represented in training programs in psychology, psychiatry, medicine, social work, nursing and other allied health professions that value evidence-based practice.[159] CT and CBT have been described as "the fasters growing and most heavily researched systems of psychotherapy on the contemporary scene". This article provides a brief overview of the conceptual, practical, and empirical aspects of CT. After highlighting some of its basic concepts and the research pertaining to Beck's cognitive theory, we discuss the general approach to treatment and review the literature in its efficacy.

COGNITIVE THEORY

Cognitive theory is based on the presumption that information processing is crucial for human adaptation and survival. Without the ability to process information from the environment, synthesize it, and formulate a plan for dealing with it, we would not survive. The cognitive (or information processing) system is intricately tied to other affective, motivational, and behavioral repertoires.[160] Each of these repertoires, or systems, serves an individual function and also operates in synchrony toward coordinated, goal-oriented strategies (e.g., approaching pleasure, avoiding pain).[161,162] The fight-flight response, for instance, arises from four systems:[161] cognitive (perception of threat), affective (feelings of anxiety or anger), motivational (the impulse to confront or feel the threatening stimulus), and behavioral (the implementation of action). In this construct, onset of a particular condition (e.g., panic disorder) is believed to occur when these different systems shift from a fairly quiescent state to a highly activated state. In the example of panic disorder,

Table 26: The cognitive profile psychological disorders[14]

Disorder	*Systematic bias in processing information*
Depression	Negative view of self, experience, and future
Hypomania	Inflated view of self and future
Anxiety disorder	Sense of physical or psychological danger
Panic disorder	Catastrophic interpretation of bodily/mental experiences
Phobia	Sense of danger in specific, avoidable situations
Paranoid state	Attribution of bias to others
Hysteria	Concept of motor or sensory abnormality
Obsession	Repeated warning or doubts about safety
Compulsion	Rituals to ward off perceived threat
Suicidal behavior	Hopelessness and deficiencies in problem solving
Anorexia nervosa	Fear of being fat
Hypochondriasis	Attribution of serious medical disorder

this might occur when the fight-flight response is activated by "false alarms" (e.g., misperceiving bodily sensations as harmful to the organism). Cognitive theory suggests that psychopathology is characterized by the activation of a conglomerate of related or contiguous dysfunctional beliefs, meanings and memories that operate in coordination with affect, motivation, behavior, and physiological responses. Different psychopathological conditions are associated with specific biases that influence how an individual incorporates and responds to new information (Table 26).

According to Beck's model[149-151,154,163,164] the cognitive appraisal of internal or external stimuli influences and is, in turn, impacted by these other systems. Thus, although cognition plays a key role in this model (i.e., the assignment of meaning is crucial to understanding maladaptive behavior), it is recognized that mental health problems involve a complex interplay among diverse and interrelated systems.[165]

Within the cognitive system are different levels of cognition, ranging from surface-level thoughts to "deeper" cognitive schemas.[166,167] Cognitive schemas are organized structures of stored information that contain individuals perceptions of self and others, goals, expectations, and memories. These elements are well organized within the cognitive structure[168] and influence the screening, coding, categorization, and interpretation of incoming stimuli and the retrieval of stored information. Schemas are adaptive insofar as they afford efficient processing of information; however, when they become negatively biased, maladaptive, rigid, and self-perpetuating, they can contribute to psychopathology.

Maladaptive cognitive schemas are believed to develop during early periods of the life span and become increasingly consolidated and organized as new experiences are assimilated into the existing belief structure.[151,163] Poor early attachment experiences and other adverse events (e.g., childhood maltreatment), for example, may contribute to the development of a maladaptive belief system. Cognitive theory is essentially a diathesis-stress model. In other words, it is possible to have a maladaptive belief system and not exhibit symptoms so long as the cognitive schema (and related systems) is not activated. Once triggered by external events, drugs, or endocrine factors, however, the cognitive schema triggers a cascade of information-processing biases.[149,152,164,166] These may be attention, memory, or interpretational biases.

The activation of maladaptive cognitive schema, along with the ensuing information processing biases, is also apparent in more surface level cognitions or what are referred to as automatic thoughts. This term refers to the stream of positive and negative thoughts that runs through an individual's mind unaccompanied by direct, conscious deliberation. Although such thoughts are more superficial and proximal to a given situation than are other levels of cognition, they are functionally related to one's deeper beliefs and schemas and seem to arise associatively as different aspects of one's core belief system are activated.

When negative cognitive schemas are activated, as in depression, they are not only identifiable but can be shown to have an influence on information processing, as manifested by cognitive biases, and have an impact on symptom development, When a depressive episode has remitted, the negative schemas are deactivated (or vice versa).

Another aspect of Beck's model is content specificity.[164,165] That is, different emotional experiences and froms of psychopathology are related to a unique cognitive profile or set of beliefs to illustrate, depression is related to thoughts and beliefs concerning personal loss, deprivation, and failure.[163] Persons with clinically signification anxiety tend to overestimate the probability of risk while simultaneously underestimating their resources for coping with potential threats. Their thoughts focus on themes of the self as vulnerable, the world as dangerous, and the future as potentially catastrophic.[154] A person with dependent personality disorder has a view of the self as weak, helpless, and incompetent.[7]

The empirical literature has provided considerable support for various aspects of Beck's cognitive theory. Hundreds of studies have demonstrated that individuals filter information and respond to stimuli in a way that is consistent with their pre-existing beliefs and assumptions. Some research has also demonstrated that negative cognitive biases precede the development of anxious[169] and depressive[170] symptoms. Supportive evidence has been obtained of the ideas that there are distinct levels of cognition that work in synchrony to impact emotional and behavioral responses and that an emotional experience or clinical disorder can be characterized by a unique set of beliefs and automatic thoughts (i.e., content specificity.[164,166] Schema organization,[166] activation,[171] and the contribution of cognitive vulnerability to the incidence of psychiatric disorders[172] have also been supported by empirical research.

COGNITIVE THERAPY

Cognitive therapy (CT) rests on three main propositions:[173,174]

1. *The access hypothesis*: With appropriate training, motivation, and attention, individuals can become aware of the content and process of their thinking.
2. *The mediation hypothesis*: The manner in which individuals think about, interpret, and construe events influences their emotional and behavioral responses.
3. *The change hypothesis*: Individuals can become more functional and adaptive by intentionally modifying their cognitive and behavioral response to the circumstances they face.

Cognitive therapy is a structured, collaborative process that helps individuals to consider both the accuracy and usefulness of their thought processes of exploration (determining one's idiosyncratic meaning system and maladaptive beliefs), examination (reviewing the evidence for and against a particular belief and considering alternative interpretations or explanations), and experimentation testing the validity of one's belief system).[175] This general approach is used early in therapy to target more proximal and surface-level cognition (e.g., automatic thoughts, dysfunctional attitudes) and in later sessions to modify deeper cognitive structures and core beliefs.

CT is not the replacement of negative thoughts with positive ones; rather, it aims to help individuals shift their cognitive appraisal from ones that are unhealthy and maladaptive to ones that are evidence-based and adaptive. Essentially, patients learn how to become scientific investigators of their own thinking to treat thoughts as hypotheses rather than as facts and to put these thoughts to the test. Framing a belief as a hypothesis provides an opportunity to test its validity, affords patients the ability to consider alternative explanations and permits them to gain distance from a thought to allow more objective scrutiny.[159] Patients learn to modify their thoughts so that they are congruent with existing evidence. When thoughts are aligned with evidence, and negative feelings exist, the cognitive therapist helps patient to deal with emotional sequels by introducing coping strategies, fostering skill development and/or problem solving.

Cognitive therapists help patients to move through the process of exploration, examination, and experimentation using collaborative empiricism, guided discovery, and socratic dialogue.[176] Collaborative empiricism means that the patient and the therapist become coinvestigators both in ascertaining the goals for treatment and investigating the patient's thoughts. Methods of guided discovery are used to help patients to test their own thinking through personal observations and experiments rather than via cajoling or persuasion. Through this process, patients are able to shift form "a conviction mode to a questioning mode". In addition, by collaboratively designing new experiences to try out (called behavioral experiments), patients are able to acquire a different perspective on themselves and their situations.[14] Socratic dialogue is a method of guided discovery in which the therapist asks a series of carefully sequenced questions to help define problems, assist in the identification of thoughts and beliefs, examine the meaning of events, or assess the ramifications of particular thoughts or behaviors.

CT is time limited. The average length of CT in outcome studies is between 12 and 24 weekly sessions, although there is more variability in clinical practice.[173] The initial sessions are often focused on enhancing the therapeutic alliance, identifying the specific problem(s) that bought the patient into treatment, socializing the patient to the cognitive understanding of psychopathology, and symptom relief via behavioral strategies. At this time, the therapist plays a more active role than the patient. As therapy progresses, the emphasis shifts from symptom amelioration to the examination and modification of the patient's patterns of thinking, and the patient assumes a more active role in identifying problems and solutions and developing homework assignments. Toward the end of therapy, sessions are usually spread apart so that the patient can consolidate gains and increase his or her confidence in the application of newly learned skills. "Booster" Sessions are frequently scheduled one or two months after the end therapy.

Homework assignments (also called action plans) are an important component of CT. Homework provides opportunities to enhance the mastery and generalization of skills learned in the weekly therapy session by applying them in the "real world", and improves treatment outcome.[177]

The specific techniques utilized in CT tend to vary depending on the disorder being treated and the case formulation. They typically include (a) establishing the therapy relationship, (b) behavioral change strategies, (c) cognitive restructuring strategies, (d) modification of core beliefs and schemas, and (e) prevention of relapse/recurrence.

The therapeutic relationship is a key ingredient of all psychotherapies, including CT. There appears to be a bidirectional relationship between the patient's perception of the therapeutic alliance and outcome: The connection between patient and therapist may facilitate change, and symptom change, in turn, enhances the bond between patient and therapist.[159] Many of the basic interpersonal variables common to other psychotherapies (e.g., warmth, accurate empathy, unconditional positive regard) serve as an important foundation for cognitive and symptomatic change. As Beck et al.[163] noted, however, these characteristics "in themselves are necessary but not sufficient to produce an optimum therapeutic effect."

Behavioral strategies are used to test and alter automatic thoughts and assumptions and to facilitate new learning. In a behavioral experiment, for instance, a patient may predict an outcome based on his or her automatic thoughts and beliefs, conduct an agreed upon behavior, and evaluate the evidenced in the context of the results of this new experiment. A related approach is hypothesis testing, which has both cognitive and behavioral components. A resident who insists. "I am not a good doctor," for example, can be asked to generate a list of characteristics or criteria that would constitute being a good physician (e.g., ability to establish rapport; knowledge base; capacity for making decision under pressure). The "experiment" would then involved collecting data by monitoring his or her behavior and seeking input from colleagues and supervisors which may help to modify this conviction (e.g., "I am a good doctor for my level of experience and training").[162] Other behavioral techniques are used to alter the patient's reinforcement schedule (therapy increasing pleasure or mastery), habituate to feared stimuli (exposure therapy), relax (Progressive muscle relaxation), or prepare for upcoming situations (behavioral rehearsal). Given that these strategies are used to foster cognitive change, the therapist routinely assesses the patient's perceptions, thoughts, and conclusions after each experiment.[14]

Cognitive restructuring strategies are also used to help patients identify and test the validity of their cognition. One important technique for eliciting and evaluating negative automatic thoughts is the Daily Record of Thoughts (DRT). A DRT entry consists of three columns representing the situation encountered, the emotion or symptoms experienced, and associated thoughts. Once patients are reliably able to identify the automatic thoughts that carry the greatest emotional charge, the process of answering back to these thoughts (or putting them on trial) can begin. This process often involves writing down the evidence that pertains to a particular belief and developing and alternative thought that incorporates the facts that bear on the belief. By writing down an activating event, the mediating thoughts, and the ensuing emotional response, the patient maintaining a DRT achieves more objectivity about and distance from his or her thoughts. The evidence pertaining to a particular belief is then examined using guided discovery and collaborative empiricism.

Specifically, patients are asked a number of questions, including: "what is the evidence for or against this believe" "What are the alternative ways to think about this situation?" "If my best friend or loved one knew that I had this thought, what would he or she say to me"? "What would it mean about me even if this particular thought was true?".[173,178-180] From this analysis of the evidence, patients are then taught to generate alternative thoughts that incorporate the evidence and lead to a shift in their emotional experience. If a given thought is inconsistent with the weight of factual evidence on the subject (e.g., "I am unlovable"), the therapist helps the patient to alter and realign the thought so that it is evidence based and, consequently, more adaptive and helpful. Sometimes collecting more information of conducting a behavioral experiment is also used to test a certain belief.

After a number of sessions using the DRT, the therapist and patient may notice a consistent pattern in the types of automatic thoughts that are elicited. This is because automatic thoughts and cognitive distortions (e.g., "If I fail at x, then I am not worthwhile") are functionally related to deeper core beliefs and schemas. The modification of these core beliefs and schemas is believed to result in the most generalizable change and the greatest prevention of relapse.[181,182] These "deeper" beliefs are tested and reconfigured using Socratic dialogue and guided discovery, role plays, behavioral experiments, and other change strategies.[159,163,173,178]

The final sessions of treatment are focused on consolidating the skills learned and on the prevention of relapse/recurrence. This includes, among other things, a gradual relation of sessions and spreading apart of their timing, reviewing the treatment strategies that were utilized and were most helpful, creating a plan for the future, discussing feelings about the termination of therapy, preparing for setbacks, identifying possible triggers of relapse and ensuring that the patient makes internal attributions for change.

EMPIRICAL EVIDENCE OF COGNITIVE THERAPY

CT/CBT is one of the most actively researched psychotherapies[183] and has received consistent empirical support for a host of mental health problems and conditions.[184,185] We focus first on the efficacy of CT for depression, as this has been most extensively studied, and also highlight findings for other psychiatric disorders and medical illness.

CT for Unipolar Depression

More than 75 clinical trials and numerous meta-analyses have been published on CT for unipolar depression.[183] For an acute episode of depression, the response achieved with CT is similar to that achieved with behavior therapy,[186] other bona fide psychological treatments,[187] and antidepressant medication, and all of these produce results superior to placebo.[175,188] Early finding[189] suggesting that CT was not effective for severe depression[190] have generated considerable controversy among researchers, and the perception that CT is not effective for severe depression has persisted despite compelling data to suggest otherwise. DeRubeis et al.[191] for example, conducted a mega-analysis in which they pooled the data from four related trials and found that CT was as effective as antidepressants (imipramine and nortriptyline) for the treatment of severely depressed individuals. More recent studies have also demonstrated that CT and pharmacotherapy (paroxetine) are equally effective for severe depression.[192,193] The weight of evidence suggests that CT/CBT is efficacious for depression, though it remains possible that the effect may be somewhat over estimated as a result of publication bias (e.g., the file-drawer effect).[194]

In addition to its efficacy for acute phase of major depressive disorder, CT also carries an advantage, relative to antidepressant medication, for the prevention of relapse. Gloaguen et al.[195] for instance, reported that the average risk of relapse (based on follow-up periods of one to two years) was 25% following CT compared to 60% following antidepressant medication. Some studies also indicated that patients who receive CT alone are one more likely to relapse after treatment than are those who continue to receive medication.[193,196] Hollon et al.[193] found equal outcomes between medication and CT in the acute phase treatment, but a lower relapse rate for CT compared to continuance medication.

Consistent with these findings are studies that have examined potential mechanisms for the prophylactic benefits of CT. It appears that CT and antidepressant medication may both change certain aspects of negative thinking (such as information Processing, automatic thoughts, and dysfunctional attitudes[170,171] but that CT may further modify some of the "deeper" cognitive structures (e.g., reduced activation of negative thinking following a negative mood manipulation in CT relative to pharmacotherapy) that give rise to relapse and recurrence.[171,181,182,197] Several studies have also assessed neuroimaging changes in cognitive therapy.[198] Goldapple et al.[199] for example, examined neurobiological responses to CT (in unmedicated depressed outpatients) and compared these finding to an independent sample of individuals treated with selective serotonin reuptake inhibitors (SSRIs). Differential pre-versus post-treatment changes in brain metabolic activity (measured by position emission tomography) were obtained in individual treated with CT compared to those treated with antidepressant medication. These researchers proposed that a top down (cortical limbic) therapeutic mechanism may have been active in CT, whereas a bottom up limbic cortical) mechanism may have been active in antidepressant treatment.

CT for Other Psychiatric Disorders

Butler et al.[183] reviewed meta-analyses of treatment outcome for CT/CBT for a number of psychological disorders. A total of 16 methodologically rigorous meta-analysis were identified from 1967 to 2004, which incorporated 9,995 research participants in 332 studies. The review focused on effect sizes found by studies the compared outcomes of CT/CBT with outcomes for control groups, providing an overview of the efficacy of CT/CBT. Large effect sizes were obtained for patients with unipolar depression, generalized anxiety, and childhood internalizing problems (the latter included depressive, anxious, and somatic disorders). Moderated effect sizes were found for patients treated for couple distress, anger, childhood somatoform disorders, and chronic pain. Small effect sizes were obtained for recidivism in sexual offenders. CBT also showed promising results as an adjunct to medication for schizophrenia.[158]

Epp and Dobson[188] recently reviewed the treatment-outcome literature for CT/CBT and summarized the meta-analytic data according to absolute efficacy (the extent to which CBT demonstrates superior outcome to no treatment, waitlist controls, or treatment as usual), efficacy relative to pharmacotherapy, and efficacy compared to other forms of psychotherapy (Table 27). Considerable empirical support has accumulated for the efficacy of CT/CBT. For some disorders (e.g., some anxiety disorders, bulimia nervosa), the evidence is compelling enough to suggest that CT/CBT should be considered the treatment of choice. The literature also suggests that CT/CBT is at least as effective as medication for a range of problems, although direct comparisons are not found for some disorders (e.g., bipolar disorder, psychosis) for which CT/CBT is used adjunctively.[173] A recent meta-analysis of CT/CBT in the treatment of schizophrenia, severe depression, and bipolar disorder was less positive,[200] suggesting that CT/CBT is no more effective than nonspecific interventions for the treatment of schizophrenia, although methodological flaws in the meta-analysis tend to vitiate the findings.[201]

CT for Medical Illnesses

CT/CBT is also effective for the treatment of anxiety and depression that are comorbid with medical problems.[202] In addition, a number of randomized controlled trials have reported benefits of CT/CBT for a wide range of physical illnesses including chronic pain, back pain, sleep disorders, fatigue and functional impairments related to cancer, health related anxiety, rheumatoid arthritis, chronic fatigue syndrome, fibromyalgia, irritable bowel syndrome, hypertension, tinnitus, headaches, sexual dysfunctions, and various neurological conditions.[202,203] CT/CBT has demonstrated efficacy for a number of psychological outcome variables (e.g., distress, attitudes, adherence to treatment regime, improved coping with pain) as well as physiological indices that are impacted by stress (e.g., lowered blood pressure, improved immune response.[202] For some illnesses, there have been a sufficient number of studies to warrant systematic review and meta-analysis. This literature demonstrates various biopsychosocial benefits of CT/CBT for back pain,[204,205] hypochrondriasis,[206] irritable bowel syndrome,[207] chronic fatigue[206,208] fibromyalgia,[209] headache,[210] insomnia,[211,212] adjustment to cancer,[213,214] and the management of diabetes.[215]

SUMMARY AND FUTURE DIRECTIONS

Considerable empirical evidence has accumulated that supports the theory and practice of CT, ant this model has been expanded over time to incorporate evidence from experimental

Table 27: Summary of efficacy findings by disorder or problem[188]

Disorder	*Treatment*	*Absolute efficacy*	*Efficacy relative to medications*	*Efficacy relative to other psychotherapies*
Unipolar depression	CBT	+	+	≃
Bipolar Disorder*	CBT	+		=
Specific phobia	Exposure and cognitive restructuring	++	+	+
Social phobia	Exposure and cognitive restructuring	++	≃	≃
Obsessive-compulsive disorder	Exposure and response prevention and cognitive restructuring	+		+
Panic disorder	Exposure and cognitive restructuring	++	≃	+
Chronic post-traumatic stress disorder	Exposure and cognitive techniques	+		=
Generalized anxiety disorder	CBT	+	+	+
Bulimia nervosa	CBT	+	+	+
Binge eating disorder	CBT	+		=
Anorexia nervosa	CBT	+	+	=
Schizophrenia*	CBT	+		+
Marital distress	CBT	+		≃
Anger and violent offending	CBT	+		
Sexual offending	CBT	+	–**	+
Chronic pain	CBT	+		≃
Borderline personality disorder	CBT	+		≃
Substance-use disorder	CBT	+		=
Somatoform disorder	CBT	+	+	+
Sleep difficulties	CBT	+	+	+

Symbols: A blank space indicates insufficient or no evidence;-, negative evidence; +, positive evidence; =, approximate equivalence; ++, treatment of choice; ≃ equivocal evidence; CBT, efficacy of specific components unknown;*, CBT is typically used as an adjunct to medication in these disorders; *, efficacy relative to physical treatment (i.e., surgical castration and hormonal treatments).

cognitive science and the neurosciences.[161,164,216] Moreover, several official reports in the United Kingdom and the United State have recommended the use of CT/CBT for a number of common psychiatric conditions.[152] Notwithstanding these treatment recommendations and the wealth of research underlying CT, it is not panacea for all mental health problems.[217] For example, more purely behavioral interventions sometimes perform as well as CT/CBT for depression and anxiety in psychotherapy outcome trials. It is important to point out, however, that the use of behavioral interventions has always been party and parcel of CT proper.[163] In addition, the theory states that whatever treatment is used so that the patient improves (or if improvement occurs via spontaneous remission), the negative belles must also normalize. Indeed, Harmer et al.[170] recently found that the administration of antidepressant medication modulated emotional processing depressed individuals prior to shifts in their mood state of symptoms. Such findings support the primacy of cognition in therapeutic change and are consistent with the idea that there are myriad ways in which to modify cognition. In addition to altering information processing however, we contend that CT also produces shifts in "deeper" levels of cognition[171,181] and that targeting this depth of change may account for reduced relapse rates in CT relative to medication.

There are a number of important future directions for the field. During the past couple of decades, we have witnessed a tremendous increase in multi wave longitudinal studies that have supported the diathesis-stress model of cognitive vulnerability.[18] Researchers are also better understanding gene environment interactions in the context of psychopathology. For example, a replicable relationship has been found between negative cognitive processing and the short version of the serotonin transporter gene.[216] Additional empirical work is necessary to further elucidate how generic, neurophysiological, environmental, and cognitive factors contribute to psychopathology and to understand the intricate relationship among cognitive, affective, motivational, and behavioral systems. Future research will no doubt also clarify the important mechanisms of change in CT. Some studies have, indeed, suggested the cognitive change is an important mediator of symptom change,[159,167,181] but additional are search is needed to ensure that these findings are robust and, if they are, to determine which strategies (and psychotherapeutic doses) produce the most stable cognitive change. Enormous strides have been made in understanding evaluating, and refining CT over the past four and a half decades.

SUMMARY POINTS

1. CT/CBT is the fastest growing and most researched contemporary system of psychotherapy.
2. The empirical literature has provided considerable support for Beck's cognitive theory and therapy.
3. Three main propositions in CT are the access hypothesis (it is possible for individuals to become aware of the content and processing of their thinking), the mediation hypothesis (the way in which individuals think about themselves and their circumstances impacts subsequent emotional and behavioral responses), and the change hypothesis (by modifying cognitive and behavioral responses, an individual can be become more functional and adaptive).
4. The main techniques used in CT focus on establishment of the therapeutic relationship behavioral change strategies, cognitive restructuring, the modification of core beliefs and schemas, and the prevention of relapse and recurrence.
5. A key advantage of CT is that it effectively treats the acute episode of psychiatric disorders (with or without medication) and provides a prophylaxis against relapse.

47.13 OCCUPATIONAL THERAPY

Sujata Malik

DEFINITION

In 1972, Susan B Fine prepared the following definition of occupational therapy for the American Occupational Therapy Association. "Occupational therapy is the application of goal directed, purposeful activity in the assessment and treatment of individuals with psychological, physical, or developmental disabilities. These services address the development and maintenance of adaptive skills and performance capacities which enable the patient to achieve optimal levels of function in such activities of daily living as work, self-care, socialization, and leisure time pursuits. The occupational therapist's functional assessments and treatment/rehabilitation methods are concerned with specific performance components which include, but are not limited to, motor, sensory-integrative, perceptual cognitive, psychological, and social interpersonal functions, as well as those environmental factors that inhibit performance."

The 'occupation' in the definition refers to "goal-directed use of time, energy, interest, and attention to foster adaptation and productivity; to minimize pathology; and to promote the maintenance of health."

Specific occupational therapy services in psychiatric settings may include, but are not limited to:

- Independent living skills, which include basic, practical and social living skills, focusing on self-care and self-maintenance.
- Task oriented treatment, using creative expressive modalities like painting, clay work, creative writing, socialization, education, leisure time activities, etc.
- Pre-vocational and work adjustment programs, which include preparation for employment and academics, home making, parenting, etc.
- Sensorimotor assessment and treatment, including neuromuscular and sensory integrative aspects.
- Therapeutic exercise to enhance functional performance.

- Discharge planning and community re-entry.
- Education and counseling of the patient and the family.

HISTORICAL ROOTS

Occupational therapy developed into an identifiable profession during the years after the First World War. At that lime, Adolf Meyer and Eleanor Clarke Slagle developed the use of carefully planned goals and methods for promoting health through the use of activities. It was in the 1920s, that Meyer restated the principles of moral treatment, and gave a context and philosophy to the development of the profession of occupational therapy. The approaches of Meyer and Slagle in the use of activities and relationships, examined in the light of today's knowledge and practice, was remarkably modern. They emphasized the developmental needs and had a sense of the importance of preparing the individual patient for functioning within the society.

William Rush Dunton Jr. a psychiatrist, simplified the categories of mental disorders and suggested the kinds of activities that could be most desirable and most therapeutic with each category. He also described the importance of the therapist's approach and attitude.

In 1930s and 1940s, psychiatric occupational therapy developed as a profession and a search for theoretical concepts began that would provide frames of reference for treatment. Occupational therapists saw their roles as closely aligned with the psychiatrists responsible for the treatment of the patients. The situation, in which they worked, involved a written prescription from the treating psychiatrist or physician, before the occupational therapist could initiate treatment.

The psychodynamic concepts, as they emerged in the sixties, emphasized a view of the activities of catalytic agents giving impetus to the development of relationships and intrapsychic experiences, which are used by the therapist and patient collaboratively to eliminate or alter pathology. The importance of nonverbal communication, with its self-expressive and interpersonal potential, remained extremely important.

MODELS FOR PRACTICE

Occupational therapists work under a myriad of theoretical approaches or conceptual models. There are a range of theories arising from the biological, psychological and social sciences which have been adapted for use in the practice of occupational therapy. Some of these theories are summarized below:

Psychoanalytical Model

The use of Freudian psychoanalytic theory in occupational therapy involves expression and exploration of inner feelings, using the symbolic and projective potential of activity. The occupational therapist learns to interpret the patient's nonverbal productions (e.g. projective use of clay, aggression, regression) and to interact to reduce the psychic conflict in a therapeutic way.

The 'Adaptive Performance Model' places the emphasis on the integration of dynamic and rehabilitative concepts.

Behavioral Model

The behavioral approach utilizes social skills training, relaxation techniques and other types of behavior therapy techniques for occupational therapy of psychiatric patients. Intelligent use of reinforcement principles and token economy is made.

The 'Occupational Behavior Therapy' is based on:

- The patient's life roles, and identification of the skills to support them.
- Providing balanced life experiences (temporal adaptation) using workplay and self maintenance.
- The fact that play is significant in development of competence and 'striving to achieve'.
- A 'systems' view in which individuals are strongly influenced by their environment (receiving stimuli and giving feedback).

Humanistic Model

The humanistic approach is concerned with the growth of the individual and self-concept, with emphasis on human potentialities, feelings, needs and relationships. Its application in occupational therapy is exemplified by creative therapies and activity used as positive experience. During therapy, self-identity and creative expression is encouraged through relationship and creative play.

Developmental Model

This model advocates step-by-step teaching of adaptive skills, with the focus usually on one area. There are two main theories using this approach.

Lloren's Theory of Facilitation of Growth and Development

Occupational theory, according to this theory, is a process of facilitating growth, as well as mastery of self and the environment through recognition of the needs, abilities and issues of the growing child. These principles have been translated into a highly successful approach for treatment with adult psychiatric patients.

Ayres' Biodevelopmental Theory

The research of Jean Ayres, into the development of sensory motor function, has led to the significant technique of sensory integration. It has gained a worldwide influence with its application to:

- Learning disordered children and mentally handicapped people.
- Schizophrenics and their perceptual and postural problems (e.g. King).
- Patients with traumatic neurological lesions.

The basic principles underlying sensory integration are three fold:

1. Early vestibular, tactile and proprioceptive experiences are important in personality development.
2. Perceptual processes are crucial for the individual to adapt to the human and nonhuman environment.
3. Lastly, carefully chosen motor and sensory activities can be effective therapy for those with deficits in their integration.

CLINICAL ISSUES

Occupational therapists work in broad range of practice areas and settings within the scope of general psychiatry, in close collaboration with other mental health professionals. Services are provided to children, adolescents, adults and elderly of all functional levels and diagnostic categories, in institutions, community based programs, day care centers, forensic programs, mental hospitals, rehabilitation centers, sheltered workshops, corrective institutions, community based mental health centers and private practice.

Upon referral or as an important member of the ongoing multidisciplinary team, occupational therapist participates in identifying problems, establishing overall treatment objectives, and developing treatment and discharge plans.

There are four basic elements, which may be considered in the psychiatric occupational therapy process:

1. The *client* (the individual who needs help)
2. The *therapist* (the individual who is the helper)
3. The *purposeful activity*, and
4. The *context* in which the helping takes place.

ASSESSMENT AND EVALUATION

Assessment is the first stage of the occupational therapy process and consists of gathering information in an effort to understand the patient and his or her situation. Since occupational therapy process is a problem-solving process primarily, it is very important to understand the problem; not only what the problem is but how it affects the person and the important others. Assessment occurs at all points during treatment; initially, subsequently and continuously.

Methods of Assessment

Basically, there are five main methods, other than general observation, of eliciting information about a patient, his or her problems, skills and the situation.

1. Interview
2. Standardized test
3. Specific observation
4. Self-rating method, and
5. Projective techniques.

Occupational therapy contributes significant information towards diagnosis, as the flexibility of the occupational therapy situation allows the patient freedom to act, freedom of choice of activity and different types of controlled group situations. If studied carefully, it can even provide a good balance to the technique of psychological assessment, in which standardized test procedures determine the functioning of the patient, in certain special task areas. Thus, the examiner-selected standardized test situations, of the clinical psychologist, can be paired-off with the flexible patient-selected task of the occupational therapist, to offer a balanced picture of the patient in somewhat different situation. This pairing-off of the occupational therapy situational observation with the psychodiagnostic methods has been used at the Hospital for Mental Diseases, Ranchi and was found highly rewarding. Occupational therapy comes closer to approximating activities of productive social nature than any other form of adjunctive treatment. It is under this context that occupational therapy can claim to be of diagnostic value in psychiatric setting.

THERAPEUTIC ISSUES

How to Plan Treatment?

Planning of treatment requires organization of information (Flow chart 3):

- Process all assessment information,
- Identify problems in functional terms,
- Identify strengths to build on, and
- Select priority problems; and establishment of aims and goals:
  - Establish overall aim,
  - Identify short-and long-term aims, and
  - Set specific goals.

Designing the Program

Therapeutic Activity

The choice of activity and its demands depend on aims, patient's preference, therapist's selection, practical constraints and overall program balance. Consider how to grade the activity in order to achieve the aim. For example, increase the complexity of task to facilitate higher learning of problem-solving skills.

Role of Therapist

The therapist's role includes the general approach to a patient and specific ways of handling behavior, and the use of self-relationship as a therapeutic tool. It depends on

Flow chart 3 A case example

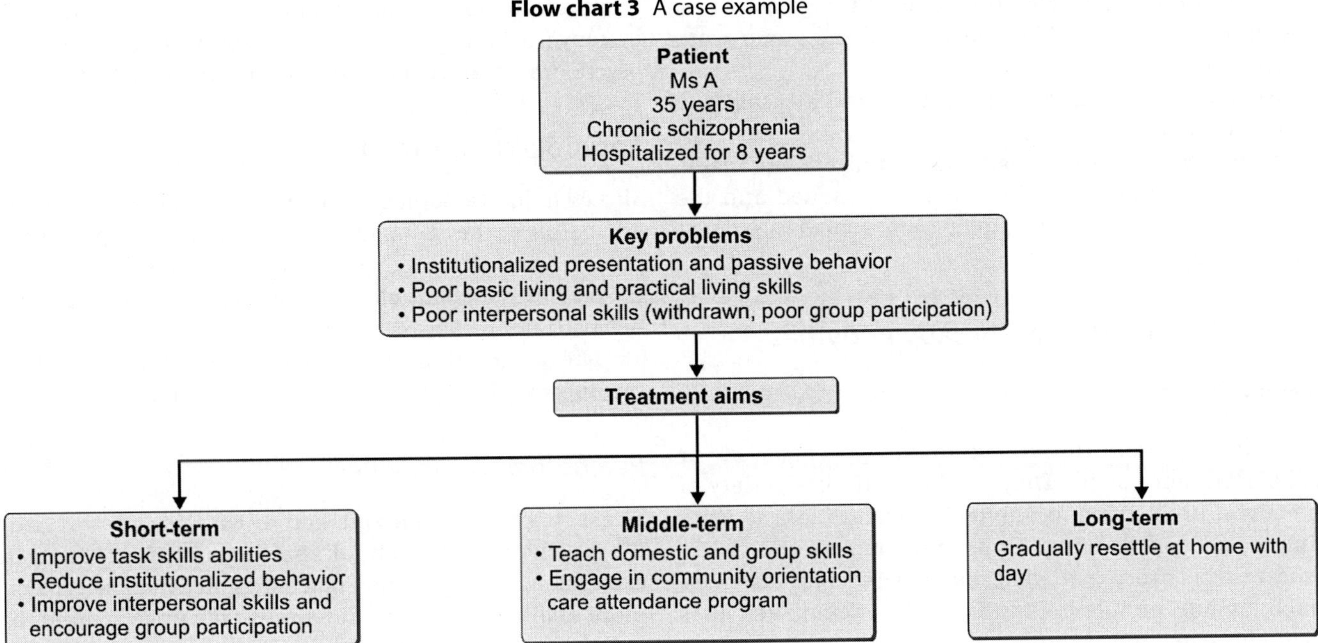

the theoretical framework, the situation, the personalities involved, etc. There is a gradation of role, in order to achieve the designed aim. For example, become less directive and reduce supports to encourage independence in the patient.

Environment

Environment includes people involved and their attitudes and physical structure. Consider how to set up the environment in order to achieve the aim. For example, reduce the amount of tools available for use, to encourage sharing among people in a group activity.

Aims

Occupational therapy aims to improve group interaction skills in particular, encourage verbal interaction with others, help to learn how to participate in a shared task, and increase awareness of the presence and needs of others.

Therapist-patient Relationship

The therapist,

1. Has to play an active and directive role.
2. Is a major source of need satisfaction.
3. Encourages trust.
4. Reinforces cooperative behavior and encourages group interaction.
5. Is responsible for organizing activities.

ACTIVITY AS TREATMENT

Purposeful activity has definitive value at different levels: applied to therapy, to ourselves and others, and to the environment. A child's use of activity in the form of play clearly illustrates how activity can be used to practice or learn new skills, and to test knowledge and perceptions.

The process of activity and its end products have the following values:

- Play and social value.
- Stimulates, activates and energizes.
- Allows exploration and expression of feelings.
- Work value; meets the needs of self-esteem, being purposeful and productive.
- Learning tools; develops skill and knowledge, competence and mastery.

Generally, the occupational therapists modify and therapeutically use activities with five main aims in mind.

1. To help the patient acquire new skills, e.g. teaching relaxation technique for improving the patient's present coping skills; teaching a new hobby to the patient for improving the future coping skills.
2. To improve the specific areas of deficit, e.g. quiz training and training of work tasks to improve deficits in the cognitive domain.
3. To raise the self-esteem of the patient, e.g. increasing confidence through achievements and increased awareness about capabilities and potentials.

4. To provide an enjoyable, social outlet through activities, spanning the range of both diversional and group-work experiences.
5. Use of activity to assess performance and measure any progress made.

In the treatment setting, grading is utilized. Gradually, one-to-one care and help in activity is lessened and the patient is encouraged to participate from a smaller group to a bigger group.

Range of Occupational Therapy Activities

Task Activities

These activities aim to improve the daily living work or task performance skills. They can be used for a variety of objectives, from trying to improve concentration, to work stimulation and training. Other common examples are wood-work, cookery, gardening; industrial therapy activities, which include stimulating factory and workshop activities (like, chalk-making, candle-making, chair-caning, book-binding and many other assembly activities); activities for reality orientation, which include group work to improve the memory and other cognitive functions, like newspaper reading and discussion (they are being commonly used for confused and disoriented elderly group of patients).

Social Activities

The wide spectrum of social activities are primarily aimed at promoting enjoyment and leisure time pursuits. They can be used at a simple level of diversion or towards a more purposeful end involving social contact and interaction. Common examples are crafts, sports, and indoor games.

Activities Involving Communication and Sharing

Communication and sharing can be either used exclusively in activity or can form an important part of nearly any activity which involves group-work. Important examples are group discussion (structured or unstructured) and drama therapy (including remedial drama, social drama, role play, psychodrama, and containing a wide range of activities).

Social Skills Education

This technique is sometimes confused with the general skills education of the mentally handicapped. In its purest use, however, it is designed as a behavioral technique to teach the patient systematic elements of social behavior, i.e. verbal behavior, nonverbal assertion, etc.

The occupational therapist works with other team members while imparting social skills training.

Psychotherapy Activities

These highly specialized activities arise mainly from the psychodynamic school and focus on facilitating the expression and exploration of feelings. Activities selected are more analytically based and are usually unstructured, e.g. painting, clay work, collage.

Thus, it is clear that the role of occupational therapy in psychiatry is now well recognized and fully developed as a technique for treatment. Besides, it has its uses in diagnosis and assessment of prognosis, and it can be used in individual or group setting. It is not just a means of diversion as many would think, nor the quality of the finish (the end product of activity) is important, as is sometimes suggested by the 'exhibitions' or 'sales' organized by day care centers or occupational therapy departments.

For example, an occupational therapist may assess a client with schizophrenia who is living in a residential hospital in order to help to determine the best placement in the community. The assessment may include standardized evaluation tools, individual interview, and observation to determine ability to function and live alone safely, and identify important roles and occupations. This information is then used to determine the skills, supports, and environmental modifications the person may need to live as independently as possible.

47.14 REHABILITATION IN PSYCHIATRY

Ashok Singhal

One of the primary problems faced by rehabilitation program planners in the past was the lack of any clear conceptualization or adequate definition of rehabilitation. Gratifyingly enough, recent authors have successfully attempted to operationalize the concept of psychiatric rehabilitation to such an extent as to make cross-cultural comparisons feasible.

Anthony et al. asserted that the main tasks of rehabilitation are to assist in reintegrating psychiatrically disabled persons into the community and to maintain their ability to function independently. Wing and Morris were more specific in their formulation. They defined rehabilitation as the process of identifying and preventing or minimizing the causes of severe social disablement accompanying psychiatric disorder, while at the same time helping the individual to develop and use his or her talents, and thus to acquire confidence and self-esteem through success in social rules.

Thus, rehabilitation can be seen to possess two distinct components: the reduction of disability, and the strengthening of individual talents and assets. These two components should, ideally, be directed towards assisting the individual to achieve a fair degree of independence and functional autonomy. In effect, rehabilitation aims at good tertiary prevention of the illness, preventing relapse and minimizing disability. Bachrach defines psychosocial rehabilitation as a therapeutic approach to the care of mentally ill individuals that encourages capacities through learning procedures and environmental supports.

A very common misconception about rehabilitation, which has unfortunate practical consequences, is the failure to distinguish between rehabilitation and resettlement. *Resettlement* is defined as placement in economic employment or domestic life. It is evident that resettlement would constitute the end point of good rehabilitation. Without rehabilitation, resettlement would not be possible, as an unprepared person with residual disability cannot be placed in either a familiar or alien environment. Rehabilitation, therefore, should prepare the person for resettlement by addressing itself to various aspects of the individual and the environment. Rehabilitation should not be restricted only to those whom it is expected to resettle, and resettlement should not be attempted without adequate rehabilitation.

In short, rehabilitation can be conceptualized as a process which comes into effect as the acute phase of the illness subsides, seeks to minimize disability and maximize assets, and strives towards resettlement and functional autonomy.

HISTORICAL ASPECTS

The origin of rehabilitation in psychiatry in the West, can be traced to the community mental health movement. Prior to the 1950s, the care of the mentally ill was primarily institution-based and custodial in approach. Much has been written about the long-term deleterious effects of such care. This led to the 'deinstitutionalization' of patients in the late 1950s and early 1960s. It was assumed that people with major mental illness should be helped to maintain themselves in the community. Although, deinstitutionalization was a positive step, it was too idealistic. It was an attempt to shift the onus of aftercare of the mentally ill on to an underprepared community. Consequently, the burden on the community of the chronically mentally ill has increased several fold. The various issues relating to deinstitutionalization have been reviewed by Lamb. However, the movement highlighted the fact that pharmacotherapy alone was inadequate. A comprehensive system of care, encompassing a variety of therapeutic approaches, is needed to enable the mentally ill patient to function optimally and live in the community.

CONCEPTUAL FRAMEWORK

Any model of psychosocial rehabilitation, in order to be effective, needs to focus not only on the impairment of the acute stage, but also on remedying disability and compensating for handicap. Following definitions are useful in clarifying the basic concepts.

Impairment

Any loss or abnormality of psychosocial, physiological or anatomical structure or function (resulting from underlying pathology). For example, the positive or negative symptoms of schizophrenia, such as delusions and hallucinations or anhedonia and apathy.

Disability

Any restriction or lack of ability to perform an activity (resulting from an impairment) in the manner or within the range considered normal, e.g. the deficient social skills seen in patients with schizophrenia.

Handicap

A disadvantage for a given individual (resulting from an impairment or a disability) that limits or prevents the fulfillment of a role that is normal for that individual (depending on age, sex, social and cultural factors) such as getting married or being gainfully employed.

It is very difficult to distinguish one from the other because impairment, disability and handicap usually merge together and coexist.

MULTIDIMENSIONAL REHABILITATION

The clinical practice of psychiatric rehabilitation joins together three major sets of factors that protect against stress and vulnerability: (1) pharmacotherapy, judiciously keyed to the type and severity of psychopathology, with doses that do not produce sedation or neuromotor and other toxic side effects that interfere with positive engagement in rehabilitation; (2) development of skills in the patient that are linked to stressors and life situation, that challenge adaptation and independence; and (3) a range of supportive social service-including housing, transitional and supported employment, financial support, and case management-that can sustain a mentally disabled person in the community.

The assumption underlying psychiatric rehabilitation is that disabled persons need maintenance medication, skills, and environmental resources and supports to fulfill the role demands of community life.

The organization of truly comprehensive psychiatric rehabilitation can be visualized on three dimensions. One dimension represents the stage of the disorder, ranging from prodromal, to acute, to residual phases. The second dimension consists of treatment and rehabilitation modalities, such as drug therapy, family and cognitive therapies, social skills training, and vocational rehabilitation. The third dimension is made up of requisite support programs, aimed at compensating for disability and minimizing handicap. These include family education and support, social service entitlements, case management, housing, and psychosocial clubs.

The psychiatric rehabilitation practitioner, following a person for many years through various phases of a disorder, is able to use the multidimensional framework to match treatments and support services to the changing needs of the patient as dictated by impairments, disabilities, and handicap, at any point in time. Rehabilitation of persons with chronic and serious mental disorders has to respond to the transition in locus and focus of care from institution to community, and from custodial care to enabling the mentally ill person to function in society. Community support programs and community mental health centers are now the hubs of psychiatric rehabilitation services, where new modes of intervention are coordinated and delivered by case managers in league with multidisciplinary teams of clinicians who assume long-term responsibility for sustaining seriously mentally ill patients in the community.

DELIVERY OF REHABILITATION SERVICES

For purposes of convenience, treatment will be dealt with in terms of the settings in which they occur: (i) inpatient, (ii) outpatient, and (iii) community. However, there are no hard and fast rules and any one or more of the treatments may be used in any of the settings.

Inpatient Setting

Pharmacotherapy

This is the main form of management in an inpatient setting, with electroconvulsive therapy being used as an adjuvant where indicated. Treatment may be directed at: (a) rapidly bringing under control the florid psychotic symptoms seen in an acute phase, (b) managing exacerbations/relapses during the long-term course, (c) treating nonresponders with standard treatment, and (d) treating depression associated with schizophrenia.

Hospitalization is an expensive form of treatment and may not always be warranted. However, it helps in deciding the optimal neuroleptic, depending on its sedative, antipsychotic and side effects profile, stabilizing or monitoring the dose required, trying out newer or alternative treatments and, finally but not the least important, giving a much needed respite to the family. In the inpatient setting, the patient, especially in the acute phase of the illness, needs time to recover from the psychosocial interventions. He would, however, benefit from a supportive relationship with the treating professional.

Depression, anxiety, grief, shame and anger are often seen in reaction to the illness or its consequences, such as loss of job or disturbed interpersonal relations with family and friends. The therapist expresses understanding, concern and acceptance of the patient and often, needs to be pragmatic and give advice on day-to-day issues.

Psychoeducation

Family members are often perceived as necessary for describing symptoms and history, but not useful in treatment. Consequently, they feel ignored. The experience of seeing a near and dear one behave in so different a manner, as is the case in a schizophrenic illness, is a bewildering and traumatic one for the family members. The inpatient setting is, therefore, an appropriate place to begin work with the family. Members of the family, especially the primary care givers, need to be provided with: (a) information regarding the nature of illness from a multifactorial view point, (b) an understanding of core symptoms, both positive and negative, (c) formal instruction with medication management, particularly in relation to side effects, and (d) guidance in practical issues that arise in the day-to-day management of a patient with schizophrenia.

Providing accurate information helps reduce distress caused by unrealistic expectations or superstitious beliefs and makes the patient and family better consumers of mental health services. Giving no information to relatives or remaining vague about the diagnosis and treatment, makes relatives feel fearful or guilty. Strachan suggests that even when the diagnosis is unclear, rather than being afraid of giving incorrect information or wrongly labeling the patient as 'schizophrenic', professionals should be clear and direct with the relatives about the lack of decisiveness, the reasons for the ambiguity and how the diagnostic decision might be clarified (e.g. further interviews, or the passing of time).

Outpatient Setting

The interventions in the outpatient setting can be essentially dealt with under two headings, depending on whether the focus is on: (a) the individual patient, or (b) the family or significant others.

Pharmacotherapy

The immediate aim of the treating professional is to ensure treatment compliance with maintenance medication. Although oral and depot neuroleptics are pharmacologically equally effective, depot preparations have been found to be more effective in preventing relapse by eliminating covert noncompliance. The efficacy of antipsychotic medication for the long-term maintenance treatment of schizophrenia has been established. However, studies are focusing on improving the benefit-to-risk ratio of long-term treatment and exploring alternative maintenance strategies. To reduce the risk of complications, such as tardive dyskinesia, the continuous low dose medication strategy has been found promising, while there is controversy as to the efficacy of targeted or intermittent medication. However, studies show that about 40% of patients relapse while on medication within the first year after discharge from hospital. Combined approaches, that employ psychopharmacologic treatment with psychosocial interventions, have been found to be effective in enhancing compliance and reducing relapse.

Functional Assessment

Functional assessment of the patient, especially in the early phases of the illness, helps to plan the treatment process and allows the professional to target interventions to the patient's specific needs and state of impairment and disability. Assessment of cognitive functions is helpful in making decisions about future educational and vocational plans. The frequency of impairment in basic cognitive functions, revealed by formal testing, is far higher than is evident on mental status examination. Test results are often useful in educating the family that failure of the patient to achieve up on their expectations, is the result of an actual disability rather than 'laziness' or lack of 'will power'. The utility of cognitive measures in the assessment and prediction of treatment effects has also been demonstrated. In general however, patients with a more malignant course in illness perform poorly on cognitive measures, particularly having impairments of attention, memory and problem solving than do patients with relatively less severe forms of the illness.

Cognitive deficits, in turn, impair the ability to function independently. Therefore, functional assessments should include an evaluation of patient's performance in other areas, especially self-care and social adjustment. A wide range of tools are available in the form of observation, interview or self-report instruments, focusing on the performance of the patient in self-care, social, family, recreational, vocational and financial domains. The user must familiarize himself with the instruments and select one which is appropriate for the setting and fits the particular needs of the patient.

Once the clinician has arrived at an understanding, either through observation or clinical interview and/or formal assessment, of the patient's day-to-day functional skills and abilities or deficits in self-care, work and leisure, he can choose interventions that will enable the patient to achieve the highest level of functioning in the desired activity. This may include not only skill building, but also environmental support for those who may require it. Thus, goal setting is a crucial stage in functional assessment. It is imperative that the professional engages in a discussion with the patient and family to set realistic/reasonable goals which are in keeping with their perceived needs. This not only emphasizes the collaborative nature of this exercise, but ensures compliance by setting individualized treatment plans.

Skill Development

Impairment in social functioning is almost characteristic of schizophrenia. However, it is not simply a by-product of positive and negative symptoms, but an independent domain of the illness. Poor social competence contributes to the impoverished quality of life and social isolation experienced by many patients. It interferes with functioning within the family or in the work place. In addition, social disability has been found to be a potent predictor of symptom exacerbation and rehospitalization.

The most promising strategy for alleviating social disability and enhancing social competence has been social skills training (SST). Social skills training is a highly structured psychosocial intervention, based on behavioral and learning principles and emphasizes modeling, role playing and social reinforcement. Goals are explicitly stated and complex social repertoires, such as going for a job interview, asking about medication, are broken down into smaller elements such as maintaining eye contact and initiating communication, which are rewarded with social reinforcement. Patients are first taught the elements and then gradually learn how to perform them smoothly in sequence. Problem solving skills are employed to enable the patient to function in real life situations.

Social skills training was introduced in the 1970s, mainly in the form of single case studies. Since then, the group format has been found to be more popular as it is not only costeffective, both in terms of time and personnel, but also enhances generalization of skills by providing a vicarious learning experience. A number of controlled studies have highlighted the efficacy of social skills training. Moreover, these studies demonstrate that the effects of training are maintained over six to twelve month periods and help in reducing relapse rates when combined with adequate pharmacotherapy. Hierholzer and Liberman recommend booster sessions to maintain skills learnt and use an open-ended, drop-in, group format.

While it is clear that social skills training is an effective strategy, more work needs to be done on issues such as generalization of skills to the natural environment, optimal frequency of sessions and direction of treatment, and patient characteristics that may contraindicate social skills training.

Cognitive Training

Patients with schizophrenia exhibit a variety of information processing deficits, particularly in attention, memory, reasoning and concept formation. It is argued that deficits in basic processes, such as attention and memory, need to be remedied before patients can learn problem solving skills, which require the ability to reason and carry out logical analysis. Cognitive training is provided on a series of tasks adapted from neuropsychological test procedures, such as card sorting and word finding (synonyms/antonyms), which focus on frontal lobe functions. However, this approach is very much in an experimental stage. Preliminary results with schizophrenia patients indicate some reasons to be optimistic about the future, yet emphasize the need to proceed with caution.

Family Focused Intervention

The need to maintain the patient in the community and at an optimal level of functioning necessitates viewing the family as an important resource in the overall management. There has been a radical shift from viewing the family as a noxious agent to including the family as a collaborative partner in the overall treatment plan. This shift is a result of three major factors: (a) the increasing acceptance of schizophrenia as a biological disease, (b) the recognition of the heavy burden on family members of caring for patient with schizophrenia, and (c) research documenting that negative family affect (referred to as *expressed emotion*) towards the patient is predictive of symptom relapses. Each of these factors are outlined below:

a. The multifactorial etiology of schizophrenia is best understood from a biopsychosocial perspective. This led to the abandoning of purely psychogenic models and consequently, the use of terms like *schizophrenogenic mother*. Blaming the family, that was prevalent in the early part of the century, led to vocal dissatisfaction expressed by many family members over how they were treated by professionals. In the West, a number of advocacy groups were formed, the largest of these being the National Alliance for the mentally ill. The group highlighted the fact that: (i) families were not to be blamed for mental illness in the individual member, (ii) families have a right to information about the illness and its treatment, and that (iii) better resources were needed for the chronic mentally ill.
b. Family members of patients with schizophrenia experience subjective distress, financial loss, risk to personal safety, etc. A number of studies, carried out in India and in the West, have documented that the burden of caring for a ill relative is high and that families are in need of support.
c. The construct of expressed emotion (EE), referred to as high levels of criticism, hostility or emotional over-involvement, was put forth by the Camberwell group. Since then, it has been demonstrated that patients suffering from schizophrenia, in contact with a relative having high expressed emotion, are more likely to relapse.

This construct has also been validated in India. In general, the authors concluded that relatives being lower in EE was a major factor in explaining the better outcome of patients in North India. A vast amount of literature is available in this area for the interested reader.

There is an increasing trend towards conceptualizing expressed emotion and family burden as interactive rather than unidirectional processes. The high EE communications are viewed as the relative's way of coping with the stress of disruptive, and often violent, patient behavior, which, in turn, exacerbate patient's symptoms and lead to the formation of a vicious cycle.

The growing acceptance of an interactive model between family stress and patient functioning has led to the development of educational/psychotherapeutic interventions. Various models and approaches to family treatment have been put forth. Prominent among these are the crisis-oriented family therapy approach of Goldstein et al., education, relatives, support group and family therapy of Leff et al.,behavioral problem solving family management by Falloon et al., and family psychoeducation and survival skills by Hogarty et al. Excellent reviews are available in this area.

The focus is on reducing the stress in the family environment and teaching family remember a problem focused coping approach. Lam identified seven common components:

i. *A positive approach and genuine working relationship between the mental health professional and the family*: Relatives are respected as individuals with their own needs, and their burden for caring for an individual with schizophrenia is acknowledged.
ii. *Provision of structure and stability*: The course of a schizophrenic illness is a fluctuating one with a certain amount of unpredictability. Maintaining regular contact with the treating team provides some structure and stability to families. Relatives are taught how to maintain a moderate interpersonal distance with the patient and at the same time set appropriate limits.
iii. *Focus on improving coping with stress in the 'here and now' rather than dwelling on the past.*
iv. *Strengthening interpersonal boundaries within the family*: Problem behaviors disrupt the functioning of the family unit as a whole and weaken generational (parent-child) or interpersonal (marital alliance) boundaries.

v. Through *education regarding the biological nature of schizophrenia*, an attempt is made to reduce the guilt of the family members and blame on the patient.
vi. *Behavioral techniques* such as assessing strengths and liabilities, and reinforcing successive approximations to desired behavior, and
vii. *Improving communication skills* using rehearsal, feedback and practice to train families to express requests in clear, simple and specific ways.

While family based approaches are labor-intensive, the interventions have been found to be cost-effective when compared to inpatient hospital treatment. Moreover, less frequent hospitalizations mean less stigmatization for patient and family, less disruption in daily routine and enhanced self-esteem for the patient. However, the existing intervention packages serve to delay rather than to prevent relapse in the long-term.

Community Setting

In addition to individual and family focused approaches, the treatment and management of chronic mental illness (such as schizophrenia) demands effective development and utilization of environmental resources. Restoration of social and vocational functioning is often limited by continuing deficits and refractory symptoms. Rehabilitation strategies are then aimed at helping the individual compensate for the disability by locating living and working environments that can accommodate to the residual deficits and symptoms. Community based care encompasses a variety of services, including day care and residential care.

Day Care

The term 'day care' in British psychiatry and the term 'partial hospitalization' in American literature are used synonymously. In effect, they refer to ambulatory treatment programs that include psychiatric, psychosocial and pre-vocational treatment modalities designed for patients with severe mental illness. Such patients require a comprehensive and multidisciplinary treatment not provided in an outpatient or inpatient setting. Partial hospitalization may include day or night hospitalization, depending on the needs of the individual patient. Day hospitalization/day care is the most common and will be dealt with briefly here.

Day hospitals and day care centers often refer to services, differing in location rather than function. While a day hospital is attached to a hospital setting, a day care center may be located in a psychiatric hospital, a general hospital, a community health center, or be free standing. Usually, the former provide for more acute short-term care, while the latter provide a more supportive, long-term management and maintenance oriented service for the chronic patient.

When there is only one facility providing day care services, it must be remembered that the treatment and management of the two categories of patients differ. The 'acute' category is likely to comprise of patients who have been recently discharged from an inpatient setting, are still symptomatic, unable to manage on their own, but not requiring 24 hour treatment or supervision.

The chronic category are symptomatically less acute and have greater long-term social or vocational problems. Day care facilities usually provide the full range of medical and psychosocial treatments, including family interventions that have been outlined earlier. However, the emphasis is on providing a social setting that is not merely concerned with reduction of disability (such as skill deficits), but also concerned with management of social disadvantage or handicap. The idea of 'normalization' is concerned with reducing the stigma and providing a culturally valued means of living.

Work has traditionally been a source of social integration. Work, in a day care setting, is used to refer to any structured, purposeful and productive activity. Ideally, there should be facilities for the assessment of work performance for training and preparation in vocational skills and placement in open or sheltered work settings. However, more often than not, in the case of chronic mental illness, individuals may not be in a position to pursue competitive, paid employment. For such persons, sheltered work provided in the form of subcontract packing and assembly jobs are useful.

Yet another subset of patients may not be able to pursue any work related activity. Such patients still benefit from a setting where they can be engaged in social, leisure and recreational activities. They can be taught basic self-help skills or domestic living skills and provided a place to meet and be with people without necessarily having to make close relationships. Patients with chronic schizophrenia do better in a nonintrusive, nondemanding social environment with more object focused activity, such as occupational therapy, than intensive interpersonal stimulation such as group therapy. Day care settings, therefore, have the tough task of balancing adequate work-oriented care and a non-threatening social environment.

Residential Care

Residential care developed initially as a transitional facility from hospital to home. 'Half-way homes', as such facilities are known, are literally just that: an intermediary point between leaving the hospital and returning to the family. Such facilities usually have the array of both individual and family based interventions, depending on the individual patient and needs of the family. While the individual focus is on developing and maintaining adequate self-help and social skills for re-entering the community, the family is prepared to receive the patient, with an emphasis on psychoeducation and reduction of expressed emotions.

However, the emphasis in residential care today is on the development of a variety of facilities providing a continuous of different levels of residential support. At one end, there is a need for hostel, like facilities for well-functioning patients who are able to hold open to sheltered employment, but have minimal or no social support. Here, the emphasis is on providing shelter, a supportive environment and supervision of medication. In the West, the growing problem of homelessness has highlighted the paucity of such services.

At the other end, there is a need for residential care of a custodial nature for patients with predominantly deficit symptoms, and who respond poorly to both pharmacotherapy and/or psychosocial interventions. Such patients may require long-term care with high levels of support even for activities of daily living, but do not need to be incarcerated in mental hospitals. Such facilities are also needed because the burden of care is often too much for the families.

THE REHABILITATION TEAM

The vast array of interventions and the wide variety of settings in which these take place, obviously necessitates a team approach. Rehabilitation efforts are most successful when a multidisciplinary team is involved comprising of psychiatrists, clinical psychologists, psychiatric social workers, psychiatric nurses and occupational therapists. In addition to professional staff, rehabilitation involves active coordination and collaboration with family members, lay volunteers and nongovernmental organizations. Team work is also essential because not only does it reduce 'burn out' on the part of the caregivers, but also reduces dependency on one therapist on the part of the patient.

STATUS OF PSYCHIATRIC REHABILITATION IN INDIA

Rehabilitation in India is still in its infancy. Although, a rehabilitation sub-program, aimed at treating and maintaining psychiatric patients in the community, was envisaged in the National Mental Health Program (1982), it could not be implemented due to a variety of reasons. At the governmental level, policy makers have been unable to devote serious attention to the development of rehabilitation services for the chronic mentally ill, primarily due to economic constraints. However, mental health professionals themselves have, to some extent, been complacent.

This has been partly due to the fact that psychoses in general, and schizophrenia in particular, have been shown to run a more benign course in the developing countries, including India. As a result, the presence of family and social support is often taken for granted.

To make the spectrum of rehabilitation services a reality in India, mental health professionals will have to actively collaborate with the nongovernmental sector.

Studies have shown that in India, families are more tolerant of deviant behavior and more willing to take care of the ill member. However, with increasing urbanization, life styles are undergoing rapid change.

The nuclear family system and shrinking social networks, combined with increasing financial strain, is making it more difficult to care for an ill relative. Studies have documented that distress and burden of caring for an ill relative are high and disruptive of daily routines. This is true for both rural and urban families.

Hospital based services are increasing being made available, especially in general hospital settings. However, it is imperative that the nongovernment or voluntary sector be actively involved in the development of a network of community based services. There is an urgent need for more day care centers that can provide the much needed respite for the family, as well as make the individual patient feel less stigmatized and more valued.

Day care centers are the cornerstone of community care. In India, there is a need to emphasize vocational training in such centers, so that patients can relearn or retrain in marketable skills. This is because the patient may often be the sole breadwinner or is at least expected to supplement the family income. In the absence of any governmental support or disability payments, as in the West, this becomes all the more important. Even in more affluent countries, as in the United States of America, the emphasis is shifting from functioning as mere social or recreational centers to more skill oriented centers. The government and private sector need to be mobilized in this regard to provide sheltered employment or at least work opportunities in the form of subcontracting routine packing and assembly kind of jobs. Work, especially paid employment, is a major factor in enhancing self-esteem and facilitating normalization. The formation of advocacy groups would also help in this regard.

At the other end of the spectrum, we are faced with the reality that a certain percentage of patients are 'non-responders' to treatment and run a downhill course. For such patients, we have to make provision for long-term residential care.

ROLE OF THE PSYCHIATRIST IN REHABILITATION

The final ingredient of a successful ACT approach, namely a psychiatrist integrated in a community team, inevitably leads to the question: what is or can be the role of a psychiatrist in rehabilitation? According to Cancro, "A properly trained psychiatrist will be able to prescribe psychosocial interventions, such as social skills training, as well as prescribe medication. This does not mean that the individual psychiatrist should be able to do everything from social skills training to vocational rehabilitation to psychoeducation to family support. It does mean, however, that the psychiatrist must know what is needed and where it can be found and must be able to play a role in directing a team of professionals who can serve these patients. Not only will the patients benefit from such an approach but so will our discipline".

Psychiatric rehabilitation is by its very nature multidisciplinary, because of the many different competencies required. It goes without saying that monitoring medication is a key task of the psychiatrist. But pharmacotherapy in psychiatric rehabilitation needs some special consideration. Symptom control does not necessarily have the highest priority, as some side effects of pharmacological treatment can weaken a person's ability to perform his or her social roles, and impair vocational rehabilitation. As such, it is no surprise that noncompliance with medication taking is one of the most serious problems in the long-term treatment of persons with serious mental illness. Many patients living in the community want to take responsibility for their medication themselves. Training in self-management of medication emphasizes patients' autonomy and increases acceptance of and responsibility for treatment. This also includes the change of medication without consultation within certain limits.

As a matter of course, most psychiatrists do not acquire all relevant skills needed in psychiatric rehabilitation during their training, which is predominantly hospital-based. Young psychiatrists today are primarily trained in diagnostic procedures and prescription of medications directed almost exclusively to symptom control, and not trained in integrating pharmacological and psychosocial interventions. Another side effect of hospital-based training is that young psychiatrists are confronted with the negative developments of difficult-to-treat patients who are frequently re-hospitalized. This is possibly one of the reasons why we found that psychiatrists in institutional settings do not hold fewer stereotypes of mentally ill people than the general population, nor display a greater willingness to closely interact with mentally ill people. Therefore, it would be beneficial if the community training of young psychiatrists could take priority over hospital based training. More training opportunities to experience the patients in the "real world" would allow psychiatrists in institutional settings to develop a more positive perspective and better understanding of persons with severe and persistent mental disorders.

OUTLOOK

Up to date, major developments in psychiatric treatment and care have evolved from psychiatric rehabilitation. This is the most visible part of psychiatric care and as such represents the link to society. The attitude of the public towards psychiatry is mostly influenced by what rehabilitation accomplishes or not. In fact, the US President's Freedom Commission on Mental Health declared that helping affected persons to achieve functional recovery is the main purpose of the mental health care system.

The refinement of psychiatric rehabilitation has achieved a point where it should be made readily available for every disabled person. But, we have to be aware that there is a long way between research and practice. Lehman and Steinwachs, for example, assessed the patterns of usual care for schizophrenic patients and examined the conformance rate with the treatment recommendations based on existing scientific evidence. The conformance rate was modest, generally below 50%. It seems to be obvious that current treatment and rehabilitation practice has to be substantially improved in the light of the rehabilitation research available.

REFERENCES

Psychoanalysis

1. Freud S. Two encyclopaedia articles. In: Strachey J. (Ed). The Standard Edition of the Complete Psychological Works of Sigmund Freud. London: Hogarth Press. [Hereafter called only SE]. 1923;18.
2. Breuer J, Freud S (1893-1895). Studies on hysteria. SE. 1955;2.
3. Freud S (1914). On the history of psychoanalytic movement. SE. 1957;14.
4. Freud S (1924). A short account of psychoanalysis. SE. 1959;19.
5. Greenson RR. The Technique and Practice of Psychoanalysis. Vol. I. New York: International Universities Press, 1967.
6. Thompson C. Psychoanalysis: Evolution and Development. London: George Allen & Unwin, 1952.
7. The New Encyclopaedia Britannica. 1979;7 and 1979;15.
8. Freud S (1915). The unconscious. SE. 1957;14:166-215.
9. Freud S (1923). The ego and the id. SE. 1961;19:12-66.
10. Freud S (1933). New introductory lectures on psychoanalysis. SE. 1964;29:5-182.
11. Freud S (1926). Inhibitions, symptoms and anxiety. SE. 1959;20:87-172.
12. Freud S (1920). Beyond the pleasure principle. SE. 1955;18.
13. Freud S (1940). Outline of psychoanalysis. SE. 1964;23.
14. Freud S (1905). Three essays on the theory of sexuality. SE. 1953;7:130-243.
15. Freud S (1915). Repression. SE. 1957;14.
16. Freud A. The Ego and the Mechanisms of Defence. London: Hogarth Press, 1937.
17. Freud S (1900). The interpretations of dreams. SE. 1953. pp. 4-5.
18. Alexander F. The Impact of Freudian Psychiatry. Chicago: Phoenix Books, 1961.
19. Sandler J, et al. Basic psychoanalytic concepts: IV. Counter-transference. Br J Psychiatry. 1970;117.
20. Woodworth. Contemporary Schools of Psychology. London: Methuen, 1949.

21. Brown JAC. Freud and the Post-Freudians. Penguin, 1978.
22. Meissner WB. Theories of personality. In: Nicholi AM (Ed). The New Harvard Guide to Psychiatry. Cambridge: Harvard, 1988.
23. Klein M. The Psychoanalytic Play Technique: New Directions in Psychoanalysis. London: Tavistock, 1971.
24. Freud S (1912-13). Totem and taboo. SE. 1953;13: XIII-162.
25. Freud S (1927). The future of an illusion. SE. 1964;21.
26. Freud S (1930). Civilization and its discontents. SE. 1964;21.
27. Kaplan HI, Sadock BJ. Modern Synopsis of Comprehensive Textbook of Psychiatry, 3rd edition. Baltimore: Williams and Wilkins, 1983.
28. Eysenck HJ. The effects of psychotherapy: an evaluation. J Consult Psychol. 1952;16:319-24.
29. Rosenzweig S. A transvaluation of psychotherapy: A reply to Hans Eysenck. J Abnorm Psychol. 1954;49:298-304.
30. Schijeilderup H. Lasting effects of psychoanalytic treatment. Psychiatry. 1955;18:109-33.
31. Radhakrishnan S. Yoga: Its meaning and functions. East and West in Religion. London: George, Allen & Unwin, 1933.
32. Neil J Smelser, Paul B Baltes. International encyclopedia of the social & behavioral sciences. Amsterdam; New York: Elsevier, 2001.
33. Nemiah JC. Foundations of Psychopathology. New York: Oxford, 2004.
34. Strachey J. The nature of the therapeutic action of psychoanalysis. Int J Psychoanal. 2004;23:107-59.
35. Spielberg CD. Encyclopedia of applied psychology. Oxford; Boston: Elsevier Academic Press, 2004.

Family and Marital Therapy

36. Murdock GP. The University of the nuclear family. In: Bell NW, Vogel EF, editors. The family. Illinois: Free press; 1960.
37. Ackerman NW. The Psychodynamics of Family Life. New York: Basic Books; 1958.
38. Vandenberg SG. Assertive mating or who marries whom? Behav Genet. 1972;2:127-57.
39. Buss OM. Marital assortment for personality disposition: assessment with three different data sources. Behav Genet. 1984;14:111-23.
40. Greene K, Bogo M. The different faces of intimate violence: implications for assessment and treatment. J Marital Fam Ther. 2002;28:455-66.
41. Brown G, Birley JLT, Wingh JK. The influence of family life on the course of schizophrenic disorder: A replication. Br J Psychiatry. 1972;121:241.
42. Beach S. Affective disorders. J Marital Fam Ther. 2003;29:247-61.
43. Diamond G, Siqueland L. Current status of family intervention science. Child Adolescent Psychiatric Clin N Am. 2001;10:641-61.
44. Johnson SM, Lebow L. The coming of age of family therapy: A decade of review. J Marital Fam Ther. 2000;26:23-38.
45. Barker P. Basic Family Therapy. III Ed. London: Collins; 1991.
46. Chanabasavanna SM, Andrade C, Rasquinha LP, et al. Family therapy at NIMHANS. Indian J Soc Psychiatry. 1987;3:368-78.
47. Bentovirn A. Forward. Applications of Systemic Family Therapy: The Milan Approach. London: Grune and Stratton; 1989.
48. Martin F. The development of systemic family therapy and its place in the field. In: Draper R. editors. Applications of Systemic Family Therapy: The Milan Approach. London: Grune and Stratton; 1989.
49. Howells JG. Theory and Practice of Family Psychiatry. Edinburgh: Oliver and Boyd; 1968.
50. Cottrell D. Family therapy influence on general adult psychiatry. Br J Psychiatry. 1989;154:473-7.
51. Bowen M. A family concept of schizophrenia. In: Jackson DO, editors. Family Therapy: Theory and Practice. New York; Gardner Press, 1976.
52. Wynne LC, Rycoff IM, Day IM, Day J, et al. Pseudomutuality in the family relations of schizophrenic patients. Psychiatry. 1958; 21:295.
53. Lidz T, Fleet S, Cornelison A. Schizophrenia and Family. New York: International Universities Press; 1965.
54. Block S, Sharpe M, Allman P. Systemic family therapy in adult psychiatry. Br J Psychiatry. 1991;159:357-64.
55. Epstein NB, Ryan CE, Bishop DS, Miller IW, Keitner GI. The McMaster model: A view of healthy family functioning. In Walsh F, editor. Normal Family Processes (3rd edition). New York: Guilford Press; 2003.
56. Sadock VA. Marital therapy. In: Kaplan HI. Sadock BJ, editors. Comprehensive Textbook of Psychiatry. III Ed. Baltimore: William & Wilkins; 1980.pp.1886-91.
57. Minuchin S. Families and Family Therapy. Cambridge: Harvard University Press; 1974.
58. Steinhauer PO, Marlin E. The family of child. In: Steinhauer PD, Rae Grant Q, editors. Psychological Problems of the Child in the Family. New York: Basic Books; 1983.
59. Varghese M, Shah A, Kumar GSU, Murali T, Paul IS. Family intervention and support in schizophrenia. A manual on family intervention for the mental health professional. Bangalore: NIMHANS; 2002.
60. Clarkin IE, Francis AS, Moodie JL. Selection criteria for family therapy. Fam Process. 1979;18:391-403.
61. Warond Skinner S. Indications and contraindication for use of family therapy. J Child Psychol Psychiatr. 1979;19:57-62.
62. Tillet R. Activity in a district psychotherapy service. Psychiatric Bull. 1994;18:544-47.
63. Esptein NB, Bishop OS, Levin S. The Mc-Master Model of family functioning. J Marriage Fam Counseling. 1978;4:19-31.
64. Steinhauer PO, Santa Barbara J, Skinner H. The process model of family functioning. Can J Psychiatric. 1984;29:77-88.
65. Sperry L. Assessment of couples and families contemporary and cutting-edge strategies. New York: Brunner-Routledge; 2004.
66. Tseng WS, McDermott JP. Triaxial family classification. J Am Acad Child Psychiatr. 1979;47:500-08.

67. Olson DH, Gorall DM. Circumplex model of marital and family systems. In Walsh F, editor. Normal Family Processes, 3rd edition. New York: Guilford Press; 2003.
68. Olson DH, Killorin E. Clinical rating scale for the circumplex model of marital and family systems. Family Social Science, University of Minnesota; 1983.
69. Olson DH, Killorin E. Clinical rating scale for the circumplex model of marital and family systems. Family Social Science, University of Minnesota; 1988.
70. Green RG. Harris RN, Forte JA. Robinson M. The wives data and FACES IV making things appear simple. Fam process. 1991;30:55-73.
71. Wilkinson A, Strauon P. The reliability and validity of a system: Family Assessment. J Fam Ther. 1981;13:73-94.
72. Avelin M. Making a psychodynamic formulation. Bull Roy Coll Psychiatr. 1980.pp.192-3.
73. Beck RL, Crawford AB. The couple assessment summary: A bridge from assessment to treatment. Am J Psychotheraphy. 2000; 54:55-66.
74. Framo J. Family origin as a therapeutic resource for adults in marital and family therapy: You can and should go home again. Family Process. 1976;15:193-210.
75. Meissner WW. The conceptualization of marriage and family dynamics from psychoanalytic perspective. In: Paolino TJ, Mc BS, editors. Marriage ad Marital Therapy. New York: Brunner/ Mazel; 1978.
76. Von Bertalanffy L. General Systems theory: Foundations, development, and application. Braziller. New York, 1968.
77. Hayes H. A reintroduction to family therapy. Classification of three schools. Aus NZ J Fam Ther. 1991;12:27-43.
78. Palazzoli MS, Boscolo L, Cecchin G, Prata G. A ritualized prescription in family therapy: Odd days and even days. J Marriage Fam Counseling. 1978;4:3-9.
79. Kempler W. Experiential psychotherapy within families Bruner/Mazel. New York, 1981.
80. Wahler RG. Deviant child behavior within the family: Developmental speculations and behavior change strategies. Handbook of Behavior Modification and Therapy. Prentice Hall, Englewood Cliffs. New Jersey.
81. Falloon I. Behavioural family therapy: systems, structures and strategies. In: Family Therapy in Britain. E Street W Dryden, editors. Milton Keynes and Philadelphia: Open University Press; 1988.
82. Howells, John G. Principles of Family Psychiatry. New York: Brunner/Mazel; 1975.
83. Howells JG. Vector therapy in family therapy. Social psychiatry and psychiatric epidemiology. 1969;4:169-72.
84. Alexander JF, Pugh C, Parsons BV, Sexton TL. Functional family therapy. In: Blueprints for Violence Prevention (Book 3), 2nd edition. In: DS Elliott, Boulder CO, editors. Center for the Study and Prevention of Violence, Institute of Behavioral Science, University of Colorado 2000.
85. Butler MH, Gardener BC, Bird MH. Not just time out: Change dynamics of prayer, religious couple in conflict situation. Fam Process. 1998;37:451-78.
86. Anderson DA, Worthen D. Exploring a fourth dimension: Spirituality as a resource for the couple therapist. Fam Process. 1998;57:451-78.
87. Weaver AJ, Koenig HG, Larson DB. Marriage and family therapists and the clergy: A need for clinical collaboration, training, and research. J Marital Fam Ther. 1997;23: 13-25.
88. Christensen A, Heavey CL. Interventions for couples. Annu Rev Psychol. 1999;50:165-90.
89. National Vital Statistics Reports, Vol. 54, No. 20, July 21, 2006.
90. Klerman GL, Weissman MM. Increasing rates of depression. JAMA. 1990;61:2229-39.
91. Emery RE. Marriage, Divorce and Children's Adjustment. Beverly Hills: Sage; 1989.
92. Wellerstein JS, Kelley JB, Surviving the Break Up: How Children Actually Cope with Divorce. New York: Basic Books; 1980.
93. Afifi TO. Brian J. Cox BJ. Enns MW. Mental health profiles among married, never-married, and separated/divorced mothers in a nationally representative sample. Soc Psychiatry Psychiatric Epidemiology. 2006;41:122-9.
94. Yaroff, Kulka RA, Douvan E. Mental Health in America: Patterns of Help Seeking from 1957 to 1976. New York: Basic Books; 1981.
95. Law DD, Crane DR. Influence of martial and family therapy on health care utilization in a health maintenance organization. J Marital Fam Ther. 2000;26:281-91.
96. Wolberg LR. Handbook of Short term Psychotherapy. New York: Thieme-Stratton; 1980.
97. Scharff JS, Scharff DE. Object relation couple therapy. Am J Psychotherapy. 1997;51:141-73.
98. Medelson C, Polonsky DC. Couples therapy. In: Kaplan HI, Sadock BJ, editors. Comprehensive Textbook of Psychiatry. V Ed. Baltimore: William & Wilkins; 1989.
99. Sager CJ. Marriage Contracts and Couple Therapy. New York: Brunner/Mazel; 1976.
100. Satir V. Conjoint Martial Therapy. Science and Behavior Books. Palo Albo. 1976.
101. Yalcin BM, Karahan TF. Effects of a couple communication program on marital adjustment. J Am Board Fam Med. 2007; 20:36-44.
102. Greene BL. Psychiatric therapy of marital problems: Modem techniques. In: Masserman J, editors Current Psychiatric Therapies. Orlando FL: Grune & Stratton; 1972;12.
103. Martin PA, Bird HW. An approach to the psychotherapy of marriage partners: The stereoscopic techniques. Psychiatry 1963;16:122-77.
104. Solomon AP, Green DL. Marital disharmony; Concurrent therapy of husband and wife by the same psychiatrist. Dis Nerv Sys. 1963;24:21-8.
105. Fitzerland RO. Conjoint marital psychotherapy: An outcome and follow-up study. Fam Process. 1969;8:260-71.
106. Bowlby J. Attachment and Loss. New York: Basic books; 1980.
107. Johnson SM, Whiffen VE. Made to measure: Adapting emotionally focused couple therapy to partners attachment style. Clinical Psychology: Sci Prac. 1999;6:366-81.

108. Johnson SM, Williams Keeler L. Creating healing relationships for couples with trauma: the use of emotionally focused marital therapy. J Mar Fam Ther. 1998;24:25-40.
109. Johnson SM. The revolution in couple therapy: a Practitioner-scientist perspective. J Marital Fam Ther. 2003;29:365-84.
110. Rogers CR. Client centered psychotherapy. Haunghton Miffin. Boston; 1951.
111. Berne E. Games people play: The psychology of Human Relationships. Castle New York: 1964.
112. Stuart RB. Helping couples change: A social learning approach to marital therapy. New York: Guilford: 1980.
113. Datillio FM. Homework assignments in couple and marital therapy. J Clin Psychol. 2002;58:535-47.
114. Gurman AS, Lebow JL. Family therapy and couple therapy. In Kaplan, Sadocks Comprehensive Textbook of Psychiatry. 7th edition B. Sadock, V. Sadock, editors. New York: Lippincott William & Wilkins; 2000. pp.215-67.
115. Siaiken K, Culler R, Pearson J. Process and outcome in divorce mediation. Mediation Quarterly. 1985;10:121-34.
116. Marlow L. Divorce mediation: Therapists in their own world. Am J Fam Ther. 1985;13:10-4.
117. Kressel K, Jaffee N, Tuchman B, Watson C, Deutsch M. A typology of divorcing couples implications for mediation and divorce process. Fam Process. 1980;19:101-16.
118. Haynes IM. The conceptual mode of the process of family mediation: implication for training. Am J Fam Ther. 1982; 10:10-6.
119. Shadish W, Baldwin S. Meta-analysis of MFT interventions. J Marital Fam Ther. 2003;29:547-70.
120. Wood N, Crane D, Schaalje B, Law D. What works for whom: a meta-analytic review of marital and couples therapy in reference to marital distress. Am J Fam Ther. 2005; 33:273-87.
121. Snyder D, Wills R, Grady-Fletcher F. Long-term effectiveness of behavioral versus insight-oriented marital therapy: a 4-year follow-up study. J Consult Clin Psychol. 1991;59:138-41.
122. Duterte E, Segraves T, Althof S. Psychotherapy and pharmacotherapy for sexual dysfunctions. In: Nathan PJ. Gorman, editors. A Guide to Treatments that Work 3rd edition New York: Oxford University Press; 2007. pp.531–69.
123. Meston C, Bradford A. Sexual dysfunctions in women. Annu Rev Clin Psychol. 2007;3:233-56.
124. Banner L, Anderson R. Integrated Sildenafil and cognitive-behaviour sex therapy for psychogenic erectile dysfunction: a pilot study. J Sex Med. 2007;4:1117-25.
125. Stith S, Rosen K. Effectiveness of couple's treatment for spouse abuse. J Marital Fam Ther. 2003;29:407-26.
126. Stith S, Rosen K, McCollum E, Thomsen C. Treating intimate partner violence within intact couple relationships: outcomes of multi-couple versus individual couple therapy. J Marital Fam Ther. 2004;30:305-18.
127. Aos S, Barnoski R, Lieb R. Watching the Bottom Line: Cost-Effective Interventions for Reducing Crime in Washington. Olympia, WA: Washington State Institute for Public Policy: 1998.
128. Klein NC, Alexander JF, Parsons BV. Impact of family systems intervention on recidivism and sibling delinquency: A model of primary prevention and program evaluation. J Consult Clin Psychol. 1977;45:469-74.
129. Byrne M, Carr A, Clarke M. The efficacy of couples based interventions for panic disorder with agoraphobia. J Fam Ther. 2004;26:105-25.
130. Renshaw K, Steketee G, Chambless D. Involving family members in the treatment of OCD. Cogn Behav Ther. 2005; 34:164-75.
131. Carr A. The effectiveness of family therapy and systemic interventions for adult-focused problems. J Fam Ther. 2009; 31:46-74.
132. O'Farrell T, Fals-Stewart W. Behavioural Couples Therapy for Alcoholism and Substance Abuse. New York: Guilford Press; 2006.
133. Pfammatter M, Junghan U, Brenner H. Efficacy of psychological therapy in schizophrenia: conclusions from meta-analyses. Schizophr Bull. 2006;32:S64–S80.
134. Kassaw K, Gabbard. The ethics of email communication in psychiatry. Psychiatr Clin N Am. 2002;25:665-74.
135. Martire L, Lustig A, Schultz R, Miller G, Helgeson V. Is it beneficial to involve a family member? A meta-analysis of psychosocial interventions for chronic illness. Health Psychol. 2004;23:599-611.
136. Jacob KS, Sharan P, Mirza I, et al. Mental health systems in countries: where are we now? Lancet. 2007;370:1061-77.
137. Samuel M, Thyloth M. Caregivers' roles in India. Psychiatr Serv. 2002; 53:346-47.
138. Verghese A. Families' participation in mental health care—The Vellore experiment. Indian J Psychiatry. 1988;30:117-21.
139. Pai S, Kapur RI. Evaluation of home care treatment for schizophrenic patients. Acta Psychiatr Scand. 1983;67:80-3.
140. Pai S, Channabasavanna SM, Nagarajaiah M, Raghuram R. Home care for chronic mental illness in Bangalore: an experiment in the prevention of repeated hospitalization. Br J Psychiatry. 1985;147:175-9.
141. Kulhara P, Chakrabarti S, Avasthi A, Sharma A, Sharma S. Psychoeducational intervention for caregivers of Indian patients with schizophrenia: a randomised-controlled trial. Acta Psychiatr Scand. 2009;119:472-83.
142. Avasthi A, Grover S. Forensic Psychiatry- clinical practice guidelines for psychiatrists in India. Jaipur: Indian Psychiatric Society; 2009. pp.148-63.
143. Fisher CB, Oran KY M. Informed consent to psychotherapy: protecting the dignity and respecting the autonomy of the patients. J Clin Psychol. 2008;64:576-88.
144. Fisher CB. Decoding the Ethics Code. A Practical Guide for Psychologists. Thousand Oaks, CA: Sage; 2003.
145. Rokeach M. The Nature of Human Values. Macmillan, New York, 1973.

146. Weyrauch KF. Malpractice, patient satisfaction and physician patient communication. JAMA. 1995;274:23-5.
147. Kassaw K, Gabbard. The ethics of email communication in psychiatry. Psychiatr Clin N Am. 2002;25:665-74.
148. American Association of Marital and Family therapy. AAMFT Code of Ethics. 2007 *http://www.aamft.org/resources/LRM_Plan/Ethics/ethicscode2001.asp.*

Cognitive Therapy: Current Status and Future Directions

149. Beck AT. Thinking and depression 0.1. Idiosyncratic content and cognitive distortions. Arch, Gen, Psychiatry. 1963;9:342-33.
150. Beck AT. Thinking and depression. 2. Theory and therapy. Arch Gen Psychiatry. 1964;10:561-71.
151. Beck AT. Cognitive Therapy and the Emotional Disorders. New York: Int. Univ. Press; 1976.p.346.
152. Beck AT. The current state of cognitive therapy: a 40-year retrospective. Arch Gen Psychiatry. 2005;62:053-59.
153. Beck AT, Resnik HLP, Lettieri DJ, editors. The Prevention of Suicide. Bowie, MD: Charles press, 1974.
154. Beck AT, Emery G, Greenberg RL. Anxiety Disorders and Phobias: A Cognitive Perspective. New York: Basic Books. 1985.
155. Beck AT, Freeman A, Davis D, et al. Cognitive Therapy of Personality Disorders. New York: Guilford, 1990.
156. Beck AT, Wright FD, Newman EF, et al. Cognitive Therapy of Substance Abuse. New York: Guilford, 1993.
157. Beck AT, Rector NA. Cognitive approaches to schizophrenia: theory and therapy. Annu Rev Clin Psychol. 2005;1:577-606.
158. Beck AT, Rector NA, Stolar N, et al. Schizophrenia: Cognitive Theory, Research, and Therapy. New York: Guilford. 2009.
159. DeRubeis RJ, Webb CA, Tang TZ, et al. Cognitive therapy. In:KS Dobson (Ed). Handbook of Cognitive-Behavioral Therapies. New York: Guilford. 2010.pp. 227-316.
160. Prochaska JO, Norcross JC. Systems of psychotherapy. In:KS Dobson (Ed). Handbook of Cognitive-Behavioral Therapies, New York: Guilford. 2010;pp. 277-316.
161. Beck AT. Beyond belief: a theory of modes, personality, and psychopathology. In: PM Salkovskis (Ed). Frontiers of Cognitive New York: Guilford. Therapy; 1996;pp.1-25.
162. Beck AT, Weishaar ME. Cognitive therapy. In: RJ Corsini, D Wedding (Ed). Current Psychotherapies; 2011.pp.276-309. Belmont: Brooks/Cole.
163. Beck AT, Rush AJ, Shaw BF, et al. Cognitive Therapy of Depression. New York: Guilford, 1979.
164. Clark DA, Beck AT, Alford BA. Scientific Foundations of Cognitive Theory and Therapy of Depression. New York: Wiley, 1999.
165. Alford BA, Beck AT. The Integrative Power of Cognitive Therapy. New York: Guilford, 1997.
166. Dozois DJA, Beck AT. Cognitive schemas, beliefs and assumptions. In: KS Dobson (Eds), Risk Factors in Depression, DJA Dozois; Oxford. UK: Elsevier/Academic. 2008.pp.121-43.
167. Garratt G, Ingram RE, Rand KL, et al. Cognitive processes in cognitive therapy: evaluation of the mechanisms of change in the treatment of depression. Clin Psychol Sci Pract. 2007;14:224-39.
168. Dozois DJA, Dobson KS. Information processing and cognitive organization in unipolar depression: specificity and comorbidity issues. J Abnorm Psychol. 2001;110:236-46.
169. Mathews A, MacLeod C. Cognitive vulnerability to emotional disorders. Annu Rev Clin Psychol. 2005;1:167-95.
170. Harmer CJ, O'Sullivan U, Massey-Chase R, et al. Effect of acute antidepressant administration on negative affective bias in depressed patients. AM J Psychiatry. 2009;116:178-84.
171. Segal ZV, Gemar M, Williams S. Differential cognitive response to a mood challenge following successful cognitive therapy or pharmacotherapy for unipolar depre sion. J Abnorm Psychol. 1999;108:3-10.
172. Alloy LB, Abramson LY, Whitehouse WG, et al. Prospective incidence of first onsets and recurrences of depression in individuals at high and low cognitive risk for depression. J Abnorm Psychol. 2006;108:3-10.
173. Dobson D, Dobson KS. Cognitive and behavioral treatment of depression. In: IH Gotlib (Ed), Handbook of Depression, CL Hammen, New York: Guilford. 2009.pp.586-603.
174. Dobson KS, Dozois DJA. Historical and philosophical bases of the cognitive-behavioral therapies. In: DS Dobson (Ed). Handbook of Cognitive-Behavioral Therapies, New York: Guilford. 2010.pp.3-38.
175. Hollon SD, Dimidjian S. Cognitive and behavioral treatment of depression. In: IH Gotlib, CL (Ed). Handbook of Depression, Hammen; New York: Guilford. 2009;pp. 586-603.
176. Padesky CA, Beck AT. Science and philosophy: Comparison of cognitive therapy and rational emotive behavior therapy. J Cogn Psyhother. 2003;17:211-24.
177. Lazantizis N, Whittington C, Dattilio F. Meta-analysis of homework effects in cognitive and behavioral therapy: a replication and extension. Clin Pshchol Sci Pract. 2010;17: 144-56.
178. Beck JS. Cognitive Therapy: Basics and Beyond. New York: Guilford. 1995.
179. Dozois DJA, Bieling PJ. Cognitive behavioral treatment of depression. In: Herbert JD, Forman EM (Eds). Cognitive Behavioral Therapy, Acceptance, Midfulness: Understanding and Applying the New Therapies. New York: Wiley. In press, 2010.
180. Greenberger D, Padesky CA. Mind over Mood: Change How You Feel by Cbanging the Way You Think. New York: Guilford, 1995.
181. Dozois DJA, Bieling PJ, Patelis-Siotis I, et al. Changes in self-schema structure in cognitive therapy for major depressive disorder: a randomized clinical trial. J Consult Clin Psychol. 2009;77:1078-88.
182. Segl ZV, Kennedy S, Gemar M, et al. Cognitive reactivity to sad mood provocation and the prediction of depressive relapse. Arch Gen Psychiatry. 2006;63:749-55.

183. Butler AC, Chapman JE, Forman EM, et al. The empirical status of cognitive-behavioral therapy a review of meta-analyses. Clin Psychol Rev. 2006;26:17-31.
184. Chambless DL, Ollendick TH. Empirically supported psychological interventions: controversies and evidence. Annu Rev Psychol. 2001;52:685-716.
185. DeRubeis RJ, Crits-Christoph P. Empirically supported individual and group psychological treatments for adult mental disorders. J Consult CLin Psychol. 1998;66:37-52.
186. Mazzucchelli T, Kane R, Rees C. Behavioral activation treatments for depression in adults: a meta-analysis and review. Clin Psychol Sci Pract. 2009;16:383-411.
187. Wampold BE, Minami T, Baskin TW, et al. A meta-(re)analysis of the effects of cognitive therapy versus "other therapies" for depression. J Affect Disord. 2002;68:383-411.
188. Epp A, Dobson KS. The evidence bases for cognitive-behavioral therapy. In: KS Dobson (Ed), Handbook of Cognitive-behavioral Therapies. New York: Guilford. 2010;pp. 39-73.
189. Elkin I, Shea MT, Watkins JT, et al. National Institute of Mental Health Treatment of Depression Collaborative Research Program. General effectiveness of treatments. Arch Gen Psychiatry. 1989;46:971-82; discussion 83.
190. Elkin I, Gibbons RD, Shea MT, et al. Initial severity and differential treatment outcome in the National Institute of Mental Health Treatment of Depression Collaborative Research Program. J Consult Clin Psychol. 1995;63:841-7.
191. DeRubeis RJ, Gelfand LA Tang TZ, et al. Medications versus cognitive behavior therapy for severely depressed outpatients: mega-analysis of four randomized comparisons. AM J Psychiatry. 1999;156:1007-13.
192. DeRubeis RJ, Hollon SD, Amsterdam JD, et al. Cognitive therapy versus medications in the treatment of moderate to severe depression. Arch Gen Psychiatry. 2005;62:409-16.
193. Hollon SD, DeRubeis RJ, Shelton RC, et al. Prevention of relapse following cognitive therapy versus medications in moderate to severe depression. Arch Gen Psychiatry. 2005;62:417-22.
194. Cuijpers P, Smit F, Bohlmeijer E, et al. Efficacy of cognitive-behavioral therapy and other psychological treatments for adult depression: meat-analytic study of publication bias. Br J Psychiatry. 2010;196:173-78.
195. Gloaguen V, Cottraux J, Cucherat M, et al. A meta-analysis of the effects of cognitive therapy in depressed patients. J Affect Disord. 1998;49:59-72.
196. Dobson KS, Hollon SD, Dimidjian S, et al. Randomized trial of behavioral activation, cognitive therapy, and antidepressant medication in the prevention of relapse and recurrence in major depression J Consult Clin Psychol. 2008;76:468-77.
197. Beevers CG, Miller IW. Unlinking negative cognition and symptoms of depression: evidence of a specific treatment effect for cognitive therapy. J Consult Clin Psychol. 2005;73: 68-77.
198. Frewen PA, Dozois DJA, Lanius RA. Neuroimaging studies of psychological interventions for mood and anxiety disorders: empirical and methodological review. Clin Psycho Rev. 2008;28:228-46.
199. Goldapple K, Segal Z, Garson C, et al. Modulation of cortical limbic pathways in major depression treatment-specific effects of cognitive behavior therapy. Arcb Gen Psychiatry. 2004;61:34-41.
200. Lynch D, Law KR, McKenna PJ. Cognitive behavioral therapy for major psychiatric disorder. Does it rally work? A meta-analytical review of well-controlled trials. Psychol Med. 2010;40:9-24.
201. Kingdon D. Over-simplification and exclusion of nonconforming studies can demonstrate absence of effect: a lynching party? Psychol Med. 2010;40:25-27.
202. Sensky T. Cognitive-behavior therapy for patients with physical illnesses. In: J Wright (Ed), Cognitive-Behavior, Therapy. Review of Psychiatry, Arlington, VA: APA publishing. 2004;23:83-121.
203. Guthrie E, Sensky T. The role of psychological treatment. In: G Lloyd, E Guthrie (Eds), Handbook of Liaison Psychiatry. Cambridge, UK: Cambridge Univ. Press. 2007.pp.795-817.
204. Raine R, Haines A, Sensky T, et al. Systematic review of mental health interventions for patients with common somatic symptoms: Can research evidence from secondary care be extrapolated to primary care? BMF. 2002;325:11.
205. Hoffman BM, Papas RK, Chatkoff DK, et al. Meta-analysis of psychological interventions for chronic low back pain. Health Psychol. 2007;26:1-9.
206. Looper KJ, Kirmyer LJ. Behavioral medicine approaches to somatoform disorders. J Consult Clin Psychol. 2002:70:810-27
207. Blanchard EB, Scharff L. Psychosocial aspect of assessment and treatment of irritable bowel syndrome in adults and recurrent abdominal pain in children. J Consult Clin Psychol. 2002;70:725-38.
208. Malouff JA, Thoresteinsson EB, Rooke SE, et al. Efficacy of cognitive behavioral therapy for chronic fatigue syndrome: a meta-analysis. Clin Psychol Rev. 2008;28:736-45.
209. Hauser W, Thieme K, Turk DC. Guidelines on the management of fibromyalgia syndrome-a systematic review. Eur J Pain. 2010;14:5 -10.
210. Holroyd KA. Assessment and psychological management of recurrent headache disorders. J Consult Clin Psych. 2002;70:656-77.
211. Wang MY, Wang SY, Tsai PS. Cognitive behavioral therapy for primary insomnia: a systematic review. J Adv Nurs. 2005;50:553-64.
212. de Niet GJ, Tiemens BG, Kloos MW, et al. Review of systematic reviews about the efficacy of non pharmacological interventions to improve sleep quality in insomnia. Int J Evidence-Based Health. 2009;7:233-42.
213. Osborn RL, Demoncada AC, Feuerstein M. Psychosocial interventions for depression, anxiety, and quality of life in cancer survivors: meta-analyses. Int J Psychiatry Med. 2006;36:13-34.

214. Hersch J, Juraskoval I, Price M, et al. Psychosocial interventions and quality of life in gynecological cancer patients: a systematic review. Psycho-oncology. 2009;18:795-810.
215. Fisher EB, Thorpe CT, Devellis BM, et al. Healthy coping, negative emotions, and diabetes management: a systematic review and appraisal. Diabetes Educ. 2007;33:1080-103; discussion 104-6.
216. Beck AT. The evolution of the cognitive model of depression and its neurobiological correlates. Ant J Psychiatry 2008;165:969-77.
217. Longmore RJ, Worrell M. Do we need to challenge thoughts in cognitive behavior therapy? Clin Psychol Rev. 2007;27:173-87.

BIBLIOGRAPHY

Psychotherapy

1. Adler A. The Education of Children. New York: Greeberg, 1930.
2. Advertisement. The Times of India. Ahmedabad Edition. March 26, 1990.
3. Aray LB, Burrows W, Grenhill JP (Eds). Dorland's Illustrated Medical Dictionary. 23rd edn. Philadelphia: Saunders, 1957.
4. Begchi BK. Mental hygiene and the Hindu doctrine of relaxation. MentHyg. 1936;20:424-40.
5. Benson H. The Relaxation Response. New York: Morroco, 1975.
6. Berne E. Transactional Analysis in Psychotherapy. New York: Grove, 1961.
7. Binswanger L. Existential analysis and psychotherapy. In: Fromm-Reichmann F, Moreno J (Eds). Progress in Psychotherapy. Vol 1. Orlando: Grune and Stratton, 1956.
8. Bloch S. Supportive psychotherapy. In: Bloch S (Ed). An Introduct-ion to the Psychotherapies. Oxford: Oxford University Press, 1979.
9. Boss M. Psychoanalysis and Daseinsanalysis. New York: Basic Books, 1973.
10. Carriel DA Scream Away From Happiness. New York: Grosset and Dunlop, 1972.
11. Conte WR. Occupational therapy. I. The psychoses. In: Masserman JH (Ed). Current Psychiatric Therapies. Vol 2. Orlando: Grune and Stratton, 1967.
12. Counselman EF, Alonso A (Eds). The ill therapist: Therapists' reactions to personal illness and its impact on psychotherapy. Am J Psychother. 1993;47:519-602.
13. Cummings J, Cummings E. Ego and Millieu: Theory and Practice of Environmental Therapy. New York: Atherton Press, 1962.
14. David-Ferdon C, Kaslow N. Evidence-based psychosocial treatments for child and adolescent depression. Journal of Clinical Child and Adolescent Psychology. 2008;37(1):62-104.
15. Eisler I, Dare C, Russell GFM, Szmuckler GA, Le Grange D, Dodge E. Family and individual therapy in anorexia nervosa: A five-year follow-up. Archives of General Psychiatry. 1997;54:1025-30.
16. Ellis A. My philosophy of psychotherapy. J Contempt Psychol. 1973;6:13-8.
17. Ellis A. Outcome of employing three techniques of psychotherapy. J ClinPsychol. 1957;13:344-50.
18. Erickson MH, Rossi E. Innovative Hypnotherapy: Collected Papers of Milton H. Erickson on Hypnosis. New York: Invington, 1980.
19. Evans FJ. The placebo response in pain reduction. In: Bonica JJ (Ed). Advances in Neurology. Vol IV. Pain. New York: Raven, 1974. pp. 289-96.
20. Eyberg SM, Nelson MM, Boggs SR. Evidence-based psychosocial treatments for children and adolescents with disruptive behavior. Journal of Clinical Child and Adolescent Psychology. 2008;37(1):215-37.
21. Fairbairn WRD. An Object Relations Theory of the Personality. New York: Basic Books, 1954.
22. Ferenczi S. Further Contributions to the Theory and Technique of Psychoanaysis. New York: Basic Books, 1952.
23. Forem J. Transcendental Meditation: Maharishi Mahesh Yogi and the Science of Creative Intelligence. New York: Dutton, 1973.
24. Frankl VE. Logotherapy and existential analysis: a review. Am J Psychother. 1966;20:252-60.
25. Freud A. The Ego and Mechanisms of Defense. London: Hogarth, 1937.
26. Fromm E. Escape from Freedom, New York: Halt, 1941.
27. Fromm E. Man for Himself. New York: Halt, 1947.
28. Glasser W, Zunin LM. Reality Therapy. In: Masserman JH (Ed). Current Psychiatric Therapies. Vol 12. Orlando: Grune and Stratton, 1972.
29. Glueck BC, Strobel CF. Biofeedback and meditation in the treatment of psychiatric illness. In: Masserman JH (Ed). Current Psychiatric Therapies. Vol. 15. Orlando: Grune and Stratton, 1975.
30. Greenblatt M, Grosser GH, Wechsler H. Differential response of hospitalized depressed patients to somatic therapy. Am J Psychiatry. 1964;120:935-43.
31. Greenwald H. Direct decision therapy. In: Herink R (Ed). The Psychotherapy Handbook. New York: New American Library, 1980.pp.152-4.
32. Gunderson JG, Will OA Jr, Mosher LR. Principles and Practice of Milieu Therapy. New York: Aronson, 1983.
33. Guralnik DP. Ed. Webster's New Word Dictionary, 2nd edn. New York: World, 1970.
34. Haun P. Recreation in medical psychiatric therapy. In: Masserman JH (Ed). Current Psychiatric Therapies. Vol 7. Orlando: Grune and Stratton, 1967.
35. Horney K. The Neurotic Personality of Our Time. New York: Norton, 1937.
36. Jacobson E. Progressive Relaxation, 3rd edn. Rev. Chicago: University of Chicago Press, 1974.
37. Janov A. The Primal Scream: Primal Therapy, The Cure of Neurosis. New York: Putnam, 1970.
38. Jaspers K. Von der Wahrheit. Munich: Piper, 1947.
39. Jung CG. Psychological Types or the Psychology of Individuation. Orlando: Harcourt, 1923.

40. Khorana AB. Concept of team functioning in the mental health field. Social Work Review. MS University of Baroda, 1973. pp.35-40.
41. Klein M. Notes on some schizoid mechanism. Im J Psychoanal. 1946;27:89-110.
42. Klein M. Our Adult World and Other Essays. New York: Basic Books, 1963.
43. Kolb LC. Modern Clinical Psychiatry. Philadelphia: Saunders, 1973.
44. Le Grange D, Binford R, Loeb KL. Manualized family-based treatment for anorexia nervosa: A case series. Journal of the American Academy of Child and Adolescent Psychiatry. 2005; 44:41-6.
45. Leichsenring F, Leibing E. Psychodynamic psychotherapy: a systematic review of techniques, indications and empirical evidence. Psychology and Psychotherapy. 2007;80(Pt 2): 217-28.
46. Levy J. Relationship therapy. Am J Orthopsychiatry. 1938;8:64-9.
47. Majumdar SK. Introduction to Yoga: Principles and Practices. New Hyde Park, NY: University Books, 1964.
48. Malhotra JC. Yoga and psychiatry: a review. J Neuropsychiatry. 1963;4:375-85.
49. Meloy JR. The Psychopathic Mind: Origins, Dynamics and Treatment. Northvale: Aronson, 1988. pp. 237.
50. Meyer A. Objective psychology and psychobiology. JAMA. 1915;65:860-3.
51. Meyer A. The Common Sense Psychiatry of Dr. Adolf Meyer. New York: McGraw-Hill, 1948.
52. Moreno JL. Ed. The International Handbook of Psychotherapy. New York: Philosophical Library, 1966.
53. Mufson L, Dorta KP, Wickramaratne P, Nomura Y, Olfson M, Weissman MM. A randomized effectiveness trial of interpersonal psychotherapy for depressed adolescents. Archives of General Psychiatry. 2004; 61(6):577-84.
54. Neufeld W. Relaxation methods in United State Navy Schools. Am J Psychiatry. 1951;108:132-7.
55. Noshpitz JD, Shapiro T, Sherman M, et al. Millieu therapy. In: Karasu TB (Ed). The Psychiatric Therapies. Washington DC: American Psychiatric Press, 1984.
56. Patanjali. Cited In: Vahia NS. Hindu philosophy and psychology. Lecture presented at the Postgraduate Centre for Mental Health, New York, 1962.
57. Pelham WE, Fabiano GA. Evidence-based psychosocial treatments for attention deficit/hyperactivity disorder. Journal of Clinical Child and Adolescent Psychology. 2008; 37(1):184-214.
58. Reich W. Character Analysis. III Ed. New York: Orgone Institute Press, 1949.
59. Rieff P. The Triumph of the Therapeutic Uses of Faith after Freud. New York: Harper and Row, 1956.
60. Rippan TS, Fletcher P. Reassurance and Relaxation. London: Routledge&Kegan Paul, 1940.
61. Rogers CR. A Way of Being. Boston: Moughton, Mifflin, 1980.
62. Rogers CR. Freedom to Learn for the 80's. Columbus: Charles E Merril, 1983.
63. Rosenzweig S. Some implicit common factors in diverse methods of psychotherapy. Am J Orthopsychiatry. 1936;6: 412-5.
64. Schachter M. Psychotherapy and Medicine. Northvale: Aronson, 1993.pp.7-16.
65. Sherwood S. Long-Term Care: A Handbook for Researchers, Planners and Providers. New York: Spectum, 1975.
66. Shor RE, Ome MT. The Nature of Hypnosis: Selected Basic Readings. New York: Halt, Reinehart and Winston, 1965.
67. Shorr JE. Psycho-imagination Therapy. New York: Stratton Intercontinental, 1972.
68. Silverman WK, Pina AA, Viswesvaran C. Evidence-based psychosocial treatments for phobic and anxiety disorders in children and adolescents. Journal of Clinical Child and Adolescent Psychology. 2008;37(1):105-30.
69. Simmons LW. Sun Chief. New Haven: Yale University Press, 1942.
70. Sullivan HS. Conceptions in Modern Psychiatry. Washington DC: William Alanson White Psychiatric Foundation, 1947.
71. Suzuki ET. Essays in Zen Buddhism. London: Rider, 1952.
72. The TADS Team. The Treatment for Adolescents with Depression Study (TADS): Long-term Effectiveness and Safety Outcomes. Archives of General Psychiatry. 2007; 64(10):1132-43.
73. Thorne FC. Principles of directive counselling and psychotherapy. Am Psychol. 1948;3:160-5.
74. Vahia NS. Hindu philosophy and psychology. Lecture presented at the Postgraduate Center for Mental Health, New York, 1962.
75. Watson G. Areas of agreement in psychotherapy. Am J Orthopsychiatry. 1940;10:698-709.
76. WHO. Expert Committee on Mental Health: Report on the first session. WHO Tech Rep Ser. 1950.pp.9-10.
77. WHO. Tenth Report of the Expert Committee on Mental Health. WHO Tech Rep Ser. 1961;36:223.
78. Wolberg LR. The Technique of Psychotherapy. 4th edn. Philadel-phia: Grune and Stratton, 1988.
79. Yalom ID. The Theory and Practice of Group Psychotherapy. New York: Basic Books, 1975.
80. Yates DH. Relaxation in psychotherapy. J Genet Psychol. 1946; 34:213-37.
81. Young HA. Rational Counselling Primer. New York: Institute for Advanced Studies in Rational Psychotherapy, 1974.

Interpersonal Psychotherapy

82. Brown GW, Harris T. Social Origins of Depression. London: Tavistock Publications; 1978.
83. Elkin I, Shea MT, Watkins JT, Imber SD, Sotsky SM, Collins JF, et al. National Institute of Mental Health treatment of depression collaborative research program: General effectiveness of treatments. Arch Gen Psych. 1989;46:971-82.
84. Fairburn CG, Jones R, Peveler RC. Three psychological treatments for bulimia nervosa: a comparative trial. Arch Gen Psych. 1991;48:436-69.

85. Frank E, Kupfer DJ, Buysse DJ, Swartz HA, Pilkonis PA, Houck PR, et al. Randomized trial of weekly, twice-monthly, and monthly interpersonal psychotherapy as maintenance treatment for women with recurrent depression. Am J Psych. 2007;164:761-7.
86. Frank E. Interpersonal psychotherapy as a maintenance treatment for patients with recurrent depression. Psychotherapy. 1991;28(2):259.
87. Henderson AS. Introduction to Social Psychiatry. Oxford: Oxford University Press; 1988.
88. Joyce PR, McKenzie JM, Carter JD, Rae AM, Luty SE, Frampton, CMA, Mulder RT. Temperament, character and personality disorders as predictors of response to interpersonal psychotherapy and cognitive-behavioural therapy for depression. The British J Psych. 2007;190: 495-502.
89. Klerman GL, Weissman MM, Rounsaville B, Chevron E. Interpersonal Psychotherapy for Depression. New York: Basic Books: 1984.
90. Luty SE, Carter JD, McKenzie JM, Rae AM, Frampton CM A, Mulder RT, Joyce PR. Randomised controlled trial of interpersonal psychotherapy and cognitive behavioural therapy for depression. The British J Psych. 2007;190:496-502.
91. Paykel ES, Weissman MM, Prusoff BA. Social maladjustment and severity of depression. Comprehensive Psychiatry. 1978;19:121-9.
92. Reynolds CF, III Frank E, Perel JM, Imber S, Cornes C, Miller MD, et al. Nortriptyline and interpersonal psychotherapy as maintenance therapies for recurrent major depression. J Am Med Assoc. 1999;281;39-45.
93. Rounsaville BJ, Chevron ES, Weissman MM, Prusoff BA, Frank E. Training therapists to perform interpersonal psychotherapy in clinical trials. Comprehensive Psychiatry. 1986;27:364-71.
94. Stuart S, Robertson M. Interpersonal Psychotherapy: A Clinician's Guide. London: Edward Arnold; 2003.
95. Weissman MM, Markowitz JC, Klerman GL. Clinician's Quick Guide to Interpersonal Psychotherapy. New York: Oxford University Press; 2007.
96. Wilfley DE, Welch RR, Stein RI, Spurrell EB, Cohen LR, Saelens BE, et al. A randomised comparison of group cognitive-behavioural therapy and group interpersonal psychotherapy for the treatment of overweight individuals with binge-eating disorder. Arch Gen Psych. 2002;59(8):713-72.

Occupational Therapy

97. American Occupational Therapy Association. Handbook for the Division of Professional Development, Mental Health. Rockville: American Occupational Therapy Association, 1981.
98. American Occupational Therapy Association. Occupational therapy: Its definition and function. Am J Occup Ther. 1972;26: 204.
99. Ayllon T, Azrin NH. The Token Economy: A Motivational System for Therapy and Rehabilitation. New York: Appleton-Century-Crafts, 1968.
100. Ayres AJ. The development of perceptual motor abilities: a theoretical basis for treatment of dysfunction. Am J Occup Ther. 1963;17:221-5.
101. College of Occupational Therapists Recovering ordinary lives: the strategy for occupational therapy in mental health services-2007-2017 a vision for the next ten years. COT, London, 2006.
102. Corrigan PW. Towards an integrated, structural model for psychiatric rehabilitation. Psychiatr Rehabil J. 2003;26(4):346-58.
103. Cowls J, Hale S. It's activity that counts: What clients value in psycho-educational groups. Can J Occup Ther. 2005;72(3): 176-82.
104. Creek J, Bullock A. Assessment and outcome measurement. In: Creek J, Lougher L (Eds). Occupational Therapy and Mental Health, 4th edn. Churchill Livingstone Elsevier, London; 2008. pp.81-107.
105. Demon P. Psychiatric Occupational Therapy. A Workbook of Practical Skills. Boston: Little Brown, 1987.
106. Duffy R, Nolan P. A survey of the work of occupational therapists in inpatient mental health services. Mental Health Practice. 2005;8(6):36-41.
107. Duncan EAS. Cognition and cognitive approaches in occupational therapy. In: J Creek, L Lougher (Eds) Occupational Therapy and Mental Health, 4th edn. Churchill Livingstone Elsevier, London: 2008;303-14.
108. Fidler GS. From crafts to competence. Am J Occup Ther. 1981; 35:567-73.
109. Fidler GS. Overview of Occupational Therapy in Mental Health. Rockville: American Occupational Therapy Association, 1981.
110. Fine SB. Occupational Therapy: The Role of Rehabilitation and Purposeful Activity in Mental Health Practice. Rockville: American Occupational Therapy Association, 1983.
111. Forsyth K, Braverman B, Kielhofner G et al. Psychometric properties of the Worker Role Interview. Work,. 2006;27(3):313-8.
112. Fortune T, Fitzgerald MH. The challenge of interdisciplinary collaboration in acute psychiatry: impacts on the occupational milieu. Australian Occupational Therapy Journal. 2009;56(1):81-8.
113. Hawkes R, Johnstone V, Yarwood R. Acute psychiatry. In: J Creek, L Lougher (Eds). Occupational Therapy and Mental Health, 4th edn. Churchill Livingstone Elsevier, London: 2008;393-408.
114. Hopkins H. An historical perspective on occupational therapy. In: Hopkins HL, Smith HD (Eds). Willard and Spackman's Occupational Therapy, 6th edn. Philadelphia: Lippincott, 1983.
115. Jenning S (Ed). Drama therapy: Theory and Practice for Teachers and Clinicians. London: Croom Helm, 1987.
116. King LJ. A sensory integrative approach to schizophrenia. Am J Occup Ther. 1974;28:529-36.
117. Lim K, Morris J, Craik C. Inpatients' perspectives of occupational therapy in acute mental health. Australian Occupational Therapy Journal. 2007;54(1):22-32.

118. Llorens L. Application of A Developmental Theory for Health and Rehabilitation. Maryland: American Occupational Therapy Association, 1976.
119. Lloyd C, Waghorn G, Williams PL, Harris MG, Capra C. Early psychosis: Treatment issues and the role of occupational therapy. Br J Occup Ther. 2008;71(7):297-304.
120. Mailloux Z, Mack W, Cooper C. Knowing what to do: the organization of knowledge for clinical practice. In: Kielhofner G (Ed). Health Through Occupation: Theory and Practice in Occupational Therapy. Philadelphia: FA Davis, 1983.
121. Mairs H. Evidence-based practice in mental health: a cause for concern for occupational therapists? Br J Occup Ther. 2003;66(4):168-70.
122. Mosey AC. Eleanor Clarke Slagle Lecture. A monistic or pluralistic approach to professional identity?Am J Occup Ther 1985;39:504-9.
123. Mosey AC. Psychosocial Components of Occupational Therapy. New York: Raven Press, 1986.
124. Mosey AC. Three Frames of Reference for Mental Health. New Jersey: Charles B Slack, 1970.
125. Patterson C. A short history of occupational therapy in psychiatry. In: Creek J, Lougher L (Eds), Occupational Therapy and Mental Health. Churchill Livingstone, Elsevier, Edinburgh. 2008;pp.3-16.
126. Prabhu G, Prabhu N. Occupational therapy in psychiatry. J Rehab Asia, 1968.
127. Reily M. Occupational therapy can be one of the greatest ideas of 20th century medicine. Am J Occup Ther. 1962;16:1-9.
128. Simpson A, Bowers L, Alexander J, Ridley C, Warren J. Occupational therapy and multidisciplinary working on acute psychiatric wards: the Tompkins Acute Ward Study. Br J Occup Ther. 2005;68(12):545-552.

Rehabilitation in Psychiatry

129. Afflec JW, McGuire RJ. The measurement of psychiatric rehabilitation status: a review of the needs and a new scale. Br J Psychiatry. 1984;145:517-25.
130. Angermeyer MC, Matschinger H. Public beliefs about schizophrenia and depression: similarities and differences. Soc Psychiatry Psychiatr Epidemiol. 2003;38:526-34. [PubMed]
131. Anthony W, Cohen M, Farkas M, et al. Psychiatric rehabilitation. 2nd edition. Boston: Center for Psychiatric Rehabilitation, Boston University; 2002.
132. Anthony WA, Liberman RP. The practice of psychiatric rehabilitation: historical, conceptual and research base. Schiz Bull. 1986;12:542-59.
133. Asarnow RF, Marder SR, Mintz J, et al: Different effect of low and conventional doses of fluphenazine on schizophrenic outpatients with good or poor information processing abilities. Arch Gen Psychiatry. 1988;45:822-6.
134. Bachrach LL. Psychosocial rehabilitation and psychiatry in the care of long-term patients.Am J Psychiatry. 1992;149: 1455-63.
135. Bachrach LL. Psychosocial rehabilitation and psychiatry in the treatment of schizophrenia-what are the boundaries? Acta Psychiatr Scand. 2000;102(Suppl. 407):6-10. [PubMed]
136. Bachrach LL. The chronic patient: Perspectives on work and rehabilitation. HospComm Psychiatry. 1992;42:890-1.
137. Barbato A, D'Avanzo B, Rocca G, et al. A study of long-stay patients resettled in the community after closure of a psychiatric hospital in Italy. Psychiatr Serv. 2004;55:67-70. [PubMed]
138. Barbato A, Monzani E, Schiavi T. Life satisfaction in a sample of outpatients with severe mental disorders: a survey in northern Italy. Qual Life Res. 2004;13:969-73. [PubMed]
139. Baronet AM, Gerber GJ. Psychiatric rehabilitation: efficacy of four models. Clin Psychol Rev. 1998;18:189-228. [PubMed]
140. Bebbington PE. The content and context of compliance. Int Clin Psychopharmacol. 1995;9(Suppl 5):41-50. [PubMed]
141. Becker T, Leese M, Clarkson P, et al. Links between social network and quality of life: an epidemiologically representative study of psychotic patients in south London. Soc Psychiatry Psychiatr Epidemiol. 1998;33:229-304. [PubMed]
142. Bellack AS, Mueser KT, Morrison RL, et al. Remediation of cognitive deficits in schizophrenia. Am J Psychiatry. 1990;147:1650-55.
143. Bellack AS. Cognitive rehabilitation for schizophrenia: Is it possible? Is it necessary? Schiz Bull. 1992;18:43-50.
144. Bennett DH. The historical development of rehabilitation services. In: Watts FN, Bennett DH. Theory and Practice of Psychiatric Rehabilitation. Chichester: John Wiley, 1983.
145. Benton MK, Schroeder HE. Social skills training with schizophrenics: A metanalytic evaluation. J Consult Clin Psychol 1990;58:741-7.
146. Bhatti RS, Janakiramaiah N, Channabasavanna SM. Family psychiatric ward treatment in India. Family Process. 1980;19: 193-200.
147. Bloch S. Supportive psychotherapy. In: Bloch S (Ed). An Introduction to the Psychotherapies. Oxford: Oxford University Press, 1986.
148. Bond GR. Supported employment: evidence for an evidence-based practice. Psychiatr Rehabil J. 2004;27:345-59. [PubMed]
149. Brenner HD, Hodel B, Roder V, et al. Treatment of cognitive dysfunction and behavioral deficits in schizophrenia. Schiz Bull. 1992;18:21-6.
150. Breslin NA. Treatment of schizophrenia: Current practice and future promise. HospComm Psychiatry. 1993;43:877-84.
151. Burns T, Catty J, Wright C. De-constructing home-based care for mental illness: can one identify the effective ingredients? Acta Psychiatr Scand. 2006;113(Suppl. 429):33-5. [PubMed]
152. Burns T, Fioritti A, Holloway F, et al. Case management and assertive community treatment in Europe. Psychiatr Serv. 2001;52:631-6. [PubMed]
153. Cancro R. The introduction of neuroleptics: a psychiatric revolution. Psychiatr Serv. 2000;51:333-5. [PubMed]
154. Cardin VA, McGill CW, Falloon IRH. An economic analysis: Costs, benefits and effectiveness. In: Falloon IRH (Ed). Family

Management of Schizophrenia. Baltimore: John Hopkins University Press, 1986.

155. Carling PJ. Housing, community support, and homelessness: emerging policy in mental health systems. N Engl J Publ Policy. 1992;8:281-95.
156. Cook JA, Lehman AF, Drake R, et al. Integration of psychiatric and vocational services: a multisite randomized, controlled trial of supported employment. Am J Psychiatry. 2008;162:1948-56.
157. Corrigan PW, McCracken SG, Holmes EP. Motivational interviews as goal assessment for persons with psychiatric disability. Commun Ment Health J. 2001;37:113-22. [PubMed]
158. Corrigan PW, Slopen N, Gracia G, et al. Some recovery processes in mutual-help groups for persons with mental illness; II: qualitative analysis of participant interviews. Commun Ment Health J. 2005;41:721-35. [PubMed]
159. Cuffel B. Comorbid substances use disorder: prevalence, patterns of use, and course. In: Drake R, Mueser K, (Eds). Dual diagnosis of major mental illness and substance disorder: recent research and clinical implications. San Francisco: Jossey-Bass; 1996.pp.93-105.
160. Cutler DL. Clinical care update. The chronically mentally ill. Commun Ment Health J. 1985;21:3-13. [PubMed]
161. Davis JM. Overview, maintenance therapy in psychiatry. I Schizophrenia. Am J Psychiatry. 1975;132:1237-45.
162. Dencker SJ, Liberman RP. From compliance to collaboration in the treatment of schizophrenia. Int Clin Psychopharmacol. 1995;9(Suppl. 5):75–78. [PubMed]
163. Eckman TA, Liberman RP, Phipps CC, et al. Teaching medication management skills to schizophrenic patients. J Clin Psychopharmacol. 1990;10:33-8. [PubMed]
164. Falloon IRH, Boyd JL, McGill CW, et al. Family management in the prevention of morbidity of schizophrenia: Clinical outcome of a two year longtudinal study. Arch Gen Psychiatry. 1985;42: 887-96.
165. Farkas M, Gagne C, Anthony W, et al. Implementing recovery oriented evidence based programs: identifying the critical dimensions. Commun Ment Health J. 2005;41:141-58. [PubMed]
166. George LK, Blazer DG, Hughes DC, et al. Social support and the outcome of major depression. Br J Psychiatry. 1989;154:478-85. [PubMed]
167. Gold JM, Harvey PD. Cognitive deficits in schizophrenia. PsychiatrClin N Am. 1993;2:295-312.
168. Goldman HH, Gattozzi AA, Taube CA. Defining and counting the chronically mentally ill. Hosp Commun Psychiatry. 1981;32:21-7. [PubMed]
169. Goldstein MJ, Rodnick EH, Evans JR, et al. Drug and family therapy in the after care treatment of acute schizophrenia. Arch Gen Psychiatry. 1978;35:169-77.
170. Gopinath PS, Chaturvedi SK. Distressing behavior of schizophrenics at home. Acta Psychiatr Scand. 1992;86:185-88.
171. Graf J, Lauber C, Nordt C, et al. Perceived stigmatization of mentally ill people and its consequences for the quality of life in a Swiss population. J Nerv Ment Dis. 2004;192:542-7. [PubMed]
172. Grove B. Reform of mental health care in Europe. Progress and change in the last decade. Br J Psychiatry. 1994;165:431-3. [PubMed]
173. Hall GB, Nelson G. Social networks, social support, personal empowerment, and the adaptation of psychiatric consumers/ survivors: path analytic models. Soc Sci Med. 1996;43:1743-54. [PubMed]
174. Harding CM, Strauss JS, Hafez H, et al. Work and mental illness. I. Toward an integration of the rehabilitation process. J Nerv Ment Dis. 1987;175:317-26. [PubMed]
175. Health PsNFCoM. Achieving the promise: transforming mental health care in America. *www.mentalhealthcommission.gov/ reports/ Finalreport/toc_exec.html.*
176. Hendrichs DW, Hanion TE, Carpenter WT Jr. The Quality of Life Scale: An instrument for rating the schizophrenic deficit syndrome. Schiz Bull. 1984;10:388-98.
177. Hierholzer RW, Liberman RP. Successful living: A social skills and problem solving group for the chronic mentally ill. Hosp Comm Psychiatry. 1986;37:913-8.
178. Hirsch SR. Medication and physical treatment of schizophrenia. In: Wing JK (Ed). Handbook of Psychiatry, Vol. 3. Psychoses of Uncertain Etiology. London: Cambridge University Press, 1982.
179. Hogarty GE, Anderson CM, Reiss DJ, et al. Family psychoeducation, social skills training and maintenance chemotherapy in the aftercare treatment of schizophrenia. I. One year effects of a controlled study on relapse and expressed emotion. Arch Gen Psychiatry. 1986;43:633-42.
180. Hogarty GE, Anderson CM, Relss DJ, et al. Family psychoeducation, social skills training and maintenance chemotherapy in the aftercare treatment of schizophrenia. II.Two-year effects of a controlled study on relapse and adjustment. Arch Gen Psychiatry. 1991;48:340-7.
181. Hogarty GE, Flesher S. Cognitive remediation in schizophrenia: Proceed with caution. Schiz Bull. 1992;18:51-7.
182. Jacobs H, Kardashian S, Kreinbring R, et al. A skills-oriented model for facilitating employment in psychiatrically disabled persons. Rehabil Counsel Bull. 1988;27:96-7.
183. Jenkins JH, Karno M. The meaning of expressed emotion: theoretical issues raised by cross-culture research. Am J Psychiatry. 1992;14:9-21.
184. Jolley AG, Hirsch SR, Morrison E, et al. Trial of brief intermittent neuroleptic prophylaxis for selected schizophrenic outpatients: Clinical and social outcome at two years. Br Med J. 1990; 301:837-42.
185. Kane JM, Marder SR. Psychopharmacologic treatment of schizophrenia. Schiz Bull. 1993;19:287-302.
186. Killaspy H, Bebbington P, Blizard R, et al. The REACT study: randomised evaluation of assertive community treatment in north London. Br Med J. 2006;332:815-20. [PMC free article] [PubMed]

187. Kopelowicz A, Liberman RP. Biobehavioral treatment and rehabilitation of schizophrenia. Harv Rev Psychiatry. 1995;3: 55-64. [PubMed]
188. Lam DH. Psychosocial family intervention in schizophrenia: a review of empirical studies. Psychol Med. 1991;21:423-41.
189. Lamb HR, et al. Treating the Long-term Mentally Ill: Beyond Deinstitutionalization. San Francisco:: Jossey-Bass; 1982.
190. Lamb HR. Deinstitutionalization at the crossroads. Hospital and Community Psychiatry. 1988;39:941-5.
191. Lauber C, Nordt C, Falcato L, et al. Factors influencing social distance toward people with mental illness. Commun Ment Health J. 2004;40:265-74. [PubMed]
192. Lauber C, Nordt C, Falcato L, et al. Public attitude to compulsory admission of mentally ill people. Acta Psychiatr Scand. 2002;105:385-9. [PubMed]
193. Leff JP, Wig NN, Ghosh A, et al. Expressed emotion and schizophrenia in North India. III. Influence of relatives expressed emotion on the course of schizophrenia in Chandigarh. Br J Psychiatry. 1987;151:166-73.
194. Lefley HP. Family Burden and family stigma in major mental illness. Am Psychol. 1989;44:556-60.
195. Left JP, Sartorius N, Jablensky A, et al. The International Pilot Study of Schizophrenia: Five year follow-up findings. Psychol Med. 1992;22:131-46.
196. Lehman AF, Steinwachs DM. Patterns of usual care for schizophrenia: initial results from the Schizophrenia Patient Outcomes Research Team (PORT) Client Survey. Schizophr Bull. 1998;24:11-20.
197. Lenzenweger MF, Dworkin RH, Wethington E. Examining the underlying structure of schizophrenic phenomenology: Evidence for a three process model. Schiz Bull. 1991;17: 515-24.
198. Liberman RP, Glick ID. Drug and psychosocial curricula for psychiatry residents for treatment of schizophrenia: part I. Psychiatr Serv. 2004;55:1217-9. [PubMed]
199. Liberman RP, Green MF. Whither cognitive-behavioral therapy for schizophrenia? Schiz Bull. 1992;18:27-35.
200. Liberman RP, Hilty DM, Drake RE, et al. Requirements for multidisciplinary teamwork in psychiatric rehabilitation. Psychiatr Serv. 2001;52:1331-42. [PubMed]
201. Liberman RP, Vaccaro JV, Corrman PW. Psychiatric Rehabilitation. In: Kaplan HI, Sadock BJ (Eds). Comprehensive Textbook of Psychiatry, 6th edition. Baltimore: Williams & Wilkins, 1995;2696-2717.
202. Liberman RP, Wallace CJ, Hassell J. Rehab rounds: predicting readiness and responsiveness to skills training: the Micro-Module Learning Test. Psychiatr Serv. 2004;55:764-66. [PubMed]
203. Link BG, Struening EL, Rahav M, et al. On stigma and its consequences: evidence from a longitudinal study of men with dual diagnoses of mental illness and substance abuse. J Health Soc Behav. 1997;38:177-90. [PubMed]
204. Linn MW, Caffey EM, Klett J, et al. Day treatment and psychotropic drugs in the aftercare of schizophrenic patients. Arch Gen Psychiatry. 1979;36:1055-66.
205. Marshall M. Case management: a dubious practice. Br Med J. 1996;312:523-4. [PMC free article] [PubMed]
206. McElroy EM. Sources of distress among families of the hospitalized mentally ill. New Dir Ment Health Serv. 1987;34: 61-72. [PubMed]
207. Mechanic D, McAlpine D, Rosenfield S, et al. Effects of illness attribution and depression on the quality of life among persons with serious mental illness. Soc Sci Med. 1994;39:155-64. [PubMed]
208. Meise U, Sulzenbacher H, Kemmler G, et al. "Not dangerous, but nevertheless frightening". A program against stigmatization of schizophrenia in schools. Psychiatr Prax. 2000;27:340-6. [PubMed]
209. Mubarak Ali R, Bhatti RS. Social support system and family burden due to chronic schizophrenia in rural and urban background. Indian J Psychiatry. 1988;30:349-54.
210. Mueller B, Nordt C, Lauber C, et al. Social support modifies perceived stigmatization in the first years of mental illness: a longitudinal approach. Soc Sci Med. 2006;62:39-49. [PubMed]
211. Mueser KT, Bellack AS, Douglas MS, et al. Prediction of social skill acquisition in schizophrenic and major affective disorder patients from memory and symptomatology. Psychiatr Res. 1991;37:281-96.
212. Murthy RS. National Mental Health Program in India (1982-1989): Mid-point appraisal. Indian J Psychiatry. 1989;31:267-270.
213. Nagaswami N, Valecha V, Thara R, et al. Rehabilitation needs of schizophrenic patients: a preliminary report. Indian J Psychiatry. 1985;27:213-20.
214. Nordt C, Rössler W, Lauber C. Attitudes of mental health professionals toward people with schizophrenia and major depression. Schizophr Bull. in press.
215. Onken SJ, Dumont JM, Ridgway P, et al. Mental health recovery: what helps and what hinders? A national research project for the development of recovery facilitating system performance indicators. *www.rfmh.org/csipmh/projects/rc10.shtm.*
216. Parker G, Hadzi-Pavlovic D. Expressed emotion as a predictor of schizophrenic relapse: an analysis of aggregated data. Psychol Med. 1990;20:961-5.
217. Pinfold V, Huxley P, Thornicroft G, et al. Reducing psychiatric stigma and discrimination-evaluating an educational intervention with the police force in England. Soc Psychiatry Psychiatr Epidemiol. 2003;38:337-44. [PubMed]
218. Priebe S, McCabe R, Bullenkamp J, et al. The impact of routine outcome measurement on treatment processes in community mental health care: approach and methods of the MECCA study. Epidemiol Psichiatr Soc. 2002;11:198-205. [PubMed]
219. Rao K, Barnabas IP, Gopinath PS. Family burden in chronic schizophrenia: The role of the day hospital. Indian J Psychol Med. 1988;10:131-5.
220. Ridgway P, Zipple AM. The paradigm shift in residential services: from linear continuum to supported housing approaches. Psychosoc Rehabil J. 1990;13:11-32.

221. Rifkin A. Pharmacologic strategies in the treatment of schizophrenia. Psychiatr Clin N Am. 1993;2:351-64.
222. Rog DJ. The evidence on supported housing. Psychiatr Rehabil J. 2004;27:334-44. [PubMed]
223. Rogers ES, Anthony W, Lyass A. The nature and dimensions of social support among individuals with severe mental illnesses. Commun Ment Health J. 2004;40:437-50. [PubMed]
224. Rogers ES, Martin R, Anthony W, et al. Assessing readiness for change among persons with severe mental illness. Commun Ment Health J. 2001;37:97-112. [PubMed]
225. Rosenfield S. Labeling mental illness: the effects of received services and perceived stigma on life satisfaction. Am Soc Rev. 1997;62:660-72.
226. Rosie JS. Partial hospitalization: A review of recent literature. HospComm Psychiatry. 1987;38:1291-8.
227. Rössler W, Loffler W, Fatkenheuer B, et al. Does case management reduce the rehospitalization rate? Acta Psychiatr Scand. 1992;86:445-9. [PubMed]
228. Rössler W, Salize HJ, Cucchiaro G, et al. Does the place of treatment influence the quality of life of schizophrenics? Acta Psychiatr Scand. 1999;100:142-8. [PubMed]
229. Royal College of Psychiatrists. Psychiatric rehabilitation. Revised. London: Gaskell; 1996.
230. Ruesch P, Graf J, Meyer PC, et al. Occupation, social support and quality of life in persons with schizophrenic or affective disorders. Soc Psychiatry Psychiatr Epidemiol. 2007;39:686-94.
231. Rusch N, Angermeyer MC, Corrigan PW. Mental illness stigma: concepts, consequences, and initiatives to reduce stigma. Eur Psychiatry. 2005;20:529-39. [PubMed]
232. Salyers MP, Becker DR, Drake RE, et al. A ten-year follow-up of a supported employment program. Psychiatr Serv. 2009;55:302-8.
233. Schwartz S, Goldfinger S, Ratener M, et al. The Young Adult Patient and the Care System: Fragmentation Prototypes. San Francisco:: Jossey-Bass; 1983.
234. Scott JE, Dixon LB. Assertive community treatment and case management for schizophrenia. Schizophr Bull. 1995;21: 657-68. [PubMed]
235. Shepherd G. Day treatment and care. In: Bannett DH, Freeman HC (Eds). Community Psychiatry: The Principles.London: Churchill Livingstone, 1991.
236. Spaniol L, ZippleAM, Lockwood D. The role of the family in psychiatric rehabilitation.Schiz Bull. 1992;18:341-8.
237. Stein LI, Test MA. Alternative to mental hospital treatment. I. Conceptual model, treatment program, and clinical evaluation. Arch Gen Psychiatry. 1980;37:392-7. [PubMed]
238. Strachan AM. Family intervention for the rehabilitation of schizophrenia: Toward protection and coping. Schiz Bull. 1986; 12:678-9.
239. Stuart H, Arboleda-Florez J, Sartorius N. Stigma in mental disorders: international perspectives. World Psychiatry. 2005;4(Suppl 1):1–62.
240. Talbott JA, Glick ID. The inpatient care of the chronically mentally ill. Schiz Bull. 1986;12:129-40.
241. Tuttman S. Protecting the therapeutic alliance in this time of changing health-care delivery systems. Int J Group Psychother. 1997;47:3-16. [PubMed]
242. Vaughn C, Leff J. The influence of family and social factors on the course of psychiatric illness. Br J Psychiatry. 1976;129: 125-7.
243. Wallace CJ, Nelson CJ, Liberman RP, et al. A review of critique of social skills training with schzophrenia patients. Schiz Bull 1980;6:42-63.
244. Wallace CJ. Functional assessment in rehabilitation. Schiz Bull 1986;12:604-24.
245. Wallace CJ. Social skills training in psychiatric rehabilitation: recent findings. Int Rev Psychiatry. 1998;19:9-19.
246. Wig NN, Menon DK, Bedi H, et al. Expressed emotion and schizophrenia in North India. I. Cross-cultural transfer of ratings of relatives' expressed emotion. Br J Psychiatry. 1987; 151:156-9.
247. Wig NN, Menon DK, Bedi H, et al. Expressed emotion and schizophrenia in North India. II. Distribution of expressed emotion components among relatives of schizophrenic patients in Aarhus and Chandigarh. Br J Psychiatry. 1987;151: 160-5.
248. Wing JK, Brown GW. Institutionalism and Schizophrenia. London: Cambridge University Press, 1970.
249. Wing JK, Brown GW. Institutionalism and Schizophrenia. London: Cambridge University Press, 1970.
250. Wing JK, Morris B. Handbook of Psychiatry Rehabilitation Practice. Oxford: Oxford University Press, 1981.
251. World Health Organization. International Classification of Functioning, Disability and Health (ICF) Geneva: World Health Organization; 2001.
252. World Health Organization. International Classification of Impairments, Disabilities and Handicaps. Geneva: World Health Organization; 1980.
253. World Health Organization. Report of the International Pilot Study on Schizophrenia. Geneva: WHO, 1973.
254. World Health Organization. Schizophrenia: An International Follow-up Study. New York: John Wiley and Sons, 1979.
255. Wykes T, Katz R, Sturt E, et al. Abnormalities of responsse processing in a chronic psychiatric group: A possible prediction of failure in rehabilitation programs? Br J Psychiatry. 1992;160: 244-52.
256. Yanos PT, Rosenfield S, Horwitz AV. Negative and supportive social interactions and quality of life among persons diagnosed with severe mental illness. Commun Ment Health J. 2001;37:405-19. [PubMed]

FURTHER READING

Psychotherapy

1. Chen E, Touyz SW, Beumont PJ, et al. Comparison of group and individual cognitive behavioral therapy for patients with

bulimia nervosa. International Journal of Eating Disorders. 2003;33(3):241-54.

2. De Mello MF, de Jesus MJ, Bacaltchuk J, Verdeli H, Neugebauer R. A systematic review of research findings on the efficacy of interpersonal therapy for depressive disorders. European Archives of Psychiatry and Clinical Neuroscience. 2005; 255(2):75-82.
3. Frank E, Kupfer DJ, Thase ME, Mallinger AG, Swartz HA, Fagiolini AM, et al. Two-year outcomes for interpersonal and social rhythm therapy in individuals with bipolar I disorder. Archives of General Psychiatry. 2005;62:996-1004.
4. Hausmann A, Hortnagl C, Muller M, Waack J, Walpath M, Conca A. Psychotherapeutic interventions in bipolar disorder: a review. Neuropsychiatry. 2007;21(2):102-9.
5. Hofmann SG, Smits JA. Cognitive-behavioral therapy for adult anxiety disorders: a meta-analysis of randomized placebo-controlled trials. Journal of Clinical Psychiatry. 2008;69(4): 621-32.
6. Linehan MM, Comtois KA, Murray AM, Brown MZ, Gallop RJ, Heard HL, et al. Two-year randomized controlled trial and follow-up of dialectical behavior therapy vs. therapy by experts for suicidal behaviors and borderline personality disorder. Archives of General Psychiatry. 2006;63(7):757-66.
7. Miklowitz DJ, Otto MW, Frank E, Reilly-Harrington NA, Wisniewski SR, Kogan JN, et al. Psychosocial treatments for bipolar depression: a 1-year randomized trial from the Systematic Treatment Enhancement Program. Archives of General Psychiatry. 2007;164(4):419-26.
8. Miklowitz DJ, Richards JA, George EL, Frank E, Suddath RL, Powell KB, Sacher JA. Integrated family and individual therapy for bipolar disorder: results of a treatment development study. Journal of Clinical Psychiatry. 2003;64(2): 182-91.
9. Perlick DA, Hohenstein JM, Clarkin JF, Kaczynski R, Rosenheck RA. Use of mental health and primary care services by caregivers of patients with bipolar disorder: a preliminary study. Bipolar Disorders. 2005;7(2):126-35.
10. Perlick DA, Rosenheck RA, Miklowitz DJ, Chessick C, Wolff N, Kaczynski R, et al. STEP-BD Family Experience Collaborative Study Group. Prevalence and correlates of burden among caregivers of patients with bipolar disorder enrolled in the Systematic Treatment Enhancement Program for Bipolar Disorder. Bipolar Disorders. 2007;9(3): 262-73.
11. Pike KM, Walsh BT, Vitousek K, et al. Cognitive behavioral therapy in the posthospitalization treatment of anorexia nervosa. American Journal of Psychiatry. 2003;160(11):2046-9.
12. Rathod S, Kingdon D, Weiden P, Turkington D. Cognitive-behavioral therapy for medication-resistant schizophrenia: a review. Journal of Psychiatric Practice. 2008;14(1):22-33.
13. Rea MM, Tompson MC, Miklowitz DJ, Goldstein MJ, Hwang S, Mintz J. Family-focused treatment versus individual treatment for bipolar disorder: results of a randomized clinical trial. Journal of Consulting and Clinical Psychology. 2003;71(3):482-92.
14. Silverman WK, Pina AA, Viswesvaran C. Evidence-based psychosocial treatments for phobic and anxiety disorders in children and adolescents. Journal of Clinical Child and Adolescent Psychology. 2008;37(1):105-30.
15. The TADS Team. The Treatment for Adolescents with Depression Study (TADS): Long-term Effectiveness and Safety Outcomes. Archives of General Psychiatry. 2007;64(10):1132-43.

Psychological Therapies

16. Anderson EM, Lambart MJ. Short term dynamically oriented psychotherapy: a review and meta-analysis. Clin Psych Rev. 1995;15:503-14.
17. Andrews G, Singh M, Bond M. The defense style questionnaire. J Ner and Ment Dis. 1993;181:246-56.
18. Azim HFA, Piper WE, Segal PM, et al. The quality of object relations scale. Bulletin of the Menniger Clinic. 1991;55:323-43.
19. Barkham M, Rees A, Shapiro DA, et al. Outcome of time-limited psychotherapy in applied settings: replicating the Second Sheffield psychotherapy Projec. Journal of Consulting and Clinical Psychology. 1996;64:1079-85.
20. Barkhman M, Guthrie E, Hardy G, et al. Psychodynamic–interpersonal therapy. Stage Beck AT 1964 Thinking and depression, H: Theory and therapy. Arch Gen Psych. 2004;10:561-71.
21. Beck AT, Emery G. Anxiety Disorders and Phobias: A Cognitive Perspective. Basic Books, New York;1985.
22. Beck AT, Freeman A. Cognitive Therapy of Personality Disorders. Basic Books, New York;1990.
23. Beck AT, Rush AJ, Shaw BF, Emery G. Cognitive Therapy of Depression. Guilford Press, New York;1979.
24. Beck AT. Cognitive models of depression. J Cog Psycho. 1987;1:5-37.
25. Beck AT. Depression: Clinical, Experimental and Theoretical Aspeacts. Harper & Row, New York;1867.
26. Blacburn IM. An appraisal of comparative trials of cognitive therapy. In: Peris G, Blackburn IM (Eds). Cognitive psychotherapy: theory and practice. Springer–Verlag, Heidelberg; 1988.
27. Blackburn IM, Davidson KM. Cognitive therapy for depression and anxiety: a practitioner's guide. Blalkwell Scientific, Oxford; 1990.
28. Bloch AL, Shear K, Markowitz JC, et al. An empirical study of defense mechanisms in dysthymia. Am J Psych. 1993;150:1194-8.
29. Bloch S (Ed.). Supportive psychotherapy. In: An introduction to the psychotherapies. Oxford Univesity Press, London; 1979.
30. Bower P, Rowland N, Mellor Clark J, et al. The Cochrane Library Issue 4, Oxford; 2002.
31. Brockman B, Poynton A, Ryle A, et al. Effectiveness of time-limited therapy carried out by trainees: comparison of two methods. British Journal of psychiatry. 1987;151:602-9.
32. Bryant RA, Harvey AG, Sackville T, et al. Treatment of acute stress disorder: a comparison of cognitive behavioural therapy

and supportive counseling. American Journal of Psychiatry. 1998;156:1780-6.

33. Busch FN, Shear K, Cooper AM et al. An empirical study of defense mechanisms in panic disorder. Journal of Nervous and Mental Disease. 1995;183:299-303.
34. Butler G, Fennel M, Robson P, Gelder M. Comparison of behaviour therapy and cognitive therapy in the treatment of generalized anxiety disorder. Journal of Consulting and Clinical Psychology. 1991;59:167-75.
35. Chambless DL, Gillis MM. Cognitive therapy of anxiety disorders. Journal of Consulting & Clinical Psychology. 1993;61:248-60.
36. Chen E, Touyz SW, Beumont PJ, et al. Comparison of group and individual cognitive behavioral therapy for patients with bulimia nervosa. International Journal of Eating Disorders. 2003;33(3):241-54.
37. Chen E, Touyz SW, Beumont PJ, et al. Comparison of group and individual cognitive behavioral therapy for patients with bulimia nervosa. International Journal of Eating Disorders. 2003;33(3):241-54.
38. Churchill R, Hunot V, Corney R, et al. A systematic review of controlled trials of the effectiveness and cost-effectiveness of brief psychological treatments for depression. Health Technology Assessments. 2001;5:35 (Executive summary).
39. Clark DM, Salkovskis PM, Hackmann A, et al. A comparison of cognitive therapy, applied relaxation and imipramine in the treatment of panic disorder. British Journal of Psychiatry 1994;164:759-69.
40. Conte HR, Plutchick R, Wild KV, Karasu TB. Combined psychotherapy and pharamacotherapy for depression. Archives of General Psychiatry. 1986;43:47-479.
41. Cooper NA, Clum GA. Imaginal flooding as a supplementary treatment for PTSD in combat vertrans: a controlled study. Behaviour Therapy. 1989;20:381-91.
42. Cottrell D, Boston P. Practitioner review: the effectiveness of systemic family therapy for children and adolescents. Journal of Child Psychiatry and Psychiatry and Allied Disciplines. 2002;43(5):573-86.
43. Coyne J, Gottlib I. The role of cognition in depression: a critical appraisal. Psychological Bulletin. 1983;94:472-505.
44. Crist-Christoph. The efficacy of brief dynamic psychotherapy: a meta-analysis. American Journal of Psychiatry. 1992;49: 151-8.
45. De Mello MF, de Jesus MJ, Bacaltchuk J, Verdeli H, Neugebauer R. A systematic review of research findings on the efficacy of interpersonal therapy for depressive disorders. European Archives of Psychiatry and Clinical Neuroscience. 2005; 255(2):75-82.
46. Department of Health 1996 NHS psychotherapy services in England: review of strategic policy. London
47. Department of Health 2000 National service framework for mental health. HMSO, London.
48. Department of Health 2001 Treatment choice in psychological therapies and counseling. HMSO, London.
49. Department of health and human Services, Public Health Service, agency for Health Care Policy and Reasearch, Rockville, MD.
50. Depression Guideliness Panel 1993 Depression in primary care: detection, diagnosis and treatment: quick rerfeence guide for clinicians. Clinical Practice Guideline No 5, AHCPR publication No 93-0552. US.
51. Diamond GS, Siqueland L. Family therapy for the treatment of depressed adolescents. Psychotherapy (special issue: Adolescent Treatment: New Frontiers and New Dimension). 1995;32:77-90.
52. Durham RC, Murphy T, Allan T. Cognititive therapy, analytic psychotherapy and anxiety management training for generalized anxiety disorder. British Journal of Psychiatry. 1991;115:315-23.
53. Durhum RC, Allan T. Psychological treatment of generalized anxiety disorder: a review of the clinical significance of outcome studies since 1980. British Journal of Psychiatry. 1993 163:19-23.
54. Elkin I 1994. The NIMH treatment of depression collaboration research program: where we began and where we are. In: Bergin AE, Garfield SL (Eds). Handbook of Psychotherapy and Behaviour Change, 4th edn. Wiley, New York.
55. Elkin I, Shea MT, Watkins JT, et al. National Institute for Mental Health Treatment Of Depression Collaborrative Research Program: general effectiveness of treatment. Archives of General Psychiatry. 1989;46:971-82.
56. Ellis A. Reason and emotion in psychotherapy. Citadel Press, Secausus, NJ. 1962.
57. Emmelkamp PM G. Behaviour therapy with adults. In: Bergin AE, Garfield SL (Eds). Handbook of Psychotherapy and Behaviour Change, 4th edn. Wiley, New York, 1994.
58. Erikson EH. Identity and the Life Cycle. International Universities press, New York, 1850.
59. Fairbairn WRD. An Objects Relation Theory of Personality: Psychoanalytic Studies of the Personality. Basic Books, New York, 1954.
60. Fairburn CG, Kirk J, O'Connor MA. Comparison of two psychological treatments for bulimia nervosa. Behaviour Research and Therapy. 1986l;24:629-43.
61. Fosbury JA. Cognitive analytic therapy with poorly controlled type 1 diabetic patients. Paper presented at the Europcan Association for the study of diabetes 27 September to 1 October, Duusseldorf, Germany, 1994.
62. Frank E, Kupfer DJ, Thase ME, Mallinger AG, Swartz HA, Fagiolini AM, et al. Two-year outcomes for interpersonal and social rhythm therapy in individuals with bipolar I disorder. Archives of General Psychiatry. 2005;62:996-1004.
63. Gaston L, Gallagher D, Couranoyer L, Gagnon R. Alliance, technique and their interactions in predicting outcome of behavioural cognitive and brief dynamic therapy. Psychotherapy Research. 1998;8:190-209.
64. Gould RA, Otto MW, Pollack MH. A meta-analysis of treatment outcome for panic disorder. Clinical Psychology Review. 1995 15(8):819-844.

65. Guntrip E, Creed F, Dawson D, Tomenson B. A controlled trial of psychological treatment for the irritable bowel syndrome. Gastroenterology. 1991;100:450-7.
66. Guthrie E, Kapur N, Mackway-jones K, et al. Randomised controlled trial of brief psychological intervention after deliberate self poisoning. British Medical Journal. 2001;323:135-8.
67. Guthrie E, Moorey J, Margison F, et al. Cost-effectiveness of brief psychodynamic-interpersonal therapy in high utilizers of psychiatric services. Archives of General Psychiatry. 1999;56:519-26.
68. Guthrip H. Schizoid phenomena, object relations, and the self. International Universalities Press, New York, 1969.
69. Hamilton J, Guthrie E, Creed F, et al. A randomized controlled trial of psychotherapy in patients with chronic fuctional dyspepsia. Gastroenterology. 2000;119:661-9.
70. Hausmann A, Hortnagl C, Muller M, Waack J, Walpath M, Conca A. Psychotherapeutic interventions in bipolar disorder: a review. Neuropsychiatr. 2008;21(2):102-9.
71. Hawton K, Salkovskis PM, Kirk DM. Cognitive Behaiourtherapy for Psychiatric Problems: A Practical Guide. Oxford University Press, Oxford, 1989.
72. Heimberg RG, Dodge CS, Hope DA. Cognitive behaviour treatment of social phobia: comparative to a credible placebo control. Cognitive Therapy and Research. 1990;14:1-23.
73. Hobson RF. Forms of Feeling. Tavistock, London, 1985.
74. Hofmann SG, Smits JA. Cognitive-behavioral therapy for adult anxiety disorders: a meta-analysis of randomized placebo-controlled trials. Journal of Clinical Psychiatry. 2008;69(4):621-32.
75. Hollon SD, Du Rubeis RJ, Evans MD, et al. Cognitive therapy and pharmacotherapy for depression: singly or in combination. Archives of general Psychiatry. 1992;49:774-81.
76. Horowitz MJ, Mibrath C, Stinson CH. Assessing personality disorders. In: Strupp HH, Horowitz LM, Lambert MJ (Eds). Measuring Patient Changes. APA, Washington, DC, 1997.pp. 401-32.
77. Horvath AO, Luborsky L. The role of the therapeutic alliance in psychotherapy. Journal of Consulting and Clinical Psychology. 1993;61:561-73.
78. Horvath AO, Symonds DB. Relationship between working alliance and outcome in psychotherapy: a meta-analysis. Journal of Counselling Psychology. 1991;38:139-49.
79. Jacobson E. Progressive Relaxation. University of Chicago Press, Chicago, 1938.
80. Kernberg O. Internal world and external reality: object relations theory applied. Aronson, New York, 1980.
81. Kessel N. Reassurance. Lancet i 1979. pp. 1128-3301.
82. Klerman GL, Weissman MM, Rounsaville BJ, Chevron ES. Interpersonal Psychotherapy of Depression. Basic Books, New York, 1984.
83. Klerman GL, Weissman MM. New Applications of Interpersonal Psychotherapy. American Psychochiatric Press, Washington, DC, 1993.
84. Kuipers L, Leff J, Lam D. Fammily Work for Schizophrenia: A Practical Guide. Gaskell, London, 1992.
85. Kupfer DJ, Frank E, Perel JM, et al. Five year outcome for maintenance therapies in recurrent depression. Archives of General Psychiatry. 1992;49:769-73.
86. Lambert MJ, Bergin AE. The effectiveness of psychotherapy. In: Bergin AE, Garfield SL (Eds). Handbook of Psychotherapy and Behaviour Change, 4th edn. Wiley, New York, 1994.
87. Ledwidge B. Cognitive behavour modification: a step in the wrong direction Psychological Bulletin. 1978;85:353-75.
88. Lichstein KL. Clinical Relaxation Strategies. Wiley, New York, 1988.
89. Liddell A, di Fazio L, Blackwood J, Ackkerman C. Long term follow-up of treated dental phobics. Behaviour Research Therapy. 1994 32:604-10.
90. Linehan MM, Comtois KA, Murray AM, Brown MZ, Gallop RJ, Heard HL, et al. Two-year randomized controlled trial and follow-up of dialectical behavior therapy vs. therapy by experts for suicidal behaviors and borderline personality disorder. Archives of General Psychiatry. 2006;63(7):757-66.
91. Luborsky L, Crits-Christoph P. Understanding transference: the CCRT (The Core Conflictual Relationship Theme) methods Basic Books, New York, 1990.
92. Lyon HM, Karle S, Bentall RP. The defensive function of persecutory delusions: evidence from attribution tasks. British Journal of Psychiatry. 1994;164:637-46.
93. Makowitz JC, Kocsis B, Fishman LA, et al. Treatment of HIV-positive patients with depressive symptoms. Archives of General Psychiatry. 1998;55:452-7.
94. Margison F, Hobson RF. A conversational model of psycholotherapy (Videotapes) Tavistock, London, 1983.
95. Marks IM, Swinson RP, Basoglu M, et al. Alphrazolam and exposure alone and combined in panic disorder with agoraphobia. Journal of psychiatry. 1993;162:776-87.
96. Martain DJ, Garske JP, Davis MK. Relation of the therapeutic alliance with outcome and other variables: a meta-analytic review. Journal of Consulting and Clinical Psychology. 2000;68: 438-540.
97. McCallum M, Piper WE (Eds) Psychological mindedness. Lawrence Erlbaum, Hillsdale, NJ, pp. 27-58.
98. Miklowitz DJ, Otto MW, Frank E, Reilly-Harrington NA, Wisniewski SR, Kogan JN, et al. Psychosocial treatments for bipolar depression: a 1-year randomized trial from the Systematic Treatment Enhancement Program. Archives of General Psychiatry. 2007;164(4):419-26.
99. Miklowitz DJ, Richards JA, George EL, Frank E, Suddath RL, Powell KB, Sacher JA. Integrated family and individual therapy for bipolar disorder: results of a treatment development study. Journal of Clinical Psychiatry. 2003;64(2):182-91.
100. Moss S, Margison F, Godberrt K. The maintenance of psychotherapy skill acquisition: a 2 years follow-up. British Journal of Medical Psychology. 1991;64:233-6.
101. Orner R, Schnyder U. Reconstruction early intervation after trauna. Oxford Univeresity Press, Oxford, 2003.

102. Ost LG. One session treatment for specific phobias. Behaviour Reasearch and Therapy, 1989;25:397-409.
103. Paris J, Zweig-Frank H, Bond M, Guzder J. Defense styles, hostility and psychological risk factors in male patients with personality disorders. 1996;184:153-8.
104. Perlick DA, Hohenstein JM, Clarkin JF, Kaczynski R, Rosenheck RA. Use of mental health and primary care services by caregivers of patients with bipolar disorder: a preliminary study. Bipolar Disorders. 2005;7(2):126-35.
105. Perlick DA, Rosenheck RA, Miklowitz DJ, Chessick C, Wolff N, Kaczynski R, et al. STEP-BD Family Experience Collaborative Study Group. Prevalence and correlates of burden among caregivers of patients with bipolar disorder enrolled in the Systematic Treatment Enhancement Program for Bipolar Disorder. Bipolar Disorders. 2007;9(3): 262-73.
106. Pike KM, Walsh BT, Vitousek K, et al. Cognitive behavioral therapy in the posthospitalization treatment of anorexia nervosa. American Journal of Psychiatry. 2003;160(11):2046-9.
107. Piper ER, Joyce AS, KcCallum M, Hassan FA. Concentration and correspondence of transference interpretation in short-term psychotherapy. Journal of Consulting and Clinical Psychology. 1993;61:586-95.
108. Pwer KG, Simpson RJ, Swanson V, Wallace CA. A controlled comparison of cognitive behaviour therapy, diazepam, and placebo alone and in combination, for the treatment of generalised anxiety disorder. Journal of Anxiety Disorders. 1990;4:267-92.
109. Quality Assurance Project. A treatment outline for depressive disorders. Australian & New Zealand journal of Psychiatry. 1983;17:129-46.
110. Rathod S, Kingdon D, Weiden P, Turkington D. Cognitive-behavioral therapy for medication-resistant schizophrenia: a review. Journal of Psychiatric Practice. 2008;14(1):22-33.
111. Rathod S, Kingdon D, Weiden P, Turkington D. Cognitive-behavioral therapy for medication-resistant schizophrenia: a review. Journal of Psychiatric Practice. 2008;14(1):22-3.
112. Rea MM, Tompson MC, Miklowitz DJ, Goldstein MJ, Hwang S, Mintz J. Family-focused treatment versus individual treatment for bipolar disorder: results of a randomized clinical trial. Journal of Consulting and Clinical Psychology. 2003;71(3):482-92.
113. Rea MM, Tompson MC, Miklowitz DJ, Goldstein MJ, Hwang S, Mintz J. Family-focused treatment versus individual treatment for bipolar disorder: results of a randomized clinical trial. Journal of Consulting and Clinical Psychology. 2003;71(3):482-92.
114. Reynolds CF, Frank E, Perel JM et al. Combined pharmacotherapy in the acute and continuation treatment of slderly patients with recurrent major depression: a preliminary report. American Journal of Psychiatry. 1992;149:1687-92.
115. Richardson, CA, Gilleard CJ, Lieberman S, Peeler R. Working with older adults and their families: a review. Journal of Family Therapy. 1994;16(3):225-40.
116. Rose S, Bisson J, Wessey S. Psychological Debriefing for Preventing Post Traumatic Stress Disorder (PTSD). The Cochrane Library, Issue 4, Oxford, 2002.
117. Royal College of General Practitioners. Prevention of psychiatric disorders in general practice. RCGP, London, 1981.
118. Ryle A. Cognitive-analytic therapy: active participation of in change. Wiley, Chichester, 1990.
119. Schnyder U, Orner R. Reconstructing early intervention Shapiro D, Firth J 1987 Prescriptive v exploratory psychotherapy: outcomes of the Sheffied Psychotherapy project. British Journal of Psychiatry. 2003;151:790-9.
120. Shapiro DA, Barkham M, Rees A, et al. Effects of treatment duration and severity of depression on the effectiveness of cognitive behavioural and psychodynamic-interpersonal psychotherapy. Journal of Consulting and Clinical Psychology. 1994;62:522-34.
121. Shapiro DA, Rees A, Barkham M, et al. Effects of treatment duration and severity of depression on the maintenance of gains following cognitive-behavioural and psychodynamic-interpersonal psychotherapy. Journal of Consulting and Clinical Psychology. 1995;63:378-87.
122. Shpiro F. Eye Movement Desensitization and Reprocessing: Basic Principles, Protocols and Procedures. Guilford Press, New York, 1995.
123. Silverman WK, Pina AA, Viswesvaran C. Evidence-based psychosocial treatments for phobic and anxiety disorders in children and adolescents. Journal of Clinical Child and Adolescent Psychology. 2008;37(1):105-30.
124. Sllivan HS. 1953 Interpersonal therapy of psychiatry. Norton, New Work Truax CB, Carkhuff RR 1967. Toward effective counseling and psychotherapy: training and practice. Aldine, Chicago.
125. Steinbruck SM, Maxwell SE, Howard GS. A meta-analysis of psychotherapy and drug therapy in the treatment of unipolar depression with adults. Journal of Consulting and Clinical Psychology. 1983;51:856-63.
126. Strupp HM. Psychotherapy research and practice-an overview. In: Bergin AE, Garfield SL (Eds). Handbook of Psychotherapy and Behaviour Change, 2nd edn. Wiley, New York, 1978.
127. Svartberg M, Stiles TC. Comparative effects of short-term psychotherapy: a meta-analysis. Journal of Consulting and Clinical Psychology, 1991;59:704-14.
128. The TADS Team. The Treatment for Adolescents with Depression Study (TADS): Long-term Effectiveness and Safety Outcomes. Archives of General Psychiatry. 2007;64(10): 1132-43.
129. Valliant GE, Bond M, Valliant O. An empirically validated hierarchy of defense mechanisms. Archives of General Psychiatry. 1986;43:786.
130. Wampold BE, Minami T, Baskin TW, Callen TS. A meta (re) analysis of the effects of cognitive therapy versus 'other therapies' for depression. Journal of Affective Disorders. 2002;68(2-3):159-65.

131. Weissman MM, Markowitz JC, Klerman GL. Comprehensive guide to interpersonal psychotherapy. Basic Behavioural Science. Basic Books, New York, 2000.
132. Weisz JR, Donenberg ER, Man SS, Weiss B. Bridging the gap between laboratories and clinic in child and adolesecent psychotherapy. Journal of Consulting and Clinical Psychology. 1995;63:688-701.
133. Wolpe J, Psychotherapy by Reciprocal Inhibition. Stanford University Press, Stanford, CA, 1958.
134. Woolfended SR, Williams K, Peat JK. Family and parenting interventions for conduct disorder and delinquency: a meta-analysis of randomized controlled trials. Journal of Pediatrics. 2002;141(5):738.

Group Psychotherapy

135. Avasthi A, Suribhatla S. Group psychotherapy. In: Textbook of Postgraduate Psychiatry. Vyas IN and Ahuja N (Eds). Jaypee Brothers Medical Publishers (P) Ltd. New Delhi, 1999.
136. Barker P. Regeneration. Penguin, Harmondsworth, 1992.
137. Beauchamp TL, Childress JF. Principles of Biomedical Ethics, 5th edn. New York: Oxford, 2001.
138. Beerer AL. Psychotherapy with schizophrenics in team groups: A systems model. Am J Psychotherapy. 1991; XLV (No.1):78-86.
139. Bernard H, Burlingame G, Flores P, Greene L, Joyce A, Kobos JC, et al. Clinical practice guidelines for group psychotherapy. Int J Group Psychotherapy. 2008;58(4):455-542.
140. Brabender V. The ethical group psychotherapist. Int J Group Psychotherapy. 2006;56:395-414.
141. Burlingame GM, Joyce SB, A MacNair–Semands, Mac-Kenzie R, Ogrodniczuk K, et al. Core battery–Revised. New York: American Group Psychotherapy Association, 2006.
142. Burlingame GM, MacKenzie KR, Strauss B. Small group treatment: evidence for effectiveness and mechanisms of change. In: MJ Lambert (Ed), Bergin and Garfield's Handbook of Psychotherapy and Behavior Change, 5th edn, New York: Wiley, 2004.pp.647-96.
143. Burlingame GM, Strauss B, Joyce AM, MacNair-Semands R, Mackenzie KR. American Group Psychotherapy Association's CORE Battery-Revised. New York: American Group Psychotherapy Association, 2006.
144. Burrow I. The group method of analysis. Psychoanalytic review. 1927;10:268-80.
145. Callahan KL, Price JL, Hilsenroth MJ. Review of Interpersonal-Psychodynamic Group Psychotherapy Outcomes for Adult Survivors of Childhood Sexual Abuse. Int J Group Psychotherapy. 2004;54(4):491-519.
146. Dies RR. Practical, theoretical and empirical foundations for group psychotherapy. In: Francis AJ, Hales RE (Eds). Psychiatry Update. American Psychiatric Association Annual Review. Washington DC: American Psychiatric Press. 1986;5.
147. Freud S. Group psychology and the analysis of the ego. In Standard edition of the Complete psychological works of Sigmund Freud, (J Strachey Ed), Hogarth Press, London. 1955;18:65-143.
148. Joyce AS, Piper WE, Ogrodniczuk JS, Klein RH. Termination in psychotherapy: A psychodynamic model of processes and outcomes. Washington, DC: American Psychological Association Press, 2007.
149. Kanas N. Group therapy for caregivers of patients with Alzheimer's disease. Int J Group Psychotherapy. 2006;56(4): 505-9.
150. Kanas N. Group therapy with schizophrenic and bipolar patients. In: Group psychotherapy of the psychoses (V Schermer, M Pines Eds). Jessica Kingsley, London, 1999.
151. Kibel HD. The evolution of the Group-as-a-Whole and Object Relations theory: From projection to introjection. Group. 2005;29:139-61.
152. Klein RH. Toward the establishment of evidence-based practices in group psychotherapy. Int J Group Psychother. 2008;58(4):441-54.
153. Kosters M, Burlingame GM, Nachtigall C, Strauss B. A meta-analytic review of the effectiveness of inpatient group psychotherapy. Group Dynamics: Theory, Research and Practice. 2006;10:146–63.
154. Melnick J, Woods M. Analysis of group composition: research and theory for psychotherapeutic and growth-oriented groups. Journal of Applied Behavioral Science. 1976;12:493-512.
155. Moreno JL. Who shall survive? Foundations of sociometry, group psychotherapy and psychodrama. Beacon House, New York, 1953.
156. Norton PJ, Philipp LM. Trans diagnostic approaches to the treatment of anxiety disorders: a quantitative review. Psychotherapy Theory, Research, Practice, Training. 2008; 45(2):214-26.
157. Ogrodniczuk JS, Piper WE, Joyce AS. Treatment compliance among patients with personality disorders receiving group psychotherapy: what are the roles of interpersonal distress and cohesion? Psychiatry. 2006;69(3):249-61.
158. Parloff M. Analytic Group Psychotherapy. In: J Marmor (Ed), Modern Psychoanalysis, New York: Basic Books, 1969.pp. 492-531.
159. Parloff MB. Group therapy and the small group field: An encounter. Int J Group Psychotherapy. 1970;20:267-304.
160. Pines M, Schlapobersky 1. Group methods in adult psychiatry. In: New Oxford Textbook of Psychiatry (Eds). Gelder MG, Lopez-Ibor JJ & Andreasen N. Oxford University Press, Oxford, 2000.
161. Pines M. Group analytic psychotherapy and the borderline patient. In: The difficult patient in the group (B Roth, W Stone, H Kibel Eds). International Universities Press, New York, 1990. pp.31-44.
162. Pratt JH. The tuberculosis class. An experiment in home treatment. Reprinted in Group psychotherapy and group function (M Rosenbaum, M Berger Eds), Basic Books, New York. 1963.pp.111-22.

163. Rapin LS. Guidelines for ethical and legal practice in counseling and psychotherapy groups. In: DeLucia-Waack JL, Gerrity DA, Kalodner CR, Riva MT (Eds), Handbook of Group Counseling and Psychotherapy. Thousand Oaks, CA: Sage. 2004. pp.151-65.
164. Red F. Group emotion and leadership. Psychiatry. 1942;5: 573-96.
165. Rickard HC. Selected group psychotherapy evaluation studies. J Gen Psychol. 1962;67:35-50.
166. Robertson M, Rushton PJ, Bartrum D, Ray R. Group-based interpersonal psychotherapy for post-traumatic stress disorder: theoretical and clinical aspects. 2004;54(2):145-75.
167. Saiger GM, Rubenfeld S, Dluhy MD (Eds). Windows into today's group therapy. Taylor and Francis group. NewYork, 2008.
168. Saiger GM. Group psychotherapy with older adults. Psychiatry. 2001;64(2):132-45.
169. Schlapobersky J, Bamber H. Rehabilitation with victims of torture. In: Refugees—the trauma of exile (D Miserez Ed), Niijhoff, The Hague. 1988.pp.206-22.
170. Schlapobersky J. Editor's Introduction and author's biography. In: Explorations with families group analysis and family therapy. Selected clinical papers of Robin Skynner. Methuen, London. Reprinted by Routledge, London, 1990.
171. Shapiro EL, Ginzberg R. Buried treasure: money, ethics and countertransference in group therapy. Int J Group Psychotherapy. 2006;56:477-94.
172. Spivack N. Subgrouping with psychiatric inpatients in group psychotherapy: linking dependency and counter dependency. Int J Group Psychotheraphy. 2008;58(2):231-51.
173. Stem MJ. Group therapy with medically ill patients. In Group therapy in clinical practice (A Alonso, HI Swiller) American Psychiatric Press, Washington, DC. 1993.pp.I85-200..
174. Thompson S, Kahn JH. The Group Process as a Helping Technique. Oxford: Pergamon Press, 1976.
175. Tyminski RF, Moore PJ. The impact of group psychotherapy on social development in children with pervasive developmental disorders. Int J Group Psychotherapy. 2008;58(3):363-79.
176. Van Ingen DJ, Novicki DJ. An effectiveness study of group therapy for anxiety disorders. Int J Group Psychotheraphy. 2009;59(2):243-51.
177. Vinogradov S, Yalorn ID. Guide to Group Psychotherapy. Washington, DC, American Psychiatric Press, 1989.
178. Wilberg T, Karterud S, Pedersen G, Irion T, Brabrand J, Haavaldsen G, et al. Outpatient group psychotherapy following day treatment for patients with personality disorders Journal of Personality Disorders. 2003;17(6):510-21.
179. Yalom I, Leszcz M. The theory and Practice of Group Psychotherapy, 5th edn. New York: Basic Books, 2005.
180. Yalom ID, Vinogradov S. Interpersonal group psychotherapy; in comprehensive Textbook of Group psychotherapy, 3rd edn, Edited by Kaplan HI, Sadock BJ. Baltimore, MD, Williams & Wilkins, 1993.pp.185-95.
181. Yalom ID. Inpatient Group Psychotherapy. New York, Basic Books, 1983.
182. Yalorn I. The Theory and Practice of Group Psychotherapy, 3rd edn. Basic Books, New York, 1985.

Current Status and Future Dirction in Couple Therapy

183. Allen ES, Atkins DC, Baucom DH, Snyder DK, Gordon KC, et al. Intrapersonal, interpersonal, and contextual factors in engaging in and responding to extramarital involvement. Clin Psychol Sci Pract. 2005;12:101-30.
184. Atkins DC, Berns SB, George W, Doss B, GAttis K, et al. 2005a. predicting success in a randomized clinical trails of marital therapy. J Consult, Clin, Psychol. In press.
185. Atkins DC, Elbridage KE, Baucom DH, et al. Christensen A. Behavioral marital therapy and infidelity: optimism in the face of betrayal. J Consult Clin Psychol. 2005b;73:144-50.
186. Atkins DC. Christensen A. Marital satisfaction and Stability for Two Years Post Treatment: Comparing the Trajectories of TBCT and IBCT. Presented at Assoc Adv Behav Ther, New Orleans, LA. 2004.
187. Baron RM, Kenny DA. The moderator mediator variable distinction in social psychological research: conceptual, strategic, and statistical considerations. J Personal Soc Psychol. 1986;51:1173-82.
188. Baucom DH, Aiken PA. Sex role identity, marital satisfaction, and response to behavioral marital therapy. J Consult Clin Psychol. 1984;52:438-44.
189. Baucom DH, Shoham V, Mueser KT, Daiuto AD, Stickle TR, Empirically supported couple and family interventions for marital distress and adult mental health problems. J Consult Clin Psychol. 1998;66:53-88.
190. Baucom DH, Station S, Epstein NB, et al. Anxiety Disorders. See Snyder & Whisman, 2003.pp.57-87.
191. Baucom DH. The active ingredients of behavioral marital therapy: the effectiveness of problem-solving/communication training, contingency contracting, and their combination. See Hahlweg & Jacobson. 1984.pp.73-88.
192. Beach SRH, Broderick JE. Commitment: a variable in women's response to marital therapy. Am J Fam, Ther. 1983;11:16-24.
193. Beach SRH Gupta M. Depression see Snyder and Whiswman, 2003.pp.88-113.
194. Bradley B, Furrow JL. Toward a mini-theory of the blamer softening event: tracking the moment-by-moment process. J Marital Fam Ther. 2004;30:1-12.
195. Byrne M, Carr A, Clark M. The efficacy of couples-based interventions for panic disorder with agoraphobia. J Fam Ther. 2004;26:105-25.
196. Chambless DL, Hollon SD. Defining empirically supported therapies. J Consult Clin Psychol. 1988;66:7-18.
197. Christensen A, Atkins DC, Berns S, Wheeler J, Baucom DH, et al. Traditional versus integrative behavior couple therapy for significantly and chronically distressed married couples. J Consult Clin Psychol. 2004;72:176-91.
198. Christensen A, Baucom DH, Vu CA, Stanton S. Methodologically sound, cost effective research on the outcome of couple therapy. J Fam Psychol. 2005;19:6-17.
199. Christensen A, Heavy CL. Interventions for couples. Annu Rev, Psychol. 1999;50:165-90.

200. Cohen J. Statistical Power Analysis for the Behavioral Sciences. Hillsdale, NJ: Erlbaum. 1987.p.474 2nd ed.
201. Cookerly JR. Does marital therapy do any lasting good? J Marital Fam Ther. 1980;6:393-97.
202. Cordova JV, Jacobson NS, Christensen A. Acceptance versus change interventions in behavioral couple therapy: impact on couples' in-session communication. J Marital Fam Ther. 1998;24:437-55.
203. Cronbach LJ, Snow RE. Aptitudes and Instructional Methods: A Handbook for Research on Interactions. Oxford, UK: Irvington. 1977.p.574.
204. Crowe MJ. Conjoint marital therapy: a controlled outcome study. Psychol Med. 1978;8:623-36.
205. Dance KA, Neufeld RWJ. Aptitude treatment interaction research in the clinical setting: a review of attempts to dispel the "patient uniformity" myth. Psychol Bull. 1988;104:1092-213.
206. Dessaulles A, Johnson SM, Denton WH. Emotion-focused therapy for couples in the treatment of depression: a pilot study. Am J Fam Ther. 2003;31:345-53.
207. Doss BD, Thum YM, Sevier M, Atkins DC, Christensen A. Improving relationships: mechanisms of change in couple therapy. J Consult Clin Psychol. In press, 2005.
208. Doss BD. Changing the way we study change in psychotherapy. Clin Psychol Sci Pract. 2004;11:368-86.
209. Dunn RL, Schwebel AI. Meta-analytic review of marital therapy outcome research. J Fam Psychol. 1995;9:58-68.
210. Dutcher TD. A meta-analytic study of marital therapy modalities and clients' presenting problems. PhD thesis. Union Inst. 1999. p. 73.
211. Fals-Stewart W, Birchler GR. A national survey of the use of couples therapy in substance abuse treatment. J Subst Abuse Treat. 2001;20:277-83.
212. Fals-Stewart W, Klostermann K, Yates BT, O'Farrell TJ, Birchler GR, 2005a. Brief relationship therapy for alcoholism: a randomized clinical trial examining clinical efficacy and cost-effectiveness. Psychol. Addict. Be hav. In press
213. Fals-Stewart W, Yates BT, Klostermann K. Assessing the costs, benefits, cost benefit ratio, and cost-effectiveness of marital and family treatments: why we should and how we can. J Fam Psychol. 2005;19:28-39.
214. Fals-Stewart W. Birchler GR, O'Farrlell TJ. Alcohol and other substance abuse. See Snyder and Whisman 2003.pp.159-80.
215. Foley SH, Rounsaville BJ, Weissman MM, Sholomaskas D, Chevron E. Individual versus conjoint interpersonal psychotherapy for depressed patients with marital disputes. Int J Fam Psychiatry. 1989;10:29-42.
216. Fruzzetti AE, Iverson KM. Intervening with couples and families to treat emotion dysregulation and psychopathology. See Snyder et al. 2006, In press.
217. Goldman A, Greenberg L. Comparison of integreated systemic and emotionally focused approaches to couples therapy. J Consult Clin Psychol. 1992;60:962-9.
218. Goottman JM. The Marriage Clinic: A Scientifically Based Marital Therapy. New York: Norton. 1999.p.456.
219. Gordon KC, Baucom DH, Snyder DK. An integrative intervention for promoting recovery from extramarital affairs. J Marital Fam Ther. 2004;30:213-31.
220. Gottman JM. Psychology and the study of marital processes. Annu Rev Psychol. 1998;49:169-97.
221. Gray-Little B, Baucom DH, Hamby SL. Marital power, marital power, marital adjustment and therapy outcome. J Fam Psychol. 1996;10:292-303.
222. Greenberg LS, Ford CL, Alden L, Johnson SM. Session change in emotionally focused therapy. J Consult Clin Psychol. 1993;61:78-84.
223. Gupta M, Coyne JC, Beach SRH. Couples treatment for major depression: critique of the literature and suggestions for some different directions. J Fam Ther. 2003;25:317-46.
224. Gurman AS. Brief integrative marital therapy: a depth-behavioral approach. In Clinical Handbook of Couple Therapy. Gruman AS, Jacobson NS (Eds) New York: Guilford. p.731, 3rd edn. 2002.pp.180-220.
225. Gurman AS. Integrative marital therapy: toward the development of an interpersonal approach. In: Forms of Brief Therapy, SH Budman (Ed). New York: Guilford p.482, 1981. pp.415-57.
226. Hahlweg K, Jacobson NS (Eds). Effectiveness of behavioral marital therapy: empirical status of behavioral techniques in preventing and alleviating marital distress. J Consult Clin Psychol. 1984;56:440-47.
227. Hahlweg K, Schindler L, Revenstorf D, Brengelmann JC. The marital therapy study. See Hahlweg and Jacobson. 1984. pp.3-26.
228. Heatherington L, Friedlander ML, Greenberg L. Change process research in couple and family therapy methodological challenges and opportunities. J Fam Psychol. 2005;19:18-27.
229. Hollon SD, Najavits L. Review of empirical studies on cognitive therapy. In: American Psychiatric Press Review of Psychiatry. Frances AJ, Hales RE (Eds) Washington, DC: Am. Psychiatr. Press. p.720, 1988;7:643-66.
230. Holtzworth-Munroe A, Marshall AD, Meehan JC, Rehman U. Physical aggression. See Snyder and Whisman, 2003.pp.201-30.
231. Hurlbert DF, White LC, Powell RD, Apt C. Orgasm consistency training in the treatment of women reporting hypoactive sexual desire: an outcome comparison of women-only groups and couples-only groups. J Behav Ther Exp Psychiatry. 1993;24:3-13.
232. Jacobson NS, Christensen A. Integrative Couple Therapy: Promoting Acceptance and Change. New York: Norton, 1996.p.283.
233. Jacobson NS, Follette WC, Pagel M. Predicting who will benefit from behavioral marital therapy. J Consult Clin Phychol. 1986;54:518-22.
234. Jacobson NS, Schmaling KB, Holtzworth-Munroe A. Component analysis of behavioral marital therapy: 2-year follow-up and prediction of relapse. J Marital Fam Ther. 1987;13:187-95.
235. Johnson SM, Hunsley J, Greenberg L, Schindler D. Emotionally focused couple therapy: status and challenges. Clin Psychol Sci Pract. 1999;6:67-79.

236. Johnson SM, Talitman E. Predictors of success in emotionally focused marital therapy. J Marital Fam Ther. 1997;23:135-52.
237. Keefe FJ, Ahles TA, Sutton L, Dalton J, Baucom DH, et al. Partner-guided cancer pain management at end of life: a preliminary study. J Pain Symptom Manage. 2005;29:263-72.
238. Keefe FJ, Caqdwell DS, Baucom DH, Salley A, Robinson E, et al. Spouse-assisted coping skills training in the management of osteoarthritis knee pain. Arthritis Care Res. 1996;9:279-91.
239. Keefe FJ, Porter LS, Labban J. Emotion regulation processes in disease-related pain: a couples-based perspective. See Snyder et al. 2006. In press.
240. Kessler RC, McGonagle KA, Zhao S, Nelson CB, Hughes M, et al. Lifetime and 12-month prevalence of DSM-III-R psychiatric disorders in the United States: results from the National Comorbidity Survey. Arch Gen Psychiatry. 1994;51:8-19.
241. Kiecolt-Glaser JK, Newton TL. Marriage and health: his and hers. Psychol Bull. 2001;127:472-503.
242. Kirby JS, Baucom DH. Treating Emotional Dysregulation in a Couples Context: a Pilot Study of a Couples Skills Group Intervention. Presented at Assoc, Adv Behav Ther. New Orleans, LA, 2004.
243. Kreider RM, Fields JM 2002. Number, timing, and duration of marriages and divorces: 1996. Current Pop. Rep. pp.70-80. Washington, DC: US Census Bur.
244. Laumann EO, Paik A, Rosen RC. Sexual dysfunction in the United States: prevalence and predictors. J Am Med Assoc. 1999;281:537-44.
245. Lebow JL, Gurman AS. Research assessing couple and family therapy. Annu Rev Psychol. 1995;46:27-57.
246. Lebow JL. What does the research tell us about couple and family therapies? J Clin Psychol. 2000;56:1083-94.
247. Leff J, Vearnals S, Brewin CR, Wolff G, Alexander B, et al. The London Depression Intervention Trial: randomized controlled trial of antidepressants vs. Couple therapy in the treatment and maintenance of people with depression living with a partner: clinical outcome and costs. Br J Psychiatry. 2000;177:95-100.
248. Lillis EA, Fruzzetti AE. DBT for Couples: A Brief Intervention for the Treatment of Couple and Individual Distress. Presented at Assoc Adv Behav Ther., New Orleans, LA, 2004.
249. Lin E, Goering P, Offord DR, Campbell D, Boyle MH. The use of mental health services in Ontario: epidemiologic findings. Can J Psychiatry. 1996;41:572-7.
250. Mohr DC, Moran PJ, Kohn C, Hart S, Armstrong K, et al. Couple therapy at the end of life Psycho oncology. 2003;12:620-7.
251. Monson CM, Stevens SP, Schnur pp. Cognitive-behavioral couple's treatment for posttraumatic stress disorder. In Focus on Posttraumatic Stress Disorder Research. TA Corales (Ed). Hauppauge, NY: Nova Sci, 290. pp. 2004.pp.251-80.
252. Murphy CM O'Leary KD. Psychological aggression predicts physical aggression in early marriage. J Consult Clin Psychol. 1989;57:579-82.
253. Osterman GP, Sher TG, Hales G, Canar WJ, Singla RM, et al. Physical illness. See Snyder and Whisman. 2003.pp.350-69.
254. O' Farrell TJ, Fals-Stewart W. Behavioral couples therapy for alcoholism and drug abuse. J Subst Abuse Treat. 2000;18:51-4.
255. O'Leary KD, Turkewitz H. A Comparative outcome study or behavioral marital therapy and communication therapy. J Marital Fam Ther. 1981;7:159-69.
256. Pearce JW, LeBow MD, Orchard J. Role of spouse involvement in the behavioral treatment of overweight women. J Consult Clin Psychol. 1981;49:236-44.
257. Raudenbush SW, Bryk AS. Hierachical Linerar Modwls: Applications and Data analysis Methods. Newbury Park, Ca: Sage, 2001.p.485, 2nd edn.
258. Regev LG, O'Donohue W, Avina C. Sexual dysfunction. See Snyder and Whisman 2003.pp.181-200.
259. Rice LN, Greenberg LS. Patterns of Change: Intensive Analysis of Psychotherapy Process. New York: Guilford, 1984.p.308.
260. Rogosa D. A longitudinal approach to ATI research: modols for individual growth and models for individual differences in response to intervention. In Improving In Inquiry in Social Science: A Volume in Honor of Lee J. Cronbach, ed. Snow RE, Wiley DE, Hillsdale, NJ: Erlbaum. 1991.pp.221-48. p.423.
261. Schmaling KB, Sher TG (Ed). The psychology of Couples and illness: Theorapy, Research and Practice Washington, DC: Am Psychol Assoc. 2000. p.407.
262. Sexton TL, Ridley CR, Kleiner AJ. Beyond common factors: multilevel-process models of therapeutic change in marriage and family therapy. J Marital Fam Ther. 2004;30:131-49.
263. Shadish WR, Baldwin SA. Effects of behavioral marital therapy: a meta-analysis of randomizes controlled trials. J Consult Clin Psychol. 2005;73:6-14.
264. Shadish WR, Baldwin SA. Meta-analysis of MFT interventions. J Marital Fam Ther. 2003;29:547-70.
265. Shadish WR, Montgomery LM, Wilson P, Wilson MR, Bright I, et al. Effects of family and marital psychotherapies: a meta-analysis. J Consult Clin Psychol. 1993;61:992-1002.
266. Sher TG, Bellg AJ, Braun L, Domas A, Rosenson R, et al. Partners for life: a theoretical approach to developing an intervention for cardiac risk reduction. Health Educ Res. 2002;17:597-605.
267. Shumway ST, Wampler RS, Derch C, Arredondo R. A Place for marriage and family services in employee assistance programs (EAPs): a survey of EAP client problems and neess. J Marital Fam Ther. 2004;30:71-9.
268. Snyder DK, Mangrum LF, Wills RM. Predicting couples' response to marital therapy: a comparison of short- and long-term predictors. J Consult Clin Psychol. 1993;61:61-9.
269. Snyder DK, Scheider WJ, Castellani AM. Tailoring couple therapy to individual differences: a conceptual approach. See Snyder and Whisman. 2003.pp.27-51.
270. Snyder DK, Simpson JA, Hughes JN (Eds). Emotion Regulation in Families: Pathways to Dysfunction and Health, Washington, DC: Am. Psychol, Assoc. In Press. 2006.
271. Snyder DK, Whisman MA (Eds). Treating Difficult Couples: Helping Clients with Co-existing Mental and Relationship Disorders. New York : Guiford. 2003.p.448.

272. Snyder DK, Whisman MA, 2004a. Comorbid Relationship and Individual Distress: Challenges for Intervention and Research. Presnted at Assoc. Adv Behav Ther. New Orleans. LA.
273. Snyder DK, Whisman MA. Treat in distressed couples with coexisting mental and physical disorders: directions for clinical training and practice. J Marital Fam Ther. 2004b; 30:1-12.
274. Snyder DK, Wills RM, Faitler SL. Distinguishing specific from nonspecific interventions in comparative outcome studies: reply to Collins and Thormpson. J Consult Clin Psychol. 1988;56:934-5.
275. Snyder DK, Wills RM. Behavioral versus insight-oriented marital therapy: effect on individual and interspousal functioning. J Consult Clin Psychol. 1989;57:39-46.
276. Snyder DK, Wills RM Grady-Fletcher A. Long-term effectiveness of behavioral versus insight-oriented marital therapy: a four-year follow-up study. J Consult Clin Psychol. 1991;59:138-41.
277. Snyder DK. Affective reconstruction in the context of a pluralistic approach to couples therapy. Clin Psychol Sci Pract. 1999;6:348-65.
278. Snyder DK. Manual for the marital satisfaction inventory-revised. Los Angeles: West Psychol. Serv. 1997. p.126.
279. Sprenkle DH (Ed). Effectiveness Research in Marriage and Family Therapy. Alexandria VA: Am Assoc Marriage Fam Ther. 2002b. p.370.
280. Sprenkle DH, 2002a. Editor's introduction. See sprinkle 2002b, pp.9-25.
281. Sprenkle DH, Blw AJ. Common factors and our sacred models. J Marital Fam Ther. 2004;30:113-29.
282. Stith SM, Rosen KH, McCollum EE, Thjomsen CJ. Treating intimate partner violence within intact couple relationships: outcomes of multi-couple versus individual couple therapy. J Marital Fam Ther. 2004;30:305-18.
283. Swindle R, Heller Km, Pescosolido B, Kikuzwa S. Responses to nervous breakdowns in America over a 40-year period: mental health policy implications. Am Psychol. 2000;55:740-9.
284. Weiedrman MW. Extramarital sex: prevalence and correlates in a national survey. J Sex Res. 2007;34:167-74.
285. Whisman MA, Dixon AE, Johnson B. Therapists' perspectives of couple problems and treatment issues in couple therapy. J Fam Paychol. 1997;11:361-6.
286. Whisman MA, Jacoboson NS. Power, marital satisfaction, and response to marital therapy. J Fam Psychol. 1990;4:202-12.
287. Whisman MA, McClelland GH. Designing, testing and interpreting interaction and moderator effects in family research. J Fam Psychol. 2005;19:111-20.
288. Whisman MA, McKelvie ML, Chatav Y. Couple distress. In Improving Outcome Behavioral Therapy. Anthony MM, Ledley DR, Heimberg RG (Eds) New York: Guilford, in press, 2005.
289. Whisman MA, Sheldon CT, Goering P. Psychiatric disorders and dissatisfaction with social relationships: Does type of relationship matter? J Abnorm Psychol. 2000;109:803-8.
290. Whisman MA, Snyder DK. Evaluating and improving the efficacy of conjoint couple therapy: In Clinical Handbook of Marriage and Couples Interventions, Halford WK, Markman HJ (Eds), 1997.pp.679-93. New York: Wiley, p.720.
291. Whisman MA, Uebelacker LA. Distress and impairment associated with relationship discord in a national sample of married or cohabiting adults. J Fam Psychol. In press, 2005.
292. Whisman MA. Maritral dissatisfaction and psychiatric disorders: results from the National Comorbidity Survey. J Abnorm Psychol. 1999;108:701-6.
293. Wilson GL. The comparative efficacy of alternative treatments in the resolution of marital dysfunction. PhD thesis. Univ. Montana. 2006.p.108.

Enduring Effects for Cognitive Behavior Therapy in the Treatment of Depression and Anxiety

294. Am. Psychiatric Assoc. Practice guideline for the treatment of patients with major depressive disorder (revision). Am J Psychiatry. 2000;157(Suppl. 4):1-45.
295. Am. Psychiatric Assoc. Practice guideline for the treatment patients with bipolar disorder (resived). Am J Psychiatry 2002;159(Suppl. 4):1-50.
296. Arntz A, Van den Hout M. Psychological treatments of panic disorder without agoraphobia: cognitive therapy versus applied relaxation. Behav Res Ther. 1996;34:113-21.
297. Ballenger JC, Davidson JR, Lecrubier Y, Nutt DJ, Marshall RD, et al. Consensus statement update on posttraumatic stress disorder from the International Consensus Group on Depression and Anxiety. J Clin Psychiatry. 2004;65(Suppl. 1):55-62.
298. Barlow DH, Gorman JM, Shear MK, Woods SW. Cognitive-behavioral therapy, imipramine, or their combination for panic disorder: a randomized controlled trial. JAMA. 2000;283:2529-36.
299. Barlow DH, Lehman CL. Advances in the psychosocial treatment of anxiety disorders. Arch Gen Psychiatry. 1996;53:727-35.
300. Barsky AJ, Ahern DK. Cognitive behavior therapy for hypochondriasis: a randomized controlled trial. JAMA. 2004;291:1464-70.
301. Beck AT, Emery G. Anxiety Disorders and Phobias: A Cognitive Perspective. New York: Basic Books. 1985.
302. Beck AT, Rush AJ, Shaw BF, Emery G. Cognitive Therapy of Depression. New York: Guilford. 1979.
303. Beck AT. Cognitive therapy: a 30 year retrospective. Am Psychol. 1991;46:368-75.
304. Blackburn IM, Eunson KM, Bishop S. A two-year naturalistic follow-up of depressed patients treated with cognitive therapy, pharmacotherapy and a combination of both. J Affect Disord. 1986;10:67-75.
305. Blomhoff S, Haug TT, Hellstrom K, Holme I, Humble M, et al. Randomized controlled general practice trial of sertraline, exposure therapy and combined treatment in generalize social phobia. Br J Psychiatry. 2001;179:23-30.
306. Borkovec TD, Costello E. Efficacy of applied relaxation and cognitive behavioral therapy in the treatment of generalized anxiety disorder. J Consult Clin Psychol. 1993;61: 611-19.

307. Borkovec TD, Newman MG, Pincus AL, Lytle R. A component analysis of cognitive behavioral therapy for generalized anxiety disorder and the role of interpersonal problems. J Consult Clin Psychol. 2002 70:288-98.

308. Borkovec TD, Ruscio AM. Psychortherapy for generalized anxiety disorder. J Clin Psychiatry. 2001;62(Suppl. 11):37-42.

309. Bouchard S, Gauthier J, LaBerge B, French D, Pelletier MH, Godbout C. Exposure versus cognitive restructuring in the treatment of panic disorder with agoraphobia. Behav Res Ther. 1996;34:213-24.

310. Bouton ME. Context, time, and memory retrieval in the interference paragigms of Pavlovian learning. Psychol Bull. 1993;114:80-99.

311. Bradley R, Greene J, Russ E, Dutra L, Westen D. A multidimensional meta-analysis of psychotherapy for PTSD. Am J Psychiatry. 2005;162:214-27.

312. Brown TA, Barlow DH, Liebowitz MR. The empirical basis of generalized anxiety disorder. Am J Psychiatry. 1994;151:1272-80.

313. Brucce TJ, Spiegel DA, Hegel MT. Cognitive-behavioral therapy helps prevent relapse and recurrence of panic disorder following alprazolam discontinuation: a long-term follow-up of the Peoria and Dartmouth studies. J Consult Clin Psychol. 1999;67:151-6.

314. Bryant RA, Harvey AG, Dang ST, Sackville T, Basten C, Treatment of acute stress disorder: a comparison of cognitive-behavioral therapy and supportive counseling. J Consult Clin Psychol. 1998;66:862-6.

315. Butler G, Cullington A, Munby M, Amies P, Gelder M. Exposure and anxiety management in the treatment of social phobia. J Consult Clin Psychol. 1984;52: 642-50.

316. Clark DM, Ehlers A, McManuas F, Hackmann A, Fennell M, et al. Cognitive therapy versus fluoxetine in generalized social phobia: a randomized placebo-controlled trial. J Consult Clin Psychol. 2003;71:1058-67.

317. Clark DM, Salkovskis PM, Hackmann A, Middleton H, Anastasiades P, Gelder M. A comparison of cognitive therapy, applied relaxation and imipramine in the treatment of panic disorder. Br J Psychiatry. 1994;164:759-69.

318. Clark DM, Salkovskis PM, Hackmann A, Wells A, Fennell M, et al. Two psychological treatments for hypochondrias: a randomized controlled trial. Br J Psychiatry. 1998;173:218-25.

319. Clarke GN, Hawkins W, Murphy M, Sheeber LB, Lewinsohn JR. Targeted prevention of unipolar depressive disorder in an at risk sample of high school adolescents: a randomized trial of a group cognitive intervention. J Am Acad Child Adolesc Psychiatry. 1995;34:312-21.

320. Clarke GN, Hornbrook MC, Lynch F, Polen M, Gale J, et al. Offspring of depressed parents in a HMO: a randomized trial of a group cognitive intervention for preventing adolescent depressive disorder. Arch Gen Psychiatry. 2001;58: 1127-34.

321. Davidson JRT, Hughes DL, George LK, Blazer DG. The epidemiology of social phobia: findings from the Duke Epidemiological Catchment Area Study. Psychol Med. 1993;23:709-18.

322. DeRubeis RJ, Crits-Christoph P. Empirically supported individual and group psychological treatments for adult mental disorders. J Consult Clin Psychol. 1998;66:37-52.

323. DeRubeis RJ, Evans MD, Hollon SD, Garvey MJ, Grove WM. Tuason VB. How does cognitive therapy work? Cognitive change and symptom change in cognitive therapy and pharmacotherapy for depression. J Consult Clin Psychol. 1990;58:862-9.

324. DeRubeis RJ, Feeley M. Determinants of change in cognitive therapy for depression Cogn Ther Res. 1990;14:469-82.

325. DeRubeis RJ, Hollon SD, Amsterdam JD, Shelton RC, Young PR, et al. Cognitive therapy vs. Medications in the treatment of moderate to severe depression. Arch Gen Psychiatry. 2005;62:409-16.

326. Devilly GJ, Spence SH. The relative efficacy and treatment distress of EMDR and a cognitive-behavior trauma protocol in the amelioration of posttraumatic stress disorder. J Anxiety Disord. 1999;13:131-57.

327. Dimidjian S, Hollon SD, Dobson KS, Schmaling KB, Kohlenberg RJ. Behavioral activation, cognitive therapy, and antidepressant medication in the acute treatment of major depression. J Consult Clin Psychol. In press, 2005.

328. Dugas MJ, Ladouceur R, Leger E, Freeston MH, Langlois F, et al. Group cognitive behavioral therapy for generalized anxiety disorder: treatment outcome and long-term follow-up. J Consult Clin Psychol. 2003;71:821-5.

329. Durham RC, Chambers JA, MacDonald RR, power KG, Major K. Does cognitive behavior therapy influence the long-term outcome of generalized anxiety disorder? An 8-14-year follow-up of two clinical trials. Psychol Med. 2003;33:499-509.

330. Eddy KT, Dutra L, Bradley R, Westen D. A multidimensional meta-analysis of psychotherapy and pharmacotherapy for obsessive-compulsive disorder. Clin Psychol Rev. 2004;24:1011-30.

331. Ehlers A, Clark DM, Hackmann A, McManus F, Fennel M, et al. A randomized controlled trial of cognitive therapy, a self-help booklet, and repeated assessments as early interventions for post-traumatic stress disorder. Arch Gen Psychiatry. 2003;60:1024-32.

332. Ehlers A, Clark DM. A cognitive model of posttraumatic stress disorder. Behav Res Ther. 2000;38:319-45.

333. Eisen JL, Goodman WK, Keller MB, Warshaw MG, DeMarco LM, et al. Patterns of remission and relapse in obsessive-compulsive disorder: a 2-year prospective study. J Clin Psychiatry. 1999;60:346-51.

334. Evans MD, Hollon SD, DeRubeis RJ, Piasecki JM, Grove WM, et al. Differential relapse following cognitive therapy and pharmacotherapy for depression. Arch Gen Psychiatry. 1992;49:802-8.

335. Fava GA, Grandi S, Rafanelli C, Ruini C, Conti S, Belluardo P. Long-term outcome of social phobia treated by exposure. Psychol Med. 2001;31:899-905.

336. Fava GA, Rafanelli C, Grandi S, Conti S, Belluardo P. Prevention of recurrent depression with cognitive behavioral therapy. Arch Gen Psychiatry. 1998;55:816-20.

337. Fava GA, Ruini C, Rafanelli C, Finos L, Salmaso L, et al. Well-being therapy of generalized anxiety disorder. Psychother Psychosom. 2005;74:26-30.
338. Feeley M, DeRubeis RJ, Gelfand LA. The temporal relation of adherence and alliance to symptom change in cognitive therapy for depression. J Consult Clin Psychol. 1999;67:578-82.
339. Foa EB, Dancu CV, Hembree EA, Jaycox LH, Meadows EA, Street GP. Comparison of exposure therapy, stress inoculation training, and their combination for reducing post-traumatic stress disorder in female assault victims. J Consult Clin Psychol. 1999;67:194-200.
340. Foa EB, Hearst-Ikeda D, Perey KJ. Evaluation of a brief cognitive-behavioral program for the prevention of chronic PTSD in recent assault victims. J Consult Clin Psychol. 1995;63:948-55.
341. Foa EB, Kozak MJ. Psychological treatment for obsessive-compulsive disorder. In: Long-Term Treatments of Anxiety Disorders. MR Mavissakalian, RF Prien (Eds), 1996.pp.285-309. Washington, DC: Am, Psychiatric Press.
342. Foa EB, Liebowitz MR, Kozak MJ, Davies S, Campeas R, et al. Randomized, placebo-controlled trial of exposure and ritual prevention, clomipramine, andheri combination in the treatment of obsessive compulsive disorder. Am J Psychiatri. 2005;162:151-61.
343. Foa EB, Rothbaum BO, Riggs DS, Murdock TB. Treatment of posttraumatic stress disorder in rape victims: a comparison between cognitive-behavioral procedures and counseling. J Consult Clin Psychol. 1991;59:715-23.
344. Frank E, Kupfer DJ, Perel JM, Cornes C, Jarrett DB, et al. Three-year outcomes for maintanence therapies in recurrent depression. Arch Gen Psychiatry. 1990;47:1093-99.
345. Frank E, Prien RF, Jarrett RB, Keller MB, Kupfer DJ, et al. Conceptualization and rationale for consensus definitions of terms in major depressive disorder: remission, recovery, relapse, and recurrence. Arch Gen Psychiatry. 1991;48:851-5.
346. Freeston MH, Ladouceur R, Gagnon F, Thibodeau N, Rheaume J, et al. Cognitive behavioral treatment of obsessive thoughts: a controlled study. J Consult Clin Psychol. 1997;65:405-13.
347. Gibbons RD, Hedeker D, Elkin I, Waternaux C, Kraemer HC, et al. Some conceptual and statistical issues in analysis of longitudinal psychiatric data: application to the NIMH Treatment of Depression Collaborative Research Program dataset. Arch Gen Psychiatry. 1993;50:739-50.
348. Gillham JE, Shatte AJ, Freres DR. Preventing depression: a review of cognitive behavioral and family interventions. Appl Prevent Psychol. 2000;9:63-88.
349. Gortner ET, Gollan JK, Dobson KS, Jacobson NS. Cognitive-behavioral treatment for depression: relapse prevention. J Consult Clin Psychol. 1998;66:377-84.
350. Greenhouse JB, Stangl D, Bromberg J. An introduction to survival analysis: statistical methods for analysis of clinical trial data. J Consult Clin Psychol. 1989;57:536-44.
351. Haug TT, Blomhoff S, Helstrom IH, Holme I, Humble M, et al. Exposure therapy and sertraline in social phobia: 1-year follow-up of a randomised controlled trial. Br J Psychiatry. 2003;182:312-18.
352. Heimberg RG, Liebowitz MR, Hope DA, Schneier FR, Holt CS et al. Cognitive behavioral group therapy vs. phenelzine therapy for social phobia: 12-weeks outcome. Arch Gen Psychiatry. 1998;55:1133-41.
353. Heimberg RG, Salzman DG, Holt CS, Blendell KA. Cognitive-behavioral group treatment for social phobia: effectiveness at five year follow-up. Cogn Ther Res. 1993;17:325-39.
354. Hellstrom K, fellenius J, Ost LG. One versus five sessions of applied tension in the treatment of blood phobia. Behav Res. Ther. 1996;34:101-12.
355. Hellstrom K, Ost LG. One-session directed exposure vs. two form of manual directed self-exposure in the treatment of spider phobia, Behav Res Ther. 1995;33:959-65.
356. Hembree EA, Riggs DS, Kozak MJ, Franklin ME, Foa EB. Long-term efficacy of exposure and ritual prevention therapy and serotonergic medications for obsessive-compulsive disorder. CNS Spectr. 2003;8:363-71.
357. Hidalgo RB, Barnett SD, Davidson JRT. Social anxiety disorder in review: two decades of progress. Int J Neuropsychopharmacol. 2001;4:279-98.
358. Hollon SD, Beck AT. Cognitive and cognitive-behavioral therapies. In: Garfield and Bergin's Handbook of Psychotherapy and Behavior Change: An Empirical Analysis. Lambert MJ (Ed). New York: Wiley. 5th edn, 2004.pp.447-92.
359. Hollon SD, DeRubeis RJ, Evans MD, Wiemer MJ, Garvey MJ, et al. Cognitive therapy and pharmacotherapy for depression: singly and in combination. Arch Gen Psychiatry. 1992a;49:774-81.
360. Hollon SD, DeRubeis RJ, Seligman MEP. Cognitive therapy and the prevention of depression. Appl Prevent Psychol. 1992b;1:89-95.
361. Hollon SD, DeRubeis RJ, Shelton RC, Amsterdam JD, Salomon RM, et al. Prevention of relapse following cognitive therapy versus medications in moderate to severe depression. Arch Gen Psychiatry. 2005;62:417-22.
362. Hollon SD, Evans MD, DeRubeis RJ. Cognitive medication of relapse prevention following treatment for depression: implications of differential risk. In: Psychological Aspects of Depression, Ingram RE (Ed), 1990.pp.117-36. New York: Plenum.
363. Hollon SD, Thase ME, Markwitz JC. Treatment and prevention of depression. Psychol Sci Public Interest. 2002;3:39-77.
364. Huppert JD, Schultz LT, Foa EB, Barlow DH, Davidson JRT, et al. Differential response to placebo among patients with social phobia, panic disorder, and obsessive compulsive disorder. Am J psychiatry. 2004;161:1485-87.
365. Iacobson NS, Dobson KS, Truax PA, Addis ME, Koerner K, et al. A component analysis of cognitive-behavioral treatment for depression. J Consult Clin Psychol. 1996;64:295-304.
366. Iacobson NS, Hollon SD. Prospects for future comparisons between drugs and psychotherapy: exchange. J Consult Clin psychol. 1996;64:104-8.

367. Imber SD, Pilkonis PA, Sotsky SM, Elkin I, Watkins JT, et al. Mode-specific effects among three treatments for depression. J Consult Clin Psychol. 1990;58:352-9.
368. Ironson G, Freund B, Strauss JL, Williams J. Comparison of two treatments for traumatic stress: a community-based study of EMDR and prolonged exposure. J Clin Psychol. 2002;58:113-28.
369. Jacobson NS, Martell CR, Dimidjian S. Behavioral activation treatment for depression: returning to contextual roots. Clin Psychol Sci Pract. 2001;8:255-7.
370. Jaycox LH, Reivich KJ, Gillham J, Seligman MEP. Prevention of depressive symptoms in school children. Behav Res Ther. 1994;32:801-16.
371. Klein DF. Preventing hung juries about therapy studies. J Consult Clin Psychol. 1996;64:74-80.
372. Klerman GL, DiMascio A, Weissman M, Prusoff B, Paykel ES. Treatment of depression by drugs and psychotherapy. Am J psychyiatry. 1974;131:186-91.
373. Klerman GL, Weissman M, Rounsavile BJ, Chevron ES. Interpersonal Psychotherapy of Depression. New York: Basic Books. 1984.
374. Koran LM, Hackett F, Rubin A, Wolkow R, Robinson D. Efficacy of sertaline in the long-term treatment of obsessive compulsive disorder. Am J Psychiatry. 2002;159:88-95.
375. Kovacs M, Rush AT, Beck AT, Hollon SD. Depressed outpatients treated with cognitive therapy or pharmacotherapy: a one year follow-up. Arch Gen Psychiatry. 1981;38:33-9.
376. Ladouceur R, Dugas MJ, Freeston MH, Leger E, Gagnon F, Thibodeau N. Efficacy of a cognitive-behavioral treatment for generalized anxiety disorder: evaluation in a controlled clinical trial. J Consult Clin Psychol. 2000;68:957-64.
377. Ladouceur R, Dugas MJ, Freeston MH, Rheaume J, Blais F, et al. Specificity of generalized anxiety disorder symptoms and processes. Behav: Ther. 1999;30:91-207.
378. Lam DH, Hayward P, Watkins ER, Wright K, Sham P. Relapse prevention in patients with bipolar disorder: cognitive therapy outcome after 2 years. Am J Psychiatry. 2005;162:324-9.
379. Lam DH, Watkins ER, Hayward P, Bright J, Wright K, et al. A randomized controlled study of cognitive therapy for relapse prevention for bipolar affective disorder: outcome of the first year. Arch Gen Psychiatry. 2003;60:145-52.
380. Liebowitz MR, Heimberg RG, Schneier FR, Hope DA, Davies S, et al. Cognitive behavioral group therapy versus phenelzine in phobia: long-term outcome. Depress. Anxiety. 1999;10: 89-98.
381. Loerch B, Graf-Morgenstern M, Hautzinger M, Schlegel S, Hain C, et al. Randomized placebo-controlled trial of moclobemide, cognitive-behavioral therapy and their combination in panic disorder with agoraphobia. Br J Psychiatry. 1999;174:205-12.
382. Lydiard RB, Brawman-Mintzer O, Ballenger JC. Recent development in the psychopharmacology of anxiety disorders. J consult Clin Psychol. 1996;64:660-8.
383. Malkoff-Schwartz S, Frank E, Anderson B, Sherrill JT, Siegel L, et al. Stressful life events and social rhythm disruption in the onset of manic and depressive bipolar episodes: a preliminary investigation. Arch Gen Psychaiatry. 1998;55:702-7.
384. Markd IM, Swinson RP, Basoglu M, Kuch K, Noshirvani H, O'Sullivan G. Alprazolam and exposure alone and combined in panic disorder with agoraphobia: a controlled study in London and Toronto. Br J Psychiatry. 1993;162:776-87.
385. Marks I, Lovell K, Noshivani H, Livanou M, Thrasher S, treatment of post-traumatic stress disorder by exposure and/or cognitive restructuring: a controlled study. Arch Gen Psychiatry. 1998;55:317-25.
386. Marks IM, Viswanathan R, Lipsedge MS, Gardner R. Enhanced relief of phobia following flooding during waning diazepam. Br J Psychiatry. 1972;121:493-505.
387. Martell CR, Addis ME, Jacobson NS. Depression in Context: Strategies for Guided Action. New york: Norton, 2001.
388. Mayou RA, Ehlers A, Hobbs M. Psychological debriefing for road traffic accident victims. Br J Psychiatry. 2000;176:589-93.
389. McLean PD, Whittal ML, Thordarson DS, Taylor S, Sochting I, et al. Cognitive versus behavior therapy in the group treatment of obsessive-compulsive disorder. J Consult Clin Psychol. 2001;69:205-14.
390. Miklowitz DJ, George EL, Richards JA, Simoneau TL, Suddarth RL. A randomized study of family-focused psycho education and pharmacotherapy in the outpatient management of bipolar disorder. Arch Gen Psychiatry. 2003;60:904-12.
391. Mowrer OH. Learning theory and the neurotic paradox. AM J Orthopsychiatry. 1948;18:571-610.
392. Mrcus SV, Maruis P, Sakal C. Controlled study of treatment of PTSD using EMDR in an HMO setting. Psychotherapy. 1997;34:307-15.
393. Mystkowski JL, Mineka S, Vernon LL, Zinbarg RE. Changes in caffeine states enhance return of fear in spider phobia. J Consult Clin Psychol. 2003;71:243-50.
394. Nathan PE, Gorman JM, (Eds). A Guide to Treatment that Work. New York: Oxford University Press, 1998.
395. Ost LG, Ferebee I, Furmark T. One session group therapy of spider phobia: direct versus indirect treatments. Behav Res Ther. 1997;35:721-32.
396. Ost LG, Westling BE. Applied relaxation vs. cognitive behavior therapy in the treatment of panic disorder. Behave Res Ther. 1995;33:145-58.
397. Otto MW, Pollack MH, Sachs GS, Reiter SR, Meltzer-Brody S, Rosenbaum JF. Discontinuation of benzodiazepine treatment: efficacy of cognitive-behavioral therapy for patients with panic disorder. Am J Psychiatry. 1993;150:1485-90.
398. Pato MT, Zohar-Kadouch R, Zohar J, Murphy DL. Return of symptoms after discontinuation of clomipramine in patients with obsessive-compulsive disorder. Am J Psychiatry. 1988;145:1521-5.
399. Paykel ES, Scott J, Teasdale JD, Johynson AL, Carland A, et al. Prevention of relapse in residual depression by cognitive therapy. Arch Gen Psychiatry. 1999;56:829-35.
400. Perlis RH, Nierenberg AA, Alpert JE, Pava J, Matthews JD. Effects of adding cognitive therapy to fluoxetine dose increase on risk of relapse and residual depressive symptoms in continuation treatment of major depressive disorder. J Clin Psychopharmacol. 2002;22:474-80.

401. Perry A, Tarrier N, Morriss R, McCarthy E, Limb K. Randomized controlled trial of efficacy of teaching patients with bipolar disorder to identify early symptoms of relapse and obtain treatment. Br Med J. 1999;318:149-53.
402. Ravizza L, Barzega G, Bellino S, Bogetto F, Maina G. Drug treatment of obsessive-compulsive disorder (OCD): long-term trial with clomipramine and selective serotonin reuptake inhibitors (SSRIs). Psychopharmacol Bull. 1996;32:167-73.
403. Resick PA, Nishith P, Weaver TL, Astin MC, Feuer CA. A comparison of cognitive-processing therapy with prolonged exposure and waiting condition for the treatment of chronic post-traumatic stress disorder in female rape victims. J Consult Clin Psychol. 2002;70:867-79.
404. Resick PA, Schnicke MK. Cognitive processing therapy for sexual assault victims. J Consult Clin Psychol. 1992;60:748-56.
405. Romano S, Goodman W, Tamura R, Gonazles J. Long-term treatment of obsessive-compulsive disorder after an acute response: a comparison of fluoxetine versus placebo. J Clin Psychopharmacol. 2001;21:46-52.
406. Roth A, Fonagy P. What Works for Whom? A Critical Review of Psychotherapy Research New York: Guilford. 2nd edn. 2005.
407. Salkovskis PM. Understanding and treating obsessive-compulsive disorder. Behav Res Ther. 1999;37(Suppl. 1): S29-52.
408. Seligman MEP, Schulman P, DeRubeis RJ, Hollon SD. 1999. December 21. The prevention of depression and anxiety. Prevent Treat 2:Article 8, retrieved July 4 2012, from http://journals.apa.org/prevention/volume2/preoo20008a.html.
409. Sharp DM, Power Kg, Simpson RJ, Swanson V, Moodle E, et al. Fluvoxamine, placebo and cognitive behavior therapy used alone and in combination in the treatment of panic disorder and agoraphobia. J Anxiety Disord. 1996;10:219-42.
410. Shea MT, Elkin I, Imber SD, Sotsky SM, Watkins JT, et al. Course of depressive symptoms over follow-up: findings from the National Institute of Mental Health Treatment of Depression Collaborative Research Program. Arch Gen Psychiatry. 1992;49:782-7.
411. Simons AD, Garfield SL, Murphy GE. The process of change in cognitive therapy and pharmacotherapy for depression. Arch Gen Psychiatry. 1984;41:45-51.
412. Simons AD, Murphy GE, Levine JL, Wetzel RD. Cognitive Therapy and pharmacotherapy for depression: sust-ained improvement over one year. Arch Gen Psychiatry. 1986;43:43-8.
413. Simpson HB, Liebowitz MR, Foa EB, Kozak MJ, Schmidt AB, et al. Post treatment effects of exposure therapy and clomipramine in obsessive-compulsive disorder. Depress. Anxiety. 2004;19:225-33.
414. Skoog G, Skoog I. A 40-year follow-up of patients with obsessive-compulsive disorder. Arch Gen Psychiatry. 1999;56:121-7.
415. Stangier U, Heidenreich T, Peitz M, Lauterbach W, Clark DM. Cognitive therapy for social phobia: individual versus group treatment. Behav Res Ther. 2003;41:991-1007.
416. Stanley MA, Beck, JG, Novy DM, Averill PM, Swann AC, et al. Cognitive-behavioral Treatment of late-life generalized anxiety disorder. J Consult Clin Psychol. 2003;71:309-19.
417. Tang TZ, DeRubeis RJ. Sudden gains and critical sessions in cognitive-behavioral therapy for depression. J Consult Clin Psychol. 1999;67:894-904.
418. Tarrier N, Pilgrim H, Sommerfield C, Faragher B, Reynolds M, et al. A randomized trial of cognitive therapy and imaginal exposure in the treatment of chronic post-traumatic stress disorder. J Consult Clin Psychol. 1999;67:13-8.
419. Taylor S, Thordarson DS, Maxfield L, Fedoroff IC, Lovell K, Ogrodniczuk J. Comparative efficacy, speed, and adverse effects of three PTSD treatments: exposure therapy. EMDR, and relaxation therapy. J Consult Clin Psychol. 2003;71:330-8.
420. Teasdale JD, Scott J, Moore RG, Hayhurst H, Pope M, Paykel ES. How does cognitive therapy prevent relapse in residual depression: evidence from a controlled trial. J Consult Clin Psychol. 2001;69:347-57.
421. Teasdale JD, Segal Z, Williams JMG, Ridgeway VA, Soulsby JM Lau MA. Prevention of relapse/recurrence in major depression by mindfulness-based cognitive therapy. J Consult Clin Psychol. 2000;68:615-23.
422. Thom A, Sartory G, Hohren P. Comparison between one-session psychological treatment and benzodiazepine in dental phobia. J Consult Clin Psychol. 2000;68:378-87.
423. Thorpe SJ, Salkovskis PM. The effect of one-session treatment for spider phobia on attentional bias, 1997.
424. Van Oppen P, de Hann E, van Balkom A, Spinhoven P, Hoogduin K, van Dyck R. Cognitive therapy and exposure in vivo in the treatment of obsessive-compulsive disorder. Behav Res Ther. 1995;33:379-90.
425. Vogel PA, Stiles TC, Gotestam KG. Adding cognitive therapy elements to exposure therapy for obsessive-compulsive disorder: a controlled study. Behav Cogn Psychother. 2004;32:275-90.
426. Warwick HMC, Clark DM, Cobb AM, Salkovskis PM. A controlled trial of cognitive-behavioral treatment of hypochondriasis. Br J Psychiatry. 1996;169:189-95.
427. Warwick HMC, Salkovskis PM. Hypochondriasis. Behav Res Ther. 1990;28:105-17.
428. Weissman MM, Klerman GL, Prusoff B, Sholomskas D, Padian N. Depressed outpatients: results one year after treatment with drugs and/or interpersonal therapy. Arch Gen Psychiatry. 1981;38:51-5.
429. Wells A, Clark DM, Salkovskis P, Ludgate J, Hackmann A, Gelder M. Social phobia: the role of in-situation safety behaviours in maintaining anxiety and negative beliefs. Bahav Ther. 1995;26:153-61.
430. Willett JB, Ayoub CC, Robinson D. Using growth modeling to examine systematic differences in growth: an example of change in functioning of families at risk of maladaptive parenting, Child abuse, or neglect. J Consult Clin Psychol. 1991;59:38-47.
431. Willett JB, Singer JD. Investigating onset, cessastion, relapse, and recovery: Why you should, and how you can, use discrete-time survival analysis to examine event occurrence. J Consult Clin Psychol. 1993;61:952-65.

432. Wilson SA, Becker LA, Tinker RH. Eye movement desensitization and reprocessing (EMDR) treatment for psychologically traumatized individuals. J Consult Clin Psychol. 1995;63:928-37.
433. Wilson SA, Becker LA, Tinker RH. Fifteen-month follow-up of eye movement desensitization and reprocessing (EMDR) treatment for post-traumatic stress disorder and psychological trauma. J Consult Clin Psychol. 1997;65:1047-56.

Behavioral Medicine

434. Ader R, Cohen N. Behaviorally conditioned immunosuppressant. Psychoses Med. 1975;37:333-40.
435. Adler NE, Smut M McEwenbs, et al. Socioeconomic status and health in industrial nations social psychological and predictability in adapting to chronic disease. J Pers. 1999;53:273-9.
436. Alberta R, Emmons ML. Your perfect right a guide to assertive living, 7th edition. Impact Publishers Sanluis Bipod. 1995.
437. Andrade AD, Bagri A, Zaw K, et al. Avatar-mediated training in the delivery of bad news in a virtual world. J Palliat Med. 2010; 13:1415-9.
438. Ane PG, Rabatin JS, Manwell LB, et al. Burden of difficult encounters in primary care: data from the minimizing error, maximizing outcomes study. Arch Intern Med. 2009;169:410-4.
439. Atkinson JH, Siater MA. Behavioral medicine approaches to chronic back pain in wisely set. Saunders Philadelphia. 1992;1961-82.
440. Back AL, Arnold RM, Tulsky JA, et al. 'Could I add something?': teaching communication by intervening in real time during a clinical encounter. Acad Med. 2010;85:1048-51.
441. Back AT. Cognitive therapy and the emotional disorders Interational Universities Press New York,1999.
442. Bosworth HB, Powers BJ, Olsen MK, et al. Home blood pressure management and improved blood pressure control: results from a randomized controlled trial. Arch Intern Med. 2011; 171:1173-80.
443. Breuner CC, Moreno MA. Approaches to the difficult patient/ parent encounter. Pediatrics. 2011;127:163-9.
444. Bruckner TA, Scheffler RM, Shen G, et al. The mental health workforce gap in low- and middle-income countries: a needs-based approach. Bull World Health Organ. 2011;89:184-94.
445. Campbell J, Prochazka AV, Yamashita T, Gopal R. Predictors of persistent burnout in internal medicine residents: a prospective cohort study. Acad Med. 2010;85:1630-4.
446. Chaudhry SI, Mattera JA, Curtis JP, et al. Telemonitoring in patients with heart failure. N Engl J Med. 2010;363:2301-9.
447. Chisholm D, Flisher AJ, Lund C, et al. Scale up services for mental disorders: a call for action. Lancet. 2007;370:1241-52.
448. Collins LG, Schrimmer A, Diamond J, Burke J. Evaluating verbal and nonverbal communication skills, in an ethnogeriatric OSCE. Patient Educ Couns. 2011;83:158-62.
449. Cuff PA, Vanselow NA, et al. Improving Medical Education. Enhancing the Behavioral and Social Science Content of Medical School Curricula. Institute of Medicine of the National Academies. Washington, DC: The National Academies Press, 2004.
450. Doherty WJ, Burge SK. Divorce among physicians. Comparisons with other occupational groups. JAMA. 1989;261:2374-7.
451. Dyrbye LN, Massie FS Jr, Eacker A, et al. Relationship between burnout and professional conduct and attitudes among US medical students. JAMA. 2010;304:1173-80.
452. Engel GM. The need for a new medical model: A challenge for biomedicine. Science. 2007;196:129-36.
453. Feldman MD, Christensen JF. Behavioral Medicine: A Guide for Clinical Practice, 3rd edn. New York: The McGraw-Hill Companies Inc., 2008.
454. Feldman MD. Role of behavioral medicine in primary care. Current Opinion in Psychiatry. 2012;25(2):121-7.
455. Fenton WS, Stover ES. Mood disorders: cardiovascular and diabetes comorbidity. Curr Opin Psychiatry. 2006;19:421-7.
456. Fletcher KE, Reed DA, Arora VM. Patient safety, resident education and resident well being following implementation of the 2003 ACGME duty hour rules. J Gen Intern Med. 2011;26:907-19.
457. Foster GD, Wyatt HR, Hill JO, et al. Weight and metabolic outcomes after 2 years on a low-carbohydrate versus low-fat diet: a randomized trial. Ann Intern Med. 2010;153:147-57.
458. Free C, Knight R, Robertson S, et al. Smoking cessation support delivered via mobile phone text messaging (txt2stop): a single-blind, randomised trial. Lancet. 2011;378:49-55.
459. Gadde KM, Allison DB, Ryan DH, et al. Effects of low-dose, controlled release, phentermine plus topiramate combination on weight and associated comorbidities in overweight and obese adults (CONQUER): a randomised, placebo-controlled, phase 3 trial. Lancet. 2011;377:1341-52.
460. Goodpaster BH, Delany JP, Otto AD, et al. Effects of diet and physical activity interventions on weight loss and cardiometabolic risk factors in severely obese adults: a randomized trial. JAMA. 2010;304:1795-802.
461. Graham AL, Cobb NK, Papandonatos GD, et al. A randomized trial of Internet and telephone treatment for smoking cessation. Arch Intern Med. 2011;171:46-53.
462. Greenway FL, Fujioka K, Plodkowski RA, et al. Effect of naltrexone plus bupropion on weight loss in overweight and obese adults (COR-I): a multicentre, randomised, double-blind, placebo-controlled, phase 3 trial. Lancet. 2010; 376:595-605.
463. Groves JE. Taking care of the hateful patient. N Engl J Med. 1978;298:883-7.
464. Hahn SR, Kroenke K, Spitzer RL, et al. The difficult patient: prevalence, psychopathology, and functional impairment. J Gen Intern Med. 1996;11:1-8.
465. Halpern J. From Detatched Concern to Empathy. New York, NY: Oxford University Press, 2001.
466. Haq C, Steele DJ, Marchand L, et al. Integrating the art and science of medical practice: innovations in teaching medical communication skills. Fam Med. 2004;36(Suppl):S43–50.

467. Harrison ME, Walling A. What do we know about giving bad news? A review. Clin Pediatr (Phila). 2010;49:619-26.
468. Heisler M, Vijan S, Makki F, Piette JD. Diabetes control with reciprocal peer support versus nurse care management: a randomized trial. Ann Intern Med. 2010;153:507-15.
469. Hinchey SA, Jackson JL. A cohort study assessing difficult patient encounters in a walk-in primary care clinic, predictors and outcomes. J Gen Intern Med. 2011;26:588-94.
470. Jackson JL, Kroenke K. Difficult patient encounters in the ambulatory clinic: clinical predictors and outcomes. Arch Intern Med. 1999;159:1069-75.
471. Kahn MW. What would Osler do? Learning from 'difficult' patients. N Engl J Med. 2009;361:442-3.
472. Katon WJ, Lin EH, Von Korff M, et al. Collaborative care for patients with depression and chronic illnesses. N Engl J Med. 2010;363:2611-20.
473. Katon WJ. Epidemiology and treatment of depression in patients with chronic medical illness. Dialogues Clin Neurosci. 2011;13:7-23.
474. Keefe FJ. Behavioral medicine: a voyage to the future. Annals of Behavioral Medicine. 2011;41:141-51.
475. Klein J, Frie KG, Blum K, von dem Knesebeck O. Psychosocial stress at work and perceived quality of care among clinicians in surgery. BMC Health Serv Res. 2011;11:109.
476. Krasner MS, Epstein RM, Beckman H, et al. Association of an educational program in mindful communication with burnout, empathy, and attitudes among primary care physicians. JAMA. 2009;302:1284-93.
477. Kreider RB, Serra M, Beavers KM, et al. A structured diet and exercise program promotes favorable changes in weight loss, body composition, and weight maintenance. J Am Diet Assoc. 2011;111:828-43.
478. Kroenke K, Theobald D, Wu J, et al. Effect of telecare management on pain and depression in patients with cancer: a randomized trial. JAMA. 2010;304:163-71.
479. Landon BE, Reschovsky JD, Pham HH, Blumenthal D. Leaving medicine: the consequences of physician dissatisfaction. Med Care. 2006;44:234-42.
480. Lea M, Feigner MJ. Guidelines for Exercise Testing and Prescription, 4th edn. American College of Sports Medicine. Philadelphia. 1991.
481. Levinson W, Roter DL, Mullooly JP, et al. Physician-patient communication. The relationship with malpractice claims among primary care physicians and surgeons. JAMA. 1997; 277:553-9.
482. Linzer M, Manwell LB, Williams ES, et al. Working conditions in primary care: physician reactions and care quality. Ann Intern Med. 2009;151:28-36; W6-9.
483. Makary MA, Clark JM, Shore AD, et al. Medication utilization and annual healthcare costs in patients with type 2 diabetes mellitus before and after bariatric surgery. Arch Surg. 2010; 145:726-31.
484. Matarazzo JD. Behavioral health and behavioral medicine: frontiers for a new health psychology. American. 2007;7:67-89.
485. McGinnis JM, Foege WH. Actual causes of death in the United States. JAMA. 1993;270:2207-12.
486. McManus RJ, Mant J, Bray EP, et al. Telemonitoring and self-management in the control of hypertension (TASMINH2): a randomised controlled trial. Lancet. 2010;376:163-72.
487. Miller NE. Behavioral medicine: symbiosis between laboratory and clinic. Annual Review of Psychology. 1983;34:1-31.
488. Neumann M, Edelhauser F, Tauschel D, et al. Empathy decline and its reasons: a systematic review of studies with medical students and residents. Acad Med. 2011;86:996-1009.
489. O'Connor PG, Spickard A Jr. Physician impairment by substance abuse. Med Clin North Am. 1997;81:1037-52.
490. Padwal R, Klarenbach S, Wiebe N, et al. Bariatric surgery: a systematic review of the clinical and economic evidence. J Gen Intern Med. 2011;26:1183-94.
491. Patel V, Weiss HA, Chowdhary N, et al. Effectiveness of an intervention led by lay health counsellors for depressive and anxiety disorders in primary care in Goa, India (MANAS): a cluster randomised controlled trial. Lancet. 2010;376:2086-95.
492. Piper ME, Smith SS, Schlam TR, et al. A randomized placebo-controlled clinical trial of 5 smoking cessation pharmacotherapies. Arch Gen Psychiatry. 2009;66:1253-62.
493. Rigotti NA, Pipe AL, Benowitz NL, et al. Efficacy and safety of varenicline for smoking cessation in patients with cardiovascular disease: a randomized trial. Circulation. 2010; 121:221-9.
494. Roberts LW, Warner TD, Moutier C, et al. Are doctors who have been ill more compassionate? Attitudes of resident physicians regarding personal health issues and the expression of compassion in clinical care. Psychosomatics. 2011;52:367-74.
495. Rock CL, Flatt SW, Sherwood NE, et al. Effect of a free prepared meal and incentivized weight loss program on weight loss and weight loss maintenance in obese and overweight women: a randomized controlled trial. JAMA. 2010;304:1803-10.
496. Roy-Byrne P, Craske MG, Sullivan G, et al. Delivery of evidence-based treatment for multiple anxiety disorders in primary care: a randomized controlled trial. JAMA. 2010;303:1921-8.
497. Satterfield JM, Adler SR, Chen HC, et al. Creating an ideal social and behavioural sciences curriculum for medical students. Med Educ. 2010;44:1194-202.
498. Shanafelt TD, Bradley KA, Wipf JE, Back AL. Burnout and self-reported patient care in an internal medicine residency program. Ann Intern Med. 2002;136:358-67.
499. Shanafelt TD, Sloan JA, Habermann TM. The well being of physicians. Am J Med. 2003;114:513-9.
500. Shanafelt TD, West CP, Sloan JA, et al. Career fit and burnout among academic faculty. Arch Intern Med. 2009;169:990-5.
501. Shield RR, Tong I, Tomas M, Besdine RW. Teaching communication and compassionate care skills: an innovative curriculum for preclerkship medical students. Med Teach. 2011;33:e408-16.
502. Sood A, Prasad K, Schroeder D, Varkey P. Stress management and resilience training among department of medicine faculty: a pilot randomized clinical trial. J Gen Intern Med. 2011; 26:858-61.

503. Spickard A Jr, Gabbe SG, Christensen JF. Mid-career burnout in generalist and specialist physicians. JAMA. 2002; 288:1447-50.
504. Stewart M, Brown JB, Boon H, et al. Evidence on patient-doctor communication. Cancer Prev Control. 1999;3:25-30.
505. Tan HD. Correlation of specific thoughts arousal and stress. Psychologist. 2009;35(9):807-17.
506. Teutsch C. Patient-doctor communication. Med Clin North Am. 2003;87:1115-45.
507. The Health Consequences of Smoking: A Report of the Surgeon General. US Department of Health and Human Services, Centers for Disease Control and Prevention, National Center for Chronic Disease Prevention and Health Promotion, Office on Smoking and Health. Atlanta, GA, 2004.
508. Vail L, Sandhu H, Fisher J, et al. Hospital consultants breaking bad news with simulated patients: an analysis of communication using the Roter Interaction Analysis System. Patient Educ Couns. 2011;83:185-94.
509. Villareal DT, Chode S, Parimi N, et al. Weight loss, exercise, or both and physical function in obese older adults. N Engl J Med 2011;364:1218-29.
510. Warnecke E, Quinn S, Ogden K, et al. A randomised controlled trial of the effects of mindfulness practice on medical student stress levels. Med Educ. 2011;45:381-8.
511. Wedding D, Stuber M. Behavior and Medicine, 5th edn. Cambridge, MA: Hogrefe Publishing, 2010.
512. Wedding, Danny. Behavior and Medicine, 3rd edn. Seattle: Hogrefe & Huber, 2001.
513. West CP, Tan AD, Habermann TM, et al. Association of resident fatigue and distress with perceived medical errors. JAMA. 2009; 302:1294-300.
514. Willett WC. Balancing life-style and genomics research for disease prevention. Science. 2002;296:695-8.
515. Yedidia MJ, Gillespie CC, Kachur E, et al. Effect of communications training on medical student performance. JAMA. 2003;290:1157-65.

Psychoanalysis, Psychoanalytic Psychotherapy, and Supportive Psychotherapy

516. Adler E. Supportive psychotherapy revisited Hillside Journal of Clinical Psychiatry. 1982;4:3-13.
517. Alstrom JE, Nordlund CL, Persson G, et al. Effects of four treatment methods on agoraphobic women not suitable for insight-oriented psychotherapy. Acta Psychiatr Scand. 1984a;70:1-17.
518. AlstrÖm JE, Nordlund CL, Persson G, et al. Effects of four treatment methods on social phobic patients not suitable for insight-oriented psychotherapy. Acta Psychiatr Scand. 1984b;70:97-110.
519. Bachrach HM, Weber JJ, Solomon M. Factors associated with the outcome of psychoanalysis (IV). International Review of Psycho-Analysis. 1985;12:379-89.
520. Baxter C, Schwartz S, Berman K, et al. Caudate glucose metabolic rate changes with both drug and behavior therapy for obsessive-compulsive disorder. Arch Gen Psychiatry. 1992;49:681-9.
521. Beck AT, Rush AJ, Shaw BF, et al. Cognitive Therapy of Depression. New York, Guilford, 1979.
522. Bellak L, Siegel H. Handbook of Intensive. Brief, and Emergency Psychotherapy. Larchmont, NY, CPS, 1983.
523. Bibring E. Psychoanalysis and the dynamic psychotherapies. J Am Psychoanal Assoc. 1954;2:745-70.
524. Bloch S. Assessment of patients for psychotherapy. Br J Psychiatry. 1979;135:193-208.
525. Blum HP. Countertransference and the theory of technique: discussion. J Am Psychoanal Assoc. 1986;34:309-28.
526. Brenner C. Psychoanalytic Technique and Psychic Conflict. New York, International Universities Press, 1976.
527. Brodaty JH. Techniques in brief psychotherapy. Aust N Z J Psychiatry. 1983;17:109-15.
528. Bruch H. Learning Psychotherapy: Rationale and Grourd Rules. Cambridge, MA, Harvard University Press, 1974.
529. Buckley P. [Supportive psychotherapy] A neglected treatment. Psychiatr Ann. 1986;16:515-7, 521.
530. Buckley P. Self-psychology, object relations theory and supportive psychotherapy. Am J Psychother. 1994;48:519-29.
531. Budman SH, Gurman AS. The practice of brief therapy Professional Psychology. 1983;14:277-92.
532. Butler SF, Strupp HH. Effects of training experienced dynamic therapists to use a psychotherapy manual. In: Psychodynamic Treatment Research Miller NE, Luborsky L, Barber JP, et al (Eds). New York, Basic Books; 1993. pp.191-210.
533. Castelnuovo-Tedesco P. The Twenty-Minute Hour: A Guide to Brief Psychotherapy for the Physician. Washingtòn, DC, American Psychiatric Press, 1986.
534. Chessick RD. Psychoanalysis: clinical and theoretical. Am J Psychiatry. 2000;157:846-8.
535. Coleman JV. Aims and conduct of psychotherapy. Arch Gen Psychiatry. 1968;18:1-6.
536. Fromm-Reichmann F. Principles of Intensive Psychotherapy. Chicago, IL, University of Chicago Press, 1950.
537. Gabbard GO. Psychodynamic Psychiatry in Clinical Practice, 3rd edn. Washington, DC, American Psychiatric Press, 2000.
538. Galatzer Levy RM, Bachrach H, Skolnikoff A, et al. Does Psychoanalysis Work? New Haven, CT, Yale University Press, 2000.
539. Gill M. The Analysis of Transference I. Theory and Technique. New York, International Universities Press, 1982.
540. Glover E. The Technique of Psychoanalysis. New York, International Universities Press, 1968.
541. Glover E. The therapeutic effect of inexact interpretation: a contribution to the theory of suggestion. Int J Psychoanal. 1931;12:397-411.
542. Gomes-Schwartz B, Hadley S, Strupp H. Individual psychotherapy and behavior therapy. Annu Rev Psychol. 1978;29:435-47.
543. Gomes-Schwartz B. Individual psychotherapy of schizophrenia. In: Schizonphrenia: Treatment, Management,

and Rehabilitation. Bellack AS, Orlando, FL, Grune & Stration (Eds); 1984. pp.307-45.

544. Greenson RR. The Technique and Practice of Psychoanalysis. New York. International University Press, 1967.
545. Grenson RR. The working alliance and the transference neurosis. Psychoanal Q. 1965;34:155-81.
546. Gunderson JE, Frank AF, Katz HM, et al. Effects of psychotherapy in schizophrenia, II: comparative outcome of two forms of treatment. Schizophr Bull. 1984;10:564-98.
547. Guthrie E, Moorey J, Margison F, et al. Cost effectiveness of brief psychodynamic-interpersonal therapy in high utilizers of psychiatric services. Arch Gen Psychiatry. 1999;56:519-26.
548. Hadley SW, Strupp HH. Contemporary views of negative effects in psychotherapy: an integrated account. Arch Gen Psychiatry. 1976;33:1291-302.
549. Hellerstein DJ, Rosenthal RN, Pinsker H, et al. A randomized prospective study comparing supportive and dynamic therapics. Outcome and alliance. J Psychother Pract Res. 1998;7:161-71.
550. Hofer MA. Relationships as regulators: a psychobiologic perspective on bereavement. Psychosom Med. 1984;46:183-97.
551. Hogarty GE, Goldberg SC, Schooler NR, et al. Drug and sociotherapy in the aftercare of schizophrenic patients, III: adjustment of nonrelapsed patients. Arch Gen Psychiatry. 1974;31:609-18.
552. Holmes J. Supportive psychotherapy. The search for positive meaning. Br J Psychiatry. 1995;167:439-47.
553. Horowitz MJ, Marmar C, Weiss DS, et al. Brief psychotherapy of bereavement reactions: the relationship of process to outcome. Arch Gen Pyschiatry. 1984;41:438-48.
554. Horowitz MJ, Marmar CR, Weiss DS, et al. Comprehensive analysis of change after brief dynamic psychotherapy. Am J Psychiatry. 1986;143:582-9.
555. Horvath A, Gaston L, Luborsky L. The therapeutic alliance and its measures Psychodynamic Treatment Research. Miller NE, Luborsky L, Barber JP, et al (Eds). New York, Basic Books; 1993. pp. 247-73.
556. House JS, Landis KR, Umberson D. Social relationships and health. Science. 1988;241:540-5.
557. Howard KI, Kopta SM, Krause MS, et al. The dose-effect relationship in psychotherapy. Am Psychol. 1986;41:159-64.
558. Kandell ER. "Biology and the future of psychoanalysis: a new intellectual framework for psychiatry revisited". Am J Psychiatry. 1999;156:505-24.
559. Kandell ER. Comment on "Biology and the future of psychoanalysis: a new intellectual framework for psychiatry revisited". Am J Psychiatry. 2000;157:839-40.
560. Kandell ER. Genes, nerve cells, and the remembrance of things past. J Neuropsychiatry Clin Neurosci. 1989;1:103-25.
561. Kandell ER. Psychotherapy and the single synapse: the impact of psychiatric thought on neurobiologic research. N Engl J Med. 1979;301:1028-37.
562. Kantrowitz JL, Katz AL, Paolitto F, et al. Changes in the level and quantity of object relations in psychoanalysis: follow-up of a longitudinal, prospective study. J Am Psychoanal Assoc. 1987;35:23-46.
563. Kantrowitz JL, Katz AL, Paolitto F. Follow-up of psychoanalysis five to ten years after termination, I: Stability of change. J Am Psychonanal Assoc. 1990;38:471-96.
564. Kantrowitz JL, Paolitto F, Sashin J, et al. Affect availability, tolerance, complexity, and modulation in psychoanalysis: follow up of a longitudinal, prospective study. J Am Psychoanal and Assoc. 1986;34:529-59.
565. Karen Horney Clinic Medical Board. Guidelines for identifying therapeutic modalities. Am J Psychonala. 1981;41:195-202.
566. Karush A, Daniels GE, O'Connor JF, et al. The response to psychotherapy in chronic ulcerative colitis, II: factors arising from the therapeutic situation. Psychosom Med. 1969;31:201-26.
567. Kates J, Rockland LH. Supportive psychotherapy of the schizophrenia patient. Am J Psychother. 1994;48:543-61.
568. Kay J. Brief psychodynamic psychotherapies. Past, present, and future challenges. J Psychother Pract Res. 1997;6:330-7.
569. Kellner R. Psychotherapy in psychosomatic disorders: a survey of controlled studies. Arch Gen Psychiatry. 1975;32:1021-8.
570. Kernberg OF, Burnstein ED, Coyne L, et al. Psychotherapy and psychoanalysis: final report of the Menninger Foundation's Psychotherapy Research Project. Bull Menninger Clin. 1972;36:1-275.
571. Kernberg OF. Affect theory. Paper presented at the annual meeting of the American Psychiatric Association, New Orleans, LA, 2001.
572. Kernberg OF. Borderline Conditions and Pathological Narcissism. New York, Jason Aronson, 1975.
573. Kernberg OF. Psychoanalysis, psychoanalytic psychotherapy and supportive psychotherapy contemporary controversies. Int J Psychoanal. 1999;80:1075-91.
574. Kernberg OF. Severe Personality Disorders. Psychotherapeutic Strategies. New Haven, CT, Yale University Press, 1984.
575. Klein DF, Zitrin CM, Woerner MG, et al: Treatment of phobias, II: behavior therapy and supportive psychotherapy: are there any specific ingredients? Arch Gen Psychiatry. 1983;40:139-45.
576. Klerman Gl., Welssman MM, Rounsaville BJ, et al. Interpersonal psychotherapy for depression, In psychiatry Update: The American Psychiatric Association Annual Review, Vol 3. In: Grinspoon L. Washington DC (Eds). American Psychiatric Press, 1984a, pp 56-67.
577. Klerman Gl., Welssman MM, Rounsaville BJ, et al. Interpersonal Psychotherapy for Depression. In: Psychiatry Update: The American Psychiatric Association Annual Review, Vol 3. In: Grinspoon L. Washington DC (Eds), American Psychiatric Press, 1984a. pp.56-67.
578. Klerman Gl., Welssman MM, Rounsaville BJ, et al. Interpersonal psychotherapy for depression, New York, Basic Book, 1984b.
579. Krupnick JL, Pincus HA. The cost-effectiveeness of psychotherapy: a plan for research. Am J Psychiatry. 1992;149: 1295-1305.
580. Langsley D, Yager J: The definition of a psychiatric: eight years later. Am J Psychiatry. 1988;145:469-75.

581. Lazar SG (Ed). Extended dynamic psychotherapy making the case in an era of managed care. Psychoanalyic Inquiry 17(special supplement), 1997.
582. Levenson H, Strupp HH. Recommendation for future of training in brief dynamic psychotherapy. J Clin Psychol. 1999;55:385-91.
583. Levinson DJ, Merrifield J, Berg K. Becoming a patient. Arch Gen Psychiatry. 1967;17:385-406.
584. Loewald HW. On the Therapeutic Action of Psychoanalysis, in Papers on Psychoanalysis, New Haven, CT, Yale University Press, 1980. pp.221-56.
585. Longorbardi PG. The impact of a brief psychological intervention on medical care utilization in an army health care setting. Med Care. 1981;19:655-71.
586. Luborsky L, Crits-Christoph P, Mintz J, et al. Who will Benefit from Psychotherapy? New York, Basic Books, 1988.
587. Luborsky L, Singer B, Luborsky L. Comparative studies of psychotherapics: is it true that "everyone has won and all must have prizes"? Arch Gen Psychiatry. 1975;32:995-1008.
588. Luborsky L. Auerbach AH. The therapeutic relationship in psychodynamic psychotherapy: the research evidence and its meaning for practice, in psychiatry update: The American Psychiatric Association Annual Review, Vol 4. Hales RE, Frances AJ (Eds). Washington DC, American Psychiatric Press, 1985. pp. 550-561.
589. Luborsky L. Critis-Christoph P. Understanding Transference. New York, Basic Books, 1990.
590. Luborsky L. Principle of Psychoanalytic Psychotherapy: A Manual for Supportive Expressive Treatment. New York, Basic Books;1984.
591. Malan DH, Heath ES, Bacal HA, et al. Psychodynamic changes in untreated neurotic patients, II: apparently genuine improvements. Arch Gen Psychiatry. 1975;32:110-126.
592. Malan DH. A Study of Brief Psychotherapy. New York, Plenum, 1975.
593. Malan DH. The Frontier of Brief Psychotherapy. New York, Plenum, 1976.
594. Malan DH. Toward the Validation of Dynamic Psychotherapy New York, Plenum, 1980.
595. Markowitz J (Ed). Interpersonal Psychotherapy. Washington DC, American Psychiatry Press, 1988.
596. Markowitz JC, Svartberg M, Swartz HA. Is IIT time-limited psychodynamic psychotherapy? J Psychother Prac Res. 1998;7:185-95.
597. Marziali EA, Sullivan JM. Methodological issues in the content analysis of brief Psychotherapy. Br J Med Psychol. 1980;53:19-27.
598. Marziali EA. Prediction of outcome of brief psychotherapy from therapist interpretive interventions. Arch Gen Psychiatry. 1984;41:304-304.
599. May PRA. Treatment of Schiophrenia: A Comparative Study of Five Treatment Methods. New York, Science House, 1968.
600. McGlashan TH. DSM-III schizophrenia and individual psychotherapy. J Nerve Ment Dis. 1982;170:752-7.
601. McNeilly CL, Howard KJ. The effects of psychotherapy: a re-evaluation based on dossage, Psychotherapy. Research. 1991;1:74-711.
602. Meany MJ. Nature, nurture, and disunity of knowledge, Ann NY Acad Sci. 2001;935:50-61.
603. Meissner WW. Neutrality, abstinence and the theurapeutic alliance. J Am Psychoanal Assoc. 1998;46:1089-128.
604. Meyer E, Derogatis LR, Miller MJ, et al. Addition of time limited psychotherapy to medical treatment in a general medical clinic: results at one-year follow-up. J Nerve Ment Dis. 1981;169:780-90.
605. Milrod B, Busch F, Cooper A, et al. (Eds). Manual of Pani-focussed Psychodynamic Psychotherapy. Washington DC. American Psychiatric Press, 1997.
606. Milrod B, Busch F, Leon AC, et al. Open trial of psychodynamic psychotherapy for panic disorder: a pilot study. Am J Psychiatry. 2000;157:1878-80.
607. Mohl PC, McLaughlin GDW. Listening to the patient in psychiatry. In: Tasman A, Kay J, Lieberman J. Philadelphia, PA, WB Saunders, 1997. pp. 3-18.
608. Mumford E, Schlesinger HJ, Glass GV, et al. A new look at evidenee about reduced cost of medical utilization folowing mental health treatment. Am J Psychiatry. 1984;141:1148-58.
609. Mumford E, Schlesinger HJ, Glass GV. The effects of Psychological intervention on recovery from surgery and heart attacks: an analysis of the literature. Am J Public Health. 1982;72:141-51.
610. Munich RL. Contemporary treatment of schizophrenia. Bell Menninger Clin. 1997;61:189-221.
611. Novalis PN, Rojee SJ Jr, Peele R. Clinical Manual of Supportive Psychotherapy. Washington, DC American Psychiatric Press, 1997.
612. Nurnberg HG. Survey of psychotherapeutic approaches to narcissistic personality disorder. Hillside Journal of Clinical Psychiatry. 1984;6:204-20.
613. O'Hara MW, Stuart S, Gorman LL, et al. Efficacy of interpersonal psychotherapy of postpartum depression. Arch Gen Psychiatry. 2000;57:1039-45.
614. Ornstein A. Supportive psychotherapy: a contemporary view. Clinical Social Work Journal. 1986;14:14-30.
615. Parloff MB, Lond P, Wolfe B. Individual psychotherapy and behavior change. Annu Rev Psychol. 1986;37:321-49.
616. Parloff MB. Psychotherapy research evidence and reimbursement decisions: Bambi meets Godzilla. Am J Psychiatry. 1982;139:718-27.
617. Perry JC, Banon E, Tanni F. Effectiveness of psychotherapy for personality disorders. Am J Psychiatry. 1999;156:1312-21.
618. Persson G, Alstrom JE. A scale for rating suitability for insight oriented psychotherapy. Acta Psychiatr Scand. 1983;68:117-25.
619. Petect JR. A closer look at the concept of support: some applications to the care of patients with cancer. Gen Hosp Psychiatry. 1982;4:19-23.
620. Pine F. [Supportive psychotherapy] A psychoanalytic perspective. Psychiatr Ann. 1986;16:526-9.

621. Pine F. On therapeutic change: perspective from a parent-child model. Pscyhonalysis and Contemporary Science. 1976;5:537-69.
622. Pinkser H. The role of theory in teaching supportive psychotherapy. Am J Psychother. 1994;48:530-42.
623. Pinsker H. A Primer of Supportive Psychotherapy. Hillsdale, NJ, Analytic Press, 1997.
624. Ponsi M. Therapeutic alliance and collaborative interaction. Int J Psychoanal. 2000;81:687-704.
625. Racker H. Meanings and uses of countertransference. Psychoanal Q. 1957;26:303-57.
626. Rea M, Strachan A, Goldstein MJ. Changes in coping style following individual and early treatment for schizophrenia. Gen Hosp Psychiatry. 1991;11:358-64.
627. Reiser MF. The dream in contemporary psychiatry. Am J Psychiatry. 2001;158:351-9.
628. Robinson MV, Flaherty JA. Self-regulationof distance in suppor-tive psychotherapy. Clinical Social Work Journal. 1982;10:209-17.
629. Rockland LH. A review of supportive psychotherapy. 1986-1992. Hosp Community Psychiatry. 1993;44:1053-60.
630. Rockland LH. Psychoanalytically oriented supportive therapy: literature review and techniques. J Am Acad Psychoanal. 1989a;17:451-62.
631. Rockland LH. Supportive Therapy: A Psychodynamic Approach. New York, Basic Books, 1989b.
632. Rosenthal RN, Muran JC, Pinsker H, et al. Interpersonal change in brief supportive psychotherapy. J Psychother Pract Res. 1999;8:55-63.
633. Rounsaville BJ, Glazer W, Wilber CH, et al. Short-term interpersonal psychotherapy in methadone-maintained opiate addicts. Arch Gen Psychiatry. 1983;40:629-36.
634. Rounsaville BJ, Grawin F, Kleber H. Interpersonal psychotherapy adapted for ambulatroy cocaine abusers. Am J Drug Alcohol Abuse. 1985a;11:171-91.
635. Rounsaville BJ, Klerman GL, Weissman MM, et al. Short-term interpersonal psychotherapy (IPT) for depression in Handbook of Depression: Treatment, Assessment and Research. Beckham EE, Leber WB (Eds). Homewood IL, Dorsey Press; 1985b. pp. 125-50.
636. Sandell R, Blomberg J, Lazar A, et al. Varieties of long-term outcome among patients in psychoanalysis and long-term psychotherapy: a review of findings in the Sto Kholim Outcome of Psychoanalysis and Psychotherpay. Project (STOPP). Int J Psychoanal. 2000;81:921-42.
637. Sandler J, Dare C, Holder A. The Patient and the Analyst: The Basis of the Psychoanalytic Process. New York, International Universities Press, 1973.
638. Sapolsky RM. Glucocorticoids and hippocampal atrophy in neuropsychiatric disorders. Arch Gen Psychiatry. 2000;57:925-35.
639. Schindler B, Shook J, Schwartz G. Beneficial effects of psychiatric intervention on recovery after coronary artery bypass graft surgery. Gen Hosp Psychiatry. 1989;11:358-64.
640. Searles HF. Collected Papers on Schizophrenia and Related Subjects. New York, International Universities Press, 1965.
641. Shapiro DA, Shapiro D. Meta-analysis of comparative therapy outcome studies: a replication and refinerment. Psychol Bull. 1982;92:581-604.
642. Sharfstein SS, Muszynski S, Myers E. Health Insurance and Psychiatric Care: Update and Appraisel. Washington, DC. American Psychiatric Press, 1984.
643. Sharpe EF. Dream Analysis. London, England, Hogarth Press, 1961.
644. Shearin E, Linchan M. Dialectical behaviour therapy for border line personality disorder: theoretical and empirical foundations. Acta Psychiatr Scand Suppl. 1994;379:61-8.
645. Sifneos PE. Is dynamic psychotherapy contraindicated for a large number of patients with psychosomatic diseases. Psychother Psychosom. 1972-1973;21:133-56.
646. Sifneos PE. Problems of psychotherapy of patients with alexithymic characteristics and physical disease. Psychother Psychosom. 1975;26:65-70.
647. Sifneos PE. Short-Term Psychotherapy and Emotional Cross Cambridge, MA, Harvard University Press, 1972.
648. Silberman EK, Certa K. Psychiatric interview settings and techniques. In: Psychiatry. Tasman A, Kay L, Lieberman J (Eds). Philadelphia, PA, WB Saunders; 1997. pp.19-39.
649. Smith ML, Glass GV, Miler TI. The Benefits of Psychotherapy Baltimore, MD. Johas Hopkins University Press, 1980.
650. Smith ML, Glass GV. Meta-analysis of psychotherapy outcome studies. Am Psychol. 1977;32:752-60.
651. Solnit AJ. Recovery and adaptation. Psychoanal Study Child. 2000;55:252-74.
652. Sonnenberg SM, Sutton L, Ursano RJ. Physician patient relationship, in Psychiatry. Tasman A, Kay J, Lieberman JA (Eds). Philadelphia, PA. WB Saunders; 1997. pp. 40-50.
653. Spiegel D, Lazar SG. The need for psychotherapy in the medically ill. Psychoanalytic Inquiry. 1997;17(Suppl):45-50.

Behavior Therapy

654. Agras WS. Eating Disorders: Management of Obesity, Bulimia, and Anorexia Nervosa. New York, Pergamon; 1987.
655. Agras WS. Understanding compliance with the medical regimen: the scope of the problem and a theoretical perspective. Arthritis Care and Research. 1989;2 (Suppl):8-16.
656. Agras WS, Rossiter EM, Arnow B, et al. Pharmacologic and cognitive-behavioral treatment for bulimia nervosa: a controlled comparison. Am J Psychiatry. 1992;149:82-7.
657. Agras WS, Telch CF, Arnow B, et al. Weight loss, cognitive-behavioral, and desipramine treatments in binge eating disorder: an additive design. Behav Ther. 1994;25:209-38.
658. Ayllon T, Azrin NH. The measurement and reinforcement of behavior of psychotics. J Exp Anal Behav. 1965; 8:357-83.
659. Ayllon T, Layman D, Kandel HJ. A behavioral-educational alternative to drug control of hyperactive children. J Appl Behav Anal. 1975;8:137-46.

660. Bandura A. Social Foundations of Thought and Action: A Social Cognitive Theory. Englewood Cliffs, NJ, Prentice-Hall; 1986.
661. Barlow DH, Craske MG, Cerny JA, et al. Behavioral treatment of panic disorder. Behav Ther. 1989;20:261-82.
662. Baxter LB, Schwartz 1M, Bergman K, et al. Caudate glucose metabolicrate changes with both drug and behavior therapy for obsessive-compulsive disorder. Arch Gen Psychiatry. 1992;49:68;1-9.
663. Becker WC, Madsen CH, Arnold CR, et al. The contingent use of teacher attention and praising in reducing classroom behavior problems. J Spec Edu. 1967;1:287-307.
664. Brent DA, Holder D, Kolko D, et al. A clinical psychotherapy trial for adolescent depression comparing cognitive, family, and supportive therapy. Arch Gen Psychiatry. 1997;54:877-85.
665. Brownell KD, Wadden TA. Behavior therapy for obesity: modern approaches and better results, in Handbook of Eating Disorders: Physiology, Psychology and Treatment of Obesity, Anorexia and Bulimia. Edited by Brownell KD, Foreyt JP. New York, Basic Books; 1986.pp.180-97.
666. Bruce TJ, Spiegel DA, Gregg SF, et al. Predictors of alprazolam is continuation with and without cognitive behavior therapy in panic disorder. Am J Psychiatry. 1995;152:1156-60.
667. Campbell M, Anderson L, Meier M, et al. A comparison of haloperidol and behavior therapy and their interaction in autistic children. J Am Aca Child Psych. 1978;17:640-55.
668. Christophersen ER, Arnold CM, Hill DW, et al. The home point system: to ken reinforcement procedures for application by parents of children with behavior problems. J Appl Behav Anal. 1972;5:485-97.
669. Christophersen ER, Barnard JD, Ford D, et al. The family training program: improving parent-child interaction patterns, in Behavior Modification Approaches to Parenting. Edited by Mash EJ, Handy LC, Hamerlynck LA. New York, Brunner/Mazel, 1976.pp.137-55.
670. Clark DM, Salkovskis PM, Hackmann A, et al. A comparison of cognitive therapy, applied relaxation and imipramine in the treatment of panic disorder. Br J Psychiatry. 1994;164:759-69.
671. Clarkin JF, Pilkonis PA, Magruder K. Psychotherapy of depression: implications for reform of the health care system. Arch Gen Psychiatry. 1996;53:717-23.
672. Cohen DJ, Shaywitz BA: Preface to special issue on neurobiological research in autism. J Autism Dev Disord. 1982; 12:103-9.
673. Craighead LW, Stunkard AJ, O'Brien R: Behavior therapy and pharmacotherapy of obesity. Arch Gen Psychiatry. 1981 38:763-8.
674. Craske MG, Maidenberg E, Bystritsky A. Brief cognitive-behavioral versus non-directive therapy for panic disorder. J Behav Ther Exp Psychiatry. 1995;26:113-20.
675. Crisp AH, Norton K, Gowers S, et al. A controlled study of the effects of therapies aimed at adolescent and family psychopa thology in anorexia nervosa. Br J Psychiatry. 1991;159:325-33.
676. de Beurs E, van Balkom AJ, Lange A, et al. Treatment of panic disorder with agoraphobia: comparison of fluvoxamine, placebo, and psychological panic management combined with exposure and of exposure in vivo alone. Am J Psychiatry. 1995;152:683-91.
677. Dumas JE, Wahler RG. Indiscrim inate mothering as a contextual factor in aggressive-oppositional child behavior: "Damned if you do and damned if you don't." J Abnorm Child Psychol. 1985;13:1-17.
678. Elkin E, Shea T, Watkins J, et al. National Institute of Mental Health Treatment of Depression Collaborative Research Program: general effectiveness of treatment. Arch Gen Psychiatry. 1989;46:971-82.
679. Epstein LH, Beck S, Figuera J, et al. The effects of targeting improvements in urine glucose on metabolic control in children with insulin dependent diabetes. J Appl Behav Anal. 1981;14:365-76.
680. Fairburn CG. A cognitive-behavioral approach to the treatment of bulimia. Psychol Med. 1981;11:707-11.
681. Fairburn CG, Jones R, Peveler RC, et al. Three psychological treatments for bulimia nervosa: a comparative trial. Arch Gen Psychiatry. 1991;48:463-9.
682. Fairburn CG, Jones R, Peveler RC, et al. Psychotherapy and bulimia nervosa: longer-term effects of interpersonal psychotherapy, behavior therapy, and cognitive-behavior therapy. Arch Gen Psychiatry. 1993;50:419-28.
683. Falloon IRH, Boyd JL, McGill CW, et al. Family management in the prevention of morbidity of schizophrenia. Arch Gen Psychiatry. 1985;42:887-96.
684. Fava GA, Zielezny M, Savron G, et al. Long-term effects of behavioural treatment for panic disorder with agoraphobia. Br J Psychiatry. 1995;166:87-92.
685. Fawzy FI, Fawzy NW Hyun CS, et al. Malignant melanoma: effects of an early structured psychiatric intervention, coping, and affective state on recurrence and survival 6 years later. Arch Gen Psychiatry. 1993;50:681-9.
686. Friedman M, Thoresen CE, Gill JJ, et al. Alteration of Type A behavior and reduction in cardiac recurrences in post myocardial infarction patients. Am Heart J. 1984;108:237-48.
687. Gadow KD. Relative efficacy of pharmacological, behavioral, and combination treatments for enhancing academic performance. Clin Psychol Rev. 1985;5:513-33.
688. Gates SJ, Colborn DK. Lowering appointment failures in a neighborhood health center. Med Care. 1976;14:263-7.
689. Heimberg RG, Barlow DH. New developments in cognitive behavioral therapy for social phobia. J Clin Psychiatry. 1991;52:21-30.
690. Heimberg RG, Salzman DG, Holt CS, et al. Cognitive-behavioral group treatment for social phobia. Cognitive Therapy Research. 1993;14:1-23.
691. Kandel ER. Genes, nerve cells, and the remembrance of things past. J Neuropsychiatry Clin Neurosci. 1989;1:103-7.
692. Kazdin AE. The Token Economy: A Review and Evaluation. New York, Plenum; 1977.
693. Kazdin AE. Conduct Disorder in Childhood and Adolescence. Newbury Park, CA, Sage, 1987.

694. Kazdin AE. Psychosocial treatments for conduct disorder in children. In: A Guide to Treatments That Work. Edited by Nathan PE, Gorman JM. New York, Oxford University Press; 1998.pp.65-89.
695. Kazdin AE, Esveldt-Dawson K, French NH, et al. Effects of parent management and problem solving skills training combined in a treatment of antisocial child behavior. J Am Acad Child Adolesc Psychiatry. 1987;26:416-24.
696. Keller M, McCullough JP, Klein DN, et al. A comparison of nefazodone, the cognitive behavioral-analysis system of psychotherapy, and their combination for the treatment of chronic depression. N Engl J Med. 2000;342:1462-70.
697. Kovacs M, Rush AJ, Beck AT, et al. Depressed out patients treated with cognitive therapy or pharmacotherapy: a one-year follow-up. Arch Gen Psychiatry. 1981;38:33-9.
698. Kozak MJ, Liebowitz MR, Foa EB. Cognitive behavior therapy and pharmacotherapy for OCD: the NIMH-sponsored collaborative study, in Treatment Challenges in Obsessive-Compulsive Disorder. Edited by Goodman WK, Rudorfer M, Maser J, Mahwah NJ, Lawrence Erlbaum, 2000.pp.501-30.
699. Lacks P, Bertelson AD, Gans L, et al. The effectiveness of three behavioral treatments for different degrees of sleep onset insomnia. Behav Ther. 1983;14:593-605.
700. Lazovik AD, Lang PJ. A laboratory demonstration of systematic desensitization psychotherapy. J Psycho Stud. 1960;11:238-47.
701. Long P, Forehand R, Wierson M, et al. Does parent training with young non compliant children have long-term effects? Behav Res Ther. 1994;32:101-7.
702. Lovaas OI. Language Development Through Behavior Modification. New York, Wiley; 1977.
703. Lovaas OI, Schreibman L, Koegel RI, et al. Selective responding by autistic children to multiple sensory input. J Abnorm Psychol. 1971;77:211-22.
704. Lovaas OI, Koegel RL, Schreibman L. Stimulus overselectivity in autism: a review of research. Psychol Bull. 1979;86:1236-54.
705. Magrab PR, Papadopoulou ZL. The effect of a token economy on dietary compliance for children on hemodialysis. J Appl Behav Anal. 1977;10:573-8.
706. Melamed BG, Siegel U. Reduction of anxiety in children facing hospitalization and surgery by use of filmed modeling. J Consult Clin Psychol. 1975;43:511-21.
707. Mitchell JE, Pyle RL, Eckert ED, et al. A comparison study of antidepressants and structured intensive group psychotherapy in the treatment of bulimia nervosa. Arch Gen Psychiatry. 1990;47:149-57.
708. Mueser KT, Sen gupta A, School NR, et al. Family treatment and medication dosage reduction in schizophrenia: effects on patient social functioning, family attitudes, and burden. J Consult Clin Psychol. 2001;69:3-12.
709. Multimodal Treatment Study of Children with ADHD (MTA) Cooperative Group: A 14-month randomized clinical trial of treatment strategies for attention-deficit/hyperactivity disorder. Arch Gen Psychiatry. 1999;56:1073-83.
710. Patterson GR. The aggressive child: victim and architect of a coercive system, In: Mash EJ, Hamerlynck LA, Handy LC Behavior Modification and Families (Eds). New York, Brunner/Mazel; 1976. pp.93-127.
711. Paul GL, Lentz RG. Psychosocial Treatment of Chronic Mental Patients: Milieu Versus Social Learning Programs. Cambridge, MA, Harvard University Press 1977.
712. Pelham WE, Carlson CL, Sams SE, et al. Separate and combined effects of methylphenidate and behavior modification on boys with attention-deficit hyperactivity disorder in the classroom. J Consult Clin Psychol. 1993;61:506-15.
713. Perri MG, McAllister DA, Gange JJ, et al. Effects of four maintenance programs on the long-term management of obesity. J Consult Clin Psychol. 1988;56:529-34.
714. Reiss M, Plotrowski WD, Bailey JS. Behavioral community psychology: encouraging low-income parents to seek dental care for their children. J Appl Behav Anal. 1976;9:387-98.
715. Rogers SJ. Empirically supported comprehensive treatments for young children with autism. J Clin Child Psychol. 1998;27:167-78.
716. Sajwaj T, Libet J, Agras WS. Lemon juice therapy: the control of life-threatening rumination in a six-month-old infant. J Appl Behav Anal. 1974;7:557-63.
717. Simons AD, Murphy GE, Levine RD, et al. Cognitive therapy and pharmacotherapy for depression. Arch Gen Psychiatry. 1986;43:43-50.
718. Spiegel D, Bloom JR, Kraemer HC, et al. Effect of psychosocial treatment on survival of patients with metastatic breast cancer. Lancet. 1989;2:888-91.
719. Stanley MA, Turner SM. Current status of pharmacological and behavioral treatment of obsessive-compulsive disorder. Behav Ther. 1995;26:163-86.
720. Steketee G, Foa EB, Gray son FB. Recent advances in the behavioral treatment of obsessive-compulsives. Arch Gen Psychiatry. 1982;39:1365-71.
721. Stunkard AF, Penick SB. Behavior modification in the treatment of obesity: the problem of maintaining weight loss. Arch Gen Psychiatry. 1979;36:801-6.
722. Taylor CB, Arnow B. The Nature and Treatment of Anxiety Disorders. New York, Free Press; 1988.
723. Wadden TA, Berkowitz RI, Sarwer DB, et al. Benefits of lifestyle modification in the pharmacological treatment of obesity: a randomized trial. Arch Intern Me. 2007;161:218-27.
724. Wahler RG. Deviant child behavior within the family: developmental speculations and behavior changestrategies, in Handbook of Behavior Modifications and Behavior Therapy. Leitenberg H. Englewood Cliffs, NJ, Prentice-Hall (Eds), 1976. pp.516-43.
725. Walsh BT, Wilson GT, Loeb KL, et al. Medication and psychotherapy in the treatment of bulimia nervosa: preliminary findings. Am J Psychiatry. 1997;523-31.
726. Wilfley DE, Agras WS, Telch CF, et al. Group cognitive-behavioral therapy and group interpersonal therapy for the

nonpurging bulimic: a controlled comparison. J Consult Clin Psychol. 1993;61:296-305.

727. Wolpe J. Psychotherapy by Reciprocal Inhibition. Stanford, CA, Stanford University Press; 1958.

728. Lazantizis N, Whittington C, Dattilio F. Meta-analysis of homework effects in cognitive and behavioral therapy: a replication and extension. Clin Pshchol Sci Pract. 2010;17:144-56.

729. Dozois DJA, Bieling PJ. Cognitive behavioral treatment of depression. In: Cognitive Behavioral Therapy, Acceptance, Midfulness: Understanding and Applying the New Therapies. JD Herbert, EM Forman(Eds). New York: Wiley; 2010.

730. Greenberger D, Padesky CA. Mind over Mood: Change How You Feel by Cbanging the Way You Think. New York: Guilford;1995.

731. Dozois DJA, Bieling PJ, Patelis-Siotis I, et al. Changes in self-schema structure in cognitive therapy for major depressive disorder: a randomized clinical trial. J Consult Clin Psychol. 2009;77:1078-88.

732. Segl ZV, Kennedy S, Gemar M, et al. Cognitive reactivity to sad mood provocation and the prediction of depressive relapse. Arch Gen Psychiatry. 2006;63:749-55.

733. Butler AC, Chapman JE, Forman EM, et al. The empirical status of cognitive-behavioral therapy a review of meta-analyses. Clin Psychol Rev. 2008;26:17-31.

734. Lazantizis N, Whittington C, Dattilio F. Meta-analysis of homework effects in cognitive and behavioral therapy: a replication and extension. Clin Pshchol Sci Pract. 2010;17:144-56.

CHAPTER 48

Geriatric Psychiatry

Late V Ramachandran

According to the 1981 census, the population of India was 665 million, and nearly 77.27% lived in rural areas. It was estimated that 6.47% of the population was aged above 60 year. In 1971, the percentage of old people was 4.5 and the population of our country was 600 million. Thus, there is a steady increase in the number and percentage of old people in our country.

In a field survey[1] carried out at Poonamallee, a suburban area 20 km from Chennai, it was found that most old people live with their spouses or some other relatives. Nearly 50% of the males and 67% of the females, above the age of 60 years, had lost their spouses. Only 12% of the old subjects were found living alone. Joint family system was common but there was a tendency for it to break down. Some elders lived separately, but were supported by their children or siblings who lived next door or nearby. Nearly 64% were illiterate, 24% had only a few years of education while 10% had completed their high school.

Nearly 50% of the aged have some physical ailment and are in need of active health care. The sensory deficits, such as visual impairment due to cataract or hearing impairment due to otosclerosis, are present in nearly 55% of the subjects aged 60 years and above.

Some of the aged are happy, actively involved in daily activities of the family or religious activities. They continue to have friends and go out to various religious centers. Some remain aloof and have very few interests; others appear disgruntled and fed up with life.[1]

EPIDEMIOLOGICAL STUDIES

There are very few studies carried out to find the prevalence of psychiatric morbidity in the aged. Most of the studies are general population surveys and the number of old subjects included are few. Further in such studies, the interview does not cover all the information one would like to have to study the elderly people.

The epidemiological studies in geriatric psychiatry should aim at:

- Finding the prevalence of psychiatric disorders in the aged,
- Identifying the disorders in their early stages of development,
- Studying the etiology of mental illnesses in late life,
- The extent of utilization of mental health facilities by elderly,
- Planning of new mental health services for the aged, and
- Studying intervention and outcome, i.e. what type of mental health services are most effective in treating the elderly mentally ill.

Many different epidemiological methods have been employed to estimate the prevalence of psychiatric disorders in the aged population. Some workers[2,3] used general practitioners as key informants. This method relies on the skill of general practitioners in identifying psychiatric cases, which varies from person to person and also depends on the quality of their record-keeping. The prevalence figures of neurotic illness found by this method have generally been much lower than those found by the direct interview methods.

The other common method used is the screening questionnaire. This is designed to detect the presence of symptoms, not to generate diagnoses. The questionnaire may consist of a checklist of symptoms which can be administered by lay interviewers.[4] At best, the screening questionnaire can identify potential cases which need to be confirmed by a clinical interview. Screening procedures may be easy but one should remember that the clinically ill population is not inevitably identical with the group which shows abnormal scores on screening questionnaires. In the absence of any objective criteria of what constitutes a psychiatric case, interview by an experienced psychiatrist becomes the ultimate method of case identification.[1,5]

Until recently, no systematic studies of the reliability of psychiatric diagnosis in the aged were made. In the epidemiological studies, different methods and definitions have been used, thus making it difficult to compare the results of one study with another.

As a part of the US/UK diagnostic project, Copeland et al[6] administered the Geriatric Mental Status (GMS) interview to a group of hospitalized patients. They were able to show that good agreement between the ratings could be achieved when the diagnoses were grouped into six main categories. These were:

1. Schizophrenia and paranoid states,
2. Affective disorders,
3. Neuroses and personality disorders,
4. Alcoholism and addictions,
5. Organic brain syndromes
6. Other diagnoses.

There is little doubt that the use of modem interview techniques with high reliability scores will be obligatory in the future.

Table 1 lists the prevalence rates of various psychiatric disorders occurring in persons aged over 60 years, in an Indian community.[1]

It can be seen that nearly 6% of the subjects, aged over 60 year, suffer from organic disorders and 27.6% of the subjects suffer from functional disorders, like depression and anxiety.

Table 2 compares the prevalence rates of various psychiatric disorders in the aged in different countries. These prevalence rates are strikingly similar, with minor differences, which can be explained away by the differences in methodology and definitions employed.

Studies of first admission rates of aged in mental hospitals reveal that it was about 5% in 1975 and 6% in 1985. Due to new admissions and aging of the chronic patients, it was found that nearly 20% of the mental hospital beds were occupied by old age subjects.

Table 1: Prevalence of psychiatric disorders in subjects aged over 60

(N=183)

Diagnosis	*Mild severity*	*Moderate to severe severity*	*Total*
Organic disorders			
Multi-infarct dementia	4	5	9
Senile dementia	0	2	2
Rate per 1000	22.0	38.7	60.8
Functional disorders			
Depression	24	14	38
Anxiety	2	0	2
Hypochondriasis	0	2	2
Personality disorder (Explosive and irritable)	3	5	8
Rate per 1000	160.0	116.0	276.2

ETIOLOGY OF PSYCHIATRIC DISORDERS

Some years ago, all psychiatric illnesses, including paranoid and affective disorders, occurring in the aged were considered as manifestations of senile psychosis, that would inevitably lead to mental deterioration and dementia. The modern era of geriatric psychiatry began at the end of the 19th century, when differentiation was made between the organic and functional disorders of old age, and their different causes, courses and outcomes were highlighted. It was gradually realized that mental illness in old age is not synonymous with senile psychosis.

Geriatric psychiatry is a sub-speciality of psychiatry, which deals with psychopathology occurring in the elderly and the various etiological factors which cause the mental disorders in old age. These factors include the following:

Cerebral Pathology

The study of mild, moderate and severe degrees of dementias and well preserved elders has led to the concept of 'threshold phenomenon' in the pathological changes relating to dementia. The senile plaques seen in senile dementia and softening of brain seen in multi-infarct dementia are also seen in normal aging process. It is suggested that there seems to be a threshold beyond which dementia occurs. Plaque count of 14 or more per field and softening of 50 ml or more of the brain are found to be associated with dementia.

The biochemical studies in Alzheimer's dementia have revealed a widespread deficit of the enzyme concerned with the synthesis and breakdown of the neurotransmitter acetylcholine.

Psychosocial Factors

Psychosocial variables, such as female sex, widowed state, unemployed condition, low educational level, low social class, nuclear family, living alone, physical illness and sensory deficit are significantly associated with depression and neuroses in old age.

Table 2: Prevalence of psychiatric disorders of old age in different countries

Country	*Study*	*Organic psychoses %*	*Functional psychoses %*	*Neurotic disorders %*
Norway	Bremer,[3] 1951	2.5	4.2	17.66
Sweden	Essen Moller,[7] 1956	5.0	1.4	12.0
England	Kay,[5] 1964	5.6	2.4	12.5
Denmark	Nielson,[8] 1963	3.1	3.7	8.7
India	Ramachandran,[1] 1980	6.4	1.7	11.6

Socioeconomic Factors

A high percentage of the aged are poor, unemployed and dependent, with a low educational level.[1] Some are physically weak, with their speed and ability limited, thus preferring not to work. Some have cataract, are afraid of getting operated and, due to the visual defect, are unable to go for work. Socioeconomic factors frequently contribute to the causation or exacerbation (or both) of mental disorders in the elderly.

Physical Illness

Poor general health, incapacity for self-care, difficulty in mobility, physical illness and presence of chronic illness correlate with depression and neuroses in old age.[1] Busse,[9] in a longitudinal study of volunteers who were aged 60 years or over, found a drop in health as a causative factor in depression. A high incidence of physical illness has been reported in geriatric psychiatric patients by many workers.[5,9,10] Post[10] remarked that the co-existence of physical illness and affective disorder in elderly is more frequent than can be explained by chance. Sainsbury[11] found that physical illness was a prominent feature of elderly suicides.

Emotional Attitudes

Attitudes of dissatisfaction with life, feeling of loneliness and self-pity have high correlation with social class and physical illness.

Social Isolation

Social isolation is found to have resulted from physical disability limiting the movement of the subject, widowed state and living alone.[1] On the other hand, Garside et al[12] reported that feeling lonely is related to emotional and personality disorders, and not to living alone and paucity of contacts. Kay et al[5] observed that the complaints of loneliness were the consequence, rather than the cause, of illness in old age. However, Ramachandran's study revealed that the feeling of loneliness is not related to the personality factors, but is related to the presence of physical disability restricting movement and widowed state.

Family Structure

This is one of the important cultural factors, which is suspected to influence the incidence of mental illness. Venkoba Rao et al,[13] in their study of mental illness in subjects aged over 50 years, paid special attention to the study of the types of patients' families in respect of the extent of their jointedness. They found a high percentage of nuclear families amongst the organic group. Family structure was cited as a major factor in the etiogenesis of geriatric psychiatric disorders.

Bereavement and Widowed State

Recent death of a close relative, such as spouse, sibling or child, was observed to be the cause of mental illness in a small percentage of subjects. There is no doubt that bereavement is a severe stressor and that some of the cultural practices, such as loud crying and other rituals, reduce the incidence of depression following bereavement.

Widowed state leads to a feeling of loneliness, lack of purpose and dissatisfaction in life. It also leads to loss of income and necessitates changes in living arrangements in some persons. Ramachandran,[1] Parkes[14] and Clayton et al[15] have reported significant association of widowed state to mental illness in old age.

Special Stressors of the Aged

In old age, the individual has to face retirement, loss of status, fall in income, loss of health, loss of loved persons and may also have to manage the failures in plans and ventures.

One has to plan ahead for the evening of his life, particularly for finance, leisure time activities, care of health, moving away of children and loss of loved persons. If done properly, the integrity of the ego will help the elderly person to handle these problems in a mature way.[16] Otherwise, suffering, despair and feeling of sadness follow. These may significantly contribute to the origin of mental disorders in that phase of life.

PSYCHIATRIC DISORDERS IN OLD AGE

Depression

There is a widespread belief that depression in the aged is much less in our country than in the West, due to the joint family system and other cultural practices which provide satisfaction and security to the aged. Elderly persons are held with reverence, are consulted in matters of marriage, festivals, property and the like, and are given prominence in all family functions. In the traditional three-generation family in the village, the elders gain satisfaction in training the youngsters in the family tradition. The aged in India have also no fear of being caste aside 'in homes for the aged'. In industrial countries, where the joint family has broken up and the nuclear family has become popular, and where higher values are attached to productiveness and attractiveness, the old age subjects are said to be at a disadvantage. This disadvantage may increase the occurrence of depression in them.

Further, it is held that depression following bereavement is less frequent in our country as the grief is thoroughly worked out by loud crying and other religious customs of mourning. Also, the Hindu philosophy prescribes asramas—the way to live at different stages of life; *brahmacharya asrama, grahastha asrama, vanprastha asrama*, and *sanyasa asrama*. In *sanyasa asrama*, the final stage of life, the individual renounces all worldly things and seeks to know, find and realize the self.[17] Due to this philosophical attitude, the aged are able to bear the losses in life without suffering from depression.

Contrary to this common belief, community surveys carried out in different parts of India have revealed that depression is the most common psychiatric disorder in late life. Nandi et al,[18] in their epidemiological survey of a rural population near Calcutta, found that 24.1% of subjects aged 60 years and above suffered from depression. Ramachandran,[1] in a geropsychiatric community survey in a suburban population near Chennai, found that 24% of the subjects aged over 60 years in the community suffered from depression, and that it is the most common psychiatric disorder in the aged. Venkoba Rao et al,[19] in their geropsychiatric morbidity survey in a semi-urban area near Madurai, found that depressive illness contributed to 67% of the total psychiatric morbidity in the aged.

Etiology

It was found that depression was more common in women than in men, and a large number of depressives were widowed and belonged to lower socioeconomic group. The death of spouse is the most stressful event, often leading to radical changes in living arrangements, loss of personal care and general loss of life-satisfaction. The elderly men suffer reduction in income either due to retirement or inability to work due to health reasons. Poor socioeconomic status results in multiple stresses, such as inadequate diet, deficient and poor medical care, and family disorganization; and all these combine to produce depression.

Comparing the family system and living conditions in depressives and normals, it was observed[1] that a higher percentage of depressives was from nuclear family system and nearly 16% of them were found to be living alone. Social isolation is one of the important factors causing depression in the elderly, and it may come on due to retirement and lack of social contact, or due to physical illness and inability to move about, or due to the children moving away from the family for reasons of employment or marriage. Depression occurring in subjects living alone and having poor family contacts is particularly dangerous, as they may not seek treatment and may attempt suicide.

Many workers have pointed out the high incidence of physical illness in elderly depressives.[5] In a study,[1] 42% exhibited physical illness of moderate to severe degree and nearly half the cases had sensory deficit due to cataract and/or deafness. Chronic illnesses, such as heart disease and arthritis, were present in 22% of the depressives.[1] On the other hand, physical illness was found in only 14% of the old subjects who were psychiatrically normal. Post[10] remarked that the coexistence of physical illness and affective disorder in the elderly person tends to be more frequent than can be explained by chance.

It is clear that a high percentage of the depressed elderly has experienced clear physical and social stress prior to the onset of the illness. It appears that in the depression of late onset (involutional depression), genetic factors are of less importance. Among depressives aged over 60 years, the morbidity rate in the relatives is only half of the depressives of the early onset.[20]

Further, it has been observed that monoamine oxidase (MAO) activity increases with age. This increase in MAO activity is more in women than in men. These biological findings may well explain why depression is more common in old age and why it is more frequent in females than in males.

Clinical Features

It is usually described that it is the rigid and obsessive type, or overanxious and sensitive type of person, who develops depression in old age. However, when the personality characteristics, such as sociability, mood swings, health concern, anxious and worrying nature, were examined, no significant difference between the normal and the depressive group was observed.[1] Chesser[21] also reported that the pre-illness personality of elderly depressives did not show any frequency of social or emotional restrictions, poverty of interests, anxiety proneness, hypochondriacal trends, mood swings or excessive religiosity. Recent workers are inclined to favor the view that the persons who develop affective disorders relatively late in life tend, if anything, to have relatively more stable pre-morbid personalities.

Major Depression (Melancholia)

Undoubtedly, a few cases of depression seen in old age can be classified as manic depressive psychosis, depressed type. In these cases, classical depressive mood, poor appetite, insomnia or hypersomnia, psychomotor agitation or retardation, loss of energy, loss of pleasure or interest in usual activities, feeling of worthlessness, self-reproach or guilt feeling, complaints of slowness of thinking, inability to take decisions, suicidal ideation, death wishes and suicidal attempts are seen. Diurnal variation of mood and early morning awakening also may be reported. There may be a clear history of previous episodes of depression or elated mood. Sometimes, depression occurring for the first time in late age may show all the above features and there may be family history of depression or manic depressive illness. In the past, involutional depression was usually described as characterized by depression, agitation, bizarre hypochondriacal and nihilistic delusions. But, such features are seen only in a small percentage of cases.[22]

Depressive Neurosis (Dysphoric Mood)

Depression occurring in the elderly is often reactive to environmental hardship, physical illness or both. It is much more common than the depression of manic depressive type described above. Depressive neurosis constitutes nearly 75% of the total neuroses of old age.[23]

The common symptoms noted are depression, sleep disturbance, anxiety, hypochondriasis, feeling of worth lessness, loss of purpose in life and suicidal ideation. The symptoms are often chronic (of more than 1 year duration).

Depression Associated with Life Stress

The symptoms are often mild and may be missed, as the elderly persons keep repeating the various hardships they have come to suffer and the symptoms of depression may get camouflaged by their description of the life stresses. Depression may be regarded as a natural reaction and not as an illness; yet they respond well to treatment with antidepressants and supportive psychotherapy.

Depression in the Physically Ill

Depression associated with physical illness needs special mention. Physical illness forms a very important cause of depression in old age. The general practitioners often miss the symptoms of depression in the physically ill. They show a blend of depression, anxiety, irritability, attention-seeking behavior and may have a number of somatic symptoms. It should be realized that these patients suffer from depressive disorder, in addition to the physical ailment.

Masked Depression

Some of the depressives present mainly with various somatic complaints, such as pains and aches of different parts of the body, and excessive preoccupation with body functions. This is called as 'masked depression'.

Organic Affective Syndrome

In these cases, depressive symptoms occur as episodes in the course of a progressive cerebral degenerative process or as a part of a well advanced metabolic disease, such as myxedema or pernicious anemia. In their most characteristic form, the depressive symptoms are of a fluctuating and fragmentary kind. Organic psychiatric features, in the form of some degree of clouding of consciousness or memory deficit, may also be found. An irregular alternation with euphoric mood may be noted.

Suicide

Suicide is more common in elderly depressives with hypochondriasis, and in depressives with chronic disabling physical illnesses.

Prognosis

Depression in old age responds well to treatment but relapses are not infrequent. Post[22] followed up 100 cases of involutional depressives for 6 years and found that 22% responded well to treatment, maintaining well throughout the follow-up period without any relapses. Another 35% took a little longer to recover but maintained well with few relapses, while 24% failed to make good recovery but deteriorated only slightly in the social arena. Affective illness became chronic in only 15% of the patients treated.

Treatment

The majority of elderly subjects with depressive illness can be treated nowadays on an outpatient basis or in a day-hospital setting. However, patients living alone, and patients exhibiting marked apathy and inertia cannot be relied upon to take medicines regularly. For such patients and patients with suicidal impulses, admission in a hospital may be necessary. As the presence of physical illnesses is a frequent contributory factor, a detailed physical examination should be carried out in every case. Routine investigations like blood counts, X-ray chest and specific tests like CT scan, when necessary, should be ordered. In some, removal from home environment, that may have been (as in the case of bereavement) a source of painful association or is a constant reminder of the problems and anxieties from which the patient has fought to extricate himself, may relieve depression to some extent. The attitude and behavior, of the hospital staff toward the patients, should be such as to make them feel wanted and arouse their sense of worth and self-respect soon, striking changes in the behavior and mood of the patient can be achieved.

Psychotherapy

Psychotherapy in the elderly needs more active involvement of the therapist. The clinician must take much greater initiative in delineating and clarifying the nature of problems, in order to rapidly evolve determinants of the current emotional problem. The clinician has to make specific enquiry into potential areas of conflicts and problems, such as the patient's health, economic status, living arrangements, current social contacts and the use of his time. He needs to enquire about recent, impending or feared losses. He must learn what the patient believes regarding what the near future holds for him. In many cases, complaints will arise from hardships which are difficult to alter. Catharsis may help him to accept the change in his life, and some practical measures may be adopted to ameliorate the worst features of the patient's environment. Psychotherapeutic measures advocated for crisis situation may be helpful.[24]

Antidepressant Drugs

Antidepressant drugs are the treatment of choice in a majority of cases of depression; the exceptions being the patients who present an immediate suicidal risk or the severely agitated. These will require electroconvulsive therapy, in addition to antidepressants. Imipramine hydrochloride is the most effective drug, particularly in endogenous depression. It can be given in doses of 25 mg thrice a day and increased later to 50 mg thrice daily. Depressives with marked anxiety respond well to amitriptyline and tri-imipramine. Both these drugs have more sedative effect, can be given in doses of 25 mg twice daily and can be increased later to 25 mg thrice daily. Presently, doxepine is advertized as a drug of choice in elderly depressives. MAO inhibitors are said to be particularly useful in reactive depression, but clinically they are found to be very mild antidepressants. The usefulness or newer antidepressants, like mianserin and trazodone, is yet to be fully studied in elderly depressives in India.

The common side-effects of tricyclic antidepressants are dryness of mouth, constipation, excessive perspiration, difficulty in starting the act of micturition, drowsiness and postural hypotension. Sudden changes in posture should be avoided as far as possible, by patients taking these drugs.

Usually, it takes 10–14 days before the depression gets lifted. Antidepressant drugs are continued for about 4–6 months or more, and then they are slowly withdrawn. Along with antidepressants, sedatives and minor tranquilizers (such as diazepam) may be used, if needed. Depressives with paranoid features and agitation respond better to a combination of antidepressants and phenothiazines.

Electroconvulsive Therapy

In patients, who present a great suicidal risk or those who are severely agitated, it is not advisable to wait for weeks for the effects of antidepressants to appear. Such patients should be given a course of electroconvulsive therapy (ECT) as soon as possible. ECT may be administered two or three times during the first week and thereafter twice weekly, up to a total of 6–8 treatments, rarely more than 10. The total number of ECTs is decided by the change in the clinical picture. ECT can be given on an outpatient basis, if needed.

High blood pressure and advanced age are not contra-indications, if ECT is justifiable on other grounds. However, it is unwise to give ECT to patients with recent myocardial infarction or with severe respiratory disease.

Psychosurgery

Although total and lasting remissions are achieved in only a small proportion of patients with depression in old age, a majority has satisfactory symptomatic improvement and social adaptation with the use of antidepressant drugs and ECT. There is, however, a minority in whom these forms of treatment fail, or only fleeting remissions can be obtained, or relapse occurs after increasingly short intervals. In these patients, prefrontal tractotomy or basofrontal tractotomy deserves consideration. Patients with severe hypertension and/or past history of myocardial infarction or stroke should not be considered for surgery. Patients with life-long history of maladjustment, or neurotic and aggressive personality are unlikely to benefit by surgery. A history of manic episode in the past precludes operation. Depressives, who do not improve with ECT and antidepressants for over 2 years, should be considered for surgery. The object is to save the patient from progressive deterioration arising from the interaction of physical and mental ill-health and risk of suicide. Sykes and Tredgold[25] have reported excellent results in involutional depressives.

Mania

Episodes of mania or hypomania constitute about 5–10% of all cases of affective disorders in old age. Nearly half of them give a history of manic attack in the earlier years; in the other half, the first attack occurs in the senium. The onset is often abrupt. During the manic episode, the patient is elated, expansive or irritable. Hyperactivity, pressure of speech, flight of ideas, inflated self-esteem, and decreased need for sleep are other features of manic episodes. The patient often exhibits grandiose delusions and sometimes persecutory delusions, arousing the suspicion of schizophrenia. The patient often becomes hostile and aggressive, if he is prevented from carrying out his grandiose and extravagant intentions.

Treatment

Manic patients are often non-cooperative for treatment and may need hospitalization. They respond well to haloperidol, 1.5 mg given thrice daily. Sometimes, they may need higher doses. Some advocate the use of lithium, if the attacks of mania occur frequently and the patient does not have cardiac failure or renal failure. The dose recommended is 600–1200 mg/day, with a blood level of 0.8–1.2 mEq/L. When lithium is administered, close monitoring of blood levels is necessary.

Neuroses

Nearly 28% of subjects, aged over 60 years, in a community suffer from neurotic disorders. Depressive neurosis is the commonest type, accounting for nearly 75% of the neuroses of old age. The second commonest is the explosive and irritable behavior. Anxiety symptoms in old age are often overshadowed by depressive symptoms. Hypochondriasis is also as common as anxiety neurosis. Histrionic behavior is commonly seen in patients suffering from physical illness. Emotional attitude, physical illness and socio-economic stresses correlate significantly with neurotic disorders in old age.[1]

Anxiety Disorder

The anxiety symptoms occurring in old age are often mixed with depression. When one feels depressed and hopeless, anxiety may occur due to anticipation of yet additional misfortunes. Guilt feelings might also arouse anxiety. If the planned ventures are not fulfilled, anxiety may occur.

Chronic neurotic anxiety is usually a carry-over from earlier years. The patient suffers from tension, agitation, and physiological concomitants of anxiety, such as restlessness, tremor of hands and poor sleep. One may find neurotic traits and maladjustment in the earlier life history.

Hypochondriasis

Hypochondriacal symptoms are also frequently associated with depression; primary hypochondriasis is seen rarely. Increasing egocentricity in old age and proneness to physical illness are possibly responsible for the occurrence of hypochondriacal complaints. Very often, the symptoms are directed to the organs of digestion and evacuation, and bones and joints. Despite the fact that cardiac illnesses are more frequent and more often fatal, the elderly person is usually much more concerned with the gastrointestinal system. Psychologically, it is believed that this concern is tied up with an unconscious expression of the person's dependency needs.

Explosive Behavior

Explosive behavior, i.e. irritability, is often seen in the elderly. Loss of status and health, neglect by other family members, increased egocentricity, and decline in brain function make them prone to irritable behavior. They may, sometimes, become verbally abusive or assaultive. The behavior may be grossly out of proportion to any precipitating psychosocial stressor. When the irritable behavior is frequent, the family members may find it hard to adjust with them.

Paranoid Disorders

Nearly 10% of the patients, aged over 60 years, seeking treatment in a mental hospital do so for paranoid disorders; 70–80% of these are females. Stressful circumstances, deafness, lack of family cohesion and feeling of loneliness are found significantly associated with paranoid disorders of late life.

The essential features are persistent persecutory delusions or delusions of jealousy. Some women complain of being observed when they are changing their dress or are taking a bath. Some have severe hypochondriacal delusions. They may have several bizarre complaints involving many organs or parts of the body. Some complain of insects crawling over their head or body and may be seen constantly trying to pick them up. Some complain of swarms moving inside their head. They are often irritable and have disturbed sleep. They may also complain of hallucinatory voices, seeing faces of people or perceiving foul smell. The intelligence is usually well preserved.

Post[26] recommended that a diagnosis of paranoid psychoses in the elderly should be made when the paranoid symptoms are not transitory, and occur in the absence of organic confusional state and affective symptomatology.

Monosymptomatic hypochondriacal delusions of insects crawling over the body are much more common in elderly.

Treatment

Many paranoiacs can be treated as outpatients, though some may need admission because of non-cooperation or nuisance to others.

These patients respond well to antipsychotic drugs. Phenothiazines and haloperidol are commonly used. It is better to start with a small dose of chlorpromazine (50 mg three times a day) or haloperidol (1.5 mg three times a day), and gradually increase the dose, if needed. Patients should be watched for the appearance of side-effects such as postural hypotension or parkinsonian symptoms. Then, the dosage may be reduced and if the patient has troublesome parkinsonian symptoms, antiparkinsonian medication may be added. Some patients may need ECTs. The patients may or may not develop insight but they stop acting on their delusional ideation. Pimozide (2 to 10 mg/day) is said to be the drug of choice for mono-symptomatic hypochondriacal psychosis.

Organic Mental Syndromes

Delirium

Delirium is an acute organic brain syndrome characterized by clouding of consciousness, disturbance of attention, perceptual disturbances, such as illusions and hallucinations, and disturbance of sleep-wake cycle. Speech is often unclear and incoherent. The patient is often restless and may be found groping or picking at the bed clothes, attempting to get out of bed and suddenly changing positions in bed. At times, the patient may be found drowsy and sluggish, becoming restless again suddenly.

Elderly are prone to delirium, particularly in the presence of any physical illness. Hence, it is most often seen by general practitioners and geriatric physicians.

It has been pointed out that the etiology of delirium is often multifactorial.[27] Age, brain damage, and impairment of vision and hearing, predispose the individual to delirium. Infection, electrolyte imbalance, cerebrovascular disorder, trauma (e.g. fracture hip) and psychosocial stressors (such as bereavement), transfer to an unfamiliar environment, or deficient sensory input may precipitate delirium. Altered pharmacokinetics in the elderly renders them susceptible to the drug-induced delirium. Anticholinergic drugs (e.g. tricyclic antidepressants and antiparkinsonian agents) and hypokalemia induced by diuretics may cause delirium.

The management of delirium involves first and foremost the investigation, identification and treatment of the underlying organic cause. Drugs that may be responsible for delirium should be withdrawn or reduced. Supportive measures include maintenance of fluid and electrolyte balance, a balanced sensory environment and a good nursing care.

Dementia

Dementia is characterized by the loss of intellectual abilities that is severe enough to impair social or occupational functioning. The other features are impairment of memory, abstract thinking and judgement, with some degree of personality change. Some patients exhibit disturbances of higher cortical functions, such as aphasia, apraxia and agnosia. The disorder may be progressive, static or reversible. It usually results from widespread cerebral damage or dysfunction.

Epidemiological studies in India reveal that nearly 6% of the subjects aged over 60 years suffer from dementia.[1] The prevalence of dementia increases with age.

The prevalence rate of dementia, as found in various surveys, is given in Table 3.

It is found that in most field surveys, about 6% of the population aged over 65 years suffers from moderate to severe dementia. The wide variation, from 2.6 to 52.7%, in the prevalence rate of mild dementia among the surveys, is attributable to the difficulties experienced in field surveys in differentiating mild cases from normal senescence.

In a study of 162 persons in an old age home, Krai[31] identified 30 persons who showed a mild memory deficit which did not worsen over the 2 years of his observations. The memory deficits were patchy and, sometimes, the patients could retrieve the former experiences correctly. He called this state as *benign forgetfulness of senescence.*

Kay[32] followed up cases diagnosed as senile and arterio-sclerotic dementia, and found that their life expectancy was reduced. The terminal event and the cause of death was difficult to determine.

These days short questionnaires, such as mental status questionnaire,[33] short portable mental status question-naire,[34] and Clifton assessment schedule[35] are used to find the presence of cognitive impairment and, when present, the degree of cognitive deficit.[36]

However, the questionnaires can only tell the degree of loss of function but not the cause.

Risk factors, which increase the chances of occurrence of dementia, can be classified into two groups: modifiable and non-modifiable. Age and sex are not modifiable, while atherogenic personal attributes, such as serum lipids, hypertension and glucose tolerance are modifiable. The cardiovascular risk factors, such as hypertension, HDL cholesterol, LDL cholesterol, triglycerides, LVH in EKG, obesity and diabetes have been studied in the aged.

The specific preventive measures, which may be of value in the elderly, are blood pressure control, weight reduction, control of HDL cholesterol, and encouragement for regular physical activity.

In the present state of our knowledge (or ignorance), the key correctable risk factor seems to be hypertension in the aged.

The various causes of dementia, particularly Alzheimer's disease and multi-infarct dementia, are discussed in detail in Chapter 4.

PLANNING MENTAL HEALTH SERVICES FOR ELDERLY

Prevention is better than cure. It is known that emotional attitudes, social stresses such as retirement, financial problems, death of the spouse, children moving away from home, and physical illness are important factors affecting the mental health of the aged. As age advances, one plans retirement and finances after retirement, takes care of health, and prepares for separation from children. After retirement, some go on pilgrimage, some spend more time in religious activities, help the family by doing day-to-day work (such as bringing milk, buying vegetables, helping grandchildren in studies, etc). Some others tend to spend more time in club activities and their hobbies. Some, with 'provident fund' money, build a house or invest in fixed deposit and ensure a good return. In some companies and private organizations,

Table 3: Epidemiological surveys of dementia

Survey	*Country*	*Age*	*Mild dementia %*	*Moderate to dementia severe %*
New York State Department of Mental Hygiene, 1961[28]	USA	65+	-	5.5
Key et al, 1964[5]	England	65+	5.7	5.6
Williamson et al,[29] 1964	Scotland	65+	15.5	5.7
Balier et al, 1964	France	65+	-	3.8
Kaneko, 1969[30]	Japan	65+	52.7	6.6
Ramachandran, 1980[1]	India	65+	2.6	6.4

the retiring persons are counseled by social welfare officers, bankers and medical officers. Such timely counseling can help them a long way. Satisfying leisure activities, financial security and good health can ensure high morale and healthy mental state in later age.

An Indian study[1] noted that even though many elderly had physical ailments, only a few were taking treatment. Many of the illnesses in the elderly, such as hypertension, diabetes, cataract, otosclerosis, can be treated and their complications can be reduced by proper care.

Pessimism, neglect of health, tendency to listen to lay advice, quacks, and old wives' tales, fear of doctors, uncomfortable and too expensive investigations, treatment the doctor may advise, and the fear of hospitals make the elderly avoid the doctors and proper treatment. Therefore, the physician must take extra care in educating and informing his aged patients.

The size of the problem, the attitude of the aged, the family and social support, and the resources that are available should be taken into consideration while planning a mental health program for the aged.

As the elderly do not generally come for treatment on their own, home visits by the health visitors and getting the sick to the primary health center appears to be the only way of ensuring early treatment. In the city, adoption of slums and certain localities by the hospital and the mobile clinics will help. Corporation health staff and primary health centers can maintain a register of the aged and organize services for the aged.

A geriatric clinic can be started in all district headquarter hospitals with the close cooperation of the physicians, psychiatrists and other specialists. The physician in-charge should be sent for in-service training in geriatric medicine and geriatric psychiatry. By organizing well-planned mother and child welfare services, we have been able to reduce maternal mortality and the incidence of diphtheria, whooping cough, tetanus and malnutrition in children. Similarly, by well-planned services for the aged, we should be able to keep the aged healthy.

It has been seen that a large percentage of elderly subjects suffering from dementia, have multi-infarct dementia. These patients come in contact with the health-care system at some point in their illness, for the treatment of giddiness, hypertension, seizures or stroke. Since multi-infarct dementia is largely preventable, it is suggested that strengthening of the present health care system and establishment of hypertension and diabetes clinics at the district headquarters' hospitals may reduce or delay the occurrence of dementia. Similarly, advanced centers for stroke and Alzheimer's disease at the tertiary care hospitals are necessary. Education of general practitioners and family physicians, for recognition of depression in the physically ill elderly, is also important.

Financial assistance to the poor elderly, increase in pension, flexible retirement policy, part-time jobs for the retired, are some of the social measures that can be taken up to improve the life of the elderly. Independence, the feeling that one is not a burden on the society, and a gainful engagement will go a long way in adding life to the years.[16]

REFERENCES

1. Ramachandran V. Psychiatric disorders in subjects aged over fifty. PhD Thesis, University of Madras, Madras; 1980.
2. Watts CAH. Walts BM. Psychiatry in General Practice. London: Churchill; 1952.
3. Bremer JA. Social and psychiatric investigations of a small community in Nonhern Norway. Acta Psychiatr Scand. 1951; (Suppl.):62.
4. Hare EH, Shaw GK. Mental Health in a New Housing Estate. New York: Oxford University Press; 1965.
5. Kay DWK, Beamish P, Roth M. Old age mental disorders in Newcastle upon Tyne. Part I: A study of prevalence. Br J Psychiatry. 1964;110:146-58.
6. Copeland JRM, Kelleher M, Duckworth G, et al. Reliability of psychiatric assessment in older patients. Int J Aging Human Dev. 1976;7:313-18.
7. Essen Moller E. Individual traits and morbidity in a Swedish rural population. Acta Psychiatr Scand. 1956;(Suppl. 100).
8. Nielson J. Geronto-psychiatric period prevalence investigation in a geographically delimited population. Acta Psychiatr Scand. 1963;38:307-12.
9. Busse EW, Blazer D. Handbook of Geriatric Psychiatry. New York: Van Nostrand; 1980.
10. Post F. The relationship to physical and mental illness in the elderly. VIII International Congress of Gerontology Proceedings, Washington DC. 1969;1:198.
11. Sainsbury P. Suicide and depression. In: Cooper A, Walk A (Eds). Recent Developments in Affective Disorders. Br J Psychiatry. 1968;(Spl.Pub.No. 3):138-52.
12. Garside RF, Kay DWK, Roth M. Old age mental disorders. In: Newcastle upon Tyne. Part III: A factorial study of medical and social characteristics. Br J Psychiatry. 1965; 111:939.
13. Venkoba Rao A, Virudhagirinathan. Menial illness in patients aged 50 and over. Indian J Psychiatry. 1972;14:319.
14. Parkes CM. Recent bereavementas cause of mental illness. Br J Psychiatry. 1964;110:198.
15. Clayton PJ, Malikas JA, Maurice WL. The depression of widowhood. Br J Psychiatry. 1972;120:71.
16. Ramachandran V. Mental health of the aged. In: Ramachandran V, Palaniappan V, Shah LP (Eds). Continuing Medical Education Programme of Indian Psychiatric Society; 1982.pp.121.
17. Prabhu PM. Hindu Social Organisation. Bombay: Popular Prakasan; 1963.pp.99.

18. Nandi DN, Ajmani S, Ganguli A, et al. Psychiatric disorders in a rural community in West Bengal: An epidemiological study. Indian J Psychiatry. 1975;38:307.
19. Venkoba Rao A, Mahadevan T. Geropsychiatric morbidity survey in a semi-urban population near Madurai. Indian J Psychiatry. 1982;24:258.
20. Stenstedt A. Involutional melancholia: An etiological, clinical and social study of endogenous depression in later life with special reference to genetic factors. Acta Psychiatr Neurol Scand. 1959;(Suppl)127:34.
21. Chesser ES. A study of some etiological factors in the affective disorders of old age. Dissertation. Institute of Psychiatry, Cited by Post F; 1968.
22. Post F. The management and nature of depressive illness in late life: a follow-through study. Br J Psychiatry. 1972;121: 393-404.
23. Ramachandran V, Palaniappan V. Depressive disorders in the aged. In: Ramachandran V, Palaniappan V, Shah LP. Eds. Continuing Medical Education Programme of Indian Psychiatric society. 1983;3:29-36.
24. Greenwood J, Bancroft J. Counselling and crisis intervention. In: Kendall RE, Zeally AK (Eds). Companion to Psychiatric Studies, IV edition. Churchill Livingstone; 1988.pp.782.
25. Sykes M, Tredgold RF. Restricted orbital under-cutting: a study of its effects on 350 patients over 10 years. Br J Psychiatry. 1964;110:669.
26. Post F. Paranoid disorders in the elderly. PG Med. 1973;53:52.
27. Lipowski ZJ. Transient cognitive disorders (delirium) in the elderly. Am J Psychiatry. 1983;140:1426.
28. New York State Department of Mental Hygiene. A Mental Health Survey of Older People. Utica: New York State Hospital Press; 1961.
29. Williamson J, Stroke IH, Gray S, et al. Old people at home: their unreported needs. Lancet. 1964;1:1117.
30. Kaneko Z. Epidemiological studies on mental disorders of the aged in Japan. Proceedings of VIII International Congress of Gerontology, Washington DC; 1969.pp.284.
31. Krai VA. Senescent forgetfulness: Benign and malignant. Can Med Assoc J. 1962;86:257-60.
32. Kay DWK. Outcome and cause of death in mental disorders of old age: A long term follow-up of functional and organic psychoses. Acta Psychiatr Scand. 1962;38:249-76.
33. Kahn RL, Goldfarb AI, Pollack M, et al. Brief objective measures for the determination of mental status in the aged. Am J Psychiatry. 1960;117:326-8.
34. Pfeiffer E. A short portable mental status questionnaire for assessment of organic brain defects in elderly patients. J Am Geriatr Soc. 1975;23:433-41.
35. Patie AH, Gilleard CJ. The Clifton assessment schedule. Br J Psychiatry. 1976;129:68-72.
36. Ramachandran V, Sathiyanathan R. Mental Health Assessment of the Aged. In: Verghese A (Ed). Continuing Medical Education Programme of Indian Psychiatric Society. 1986;6:53-8.

SUGGESTED READING

1. Anderson R. The unremitting burden on carers. Br Med J. 1987;294:73-4.
2. Arie T. Ed. Recent Advances in Psychogeriatrics. Edinburgh: Churchill Livingstone; 1985.
3. Berenger M. Psychogeriatrics: An International Handbook. New York: Springer Verlag; 1987.
4. Blessed G, Wilson ID. The contemporary natural history of mental disorderin old age. Br J Psychiatry. 1982;141:59-67.
5. Brocklehurst JC. Textbook of Geriatric Medicine and Gerontology. Edinburgh: Churchill Livingstone; 1985.
6. Busse EW, Blazer DG. Geriatric Psychiatry. Washington DC: American Psychiatric Press; 1989.
7. Butler RN, Lewis MI. Love and Sex Over Sixty. II Ed. New York: Harper and Row; 1988.
8. Clark ANG, Mankikar I. Diogenes syndrome: A clinical study of gross neglect in old age. Lancet. 1975;1:366-68.
9. Goldstein MZ. Family Involvement in the Treatment of the Frail Elderly. Washington DC: American Psychiatric Press; 1990.
10. Greengross S. The Law and Vulnerable Elderly People. Age Concern. Mitcham: Surreys; 1986.
11. Horrocks P. The components of a comprehensive district health service for the elderly people: A personal view. Age and Ageing. 1986;15:321-42.
12. Israel L, Kozarevic D, Sartorius N. Source Book of Geriatric Assessment. New York: Karger; 1984:Vols I, II.
13. Jarvik L, Small G. Parent Care: A Commonsense Guide for Adult Children. New York: Crown; 1988.
14. Kiloh LG. Pseudodementia. Acta Psychiatr Scand. 1961;37:336-51.
15. Murphy E. Social origins of depression in old age. Br J Psychiatry. 1982;141:135-42.
16. Rabin DL, Stockton P. Long-Term Care for the Elderly: A Fact-Book. New York: Oxford University Press; 1987
17. Reisberg B. Brain Failure: An Introduction to Current Concepts of Senility. New York: Free Press; 1981.
18. Roth M, Huppert FA, Tym E, Mountjoy CQ. The Cambridge Examination for Mental Disorders of the Elderly (CAMDEX). Cambridge: Cambridge University Press; 1988.
19. Roth M. The natural history of mental disorder in old age. J Ment Sci. 1955;101:281-301.
20. Tobias CR, Lippmann S, Pary R. Dementia in the elderly. Postgrad Med. 1989;86:97-108.
21. Wattis JP, Church M. Practical Psychiatry of Old Age. London: Croom Helm; 1986.

CHAPTER

49 Life Stress and Psychiatric Disorders

Indira Sharma, Abhishek Pathak

INTRODUCTION

Life without stress cannot be imagined. Psychological stress forms an inseparable part of life and, up to a degree, may be essential for normal personality development. However, if these stresses become too severe or too numerous, they may affect the psychiatric equilibrium, producing maladaptive patterns of behavior and possibly mental disorders. It is recognized that stress can be one of the components of any disease, not just those designated as psychosomatic. The diseases of our times are etiologically linked with excessive stress and, in turn, this stress is a product of specifically structured social situations inherent in the organization of modern technological societies[1].

Selye,[2] in his classical work, postulated that any type of life change could act as a stressor, causing physiological arousal and enhanced susceptibility to illness. Stress operates via the autonomic nervous system and endocrine glands; though the precise relationship between neurogenic and hormonal regulation in normal and pathological conditions is not very clear. Stress is not necessarily unpleasant. Essentially, stress can be of two types: pleasant stress called as eustress; and unpleasant stress called as distress. There may also be some life events which simply act to help maintain the internal steady state or to keep the individual interested in undertaking appropriate activities. Such stress may be called 'Neustress'.[3]

The term "stress" has been defined in different manners throughout the literature, different models of stress like medical, environmental, and psychological have been proposed.[4]

Medical model of stress: According to the medical model, stress is a state of distress in an individual in response to an environmental precipitant. This physiological response of an organism can be measured by increased heart rate, elevated blood pressure, and the presence of hormones and neurotransmitters (i.e. cortisol, adrenaline, norepinephrine) that heighten the arousal of the organism.[5] Distress, occurring within a normal range, is adaptive in nature; this heightened arousal prepares an organism to effectively deal with stress. However, chronic stimulation of the stress-response system has been linked to depressed immune functions and diminished life satisfaction.[6]

Environmental model of stress: According to the environmental model, stress is defined as external to an organism, including threats of immediate harm or aversive conditions. Stress of this type is typically measured using stress inventories, which are checklists of events believed to be taxing to an individual.[7]

Psychological model of stress: The Psychological model focus on the concept of perceived stress, which refers to interactions between an environmental precipitant (external stress); the physiological reactions of the body (distress); and a person's cognitive, emotional, and behavioral response to this interaction. Stress is perceived when an external event causes aversive physiological and cognitive distress in an individual that exceeds his or her emotional and behavioral repertoire designed to negate the harmful effects of external stressors. This model of stress[8] has come to be regarded as the most widely accepted and cited definition of stress.[9,10]

CONCEPTUAL MODELS

The exact nature of the causal link between life stress and psychiatric disorders is largely a matter of speculation. These models consider the impact of stress in both physiological and psychological spheres. Various conceptual models have been proposed, some of which are as follows:

- *Principle of optics*: Rahe et al.[11] gave a model by using the principle of optics. A series of lenses and filters are employed to indicate the various steps along the pathway between the subject's exposure to recent life stress and his subsequent illness. A subject's past experience may alter the significance of his recent life change. Defense mechanisms are employed which diffract away some of the life change events. Those not diffracted away stimulate a multitude of physiological processes. The subject may then 'absorb' some of his physiological reactions, e.g. lower blood pressure by relaxing large muscle groups.

Prolonged, unabsorbed psychophysiological activations eventually lead to organ system dysfunction and bodily disease.

- *Crisis theory*: The 'crisis theory,' proposed by Lindenmann and elaborated by Satin,[12] maintains that when an individual is faced with a new situation (stress), he goes into a period of disequilibrium (crisis). The outcome of crisis may be adaptive in terms of the enlargement of the individual's experience and coping resources, and thus may be a part of maturation. It may be maladaptive in terms of the development of a pathological state of avoidance of the adjustment problem, the development of displaced problem (such as a physical illness), or the exhibition of symptoms of strain (emotional illness or reduced functional capacity).
- *Differential effect*: Brown, et al.[13] have suggested two extreme positions regarding the causal role of events. The first emphasizes the importance of predispositional factors and, at most, the events are seen as triggering an illness, which may at the most bring the onset forward by a short period of time and perhaps makes it more abrupt. The opposing position is that the events play an important formative role and the onset is either substantially advanced in time by the event or brought about by it altogether. Both triggering and formative effects may be either short-term or long-term. Triggering and formative effects are the opposite ends of a continuum rather than qualitatively different processes.

  The estimate of the average time from an onset produced by an event to the time when a spontaneous onset would have occurred, had not the events intervened, has been called 'brought forward time'. This can be used as an index of the etiological significance of a class of events. If brought forward time is large, for example 12 months or more, one can conclude that the effect is formative; if it is too small, we conclude that the effect may be triggering, leaving open the possibility that the formative effect may be operative. Thus, the length of time allows one to choose between the two rival hypotheses.
- *Cybernetic model*: Kagan and Levi[14] have proposed a model in which the sequence of interactions is not a one-way process, but constitutes a part of a cybernetic system with continuous feedback. The combined effect of psychosocial stresses and psychobiological program (genetic factors and earlier environmental influences) determine the psychological or physiological reactions which may lead to precursor of disease and/or disease itself. The sequence of events can be promoted or counteracted by intervening variables.
- *Diathesis or vulnerability models*: The initial one was proposed by Meehl[15] and it was later modified by Rosenthal.[16] Vulnerability models assume that people have varying degrees of vulnerability for development of a mental disorder and that the likelihood to develop an illness is a function of both the extent of the biologically influenced vulnerability and the magnitude of stress that the individual is encountering. Vulnerability approach postulated that a balance and counter balance is maintained between vulnerability and the amount of stress that can be tolerated before the symptoms appear. This model is used essentially to explain schizophrenia.[17]
- *Psychodynamic theories*: According to the theories of Freud, Jung and Sullivan, psychological stress results in regression and triggers a sequence of internal changes whose outward expression is the manifestation of psychological symptoms. The stress itself may be more of prolonged conflict than a single disturbing experience or it may be objectively minor but have special psychological implications for the individual or it might exert its effect by virtue of acting on an already abnormal personality structure.

MEASUREMENT OF STRESS

There have been numerous attempts at quantification of life stress.

Social Readjustment Rating Scale (SRRS): Holmes and Rahe[18] constructed the Social Readjustment Rating Scale (SRRS), on the premise that events cause life changes of such magnitude and intensity as to initiate a later onset of disease. The effect of events, desirable or undesirable, is cumulative. The scale consisting of 43 items, rated from 0 to 100, was standardized on 394 Americans and has been most widely used. Each item has a "life change unit" (LCU). The more severe the item, the greater change it calls for, and so the greater is its LCU. An important limitation of the scale is the lack of flexibility for subjective quantification of events. Besides, it has been reported that 29 out of the 43 items may be symptoms or consequences of illness, and this has been a major source of error in life event research.

Schedule for life events: Developed by Paykel et al.[19] this covers 64 defined life events, rated from 0 to 20 which are again divided into nine categories—work, education, finance, health, bereavement, migration, family and social relationship. It is administered in the form of a semi-structured interview, where each event is enquired for until it clearly does not apply covering a period of one year prior to the interview. It is preferred by some because of its greater reliability and scores for subjective evaluation of events. These workers have also used qualitative categorization of events into exit and entrance events, desirable and undesirable events, and events in relation to health, employment, family, marriage and law.[20,21]

Life event scale: Tenant and Andrews[22] evolved an inventory incorporating the concepts of life change and distress.

Bedford College Life Events and Difficulties Schedule (LEDS): This schedule was developed by Brown and Harris[23] and is the most widely used personal interview method. It is a semi-structured survey instrument that assesses a wide variety of stressors and is appropriate for use in community samples as well as on an individual basis with patients. The interview consists of a series of questions asking whether certain types of events had occurred over the past 12 months (or larger period) and a set of guidelines for probing positive responses. Dichotomy of events is into those definitely and those only possibly independent of the illness. The severity of the threatening implications is rated on a 4-point scale (marked, moderate, little, and none) for severity of the threat, one week after the immediate effects were over.

Structured Event Probe and Narrative Rating Method (SEPRATE): The method was developed by Dohrenwend et al.[24] It is an alternative life events interview and rating system using a magnitude of "life change" rating system. It consists of a series of yes/no questions regarding 84 types of events or difficulties that may have occurred and been severely stressful.

British Life Events Inventory for Children: The inventory was developed by Monaghan et al.[25] and is specially designed to assess life events of children.

Presumptive Stressful Life Events Scale (PSLE): In view of the limitations of the western scales and their indiscriminate use, with local translations and modifications, Singh et al[26] developed the Presumptive Stressful Life Events Scale[26] consisting of 51 items drawn by an open ended enquiry from 200 adult subjects, with Holmes and Rahe's list as the base. It has been standardized on Indian population. Many events are culture specific. Events included in the western lists, like 'change in church activities' or 'change in recreational activities', may not be relevant for Indian population.

Life event research is beset with a number of methodological problems which have been reviewed.[27-30] Only some of these methodological problems have been addressed to.

LIFE EVENTS AND ILLNESS

Life events can occur in a variety of domains (family, health, and work) and may be age graded (school, marriage and retirement), history graded (war and depression), or non-normative (illness and divorce). A large number of published reports attest to the association of life stress and a wide range of disorders and distress. According to Settersten and Mayer,[31] "A life event is a significant occurrence involving a relatively abrupt change that may produce serious and long lasting effects". It has been suggested that life stresses have generalized effects which may be expressed in varying symptomatology, depending upon the characteristics of the individual.[32]

The review of epidemiological studies of life events and psychiatric disorders has shown that 32% of the psychiatric cases (among females, 41%) can be attributed to stressful life events.[33] An 18 months prospective study on a group of psychiatric patients found undesirable and uncontrollable events related positively, and desirable events related negatively, to the symptoms. Dysphoric and somatic symptoms were most commonly related to event change.[34] From India, Saxena et al.[35] in an outpatient psychiatric population, reported life events (desirable and undesirable) from all areas of functioning, significantly more in patients as compared to controls.

Reactions to Major National Events

In India, no systematic research has been carried out on the psychiatric sequelae of national disasters like droughts, floods, financial indebtedness of the farming community, earthquakes and accidents, and major national events.

Political assassination is one such happening known to evoke a variety of emotional responses in different individuals. The National Opinion Research Centre Survey of public reaction to President Kennedy's death found that a sizeable proportion of the national sample of adults experienced a variety of symptoms,[36] four days following President's assassination, such as headache (62%), insomnia (45%), rapid heart-beat (26%) and perspiration (17%). All the percentages were substantially above the normal prevalence of such signs of distress. Four out of five Americans felt the loss as of someone very close and dear. Intense emotion was felt by Kennedy's opponents as well as supporters. Indeed, the former were sometimes taken aback at the intensity of their own responses. Comparable public responses have been observed after the death of Lincoln, Roosevelt, McKinley Garfield and even Harding, all of whom died while in office.[37]

The psychological impact of the assassination of Prime Minister Indira Gandhi on psychiatric inpatients was studied by a semistructured interview by Varma et al.[38] The results indicated faulty perception and inappropriate reaction to the event in the patients, often colored by their background and illness. There was a significant rise in score the modified BPRS soon after the event. The controls reacted to the event in a unique and individual manner, and in them a general pattern of adaptation could be discerned. The study supported the theory that psychiatric patients show more frequent and severe cognitive responses to a cataclysmic event than control subjects because of reduced capacity of cognitive control and/or heightened susceptibility to enter a state of stress.

Physical Illness

Research shows that almost every system in the body can be influenced by chronic stress. When chronic stress goes unreleased, it suppresses the body's immune system and ultimately manifests as illness.

A host of studies have suggested a positive relationship between stressful life events, single or in series, and subsequent illness, like multiple sclerosis,[39] myocardial infarction,[40] congestive heart failure,[41] and hypertension.[41] It has been shown that the incidence of life stress prior to the onset of illness is significant and also that the severity of illness is related to the severity of stress.[42] Death of a close family member, change in financial state and increased job responsibilities, seem to play a significant role in the onset of myocardial infarction.[43]

Myocardial infarction patients experience more number of stressful events and have a higher distress score as compared to controls. Clustering of events was not evident, suggesting life-long distress.[44] Alcoholics have been reported to experience more life stress, particularly undesirable and related to personal life, than controls one year prior to addiction.[45] The INTERHEART study[46] revealed that people with myocardial infarction reported higher prevalence of four stress factors: stress at work and at home, financial stress and major life events in the past year. As blood pressure and serum cholesterol increase during stress, a relationship between stress and hypertension has long been suspected. Emotional stress is generally regarded as a major factor in the etiology of hypertension.[47]

Gastrointestinal diseases such as peptic ulcer and ulcerative colitis are known to be greatly influenced by stress. Early life stress in the form of abuse also plays a major role in the susceptibility to develop functional gastrointestinal disorders as well as irritable bowel disease later in life.[48] There is also evidence that emotionally stressful experience is associated with endocrine disorder such as diabetes mellitus.[49]

Mental Illness

Schizophrenia

The etiology of schizophrenia is multifactorial, which includes psychosocial factors as well. In a review of major social stresses such as war, it was concluded that there was no apparent effect on admission rates for psychosis, while increase in rates for neuroses, psychosomatic, conditions, depression and suicide was demonstrated.[50] However, a study of inductions into the army found a higher incidence of admission for schizophrenia in the first month of basic training, diminishing thereafter.[51] Similar observations were made with regard to British Navy personnel,[52] suggesting that intensive need for social adaptation is an effective precipitant for acute schizophrenic symptoms in predisposed individuals.

The work on acute schizophrenics (i.e. onset occurring within 13 weeks of admission) by Brown and Birley[53,54] suggest that most life events serve to trigger the onset of illness in those who are predisposed (and are experiencing tense and difficult situations, either at home or at work with some key relationships). Causal period of 3 weeks and brought forward time of 10 weeks was found in the group of patients studied. However, for markedly threatening events in the 12 weeks before illness, the frequency was 3 times than the expected number and the brought forward time 7 months. Thus, a formative effect might well be present for some. Further work is needed as the numbers in the sample were small. It was also observed that all patients, who relapsed while taking phenothiazines, had experienced a disturbing life event.

Schizophrenics have been reported to experience significantly more life events in the 3 weeks,[53,54] 6 months,[55] and 1 year[56] prior to the onset of illness than controls in areas of work, health and social relations.[55] Non-independent life events such as being fired from a job, divorce, failing in an exam, may reflect the prodromal period of the illness or an ongoing schizophrenic process. Zubin and Spring[17] have labeled the processes by which schizophrenic patients often bring an excess of life events upon themselves as "stress prone patterns of living". In a study of schizophrenics and normals, Serban[57] concluded that chronic schizophrenics experienced maximum stress, acute schizophrenics medium amount, while normal had a minimum level of stress in their daily lives. The highest stressors for acute and chronic schizophrenics were related to interpersonal relationships and social performance. Das et al.[58] reported higher number of life events in the one year preceding relapse in relapsed schizophrenics as compared to those with stable schizophrenia. Ventura et al.[59] reviewed the studies on life events and concluded that both vulnerability and stress factors, and not just the latter, contribute to the onset and course of schizophrenia.

Life events have been found to exert their greatest influence on nonpsychotic symptoms, such as anxiety, depression and somatic concern than on psychotic symptoms.[60,61]

Mania

Meynert[62] and Westphal[63] have suggested that exogenous factors can play a part in the precipitation of mania. Most commonly, romantic and psycho-reactive factors were taken into account. However, these references are based on impressions rather than on systematic study. It has been reported that 60% of the manic patients experience life events in the 3 months period preceding onset. Compared to women, men more often report work and interpersonal difficulties.[64,65] Life event in the form of loss or threat was found to be a common precipitant of mania.[66] Kennedy et al.[67] demonstrated a two-fold increase in life events of 20 manic patients during the 4 months period before admission to hospital. Life events independent of affective illness and having significant negative impact were significantly more common. In a study from India involving 30 persons with mania and 30 matched controls, death of close relatives, financial difficulties, death of spouse, and disappointment due to defeat in election turned out to be major life events contributing to manic pathology.[68]

Depressive Illness

The typical precipitating stresses in severe depression fall into 3 general categories: death of a loved one, failure in an important interpersonal relationship (usually with one's spouse), and a severe setback in work or other goals to which an individual has been devoted).[69] In a controlled study on 185 depressives, Paykel et al.[20] concluded that patients with depression report almost 3 times as many events as the controls in the period of 6 months immediately prior to onset of depression.

Events involving 'loss', 'separation' or 'hazard',[70] 'exits' and 'interpersonal argument'[71] have been shown to precede the inception of depressive illness. Loss is interpreted in a general term, ranging from loss from death, separation, loss of organs or limbs, and loss of self-esteem.

Brown et al.[23] have reported interesting information on the significance of life events in depressive illness. When all events were considered, a real increase in the frequency of moderately threatening events was observed in the 3 weeks before onset, and the brought forward time being 3 months, suggesting a triggering effect of these life events. However, when the data was analyzed for markedly threatening events with causal period of 1 year, a 5-fold increase in life events was observed for the one year before onset, with a brought forward time of two years, suggesting that such events have a formative role to play. Minor events do not play any causal role in depression. Thus, the results indicate that over 1/3rd, and perhaps more, cases of depression are as a result of formative environmental influences.

Suicide attempters reported 4 times as many events as were reported by the general population controls and 1½ times as many as were reported by patients with depression, 6 months prior to the illness onset.[21]

Many investigations have documented the role of bereavement in the causation of depressive illness. Parkes[72] observed that the number of patients, whose illness followed the loss of a spouse, was 6 times greater than expected otherwise. In a prospective epidemiological study, it was noted that 35% of widows and widowers widowed 18 months earlier suffered from depression.[73] Subsequently, the same authors noted that younger people who lost a spouse, tended to show more physical depressive symptoms, than either matched married controls or older widows and widowers at one year.[74]

Brown et al.[75] noted that all types of past losses by death were associated with psychotic-like depressive symptoms, while other types of past losses with neurotic-type depressive symptoms. In addition, among women, loss of mother before the age of 11 was associated with greater risk of depression. Paykel and Tanner[76] found life events to precede relapses in cases of relapsing depression.

Studies have shown clustering of life events during the 1 month,[77] 6 months,[19] and 2 year period[78] before the onset of illness. However, in the latter study, the life event inventory was administered in the depressive phase. Venkoba Rao and Nammalvar[78] opined, that given a pause between the events, the individuals may have adapted to the event, but a quick succession of events prevented coping. Similar observations were made by Birley and Brown[54] and Paykel et al.[19]

Psychotherapeutic and social interventions for those, who face a clustering of events as a form of primary prevention, has been suggested.[78] A trial of antidepressants is also recommended in such cases. However, such an intervention was not found to prevent recurrences in elderly depressives.[79]

Indian workers have observed an association between early parental deprivation and later onset of depression.[80] One out of every three patients, suffering from a severe affective illness, gave a history of having lost one or both parents before reaching the age of sixteen years. However, early parental loss did not figure significantly in the sample of Venkoba Rao and Nammalvar.[81,82]

Depressives have been found to experience numerically more number of events than schizophrenic controls, and the events pertain to the death of the family members.[83] Other workers[84] also observed clustering of events in depressives. Common events in their sample were medical and surgical illnesses and obstetric events. Bereavement, interpersonal and social events followed in numerical order. A significant correlation between the number of life events and severity of depression has also been noted.

None of the depressives in Indian studies suffered a 'single' event or 'no event'. The studies from India generally indicate that 2 events within a year are held tolerable and clustering of events is the rule in the predepressive state.[85]

The role of life events in first-episode depression in old age has been investigated. Depressives reported higher incidence of life events as compared to controls. Life events relating to financial problems occurred with greatest frequency, followed by life events pertaining to bereavement, like death of spouse or death of close family member, and marital and family conflicts. Other life events were unemployment and property damage. These are important as they have financial implications.[86]

Few investigators have investigated the relevant 'non-stress' factors in depressive illness. In a large community sample of Los Angeles bounty adults, life events, losses and perceived strain were positively related to depressive symptomatology while close relationships and perceived support were negatively related to these symptoms. Thus, social support, while protecting the individual against the negative impact of stress, may itself be important in the amelioration of depressive symptoms.[87] Flaherty et al.[88] in a study of 44 out-patients, observed that patients with good social support had significantly better scores on the Hamilton Rating Scale of Depression and Social Readjustment Rating Scale self-report.

The data from 2 longitudinal studies of community residents (urban 235 and rural 531) from Middle Tennessee showed the buffering effects of personal coping resources, in that those high in personal competence had lower levels of depression and showed less vulnerability to medical problems.[89]

The evidence to date from various studies indicates that disturbing life events, particularly 'losses', precede the onset of unipolar and bipolar illness and act as risk factors for these conditions. Available social support and coping resources are the major nonstress factors which modify the effect of the stressful life events on the individual.

Anxiety Disorders

Life event research in anxiety and related disorders may be particularly relevant since psychosocial factors are more likely to be of etiological significance. Individual differences in experiencing events may be due to the cognitive appraisal.[90] Neurotics have very high drive, react with more sense of personal injury and without the possibility of inner control; hence, become more concerned with undesirable events.[91]

Neurotic patients have been found to experience significantly more life events, particularly serious and threatening ones, during the period of 3 months,[92,93] 6 months[94] and 1 year prior to onset of illness, and during life time.[95] Cooke and Hole[33] could explain 3/4th of the cases of anxiety neuroses directly by 'danger' events. In another study on 863 neurotics, it was found that it is indeed the distressing quality of life events and not merely the change they produce that is associated with neurotic impairment.[96]

Barrett[97] observed that certain types of events, those having to do with performance, were experienced as more stressful by those with anxiety disorders, as compared to those with depressive disorders. In the study of Bhatti and Channabasavanna[95] on neurotics, stress in the area of education, important academic failure, and preparation for or taking an important examination, was found to have a definite relationship with anxiety neurosis. Likewise, Sharma and Ram[98] observed academic failure in examination and appearing for interview to be significantly more in anxiety neurotics than in controls, during the 6 months prior to the onset of illness.

Symptom intensity has been found to be directly related to the amount of recent life stress.[99] Stress, however, did not appear to be differentially related to any particular symptom constellations. The number of threatening events experienced in the past 3 months has been found to be strongly related to the severity of psychological symptoms (anxiety, depression, tiredness and irritability) and only weakly, if at all, to the severity of the physical symptoms (backache, palpitations, dizziness and breathlessness). People with few friends tended to have high symptom levels.[93]

Life change (adjustment) and emotional distress (undesirability) have been clearly conceptualized as distinct. Despite this, these measures have been confounded in earlier work. In a retrospective study, life change measures were more powerful indicators of adult neurotic impairment than undesirability.[100] However, in a subsequent 5 years prospective study, undesirability measures were found to be more powerful predictors of disturbed childhood behavior.[101]

One study found a significant relationship between life events and panic disorder.[102] Epidemiological and clinical data are consistent with the view that panic disorder is significantly and strongly associated with both parental death and separation in childhood.[103] In an investigation of 157 patients with panic disorder, Servant and Parquet[104] found that 53 patients (33.7%) had experienced a major loss or separation before the age of 15 years, and it was also noticed that the panic group with early life events showed a significantly higher life time prevalence of major depression than panic group who did not experience early life events. Loss of social support was a more common life event in panic patients compared to normal; the patients tended to use coping skills judged as ineffective. Other workers have reported a history of childhood physical or sexual abuse to positively correlate with clinical severity in patients with panic disorder.[105]

Khanna et al.[106] reported an excess of life events in the preceding two months in the Obsessive Compulsive Disorder sample. These events were identified to be more independent, to have significantly higher negative impact and to be more uncontrolled.

NEUROBIOLOGY OF STRESS

The immune system is susceptible to stress. Psychoneuroimmunology is the study of the intricate interaction of consciousness (psycho), brain and central nervous system (neuro), and the body's defense against external infection and aberrant cell division (immunology).[107] Several studies have shown that chronic stress exerts a general immunosuppressive effect that suppresses or withholds the body's ability to initiate a prompt, efficient immune reaction.[108] This has been attributed to the abundance of corticosteroids produced during chronic stress, which produces an imbalance in corticosteroid levels and weakens immunocompetence. This weakening of immune function is thought to be associated with general strain on the various body parts associated with the production and maintenance of the immune system. The longer the stress, the more the immune system shifted from potentially adaptive changes (such as those in fight-or-flight response) to potentially detrimental changes, at first in cellular immunity and then in broader immune function. Immune systems of people who are older or already sick are more prone to stress-related change.[109] Both clinical and experimental studies indicate that stress and depression are associated with increased circulating concentrations of cytokines such as IL-1β, IL-6 and γ-IFN and positive acute phase proteins, and hyperactivity of the HPA-axis. In addition, it has been reported that immunological activation induces "stress-like" behavioral and neurochemical changes in laboratory animals. In addition, increased monocyte phagocytosis has been observed in depressed patients, an effect that is reversed upon successful antidepressant treatment, suggesting that increased monocyte phagocytosis is a state marker of stress and depression.[110]

Hypersecretion of corticotropin-releasing factor (CRF) has been previously implicated to play a role in the pathophysiology of depressive illness.[111] In addition, HPA-axis activation and consequently hypercortisolemia is a common abnormality reported in a large proportion of depressed patients.[112] Interestingly, in depression there seems to be a defect in the inhibitory feedback mechanism of cortisol on CRF secretion, thereby facilitating the maintenance of elevated cortisol levels. Positive correlation between monocyte production of IL-1β and increased serum cortisol concentrations has also been reported. It is well established that HPA axis activation is elicited by exogenous cytokine (IL-1, IL-6 and TNF-α) administration to rodents.[112,113]

LIFE EVENTS AND INTERVENING VARIABLES

Several investigators have drawn attention to the fact that the relationship between stressful life events and onset of psychiatric illness is not a simple one. There are several intervening variables which greatly modify the effect of life events on the individual. Rabkin and Struening[107,114] described them as:

- Characteristics of the stressful situation,
- Individual biological and psychological attributes; specific vulnerability and strengths of the individual personality, and
- Characteristics of the social support available to the individual.

The individual social support ties and coping resources have been singled out as the most important mediating factors which prevent the onset of psychological problems as a result of stressful events.[89]

Coping has been defined as the cognitive and behavioral efforts made to master, tolerate or reduce external demands and conflicts.[108,115] It is seen as having two main constituents: intrapsychic mechanisms and behavior. A number of coping strategies are usually employed: rejection, control, resignation, dependency, avoidance and minimization.[109,116] Interest in the individual coping resources such as self-esteem, mastery, personal competence and control has been forthcoming for their role in alleviating stress.[89]

Social support of an individual has been defined by Caplan as 'enduring interpersonal ties to a group of people who can be relied upon to provide emotional sustenance, assistance and resource in times of need, who provide feedback and who share standards and values'.[110,117] The social support system can act as a cushion against crisis.[111,118] Furthermore, lack of social support is postulated to be causative for psychiatric disorders.[112,119] This was clearly demonstrated by Swank's[113,120] observation that breakdown did not necessarily occur in soldiers exposed to stressful combat, but tended to occur when they experienced loss of social support system, i.e. when about 65% of their companions became casualties.

While Henderson et al.[114,121] have considered 'primary group' as the major source of support, Indian workers have reported that the joint family, rather than a unitary family, is a better source of security and support for vulnerable individuals, especially in adversity as it perpetuates greater emotional stability and has strong in-built resistance which ensures lesser vulnerability towards development of neurotic illness.[114,121] Since the primary group is composed of all nominated friends, work associates and neighbors, the family automatically becomes a part of the primary group.

Andrews et al.[115,122] studied life events, social support, coping style and risk of psychological impairment in neurotic patients. Persons with low events, good support and good coping had an illness risk of 12.8%, while persons with high events, poor coping and poor support had an illness risk of 43.3%, and persons with intermediate combination of the predisposing factors had intermediate risk.

Studies of the correlation of life events with severity of neurotic presentation have reported correlation coefficients which were typically below 0.3, suggesting that life events may account at best for 9% of the variance in illness.[107,114]

Sharma and Ram[116,123] investigated the relationship between life events, social and family support, and magnitude of illness in 87 patients of anxiety neurosis and 47 controls. In comparison to controls, anxiety neurotics had less social and family support. Life time stress score of patients correlated positively with Hamilton, Anxiety Score (r=0.55) while family jointness, social support, and socioeconomic status correlated negatively with the intensity of symptoms. Life time stress and family jointness alone accounted for 30% and 27%, respectively, of the variability in the intensity of symptoms.[98] These findings provide further support for the buffering model of support system. In addition, the findings highlight the significance of experience of stresses over life time in the etiology of anxiety disorder. When the combined effect of these variables (5 variables) were studied,[116,123] life time and recent stress score, economic and socioeconomic status and family jointness turned out to be significant, and accounted for 50% of variability in the intensity of symptoms. Amongst these, life time stress score and family jointness turned out to be highly significant predictors of the level of anxiety, their partial correlation coefficients being 0.51 and 0.45, respectively. The findings suggest that the joint family is the major support system for Indian patients, which dilutes the effect of stressful life events on the individual.

CONCLUSION AND FUTURE RESEARCH

A large body of research, accumulated over the past three decades, indicates that life events are associated with a wide range of disorders and distress, but do not provide a clear picture of the nature and strength of this relationship. Stressful situations act as general precipitants, which may be expressed in varying symptomatology or behavioral disturbances, depending upon the characteristics of the individual and the resources at his disposal to cope with stress. There is also some evidence to suggest that specific stressful events may lead to the eruption of specific psychiatric disorders.

Future research must address the major methodological issues that have been ignored.

Life event research is difficult and requires meticulous methodology. By its very nature, it is retrospective and subject to errors of omission, distortion and falsification. It is often hard to define a clear onset and whether the events that occur are independent of the patient's mental condition. Certain qualitative aspects of stressful life events have not received sufficient attention. These are dependent versus independent life events, lack of control versus under control, experienced versus imagined, anticipated versus unanticipated, novel versus old experience, acute versus chronic, etc. Summation of life event scores has been used which appears to be an over-simplification and may not be valid.

There is an urgent need to determine the strength of the relationship between the life events and health and illness, and the specific conditions that control the strength, in order to assess realistically the risk of stress-induced illness and its prevention at different levels. Biological correlates of life stress and their role as intervening variables need to be studied in depth.

REFERENCES

1. Dodge D, Martin W. Social Stress and Chronic Illness. Notre Dame: University of Notre Dame Press; 1970.
2. Selye H. Stress and psychiatry. Am J Psychiatry. 1956;111:276.
3. Bemad J. The endaemonists. In: Klausher SZ (Ed). Why Man Takes Chances. New York: Garden City; 1968.
4. McNamara S. Stress in young people: What's new and what can we do? New York: Continuum; 2000.
5. Selye H. History of the stress concept. In: Goldberger L, Breznitz S (Eds), Handbook of Stress: Theoretical and Clinical Aspects, 2nd edn. New York: Free Press. 1993.pp.7-17.
6. Stein M, Miller AH. Stress, the immune system, and health and illness. In: Goldberger L, Breznitz S (Eds), Handbook of Stress: Theoretical and Clinical Aspects. New York: Free Press. 1993. pp.127-41.
7. Jaser SS, Langrock AM, Keller G, Merchant MJ, Benson MA, Reeslund K, et al. Coping with the stress of parental depression II: Adolescent and parent reports of coping and adjustment. Journal of Clinical Child and Adolescent Psychology. 2005;34:193-205.
8. Lazarus RS, Folkman S. Stress, Appraisal and Coping. New York: Springer; 1984.
9. Grant KE, Compas BE, Stuhlmacher AF, Thurm AE, McMahon SD, Halpert JA. Stressors and child and adolescent psychopathology: Moving from markers to mechanisms of risk. Psychological Bulletin. 2003;129:447–66.
10. Hess RS, Copeland EP. Stress. In: Bear G, Minke K (Eds), Children's needs III: Development, prevention,and correction. Bethesda, MD: National Association of School Psychologists. 2006.pp.255-65.
11. Rahe RH, Floistad J, Bergon T, et al. A model for life changes and illness research. Arch Gen Psychiatry. 1974;31:172.
12. Sating DC. Life stress and psychological problems in the hospital emergency unit. Soc Psychiatry. 1973,8.
13. Brown GW, Sklair F, Hams TO, et al. Life events and psychiatric disorders. Part I: Some methodological issues. Psychol Med. 1973;3:74-87.
14. Kagan A, Levi L. The concept of normality: Male/female roles and relationships. In: Levi O (Ed). Society, Stress and Disease. New York: Oxford University Press. 1974.pp.3-7.
15. Meehl PE (1962). Schizotaxia, schizotypy, schizophrenia. American Psychologist, 17,827-838. In: Joseph P Anto (1995). Life events in first episode depression, mania and schizophrenia.
16. Rosenthal D (1970). Genetic theory and abnormal behaviour. New York: McGraw hill. In: Joseph P Anto (1995). Life Events in First Episode Depression, Mania & Schizophrenia.
17. Zubin J, Spring B. Vulnerability – A new view of schizophrenia. Journal of Abnormal Psychology. 1977; 86:103-26.
18. Holmes TH, Rahe RH. Life changes: Do people really remember? Arch Gen Psychiatry. 1967;36:379-384.
19. Paykel ES, Prussoff BA, Uhlenhuth EM. Scaling of life events. Arch Gen Psychiatry. 1971;25:340.
20. Paykel ES, Dienelt MN, Lindenthal JJ. Life events and depression: A controlled study. Arch Gen Psychiatry. 1969;21: 753.
21. Paykel ES, Prussof BA, Myers JK. Suicide attempts and recent life events: A controlled comparison. Arch Gen Psychiatry. 1975;32:32.
22. Tenant C, Andrews G. A scale to measure the stress of life events. ANZ J Psychiatry. 1976;10:27.
23. Brown GW, Harris TO, Peto T. Life events and psychiatric disorders. Part 2: Nature of causal link. Psychol Med. 1973; 3:159-76.
24. Dohrenwend BP, Raphael KG, Schwartz S, Stueve A, Skodol A. The structured event probe and narrative rating method for measuring stressful life events. In: Goldberger L, Breznitz S (Eds). Handbook of Stress. New York: Free Press. 1993. pp.174-99.
25. Monaghan (1978) British life event inventory for children. In: Malhotra S, Kaur S, Nehara K. Life events in psychiatrically ill children. Indian Journal of Psychiatry; 1992.

26. Singh C, Kaur D, Kaur H. Presumptive stressful life events scale (PSLES). Indian J Clin Psychol. 1981;8:173.
27. Murthy RS. Methodological problems in the study of life stress and psychiatric illness: A review. Indian J Psychiatry. 1975;50:1-10.
28. Dohrenwed BS, Dohrenwend BP. Some issues on research on stressful life events. J Nerv Ment Dis. 1978;166:7-15.
29. Hirschfeld RMA, Cross CA. Epidemiology of affective disorders. Arch Gen Psychiatry. 1982;39:35-46.
30. Saxena S, Mohan D. Life events research: A review of methodology with special reference to India. Indian J Psychiatry. 1982;24:322-8.
31. Settersten RA, Mayer LU (1997). The measurement of age, age - structuring and the life course. Annual Review of Sociology, 1997;23:233-61. In: Hutchison ED (2003) Dimensions of Human Behaviour: The Changing Life Course, 2nd edn. Sage Publications Inc. USA.
32. Eisler M, Polak PR. Social stress and psychiatric disorder. J Nerv Ment Dis. 1971;153:227.
33. Cooke DJ, Hole DJ. An etiological importance of stressful life events. Br J Psychiatry. 1983;143:397.
34. Grant I, Sweetwood HL, Yager J, et al. Quality of life events in relation to psychiatric symptoms. Arch Gen Psychiatry. 1981;38:335.
35. Saxena S, Mohan D, Dube S, et al. Stressful life events in psychiatric outpatients: A controlled study. Indian J Psychiatry. 1983;25:120.
36. Sheatsiey RB, Feidman JJ. The assassination of President Kennedy: A preliminary report on public reaction and behavior, Pub Opin Q. 1965;28:189-215.
37. Orlansky H. Reactions to the death of President Roosevelt. J Soc Psychol. 1949;26:235-66.
38. Varma VK, Chandiramani K, Rao G, et al. Assassination of Indira Gandhi: Impact on psychiatric patients. Am J Psychother. 1989;XLIII:77-85.
39. Antonovsky A, Kats R. The life crises history as a tool in epidemiological research. J Health Behav. 1967;8:15-21.
40. Theorell T, Rahe RH. Psychosocial factors and myocardial infarction. J Psychosom Res. 1971;15:25.
41. Peatman LV, Ferguson S, Bergua K, et al. Precipitation of congestive heart failure: Social and emotional factors. Ann Indian Med. 1975;75:1.
42. Wyler AK, Masuda M, Holmes TH. Magnitude of life events and seriousness of illness. J psychosom Med. 1971;33:115-22.
43. Singh SB, Mishra S. Stressful life events and myocardial infarction. Indian J Clin Psychol; 1987.
44. Lal N, Ahuja R. Perception of distress by patients of myocardial infarction. Indian J Psychiatry. 1987;29:259-62.
45. Rangaswami K. Personality, life events and alcoholism. Indian Clin Psychol 1983;10:179-82.
46. Rosengren A, Hawken S, Ounpu S, Silwa K, Zubaid M, Akmahemeed WA, et al. Association of psychosocial risk factors with risk of myocardial infarction in 11,119 cases and 13,648 control from 52 countries (INTERHEART study): case control study .The Lancet. 2004;364:953-63.
47. Dunbar F. Psychosomatic diagnosis. New York:Harper; 1943.
48. Drossman DA, Sandler RS, Mckee DC. Bowel patterns among subjects seeking treatment. Health Care. 1982,83:529-34.
49. Stenstrom U, Wikby A, Hornquist JO, Andersson PO. Recent life events, gender and the control of diabetes mellitus. Gen Hosp Psychiat. 1993,15:82-8.
50. Reid DD. Precipitating proximal factors in the occurrence of mental disorders: Epidemiologic evidence. In: Causes of Mental Disorders: A Review of Epidemiologic Knowledge. New York: Milbank Memorial Funds; 1961.
51. Sleinburg HR, Durell J. Stressful social situation as a precipitant of schizophrenic symptoms: An epidemiological study. Br Psychiatry. 1968;114:1097.
52. Wallis GC. An epidemiological and follow-up study of schizophrenia in Royal Navy. MD Thesis. University of London. Cited in 44, 1965.
53. Brown GW, Birley JLT. Crisis and life changes and the onset of schizophrenia. J Health Soc Behav. 1968;9:203-14.
54. Birley JLT, Brown GW. Crises and life changes preceding the onset or relapse of acute schizophrenia. Br J Psychiatry. 1970;116:327-33.
55. Canton C, Francon IG. Life events and schizophrenia. Acta Psychiatr Scand. 1985;71:221.
56. Jacob S, Myers J. Recent life events and acute schizophrenic psychosis. J Nerv Ment Dis. 1976;162:75-87.
57. Serban G. Stress in schizophrenics and normals. Br J Psychiatry. 1975;126:397.
58. Das MK, Kulhara PL, Verma SK. Life events preceding relapse of schizophrenia. International Journal of Social Psychiatry. 1997;43:56-63.
59. Ventura J, Nuechterlein KH, Lukoff D. A prospective study of stressful life events and schizophrenic relapse. Journal of Abnormal psychology. 1989;98:407-11.
60. Carol CS, Myers JK. Life events and schizophrenia. I: Comparison of schizophrenics with a community sample. Arch Gen Psychiatry. 1977;34:1242.
61. Carol CS, Myers JK. Life events and schizophrenia. II: Impact of life events on symptom configuration. Arch Gen Psychiatry. 1977;34:1242.
62. Meynen TH. Cited in 53, 1890.
63. Westphal A. Cited in 53, 1911.
64. Patrick V, Dunner DL, Fieve RR. Life events and primary affective illness. Acta Psychiatr Scand. 1979;58:48.
65. Dunner DL, Patrick V, Fieve RR. Life events at the end of bipolar affective illness. Am J Psychiatry. 1979;136:508.
66. Ambelas A. Psychologically stressful events in the precipitation of manic episodes. Br J Psychiatry. 1978;135:15.
67. Kennedy S, Thompson R, Slander HC, et al. Life events precipitating mania. Br J Psychiatry. 1983;142:398.
68. Singhal AK, Agrawal SC, Nathawat SS. Role of stressful life events in mania. Indian J Psychiatry. 1984;26:219.

69. Arieti S. Manic depressive psychosis. American Handbook of Psychiatry. New York: Basic Books; 1959.
70. Beck JC, Worthen K. Precipitating stress crisis theory and hospitalization in schizophrenia and depression. Arch Gen Psychiatry. 1972;26:123.
71. Jacob SC, Prusoff BA, Paykel ES. Recent life events in schizophrenia and depression. Psychol Med. 1974;4:444.
72. Parkes M. Recent bereavement as a cause of mental illness. Br J Psychiatry. 1964;110:198.
73. Clayton PJ, Desmarais L, Winokur G. A study of normal bereavement. Am J Psychiatry. 1968;125:168.
74. Clayton PJ. The effect of living alone on the bereavement symptoms. Am J Psychiatry. 1975;132:133.
75. Brown JR, Harris TO, Copeland JR. Depression and loss. Br J Psychiatry. 1977;130:1.
76. Paykel ES, Tanner J. Life events, depressive relapse and maintenance treatment. Psychol Med. 1976;67:481.
77. Leff MJ, Roatch JF, Bunney WE. Environmental factors preceding the onset of severe depression. Psychiatry. 1970,33: 298.
78. Venkoba Rao A, Nammalvar N. Life events and depressive disease. Indian J Psychiatry. 1976;18:293.
79. Post F. The management and nature of depressive illness in late life: A follow through study. Br J Psychiatry. 1972;121:393.
80. Wig NN, Verma HD, Shah DK. Parental deprivation and mental illness: A study of incidence of parental death in.childhood in 2000 psychiatric patients. Indian J Psychiatry. 1969;11:1.
81. Venkoba Rao A. Broken home in particular reference to parental death and its relationship to depressive illness. Indian J Psychiatry. 1970;12:23.
82. Venkoba Rao A, Nammalvar N. Life events and depression: possible prevention by psychological and psychiatric methods. In: Falberg A (Ed). Proceedings of IX International Congress on Suicide Prevention and Crisis Intervention. Helsinki; 1977. pp.499-505.
83. Prakash R, Trivedi JK, Sethi BB. Life events in depression. Indian Psychiatry. 1980;22:56.
84. Chatterjee RN, Mukherjee SP, Nandi DN. Life events and depression. Indian J Psychiatry. 1981;23:333-37.
85. Venkoba Rao A. Depressive Disease. Madras: ICMR; 1986.
86. Sharma DK, Satija DC, Nathawat SS. Psychological determinants of depression in old age. Indian J Psychiatry. 1985;27:83-90.
87. Aneshensel CS, Stone JD. Stress and depression: A test of the buffering model of social support. Arch Gen Psychiatry. 1982;39:1392.
88. Flaherty JA, Gaviria FM, Black EM, et al. The role of social support in the functioning of patients with unipolar depression. Am Psychiatry. 1983;140:473.
89. Husaini BA, Garylin J, Willenstovall R. Stress and depression in rural and American communities: Longitudinal studies. Indian J Soc Psychiatry. 1986;2:311-4.
90. Ax AF. Goals and methods of psychophysiology. Psychophysiology. 1964;1:8-25.
91. Chattopadhya PK, Das M. Stressful life events and psychopathological episodes. Indian J Clin Psychol. 1983;10.
92. Cooper B, Sylph J. Life events and onset of neurotic illness: An investigation in general practice. Psychol Med. 1973;3:421.
93. Miller P, Mc C, Indham JG, et al. Life events, symptoms and social support. I Psychosom Res. 1976;20:515-22.
94. Sharma I, Ram D. Life events in anxiety neurosis. Indian J Psychiatry. 1985;27:127-37.
95. Bhatti RS, Channabasavanna SM. A study of neurosis. I. Life events and personality dimensions. Indian J Psychiatry. 1985;27:127-37.
96. Tenant S, Andrews G. The pathogenic quality of life events stress in neurotic impairment. Arch Gen Psychiatry. 1978;35:859.
97. Barrett JE. The relationship of life events to the onset of neurotic disorders. In: Barett JE, Rose RM, Klerman CL (Eds). Stress and Mental Disorders. New York: Raven Press; 1979.
98. Sharma I, Ram D. Life events and support systems in anxiety state. Indian J Psychiatry. 1986;2:357-67.
99. Uhlenhuth EH, Paykel ES. Symptom intensity and life events. Arch Gen Psychiatry. 1973;28:473.
100. Dohrenwend BS. Life events as stressors: A methodological enquiry. J Health Soc Behav. 1973;14:167.
101. Gersten JC, Langer TS, Eisenberg JC, et al. Child behavior and life events: undesirable change or change per se? In: Dohrenwend BS, Dohrenwend BP (Eds). Stressful Life Events: Their Nature and Effects. New York: Wiley; 1974.
102. Faravelli C, Pallti S. Recent life events and panic disorder. American Journal of Psychiatry. 1989;146:622-6.
103. Servant D, Parquent PJ. Life events and anxiety. Encephale. 1994b;20:333-7.
104. Servant D, Parquet PJ. Early life events and panic disorder. Course of illness and comorbidity. Neurophychopharmacological Biological Psychiatry. 1994a;18:272-379.
105. Friedman S, Smith L, Fogel D, Paradis C, Vishwanathan R, Ackerman R, Trappler B. The incidence and influence of early traumatic life events in patients with panic disorder: a comparison with other psychiatric outpatients. Journal of Anxiety Disorders. 2002;16(3):259-72.
106. Khanna S, Rajendra PN, Channabasavanna SM. Life events and onset of obsessive compulsive disorder. International Journal of Social Psychiatry. 1988;34:305-09.
107. Pelletier KR. Mind as healer, mind as slayer. New York: Dell Publishing Co.; 1977.
108. Hafen BQ, Frandsen KJ, Karren K, Hooker KR. The health effects of attitudes, emotions and relationship. Provo UT: EMS Associates; 1991.
109. Segerstrom SC, Miller GE. Psychological stress and the human immune system: A meta-analytic study of 30 years of inquiry. Psychol Bull. 2004;130:601-30.
110 McAdams C, Leonard BE. Neutrophil and monocyte phagocytosis in depressed patients. Prog Neuro Psychopharmacol, Biol Psychiat. 1993;17;971-84.
111. Owens MJ, Nemeroff CB. Physiology and pharmacology of corticotropin releasing factor. Pharmacol. Rev. 1991;4:425-73.

112. Butler LD, Layman NK, Riedl PE, Cain RL, Shellhaas J, Evans GF, Zukerman SH. J of Neuroimmunology. 1989;24:143-53.
113. Dunn AJ. The role of interleukin-I and tumor necrosis factor-α in the neurochemical and neurocrine responses to endotoxin. Brain Res Bull. 1992;29:807-12.
114. Rabkin JA, Struenuig EL. Life events, stress and illness. Science. 1976;194:1015.
115. Cohen, Lazarus. Cited in 93, 1985.
116. Pullela S. Concept of coping. Indian J Psychiatry. 1985: 27:106-7.
117. Caplan J. Support System and Community Mental Health. New York: Behavioral Publication; 1974.
118. Cassel J. Handbook of Evaluation Research. Struening E, Gultenland M (Eds). California: Serge; 1975.
119. Henderson S, Dunchan Jones P, McAuley M, et al. The patient's primary groups. Br J Psychiatry. 1978;132:74.
120. Swank RL. Combat Exhaustion. J Nerv Ment Dis. 1949;109: 475-508.
121. Selhi BB, Sharma M, Srivastava A. Social interaction and neurosis (the family and primary group): A pilot study. Indian J Psychiatry. 1981:23:33.
122. Andrews G, Tennant C, Hewson D, et al. Life events stress, social support, coping style and risk of psychological impairment. Nerv Men Dis. Cited in 85, 1978.
123. Sharma I, Ram D. Life events in anxiety neurosis. A study of the effect of intervening variables. Indian J Psychiatry. 1987;29:181-7.

FURTHER READING

1. Gamefski N, van Egmond M, Straalman A. The influence of early and recent life stress on severity of depression.Acta Psychiatr Scand. 1990;81:295-301.
2. Swann AC, Secunda SK, Stokes FE, et al. Stress, depression, and mania: relationship between perceived role of stressful events and clinical and biochemical characteristics. Acta Psychiatr Scand. 1990;81:389-97.
3. Sciare P, Creed F. Life events on the onset of mania. Br J Psychiatry. 1990;156:508-14.
4. Rodgers B. Adult affective disorder and early environment. Br J Psychiatry. 1990;157:539-50.
5. Ellicott A, Hammen C, Gitlin M, et al. Life events and the course of bipolar disorder. Am J Psychiatry. 1990;147:1194-98.
6. Ganzini L, McFarland BH, Cutler D. Prevalence of mental disorders after catastrophic financial loss. J Nerv Ment Dis. 1990;178:680-85.
7. Venture J, Nuechterlein KH, Lukoff D, Hardesty JP. A prospective study of stressful life events and schizophrenic relapse. Journal of Abnorm Psychol. 1989;98:407-11.
8. Yacoubian W, Hacker FJ. Reactions to disaster at a distance. Bull Menninger Clin. 1989;53:331-9.
9. Gautam S, Kamal P. A study of impact of stresstul life events in neurotic patients. Indian J Psychiatry. 1990;32:356-61.
10. Liu LY, Coe CL, Swenson CA, Kelly EA, Kita H, Busse WW. School examination enhances airway examination to antigen challenge. Am J Resp Crit Care Medicine. 2002;165:1062-7.
11. Drossman DA, Sandler RS, Mckee DC. Bowel patterns among subjects seeking treatment. Health Care. 1982;83:529-34.
12. Greenberg JS. Comprehensive Stress Management, 7th edn. New York: McGraw-Hill; 2002.
13. European Helicobacter pylori study group. Current European concepts in the management of H. pylori information: The Maastricht Consensus. Gut. 1997;41:8-13.
14. Chockalingam A, Venkatesan S, Dorairajan S, Mooorthy C, Chockalingam V, Subramaniam T. Estimation of subjective stress in acute myocardial infarction. J Postgrad Med. 2003; 49:207-10.
15. Tennant C. Life stress, social support and coronary heart disease. Aust NZ J Psychiat. 1999;33:636-41.
16. Rosengren A, Orth Gomer K, Wedel H, Wihelsem L. Stressful life events, social support and mortality in men born in 1933. Brit Medi J. 1993,307:1102-5.
17. Rosengren A, Hawken S, Ounpu S, Silwa K, Zubaid M, Akmahemeed WA, et al. Association of psychosocial risk factors with risk of myocardial infarction in 11,119 cases and 13, 648 control from 52 countries (INTERHEART study): case control study. The Lancet. 2004,364:953-63.

CHAPTER

50

Sociology and Psychiatry

Indira Sharma, Abhishek Pathak

INTRODUCTION

Mental health can only be achieved in an environment which provides opportunities for self expression, social usefulness, and the attainment of human satisfaction. Psychiatry became a well established branch of medicine by the mid-nineteenth century Sociology, by comparison, achieved some form of general recognition only in the 1960's. The initial association of sociology with the medical profession has been through psychiatry, which stimulated much sociological research in mental disorders. It is only recently that we can legitimately talk of sociological contributions to psychiatry.

In India, mental health services over the years have shown significant changes, with early emphasis on mental hospital custodial care, followed by treatment in general hospitals, and then outpatient care in the community. These changing trends have brought greater awareness regarding the social aspects of mental disorders. Mental disorders in relation to society, groups of mentally ill persons and their major societal processes have been the focus of attention of sociologists.

SOCIOLOGICAL THEORY AND MENTAL DISORDER

There have been two major sociological approaches to understand mental illness and mentally ill. The first, 'macro approach', is directed towards an understanding of human behavior from the standpoint of the society as a whole. The other 'micro' approach focuses on the interpersonal interaction that takes place between individuals as they participate in collective life.

No review of social science in relation to psychiatry can be complete without a reference to the pioneering work of Emil Durkheim (1858–1917), a French sociologist. In his published classic monograph on suicide, rising suicide rates were considered indicators of anomie or normlessness, a state in which people felt a loss of purpose and direction. Anomie literally means 'de-regulation' or 'normlessness'; it represents situations where the individuals sense that their own norms and values are no longer relevant, leading to the weakening or loss of socialities. The typology of absent developed and confused personal identity produced three different types of suicide: altruistic, in which suicide was committed for the sake of the group; egoistic, when the sense of individuality was excessive; and anomic, when the sense of purposelessness to life produced self destruction. Durkheim applied these models to contemporary suicide data to show, for example, how war or marriage increased the feeling of solidarity and decreased the modern epidemic of egoistic and anomic suicide. Durkheim emphasized that people behave in accordance with the values and norms of their society. The word 'anomie' was used extensively to explain social order and deviant behavior-crime, delinquency, mental disorder, alcoholism or drug addiction. Anomie, as Durkheim conceived, had three characteristics: (a) a painful uneasiness or anxiety, (b) a feeling of separation from the group of the individual, and (c) a feeling of pointlessness that no certain goal exists. Individuals are anomic, when (a) their lives are powerless in the absence of value, (b) they pursue means, such as power, for their own sake, and (c) they are isolated from meaningful human relations. Cohen said that anomie exists when either the rules governing behavior in a specific situation are unclear or no rules apply to a situation that arises. Deterioration of heroes has been considered as an important indicator of suicide. Deviant behaviors are heroized and conventional heroes are mocked.

Channabasavanna and Bhatti in a group of 75 postgraduate students studied the extent of anomie that students perceived in the society and its relationship with sociodemographic factors. Higher percentage of anomie was found in nonmedical postgraduates, second divisioners, in those who have dissimilarities in the level of aspirations, in the lower income group, in females, and in the urban respondents. They explained that the role of nonmedical professionals is ill-defined as well as there is conflict for hierarchy, and job prospects are less bright as compared to medical postgraduates. Second divisioners and those with dissimilarities in the level of aspirations are also more likely to be frustrated. All these could account for the higher perception of anomie.

Without externally imposed restraints to his passions, Durkheim claims that man's desires would know no limit. Chronic overeating can be seen as an anomie of will. Hughes showed how anomie contributed to schizophrenia, among selected lonely bachelor farmers in rural Ireland. There is evidence to suggest that major societal processes correlate with rates of psychiatric morbidity. Brenner provided data to support his major hypothesis that mental hospitalizations increase during economic downturns and decrease during upturns. Accordingly, he proposed: (i) the provocation hypothesis, i.e. an economic downturn causes vulnerable people to become mentally ill, and (ii) the uncovering hypothesis, i.e. 'borderline' cases are uncovered during an economic downturn. His data favored the former hypothesis.

Another example is the fundamental hypothesis that a community's degree of integration is related to the mental health of its inhabitants and that disintegration fosters psychiatric disorder. The researchers established criteria for rating communities on an integration-disintegration continuum.

The 'Road', a small community in Sterling County, which is a predominantly rural county in Nova Scotia, had considerably disintegrated in the 1950's. A marked decrease in the prevalence of mental disorder between 1950's and 1960's was observed. This community was restudied in the 1960's when, with the advent of increased economic and educational opportunities, it had changed dramatically; it was then rated as somewhat integrated. The other disintegrated communities, that had not changed as much during the years, had a much higher frequency of mental disorder in 1962 than did the 'Road'.

Subsequent work by the same authors was done in Algeria in the Yoruba tribe.

They categorized their villages into four types: (i) changing and integrated, (ii) changing and disintegrated, (iii) traditional and integrated, and (iv) traditional and disintegrated. The mental health risk was lowest in the changing and integrated, and highest in the traditional and disintegrated villages. The results of both these studies confirmed the above hypothesis and showed that the community 'integration-disintegration' frame of reference could be applied to vastly different cultures. They noted that social and cultural change leads to higher risk only when the social system becomes disintegrated. This schema can be compared with that of Marx who had a different concept of human nature. In an important sense identity was pre-given for Marx; it was socialization which—at least in its nonsocialist forms—produced a sense of estrangement which Marx called alienation. Thus the two key sociological concepts of alienation and anomie are similar in their apparent psychological effect on people, but very different in their origins: alienation being produced, in effect, by too much (of the wrong) socialization; anomie, brought about by too little.

Freud would seem to fit more in the Durkheimian camp than the Marxist, believing that individual identity was a product of socialization; restraining the biological and mysterious 'id'. Perhaps this helps to explain the dominance in psychiatry of models based on anomie rather than alienation. It is essentially the effect of social disintegration on the sense of identity—and hence on psychiatric morbidity—which has provided the principal framework for social psychiatric studies from Leighton's post-war Sterling County study to the recent work of Brown and his colleagues in London.

These studies illustrate how large scale social processes, beyond an individual's control, can predict indices of mental morbidity.

SOCIOLOGY OF PSYCHIATRY

Whereas sociology in psychiatry accepts the legitimacy and validity of what psychiatry is trying to do, the sociology of psychiatry wishes to examine and challenge precisely those assumptions. It is therefore inherently more critical, and has been accordingly less acceptable to many psychiatrists. Yet while certain elements of sociology of psychiatry fit into an 'antipsychiatry' framework, it is not necessarily part of that broad alliance. Three related strands can be identified.

Labeling Theory

Labeling theory is derived from the interactionist perspective in psychiatry and is considerably influenced by the work of Mead, a social psychologist. All human behavior, according to him, is self-directed on the basis of the symbolic meanings, shared, communicated and manipulated by people through the process of social interaction. Reality is, therefore, socially constructed. Whether an act is deviant or not would depend on how it is defined by the group. Becker maintains that social groups create deviance by making rules whose violation constitutes deviance. A form of 'residual rule breaking' has been described in acts of mental disorder, wherein the behavior is clearly unnatural and violates basic social norms of behavior. Scheff states that virtually everyone, at sometime or other, commits acts or behaves in a way that could be seen as being mentally abnormal. In a similar vein, Szasz says that the root of the matter, when a person is diagnosed mentally ill, is our intolerance for certain kinds of behavior. Laing insists that society is irrational and that the schizophrenic's 'disturbed' behavior is appropriate. Accordingly, the behavior that gets labeled as schizophrenic is a special strategy that a person invents in order to live an unlivable situation.

Labeling theory explains the social mechanisms through which mental patients or former mental patients are stigmatized as a result of their mental illness and also explains how labeling places a person in certain circumstances. However, it tends to ignore the motives and intentions of the deviant. Labeling can have a negative impact on one's income, employment and other areas of life. For example, an ex-convict may not be able to get an honest job because of the label and thus be forced to return to crime.

Apart from this, labeling can continue to exert a deleterious effect on the person since he incorporates a sense of illness and deficiency in his self-concept. However, although labeling may be unavoidable, when people observe former patients behaving normally they may in due course discard the label. Gove sides with the labeling theorists. According to him the societal reaction approach, by Szasz and other proponents of anti-psychiatry, is incorrect, for hospitalization occurs in most cases because the individual has a psychiatric disturbance, not simply because of societal reaction.

Rosenhan reported on 8 subjects who gained voluntary admission in 12 different mental hospitals by faking symptoms of schizophrenia. Although they reverted to their usual normal behavior soon after admission, the hospital staff could not detect them as pseudo-patients and released them as cases of schizophrenia in remission. The patients of the hospitals, however, enquired from the pseudo-patients over their note taking, asking whether they were investigating journalists. The study well illustrates the power of labeling in psychiatric evaluation. Many psychiatrists would acknowledge that there are instances when people with marginal problems become patients through contact with psychiatric services, as Rosenhan tried to show. A diagnostic label may exacerbate the underlying problem or engender a dysfunctional dependency on the psychiatric services. The detrimental effects of labeling, can be seen, in its most florid form, in large psychiatric hospitals. Goffman's books Stigma and Asylums, which documented the internal psychological changes induced by a label and the subsequent reaction of others in the context of 'total institutions', can firmly claim to have had an important influence on the development of the idea of 'institutionalization' and hence on psychiatric policy in the last two decades.

Numerous extra-psychiatric factors such as socio-economic status, and socially-shared expectations and beliefs can affect the labeling process and influence psychiatric outcomes. Generally, these favor the more affluent persons allowing them greater control over whether they are admitted or released. Fewer West Indians would be admitted to mental hospitals in Britain, if their subculture was better understood. Besides for some psychiatrists, the 'social distance' between the lower class patients and themselves may be too great, more so when they practice in an alien culture. This increases the probability that a patient may be labeled as 'schizophrenic'.

Social Control

Sociologists believe that psychiatrists are agents of social control, perhaps because of the element of implied coercion. Psychiatrists do have coercive powers, but use them only rarely; most of their work is therapeutic and not concerned with 'coercion'.

Psychiatry is an agency of social control because it is concerned with identifying and regulating illness—an important form of social deviance. Role of psychiatry is to identify sickness and to treat it in such a manner so that it no longer poses a threat to social order, nor leaves the sufferers on the deviant margins of society. Thus psychiatry fits very well into this model of social control.

Another common formulation of this model of social control is social class analysis. The dominant social class or ruling elite maintain their supremacy through institutions, like psychiatry, which implicitly support the existing social order. Scull, for example, has argued that the emergence of the lunatic asylum in the 18th and 19th centuries was related to controlling itinerant labor and the work shy, and the demise of the large asylum in the late 1960s was the product of an economic crisis brought about by the inability of capital to pay for such 'welfare' services.

Social Constructionism

Durkheim's final major work, Elementary Forms of the Religious Life, argued that the categories of human thought have their origins and patterning in social life. Extended to medicine, this position holds that there are no diseases existing in nature (either organic or psychiatric); they only exist as artefacts of human classifications.

If psychiatric diagnostic categories somehow correspond or relate to socially significant patterns, then for the sociologist the study of psychiatric labels will afford a valuable way of 'reading' society. For example, the shift from the major problem of insanity at the end of the 19th century to the generalized problems of the neuroses might be explained by the fact that insanity was underpinned by the importance of rationality in the 19th century and the neuroses by our 20th century preoccupation with individual coping.

SOCIAL EPIDEMIOLOGY

Socio-economic and cultural factors have always attracted widespread attention and a search is on to link them, in a precise manner, with psychiatric conditions. Any review of sociological studies in the Indian context would be incomplete without a consideration of various social factors prevailing in this culture. India has a long history of ancient civilization and traditions. Perhaps, the most important feature is the immensity of its size and diversity of its population in terms of ethnic background, language, customs, food habits and religious practices.

Several studies have been conducted in an attempt to identify the relationships between mental disorders and certain socio-demographic variables. Dohrenwend, while reviewing 80 studies concerning the prevalence of mental disorders in different communities in the West since 1900, observed certain consistent trends. Mental disorder was significantly related to social class position and domicile. This was despite the wide differences in cultures, methodologies, time periods covered and definitions of mental disorder. Some of the well known pioneering investigations are described here.

Social Class

The relationship between social/socio-economic class and mental disorder is one of the strongest associations in epidemiology.

An important issue is the definition of social class. The British Registrar General considers the occupation of the head of the household to be sufficient for determining social class. In comparison, many sociologists, including Hollingshead and Redlich, have given differential weightage to each of the factors including income, occupation, education, religion, and locality and type of residence. Most Indian authors have determined socioeconomic status by the total family income. Sethi et al, in addition, gave equal weightage to education and occupation in determining socio-economic status. Despite these difficulties, some consistent trends have emerged.

Faris and Dunham's study, in Chicago, supplied a tremendous impetus for the investigation of social correlates for mental illness. They studied private and public mental hospital patients and found that a person living in the central slum areas is 15 times more likely to be committed to a mental hospital than a person living in the outskirts.

Eaton and Weils studied a distinct group, the Hutterites, which had maintained its distinct cultural heritage for over 400 years. The Hutterite way of life, despite the good mental health reputation of its members, did not provide immunity from severe psychiatric disturbances. Thus, the authors stated poignantly that genetic and organic factors predispose some individuals to mental disorder, no matter how stable and stress-free the social system is, and mental health utopia is probably impossible. The findings of this study diminish the importance of the role of social class in the production of mental disorders.

The most influential to date is the study by Hollingshead and Redlich in New Haven, Connecticut, which is cited all over the world. They compared public and private mental patients, both inpatients and outpatients, to a sample of the general nonpatient population. The first major finding was a definite inverse relationship between social class and being a psychiatric patient. The other major findings were that the types of mental illness varied with class position, and real differences existed in 'where', 'how' or 'how long' persons in different classes were cared for by psychiatrists. Lower the class, greater was the prevalence of schizophrenia and poorer was the prognosis. It is, however, possible that the higher prevalence rates for schizophrenia among the poor might only reflect inadequate treatment, leading to chronicity. Higher the social class, greater was the tendency towards anxiety disorders. Almost all class I and II neurotics were treated by private practitioners in private hospitals, whereas almost all class V neurotics were treated in public clinics, Military Veterans' Administration Hospitals or State Hospitals. Similar relationships were found for where the psychotics received care. How patients were treated, also followed class lines. Many class I and II patients received psychotherapies; in contrast, many class IV and V patients received organic therapies or custodial care. How long patients were treated, also varied with social class status. The mean length of treatment of neurotic patients in class I and II was almost 3 years, but for class V psychotics it was about 10 years.

Motivated by investigations, Srole and co-workers conducted the largest and the most ambitious investigation in the USA. They determined the true prevalence of mental disorder in 1660 noninstitutionalized persons living in Manhattan area of New York City. Both treated and untreated cases were included. Mental disorder was more prevalent among the lower class and was seen as a possible product of greater stress of lower class life with limited coping resources.

Goldberg and Morrison found that schizophrenics were in lower status occupations than their fathers, who were normally representative of all the classes, and had drifted downwards long before they were diagnosed. These findings settle the debate between the 'drift' and 'generation' hypotheses.

Subsequently, Leighton and co-workers conducted a thorough survey in Sterling County, a rural county in the Canadian province of Nova Scotia. The county had a population of less than 20,000. Fishing, timbering and farming were the three principal occupations, and the people had maintained for long their distinctive cultural traditions and identities. Mental disorder was most common amongst the lowest socioeconomic group.

Epidemiological surveys in Britain and the USA have shown markedly higher rates for most forms of mental disorder among the lower classes. A review of studies from different parts of the world, by Cockerham, indicates that the lowest social class had a greater prevalence of mental disorders in general, and schizophrenia and personality disorders in particular, while affective disorders and anxiety disorders tend to be more common among the upper and middle classes.

Numerous explanations have been advanced to account for the relationship between social class and mental illness. Some of these are enumerated below:

- There is greater genetic predisposition towards mental disorders among the lower class. Although this may be true, some environmental factors may also be contributory.
- The 'social stress' hypothesis maintains that greater mental disorder in the lower class is the result of greater stress as a result of living in poverty (leading to seclusion, social isolation and impaired communication) with limited coping resources.

- The 'social selection' hypothesis has the 'drift' and 'residue' hypotheses as its components. According to the 'drift' hypothesis, mentally ill persons tend to drift downwards in society where social demands are less. On the other hand, the residue hypothesis contends that the mentally healthy individuals in the lower class tend to be upwardly mobile, thus leaving behind a residue of mentally ill persons.
- The 'differential tolerance' hypothesis postulates that various communities have different levels of tolerance for schizophrenics. Many schizophrenics; therefore, move into areas that are more tolerant towards their behavior. In the same line, Hare advanced the thesis that the uneven distribution of schizophrenics in large cities could be explained, in part, by 'voluntary segregation', i.e. individuals with schizoid personalities or incipient schizophrenia actively self-locate (not merely drift) in poor sections of cities (where there are fewer manifest pressures to conform to the expectations of the social group, particularly the middle class) to secure social isolation a factor in the development of schizophrenia. It may be that genetic, social stress, and social selection factors may all be involved in varying degrees in the greater occurrence of mental illness among the lower class.
- Clausen and Kohn's 'small city hypothesis' suggested that geographic schizophrenic rate differentials could be found only after a city attained a certain size, since small cities simply did not contain collecting areas in which the mentally ill could find suitable lodgings. Also, there is less social isolation in small, stable cities as 'everybody knows everybody'.

Several surveys of mental morbidity have been conducted around all areas of our country. There are wide differences in the figures of morbidity reported by different workers. Some of the disagreement in the reports appears to be a product of variations in the methodology. For example, the psychiatric morbidity rate of the Agra survey was significantly less than that observed in the Lucknow and the Vellore surveys, possibly because the Agra investigators were primarily concerned with only 'severe' cases and had not included 'moderately' sick cases, which would undoubtedly form a vast majority of cases. In most of the studies, the rates of schizophrenia and organic psychosis are considerably similar. Wide differences, however, exist in regard to all other disorders, especially neurotic depression, hysteria, mental retardation and miscellaneous category. In spite of these differences, some useful data has enriched our knowledge of the morbidity in India, based on socio-demographic factors.

When comparisons are made between the incidence of depressive illness in our country and the West, one is impressed by the fact that while affective psychosis is more common in the Indian setting, depressive neurosis is more frequently diagnosed in the UK and the USA, possibly because of diagnostic bias. Of particular interest is the finding of 3–5 times higher incidence rates of depressive illness from North India, than that reported from centers in the South. Two explanations have been advanced to account for this finding. First, there exists probably a greater tolerance of depressive symptoms in Southern and Western India, than in Northern India. If this was so, the prevalence rate of depression should have been much higher in the population surveys in the South. This has not been found. Secondly, North Indians have a different genetic pool from South Indians and because Punjabis tend to marry Punjabis, the incidence of a genetically determined illness would be expected to be higher in North-West India. These hypotheses need confirmation.

Some Indian studies, on the natural history of mental disorders in-rural communities, have shown that the prevalence rates did not change appreciably after intervals of one and ten years, suggesting that community maintains a dynamic equilibrium in its morbidity. The factors maintaining equilibrium are divisible into two categories: one, increasing the morbidity rate (incidence of new cases and migration of morbid people into the village) and the other, decreasing the morbidity rate (recovery of cases, death of cases, migration of morbid people from the village and rise in the number of healthy persons). The popular notion, that mental morbidity is on the increase, has not been borne out by these surveys.

Social class in relation to mental illness had attracted the attention of investigators in India nearly three decades ago. These investigators did not report the relationship of the incidence of neurosis with higher social level or of psychosis with a lower level. While Mohan reported the majority of patients to be in lower and middle class, Thacore et al found higher morbidity in the middle and upper social classes. Except for two studies that linked lower income with psychiatric morbidity, significant relationship of income with psychiatric disorders has not been reported. In these studies, income was used as an index of social status.

Some interesting data has been provided by Nandi and co-workers. Four times higher mental morbidity was observed in an urban community of higher socioeconomic status, in comparison to that in an urban slum area in Kolkata. The prevalence of schizophrenia was, however, much higher in the latter sample. In this study, higher rates of affectivity were observed in the families of lower socioeconomic status. It was further observed that the differences in the prevalence rate of neurosis, in the upper and lower socioeconomic classes, was at the root of the wide divergence in the rates of total morbidity of different socioeconomic classes. Later, the same authors reported that people in the highest class had the highest risk of developing mental illness. This was a stable characteristic of the rural community studied by them, being maintained during a course of time. The earlier finding of Hagnell that people in the lowest social class have least risk of developing mental disorder was thus corroborated. These findings are strikingly in contrast with those reported from the West that has linked psychiatric morbidity to lower social class. It may be mentioned that our social classes are not strictly comparable with the West. In the absence of suitable system for classifying social class, a precise relationship between social class and mental illness may not be possible. Further studies, in the other slum areas in other major cities in India, are needed before a final answer can be provided.

Sex

Most studies in the West have observed no consistent sex differences with regard to schizophrenia. Affective disorders, anxiety disorders and primary degenerative dementia are significantly more common in women, while personality disorders and substance abuse disorders are more common in men. These differences are probably due to biological and sociocultural factors, particularly differences in sex role expectations. It has been observed that younger boys have higher rates than girls until they reach puberty, because even though their intellectual and physical development was slower, they were expected to perform as well as girls. Girls, on the other hand, showed higher rates of morbidity after adolescence because of the increased social pressure to adopt traditional female role, such as submission and dependency on males, motherhood and family responsibilities, over career interests.

Research has shown that roles of adult women, whether at home or in job, predispose them to anxiety and depression. The house-wife's role is such that the household duties are unstructured; more or less isolating her from the outside environment, and are greatly limited as a source of gratification. Working women, in comparison to men, are disadvantaged in salaries and promotions, and are faced with conflicts of family aspirations versus professional interests. Besides, for men, the society is more permissive and traditional roles provide more alternatives.

It is interesting to note that when both men and women perform acts indicative of a mental disorder, men are more likely to be perceived s mentally ill or admitted for longer periods to mental hospitals, presumably because symptoms of distress and hospitalization are considered to be common among females.

From India, it has been repeatedly reported that higher percentage of male population register at the psychiatric facilities. This is by no means indicative of a higher morbidity in males. Rather, this may be due to lack of education, presence of superstitions, reluctance on the part of the women folk because of the social stigma and bleak chances of matrimonial placement in our culture. Besides, a large number of male beds in hospitals are indicative of society's neglect of his fair sex in our culture.

The female has for long in the Indian culture, being forced to be the feeder and breeder, and following the leader who is the male. Often, she has no voice, particularly in the orthodox families. No wonder that she falls prey to neurosis (particularly hysteria). Numerous reports show that housewives are highly prone to develop neurosis and depression. The social roles played by women in the East (and in India), though different from those in the West, are similarly responsible for a greater vulnerability to psychiatric disorders.

Some population surveys, however, have shown varying results with regard to sex and mental illness by the same investigators. No significant sex difference in the mental morbidity in an urbanized tribal community was observed. The women in tribal communities are less vulnerable, than in other communities, might be a reflection of their gender role characteristics in their societies. Greater affectivity in women has been reported in urban and rural surveys. Furthermore, the finding in 1972 was replicated 10 years later, suggesting that greater vulnerability of women to mental illness is a stable feature which cuts across cultures and persists in time in a given culture.

Domicile

Domicile has also attracted the attention of mental health investigators. They have favored the popular speculation linking urbanized technologically oriented social settings to psychiatric disorders. From a review of several reports from all over the world, it has been concluded that urban areas have a higher morbidity. Hospital admissions in Jerusalem and India have also indicated a higher rate of admissions for persons in urban than in rural areas. In addition, it has been reported that while schizophrenia, anxiety and personality disorders are more common in urban centers, manic depressive rates are higher in rural areas.

A perusal of the Indian literature reveals some inconsistencies. Some rural surveys have found very high psychiatric morbidity, 102.8 and 369.0/1000 population respectively, much higher than that reported in any other survey in India, except morbidity of 207/1000 population reported in an urban community of high socioeconomic status from Kolkata. However, most studies have reported higher rates in the urban as compared to the rural population.

In different field surveys of mental morbidity conducted by Nandi and associates in rural and urban areas of West Bengal, mental illness was either unrelated to socioeconomic class or persons belonging to the urban population had higher rates. These diametrically opposite findings suggested consideration of some psychological attributes of the community. Thus, they investigated morbidity in two communities, both of lower status, but one, an uprooted community, had higher level of aspiration than the other neighboring community. The community having a high level of aspiration showed a higher rate of stress-dependent mental disorders (neurosis, psychosomatic illness and depression) than the native-born community with lower level of aspiration. Further work involving uprooted communities living in camps, which do not strive to improve their status, would provide useful information.

The stress of urbanization, competitive life of cities and overcrowded housing, leading to strained relations, have often been implicated in causation of mental disorders. It is not clear whether these factors contribute to mental disorders that are most common in cities. It is possible that a set routine of an isolated life, with limited stimulation in villages, may contribute towards greater prevalence of manic depressive symptoms among rural folk. The fact that the urban population has an easy approach to psychiatric facilities, while the rural population at large, cannot reach the benefit of the same, may account only in part for the rural-urban differences.

Marriage

A reasonable assumption is that married persons should have better mental health than unmarried people because marriage is believed to offer the partners a lifelong security and happiness. In the West, while this is true for males, among females, particularly from the lower status, marriage is not associated with lower prevalence of mental illness. In India, higher morbidity in the married as compared to single, divorced/widowed has been observed. Of the married, the housewives are more prone to develop neurosis. Early marriage, being common, carries the risk of early pregnancy and the responsibilities of rearing children, in addition to the multiple chores of a housewife. Further, old orthodox customs in certain parts of India cause a wife to take her life on the funeral pyre of her husband, referred to as 'Sati.' Such life situations make her more vulnerable to stress conditions.

Family

In India, family is the most important part of the social orbit. Families are the primary transmitters of the cultural patterns from one generation to the other. Eight out of the ten studies, reviewed by Sethi and Manchanda, have shown a greater vulnerability amongst those belonging to a unitary family structure. Hysteria, however, was more prevalent in the joint families. Restriction of independence in women, dominance of elders and resultant interpersonal maladjustments in joint families seem to breed hysterical manifestations. Despite this, Sethi and coworkers believe that joint family system provides some safety measures which are usually missing in unitary families.

An interesting finding emerged from a rural survey in Kota consisting of three caste groups—Brahmins, Mogers and Bants, in relation to family inheritance. Matrilineal families, which were in the process of changing over to the patrilineal system, had a higher case rate than those families where the change had already been effected.

Earlier authors had taken residentially as the sole criterion for categorizing the family type. However, this did not provide convincing evidence of actual functioning or integration of the family. Agarwal et al adopted an objective and rational criterion of measuring 'family jointness' in terms of financial jointness and jointness in living and decision making. The degree of jointness was found to have an inverse relationship with neurotic manifestations in the wives of male neurotics.

The eldest son in the Indian society has the most privileged position with regard to inheritance and receives preferential treatment from all the family members. But, after the demise of the father, he is expected to provide education and occupation to his brothers and to settle marriage of his sisters, with the dowry system prevailing in India. Likewise, the eldest daughter is expected to share the responsibilities of the mother and household in general. Thus, the eldest sibling goes through severe tension and stress. No wonder that the eldest or early born siblings have been over-represented in most of the psychiatric groups in several studies in India.

Race

Significant differences in the rates of major mental disorders among different cultural and ethnic groups have been reported. The findings of Pasamanick however, have not supported this stand. No differences occur in the rates of mental disorders between blacks and whites in the USA, nor do Spanish-speaking persons or American Indians have high prevalence rates. Asian Americans, however, have exceedingly low rates of mental disorder. Real differences, if at all exist, are possibly because the racial minorities are also lower in the social class.

Religion

Religion may be an important determinant of mental health. Different religions again cause barriers, with nonintegration of people with different faiths. In the West, there seems to be a general consensus that Catholics have rates similar to those seen in the general population. Protestants have lower rates, while Jews are over-represented.

India is diversified by the, different religions and languages. The different religions and groups among the population are Hindus (82.7%), Muslims (11.2%), Christians (2.6%), Scheduled Caste and Tribes (21.9%) and others (0.84%). The caste system followed by different religions, in different areas results in segregation and denial of equal opportunities. Untouchability, with regard to Harijans, still prevails in India. Religion forms an important part of life of most Indians.

Few workers have studied the role of religion on mental health. Carstairs and Kapur reported the findings of a systematic survey, which they conducted on 9000 inhabitants of Kota, a village on the western coast of India. Brahmins had a much lower 'case rate' than the 'Bants' and 'Mogers.' The Brahmins, however, also had a higher socioeconomic and educational level, so that caste may have played only a minimal role.

Primitive Societies

Eminent pioneers, such as Freud and Maudsley, share the view that mental disorder in the primitive society was a result of the restriction and stresses of modern civilization and, thus, would be rare in persons not yet affected by industrialization. However, subsequent research has shown that mental disturbance occurs in every society without exception, but varies in its frequency of occurrence in different societies.

Some studies have brought to light two very vital facts. First, a large scale survey, among the Yoruba tribe in Africa, established the validity of standard psychiatric concepts in tribal settings, Secondly, among tribals, there is evidence that there is more psychosis among those who have been exposed to the conditions of life in the alien and largely urban environment.

Nandi et al conducted a rural field study in two tribal communities, 'Lodha' and 'Munda', living in the tribal belt of the district of Midnapore in West Bengal and a neighboring Brahmin community. The two tribes had settled themselves for generations in agricultural life and were still free from the impact of technological change. The rate of mental morbidity amongst the Brahmins was four times that amongst the tribals. This cross-cultural difference in the rate of morbidity cannot be brushed aside. It should attract more studies in ethno-psychiatry.

Although the Brahmins and tribals differed widely in their rates of morbidity they differed little in their clinical picture. Of particular interest was the absence of neurotic disorders, like anxiety and depression, amongst the tribals, which were frequently observed amongst the Brahmins. Another outstanding fact was that the total morbidity reached its peak, a decade earlier in the tribals as compared to that in the Brahmins. This earlier shift was possibly related to the early assumption of family responsibility amongst the tribals. An additional contributory factor was the lack of psychological support of the joint family, as most of the tribals had nuclear families. Many Brahmins, on the other hand, had the benefit of joint families. Another important finding was that hysteria was confined to females amongst the Brahmins, but tribal hysterics were distributed in both sexes. This study corroborated the earlier reports on Zulu disorders of the existence of hysteria ('crying fit') amongst both males and females.

Bannerjee et al studied psychiatric morbidity in an urbanized tribal community in West Bengal. The latter was selected as it could more faithfully represent the effect of urbanization in having no intermediate exposure to an alien culture. The people under study had settled down in an urban set-up with the active support of the Government and a philanthropic society. From the results of this study, it was concluded that urbanization *per se* exerts no adverse effect on the mental health of a tribal community, provided it is allowed to preserve its ethnicity and basic cultural pattern. The stress of urbanization had not affected the basic personality structure and the cultural mould of the tribes, as obsessions and phobias were still absent in this community. Wintrobe and Wittkower suggested that the disease of super-ego conflict (obsession) is likely to be rare in tribal culture. Studies of psychiatric morbidity in tribal communities urbanized through generations would be of much interest.

India is a land of different languages. About 25 million people (4.5% of the total population) speak their mother tongue, other than the 15 languages listed in the constitution. Language gives extraordinary mastery to man over his physical surroundings. It also serves to divide, rather than unite people and can form the basis for the development of paranoid disorder. This area needs investigation.

Age

In the West, mental illness increases proportionately with age and there is a steep rise in the first hospital admissions after middle age. Dohrenwend and Dohrenwend, after an extensive review of the western literature, concluded that age shows no consistent relationship with morbidity in most studies. Most reports from India indicate an increase in the morbidity after 30 and a fall after 50 years of age. Further, it has been observed that, over a span of 10 years (1957–67), the number of psychiatric admissions of patients over 60 years in a general hospital, continued to be small. Several explanations can be offered. First, there is a shorter life span in our country. Second, physical problems are common after 50, so that psychiatric problems are likely to be overlooked. Third, joint families are still widely prevalent, accepting greater responsibility for the aged. Finally, old age symptoms may be considered as 'normal' manifestations of old age. A few investigators have found increasing mental morbidity with advancing age. Others observed similarly, except that there was a drop in the 35 to 44 years category. In an industrial population, Ganguly observed no variations related to age. Increasing dissolution of the traditional joint families and the adoption of Western values could account for some of the discrepant findings.

Migration

Extensive movement of persons has been a prominent feature of the 20th century life. The mental health of immigrants has long been a matter of concern to governments in defining immigration policies. Stresses of settling in a foreign culture can affect mental health.

In 1885, when immigration to the USA was not legally restricted, the ratio of mentally ill was higher in the foreign population in Massachusetts than in the native population, but mental deficiency was much less common among the foreigners than among the native born.

It was convincingly demonstrated that Norwegians settling in Minnesota had higher rates of schizophrenia than either their native or adoptive populations. However, the results were attributed to constitutional factors, rather than to the hardships of migrant life. Subsequently, the rates of admission to New York institutions were reported to be higher for the immigrants than for the native born.

Murphy's study, of World War II refugees to Britain, shows that they had higher rates of mental hospitalization, but the refugees had been subjected to persecution and deportation. Murphy's subsequent review of studies of immigrants indicates that those from Asia-Africa had higher mental hospitalization rates than the local Jewish population. Jewish immigrants from Europe (whose status was similar) did not have higher hospitalization rates. Higher rates of all forms of mental illness were found in English migrants, in the French speaking province of Ontario, than in the English speaking province.

Among migrants to Victoria, two groups were identified. One group was of unstable single men from Western Europe, who broke down soon after emigration and was probably schizophrenic before emigration. The other group included migrants from Southern and Eastern Europe, who broke down after a year or more, because of stresses relating to their lack of acceptance by the host culture.

A few workers have, however, observed that migration is not always associated with high-risk of mental illness. Kaila et al found that immigrant refugees in Finland did not have significantly higher mental illness rates than the general population. They concluded that overseas migration is associated with greater risk for mental illness, while internal migration is associated with lower risk. In Swede and Dane migrants to rural areas in Norway, Astrup and Odegaard found lower first admission rates than in nonmigrant Norwegians. From a study of Hungarian refuges. Mezey concluded that 'selective migration' of the mentally ill took place.

Srole et al. and most others have concluded that it is the low status and poverty of immigrants which is responsible for the poor mental health of immigrants.

Murphy presented three postulates to explain the relationship between migration and mental illness:

- Persons with incipient mental disorders, who are unable to adjust to the conditions of life in their homeland, tend to migrate.
- Hardships of migration precipitate mental disorders.
- Migration, as a unitary variable, is not directly related to increased mental illness rates; it is one of the several factors that combine to produce high rates.

The results of studies on migration and mental illness lack uniformity because of methodological differences. Besides, majority of the studies have been reported from the West. Momore people migrate to other countries from India as it is developing nation. However, there have been large scale population shifts to India on at least four occasions. One was from West Pakistan to India at the time of our independence in 1947, the second forced migration was during the formation of Bangladesh involving 90 million people, and the third was of Tamil refugees from Sri Lanka to southern parts of India, while the fourth was of Afghan refugees from Afghanistan. Although these populations faced threats to their survival, they are in the process of rehabilitating themselves.

Of particular interest are the results from the study of Sethi et al. on migrants from West Pakistan. People displaced 30 years earlier and their offspring, born in the 10 years following displacement, still showed higher frequency of mental disorder than their urban neighbors. Similar findings in Punjabi refugees were reported by Dube. In addition, he observed that the excess rates applied to Punjabi refugees who had a difficult time during migration, but not Sindhi refugees who had an easier time during migration. Psychiatric morbidity was observed in 35% of a migrated industrial population.

There are few studies of Indian immigrants settled elsewhere. A higher prevalence rate for all diagnostic entities, particularly of schizophrenia, was observed in the Asian immigrants than English patients.

Majority of the studies from India and abroad provide evidence that migration, for various reasons, is associated with increased rates of psychiatric morbidity. Migration in relation to mental illness is a huge and, complex problem. Each passing day evidences a drift from the village to the city in search of employment, stability and money. It remains to be seen whether this social drift assists in stability or causes tension and increase in the quantum of psychiatric illness in cities.

BIBLIOGRAPHY

1. Abraham A, Subramaniam K, Verghese A. Birth order and psychiatric disturbances. Indian J Psychiatry. 1973;15:11-16.
2. Agarwal AK, Mehta UK, Gupta SC. Joint family and neurosis. Indian J Psychiatry. 1978;20:232-36.
3. Armstrong D. Madness and coping. Sociology of Health and Illness. 1979;2:293-316.
4. Armstrong D. The contribution of sociology to psychiatry: a review Journal of the Royal Society of Medicine. 1988;81:161-3.
5. Astrup C, Odegaard O. Internal migration and mental disease in Norway. Psychiatr Quart. 1960;34(Suppl):166-80.
6. Bannerjee T, Mukerjee SP, Nandi DN, et al. Psychiatric morbidity in an urbanized tribal (Santal) community: A field survey. Indian J Psychiatry. 1986;28:243-48.
7. Bhaskaran K, Sethi RC, Yadav SN. Migration and mental health in industry. Indian J Psychiatry. 1970;12:102-9.
8. Brenner MH. Mental Illness and the Economy. Cambridge: Harvard University Press, 1973.
9. Brown GW, Harris T. Social origins of depression. London: Tavistock; 1978.
10. Canard BM. Anomie and Deviant Behaviour: A Discussion and Critique. New York: Free Press; 1964.p.2.
11. Carstairs GM, Kapur RL. The Great Universe of Kota: Stress, Change and Mental Disorder in an Indian Village. London: Hogarth Press, 1976.

12. Carstairs GM. Medicine and faith in rural Rajasthan. In: Paul BD (Ed). Health, Culture and Community New York: Russell Sage, 1955.
13. Channabasavanna SM, Bhatti RS. Student perception of anomie. Indian J Psychiatry. 1977;19:17-23.
14. Clausen JA, Kohn ML. Relation of schizophrenia to the social Structure of a small city. In: Pasamanick B (Ed). Epidemiology of Mental Disorder. Washington DC: Am Assoc Adv Sci. 1959. pp.69-94.
15. Cockerham WC. Sociology and Psychiatry In: Kaplan HI, Sadock BJ (Eds). Comprehensive Textbook of Psychiatry, 4th Edn. Baltimore: Williams & Wilkins, 1985.
16. Cohen K. The study of social disorganization and deviant behaviour. In: Menon, Broom, Cortell (Eds). Sociology Today. New York: Basic Books; 1959.p.461.
17. DeSousa A, DeSousa D. My India, Our India. In: DeSousa A, DeSousa D (Eds). Psychiatry in India. Bombay: Bhalani Book Depot; 1984.
18. Dohrenwend BP, Dohrenwend BS. Psychiatric disorders in urban settings. In: Arieti SA (Ed). American Handbook of Psychiatry, 2nd edition. New York: Basic Books, 1974.
19. Dohrenwend BP. Sociocultural and social-psychological factors in the genesis of mental disorders. J Health Soc Behav. 1975;16:365-8.
20. Dube KC. A study of prevalence and biosocial variables in mental illness in a rural and an urban community in Uttar Pradesh. Acta Psychiatr Scand. 1970;46:327-32.
21. Dube KC. Mental disorder in Agra. Soc Psychiatry. 1968;3:179.
22. Durkheim E. Suicide: A Study of Sociology. New York: Free Press; 1951.p.249. (Reprint of 1857).
23. Durkheim E. The elementary forms of the religious life. London: Allen and Unwin; 1915.
24. Eaton JW, Weils RJ. Culture and Mental Disorders. New York: Free Press; 1955.
25. Elanger MN, Maittre P, Rao MN. Mental health in an Indian rural community. Br J Psychiatry. 1971;1438:499.
26. Faris REL, Dunham HW. Mental Disorders in Urban Areas: An Ecological Study of Schizophrenia and Other Psychoses. Chicago: Chicago University Press; 1939.
27. Fotes M, Mayer DY. Cited in Hsu FLK (Ed). Psychological Anthropology. Cambridge: Schenkman, 1972.pp.108.
28. Ganguli HC. Prevalence of psychological disorders in an Indian industrial population. I-Ill. Indian J Med Res. 1968;56:754.
29. Gershon ES, Liebowitz JH. Sociocultural and demographic correlates of affective disorders in Jerusalem. J Psychiatry Res. 1975;12:37-42.
30. Goldberg EM, Morrison SL. Schizophrenia and social class. Br J Psychiatry. 1963;109:785-802.
31. Gove W, Tudor JF. Adult sex role and mental illness. Am J Sociology. 1973;78:812-17.
32. Gove WR. Who is hospitalized: A critical review of some sociological studies. J Health Soc Behav. 1970;11:294-303.
33. Hangnell O. A Prospective Study of the Incidence of Mental Disorder. Stockholm: Svenska-Bokforlaget Nortedts Bonniers, 1996.
34. Hare EG. Mental illness and social conditions. J Ment Sci. 1956;102:349-62.
35. Hollingshead AB, Redlich FC. Social Class and Mental illness. New York: John Wiley; 1958.
36. Jarvis E. Report on Insanity and Idiocy in Massachusetts: By the Commission on Lunacy, under resolve of the legislature of 1854. Boston: William White, 1855.
37. Jones K, Fowles AJ. Ideas on institutions. London: Routledge and Kegan Paul, 1984.
38. Kala A, Kala R, Bhatia K. Changing socio-demographic and clinical profile of patients attending a general hospital psychiatric clinic: Some indications of community acceptance. Indian J Psychiatry. 1981;23:86-9.
39. Kimmich. Ethnic aspects of schizophrenia in Hawaii. Psychiatry 1960;23:97-9.
40. Klapp OE. Heroes, Villians and Fools. Englewood Cliffs. S: Prentice Hall; 1962.
41. Krupinske J. Sociological aspects of mental health in migrants. Soc Sci Med. 1967;1:267-81.
42. Laing RD. Cited: Holt H. Existential psychoanalysis. In: Freedman AM, Kaplan HI, Sadock BJ (Eds). Comprehensive Textbook of Psychiatry, 2nd edition. Baltimore: Williams & Wilkins; 1975.pp.665-6.
43. Laing RD. The Politics of Experience and the Bird of Paradise. London: Penguin; 1967.
44. Lee SC. Some Zulu concepts of psychogenic disorder. J Soc Res Pretoria. 1950;1:9.
45. Leighton AH, Lambo TA, Hughes CC, et al. Psychiatric Disorder Among The Yoruba. Ithaca, NY: Comell University Press, 1963.
46. Leighton AH. My name is legion. The Stirling County Study. New York: Basic Books; 1959;1.
47. Leighton AH. Poverty and social change. Si Am. 1965;212:21-7.
48. Leighton DC, Harding JS, Mackim DB, et al. The character of danger: Psychiatric symptoms in selected communities. The Stirling County Study of Psychiatric Disorder and Sociocultural Environment. New York: Basic Books. 1963;3.
49. Leighton DC, Harding JS, Macklin DB, et al. The character of danger. New York: Basic Books, 1963 Brown GW, Harris T. Social origins of depression. London: Tavistock; 1978.
50. Littlewood R, Lipsedge M. Acute psychotic reactions in Carribean-born patients. Psychol Med. 1981;11:303-18.
51. Lukes S. Alienation and anomie. In: Laslett P, Runciman WG (Eds). Philosophy, politics and society. Oxford: Blackwell; 1967.
52. Mac-Iver RM. The Ramparts We Guard. New York: Macmillan; 1950.
53. Maltzberg B. Internal migration and mental disease among the white population of New York State. 1960-61. Int J Soc Psychiatr. 1967.pp.184-91.
54. Maltzberg B. Mental disease in New York State according to nativity and parentage. Mental Hygiene. 1935;19:635-60.
55. Marfatia JC. A survey of 2000 private adult patients. Indian J Psychiatry. 1973;15:279-82.
56. Mezey AS. A study of mental disease among Norwegian-born population in Minnesota. Acta Psychiatr Scand. 1960(Suppl 4).

57. Mohan B. Sociology of mental illness in India. Indian J Psychiatry. 1970;12:278-86.
58. Murphy HBM. Flight and Resettlement. Paris: UNESCO, 1955.
59. Murphy HBM. Migration and major mental disorders: A reappraisal. In: Kanter MB (Ed). Mobility and Mental Health. Springfield: Thomas; 1965.pp.5-29.
60. Murphy JM. A cross-cultural comparison of psychiatric disorders: Eskimos of Alaska, Yorubas of Nigeria, and Nova Scotians of Canada. In: Lebra WE (Ed). Transcultural Research in Mental Health. Honolulu: University Press of Hawaii; 1972. pp.213-26.
61. Nandi DN, Ajmany S, Ganguli H, et al. Psychiatric disorders in a rural community in West Bengal: An epidemiological study. Indian J Psychiatry. 1975;17:87-98.
62. Nandi DN, Bannerjce G, Ganguli H, et al. The natural history of mental disorders in a rural community: A longitudinal field survey. Indian J Psychiatry. 1978;20:12.
63. Nandi DN, Bannerjee G, Mukerjee SP, et al. A study of psychiatric morbidity of a rural community at an interval of ten years. Indian J Psychiatry. 1986;28:179-94.
64. Nandi DN, Das NM, Chaudhuri A, et al. Mental morbidity and urban life: An epidemiological study. Indian J Psychiatry. 1980;22:234-9.
65. Nandi DN, Mukerjee SP, Boral GC, et al. Prevalence of psychiatric morbidity in two tribal communities in certain villages of West Bengal: A cultural study. Indian J Psychiatry. 1977;19:2-12.
66. Neki JS, Kapoor RK. Social stratification of psychiatric patients. Indian J Psychiatry. 1963;5:76-85.
67. Odegaard O. A study of mental disease among Norwegian born population in Minnesota. Acta Psychiatr Scand. 1932 (Suppl 4).
68. Owen MB. Alternative hypothesis for the explanation of some of Faris and Dunham's results. Am J Sociology. 1941;4:48-52.
69. Pasamanick B. A survey of mental disease in an urban population. VII. An approach to total population by rear. Am J Psychiatry. 1962;99:299-304.
70. Pinto R. Psychosocial variables associated with mental illness in patients of Asian origin. Indian J Psychiatry. 1974;16:203-6.
71. Prabhu GG, Ramchandran K. Birth order and schizophrenia. Indian J Psychiatry. 1973;15:1-6.
72. Rao S. Birth order and schizophrenia. J Nerv Ment Dis. 1964;139:87-9.
73. Ray SD. Social stratification of mental patients. Indian J Psychiatry. 1962;4:3-11.
74. Rennie TAG, Woodward LE. Mental Health in Modern Society. New York: Commonwealth Fund; 1948.p.385.
75. Rosenhan DL. On being sane in insane places. Science. 1973;173:250-58.
76. Scheff TJ. Being Mentally ill. London: Weidnefied & Nicholson, 1966.
77. Scull A. Decarceration. Englewood Cliffs: Prentice-Hall; 1977.
78. Scull A. Museum of madness. London: Allen Lane; 1979.
79. Sethi BB, Gupta SC, Kumar R. 300 families: A psychiatric study. Indian J Psychiatry. 1967;9:280-89.
80. Sethi BB, Gupta SC, Kumar RN, et al. A psychiatric survey of 500 rural families. Indian J Psychiatry. 1972;14:183-88.
81. Sethi BB, Gupta SC, Mahendru RK, et al. Mental health and urban life: A study of 850 families. Br J Psychiatry. 1974;124: 243-47.
82. Sethi BB, Gupta SC, Mahendru RK, et al. Migration and mental health. Indian J Psychiatry. 1972;14:115-19.
83. Sethi BB, Gupta SC. Sibling position in India. Am J Psychotherapy. 1973;27:61.
84. Sethi BB, Manchanda R. Socioeconomic, demographic and cultural correlates of psychiatric disorders with special reference to India. Indian J Psychiatry. 1978;20:199-211.
85. Singh G. Depression in India: A cross-cultural perspective. Indian J Psychiatry. 1979;21:235-39.
86. Slater E, Roth M, Mayer-Gross. Clinical Psychiatry, 3rd edition. London: Cassel; 1969.
87. Sren B, Nandi DN, Mukeijee SP, et al. Psychiatric morbidity in an urban slum-dwelling community Indian J Psychiatry. 1984;26:185-93.
88. Srole L, Langner TS, Michael ST, et al. Mental Health in the Metropolis: The Mid-town Manhattan Study. NewYork: McGraw-Hill. 1962;1.
89. Sundaraj N, Rama Rao BS. Order of birth and schizophrenia. Br J Psychiatry. 1966;112:1127-9.
90. Szasz T. What psychiatry can and cannot do? In: Szasz T (Ed). Ideology And Insanity. London: Pelican; 1974.pp.78-85.
91. Teja JS, Narang RL. Pattern of incidence of depression in India. Indian J Psychiatry. 1970;12:23-6.
92. Teja JS. Birth order and schizophrenia. Indian J Psychiatry. 1967;9:203-8.
93. Thacore VR. Gupta SC. Suraiya M. Psychiatric clinic at the urban centre, Alambagh, Lucknow. Indian J Psychiatry. 1971;13:253-7.
94. Thacore VR. Mental illness in an Urban Community. Allahabad: United Publishers, 1973.
95. Verghese A, Beig A, Abraham A. Social class and psychiatric disturbance: A community study. Indian J Med Res. 1976;64: 1672-4.
96. Verghese A, Beig A, Senseman LA, et al. A social and psychiatric study of a representative group of families in Vellore town. Indian J Med Res. 1973;61:618-20.
97. Verghese A, Beig A. Neurosis in Vellore town: An epidemiological study. Indian J Psychiatry. 1974;16:1-11.
98. Wig NN, Verma VK, Khanna BC. Diagnostic characteristics of a general hospital psychiatric adult outpatient clinic. Indian Psychiatry. 1978;20:262-5.
99. Wintrobe R, Wiltkower ED. Magic and Witchcraft in Liberia: Their psychiatric implications. Transcult Psychiatric Res Rev. 1966;3:149.

CHAPTER

51 Sociology, Psychiatry and Mental Health

JN Vyas, Veena Vyas

INTRODUCTION

Sociological contribution to psychiatry have tended to reflect divergent theoretical and methodological orientations: social causation, interpretive microsociology, structuralism and poststructuralism. Social causationism, which is the oldest tradition, focuses on the social causes of mental illness and accepts the legitimacy of psychiatric nosology (treating diagnostic categories like 'depression' or 'schizophrenia' and the scientific method as unproblematic). A close association between sociology and medicine is evident within this tradition, traceable to 19th century social medicine. The approach has largely spawned epidemiological surveys of community populations or hospital admissions.

The social causation thesis peaked in popularity in the 1950s. During the 1960s, versions of *microsociology* appeared, which challenged the methodological dominance of epidemiology and structural functionalism (which tended to view society as a functional whole made up of interlocking and compatible subsystems). Its theoretical roots were to be found mainly in symbolic interactionism and social phenomenology which focused on interpreting phenomena in the social world (Goffmann 1961, Lemert 1967, Scheff 1966). The methodological emphasis was on ethnographic or naturalistic studies of institutional life and everyday rule enforcement. This approach allowed sociologists access to the fine grain of the mentally ill, beyond what could be described by epidemiology. Symbolic interactionism allowed a perspective to emerge from the 'underdog'. In particular, a voice could be given to the 'unofficial', side of the hospital and being 'mentally ill' which countered uncritical structural-functionalist accounts of medical life (e.g. Parsons 1951). This interpretive sociology also subsumed the emergence of ethnomethodology. This described how individuals make sense of social situation, and at times it shaded into philosophical inquiry. Contra the social causationists, the focus turned towards the relativity of concepts of mental health and illness and the notion that both are socially negotiated.

During the 1970s doubts began to emerge about sociology setting into an interpretive scheme. In particular Marxian critiques tried to set the organization and activities of psychiatry into a macroeconomic context. For example, Scull (1979) was guided in the main by economic notions, backed up by documentary evidence analyzing the emerging social control role of psychiatry in the 19th century and the functional value it held for the capitalist state. Scull (1977) also sought to explain the emergence of deinstitutionalization in response to fiscal pressures after the second world war. A political economy approach to evaluating schizophrenia and its treatment also started to emerge in the work of some social psychiatrists (e.g. Warner1985).

Over the past three decades the influence of Foucault on psychiatry has been apparent. Overall Foucauldian work stands separately from both microsociology and structuralism in relation to psychiatry. At the outset, in the 1960s, Foucault's own work centerd on the emergence of the asylum (Foucault 1965). The methodological implications of Foucauldian research are novel-empirical knowledge claims are of interest not (only) to produce knowledge in itself but also to read and reread or deconstruct that knowledge. This task is near to interpretive sociology (both can be placed in a hermeneutic framework) but focuses on discourses rather than social actors. Moreover, it does not accept the presuppositions of humanism, such as a coherent or stable subjectivity, nor does it privilege individual agents in sociological enquiry; instead it opposes or seeks to transcend the personalistic' or 'homocentric' feature of the older interpretive tradition. On a second front, the over-determining role of the state or political economy is rejected. While this influence or role is conceded, stable or predictable causal patterns are not.

In the 1980s sociology in this poststrucuralist mode issued a set of discourses on discourses. It opened up the inevitability of plural social realities regarding the precarious nature of knowledge claims. Foucault's own work on institutional psychiatry was categorized by his followers as scene setting-documenting the prehistory of the discipline or the conditions which made it possible. New formations of psychiatric work were subsequently the focus of deconstructions. Twentieth century psychiatry was described as eclectic, and its ambit was now seen to extend beyond the boundaries of both the asylum and madness. In particular, psychological as well as biodeterministic features of psychiatry were highlighted. For example, the deconstruction of the emergent 'shell shock' problem of the first world war by Stone (1985) shows the eugenic discourse about 'England's finest blood' -officers and gentlemen and working class volunteers were breaking down under the strain of a war of unprecedented attrition and stalemate.

Poststructuralist also rejected the antipsychiatric emphasis on the destructive and oppressive features of modern psychiatry. Miller and Rose (1988) put this succinctly: 'We argue that it is more fruitful to consider the ways that regulatory systems have sought to promote subjectivity than to document the way in which they have crushed it'. Consequently their focus has been on new psychological discourses in contemporary society rather than on the legacyof Victorian biological psychiatry. A similar emphasis on the changing discursive forms of psychiatry can be found in the recent work of de Swaan, who draws attention to the particular features associated with neurosis and psychological therapies. de Swaan (1990) talks of clients now being proto-professionalized because they develop a cognitive set within which to see their personal difficulties in professional terms. Thus, it can be seen that recently an eclectic sociology has emerged, which embraces both the causal emphasis of Durkheim and Marx and the hermeneutic or interpretive emphasis from Weber. These have been supplemented further by deconstruction.

Having provided a general overview of dominant sociological positions in relation to psychiatry, we now explore in more detail the way in which society and mental health can be understood. The relationship between society and mental health care be broadly understood in three ways by sociologist, each with a different notion of the 'social'.

1. The mental health of people is partially or wholly caused by societal influences (**Social causationism).**
2. The mental health of people is socially negotiated (**Labeling theory**).
3. Mental health and illness are socially constructed (**Social constructionism**).

THREE PERSPCETIVES OF THE SOCIAL

Social Causationism

Mental health is socially patterned, and there is a large body of knowledge about the various ways in which membership of particular social groups, makes people vulnerable to mental health problems. A groundbreaking example of this approach was Durkheim's scientific approach to the study of sociology, which to a significant extent, was based on his exploration of the types of social conditions which could be expected to generate high rates of suicide. Durkheim (1952) argued that the type of explanations of suicide which focused only upon inner emotional experiences or personal reasons were inadequate. Since suicide rates remained relatively stable in any given society from year to year, he concluded that suicide had an existence external to anyone instance of it. It was therefore possible to think of suicide as a social fact which needed to be explained in terms of other social facts.

Other more recent examples of the social causationist approach, which have used key social variables, include:

- *Social class:* Mental health is positively correlated with social class. The poorer people are, the greater the chances that they will be diagnosed as being mentally ill. The correlation indicates the increased probability of mental health problems with decreasing socio-economic status. The direction of causality in this association between poverty and severe mental health problems has been the subject of particular controversy. Social causationists argue that greater exposure to the environment and social stressors associated with poverty increases the incidence of mental health problems. By contrast, the social selection theory suggests that social class is affected by mental disorder. That is, mentally ill people 'drift' into poverty because their illness makes them socially incompetent. Some evidence of mental health problems. By contrast, the social selection theory suggests that social class is affected by mental disorder. That is, mentally ill people 'drift' into poverty because their illness makes them socially incompetent. Some evidence suggest that the validity of the different causal explanations may vary according to the type of mental health problem under investigation. Social causation may be stronger than social selection in explaining the inverse association of socioeconomic status to severe depression in women, substance abuse and antisocial personality in men; but, for those who carry a diagnosis of schizophrenia, social selection may be a more relevant explanation (Dohrenwend et al1992).
- *Gender:* The findings of community studies have been used to suggest that women experience relatively high rates of depression and other psychiatric disorders compared with men. Walter Gove and his colleagues focused on the higher rates among married women than men, and a number of studies since have identified difference in female rates compared with male (Kessler et al 1994). Gender differences have been attributed to a range of social, familial, personal and measurement artifact explanations. One of the most consistent findings is of a greater female prevalence of depressive disorder and 'nonspecific' psychological distress which has been explained with reference to adverse experiences in childhood and adolescence, sociocultural roles and psychological attributes with predispose individuals to negative life events (Nazroo at al 1998).

- *Race:* Mental health is racially patterned. Estimates from the UK suggest that the annual prevalence of hallucinations is higher in Caribbean than South Asian or White populations. This variation is accounted for with reference to cultural differences in experience and is not seen as invariably associated with psychosis (Johns et al 2002). In general terms, the racialization of psychiatric provision reflects continuing disadvantages that were rooted in slavery, enforced migration, colonialism and racial discrimination. For example in Australia aboriginal people are over represented in psychiatric populations. In the USA Black, Hispanic and Native American groups are over represented. In England Irish and Afro-Caribbean people are more likely to have mental health problems.
- *Age:* Certain problems emerge at different points in the lifespan. In old age, dementia increase in probability with time. A greater problem, though is depression. Twice as many old people are depressed than are dementing. The raised incidence of dementia is generally deemed to reflect an amplification of neurological deterioration that occurs with the ageing process. However, social factors are also implicated. The severity of symptoms in dementia is correlated with both social stimulation and with earlier educational experience. With regard to depression in old age, this has been accounted for by one or more combination of the following stressors; poverty, the distress of multiple physical illness, aggregating grief as peers die around survivors; under stimulating living conditions; and loss of control of the latter with enforced moves to hospitals, nursing homes or residential facilities. Severe mental health problems are also more likely to occur in young adulthood and late adolescence than in childhood and middle and later adulthood.
- *Victims of trauma:* People who have been sexually abused (in either childhood or later years) are more likely to develop mental health problems than those who are not sexually assaulted. Problems can emerge both in the immediate wake of the abuse and many years later. The correlation with diagnosis is important to note here. The over-representation of survivors of sexual abuse in a psychiatric population is accounted for by all diagnoses except schizophrenia, manic-depression and obsessive-compulsive disorder. Other sources of trauma that increase the probability of suffering from mental health problems include warfare, domestic violence, being a victim of urban crime, physical injury from accidents, and bereavement.

Because the above social groupings are not mutually exclusive, the social caustionist position inevitably leads to complex, multifactorial models of causation. Among other things, it would imply that the mental health of individuals and groups would be facilitated and maintained by interpersonal support throughout the lifespan and the avoidance of stressors such as poverty, sexism, trauma and racism.

Much of the research exploring social causes social causes has focused on factors external to the individual which emanate from the environmental or social context. This body of knowledge has emphasized mental ill health as a product of various forms of social stress, pressure or trauma, which have been accounted for by tracing antecedent social conditions. There is also interest in the reverse of this, i.e. the type of social conditions which protect, enhance or maintain positive mental health. Thus the social causationist position provides a framework for understanding the promotion of mental health in society, which is discussed in more detail below.

Structural Levels of Analysis in Social Causation

Causal factors and their relevant mechanisms are seen to operate at different levels. The more common analytical method associated with social causationism is some version of social or psychiatric epidemiology. Population or subpopulations (social groups) are studied in order to discover the distribution of first cases of mental ill health (incidence) and the aggregate of all diagnosed cases at a point in time (prevalence). In addition, the causal factors involved in variations in incidence or prevalence are proffered by researchers using this perspective.

Two broad conceptualization have underpinned structural approach to the study of social inequalities and mental health:social stratification and social class (Muntaner et al. 2000). Social stratification studies use measures of inequalities, which focus on disparities in social resources such as years of education, occupation and income (Bartley et al 1998). Social class tends to refer to people's class locations originating from ownership and control over different types of assets (e.g. property organization and credentials). Registrar General's classification of occupations using a classification of:

- Higher professional and managerial
- Lower professional technical and managerial
- Skilled-nonmanual workers and clerical workers
- Semi-skilled workers
- Unskilled workers.

Traditional 'Structural' approaches to mental health inequalities such as the community studies of the impact of the environment on mental health conducted in the 1950s and 1960s (e.g. Hollingshead & Redlich 1958, Myers & Bean 1968) suggested links between social conditions and disadvantage (e.g. unemployment, poverty and racism) and psychiatric morbidity. At the outbreak of the second world war, a prominent study based on social ecology (mental disorders in urban areas) was published by members of the Chicago School (Faris & Dunham 1939). In exploring the influence of poverty and deprivation, the authors contrasted the prevalence of manic-depressive psychosis, which appeared to be randomly distributed across the city of Chicago, with that of people diagnosed with schizophrenia, who were found predominantly in poorer areas.

More recent research has extended interest into exploring other dimensions and conditions produced by the social structure. The prevalence of mental disorder among women, and the impact of employment, unemployment and standard of living, point to the importance of macrostructural variables and environmental variables and environmental causes in determining mental health (Paykel 1991, Lewis 1998). There is some evidence which demonstrates that improvements in mental health can be achieved by changing the socio-structural environment. One of most obvious examples is the impact of employment and unemployment on mental health. Overall unemployment has been shown to have a negative effect on mental health at least in terms of depression. Suicide rates are higher among the unemployed (Platt et al 1992). There is also some indication that the mental health of the population can be improved by improvements to housing and the local area. For example, rehousing on the grounds of mental health has been shown to impact favorably on anxiety and depression (Elton & Packer 1986). Provision of financial resources and reconstruction of housing has been found to make a critical difference to recovery from mental health emergencies that arise from major disruption to or destruction of living environments (Wang et al 2000).

Psychosocial Level of Analysis

The psychosocial perspective refers to a number of related approaches which place greater emphasis on precipitating than on predisposing factors, and upon attempting a reduction of the prevalence rather than the incidence of mental health problems. The concept of stress provides a means of linking aspects of an individual's social situation with the occurrence or reoccurrence of mental ill health. The term 'stress' refers both to the characteristics of a person's circumstances (e.g. 'stressors', life events', 'stress situations') and responses that people make to those circumstances (stress reactions). Social stress theorists are also concerned with the distribution and deployment of coping resources (social support, self-esteem, a personal sense of control) and strategies (behavioral and cognitive devices to manage external and situational demands) among different groups in the populatin. Within this tradition, it is possible to distinguish between approaches which examine direct influences on psychological distress versus those where the focus is more indirect, e.g. when stress is expressed in health-damaging behavior such as violence or excessive consumption of alcohol and drugs (Elstad 1998). One of the most sophisticated developed theories of negative stressors in the life events model which encompasses the work of George Brown and his colleagues in relation to depression (Brown & Harris 1978). In mapping the social origin of depression, attention is drawn to three groups of interacting factors that produce depression: vulnerabiltity factors, provoking agents and symptom formation factors.

This research focuses on ongoing circumstances which were successful, and their model of depression incorporates the importance of both long-term difficulties and more temporary time-limited events.

While there has been a tendency in the past for researchers to focus on either the impact of macrostructural factors or the coping and responses of individuals to adverse events, there is a growing recognition of the need to view psychosocial influences as embeded in rather than separated out from material influences (Stansfield et al 1999). A link between agency and wider structural determinants of mental health is evident in a self-efficacy approach characterizing the work of a number of social sceientists interested in mental health (Mirowsky & Ross 1984, Pearlin 1989, Aneshensel 1992, Thoits 1995). Such studies have explored people's responsiveness to specific environmental opportunities and highlighted the effect of achievement of, or blocking of, personal goals on mental health. Thus, rather than viewing people as passive recipe-seeking and perceived control of the environment and opposite notions such as fatalism and powerlessness are viewed as important in relation to changing opportunity structures.

Labeling Theory

As mentioned above, most studies tracing the relationship between social disadvantage and mental illness implicitly accept the legitimacy of psychiatric knowledge, treating diagnostic categories, like 'depression' or 'schizophrenia'; as unproblematic and focusing on their links to social conditions. Labeling theorists and social constructionists on the other hand emphasize that mental health is negotiated and thus cannot be understood simply in terms of cause and effect relationships. Labeling theorists have tended to ignore the issue of cause altogether, while the constructionists have explored the epistemological assumptions of bodies of scientific knowledge and linked them to the way in which knowledge is constructed and shaped by a number of social influences and factors.

Labeling theory emanates from a version of sociology called 'symbolic interactionism', which is concerned with mapping ways in which social reality is negotiated. Emphasis is placed on the roles people take up and the meanings that are exchanged with others when occupying different roles. A failure to act appropriately in a role then becomes a critical point of understanding for those involved. Labeling theory has been adapted and applied to a wide set of social situations and social groups (e.g. schooling and education, crime and criminology) but it was developed most fully in relation to mental illness by Thomas Scheff in his book Being Mentally III (1966).

According to those emphasizing societal reaction (labeling theorists), mental health can have a variety of influences, including biological, psychological and social factors. However what labeling theorists are then keen to emphasize is that in certain situations rule breaking is accepted, ignored or 'normalized'; whereas at other times it is labeled as deviant. Once action is taken in the wake of this labeling it sets in chains, a process of negotiation about a deviant role. Under these circumstances, the labeled person starts to take on the role of being a mentally ill person. This role is maintained by the views of others and the new identity that the mentally ill person ascribes to herself.

The methodological emphasis of labeling theorists, as their name implies, is on investigating the process and consequences of labeling. Rather than what caused people to act oddly in the first place (primary deviance). The answer given is in terms of contingencies. That is the same behavior will be ignored in some circumstances, whereas in other circumstances it will provoke concerns and the need for expert help. The transition between these two sets of circumstances can be linked to either a one off crisis or a series of gradual shifts.

Labeling theorists have pointed out that a deviant role can emerge either rapidly or following a lengthy period when oddity is present but a problem is denied. More recent evidence suggests that auditory hallucinations are widespread in community samples, and that voice hearers who have not been diagnosed as suffering from schizophrenia have various ways of living with the experience (Epstein et al 2002, Jones et al 2003).

Of great interest to labeling theorists are the circumstances under which primary deviance is confirmed and amplified by contact with professionals and lay people. Relatives or other 'significant others' change from tolerating, denying or ignoring problem behavior and begin to acknowledge its existence. Those who are more relationally distant are more willing to identify and attach a label of mental illness. Mental illness is recognized in families before professionals are invited to rubber stamp this lay decision-making. The combination of labeling from professional and significant others defines the deviant person in a new role: of psychiatric patient. The final phase of the process entails the labeled person accepting or internalizing the ascribed deviant identity. Mental hospitalization strips them of their old identity in what Goffmann calls a 'status degradation ceremony' and is replaced by a new identity and social role. Being a patient can then become a 'Career'.

While generally a deviant role takes a while to emerge and to be confirmed and internalized, there has been some experimental evidence that it can occur very rapidly. For example, in one study, confederate 'pseudopatients' were admitted to psychiatric facilities by presenting with isolated auditory hallucinations. In all other respects, the confederates did not act oddly once admitted. Despite this, the psychiatric staff treated them as if they were mentally ill and reframed their actions in this light. For example, when the confederates were seen keeping field notes, their actions were recorded as 'indulges in writing behavior' (Rosenhan 1973).

Modified Labeling Theory

A more recent derivative of these original ideas is modified labeling theory, which emphasizes a causal role for sigma in the 'relapse' of episodes of mental distress, linked to negative outcomes in employment and social functioning. Stigma can be defined as constituting three elements.

1. A label that separates a person from others.
2. The linking of the marked person to undesirable characteristics.
3. The rejection and avoidance of the stigmatized person by others.

Rejection may be experienced in a range of areas such as employment and housing, through to everyday slights and minor insults. Stigma has been found to be highly prevalent among people labeled with a serious mental health problem living in the community (Link et al 1997). The effects of labeling are mediated by social psychological mechanisms in which both former psychiatric patients and members of the general population internalize negative cultural conceptions and attitudes about people who have been diagnosed with a mental illness, leading to personal discrimination. For many fomer psychiatric patients a negative self concept emerges from a combination of their primary disability and from the cumulative reaction of others. Social rejection is an ongoing and recursive experience in the community setting and a persistent form of social stress for discharged patients. Experiences of social rejection increase feelings of self-deprecation, which act to weaken a sense of mastery and self control (Barham & Haywood 1991) and exposure to stigmatizing everyday experience from postinstitutional living (e.g. negative or avoidance attitudes from others) constitutes a source of significant and recurrent stress. This has long-term implications a source of significant for a person's ability to function fully in society. An ethnographic study has showng how the expectations and avoidance of stigma leads to restricted social networks among former psychiatric patients (Estroff 1981).

Social Constructionism

One of the most influential theoretical positions evident in the sociology of health and illness in recent years has been social constructionism. Three main current within social constructionism can be identified:

1. The first approach has most affinity with labeling theory as it not concerned with demonstrating the reality or otherwise of social phenomena but with the social forces which define them. This might involve investigation of a social problem, such as drug abuse or mental illness, in terms of exploring the lived experience of social actors in 'deviant' communities or those working with and labeling them.

2. The second approach is more influenced by the post-structuralism of Foucault and is concerned with deconstruction, which is the critical examination of language and symbols in order to illuminate the creation of knowledge, its relationship to power and the unstable varieties of reality which attend human activity-discursive practices.
3. The third approach is concerned with understanding the production of scientific knowledge and the pursuit of individual and collective professional interests (Latour 1987) or interest work. In contrast to the poststructuralist emphasis upon idea, emphasis is placed more on action and negotiation.

Despite their difference, certain core themes can be detected across these three types:

1. Reality is problematized to some degree.
2. Scientific and other realities are viewed wholly or partly as a product of human activity.
3. Power relationships are inextricably bound up with the ways in which reality is defined.

In relation to the field of mental health, the social constructionist position goes further than that put forward by the labeling theorists. It also interested in the categories used to describe or account for primary deviance. It is concerned with understanding the ways in which concepts, constructs or representations about mental health emerge as products of communal exchange between social groups. There is a particular emphasis within this approach on analyzing dominant professional representations and the interest that are served by them. Thus, the method of investigation associated with social constructionism is deconstruction or discourse analysis. Accordingly, social constructionists emphasize that reality (about mental health or anything else) is socially constructed and thus bound up with the material and cognitive interests of social groups. This contrasts with the position of social causationists, which is that there is a stable reality that exists independently of the investigator (*Realism or Positivism)*. The social constructionist is interested in examining how variations in human experience and conduct come to be represented as illness categories and how diagnoses inscrible a version of some people but not others.

Some Examples from Social Constructionism

Social constructionists researching mental health have made two main critical points. The first is that concepts (or constructs) that are fragile, incoherent, illogical or invalid may still survive or may even be actively promoted in society. The second point they make is that constructs serve the interests of the social groups utilizing them (e.g. mental health professionals, relatives of identified patients, drug companies). Here are some examples from the field of mental health:

- Constructionists problematize the factual status of mental illness (e.g. Szasz 1961). They analyze the ways in which mental health work has been linked to the production of psychiatric knowledge. Schizophrenia has the status of an illness and yet the diagnosis lacks both conceptual validity and reliability. Two people with different symptoms can both be diagnosed as schizophrenic–it is a disjunctive construct. Despite large amounts of research funding over the past hundred years for investigations that have tested a variety of environmental and biological hypotheses, the etiology of the disease remains highly contested. There is no biological marker (analogs to a blood test to diagnose diabetes) for schizophrenia. One possible explanation for the continuation of a weak construct is the role its play in supporting the mandate of psychiatry in society and the comfort it gives to the relatives of mad people.
- Agoraphobia emerged at the time when the social emancipation of women became a possibility. For this reason, the meaning of the condition can be understood as part of a context that problematized the use of public space, not just as a set of symptoms within its individual sufferers. Here de Swann (1990:144) makes this points.
- The way in which psychiatric knowledge about women is generated is, according to some feminist scholars, imbued with sexual role stereotypes and notions of female inferiority. These points are made contentiously in the work of Ehrenreich and English. Their key argument is that male doctors have historically defined women's problems as illness or sickness and have promoted a notion of femininity which itself is viewed as pathological. This combination has resulted in female dependence on male experts and in lives of inactivity.
- Like schizophrenia, the concept or psychopathy is incoherent because it covers so many people who have different symptoms but can share the same label and has no biological marker. The definition is invevitably circular. People are deemed to be psychopathic because of their antisocial acts and their antisocial acts are explained by the actor's psychopathy. As a consequence, there is no independent way of validating the diagnosis. It has the same explanatory value as the notion of evil. Given the evil has been medicalized, the deconstructionist would be interested in the social history of this professional interest in certain types of antisocial action.
- Depression seems to be a straightforward description of depressed mood. However, ascriptions of helplessness, powerlessness and worthlessness can only be made in relation to interpersonal processes. Thus depression cannot be understood simply as a set affective and cognitive characteristics of suffering individuals – it is defined and constituted by social processes.

These are some specific examples of how psychiatric diagnoses might be understood within a social constructionist framework. Some deconstructionists, like Szasz, have argued that the whole body of knowledge that follows from a commitment to the notion of mental illness has arisen in order to ensure t he individual and collective advancement of psychiatric professionals and to protect the social order. In this way, he argues, professional knowledge, professional advancement, and social control are intimately entwined. Other deconstructionists, such as Rose, extending the work of Foucault, go further and argue that voluntary therapies that are anxiously sought and gratefully received by clients also contribute to social order via self-surveillance and the individualization of distress.

Mental Health in Society

Having outlined the three perspectives on the social in discussions about mental health, we will now discuss some wider issues about mental health in society.

Mental Health or Mental Illness?

Both professionals and lay people have a disproportionate interest in mental abnormality or illness. This in itself is a social phenomenon. The term 'mental health' in recent years has come to be used throughout western societies as a substitute for its opposite (mental illness). For example, it is common place now to hear terms such as mental health policy' or mental health facilities; which are actually euphemisms that refer to the management of mental abnormally in society.

Difficulties in Articulating Mental Healthiness

While the term 'mental health' has become a more acceptable substitute for 'mental illness' it has remained relatively under developed as a concept (Jahoda1958). Neither professional nor lay people have a well-proven facility for discussing mental health.

Sociologists point out that we are generally asked to produce accounts for others when things go wrong. We tend not to explain how things go right. For example, if a rule is broken, a convention breaks down, or a person acts out of character or out of role, explanations are expected. These explanations may be invited from the people acting in an odd way, those who witness the events, or those who are responsible for formally recognizing and managing their consequence. By contrast, when life goes smoothly with no rule infraction and people acting in the way they expert of others and themselves, there are few calls for explanation. As a consequence of this difference between the two conditions, we become much more skilled at articulating reasons for abnormal than for normal phenomena in everyday life. It seems that people expect negative emotions to be part of everyday life, and separating, the negative from the positive aspects of mental health does not relate easily to everyday experience. Additionally, while the 'mind' is meaningful to people, it is not as readily described as the body (Rogers & Pilgrim 1997).

Professionals and Interprofessional Relationships

Attempts to understand mental health professionals have drawn upon a number of theoretical strands from within the sociology of the professions.

Durkheimian Tradition

Durkheim and structural functionalists (e.g. Talcott Parsons) have viewed professional groups as providing a disinterested and integrative societal function which counter balanced the tendency of egotistical individuals to fragment society. From this perspective professions are a source of community for one another and stability for the wider society they serve. They regulate their own practices and practitioners (through, e.g. 'peer review') and ensure good practice though the setting of codes of conduct and punishing errant colleagues. Following of this approach to the sociology of profession have tended to take claims of special knowledge and altruism at face value and have focused on categorizing professions in terms of traits and descriptions of their work.

Weberian Tradition

The Weberian framework stresses the development of professional strategies to advance their own social status, persuade clients about the need for the service they offer and corner the market in a service sector in away that excludes competitors. From this perspective two aspects are particularly noteworthy: collective social advancement rests upon social closure, and professionals exercise power over others through *professional dominance.* Social closure refers to a situation where a monopoly is gained to work in a specialized way with a particular group so that other occupational groups seeking a similar role are excluded. In order for professionals to maintain their social status they must convince those outside their boundaries that they are offering a unique service, and as a consequence they develop various rhetorical devices to persuade the outside world of their unique and special qualities. To do this, they need to justify a peculiar knowledge-base that has a technical rationality that is not easily understood or deployed by competitors.

Professional dominance refers to the exercising of power over others in three senses:

1. Professions have power over their clients. An imbalance of specialized knowledge keeps the user in a state of ignorance, insecurity and vulnerability. This imbalance is reinforced by professionals to operate within their own

territory rather than that of their clients (e.g. treatment in hospital rather than in the client's own home).

2. Professionals exercise power over their new recruits (e.g. trainers are dependent on their superiors for career progression).
3. Professionals seek to establish a dominant relationship of other occupational groups with the same client group.

Interprofessional Relations

The shifting location of mental health services has had a major impact on how professionals organize their work and the way in which they relate to patients and each other. The territorial base of the asylum and hospital has to a large extent been replaced by the need to negotiate one-to-one relationships in a domestic or community context. Mental health workers have been faced with the need to change their working practices and the way in which they interact. In particular, work outside the hospital has brought with it a philosophy of multidisciplinary working, which had already operated, in theory at least, in inpatient setting. The basic tenets of multidisciplinary working are:

- That each member of the mental health team has special skill to contribute to the management to patients.
- That these are contributed in co-operation and liaison with other mental health workers
- That this leads to the establishment of corporate consensual goals in delivering a service.

Difficulties in ensuring multidisciplinay co-operation and corporate goal achievement stem from the differing secondary socalisation and training of mental health workers. Unidisciplinary groupings tend to emphasize the status, training levels and accreditation of their own group as their contribution to improving service quality, whereas multidisciplinary commitment to practice guidelines to standardize best practice and outcome tends to be less supported.

Team work poses a problem for professionals around role and identity once they have been fully socialized into distinct professional groupings, as suggested by Onyett et al (1994). The concentration of practitioner into teams places professional workers in a special dilemma. They become members of two groups: their profession and their team. As a result they may find themselves torn between the aims of a community mental health movement that explicitly values egalitarianism, role blurring and a surrender of power to lower status workers and service users on the one hand, and a desire to hold on to tradionally, socially valued role definitions and practice on the other (Onyett et al 1994). As well as competing professional interests, knowledge claims about mental health are varied and to some extent reflect different ideologies and values.

Social and Cultural Influences on Models of Illness and Management of Mental Health Problems

Cross-cultural and historical evidence suggests that notions of mental distress and madness are prevalent in all societies. The following points can be made to support this conclusion.

- In the prepsychiatric times of ancient Rome and Athens, madness was documented as being associated with aimless wandering and violence.
- In more recent times, people living in societies such as Laos, which had neither mental hospitals nor psychiatric professionals, still provided accounts of madness.
- In localities without mental institutions, very clear conceptual distinctions are made by lay people about sanity and insanity.
- Whereas there are differences between cultures about how sadness, fear and madness are represented and explained, all societies, now and in the past, have provided descriptions of these emotional and behavioral phenomena, put differently, anxiety, depression and psychosis may be products of modern western psychiatry, but fear, sadness and madness are not.

Nonetheless, criteria used to judge both the cause and presence of mental illness can be rendered problematic, if understood in their social context. Turning to mental health, social relativism appears immediately. Some notions in everyday use about mental health are only meaningful to people in cultures that contain and appreciate psychoanalysis or humanistic psychology. Resistance to stress is superficially appealing as a definition of mental health but what of those people who are unperturbed by stress? Many psychiatrists would describe these as 'primary psychopaths'. As for autonomy, what of people who are compulsively independent and avoid social relationships? Competence is not an invariant capacity but relies for its definition on value judgments made in a specific social setting about conformity to expectations of roles and rules. The social context also determines whose judgment prevails about the competence of others. Finally judgements about accurate perception of reality are social judgments. Hearing voices, or seeing things others cannot, may be deemed to be symptomatic of schizophrenia in another.

Mental Health Services in the Social Context

The discussion above has mainly focused on the relationship between society and forms of knowledge about mental health. Societal influences are also relevant when we come to understand the provision of mental health services. The notion of 'mental health services' is actually quite recent. Up until the first part of the 20th century, there were only hospitals, clinics and asylums. The notion of 'services' has replaced these individual descriptions of facilities in the last fifty years.

The way in which the modern general hospital has been depicted provides a benchmark with which both the old asylum system and the new arrangements for delivering psychiatric services in a postasylum era can be compared. The modern hospital, with its high technology equipment, elaborate procedures and specialized skills has frequently been viewed as an outcome of 'scientific developments' and medical progress over the last century (Tuckett 1976). This assumption has led a number of sociologists to comment that the modern hospital is an example of Max Weber's notion of a 'bureaucratic organization'. Sociologists of organizations have identified characteristics of the 'typical' modern hospital that have been influenced by Webers ideal type. Perrow (1995), a systems analyst, identified three factors which determine the way in which organizations functions.

- The cultural system which sets the legitimate or formal goals
- Technology which is the means of achieving these goals in the hospital this includes the types of therapeutic techniques in use
- The structure of organization in which techniques are embedded and person power is organized as a means of achieving the set goals.

Asylum System

During the 19th century in western Europe and North America, most countries developed centrally regulated asylum systems. The emergence of large asylums in most localities was associated with the need to control non-productive deviance in increasingly urbanized and complex capitailist societies. In other words, economic life was disrupted or impaired by madness ('lunatics' or 'dements') and by those with learning difficulties ('aments'). Both of these groups were 'warehoused' in asylums to remove their negative impact on socio-economic order and efficiency, just as orphans, the physically sick and the elderly were placed in poor houses. Professionals at that time took little or no interest in sane people who were frightened or sad (the neuroses). This changed after the first world war, when the 'shell shock' problem altered the focus of professional interest. Warfare ensured that stress-induced problems, later to be called 'battle neurosis' or 'post-traumatic stress disorder', recurringly shifted professional attention away from madness and toward neurosis during the 20th century. This also expanded the range of interventions offered or preferred by professionals to include talking treatments. As result, psychiatric treatment became more eclectic, although it remained dominated by biomedical interventions.

During periods of peacetime, the focus on madness returned, along with biological treatments in institutional settings. After the second world war, the old asylum system came into crisis for a number of reasons.

- The expansion of the remit of psychiatry and its associated professions to include talking treatments with neurotic patients in community settings, increased expectations that mental health services should shift away from biomedical treatments inside institutions.
- In the wake of the widespread cultural shuck of the Nazi concentration camps, western liberal democracies witnessed a popular disquiet about segregation. Also, lessons about the disabling impact of institutionalization (institutional neurosis) were drawn from observation in the camps of ritualised, rigid and stereotyped behavior of their inmates.
- Large institutions were expensive and placed a large fiscal burden upon government budgets. Deinstitutionalization offered itself as a cost-cutting exercise.
- Doubts about institutional life were reinforced by researches its negative impact from social psychiatry, sociology, and from dissent within clinical psychiatry (antipsychiatry).
- A new social movement of mental health service users that was critical of hospital based biomedical regimens emerged internationally.

Contemporary Organization of Psychiatry

At the end of the 20th century, deinstitutionalization had become a dominant mental health policy goal in most western democracies. However, this formal goals has become clouded by evidence that the gradual reduction of large institutions has been replaced by a scattering of smaller ones 'in the community'. Also, most countries still have legal statutes to coercively remove madness from community settings. The extent of this continued coercive control varies from one country to another. For example, more conformist or authoritarian cultures such as Japan or Russia have higher rates of involuntary detention in psychiatric facilities. What is clear is that a policy of deinstitutionalization and one of genuine community care are not the same. Currently, it may be more accurate to talk of 'reinstitutionalization' as the actual outcome of large hospital closures rather than 'community care'.

There has been greater attention paid to considering the cause and solution of mental health problems within a public health context in which problem management stretches beyond the structural and organizational arrangements of traditional health services. A multisectoral approach to mental health is outlined in the Government's Green paper *our Healthier Nation* (1998) in which effective policy responses to mental health problems are viewed as implicating local and central players, community resources, the environment and individual action. Thus the focus has moved, at the level of policy at least, to incorporating aspects of employment and individual action. Thus the focus has moved, at the level of policy at least, to incorporating aspects of employment, social community and voluntary organizations in the prevention and management of mental health problems. New technologies and information systems have also led to fundamental changes and diversification in the availability of mental health technologies. For example, self-management for mental health problems is increasingly being seen as a means of making psychological therapies more widely available to those with mind mental stress. A key aspect of the philosophy of such therapy relates to increasing the patient's self-efficacy, and the locus of facilitation is on increasing patients feelings of confidence in using the technology of self-help. Much of self-management takes place within the person's own environment and is increasingly distanced from the place of professionally delivered services. One of the most important consequences of new technologies such as the internet is the rapid increase it allows in mutual non-professional support. The anonymous helper in an electronic conference or the support group on the web provides the basis of a revolution in mental health support that has emerged as an unpredicted and major element in the global organization of mental healthcare.

Gradient of Coercion Operating in Mental Health

The growing eclecticism of psychiatric provision is accompanied by differentiation in levels of coercion. The coercive role of psychiatric service in response to certain types of social crisis and deviance has been a salient feature of sociological analysis about psychiatry (e.g. the work of Szasz, Laing, Scull and Goffmann). Collectively, this body of work suggests that the function of psychiatry is different from other branches of medicine. In psychiatric services, the over representation of people from a lower social class and some ethnic minorities in coercive contexts is not about meeting need in the same way that health services respond to physical problems. In other words, the assumptions of the 'inverse care law' (Tudor Hart 1971) are not directly applicable. (The law is the notion that access to care has a tendency to increase with increasing class status, with the poorest people tending to get the poorest health care).

In psychiatric services, involuntary detention and treatment are explicit and operational features. A proportion of patients are forcibly detained and treated by the use of therapeutic law; some are notionally voluntary but de facto detainees, and others are genuinely voluntary patients but are in a service context where the threat of coercion is ever present. In the light of these peculiar features about psychiatry, mental health management can be conceptualized as part of a wider state apparatus which controls the social problems associated with poverty and the underclass. Once conceived in this way, a unitary view of service contact as necessarily aiming for or achieving a gain in the mental health status of service recipients is rendered problematic.

Of course not all service provision is coercive to the same degree, but a graduated system of control operating in services is a relevant consideration in making judgements about the extent to which services meet need (Rogers & Pilgrim 2003). For example, some wards are locked in open psychiatric units (intensive care units) and some hospital hold patients in conditions of 'medium security'. Others contain mentally diorderd offenders in high security conditions. Outside of acute inpatient provision and forensic services the coercive/ social control function is lessened and the use of services is more akin to those for patients with physical conditions. However, even in primary care, the GP acts as a second option 'medical practitioner in supporting applications for involuntary detention in hospital. This may mean that the possibility of compulsion and the stigma attached to secondary services may impact on the willingness to access and utilize primary-care services (Rogers et al 2001).

Nevertheless, overall, primary care is less coercive than other parts of the mental health system and is principally influenced by patients' decision-making about when and how to access services. It is also the area where the social contract in providing a national health service free at the point of need in most meaningful, given the direct access that it, permits to citizens. The emergence of voluntary organizations, the increase of private practice and user led services and self-management are significant changes in the pattern of service provision. The utilization of nonstate employees in the delivery of services also changes the nature of service delivery. The rise of self-employed primary-care counselors trained outside mainstream. State provided higher education for health professionals in an example here. Users have taken on roles previously monopolized by mental health professional both in the provision of user-led schemes (e.g. crises houses) and in increasingly using self-care options which is as discussed in the previous section, emphasize the centrality of self efficacy and the patient as change agent.

The impact of the entanglement of control and coercion in mental health care is compounded when psychiatric service contact with key marginal social groups is involved.

Racism and Contact with Psychiatry

Cultural analysis (analysis of differences in language, values, norms and beliefs) focuses on the individual or their culture and is concerned mainly with examining the role of prejudice and discrimination in determining differences in health behavior and the use of services. 'Prejudice' implies a psychological concept in that it refers to a set of personal attitudes. Transcultural psychiatry, e.g. is concerned with how different ethnic groups are treated by mental health workers socialized in the ways of the 'dominant culture' (Rack

1982, Fernando 1988). This position advocates initiatives aimed at challenging and changing prejudices through 'race awareness' training. This works on the premise of challenging the stereotypical and negative views about minority ethnic groups held by powerful individuals, like professionals. However, what tends to be missing from analyses based on prejudice is a consideration of the impact of inequality how the latter is manifested in mental illness rates, services and professional responses to black and other minority groups. In contrast to prejudice, racism implies a sociological rather than a psychological analysis and emphasizes the roles of institutions in perpetuating disadvantage and the need to combat institutional racism through antiracism measures.

Afro-Caribbean people are much more likely than white people to make contact with mental health service via the police, courts and prison and once contact has been made, there is evidence of their over-representation in compulsory admission and in receiving a diagnosis of schizophrenia compared with white people (Bhui et al. 1995). At the other end of the spectrum, there is evidence to suggest that black people are under-represented in outpatient and self referred services ands less likely than other groups to be referred by general practitioners (e.g. Harrison et al. 1988).

The pathways by which young black men come to the attention of mental health services have led some commentators to suggests that the 'criminalization' and medicalization of black people are closely connected processes which implicate psychiatry as part of a larger social control apparatus which regulates and overses the lives of black people (Francis 1988). The multiple contacts, judgments and processes which are involved in referral to psychiatric services may also imply a process of 'transmitted discrimination' in which contingencies and the subtle discriminatory acts and views may be transferred from one agency to another. Differences in the processes of referral, labeling and help-seeking are all likely to be implicated. Black people may express their distress at times in a culturally idiosyncratic way. Much of the psychiatric literature suggests that the manifestation of 'mental illness' predisposes Afro-Caribbeans towards police arrest because they present in a particularly disturbed way, and the place in which behavior takes place is also deemed to be important. Bean (1986) suggests that if a greater part of young Afro-Caribbean social life takes place in public, then 'mad' behavior is more likely to be detected and dealt with by agents such as the police, than is the case of white people, who have more of an 'indoor culture'. The tendency to label a person mentally ill increases with the cultural distance between the labeler and labeled, suggesting that members of minority ethnic groups are more likely to be labeled mentally ill than dominant indigenous groups by members of the public as well as by professionals.

Gender and Sexuality

The psychiatric response of sexuality has changed according to changes in treatment philosophies and norms and values associated with homosexuality. In the 19th century the assumed biological determination of homosexuality led not to active physical intervention (as with other types of madness) but with fatalism to a 'problem behavior' which prompted little therapeutic interest (Diamont 1987). It was only when psychoanalytical and the behavioral therapeutic methods were introduced during the 20th century that psychiatrists began to interfere with homosexuality and aspire to 'cure' the condition. The optimism of these newer environment/psychological theories prompted professionals to be more interventionist. In relation to contemporary treatments and contact with services, a recent study of therapist attitudes to gay clients suggests that many therapists do not see social and gay and lesbian identity as relevant to the therapeutic process and that gay and lesbian mental health users may still encounter overt and covert bias which includes the pathologization of homosexuality (Bartlett et al 2001).

It is likely that internalized stigmatized identities reinforce the biases of mental health professionals and therapies. For example, if gay and lesbian people have been socialized into accepting the bias in society against them, they may be more inclined to collude with ill advised therapeutic efforts to modify sexual orientation. Negative stereotypes about sexuality may then be reinforced by therapists who share them and who fail to acknowledge them as indications of homophobia. However, it is also the case that changing norms about the acceptability of homosexuality in wider society are also reflected in psychiatry. For example the Royal College of Psychiatrists established a Gay and Lesbian Mental Health Special Interest Group in 2001.

SUGGESTED READING

1. Dohrenwend BP. A psychosocial perspective in the past and future of psychiatric epidemiology. American Journal of Epidemiology. 1998;147(3):222-9.
2. Dohrenwend BP, Dohrenwent BS. Perspectives on the past and future of psychiatric epidemiology. American Journal of Public Health. 1982;72:1271-9.
3. Dohrenwend BP, Brice P, Levar I, et al. Socioeconomic status and psychiatric disorders: the causation selection issue. Science. 1992;255:946-51.
4. Durkheim E. Suicide: A Study in Sociology. Routledge & Kegan Paul, London, 1952.
5. Elstad JI. The Psycho-social perspective on social inequalities in health. Sociology of Health and Illness. 1998;20(5):598-618.
6. Elton PJ, Parker JM. A prospective randomised trial of value of re-housing on the grounds of mental ill-health. Journal of Chronic Disease. 1986;39:221-7.

7. Enhrenreich B, English D. For her own good: 150 years of the experts advice to women, Pluto, London, 1978.
8. Eptein RM, Bonell F, Visser A. Hearing voices: patient centred care with diverse populations. Patient Education & Counselling. 2002;48:1-3.
9. Estroff S. Making it crazy: an ethnography of psychiatric clients in an American community. University of California Press, Berkeley, 1981.
10. Faris RE, Dulnham HW. Mental disorders in urban areas: an ecological study of schizophrenia and other psychoses. University of Chicago Press, Chicago, 1939.
11. Fernando S. Race and culture in psychiatry. Tavistock / Routledge, London, 1988.
12. Foucault M. Madness and civilization. Random House, New Work, 1965.
13. Francis E. Black people, dangerousness and psychitric compulsion. In: Brackx A, Grimshow C (Eds). Mental health care in crisis, Pluto, London, 1988.
14. Goffmann E. Asylums. Penguin, Harmondsworth, 1961.
15. Goldberg D, Huxley P. Mental Illness in the Community. Tavistock, London, 1980.
16. Gove W. The relationship between sex roles, marital status and mental illness; Social Forces. 1972;51:33-44.
17. Gove W, Tudor JF. Adult sex roles and mental illness. American Journal of Socialogy. 1972;78:812-35.
18. Harrison G, Owens D, Holton A, et al. A prospective study of severe mental disorder in Afro-Caribbean patients. Psychological Medicine. 1988;11:289-302.
19. Hollingshead A, Redlich RC. Social Class and Mental Illness. Wiley, New York, 1958.
20. Huxley P, Rogers A. Urban regeneration and mental health. Health Variations. 2001;7(April):8-9.
21. Jahoda M. Current Concepts of Positive Mental Health. Basic Books, New York, 1985.
22. Johns LC, Nazroo JY, Bebbington P, Kuipers E. Occurrence of hallucinatory experiences in a community sample and ethnic variations. British Journal of Psychiatry. 2002;180:174-8.
23. Jones S, Guy A, Pramod JA. A methodological study of hearing voices: a preliminary exploration of voice hearers and understanding of their experiences. Psychology & Psychotherapy. 2003;76:189-209.
24. Kessler RC, McGonagel KA, Zhai S, et al. Lifetime and 12 month prevalence of DSM-III – R psychiatric disorders in the United States. Archives of General Psychiatry. 1994;51:8-19.
25. Latour B. Science in action: how to follow scientist and engineers through society. Cambridge, MA: Harvard University Press, 1987.
26. Lemert E. Huan deviance, social problems and social control. Prentice Hall, Englewood Cliffs, NJ, 1967.
27. Lewis G, Bebbington P, Brugha T, et al. Socioeconomic status standard of living and neurotic disorder. Lancet. 1998;352: 605-9.
28. Link BG, Struening EL, Rahav M, et al. On stigma and its consequences: evidence from a longitudinal study of men with dual diagnoses of mental illness and substance abuse. Journal of Health and Social Behaviour. 1997;38:177-90.
29. Miller P, Rose N. The Tavistock programme: the government of subjectivity and social life. Sociology. 1988;22(2):171-92.
30. Mirowsky J, Ross CE. Mexican culture and is emotion contradictions. Journal of Health and Social Behaviour. 1984; 25(1):2-13.
31. Muntaner C, Eaton WW, Chamberlam CD. Social inequalities in mental health: a review of concepts and underlying assumptions. Health. 2000;4(1):89-109.
32. Myers J, Bean L. A decade later: a follow up social class and mental illness. Wikey, New York, 1968.
33. Nazroo JV, Edwards AC, Brown GW. Gender differences in the prevalence of depression: artefact, alternative disorders, biology or roles? Sociology of Health and Illness. 1998;20(3): 312-30.
34. Onyett S, Heppleston T, Bushnell D. A national survey of community mental health team structure and process. Journal of Mental Health. 1994;3:175-94.
35. Parsons T. The social system. Routledge & Kegan Paul, London, 1951.
36. Paykel ES. Depression in women. British Journal of Psychiatry. 1991;158(Suppl 10):22-9.
37. Pearlin LI. The sociological study of stress. Journal of Health and Soacil Behavior. 1989;30(3):241-56.
38. Perrow C. Hospitals: technology, structure and goals. In: March JG (Ed). Handbook of Organisations. Rand McNally, Chicago, 1965.
39. Pilgrim D, Rogers A. A Sociology of Mental Health and Illness, 2nd edn. Open University Press, Milton Keynes, 1999.
40. Platt S, Micciolo R, Tansella M. Suicide and unemployement in Italy: description analysis and interpretation of recent trends. Social Science and Medicine. 1992;34(11):1191-1201.
41. Rack P. Race, culture and mental disorder. Tavistock, London, 1982.
42. Rogers A, Pilgrim D. The contribution of lay knowledge to the understanding and promotion of mental health. Journal of Mental Health. 1997;6(1):23-5.
43. Rogers A, Pilgrim D. Mental health policy Britain, 2nd edn. Palgrave, Basingstoke, 2001.
44. Rogers A, Pilgrim D. Mental Health and inequality. Palgrav, Basingstoke, 2003.
45. Rogers A, May C, Oliver D. Experiencing depression, experiencing the depressed: the management of depression in primary care. Journal of Mental Health. 2001;10(3):317-33.
46. Rose N. Governing the soul. Routledge, London, 1990.
47. Rosenhan DL. On being sane in insane places. Science. 1973; 179:250-8.
48. Scheff T. Being mentally ill: a sociological theory. Aldine, Chicago, 1966.
49. Scull A. Decareeration: community treatment and the deviant – a radical view. Prentice – Hall, Englewood Cliffs, NJ, 1977.
50. Scull A. Museums of madness, Penguin, Harmondsworth, 1979.

51. Stansfield S A, Fuhrer R, Cattell V, et al. Psychosocial factors and the explanation of socio-economic gradients in common mental disorders. Health variations 4: 4-5. ESRC, Lancaster, 1999.
52. Stansfield SA, Marmot MG. Social class and minor psychiatric disorders in British Civil service: a validated screening survey using the General Health Questionnare. Psychological Medicine. 1992;22:739-49.
53. Stone M. Shell shock and the psychologists. In Bynum WF, Porter R (Eds). The anatomy of madness. Tavistock, London, 1985.
54. Szasz TS. The uses of naming and the origin of the myth of mental illness. American Psychologist. 1961;16:59-65.
55. Thoits PA. Self-labeling process in mental illness: the role of emotional deviance. American Journal of Sociology. 1995;91:221-49.
56. Thoits PA. Stress, coping and social support processes: where are we - what next',. Journal of Health and Social Behaviour. 1995;(extra issuse): 53-79.
57. Tuckett D. The organisation of hospitals. In: Tuckett D (Ed). An introduction to medical sociology. Tavistock, London, 1976.
58. Tudor - Hart J. The inverse care law. Lancet. 1971;(7696): 405-12.
59. Wang X, Gao L, Shinfuku N, et al. Longtitudinal study of eartquake related PTSD in a randomly selected community sample in North China. American Journal of Psychiatry. 2000;157(8):1260-6.
60. Warner R. Recovery from schizophrenia. Psychiatry and Political Economy. Routledge, London, 1985.
61. Wilkinson RG. Unbealthy societies: the afflictions of inequalities. Routledge, London, 1996.
62. Yarrow MJ, Schwartz G, Murphy H, Deasy I. The psychological meaning of mental illness. Journal of Social Issues. 1955;11: 12-24.
63. Aneshensel CS. Social stress theory and research. Annual Review of Sociology. 1992;18:15-38.
64. Barham P, Haywood R. From the mental patient to the person. Routledge, London, 1991.
65. Bartlett A, King M, Philips I. Straight talking: an investigation of the attitudes and practice of psychoanalysts and psychotherapists in relation to gays and lesians. British Journal of Psychiaatry. 2001;179:545-9.
66. Hartley M, Blane' D, Davey-Smith G. Beyond the Black Report. Sociology of Health and Illness. 1998;20(5):563-77.
67. Bean P. Mental disorder and social control. Cambridge University Press, Cambridge. 1986.
68. Bhaskar R. Reclaiming reality. Verso, London, 1989.
69. Bhui K, Chirstie Y, Bhugra D. The essential elements of culturally. Sensitive psychiatric services. International Journal of Social Psychiatry. 1995;41(4):246-56.
70. Brown GW, Harris TO. Social origins of depression: a study of Psychiatric disorder in women. Tavistock, London, 1978.
71. Clegg SR. Modern organisations. Sage, London, 1990.
72. De Swann A. The management of normality. Routledge, London Diamont L. 1987 Male and female homosexuality: psychological approches. Hemisphere, New York, 1990.

CHAPTER 52

Mental Health Issues in Women

SC Malik

'If you want to know more about femininity, enquire from your own experiences of life or turn to the poets or wait until Science can give you deeper and more coherent information'.[1]

The far-reaching differences between men and women have inspired curiosity, poetry, romance and polemics for centuries, but only recently have they been the subject of scrutiny by medical and social scientists. Earlier, social lives of men and women used to be more predictable, fitted as they were in stereotyped roles. With society in transition, options expanded for both sexes, and men and women began to vary more in their roles, attitudes and behaviors.

What are women's health issues? The following definition was developed by Public Health Task Force on Women's health in USA.[2]

- Diseases or conditions unique to women or some subgroups of women.
- Diseases or conditions more prevalent in women or some subgroups of women.
- Diseases or conditions more serious among women or some subgroups of women.
- Diseases or conditions, for which the risk factors are different for women or some subgroups of women.
- Diseases or conditions, for which the interventions are different for women or some subgroups of women.

Women live longer than men. At every point of development, females live longer and maintain a biological advantage over males. Mortality is higher for males at all ages and there are more men in all leading causes of death. However, health statistics regarding morbidity show higher rates for acute conditions and nonfatal chronic diseases for women. They also have more short-term disability, medical service use and medical drug use.

While mortality is higher in men, chronic conditions like rheumatoid arthritis, SLE, autoimmune liver disease and minor psychiatric morbidity are more prevalent in women. Further, perhaps due to their close contact with children and their roles as health workers and care-takers, they experience more respiratory and digestive conditions. Men have higher injury rates, partly because of occupational and recreational exposure to dangerous situations. As roles change in our society as well, the emerging picture is likely to be different.

Some long-term disabilities are more prevalent among women. More women in middle and older ages report trouble carrying out their secondary activities, like shopping and recreation, due to chronic health problems than men of the same age. Sex difference in health service use is largest for young adults and narrows as age advances.

In our country, women tend to somatize or develop 'fits' for which they may seek help. Some senior psychiatrists from our country, like VenkobaRao, Nandi, Neki and Wig, were perceptive early enough to report on these aspects. Women have more frequent illness and disability but the problems are typically not serious or life-threatening ones. In contrast, men suffer from more life-threatening diseases and these cause more permanent disability and earlier death for them. One sex is sicker in the short run; the other in the long run.

Only a small part of the 'iceberg of morbidity' is visible in health statistics or clinical practice.[3] It's gender hue varies, most likely being deeply feminine at the bottom and gradually fading until it is intensely masculine at the very top. The bulk of the iceberg is of a feminine shade.

BIOLOGICAL RISKS IN WOMEN

There are intrinsic differences between males and females based on their genes or reproductive physiology which confers differential risks of morbidity. It is generally thought that males are less durable biologically than females, offset only during females' reproductive years by pregnancy related and breast-genital tract morbidity.

The specific hypotheses are:

- Women have greater genetic resistance to infectious diseases and also some rare X-chromosome linked disease.
- Women are protected from cardiovascular morbidity by sex hormones up to menopause.

- The reproductive events of pregnancy, childbirth and puerperium give women unique morbidity risks not experienced by men. In addition, they have female specific disorders such as those related to breast, genital, genitourinary areas (e.g. cervicitis, menstrual or menopausal symptoms).
- The pathology of some diseases, their symptoms and developmental course may differ for men and women.

ACQUIRED RISKS IN WOMEN

Men have more risks from their jobs, household tasks, life style behaviors, self-imposed stress, social ties and reaction to stresses over a life time. Women have more risks in two respects-from more contact with young children and from more emotional distress.

- Men encounter more risks of serious injury than women.
- Men's choice of hobbies and sports boosts their risks of injury.
- Men tend to drink, smoke and drive more than women—these behaviors elevate their risks of some chronic diseases and injuries.
- Women adopt more preventive health practices—vitamin supplements, drug prescriptions, less alcohol consumption and frequent consultations for minor symptoms.
- Women feel more psychological distress (anxiety, depression, guilt, conflicting demands) on a day-to-day basis and over their life-times than men do, and this may decrease their physiological resistance to acute and chronic conditions.
- Women tend to be less delighted about life than men and this may make them more vulnerable to stress-related illnesses, but women also buffer the route from stress to disease by reacting to disrupting life events and upsets in more benign ways. They turn to other people and to medical drugs for relief whereas men opt for quiet brooding or resort to alcohol, cigarettes and illicit drugs.
- Over their lifetime, women maintain stronger emotional ties with more people. Intimate ties with friends, colleagues and neighbors offer social support and deter loneliness. This may act as a buffer for disease-reducing its occurrence, severity and especially, its duration.

The most popular reason offered for greater female distress concerns women's social roles in traditional cultures. Home-makers of this era are thought to feel unchallenged, bored and undervalued, whereas employed women are believed to have excessive demands on their time and attention, since they relinquish few responsibilities for child care or home-management when they work. It is thus argued that contemporary women have more stressed lives than men, no matter what they do.

EATING

Obesity in women is generally defined as body fat greater than 30%. Obesity is a health hazard because it is linked to an increased likelihood of hypertension, atherosclerosis and diabetes, which are major risk factors for coronary artery disease.

Exercise and dieting are the common means of weight reduction, but calorie restricted diets that do not account for a woman's nutritional needs, coupled with excessive exercise, pose serious health risks to women.[4,5] The antiobesity clinics in many cities are being run by unqualified persons and more on a commercial basis.

ALCOHOL AND DRUG ABUSE

Alcohol is consumed in lesser quantities by women in our country as compared to others, but in those who drink, fetal alcohol syndrome is of significant concern. Prescription drugs and over the counter drugs are consumed more by women. Two thirds of prescriptions for psychotropic drugs, such as diazepam and alprazolam are for women. Multi-centered sample surveys in schools and colleges carried out by Mohan and others have, over the last two decades, found similar trends.

DRUG TRIALS

Women subjects are conspicuously absent or under-represented in drug trials. Thus, the possible gender differences in therapeutic response do not receive adequate attention.

ILLNESS BEHAVIOR

Hypotheses of psychological differences proposed are:

- *Perception*: Women are more sensitive to bodily discomforts than men are. This may be because of childhood socialization—discouragement for boys to complain about bumps and bruises; and in girls, more attention given to menarche and puberty, and the body awareness that menstruation and reproduction provoke.
- *Evaluation*: Women are more apt to label their symptoms as physical illness and after such labeling, assess their illnesses and injuries as more severe and serious than men. On the other hand, it is not 'masculine' to be ill and men ignore the implication of symptoms for their usual activities.
- *Behavior*: Women take action by adopting a sick-role. This occurs through both their willingness and ability, and may have numerous factors, some of which may be that it is more socially acceptable. They also have more

dependent and help-seeking behavior and have more trust in authority.

The concept of learned helplessness is more typical of women than men.

In addition, bed rest, activity restriction and turning to others/medical attention is believed by them to be helpful.

Looking at ability factors, women have more flexible time schedules and fewer time constraints to accommodate health problems. They may even drop out of a job while men continue to work more often even when ill.

Whereas response to serious or life-threatening illness is of a uniform pattern in terms of hospitalization and medical care, the minor psychiatric morbidity seen more often in women offers a variety of possible responses. This may be in the form of neglecting it, talking about it to neighbors and friends, turning to faith healers and traditional health care systems, visiting religious places or seeking professional help. This provides plenty of discretion to the individual and family members. The more discretionary a health action is, the more it allows psychosocial factors to operate, leading to gender differences in help seeking behavior.

HEALTH REPORTING BEHAVIOR

Women are more willing to talk about their symptoms to others, whether they are friends, employees, interviewers or physicians.

Women recall minor health problems and minor health actions better than men do. A presumed reason is that women are more interested in health matters and also more often involved in them as a health helper for children and kin, and this greater salience enhances their memory.

Vocabulary of illness differs for women and men. They may elaborate more and their presentation includes both somatic and psychological content more often.

VIOLENCE AGAINST WOMEN

The scope of violence against women is of a stunning magnitude when crimes by intimate perpetrators and strangers are considered.

They do not come to public attention because of 'cover ups' facilitated by forced secrecy demanded by perpetrators of abuse, or due to closed family boundaries.

Family members committed 90% of the physical and sexual assaults recalled by psychiatric patients.[6] We have no figures from India, but are we enquiring about them in our case histories?

Exposure to sexual violence fails to be included in standard sexual history in clinical medicine, even in the developed countries. Standard psychiatric assessments routinely fail to detect histories of sexual assault among inpatients. Thus, when psychological variables are ignored in diagnosis, somatic complaints which are the ticket of admission to a medical system may be inaccurately or inappropriately diagnosed as organic in etiology. While somatic complaints place a burden on the health service delivery system, opportunities are missed to facilitate simple confiding in a caring person who has a demonstrated therapeutic response on the immune system. Furthermore, the psychiatric aspects of the perpetrators and victims of dowry deaths also need to be explored.

GENDER DIFFERENCES IN TREATMENTS RENDERED AND RECEIVED

Physicians distinguish the characteristics of 'difficult patients' along gender lines.[7] Physicians' perception of difficult patients mainly involves two factors:

1. Medical uncertainty (vague, difficult to describe symptoms—frequently changing symptom picture).
2. *Interpersonal difficulty:* Difficult physician-patient relationships result in poor health care delivery as well as in patient dissatisfaction.

OCCUPATIONAL STRESS

A working woman performs multiple roles in life, including that of a wife, mother, employee, maintainer of extended family ties and caretaker of elderly relatives. This trend has raised questions even in the West whether the prevalence of heart disease amongst women would begin to rise as a response to occupational stress and multiple role tensions. However, data from Western countries indicates that working women have a slight health advantage over housewives. The changing scene of Indian society provides a good opportunity for studying this phenomenon and its mechanisms.

Contrary to the notion that executive jobs produce high stress, heart disease is more common among women in clerical or low status jobs. In an eight year prospective study reported by Eaker (1989),[8] clerical workers, who reported having an unsupportive boss, were at increased risk of developing coronary artery disease. Also, meta-analysis studies of job involvement among women have indicated that it is unrelated to a type A personality—a constellation of personality traits that have been linked to heart disease in men.[9]

Women who smoke have two or four times the risk of heart attack of nonsmoking women. Further, the risk factors for coronary artery disease (lipid disorders, hypertension, diabetes and smoking) tend to cluster in the same patients. In our country, even though women commonly do not smoke, they are subjected to passive smoking due to constraints of living space and traditional subservience.

SEX DIFFERENCES IN THE BRAIN

The bulk of the evidence, as reviewed by Kumra (1992),[10] suggests that the effect of sex hormones on brain organization occurs so early in life that, from the start, the environment is acting on different wired brains in girls and boys.

Major sex differences in intellectual functions seem to lie in patterns of ability rather than in overall IQ. In laboratory experiments, researchers have found that women tend to remember landmarks such as a well on the lower right or a tree at an intersection. Men appear to learn routes faster but cannot recall landmarks as readily. They may rely preferentially on spatial cues such as distance or direction.

Men on an average perform better than women on certain spatial tasks. In particular, men have an advantage in tests that require the subject to imagine rotating an object or manipulating in some other way. They outperform women in mathematical reasoning tests and in navigating their way through a route. Further, men are more accurate in tests of target directed motor skills; that is, in guiding or intercepting projectiles. Women tend to do better at rapidly identifying matching items—a skill called perceptual speed. They have greater verbal fluency, including the ability to find words that begin with a specific letter or fulfil some other constraint. Women also outperform men in arithmetic calculation and recalling landmarks from a route. Moreover, women are faster at a certain precision manual tests such as placing pegs in designated holes on a board.

Marion Eals and Irwin Silverman of York University, USA, studied the ability to recall objects and their location within a confined space—such as in a room or a table top. Women were better able to remember if an item was displaced or not. They also were able to replace them in their exact position more accurately than men.

The life-long effects of early exposure to sex hormones ore characterized as organizational because they appear to alter brain function permanently during a critical period. Administering the same hormone at a later stage has no such effect. Hormonal effects are not limited to sex or reproductive behavior but to all known behavior in which males and females differ. For example, Michael Meaney of McGill University found that dihydrotestosterone working through the amygdala rather than the hypothalamus gave rise to play-fighting behavior in juvenile male rodents. However, the area in the brain that organizes female and male reproductive behavior is the hypothalamus. Roger Gorki and his colleagues at University of California at Los Angeles have shown that a region of the preoptic area in the hypothalamus is visibly larger in male rats than female rats. Laura Allen in Gorki's lab has found a similar sex difference in human brain.

In 1991, Simon LeVay of the Salk Institute for Biological Studies in San Diego reported that the interstitial nucleus of the anterior hypothalamus is larger in human males than females and smaller in homosexual men. Sexual preference may thus have a biological substrate. It is a well-documented fact that exposure to androgens in girls makes them grow tomboyish .

In 1991, DeLacoste and her colleagues reported that the right cortex was thicker than left in men. Jane Stewart of Concordia University in Montreal, working with Bryan Kolb in Alberta postulate that androgens appear to suppress the left cortex. It is widely assumed that two hemispheres are more asymmetrically organized for speech and spatial function in men as compared to women.

MENTAL DISORDERS AND WOMEN

Psychosis

A review of literature on sex differences reveals that the psychiatric focus has swung from questionable assertions of 'anatomy' (or perhaps evolution) as destiny to a relative neglect of sex as relevant at all. The vast majority of follow-up studies of schizophrenic patients since 1980, continue to ignore the gender factor. Perusal of the literature on sex differences in affective and schizoaffective disorders reveals even less recognition of the issue.

Schizophrenia

Strenuous attempts to define onset have been made by some authors.[11] Others have chosen to record the age at first psychiatric contact, admission or treatment. Whichever way onset is defined, the earlier appearance of symptoms in men than women is a well replicated finding. This was found in early studies (reviewed by Lewine et al, 1981)[12] and has been reported across several cultures,[13] and with different diagnostic systems. Typical findings are that 50–60% of men but only about a third of women have their first admission by the age of 25. Goldstein et al (1989)[14] studied the age of onset and found that the mean age was 24.3 for males, and 27.9 for females. Onset at age forty occurred in 8% of females and only 1% of males.

Differences in age at first admission do not seem to reflect sex differences in illness behavior nor greater social tolerance of bizarre behavior for females.[11,12] Other aspects of onset may also show sex differences; life events heralding onset seem to be more commonly reported by females.[15] The season of onset may also differ; Takei et al (1992),[16] found that schizophrenic females, like male and female manic patients, showed a significant seasonality of first admission with a peak of July. In contrast, schizophrenic men showed an admission peak in January. A winter peak was most pronounced for males with early onset schizophrenia (first admission before the age of 25).

Course and Outcome

Angermeyer et al (1990) reviewed the world literature on the effect of gender on the course of schizophrenia. There is a tendency for attenuation of these gender differences in very long outcome studies. Almost all studies found the outcome of schizophrenia to be better in females, at varying lengths of follow-up. Thara and Rajkumar (1992)[17] from SCARF, Madras, have also reported a better outcome in females. McGlashan and Bardenstein (1990)[18] found that the gender differences in outcome were more pronounced in schizophrenia than schizoaffective and affective disorders.

Suicide in schizophrenia is more common in men.[19] Part of the better outcome in females in the short and mid-term may be explained by a better response to both drug treatment and family interventions.[20,21]

Premorbid Function

There is now good evidence that, on a range of measures, antecedent deficits are more common and more severe in boys going on to develop schizophrenia than in girls. If we accept Kraepelin's views that childhood behavior deficits are really the first evidence of a continuous disorder, these results suggest the gender effect at onset not only for psychotic symptoms, but for prepsychotic signs as well.[22]

Incidence

Conventionally, men and women are at equal risk of developing schizophrenia. The introduction of operationalized criteria has changed all this. The life time morbid risk of schizophrenia does appear to be slightly higher in men even when broad RDC criteria are used.

Phenomenology

Several studies and reviews[15,21] have concluded that there are differences in the nonnuclear symptoms of schizophrenia between the two sexes. Overall, men are more prone to express negative defect symptoms such as social withdrawal and blunted affect. Females are more likely to present with dysphoria and depressive symptoms. Substance abuse and antisocial behavior are more common in schizophrenic men.[15]

These sex differences in symptoms could imply differences in neuropsychology.

Familial Risk

Goldstein et al. (1990)[23] found that the age corrected life-time risk of DSM-III schizophrenic men was 2.2% compared with 5.2% in relatives of schizophrenic women—a significant and surprising difference. Relatives of schizophrenic men were significantly more likely to show schizotypal personality disorder. Interestingly, both male and female relatives of female probands had a higher risk of schizophrenia. This is not explainable on any known genetic models.

Interestingly, increased risk to relatives of female probands in also found in neurodevelopmental disorders, such as stuttering and epilepsy. Goldstein et al.[23] interpret these findings as support for the existence of a subgroup of severe, poor prognosis schizophrenia arising predominantly out of nongenetic factors—a subtype which appears mainly in men.

Brain Structure

There is evidence that schizophrenic men more often show structural brain abnormalities which are more clearly of neurodevelopmental origin. Studies using MRI have reported reduced coronal brain area, enlarged ventricles, and small left hippocampal formation in men with schizophrenia, but not women. Other studies have found ventricular enlargement in both schizophrenic men and women.[24]

To conclude, these differences are already being used to try and tease out possible subtypes of schizophrenia.

The advantage of using gender as a subdividing variable with which one can look for heterogeneity is that it is completely reliable, stable and valid in its definition-what Lewine (1988)[12] has called an immutable sociodemographic variable.

Thus, men are more likely to have early onset, negative, process, sporadic schizophrenia. In addition, women schizophrenic patients are different in terms of treatment response: antipsychotics, family interventions, as well as increased compliance with treatment.[25] Goldstein et al.[26] reported that there was a subtype twice as common in men with poor premorbid history, blunted affect and winter birth (early neural damage). Furthermore, these men had the fewer relatives with schizophrenia.[26]

Affective Disorders

Male bipolar patients have worse outcomes than male unipolar patients, whereas outcomes for female unipolar and bipolar patients are comparable.[27] Such evidence warrants consideration of each subtype separately.

Bipolar Disorder

This disorder seems to occur at a similar age and rate in men and women. Schizophrenia-like symptoms, if present, are equally distributed. By the lime they are hospitalized, female patients have had more episodes and less precipitating factors. The outcome scenario is somewhat equivocal and even contradictory. On the one hand, bipolar women are rehospitalized less frequently, are healthier at last contact, and less episodic postdischarge. They also control drug and alcohol abuse better than their male counterparts. At outcome, bipolar women function better with respect to occupation, living situation, and global recovery. On the other hand, studies show that bipolar women commit suicide more often, remit less frequently, die earlier, and comprise a majority of the 'rapid cyclers' who have the worst outcomes. Compared to schizophrenic cohorts, bipolar men and women are comparable premorbidly and exhibit more differences at outcome.

Unipolar Disorder

Most unipolar sex differences concern premorbid and baseline characteristics. A female to male prevalence ratio of 2:1 is consistently noted in epidemiological surveys. Current discussions of gender and unipolar disorder focus on hypothesized male equivalents of depressive symptoms which may skew results, especially the possibility that depression is expressed in men as antisocial behavior or alcoholism. Including such depressive equivalents when determining prevalence would more than even the male/female ratio of 1:2.

Suicide

In India, the pioneering work by VenkobaRao on depression and suicide is worthy of note. He has highlighted not only the gender differences but also the transcultural aspects. In Nepal, suicide was the leading individual cause of death for women of reproductive age in both the 1998 and 2008/09 MMM studies, with the percentage of deaths attributable to suicide increasing from 10 to 16%. The rates give an indication of the severity of the problem, at 22 per 100,000 in 1998 and 28 per 100,000 in 2008/09. Females are still remain psychologically and emotionally suppressed in our society which may be the reason of being suicide more common on them. According to the Metropolitan Police Range, Hanumandhoka, girls committed 90 percent of total child suicide cases in Kathmandu. It was reported that nine out of 10 suicide cases were committed by girls and all these children were found hanged themselves. A cross sectional study of 100 patients of self-harm coming to Emergency Department of Tribhuvan University Teaching Hospital found female (71%) more than male (29%). Among female,16–30 years age group to be the largest (76%) and Metacid ingestion (29%) was found to be the most common cause for self-harm.[28]

Schizoaffective Disorders

In the Chestnut Lodge Follow-up Study,[18] the schizoaffective cohort weakly echoed the findings in the schizophrenic probands; namely, gender differences in the same direction but in fewer categories. Schizoaffective women were married more often than the men at index hospitalization. Schizoaffective males presented with higher IQs and greater antisocial behavior; in contrast to the schizophrenic cohort, schizoaffective men displayed greater affect than women. The study also found no differences in global outcome, although the males achieved more education than the females. Marital rates were not found to differ in another study. Additional differences noted are a higher prevalence, older age of onset and greater suicidal tendencies in women.

Postpartum Psychiatric Disorders

Pitt in 1908 alerted psychiatrists that 1 in 10 postnatal women experience clinical depression. Most research on postpartum depression has been done in Greet Britain and Scandinavia, and only recently (after 1980) in North America and Europe. Scientific studies from developing countries are lacking.

Several prospective studies have found that postpartum period is a time of greater risk for depression than pregnancy. Postpartum depression, when it does occur, interferes with the developing mother-infant relationship and causes disruption of family life.[29] Cox et al.[29] have developed the Edinburgh postnatal depression scale to study postnatal depression. At any rate, depression is very common in the child-bearing age and it has been postulated that etiology of postnatal depression may well be biological (hormonal). The incidence of postpartum psychosis has been reported as 1-2/1000 deliveries. Kendell and colleagues (1987)[30] have noted that for primipara, the relative risk in the first month for psychotic breakdown is very high. Perplexity and confusion are very frequently encountered symptoms in phenomenology. Our findings from Lady Hardinge[31] are also similar. Those with a past history of bipolar depressive illness are at greater risk of postpartum breakdown than unipolar depressives.

Menopause and Mental Disorders

For many years, it was believed that there was a specific depressive syndrome occurring in perimenopausal years. However, articles over the past 25 years show a paucity of evidence for any separate depressive entity occurring in the menopausal years. Milder psychiatric syndromes may occur between the ages of 45 and 49, although there may be no association between these syndromes and biological menopause.

The only comparative recent evidence, suggesting that major mood symptoms may be linked to menopausal years, comes from studies demonstrating a decrease in serotonin measures (either plasma free tryptophan or platelet serotonin) in the perimenopausal and menopausal years. This time period correlates with peak suicide rates for women—a peak not found in men. It has been suggested that low 5 HIAA, the final by-product of the tryptophan-indoleamine pathway, may be low in suicidal patients, particularly those who commit violent suicide. Although purely speculative at this point, it is possible that decreased serotonin during menopause temporarily causes a greater susceptibility to suicides in vulnerable women who may also be depressed.

Hysterectomy and Mental Disorders

Based on the more recent well designed studies, there is a little evidence that hysterectomy is followed by a higher rate of postoperative psychopathology or depression. The subgroup at a higher risk is composed of women with pre-operative psychopathology. Recently, Indian studies on Family Planning and Mental Health have been reviewed by Bhatia and Malik (1990)[32] and they point out that the physical and psychological symptoms that appear show a decline with passage of time. There is also a need for preoperative counseling in this area.

Mental Disorders in Gynecological Patients

Most of the studies on gynecological patients,[33-35] show that (a) patients with gynecological disorders had a high rate of emotional disorders, and (b) the highest proportion of emotional disorders were found in patients with uterine bleeding.

VULNERABILITY FACTORS AND SOCIAL SUPPORT

In a community study, Brown and Harris (1978)[36] described four vulnerability factors, which increased the chances of a woman developing stress in the form of depression in the presence of a life-event or difficulty. They were:

- Lack of good marital relationship,
- Lack of full-time or part-time employment,
- The presence of three or more children under fourteen years at home
- Parental loss before seventeen years of age.

Women's status and reality in the authoritarian patriarchal society of India may further exacerbate life-stresses, anxiety or depression. In India, Agarwal et al. have drawn attention to the fact that women staying with psychiatrically ill husbands in nuclear families show more psychiatric disturbance. In an Indian study by Mayamma and Sathyavathi (1987),[37] it was seen that neurotics and their spouses appeared to have more conflicts with regard to finance, household tasks and companionship, and to a lesser extent with child rearing. This probably highlights the clash between traditional and modern values as women take up careers and increasingly emerge as individuals in their own right. Points of conflict may arise in various circumstances, if the norms and personal preferences of the husband are opposing those of the wife or vice-versa. Such findings are usually interpreted in two ways: firstly, maritally distressed individuals may produce such marked discrepancies primarily as the function of their unrealistic attitudes, needs and expectations. Secondly, distressed and nondistressed individuals may differ only in the degree to which similarly held expectations are actualized, which in turn may be related to differences in personality traits, communication abilities or social skills repertoire. The marriages of normal couples on the other hand are characterized by a relative absence of conflicts and discrepancies between expectations and performances of both spouses.

In a study of 120 women by AvinashVirk (1990),[38] it was found that the number of desirable and undesirable events experienced by a single woman is almost the same but a trend towards an increase in undesirable events is seen with marriage. He also found that personal events contributed towards greater stress in married women. Marriage contributed to the development of greater symptoms in women. Work appeared to have a protective effect, but to a small extent.

Bernard (1976)[39] suggests that women are dependent for satisfaction of affiliative needs on their husbands who lack training in being expressive. Dependence is related to helplessness. It could also mean that dependent women relate to their husband in a child-parent way or remain excessively involved in their families of origin to the detriment of their marriages. The picture gets complicated because dependency may become worse by a depressive illness. Seligman believes that cognitions of helplessness to be the core cause.

Brown (1973)[40] emphasizes the protective function of the ability to have confiding and intimate relationship with spouse/boyfriend against developing depression. This however, may itself be a function of a stable personality. The role of a housewife played by married women is relatively unskilled, undemanding, boring and low in status. In addition, this role is invisible, unstructured and allows the occupant to brood and become involved in personal problems in a way that working women in a more structured role cannot. The 'daily hassles' of a housewife may have a cumulative effect; similarly, frustrations or strains from on-going problematic situations at work, e.g. with a coworker.

Van Fossen (1981)[41] has emphasized the role of affirmation and support received from their husbands as important regarding their work. Researchers have pointed out that even among professional women, who perceived their careers as being just as salient or integral to their lives as their spouse, their family interests superseded their career concerns.[42]

The housewife's role identity is particularly dependent on family responses because she has no external evaluators to turn to for contrary opinion when her husband and/or children do not perceive her work as worthwhile. Unfortunately, a negative evaluation of her role by her family is quite frequently the case, since the status of a housewife in our society is relatively low. In a money-based economy, a job that engenders no income has a lessened status value.

"Our definitions of work", writes David Reisman, "also mean that the housewife, although producing a social work-product does not find her work explicitly defined and totalled either as an hour product or as a dollar product in the national census or in people's minds. And since her work is not defined as work, she is exhausted at the end of the day without feeling any right to be, insult thus being added to injury".

It is high time that the medical profession in our country became more aware about women's health issues. Psychiatrists can take a lead by impressing upon the government and other scientific bodies like the ICMR to conduct scientific studies in the form of a Task Force on Women's Mental Health. This will be quite befitting in the 'Decade for the Woman' as declared by the SAARC countries.

WOMEN'S MENTAL HEALTH: RECENT FACTS ACCORDING TO WORLD HEALTH ORGANIZATION

Depressive disorders account for close to 41.9% of the disability from neuropsychiatric disorders among women compared to 29.3% among men. Leading mental health problems of the older adults are depression, organic brain syndromes and dementias. A majority are women. An estimated 80% of 50 million people affected by violent conflicts, civil wars, disasters, and displacement are women and children. Lifetime prevalence rate of violence against women ranges from 16 to 50%. At least one in five women suffer rape or attempted rape in their lifetime.[43]

Depression, anxiety, psychological distress, sexual violence, domestic violence and escalating rates of substance use affect women to a greater extent than men across different countries and different settings. Pressures created by their multiple roles, gender discrimination and associated factors of poverty, hunger, malnutrition, overwork, domestic violence and sexual abuse, combine to account for women's poor mental health. There is a positive relationship between the frequency and severity of such social factors and the frequency and severity of mental health problems in women. Severe life events that cause a sense of loss, inferiority, humiliation or entrapment can predict depression.[43]

Up to 20% of those attending primary health care in developing countries suffer from anxiety and/or depressive disorders. In most centers, these patients are not recognized and therefore not treated. Communication between health workers and women patients is extremely authoritarian in many countries, making a woman's disclosure of psychological and emotional distress difficult, and often stigmatized. When women dare to disclose their problems, many health workers tend to have gender biases which lead them to either over-treat or under-treat women.[44]

Research shows that there are 3 main factors which are highly protective against the development of mental problems especially depression.[43] These are:

1. Having sufficient autonomy to exercise some control in response to severe events.
2. Access to some material resources that allow the possibility of making choices in the face of severe events.
3. Psychological support from family, friends, or health providers is powerfully protective.

WHO'S[43] FOCUS IN WOMEN'S MENTAL HEALTH

- Build evidence on the prevalence and causes of mental health problems in women as well as on the mediating and protective factors.
- Promote the formulation and implementation of health policies that address women's needs and concerns from childhood to old age.
- Enhance the competence of primary health care providers to recognize and treat mental health consequences of domestic violence, sexual abuse, and acute and chronic stress in women.

REFERENCES

1. Freud S. Femininity. In: Complete Psychological Works. Standard Edition. Vo1. 22. I Ed & Transl. J. Strachey London: Hogarth Press; 1933.pp.112-35.
2. DHHS. US Public Health Service.Report of US Public Health Service Task Force on Women's Health Issues. DHHS Publication No. PHS 85-50206. Washington DC: Govt. Printing Office; 1985.
3. White KL. The ecology of medical care. N Engl J Med. 1961;265:885-92.
4. Dazzi A, Dwyer J. Nutritional analysis of popular weight reduction diets in books and magazines. Int J Eating Dis. 1984;3:61-79.
5. DHHS. US Public Health Service. Women's Health (Supplement). Public Health Reports. Washington DC: Govt. Printing Office; 1981.
6. Carmen EH. Victims of violence and psychiatric illness. Am J Psychiatry. 1984;141:378-83.
7. Schwenk TL. Physician and patient determinants of difficult physician-patient relationships. J Family Practice. 1989;28: 59-63.
8. Eaker ED. Psychosocial factors in the epidemiology of coronary heart disease in women. Psychiatr Clin N Am. 1989;12:167-73.
9. Booth F. Psychological predictors of heart disease: A quantitative review. Psychol Bull. 1987;101:343-62.
10. Kumra D. Sex differences in the brain. Sci Am (Mind and Brain Spl. Issue). 1992;118-26.
11. Hafner K. How does gender influence age at first hospitalization for schizophrenia? A transnational case register study. Psychol Med. 1989; 19:903-18.
12. Lewine RJ. Gender and schizophrenia. In: Nasrallah HA (Ed). Handbook of Schizophrenia. Vol. 3. Amsterdam: Elsevier; 1988.
13. Sartorius NK. Early manifestations of first contact incidence of schizophrenia in different cultures. Psychol Med. 1986;16: 609-28.

14. Goldstein JM. Gender and schizophrenia: Implications for understanding the heterogeneity of the illness. Psychiatry Res. 1989;28:243-53.
15. Bardenstein, McGlashan B. Gender differences in affective, schizo-affective and schizophrenic disorders: A review. Schizophr Res. 1990;3:159-72.
16. Takei N. Seasonality of admission rates in psychosis: Effects of diagnosis, sex and age at onset. Br J Psychiatry. 1992;161: 506-11.
17. Thara K, Rajkumar S. Gender differences in schizophrenia: Results of a follow up study from India. Schizophr Res. 1992;7:65-70.
18. McGlashan B, Bardenstein. Gender differences in affective, schizo-affective and schizophrenic disorders. Schizophr Bull. 1990;16:205-10.
19. Breier A, Astrachan B. Characteristics of schizophrenic patients who commit suicide. Am J Psychiatry. 1984;141:206-9.
20. Seeman, Lang S. The role of estrogen in schizophrenia: Gender differences. Schizophr Bull. 1990;16:185-95.
21. Haes N. Gender and schizophrenia outcome: A clinical trial of an inpatient family intervention. Schizophr Bull. 1990;16:277-92.
22. Castle, Murray C. The neurodevelopmental basis of sex differences in schizophrenia. Psychol Med. 1991;21:565-75.
23. Goldstein JM. Sex differences in the familial transmission of schizophrenia. Br J Psychiatry. 1990;156:819-26.
24. Lewis S. Sex and schizophrenia: vive la difference. Br J Psychiatry. 1992;161:445-50.
25. Zito GJ. Clinical characteristics of hospitalized psychotic patients who refuse anti-psychotic drug therapy. Am J Psychiatry. 1985;142:822-6.
26. Goldstein JM. The role of gender in identifying subtypes of schizophrenia: A latent class analytic approach. Schizophr Bull. 1990;16:263-75.
27. Loyd KN. Are there sex differences in the long term outcome of schizophrenia? Comparison with mania, depression and surgical controls. J Nerv Ment Dis. 1985;173: 643-9.
28. YL Shakya, Acharya R, Gupta MP, Banjara MR, Prasad PN. Factors determining self-harm. Journal of Institute of Medicine. 2010;32:3:14-7.
29. Cox JL, Paykel ES, Paage ML. Current Approaches: Childbirth as a Life-event. Southampton: Duphar Medical; 1989.
30. Kendell RE. Epidemiology of puerperal psychosis. Br J Psychiatry. 1987;150:662-73.
31. Agarwal P, Bhatia MS, Malik SC. Post-Partum Psychosis: A study of indoor cases in a general hospital psychiatric clinic. Acta Psychiatr Scand. 1990;81:571-5.
32. Bhatia MS, Malik SC. Family planning and mental health: A review of Indian Studies. Indian Practitioner. 1990;1103-5.
33. Agarwal P, Malik SC, Padubidri V. A study of psychiatric morbidity in gynecology outpatient clinic. Indian J Psychiatry. 1990;32:57-63.
34. Agarwal P, Malik SC, Padubidri V. Psychiatric morbidity in patients suffering from menstrual disturbances. Indian J Psychiatry. 1989;31:173-6.
35. Bhatia MS, Bohra N, Malik SC. A study of psychiatric referrals from gynecology and obstetrics department. Indian Med Gazette. 1989;123:55-7.
36. Brown GW, Harris TO. Social Origins of Depression: A Study of Psychiatric Disorder in Women. London: Tavistock; 1978.
37. Mayamma S. Marital role conflicts in neurotics. Indian J Clin Psychol. 1987;14:65-7.
38. Virk A. Women, marriage and work: A study of relative role of stress, social support and mental health. MD Thesis, Punjab University, Patiala, India; 1990.
39. Bernard. Homosociability and female depression. J Soclssues. 1976;32:213-38.
40. Brown GW. Life events, vulnerability and onset of depression. Br J Psychiatry. 1987;150:30-42.
41. Van Fossen BE. Sex differences in the mental health effects of spouse support and equity. J Health Soc Behav. 1981;22:130-43.
42. Hardesty SA, Betz NE. The relationships of career salience, attitudes towards women and demographic and family characteristics to marital adjustments in dual career couples. J Vocational Behav. 1980;17:242-50.
43. WHO, Gender and Womens Mental Health. 2013. Viewed 7 October. 2013. <http://www.who.int/mental_health/prevention/genderwomen/en/>
44. Sarah B. Mental Health Concerns for Indian Women. Indian Journal of Gender Studies. 2012;19:127-36.

CHAPTER

53

Mental Health Issues in Indian Minorities

RC Jiloha

Human behavior is conceived of as the outcome of genetic and biochemical characteristics, past learning experiences, motivational states, psychosocial antecedents and cultural context in which it unfolds.[1] Culture plays an important and complex role in the natural history and psychosocial development of human behavior[2] which comprises of customs, beliefs, values, knowledge and skills.[3] Social norms and shared rules that specify appropriate and inappropriate behavior,[4] mores that people consider vital to their well-being and to their most cherished values,[5] and the sanctioned socially-imposed rewards and punishments that compel people to comply with norms constitute important ingredients of culture.

Culture is defined[6] as shared values, norms, traditions, customs, art, history, folklores and institutions of a group of people.[2] Within this perspective and form, Indian society cannot be regarded as having a "cultural homogeneity" as described by sociologists, because shared beliefs, customs and values of different communities in India are different and identify themselves with their different caste-groups. Caste-system is peculiarly fitted in Indian society, to hand on cultural patterns and particular items of the culture. Stigma of caste and its polluting effect is not just confined to the realm of ritual but has its ramifications in economic, social, and political position though enforcement of certain social laws and physical segregation of minority groups.[7]

Indian subcontinent has been likened to be a deep net into which various races and people have drifted and been caught[8] and their diverse origin has dictated variety. Geographical conditions forced these varied people to stay together in a "multiple" society, imposing on them what has been described by historians as *"unity in diversity"*, meaning complete harmony, peace and adjustment among different cultural elements. This arises from a view of accepting the textual position of Hindu social system and explaining as well as justifying empirical social reality in terms of *Vedic Scriptures*[9] based on consensus model. But contrary to this belief, there is dialectical inter-relationship between those caste-groups who have monopolized the scarce goods of power and privilege and those who lack these resources. Deprivation plays an important role in unfolding of behavior in Indian society.

These deprived masses, which constitute the minorities of the Indian society, are described compendiously in the Constitution of India as Scheduled Castes (SC) and Scheduled Tribes (ST). They are in fact low castes in the traditional Hindu social order, generally treated as 'casteless', 'outcasts' and 'untouchables'. They have often been subjected to deprivation and discrimination for centuries. Historically, they spring from the aboriginal inhabitants, conquered and enslaved by Aryan invaders.

For the first-time in the history, these minorities came to be accepted as equal to other citizens in the independent India. With the desire to bring these communities in step with the mainstream communities of Hindu society, a reservation policy was introduced, offering them the benefit of education and jobs. As a result, there has been a massive social mobility and transformation, as well as the emergence of "educated" among these minority groups, looked down upon with contempt by larger society for their mobility on crutches of reservations.

With the advent of education, members of low caste groups have also started realizing that the deprivation they are subjected to is for no fault of theirs. There is an increasing resolve on their part to assert for their due share in the national resources that speaks of their resentment and frustration.

In Indian society, where social diversity, stratification, deprivation, social mobility, contempt and frustration are operating in a complex manner, mental health assures greater significance. Mental health is not simply the absence of mental illness but a positive concept[10] of displaying ability for adaptive social and interpersonal relationships and ability to reach a harmonious relationship with the society.[11] A stable society has a clear role definition while social change burdens the individual with new role demands. When the individual is unable to cope with the sociotechnological changes, it not only affects the social roles but also is instrumental in disturbing the psychosocial homeostasis.[12] As such, the ethnic minorities are subjected to mental health strains.[11] The subject of mental health becomes more important when sociotechnical changes operate in a diverse and complex manner to influence human behavior. Our existing conceptual framework of comprehending it is inadequate[13] and multidisciplinary approach is needed to understand this complex social phenomenon.

MINORITY CHILDREN AND THEIR DEVELOPMENT

Early environmental influences of stimulation or isolation have a marked effect on measurable cognitive development.[14] Social class differences affecting language development emerge during the first year of life. A child born in a traditionally low caste poor family suffers from protein-calorie malnutrition which may retard his intellectual growth.

A child from lower community, when he grows up, becomes aware of his minority status early in life.[11] Between the age of 3–6 years, incipient attitudes of his social group show systematic development,[15] which get correctly categorized around 8 years of age.[16-18] Such a child would emerge out with a checkered personality,[14] ill equipped to face the divergent ways of society and culture at large.

MINORITY CHILDREN AND THEIR SCHOLASTIC DIFFICULTIES

Spread of education in Indian low castes has been relatively slower[19] because of their poverty, ignorance[20] and other hindering factors. It is pointed out that high percentage of irregular attendance, drop out from schools[21] and internal administrative and academic problems[22] are the causes of their disinterest in studies and these students become the source of irritation, heartburn and intercommunity tension in the educational institutions.

Capacity to respond to and benefit from education depends upon child's intellect, language and emotional maturity.[23] Another equally important factor is the availability of role model[11] for educational achievement which is generally lacking in traditional low caste families. Studies reveal that these children carry very low aspiration[24] for money, material, occupational status, etc. They have very low self-concept, low self-esteem and lower need for achievement.[25] They have a overwhelming concern for immediate needs for sustenance, with a static level of aspiration. They are extremely cautious and avoid taking risk when possibility of failure is there.[26] They are vague and fantasy-oriented in their future planning. In a study of low achievers, it was found that they are comparatively older, have poor academic background, come from less educated or illiterate parents, are complacent and have poor emotional integration.[27] It is felt that parent's poor occupational status is responsible for child's poor emotional stability.[28] Indifference of teachers and parents is also contributory.[29]

India's low caste illiterate parents, engaged in repugnant and defiling occupations, breed emotionally less stable children, destined to low achievement because of lack of qualitative interaction and inadequate development of cognitive and linguistic skills. The belief, that formal education itself could bring about the desired changes, has been found to be unrealistic in the light of our understanding of low castes. An intervention program, devised to educate parents to bring up their children, could be of help to improve linguistic and cognitive skills.[23] Concurrent maternal participation leads to substantial improvement.[30-32] It is expected that with the spread of education, the following generation of educated parents will interact qualitatively with their children to avail the fruits of education.

PERSONALITY PROFILE OF MINORITY STUDENTS

Various studies reveal that these students have a strong tendency to refer their success to external factors, like kindness of their teacher, mercy of God and their good luck,[20] rather than attributing their success to their own efforts and thus taking pride in their accomplishment and experience a sense of fulfilment which would be reinforcing to their success behavior.[33] This tendency leads to superstitious behavior, perpetuation of fatalistic outlook, ritualism and ingratiation of the significant others. On the other hand, failure is often ascribed to oneself.[34] These students have harsh self-criticism, less favorable self-concept and rigid standards to evaluate one's own performance.[22] This builds up an ego-damaging and self-discouraging internalized mechanism.

According to the "cognitive approach hypothesis", negative self-evaluation leads to social anxiety.[35] This anxiety leads to avoidance behavior in certain social situations which demand their attention and decision making.[36] In these situations, which demand their attention, they are found to be more tense and anxious for the year of things going wrong.[37] A scheduled caste student is generally more cautious, careful and guarded as compared with the upper caste Hindu student.

"Memory for self-relevant information" research suggests that once a person views himself and his performance negatively, he is more likely to recall incidents in which he performed poorly.[38] There easily accessed negative memories serve to precipitate social anxiety when future encounters are contemplated.

Generally, a person is more highly motivated to seek others' approval, acceptance and affection than to seek others' disapproval and rejection.[39] Where need for approval is high, a person tries to manage a better impression.[40] Therefore, the factors which heighten people's motivation to seek approval are associated with increased social anxiety[41] and that is why a person's feelings of self-work are partially dependent upon other's evaluation.[42-44] Low-caste students, who are in want of social approval and acceptance, carry higher levels of social anxiety as compared to general population of students. This anxiety interferes with their work efficiency, resulting in poor performance.

The low caste students have low and unrealistic motivation, external locus for success, personal inadequacies for failures, harsh and rigid self-evaluation, and extreme anxiety for outcome of personal performance. They exhibit avoidance behavior, lack decision making capacity, tend to have negative memory of past experiences, carry very low self-concept and need social approval. Success is not as re-enforcing as it should be and failure is extremely discouraging. It is found that they experience the fear of failure because of internalization of personal inadequacies, negative memories, low perception of self and heightened social anxiety.[36]

The entire mechanism is motivationally damaging and that is why low caste students account for largest population of failures and dropouts.

SOCIAL STIGMA AND MINORITIES

Social stigma refers to "defect in person's social identity," a negative information about a person that is known by others.[45] Because a stigmatized person is highly self-conscious, he is sensitive to others comments, real or imagined evaluation, highly motivated to make as good an impression as possible and likely to feel socially anxious, especially when under observation.[41] Not only does the possession of social stigma induce public self-awareness, it also makes him doubt that others will evaluate him favorably, which further leads to social anxiety and thus reduction in his performance.

According to "self-preservation theory", social anxiety arises when a person is motivated to make a particular impression on the others but doubts that he will be able to do so because of negative social experience.[40] Viewed from social learning principle, classical conditioning occurs when people associate certain situations with positive or negative outcome.[46] When the past has been unsuccessful, punitive, awkward and otherwise aversive, the future too is perceived the same way and a doubt arises in the mind whether he will be able to create a desirable impression in the larger society.

EDUCATED MINORITIES IN NEW ROLE

The role is the part that a person plays within the given social context.[47] Associated with each role, is a set of expectations regarding the appropriate behavior for the occupant of that role to perform.[48] Role novelty occurs when a person finds himself in a position he has not previously occupied and, while playing the new role, he may be unaware which behavior he perceives to be appropriate.[49] This is a common source of self-presentational uncertainty and triggers social anxiety.[39]

In independent India, where urbanization, modern education and new technologies[12] have created occupational mobility from traditional repugnant occupations to newly created white-collar positions, an educated member from low caste finds himself in a new role. This sudden change in role in the same given social context has created many psychological difficulties.

CHILDREN OF EDUCATED MINORITY PARENTS

Public self-consciousness is a related phenomenon if people of different hierarchy are considered. Development of public self-consciousness starts right from childhood experiences. Children of publicly self-conscious parents may learn to be publicly self-conscious through 'modeling process'. Children who observe that their parents are much concerned how they are evaluated by others are likely to learn to adopt greater self-scrutiny than the children from larger society parents. When parents often express concern with what neighbors, friends, family and co-workers think about the prestige of parents' background, children may come to believe that it is important to consider others' perception and evaluation of themselves. No wonder that then the children born of educated *'dalits'*, after independence, are excessively self-conscious, extremely shy, oversensitive to reference to caste and have tendency towards isolation. Heightened self-consciousness further adds to their already existing tendency towards isolation, defeating the efforts of their government to resolve the problem of their isolation. They do not feel secure and comfortable in larger groups.

Of course, no environment guarantees high achievement, whether one's own or larger, yet a much higher proportion with unrealized potential will be found among certain economic sections, social classes, ethnic groups and geographical areas.

India's minorities perceive outside world to be hostile and they live in constant fear under the shadow of violence to their person and property. Everyday, two members of low castes are murdered and three females are raped.[50] Under such conditions, they find themselves unable to achieve their specific goals and true integration with the main stream.

India's deprived castes present a number of problems related to mental health. Their developmental process to assume psychological maturity and to achieve mental health is retarded by a number of factors, like deprivation of childhood experiences, lack of qualitative interaction required for health, development of cognitive and linguistic skills, unrealistic motivation, external locus for success, harsh and rigid self-evaluation, high levels of social anxiety, avoidance behavior and so on. They are exposed to multiple psychological strains and may be vulnerable to develop certain psychological aberrations. Though there are no systematic studies in this regard, it is implicit from the observations that they need more attention is the form of praise and recognition, which are almost lacking.[51] This need is more readily satisfied in case of members of larger group. In contrast, minority group members get far less, if any, praise and recognition; yet their needs are immeasurably greater. Whatever small success they achieve, inevitably demands far more efforts and perseverance; yet they receive no regard. Rather, they are ridiculed for achieving less despite of benefit of reservations.[52]

Cultural Competence in the Treatment of Ethnic Minority Populations

The call for cultural competence in mental health practice has been a frequent theme voiced by the four major ethnic minority psychological associations (Asian American Psychological Association, Association of Black Psychologists, National Latin Psychological Association, and the Society of Indian Psychologists).[51] In an effort to address concerns and provide assistance to service providers, these four associations have produced this booklet to:

- Produce a highly readable brochure summarizing in broad terms the mental health issues of greatest concern to the four ethnic minority psychological associations
- Increase awareness regarding the need for balance between culturally universal modes of helping with the increasing recognition of the effectiveness of culture-specific and indigenous healing approaches
- Provide culturally relevant mental health practice recommendations to practitioners and students who work with ethnic minority populations.

REFERENCES

1. Sutker P. Drug and Psychopathology. Research Issue 19. Maryland: National Institute of Drug Abuse Research; 1977.
2. Orlandi MA. Cultural Competence for Evaluators. US Department of Health and Human Services. Rockvile, Maryland: OSAP Production and Editing office; 1992.
3. Linton R. The study of Man. New York: Appleton; 1947.
4. Berne E. Games People Play: The Psychology of Human Relationship. New York: Newtor Books; 1964.
5. Bellah RN, et al. Habits of the Heart. New York: Harper and Row; 1985.
6. Light D, Keller S. Sociology. New York: Knopf; 1985.
7. Sachchidanand. The Harijan Elites. Faridabad: Thompson Press; 1977.
8. Hutton JH. Caste in India. Bombay: Oxford University Press; 1961.
9. Dumont L. Homo-Hierachicus. Delhi: Vikas Publications; 1970.
10. WHO. Concept of Health Behavioral Research. SEARO Regional Health Papers No. 13, 1986
11. Varma VK. Social disadvantage, mental health and social justice. Indian J Soc Psychiatry. 1992;8:8-12.
12. Sharma SD. Impact of social change on mental health. Presidential address. Indian J Soc Psychiatry. 1987;3:3-17.
13. Sethi BB. Socio-technological changes and behaviour. Editorial. Indian J Soc Psychiatry. 1987;3.
14. Jaya-Nagaraja. Effect of family and culture on development of a child. Child Psychiatr Quart. 1986;14:52-5.
15. Clark KB, Clark MP. Racial identification and performance in Negro children. In: Newcomb TM, Hartly EL (Ed). Readings in Social Psychology. New York: Hold; 1947.
16. Goodman N. Race Awareness in Young Children, 2nd edition. New York: Crowell Collier; 1994.
17. Morland JK. A comparison of race awareness in northern and Southern children. Am J Orthopsychiatry. 1966;36:410-21.
18. Porter J. Black Children, White Children: The Development of Racial Attitude. Cambridge, Mass: Harvard University Press; 1971.
19. Naik JP. Education of the Scheduled Castes. ICSSR Sponsored Study. 1965-66. New Delhi, 1971.
20. Pimpley PN. Problems of non-attendance of school among scheduled caste children. In: Sharma SK (Ed). Reform Protest and Social Transformation. Delhi: Ashish Publication; 1987.
21. Chitnis S. Education for equality: Case of scheduled castes. Economic and Political Weekly, 1977;7.
22. Sinha D. Cognitive and motivational correlates of deprivation and their implication for the education of scheduled caste children. J Person Clin Stud. 1985;1:11-6.
23. Pringle MK. The Needs of the Children. London: Hutchinson; 1974.
24. Rath R. Teaching and learning problems of disadvantaged tribal children. XII Annual Conference of Indian Academy of Applied Psychology. Bhubaneshwar: Utkal University; 1976.
25. Gokulnath PP, Mehta CP. Achievement motive in tribal and non-tribal Assamese secondary school adolescents. Indian Educat Rev. 1972;1:67-90.
26. Sinha D. Indian Villages in Transition: A Motivational Analysis. New Delhi: Associated Publishers; 1969.
27. Wg NN. Why students fail: A psychological study of low achievers. Indian J Psychiatry. 1972;2:31-2.
28. Davis R. The behavior and adjustments in school of seven years and sex and social class differences. Early Child Development and Care. London: Hutchinson; 1977.
29. Burt C. The gifted child. Year Book of Education. 1962;24-58.
30. Bronfern-Brenner. Development research, public policy and ecology of childhood. Annual Meeting of the Society for Research in Child Development, Philadelphia; 1973.
31. Halsey AH. Problems and Policies: Educational Priority. Vol. 1. HMSO; 1973.
32. Mid-Winter AE. Projections: An Educational Priority. London: Wardlock Educational Society; 1972.
33. Sharma SK. Reform Protest and Social Transformation. New Delhi: Ashish Publishing House; 1987.
34. Videback R. Self-concept and Reaction of Others. Vol. 23. London: Society; 1960.pp.251-9.

35. Clark JV, Arkowitz H. Social anxiety and self-evaluation of interpersonal performance. Psychol Report. 1975;36:211-21.
36. Pandey N, Tripathi RC. Scheduled caste children in high caste schools. Sinha D (Ed). New Delhi: Concept Publishing; 1982.
37. Yurlova SE. Scheduled Castes in India. New Delhi: Patriotic Publication; 1990.
38. Schlenker B, Leary MR. Social anxiety and self-presentation. A conceptualisation and model. Psychol Bull. 1982;92:641-69.
39. Marc R, Learn MR. Understanding Social Anxiety: Social Personality and Clinical Perspectives. London: Sage Publication; 1963.
40. Schlenker B. Impression Management: The Self-concept and Social Identity and Interpersonal Relations. California: Monterey Books; 1980.
41. Markas H. Self-scheme and processing information about the self. J Person Soc Psychol. 1977;35:69-78.
42. Cooley CH. Human Nature and The Social Order. Rev. Ed. New York: Scriber; 1922.
43. Coppersmith S. The Antecedents of Self-esteem. San Francisco: WH Feeman; 1967.
44. Mead GW. Mind, Self and Society. Chicago: University of Chicago Press; 1934.
45. Leary MR. The social psychology of shyness: Testing a self-presentation model. Unpublished doctoral dissertation, University of Florida; 1980.
46. Bandura A. Principles of Behavior Modification New York: Hold; 1969.
47. Feingstein A. Self-consciousness, self-attention and social integration. J Person Soc Psychol. 1979;1:100-5.
48. Hass HT, Maehr ML. Two experiments in the concept of self and the reactions of others. J Person Soc Psychol. 1969;1:92-9.
49. Goodenough WH. Co-operation in change: An anthropological approach to community development. New York: Russel Sage Foundation; 1963.
50. Biswas S. Social Justice.Letter to the Editor. The Times of India, Delhi, 1994;19.
51. American Psychological Association. Psychological Treatment of Ethnic Minority Populations. Viewed 8 October 2013, <http://www.apa.org/pubs/info/brochures/treatment-minority.aspx>
52. Bhui K, Warfa N, Edonya P, et al. Cultural competence in mental health care: a review of model evaluations. BMC Health Services Research. 2007;7:15.

FURTHER READING

1. Bhui K, McKenzie K. Rates and risk factors by ethnic groups for suicides within a year of contact with mental health services in England and Wales. Psychiatric Services. 2008;59:414-20.
2. Crawford MJ, Nur U, McKenzie K, et al. Suicidal ideation and suicide attempts among ethnic minority groups in England: results of a national household survey. Psychological Medicine. 2005;35:1369-77.
3. Commission for Racial Equality. Employment and Ethnicity (Factfile 1). CRE .2006.(http://www.equalityhumanrights.com/Documents/CRE/PDF/factfile01_employment_and_ethnicity.pdf).
4. Grewal I, Lloyd K. Use of services. Ethnic Differences in the Context and Experience of Psychiatric Illnesses: A Qualitative Study W. O'Connor & J. Nazroo (Eds) 2002; 51-60. TSO (The Stationery Office).
5. Hunt I, Robinson J, Bickley H, et al. Suicides in ethnic minorities within 12 months of contact with mental health services. British Journal of Psychiatry. 2003;183:155-60. Abstract/FREE Full Text.
6. Karlsen J Nazroo, K, McKenzie K, et al. Racism, psychosis and common mental disorder among ethnic minority groups in England. Psychological Medicine. 2005;35:1795-803.
7. McKenzie K, Bhui K. Institutional racism in mental health care. 2007;BMJ:334:649–50.
8. O'Connor W, Nazroo J. Ethnic Differences in the Context and Experience of Mental Illness: A Qualitative Study. TSO (The Stationery Office); 2002.
9. Sproston K, Nazroo J. Ethnic Minority Psychiatric Illness Rates in the Community (EMPIRIC) – Quantitative Report. UK Department of Health; 2002.

CHAPTER 54

Women and Aggression

Jayati Simlai, Swarnali Bose, Sourav Khanra, CRJ Khess

'Violence against women is a global health problem of epidemic proportions'

—Margaret Chan

INTRODUCTION

Women have been kept in the background by the society worldwide, since time immemorial. Rules framed by the society have deprived them of certain rights and privileges. They have subtly been hinted as being inferior to men by narrating legends of self-sacrifice, self-effacing pure image of women and by their day to day ritual practices in India. These rituals project women as a faithful wife or a devout mother. The famous Laws of Manu insist on the worship of the husband by the wife as God in spite of a lack of character and she is made dependent on the husband without trying to break the bond of control. The salvation and happiness revolves around her virtue and chastity as daughter, wife and widow.

In the Indian context, women have a dual concept in the Hindu philosophy. On one hand she is fertile, benevolent and bestows prosperity like goddess Parvati, Lakshmi and Saraswati. On the other hand she is aggressive, malevolent and destructive, depicted in goddess Durga and Kali.

The problem of violence against the 'fair sex' in India is age old. In the West, the term 'fairer sex' in recent times is taken to be derogatory, while in the colonial times in India, women were often complimented as the 'fair sex' and it was acknowledged well. Violence was never an issue in India probably because of religious values and socio-cultural attitudes. The early reports of violence against women came in the late 1960s in India and it gained the image of public problem rather than a private one, in early 1970s.

There is probably no woman who has not suffered harassment, humiliation, exploitation and violence at any point of time, just because she is a female. Woman, on one hand, has the pleasure and danger, on the other, of being what she is. They are routinely defined by their sex in their day to day life and even if not all men are dangerous as kidnappers, rapists, molesters, batterers, all women are potential victims.

If we look into the facts and figures on violence against women, we can sense the severity of the issue and the urgency of steps to be taken to fight this, not only as medical but as a burning psychosocial, socio-political and legal problem of our country.

Prevalence studies of violence against women report wide variations in levels of violence within and between health care settings. The reported lifetime prevalence of physical or sexual violence, or both, varied from 15% to 71% among the countries studied in the World Health Organization (WHO) multi-country study. According to a recent full report by WHO (2013), the total prevalence of intimate partner violence in South-East Asia region is 27.99% (23.7 to 32.2, 95% CI). At the same time total prevalence of non-partner sexual violence in same region is found to be 5.28% (0.94 to 9.61, 95% CI). Violence against women has been estimated by the World Health Organization (WHO) to account for between 5% and 20% of healthy years of life lost in women aged 15 to 44 (WHO 1997). Violence by an intimate partner affects about 30% of women worldwide. 38% of all murdered women were killed by their intimate partners and 42% of women who experienced physical or sexual violence by a partner and sustained injuries as a result. In India the National Crime Records Bureau (NCRB) reported a total of 244270 cases of crime against women under Indian Penal Code (IPC) and Special Local Laws (SLL) for the year 2012, which was 6.4% increase from the previous year. Violence against women has increased by 4.3% to 17.4% within last 20 years. Followings are relevant information for an overview of the diversity of aggression, violence and crimes against women. Cases under dowry prohibition act have increased by 2.7% during the year 2011. In the same year torture cases in the country was increased by 5.4%. Cases of molestation was increased by 5.8%. Apart from these importation of girls was observed to be increased by 122.2%. A total of 2, 28,650 incidents of crime against women (both under IPC and SLL) were reported in the country during the year 2011. The demographic distribution revealed a total of 33,789 cases of crimes against women during the year 2011 took place in metro cities.

Worldwide, domestic violence is as serious cause of death and incapacity among women aged 15 to 49 years as cancer and a greater cause of ill health than traffic accidents and malaria combined (The World Bank 1993). In addition to causing injury, violence increases women's long-term risks of a number of other health problems, including chronic pain, physical disability, drug and alcohol abuse, and depression.

FORMS OF AGGRESSION, VIOLENCE AND CRIME AGAINST WOMEN

One of the main difficulties, international researchers face on violence against women, is to develop clear operational definitions of different types of violence and tools for measuring violence that permit meaningful comparisons among diverse settings. In the World report on violence and health, World Health Organization adopted a typology that categorizes violence in three broad categories, according to those committing the violent act: self-directed violence, interpersonal violence and collective violence. These categories are each divided further to reflect specific types of violence. Self-directed violence may be self-abuse or suicidal behavior. Interpersonal violence may be at either family/partner or community level. Lastly collective violence may be social, political or economical.

Violence is also known as abuse and includes any sort of physical aggression or misbehavior. When violence is committed at home it becomes domestic violence and involves family members such as children, spouse, parents or servants. Domestic violence may involve different means such as hitting, kicking, biting, shoving, restraining and throwing objects. In broad terms, it includes threats, sexual abuse, emotional abuse and controlling or domineering behavior. The classification of modes of violence and/or aggression against women varies across literature. It usually depends on the country, ethnicity and local tradition prevailing at a particular place and hence is often under reported. This section would focus on classification which have been found to be discussed across most literatures. Readers would have to keep in mind that new mode of violence may emerge in future if not in recent times.

Violence or aggression against women may involve more than one area of a woman's life. These include physical, psychological, emotional, economic, etc. The various kinds of atrocities against women need special mention.

Rape as a war crime is a form of torture but warrants mention because of its unique characteristics. Prostitution enforced on a large scale by government officials or armed opposition forces on detainees are considered to be a crime against humanity and deserve intervention by the country's courts' jurisdiction.

Incest of girl child is imposition of any sexual behavior on her by a family member including extended family members like teachers, etc. Sexual contact in incest is defined by a variety of verbal and or physical behaviors and penetration is not necessary to define it.

In India, dowry deaths and bride burning accounts for 5000 deaths each year. The demand for the obligatory marriage dowry is heavy and prolonged and persists for few years till after the marriage. Greed causes murder of the bride which is usually depicted as a household accident and all the family members go scot free. In ancient times in India, child marriage was rampant. The Sati or Jowhar was the act of self-immolation on death of the husband, which was a compulsory Hindu ritual, where widows were forced to sit in their husband's pyre.

Acid attack is a very common form of showing aggression towards women with very serious outcomes. The rate of attack was so high in Bangladesh that a foundation for the survivors was established in May 1999. Simple reasons like rejection of a marriage proposal or delayed meal were enough justification. The most commonly used chemical is sulfuric acid which is easily available.

Honor killing is another form of brutality where a girl of higher cast is killed by her family members if she is either attracted or engaged to a boy of lower cast. In the ancient times men killed their female relatives in India, in the pretext of family honor for forced or sexual activity outside marriage including rape. The offenders were often reported to be below 18. It was common in India, Pakistan, Jordan, Yemen, Lebanon, Egypt, etc.

Female feticide and infanticide are common forms of crime, committed on the unborn and newly born female fetus. Gender identification during pregnancy by way of ultrasound imaging and amniocentesis in India led to many abortions as families did not want a girl child. The boy child is valued socially and economically above the girl child. Many inhuman forms of infanticide are practiced in rural parts of India, leading to death of pregnant mothers. The newborn girl child in many parts of India is suffocated to death by smothering or drowning. Medical sex identification techniques have been banned in India, China and Republic of Korea but the business seems to be booming everywhere.

Female Genital Mutilation (FGM) consists of three main varieties—'Sunna' or circumcision, clitoridectomy and infibulation. Sunna means 'traditional' and it consists of the removal of prepuce (the fold of skin covering the clitoris) and or the tip of the clitoris. Clitoridectomy or excision is removal of the entire clitoris and the removal of the adjacent labia. Infibulation or "pharaonic" circumcision is the most extreme form. It consists of the removal of the clitoris, the entire labia and joining of the scraped sides of the vulva across the vagina, where they are secured with thorns or sewn with catgut and thread. A small opening is kept to allow passage of urine and menstrual blood. An infibulated woman during intercourse is cut open on the wedding night and closed again afterwards in order to secure fidelity to the husband. This procedure has no health benefits to women and can cause severe bleeding. It can lead to cysts and infertility in future. According to a recent report by WHO, 140 million girls and women are living with the consequences of FGM. The practice is mostly carried out by traditional circumcisers who often play a central roles in communities. It is mostly prevalent in communities in Africa, in some countries in Asia and Middle East.

Kidnapping and abduction is a fairly common happening in India. Girls and women are usually abducted with the intention of sexual gratification and or marriage. Economic reason in the form of ransom is accountable in a small number of cases.

Eve teasing and stalking are very common in day-to-day life. Young girls and women are victim of both these forms of atrocities. Eve teasing is in the form of whistling and passing verbal comments, usually obscene that humiliates the female passerby. It is common in young and adolescent groups. Stalking is repeated visual or physical proximity, non-consensual communication, verbal, written or implied threats, severe enough to cause a high level of fear in a reasonable person. It is common in the West and gradually appearing in some parts of urban India.

Sexual harassment is seen to be on the rise in India as more and more women are moving out of homes to have a career. Unwelcomed sexual advances, subtle or overt pressure for sexual favors, suggestive, insulting or obscene comments or gestures, repeated advances or propositions, verbal abuse of sexual nature, graphic comments about an individual's body, sexual prowess or sexual deficiencies are made. Leering, whistling, touching, pinching in a suggestive or sexual manner, coerced sexual acts, and display of objects or pictures of sexual nature, all suggest sexual harassment.

Sexual assault and battering is a visible form of violence inflicted on women worldwide. It may be threatened, attempted or actually inflicted physical harm, like simple slapping and hitting to the use of gun in the West.

Sexual slavery in the form of trafficking of women and children is on the rise as reported in March 2001. Women and children from poor and backward countries are moved to countries like US, Canada, Belgium Netherlands and France and forced into prostitution.

Domestic violence in India is a well-known and raging problem in India. It includes harms and injuries which endangers women's health, safety, life, limb or well-being inside households, which is either mental or physical. It is in the form of physical, sexual, verbal, emotional and economical abuse. Surveys indicate that 10 to 58% of women have experienced physical abuse by an intimate partner in their lifetimes. Preliminary results from a World Health Organization (WHO) Multi-Country Study on Women's Health and Domestic Violence indicate that in some parts of the world as many as one half of women have experienced domestic violence.

THEORIES OF AGGRESSION

Aggression and victimization are correlated. Men are socialized to be aggressive and women to be victims. Support for the theory that aggressive behavior is instinctual comes from 1) Ethologists such as Desmond Morris, Conard Lorens, Robert Ardey; 2) Research on electrical and chemical brain stimulation; 3) Psychoanalytic theory. The ethologists propose that our animal ancestors were instinctively violent beings and that our violent behaviors are products of these inherited instinctual drives. An intriguing theory is that violence is not an instinctual behavior but learned one. The expression of such learned aggression may be as varied as the environments in which it is learned. Freud and his contemporaries held that aggression is instinctive. Goldstein, viewing aggression as a learned behavior, proposes that there are long-term and situational factors that facilitate either aggressive or non-aggressive behavior. Long-term factors include the process of socialization. Interestingly, several of these studies find that males are more prone to aggression than females. Kagan and Moss (1962) found that aggressive behavior was learned through childhood, especially for males. Eric Fromm's analysis has addressed the errors and limitations in explaining the causes and origins of human aggression from bevioral schools of psychology. The observable difference between male/female aggressions has been ignored. From specifically includes women in his definition of mankind as it relates to human destructiveness. According to him it would be wrong to assume that the male is innately more violent than women. Ahuja (1987:166-185) identifies fourteen theories for understanding violence committed by an individual. Theories range from intrapsychic theories to macro-sociological theories. He decides those theories on the basis of three (theoretical) level of analysis. They are psychiatric or psychopathological analysis, socio-psychological analysis and sociological or socio-cultural analysis.

The Psycho-pathological Model

This focuses on the offender's personality characteristics as the chief determinants of criminal violence. This model includes analysis that links mental analysis with act of violence. The determinants leading to the ultimate act is assumed to be arising from psychopathologies or personality traits which makes the offender vulnerable to commit violence.

The Socio-psychological Model

According to this model examination of external environment is necessary to understand the impact on the individual offender. It also takes interpersonal factors, which are determinants of violence, into account. Many theories, such as the Frustration-Aggression theory, the Perversion theory, the Self-Attitude theory and the Motive Attribution theory, have emphasized on these in their approach to criminal violence.

The Sociological or Socio-cultural Model

In contrast to socio-psychological model, which is based on micro level analysis, socio-cultural model talks about macro-level analysis. This model views criminal violence in respect to socially structured inequality and social and cultural attitudes and norms regarding anti-social behavior and interpersonal relations. Besides the two well-known theories, viz., the structural–functional theory and the theory of sub-culture of violence, the learning theory, the exchange theory, the anomic theory and the resource theory, etc. also come under a socio-cultural analysis.

Ahuja (1987) examines his own Social Bond Theory to explain crime against women. Social Bond Theory based on adjustment, commitment and attachment and the relative feeling of deprivation is different from the Frustration Aggression Theory in the sense that frustration are the consequences of interpersonal relations and the functioning of sub-systems in the society.

The dominant view holds that female victimization is a complex phenomenon having deep roots in the male dominated socioeconomic, legal and political order. It is an expression of imbalance in the power structure that regulates women to a secondary social position, thereby making them vulnerable to various forms of oppression, exploitation and abuse.

Biological Models of Aggression

Hormones are chemicals that regulate and control bodily functions. Two of these have been implicated in aggressive behavior, namely testosterone and cortisol. Males produce testosterone in the testes. Women also produce testosterone, but in smaller amounts, by converting dehydroepiandrosterone (DHEA) in the adrenal glands. There are several findings which have linked testosterone with aggression. For example, castration leads to a marked decrease in aggression in both nonhumans and humans, and replacement testosterone (in castrated mice) restores aggression levels, but only if the replacement occurs within ten days of birth. The problem with many studies, on the relationship between testosterone and aggression, is that they are correlational, and the big weakness of correlational studies is that just because two things are correlated, it does not necessarily mean that a change in one causes a change in the other. However, if we were to administer testosterone to a person and they behaved more aggressively, this would be good evidence that testosterone causes aggression. Tomaszewski, et al (2009) found no difference in testosterone levels in 933 healthy young men, even though some were much more aggressive than others. Similarly, Bain, et al. (1987) found no significant differences in the testosterone levels of men who had been charged with murder or violent assault and men who had been charged with nonviolent crimes such as burglary. Although there seems to be strong evidence for a clear link between testosterone and aggression in nonhumans, the studies described above indicate that the link in humans is less clear. Indeed, according to Sapolsky (1997) it is also worth noting that the majority of these researches have concentrated on male aggression. Some researches have found that 'high testosterone' women are more likely to report dominating behavior, but other studies have found no such relationship. It has been suggested that women may respond to challenging situations with increased testosterone, and so display characteristics such as aggressiveness and dominance. However, enough research has not yet been done on female aggression.

Cortisol is produced by the adrenal medulla, and is an important part of the body's response to a stressor. It has been suggested that lower levels of cortisol are correlated with higher levels of aggression. There could be two reasons for this. First, it could be that some people are born with an under-reactive autonomic nervous system (ANS). So, in order to increase their arousal level (because a low level of arousal is aversive or unpleasant), these people would behave aggressively to create stress, which would increase both ANS activity and cortisol release. If true, this would indicate that cortisol is a consequence of aggression rather than a cause of it. The second possibility is that cortisol is directly or indirectly involved in the causation of aggression, and that it actually inhibits aggressive behavior. Two findings suggest that cortisol may be involved in aggression. First, lower levels of cortisol have been found in habitually violent offenders and aggressive school children. This would suggest a direct causal link. Second, people with low cortisol levels and high testosterone levels behave more aggressively than people with high cortisol levels and high testosterone levels. This finding suggests that testosterone can only exert its effects when cortisol levels are low. Cortisol may therefore be controlling the increase in aggression associated with testosterone. This would mean it is indirectly linked with aggression. The problem is that the findings are not consistent in this area of research. Many studies have found no differences between the cortisol levels of aggressive and non-aggressive people, whilst others have even found higher cortisol concentrations in aggressive participants. This may be because of methodological issues: cortisol levels vary in a circadian way, so how much cortisol production is observed may depend on when the measurement is taken.

FACTORS RELATED TO AGGRESSION AGAINST WOMEN

Violence against women is shaped by attitudes and social norms, gendered inequalities of power, and a wide variety of other social factors. The incidents of aggression towards women have increased significantly in South Asia. There are different socioeconomic, political, cultural and religious factors contributing to violence against women. These are enumerated here:

- *Gender roles and relations:* Gender role is an important factor related to aggression and/or violence. One key factor here is men's gender-role attitudes and beliefs. Men's predilection with sexist, patriarchal, or sexually hostile attitudes is an important predictor of their present and future use of violence against women. On the other hand, in many ways, violence is part of 'normal' sexual, intimate, and family relations. For example, for many young people, male aggression is expected and normalized. Girls are compelled and obliged to accommodate male 'needs' and desires.
- *Male dominated society:* In a male dominated society, like India, men in all sphere of their life dominate women. Men play important figures in the whole life of a woman. The figure can be of a father or of a brother or of a husband and lastly of a son. Owing to such dependency, the male members think that they always direct women and all services should be centered to the interest of the male.
- *Socioeconomic factors:* A nonparallel change has been observed through the last decade or so, in traditional rural economic pattern with respect to areas like health, education social security, etc. On the other hand, traditional socio-cultural practices, low rate of education, lack of employment opportunity, and low nutritional and health status, etc. have persisted. This has had an adverse effect on women and has become responsible for increased stress and tension in male-female relations, poor households and has given rise to aggression and violence.
- *Devaluation of moral character:* Prevailing socio-economic conditions like poverty, unemployment, etc. and political turmoil pushed young people to be involved in criminal activities, drug addiction, hijacking, illegitimate sex and other anti-social behaviors. Thus dislocated from moral courage, they liked to get involved in rape, violence as an thrill or adventure.
- *Access to resources and systems of support:* Increasing portrayal of violence through popular reading, theaters, film and TV shows, satellite culture, etc. directly or indirectly encourage men to commit offences like rape or other violence. Simultaneously, social isolation leads men to commit crime. Among young women, rates of domestic violence were found to be higher in those who are not involved in schools or do not experience positive parenting and supervision in their families. In adult couples, social isolation is both a cause and a consequence of wife abuse. Women with strong family, friends and social networks experience lower rates of violence. Particular personality characteristics are predisposing factors in men's perpetration of partner violence. Spouse abusers tend to have more psychological problems than nonviolent men, including borderline, mood disorders, and depression. Adolescent delinquency—antisocial and aggressive behavior committed during adolescence—is a predictor of men's later perpetration of sexual assault. Men's abuse of alcohol or drugs is another risk factor.
- *Other influential factors:* Besides these, other influential components are responsible for the rape occurrence in the country. Lack of education and awareness in case of women, poverty, practice of power, illicit love affair, opposing second marriage are directly or indirectly associated with criminal activities including women violence.

IMPACT OF AGGRESSION ON HEALTH OF WOMEN

Impact of violence and aggression on women are observed not only in physical and medical consequences but also in psychological morbidities also. Often, the women suffer from these morbidities through indirect way. Though physical consequences drag psychological morbidities along with it and vice-versa, for the ease of discussion, physical followed by psychological impact would be focused on separately.

Physical/Medical Consequences

Numerous ill effects of intimate partner violence in terms of health outcomes have been reported. Some of these are HIV infection, sexually transmitted infections (STIs), induced abortion, low birth weight, premature birth, growth restriction in utero and/or small for gestational age, alcohol use, depression and suicide, injuries, and death from homicide.

Women with a history of intimate partner violence (IPV) are more likely to report HIV risk factors. They indulge in unprotected sex, injection drug use and alcohol abuse. Also, they are less likely than other women to display high levels of self-efficacy for HIV prevention. They are associated with less use of antiretroviral medication, decreased medication adherence, and increased risk of death. HIV infection may trigger or augment physical violence, particularly against women. One large study reported that over one in five HIV positive women reported physical harm since HIV diagnosis. Half of these was attributed to their HIV positive status. On the other hand, genital tract injury associated with sexual violence can increase the risk for HIV infection. Research suggests a different type of synergistic relationship, referred to as "syndemic" relationship between violence and HIV, that results in health outcomes worse than either condition alone. Many other physical, mental and sexual and reproductive health effects have been linked with intimate partner violence. These include adolescent pregnancy, unintended pregnancy in general, miscarriage, stillbirth, intrauterine hemorrhage, nutritional deficiency, abdominal pain and other gastrointestinal problems, neurological disorders and chronic pain.

Over the past decade, there has been growing recognition that intimate partner violence is an important contributor to women's vulnerability to HIV and STIs. Women in violent relationships, or who live in fear of violence, have limited control over the timing or circumstances of sexual intercourse, or their ability to negotiate condom use. Separation due to partner violence may also be an important determinant which may increase a woman's risk of HIV if she acquires a new partner. Furthermore, there is behavioral evidence that men who use violence against their female partners are more likely than nonviolent men to have a number of HIV-risk behaviors. They have multiple sexual partners, frequent alcohol use, visit sex workers, and have a STI, all of which can increase women's risk of HIV.

Women's reproductive and sexual health is clearly affected by gender-based violence. A US study found that women who experienced intimate partner violence, were three times more likely to have a gynecological problem than those who were nonabused. These problems include chronic pelvic pain, vaginal bleeding or discharge, vaginal infection, painful menstruation, sexual dysfunction, fibroids, pelvic inflammatory disease, painful intercourse, urinary tract infection, and infertility. In addition to damage to the urethra, vagina, and anus, abuse can result in sexually transmitted infections (STIs), including HIV/AIDS. Women who disclose that they are infected with HIV also may be subjected to violence. Apart from these, early childbearing, often a consequence of early and forced marriage, can result in a range of health problems, including effects of unsafe abortion. It has been reported that girls under 15 years of age are five times more likely to die in childbirth than women in their twenties. They also are more vulnerable to obstetric fistula, which can result from prolonged and obstructed labor. Women who have been sexually abused are more likely to have a partner, who refuse to use a condom to prevent disease. Violent relationships are frequently marked by fear and controlling behaviors by partners, eventually, women in these relationships report more adverse sexual and reproductive health outcomes. The higher rates of adverse reproductive events can be explained by direct consequences of sexual violence and coercion, as well as by more indirect pathways affecting contraceptive use, such as sabotage of birth control, disapproval of birth control preventing use of contraception, or inability to negotiate condom use for fear of violence. As a result, women in abusive relationships have more unintended pregnancies. Of the estimated 80 million unintended pregnancies each year, at least half are terminated through induced abortion and nearly half of those take place in unsafe conditions. While unintended pregnancies carried to term have been associated with health risk to mothers and infants, illegal and unsafe abortions place women's health at even greater risk. Low birth weight can result from either preterm birth or growth restriction in utero, both of which can be directly linked to stress. Living in an abusive and dangerous environment marked by chronic stress can therefore be an important risk factor for maternal health, as well as a factor affecting birth weight.

Besides these, nonfatal injuries are often associated with violence against women. Unlike other consequences mentioned above, these are the most direct effects and needs mentioning in this section. The head, neck and face are the most common locations of injuries related to partner violence, followed by musculoskeletal injuries and genital injuries.

Psychological Consequences

Experiences with violence can have various impacts on women's physical and psychological health, including their levels of mental health and substance use. Evidence suggests that women's health is severely impacted by violence, mental health and substance use and the co-occurrence of these three conditions can adversely impact the outcome of each. There is strong evidence to draw conclusion that women's experiences of violence precede their substance use and/or mental health issues. In fact, according to some researchers, causal relationship between violence against women and mental health and substance use might not be denied. For example, approximately two-thirds of women accessing antiviolence services report that they began their problematic substance use following experiences of violence in their relationships. At the same time, there is evidence that substance use and/or mental health concerns can create a vulnerability to violence and that the pre-existence of these conditions may exacerbate the effects of abuse. The association between these three issues is, therefore, both complex and multidirectional.

Violence and Mental Health

Experiences with violence can have significant impacts on women's mental health. Systematic reviews examining the link between violence against women and depression have found significantly higher rates for women who had experienced violence in their lives compared to general population of women. For example, Cascardi, O'Leary & Schlee reviewed 14 studies and found prevalence rates of depression to be between 38 and 83%, while Golding found an average prevalence rate of 47.6% for women impacted by violence. It has been found that women's compromised level of mental health may directly or indirectly interact with their partner's behavior and attitudes towards them. If a woman is having psychological morbidity, her partner is found to more likely keep medications away from her or over medicate her; to take advantage of changes in her symptoms or feelings (i.e. encouraging suicidal thoughts); to claim that she is an unfit mother, and/or to minimize her credibility. For many women mental health concerns develop in response to the violence and feelings that arise from those experiences of violence. As Morrow and Chappell argue, "For many women social conditions of inequity, in particular experiences of violence, precipitated their entry into the mental health system". As a result, many researchers and service providers believe that it would be rare for women to experience violence without having some kind of mental health consequence. Therefore, researchers and women themselves believe that many mental health concerns are natural responses to the violence women experience and should be attended to as such. A trend has been noted in which health and mental health professionals have been increasingly diagnosing women, who have experienced violence, with mood disorder such as depression and borderline personality disorder, with little or no consideration for the social context that may be precipitating their illness. Subsequently these can be stigmatizing and may create barriers to services. Finally, women are prescribed medications by physicians for mental health concerns, including depression and anxiety but the underlying psychosocial issues remain unaddressed. On the other hand many of these medications have abuse potential and may lead to dependence.

Violence and Suicide

In the WHO Multi-Country Study (MCS) on women's health and domestic violence against women, a survey of 15 sites in 10 mostly low and middle income countries, the self-reported lifetime prevalence of ever attempting suicide ranged from less than 1% of women up to 12.0% of women. It would be worthwhile to note that when exposures to violence occur during childhood, there is alteration in the ability to cope with exposure to subsequent stressors. This has been replicated in many other longitudinal and twin studies. Besides this, mothers who are experiencing chronic fear and stress and consequent physiological changes as a result of partner violence are less likely able to provide the same kind of caring and supportive environment that will enable children to develop healthy attachments and internal regulation processes. Adult exposures to violence and other traumatic events could also increase the risk of suicide in a similar way. The stress response, and the ongoing fear and isolation that can result from experiences of physical, sexual and psychological violence, can increase feelings of hopelessness and helplessness and biological responses that often precede suicidal behavior. Indirectly, many of the other sequelae of severe physical and sexual abuse like anxiety, depression, and post-traumatic stress disorder may also contribute independently to suicidality.

Violence and Substance Abuse

A large proportion of women who use substances have experienced violence in their relationships. They also had acknowledged incest, rape, sexual assault and child physical abuse in their early life. The United Nations has recognized that experiences of relationship violence lead to increased alcohol and drug dependency in women. Women impacted by violence are more likely to smoke cigarettes, use alcohol heavily, misuse prescription drugs, and use illegal drugs. Alcohol dependency has been found to be up to 15 times higher for women impacted by violence than in the general public. Moreover, those who misuse substances are more likely to use multiple types of substances and to use higher levels of substances than those who have not experienced violence. Approximately 40% of women, who use substances, have a co-occurring major mental health disorder, up to 67% have a history of abuse, and almost 50% are in a currently abusive relationship. In another systematic review, Najavits, Weiss and Shaw found that 36–51% of women in community samples reported a lifetime history of physical and sexual violence compared to 55–99% of women with substance use issues. In this study, women reported being a victim of adult physical violence (56.1%), childhood sexual violence (56.3%), childhood physical violence (56.1%) and adult sexual violence (45.4%). Despite this evidence, many services fail to respond to these connections when serving women. When asked about reason of using substances, it was found that many of them used substances to cope with the violence and the resulting effects on their physical and mental health or other stressors in their lives (poverty, lack of safe, affordable housing, etc.). The researchers also found that supporting women around their experiences of violence and other stressors can reduce stress and, in turn, help reduce levels of substance use.

Women as Aggressors

Reports have appeared in recent years concluding that women are just as violent as men. These reports often cite many studies of self-reported physical aggression based on data from the Conflict Tactics Scale (CTS), a widely used measure of physical aggression between intimate partners. A meta-analysis of gender differences in rates of physical abuse found that women were slightly more likely than men to use physical aggression against intimate partners. These findings have generated a great deal of controversy, in part because there has been no evidence based theoretical ground to explain women's violence. Following points would be important to keep in mind while discussing about when women use violence—(a) women's violence in the context of their victimization by male partners; (b) factors that influence women's violence and victimization, namely, women's motivations for violent behavior and the coping strategies women utilize in response to relationship problems; (c) the historical context of women's experiences of childhood trauma; and (d) outcomes of depression, anxiety, post-traumatic stress disorder (PTSD), and substance use. Swan and Snow (2002) found that women in their sample used equivalent levels of emotional and/or verbal abuse (e.g. yelling and screaming, name calling) as their partners used against them. Women also committed significantly more moderate physical violence (e.g. throwing something, pushing and/or shoving) than their partners used against them. However, women were more often victims of quite serious types of abuse, including sexual coercion, injury, and coercive control behaviors (e.g. restricting social contact, controlling the partner's activities and decisions). There is bidirectional path between the woman's violence and her partner's violence. This supposes that is, if there is violence of one partner, the violence of the other partner is more likely as well. A study demonstrated a path model to describe bidirectional relationship between women's violence and their male partners' violence against them.

- *Self-defense:* Research suggests that the motivations for women's violent behavior in intimate relationships are often quite different from those for men. In case of women, self-defense is reported as a motivation for violence more frequently than men. For example, one study found that 36% of women listed self-defense as a motivation compared to 18% of men. In an analysis of women's motivations for violence, self-defense was the most frequently endorsed motive, with 75% of participants stating that they had used violence to defend themselves.
- *Fear:* Women also are more likely to report fear in domestic violence (DV) situations. In a study of men and women court ordered to a DV treatment program and women residing in a DV shelter, both samples of women reported greater fear of their partner's violence than the male sample. In DV situations, women are much more likely than men to be injured, and injured severely. In a study of 199 military couples mandated to DV treatment, 33% of the husbands reported injuries compared to 65% of wives. Also, wives reported feeling significantly more fearful of their partners than husbands. Thus, fear of assault from their partners and the need to protect themselves from physical harm is an important determinant for women's violent behavior.
- *Defense of children:* It has been estimated that 30–60% of children whose mothers are battered are themselves victims of abuse. Children living with an abused mother have been found to be 12–14 times more likely to be sexually abused than children whose mothers were not abused. The effects of partner or family violence on children in terms of actual physical abuse of children and what children witness, modulate how women behave in violent relationships. Some women behave violently toward their partners to protect their children and themselves.
- *Control:* Studies consistently show that men are more likely than women to use violence to regain control of the relationship or a partner who is challenging their authority. Swan and Snow (2006) found that 38% of women stated that they had threatened to use violence at least sometimes to make their partner do the things they wanted him to do. Among them, 53% stated that the threats were effective at least some of the time.
- *Retribution:* Finally, several studies suggest that retribution for real or perceived wrong doing is a common motivator of women's and men's violent behavior. Forty-five percent of the women in the Swan and Snow (2003) study stated that they used violence to get even with their partners for something they had done. Women stated they used violence in retribution for the partners' emotionally abusive behavior (e.g. "punishment for his insults"), while men did not. This was replicated in an another study among dating college students, where, 56% of women who used violence did so in retaliation for being emotionally hurt, as compared to 25% of men.

In summary, the motivations described above fall under two categories. Some of them are defensive motivations (self-defense, protecting children, and fear). These deals with defending oneself and one's children from physical harm. Rest are active motivations (control and retribution) which refer to motivations that go beyond self-defense and encompass anger, revenge, and a desire to control the partner.

WOMEN'S COPING WITH VIOLENCE AND AGGRESSION

The issue of how women cope with violence and/or aggression against them has received some attention. In the general literature, coping is usually of three types: avoidant, problem solving, and support seeking. Evidence typically suggests that avoidant strategies are related to poorer outcomes, and problem solving and support seeking are related to positive outcomes. Among victims of DV, avoidant coping strategies have been associated with the development of psychological problems such as depression. Problem-solving coping, on the other hand, has been found to be related to well-being. Several studies document the variety of active coping strategies battered women use in response to abuse. Social attachment has also been found to be related with reduced symptoms of PTSD and depression. The extent to which three types of coping were utilized in relation to a recent problem or conflict in women's relationships was assessed by Swan (1999). Problem-solving coping was negatively correlated with women's violence, indicating that the more problem-solving strategies women employed, the less violence they used. Avoidance coping was positively correlated with violence.

SERVICE PROVISIONS FOR VICTIMIZED WOMEN–INDIAN SCENARIO

Women's political participation is now institutionalized and incorporated in many regional and national plans of action. The Government of India had declared the year 2001 as the year for the empowerment of women. Many steps had been taken legally including creating new laws to protect women from violence or crime. We can classify them into three types as Constitutional Empowerment, Protection through IPC and Protection through the SLL.

Constitutional Provisions to Secure and Empower the Women

The constitution of India guarantees formed equality to all its citizen. The directive principles have been formulated to attain justice, liberty and equality for men as well as for women. Several legal measures have been introduced in order to improve the position of women. All these steps have been taken by the government to wipe out the ravages of hundreds of years of effacement of women by our society. Directive principle of the constitution also directs the state to make laws to secure women. Constitution of India makes special protection on the form of Right to equality, Right to life and personal liberty, Protection against traffic in human beings (prostitution) and forced labor. Constitution also makes moral liability on the state to ensure equal right for men and women regarding livelihood, Equal pay for equal work, and health and strength of women shall not be abused, to provide equal justice and free legal aid. Constitution also provides many directions through Article 21 and an important duty has been imposed on all the citizen of India to maintain and ensure dignity of women through fundamental duties. Apart from this Article 15, prohibits, discrimination against any citizen on grounds of religion, race, caste, sex, etc. Article 16, provides for equality of opportunities, matters relating to employment or appointment to any office under the state. Article 39(a), (d), mentions policy security of state equality for both men and women the right to a means of livelihood and equal pay for equal work for both men and women. Article 42, directs the State to make provision for ensuring just and humane conditions of work and maternity relief.

Legal Provisions for Women are as Under

- *Child Marriage Act, 1929:* The Child Marriage Act was enacted in 1929 to stop the customary practices of child marriage, since the introduction of the act it has gone through various changes. The main purpose of this law is to create a check on population growth. It was also passed to eliminate potential danger to the life and health of female children who cannot withstand the stress and strains of married life and to avoid early deaths of minor mothers. Under this act child means, below 21 year of age and female below 18 years and a minor as a person of either sex who is below 18 years of age. Beside this, some other state also enacted laws to prevent the custom of Devdasis, for instance The Karnataka Devdasis (prohibition of dedication) Act 1982 and Andhra Pradesh Devdasis prevention and dedication act 1947, banned the practice of marrying young girls to a deity.
- *Factories Act, 1948:* This act is applicable to the factories or establishment, where workers are working with power. Similar provisions are also provided to mines under mines act and some other welfare labor laws. No women shall be allowed to clean, lubricant or adjust any part of a prime mover or of any transmission machinery while the prime mover or transmission machinery is in motion. Under this Act, a woman cannot be forced to work beyond 8 hours and employment of women except between 6 A.M. and 7 P.M is prohibited.
- *The Immoral Traffic Prevention Act, 1956:* The government has enacted this special law in 30th December 1956. The objective and reason of the act was to make punishable acts such like:
  - Keeping a brothel or allowing premises to be used as a brothel
  - Living on the earning of prostitution
  - Procuring, inducing or taking person for the sake of prostitution

  Besides these this act prohibits many other activities related to brothel. All offences under this act are cognizable. This act provides the procedure for arrest and constitution of separate court for offences under this act. One defect of this act is that prostitutes are also treated as offenders and made punishable whereas they are the victim of the society.
- *Probation of Offenders Act, 1958:* It describes Power of court to release certain offenders after admonition. When any person is found guilty of having committed an offence punishable under section 379 or section 380 or section 381 or section 404 or section 420 of the Indian Penal Code or any offence punishable with imprisonment for not more than two years, or with fine, or with both, under the Indian Penal Code or any other law, and no previous conviction is proved against him and the court by which the person is found guilty is of opinion that, having regard to the circumstances of the case including the nature of the offence and the character of the offender, it is expedient so to do, then. Notwithstanding anything contained in any other law for the time being in force, the court may, instead of sentencing him to any punishment or releasing him on probation of good conduct under section 4, release him after due admonition. But, women for death sentences or imprisonment for life are not punishable for more than seven years of imprisonment. They are entitled to be released on admonition or on probation.
- *Maternity Benefit Act, 1961*: A Woman is entitled 12 weeks maternity leave with full wages. This act facilitates to women to take rest for a certain period before and after child-birth and provides for maternity benefit. It came into force on 1st November 1963. Under this act women' means a women employed whether directly or through any agency for wages in any establishment .This act empowers the women to avail twelve weeks paid maternity leave at the time of each delivery. This benefit is also applicable

at the time of adoption of a child, before the maternity period. Pregnant women are entitled to work in favorable condition, besides the regular payment she is entitled for maternity bonus fixed by the government.

- *The Dowry Prohibition Act, 1961:* Under the provisions of this Act demand of dowry either before marriage, during marriage and/or after the marriage is an offence. It came in force from July 1, 1961. This aims to secure the women from social evil. This act provides penalty for illegal transaction of dowry. If any dowry is given it shall be transferred to the women in marriage and if not transferred, such person will be punishable. Offences under this act are cognizable for certain purpose even nonbailable and noncompoundable.
- *The Equal Remuneration Act of 1976:* This act provides equal wages for equal work: It provides for the payment of equal wages to both men and women workers for the same work or work of similar nature. It also prohibits discrimination against women in the matter of recruitment. This act provides for payment of equal wages for work of same and similar nature to male and female workers and for not making discretion against female employee in the matter of transfer, training and promotion, etc. Central government is the appropriate government in respect of industries/establishment under the Industrial Disputes Act 1947. The objective of the act is to provide for the payment of equal remuneration to men and women workers and for the prevention of discrimination on the ground of sex, against women in the matter of employment and for matters, connected therewith or incidental.
- *The Child Marriage Restrain Act of 1976:* This act raises the age for marriage of a girl to 18 years from 15 years and that of a boy to 21 years.
- *Indian Penal Code:* Section 354 and 509 safeguards the interests of women.
- *The Medical Termination of Pregnancy Act of 1971:* The Act safeguards women from unnecessary and compulsory abortions. It was enacted on 10th of August 1971. The objective of the act was to provide legal restrictions for termination of certain pregnancies by registered medical practitioners and for matters connected there with and made sure the pregnancy termination by unregistered practitioner would be an offence, punishable under Indian penal code.

  Amendments to Criminal Law 1983, which provides for a punishment of 7 years in ordinary cases and 10 years for custodial rape case.
- *73rd and 74th Constitutional Amendment Act:* It reserved 1/3rd seats in Panchayat and Urban Local Bodies for women.
- *The Commission on Sati (Prevention) Act, 1987:* This provides more effective prevention of the commission of sati and its glorification and for matters connected therewith or incidental thereto. Some powers are given to the collector or district magistrate to prevent offences relating to sati, for this purpose special court are constituted. Offences under this act is A. attempt to commit sati B. Abetment of sati and C. Glorification of sati.
- *The National Commission for Women Act, 1990:* The Commission was set up in January, 1992 to review the Constitutional and legal safeguards for women.
- *The protection of Human Rights Act, 1993:* This act is responsible for the protection and promotion for human rights, defined by the Act as "rights relating to life, liberty, equality and dignity of the individual guaranteed by the Constitution or embodied in the International Covenants".
- *The Pre-conception and Pre-natal Diagnostic Techniques (Regulation and Prevention of Misuse) Act, 1994:* It was brought into operation on 1st of January 1996 and was intended to regulate the use of prenatal diagnostic techniques to detect genetic and metabolic disorders, chromosomal abnormalities, certain congenital malformation and/or sex linked disorders. In practice the techniques for prenatal determination of sex of the fetus led to female feticide and reinforced the gender bias. It was also amended in the year 2002 for proper implementation. It has provisions like quick hearing, fast remedy, etc.
- *Protection of Women from Domestic Violence Act, 2005:* This Act protects women from any act/conduct/omission/commission that harms, injures or has potential to harm. All these are to be considered as domestic violence. It protects the women from physical, sexual, emotional, verbal, psychological and economic abuse.
- *Protection of Women against Sexual Harassment at Workplace Bill, 2010:* On November 4, 2010, the Government introduced protection of Women against Sexual Harassment at Workplace Bill, 2010, which aims at protecting the women at workplace, not only to women employees but also to female clients, customer, students, and research scholars in colleges, universities and patients in hospitals. The Bill was passed in Lok Sabha in 2012.

CONCLUSION

Clinicians must be well trained in how to enquire and respond to abuse, and they should be prepared to help survivors of abuse with treatment and referral. The high prevalence rates of violence experienced by women suggest that clinicians practicing in all areas of medicine need to recognize and explore the potential relevance of violence issues when considering women's reasons for presenting with ill health. In parallel, sensitization to the problem of domestic violence should be incorporated not only in medical training, but also into governmental, legal, and judicial organizations. Much more work needs to be done to acknowledge and understand the needs of women. More research is required to have a comprehensive understanding of the impact, violence has on women's mental health. Implementation of legal and policy frameworks must be strengthened with accountability. Also, structural and underlying causes and risk factors should be addressed in order to prevent violence against women. Multisectoral services, programs and responses to violence against women must be prompt.

BIBLIOGRAPHY

1. Abrahams N, et al. Sexual violence against intimate partners in Cape Town: prevalence and risk factors reported by men. Bulletin of the World Health Organization Bulletin. 2004;82(5):330-7.
2. Ad Hoc Working Group on Women, Mental Health, Mental Illness and Addictions. Women, Mental Health and Mental Illness and Addiction in Canada: An Overview. 2006 Retrieved March 30, 2010 from *http://www.cwhn.ca/PDF/womenMentalHealth.pdf*
3. Ahuja R. Crime against Women. Jaipur. Rawat Publication, 1987. Available: *http://opac.tiss.edu/cgi-bin/koha/opac-detail.pl?biblionumber=215713*
4. Amirkhan JH. A factor analytically derived measure of coping: The coping strategy indicator. Journal of Personality and Social Psychology. 1990;59:1066-74.
5. An update on WHO's work on female genital mutilation, World Health Organization, 2011.
6. Anderson T, Aviles A. Diverse faces of domestic violence. ABNF Journal. 2006;17(4):129-32.
7. Andersson N, Cockcroft A, Shea B. Gender-based violence and HIV: relevance for HIV prevention in hyperendemic countries of Southern Africa. AIDS. 2008;22(Suppl 4):S73-S86.
8. Archer J. Sex differences in aggression between heterosexual partners: A meta-analytic review. Psychological Bulletin. 2000;126:651-80.
9. Bain J, Langevin R, Dickey R, Ben-Aron M. Sex hormones in murderers and assaulters. Behav Sci Law. 1987;5:95-101.
10. Barnett OW, Lee CY, Thelen RE. Gender differences in attributions of self-defense and control in interpartner aggression. Violence Against Women. 1997;3:462-81.
11. Campbell JC, et al. The intersection of intimate partner violence against women and HIV/AIDS: a review. International Journal of Injury Control and Safety Promotion. 2008;15(4):221-31.
12. Cascardi, et al. Co-occurrence and correlates of post-traumatic stress disorder and major depression in physically abused women." Journal of Family Violence. 1999;14(3):227-49.
13. Coker AL. Does physical intimate partner violence affect sexual health? A systematic review. Trauma Violence and Abuse. 2007;8(2):149-77.
14. Cory J, Godard L, Abi-Jaoudé A, Wallace L. Building Bridges: Linking Woman Abuse, Substance Use and Mental Ill Health Summary Report. 2010. *http://www.bcwomens.ca/NR/rdonlyres/C1AA97BC-FAAB-40E9-972DF377EE729080/45188/BB_summaryreport.pdf*
15. Das Dasgupta SD. A framework for understanding women's use of nonlethal violence in intimate heterosexual relationships. Violence Against Women. 2002;8:1364-89.
16. Devries KM, Seguin M. Violence against Women and Suicidality: Does Violence Cause Suicidal Behaviour? In: García-Moreno C, Riecher-Rössler A (Eds), Violence against Women and Mental Health. Key Issues Ment Health. Basel, Karger. 2013;178:148-58.
17. Dunkle KL, et al. Perpetration of partner violence and HIV risk behaviour among young men in the rural Eastern Cape, South Africa. AIDS. 2006;20(16):2107-14.
18. Fernandez-Botran R, et al. Correlations among inflammatory markers in plasma, saliva and oral mucosal transudate in post-menopausal women with past intimate partner violence. Brain, Behavior, and Immunity. 2011;25(2):314-21.
19. Foa EB, Cascardi M, Zoellner LA, Feeny NC. Psychological and environmental factors associated with partner violence. Trauma, Violence, & Abuse. 2000;1:67-91.
20. Follingstad DR, Wright S, Lloyd S, Sebastian JA. Sex differences in motivations and effects in dating violence. Family Relations. 1991;40:51-7.
21. Freeman R, Collier K, Parillo K. Early life sexual abuse as a risk factor for crack cocaine use in a sample of community recruited women at high risk for illicit drug use. Am J Drug Alcohol Abuse. 2002;28(1):109-31.
22. García-Moreno C, Watts C. Violence against women: its importance for HIV/AIDS. AIDS. 2000;14(Suppl. 3):S253-65.
23. Gerra G, Zaimovic A, Avanzini P, Chittolini B, Giucastro G, Caccavari R, et al. Neurotransmitter-neuroendocrine responses to experimentally induced aggression in humans: influence of personality variable. Psychiatry research. 1997;66(1):33-43.
24. Gilbert L, et al. Intimate partner violence and HIV risks: a longitudinal study of men on methadone. Journal of Urban Health. 2007;84(5):667-80.
25. Global and regional estimates of violence against women: prevalence and health effects of intimate partner violence and non-partner sexual violence, WHO Library Cataloguing – in – Publication Data, World Health Organization. 2013.
26. Golding J. Intimate partner violence as a risk factor for mental disorders: a meta analysis. Journal of Family Violence. 1999;14(3):99-132.
27. Goldstein Jeffrey H. Aggression and crimes of violence. Oxford, England: Oxford U press. 1975;14:192.
28. Goodwin MM, et al. Pregnancy intendedness and physical abuse around the time of pregnancy: findings from the pregnancy risk assessment monitoring system, 1996–1997. Maternal and Child Health Journal. 2000;4(2):85-92.
29. Gundappa A. Violence Against Women in India: Preventive Measures. Indian Streams Research Journal. 2012;2(12):1-4.
30. Hamberger LK, Guse CE. Men's and women's use of intimate partner violence in clinical samples. Violence Against Women. 2002;8:1301-31.

31. Heise L, et al. Ending violence against women. Population Reports, Series L, No. 11. Baltimore: Johns Hopkins University School of Public Health, Population Information Program. 1999.
32. Hendy HM, Weiner K, Bakerofskie J, Eggen D, Gustitus C, McLeod K. Comparison of six models for violent romantic relationships in college men and women. Journal of Interpersonal Violence. 2003;18:645-65.
33. Indian Penal Code. Available: *https://www.childlineindia.org.in/.../Indian%20penal%20code%201860.pdf.*
34. Kegan J, Moss HA. Birth to maturity: a study in psychological development. New York: Wiley; 1962. p. 381.
35. Krug EG, et al. World report on violence and health. Geneva, World Health Organization, 2002.
36. Makepeace JM. Gender differences in courtship violence. Family Relations.1986;35:383-8.
37. Maman S, et al. The intersections of HIV and violence: directions for future research and interventions. Social Science and Medicine. 2000;50(4):459-78.
38. Mangoli RM, Tarase GM. Crime against Women in India: A Statistical Review; International Journal of Criminology and Sociological Theory. 2009; 2(2):292-302.
39. Ministry of Law and Justice. Indian Constitution 1950. Availabe: *https://www.google.com.np/?gws_rd=cr&ei=lbQpVo_GApK0uATq-ZfoBQ#q=indian+constitution+1950+pdf.*
40. Moore AM, Frohwirth L, Miller E. Male reproductive control of women who have experienced intimate partner violence in the United States. Social Science and Medicine. 2010;70(11):1737-44.
41. Morrow M, Chappel M. Hearing Women's Voices: Mental Health Care for Women. Vancouver, BC: BC Centre of Excellence for Women's Health, 1999.
42. Najavits LM, Weiss RD, Shaw SR. The link between substance abuse and post-traumatic stress disorder in women: A research review. American Journal on Addictions. 1997;6:273-83.
43. Pallitto CC, Campbell JC, O'Campo P. Is intimate partner violence associated with unintended pregnancy? A review of the literature. Trauma, Violence, and Abuse. 2005;6(3):217-35.
44. Raj A, et al. Perpetration of intimate partner violence associated with sexual risk behaviors among young adult men. American Journal of Public Health. 2006;96(10):1873-8.
45. Report on Violence Against Women, Mental Health and Substance Use, Canadian Women's Foundation, 2011.
46. Santana MC, et al. Masculine gender roles associated with increased sexual risk and intimate partner violence perpetration among young adult men. Journal of Urban Health. 2006;83(4):575-85.
47. Sapolsky, Robert M. "Testosterone Rules." The Gendered Society Reader, 3rd edn, In: MS Kimmel, Aronson A (Eds). New York: Oxford University Press; 1997.pp.26-31.
48. Sedgh G, et al. Induced abortion: incidence and trends worldwide from 1995 to 2008. The Lancet. 2012;379(9816):625-32.
49. Siegel JA. Aggressive behavior among women sexually abused as children. Violence and Victims. 2000;15:235-55.
50. Silverman JG, et al. Intimate partner violence and unwanted pregnancy, miscarriage, induced abortion, and stillbirth among a national sample of Bangladeshi women. BJOG: An International Journal of Obstetrics and Gynaecology. 2007;114(10):1246-52.
51. Singh S. Abortion worldwide: a decade of uneven progress. New York, Guttmacher Institute, 2009.
52. Straus MA. The controversy over domestic violence by women: A methodological, theoretical, and sociology of science analysis. In: Arriaga XB, Oskamp S (Eds), Violence in intimate relationships. Thousand Oaks, CA: Sage;1999.pp.14-44.
53. Sullivan TP, Meese KJ, Swan SC, Mazure CM, Snow DL. Precursors and correlates of women's violence: Child abuse traumatization, women's victimization, avoidance coping and psychological symptoms. Psychology of Women Quarterly. 2005;29:290-301.
54. Swan SC, Snow DL. A typology of women's use of violence in intimate relationships. Violence Against Women. 2002;8: 286-319.
55. Swan SC, Snow DL. Behavioral and psychological differences among abused women who use violence in intimate relationships. Violence Against Women. 2003;9:75-109.
56. Swan SC. The Development of a Theory of Women's Use of Violence in Intimate Relationships; Violence Against Women. 2006;12(11).
57. Swan SC. When battered women use violence: Implications for health outcomes. Paper presented at the Meeting of the Division of Prevention and Community Research, New Haven, CT. 1999.
58. Tolman D, Spencer R, Rosen-Reynoso M, Porche M. Sowing the Seeds of Violence in Heterosexual Relationships: Early adolescents narrate compulsory heterosexuality. Journal of Social Issues. 2003;59(1):159-78.
59. Tomaszewski, et al. Association between lipid profile and circulating concentrations of estrogens in young men; Atherosclerosis. 2009;203(1):257-62.
60. Vezina J, Hebert M. Risk Factors for Victimization in Romantic Relationships of Young Women: A Review of Empirical Studies and Implications for Prevention. Trauma Violence Abuse. 2007;8(1):33-66.
61. Wallace L. The Harms of Help: Exploring Women's Experiences with Anti-Violence, Addictions and Mental Health Services Within British Columbia. Master's Thesis. Simon Fraser University, 2010.
62. Warshaw C, Moroney G. Mental health and domestic violence: collaborative initiatives, service models and curricula. The National Center on Domestic Violence, Trauma & Mental Health. 2002. *http://www.nationalcenterdvtraumamh.org/lib/File/Model%20Collab%2011.6.02.pdf.*
63. Wingood GM, DiClemente RJ. The effects of an abusive primary partner on the condom use and sexual negotiation practices of African-American women [see comments]. American Journal of Public Health. 1997;87(6):1016-8.

CHAPTER 55

Psychiatry and Reproduction

Jayati Simlai, Swarnali Bose, Umesh S, CRJ Khess

INTRODUCTION

Women are affected by various mental health related problems across their lifespan, right from childhood, adolescence, adulthood, reproductive age and old age. The reproductive age group consists of more than one-third of the lifespan of a woman. Reproductive events and processes have both physiological and psychological concomitant. Psychological states of a woman not only affect her reproductive physiology but also modulate reproductive events and exert bidirectional relationships. Many psychiatric disorders have onset during the reproductive age. Apart from this, psychiatric disorders during this period not only have devastating effects on women's mental health, but also on her immediate environment and more specifically on her offspring. Hence, psychiatric problems that arise during this childbearing age are important because optimal care has to be provided for the women in need, especially during this period.

REPRODUCTIVE DEVELOPMENT AND PHYSIOLOGY

Development of Female Gonads

During embryogenesis, sex differentiation occurs that involve a complex process and interplay of many genes. The key component to sexual dimorphism is the Y chromosome that is donated by sperm, which contains the master gene SRY (sex-determining region on Y) on its short arm.[1] The protein product of this gene (SRY protein; testis determining factor) initiates a cascade of downstream genes which influences steroidogenesis factor 1 (SF1) to induce differentiation of Sertoli and Leydig cells. Sertoli cells then produce müllerian inhibiting substance (MIS, also called antimüllerian hormone) that causes regression of the müllerian ducts and influences the development of male genitals. Sexual differentiation in females was once thought to be a default mechanism that occurred in the absence of a Y chromosome, but it now appears that there are specific genes like *DAX1* gene located on the short arm of the X chromosome which plays a pivotal role in the development of female genital system. DAX1 down-regulates steroidogenesis factor 1 (SF1) activity, thereby preventing differentiation of Sertoli and Leydig cells. In the absence of MIS production by Sertoli cells, the müllerian ducts are formed and are stimulated by estrogens to form the uterine tubes, uterus, cervix and upper vagina.[2] Estrogens also act on the external genitalia at this stage to form the labia majora, labia minora, clitoris and lower vagina. In female fetus, ovary develops at around four weeks from the germinal epithelium and the peak number of germ cells is attained at around twenty weeks of gestation; this results in the development of primordial follicles and later followed by primary follicles. Majority of follicles undergo atresia and rest remain dormant till puberty. During puberty, follicular growth occurs and oocyte enlarges and matures to form ovum that is shed during the process of ovulation.

Puberty in Females

Puberty typically begins in girls between the ages of nine and fourteen years. It is initiated by the release of gonadotropin releasing hormone which is produced by the hypothalamus in a pulsatile and synchronous manner. This mechanism of release is active in fetus and neonate but then remains dormant until puberty. There appears to be genetic expression of the *KiSS1* gene (a gene that encodes a family of neuropeptides called kisspeptins) for these physiological processes.[3] Between the ages of eight and thirteen years, breast buds appear, and pubic hair begins to develop. Later on, when the breast areolae and nipples begin to form, onset of menstruation occurs which is known as menarche.[4] These initial menstrual cycles are usually painless as they are not accompanied by ovulation. During this time, asymmetry of breast development is common and vaginal secretions also increase, both of which cause concern in some girls. Growth rate slows after the onset of menstruation, and most girls have significant weight gain during this period.

This biological shift and timing of maturation in girls also has effects on cognitive, psychosocial and sexual behaviors. There are major social changes as well as expectations in roles during this period. Finally, there are major psychological changes that are linked to enhanced social and cognitive maturity. These rapid changes or transitions become a heightened potential for both positive and negative outcomes and make them vulnerable to various stressors. Puberty is all about the emergence of sexuality and physical changes of puberty increases the individual's interest in sex. These changes can have a profound impact on development and harbors risk of pregnancy and sexually transmitted diseases. However, both the frequency and long-term consequences of these behaviors differ across various cultural groups.[3]

The Menstrual Cycle

The menstrual cycle is a normal physiological process occurring in women that makes reproduction possible. The menstrual cycle starts in adolescence (menarche), temporarily ceases during pregnancy, breast-feeding and illness (e.g. anorexia nervosa) and permanently ceases in late adulthood (menopause). A regular menstrual cycle is considered to be a sign of good health, represents biological maturity, signifies ability to bear children and also indicates pregnancy. The cycles are regulated primarily by the actions of gonadotropin releasing hormone (GnRH) in hypothalamus, follicle-stimulating hormone (FSH) and luteinizing hormone (LH) in anterior pituitary, estrogen and progesterone in the ovary. Follicular development is initiated by the pulse release of GnRH that stimulates the release of the pituitary gonadotropins luteinizing hormone (LH) and follicle-stimulating hormone (FSH). LH in turn stimulates ovarian theca cells to synthesize and secrete androgens whereas FSH induces granulosa cell development, including the synthesis of enzyme aromatase, which converts the thecally produced androgens to estrogens. In the presence of a constant GnRH pulse frequency of one pulse each 90 minutes, the secretion of LH and FSH in the follicular phase occurs and is regulated primarily by estrogen feedback at the level of the pituitary.[3] Rising estrogen levels suppress FSH, thereby limiting the number of follicles that become mature oocytes capable of ovulating. Thereafter, granulosa cells are transformed into progesterone-secreting luteal cells and the ovulated follicle is then referred to as the corpus luteum, which secretes progesterone. The average length of the menstrual cycle is 28 to 30 days.

There are several mechanisms by which psyche and soma interact with each other and has effects on both physiological and psychological health at different periods of menstrual cycle. As in cases of premenstrual dysphoric disorder (PMDD), the mood, cognitive and behavioral changes occurs in association with the phases of menstrual cycle whereas significant stressors can lead to menstrual abnormalities. These conditions exemplify a somatopsychic interplay in which biological changes occurring in the soma trigger changes in the psychological state and vice-versa in predisposed women.[3]

Physiology of Female Sexuality

Female sexual response is divided into four successive phases; excitement, plateau, orgasm and resolution (The EPOR model) as per Master and Johnson.[5] During sexual arousal, the clitoris and labia minora become engorged with blood causing increase in their length and diameter. Kaplan[6] proposed the aspect of *desire* in the three-phase model, consisting of desire, arousal, and orgasm. In this model, desire is the factor that provides momentum to the overall response cycle.

There are various neurogenic mediators of female sexual responses within the central nervous system including the medial preoptic, anterior hypothalamic region and related limbic-hippocampal structures which mediates by activating parasympathetic and sympathetic nervous systems. Immunohistochemical studies have found rich network of nerve fibers in human vaginal tissues which secretes neuropeptide-Y (NPY), vasoactive intestinal peptide (VIP) and nitric oxide synthase (NOS) that are involved in modulating vaginal relaxation and secretory processes. It also plays a role in regulating vaginal and clitoral NOS expression.[7] Phosphodiesterase type 5, the enzyme responsible for degradation of cGMP, is present in human clitoral, vestibular bulb and vaginal smooth muscles and is inhibited by sildenafil citrate. Alpha-1 and alpha-2 adrenergic mediators also appear to play a physiological role in female sexual arousal in modulating smooth muscle tone. Hormone like estrogen plays a significant role in regulating female sexual functions. Estrogens have vasoprotective and vasodilatory effects, which result in increased vaginal, clitoral and urethral arterial flow, resulting in maintenance of the female sexual response.[7]

PHYSIOLOGY OF PREGNANCY

A normal pregnancy invites many systemic changes in the mother. Those changes affect systems like cardiovascular system, endocrinal system, nervous system, etc. This section deals with an overview of changes and response of the maternal physiology to pregnancy. In pregnancy, large amount of human chorionic gonadotropin, estrogens, progesterone and human chorionic somatomammotropin are synthesized by placenta that are essential for a normal pregnancy. These sex hormones prevent menstruation and cause the endometrium to grow and store large amounts of nutrients rather than being shed in the menstruum. Under the influence of human chorionic gonadotropin, the corpus luteum secretes estrogens and progesterone which maintains the decidual nature of the uterine endometrium, necessary for the early development of the fetus. Besides this, large quantities of estrogen secreted by placenta causes (1) enlargement of the mother's uterus, (2) enlargement of the mother's breasts and growth of ductal structure, and (3) enlargement of the mother's female external genitalia. The estrogens also relaxes the pelvic ligaments and the symphysis pubis becomes elastic. These changes allow easier passage of the fetus through the birth canal.[8]

Another important hormone secreted by corpus luteum initially and by placenta later is progesterone. Its importance lies in following areas: (1) Progesterone causes decidual cells to develop in the uterine endometrium, and these cells play an important role in the nutrition of the early embryo. (2) Progesterone decreases the contractility of the pregnant uterus, thus preventing uterine contractions from causing spontaneous abortion. (3) Progesterone contributes to the development of the conceptus even before implantation by providing appropriate nutritive matter from the fallopian tube secretions to the developing morula and blastocyst. (4) The progesterone secreted during pregnancy helps the estrogen prepare the mother's breasts for lactation.

Due to effect of placental hormones on pituitary gland and increased metabolic demand during pregnancy, almost all other nonsexual endocrine glands react to the pregnant state. The anterior pituitary gland of the mother enlarges at least 50% during pregnancy and increases its production of corticotropin, thyrotropin, and prolactin. The rate of adrenocortical secretion of the glucocorticoids is moderately increased throughout pregnancy.[8] The mother's thyroid gland ordinarily enlarges up to 50% during pregnancy and increases its production of thyroxine. The increased thyroxine production is caused partly by a thyrotropic effect of human chorionic gonadotropin secreted by the placenta.

Not only endocrinal glands react to pregnancy, there are various changes noted in mother's body in response to the same. For instance, the uterus increases from about 50 g to 1100 g, and the breasts approximately double in size. At the same time, the vagina enlarges and the introitus opens more widely. Also, the various hormones can cause marked changes in a pregnant woman's appearance, sometimes resulting in the development of edema, acne etc. The average weight gain during pregnancy is about 6–10 kg, most of which occurs during the last two trimesters. There is also increase in basal metabolic rate to about 15% during the latter half of pregnancy.[8]

REPRODUCTIVE AND DEVELOPMENTAL TOXICOLOGY

Reproductive toxicology deals with the causes, mechanisms, effects and prevention of disturbances throughout the reproductive cycle that are induced by chemicals. Teratology is the science concerned with the birth defects of a structural or functional nature. Embryo/fetotoxicity involves any toxic effect on the conceptus resulting from prenatal exposure, including the structural and functional abnormalities and postnatal manifestations of such effects. A wide variety of responses characterizes developmental toxicity that include chromosomal and genetic disorders, spontaneous abortion, intrauterine death, prematurity, low birth weight, birth defects and functional disorders that are the effects of such drug interference with the developmental processes. A critical phase for the induction of structural malformations usually occurs during the period of organogenesis. In humans, this critical period extends from about 20 to 70 days after the first day of the last menstruation period. Therefore, this is the susceptible period for the induction of insults that may lead to structural or functional deficits which is later manifested as abnormalities in behavior, cognition and various other psychological disturbances. When considering the use of a psychotropic medication during pregnancy, the clinician must address four primary types of risk with respect to the developing fetus: (1) risk of pregnancy loss or miscarriage, (2) risk of organ malformation or teratogenesis, (3) risk of neonatal toxicity or withdrawal syndromes during the acute neonatal period, and (4) risk of long-term neurobehavioral sequelae.[9]

To provide guidance to physicians seeking information on the reproductive safety of various prescription medications, the FDA established a system that classifies medications into five risk categories (A, B, C, D, and X) based on data derived from human and animal studies. Category A medications are designated as safe for use during pregnancy, while category X drugs are contraindicated and are known to have risks to the fetus that outweigh any benefit to the patient. Most psychotropic medications are classified as category C, agents for which human studies are lacking and for which "risk cannot be ruled out." Category D indicates "positive evidence of risk." No psychotropic drugs are classified as safe for use during pregnancy (category A).[9]

PSYCHIATRIC DISORDERS DURING REPRODUCTIVE CYCLE

Premenstrual Dysphoric Disorders

Interestingly, various reproductive hormones like estrogen and progesterone bear effects on emotion, cognition and behavior. These ovarian hormones have influence on central serotonergic system, their receptors and influence their metabolism. Menstrual cycle is accompanied by substantial changes of hormonal levels and is associated with changes in mood or development of mood symptoms. One well-studied mood disorder with respect to the influence of ovarian steroids on mood is premenstrual dysphoric disorder (PMDD). According to DSM-5[10] PMDD is diagnosed if most menstrual cycles in one year are manifested with one essential symptoms of anger/irritability, depressed mood, anxiety or emotional lability present for most of the time during the last week of the onset of menses and begin to remit within a few days after the onset of menses and become minimal or absent in the week postmenses. This is usually accompanied by symptoms like anhedonia, lack of energy, change in appetite, sleep, sense of feeling overwhelmed and other physical symptoms like breast tenderness, bloating sensation and weight gain. There is usually significant functional impairment during these periods. Premenstrual syndrome (PMS) is considered to be less severe than PMDD as there is no stipulation of affective symptoms and does not require multiple physical and psychological discomforts. Functional impairment is usually not seen in PMS. PMS may affect up to 80% of reproductive-aged women whereas the incidence of PMDD is approximately 6%.[10]

In women with PMDD, the ovarian axis is apparently functioningandhasbalancedestrogenandprogesteronelevels. However, there is a definitely compromised psychological health. These findings have made researchers curious and have encouraged them to investigate the neuroendocrine-modulated central neurotransmitters and the role of the Hypothalamic-Pituitary-Gonadal (HPG) axis in PMDD. There is an increasing attention drawn towards metabolite of progesterone that is allopregnanolone in the manifestation of premenstrual symptomatology. Allopregnanolone is thought to modulate GABA (γ-amino-butyric acid) receptor functioning and produce an anxiolytic effect. Withdrawal of progesterone during the premenstrual phase cause changes in the sensitivity of GABA receptors resulting in manifestation of symptoms.[11] An inverse relationship also exists between androgens and serotonin level in the brain. An increased androgen level during this period reduces serotonin activity and thereby results in irritability, depression, impulsive behavior and decreased libido.

Current literatures in the management of PMDD recommends for effective and interdisciplinary treatments. Life style modification that includes dietary routines (reduction of caffeine, salt, alcohol and smoking), regular physical activity, relaxation, hypnosis and psychotherapy have been recommended. Other modes of treatment includes, hormonal contraceptives, vitamin supplementation, use of antidepressant like SSRIs (sertraline, fluoxetine, paroxetine), GABA agonist alprazolam is considered to be an adjuvant treatment. Other medication like 5-HT_{1A} agonists (buspirone) has shown good results in PMDD.[11]

PSYCHIATRIC DISORDERS DURING PREGNANCY AND PERIPARTUM PERIOD

Pregnancy and the postpartum period are considered to be period when women are vulnerable to many psychiatric disorders. Psychiatric disorders during pregnancy are associated with poor maternal health status and inadequate antenatal care. Maternal psychiatric disorders during pregnancy and the postpartum period are also associated with numerous adverse outcomes for the offspring that includes maladaptive fetal growth and development, poor cognitive development and behavioral problems during childhood and adolescence. For these reasons, accurate information about the mental health status of women during pregnancy and the postpartum period should be understood properly for optimal care. According to World Health Organization the perinatal period is defined as commencing "at 22 completed weeks (154 days) of gestation (the time when birth weight is normally 500 g) and ends seven completed days after birth.[12]" This is a period when the women are particularly vulnerable due to hormonal imbalances, high expectation in society, stressors and physical complications. Despite these conditions, majority of the women sail through this period without undue complications, but some of them suffer from mild to severe forms of psychiatric illnesses. Women who are particularly at risk include those who lack support of the partner, family members, previous history of psychiatric disorder and lifetime exposure to traumatic events.[12] They are prone to develop mood disorders, psychosis, anxiety disorders and few become victims of suicide while some others commit homicide of newborn.

Antenatal Depression

Depression is prevalent in pregnant women, affecting 10 to 25% of them.[13] Pregnancy itself can be a risk factor for depressive episodes. Depression during pregnancy or a previous history of depression outside of pregnancy is also significant predictors of postnatal depression. Other risk factors for antenatal depression include marital discord or dissatisfaction, inadequate psychosocial supports, recent adverse life events, lower socioeconomic status, and unwanted pregnancy. Prenatal depression increases in severity from the first to the second trimester, negatively affecting fetal development and neonatal outcome. Prenatal depression is associated with higher rates of pre-eclampsia, placental abnormalities, spontaneous abortion, premature delivery as well as low birth weight in neonates. Depressed mothers exhibit a number of physiological changes that may influence fetal development and include increased and prolonged cortisol production that may further impact the offspring's own stress hormone and neurotransmitter regulation.[13] Despite these known risks, depression during the antenatal period is often not recognized and treatment rates are lower in pregnant than in nonpregnant women.

Pregnancy and Psychosis

The fertility rate among women suffering from schizophrenia and other severe forms of psychotic disorders have increased over the past few decades.[14] This may be a direct result of the concurrent changing attitudes towards conception among those with serious mental illnesses. Unfortunately, unplanned and unwanted pregnancies occur more frequently in women with psychosis than in the general population. Although it is described that improvement of psychotic symptoms in some women with chronic psychotic illnesses occurs during pregnancy, the data also suggest that maternal and neonatal morbidity associated with such illnesses are significant. Studies show that women with chronic psychotic disorders are at increased risk for poor fetal outcome, including stillbirth, preterm delivery, low birth weight, and infant death. Acute psychosis during pregnancy is both an obstetric and a psychiatric emergency. Psychosis during pregnancy may inhibit a woman's ability to obtain appropriate and necessary prenatal care and may impede her ability to cooperate with caregivers during delivery. Furthermore, psychosis during pregnancy predicts an increase in the risk of postpartum psychotic exacerbation.

Pregnancy and Bipolar Disorders

Bipolar disorders usually overlap with a woman's prime childbearing age. Pregnancy has traditionally been considered protective against the risk of relapse of bipolar disorder. However, new evidence is emerging that in any case, pregnancy is not protective for all women with bipolar disorder and management of the illness in pregnancy is most difficult when the pregnancy is unanticipated. Although recurrence rates among the pregnant women were similar to the rates in the nonpregnant control subjects, recurrences of illness is 2.9 times more frequent in the postpartum period compared with nonpregnant women.[15] These findings suggest that risk of recurrent illness increases sharply during the postpartum period. It is also important for clinicians to be knowledgeable about approaches to and risks associated with medication treatment during pregnancy. Close monitoring of these patients is necessary. Rapid intervention can significantly reduce morbidity and improve overall prognosis of such patients. Since many pregnancies are unplanned in women with bipolar disorder, it is important to carefully plan pregnancy which can benefit the mother and minimize the risks to the fetus.[15]

Postpartum Depression

The postpartum period has typically been considered a time of risk for the development of mood disorder. Postpartum depression (PPD) is defined in the psychiatric nomenclature as a major depressive disorder (MDD) with a specifier of postpartum onset within 1 month after child birth. However, depression in women during the postpartum period may start during pregnancy or may have onset beyond the first postpartum month. Women who meet criteria for MDD i.e. depressed mood or loss of interest or pleasure in activities must be present for at least 2 weeks. In addition, symptoms of sleep disturbance, appetite disturbance, loss of energy, feelings of worthlessness or guilt, diminished concentration, and thoughts of suicide may be present. However, the diagnosis of PPD is challenging because of changes in sleep patterns, changes in appetite, and excessive fatigue being routine for women after delivery. Majority of the cases seen during the routine mental health consultation of postpartum women includes those suffering from postpartum blues, those with 'new' onset nonpsychotic postpartum depression, third being women with past history of major depression and fourth one, suffering from postpartum psychosis.[16]

- *Postpartum blues:* Postpartum 'blues' is considered the mild form of the postpartum mood disturbances; its prevalence has been reported to be varying from 26 to 85%.[16] The symptoms of this syndrome typically begin within the first week following childbirth, peak on the fifth day and resolve by the twelfth day postpartum. Symptoms include dysphoria, mood lability, weeping spells, anxiety, insomnia, poor appetite and irritability. The mood disturbance characterizing postpartum blues is considered transient and insufficient to cause serious impairment of a woman's functioning. In at least 25% women, however, the disturbance may persist beyond the initial postpartum period, leading to more serious postpartum depression (PPD). In these subgroup of women, particularly those with a history of recurrent depression, may display a heightened sensitivity to changes in reproductive hormone levels, such as those occurring premenstrually, as well as to changes that occur during postpartum reproductive transitions. It is also important to note that chronic psychosocial stressors may sensitize the brain to subsequent metabolic or hormonal changes and vice versa and makes them more vulnerable to postpartum blues or postpartum depression.
- *The 'new' onset nonpsychotic postpartum depression:* The first episode of depression in this group of women occurs in the early postpartum period, often within the first 2 to 4 weeks after delivery. There is usually family history of depression but the women herself has not experienced any prior episodes of depression. Women with a history of postpartum depression are at significant risk with rates of postpartum recurrence as high as 50%.[16] There appears to be a strong biological vulnerability in such women and they definitely have chances of recurrence even beyond the postpartum period. The onset is usually acute and often severe illness is documented. These women tend to respond well to antidepressants, preferably SSRIs combined with psychoeducation, supportive therapy and interpersonal therapy. Such patients are also treated with electroconvulsive therapy if they fail to respond to the treatment.
- *Women with past history of major depression:* These groups of women with postpartum depression often have past history of major depressive episode and/or history

of dysthymia. There is often a family history of mood disorder. Onset is usually acute or insidious and severe. An important and frequently misdiagnosed presentation is the women in depressed phase harboring bipolarity which may be confused with postpartum depression.[16]

- *Postpartum psychosis:* The onset of postpartum psychosis occurs at a rate of approximately 1 in 1000 births.[16] The onset is usually acute and presents during the first two weeks to four weeks postpartum. The course is often fluctuating, changing rapidly throughout the day and throughout the postpartum period. In women with postpartum psychosis, it is more likely that at least 70% might have recurrence of episodes in the subsequent pregnancies. Current evidence indicates that postpartum psychosis is most commonly associated with the diagnosis of bipolar disorder. Risk factors include a previous episode of postpartum psychosis, previous hospitalization for a manic or psychotic episode, recent discontinuation of mood stabilizers, primiparity, obstetric complications, sleep deprivation, and a family history of bipolar disorder or postpartum psychosis. The clinical presentation may be varied from restlessness, insomnia, agitation to auditory or visual hallucinations, paranoid or grandiose delusions, elements of delirium or disorientation, mutism and/or stupor and extreme deficits in judgment accompanied by high levels of impulsivity that may contribute to increased risks of suicide or infanticide (5% of psychotic women). Postpartum psychosis carries a relatively good prognosis with early detection and vigorous treatment, but if left untreated may progress to the second postpartum year and become more refractory to treatment.[16]
- *Issues on infanticide:* Infanticide is one of the most serious risks of postpartum psychosis. Sadly, it is difficult to predict which women with postpartum psychosis will commit infanticide. Symptom exacerbation, command hallucinations, and the stressor of new infant care can increase the risk of infanticide after delivery in a mother with psychosis. Infanticide may also occur in the context of severe PPD, caused by neglect and abuse, because of the child being unwanted or as revenge against the infant's father. Between 16% and 29% of mothers who kill their children end committing suicide themselves. However, more studies are needed to identify risk factors for neonaticide and infanticide.[17]

There are robust evidences from various open label trials and randomized control trials which have shown various medications to be efficacious in the treatment of postpartum depression. Tricyclic antidepressants (TCAs) like nortriptyline and selective serotonin reuptake inhibitors (SSRIs) like fluoxetine, sertraline, paroxetine, serotonin nor-epinephrine reuptake inhibitors (SNRIs) like venlafaxine are found to be effective in postpartum depression. Several open-label trials have also found nefazodone, fluvoxamine and bupropion to be effective. Others include omega-3 fatty acid as dietary supplementation which has been found to be controversial in PPD.[16]

Postpartum Bipolar Disorder

Women with a history of bipolar disorder are at exceptionally high risk for episode recurrence during the postpartum period. There is nearly twofold higher risk for a recurrent episode in puerperal women, compared with nonpostpartum and non-pregnant women. Symptom emergence is often rapid and may commence a few weeks before or within the first few days to weeks after parturition. Although the cause of this heightened recurrence risk during postpartum is unknown, it may be associated with abrupt changes in estrogen and progesterone, perturbation of the hypothalamic–pituitary–thyroid axis, decreased or erratic sleep patterns, increased psychosocial stress associated with motherhood and young infant care, or any combination of these factors. Indeed, research indicates that disruptions in biological and social causes increases risk of relapse among bipolar patients.[18] Hence, close clinical monitoring and efforts to enlist the aid of social supports to prevent sleep disruption and stabilize social rhythms in the new mother with a history of bipolar disorder may be particularly important. It is advisable to maintain the woman on mood stabilizers within 24 hours of delivery in severe cases to prevent the high risk of relapse that occurs during the postpartum period.

PHARMACOLOGICAL TREATMENT OF MOOD AND PSYCHOTIC DISORDERS DURING PREGNANCY AND LACTATION

Psychiatric disorders of reproductive age can cause devastating effects on both mother and infant. Despite the morbidity associated with these disorders, practitioners are usually reluctant to start psychotropic medications considering its possible anticipated teratogenic effects. Teratogens are the substances or environmental agents that cause abnormal embryonal or fetal growth resulting in congenital birth defects. It is worth mentioning that all the psychotropic medications cross the placental barrier. However, there has been a recent dearth of literature about risk and benefits of these medications and has made the practitioner confident in providing rationale for prescribing various psychotropic medications during pregnancy and lactation.[19]

Antipsychotics in Pregnancy

- *Amisulpride:* Despite there being no evidence of teratogenicity in embryofetal developmental studies in mice and rabbits following oral doses up to 4 times the maximum recommended human dose, no published information on human pregnancy is available.

- *Aripiprazole:* Aripiprazole is rated as FDA Pregnancy Category C drug. Despite the risk in animal studies that demonstrated teratogenicity and developmental toxicity, few case reports have considered it to be safer in human pregnancies.
- *Clozapine:* Clozapine is rated as FDA Pregnancy Category B, despite paucity of data. Reproductive studies performed in rats and rabbits at doses of approximately 2 to 4 times the human dose revealed no harm to the fetus. In humans, single cases of major malformations, gestational metabolic complications, poor pregnancy outcome and perinatal adverse reactions associated with exposure to clozapine during various stages of pregnancy have been subsequently reported in few case reports. However, clozapine overdose during pregnancy may cause fatal poisoning of the newborn.
- *Olanzapine:* Olanzapine is rated as FDA Pregnancy Category C drug and reports no evidence of fetal harm in animals. Till date olanzapine is not carrying increased risk of major fetal malformations, nonetheless, sporadic cases of olanzapine-associated fetal malformations, gestational metabolic complications associated with being large for gestational age and neonatal adverse reactions are mentioned in the literature.
- *Quetiapine:* Quetiapine is rated as FDA Pregnancy Category C drug. Preclinical safety report no teratogenic effects in animals. In human studies, Quetiapine showed the lowest amount of placental passage when compared with both FGAs (haloperidol) and SGAs (risperidone and olanzapine) and was considered to be a safer option in pregnancy.
- *Risperidone:* Risperidone is rated as FDA Pregnancy Category C and has not shown direct teratogenic effects in animal studies, however human studies are limited. Only sporadic clinical observations have described fetal malformations and complicated pregnancy outcomes.
- *Ziprasidone:* Ziprasidone is rated as FDA Pregnancy Category C. Animal studies have demonstrated developmental toxicity, including possible teratogenic effects (mainly ventricular septum defects and kidney malformations), at doses similar to the human therapeutic dose. At present, no human data are available.
- *Haloperidol:* Haloperidol is FDA as Pregnancy Category C drug. In animal studies, haloperidol rarely induced fetal malformations. Information describing congenital anomalies (most frequently, limb defects) in neonates is available since 1966. However, these clinical observations remain controversial. Neonates exposed *in utero* to haloperidol have shown congenital malformation rates within the expected baseline risk for the general population.
- *Chlorpromazine:* Chlorpromazine is rated as FDA Pregnancy Category C. In animal studies, chlorpromazine has been associated with an increased risk of congenital malformations (including low birth weight, skeletal malformation, cleft palate, intrauterine death) but at doses many times higher than the human-recommended dose. In humans, chlorpromazine might be associated with an increased risk of neonatal respiratory distress if used at daily doses higher than 500 mg. Until now, only one case of fetal malformation or gestational diabetes has been reported, whereas perinatal complications seem to be relatively common when the drug is used in late pregnancy. As thought earlier that chlorpromazine is a teratogen that carries possible increase risk of fetal malformations, recent reviews emphasize that the molecule is relative safer during pregnancy.[19]

Mood Stabilizers and Pregnancy

- *Lithium:* Lithium is category D drug and has evidence for human fetal risk. Prenatal lithium exposure can cause 400-fold higher rate of cardiovascular malformations, most notably Ebstein's anomaly, as compared with the general population. Lithium-exposed infants were found to weigh significantly more than normal subjects. The most common toxicity effect in offspring exposed to lithium during labor is the "floppy baby" syndrome, characterized by cyanosis and hypotonicity. Cases of neonatal hypothyroidism and nephrogenic diabetes insipidus have also been described. Hence, close monitoring of lithium levels in the mother during pregnancy is done. In the case of first-trimester exposure, anomalies can be identified with prenatal screening with a high-resolution ultrasound examination and fetal echocardiography at 16–18 weeks gestation.[20] This procedure aids parents in decisions regarding pregnancy termination and perinatal interventions after delivery.
- *Carbamazepine:* Carbamazepine is a category D drug and should be avoided during pregnancy. Prenatal exposure to carbamazepine during the first-trimester increases the risk of craniofacial defects, fingernail hypoplasia, developmental delay, low birth weight and reduced head size. The rate for neural tube defects ranges between 0.5% and 1%. It is also associated with transient hepatic toxicity (cholestatic hepatitis and direct hyperbilirubinemia) in neonates exposed *in utero*. Carbamazepine can also cause fetal vitamin K deficiency. Since adequate levels of vitamin K are necessary for normal mid-facial growth and for the functioning of clotting factors, carbamazepine exposure *in utero* could increase the risk of neonatal bleeding and mid-facial abnormalities.[20]
- *Valproate:* Valproate has a FDA pregnancy category rating of D. It is considered a human teratogen and use of this compound during the first-trimester is associated with

neural tube defect rates of about 5 to 14%. The effect of the drug on neural tube development is related to its use 17 to 30 days postconception, and risk is dose related. This defect is more likely to be lumbosacral rather than anencephalic, which suggests a drug effect on neural crest closure. Some researchers have suggested that intrauterine growth retardation and mild mental retardation as a part of the "fetal valproate syndrome." Neonatal complications associated with valproate use near the time of delivery include heart rate decelerations and withdrawal symptoms of irritability, jitteriness, feeding difficulties, and abnormal tone. Other complications among neonates include liver toxicity and hypoglycemia. Reductions in neonatal fibrinogen levels have also been reported. Folate supplementation during pregnancy reduces the risk of neural tube defects generally, but it has not been tested as prophylaxis in pregnant women undergoing valproate treatment.[20]

- *Lamotrigine:* Lamotrigine is classified as pregnancy category C. Although to date teratogenicity has not been definitively demonstrated in animals or humans, the ability of lamotrigine to inhibit dihydrofolate reductase *in vitro* has raised concerns regarding the risk of malformations. The rate of malformation with lamotrigine is similar to that of general population. The risk of neonatal rashes should be monitored.

Mood Stabilizers and Breastfeeding

- *Lithium:* Lithium is secreted into breast milk and levels achieved are nearly half of maternal serum levels. The diminished renal clearance in neonates can elevate serum levels of lithium. It is reported that lithium concentrations in breast milk ranges from 0.1 mmol/liter to 0.6 mmol/liter).[21] One concern regarding appreciable lithium levels is the propensity for rapid dehydration in neonates with febrile illnesses. Another concern is that the longer-term effects on the infant of sustained lithium levels are not known. It is recommended that breastfeeding should be undertaken with caution by women undergoing lithium treatment. In a breastfed infant exposed to lithium, serum lithium concentrations should be monitored.
- *Valproate:* There are no adverse effects reported among infants whose mothers were treated with valproate solely during breastfeeding. However, human breast milk concentrations are approximately 1 to 10% of maternal serum levels.[21] Some experts recommend avoiding valproate because of increased risk of hepatotoxicity, thrombocytopenia and anemia in the neonates.
- *Carbamazepine:* Concentrations of carbamazepine in breast milk are detectable but low. Human breast milk concentrations of approximately 7 to 95% of maternal serum levels and serum carbamazepine levels in the infant are usually <1 μg/mL. It is recommended that the neonates should be monitored if they develop drowsiness, poor feeding, seizure-like activity, irritability, and high-pitched cry and also monitor for hepatotoxicity and hematological toxicity.[21]
- *Lamotrigine:* Lamotrigine is excreted into human breast milk with a milk/plasma ratio of 0.61. Serum concentrations in nursing infants are approximately 30% of maternal serum concentrations. No adverse effects have been documented but it is recommended that the baby be monitored for rash.

Antidepressants during Pregnancy

Classes of antidepressant drugs for use during pregnancy include the tricyclic antidepressants, selective serotonin-reuptake inhibitors (SSRIs), and serotonin–norepinephrine reuptake inhibitors (SNRIs). Although none of these agents have been proved absolutely safe in pregnant women, there are more reassuring data on the SSRIs than on the other two classes of drugs. Most malformations were cardiac septal defects that were associated with maternal use of tricyclic antidepressants (primarily clomipramine). There is often an association between the use of paroxetine and congenital cardiac defect and persistent pulmonary hypertension. Very few studies have reported the same with SSRIs like fluoxetine and sertraline. Low birth weight, preterm delivery, fetal hypoglycemia, jaundice, respiratory problems and low Apgar score are associated with tricyclics. A "neonatal adaptation syndrome" has been described in 15 to 30% of newborns exposed to tricyclics and SSRIs in late pregnancy and might be a result of withdrawal effects.[22] The symptoms and signs include irritability, weak crying, tachypnea, temperature instability and hypoglycemia and occasionally seizures; these symptoms and signs typically resolve within 2 weeks after birth.

Antidepressants and Breastfeeding

The breastfeeding woman with PPD must weigh the potential efficacy of antidepressant medication for her depression, the potential risks of exposure of her infant to antidepressant medication through breastfeeding and the known negative effects of not treating her depression on child development. However, it is important that neonates and infants are especially vulnerable to potential drug effects due to their immature hepatic and renal systems, immature blood–brain barriers, and developing neurological systems. When an antidepressant is started in the woman after delivery, it is recommended to start with low doses and to titrate the dose up slowly while monitoring the infant for adverse effects. Possible adverse effects in the breastfeeding infants include irritability, sedation, poor weight gain or a change in feeding patterns. Several reviews on the safety of selective serotonin reuptake inhibitors (SSRIs), tricyclic antidepressants

(TCAs), and newer antidepressants like mirtazapine and venlafaxine with breastfeeding have been conducted. SSRIs like sertraline, paroxetine and TCAs like nortriptyline usually yield undetectable infant serum levels and that elevated infant levels are more likely with fluoxetine and citalopram. Sertraline has been reported to have minimal or no effect on the infant. Adverse events are most likely to occur in newborn infants up to 8 weeks of age and infants who are born prematurely or with medical problems may be at increased risk. Infant exposure to antidepressants can be minimized by avoiding breastfeeding at the time of peak antidepressant concentration in the breast milk. If adverse effects are noted in the infants, options include decreasing the dose, changing to partial or full bottle feeding, or changing the medication. Even if there are no adverse effects in infants, the long-term effects of antidepressant exposure through breast milk on child cognitive, motor, neurological and behavioral development are unclear.[22]

Electroconvulsive Therapy during Pregnancy

The use of electroconvulsive therapy (ECT) during pregnancy usually raises considerable anxiety on the part of clinicians and patients despite safety records being well documented over the last 50 years. ECT is imperative in instances of severe mania or psychotic depression with suicidal thoughts and disorganized thinking during pregnancy. Such clinical situations are associated with a danger from impulsivity or self-harm. The safety and efficacy of ECT in such settings are well described, particularly when the ECT is instituted in collaboration with a multidisciplinary treatment team, including an anesthesiologist, a psychiatrist, and an obstetrician. A limited course of treatment may be sufficient followed by institution of treatment with one agent or a combination of agents, such as antidepressants, neuroleptics, benzodiazepines, or mood stabilizers. ECT during pregnancy tends to be underused because of concerns that treatment will harm the fetus. Despite one report of placental abruption associated with the use of ECT in pregnancy considerable experience supports its safe use in severely ill gravid women. Thus, it becomes the task of the psychiatrist to decide and facilitate the most clinically appropriate intervention whenever necessary.[23]

Nonpharmacological Interventions during Pregnancy

Until recently, there were few data on the role of non-pharmacological treatments for depression during pregnancy. For women with mild to moderate depressive symptoms, nonpharmacologic interventions, including interpersonal therapy (IPT), cognitive behavioral therapy (CBT), and supportive psychotherapy, may be attractive alternatives to medication during pregnancy. In women, who are receiving maintenance antidepressant treatment, nonpharmacologic interventions may potentially facilitate tapering of medication or may allow for use of lower dosages of medication. IPT is a short-term, manual-driven psychotherapy that deals primarily with four major problem areas: grief, interpersonal disputes, role transitions and interpersonal deficits. Given the importance of interpersonal relationships in couples expecting a child and the significant role transitions that take place during pregnancy and subsequent to delivery, IPT is ideally suited for the treatment of depressed pregnant women.[23]

Anxiety Disorders during Pregnancy and the Postpartum Period

Although anxiety disorders during pregnancy and postpartum period are associated with adverse fetal and developmental consequences, researches in this area have received lesser emphases as compared to depression. The peak age at onset for anxiety disorders in women occurs in the third decade which is peak childbearing years. Considering the high prevalence of mood and anxiety disorders in women, it follows that substantial numbers of women will exhibit symptoms and, therefore, benefit from treatment for anxiety disorders during pregnancy and the postpartum period.[23]

Apart from the increased neuroendocrine demands of pregnancy and postpartum period, over activity due to stress and anxiety has been implicated in negative health outcomes in fetuses born to such mothers. The catecholamine's released during stress causes adverse effects to the developing fetus as it causes compromised blood flow and oxygen due to vasoconstriction. Anxiety disorders also contribute to elevated cortisol levels in pregnancy and causes premature labor and delivery. The exposure of the fetus to maternal stress and increased levels of adrenal hormones, therefore has possible consequences for fetal central nervous system development and specifically glucocorticoid brain receptor development. Hence, it appears clear that anxiety disorders in pregnancy and postpartum needs to be understood in greater details considering the lasting effects. The subsequent section deals with perinatal panic disorder, obsessive-compulsive disorder, post-traumatic stress disorder and generalized anxiety disorder.

- *Impact of untreated anxiety disorder in pregnancy:* There are few data regarding the long-term risk to the fetus of untreated psychiatric illness during pregnancy. Overall, the clinical and laboratory data indicate that untreated maternal anxiety during pregnancy can cause lower infant birth weight, lower gestational age, altered Apgar scores, and impairment of fetal hemodynamic and fetal movement. Anxiety symptoms early in pregnancy are also associated with a 3-fold increase in pre-eclampsia and association with premature rupture of the membranes, cervical dyskinesia, and higher incidence of caesarean section.[23] Panic attacks during pregnancy can cause placental abruption, fetal distress, decreased nutrition, and use of potentially harmful substances for self-medication. Agoraphobia in addition to panic disorder is assumed to impair prenatal care and adversely affect the outcome of pregnancy.[23]

Panic Disorder

Panic disorder is characterized by sudden, recurrent and unpredictable panic attacks, associated with persistent worry about the possibility of having future panic attacks. Symptoms of panic attacks typically include shortness of breath, heart palpitations, chest pain, dizziness, and fear of losing control or dying. There has been a relatively consistent prevalence rates ranging from 1.3% to 2% with a typical age at onset in late adolescence to the mid-30s reported for panic disorder during the perinatal period.[24]

- *Clinical presentation, predictors, course and differential diagnosis of panic disorder:* Although symptoms of panic during the perinatal period are typical of symptoms in the general population, they are often interpreted in the context of the perinatal state. For example, women may interpret panic attacks during pregnancy as an indication that something is wrong with the fetus. Postpartum women typically worry about the future anticipated attacks and hence try to avoid the social situations. Although there is paucity of literature for predicting of perinatal panic disorder, there is some evidence from retrospective studies that provide relationship between lactation/weaning and panic symptoms. A woman who does not breastfeed their babies have panic attacks during postpartum period. Weaning is also associated with new onset or exacerbation of panic. However, these results are yet to be confirmed by controlled prospective studies. New onset panic disorder occurs in postpartum period during the first 12 weeks.[23] It could be assumed that childbirth occupies a significant area in the memory as a major life event. Despite limited literature, it is clear that many women experience pregnancy following the onset of panic disorder. Although there are conflicting findings, a general pattern of improvement in panic symptoms during pregnancy, followed by worsening during the postpartum period has been reported in retrospective studies whereas few studies found no change in symptom severity during the perinatal period. Panic symptoms closely resemble anemia, hyperthyroidism, pre-eclampsia and pheochromocytoma and should be ruled out in case of suspicion.
- *Treatment of perinatal panic disorder:* Research evidence to guide treatment of perinatal panic disorder is extremely limited, as no controlled or uncontrolled studies have been published. However, few researches have described successful treatment with antipanic medications, particularly imipramine, SSRIs and cognitive-behavioral therapy. SSRIs are the first-line treatment for anxiety disorders because of data supporting their efficacy, their minimal need for dose titration, and their overall favorable side effect profile with no risk of teratogenicity. Newer antidepressants, such as venlafaxine and mirtazapine are options for patients unresponsive to, or intolerant of, SSRIs. Benzodiazepines are associated with oral cleft and may cause physiological dependence and withdrawal in the newborn, so they should be avoided if alternative treatments are available. Other self-care strategies, such as elimination of caffeine, reduction of sleep deprivation, and relaxation techniques have been recommended if avoidance of pharmacotherapy is desired and possible. Women who have avoided medications during pregnancy should consider resumption during postpartum because the postpartum period is a time of high-risk for relapse. The clinician should give the patient as much information as possible to facilitate the decision-making process.[24]

Obsessive-compulsive Disorder

Obsessive-compulsive disorder (OCD) is characterized by repetitive, intrusive thoughts or images, known as obsessions, and/or repetitive or ritualistic behaviors, known as compulsions. Typically, obsessions are anxiety provoking, whereas compulsions reduce anxiety for a short time, particularly when triggered by obsessions. OCD, more than other anxiety disorders, is thought to have a strong neurobiological basis. Guided by the well-known "serotonin hypothesis" it is generally implicated that there is a dysregulation of the serotonin system in the generation of obsessional thoughts and compulsive behavior. In particular, there is some evidence to suggest that fluctuations in estrogen, progesterone levels (as observed in late pregnancy) may alter serotonergic transmission, reuptake and binding. There is also association of OCD with cortico-striatal-thalamic-cortical circuits in the pathophysiology. Perhaps as a result of this neurobiological basis, OCD is notable in that its symptoms vary little across time, culture, sex and age estimated lifetime prevalence of OCD in the general population of 2.5% and 1-year prevalence is 1.5 to 2.1%. However, the prevalence of OCD may be lower during pregnancy (0.2–1.2%) than during the postpartum period (2.7–3.9%).[24]

- *Clinical presentation, predictors and course of perinatal OCD:* It has been extensively reported that obsessions in perinatal women often include fears of intentionally or accidentally harming the fetus or infant. Obsessional thoughts about harming the infant are not specific to OCD as they have been reported by over 40% of women with postpartum depression and from 34% to 65% of new parents in volunteer community samples.[23] Evolutionary theories propose that these thoughts may be adaptive in that they may cause the parent to be vigilant in protecting the infant from potential harm. These adaptive behaviors may trigger or increase obsessional symptoms in women with pre-existing OCD or a genetic, neurologic, or cognitive vulnerability to OCD. It is important that OCD-related obsessions of infant harm be carefully differentiated from infanticidal ideation characteristic of postpartum psychosis and severe postpartum depression. The primary difference in clinical presentation relates to insight. In contrast to obsessions, compulsive behaviors like hand washing or cleaning behavior are common in postnatal period and often attribute to concerns that the infant would get exposed to contamination.

Several studies have investigated the extent to which women with OCD report the onset of their illness to be associated with pregnancy or childbirth. These results suggest that, as many as 40% have onset during pregnancy and up to 30% have onset during the postpartum period. In the cases of those women with preexisting OCD, up to 69% report no change in their symptoms during pregnancy but rest have symptom exacerbation during postpartum period.[24]

- *Treatment of perinatal OCD:* As with panic disorder, no controlled studies have been conducted to examine effectiveness of treatment methods for perinatal OCD. However, preliminary evidence supports SSRIs like fluoxetine and cognitive behavioral therapy, either independently or in combination, as most effective. Research on cognitive-behavioral therapy may be especially important for this particular OCD subgroup since the use of SSRI pharmacotherapy in breastfeeding women must be considered carefully.

Post-traumatic Stress Disorder

Post-traumatic stress disorder (PTSD) is an anxiety disorder characterized by exposure to a traumatic event appraised by the individual to actual or threatened death or serious injury or a threat to the physical integrity of self or others. Moreover, the person's response to the stressor involves intense fear, helplessness or horror. Symptoms of PTSD include re-experiencing of the traumatic event, such as intrusive recollections or recurrent and distressing dreams of the event, avoidance of stimuli associated with the trauma and numbing of emotional responsiveness and hyperarousal, such as difficulty sleeping and concentrating and irritability. Although DSM-5[10] does not specifically identify childbirth as an example of an extreme stressor, reports suggest that childbirth can qualify as a traumatic event that results in PTSD in some women. PTSD has been recognized as occurring after stressful medical and surgical procedures that involve intense pain, invasive obstetric and gynecologic procedures, suggesting that it is also relevant to consider traumatic labor and birth experiences as potential stressors for PTSD symptoms. There is inconsistency in assessment measures, and in particular, the absence of differentiation between clinical PTSD and PTSD symptoms that may in part explain the wide range of prevalence rates (0–6.9%) reported.[23]

- *Clinical presentation, predictors and course of perinatal PTSD:* Perinatal PTSD has been associated with some distinct clinical features, including avoidance of the baby/impaired mother-infant relationship, sexual dysfunction and avoidance of future childbearing. PTSD occurring after childbirth may lead to postponement or avoidance of future childbearing or requests for planned Cesarean sections in an attempt to avoid re-traumatization by childbirth. Requests for termination of an unplanned pregnancy and sterilization have also been documented. Childhood or adulthood sexual assault can also be associated with perinatal PTSD. Women with a history of sexual abuse may experience triggering of memories of abuse in response to childbirth procedures. Finally, maternal and infant complications like pre-eclampsia and hypoxic injuries to newborn have been associated with perinatal PTSD. Till date, no studies have reported on the course of PTSD in perinatal women with pre-existing disorder.
- *Treatment of perinatal PTSD:* There are no published studies which have evaluated treatment intervention for perinatal PTSD. However, some efforts have been made to prevent PTSD among women assessed as having had a traumatic childbirth using critical event debriefing. This prevention strategy involves talking about the traumatic experience with a trained professional; both validation and accommodation of the traumatic event may be facilitated. A more recent study found that a debriefing-modeled counseling intervention was effective in reducing risk of trauma symptoms and depression at 3 months postpartum. This recent promising result suggests that further research is warranted to examine the potential for prevention of perinatal PTSD using debriefing-style counseling interventions.

Generalized Anxiety Disorder

Generalized anxiety disorder (GAD) is a chronic condition characterized by at least 6 months of frequent worry, together with additional symptoms including poor concentration, muscle tension, fatigue, and restlessness. GAD affects approximately 5% of the general population. Only one study has estimated the prevalence of perinatal GAD reporting a rate of 8.5% during the third trimester of pregnancy.[23]

- *Clinical presentation, predictors and course of perinatal GAD:* It can be difficult to differentiate GAD from normal, nonpathologic anxiety, since worries about the health of the fetus or anticipation of a painful delivery are common among healthy perinatal women. No studies to date have compared the content and nature of worry in women with GAD to that in healthy perinatal women. In the general population, GAD is distinguished from normal worry on the basis of 3 characteristics; in GAD, worry is excessive and interferes with daily functioning; worry is widespread, usually to multiple domains of the person's life; and worry can occur without any identifiable trigger. These same characteristics may be helpful in differentiating perinatal GAD from normal anxiety as well. It has been recommended that perinatal worry be further investigated when a woman is worrying more than other perinatal women, when she cannot be reassured or cannot control the worry, or when excessive and uncontrollable worry has persisted for 6 months or more. No studies have reported on risk factors or predictors of GAD in the perinatal period. Further, no studies have examined the course of pre-existing GAD across the perinatal period.

- *Treatment of perinatal GAD:* No studies have investigated treatment of perinatal GAD; however, there is evidence for the effectiveness of cognitive-behavioral therapy, SSRIs, and benzodiazepines in the general population of GAD patients. As with panic disorder, careful assessment is required to rule out potential medical causes of anxiety symptoms before treatment is initiated. If pharmacotherapy is used, antidepressant medications are preferred over the benzodiazepines due to their better safety profile for the developing fetus and/or breastfeeding infant.[24]

Pseudocyesis

When a woman believes herself to be pregnant and develops symptoms and signs of pregnancy, this condition is called pseudocyesis. The clinical features include, a firm belief in the pregnancy, amenorrhea, morning sickness and/or pica, breast enlargement and pigmentation of nipples, discharge of colostrum, abdominal enlargement, assumed fetal movements caused by muscular contraction, fat, retained feces. The psychological basis is usually an intense desire for children. In some cases, however, a guilt or fear of pregnancy has been the background. Pseudocyesis is a demonstration of the influence of psyche over soma, mediated by hormonal secretion. It occurs in at least a dozen other mammals. Persistence of the corpus luteum would explain breast changes, moderate uterine enlargement and secretory endometrium, but does not explain the whole phenomenon. Hormonal measurements are found to be having chronic anovulatory states, hyperprolactinemia or androgen excess.[3] Simply revealing the diagnosis is unsatisfactory because the patient may misinterpret the advice, consult another doctor or develop a recurrence. The underlying conflicts must be explored, helping the patient to accept that she is not pregnant. Psychotherapy is recommended during or after a presentation of pseudocyesis to evaluate and treat the underlying psychological dysfunction.[16] The differential diagnosis of pseudocyesis includes delusions of pregnancy occurring in women (also men) with a variety of psychoses, but without the somatic changes of pregnancy.

SEXUAL DYSFUNCTION IN WOMEN

Sexuality is a complex process and is coordinated by the neurologic, vascular, endocrine systems and psychological conditions. Sexuality not only incorporates the biological aspects but also concerns family, societal and religious beliefs, aging, health status and personal experience. Increased risk factors for female sexual dysfunction include neurologic disease, genital atrophy, genital surgery, endocrinopathies, peripheral vascular disease, sexual abuse, psychological factors, interpersonal relationships, etc.[6] In addition, sexual activity incorporates interpersonal relationships, each partner bringing unique attitudes, needs and responsibilities of couples. A breakdown in any of these areas may lead to sexual dysfunction. Sexual disorders in females can be lifelong or acquired, generalized or situational, drug induced, organic, psychogenic or mixed and at times idiopathic.

- *Hypoactive sexual desire:* It is among the common complaints of women who seek expert's consultation. This can be defined as a "persistent or recurring deficiency (or absence) of sexual thoughts, desire, or fantasies, and the lack of receptivity for sexual activity leading to personal distress." Sexual desire is a subjective in nature and lacks absolute standards. With one woman's perception of lack of desire being another's concept of normal or even excess desire. This complaint may be triggered by a mismatch with the desire of the partner. A noticeable and disturbing change in level of libido also triggers consultation in women. This disorder may be caused by insufficient or ineffective stimulation (not only physical but also emotional), hormonal imbalance, dysphoria, depression, stress, medical disorders, body image issues (e.g. mastectomy) or partner-related issues. Some women find their enjoyment in alternative sexual fantasies or practices thereby creating a lack of desire for sexual intercourse.[6]
- *Sexual arousal disorder* is an inability to reach or maintain a satisfactory sexual excitement resulting in personal distress. These disorders are predominantly caused by failure to obtain adequate vaginal lubrication or vaginal smooth muscle relaxation. This condition is usually associated with inadequate pelvic blood flow or local trauma. It may also be expressed as lack of subjective excitement that can be triggered by physiologic problems.[7]
- *Orgasmic disorder* is a recurrent or persistent difficulty or inability to experience orgasm or prolonged delay in reaching orgasm, occurring in the presence of adequate stimulation and arousal, and results in personal distress. Primary orgasmic disorder is when a woman has never experienced orgasm and may be caused by insufficient

stimulation, lack of experience (for one or both partners) and the backdrop of sexual abuse. Secondary anorgasmia occurs when the woman has previously been orgasmic, but that ability is diminished or has ceased. Local trauma, hormone imbalance, medical disorders, psychiatric disorders, medications (selective serotonin reuptake inhibitors), substance abuse and psychological or social factors are some causes of orgasmic disorder.[7]

- *Dyspareunia* is a common sexual pain disorder. It is defined as "recurrent or persistent pain during sexual intercourse." Insufficient lubrication is the usual cause with prevalence rates as high as 45%. Local vaginal infections, endometriosis, pelvic adhesions, and cystitis may also be associated with dyspareunia. Women with a retroverted uterus occasionally have pain during intercourse. In menopausal women who have not had intercourse for sometime, the vagina does 'shrink' and combined with loss of lubrication, may result in pain on penetration. Psychological factors depressive symptoms, somatic complaints, other sexual dysfunction, and increased marital distress can also lead to pain on intercourse.
- *Vaginismus* is defined as "involuntary contractions of the pubococcygeal muscle and the muscles of the outer third of the vagina, making it impossible to penetrate the introitus, or extremely painful during the act of penetration.[3] The cause of vaginismus is unknown, and it may also be associated with conditioned aversion to previously painful penetration of the vagina. The emotional sequelae of pain, such as anxiety, depression, relationship problems can also lead to additional sexual dysfunctions. Medical conditions like genital infections, endometriosis, prior genital mutilation, chronic pelvic pain (vulvodynia), vestibulitis and interstitial cystitis may also cause vaginismus.[7]
- *Sexual aversion disorder* is the active avoidance of sexual contact leading to personal distress. In some cases, it can occur in a relationship because of performance anxiety or fear, alternatively because of the partner's behavior before or during intercourse. Prolonged sexual aversion is usually related to prior noxious events, such as incest, rape or abuse or underlying psychiatric disorders.[3]
- *Treatment of female sexual dysfunction:* Treatment of sexual dysfunctions depends on appropriateness of diagnosis. Both medical treatment and psychotherapy remains the mainstay in management. Organic or anatomical causes must be considered and may require medical or surgical remedies. Behavioral therapies, such as sensate focus exercises, sex therapy, desensitization strategies for anxiety, relaxation training and assertiveness training have been successful alone or in combination.[3]Depending on the circumstances, couple counseling and therapy may be recommended. The outcome of treatment depends on the diagnosis and is variable across individuals.[3]

INFERTILITY AND RELATED PSYCHOSOCIAL ISSUES

Approximately 1 in 10 couples experience either primary or secondary infertility worldwide. Infertility is defined as the inability of a couple to achieve pregnancy after at least one year of unprotected intercourse. Women experiencing infertility report high level of psychological distress, dysphoria, a decline in their sexual functioning and a feeling of lowered self-worth. In many cases, infertile women feel that the issue of their infertility has become so all important to them that they are less interested in other aspects of their lives.[25] When a couple faced with infertility, women tend to be more emotionally affected than their male counterparts. Infertility is universally described as a stressful experience for females affecting all aspects of their lives: marital, social, physical, emotional, financial and spiritual. In a comparison to patients with other medical conditions, psychological symptoms associated with infertility are similar to those related to cancer, hypertension and cardiovascular illness. Infertile women, in comparison with control group, showed higher scores on depression and anxiety scales.[26] Infertile stress impacts the marital relationship by depleting sexual intimacy. It is important to note that 26.8% of the women undergoing artificial reproductive technology (ART) met criteria for a mood disorder, 17% for major depression and 9.7% for dysthymia. Another study showed that those who had 2 to 3 years infertility had more depression and anxiety than those who had this problem for a year or more than 6 years.[26] Some individuals experience exacerbations of pre-existing psychiatric disorders due to infertility. At the same time, infertile individuals undergoing assisted reproduction do appear to be at greater risk for psychological distress, like anxiety, distress and grief particularly if treatment is unsuccessful. Other factors that also contribute to grief reaction include unsuccessful *in vitro* fertilization (IVF) in over-optimistic couples. Research indicates that mood (anxiety, depression, or distress) fluctuates in men and women over the course of assisted reproduction treatment cycles with the severity of emotional distress diminishing with repeated cycles.

Pharmacological agents used to treat disorders of ovulation or to hyperstimulate the ovaries may alter mood and cognition. These agents include clomiphene citrate, antiestrogens, GnRH analogs, human gonadotropins, progesterone and so on.[27] Most of the agents do alter estradiol and progesterone levels and the resultant hormonal fluctuations may trigger mood lability and depression in sensitive individuals. Such individuals should be informed about the medications and adverse effects to mood and preferably should be treated by psychotherapeutic procedures rather than prescribing antidepressants or anxiolytics as they improve spontaneously on withdrawing the causative medication. With the advent of assisted reproduction, the role of the mental health professional in the treatment of infertility has shifted from curative to a more complex and comprehensive role that includes provision of patient education, screening, guidance, preparation for medical treatments, advice, support and assistance for decision making, assessment of current mental health, treatment of pre-existing or ongoing psychiatric diagnosis, sexual problems, marital problems, bereavement therapy and handling emotional crisis of infertility.[3]

PERIMENOPAUSE AND RELATED ISSUES

The transition into menopause is a major hormonal event and is associated in many women with both physical and psychological symptoms. The term "perimenopause" describes the period immediately before the menopause, i.e. from the time when the hormonal and clinical features of approaching menopause commence until the end of the first year after menopause. Changes most commonly associated with estrogen depletion or fluctuations that causes vasomotor symptoms such as hot flushes and night sweats, urogenital dryness/atrophy causing dyspareunia as well as an increased risk of osteoporosis and cardiovascular disease are frequent.[3]

The relationship between the perimenopause/menopause and mood disorders is less well understood. However, some epidemiological data indicates that a higher than expected prevalence of depressive-like symptoms are observed in peri and postmenopausal women attending gynaecological clinics.[28] The most prevalent mood symptoms during the perimenopause includes irritability, tearfulness, anxiety, depressed/labile mood, lack of motivation/energy, poor concentration and interrupted sleep.[29] These symptoms have been linked to fluctuations in estradiol levels in blood, especially abrupt withdrawal from very high erratic levels, rather than to times when levels are slowly and gradually declining.

Management of Perimenopausal Mood Symptoms

There has been an interesting convergence of hormonal, antidepressant and insomnia pharmacotherapies for perimenopausal symptoms over the last decade. The replacement of perimenopausally declining estradiol and progesterone is with exogenous hormones. Antidepressant drugs are increasingly prescribed for hot flashes based on clinical trials that show benefit with low-dose serotonin/serotonin-norepinephrine reuptake inhibitors (escitalopram, venlafaxine, and duloxetine).[30] It is proposed that antidepressants may improve distress tolerance of hot flashes via symptomatic improvement of coexisting mild insomnia, anxiety, dysphoria, and/or irritability. Sleep disturbance affects nearly 50% of perimenopausal women and significantly contributes to reduced quality of life. Perimenopausal insomnia is variably attributed to vasomotor symptoms, night sweats, and mood disturbance. Targeting the sleep symptoms with sleep hygiene interventions may result in sleep and quality-of-life improvement of similar magnitude to that provided by hormone replacement therapy (HRT). Conversely, estradiol has proven to be useful in the treatment of minor and major depression. Women with endocrinologically confirmed perimenopause and with structured interview–based diagnosis of depression experienced a 70 to 80% rate of remission during treatment with 50 to 100 μg per day of 17β-estradiol.[3]

CONCLUSION

Women mental health and reproduction is a dynamic biological and psychosocial interface that is complex in nature and varies across age, ethnic and racial groups. Misdiagnosis or under-diagnosis continues to be a critical issue in women's mental health and the same carries for women who suffer from psychiatric problems during child-bearing age. Future researches should emphasize on understanding the relationship of reproduction with women mental health and thorough understanding of biological underpinnings as well as women's social roles and position in society during this period is essential. Also, we must remember that, medications should be properly prescribed and monitored in these women to prevent adversities in future offspring.

REFERENCES

1. Haqq CM, et al. Molecular basis of mammalian sexual determination: activation of mullerian inhibiting substance gene expression by SRY. Science. 1994;266:1494.
2. Sadler TW. Langman's medical embryology, 11th edition. Philadelphia: Lippincott Williams & Wilkins, 2010.
3. Berga SL, Parry BL, Moses-Kolko EL. Psychiatry and reproductive medicine. In: Kaplan HI, Sadock BJ. Comprehensive Textbook of Psychiatry, 9th edition. Philadelphia: Lippincott Wiliams & Wilkins, 2009.pp.2539-62.
4. Tanner JM. Normal growth and techniques of growth assessment. Clin Endocrinol Metab. 1986;15:411.
5. Masters WH, Johnson V: Human Sexual Response. Boston, MA, Little, Brown, 1966.
6. Kaplan HS: The New Sex Therapy: Active Treatment of Sexual Dysfunctions. New York, Brunner/Mazel, 1974.
7. Bhasin S, Basson R. Sexual Dysfunction in Men and Women. In: Kronenberg H, Larsen R, Melmed S, Polonsky K (Eds). Williams' Textbook of Endocrinology, 9th edition. Philadelphia, PA: Elsevier, 2011.

8. Guyton AC, Hall JE. Textbook of Medical Physiology, 11th edition. Philadelphia: Saunders; 2006.pp.1027-34.
9. Cohen LS, Altshuler L. Pharmacologic management of psychiatric illness during pregnancy and the postpartum period, in Psychiatric Clinics of North America Annual of Drug Therapy. Dunner D, Rosenbaum J (Eds). Philadelphia, PA, WB Saunders; 1997.pp.21-60.
10. American Psychiatric Association. Diagnostic and statistical manual of mental disorders, (5th edition). Arlington, VA: American Psychiatric Publishing, 2013.
11. Zukov I, Ptácek R, Raboch J, Domluvilová D, Kuzelová H, Fischer S, Kozelek, P. Premenstrual dysphoric disorder–review of actual findings about mental disorders related to menstrual cycle and possibilities of their therapy. Prague Med. Rep. 2010; 111(1):12-24.
12. Buist A. Managing depression in pregnancy. Aust Fam Physician. 2000;29(7):663-7.
13. Cohen LS, Wang B, Nonacs R, Viguera AC, Lemon EL, Freeman MP. Treatment of mood disorders during pregnancy and postpartum. Psychiatr Clin North Am. 2010;33: 273-93.
14. Pugh TF, Jerath BK, Schmidt WM, Reed RB. Rates of mental disease related to childbearing. N Engl J Med. 1963;268: 1224-8.
15. Yonkers KA, Wisner KL, Stowe Z, et al. Management of bipolar disorder during pregnancy and the postpartum period. Am J Psychiatry. 2004;161:608-20.
16. Pearlstein T, Howard M, Salisbury A, Zlotnick C. Postpartum depression American Journal of Obstetrics and Gynecology. 2009;200(4):357-64.
17. Fairbrother N, Woody SR. New mothers'thoughts of harm related to the newborn. Arch Womens Ment Health. 2008; 11:221-9.
18. Leibenluft E. Women with bipolar illness: clinical and research issues. Am J Psychiatry. 1996;153:163-73.
19. Gentile S. Antipsychotic therapy during early and late pregnancy. A systematic review. Schizophr Bull. 2010;36:518-44.
20. Fortinguerra F, Clavenna A, Bonati M. Psychotropic drug use during breastfeeding: a review of the evidence. Pediatrics. 2009;124(4).
21. Burt VK, Rasgon N. "Special considerations in treating bipolar disorder in women." Bipolar disorders. 2004;6(1):2-13.
22. Spinelli M. Antidepressant treatment during pregnancy. Amer J of Psychiatry. 2012;169(2):121-4.
23. Cohen LS, Nonacs RM. Mood and Anxiety Disorders During Pregnancy and Postpartum. Oldham JM, Riba MB (Eds). Washington, DC, American Psychiatric Publishing, 2005.
24. Ross LE, McLean LM. Anxiety disorders during pregnancy and the postpartum period: a systematic review. J Clin Psychiatry. 2006;67:1285-98
25. Anderson KM, Sharpe M, Rattray A, Irvine DS. Distress and concerns in couples referred to a specialist infertility clinic. [Comparative Study]. J Psychosom Res. 2003;54(4):353-5.
26. Domer AD, Zutter meister PC, Seibel M, Friedman R. The psychological impact of infertility: a comparison with patients of other medical condition. J Psychosom Obstet Gynaecol; 1993.pp.45-52.
27. van Wely M, Westergaard LG, Bossuyt PM, et al. Human menopausal gonadotropin versus recombinant follicle stimulation hormone for ovarian stimulation in assisted reproductive cycles. Cochrane Database Syst Rev, 2003.
28. Freedman RR. Hot flashes revisited. Menopause. 2000;7:3-4.
29. van Amelsvoort TA, Abel KM, Robertson DM, et al. Prolactin response to d-fenfluramine in postmenopausal women on and off ERT: comparison with young women. Psychoneuroendocrinology. 2001;26:493-502.
30. Soares C, Almeida OP, Joffe H, Cohen LS. Efficacy of estradiol for the treatment of depressive disorders in perimenopausal women: a double blind randomized placebo-controlled trial. Arch of Gen Psychiatry, 2001.

CHAPTER 56 Culture and Psychiatry

PB Behere, M Behere, A Das

DEFINING CULTURE

There are as many definitions of culture as given by many scholars. The aggregate of all the beliefs, customs, technologic achievements, language, and history of a people would constitute a culture—although this is only one of many definitions of the word culture. Kroeber and Kluckhohn (1952) apply the term to too many different aspects of social organization.[1]

A culture comprises all of the beliefs, laws, customs, morals, capabilities, and habits of people who cooperatively work and live in an identified social unit (Tribes, cities, nations, etc.) or in institutions (armed forces, religious orders, hospital staffs, etc.). A traditional survey of the culture of physicians would include descriptions of their scientific beliefs, the varieties of medical and surgical subspecialty practice, the work settings, and the economic exchanges and other customs that are features of the delivery of health care. Thus culture in a nutshell can be best conceptualized as a totality, a complex system of symbols possessing subjective drives such as values, feelings or ideals.[2]

The term "culture" may be applied to the social heritage-myths of origin, traditions, etc.—in a society, transmitted from each generation to the next. A historical resume of the culture of medicine would trace the earliest records of healing procedures, the developments in medical and surgical treatment up to the present time, and the ways in which theories of disease and actual practices have been transmitted through apprenticeships formal education, and literary records.[3]

Culture includes or influences dress, language, religion, customs, food, laws, codes of manners, behavioral standards or patterns, and beliefs. It plays an important role in how people of different backgrounds express themselves, seek help, cope with stress and develop social supports. Culture affects every aspect of an individual's life, including how we experience, understand, express, and address emotional and mental distress. Culture is manifested in the core of behavior and the various ways in which life is regulated, such as rituals, customs, etiquette, taboos, and laws. It is reflected in such things as common sayings, legends, drama, art, philosophical thought, and religions. Culture shapes people's behavior, but at the same time it is moulded by the ideas and behavior of the members of the culture. Thus, culture and people influence each other reciprocally.[4]

*Culture is **learned** through active teaching, and passive acting, **shared** among its group members, **patterned** as having definite sets of beliefs and practices that guide different areas of individual and social life, **adaptive,** through change across variable environments and **symbolic** with many arbitrary signs that represent something special to the group.*

CULTURAL COMPETENCE

It is the ability to relate effectively to individuals from various groups and backgrounds. Competency means to respond to the unique needs of members of minority populations. Cultural competence must be a guiding principle, so that services are culturally sensitive and provide culturally appropriate prevention, outreach, assessment and intervention. The dimensions of cultural competency include:

- Race
- Ethnicity
- Language
- Sexual orientation
- Gender
- Age
- Disability
- Class/socioeconomic status
- Education
- Religious/spiritual orientation.

Culture competence has got certain components. This was explained by Tseng et al.[5]

These are:

Cultural Sensitivity

Cultural sensitivity refers to recognition of the diversity of viewpoints, attitudes, and lifestyles among human beings. It includes the recognition that groups of people may tend to experience different types of stress in living and to utilize relatively distinctive coping patterns.

Cultural Knowledge

However, it is desirable to have some basic anthropological knowledge about how human beings vary in their habits, customs, beliefs, value systems, and especially illness behavior. This basic knowledge should be extended with regard to the cultural systems of patients, so that culturally relevant assessment and care can be delivered.

Cultural Empathy

An intellectual understanding about a patient's culture is often not sufficient for effective treatment. There is another quality needed: the ability to feel and understand, on an emotional level, the patient's own cultural perspective.

Cultural Guidance

Specific treatment models for particular ethnic groups are unlikely to be useful in clinical practice. There are so many kinds of problems within any given ethnic group that different therapeutic approaches must be applied accordingly. However, a certain general approach might be better suited to a specific ethnic group because of varying ways to relate to a doctor, cope with mental problems, and understand the role of psychiatric services.

CULTURE AND MEDICINE

In medicine, culture has got three dimensions. An appropriate understanding of these three cultural dimensions is essential to the comprehension and performance of culturally competent clinical work. As explained by Tseng WS et al[4] they are as follows:

The culture of the patient: In addition to individual factors—such as level of education, medical knowledge, and personal life experiences—culture will contribute to the patient's understanding of illness, perception and presentation of symptoms and problems, and reaction and adjustment to illness. The patient's expectations of the physician, motivation for treatment, and compliance with treatment recommendations are also influenced by culture.

The culture of the physician: The culture of the physician will shape the pattern of interaction and communication with the patient. The culture of the physician explicitly or implicitly affects his or her attitude toward the patient, understanding of the patient's problems, and approach to caring for the patient.

The medical culture: Medical culture includes traditions, regulations, customs, and attitudes that have developed within the medical service setting beyond medical knowledge and theory. The practice of general psychiatry is strongly embedded in the medical culture that has developed within the medical system.

CULTURE AND PSYCHIATRY

The term cultural psychiatry is synonymous to transcultural psychiatry because as it avoids some negative aspects of ethnocentrism, nevertheless has the disadvantage of minimizing the comparative, "trans" aspect of the subject. Undoubtedly sociocultural psychiatrists, like most anthropologists, are intrigued by the differences across ethnic, national, racial and most important sub-cultural boundaries but the vital legacy of the anthropologist-psychiatrists collaboration of the early part of this century by people such as Margaret Mead, Malinowski and Ruth Benedict has been to highlight cultural relativism. There are differences of family structure, courtship patterns, and baptism and funeral rituals between cultures but a value judgment about their appropriateness success from someone outside the sub-culture is rarely constructive and can be deeply offensive.

Cross-cultural psychiatry, transcultural psychiatry, or cultural psychiatry is a branch of *psychiatry* concerned with the *cultural* context of *mental disorders* and the challenges of addressing *ethnic* diversity in psychiatric services. It emerged as a coherent field from several strands of work, including surveys of the *prevalence* and form of disorders in different cultures or countries; the study of *migrant* populations and ethnic diversity within countries; and analysis of psychiatry itself as a cultural product.

Transcultural psychiatry is defined as the study and comparison of mental illness in different cultures. Its focus generally has been the role of socio cultural factors on behavior. Even in cases of well defined organic conditions, the focus is on the perceptions of behavior and contents of psychiatric symptoms such as hallucinations and delusions.[6] As defined by Fabrega in 2001[7] "Psychiatry may outline a science of the psyche and its disturbances but it also reflects a cultural interpretation about personal experience, responsibility, social behavior, and the requirements for social order. The cultural character of the psychiatric enterprise itself, just as much as the characteristics of its disorders constitute the subject matter of cultural psychiatry."

The very definition of the disease is that it is a product of social happening and hence conceptualization about diseases has important social implications. Most diseases have also a biological base but psychiatric illness occupies an anomalous position. Its defining characteristics involve concepts related to the mental realm as well as social relationships. Its manifestations are abnormal behavior. Thus, a set of behavioral indicators can represent a disease and the diagnosis depends on inferences about the behavior. As psychiatric symptoms are the product of social, cultural and biological relationships, culture has some etiological or modifying role in the manifestation of mental illnesses.[6]

Is the mental illness the same all over the world? Kraepelin (1921) traveled to South East Asia and other parts of the world to find answer to the question.[8] He concluded that the mental illness was the same all over the world and even Latah and the catatonia were similar in nature, making them universal. The finding that psychopathology is a universal phenomenon would give support to the view that it is part of human nature and that some cultural context may only influence the threshold of manifestations rather than eliminate them completely. Psychopathology may express in culture bound syndromes bearing the marks of culture and, are closely associated with the cultural context.

Cultural Barriers to Mental Health Care

Cultural barriers that prevent members of minority populations from receiving appropriate care include:[9]

- Mistrust and fear of treatment.
- Alternative ideas about what constitutes illness and health.
- Language barriers and ineffective communication.
- Access barriers, such as inadequate insurance coverage.
- A lack of diversity in the mental health workforce.

Tseng[10] proposes three levels of approach for cultural psychiatry:

1. *Clinical level:* It aims to promote culturally competent mental health care for patients of diverse ethnic and cultural backgrounds, viz., culturally relevant assessment and culturally appropriate care.
2. *Research level:* It is the exploration of how ethnic or cultural factors influence behavior and psychopathology as well as the process of healing (ethnopharmacology).
3. *Theoretical level:* It aims to expand our knowledge of human behavior and mental problems transculturally to facilitate the development of more universally applicable and cross-culturally valid theories of psychopathology.

IMPORTANT TERMS IN CULTURAL PSYCHIATRY

Cultural system may be defined as the interaction of different elements of culture with the individual or groups. It is a dynamic process and different from social system. Sometimes both systems together are referred as sociocultural system.

Enculturation: The process by which a person learns the requirements of his/her own culture, and acquires values and behaviors that are appropriate or necessary in that culture.[11] The process of enculturation is related to socialization. It is a learning process from parents, family members, neighbors, friends, school, social events, traditional literature and media.

Acculturation: The process in which members of one cultural group adopting the cultural traits or social patterns of another group. Acculturation is an important process of cultural change in immigrated population[12] and influences their mental health.[13]

Acculturative stress: It refers to the psychological, somatic, and social difficulties that may accompany acculturation processes. This was first described by Redfield et al.[14] as, "psychic conflict" that may arise from conflicting cultural norms.

Assimilation: It is the process whereby a minority group gradually adapts to the customs and values of the prevailing culture. It is a two way process—firstly, an individual or a group of diverse ethnic and racial minority or immigrant individuals comes to adopt the beliefs, values, attitudes, and the behaviors of the majority or dominant culture and secondly, at the same time, they relinquishes the value system of their cultural tradition and becomes a member of the dominant society.

Cultural identity: It is the identity of a group or culture or of an individual as far as one is influenced by one's belonging to a group or culture. The usual cultural identifiers are place, gender, history, nationality, ethnicity, language, religious faith, and esthetics.[15]

Deculturation or cultural uprooting: Deculturation results when members of nondominant cultures become alienated (either by accident or by force) from the dominant culture and from their own minority society.[12] Deculturation is the loss of one's traditional culture without integration into a new culture. The consequence of deculturation may result in increased stress and psychopathology[16] and cultural bereavement.[17]

Cultural diffusion: It is the spreading of ideas or products from one culture to another. This concept was first introduced by Krober.[18] There are three categories of cultural diffusion: *Direct diffusion* is when two cultures are very close to each other, resulting in intermarriage, trade, and even warfare. *Forced diffusion* occurs when one culture subjugates (conquers or enslaves) another culture and forces its own customs on the conquered people. *Indirect diffusion* is when cultural ideas are spread through a middleman or even another culture.

Diaspora: It is the movement, migration, or scattering of people away from an established or ancestral homeland. The term *Diaspora* carries a sense of displacement and a sense of hidden hope or desire to return to homeland.

Cultural paranoia: The concept was introduced by Grier and Cobbs[19] in their book 'Black Rage', where they said that Black clients may not disclose personal information to White therapists for fear that they may be vulnerable to racial discrimination and this condition was regarded not a form of psychopathology but a healthy and adaptive response by African Americans towards the white Americans. Culture deeply influence our cognitive reference, perceptual experiences and belief system and thus have strong influence on persecutory ideas, shared delusions[20] and even treatment seeking and hospitalization.[21]

Culture shock: It is the difficulty people have adjusting to a new culture that differs markedly from their own, usually occurs during visiting a new place or during a short-term sojourn (international students). Thorough phases of initial excitement and then negotiation and adjustment, people usually master the new environment. There are many symptoms and signs of culture shock, including general unease with new situations, irrational fears, difficulty with sleeping, feeling sick, anxiety and depression, preoccupation with health, and homesickness.

Cultural confusion results from a growing lack of consensus about what is proper or appropriate in a given circumstances. It is the initial phase of culture shock when people become confused, tired and disoriented in a new foreign environment.

Cultural accommodation: It is the process by which individuals may take on values and beliefs of the host culture and accommodate them in the public sphere, while maintaining the parent culture in the private sphere.

CULTURE AND PSYCHOPATHOLOGY

Tseng[5] gave seven types of relation between culture and psychopathology.

Pathogenic effects: Refers to situations where culture is a direct causative factor in forming or generating psychopathology, e.g. *stress* can be created by culturally formed anxiety, culturally demanded performance or culturally prescribed roles and duties. So culture is considered to be a causative factor, because culture-specific beliefs and ideas contribute directly to the formation of particular stress inducing certain type of psychopathology. Culture-bound Syndromes are the example.

Pathoselective effects: Cultural choice to stress reaction that shapes the nature of psychopathology, e.g. Running amok in Malaysia, familial suicide in some cultures.

Pathoplastic effects: The ways in which culture contributes to modeling or plastering of the manifestation of psychopathology.

Pathoelaborating effects: Certain behaviors (either normal or pathological) may become exaggerated to the extreme by *cultural reinforcement*:
Hara-kiri – formal way of suicide by a soldier in Japan to avoid capture or humiliation by enemy is an honorable way of ending one's life.

Pathofacilitative effects: Many psychiatric disorders are intimately tied to psychological and socio cultural variables in their development. Unemployment leading to substance abuse.

Pathodiscriminating effects: Socio cultural labeling of behavior as normal or abnormal-several mental conditions or behaviors, e.g. personality disorder, sexual deviation and substance abuse are accepted or rejected as per the social discrimination according to cultural factors.

Pathoreactive effects: Culture influences how people label a disorder and how they emotionally react to it. Prognosis of schizophrenia is better in less developed, rural, farming societies than industrialized nations. The social environment, attitudes of family and community determine how well the person will rehabilitate into social and family life, thus affecting the prognosis.

CULTURAL INFLUENCES ON CLASSIFICATION OF MENTAL DISORDERS

The taxonomy of mental and behavioral disorders is derived from combinations of descriptive, etiologic, pathophysiologic, and psychological criteria This process has been going on since antiquity in the attempt to "explain" human behavior and misbehavior and continues today in the ongoing effort to apply medical, psychological, and sociologic criteria to these problems. Many attempts at systematic classification (including "folk taxonomies") emphasize differences between psychotic and nonpsychotic disorders. Even allowing for cultural variability, Murphy (1976) found that systematic classifications worldwide define the symptom clusters of schizophrenic disorders as psychotic. Most societies classify less socially disruptive disorders as nonpsychotic. From a cross-cultural perspective these nonpsychotic conditions, although they show great variation, can be informally subclassified into (1) moderate maladaptations and abnormalities (e.g. "dysthymic disorder," "conversion disorder"); (2) characteristics abnormalities (e.g. paranoid personality, "narcissistic personality"); or (3) abnormalities of adjustment (e.g. "conduct disorder," "situational crisis").[22]

Although some sources of stress (e.g. puberty, bereavement) are universal, the meanings of such stresses and the ceremonial resources for dealing with them vary widely in different cultures. Thus, the processes of diagnosis and treatment may differ in different cultures in 4 ways: (1) in the definitions of what constitute symptoms of disease; (2) in the interpretation and presumed causes of such symptoms; (3) in the classification of symptoms into syndromes; and (4) in perceptions about what constitutes an acceptable method of treatment. Regardless of their utility and validity, all classifications of psychiatric syndromes are affected by cultural variables.

It has been a general assumption that cultural difference has a significant effect on the determination of diagnostic categories. These axiom sterns at least partly from the observation that different cultures are often in disagreement as to what behavior they label normal or abnormal. Wig (1983), when suggesting that culture has powerfully influenced diagnostic classification systems, noted that current American and European Classification systems have elevated emotions such as anxiety and depression to the level of specific disorders. However, he wondered why other emotions such as jealousy or hatred have not been treated in the same way. Wig was making the point that jealousy and hatred might be treated with much more emphasis in other cultures and therefore in a nonEuroAmerican system could be considered worthy of consideration as specific disorders.[23]

Significant cultural variability exists in the manner in which an individual is able or chooses to express inner turmoil. Many workers[24-26] have noted that the phenomenon of expressing distress verbally and emotionally, seen predominantly in North American and Western European societies, is not a cultural given for the rest of the world. The experience and expression of distress not only as a mental but also as a bodily dysfunction, dubbed somatization by Western cultures, seems to be the global rule, not the exception. "Psychologization," or the experience and expression of distress in primarily mental or psychological terms, seems to be a culture-bound phenomenon in the West, perhaps a vestige of outdated theories of mind-body duality.[27]

COMMUNICATION

Language, as a subset of culture, has a more concrete influence on diagnosis in psychiatry. For example, questions have been raised about the existence of depression as a concept in some languages. Some cultures facilitate the expression of complaints, whereas other cultures may inhibit the communication of inner feelings to health professionals. In a transcultural context, language is also thought to have another special influence. This occurs when a health professional assesses a patient whose language is different from that of the clinician. Marcos (1975) found marked distortion when evaluations of patients were conducted through interpreters, even when such interpreters were proficient.[28]

Psychiatry, more than any other branch of medicine, depends on communication for both diagnosis and therapy. A method of microanalysis of therapeutic conversation has recently been developed by Labov and Fanshell.[29] The psychiatrist must be attentive not only to what a patient says and does but also to the cultural context of the patient's communication.

Few would dispute the proposition that culture makes a difference, whether in relation to detecting mental disorders, searching for their causes, or providing care for patients and their families. However, building a bridge from proposition to culturally competent actions requires conceptualizing intersections between culture and health that are not always immediately apparent and grounding research, practice system planning, and advocacy in principles that do not translate easily into operational terms.[30]

For a better communication a doctor should:

- Be aware that a person's culture will shape how they understand health and ill-health.
- Learning about the specific cultural beliefs that surround mental illness in the person's community.
- Know what is normal, and what is not, in the person's culture.
- Know what culturally appropriate communication is.
- Learning how mental illness is described in the person's community (knowing what words and ideas are used to talk about the symptoms or behaviors).
- Be aware of what concepts, behaviors or language are taboo (knowing what might cause shame).

SOCIOCULTURAL INFLUENCES ON THE ETIOLOGY OF MENTAL DISORDERS

The incidence of mental disorders, particularly of behavioral disturbances such as attempted suicide, drug abuse, and alcoholism, is closely associated with social, situational i.e. related to certain phases of life and cultural factors. These factors influence not only the genesis and course of mental disorders but also the perception of symptoms and help-seeking and, utilization-of-services behavior. Severe mental disorders, such as depression, dementia and schizophrenia, are far less influenced by socio cultural factors than are minor mental disturbances. This is probably one of the reasons why transcultural psychiatry has lost more and more ground since Kraepelin's days.

How slight the influence of sociocultural factors is even on the manifestation of psychotic illnesses is shown by the findings of the WHO International Pilot Study of

Schizophrenia[31,32] and two later studies.[33,34] Starting in 1966 in nine countries differing widely in socio cultural characteristics, the study showed that schizophrenic patients with similar characteristics could be identified in all the nine centers in which the study was conducted, and that the degree of similarity among them could he specified by applying standardized assessment methods ensuring cross-cultural comparability. Furthermore, in all the cultures studied, patients diagnosed as suffering from schizophrenia could be distinguished clearly, in terms of clinical symptoms, from, patients with a diagnosis of affective psychosis or another functional mental disorder. It seemed also that a precise and narrow definition of schizophrenia led to quite identical incidence rates in representative first-admission samples across the participating centers.[34]

Unlike functional psychoses and mental disorders of organic origin, minor mental disorders vary from culture to culture to a far greater extent. The outcome of the latter disorders and of schizophrenia varies greatly between developing and developed countries, and hence so does their prevalence.[31,32]

The symptoms of psychiatric disorders are frequent topics of investigations in anthropology, psychology and psychiatry. In studies of this type, the researcher contends that cultural factors might be operative in the way a person who is ill behaves. Employing approaches of social sciences, most of these studies therefore have viewed behavior in a social and psychological point of view. Emphasis is frequently placed on thought content emotional expression, perceptions and social relations.[6]

DSM-IV AND THE CULTURAL CONTEXT

An important result of these efforts has been the cultural formulation, devised as a way of integrating an individual's culture and experiential context into the scope of diagnosis[35] explanatory outline for deriving the cultural formulation can be found in Appendix I of DSM-IV. It focuses the diagnostician's attention of five components of cultural data, the synthesis of which then produces a more complete view of the individual within the cultural context. These five components include the following:

1. The cultural identity of the individual, including the contrast between culture of origin and host culture in immigrant or ethnic minority individuals.
2. Cultural explanations of the individual's illness, such as idioms of distress, culturally based meaning of symptoms, and perceived causes or models of illness.
3. Cultural factors related to psychosocial environment, including culturally informed interpretations of problems with social support and environmental stressors.
4. Cultural aspects of the relationship between individual and clinician, including potential barriers to understanding and assessing the meaning of symptoms.
5. An overall assessment of how the cultural context influences the diagnosis and the approaches to treatment.

Agrawal et al (1993) highlighted influence of culture in field trial of WHO ICD-10 in India.[36]

DSM-5 AND CULTURAL CONTEXT

In an effort to improve diagnosis and care to people of all backgrounds, the fifth edition of the *Diagnostic and Statistical Manual of Mental Disorders* (DSM-5)[37] incorporates a greater cultural sensitivity throughout the manual. Rather than a simple list of culture-bound syndromes, DSM-5 updates criteria to reflect cross-cultural variations in presentations, gives more detailed and structured information about cultural concepts of distress, and includes a clinical interview tool to facilitate comprehensive, person-centerd assessments.

Different cultures and communities exhibit or explain symptoms in various ways. Because of this, it is important for clinicians to be aware of relevant contextual information stemming from a patient's culture, race, ethnicity, religion or geographical origin.

Cultural Considerations in Clinical Practice

Throughout the DSM-5 development process, the work Groups made a concerted effort to modify culturally determined criteria so they would be more equivalent across different cultures. In Section II, specific diagnostic criteria were changed to better apply across diverse cultures. For example, the criteria for social anxiety disorder now include the fear of "offending others" to reflect the Japanese concept in which avoiding harm to others is emphasized rather than harm to oneself.[37]

The new manual also addresses cultural concepts of distress, which detail ways in which different cultures describe symptoms. It helps clinicians in recognizing how people in different cultures think and talk about psychological problems.

Finally, the cultural formulation interview guide will help clinicians to assess cultural factors influencing patients' perspectives of their symptoms and treatment options. Cultural formulation is a set of 14 questions in 4 domains. These are:

- Cultural definition of the problem
- Cultural perceptions of cause, context, and support
- Current help seeking
- Cultural factors affecting self coping and past help seeking.

GLOBALIZATION AND IMPACT ON CULTURAL PSYCHIATRY

Globalization means crossing borders. All of the social and economic forces driving globalization relate to the opening or dismantling of borders: instant communication, easy travel, deregulation of commerce and widened access to information and technology.[38]

Key features of globalization are:[38]

- Instant communication (e.g. by the internet)
- Fast, efficient means of travel
- Deregulation of commerce
- Widened access to technology
- Supranational political bodies
- Cross-border cultural interaction.

Globalization has led to a significant increase in migration. People are now moving further, faster and in greater numbers than ever before. Migration is known to have significant effects on health, with migrants showing higher rates of both physical[39] and mental illness.[40]

Most of the immigrants suffer from depression, social anxiety, adjustment problems, abuse and discrimination. Social isolation can lead to increased rate of suicide and substance abuse.

CULTURAL CONSIDERATIONS IN VARIOUS PSYCHIATRIC DISORDERS

Schizophrenia and Related Psychotic Disorders

Schizophrenia, the most important and troublesome psychiatric illness, is expressed differently in various cultures. It may be the same psychosis but the conflict the illness creates is manifested in differential patterns. Such an assumption is supported by the finding of a study which indicates that in people of the same genetic origin who live in different social settings, there can be considerable variation in the course of schizophrenia. In UK, the schizophrenic patients from St. Thomas showed a different pattern from those patients from Mauritius in spite of their common genetic origin. In Canada, the old and new French people were different in response an outcomes.[41] Leong (1989) noted in a Hawaiian study that Caucasian schizophrenic patients were more likely than the Asian patients to have suicidal thoughts and acts, anxiety, depressed mood, grandiosity and inappropriate affect.[42] Enright and Jaeckle (1963) compared the pattern of manifest symptoms and social behavior of paranoid schizophrenics of Japanese and Filipino extraction in Hawaii. The differences found in these groups were striking. The Japanese were seclusive and the Filipino was manic like and belligerent.[43]

In a house to house survey of 1158 people, Venkataramaiah et al (1981) found that 4 to 3 cases of possession syndrome. Possession by the spirit and god was the most common.[44] Some of the possessed obtained a special social status in the rural community and hence, most of the cases were from the rural community. Many healers benefited from being possessed in order to drive the evil out. Hence, it serves to increase social prestige and to help someone to become a healer. These would have been diagnosed by the Western psychiatrists as schizophrenia.

Singh and Sachdev (1981) indicated that acute schizophrenic episodes in India did not represent this category at ICD8 and ICD9 were not useful in making this diagnosis.[45] In India, the clinical picture of acute schizophrenic episode may be manifested by nutritional deficiency and other processes indicating that socio cultural factors play a role in the manifestation of the disease. UK Cross National Study, a bicultural study of schizophrenia indicated that even though there were minimal differences between the actual patient populations, there was predilection of American Psychiatrists to diagnose schizophrenia more often than British psychiatrists.[46] The similar finding was noted in a comparison of Dutch and American patients.[47] The over-diagnosis of schizophrenia is particularly disturbing as labeling being a stigma can prevent the proper treatment[48,49] what remains to be understood are the cultural factors responsible for the over-diagnosis of schizophrenia. Another multicultural study by the transcultural group of the McGill University concluded that a core pattern of schizophrenic symptomatology was universal in all cultures. Yet, schizophrenic symptoms and subtypes varied from culture to culture. The World Health Organization Study[50-52] indicated that there was a high degree of similarity with regard to the psychopathology of schizophrenics in different cultures. However, the problem of cross-cultural variation was not addressed in this study leaving the controversy open. Cultural context and other methodological variables make it difficult to conduct cross-cultural studies but at the same time provide a challenge for the investigators.

Course of Schizophrenia

The cross-cultural presentation and course of schizophrenia are among the best-studied aspects of cultural psychiatry. Research has revealed both cross-cultural similarities and differences, both of which are important for elucidating the biological and environmental bases of the disease. A "spectrum" of schizophrenic syndromes-consisting of combination of certain positive and negative psychotic symptoms-has been found nearly everywhere, although the specific content of hallucinations and delusions as well as the prevalence of visual and other nonauditory hallucinations varies.[53,54] Significant cross-cultural variation has been found, however, in several features of the syndrome. Its distribution is not uniform, ranging from 1 in a 1,000 in the nonwestern societies to more than 1% in the West; its highest prevalence is displayed in economically and technologically advanced, urbanized, and bureaucratized societies.[55,56] Its phenomenology varies with cultural setting, with much higher rates of catalonia in India and of hebephrenic in Japan than in the West. Most important, the course and outcome of schizophrenia are markedly better in non industrialized countries, even when cultural differences in outcome assessment and in acuteness of presentation are taken into account.[57-59] Variations in outcome are thought to be related in part to different attitudes toward persons with the disorder, a set of culturally patterned interactions studied under the rubric of expressed emotion.[60]

Cross-cultural differences have also been detected in emotional processing among the German, American, and Indian subjects with schizophrenia Face discrimination performance was most impaired in the Indian subgroup.[61]

Outcome: The work by Murphy and Raman[62] is a striking example of the cultural influences in the treatment of schizophrenia. In a study of the same genetic group of patients living in Britain and Mauritius, it was noted that those needing continuous hospitalization were similar in number and yet the percent of patients with intermittent or semi chronic course were very different. Similarly, the WHO study indicated that the percentage of chronicity among Indian psychiatric schizophrenic patients was lower than that in the Western population. If it is assumed that the same genetic disorder was treated in both places, should it be then that socio cultural factors play a role in the outcome? A number of investigators have indicated that[63,64] severe and chronic forms of schizophrenia were less frequent in India thereby indicating a favorable outcome this was warm out in WHO study in 1979.[32]

Several studies have shown that the outcome of schizophrenia is more favorable in developing countries, such as India, than in developed countries, such as the United States. Murphy and Raman[62] were the first to examine possible differences in outcome between Western developed nations and other developing or undeveloped nations. Comparing the nonwhite schizophrenic population of Mauritius with European populations, they found that the subjects from Mauritius were relatively symptom free at follow-up and were functioning normally in virtually every aspect of their lives. These subjects also had fewer relapses and overall better outcome at 12 year follow-up. In fact, 60% were found to be leading 'normal' lives at follow-up. Nancy Waxler[65] in her landmark study in a Sri Lankan population reported significantly good outcome.

The modern research in transcultural aspects of schizophrenia started with the famous Cooper-Carpenter UK-USA study in the late 1960s comparing schizophrenia on the two sides of north Atlantic.[66]

As stated earlier in this chapter; in the 1960s, the WHO launched an important study, the International Pilot Study of Schizophrenia (IPSS), a transcultural comparison of over 1200 patients in nine countries, using rigorous and comparable methodologies. The main findings of IPSS were presented in monographs.[31,32] Later publications reported on 5 year and longer follow-ups of the study cohort.[66-70]

The WHO researchers concluded that there were clear differences in the course and outcome of schizophrenia, with patients indeveloping countries on the average having a better course and outcome than those in centers in the developed countries. The outcome may be more favorable in settings characterized by agricultural economy, little vertical mobility, extended families, psychiatric services which include the active participation of the family and the absence of specific community stereotypes of the mentally ill.

A subsequent study, the Determinants of Outcome of Severe Mental Disorder study (DOSMeD) was carried out in which I was one of the research assistants from Chandigarh Center.

DOSMeD was carried out at 12 centers in, 10 countries representing both the developing and the developed world. There were 8 centers in developed countries, i.e. Aarhus (Denmark), Dublin (Ireland), Honolulu and Rochester (USA), Moscow (USSR), Nagasaki (Japan), Nottingham (UK), and Prague (Czechoslovakia). The developing countries were represented by Agra and Chandigarh (India), Cali (Colmbia) and Ibadan (Nigeria). Chandigarh, India was actually represented by two subcenters, a rural and an urban.

The incidence study conducted in India as part of WHO studies reported annual incidence Rate were 4.4 and 3.8 per 10,000 for rural and urban area respectively.[71] Influence of culture in schizophrenia is extensively reviewed elsewhere.[72]

However one needs to be conscious of two possible dangers: the first is that of ethnocentricity or the belief that is my culture is the best and second is the likelihood of mental health becoming a movement away from science which is at present the basis of medicine and health.[73]

Mood Disorders

Contemporary cross-cultural research on mood disorder has focused on unipolar depression syndromes, revealing extensive cultural patterning as well as significant similarities. For example, the World Health Organization Collaborative Study on Depression found a core depressive syndrome in the five countries studied, but it also revealed substantial cross.

Cultural differences in symptom presentation affect conceptualization, level of severity, and influence of acculturation, despite a methodology that tended to accentuate similarities at the expense of local differences.

Culture and other social factors, such as class and gender, influence the interpretation of and exposure to stressors that predispose to depression.[74]

In addition, most cross-cultural studies have found a significantly higher rate of somatic complaints associated with depression (and anxiety) among the non-Western groups than in the Western settings, including the presence of unique symptoms [e.g. "heat or water in the head" and "crawling sensation of worms and ants" in the Nigerian cultures].[75] Emotional complaints are often present as well but may not be considered the source of distress or impairment.

The substantial overlap of depression with anxiety, somatoform, and dissociative disorders implies a higher probability of under-recognition or misidentification of affective disorders in many ethno cultural groups.[76]

Depression

Much of the research in depression however, has produced findings that ignore the role of culture in identifying and shaping the form and meaning of antecedent risk factors, the consequences attributed to illness, and the very conceptualization of depressive disorder. We can expect cross-cultural comparative research not only to elucidate both similarities and differences across cultures, but also to enable us to recognize and question previously unconscious assumptions within our own culture about the nature of illness, its antecedents and effects, and their practical implications. Culture and depression was reviewed extensively recently.[77]

One must recognize the impact of local beliefs, practices, and institutions in relationships with stressors, supports, and social power if research is to generate information that is reliable by current epidemiological standards, valid, and suitable as a practical guide for applications in a particular culture.[78]

Current research, along with clinical descriptions and artistic renderings of depression and melancholia in literature, painting, and sculpture throughout history, strongly suggest that core features of depressive disorder are relevant across cultures.[79-81] Culture may influence the incidence and prevalence of depression as well as the patterning of distress and a patient's recognition of it as illness.

Culture also affects a clinical presentation of the illness, its relationship to local idioms o distress, the names by which it is known, the local models that persons construct to explain it, patterns of help-seeking in response to it, and its course and outcome. Consequently, Marsella et al. (1985) concluded, "Studies of the epidemiology of depression, although numerous, have yielded few firm conclusions about ethno cultural variations in the frequency and distribution of depressive disorders".[82]

Current research has revised our understanding of the epidemiology of depression; it shows that unipolar depression, the modern analog of melancholia, and depressive symptoms in community surveys are more prevalent among lower socioeconomic classes.[83]

Neurasthenia remains a particularly important presentation for Chinese patients with depressions,[84] and for other patients in developing countries as well, somatization is a common clinical problem throughout the world. Although somatization (i.e. somatic symptoms without sufficient organic pathology to account for them) occurs frequently among depressed patients in primary health settings of developed countries.[85,86] The absence of spontaneous reports of mood dysphoria as a symptom of depression has been both striking and confusing for Western clinicians working in developing countries.

Much of the literature of cross-cultural psychiatry holds that Western patients, unlike patients, elsewhere, typically report guilt and self-reproach as features of depression. Kraepelin (1921) found his experience in Java remarkable for the absence of feelings of guilt and sinfulness, which, according to his report, did not accompany depression there.[87] Murphy and his colleagues suggested that finding guilt associated with depression may reflect the influence of the Judeo-Christian heritage.[88]

Despite substantial findings of guilt in India,[89-91] discussions in the Indian literature minimize its significance or explain it away unconvincingly as a milder or different kind of guilt. Kulhara and Varma (1985) distinguish covert and overt types of guilt to account for more frequent reports of guilt with depression in India than they could explain otherwise,[92] Venkoba Rao (1973) studied two kinds of guilt, distinguishing the type related to deeds in a previous life (karma) from a focus on the present life. He argued, however, that a belief in karma was protective against guilt.[91]

Venkoba Rao (1984) recognized that it is especially difficult for those not familiar with a particular culture, despite their clinical training to identify dysphoric affect, and such clinicians, therefore, might easily miss this cardinal feature of depression. Among Indian patients, he argued that although depressed mood is rarely the chief complaint motivating the clinical consultation, a skillful clinician with a sensitive interview technique can invariably elicit it as a sign, if not a symptom, of depressions.[81]

While suicidal ideation is commonly reported among Indian patients, as often as among Western patients, completed suicides are distinctly less frequently reported for third world patients than for Western patients. While this may be an artifact of reporting Venkoba Rao argued that a number of cultural factors in India may protect against suicide. For example, the emphasis on obligations to the family rather than rights of the individual enhances a sense of responsibility. The question "Who will marry my child if I commit suicide is especially compelling the socially sanctioned ritual suicide of the devoted Hindu widow (sati) however, demonstrates that cultural factors do not always deter one from suicide;[93] in fact, they may have the opposite effect. The concept of Karma, which implies an individual will be reborn into a less desirable birth as a result of suicide (though not in the case of the sati), may also function to protect against suicidal behavior.

Although there is no conclusive epidemiological evidence to support the view that some cultures cause depression, ethnographers and clinicians have considered several factors to be protective. These include certain rituals and beliefs that facilitate mourning,[94] an extended family system, provision of status for the elderly, permissive child-rearing practices, and less inhibition of aggression. Most of the evidence is anecdotal, however, and has been offered within the contextual framework of contemporary cosmopolitan

Western psychological and social theories with little regard for indigenous conceptualizations.[95]

One may consider the experience of depressive illness with reference to the cosmological, moral, and religious ideologies of a particular culture. For example, the relationship between normal suffering and clinical depression may be different in Buddhist societies, where suffering is often considered an intrinsic feature of the human condition rather than an indication of disorder.

Lambo (1956), of Nigeria, thought that the rarity of depression observed by many workers in African countries might be due to erroneous diagnosis, and that most of the cases remain concealed by the label of 'neurasthenia'.[96]

The absence of delusions of sin in Chinese as well as in Japanese depressives has also been noted by Yap (1958).[97] On the other hand, Eaton and Weil (1955), in a study concerning the Hutterites, have reported a high incidence of guilt-ridden depression.[98]

In an analysis of south Indian depressive patients, Venkoba Rao (1966) reported[99] that symptoms of anxiety, agitation, somatic complaints and suicidal tendency were found to be common, while feelings of sin, guilt and self reproach were present only in one fourth of the cases. As a possible explanation for the low incidence of depression in South India, this author has put forward the hypothesis of prolonged mourning rituals with diminished sense of guilt among the Hindus. Teja and Narang (1970), however, contest this in view of their findings of a high incidence of depression among the North Indians, although the Hindus they have similar mourning rituals to those in south India.[100] Bagadia et al. (1970), found a low percentage of agitation (27%) hypochondriasis (15%) and guilt feelings (5.3%) in their 233 depressives from Bombay in west India.[101] Murphy et al (1967) have also reported that guilt feelings and diurnal variation are uncommon among the Hindus.[102]

In a number of reports the incidence of depression is reported to be less in south India and comparatively high in north India.[100]

Guilt, late insomnia and retardation were significantly more in Carney's group of depressives, while depression, suicide, diurnal variation and especially somatic symptoms were significantly more in Rao's group.

Again, in spite of this the obsessional symptoms were significantly more frequent in Western depressives. Somatic symptoms are present in both north and south Indian depressives in an outstandingly greater frequency in comparison to the British depressives; there being no significant difference in the frequency of these symptoms among the two Indian groups.

The Indian patient, therefore, uses the medium of the body more often for expressing inner tensions. Indian depressives are significantly more often agitated and anxious than the Western cases. The relatively less frequent occurrence of guilt feeling among the Eastern patients has been commented on by a number of workers.

It was seen that somatic symptoms, hypochondriasis, anxiety and agitation were present in a significantly larger percentage of Indian depressives.[90]

The cross-national research on mental disorders was conducted including the International Pilot Study of Schizophrenia and the WHO study of Depressive Disorders in Different Cultures,[103] these studies reflected a much narrower approach to cultural comparisons. They were limited for the most part to questions of whether rates of these disorders differed in different countries, rather than more fundamental consideration, as Sartorius himself had advocated, of the role of socio cultural contexts and the local cultural experience of these conditions, their meaning, and how these were related to behaviour.[104]

Anxiety Disorders

The effect of culture on anxiety is similar to that on depression, especially since cross-cultural studies have shown a marked tendency for anxiety and depression to overlaps.[105] Cultural factors affect the precipitants, symptom presentations, pathological thresholds, and specific syndrome criteria of the anxiety disorders.[106]

Cultural and ethnic elements have been invoked to explain local differences in anxiety disorder prevalence that persist after controlling for other social factors. For example, the higher rate of simple phobia, social phobia, and agoraphobia among the African-Americans, as compared to whites,[107] has been attributed to the stress resulting from racial discriminations.[108]

Somatoform Disorder

Many nosologies around the world do not distinguish between mood, anxiety, somatoform disorders, and dissociative disorders, because sufferers report single syndromes that run across boundaries of the diagnostic categorizes.[109] This is similar to the situation with depression, where a single description of the disorder has led to under-recognition and misidentification of depressive syndromes in many ethno cultural groups.[76]

In most of the world, the degree to which symptoms are medically unexplained is difficult to ascertain owing to the marked limitation of diagnostic tests and medical personnel. Moreover, the high prevalence of endemic disease in the underdeveloped countries, often with protean and inchoate manifestations, may also confound the assessment of the somatoform disorders. This may result in over diagnosis if organic causes are not identified or under diagnosis if organic explanations are uncritically accepted for systemic illness.[110]

Dissociative Disorders

A study performed in an outpatient psychiatric clinic in India found that more that 90% of dissociative disorder cases did not fulfill criteria for the specified categories, ironically receiving instead diagnosis of atypical dissociative disorder. Distressing trance states and possession trance episodes constituted most of these cases.[111] These instances of misdiagnosis again call to question the usefulness of some of the standard diagnostic categories of the North American psychiatry.[76]

Some of these syndromes are characterized by involuntary possession trance - dissociative alterations in identity attributed to the invasion by external spirits or agents-distinguished from dissociative identity disorder by their episodic and remitting course, the nature and number of their alternative identities, and their gradual response to treatment. These syndromes have been identified in India, Western Africa, China, Malaysia, Brazil and the Caribbean, among many others settings.[112-114]

In fact, extensive cross-cultural research reveals that most dissociative experiences around the world are completely normal usually forming part of religious and ritual events.[112]

Culture and Alcohol and Substance Use Disorder

Since prehistoric times alcohol has been the most important means of conserving beverages. As beverages containing alcohol are very easy to produce and are germ free, they have in many cases replaced infected drinking water. Hence, almost all cultures have been confronted with the problem of alcohol for thousands of years.

According to the status that alcohol has in a culture, we can distinguish three type of culture: abstaining, ambivalent, and permissive.[115] Societies in which the prohibition of alcohol and individual abstinence are religiously motivated are capable of maintaining the individual risk at a minimum level. In the so-called ambivalent cultures, e.g. in the sphere of Anglo-American Protestantism and the Scandinavian countries, the distribution of alcohol is often subject to temporal and regional restrictions.

There is also a relationship between social tolerance of alcohol and its availability. It is therefore the right approach to restrict the availability of alcohol as the first step in global preventive programs.[116] As the example of Denmark shows, where the availability of alcohol has been restricted by raising the tax on alcoholic liquor proportionally to its level of pure alcohol, preventive programs have a considerable chance of succeeding. The introduction of the system of taxing alcohol led to a four-to six fold decrease in per capita consumption, to an eight fold decrease in deaths caused by cirrhosis of the liver, and to a 16-fold drop in the incidence rate of alcoholic delirium.[117] The conclusion that can be drawn from these results is the efficacy of preventive measures that make more difficult the consumption of alcoholic drinks that easily and quickly feed the organism a large amount of alcohol.

The effects of the abolition of existing regulations also serve to illustrate the effectiveness of preventive measures. The lowering of the age limit for the purchase of alcohol from 21 to 18 years in the United States, e.g. led, in the year following this legislation, to a rise in alcohol-related accidents by 80 to 300% in the age group 18 to 21, even though the age restriction had not been strictly observed.

When we focus on that meaning of the term culture that embraces the entire way of life of a people, it is noteworthy, that alcohol impinges on virtually every aspect. It is for this reason that it is spoken of alcohol as providing a "window on culture".[118] As Duster[119] said, "Alcohol is to social science what dye is to microscopy (allowing us) to penetrate the structure". Any culture is a complex system of interrelated things, ideas, institutions, and processes, all of which can be classified in myriad ways. Volumes have been written about each, but within the limited scope of this chapter, it seems appropriate simply to refer to some of the universal aspects of culture in alphabetic order under the categories of arts and literature, economics, history, recreation and entertainment, religion and ideology, and social and political relations. Other aspects, such as technology, conflict management, and science, are beyond it scope of so brief a summary.

Socio cultural factors exert considerable influence over some aspects of substance use disorders and not others. The prevalence rates of alcohol and drug abuse and dependence vary significantly across cultures. Lifetime rates for alcoholism, for example, range from 23% among the American Indians to 0.45% among the population of Shanghai Helzer and Canino 1992.[120] In our own study in dry district of Wardha, abstinent from work secondary to alcoholism is the dominating social problem in 67% of subjects.[121]

Cultural Variation in Suicide Rates

Suicidal acts—including both completed and attempted suicide—are forms of individual behavior and thus, like other behavior, subject to judgment by normative and cultural criteria on the part of society.

In some strongly Catholic countries and regions, suicide and attempted suicide used to be liable to punishment by the Church or law, up to as recently as the mid-twentieth century. Among Muslims, too, suicide is regarded as an act of disobedience and resistance to the will of God. In spite of suicides having now ceased to be a social taboo in most countries and its recognition as a behavior disorder, suicide rates still continue to be lower among Catholics and in mainly Catholic countries than among Protestants. In the Western countries, depressions, of all mental disorders, entail the highest risk for a successfully committed suicide or a suicide attempt of very serious intent.[122]

Cultural factors may also cause an elevated suicide rate, as the example of Japan shows. Suicides committed in order to restore lost personal honor are neither related to illness nor are they the result of deviant behavior in countries where suicide has been considered a moral obligation. Because of its conformity with cultural norms, Durkheim[123] termed this altruistic suicide, as opposed to anomic and egoistic suicide. Even today in countries where suicide used to be a custom or at least more or less tolerated, suicide rates are higher than in cultures that have always disapproved of it.

CULTURE-BOUND SYNDROMES IN INDIA

According to DSM-IV culture-bound syndrome denotes recurrent, locality-specific patterns of aberrant behavior and troubling experience that may or may not be linked to a particular DSM-IV diagnostic category. Many of these patterns are indigenously considered to be 'illnesses', or at least afflictions and most have local names. Although presentations conforming to the major DSM-IV categories can be fòund throughout the world, the particular symptoms, course, and social response are very often influenced by local cultural factors. In contrast, *culture-bound syndromes* are generally limited to specific societies or culture areas and are localized, folk, diagnostic categories that frame coherent meanings for certain repetitive, patterned, and troubling sets of experiences and observations.

Culture-specific syndrome or culture-bound syndrome is a combination of psychiatric and somatic symptoms that are considered to be a recognizable disease only within a specific society or culture.[124] The term "culture-bound" was used to describe a certain number of psychiatric disorders whose phenomenologies made them distinct from the Western categories and the theoretically could be singled out as unique to a particular cultural setting.[125] The clear implication was that the Western categories were not culture-bound but rather universal, and that proper characterization would disclose a translation key for specific non-Western syndromes.

In this modern sense, "cultural-bound syndrome" is an inherited and controversial term that is used in practice to describe psychiatric categories, whether they are part of the Western or non-Western nosologies, on whose emergence, manifestation, or course culture is thought to, exert a particularly strong influences.[126,127] The term continues to refer to relatively consistent illness categories with characteristic courses ("syndromes") and specific labels. The organizing principle that unifies a syndrome conceptually can be (1) a collection of symptoms, which can follow diverse classificatory schemes (descriptive); (2) a cause, including an immediate precipitating context (etiological); or (3) a response to treatment.[128]

Contemporary use of this terminology allows us to understand certain difficulties in the integration of the Western and non-Western categories of psychiatric illness and their original.[129-131]

Dhat Syndrome

Dhat syndrome is a clinical entity recognized both by general public as well as medical practitioners characterized by nocturnal emissions of semen leading to sever anxiety and hypochondriasis, often associated with sexual impotence. Various somatic, psychological and sexual symptoms are present. Patient also attributes it to the passing of whitish discharge, believed to be semen (Dhat), in urine. 'Dhatu' meaning precious fluid. Dhatus in Sanskrit are elixir of the body. Semen is considered to be the most precious elixir. This gives rise to belief that loss of excessive semen in any form e.g. masturbation, nocturnal emissions etc. is harmful. On the other hand its preservation will lead to health and longevity. Thus the belief in precious and life-preserving properties of semen is deeply ingrained in Indian culture.

The term was first used by Wig in 1960. The physical and mental symptoms which patient suffer from are:

- Generalized weakness
- Aches and pains all over body
- Easy fatigue
- Loss of appetite, weight loss
- Excessive worrying
- Sadness of mood
- Feelings of guilt (especially towards masturbation during adolescence)
- Sexual complaints are that of premature ejaculation and erectile dysfunction. The syndrome is seen usually in people from lower socioeconomic strata. Also seen in surrounding countries like Sri Lanka (Sukra Prameha), Pakistan and even Bangladesh and in China (Sen-k'uri). Treatment mainly consists of dispelling of myths by psycho education, reassuring the patient, treating any underlying psychiatric disorder.[132,133]

Possession Syndrome

Patient is possessed usually by 'spirit/soul' of deceased relative or a local deity. Usually seen in rural areas or in migrants from rural areas. Majority of these patients are females who have repressed emotions. Treatment includes careful exploration of underlying stress which precipitated the possession attack. Also precautions are taken to decrease any secondary gains patient may be getting from this behavior. Included in ICD-10 under Dissociative Disorders.

Antidepressants and anxiolytics are helpful in certain cases.

Koro

There is intense fear of genitalia retracting into abdomen leading ultimately to death. It is seen in both sexes. Person applies external retractors to the genitalia in form of clamps, chains etc. to avoid it retracting back. It may occur as an epidemic.

Culture-bound Suicide

Sati is a form of culture-bound suicide in which there is self-immolation by a widow on her husband's pyre. Sati the wife of Dakhsha was so overcome at the demise of her husband that she immolated herself on his funeral pyre and burnt herself to ashes. It was seen mostly in Upper Castes notably Brahmins and Kshatriyas. Ultimately it was banned in India.

Ascetic Syndrome

It was first described by Neki in 1972. Mostly appears in adolescents and young adults. Characterized by social withdrawal, severe sexual abstinence, practice of religious austerities, lack of concern with physical appearance and considerable loss of weight.[134]

Jhin Jhinia

It occurs in epidemic from in India. Characterized by bizarre and seemingly involuntary contractions and spasms.

Bhanmati Sorcery

This is seen in South India. It is believed to be due to psychiatric illness, i.e. conversion disorders, somatization disorders, anxiety disorder, dysthymia, schizophrenia, etc.

Suudu

It is a culture specific syndrome of painful urination and pelvic "heat" familiar in south India, especially in the Tamil culture. It occurs in males and females. It is popularly attributed to an increase in the "inner heat" of the body often due to dehydration.

INFLUENCE OF CULTURE ON MENTAL HEALTH

Study of the influence of culture and related socioeconomic factors on mental health is a complex task. It is advisable to investigate the influence of cultural factors not only on individual behavior and the distribution of risk factors but also on attitudes toward mental illnesses, their definition, and treatment. Besides socio-cultural differences, on which attitudes toward mental illnesses and their definition depend, the structure and capacity of mental health services largely determine who utilizes such services and, consequently, who is regarded as ill in need of treatment.

Although many developing countries have specialist psychiatric services, they frequently lack larger components of a modern community-based psychiatric service network, such as outpatient, complementary, and rehabilitation facilities and specialized services for particular risk groups (alcoholics, etc.). Developing countries often have neither enough trained personnel nor the financial resources to implement extended mental health care programs, though the proportion of the population with mental disorders is the same as that in developed countries.

THERAPIES

Culture plays an important role on various types of therapies.

Psychopharmacology

The relation between culture and psychopharmacology is as fascinating as it is complex. To complete the picture, the clinician and researcher must consider additional factors such as the patients culturally based expectations of optimum psychiatric treatment (pharmacotherapy or psychotherapy), expected rate of recovery (fast or slow), target symptoms, and threshold and tolerance for adverse effects.

Antipsychotic

Clinical lore has it that Asian patients require lower dosages of dopamine receptor antagonist (typical antipsychotic) medications than comparable white patients to achieve a similar clinical outcome and that when treated on a fixed-dosage schedule. Asians seem to develop significantly greater extra pyramidal adverse effects. These reports were corroborated by Potkin S. (1983) study, that found a 52% higher plasma concentration of haloperidol in Chinese schizophrenia patients living in China than in non-Asian schizophrenia patients residing in the United States when both groups received treatment on a fixed-dosage schedule.[134]

Dosages above 30 mg a day might not be necessary in Chinese patients to obtain the 20 mg/mL to 25 mg/mL currently considered the upper therapeutic plateau for haloperidol plasma concentration. Dosages above 50 mg to 60 mg a day might not be needed in non-Chinese patients.

Tricyclic Drugs

As is the case with neuroleptics, studies with tricyclic drugs have shown that average dosage prescribed for Asians are significantly lower (up to 50% lower) than dosage prescribed in the United States for non-Asians, results that cannot be explained by ethnic differences in protein binding alone.

Lithium

As with tricyclic drugs, antipsychotics, and benzodiazepines, Asians seem to achieve clinical response comparable to those of non-Asian patients using significantly lower dosages and serum concentrations of lithium; 0.5 mEq/L to 0.7 mEq/L versus the 0.8 mEq/L to 1.2 mEq/L generally required by white populations.[135]

Psychotherapy

A doctor can give penicillin to any patient who has certain kind of infections and the patient will get well. The penicillin does not depend upon a common language or a shared world view. Communication is even not necessary. This is not true for psychotherapy communication as its essence. Real communication presupposes not only a shared language but a shared world view as well.

Since in India majority is of illiterate and belongs to extended nuclear family, hence; family member bringing in picture will rather ensure continuation of therapy and more successful techniques.

Thus therapies should be tuned and modified according to their cultures, most important problems are of psychological sophistication, dependence, social distance in therapist and patient, philosophical and religious beliefs. Hence unlike surgeries, psychotherapy cannot expect to have universally uniform techniques. Therefore, western model of psychotherapy needs modification for Indian culture.

Psychotherapy should be shorter crisis oriented,[136] Religious concept should be used especially from *Bhagawat Geeta.*[137] More important is attitude understanding of people regarding causation of illness.[138-140] Model of Psychotherapy which will widely be acceptable to Indian Patients could be found in the traditional concept of relationship between Guru and Chela.[141,142] Privacy is no more considered as obligatory for psychotherapy. Even Mauna (silent) can be tried instead of talk therapy.[143] Hoch (1977) Suggested *'hamdardi'* (Sympathy) for illiterates.[139]

Parikh (1984)[144] highlighted psychotherapy based on Hindu philosophy, using principles of Karma, role of nature and goal of life, etc. Nandi (1985)[145] suggested modification of Psychotherapy for Indian culture.

Even Ancient Indian physician Charaka has described principles of Psychotherapy in Ayurveda in chapter of Cikitsasthanarm. It is highlighted that the patient should be consoled by friends with religions and moral statements. The effectiveness of "traditional mental health promoting practices" was identified as health regimens (swasthvrtt), correct behavior (sadvrtt), and yoga. Sattvavajaya as psychotherapy, is the mental restraint, or a "mind control" as referred by Caraka, is achieved through "spiritual knowledge, philosophy, fortitude, remembrance and concentration". According to Ayurveda, "volitional transgression (Prajnaparadha)" is "the main etiopathological factor" in mental illness, and can be corrected through psychotherapy or Sattvavajaya. Sattvavajaya is that method of treatment through which one tries to bring the intellect (dhi), fortitude (dhrti) and memory (smrti) of the patient into a proper condition. Two methods of Sattvavajaya:

1. Assurance to the patient of the return of lost objects or persons.
2. Inducement of emotions opposite to those associated with patient's distress.[146]

The technique of replacement of emotion is compared to shuttling in Gestalt therapy, while refraining of ideas is compared to Ericksonian hypnosis. Since Sattvavajaya literally means "winning the mind" the single reference to Sattvavajaya from which Ayurvedic therapy has been (re)constituted could easily be interpreted to mean not a relationship between doctor and patient, but rather a mental discipline. It is therapy that can be administered by oneself or by one's family or community or by a practitioner who specializes in mediations with unseen realms.

When we integrate the contemporary art of psychotherapy with the ancient science of Ayurveda, it becomes a powerful combination that is called Psycho Veda.[146] Other types of psychotherapy are Yuktivyapashraya which is rational therapy and Daivyapashray which is faith therapy.

RELIGION AND SPIRITUALITY IN MENTAL ILLNESS

Religion is an organized system of beliefs, practices, rituals, and symbols designed to facilitate closeness to the sacred or transcendent (God, higher power, or ultimate truth/reality).

Spirituality is the personal quest for understanding answers to the ultimate questions about life, about meaning, and about relationship with the sacred or transcendent, which may (or may not) lead to or arise from the development of religious rituals and the formation of a community.

Religion usually refers to socially based beliefs and traditions, often associated with ritual and ceremony, whereas spirituality generally refers to a deep-seated individual sense of connection through which each person's life is experienced as contributing to a valued and greater 'whole', together with a sense of belonging and acceptance. Spirituality is expressed through art, poetry and myth, as well as religious practice. Both religion and spirituality typically emphasize the depth of meaning and purpose in life.

Spike et al. (1985)[147] suggested four general types of effects of religion on mental illness:

1. Religion allows and fosters mental illness, e.g. by encouraging guilt.
2. Religion controls or suppresses mental illness, e.g. by encouraging happiness.
3. Religion may protect from stress or its effects, e.g. by raising self-esteem.
4. Religion may be therapeutically useful, e.g. by providing sympathetic counselors.

All the major religions have many different forms of denominations often with considerable variation in belief and practice, but there are some similarities across religion.

Beliefs about mental illness and its treatment may be closely tied to beliefs about sin and suffering, and quite wide spreads are views that mental illness may result from the divine or even possession by evil.

It is interesting that in Britain the Lunacy Act of 1890 ordered a church in every asylum, which the inmates had to attend twice a day, while in France by contrast; Pinel insisted that the mentally ill should not be exposed to religious practices as it was felt that these might encourage delusions and hallucinations.

Larson et al. (1998)[148] in their study of persons who were more spiritually or religiously involved found

- Higher rates of overall well-being and life satisfaction.
- Lower rates of depressive symptoms and suicide.
- Lower rates of diverse and higher rates of marital satisfaction.
- Lower rates of alcohol abuse and other drug abuse, including cigarette smoking and recreational drug use.

Suicide is far less common in Catholic countries than in Protestants. Professor Ringel the founder President of International Association for Suicide Prevention remarked that a sure method of preventing suicide by becoming a Catholic. On the other hand in Japan where Buddhism is practiced suicide is socially sanctioned among Islamic nations suicide is relatively rare. These indicate that there are religious "built in" "counters" within the individual and culture against suicide act.[149]

Pseudo philosophical and a pseudo religious ideas and delusion mark hebephrenic schizophrenia Religious murder is not uncommon among the paranoids. Recent psychopathological researches in Africa have tended to confirm the dominant supernatural dimension of Psychiatry overriding the biochemical.

In diagnostic and Statistical Manual-IV sub category (V 62.89) of "Religious or Spiritual Problems" was included. The new category could help to promote a new relationship between psychiatry and the fields of religion and spirituality that will benefit both mental health professionals and those who seek their assistance.

Behere (1990) emphasized the role of traditional beliefs and religion of presentation of outcome of schizophrenia. In India which is a land of many religions and the people here speaks so many languages and are illiterate and suffer from economic poverty, the tendency for psychiatric patients to seek refuge and cure in occult healing practices, and submit to pseudo religious and magical traditional healers would be expected.[150]

According to the Harvard psychologist Gordon Allport a persons' religious orientation may be intrinsic and/or extrinsic: [151]

Extrinsic orientation: Persons with this orientation are disposed to use religion for their own ends. May find religion useful in a variety of ways—to provide security and solace, sociability and distraction, status and self-justification. The embraced creed is lightly held or else selectively shaped to fit more primary needs. [151]

Intrinsic orientation: Persons with this orientation find their master motive in religion. Other needs, strong as they may be, are regarded as of less ultimate significance, and they are, so far as possible, brought in harmony with the religious beliefs and prescriptions. Having embraced a creed the individual endeavors to internalize it and follow it fully.[151]

Usually, the intrinsic orientation is associated with healthier personality and mental status, while the extrinsic orientation is associated with the opposite. Extrinsic religiosity is associated with dogmatism, prejudice, fear of death, and anxiety, it "does a good job of measuring the sort of religion that gives religion a bad name. This very important and consistent finding totally contradicts Ellis who argued that one way that religiosity sabotaged" mental health was a lack of self-interest rather than be primarily self-interested, devout deity-oriented religionists put their hypothesized god(s) first and themselves second—or last. It is exactly this behavior that has been most consistently associated with better mental health.

How Religion could Influence Mental Health?

- *Healthy behaviors and lifestyle*: Several illnesses are related to behavior and lifestyle. The way we eat, drink, drive our automobile, have sex, smoke, use drugs, follow medical prescriptions, exam ourselves for prevention have important influences in our health. Most religions prescribe or prohibit behaviors that may impact health. The biblical teachings, 3000 years ago, about diet, ways to handle food, cleaning and purity, circumcision, sexual behavior were important for preventing disease. Today other illnesses are more relevant. Prescriptions about keeping a day of rest, the body as a sacred temple, monogamous sex, moderation on eating and drinking, peaceful relationships are doctrines that might be also helpful for contemporary health problems (related to stress, competition, individualism, narcissism, anger, shame etc.)[152]
- *Social support*: Belonging to a group brings psychosocial support that can promote health. Religion might provide social cohesion, the sense of belonging to a caring group, continuity in relationships with friends and family and other support groups. Social support can influence health by facilitating adherence to health promotion programs, offering fellowship in times of stress, suffering and sorrow, diminishing the impact of anxiety and other emotions and anomie.[152]
- *Belief systems, cognitive framework*: Beliefs and cognitive processes influence how people deal with stress, suffering

and life problems. Religious beliefs can provide support through the following ways: enhancing acceptance, endurance and resilience. They generate peace, self-confidence, purpose, forgiveness to the individuals own failures, self-giving and positive self-image. On the other hand, they can bring guilt, doubts, anxiety and depression through an enhanced self-criticism.[151]

- *Religious practices*: Public and private religious practices can help to maintain mental health and prevent mental diseases. They help to cope with anxiety, fears, frustration, anger, anomie, inferiority feelings, despondency and isolation.[151]
- *Spiritual direction*: Described as a special relationship between two human beings to help the development of the spiritual self. Its aims are to develop a relationship with God, to find meaning in life, and to promote personal growth. Several religious and psychological techniques may be used, and great similarities with psychotherapy can be found, as the same themes are discussed. The psychotherapy and its Indian adaptation are discussed in different article elsewhere.[151]
- *Idiom to express stress*: In times of stress and social disorganization certain religious rituals by means of techniques that elicit altered states of consciousness, can produce catharsis, dissociative states and a special milieu to express problems and suffering.

CONCLUSION

Culture is a holistic concept whose utility goes far beyond the study of exotic tribes in distant locals. Cultural anthropology is pertinent to the study of industrial society in general and the subcultures of modern society in particular. We believe that cultural psychiatry is a concept that has finally arrived and one that will share a central position in the mainstream of psychiatry.

Cultural psychiatry promises no millennium, no bold new approach. Rather, we saw the inclusion of the cultural dimension as an essential integrative component of scientific psychiatry.[153] As an application of knowledge from many disciplines, cultural psychiatry has much in common with psychological anthropology, comparative sociology, and cross-cultural psychology, but its ultimate raison d'etre is medical to further our understanding of mental health and to make more effective our efforts to promote health, to alleviate suffering, and to prevent, diagnose, and treat illness.

Few would dispute the proposition that culture makes a difference, whether in relation to detecting mental disorders, searching for their causes, or providing care for patients and their families. However, building a bridge from proposition to culturally competent actions requires conceptualizing intersections between culture and health that are not always immediately apparent and grounding research, practice system planning and advocacy in principles that do not translate easily into operational terms.[154]

However, future studies must evolve to include psychological and psychiatric measures that are relevant and appropriate for distinct cultural groups, since many cross-cultural studies utilize the Western concepts to explain the modes of expression of psychopathological manifestations,[155] ways of seeking aid, use of mental health services, or treatment outcome, without taking into account their close relationship with cultural factors.[156]

Cultural formulation will be an integral part in DSM-5. Thus culture plays an important role not only in epidemiological studies but also symptomatology, presentation, classification, treatment and outcome of mental disorders.

REFERENCES

1. Kroeber AL, Kluckhohn C. Culture. Vintage Books, 1952. Manual of the International Statistical Classification of Diseases, Injuries and Causes of Death (ICD- 9), 9th edition. World Health Organization; 1977.
2. Gautam S, Jain N. Indian Culture and Psychiatry. Indian Journal of Psychiatry. 2010;52:301-13.
3. Johnson FA. Contributions of Anthropology to Psychiatry. In Review of General Psychiatry. Goldman HH, (Ed). Lange Medical Publication, USA; 1984.
4. Wen-Shing Tseng, Jon Streltzer. Introduction: Culture and Psychiatry. FOCUS. 2006;4:81-90.
5. Tseng WS. The Clinician's Guide to Cultural Psychiatry. San Diego, CA, Academic Press; 2003.
6. Jambur A. Culture and Mental Illness. Psychiatric Research in Asian Countries; 1989.
7. Fabrega H Jr. Culture and history in psychiatric diagnosis and practice. Psychiatric Clinics of North America. 2001;24(3): 391-405.
8. Kraepelin E. Manic-depressive insanity and paranoia CR. M Barclay, Trans.; Robertson GM, (Ed.). Edinburgh: Livingstone; 1921.
9. Cultural competence. *www.upennrrtc.org.*
10. Tseng WS. Handbook of cultural psychiatry. Academic Press, ISBN 0-12-701632-5, San Diego; 2001.
11. Grusec JE, Hastings PD. Handbook of Socialization: Theory and Research. Guilford Press, ISBN 9781593853327, New York; 2007.pp.547.
12. Berry JW. Immigration, acculturation and adaptation. Applied Psychology: An International Review. 1977;46(1):5-68.
13. Bhui K, Stansfeld S, Head J, Haines M, Hillier S, Taylor S, Viner R, Booy R. Cultural identity, acculturation, and mental health among adolescents in east London's multiethnic community. Journal of Epidemiology and Community Health. 2005;59:296-302.
14. Redfield R, Linton R, Herskovits MJ. Memorandum for the study of acculturation. American Anthropologist. 1936;38(1): 149-52.

15. Groen S. Recognizing cultural identity in mental health care: Rethinking the cultural formulation of a Somali patient. Transcultural Psychiatry. 2009;46(3):451-62.
16. Cheetham RW, Edwards SD, Naidoo LR, Griffiths JA, Singh, VG. Deculturation as a precipitant of parasuiside in an Asian group. South African Medical Journal. 1983;63(24):942-5.
17. Bhugra D, Bhui K. Cross-cultural psychiatric assessment. Advances in Psychiatric Treatment. 1997;3:103-10.
18. Kroeber AL. Stimulus diffusion. American Anthropologist, 1940;42(1):1-20.
19. Grier WH, Cobbs PM. Black Rage. Basic Books, ISBN 13: 9780465007035, New York; 1968.
20. Sen P, Chowdhury AN. Culture, ethnicity and paranoia. Current Psychiatric Reports. 2006;8:174-8.
21. Whaley AL. Ethnicity/race, paranoia, and hospitalization for mental health problems among men. American Journal of Public Health. 2004;94(1):78-81.
22. Murphy JM. Psychiatric labelling in cross-cultural perspectives. Science. 1976;191:1019.
23. Wig NN. DSM-III: a perspective from the third world, in International Perspectives on DSM-III. Edited by Spitzer RI, Williams JBW, Skodol AE. Washington, DC, American Psychiatric Press; 1983.pp.79-89.
24. Florsheim P. Cross-cultural views of self in the treatment of mental illness: disentangling the curative aspects of myth from the mythic aspects of cure. Psychiatry. 1990;53: 304-15.
25. Katon W, Kleinman A, Rosen G. Depression and dramatization review. Am J Med. 1982;72:127-35.
26. White GM. The role of cultural explanations in 'somatization' and 'psychologization.' Soc Sci Med.1982;16:1519-30.
27. Goodman A. Organic unity theory: the mind-body problem revisited. Am J Psychiatry. 1991;148:553-63.
28. Marcos LR. Effects of interpreters on the evaluation of psychopathology in non-English-speaking patients. Am J psychiatry. 1975;136:171-4.
29. Labov W, Fanshell D. Therapeutic Discourse. New York, Academic Press; 1977.
30. Heiser M. Culture and Psychiatry, or 'The tale of the Hole and the Cheese'. The Canadian Jn Psychiatry. 2003;40:3.
31. WHO, Report of the International Pilot study of Schizophrenia World Health Organization: Geneva; 973.
32. WHO, Report of the International Follow-up study of Schizophrenia John Wiley and Sons, New York; 1979.
33. Jablensky A, Schwarz R, Tomov J. ~WHO - collaborative study on impairments and disabilities associated with schizophrenic disorders. Acta Psychiatrica Scandinavica, Suppl. 1980;285: 152-63.
34. Jablensky A. Multicultural studies and the nature of schizophrenia: a review. Journal of the Royal Society of Medicine. 1987;80:162-7.
35. Mezzich JE, Good BJ. On culturally enhancing the DSM-IV multiaxial formulation, in DSM-IV Sourcebook, Vol 3. Edited by Widiger TA, Frances AJ, Pincus HA, et al. Washington, DC, American Psychiatric Press; 1997.pp.983-9.
36. Agrawal AK, Abuja N, Awasthi A, Bandopadhyay G. Behere PB, et al. ICD-10 field trials in India - A WHO sponsored reference study. Supplement. Indian J Psychiatry. 1993;35:198-222.
37. Culture and psychiatry. *www.dsm5.org.*
38. Brendan D. Kelly. Globalisation, psychiatry and human rights: new challenges for the 21st century. Published by RC Psych Publications, 2010; ISBN: 978-1-904671-82-4.
39. Gleize L, Laudon F, Sun LY, et al. Cancer registry of French Polynesia: results for the 1900–1995 periods among native and immigrant population. European Journal of Epidemiology. 2000;16:661-7.
40. Gavin BE, Kelly BD, Lane A, et al. The mental health of migrants. Irish Medical Journal. 2001;94:229–30.
41. Murphy HBM. Chronicite Communaute et Culture in Chiland C Bequant P (Ed) Traitements au long coursdes etats psychotiques Toulouse Privat, 1974.
42. Leong FTL. Cultural variations in the treated prevalence rate and symptomatology among Chinese, Japanese, Filipino and Caucasian schizophrenic patients in Hawaiii. Schulz S, C Tamminga (Eds). In: Schizophrenia: Scientific Progress New York Oxford University Press; 1989.pp.36-40.
43. Enright J, Jaeckle W. Psychiatric symptoms and diagnosis in two subcultures. Int J Soc Psychiatry, 1963;9:12-17.
44. Venkataramaiah V, Mallikarjunaiah M, Chandrashekhar CR, Vasudeva Rao CK, Narayana Reddy GN, Possession Syndrome: An epidemiological study in west Karnataka. Indian J Psychiatry. 1981;23:213-8.
45. Singh G, Sachdev JS. Acute Schizophrenic episodes. Indian J Psychiatry. 1981;23:200-05.
46. Cooper JE, Kendell RE, Garland BJ. Psychiatric diagnosis in New York London: Oxford University Press. Maudsley Monograph Series No. 20, 1972.
47. Saenger G. Psychiatric outpatients in America and the Netherlands: A transcultural comparison. Social Psychiatry. 1968;3:149-64.
48. Levine HI. Acute schizophrenia: clinical aspects of labeling process. Arch Gen Psychiatry. 1971;25:215-22.
49. Wing JK, Brown GW. Institutionalism and schizophrenia New York, Cambridge University Press; 1970.
50. World Health Organization: Schizophrenia: A multinational study Geneva; 1975.
51. Lin T, Standley CC. The scope of epidemiology in psychiatry WHO Public Health Paper No 16 Geneva World Health Organization, 1962.
52. Reid DD. Epidemiological methods in the study of psychiatric disorders. Geveva: World Health Organization Public Health Papers No. 2, 1960.
53. Krassoievitch M, Perez-Rincon H, Suarez P. Correlation entreles hallucinations visuelles et auditives dans une population de schizophrenes mexicains. Conront Psychiatr. 1982;15: 149-62.

54. Ndetei DM, Vadher A. A comparative cross-cultural study of the frequencies of hallucination in schizophrenia. Acta Psychiatr Scand. 1984;70:545-9.
55. Kleinman A. Rethinking Psychiatry. Free Press, New York; 1988.
56. Warner R. Recovery from Schizophrenia: psychiatry and Political Economy. Routledge & Regan Paul, New York; 1985.
57. Sartorius N, Jablensky A, Korten A, et al. Early manifestations and first-contact incidence of schizophrenia indifferent cultures. Psychol Med. 1986;16:909-28.
58. Lin KM, Kleinman A. Psychopathology and clinical course of schizophrenia: A cross-cultural perspective. Schizophr Bull. 1988;14:555-67.
59. Kulhara P, Chakrabarti S. Culture and schizophrenia and other psychotic disorders. Psychiatr Clin N Am. 2001;24(3):449-64.
60. Jenkins JH, Karno M. The meaning of expressed emotion: Theoretical issues raised by cross-cultural research. Am J Psychiatr. 1992;149:9-21.
61. Habel U, Gur RC, Mandal MK, et al. Emotional processing in schizophrenia across cultures: Standardized measures of discrimination and experience. Schizophr Res. 2000;42:57-66.
62. Murphy HBM, Raman AC. The Chronicity of schizophrenia in indigenous tropical peoples. Brit J Psychiatry. 1971;118:489-97.
63. Sartorius N, Jablensky A, Shapiro R. Two year follow up of the patients included in the WHO international study of schizophrenia. Psychological Medicine. 1977;7:529-41.
64. Verghese A, Dube KG, John J, Menon D, Sarda Menon K, Rajkumar M, Richard S, Sethi BB, Trivedi JK, Wig NN. Factors associated with the course and outcome of schizophrenia I: Objectives and methodology, Indian Journal of Psychiatry. 1985;27:201-6.
65. Waxier N. Is outcome for schizophrenia better in no industrial societies? The case of Sri Lanka, Journal of Nervous and Mental Disease. 1979;167(3):144-58.
66. Carpenter WT, Strauss JS. The prediction of outcome in schizophrenia: IV. Eleven year follow-up of the Washington IPSS cohort. Journal of the Nervous and Mental Disease. 1991;179:517-25.
67. Dube KC, Kumar N, Dube S. Long-term course and outcome of the Agra cases in the International Pilot Study of Schizophrenia Acta Psychiatrica Scandinavica. 1984,70(2):170-79.
68. Leon C. Clinical course and outcome of schizophrenia in Cali. A 10 year follow-up study (Spanish). Acta psiquitrica Y Psicologica de America Latina. 1986;32(2):95136.
69. Leon CA. Clinical course and outcome of schizophrenia in Cali. A 10 year followup study. Journal of Nervous and Mental Disease. 1989;177:593-606.
70. Leff J, Sartorius N, Jablensky A, Korten A, Ernberg G. The International Pilot Study of Schizophrenia: five-year follow-up findings. Psychological Medicine. 1992;22(1):131-45.
71. Wig NN, Varma VK, Mattoo SK, Behere PB, Phookan HR, Misra AK, Murthy RS, Tripathi BM, Menon DK, Khandelwal SK, Hedi H. An incidence study of schizophrenia in India. Indian Journal of Psychiatry. 1993;35:11-7.
72. Behere PB, Behere M. Influence of culture in schizophrenia In: Current Developments in Schizophrenia. Mandal MK, Nigamie SH (Eds). Allied Publishers Pvt. Ltd. Hyderbad; 2004.
73. Wig NN. Mental health and spiritual values. A view from the East. International Review of Psychiatry. 1999;11:92-6.
74. Marsella AJ, Sartorius N, Jablensky A, Fenton FR. Cross-cultural studies of depressive disorders: An overview. In: Culture and Depression: Studies in Anthropology and Cross-Cultural Psychiatry of Affect and Disorder. Kleinman A, Good BJ (Eds). University of California Press, Berkeley; 1985.pp.299-324.
75. Ebigbo PO. Development of a culture specific (Nigeria) screening scale of somatic complaints. Cult Med Psychiatr. 1982;6:29-44.
76. Kirmayer LJ, Groleau D. Affective disorders in cultural context. Psychiatr Clin N Am. 2001;24(3):465-78.
77. Behere PB, Behere M. Culture and Depression in proceedings of 13th Mid Term CME of W.Z. of Indian Psychiatry Society. Nasik; 2004.
78. Kleinman A, Good BJ. (Eds.). Culture and depression. Berkeley: University of California Press; 1985.
79. Klibansky R, Panofsky E, Saxl F. Saturn and melancholy: Studies in the history of natural philosophy, religion and art. New York: Basic Books; 1964.
80. Sartorius N, Davidian H, Ernberg, G, Fenton FR, Fujii I, Gastpar M, Gulbinat W, Jablensky A, Kielholz P, Lehman HE, Naraghi M, Shimizu M, Shinfuku N, Takahashi R. Depressive disorders in different cultures: Report on the WHO collaborative study on standardized assessment of depressive disorders. Geneva: World Health Organization; 1983.
81. Venkoba Rao A. Depressive illness in India, Indian Journal of Psychiatry. 1984;26,301-11.
82. Bebbington PE. The epidemiology of depressive disorder. Culture, Medicine and Psychiatry. 1978;2:297-341.
83. Kleinman A. Neurasthenia and depression: A study of somatization and culture in China Culture, Medicine and Psychiatry. 1982;6:117-90.
84. Krimayer LJ. Culture, affect and dramatization Parts I and II. Transcultural Psychiatric Research Review. 1984;21:159-88, 237-62.
85. Schurman RA, Kramer PD, Mitchell JB. The hidden mental he lathnetwork. Archives of General Psychiatry. 1985;42: 89-94.
86. Kraepelin E. Manic depressive Insanity and Paranoia. (Translated by M Barclay), Edinburgh: ES Livingstone, 1921.
87. Murphy HBM, Wittkower ED, Chance NA. 'Cross cultural inquiry into the symptomatology of depression.' International Journal of Psychiatry. 1967;3:6.
88. Ansari SA. Symptomatology of Indian depressives. Transactions of All India Institute of Mental Health. 1969;9:1-18.
89. Teja JS, Narang RL, Agrawal AK. Depression across Culture. Brit J Psyciat. 1971;119:253-60.
90. Venkoba Rao A. Depressive illness and guilt in Indian culture. Indian Journal of Psychiatry. 1973;15:231-6.

91. Kulhara P, Varma VK. Phenomenology of schizophrenic and affective disorders in India: A review. Indian Journal of Social Psychiatry. 1985;I:148-67.
92. Peggs J. Cries of agony: An historical account of suttee, infanticide, ghat murders and slavery in India. Rpt. Delhi: Discovery; 1984.
93. Eisenbruch M. Cross-cultural aspects or bereavement. Culture, Medicine and Psychiatry. 1984;8:283-309,315-47.
94. Singer K. Depressive disorders from a transcultural perspective. Social Science and Medicine. 1975;9:289-301.
95. Lambo TA. Neuropsychiatric observations in the Western region of Nigeria. British Medical Journal. 1956;ii:1388-94.
96. Yap PM. Suicide in Hong Kondg, London; 1958.
97. Eaton JW, Well RJ. Culture and Mental Disorders, New York, 1955.
98. Venkoba Rao A. 'Depresion—a psychiatric analysis of thirty cases.' Indian Journal of Psychiatry. 1966;8:143-54.
99. Teja JS, Narang RL. 'Pattern of incidence of depression in India' India Journal of Psychiatry. 1970;12:33-9.
100. Bagadia VN, Jeste DV, Dave KP, Dosm SU, Shah LP. A prospective epidemiological study of 233 cases of depression. Indian Journal of Psychiatry; 1970.
101. Murphy HBM, Wittkower ED, Chance NA. 'Cross cultural inquiry into the symptomatology of depression' International Journal of Psychiatry. 1967;3:6.
102. World Health Organisation (WHO). Depressive Disorders in Different Cultures: Report on the WHO Collaborative Study on Standardized Assessment of Depressive Disorders Geneva: WHO; 1983.
103. Santorius N. Culture and epidemiology of depression. Psychiatric neurologia Neurochirugia. 1973;76:479-87.
104. American Psychiatric Association. Diagnostic and Statistical Manual of Mental Disorders, 4th edition. APA, Washington DC; 1994.
105. Good BJ, Kleinman A. Culture and anxiety: Cross-cultural evidence for the patterning of anxiety disorders. In anxiety and the anxiety disorders. Tuma A, Maser J (Eds). Erlbaum, Hillsdale, NJ, 1985.
106. Neal AM, Turner SM. Anxiety disorders research with African Americans: Current status. Psychol Bull. 1991;109: 400-10.
107. Brown DR, Eaton WW, Sussman L. Racial differences in prevalence of Phobic disorders. J Nerv Ment Dis. 1990;178: 434-41.
108. Lewis-Fernandez R. The proposed DSM-IV trance and possession disorder category: Potential benefits ad risks. Transcult Psychiatr Res Rev. 1992;29:301-17.
109. Krimayar LJ, Weiss M. On cultural considerations for somatoform disorders in DSM-IV. In: Sourcebook for DSM-IV, Widiger T, Frances AJ, Pincus HA, et al (Eds). American Psychiatric Press, Washington DC; 1997.pp.933-42.
110. Saxena S, Prasad KVSR. DSM-III classification of dissociative disorders applied to psychiatric outpatients in India. Am J Psychiatr. 1989;145:261-2.
111. Lewis-Fernandez R. Culture and dissociation: A comparison of ataque de nervios among Puerto Ricans and possession Syndrome' in India. In Dissociation: Culture, Mind, and Body. Spiegel D (Ed). American Psychiatric Press, Washington DC; 1994.pp.123-7.
112. Ward CA. Editorial Altered States of Consciousness and Mental Health: A Cross Cultural Perspective. Sage, Newbury Park; 1989.
113. Spiegel D, Crdena E. Disintegrated experience: The dissociative disorders revisited. J Abnorm Psychol. 1991;100:366-78.
114. Pittman BJ. International overview: Social and cultural factors in drinking patterns. In: Alcoholism BJ Pittman (Ed.). New York, Harper & Row; 1967.
115. Bruun K, Edwards G, Lumio M. Alcohol control policies in public health perspective. The Finnish Foundation for Alcohol Studies; 1975.p.25.
116. Nielsen J, Sorensen K. Alcohol Policy. Alcohol consumption, alcohol prices, delirium tremens and alcoholism as cause of death in Denmark. Social Psychiatry. 1979;14:133-8.
117. Heath DB. Anthropology. In: Recent Developments in Alcoholism (Ed). Galanter M Vol I I. New York: Plenum; 1993.
118. Duster T. Commentary. In: Alcohol and Disinhibition: Nature and Meaning of the find. R Room, G Collins (Eds). Research Monograph 12. Rockville, Md.: National Institute on Alcohol Abuse and Alcoholism; 1983.
119. Helzer Je, Canino GJ (Eds.). Alcoholism - North America, Europe, and Asia: A coordinated analysis of population data from ten regions, Oxford, London; 1992.
120. Jain AP, Behere PB, Gupta P. Neurological complication in alcohol abusers in dry district. The Indian Practitioner. 2003; 56:170-72.
121. Haifner H, Welz R, Gorenc K, Kleff F. Selbstmordversuche und depressive Storungen, Schiwiezer Archiv fuir Neurologie, Neurochirurgie and Psychiatric. 1983;133:283-94.
122. Durkheim E. New York, The Free Press of Glencoe; 1951.
123. Chhabra V, Bhatia MS, Gupta R. Cultural Bound Syndromes in India. Delhi Psychiatry Journal. 2004;11(1):15-8.
124. Hughes CC, Simons RC, Wintrob RM. The 'culture-bound syndromes' and DSM-IV. In: Sourcebook for DSM-IV, Widiger T, Frances AJ, Pincus HA, et al (Eds.). American Psychiatric Press, Washington DC; 1997.pp.991-1000.
125. Hahn RA. Culture-bound syndromes unbound. Soc Sci Med. 1985;21:165-71.
126. Guamaccia PJN, Rogler LH. Research on culture-bound syndromes: new directions. Am J Psychiatr. 1999;156(9): 1322-7.
127. Good BJ, Kleinman A. Toward a meaning-centered analysis of popular illness categories: 'Fright-illness' and 'heart distress' In Iran. In: Cultural Conceptions of Mental Health and Therapy, Marsella AJ, White GM (Eds.). Reidel, dordrecht. 1982. pp.141-66.
128. Wig NN. DSM-III: A perspective from the third world, in International Perspectives on DSM-III. Spitzer RI, Williams JBW, Skodol AE (Eds.). American Psychiatric Press, Washington DC; 1983.pp.79-89.

129. Behere PB, Natraj GS. Dhat syndrome: The phenomenology of a culture bound sex neurosis of the orient. Ind J Psychiat. 1984;26:76-8.
130. Behere PB, Wig NN, Behere M. Ancient Indian concept of Dhat syndrome: A cultural bound sex neurosis of the orient. Ind J Psychol Med. 1991;14:85-7.
131. Bhatia MS, Malik SC. Dhat syndrome—a useful diagnostic entity in Indian Culture. Br J Psych. 1991;159:691-5.
132. Singh G. Dhat syndrome revisited. Ind J Psych. 1985;27: 119-22.
133. Neki JS. The Ascetic syndrome. Mimeographed. New Delhi: All India Institute of Medical Sciences; 1972.pp.1-5.
134. Potkin SG, Sheu Y, Pardes H. Haloperidol concentrations elevated in Chinese patients. Psychiatry Res. 1984;12:167.
135. Okpaku S, Frazier A, Mendel J. A pilot study of racial differences in erythrocyte lithium transport. Am J Psych. 1980;137:120.
136. Varma VK, Ghosh A. Psychotherapy as practiced by Indian Psychiatrists, Ind J Psych. 1976;18:177.
137. Venkoba Rao A, Parvathi Devi. Psychotherpy and Bhagwat Geeta. Ind J Psych; 1974.
138. Hoch E. "Pir, faquir and psychotherapist". The human Context VI No. 3:668, 1974.
139. Hoch E. Psychotherapy for the illiterate' in New Dimension in Psychiatry—a World view. Ariety S (Ed). John W'ley and Sons, New York; 1977.
140. Hoch E. 'Process in Instant Cure' in Psychotherapeutic processes. Kapur M, Murthy VN, Sathyavathi K, Kapur RL (Eds.). NIMHANS Bangalore; 1978.
141. Neki JS. 'Psychiatry in South East Asia. Brit J Psych. 1973;123: 157.
142. Neki JS. Psychiatry in India. Ind J Psych. 1977;19(2):1-10.
143. Neki JS. "Psychotherapy in India past, present and future". Am J Psycho. 1976;75:92.
144. Parikh MD. Psychotherapy based up on Hindu Philosophy CME. Ind Psych Soc; 1984.
145. Nandi D. Psychotherapy in India. CME Ind Psych Soc; 1985.
146. Jean M Langford. Ayurvedic Psychotherapy: Transposed Signs, Parodied Selves. 1989.
147. Spika B, Hood RW, Gorsuch RL. The psychology of religion: an empirical approach. Prentice Hall, Englewood Cliffs, NJ; 1985.
148. Khurana PS, Malhotra A. Religion and Psychiatry. Indian J Social Psychiatry. 2001;17:50-57.
149. Behere PB. The influence of traditional beliefs and religion on mental illness in India. In the proceedings of Third International Congress on Traditional Asian Medicine Bombay; 1990.
150. Alexander Moreira-Almeida; Francisco LotufoNeto; Harold G Koenig. Religiousness and mental health: a review. Rev. Bras. Psiquiatr. vol. 28 no. 3 São Paulo Sept. 2006 Epub Aug 10, 2006.
151. Behere A. Treatment seeking pattern of psychiatric patients for current problems. Project report submitted to ICMR as short term research studentship; 2002.
152. Kennedy JG. Cultural psychiatry, in Handbook of Social and Cultural Anthropology. Honigman JJ (Ed.). Chicago Rand McNally; 1973.pp.1119-98.
153. Heiser M. Culture and Psychiatry or "The tale of the Hole and the Cheese". The Canadian in Psychiatry, 2003;40:3.
154. Alarcon AD, Becker AB, Lewis-Fernandez R. Issues for DSM-V: the role of culture in psychiatric diagnosis. J Nerv Ment Dis. 2009;197:559–6.
155. Kendler KS, Zachar P. The incredible insecurity of psychiatric nosology. In: Kendler KS, Parnas J, editors. Philosophical issues in psychiatry. Explanation, phenomenology and nosology. Baltimore: Johns Hopkins University Press; 2008. pp.369-85.
156. Angst J. Psychiatric diagnosis: the weak component of modern research. World Psychiatry. 2007;6:94-5.

CHAPTER 57

Culture-bound Syndrome

Sandeep Grover, Alakananda Dutt, Ajit Avasthi

INTRODUCTION

Psychiatry deals with pathology of cognition, feelings and self-concept and hence cannot remain uninfluenced by man's sociocultural and religious background. Culture is an important determinant of manifestations of various psychiatric disorders and has been defined in various ways. The most accepted definition of culture is given by the National Institute of Mental Health and Diagnosis Group which describes it as "meanings, values and behavioral norms that are learned and transmitted in the dominant society and within its social groups". Cultural influences on psychiatric syndromes can occur in at least six distinct ways: (1) pathogenic effect (cultural influence on the formation of a disorder); (2) psychoselective effect (culture selecting certain coping patterns to deal with stress); (3) psychoplastic effect (culture modifying the clinical manifestation); (4) pathoelaborating effect (culture elaborating mental conditions into a unique nature); (5) psychofacilitating effect (culture promoting the frequency of occurrence); or (6) psychoreactive effect (culture shaping folk responses to the clinical condition) (Tseng, 2001). The psychoreactive effect is nonspecific and only effects the interpretation and labeling of phenomenon and does not result in the development of any unique pathological condition. The recognition of this unequivocal influence of culture on psychiatric disorders have led to the development of concept of *Culture-bound Syndromes*.

Culture bound syndromes denote a specific array of behavioral and experiential phenomena that tend to present themselves preferentially in particular sociocultural contexts and are readily recognized as illness behavior by people of that culture. They are commonly assigned culturally sanctioned explanations and interpretations that, in turn, generate a set of remedies congruent to that culture. Their clinical manifestations tend to be different from those of psychiatric disorders that fit within existing psychiatric classifications. Over the years various culture bound syndromes have been described from various cultures. The DSM-IV glossary includes descriptions of 25 syndromes that cultural experts identified as particularly relevant to psychiatry.

EVOLUTION OF THE CONCEPT

The 20th century heralded a period during which due to the zeal of Western societies for colonization, Western missionaries and physicians came in contact with cultures foreign to their own. Under these circumstances they encountered unique behaviors and psychiatric conditions which appeared incomprehensible to them. These unique behaviors occurred in the specific native populations, had local explanations for the symptom manifestations and required interventions and these were labeled differently. Therefore, they labeled latah, amok, and koro conditions indigenous to these "foreign lands" as 'peculiar' phenomena by some (Yap, 1951) and 'uncommon,' 'extraordinary,' or 'unclassifiable' mental disorders by others. This was further enhanced by the tendency to consider anything that is inexplicable on the basis of the Anglo-Saxon prototype on which the psychiatric classifications were originally based, as unusual or atypical. After reviewing the literature on some of the 'peculiar' disorders from the perspective of comparative psychiatry, Yap (1962) initially suggested the term 'atypical, culture-bound, psychogenic psychosis', but later in order to cover the various psychopathologies or atypical syndromes that seem to be bound to certain cultures and occur as a result of psychological reactions, Yap (1967), later on used the term 'culture-bound, reactive syndrome' and then 'culture-bound syndrome'. The use of the term 'bound' highlighted that these psychiatric syndromes were 'bound' to a particular cultural group or setting, such as amok among Malay people, koro among the Southern Chinese, and Dhat syndrome among people in India.

CLASSIFICATION OF CULTURE-BOUND SYNDROMES

Yap (1967), attempted to classify the culture-bound syndromes on the basis of the cardinal symptoms as primary fear reactions (malignant anxiety, latah, psychogenic or magical death), morbid rage reaction (amok), specific culture-imposed, nosophobia (koro) and trance dissociation (windigo psychosis). Later on Simons and Hughes (1985) categorized culture-related syndromes by a common factor, that is, 'taxon'. This included the startle-matching taxon (including latah, imu), the sleep-paralysis taxon and the genital-retraction taxon. Recently Tseng (2001) divided specific syndromes into several groups based on the different ways that culture impacts psychopathology. These are culture-related beliefs as causes for the occurrence (such as koro or Dhat syndrome), culture-patterned specific stress-coping reactions (such as amok or family suicide), culture-shaped variations of psychopathology (such as taijinkuofusho or brain fag syndrome), culturally elaborated unique behavior reactions (such as latah), culture-provoked frequent occurrences of pathological conditions (such as mass hysteria or substance abuse), and cultural interpretations and reactions to certain mental conditions (such as hwabyung or susto). It has been suggested that this is a more meaningful approach for addressing and understanding these disorders from a cultural perspective.

Difficulty arises when one attempts to fit such culture-related specific syndromes into the categories of the existing classification system, or to create new categories of disorders within the current classification system. These syndromes will invariably be classified as NOS (not otherwise specified) or, at best, as 'variations' of presently recognized disorders within the current classification system. According to some of the researchers such efforts would lead to the loss of the unique meaning of these syndromes, from a cultural perspective. It has also been suggested that addition of such mental conditions into the present classification system would not be very useful from a practical point of view as they are rarely observed (Tseng, 2006).

PHENOMENOLOGY OF CULTURE-BOUND SYNDROMES

Dhat Syndrome

Although the term Dhat syndrome was used for the first time by Wig (1960), Still (1940) first made remarks about the etiology and symptoms of the Dhat syndrome observed among young (male) Indian men in the Indian Medical Gazette. The term was first used by Wig in 1960 to describe a culture bound sexual neurosis, for patients preoccupied with the excessive loss of semen by nocturnal emissions or in urine although there was no objective evidence for the same. Further, this preoccupation led to guilt and undue concern with the debilitating effect of loss of semen on physical and psychological health (Wig, 1960). In the later description, further elaboration of phenomenology was done by various researchers. It was reported that these patients present with vague and multiple somatic and psychological symptoms like lack of physical strength, fatigue, listlessness, poor concentration, forgetfulness, etc. (Avasthi and Nehra, 2001). It is now understood that the core feature of Dhat syndrome is the undue concern of passage of semen during micturition or while straining to pass stools, although there is no objective evidence of semen in urine or its passage otherwise. The belief may also be accompanied by anxiety or depressive symptoms and the patient may present with or without sexual dysfunction. Accordingly, some researchers have described subgroups of Dhat syndrome, viz. Dhat syndrome alone, Dhat syndrome with anxiety or depressive symptoms and Dhat syndrome with sexual dysfunction.

Dhat syndrome is usually described in subjects of younger age (16–25) from lower socioeconomic classes (Behere and Nataraj, 1984; Malhotra and Wig, 1975). It is often comorbid with depressive and anxiety disorders (Singh, 1985). It has been noted that the symptoms usually disappear if the misconceptions about semen loss are effectively dealt with and by increasing knowledge about sex the syndrome would become less common.

The concept of Dhat syndrome has also been extended to include Indian women presenting with somatic symptoms associated with leukorrhea, and explained as due to loss of a 'vital fluid'(Singh et al, 2003).

Besides being studied in India, Dhat syndrome has also been studied in other South-Asian countries. Mumford (1996) studied men attending medical clinics in Lahore and reported that about 30% of the subjects complained of Dhat and the prevalence of Dhat was equal in patients with 'functional' and 'organic' diagnosis. In another study, Khan (2005) studied the treatment seeking pattern of subjects with Dhat syndrome in Lahore and found that about 50% of the subjects sought help from Hakims; only 1.6% consulted psychiatrist. In studies from Sri Lanka, De Silva and Dissanayake (1989) and Dewaraja and Sasaki (1991) studied men with sexual dysfunction and they reported that in many cases the subjects attributed their dysfunction to semen loss. Half of the patients also had somatic symptoms.

Koro

Koro is also known as suo-yang (or shook-yang in Cantonese), which literally means 'shrinking penis'. The first known reference of suo-yang is available from northern China reportedly in 7000 BC. However, the first well-developed concept of suo-yang was described sometime between 476 and 221 BC, in the first textbook of Chinese medicine, the Yellow Emperor's Classic Text of Internal Medicine, or Nei

Ching. The two fundamental ideas were given to explain suo-yang. It is the dual power of 'Yin' (literally, 'the shady side of the hill') and 'Yang' (literally 'the sunny side of the hill') that unites cosmology and astrology, and that serves as the basis for an understanding of basic worldly contrasts. In the recent literature, van Wulfften Palthe (1934) reported on *koro* in a European journal.

Koro begins with the perception that a protruding organ, most often the male genitalia, but possibly the female breasts or the tongue, is retracting into the body and the belief that a complete retraction of the organ will lead to death. Hence, this experience is accompanied by emotions of fear, anxiety and panic. Injuries and even death occur mainly due to the attempts made by patients and other male family members, friends and neighbors to grasp and prevent the penis from retracting. The syndrome is commonly seen in young, mentally healthy people who have knowledge of the existence of Koro. Sometimes the victim is identified by the surrounding persons and treated without consent. It is commonly seen in Asian countries. It is divided into two types—epidemic and isolated. The epidemic type usually has a cultural basis, affects hundreds of people at once, is predominately found in Southeast Asia, presents and resolves acutely. Several such epidemics have been reported, in Singapore, Thailand and India. In contrast, isolated Koro occurs in a variety of places, have little cultural basis, is associated with medical or psychiatric abnormalities and often persists despite treatment. The etiological or predisposing factors include psychosexual conflicts, personality factors, cultural beliefs, sexual conflicts and guilt feelings. In epidemics, rumors and suggestibility, commonly shared beliefs, social crisis as well as geographic seclusion, mostly young poorly educated men susceptible to superstitious beliefs, suggestions, belief and previous knowledge of Koro, immature personality and lack of sexual confidence, poor body image, history of venereal disease and preoccupation with genitals are often considered as risk or etiological factors.

Koro has also been described in India as "jhinjhini bimari" (tingling disease) as the first symptoms can start with a tingling sensation. A study in Indians during the Koro epidemic revealed that majority of those with Koro were suffering from venereal diseases or scrotal filaria at the onset of a Koro attack as compared to the control population (Chowdhury, 1989).

Latah

In the recent literature, W Gilmore Ellis (1893, 1897), the British medical superintendent of the Government Asylum in Singapore, described latah as a mental malady of the Malays, in the Journal of Mental Science. The term latah is of Malaysian or Indonesian origin, but the syndrome has been found in many parts of the world. Other terms for this condition are amurakh, irkunii, ikota, olan, myriachit, and menkeiti (Siberian groups); bah tschi, bah-tsi, and baah-ji (Thailand); imu (Ainu, Sakhalin, Japan); and mali-mali and silok (Philippines). It presents with a sudden fright in an individual resulting in imitative behaviors that appear beyond control, including imitation of movements and speech, following commands leading to enactment of acts against his or her wish (e.g. verbal repetition of obscenities). In Malaysia, it is more frequent in middle-aged women. Some authors have argued that the predominant feature of latah is the cultural elaboration of the neurophysiological startle reflex, while others attribute the genesis of latah to the difficult social status of being an older woman past childbearing age which violate the cultural norms of order, self-control, and courtesy.

Amok

In the recent literature, W Gilmore Ellis (1893, 1897), the British medical superintendent of the Government Asylum in Singapore, for the first time reported the phenomenon of *amok* observed among the Malays. It is described as a dissociative episode characterized by a period of brooding followed by an outburst of violent, aggressive, or homicidal behavior directed at people and objects usually precipitated by a perceived slight or insult. The episode is often accompanied by persecutory ideas, automatism, amnesia, exhaustion, and a return to a premorbid state after the episode. It is seen mostly in men. Some instances of amok may occur during a brief psychotic episode or constitute the onset or exacerbation of a chronic psychotic process. Though originally reported from Malaysia, similar behavior pattern has been reported from Laos, Philippines, Polynesia, Papua New Guinea, and Puerto Rico.

Ataque De Nervios

It is an idiom of distress characterized by uncontrollable shouting, attacks of crying, trembling, heat in the chest rising into the head, and verbal or physical aggression. Dissociative experiences, seizure-like or fainting episodes, and suicidal gestures are prominent in some attacks. It is mainly reported among Latinos from the Caribbean but recognized among many Latin American and Latin Mediterranean groups as a direct result of a stressful event relating to the family (e.g. news of the death of a close relative, a separation or divorce from a spouse, conflicts with a spouse or children, or witnessing an accident involving a family member). People may experience amnesia for what occurred during the attack, but tend to rapidly return to their usual level of functioning. It differs from the DSM-IV description of panic attacks by the presence of a precipitating event and the frequent absence of the hallmark symptoms of acute fear or apprehension. High rates of comorbidities with DSM-IV anxiety and affective disorders are common. It has been suggested that presence of specific symptoms like prominent presence of fear (and associated bodily sensations) and overt anger and aggressive behavior predicts comorbidity with anxiety and panic disorders and affective disorders respectively.

Bilis and Colera (Also Referred to as Muina)

It is characterized by acute nervous tension, headache, trembling, screaming, stomach disturbances, and in more severe cases, loss of consciousness due to strongly experienced anger or rage. Chronic fatigue may result from the acute episode.

Bouffee Delirante

It usually presents with a sudden outburst of agitated and aggressive behavior, marked confusion, and psychomotor excitement. It may sometimes be accompanied by visual and auditory hallucinations or paranoid ideation. These episodes may resemble an episode of brief psychotic disorder. It is commonly observed in West Africa and Haiti.

Brain Fag

It is characterized by difficulties in concentrating, remembering and thinking in high school or university students in response to the challenges of schooling. Students often state that their brains are fatigued. Additional somatic symptoms are usually centered around the head and neck and include pain, pressure or tightness, blurring of vision, heat, or burning. It was initially reported from West Africa but has been now reported from various parts of the world.

Falling Out or Blacking Out

Characterized by episodes of falling out or blacking out that occur primarily in the southern United States and in Caribbean groups. They are characterized by a sudden collapse, which sometimes occurs without warning but sometimes is preceded by feelings of dizziness or swimming in the head. The individual's eyes are usually open, but the person claims an inability to see although the affected person usually hears and understands what is occurring around him or her. This may correspond to a diagnosis of conversion disorder or a dissociative disorder.

Ghost Sickness

A preoccupation with death and the deceased (sometimes associated with witchcraft) characterized by various symptoms including bad dreams, weakness, feelings of danger, loss of appetite, fainting, dizziness, fear, anxiety, hallucinations, loss of consciousness, confusion, feelings of futility, and a sense of suffocation generally attributed to ghosts are seen frequently among members of many American Indian tribes.

Hwa-Byung (Also known as Wool-Hwa-Byung)

Hwa-byung is a Korean folk syndrome that is literally translated into English as anger syndrome and is attributed to the suppression of anger. The symptoms include insomnia, fatigue, panic, fear of impending death, dysphoric affect, indigestion, anorexia, dyspnea, palpitations, generalized aches and pains, and a feeling of a mass in the epigastrium.

Locura

It is a term used by Latinos in the United States and Latin America in reference to a severe form of chronic psychosis. The condition is attributed to an inherited vulnerability, the effect of multiple life difficulties, or a combination of both factors. Symptoms exhibited by persons with locura include incoherence, agitation, auditory and visual hallucinations, inability to follow rules of social interaction, unpredictability and possible violence.

Mal De Ojo

It is a concept widely found in Mediterranean cultures and elsewhere in the world. Mal de ojo is a Spanish phrase translated into English as evil eye. Children are especially at risk of symptoms like fitful sleep, crying without apparent cause, diarrhea, vomiting, and fever due to the evil eye. Sometimes adults (especially women) have the condition.

Nervios

Nervios refers to a general state of vulnerability to stressful life experiences and to a syndrome brought on by difficult life circumstances. Common symptoms include headaches and brain aches, irritability, stomach disturbances, sleep difficulties, nervousness, easy tearfulness, inability to concentrate, trembling, tingling sensations, and mareos (dizziness with occasional vertigo-like exacerbations). It is a common idiom of distress among Latinos in the United States and Latin America but also reported among Greeks in North America. It is a broad syndrome ranging from cases free of a mental disorder to presentations resembling adjustment, anxiety, depressive, dissociative, somatoform, or psychotic disorders.

Pibloktoq

It is characterized by abrupt dissociative episode accompanied by extreme excitement, convulsive seizures and coma lasting up to 12 hours. During the attack, the individual may tear off his or her clothing, break furniture, shout obscenities, eat feces, flee from protective shelters, or perform other irrational or dangerous acts. This is observed primarily in arctic and subarctic Eskimo communities, although regional variations in name exist.

Qi-gong

It is a term used to describe an acute, time-limited episode characterized by dissociative, paranoid, or other psychotic or nonpsychotic symptoms that may occur after participation in the Chinese folk health-enhancing practice of qi-gong (meaning exercise of vital energy).

Rootwork

It involves cultural interpretations ascribing illness to hexing, witchcraft, sorcery, or the evil influence of another person. Symptoms may include generalized anxiety and GI complaints (e.g. nausea, vomiting, and diarrhea), weakness, dizziness, the fear of being poisoned, and, sometimes, the fear of being killed (voodoo death). Rootwork is found in the southern United States among African-American and European-American populations and in Caribbean societies. It is also known as mal puesto or brujeria in Latino societies.

Sangue Dormido (Sleeping Blood)

Sangue dormido is found among Portuguese Cape Verde Islanders (and immigrants from there to the United States) and includes pain, numbness, tremor, paralysis, convulsions, stroke, blindness, heart attack, infection, and miscarriage.

Shenjing Shuairuo (Neurasthenia)

In China, shenjing shuairuo is a condition characterized by physical and mental fatigue, dizziness, headaches, other pains, concentration difficulties, sleep disturbance and memory loss. Other symptoms include gastrointestinal problems, sexual dysfunction, irritability, excitability, and various signs suggesting disturbance of the autonomic nervous system. In many cases, the symptoms would meet the criteria for a DSM-IV-TR mood or anxiety disorder.

Shen-K'uei (Taiwan); Shenkui

Shen-k'uei or shenkui is a Chinese folk label used to describe marked anxiety or panic symptoms with accompanying somatic complaints including dizziness, backache, fatigability, general weakness, insomnia, frequent dreams, and complaints of sexual dysfunction (such as premature ejaculation and impotence) for which no physical cause can be demonstrated. Symptoms arise because of the belief that excessive semen loss from frequent intercourse, masturbation, nocturnal emission, or passing of white, turbid urine lead to loss of one's vital essence and can thereby be life-threatening.

Shin-Byung

Shin-byung is a Korean folk label for a syndrome in which initial phases are characterized by anxiety and somatic complaints (general weakness, dizziness, fear, anorexia, insomnia, and GI problems), with subsequent dissociation and possession by ancestral spirits.

Spell

A spell is a trance state in which individuals communicate with deceased relatives or with spirits seen among African-Americans and European-Americans from the southern United States. Spells are not considered to be medical events in the folk tradition but may be misconstrued as psychotic episodes in clinical settings.

Susto (Fright or Soul Loss)

Susto is a folk illness attributed to a frightening event that causes the soul to leave the body and results in unhappiness and sickness characterized by appetite disturbances, inadequate or excessive sleep, troubled sleep or dreams, a feeling of sadness, lack of motivation to do anything, and feelings of low self-worth or dirtiness. It is also accompanied by somatic symptoms like muscle aches and pains, headache, stomach ache, and diarrhea. It is associated with significant strains in key social roles and is commonly reported by Latinos in the United States and among people in Mexico, Central America, and South America.

Taijin Kyofusho

It is a culturally distinctive phobia in Japan presenting with intense fear that one's body, or its parts, or its functions displease, embarrass, or are offensive to other people in appearance, odor, facial expressions or movements.

Zar

Zar is a general term applied in Ethiopia, Somalia, Egypt, Sudan, Iran, and other North African and Middle Eastern societies to describe the experience of spirits possessing an individual and presents with dissociative episodes that may include shouting, laughing, hitting the head against a wall, singing, or weeping. Individuals may show apathy and withdrawal, refusing to eat or to carry out daily tasks, or may develop a long-term relationship with the possessing spirit. Such behavior is not considered pathological locally.

NEW CONCEPTS

Recent findings suggest that disorders like amok, koro, latah, Dhat to name a few are not 'bound' to specific cultures and core features are seen across culture over various time periods. Hence, the relevance of these syndromes in a particular culture tends to vary over time. This is exemplified by the findings that Dhat syndrome had been reported earlier from various parts of Europe but currently it has become limited to South-East Asia. This can be attributed to the changes in culture that occur over time. Therefore, it has been suggested that instead of the term 'culture-bound' terms like 'culture-related specific psychiatric conditions' (Tseng and McDermott, 1981) or 'culture-related specific syndromes' (Tseng, 2001) or 'culture-related syndromes' (Jilek, 2000) should be used to describe these disorders as such terms may more accurately describe a syndrome that is closely related to certain cultural traits or cultural features. This term takes into consideration the changeability of culture and hence its impact on human behavior and psychopathology is dynamic. This is highlighted by historical evidence that amok originally referred to the war cry of Malay pirates which was socially honored and considered "normal". Over time it became sudden and unpremeditated resulting in mass killings occurred in a dissociated state, with subsequent amnesia. Finally, because of the high frequency of amok, legislation was passed in 1893 by the British colonial government ruling that all amok subjects should be apprehended and tried in court. This clearly demonstrates how changes in cultural acceptance render a particular behavior "abnormal". Similarly brain fag has now been reported in people apart from students and those who are sophisticated tend to explain their symptoms in more psychologically-oriented terms and not the somatic symptoms associated with brain fag. Many controversies surround the concept of Dhat syndrome. Raghuram et al (1994) argued that semen is one of the seven dhatus, hence use of term Dhat is over inclusive and it should be discarded. Authors from various parts of the world do not agree with the concept of Dhat syndrome as a culture bound syndrome. Mumford (1996) argues that 'Dhat' should be primarily regarded as a culturally determined symptom associated with depression rather than a separate culture-bound syndrome. Other authors like Sumathipala et al (2004) and Jadhav (2004) also argue that the symptoms of semen loss anxiety are reported from various cultures and it should be considered as a culture related rather than culture-bound disorder. Others have opined that no single nosological entity encompasses the clinical presentation of Dhat syndrome–anxiety, phobic, affective symptoms, obsessive, hypochondriacal, body dysmorphic symptoms and uncommonly delusional beliefs are the presenting clinical entities. The underlying belief is dimensional and hence the presentation of symptoms needs to be seen from a clinical prospective rather than viewing it as a neurotic disorder alone.

In recent years, there is increased recognition by cultural psychiatrists of syndromes in Western cultures that are heavily culture related, including: anorexia nervosa, obesity, drug-induced dissociative states, multiple personality and even premenstrual syndrome. Since these conditions are already recognized in the existing Western nosological system as 'ordinary' disorders, they are in a sense, not viewed as 'specific' syndromes. However, they can be viewed as 'culture-related' psychiatric conditions that are influenced by various aspects of Western culture.

It has also been suggested that social changes contribute to the fading of such syndromes as exemplified by the decline of family suicide and Taijinkuofusho in Japan due to changes in social demands. Similarly, latah has become restricted mainly to old ladies who have known of the phenomenon since they were young.

The importance of these syndromes lie in the risk of misunderstanding in attempts to identify and explain culture-related specific disorders based exclusively on individual psychodynamics and culture-specific personality traits without taking into consideration the total geopolitical, socioeconomic, and ideological circumstances of the society in which the phenomena occur. However, there is also a risk in interpreting culture-related specific syndromes solely from the perspective of social or behavioral sciences, without adequate clinical knowledge and psychiatric insight.

MANAGEMENT

Assessment should be done considering patient's cultural identity, the perceived causes or explanatory models that the individual and the reference group use to explain illness and to seek its treatment. Additionally, one must take into account the cultural factors related to psychosocial environments and levels of functioning, and most importantly, the cultural elements of the relationship between the individual and the clinician as highlighted by requirement of the cultural formulation proposed by the DSM-IV-TR. Tools like Tell-Me-A-Story (TEMAS) has been developed for Hispanics by Giuseppe Constantino to assess conflict in urban situations. The test achieves significant interrater reliability, internal consistency, and predictive validity. In the absence of ethnicity-specific validated tests, such systems may encourage the use of relatively culture-free instruments (Bender-Gestalt and Porteus-Maze, for example) and widely translated self-rating scales, such as the symptom checklist-90 and the Zung Self-Rating Depression Scale. Westermeyer, among others, has demonstrated that self-rated scales and psychiatrist-rated scales have shown strong reliability cross-culturally.

Pharmacological

Pharmacological management should take into account the differential pharmacogenomics and pharmacodynamics and the impact of giving or withholding medications. Expectations about the use of medications, as well as the parallel use of traditional herbs, which is widespread in many cultures, should also be considered.

Nonpharmacological Management

The greatest challenge lies in the development of culture-specific therapies empirically derived from culture-specific behavioral features. This is exemplified by the work done with patients with Dhat syndrome. The most important aspect of treatment of such patients includes providing adequate sex knowledge and clarifying sexual myths. Sex education should mainly focus on anatomy and physiology of sexual organs and their functioning with reference to masturbation, semen formation, nocturnal emissions and their functioning with genitourinary system independent of gastrointestinal tract, etc. Relaxation therapy including Jacobson's Progressive Muscular Relaxation Technique combined with biofeedback (as to facilitate objective evidence and mastering of anxiety by the patient) can be practiced 2–3 times/day regularly, especially after therapy sessions are over (Avasthi et al, 2006). Further it is suggested that, initially the patients with Dhat syndrome should be evaluated for the presence of comorbid sexual dysfunction, psychiatric disorders, urinary tract infections, and sexually transmitted diseases. If the patient has associated psychiatric disorders, then it should be addressed prior to the treatment of Dhat syndrome with appropriate pharmacotherapy and psychotherapy. However, if the patient has associated sexual dysfunction, then the Dhat syndrome must be addressed before the treatment of associated sexual dysfunction. If the patient has associated urinary tract infections and/or sexually transmitted diseases, it should be treated adequately in liaison with other specialists and after adequate treatment, patient should be re-evaluated for the diagnosis of Dhat syndrome.

FUTURE DIRECTIONS

There is a need for studies that focus on the cultural dimensions and the impact of culture on such syndromes as majority of the work carried out in the past are demographic surveys and clinical descriptions. This should also include intensive studies of individual cases in order to understand the psychological and social dynamics of the disorders. Till date well-designed questionnaire surveys to test hypotheses about the specific ways in which culture may contribute to a particular disorder are rare. This calls for more comprehensive culture-focused clinical studies, including comparative studies of different groups to solicit and verify cultural variables that contribute to the occurrence of culture related specific syndromes among certain groups of people. Because cases of culture-related syndromes are rare, it is relatively difficult to design and conduct a survey, unless it occurs as an epidemic or at least in an endemic way. However, survey of nonpatient groups in communities where a specific syndrome tends to occur, followed by comparison of their responses with individuals in communities where the syndromes seldom occur may reveal differences in views, understandings, and attitudes toward the disorder.

SUGGESTED READING

1. American Psychiatric Association. Diagnostic and Statistical Manual of Mental Disorders: DSM-IV. Washington, DC: American Psychiatric Press; 1994.
2. Avasthi A, Grover S. Dhat syndrome: A sexual disorder of Indian Sub-continent. Culture and Mental Health. AK Kala, R Kala, D J Singh (Eds), Pradipika Publishers, Ludhiana, India; 2008.
3. Avasthi A, Rao TSS, Grover S, Biswas PS, Kumar S. Indian Psychiatric Society: Clinical Practice Guidelines for management of sexual dysfunctions. In: Shiv Gautam Ajit Avasthi (Eds). Published by Indian Psychiatric Society. 2006;2:144-231.
4. Fernandez RL, Guarnaccia PJ, Ruiz P. Culture Bound Syndrome. Comprehensive Textbook of Psychiatry. In: B J Sadock, VA Sadock, P Ruiz (Eds), 9th edition. Lippincott Williams and Wilkins, Philadelphia; 2009.pp.2519-539.
5. Simons RC, Hughes CC. The Culture-Bound syndromes: Folk Illnesses of Psychiatric and Anthropological Interest. Dordrecht, the Netherlands, D Reidel; 1985.
6. Tseng WS. From peculiar psychiatric disorders through culture-bound syndromes to culture-related specific syndromes. Transcult Psychiatry. 2006;43:554-76.
7. Tseng WS. Handbook of cultural psychiatry. San Diego, CA: Academic Press; 2001.
8. Wig NN. Problem of mental health in India. J Clin Social Psychiatry (India). 1960;17:48-53.
9. Yap PM. Classification of the culture-bound reactive syndromes. Australia and New Zealand Journal of Psychiatry. 1967;1:172-9.
10. Yap PM Koro. A culture-bound depersonalization syndrome. Br J Psychiatry. 1965;111:43-50.
11. Yap PM. Mental diseases peculiar to certain cultures: A survey of comparative psychiatry. Journal of Mental Science. 1951;97:313-27.
12. Yap PM. Words and things in comparative psychiatry, with special reference to the exotic psychoses. Acta Psychiatrica Scandinavica. 1962;38:163-9.

CHAPTER

58 Transcultural Psychiatry

VK Verma

During the past decades, along with advances in the understanding and treatment of mental illness, transcultural psychiatry has undergone a conceptual reformulation. Broadly speaking, transcultural psychiatry deals with how social and cultural factors create, determine or influence mental illness. In doing so, new and innovative treatment strategies are created. Despite influences of human and social sciences, transcultural psychiatry is rooted in medicine, especially in the biopsychosocial model. Contemporary developments such as globalization, massive migrations and the uprooting of populations (Kirmayer and Minas, 2000) put into focus questions of mental health of minorities. This has become a major focus of concern in the United States as well in other countries.

It has been increasingly recognized that simply looking at the individual variables in the etiology and manifestations of psychopathology is not enough. If a certain psychopathology is largely distributed in the society, it would be more worthwhile to look for the factors in the society and culture which may have been responsible, partly or wholly, in the causation of the malady and in modifying its nature and course.

The above point has been recognized over a long period of time, and subsequent to the increasing emphasis on individual factors in the last several decades, there has been a resurgence of interest in the social correlates of mental illness.

Transcultural psychiatry need not be only of esoteric interest but may be of relevance and importance to all psychiatrists and other mental health professionals. As the phenomenology, course and outcome of mental disorders may be dependent to a great extent on sociocultural factors, an analysis of the transcultural differences in the phenomenology and natural history of illness may be helpful in distinguishing the culturally generated features from others. If we look crossculturally, the transcultural differences may be alluded to the pathoplastic influence of the culture, whereas the commonalities may represent the real 'core' nature of the illness. Thus, transcultural psychiatry may be helpful in facilitating greater insight into the concept of mental illness and its treatment.

Transcultural psychiatry may be taken to include the following topics:

- Differences across cultures in the incidence, typology, and symptomatology of mental illness.
- Transcultural differences in the course and outcome of the various mental illnesses.
- Culture and personality issues.
- Relationship of cultural variables to mental illness.
- Culture and its relationship with language and cognition.
- Culture and positive mental health, including the concept of culture defenses.
- The transcultural factor applicable to the practice of psychotherapy and other treatments.
- The relationship of culture, personality, language and cognition, with coping mechanisms and mental illness.

HISTORICAL BACKGROUND

Emil Kraepelin travelled in the early twentieth century (1904) to Java to ascertain whether mental illness was at all to be found there. This interest in a very different culture was possibly the result of the conception that mental illnesses were a product of civilization and that the apparently primitive people were immune to mental illness. Kraepelin's visit to Java can be said to be the beginning of transcultural psychiatry as a pursuit of the psychiatrists. It followed the development of cultural anthropology, a discipline to which it owes a great deal.

Starting around the last decades of the 19th century, social scientists became increasingly aware of and interested in cultures elsewhere in the world, and started a systematic analysis into how such cultures functioned and what holds them together. This followed the increased awareness into other cultures as an offshoot of the exploration, exploitation and subjugation of the rest of the world by certain Western European powers. The American brand of cultural anthropology followed a few decades later.

In the beginning, there was an idle curiosity into the affairs of other cultures, the interest mostly on account of their being peculiar, quaint, exotic, alien and different.

Thus were described the Samoa, Trobriand, Alor Kwakiutl, Hopi, Zuni, Arapesh and other cultures in the different parts of the world. It was only later that anthropologists started looking at these different cultural forms as comprehensive, viable solutions to the problems of human existence. Some of the earlier contributions in this direction were by Tylor,[1] who is considered to be the father of social and cultural anthropology, Sir John Frazer and WRH Rivers, who were all Englishmen. Their work was followed by that of Franz Boas,[2] originally a German who is considered to be the father of American anthropology, and then his students and followers, notably Ruth Benedict[3,4] and Margaret Mead.[5] As Ruth Benedict stated, "is it not wonderful that there can be so many different solutions to the problem of human existence, and is it not great that all seem to work, more or less". This led to the concept of cultural relations and the theory of functionalism which states that each of the cultural forms, norms and institutions, roles and expectations, that hold a culture together, fit with each other to produce the culture as a functional whole, just like pieces of a jigsaw puzzle.

The early development in transcultural psychiatry followed a parallel pattern. After Kraepelin was able to document the incidence of mental illness in a 'primitive' country, namely Java, Western psychiatrists became aware of the apparently unusual and peculiar presentations of psychopathology in the non-Western societies. A number of so-called culture-bound syndromes were identified and described, and specific names were applied to them. Thus, syndromes like Amok, Latah, Koro and Piblokto were identified. It has been only much later that the appreciation is dawning upon the scientific community that the so-called culture bound syndromes do not represent any specific entities but illustrate the influence of cultural factors in modifying the manifestations of psychological upheavals—the pathoplastic influence of culture—and that there may be nothing about them, qualifying them as clearly different clinical entities. In the same way, the various so-called 'primitive' societies do not necessarily represent different points in an evolutionary scheme, but present the various functional integrations possible of human conglomerations.

The world is literally shrinking now, with increasing interest in and awareness of other cultures, and ease of travel resulting in a larger proportion of the world population developing direct knowledge of other societies. A number of studies have been carried out in a number of areas pertaining to mental illness. These included the elucidation of the so-called culture bound syndromes, studies in the incidence of major and common mental illnesses like schizophrenia, depression and neuroses, and of their course and outcome in different parts of the world.

To a large extent, however, the model of transcultural psychiatry, as it has emerged, has remained basically at the descriptive and phenomenological level. It has been suggested[6] that there is a great need to correlate the transcultural variables in mental illness with the differences in the cultural variables, so as to arrive at a dynamic model of transcultural psychiatry. The role of sociocultural factors in the transcultural differences in mental illnesses must be understood and correlated with each other. The relationship between the two must be visualized, not as a static but as an on-going dynamic interchange.

CULTURE AND MENTAL ILLNESS

Influenced by the social philosophy of Rousseau, primitive man was believed to be free of the anguish and discontentment of 'mental illness'; the idea of the 'good savage' or 'happy savage'. The concept that civilization produces insanity is not of recent origin, but dates as far back as Kraepelin who linked technology to mental illness. Freud believed that culture creates repression. Schizophrenia was thought to be absent and neuroses rare among Papero-Melanesians.[7] How culture and cultural situations might exert causal or determining influences on psychiatric disorders was described by Leighton and Murphy,[8] and Murphy and Leighton.[9] Culture may be thought to:

- Determine the pattern of certain specific disorders
- Produce basic personality types, some of which are especially vulnerable to psychiatric disorders
- Produce psychiatric disorders through certain child-rearing practices
- Have selective influences through types of sanction and whether 'shame' or 'guilt' is engendered
- Precipitate disorder by rewarding it in prestigious roles such as holy man, witch doctor or shaman
- Precipitate disorder by changing more rapidly than personality systems are able to tolerate
- Produce disorder through inculcation of sentiments damaging to the mind such as fears, jealousies, and unrealistic aspirations
- Affecting the distribution of some kinds of disorder through breeding pattern
- Influencing the amount and distribution of disorder through patterns of poor hygiene and nutrition.

Likewise, there are certain types of cultural change that are hazardous to personality and psychic equilibrium. Change is likely to be stressful:

- When the tempo is accelerated and especially when major dimensions of the change occur within the life span of a single generation
- When it involves pervasive reorientation about basic values and assumptions
- When it is experienced at the outset of a cycle when few guides and models exist
- When there has been little formal training and preparation in the skills and techniques necessary to accomplish the new tasks
- If there are serious ambiguities about what change is leading to

- If it involves new roles or values that are imperfectly integrated into or are incompatible with the rest of the sociocultural system
- If it involves expectations that are prone to be frustrated, given the pre-existing pattern of life
- If it involves expansion rather than substitution and creates a sense of overloading.

Given the changing nature of almost every culture known in the twentieth century, this is a factor of considerable moment in comparative studies of mental health.

Crosscultural Epidemiology of Mental Illness

Schizophrenia

Many reviews of the cross-cultural prevalence of schizophrenia have appeared in recent times, the most significant being that of Leff,[10] detailing information about 47 studies (1931–1980). There have been numerous methodological differences in these studies but the range of prevalence rates is approximately 1 to 10 per 1000. Torrey et al[11] interpret the evidence as indicating that schizophrenia may be more common among societies that have had greater exposure to Western influences. They suggest that "as civilization makes inroads, schizophrenia follows in its footsteps". They take support from the existing evidence of differences in the rates of occurrence of the disorder reported in populations of particular epidemiological interest (for example, ecological or genetic isolates, junctions between different cultural influences), like, the fact that some of the lowest rates are for the aborigines such as the Taiwanese (0.9/1000) or religious enclave groups such as the Hutterites (1.1/1000), while some of the highest rates are in the developed countries such as Sweden (9.5/1000).

Leff,[10] on the other hand, agrees with most earlier reviewers in concluding that the prevalence rates in developing countries "vary within relatively narrow limits" and are quite comparable to rates for developed countries. In a series of Asian studies, he points out a range of 3.3 to 8.0, with a mean of 4.9/1000, comparing it with that of an urban district of London which is 4-5/1000. Similarly, Warren Dunham[12] has compared prevalence rates from 19 surveys in Europe, Asia and North America (Table 1) and concluded that the prevalence rates are quite comparable. Murphy and Raman,[13] in a study of first admission for schizophrenia in Mauritius, found the age-specific incidence reported in England and Wales. Murphy,[14] quoting rates of non-hospitalized schizophrenics in two Western and two non-Western samples, concludes that the "non-Western way of life does not offer protection against mental illness to a point of making a marked difference in frequency".

Table 1: Prevalence rates (per 1000)

Swedish	5.7	Eskimo	4.4
Canadian	5.6	Yoruba	6.8

Neurotic Disorders (Including Depression)

The prevalence of neurotic disorders shows a much greater amount of variability than that of schizophrenia, as is demonstrated by Leff's comparison of 16 studies in non-Western areas.[10] The lowest prevalence rate is 0.8/1000 for Taiwanese natives, while the highest rates come from Uganda (269/1000), and Argentina (287/1000). But, the methods of data collection have also been varied in these studies.

Two studies, where comparable structured schedules were used to gather data, were conducted in the United States[9] and in the UK (Table 2).[15]

It was noted that the rate in Uganda was more than twice that in Nigeria, both traditional African societies; thus suggesting some factors in the local culture of Uganda which might foster neurotic disorders. Secondly, depression was more common than anxiety, and the difference in the rates was also more for depression. This would suggest that depression varies more than anxiety in terms of cultural setting and is more responsive to social circumstances. Orley[16] points out that depressed women in Uganda are more likely to blame themselves than depressed women in London, who are more prone to irritability, emphasizing the contrast between 'intraprimitive' and 'irritability' depression. This is similar to Kleinman's[17] view that some cultures may shape depression into a 'somatization' syndrome explained on the basis of the absence of Cartesian (body-mind) dualism. For example, a diagnosis of neurasthenia is more comparable with the Chinese orientation than is depression, and in a consecutive series of outpatients, one-third of the patients were given a diagnosis of neurasthenia while only 1% received a diagnosis of depression. A comparative study with the West is important because Western patients also somatize, as is evident by the diagnosis of 'masked depression' and complaints of suffering from 'nerves' rather than from depression.

Table 2: US Study vs. UK Study

US Study	*UK Study*
Alaska 14%	Uganda 22%
Nigeria 10%	London 10%
Canada 12%	(Camberwell district)

Culture and Mental Symptoms

The system of behavioral, attitudinal and conceptual norms differs from culture to culture, and it is these differences that a cross-cultural comparison of 'normal' and 'abnormal' states of mind has to take into account. Some cultures are more stressful than others, and cultural pressures and stresses may differentially dispose individuals towards mental illness. Thus, symptoms may be expected to occur with different frequencies or to constellate into different patterns of syndromes in various cultures. There are, however, mental conditions, the abnormal character of which is recognized across cultures, such as mental retardation, dementia, agitated delirium, etc. Nevertheless, there can be little doubt that in the great majority of psychiatric conditions, culture plays an important role. This role has been found to be both *pathogenic* (i.e. causing pathology) and *pathoplastic* (i.e. shaping pathology).

Schizophrenia

Cultural factors inherent in modern Western society have been held responsible for schizophrenia by Devereux.[18] He calls it an 'ethnic psychosis' characteristic of modern Western society. He sees schizophrenic thinking and behavior as 'taught' and 'inculcated' by modern civilization. Early studies claimed that schizophrenia is nonexistent in some non-Western cultures. Later studies, however, showed that the incidence of schizophrenia is almost universal.[19] But, there is a good deal of evidence that symptoms might occur with different frequencies or constellate into different patterns in various cultures. For instance, it is reported that catatonic rigidity, negativism and stereotypy are more common in India than in other countries.[19] Patients appear to be quieter in Africa, displaying more features which suggest deterioration such as blunting of affect or bizarreness of behavior.[20] African schizophrenia is claimed to be a 'poor imitation of the European forms', showing less violence and aggression than in the West.[21] Schizophrenic patients in Iraq and Italy appear to show the opposite trends. They are more expressive and more aggressive than patients in the United States and other Western countries, and rarely show social withdrawal.[19]

Enright and Jaeckle[21] found Japanese paranoid schizophrenics to have ideas of reference and disturbances of thinking more frequently than their Filipino counterparts. They also showed more apathy, social isolation and loss of interest in their surroundings. Unlike Western patients, the Hutterite schizophrenic does not show severe regression, excitement or any extreme antisocial acts.[22]

In an extensive cross-cultural study,[13] data was collected through questionnaires sent to psychiatrists from different cultures. Symptoms such as social and emotional withdrawal, auditory hallucinations, general delusions and flatness of affect appear to occur frequently in all their samples. Delusions of destructiveness and religious nature are frequently reported only among Christians and Muslims. Delusional jealousy is most frequent among Asians while social hallucinations are reported most often in Africa and the Near East. While depersonalization is most frequent among urban patients, delusions of grandeur are common in the rural patients.

Another cross-cultural study[23] comparing Japanese and American schizophrenics found greater disruption of reality testing, hallucinations and bizarre ideas in American patients. Physical assaultiveness was more prevalent among the Japanese.

Non-Western patients sometimes show the familiar Western symptoms, but they may differ in their onset and duration, e.g. the transitory psychotic states, reported by Collomb (1966) in the Senegal, precipitated by stress; or catatonia among the Eskimos as a result of fear of spirits.

In the West, Opler[24] reported that there are subcultural differences in symptomatology. There is more hostility, acting out, elation, and bizarre mannerisms among Italian paranoid schizophrenics than among their Irish counterparts. Further, while Irish patients had guilt preoccupations concerning sexuality, Italians had no feelings of sin or guilt in this area. From the various studies, it appears that it is the hebephrenic or catatonic, rather than the paranoid type, that is found by investigators in non-Western cultures.[23-26]

This variation in symptomatology is attributed to several factors. It was found that formal thought disorder and flatness of affect were significantly higher in illiterates while paranoid delusions were not related to literacy. Literacy affects the contents of the patients' delusions, e.g. literate African patients were more apt to have grandiose delusions of identification with God or influences through electricity or wireless.[27] The quiet behavior in the Indian patients has been explained on the basis of cultural values, like cultural control of anger and aggression; the opposite behavior in the Italian and the Iraqi patients, a result of cultural encouragement of aggression and the lack of strong feeling of guilt. More hallucinations and delusions among Black than among White patients were attributed to the Black patient's delay in coming to the hospital, i.e. the apparently different symptoms were actually present due to a more severe presenting illness, resulting from a delay in receiving treatment.

International Pilot Study on Schizophrenia (IPSS)

In this study,[28] nine field centers in nine countries were selected to represent the major contrasting cultures of the world at different levels of social and industrial development, namely Aarhus (Denmark); Agra (India); Cali (Columbia); lbadan (Nigeria); London (England); Moscow (USSR); Taipai (Taiwan); Washington (USA); and Prague (Czechoslovakia). Of the 1202 cases studied, 811 received a clinical diagnosis of schizophrenia. The largest diagnostic subgroup was paranoid (318), and it was the largest group in all the centres except for Agra, Cali and Moscow. The second largest subgroup was schizoaffective schizophrenia (107), most strongly represented in Agra, lbadan and Prague. There were 86 hebephrenics and 56 catatonics. In Agra, the largest individual group was unspecified schizophrenia. Apart from this, the patients were classified using two other methods: a computer diagnosis of schizophrenia (CATEGO S), based on the presence of a few important typical symptoms, and cluster analysis. 563 and 550 patients respectively, out of 811, were diagnosed as schizophrenic by the two methods.

A two-year follow-up[28] reported two important findings: (i) a very marked variability of course and outcome among the schizophrenic patients whose diagnoses were based on strict symptomatology criteria, and (ii) the consistent differences between the groups of schizophrenic patients in different cultural settings, with patients in developing countries having a more favorable course and outcome (Table 3). The observed variability of course and outcome can support both the view that many schizophrenic patients do surprisingly well in later life, and the view that many patients have a very poor prognosis. A clinical diagnosis of schizophrenia alone does not say much about the likely pattern of course.[29]

The best predictors of outcome in general were social isolation, length of the episode before the initial evaluation, past history of treatment, marital status, and history of behavior disorder in adolescence. In developing countries, education level, and in developed countries, occupational level were additional predictors.

The WHO researchers concluded that there were "clear differences in the course and outcome of schizophrenia, with patients in developing countries on the average having a better course and outcome than those in centers in the developed countries. The outcome may be more favorable in settings characterized by agricultural economy, little vertical mobility, extended families, psychiatric services which include the active participation of the family, and the absence of specific community stereotypes of the mentally ill".[28] The overall outcome varied from an index of 0.71 (lbadan), 0.61 (Agra), to 0.37 (Aarhus), 0.40 (Prague), 0.43 (London), and 0.44 (Washington DC).

From the work completed in phases I and II of the IPSS, three major conclusions can be drawn:[30]

1. It has been possible to carry out a large scale international psychiatric study involving workers from different countries with diverse cultures, socioeconomic conditions and psychiatric teaching.
2. Similar groups of schizophrenics can be identified in every one of the nine countries involved.
3. It is possible to develop valid and reliable research instruments for practical use in international studies.

Table 3: Comparative outcome of schizophrenic patients in developed and developing countries

	Best outcome	*Poorest outcome*
Developing countries	40%	24%
Developed countries	15%	25%

A five-year follow-up study in Sri Lanka reports good prognosis of schizophrenic patients, which cannot be explained by artifacts of sampling or diagnostic methods or by the family's willingness to tolerate deviance.[31] It could be attributed to "cultural factors such as the traditional system of beliefs, structure of the treatment system, and family norms".[31] Beliefs and practices in nonindustrialized societies encourage short-term of illness and quick return to normality.

Manic Depressive Psychosis

Manic depressive psychosis does occur in the non-Western cultures but its depressive type has been thought to be rare.[32] It has been the observation that feelings of guilt, self-accusation or ideas of unworthiness do not occur in these cultures and suicide also seems to be rare. Studies on Jewish and Negro patients have shown that hostility is directed more towards the environment than the self. Murphy and Leighton[9] conducted an extensive cross-cultural study of depression, in which they found that depressive mood, dejection, diurnal mood change, insomnia with early morning awakening, and decreased social interests were almost universal across cultures. Self-neglect and semimutism were rare among Europeans in contrast to members of other cultures. There was a definite association between religion and the feeling of guilt, the Christians showing a positive correlation between the intensity of belief and guilt, and self-depreciation. This was not seen in Hindus and Muslims. The Muslim patients showed less guilt feelings and suicide, but had unusual symptoms like ideas of influence and possession. The Japanese showed a higher frequency of despondency and thought retardation, but decreased religious preoccupation, loss of sexual interest, excitement and theatrical grief.

The rarity of depression or self-reproach in primitive societies has been attributed by Opler[33] to the individual's tendency to minimize free will, and to shift responsibility from personal level to groups or to shift grief from isolated to group ritual. Tooth[27] explained the rare incidence of depression by describing the cultural provision of institutionalized grief after death. Among the Hutterites, depression occurs without feelings of shame and guilt because of the belief that the illness is a spiritual or religious trial by God to test the sincerity of man's belief in him.[22] Similarly, suicide is condemned in the Hutterites and the Muslims as a serious sin.

In Africa, depression is milder and of shorter duration. There is an absence of guilt in the ideas and of suicide, but confusional symptoms are present.[34] Among the Chinese depressives, there is presence of a tendency towards somatization with absence of delusions of sin. The high incidence of the manic form of manic-depressive psychosis is attributed to the diagnoses of states of excitement and confusion. Psychiatrists may confuse mania with catatonic excitement or schizoaffective states.

Neuroses

Although all the traditional psychoneurotic disorders appear to occur in the non-Western cultures, they may take different forms than their Western counterparts.

- *Anxiety*: Acute anxiety states of short duration appear to be more common in the primitive than in the advanced societies. Severe anxiety may be precipitated by disturbing events such as migrating to a city or passing through a place believed to be habituated by spirits, and may reach a panic state with incoherent thoughts, confusion, delusions, and hallucinations. These attacks have been reported from Africa,[35] China,[36] and Zurkese society.
- *Depression:* Among the Hutterites, neurotics react to the most stressful situations with depressive rather than with anxiety, paranoid or obsessive tendencies as patients often do in the American culture. This was explained by Eaton and Weil[22] to be the result of the close interpersonal relationship, and the great social and psychological support a Hutterite receives from his family and the community.
- *Obsessive-compulsive neurosis:* This was rarely found in the studies from Kenya,[35] Nigeria,[27] or among the Hutterites.[22] One reason given for this low incidence was that these cases are unrecognized because the symptoms resemble the characteristics of the cultural background. Persons may seem compulsive in a loosely organized social system, but would be more normal in a rigid culture where life is very much rated by tradition.
- *Hysteria:* Hysteria seems more common among the primitive people than in the West. Mass hysteria, which used to occur in Europe in the middle ages, can be found in Africa and Asia today. In its dramatic form, hysteria is more common among the illiterate and less sophisticated members of the community.[37] It appears that the neurotic problems find expression in somatic rather than psychological complaints like vague aches and pains, strong painful sensations of head, and functional visceral disorders.
- *Sexual deviations:* Two observations are widely emphasized in the cross-cultural studies of sexual behavior. One is that societies show striking contrasts in the amount of permissiveness regarding sexual behavior. The other is that some deviant sexual behavior in the West may be regarded as normal in other cultures.
  - There is a difference among societies in attitudes and practices in the spheres of extramarital sexual relations, sex-play among children, sex among adolescents, acceptance of transvestites, tolerance of nudity and homosexuality. That different attitudes towards sex may result in contrasted sexual behavior is demonstrated by Carstairs[38] in his study of the high-caste Hindus and the *Bhil* tribes who live in the same area of the North-West India. The high caste Hindus regard sex as degrading and tend to punish sex interest or activities of their children. The *Bhil* tribe are more tolerant towards sex play or sex adventures. One consequence of these contrasted attitudes is the widespread preoccupation with impotence in Hindus which is unknown among the *Bhil* people.
  - In their study of 76 primitive societies, Ford and Beach[39] concluded that homosexuality exists all over the world. They also found that in approximately two-thirds of these societies, homosexuality is regarded as normal and acceptable.
- *Alcoholism:* The main finding in the cross-cultural studies of alcoholism is that alcoholism as a problem tends to be associated with the attitudes of the amount of alcohol consumed by the individuals. Studies of American Indians, Italians and Jewish groups reveal a low rate of alcoholism. In the American Indians, alcohol drinking seems to bring about social participation. Similarly, the rate of alcoholism among Italians is about one eighth the rate in the United States because of integration of alcohol consumption into the Italian daily life. Among the Jews, alcohol drinking is integrated into religion and family life. But, drinking becomes a serious problem when members of such cultures migrate to less tolerant cultures.[40]
  - In contrast, the high rate of alcoholism among the Irish is explained in terms of the use of alcohol by the individual.
  - Culture seems to be an important variable in determining the pattern of alcoholism. Gamma alcoholism, which involves the loss of control, is more prevalent in the Anglo-Saxon countries in which whisky consumption predominates; delta alcoholism, which involves an inability to abstain, is more prevalent in the Latin countries in which wine consumption predominates. In the Middle-East, public prohibition of alcohol consumption seems to reduce the incidence of alcoholism, despite the fact that individuals tend to drink heavily in private, given the opportunity. In China, cultural sanctions against solitary drinking account for the low incidence of alcoholism.
- *Psychosomatic disorders:* Since these are assumed to be the result of tensions and anxieties in modern living, they are expected to be less frequent in non-Western cultures. But, despite the variations in incidence, all psychosomatic disorders have been reported from the non-Western cultures.[41] Although coronary artery disease, peptic ulcer, and hypertension seem to occur less frequently in India than in Germany, all other 'diseases of civilization' occur as frequently. Collomb (1965) found that, vascular disorders, hypertension, gastrointestinal ulcers, bronchial asthma, skin diseases, and diabetes mellitus were as frequent in the Senegal as in Europe. London (1959)

found that duodenal ulcer, asthma and psoriasis were rare among the African Bantu.

- Rin and Lin[42] investigated the relationship between social class and the choice of symptoms in Taiwan. The findings showed that the lower class tended to have illnesses more frequently of the musculoskeletal and cardiovascular systems, while the upper class group tended to 'choose' respiratory, skin and gastro-intestinal systems.

Culture-bound Syndromes

Apart from cultural variations in the symptomatology familiar in the West, certain atypical psychiatric symptomatology has been reported in the non-Western cultures. Most students of these syndromes agree that they are not uniquely 'culture-bound,' that is, they occur in a variety of cultures including quite dissimilar ones separated by considerable distances. In addition, the subsequents of these syndromes are not unique but include such common manifestations as fear, anxiety, anhedonia, aimless escape, psychophysiological symptoms, social withdrawal, behavioral deviance, and nondirected violence. Nonetheless, it is remarkable that these syndromes do occur with much greater frequency in some societies than in others.

The concept of culture-bound syndromes originated with PowMeng Yap, a pioneer of transcultural psychiatry. In 1962, he suggested the term 'Atypical Culture-Bound Psychogenic Psychosis' for conditions like latah, amok, and koro, which he considered to be atypical with reference to psychiatric nomenclatures, due to the overriding influence of specific cultural traits in the formation of these conditions. Later on, he substituted 'reactive' for psychogenic and 'syndrome' for psychosis and devised a classification of so-called 'culture-bound reactive syndromes'. He emphasized that these syndromes are not independent disease entities; rather, he held them to be culture-bound variations of the universal clinical prototypes, variations resulting from the effect of culture-specific factors operant in a given society. Pfeiffer[26] defined the cultural influences involved in the causation and in the shaping of culture-bound syndromes in terms of four dimensions:

1. Culture-specific areas of stress
2. Culture-specific shaping of conduct
3. Culture-specific interpretations
4. Culture-specific interventions.

He classified the culture-bound syndromes according to culture-specific pathogenic and pathoplastic factors.

Yap[43] defined such syndromes as "culture-bound in that certain symptoms of implicit values, social structures, and obviously shared beliefs produce unusual forms of psychopathology that are confined to special areas". These syndromes often wax and wane over time and can occur in sudden widespread 'epidemics' such as outbreaks of koro, bulimia and amok. They do not accompany any single psychiatric diagnosis but may be associated with any disorder. Some students of these phenomena (mostly social scientists) stress the cultural uniqueness of these syndromes and insist that they can or should be considered only within their own sociocultural context. Others (usually clinicians) argue that we can learn by studying and comparing the biopsycho-sociocultural concomitants of these disorders, wherever they occur. This controversy arises from the differences in the research tools of the two groups, i.e. the sociologically and the medically oriented.

1. *Amok*: Originally reported by the English from India around 1600 AD, this condition used to be almost exclusively associated with Malayan people, occurring only among men. But, recently it has also been reported, occasionally, from other tropical cultures like Africa, and Papua, New Guinea. The word 'amok' means 'to engage furiously in battle.'[44] In this syndrome, the affected person displays sudden unprovoked outbursts of wild rage, runs about madly, armed with a knife or firearm. He attacks and maims or kills indiscriminately any people and animals in his way before being overpowered or killed himself, the number of victims being about ten on an average. A period of preoccupation, brooding and mild depression usually precedes the attack, which lasts a few hours and is followed by exhaustion, amnesia and often suicide. The only immediate treatment consists of physically overpowering and controlling the patient.
   - The nature and purpose of this behavior has been changing over time.[45] In the 15th century, it was considered an understandable reaction to frustration or humiliation and served as a means of suicide in the face of intolerable stress. Later, it occurred in people with chronic physical ailments who later pleaded amnesia for the event, claiming possession by the devil after the attack. The incidence has remarkably decreased in the 20th century, the disease occurring usually in patients with either acute toxic or delusional psychoses. The treatment of the underlying cause may relieve the person of this behavior.
   - Several reasons have been proposed for the development of these symptoms in the Malayan people, like belief in magical possession by demons, easy availability of lethal weapons, excessive cultural restriction on emotional reactions, shame,[46] separation, loss, alcoholic intoxication, and role crises.[44] Preventive measures would, therefore, focus on changing those social norms which facilitate such behavior.
   - Such cases have been reported in psychiatric literature from India also. Gautam, Venkataramiah and Pushpam (1979) reported such a case in a 29-year old man after the funeral of his younger brother. He obtained average scores on intelligence and memory

tests but some signs of underlying psychosis were found on Rorschach test.

2. *Koro:* This syndrome occurs almost exclusively among the people of the Malay archipelago and among the South Chinese (Cantonese) where it is called '*sukyeorg*.' Occasional cases have been reported in the West as a part of another illness, e.g. among the hypochondriacal delusions of a manic depressive (Kraepelin), amphetamine intoxication and frontotemporal brain tumor.
   - The clinical picture is that of an acute anxiety reaction, characterized by the patient's desperate fear that his penis is shrinking and may disappear into his abdomen, resulting in death. He, therefore, secures a strong physical hold on his penis, by tying a ribbon around it or by clamping it into a wooden box. In females, the person complains of shrinkage of her vulval labia and breasts. This psychogenic disorder results from cultural, social and psychodynamic influences upon predisposed personalities. Such patients are preoccupied with fears about nocturnal emission, masturbation, sexual excesses and virility. Yap[47] considered this a unique type of depersonalization syndrome where insight is also impaired. He described precipitating factors like coitus, exposure of genitalia to cold air or water, and hearing about people dying from koro.
   - Koro has recently been reported as an epidemic in the lower parts of Assam (June-September, 1982). In a survey of 83 cases, that included 19 females also, Datta (1983) and Dutta, Phooken and Das (1982) reported that the illness affected mostly males, below 30 years of age, belonging to Hindu, lower class, Assamese community. Marriage, education and skill in occupation did not offer any immunity to the victims; relapses were few and fatality absent. Cases of Koro have been reported from Ahmedabad (Chakraborty, 1982) and Jhansi (Shukla and Mishra, 1981) also.
   - The treatment in such cases would include psychotherapy, tranquilizing drugs, modified insulin coma therapy and electroconvulsive therapy, and treatment of the underlying psychiatric illness, if any.
3. *Latah:* This disorder is found among the Malaysian people, especially the Javanese, and is seen more often in the women. Similar conditions have been reported in other cultures like Africans, aboriginal Siberians, Laplanders, and North Americans.
   - The syndrome occurs clinically in two different forms. One is the 'startle reaction' in which a sudden stimulus provokes the suspension of all normal activities and triggers a set of unusual and inappropriate motor and verbal manifestations over which the affected person has no voluntary control. The other type of latah is a 'mimetic' or 'echo reaction' in which a sudden stimulus compels the affected person to imitate any action or words to which he is exposed. He exhibits sustained and complete echopraxia, echolalia, and often automatic obedience. The affected person is aware of his peculiar behavior, although has no control over it. Because he is compelled to carry out ridiculous actions, he may sometimes be the butt of practical jokes. Two variants of this disorder may be a 'brief startle reaction with echo symptoms' in which the person may utter obscenities, and a chronic disease which over time leads to permanent automatic obedience, echo reactions and personality deterioration.
   - Yap[48] considered latah to involve disorganization of the ego and ego boundaries. It is an intense fright reaction which causes inhibition of the proper perceptuomotor integration and renders the patient vulnerable to any stimulus in the environment. Murphy[49] likened it to posthypnotic behavior, where disinhibition may result in symptoms like automatic obedience, and cultural factors, like belief in possession states, may influence the symptomatology.
4. *Piblokto*: This is a hysterical state of dissociation occurring among the Eskimos and sometimes referred to as 'Arctic hysteria.' It is characterized by attacks lasting 1–2 hours, during which the patient, usually a woman, begins to scream, imitating the cry of some animal or bird. She may tear off and destroy her clothing, throw herself on the snow or run wildly about on the ice, despite the very low temperatures. After the attack, the person appears quite normal and usually has amnesia for the event. The Eskimos are reluctant to touch any afflicted person during the attack because they think that it has something to do with evil spirits.
   - The frequency of this syndrome is low while other common forms of hysterical reactions may more often be seen among the female Eskimo patients.
5. *Wihtigo:* Wihtigo or Windigo psychosis is confined to the Gee, Ojibway and Satteaux Indians of North America, though extremely rare in the present times. There is a prevailing belief in the Wihtigo, a giant monster that eats human flesh, in witchcraft and the possibility of the transformation of man into this monster. During times of starvation, symptoms concerning the alimentary tract, such as loss of appetite or nausea from trivial causes, may sometimes cause the patient to become greatly excited for the fear of being transformed into a wihtigo. He may develop the delusion that this transformation has taken place. Yap[43] considered this illness to be essentially hysterical in nature, the clinical picture being influenced by the mythology and cultural beliefs.
6. *Voodoo death* or *Thanatomania:* This voodoo cult is practised in African societies and among native

West Indians. The psychiatric significance of this is multifold. The typical voodoo ceremony includes short-lasting, voluntary, ritual-induced hysterical or psychotic states, trance-like states, convulsions, excitement and twilight states. Further, the belief in the possibility of being involuntarily possessed by evil spirits induces chronic hysterical and psychosomatic symptoms. There are the voodoo deaths or fatal consequences of the patients' belief that he is the victim of black magic and of an evil spell cast upon him. The apparent reason may be taboo violation (Africa), shame (Polynesia), or sorcery (Australia). The underlying cause of death may be a state of shock produced by overstimulation of the sympathetic or parasympathetic systems. Many deaths may be due to poison, organic illness, or the victims' refusal of food and water. The anthropologist Lester (1972) compared the voodoo death to Engel's giving up-given up complex,[50] a psychological state in which a person is highly susceptible to serious physical illness.

7. *Atypical hysterical reaction*: This type of reaction is seen in the New Guinea Highlands. This has a sudden onset, occurring when the patient is hit by a wave of coldness and is followed by complete or partial deafness. He loses muscular control, shivers, and tends to exhibit sudden violence. These attacks seem to be a breakaway from facing frustrating social situations.[51] The abnormal behavior lasts about 48 hours and sleep usually brings about recovery.
8. *Susto*: This is more similar to depression, and is characterized by restlessness during sleep, listlessness, and loss of appetite and weight.[52] Sincesusto is usually precipitated by stressful situations, it is more like reactive depression. It is seen in Hispanic Americans, particularly in women.
9. *Malignant anxiety:* Acute anxiety reactions resembling hysterical panic states with paranoid features center around a delusion of bewitchment.[48,53] The acute, brief psychotic reaction is accompanied by aggressive, often homicidal, behavior precipitated by fears of bewitchment.

CULTURE AND PERSONALITY

Definition of Culture

The term culture has a number of definitions. It has been said that the English language has as many as 160 definitions of culture. Since including all these definitions is not possible, and since presenting an extensive survey of the concept and definition of culture is not the objective here, only a few representative definitions shall be quoted.

An oft repeated and perhaps the most famous one is by Tylor, considered to be the father of cultural anthropology. Culture, according to him "...is that complex whole which includes knowledge, belief, art, morals, law, customs, and any other capabilities and habits acquired by man as a member of the society".[1]

Ralph Linton,[54] who along with Abram Kardiner, was the moving force behind the famous Columbia University project, defined culture as "the configuration of learned behavior and results of behavior whose component elements are shared and transmitted by the members of a particular society". Two quite similar definitions of Kroeber and Wallace emphasize upon the learned patterns of behavior. Kroeber[55] said that culture consists of "patterns, explicit and implicit, of and for behavior acquired and transmitted by symbols, constituting the distinctive achievement of human groups, including their embodiment in artefacts; the essential core of culture consists of traditional ideas and especially their attached values; culture systems may on one hand be considered as products of action, on other as conditioning elements of further action."[55] Wallace[56] conceptualized it as "those ways of behavior or techniques of solving problems which, being more frequent or more closely approximated than other ways, can be said to have a high probability of use by individual members of the society".

Simpler definitions also exist. Going by Murphy, culture is simply a "way of life".[9] An elaboration of the same is offered by Barnouw:[57] "A culture is a way of life of a group of people, the configuration of all of the more or less stereotyped patterns of learned behaviors which are handed down from one generation to the next through the means of language and imitation". Levine[58] feels it to consist of "both the distinctively human forms of adaptation and the distinctive ways in which different human populations organize their lives on earth".

All these definitions, thus, help us to form some idea of the term culture. One point, however, needs mention. Culture, here, does not mean sensitivity into the so-called finer things in life, such as ability to perceive and appreciate music, painting, literature, etc. Rather, it means the sum of distinctive characteristics of a society, which are common to all its members and which determine their adaptation and reaction to familiar situations and demands. These are handed over from one generation to the other and are shared by most members of that culture. Thus, taken together they help in distinguishing one society from another.

Culture and Personality Approach

Personality, here, refers to distinctive patterns of behavior (including thoughts and emotions) that characterize each individual's adaptation to his or her life. As culture involves conglomeration of individuals, similarity between the objective and concern of the culture may be quite understandable. Ruth Benedict's statement,[3] that "a culture, like an individual, is more or less consistent pattern of thought and action, governed by its own characteristic purposes," sums this up quite aptly.

The history of this relationship between culture and personality, however goes back much further, to Hippocrates (460-377 BC) and Galen (130-200 AD), who used the notion of a temperament, and the Arab social scientist IbnKhaldun (1332-1406 AD) who discerned common patterns of feelings in races. Later, others like Wilhelm Humboldt (1767-1835), Emile Durkheim and Gustav le Bon carried this relationship further.

William Dithley understood cultures in terms of purposefulness of human beings and alluded to the driving attitudes and motives in the culture's philosophy. Oswald Spengler characterized classical Western world as Apollonian and the modern culture as Faustian. George Devereux considered that "...cultural influences may have their greatest effect during the Oedipal period, at least with regard to the formation of the socially most relevant segment of personality..."[54] CP Snow, the British intellectual, talking about a culturally determined personality pattern, put it simply as "without thinking about it, they respond alike. That is what a culture means".[9]

The scientific study of culture and personality began with Franz Boas, who influenced a number of later authors including Mead, Benedict and Sapir. Margaret Mead[5] emphasized on the different traits of different cultures, e.g. the Arapesh manifested passive growth whereas the Tchambuli were more artistic and creative. Ruth Benedict[3] pointed out similar differences while considering Zuni (Pueblo) Indians to be Apollonian and the Dobuans paranoid. She believed in the underlying idea of wholeness in cultures and developed the idea of cultural configurations, namely that "cultures... are individual psychology thrown large upon the screen, given gigantic proportions and a long time span". Thus to her, the cultural pattern meant a configuration, gestalt or an integrated whole, and she felt that culture's wholeness and its distinctive purposes emerge from "emotional and intellectual mainstreams". Later, interest was focused more on the study of a basic personality, what was also called a 'modal personality' or 'national character'. This will be discussed a little later.

Coming back again to the culture and personality approach, we consider Linton's comment of similarities and dissimilarities within a culture. He argued[54] that the societies are people, while cultures exist on a psychological and behavioral level. He further said[54] that "since there are no identities anywhere in the universe, no two situations, no two behaviors, etc. are identical. Yet even though there is no real identity anywhere, neither is there infinite variety.... Briefly stated, while the behavior of the members of a society will vary with respect to a particular type of situation, these variations will be within a definite and finite range. This range is what we call the real culture pattern..."

Many people have tried to find out what is the basic thing that differentiates one culture from another. As has been pointed out by Wallace,[56] the national character should include at least three things, namely the statements about genius, the world-view, and the values. Honigman[59] cites five basic aspects of culture and personality relationship. They are:

- What is the character of innate human nature?
- What relationship connects man to nature?
- What time dimension is most significant: past, present or future?
- What is the significant end of human activity?
- How are men related to one another?

Abram Kardiner identifies the following key ingredients of the personality in the cultural content:

- Family organization
- Disciplines applied to sex, anal behavior, dependence and aggression
- Experience gained in coping with things and with people
- Rules, values, taboos and myths.

According to Ralph Linton,[54] a culture is made of the range of variations at a point of maximum frequency. The content of the culture of any homogeneous society can be divided into three categories, viz.

1. Universals-common to all
2. Specialities-shared by members of a social category
3. Alternatives, while individual peculiarities is the final variable.

With regard to influence of the society on the individual, Linton[54] mentions three basic areas. First is what other people do to the individual, followed by what other people consciously teach him, and finally, the behavior of other people as observed by the individual.

Finally, Spiro in an overview of the culture, personality approach and the modal personality commented:

"However much societies may differ, they must all cope with man's common biological features, especially his prolonged infantile dependency, the adaptively viable means for coping with the latter condition exhibit common social and cultural features across a *narrow range of social and cultural variability;* these common biological, social and cultural features are a set of constants which, in their interaction, produce a universal human nature" (Spiro, 1978; italics added by the present author).

Similarly, VK Varma[60] has identified three major sources of differentiation across cultures. These are:

1. Our attitude towards biological functions
2. The social inter-relationships
3. The religious and cosmological values.

These will be discussed later. Before proceeding further, a few pitfalls of the culture-personality approach have to be mentioned. David Hume (1741), writing on the national character, had cautioned, "the vulgar are apt to carry all national characters to extremes, and having once established it as a principle that any people are knavish, or cowardly, or ignorant, they will admit of no exception, but comprehend every individual under the same censure. Men of sense condemn these undistinguished judgements; though at the same time, they allow that each nation has a peculiar set of manners, and that some particular qualities are more frequently to be met with among one people than among their neighbors" (cited by Sir Aubrey Lewis, 1965, Ciba symposium).

VK Varma, before proceeding on a discussion of the Indian and the Euro-American personality types, also concedes that "it would be a folly to lump together all developing pro-industrial societies in one basket and ignore the considerable differences across them". Many such societies may represent what he has labeled as 'island culture' with lesser tradition rootedness and being more easily swayed by all external influences. Criticisms and cautions apart, this approach has nevertheless generated a lot of interest.

Concept and Definitions of Modal Personality

One area of the culture and personality approach has been the identification and description of a personality confined to a particular culture. This has been given different names by various authors such as 'ethnic personality' by Devereux, 'national character' by Mead, 'social character' by Eric Fromm, 'basic personality' by Linton, 'modal personality' by Cora Dubois, and so on.

The foundations of this field were laid by Margaret Mead who, in her books 'Coming of Age in Samoa'[5] and 'Sex and Temperament', did most to refurbish the ancient idea of a social personality. Her work was carried on further by Ruth Benedict and Edward Sapir, who explored the psychological attributes of cultures, thus identifying the basic personality type. Simultaneously, another important development took place, namely the famous Columbia University Project. Here, a group of professionals under Ralph Linton, an anthropologist, and Abram Kardiner, a psychoanalyst, held discussions on a number of issues pertaining to culture, personality and mental illness. They also identified a basic or ethnic personality.

In 1942, in the publication of 'People of Alor', Cora Dubois gave the concept of modal personality as a statistical norm. Later, sociologists like Inkeles and Levinson in 1954, formulated a definition of national character. Except for a few works, e.g. Tocqueville's description of American society, the initial descriptions of a modal personality were confined to small primitive, preliterate societies in different parts of the world. Later, the focus shifted to complex and modern societies such as American (Mead, Geoffery, Hsu), Japanese (Caudill, Benedict), Chinese (Hsu), Indian (Neki, Varma), and others. This concept was also not free from faults. As pointed out by Varma,[6]... "it obscures intrasocietal differences and gives rise to stereotypes, often with pejorative and prejudicial connotations". However, he adds[6] that "this is not meant to obscure individual differences within a culture but to highlight how cultures generally seem to differ from each other... Furthermore, such categorization should not give rise to value judgements or discrimination".

Definitions

Definitions of modal personality or basic personality of a culture seem as numerous as the definitions of culture itself. A few key features, however, can be identified in all the definitions.

For example, Honigman,[59] while defining social personality, feels that it "... refers to a set of broad regularities running through behavior manifested by an organized aggregate of people in a wide range of situations, as well as being reflected in things they make and use".

The basic personality has been defined by Linton[54,61] variously as "the personality configuration of maximum frequency in a particular society at a particular time", or "the basic personality type for any society is that personality configuration which is shared by the bulk of the society's members as a result of early experiences which they have in common".

Major Studies in National Characters

The description of various national characters and modal personalities provide interesting reading. An early description of the *German character* was provided by Kant. He said that "the German,.. ishomeloving; solid but not brilliant; industrious, thrifty, clearly without much flash of genius,... persistent in reasoning; intelligent, capable, but lacking in wit or taste;...imitative; overmethodical, pedantic;...docile under government, accepting depotism rather than resisting or altering the established order of authority"[59]

Early descriptions of the *Japanese character*, such as those by Weston La Barre, are available.[59] The author considered the Japanese as pervasively compulsive with high tyrannical conscience. The major Western publication, however, is Ruth Benedict's 'The Chrysanthemum and the Sword'.[4] William Caudhill extracts the following common themes relating to Japanese character, nearly all of which appear in Benedict's work:

- A sense of the group of communality as being of central importance.
- A strong sense of obligation and gratitude.
- A sense of sympathy and compassion (*ringo*) for others.
- A strong sense of 'we' versus 'they'.
- An underlying emotionality and excitability which is controlled by a somewhat compulsive attention to details, plans and rules.
- A willingness to work hard, and to persevere towards long range goals.
- Devotion to parents, and an especially long enduring tie to the mother persisting in almost its childhood form.
- An emphasis on self-effacement and a tendency to avoid taking responsibility for actions of oneself and others.

- A tendency towards understatement and an emphasis on nonverbal communication.
- A great pleasure in simple things of life such as being in beautiful surroundings, playing with children, bathing, drinking, eating and sex.

The chief criticism of this study was that it presented a static picture of the ideal patterns of a time long gone by, and ignored distinctions of social class and changes through time. Jean Stoetzel's post-war study of attitudes and values, 'Without the Chrysanthemum and the Sword,' also indicated that much of what Benedict describes did not apply at least to the youthful Japanese of mid-1950s. But, the study stimulated interest in the Japanese character and was followed by a number of other studies. T. Kawashima (1951) studied the modes and differences in conceptions of values in interpersonal relations. In 1953, the Human Relations Research Group under TsureoMuramatsu, began a large project to determine both the national modes and the regional differences in cultural values as these are related to types of personality.

Robert Munroe, Ruth Munroe and Robert Levine have attempted to study personality characteristics of Sub-Saharan African people. Because of the vast population and scant literature, their task has been difficult.[62] Nevertheless, they succeeded in compiling a list of what they thought to be distinctively *African cultural characteristics*. These include:

- Pastoralism
- Highly developed prestige economy and acquisitive culture patterns
- Centralized political institutions and institutionalized leadership
- Unilineal descent groups
- Polygyny and mother-child households
- Initiation rites and genital operations
- Bridewealth
- Witchcraft and sorcery
- Ancestor cults
- Structural peculiarities of certain language
- Importance of proverbs in folklore
- Separatist offshoots of Christian churches.

They added some other psychologically relevant conditions to the list, including:

- Both extremely high and extremely low population densities
- A high malnutrition rate
- Societies arbitrarily divided by Europeans and subjected to different colonial rules, with the arbitrary boundaries retained after independence
- Rapid emergence of elites.

The American culture has also generated a lot of interest among anthropologists. The earliest description is by the famous French explorer Tocqueville. After a comprehensive sampling of literature down to 1940, Lee Coleman listed the following as the 'American traits': "associational activity, democracy and belief and faith in it, belief in the equality of all as a fact and as a right, freedom of the individual in ideas and in fact, disregard of law, direct action, local government, practicality, prosperity and general material well-being, puritanism, emphasis on religion and its great influence in national life, uniformity and conformity".[62] Cuber and Harper, writing about ten years later, reduced the total number of American values. In their book 'Problems of American Society: Values in Conflict', they list the following: "monogamous marriage, freedom, acquisitiveness, democracy, education, monotheistic religion, freedom and science".[62]

Over the years, the analysis of American values remained stagnant. Thus, Robin Williams in 1951 gives us a very similar list as the earlier ones.[62] These values are 'achievement' and 'success', 'activity' and 'work', 'moral orientation', 'efficiency and practicability', 'progress', material 'comfort', 'equality', 'freedom', 'external conformity', 'science', 'secular rationality', 'nationalism-patriotism', 'democracy', 'individual personality', 'racism' and related 'group superiority' themes. However, Williams does take a step further and classifies the values to emphasize some and de-emphasize others.

- Quasi-values or gratifications; such as material comforts.
- Instrumental interests or mean values; such as wealth, power, work and efficiency.
- Formal universalistic value of Western tradition; rationalism, impersonal justice, universalistic ethics, achievement, democracy, equality, freedom, certain religious values of individual personality.
- Particularistic, segmental or localistic values; best exemplified in racist-ethnic superiority doctrines and in certain aspects of nationalism.

David Reisman (1950), in his book 'The Lonely Crowd', attempts to characterize the *American national character* as having changed from inner-direction to other-direction. However, this does not answer such basic contradictions in the American values, e.g. existence of racist attitudes in the South with belief in democratic values at the same time. Some authors thus characterize the American culture as 'schizoid' (Bain, 1935); 'dualistic', that is to say full of opposites (Harold J. Laski, 1948); and some just leave it as such, e.g. Gunnar Myrdal whose book 'An American Dilemma' (1944) summarizes his conclusion about this problem peculiar to America. This produces a sense of frustration even in eminent scholars like Henry Steele Commanger who notes: "All this presented to the student of American character a most perplexing problem. It was the business of advertisers to know that character and their resources enabled them to enlist in its study the aid of most perspicacious sociologists and psychologists. Yet, if their analysis was correct, the American people were decadent and depraved. No other evidence supported this conclusion. Advertisers appealed to fear, snobbery, and self-indulgence, yet no one familiar with the American character would maintain that these were indeed its predominant motivations, and Statesmen who knew the American people appealed to higher motives and not in vain. The problem remained a fascinating one, for it was clear that advertizers libeled the American character; it was equally clear that Americans tolerated and even rewarded those who libeled them".[62] No discussion on this subject would be complete without mentioning the famous anthropologist, Frances Hsu. Hsu has been studying the differences between current American culture and certain traditional Asian cultures, especially the Chinese and the Indian. In his work 'Class, Club and Caste',[63] he contrasts American, Indian and Chinese basic personality and social configuration. Some of his main findings are summarized in Table 4.

Hsu[62] stresses on the American core value of self-reliance, and says that the most persistent psychological expression is fear of dependence. All American values enumerated in literature, both good and bad, are in some way connected to self-reliance. But, this is a militant ideal, according to Hsu, and leads to such a great fear of dependence that anyone who is not self-reliant is considered a misfit. Since the very foundation of human life is man's dependence on his fellow beings, the basic American value orientation of self-reliance, by its denial of the other man's importance, creates contradictions for the person. Some contradictions mentioned by Hsu are:

- Christian love and bigotry.
- Emphasis on science, progress, humanitarianism, with parochialism, group superiority themes and racialism.
- Puritan ethics with increasing laxity in sex mores.
- Democratic ideals of equality and freedom with totalitarian tendencies and witch hunting.

There is, thus, a direct relationship between self-reliance and individual freedom on one hand, and submission to organization and conformity on the other. These inherent contradictions create a number of problems for the American people, the most ubiquitous of which, according to Hsu, is insecurity. Hsu then goes on to discuss the various American values and their uses.

All this is summed up in a very succinct and prophetic ending which says:[62]" the purpose of this paper...is to place the much lauded American values in their proper genetic perspective. When this is done, we find the best of America is directly linked with her worst, like Siamese twins. The way out of the worst is not to deny it but to recognize it for what it is".

In India, authors like Neki and Varma have done a lot of work in attempting to formulate a *modal personality for the Indian culture.* In his important work on the differences between the Indian and the Euro-American personalities, Varma[6] has argued for the use of a statistical model, e.g. analysis of variance. This is a step in the direction towards a more scientific analysis of the data, which till now, has largely relied on phenomenological and descriptive approaches. More about this is discussed later.

CULTURAL VARIABLES RELEVANT TO MENTAL ILLNESS

The relationship between culture, personality and mental illness has been commented upon by various authors. VK Varma[6] has tried to evolve a model to link these variables and show that transcultural differences in mental illness need to be explained and understood in terms of culture and personality variables. He identifies six cultural variables related to psychopathology, namely:

1. Dependence versus autonomy
2. Linguistic competence
3. Cognitive style
4. Social support system
5. Material culture
6. Psychological sophistication.

Dependence versus Autonomy

The major contribution of the author[6] is the concept of dependence versus autonomy.

Dependence as an important transcultural personality variable has been pointed out by earlier workers in different cultures. In India, early writings such as those by Neki[64-66] and Varma[67,68] mention the importance of dependence. The Indian, as has been pointed out, is more dependent on others than his Western counterpart. As children we depend on parents, as youth on peer groups, as husbands on spouses, and as older people depend on children, thus completing the circle. A beautiful system of *interdependence* is created with everyone leaning on the other. This is reflected in colloquial language, idioms and folklore. All such forms revolve around a theme of giving and receiving, a sense of piety, sacrifice, submission and gratitude, and ideas with reference to oral

Table 4: Basic personality

Hindu	*American*	*Chinese*
Supernatural centredness	Individual centredness	Situation centredness
Unilateral dependence	Self-reliance, abhorrence of dependence	Mutual dependence
Remarkable degree of internal dynamism that leads to no real change	Dynamic, great impetus for change	Static, lacking impetus for change
Impediment-expressed ineffusion, passivity and irascibility	Repression	Supression

activities, e.g. he ate up the money. The Indian variable of dependence is more of a unilateral one and more one-sided, with the dependent person not always expected to extend reciprocal support. This differs from the other Asian cultures, e.g. the Chinese, where there is more give-and-take dependence.[69-72]

This concept of autonomy and dependence is very similar to the Eriksonian one. The concept of autonomy in the Eriksonian sense means that a person has control over his own body. Thus, this is 'me' and this is 'my corpus' and I do have or I should have complete control over my corpus; over its feelings, emotions and actions. The initial manifestation of this autonomy is in the control of one's sphincters. Accordingly, the autonomous person develops a sense of control and responsibility over himself, and expects others to do the same with their bodies. In contrast, the dependent individual has a number of related features, such as a strong sense of identity with the primary filial group. Much of his life seems to evolve around this group and one's responsibilities and obligations towards it. Accordingly, codes of conduct differ between those within the primary group and those outside it. To illustrate, although Indian hospitality has been highly praised, it applies only to members of the primary group, or those who can be brought into it. The Indian can be strangely rude and callous to a stranger, and the Western value of according respect and consideration to somebody, simply because he is human, is relatively lacking. The concept of dependence or autonomy governs one's interpersonal and social relationship. There is a greater ability to both accept and accord dependence, and to be able to accept and receive it. A number of related traits of dependence can be thought of, namely:

Concept of Ego Boundaries

This concept, developed mainly by Marriot,[70-72] emphasizes a sense of personal identity and requires that the person is able to distinguish himself and others, i.e. 'me' versus 'not me'. As pointed out by Marriot,[70] in contrast to the generally closed homogenous mental integrations attributable to adult persons in the West, the Hindus are posited as persons "who are open, composed of exogenous elements, substantially fluid,...and thus necessarily changing and interchanging in their nature... given the vulnerability of open Hindu person to a cosmos of interpersonal flow, persons as... cannot be thought of enduring or bounded 'egos' in Western sense". In a general sense, we can see that in Eastern-Indian and other Asian cultures, there is more of an ongoing interaction across individuals. Individuals consider themselves as an integral part of the social system and the differentiation between 'me' and 'not me' is not so great. The responsibilities are often viewed as common and communal, rather than individual and specific.

Empathy versus Rules

Dependence gives rise to empathy. Much of the social interrelationship is governed by the principle of empathy in a dependence oriented society. As the Sanskrit saying goes *"Atma vat sarvabhootanm"*, everybody is like myself and if you can do that and if you can empathize with the other person, the rules can come to you automatically. There are 'thus' no wrong rules. In contrast, autonomy-oriented societies abound in specific and wrong rules. Unfortunately, the rules do not apply in all situations and that gives rise to various problems.

Friendship versus Fairplay

In a dependence oriented society, the concept of friendship is very important. Hence, friend has always been eulogized in Indian literature and art forms. Friendship is viewed as an all-out kind of interaction and people are supposed to do everything for a friend. This might not be true in all real life situations, nevertheless the concept is totally different from the limited concept of friendship in an autonomy-oriented Western society. Consequently, the concept of fairplay, 'let the best man win', exists in the West but not in India. In dependence-oriented societies, friendship has no such restraints as fairplay. 'Either I am your friend or I am not, if I am I must do everything whether fair or foul for you'.

Autonomy and Self-reliance

The key attribute of autonomy is self-reliance. An autonomous individual is self-reliant, responsible for his actions and expects others to be self-reliant like him. This makes him more acutely aware not only of his responsibilities but also of his rights and prerogatives on an individual basis. As already mentioned, this rigid concept of self-reliance is not without its problems. Neither total autonomy nor total dependency is possible in any society. Total dependence results in total submission and converts the person into a nonentity, whereas total autonomy breeds fear of dependence and leads to insecurity. There are other dangers of autonomy. In the Western situation, the pressure to achieve autonomy is so great that children from a young age start looking for sources of income. This leads to the death of childhood. Further in life, autonomy interferes with a much needed open and confiding relationship with friends and spouses, because every relationship is being constantly evaluated, leaving no room for unquestionable or unqualified acceptance. As the Urdu poet SahirLudhianvi lamented: "No friendship, no love, no etiquettes, no consideration, nobody belongs to anybody, all men are lonely now!". The effect of this loneliness is felt by the elderly in the West, who can not or will not accept help from their grown-up children. The effect on the married couple is that it remains a virtual two person system from the wedding to death or separation. Each partner, thus, is expected to fulfil all the needs of the other-a stupendous task! No wonder there are frequent breakdowns of the unitary husband-wife pair as well as the unitary family system. In a dependence-oriented society like India, on the other hand, many roles are fulfilled by various persons in a large family, starting from surrogate parenthood to the care of the aged. The dependent individual, on account of the richness of the social inter-relationships, feels more secure in the sanctity and security of the social network.

Another aspect of autonomy is the sense of responsibility that accompanies it. This leads to the notion that each and every failure must be accounted for and punished appropriately. The punishment may appear out of context or beyond limits; it is nevertheless administered with regularity for every lapse since an autonomous person by principle is not allowed lapses. This has gradually given birth to the rigid calvinistic, puritanical Western superego. The grotesque limits to which this punishment and responsibility can be carried out is easily seen in the rise of litigations in the West.

Impersonalization of Friendship and Foeship

Since the Western concept of friendship is too limited, all friendships in the West are only relative. Friends only come together for specific purposes. Friendship becomes an impersonal rather than a personal relationship. This is manifested in the West as egalitarianism, a highly prized value, or by the conversion of a purely social relationship into a formal one. You do not meet a friend to talk with him, rather you meet him to play poker which is not much different from meeting a business associate for a contract. Of course, occasions, such as poker games, do subserve or fulfil in varying degrees the need for socialization. But more importantly, they lead to denial and negation of our social needs to a large extent. Like friendship, foeship also becomes impersonal. You do not know your enemy, you have not seen him, you do not particularly hate him, but still you kill him and perhaps more ruthlessly than before. The aggression is no longer direct, as in the earlier dependence-oriented societies. However, millions of people slaughtered in the Second World War, stand testimony to the fact that indirect aggression is more barbarous, more inhuman and certainly more evil than any form of direct aggression. This brings us back to the start, that there can be no society, which is either totally autonomous or totally dependent. The societies have to be organized in a dependence-autonomy continuum, with some being relatively more autonomous and some relatively more dependent.

One advantage of the system of autonomy and dependence is that it is a nonhierarchical system, in the sense that it does not try to organize societies in the evolutionary sense of the term. Autonomy or dependence is simply one of the variables before a society and one society is not ahead of the other in evolutionary terms. On account of this, certain people have tried to correlate the autonomy or dependence in terms of technological stage of the society. Neki[65] has pointed out that dependence was more suited to an agrarian society where people have to work together in an informal way. On the other hand, autonomy is more suited to the industrial society where people have to be responsive to their own little bits of responsibility. If one looks at the typical assembly line situation of the industrial society, one sees how the system works well in that every person does his bit and fulfils his needs as an autonomous and responsible individual. Also, in such a system an individual lapse has a much greater consequence on the total system than in the case of an agrarian society. However, it seems that the differences across societies in terms of autonomy and dependence may not be simply a function of technological or industrial development. A review of the popular literature (some of which has been written in the present century, speculating on the situation in earlier times) shows that the European society was probably much more autonomy-oriented even before what went off as the industrial revolution. Thus, it is very dangerous to historically view this phenomenon and to offer offhand explanations or conclusion.

Other Variables

The Indian and Western cultures differ on certain other variables, such as:

- *Social ethos and communal responsibility*: In certain ways, the Indian seems to be more selfish, e.g. personal cleanliness is highly valued among Indians, whereas concern about public cleanliness is lacking. The rules of social interaction in the Indian context are defined largely in an egocentric and intuitive way. Codes are simple in contrast to other codes (e.g. Jewish codes).
- *Obsessionality*: The lack of compulsivity in performing a job, the casual attitude, and the lack of pride in doing a job well, are certain characteristics of Indian culture which contrast sharply with the Western work ethic, compulsivity, meticulousness and thoroughness.
- *Preoccupation with peace and fear of aggression:* This is another characteristic Indian trait, which probably reflects decadence rather than development.
- *Tradition-orientation:* Traditionalism, not surprisingly, is quite dominant in the Indian culture. Though it might be an impediment to change, it does provide a stability to the social structure.
- *Duality:* Duality in value system, omnipotence and a sense of narcissism are present in the Indian culture as well as other cultures, in varying degrees.

Before ending this comparison, a word of caution is necessary. The prototype for the Eastern culture in this discussion is Indian and that of the West, America. This does not, however, mean that these two represent personality configurations in different societies in the world, nor do they represent all configurations found in the 'East' or 'West'. The fact remains, that such a comparison can be used to contrast the developing and traditional countries, and the developed, industrialized and urbanized countries of the West.

Basic Needs

In the larger sense, the transcultural differences in personality configurations can be understood in terms of the basic needs. They are:

- *Biological needs:* All men are born with certain undeniable basic biological needs, such as nutritional, eliminative and sexual needs. Denial, projection, or reaction formation may characterize the attitude towards these needs or there may be ready acceptance or sublimation of these. Denial seems characteristic of the Indian mind. So, we have traditions such as fasting to deny nutritional needs, and the traditional 'modesty' in sexual and eliminative matters which is actually a denial of these needs. Surprisingly, the attitudes in West are quite similar. The present apparent permissiveness in matters of sexuality does not represent a basic change. Rather, it is a facade maintained at a tremendous emotional cost of guilt and anxiety. It is perhaps the Chinese or Japanese who have truly accepted these biological needs. Thus, so far, the average human is still seeking fulfilment of his biological needs, in different cultures over the world. It is hoped that with time he will be able to achieve the level of, what has been called by Erikson as, creative, integrative and generative personalities.
- *Social relationships and needs:* One aspect of the social relations is the nature and configuration of the superego, since it reflects 'internalization'. In an autonomous society, group dominance is more, independence is emphasized, and internalization is to a great extent leading to a guilt-orientation.[73] Interdependence, on the other hand, leads to control of behavior in the form of interpersonal surveillance leading to shame-orientation.[65]
- *Cosmic, existential and religious needs:* Societies vary in terms of these needs. Cosmology seems to be the only true universal need, whereas religious concepts vary in their level of abstraction in different cultures.

Linguistic Competence

Language, despite being a species-specific attribute of Homo sapiens, differs widely across cultures. The difference may be in basic things such as classification of words and rules of syntax, or complex temporal and spatial relationships such as a static versus flowing concept of time. Benjamin Whorf,[74] who formulated the Whorfian hypothesis, said that language "is itself the shaper of ideas, the programs and guide for individual mental activity". Later, authors like Brown and Lennenberg[75] confirmed that language determines the concept of reality, and that language and thought develop together.

Based on transcultural differences in phenomenology and outcome of mental illness and language as well, Varma[76] proposed that the two are interrelated. He proposed that a high level of linguistic competence leads to binding of intense anxiety found in initial stages of schizophrenia,[77] leading to elaborate delusions that are less amenable to treatment. A low level of competence leaves the anxiety unbound and results in catatonic and somatic symptoms. A study using a specially constructed linguistic competence scale found that paranoid schizophrenics and obsessional anxiety neurotics had a higher level than chronic schizophrenics and manics.[78] So, it suggested that the above illnesses may be phenomenological correlates of high and low linguistic competence, thus supporting the theory that linguistic competence may determine manifestations of psychopathology.

Cognitive Styles

Cognitive styles represent ways in which the mind perceives the environment, interprets and draws conclusions about it. Cognitive styles can be 'analytic', i.e. understanding by breaking things into parts; and 'synthetic', i.e. understanding by considering a phenomenon in totality and relating it to others. The Western mind, shaped by Aristotelian logic, is classically analytical, and hence suits science and technology well. However, it fails to suffice in certain fields, e.g. human behavior. The Indian mind, in contrast, is synthetic in its cognitive style. This is more conducive to the development of unitary and holistic concepts; and the ability to deal with several things simultaneously. Cognitive styles may also be related to the dependency-autonomy continuum. Thus, synthetic styles are consistent with dependence and loose ego boundaries in relationship of the individual to the society, whereas analytical approaches prevail in autonomy oriented societies.

Social Support System

With increasing transcultural research, the differences across cultures in social support system have been correlated with course and outcome of illness. Studies have shown that traditional, developing societies, richer in social support network, have better prognosis for severe mental illness.[28] In a related area, such as relationship of joint versus nuclear families with outcome, the conclusions are rather ambiguous.[79] However, study areas such as 'expressed emotions' and outcome have yielded fruitful results.

Material Culture

Since definitions of cultures include artefacts as well as subjective beliefs, norms, etc. it can be quite safely assumed that material culture will influence psychopathology. Thus, we have possession by ghosts and evil spirits in a developing society, whereas in a technologically advanced one, the same is attributed to Martians and UFOs.

Psychological Sophistication and the Nature of Guilt versus Shame

VK Varma has analyzed and pointed out a number of variables which might be important in mediating cross-cultural differences between Western and Indian models of psychotherapy;[67,73,80] some of these are dependence versus autonomy, personal responsibility, and social and religious beliefs. Two other important variables are psychological sophistication and the nature of guilt versus shame.

'Psychological sophistication' can be perceived as the ability to see conflicts in intrapsychic terms as required in psychotherapy. It involves introspection and the ability to translate one's emotions into words. Since these have been shown to differ widely across cultures, they need to be taken into account during psychotherapy.

Operating intrapsychically, psychotherapy is more suited for guilt-prone societies rather than shame-prone ones. As VK Varma has pointed out, "it is possible that whereas societies following the Judeo-Christian religions are guilt-prone on subscribing to the view that man was created in sin..., the Eastern religions do not subscribe to guilt as a prerequisite to human existence".[80] Cross-cultural differences arising thus are important considerations in psychotherapy.

Ages of Mankind

As society is a conglomeration of individuals, it can be argued that the needs of the society should be comparable to the needs of the person. Dynamically speaking, the problems of human existence can be understood in terms of man's coming to terms with, adequately mastering as it were, his drive in harmonious relationship with the environment, including people in it. Just as the individual personality develops, the society also develops in an attempt to fulfil the same biological and psychological needs of its members, as well as additional socially generated needs.

Depending upon the major biological concerns, societies manifest variable degrees of 'oral', 'anal' and 'genital' traits which may find reflection in the individual personality. So, the day men are able to adequately fulfil or master their needs, so will be the society.

CULTURE AND POSITIVE MENTAL HEALTH

Man lives in an intimate relationship with the society. The important relationship between man and society has been extensively studied and variously interpreted. Mental health and illness are just as dependent upon sociocultural factors as upon individual psychological variables. The culture may exercise powerful pathogenic and pathoplastic, as well as health sustaining, influences. On the one hand is the view that culture is constraining and limiting, having a generally undesirable and deleterious effect. In a way, this can be linked to the increasing complexity of life, especially since the industrial revolution, thus leading to viewing 'cultivation' as bad and holding a fond wish of the return of the primitive, 'the happy savage' (Rousseau). Even Freud was not immune to this bias and "when he turned his attention to social phenomena, it seems to have been with the intention of indicting society for its deleterious influences on personality."[81]

However, not everyone has taken a negative view of culture, which evolves as a group solution to the problems of human existence and should thus be something positive and beneficial to mankind. Civilization can be viewed as reducing sources of acute fear, disgust and anger; reducing variability in the environment and making it more predictable and manageable.[82] Fromm[83] viewed this issue in a larger perspective: "It is the belief of the progressive forces in society that such a realization is possible, that the interest of society and of individual need not be antagonistic forever."

Conflict is an integral part of human existence, and can be said to exist intrapsychically when a particular wish or impulse can not be readily realized in a harmonious relationship with one's superego and the external reality, including the people in it. In such a situation, the individual brings into play certain mental defense mechanisms, genetically determined and unconsciously operating, to reduce the anxiety and the guilt, and permit partial gratification of the wish.

It is proposed[84] that, similar to individual defenses, there exist a number of '*cultural defenses*' which are the culturally determined mechanisms of allaying anxiety. These are available in a readymade form for all members of the society to utilize them in appropriate situations. Cultural defense has been defined as a "psychological defense mechanism, genetically determined and unconsciously operative, which allays anxiety and enables partial gratification and where the mechanism is provided in the form of institutions, customs, traditions, rituals, sanctions, prohibitions, folkways and symbolisms; and is available for use of all members of the society in appropriate situations."

Cultural defenses are similar to the individual defense mechanisms in that these are brought into play to alleviate anxiety and permit gratification. However, rather than the individual using his ingenuity to fabricate, as it were a defense mechanism, he utilizes one, readymade, provided by the society for use of its members in similar situations.

Culturally determined filters, perceptual as well as cognitive, serve such defensive functions. The child is taught early in life that it is wrong to see, think, or know about certain things. In this way, the individual is spared the anxiety which can be invoked by such conflictual areas. Social institutions like marriage, family, school, church, caste and class systems reduce uncertainties and channelize gratifications in an acceptable form, and hence can be considered to be subserving defensive functions.

A study of the customs and rituals is a rich source of understanding defenses. Although some customs and rituals are understandable as serving realistic, useful functions, many other rituals and customs do not appear meaningful and useful. The question arises then as to why are they practised. The thesis is put forward that, in addition to serving realistic functions, they also operate at a symbolic level to serve as defense mechanisms. In so far as these are available to be shared by all members of society, these can be called 'cultural defenses.'

A simple example of the defensive functions of the customs is illustrated by the ritualized group mourning process associated with the death of a family member. Elaborate customs prevail in practically all cultures to permit this communal mourning. In India, the process in Hindus lasts for about thirteen days, with specific rituals and activities to be performed on the various days. This permits members of the family to come together, to talk about the deceased, to relive their life with him, and thus to relinquish him. This is precisely the treatment of grief reaction, and the death ritual permits this treatment at a group level to permit an optional resolution of the bereavement.

Similarly, there are other customs and rituals practised in different societies which serve defense functions. One such example is that of initiation ceremonies common in many cultures. Amongst boys, this often involves torture and fear inflicted upon him; a haircut or shaving the head or expectation of the display of proof of his strength and fearlessness. This symbolic castration, as it were, serves to reduce anxiety aroused by sexuality, by undoing or expiating for the guilt of sexual desire. The display of strength may be analogous to the sadist's display of strength before he is able to enjoy sexuality. "I do not have to fear castration, I can, myself, castrate". Similarly in girls, at menarche and menstruation, isolation is resorted to on grounds of uncleanliness. This apparently meaningless custom can be understood as a perceptual filter to keep out of awareness an embarrassing matter, namely that women have been mutilated (castrated).

With regard to sex and marriage, the custom of incest taboo has been shown to be universal. Elaborate rules exist in different cultures in this matter and with regard to the interaction between the two sexes. "A great many cultures with preadolescent sexual license require marital fidelity and a great many which value premarital virginity in either male or female arrange their marital life with great license" (Benedict, 1959). This, as well as the institution of marriage, regulates the gratification of the sexual need and removes uncertainties about the process. In many cultures, including our own, self-sacrifice and privation are associated with the rituals of marriage. Fasting for several days before the wedding in Hindus and voluntary abstinence in some other societies serve to reduce guilt associated with sex.

The naming of an infant is an important activity. Many cultures practice '*teknonymy*' namely, calling someone not by his given name but as so-and-so's father, mother, son, daughter, etc. It has been suggested[6] that teknonymy can foster identification between members of a family and facilitate identification of a parent with his or her child.

The reaction to illness also illustrates defensive functions of the customs. Ascribing illness to external malevolent influences or projection is very common in many cultures, including India. It often leads to aggression towards an animal or a human, resulting from projection. Introjection, i.e. blaming oneself for the illness, and deliberate acts to deflect illness, is also common.

It is in the rituals related to death that the cultural defenses are brought to full force. The defensive functions of the rituals can be considered under two major headings:

1. Denial
2. Introjection and projection.

Denial consists of such things as refusing to utter the name of the deceased, dressing up the corpse and providing it with food and other articles of everyday life. It is also manifested by the belief in after-life. Such denial may take the shape of belief in transmigration of souls, like amongst Hindus; or belief in a final resting place of the soul, the Valhalla of the early Nordics, and heaven and hell of Christianity and Islam. How can something as important as human life just simply disappear? It is frustrating that mankind, having developed as far intellectually, morally, aesthetically and religiously, should end entirely with death. "For, we are not born or created idly or fortuitously, but doubtless there is some power which takes thought for the race of men and which was not likely to create and foster what-when it had accomplished all its toils-would sink into everlasting misery in death."[85]

Introjection and projection following death are manifested by such things as shaving or haircut, and other forms of self-inflicted injuries, including the *Suttee* system. In many societies, the family members carry out acts of actual or symbolic torture and self-injury, viewed as symbolic castration to undo one's assumed responsibility in the death. Projection is manifested by such things as fear of ghosts, blaming others for the death, and taking steps to expiate the passage of the spirit. As Ruth Benedict[3] comments, in many cultures burial is an orgy of terror. In Australian tribes, the nearest of the kin fall upon the skull and pound it to bits, so that it may not subsequently trouble them.[3] To reduce the danger of the ghosts, steps include carrying out one's duties during the process of the mourning and attempting to appease and expedite the passage of the spirit. In Hindus, the spirit is believed to be in an intervening period between death and rebirth for 13 days, during which fasting and offerings are made to expedite its passage.

A most striking and intriguing aspect of the rituals associated with the death is the institution of death feasts, which appears to be widespread. Although it seems incongruous that a period of mourning after death should be marked with feasting that generally goes with joyous occasions, it may be explained in these terms that death feast may serve the purpose of incorporation of the person, a symbolic cannibalism, so to say.

Culturally determined rituals and customs serve defensive functions. The defense mechanisms illustrated include denial (e.g. of death or castration), repression and sublimation (e.g. of sexual drive), projection (e.g. by blaming others for illness or death), incorporation (e.g. death feasts), introjection (e.g. self-punitive behavior following death), identification (e.g. teknonymy), and undoing (e.g. personal suffering and privation associated with sex and marriage).

It may be noticed that most of the examples given pertain to the less developed societies. By comparison, it can be said that the developed societies make lesser use of rituals. Some rituals may become victim to the scientific advancement, making them no longer tenable. But what about their defensive role? Would giving up one set of rituals give rise to another set, better camouflaged and appearing rational? Wittkower and Dubreuil[86] have expressed concern that "inhibition of these cultural strategies for the sake of the highly valued social conformity, especially in North America, may have reduced the beneficial effects of these institutionalized emotional outlets". By denuding societies of the protection of cultural defenses, are we not exposing them to the possibility of cataclysmic and irrational outbursts of human drives-sexual, aggressive and others? The answer to this question may have very important and far-reaching consequences for human society and implications for those interested in futuristic social engineering and control.

TRANSCULTURAL ASPECTS OF PSYCHOTHERAPY

Psychotherapy has been defined in numerous ways, the common concept of which means those maneuvres which can be called psychological (as opposed to organic) in the treatment of problems of an emotional or psychological nature. "As psychotherapy is predicated upon a linguistic system of thoughts and emotions, it is inevitable that cross-cultural differences in these... must be taken into account in ascertaining suitability of and in adapting psycho-therapy for a particular culture."[80] People around the world are not alike, and those of one culture differ from those of other cultures in many important ways which may have direct relevance to psychotherapy; such as the religious philosophical background, the experimental repertoire, language, modes of affective expression, moral and social norms, mores, the culturally determined conflicts, and defenses. Wittkower and Warnes[87] have emphasized that to be popular, psychotherapy must be consistent with the socio-philosophical background of the people. "Psychoanalysis became popular in the USA because of emphasis on individualism, rational thinking, free expression and tolerance of dissent. So became work therapy in the Soviet Union, autogenic training in Germany and Morita therapy in Japan, in each case because it was consistent with the respective values".[84]

Comments and reservations are often expressed, formally and informally, by Indian psychiatrists and other mental health professionals regarding the place, the relevance for India, of psychotherapy, as it is understood in the West. For example, Neki[64] feels that "Western psychotherapy, as it is, is hardly applicable to the multitudes in India except for a handful of Westernized Indians living in large cosmopolitan cities". Surya and Jayaram,[88] among other authors, have also voiced reservations regarding practicability of transposing psychotherapy developed in one culture to some other culture.

There are certain cross-cultural differences in personality configurations which are important in deciding which type of psychotherapy would be best relevant to a given culture.

- *Fulfilment of biological needs*: Denial, projection and reaction formation, as opposed to due acceptance, may characterize handling of needs, such as nutritional, eliminative and sexual. The truly oriental cultures, namely the Chinese and the Japanese, seem to have more open, accepting and realistic attitudes towards the fulfilment of eliminative and sexual needs.[6]
- *Social relationships and needs:* The interrelationships between individuals in a society can be understood as interdependence, on a dependence-autonomy continuum, and also as the internalization of the social and moral values into the superego. Different societies differ in the amount of dependency or autonomy as well as the degree of internalization of the superego into the psyche.
- *Cosmic, existential and religious values, and needs:* The concepts of the nature and meaning of one's existence, transcendence, continuity of life after death and of God, vary from culture to culture, and may represent varying degrees of abstraction.
- *Cognitive styles:* Cultures differ from each other in cognitive style, ranging from 'analytical' to 'synthetic'. Analytical thinking may be more conducive to scientific and technological progress, whereas the synthetic approach may be more applicable to societies with high dependence and loose ego boundaries.[80]
- *Linguistic competence*: Related to the above, cross-cultural differences in linguistic competence[76] result in differing emphasis upon the experiencing of an event as opposed to recording and chronicling it by translating it into words.

Individuals vary, both within and across cultures, in personality structure and psychological mechanisms. However, in so far as the interculture differences appear greater than the intracultural variations, the role of culture can be said to be significant.

There have been several attempts to understand the common factors involved in different forms of psychotherapy around the world, which are instrumental in the healing process. Frank (1968) and Abrams (1968) have emphasized the role of persuasion as a therapeutic ingredient. "We must assume that most, if not all, psychiatric patients are influenced to some extent by the demand character of the therapy situation and the implicit or explicit expectation of the therapist..." (Frank, 1968). Torrey[89] has named four ingredients common to all psychotherapies. These are:

- A shared world-view, and the therapist's ability to name the offending agent. (The principle *of Runpel-stiltskin).*
- The personal qualities of the therapist.
- The high expectations with which the patient approaches the apparently exalted position of the therapist, which he calls the 'edifice complex'.
- *The technique:* He feels that the contribution of the so-called technique in the Western psychotherapy towards a favorable outcome has been overemphasized.

To apply the conventional Western model psychotherapy for another culture like India, a number of sociocultural variables must be taken into account to ascertain its applicability. Certain attributes of the Indian personality can be pointed out in contrast to the Western personality and can be identified as having relevance to the applicability of the Western-model psychotherapy for India. The more important of these are as follows:

- *Dependence vs autonomy*: As compared to Western societies, the individual in a traditional developing society like India develops a greater amount of dependence. It is questionable how far Western psychotherapy with its high emphasis on autonomy and individual responsibility can be prescribed for members of such a society.
- *Psychological sophistication, introspective and verbal abilities*: Defining psychological sophistication as "the ability to understand one's emotions and actions, conflicts and difficulties in intrapsychic rather than environmental terms,"[6,80] the Indian mind lacks such sophistication and tends to perceive conflicts and difficulties in extrapsychic terms.
- *Need for confidentiality and the nature of dyadic relationship*: In the primary, group-oriented, 'open' societies like India, confidentiality may figure less as a need and prerogative. Patients often actually welcome the participation of family members and friends in the therapeutic process. This raises a question regarding the relevance for confidentiality and the one-to-one relationship that are the hallmarks of conventional psychotherapy in the West.
- *Personal responsibility and decision making*: Coming from a society with a strong primary identification and rich network of social interactions, the Indian mind is less able to develop a strong sense of personal responsibility. In the conventional Western psychotherapy, the patient is regarded as a responsible individual with whom lies the final decision. In the Indian setting, the patient may require a more assertive and protective role of the therapist.
- *Nature of guilt and shame*: Operating intrapsychically, psychotherapy can be considered to be more suited for guilt-prone societies. The Indian mind can be said to be more shame-oriented, requiring the surveillance of other people for it to operate.
- *Religious and social belief systems*: Most societies and religions around the world indicate an ambivalence between the concept of free-will and determinism. The Indian mind is more tuned to the concept of determinism and fatalism, with a belief in reincarnation.
- *Patients' expectations*: Coming from a more dependence-prone society, the Indian mind approaches the therapist with greater expectation and submission, leading to greater faith and trust, and hence requiring a more dominating role of the therapist.
- *Social distance between the patient and the therapist*: Indian society, being more traditional and class-oriented, has resulted in greater acceptance of social distance between individuals. The patient identifies his doctor with the superior class, and assumes an obsequious and submissive position in relation to him. There is also a tendency to replace a purely professional relationship by a filial relationship.

In view of the relationship between culture, personality and psychotherapy, it is important that the Western-model psychotherapy be adapted for use in a non-Western culture. In a survey of psychotherapy practice by Indian psychiatrists,[90] the following adaptations to therapy, considered necessary for India, were suggested:

- *Use of lesser-trained professionals*: The limited number of psychiatrists and other highly qualified professionals necessitates that a simplified version be imparted to those basically less educated or qualified. Lesser-trained professionals can be used as vehicles of psychotherapy.
- *Greater activity on the part of the therapist*: In view of the differences in personality structure, the Indian patient demands and welcomes a more active role on the part of the therapist as compared with his Western counterpart.
- *Making it briefer, crisis-oriented, supportive, flexible and eclectic, and tuned to the cultural and social conditions*: There are several reasons for this, like manpower limitations, rich social support available, and the prevailing medical model of psychiatric illness which makes it easier for patients to receive directive guidance. A flexible approach helps to deal with patients from different social backgrounds and literacy levels.
- *Adoption of a more 'activist' model*: Social system psychotherapeutic models have been elucidated by Pattison (1973) as a multiperson, multirelational interaction, an 'open' model psychotherapy. The patient seeks return to the social system which is the venue of the

psychotherapy and on which it is focused. Hence, a more activist model to the social milieu could be more relevant to psychotherapy in India.

- *Greater use of suggestion and reassurance*: The Indian patient more clearly needs reassurance from the therapist. He also desires and requires direct suggestions and guidance on how to handle his problems. Rather than giving elaborate explanations and pursuit of insight, the patients expect to be more explicitly reassured and clearly given the specific directions in resolving their emotional and situational problems.
- *Lesser use of dynamic interpretation*: The Indian patient may be less able to understand and accept interpretation based in terms of intrapsychic conflicts and exchanges. Hence, to be acceptable, the interpretation should be given in more clearly understandable terms, often relating it to the social realities so as to make it more acceptable.
- *Blending it with the religious beliefs*: Certain religious beliefs can be clearly exploited in psychotherapy. For example, relating the illness and difficulties to the events of previous birth can certainly be comforting. In the same way, mythology and folklore can be utilized to therapeutic advantage. The *Hanuman complex*[91] can be utilized. Hanuman, the monkey god and the trusted aide of Lord Rama, was himself unaware of his great powers and capabilities until he was made aware of them. In this way, the psychiatric patient needs to be made aware of his underlying potential.

Hence, psychotherapy cannot divorce itself from the psychosocial variables and cultural-religious milieu of the patients. These must be taken into account and interwoven, both in its theoretical base and also in its practical considerations.

OVERVIEW OF CULTURE, PERSONALITY, AND MENTAL ILLNESS

Personality, Coping Mechanisms, and Mental Illness

In the context of schizophrenic psychoses, Manfred Bleuler[92] comments: "...unhappiness can reach a threshold... when the patient autistically withdraws from reality under overwhelming stress, when he thinks, acts, feels as if he is not in the real world but in a world...adapted to...the disharmony between his needs and reality". However, referring to his illustrious father, he comments[92] that "he did not answer the question of why the schizophrenic individual tries to defend his ego in the schizophrenic way and not in the way of a neurotic or healthy way."

It is possible that the culturally determined personality attributes may importantly influence coping mechanisms and mental illness. When faced with emotional conflict, a passive dependent person may be likely to more easily 'give up', throw in the towel, so as to say. He may, thus, be more prone to break with reality and develop psychotic coping behavior. On account of close ties with the society, he can more easily turn to them to be taken care of. He may also develop hysterical and somatoform disorders, so as to involve other members of the society in its resolution. On the other hand, an autonomous individual, on account of his abhorrence of loss of control and rejection of his dependency needs, may try to resolve his conflicts himself, at the intrapsychic level. He may keep on battling with the anxiety, unbound, or may convert it into a development of neurotic-type distress.

There are clear limitations in the ways in which a person can react when faced with an emotional conflict. The total repertoire of human behavior, normal as well as abnormal, clearly does not exhaust all that can be theoretically possible. The person can continue to battle with the conflict and the resultant anxiety. Alternatively, (a) the anxiety can be channelized into neurotic symptoms which magically or expediently control it (e.g. phobia, obsession, somatization, or depression); or (b) the anxiety can lead to avoidance of really or potentially anxiety-provoking situations (e.g. constraints in interaction as exemplified by personality disorders); or (c) it can be resolved by renunciation of reality. It is possible that the personality configuration, either individually or culturally shaped, may influence the choice made. The subsequent elaboration and proliferation of the symptomatology may depend to a certain degree, upon the various sociocultural factors as earlier discussed.

REFERENCES

1. Tylor E. Primitive Cultures. London; 1971.
2. Boas F. The Mind of Primitive Man. New York: Free Press; 1965.
3. Benedict R. Patterns of Culture. London: Routledge&Kegan Paul; 1935.
4. Benedict R. The Chrysanthemum and the Sword. Boston: Houghton Mifflin; 1961.
5. Mead M. Coming of Age in Samoa. New York: Morrow; 1935.
6. Vanna VK. Cultural psychodynamics in health and illness. Indian J Psychiatry. 1986;28:177-86.
7. Seligman CG. Temperament, conflict and psychosis in a stone age population. Br J Med Psychol. 1926;9:196-202.
8. Leighton AH, Murphy JM. Psychiatric Disorders among the Yoruba. Ithaca: Cornell University Press; 1963.
9. Murphy JM, Leighton AH. Approaches to Cross-cultural Psychiatry, Ithaca: Cornell University Press; 1965.
10. Leff J. Psychiatry Around the Globe: A Transcultural View. New York: Marcel Dekker; 1981.
11. Torrey EF, Torrey BB, Burton-Bradley BG. The epidemiology of schizophrenia in Papua New Guinea. Am J Psychiatry. 1974;131:576-8.
12. Dunham HW. Community and Schizophrenia: An Epidemiological Analysis. Detroit: Wayne State University Press; 1965.

13. Murphy HBM, Raman AC. The chronicity of schizophrenia in indigenous tropical people. Br J Psychiatry. 1971;118:489-97.
14. Murphy HBM. Comparative Psychiatry: The International and Intercultural Distribution of Mental Illness. Berlin: Springer; 1982.
15. Wing JK, Brown GW. Institutionalism and Schizophrenia. Cambridge: University Press; 1970.
16. Orley JH. Culture and Mental Illness. East African Publishing House; 1970.
17. Kleinman A. Major conceptual and research issues for cultural (and anthropological) psychiatry. Cult Med Psychiatry. 1980;4:3-13.
18. Devereux G. Cultural thought models in primitive and modern psychiatric theories. Psychiatry. 1958;21:359-74.
19. Wittkower ED, Rin H. Transcultural psychiatry. Arch Gen Psychiatry. 1965;13:387-94.
20. Benedict PK, Jacks I. Mental illness in primitive societies. Psychiatry. 1954;17:377-89.
21. Enright JB, Jaeckle WR. Psychiatric symptoms and diagnosis in two sub-cultures. Inter J Soc Psychiatry. 1963;9:12-17.
22. Eaton JW, Weil RJ. Culture and Mental Disorder. Glencoe: Free Press. 1955.
23. Schooler E, Caudill W. Symptomatology in Japanese and American schizophrenics. Ethnology. 1964;3:172-8.
24. Opler M (Ed). Culture and Mental Health. New York: MacMillan; 1959.
25. Kline NS. Psychiatry in Indonesia. Am J Psychiatry. 1963:119:809.
26. Pfeiffer WM. TranskulturellePsychiatrie-Ergebnisse and probleme. Stuttgart: Verlag; 1970
27. Tooth E. Studies in Mental Illness in Goldcoast. Colonial Research Publication. London: Her Majesty's Stationary Office. 1950;6.
28. World Health Organization. Schizophrenia: An International Follow-up Study. Chicester: Wiley; 1979.
29. Sartorius N, Jablensky A, Shapiro R. Cross-cultural differences in short term prognosis of schizophrenic psychoses. Scliizophr. Bull. 1978;4:102-13.
30. Tsuang M. Schizophrenia around the world. Compr Psychiatry. 1976;17:477-81.
31. Waxler NE. Is mental illness cured in traditional societies? A theoretical analysis.Cult Med Psychiatry. 1977;1:233-53.
32. Carothers JC. A study of mental derangement in Africa and an attempt to explain its peculiarities more especially in relation to African attitude to life. Psychiatry. 1948;11:47-85.
33. Opler MK. Culture, Psychiatry and Human Values. Springfield: Charles C Thomas; 1956.
34. Lin TY. A study of the incidence of mental disorder in Chinese and other cultures. Psychiatry. 1953;16:313-36.
35. Carothers JC. The African mind in health and disease: A study in ethnopsychiatry. WHO Monograph Series. No. 17. Geneva: World Health Organization; 1953.
36. Carpenter ES. Witch fear among the Aivilik Eskimos. Am J Psychiatry. 1953;110:194.
37. Al-Issa I. Culture and Psychopathology. Baltimore: University Park Press; 1982.
38. Carstairs GM. The Twice Born: A study of a community of high caste Hindus. Bloomington: Indiana University Press; 1957.
39. Ford CS, Beach FA. Patterns of Sexual Behaviour. New York: Harper and Row; 1951.
40. Fried J. Acculturation and mental health among Indian migrants in Peru. In: Opier M (Ed). Culture and Mental Health. New York: Macmillan; 1959.
41. Pflanz M, Lambelet L. Zivilisationskankheiten and psychosomatischeproleme. I. LandlichenIndien. Munich Med Wschr; 1965.pp.1493-502.
42. Rin H, Lin TY. Mental illness among Formosan aboriginees as compared with the Chinese in Taiwan. J Ment Sci. 1962;108:134-46.
43. Yap PM. Words and things in comparative psychiatry, with special reference to the exotic psychoses. Acta Psychiatr Scand. l962;38:163.
44. Westermeyer J. On the epidemiology of amok violence. Arch Gen Psychiatry. 1973;28:873-6.
45. Murphy G. Human Potentialities. Baltimore: Penguin; 1975.
46. Weidman HH, Sussex JN. Cultural values and ego functioning in relation to the atypical culture-bound reactive syndromes. Paper presented at the II International Congress Society of Psychiatry, London; 1969.
47. Yap PM. Koro: A culture-bound depersonalization syndrome. Br J Psychiatry. 1965;111:43.
48. Yap PM. The Latah reaction: Its psychodynamics and nosological position. J Ment Sci. 1952;98:515.
49. Murphy HBM. History and evolution of syndromes: The striking case of latah and amok. In: Hammer M (Ed). Psychopathology. New York: Wiley; 1973.
50. Scchmale A, Engel GL. The giving up-given up complex. Arch Gen Psychiatry. 1967;17:135-45.
51. Newman PL. 'Wild man' behaviour in a New Guinea highlands community. Am Anthropol. 1964;66:1-19.
52. Rubel AJ. The epidemiology of a folk illness: Susto in Hispanic America. Ethnology. 1964;3:268-83.
53. Lambo TA. Neuropsychiatric observations in the Western Region of Nigeria. Br Med J 1956; ii: 1388.
54. Linton R. Culture and Mental Disorders. Springfield: Charles C Thomas; 1956.
55. Kroeber AC, Kluckhon C. Critical Review of Concepts and Definitions. New York: Vintage; 1952.
56. Wallace AFC. Culture and Personality. Homewood: Dorsey Press; 1961.
57. Barnouw V. Culture, Behaviour and Personality. Homewood: Dorsey Press; 1973.
58. Levine RA. Culture, Behaviour and Personality. Chicago: Aldine; 1973.
59. Honigman JJ. Personality in Culture. New York: Harper and Row; 1967.
60. Varma VK. The epistemology of 'mental' phenomena.Indian J Psychiatry. 1989;31:3-21.

61. Kardiner A, Linton R, Dubois C, et al. The Psychological Frontiers of Society. New York: Columbia University Press, 1945.
62. Hsu FLK. Psychological Anthropology: Approaches to Culture and Personality. Homewood: Dorsey Press, 1961.
63. Hsu FLK. Clan, Caste, Club. Princeton: Van Nostrand, 1963.
64. Neki JS. Psychotherapy in India: Past, present and future. Am J Psychother. 1975;29:92.
65. Neki JS. An examination of cultural relativism of dependence as a dynamic of social and therapeutic relationship. I. Socio-developmental. Br J Med Psychol. 1976;49:1-10.
66. Neki JS. An examination of cultural relativism of dependence as a dynamic of social and therapeutic relationship. II. Therapeutic. Br J Med Psychol. 1976;49:11-22.
67. Varma VK. Present state of psychotherapy in India. Indian J Psychiatry. 1982;24:209-26.
68. Varma VK. The Indian mind and psychopathology. Integr Psychiatry. 1985;3:290-6.
69. Hsu FLK. Americans and the Chinese. Garden City: Natural History Press; 1970.
70. Marriot M. Interpreting Indian society: A monistic alternative to Dumont's dualism. J Asian Stud. 1976;36:189-95.
71. Marriot M, Inden RB. Towards an ethnosociology of South Asian caste system. In: David K (Ed). The New Wind: Changing Identities in South Asia. The Hague: Mouton, 1977.
72. Marriot M. The open Hindu person and human sciences. Unpublished paper.
73. Vaima VK. Culture, personality and psychotherapy. Paper presented at the XIII International Congress of Psychotherapy, Opatija, Yugoslavia, October, 1985.
74. Whorf BL. Four Articles on Metalinguistics. Washington: Foreign Service Institute, 1950.
75. Brown R, Linnenberg EH. A study in language and cognition. J Abnorm Soc Psychol. 1954;49:254.
76. VarmaVK. Linguistic competence and psychopathology: A cross-cultural model. Indian J Psychiatry. 1982;24:107-14.
77. Arieti S. Interpretation of Schizophrenia. New York: Brunner; 1955.
78. Varma VK, Das K, Jiloha RC. Correlation of linguistic competence with psychopathology. Indian J Psychiatry. 1985;27:193-9.
79. Sethi BB, Sharma M. Family factors in psychiatric illness. In: Kiev A, VenkobaRao A (Ed). Readings in Transcultural Psychiatry. Madras: Higginbothams; 1982.
80. Varma VK. Psychosocial and cultural variables relevant to psychotherapy in developing countries. In: Psychiatry: The State of Art. No. 14. New York: Plenum; 1985.pp.159-65.
81. Hall CS, Lindzey G. The relevance of Freudian psychology and related viewpoints for the social sciences. In: The Handbook of Social Psychology. No. 1. Addison-Wesley; 1968.pp.245-319.
82. Lindgren HC. An Introduction to Social Psychology. New York: Wiley, 1969.
83. Fromm E. Individual and social origins of neurosis. In: Kluckhon C, Murray HA (Eds). Personality in Nature, Society and Culture. New York: Knopf; 1959.
84. Varma VK. Toward a theory of cultural defence. In: Kiev A, VenkobaRao A (Ed). Readings in Transcultural Psychiatry. Madras: Higginbothams; 1982.
85. Cicero. Cited in Encyclopedia Britannica. No. 1. 12. University of Chicago; 1964.pp.109.
86. Wittkower ED, Dubreuil. Reflections in the interface between psychiatry and anthropology. In: Gladston I (Ed). Interface between Psychiatry and Anthropology. New York: Brunner/Mazel, 1971.
87. Wittkower ED, Warnes H. Cultural aspects of psychotherapy. Am J Psychother. 1974;28:566.
88. Surya NC, Jayaram SS. Some basic considerations of psychotherapy in the Indian setting. Indian J Psychiatry. 1964;6:154.
89. Torrey EF. The Mindgame: Witchdoctors and Psychiatrists. New York: Emerson Hall; 1972.
90. Varma VK, Ghosh A. Psychotherapy as practiced by the Indian psychiatrists. Indian J Psychiatry. 1976;18:177-86.
91. Wig NN. Personal communication on transcultural psychiatry. Transcultural Psychiatric Research Review. 1975;7:37-39.
92. Bleuler M. On schizophrenica psychoses. Am J Psychiatry. 1979;136:1403-9.

FURTHER READING

1. American Psychiatric Association. Culture and psychiatry. Available fromwww.dsm5.org.
2. Behere PB, Behere M. Culture and Depression in proceedings of i 3th Mid Term CME of W.Z. of Indian Psychiatry Society. Nasik. 2004.
3. Brendan D. Kelly. Globalisation, psychiatry and human rights: new challenges for the 21st century. Published by RCPsych Publications. 2010; ISBN: 978-1-904671-82-4.
4. Gavin BE, Kelly BD, Lane A, et al. The mental health of migrants. Irish Medical Journal. 2001;94:229–30.
5. Gleize L, Laudon F, Sun LY, et al. Cancer registry of French Polynesia: results for the 1900–1995 periods among native and immigrant population. European Journal of Epidemiology. 2005;16:661-7.
6. Habel U, Gur RC, Mandal MK, et al. Emotional processing in schizophrenia across cultures: Standardized measures of discrimination and experience. Schizophr Res. 2000;42:57-66.
7. Jenkins JH, Karno M. The meaning of expressed emotion: Theoretical issues raised by cross-cultural research. Am J Psychiatr. 1992;149:9-21.
8. Kirmayer LJ, Groleau D. Affective disorders in cultural context. Psychiatr Clin N Am. 2001;24(3):465-78.
9. Kulhara P, Chakrabarti S. Culture and schizophrenia and other psychotic disorders. Psychiatr Clin N Am. 2001;24(3) (Sept.):449-64.

CHAPTER

59 Anthropology and Psychiatry

M Behere, PB Behere, A Das

INTRODUCTION

The term anthropology originates from the Greek word anthropos “man” (understood to mean humankind or humanity), and -logia "word" or "study." The term anthropology was coined by German university professors in 16th century. At that time it was not studied as a separate branch, rather it was seen as a systemic observation and examination of evolution of human mankind. The first use of the term "anthropology" in English to refer to a natural science of humanity was apparently in 1593, the first of the "logies" to be coined.[1] Anthropology is defined as the study of human beings, in particular the study of their physical character, evolutionary history, racial classification, historical and present-day geographic distribution, group relationships, and cultural history. Anthropology can be characterized as the naturalistic description and interpretation of the diverse peoples of the world. Modern-day anthropology consists of two major divisions: cultural anthropology, which deals with the study of human culture in all its aspects; and physical anthropology, which is the study of human physical character, in the past and present.[2]

Encyclopedia Americana defines it as the study of man from both a biological and a cultural perspective. There are various subtypes in anthropology depending on which part is defined. That part of anthropology concerned with man as an animal species is called physical anthropology. The portion concerned with the ways of life devised by human beings living in societies is called cultural anthropology. Ethnology (from the *Greek ethnos* meaning "nation") is the branch of *anthropology* that compares and analyzes the characteristics of different *peoples* and the relationship between them. *Social anthropology* is now defined as the study of social organization in nonstate societies and is sometimes referred to as socio cultural anthropology in the parts of the world that were influenced by the European tradition.[3] No single anthropologist can possibly cover all the ground marked out by this definition; however, man in his entirety is the central focus of all anthropological research.[4] Of late anthropology has been central in the development of several new (late 20th century) interdisciplinary fields such as *cognitive science,*[5] *global studies*, and various *ethnic studies*. Current modern anthropology also consists of biological anthropology, anthropological linguistics and applied anthropology.

Anthropology differs from history, as commonly understood, not by excluding historical studies of peoples, institutions, beliefs, or customs, but by using as far as possible direct observation of human beings, their activities and their products rather than documentary accounts; and also by viewing the results of any such study as part of the total human record and as a contribution to the better understanding of the complex processes involved in the biological and cultural development of mankind. Similarly, it differs in approach from physiology or psychology in concerning itself with variations and collective differences in human physique and mentality. Thus anthropologists seek to study and interpret the special characteristics of any particular population or activity in terms of its time and place in the total history of mankind.[6]

ANTHROPOLOGY AND MEDICINE: PSYCHOLOGICAL PERSPECTIVE

Medical anthropology studies “human health and disease, health care systems, and biocultural adaptation”. It views humans from multidimensional and *ecological* perspectives. It is one of the most highly developed areas of *anthropology* and *applied anthropology* and is a subfield of *social* and *cultural anthropology* that examines the ways in which culture and society are organized around or influenced by issues of *health, health care* and related issues. The term "medical anthropology" has been used since 1963 as a label for *empirical research* and theoretical production by anthropologists into the social processes and cultural representations of health, illness and the nursing care practices associated with these.[7]

The discipline draws upon the four fields of anthropology to analyze and compare the health of regional populations and of ethnic and cultural enclaves, both prehistoric and contemporary. There are three major domains in medical anthropology. Medical ecology views populations as biological as well as cultural units and studies interactions among ecological systems, health, and human evolution. Ethnomedical analysis focuses on cultural systems of healing and the cognitive parameters of illness. Applied medical anthropology deals with intervention, prevention, and policy issues and analyzes the socioeconomic forces and power differentials that influence access to care.[8] Culture is almost always associated with the three domains. Among medical anthropology psychological aspect is strongly inter-related to culture and society. Psychological anthropology is an interdisciplinary subfield of anthropology that studies the interaction of *cultural* and *mental processes.* This subfield tends to focus on ways in which humans' development and *enculturation* within a particular cultural group—with its own history, language, practices, and conceptual categories—shape processes of human *cognition, emotion, perception, motivation,* and *mental health.* It also examines how the understanding of cognition, emotion, motivation, and similar psychological processes inform or constrain our models of cultural and social processes. Each school within psychological anthropology has its own approach.

Medical anthropology is a robust expanding subfield of social anthropology. It includes comparative study of healing systems and the social, economic, political and cultural context of health and health care. The field also encompasses the study of how social processes produce health effects and how cultural processes construct illness experience.

The fields contribution of general medicine in domains of infectious diseases, chronic medical disorders, disability and public health have arguably become increasingly visible and relevant since late 1970s, where as the recently emerging paradigm of neurobiological psychiatry increasingly locates mental illness in the brain and favors universalizing theory of psychiatric illness, anthropology engages the diversity of human experience.

PSYCHIATRIC ANTHROPOLOGY

Anthropology and psychiatry have been historically linked since the late nineteenth century when WHR. Rivers, a psychiatrist, was joined by several other physicians on an expedition to the Torres Strait. That research trip to the South Pacific was the source of much empirical research in British social anthropology. Rivers' ethnographic and clinical expertise converged not only in his cross-cultural studies on religious healing and on pain sensation but also in the form of psychotherapy that he later developed to treat soldiers with shell shock during World War I.

The relation between anthropology and psychiatry dates back to the 1904 when Kraepelin wrote its relation in the essays of *Comparative Psychiatry.* However, the observation of ethnic differences in mental illness was found as early as the 18th century. In 19th and 20th century, the physicians working in colonies described the symptoms which seemed strange from the European-American point of view, i.e. from the viewpoint of western culture and civilization. These culture specific symptoms were referred to as culture bound syndromes.[9,10] In 1978, American cultural psychiatrists AR Favazza and M Oman proposed the term cultural psychiatry.

Anthropology and psychiatry are both concerned with the understanding of human behavior. Anthropology is study of culture, which is the external expression of individual mental life as represented by manners, customs, skills, language, parent-child interactions, beliefs, and social life. Cultures differ in their definitions of health, illness, and healing and also vary greatly in child-rearing patterns, social models and opportunities, and other variables. Anthropology also includes cross cultural studies, which are used in the field of comparative psychiatry to describe and analyze cross-cultural variations in the incidence and prevalence of syndromes. Disorders are compared from one culture to another to see if there are universal characteristics that transcend cultural differences. Classic examples include the state of trance and obsession which are usual and normal in many nonwestern cultures. The manner a person accepts and experiences illness, deals with it, understands it and lives with it are—from anthropologists' viewpoint is crucial for the understanding and treatment of illness. That is the reason why anthropologists speak of the social course of an illness, which means that the local environment shapes the progress of an illness to the extent that in different surroundings it follows a different course.

Mihanovic, et al[11] have described the contributions of anthropology in psychiatry.

- Anthropology gives importance to the relevance of social environment in the diagnosis, treatment and prognosis as well as in creating concepts and methods that psychiatrists are able to apply.
- Anthropology helps in contributing to socially optimal psychiatric programs.
- It differs from neurobiological approach to psychiatry, anthropology offers a transnational and transethnic approach (Fig. 1).
- Anthropology secures the development of politics and programs implying close interconnectedness of social conditions and mental health.
- Anthropology helps in better adaptation to the local cultural environment for psychiatric knowledge and practice.

The relevance of anthropological contributions to psychiatry is most apparent in three critical areas.

First, from a theoretical standpoint, the documentation of particular mental disorders in different sociocultural contexts provides evidence for their syndromes significance and integrity in the absence of biological markers.

Second, from a clinical standpoint, the elicitation of explanatory models from and the engagement of the growing number of patients from culturally and ethnically diverse backgrounds play an essential role in formulating illness and responding to it in culturally appropriate ways.

Third, from a public health perspective, understanding the social production and social course of mental illness suggests means of improving outcome of even preventing illness.

ETIC AND EMIC CONSTRUCTS

In the study of cognition in organizations, and in social science more broadly, there are two approaches to understanding the role of culture and its impact on mental illness: (1) the inside perspective of ethnographers, who strive to describe a particular culture in its own terms, and (2) the outside perspective of comparativist researchers, who attempt to describe differences across cultures in terms of a general, external standard.[12] Pike (1967) designates these approaches as the *emic* and *etic* perspectives. Mental illness can be described in both the constructs. To minimize the risk of creating a category fallacy, it is helpful to draw from the anthropological concepts of etic and emic levels of analysis in investigating psychiatric disorders transculturally. Etic, in this case refers to the application of Western categories to another cultural context, whereas emic refers to the use of locally meaningful categories.[13]

- An '*emic*' account is a description of behavior based on one's own cultural influences; i.e. an *emic* account comes from a person within the culture. Almost anything from within a culture can provide an *emic* account (Fig. 2).
- An '*etic*' account is a description of a behavior or belief based on influences of another culture (Fig. 3).

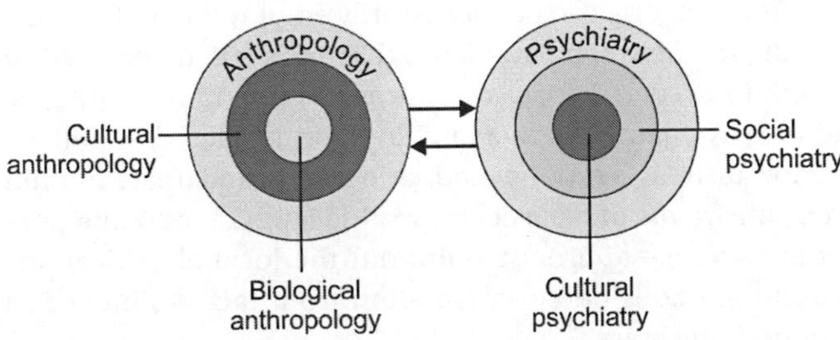

Fig. 1: Mihanovic, et al[11] relation of anthropology and psychiatry

SOCIAL FACTORS INFLUENCING MENTAL HEALTH

Environmental Factor

- Poverty
- Racial discrimination
- Poor housing
- Poor health care.

Social Change

- Unemployment
- Migration
- Urbanization.

The contribution of anthropology has been to define the influence of culture on views of causation and appropriate treatment of mental disorders. When the cultural backgrounds of the patient and the clinician are divergent, they might not share basic assumptions about the probable origin, nature and treatment of mental disorders.[14]

CULTURAL INFLUENCES

Culture has been defined by Cecil Helman as a set of guidelines by which the individuals of a particular society

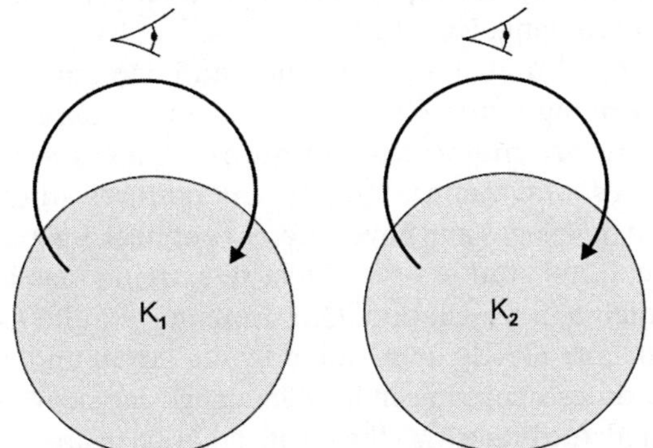

Fig. 2: Mihanovic, et al[11] Emic approach to comprehension and interpretation of a mental disorder. Cultures (K1, K2) are observed from within, i.e. they are their own reference systems

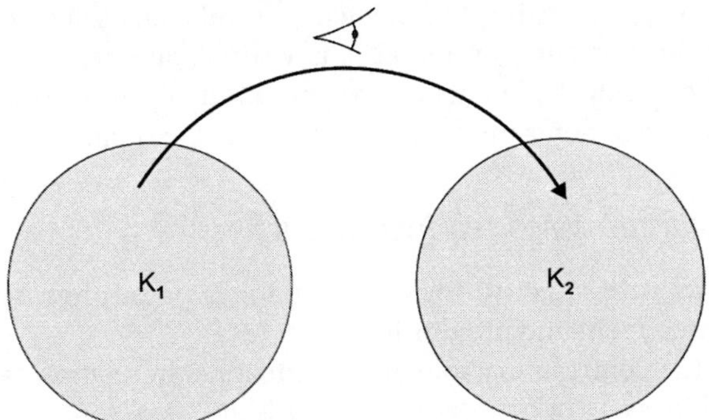

Fig. 3: Mihanovic, et al[11] Etic approach to comprehension and interpretation of a mental disorder. The culture (K1) from which is observed is taken as a system of reference

view the world, experience it emotionally and behave in relation to other people, to the supernatural and to nature.

Culture means the total way of life of a given group of people. If refers to an organized group of ideas, habits conditions and, emotional responses shared by the members of a social group. The technology economic system, family structure, religious beliefs and value system are implied in concept of culture.

Definition of what is normal and abnormal behavior vary widely from culture to culture and, within any given group, are dependent on demographic factors such as age and sex, social class, and occupation. Behaviors that may be perceived as abnormal at one time may be regarded as normal at other times, such as during carnivals. At these times, it is culturally acceptable for men to dress as women or animals.[15] Western doctors may encounter behaviors that in other societies are acceptable, at least some times, but that could be interpreted as signs of mental illness.

Culture is transmitted down the generations by language, symbols and rituals; neither static not homogeneous, nor the differences between members of one cultural group can be as great as the differences between members of different cultural groups. It is important not to blame culture for economic and social hardship and racial discrimination. Thus overcrowding might be due to poverty and/or discrimination in housing, rather than to the extended family.

The influences of culture include:

- Patients' illness behavior
- The content of delusions and hallucinations
- Attitudes of the family and community
- Assumptions regarding the recognition and etiology of illness
- The appropriateness of treatment.

Arthur Kleinman[16] has developed the concept of Explanatory Models in order to understand the cultural influences each person brings to his or her illness. In non-industrialized small-scale societies, social causes of both mental and physical illness (e.g. envy, the evil eye, witchcraft) and supernatural causes (e.g. malign spirit possession) are common explanations for sickness. In Western societies, etiologies tend to be physiological (e.g. imbalance, deficiency, heredity) or environmental (e.g. viruses, allergens). These and etiological explanations are not mutually exclusive, and for many patients the explanation is multifactorial.

Explanatory Models Incorporate

- Culture-specific ideas of etiology, pathophysiology, treatment and prognosis.
- The contributory role of the individual in relation to the illness.
- The contributory role of the individual's social milieu in relation to the illness.

Somatization

This is the cultural patterning of psychological discomfort ('dysphoria') into the language of bodily distress which employs the idiom of physical ill health, especially pain, weal mess and fatigue. It cannot be regarded as a purely not Western phenomenon, since it is commonly found in those who have rule ability to 'psychologize', i.e. to express worry, depression and anxiety verbally. The expression of psychological distress in Western cultures depends much upon the language of the mind/body split. Where the relationship between mind and body is conceived differently (as in the Indian subcontinent), a different, usually somatic, language is employed to express psychological distress.[14] In India, there is somatization of psychological stress as compared to 'Psychologize' of somatic symptoms in westerns culture.

The relationship between psychopathology and culture remains a vexed question. Whilst organic reactions (and by extension the functional psychoses) can be conveniently coded in terms of an invariate biologically determined form and a culturally variable content, the same is not true of those reactions which we might feel are characteristic of Western society: agoraphobia, anorexia nervous, self-poisoning, Briquet's syndrome or the chronic pain syndromes. Hence cultural explanations are offered, however, they usually employ nave and implicit anthropological assumptions, and it is perhaps only the phenomenon of conversion hysteria in the nineteenth century which has been adequately related to its social context.[17]

As lay theories do not necessarily employ the professional distinction between psychiatric disorders and other medical conditions, such medical classifications offer much of interest to the psychiatrist, particularly in their detailed descriptions of how distress is experienced, recognized, and treated within the constraints of a particular world view. Critics of the pure ethno science approach point out the local classifications cannot be considered in isolation from tacit political and cultural processes.[18]

Medical anthropology offers psychiatry a fresh approach to the question of biology and culture which does not employ the form/content distinction.

Cross-cultural studies examine and compare different cultures along a number of parameters: attitudes, beliefs, expectations, memories, opinions, roles stereotypes, prejudices, and values. Usually, the cultures studied use different languages and have different political organizations. Cross-cultural studies are subject to extreme bias because of problems in translation. Questions have to be asked in ways that are clearly understood by the group under study. Many a times symptoms in local language can not exactly be translated into English. At the most, it may be nearest possible translation. At times is process of translation the meaning and originality changes.

Diagnoses of mental disorders have been conducted among various cultures by the World Health Organization. The International Pilot Study of Schizophrenia[19] confirmed that schizophrenia exists among all groups studied (e.g. Nigerians, Danes, Laotians, Celts, Croatians, Hutterites, Indian, South Pacific Tongans, and Taiwanese) and is constant across cultures. Outcome studies of patients with schizophrenia, however, are not reliable because some societies (in contrast to the United States) do not stigmatize persons with mental illness, who are quickly reintegrated into the society. A major difficulty in cross-cultural diagnosis is the bias arising from the researcher's cultural background.

Certain symptoms exist in all societies: Anxiety, mania, depression, suicidal ideation, somatization, paranoia (persecutory delusions), and thought disorder. Although different labels may be applied in different cultures, recognition of deviant behavior and agreement that conditions are treatable (whether by the psychiatrist in one culture or the shaman in another) are universal.[20]

CULTURAL ASPECTS OF DISEASE

Ethnic origin plays a great role in the way an illness is perceived. Doctor patient relationship, treatment and prognosis are all dependent on the ethnicity. It is important, however, to avoid generalizations. The patients must be understood in terms of the specific culture of ethnic group to which he or she belongs. Mexican Americans and Puerto Rican Americans, e.g. share as many group cultural differences as they do commonalities. Different cultures—Haitians, West Indians, Puerto Ricans, and Christian faith healers—incorporate shamans, persons who follow a divine call to healing. The clinician must find out how acculturated the patient is to the cultural mainstream of life. The influence of culture on the reporting and presentation of symptoms must be considered.[21] A reluctance to discuss certain topics may stern from the patient's individual psychology or from adherence the customs and etiquette of the social group.

Conversion disorder is seen much less frequently in America today compared with 19th century European society. The symptoms of anorexia nervous are related to the cultural expectations of weight and body image in modern Western industrial society. The conversion dissociation disorders are frequently seen in India.

Numerous studies have sought to demonstrate the cross-cultural epidemiology of major mental illness, both, to demonstrate the universality of particular syndromes and to investigate how prevalence and phenomenology may differ relative to cultural context. The interpretation of findings, however, has been limited by major methodological pitfalls in conducting transcultural research and a persistent tendency to interpret data as evidence of universality rather than of heterogeneity of disorders.

Anthropologists have argued that emotions, such as a depressed or anxious mood, are themselves culturally constituted and that the ways in which feelings are experienced, processed, and communicated are constrained and evolved by the cultural milieu.[22]

These problems are somewhat attenuated when local ethno psychological or ethno medical theories are used to establish illness or emotional categories relevant to the cultural group being studied. For example, the revised second edition of Chinese Classification of Mental Disorders (CCMD-2-R) represents an attempt to include Chinese mental illness nosology within a Western psychiatric nosology. The CCMD-2-R includes such illness categories as shelving shuairuo (neurasthenia) and quigong-induced mental disorder and train or travel psychosis is a candidate diagnosis while excluding certain Western disorders that hold no local relevance, such as somatoform disorders, pathological gambling, and some personality disorders.

The bias in cross-cultural epidemiological research in investigating and reporting universals rather than the heterogeneity of illness presentations is exemplified in the International Pilot Study of Schizophrenia (IPSS)[19] and the Determinants of Outcome Study sponsored by the World Health Organization.[23] The IPSS attempted to document core schizophrenic symptoms in diverse cultural contexts. Although it succeeded in establishing clusters of similar symptoms across a variety of Western and nonwestern contexts, its rigorous inclusion and exclusion criteria effectively selected for homogeneity and against heterogeneity across cases. Despite this selection bias, the IPSS documented that the course of schizophrenia differed cross-culturally. However, this finding was deemphasized relative to the demonstration of core schizophrenic symptoms across cultures. Similarly, although data generated from the Determinants of Outcome Study showed impressive variation in the cross-cultural prevalence of subtypes of schizophrenia, the authors of the study chose to highlight cross-cultural similarities.[24]

The WHO (1979) researchers concluded that there were "clear differences in the course and outcome of schizophrenia, with patients in developing countries on the average having a better course and outcome than those in centers in the developed countries". The outcome may be more favorable in settings characterized by agricultural economy, little vertical mobility, extended families, psychiatric services which include the active participation of the family, and the absence of specific community stereotypes of the mentally ill.[23]

Cultural differences in psychiatric illness have been commonly understood as superimposed on biological substrates. Within this model of biological primacy, culture has been conceptualized as contributing only to the particular local manifestations of an underlying disorder. Anthropological research challenges this perspective by providing data on the dialectical interplay of psychobiological and sociocultural processes in the prevalence, phenomenology, course, and outcome of mental illness.[25]

CLASSIFICATION

Due to influence of culture in psychopathology, various authors tired to put cultural component in classification of psychiatric disorders.

It has been frequently observed that symptoms of patients can be more meaningfully related to their sociocultural background than to their diagnoses; further the prevailing cultural and social beliefs and values influence the content of various psychopathological patterns.[26]

Attempts were made at evolving an Indian classification of psychiatric disorders (Wig and Singh, 1967;[27] Teja 1971[28]) Wig and Singh (1967)[27] proposed a classification of psychiatric disorders. Teja (1971)[28] further proposed a classification of "Other Psychoses" for use in India.

In one of the WHO multifaceted collaborative studies across countries, it was found that the existing classification of mental disorders needs modification which is more culturally relevant (Agrawal et al. 1993).[29] A question was raised to what extent are local conceptualizations of distress actually part of the symptomatology. It was even suggested to include introductory cultural statement in DSM IV together with a provisional appendix with some such title, at the beginning of preparation of DSM IV (APA, 1994).[30]

The Dhat syndrome in the context of culture has been included in ICD-10 in other neurotic disorders.[31,32] The outcome of schizophrenia differs in various countries due to influence of culture. Explanatory model of mental disorders in Indian psychiatric patients was further put forward to elicit the culture models of illness, pattern of help seeking and their determinants.[33]

There are so many social factors which relate to income level to the incidence and prevalence to mental illness. Studies of suicide are often quoted as evidence for the influence of economic factors since suicide and unemployment are undoubtedly linked.[34] A lot of written about spiritual values and mental health.[35] Religious contents of various symptomatology is reported by Behere.[36,37]

Behere (1993) emphasized the value of patients and their key relatives own explanation of mental illness, like dietary restriction, etc. help us in understanding symptomatology and improve outcome or follow-up.[33]

Ujalambkar and Behere (1998) extensively reviewed cultured correlates of maintenance therapy for schizophrenia.[38]

The one of the important factors in better outcome in developing countries including India was, community care of schizophrenia with strong family support and schizophrenia are better care in community.[39]

Finally the cultural anthropology contributes to Medicine and Psychiatry in 3 principal ways:

1. The first is by providing descriptions of cultures and sub cultural groups and their customs, communications and beliefs. Such understanding have broad implications for the incidence and prevalence of disease, behavior during illness, and the nature of cooperation with health care specialists in preventing or treating disease.
2. A second major contribution of cultural anthropology to medicine and psychiatry consist of the rich body of information that has increased our understanding of certain universal characteristics of individuals, families and groups.
3. The third contribution lies in cross-cultural methods of research that have been applied to clinical studies in medicine and psychiatry. These methods have been fruitful in defining both variations and shared features in the experience of disease among various ethnic and national groups. For example, the incidence of gastric carcinoma, hypertension, and myocardial infarction among some descendants of Japanese immigrants who settled in the USA and Brazil has been compared with the incidence observed in cousin cohorts in Japan. Results showed lower rates of cardiovascular disease among Japanese who did not emigrate but higher rates of gastric carcinoma. Since the hereditary factors are relatively invariant in both groups, some combination of dietary, environmental, and stress factors must be sought in an effort to explain the differences in incidence of these diseases.[40]

The culture and depression[41] and culture and psychiatry[42] is dealt extensively elsewhere in this book in different chapter.

FUTURE OF ANTHROPOLOGY AND PSYCHIATRY

According to Klienman[43] psychiatry and mental health has almost turned its back on anthropology and has moved away from sociocultural sciences. It has become more oriented and focused in the study of genetics, neuroimaging and neurobiology. On the contrary, anthropology has much to offer to psychiatry and mental health. Development of new anthropologically-informed research approaches should be the focus in coming years.

The term "social suffering" was coined by Veena Das, Margaret Lock and Kleinman[43] to emphasize how ordinary social life everywhere is experienced as pain and suffering at least as much as joy and happiness, and that such collective pain and suffering is normative and normal. Social suffering also referred to extraordinary human experience from the social consequences of individual catastrophes to collective disasters. Anthropology and psychiatry and public health, will not be on the classical order of the normal and the abnormal; but rather will involve a much deeper phenomenology of the forms of social suffering; an epidemiology of the causes and consequences of social suffering; and the implementation science of policy and programs for that subset of social suffering that is represented by psychiatric disorder as well as for psychiatric conditions that are not tied to social suffering.

Social death refers to the stigma attached to mental disorders. Anthropological research should be implemented to remove this social death.

There is a huge ethnographic imbalance in the way treatment is provided to mentally ill. Studies have found that the underprivileged class of society are always under diagnosed and under treated; whereas the upper class are always over diagnosed and over treated with unnecessary poly pharmacy. Anthropological studies can help to protect the mentally ill by providing health care services such as appropriate psychopharmaceuticals, and also including resources that support families who are placed under the greatest financial, social and moral pressure. This research is urgently needed to balance the ethnographic picture.[43]

The current age is what is called golden age of neurobiology. New neurobiology is recasting both cultural common sense and scientific logic about cognition, affect and abnormality. Anthropological research should be merged along with new neurobiological studies to better understand human behavior.

REFERENCES

1. "Four-Field Commentary:" in Anthropology Newsletter. American Anthropological Association (Washington, DC). 1992;33(9):3.
2. Encyclopaedia Britanica CD, 2002.
3. Layton, Robert. An Introduction to Theory in Anthropology. Cambridge: Cambridge University Press; 1998.pp.40-3.
4. Encyclopaedia Americans. American Corporation, New York. 1970;2:43-52.
5. Bloch Maurice. "Language, Anthropology and Cognitive Science". Man (London School of Economics and Political Science). 1991;26(2):183-98.
6. The New Encyclopaedia Britannica. The Encyclopaedia Britannica, Inc. Chicago. 1989;1:446-7.
7. Bibeau, Gilles. Cultural Psychiatry in a Creolizing World. Questions for a New Research Agenda, Transcultural Psychiatry. 1997;34(1):9-41.
8. A McElroy, D Levinson, M Ember. Medical Anthropology. Encyclopaedia of Cultural Anthropology, New York. 1996;26: 44-6.
9. Wittkower DR. Prince: A review of transcultural psychiatry. In: Arieti S (Ed): American Handbook of Psychiatry. Vol. 1, 2nd edn. (New York: Basic Books, 1974)—2.
10. Tseng WS. Handbook of Cultural Psychiatry. (Academic Press, San Diego, 2001).
11. M Mihanovic, et al. Anthropology and Psychiatry. Coll Anthropology. 2005;29(2):747-51.
12. Michael Morris, et al. Views from inside and outside: integrating emic and etic insights about culture and justice judgment. Academy of Management Review. 1999;24(1):781-96.
13. Eisenberg L. Psychiatry and health I low-income populations. Comprehensive Psychiatry. 1997;38:69.
14. Rees R, Lipsedge M, Chris B. Textbook of Psychiatry Oxford University Press, 1997.
15. Dein S. Mental Health in multiethnic society. In ABC of mental health Eds. Davies T, Craig TKG. London: BMJ Books publications, 1998.
16. Kleinman. A patients & Healers in the context of culture, University of California Press, Berkeley, 1980.
17. Ellenberger HB. The Discovery of the Unconscious: The History and Evolution of Dynamic Psychiatry: London: Allen Lane, 1970.
18. Good BJ. The heart of what's the matter: The semantics of illness in Iran. Culture, Medicine & Psychiatry. 1977;1:25-8.
19. World Health Organisation. The Report of the International Pilot Study of Schizophrenia. Geneva, 1973, WHO.
20. Kaplan H, Sadock. Synopsis of Psychiatry Williams and Wilkins, Baltimore, USA, 1991.
21. Behere PB, Behere M. Influence of culture in Schizophrenia. In current developments in schizophrenia. Mandel, M and Nizamie H (Ed). Allied Publishers Pvt. Ltd., 2004.
22. Good BJ. Medicine, Rationality, and Experience: An Anthropologic Perspective. Cambridge University Press, Cambridge, 1994.
23. World Health Organisation. Schizophrenia: An international follow up study. Chicester, Welley. 1979.
24. Kirmayer LJ, Young A. Culture and somatization: Clinical, epidemiological and ethnographic perspectives. Psychosomatic Medicine. 1998;60:420.
25. Kleinman A, Becker AE, Dimsdale J. "Sociosomatics:" The contributions of anthropology of psychosomatic medicine. Psychosomatic Medicine. 1998;60:389.
26. Kulhara P, Matto SK, Chandiramni K. Diagnostic symptoms for schizophrenia—A cross sectional study of concordance from India. Acta Psychiatric Scandinavica. 1986;74:55-61.
27. Wig NN, Singh G. A proposed classification of psychiatric disorders for use in India. Indian Journal of Psychiatry. 1967; 9:158-67.
28. Teja JS. Proposed classification of other psychoses for use in India. Indian Journal of Psychiatry. 1971;13:7-10.
29. Agrwal AK, Abuja N, Awasthi A, Bandopadhyay G, Behere PB, et al. ICD-10 field trials in India—A report, WHO sponsored study. Supplement. Indian Journal of Psychiatry. 1993;35:198-222.
30. American Psychiatric Association Diagnostic and statistical manual of mental disorders Washington DC: American Psychiatric Association, 1994.
31. Behere PB, Natraj GS. Dhat syndrome: The phenomenology of culture bound sex neurosis of the orient. Indian J Psychiat. 1984;26:76-8.

32. Behere PB, Wig NN, Mehere M. Ancient Indian concept of Dhat syndrome: A cultural bound sex neurosis of the orient. Indian J Psychological Medicine. 1991;14:85-7.
33. Behere PB. Explanatory model of mental disorders in Indian psychiatry patients. Central Zone Oration. Indian J Behan Sc. 1993;1:11-4.
34. Dublin L. Suicide: A serological and statistical study, New York, Ronald Press, 1963.
35. Wig NN. Mental Health and Spiritual values. A view from the east. International Review of Psychiatry. 1999;11:92-6.
36. Behere PB, Behere M. The influence of traditional beliefs & religion on mental illness psychopathologyin India. Transcultural Psychiatry Bulletin (In press), 2000.
37. Behere PB. The influence of traditional beliefs and religion on mental illness in India In the proceedings of Third International Congress on Traditional Asian Medicine, Bombay, 1990.
38. Ujalambakar, Behere PB. Maintainance therapy of schizophrenia Journal of CI. Psychiatry, India. 1998;3:11-6.
39. Behere PB, Ujalambkar S. Community care of schizophrenia: Indian scene. Schizophrenia Bulletin. 1999;2:18-21.
40. Johnson FA. Contributions of Anthropology to Psychiatry. In Review of General Psychiatry. Goldman HH (Ed), 1984; Lange Medical Publication USA.
41. Behere PB, Behere M. Culture and Depression. Proceedings of 13th Mid Term CME of West Zone of Indian Psychiatric Society 2004, at Nasik, 29–30 May.
42. Behere PB, Behere M. Culture and psychiatry. In: Textbook of Postgraduate Psychiatry. 2005; Pars Medical Pub. Hyderabad.
43. Arthur Kleinman. Medical Anthropology and Mental Health: Five Questions for the Next Fifty Years. 2005. pp.178-96.

CHAPTER

60

Psychiatry and Spirituality

CRJ Khess, Sourav Khanra, Swarnali Bose, Jayati Simlai

"Spirituality is not necessarily exclusive; it can be and in its fullness must be all-inclusive."

—Sri Aurobindo (The Renaissance in India, 1918)

INTRODUCTION

Though rooted in ancient times in history of human civilization, spirituality has only recently gained attention in the field of mental health care. Even after full and comprehensive effort to conceptualize and comprehend mental illness from various aspects like psychology, sociocultural view, biology, etc. had been made, culture had always been found to modify mental illness in terms of etiopathogenesis or course or both. Spirituality, a key component of culture is much broader and ever growing concept. The word 'spirituality' comes from the Latin word *'spiritus'*. The word *'spiritus'* itself is a translation from a Greek word *'pneuma'* which is originated from a Hebrew word meaning 'breeze', 'wind', 'breath', the 'life principle' or 'breath of life'. It provides a reason to live for many people. Spirituality being a principal component of culture has drawn attention of many researchers. It would not be illogical to mention here that spirituality is often associated with religion and used interchangeably. The spiritual and/or religious practices as a means of cure for mental illness can be dated back in 13th century.

Historically, in medieval Europe, the shrines of St Maturin and St Aquarius in France, St Dymphna in Flanders drew attention for miraculous cure for people with mental illnesses. In 1247 the priory of St Mary of Bethlehem was founded in Kent, England, for the care of the insane. But, those institutes had been criticized for the inhumanities that arose there and elsewhere and the so-called 'moral approach' to the care of the insane gradually became dominant in the then mental health care. In the late 18th-century, this movement was led by William Tuke, a Quaker, who established the Retreat at York for the humane care of people with mental disorders. In parallel with this, there were remarkable developments in brain localization and neurohistology during the 19th century in Germany. Wilhelm Griesinger regarded 'mental illnesses' as 'illnesses of the nerves and brain' (1867). As far as interlink between religion and psychiatry was concerned, these discoveries fueled an attitude of reductionism. Meanwhile, French psychiatrists started to think complex behavior to be occurring as a result of unconscious mechanisms, ultimately influenced by the state of the brain. Jean-Martin Charcot and Pierre Janet had initiated the beginnings of psychotherapy by the end of the 19th century. Religion and faith were not seen as exclusively necessary for explaining human activity. Another development in this area was Charles Darwin's Origin of the Specie, the concepts of 'natural selection' and 'survival of the fittest' had impact for the care of the mentally ill. His work led to the subsequent interest in 'somatology', which discounted everything about man. To add with this, hypothesis of 'degeneration' postulated that all psychiatric illness was to be inherited and to become more severe in later generations. Putting them all together these theories and developments ushered therapeutic nihilism over several decades in psychiatry, which inhibited the search for new, effective methods of treatment. The whole scenario became more colored and conflicting with arrival of Sigmund Freud. He had asserted that belief in a single God was delusional and that all religions are mass neurosis. Psychoanalysis was in conflict with traditional religious attitudes and many churches identified Freud, psychoanalysis and by association the whole of psychiatry, to be antagonistic to religion and a challenge. By the 1960s, there was no sense that the patient's religious beliefs contributed significantly to the psychiatric history, formulation or planning of treatment. Spiritual aspects of the patient's mental health problem were usually started to be ignored. In 1968, the Committee on Psychiatry and Religion of the Group for the Advancement of Psychiatry published a report where they reported the positive as well as the negative influences of religion on mental health. In 1986, a seminal review article by Larson and colleagues documenting the lack of adequate literature on the mental health effects of religion, was published in the American Journal of Psychiatry. The Scientific and Medical Network was set-up in 1974, encouraging the exploration of the interface between spirituality, consciousness and mind. In 1994, the newly published revision of the Diagnostic and Statistical Manual of the American Psychiatric Association (DSM-IV) included for the first time a category of 'religious or spiritual problem.' In 1997, the Archbishop of Canterbury addressed a joint annual meeting of the Royal College of Psychiatrists and the Association of European Psychiatrists. Religious belief was still not regarded as respectable by the rest of the profession but there was less agitation and animosity. Psychiatry, as a profession, became more accepting of the spiritual and religious concerns of patients and more interested in the relationship between psychiatry and religion. Research in the area of mental illness and religious belief developed during the 1990s from almost none to an accepted and significant area of enquiry with research funding. Correspondingly, publications on spirituality in the psychological and health care literature increased exponentially.[1]

WHAT IS SPIRITUALITY?

As mentioned earlier the meaning of spirituality and religion are overlapping but distinctively different. Spiritual persons may neither participate in a religion nor possess religiosity, or they may participate in a religion but lack religiosity, or they may participate and have religiosity. In some instances people who attend church may be spiritual but lack religiosity, or people may possess religiosity but not attend church, and so on. Mentioning all possible and available definition would be beyond the scope of this chapter, but to begin with, following working definitions can be considered for their specific relevance to psychiatry.

"Spirituality is a distinctive, potentially creative and universal dimension of human experience arising both within the inner subjective awareness of individuals and within communities, social groups and traditions. It may be experienced as relationship with that which is intimately 'inner,' immanent and personal, within the self and others, and/or as relationship with that which is wholly 'other,' transcendent and beyond the self. It is experienced as being of fundamental or ultimate importance and is thus concerned with matters of meaning and purpose in life, truth and values" (Cook, 2004a: pp. 548–549).[2]

Noteworthy from the above definition are universality of spirituality as a subjective dimension of the experience of being human, at the same time an attempt to recognize that this is still, nonetheless, a socially situated phenomenon.

"Spirituality...is a way of being and experiencing that comes through awareness of a transcendental dimension and that is characterized by certain identifiable values in regard to self, others, nature, life and whatever one considers to be ultimate"(Elkins et al. 1988).[3]

Here spirituality is an intra, inter and transpersonal experience that is shaped and directed by the experiences of individuals and of the communities within which they live out their lives. It is intrapersonal in that it refers to the voyage for inner connectivity. It is interpersonal in that it relates to the relationships between people and within communities. It is transpersonal in as it reaches beyond self and others into the consummate dominion of experience that move beyond that which is available at a prosaic level.[4]

Religion is also susceptible to widely varying definitions—the emphasis varies from one definition to another including personal, social, belief and others behavior, tradition and others function, and so on. For the purpose of discussion we have to keep in mind that religion is concerned with socially and traditionally shared beliefs and experience, and while doing so we must not forget of its personal and subjective dimension.[5]

For current purposes, spirituality can be categorized into two types: 'nonreligious' and 'religious.' While human spirituality is institutionalized and ritualized within particular religious traditions, it is not defined as a specifically religious concept. Formal, organized religion is viewed as one of a number of ways for the expression of human spirituality. This broader understanding views spirituality as a common human experience that forms an integral part of every person's striving to make sense of the world and their life within it. Such understanding incorporates humanistic, existential and philosophical perspectives as well as religious ones. Larson, Swyers and McCullough[6] define the criterion for such a wider understanding of spirituality thus:

- The feelings, thoughts, experiences, and behaviors that arise from a search for the sacred. The term 'search' refers to attempts to identify, articulate, maintain, or transform. The term 'sacred' refers to a Divine Being or Ultimate Reality or Ultimate Truth as perceived by the individual...
- The means and methods (e.g. rituals or prescribed behaviors) of the search that receive validation and support from within an identifiable group of people.

Understanding of spirituality manifests itself in various forms and includes perspectives drawn inter alia from religious, humanistic, atheistic and agnostic conceptions of spirituality. Below given some of the central features of this expanded definition of spirituality.

- Meaning the ontological significance of life; making sense of life situations; deriving purpose in existence.
- Value beliefs and standards that are cherished; having to do with the truth, beauty, worth of a thought, object or behavior; often discussed as 'ultimate values.'
- Transcendence experience and appreciation of a dimension beyond the self; expanding self-boundaries.
- Connecting relationships with self, others, God/higher power, and the environment.
- Becoming an unfolding of life that demands reflection and experience; includes a sense of who one is and how one knows.[7]

One may notice that spirituality's definition is more subjective, less measurable. From a clinical perspective, having a term that is broad and diffuse is good because this allows patients to define what it means for them. As noted earlier the term is often used to denote the experiential and personal side of our relationship to the eternal or sacred. Those who use the term in this way typically contrast it with religion, which they define narrowly as the organizational structures, practices, and beliefs of a religious group. Theologians and religious practitioners, on the other hand, tend to prefer definitions that draw less of a strict division between religion and spirituality. In their views, spirituality is the living reality of religion as experienced by an adherent of the tradition. Roof (1999)[8] argues that spirituality encompasses 4 themes: (1) a source of values and ultimate meaning or purpose beyond the self, including a sense of mystery and self-transcendence; (2) a way of understanding; (3) inner awareness; and (4) personal integration. The theme of personal integration is particularly important. Spirituality has an integrative and harmonizing function that involves (a) our inner unity and (b) our relationship and connectedness with others and to a broader reality that powers our ability to be transcendent. Thus, the fact that we are spiritual is not a separate nature or characteristic that we have but an inseparable part of all we are and do. What is clear from available literature is that spirituality is much more inclusive than religiosity and it is a human dimension which is understandably universal. Spirituality does not follow set of assumptions or beliefs or practices.

FORMS OF SPIRITUALITY

The definitions of spirituality are over-inclusive rather than exclusive, as we have noted, there are many ways people follow to lead and achieve spiritual life. What is a spiritual life to a person may not be so to other persons. This section describes some of those ways people choose to attain spirituality.

- *Prayer and meditation:* Prayer and meditation are perhaps the most important spiritual practices. Prayer is a central feature of many religious traditions.[9] Though it is typically associated with Christianity, many people in the devotional traditions of Hinduism and Buddhism also practice it. It can be expressive or introspective type. Meditation has a different emphasis than prayer, although in practice the two overlap to some extent. Prayer usually has a conversational or discursive aspect in which thoughts and feelings are directed out of us toward someone or something (God, in theistic traditions). On the other hand, meditation involves nondiscursive procedures aimed at altering attention, establishing a more receptive mode of consciousness. It is often thought of as a practice of Eastern religions like Hinduism or Buddhism rather than Christianity, but activities like meditation can be found in all three traditions.[10] While prayer and meditation are definitely not synonymous they share many similarities. Meditation is known as a technique for control of attention, but many versions of prayer also emphasize this;[11] prayer is known as a way of seeking transfiguration, but meditation is also potentially a trans figurative experience, broadening our consciousness to new perceptions of the world. Eastern traditions do not always use the word meditation, but when they do, it typically refers to a practice designed to develop voluntary control over concentration and awareness.[12] The Christian concept of contemplation is probably closer to the Eastern idea of meditation as both offer access to a kind of transitional space, although there are important differences as well. An important concept in Buddhist psychology is mindfulness (sati). Mindfulness actually refers to a number of related concepts.[13] First, like concentration, mindfulness is an important mental ability. It involves full awareness and attentiveness to the present and assists the spiritual seeker in many ways.[14] Second, mindfulness refers to a steady guarding of the mind that provides a foundation for moral development. At the level of virtue, mindful awareness helps persons exercise mental restraint so that they do not attend to things that may become objects of craving, freeing them to develop the concentration and other kinds of skills necessary for advanced meditation. Third, mindfulness is a technique of meditation in which the individual enters directly into the mindful contemplation of the changing mental and material processes in his own experience.[15] It produces a mental state that stands between total concentration, on the one hand, and daydreaming, on the other. Mindfulness is accompanied by enhancing control over attention and balance of mental and emotional factors, and can lead to important insights about the nature of reality.
- *Transcendental meditation:* Transcendental Meditation (TM) was developed by Maharishi Mahesh Yogi and brought to the West in the 1950s. Based on the Hindu tradition, TM is supposedly neither a contemplative nor concentrative exercise but a developmental technology. The crude difference from other forms and practices of spirituality lies in the fact that it advocates claim that it requires no change in lifestyle or belief system. It involves an effortless 15–20 minutes practice of meditation during the day with eyes closed while reciting a sound or mantra. This procedure acts to accelerate the development of consciousness.[16,17] TM is based upon a seven-stage model of consciousness and organization drawn from the Hindu Vedic tradition.[18] The first three stages are everyday temporary ones: waking, dreaming, and dreamless sleep. Above these stages are higher levels of transcendental or purse consciousness, which allow contact with the true Self and are the immediate goal of TM practice. These stages are characterized by an equable state of pure consciousness during daily activities, refinement of personality or emotional qualities, and increasing unity between subject and object. Though researches on TM had been criticized for their design and sampling error, those

researches suggest TM exerts some psychophysiological effects.[19,20] Firstly, there are changes in brain wave activity including increased intensity/amplitude of slow alpha, bursts of high voltage theta, and higher EEG coherence/ synchrony in frontal areas, most frequently in regular practitioners; along with this, increased blood flow in frontal areas suggesting alertness. Secondly, physiological changes similar to a relaxed state of decreased autonomic activity and metabolism such as decreased blood pressure and oxygen consumption have been noticed following TM. In addition, there are possible changes in body chemistry including reduction in cholesterol and lipid levels or lowered adrenocortical activity, suggesting decreased levels of stress. Thirdly, increased assemblage in surrounding consciousness is noted, affecting crime rates and other social phenomenon which is referred to as the Maharishi effect.[21] Fourthly, there are increased self-actualization, positive emotions, cognitive performance, and psychological health, in part through reduction of anxiety, depression, anger, impulsivity, aggressiveness, and substance abuse.[22]

- *Samadhi:* Samadhi is a process of meditation mentioned in Hinduism. It involves a trance state. It ultimately leads to detachment from one's on ego. The mediator may achieve the deepest moment of self-actualization and there might be a realization of unity of the Universe.[23]
- *Zen:* Its origin lies in the word 'zazen'. It means seated meditation in Japanese language. Koans which are used in practice of zen are seemingly meaningless dialogues. The goal of zazen is an epiphany or lasting enlightenment about the true nature of creation.[23]
- *Mysticism:* Mysticism is a well-known in Christian tradition, Hindu tradition/Tantric culture. It is characterized by intense altered state of consciousness. It refers to reaching out and "nonconceptual knowing of God" accomplished through experiences of union.[24] During the experience the mystic feel totally absorbed by the awe of the unity of the universe. They feel a unique joy and elation. As the experience ends, the mystics return to normal life but transformed to a state somewhat between God and humankind.[23] William James[25] (1961) identified the following as central features of mystical experience: Ineffability: a felt inability to describe the experience, Noetic quality: a sense that something fundamental was learned, transiency: the experience lasts for a brief period of time, passivity: a sense that the experience was not under the person's control. Mystical experiences can be negative (apophatic) or positive (kataphatic).[26] Central to this type of experience is a unitive experience—a sense of union with God or Universe.[27] They involve both a feeling of underlying unity and a sense of participation to such an extent that the self is lost and metamorphosed.[28]
- *Spirit possession:* Spirit possession is found from ancient times. The belief behind this remains that a supernatural entity enters into one's body and starts to control its activity. The effect of possession may be both towards a sick or a prophet. It is mentioned in Qur'an and prevalent in various cultures including in Egypt, Sudan, Ethiopia and India etc.[23]

HUMAN DEVELOPMENT AND SPIRITUALITY

Development of spirituality across life span has been mentioned in various discussions of many disciplines. They differ significantly in ways regarding how spirituality is developed in a person. Spirituality has been thought of not only arising from a religious journey but also from genetic and cognitive development. This section describes some of these approaches.

Religious Perspective

Christian Perspective

Writers from this early period such as Evagrius Ponticus (345–399) believed that if a person was willing to open themselves to God through physical and mental effort, they could gradually become like God in a process of transformation known as theosis or divination. The concept of theosis was especially developed in the thought of Maximus Confessor (c. 580–662). According to his view that theosis is a lifelong process involving all aspects of the person. In his writings four aspects of process of theosis have been mentioned:

1. *Effort and noneffort:* In the process, we need to engage in the kind of lifestyle and practices that make the process possible. The nature and kind of challenges in the process are ever-changing and the more new challenges would come the more old challenge would fade. One can overcome those challenges only with due effort in the developmental process.
2. *Transformation:* As the process of theosis progresses, deification makes us into a likeness of God through an on going personal encounter and imitation, which leads to new knowledge and the imitation of divine virtues like love. As a result, God is manifested through us in our virtues so that eventually our body and soul become 'the clearest of mirrors' reflecting God.[29]
3. *Unification:* For maximus, divinization is the uniting with God of those who have become like him. This union is a kind of mutual phenomenon (perichoresis) that respects the nature of each. It provides ultimate meaning of life.
4. *Love and freedom:* The evidence and result of theosis is the growth of love and freedom in our lives. As we become like God, we become united in love with the Divine and develop love and compassion for all other things that are also loved by God. Love thus promotes unity. This compassion helps us fight the problem of arrogance, which is always a temptation as we reach higher levels of development. Through these, Theosis leads to spiritual

freedom, a state of rest and satisfaction of desire. Life without this freedom is incomplete; with it, we can use our gifts to their full potential.[30,31]

On the other hand Western Christians approached differently than their counterpart from Eastern world. They divided the journey to God into three to four stages. Central to these theories were three modes or 'ways' of the spiritual life: the Via Purgativa (purgation), Via Iluminativa (illumination) and Via Unitiva (union). Purgation is defined when one is purified and develops the underlying character, personal habits, and mental attitudes necessary for progress in spiritual life. Illumination is an increasing sense of God's presence, as well as feelings of love and unity toward all things. In the final stage of development, there is an increasing sense of union with God. The highest stage of development is described by many Christian writers in metaphorical terms using a variety of images such as '*a beatific vision*,' '*the intimacy of mutual love between bride and bridegroom*,' '*becoming like God*,' '*a boiling over of God within*,' '*a state of ecstasis or going out of oneself*,' and '*a state of epectasis*' or '*increasing desire for God and penetration into the divine light*'. The rich use of metaphors to describe the highest stage might be due to ineffable nature of the experience.[32-34]

Hinduism and Buddhism Perspective

Traditional Hindu thought sees spiritual development in the context of the human life span. For instance, the Laws of Manu[35] divide the life of the upper caste Hindu worshipper into four stages or Ashrama. The process begins during Bramacharya when the child or adolescent works as a student and family member. They try to master the basic skills and cultural abilities necessary for life and study the Vedas under a teacher. In the second stage or Grihastha, one marries after completing his study and becomes a productive householder. The individual continues their spiritual study and observes traditional religious rituals and requirements for offerings. After the birth of grandchildren and around midlife one moves into Vanaprastha or simple retirement and becomes a forest inhabitant. This stage marks the beginning of more intensive spiritual seeking, reciting the Vedas and practicing benevolence. Finally at the end of life, one enters Saanyasa and experiences a renunciation, taking up a reclusive lifestyle and engaging in deep meditation. In practice, these last two stages are not sequential but represent different end paths of development. The stages refer to both a place of residence for religious exertion and also a mode of life.

On the contrary in Buddhism spirituality development happens in relation to meditation practice. Example of spiritual development in the Zen Buddhist tradition is provided in the Ten Oxherding Pictures.[36] This series of pictures depicts the journey toward the Buddhist goal of discovering the emptiness of the false self and leaving it behind for our true self and a state of nondualism. It is a journey that begins with a state of emptiness and ends with a different experience of it.

Genetic Perspective

Among many theories of psychological development, theories on moral development overlap with spiritual and religious formation. Moved away from a philosophical analysis of adult thought, those theories began to look at the genesis or source of mental life, how our abilities emerge or derive from their earliest beginnings in childhood. This emphasis on genesis led to the development of genetic psychology which focused not on heredity but on the developmental sources and processes behind the psyche. Among many contributors we may discuss the contribution of G Stanley Hall, James Mark Baldwin and Jean Piaget.

G Stanley Hall

Hall proposed a theory of development which had given an important place to religion. According to this, the various states of development in the individual (ontogeny) recapitulate or repeat the stages in evolution or development of the species (phylogeny). The time period of adolescence is supposed to be the key time for religious development. According to his views teenage years is a time of turmoil when unconscious materials from our racial past become available to us, and the psyche attempts to establish a new balance and mental unity. Adolescence is responsible for development of sexuality and increased capacity for love, which permits us to make connections with others and with our past. Hall argued that the adolescent transition should include a change in one's attitude toward religion, which can help us achieve our true place in the world.[37]

James Mark Baldwin

Baldwin's theory was an appraisal about how we go about thinking and give meaning to experience. Several key ideas underlie Baldwin's genetic theory. Firstly, he accepted the concept of recapitulation as found in Hall. This means that ways of interpretation of things are modified in the way they were interpreted in early human societies. Secondly, development had a social dimension, where growth in the real self occurs in dialectical social relationships between the individual and others. He argued that the individual is not only a passive recipient of information from the environment but also actively reacts. Baldwin thought that religious development proceeded through a number of stages. He named those stages as prelogical, logical hyperlogical and finally extralogical. At the earliest stage or prelogical stage, thinking is spontaneous and thoughts of emotional or practical or intellectual nature are not differentiated. Religious dependence emerges only when a sense of trust in the environment and one's caretakers is built up. However, after emotional, practical, and intellectual thinking becomes separated from each other in the logical stage, religious freedom becomes compromised. Then discursive and critical intellectual thought gain predominance. Logical thought always tends to ignore certain kinds of experiences that do not fit within it. This leads to a dualism between subject and object, mind and body. This stage is followed by hyperlogical stage. A hyperlogical stage is marked by introspective intuition and immediate perception of knowledge and value. At this level, the person is able to defer his practical and intellectual reasons and can directly perceive and interpret objects. Lastly the highest level was defined by the extralogical or moral and ethical stage of development. Development of an ethical self is hallmark of this stage. The ethical self is conscious of its ability to do right or wrong. It is driven by sentiment and a sense of obligation to go beyond habit. It struggles to achieve an ethical ideal.[37]

Before we move to discuss the cognitive approaches it is noteworthy that a key characteristic of early psychological theories of religious development is that they primarily focused on childhood and adolescence.[37]

Cognitive–structuralist Approaches

These theories attempted to understand the human person by trying to identify underlying organized structures or schemas of mental activity. Cognitive-structural theories of moral development have been particularly popular, because morality is central to most religious traditions, even though it has features that are developmentally unique.[37]

Jean Piaget

Apart from this well-known stage of cognitive development, Piaget discussed about moral development also in his early work. He was concerned about rational base of morality rather than its affective aspect. He referred those rules as 'the deepest functional constant of human nature' which form the basis of moral nature. According to his view two types of morality evolve during development. He named those as heteronomous and autonomous types of morality. Heteronomous form of morality involves deals with egocentric needs. As the child grows up and his experiences become enriched, his moral reasoning would eventually change. This leads to a superior system of autonomous morality and justice reasoning based on mutual respect and reciprocity. According to Piaget an ideal religion would be an individualistic one which adjusted religion to modern thought. Piaget[38] associated mystical experience and religious orthodoxy with immature and egocentric thought. He viewed that mysticism comes from feelings of unilateral respect for parents and adults and is associated with imposed rules of ritual, taboo, and moral realism. He also thought that mysticism is connected with egocentrism in which individuals confuse their own wishes with those of God. This means that feelings of transcendence and the myths associated with them are irrational and have no value as beliefs. In more advanced stages of development, we should abandon these myths and substitute rational experiment and naturalistic explanations for supernatural mysticism. This development should climax in adolescence with the integration of a new rational religion into our life system and plans in which God and individual cooperate with each other.[32, 36]

Lawrence Kohlberg

Discussion on cognitive—structuralist approaches would be incomplete without mentioning Kohlberg's stages of moral development. Although Kohlberg wrote primarily about the development of moral reasoning, he also wrote about religious development and attempted to relate his theory to it. In his view, religious development may parallel but also differs from moral development as it deals with different kinds of questions. He argued that morality is concerned with the nature of the good life and the good person, while religion searches answers of fundamental questions about human nature and the human condition. Kohlberg believed that morality was a 'logically independent realm' from religion because (1) moral development occurs in people with no religious beliefs, and (2) individuals at a high stage of moral development can have very different religious views. As in the case of morality, Kohlberg assumed that there are universal issues like our relationship to the eternal, which people try to answer through their religious reasoning in an attempt "to affirm life and morality as related to a transcendent or infinite ground or sense of the whole".[37]

James Fowler and Faith Development

Fowler is a theologian who worked at Harvard and defined faith as an evolving sense of sprit and relatedness to others that provides meaning and coherence and allows participation in 'an ultimate environment'. In his view, faith is a more fundamental category than religion, which involves beliefs, practices and images that express and inform faith.[39] Faith involves patterns of (1) knowing or belief, (2) valuing or commitment, and (3) meaning construction, typically expressed through narrative. According to Fowler, faith is based in our sense of self that develops on several levels: an emergent self in infancy that forms the basis of imagination, a core or embodied self that appears in physical rituals, and an intersubjective self that allows us to develop shared frameworks and fantasies. This faith creates triadic relationships between ourselves, others and "shared centers of value and power". In this view, different kinds of personal identities in people can be thought of as coming from various sorts of relations with potential centers of value. Some people have multiple centers of value with no specific center; they have many compartmentalized identities and move between different interests and situations. Fowler called these people 'polytheists'. This pattern is often found in contemporary culture, particularly in people who suffer from personality disorders. Others are 'henotheists', who have an identity unified around a single center of power that is not of ultimate concern, such as money or status. The last group is made up of 'radical monotheists', who have "loyalty to the principle of being and to the source and center of all value and power". Fowler's theory has been widely influential. It has all the advantages of a structural approach. It helps us understand universal features of faith and ways of knowing, allowing for comparisons between diverse groups and among individuals within.[37]

Fritz Oser and Religious Judgment

A different perspective on cognitive development and religion is provided by Fritz Oser and his colleagues,[37] who have developed a theory of religious judgment. According to their definition, religious judgment is how the individual deals subjectively with the process of meaning making, coping with contingencies, and creating subjective security in a world of objective insecurity. It also involves how people think about their relation with the Ultimate. It provides a deep reflective or 'mother-structure' that operates in the background most of the time but can be seen when crises challenge the way we understand the meaning of events. Oser describes the differences between Piaget, Kohlberg, and himself in terms of how subject and object relations are handled. In Piaget, the emphasis is on intellectual development and the relation between subject and object. Kohlberg, on the other hand deals with social development and the subject-subject relation. Oser's theory differs from both as he deals with religious development and the relation of subjects to the Ultimate and thus to each other. Oser sees that development is a process where the individual seeks equilibrium on seven bipolar dimensions that are important for religious judgment: transcendence versus immanence, freedom versus dependency, trust versus fear or anxiety, sacred versus profane, hope versus absurdity, eternity versus ephemerality, and functional transparency (seeing how things work) versus opaqueness (having a hidden or magical quality). During different stages of growth, these dimensions are balanced in various ways, but development seeks a complex equilibrium that is finally achieved in the last stage. Stage transitions are often triggered by important life experiences or changes that cannot be dealt with adequately within existing cognitive structures and call for the integration of new elements of thought. Each contains a new worldview and way of interpreting experience, and with it a new subjective perception of our relationship with God. The outcome of each stage produces a set of competencies, which may or may not translate into action.[40]

Integrative Approaches

Ken Wilber

One of the most sophisticated integrations of Eastern perspectives with modern psychology can be found in the work of Ken Wilber. Spiritual development happens through a stage-like progression. According to Wilber all of us have a drive towards Spirit. He has outlined a stage model describing the path of personal evolution. Each stage shares a similarity in term of creation of basic structures such as sensorimotor abilities or formal operational reasoning. These structures remain available to the person in all stages subsequent to their emergence. At each stage, transition structures are developed. These structures are specific for that stage but will disappear when the person moves on to a new level of development. He argued that our experience of the self is an example of a transition structure, as it changes to new unique forms as we move from one stage to another. To describe development of an individual he coined terms like 'outward arc' and 'inward arc'. An 'outward arc' of development of subconscious and conscious awareness of self and environment is predominant in the prepersonal and personal phases. This is followed in some individuals by a transpersonal phase, an 'inward arc' that involves development of higher states of consciousness. The outward arc involves a series of stages at the gross level of development and perception that include many of the cognitive, emotional, motivational, and experiential changes discussed by Piaget and other developmental psychologists. The peak of the arc is the 'centauric stage', which is a creative, spontaneous way of being that has characteristics similar to the state of self-actualization described by Maslow. Following this in the inward arc are a series of subtle and causal stages that are marked by increasing experiences of connectedness with the world and others, including paranormal experiences. The final goal of development is an experience of unity with the world in which the self dissolves.[37]

James Loder

The work of James Loder is important because he offers one of the few models of development that has both theological and psychological elegance. He believed that theological as well as psychological perspectives were necessary to understand human development. Loder's theory is based on the idea that human development is shaped by spiritual transformation. In his view, development takes place in two orders, 'divine' and 'contingent', with the former surrounding the latter. The divine order can remake human life and the environment within which development occurs, on the other hand, changes in the body, soul (psychological ego), and sociocultural contexts lie within the contingent order. Spiritual development takes place on the boundary between the two and thus is affected by both divine and contingent orders. The divine order has the potential to affect the contingent order when surprise intrudes upon the fixed patterns of contingent time, providing the potential for transformation.[37]

SPIRITUAL MODEL OF MENTAL HEALTH

The relationship between religion or spirituality and mental health has always been complex. An important connection between religious activities, mental health, and spiritual wellness can be well appreciated though the nature of connection which may not be easy to delineate. Freud had blamed religion as a kind of psychological pathology. But more recent work has often suggested that religion has a positive effect on mental health and that good mental health is an important necessity for spiritual development. Spiritual problems might involve issues of balance more than a specific and predictable set of psychological problems. So, one can experience that spirituality, on occasions, may be cause for exacerbation of pathology.

Though religious and spiritual authors tried to explain mental illness for long, the medical model is most prominent and is used across diagnostic systems. Medical model has its own issues which are raised by religious and spiritual authors. Firstly, a definition of health as absence of illness is negative and ignores the presence or absence of human strengths. Furthermore, terms like 'normal' lacks precision. For example, we may find difficult to find a firm line between delusional, spiritual, and 'normal' experiences or beliefs. Secondly, people without psychiatric diagnoses endorse many unusual beliefs, and those with mental illness have largely typical ideas about the world, which are overlapping with those who do not have mental illness according to diagnostic systems. Thirdly, in medical model individualistic and biological views of mental disorder and treatment are unnecessarily over emphasized, in turn under recognizing personal choices or social and relational factor. Fourthly, it also ignores the moral component and consequences involved in many forms of mental disorders. In summary, the definition of mental health is based on adaptiveness, flexibility, and lack of distress and is reluctant to include spiritual and religious concerns.[37]

After the work of a group of transpersonal psychiatrists, recent revisions of medical model, it encourages modifications toward greater cultural sensitivity in diagnosis and treatment. In the new category, religious problems are conceptualized as difficulties related to institutional practices, while spiritual problems are related to our relationship with a higher power or transcendence. Spiritual problems could include spiritual experiences or dealing with problems that have a spiritual component such as a terminal illness or an addiction. Some transpersonal authors also distinguish between a spiritual crisis—a life event with a spiritual component—and a spiritual emergency which is distress related to a spiritual experience or the outcome of spiritual practices. It is now believed that there is a small positive correlation between religiosity and good mental health. This relationship is especially true among individuals who are both spiritual and religious compared with those who identify themselves as neither. Studies differ in their conclusions on relationship between spirituality and mental health. Those that define mental health as an absence of illness generally find a small positive relationship between health and religious involvement, while researches that include self-actualization, personal integration or existential well-being in their definition of mental health find stronger positive relationships. One should also be aware about negative effect of religion and/or spirituality on mental health. Studies indicate following possibilities. (1) interpersonal problems or religious struggles related to beliefs, community participation or the effects of religious practices; (2) unbalanced beliefs, such as stress on sinfulness leading to excess guilt; and (3) spiritual abuse, "the misuse of social or political power in a spiritual context". Presumably, religious or spiritual activities performed out of a sense of obsessive need rather than free choice will also have less desirable outcomes.

Dissatisfaction with the negative medical model approach to mental health has led many psychologists to consider other alternatives. In these new approaches, human health is conceptualized as more than an absence of illness. It tries to have a broader vision of what the 'good life' or goal of human existence is like and how it should be achieved. Ryan and Deci[41] have noted that positive models of mental health tend to follow two different approaches that have different visions for the goal of human life. In the 'hedonic approach', positive mental health is in parallel with happiness, the short term experiences of pleasure and avoidance of negative emotions or subjective well-being (SWB), which is the individuals' evaluation of the quality of their lives. In the 'eudaimonic approach', mental health is thought of as a dynamic process rather than an end state of pleasure, and is described in somewhat broader terms as psychological well-being (PWB), the position of a fully functioning individual who (a) engages life, seeking to actualize their potential and find meaning; (b) develops quality relationships; and (c) develops competence and seeks to master the environment. Dimensions of religion related to SWB include intrinsic religious motivation; individual beliefs, religious experiences, and devotional practices that generate positive feelings; participation in organized activities, and identification with a supportive community. In an important study, Wink and Dillon (2003) found that religiousness was related to relational aspects of well-being through service, generative, and creative activities, while spirituality was related more to self-perceived personal growth.[42]

Here we can look into the relationship between positive psychology and religion. Firstly, religion can be seen as a source of moral inspiration and a dialogue partner that helps to provide more sophisticated and useful definitions of concepts. Secondly, religion or spirituality can be seen as a kind of goal-directed activity or striving for the sacred that can have positive benefits. Emmons[43] refers to the pursuit of meaning as spiritual striving and sees it as an inherent part of the personality that brings inner unity, minimizing conflicts between goals and making painful experiences comprehensible. This lack of meaning is important according to other authors. Maddi[44] has referred it as existential sickness. It has three components: (1) vegetativeness—loss of interest, apathy, and boredom; (2) nihilism—a need to disconfirm the possible positive meanings of others and along with it anger, distrust, and cynicism; competitiveness and combativeness; and (3) adventurousness—attempting to counter lack of meaning and boredom through high-risk activities.

Apart from effects in hedonic or eudaimonic approaches, some authors argue that religion also produces a kind of well-being that is different from those approaches, described above. Craig Ellison[45] has developed the concept of spiritual well-being to describe this unique effect. In his view, in addition to desires for pleasure or self-fulfillment, need for transcendence cannot be neglected as far as needs for human are concerned. To him transcendence is "the sense of well-being that we experience when we find purposes to commit ourselves to that which involve ultimate meaning for life". This type of well-being provides integration, harmony, and freedom within the personality. He also elaborated about nature of transcendence human should achieve. First, it involves a vertical relation or well-being in connection to God, which he calls religious well-being. Second, it includes a horizontal relation to the world around us, including a sense of life purpose and satisfaction, or existential well-being. According to him, spiritual well-being can be an expression of spiritual health but is not identical with them. It is different than psychosocial well-being because it does not remain confined to material aims. It does not focus much on goal-directed striving and has less of a set pattern of development. Spiritual well-being is associated with better physical and psychological well-being, lower anxiety, and less depression. It is also related to self-realization, as individuals who have higher levels of self-realization have greater spiritual well-being. Development of spiritual well-being is related to positive relations with parents, personality characteristics like conscientiousness or agreeableness. Moreover, presence of religious experiences is influenced by spiritual well-being.

Discussion of mental illness is commonly found in literature of Christian and Islamic religion. Models of soul care like that of Evagrius or Western authors like Gregory the Great dominated spiritual and emotional healing until the rise of medical psychiatry in the 19th century. The decline of a distinctively Christian perspective was due to several reasons, including (1) fascination with secular approaches which led to neglect of wisdom in the religious tradition, and (2) the separation between psychological and spiritual aspects of care. However, recently there has been a resurgence of interest in formulating a distinctively Christian view of psychopathology that takes into account modern scientific knowledge. The recent work of Yarhouse et al.[46] is an excellent example that has parallels to other work in Christian psychology and theology. They argue that a Christian view of mental illness will contain personhood and a set of values defining means to be healthy. That should also include the possible causes of human suffering along with a view of the helping process. An integrated view of the person is emphasized. The individual exists in relationship to God and as part of a community with mutual responsibility to others. He is not viewed as isolated. He also argued that religious and spiritual development are related to psychological wholeness but not necessarily connected with mental health. In contrast to a hedonic view of the human person that sees depression (unhappiness) as the ultimate human suffering; modern Christian authors have tended to see anxiety as the central psychological problem. They classified anxiety into neurotic anxiety and existential anxiety. According to them, neurotic anxiety arises from psychological problems, while, existential anxiety generates from our fundamental limitations and separation from God and others. Unlike existential anxiety, neurotic anxiety is problematic and a mental health issue. On the other hand existential anxiety may be positive if it helps us to progress, identify with others in need, or is a sign that we do not fit in with a modern society that pursues dysfunctional aims—adaptation is not always good. It may be negative if it leads to loss of hope or isolation. This latter kind of anxiety is conquered through spiritual awareness but not through psychology.

On the other hand the Islamic psychology movement chose to formulate a psychology that is based on Islamic fundamentals. Scholars working to construct an Islamic psychology argue that it must be based on ideas about truth which can be found in the religion. In Islamic thought, true knowledge can be gained only through the use of all our faculties. To serve our nature both as intellectual and spiritual, the search for truth cannot be based upon just intellectual or scientific knowledge but must include a spiritual dimension. There are four levels of the search for truth: (1) knowledge and principles from the *Quran*, (2) the *Sunnah* or sayings of Mohammed, (3) *inma* or consensus opinion of Muslims, and (4) quays, deduction within the framework of Islamic law.[37] It is to be kept in mind that Islam does not view a person through cognitive or biological perspective. Rather according to them, each person comprises four parts. They are heart (*qalb*), intellect (*aql*), spirit (*ruh*) and self (*naf*). The heart (*qalb*) and intellect (*aql*) allow us to under-stand knowledge as given to us in the *Quran* and other sources. The heart in particular is critical, as it is the essence of our spirit and the place where we meet God, a mirror which can be polished to reflect the Divine. These help us follow the spirit (*ruh*) given by God to each person that contains a template of potential for that person, and the self (*nafs*) which encompasses the biological and psychic aspects of the individual, our animal nature.[37]

SPIRITUALITY IN PSYCHIATRIC DISORDERS

A vast literature exists on the relationship between religion and spirituality and many specific psychiatric disorders.

Spirituality and Addiction

It has long been thought that religion and spirituality are very helpful in the understanding and treatment of addictive disorders. Virtually all studies on alcohol use or abuse and other drug problems have found that religiousness—especially intrinsic religiosity—is associated with fewer problems. However, the relationship is not a straightforward one. It depends upon a number of factors, including childhood religion and current religious affiliation of self and spouse, level of commitment or participation, and how the person interprets his or her religious tradition. Religion seems to have its biggest effect in preventing initial problems rather than helping after a problem with addiction has developed.[47] It does this through modifying various other factors. It provides a community environment, social norms and beliefs that reduce opportunities for use. It helps to provide nondrug related ways of coping. People who are successful in treatment have higher levels of religious faith and spirituality, which is related to a number of helpful factors such as optimistic life orientation, greater perceived social support, better resilience in response to stress, and lower anxiety.[48-50] Qualitative studies also found that spirituality plays an important role in therapeutic program on alcohol use like in Alcoholic Anonymous (AA). Through the spiritual aspect of the program, members move towards accepting help from something outside the self. They also frequently report spiritual awakenings.[51] They do change their perception about self and the world.[52]

The most thoroughly worked out theory of the relationship between spirituality and addiction is that of contemplative psychiatrist Gerald May (1982). According to May,[53] there are several ways to deal with addiction including a spiritual one. One way is to avoid the emptiness of freedom and to fill it up with another less damaging addiction. But, this does not really solve the underlying problem. A second way or possibility is to use psychological techniques or even spiritual techniques like meditation to decrease the negative effects of addictions. This can also be positive, but meditation when used in this way is no longer a spiritual technique because it does not deal with the underlying spiritual issue. The third approach is a spiritual one: to give up false security and detach from addictive behaviors or objects. Other than May's views, another important technique involving spirituality to deal with addiction is Transcendental Medicine (TM) and mindfulness. Details of these are given in a further section of this chapter.

Spirituality and Depression

Depression is a condition that can involve sadness, loss of interest in activities, changes in cognition such as negative thoughts, and a number of physical problems such as disturbed sleep. It is also associated with problems in mood regulation such as a tendency toward automatic, stronger, and persistent responses to negative stimuli.[54] It is associated with increased mortality, as well as decreased quality of life and productivity.[55] Overall, religious involvement and affiliation appears to be related to fewer problems with depression, higher levels of well-being, and quicker recovery from depressive episodes when problems occur, especially in those with an intrinsic religious motivation.[56,57] There is even stronger evidence for a relationship between religiousness and suicide. Higher rates of suicide are observed in countries with lower rates of religious participation, and lower rates of suicide may be associated with specific religious beliefs and prohibitions.[58] Though from the above discussion it seems religion has only protective effects on depression, this is not consistent across literature. Religious problems can be associated with higher rates of depression, and some religious groups such as Pentecostal Christians appear to have more problems.[59] Exline et al found that college students reporting religious strain, such as religious doubts or disagreements with family over religious issues, reported higher levels of depression and suicidality independent of religiousness and the degree of comfort provided by religion. In these students, depression was associated with alienation from God. Those with higher levels of strain were also more interested in discussing religious issues in counseling.[60] Thus, the presence of positive religiousness does not mean that a person may not have religious problems that are negatively impacting his mental health. Authors have tried to understand the mechanisms for the relation between religiosity and depression. Three commonly discussed possibilities are:

1. Religiousness may have a buffering mechanism. It may both act as a suppressor or moderator, and providing positive coping or appraisal mechanisms. In the suppressor model, religious practices increase in response to stress and act to buffer its potential to trigger depression. In the moderator model, religious practices do not increase, but they become more effective at higher levels of stress, buffering against the possibility of depression.
2. Religiousness may help the person to cope with the emotional effects of depression, perhaps providing a way of seeking comfort or avoiding distress.
3. Religiousness may help to prevent depression by discouraging behaviors that increase the risk of stress or depression, such as substance use.

Most research has suggested that the main helpful effect comes from long-term involvement in beliefs, practices, and community, which buffers the negative effects of stress on mental health and psychological well-being.[61] Spirituality when separated from religion does not have the same effect. There is support for both suppressor and moderator models, as the negative correlation between religion and depression are stronger in high stress situations.[62] Some specific factors that buffer, provide comfort or prevent depression include the following:

- Specific beliefs, including (a) after life beliefs, which may reduce depression and anxiety particularly among the bereaved;[63,64] (b) God image beliefs, with a stern God image related to higher levels of depression in men; or (c) beliefs that reduce hopelessness.
- The use of positive religious coping such as seeing God as a partner and not feeling isolated.
- Social support from others in a religious community, or spiritual support, a sense that a person is loved by God and can love in return. Both kinds of support are related to protective effects against stress, lower levels of depression, and higher levels of life satisfaction.[37]

Spirituality and Psychosis

Patients' narratives of the experience of psychosis as well as accounts by psychiatrists give good descriptions from both subjective and objective perspectives and are recommended reading for all who want to understand their patients and the inner world of psychosis. In psychosis, meaning and purpose may become distorted. Delusions are common in a psychotic experience. The elaboration of delusional beliefs into systems, in which it is possible for the person to reconfigure their identity, is often significantly accompanied by a subjective experience of meaning and purpose—the 'comforts of madness.'[65] Many patients present with delusions of a religious nature (even if they themselves do not practice a religion) and religious patients when they develop psychosis are very likely to express themselves through the language and imagery of their beliefs. Psychiatrists should be aware of these issues and should refrain from making assumptions about religious beliefs. The psychiatrist should be prepared to investigate the background relevant to each individual case. Many scholars, Freud (1927) and Dawkins[57] included, have regarded religious beliefs as delusions, on the basis that religion is inherently fabricated and therefore beliefs associated with it are also false. But current psychiatric convention is that beliefs shared by people with a similar religious or cultural background are not delusions, although they may be accompanied by the same phenomenological characteristics as delusion—'a belief firmly held on inadequate grounds ... not arrived at through normal processes of logical thinking'.[66]In the case of psychotic religious delusions, the beliefs are not generally shared with the religious or cultural group. Particular difficulties may arise, however, where the origin and resolution of the delusional beliefs held by an individual and their religious community are in conflict with conventional psychiatric practice and will need sensitive handling. Mystical experiences are to be mentioned in discussion of interface between psychosis and spirituality. Mystics of different religious faiths have long been known to have psychotic experiences; this neither confirms nor invalidates their spiritual standing. Mystical experiences are not uncommon in the population and they may be reported more frequently by people with certain abnormalities of personality, notably schizotypy. A number of studies[67-69] have found it impossible to differentiate between mystical experiences and psychosis solely on the basis of phenomenological description. Jackson and Fulford (2002)[70] acknowledge the limitations of traditional descriptive diagnostic criteria in distinguishing pathological from non-pathological psychotic experiences. They stress the need for an additional evaluative criterion, one that will distinguish medical value from values of other kinds. Buckley[71] who compared autobiographical accounts of acute mystical experience and schizophrenia, found that the appearance of a powerful sense of noesis, heightening of perception, feelings of communion with 'the divine', and exaltation may be common to both states. Distress and unwanted preoccupations characterize psychosis, whereas spiritual experiences may be sought after and are more often associated with positive life changes.[72,73] Jackson, however, observes that the distinction based on whether the experience is life-enhancing or overwhelming and isolating becomes blurred in the longer term. Though the interplay between psychosis and spirituality is exceedingly complex certain issues have to be kept in mind when dealing with a mentally ill person with psychosis. A recent study[74] suggests that there may be a relationship between the stage of the patient's recovery and the importance they place on spirituality in their lives. Finding out about patients' religious and spiritual background may help us to avoid making premature assumptions. This collaborative exploration of the religious and spiritual is a dynamic process; meanings may change depending on the severity or stage of the disorder. Role of spirituality in the journey to recovery from psychotic experience is described in Peter Chadwick's writing. Chadwick refers to the spiritual dimension of his illness as reenergizing and enriching of creative and emotional life and states that 'the recognition of the spiritual side of my illness and the taking of it seriously by clinicians and social workers were extremely important in my recovery.'[75] A practical, grounded, 'recovery oriented' spirituality that incorporates humanity and compassion while accepting the integrity of personal experience is necessary. This should be more a matter of:

- Values than visions
- Love, compassion and kindness than beliefs
- Humility and tolerance than knowingness
- Spiritual life than religious conformity

- The pursuit of wellness than possessing 'the truth'
- The deep experience of common humanity than allowing unusual experience to separate us.

Spirituality and Anxiety Disorders

Religious and spiritual intervention when combined with traditional psychotherapy can alleviate symptoms in generalized anxiety disorder and panic disorder. This finding is not consistent in obsessive compulsive disorder. Patients with religious obsession are found to have worse prognosis than those who do not have them. Religious beliefs and practices are often inversely correlated with anxiety symptoms or disorders, but not always so. Religion helps many patients with anxiety disorders to cope with their symptoms, and religious therapies are effective in reducing symptoms of anxiety. Religion may also exacerbate anxiety disorder; patients with anxiety disorders may manipulate or distort religion; and patients may use religion defensively to avoid healthy change. Clinicians with appropriate training can use the religious beliefs of patients to help treat anxiety disorders by supporting, encouraging, or directly using those beliefs in therapy.[76]

Spirituality and the Brain

Serotonin and dopamine have mostly been studied in terms of spirituality.[77] Drugs like LSD, Psilocybin, which are known to act on 5-HT system in brain, can lead to spiritual like experience. Perceptual distortions, illusions and hallucinations, and sometimes a sense of insight and spiritual awareness, mystical experiences, and religious ecstasy are reported after overdose or intoxication from these drugs. These effects resemble the perception and ideation described by those persons experiencing spirituality. On the other hand Dopamine is the primary neurotransmitter involved in the reward pathways and is commonly associated with the pleasure system of the brain. Being proven its involvement in many personality traits or dimensions such as anger-related traits and the main role of this neurotransmitter in the function of the frontal lobes, dopamine has also been investigated in spirituality. Moreover, from a psychiatric point of view, derangement of dopaminergic systems has been suggested in psychiatric disorders including schizophrenia, Parkinson's disease, and drug and alcohol dependence. Of note, dopaminergic neurons are also under the control of the 5-HT system. Newberg found several regions and pathways involved in meditative actions. The frontal lobe is one of the regions that has been most implicated in religious activity. Newberg[78-80] focused on the prefrontal cortex and its connections with the thalamus, posterior superior parietal lobe, and limbic system (mainly the amygdala and hippocampus). By measuring cerebral blood flow, he suggested that the more deeper people enter into meditation or prayer, the more active the frontal lobe and the limbic system.[81-84] To a lesser extent, the medial temporal lobe has also been involved in religious activity, and individuals who were more spiritual have reported stronger beliefs in paranormal phenomena[85-88] Apart from neurotransmitter and anatomical areas found to be associated with spiritual and religious practices, studies also found involvement of autonomic nervous system. Activation of the autonomic system creates a reduction in heart and respiratory rates, which in turn brings about a sense of relaxation. Couples of neurotransmitter receptor have been hypothesized to influence spirituality. Examples are the serotonin receptor 1A (5-HT1A), insertion-deletion in the promoter region of the serotonin transporter gene (5-HTTLPR), single nucleotide polymorphisms in the 5-HT Receptors, dopamine transporter and the activating protein-2 (AP-2), polymorphisms in the dopamine receptor 4 gene (DRD4), the cytochrome P450 2C19 (CYP2C19) polymorphism. Over all researches suggest that a high degree of spirituality is linked to 5-HT and dopaminergic systems. The above studies of 5-HT and dopaminergic genes suggest higher levels of activity in both systems, not only in individuals with a high sense of spirituality but also during religious activities such as meditation. It can be speculated that, during the development of the mid-brain neurotransmitter systems, early genetically driven modulation of the 5-HT and dopamine systems participate in the formation of spirituality in adults.[77]

ASSESSMENT OF SPIRITUALITY

In clinical setting assessment of a mentally ill person through biopsychosocial approach does not suffice if we do not take cultural aspect into account. A cultural formulation is incomplete without assessment of spirituality. Apart from discovering personal and environmental strengths, assessment of spiritual needs of patients in clinical settings would serve the following purposes like

- The very nature of spirituality as a source of vitality, motivation and a healthy sense of belonging and being valued.
- The patients' wishes as well as those of carers.
- The epidemiology of spirituality/religion and mental health.
- The influence of spirituality/religion on the attitudes and decisions of psychiatric staff.[89]

The most common and possibly most useful method of assessing spiritual needs is 'taking a spiritual history'. It involves engaging with people (who happen, for the time being, to be patients) as equals in enquiry and discussion, using their own words about what—at the deepest level—makes sense to them, what motivates them and what holds them back. This is the most direct way to get quickly to the heart of whatever is troubling the patient. It coincides with good medical practice: two people, doctor and patient, engaged in genuine and meaningful communication about what matters most in terms of physical, mental and spiritual health. Unlike assessment in other areas, it seems worth noting that both may gain from the encounter.

For clinicians, taking a spiritual history is clearly indicated when a mentally ill person present with chief complaints regarding religious and/or spiritual issues, for example in religious delusions, feelings of rejection (by God or a faith group) and excessive guilt or shame.[89]

Quantitative Methods

Quantitative methods for assessment of spirituality have been criticized due to its inability to capture human's subjective experience which is essence of the same. Several clinically tested instruments are available for spiritual assessment, including the Royal Free Interview for Religious and Spiritual Beliefs,[90] the Spiritual Involvement and Beliefs Scale,[91] the multi-dimensional instrument developed by the Fetzer Institute[92] and Hill & Hood's Measures of Religiosity.[93] As like in other quantitative approaches in measurement here also it may encourage unnecessarily intrusiveness and patient may feel and be valued insufficiently as an individual. For these reasons, and because such methods are usually too detailed, they are more suitable for research and audit projects than for clinical use.

Standard et al. (2000)[94] have reviewed the following quantitative instruments

- Spiritual Assessment Inventory (SAI; Hall and Edwards, 1996)
- The Index of Core Spiritual Experiences (INSPIRIT; Kass, Friedman, Leserman, Zuttermeister and Benson, 1991)
- Spiritual Well-Being Scale (SWBS; Ellison, 1983)
- Spiritual Health Inventory (SHI; Veach and Chappel, 1992)
- Brown-Peterson Recovery Progress Inventory (B-PRPI; Brown and Peterson, 1991)
- Spirituality Scale (SS; Jagers, Boyking, and Smith)
- Spirituality Assessment Scale (SAS; Howden, 1992).

Qualitative Methods

In the clinical setting, where richness and the emotional tone of information can be of special importance, qualitative methods of enquiry into spirituality work better. These get closer to patients' experience of reality by being person-centered, open-ended and process (rather than structure) orientated.

The principal qualitative method of spiritual needs assessment in clinical practice involves taking a spiritual history. It is a skill that requires empathic engagement with the patient, and which therefore sanctions the judicious use of both intuition and initiative by the assessor. It is therefore important to be reasonably systematic and thorough.

It may be noted in a developing country like India where there is shortage of mental health professional; clinicians may be required to carry out rapid or brief assessment. At such times two types of questions are useful.

1. What helps you most when things are difficult, when times are hard (such as when you are facing big problems, major losses or other important challenges)?[89]
2. Do you think of yourself as being either religious or spiritual?[89]

This second question may explore further information about whether the person is familiar with and identifies with being one of the following: atheist, agnostic, unsure, religious, or spiritual.

- *Atheist:* To be atheist is to deny emphatically the existence (even the possibility) of a sacred being, supreme reality, God or other deity.
- *Agnostic:* To be agnostic is to assert that we cannot truly know about the existence or otherwise of a sacred being, supreme reality, God or other deity.
- *Unsure:* To be unsure means the person does not know what he or she believes about a sacred being, supreme reality, God or other deity.
- *Religious:* To be religious is to believe and have faith in a sacred being, supreme reality, God or other gods, and/or to belong to and practice within an organized religion.
- *Spiritual:* To be spiritual is to experience awareness of relationship with a sacred reality, whether or not also belonging to or practicing within an organized religion.

Indicators for a full spiritual assessment are when: (1) "client declares that religious/spiritual issues are important in his or her life; (2) a spiritual issue or concern is evident in the presenting complaint; (3) the clinical issue involves morality and guilt; or (4) persistent concern regarding meaning or purpose in life are noted".[95]

Followings are some of the guidelines available for detailed assessment.[89]

- The first approach, outlined in the guide published by the Spiritual Competency and Resource Centre (*http://www.spiritualcompetency.com/assess_spirit/ASrshx.asp*), focuses on religious background and beliefs as well as spiritual meaning and values.
- In a guide to the assessment of spiritual concerns in mental healthcare, Eagger (2006) lists some simple, nonintrusive questions that can inform the care team's approach.[96] These look, for example, at the place of spirituality or religion in the patient's past or present, the nature of its influence (positive or negative, supportive or excluding) and whether it affects the patient's acceptance of and engagement in treatment.
- The leaflet Spirituality and Mental Health (Royal College of Psychiatrists, 2006) suggests five broad areas of questioning: setting the scene, the past, the present, the future, and remedies.[97] These gather a picture of how patients see themselves, their place and purpose in life

and their future, and ask whether spirituality or religion might be part of the problem or could be the solution.

- In an article aimed at health care professionals, Puchalski and Romer's (2000) guide to taking a spiritual history uses the mnemonic FICA:[98]
  - Faith and belief (what gives the patient's life meaning)
  - Importance (how important is this to their situation)
  - Community (their place in any social or religious group)
  - Address in care (how they would like their personal spirituality addressed in health care).
- A fifth tool for spiritual assessment involves the HOPE questions (Anandarajah and Hight, 2001). The mnemonic HOPE[99] directs the assessor's attention to four areas of the patient's life:
  - Sources of Hope, meaning, comfort, strength, peace, love and connection
  - Organized religion
  - Personal spirituality and practices
  - Effects on medical (psychiatric) care and End-of-life issues.
- Finally, another useful mnemonic is SPIRIT (Maugans, 1996):[100]
  - Spiritual belief system
  - Personal spirituality
  - Integration/Involvement in a spiritual or religious community
  - Ritualized practices and restrictions
  - Implications for medical care
  - Terminal events planning.

Apart from qualitative and quantitative methods discussed clinicians may supplement assessment procedure with diagrammatic approach like spiritual ecomaps, spiritual genograms and spiritual maps, etc.

Spiritual Timelines

Spiritual timeline is a simple graph or chart which chronologically places a client's religious or spiritual experiences. It allows to viewing a client's spiritual journey over long period of time, thus placing everything in perspective.[101] Clients are asked to draw a time line of their religious experiences, using an elaborate or simple graph or chart to chronologically depict their beginning spiritual experiences, principle spiritual events, and current experiences.

Spiritual Lifemaps

Spiritual lifemaps include much of the same information as a spiritual genogram, but depict it in terms of the spiritual journey the client has traveled. They illustrate the contours of the spiritual journey. They accomplish in geographic analogy what spiritual genograms accomplish in genetic analogy, and can be as varied as those depicting their journeys.[101]

Spiritual Eco-maps

Spiritual eco-maps may be useful where more present-focused assessment approaches better suit clients' desires due to the here and now orientation and their relatively rapid construction.[101]

Spiritual Genograms

Spiritual genograms depict the spiritual heritage of clients. It resembles family genogram recorded in family history of a client. It is a diagram of the important spiritual persons and influences in the client's family over three generations. It should include religious affiliations, religious beliefs, spiritual events, and notable spiritual relationships, flow of spiritual resources, and spiritual conflicts—persons, places, ideas, and experiences that have formed a client's current spiritual identity or a perceived lack of the same.[101] The genogram also should be able to convey about how these key persons, ideas, and events have changed, modified, or negated earlier spiritual positions.

SPIRITUALITY AS AN INTERVENTION

Spiritual approaches in mental health care are still in their infancy. Due to concerns about harmful effects, a controversy is ongoing regarding whether or not to integrate spiritual elements into the treatment of persons suffering from mental illness. At the same time, a growing body of evidence shows beneficial outcomes of religious and spiritual approaches to psychiatric disorders with regard to the following aspects: seeing spirituality as a unique human dimension, making life sacred and meaningful, being an essential part of the physician-patient-relationship, and the recovery process. Religion and spirituality constitute an additional, distinct, and independent dimension, interacting with biological, psychological, and social factors creating an extended bio-psycho-social model. Religion and spirituality can be causing, mediating, or moderating factors on mental health and disease in the same way as biological, psychological, and social factors. Given the fact that people with serious mental illnesses already struggle against widespread prejudice and discrimination, it would seem important to maintain or strengthen people's existing religious affiliations and support systems as part of their treatment or rehabilitation plan. Rebecca Proust from the Department of Counseling Psychology, Portland, Oregon, conducted a comparative study of the efficacy of religious and nonreligious cognitive-behavioral therapy with religious and nonreligious therapists on religious patients with clinical depression. She hypothesized that religious cognitive-behavioral therapy (RCT) might be more effective for religious patients than standard cognitive-behavioral therapy (CBT) because of higher consistency of values and frameworks. Recent studies also emphasized that partnerships between mental health providers and faith-based communities may be a particularly effective strategy for meeting the mental health service needs of populations that are underserved by the mental health system, such as persons with low incomes, ethnically diverse communities, and recent immigrants. Patients with anxiety disorders often have problems with attachment rooted in their early developmental experiences and relationships with parents. Religious IPT may facilitate healing of these early relationships by focusing on the person's image of God and substituting a relationship with God for missing or disordered parental attachments. Likewise importance of incorporation of spirituality in psycho educational group meeting are developing life perspectives despite illness and limitations, coping with fear and depression, attaining personhood, spiritual identity ("I called you by your name"), understanding healthy and unhealthy religiosity and spirituality.[102]

SPIRITUALITY IN INDIAN CONTEXT

Spirituality is rooted in Indian culture in ancient times. India's emphasis on spirituality can be ascertained from the productive constellations reported in Kroeber's (1944) work; it received the singular distinction of being a culture that has the longest duration of evolution of philosophy, from AD 100–500, and 600–1000. If we add the period of Buddha, Mahavira, and Samkhya around 500 BC, and the period of medieval Bhakti Movement from1100–1800, we can see that India has emphasized spirituality for almost 2000 years, which is more than any other culture. These spiritual gurus came from all castes, and were not limited to the caste of Brahmin only, the caste that had the privilege of being a teacher or a guru. They also came from many religions, e.g. Hinduism, Buddhism, Jainism, Sikhism, Islam, and Sufism. Also, they were not limited to any particular part of the country; they came from east, west, south, and north. Therefore, it could be argued that spirituality is a cultural phenomenon for India. Spirituality is valued in India even today, and spiritual masters are making innovations that reflect cultural configurations.

Ramakrishna's unique spiritual journey, and what he was able to do in a short life of 50 years (February 18,1836–August 16, 1886), what has perhaps never even been attempted in human history, points to his contribution to the field of spirituality. Ramakrishna learned about the Advaita Vedanta philosophy under another guru, Tota Puri, sometime around the end of 1865. Nirvikalpa samadhi, the highest state of meditation, was not easy even for Ramakrishna. He achieved a unique distinction of successfully following the two major spiritual traditions of Hinduism, the path of devotion and the path of knowledge. He extended it further in the next 10 years by practicing other religious faiths.

Mahesh Prashad Varma, who later became Maharishi Mahesh Yogi dedicated himself to the service of his spiritual master, and spent many years in the Himalayas, where the atmosphere is conducive to meditation. The Maharishi had his first public appearance in October 1955 at a conference, and he made his impact by connecting science and spirituality. According to him the energy of the electrons and protons is due to the Agni-tatva and motion in them is due to Vayu-tatva. The Maharishi explained the other Tatvas (elements) as *Agni* (fire), *Vayu* (air), *Akash* (sky), *Aham* (self), *Mahat* (soul), and *Prakriti* (nature); and Brahma (formless God)-tatva as the very cause of all these Tatvas. He argued that the meditation technique that his guru presented would help achieve Sat-Chit-Anandam, and implied that spirituality was superior to science, which dealt with the lower level of Tatvas. The Maharishi's genius lay in starting a worldwide spiritual movement by keeping the individual at the center stage. The Maharishi might be the first person to bridge science and spirituality. In 1964, 'deep meditation' became 'transcendental deep meditation' or simply transcendental meditation (TM). Of all the Indian traditions of spirituality, TM is the closest to being a science, and that is clearly the Maharishi's most significant contribution.

Osho Rajneesh was one of the most controversial spiritual masters that India has seen in this century. Rajneesh started by lecturing about Mahavir, the Jain prophet, in the business circles of India, which grew in popularity over the years. He continued to appreciate Mahavir and Buddha as spiritual masters in his later years. Rajneesh shocked the Indian populace by linking sex to super consciousness in1968. He became an instant star following his declaration that sex was not to be repressed, and through it people could get into Samadhi, the highest state of being in yoga. In 1969, Rajneesh prescribed a new method of meditation to his disciples called Dynamic Meditation. Rajneesh's philosophy emerged from the ancient culture of India, but his expressions were shaped by the contemporary Indian and international cultures, i.e. by the global Zeitgeist.[103]

CONCLUSION

A growing scientific literature based on spirituality and psychiatry has allowed rapid progress in the integration of religion into psychiatry. Despite this progress, the integration of relevant religious and spiritual issues into clinical practice will likely meet resistance for many years to come. There is some question, however, about whether concepts such as well-being, meaning, or even recovery belong exclusively to the domain of conventional psychiatry. Despite a certain level of subjectivity, the diversity of approaches expressed here has at least exposed readers to the multidisciplinary nature of this interaction between religion and mental health care. In the case of the treatments described, clinicians should know that these approaches exist so that they can formulate appropriate treatment for the patients when necessary or be able to answer patients when they ask for advice about participating in such treatments.

REFERENCES

1. Sims A, Cook CCH. Spirituality and psychiatry, RCPsych Publications; 2009
2. Cook CCH. Addiction and spirituality. Addiction. 2004a;99: 539-51.
3. Swinton J. Spirituality and Mental Health Care—Rediscovering a 'Forgotten' Dimension. Jessica Kingsley Publishers. London and Philadelphia, 2003
4. Elkins DN, Hedstrom JL, Hughes LL, Leaf JA, Saunders C. 'Toward a Humanistic-Phenomenological Spirituality: Definition, Description and Measurement.' Journal of Humanistic Psychology. 1988;4:5-18.
5. Bowker J. Oxford dictionary of World Religions. Oxford University Press; 1997.
6. Larson DB, Swyers JP, McCullough M. Scientific Research on Spirituality and Health: A Consensus Report. National Institute for Healthcare Research. 1997.
7. Martsolf DS, Mickley JR. 'The Concept of Spirituality in Nursing Theories: Differing World-Views and Extent Focus.' Journal of Advanced Nursing. 1998;27:294-303.
8. Roof WC. Spiritual marketplace: Baby boomers and the remaking of American religion. Princeton, NJ: Princeton University Press; 1999.
9. Putt BK. "Too deep for words:" The conspiracy of divine "soliloquy." In: B Benson, N Wirzba (Eds). The phenomenology of prayer. New York: Fordham University Press; 2005.pp.142-53.
10. Andresen J. Meditation meets behavioural medicine: The story of experimental research on meditation. In: J Andresen, RKC Forman (Eds). Cognitive models and spiritual maps: Interdisciplinary explorations of religious experience. Thorverton, UK: Imprint Academic; 2000.pp.17-73.
11. Kadloubovsky E, Palmer GEH (Trans.). Writings from the 'Philokalia' on prayer of the heart. London: Faber and Faber. (Original work published 1951); 1992.
12. Walsh R, Shapiro SL. The meeting of meditative disciplines and Western psychology: A mutually enriching dialogue. American Psychologist. 2006;61:227-39.
13. Flood G. The ascetic self: Subjectivity, memory and tradition. Cambridge: Cambridge University Press; 2004.
14. Newman JW. Disciplines of attention: Buddhist insight meditation, the Ignatian spiritual exercises, and classical psychoanalysis. New York: Peter Lang; 1996.
15. Anuruddha A. A comprehensive manual of Abhidhamma B Bodhi, M Narada (Eds) (Trans.). Seattle: BPS Pariyatti; 2000.
16. Orme-Johnson D, Zimmerman E, Hawkins M. Maharishi's Vedic psychology: The science of the cosmic psyche. In: H Kao, Sinha D (Eds), Asian perspectives on psychology. New Delhi: Sage; 1997.pp.282-308.
17. Alexander CN, Druker S, Langer E. Introduction: Major issues in the exploration of adult growth. In: Alexander C, Langer E (Eds). Higher stages of human development. New York: Oxford University Press; 1990.pp. 3-32.
18. Dillbeck MC, Alexander CN. Higher states of consciousness: Maharishi Mahesh Yogi's Vedic psychology of human development. The Journal of Mind and Behaviour. 1989;10: 307-34.
19. Jiving R, Wallace RK, Bieidebach M. The physiology of meditation: A review. A wakeful hypometabolic integrated response. Neuroscience and Biobehavioural Reviews. 1992;16: 415-24.
20. Walton K, Schneider RH, Nidich SI, Salerno JW, Nordstrom CK, Bairey Merz CN. Psychosocial stress and cardiovascular disease part 2: Effectiveness of the transcendental meditation program in treatment and prevention. Behavioural Medicine. 2002;28:106-23.
21. Orme-Johnson D, Zimmerman E, Hawkins M. Maharishi's Vedic psychology: The science of the cosmic psyche. In: Kao H, Sinha D (Eds). Asian perspectives on psychology. New Delhi: Sage; 1997.pp.282-308.
22. Gelderloos P, Hermans H, Ahlscruom H, Jacoby R. Transcendence and psychological health: Studies with long-term participants of the transcendental meditation and TM-Sidhi program. The Journal of Psychology. 2001;124:177-97.
23. Favazza AR. Comprehensive Textbook of Psychiatry. Lippincott Williams and Wilkins; 2009.
24. Vergote A. Plying between psychology and mysticism. In: Belzen J, Geels A (Eds). Mysticism: A variety of psychological perspectives. Amsterdam: Rodopi; 2003.pp.81-7.
25. James W. The varieties of religious experience. New York: Collier. (Original work published 1902); 1961.
26. Turner D. The darkness of God: Negativity in Christian mysticism. New York: Cambridge University Press; 1995.
27. Vergote A. Psychoanalysis, phenomenological anthropology and religion (J Corveleyn and D Hutsebaut, Eds), Leuven: Leuven University Press; 1998.
28. Hood RW Jr. Dimensions of mystical experiences: Empirical studies and psychological links. Amsterdam: Rodopi; 2001.
29. Louth A. Maximus the Confessor. London: Routledge; 1996.
30. Welch J. The Carmelite way: An ancient path for today's pilgrim. New York: Paulist Press; 1996.
31. Theophan St. The spiritual life and how to be attuned to it (A Dockham, Trans.). Platina, CA: St Herman of Alaska Brotherhood; 1995.
32. Underhill E. Mysticism. New York: Image. (Original work published 1911); 1990.
33. Aumann J. Spiritual theology. London: Sheed and Ward; 1980.
34. Merton T. Pre-Benedictine monasticism: Initiation into the monastic tradition 2 (P O'Connell, Ed.), Kalamazoo, MI: Cistercian Press; 2006.
35. Olivelle P (Trans.). The law code of Manu. New York: Oxford University Press; 2004b.
36. Loori JD. Riding the ox home: Stages on the path of enlightenment. Boston: Shambhala; 1999.
37. Nelson JM. Psychology, religion and spirituality. Springer; 2009.

38. Piaget J. The moral judgment of the child (M Gabain, Trans.). New York: Free Press. (Original work published 1932); 1997.
39. Fowler JW, Dell ML. Stages of faith and identity: Birth to teens. Child and Adolescent Psychiatric Clinics of North America. 2004;13(1):17-33.
40. Oser F. Toward a logic of religious development: A reply to my critics. In: Fowler J, Nipkow K, Schweitzer F (Eds). Stages of faith and religious development: Implications for church, education, and society. New York: Crossroad; 1991. pp.37-64.
41. Ryan R, Deci E. On happiness and human potentials: A review of research on hedonic and eudaimonic well-being. Annual Review of Psychology. 2001;52:141-66.
42. Dillon M, Wink P. Religiousness and spirituality: Trajectories and vital involvement in late adulthood. In: Dillon M (Ed). Handbook of the sociology of religion. Cambridge: Cambridge University Press; 2003.pp.179-89.
43. Emmons RA. The psychology of ultimate concerns: Motivation and spirituality in personality. New York: Guilford Press; 1999.
44. Maddi S. Creating meaning through making decisions. In: Wong P, Fry P (Eds). The human quest for meaning: A handbook of psychological research and clinical applications. Mahwah, NJ: Lawrence Erlbaum Associates; 1998.pp.3-26.
45. Ellison CW. Spiritual well-being: Conceptualization and measurement. Journal of Psychology and Theology. 1983;11: 330-40.
46. Yarhouse M, Butman R, McRay B. The modern psychopathologies: A comprehensive Christian appraisal. Downers Grove, IL: InterVarsity Press; 2005.
47. Gorsuch RL. Religious aspects of substance abuse and recovery. Journal of Social Issues. 1995;51(2):65-83.
48. Booth J, Martin J. Spiritual and religious factors in substance use, dependence, and recovery. In: Koenig H (Ed). Handbook of religion and mental health. San Diego, CA: Academic Press; 1998.pp.175-200.
49. Plante T, Sharma N. Religious faith and mental health outcomes. In: Plante T, Sherman A (Eds). Faith and health: Psychological perspectives. New York: Guilford; 2001. pp.240-64.
50. Pardini DA, Plante TG, Sherman A, Stump JE. Religious faith and spirituality in substance abuse recovery: Determining the mental health benefits. Journal of Substance Abuse Treatment. 2000;19:347-54.
51. Sommer SM. The experience of long-term recovering alcoholics in alcoholics anonymous: Perspectives on therapy. Alcoholism Treatment Quarterly. 1997;15:75-80.
52. Kaskutas LE, Turk N, Bond J, Weisner C. The role of religion, spirituality and Alcoholics Anonymous in sustained sobriety. Alcoholism Treatment Quarterly. 2003;21:1-16.
53. May G. Care of mind, care of spirit. San Francisco: HarperSanFrancisco; 1992.
54. Larson C, Nitschke J, Davidson R. Common and distinct patterns of affective response in dimensions of anxiety and depression. Emotion. 2007;7:182-91.
55. Murphy JM, Nierenberg AA, Laird NM, Monson RR, Sobol AM, Leighton AH. Incidence of major depression: Prediction from subthreshold categories in the Stirling County Study. Journal of Affective Disorders. 2002;68:251-9.
56. McCullough ME, Smith T. Religion and health: Depressive symptoms and mortality as case studies. In: M Dillon (Ed). Handbook of the sociology of religion. Cambridge: Cambridge University Press; 2003.pp.190-204.
57. Koenig HG, Larson DB. Religion and mental health: Evidence for an association. International Review of Psychiatry. 2001;13:67-78.
58. Koenig HG. Religion and medicine II: Religion, mental health, and related behaviours. International Journal of Psychiatry in Medicine. 2001a;31:97-109.
59. Meador K, Koenig H, Hughes D, Blazer D. Religious affiliation and major depression. Hospital and Community Psychiatry. 1992;43;1204-08.
60. Exline JJ, Yali AM, Sanderson WC. Guilt, discord, and alienation: The role of religious strain in depression and suicidality. Journal of Clinical Psychology. 2000;56:1481-96.
61. Wink P, Dillon M, Larsen B. Religion as moderator of the depression-health connection: Findings from a longitudinal study. Research on Aging. 2005;27:197-220.
62. Smith TB, McCullough ME, Poll J. Religiousness and depression: Evidence for a main effect and the moderating influence of stressful life events. Psychological Bulletin. 2003;129:614-36.
63. Flannelly KJ, Weaver AJ, Smith WJ, Handzo GF. Psychologists and health care chaplains doing research together. Journal of Psychology and Christianity. 2003;22:327-32.
64. Patrick J, Kinney J. Why believe? The effects of religious beliefs on emotional wellbeing. In: McFadden S, Brennan M, Patrick J (Eds). New directions in the study of late life religiousness and spirituality. Binghampton, NY: Haworth Pastoral Press; 2003. pp.153-70.
65. Roberts GA. Delusional belief systems and meaning in life: a preferred reality? British Journal of Psychiatry; 1991;159(suppl. 14):19-28.
66. Dawkins R. The God Delusion. Bantam Press; 2006.
67. Gelder M, Gath D, Mayou P, et al. Oxford Textbook of Psychiatry (3rd edition). Oxford University Press; 1996.
68. Greenberg D, Witztum E. Buchbinder JT. Mysticism and psychosis: the fate of Ben Zoma. British Journal of Medical Psychology. 1992;65:223-35.
69. Jackson M, Fulford KWM. Spiritual experience and psychopathology. Philosophy, Psychiatry and Psychology. 1997;4:41-65.
70. Saver JL, Rabin J. The neural substrates of religious experience. Journal of Neuropsychiatry and Clinical Neurosciences. 1997;9:495-510.
71. Buckley P. Mystical experience and schizophrenia. Schizophrenia Bulletin. 1981;7:516-21.
72. Lukoff D. Transpersonal perspectives on manic psychosis: creative visionary and mystical states. Journal of Transpersonal Psychology. 1985;20:111-39.

73. Greenberg D, Witztum E, Buchbinder JT. Mysticism and psychosis: the fate of Ben Zoma. British Journal of Medical Psychology. 1992;65:223-35.
74. Dinniss S, Roberts G, Hubbard C, et al. User-led assessment of a recovery service using DREEM. Psychiatric Bulletin. 2007;31:124-7.
75. Chadwick PK. Sanity to supersanity to insanity: a personal journey. Psychosis and Spirituality: Exploring the New Frontier (I Clarke Ed). Whurr; 2001.pp.75-89.
76. Koenig HG. Religion and Spirituality in Psychiatry. Cambridge University Press; 2009
77. Perroud N. Religion and Spirituality in Psychiatry. Cambridge University Press; 2009.
78. Newberg A, Alavi A, Baime M, Pourdehnad M, Santanna J, d'Aquili E. The measurement of regional cerebral blood flow during the complex cognitive task of meditation: a preliminary SPECT study. Psychiatry Res. 2001;106 (2): 113-22.
79. Newberg A, Pourdehnad M, Alavi A, d' Aquili EG. Cerebral blood flow during meditative prayer: preliminary findings and methodological issues. Percept Mot Skills. 2003;97(2): 625-30.
80. Newberg AB, Iversen J. The neural basis of the complex mental task of meditation: neurotransmitter and neurochemical considerations. Med Hypotheses. 2003;61(2):282-91.
81. Aftanas LI, Golocheikine SA. Human anterior and frontal midline theta and lower alpha reflect emotionally positive state and internalized attention: high-resolution EEG investigation of meditation. Neurosci Lett. 2001;310(1): 57-60.
82. Jevning R, Anand R, Biedebach M, Fernando G. Effects on regional cerebral blood flow of transcendental meditation. Physiol Behav. 1996;59(3):399-402.
83. Lehmann D, Faber PL, Achermann P, Jeanmonod D, Gianotti LR, Pizzagalli D. Brain sources of EEG gamma frequency during volitionally meditation-induced, altered states of consciousness, and experience of the self. Psychiatry Res. 2001;108 (2):111-21.
84. Azari NP, Nickel J, Wunderlich G, et al. Neural correlates of religious experience. Eur J Neurosci. 2001;13(8):1649-52 Persinger MA. Preadolescent religious experience enhances temporal lobe signs in normal young adults. Percept Mot Skills. 1991;72 (2):453-4.
85. Persinger MA. Preadolescent religious experience enhances temporal lobe signs in normal young adults. Percept Mot Skills. 1991;72(2):453-4.
86. Persinger MA. People who report religious experiences may also display enhanced temporal-lobe signs. Percept Mot Skills. 1984;58(3):963-75.
87. Britton WB, Bootzin RR. Near-death experiences and the temporal lobe. Psychol Sci. 2004;15(4):254-8.
88. MacDonald DA, Holland D. Spirituality and complex partial epileptic like signs. Psychol Rep. 2002;91(Pt 1):785-92.
89. Larry Culliford, Sarah Eagger. Spirituality and Psychiatry. RCPsych Publication; 2009.
90. King M, Speck P, Thomas A. The royal free interview for religious and spiritual beliefs: development and standardisation. Psychological Medicine. 1995;25:1125-34.
91. Hatch RM, Burg MA, Naberhaus DS, et al. The Spiritual Involvement and Beliefs Scale: development and testing of a new instrument. Journal of Family Practice. 1998;46:476-86.
92. Fetzer Institute/National Institute on Ageing Working Group. Multidimensional Measurement of Religiousness/Spirituality for Use in Health Research. Fetzer Institute; 1999.
93. Hill P, Hood R. Jr Measures of Religiosity. Religious Education Press; 1999.
94. Standard R, Sandhu D, Painter L. Assessment of spirituality in counseling. Journal of Counseling and Development. 2000;78(2):204-11.
95. Sperry L. Spirituality in Clinical Practice. Ann Arbor, MI: Sheridan Books; 2001.
96. Eagger S. A Short Guide to the Assessment of Spiritual Concerns in Mental Healthcare. Royal College of Psychiatrists (*http://www.rcpsych.ac.uk/PDF/DrSEaggeGuide.pdf*). 2006.
97. Royal College of Psychiatrists. Spirituality and Mental Health (Help is at Hand Series leaflet). Royal College of Psychiatrists; 2006.
98. Puchalski C, Romer A. Taking a spiritual history allows clinicians to understand patients more fully. Journal of Palliative Medicine. 2000;3:129-37.
99. Anandarajah G, Hight E. Spirituality and medical practice: using the HOPE questions as a practical tool for spiritual assessment. American Family Physician. 2001;63:81-92.
100. Maugans TA. The spiritual history. Archives of Family Medicine. 1996;5:11-6.
101. Bullis RK. Spirituality in social work practice. Washington, DC: Taylor & Francis; 1996.
102. Rene Hefti. Religion and spirituality in psychiatry. Cambridge University Press; 2009.
103. Bhawuk DPS. Culture's influence on creativity: the case of Indian spirituality. International Journal of Intercultural Relations. 2003;27:1-22.

CHAPTER 61 Community Psychiatry

Suresh Bada Math, Naveen Kumar C, CR Chandrashekar

INTRODUCTION

Mental health problems are seen worldwide. The psychiatry morbidity shown by different Indian studies pointed out a major problem as in other countries.[1-19] They affect all sections of the society irrespective of age, class, religion, ethnicity, rural or urban domicile. They constitute a wide spectrum ranging from sub-clinical states to very severe forms of disorders. Mental health problems can attain the disorder/syndrome or disease levels which are considered easy to recognize, define and diagnose. Hence, they can be called as *'Visible Mental Health Problems'* in the community. These visible mental health problems can again be classified into *Major mental disorders* (Schizophrenia, mania, depression and bipolar disorders and so forth) and *minor mental disorders* (Anxiety disorders, somatoform disorders, stress-related disorders, dissociative disorders, insomnia and so forth). Major mental disorders are commonly encountered in hospitals; minor mental disorders however are commonly seen in the community. Another group of mental health problems remain at sub-clinical/non-clinical/sub-syndromal level. They are difficult to recognize, define or diagnose. These are called as *'Invisible Mental Health Problems'* in the community.[2] There also exists an argument not to pathologize these problems which are faced by most of the individuals on day to day basis secondary to common life stressors. Mental health problems affect the normal functioning of the individuals and have direct effect on the quality of life as well. Not only individuals suffer, but also the family and society at large. These have direct effects on the productivity and economic growth of the society.

Community psychiatry as a term was originally meant to denote 'deinstitutionalization' in the western countries. As the specialty developed, so did the concept and as it stands now means any activity related to mental health that happens outside the premises of a mental hospital.[6] The true essence of community psychiatry is to make sure that care reaches each one of the deserved patients at their doorsteps and includes all such approaches that contribute towards this goal. This goal is supposed to be achieved through various means such as *outpatient mental health services, mobile outreach treatment units, intensive outpatient services, case management and assertive community treatment, community rehabilitation centers* and *support groups* who are in need of psychiatric services.

Community outpatient mental health services are designed to serve patients who are discharged from the psychiatry inpatient units who require a higher level of care at their residential places. *The community mobile treatment units* travel to interior places and then services are delivered in the patient's home or in appropriate community settings on regular basis. *The Case Management and Assertive Community Treatment* involves individualized services for those having chronic major mental illnesses, homeless persons with mental illnesses and persons with mental illnesses requiring assistance for general medical conditions. These units provide education, crisis intervention, community support, needs assessments, personalized service plans (such as money management, assistance in daily living), consumer advocacy and facilitate/coordinate individuals' access to psychiatric care, emergency care, etc. *Home visit services* by the community team is done to assess and manage the patients at home and it also enables the professionals to better understand the patient's social circumstances so that the appropriate assistance can be rendered to the patient and his family. This is particularly useful for elderly with dementia, individuals with mental retardation, autism, organic brain disorders and so forth. Vocational rehabilitation at the community enables the occupational therapist to assess the patient's ability to cope with his activities of daily living at home and provides suitable therapy. *Community rehabilitation centers* are important to enable the mentally ill to integrate back into society. Day care centers, sheltered workshops, day support, respite care, and vocational rehabilitation centers endure to optimize functional levels of patients and help them prepare for employment. *Community Support Groups* (such as family support groups, spouse support group, self help groups and voluntary lay counselors groups) enable net working, crisis management, socialization, recreational and educational activities of the mentally ill. These support groups bring together care-givers and significant others to share their experiences and learn from one another about looking after the mentally ill in the family and community at large. At times, combination of the above services is provided by the group of trained professionals after liaising with the local leaders of the community. Some of the above mentioned services are not yet active in India as they are not economically feasible. In India, any mental health related activity that occurs outside the premises of hospitals can be brought under the purview of community psychiatry. These include activities such as those carried out by non-governmental organizations, rehabilitation centers, lay counselors, alternative systems working towards mental health care, the role of families in caring for the mentally ill, mental health care that occurs in primary health centers, national programs of mental health, research that occurs in communities, psychiatric epidemiology, etc.

To cover the entire gamut of community psychiatry is beyond the scope of this chapter. In this chapter, we touch upon the three important dimensions of community psychiatry viz: community studies in India, the National Mental Health Program and the research in the area of community psychiatry focusing on severe mental disorders. At the outset, the authors wish to state that the information contained herein is by no means comprehensive. Issues such as child and adolescent psychiatry, geriatric psychiatry or addiction psychiatry have not been discussed. Authors have attempted to summarize the research done in the area of community psychiatry specifically focusing on those studies in which sampling frames include rural areas. This is because India is a predominantly rural country and about 70% of the population lives in village communities. This makes the findings relatively generalizable.

FREQUENCY OF MENTAL DISORDERS IN THE COMMUNITY

Community psychiatry not only focuses on available treatment resources, but also on the aim of understanding and controlling the occurrence of mental illness. The patients from community settings differ from those of hospitals because of the following reasons: a) community samples contain patients who are usually mildly ill, b) they are not treatment seekers, c) course and outcome of the community sample and d) biological, occupational and social dysfunction associated with community samples may be different from those encountered in hospitals. This can be further explained by the pathways to care pyramid as shown in Figure 1.[2]

In countries such as ours, only minority of the psychiatric patients receive treatment. Majority of the patients approaching primary care physicians, family physicians and alternative complimentary medicine do not receive adequate psychiatric treatment. They receive nonspecific treatments because the knowledge about mental health in these service providers is very poor. Religious and faith healers also contribute to this group. At the bottom of the pyramid remains a huge population who may not receive treatment at all. Reasons for this can be extremely complex and needs to be addressed urgently. In this background, a recent qualitative study done by Reddy et al (in press)[14] systematically studied the factors that kept rural community patients out of the treatment ambit. Hierarchy of these factors were as follows: Patients'/family member's knowledge and

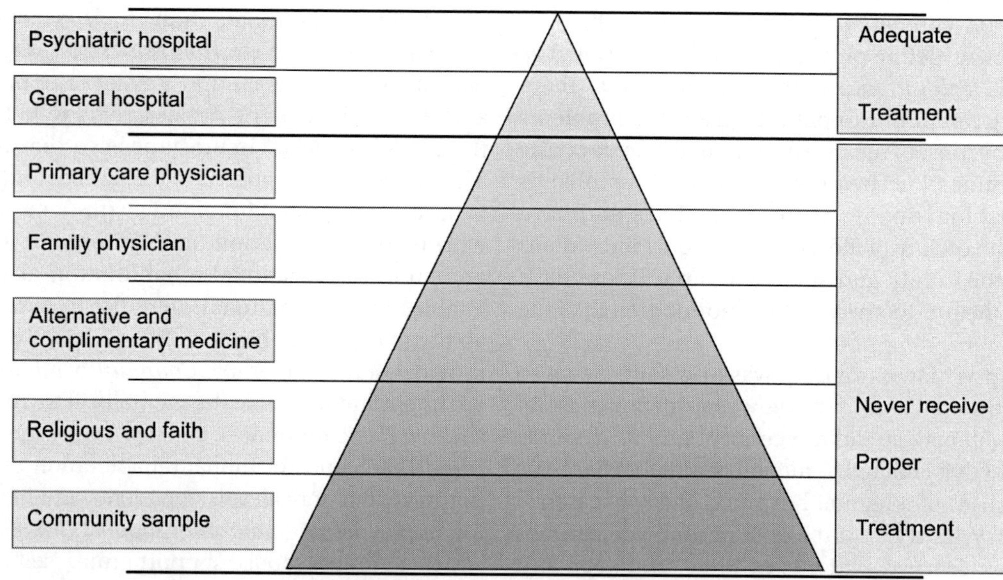

Fig. 1: Pathways to mental healthcare pyramid in developing countries

attitude towards illness; family support; patients'/family members' attitude towards the need for treatment; family dynamics; family's tolerance and acceptance of illness and related disability; financial constraints; lack of insight and active non-cooperation from the patient; family's resilience towards symptoms and disability; community's attitude and beliefs; gender; community's acceptance and support for the patient; accessibility of treatment centers; age of the patient; stigma and medical illnesses/ conditions.

Across the globe, community sampling is advocated in order to get a complete and comprehensive understanding of morbidity experiences. This is even more so in countries such as India.[2] In the *community survey* approach, each member of the study sample is individually investigated to accurately classify his/her disease status. These types of studies may be accurate when compared to hospital sampling studies but are difficult to conduct and requires huge amount of resources. Providing accurate prevalence data on mental disorders though essential in policy making and providing care in the community, one needs to keep in mind the variability of the prevalence rates both within the community over time and also across populations during the same time.

ECONOMIC COST INCURRED BY THE PERSON WITH MENTAL ILLNESS FOR TREATMENT

Most of the community based Indian studies are on point prevalence. Table 1 summarizes the prevalence of psychiatric morbidity in community surveys. Studies summarized cover all psychiatric disorders or at least priority/major mental disorders covering all age groups. These studies report varying prevalence rates, ranging from 9.5[1] to 102[11] per 1000 population.

Table 1: Prevalence of psychiatric morbidity in general population

Investigator	*Year*	*Center*	*Location*	*Sampling*	*Tool*	*Pop*	*Prevalence/ 1000*
Surya[1]	1964	Pondicherry	U	H-H	MHSQ(P)	2731	9.5
Sethi et al[3]	1967	Lucknow	U	H-H	QAPF	1733	72.7`
Dube[4]	1970	Agra	M	H-H	DCP	29.468	18
Elnager et al[5]	1971	Hoogly	R	H-H	CHM & DCP (2)	1393	27
Sethi et al[6]	1972	Lucknow	R	H-H	CHQ & CHM	2691	39.4
Verghese et al[8]	1973	Vellore	U	SRS	MHIS & DCP as per ICD (1965)	1887	66.5
Sethi et al[9]	1974	Lucknow	R	3SPS	PSQ & DCP as per DSM-II (1968)	4481	67.0
Thacore et al[10]	1975	Lucknow	U	H-H	PHQ & DCP	1977	81.6
Nandi et al[11]	1975	West Bengal	R	H-H	HS, QS & CRS as per ICD (1965 R)	1060	102.8
Nandi et al[12]	1979	West Bengal	R	H-H	HS, SESS, CDS & CRS	3718	102
Shah et al[13]	1980	Ahmedabad	U	H-H	MHSQ & DCP	2712	47.2
Mehta et al[15]	1985	Vellore	R	S-S	IPSS & DCP	5941	14.5
Sachdeva et al[16]	1986	Faridkot	R	H-H	HS, SESS & CDS	1989	22.12
Premrajan et al[17]	1993	Pondichery	U	RS	IPSS & DCP as per ICD-9R	1115	99.4
Shaji et al[18]	1995	Ernakulam	R	H-H	IPSS, SESS, CRS & DCP, ICD-10	5284	14.57
Sharma and Singh[19]	2001	Goa	M	SRS	RPES & DCP as per ICD-9	4022	60.2

Source: Math et al 2007, IJMR, 183-192

Abbreviations:

U-urban; R-rural; H-H- house to house survey; S-S - systematic sampling; SRS - stratified random sampling 3SPS- 3 stage probability sampling; RS- random sampling, ICD- international classification of diseases DSM-II- diagnostic and statistical manual of mental disorders.

Tools:

MHSQ= Mental health Screening Questionnaire
QAPF=Questionnaire for the assessment of psychiatric state of the family
DCP = Diagnosis confirmed by a psychiatrist(s)
CHQ = Case history questionnaire
SFQ=Social functioning questionnaire
PSQ=Psychiatric screening questionnaire
HS=Household schedule
CRS=Case record schedule
SESS=Socio-economic status schedule
CHM = Case history method
IPSS=Indian Psychiatric Survey Schedule
MHIS=Mental health item sheet
PHQ=Psychiatric health questionnaire
QS=Questionnaire schedule
CDS = Case detection schedule
RPES= Rapid psychiatric examination schedule

Table 2: Reasons for wide variations in reported in Indian epidemiological studies[2]

- Inherent nature of the psychiatric disorders
- Diagnostic methods
- Definition used to define a 'case'
- Systematic under-reporting
- Recall bias
- Single informant
- Need for treatment
- Screening instrument
- Diagnostic methods used (clinical interview, structured interview or semi-structured interview)
- Sampling procedure
- Sampling bias

Table 3: Conservative estimate of treating mentally ill patients

Cost for mental health care for an individual	*Per month*
Medication cost per month for an individual suffering from mental illness	₹ 300
Traveling cost to meet the mental health professionals	₹ 100
Doctors fees (mental health professionals) Loss of daily wages (for two people) Miscellaneous expenditure during travel (such as food, water, etc.)	₹ 200 ₹ 300 ₹ 100
Total	**₹ 1000**
Cost for mental health care for the whole country per month Considering prevalence to be 50–60/1000 population, 6 crore population requires professional help. (Total cost = 6 crores × ₹ 1000)	6000 crores

Reasons for such wide variations in prevalence rates are summarized in the Table 2.[2]

A meta-analysis of 13 epidemiological studies by Reddy and Chandrasekar in (1998),[20,21] reported a total morbidity of 58.2 per 1000. Another meta-analysis of epidemiological studies by Ganguli (2000)[22] reported a total morbidity of 73 per 1000. Macro-economic commission report of 2005 considered prevalence rate of 65/1000 population (average of two meta-analysis).[23] In simple words, approximately 5-6 crore persons in India require professional help for their mental morbidity. If we consider that each patient requires ₹ 1000 per month for his/her mental health care (including medication costs, doctor's fees and traveling costs to meet the doctor), the approximate total cost required per month will be a mind-boggling 6000 crores rupees (Table 3). To address this costly issue, India adopted National Mental Health Program (NMHP) to provide services at the doorsteps by integrating mental health care into the primary health care system. This integrative model was first successfully tested in Bellary district of Karnataka State in 1985.

Unfortunately, mental illness requires medication for longer durations. Most of them require medications from several months to years. Many of these disorders if not detected early and treated may become chronic and require medication for life. If we do not address this issue, then the indirect costs in terms of loss of wages, disability, absenteeism and substance use is unimaginable. Above all, these families face social isolation, burden, stigma, poor quality of life and an enormous psychological strain.

Community psychiatry is based on the strong principle that person with mental illness can be effectively treated in their local environment using the community resources rather than in a mental hospitals. This model of approach is cost-effective, reduces stigma and provides an excellent opportunity to the community members in raising awareness and also patients get integrated back to the community at the earliest. The patient and family members seek psychiatric help if it is available within the community, thus enabling early detection and treatment. It is also essential that community psychiatric services are affordable, comprehensive and accessible. This can be achieved by integrating mental health service with the primary care. It is essential to invest in mental health by the government for providing care at the door steps which is actually the fundamental goal of community psychiatry. In order to achieve this goal, Government of India implemented the National Mental Health Program (NMHP).

DISTRICT MENTAL HEALTH PROGRAM

District Mental Health Program (DMHP) is the vehicle through which the goals and objectives of the National Mental Health Program (NMHP) are supposed to be met.[24] The DMHP was started based on the successful model demonstrated in Bellary district of Karnataka state way back in 1985. Government of India has till now operationalized DMHP in many districts of the country and envisages extending this program to all districts of the country in the coming years. In summary, the objectives of the DMHP include:

- Provision of basic mental health care in the community by integrating mental health system into the general health care delivery system (Primary Health Centers). Identification and treatment of persons with mental disorders to be done by the health workers and primary care physicians
- To launch extensive information and communication activities about the nature, course and the availability of treatment for mental disorders
- To facilitate adequate psychosocial care of the recovered mentally ill in the community by making linkages with non-governmental organizations locally
- Initiate mental health promotional activities in schools and colleges
- To develop active public-private partnerships.

Over a period of time, the NMHP has undergone a complete review and reorientation and a major achievement has been the increase in funds. Various innovative approaches adopted in the current NMHP include rural and urban mental health, school mental health, adolescent mental health, suicide prevention and public private partnership. Following are the salient features of the revised NMHP:

- *The District Mental Health Program:* The DMHP was developed as an approach to deliver mental health care through primary health care for the entire district. Based on the mid-term review and two national consultative meetings, the existing DMHP is being strengthened by adding the adolescent mental health programme that includes health promotion for high school students, intervention for students with emotional problems, counseling for out of school children and college based counseling services. Urban Mental Health Programme (UMHP) is a new addition to the NMHP.
- *Preparatory phase:* This is a new concept, in which each state should map the mental health resources in the private and public sectors before applying for the project. The state has to identify the nodal officer and programme officer and get their written consent. They should undergo sensitization and the programme officer should undergo training for three months before the total grants are released.
- *Adolescent and School Mental Health Program:* This involves health promotion through life skills education for development of psychosocial competence. This model, using teachers as trained resource staff has been approved as an accepted strategy internationally both in developing and developed countries. It is envisaged that 500 rural blocks and 100 urban blocks will be taken up for the adolescent mental health programme that includes life skills education for adolescents and intervention for emotional problems. Adolescents' mental health programme for out of school adolescents in both rural and urban districts in the country is also envisaged. Networking with department of youth and sports, NGOs and other voluntary organizations will be established to provide appropriate interventions for this population. This programme will cater to 30,000 schools covering 1,00,00,000 adolescents.
- *College Mental Health Program:* Emotional distress, adjustment and substance use problems are significant issues in college students that need attention. Trained teachers can effectively handle such problems within the context of the college. It is planned to cover all the pre-university and degree colleges in all the districts in the country. One hundred college teachers in each of the 500 rural districts and 300 college teachers in each of the 50 urban districts will be trained to provide counseling services in the college.
- *Improvement in health manpower status:* It is envisaged to support the development of 11 regional Institutes of Mental Health with a one time grant of ₹ 30 crores for infrastructure development. It is also proposed to equip 30 medical colleges to start/strengthen their post-graduate programme in mental health. The running cost for 5 years will be met in addition to the initial support for infrastructure development.
- *Research and mental health:* This may be implemented under the following headings:
  - Biology of mental disorders
  - Early intervention for mental disorders
  - Improving long term outcomes in drug and alcohol dependence
  - Social factors/support systems to minimize disability in chronic psychosis.
  - Health behavior research
  - Psychological and social factors contributing to mental disorders and disability
  - Interventions to improve functional outcome, reduce disability and stigma
  - Interventions for prevention of illness and promotion of mental health.
  - Levels and limits of mental health care by primary care doctors.
  - Outcome of mental disorders treated in primary care settings.
- *IEC activities:* Under this head, the following issues require to be addressed:
  - Development of public awareness material such as video clippings, posters radio/TV messages and wall writings. Projects may be awarded for developing such material with an incentive of a cash prize for the best product. Scientific methods to evaluate the impacts of these on the public have to be initiated.
  - Training material for undergraduate/post graduates in the form of videos, interactive CDs for use on the net/distant education have to be developed.
- *Support money for implementation of the Mental Health Act 1987:* It is proposed to allocate separate funds to assist both the central and the state Mental Health Authorities.
- *Public-Private-Partnership:* This is a key concept. Efforts of government alone are inadequate to realize all the goals of NMHP. The role of NGOs and related organizations in all components of NMHP has been recognized. Appropriate linkages between NGO activities as well as NMHP components by matching them can increase efficiency. A substantial part of the NMHP can be contracted to well-established NGOs/private bodies. For example, the entire life-skill programme (school mental health) can be run by NGOs with checks and balances and monitoring from the professionals; this would also apply to the components of IEC. NGOs can be involved in spreading awareness about mental disorders, organization of self help groups, day care centers, support for families and conduct of mental health camps.

- *Monitoring:* Monitoring the implementation of DMHP in the country is very critical to plan mid-course correction. It is proposed that a central and state level monitoring committee be formed to monitor the DMHP on a monthly basis.
- *Suicide prevention:* Suicide is a growing cause of premature mortality. The causes include psychiatric disorders as well as socioeconomic reasons. Recognition of any underlying psychiatric disorder and early treatment has the potential to prevent suicide. Several vulnerable populations require life skills training and/or counseling to prevent suicides—school and college populations are two examples. Varied social factors need to be addressed that are regionally relevant. Several other sectors have to be linked for networking resources for suicide prevention. Special IEC activities will target specific populations. Each state's nodal officer will be responsible in implementing suicide prevention programme in one or two chosen districts. The budget is proposed for 50 districts (one or two in each state). If the state needs to implement this in more districts, the same may be done through grants for NGOs or state's own resources.
- *Stress management:* Stress is a physiological response of the body to changes within and outside an individual. It is important to recognize that stress responses are an inevitable part of human existence. Stress affects people irrespective of their age, gender, socioeconomic, occupational and educational status. Many empirical studies have established the relationship between stress and illness. Studies based in the United States report that 80–90% of all illnesses are stress related. It is also estimated that 7–8 out of every 10 individuals who consult general practice doctors, do so because of stress and anxiety related symptoms. Studies conducted in India regarding prevalence of psychological distress suggests that nearly one-third to one half of executive officers report symptoms of psychological distress and nearly one in four of them suffer from stress related disorders like diabetes, hypertension, arthritis, various skin and respiratory disorders. It is important to note that prevalence of psychological distress is distinctly more in women compared to men. This difference in psychological distress seems to be related to cultural factors, ability to verbalize emotions, willingness to reliably report symptoms rather than differential vulnerability. It is encouraging to find that a small proportion of individuals have made initiatives to start incorporating life style changes to limit damages due to stress. Most often, the individual makes life style changes after the onset of illness but not before it. Hence, it is clear that the need for stress management is beyond doubt but the crucial question is the conviction to incorporate and to adopt necessary specific life style changes.

Realizing the Goals of the NMHP

In India, the number of formal treatment facilities is far too few. The current development of implementing national mental health programme in a phased manner is indeed very positive. Developing a mechanism to monitor the programme and institutionalize the process so that the local district authorities carry on the task is an important outcome of this activity. DMHP seeks to implement mental health care using the public health approach. The most important aspect of the DMHP is to train doctors, multipurpose workers and other functionaries in task oriented mental health skills. The doctor is expected to evaluate patients attending his/her clinic, diagnose and treat the referred cases from the field. The multi-purpose workers are expected to follow-up the treated patients, monitor the side effects of medication as the case may be, educate the families about the nature of the illness and to support the family during crisis. The doctor is expected to actively support and encourage the multipurpose workers to visit the field and carryout the above mentioned tasks. The District Mental Health Programme officer is available to provide clarification and support to the primary care physician. The primary care physician can refer a case for opinion or inpatient care to the district psychiatrist. Thus, a paradigm shift in strategy from institutional treatment to a holistic community approach has been adopted in the NMHP keeping the aims of promotion, prevention, early detection and treatment. Such an approach would also minimize disability.

Regarding research related to DMHP, Waraich et al (2003)[25] in their study highlighted the huge treatment gap with respect to psychiatric disorders in the country and showed that the follow-up rates can be improved by making treatments available at patients' doorsteps. This study was conducted in a place where DMHP was initiated and in a way gave a glimpse of DMHP activity.

Murthy (1989)[26] in an editorial reported that the main problem was that the targets were not achieved. Delay in formation of advisory groups, limited funding, lack of administrative mechanisms for monitoring the program and variable enthusiasm at the state/union territory levels to include mental health as part of the primary health care level were the causes for this deficit. Similarly, Agarwal (1991)[27] has noted that the program failed to have significant impact in majority of states. Poor infrastructure and lack of political will were some of the possible reasons for its failure. Very recently, Jacob has observed that the national mental health program has failed despite its good intentions. Failure of the recent compilation of evidence (regarding evaluation of magnitude of the burden of mental illnesses and the scientific evidence for their treatment) to acknowledge the reality of the primary care delivery system, poor infrastructure, overburdened systems, inappropriate training, professional apathy, very low spending and utilization on mental health issues and finally the low technical inputs and guidance to revive community psychiatry programs at national levels are among the important reasons for this failure.[28]

CONTRIBUTIONS FROM RESEARCH TOWARDS THE DEVELOPMENT OF COMMUNITY PSYCHIATRY IN INDIA

Research in community psychiatry has dealt with a number of issues such as models for mental health care delivery in rural community, course and outcome of severe mental disorders, evaluation of the district mental health programs, community based rehabilitation (CBR) approaches, training, evaluation of various screening tools and telemedicine approaches. While doing so, the authors have focused on studies on severe mental disorders as they are the most burdensome and consequently, have received largest research attention. This does not in any way mean that other disorders are any less important. Elegant studies for example have been done in communities on suicide, alcohol use disorders, disability, life skills, high-risk groups, disaster and so forth. Hence, keeping in mind the constraints of space and time, only selective review of studies are done.

Chandrashekar et al in (1981)[29] showed that severe mental disorders can be detected and managed in homes if the doctor-cum health worker team of primary health centers (PHCs) are sufficiently trained and if persistent efforts are put into make patients accept long-term regular medications. Similarly, Isaac et al in (1982)[30] reported the successful development and evaluation of a training program for PHC doctors and ground level health workers which aimed at delivering mental health through rural primary care. A community outreach program providing psychotropic medications and basic psychosocial support can be effective in improving a host of outcomes in patients with untreated schizophrenia including disability, symptom severity, family burden and functioning.[31] Recent studies not only have looked into clinical outcomes and functional outcomes from clinician perspective but also from the patient and care-givers perspectives. Both patient and care-givers groups desired, symptom control; employment/education; social functioning; activity; fulfillment of duties and responsibilities; independent functioning; cognitive ability; management without medication; reduced sideeffects; self-care; and self-determination as their desired outcomes.[32] Further, studies have also looked into filling the gap of scarce mental health human resources through systematic development of a lay worker deliverable community based interventions for persons with schizophrenia. These lay workers provide interventions that contain basic components such as psycho-education, adherence management, rehabilitation, referral to community agencies and health promotion supervised by specialists.[33]

In the past decade, innovative community intervention programs are underway in two rural taluks of Karnataka state. The aims of these programs are to identify, treat and follow-up all patients with schizophrenia. The key-informant method is employed for case-identification. Though psychiatrists are involved in confirming the diagnosis, their role is limited in the overall care of patients as they visit these sites only periodically. Social workers are involved in coordinating the entire program by taking part in each and every step of the program implementation including case-identification, involving and training the local health workers including ASHA workers (Accredited Social Health Activist), coordinating follow-up visits, visiting patients' homes in times of need, acting as first contact to patients/families and guiding them at times of emergencies and coordinating with the local health administration (for example, ensuring endless supply of antipsychotic medications in the PHC) in order to run the program smoothly. In a way, one social worker is responsible for the care of most patients with schizophrenia of the entire taluk. Psychotropic medications is being provided free of cost. Basic psychoeducation about the nature and course of severe mental disorders and need for long-term medications are being provided on a regular basis.[34] Studies that have emanated from these intervention programs have given results of considerable public health significance. For example, those patients on regular medications had significantly less disability when compared to those who were not taking antipsychotic medications.[35] Adhering to antipsychotic medications alone in the community can result in considerable reduction of disability and also enhanced work performance.[34,36,37] Another important area which has been studied is the metabolic syndrome. When compared to the urban samples, rates of metabolic syndromes are low among rural patients.[38-40] The complex interactions between genetic and environmental factors are responsible for the manifestation of metabolic syndrome in patients with schizophrenia.

Regarding Community Based Rehabilitation (CBR) approaches, there have been two elegant studies which have shown that even for severe mental disorders, CBR could be feasible and successful and better than routine out-patient care. Chatterjee et al in their study (2003), showed that within the CBR group, compliant participants had significantly better outcomes compared with partially compliant or non-complaint participants.[41] Another study by the same group, showed that disability levels reduce to very low levels after four years of follow-up among those who engaged actively in the CBR program.[42] The utilization of community care by chronic mentally ill depends directly on financial constraints, limited accessibility, lack of awareness and lack of support from the families and communities. Community based initiatives in the management of mental disorders may not be sustainable unless the family and the community are actively and continuously involved with support from mental health professionals.[43]

CHALLENGES AND FUTURE DIRECTIONS IN COMMUNITY PSYCHIATRY

Barriers in successfully implementing mental health services at the community level include following; lower priority in comparison with physical health needs; the stigma associated with mental disorders results in failure to seek appropriate care; poor funding towards mental health; lack of trained man-power, scarcity of public-health perspectives in mental health leadership, lack of consumer movements and vertical nature of community health programs with different programs competing for the health worker's time and expertise and the enlarged scope of mental health programs being beyond the scope of the available resources and expertise.[44,45]

There is a need to improve mental health care delivery, restructure medical and nursing education into skill based courses, revamping of psychiatric training by enabling professionals to recognize and manage psychiatric disorders at the primary health care level, revitalizing primary care by strengthening the general health infrastructure, transforming the overburdened and demoralized primary care systems, generation of political will towards organization of mental health care, shifting the immediate goal to be restricted to the identification and treatment of priority disorders (psychoses, depression and substance use disorders), bridging mental health issues with existing public health priorities by shifting community psychiatry to the field of community medicine, seeking active cooperation from private health systems and traditional health system workers, faith-healers, overcoming resistance to decentralization of resources, development of community mental health services including continuous support for primary health care workers and finally harnessing all available media resources to enhance awareness regarding mental disorders and their treatment.[28,45-48]

In contemporary world, the role of telepsychiatry has been widely discussed in community psychiatry. Thara (2013) gives glimpses of a mobile telepsychiatry unit in the Tamil Nadu state.[49] The services are provided on a custom-built bus that contains a consultation room and a pharmacy. The communication takes place between the patient/care-givers inside the bus and the mental health professional elsewhere. The program has largely been successful and has demonstrated the feasibility of service delivery. The author concludes by stating that with the recent advances in telecommunication facilities in India, this could be the ideal time to exploit the immense potential of telepsychiatry. However, telemedicine has disadvantages also. This is exemplified by a study by Holla et al (in press).[50] They described the utilization pattern and challenges of the telemedicine network project of the Karnataka state. They reported that though services were operational in 25 district hospitals, its utilization was not optimal: quality of satellite connection was acceptable in 18 (72%) center. Teleconsultation advices from nodal centers were carried out completely in only 9 (36%) centers. Only in 13 (52%) client centers, did doctors keep up with appointment regularly. All technicians reported that the training they received was inadequate. 16 (64%) technicians were asked to do works that were not pertaining to telemedicine. The researchers concluded that the service is largely under-utilized and has failed to deliver the promise. Tele-medicine approach if properly implemented can inject much needed support to community psychiatry.

CONCLUSION

Community care of persons with mental illness has moved a long way from the institution to community settings. This has been possible because of the commitment on the part of the Government, professionals, institutional policies and legislations. Community is not a cheap alternative to hospital but a realistic alternative to fill the wide treatment gaps that exists. Community care has been accepted as the most suitable and realistic alternative. Treating patients at their doorsteps is cost-effective, can reduce stigma and can provide an excellent opportunity to community to raise awareness. Also patients can get integrated to the community at the earliest. Community care has its merits even from the human rights perspective. The DMHP promises to provide easy access to mental health care without any discrimination. Realized into action, it will reduce disability, lowers family distress and burden and reduces the stigma of mental illness. Ultimately, it will integrate mental health care with primary health care, which is the main objective of the National Mental Health Program. Taking basic and free mental health care to the doorstep of every member in our society will realize the vision of Health as a Fundamental Right.

REFERENCES

1. Surya NC. Mental morbidity in Pondicherry. Transaction-4, Bangalore: All India Institute of Mental Health. 1964.
2. Math SB, Srinivasaraju R. Epidemiology of psychiatric disorders in India. Indian J Psychiatry. 2010;52:95-103.
3. Sethi BB, Gupta SC, Rajkumar S. Three hundred urban families-a psychiatric study. Indian J Psychiatry. 1967;9:280-302.
4. Dube KC. A Study of prevalence and biosocial variables in mental illness in rural and urban community in Uttar Pradesh, India. Acta Psychiatr Scand. 1970;46:327-59.
5. Elnager MN, Maitra P, Rao MN. Mental health in an Indian rural community. British Journal of Psychiatry. 1971;118:499-503.
6. Thara R, Ramesh Kumar S, CG M. Publications on community psychiatry. Indian J Psychiatry. 2010;52 (Suppl 1):274-7.
7. Sethi BB, Gupta SC, Mahendru RK, Kumari P. A psychiatric survey of 500 rural families. Indian J Psychiatry. 1972;14:183-96.
8. Verghese A, Beig A, Senseman LA, Sundar Rao PSS, Benjamin V. A social and psychiatric study of a representative group of families in Vellore town. Indian J Med Res. 1973;61:608-20.

9. Sethi BB, Gupta SC, Mahendru RK, Kumari P. Mental Health and urban life: A study of 850 families. British Journal of Psychiatry. 1974;124:243-6.
10. Thacore VR, Gupta SC, Suriya M. Psychiatric Morbidity in North Indian Community. British Journal of Psychiatry. 1975;126:364-9.
11. Nandi DN, Ajmany S, Ganguly H, Banerjee G, Boral GC, Ghosh A, et al. Psychiatric disorders in a rural community in West Bengal - an epidemiological study. Indian Journal of Psychiatry. 1975;17:87-99.
12. Nandi DN, Ajmany S, Sachder S, Ganguli H, Banerjee G, Boral GC, et al. Socio-economic status and prevalence of mental disorders in certain rural communities in India. Acta Psychiatr Scand. 1979;59:276-93.
13. Shah AV, Goswami UA, Maniar RC, Hariwala DC, Sinha BK. Prevalence of psychiatric disorders in Ahmedabad: an epidemiological study. Indian Journal of Psychiatry. 1980;22:384-8.
14. Reddy KS, Kumar CN, Thirthalli J, Renuka Devi NR, Rawat V, Bijjal S, et al. Factors Influencing Access to psychiatric treatment in Persons with Schizophrenia: A Qualitative Study In A Rural Community. Indian J Psychiatry (in Press). 2013.
15. Mehta P, Joseph A, Verghese A. An epidemiological study of psychiatric disorders in a rural area in Tamil Nadu. Indian Journal of Psychiatry. 1985;27:153-8.
16. Sachdeva JS, Singh S, Sidhu BS, Goyal RKD, Singh J. An epidemiological study of psychiatric disorders in rural Faridkot (Punjab). Indian Journal of Psychiatry. 1986;28:317-23.
17. Premrajan KC, Danabalan M, Chandrasekhar R, Srinivasa DK. Prevalence of psychiatric morbidity in an urban community of Pondicherry. Indian Journal of Psychiatry. 1993;35:99-102.
18. Shaji S, Verghese A, Promodu K, George B, Shibu VP. Prevalence of priority psychiatric disorders in a rural area of Kerala. Indian Journal of Psychiatry. 1995;37:91-6.
19. Sharma S, Singh MM. Prevalence of mental disorders: An epidemiological study in Goa. Indian Journal of Psychiatry. 2001;43:118-26.
20. Math SB, Chandrashekar CR, Bhugra D. Psychiatric epidemiology in India. Indian J Med Res. 2007;126(3):183-92. PubMed PMID: 18037711. Epub 2007/11/27. eng.
21. Reddy MV, Chandrasekar CR. Prevalence of mental and behavioural disorders in India : A meta-analysis. Indian Journal of Psychiatry. 1998;40:149-57.
22. Ganguli HC. Epidemiological finding on prevalence of mental disorders in India. Indian Journal of Psychiatry. 2000;42:14-20.
23. Gururaj G, Girish N, Isaac MK. Mental, neurological and substance abuse disorders: Strategies towards a systems approach, NCMH Background Papers-Burden of Disease in India; Available from: http://whoindia.org/en/section102/section201_888.htm. New Delhi: Ministry of Health & Family Welfare. 2005.
24. District Mental Health Program. National Institute of Mental Health and Neurosciences. Operational Manual for the District Mental Health Program.Available online at http://nimhans.kar.nic.in/dmhp/manuals/man5.pdf accessed on 25 September 2013.
25. Waraich BK, Lok Raj, Chavan BS, Badhan R, Panda SN. Decentralization of Mental health services under DMHP. Indian J Psychiatry. 2003;45:161-5.
26. Murthy RS. National Mental Health Program in India (1982-1989). Mid-point appraisal. Indian J Psychiatry. 1989;31:267-70.
27. Agarwal AK. Mental Health Programme: Need for redemption. Editorial. Indian J Psychiatry. 1991;33:85-6.
28. Jacob KS. Repackaging mental health programs in low- and middle-income countries. Indian J Psychiatry. 2011;53:195-8.
29. Chandrashekar CR, Isaac MK, Kapur RL, Parthasarathy R. Management of priority mental disorders in the community. Indian J Psychiatry. 1981;23:174-80.
30. Isaac MK, Kapur RL, Chandrashekar CR, Kapur M, Parthasarathy R. Mental health delivery through rural primary care-development and evaluation of a training programme. Indian J Psychiatry. 1982;24:131-8.
31. Murthy RS, Kumar KKV, Chisholm D, Thomas T, Sekar K, CR C. Community outreach form untreated schizophrenia in rural India: a follow-up study of symptoms, disability, family burden and cost. Psychol Med. 2005;35:341-51.
32. Balaji M, Chatterjee S, Brennan B, Rangaswamy T, Thornicroft G, Patel V. Outcomes that matter: a qualitative study with persons with schizophrenia and their primary caregivers in India. Asian J Psychiatry. 2012;5:258-65.
33. Balaji M, Chatterjee S, Koschorke M, Rangaswamy T, Chavan A, Dabholkar H, et al. The development of a lay health worker delivered collaborative community based intervention for people with schizophrenia in India. BMC Health Serv Res (in press). 2012.
34. Thirthalli J, Venkatesh BK, Kishorekumar KV, Arunachala U, Venkatasubramanian G, Subbakrishna DK, et al. Prospective comparison of course of disability in antipsychotic-treated and untreated schizophrenia patients. Acta Psychiatr Scand. 2009;119:209-17.
35. Thirthalli J, Venkatesh BK, Naveen MN, Venkatasubramanian G, Arunachala U, Kishore Kumar KV, et al. Do antipsychotics limit disability in schizophrenia? A naturalistic comparative study in the community. Indian J Psychiatry. 2010;52:37-41.
36. Kumar CN, Suresha KK, Thirthalli J, Venkatesh BK, Bijjal S, Arunachala U, et al. Four-year follow-up of schizophrenia in a rural community: Good outcome and public health implications. Paper presented at the annual national conference of the Indian Psychiatric Society, New Delhi. 2011.
37. Suresha KK, Kumar CN, Thirthalli J, Bijjal S, Venkatesh BK, Arunachala U, et al. Work Functioning of Schizophrenia Patients in a Rural South Indian Community: Status at 4 years Follow-up. Soc Psychiatry Psy Epidemiol. 2012;47(11):1865-71.
38. Rawat V. Point prevalence of metabolic syndrome in schizophrenia patients living in a rural south Indian community. MD thesis submitted to National Institute of Mental Health and Neurosciences (Deemed University), Bangalore, India, 2010.

39. Kumar CN, Thirthalli J, Suresha KK, Arunachala U, Gangadhar BN. Metabolic syndrome among schizophrenia patients: Study from a rural community of south India. Asian J Psychiatry (In press). 2013.
40. Padmavati R, McCreadie RG, Tirupati S. Low prevalence of obesity and metabolic syndrome in never-treated chronic schizophrenia. Schizophrenia Research. 2010;121:199-202.
41. Chatterjee S, Patel V, Chatterjee A, Weiss HA. Evaluation of a community-based rehabilitation model for chronic schizophrenia in rural India. British Journal of Psychiatry. 2003;182:57-62.
42. Chatterjee S, Pillai A, Jain S, Cohen A, Patel V. Outcomes of people with psychotic disorders in a community-based rehabilitation programme in rural India. British Journal of Psychiatry. 2009;195:433-9.
43. Thara R, Padmavati R, Aynkran JR, John S. Community mental health in India: A rethink. Int J Ment Health Syst. 2008;2:11.
44. Jacob KS. Community care for people with mental disorders in developing countries: Problems and possible solutions. British Journal of Psychiatry. 2001;178:296-8.
45. Jacob KS, Sharam P, Mirza I, Garrido-Cumbrera M, Seedat S, Mari JJ, et al. Mental health systems in countries: where are we now? Global Mental Health. Lancet. 2007;370: 1061-77.
46. Saraceno B, Ommeren M, Batniji R, Cohen A, Gureje O, Mahoney J, et al. Barriers to improvement of mental health services in low-income and middle-income countries. Lancet. 2007;370:1164-74.
47. Saxena S, Thornicroft G, Knapp M, et al. Resources for mental health: scarcity, inequity, and inefficiency. Lancet. 2007;370:878-9.
48. Chandrashekar CR, Math SB. Psychosomatic disorders in developing countries: current issues and future challenges. Current Opinion in Psychiatry. 2006;19:201-6.
49. Thara R. Mobile telepsychiatry in India. World Psychiatry. 2013;12:84.
50. Holla B, Viswanath B, Neelaveni S, Harish T, Kumar CN, Math SB. Karnataka state Telemedicine project - utilization pattern, current and future challenges. Indian J Psychol Med (in press). 2013.

CHAPTER 62

Psychiatric Nursing

Raminder Kalra, Sarita Parajuli

Nursing is an essential, evolving part of society that has always been directed to serving healthcare needs. Nursing did not begin with Florence Nightingale, since nursing is as old as Medicine. Throughout history, nursing and medicine have had an interdependent relationship. Today, nursing has developed as a profession, which is complex and multifaceted. The diverse education prepares the nurse to function in a multidimensional role as that of caregiver, teacher, counselor, advocate and researcher. Conceptual and theoretical nursing models provide knowledge to improve practice, guide research and nursing curricula, and identify the domain and goals of nursing practice. The standards of practice set forth by professional nursing associations provide guidelines for competent, safe and professional practice.

In mental health settings, a team of workers work together to provide quality care for the clients. Collaborate efforts of the team need to be directed towards improving the mental health services delivered. Each member of the mental health team needs to cooperate and respect the position and role of others. All members need to work in collaboration by sharing the information to improve the quality of health services provided. Psychiatric mental health team includes psychiatrists, clinical psychologists, psychiatric social workers, psychiatric nurses, technicians and occupational, art, musical, psycho-drama, recreational, play and speech therapists.

PRINCIPLES OF PSYCHIATRIC NURSING

Psychiatric nursing is the process whereby the nurse assists persons, as individuals or in group, in developing a more positive self-concept, a more harmonious patterns of interpersonal relationships, and a more productive role in society.[1]

Psychiatric mental health nursing has evolved into a unique discipline. It now combines the knowledge, experience and skills of nursing and mental health. In actuality, the name 'psychiatric mental health nursing' implies two different areas of nursing that often interact and overlap. Psychiatric nursing focuses on the care and rehabilitation of those with identifiable emotional disorders.

Psychiatric nurse is a registered nurse who specializes in mental health nursing by employing theories of human behavior and therapeutic use of self. The principles of psychiatric nursing are described here.

In caring for the clients, the nurse should attempt to:

- Accept and respect people as individuals, regardless of their behavior.
- Limit or reject the individual's inappropriate behavior without rejecting the individual.
- Recognize that all behavior has meaning and is meeting the needs of the performer, regardless of how distorted or meaningless it appears to others.
- Accept the dependency needs of individuals while supporting and encouraging moves towards independence.
- Help individuals set appropriate limits for themselves or set limits for them when they are unable to do so.
- Encourage individuals to express their feelings in an atmosphere free of reprisal or judgment.
- Recognize that individuals need to use their defenses until other defenses can be substituted.
- Recognize how feelings affect behavior and influence relationship.
- Recognize that individuals frequently respond to behavioral expectations of others, including family, pears, and authority (staff).
- Recognize that all individuals have a potential for movement toward higher levels of emotional health.

DEVELOPMENT OF PSYCHIATRIC NURSING

Mental illness was always associated with ignorance, superstition and fears.

Through the age, psychiatric care has been the product of two different traditions: one stressing a need to appease magical or supernatural forces and other attempting to understand through rational methods, the causes and cure of the disease.

Psychiatric nursing and nursing in general developed from the need for the hospitals to provide socially acceptable levels of care for the patients. The training of psychiatric nurses has changed from experience acquired solely in mental hospital to enrolment in colleges and universities to study nursing.

In 1873, Linda Richards developed better nursing care in psychiatric hospitals and organized nursing services and educational programs in state mental hospitals for these activities. She is known as the first American Psychiatric Nurse.

The first training school for mental health nurses started at McLean Hospital, Waverly, Massachusetts in 1882.[2] In England, preparation of mental health nurses and their certification by the Medical Psychological Association began in 1891. 'Nationally recognized qualification' of general nurses in Britain started in 1925.

The two world wars provided important clinical understanding about short-term treatment, as a result of treating soldiers who were experiencing battle fatigue, as well as post-traumatic stress disorder. After World War II, the need for more psychiatric nurses and more educational programs became increasingly clear. The National Mental Health Act (UK) of 1946 changed nursing practice to include more direct involvement of the nurses in communication with mentally ill clients and other therapies.

The role of psychiatric nursing was widened in caring for mentally ill patients with Maxwell Jones' concept of 'therapeutic community'. He emphasized the important role of a psychiatric nurse in the early recovery of patient. The first doctoral program in psychiatric nursing was started in Boston in 1960.

In 1963, the Community Mental Health Act authorized funding for the establishment of community health centers. This act played an important part in the specialization of psychiatric nursing services. During the present century, psychiatric nursing also began to evolve as a clinical specialty. Previously, the nurses provided therapeutic care based on the medical model. By advanced study and clinical practice experienced in a master's program in psychiatric nursing, clinical specialists and nurse practitioners are able to gain expert knowledge in the care and prevention of psychiatric disorders.

DEVELOPMENT OF PSYCHIATRIC NURSING IN INDIA

In the nursing curriculum in India, there was earlier no component of psychiatric nursing. The Health Survey Committee's Report in 1946 recommended preparation of nursing personnel in psychiatric nursing. The committee also recommended that the existing institutions like the Bangalore Mental Hospital and Ranchi Mental Hospital should start with the training of nursing personnel.

Based on the Committee's recommendations, a one year post certificate course in psychiatric nursing was started in 1956 at the All India Institute of Mental Health, Bangalore, now called National Institute of Mental Health and Neurosciences (NIMHANS). Based on the recommendations of the Mudaliar's Committee (1964) to prepare a large number of psychiatric nurses, the Indian Nursing Council (INC) included psychiatric nursing as a compulsory course in the BSc Nursing programme. In 1965–66, psychiatric nursing component was added in General Nursing and Midwifery course also. In 1975, psychiatric nursing was offered as an elective subject in MSc. Nursing at the Rajkumari Amrit Kaur College of Nursing, New Delhi. Now, there are many colleges of nursing offering postgraduation in psychiatric nursing.[3]

In February 1991, psychiatric nursing experts formed an association known as the Indian Society of Psychiatric Nurses. Today, psychiatric nurses work not only in mental hospitals, but also in child guidance centers, deaddiction centers, half-way homes, old age homes, and in foster homes for the destitute and mentally retarded.

THERAPEUTIC COMMUNICATION

Like everyone else, nurses are affected by the behavior of the people around them. When nurses work with clients having psychiatric problems, they may encounter various forms of disturbed behavior (bizarre, aggressive, hostile, suspicious, dependent and violent). Their reactions to these behaviors are likely to reflect the range of their experiences and values. There is no one 'right way' to intervene therapeutically in disturbed behavior. Mental healthcare providers explore their thoughts and feelings, follow certain broad guidelines, and experiment with what works for them. Nurses and other care providers cannot impart wisdom to anyone, but they can give of themselves their caring and hopes to the others.

When the nurse works with patients or families who seek help for their physical or emotional problems, two types of interactions may occur, i.e. social and therapeutic. Social interactions occur daily when the nurse and patient greet each other or have a small talk.

During a therapeutic interaction, the nurse helps or encourages the patient to communicate his feelings, anxieties and share his thoughts, perceptions, expectations and frustrations. An understanding of the principles of effective communication is essential for the psychiatric nurse because her ability to intervene therapeutically with the clients is highly related to the effectiveness of her communication skills.

Shives[4] gives the following suggestions to enable one to develop good communication skills for effective therapeutic interactions:

- *Know yourself:* Identify your emotional needs, so that they do not interfere with the ability to relate to others.

- *Be honest with your feelings:* Your nonverbal communication may contradict your spoken word, if you are not honest with the patient.
- *Be secure in your ability to relate to people:* Do not allow the behavior of others to threaten or intimate you.
- *Be sensitive to the needs of others:* Use tact and diplomacy while conversing with others.
- *Be consistent:* Consistency in what you say and do encourages the development of trust.
- *Recognize symptoms of anxiety:* Anxiety impairs communication.
- *Watch your nonverbal reactions:* Be aware of your body language because it punctuates and modifies verbal messages.
- Recognize and evaluate your own actions and responses.

THERAPEUTIC RELATIONSHIP

The therapeutic relationship is the cornerstone of psychiatric/mental health nursing. The therapeutic nurse-client relationship is the interpersonal process between a professional nurse and a client that helps the client. The purpose of the relationship is to foster and promote growth of the personality to help the client improve in constructive and productive ways of living.

Rogers (1961)[5] lists eight conditions essential for a therapeutic relationship to occur. They include:

1. *Empathy:* To "walk in another's shoes" describes empathetic understanding because such an action enables one to experience the feelings of another and respond to them.
2. *Respect:* The helper considers the person to be deserving of high regard and cares deeply for the person as a human body. Consistency on the part of the helper conveys respect.
3. *Genuineness:* The helper is sincere, honest and authentic in responses.
4. *Self-disclosure:* Exposing a view of one's attitudes, feelings and beliefs in self-disclosure.
5. *Concreteness and specificity:* The ability to identify feelings by skillful listening requires the helper to be realistic, not theoretical while assisting the person in expressing specific feelings. She/he should not expect a patient to be a textbook picture of an illness and stereotype or label symptoms.
6. *Confrontation:* Discussing discrepancies in the person's behavior must be done in an accepting manner after the helper has established a good rapport with the person.
7. *Immediacy of relationship:* Recognizing one's own feelings and sharing them with the patient is essential. Once a relationship exists, the helper shares spontaneous feelings, when she feels the patient will profit from such a discussion.
8. *Self-exploration:* The patient needs to be encouraged in self-exploration. The more patient investigates his feelings, the more he learns to cope and adapt.

Confidentiality is essential in a therapeutic relationship. The patient has a right to privacy.

Phases of Therapeutic Relationship

The therapeutic relations consists of 3 phases.

1. Initiating or Orientation or Introductory Phase

During this phase, the patient and the nurse both get acquainted with each other. Both the nurse and the patient may experience anxiety when they first meet. The tasks accomplished during this phase include:[4]

- Building trust and rapport.
- Establishing a therapeutic environment.
- Formation of pact-establishing a contract regarding time, place and duration for each meetings, as well as length of time the relationship will be existing.
- Assessing the patient's strengths and weaknesses.

2. Working Up-phase or Phase of Emerging Identifies

Once the contract is established, the second phase begins. The patient trusts the nurse, feels relaxed and is able to discuss mutually decided-on goals with the nurse. Therapeutic tasks accomplished during this phase includes:

- Exploring perception of reality.
- Developing positive coping behaviors.
- Identifying available support systems.
- Promoting a positive self-concept.
- Encouraging verbalization of feelings.
- Developing a realistic plan of action, implementing it and evaluating the results.
- Promoting independence.

3. Terminating Phase or End or Resolution Phase

The end phase of therapeutic relationship is characterized by termination of contact between psychiatric nurse and client. This phase is as important as the previous two.

The course of the nurse-client relationship progresses through various states, each with tasks, difficulties and potential rewards. The ultimate goal of the nurse-client relationship is independent functioning of the client.

ROLE OF THE NURSE

Historically, when nurses first became involved in the care of psychiatric patients, they were primarily responsible for the patient's physical well-being. Their responsibilities mainly included administering drugs prescribed by the physician and caring for patients undergoing somatic treatments such as ECT, insulin shock.

The nurse coordinates the patient's healthcare experiences. She elicits his needs and when necessary, interprets these needs to other mental health team members. She applies her knowledge of nursing theory and biological and social sciences to the patient's health problems and utilizes this knowledge to device a sophisticated plan of care. She is also responsible to be sure that the patient understands this plan. If he seems puzzled or is non-complaint, the nurse explores his understanding and explains the nursing care plan as needed.

Most important, the nurse cares for the patient, in the fullest sense of caring. She listens to his problems non-judgmentally. She empathizes and helps him to identify and articulate his feelings. She is accessible at the time a need arises and conveys a sense of availability to the patient. She engenders trust by being consistent and reliable and by maintaining confidentially. She encourages the patient to be as independent as possible but also allows dependency when this is necessary. Through the application of psychomotor and interpersonal skills, the nurse assists the patient to grow and to reach his maximal functional capabilities.[6]

Gary (1991)[7] describes nine therapeutic roles assumed by nurses in applying psychiatric nursing principles to patient's needs: healthy role model, nurturing parent, reality base, technician, socializing agent, manager, teacher, patient advocate and counselor. Each role is applicable in varying degrees to all the areas and levels of nursing practice. Personal characteristics that facilitate the therapeutic process include: genuine concern and caring, commitment, an analytical mind, a therapeutic use of self, and awareness and acceptance of self and others.

Consultation in the General Hospital

The role of the psychiatric nursing consultant in the general hospital has evolved from the humanistic view that the mind is invisibly connected with the body. There is a wide variability in individual perceptions of stressful events. Some of the common situations that the consultant deals within practice are: demanding patients, patients in pain, dependent patients, 'problem' families, patients in intensive care units, patients who act out sexually and dying patients.[8]

STANDARDS OF PSYCHIATRIC MENTAL HEALTH NURSING CARE

Nursing is involved and concerned with the provision of quality care. In 1973, the American Nurses Association developed 14 standards of psychiatric mental health nursing practice. Standards represent agreed upon levels of practice; they have been developed to characterize, to measure and to provide guidance in achieving excellence in care. Considering the status of nursing practice in India, to reach the American Psychiatric and mental health nursing standards, it will require continuous effort on the part of policy makers, nursing educators, nursing administrators and nurses. These efforts would no doubt make the formulation of Indian Standards of psychiatric and mental health nursing practice a reality to be attainable in near future.[9]

MENTAL HEALTH NURSING IN THE COMMUNITY

Many people consider the 1960s as a pivotal time for community mental health nursing. The chronically mentally ill are generally considered to have the highest priority in public mental health care, with heightened attention given to creating better support programs for de-institutionalized patients and attacking the issue of homelessness.

Nursing roles in community mental health are centered around the basic elements of community nursing: health promotion, prevention of disease and evaluation and research.[7]

Special attention is given to high-risk populations, which include the elderly, the abused, the homeless and individuals at high risk for AIDS. The nurse assumes direct and indirect practice roles in the community. Nurses bring about changes in the community through use of various treatment modalities such as self-help groups. Nurses also make a contribution to the mental health of the community by sharing their knowledge and clinical expertise with other health care providers.[10]

The psychiatric home care nurse plays a pivotal role in assisting patients to more readily adapt to the community setting. The nurse needs to be sensitive to changes in behavior that signal that the patient is decompensating psychiatrically and or medically and possibly arrange for earlier re-hospitalization. Working collaboratively with the psychiatrist in providing in-depth psychiatric home care can be a rewarding experience. The nurse and the physician can learn from each other in terms of scope of practice, medication actions and responses, and behavioral management.[11]

Psychiatric mental health nursing is in transition, a transition influenced by aging client population, advances in technology, biological psychiatry and a decline in new graduates entering the specialty.[12-14] Psychiatric nurses need to understand the psychosocial connection in psychiatric disorders and the influence of a biological psychiatry model that integrates the relationship between brain and behaviors. Lowery[13] stresses that Psychiatric Mental Health nurses of the future need to rethink the way they are to deliver care, educate and research the care provided to mentally ill.[15]

REFERENCES

1. Taylor CM. Mereness' Essentials of Psychiatric Nursing, 11th edn. Toronto: CV Mosby; 1982.
2. Johnson BS. Psychiatric Mental Health Nursing: Adaptation and Growth, 2nd edition. Philadelphia: JB Lippincott; 1989.
3. Kapoor B. A Textbook of Psychiatric Nursing. New Delhi: Kumar Publishing House; 1991.
4. Shives LR. Basic Concepts of Psychiatric Mental Health Nursing, 2nd edn. Philadelphia: JB Lippincott; 1990.
5. Rogers C. On Becoming a Person. Boston: Houghton, Miffin; 1961.
6. Stuart GW, Sundeen SJ. Principles and practice of psychiatric nursing. Toronto: CV Mosby; 1979.
7. Gary F, Kavanagh CK. Psychiatric Mental Health Nursing. Philadelphia: JB Lippincott; 1991.
8. Wilson H, Kneil CR. Psychiatric Nursing. California: Addison Weseley Publishing; 1979.
9. Lalitha K, Pereira. Standards of psychiatric nursing: A myth or reality in India. Nurs J India. 1991;82:324-6.
10. Beck CK, et al. Mental Health Psychiatric Nursing: A Holistic Life Cycle Approach, 2nd edition. Philadelphia: Mosby Year Book; 1988.
11. Hellwig K. Psychiatric home care nursing: managing patients in the community setting. J Psychosoc Nurs Soc Serv. 1993; 31(12).
12. Abbondanza DM, et al. Psychiatric mental health nursing in a psychosocial era. Perspec Psychiatr Care. 1994;30(3).
13. Lowery B. Psychiatric nursing in the 1990's and beyond. J Psychosoc Nurs Soc Serv. 1994;30(1).
14. Hoekstra HJ, van Meijel BB, van der Hooft-Leemans TG. A nursing career in mental health care: Choices and motives of nursing students. Nurse Educ Today. 2010;30:4-8.
15. Khadria B. International nurse recruitment in India. Health Serv Res. 2007;42:1429-36.

FURTHER READING

1. Arnold SA, Deans C, Munday J. University and service sector collaboration for undergraduate psychiatry nursing education. Int J Ment Health Nurs. 2004;13:61-6.
2. Balon R, Franchini G, Freeman P, Hassenfeld I, Keshavan M, Yoder E. Medical students' attitudes and views of psychiatry. Academic Psychiatry. 1999;23:30-6.
3. Beck CK, et al. Mental Health Psychiatric Nursing: A Holistic Life Cycle Approach, 3rd edition. Philadelphia: Mosby Year Book, 1993.
4. Clinton M, Hazelton M. Towards a Foucauldian reading of the Australian mental health nursing workforce. Int J Ment Health Nurs. 2002;11:18-23.
5. Curtis J. Working together: A joint initiative between academics and clinicians to prepare undergraduate nursing students to work in mental health settings. Int J Ment Health Nurs. 2007;16:285-93.
6. DeKeyser Ganz F, Kahana S. Perceptions of Israeli student nurses regarding clinical specialties and factors that influence these perceptions. J Adv Nurs. 2006;56:88-98.
7. Geneva: World Health Organization. WHO. Atlas Country Profiles of Mental Health Resources; 2001.
8. Geneva: World Health Organization; 2005. WHO. Mental Health Atlas; 2005.
9. Goodwin V, Happell B. Psychiatric nurses' attitudes toward consumer and carer participation in care: Part 2: Barriers to participation. Policy Polit Nurs Pract. 2008;9:249-56.
10. Gouthro TJ. Recognizing and addressing the stigma associated with mental health nursing: A critical perspective. Issues Ment Health Nurs. 2009;30:669-76.
11. Halter MJ. Perceived characteristics of psychiatric nurses: Stigma by association. Arch Psychiatr Nurs. 2008;22:20-6.
12. Happell B, Robins A, Gough K. Developing more positive attitudes towards mental health nursing in undergraduate students: Part 1: Does more theory help? J Psychiatr Ment Health Nurs. 2008;15:439-46.
13. Happell B, Robins A, Gough K. Developing more positive attitudes towards mental health nursing in undergraduate students: Part 2-The impact of theory and clinical experience. J Psychiatr Ment Health Nurs. 2008;15:527-36.
14. Happell B. Can education make a difference to undergraduate nursing students' attitudes to psychiatric nursing? Contemp Nurse. 2000;9:40-50.
15. Happell B. Influencing undergraduate nursing students' attitudes toward mental health nursing: Acknowledging the role of theory. Issues Ment Health Nurs. 2009;30:39-46.
16. Happell B. Psychiatric nursing education: Can it make a difference? Int J Psychiatr Nurs Res. 2000;6:657-69.
17. Happell B. Who wants to be a psychiatric nurse. Novice student nurses' interest in psychiatric nursing? J Psychiatr Ment Health Nurs. 1999;6:479-84.
18. Harborne G, Jones A. Supplementary prescribing: A new way of working for psychiatrists and nurses. The Psychiatrist. 2008;32:136-9.
19. Hoencamp E. 'Yes doctor, no doctor': What do patients want from you? Acta Psychiatr Scand. 1999;100:319-20.
20. Kaslow FW, et al. Supervision Consultation and Staff Training in the Helping Professions. San Francisco: Jossey-Bass; 1977.
21. Laugharne R, Appiah-Poku J, Laugharne J, Shankar R. Attitudes toward psychiatry among final-year medical students in Kumasi, Ghana. Acad Psychiatry. 2009;33:71-5.
22. Madianos MG, Priami M, Alevisopoulos G, Koukia E, Rogakou E. Nursing students' attitude change towards mental illness and psychiatric case recognition after a clerkship in psychiatry. Issues Ment Health Nurs. 2005;26:169-83.
23. McCann TV, Clark E, Lu S. Bachelor of Nursing students career choices: A three-year longitudinal study. Nurse Educ Today. 2010;30:31-6.
24. Mullen A, Murray L. Clinical placements in mental health: Are clinicians doing enough for undergraduate nursing students? Int J Ment Health Nurs. 2002;11:61-8.

25. Pailhez G, Bulbena A, Coll J, Ros S, Balon R. Attitudes and views on psychiatry: A comparison between Spanish and US medical students. Acad Psychiatry. 2005;29:82-91.
26. Potter PA, Perry AG. Fundamentals of Nursing, 2nd edition. Toronto: CV Mosby; 1989.
27. Pye SA, Whyte LA. Factors influencing the branch choice of students on a nursing undergraduate programme. Nurse Educ Today. 1996;16:432-6.
28. Romem P, Anson O, Kanat-Maymon Y, Moisa R. Reshaping students' attitudes toward individuals with mental illness through a clinical nursing clerkship. J Nurs Educ. 2008;47: 396-402.
29. Rushworth L, Happell B. Psychiatric nursing education: Doing the impossible? Arch Psychiatr Nurs. 1998;12:319-25.
30. Stevens JA, Dulhunty GM. New South Wales Nursing Students' attitudes towards a career in mental health. Australian Journal of Mental Health Nursing. 1992;2:59-64.
31. Surgenor LJ, Dunn J, Horn J. Nursing student attitudes to psychiatric nursing and psychiatric disorders in New Zealand. Int J Ment Health Nurs. 2005;14:103-8.
32. Wynaden D, Orb A, McGowan S, Downie J. Are universities preparing nurses to meet the challenges posed by the Australian mental health care system? Aust N Z J Ment Health Nurs. 2000;9:138-46.
33. Yamauchi T, Semba T, Sudo A, Takahashi N, Nakamura H, Yoshimura K, et al. Effects of psychiatric training on nursing students' attitudes towards people with mental illness in Japan. Int J Soc Psychiatry. 2011;57:574-9.

CHAPTER 63 Computers in Psychiatry

Chittaranjan Andrade, Shashi Kiran, N Sanjay Kumar Rao

Computers have been of use in science for over half a century; initially, in frontier fields of research and later, in high-technology instrumentation situations. During the present decade, there have been rapid advances, leading to the development of more powerful computer hardware; this in turn has led to the development of more powerful software. Additionally, operating environments and computer programs have become more user-friendly. Accompanying these changes, computers have become available and affordable even to the common man. Mental health scientists and professionals consequently need to seriously consider the extent to which they can take advantage of computers to provide assistance in work that ranges from routine administrative activities to esoteric scientific applications.

This chapter briefly examines the relevance of computers to mental health professionals, focusing on academic developments as well as on matters that are of relevance to practicing clinicians. The chapter is organized into the following sections:

- Applications of computers in assessments and investigations
- Applications of computers in therapy
- Modeling of cognition, physiology and behavior
- The Internet and psychiatry
- Applications of computers in administrative psychiatry
- Miscellaneous applications of computers in psychiatry.

APPLICATIONS OF COMPUTERS IN ASSESSMENTS AND INVESTIGATIONS

Computers find application in both clinical and laboratory assessments of patients. In clinical assessments, computers may be used to assist in diagnosis, to rate the severity of psychopathology, and to evaluate clinical progress. In the laboratory setting or in the context of investigations, computers are used for a host of purposes ranging from electroencephalography to brain imaging. Certain of these applications are discussed in this section.

Computerized Diagnostic Assessments

Structured diagnostic interviews are important in research situations because they offer reliable and valid diagnoses for psychiatric research in general, and for epidemiological studies in particular. Structured diagnostic interviews are also important in routine clinical care because such interviews ensure that no aspect of the patient's clinical state is missed (too often do busy clinicians pounce upon some obvious psychopathology and focus upon it, not realizing that comorbidity is present). Unfortunately, structured interviews suffer from several disadvantages; they require much staff training, and much time for administration; their administration is seldom time-cost effective, particularly in routine clinical contexts; their administration may be compromised by staff fatigue effects; their results may be biased by staff expectations.

To reduce or eliminate such problems, a number of diagnostic interviews in psychiatry have been computerized. The patients' responses are directly keyed into the computer; usually, subsequent questions are asked depending upon the responses to previous questions. In effect, the interview follows a decision-making tree. Computerized versions of such interviews are often self-cleaning; that is, they do not accept out of range entries, and provide for some logic checks across questions. Thus, errors due to incorrect probing, or the entry of inappropriate values, are minimized. The computer assigns a diagnosis when the response set received matches the response set expected for a particular diagnosis. If no diagnosis is warranted, this too is indicated.

By way of example, the Diagnostic Interview Schedule (DIS), used to generate DSM diagnoses, has been computerized to the extent that the patients' responses are fed into the computer and the diagnosis is made by the computer. An abbreviated version of the DIS, known as the DIS Screening Interview (DISSI), has also been constructed and computerized. Limitations in DISSI have led to the development of a Quick DIS-IIIR (Q-DIS) computerized interview which enquires after symptoms (related to diagnostic criteria) in logical sequence. An important difference between DIS and Q-DIS is that the former sets every question before the respondent while the latter presents only as many questions as are required to ascertain whether a patient meets or will not meet the diagnostic criteria for a particular disorder. Another important difference is that DIS must be interviewer-administered, while Q-DIS can be answered by the patient himself, directly into the computer.[1]

Q-DIS was found to have high sensitivity and specificity, and excellent diagnostic agreement with DIS for most psychiatric disorders. It was more convenient to administer, and required less time. The limitations of DIS, such as missing patients with generalized anxiety disorder, or misclassifying cases of post-traumatic stress disorder, arose more from the content of the interview than from the computerization thereof.[1]

Similarly, computerized screening for psychiatric disorders in an outpatient setting has been described, using an instrument known as PRIME-MD (Primary Care Evaluation of Mental Disorders). This instrument is available in both desktop computer and interactive computerized voice response versions. Using the Structured Clinical Interview for DSM-IV (SCID-IV) as the gold standard criterion, PRIME-MD was found to have high sensitivity, specificity and positive predictive value for most diagnoses. No significant difference was found in how well patients liked the two forms of the computerized interview.[2]

The Composite International Diagnostic Interview (CIDI-auto) has also been computerized and studied in the contexts of major depression and anxiety disorders; the computerized version showed generally high sensitivity (except for generalized anxiety disorder) but low specificity; overall, only modest agreement was observed with clinician-obtained assessments.[3] While these results indicate that there is much scope for improvement of the computerized version of the interview, the general conclusion that was drawn is that computerization of the CIDI-auto can be of much assistance in many research and epidemiological contexts. The application of computerized diagnostic interviews in psychiatry has recently been discussed elsewhere.[4,5]

For the assessment of psychopathology in children, a self-administered, computerized version of the Diagnostic Interview for Children and Adolescents (DICA-R) was developed, with separate versions for children aged 6–12 years, for children aged 13–18 years, and for parents of children aged 6–18 years. The test-retest reliability of the computerized interview was found to be modest, and comparable with reliability coefficients reported with clinician-conducted interviews. Acceptance of the computerized interview was high.[6]

Computerized Ratings of Psychopathology

The use of rating scales is essential in research settings to provide a quantitative estimate of the psychopathology under study. Ratings scales are increasingly finding application in routine clinical care as well, to provide an objective measure of the progress of the patient. In recent years, computerized interviews have been developed to obtain clinical ratings such as for depression, using the Hamilton Rating Scale for Depression,[7] for obsessive-compulsive disorder (OCD), using the Yale-Brown Obsessive Compulsive Scale (YBOCS),[8] for anxiety, using the Hamilton Anxiety Scale,[9] and for social phobia, using the Leibowitz Social Anxiety Scale.[10]

Computer-administered ratings are time-cost-energy efficient. Their availability and the rate, at which they are administered, do not depend on the clinician's time constraints. Total and subscale scores can immediately be obtained. Such computerized interviews for the rating of the severity of psychopathology have been found to compare very favorably with interviews administered by human raters; for example, the computerized version of YBOCS has been reported to have had a good acceptance, and a high correlation of 0.88 with clinician-obtained ratings in a sample of 31 patients with OCD.[8]

A computer-assisted telephone administration system has been developed for YBOCS.[11] Using digitized human speech, 18 patients with OCD were interviewed by the computer over the telephone. There was a near perfect agreement between ratings obtained through computer-assisted telephone enquiry, human telephone enquiry and self-ratings. However, no patient preferred the computer as the interview method of choice. This study has far-reaching implications. For research purposes, when follow-up data are required, and when such cannot be conveniently obtained or when the risk for drop-outs is high, computer-assisted telephonic ratings can be a convenient, time-cost-energy effective and reliable method of acquiring data.

Palmtop computers have been used to beep patients into making entries about their behavior at different times of day. These entries can be used in the compilation of data about clinical events and behavior.[4]

Computerized Ratings of Clinical Progress

Software for the assessment of the progress of the patient and the provision of cost-benefit analyses has been available since 1989. These systems computerized a proven paper and pencil method.[12,13] A more elaborate program has recently been developed. Known as CORM (Clinical Outcome and Resource Measure), the program allows clinicians and patients to use a computer to rate any outcome for which there is a measure. Various measures are built into the software; these are general, syndromal or patient-specific. General measures include assessments of social disability and global ratings of severity of illness. Syndromal measures include specific rating instruments such as YBOCS. Patient-specific measures address problems and goals that are peculiar to individual patients. CORM also provides entries for time and financial costs. The program generates charts that map a patient's progress, and the rough cost of obtaining that progress. Such data are of value in audits of clinical practice.[14]

Acceptance of Computerized Interviews

How do patients react to computerized interviews? In general, reactions have been positive. Patients with social phobia, and those who have attempted suicide, prefer being interviewed by a computer while those with affective disorder, panic disorder and generalized anxiety disorder prefer clinician-administered interviews. Patients with OCD and control subjects express no particular preference between computers and clinicians. Of note, patients are more likely to disclose sensitive information, such as suicidal ideation, sexual difficulties and alcohol-related behavior, to the computer.[2,4,15] As already mentioned, computerized telephone interviews are not preferred by patients with OCD.[11]

Children show high acceptance of computer-administered interviews. They enjoy the colors, the graphics, and the active involvement through punching keys or typing in information. Children were found to be more than twice as likely to prefer a computer to a human interviewer, and nearly twice as likely to tell the computer things that they would not tell a person.[6]

Computerized Interviews: Caveats

Some cautions must be exercised in evaluating computer-obtained clinical ratings. An obvious caveat is that normative data may differ between clinician-administered and computer-administered versions of the same instrument. Computer interviews must, therefore, be standardized just as clinical interview are standardized. Reliability and validity data need to be obtained across diagnoses and across situations. It must be remembered that computers do not have the power to observe the patient's behavior during the interview, to tailor the questions to the patients' comprehension, or to draw intuitive conclusions based upon a variety of factors. Clinicians also need to ensure that their personal inputs to the patient do not decrease because the computer has taken over certain of their responsibilities.[15]

Applications of Computers in Other Assessments and Investigations

Computers find application in a plethora of investigations and assessments that are of direct or indirect application in psychiatry. These include:

- Radiological procedures, such as computerized tomography (CT), magnetic resonance imaging (MRI), positron emission tomography (PET) and other imaging techniques.
- Electrophysiological procedures, such as electroencephalography (computerized EEG), evoked potentials, electrophysiological brain mapping, etc.
- Clinical laboratory procedures, such as chromatography and assays for estimation of drug, hormone, neurotransmitter and other levels.
- Experimental laboratory procedures, such as those which involve the use of sophisticated equipment for the assessment of animal behavior, for the modeling of operant conditioning, etc.

While the need for computers in all four categories will be apparent to all clinicians, special examples of the second and fourth categories are presented briefly.

Since electroconvulsive seizures that are comparable in duration may be disparate in efficacy, it becomes necessary to devise means of differentiating less adequate from more adequate seizures. At present, it appears that on-line electroencephalographic seizure assessments during ECT may offer the best indices of adequacy. Somatics, Inc., USA, has introduced an electroconvulsive therapy (ECT) device (Thymatron) with technology built in for the computerized assessment of seizure quality. These assessments are based on an analysis of the EEG during and after the ECT seizure, and are computed using algorithms run by preprogrammed computer chips. Three seizure quality measures are presented in the Thymatron device: the seizure energy index, the postictal suppression index, and the seizure concordance index. Desirable values for each have been recommended; however, the indices and the recommendations based thereon need to be prospectively validated in depressive and other disorders for which ECT is prescribed, as well as in demographically distinct populations. For the moment, these indices represent a promising start in the development of modern measures of seizure adequacy.[16-18]

Motility of experimental rats frequently requires to be assessed because this motility is influenced by agonist or antagonist drugs at various neuroreceptor sites, by somatic therapies such as ECT, by induced emotional states, by stereotactically-induced lesions in the brain, etc. Motility monitoring can be effected by placing the animal in an enclosed chamber crisscrossed by infrared beams. As the animal moves, it interrupts these beams. Interruptions in the beams can be detected by sensors, sampled at a specified frequency by an interfaced computer, and analyzed to provide information on several measures of motility. Possible measures that may be obtained are the distance that the rat travels during the period of monitoring, the sum total duration of movement periods, the sum total duration of resting periods, the number of occasions of behavioral stereotypies, the number of vertical movements, the number of clockwise rotations, and the number of anticlockwise rotations.[19] These data can be appropriately interpreted in the context of the status of the brain in response to the experimental situation.

APPLICATIONS OF COMPUTERS IN THERAPY

Computer software has recently been developed with the potential to provide psychotherapy to the patient with limited or no human supervision. Such software principally employs cognitive behavior therapy or other behavior therapy principles. This is because behavior therapy is highly structured, comprises well-delineated procedures that may need to be repetitive, targets specific symptoms and behavior, and proceeds in a systematic fashion. While such nonhuman interventions will never have the flexibility, the intuitiveness and the innovativeness of a human therapist, nor ever be able to provide the nonspecific benefits deriving from such a person to person therapeutic relationship, it should be acknowledged that the use of computers in therapy does promise several advantages; these are listed in Table 1.

Advantages notwithstanding, it must be kept in mind that the use of computers in therapy is fraught with limitations or even dangers. The disadvantages associated with the use of computers in therapy are listed in Table 2. Although these advantages and disadvantages are pointed out in the context of the use of computers in therapy, it must be understood that most of these advantages and disadvantages apply to the use of computers in other clinical contexts as well (such as for screening or rating patients). Certain pros and cons of computer-assisted therapy have also been discussed elsewhere.[4,20]

There are several situations in which the computer can partly or entirely replace a human therapist. Several widely different situations are discussed, such as the cognitive therapy of depression, the cognitive therapy of anxiety, behavior therapy of phobic disorders, and cognitive retraining of brain-damaged persons.

Table 1: Advantages arising from delivery of psychotherapy through use of appropriate computer software
• Patients who intellectualize, or who are sensitive to the examination of their weaknesses, may find the impersonal computer a more acceptable therapist than a human
• The novelty of being a self-therapist through the medium of computer instruction may be a nonspecific therapeutic factor for some patients
• Since clients are responsible for their own treatment, the process encourages a sense of mastery and control
• The therapeutic load on the clinician is reduced
• The administration, the conduct and the assessment of homework assignments in therapy can conveniently be conducted (by the computer program). The software can be programmed to beep the patient at appropriate times to indicate that an assignment is due. The assignment is date stamped by the computer; this prevents patients from completing all assignments at one go just before the therapy session
• Progress in therapy can periodically be assessed by the program, and the course of therapy can automatically be modified depending upon the results
• Patients (and the human supervisor) can conveniently review material of importance as this material would have been stored on disk. Such review is not easy in interpersonal therapy
• Patients can move at their own pace, instead of at the pace set by the (human) therapist
• The therapeutic approach is replicable; this is of value in research, where therapeutic interventions need to be tightly controlled
• Details of the patient-computer interactions can be recorded and analyzed in minute detail; this can be helpful for the identification of therapeutic components of the package
• The structured nature of therapy permits a systematic study of the treatment process and its relationship to outcome
• Computers do not forget, ignore or otherwise miss out any aspect of therapy
• The availability of computer-assisted therapy does not depend on the availability and the time constraints of the human therapist
• Computers, unlike human therapists, do not suffer from fatigue effects, nor do they have 'bad' days
• Computer-based analyses can be made instantly available, depending upon the facilities offered in the program.

Computer-directed Cognitive Therapy for Depression

A computer program, called Overcoming Depression, has been available since 1991.[21] The program is designed to provide cognitive therapy for patients suffering from mild-to-moderate depression. According to Colby, the author of the program, the program is not intended to represent a computer simulation or imitation of a human psychotherapist; rather, it introduces a new therapeutic style with its own strengths and weaknesses.

The program consists of a text mode interwoven with a dialogue mode. The text mode is instructive and self-educative. It provides facts and explanations about depression along with cognitive strategies for alleviating the disorder and preventing its recurrence.

The dialogue mode permits the program and the patient to interact in everyday language. This unique feature encourages free expression, helps the patient to put his innermost thoughts and feelings into words that can be looked at and thought about, provides support, arouses hope, individualizes therapeutic learning and promotes cognitive action.

There are seven lessons: Negative Self-comparisons, Mood Balance and Values, Ideal Standards, Reprogramming Yourself, Obstacles to Overcoming Depression, Changing Values, and Suicide and Antidepressant Medication. Overcoming Depression comes in a home-user version, designed for the use of one person, and a professional version, which can handle multiple users, has special printout features and can serve as a therapeutic adjunct for the mental health professional.

A large proportion of depressed patients never seek help; a variety of reasons may be responsible, such as unavailability or unaffordability of a therapist, unwillingness to admit the existence of psychological dysfunction, unwillingness to face the stigma of requiring psychiatric assistance, etc.

Table 2: Disadvantages arising from delivery of psychotherapy through use of computer software

• Patients assigned to computer-directed therapy may have difficulties unless they are at least minimally computer literate
• Patients may not feel comfortable with the use of an inanimate, unfeeling and unempathetic object in the treatment of their very human problems
• Many patients with problems of living already feel alienated from the mainstream of society. The computer cannot form a meaningful clinical relationship with the patient as can a human therapist. The use of a computer in therapy may, therefore, reinforce the patient's alientation
• Computers do not have the capacity to handle the great variety of problems that arise in clinical contexts, nor can they address the complexity associated with these issues
• Computer software can assist behaviorally-oriented therapy but is less capable, or totally incapable, of promoting psychotherapies derived from other schools of psychology.
• Human therapists have the flexibility to change a therapeutic approach depending upon the need of the circumstances. Computers can have decision-making trees built into the program, but cannot of themselves initiate a therapeutic change
• Human therapists have varying degrees of intuitiveness that guide them in their therapeutic approach. Computers lack intuitiveness altogether
• Human therapists have the innovativeness to incorporate unusual therapeutic approaches, depending upon circumstances. Computers have no innovativeness
• Computer-directed therapy cannot provide the nonspecific factors in psychotherapy that are associated with interpersonal therapeutic interactions
• Computer-directed therapy will need to be supervised by a human therapist to ensure that no untoward situation is developing
• No computer program can be as naturally and comprehensively interactive as can a human therapist
• Interactions with a computer are restricted to a keyboard and screen format; this is unnatural. While voice recognition software is being developed, and while soundcards and speakers are capable of delivering simulations of the human voice, oral transactions between computers and humans in therapy are currently unavailable
• No computer program can ever understand the needs of a patient to the extent that a therapist can

The availability of a computer program to help such persons handle their problems is akin to the availability of self-help books—with the difference that this computer program is *individually interactive*. Such an availability of a surrogate therapist may be a nonspecific therapeutic factor of sorts.

Selmi et al.[22] reported their evaluation of a computer-administered cognitive-behavioral therapy program for depression. Three groups were compared: a group assigned to the computer, a group assigned to a human therapist who used similar intervention principles, and a waiting list control group. There were 12 patients in each group. The computer program provided session to session instructions to the patients, assigned homework and evaluated progress; the component of interactiveness, developed in the Colby software, was however absent. After a 6-sessions treatment phase and at 2-months' follow-up, both active therapy groups experienced a comparable degree of improvement on several outcome measures; the improvement was significantly superior to that in the waiting list controls.

While Colby[21] reported a 96% satisfaction rating from 142 users, it goes without saying that controlled trials are necessary before concluding that such programs are helpful. Computer-based cognitive psychotherapy may have certain advantages, such as convenience, but it also has very many limitations, such as the impossibility of perfect interactiveness. No program can understand a patient and his problems, and thereby develop an intervention package exactly tailored for individual requirements.

Nevertheless, if the utility of such computer programs can indeed be demonstrated, several axioms of psychotherapy may require to be examined-such as the need for a human therapist, the role of nonverbal communication in therapeutics, etc.

Computer-assisted Cognitive Behavior Therapy for Generalized Anxiety Disorder

Newman et al.[4] have outlined a computer therapy program for generalized anxiety disorder (GAD). The program comprises four modules: assessment, cognitive therapy, relaxation training and exposure.

The assessment module evaluates the patient's signs and symptoms along several different measures, at different times of day, and at different stages of therapy. Patients are asked about the outcome of the events about which they worried, and the strength of their coping. Patients are offered more appropriate self-coping statements.

The cognitive therapy module facilitates the recognition of anxiety triggers and the content of anxiety-inducing thoughts. It encourages users to see their thoughts as hypotheses and to put these thoughts into perspective. It helps users identify and redress logical errors by providing definitions and examples of coping statements. It evaluates levels of anxiety before and after the application of cognitive therapy.

The relaxation module instructs the user on diaphragmatic breathing, progressive muscle relaxation and pleasant imagery. It evaluates levels of anxiety before and after relaxation.

The exposure module prompts users to imagine themselves exposed to forthcoming situations that are likely to induce anxiety. It encourages them to think about the situation for long enough for the anxiety to subside as a result of the employment of coping strategies. It evaluates levels of anxiety before and after the application of exposure.

Pilot data on this program suggest that the program is effective, and that clinical gains are maintained at 6-months follow-up.

Computer-based Cognitive Restructuring of Self-esteem

Horan[23] examined the effects of a computer-based cognitive restructuring program on rationally-mediated self-esteem in 28 male and 28 female students aged 16–19 years. These students were selected from the bottom half of a sample of 108 students who completed an assessment of self-esteem; that is, these students had below median self-esteem. Selected students were randomized to receive either the computer-based therapy or a control program comprising audio tapedriven relaxation exercises.

The computer therapy involved the use of Authorware, Version 2 (1995), which is a multimedia program containing components of 13 separate cognitive restructuring modules which focus on specific irrational cognitive beliefs. The modules were delivered in 50 minutes sessions, conducted on consecutive days. Seven modules were scheduled for the first day, and 8 for the second. Each module began with a video clip of a screen student expressing an emotional, personal or social problem. The computer then enquired whether the subject experienced similar problems. If yes, the program took the subject through a series of discussions on irrational cognitions related to that theme, seeking the subject's response at each step. Subjects were provided the opportunity to recycle through the discussions. Music and graphics were interspersed throughout. The next module began after completion of the previous one.

Experimental subjects recorded small gains in measures of self-esteem. It is unclear whether the modest results were due to the limitations of the program, the rapidity with which it was administered, or factors such as the sourcing of subjects from a population without low self-esteem, as might be seen in clinical contexts.

The Computer as a Therapist for Phobic Disorder

It is generally accepted that exposure therapy is the intervention of choice for patients with phobias; thus, for example, a patient who fears spiders may be exposed to pictures of spiders, or to a video of spiders, or to live spiders. This exposure may be effected in a systematic desensitization (graded exposure) hierarchy and may be conducted in the presence of a clinician who guides the patient through his experience. The therapist's behavior during the exposure serves as a model to the patient and may help the patient develop a coping style that facilitates mastery over his fear.

A computer might be employed in such therapy in one or more of several ways. If the patient is given the responsibility for constructing his graded exposure program, computer software can be designed to define appropriate steps or tasks for the exposure program; the software can also assist the patient in assessing his progress, and in modifying the exposure program depending upon the progress. One such application of the computer has already been field-tested. Ghosh et al.[24] assigned patients with simple and social phobia, and with agoraphobia, to receive assistance from a human therapist, from a self-help manual or from a computer, for the construction of homework exercises for self-exposure. All three groups shows significant and comparable improvement up to a six-month follow-up.

The computer can also serve as a tool for the presentation of still or video images of the object of the fear. A recent study[25] used a computerized hierarchy of images of spiders, ranging from simple drawings to a video clip with a sound track. Patients with spider phobias were assigned to therapy with this computer approach, or to exposure therapy *in vivo*, or to live modeling with guided participation. All three groups of patients showed statistically and clinically significant improvement, while patients assigned to a waiting list did not improve.

Of greater interest, however, is the use of the computer in generating virtual reality environments that are relevant to the patient's phobia. Virtual reality refers to the production of a three dimensional image through which the individual 'moves'. In nonimmersive virtual reality, the image is confined to the screen and the individual explores the image with the help of a computer mouse much as he might explore a real environment. In immersive virtual reality, the individual wears a headset that permits the computer to generate a virtual reality field that seems to surround the patient; in effect, the individual experiences himself to be within the simulated environment.

Therapist-guided immersive virtual reality therapy has already been used with success in the treatment of acrophobia (fear of heights); the task comprised graded exposure to heights using a virtual reality simulation of a glass elevator, and of bridges of different heights. Ten subjects who completed an 8-week program involving the virtual reality therapy were significantly improved while 7 subjects on a waiting list were unchanged.[26]

Kirkby et al.[27,28] developed a different approach using nonimmersive virtual reality. In this program, an imaginary phobic patient is depicted (on the computer screen) in a house that includes a room containing the phobic object. The actual patient, using the computer mouse, moves the screen patient through the house. The anxiety response of the screen patient is depicted on the computer monitor, as also the amount of exposure the screen patient has to the phobic object. The actual patient endeavors to 'habituate' the screen patient to the phobic object using the technique of exposure. Thus, this program models the treatment process and the consequence of initial and cumulative exposure, on the anxiety response.

The therapeutic skills that the actual patient develops using this program are applied to his or her own phobia.

What is now necessary is to determine the advantages of such computer programs over real life exposure situations, and the relative merits of the different computer-assisted approaches.

Computer-assisted Self-analysis

Self-analysis through a psychoanalytically-based approach has long been mooted. Recently, Jerome[29] suggested possible applications of a computer in self-analysis. Although the software cannot possibly have an impact similar to that in behaviorally-oriented therapies, it can assist in ironing out possible blind spots, in recording information, and in retrieving information for later analysis.

Using Computers to Treat Cognitive Deficits

Patients, who have experienced brain damage due to a head injury or any other cause, usually manifest a variety of cognitive deficits. The nature of these deficits depends on the characteristics of the individual (age, sex, hemispheric dominance, premorbid level of functioning, etc.) as much as they depend on the characteristics of the lesion (number, site, depth, nature, etc.).

Just as physical rehabilitation is undertaken to treat motor deficits resulting from neurological disorders, so too is cognitive rehabilitation undertaken to treat cognitive deficits resulting from brain damage. The computer is an ideal tool for the process, and several programs have already been written towards this end. One such program is the *PSS CogReHab v.95*. The program is a multimedia cognitive rehabilitative software system, which operates through Microsoft Windows. It requires a 386 or higher IBM compatible microcomputer with certain other hardware and software specifications.

There are eight packages: Foundations I and II; Visuospatial I and II; Memory I and II; and, Problem Solving I and II. Essentially, the programs present a series of exercises to the patient. The patient's responses are measured and an immediate feedback is given so that the patient can reset his responses to the pattern desired by the program. Examples of variables assessed are the correctness of perception, the speed of thinking, the correctness of movement, the speed of movement, etc.

Initially, therapy focuses on visual and auditory attention, re-establishing awareness of the full visual field, improving visual tracking, scanning and searching, shifting attention and attending to multiple stimuli simultaneously, etc. Initiation and inhibition skills are addressed by requiring quick responses, and by setting up situations where stopping a response or making no response is desired. By changing orientations and reversing the demands placed upon the individual, cognitive flexibility is brought about along with the ability to orient and reorient.

The tasks are set for different cognitive processes, the selection of which depend on the nature of the deficits experienced by the patient. The tasks are graded in difficulty, increasing in complexity and demands as the patient masters each increment in difficulty.

A more modest cognitive rehabilitation software package, *Brain Function Therapy*, has been developed by the Clinical Neuropsychology Unit of the Department of Clinical Psychology at the National Institute of Mental Health and Neurosciences (NIMHANS), Bengaluru, Karnataka, India.

When evaluating cognitive rehabilitation software, clinicians need to ask two questions: is there empirical evidence that cognitive gains result from the use of such programs? And, are the gains manifest on the computer screen generalized to gains in activities of daily life? Obviously, results from appropriately designed prospective, randomized controlled trials are required before conclusions are drawn.

Using Computers to Plan Therapy

Computer software can be used to analyze patient characteristics and responses in order to gain insights into the form of therapy ideal for individual patients. By way of example, Lieberman et al.[30] discussed the use of multimedia software in the rehabilitation of psychiatric patients. Known as *Making Choices*, the software identifies the needs and preferences of patients for their rehabilitation program. The software was found to have good acceptance amongst patients and their clinicians alike.

The Future

The use of computers has been examined in the therapy of very few disorders in psychiatry. Numerous situations lend themselves to computer-assisted or computer-directed therapy. Educational packages, considered to be of great importance in the family therapy of schizophrenia and several other disorders, can be delivered through computers. Marital therapy is a hitherto untouched area: problems can be identified on-screen and, through a decision-making tree, a hierarchy of solutions can be presented. Progress can be assessed periodically, and treatment approaches can be altered depending upon the progress. The applications of computers are limited only by the knowledge, the skills and the imaginativeness of the therapist and his team of computer programs.

Software can be developed to create a simulated patient. The behavior of this simulated patient can be used to model psychiatric disorders, and the response to various treatment interventions.

Rigorously designed controlled trials are necessary to confirm the therapeutic utility of different computer programs in different situations. The problems associated with and the benefits accruing from such programs need to be identified and compared. Indications and contraindications for computer-based therapy need to be developed. Predictors of benefit from computer-based therapy require to be identified. The shortcomings of existing studies include restricted situations of study, small sample sizes, inadequate control groups, inadequate follow-up assessments, etc. these have recently been reviewed.[4]

Cost-efficacy analyses need to be conducted. On the surface, it appears that computers may be able to serve a larger number of persons because therapy can be conducted in a variety of settings ranging from the clinic to the home, and can progress even in the relative absence of a therapist; this frees the therapist for other tasks as well as provides the patient with greater independence and flexibility. However, computer hardware and software costs need to be reckoned, as well as the costs associated with identifying and removing bugs in the program.

The use of computers in therapy is likely to gain ground as hardware and software technology improves. For example, computer software with voice recognition capacity is already commercially available; since multimedia computers have long been able to produce voice output, at sometime in the future, verbal patient-computer interactions may become feasible. This will eliminate the need for keyboard and screen-based interactions, which are currently a major disadvantage of computer-directed therapy.

MODELING OF COGNITION, PHYSIOLOGY AND BEHAVIOR

The brain has often been likened to a computer; neurons are wires that are connected to each other through switches known as synapses. Neurons receive inputs from external sources (e.g. glands) through more switches and, in turn, influence such external sources through still more switches.

There are several issues that magnify the complexity of this description:

- The number of 'wires' and 'switches' in a computer chip is tiny in comparison with the number of neurons and synapses in the brain. It is estimated that the brain is made up of a hundred billion neurons interconnected through a hundred thousand billion synapses.[31]
- The circuitry in a computer chip is predetermined, and the failure of a few connections or switches may make the chip substantially or entirely dysfunctional. While neurons may fail, even in large numbers, they also have the potential to recover from injury. And, neurons can branch out and establish new synapses in order to improve upon existing function or compensate for neurons that have failed (plasticity).
- A neuron is not merely a wire which conducts an electrical impulse; it is a living structure which has the capacity to modulate the input signal as a function of the factors that operate upon its receptors, its membrane, its second messenger chemistry, etc. The modulation that is effected is nonlinear; that is, the effect of the stimulus is not related in a linear fashion to the nature and magnitude of the stimulus, but depends upon all the internal and external factors operating on the neuron.
- A synapse is not merely an on/off switch. It has the potential to amplify or diminish the input signal in a nonlinear fashion, depending on neurotransmitter availability, the status of the different receptor subtypes on the presynaptic and postsynaptic membranes, the status of other neuronal systems with which the synapse interacts, etc.
- The complexity of parallel connections in the brain is staggering, and far exceeds that built into a computer; a single neuron may receive inputs from several neurons, and may itself project through synapses to several more neurons.
- On the flip side, neurons are far slower and far more prone to occasional idiosyncratic malfunction than the circuitry on silicon chips.

While wires, switches, parallel connections, randomness, and even nonlinear responses can be programmed into a computer, the simulations achieved as of today are very far below the complexity that is built into the human brain. All these and more issues need to be kept in mind in any discussion on *artificial intelligence*, or on the similarities between computers and the human brain.

It must also be considered that computers lack self-direction, intuitiveness, innovativeness, imaginativeness, metaphoricality, creativity, flexibility, versatility, emotionality, irrationality, inconsistency, subjectivity, consciousness and other 'mind' characteristics, unless they are preprogrammed to exhibit responses that simulate these characteristics. The use of the word 'simulate' itself suggests that artificial intelligence is truly 'artificial', not 'genuine'. *Deep Blue*, the chess-playing computer which made history, used its awesome computing capacities to defeat Gary Kasparov by laboriously analyzing an enormous range of combinations before arriving at the move which offered the best probability of a favorable outcome; brute computing power rather than an intelligent or intuitive choice of options governed its play.

Again, computers handle only issues concerning which they have been programmed. A computer programmed to play chess and learn from its mistakes cannot learn or play bridge; a computer programmed to recognize voice patterns and to update its memory banks based upon its recognitions cannot solve mathematical problems. Thus, programs that 'think' do so because they are programmed to do so in ways in which the programs devised beforehand. The 'thinking' processes follows the 'rules' laid down in the program. Idiosyncratic, nonlinear or chaotic responses occur only if they are built into the program.

Programs that 'learn', however, move one step closer towards a definition of intelligence; modeling of learning is examined later in this section. Artificial intelligence is the subject of hot debate, and arguments hinge on issues such as the definition of intelligence, or of consciousness. The field has advanced to the point where it is now an independent science in its own right. An appealing, nontechnical discussion on the subject has been provided by Lenat.[32] A discussion on artificial intelligence *per se* is out of the scope of this chapter; however, certain issues related thereto are considered.

Computers can be used to simulate a variety of physiological or behavioral processes such as memory, language, perception and related functions. The simulation involves the creation of artificial neurons in neural network models; these neurons behave in accordance with mathematical rules that are programed into the network. Such artificial networks have been used to model not only physiological states but also pathological states, such as Alzheimer's disease, aphasia, dyslexia, epilepsy, stroke, Parkinson's disease, schizophrenia, depression and related problems.[33]

Neural modeling was a dynamic field of investigation in the early 1960s. Over the next 15 years, interest in the field languished. From the mid-1980s onwards, there was a tremendous resurgence of activity in the area. Today, mathematicians, physicists, computer scientists, engineers, neuroscientists and cognitive psychologists are actively engaged in the examination of neural models; such models are considered as major theoretical tools. A few studies of interest are considered in this section.

Simulations of Impaired Cognition

Several studies have used computer programs that model the neuronal basis of memory using the principle of *attractor neural networks*. These neural networks are imaginary assemblies of model neurons that synapse with each other and with external structures. When a neuron fires, its output, weighted by synaptic strengths, is communicated to the neurons to which it is connected. These neighboring neurons may fire in response.

By using specific learning rules that govern the way synaptic strengths in the network are established, a specific set of input patterns can be memorized or stored in the network. These stored patterns are known as 'attractors'. The term attractor means that if a pattern which is sufficiently similar to one of the stored memory patterns is presented as input to the network, the state of the network will gradually evolve until it converges to the state representing that memory pattern. Since the state of the network is in this manner repeatedly updated, the *attractor network may therefore be regarded as an associative memory system.*

In attractor neural networks, stored memories are not represented locally at specific neurons, but their corresponding representations are distributed; many neurons participate in a given memorized pattern, and a particular neuron participates in several different patterns. Learning in this system is not a 'one-shot' process; a pattern to be stored must be presented to the system several times before it becomes engraved, as a memory, with sufficient strength upon the synaptic matrix.[34] Interested readers may refer to the description provided by Hinton et al[35] this is a less technical but more detailed explanation of the concepts involved in the use of neural networks to model learning, memory and the consequences of brain damage.

Carrie[36] conducted a series of computer simulations with lesioned attractor neural networks and concluded that such models show a gradual degradation in memory retrieval performance as the number of viable neurons (and their synapses) decreases. Carrie, however, found that the degree of modeled amnesia was linear to the neuronal loss instead of arising only after a critical stage of neuronal loss was attained with progressive lesioning; furthermore, no differences between recent (memories stored after lesioning) and remote (memories stored before lesioning) memories was detected.

In a series of experiments, Ruppin and Reggia[34] used a more complex variant of the attractor neural network and demonstrated progressive amnesia with increasing lesion severity. The impairment was gradual and not linear; this was accomplished by modeling synaptic compensatory changes as an accompaniment to the neuronal loss (thus, Alzheimer's disease was modeled as a failure of the synaptic compensatory responses to keep pace with the ongoing accelerated synaptic deletion). A temporal gradient of amnesia was demonstrated, with recent memories more affected than remote memories. Also similar to observations in clinical contexts, distractor patterns produced the equivalent of false positive recognitions. In this model, the synapse to neuron ratio was found to be an important determinant of the performance of the neural network. Overall, a close resemblance to performances in Alzheimer's patients was demonstrated.

Attractor networks are not the only models used to study cognition. *Synaptic runway models* have also been employed. These are pathological, exponential growths of synaptic connections occurring when previously stored memory patterns interfere with the storage of new patterns in the neural network model. The interference is proactive; it occurs because when a new memory pattern is stored in the network, the resultant network activity is guided not only by the new pattern but also by all the previous memory patterns engraved in the synaptic matrix. Thus, previous memories bias the activation in their direction during new storage. This reinforcement leads to a pathological increase in the number of synapses. Synaptic runway has been hypothesized to comprise one pathological process in Alzheimer's disease; the metabolic or excitotoxic stress in establishing new connections leads to neuronal degeneration. This model has even been used to explain the location, development and progress of the neuropathological lesions characteristic of Alzheimer's disease.[37]

A useful overview of the use of neural networks in the modeling of cognitive function and dysfunction has been presented by Reggia et al.[33]

Simulations of Schizophrenic and Manic Symptoms

Hoffman used a learning paradigm to model associative memory and gestalt seeking during cognition. Perturbations imposed on such computer simulations caused catastrophic breakdowns of neural network functioning. The resulting cognitive disturbance assumed two forms. One form was induced by memory overload; it resulted in misperceptions, loose associations, and also parasitic processing states that pathologically controlled the flow of associations. This form was suggested to model schizophrenic symptomatology. The other form was induced by increased randomness of neural activity, which occasioned jumps from one gestalt to another; this form was suggested to model manic symptomatology. While the earlier described models of cognitive impairment due to neuronal loss mimicked the clinical etiopathogenesis of the disorder,[34-36] the weakness of Hoffman's modeling is that the processes whereby the schizophrenic or manic dysfunctional systems are induced have not been proven to represent the manner in which schizophrenia and mania clinically develop.[38]

Hoffman[39] discussed reduced corticocortical connectivity simulations to model schizophrenia. He demonstrated that such models become functionally fragmented, suggesting loose associations. The models produced recurrent, intrusive representations suggesting delusions. Pruning of back propagation simulations of speech perception produced spontaneous output which modeled hallucinated speech. The model also suggested how dopamine blockade might reduce positive symptoms, and why negative symptoms arise in the wake of positive symptoms.

Simulations of Delusions

Spitzer[40] provided a cogent account of the manner in which computer-modeling of neuronal functioning is effected. In a detailed yet simply written article, he described how such neural network models can be used to generate a computational surface that creates and maintains memory maps for the representation of important sensorimotor and cognitive events. Such maps can be shown to change dynamically according to the salience and the frequency of the inputs into the neural network; this feature models neuroplasticity. General operational characteristics of such maps can be fine-tuned according to specific processing needs; this feature models neuromodulation.

Spitzer used these principles of neuromodulation to model acute delusions, and these principles of neuroplasticity to model chronic delusions. He argued, for example, that a high signal to noise ratio could be cognitively counterproductive because it could lead to over attention to irrelevant stimuli, and hence an attachment of unwarranted significance to these stimuli; the result is a delusional belief. Delusions comprise distortions of the cortical maps; once established, such delusions are easier to reinforce (through subsequent stimuli and experiences) than remove (through normalizing processes); this is possibly because the reinforcing processes recur while the normalizing processes are undefined.

Spitzer's operational concepts of acute and chronic delusions do not necessarily agree with those held by experts in psychopathology. A high signal to noise ratio may certainly result in irrelevant stimuli becoming etched into memory maps in neural networks, and these irrelevant details may certainly assume a delusional salience in the network that rivals the salience with which relevant stimuli are treated; nevertheless, there is little evidence to claim that a similar process generates delusional beliefs in psychotic individuals. However, Spitzer's arguments are valuable because they generate predictions that can be addressed in phenomenological approaches to psychopathology and its treatment. Thus, for example, Spitzer suggested that a psychosocial environment with restricted sensory and cognitive input is associated with a high signal to noise ratio; such an environment will generate and reinforce delusional beliefs; in contrast, the provision of an environment that is rich and stimulating will have an opposite effect and might hence be therapeutic in patients with delusions.

Simulations of Epilepsy

Several important neural models of epileptic abnormalities have been developed. For example, by simulating a blockade of inhibitory neurotransmission, insights are obtained into the mechanisms underlying abnormal neuronal bursting and after-discharges.

Kindling in neural networks has been modeled as the formation of a large number of excitatory synapses through a learning process which is similar to that described in an earlier section. The model demonstrates several experimentally observed phenomena, such as the initial rapid growth and eventual saturation of the amplitude and duration of the after-discharge, the insensitivity of the rate of kindling to the amplitude of the stimulus, the drop in the after-discharge threshold due to repeated stimulations, the frequency dependence of the kindling rate, etc. The model predicts that one of the reasons for the termination of epileptic after-discharges is that the neuronal network gets trapped in 'normal', low activity attractors of network dynamics.[41,42]

Other Simulations

Neural network simulations have also been used to model and/or explain the phantom limb syndrome,[43] cortical map reorganization after a stroke,[44] structural versus functional damage in multi-infarct dementia,[45] movement disturbance in Parkinson's disease and Huntington's disease,[46] functioning of the prefrontal cortex in affective, memory and behavioral dimensions,[47] etc.

Evaluation

Computer modeling of physiological and behavioral processes suffer from at least two important disadvantages:

1. Neural networks necessarily (markedly) simplify the biological phenomena that occur in the nervous system.
2. Neural networks are severely constrained in size.
3. There is no assurance that the theoretical rules programmed into the behavior of the network validly represent the rules that govern physiological processes.

Nevertheless, such computer-based models assist traditional methods of brain study in several ways:

- Neural networks can be studied in experimental contexts to examine issues and test hypotheses that cannot be ethically studied in humans.
- Lesion size and location can be precisely controlled; lesion size and location can also be systematically varied over a large number of hypothetical subjects and information processing tasks. Potentially valuable information leads can thus be obtained.
- Changes following a simulated lesion can be subjected to a detailed inspection, and processes in the evolution of these changes can be scrutinized. Theories of etiology and pathophysiology can subsequently be developed, some of which may be clinically testable. Ruppin and Reggia,[34] for example, used computer simulations to make specific predictions about patterns of cognition in patients with Alzheimer's disease, while Spitzer[40] used a neural network model to predict the genesis and behavior of delusions in the context of cortical maps.
- Responses of the system to external therapeutic or noxious influences can be modeled; this too has obvious practical significance.

THE INTERNET AND PSYCHIATRY

What is the Internet? It is the linking of computers across geographical boundaries. In 1967, about 20 computers were networked across the USA. By 1986, the number had increased, but had not crossed 10,000. Today, the Internet links millions of computers all over the world. Thus, resources such as files and programs on any of these computers can be made available to the remaining computers.[48]

Each computer on the Internet is fitted with a gadget known as a *modem*; this enables the computer to send and receive messages through telephone lines. Interlinking of individual computers is effected through agencies known as *service providers*. These service providers house many networked mainframe computers at a single location, and provide two important services: the software necessary for individual computers to access facilities on the Internet, and the actual linking through cables or satellite to other service providers elsewhere in the world. The service provider's resources thus act as an extension for the individual computers served by the provider. Each computer/user on the Internet has a unique name/address. This identifies not only the individual but also the Internet service to which he is attached.[48,49]

The Internet permits individuals to communicate computer to computer; this is known as *electronic mail (e-mail)*. E-mail is fast; most messages reach the day they are sent. E-mail is inexpensive, costing the equivalent of a local telephone call. The same message can be sent to several receivers. The receiver does not have to be present at time the message arrives, nor does his computer need to be on all through the day to receive messages. A response to a message is automatically addressed to the sender, and is accomplished through a single keystroke.[48] A disadvantage of e-mail, however, is that messages are not private: they can be read, monitored, recorded and/or stored by third parties.

Through the e-mail, automatic software known as *LISTSERV* can be utilized to receive and dispatch letters amongst members of a group; thus, the group can pool its information, share its experiences, clarify doubts, etc.[48]

The Internet provides access to *software*. It permits individuals to access technical and nontechnical medical and nonmedical *information*. An especially useful facility for medical professionals is the accessibility of electronic databases such as MEDLINE; many leading journals are also available, either in part or in whole on the Internet. Nonprofessionals can benefit from support groups, self-help groups and discussion groups, as well as from nontechnical medical information. Users of the Internet can select channels featuring conversations of interest, and thereby participate in real-time, on-line, group discussions on *Internet Relay Chat* channels; this is like a conference call, except that the dialogue is typed onscreen.[50]

The Internet also enables the *World Wide Web (WWW)*. This is an enormous collection of text, graphics and sound which provides information on different subjects. Individuals read pages on and navigate through the Web using a graphical interface known as a browser; examples of browsers are Netscape and Mosaic. Web pages have *hypertext links* which are highlighted; these allow the individual to move from one page on one computer to another page on another computer (on the Internet) in another part of the world. Thus, reading is nonlinear; it does not follow any preset sequence, nor is there any numbering or ordering of pages. The number of Web home pages is growing at a tremendous rate: there were fewer than 100 sites in 1993; by October, 1995, the number had expanded to 48,000. In February, 1996, there were an estimated two and a half million Websites.[48]

Users of the Internet can employ powerful software known as *search engines* (e.g. Yahoo, Lycos) to identify Web pages that contain information on the subject of the search, and can, thereafter, move from page to page, or site to site, through selected hypertext links that they consider relevant or interesting.[48,49]

The Internet is awesome not merely because it has revolutionized communication through e-mail but because it has opened a highway to more information than an individual can hope to access in a lifetime. The on us, therefore, lies on the user to filter out the unnecessary and identify the useful. The principle of caveat emptor will also apply: *there are no guarantees about the reliability/fidelity of any service/ information accessed through the Internet.*

Sites on the Internet cover virtually every medical topic; some are informative, some are educative, and some serve as a forum for discussion. By way of example, Galanter, et al.[51] developed a course on network therapy for substance abuse and put it on the Internet; they subsequently examined and presented their experiences in a discussion on the use of the Internet for clinical training.

The Internet offers other facilities. *Gopher* refers to a set of preorganized links (on different computers) that are offered to the user. *File transfer protocol* refers to the acquisition of data or software through telephone lines. *Telnet* is a way of connecting to remote computers and using them as though the user were on site. *News groups*, also called USENET groups, allow communication between persons with similar interests; users can sign onto news groups to receive the latest messages posted to the group, and can also send messages back to the group; over 11,000 USENET groups exist.[48]

Clinicians may note that the Internet offers them facilities not only to access services but also to provide these services themselves, to other clinicians or to the lay public. The Internet offers great potential to revolutionize the face of education, clinical care, research and administration in psychiatry; future scenarios have been considered by Huang and Alessi.[50] Technical information, practical information, and useful Internet addresses for clinical information, training and research have been published.[48,50,52] Further information on the Internet has been provided by Hancock.[53]

APPLICATIONS OF COMPUTERS IN ADMINISTRATIVE PSYCHIATRY

At the risk of stating the obvious, it must be affirmed that the greatest assistance that a computer can afford a clinician lies in his routine activities. These include the following:

The Storage of Patient Records in a Suitably Constructed Database

This requires the use of database software. Using these programs, information can be stored so that individual records can be conveniently retrieved. More usefully, at the time of storage the data can be classified into appropriately constructed storage fields such that records can later be extracted thematically; this can permit, by way of example, the instantaneous retrieval of the records of all male schizophrenic patients in the database, aged 31–40 years, who had been treated with clozapine and who had required withdrawal of the drug because of the development of a fall in white blood cell counts.

A further advantage of using computerized databases is that these eliminate the need for paper-based records. Finally, confidentiality and security of records can be maintained with greater efficiency.

These applications are considerably useful in hospital-based environments, and in research settings. However, they can be advantageous in individual practice as well. Common database programs include DBase, Foxbase, FoxPro, Access and Approach; for special settings, and in institutional practice, special software may need to be developed to cater to idiosyncratic requirements.

Processes involved in the computerization of psychiatric case records and descriptions of the usefulness thereof have been provided in literature.[54-56] Computerized records can save time by automatically issuing reports and discharge summaries. Computerized records can improve clinical practice, simplify quality assurance, and ease the collection and analysis of data for statistical purposes or research. Computerized records are also useful for case audits and accounting. Treatment plans and medication orders can be entered on-line. Electronic communication of case and treatment material within and outside the hospital can be conveniently effected.

The Production of Reports, Certificates and Other Documents

The typewriter is today obsolete because very little amendment of text is possible once letters have been typed upon a page. In its place, word processing software permits the user to make corrections in his document as he is typing. He can move sections or parts thereof within or between documents. He can, with minimum additional effort, individually address or otherwise customize the same document to scores of persons on a mailing list. He can change the formatting of the document to suit the need, and increase the attractiveness of presentation by altering fonts and style, or by including graphics or even sound (this facility is applicable only to material that is transmitted in an electronic and not printed format). He can maintain his records for convenient, paperless retrieval at any time in the future.

Likewise, the computer permits the user to prepare charts, tables, graphs, figures and other presentation material with effortless convenience. Intercompatibility of programs permits data stored in one program to be imported into another program for use. Common word processing programs include WordStar, Word Perfect, Word, and Word Pro. Common graphics programs include Harvard Graphics, Freelance Graphics and Power Point.

The Computation of Statistics and Accounting Data

Data collected frequently needs to be examined in sets. Accounts need to be computed. Means, standard deviations, and frequency counts need to be generated. Data need to be compared across groups. Forecasts need to be made.

Almost everybody will have need for the generation of descriptive statistics; these can be more easily and more reliably extracted from computerized than from manual records. It goes without saying that in research the analysis of data is rendered ridiculously easy with the help of a computer, and computations, that might otherwise have taken weeks or months, can be completed within hours or less using appropriate statistical software.

Common spreadsheet and statistical packages include Lotus 123, Excel, Statistical Package for Social Sciences (SPSS), StatGraf, and Systat.

Online Monitoring of Drug Utilization Patterns

Implemented in certain states in the USA, computerized online monitoring of drug utilization patterns seeks to identify overuse or underuse of drugs; inappropriate prescriptions in drug dosage, drug combination or duration of therapy, and problems of a similar nature. The service also seeks to provide long-term audits of drug-utilization patterns which might be used to provide a feedback to clinicians in order to beneficially alter prescription patterns.[57] It is acknowledged that such facilities have been criticized; however, the criticism is more about the construction of the audit and the interpretation of the data than the computerization *per se*. If these matters can be satisfactorily resolved, the data so generated can be immensely valuable. Computerization is the most efficient means of compiling such data.

Monitoring of Healthcare Delivery

The British government has decreed that within the next few years, every mental health unit in Britain should install a computerized clinical information system. Such a change could revolutionize the monitoring of healthcare delivery in the field of psychiatry, facilitate the compilation of statistics, and help identify untoward or unusual situations. However, the government notification has met with a reserved response from the clinical community; possible concerns include fears that information technology through computers wastes time instead of saving time, that computer software is more suited to financial and accounting situations than to clinical situations, that computers do less than they have been claimed to do (and may be less efficient, or even more fallible, at times, than human processes), that confidentiality may be difficult to maintain if records are computerized, that computerized data may not be as easily accessible as paper-based data, etc. These and other concerns have been discussed by Briscoe,[58] and solutions have been proposed.

MISCELLANEOUS APPLICATIONS OF COMPUTERS IN PSYCHIATRY

Education

Computer software is available to explain the working of the human body, to detail human anatomy, to display surface relations or sections of the body at various levels and so on. These programs are educative in nature and target the lay public as well as medical students. For the neurosciences, computerized brain maps and atlases have been developed to facilitate learning, neuroimaging procedures, and surgical procedures requiring neuroimaging.[31,59]

Computerized brain atlases are advantageous for several reasons. They provide three dimensional representations; the structures depicted can be deformed so as to fit the sizes and shapes of individual brains. The atlases can be used to compensate for the shrinkage and distortions during sectioning and embedding of postmortem brains, to study structural-functional relationships in the human brain at both the macroscopic and microscopic levels, to study variations in gross morphology and microstructure, to develop a three dimensional human brain database, and to assist generalizations about localization of function and structure at both macroscopic and microscopic levels. A detailed discussion on the subject has been provided by Roland and Zilles.[60]

At present, with the exception of software on the anatomy and the physiology of brain mechanisms, there may not be much of a role for similar software in psychiatry. However, programs can be developed that demonstrate phenomena or test a student's skills. For example, a program known as *Racter* provides excellent samples of formal thought disorder in response to a clinical interview conducted by the student via a keyboard. Likewise, subject-specific software (while currently unavailable) can be prepared to test a student's knowledge or help him prepare for an examination. Continuing Medical Education (CME) programs can be similarly formulated.

Literature Searches

Computerized databases are today the ideal resource for conducting literature searches. Several such databases are available, such as Medline, Embase and Psyclit. Using specific key words that define the scope of the search, all articles published in specified journals during a specified period can be rapidly and conveniently identified and extracted. This method eliminates the laborious physical searches through the indexes of each volume of each journal, the luck of the draw in identifying relevant articles, the biases associated with snowball literature searches (based on cross-references cited in identified articles), etc. Major databases, journals and textbooks are now available on disk as an alternative to the paper hardcopy and, very recently, societies such as the Society of Biological Psychiatry have also published conference proceedings in disk form for easy storage and retrieval.

Elaborate computerized databases on the brain are also being developed; these are more than just a list of articles published on a topic. Such databases are intended to provide users with structural, functional and other data on aspects related to the brain; these data will be accessible through appropriate menus built into the software. Such databases will facilitate the integration of the activities of neuroscientists with differing superspecializations; scientists working in one field will have the opportunity to obtain insights into their work arising from research published in other fields; to employ the famous metaphor, scientists will be able to examine the whole elephant, and not just parts thereof.[61]

CONCLUDING NOTES

When using computers, certain obvious practical precautions need to be kept in mind; these include the need for uninterrupted power supply, for adequate backups of software and data on diskettes or magnetic tape (stored in suitable locations), etc.

Clinical precautions need to be considered. Computers can not replace the human touch; clinicians, therefore, should not be tempted to surrender their clinical responsibilities to the computer.

Conceptual precautions need to be exercised. For example, computer-patient interactions may elicit different patient responses than clinician-patient interactions. This means that the interpretation of processes arising out of computer-directed therapy, or the interpretation of computer-obtained clinical ratings, should consider the source of the data.

The software should be critically evaluated. Computer programs and manufacturers are not mental health professionals, and may make errors during the software design. Reliability and validity data reported by the manufacturer may not be applicable to the specific contexts in which the clinician is using the software.

The American Psychological Association[62] has developed guidelines for the ethical use of computer-based tests, including guidelines for authors and publishers of tests, professionals using these tests, test subjects and test administrators. The Ethics Committee of the American Psychological Association[63] has expressed concerns that interventions over the telephone or the Internet may not allow the therapist to adequately assess the patient, develop a relationship or otherwise provide satisfactory standards of care; similar concerns surely need to be considered in the context of computer-based therapies.

The advent of the computer has revolutionized the field of medicine and psychiatry. On the one hand, computers can relieve the clinician of the responsibility for clinical chores, giving him greater scope to focus on therapeutic relationships and issues arising therefrom. On the other hand, newer and newer applications for computers are being conceived and developed, enabling clinicians to do more than they earlier did, with greater efficiency, and in less time. In the foreseeable future, clinicians' reliance on computers will increase to the point at which computers become a necessity; this situation will, hopefully, idealize the balance between demands and resources in clinical care.[64]

Finally, there is a such a wealth of literature on computers in psychiatry that a comprehensive review of the subject is impossible; indeed, a special journal *Computers in Human Behavior* is dedicated to the field; this journal is in its fourteenth year of publication. Furthermore, applications of computers in psychiatry is a field that is advancing on an almost day to day basis; any article on the subject will probably become outdated on the day after it is written. Accordingly, this chapter is written to provide an overview of the subject, and is, therefore, a sampler of the tremendous potential that computers have to augment research and practice in psychiatry.

REFERENCES

1. Bucholz KK, Marion SL, Shayka JJ, Marcus SC, Robins LN. A short computer interview for obtaining psychiatric diagnoses. Psychiatr Serv. 1996;47:293-7.
2. Kobak KA, Taylor LVH, Dottl SL, Griest JH, Jefferson JW, Burroughs JW, Katzelnick DJ, Mandell M. Computerized screening for psychiatric disorders in an outpatient community mental health clinic. Psychiatr Serv. 1997;48:1048-57.
3. Peters L, Andrews G. Procedural validity of the computerized version of the Composite International Diagnostic Interview (CIDI-Auto) in the anxiety disorders. Psychol Med. 1995;25:1269-80.
4. Newman MG, Consoli A, Taylor CB. Computers in assessment and cognitive behavioral treatment of clinical disorders: anxiety as a case in point. Behav Ther. 1997;28:211-35.
5. Issac M. Diagnostic assessment in psychiatry: Current Status. NIMHANS Journal 1997 (in press).
6. Reich W, Cottler L, McCallum K, Corwin D, VanEerderwegh M. Computerized interviews as a method of assessing psychopathology in children. Compr Psychiatry. 1995;36:40-5.
7. Kobak KA, Reynolds WM, Rosenfeld R, Griest JH. Development and validation of a computer-administered version of the Hamilton Depression Rating Scale. Psychol Assess. 1990;2:56-63.
8. Rosenfeld R, Dar R, Anderson D, Kobak KA, Griest JH. A computer-administered version of the Yale-Brown Obsessive Compulsive Scale. Psychol Assess. 1992;4:329-32.
9. Kobak KA, Reynolds WM, Griest JH. Development and validation of a computer-administered version of the Hamilton Anxiety Scale. Psychol Assess. 1993;5:487-92.
10. Katzelnick DJ, Kobak KA, Griest JH Jefferson JW, Mantle JM, Serlin RC. Sertraline in social phobia: a double-blind,

placebo-controlled crossover study. Am J Psychiatry. 1995;152:1368-71.

11. Baer L, Brown-Beasley MW, Sorce J, Henriques AI. Computer-assisted telephone administration of a structured interview for obsessive-compulsive disorder. Am J Psychiatry. 1993;150:1737-8.
12. Marks IM, Blanes T, McKenzie N. Computerized clinical benefit-cost audit of mental health care, Ist edition. Theoretical and practical issues. J Ment Health. 1995;1:63-9.
13. McKenzie N, Blanes T, Marks IM. Computerized clinical benefit-cost audit of mental health care, 2nd edition. Case examples. J Ment Health. 1995;1:71-8.
14. Marks I. A computerized system to measure treatment outcomes and cost. Psychiatr Serv. 1995;47:811-2.
15. Kobak KA. Computer-administered symptom-rating scales. Psychiatr Serv. 1996;47:367-9.
16. Swartz CM, Abrams R. ECT Instruction Manual. Lake Bluff, Illinois: Somatics, Inc., 1994.
17. Andrade C. ECT devices and measures of seizure adequacy. Psychiatry Update. 1997;3:36-7.
18. Andrade C. Assessment of the therapeutic adequacy of the ECT seizure: Current status. NIMHANS Journal 1997 (in press).
19. Andrade C, Gangadhar BN, Meena M, Pradhan N. Dopamine post-synaptic receptor effects of restricted schedules of electroconvulsive shock. Indian J Psychiatry. 1990;32:297-301.
20. Colby KM, Gould RL, Aronson G. Some pros and cons of computer-assisted psychotherapy. J Nerv Ment Dis. 1989;177:105-8.
21. Colby KM. A computer program using cognitive therapy to treat depressed patients. Psychiatric Services. 1995;46:1223-5.
22. Selmi PM, Klein MH, Greist JH, Sorrell SP, Erdman HP. Computer-administered cognitive-behavioral therapy for depression. Am J Psychiatry. 1990;147:51-6.
23. Horan JJ. Effects of computer-based cognitive restructuring on rationally mediated self-esteem. J Counsel Psychol. 1996;43:371-5.
24. Ghosh A, Marks IM, Carr AC. Therapist contact and outcome of self-exposure treatment for phobias. Br J Psychiatry. 1988;152:234-8.
25. Hasan AAM. A comparison of computer-based symbolic modelling and conventional methods in the treatment of spider phobia. Doctoral dissertation, University of Leeds, England; 1992.
26. Rothbaum BO, Hodges LF, Kooper R, Opdyke D, Williford JS, North M. Effectiveness of computer-generated (virtual reality) graded exposure in the treatment of acrophobia. Am J Psychiatry. 1995;152:626-8.
27. Kirkby KC. Computer-assisted treatment of phobias. Psychiatr Serv. 1996;47:139-40.
28. Kirkby KC, Daniels BA, Watson PJ. An interactive computerized teaching program for self-exposure therapy of avoidant behavior in phobic disorders. In: Sanders MR, Halford WK (Eds). Fourth World Congress on Behavior Therapy, Program and Abstracts. Bowen Hills, Queensland: Australian Academic Press; 1992.
29. Jerome C. Self-analysis: Structure, extension, and computerization. J Nerv Ment Dis. 1995;183:472-7.
30. Lieberman HJ, Goldberg F, Kaplan G. The CD-ROM as a multipurpose clinical and management tool. Psychiatr Serv. 1997;48:1014-6.
31. Swanson LW. Mapping the human brain: past, present and future. Trends In Neurological Sciences. 1995;18:471-4.
32. Lenat DB. Artificial intelligence. Sci Am. 1995.pp.62-4.
33. Reggia JA, Ruppin E, Berndt RS. Modeling brain and cognitive disorders. In: Reggia JA, Ruppin E, Berndt RS (Eds). Neural Modeling of Brain and Cognitive Disorders. Singapore, World Scientific Publishers; 1996.pp.3-39.
34. Ruppin E, Reggia JA. A neural model of memory impairment in diffuse cerebral atrophy.Br J Psychiatry. 1995;166:19-28.
35. Hinton GE, Plaut DC, Shallice T. Simulating brain damage. Scientific American; 1993.pp.76-82.
36. Carrie JR. Evaluation of a neural network model of amnesia in diffuse cerebral atrophy. Br J Psychiatry. 1993;163:217-22.
37. Hasselmo ME, Wyble BP. Does the spread of Alzheimer's disease neuropathology involve the mechanisms of consolidation? In: Reggia JA, Ruppin E, Berndt RS (Eds). Neural Modeling of Brain and Cognitive Disorders. Singapore: World Scientific Publishers; 1996.pp.43-62.
38. Hoffman RE. Computer simulations of neural information processing and the schizophrenia-mania dichotomy. Arch Gen Psychiatry. 1987;44:178-88.
39. Hoffman RE. Neural networks, cortical connectivity and schizophrenia psychosis. In: Reggia JA, Ruppin E, Berndt RS (Eds). Neural Modeling of Brain and Cognitive Disorders. Singapore: World Scientific Publishers; 1996.pp.441-56.
40. Spitzer D. A neurocomputational approach to delusions. Compr Psychiatry. 1995;36:83-105.
41. Metha MR, Dasgupta C, Ullal GR. A neural network model for kindling of focal epilepsy: basic mechanism. Biol Cybern. 1993;68:335-40.
42. Metha MR, Dasgupta C, Ullal GR. A neural network model for kindling of focal epilepsy. In: Reggia JA, Ruppin E, Berndt RS (Eds). Neural Modeling of Brain and Cognitive Disorders. Singapore: World Scientific Publishers; 1996.pp.347-75.
43. Spitzer M. Phantom limbs, self-organizing feature maps and noise-driven neuroplasticity. In: Reggia JA, Ruppin E, Berndt RS (Eds). Neural Modeling of Brain and Cognitive Disorders. Singapore: World Scientific Publishers; 1996.pp.273-82.
44. Reggia J, Goodall S, Chen Y, Ruppin E, Whitney C. Modeling post-stroke cortical map reorganization. In: Reggia JA, Ruppin E, Berndt RS (Eds). Neural Modeling of Brain and Cognitive Disorders. Singapore: World Scientific Publishers; 1996. pp.283-302.
45. Ruppin E, Reggia JA. Functional versus structural damage in multi-infarct dementia: A computational study. In: Reggia JA, Ruppin E, Berndt RS (Eds). Neural Modeling of Brain and Cognitive Disorders. Singapore: World Scientific Publishers; 1996.pp.303-25.
46. Contreras-Vidal JL, Teulings HL, Stelmach GE. A neural network model of movement production in Parkinson's disease

and Huntington's disease. In: Reggia JA, Ruppin E, Berndt RS (Eds). Neural Modeling of Brain and Cognitive Disorders. Singapore: World Scientific Publishers; 1996.pp.377-92.
47. Levine DS. Modeling dysfunction of the prefrontal executive system. In: Reggia JA, Ruppin E, Berndt RS (Eds). Neural Modeling of Brain and Cognitive Disorders. Singapore: World Scientific Publishers; 1996.pp.413-39.
48. Lim RF. The Internet: Applications for mental health clinicians in clinical settings, training and research. Psychiatr Serv. 1996;47:597-9.
49. Robinson D. Surfing the Internet: Challenges for health-care. Psychiatr Care. 1997;4:124-6.
50. Huang MP, Alessi NE. The Internet and the future of psychiatry. Am J Psychiatry. 1996;153:861-9.
51. Galanter M, Keller DS, Dermatis H. Using the Internet for clinical training: A course on network therapy for substance abuse. Psychiatr Serv. 1997;48:999-1000, and 1008.
52. Glowniak JV, Bushway MK. Computer networks as a medical resource: Accessing and using the Internet. JAMA. 1994;271:1934-9.
53. Hancock L. The Physician's Guide to the Internet. Philadelphia: Lippincott-Raven; 1996.
54. Modai I, Rabinowitz J. Why and how to establish a computerized system for psychiatric case records. Hosp Comm Psychiatry. 1993;44:1091-5.
55. Rabinowitz J, Modai I, Valevski A, Zemishlany Z, Mark M. Benefits of a structured format for paper and computerized psychiatric case records. Hospital and Community Psychiatry. 1993;44:1095-7.
56. Weiss KM, Chapman HA. A computer-assisted inpatient psychiatric assessment and treatment planning system. Hosp Comm Psychiatry. 1993;44:1097-100.
57. Soumerai SB, Lipton HL. Computer-based drug-utilization review-risk, benefit, or boondoggle? N Engl J Med. 1995;332: 1641-5.
58. Briscoe M. Obstacles to the use of computers in British Mental Health Services. Psychiatr Serv. 1997;48:329-30.
59. Greitz T, Bohm C, Holte S, Eriksson L. A computerized brain atlas: construction, anatomic content, and some applications. J Computer Assisted Tomography. 1991;15:26-38.
60. Roland PE, Zilles K. Brain atlases: a new research tool. TINS. 1994;17:458-67.
61. Gibbons A. Databasing the brain. Science. 1992;258:1872-3.
62. American Psychological Association. Guidelines for computer-based tests and interpretations. Washington, DC: American Psychological Association; 1986.
63. American Psychological Association, Ethics Committee. Report of the ethics committee, 1995. Am Psychol. 1996;51:1279-86.
64. Govender T, Adebajo O. Computers in Psychiatry. The British Journal of Psychiatry. 2008;192:479-80.

CHAPTER 64

Amnesic Disorders

JN Vyas, Anushul Khichy, Jayati Simlai, Christoday RJ Khess

Memory disturbances frequently occur after brain damage, but can be associated with psychiatric illnesses as well. Amnesia—the most severe form of memory impairment has several variants, including anterograde and retrograde amnesia, material-specific and modality-specific amnesia, and transient global amnesia. Research into amnesia has increased exponentially, probably because of the availability of modern brain-imaging techniques. In line with the view that memory is not a unity but is organized into several systems, amnesia is described as a multifaceted disease with a frequently poor prognosis.

INTRODUCTION

The term amnesia is mainly used in two ways. First, it is generally used to describe any severe memory impairment or deficit, irrespective of the cause. Second, it is used in line with the traditional view that amnesia is a memory impairment that occurs in the absence of other substantial cognitive impairments, and is restricted to specific disorders. These disorders-referred to as either amnesic or amnestic disorders according to different international classifications - have as a core feature a memory impairment that is not due to dementia or delirium and represents a decline from a previously attained functional level. This decline in function differentiates them from infantile amnesia or neuro-developmental disorders.

In this chapter we outline the classification of memory systems and summarize relevant aspects of what causes amnesic disorders, their neurobiology, epidemiology, diagnosis, and management. We discuss neuroimaging and genetic studies and emphasize the need for methodological rigor with respect to memory-testing paradigms.

MEMORY SYSTEMS AND MEMORY PROCESSES

Although the term amnesia was used rather loosely until the 1980s[1]—often to describe total memory loss, we now know that memory impairment in amnesic disorders is likely to be restricted to specific kinds of memory. This view is supported by the existence of several distinct memory systems, each with different neuroanatomical substrates. In addition to the division into short-term and long-term memory the work of Tulving,[1-4] especially, led to a content-based classification of long-term memory into five systems, which are hierarchically organized according to their assumed ontogenetic and phylogenetic development.

A distinction is made between episodic-autobiographical memory (EAM-e.g. remembering your dinner from the previous night) and semantic autobiographical memory (e.g. memory or knowledge of your date of birth). Semantic autobiographical memory might be impaired in dissociative amnesia, but is usually preserved in other amnesic disorders; to know a fact is assumed to need less contextual and associational information than to remember a personal event.

The inability to store new information long-term is named anterograde amnesia and the inability to recall stored information is termed retrograde amnesia. Retrograde memory impairment usually follows Ribot's law of regression,[5] i.e. recent memories are more affected than earlier ones. Isolated retrograde amnesia is reported to occur after neurological or psychological incidents. Some investigators argue that even with clear evidence of pathological changes within the brain, psychological factors substantially contribute to persistence of retrograde EAM impairment.[6]

EAM serves both retrospective and prospective functions. The ability to remember to do a future action in response to a prespecified cue (prospective memory) might be impaired in amnesic disorders as a result of disruptions to EAM, semantic memory, or executive functions.[7]

Memory processing is implicit (subconscious) or explicit (conscious). Implicit processing is typically coupled with procedural and priming memory systems and explicit memory is generally associated with perceptual and semantic memory and EAM. EAM is state-dependant; optimum retrieval of memories occurs when the environmental and mood conditions match those that were present when the memory was encoded. Panel 1 shows various kinds of amnesia (see appendix for the psychological processes associated with memory).

NEUROANATOMY AND NEUROBIOLOGY OF MEMORY

The debate about whether the brain contains functionally specialized regions or acts Gestalt-like[1] (as a whole) took on a new dimension with the advent of functional imaging, which sometimes points towards a high degree of cortical specialization.[8] Amnesias arise after damage to bottleneck structures through which information has to pass before it is stored long-term[9] but can also take place after widespread cortical damage (Panel 2). Panel 3 presents brain regions whose (bilateral) damage is most frequently implicated in amnesia.

Some amnesic disorders occur without evidence of substantial brain damage on conventional structural imaging. These disorders include those that are etiologically linked to psychosocial mechanisms, such as dissociative or psychogenic amnesias or mnestic block syndrome,[10] and amnesic disorders with an unknown cause (functional amnesias; see Panel 1)[11] After research by HJM[11] and colleagues, was reported, several studies identified changes in brain function affecting regions with crucial roles in memory processing in amnesic disorders that do not show evidence of structural brain damage.[10,12,13] Investigators have analyzed data obtained with glucose PET from 14 patients at rest with dissociative amnesia and severe retrograde EAM impairments and reported hypometabolism in the right temporofrontal regions, especially in the inferolateral prefrontal cortex.[10]

Processing in various memory systems is associated with similar mechanisms and molecular steps across many species, especially during encoding, consolidation, and storage. Several types of synaptic plasticity subserve memory formation, such as long-term potentiation and depression, synaptogenesis, and synapse remodeling. The cellular and molecular mechanisms underlying long-term memory acquisition consist of various signaling pathways, gene transcription, protein synthesis, and synaptic morphological changes.[14,15] Long-term storage of memories might need active self-sustaining molecular mechanisms (e.g. a functional prion protein).[16]

Environmentally driven changes in long-term memory formation and synaptic plasticity might arise as a result of changes in gene transcription and protein synthesis via epigenetic mechanisms (DNA methylation, post-translational histone chemical modifications, or micro RNAs).[16,17] Some epigenetic modifications might be reversible via pharmacological manipulation.[17]

INTERNATIONAL CLASSIFICATIONS OF AMNESIC DISORDERS

The International Statistical Classification of Diseases and Related Health Problems, tenth revision (ICD-10)[18] and the Diagnostic and Statistical Manual of Mental Disorders, fourth edition, text revision (DSM-IV-TR)[19] classify amnesic disorders on the basis of their strong etiological link to general medical disorders, the direct effects of psychoactive substances in the patient's body persisting beyond the intoxication or withdrawal period, or psychological factors. Although the terms dissociative, psychogenic, and functional amnesia are often used interchangeably, differences exist between them.

Several medical disorders can lead to amnesic disorders (Panel 2), In most cases, EAM is solely or predominantly affected. A new form of substance induced memory impairment is emerging that has therapeutic aims-namely, to weaken traumatic memories by hampering their consolidation or postretrieval reconsolidation.[20] Electroconvulsive therapy has received much attention with respect to the extent and persistence of retrograde memory loss that it can cause.[21] Most research with objective measures showed that EAM loss in patients who had undergone electroconvulsive therapy was short-term, but in a prospective, naturalistic, non-randomized study, some patients still had EAM impairments after 6 months.[22]

BRAIN DAMAGE OF THE LIMBIC SYSTEM AND AMNESIA

Data for amnesia come from case reports and group studies. These group studies frequently combine patients whose amnesia has different causes, but who presumably have the same main locus of brain damage. Three main forms of amnesia have been classically described on the basis of the locus of brain damage: hippocampal or medial temporal lobe (MTL) amnesia, diencephalic amnesia, and basal forebrain amnesia. Despite some differences (Table 1), they share many features. Various portions of the limbic system can easily be arranged in a Gestalt-like way, which is supported by findings that severe amnesia can result from brain damage at the intersection between the MTL and the diencephalon. Using diffusion tensor imaging, Papanicolaou and colleagues[23] provided evidence that bilateral damage to fornix—the fiber bundle projecting from the hippocampal formation (HF; part of the MTL) to the mammillary bodies (part of the diencephalon)—was underlying a case of severe amnesia.

The amygdaloid complex—a region whose contribution to amnesic disorders has been debated—is situated within the MTL and, concomitantly, is part of the basolateral limbic circuit with connections to diencephalon and basal forebrain.[24] The amygdala is implicated in emotional tagging of EAM. Activation of right amygdala was recorded during retrieval of old emotional EAM[25] and association of faces with emotional judgments (social memory).[26] Hurlemann[15] emphasized that both hypermnesia and periemotional amnesia (diminished memories of neutral events during simultaneously enhanced encoding of an aversive event) are amygdale-dependant, varying as a function of noradrenergic-glucocorticoid input to the amygdala. Rutishauser and colleagues[27] reported that

Table 1: Characteristics of amnesias related to medial temporal lobe (MTL), diencephalic (D), and basal forebrain (BF) damage

	MTL	*D*	*BF*
Abilities of conscious reflection and self-awareness	+	+/–	–/+
Tendencies of disinhibition and perseveration	–	+/–	–/+
Anosognosia	–	–/+	+
Initial loss of the sense of time (chronotaraxis)	–	–/+	–
Disproportional impairment of recall as opposed to recognition	–	–	+
Tendency to confabulate	–	–/+	+
Deficits in tasks needing executive functions	–	+/–	+
Emotional instability and mood disorders	–	–/+	+
Difficulties with attention and concentration	–	–	+
Damage to the region is (+) associated; (–) not associated; (+/–) often associated; or (–/+) occasionally associated with this characteristic			

single-unit activity in hippocampus and amygdala correlated positively with successful recollection of previously perceived stimuli. EAM impairments might accompany Urbach-Wiethe disease, a genetic disorder associated with bilateral amygdala calcifications.[28]

Evidence that the MTL-particularly the HF-played a major part in memory first appeared in about 1900,[1] however, no-one focused on MTL's association with memory until 1957 when Scoville and Milner reported patients with bilateral MTL surgery secondary to intractable epilepsy.[29] Within this series, the case of one patient known as HM - became famous. HM was operated on in 1953 and died in 2008. At the time of surgery, he had normal intelligence and memory function. After surgery he lost his ability to consciously form new, stable long-term memories, although his preoperative semantic and procedural memories remained largely intact. Initial descriptions suggested that he could retrieve most of his old autobiographical events. Later studies revealed that he could still acquire information that was processed at the levels of conditioning, priming, and procedural memory. Imaging that was undertaken almost four decades after surgery revealed that HM had undergone bilateral removal of the amygdala, parahippocampal-entorhinal cortex, and anterior hippocampus.

Since the first reports of HM's memory deficits, HF (including hippocampus proper, dentate gyrus, and subiculum) was thought to be the major hub for transmission of information from short-term to long-term storage, and this view received support from subsequent work in people and animals. Pathological changes to HF were thought to underlie amnesic disorders caused by MTL epilepsy viral infections, hypoxia, or carbon monoxide poisoning.[30] However, investigators have questioned how selective patients' brain damage is after they have had these disorders.[31,32] For example, herpes simplex encephalitis might lead to degeneration of the anterior and medial temporal lobes and orbitofrontal cortex.[32]

HF atrophy generally accompanies early Alzheimer's disease, but was also noted in nondemented elderly people.[33] For the past few years, researchers have attempted to differentiate, within the HF, activations during encoding from activations during retrieval[32] and different forms of memory (semantic memory, EAM, and spatial memory).[33] Studies reporting that patients with damage to the HF find it difficult to imagine new experiences[34] or re-experience old EAMs ignited much interest;[35] however, subsequent investigations into imagination of future experiences in patients with HF damage did not yield uniform results, perhaps because there were differences in the extent and onset of the damage, selectivity of lesions, and testing methods.[36]

Several studies of patients with MTL amnesia or diencephalic amnesia have focused on the possibility that recollection and familiarity processes are neuroanatomically separate. Recollection is the process needed to recall associative elements of knowledge and specific contextual details of a previous event so that the past can be re-experienced or relived. The feeling of familiarity is based on the matching of processes between retrieval cues and memory representations, in the absence of recollective experience. Shortcomings of studies attempting to discover which brain regions are implicated in specific processes include the small number of study patients and the low selectivity of their lesions.

Gilboa and colleagues' article,[37] reportedly on hippocampal contributions to recollection, stemmed from findings from two patients-one with "bilateral fornix and septal nuclei lesions" and mild "cortical and hippocampal atrophy" (the hippocampus is in fact a component of the cerebral cortex), and the other with traumatic brain injury with widespread limbic and neocortical damage of all cortical lobes. Despite the low number of cases and the nonselectivity of the brain damage, the investigators still concluded that the "extended hippocampal system is required to support recollection".[37]

In a thoughtful theoretical analysis based on quantitative modeling, Shimarnura[38] concluded that retrieval of EAM is a whole-brain experience in which the hippocampus proper can be viewed as sitting at the top of a hierarchy of MTL structures, all of which are dependent on further sensory and emotional information processing regions. This view is the same as the one proposed of HJM's report of psychogenic amnesia.[39] Differing theories exist about whether the retrieval of old auto-biographical memories occurs independently from MTL structures such as the HF, or whether these structures are engaged in addition to neocortical networks.[40] The standard model assumes that newly consolidated information becomes independent of the hippocampus after sometime, whereas the multiple-trace model[41] assumes that hippocampal regions remain engaged during retrieval for the duration of that person's life. Winocur and colleagues[42] formulated a compromise by suggesting that less integrated, schematic versions of original EAMs become independent of the hippocampus, whereas those with contextual details remain dependent on the hippocampus.

A special variant of MTL amnesia is developmental amnesia, which is thought to be caused by selective damage to hippocampi due to neuronal loss (usually leading to at least a 30–40% reduction in bilateral volume of hippocampi compared with controls). It might follow episodes of ischemic hypoxia, occurring perinatally or in childhood. Children with developmental amnesia can acquire and retrieve facts, but their acquisition and retrieval of EAMs is greatly impaired. These findings emphasize that HF is a key structure in the formation of lasting EAMS.

Studies of young adults with developmental amnesia have explored the ability of these patients to imagine the future[43,44] and differences between recognition/familiarity versus recall/recollection.[45,47] With respect to imagination of future episodes, only one[43] of the two studies[43,44] identified deficits, despite similar hippocampal volume reductions (50%). This finding warrants the need for additional investigations into the contribution of residual hippocampal tissue in the imagination of future events compared with the contribution of other structures. Besides hippocampal abnormalities, older studies of developmental amnesia described some changes to the putamen, thalamus, and right retrosplenial cortex.[45] With respect to recognition/familiarity versus recall, a disproportionally high impairment in free recall was consistently reported,[46,47] which is a result not always[48] described in hippocampal damage of adult onset. Patients with developmental amnesia seem therefore to have deficit patterns that partly overlap with those of patients who acquired their hippocampal abnormalities in adulthood, suggesting that hippocampal damage might lead to specific variations in phenotype, dependent on the onset of the damage.

The prototype of diencephalic amnesia is Wernicke-Korsakoffs syndrome, which is characterized by both anterograde and retrograde impairments of EAM, and occasionally by impairments of semantic memory, and confabulations.[49,50] The syndrome typically occurs in individuals with chronic alcohol misuse and concurrent thiamine deficiency, or with other disorders associated with thiamine deficiency,[49] Because patients with chronic alcoholism might also display EAM impairments and deficits in working memory, metamemory, and executive functions,[51] there might be a continuum between symptoms of alcoholism and Korsakoffs syndrome.[51] Brain abnormalities in patients with Korsakoffs syndrome might seem to be more widespread (including the middle cingulate gyrus) when measured by changes in brain glucose metabolism[51] than when assessed by postmortem analyses. Postmortem findings mainly point to the degeneration of midline diencephalic structures, but do not confirm whether, in addition to the usually affected mammillary bodies, degeneration occurs in the mediodorsal thalamic nucleus (or just its medial, magnocellular portion) or the parataenial nuclei situated medially to the mediodorsal nucleus.

Studies of patients with more selective bilateral mediodorsal or anterior thalamic nuclear damage have pointed to the association of these parataenial nuclei with memory.[52] Furthermore, several reports have provided evidence that bilateral damage to the mammillary bodies or the mammillothalamic tract (or even to the tegmental nuclei of Gudden with bidirectional connections with the mammillary nuclei) is sufficient to cause amnesia.[53] Earlier predictions linking different aspects of memory processing (familiarity versus recollection) to the anterior or mediodorsal thalamus were not confirmed.[52] However, investigators have now proposed that mammillothalamic or anterior nuclei damage probably leads to deficits in recollection, whereas damage to the ventral amygdalofugal pathway or mediodorsal nucleus affects familiarity processing.[54] Thalamic damage is most common after stroke. Four arterial branches vascularize different thalamic regions and can be affected either in combination or individually, leading to distinct symptoms.[55]

The basal forebrain is composed of three major nuclear complexes made up of neurons containing acetylcholine (and y-aminobutyric acid): basal nucleus of Meynert, diagonal band of Broca, and septal nuclei. These nuclei proiect to the HF and other cortical areas. The (medial) septal region is connected to the amygdaloid complex. The amygdaloid complex enhances the emotional relevance of information while the septal nuclei are thought to exert an opposite, dampening effect. Basal forebrain amnesia can occur after rupture and surgery of aneurysms of the anterior communicating artery and tumors. Clinical differences between basal forebrain amnesia and MTL or diencephalic amnesia mainly arise because of the location of the basal forebrain nuclei in the penumbra of the ventral prefrontal cortex. In basal forebrain amnesia, executive dysfunctions are common, and recall-requiring active effort-is more impaired than recognition of information.[56] If the damage extends to upper portions of the frontal lobes, source amnesia (failure to remember where information came from) might occur.[57] Damage to basal forebrain associated with aneurysms of anterior communicating arteries can lead to enhanced vulnerability to provoked confabulations and false recognition in procedural memory (Table 1).[58]

WHITE-MATTER DAMAGE AND AMNESIA AS A DISCONNECTION SYNDROME

The occurrence of amnesia after fiber tract damage was first reported some time ago.[1] Several fiber bundles are of special interest in memory processing because they interconnect relevant bottle neck structures.[9,59,60] The fornix connects all three major regions that are important for memory consolidation and transfer into long-term memory (MTL, diencephalon, and basal forebrain). In a study of 38 patients who had undergone colloid cyst removal, significant negative correlations were reported between fornix volume and recall in standardized memory tests.[61] Fibers passing through the internal and external capsules (especially thalamocortical connections) and temporal stem (especially the uncinate fascicle connecting prefrontal, amygdala, and temporal areas) provide important links that complete the network of limbic and paralimbic regions (prefrontal and temporal lobes, and diencephalon), and their damage can lead to memory deficits.[62]

Mesulam[63] and others reported the existence of large scale networks for mnemonic processing. Functional neuroimaging enabled the characterization of large-scale brain systems, such as the default mode network, which has functions in prospection and EAM.[64] Abnormal default mode network activity was reported in amnestic mild cognitive impairment and early Alzheimer's disease.[64]

White matter ensures proper flow of information in brain networks. Structural imaging techniques, such as diffusion tensor imaging and magnetization transfer ratio measurement, improved the ability to estimate the integrity of white matter in memory-impairing disorders. Investigators using magnetization transfer imaging in a patient with functional amnesia recorded subtle changes in white matter in the right prefrontal area.[65] White-matter damage occurs in several illnesses, such as multiple sclerosis (in which memory difficulties are common). Sepulcre and colleagues[66] identified damage to many fiber tracts, especially those running through the temporal stern and internal capsule, in a large sample of patients with multiple sclerosis. White-matter damage is common in patients who have had a stroke. Stroke is the only cause of amnesia that can affect all memory-processing structures of the limbic system.[67]

Traumatic brain injuries resulting in diffuse (multifocal) axonal injury might also lead to disturbances in anterograde and retrograde memory.[6] One topic of continuing interest is the relation between traumatic brain injury, in particular (concussive) mild head injury, and psychogenic or functional amnesia.[11,65] To what extent the rupture of fine connections between synapses and dendrites might cause widespread cerebral dysfunction is unresolved, and whether the traumatic experience itself can lead to a psychological shock disorder, which then might result in severe and persistent amnesia and other cognitive disturbances, is also unknown.[13] Incidentally, brain concussions at various locations along the skull can lead to amnesia that is mainly retrograde.[6]

AMNESIAS WITH MIXED PSYCHOLOGICAL AND PHYSIOLOGICAL CAUSES

Transient global amnesia happens suddenly, usually in adults older than 60 years, and is triggered by physiological or psychological factors.[68] Its course is benign because it (typically) disappears within a day. Slight memory deficits might, however, persist for months, especially if patients continue to have anxiety or depression.[69] Transient global amnesia affects mostly anterograde memories, but can partly affect retrograde memories as well.[70] The cause of transient global amnesia is still elusive, although hypotheses have suggested that small thrombi in deep cerebral veins[71] or internal jugular vein valve incompetence[72] might be to blame. Bartsch and Deuschl[70] emphasized that the vulnerability of the cornu ammonis (CA1) neurons of the hippocampus to metabolic stress is pivotal in the pathophysiological cascade underlying transient global amnesia. The transient global amnesia recurrence rate is substantial (6–10% per year).[70]

Differential diagnoses of transient global amnesia include the recurrent shorter-lasting episodes of transient epileptic amnesia, which can occur on awakening in individuals of middle and old age (mean age of 57 years). Patients with transient epileptic amnesia often complain of persistent inter episodic memory deficits. Although objective measures on standard tests of anterograde memory can be normal, accelerated long-term forgetting for days to weeks and deficits of remote EAM were docummented.[73]

Functional, psychogenic, or dissociative amnesias might be associated with psychological factors co-occurring with a (minor) physical injury. They are generally diagnosed in people aged 20–40 years and characterized by retrograde EAM impairments. Occasionally, anterograde amnesia in the absence of retrograde EAM impairment might take place.[13]

The mechanism of dissociation underlies dissociative amnesia,[19] which is linked to psychological stress in various cultures.[13] Psychogenic amnesia consists of disorders with various psychological mechanisms.[13] Not all functional amnesias are diagnosed with a definite background of psychological factors.[13]

EPIDEMIOLOGY AND GENETICS

Epidemiological data are available for only specific amnesic disorders. The incidence of transient global amnesia is 3–8 per 100000 people per year.[70] Head trauma is the most probable cause of amnesic disorders that are due to a general medical disorder. Although decreases in the incidence of thiamine-related disorders were reported in several countries after fortification of bread with thiamine, an increase in the incidence of Korsakoffs syndrome was described in some European countries.[49] For dissociative amnesia, a 12 month prevalence of 1–8% was reported in a US community of 658 adults,[74] the genetic underpinnings of human amnesia are still unknown. Studies of the genetics of Korsakoff's syndrome and transient global amnesia yielded no conclusive results.[49,75] Although EAM impairments could be regarded as an intermediate phenotype[76] in amnesic disorders, which might be proximal to their underlying genetic risk, data about how genetics affect EAM are inconclusive, several researchers state that about 50% of the interindividual variability in memory ability is attributable to genetic factors;[76] this assertion is, however based on results of behavioral genetic twin studies[77] that did not use EAM testing paradigms in accordance with the present definition of EAM.[3]

Work in animals prompted several hypothesis-driven behavioral and imaging genetic studies that investigated the association between memory performance in different populations and variants of several candidate genes.[76-78] Several researchers have done genome-wide association studies to try to find associations between variations of different genes and episodic memory performance.[76,79,80] However, apart from one minor exception,[81] most studies that reported to have investigated an association between one of the described gene variants and episodic memory did not use EAM testing paradigms that were congruent with EAM's definition. [76,79,80,82]

Because EAM is a complex neurocognitive system, it is probably affected by genes, environment, and their interplay. Technological improvements and the use of methodological rigor with respect to EAM testing paradigms might help us to better understand EAM's genetic foundation.

ASSESSMENT OF AMNESIA DISORDERS

Assessment of amnesic disorders includes anamnesis and medical, laboratory, and occupational-therapy evaluations. Neuropsychological testing is invaluable to objectively establish the nature and severity of the memory impairment, to quantify longitudinal changes, and to distinguish between amnesias of different causes and feigned amnesia. Cognitive disturbances due to infarct or closed head injury can change over time. Furthermore, studies sometimes report discrepancies between subjective complaints and objective measurement[21] or suggest exaggeration or reduced effort.[56]

Various approaches attempt to differentiate feigned from true amnesia. Many are based on testing with concealed levels of difficulty and use effort measures, recognition (forced-choice paradigms), or calculation abilities.[83-85] The idea is to provide the potential feigner with a substantial amount of simple information and to convey the impression of a difficult memory task, when in reality it is not difficult (healthy people perform at the upper limit).[84] Results from psychological experiments show that we are easily able to recognize an enormous number of pictures and are typically much better at item recognition than at item (free) recall. Furthermore, we perform during free recall in a typical pattern-namely, in a learning curve with a primacy and a recency effect. However, feigners might show atypical or inconsistent performance on systematic testing. Structured inventories can aid with detection of malingering in forensic or litigation cases.[84] Functional neuroimaging can be used to investigate neural correlates of false memories and feigning.[86] Results are still divergent, and designs that are more ecologically valid are being tested.[87]

In amnesic disorders, the acquisition of a multi-dimensional profile is advisable. Usually, left-hemispheric damage mainly leads to verbal memory impairments, whereas right-hemispheric damage affects nonverbal memory deficits. Short-term memory is only rarely affected.

The patient's intelligence should always be measured or at least estimated. Because low levels of attention and concentration can impair the acquisition of new information, their measurement is essential. Differentiation between memory measures of free recall (active information generation), cued recall, and recognition is important. Patients, especially those with frontal lobe damage, might show a discrepancy between recognition and free recall.[56]

PROGNOSIS AND TREATMENT OF AMNESIC DISORDERS

A few amnesic disorders (such as transient global amnesia) have good prognosis, others partly improve, and for some disorders-especially those with complete bilateral damage to MTL, diencephalon, or basal forebrain-prognosis remains poor. Traditionally, most cases of dissociative amnesia were reported to resolve spontaneously; however, reports have since suggested that chronic forms exist.[10,13]

Parental thiamine given routinely to patients at risk decreases their likelihood of developing Wernicke-Korsakoff syndrome.[49] Memory impairments related to electroconvulsive therapy might be reduced by unilateral electrode placement, titration of the electrical current according to the patient's seizure threshold,[21,22] and ultra brief pulses.[88]

Pharmacological treatment data for amnesic disorders are scarce and come from studies with small numbers of cases that often do not have a placebo-control group. An open-label, nonrandomized study of 11 patients with basal forebrain amnesia after aneurysm rupture noted verbal memory improvements after a 12 week trial of 5–10 mg donepezil per day.[89]

A few placebo-controlled studies suggested that cholinesterase inhibitors could be used to address chronic post-traumatic memory impairments in patients with traumatic brain injury.[90,91] No controlled studies addressed the psychopharmacological (or psychotherapeutic) treatment of dissociative amnesia.[12] Studies have looked at novel drugs (histone deacetylase inhibitors)[17] and somatic (brain stimulation) interventions that might aid memory improvement.[92]

Thus, no evidence-based psychopharmacological or somatic treatments are known to be definitively effective at reversing memory impairments or deficits in amnesic disorders. The increase in group studies and rapid advances in the biological understanding of memory give hope to the development of effective psychopharmacological and somatic interventions for amnesic disorders.

Ideally, rehabilitation should address cognitive, emotional, and psychosocial functioning and prospective memory.[93] Generally it consists of training strategies aiming to establish previous levels of functioning and compensatory strategies. Implicit training strategies with procedural and priming tasks have been successfully used for patients with severe forms of amnesia.[94] Emphasis is laid on errorless learning procedures[95] and semantic strategies.[96] Success with implicit and errorless learning is not that common and cannot be generalized.

Supportive psychotherapy can enhance rehabilitation outcomes for patients with preserved insight. Besides computer-aided training,[97] virtual-reality environments are used for memory training,[98] and even noninvasive cortical stimulation has been applied.[99] Reliance on external memory aids and support from modem computer-based equipment is increasing.

Evidence-based data for memory rehabilitation are scarce.[100] Cicerone and colleagues[100] reviewed class la studies that provided evidence that visual imagery is better than standard memory training; the same was true for self-instructed training, at least for patients with mild memory impairment. The use of portable pagers was also effective.

However, a detailed review on cognition-based interventions in older people, including memory training and transfer of training effects, stated that "immediate and delayed verbal recall improved significantly through training compared to a no-treatment control condition, but the improvements did not exceed the improvement in the active control condition".[101]

FUTURE DIRECTIONS

Amnesia in the strict sense, i.e. a total and exclusive loss of the ability to store new information consciously and long-term, or to retrieve long-term stored information consciously—is rarely found. In fact, proposals were made by the DSM-5 neurocognitive disorders work group to replace the DSM-IV-TR category of delirium, dementia, amnestic and other geriatric cognitive disorders with a new category called neurocognitive disorders. Longitudinal studies of (dissociative) amnesia might be needed to quantify possible cognitive deteriorations over time.[102] The identification of neural correlates of various amnesias and predictors for effective rehabilitation might benefit from combined use of functional and structural imaging. An understanding of the (epi) genetics of memory processes might help with the design of novel treatments for amnesias in the future.

Panel 1: Variants of Amnesia and Forms of Associated Diseases or Behavioral Disorders

Global Amnesia

An outdated diagnosis that implies total memory loss (it is outdated because in most amnesiacs implicit processing via the procedural and priming systems is usually preserved).

Anterograde Amnesia

Inability to acquire, store, or retrieve new information long-term and consciously after a memory-impairing incident.

Retrograde Amnesia

Inability to consciously re-activate information that was stored long ago.

Partial Amnesia (Lacunar Amnesia)

Memory loss restricted to particular kinds of information or life epochs.

Material-specific Amnesia

Naming impairment with respect to objects or materials.

Autobiographical Amnesia

Inability to recall events (and to a minor degree personal knowledge) from own life.

Semantic Amnesia

Inability to reactivate general facts, or (less often) linguistic expressions (as in semantic dementia).

Topographical Amnesia

Disturbance of memory for locations and space.

Reduplicative Paramnesia

Disturbed sense of familiarity; the patient is convinced that a person, place, or object exists twice (repeatedly) usually caused by organic brain damage (i.e. neurologically based).

Capgras (Delusion) Syndrome

Disturbed sense of familiarity; the patient assumes that a close friend or relative has been replaced by an impostor, or double; usually no hallucinatory symptoms, but subsumed under psychiatric diseases.

Infantile/Childhood Amnesia

Inability to consciously retrieve events from the first 3–4 years of life (probably caused by insufficiently developed brain, self, and language and by the existence of state-dependent memory retrieval).

Developmental Amnesia

Episodic-autobiographical amnesia with presented semantic memory after hypoxic-ischemic events sustained usually within the hrst year of life.

Korsakoff's Syndrome/Amnesia

A symptom agglomerate with severe anterograde amnesia, variable retrograde amnesia, confabulations, and a disorientation with respect to time and place; intelligence and short-term memory are frequently presented; usually caused by severe and long-term alcohol misuse, but mainly a disorder of malnutrition with a distinct pattern of mainly medial diencephalic brain degeneration.

Pseudodementia

Amnesia-like symptoms might be apparent, but the primary cause of the disorder is based on a depressive illness.

Mnestic Block Syndrome

Memory block, caused by psychological factors such as severe stress or psychological trauma.

Dissociative Amnesia

Psychiatric disorder characterized by an inability to recall personal information that is underlain by the psychological mechanism of dissociation.

Dissociative Fugue

Form of dissociative amnesia that is characterized by the patient leaving their place of living (their home).

Dissociative Identity Disorder (Multiple Personality Disorder)

Existence of two or more personalities or personality states; amnesia for everyday events is a common feature and personalities are usually amnesic towards each other.

Ganser Syndrome

Dissociative disorder solely detined when a patient gives approximate answers to questions; its original description also included hysterical semitrance, amnesia, and hallucinations.

Psychogenic Amnesia

Broad term that refers to amnesic disorders that are linked to psychological factors; it makes no a-priori assumption about the nature of the associated psychological mechanisms.

Functional Amnesia

Amnesia usually without evidence of brain damage on conventional structural imaging, and of an unsure cause.

Posthypnotic Amnesia

Inability to recall events that occurred during hypnosis.

Transient Global Amnesia

Massive anterograde and partial retrograde amnesia, usually of elderly people (>60 years), lasting less than 24 hours; it is thought to be benign and is usually triggered by physical or psychological stress factors.

Transient Epileptic Amnesia

Recurrent, transient episodes of isolated memory loss usually lasting less than 1 hour; a subtype of temporal lobe epilepsy.

Amnestic Mild Cognitive Impairment

Subtype of mild cognitive impairment characterized by a decline in memory beyond age-correlated benign forgetfulness and with a higher likelihood of progression to Alzheimer's disease than other forms of mild cognitive impairment.

Post-traumatic Amnesia

Term used in publications about traumatic brain injury; sometimes it describes the phase after the resolution of delirium that is characterized mainly by memory impairments;

sometimes the term overlaps with delirium, encompassing a period from injury until recovery of full consciousness and memory.

Feigned Amnesia

Feigned memory impairments or intentional exaggeration of existing memory impairments, possibly motivated by external incentives (in the case of malingering) or the intrapsychic need to assume the sick role (such as in factitious disorder).

Panel 2: Medical, Substance-related, Psychiatric, and Iatrogenic Causes of Amnesic Disorders

Medical

- Head injury (closed or penetrating)
- Stroke (ischemic or hemorrhagic)
- Aneurysmal bleeding (subarachnoid hemorrhage) or aneurysm surgery
- Medial temporal lobe epilepsy
- Intracranial tumor
- Limbic encephalitis due to infections (herpes simplex virus 1 and 2, herpes zoster virus, and human herpes virus 6 in transplant recipients), of paraneoplastic origin, or associated with autoimmune diseases (e.g. systemic lupus erythematous, voltage-gated potassium channel antibody-associated encephalitis, or encephalitis associated with antibodies against N-methyl-D-aspartate receptor)
- Neurosyphilis
- Vitamin deficiencies (vitamin B_1 deficiency)
- Transient global amnesia
- Transient epileptic amnesia.

Substance-related

- Chronic alcohol misuse/vitamin B_1 defciency (Korsakoff's syndrome)
- Drug misuse; anxiolytics (benzodiazepines), sedative-hypnotics (barbiturates, zolpidem)
- Anticholinergics.

Psychiatric

- Dissociative amnesia
- Dissociative fugue
- Dissociative identity disorder (multiple personality disorder)
- Dissociative trance disorder.

Latrogenic

- Drug side-effects, e.g. of anticholinergic drugs including antidepressants (tricyclic and tetracyclic antidepressants), antipsychotics, or antiparkinsonian agents with anticholinergic properties (e.g. benztropine), and anesthetics
- Surgical procedures on brain
- Electroconvulsive therapy.

Panel 3: Brain Regions whose (Bilateral) Damage is Followed by Characteristic Memory Disturbances

Medial Temporal Lobe (Especially Hippocampal Formation and Surrounding Structures)

Encoding and consolidation of EAM and semantic memory into the long-term store; spatiotemporal integration.

Amygdaloid Complex

Assessment of biological and social significance; emotional tagging of memories, especially of episodic-autobiographical memory.

Prefrontal Cortex

Short-term memory (dorsolateral prefrontal cortex); encoding and recall of episodic and semantic information (especially effortful recall).

Orbitofrontal Cortex; Basal Forebrain

Encoding and emotional connections to information; control and suppression of confabulatory tendencies.

Limbicthalamic Nuclei; Fornix; Mammillary Bodies

Binding and association processes for transfer into long-term storage; consciousness.

Pulvinar

Processing, especially of language-related information, attention, and somatic memory.

Cingulate Gyrus

Processing of components of memory related to attention and wilful acts.

Retrosplenial Cortex; Precuneus

Imagination; representation of memories; familiarity.

Lateral Parietal Cortex (Especially Left)

Short-term memory; mediation of mnemonic processing by attention.

Basal Ganglia

Procedural memory processing.

REFERENCES

1. Markowitsch HI. Intellectual functions and the brain: an historical perspective. Toronto: Hogrefe & Huber Publishers, 1992.
2. Tulving E. Episodic memory from mind to brain, Annu Rev Psychol. 2002;53:1-25.
3. Tulving E. Episodic memory and autonoesis: uniquely human? In: Terrace H, Metcalfe J (Eds). The missing link in Cognition; origins of self reflective consciousness, New York: Oxford University Press; 2005. pp.3-56.
4. Markowitsch HJ. Anterograde memory. In: Goldenberg G, Miller BL (Eds). Handbook of clinical neurology, neuropsychology and behavioral neurology. Amsterdam: Elsevier. 2008;88: 155-83.
5. Ribot T. Diseases of memory. New York: D Appleton & Company, 1882.
6. Kopelman MD. Retrograde memory loss, In: Goldenberg G, Miller BL (Eds). Handbook of clinical neurology, neuropsychological and behavioral neurology Amsterdam: Elsevier. 2008;88:185-202.
7. Eustache F, Desgranges B, MNESIS: Towards the integration of current multisystem models of memory Neuropsyghal Rev. 2008;18:53-69.
8. Kanwisher N. Functional specificity in the human brain: A window into the functional architecture of the mind. Proc Natl Acad Sci USA. 2010;107:11163-70.
9. Brand M, Markowitsch HJ. The principle 0f bottleneck structures. In: Kluwe RH, Luer G, Rosler F (Eds). Principles of learning and memory. Basel: Birkhauser; 2003.pp.171-84.
10. Brand M, Eggers C, Reinhold N, et al. Functional brain imaging in 14 patients with dissociative amnesia reveals right inferolateral prefrontal hypometabolism. Psychiatry Res. 2009;174;32-9.
11. Markowitsch HJ. Functional retrograde amnesia-mnestic block syndrome. Cortex. 2002;38:651-54.
12. Markowitsch HJ, Kessler 1, Weber-Luxenburger G, Van der Ven C, Heiss WD. Neuroimaging and behavioral correlates of recovery from 'mnestic block syndrome' and other cognitive deteriorations. Neuropsychiatry Neuropsychol Behav Neurol. 2000;13:60-66.
13. Staniloiu A, Markowitsch HJ. Searching for the anatomy of dissociative amnesia. J Psychol. 2010:218;96-108.
14. Gold PE. Protein synthesis inhibition and memory: Formation vs amnesia, Neurobiol Learn Mem. 2008;89:201-41.
15. Hurlemann R. Noradrenergic-glucocorticoid mechanisms in emotion-induced amnesia; from adaptation to disease. Psychopharmacology. 2008;197:13-23.
16. Kandel ER. The biology of memory: 3 forty-year perspective. J Neurosci. 2009;29:12748-56.
17. Zhang T-Y, Meaney My. Epigenetics and me environmental regulation of the genome and ns function. Annu Rev Psychol. 2010;61:419-66.
18. WHO: The ICD-10 Classification Of mental and behavioral disorders: clinical descriptions and diagnostic guidelines. Geneva; WHO, 1992.
19. American Psychiatric Association: Diagnostic and statistical manual of mental disorders, 4th edition, text revision (DSM-IV-TR). Washington, DC: American Psychiatric Publishing, 2000.
20. Brunei A, Orr SP, Tremblay J, et al. Effect of post-retrieval propranolol on psychophysiologic responding during subsequent script-driven traumatic imagery in post-traumatic stress; disorder. j Psychiatr Res. 2008;42:503-06.
21. Fraser LM, O'Caroll RE, Ebmeier KP. The effect of electroconvulsive therapy on autobiographic memory: a systematic review. J ECT. 2008;24:10-17.
22. Sackeim HA, Prudic J, Fuller R, et al. The cognitive effects of electroconvulsive therapy in community settings. Neuropsychopharmacology. 2007;32:244-54.
23. Papanicolaou AC, Hasan KM, Boake C, EluvathingalTJ, Kramer L. Disruption of limbic pathways in a case of profound amnesia. Neurocase. 2007;13:226-28.
24. Markowitsch HJ, Staniloiu A. Amygdala in action; relaying biological and social Significance so autobiographical memory Neuropsychologia. 2011;49:718-33.
25. Buchanan TW mnel D, Adolphs R. Emotional autobiographical memories in amnesic patients with medial temporal lobe damage. J Neurosci. 2005;25:3151-60.
26. Somerville LH, Wig GS, Whalen PJ, Kelley WM. Dissociable medial temporal lobe contributions to social memory. J cogn Neurosci. 2008;18:1253-65.
27. Rutishauser U, Schuman EM, Mamelak AN. Activity of human hippocampal and amygdala neurons during retrieval of declarative memories, Proc Natl Acad Sci USA. 2008;105: 329-34.
28. Hurlemann R, Wagner M, Hawellek B, et al. Amygdala control of emotion-induced forgetting and remembering: evidence from Urbach-Waethe disease. Neuropsychalogia. 2007;45:877-84.
29. Scoville WB, Milner B. Loss of recent memory after bilateral hippocampal lesions. J New Neurosurg Psychiatry. 1957;20: 11-21.
30. Bird CM, Shallice T, Cipolotti L. Fractionation of memory in medial temporal lobe amnesia. Neuropsychologia. 2007;45:1160-71.
31. Schon K, Quiroz YT, Hasselmo ME, Stem CE. Greater working memory load results in greater medial temporal activity at retrieval. Cereb Cortex. 2009;19:2561-71.
32. Greenberg DL, Keane MM, Ryan L, Vefaellie M. Impaired category fluency in medial temporal lobe amnesia; the role of episodic memory. J Neurosci. 2009;29:10900-08.
33. Knoops AJG, van der Graaf Y, Appelman APA, et al. visual rating of the hippocampus in non-demented elders: does it measure hippocampal atrophy or other indices of brain atrophy? The SMART-MR study. Hippocampus. 2009;19:1115-22.

34. Hassabis D, Kumaran D, Vann SD, Maguire EA. Patients with hippocampal amnesia cannot imagine new experiences. Proc Natl Acad Sci USA. 2007;104:1726-31.
35. Steinvorth S, Levine B, Corkin S. Medial temporal lobe structures are needed to re-experience remote autobiographical memories evidence from H.M. and w.R. Neuropsychologia. 2008;45:479-96.
36. Squire LR, van der Horst AS, McDuff SGR, et al. Roll of the hippocampus in remembering the past and imagining the future. Proc Natl Acad Sci USA. 2010;107:19044-48.
37. Gilboa A, Winocur G, Rosenbaum RS, et al. Hippocampal contributions to recollection in retrograde and anterograde amnesia. Hippocampus. 2008;16:966-80.
38. Shimamura AP. Hierarchical relational binding in the medial temporal lobe: the strong get stronger Hippocampus. 2010;20:1206-16.
39. Markowitsch HJ, Psychogenic amnesia. Neuroimage. 2003;20 (Suppl 1):S132-38.
40. Squire LR, Bayley PJ. The neuroscience of remote memory, Curr Opin Neurobiol. 2007;17:185-96.
41. Moscovitch M, Nadel L, Winocur G, Gilboa A, Rosenbaum RS. The cognitive neuroscience of remote episodic, semantic and spatial memory. Curr Opin Neurobiol. 2006;16:179-90.
42. Winocur G, Moscovitch M, Bontempi B. Memory formation and long-term retention in humans and animals: convergence towards a transformation account of hippocampal-neocortical interactions. Neuropsychologia. 2010;48:2329-56.
43. Kwan D, Carson N, Addis DR, Rosenbaum RS. Deficits in past remembering extend to future imagining in a case of developmental amnesia. Neuropsychologia. 2010;48: 3179-86.
44. Maguire EA, Vargha-Khadem F, Haassabis D. Imaging fictitious and future experiences: evidence from developmental amnesia. Neuropsychologia. 2010;48:3187-92.
45. Vargha-Khaden F, Salmond CH, Watkins KE, et al. Developmental amnesia: effect of age at injury. Proc Natl Acad Sci USA. 2001;100:10055-60.
46. Brandt KR, Gardiner JM, Vargha-Khadem F, Baddeley AD, Mishkin M. Impairment of recollection but not familiarity in a case of developmental amnesia. Neurocase. 2008;15:60-65.
47. Adlam A-LR, Malloy M, Mishkin M, Vargha-Khadem F. Dissociation between recognition and recall in developmental amnesia; Nauropsychologia. 2009;47:2207-10.
48. Jeneson A, Kirwan BC, Hopkins RO, Wixted JT, Squire LR. Recognition memory and the hippocampus: a test of the hippocampal Contribution to recollection and familiarity. Learn Mem. 2010;17:63-70.
49. Zahr NM, Kaufman KL, Harper co. Clinical and pathological features of alcohol-related brain damage. Nat Rev Neurol. 2011;7:284-94.
50. Borsutzky S, Fujiwara E, Brand M, Markowitsch HJ. Confabulations in alcoholic Korsakoff patients. Neuropsychologia. 2008;46:3133-43.
51. Pitel AL, Beaunieux H, Witkowski T, et al. Episodic and working memory deficits in alcoholic Korsakoff patients: the continuity theory revisited. Alcohol Clin Exp Res. 2008;32:1229-41.
52. Cipolotti L, Husain M, Crinion J, et al. The role of the thalamus in amnesia; a tractography, high-resolution MRI and neuropsychological study Neuropsychologia. 2008;46:2745-58.
53. Vann SD. Re-evaluating the role of the mammillary bodies in memory. Neuropsychologia. 2010;48:2316-27.
54. Carlesimo GA, Lombardi MG, Caltagirone C. Vascular thalamic amnesia: a reappraisal. Neuropsychologia. 2011;49:777-89.
55. Perren F, Clarke S, Bogousslavsky J. The syndrome of combined polar and paramedian thalamic infarction. Arch Neurol. 2005;62:1212-16.
56. Jetter J, Poser U, Freeman RB Jr, Markowitsch HJ. A verbal long term memory deficit in frontal lobe damaged patients. Cortex. 1986;22:229-42.
57. Lakhan SE. Neuropsychological generation of source amnesia; an episodic memory disorder of the frontal brain. J Med Biol Sci. 2006;1:1-13.
58. Borsutzky S, Fujiwara E, Brand M, Markowitsch HI. Susceptibility to false memories in patients with ACOA aneurysm. Neuropsychologia. 2010;48:2811-23.
59. Kier EL, Staib LH, Davis LM, Bronen RA. MR Imaging of the temporal stem: anatomic dissection tractography of the uncinate fasciculus, inferior occipitofrontal fasciculus, and Meyer's loop of the optic radiation. AJNR Am J Neuroradial. 2004;25:677-91.
60. Schmahmann JD, Smith EE, Eichler FS, Filley CM. Cerebral white matter: neuroanatomy, clinical neurology, and neurobehavioral correlates. Ann NY Acad Sci. 2008;1142:266-309.
61. Tsivilis D, Vann SD, Denby C, et al. A disproportionate role for the fornix and mammillary bodies in recall-versus recognition memory. Nat Neurosci. 2008;11:834-42.
62. Gerber DJ, Weintraub AH, Cusick CP, Ricci PE, Whiteneck GG. Magnetic resonance imaging of traumatic brain injury: relationship of T2 SE and T2'GE to clinical severity and outcome. Brain lnj. 2004;18:1083-97.
63. Mesulam MM. Behavioral neuroanatomy: large-scale networks, association cortex, frontal syndromes, the limbic system, and hemispheric specialization. In: Mesulam MM (Ed). Principals of behavioral neurology. New York: Oxford. University Press; 2000.pp.1-120.
64. Buckner RL, Andrews-Hanna JR, Schacter DL. The brain's default network: anatomy, function, and relevance to disease. Ann NY Acad Sci. 2008;1124:1-38.
65. Tramoni E, Albert-Khalfa S, Guye M, et al. Hypo-retrieval and hyper-suppression mechanisms in functional amnesia. Neuropsychologia. 2009;47:611-24.
66. Sepulcre J, Masdeu JC, Sastre-Garriga J, et al. Mapping the brain pathways of declarative verbal memory: evidence from white matter lesions in the living human brain. Neuroimage 2008;42:1237-43.
67. Lim C, Alexander MP. Stroke and episodic memory disorders. Neuropsychologia. 2009;47:3045-58.

68. Markowitsch HJ (Ed). Transient global amnesia and related disorders. Toronto: Hogrefe & Huber Publishers; 1990.
69. Noel A, Quinette P, Dayan J, et al. Influence of patients' emotional state on the recovery processes after a transient global amnesia. Cortex. 2011;47:981-91.
70. Bartsch T, Deuschl G. Transient global amnesia: functional anatomy and clinical implications. Lancet Neurol. 2010;9:205-14.
71. Solheim O, Skeidsvoll T. Transient global amnesia may be caused by cerebral vein thrombosis. Med Hypotheses. 2005;65:1142-19.
72. Cejas C, Fernandez Cisneros L, Lagos R, Zuk C, Ameriso SF. Internal jugular vein valve incompetence is highly prevalent in transient global amnesia; Stroke. 2010;41:67-71.
73. Butler CR, Graham KS, Hodges JR, et al. The syndrome of transient epileptic amnesia. Ann Neurol. 2007;61:587-98.
74. Johnson JG, Cohen P, Kasen S, Brook JS. Dissociative disorders among adults in the community, impaired functioning, and axis I and II comorbidity. J Psychiatr Res. 2006;40:131-10.
75. Segers-van Rijn J, de Bruijn SF. Transient global amnesia; a genetic disorder? Eur Neurol. 2010;63:186-82.
76. Rascla B, Papassotiropoulos A, de Quervain DF. Imaging genetics of cognitive functions: focus on episodic memory, Neuroimoge. 2010;53:870-77.
77. McClearn GE, Johansson B, Berg S, et al. Substantial genetic influence on cognitive abilities in twins so or more years old. Science. 1997;276:1560-63.
78. Papassotiropoulos A, Stefanova E, Vogler C, et al. A genome-wide survey and functional brain imaging study identify CTNNBL1 as a memory-related gene. Mol Psychiatry 2011; published online Nov 22. DOI:10.1038/mp.2011.148.
79. Papassotiropoulos A, Stephan DA, Huentelman MI, et al. Common Kibra alleles are associated with human memory performance. Science. 2006;314:475-78.
80. Preuschhof C, Heekeren HR, Li SC, et al. KIBRA and CLSTN2 polymorphisms exert interactive effects on human episodic memory. Neuropsychologia. 2010;48:402-08.
81. Lemogne C, Bergouignan L, Boni C, et al. Genetics and personality affect visual perspective in autobiographical memory. Conscious Cogn. 2009;18:823-30.
82. Wisdom NM, Callahan JL, Hawkins KA. The effects of apolipoprotein E on non-impaired cognitive functioning: a meta-analysis. Neurobiol Aging. 2011;32:63-74.
83. Taylor JA, Krentzer JG, West DD. Evaluation of malingering cut-off scores for the Rey 15-item test; a brain injury case study series. Brain lnj. 2003;17:295-308.
84. Greiffenstein MF, Greve KW, Bianchini KJ, Baker WJ. Test of memory malingering and word memory test: a new comparison of failure concordance rates. Arch Clin Neuropsychol. 2008;23:801-07.
85. Yochim BP, Kane KD, Horning S, Pepin R. Malingering or expected deficits? A case of herpes simplex encephalitis. Neurocase. 2010;16:451-60.
86. Abe N, Okuda J, Suzuki M, et al. Neural correlates of true memory, false memory, and deception. cereb Cortex. 2008;18:2811-19.
87. Mohamed FB, Faro SH, Gordon NJ, et al. Brain mapping of deception and truth telling about an ecologically valid situation: functional MR imaging and polygraph-initial experience. Radiology. 2006;238:679-88.
88. Sackeim HA, Prudic J, Nobler MS, et al. Effects of pulse width and electrode placement on the efficacy and cognitive effects of electroconvulsive therapy Brain; Slimul. 2008;1:71-83.
89. Benke T, Koylu B, Delazer M, Trinka E, Kemmler G. Cholinergic treatment of amnesia following basal forebrain lesion due to aneurysm rupture - an open-label pilot study. Eur J Neurol. 2005;12:791-96.
90. Writer BW, Schillerstrom JE. Psychopharmacological treatment for cognitive impairment in survivors of traumatic brain injury; a critical review. J Neuropsychiatr Clin Neurosci. 2009;21:302-70.
91. Silver JM, Koumaras B, Meng X, et al. Long-term effects of rivastigmine capsules in patients with traumatic brain injury Brain Injury. 2009;23:123-32.
92. Laxton AW Tang-Wai DF, McAndrews MP, et al. A phase I trial of deep brain stimulation of memory circuits in Alzheimer's disease, Ann Neurol. 2010;68:521-34.
93. Cheng H, Tian Y, Hu P, Wang J, Wang K. Time-based prospective memory impairment in patients with thalamic stroke. Behav Neurosci. 2010;124:152-58.
94. Dewar B-K, Patterson K, Wilson BA, Graham KS. Re-acquisition of person knowledge in semantic memory disorders, Neuropsychol Rehab. 2009;19:383-421.
95. Laffan AJ, Metzler-Baddeley C, Walker I, et al. Making errorless learning more active; self-generation in an error free learning context is superior to standard errorless learning of face-name associations in people with Alzheimer's disease. Neuropsychol Rehab. 2010;20:197-211.
96. Moses SN, Ostreicher ML, Rosenbaum RS, Ryan ID. Successful transverse patterning in amnesia using semantic knowledge. Hippocampus. 2008;18:121-24.
97. Gaggioli A, Meneghini A, Morganti F, Alcaniz M, Riva G. A strategy for computer-assisted mental practice in stroke rehabilitation. Neurorehabil Neural Repair. 2006;20: 503-07.
98. Crosbie JH, Lennon S, Basford JR, McDonough SM. Virtual reality in stroke rehabilitation: still more virtual than real. Disabil Rehabil. 2007;29:1139-46; discussion 1147-52.
99. Floel A, Cohen LG. Contribution of noninvasive cortical stimulation to the study of memory functions. Bruin Res Rev. 2007;53:250-9.
100. Cicerone KD, Dahlberg C, Malex JF, et al. Evidence-based cognitive rehabilitation: updated review of the literature from 1998 through 2002. Arch Phys Med Rehabil. 2005;86:1681-92.
101. Martin M, Clare L, Altgassen AM, et al. Cognition-based interventions for healthy older people and people with mild cognitive impairment. Cochrane Database Syst Rev. 2011;1:CD006220.
102. Yaffe K, Vittinghoff E, Lindquist K, et al. Post-traumatic stress disorder and risk of dementia among Us veterans, Arch Gen Psychiatr. 2010;67:608-13.

CHAPTER 65 Medically Unexplained Symptoms in the Patients Attending Medical Clinics

Neena Bohra, NK Bohra

Patients commonly present to doctors with symptoms, and the doctors seek disease to explain these symptoms. However, in about one-third of medical outpatients the symptoms remain inadequately explained by disease, even after exhaustive assessment. The size of the problem of medically unexplained symptoms, their cost to services, and public health importance are all becoming increasingly clear.

Medically unexplained symptoms may be described as due to somatization, or as somatoform or functional symptoms—common examples being pain, fatigue, and weakness. They may also be described in terms of a functional somatic syndrome diagnosis such as irritable bowel syndrome, fibromyalgia, or chronic fatigue syndrome.

Clinical approach—patients with medically unexplained symptoms may have substantial disability, distress, and a poor prognosis. Most doctors still regard such symptoms as purely mental in origin, but it has become increasingly obvious that such an approach is both scientifically inadequate and practically unhelpful. Patients regard a purely mental explanation as dismissive and stigmatizing, and physicians find it frustrating as it does not help them manage the patient. The evidence favors a more complex understanding of etiology in which genetic vulnerability, early experience, and life stress interact to produce symptoms that are associated with reversible changes in the nervous system and associated function. Developments in neuroscience combined with increasing consumerism amongst patients require that we take a more positive approach to this neglected area of medical research and practice.

Management—to be effective, this requires more than simply the exclusion of disease:[1] the patient needs their symptoms to be taken seriously;[2] it is important to seek other symptoms of depression and anxiety that are commonly associated;[3] a positive diagnosis needs to be made (often as a functional somatic syndrome with or without associated depression or anxiety) and appropriate explanation for the symptoms (in terms or reversible changes in bodily function) given to the patient;[4] a practical management plan is required, including education about the symptoms and a gradual return to normal activity. The so-called antidepressants drugs may be effective even if the patient is not depressed;[5] some patients may require referral for specialist treatment, there being most evidence of efficacy for cognitive behavioral therapy (CBT).

DEFINITION AND TERMINOLOGY

Various terms have been used to describe symptoms unexplained by identifiable disease. These include:

- *Medically unexplained:* A useful and simple operational term, but a negative one with the potential disadvantage of suggesting that psychophysiological explanations are not 'medical'.
- *Functional:* Originally meaning a disturbance of bodily function rather than of bodily structure, it is unfortunate that this term is now used pejoratively by some doctors to mean 'all in the mind', although it appears to be acceptable to patients who understand it in its original meaning.
- *Somatization:* A widely used term implying a psychological problem that has become expressed somatically. It should arguably be restricted to cases where the somatic symptoms are plausibly understood as an expression of emotional disorder.
- *Conversion:* Used specifically to refer to loss of function such as weakness of a limb. Embodies the (unproven) assumption (as for somatization) that the symptoms are due to a 'conversion' of psychological problems into somatic symptoms.
- *Somatoform:* A diagnostic category in the psychiatric classifications. Intended to be a theoretical but obviously linked to the idea of somatization and implying a mental disorder in physical form.

There is no entirely satisfactory term: the best term for scientific use is probably 'medically unexplained', or perhaps better 'unexplained by identifiable disease'. However, most textbooks and computer databases use the terms 'somatoform' and 'somatization', and patients prefer 'functional'.

SYMPTOMS

Almost any symptom can remain medically unexplained, even after exhaustive medical assessment. Common examples include pain (including back pain, chest pain, abdominal pain, and headache); fatigue and weakness; dizziness; 'fits' and funny turns.

SYNDROMES

Unexplained symptoms have been grouped into syndromes. Each medical specialty has at least one of these (Table 1): rheumatologists label prominent muscle pain and tenderness as fibromyalgia; gastroenterologists describe abdominal pain with altered bowel habit as irritable bowel syndrome; and infectious disease specialists refer to chronic fatigue and myalgia as postviral or chronic fatigue syndrome. It has been argued that these 'functional syndromes' are not really separate conditions but merely a reflection of the tendency of specialists to focus only on those symptoms that relate to their (organ based) specialty. The research literature offers support for this hypothesis by revealing substantial overlap between these syndromes in their constituent symptoms, proposed etiological factors, and response to treatment.

The Significance of Medically Unexplained Symptoms and Syndromes

Medically unexplained symptoms are a common and important, but remarkably neglected, medical problem. They account for a substantial proportion of the work of most doctors and are the reason for approximately a third of new medical outpatient consultations. Although sometimes dismissed as merely the 'worried well', these patients often suffer more disability and distress than patients whose symptoms are explained by disease. They are also expensive to the health care system because they attend multiple specialist services where they receive extensive but unproductive investigation and treatment. Doctors working in these services not surprisingly find them 'difficult to help'. The size and importance of this clinical problem makes it all the more curious so that few doctors take any special interest in it.

Table 1: Functional somatic syndrome by medical specialty

Specialty	Syndrome
Gastroenterology	Irritable bowel syndrome, nonulcer dyspepsia
Gynecology	Premenstrual syndrome, chronic pelvic pain
Rheumatology	Fibromyalgia
Cardiology	Atypical or noncardiac chest pain
Respiratory medicine	Hyperventilation syndrome
Infectious diseases	Chronic (postviral) fatigue syndrome
Neurology	Tension headache, non-epileptic attacks
Dentistry	Temporomandibular joint dysfunction, atypical facial pain
Ear, nose, and throat	Globus syndrome
Allergy	Multiple chemical sensitivity

Historical Perspective

Throughout the history patients have presented with somatic symptoms that their doctors could not explain in terms of objectively identifiable disease. Modern medical advances have improved the precision with which disease can be identified, but have not solved the problem. Many patients still present with symptoms that remain unexplained by disease even after state of the art investigation and they still present a challenge to doctors.

The explanations that have been proposed for medically unexplained symptoms have varied over time. The early ideas located their cause in a disturbance of a bodily organ, often the uterus. Attention then moved to the peripheral nervous system, later the central nervous system, and more recently the mind. These changing etiological theories have been reflected in the terms used to describe the symptoms: the organ theory gave rise to 'hysterical' (referring to the uterus) and 'hypochondriacal' (below the ribs); the nervous system theory to 'nervous', 'functional nervous' (malfunctioning nerves), and neurasthenic (weak nerves); and the mental theory to 'psychological,' 'psychogenic', and somatization (mental problems made somatic).

The changing theories have produced changing approaches to management. Early treatments focused on the organ believed to be giving rise to the symptoms. Consequently, manipulations of, and even removal of, the female reproductive organs were carried out. When the proposed explanation shifted to the peripheral nervous system the preferred treatments became nerve tonics, electrical stimulation, and other methods that were intended to regenerate nervous energy. As interest shifted to the central nervous system, hypnosis became a favored treatment and was used by famous physicians such as Charcot. It was only in the 20th century, following the work of Freud and the rise in popularity of psychoanalysis, that medically unexplained symptoms came to be seen as a 'mental' problem requiring psychiatric rather than medical treatment. This view persisted for most of the 20th century.

Most doctors still regard medically unexplained symptoms as purely mental in origin, but it has become increasingly obvious that such an approach is both scientifically inadequate and practically unhelpful. Developments in neuroscience have supplemented previous studies demonstrating a variety of associated physiological changes and indicate that many so called unexplained symptoms have a basis in the functioning of the nervous system. In practice, patients regard a purely mental explanation as dismissive and stigmatizing, and physicians find it frustrating as it does not help them manage the patient. A better approach is required, and one that sees such symptoms as not only psychological but also having a basis in changed nervous system functioning offers both a new research paradigm and better ways of talking to patients about their symptoms. Although offering new opportunities this idea is in fact a rediscovery of the concept of functional disorders that was in common usage in the 1890s.

ETIOLOGY AND PATHOPHYSIOLOGY

The precise etiology of many medically unexplained symptoms is unknown, but there is evidence of an etiological role for biological, psychological, and interpersonal factors. For any given case, rather than seeking a single cause for the patient's symptoms, it is probably better to consider the relative contribution of these factors. They may be conveniently considered as having predisposing, precipitating, or perpetuating influences on the symptoms (Table 2). Perpetuating factors are especially important to identify as they offer targets for treatment. For example, a person may be predisposed by virtue of genetics or childhood experience to develop irritable bowel syndrome. This may have been precipitated by a combination of infection and psychological stress. The symptoms are then perpetuated by a vicious circle of changed bowel motility, fear of gastrointestinal disease, and iatrogenic overinvestigation. Effective management addresses these perpetuating factors.

Although the physiological mechanisms of symptom production are not fully understood, many putative mechanisms have been identified. These interact with psychological and interpersonal factors to perpetuate the illness. Hence, overbreathing gives rise to paresthesiae and dizziness (by lowering plasma carbon dioxide). These symptoms may be interpreted by the patient as indicating a 'stroke' and lead to increased lead to anxiety and the seeking of medical care. Medical attention may inadvertently increase the fear about stroke and consequently the anxiety, leading to further hyperventilation, more symptoms and so on. A number of putative physiological mechanisms are listed in Table 3.

EPIDEMIOLOGY

Medically unexplained somatic symptoms are extremely common in the general population of all countries. However, only some of the people experiencing them will seek medical attention, usually because of concern about the cause or because of severe discomfort or disability.

- Primary care: Medically unexplained symptoms are the principal reason for a quarter to a half of all consultations in primary care, but only a few are referred to hospital clinics.
- Hospital outpatient care: At specialist outpatient clinics a third of all new patients have symptoms that remain inadequately explained by disease, even after exhaustive assessment. Some are admitted to hospital.
- Hospital inpatient care: While only a few patients with medically unexplained complaints become inpatients, these can be particularly costly to the service and are at high risk of iatrogenic harm, e.g. from unnecessary surgery.

Prevention

We do not know enough about the etiology of medically unexplained symptoms to know which primary preventive strategies are effective. However, there is increasing evidence that while genetic factors play a part, the interpersonal and economic factors of parenting, the stigma of psychiatric

Table 3: Examples of possible physiological mechanisms for medically unexplained physical symptoms that are supported by evidence

Noncardiac chest pain	Chest wall pain and paresthesiae from over breathing
Localized chronic pain	Neuronal plasticity
Fibromyalgia	Changed overall CNS pain sensitivity
Chronic fatigue	Neuroendocrine changes
Irritable bowel	Changed neuronal control of bowel motility

Table 2: The etiology of medically unexplained symptoms

	Predisposing	*Precipitating*	*Perpetuating*
Biological	Genetic	Acute illness or injury	Neuro-physiological mechanisms
			Effects of reduced activity
Psychological	Childhood abuse	Stresses	Fears and beliefs about symptoms
			Anxiety or depression
			Adoption of a disabled lifestyle
Interpersonal	Childhood experience of illness	Conflicts, e.g. at work	Iatrogenesis and lack of effective treatment
			Financial and other gain from being ill
			Behavior of family, doctors, and others

illness, and the nature of our current benefit and litigation systems are relevant and reversible influences. For secondary prevention, effective early management probably reduces the risk of chronicity, whereas poor explanation, overinvestigation, and inappropriate medical treatment probably increase it. Tertiary prevention can be achieved by effective management of the patient with chronic established symptoms and by limiting iatrogenic harm.

Clinical Features

Pointers to a patient having medically unexplained complaints may be apparent even before the initial consultation. The referral letter and medical notes may record frequent attendance at medical services, numerous negative (and often repeated) investigations, and a previous history of repeated unsuccessful surgery. At the consultation the presentation of multiple symptoms is strongly suggestive. However, the only way of confidently diagnosing complaints as medically unexplained is to complete the appropriate history, examination, and investigation. It should also be remembered that patients may have some symptoms that are explained by disease and others that are unexplained, for example the co-occurrence of epilepsy and nonepileptic attacks.

It is important to remember that many (but not all) unexplained medical complaints are somatic symptoms of depression or anxiety, most medically unexplained complaints reflect genuine suffering and disability, and the deliberate manufacturing of complaints is uncommon in ordinary (non-medico-legal) medical practice.

Differential Diagnosis

The main medical differential diagnosis for medically unexplained symptoms is from symptoms due to disease. Diagnostic difficulties are likely to occur with unusual presentations of common diseases and with rare diseases. While missing diagnosis of serious disease is an appropriate concern, the evidence indicates that once a patient has been carefully assessed the emergence of a 'missed' disease at a later date is uncommon.

Patient Assessment

When assessing the patient the main tasks are to:

- Make it clear that you are taking the symptoms seriously.

Clarify the nature of the presenting symptoms. For example, what does the patient really mean by fatigue? Is it lack of energy (nonspecific), sleepiness (suggesting a sleep problem), or lack of motivation or depression.

- Find out what other symptoms the patient has. It is worth asking for an exhaustive list: the more symptoms, the more likely it is that they will all be medically unexplained.
- Ask the patient what they think or fear is wrong with them. This can reveal why they have presented (e.g. 'I am worried that it could be cancer').
- Ask about life 'stresses'. This may be why the patient is presenting now.
- Seek evidence of depression and anxiety. This is often best done towards the end of the consultation so that the patient does not feel they are being dismissed as 'just psychiatric'. Stigma can be minimized by linking depression and anxiety with 'understandable' causes such as stress or the symptoms themselves.
- Physically examine the patient. This may reveal unsuspected signs of disease. It also helps to convince the patient that they have been taken seriously and properly assessed.
- Do not omit reasonable investigations. Misdiagnosis is relatively uncommon, but more likely when the patient looks 'psychiatric'. A balance must be struck between the risk of missing disease and the iatrogenic psychological harm from

Management

The general principles of management are outlined in Box 1.

GIVING REASSURANCE, EXPLANATION, AND ADVICE

As well as being reassured that there is no evidence they have an unpleasant disease, patients require a positive diagnosis and a credible explanation for their symptoms. They also need practical advice on what to do.

REASSURANCE

The provision of appropriate reassurance is an important part of the medical consultation. To be effective it must be based on the patient's concerns, not just on those of the doctor. Hence, it is important to ask the patient what they are worried they have, before reassuring them that they do not.

Box 1: Principles of general management of medically unexplained symptoms

- Exclude disease, but avoid unnecessary investigation or referral
- Seek specific treatable psychiatric syndromes
- Demonstrate to the patient that you believe their complaint(s)
- Take a full and sympathetic history
- Give the patient a diagnosis of a functional symptom or syndrome
- Give the patient a positive explanation, including but not overemphasizing psychological factors
- Encourage a return to normal functioning
- Consider prescribing antidepressant drugs

Many patients report the physical examination as particularly reassuring. A detailed explanation of what any investigations show can also help. Clearly it is unwise to state categorically to any patient that they have no disease, but appropriate to explain that the probability they have the disease they fear is very low and why. Beware of the patient who repeatedly asks for reassurance about the same disease—they may have health anxiety (hypochondriasis). This is considered further here.

GIVING A DIAGNOSIS AND EXPLANATION

Patients benefit from a positive diagnosis, and the failure to offer one may set them off on an unhelpful search. Clearly the diagnosis must be appropriate; it may be 'functional symptoms' or a named functional syndrome (such as irritable bowel syndrome). This diagnosis should then be elaborated with an explanation of why the patient has the symptoms. While our understanding is imperfect, we do have some evidence about etiology as described above. Explanations that include both psychological and biological factors and emphasize their reversibility helpfully set the scene for treatment. Some explanations are probably unhelpful. Dismissing the symptoms as 'just psychological' or 'all in the mind' is likely to reduce the patient's confidence in the doctor and reduce the value of their reassurance. Colluding with the patient's belief that their symptoms are explained by an untreatable disease (such as myalgic encephalopathy or chronic Lyme's disease) when they are not is likely to make them less willing to accept appropriate treatment and to encourage invalidity.

GIVING PRACTICAL ADVICE

After diagnosis and explanation, a positive plan of action that specifies both what the patient can change and what the doctor will do is required. The patient can be advised how to overcome the illness perpetuating factors, e.g. by becoming more active or by addressing stress. The doctor can provide accurate information about the illness, review progress, prescribe (e.g. an antidepressant drug), and if appropriate refer (e.g. to physiotherapy or psychology).

Writing to the patient as well as to the general practitioner to summarize the conclusions of the medical assessment and the proposed plan of action usefully reinforces messages that may otherwise be easily forgotten.

PRESCRIBING ANTIDEPRESSANT DRUGS

The so-called antidepressant drugs are most likely to be of benefit when the patient is depressed or anxious, but they can also reduce symptoms in patients who are not depressed or anxious. A systematic review of their use in patients with functional syndromes found them to be moderately effective. The odds ratio for improvement with antidepressant drug treatment compared with placebo was 3.4, but a high dropout rate from treatment was also noted, emphasizing the need for careful explanation and follow-up to ensure adherence.

For these drugs to be accepted by the patient, a clear explanation that minimizes stigma of why they are being prescribed is required. One of the following two approaches is suggested: the first is to explain that the term 'antidepressant' is a misnomer and that the drugs are actually broad-spectrum 'nerve tonics' of proven value for symptoms such as difficulty sleeping and pain, as well as for depression; the second is to be explicit that they are being prescribed for depression or anxiety, but to emphasize that these emotional problem are an understandable reaction to the somatic symptoms.

REFERRAL FOR PSYCHOLOGICAL OR PSYCHIATRIC MANAGEMENT

A referral for specialized psychological treatment may be required when simple measures and antidepressant drugs are insufficient to relieve the patient's symptoms. The most widely used are behavioral or cognitive behavioral therapy (CBT), which aims to help the patient change thinking (cognitions) and ways of coping (behavior) that are perpetuating symptoms. A systematic review of CBT for medically unexplained symptoms found that it was significantly superior to nonspecific treatment or no treatment in 70% of trials. Individual behavioral components of CBT, such as graded exercises, are less studied but also of value.

The decision to refer to specialist services will be based on the physician's assessment of the patient and on knowledge of what services are available. While ideally all medical clinics would have dedicated specialist psychiatric or psychology services, in practice this is rarely the case. Consequently, it is wise to find out before the need to refer arises which local practitioners are interested in physical symptoms and willing to accept referrals. If the options are few it may be necessary to make the case for better services.

Reasons to refer to include: to psychology for specialist CBT; to psychiatry if the patient is judged to be at risk of self-harm; to psychiatry or psychology if the patient has severe emotional distress; to a specialist service, e.g. for chronic pain or chronic fatigue syndrome (CFS). When explaining the referral to the patient, it is wise to be positive about the service you are referring to and to emphasize that the referral does not mean you regard the patient's symptoms as 'all in the mind.'

A patient is more likely to attend for a referral if you have said: 'I see you have real and troublesome symptoms. I am pleased to tell you that you do not have serious disease but I am sorry to say that I do not have a simple cure that I can prescribe. However, I can recommend and refer you to a specialist service for your problem,' than if you have told them: 'There is clearly nothing wrong with you; it must all be in your mind. There is nothing to do now but to refer you to the shrinks.'

MANAGEMENT OF THE CHRONIC COMPLEX PATIENT

Advice for the management of patients with chronic persistent symptoms is shown in Box 2.

WHAT HAPPENS IN PRACTICE?

In practice, management of medically unexplained symptoms is frequently suboptimal, and iatrogenic psychological and physical harm from unhelpful explanations, unnecessary tests, and ineffective medical and surgical treatments is probably common. The evidence based treatments of antidepressant drugs and CBT are rarely offered and frequently refused by patients. Specific services such as psychological services for chronic pain are often not available. We surely could do better.

PROGNOSIS

The prognosis for those patients whose symptoms are sufficiently severe and persistent to lead to referral to a specialist service is often poor. It is not uncommon for symptoms and disability to persist for years, but this reflects in part a failure to provide treatment. The prognosis is best for those patients who were well before the onset of symptoms and who have clear depressive and anxiety disorders. It is worst for those patients with long-standing multiple symptoms.

SPECIFIC SYNDROMES

Classification

There are parallel medical and psychiatric classificatory schemes for medically unexplained symptoms, which is confusing. The former emphasizes the nature of the symptom and lists functional syndromes by organ system as in Table 1; the latter emphasizes the number of symptoms and associated psychological factors and is shown in Table 4.

The implication of these parallel, overlapping classifications is that most patients will qualify for both a medical and a psychiatric diagnosis. Both may be useful in guiding management and prognostication, hence a combined medical/psychiatric diagnosis such as 'irritable bowel syndrome/anxiety disorder' is probably more useful than either alone. An alternative multidimensional classification system that unifies the medical and psychiatric approach would be preferable: an example is shown in Box 3.

Common Syndromes

This section addresses specific aspects of the main psychiatric diagnoses for medically unexplained symptoms listed in Box 3.

Predominant Worry About Disease: Health Anxiety or Hypochondriasis

The central feature of hypochondriasis is a persistent preoccupation with the possibility that one has a serious or progressive medical condition. These fears persist despite

Box 2: Management of patients with chronic, persistent symptoms

- Try to be proactive, not reactive; see the patient at regular, fixed intervals, not on demand
- Aim to broaden the agenda with the patient to include nonmedical problems
- Reduce or taper unnecessary drugs
- Minimize the contact the patient has with other specialists or practitioners
- Try to coopt a relative as a therapeutically to implement your management goal
- Aim for containment of demands, damage limitation, and avoidance of iatrogenic harm
- Encourage the patient (and yourself) to think in terms of coping rather than curing

Table 4: The main psychiatric diagnostic categories of medically unexplained symptoms

Main feature	*Diagnosis*
Predominantly worry about disease	Hypochondriasis
Predominantly concern about symptoms	Somatization (somatic presentation of depression and anxiety)
Small number of symptoms	Simple somatoform disorders
Chronic multiple symptoms	Somatization disorder (Briquet's syndrome)
Loss of function	Conversion disorder
Dislike of body parts	Body dysmorphic disorder
Other unusual presentations	
Deliberate deception	Factitious disorder and malingering (including Münchausen's syndrome)

Box 3: A multidimensional classificatory scheme of medically unexplained symptoms

- Duration of illness
- Number of symptoms
- Degree of disability
- Severity of depression/anxiety
- Patients fears/beliefs

the fact that repeated investigations and examinations have identified no such condition, and appropriate reassurance has been given.

Predominant Concern about Symptoms: Somatic Presentation of Depression and Anxiety

One of the most common causes of medically unexplained somatic symptoms is undiagnosed depressive and anxiety disorders. Because depression is (erroneously) thought of as a purely 'mental illness', it is readily forgotten that it also has prominent somatic symptoms. These include fatigue, pain (often of chronic widespread nature), and loss of weight and appetite.

Somatic symptoms of anxiety in generalized form (generalized anxiety disorder) or episodic severe form (panic disorder) include fatigue, dizziness, paresthesias, chest pain and palpitations, and shortness of breath (especially 'getting enough breath in').

Predominant Concern about Symptoms: Simple Somatoform Disorders

This diagnosis refers to the patient with a single or small number of somatic complaints that do not appear to be expressions of depressive or anxiety disorders. It includes so-called undifferentiated somatoform disorder and somatoform pain disorder. The most commonly encountered clinical problem in this category is chronic medically unexplained persistent pain, such as chronic back pain or chronic headache. The physical symptoms may have commenced after a trivial injury or accident, but the subsequent disability is out of proportion to the objective finding.

Chronic Multiple Symptoms: Somatization Disorder (Briquet's Syndrome)

Somatization disorder, or Briquet's syndrome, is a term used to describe patients—mostly women—who have a lifelong history of multiple recurrent somatic complaints referable to multiple bodily systems. Such patients are relatively easy to identify as although the current presenting complaint may be of only one or two symptoms, scrutiny of the past medical notes reveals a long history of outpatient visits to different clinics with medically unexplained symptoms such as abdominal pain and bloating, diffuse muscular pains and tenderness, and chronic lassitude. A history of childhood abuse and unnecessary surgery is common.

Example 1

The patient is a young woman. Her urgent referral is faxed to you by her general practitioner (GP). She has attended the general practice clinic daily for the last 2 weeks with headache. The history reveals that her father died of a brain tumor 2 years ago and when he presented to the GP was told it was only a 'tension headache'. Examination is normal but she is very anxious indeed and repeatedly asks for your reassurance that she does not have a brain tumor. She wants a brain scan.

Management and Prognosis: Assessment should aim to clarify the patient's fears. A useful question is: 'what is your worst fear?' The patient's fear makes their anxiety and behavior understandable. For example, if the patient thinks, 'I have a brain tumor', she will be understandably anxious and keen to seek urgent medical attention. The symptom (headache) leads to thoughts ('I have a brain tumor') that in turn lead to anxiety, to certain coping behaviors (visiting doctors and requesting a scan). The more she seeks reassurance the stronger the worry she has a brain tumor becomes and so on in a vicious circle. Eliciting this sequence from the patient, and describing it to them, perhaps using a diagram, aids explanation. While is it is appropriate to reassure them that they do not have a tumor, responding to requests for repeated reassurance or investigations can paradoxically worsen the patient's worry. In this circumstance the patient can be told, 'I have already reassured you a number of times; every time I do this it makes you feel better for a short period. But we know if I keep doing this it will make your worries stronger and make you want yet more reassurance and more tests. So I am not going to reassure you again or do any more tests'.

Depressive disorder is common in such patients, in which case effective treatment of depression may resolve the problem. There is also some evidence for the effectiveness of CBT in health anxiety. While most acute cases resolve, the condition can become chronic. In a few patients the concern with disease is delusional in intensity, and these should be referred to a psychiatrist.

Example 2

The patient is a middle-aged woman, referred to as a 'heart-sink' patient by the referring GP. She presents with dizziness, bloating of her stomach, and generalized weakness. She has three volumes of medical notes documenting her previous presentations with a range of symptoms including pain in various places, irritable bowel, menstrual problems, and transient loss of sight. She has had many investigations, as well as a hysterectomy and three laparotomies. She is taking a long list of prescribed medications including oral opioids, but review of her notes does not reveal any convincing evidence of disease. Examination reveals only a number of operation scars.

Management and Prognosis: If possible, it is desirable to review the case notes before seeing the patient. It is also worth considering why the patient, who has a chronic condition, has been referred now. The GP may be feeling more frustrated or helpless than usual in the face of repeated complaints, the patient may have seen a different GP who was unaware of her history, or the patient's presentation may have changed, raising concern about disease. If the presentation justifies it, reasonable efforts must be made to exclude disease—but also noting what investigations have already been done. The general approach should be one of helping patient and GP to cope with a chronic illness, rather than investigation and cure. Some practical management strategies are listed in Box 2. Depression is common in such patients, makes symptoms worse and should be treated. Long-term but infrequent follow-up (by a hospital doctor, GP, psychiatrist, or a combination of these) is desirable to prevent iatrogenic harm. The condition is very likely to persist.

Example 3

A 40-year-old man presents to the Emergency Department with acute chest pain and breathlessness with fatigue. Examination and investigations are negative. Only after admission to hospital does a junior doctor examine the patient's mental state and find that he has symptoms of both depression and severe episodic anxiety associated with overbreathing and many other somatic symptoms. The diagnosis is depressive disorder with associated panic disorder.

Management and Prognosis: Treatment is by making a positive diagnosis, providing reassurance and explanation, and treating the depression and anxiety. This can be achieved most simply by prescribing an antidepressant agent with appropriate explanation and active follow-up to ensure adherence. In some cases psychological treatment may also be required. The prognosis for recovery within 6 months is good, although there is a risk of relapse. Patients should continue to take the antidepressant drug for at least 6 months after they have recovered in order to prevent early relapse. Antidepressant drugs can initially make anxiety worse, and short-term prescription of benzodiazepines may also be required.

Loss of Function: Conversion Disorder: Conversion disorder refers to the loss of function of a body part or to abnormal body movements. Examples are transient medically unexplained blindness, paralysis of a limb, or nonepileptic attacks. These symptoms are regarded as not being produced intentionally (in distinction to factitious disorder and malingering—see here), but rather 'subconsciously'. In practice this distinction can be difficult to make. Persistence of functional impairment even when the patient believes they are not being observed suggests that the symptoms are not deliberately feigned. Other often quoted signs of conversion disorder such as 'belle indifference' (smiling indifference to disability) are unreliable. Acute presentations may have arisen in the context of severe interpersonal stress, conflict, or physical injury. The patient may have experienced a family member with similar symptoms.

Example 4

A middle-aged man presents with pain in his back. He believes that his symptoms are a result of lifting heavy items at work and is engaged in litigation against his former employer. There is a history of depression some 12 months ago, but this has largely resolved. Physical examination is normal. The patient walks with a stick and seems concerned to demonstrate to you how ill he is.

Management and Prognosis: As well as diagnosis explanation and symptomatic treatment (including pain management programs), antidepressant drugs may be tried on an empirical basis. There is a role for CBT. Improvement may occur over many months. The prognosis for acute problems is fairly good, but for established symptoms with associated disability is poor. Legal proceedings complicate management and probably worsen prognosis.

Example 5

A young woman is referred for sudden onset of weakness of her left side and a stroke is suspected. She reports being unable to move her left arm and leg. Enquiry reveals that she was sexually assaulted the week before her symptoms began. She herself offers no explanation for the symptoms. On examination her left arm and leg appear weak, with a 'collapsing' pattern, but there are no abnormalities of reflexes. An MRI brain scan is normal.

Management and Prognosis: An acute case of conversion disorder such as this needs to be given a diagnosis, a positive explanation that describes how reversible brain malfunction causes the symptoms, and a plan of gradual return to normal function. However, there have been very few clinical trials of treatment. Physiotherapy may be useful. Depression should be sought and treated if present. The prognosis is good for cases of acute onset, but in established cases it is poor and long-term invalidism with dependence on state benefits is common, although referral to a physical rehabilitation service may be helpful.

Dislike of a Body Part: Body Dysmorphic Disorder: Patients who are dissatisfied with some aspect of their bodily appearance or shape may find their way into the clinics of physicians and surgeons. Some of these patients are preoccupied with a perceived defect in appearance, such as a large nose. Others have more substantial concerns, such as disliking a limb sufficiently to request its amputation. Even in the presence of a minor physical abnormality, the person's concern appears to be markedly excessive (see Example 6).

Example 6

A 30-year-old woman complains about the shape of her nose and blames this for her inability to find a partner and for many other difficulties in her life. She requests plastic surgery.

Management and Prognosis: In the absence of a conspicuous physical abnormality or deformity, it is usually prudent to seek a psychiatric opinion. There is some evidence for the effectiveness of CBT. Surgery may have good psychological results where there is a single clear abnormality to correct, but should only be carried out after careful assessment.

OTHER UNUSUAL PRESENTATIONS

Atypical Eating Disorders

Some patients who attend with symptoms of abdominal pain after food, vomiting, anorexia, or constipation may have a covert eating disorder. Judicious enquiry about weight loss, amenorrhea, and laxative use may help to establish the correct diagnosis.

Chronic Constipation that has not Responded to Conventional Treatment

Patients may present with a history of constipation for two or three decades that has proved unresponsive to all treatment. In such cases there is often no identifiable medical cause, but they may be referred to surgeons for colectomy. All require a thorough psychiatric assessment before major decisions about treatment are implemented. Treatment with biofeedback may benefit some patients, but is not generally available.

Loin Pain Hematuria Syndrome

This is a rare syndrome that is poorly understood but thought to be a somatoform disorder. Patients may abuse opioid analgesics, and some are thought to simulate their pain. It is unwise to carry out renal autotransplantation because it often fails to cure the pain, which may recur on the opposite side of the body, and puts the patient at risk of the complications of surgery.

DELIBERATE DECEPTION

Factitious Disorder

Patients with factitious disorder deliberately feign or simulate illness in order to obtain medical attention. The term 'factitious disorder' is preferable to the eponym Munchausen's syndrome, because this stereotype is often misleading. The label of 'Munchausen's syndrome' is generally applied to wandering, untreatable, male sociopaths, whereas most patients with factitious disorders are women working in medically related occupations. They often report a large number of childhood illnesses and operations. High rates of substance abuse, mood disorder, and personality disorder have been reported. Some patients exaggerate genuine disease (usually chronic) to create dramatic medical emergencies (see Example 7).

Example 7

A student nurse is repeatedly admitted to hospital with breakdown of an abdominal surgical wound. She is observed rubbing feces into the wound. When confronted with this she discharges herself immediately.

Management and Prognosis: A 'supportive confrontation' is generally recommended, but there have been few systematic studies of management. This means presenting the patient with the evidence that they have been manufacturing symptoms and signs, while suggesting that they have an emotional problem for which help and support is offered. Ideally, the physician and psychiatrist do this jointly. There is some evidence that psychological support following hospital discharge may be associated with an improved outcome. Patients with stable, social networks have a better prognosis.

Malingering: The term malingering is not a medical diagnosis. It refers to the behavior of the deliberately simulating or exaggerating symptoms for obvious and understandable gain, e.g. monetary compensation, disabled status, avoidance of criminal prosecution, or conscription. It is differentiated from factitious disorder in which the aim of simulation is simply to get medical attention. Doctors are often reluctant to describe a patient as malingering lest it adversely affect their health care, occupation, or legal case. However, malingering does occur, especially in medicolegal contexts. It can be hard to detect reliably in a medical consultation and is often detected by covert video surveillance that reveals the patient vigorously engaging in an activity (such as playing sport) that they have reported they are unablex to do. There is probably a continuum of behavior from the minor embellishment of symptoms to frank malingering (see Example 8).

Example 8

A 30-year-old man is seen in order to produce a legal report in relation to his claim for compensation. He reports severe back pain following a car accident 2 years ago and presents in a wheelchair. There are no neurological signs and no muscle wasting. He is later seen walking to his car and lifting his wheelchair into the boot.

Management and Prognosis: Malingering is a behavior, not a medical diagnosis. If management is required, it is by confrontation. Often the identification of malingering ends the behavior (and the legal case).

Areas of Uncertainty and Controversy: Many aspects of the nature and management of medically unexplained somatic symptoms are controversial. The core issue is whether they are best regarded as a psychiatric/psychological problem or as a medical condition. This issue has been played out particularly prominently in the debate over the chronic fatigue syndrome/myalgic encephalomyelitis. A consideration of the changing medical fashions for the explanation of such symptoms over the last few hundred years should encourage humility and suggests that current controversies may tell us more about the inadequacies of our conceptualization of illness and our health services than they do about the patients.

Likely Developments Over the Next Few Years

The size of the problem of medically unexplained symptoms, its cost to services, and its public health importance is becoming increasingly clear. A likely scientific development that will come from brain imaging studies is the better understanding of the neuropsychological mechanisms of symptom production, both medically unexplained and associated with disease. Better drugs for a variety of symptoms are a likely development, although psychological treatments are likely to remain important. A more consumerist attitude from symptomatic patients who will be less willing to be told that 'there is nothing wrong with them' is to be expected. These factors will drive better management and better services for symptoms in general. We can expect the development of more symptom treatment programs that coexist with current disease oriented disease management, as exemplified by some existing pain and palliative care services.

FURTHER READING

1. Barsky AJ, Borus JF. Functional somatic syndromes. Ann Intern Med. 1999;130:910-21.
2. Barsky AJ. A comprehensive approach to the chronically somatizing patient. J Psychosom Res. 1998;45:301-6.
3. Bass C, Gill D. Factitious disorders and malingering. In: Gelder M, et al. (Eds) New Oxford Textbook of Psychiatry. 2000. pp. 1126-32. Oxford University Press, Oxford.
4. Bass C, May S. Chronic multiple functional somatic symptoms. BMJ. 2002;325:323-26.
5. Drossman DA. Diagnosing and treating patients with refractory functional gastrointestinal disorders. Ann Intern Med. 1995;123:688-97.
6. Henningsen P, Zipfel S, Herzog W. Management of functional somatic syndromes. The Lancet. 2007;369:946-55.
7. Hotopf M. Preventing somatization. Psychol Med. 2004;34:195-98.
8. Kroenke K, Swindle R. Cognitive-behavioral therapy for somatization and symptom syndromes: a critical review of controlled clinical trials. Psychother Psychosom. 2000;69:205-15.
9. Mayou R, et al. Somatoform disorders: time for a new approach in DSM-5. Am J Psychiatry. 2005;162:847-55.
10. Mayou RA, Bass C, Sharpe M. Treatment of functional somatic symptoms. Oxford University Press, Oxford. 1995.
11. O'Malley PG, et al. Antidepressant therapy for unexplained symptoms and symptom syndromes. J Fam Pract. 1999;48:980-90.
12. Royal College of Physicians, Royal College of Psychiatrists. The psychological care of medical patients: a practical guide. Royal College of Physicians, London. 2003.
13. Smith RC. Somatization disorder: defining its role in clinical medicine. J Gen Intern Med. 1991;6:168-75.
14. Veale D. Body dysmorphic disorder. Postgrad Med J. 2004;80:67-71.
15. Wessely S, Nimnuan C, Sharpe M. Functional somatic syndromes: one or many? Lancet. 1999;354:936-9.

CHAPTER

66

Erectile Dysfunction

JN Vyas, SK Pandey

INTRODUCTION

Erectile dysfunction (ED) is defined as "the persistent inability to achieve or maintain an erection sufficient for satisfactory sexual performance". ED is highly prevalent, currently affecting around 30 million men in the United States and is also believed to be more in other part of the world. As the male population ages and awareness of the problem increases, this number is expected population ages and awareness of the problem increases, this number is expected to at least double by 2025. Several emotional, physical, and medical factors contribute to ED, and this condition may also be a symptom of various chronic diseases. ED may affect total health, relationships, and overall quality of life. Although the majority of patients with the condition remain undiagnosed and untreated, the number of patients seeking treatment for ED has increased dramatically in the past three years.

EPIDEMIOLOGY

A 1990 meta-analysis, which summarized 23 community based studies published in English over the previous 50 years, found an ED prevalence range of 3-9% for all male ages. The most frequently cited modern surveys reporting prevalence data on ED in the United States are the National Health and Social Life Survey (NHSLS) was a national probability study of men and women between 18 and 59 years of age living in the United States in 1992. The study included 1410 men. The ED prevalence rates were as follows: 7% for ages 18–29 years, 9% for ages 30–39 years, 11% for ages 40–49 years, and 18% for ages 50–59 years.

The MMAS included 1709 noninstitutional men between the ages of 40 and 70 years living in the greater Boston area. Some degree of ED was reported by 52% of all men. Between ages 40 and 70, the probability of complete ED increased from 5% to 15% and the probability of moderate ED from 17% to 34%, based on self-reported ED status on a questionnaire. An update on this study was published in 2000, in which data from 847 men of the initial study were available for analysis. The study prevalence of ED for the age groups 40–49, 50–59, and 60–69 was 0.08, 0.16, and 0.37, respectively. The crude incidence rate for ED was 25.9 cases per 1,000 man years and the annual rate increased with each decade of age, reaching 46.4 cases for men 60–69 years old. The age adjusted risk of ED was higher for men lower education, diabetes, heart disease, and hypertension. The study suggested that 617, 715 new cases are expected annually among white males in the United States. Recently, several studies have attempted to determine the prevalence of ED in the Netherlands, Spain, the United Kingdom, Germany, and Australia. Results overall indicated an ED prevalence between 11% and 33.9% (Table 1). Higher prevalence rates were found in community and practice based studies that used validated questionnaires and quantitative assessments to establish the presence of ED. Differences among the studies in patient demographics and inclusion criteria accounted for some variability in the findings.

Table 1: Prevalence of erectile dysfunction (ED): sampling of worldwide results

Population	*Age (years)*	*(%) ED*
Cologne, Germany	30–80	19.2
Iberian Peninsula, Spain	25–70	18.9
Perth, Australia	40–69	33.9
Krimpen, Netherlands	50–78	11.0
London, UK	16–78	19.0
Boston, MA, USA	40–70	52.0
NHSLS, USA	50–59	18.0

PHYSIOLOGY OF ERECTION: NEUROANATOMY

Animal studies have identified several brain regions as important to penile erection. The medial preoptic area (MPOA) of the hypothalamus may be the integration point for the central control of erection. It receives sensory impulses from the amygdala that have inputs from cortical association areas. These include norepinephrine mediated inhibitory signals and dopamine-mediated proerectile stimuli. The para-ventricular nucleus (PVN) of the hypothalamus, which receives neural input from the MPOA, may have a proerectile action through oxytocin-mediated descending pathways.

Periaqueductal gray matter, which provides neural connections between the MPOA and the brain stem, may also have proerectile activity; neurons from the PVN are known the project through it to thoracic and lumbosacral nuclei concerned with erection. Reflex erections originate in the erection generating center of the spinal cord (T12-S3).

The penis is innervated by the sympathetic (T11-L2), parasympathetic (S2-S4), and somatic (S2-S4) nervous systems. Sympathetic input is antierectile, whereas parasympathetic and somatic input is proerectile. Both sympathetic and parasympathetic fibers reach the pelvic or inferior hypogastric plexus where autonomic input to the penis is integrated; the cavernous nerves originate from this plexus. The sacral reflex arc, another pathway, conveys stimuli from the perineum and the lower urinary tract mucosa.

The lesser cavernous nerves originate from the pelvic plexus and travel along the penis to supply the penile urethra and the erectile tissue of the corpus spongiosum. The greater cavernous nerves also originate in the pelvic plexus. They innervate the helicine arteries and erectile tissue.

Intracavernous nerves are encased in fibrous tissue, which prevents their compression during an erection. Their branches travel with prostatovesicular artery branches, which provide a visual landmark during nerve sparing radical prostatectomy. The dorsal penile nerves, branches of the pudendal nerves, and the ilioinguinal nerve also innervate the penis. These nerves provide sensory input from the glans penis and skin, and penile root.

ERECTION: A NEUROVASCULAR REFLEX

An erection is a hemodynamic event determined by the contractile state of penile smooth muscle. When a penis is in its flaccid state, sympathetic neural activity predominates;this minimizes blood flow into the sinuses of the corpora cavernosa. With sexual stimulation, parasympathetic neural activity predominates; this leads to increased blood flow into the sinuses and achievement of erection due to smooth muscle relaxation in the corpora cavernosa. The maintenance of the intracorporal muscle in a semicontracted state during flaccidity results from intrinsic myogenic activity, adrenergic neurotransmission, and endothelium-derived contracting factors such as prostaglandin F2 and endothelins. Several factors are required for penile smooth muscle cells to contract, including the following: adequate local levels of neurotransmitter, adequate expression of receptors, integrity of the transduction mechanism, i.e. channel homeostasis, interactions between contractile proteins, and effective communication between smooth muscle cells over gap junctions.

The main neurotransmitter mediating penile erection in nitric oxide (NO), which is released from the endothelium of the corpora cavernosa during nonadrenergic, noncholinergic neurotransmission. Within the muscle cell, NO activates a soluble guanylyl cyclase, which raises the intracellular concentration of cyclic guanosine monophosphate (cGMP). cGMP in turn activates a specific protein kinase, which phosphorylates certain proteins and ion channels. This results in the opening of potassium channels and hyperpolarization of the muscle cell membrane, sequestration of intracellular calcium by the endoplasmic reticulum, and blocking of calcium influx by calcium channel inhibition. The consequence is a drop in cytosolic calcium concentration and relaxation of the smooth muscle, resulting in dilation of arterial vessels and increased blood flow into the sinuses of the corpora cavernosa.

RISK FACTORS AND PATHOPHYSIOLOGY

Major risk factors for ED include advancing age, the presence of chronic illness (e.g. heart disease, hypertension, diabetes mellitus, depression), smoking, stress, alcohol and drug abuse, and sedentary life style. The causes of ED are organic (vascular, neurogenic, hormonal, anatomical/structural, drug induced), psychogenic, or, most commonly, mixed. Although in the past ED was thought to be primarily due to psychogenic factors, it is now generally acknowledged that organic causes are present in most patients. Causes can be acquired or congenital, and psychogenic causes can be either generalized or situational.

Psychogenic causes of ED include depression, performance anxiety, relationship problems, and psychosocial distress. Organic causes are subdivided into vascular, neurogenic, hormonal, penile injury or disease, drug induced, and those related to other systemic diseases. Among organic ED causes, 40% involve vascular problems and 30% relate to diabetes. A combination of factors is not uncommon.

Aging constitutes an independent risk factor for ED. As men age, physiologic changes cause a progressive decline in sexual function. The incidence of chronic disease also increases with age. Because ED is a marker of serious medical conditions such as hypertension, diabetes mellitus, cardiovascular disease, or depression, it is an important factor in "men's health". The role of androgens in erectile function is controversial.

PATIENT EVALUATION

The First International Consultation on Erectile Dysfunction, co-sponsored by the World Health Organization (WHO), convened in 1999 in Paris, France. Its mission was to develop recommendations for the diagnostic for the evaluation of the ED patient, the tests in use were stratified as highly recommended (should be done on every patient),

Table 2: World Health Organization recommendation for the diagnosis evaluation of erectile dysfunction (ED)

- Highly recommended evaluation and tests
  - *Comprehensive sexual, medical and psychosocial history:* Medical and sexual history, including erectile insufficiency (onset, duration, progression, severity, nocturnal, self-stimulatory, and visual erotic-induced erections), altered sexual desire, ejaculation, orgasm, sexually induced genital pain, partner sexual function, lifestyle factors, smoking, chronic medical illnesses, pelvic/perineal/penile trauma and surgery, medications, recreational drug use, pelvic radiotherapy, neurological disease, endocrine disease, psychiatric illness, current psychological state, depression ED intensity and impact scales, e.g. ED intensity scale, ED impact scale
  - *Focused physical examination:* Assessment of body habitus and cardiovascular, neurological, and genitourinary system, including penile, testicular, and rectal examination, blood pressure, heart rate
- Recommended diagnostic tests
  - Fasting glucose or glycosylated hemoglobin (Hba1c) and lipid profile
  - Evaluation of the hypothalamic-pituitary-gonadal axis with a testosterone assay
- Optional diagnostic tests
  - Psychological and/or psychiatric consultation
  - Laboratory investigations: Serum prolactin, luteinizing hormone, complete blood count, urinalysis
- Specialized evaluation and diagnostic tests
  - In depth psychosexual and relationship evaluation
  - Psychiatric evaluation
  - Nocturnal penile tumescence and rigidity assessment
  - Vascular diagnostics (penile injection pharmacotesting, penile Doppler ultrasound, pharmacocavernosometry and pharmacocavernosography, penile arteriography, computed tomography/magnetic resonance imaging, nuclear imaging)
  - Specialized endocrinological testing (thyroid function studies, hypothalamic-pituitary-gonadal function studies, magnetic resonance imaging of sella turcica)
  - Neurophysiologic testing (vibrometry, bulbocavernosus reflex latency, cavernosal electromyogram, somatosensory evoked potential testing, pudendal and sphincter electromyogram)

recommended (test of proven value in most patients, strongly encouraged during initial evaluation), optional (test of proven value in specific profiles), and specialized (test of value in selected patient profiles in specialized settings). The recommended tests are shown in Table 2. Recent diagnostic criteria of ED according to DSM-5 is listed below:

DSM-5 Diagnostic criteria for erectile disorder (F52.21)

- At least one of the three following symptoms must be experienced on almost all or all (approximately 75–100%) occasions of sexual activity (in identified situational contexts or, if generalized, in all contexts):
  - Marked difficulty in obtaining an erection during sexual activity
  - Marked difficulty in maintaining an erection until the completion of sexual activity
  - Marked decrease in erectile rigidity.
- The symptoms in Criterion A have persisted for a minimum duration of approximately 6 months.
- The symptoms in Criterion A cause clinically significant distress in the individual.
- The sexual dysfunction is not better explained by a nonsexual mental disorder or as a consequence of severe relationship distress or other significant stressors and is not attributable to the effects of a substance/medication or another medical condition.

Specify whether:

Lifelong: The disturbance has been present since the individual became sexually active.

Acquired: The disturbance began after a period of relatively normal sexual function.

Specify whether:

Generalized: Not limited to certain types of stimulation, situations, or partners.

MANAGEMENT

The step-care approach to ED management ranges from life style medication and counseling to survey. The patient progresses through this staged therapy, choosing the therapeutic options with which he, his partner, and the clinician are most comfortable. Table 3 the therapeutic options of the first, second, and third line therapy. This review emphasizes androgen replacement and oral agents in the first line therapy section, transurethral and intracavernous therapy in the second line therapy section, and penile prosthesis in the third line therapy section.

FIRST-LINE THERAPY

Lifestyle modifications are an integral part of first line therapy. WHO recommendations include smoking

Table 3: Step-care approach to management of erectile dysfunction: therapeutic options

First-line therapy
- Lifestyle/drug therapy modification
- Psychosocial counseling
- Androgen replacement therapy
- Oral therapy

Second-line therapy
- Vacuum construction device
- Intracavernosal injection
- Transurethral therapy

Third-line therapy
- Penile prosthesis
- Revascularization

cessation, avoidance of alcohol and drug abuse, healthy diet, exercise, and adequate sleep. In addition, drug therapy associated with ED should be avoided or therapeutic regimens modified whenever possible. Psychosocial therapy addresses anxiety reduction and desensitization, cognitive behavioral interventions, increased sexual stimulation, and interpersonal assertiveness through couples communication training.

Androgens

Although endocrine factors comprise only around 3% of organic ED factors, androgens and their role in ED therapy have recently attracted interest. Types of androgen replacement therapy include transdermal testosterone in the form of a gel or nonscrotal patch, intramuscular injection of testosterone cypionate, or a subcutaneous implant. Testosterone is thought to primarily stimulate libido at the level of the central nervous system. The role of androgens in ED, however, remains controversial. Although rat studies show that penile cavernosal and spongiosal cells undergo apoptosis in response to castration, which is reversible after testosterone supplementation, in human studies about 50% of castrated sex offenders could achieve and sustain an erection. Although nocturnal penile tumescence is inhibited by androgen deficiency, erections in response to visual erotic stimuli may be partially androgen independent. Korenman et al. found no difference in serum bioavailable testosterone levels between impotent and potent older men. They therefore proposed that ED and secondary hypogonadism are two common independent disorders in the aging male. Data from animal and human studies indicate that low normal range concentrations of testosterone are sufficient to maintain sexual activity, and above a threshold level of testosterone there is no further improvement in response to therapy. Administration of testosterone to eugonadal men enhances the rigidity but does not change circumference or frequency of erections during nocturnal penile tumescence. In hypogonadal men, however, it improves libido and sexual performance. Guay et al. investigated the impact of raising endogenous testosterone levels in hypogonadal men with ED by administering clomiphene citrate, which binds to estrogen receptors to produce estrogenic and antiestrogenic effects. They found no clear improvement of sexual function as monitored subjectively by questionnaires and objectively by nocturnal penile tumescence and rigidity testing. In addition, unless testosterone deficiency was severe (free testosterone <7 to 8 pg/mL), testosterone replacement therapy did not significantly improve the success rate of sildenafil therapy in patients with ED and hypogonadism. Androgen deficiency, especially in elderly men, is not the most common cause of ED. Other common vascular, neurological, and psychological iatrogenic factors are very likely to coexist with androgen deficiency and therefore prevent beneficial effects of androgen replacement therapy.

PDE5 Inhibitors

Sildenafil is an approved, orally active, potent, and selective inhibitor of cGMP specific phosphodiesterase type 5 (PDE5), which is the predominant isoform in human penile tissue. Sildenafil enhances the relaxant effect of the no released into the corpora cavernosa from the nonadrenergic-non-cholinergic (NANC) autonomic nerves of the parasympathetic system and the vascular endothelium during sexual stimulation.

Because sildenafil potentiates the hypotensive effects of nitrates, it is contraindicated in patients who are using organic nitrates or other nitric oxide donors. It may be hazardous for patients with active coronary ischemia, congestive heart failure and borderline low blood pressure, borderline low cardiac volume, or a complicated multidrug antihypertensive program, or for patients on a drug regimen that can prolong the half-life of sildenafil. The efficacy of various sildenafil doses in improving erectile function was demonstrated in more than 3000 patients in 21 American and European randomized, double-blind, placebo-controlled phase III trials lasting up to 6 months. In long-term follow-up at 1 year (n = 2482), 2 years (n = 900), and 3 years (n = 245), more than 95% of men have maintained efficacy (improved erections) and an improved ability to engage in sexual activity. The most common adverse events in clinical trials included headaches, flushing, nasal congestion, dyspepsia, abnormal vision, diarrhea, and dizziness.

The success of sildenafil has resulted in growth in the field of oral drug therapy for ED. In addition to sildenafil, two other highly potent and selective PDE5 inhibitors, tadalafil and vardenafil have been proven effective in men with a broad range of severity of ED in multicenter, double-blind, placebo-controlled studies and have been submitted for approval in US market. Although mechanism of action is similar for all three agents, there are several pharmacologic differences between them. Pharmacokinetic studies in healthy adults demonstrated that, in contrast to sildenafil, the plasma concentration of tadalafil was unaffected by food or alcohol consumption. These findings suggest that tadalafil can be administered at any time with or without food. The effect of food on plasma concentration of vardenafil has not been reported. Sildenafil has a median plasma half life of 3–5 hours and vardenafil has a mean half-life 4 hours, whereas tadalafil has a median half-life of 17.5 hours. The 17.5 hours half-life of tadalafil supports results from clinical trials that indicated a period of responsiveness for up to 24 hours after administration. Finally, relative to sildenafil, vardenafil and tadalafil are poor inhibitor of PDE, which is predominant in the retina. Thus, one would expect fewer visual side effects with the use of tadalafil.

Cardiovascular Effects

Without sildenafil, the relative risk of myocardial infarction (MI) occurring 2 hours after sexual activity is low: 2.5 in those with no prior cardiac disease and 2.9 in those with prior MI. After correction for chance occurrence, sexual activity was a likely contributor to the onset of MI in ~0.9% of cases in a case-crossover trial of sexually active men and women with a history of MI within the previous 30 days. In order to examine the relationship between sildenafil use and adverse cardiovascular events in men with coronary artery disease, Arruda-Olson et al. evaluated cardiovascular effects of sildenafil during exercise in men with coronary artery disease and ED. They found that in men with stable coronary artery disease, sildenafil had no effect on symptoms, exercise duration, or the presence or extent of exercise induced ischemia, as assessed by exercise echocardiography. The incidence of any cardiovascular adverse event was 3.0% in the sildenafil group and 3.5% in the placebo group in clinical trial database of 18 placebo controlled studies. Long-term efficacy and safety of sildenafil were assessed recently in 1008 ED patients enrolled in four flexible dose (25–100 mg), open-label, 36- or 52-weeks extension studies. After 36 and 52 weeks, respectively, 92% and 89% of patients felt that treatment with sildenafil had improved their erections. The occurrence of treatment related cardiovascular adverse events, such as hypertension, tachycardia, and palpitation, was <1% and discontinuations due to treatment related adverse events were low (2%). In a prescription event monitoring study from England, questionnaires from 5601 sildenafil patients were analyzed using indirect standardization to compare mortality from ischemic heart disease in the cohort with that in the general population. No evidence of higher incidence of fatal MI or ischemic heart disease among men taking sildenafil was reported. In summary, long-term therapy does not diminish the safety or efficacy of sildenafil in patients with ED.

Optimizing PDE5 Inhibitor Therapy

Incorrect use of a PDE5 inhibitor may lead in treatment failure. Patient education is important in order to optimize treatment outcome and patient satisfaction. Patients should be advised that adequate sexual stimulation is needed to trigger the cascade of drug induced events leading to erection. Although the majority of patients respond to treatment after 1 or 2 doses of medication, some patients may need 7 or 8 attempts before they are successful. In the case of sildenafil, the drug should be taken on an empty stomach and excessive use of alcohol should be avoided. Addressing possible comorbid conditions, cultural issues, and confidently are also important in finding the optimal medical therapeutic solution for the ED patient and his partner. The patient's partner should be evaluated, since the partner's expectations, history, upbringing, religion, and culture can contribute to sexual and relationship difficulties.

Future Uses of PDE5 Inhibitors

PDE5 inhibitors are being investigated for a variety of other uses, including female sexual dysfunction, pulmonary hypertension, and diabetic gastropathy.

APOMORPHINE SL

Apomorphine is a D1/D2 dopamine receptor agonist from the aporphine (nonopiate) drug class. In rodents, apomorphine has been demonstrated to activate *c-fos* gene expression specifically in the paraventricular and supraoptic nuclei of the hypothalamus, resulting in stereotypical behavior of erection and yawning. In humans, apomorphine produces nonsexual erections that are enhanced by erotic stimulation without changes in libido; however, significant side effects, especially nausea, can occur. A sublingual formulation of apomorphine (apomorphine SL 2 and 4 mg) with a rapid onset of action (15–25 m) was shown to be efficacious in ED patients with controlled diabetes, hypertension, begin prostatic hypertrophy, or coronary vascular disease. Adverse effects included nausea, dizziness, and somnolence.

OTHER ORAL AGENTS

Substances that either enhance or block various neurotransmitters may act centrally to initiate erection or peripherally by relaxing corporate smooth muscle.

Yohimbine is a centrally acting a adrenergic blocker that is thought to act on the brain centers involved in libido and erection. A recent meta-analysis of 7 randomized, controlled trials in men with ED found yohimbine superior to placebo, especially for nonorganic ED. Side effects include palpitation, tremor, elevated blood pressure, and anxiety.

Peripherally acting agents include arginine and phentolamine. A double-blind, placebo-controlled, three-way crossover, randomized clinical trial compared the efficacy and safety of the combination of 6 g of L-arginine glutamate and 6 mg of yohimbine hydrochloride with that of 6 mg of yohimbine hydrochloride alone and that of placebo alone, for the treatment of ED in 45 patients. The study showed that the on-demand oral administration of the arginine-yohimbine combination was effective in improving erectile function in patients with mild to moderate ED. The differences in the Erectile Function Domain score of the International Index of Erectile Function (IIEF) between the combination group and the placebo group were statistically significant. Oral phentolamine has been proven to improve mild ED. It has not been approved by the FDA, although it is available in several South American countries.

Over the counter herbal agents such as ginseng and Ginkgo biloba have received considerable attention in the media as ED remedies. Their mechanism of action is unknown.

SECOND-LINE THERAPY

Intracavernosal Injection Therapy

The first clinically effective pharmacologic treatment for ED was intracavernosal papaverine injections. Papaverine is a nonspecific phosphodiesterase inhibitor that causes an increase in intracellular cAMP and cGMP, leading to corporal smooth muscle relaxation and penile tumescence. In the corpora cavernosa, prostaglandin E_1 (PGE_1) modulates adnyl cyclase to increase cAMP concentrations. This response leads to a decrease in intracellular free calcium, which induces smooth muscle relaxation of the arterioles and sinusoids of the corpora, resulting in erection. Intracavernous alprostadil relaxes arterial smooth muscle, producing vasodilation. It is effective in men who fail initial oral therapy with a PDE5 inhibitor, as demonstrated in an open label, multicenter study. When compared to intraurethral alprostadil, a randomized, crossover, multicenter study demonstrated that intracavernous therapy was more efficacious, better tolerated, and preferred over the transurethral application. A combination therapy using a mixture of papavaerine, phentolamine, and PGE_1 has become popular owing to its high efficacy, lower incidence of pain, and lower cost per dose. Many clinicians reserve the trimixture regimen for men with vascular ED who fail therapy with PGE_1 or the papaverine/phentolamine combination, or for patients who experience severe penile pain with PGE_1 injection. In addition to priapism, side effects of intracavernosal therapies include burning sensations, penile pain, penile hematoma, penile edema, and fibrotic changes within the tunica albuginea in the form of palpable nodules or plaques.

Intraurethral Therapy

Although the intracoroporal injection of vasoactive substances remains a very effective pharmacologic therapy for ED, long-term follow-up reveals a high dropout rate. Reasons for patient discontinuance include penile pain, high cost, concomitant illness, and fear of self-injection with a needle. Transurethral drug delivery, delivered retrogradely, allows the transfer of drugs from the urethra directly into the corpora cavernosa, enabled by vascular communications from the corpora spongiosa (urethra) to the cavernosal spaces. In initial studies, 66% of patients had a maximal penile erection response sufficient for intercourse. Another multicenter study has reported a success rate of 49%, including at home treatment. Although alprostadil is a vasodilatory agent, it has few systemic effects. The most common side effect of intraurethral alprostadil is local penile pain (29–41%). Other side effects include urethral bleeding (4–5.5%), dizziness (1.9–14%), and urinary tract infection (0–0.2%). Intraurethral alprostadil is contraindicated in men with acute and chronic urethritis or abnormal penile anatomy, proclivity for priapism, and conditions that make sexual activity unadvisable, such as acute MI.

Although oral medications have significantly improved ED therapy, there will always be patients who fail to respond to all nonsurgical therapies. For this group with severe, pharmacotherapy refractory end organ failure, penile prosthetic survey will continue to play an important role. Penile implants are indicated in patients with organic causes of ED, who have failed to respond to, do not tolerate, or are unwilling to consider conservative options. Patients with severe ED due to diabetes mellitus or radical pelvic survey have a high chance of failing oral therapy. Patients with Peyronie's disease associated with ED, severe penile fibrosis (e.g., after injection therapy), or conditions after priapism should also be considered for implantation of penile prostheses.

Several major long-term studies have demonstrated mechanical reliability and excellent overall patient satisfaction rates of >85% in patients with penile prostheses. Intraoperative problems of penile prosthetic surgery include cross dilation, proximal perforation of the corpora cavernosa, difficult distal dilatation and perforation, difficult closure of corporotomy, urethral trauma, and migration or malfunction of the prosthesis. Postoperative complications include infection, mechanical failure, penile curvature, corporal fibrosis, penile necrosis, erosion/migration, hypermobile/flaccid glans, perineal pain, and hematoma infection is one of the most serious possible complications of the procedure. The incidence varies from 0.7% to 16.7%, with most series finding infection rates in the range of 2–3%. Large implantation studies have described spinal cord injury and use of immunosuppressants as predisposing factors for infection. Despite the availability of less invasive therapeutic options in patients with ED, penile prosthesis survey has matured into an effective, and satisfying treatment modality.

CONCLUSION

The treatment of ED has changed significantly in the past few years. Revolutionary advances in oral treatment have replaced invasive modalities in many case. Furthermore, basic and clinical research have revealed new, interesting aspects of the physiology and pathology of this common, often undertreated disorder. Guidelines regarding the diagnostic and therapeutic approach for men with ED have been developed.

Because ED can be associated with serious medical conditions, a multidisciplinary approach using evidence based guidelines is key for thorough evaluation and effective treatment of the ED patient. New oral therapies are expected in the near future, and long-term studies will provide further data on efficacy, safety, and adverse events of the different compounds.

BIBLIOGRAPHY

1. Araujo AB, Durante R, Feldaman HA, et al. The relationship between depressive symptoms and male erectile dysfunction: cross sectional results from the Massachusetts Male Aging Study. Psychosom Med. 1998;60:458-65.
2. Araujo AB, Johannes CB, Feldman HA, et al. Relation between psychosocial risk factors and incident erectile dysfunction: prospective results from the Mass-achusetts Male Aging Study. Am J Epidemiol. 2000;152:533-41.
3. Arruda-Olson AM, Mahoney DW, Nehra A, et al. Cardiovascular effects of sildenafil during exercise in men with know or probabale coronary artery disease: a randomized crossover trial. JAMA. 2002;287:719-25.
4. Aytac IA, McKinlay JB, Krance RJ. The likely worldwide increase in erectile dysfunction between 1995 and 2025 and some possible policy consequences. BJU Int. 1999;84:50-56.
5. Benet AE, Melman A. The epidemiology of erectile dysfunction. Urol Clin North Am. 1995;22:699-709.
6. Berman JR, Berman LA, Lin H, et al. Effect of sildenafil on subjective and physiologic parameters of the female sexual response in women with sexual arousal disorder. J Sex Marital Ther. 2001;27:411-20.
7. Bhasim S. The does dependent effects of testosterone on sexual function and on muscle mass and function. Mayo Clin Proc 2000;75(Suppl.):70-5.
8. Blanker MH, Bohnen AM, Groeneveld FP. et al. Correlates for erectile and ejaculatory dysfunction in older Dutch men: a community based study. J Am Geriatr Soc. 2001;49: 436-42.
9. Boolell, Allen MJ, Ballard SA, et al. Sildenafil: an orally active type 5 cyclic GMP-specific phosphodiesterase inhibitor for the treatment of penile erectile dysfunction. Int J Impot Re-s. 1996;8:47-52.
10. Braun M, Wassmer G, Klotz T, et al. Epidemiology of erectile dysfunction: results of the 'Cologne Male Syrvey.' Int J Impot Res. 2000;12:305-11.
11. Burchardt M, Burchardt T, Anastasiadis AG, et al. Erectile dysfunction is a market for cardiovascular complications and psychological functioning in men with hypertension. Int J Impot Res. 2001;13:276-81.
12. Carani C, Scuteri A, Marrama P, Bancroft J. The effects of testosterone administration and visual erotic stimuli on nocturnal penile tumescence in normal men. Horm Behav. 1990;24:435-41.
13. Carson CC, Mulcahy JJ, Govier FE. Efficacy, safety and patient satisfaction outcomes of the AMS 700CS inflatable penile prosthesis: results of a long term multicenter study. AMS 700CX Study Group. J Urol. 2000;164:376-80.
14. Chan P, Korenman SG, Morley JE, Mooradian AD, et al. Secondary hypogonadism in older men: its relation to impotence. J Clin Endocrinol Metab. 1990;86:2391-94.
15. Chew KK, Earle CM, Stuc key BG, et al. Erectile dysfunction in general medicine practice: prevalence and clinical correlates. Int J Impot Res. 2000;12:41-5.
16. Chiang HS, Wu CC, Wen TC. 10 years of experience with penile prosthesis implantation in Taiwanese patients. Urol. 2000;163:476-80.
17. Choi YD, Choi YJ, Kim JH, Choi HK. Mechanical reliability of the AMS 700-CXM inflatable penile prosthesis for the treatment of male erectile dysfunction. J Urol. 2001;165:822-24.
18. Chun J, Carson CC. Physician patient dialogue and clinical evaluation of erectile dysfunction. Urol Clin North Am. 2001;28:249-58.
19. Ernst E, Pittler MH. Yohimbine for erectile dysfunction: a systematic review and meta analysis of randomized clinical trials. J Urol. 1998;159:433-6.
20. Evans C. The use of penile prostheses in the treatment of impotence. Br J Urol. 1998;81:591-8.
21. Feldaman HA, Godstein I, Hatzichristou DG, et al. Impotence and its medical and psychosocial correlates: results of the Massachusetts Male Aging Study. J Urol. 1994;151:54-61.
22. Goldmeier D, Keane FE, Carter P, et al. Prevalence of sexual dysfunction in heterosexual patients attending a central London genitourinary medicine clinic. Int J Sex Transm Dis. AIDS. 1997;8:303-6.
23. Goldstein I. The Working Group for the Study of Central Mechanisms in Erectile Dysfunction. Male sexual circuitry. Sci Am. 2000;283:70-5.
24. Grimm RH Jr, Grandits GA, Prineas RJ, et al. Long term effects on sexual function of five antihypertensive drugs and nutritional hygienic treatment in hypertensive men and women. Treatment of Mild Hypertension Study (TOMHS). Hypertension. 1997;29:8-14.
25. Guay AT, Bansal S, Heatley GJ. Effect of raising endogenous testosterone levels in impotent men with secondary hypogonadism: double blind placebo controlled trial with clomiphene citrate. J Clin Endocrino Metab. 1995;80:3546-52.
26. Guay AT, Perez JB, Jacobson J, Newton RA. Efficacy and safety of sildenafil citrate for treatment of erectile dysfunction in a population with associated organic risk factors. J Androl. 2001;22:793-97.
27. Hasler WL. Are things looking up for the treatment of gastroparesis? Sildenafil in animal models of diabetic gastropathy. Gastroenterology. 2001;120:576-8.
28. Hasler WL. Are things looking up for the treatment of gastroparesis? Sildenafil in animal models of diabetic gastropathy. Gastroenterology. 2001;120:576-8.
29. Hatzichristou DG. Sildenafil citrate: lessons learned from 3 years of clinical experience. Int J Impot Res. 2002;14(Suppl.1): 43-52.

30. Heim N. Sexual behaviour of castrated sex offenders. Arch Sex Behav. 1981;10:11-9.
31. Hellstrom WJ, Bennett AH, Gesundheit N, et al. A double blind, placebo controlled evaluation of the erectile response to transurethral alprostadil. Urology. 1996;48:851-6.
32. Jain S, Bhojwani A, Terry TR. The role of penile prosthetic survey in the modern management of erectile dysfunction. Postgrad Med J. 2000;76:22-25.
33. Jardin A, Wagner G, Khoury S, et al. Recommendations of the 1st International Consultation on Erectile Dysfunction. In: Jardin A, Wagner G, Khoury S, et al. (Eds). Erectile Dysfunction Plymouth:Plymbridge Distrib. 2000;pp. 711-26.
34. Johannes CB, Araujo AB, Feldaman HA, et al. Incidence of erectile dysfunction in men 40 to 69 years old: longitudinal results from the Massachusetts Male Aging study. J Urol. 2000;163:460-63.
35. Jonler M, Moon T, Brannan W, et al. The effect of age, ethnicity and geographical location in impotence and quality of life. Br J Uro-l. 1995;75:651-55.
36. Kaufman JM, Kaufman JL, Borges FD. Immediate salvage procedure for infected penile prosthesis. J Urol. 1998;159:816-8.
37. Kloner RA. Erectile dysfunction and cardiovascular risk factors. Hosp Pract. 2001;36:41-51.
38. Korenman SG, Morley JE, Mooradian AD, et al. Secondary hypogonadism in older men: its relation to impotence. J Clin Endocrinol Metab. 1990;71:963-69.
39. Laumann EO, Paik A, Rosen RC. Sexual dysfunction in the United States: prevalence and predictors. JAMA. 1999;281:537-44.
40. Laumann EO, Paik A, Rosen RC. Sexual dysfunction in the United States: prevalence and predictors. JAMA. 1999;281:537-44.
41. Lebret T, Herve JM, Gorny P, et al. Efficacy and safety of a novel combination of L-arginine glutamate and yohimbine hydrochloride: a new oral therapy for erectile dysfunction. Eur Urol. 2002;41:608-13.
42. Leugwattanakij S, Flynn V Jr, Hellstrom WJG. Intracavernosal injection and intraurethral therapy for erectile dysfunction. Urol Clin No Am. 2001;28:343-54.
43. Linet OI, Ogrinc FG. Efficacy and safety of intracavernosal alprostadil in men with erectile dysfunction. N Engl J Med. 1996;334:873-7.
44. Lue TF. Erectile dysfunction. N Engl J Med. 2000;342:1802-13.
45. Martin-Morales A, Sanchez-CruzJJ, Saenz de Tejada I, et al. Prevalence and independent risk factors for erectile dysfunction in Spain: results of the Epidemiological de la Disfunction Erectil Masculina Study. J Urol. 2001;166:569-75.
46. Mc Vary K, Carrier S, Wessells H. The Subcommittee on smoking and Erectile Dysfunction, Socioeconomic committee, Sexual Medicine Society of North America. Smoking and erectile dysfunction: evidence based analysis. J Urol. 2001;166:1624-32.
47. McKinley JB. The worldwide prevalence and epidemiology of erectile dysfunction. Int J Impot Res. 2000;4(Suppl.) 6-11.
48. Melis MR, Succu S, Argiolas A. Dopamine agonists increase nitric oxide production in the paraventricular nucleus of the hypothalamus: correlation in penile erection and yawning. Eur J Neurosci. 1996;8:2056-63.
49. Montorsi F, Rigatti P, Carmignani et al. AMS three-piece inflatable implants for erectile dysfunction: a long term multi institutional study in 200 consecutive patients. Eur Urol. 2000;37:50-5.
50. Morales A, Gingell C, Collins M, et al. Clinical safety of oral sildenafil citrate (VIAGRA) in the treatment fo erectile dysfunction. Int J Impot Res. 1998;10:69-73.
51. Morales A, Gingell C, Collins M, et al. Clinical safety of oral sindenafil citrate (VIAGRA) in the treatment of erectile dysfunction. Int J Impot Res. 1998;10:69-73.
52. Morales A, Johnston B, Heaton JP, London M. Testosterone supplementation for hypogonadal impotence: assessment of biochemical measures and therapeutic outcomes. J Urol. 1997;157:849-54.
53. Moyad MA, Hathaway S, Ni HS. Traditional Chinese medicine, acupuncture, and other alternative medicines for prostate cancer: an introduction and the need for more research. Semin. Urol Oncol. 1999;17:103-10.
54. Mulcahy JJ. Surgical management of penile prosthesis complications. Int J Impot Res. 2000;12(Suppl.):108-11.
55. Muller JE, Mittleman A, Maclure M, et al. Triggering myocardial infraction by sexual activity. Low absolute risk and prevention by regular physical exertion. Determinants of Mycardial Infarction Onset Study investigators. JAMA. 1996;275: 1405-9.
56. NIH Consensus Development Panel on Impotence. NIH Consensus Conference: Impotence. JAMA. 1992;270:83-90.
57. Padma-Nathan F, Giuliano F. Oral drug therapy for erectile dysfunction. Urol Clin No Am. 2001;28:321-34.
58. Padma-Nathan H, Hellstrom WJ, Kaiser FE, et al. Treatment of men with erectile dysfunction with transurethral alprostadil. Medicated Urethral System for Erectile (MUSE) Study Group. N Engl J Med. 1997;336:1-7.
59. Padma-Nathan H, Rosen RC, Shabsigh R, et al. CialisTM (IC351) provides prompt response and extended period of responsiveness of rthe treatment of men with erectile dysfunction (ED). J Urol. 2001;165:923 (Abstract).
60. Perelman MA. FSD partner issues: expanding sex therapy with sildenafil. J Sex Martal Ther. 2002;28(Suppl.):195-204.
61. Perelman MA. The impact of the new sexual pharmaceuticals on sex therapy. Curr Psychiatry Rep. 2001;3:195-201.
62. Porst H. IC351 (tidalafil, Cialis): update on clinical experience. Int J Impot-Res. 2002;14(Suppl. 1):57-64.
63. Porst H. The rationale for prostaglandin E1 in erectile failure: a survey of worldwide experience. J Urol. 1996;155:802-15.
64. Rajfer J, Aronson WJ, Bush PA, et al. Nitric oxide as a mediator of relaxation of the corpus cavernosum in response to nonadrenergic, noncholinerigic neurotransmission. N Engl J Med. 1992;326:90-4.

65. Riley A. The role of the partner in erectile dysfunction and its treatment. Int J Impot Res. 2002;14(Suppl-1):S105-S109.
66. Rosen RC, Lane RM, Menza . Effects of SSRIs on sexual function: a critical review. J Clin Psychopharmacol. 1999;19: 67-85.
67. Rosen RC. Psychogenic erectile dysfunction. Classification and management. Urol Clin North Am. 2001;28:269-78.
68. Sadovsky R, Miller T, Moskowitz M, Hackett G. Three year update of sildenafil citrate (Viagra) efficacy and safety. Int J Clin Pract. 2001;55:115-28.
69. Saenz de Tejada I. Anatomy, physiology and pathophysiology of ED. In: A Jardin, G Wagner, S Khoury, et al. (Eds). Erectile Dysfunction Plymouth, UK: Plymbridge Distrib. 2000;pp. 65-102.
70. Segraves RT, Bari M, Segraves K, Spirnak P. Effect of apomorphine on penile tumescence in men with psychogenic impotence. J Urol. 1991;145:1174-5.
71. Seidman SN, Roose SP, Menza MA, et al. Treatment of erectile dysfunction in men with depressive symptoms: results of a placebo controlled trial with sildenafil citrate. Am J Psychiatry. 2001;158:1623-30.
72. Shabsigh R Raymond JF, Olsson CA, et al. Androgen induction of DNA synthesis in the rat penis. Urology. 1998;52: 723-28.
73. Shabsigh R, Padma-Nathan H, Gittleman M, et al. Intracavernous alprostadil alfadex is more efficacious, better tolerated, and preferred over intraurethral alprostadil plus optional actis: a comparative, randomized, crossover, multicenter study. Urology. 2000;55:109-13.
74. Shabsigh R, Padma-Nathan H, Gittleman M. et al. Intracavernous alprostadil alfadex (EDEX/VIRDAL) is effective and safe in patients with erectile dysfunction after failing sildenafil (Viagra). Urology. 2000;55:477-80.
75. Shakir SA, Wilton LV, Boshier A, et al. Cardiovascular events in users of sildenafil: results from first phase of prescription event monitoring in England. BMJ. 2001;322:651-2.
76. Spector IP, Carey MP. Incidence and prevalence of sexual dysfunctions: a critical review of the empirical literature. Arch Sex Behav. 1990;19:389-408.
77. Stark S, Sachse R, Liedl T, et al. Vardenafil increases penile rigidity and tumescence in men with erectile dysfunction after a single oral dose. Eur Urol. 2001;40:181-90.
78. Steers W, Guay AT, Leriche A, et al. Assessment of the efficacy and safety of Viagra (sildenafil citrate) in men with erectile dysfunction during long-term treatment. Int J Impot Res. 2001;13:261-67.
79. Tiefer L, Schuetz Mueller D. Psychological issues in diagnosis and treatment of erectile disorders. Urol Clin North Am. 1995;22:767-73.
80. Usta MF, Erdogru T, Tefekli A, et al. Honeymoon impotence: psychogenic or organic in origin ? Urology. 2001;57:758-62.
81. Wallen K. Sex and context: hormones and primate sexual motivation. Horm Behav 2001;40:339-57.
82. Wang C, Swedloff RS, Iran Manesh A, et al. Transdermal testosterone gel improves sexual function, mood, muscle strength, and body composition parameters in hypogonadal men. Testosterone Gel Study Group. J Clin Endocrinal Metab. 2000;85:2839-53.
83. Wespes E, Amar E, Hatzichristou D, et al. Guidelines on erectile dysfunction. Eur Urol. 2002;41:1-5.
84. Wilson SK, Delk JR II. Inflatable penile implant infection: predisposing factors and treatment suggestions. J Urol. 1995;153:659-61.
85. Zhao L, Mason NA, Morrell NW, et al. Sildenafil inhibits hypoxia induced pulmonary hypertension. Circulation. 2001;104:424-28.

CHAPTER

67

Suicide in Young Men

Neena Bohra, NK Bohra

INTRODUCTION

Suicide risk has historically been described to increase with age, with older men being identified as the group at highest risk. However, in the 1970s in some high-income countries, suicide became increasingly common in young adults, especially in young men.[1] Although the focus of concerns is now shifting to middle-aged men, who are the group at highest risk in many countries, the lower life expectancy of working-age men remains a major problem.[2] In the context of the global financial crisis and the propagation of new suicide methods, such as charcoal burning, policy responses are needed. In this review we aim to provide an updated perspective on the burden of suicide in young men, specific risk factors, and evidence-based interventions, using published international evidence from 2000–2011. We chose to focus on data for men aged 19–30 years, which is the most common age group used for young men in population research.

HISTORICAL PATTERNS OF SUICIDE IN YOUNG MEN

Fifty years ago suicide accounted for 10% of deaths of people aged 10–24 years in countries in the Organisation for Economic Cooperation and Development (OECD) countries, against a backdrop of 2% or fewer globally.[3] By the mid-1980s suicide had become a leading cause of death in men aged 25–34 years in high-income countries, accounting for up to a third of mortality in young men.[1] Until this point elderly men had been regarded as the group at highest risk of death by suicide. However, between 1950 and 1999 the highest suicide rates shifted from elderly people towards middle-aged people (those aged 35–45 years), and in some countries to younger age groups (those aged 15–25 years).[4] Concerns about suicide at the turn of the 21st century related not only to WHO's report of a 60% global increase in recorded suicide mortality during the previous 45 years,[4] but specifically a 7% global increase in death by suicide in men from 1960–1999.[5] This increase was attributed to an increase in suicide in young men accompanied by a decrease in suicide in older men.[5] Also, suicide became increasingly more common in men than in women in people aged 15–29 years in Europe, the USA, Asia, Australasia, and some Latin American countries.[1] Comparison of 1970 and 1985–1986 WHO data show that although the highest rates were seen in men older than 60 years, suicide rates in men aged 15–29 years in Australia, New Zealand, Mexico, Canada, the USA, and Ireland had reached panty with (or in some cases surpassed) those in men aged 30–59 years.[1] These international patterns seemed to suggest that suicide, although a rare event, had become a serious problem in young men in some parts of the world.

GLOBAL PATTERNS IN SUICIDE IN YOUNG MEN

The number of suicide deaths in young men is probably substantially underestimated. Wide international variations in the quality of suicide data are explained by under-reporting and misclassification of suicide (partly related to legal and cultural factors), inconsistent conventions and discontinuities in the coding of deaths, and differing categories of death included in suicide analyses.[6] WHO has little suicide mortality data for many low-income and middle-income countries (LMICs), and a proportion of accidental death and undetermined death registrations internationally should be assumed to be suicide deaths. This potential is increased in young men, in view of their high rates of accidental death.[2,7]

Findings from studies done since 2000 show that suicide is among the top three to five causes of mortality in young men in most high-income and middle-income countries sampled,[2] and that accidental death remains the leading cause of death in young men for countries at all levels of economic development.[8] Analysis of mortality patterns in 44 countries across all continents (with data for 1997–2003) shows that suicide was among the top three causes of death for young men (aged 15–44 years) in 25 of those countries, and accidents were the leading cause of death in 38 countries.[2] Suicide accounts for a much greater proportion of total deaths in young men in high-income countries than it does for those in LMICs, but absolute rates of suicide in young men are about the same in high-income countries and LMICs, because of the greater contribution of violence and traffic accidents in LMICs.[8]

Temporal trends since the 1990s show a suicide rates in young men have decreased in countries such as Australia,[9] New Zealand,[10] China,[11] Thailand,[12] the USA,[13,14] Italy,[15] Austria,[16] the Czech Republic,[17,18] Scotland,[19] England and Wales,[20] and other western European countries.[17,21,22] Meanwhile, rates have risen in countries such as Brazil,[23] Singapore,[24] South Korea,[25] Lithuania,[26] Ireland,[27] and Northern Ireland.[28,29] However, this division is a potentially misleading oversimplification of a complex public health problem, involving a very different evolution of risk and protective factors in each country. The dichotomy also erroneously implies that suicide in young men is no longer a problem in countries where rates have fallen. Apparent decreases in suicide rates in young men at a national level mask rising suicide rates in young men at the sub-national level. This difference is apparent by region[30] and by remote residence in the UK,[30] by socioeconomic status in Australia,[30,31] and by ethnic origin in South Africa.[32,33] Additionally decreases in the number of suicides in young men in New Zealand are only moderate progress towards the low rates seen in the mid-1960s.[1,10,17]

The economic and social cost of suicide in younger age-groups is rarely reported, despite the greater contribution deaths in young people make to life-years lost. The cost of each young man dying by suicide in England has been valued as £1.67 million (2009 prices),[34] but has not yet been calculated in any LMICs. Despite their ageist bias, measures such as potential years of life lost (PYLL) are sensitive to changes in the demographic structure, revealing the wider effect of suicide even when the youth suicide rate is low or falling, In south India, local surveillance data show that suicides of men aged 15–29 years account for the greatest proportion of PYLL when compared with men in all other age groups, exceeded by only women aged 15–29 years.[35] Taiwanese national mortality statistics show that the greatest proportion of PYLL due to suicide is seen in men and women aged 25–39 years , although the greatest number of suicide deaths occur between the ages of 40 years and 59 years.[36]

Economic data also show that although media reports have tended to focus on suicides in young men, the burden of suicide in young women and middle-aged men are serious public health problems. In Taiwan, during the period 1997–2007 the greatest increases in PYLL were seen in men aged 40–59 years.[36] Other epidemiological studies show that although Sri Lanka and Russia rank highest internationally for suicide rates in young men,[37] the greatest total numbers of suicides in Sri Lanka are seen in men aged 41–55 years and women aged 21–45 years,[38] and in Russia are seen in men aged 45–54 years.[19]

The historical pattern of suicide risk increasing with age (but representing a decreasing proportion of total deaths) still applies in many LMICS and high-income countries in Europe, the Americas, Israel, India, and the far east.[7,10,11,24,35,40-52] International comparisons of the most up-to-date data from 44 high-income and middle-income countries show median suicide rates rising through successive age-groups:14.4 per 100000 men aged 15–24 years, 21.9 per 100000 men aged 25–34 years, and 24.7 per 100000 men aged 35–44 years.[2] Similarly, although an excess of suicide deaths in men holds true in young people globally,[2,50] the ratio is reversed for young women in two of the most populous countries: China[37,40,44,53-56] and India.[35,57,58] This occurrence is likely to be a consequence of high rates of suicide in women in rural areas,[54] but does draw attention to the importance of exploring sub-national trends and of comparing mortality indicators across all age groups in both sexes. Indeed, one of the most striking characteristics of the studies reviewed was the restricted range of mortality indicators presented and the substantial variability in the comparison groups used. Such restriction hampered an assessment of the suicide burden in young men compared with other groups. Future epidemiological studies will have greater use for policy makers, if they present national suicide rates in the context of other mortality indicators, to identify groups at highest risk of suicide.

SUICIDE METHODS USED BY YOUNG MEN

International variations in the frequency of suicide methods relate generally to local data availability. The WHO databank does not specify method-specific suicides, which means that global patterns in suicide methods have to be derived from individual countries' data.[21] Unfortunately, few studies disaggregate data by age group and sex. Hanging is the leading method in young men in Europe and Australia, and patterns of its use are closely associated with changes in suicide rates for this group,[9,19-21,59-62] Exceptions are New Zealand, where the proportion of men aged 15–24 years using hanging has been rising (despite concurrent falls in this group's suicide rate),[10] and Italy, where suicide rates for men aged 15–24 years and 25–44 years decreased from the mid-1990s despite a rise in hanging and jumping from a height in young men.[15] Japanese data for 1999 show that hanging accounted for 63% of suicides in men aged 20–39 years, and jumping from height accounted for 14%.[47] In the USA, however, firearms (followed by hanging or suffocation) is the most common method of suicide in men aged 15–24 years,[14] accounting for 55% of suicides in men aged 20–39 years; hanging accounts for 26%.[47] Patterns at the sub-national level show that young men in specific indigenous groups prefer specific suicide methods: firearms in the USA, hanging or asphyxiation in Canada, and hanging in Australia.[63]

In South Africa, hanging and firearms are the most-used methods in men aged 15–34 years.[33] High case-fatality ratios for intentional self-harm are seen in many Asian countries. For example, in China an estimated 82% of suicide deaths are clue to poisoning, although data are not specific to young men.[64] In India pesticide poisoning is the leading method of suicide for young men, accounting for 58% of suicides in men (and 25% in women) aged 21–30 years.[65] In Sri Lanka, acute poisoning (including pesticides) is the leading method used by men (and women) in all age groups.[38] New and highly lethal suicide methods have emerged in east Asia, including home-manufactured hydrogen sulphide[66] and other chemical suicide methods. Charcoal-burning has rapidly increased as a new method in Taiwan and Hong Kong, especially in men (and women) aged 24–39 years, with little evidence for substitution of older methods.[67] In Taiwan, charcoal-burning suicide rates during 2001–2006 rose most sharply in the age group 25–44 years, With an odds ratio of 1.3 (95% CI 1.2–1.4) for men dying by this method compared with women.[68] Overall it accounted for 34% of suicide deaths in Taiwan during 2006.[68] There are concerns about the proliferation of new media driving the popularity of new methods,[66] especially in young people.[66,69]

INDIVIDUAL–LEVEL RISK FACTORS FOR SUICIDAL IN YOUNG MEN

Several suicide risk factors that are well established in the wider population have not been investigated specifically in relation to young men.[71-75] The absence of such investigation is because large sample sizes of young men are needed to achieve adequate statistical power, and risk factors cannot necessarily be inferred from wider studies that treat age group and sex as separate variables. A meta-analysis of international psychological autopsy studies, in which men had a mean age of 28.5 years (SD 12.8), showed higher odds of childhood disorders (odds ratio=4.95 [95% CI 2.7 to 9.3), substance-related problems (3.58 [2.8–4.6]), and personality disorders (2.01 [1.4–3.0]) for suicides in men, but lower odds of any affective disorders (0.6 [0.5–0.8]).[70]

The relative risk of suicide in men younger than 35 years with a psychiatric disorder has been estimated from meta-analysis of studies in high-income and middle-income countries, and ranked as follows: schizophrenia (relative risk = 13.66 [95% CI 5.18–36.04]), affective disorders (9.26 [4.99–17.19]), substance use disorders (5.09 [2.81–9.25]), personality disorders (4.14 [2.81–9.25]), and anxiety disorders (3.31 [1.53–7.18]).[72] Population attributable risk (PAR) of suicide for each psychiatric disorder (but for men of all ages) show slightly different rankings: 26% for affective disorder, 19% for substance abuse, 15% for personality disorder 7% for schizophrenia, and 5% for anxiety disorder.[72] This conveys the public health importance of addressing untreated depression, although psychiatric illness, particularly depression, has been suggested to make a greater contribution to suicide risk with increasing age, especially in individuals older than 45 years.[73] International studies of help-seeking patterns suggest that male sex and age below 45 years predict lower help-seeking in depression.[74]

Only one study has investigated risk of suicide following self-harm, finding that in England men aged 10–24 years are at lower risk of suicide following self-harm than are older men after self-harm.[73] Ecological data describe the effect of population-level alcohol consumption on suicide rates in men aged 15–29 years, finding that (after controlling for macro-socioeconomic variables) national alcohol consumption was not related to suicide rates in young men.[22] However, an association absent at an aggregate level might exist at the individual level.

Evidence that homosexuality is a ns actor for suicide in men in men derives from Danish data showing that men in same-sex, legalized partnerships had a suicide risk nearly eight times greater than men in heterosexual marriages, and double that of men who had never married.[76] Studies specific to young men who have sex with men are needed, notwithstanding difficulties in establishing sexual orientation. In the wider population, specific occupational groups (doctors, farmers) and unemployed individuals are cited as higher-risk groups for suicide. A study of doctors in England and Wales recorded suicide rates for male doctors in all age groups to be two-thirds that of men in the general population, but showed increased rates in their female counterparts.[77]Although suicide risk in young male farmers is often mentioned in newspaper reports from the Indian subcontinent and suicide risk in young male farmers is often mentioned in newspaper reports from the Indian subcontinent and West Africa, no quantitative epidemiological studies have addressed this group. Australian studies, however, show high rates of suicide in young male agricultural workers.[78,79] In the USA, Britain, and France, there are conflicting findings in relation to the risk of suicide in young men in the army depending on which age groupings are assessed.[80-82] Data from the USA show an increased risk in male army veterans aged 18–34 years, with suicide rates twice that of the general population,[80] whereas data from the UK show a reduced suicide risk for men in the armed forces in all age groups older than 20 years.[81] In France, men in the army have a reduced risk of suicide compared with the general population, but the suicide incidence rate ratio for those younger than 25 years is twice that for men aged 25–29 years.[82]

Ethnic origin and indigenous group also predict suicide risk in young men. Worldwide, the highest suicide rates in young men are seen in white men in South Africa;[32,33] first-generation Eastern European and Caribbean immigrants to England and Wales,[83] indigenous Sami in Arctic Norway,[84] Maori men aged 15–34 years in New Zealand,[10] indigenous men aged 15–34 years in Australia,[63,85,86] Inuit men aged 15–24 years in Canada,[87] and Native American men aged 15–24 years[88] and 20–39 years[47] in the USA. There is also evidence suggesting that young Aboriginal men in Canada[89] and Ethiopian immigrants to Israel[90] might be high-risk groups although more data specific to this sex and age group are needed. Interpretation of all studies of ethnic minority groups should take into account the possible under-estimation of youth suicide owing to differential misclassification.[63,88,91] Although suicide rates might be higher in some minority ethnic groups; this minority status could actually be protective in neighborhoods with large minority populations. This so-called relative misery hypothesis has been used to explain higher suicide rates in young Aborigines and Torres Strait Islanders compared to their white peers in mainstream Australian schools.[63]

Rural or remote residence is shown to increase the risk of suicide in young men in Australia,[92-95] China,[92] Denmark,[96] Austria,[97] and England and Wales.[30,98] The overall decline in suicide rates for Australian men aged 20–34 years (from 40 per 100000 in 1997–98 to 20 per 100000 in 2003[9]) masks the continued rise in suicide rates in young men in remote areas[93] as well as in lower socioeconomic groups.[31] Explanations relate to the migration of healthy workers to cities, and the increasing economic disparity between men in rural and urban areas. In relation to marital status, evidence from high-income countries shows that marital status in men interacts with age, such that being separated increases suicide risk in young men to a greater extent than in older men.[99] In high-income countries, young men who are divorced,[99] have never married[100] or are widowed[101-103] are at higher risk of suicide than if married. Good academic performance in school has been shown to protect against suicide in young men (but not young women) in Swedish record linkage studies.[104]

POPULATION-LEVEL EFFECTS ON SUICIDE IN YOUNG MEN

Cultural and socioeconomic variables, such as rising unemployment, are suggested as area-level effects on suicide in young men, and are likely to mediate individual-level risk factors.[105-114] A pan-European study has shown a nonsignificant negative association between a 1% rise in unemployment and suicide in men aged 15–29 years, but a significant positive association for women of the same age.[105] At the national level, a positive association between unemployment and suicide applies to young men in England and Wales,[106] Ireland,[106] and Asia.[108] In Australia, this positive association seems to be more pronounced in younger men than it is in oldermen,[109] as does the association between lower socioeconomic status and suicide risk.[110] In England, social deprivation is positively associated with suicide risk for men aged 10–29 years.[11] Evidence from England and Wales suggests that suicide risk for men age 15–44 years is highest in the most socially fragmented areas,[112,113] but this effect might be more pronounced in men aged 45–64 years.[114] Such studies might not be generalizable to low-income countries.

Period effects in the past three decades likely to have affected suicide rates in young men internationally include war, natural disasters, the introduction of new means of suicide,[67,68] and new substances of misuse, policies restricting specific means of suicide, specific youth suicide prevention policies, the expansion of new media (and its effect on suicide contagion), and economic downturn. Cohort effects affecting suicide rates in young men will derive from the relative size of that birth cohort in each country; exposure to childhood trauma (e.g. civil war); psychotropic prescribing patterns; and the effect of the media (on young people's attitudes to the social acceptability of suicide, in raising their expectations unrealistically and affecting preference for specific suicide methods). The media has been implicated in the social modeling of suicidal behavior in young people and the spread of new means of suicide. In Taiwan, for example, extensive news reporting of a 59-year-old male celebrity's suicide was associated with an increase in suicides in men younger 35 years.[115]

INTERVENTIONS TO REDUCE SUICIDES IN YOUNG MEN

As with risk factor studies, research specifically assessing the effect of interventions on young men is restricted. Population-based strategies with the potential to reduce suicides in young men are those that reduce the proportion of young men with suicide risk factors, and those that reduce the availability of methods often used by this group. Unfortunately, the methods common in high-income countries (especially hanging) are also the hardest to restrict.[73] Nonetheless, a decrease in poisoning deaths, predominantly in men and younger age groups, followed the withdrawal of co- proxamol in Scotland.[116] Legislation to restrict Firearms has not been associated with a reduction in firearm suicides in young men in the USA,[117] but is associated with statistically significant declines in Canadian men aged 15–34 years.[118] Falls in firearm suicides in young Australian men, and concurrent increases in suicides by hanging in this age group, preceded firearm legislation, suggesting cultural explanations for method substitution rather than solely the effects of the intervention.[119] Controls on pesticide imports to Sri Lanka have been followed by substantial declines in suicide in men aged 17–35 years.[120]

Untreated depression is another target for intervention, especially in view of the high PAR associated with affective disorder.[72] However, the evidence for antidepressant treatment remains mixed as to the appropriate balance of risks in young people. A Swedish ecological study covering 1977–1987 detected an association between increased sales of selective serotonin reuptake inhibitors (SSRIs) and a decrease in suicide rates in both men and women, with the largest reduction in 15–44 year-old individuals of both sexes.[121] A US cohort study measuring nonfatal suicide attempts in a veterans sample (where only 8% were women) recorded a protective effect of SSRI monotherapy compared with no antidepressant, with the caveat that these results might not hold for completed suicides.[122] The US Food and Drug Administration (FDA) has published a meta-analysis of antidepressant trials showing a nonsignificantly increased risk of suicide in adults under 25 years prescribed antidepressants for any indication.[123]

Labeling of antidepressants in the USA has been amended to draw attention to the strong age-related risk in individuals younger than 25 years, which seems to be neutralized between the ages of 25 years and 64 years.[123]

Young men feature as a high-risk group in many nations' suicide prevention strategies, but evidence is scarce as to which interventions reduce this risk. The 1995–1997 Australian National Youth Suicide Prevention Strategy (NYSPS) sought to reduce risk factors in young men through a comprehensive set of targeted and population—level interventions, but a controlled study showed no effect on suicide rates in men (or women) aged 20–34 years.[124] Novel targeted approaches are based on the theoretical effect of efforts to change young men's help-seeking behavior, often involving sporting role models and outreach to sports clubs, pubs, and workplaces. Their effect on suicides in the target group has not yet been assessed. There is also potential for media guidelines on suicide reporting and supportive internet sites to reduce suicides in young men, but se again will need specific investigation.

IMPROVING RESPONSIVENESS TO EMERGING RISK GROUPS

An improved understanding of how the burden of suicide compares between age groups for each sex can be provided by studies that define narrower and more consistent age ranges than has previously been done, especially in view of the different suicide patterns seen in adolescents and young adults.[10] WHO might consider establishing minimum standards on the range of descriptive statistics presented in published studies for every group investigated: suicide rates (both crude and age-adjusted), absolute numbers of suicides, proportional mortality ratios (PMRs), the ranking of suicide as a cause of death, and PYLL. This multidimensional picture would improve research cost-effectiveness and allow a more responsive approach to suicide prevention, in view of the fact that high-risk groups are constantly evolving.

Other areas for improving future research on the burden of suicide in any group include the avoidance of presenting confounded associations and group-level associations. Studies investigating risk factors would be more useful if they explored associations in specific groups, where sufficient power permitted this. Case control studies are probably the best means of investigating rare outcomes such as suicide but they will always be subject to residual confounding. Cohort studies that quantify the PAR of specific risk factors for completed suicide in different age groups and sexes in local settings are likely to be most helpful in planning interventions. WHO might also consider commissioning rapid analysis of its datasets to reduce the substantial time lag between suicide data collection and its translation into evidence based preventive interventions.

Panel 1: Evidence-based risk factors for suicide in young men

Individual-level
- Psychiatric disorder
- Substance misuse
- Occupational group (agricultural workers in Australia; army veterans in the USA)
- Ethnicity and indigenous group
- Rural or remote residence (in Australia, China, Denmark, Austria, England, and Wales)
- Lower socioeconomic status (Australia)
- *Single marital status*: Separated, divorced, never married, or widowed (high-income countries)

Population-level
- Unemployment (England and Wales, Ireland, Asia, Australia)
- Social deprivation and social fragmentation (England and Wales)
- Media influences, e.g. reporting of suicides (Taiwan)

CONCLUSION

In this review, we have drawn attention to wide socio-geographic variations in the epidemiology of suicide, and a rapidly changing picture in relation to the direction of temporal trends. In countries where decreases in suicides in young men have been seen, studies investigating suicide risk at a sub-national level have shown rates to be rising in specific sub-groups defined by geography, ethnic origin, and socioeconomic status,[30-33] Comparisons of suicide rates in young men at the national level might therefore be misleading, conveying little of the variations apparent at a local level. Several studies suggest that in some parts of the world suicides in middle-aged men or young women could outnumber those in young men.[37] Suicide risk factors specific to young men (Panel 1) include psychiatric illness, substance misuse, ethnic origin, lower socioeconomic status, rural residence, and single marital status. Population-level factors shown to affect rates of suicide in young men in specified parts of the world include unemployment, social deprivation, and the media's reporting of suicide. This review underlines the importance of the development of regionally and nationally tailored approaches to reducing suicide, and remaining abreast of key mortality indicators to identify he groups at highest risk of premature death.

REFERENCES

1. Diekstra RFW. Suicide and the attempted suicide: an international perspective. Arm Psychiatr Scand. 1939;80:1-24.
2. White A, Holmes M. Patterns of mortality across 44 countries among men and women aged 15–44 years. J Mens Health. 2006;3:139-51.
3. Viner RM, Coffey C, Mathers C, et al. 50-year mortality trends in children and young people: a study of 50 low-income, middle-income, and high-income countries. Lancet. 2002;377:1162-74.

4. WHO. WHO multisite Interventions Study on Suicidal Behaviours-SUPRE-MISS: protocol of SUPRE-MISS. Geneva: World Health Organization, 2002.
5. De Leo D, Evans R. International suicide rates and prevention strategies. Cambridge. MA: Hogrefe and Huber, 2004.
6. Jacob KS, Sharan P, Mirza I, et al. Mental health systems in countries: where are we now? Lancet. 2007;370:1061-77.
7. Pritchard C, Hean S. Suicide and undetermined deaths among youths and young adults in Latin America: comparison with the 10 major developed countries: a source of hidden suicides? Crisis. 2008;29:145-53.
8. Patton GC, Coffey C, Sawyer S, et al. Global patterns of mortality in young people: a systematic analysis of population health data. Lancet. 2009;374:881-92.
9. Morrell S, Page AN, Taylor RJ. The decline in Australian young male suicide. Soc Sci Med. 2007;64:747-54.
10. Beautrais A. Suicide in New Zealand l: time trends and epidemiology. NZ Med J. 2003;116: U460.
11. Yip PSF, Liu KY, Hu J, Song XM. Suicide rates in China during a decade of rapid social changes. Soc Psychiatry Psychiatr Epidemiol. 2005;40:792-98.
12. Lotrakul M. Suicide in Thailand during the period 1998–2003. Psychiatry Clin Neurosci. 2006;60:90-5.
13. Hu G, Wilcox HC, Wissow L, Baker SP. Mid-life suicide: an increasing problem in US whites, 1999-2005. Am J Prev Med. 2008;35:589-93.
14. Lubell KM, Kegler SR, Crosby AE, Karch D. Suicide trends among youths and young adults aged 10-24 years-United States, 1990-2004. MMWR Morb Mortal Wkly Rep. 2007;56: 905-9.
15. Vichi M, Masocco M, Pompili M, Lester D, Tatarelli R, Vanacore N. Suicide mortality in Italy from 1980 to 2002. Psychiatry Res. 2010;175:89-97.
16. Etzersdorfer E, Voracek M, Kapusta N, Sonneck G. Epidemiology of suicide in Austria 1990–2000: general decrease, but increased suicide risk for old men. Wiener Klinischc Wochenschrift. 2005;117:31-5.
17. Levi F, La C, Lucchini F, et al. Trends in mortality from suicide, 1965-99. Acta Psychiatrica Scandinavian. 2003;108:341-9.
18. Dzurova D, Vevera J, Motlowa L, Dragomirecka E. Analysis of parasuicide, psychiatric care and completed suicides, implications for intervention strategy (Czech Republic, 1996-2000). Int J Public Health. 2008;53:139-49.
19. Stark C, Stockton D, Henderson R. Reduction in young male suicide in Scotland. BMC Public Health. 2008:8:49.
20. Biddle L, Brock A, Brookes ST, Gunnell D. Suicide rates in young men in England and Wales in the list century: time trend study. BMJ. 2008;336:539-42.
21. Varnik A, Kolves K, Allik J, et al. Gender issues in suicide rates, trends and methods among youths aged 15–24 in 15 European countries. J Affect Disord. 2009;113:216-26.
22. Innamorati M, Lester D, Amore M, Girardi P, Tatarelli R, Pompili M. Alcohol consumption predicts the EU suicide rates in young women aged 15–29 years but not in men: analysis of trends and differences among early and new EU countries since 2004. Alcohol. 2010;44:463-9.
23. de Mello-Santos C, Bertolote JM, Wang YP. Epidemiology of suicide in Brazil (1980–2000): Characterization of age and gender rates of suicide. Revista Brasileira de Psiquiatria. 2005;27:131-4.
24. Ng DW Lau G. Suicide trends in Singapore: two decades down the road. Med Sci Law. 2003;43:141-7.
25. Kwon JW, Chun H, Cho SI. A closer look at the increase in suicide rates in South Korea from 1936–2005, BMC Public Health. 2009;9:72.
26. Tamosiunas A, Reklaitiene R, Virviciute D, Sopagiene D. Trends in suicide in a Lithuanian urban population over the period 1984–2003. BMC Public Health. 2006;6:184.
27. Walsh B, Walsh D. Suicide in Ireland: the influence of alcohol and unemployment. Econ Soc Rev (Irel). 2011;42:27-47.
28. Largey M, Kelly CB, Stevenson M. A study of suicide rates in Northern Ireland 1984–2002. Ulster Med J. 2009;78:16-20.
29. Northern Ireland Statistics and Research Agency. Statistical bulletin: deaths in Northern Ireland (2010). *http://www,nisra.gov.uk/archive/demography/publicatinns/births_deaths/deaths_2010. pdf* (accessed Sept 30, 2013).
30. Grinnell D, Wheeler B, Chang SS. Thomas B, Sterne JAC, Dorling D. Changes in the geography of suicide in young men: England and Wales 1981–2005. J Epidemiol Community Health. 2012;6:536-43.
31. Page A, Morrell S, Taylor R, Carter G, Dudley M. Divergent trends in suicide by socio-economic status in Australia. Soc Psychiatry Psychiatr Epidemiol. 2006;41;911-7.
32. Burrows S, Laflamme L. Living circumstances of suicide mortality in a South African city: an ecological study of differences across race groups and sexes. Suicide Life Threat Behav. 2005;35:592-603.
33. Burrows S, Vaez M, Laflamme L. Sex-specific suicide mortality in the South African urban context: the role of age, race, and geographical location. Scand J Public Health. 2007;35:133-9.
34. Knapp M, McDaid D, Parsonage M. Mental health promotion and prevention: the economic case. London UK: Personal Social Services Research Unit, London School of Economics and Political Science, 2011.
35. Bose A, Konradsen F, John J, Suganthy P, Muliyil J, Abraham S. Mortality rate and years of life lost from unintentional injury and suicide in South India. Trop Med Int Health. 2006;11:1553-6.
36. Law C-K, Yip P, Chen Y-Y. The economic and potential years of life lost from suicide in Taiwan, 1997–2007. Crisis. 2011;32:152-9.
37. Apter A, Bursztein C, Bertolote JM, Fleischmann A. Wasserman D. Suicide on all the continents in the young. In: Wasserman D, Wasserman C (Eds). Oxford Textbook of Suicidology and Suicide Prevention: a global perspective. Oxford: OUP; 2009. pp.621-8.
38. Jayasinghe NRA, Faster JH. Delibrate self-harm/poisoning, suicide trends: the link to increased alcohol consumption in Sri Lanka. Arch Suicide Res. 2011;15:223-37.

39. Sakharova O, Gurovich l, Wahlbeck K. Mental health indicators in Russia. A study of the availability of European indicators for the MINDFUL project. Helsinki, Finland: STAKES, 2007.
40. Qin P, Mortensen PB. Specific characteristics of suicide in China. ACM Psychiatrica Scandinavina. 2001;103:117-21.
41. Prasad J, Abraham VJ, Minz S, et al. Rates and factors associated with suicide in Kaniyambadi Block, Tamil Nadu, South India, 2000–2002. Int J Soc Psychiatry. 2006;52:65-71.
42. Kapusta ND, Sonneck G. Suicides of men in Austria: an epidemiological analysis over a 30-year period. J Mans Health. 2004;1:197-202.
43. Zacharakis CA, Hadjivassilis V, Madianos MG, Papadimitriou GN. Stefanis CN. Suicide in Cyprus 1988-1999. Eur Psychiatry. 2005;20:110-14.
44. Yip PSF. An epidemiological profile of suicides in Beijing, China, Suicide Life Threat Behav. 2001;31:62-70.
45. Hong JP, Bae MJ, Suh T. Epidemiology of suicide in Korea. Psychiatry Invstig. 2006;3:7-14.
46. lm JS, Choi SH, Hong D, Seo HJ, Park S, Hong JP. Proximal risk factors and suicide methods among suicide completers from national suicide mortality data 2004–2006 in Korea. Compr Psychiatry. 2011;52:231-7.
47. OJima T, Nakamura Y, Detels R. Comparative study about methods of suicide between Japan and the United States. J Epidemiol. 2004;14:187-92.
48. Rodrigues NC, Werneck GL. Age-period-cohort analysis of suicide rates in Rio de Janeiro, Brazil, 1979–1998. Soc Psychiatry Psychiatr Epidemiol. 2005;40:192-6.
49. Lubin G, Glasser S, Boyko V, Barell V. Epidemiology of suicide in Israel: a nationwide population study. Soc Psychiatry Psychiatr Epidemiol. 2001;36:123-7.
50. Pritchard C, Amanullah S. An analysis of suicide and undetermined deaths in 17 predominantly Is LMIC countries contrasted with the UK. Psychol Med. 2007;37:421-30.
51. Centers for Disease Control and Prevention Web-based Injury Statistics Query and Reporting System (WISQARS). Suicide: facts at a glance. *http://www.cdc.gov/Violenceprevention/suicide/ statistics/aag.html* (accessed Sept 30, 2011).
52. Hempstead K. The geography of self-injury: spatial patterns in attempted and completed suicide. Soc Sci Med. 2006;62: 3186-96.
53. Schmidtke A, Weinacker B, Apter A, et al. Suicide rates in the world: update, Arch Suicide Res. 1999;5:81-89.
54. Yip PSF, Liu KY. The ecological fallacy and the gender ratio of suicide in China. Br J Psychiatry. 2006;189:465-6.
55. Phillips MR, Li X, Zhang Y. Suicide rates in China, 1995–99. Lancet. 2002;359:835-40.
56. Law S, Liu P. Suicide in China: unique demographic patterns and relationship to depressive disorder: Curr Psychiatry Rep. 2008;10:80-86.
57. Joseph A. Abraham S, Muliyil JP, et al. Evaluation of suicide rates in rural India using Verbal autopsies, 1994–99. BMJ. 2003;326:1121-2.
58. Soman CR, Safrai S, Kutty V, Vijayakumar K, Ajayan K. Suicide in South India: a community-based study in Kerala. Indian J Psychiatry. 2009;51:261-4.
59. Gunnell D, Wehner H, Frankel S. Sex differences in suicide trends in England and Wales. Lancet. 1999;353:556-7.
60. Stark C, Hopkins P, Gibbs D, Rapson T, Belbin A, Hay A. Trends in suicide in Scotland 1981–1999: age, method and geography, BMC Public Health. 2004.pp.4-49.
61. Beautrais AL. Methods of youth suicide in New Zealand: trends and implications for prevention. Aust NZJ Psychiatry. 2000;34:413-9.
62. Starkuviene S, Kalediene R, Petrauskiene J. Epidemic of suicide by hanging in Lithuania: does socio-demographic status matter? Public Health. 2006;120:769-75.
63. Hunter E, Harvey D. Indigenous suicide in Australia, New Zealand, Canada, and the United States. Emerg Med (Fremantle). 2002:14:14-23.
64. Li XY, Phillips MR. Zhang YP, Xu D, Yang GH. Risk factors for suicide in China s youth: a case-control study. Psychol Med. 2008;38:397-406.
65. Sharma BR. Sharma V, Harish D, Vij K. Suicides in Northern India: causes, methods used and prevention. Med Sci Law. 2003;43:221-9.
66. Morii D, Miyagatani Y, Nakamae N, Murao M, Taniyama K. Japanese experience of hydrogen sulfide: the suicide craze in 2008. J Occup Med Toxicol. 2010;5:28.
67. Liu KY, Beautrais A, Caine E, et al. Charcoal burning suicides in Hong Kong and urban Taiwan: an illustration of the impact of a novel suicide method on overall regional rates. J Epidemiol Community Health. 2007;61:248-54.
68. Pan YJ, Liao SC, Lee MB. Suicide by charcoal burning in Taiwan, 1995-2006. J Affect Disord. 2010;120:254-52.
69. Chen Y-Y, Liao S-F, Teng P-R, et al. The impact of media reporting of the suicide of a singer on suicide rates in Taiwan. Soc Psychiatry Psychaitr Epidemiol. 2012;47:215-21.
70. Arsenault-Lapierre G, Kim C, Turecki G. Psychiatric diagnoses in 3275 suicides: a meta-analysis. BMC Psychiatry. 2004;4:37.
71. Kim C, Lesage A, Seguin M, et al. Patterns of co-morbidity in male suicide completers. Psychol Med. 2003;33:1299-309.
72. Li Z, Page A, Martin G, Taylor R. Attributable risk of psychiatric and socio-economic factors for suicide from individual-level, population-based studies: a systematic review. Soc Sci Med. 2004;72:608-16.
73. Beautrais A. Suicide in New Zealand Il: a review of risk factors and prevention. NZ Med J. 2003;116:461.
74. Moller-Leimkuhler A-M. Barriers to help-seeking by men: a review of sociocultural and clinical literature with particular reference to depression. J Affect Disord. 2002:71:1-9.
75. Hawton K, Zahl D, Weatherll R. Suicide following deliberate self-harm: long-term follow-up of patients who presented to a general hospital. Br J Psychiatry. 2003;182:537-42.
76. Mathy R, Cochran S, Olsen J, Mays V. The association between relationship markers of sexual orientation and suicide:

Denmark, 1990–2001. Soc Psychiatry Psychiatr Epidemol. 2011;46:111-7.

77. Hawton K, Chements A, Sakarovitch C, Simkin S, Deeks JJ. Suicide in doctors: a study of risk according to gender: seniority and specialty in medical practitioners in England and Wales, 1979–1995. J Epidemiol Community Health. 2001;55:296-301.
78. Page AN, Fragar LJ. Suicide in Australian farming, 1988–1992. Aust NZJ Psychiatry. 2002;36:81.
79. Andersen K, Hawgood J, Klieve H, Kolves K, De D. Suicide in selected occupations in Queensland: evidence from the State suicide register. Aus NZJ psychiatry. 2010;44:243-50.
80. Kaplan MS, McFarland BH, Huguet N. Firearm suicide among veterans in the general population: Findings from the national violent death reporting system. J Trauma. 2009;67:503-7.
81. Fear NT, Ward VR, Harrison K, Davison L, Williamson S, Blatchley NF. Suicide among male regular UK Armed Forces personnel, 1984–2007. Occup Environ Med. 2009;66:438-41.
82. Desjeux G, Labarere J, Galoisy-Guibal L, Ecochard R. Suicide in the French armed forces. Eur J Epidemiol. 2004:19:823-9.
83. Shah A, Lindesay J, Dennis M. Suicides by country of birth groupings in England and Wales: age-associated trends and standardised mortality ratios. Sac Psychiatry Psychiatr Epidemiol. 2011;46:197-206.
84. Silviken A, Haldorsen T, Kvernmo S. Suicide among indigenous Sami in Arctic Norway 1970–1998. Eur J Epidemiol. 2006;21:707-13.
85. Cantor C, Neulinger K. The epidemiology of suicide and attempted suicide among young Australians. Aust NZJ Psychiatry. 2000;34:370-88.
86. Krysinska K, Martin G, Sheehan N. Identity voice, place: suicide prevention for indigenous australians: a social and emotional wellbeing approach. Queensland: Centre for Suicide Prevention Studies. The University of Queensland, 2009.
87. Boothroyd LJ, Kirmayer LJ, Spreng S, Malus M, Hodgins S. Completed suicides among the Inuit of northern Quebec, 1982–1996: a case-control study. CMAJ. 2001;165:749-55.
88. EchoiHawk M. Suicide prevention efforts in one area of Indian Health Service, USA. Arch Suicide Res. 2006;10:169-76.
89. Kirmayer L, Brass GM, Holtonli T, Paul K, Simpson C, Tait C. Suicide among aboriginal people in Canada, Ottawa, Canada: Aboriginal Healing Foundation, 2007.
90. Shoval G, Schoen G, Vardi N, Zalsman G. Suicide in Ethiopian immigrants in Israel: a case for study of the genetic-environmental relation in suicide. Arch Suicide Res. 2007;11:247-53.
91. Rockett IR, Wang S, Stack S, et al. Race/ethnicity and potential suicide misclassification: window on a minority suicide paradox? BMC Psychiatry. 2010;10:35.
92. Yip PSF, Callanan C, Yuen HP, Urban/rural and gender differentials in suicide rates: east and west. J Affect Disard. 2000;57:99-106.
93. Page A, Morrell S, Taylor R, Dudley M, Carter G. Further increases in rural suicide in young Australian adults: secular trends. 1979–2003. Soc Sci Med. 2007;65:442-54.
94. Taylor R, Page A, Morrell S, Harrison J, Carter G. Social and psychiatric influences on urban-rural differentials in Australian suicide. Suicide Life Threat Behav. 2005;35: 277-90.
95. Wilkinson D, Gunnell D. Youth suicide trends in Australian metropolitan and non-metropolitan areas, 1988–1997. Am NZJ Psychiatry. 2000;34:822-8.
96. Qin P. Suicide risk in relation to level of urbanicity: a population-based linkage study. Int J Epidemiol. 2005;34:846-52.
97. Kapusta ND, Zorman A, Etzersdorfer E, Ponocny-Seliger E, Jandl-lager E, Sonneck G. Rural-urban differences in Austrian suicides. Soc Psychiatry Psychiatr Epidemiol. 2008;43:311-8.
98. Middleton N, Gunnell D, Frankel S, Whitley E, Dorling D. Urban-rural differences in suicide trends in young adults: England and Wales, 1981–1998. Soc Sci Med. 2003;57:1183-95.
99. Wyder M, Ward P, De D. Separation as a suicide risk factor. J Affect Disord. 2009;116:208-13.
100. Masocco M, Pompili M, Vichi M, Vanacore N, Lester D, Tatarelli R. Suicide and marital status in Italy. Psychiatr Q. 2008;79:275-85.
101. Luoma JB, Pearson JL. Suicide and marital status in the United States, 1991–1996: is widowhood a risk factor? Am J Public Health. 2002;92:1518-23.
102. Yip PS, Thorburn J. Marital status and the risk of suicide: experience from England and Wales, 1982–1996. Psychol Rap. 2004;94:401-7.
103. Griffiths C, Ladva G, Brock A, Baker A. Trends in suicide by marital status in England and Wales. 1982–2005. Health Stat Q. 2008;37:8-14.
104. Gunnell D, Lofving S, Gustafsson JE, Allebeck P. School performance and risk of suicide in early adulthood: follow-up of two national cohorts of Swedish school children. J Affect Disord. 2011;131:104-12.
105. Stuckler D, Basu S, Suhrcke M, Coutts A, McKee M. The public health effect of economic crises and alternative policy responses in Europe: an empirical analysis. Lancet. 2009;374:315-23.
106. Gunnell D, Lopatatzidis A, Dorling D, Wehner H, Southall H, Frankel S. Suicide and unemployment in young people: analysis of trends in England and Wales, 1921–1995. Br J Psychiatry. 1999;175:263-70.
107. Corcoran P, Arensman E. Suicide and employment status during Ireland's Celtic Tiger economy. Eur J Public Health. 2011;21:209-14.
108. Chang SS, Gunnell D, Steme JA, Lu TH, Cheng AT. Was the economic crisis 1997–1998 responsible for rising suicide rates in East/Southeast Asia? A time-trend analysis for Japan, Hong Kong, South Korea, Taiwan, Singapore and Thailand. Soc Sci Med. 2009;68:1322-31.
109. Berk M, Dodd S. Henry M. The effect of macroeconomic variables on suicide. Psychol Med. 2006;36:181-9.
110. Taylor R, Page A, Morrell S, Harrison I, Cartier G. Mental health and socioeconomic variations in Australian suicide. Soc Sci Med. 2005;61:1551-60.

111. Rezaeian M, Dunn G, St Leger S, Appleby L. The ecological association between suicide rates and indices of deprivation in English local authorities. Soc Psychiatry Psychiatr Epidemiol. 2005;401785-91.
112. Evans J, Middleton N, Gunnell D. Social fragmentation, severe mental illness and suicide. Soc Psychiatry Psychiatr Epidemiol. 2004;39:165-70.
113. Middleton N, Sterne JAC, Gunnell D. The geography of despair among 15-44-year-old men in England and Wales: putting suicide on the map. J Epidemiol Community Health. 2006;60:1040-8.
114. Middleton N, Whitley E, Frankel S, Dorling D, Sterne J, Gunnell D. Suicide risk in small areas in England and Wales, 1991-1993. Soc Psychiatry Psychiatr Epidemiol. 2004;39:45-52.
115. Cheng ATA, Hawton K, Lee CTC, Chen THH. The influence of media reporting of the suicide of a celebrity on suicide rates: at population-based study. Int J Epidemiol. 2007;36: 1229-34.
116. Sandilands EA, Bateman DN. Co-proxamol withdrawal has reduced suicide from drugs in Scotland, Br J Clin Pharmacol. 2008;66:290-3.
117. Ludwig J, Cook PJ. Homicide and suicide rates associated with implementation of the Brady handgun violence prevention act. JAMA. 2000;284:585-91.
118. Gagne M, Robitaille Y, Hamel D, St-Laurent D. Firearms regulation and declining rates of male suicide in Quebec. Inj Prev. 2010;161:247-53.
119. Klieve H, Barnes M, De Leo D. Controlling firearms use in Australia: has the 1996 gun law reform produced the decrease in rates of suicide with this method? Soc Psychiatry Psychiatr Epidemiol. 2009;44:285-92.
120. Gunnell D, Fernando R, Hewagama M, Priyangika WDD, Konradsen F, Eddleston M. The impact of pesticide regulations on suicide in Sri Lanka. Int J Epidemiology. 2007;36:1235-42.
121. Carlsten A, Waern M, Ekedahl A, Ranstam J. Antidepressant medication and suicide in Sweden. Pharmacoepidemiol Drug Saf. 2001;10:525-30.
122. Gibbons RD, Brown CH, Hur K, Marcus SM, Bhaumik DK, Mann J. Relationship between antidepressants and suicide attempts: an analysis of the veterans health administration data sets. Am J Psychiatry. 2007;164:1044-9.
123. Stone M, Laughren T, Jones ML, et al. Risk of suicidality in clinical trials of antidepressants in adults: analysis of proprietary data submitted to US Fond and Drug Administration. BMJ. 2009;339:339.
124. Page A, Taylor R, Gunnell D, Carter G, Morrell S, Martin G. Effectiveness of Australian youth suicide prevention initiatives. Br J Psychiatry. 2011;199:423-9.

CHAPTER

68 Mechanisms of Disease: Drug Addiction

JN Vyas

Drug addiction is a chronic, relapsing disorder in which compulsive drug-seeking and drug taking behavior persists despite serious negative consequences. Addictive substances induce pleasant states (euphoria in the initiation phase) or relieve distress. Continued use induces adaptive changes in the central nervous system that lead to tolerance, physical dependence, sensitization craving, and relapse (Table 1). The addictive drugs discussed here are opioids, cannabinoids, ethanol, cocaine, amphetamines, and nicotine.

The World Health Organization and the American psychiatric association use the term "substance dependence" rather than "drug addiction." "Drug addiction," however, emphasizes the behavioral connotation of the term and is less likely to be confused with physical dependence. The American Psychiatric Association's definition of substance dependence requires a patient to meet at least three of the seven criteria listed in Table 1. Tolerance and physical dependence reflect physiological adaptation to the effects of a drug, whereas the remaining criteria define uncontrollable drug consumption. However tolerance and physical dependence are neither necessary nor sufficient for a diagnosis of substance dependence. Substance abuse of harmful use, a less severe disorder, may result in dependence.

Theories of addiction have mainly been developed from neurobiologic evidence and data from studies of learning behavior and memory mechanisms. They overlap in some aspects and are not mutually exclusive. None of them alone can explain all aspects of addiction. Generally, addictive

Table 1: Definition of term used in drug addiction
Craving (formerly called **psychological dependence**) is and intense desire to re-experience the effects of a psychoactive substance. Craving is the cause of relapse after long periods of abstinence.
Physical or physiological dependence is an outdated term refers to physical tolerance and the withdrawal and the withdrawal syndrome.
Priming refers to a new exposure to a formerly abused substance. This exposure can precipitate rapid resumption of abuse at previous levels or at higher levels.
Relapse is a resumption of drug-seeking or drug-taking behavior after a period of abstinence. Priming, environmental cues (people, places, or things associated with past drug use), and stress can trigger intense craving and cause a relapse.
Reward is a stimulus that the brain interprets as intrinsically positive or as something to be attained.
Sensitization is the increase in the expected effect of a drug after repeated administration (e.g. increased locomotor activation after the administration of psycho stimulants). Sensitization also refers to persistent hypersensitivity to the effect of a drug in a person with a history of exposure to that drug (or to stress). Sensitization is one of the neurobiologic mechanisms involved in craving and relapse.
Substance abuse is characterized by recurrent and clinically significant adverse consequences related to the repeated use of substances, such as failing to fulfill major role obligations, use of drug in situations in which it is physically hazardous, occurrence of substance-related legal problems, and continued drug use despite the presence of persistent or recurrent social or interpersonal problems.
Substance dependence is cluster of cognitive, behavioral, and physiological symptoms indicating that a person in continuing to use a substance despite having clinically significant substance-related problems. For substance dependence to diagnosed, at least three of the following must be present: symptoms of tolerance; symptoms of withdrawal; the use of a substance in larger amounts or for longer periods than intended; persistent desire of unsuccessful attempts to reduce or control use; the spending of considerable time in efforts to obtain the substance; a reduction in important social, occupational or recreational activities because of drug use; and continued use of a substance despite attendant health, social, or economic problems.
Withdrawal syndrome is a constellation of signs and symptoms that follows the abrupt discontinuation or reduction in the use of a substance or after blockage of the actions of a substance with antagonists (e.g. naltrexone in heroin addiction). The syndrome can also be produced by cues associated with substance use (**conditioned withdrawal**) symptoms tend to be the opposite of those produced after short-term exposure to a drug. Withdrawal in one of the causes of compulsive drug-taking behavior and short-term relapse.

drugs can act as positive reinforces (producing euphoria) or as negative reinforces (alleviating symptoms of withdrawal or dysphoria). Environmental stimuli (cues) associated in the absence of the drug.

Koob and Le Moal have proposed that the organism tries to counteract the effects of a given drug through a vicious circle in which the hedonic set point (the point at which pleasure in achieved) continually changes in response to the administration of the substance. They argue that drug addiction result from dysregulation of the reward mechanism and subsequent allostasis, the ability to achieve stability through change. Robinson and Berridge emphasize the dissociation between the incentive value of the drug (wanting) and its pleasurable or hedonic effects (liking), so that the brain system involved in the reward mechanism becomes hypersensitized to both the direct effects of the drug and associated stimuli that are not directly attributable to the drug. This hyper-sensitization causes pathologic wanting, or craving, independently of the presence of withdrawal symptoms and leads to compulsive drug-seeking and drug-taking behavior. Although liking progressively decreases, drugs become pathologically wanted (craving). Complementary to this incentive-sensitization theory compulsive drug-seeking and drug-taking behavior is facilitated by difficulties in decision making and the ability to judge the consequences of one's own action. These cognitive difficulties have been linked to deficits in the activation of areas in the prefrontal cortex.

FACTORS INFLUENCING DRUG ABUSE AND DEPENDENCE

Pharmacologic and Physiochemical Properties of Drugs

Pharmacologic and physiochemical properties of drugs are important factors in how drugs are consumed. Liposolubility increases the passage of a drug through the blood-brain-barrier, water solubility facilitates the injection of a drug, volatility favors the inhalation on drugs in vapor form, and heat resistance favors smoking of the drug. Characteristics such as rapid onset and intensity of effect increase the potential for abuse; therefore, substances that rapidly reach high levels in the brain are usually preferred (e.g. flunitrazepam is preferred over triazolam, and smoking "crack" cocaine is preferred to intranasal administration). A short half-life (e.g. that of heroin) produces more abrupt and intense syndromes of withdrawal that does a long half-life (e.g. that of methadone).

Personality and Psychiatric Disorders

Personality traits and mental disorders are major conditioning factors in drug addiction. Risk-taking or novelty-seeking traits favor the use of addictive drugs. Polydrug use is frequent among those with drug addiction, and many fulfill the criteria for dependence on or abuse of (or both) more than one substance. Psychiatric disorders, particularly schizophrenia, bipolar disorder, depression, and attention-deficit-hyperactivity disorder, are associated with an increased risk of abuse. A dual diagnosis (substance abuse and mental disorder) has unfavorable implications for management and outcome.

Genetic Factors

Genetic factors that influence the metabolism and the effects of drugs contribute to the risk of addication. Men whose parents were alcoholics have an increased likelihood of alcoholism even when they were adopted at birth and raised by parents who were not alcoholic, and they also have reduced sensitivity to alcohol that predicts the development of alcoholism. Carriers of an allele of aldehyde dehydrogenase that encodes an isoenzyme with reduced activity are less likely to abuse alcohol owing to the presence of increased level of acetaldehyde, which is responsible for aversive affects. A Leu 7 pro polymorphism of the neuropeptide Y gene has been correlated with increased alcohol consumption, and single-nucleotide polymorphisms of the gene encoding the μ opioid receptor correlates with an increased likelihood of heroin abuse. A deficiency in the cytochrome p-450 2D6 gene blocks the enzymatic conversion of codeine to morphine, thereby preventing codeine abuse.

With regard to nicotine dependence, subjects with defective cytochrome 9-450 2A6 *2 and *4 alleles, which impair the metabolism of nicotine, smoke fewer cigarettes and are less likely to be dependent than subjects who are homozygous for these alleles. A single-nucleotide polymorphism in the gene encoding fatty acid amide hydrolase, a major endocannabinoid-inactivating enzyme, has recently been associated with both an increased likelihood of recreational use of illegal drug and problem use of drugs or alcohol. The minor (A1) allele of the TaqIA D2 dopamine receptor gene has been linked to severe alcoholism; polysubstance, psycho-stimulant abuse or dependence; and opioid and nicotine dependence. Advances in genomic scanning (for quantitative trait loci) will allow the identification of allelic variants that contribute to the vulnerability to addiction.

DRUG EFFECTS AND MECHANISMS ACTION

Opioids

Short-term administration of heroin or morphine produces euphoria, sedation, and a felling of tranquility. Repeated administration rapidly produces tolerance and intense physical dependence. Over-dose can cause lethal respiratory depression. Numerous reports have documented impairments in health related to long-term heroin use.

Opioids activate specific receptors (μ, δ, and κ) that couple the G protein. Knockout mice lacking the μ receptor neither exhibit the behavioral effects induced by opioids nor become physically dependent when given opioids. The μ receptor has also been implicated in mediating or modulating the rewarding effect of other drugs of abuse (e.g. cannabinoids). Mice in which different receptors (CB_1 cannabinoid and D2 dopamine receptors) and transporters (dopamine) have been knocked out, have been used to demonstrate the effect of systems other than the opioid on opioid-induced pharmacologic responses.

Cannabinoids

The use of marijuana or hashish produces feelings of relaxation and well-being and impairs cognitive function and performance of psychomotor tasks. Overdose can induce panic attack and psychosis. A high incidence of cannabis consumption has been reported among patients with schizophrenia. Symptoms of withdrawal—restlessness, irritability, and insomnia—are subtle and appear in heavy consumers. The long-term effects of high doses of cannabinoids is a complex and controversial subject. Although there is evidence that long-term use of cannabis impairs memory, the cause of the marijuana amotivational syndrome—loss of energy and drive to work—remains unclear.

G-protein-coupled cannabinoid CB_1 receptors which are richly distributed in basal ganglia and cerebral-cortex regions, are implicated in cannabinoid abuse and addiction. In contrast to other neurotransmitters, endocannabinoids act as retrograde messengers at many central synapses. They are released from postsynaptic neurons and activate CB_1 receptors on presynaptic neurons, inhibiting the release of neurotransmitters. Natural ligands of CB_1 receptors have a shorter period of action than synthetic or plant-derived cannabinoids. Selective synthetic agonists and antagonists of CB_1 receptors are currently being developed for medical purposes.

Ethanol

When ethanol is given at low doses or initially during acute ethanol intoxication, it is perceived as a stimulant owing to the suppression of central inhibitory systems, but as the plasma levels of ethanol increase, sedation, motor incoordination, ataxia, and impaired psychomotor performance appear. The withdrawal syndrome (seizures and delirium tremens) may be severe and clinically challenging. The long-term effects of ethanol consumption have been extensively reviewed elsewhere.

Ethanol modifies the activity of serotonin (5-hydroxytryptamine-3 [5-HT_3]) receptors, nicotinic receptors, γ-aminobutyric acid type A ($GABA_A$) receptors, and the N-methyl-D-aspartate (NMDA) subtype of glutamate receptors. Ethanol acutely inhibits binding to the δ-opioid receptor, and long-term exposure to ethanol increases the density of μ and δ receptors. Its action on nearly all receptors are the results of a direct interaction with the receptor protein.

Cocaine and Amphetamines

Short-term administration of psychostimulants such as amphetamine produces euphoria, a feeling of well-being, and alertness as well as increased arousal; concentration, and motor activity. These substances increase blood pressure and the pulse rate and induce the release of corticotropin-releasing factor, corticotropin, and cortisol. Long-term use may cause irritability, aggressive and stereotyped behavior, and paranoid-like psychosis. Where as signs of withdrawal can be mild (depression, lack of energy, and insomnia), craving is very intense. So-called designer derivatives of amphetamine (3,4-methylene-dioxy-meth-amphetamine) [MDMA], or "ecstasy") produce euphoria and increased empathy (an "entactogenic" effect),but some derivatives have hallucinogenic effects. Acute intoxication with a psychostimulant can cause cerebral hemorrhage, hyperthermia and heat stroke, the serotonin syndrome, panic, and psychosis. The serotonin syndrome is characterized by altered mental status, autonomic instability, and neuromuscular abnormalities resulting in hyperthermia. So-called designer derivatives of amphetamine may have toxic effects in dopamine and serotonin neurons.

Cocaine is a potent blocker of the dopamine, norepinephrine, and serotonin-uptake transporters. Amphetamines have a more complex mechanism of action. Amphetamines cause neuronal storage vesicles in the cytoplasm to release neurotransmitters to the synapse; inhibit the uptake of dopamine, norepinephrine, and serotonin by membrane transporters; and act as mild inhibitors of monoamine oxide. Amphetamine and methamphetamine seem to be more selective for dopamine and norepinephrine than for serotonin transporters, but MDMA and designer amphetamines are more selective for the serotonin transporter.

Other Addictive Substances

Nicotine binds to neuronal nicotine acetylcholine receptors, and barbiturates and benzodiazepines bind and modulate the ion-channel-gated $GABA_A$ receptors. The psychotomimetic actions of dissociative anesthetics (phencyclidine and ketamine) are mediated by their noncompetitive antagonism at the NMDA-sensitive glutamate receptor (ligand-gated ion channel). LSD or mescaline (classic hallucinogens) are partial agonists at 5-HT_{2A} receptors, whereas salvinorin A induces their effects through the activation of k-opioid receptors.

NEUROBIOLOGY

Animal Model

Various animal behavioral paradigms have been used to study the neuronal substrates involved in addiction, especially euphoria and rewarding effects, including self-stimulation, self-administration, and conditioned place-preference models. In the place-preference model, the rewarding properties of a compound are associated with the particular characteristics of a given environment (place): after conditioning, the animal prefers to spend more time in the environment associated with the drug. Molecular studies have identified regulatory processes that occur after drug administration at the level of receptors membrane transporters, and their associated signaling proteins. Useful stains of mice have been developed by genetically disrupting drug targets (receptors and transporters) or proteins in the pathways of these targets. Genetic alterations are generally presents throughout development in these mice. Therefore, when the phenotypes of interest are absent, the effect of a drug could actually reflect compensatory changes in other neurobiologic system. To avoid this limitation, conditioned and tissue-specific knockout animal have been developed.

For some drugs, the risk of abuse in humans can be predicated with the use of tests based on behavioral paradigms in animals. These methods, however, are not systematically used during the development of centrally acting drugs, probably because the methods are not required by regulatory agencies.

Neuroanatomical Substrates

The neuronal pathways of drug addiction are components of the mesocorticolimbic dopamine systems that originate in neurons in the ventral tegmental area. All drugs of abuse act on this system at different levels. The mesolimbic circuit includes projections from cell bodies of the ventral tegmental area to limbic structures, such as the nucleus accumbens, amygdale, and hippocampus. This circuit has been implicated in acute reinforcing effects, memory, and conditioned responses linked to craving and the emotional and motivational changes of withdrawal syndrome. The mesocortical dopamine circuit includes projections from the ventral tegmental area to the prefrontal cortex, orbitofrontal cortex, and anterior cingulated. It is involved in the conscious experience of the effects of drugs, drug craving and the compulsion to take drugs. The mesolimbic and the mesocortical dopamine circuits operate in parallel and interact with each other and with other areas-forming the so-called extended amygdale—by means of projections from the GABA neurons of the nucleus accumbens to the ventral tegmental area and prefrontal cortex and glutamatergic projections from the prefrontal cortex to the nucleus accumbens and ventral tegmental area.

The Leading Role of the Dopamine Pathway

Both natural rewards (food, drink, and sex) and addictive drugs stimulate the release of dopamine from neurons of the presynaptic ventral tegmental area into the nucleus accumbens, causing euphoria and reinforcement of the behavior. In the case of natural rewards, there is a very rapid adaptive change, or habituation, after a few experiences, and the novelty or unexpectedness of the reward seems to play a major part in the initial response. The response to addictive drugs is not influenced by habituation, and each dose of the drug stimulates the release of dopamine. Moreover, dopamine mediates the hedonic consequences of a learning about the stimulus or anticipating its rewarding effects. During the withdrawal syndrome associated with opioids, cannabinoids, ethanol, psychostimulants, and nicotine, there is a substantial decrease in dopamine levels in the nucleus accumbens.

Dopamine binds to a G-protein-coupled receptor with two main subtypes, D1-like receptors (D1 and D5) and D2-like receptors (D2, D3, and D4). D1-like receptor activate adenylyl cyclase, whereas D2-like receptor inhibit the enzyme. A membrane dopamine transporter moves the released neurotransmitter from the extracellular space back into the presynaptic neuron (uptake). Animals can be taught to self-administer D1-like and D2-like receptor agonists.

Dopamine and Opioids

Opioids release dopamine mainly by an indirect mechanism that decreases the activity of GABA-inhibitory interneurons in the ventral tegmental area. Rodents can be taught to self-administer μ-receptor agonists into both the ventral tegmental area and the nucleus accumbens. Stimulation of k receptors decreases dopamine levels on the nucleus accumbens and produces aversive responses. Rodents will continue to self-administer opioid into the nucleus accumbens even in the presence of dopaminergic lesions or after a dopamine antagonist has been given. Reward and physical dependence on opioids are mediated by the activation of μ receptors, since reinforcement is blocked by selective receptor antagonists. Mice in which the μ-receptor has been knocked out do not exhibit place preference or withdrawal sings after the administration of morphine.

Dopamine and Cannabinoids

Cannabinoids increase the efflux of dopamine in the nucleus accumbens and cell firing in the ventral tegmental area by their actions on CB_1 receptors in glutamatergic and GABA-ergic neurons associated with the nucleus accumbens and ventral tegmental area. Highly potent, short-acting synthetic cannabinoid agonists (e.g. Win 55,212-2) induce self-administration behavior in rodents. Selective cannabinoid antagonists (e.g. SR 141716A) precipitate a withdrawal syndrome in cannabinoid-dependent animals, but at doses that are difficult to extrapolate to the consumption of plant-derived cannabis in humans.

Dopamine and Ethanol

Ethanol raises dopamine levels in the nucleus accumbens by an indirect mechanism: it increases the firing of dopamine neurons in the ventral tegmental area by activating $GABA_A$ receptors or by inhibiting NMDA receptor. Alcohol administration induces specific, long-lasting adaptive changes in the composition of NMDA receptor subunits, which enhances the function of NMDA receptors. These findings are the basis of the experimental and clinical use of NMDA antagonists for treating the ethanol-withdrawal syndrome and reducing alcohol intake and relapse rate. Opioid and serotonin receptors seem to have a role in the reinforcing effects of ethanol. In rats, naltrexone decreases the rate of self-administration of ethanol, and selected 5-HT_3 antagonists block the release of dopamine induced by ethanol and reduce alcohol consumption.

Dopamine, Cocaine and Amphetamines

Cocaine and amphetamines increase synaptic dopamine levels by inhibiting the activity of dopamine transporters. Imaging of the brain has shown that cocaine and amphetamines increase extracellular dopamine levels in the striatum and that euphoria is related to the occupancy of dopamine transporters by cocaine and amphetamines. Lesions in dopamine pathways, inhibition of dopamine synthesis, and dopamine antagonists markedly attenuate the rate of self-administration of cocaine in rats. Dopamine-transported-knockout mice are insensitive to the locomotor stimulatory effects and are less sensitive than normal mice to the behavioral effects of psychostimulants, but they will still self-administer cocaine and amphetamine. This effect may indicate a contribution of the serotonin and norepinephrine systems to the maintenance of the rewarding properties of cocaine.

Dopamine and Nicotine

Nicotine exerts its positive reinforcing effects by acting on α4β2 nicotinic acetylcholine receptors located on the somatodendritic membranes of the dopamine cells of the ventral tegmental area and possibly by sensitizing α7 nicotinic acetylcholine receptors located on glutamate terminals. Experiments with mutant mice lacking β2 nicotinic acetylcholine receptors confirm the primary role of this receptor in promoting the self-administration of nicotine.

THE OPIOID PATHWAY

The opioid system is another pathway in the brain involved in the rewarding effects of addictive drugs. The importance of this system in addiction to cannabinoids was brought out by studies in which opioid-receptor antagonists were found to attenuate the self-administration of cannabinoids and precipitate behavioral signs of withdrawal in rats treated with cannabinoid agonists for long periods. Opioid antagonists reduce the consumption and self-administration of ethanol in animals, but naltrexone does not reduce the rate of relapse or alcohol consumption in patients with alcoholism. By contrast, μ-receptor-knockout mice cannot be induced to self-administer alcohol. The opioid system also inhibits the self-administration of nicotine in animals. Indeed, naltrexone precipitates withdrawal in rats that receive nicotine for long periods and reduces cigarette consumption in smokers. In addition, nicotine-induced conditioned place preference is abolished in μ-receptor-knockout mice.

LONG-TERM DRUG USE AND NEUROADAPTATION

Tolerance and Withdrawal

Tolerance leads to modifications of drug use to obtain desired effects, by increasing the dose, reducing the intervals between doses, or both. Withdrawal compels addicts to resume drug use to prevent or reduce physical symptoms and dysphoria. Both tolerance and withdrawal increase compulsive drug-seeking and drug-taking behavior and are essential in maintaining the addiction. Sensitization, however, is also important. Molecular adaptations related to tolerance and dependence have been studied extensively in animals models of opioid and cocaine addiction.

Opioid Tolerance

Short-term administration of opioid activates the μ-opioid G-coupled receptor, which inhibits adenylyl cyclase, lowers cyclic adenosine mono-phosphate (cAMP) levels, decreases cAMP-dependent protein kinase A activity, and reduces phosphorylation of cytoplasmic and nuclear targets, including cAMP-responsive element-binding protein (CREB), a transcription factor. Activation of μ-receptors can also cause the phosphorylation of some mitogen-activated protein kinases, which in turn phosphorylate CREB and other transcription factors. Decrease in the number of opioid receptors have been related in some reports to the development of opioid tolerance. Continuous stimulation desensitizes opioid receptors, which become phosphorylated by G-protein-coupled receptor kinases; β-arresting then bind to the receptors causing them to be internalized by the neuron. Other studies, however, have found that opioids that cause internalization of the opioids receptors are inefficient in initiating tolerance.

Opioid Withdrawal

Chronic activation of opioid receptors produces effects opposite to those of acute activation. It up-regulates cAMP signaling pathways by increasing the activity of adenylyl cyclases (subtypes I and VII), cAMP-dependent protein kinase A, and tyrosine hydroxylase. In addition, chronic activation of opioid receptors increase the phosphorylation of CREB and FosB, factors regulating gene transcription.These changes correlate with the manifestations of the withdrawal syndrome.

Up-regulation of cAMP is a homeostatic response to the inhibition of the locus ceruleus by opioids and a key mechanism in withdrawal. The locus ceruleus is a noradrenergic nucleus that regulates arousal, responses to stress, and the activity of the autonomic nervous system. Tolerance to the inhibitory effects of opioids occurs in the locus ceruleus during long-term administration. When opioid levels fall, the firing rates of neurons in the locus are unopposed and lead to adrenergic over activation. A direct relation between overactivity of the locus ceruleus neurons and the somatic expression of opioid withdrawal has been demonstrated. Mechanisms other than noradrenergic neurons may also participate in opioid withdrawal because destruction of the locus ceruleus does not alter naloxone-precipitated or spontaneous opioid withdrawal.

In the nucleus accumbens, a similar up-regulations of the cAMP pathway, including activation of CREB, occurs after long-term administration of opioids, ethanol, or cocaine. CREB increase the production of dynorphin, which activates *k* receptors in the neurons of the ventral segmental area and decrease the release of dopamine in the nucleus accumbens. These changes contribute to the negative emotions (dysphoria and anhedonia) present during the early phase of abstinence.

Stress Systems

Drug administration and withdrawal activate central and peripheral stress systems. Short-term administration elevates peripheral glucocorticoid levels and central corticotropin-releasing factors levels. These hormonal elevations have been related to the rewarding properties of drug use. During withdrawal, an increase in corticotropin-releasing factor in the amygdale has been related to stress and negative effects of abstinence.

MOLECULAR MECHANISMS OF SENSITIZATION AND RELAPSE

Long-term administration of addictive drugs produces alterations in the brain that increase vulnerability to relapse and facilitate craving even months or years after successful detoxification. Factors involved in relapse and craving include acute re-exposure to the drug or drug-priming, exposure to environmental stimuli previously paired with drug use or conditioned drug cues, and exposure to environmental stressors. The extent of sensitization varies with different drugs and is responsible for responses, craving, and relapse.

Functional Changes

Repeated administration of opioids, psychostimulants, or nicotine sensitizes laboratory animals to the stimulant or rewarding effects, or both, of these addictive substances. Behavioral sensitization is associated with marked and long-lasting alterations in the functional activity of the mesocorticolimbic dopamine transmission in the nucleus accumbens. Elevated levels of the R1 subunit of AMPA subtype of glutamate receptors seems to be involved in sensitization and relapse. Stress or a single dose of addictive substances with different molecular mechanisms of action (cocaine, amphetamine, morphine, ethanol, or nicotine) produces similar degrees of enhancement in the strength of glutamate excitatory synapses (AMPA-sensitive glutamate receptors) on dopamine neurons in the ventral tegmental area. The administration of a glucocorticoid antagonist blocked the actions of stress but not those of addictive substances. These changes can have a role in behavioral sensitization.

Sensitization is associated with long-lasting adaptive changes in the patterns of expression of genes of the terminal mesolimbic dopamine systems, in particular the activations of proteins belonging to the family of transcription factors activator protein 1, such as Fos proteins. In self-administration models, long-term treatment with morphine, cocaine, or nicotine increases the expression of the family of Fos-related transcription factors, particularly the extremely stable isoforms of FosB. The persistent increase in the expression of Fos genes in mesolimbic structures is in part, a consequence of the activation of the cAMP cascade through D1 dopamine receptors in the ventral tegmental area.

Structural Changes

Exposure to addictive drugs can cause long-lasting structural changes in neurons. Opioids decrease the size and the caliber of dendrites and soma of dopamine neurons of the ventral tegmental area. Repeated use of cocaine or amphetamine increase the number of dendritic branch points and spines on both medium spiny neurons in the medial prefrontal cortex. Neurotrophic factors seems to be responsible for these changes. Notifications in the density of dendritic spines and neurotrophic factors have been implicated in long-term potentiation and long-term depression by AMPA-sensitive glutamate receptors.

The glutamate systems of the brain is responsible for the long-term plasticity associated with learning and memory.

It is therefore not surprising that the same glutamatergic mechanisms also underlie addiction-related behavior. Behavioral sensitization can persist for weeks or months and augmented by environmental cues (e.g. people, places, or paraphernalia associated with past drug use). These cues and sensitization contributes to pathways involved in the rewarding properties of drug abuse.

BIBLIOGRAPHY

1. Abraham HD, McCann UD, Ricaurte GA. Psychedelic drugs. In: Davis KL. Charchopharmacology: The Fifth Generation of Progress. Philadelphia: Lippincott Williams and Wilkins, 2002. pp.1545-56.
2. American Psychiatric Association. Diagnostic and Statistical Manual of Mental Disorders, 4th edition, text revision: DSM-IV-TR. Washington, D.C.: American Psychiatric Association, 2000.
3. Balster RL. Drug abuse potential evaluation in animals. Br J Addict. 1991;86:1549-58.
4. Berke JD, Hyman SE. Addiction, dopamine, and the molecular mechanisms if memory. Neuron. 2000;25:515-32.
5. Berrendero F, Kieffer BL, Maldonado R. Attenuation of Nicotine-induced antinociception, rewarding effects, and dependence in mu-opioid receptor knock-out mice. J Neurosci. 2002;22:10935-40.
6. Bolla KI, Brown K, Eldreth D, Tate K, Cadet JL. Dose-related neurocognitive effects of marijuana use. Neurology. 2002;59:1337-43.
7. Budney AJ, Hughes JR, Moore BA, Novy PL. Marijuana abstinence affects in marijuana smokers maintained in their home environment. Arch Gen Psychiatry. 2001:58:917-24.
8. Caille S, Espejo EF, Eneric JP, Cador M, Koob GF, Stinus L. Total neurochemical lesion of noradrenergic neurons of thelocus ceruleus does not alter either naloxone precipitated of spinataneous opiate withdrawal nor does it influence ability of clonidine to reverse opiate withdrawal . J Pharmacol Exp Ther. 1999;290:881-92.
9. Cami J, Farre M, Mass M, et al. Human Pharmacology if 3,4 Methylenedioxymethamphetamine (ecstasy): Psychomotor Performance and subjective effects. J Clin Psychopharmacil. 2000;20:455:66.
10. Cami J, Gilabert M, San L, de LaTorre R. Hypercortisolism after opioid discontinuation in rapid detoxification of heroin addicts. Br j Addict. 1992;87:1145-51.
11. Cami J. Human drug abuse liability. Testing times ahead. Br J Addict. 1991;86:1525-6.
12. Carlezon WA JR, Nestler EJ. Elecated levels of GuluR1 in the midbrain: a trigger for sensitization to drugs of abuse? Trends neurosci. 2002;25:610-5.
13. Crabbe JC. Genetic contributions to addiction. Annu Rev Psychol. 2002;53:435-62.
14. De Vries TJ, Shippenbreg TS. Neural systems underlying opiate addiction. J Neurosci. 2002;22:3321-5.
15. Di Chiara G. Drug addiction as dopamine-dependent associative learning disorder. Eur J Pharmacol. 1999;375:13-30.
16. Duman RS, Melberg j, Nakagawa S. Regulation of adult neurogenesis by psychotropic drugs stress. J Pharmacol Exp Ther. 2001;299:401-7.
17. Ernst T, Chang L, Leonido-yee M, Speek O. Evidence for long-term neurotoxicity associated with methamphetamine abuse: a 1H MRS study. Neurology. 2000;54:1344-9.
18. Everitt BJ, Wolf ME. Psychomotor stimulant addiction: a neural systems perspective. J Neurosci. 2002;22:1a.
19. Farre M, Cami J. Pharmacokinetic considerations in abuse liability evaluation. Br J Addict. 1991;86:1601-6.
20. Farre M, de la Torre R, Gonzalez ML, et al. Cocaine and alcohol interactions in humans: neuroendocrine effects and cocaethylene metabolism. J Pharmacol EXP Ther. 1997;283:164-76.
21. Farre M, Mas A, Torrens M, Moreno V, Cami J. Retention rate and illicit opioid use during methadone maintenance interventions: a meta-analysis. Drug Alcohol Depend. 2002;65:283-90.
22. Farre M, Teran MT, Roset PN, Mas M, Torrens M, Cami J. Abuse liability of flunitrazepam among methadone-maintained patients. Psychopharmacology (Berl). 1998;140:486-95.
23. Fattore L, Cossu G, Martellotta CM, Fratta W. Intravenous self-administration of the cannabinoid CB1 receptor agonist WIN 55,212-2 in rats. Psychopharmacology (Berl). 2001;156:410-6.
24. Fiellin DA, O'Connor PG. Office-based treatment of opioid-dependent patients. N Engl J Med. 2002;347:817-23.
25. Franklin TR, Acton PD, Maldjian JA, et al. Decreased try matter concentration in the insular, orbitofrontal, cingulated, and temporal cortices of cocaine patients. Boil Psychiatry. 2002;51:134-42.
26. Fudala PJ, Bridge TP, Herbert S, et al. Office-based treatment of opiate addiction with a sublingual-tablet formulation of buprenorphine and naloxone. N Engl J Med. 2003;349:949-58.
27. Goldstein RZ, Volkow ND. Drug addiction and its underlying neurobiological basis: neuroimaging evidence for the involvement of the frontal cortex. Am J Psychiatry. 2002;159:1642-52.
28. Gonzalez G, Oliveto A, Kosten TR. Treatment of heroin (diamorphine) addiction: current approaches and future prospects. Drugs. 2002;62:1331-43.
29. Hall W, Solowji N. Adverse effects of cannabis. Lancet. 1998;352:1611-6.
30. Harris DS, Baggott M, Mendelson JH, Mendelson JE, Jones RT. Subjective and hormonal effects if 3-4 methylenedioxymeth-amphetamine (MDMA) in humans. Psychopharmacology (Berl). 2002;162:396-405.
31. Hatsukami DK, Fischman MW. Cack cocaine and cocaine hydrochloride: are the differences myths or reality? JAMA. 1996;276:1580-8.
32. He L, Fong J, von Zastrow M, Whistler JL. Regulation of opioid receptor trafficking and morphine tolerance by receptor oligomerization. Cell. 2002;108:271-82.

33. Helmus TC, Downey KK, Artken CL, Henderson MJ, Schuster CR. Novelty Seeking as a predictor of treatment retention for heroin dependent cocaine users. Drug Alcohol Depend. 2001;61:287-95.
34. Holdstock L, de Wit H. Individual differences in the biphasic effects of ethanol. Alcohol Clin Exp Res. 1998;22:1903-11.
35. Hyman SE, Malenka RC. Addiction and the brain: the neurobiology of compulsion and its persistence. Nat Rev Neurosci. 2001;2:695-703.
36. Idem. Addiction. Annu Rev Psychol. 2003;54:25-53.
37. Idem. Drug addiction, dysregulation of reward, and allostatis. Neuropsychopharmacology. 2001;24:97-129.
38. Johnson RE, Chutuape MA, Strain EC, Strain EC, Walsh SL, Stitzer ML, Bigelow GE. A comparison of levomethadyl acetate, buprenorphine, and methadone for opiod dependence. N Engl J Med. 2000;343:1290-7.
39. Kalivas KL, Charney D, Coyle JT, Nemeroff C (Eds). Neuropsychopharmacology: The Fifth Generation of Progress. Philadelphia: Lippaincott Williams & Wilkins, 2002.pp.1357-66.
40. Kathiramalainathan K, Kaplan HL, Romach MK, et al. Inhibition of cytochrome P450 2D6 modifies codeine abuse liability. J Clin Psychopharmacol. 2000;20:435-44.
41. Kavangh DJ, McGrath J, Sunders JB, Dore G, Clark D. Substance misuse in patients with schizophrenia: epidemiology and management. Drugs. 2002;62:743-55.
42. Kelz MB, Nestler EJ. Delta fosB: a molecular switch underlying long-term neural plasticity. Curr Opin Neurol. 2000;13:715-20.
43. Kieffer BL, Gaveriaux-Ruff C. Exploring the opioid system by gene knockout. Prog Neurobiol. 2002;66:285-306.
44. Konipsky KL, Hyman SE. Molecular and cellular biology of addiction. In: Davis KL, Charney D, Coyle JT, Nemeroff C (Eds). Neuropsychopharmacology: The Fifth Generation of Progress. Philadelphia: Lippincott Williams and wilkins, 2002:1367-79.
45. Koob GF, Le Moal M. Drug abuse: hedonic homeostatic dysregulation. Science. 1997;278:52-8.
46. Kreek MJ, LaForge KS, Butelman E. Pharmacotherapy of addictions. Nar Rev Drug Discov. 2002;1:710-26.
47. Kreek MJ. Drug addiction: molecular and cellular endpoints. Ann N Y Acad Sci. 2001;937:27-49.
48. Krystal JH, Cramer JA, Krol WF, Kirk GF, Rosenheck RA. Naltrexone in the treatment of alcohol dependence. N Engl J Med. 2001;345:1734-9.
49. Laakso A, Mohn AR, Gainetdinov RR, Caron MG. Experimental genetic approaches to addiction. Neuron. 2002;36:213-28.
50. Lappalainen J, Kranzler HR, Malison R, et al. A functional neuropeptide Y leu7Pro polymorphism associated with alcohol dependence in a large population sample from the United States. Arch Gen Psychiatry. 2002;59:825-31.
51. Leri F, Bruneau J, Stewart J. Understanding polydrug use: review of heroin and cocaine co-use. Addiction. 2003;98:7-22.
52. Maddux JF, Desmond DP. Addiction or dependence? Addiction. 2000.pp.661-5.
53. Maldonado R, Rodriguez de fonseca F. Cannabinoid addiction: Behavioral models and neural correlated. J Neurosci. 2002;22:3326-31.
54. Maldonado R. Study of cannabinoid dependence in animals. Pharmacol ther. 2002;95:153-64.
55. Mansvelder HD, McGehee DS. Cellular and synaptic mechanisms of nicotine addiction. J Neurobiol. 2002;53:606-17.
56. Mantamadiotis T, Lemberger T, Bleckmann SC, et al. Disruption of CREB function in brain leads to neurodegeneration. Nat Genet. 2002;31:47-54.
57. Martin BR. Indentification of the endogenous cannabinoid system through integrative pharmacological approaches. J Pharmacol EXP Ther. 2002;301:790-6.
58. McLellan AT, Lewis DC, O' Brien CP, Klber HD. Drug dependence, a chronic medical illness: implications for treatment, insurance, and outcomes evaluation. JAMA. 2000; 284:1689-95.
59. Mello NK, Mendelson JH. Cocaine's effects on neuroendocrine systems: Clinical and preclinical studies. Pharmacol Biochem Behav. 1997;57:571-99.
60. Mendelson JH, Mello NK. Management of cocaine abuse and dependence. N Engl J Med. 1996;334:965-72.
61. Merlo E, Deidbreder C, Mugnaini M, Teneggi V. Molecular and behavioral aspects of nicotine dependence and reward IN: Maldonado R (Ed). Molecular biology of drug addiction. Totowa, N.J.: Humana Press, 2002;315:38.
62. Mumford GK, Evans SM, Fleishaker JC, Griffiths RR. Alprazolam absorption kinetics affects abuse liability. Clin Pharmacol Ther. 1995;57:356-65.
63. Navarro M, Chowen J, Rocio A, et al. CB1 cannabinoid receptor antagonist induced opiate withdrawal in morphine-dependent rats. Neuroreport. 1998;9:3397-402.
64. Nestler EJ, Earrot M, Self DW. Delta Fos:a sustained molecular sitch for addiction. Proc natl Acad Sci USA. 2001;98:11042-6.
65. Nestler EJ, Landsman D. Learning about addiction from the genome. Nature. 2001;409:834-5.
66. Nestler EJ. Genes and addiction. Nat Genet. 2000;26:277-81.
67. Nestler EJ. Molecular basis of long-term plasticity underlying addiction. Nat Rev Neurosci. 2001;2:119-28.[Erratum, Nat Tev Neurosci. 2001;2:215].
68. Nestler EJ. Molecular neurobiology of addiction. Am J Addict. 2001;10:201-17.
69. Netler EJ, Aghajanian GK. Molecular and cellular basis of addiction. Science. 1997;278:58-63.
70. Noble EP. D2 dopamine receptor gene in psychiatric and neurologic disorders and its phenotypes. Am J Med Genet. 2003;116B:103-25.
71. O'Connor PG, Schottenfeld RS. Patients with alcohol problems. N Engl J Med. 1998;338:592-602.
72. Picciottp MR, Corrigall WA. Neuronal systems underlying behaviors related to nicotine addiction: neural circuits and molecular genetics. J Neurosci. 2002;22:3338-41.

73. Rao Y, Hoffmann E, Zia M, et al. Duplications and defects in the CYP2A6 gene: identification, genotyping, and in vivo effects in smoking. Mol Pharmacol. 2000;58:747-55.
74. Rasmussen K, Beitner-Johnson DB, Krystal JH, Aghajanian GK, Nestler EJ. Opiate withdrawal and the rat locus coeruleus: behavioral, electrophysiological, and biochemical correlates. J Neurosci. 1990;10:2308-17.
75. Ricaurte GA. Yuan J, Hatzidimitrious G, Cord BJ. McCann UD. Severe dopaminergic neurotoxicity in primates after a common recreational dose regimen of MDMA (ecstasy). Science. 2002;297:2260-3.
76. Robbe D, Alonso G, Duchamp F, Bockaert J, Manzoni OJ. Localization and mechanisms of action of cannabinoid receptors at the glutamatergic synapses of the mouse nucleus accumbens. J Neurosci. 2001;21:109-16.
77. Robinson TE, Berridge KC. Incentive sensitization and addiction. Addiction. 2001;96:103-14.
78. Robison TE, Gorny G, Mitton E, Kolb B. Cocaine self-administration alters the morphology of dendrites and dendritic spines in the nucleus accumbens and neocertex. Synapse. 2001;39:257-66.
79. Roset P, Farre M, de la Torre R, et al. Modulation of rate of onset and intensity of drug effects reduces abuse potential in healthy males. Drug Alcohol Depend. 2001;64:285-98.
80. Roth BL, Baner K, Westkaemper R, et al. Salvinorin A: a potent naturally occurring nonnitrogenous kappa opioid selective agoinst. Proc Natl Acad Sci USA. 2002;99:1193-9.
81. Saal D, Dong Y, Bonci A, Melenks RC. Drugs of abuse and stress trigger a common synaptic adaptation in dopamine neurons. Neuron. 2003;37:577-82 [Erratum. Neuron 2003;38:359]
82. Sarnyai Z, Shaham Y, Heinrichs SC. The role of corticotrophin-releasing factor in drug addiction. Pharmacol Rev. 2001; 53:209-43.
83. Schukit MA, Edenbreg HJ, Kalmijn J, et al. A genome-wide search for genes that relate to a low level of response to alcohol. Alcohol Clin Exp Res. 2001;25:323-9.
84. Shalev U, Grimm JW, Shaham Y, Neurobiology of relapse to heroin and cocaine seeking: a review. Pharmacol Rev. 2002;54:1-42.
85. Sipe JC, Chiang K, Gerber AL, Beuder E, Cravatt BF. A missense mutation in human fatty acid amide hydrolase associated with problem drug use. Proc Natl Acad Sci USA. 2002;99:8394-9.
86. Sklait-Tavron L, Shi WX, Lane SB, Harris HW, Bunney BS, Nestler EJ, Chronic morphine induces visible changes in the morphology of mesolimbic dipamine neurons. Proc Natl Acal Sci USA. 1996;93:11202-7.
87. Smith DE, Wesson DR. Benzodiazepines and other sedative-hypnotics. In: Galanter M, Kleber HD (Eds). The American Psychiatric press textbook of substance abuse treatment. 2nd edition. Washington, D.C.: American Psychiatry press, 1999;239-50.
88. Solowij N, Stephens RS, Roffman RA, et al. congnitive functioning of long-term heavy cannabis users seeking treatment. JAMA. 2002;287:1123-31. [Erratum, JAMA. 2002; 287:1651.]
89. Spanagel R, Weiss F. The dopamine hypothesis of reward: past and current status. Trends Neurosci. 1999:22:521-7.
90. Spanagel R. Behavioral and molecular aspects of alcohol craving and relapse. In: Maldonado R (Ed). Molecular biology of drug addiction. Totowa, N.J.: Humana Press, 2002. pp.295-313.
91. Stolerman I. Drugs of abuse: behavioural principles, methods and terms. Trends Pharmacol Sci. 1992;13:170-6.
92. Swift RM. Drug therapy for alcohol dependence. N Engl J Med. 1990;340:1482-90.
93. Taylor DA, Fleming WW. Unifying perspectives of the mechanisms underlying the development of tolerance and physical dependence to opioids. J Pharmacol Exp Ther. 2001;297:11-8.
94. Uhl GR, Liu QR, Naiman D. Substance abuse vulnerability loci: converging genome scanning data. Trends Genets. 2002;18:420-5.
95. Volkow ND, Fowler JS. Application of imaging technologies in the investigation of drug addiction. In: Davis KL, Charney D, Coyle JT, Nemeroff C (Eds). Neuropsycho-pharmacology: the fifth generation of progress. Philadelphia: Lippincott Williams and Wilkins, 2002.pp.1475-90.
96. Watts VJ. Molecular mechanism for heterologous sensitization of adenylate cyclase. J Pharmacol Exp Ther. 2002;302:1-7.
97. Weiss F, Porrino LJ, Behavioral neurobiology of alcohol addiction: recent advances and challenges. J Neurosci. 2002;23:3332-7.
98. Wilson RJ, Nicoll RA. Endocannabinoid signaling in the brain. Science. 2002;296:678-82.
99. World Health Organization. The ICD-10 classification of mental and behavioral disorders: clinical descriptions and diagnostic guidelines. Geneva: World Health Organization, 1992.
100. Zammit S, Allebeck P, Andreassin S, Lundberg I, Lewis G. Self-reported cannabis use as a risk factor for schizophrenia in Swedish conscripts of 1969: historical cohort study. BMJ. 2002;325:1199.
101. Zhang L, Hosoi M, Guzuzawa M, Sun H, Rawling RR, Weight FF. Distinct molecular basis for differential sensitivity of the serotonin type 3A receptor to ethanol in the absence and presence of agonist. J Biol Chem. 2002;277:46256-64.

CHAPTER

69

Schizophrenia: New Pathological Insights and Therapies

JN Vyas

INTRODUCTION

Schizophrenia is widely considered a neurodevelopmental disorder that stems from interactions among genetic and environmental factors. Although the contribution of any single gene appears to be quite small, the combined influence of multiple susceptibility genes contributes substantially to the risk of developing schizophrenia.[1] Epidemiological studies have also identified a number of environmental factors that confer additional risk, including early life exposure to infection, trauma, and hypoxia.[2] Despite the influence of multiple genetic and environmental factors on brain development, however, the clinical symptoms of psychosis typically remain dormant until adolescence or early adulthood. It has been postulated that the delayed onset of symptoms may be due to maturational processes such as puberty, cortical synaptic pruning, and myelination, which 'unmask' pre-existing deficits.[3] Whereas the neurodevelopmental hypothesis posits a static lesion based on the presence of fixed deficits established in early development, recent studies indicate that new-onset schizophrenia is often characterized by a period of clinical and functional decline accompanied by progressive neurostructural changes, which suggests that a limited neuroprogressive process may also be involved.[3]

Converging evidence from neuroimaging, neurocognitive, gene array, and postmortem neuropathological studies indicate that the pathophysiology of schizophrenia involves disrupted synaptic connectivity that affects both inhibitory and excitatory circuits. These findings are consistent with emerging evidence of cortical hypofrontality that has prompted revisions to the traditional dopamine hypothesis, i.e. that schizophrenia stems from subcortical hyperdopaminergia. The most recent neurochemical hypothesis implicates a primary cortical hyperdopaminergia and cortical hypodopaminergia.[4] This hypothesis provides a more nuanced and unifying explanation for the clinical presentation of schizophrenia. It accounts for positive symptoms (e.g. delusions, hallucinations), negative symptoms (e.g. apathy), and cognitive symptoms (e.g. disorganization), and it provides the basis for novel treatment approaches that extend beyond dopamine subtype-2 (D_2) receptor antagonism.

NEUROPATHOLOGY

Neuronal and Glial Density

Unlike many classic neurodegenerative disorders, schizophrenia is not characterized by large-scale neuronal loss. One of the few studies to have examined total cortical neuronal number found no difference between schizophrenics and controls.[5] In dorsolateral prefrontal cortex (DLPFC), several studies found increased neuronal density in schizophrenia due to slight reductions in cortical neuropil, but overall neuronal numbers were not changed.[6] Other studies identified reductions in the densities of neuronal subpopulations, including interneuron in layer II of DLPFC and in layers II-VI of anterior cingulated cortex (ACC).[7,8] Several studies,[9,10] though not all,[11] found that in contrast to cortical areas, neuronal density in mediodorsal thalamus was reduced. In hippocampus, most studies have not demonstrated an overall loss of neurons;[12] however, several studies have identified reductions in GABAergic (gamma amino butyric acid) interneuron subpopulations.[13]

Also in contrast to classic neurodegenerative disorders, schizophrenia is characterized by and absence of glial proliferation,[14] and recent data even suggest that cortical glial density is decreased.[15] The absence gliosis strongly suggests the absence of a classic neurodegenerative process, providing general support for schizophrenia as a disorder of neurodevelopment. However, the absence of gliosis does not rule out a more limited degenerative process.

Synapses and Dendrites

Many lines of evidence suggest that schizophrenia is a disorder of synaptic connectivity and involves a reduction in cortical neuropil.[6] This is supported by evidence of reduced density of dendritic spines and dendritic length in DLPFC in schizophrenia.[16] Furthermore, reduced expression in DLPFC of Cdc42 and Duo, two members of the RhoGTPase family involved in regulating spine dynamics, could contribute to the underlying mechanism of altered spine density.[17] Reduced neuropil is also consistent with decreased levels of the presynaptic marker synaptophysin in DLPFC.[18] Synaptic pathology is similarly suggested in hippocampus, where investigators have found reduced levels of synaptophysin[19] and the dendritic spine marker spinophilin.[20] Altered synaptic connectivity in schizophrenia is also supported by a gene array study showing reductions of multiple genes that code for synaptic gene products in DLPFC.[21] Finally, reductions in pyramidal neuronal size in DLPFC have been reported.[22] This may not be surprising, since the extent of dendritic and axonal arborization contributes to somal size.[23]

GABAergic Deficits

Deficits in GABAergic interneurons in DLPFC are among the best-replicated neuropathological findings in schizophrenia. Because of the importance of GABAergic inhibition in circuits of normal brain function-including working memory-deficits in GABAergic neurons are likely to make important contributions to cognitive and other clinical dimensions of schizophrenia.[24] For example, glutamic acid decarboxylase (GAD)—the GABA-synthesizing enzyme is substantially reduced in DLPFC.[25] Similarly, $GABA_A$ receptor binding is increased in ACC and DLPFC,[26] representing a potential compensatory up-regulations in response to lower GABA levels.[27] Furthermore, studies have found fewer GABA membrane transporters (GAT-1) cartridges in the GABAergic chandelier neurons of DLPFC.[28] GAT-1 cartridges reflect the vertical arrangement of axon terminals of chandelier cells that synapse at the axon initial segment of layer 3 pyramidal neurons in DLPFC and are thought to modulate excitatory output from pyramidal neurons.

Investigators have also examined parvalbumin (PV) expression, a calcium-binding protein present in subpopulation of interneurons. Several studies found that PV-immunoreactive (IR) neurons were reduced in DLPFC in schizophrenia[29] whereas another study found no difference.[30] Reduced PV-IR varicosities have also been reported in layer III of DLPFC,[31] but although PV mRNA was also reduced, this reduction was per neuron rather than an overall reduction of PV mRNA-containing neurons.[32] In summary, although total interneuron numbers do not seem to be altered, deficits in GABAergic neuron subpopulations are evident in schizophrenia.

Evidence of Progressive Neuropathological Changes

Cross-sectional structural neuroimaging studies have demonstrated consistent brain abnormalities in schizophrenia. These include enlarged lateral and third ventricles and reduced cortical gray matter volume in whole cortex and in cortical subregions, especially prefrontal and temporal areas.[33] Evidence for modest but significant volume reduction in hippocampus has also been established.[34] The finding of reduced cortical gray matter even in the first episode of psychosis[35] suggests that the loss of gray matter at least in part predates the onset of clinical symptomatology. Because cross-sectional studies cannot demonstrate whether these changes incorporate a progressive component, recent studies have applied longitudinal neuroimaging strategies.

Interestingly, progressive loss of gray matter has been identified in several cortical and subcortical regions in prodromal patients who later developed psychosis.[36] In childhood-onset schizophrenia, excess cortical gray matter loss compared to normal controls was observed in frontal, temporal, and parietal cortices.[37,38] Likewise, in new onset schizophrenia, progressive volume loss has been reported globally and in multiple cortical subregions.[39,40] These data suggest that the onset of schizophrenia is associated with a progressive loss of cortical gray matter and provide *in vivo* support for the hypothesis that there may be active loss of neuropil and synaptic elements in the early stages of psychosis.[41]

One challenge in understanding the basis of the progressive neurostructural changes relates to the potential confounding effects of antipsychotic treatment. A recent two-year longitudinal study of first-episode schizophrenia found that only patients randomized to haloperidol experienced significant cortical gray matter loss, whereas patients who received olanzapine had no gray matter loss.[42] Although this study could not distinguish underlying pathophysiology from medication effects, it is clear that antipsychotic medications can influence longitudinal neuroimaging data. A recent postmortem analysis of monkeys treated chronically with haloperidol, olanzapine, or placebo supports the conclusion that antipsychotic may contribute to gray matter loss.[43] A longitudinal neuroimaging study of antipsychotic and placebo-treated monkeys would help disentangle the relative contributions of medications and pathophysiology.

Genetic Associations

A recent meta-analysis of twin studies demonstrated that the genetic contribution to the etiology of schizophrenia is upward of 80%.[44] A handful of genes are now beginning to emerge as likely to be implicated in schizophrenia, including neuregulin-1 (NRG1), Disrupted-in-schizophrenia-1 (DISCI), Regulator of G-protein signaling 4 (RGS-4), Catechol-O-methyl-transferase (COMT), and Dysbindin (DTNBP1).[45] These associations have been verified in multiple cohorts, and each also has at least reasonable biological plausibility (1). For example, one elegant study[46] showed that DISC1 is involved in critical aspects of normal microtubular dynamics and that loss of normal DISC1 function recapitulates several aspects of the neuropathology of schizophrenia, including stunted neurite outgrowth and subtle migration abnormalities. It is important to note that individual genes, rather than being causative, appear to confer risk of developing the disorder. The current iteration of the neurodevelopment hypothesis suggest that the etiology of schizophrenia involves a complex interplay among risk genes and protective genes in the setting of particular environmental factors during early development. These environmental factors modify the genetic risk, and gene-environment interactions ultimately determine whether a given individual will develop psychosis.[1] As larger populations are examined and more sophisticated experimental approaches are undertaken, some of the current list of promising genes may not stand the test of replication, and new genes of risk are likely to be identified.

ANTIPSYCHOTIC TREATMENTS

Typical Antipsychotic Drugs and their Limitations

The era of pharmacological treatment for schizophrenia began with the discovery of the antipsychotic properties of chlorpromazine in 1952, and since then other typical (first generation) antipsychotic drugs (APD_S) such as haloperidol and perphenazine have been developed. All were based on the hypothesis that schizophrenia reflected a disorder of stratial hyperdopaminergia, with the D_2 receptor most strongly associated with antipsychotic response.[47] Although typical APD_S are often effective for treating positive psychotic symptoms, up to two-thirds of patients remain symptomatic and are labeled either treatment-refractory or partially responsive.[48] In addition, typical APD_S have little impact on negative symptoms or cognitive impairments, which are closely associated with functional outcome in schizophrenia.[49] D_2 antagonists also produce a variety of side effects, including acute extrapyramidal side effects (EPS) and hyperprolactinemia as well as tardive dyskinesia associated with long-term exposure.[50] These side effects may reduce medication compliance, which in turn leads to psychotic relapse and rehospitalization.

Pharmacological Basis of Atypical Antipsychotic

The reintroduction of clozapine in 1990 represented a breakthrough in the pharmacotherapy of schizophrenia. Clozapine was found superior to typical APD_S in treatment-resistant schizophrenia,[51] although its potential has never been fully realized because of the elevated risk of agranulocytosis. Other atypical (second-generation) antipsychotic drugs, including risperidone, olanzapine, quetiapine, and ziprasidone, have since been introduced in efforts to match the therapeutic benefits of clozapine without the associated risk of blood dyscrasias. Although the efficacy of clozapine in treatment-resistant patients is still unique, the newer atypical agents have a better overall safety profile, and they also produce fewer neurological side effects (reduced EPS and tardive dyskinesia) and appear to offer some advantages in cognition, relapse prevention, functional capacity, and quality of life compared with typical APDs. Accordingly, the newer atypical APDs have, in most settings, become first-line agents for acute and maintenance therapy.[53]

Although there is debate as to what constitutes atypicality, one defining feature of this class of agents is a wider separation between the dose that results in an antipsychotic effect and the dose that increases the risk of EPS.[54] To date, two major theories have been proposed to account for an atypical profile: (a) The high $5\text{-}HT_{2A}$ receptor affinity of many atypical APDs is thought to mitigate EPS side effects associated with D_2 antagonism,[48] and (b) lower mean levels of D_2 receptor occupancy (<80%) are associated with therapeutic doses of atypical APDs.[55] Although both of these theories offer insight into the potential mechanisms of action of antipsychotic medications, neither fully accounts for the unique efficacy of clozapine.

The wide range of other receptor binding activities shown by atypicals, in binding dopamine (D_1, D_3, D_4), serotonin ($5\text{-}HT_{1A}$, $5\text{-}HT_{2c}$, $5\text{-}HT_6$, $5\text{-}HT_7$), muscarinic cholinergic, noradrenergic (α_1, α_2), and histamine families, suggests that other receptor systems also contribute to the activity of these drugs (Table 1). In addition, *in vitro* and *in vivo* evidence suggests that atypical APDs have neuroprotective effects, including production of neurotrophic factors,[57] prevention of glutamate excitotoxicity, oxidative stress and apoptosis,[58] and enhancing neurogenesis and connectivity,[59] which could also contribute to the antipsychotic mechanism of action.

Revised Dopamine Hypothesis of Schizophrenia and Dopamine Partial Agonism

The original dopamine hypothesis, which posited that schizophrenia, is associated with subcortical hyperactivity at the D_2 receptor, has been validated using positron emission tomography (PET).[60] This hypothesis has also been substantially updated. Imaging studies point to a dopaminergic imbalance involving a primary mesocortical hypodopaminergic state associated with hypofunctioning glutamate signaling, which results in hypostimulation of prefrontal D_1 function may lead to negative and cognitive symptoms, and a later-developed episodic hyperactivity of the mesolimbic dopamine system in turn leads to hyperstimulation of postsynaptic D_2 receptors and emergence of positive symptoms.[4]

The use of partial dopamine agonists is a novel strategy to normalize dopaminergic deregulation without the adverse effects of full D_2 antagonists.[61] This class of compounds has lower intrinsic activity at D_2 receptors than full agonists have, allowing them to act as either an agonist or antagonist depending on the synaptic dopamine levels.[62] In schizophrenia, an effective partial D_2 agonist is thought to act as a functional antagonist in the mesolimbic dopamine pathway to control positive symptoms and as a functional

Table 1: Relative neurotransmitter receptor affinities for antipsychotics at therapeutic doses[52]

Receptor	*Haloperidol*	*Perphenazine*	*Clozapine*	*Risperidone*	*Olanzapine*	*Quetiapine*	*Ziprasidone*	*Aripiprazole*
D_1	+		+	+	++	–	+	+
D_2	++++	++++	++	++++	+++	+	+++	++++
D_3	+++		+	++	+	–	++	++++
D_4	+++	+	++	+++	++	–	++	++
$5\text{–}HT_{1A}$	–		+	–	–	–	+++	+++
$5\text{–}HT_{1D}$	–		–	+	–	–	+++	
$5\text{–}HT_{2A}$	+	+++	+++	++++	+++	+	++++	++
$5\text{–}HT_{2C}$	–		++	++	++	–	++++	++
$5\text{–}HT_6$	–		++	–	++	–	+	+
$5\text{–}HT_7$	–		++	+++	–	–	+++	++
α_1	+++	++	+++	+++	++	+++	++	+
α_2	–	–	+	++	+	–	–	–
H_1	–		+++	+	+++	++	+	+
M_1	–	–	++++	–	+++	+	–	–
DA Transporter			++		++			
NA Transporter			+		++		++	
5-HT Transporter							++	
– = minimal to none; + = low; ++ = moderate; +++ = high; +++++ = marked								

agonist in the mesocortical pathway to improve negative and cognitive symptoms. In addition, it maintains dopaminergic tone in the nigrostriatal and tuberoinfudibular pathways, avoiding the EPS and hyperprolactinemia associated with complete D_2 antagonism. Thus, partial D_2 agonist activity could stabilize the dopamine system in different areas of the schizophrenic brain.[62]

Aripiprazole is the first partial dopamine agonist approved for use in treating schizophrenia.[63] It has a very high affinity for D_2 and D_3 receptors (Table 1) and acts on both postsynaptic D_2 receptors and presynaptic autoreceptors. In addition, it displays partial $5\text{-}HT_{1A}$ agonism and $5\text{-}HT_{2A}$ antagonism, which could imply efficacy in anxiety, mood disturbances, cognitive deficit, and negative symptoms. PET studies in healthy volunteers indicate that although the agent occupies up to 90% of striatal D_2-like dopamine receptors at clinical doses, it does not cause EPS. This finding suggests that its inherent agonism may provide a mechanism that protects against excessive blockade of the D_2 system.[64]

Comparison of Clinical Profiles of Atypical Antipsychotics

There has been considerable debate as to the clinical superiority of atypical APDs. Leucht et al.[65] performed a meta-analysis of the atypical APDs risperidone, olanzapine, sertindole, and quetiapine compared with placebo and typical APDs. They suggested minor efficacy advantages for olanzapine and risperidone, moderate overall tolerability advantages for quetiapine and olanzapine, and lower EPS liability (as reflected in lower antiparkinsonian medication use) for all the atypical APDs compared to haloperidol. However, in a second meta-analysis comparing atypical APDs only to low-potency typical, Leucht et al.[66] reported no advantage on EPS liability for the atypicals (other than clozapine), although a moderate superiority in efficacy was documented for the atypicals. The studies by Leucht et al. have been generally consistent with other recent meta-analysis, with several qualifications. Geddes et al.[67] asserted that the atypicals are equally efficacious as a homogeneous group, and Davis et al.[68] concluded that some atypicals (clozapine amisulpiride, risperidone, and olanzapine) are superior to other atypicals (sertindole, quetiapine, ziprasidone, and remoxipride).

It should be noted that these meta-analyses lack data currently available to evaluate other relevant clinical dimensions (e.g. cognition, affect, quality of life). Moreover pharmaceutical company sponsorship of studies, limited types of assessment measures used (e.g. last-observation-carried-forward analyses), and relatively short durations of trials could limit the generalizability of the results of previous efficacy studies for atypical APDs.

Primary Outcomes of the CATIE Schizophrenia Trial

The Clinical Antipsychotic Trials of Intervention Effectiveness (CATIE) study sponsored by the National Institute of Mental Health was developed to determine whether the overwhelming use of atypical APDs represents a rational and appropriate approach to treating schizophrenia.[69] CATIE was the largest, longest, and most comprehensive independant trial ever performed to examine exiting therapies for schizophrenia. This double-blind randomized study compared the effectiveness of the atypical APDs olanzapine, quetiapine, resperidone, and ziprasidone, and one typical APD, perphenazine , for up to 18 months in 1493 patients with chronic schizophrenia.[70] The study demonstrated that overall, all of the medications were comparably effective. The mean rate of all-cause discontinuation (i.e. discontinuation due to poor efficacy, side effects, or other reasons) was 74% prior to 18 months; the individual discontinuation rates were 64% for olanzapine, 74% for risperidone, 75% for perphenazine, 79% for ziprasidone, and 82% for quetiapine. Olanzapine had the lowest rate of all-cause discontinuation and also the lowest rate of discontinuation due to lack of efficacy. However, olanzapine was also associated with greater weight gain and metabolic side effects than were other medications. Somewhat surprisingly perphenazine was similar in efficacy and tolerability to the other atypical APDs, suggesting that typical APDs remain a viable treatment option in chronic schizophrenia. Future reports from the CATIE study will address questions regarding the cost-effectiveness of the drugs, their effects on cognitive functioning, rates of recovery, the effectiveness of clozapine for patients with persistent symptoms, and the reversibility of drug-induced side effects (e.g. weight gain). Although the contribution of antipsychotics to longitudinal brain change also remains an important area of investigation, the CATIE study could not include a neuroimaging component owing to funding constraints.

Novel Pharmacotherapeutic Approaches

In the United States, several novel antipsychotic compounds, including asenapine, bifeprunox, iloperidone, paliperidone, and bifeprunox, are currently in phase II or III FDA clinical trials. Asenapine, iloperidone, paliperidone, and ocaperidone have serotonin-dopamine (5-HT_{2A}/D_2) antagonist properties; bifeprunox is a partial dopamine agonist/antagonist, as well as 5-HT_{1A} agonist.

With the emerging evidence for glutamatergic dysregulation in schizophrenia, a number of agents with direct or indirect activity in the glutamate system are being investigated, especially for their potential impact on cognitive and negative symptoms. Glutamate-based agents in various stages of development include agonists at the glycine site of the NMDA receptor, glycine reuptake inhibitors, glutamate release inhibitors, AMPA agonist, and antagonists, and ampakines.[56] The glycine site agonists appear to reduce negative symptoms and cognitive deficits in schizophrenia when used to augment antipsychotic treatment. In the case of AMPA ligands, it remains unclear whether agonists, antagonists, or partial agonists/modulators will be most successful.

It has also been suggested that the central cholinergic system is involved in the cognitive deficits observed in schizophrenia, and enhanced cholinergic activity may improve these deficits. Currently available treatments that may suit this purpose include acetylcholinesterase inhibitors (e.g. galantamine), muscarinic partial agonists (e.g. xanomeline), nicotinic agonists, and allosteric potentiators of nicotinic receptor function.[71] Other potential cognitive enhancers for the treatment of schizophrenia include memantine (an NMDA receptor antagonist), modafinil (a wake-promoting agent currently used to treat narcolepsy), talnetant (a neurokinin-3 antagonist), and tolcapone (a catechol-O-methyltransferase inhibitor), all of which are currently in phase II FDA clinical trials.

SUMMARY

- Synaptic dysconnectivity has emerged as a core neuropathological deficit in schizophrenia.
- Recent data indicate that some of these deficits are progressive, at least around the onset of psychosis.
- APDs appear to affect the progressive structural changes. Atypical APDs, but not typical APDs, exert a potential neuroprotective effect.
- New developments in antipsychotic treatments include partial dopamine agonists and agents that target non-dopamine-based neurotransmitter systems. These offer the potential for improving dimensions of the illness, such as cognitive and negative symptoms, which are not adequately treated with currently available medications.

REFERENCES

1. Harrison PJ, Weinberger DR. Schizophrenia genes, gene expression, and neuropathology: on the matter of their convergence. Mol Psychiatry. 2005;10:40-68.
2. Cannon M, Jones PB, Murray RM. Obstetric complications and schizophrenia: historical and meta-analytic review. Am J Psychiatry. 2002;159:1080-92.
3. Lieberman JA, Perkins D, Belger A, et al. The early stages of schizophrenia: speculations on pathogenesis, patho-physiology, and therapeutic approaches. Biol Psychiatry. 2001; 50:884-97.
4. Laruelle M, kegeles LS, Abi-Dargham A. Glutamate, dopamine, and schizophrenia: from pathopysiology to treatment. Ann NYAcd Sci. 2003;1003:138-58.
5. Pakkenberg B. Total nerve cell number in neocortex in chronic schizophrenics and controls estimated using optical dissectors. Biol Psychiatry. 1993;34:768-72.
6. Selemon LD, Goldman-Rakic PS. The reduced neuropil hypothesis: a circuit based model of schizophrenia. Biol Psychiatry. 1999;45:17-25.
7. Benes FM, McSparren J, Bird ED, et al. Deficits in small interneuron in prefrontal and cingulate cortices of schizophrenic and schizoaffective patients. Arch Gen Psychiatry. 1991;48:996-1001.

8. Benes FM, Vincent SL, Todtenkopf M. The density of pyramidal and nonpyramidal neurons in anterior cingulated cortex of schizophrenic and bipolar subjects. Biol Psychiatry. 2001; 50:395-406.
9. Byne W, Buchsbaum MS, Mattiace LA, et al. Postmortem assessment of thalamic nuclear volumes in subjects with schizophrenia. Am J Psychiatry. 2002;159:59-65.
10. Popken GJ, Bunney WE Jr, Potkin SG, et al. Subnucleus-specific loss of neurons in medial thalamus of schizophrenics. Proc Natl Acad Sci USA. 2000;97:9276-80.
11. Dorph-Petersen KA, Pierri JN, Sun Z, et al. Stereological analysis of the mediodorsal thalamic nucleus in schizophrenia: volume, neuron number, and cell types. J Comp Neurol. 2004; 472:449-62.
12. Heckers S, Heinsen H, Geiger B, et al. Hippocampal neuron number in schizophrenia. A stereological study. Arch Gen Psychiatry. 1991;48:1002-8.
13. Benes FM, Kwok EW, Vincent SL, et al. A reduction of nonpyramidal cells in sector CA2 of schizophrenics and manic depressive. Biol. Psychiatry. 1998;48:88-97.
14. Arnold SE, Trojanowski JQ, Gur RE, et al. Absence of nurodegeneration and neural injury in the cerebral cortex in a sample of elderly patients with schizophrenia. Arch Gen Psychiatry. 1998;55:225-32.
15. Stark AK, Uylings HB, Sanz-Arigita E, et al. Glial cell loss in the anterior cingulated cortex, a subregion of the prefrontal cortex, in subjects with schizophrenia. Am J Psychiatry. 2004;161:882-8.
16. Glantz LA, Lewis DA. Decreased dendritic spine density on prefrontal cortical pyramidal neurons in schizophrenia. Arch Gen Psychiatry. 2000;57:65-73.
17. Hill JJ, Hashimoto T, Lewis DA. Molecular mechanisms contributing to dendritic spine alterations in the prefrontal cortex of subjects with schizophrenia. Mol Psychiatry. 2006; 11:557-66.
18. Glantz LA, Lewis DA. Reduction of synaptophysin in the prefrontal cortex of subjects with schizophrenia. Regional and diagnostic specificity. Arch Gen Psychiatry. 1997;54:660-69.
19. Eastwood SL, Harrison PJ. Decreased sunaptophsysin in the medial temporal lobe in schizophrenia demonstrated using immunoautoradiography. Neuroscience. 1995;69:339-43.
20. Low AJ, Weickert CS, Hyde TM, et al. Reduced spinophilin but not microtubule-associated protein 2 expression in the hippocampal formation in schizophrenia and mood disorders: molecular evidence for a pathology of dendritic spines. Am J Psychiatry. 2004;161:1848-55.
21. Mirnics K, Middleton FA, Marquez A, et al. Molecular characterization of schizophrenia viewed by microarray analysis of gene expression in prefrontal cortex. Neuron. 2000; 28:53-67.
22. Pierri JN, Volk CL, Auh S, et al. Somal size of prefrontal cortical pyramidal neurons in schizophrenia: differential effects across neuronal subpopulations. Biol Psychiatry. 2003;54:111-20.
23. Jacobs B, Driscoll L, Schall M. Life-span dendritic and spine changes in areas 10 and 18 of human cortex: a quantitative Golgi study. J Comp Neurol. 1997;386:661-80.
24. Lewis DA, Lieberman JA. Catching up on schizophrenia: natural history and neurobiology. Neuron. 2000;28:325-34.
25. Volk DW, Austin MC, Pierri JN, et al. Decreased glutamic acid decarboxylase67 messenger RNA expression in a subset of prefrontal cortical gamma-aminobutyric acid neurons in subjects with schizophrenia. Arch Gen Psychiatry. 2000;57:237-45.
26. Benes FM, Vincent SL, Alsterberg G, et al. Increased GABA-A receptor binding in superficial layers of cingulated cortex in schizophrenics. J Neurosci. 1992;12:924-29.
27. Benes FM, Vincent SL, Marie A, et al. Up-regulation of GABA-A receptor binding on neurons of the prefrontal cortex in schizophrenic subjects. Neuroscience. 1996;75:1021-31.
28. Woo TU, Whitehead RE, Melchitzky DS, et al. A subclass of prefrontal gamma-aminobutyric acid axon terminals are selectively altered in schizophrenia. Proc Natl Acad Sci USA. 1998;95:5341-6.
29. Beasley CL, Reynolds GP. Parvalbumin-immunoreactive neurons are reduced in the prefrontal cortex of schizophrenics. Schizophr Res. 1997;24:349-55.
30. Woo TU, Miller JL, Lewis DA. Schizophrenia and the parvalbumin-containing class of cortical local circuit neurons. Am J Psychiatry. 1997;154:1013-5.
31. Lewis DA, Cruz DA, Melchitazky DS, et al. Lamina-specific deficits in parvalbumin-immunoreactive varicosities in the prefrontal cortex of subjects with schizophrenia: evidence for fewer projections from the thalamus. Am J Psychiatry. 2001; 158:1411-22.
32. Hashimoto T, Volk DW, Eggan SM, et al. Gene expression deficits in a subclass of GABA neurons in the prefrontal cortex of subjects with schizophrenia. J Neurosci. 2003;23:6315-26.
33. Shenton ME, Dickey CC, Frumin M, et al. A review of MRI findings in schizophrenia. Schizophr Res. 2001;49:1-52.
34. Nelson MD, Saykin AJ, Flashman LA, et al. Hippocample volume reduction in schizophrenia as assessed by magnetic resonance imaging: a meta-analytic study. Arch Gen Psychiatry. 1998;55:433-40.
35. Gur RE, Cowell P, Turetsky BI, et al. A follow-up magnetic resonance imaging study of schizophrenia. Relationship of neuronatomical change to clinical and neurobehavioral measures. Arch Gen Psychiatry. 1998;55:145-52.
36. Pantelis C, Valakoulis D, McGorry PD, et al. Neuroanatomical abnormalities before and after onset of psychosis: a cross-sectional and longitudinal MRI comparison. Lancet. 2003; 361:281-88.
37. Gogtay N, Sporn A, Clasen LS, et al. Comparison of progressive cortical gray matter loss in childhood-onest schizophrenia with that in childhood-onset atypical psychoses. Arch Gen Psychiatry. 2004;61:17-22.
38. Thompson PM, Vidal C, Giedd JN, et al. Mapping adolescent brain change reveals dynamic wave of accelerated gray matter loss in very early-onset schizophrenia. Proc Natl Aced Sci USA. 2001;98:11650-55.
39. Cahn W, Pol HE, Lems EB, et al. Brain volume changes in first-episode schizophrenia: a 1-year follow-up study. Arch Gen Psychiatry. 2002;59:1002-10.

40. Kasai K, Shenton ME, Salisbury DF, et al. Progressive decrease of left superior temporal gyrus gray matter volume in patients with first-episode schizophrenia. Am J Psychiatry. 2003; 160:156-64.
41. Glantz LA, Gilmore JH, Lieberman JA, et al. Apoptotic mechanism and the synaptic pathology of schizophrenia. Schizophr Res. 2006;81:47-63.
42. Lieberman JA, Tollefson GD, Charles C, et al. Antipsychotic drug effects on brain morphology in first-episode psychosis. Arch Gen Pschiatry. 2005;62:361-70.
43. Dorph-Petersen KA, Pierri JN, Perel JM, et al. The influence of chronic exposure to antipsychotic medication on brain size before and after tissue fixation: a comparison of haloperidol and olanzapine in macaque monkeys. Neuropsyhopharmacology. 2005;30:1649-61.
44. Sullivan PF, Kendler KS, Neale MC. Schizophrenia as a complex trait: evidence from a meta-analysis of twin studies. Arch Gen Psychiatry. 2003;60:1187-92.
45. Sullivan PF. The genetics of schizophrenia. PLoS Med. 2005; 2:e212.
46. Kamiya A, Kubo K, Tomoda T, et al. A schizophrenia-associated mutation of DISC1 perturbs cerebral cortex development. Nat Cell Biol. 2005;7:1167-78.
47. Creese I, Burt, DR, Snyder SH. Dopamine receptor binding predicts clinical and pharmacological potencies of antischizophreninc drugs. Science. 1976;192:481-3.
48. Miyamoto S, Duncan GE, Mailman RB, et al. Developing novel antipsychotic drugs: strategies and goals. Curr Opin CPNS Invest Drugs. 2000;2:25-39.
49. Green MF, Kern RS, Braff DL, et al. Neurocognitive deficits and functional outcome in schizophrenia: Are we measuring the right stuff? Schizophr Bull. 2000;26:119-36.
50. Fleischhacker WW. New drugs for the treatment of schizophrenic patients. Acta Psychiatr. Scand Suppl. 1995; 388:24-30.
51. Kane J, Honigfeld G, Singer J, et al. Clozapine for the treatment-resistant schizophrenic. A double-blind comparison with chlorpromazine. Arch Gen Psychiatry. 1988;45:789-96.
52. Miyamoto S, Lieberman JA, Fleischhacker WW, et al. Antipsychotic drugs. In: Psychiatry (Ed). A Tasman, J Kay, JA Liaberman, Chichester, UK: John Wiley & Sons. 2003; pp. 1928-64.
53. Kane JM, Leucht S, Carpenter D, et al. Expert consensus guideline series. Optimizing pharmacologic treatment of psychotic disorders. Introduction: methods, commentary, and summary. J Clin Psychiatry. 2003;64(Suppl. 12):5-19.
54. Meltzer HY, Matsubare S, Lee JC. Classification of typical and atypical antipsychotic drugs on the basis of dopamine D-1, D-2 and serotonin2 pKi values. J Pharmacol Exp Ther. 1889; 251:238-46.
55. Seeman P. Atypical antipsychotics: mechanism of action. Cen J Psychiatry. 2002;47:27-38.
56. Miyamoto S, Duncan GE, Marx CE, et al. Treatments for schizophrenia: a critical review of pharmacology and mechanisms of antipsychotic drugs. Mol Psychiatry. 2005; 10:79-104.
57. Bai O, Chlan-Fourney J, Bowen R, et al. Expression of brain-derived neurotrophic factors mRNA in rat hippocampus after treatment with antipsychotic drugs. J Neurosci Res. 2003; 71:127-31.
58. Farber NB, Foster J, Duhan NL, et al. Olanzapine and fluperlapine mimic clozapine in preventing MK-801 neurotoxicity. Schizophr Res. 1996;21:33-37.
59. Wakade CG, Mahadik SP, Waller JL, et al. Atypical neuroleptics stimulate neurogenesis in adult rat brain. J Neurosci Res. 2002; 69:72-79.
60. Abi-Dargham A, Rodenhiser J, Printz D, et al. Increased baseline occupancy of D2 receptors by dopamine in schizophrenia. Proc Natl Acad Sci USA. 2000;97:8104-9.
61. Abi-Dargham A, Moore H. Prefrontal DA transmission at D1 receptors and the pathology of schizophrenia. Neuroscientist. 2003;9:404-16.
62. Lieberman JA. Dopamine partial agonists-a new class of antipsychotic. CNS Drugs. 2004;18:251-67.
63. Potkin SG, Saha AR, Kujawa MJ, et al. Aripiprazole, an antipsychotic with a novel mechanism of action, and risperidone vs placebo in patents with schizophrenia and schizoaffective disorder. Arch Gen Psychiatry. 2003;60:681-90.
64. Yokoi F, Grunder G, Biziere K, et al. Dopamine D2 and D3 receptor occupancy in normal human treated with the antipsychotic drug aripiprazole (OPC 14597): a study using positron emission tomography and [11C] raclopride. Neuropsychopharmacology. 2002;27:248-59.
65. Leucht S, Pitschel-Walz G, Abraham D, et al. Effcacy and extrapyramidal side-effects of the new antipsychotics olanzapine, quetiapine, risperidone, and sertindole compared to conventional antipsychotics and placebo. A meta-analysis of randomized controlled trials. Schizophr Res. 1999;35:54-68.
66. Leucht S, Wahlbeck K, Hamann J, et al. New generation anti-psychotics versus low-potency conventional antipsychotics: a systematic review and meta-analysis. Lancet. 2003;361:1581-89.
67. Geddes J, Freemantle N, Harrison P, et al. Atypical antipsychotics in the treatment of schizophrenia: systematic overview and meta-regression analysis. BMJ. 2000;321:1371-76.
68. Davis JM, McEvoy JP, Swartz MS, et al. A meta-analysis of the efficacy of second-generation antipsychotic. Arch Gen Psychiatry. 2003;60:553-64.
69. Stroup TS, McEvoy JP, Swartz MS, et al. The National Institute of Mental Health Clinical Antipsychotic Trials of Intervention Effectiveness (CATIE) project: schizophrenia trial design and protocol development. Schizophr Bull. 2003;29:15-31.
70. Lieberman JA, Stroup TS, McEvoy JP, et al. Effectiveness of antipsychotic drugs in patients with chronic schizophrenia. N Engl J Med. 2005;353:1209-23.
71. Friedman JI. Cholinergic targets for cognitive enhancement in schizophrenia: focus on cholinesterase inhibitors and muscarinic agonists. Psychopharmacology (Berl). 2004; 174:45-53.

CHAPTER

70 Borderline Personality Disorder

JN Vyas

INTRODUCTION

Borderline personality disorder is a common mental disorder associated with high rates of suicide, severe functional impairment, high rates of comorbid mental disorder, intensive use of treatment, and high costs to society.[1-5] In recent years, research findings have contributed to an improved understanding and therapy of these difficult-to-treat patients.

EPIDEMIOLOGY

In epidemiological studies of adults in the USA, prevalances for borderline personality disorder were between 0.5% and 5.9% in the general US population[6,7] with a median prevalence of 1.35 as assessed by Torgersen and colleagues.[8] There is no evidence that borderline personality disorder is more common in women.[7,9] In clinical populations, borderline personality disorder is the most common personality disorder, with a prevalence of 10% of all psychiatric outpatients and between 15% and 25% of inpatients.[9,10] In a study of a non-clinical sample,[7] a high rate of borderline personality disorder was reported (5.9%), indicating that many individuals with this disorder do not seek psychiatric treatment. In primary care, the prevalence reported for borderline personality disorder was four-times higher than that in the general population, suggesting that individuals with this disorder are frequent users of general medical care.[11]

DIAGNOSIS

According to the current psychiatric classification system in the fourth edition of the Diagnostic and Statistical Manual of Mental Disorders (DSM-IV), borderline personality disorder is characterized by a pervasive pattern of instability in interpersonal relationships, identity, impulsivity, and affect (panel).[12] For a diagnosis of borderline personality disorder, at least five of the nine criteria must be met. However, suicidal tendency or self-injury are the most useful indications for a correct diagnosis,[11] whereas suicidal tendency or self-injury and unstable relationships have been the most predictive features in follow-up studies.[13,14] Accordingly, the rank ordering of criteria as most prototypical of this disorder in DSM-IV was not supported by the evidence. Further research is needed to establish whether some criteria should be given more emphasis than others.[5] The nine DSM-IV criteria of borderline personality disorder seem to indicate a statistically cohererent construct.[15] Because factor analyses have established both a one-factor model and a three-factor model (disturbed relatedness, behavioral dysregulation, affective dysregulation), an underlying multidimensional structure of borderline personality disorder consisting of three homogeneous components might exist.[5,15] With nine DSM-IV criteria and a threshold for five positive criteria of a diagnosis of borderline personality disorder, however, there are 151 theoretical possible ways of diagnosing this disorder.[2,3] Thus, despite conceptual coherence, borderline personality disorder seems to be a heterogeneous diagnostic category, which can include subtypes of patients, such as those with or without stress-related paranoid ideations or chronic feelings of emptiness.[3] DSM-5 diagnostic criteria for borderline personality disorder is listed below.

DSM-5 Diagnostic criteria for borderline personality disorder

A pervasive pattern of social and interpersonal deficits marked by acute discomfort with, and reduced capacity for, close relationships as well as by cognitive or perceptual distortions and eccentricities of behavior, beginning by early adulthood and present in a variety of contexts, as indicated by five (or more) of the following:

- Frantic efforts to avoid real or imagined abandonment. (Do not include suicide or self-mutilating behavior covered in criteria 5)
- A pattern of unstable and intense interpersonal relationships characterized by alternating between extremes of idealization and devaluation.
- Identity disturbance: markedly and persistently unstable self-image or sense of self.
- Impulsivity in atleast two areas that are potentially selfdamaging (e.g. spending, sex, substance abuse, reckless driving, binge ating). (Note: Do not include suicide or self-mutilating behavior covered in criteria 5).

Contd...

Contd...

- Recurrent suicidal behavior, gestures, or threat, or self-mutilating behavior.
- Affective instability due to a marked reactivity of mood (e.g. intense episodic dysphoria, irritability, or anxiety usually lasting a few hours and only rarely more than a few days.
- Chronic feelings of emptiness.
- Inappropriate intense anger or difficulty controlling anger.
- Transient, stress-related paranoid ideation or severe dissociative symptoms.

COURSE

Although more stable than more depressive disorder, borderline personality disorder seems to be less stable over time than expected for personality disorder.[5,36,17] High rates of remission were reported in both short-term and long-term follow-up studies.[16] The rate of remission does not seem to be affected by major depressive. By contrast, the rate of remission of major depressive disorder does seem to be significantly reduced by co-occurring borderline personality disorder.[25] Affective features (e.g. anger, anxiety, depression) and interpersonal features indicative of abandonment and dependency were the most prevalent and stable,[18] whereas impulsive symptoms (e.g. suicide efforts, self-injury) and interpersonal features indicative of treatment regressions were the least prevalent and consistent.[19] Features of this disorder decline over time and this process seems to be party affected by temperament.[19] With fewer features over time, personality disorders such as borderline personality disorder become more correlated with each other and less distinct as individual disorder.[20] Changes in personality traits (defined by the five-factor model) seem to be followed by changes in the personality disorder psychopathology of borderline personality disorder, but not vice versa.[21] Traits were more unstable in patients with borderline personality disorder than in patients with other personality disorders indicating a "stable instability",[22] a term introduced by Schmideberg.[23] Data from most studies show that patients with borderline personality disorder are not at higher than average risk for schizophrenia or bipolar disorder.[24, 25]

COMORBIDITY

Borderline personality disorder is regularly associated with comorbid axis I and axis II disorders.[5-7] 84.5% of patients with borderline personality disorder met criteria for having one or more 12 month axis I disorders, and 73.9% met criteria for another lifetime axis II disorder.[6,7] Borderline personality disorder is most frequently associated with mood disorders, anxiety disorders, and disorders associated with substance misuse.[5-7] With a lifetime prevalence of 39.2% post-traumatic stress disorder is common but not universal in patients with borderline personality disorder,[7] which questions the view of borderline personality disorder as a complex form of post-traumatic stress disorder.[26] With respect to comorbid mental disorders, differences between female and male patients with borderline personality disorder have been reported, with disorders associated with substance misuse being more common in men and eating disorders being more common in woman.[7]

Borderline personality disorder is associated with severe and stable functional impairment[5-7,27] and characterized by a high risk of suicide.[3,28] The mortality rate from suicide is between 8% and 10%, which is 50 times higher than in the general population.[3,28] However, there are reports of lower rates.[29] Patients with borderline personality disorder have more functional impairment and higher use of treatment than do patients with major depressive disorder.[1,30] However, some patients with borderline personality disorder have good psychosocial functioning (25.9%), but most of them (80%) lose this level of functioning over time and do not regain it.[31] Personality disorders have a negative effect on the treatment outcomes of various axis I disorders.[2]

PSYCHOSOCIAL FACTORS IN THE DEVELOPMENT OF BORDERLINE PERSONALITY DISORDER

Patients with borderline personality disorder report many negative events (e.g. trauma, neglect) during childhood[32] and substantially more adverse events than do patients with other personality disorder.[33] However, no close association between these experiences and the development of psychopathological changes in adulthood has been identified.[34,35] For this reason, an interaction between biological (e.g. temperamental) and psychosocial factors (e.g. adverse childhood events) will probably provide the best explanation of how the condition develops,[36] consistent with results from recent studies of gene/environment interaction in this disorder.[37,38]

GENETIC FACTORS AND NEUROBIOLOGY

Evidence has emerged that genetic factors contribute to the development of borderline personality disorder,[39-41] however, no specific genes have yet been clearly identified as causative. For dimensional representations of borderline personality disorder traits (i.e. their quantitative intensity), a moderate heritability has been reported.[40] In studies of twins, heritability scores for the full diagnosis were 0.65 to 0.75,[42] consistent with heritability estimates for personality disorders in general (40–60%).[43] Impulsive aggression, common in patients with borderline personality disorder, is associated with reduced serotonergic responsiveness,[44] and some genes that might be linked to psychopathological changes in the disorder are involved in the serotonergic system.[42] Thus, the serotonin system is the neurotransmitter system of greatest interest in these patients, and is the assumed site of action for specific selective serotonin-reuptake inhibitors.[42,45] Data from a candidate gene (the serotonin–transporter-linked promoter region [5-HTTLPR] in SLC6A4) and development of borderline personality disorder, however, no association between polymorphisms in 5-HTTLPR and this disorder were reported in another study.[46] Presence of the short allele of 5-HTTLPR can also indicate a poor treatment response to fluoxetine in patients with borderline personality disorder.[47] Polymorphisms in 5-HTTLPR might also modulate the association between serious life events and the development of impulsivity in patients.[37]

In a study of gene-gene interactions,[48] an interaction between the Met158 allele of the catecholamine-O-methyltransferase gene (COMT) and the short allele of 5-HTTLPR was reported in patients with borderline personality disorder, but no association between the 5-HTTLPR genotype alone and development of this disorder was reported. Although the results of these studies suggest a role for polymorphisms in 5-HTTLPR in these patients, there are undoubtedly complex gene-gene and gene–environment interactions, thus making the results inconclusive.[42]

Another gene that has been implicated in impulsive aggression and suicidal behavior is the tryptophan hydroxylase gene (TPH), which encodes the first enzyme in serotonin biosynthesis. Two isoforms are known TPH-1 and TPH-2. Patients with borderline personality disorder have a higher frequency of two of eight polymorphisms in TPH-2 than do controls.[49]

Finally, in a recent case-control study,[50] patients with borderline personality disorder had a greater frequency of polymorphisms in the variable number tandem repeat of the high-activity monoamine oxidase. A gene promoter allele than did healthy volunteers. Taken together, the published evidence suggests that this defect might be associated with specific genetic risk factors, but the precise molecular nature of this abnormality is not yet clear. Data from early studies of dexamethasone suppression tests[51,52] have suggested that this disorder was associated with excessive production of cortisol and hypothalamic-pituitary-adrenocortical hyperactivity, although this finding was reported in many patients who had post-traumatic stress disorder with severe histories of trauma. However, in more recent studies that investigated borderline personality disorder without comorbid post-traumatic stress disorder, there was evidence of hypersuppression of cortisol, interpreted as increased feedback inhibition of the hypothalamic-pituitary-adrenocortical axis.[53]

Panel: DSM-IV-TR diagnostic criteria for 301. 83 borderline personality disorder

The essential feature of borderline personality disorder is that it has a pervasive pattern of instability of interpersonal relationships, self-image, and affect, with notable impulsivity that begins by early adulthood and is present in various contexts, as indicated by five (or more) of the following:

- Frantic efforts to avoid real or imagined abandonment*
- A pattern of unstable and intense interpersonal relationships characterized by alternating between extremes of idealization and devaluation
- Identity disturbance: notably and persistently unstable self-image or sense of self
- Impulsivity in at least two areas that are potentially self-damaging (e.g. spending, sex, substance misuse, reckless driving, binge eating)*
- Recurrent suicidal behavior gestures, or threats or self-mutilating behavior
- Affective instability cause by a distinct reactivity of mood (e.g. intense episodic dysphoria, irritability, or anxiety usually lasting a few hours and only rarely more than a few days)
- Chronic feelings of emptiness
- Inappropriate intense anger or difficulty controlling anger (e.g. frequent displays of temper, constant anger, recurrent physical fights)
- Transient, stress-related paranoid ideation or severe dissociative symptoms

**Note:* Does not include suicidal or self-mutilating behavior covered in criterion 5. DSM-IV=Diagnostic and Statistical Manual of Mental Disorders, fourth edition.

NEUROIMAGING

Anatomical MRI Findings

Although CT studies of the brain did not detect any morphological changes in patients with borderline personality disorder, reduced volume in the amygdala has been reported in some studies with structural MRI.[54, 55] Excitotoxicity in the course of this disorder was discussed as a possible cause of reduced amygdala volume. Similar to these findings, no morphological changes in the amygdala were reported after the first appearance of symptoms in teenagers.[56] Reduced hippocampal volumes,[57] but no reductions in the amygdala volume, were observed in patients with post-traumatic stress disorder.[58] Although results from a recent meta-analysis[59] indicated that the amygdala volume in patients with borderline personality disorder was smaller than that in healthy controls, data from studies not included in that analysis,[60-63] including some with hand-tracing of the amygdala, did not show a reduced amygdala volume in these patients. Data from these subsequent studies also highlight the importance of taking into account the effect of comorbid post-traumatic stress disorder on amygdala volume, because patients with borderline personality disorder without post-traumatic stress disorder might not have reduced amygdala volumes.[60] Thus, evidence about the specificity of reductions in amygdala volume in patients with borderline personality disorder is inconsistent.

Although there were no volumetric differences in the pituitary gland between patients with early-stage borderline personality disorder and controls,[64] the pituitary gland volume in teenagers with first-presentation borderline personality disorder was positively correlated with the number of parasuicidal actions.[65] In psychosis, the volume of the pituitary gland seems to be positively correlated with the extent of activation of the hypothalamic-pituitary-adrenocortical axis.[66] Thus, an increased volume of the pituitary gland in patients with borderline personality disorder might be an indicator of increased activity of this axis.[65] Several reports have revealed morphological changes in other neuroanatomical structures in patients with borderline personality disorder. A reduction in gray matter volume in the anterior cingulated gyrus, posterior cingulated gyrus,[63] or hippocampus,[55,67] and a reduced size of the right parietal cortex in these patients[67] have been reported. Moreover, size abnormalities of the superior parietal cortices were correlated with dissociation in these patients.[68] Reduced gray matter volumes in the dorsolateral cortex and in the left orbitofrontal cortex were reported in an early stage of borderline personality disorder.[69]

PET

Results from most PET studies detected changes in frontal glucose metabolism in patients with borderline personality disorder. In theses studies, a hypometabolism was more often reported than a hypermetabolism,[70] which lends support to the assumption of a frontolimbic dysfunction in these patients. Moreover, autobiographical memories of abuse events in traumatized woman without borderline personality disorder were accompanied by large increases in blood flow of the prefrontal cortex (right anterior cingulated, left orbitofrontal, right dorsolateral prefrontal cortex) and a decrease in the left dorsolateral prefrontal cortex compared with traumatized woman with borderline personality disorder.[60] These findings might be indicative of dysfunctions in prefrontal areas in this disorder. In a recent PET study[71] of aggression provocation, patients with borderline personality disorder activated orbital cortex more than did controls, whereas controls activated regions of prefrontal cortex more typically associated with emotion control than did those with borderline personality disorder. This result lends further support to the view that there is an abnormality in prefrontal brain regions associated with emotional control function in borderline personality disorder.

Functional MRI Findings

The most consistent finding in patients with borderline personality disorder is increased amygdala activation compared with control individuals when viewing aversive emotion-inducing slides[72] or when viewing pictures of human emotional facial expressions.[73] During the recall of an unresolved life event, only patients with borderline personality disorder (vs healthy controls) showed bilateral activations of the amygdala.[74] The amygdala is assumed to function as a key structure during the processing of anxiety and other affective states. As expected, there was no activation of the amygdala in patients with borderline personality disorder or in healthy individuals when positive visual material was presented.[75] Furthermore, activation of the prefrontal cortex was reported for patients with borderline personality disorder after including negative emotions, possibly indicating an attempt to control intensive emotions.[74,76] When asked to use a cognitive strategy to control their responses to unpleasant pictures by distancing themselves from the image, those with borderline personality disorder had less blood-oxygen-level dependent (BOLD) signal changes in the anterior cingulated and had greater activation in the superior temporal sulcus and superior frontal gyrus than did controls. Thus, patients with borderline personality disorder do not seem to engage the cognitive control regions to the extent that healthy individuals do, which might contribute to the affective instability of this disorder.[75] Further findings from functional MRI studies indicate different neuronal patterns of traumatic memory in patients with and without post-traumatic stress disorder.[77] Only in patients with post-traumatic stress disorder did a thermic pain induction evoke a decreased amygdala activation.[78] These results might indicate the existence of different neural networks in subgroups of patients with borderline personality disorder.

These reports lend support to the assumption of a dysfunctional frontolimbic network in borderline personality disorder. This network seems to involve the anterior cingular cortex, the hippocampus, and the amygdala. However, future studies are needed, including with individuals who do not have borderline personality disorder, including healthy controls, patients with axis I disorders or patients with other personality disorders to investigate the specificity of these findings.

TREATMENT

The American Psychiatric Association's practice guideline recommends psychotherapy as the main treatment of borderline personality disorder, with pharmacotherapy as an adjunctive component of treatment that targets state symptoms during periods of acute decompensation and trait vulnerabilities.[28] This guideline is a set of evidence-based practice recommendations. The pharmacotherapy algorithms are direct towards three clusters of symptoms: cognitive-perceptual symptoms (with neuroleptics), affective symptoms (with selective serotonin-reuptake inhibitors), and impulsive-behavioral dyscontrol (with selective serotonin-reuptake inhibitors and low-dose neuroleptics).[28]

Pharmacotherapy

Following the Cochrane criteria, evidence for the pharmacological treatment of BPD was reviewed in 2006;[79]

only ten small randomized controlled trails (RCTs) were identified.

The antidepressants amitriptyline and imipramine were more effective than placebo for some symptoms of depression, but not for other symptoms of borderline personality disorder.[84] Few differences between monoamine oxidase inhibitors (phenelzine) and placebo were reported.[72-85] Phenelzine reduced hostility, but not depression.[83] In one RCT, fluoxetine was not clearly more effective than placebo for depression, but a beneficial effects of fluvoxamine on mood shifts were reported, but not on aggression or impulsivity.[86,105,106]

In some studies, the typical antipsychotic haloperidol was more effective than placebo for several symptoms, but results vary.[83,84,87] By contrast with their previous results,[84] Soloff and colleagues[83] did not find haloperidol more effective than placebo for most outcome measures. Haloperidol seems to be more effective than tricyclic antidepressants (amitripityline) for hostility and schizotypal symptoms.[84] Phenelzine was more effective than haloperidol for some symptoms (e.g. depression, anxiety, schizotypal symptoms), but not for others (e.g. impulse control).[83] At present, there is no evidence that one typical antipsychotic is more effective than another (i.e. loxapine vs chlorpromazine or tiotxene vs haloperidol).[79, 88]

In two RCTs, the atypical antipsychotic olanzapine was more effective than placebo for several, but not all, symptosms,[89,90] however, in another RCT, no superiority of olanzapine over placebo was reported.[97] Olanzapine monotherapy and olanzapine combined with fluoxetine were more effective than fluoxetine alone for depression and impulsive aggression.[91-98] This combination had no advantage over olanzapine monotherapy.[91] Ziprasidone had no superiority over placebo.[100]

The mood stabilizer carbamazepine had no superiority over placebo.[92] No effects of sodium valproate were reported on depression.[82,93,94] Beneficial effects of lamotrigine on affective instability and impulsivity were reported in one RCT.[96] Improvements were reported for an omega-3 fatty acid treatment[95] in one small RCT of 30 patients with borderline personality disorder, and for clonidine in 18 patients in another small RCT.[99]

In summary, evidence for pharmacotherapy in borderline personality disorder varies. Beneficial effects on depression, aggression, and other symptoms were reported in some RCTS, but not in others. Many of the findings are based on single RCTs or on small samples of patients. Some studies (e.g. of olanzapine) included only female patients. Only a few studies included long-term follow-ups.[105] As stressed by the NICE group, some of the drugs are potentially harmful—e.g. valproate semisodium, which is dangerous for woman of child-bearing age.[106] Antipsychtics have many neurological side-effects and metabolic effects leading to weight gain and increased risk of diabetes.[106] Thus, more evidence is needed before definitive recommendations can be made about the pharmacological treatment of any symptoms of borderline personal disorder.

Psychotherapy

Several methods of psychotherapy are available for patients with borderline personality disorder—e.g. cognitive-behavioral, interpersonal, or psychodynamic treatments. Two formal reviews on the efficacy of psychotherapy for the disorder exist.[107,108] Following Cochrane criteria, Binks and colleagues[107] indentified only seven RCTs published up to 2002.[109-115] Brazier and colleagues[108] included two additional RCTs.[116,117] In their review on borderline personality disorder, Lieb and colleagues,[4] indentified 11 RCTs. Since 2006, several RCTs on psychotherapy have been published. Following the Cochrane criteria used by Binks and colleagues,[107] 24 RCTs on psychotherapy alone in borderline personality disorder were indentified.

For cognitive behavior therapy, the results can be summarized as follows. In studies comparing dialectical behavior therapy with treatment as usual, dialectical behavior therapy was more effective in several outcome measures (e.g. self harm, parasuicidal behavior, suicidal ideation).[110-112,114,128,131] However, the number of patients still meeting the diagnostic criteria of borderline personality disorder did not differ. For depression, anxiety, admission to hospital, or drop outs, only two trails also reported superiority of dialectical behavior therapy.[118-121,128] In another RCT,[131] dialectical behavior therapy was more effective than treatment as usual in reducing self-mutilating behaviors and self-damaging impulsive acts, but not in reducing suicidal behavior. The skills training component for dialectical behavior was superior to a nonmanualized standard group therapy in several measures (e.g. depression, anxiety).[130] Furthermore, dialectical behavior therapy superior to a community treatment by experts (not further specified noncognitive behavior therapy) with respect to remission of co-occurring substance-dependence disorders.[126,127] No clear differences were reported between dialectical behavior therapy focusing on substance misuse and comprehensive validation therapy plus a 12-step substance misuse program.[111] Compared with client-centred therapy, dialectical behavior therapy was superior in reducing parasuicidal behavior, suicidal ideation, and general psychiatric severity.[115] No superiority of dialectical behavior therapy over client-centerd therapy was identified for anxiety.[115] In the most recent RCT,[129] which was sufficiently powered to detect a medium effect size (sample sizes of 90 for both gropus), both dialectical behavior therapy and a well specified and psychodymanically informed clinical management provided significant improvements with no differences between treatments. Results from another RCT indicated that schema-focused therapy was superior to transference-focused psychotherapy.[125,132] However, differences in therapist competence ratings indicate that transference-focused psychotherapy might have been less competently implemented than schema-focused therapy. Thus, replications are needed. Adding an 8 month schema-focused therapy group to treatment as usual was more effective than just treatment as usual.[124] Adding availability of a therapist by telephone outside office hours to schema-focused therapy did not lead to extra effects.[134] Client-centred therapy was as effective as cognitive behavior therapy with respect to the response criterion, although cognitive behavior therapy was superior in some other outcome measures.[123] Brief cognitive behavior therapy was not superior to treatment as usual, but was more cost-effective.[117] In three studies, new and brief cognitive-behavioral treatments for patients with borderline personality disorder were tested in an add-on design.[119,120,133] When added to treatment as usual, these strategies were superior to treatment as usual alone in some, but not in all, outcome measures.[119,120,133]

In summary, dialectical behavior therapy and specific forms of psychodynamic psychotherapy seem to be superior to treatment as usual in some clinically relevant problems of borderline personality disorder. Adding brief cognitive behavior therapy to treatment as usual seems to be superior to treatment as usual alone. According to follow-up studies, effects of psychotherapy are stable over time.[111,112,116,119,120,124,127,128,136-138] At present, there is no clear evidence that one specific form of psychotherapy is superior to another.[139] In several studies comparing specific forms of psychotherapy, however, power was not sufficient to detect possible differences.[111,116,122] In summary, there is evidence that psychotherapy is beneficial with respect to some clinically relevant problems of patients with borderline personality disorder. However, the available forms of psychotherapy do not yet lead to remission of borderline personality disorder for most patients (i.e. no longer fulfilling the criteria of a diagnosis of borderline personality disorder). Thus, further research is needed.

Pharmacotherapy with Psychotherapy

The benefit of a combination of pharmacotherapy and psychotherapy in borderline personality disorder is unclear. Fluoxetine combined with dialectical behavior therapy provided no additional benefit compared with dialectical behavior therapy plus placebo.[102] In one study,[103] olanzapine added to dialectical behavior therapy provided an additional benefit compared with dialectical behavior therapy, although no differences were reported in another study in favor of the combined treatment.[104] The combination of interpersonal therapy and fluoxetine was superior to fluoxetine plus clinical management.[101]

FUTURE PERSPECTIVES

Although much has been learned about borderline personality disorder in recent years, several questions remain. Despite conceptual coherence, borderline personality disorder seems to be a heterogeneous diagnostic category that is less stable and distinct over time than expected. These findings raise questions of both how to conceptualize this disorder and how to implement it in future versions of DSM as a form of personality pathology that is both enduring and distinct from other personality disorders.[20] Furthermore, the discussion on whether a categorical or a dimensional model best suits personality disorders is ongoing.[140,141] The results of the Collaborative Longitudinal Personality Disorder Study (CLPS)[5,142] suggest reconceptualizing personality disorders as hybrids of stable personality traits and as intermittently expressed symptomatic behaviors that are attempts to cope with of defend against or compensate for these pathological traits (e.g. self-harm to reduce affective tension). Further research is needed on the association between personality traits and personality disorder psychopathological changes as well as on the relation between personality disorders and personality functioning.[21,143] Personality might function differently as different ages and in response to different needs.[143] Future research on the causes of this disorder should investigate how genetic and psychosocial factors interact with neurotransmitter function to led to cognitive and emotional regulations and specific traits.[144-145] The available findings of neuroimaging studies lend support to the assumption of a dysfunctional frontolimbic network in borderline personality disorder.

REFERENCES

1. Bender DS, Dolan RT, Skodol AE, et al. Treatment utilization by patients with personality disorders. Am J Psychiatry. 2001;158:295-302.
2. Skodol AE, Gunderson JG, Pfohl B, Widiger TA, Livesley WJ, Siever LJ. The borderline diagnosis I: psychopathology, Comorbidity, and personality structure. Boil Psychiatry. 2002;51:36-50.
3. Oldham JM. Borderline personality disorder and suicidality. Am J Psychiatry. 2006;163:20-26.
4. Lieb K, Zanarini MC, Schmahl C, Linehan MM, Bohus M. Borderline personality disorder. Lancet. 2004;364:453-61.
5. Skodol AE, Gunderson JG, Shea MT, et al. The Collaborative Longitudinal Personality Disorders Study (CLPS): overview and implications. J Pers Disord. 2005;19:487-504.
6. Lenzenweger M, Lane M, Loranger A, Kessler R. Personality disorders in the National Comorbidity Survey Replication. Boil Psychiatry. 2007;62:553-64.
7. Grant BF, Chou SP, Goldstein RB, et al. Prevalence, correlates, disability, and Comorbidity of DSM-IV borderline personality disorder: results from the Wave 2 National Epidemiologic Survey on Alcohol and Related Conditions. J Clin Psychiatry. 2008;69:533-45.
8. Torgarsen S, Kringlen, E, Cramer V. The prevalence of personality disorders in a community sample. Arch Gen Psychiatry. 2001;58:590-6.
9. Torgen J. Epidemiology. In: Oldham J, Skodol AE, Bender, DS, eds. Textbook of personality disorders. Washington, DC: American Psychiatric Publishing; 2005.pp.129-41.

10. Gunderson JG. Borderline personality disorder: ontogeny of a diagnosis. Am J Psychiatry. 2009;166:530-39.
11. Gross R, Olfson M, Gemeroff M, et al. Borderline personality disorder in primary care. Arch Intern Med. 2002;162:53-60.
12. American Psychiatry Association. Diagnostic and Statistical manual of Mental Disorders, fourth edn. Washington, DC: American Psychiatry Association, 1994.
13. Grilo CM, Becker DF, Anez LM, McGlashan TH. Diagnostic efficiency of DSM-IV Criteria for borderline personality disorder: an evaluation in Hispanic men and women with substance use disorders. J Consult Clin Psychol. 2004;72:126-31.
14. Grilo CM, Sanislow CA, Skodol AE, et al. Longitudinal diagnostic efficiency of DSM-IV criteria for borderline personality disorder: a 2-year prospective study. Can J Psychiatry. 2007;52:357-62.
15. Sanisslow CA, Grilo CM, Morey LC, et al. Confirmatory factor analysis of DSM-IV criteria for borderline personality disorder: findings from the collaborative longitudinal personality disorders study. Am J Psychiatry. 2002;159:284-90.
16. Zanarini MC, Frankenburg FR, Hennen J, Reich DB, Silk KR. Prediction of the 10-year course of borderline personality disorder. Am J Psychiatry. 2006;163:827-32.
17. Gunderson JG, Bender D, Sanislow C, et al. Plausibility and possible determinants of sudden "remissions" in borderline patients. Psychiatry. 2003;66:111-9.
18. Gunderson JG, Morey LC, Stout RL, et al. Major depressive disorder and borderline personality disorder revisited: longitudinal interactions. J Clin Psychiatry. 2004;65: 1049-56.
19. Zanarini MC, Frankenburg Fr, Reich DB, Silk KR, Hudson JI, McSweeney LB. The subsyndromal phenomenology of borderline personality disorder: a 10-year follow-up study. Am J Psychiatry. 2007;164:929-35.
20. Sanislow CA, Little TD, Ansell EB, et al. Ten-year stability and latent structure of the DSM-IV schizotypal, borderline, avoidant, and obsessive-compulsive personality disorders. J Abnorm Psychol. 2009;118:507-19.
21. Warner MB, Morey LC, Finch JF, et al. The longitudinal relationship of personality traits and disorders. J Abnorm Psychol. 2004;113:217-27.
22. Hopwood CJ, Newman DA, Donnellan MB, et al. The stability of personality traits in individuals with borderline personality disorder. J Abnorm Psycho. 2009;118:806-15.
23. Schmideberg M. The borderline patient. In: Arieti S, ed. American Handbook of Psychiatry New York: Basic Books; 1959.pp.398-416.
24. Carpenter WT Jr, Gunderson JG. Five year follow-up comparison of borderline and schizophrenic patients. Compr Psychiatry. 1977;18:567-71.
25. Paris J, Gunderson J, Weinberg I. The interface between borderline personality disorder and bipolar spectrum disorders. Compr Psychiatry. 2007;48:145-54.
26. Lewis KL, Grenyer BF. Borderline personality or complex posttraumatic stress disorder? An update on the controversy. Harv Rev Psychiatry. 2009;17:322-8.
27. Skodol AE, Pagano ME, Bender DS, et al. Stability of functional impairment in patients with schizotypal, borderline, avoidant, or obsessive-compulsive personality disorder over two years. Psycho Med. 2005;35:443-51.
28. American Psychiatric Association Practice Guidelines. Practice guideline for the treatment of patients with borderline personality disorder. Am J Psychiatry. 2001;158:1-52.
29. Zanarini MC, Frankenburg FR, Vujanovic AA, Hennen J, Reich DB, Silk KR. Axis II comorbidity of borderline personality disorder: description of 6-year course and prediction to time-to-remission. Acta Psychiatr Scand. 2004;110:416-20.
30. Skodol AE, Gunderson JG, McGlashan TH, et al. Functional impairment in patients with schizotypal, borderline, avoidant, or obsessive-compulsive personality disorder. Am J Psychiatry. 2002;159:276-83.
31. Zanarini MC, Frankenburg FR, Reich DB, Fitzmaurice G. the 10 year course of psychosocial functioning among patients with borderline personality disorder and axis II comparison subjects. Acta Psychiatr Scand. 2010;122:103-9.
32. Zanarini MC, Yong L, Frankenburg FR, et al. Severity of reported childhood sexual abuse and its relationship to severity of borderline psychopathology and spychosocial impairment among borderline inpatients. J Nerv Ment Dis. 2002;190:381-7.
33. Yen S, Shea MT, Battle CL, et al. Traumatic exposure and post-traumatic stress disorder in borderline, schizotypal, avoidant, and obsessive-compulsive personality disorders: findings from the collaborative longitudinal personality disorders study. J Nerv Ment Dis. 2002;190:510-8.
34. Fossati A, Madeddu F, Maffei C. Borderline personality disorder and childhood sexual abuse: a meta-analytic study. J Personal Disord. 1999;13:268-80.
35. Paris J. The nature of borderline personality disorder: multiple demensions, multiple symptoms, but one category. J Pers Disord. 2007;21:457-73.
36. Gabbard GO. Mind, brain, and personality disorders. Am J Psychiatry. 2005;162:648-55.
37. Wanger S, Baskaya O, Lieb K, Dahmen N, Tadic A. The 5-HTTLPR polymorphism modulates the association of serious life events (SLE) and impulsivity in patients with borderline personality disorder. I Psychiatr Res. 2009;43:1067-72.
38. Wanger S, Baskaya O, Lieb K, Dahmen N, Tadic A. Modulatory role of the brain-derived neurotrophic factor Val66Met polymorphism on the effects of serious life events on impulsive aggression in borderline personality disorder. Genes Brain Behav. 2009;9:97-102.
39. Siever LJ, Torgersen S, Gunderson JG, Livesley WJ, Kendler KS. The borderline diagnosis III: identifying endophenotypes for genetic studies. Boil Psychiatry. 2002;51:964-8.
40. Torgersen S, Czajkowski N, Jcobson K, et al. Dimensional representations of DSM-IV cluster B personality disorders in a population-based sample of Norwegian twins: a multivariate study. Psychol Med. 2008;38:1617-25.
41. Skodol AE, Siever LJ, Livesley WJ, Gunderson JG, Pfohl B, Widiger TA. The borderline diagnosis II: biology, genetics, and clinical course. Boil Psychiatry. 2002;51:951-63.

42. New AS, Goodman M, Triebwasser J, Siever LJ. Recent advances in the biological study of personality disorders. Psychiatr Clin North Am. 2008;31:441-61.
43. Cloninger CR. Genetics. In: J. Oldham JM, Skodol AE, Bender DS, eds. Textbook of Personality Disorders. Washington, DC: American Psychiatric Publishing; 2005.pp.143-54.
44. Coccaro EF, Siever LJ. Neurobiology. In: Oldham JM, Skodol AE, Bender DS, eds. Textbook of personality disorders. Washington, DC: American Psychiatric Publishing; 2005.pp.155-69.
45. Ni X, Chan K, Bulgin N, et al. Association between serotonin transporter gene and borderline personality disorder. J Psychiatr Res. 2006;40:448-53.
46. Pascual JC, Soler J, Barrachina J, et al. Failure to detect an association between the serotonin transpoter gene and borderline personality disorder. J Psychiatr Res. 2008;42: 87-88.
47. Silva H, Iturra P, Solari A, et al. Serotonin transporter polymorphism and fluoxetine effect on impulsiveness and aggression in borderline personality disorder. Actas Esp Psiquiatr. 2007;35:387-92.
48. Tadic A, Victor A, Baskaya O, et al. Interaction between gene variants of the serotonin transporter promoter region (% - HTTLPR) and catechol O-methyltransferase (COMT) in borderline personality disorder. Am J Med Genet B Neuropsychiatr Genet. 2009;150B:487-95.
49. Ni X, Chan D, Chan K, McMain S, Kennedy JL. Serotonin genes and gene-gene interactions in borderline personality disorder in a matched case-control study. Prog Neuropsychopharmacol Biol Psychiatry. 2009;33:128-33.
50. Ni X, Sicard T, Bulgin N, et al. Monoamine oxidase a gene is associated with borderline personality disorder. Psychiatr Genet. 2007;17:153-7.
51. Lahmeyer HW, Reynolds CF 3re, Kupfer DJ, King R. Biologic markers in borderline personality disorder: a review. J Clin Psychiatry. 1989;50:217-25.
52. Grossman R, Yehuda R, Siever L. The dexamethasone suppression test and glucocorticoid receptors in borderline personality disorder. Ann NY Acad Sci. 1997;821:459-64.
53. Zimmerman DJ, Choi-Kain LW. The hypothalamic-pituitary-adrenal axis in borderline personality disorder: a review. Harv Rev Psychiatry. 2009;17:167-83.
54. Schamahl CG, Vermetten E, Elzinga BM, Bremnr DJ. Magnetic resonance imaging of hippocampal and amygdala volume in women with childhood abuse and borderline personality disorder. Psychiatry Res. 2003;122:193-8.
55. Weniger G, Lange C, Sachsse Sachsse U, Irle E. Reduced amygdala and hippocampus size in trauma-exposed woman with borderline personality disorder and without post-traumatic stress disorder. J Psychiatry Neurosci. 2009;34:383-8.
56. Chanen AM, Velakoulis D, Carison K, et al. Orbitofrontal, amygdala and hippocampal volumes in teenagers with first-presentation borderline personality disorder. Psychiatry Res. 2008;163:116-25.
57. Kitayama N, Vaccarino V, Kutner M, Weiss P, Bremner JD. Magnetic resonance imaging (MRI) measurement of hippocampal volume in posttraumatic stress disorder: a meta-analysis. J Affect Disord. 2005;88:79-86.
58. Bremner JD, Radall P, Vermetten E, et al. Magnatic resonace imaging-based measurement of hippocampal volume in posttraumatic stress disorder related to childhood physical and sexual abuse-a preliminary report. Boil Psychiatry. 1997;41:23-32.
59. Nunes PM, Wenzel A, Borges KT, Porto Cr, Caminha RM, de Oliveira IR. Volumes of the hippocampus and amygdala in patients with borderline personality disorder: a meta-analysis. J Pers Disord. 2009;23:333-45.
60. Schmahl C, Berne K, Krause A, et al. Hippocampus and amygdala volumes in patients with borderline personality disorder with or without posttraumatic stress disorder. J Psychiatry Neurosci. 2009;34:289-95.
61. Chanen AM, Velakoulis D, Carison K, et al. Orbitofrontal, amygdala and hippocampal volumes in teenagers with first-presentation borderline personality disorder. Psychiatry Res. 2008;163:116-25.
62. New AS, Hazlett EA, Buchsbaum MS, et al. Amygdala-prefrontal disconnection in borderline personality disorder. Neuropsychopharmacology. 2007;32:1629-40.
63. Minzenberg MJ, Fan J, New AS, Tang CY, Siever LJ. Frontolimbic structural changes in borderline personality disorder. J Psychiatr Res. 2008;42:727-33.
64. Garner B, Chanen AM, Phillips L, et al. Pituitary volume in teenagers with first-presentation borderline personality disorder. Psychiatry Res. 2007;156:257-61.
65. Joven M, Garner B, Phillips L, et al. An MRI study of pituitary volume and parasuicidal behaviour in teenagers with first-presentation borderline personality disorder. Psychiatry Res. 2008;162:273-7.
66. Garner B, Pariante CM, Wood SJ, Velakoulis D, Phillips L, Soulsby B. Pituitary volume predicts future transition to psychosis in individuals at ultra-high risk of developing psychosis. Boil Psychiatry. 2005;58: 417-23.
67. Irle E, Lange C, Sachsse U. Reduced size and abnormal asymmetry of parietal cortex in woman with borderline personality disorder. Boil Psychiatry. 2005;57:173-82.
68. Irle E, Lange C, Weniger G, Sachsse U. Size abnormalities of the superiar parietal corties are related to dissociation in borderline personality disorder. Psychiatry Res. 2007;156: 139-49.
69. Brunner R, Henze R, Parzer P, et al. Reduced prefrontal and orbitofrontal gray matter in female adolescents with borderline personality disorder: is it disorder specific? Neuroimage. 2010;49:114-20.
70. Juengling FD, Schmahl C, Hesslinger B, et al. Positron emission tomography in female patients with borderline personality disorder. J Psychiatr Res. 2003;37:109-15.

71. New AS, Hazlett EA, Newmark RE, et al. Laboratory induced aggressive individuals with borderline personality disorder. Boil Psychiatry. 2009;66:1107-14.
72. Koenigsberg HW, Siever LJ, Lee H, et al. Neural correlates of emotion processing in borderline personality disorder. Psychiatry Res. 2009;172:192-9.
73. Minzenberg MJ, Fan J, New AS, Tang CY, Siever LJ. Fronto-limbic dysfunction in response to facial emotion in borderline personality disorder: an event-related fMRI study. Psychiatry Res. 2007;155:231-43.
74. Beblo T, Driessen M, Mertens M, et al. Functional MRI correlates of the recall of unresolved life events in borderline personality disorder. Psycho Med. 2006;36:845-56.
75. Koenigsberg HW, Fan J, Ochsner KN, et al. Neural correlates of the use of psychological distancing to regulate responses to negative social cues: a study of patients with borderline personality disorder. Boil Psychiatry. 2009;66:854-63.
76. Herpertz SC, Dietrich TM, Wenning B, et al. Evidence of abnormal amygdala functioning in borderline personality disorder. A functional MRI study. Boil Psychiatry. 2001;50:292-8.
77. Driessen M, Beblo T, Mertens M, et al. Posttramatic stress disorder and fMRI activation patterns of traumatic memory in patients with borderline personality disorder. Boil Psychiatry. 2004;55:603-11.
78. Kraus A, Esposito F, Seifritz E, et al. Amygdala deactivation as a neural correlate of pain processing in patients with borderline personality disorder and co-occurrent posttaumatic stress disorder. Boil Psychiatry. 2009;65:819-22.
79. Binks CA, Fenton M, McCarthy L, Lee T, Adams CE, Duggan C. Pharmacological interventions for people with borderline personality disorder. Cochrane Database Syst Rev. 2006;1: CD005653.
80. Nose M, Ciprani A, Biancosino B, Grassi L, Barbui C. Efficacy of pharmacotherapy against core traits of borderline personality disorder: meta-analysis of randomized controlled trails. Int Clin Psychopharmacol. 2006;21:345-53.
81. Leib K, Vollm B, Rucker G, Timmer A, Stoffers JM. Pharmacotherapy for borderline personality disorder. Cochrane systematic review of randomized trails. Br J Psychiatry. 2010;196:4-12.
82. Frankenburg FR, Zanarini MC. Divalprox sodium treatment of woman with borderline personality disorder and bipolar II disorder: a double-blind placebo-controlled pilot study. J Clin Psychiatry. 2002;63:442-6.
83. Soloff PH, Cornelius J, George A, Nathan S. Perel JM, Ulrich RF. Efficacy of phenelzine and haloperidol in borderline personality disorder. Arch Gen Psychiatry. 1993;50:377-85.
84. Soloff PH, George A, Nathan S, et al. Amitriptyline versus haloperidol in borderlines: final outcomes and predictors of response. J Clin Psychopharmacol. 1989;9:238-46.
85. Salzan C, Wolfson AN, Schatzberg A, et al. Effect of fluoxetine on anger in symptomatic volunteers with borderline personality disorder. J Clin Psychopharmacol. 1995;15:23-9.
86. Rinne T, van den Brink W, Wounters L, van Dyck R. SSRI treatment of borderline personality disorder: a randomized, placebo-controlled clinical trial for female patients with borderline personality disorder. Am J Psychiatry. 2002;159: 2048-54.
87. Goldberg SC, Schulz PM, Resnick RJ, Hamer RM, Friedel RO. Borderline and schizotypal personality disorders treated with low-dose thiothixene vs placebo. Arch Gen Psychiatry. 1986;43:680-6.
88. Leone NF. Response of borderline patients to laxapine and chlorpromazine. J Clin Psychiatry. 1982;43:148-50.
89. Bogenschutz MP, George Nurnberg H. Olanzapine versus placebo in the treatment of borderline personality disorder. J Clin Psychiatry. 2004;65:104-9.
90. Zanarini MC, Frankenburg FR. Olanzapine treatment of female borderline personality disorder patients: a double-blind, placebo-controlled pilot study. J Clin Psychiatry. 2001;62: 849-54.
91. Zanarini MC, Frankenburg FR, Parachini EA. A Preliminary, randomized trial of fluoxetine, olanzapine, and the olanzapine-fluoxetine combination in woman with borderline personality disorder. J Clin Psychiatry. 2004;65:903-7.
92. De la Fuente JM, Lotstra F. A trial of carbamazepine in borderline personality disorder. Eur Neuropsychopharmacol. 1994;4:479-86.
93. Hollander E, Allen A, Lopez RP, et al. A preliminary double-blind, placebo-controlled trial of divalproex sodium in borderline personality disorder. J Clin Psychiatry. 2001;62:199-203.
94. Hollander E, Swann AC, Coccaro EF, Jiang P, Smith TB. Impact of trait impulsivity and state aggression on divalproex versus placebo response in borderline personality disorder. Am J Psychiatry. 2005;162:621-4.
95. Zanarini MC, Frankenburg FR. Omega-3 fatty acid treatment of woman with borderline personality disorder: a double-blind placebo-controlled pilot study. Am J Psychiatry. 2003;160:167-9.
96. Reich DB, Zanarini MC, Bieri KA. A preliminary study of lamotrigine in the treatment of affective instability in borderline personality disorder. Int Clin Psychopharmacol. 2009;24:270-5.
97. Schulz SC, Zanarini MC, Bateman A, et al. Olanzapine for the treatment of borderline personality disorder: variable dose 12-week randomized double-blind placebo-controlled study. Br J Psychiatry. 2008;193:485-92.
98. Shafti SS, Shahveisi B. Olanzapine versus haloperidol in the management of borderline personality disorder: a randomized double-blind trial. J Clin Psychopharmacol. 2009;29:170-3.
99. Ziegenhorn AA, Roepke S, Schommer NC, et al. Clonidine improves hyperarousal in borderline personality disorder with or without comorbid posttraumatic stress disorder: a randomized, double-blind, placebo-controlled trial. J Clin Psychopharmacol. 2009;29:170-3.
100. Pascul JC, Soler J, Puigdemont D, et al. Ziprasidone in the treatment of borderline personality disorder: a double-blind,

placebo-controlled, randomized study. J Clin Psychiatry. 2008;69:603-8.
101. Bellino S, Zizza M, Rinaldi C, Bogetto F. Combined treatment of major depression in patients with borderline personality disorder a comparison with pharmacotherapy. Can J Psychiatry. 2006;51:453-60.
102. Simpson EB, Yen S, Costello E, et al. Combined dialectical behavior therapy and fluoxetine in the treatment of borderline personality disorder. J Clin Psychiatry. 2004;65:379-85.
103. Soler J, Pascual JC, Campins J, et al. Double-blind, placebo-controlled study of dialectical behavior therapy plus olanzapine for borderline for borderline personality disorder. Am J Psychiatry. 2005;162:1221-4.
104. Linehan MM, McDavid JD, Brown MZ, Sayrs JH, Gallop RJ. Olanzapine plus dialectical behavior therapy for woman with high irritability who meet criteria for borderline personality disorder: a double-blind, placebo-controlled pilot study. J Clin Psychiatry. 2008;69:999-1005.
105. Borderline personality disorder. The NICE guideline on treatment and management. The British Psychological Society and The Royal College of psychiatrists. http://www.nice.org.uk/nicemedia/live/12125/43045/43045.pdf:p218(accessed Aug 30, 2011).
106. Kendall T, Burbeck R, Bateman A. Pharmacotherapy for borderline personality disorder. NICE guideline. Br J Psychiatry. 2010;196:158-9.
107. Bink CA, Fenton M, McCarthy L, Lee T, Adams CE. Duggan C. Psychological therapies for people with borderline personality disorder. Cochrane Database Syst Rev. 2006;1:CD005652.
108. Brazier J, Tumur I, Holmes M, et al. Psychological therapies including dialectical behaviour therapy for borderline personality disorder: a systematical review and preliminary economic evaluation. Health Technol Assess. 2006;10:1-117.
109. Bateman A, Fonagy P. Effectiveness of partial hospitalization in the treatment of borderline personality disorder: a randomized controlled trial. Am J Psychiatry. 1999;156:1563-9.
110. Linehan MM, Armstrong HE, Suarez A, Allmon D, Heard HL. Cognitive-behavioural treatment of chronically parasuicidal borderline patients. Arch Gen Psychiatry. 1991;48:1060-4.
111. Linehan MM, Dimeff LA, Reynolds SK, et al. Dialectical behavior therapy versus comprehensive validation therapy plus 12-step for the treatment of opioid depended woman meeting criteria for borderline personality disorder. Drug Alcohol Depend. 2002;67:13-26.
112. Linehan MM, Schmidt H, Dimeff LA, Craft JC, Kanter J, Comtois KA. Dialectical behaviour therapy for patients with borderline personality disorder and drug-dependence. Am J Addict. 1999;8:279-92.
113. van den Bosch LM, Verheul R, Schippers GM, van den Brink W. Dialectical behaviour therapy of borderline patients with and without substance use problems. Implementation and long-term effects. Addict Behav. 2002;27:911-23.
114. Koons CR, Robins CJ, Tweed JL, et al. Efficacy of dialectical behaviour therapy in woman veterans with borderline personality disorder. Behavior Therapy. 2001;32:371-90.
115. Turner R. Naturalstic evaluation of dialectical behaviour therapy-oriented treatment for borderline personality disorder. Cognitive and Behavioral Practice. 2000;7:413-9.
116. Munroe-Blum H, Marziali E. A controlled trial of short-term group treatment for borderline personality disorder. J Pers Disord. 1995;9:190-8.
117. Tyrer PTS, Schmidt U, Jones V, et al. Randomized controlled trial of brief cognitive behaviour therapy versus treatment as usual in recurrent deliberate self-harm: the POPMACT study. Psycho Med. 2003;33:969-98.
118. Bateman A, Fonagy P. Randomized controlled trial of outpatient mentalization-based treatment versus structured clinical management for borderline personality disorder. Am J Psychiatry. 2009;166:1355-64.
119. Davidson K, Norrie J, Tyrer P, et al. The effectiveness of cognitive behavior therapy for borderline personality disorder study of cognitive therapy (BOSCOT) trial. J Pers Disord. 2006;20:450-65.
120. Blum N, St John D, Pfohj B, et al. System training for Emotional Predictability and Problem Solving (STEPPS) for outpatients with borderline personality disorder: a randomized controlled trial and 1-year follow-up. Am J Psychiatry. 2008;165:468-78.
121. Bohus M, Haaf B, Simms T, et al. Effectiveness of inpatient dialectical behavioral therapy for borderline personality disorder. A controlled trial Behave Res Ther. 2004;42:487-99.
122. Clarkin JF, Levy KN, Lenzenweger MF, Kernberg OF. Evaluating three treatments for borderline personality disorder: a multiwave study. Am J Psychiatry. 2007;164:922-8.
123. Cottraux J, Note ID, Boutitie F, et al. Cognitive therapy versus rogerian supportive therapy in borderline personality disorder. Two-year follow-up of a controlled pilot study. Psychother Psychosom. 2009;78:307-28.
124. Farrell JM, Shaw IA, Webber MA. A schema-focused approach to group psychotherapy for outpatients with borderline personality disorder: a randomized controlled trial. J Bhav Ther Exp Psychiatry. 2009;40:317-28.
125. Giesen-Bloo J, van Dyck R, Spinhoven P, et al. Outpatient psychotherapy for borderline personality disorder: randomized trial of schema-focused therapy vs transference-focused psychotherapy. Arch Gen Psychiatry. 2006;63:649-58.
126. Gregory R, Chlebowski S, Kang D, et al. A controlled trial of psychodynamic psychotherapy for co-occurring borderline personality disorder and alcohol use disorder. Psychotherapy: Theory/Research/Practice/Training. 2008;45:28-41.
127. Harned MS, Chapman AL, Dexter-Mazza ET, Murray A, Comtois KA, Linehan MM. Treating co-occurring axis I disorders in recurrently suicidal woman with borderline personality disorder: a 2-year randomized trial of dialectical behavior therapy versus community treatment by experts. J Consult Clin Psychol. 2008;76:1068-75.

128. Linehan MM, Comstois KA, Murray AM, et al. Two-year randomized controlled trial and follow-up of dialectical behavior therapy vs therapy by experts for suicidal behaviors and borderline personality disorder. Arch Gen Psychiatry. 2006;63:757-66.
129. McMain SF, Links PS, Gnam WH, et al. A randomized trial os dialectical behavior therapy versus general psychiatric management for borderline personality disorder. Am J Psychiatry. 2009;166:1365-74.
130. Soler J, Pascual JC, Tiana T, et al. Dialectical behaviour therapy skills traing compared to standard group therapy in borderline personality disorder: a 3-month randomized controlled clinical trial. Behave Res Ther. 2009;47:353-8.
131. Verheul R, Van Den Bosch LM, Koeter MW, De Rider MA, Stijnen T, Van Den brink W. Dialectical behaviour therapy for woman with borderline personality disorder:12-month, randomized clinical trial in The Netherlands. Br J Psychiatry. 2003;182:135-40.
132. Doering S, Horz S, Rentrop M, et al. Transference-focused psychotherapy v. treatment by community psychotherapists for borderline personality disorder: randomized controlled trial. Br J Psychiatry. 2010;196:389-95.
133. Weinberg I, Gunderson JG, Hennen J, Cutter CJ Jr. Manual assisted cognitive treatment for deliberate self-harm in borderline personality disorder patients. J Pers Disord. 2006;20:482-92.
134. Nadort M, Arntz A, Smit JH, et al. Implementation of outpatient schema therapy for borderline personality disorder with versus without crisis support by the therapist outside office hours: a randomized trial. Behav Res Ther. 2009;47:961-73.
135. Levy KN, Meehan KB, Kelly KM, et al. Change in attachment patterns and reflective function in a randomized control trial of transference-focused psychotherapy for borderline personality disorder. J Consult Clin Psycho. 2006;74;1027-40.
136. Baterman A, Fonagy P. Treatment of borderline personality disorder with psychoanalytically oriented partial hospitalization: an 18-month follow-up. Am J Psychiatry. 2001;158:36-42.
137. Linehan MM, Haard HL, Armstrong HE. Naturalistic follow-up of a behavioural treatment for chronically parasuicidal borderline patients. Arch Gen psychiatry. 1993;50:971-4.
138. Bateman A, Fonagy P. 8-year follow-up of patients treated for borderline personality disorder: mentalization-based treatment versus treatment as usual. Am J Psychiatry. 2008;165:631-8.
139. Zanarini MC. Psychotherapy of borderline personality disorder. Acta Psychiatr Scand. 2009;120:373-7.
140. Skodol AE, Oldham JM, Bendar DS, et al. Dimensional representations of DSM-IV personality disorders: relationships to functional impairment. Am J Psychiatry. 2005;162:1919-25.
141. Widiger TA. Current controversies in nosology and diagnosis of personality disorders. Psychiatric Annals. 2007;32:93-9.
142. McGlashan TH, Grilo CM, Sanislow CA, et al. Two-year prevalence and stability of individual DSM-IV criteria for schizotypal, borderline, avoidant, and obsessive-compulsive personality disorders: toward a hybrid model of axis II disorders. Am J Psychiatry. 2005;162:883-9.
143. Tyrer P, Coombs N, Ibrahimi F, et al. Critical developments in the assessment of personality disorder. Br J Psychiatry Suppl. 2007;49:s51-9.
144. American Psychiatric Association. DSM-5: The future of psychiatric diagnosis. http://www.dsm5.org (accessed Aug 30, 2012).
145. American Psychiatric Association. Desk Reference to the Diagnostic Criteria from DSM-5. Washington DC. 2013.

CHAPTER 71

Advancements in the Treatment of Epilepsy

VS Chadda

INTRODUCTION

Epilepsy, operationally defined as having or being at risk of having recurrent unprovoked seizures. The diagnosis of epilepsy confers a greater likelihood of injury and sudden unexplained death, as well as a loss of independence and perceived stigmatization. Patients with epilepsy report poorer overall health-related quality of life, and exhibit activity limitations, psychiatric comorbidities, increased unemployment rates, and lower educational attainment and income than those without seizures.[1-3] The goal of treatment is to attain seizure freedom without side effects and return patients to normal, healthy lifestyles.

The past several years have brought new diagnostic aids, medication options, and devices for the treatment of seizures. It is not just the armamentarium that has changed but also the way it is used. Imaging techniques once confined to research laboratories are now routinely used in clinics. Medications that were new and unfamiliar a few years ago are now first-line treatments. Patients and physicians push for earlier surgical intervention to treat refractory seizures and actively seek alternatives in diets and implantable devices. This is an exciting time in epileptology, and below we share some of the recent developments.

DIAGNOSIS

Successful treatment requires a precise diagnosis. Recent advances in imaging technology help to identify subtle lesions that my represent epileptogenic foci. Magnetic resonance imaging, for example, now with phased array surface coils (PA MRI) and field strengths of 3 Tesla (3T), has signal-to-noise ratios 6 to 8 times that of conventional 1.5T scans. PA MRI better defines the gray-white junction and creates a more uniform signal intensity of normal cortex, allowing better visualization of abnormalities such as cortical dysplasias. A study of 3T PA MRI detected brain lesion in 65% of patients with focal epilepsy and reportedly normal standard 1.5T scans. In addition, in 33% of patients with lesions revealed by 1.5T scans, abnormalities were better defined on the 3T images.[4] A greater ability to detect or characterize subtle lesions may alter treatment strategies.

Although still largely a research tool concurrent EEG and functional MRI (EEG/fMRI) is now used for clinical purposes at some centers. Functional MRI uses blood oxygenation level dependent (BOLD) pulse sequences, which map cerebral blood flow with millisecond temporal resolution.[5] With simultaneous EGG, it is possible to correlate areas of altered blood flow with the occurrence of interictal or ictal discharges.[6] This may help to identify foci or networks that are functionally abnormal during spikes and sharp waves; although they may not be recognized as structural lesions on standard MRI scans.[7]

Whereas EGG detects electrical potentials, magnetoencephalography (MEG) senses magnetic fields created by activity of apical dendrites, providing a novel technique for the localization of ictal and interictal epileptiform activity.[8] An advantage of MEG is the relative lack of signal attenuation by the skull and scalp compared with EEG. MEG, however, only measures those fields tangential to the scalp. It is most sensitive to discharges in the neocortical convexities and relatively poor at detecting more mesial sources. Although MEG may identify epileptiform discharges missed by routine scalp EEG, its utility continues to be debated.

Nuclear imaging modalities have also gained popularity, as a growing number of centers now have access to this technology. Positron emission tomography (PET) scanning, for example, is commonly used to aid in localization of seizure foci. Interictal injection with a radio-labeled tracer, most often fluorodeoxyglucose-18 (FDG), may reveal regions of cellular hypometabolism that signify underlying abnormal, potentially epileptogenic, brain tissue. In contrast, ictal single-photon emission computed tomography (SPECT) uses injection of technetium-99-labeled tracer at the start of a seizure. This lipophilic tracer is 90% extracted on first pass into lipid-rich tissue, including brain, in proportion to local perfusion. Uptake of the tracer by a brain region with actively firing cells, evident on the scan as focal area of hyperperfusion, may indicate the region of seizure onset. SISCOM, a technique in which SPECT images obtained during ictal and interictal periods are subtracted and coregistered with MRI, further improves localization. The utility of ictal SPECT may be limited, however, by the logistic is appropriately timing the injection and by the sensitivity of various tracers. Nevertheless, this method is often useful in settings in which the MRI is unrevealing.[9]

The availability of minimally invasive techniques provides additional tools for seizure localization. Older methods for focus identification, such as foramen ovale electrodes and epidural pegs, have seen resurgence. Foramen ovale electrodes are placed percutaneously through the foramen so that they lie along the inferomesial aspect of the temporal lobe. This allows recordings to be obtained from deep medial structures without the need for surgical placement of depth electrodes into brain tissue. Epidural pegs provide a method for obtaining recordings over the convexities through small burr holes, which eliminates the muscle artifact that may contaminate scalp leads. This technique may be used to plan for the optimal placement of grids of strips, or it may potentially obviate the need for further invasive recording. These methods, either separately or in conjunction, have been helpful in many cases in which scalp EEG data have been inconclusive.[8]

MEDICATIONS

Historically, treatment options for epilepsy have been limited. Major pharmacologic options included carbamazepine, phenobarbital, phenytoin, primidone, ethosuximide, and valproic acid. Though often effective, relatively affordable and familiar, these older medications carry the risk of hepatic dysfunction, drug interactions, and other significant side effects. Between 1978, when valproic acid was introduced and 1993, when felbamate was approved, on new anticonvulsants were approved by the US Food and Drug Administration (FDA). In contrast, in the past decade, eight new anticonvulsants were approved in The United States. These agents typically offer equal efficacy but may have fewer adverse effects and drug interaction than the older generation of medications.[9a,9b] Newer anticonvulsants (listed in reverse order of FDA approval) include pregabalin, oxcarbazepine, zonisamide, levetiracetam, tiagabine, topiramate, lamotrigine, gabapentin and felbamate (Table 1).

What may be more striking than the number of new medications, however, is how quickly these drugs have become first-line therapies. In 2005, Karceski et al.[10] surveyed 43 epileptologists regarding their prescribing practices. Lamotrigine was considered a first-line treatment for idiopathic primary generalized tonic-clonic, absence, simple partial, and secondarily generalized tonic-clonic seizures, and it was the treatment of choice for complex partial seizures. Topiramate was a first-line medication for treatment of idiopathic primary generalized tonic-clonic seizures. Oxcarbazepine had become the treatment of choice for simple partial and secondarily generalized tonic-clonic seizures, and levetiracetam was also an acceptable initial option for treatment of these partial-onset seizure types. The survey also marked a shift in thinking from as little as five years earlier, when lamotrigine, topiramate, and levetiracetam were often considered to be second-line agents.

With new treatments, however, often comes confusion and a lack of consensus regarding prescribing practices. The American Academy of Neurology (AAN) and American Epilepsy Society (AES) have published recommendations for use of many of the newer medications.[11-13] The choice in a given patient, however, continues to be guided by seizure type, patient characteristics and side effect profiles. Below we summarize the indications, associated adverse events, mechanisms and pharmacokinetic properties of the more recently approved anticonvulsants. These drugs are discussed in the reverse order of their approval in the United States (Table 2).

Pregabalin

Pregabalin is the newest anticonvulsant. It is structurally similar to gabapentin but has a slightly longer half-life. Although structurally related to gamma-aminobutyric acid (GABA), the drug does not have GABA-ergic activity. Pregabalin binds to the alpha2-delta subunit of voltage-gated calcium channels, reducing calcium influx and thereby decreasing release of several neurotransmitters, including glutamate.

Clinical experience with pregabalin is limited because it was only approved by the FDA in June, 2005. The drug is currently indicated for adjunctive treatment of partial onset seizures in adults, on the basis of studies demonstrating seizure frequency reduction up to 47.8–54% in this population.[14-16] Most clinicians' experience suggests that pregabalin may worsen idiopathic generalized epilepsy.

Initial studies suggest a few potential advantages of pregabalin. The drug is reasonably well tolerated at starting doses up to 600 mg/day.[14] although many patients complain of dizziness at initial doses above 100–150 mg/day. In urgent situations, steady state can be achieved in as little as 48 hours. Pregabalin is renally excreted, so it is suitable for parents with hepatic disease. A lack of hepatic enzyme induction of inhibition is also advantageous in that the drug poses little risk for interaction with other medications.

In addition, pregabalin is generally safe. Serious adverse events included a maculopapular rash in one patient, which resolved after discontinuation of the drug, as well as isolated reports of cholestatic jaundice. There is no know association of pregabalin with cardiovascular dysfunction; cases of peripheral edema have been reported, but detailed cardiac testing of those patients has not been described.[16] These adverse events are typically dose-related. They tend to occur

Table 1: FDA-approved indication for new anticonvulsants

Medication	*Use in partial seizures (simple, complex, secondarily generalized)—adjunctive*	*Use in partial seizures (Simple, complex, secondarily generalized)—monotherapy*	*Use in absence seizures—monoth-erapy*	*Use in primary generalized conic-clonic seizures—adjunctive*	*Use in primary generalized tonic-clonic seizures—monotherapy*	*Use in Lennox Gastaut (Tonic/atonic and tonic-clonic seizures)—adjunctive*	*Use in myoclonic seizures of JME—adjunctive*
Pregabalin	Adults						
Oxcarbazepine	Adults, children ≥2 years of age	Adults, children ≥4 years of age					
Zonisamide	Adults						
Levetiracetam	Adults, children ≥4 years of age			Adults, children ≥6 years of age			Adults, children ≥12 years of age
Tiagabine	Adults, children ≥12 years of age						
Topiramate	Adults, children ≥2 years of age	Adults, children ≥10 years of age		Adults, children ≥2 years of age	Adults, children ≥10 years of age	Adults, children ≥2 years of age	
Lamotrigine	Adults, children ≥2 years of age	Adults	Children	Adults, children ≥2 years of age	Adults	Adults, children ≥2 years of age	
Gabapentin	Adults, children ≥3 years of age, ≥12 years of age if secondary generali-zation	Adults and adolescents					
Felbamate	Adults	Adults				Adults, children ≥2 years of age (≥4 years per AAN)	

shortly after the medication is started, often within one week of initiation, and are generally self-limited, even if the drug is continued. Weight gain has been reported in substantial fraction of patients chronically treated with pregabalin.

Oxcarbazepine

Oxcarbazepine is FDA approved for use as monotherapy and adjunctive treatment in children[17,18] and adults[19-21] with partial seizures. Oxcarbazepine has rapidly become a first-line agent for those with partial seizures and is often preferred in patients with psychiatric comorbidities because of its apparent mood-stabilizing effects. Studies comparing oxcarbazepine monotherapy with phenytoin,[22,23] valproic acid,[24] and carbamazepine[25] demonstrate equivalent rates of seizure freedom in populations with both partial-onset and primary generalized tonic-clonic seizures. The ANN/AES guidelines suggest that although oxcarbazepine monotherapy is appropriate in populations that include patients with newly diagnosed partial and/or generalized seizure disorders there is insufficient evidence to determine efficacy for those with primary generalized seizures alone.

The drug was developed as a structural variant of carbamazepine, designed to eliminate the carbamazepine epoxide metabolite thought to cause side effects. Carbamazepine and oxcarbazepine are distinct drugs, with separate metabolic pathways and somewhat different modes of action and side effect profiles.[26]

Oxcarbazepine exerts much of its effect through 10-monohydroxy metabolite (MHD), an active metabolite not present with carbamazepine. Oxcarbazepine blocks voltage-sensitive sodium channels, stabilizing neuronal membranes and inhibiting repetitive firing at lower concentrations than that required by carbamazepine. Increased potassium conductance and modulation of voltage-activated calcium channels may also play a role in its anticonvulsant effect. The interaction occurs at the N-, P- and R- type calcium channels rather than the L-type channels affected by carbamazepine.

Metabolites of oxcarbazepine, unlike those of carbamazepine, are excreted in the urine, so dosing must be

Table 2: Properties of new anticonvulsants

Medication	*Half-life*	*Mechanism*	*Clearance*	*Hepatic enzyme effects*	*Notable drug interactions*	*Cautions*
Pregabalin	6 hours	Likely related to effects at voltage-gated calcium channels	Renal	None	None	None
Oxcarbazepine	4–9 hours	Sodium channel blockade; possible contribution of effect on potassium and calcium channels	Renal and hepatic	Minimal induction and inhibition of subtypes	Decreases levels of: carbamazepine dihydropyridines oral contraceptives lamotrigine (?) Increases level of: Phenobarbital phenytoin MHD decreased by: verapamil carbamazepine Phenobarbital phenytoin valproate	Cross-reactivity of hypersensitivity to carbamazepine; risk of hyponatremia
Zonisamide	24–60 hours	Sodium and calcium channel blockade	Hepatic more than renal	None	Levels decreased by hepatic enzyme-inducing medications: carbamazepine phenytoin Phenobarbital	Do not use if patient has sulfa allergy or history of nephrolithiasis
Levetiracetam	6–8 hours	Binding at SV2A synaptic vesicle protein and high-voltage calcium channels, modulation of GABA and glycine receptors	Renal, hydrolysis	None	None	Risk of psychiatric side effects
Tiagabine	4–9 hours	Inhibition of GABA reuptake	Hepatic	None	Levels decreased by hepatic enzyme-inducing medications: carbamazepine phenytoin Phenobarbital	Risk of "spike-wave" stupor
Topiramate	15–23 hours	Blockade of voltage-dependent sodium channels, inhibition of carbonic anhydrase, antagonizes AMPA/ Kainate glutamate receptors, and modulates GABAa-mediated chloride activity	Renal more than hepatic	Induction and inhibition	Decreases levels of: oral contraceptives (no effect with topiramate doses <200 mg/d), lithium, digoxin, valproate Increases levels of: haloperidol, phenytoin Levels decreased by hepatic enzyme-inducting medications: carbamazepine, phenytoin, valproate	Don't use if patient has sulfa allergy or history of nephrolithiasis. Potential side effects include cognitive impairment, open-angle glaucoma, metabolic acidosis, weight loss
Lamotrigine	15–35 hours	Likely related to inhibition of voltage-sensitive sodium channels	Hepatic	Minimal induction	Decreases levels of: valproate, oral contraceptives Levels decreased by: phenytoin, oral contraceptives Levels increased by: valproate	Risk of rash, particularly with concurrent use of valproate

Contd...

Contd...

Medication	*Half-life*	*Mechanism*	*Clearance*	*Hepatic enzyme effects*	*Notable drug interactions*	*Cautions*
Gabapentin	4–6 hours	Unknown; may be related to voltage-activated calcium channels	Renal	None	Levels decreased by: Maalox-TC	None
Felbamate	20–23 hours	Antagonist of glycine recognition site of NMDA receptor	Renal and hepatic	Induction and inhibition	Increases levels of: valproate, phenytoin, carbamazepine, epoxide, phenobarbital Decreases levels of: carbamazepine, oral contraceptives Levels increased by: valproate Levels decreased by: phenytoin, carbamazepine	Risk of aplastic anemia, hepatic failure, and rash.

adjusted in patients with renal disease. The effect on P-450 hepatic enzyme subtypes in minimal, causing only limited drug interactions. Of particular concern, however, is the induction of CYP3A4 and CYP3A5 enzymes, which may reduce concentrations of oral contraceptives. Nevertheless, oxcarbazepine is associated with fever hepatic enzyme and drug interactions than carbamazepine of other older agents.

In general, oxcarbazepine carries lower risk of adverse events than the prior generation of anticonvulsants. Clinical experience, however, suggest that oxcarbazepine does have adverse effects, often causing headache.[26a] Side effects are typically dose-related, and slow titration is recommended to minimize risk. Serious side effects include rash and hyponatremia. Rash, when it occurs, generally appears within one month of use. Because cross reactivity of allergic reaction occurs in up to 27% of patients, those with exfoliative dermatitis from use of carbamazepine should not receive oxcarbazepine. The incidence of hyponatremia is greater with oxcarbazepine than with carbamazepine, and is of particular concern in the elderly and those on sodium wasting agents. The hyponatremia is most often chronic and asymptomatic, developing gradually over the first six weeks of treatment. Sodium levels typically normalize with reduction or cassation of oxcarbazepine treatment and may respond to fluid restriction. Sodium levels should be obtained prior to initiating treatment and should be monitored during the first three months of use in those at risk. No consensus exists as to a threshold for discontinuation of the drug, although levels less than 128 mEq/L and a continuing downward trend are worrisome.

Zonisamide

Zonisamide is FDA approved for adjunctive treatment of partial seizures in patients 16 years of age and older.[27,28] Although some studies demonstrate efficacy in children with partial and generalized epilepsy,[29] including infantile spasms[30] and myoclonic seizures,[31] AAN/AES guidelines caution that there is insufficient evidence to recommend use of zonisamide in children or patients with primary generalized seizures. Further data are also required to confirm utility as monotherapy, although zonisamide is often used as such for treatment of partial seizures in adults.

Zonisamide contains a sulfonamide chemical structure, precluding its use in patients with a sulfa allergy. It produces its anticonvulsant effect by blockade of sodium and T-type calcium channels, thereby stabilizing neuronal membranes. Zonisamide also has weak carbonic anhydrase-inhibiting activity, but this does not appear to substantially contribute to its antiseizure properties.

The medication offers several advantages. First, although the drug undergoes primarily hepatic elimination, it does not alter hepatic metabolism. Hence, zonisamide has fewer drug interactions than older medication do. Second, estimates of the half-life are as great as 24–60 hours. This long duration enables once-per-day administration, improving compliance. Third, the drug may cause weight loss, as opposed to weight gain caused by many alternative medications. The drug is now available as a generic formulation, potentially making it more affordable. Finally, open-label data and anecdotal experience suggest the zonisamide may have antimigraine properties, providing a reasonable option for those with comorbid headaches.

Adverse reactions are typically dose-dependent. Most commonly, patients report cognitive clouding. Nephrolithiasis may be associated with zonisamide use. Concomitant administration of other carbonic anhydrase inhibitors, such as acetazolamide or topiramate, may increase the risk for renal stone formation. The drug should be avoided in patients with a history of nephrolithiasis, and those taking the medication should be encouraged to drink sufficient amounts of water. Another serious risk is that of hypohydrosis with resultant hyperthermia, a rare side effect that occurs primarily in children. Zonisamide may also cause a rash and, rarely, Stevens-Johnson syndrome.

Levetiracetam

Levetiracetam is indicated for adjunctive treatment of partial epilepsy in adults[32,33] and children aged 4 years and older[34,35] with refractory seizures. Data also support conversion to monotherapy in patients with refractory partial epilepsy.[36] In clinical practice, levetiracetam is often prescribed as monotherapy on the basis of its success as an add-on treatment. Use as monotherapy, however, is not currently FDA approved or ANN/AES recommended owing to insufficient data regarding efficacy. Levetiracetam is indicated for add-on therapy of myoclonic seizures in patients aged 12 years and older with juvenile myoclonic epilepsy.[37,38] Most recently, levetiracetam also received FDA approval for adjunctive treatment of primary generalized tonic-clonic seizures in adults and children aged 6 years and older with idiopathic generalized epilepsy.

Levetiracetam has rapidly gained popularity owing to its ease of administration. Taken orally twice per day, the drug is at steady state within three does and can be rapidly titrated to therapeutic levels. A new intravenous formulation is available, indicated for adjunctive treatment of partial seizures in adults and as an alternative when oral administration is temporarily prohibited. Access to intravenous levetiracetam may increase its off-label use in acute situations, as case reports have indicated benefit in status epilepticus.[39] Because it has no hepatic effects, levetiracetam is a first-line medication for those with liver dysfunction. The lack of hepatic effects also minimizes the potential for drug interactions, making levetiracetam a preferred agent for patients taking multiple medications, such as those who are elderly, HIV-positive, or on chemotherapy.

Levetiracetam's mechanism of action is unknown. It does not act at the receptors typically affected by antiepileptic medications. The drug binds to a presynaptic protein, SV2A, located on synaptic vesicle. The protein is probably involved in vesicle fusion to the presynaptic membrane and may reduce neurotransmitter release, but the relationship between SV2A binding and anticonvulsant properties are unclear. The anticonvulsant effect of levetiracetam may also be related to other atypical mechanisms, such as reduction of current through neuron-specific high voltage-activated calcium channels and modulation of the effects of zinc and beta-carbolines on inhibitory GABAa and glycine receptors.

No serious adverse reactions to levetiracetam have been reported. Common side effects include irritability and behavioral changes, and in some patients these adverse effects may be treatment limiting.

Levetiracetam has a particularly wide therapeutic range. Hence, levetiracetam levels are typically not clinically useful, except to determine compliance.

Tiagabine

Tiagabine exerts its anticonvulsant effect via a novel mechanism involving inhibition of GABA reuptake into neurons and glia. The medication is indicated as adjunctive therapy in patients aged 12 years and older for the treatment of partial seizures.[40-42] However, little evidence supports its use as monotherapy, in younger children, or for treatment of generalized-onset seizures.

There are four reasons why tiagabine is not commonly prescribed. First, the drug may not be as effective as other.[40-42] Although it is not possible to directly compare trials owing to differences in study populations, dosages, and design, tiagabine seems to have somewhat lower responder rates than the other newer medications. Second, tiagabine undergoes hepatic elimination. This makes it a less desirable option for patients with liver disease. Tiagabine itself does not alter hepatic enzyme function, but its metabolism may be affected by enzyme inducers and inhibitors, which raises concern about drug interactions. Third, the medication takes several weeks to titrate to a therapeutic dosage. Fourth and most important, the drug carries the potential for serious side effects.

Use of tiagabine may cause a paradoxical increase in seizure activity. New seizure types may develop, along with an increased incidence of nonconvulsive status epilepticus (NCSE) or so-called spike-wave stupor. In a recent retrospective study of patients with refractory partial seizures, 7.8% of those treated with tiagabine experienced episodes of NCSE, confirmed by spike-and polyspike wave discharges on EEG that resolved after discontinuation of the drug.[43] In fact, the FDA has issued a safety alert in response to reports of new-onset seizures and status epilepticus in patients without epilepsy who were prescribed tiagabine for other indications. Some patients on tiagabine have developed an encephalopathy that is probably related to seizure activity. These effects do not appear to be dose-related and may develop more than three months after treatment is initiated. Assertions that frontal lobe epilepsy increases these risks are controversial and not well documented in the literature. The mechanism for development of encephalopathy is uncertain, but is probably related to GABA-mediated pathways.

Topiramate

Topiramate blocks voltage-dependents sodium channels, inhibits carbonic anhydrase, acts as an antagonist of 2-(aminomethyl) phenylacetic acid (AMPA)/kainate glutamate receptors, and modulates GABAa-mediated chloride activity. The mode of action underlying its anticonvulsant effect, however, remains unknown.

Topiramate is approved by the FDA as initial monotherapy for partial-onset or primary generalized tonic-clonic seizures in patients 10 years of age and older. Studies supporting this indication have shown that patients with partial[44] and primary generalized tonic-clonic[45] seizure randomized to higher doses of topiramate had significantly greater rates of seizure freedom than those on lower doses of the drug. Topiramate is also approved as adjunctive therapy for patients 2 years of age and older with refractory partial seizures, primary generalized tonic-clonic seizures, and Lennox-Gastaut syndrome. Randomized double-blind add-on studies support its use in these populations, demonstrating greater reduction in partial-onset seizures,[46] primary generalized tonic-clonic seizures,[47] and drop attacks[48] compared to placebo. Efficacy and safety of conversion from another antiepileptic medication to topiramate monotherapy have not been adequately studied.

Topiramate is advantageous in its broad range of efficacy. It may also help prevent migraines and is at times favored for patients with comorbid headaches and seizures. The medication also has mood-stabilizing effects. Topiramate may be less preferable as a first-line agent, however, owing to its long list of potential side effects.

Common adverse reactions to topiramate include cognitive dysfunction, often associated with word-finding difficulties. Paresthesias of fingertips and toes may occur shortly after the medication is initiated, probably related to carbonic anhydrase inhibition. Paresthesias are typically self-limited, resolving over weeks. If bothersome or prolonged, isolated case reports indicate that potassium supplementation at 20–40 mEq per day may be helpful,[49] although no placebo-controlled trials have been published to date. Serious side effects include nephrolithiasis in 1–5% of patients, and the drug should be avoided in those with a history of renal stones. The acute onset of diminished visual acuity of ocular pain should prompt concern about open-angle glaucoma associated with topiramate use, typically occurring within the first month of treatment. Other possible side effects include hypohydrosis, particularly in children, and a hyperchloremic, nonanion gap metabolic acidosis. Transient but significant weight loss may also occur. The risk of the above side effects appears to be dose-related and may be minimized by slow titration. Despite the mood-stabilizing properties of topiramate, there are reports of rare topiramate induced suicidality. In addition, the drug is a sulfa derivative and is contraindicated in patients with sulfa allergies.

Lamotrigine

Lomotrigine has rapidly become a first-line agent for many seizure types and patient populations. It is currently FDA approved as adjunctive therapy for partial[50-53] and primary generalized tonic-clonic[54] seizures, as well as generalized seizures of Lennox-Gastaut syndrome,[55] in patients 2 years of age and older. Lamotrigine is also indicated for conversion to monotherapy in adults with partial seizures receiving treatment with carbamazepine, phenytoin, phenobarbital, primidone, or valproate.[56] Conversion to monotherapy from other anticonvulsants or from multiple anticonvulsants is not currently approved. Nor is the drug approved for initial monotherapy, although there is evidence of efficacy in this situation.[57-59] In practice, lamotrigine is often used as initial monotherapy for partial-onset and primary generalized tonic-clonic seizures. The AAN/AES guidelines also indicate that lamotrigine is effective for newly diagnosed absence seizures in children,[60] although it is not FDA approved for this indication. Anecdotal reports suggest that in some patients, lamotrigine may worsen myoclonic jerks.[61]

Lamotrigine has become a preferred agent for women planning pregnancy. In multiple pregnancy registries, the rate of fetal malformations in children born to mothers on lamotrigine monotherapy has been low, 2.5–2.9%. A single report suggests that within that rate, there may be an over-representation of a specific malformation, cleft lip or palate.[62] Because this finding has not been confirmed in other pregnancy registries, many epileptologists consider lamotrigine to be first-line agent in pregnancy. This issue is likely to generate further discussion as additional data become available.

Lamotrigine offers several advantages. The drug is considered to be effective and generally well tolerated. Although it is metabolized by the liver, lamotrigine elicits little hepatic enzyme induction and no enzyme inhibition. Hence, there are relatively few drug interactions, making lamotrigine a reasonable option for the elderly, patients with HIV, and patients with other underlying medical problems in whom polypharmacy is an issue. Owing to its mood-stabilizing effects, the drug has also become a popular choice for patients with comorbid depression or bipolar disorder. Lamotrigine is a first-line agent of patients with renal or hepatic dysfunction, as well. Although its metabolism may be affected by hepatic disease, the drug itself causes little renal or hepatic toxicity.

A few notable drug interactions, however, do exist. Lamotrigine causes a modest reduction in levonorgestrel levels, and ethinyl estradiol may decrease lamotrigine levels. Adequate lamotrigine levels may be difficult to attain in the presence of phenytoin, as this drug induces the metabolism of lamotrigine. Very high dosages of lamotrigine may be required to yield therapeutic blood levels with concomitant phenytoin use. In contrast, valproate may significantly increase lamotrigine blood levels. When converting to lamotrigine monotherapy from these anticonvulsants. Lamotrigine levels should be monitored carefully. The therapeutic range begins at 4–6 mcg/mL. Some patients may benefit from higher levels, although our clinical experience suggests that levels in the teens pose a greater risk for side effects.

Although the drug is typically well tolerated, a few potential side effects deserve mention. Use of lamotrigine carries a risk of rash. The risk appears similar to that associated with phenytoin and carbamazepine, but if a lamotrigine-associated rash occurs, it may be very serious and patients should be encouraged to contact a physician immediately. Cases of Stevens-Johnson syndrome and toxic epidermal necrolysis have been reported. The risk is highest for children and those on concurrent valproate. Uncommon side effects also include cough and insomnia.

Risks are minimized by slow titration. It takes several weeks to properly attain a therapeutic dosage; the titration schedule may be confusing for some patients, and various blister starter packets are available to simplify the regimen. An even slower titration schedule should be employed for those also taking valproate, and separate starter packets are available for the purpose.

The chemical structure of lamotrigine is unrelated to those for the other anticonvulsants. The mechanism underlying lamotrigine's anticonvulsant effect is uncertain. The drug is postulated to act by inhibiting use-and voltage-sensitive sodium channels, thereby stabilizing neuronal membranes and modulating release of excitatory neurotransmitters such as glutamate.

Gabapentin

Although gabapentin is structurally related to GABA, the drug does not act via GABA-ergic mechanisms. The mechanism of its anticonvulsant activity is unknown. Animal data suggest that it binds to a subunit of voltage-activated calcium channels, but the functional importance of this is unclear.

Gabapentin is FDA approved as adjunctive therapy for partial seizures in patients aged 3 years and older and for seizures with secondary generalization in those aged 12 years and older. These indications are supported by double-blind randomized placebo-controlled studies.[63-65] According to the AAN/AES evidence-based guidelines, gabapentin is also a reasonable option as initial monotherapy for adolescents and adults with newly diagnosed partial-onset seizures.[66] Although it is not yet FDA approved for this indication. Insufficient evidence exists to support its use as monotherapy in those with refractory partial seizures. The drug has not been shown to be effective for primary generalized epilepsies and may in fact worsen myoclonic jerks,[67] absence, and primary generalized tonic-clonic seizures.

Gabapentin is typically quite well tolerated with few drug interactions. Our clinical experience suggests, however, that it is less efficacious than other available anticonvulsants.

Felbamate

Felbamate, an N-methyl-D-aspartate (NMDA) receptor antagonist, was approves by adjunctive treatment[68] or monotherapy[69-71] in adults with partial-onset seizures and as adjunctive treatment for seizures associated with Lennox-Gastaut syndrome in patients 2 years of age and older.[72] In addition, limited data suggest efficacy as add-on treatment for typical and atypical absence seizure,[73,74] partial seizures in children,[75] and generalized tonic-clonic seizures in adults.[76] Although one study demonstrated efficacy as monotherapy or adjunctive treatment for myoclonic, typical absence, and generalized tonic-clonic seizures associated with juvenile myoclonic epilepsy in adolescents and adults,[77] the results must be interpreted with caution given the small sample size.

The drug appeared to be well tolerated and to cause less sedation than other anticonvulsants. In 1994, however, a "Dear Doctor" letter proposed that physicians discontinue use of the drug owing to cases of aplastic anemia, with recent estimates suggesting a prevalence of 27–209 cases per million. The course of aplastic anemia depends on the severity of bone marrow suppression. Reports also identified instances of hepatic failure and rash, including Stevens-Johnson syndrome and toxic epidermal necrolysis, associated with felbamate use. Although rare, these reactions were serious and prompted many physicians to discontinue felbamate therapy in their patients.

In light of these findings, the AAN issued a guideline for felbamate use.[78] The guideline suggests that felbamate may be an appropriate choice for patients over age 4 with Lennox-Gastaut syndrome, and for patients over age 18 with partial seizures refractory to first-line anticonvulsants. One may also consider use of felbamate in certain situations for children with partial of generalized epilepsies and patients with Lennox-Gastaut syndrome under age 4 who are unresponsive to or intolerant of first-line agents. Data suggested a better risk/benefit ratio for treatment with monotherapy and for continuation in patients who have taken the drug for more than 18 months.

The AAN guideline notes that the risk/benefit ratio should be examined carefully in each patient, however, and that patients should be counseled regarding possible side effects and the recommendations for monitoring. Routine laboratory studies had not been shown to be useful, but the manufacturer and FDA do recommend liver function test and blood counts. Because the risk of aplastic anemia declines after one year of treatment, the value of routine monitoring after this time period is less clear. The drug should not be used in patients with a history of hematologic abnormalities, liver disease or systemic lupus erythematosus, patients who cannot comply with close follow-up, or patients and guardians unable to provide informed consent. Should physicians choose to prescribe felbamate, they are encouraged to register their patients in the Felbatol Registry.[78a]

Vigabatrin

Vigabatrin is a derivative of the inhibitory neurotransmitter GABA and irreversibly inhibits GABA transaminase, preventing breakdown of the neurotransmitter. The drug was initially intended to treat partial seizures in adults. Used in Europe since the late 1980s, it was found to be effective, particularly as adjunctive therapy for complex partial seizures and partial seizures with secondary generalization.[79,80] The medication appeared to be relatively well tolerated with minor side effects. After several years on the market in Europe, however, it was discovered that vigabatrin caused visual field defects in up to nearly 50% of adult,[81] with additional case reports in children.[82] Some patients also developed diminished visual acuity, deficits in color vision, and other retinal abnormalities.[81] When FDA approval was sought in 2004, it was denied because of these potential visual effects. As a recent AAN practice parameter suggests, however, the drug may be effective for treatment of infantile spasms, including spasms in the setting of tuberous sclerosis, for which there are few other treatment options.[83] Many physicians and parents of these patients obtain the drug from outside the United States despite the potentially serious side effects.

Drugs in Development

Several new compounds are currently in development, and the following drugs are quickly moving along the pipeline.[84] Brivaracetam, an SV2A ligand related to levetiracetam, recently acquired orphan drug status for symptomatic myoclonus and is undergoing evaluation for add-on treatment of partial seizures and Unverricht-Lundborg disease. Eslicarbazepine acetate, structurally related to carbamazepine and oxcarbazepine, is in phase III clinical trials for the adjunctive treatment of partial seizures in adults, with results expected this year. Lacosamide, in both intravenous and oral formulations, is under phase III investigation for the treatment of partial seizures. Thought to be effective in partial-onset seizures, retigabine and carisbamate are also in phase III trials.[85] A New Drug Application has been submitted to the FDA for rufinamide, a compound believed to be efficacious for adults and adolescents with refractory partial seizures as well as for adults and children with Lennox-Gastaut syndrome. Each new drug provides additional hope for seizure freedom in patients with epilepsy.

Drug Monitoring

Routine monitoring for anticonvulsant levels is not recommended except during pregnancy, when an increased volume of distribution causes levels to fall and changes in dosage are often required. Levels should be used to address specific concerns, e.g. to document compliance, assess for toxicity, or aid in management when changing drug regimens or when breakthrough seizures occur.

ALTERNATIVES TO PHARMACOLOGIC MANAGEMENT

A 2001 study of patients with newly diagnosed epilepsy found that 47% become seizure-free with the first anticonvulsant prescribed.[86] The probability of successful treatment diminishes with successive trials of different medications. Typically patients are considered to be refractory to medications when they have failed three or more anticonvulsants. Failure is defined as breakthrough seizures of any frequency, often quantified in the literature as at least one seizure within the past year. For these patients, ~30% for those with epilepsy alternative to pharmacologic management should be considered.

The utilization of surgical approaches for refractory epilepsy has increased. Resection is an effective treatment with little associated morbidity. In the first randomized controlled trial of epilepsy surgery, 64% of those who underwent anteromesial temporal lobectomy for refractory complex partial seizures were free of seizures that impaired consciousness compared to 8% of those who received medical management alone. Moreover, 42% of the surgical patients were completely seizure-free.[87] A review of the literature regarding anteromesial temporal lobectomy and neocortical resections yielded similar result.[88] On the basis of these data, the practice parameter set by the AAN and AES in 2003 states that referral to a surgical center should be considered for patients with refractory, disabling, complex partial temporal lobe seizures. A more recent report demonstrate event more impressive statistics, with 73% of those undergoing resection for mesial temporal lobe epilepsy rendered seizure-free.[89] Unfortunately, many potential surgical candidates are not referred for evaluation or are referred after long delays.

The appropriate timing of surgical intervention remains in question. A trial to assess outcomes of early surgery (the Early Randomized Surgical Epilepsy Trial, or ERSET) was unable to recruit a sufficient number of subjects. Anecdotal reports and small case series suggest a role for urgent resection in refractory status epilepticus, although randomized controlled trials have not been performed. This highlights the need for studies of treatment strategies for medically refractory seizure.

Implantable devices are an alternative for patients who are not candidates for, or do not desire, resection. Vagus nerve stimulation (VNS) was the first implantable device developed for treatment of seizures. Its mechanism of action remains unknown. Electrodes wrap around the left vagus never and connect to a generator placed subcutaneously in the chest wall. The stimulator delivers preprogrammed intermittent electrical pulses to the vagus nerve. It may also be activated by the swipe of a magnet to abort a seizure. During stimulation, however, patients may experience cough, hoarseness, or throat pain. Moreover, VNS requires surgical implantation, a costly procedure that poses a risk of injury to the nerve and carotid sheath. Very few adult patients (only isolated case reports) are rendered seizure-free by the device, and the risk must be weighed against the low probability of significant benefit. Overall, VNS is not believed to be useful in adults, although some success has been reported in children with refractory seizures. The AAN practice guidelines state that VNS is indicated for those aged 12 years and older with refractory partial seizures who are not candidates for resection.[90]

VNS has, however, paved the way for new device-driven therapies. A trial is under way to assess the efficacy of responsive or "closed loop" stimulators. These devices, implanted in the epileptogenic focus, detect epileptiform activity. They then deliver electrical stimulation to abort the abnormal discharges, thereby preventing the evolution of a clinical seizure. Some centers are also investigating use of deep brain stimulation for the treatment of epilepsy. Deep brain stimulation delivers "scheduled" or "open loop" stimulation to structures such as the thalamus, cerebellum, and hippocampus.[91]

The implantation of any device poses a small risk of infection and hemorrhage. It also requires rigorous workup, as would a surgical resection. For example, one must know the precise location of seizure onset in order to plan the placement of a closed-loop stimulator. This may require invasive EEG monitoring with recording grids, strips, or depth electrodes.

Dietary treatments provide an alternative, noninvasive approach for patients with refractory seizure disorders. The classic ketogenic diet, developed in the 1920s, recently gained popularity.[92] It involves low carbohydrate and high fat intake, with resultant ketosis. The mechanism of action underlying its efficacy, however, remains unclear. Approximately 20% of children on the diet have a >90% reduction in seizure frequency, with 7% seizure-free at one year. Although the diet is most effective in children, adults have also attained good results. It is typically used for treatment of generalized seizures of multiple seizure types but may also be considered for any patient with refractory seizures of intolerance of medications. The diet requires monitoring of weight, lipid profiles, electrolytes, urinalyses, urine calcium, and creatinine every 3–6 months. The risk of hyperlipidemia, however, is relatively low. More common side effects include weight loss, gastrointestinal upset, and acidosis.

Unfortunately, the diet also tends to be restrictive and unpalatable. A low-glycemic-index diet, allowing more carbohydrates and less fat, provides a less restrictive alternative. The diet is limited to foods that produce relatively little increase in blood glucose levels. In a study of 20 patients, 50% of those treated with this diet had a >90% reduction in seizure frequency.[93] A modified Atkins diet offers another less restrictive option. This diet yields seizure reduction rates comparable to that of the ketogenic diet but without the limitations on calories, fluid, and protein. At six months, 35% of 20 patients placed on the modified Atkins diet had a >90% improvement in seizure frequency, and particular efficacy was noted for absence seizures.[94] Some suggest that this diet may be appropriate for parents with more recent-onset, less refractory seizures than those treated with the ketogenic diet. Overall, dietary therapies are good options for those resistant to or intolerant of anticonvulsants, with the goal of discontinuing or reducing medications.

OTHER TREATMENT ISSUES

Patients with epilepsy often demonstrate subtle or transient cognitive dysfunction in areas such attention, language, and memory, despite otherwise normal intelligence. Factors that may contribute to cognitive difficulties include seizure type, frequency, severity, and age of onset; side effects of treatment; and perhaps most important, psychosocial and psychiatric comorbidities.[95-97] Patients with seizures have a greater incidence of anxiety, depression, and bipolar disorder, with suicide rates ten times higher than that of the general population.[3] These cognitive and emotional symptoms may be the most troublesome aspects of epilepsy for patients. It has become increasingly clear in recent years that those with epilepsy should be screened for concurrent cognitive and psychiatric disorders.

FUTURE DIRECTIONS

Further advancements in the diagnosis and treatment of epilepsy may stem from the study of genetics. It has long been accepted that many of the primary generalized epilepsies have a genetic basis. A recent trend in genetic studies of epilepsy has been the finding of gene mutations resulting in channelopathies. Mutations in genes encoding sodium channel subunits were found to underlie various epileptic syndromes of infancy, including generalized epilepsy with febrile seizures plus (GEFS4), severe myoclonic epilepsy of infancy, and benign familial neonatal-infantile seizures. The syndrome of benign familial neonatal convulsions has been traced to gene mutations causing aberrant voltage-dependent potassium channels, and mutations that alter voltage-gated chloride channels have been linked to childhood absence epilepsy, juvenile absence epilepsy, juvenile myoclonic epilepsy, and epilepsy with grand-mal seizures on awakening.[98]

Recent studies have also revealed a genetic basis to various focal epilepsies. It is an intriguing notion that such a diffuse process results in a focal brain abnormality, as seen with nicotinic acetylcholine receptor gene mutations in autosomal dominant nocturnal frontal lobe epilepsy and LGI-1 mutations in familial lateral temporal lobe epilepsy.[99]

The importance of these studies may lie in their implications for optimizing future treatment. For instance, genetic markers that predict anticonvulsant response would be invaluable. Genetic testing might also identify patients at risk for seizure recurrence, allowing more rapid initiation of treatment. Many of the genetic tests are now commercially available, although interpretation of results may be complicated by possible polygenetic mechanisms or variable penetrance. Currently such testing does not typically play a role in clinical management. If patients or their families desire such testing, referral to a genetic counselor should be considered.

SUMMARY

Recent years have brought new tools for the diagnosis of epilepsy, with advances in MRI techniques, the advent of MEG, increased availability of PET and SPECT, and use of multimodal imaging studies such as EEG/fMRI. Minimally invasive means of intracranial EEG monitoring are more commonly employed, such as epidural pegs and foramen ovale electrodes. A wider range of treatment options also exists, including new anticonvulsants, dietary therapies, implantable devices, and earlier surgical interventions. Great strides have been made in the management of epilepsy, as many of today's standard diagnostic procedures and first-line therapies were not available just a few years ago.

REFERENCES

1. Centers for Disease Control. Revalence of epilepsy and health-related quality of life and disability among adults with epilepsy-South Carolina, 2003 and 2004. MMWR Weekly. 2005; 54:8080-2.
2. Kobau R, DiIorio CA, Price PH, et al. Prevalence of epilepsy and health status of adults with epilepsy in Georgia and Tennessee: Behavioral Risk Factor Surveillance System, 2002. Epilepsy Behav. 2004;5:358-66.
3. Strine TW, Kobau R, Chapman DP, et al. Psychological distress, comorbidities, and health behaviors among U.S. adults with seizures: result from the 2002 National Health Interview Survey. Epilepsia. 2005;46:1133-9.
4. Knake S, Triantafyllou C, Wald LL, et al. 3T phased array MRI improves the presurgical evaluation in focal epilepsies: a prospective study. Neurology. 2005;65:1026-31.
5. Ogawa S, Lee TM, Kay AR, et al. Brain magnetic resonance imaging with contrast dependent on blood oxygenation. Proc. Natl. Acad. Sci. USA. 1990;87:9868-72.
6. Salek-Haddadi A, Friston KJ, Lemieux L, et al. Studying spontaneous EEG activity with fMRI. Brain Res. Brain Res Rev. 2003;43:110-33.
7. Salek-Haddadi A, Merschhemke M, Lemiexu L, et al. Simultaneous EEG-correlated ictal fMRI. Neuroimage. 2002; 16:32-40.
8. Knowlton RC, Shih J. Magnetoencephalography in epilepsy. Epilepsia. 2004;45(Suppl. 4):61-71.
9. Van Paesschen W. Ictal SPECT. Epilepsia. 2004;45(Suppl 4): 35-40.

9a. Brunbech L, Sabers A. Effect of antiepileptic drugs on cognitive function in individuals with epilepsy: a comparative review of newer versus older agents. Drugs. 2002;62:593-604.

9b. Asconape JJ. Some common issues in the use of antiepileptic drugs. Semin Neurol. 2002;22:27-39.

10. Karceski S, Morrell MJ, Carpenter D. Treatment of epilepsy in adults: expert opinion, 2005. Epilepsy Behav. 7 (Suppl. 1) S1, 2005;64; quiz S65-67.
11. French J, Smith M, Faught E, et al. Practice advisory: the use of felbamate in the treatment of patients with intractable epilepsy. Report of the Quality Standards Subcommittee of the American Academy of Neurology and the American Epilepsy Society. Neurology. 1999;52:1540-5.
12. French JA, Kanner AM, Bautista J, et al. Efficacy and tolerability of the new antiepileptic drugs I: treatment of new onset epilepsy. Report of the Therapeutics and Technology Assessment Subcommittee and Quality Standard Subcommittee of the American Academy of Neurology and the American Epilepsy Society: Neurology. 2004;62:1252-60.
13. French JA, Kanner AM, Bautista J, et al. Efficacy and tolerability of the new antiepileptic drugs II: treatment of refractory epilepsy. Report of the Therapeutics and Technology Assessment Subcommittee and Quality Standards Subcommittee of the American Academy of Neurology and the American Epilepsy Society: Neurology. 2004;62: 1261-73.
14. French JA, Kugler Ar, Robbins JL, et al. Dose-response trial of pregabalin adjunctive therapy in patients with partial seizures. Neurology. 2003;60:1631-7.
15. Beydoun A, Uthman BM, Kugler AR, et al. Safety and efficacy of two pregabalin regimens for add-on treatment of partial epilepsy. Neurology. 2005;64:475-80.
16. Arroyo S. Anhut H, Kugler AR, et al. Pregabalin add-on treatment: a randomized, double-blind, placebo-controlled, dose-response study in adults with partial seizures. Epilepsia. 2004;45:20-7.
17. Glauser TA, Nigro M, Sachbdeo R, et al. Adjunctive therapy with oxcarbazepine in children with partial seizures. The Oxcarbazepine Pediatric Study Group. Neurology. 2000; 54:2237-44.
18. Kothare SV, Khurana DS, Mostofi N, et al. Oxcarbazepine monotherapy in children and adolescents: a single-center clinical experience. Pediatr. Neurol. 2006;35:235-9.
19. Beydoun A, Sechdeo RC, Rosenfeld WE, et al. Oxcarbazepine monotherapy for partial-onset seizures: a multicenter, double-blind, clinical trial. Neurology. 2000;54:2245-51.
20. Sachdeo R, Beydoun A, Schachter S, et al. Oxcarbazepine (Trileptal) as monotherapy in patients with partial seizures. Neurology. 2001;57:864-71.
21. Barcs G, Wlaker EB, Elger CE, et al. Oxcarbazepine placebo-controlled, dose ranging trial in refractory partial epilespsy. Epilepsia. 2000;41:1597-607.
22. Bill PA, Vigonius U, Pohlamann H, et al. A double-blind controlled clinical trial oxcarbazepine versus sodium valproate in adults with newly diagnosed epilepsy. Epilepsy res. 1997; 26:451-60.

23. Guerreior MM, Vigonius U, Pohlamann H, et al. A double-blind controlled clinical trial of oxcarbazepine versus phenytoin in children and adolescents with epilepsy. Epilepsy res. 1997; 27:205-13.
24. Christe W, Kramer G, Vigonius U, et al. A double-blind controlled clinical trial: oxcarbazepine versus sodium valproate in adults with newly diagnosed epilepsy. Epilepsy Res. 1997;26:451-60.
25. Dam M, Ekberg R, Lyning Y, et al. A double-blind study comparing oxcarbazepine and carbamazepine in patients with newly diagnosed, previously untreated epilepsy. Epilepsy Res. 1989;3:70-6.
26. Schmidt D, Elger CE. What is the evidence that oxcarbazepine and carbamazepine are distinctly different antiepileptic drugs? Epilepsy Behav. 2004;5:627-35.
26a. Palmiri A. Oxcarbazepine-induced headache. Cephalalgia 2007;27:91-3.
27. Faught E, Ayala R, Montouris GG, et al. Randomized controlled trial of zonisamide for the treatment of refractory partial-onset seizures. Neurology. 2001;57:1774-9.
28. Schmide D, Jacob R, Loiseau P, et al. Zonisamide for add-on treatment of refractory partial epilepsy: a European double-blind trial. Epilepsy Res. 1993;15:67-73.
29. Kothare SV, Kaleyias J, Mostofi N, et al. Efficacy and safety of zonisamide monotherapy in a cohort of children with epilepsy. Pediatr Neurl. 2006;34:351-4.
30. Yanai S, Hanai T, Narazaki O. Treatment of infantile spasms with zonisamide. Brain Dev. 1999;21:157-61.
31. Kyllerman M, Ben-Menachem E. Zonisamide for progressive myoclonus epilepsy long-term observations in seven patients. Epilepsy Res. 1998;29:109-14.
32. Shorvon SD, Lowenthal A, Janz D, et al. Multicenter double-blind, randomized, placebo-controlled trial of levetiracetam as add-on therapy in patients with refractory partial seizures. European Levetiracetam Study Group. Epilepsia. 2000;41:1179-86.
33. Careghino JJ, Biton V, Abou-Khalil B, et al. Levetiracetam for partial seizures results of a double-blind, randomize clinical trial. Neurology. 2000;55:236-42.
34. Glauser TA, Ayala R, Elterman RD, et al. Double-blind placebo-controlled trial of adjunctive levetiracetam in pediatric partial seizures. Neurology. 2006;66:1654-60.
35. Glauser TA, Pellock JM, Bebin Em, et al. Efficacy and safety of levetiracetam in children with partial seizures: an open-label trial. Epilepsia. 2002;43:518-24.
36. Ben-Menachem E, Falter U. Efficacy and tolerability of levetiracetam 3000 mg/d in patients with refractory partial seizures: a multicenter, double-blind, responder-selected study evaluating monotherapy. European Levetiracetam Study Group. Epilepsia. 2000;41:1276-83.
37. Specchio LM, Gambardella A, Giallonardo AT, et al. Open label, long-term, pragmatic study on levetiracetam in the treatment of juvenile myoclonic epilepsy. Epilepsy Res. 2006;71:32-9.
38. Labate A, Colosimo E, Gambardella A, et al. Levetiracetam in patients with generalized epilepsy and myoclonic seizures: an open label study. Seizure. 2006;15:214-8.
39. Patel NC, Landan IR, Levin J, et al. The use of levetiracetam in refractory status epilepticus, Seizure. 2006;15:137-41.
40. Sachdeo Rc, Leroy RF, Krauss GL, et al. Tiagabine therapy for complex partial seizures. A dose-frequency study. The Tiagabine Study Group. Arch Neurol. 1997;54:595-601.
41. Uthman BM, Rowan AJ, Ahmann PA, et al. Tiagabine therapy for complex partial seizures: a randomized, add-on, does-response trial. Arch. Neutrol. 1998;55:56-62.
42. Richens A, Chadwick DW, Duncan Js, et al. Adjunctive treatment of partial seizures with tiagabine: a placebo-controlled trial. Epilepsy Res. 1995;21:37-42.
43. Koepp MJ, Edward M, Collins J, et al. Status epilepticus and tiagabine therapy revisited. Epilepsia. 2005;46:1625-32.
44. Gilliam FG, Veloso F, Bomhof MA, et al. A dose-comparison trail of topiramate as monotherapy in recently diagnosed partial epilepsy. Neurology. 2003;60:196-202.
45. Arroyo S, Dodson We, Privitera MD, et al. Randomized dose-controlled study of topiramate as first-line therapy in epilepsy. Acta Neurol, Scand. 2005;112:214-22.
46. Ben-Menachem E, Henriksen O, Dam M, et al. Double-blind, placebo-controlled trial of topiramate as add-on therapy in patients with refractory partial seizures. Epilepsia. 1996; 37:539-43.
47. Biton V, Montouris GD, Ritter F, et al. A randomized, placebo-controlled study of topiramate in primary generalized tonic-clonic seizures. Topiramate YTC Study Group. Neurolog. 1999;52:1330-7.
48. Sachdeo RC, Glauser TA, Ritter F, et al. A double-blind, randomized trial of topiramate in Lennox-Gastaut syndrome. Topiramate YL Study Group. Neurology. 1999;52:1882-7.
49. Silberstein SD. Control of topiramate-induced paresthesias with supplemental potassium. Headache. 2002;42:85.
50. Matsuo F, Bergen D, Faugh E, et al. Placebo-controlled study of the efficacy and safety of lamotrigine in patients with partial seizures. U.S. Lamotrigine Protocol 0.5 Clinical Trial Group. Neurology. 1993;43:2284-91.
51. Messenheimer J, Ramsya RE, Willmore LJ, et al. Lamotrigine therapy for partial seizures: a multicenter, placebo controlled, double-blind, cross-over trial. Epilepsia. 1994;35:113-21.
52. Schapel GJ, Beran RG, Vajda FJ, et al. Double-blind, placebo controlled crossover study of lamotrigine in treatment resistant partial seizures. J Neurol Neurosurg Psychiatry. 1993;56: 448-53.
53. Duchowny M, Pellock Jm, Graf Wd, et al. A placebo-controlled trial of lamotrigine add-on therapy for partial seizures in children. Lamictal Pediatric Partial Seizure Study Group. Neurology. 1999;53:1727-31.
54. Biton V, Sackellares JC, Vuong A et al. Double-blind, placebo-controlled study of lamotrigine in primary generalized tonic-clonic seizures. Neurology. 2005;65:1737-43.

55. Motte J, Trevathan E, Arvidsson JF, et al. Lamotrigine for generalized seizures associated with the Lennox-Gastaut syndrome. Lamictal Lennox-Gastaut Study Groupl. N Engl J Med. 1997;337:1807-12.
56. Gilliam F, Vazquez B, Sackellares JC, et al. An active-control trial of lamotrigine monotherapy for partial seizures. Neurology. 1998;51:1018-25.
57. Steinhoff BJ, Ueberall AM, Siemes H, et al. The LAM-SAFE study lamotrigine versus carbamazepine or valproic acid in newly diagnosed focal and generalized epilepsy in adolescents and adults. Seizure. 2005;14:597-605.
58. Steiner TJ, Dellaportas CI, Findley LJ, et al. Lamotrigine monotherapy in newly diagnosed untreated epilepsy: a double-blind comparision with phenytoin, Epilepsia. 1999;40: 601-7.
59. Brodie MJ, Richens A Yuen AW. Double-blind comparison of lamotrigine and carbamazepine in newly diagnosed epilepsy. UK Lamotrigine/Carbamazepine Monotherapy Trial Group. Lancet. 1995;345:476-9.
60. Frank LM, Enlow T, Holmes GL, et al. Lamictal (lamotrigine) monotherapy for typical absence seizures in children. Epilepsia. 1999;40:973-9.
61. Janszky J, Rasonyi G, Halasz P, et al. Disabling erratic myoclonus during lamotrigine therapy with high serum level-report of two case. Clim Neuropbarmacol. 2000;23:86-9.
62. Homes LB, Wyszynski DF, Baldwin EJ, et al. Increased risk of nonsyndromic cleft palate amongst infants exposed to lamotrigine during pregnancy. Birth Defect Res Part A. 2006;76:318.
63. Appleton R, Fichtner K, LaMoreaux L, et al. Gabapentin as add-on therapy in children with refractory partial seizures: a 12-week, multicenter, double-blind, placebo-controlled study. Gabapentin Paediatric Study Group. Epilepsia. 1999;40:1147-54.
64. UK Gabapentin Study Group. Gabapentin in partial epilepsy. Lancet. 1990;335:1114-1.
65. Anhut H, Ashman P, Feuerstein TJ, et al. Gabapentin (neurontin) as add on therapy in patients with partial seizures: a double-blind, placebo-controlled study. The International Gabapentin Study Group. Epilepsia. 1994;35: 795-801.
66. Chadwick DW, Anhut H, Greiner MJ, et al. A double-blind trial of gabapentine monotherapy for newly diagnosed partial seizures. International Gabapentin Monotherapy Study Group 945-77. Neurology. 1998;51:1282-8.
67. Asconape J, Diedrich A, DellaBadia J. Myoclonus associated with the use of gabapentin. Epilepsia. 2000;41:479-81.
68. Leppik IE, Dreifuss FE, Pledger GW, et al. Felbamate for partial seizures: result of a controlled clinical trial. Neurology. 1991;41:1785-9.
69. Faugth E, Sachdeo RC, Remler MP, et al. Felbamate monotherapy for partial onset seizures: an active-control trial. Neurology. 1993;43:688-92.
70. Sachdeo R, Kramer LD, Rosenberg A, et al. Felbamate monotherapy controlled trial in patients with partial onset seizures. Ann Neurol. 1992;32:386-92.
71. Devinsky O, Faught RE, Wilder BJ, et al. Efficacy of felbamate monotherapy in patients undergoing presurgical evaluation of partial seizures. Epilepsy Res. 1995;20:241-46.
72. The Felbamate Study Group in Lennox-Gastaut syndrome. Efficacy of Felbamate in childhood epileptic encephalopathy (Lennox-Gastaut Syndrome). N Engl J Med. 1993;328:29-33.
73. Devinsky O, Kothari M, Rubin R, et al. Felbamate for absence seizure. Epilepsia. 1992;33:84.
74. Kuzniecky R, Thompson G, Faught E, et al. Felbamate add-on therapy in intractable atypical absence. Epilepsia. 1991;32:10.
75. Carmant L, Homes GL, Sawyer S, et al. Efficacy of felbamate in therapy for partial epilepsy in children. J Pediatr. 1994;125:481-6.
76. Leroy RF, Castain T. Pilot study of felbamate in adult medically refractory primary generalized seizure patients. Epilepsia. 1991;32:13.
77. Sachdeo RC, Wagner ML. Felbamate in generalized tonic-clonic seizures. Epliepsis. 1991;32:54.
78. French J, Smith M, Faught E, et al. Practice advisory: the use of felbamate in the treatment of patients with intractable epilepsy. Report of the Quality Standards subcommittee of the American Academy of Neurology and the American Epilepsy Society. Neurology. 1999;52:1540-5.
78a. Pellock JM, Faught E, Leppik IE, et al. Felbamate: consensus of current clinical experience. Epilepsy Res. 2006;71:89-101.
79. Dean C, Mosier M, Penry K. Dose-response study of vigabatrin as add on therapy in patients with uncontrolled complex partial seizures. Epilepsa. 1999;40:74-82.
80. Bruni J, Guberman A, Vachon L, et al. Vigabatrin as add-on therapy for adult complex partial seizures: a double-blind, placebo-controlled multicenter study. The Canadian Vigabatrin Study Group. Seizure. 2000;9:224-32.
81. Miller NR, Johnson MA, Paul SR, et al. Visual dysfunction in patients receiving vigabatrin: clinical and electrophysiologic finding. Neurology. 1999;53:2082-7.
82. Iannetti P, Spalice A, Peral FM, et al. Visual field constriction in children with epilepsy on vigabatrin treatment. Pediatrics. 2000;106:838-42.
83. Mackay MT, Weiss SK, Adams-Webber T, et al. Practice parameter: medical treatment of infantile spasms. Report of the American Academy of Neurology and the Child Neurology Society. Neurology. 2004;62:1668-81.
84. Bailer M, Johannessen SI, Kupferberg HJ. Progress report on new antiepileptic drugs: a summary of the eighth Eilat Conference (EILAT VIII). Epilepsy Res. 2007;73:1-52.
85. Porter RJ, Partiot A, Sachdeo R, et al. Randomized, multicenter, dose-ranging trial of retigabine for partial-onset seizures. Neurology. 2007;68:1197-204.
86. Kwan P, Brodie MJ. Effectiveness of first antiepileptic drug, Epilepsia. 2001;42:1255-60.

87. Wiebe S, Blume WT, Girvin JP, et al. A randomized, controlled trial of surgery for temporal-lobe epilepsy. N Engl J Med. 2001; 345:311-8.
88. Engel J Jr, Wiebe S, French J, et al. Practice parameter: Temporal lobe and localized neocortical restriction for epilepsy. Epilepsia. 2003;44:741-51.
89. Engle J Jr, Tedeschi H, Oliveira EL, et al. Comparison of short-term outcome between surgical and clinical treatment in temporal lobe epilepsy: a prospective study. Seizure. 2006; 15:35-40.
90. Fisher RS, Handforth A. Reassessment: vagus nerve stimulation for epilepsy. A report of the Therapeutics and Technology Assessment Subcommittee of the American Academy of Neurology. Neurology. 1999;53:666-9.
91. Morrell M. Brain stimulation for epilepsy: Can scheduled or responsive neurostimulation stop seizures? Curr Opin Neurol. 2006;19:164-8.
92. Sinha SR, Kossoff EH. The ketogenic diet. Neurologist. 2005; 11:161-70.
93. Pfeifer HH, Thiele EA. Low-glycemic-index treatment: a liberalized ketogenic diet for treatment of intractable epilepsy. Neurology. 2005;65:1810-2.
94. Kossoff EH, McGrogan JR, Blumi RM, et al. A modified Atkins diet is effective for the treatment of intractable pediatric epilepsy. Epilepsia. 2006;47:421-4.
95. Pavone P, Bianchini R, Trifiletti RR, et al. Neuropsychological assessment in children with absence epilepsy. Neurology. 2001;56:10487-51.
96. Motamedi G, Meador K. Epilepsy and cognition. Epilepsy Behav. 2003;4(Suppl 2):S25-38.
97. Meador KJ. Cognitive outcomes and predictive factors in epilepsy. Neurology. 2002;58:S21-6.
98. Gardiner M. Genetics of idiopathic generalized epilepsies. Epilepsia. 2005;46(Suppl 9):15:20.
99. Andermann F, Kobayashi E, Andermann E. Genetic focal epilepsies: state of the art and paths to the future. Epilepsa. 2005;46(Suppl 10):61-7.

CHAPTER

72

Psychological Adjustment to Chronic Disease

JN Vyas

INTRODUCTION

Chronic illnesses are disorders that persist for an extended period and affect a person's ability to function normally. Some chronic diseases (e.g. rheumatoid arthritis) need long-term pharmacological treatment and are often characterized by progressive physical disability and pain. Other (e.g. diabetes) can be medically controlled, but only at the cost of strict adherence to disease management regimens. Thus, a chronic illness has the potential to induce profound changes in a person's life, resulting in negative effects on quality of life and wellbeing.[1]

After the medical diagnosis of chronic illness, patients are confronted with new situations that challenge their habitual coping strategies. As a result, they must find new ways of coping to adjust to their altered condition.[2] We use the terms adjustment and psychological adjustment interchangeably to refer to the healthy rebalancing by patients to their new circumstances. Most patients eventually reach a state of good psychological adjustment, but for about 30% of patients, the adjustment phase is prolonged and sometimes unsuccessful.[2]

At least five key elements of successful adjustment to a chronic illness have been identified: the successful performance of adaptive task (e.g. adjustment to disability, maintained emotional balance, and preservation of healthy relationships),[3] the absence of psychological disorders, the presence of low negative affect and high positive affect, adequate functional (e.g. work) status, and the satisfaction and wellbeing in various life domains.[4] Several models have been proposed on how patients could achieve these outcomes, including: the model of cognitive adaptation, which emphasizes acceptance and perceptions of control over illness,[5] the personality model that emphasizes the role of personality factors (such as optimism or neuroticism) in adjustment; and the stress and coping model that emphasizes strategies used by patients to deal with adaptive tasks imposed by disease.[6] The authoritative stress and coping model acknowledges the chronic illness consists of several challenges, but at the same time, it highlights-more than other models of adjustment-processes of appraisal and coping the explain why some patients successfully identify and act to opportunities to manage these tasks whereas others might fail to do so. More recently, the stress and coping model has been extended with the model of self-regulation, which allows patients to deal with illness more proactively.[7] Both models show the active role that patients may have in adjusting to the challenges posed by their condition, and they have been used to study processes of adjustment in diverse chronic conditions including cancer, diabetes, HIV-infection, asthma, and rheumatoid arthritis.[8,9]

THE CHALLENGE OF PATIENTS REMAINING ACTIVE DESPITE CYTOKINE ACTIVITY

Infectious and inflammatory process and induce a constellation of nonspecific symptoms, often called sickness behavior, including weakness, malaise, inability to concentrate, depressed mood, lethargy, anhedonia, and anorexia.[10] Therefore, in addition to dealing with the behavioral, cognitive, and emotional challenges of disease, patients must also cope with these physiologically-induced symptoms to preserve an active life.

The psychological effects of these pathophysiological processes are mediated by cytokines. Several studies have shown that proinflammatory cytokines such as tumor necrosis factor α (TNFα) and interferon alfa seem to promote the psychological symptoms seen with several chronic diseases. Proinflammatory cytokines contribute to the vital exhaustion (loss of energy, increased irritability, and feeling of demoralization) seen with acute myocardial infarction.[11] In diabetes, increased concentrations of proinflammatory cytokines are produced by adipose tissue, and by monocytes and macrophages seen with increasing age, and could contribute to depression and so-called sickness behavior.[12] In cancer, these cytokines contribute to fatigue, memory and concentration problems, depression, and anxiety.[13]

Immunotherapy with cytokines has also been shown to promote these symptoms. In uncontrolled prospective trials with interferon-alfa infusions, patients frequently report fatigue (70–100%), depressive symptoms (21–58%), and depression according to diagnostic criteria (9–45%) as well as anorexia, pain, cognitive slowing, confusion, lethargy, mania, inner tension, anxiety, and reduction in goal-directed bahavior.[14-17]

Evidence suggests the cytokines mediate disease-induced inactivity and distress. In patients with rheumatoid arthritis who do not respond to conventional disease-modifying antirheumatic drugs, reduced disease activity can be achieved by blockade of proinflammatory cytokines. Immediately after blocked of TNFα, a substantial improvement of physical functioning, quality of life, and fatigue can be seen (Panel 1). The finding that proinflammatory cytokines can promote-and by blockade reduce-these symptoms shows that physiological factors are a real obstacle to the psychological adjustment to chronic illness.

The malaise and behavioral inactivation associated with illness is generally regarded as adaptive, especially during acute infection and inflammation. By inducing rest, this response conserves energy and promotes healing, and thus stimulates adjustment similar to the desire for food in response to hunger, pain in response to injury, and the fight-or-fight response can endanger patients with cardiovascular disease. Thus, symptoms (such as fatigue and pain) that are beneficial during an acute illness can become obstacles to psychological adjustment in chronic disease.

Panel 1: Effects of blockade of proinflammatory cytokines on psychological adjustment in patients with rheumatoid arthritis, as shown in relevant studies

- *Disability in daily activities*: Disability scores have been shown to improve after the first week of medication.[18-29] This improvement was sustained with prolonged drug use (up to 5 years).[19] Effect size was about 0.6 SD units,[20,25] regrade as a moderate change; percentage change varied between 40%[22,23,26,29] and 80%.[25]
- *Quality of life*: Summary scores of the short form 36, measuring physical functioning, improved.[18,20-22,24,25,28,29] Effect size was more than 0.5 SD units,[20,25] regarded as a moderate change; percentage change was about 40%.[22,25] Improvement on the summary score of the short from 36, measuring mental wellbeing (which did not differ greatly form the general population at baseline),[21] was generally small (about 15%).[20-22,24,25,28,29]
- *Fatigue and vitality*: Substantial improvement was seen on the fatigue scale of the Functional Assessment of Chronic Illness Therapy questionnaire.[29] Change on the vitality scale of the short form 36 was as large as the change seen on physical functioning scales.[18,20]

Chronic pain has been suggested not only to lead to pain-avoidance behavior but also to persistence of even overuse of activities, both of which can lead to disability.[30] Furthermore, patients with other chronic diseases are faced with the challenge to pace their activity and find a new balance in their lives. Only a few decades ago, the common recommendation given to patients with chronic inflammatory diseases such as rheumatoid arthritis was to rest.[31] Nowadays, graded exercise tailored to the patients' abilities and disease severity is thought to lead to improved physical, functional, and emotional outcomes.[32,33] Inactivity in response to acute illness is natural and often beneficial. But one of the challenges facing patients with chronic illness is to engage in those activities that can improve functional ability and emotional status in the face of real cytokine-related symptoms that make activity difficult.

EMOTIONAL REGULATION: TO FEEL OR NOT TO FEEL

Patients with chronic illness typically have anxiety, depression, and other negative emotions.[2] How these individuals cope with these emotions can affect how well they adjust to their illness. Emotion regulation is a term encompassing several conscious or unconscious styles of experiencing, processing, and modulation emotions.[34] Two main categories of emotion regulation have been distinguished: avoidance and inhibition of emotions, and expression and acknowledgment of emotions. Although the fires category—when generally applied—is associated with maladaptive outcomes such as an increase in disease occurrence and risk of disease progression, increasing evidence has shown that the habitual acknowledgment and expression of emotions can promote good adjustment.[35]

In cross-sectional studies, maladjustment to chronic illness is commonly related to styles of emotion regulation characterized by avoidance and nonexpression. Examples include patients having difficulty identifying and describing emotions (alexithymia), being unaware of emotions (repression), avoiding the expression of emotions (emotional control, suppression, antiemotionality), and being ambivalent about expressing emotions.[36] Although patients are often advised to face and express emotions, cross-sectional relations between adjustment and the acknowledgment and expression of emotions have been inconsistent.[37] However, these cross-sectional findings do not prove that emotion regulation affects adjustment; it is equally possible that the distressing emotions experienced during chronic illnesses after emotion regulation.

Prospective studies examining which types of emotion regulation affect adjustment show that, at least in the North American and western European cultures, the regular use of avoidant nonexpressive styles of emotion regulation is disadvantageous for psychological adjustment and survival. In less emotionally expressive Asian cultures, nonexpressive emotion regulation styles have proven advantageous, suggesting that the congruence between one's general style to handle emotions and the style advocated in one's cultural system determines whether the emotion regulation style is adaptive or maladaptive.[38] Acknowledgment and intense experience of emotions are suggested to be beneficial for adjustment as long as those emotions are expressed and

Panel 2: Prospective and experimental studies of associations between emotion regulation and adjustment to chronic illness

Prospective studies

Psychological adjustment

- Emotional control before diagnosis of breast cancer predicted increased psychological distress after diagnosis.[39] Control did not predict increased distress 15 months later in rheumatoid arthritis.[40]
- Emotional processing and affect intensity not only predicted positive affect scores in rheumatoid arthritis,[41] but also negative affect [41] and increased distress in patients with breast cancer and rheumatoid arthritis after 3–15 months[40,42]
- Mood repair and mood clarity predicted reduced pain-related psychological distress in rheumatoid arthritis and osteoarthritis.[42,43]
- Expression of emotion predicted reduced distress after diagnosis of breast cancer and 3 months after diagnosis,[39,42] and did not predict distress in rheumatoid arthritis after 15 months.[40]

Physical adjustment

- Alexithymia and ambivalence over expression of emotions predicted an increase in self-reported disease activity in rheumatoid arthritis after 15 months[40]
- Nonexpression of emotions predicted rapid disease progression in HIV after 6 months to 9 years [44]
- Repression of emotions[45] and emotional control[46,47] predicted increased mortality in cancer, whereas other studies showed no association with survival, [48-50] and one study in Japan showed moderate antiemotionality to predict survival[38]
- Emotional expression resulted in improved self-perceived health status and reduced number of medical visits in breast cancer after 3 months,[42] and on change in perceived health in rheumatoid arthritis after 15 months[40]
- Emotional expression predicted survival in breast cancer[46]

Experimental studies

Psychological adjustment

- Emotional expression in several chronic diseases led to decreased distress, mood improvement, or reduced intrusions up to several months after the intervention,[51-55] or resulted in no change or change in only one minor outcome variable[56-60]

Physical adjustment

- Emotional expression in several chronic diseases led to a reduction in health-care use, improved physical functioning, fewer symptoms reported, or reduced self-perceived disease activity up to several months after the intervention,[51-54,57,59,60] or resulted in no change[56]
- Emotional expression led to improvements in clinical and laboratory observations (e.g. pulmonary function in asthma, joint score in rheumatoid arthritis, CD4+ lymphocyte counts in HIV) up to several months after the intervention,[51,57,61,62] or result in no change.[53,54,56,58,59,63]

processed; the mere uncontrolled expression of emotions without processing can be maladaptive (Panel 2).

Physiological and psychological mechanisms have been proposed to explain the negative effect of avoidant and nonexpressive emotion regulation styles on adjustment.[65] Although denial and nonexpression of emotions can be a useful initial coping strategy to deal with the stress the accompanies the diagnosis of a chronic disease,[66] failure to acknowledge and express emotions can leave these emotions unresolved. These unresolved emotions can affect patients' health negatively by, for example, chronic raised activity of the sympathetic nervous system.[67] The inhibition of emotions can also delay help-seeking behavior. When it hampers symptom recognition and, when help is sought, compromise the communication with healthcare providers. Such inhibition can also lead to patients failing to practice health-protective behaviors and adhere to treatment.[66]

Alternatively, different mechanisms have been proposed to explain why acknowledgment and expression of emotions are beneficial for patients.[68] Although the acknowledgment and experience of negative emotions can be adaptive because they focus attention toward threats, elicit action, and provide feedback on progress toward important goals,[66] repeated reflection on or rumination about negative feelings without emotions will make their experience less intensive and invasive (habituation), whereas it can also increase insight into why emotions are experienced and how their effect can be reduced (cognitive reappraisal). Furthermore, expression of emotions can decrease emotional distress and restore psychophysiological balance, and create opportunities for social support and enhanced closeness with others, benefit finding, and improve self-regulation.[35,69]

Overall, when confronted with chronic illness it seems better for patients to generally express than to deny or inhibit emotions, as long as this strategy surpasses the unbridled spouting of emotions and helps to achieve mort insight. Evidence on the role of emotion regulation in adjustment to chronic illness implies that patients acknowledging and dealing with the negative emotions surrounding chronic illness is not necessarily bad for adjustment. Although styles of emotion regulation are a stable characteristic of a person and can be difficult to change, interventions that aim to teach more effective styles to regulate emotions have proven beneficial for individuals who consistently use ineffective emotion regulation styles in adjusting to their chronic condition.[64]

SELF-MANAGEMENT: IMPROVEMENT OF MOOD AND HEALTH BEHAVIOR

Management of chronic illness is characterized by many responsibilities regarding medication use, lifestyle changes, and behavior to prevent long-term complications-generally referred to as self-management of disease.[70] May studies have shown that patients who engage in healthy diet, exercise, or other aspects of self-management have physical benefits in terms of fewer symptoms, better functional capability, and fewer complications than those who do not in various diseases (e.g. HIV/AIDS,[71] rheumatoid arthritis,[72] asthma or chronic obstructive pulmonary disease,[73] diabeties,[74] and heart failure[75]). However, the extent to which self-management can also affect psychological adjustment is much less understood. Studies have shown a low adherence to self-management regimens; only about 15–25% of patients improve their health practices after diagnosis,[76] suggesting that they find disease management difficult to integrate into their lives. Indeed, many patients have a great fear of lifestyle changes[77,78] and report more nonadherence to diet and exercise than to medication use or check-up appointments and symptom monitoring.[69,79] An explanation for the nonuse of self-management might be the large amount of time and effort needed,[80] and patients might not always have immediate benefits in terms of symptom improvement or a sense of improved wellbeing.[75] The burden of self-management could be the reason why patients who show signs of poor psychological adjustment face particular difficulties in self-management.

Many studies on adjustment and self-management have highlighted the role of major depression as a risk factor of nonadherence to self-management recommendations, with depressed patients frequently reporting indecisiveness and reduced self-confidence about self-management.[81] The presence of clinical depression has been shown to disrupt adequate self-treatment in diabetes,[79,82] COPD,[83] and HIV.[84] Although depression is thought to precede poor self-management instead of the other way around, the cross-sectional design used in such studies precludes conclusions about the causal link between self-management and psychological adjustment. Symptoms of depression, such as reduced energy or motivation, can clearly interfere with self-management can also lead to feelings of helplessness and hopelessness.[85] Major depression and poor self-management can even be regarded as independent outcomes resulting from cytokines and other pathophysiological mechanisms.[86] Clinical forms of anxiety have also been suggested to compromise self-management, but this association has not been studied extensively.[82]

Even when patients do not meet criteria for clinical diagnosis of depression (or anxiety), they can have some form of psychological distress,[87] which could be regarded a signal of poor adjustment. Some of the most frequently reported sources of distress include worries about long-term complications, guilt or anxiety when problems in self-management occur, and fear about other potential negative effects of the disease.[88] Like major depression, mild forms of distress have been associated with reduced self-management in cross-sectional studies of different chronic conditions, including COPD,[89] diabetes,[90] HIV,[72] and asthma.[91] Notably, the few available prospective studies of distress and self-management suggest a different pathway than assumed in studies of depression and self-management, and lend support to the assumption that poor self-management could precede decreased adjustment. For example, a cancer study showed that patients with decreased self-management predicted a reduced quality of life and increased mood disturbance after 8 months,[92] whereas a study of individuals with rheumatoid arthritis showed that a decline in the ability to perform self-management activities predicted the subsequent onset of depressed feelings.[93]

Most relevant studies have examined the association between poor adjustment and poor self-management. However, other studies have investigated the connection between good adjustment and engagement in self-management practices. These studies are rare, although their prospective design allow for an interpretation of the direction of the connection. Importantly, these studies show evidence of a bidirectional association between wellbeing and adherence to self-management regimens. Patients who can maintain good moods seem to be more willing to engage in lifestyle changes, and those who practice self-management behaviors also report improved wellbeing (Panel 3).

These studies suggest a different connection between self-management and adjustment than has been assumed so far. Research on the association between depression and self-management has been driven by the assumption that depression precedes poor self-management, but the available cross-sectional studies can neither support nor refuse this assumption. Moreover, the role of mild forms of psychological discomfort needs more research since such low levels of mood disturbance could impair self-management to the same extent as clinical manifestations of poor

Panel 3: Positive moods and self-management

Not only can positive mood benefit self-management, but adequate self-management can also promote wellbeing. In patients with diabetes who reported increased levels of perceived competence and autonomous motivation for self-management, improved life satisfaction[94] and self-management behavior were reported, which in turn increased glycemic control after 1 year.[74] Engagement in self-management could also benefit psychological adjustment, both in the short-term and long-term, as shown in several prospective studies in cancer. Such results indicated that patients with head and neck cancer who took appropriate self-management measures after surgery were less anxious the next day,[95] and women with cancer who exercised at least 90 min per week on 3 or more day reported less fatigue and emotional distress as well as higher functional ability and quality of life than less active women during treatment.[96] Similar effect of self-management on psychological adjustment have been shown in prospective studies of patients with heart failure[97] and patients who had cardiac surgery.[98] Only a few self-management interventions have also examined adjustment; although patients increase efforts in self-management. When participating in the intervention, they have mixed findings regarding the effect on adjustment. Some studies show that self-management does not necessarily benefit adjustment [75,97] whereas others report improved quality of life and mood after some time.[69,72,92] These findings suggest that patients can learn to appreciated the need of self-management as a result of participating in interventions, but that such benefits of improved wellbeing could takes some time.

adjustment in terms of (major) depression. Perhaps even more important is the finding that good adjustment predicts increased participation in self-management and vice versa. This association could have important implications for self-management interventions, which vary greatly in approach (from education to cognitive-behavioral treatment)[72] but share and emphasis on improving skills such as problem-solving and goal-setting.[99] These self-management skills are recognized and appreciated by many patients, including those form ethnic group,[100] suggesting that they are valuable ingredients of self-management interventions. However, although good mood seems to promote engagement in self-management of illness, improvement of moods could prove valuable to self-management interventions since many patients report feelings of discomfort about disease, sometimes only after they have been dealing with disease for several years.[101]

COGNITIVE PROCESSING: BEYOND NEGATIVE OUTCOMES

Although health-related quality of life of patients with chronic conditions is generally lower than that of healthy controls,[1] this difference is less pronounced or even absent in aspects of mental health.[1,102] Individuals can use various cognitive strategies to counteract the negative effect of illness on their wellbeing. Much research has addressed Howard Leventhal's model of illness representations,[103] showing that patients' beliefs (e.g. about the course and consequences of their illness) can affect adjustment in chronic conditions such as diabetes.[104] Only recently, attention has been paid to post-traumatic growth and benefit finding,[105-107] as well responsed shift.[108]

The experience of dealing with illness is not all negative. individuals have reported positive outcomes form various diseases (e.g. breast, [52,69,109-113] cancer,[115,116] rheumatoid arthritis,[116] multiple sclerosis,[111] myocardial infarction,[111] HIV/AIDS,[118] and fibromyalgia[105]), such as an improved appreciation of life, enhanced sense of purpose, changes in life priorities, and improved personal relationships. About 60–85% of patients with breast cancer,[111,112] 83% of HIV-positive women,[118] 73% of patients with rheumatoid arthritis,[116] and 58% of individuals with myocardial infarction[111] have reported at least one positive change as a result of their illness. With multi-item scales used to measure benefit, patients have generally reported a small-to-moderate degree of perceived positive change.[69,109,110,112,115,117] Moreover, survivors of breast cancer have reported more positive growth experiences than matched controls (who reported on a stressful event in the same period), even though the survivors have reported either similar [119,120] or increased levels of distress, [114] worsened physical functioning,[114,119] or more negative changes as a result of the experience.[120]

Some patients with chronic illness are more likely to report positive experiences than are other patients. Report of positive changes are correlated with demographic variables such as young age[69,11,115,121,122] and, perhaps counter-intuitively, minority status,[110,113] but generally not with sex,[115-117,121,122] and inconsistently with socioeconomic status and education.[110,112,113,115] Consistent with the theoretical assumption that an event should be intense to provoke growth of benefit finding,[106,107] some cancer studies have suggested that heightened physical threat (i.e. poor disease stage or increased physical symptoms)[110,113] and raised perceived stress[13] are related to an increased report of positive changes. However, a study exploring the curvilinear association between cancer stage and post-traumatic growth showed that very high levels of threat (stage IV breast cancer) resulted in reduced perceived benefit.[122] With respect to time since diagnosis, findings are inconsistent.[110,116,122] Theoretically, a positive correlation would be expected because time is needed to work through the event to experience growth.[112,18,121] One prospective study[69] showed that post-traumatic growth in patients with breast cancer increased consistently during the first 18 months after diagnosis. Benefit finding and growth have also been related to personality characteristics such as trait optimism,[112,121] dispositional hope,[105,112] and extraversion.[121]

Prospective studies examining the relation between growth of benefit finding and psychological adjustment have shown mixed result (Panel 4). Research suggests that effects could depend on the time of assessment and length of follow-up. Positive effects on adjustment were recorded in samples in which benefit finding was assessed some time after diagnosis[110,111] or with an extended follow-up.[123] Benefit finding that is early in the adjustment process could represent a form of avoidance,[129] or early benefit finding could be qualitatively different from benefit finding later on.[113] Research shows that benefit finding that is induced[52] or that is a result of an intervention[109] shortly after diagnosis does lead to positive outcomes, including positive effects on physical adjustment.

Finding benefit of growth could be one of the cognitive strategies used to offset the negative effect of illness and could be viewed as part of a so-called response shift process.[108] When diagnosed, individuals may change their internal standards of what constitutes health or other aspects of quality of life (recalibration), adjust their values and priorities (repritization), or redefine what they think is important (reconceptualization) to maintain an acceptable quality of life in the face of declining health.[108] Most research has focused on recalibration and supports the assumption that individuals change their internal standards of aspects of quality of life over time or as a result of medical treatmemt.[115,130-132] Evidence has also shown the occurrence of reconceptualization[131,133] and reprioritization.[133,134]

Panel 4: Prospective and experimental studies examining relations between benefit finding or growth and adjustment

Prospective studies

Positive affect

Benefit finding in survivors with breast cancer (1–5 years after diagnosis)[110] and rheumatoid arthritis and multiple sclerosis (on average 10 years after diagnosis)[110] and rheumatoid arthritis and multiple sclerosis (on average 10 years after diagnosis)[121] predicted increased positive affect after 5 years and 1 year, respectively. Two studies in patients recently diagnosed with breast cancer (4 months postdiagnosis[113] and post-treatment completion[112]) showed on relation with positive after 3–12 months.

Negative affect, depression and mental functioning

Benefit finding in patients with breast cancer (3, 6, and 12 months after diagnosis) predicted decreased negative affect and depression after 4–7 years,[123] In patients recently diagnosed with breast cancer (4 months after diagnosis),[133] benefit finding predicted increased negative affect after 3–9 months and worsened mental functioning after 3 months for women with more severe stages of disease (relations were weak of absent for women with less sever stages). Other studies of breast cancer (1–5 years after diagnosis[110] and post-treatment completion,[132] respectively) showed that rheumatoid arthritis[116,121] and multiple sclerosis[122] showed no effects on negative affect,[110,121] mental functioning,[111] or psychological distress.[117]

Disability, physiology, and mortality

In patients with rheumatoid arthritis (average 10–16 years after diagnosis) benefit finding was related to reduced disability in one study[116] but not in another.[121] Studies of breast cancer did not find relations between benefit finding and self-reported physical functioning[110,113] or perceived health.[112] In HIV-positive men (on average 8 months after bereavement), benefit finding was related to a more favorable immune status (CD4 to cells) after 2–3 years and decreased AIDS-related mortality after a follow-up of 4–9 years.[124] In the only prospective study before 1996, benefit finding in patients with heart attacks (7 weeks after the attack) was related to a reduced likelihood of heart attack recurrence and morbidity at 8 years of follow-up.[125]

Experimental studies

A cognitive-behavioral stress management intervention for recently diagnosed patients with breast cancer led to increased benefit finding at 9-month follow-up.[109] At 3-month follow-up, increased benefit finding was related to improved immune status (lymphocyte proliferation)[126] and reduced concentration of testosterone[127] and serum cholesterol[128] immediately after intervention.

Benefit finding that is induced experimentally (i.e. patients writing about positive thoughts and feelings regarding the experience of having breast cancer) reduced medical visits for cancer-related morbidities at 3 months' follow-up in patients recently diagnosed with breast cancer.[52] Benefit finding reduced psychological distress in women with high cancer-related avoidance. No effects were seen on perceived quality of life or physical symptoms.

These finding are relevant to psychological interventions such as cognitive-behavioral therapy. Cognitive-behavioral therapy includes various strategies that promote a realistic but optimistic attitude to illness, but few attempts have incorporated element of response shift of benefit finding into the approach. Encouragement for patients of identify advantages after the development of illness or to shift from a state of compromised function to improved function could prove to be valuable ingredients of cognitive behavioral therapy.[7] Although chronic illnesses are undoubtedly stressful, traditional research focusing on the negative aspects provides an incomplete picture since many patients can find a new equilibrium by focusing to the positive aspects of illness.

DISCUSSION

Psychological adjustment to chronic illness is tremendously important. An estimated 50% of people have a chronic physical condition, needing some form of medical intervention.[135] About 35% of young adults report at least one chronic condition[2] and more chronic illness occur in older adults. While the average age of the population increases, so does the occurrence of chronic Illness.[136] Moreover, the rapid developments in medical knowledge have resulted in a growing number of chronic diseases that previously were considered immediately life-threatening (cancer, AIDS) or characterized by rapid deterioration (asthma, diabetes).

This review addresses how chronic illnesses challenge adjustment, by the possible malaise imposed by physiological processes, avoidant styles of emotion regulation, problems faced by patients attempting to change their lifestyle, or difficulties in accepting adverse consequences of disease. Although previous research has focused on explaining poor adjustment, recent developments have shifted to understanding the conditions under which patients can maintain their lives under favorable conditions. Many patients will eventually succeed in adapting to the changes imposed by chronic disease, especially if they can recognize the long-term demands needed for adjustment of chronic illness and the difference in dealing with acute illness. Appreciation of such long-term adaptive demands helps patients to resist the appeal of reducing activities. Long-term task of adjustment can also help individuals to confront and work through the negative feelings induced by illness and to engage in the demanding self-management behaviors that many improve their condition. Patients who can overcome the serious negative consequences of disease can eventually come to terms with disease and find benefit.[130-138]

Of course, psychological adjustment cannot be enforced. Interventions advocating tyrannical positive thinking could bear a serious risk for maladjustment if patients deny the limitations imposed by disease.[137] Additionally, the current focus on patients' autonomy and active participation in illness management should not lead to an overestimation of the patient's responsibility.[138] Finally, most studies on adjustment to chronic illness have been done in white, middle-class populations and in specific chronic diseases, thus limiting the generalization of findings to ethnic groups, patients with low socioeconomic status, and other chronic conditions.[139]

Although studies have shown that psychological adjustment to chronic illness is possible, treatment could increase the burden for patients in the short-term. To achieve psychological adjustment, patients need to face the reality of being chronically ill and make efforts to change their lives to adjust to the new circumstances imposed by their illness. In the small proportion of patients who have serious psychological problems, professional help should be considered. Psychosocial interventions have been designed to assist patients who have difficulty in adjustment.[140,141] For the remainder of patients, healthcare practitioners should consider encouraging them to engage in pleasant activities, acknowledge the emotions they have about the disease, challenge the barriers for engaging in self-management, and find meaning in small things.

REFERENCES

1. Sprangers MAG, de Regt EB, Andries F, et al. Which chronic conditions are associated with better or poorer quality of life? J Clin Epidemiol. 2000;53:895-907.
2. Taylor SE, Aspinwall Lg. Psychosocial aspects of serious illness: chronic conditions, fatal diseases, and clinical care. Washington, DC: American Psychological Association; 1996. pp.7-60.
3. Maes S, Leventhal H, de Ridder D. Comping with chronic disease. In: Zeidner M, Endler N (Eds). Handbook of coping: theory, research applications. New York: Wiley; 1996. pp.221-51.
4. Stanton AL, Collins CA, Sworowski LA. Adjustment to chronic illness: theory and research. In: Baum A, Revenson TA, Singer JE (Eds). Handbook of health psychology. Mahwah, NJ: Erlbaum; 2001.pp.387-403.
5. Taylor SE. Adjustment to threatening events: a theory of cognitive adaptation. Am Psychol. 1983;38:1161-73.
6. Adler N, Matthews K. Health psychology. Why do some people get sick and some stay well? Annu Rev Psychol. 1994;45:229-59.
7. Cameron LD, Leventhal H. Self-regulation, health, and illness. An overview. In: Cameron LD, Leventhal H (Eds). The self-regulation of health and illness behaviour. New York: Routledge; 2003.pp.1-13.
8. Sharpe L, Curran L. Understanding the process of adjustment to illness. Soc Sci Med. 2006;62:1153-66.
9. Walker JG, Jackson HJ, Littlejohn GO. Models of adjustment to chronic illness: using the example of rheumatoid arthritis. Clin Psychol Rev; 2004.pp.461-88.
10. Dantzer R. Cytokine-induced sickness behavior: mechanisms and implications. Ann NY Acad Sci. 2001;933:222-34.
11. Janszky I, Lekander M, Blom M, Georgiades A, Ahnve S. Self-rated health and vital exhaustion, but not depression, is related to inflammation in women with coronary heart disease. Brain Behav Immun. 2005;19:555-63.
12. Musselman DL, Betan E, Larsen H, Phillips LS. Relationship of depression to diabetes types 1 and 2: epidemiology, biology, and treatment. Bio Psychiatry. 2003;54:317-29.
13. Lee BN, Dantzer R, Langley DE, et al. A cytokine-based neuroimmunologic mechanism of cancer-related symptoms. Neuroimmunomod. 2004;11:279-92.
14. Malik UR, Makower DF, Wadler S. Interferon-mediated fatigue. Cancer. 2001;92:1664-68.
15. Raison CL, Demetrashivili M, Capuron L, Miller AH. Neuropsychiatric adverse effects of interferon-alpha. Recognition and management. CNS Drugs. 2005;19:105-23.
16. Schaefer M, Engelbrecht MA, Gut O, et al. Interferon alpha (IFN alpha) and psychiatric syndromes. A review. Prog Neuropsychopharmacol Biol Psychiatric. 2002;26:731-46.
17. Trask PC, Paterson AG, Esper P, Pau J, Redman B. Longitudinal course of depression, fatigue, and quality of life in patients with high risk melanoma receiving adjuvant interferon. Psycho-Oncol. 2004;13:526-36.
18. Durez P, Toukap AN, Lauwerys BR, et al. A randomized comparative study of the short term clinical and biological effects of intervenous pulse methylprednisolone and infliximab in patients with active rheumatoid arthritis despite methotrexate treatment. Ann Rheum Dis. 2004;63:1069-74.
19. Genovese MC, Bathon JM, Fleischmann RM, et al. Long term safety, efficacy, and radiographic outcome with etanercept treatment in patients with early rheumatoid arthritis. J Rheumatol. 2005;32:1232-42.
20. Heiberg MS, Nordvag BY, Mikelsen K, et al. The comparative effectiveness of tumor necrosis factor-blocking agents in patients with rheumatoid arthritis and patients with ankylosing spondylitis. A six-month, longitudinal, observational, multicenter study. Arthritis Rheum. 2005;52:2506-12.
21. Kosinski M, Kujawski SC, Martin R, et al. Health-related quality of life in early rheumatoid arthritis: impact of disease and treatment response. Am J Manag Care. 2002;8:231-40.
22. Lipsky PE, van der Heijde DMFM, St Clair EW, et al. Infliximab and methotrexate in the treatment of rheumatoid arthritis. N Engl J Med. 2000;343:1594-602.
23. Main RN, Breedveld FC, Kalden JR, et al. Sustained improvement over two years in physical function, structural damage, and signs and symptoms among patients with rheumatoid arthritis treated with infliximab and methotrexate. Arthritis Rheum. 2004;50:1051-65.
24. Moreland LW, Schiff MH, Baumgartner SW, et al. Etanercept therapy in rheumatoid arthritis. A randomized, controlled trial. Ann Intern Med. 1999;130:478-86.
25. Quinn MA, Conaghan PG, O'Connor PJ, et al. Very early treatment with infliximab in addition to methotrexate in

early, poor-prognosis rheumatoid arthritis reduces magnetic resonance imaging evidence of synovitis and damange, with sustained benefit after infliximab with drawal. Results forn a twelve-month randomized, double-blind, placebo-controlled trial. Arthritis Rheum. 2005;52:27-35.
26. Russell AS, Conner-Spady B, Mintz A, Mallon C, Maksymowych WP. The responsiveness of generic health status measures as assessed in patients with rheumatoid arthritis receiving infliximab. J Rheumatol. 2003;30:941-47.
27. Sany J, Kaiser MJ, Jorgensen C, Trape G. Study of the tolerance of infliximab infusions with or without betamethasone premedication in patients with active rheumatoid arthritis. Ann Rheum Dis. 2005;64:1647-49.
28. St Clair Ew, van der Heijde DMFM, Smolen JS, et al. Combination of inflimab and methotrexate therapy for early rheumatoid arthritis. A randomized, controlled trial. Arthritis Rheum. 2004;50:3432-43.
29. Weinblatt ME, Keystone EC, Furst DE, et al. Adalimumab, a fully human anti-tumor necrosis factor and monoclonal antibody, for the treatment of rheumatoid arthritis in patients taking concomitant metotrexate. The ARMADA trial. Arthritis Rheum. 2003;48:35-45.
30. Vlaeyen JW, Morley S. Active despite pain: the putative role of stop-rules and current mood. Pain. 2004;110:512-16.
31. Smith RD, Polley HF. Rest therapy for rheumatoid arthritis. Mayo Clin Proc. 1978;53:141-45.
32. de Jong Z, Munneke M, Zwinderman AH, et al. Is a long-term high-intensity exercise program effective and safe in patients with rheumatoid arthritis? Results of a randomized controlled trial. Arthritis Rheum. 2003;48:2415-24.
33. Smidt N, de Vet HCW, Bouter LM, Dekker. Effectiveness of exercise therapy: a best-evidence summary of systematic reviews. Aust J Physiother. 2005;51:71-85.
34. Gross JJ. The emerging field of emotion regulation: an integrative review. Rev Gen Psychol. 1998;2:271-99.
35. Austenfeld JL, Stanton AL. Coping through emotional approach: a new look at emotion, coping, and health-related outcomes. J pers. 2004;72:1335-64.
36. Garssen B. Repression: finding our way in the maze of concepts. J Behav Med. 2007;30:471-81.
37. Solano L, Montella F, Salvati S, et al. Expression and processing of emotions: relationships with CD4+ levels in 42 HIV-positive asymptomatic individuals. Psychol Health. 2001;16:689-98.
38. Hirokawa K, Nagata C, Takatsuka N, Shimizu H. The relationships of a rationality/antiemotionality personality scale to mortalities of cancer and cardiovascular disease in a community population in Japan. J Psychosom Res. 2004;56:103-11.
39. Iwamitsu Y, Shimoda K, Abe H, Tani T, Okawa M, Buck R. Anxiety, emotional suppression, and after breast cancer diagnosis, Psychosomatics. 2005;46:19-24.
40. van Middendorp H, Geenen R, Sorbi MJ, Van Doornen LJP, Bijlsma JWJ. Emotion regulation predicts change of perceived health in patients with rheumatoid arthritis. Ann Rheum Dis. 2005;64:1071-74.
41. Hamilton NA, Zautra AJ, Reich JW. Affect and pain in rheumatoid arthritis: do individual differences in affective regulation and affective intensity predict emotional recovery form pain? Ann Behav Med. 2005;29:216-24.
42. Stanton AL, Danoff-Burg S, Cameron CL, et al. Emotionally expressive coping predicts psychological and physical adjustment to breast cancer. J Consult Clin Psychol. 2000;68: 875-82.
43. Zautra A, Smith B, Affleck G, Tennen H. Examinations of chronic pain and affect relationships: applications of a dynamic model of affect. J Consult Clin Psychol. 2001;69:786-95.
44. Solano L, Costa M, Temoshok L, et al. An emotionally inexpressive (type C) coping style influences HIV disease progression at six and twelve month follow-ups. Psychol Health. 2002;17:641-55.
45. Weihs KL, Enright TM, Simmens SJ, Reiss D. Negative affectivity, restrication of emotions, and site of metastases predict mortality in recurrent breast cancer. J Psychosom Res. 2000;49:59-68.
46. Reynolds P, Hurley S, Torres M, Jackson J, Boyd P, Chen VW. Use of coping strategies and breast cancer survival: results from the Black/White Cancer Survival Study. Am J Epidemiol. 2000;152:940-40.
47. Tijhuis MAR, Elshout JRAF, Feskens EJM, Janssen M, Kromhout D. Prosopective investigation of emotional control and cancer risk in men (the Zutphen Elderly Study) (The Netherlands). Cancer Cause Control. 2000;11:589-95.
48. Giraldi T, Rodani MG, Cartei G, Grassi L. Psychosocial factors and breast cancer: a 6-year Italian follow-up study. Psychother Psychosom. 1997;66:229-36.
49. Good win PJ, Ennis M, Bordeleau LJ, et al. Health-related quality of life and psycosocial status in breast cancer prognosis: analysis of multiple variables. J Clin Oncol. 2004;22:4184-92.
50. Watson M, Haviland JS, Greer S, Davidson J, Bliss JM. Influence of psychological response on survival in breast cancer: a population-based cohort study. Lancet. 1999;354:1331-36.
51. Kelley JE, Lumley MA, Leisen JC. Health effects of emotional disclosure in rheumatoid arthritis patients. Health Psychol. 1997;16:331-40.
52. Stanton AL, Danoff-Burg S, Sworowski LA, et al. Health effects of written emotional disclosure in adolescents with asthma: a randomized, controlled trial. J Clin Oncol. 2002;20:4160-68.
53. Warner LJ, Lumley MA, Casey RJ, et al. Health effects of written emotional disclosure in adolescents with asthma: a randomized, controlled trial. J Pediart Psychol. 2006;31:557-68.
54. Wetherell MA, Byrne-Davis L, Dieppe P, et al. Effects of emotional disclosure in psychological and physiological outcomes in patients with rheumatoid arthritis: and exploratory home-based study. J Health Psychol. 2005;10:277-85.
55. Zakowski SG, Ramati A, Morton C, Johnson P, Flanigan R. Written emotional disclosure buffers the effects of social

constraints on distress among cancer patients. Health Psychol. 2004;27:50-59.

56. De Moor C, Sterner J, Hall M, et al. A pilot study of the effects of expressive writing on psychological and behavioral adjustment in patients enrolled in a Phase II trial of vaccine therapy for metastatic renal cell carcinoma. Health Psychol. 2002;21:615-19.
57. Hockemeyer J, Smyth J. Evaluating the feasibility and efficacy of a self-administered manual-based stress management intervention for individuals with asthma: results from a controlled study. Behaw Med. 2002;27:161-72.
58. Rosenberg HJ, Rosenberg SD, Ernstoff MS, et al. Expressive disclosure and health outcomes in a prostate cancer population. Int J Psychiart Med. 2002;32:37-53.
59. Taylor LA, Wallander JL, Anderson D, Beasley P, Brown RT. Improving health care utilization, improving chronic disease utilization, health status, and adjustment in adolescents and young adults with cystic fibrosis: a preliminary report. J Clin Psychol Med Settings. 2003;10:9-16.
60. Walker BL, Nail LM, Croyle RT. Dose emotional expression make a difference in reactions to breast cancer? Oncol Nurs Forum. 1999;26:1025-32.
61. Petrie KJ, Fontanilla I, Thomas MG, Booth RJ, Pennebaker JW. Effect of written emotional expression on immune function in patients with human immunodeficiency virus infection: a randomized trial. Psychosom Med. 2004;66:272-75.
62. Smyth JM, Stone AA, Hurewitz A, Kaell A. Effects of writing about stressful experiences of symptom reduction in patients with asthma or rheumatoid arthritis: a randomized trial. JAMA. 1999;281:1304-09.
63. Harris AH, Theoresen CE, Humphreys K, Faul J. Does writing affect asthma? A randomized trial. Psychosom Med. 2005;67:130-36.
64. Giese-Davis J, koopman C, Butler LD, et al. Change in emotion-regulation strategy for women with metastatic breast cancer following supportive-expressive group therapy. J Consult Clin Psychol. 2002;70:916-25.
65. Pennebaker JW. Health effects of the expression (and non-expression) of emotions through writing. In: Viagerhoets A, van Bussel F, Boelhouwer J (Eds). The (non) expression of emotions in health and disease, Tilburg University Press; 1997.pp.267-78.
66. Wiebe DJ, Korbel C. Defensive denial, affect and the self-regulation of health threats. In: Cameron LD, Leventhal H (Eds). The self-regulation of health and illness behaviour. New York: Routledge; 2003.pp.184-203.
67. Mauss IB, Gross JJ. Emotion suppression and cardiovascular disease: is hiding feelings bad for your heart? In: Temoshok LR, Nyklicek I, Viingerhoets A (Eds). Emotions in health promotion and disease. London. Harwood Academic Press; 2004.pp.61-81.
68. Lutgendorf SK, Ullrich P. Cognitive processing, disclosure, and health: psychological and physiological mechanisms. In: Lepore SJ, Smyth JM (Eds). The writing cure: how expressive writing promotes health and emotional well-being. Washington, DC: Americna Psychological Association; 2002. pp.177-96.
69. Manne S, Ostroff J, Winkel G, Goldstein L, Fox K, Grana G. Post-traumatic growth after breast cancer: patient, partner, and couple perspectives. Psychosom Med. 2004;66:442-54.
70. Barlow J, Wright C, Sheasby J, Turner A, Hainsworth J. Self-management approaches for people with chronic conditions: a review. Patient Educ Couns. 2002;48:177-87.
71. Collins RL, Kanouse DE, Gifford AL, et al. Changes in health-promoting behavior following diagnosis with HIV: prevalence and correlates in a national probability sample. Health Psychol. 2001;20:351-60.
72. Riemsam RP, Taal E, Kirwan JR, Rasker JJ. Systematic review of rheumatoid arthritis patient education. Arthritis Rheum. 2004;51:1045-59.
73. Bailey WC, Kohler CL, Richards JM, et al. Asthma self-management. Do patient education programs always have an impact? Arch Intern Med. 1999;159:2422-28.
74. Williams GC, McGregor HA, Zeldman A, Freedman ZR, Deci EL. Tasting a self-determination theory process model for promoting glycemic control through diabetes self-management. Health Psychol. 2004;23:58-66.
75. Jaarsma T, Halfens R, Tan F, Abu-Saad HH, Dracup K, Diederiks J. Self-care and quality of life in patients with advanced heart failure: the effect of a supportive educational intervention. Heart Lung. 2000;29:319-30.
76. Dunbar-Jacob J, Mortimer-Stephens MK. Treatment adherence in chronic disease. J Clin Epidemiol. 2001;54:S57-60.
77. Gillibrand W, Flynn M. Forced externalization of control in people with diabetes: a qualitative exploratory study. J Adv Nurs. 2001;34:501-10.
78. Weijman I, Ros WJG, Rutten GEHM, Schaufeli WB, Schabracq MJ, Winnubst JAM. Frequency and perceived burden of diabetes self-management activities in employees with insulin-treated diabetes; relationship with health outcomes. Diabetes Res Clin Pract. 2005;68:56-64.
79. Lin EHB, Katon W, von Korff M, et al. Relationship of depression and diabetes self-care, medication adherence, and preventive care. Diabetes Care. 2004;27:2154-60.
80. Safford MM, Russell L, Suh DC, Roman S, Pogach L. How much time do patients with diabetes spend on self-care? J Am Board Fam Pract. 2005;18:262-70.
81. DiMatteo MR, Lepper HS, Croghan TW. Depression is a risk factor for noncompliance with medical treatment. Meta-analysis of the effects of anxiety and depression on patient adherence. Arch Intern Med. 2000;160:2101-07.
82. Peyrot M, Rubin RR. Levels and risk of depression and anxiety symptomatology among diabetic adults. Diabetes Care. 1997;20:585-90.
83. Dowson CA, Town GI, Frampton C, Mulder RT. Psychopathology and illness beliefs influence COPD self-management. J Psychosom Res. 2004;56:333-40.

84. Fehr JS, Nicca D, Sendi P, et al. Starting or changing therapy. A prospective study exploring antiretroviral decision-making. Infection. 2005;33:249-56.
85. Lustman PJ, Freeland KE, Griffith LS, Clouse RE. Fluxetine for depression in diabetes. A randomized double-blind placebo-controlled trial. Diabetes Care. 2000;23:618-23.
86. Lustman PJ, Clouse RE, Ciechanowski PS, Hirsch IB, Freedland KE. Depression-related hyperglycemia in type 1 diabetes: a meditational approach. Psychosom Med. 2005;67:195-99.
87. Polonsky WH. Understanding and assessing diabetes-specific quality of life. Diabetes Spectrum. 2000;13:36-41.
88. Polonsky WH, Anerson BJ, Lohrer PA, et al. Assessment of diabetes-related distress. Diabetes Care. 1995;18:754-83.
89. Katz PP, Eisner MD, Yelin EH, et al. Functioning and psychological status among individuals with COPD. Qual Life Res. 2005;14:1835-43.
90. Lloyd CE, Dyer PH, Lancashire RJ, Harris T, Daniels JE, Barnett AH. Association between stress and glycemic control in adult with type 1 (insulin-dependent) diabetes. Diabetes Care. 1999; 22:1278-83.
91. Main J, Moss-Morris R, Booth R, Kaptein AA, Kolbe J. The use of reliever medication in asthma: the role of negative mood and symptom reports. J Asthma. 2003;40:257-65.
92. Lev EL, Paul D, Owen SV. Age, self-efficacy, and change in patients adjustment to cancer. Cancer Pract. 1999;7:170-76.
93. Katz PP, Yelin EH. Activity loss and the onset of depressive symptoms. Do some activities matter more than others? Arthritis Rheum. 2001;44:1194-202.
94. Senecal C, Nouwen A, White D. Motivation and dietary self-care in adults with diabetes: are self-efficacy and autonomous self-regulation complementary of competing constructs? Health Psychol. 2000;19:452-57.
95. Dropkin MJ. Anxiety, coping strategies, and coping behaviours in patients undergoing head and neck cancer surgery. Cancer Nurs. 2001;9:119-27.
96. Mock V, Pickett M, Ropka ME, et al. Fatigue and quality of life outcomes of exercise during cancer treatment. Cancer Pract. 2001;9:119-27.
97. Jaarsma T, Halfens R, Abu-Saad HH, Dracup K, Stappers J, van Ree J. Quality of life in older patients with systolic and diastolic heart failure. Eur J Heart Fail. 1999;1:151-60.
98. Ai AL, Dunkle Re, Peterson C, Saunders DG, Bolling SF. Self-care and psychosocial adjustment of patients following cardiac surgery. Soc Work Health Care. 1998;27:75-95.
99. de Ridder D, Schreurs K. Developing interventions for chronically ill patients: is coping a helpful concept? Clin Psycho Rev. 2001;21:205-40.
100. Walker C, Weeks A, McAvoy B, Demetrious E. Exploring the role of self-management programmes in caring for people form culturally and linguistically diverse backgrounds in Melbourne, Australia. Health Expect. 2005;8:315-23.
101. Polonsky WH. Diabetes burnout. Alexandria, VA: American Diabetes Association; 1999.
102. Van't Spijker A, Trijsburg RW, Duivenvoorden HJ. Psychological sequelae of cancer diagnosis: a meta-analytical review of 58 studies after 1980, Psychosom Med. 1997;59:280-93.
103. Leventhal H, Brisette I, Leventhal EA. The common-sense model of self-regulation of health and illness. In: Cameron LD, Leventhal H (Eds). The self-regulation of health and illness behaviour. London: Routledge; 2003.pp.42-65.
104. Skinner TC, Hampson SE, Fife-Schaw C. Personality, personal model beliefs, and self-care in adolescents and young adults with Type 1 diabetes. Health Psychol. 2002;21:61-70.
105. Affleck G, Tennen H. Construing benefit from adversity: adaptatinal significance and dispostional underpinnings. J Pers. 1996;64:899-992.
106. Janoff-Bulman R. Post-traumatic growth: three explanatory models. Psychol Inq. 2004;15:30-4.
107. Tedeschi RG, Calhoun LG. Post-traumatic growth: conceptual foundations and empirical evidence. Psychol Inq. 2004;15:1-18.
108. Sprangers MAG, Schwartz CE. Integrating response shift into health-related quality of life research: a theoretical model. Soc Sic Med. 1999;48:1507-15.
109. Antoni MH, Lehman JM, Kilbourn KM, et al. Cognitive-behavioral stress management intervention depresses the prevalence of depression and enhances benefit finding among women under treatment for early-stage breast cancer. Health Psychol. 2001;20:20-32.
110. Bower JE, Meyerowitz BE, Desmond KA, Bernaards CA, Rowland JH, Ganz PA. Perceptions of positive meaning and vulnerability following breast cancer: predictors and outcomes among long-term breast cancer survivors. Ann Behav Med. 2005;29:236-45.
111. Patrie KJ, Buick DL, Weinman J, Booth RJ. Positive effects of illness reported by myocardial infarction and breast cancer patients. J psychosom Res. 1999;47:537-43.
112. Sears SR, Stanton AL, Danoff-Burg S. The yellow brick road and the emerald city: benefit finding, positive reappraisal coping, and post-traumatic growth in women with early-stage breast cancer. Health Psychol. 2003;22:487-97.
113. Tomich PL, Helgeson VS. Is finding something good in the bad always good? Benefit finding among women with breast cancer. Health Psychol. 2004;23:16-23.
114. Andrykowski MAA, Bishop MM, Hahn EA, et al. Long-term health-related quality of life, growth, and spiritual well-being after hematopoietic stem-cell transplantation. J Clin Oncol. 2005;23:599-608.
115. Widows MR, Jacobsen PB, Booth-Jones M, Fields KK. Predictors of post-traumatic growth following bone marrow transplantation for cancer. Health Psychol. 2005;24:266-73.
116. Danoff-Burg S, Revenson TA. Benefit-finding among patients with rheumatoid arthritis: positive effects on interpersonal relatioinships. J Behav Med. 2005;28:91-103.
117. Pakenham KI. Benefit finding in multiple sclerosis and associations with positive and negative outcomes. Health Psychol. 2005;24:123-32.

118. Siegel K, Schrimshaw EW. Perceiving benefits in adversity: stress -related growth in women living with HIV/AIDS. Soc Sci Med. 2000;51:1543-54.
119. Andrykowski MA, Curran SL, Studts JL, et al. Psychosocial adjustment and quality of life in women with breast cancer and ben benign breast problems-a controlled comparison. J Clin Epidemiol. 1996;49:827-34.
120. Tomich PL, Helgeson VS, Nowak Vache EJ. Perceived growth and decline following breast cancer: a comparison to age-matched controls 5-years later. Psycho-Oncol. 2005; 14:1018-29.
121. Evers AWM, Kraaimaat FW, van Lankveld W, Jongen PJH, Jacobs JWG, Bijlsma JWJ. Beyond unfavorable thinking: the illness cognition questionnaire for chronic disease. J Consult Clin Psychol. 2001;69:1026-36.
122. Lachner SC, Zakowski SG, Antoni MH, Greenhawt M, Block K, Block P. Do socio-demographic and disease-related variables influence benefit-finding in cancer patients? Psycho-Oncol. 2003;12:491-99.
123. Carver CS, Antoni MH. Finding benefit in breast cancer during the year after diagnosis redicts better adjustment 5 to 8 years after diagnosis. Health Psychol. 2004;23:595-98.
124. Dower JE, Kemeny ME, Taylor SE, Fahey JL. Cognitive processing, discovery of meaning, CD4 decline, and AIDS-related mortality among bereaved HIV-seropositive men. J Consult Clin Psychol. 1998;66:979-86.
125. Affleck G, Tennen H, Croog S, Lvine S. Causal attribution, perceived benefits, and morbidity after a heart attack: an 8-year study. J Consult Clin Psychol. 1987;55:29-35.
126. McGregor BA, Antoni MH, Boyers A, Alferi SM, Bolmberg BB, Carver CS. Cognitive-behavioral stress management increases benefit finding and immune function among women with early-stage breast cancer. J Psychosom Res. 2004;56:1-8.
127. Cruess DG, Antoni MH, Kumar M, et al. Effects of stress management on testosterone levels in women with early-stage breast cancer. Int J Behav Med. 2001;8:194-207.
128. Cruess DG, Antoni MH, McGregor BA, et al. Cognitive-behavioral stress management reduces serum cortisol by enhancing benefit finding among women being treated for early stage breast cancer. Psychosom Med. 2000;62: 304-08.
129. Stanton AL, Bower JE, Low CA. Post-traumatic growth after cancer. In: Calhoun LG, Tedeschi RG (Eds). Handbook of post-traumatic growth: research and practice. Mahwah, NJ: Erlbaum; 2006.
130. Ahmed S, Mayo NE, Corbiere M, Wood-Dauphinee S, Hanley J, Cohen R. Change in quality of life of people with stroke over time: true change or response shift? Qual Life Res. 2005;14: 611-27.
131. Scwartz CE, Sprangers MAG, Carey A, Reed G. Exploring response shift in longitudinal data. Psychol Health. 2004; 19:51-69.
132. Sprangers MAG, van Dam FSAM, Broersen J, et al. Revealing response shift in longitudinal research on fatigue. The use of the thentest approach. Acta Oncol. 1999;38:709-18.
133. Oort FJ, Visser MRM, Sprangers MAG. An application of structural equation modeling to detect response shifts and true change in quality of life data from cancer patients undergoing invasive surgery. Qual Life Res. 2005;14:599-609.
134. Bernhard J, Lowy A, Mathys N, Hermann R, Hurny C. Health related quality of life: a changing construct? Qual Life Res. 2004;13:1187-97.
135. Epping-Jordan J, Bengoa R, Kawar R, Sabate E. The challenge of chronic conditions: WHO responds. BMJ. 2001;323:947-48.
136. Rotheberg RB, Koplan JP. Chronic disease in the 1990s. Ann Rev Public Health. 1990;11:267-96.
137. Holland JC, Lewis S. The human side of cancer, living with hope, coping with uncertainty. New York: Harper Collins; 2000.
138. Holman H, Lorig K. Patients as partners in managing chronic disease. Partnership is a prerequisite for effective and efficient health care. BMJ. 2000;320:526-27.
139. Baumann LC. Culture and illness representation. In: Cameron LD, Leventhal H (Eds). The self regulation of health and illness behavior. New York: Routledge; 2003.pp.242-53.
140. Roesch SC, Adams L, Hines A, et al. Coping with prostate cancer; a meta-analytic review. J Behav Med. 2005;28:281-93.
141. Newman S, Steed L, Mulligan K. Self-management interventions for chronic illness. Lancet. 2004;364:1523-37.

CHAPTER 73

Delirium in Older Person

JN Vyas

Delirium, an acute decline in attention and cognition, is a common, life threatening, and potentially preventable clinical syndrome among persons who are 65 years of age or older. The development of delirium often initiates a cascade of events culminating in the loss of independence, an increased risk of morbidity and mortality, and increased health care costs.[1-6] Delirium in hospitalized older patients has assumed particular importance because the care of such patients accounts for more than 49% of all hospital days.[7]

EPIDEMIOLOGY AND DIAGNOSTIC CRITERIA

In direct contrast to dementia, which is a chronic confusional state, delirium is an acute confusional state. Rates of delirium are highest among hospitalized older patients, and the rates vary depending on the patients' characteristics, setting of care, and sensitivity of the detection method.[8-10] The prevalence of delirium at hospital admission ranges from 14% to 24%, and the incidence of delirium arising during hospitalization ranges from 6% to 56% among general hospital populations.[11,12] Delirium occurs in 15–53% of older patients postoperatively[11] and in 70–87% of those in intensive care.[13] Delirium occurs in up to 60% of patients in nursing homes or postacute care settings[14,15] and in up to 83% of all patients at the end of life.[16,17] Although the overall prevalence of delirium in the community is only 1-2%,[18,19] the prevalence increases with age, rising to 14% among those more than 85 years old. Moreover, in 10–30% of older patients presenting to emergency departments have delirium. Delirium is a symptom[11] that often heralds the presence of life threatening conditions. The mortality rates among hospitalized patients with delirium range from 22% to 76%,[20] as high as the rates among patients with acute myocardial infraction or sepsis. The one year mortality rate associated with cases of delirium is 35–40%.[21-23]

The diagnosis of delirium is primarily clinical and is based on careful bed side observation of key features. Delirium is often unrecognized by the patients, physicians and nurses,[1,24] in part because of its fluctuating nature, its overlap with dementia, lack of formal cognitive assessment, under appreciation of its clinical consequences, and failure to consider the diagnosis important.

DSM-5 Diagnostic Criteria for Delirium

- A disturbance in attention (i.e. reduced ability to direct, focus, sustain, and shift attention) and awareness (reduced orientation to the environment).
- The disturbance develops over a short period of time (usually hours to a few days), represents a change from baseline attention and awareness, and tends to fluctuate in severity during the course of a day.
- An additional disturbance in cognition (e.g. memory deficit, disorientation, language, visuospatial ability, or perception).
- The disturbances in Criteria A and C are not better explained by another preexisting, established, or evolving neurocognitive disorder and do not occur in the context of a severely reduced level of arousal, such as coma.
- There is evidence from the history, physical examination, or laboratory findings that the disturbance is a direct physiological consequence of another medical condition, substance intoxication or withdrawal (i.e. due to a drug of abuse or to a medication), or exposure to a toxin, or is due to multiple etiologies.

Specify whether:
Substance intoxication delirium: This diagnosis should be made instead of substance intoxication when the symptoms in Criteria A and C predominate in the clinical picture and when they are sufficiently severe to warrant clinical attention. *Coding note:* The ICD-9-CM and ICD-10-CM codes for the [specific substance] intoxication delirium are indicated. Note that the ICD-10-CM code depends on whether or not there is a comorbid substance use disorder present for the same class of substance. If a mild substance use disorder is comorbid with the substance intoxication delirium, the 4th position character is " 1," and the clinician should record "mild [substance] use disorder" before the substance intoxication delirium (e.g. "mild cocaine use disorder with

cocaine-induced intoxication delirium"). If a moderate or severe substance use disorder is comorbid with the substance intoxication delirium, the 4th position character is "2," and the clinician should record "moderate [substance] use disorder" or "severe [substance] use disorder," depending on the severity of the comorbid substance use disorder. If there is no comorbid substance use disorder (e.g., after a one-time heavy use of the substance), then the 4th position character is "9," and the clinician should record only the substance intoxication delirium.

CLINICAL CHARACTERISTICS

Because delirium remains a bedside diagnosis, understanding its clinical features (Table 1) is crucial to the diagnosis of delirium. Delirium has hypoactive and hyperactive forms (Table 1). The hypoactive form of delirium is more common among older persons and often goes unrecognized.

Table 1: Clinical features of delirium

Acute onset	Occurs abruptly, usually over a period of hours or days Reliable informant often needed to ascertain the time, course of onset
Fluctuating course	Symptoms tend to come and go or increase and decrease in severity over a 24-hour period Characteristic lucid intervals
Inattention	Difficulty focusing, sustaining, and shifting attention Difficulty maintaining conversation or following commands
Disorganized thinking	Manifested by disorganized or incoherent speech Rambling or irrelevant conversation or unclear or illogical flow of ideas
Altered level of consciousness	Clouding of consciousness, with reduced clarity of awareness of the environment
Cognitive deficits	Typically global or multiple deficits in cognition, including disorientation, memory deficits, and language impairment
Perceptual disturbances	Illusions or hallucinations in about 30% of patients
Psychomotor disturbances	Psychomotor variants of delirium *Hyperactive:* Marked by agitation and vigilance *Hypoactive:* Marked by lethargy, with a markedly decreased level of motor activity Mixed
Altered sleep-wake cycle	Characteristics sleep-cycle disturbances Typically daytime drowsiness, night time insomnia, fragmented sleep, or complete sleep-cycle reversal
Emotional disturbances	Common

Etiologic and Risk Factors

The cause of delirium is typically multifactorial.[25] In fact, the development of delirium involves the complex interrelationship between a vulnerable patient (one with predisposing factors) (Table 2) and exposure to precipitating factors or noxious insults (Table 3).[26,27] Thus, in patients who are highly vulnerable to delirium, such as those with dementia and multiple coexisting conditions, it may develop as a result of relatively benign insults, such as one dose of a sleeping medication. Conversely, in patients who are not vulnerable to delirium, it develops only after exposure to multiple noxious insults, such as general anesthesia, major surgery, and psychoactive medications. Addressing just one contributing factor is unlikely to resolve delirium in an older person; they should all be addressed when possible.

Table 2: Predisposing factors for delirium

Demographic characteristics	Age of 65 years or older Male sex
Cognitive status	Dementia Cognitive impairment History of delirium Depression
Functional status	Functional dependence Immobility Low level of activity History of falls
Sensory impairment	Visual impairment Hearing impairment
Decreased oral intake	Dehydration Malnutrition
Drugs	Treatment with multiple pychoactive drugs Treatment with many drugs Alcohol abuse
Coexisting medical conditions	Severe illness Multiple coexisting conditions Chronic renal or hepatic disease History of stroke Neurologic disease Metabolic derangements Fracture or trauma Terminal illness
Infection with human immunodeficiency virus	

Table 3: Precipitating factors or insults that can contribute to delirium
Drugs:
Sedative hypnotics
Narcotics
Anticholinergic drugs
Treatment with multiple drugs
Alcohol or drug withdrawal
Primary neurologic diseases:
Stroke, particularly nondominant hemispheric
Intracranial bleeding
Meningitis or encephalitis
Intercurrent illnesses:
Infections
Iatrogenic complications
Severe acute illness
Hypoxia
Shock
Fever or hypothermia
Anemia dehydration
Poor nutritional status
Low serum albumin level
Metabolic derangements (e.g. electrolyte, glucose, acid-base)
Surgery
Orthopedic surgery
Cardiac surgery
Prolonged cardiopulmonary bypass
Noncardiac surgery
Environmental
Admission to an intensive care unit
Use of physical restraints
Use of bladder catheter
Use of multiple procedures
Pain
Emotional stress
Prolonged sleep deprivation

PATHOGENESIS

The pathophysiology of delirium remains poorly understood. Electroencephalographic studies have demonstrated diffuse slowing of cortical background activity, which does not correlate with underlying causes.[28] Neuropsychological and neuroimaging studies reveal generalized disruption in higher cortical function, with dysfunction in the perfrontal cortex, subcortical structures, thalamus, basal ganglia, frontal and temporoparietal cortex, fusiform cortex, and lingual gyri, particularly on the nondominant side.[29,30] The leading hypotheses for the pathogenesis of delirium focus on the roles of neurotransmission, inflammation, and chronic stress.

Extensive evidence supports the role of cholinergic deficiency. Administration of anticholinergic drugs can induce delirium in humans and animals, and serum anticholinergic activity is increased in patients with delirium. Physostigmine reverses delirium associated with anticholinergic drugs, and cholinesterase inhibitors appear to have some benefit even in cases of delirium that are not induced by drug(s).[15,29,31]

Dopaminergic excess also appears to contribute to delirium, possibly owning to its regulatory influence on the release of acetylcholine.[29] Dopaminergic drugs (e.g. levodopa and bupropion) are recognized precipitants of delirium, and dopamine antagonists (e.g. antipsychotic agents) effectively treat delirium symptoms. Perturbations of other neurotransmitters, such as norepinephrine, serotonin, γ-aminobutyric acid, glutamate, melatonin, may also have a role in the pathophysiology of delirium, but the evidence is less well developed.[1,29,32] These neurotransmitters may exert their influence through interactions with the cholinegic and dopaminergic pathways.

Cytokines including interleukin-1, interleukin 2, interleukin 6, tumor necrosis factor a (TNF), and interferon, may contribute to delirium [1,29,33] by increasing the permeability of the blood brain barrier and altering neurotransmission. Finally, chronic stress brought on by illness or trauma activates the sympathetic nervous system and hypothalamic pituitary adrenocortical axis, resulting in increased cytokine levels and chronic hypercortisolism.[34] Chronic hypercortisolism (5-hydroxytryptamine [5-HT]) 5HT-1A receptors, which may contribute to delirium.[29,35,36] Given the clinical heterogeneity and multifactorial nature of delirium, it is likely that multiple pathogenic mechanisms contribute to the development of delirium.

APPROACH TO EVALUATION

The approach, based on current clinical guidelines and expert opinon,[9,20] must be guided by the individual patient's medical history, findings on physical and neurologic examination, and clinical setting. When a patient with confusion is admitted, determining the acuity of the change in mental status is the essential first step. Neglecting this step is the leading reason for missing the diagnosis of delirium. If no history can be obtained, then the patient should be assumed to be delirious until proved otherwise. Every older hospitalized patient should undergo brief but formal cognitive testing with the use of instruments such as the Mini Mental State Examination and the Confusion Assessment Method, since subtle delirium is often missed. Older patients should be aroused during rounds and evaluated daily for the hypoactive form of delirium, which is often overlooked.

When clinicians search for the underlying cause of delirium, they need to be aware of the possibility of occult or atypical presentations of many diseases in the elderly, including myocardial infraction, infection, and respiratory failure, because delirium is often the sole manifestation of serious underlying disease. All pre-admission and current medications should be reviewed; even long standing medications can contribute to delirium and should be reevaluated. If changes in long-term medications are appropriate after the indications and risk benefit ratios have been carefully weighed, the hospital represents the ideal venue for making these changes. A medical history must be meticulously obtained to detect occult alcohol or benzodiazepine use, which can contribute to delirium.[37]

Electroencephalography has a limited role in the diagnosis of delirium, because of its false negative rate of 17% and false positive rate of 22%;[12] it is most useful for detecting occult seizures and differentiating delirium from psychiatric disorder. Neuroimaging studies have a low clinical yield (the number of positive results divided by the total number of studies performed) in the evaluation of delirium and should be reserved for patients with new focal neurologic signs, those with a history or signs of head trauma, those with fever and acute changes in mental status in whom encephalitis is suspected, or those with no other identifiable cause of the delirium.[12] However, neuroimaging should be considered when the history cannot be obtained or the neurologic examination cannot be completed (e.g., when the patient is combative) so as not to miss uncommon conditions that are life threatening but treatable, such as subarachnoid hemorrhage and encephalitis.

PREVENTION AND MANAGEMENT

Preventing delirium is the most effective strategy for reducing its frequency and complications. Successful preventive strategies include multi-component approaches to reduce risk factors. Because delirium has many causes, multicomponent approaches represent the most effective and clinically relevant ones. The Yale Delirium Prevention Trial[8] demonstrated the effectiveness of intervention protocols targeted toward six risk factors: orientation and therapeutic activites for cognitive impairment, early mobilization to avert immobilization, nonpharmacologic approaches to minimize the use of psychoactive drugs, interventions to prevent sleep deprivation, communication methods and adaptive equipment (particularly eye-glasses and hearing aids) for vision and hearing impairment, and early intervention for volume depletion. A randomized clinical trial involving patients who had hip fractures demonstrated the effectiveness of a multicomponent strategy for geriatric consultation targeted towards 10 domains:[38] oxygen delivery to the brain, fluid and electrolyte balance, pain management, reduction in the use of psychoactive drugs, bowel and bladder function, nutrition, early mobilization, presentation of postoperative complications, appropriate environmental stimuli, and treatment of symptoms of delirium.

Once delirium occurs, the key steps in management are to address all evident causes, provide supportive care and prevent complications, and treat behavioral symptoms. Because delirium can be a medical emergency, the first aim of management is to address predisposing and precipitating factors promptly. Supportive care should include protecting the patient's airway, maintaining hydration and nutrition, positioning and mobilizing the patient to prevent pressure sores and deep venous thrombosis, avoiding the use of physical restraints, and supporting the patient's daily care needs. Nonpharmacologic approaches to managing symptoms of delirium should be instituted in every patient. These approaches includes creating a calm, comfortable environment with the use of orienting influences, such as calendars, clocks, and familiar objects from home; regular reorienting communication with staff members; involving family members in supportive care; limiting room and staff changes; coordinating schedules for administering drugs, obtaining vital signs, and performing procedures to allow the patient an uninterrupted period for sleep at night with low levels of noise and lighting; and encouraging normal sleep wake cycles by opening blinds and encouraging wakefulness and mobility during the daytime. Since delirium may take weeks months to resolve, patients must be cared for in supervised settings. Close clinical follow-up after discharge is needed, especially because of the poor long-term prognosis associated with delirium.

Pharmacologic management should be reserved for patients whose symptoms of delirium would threaten their own safety or the safety of other persons or would result in the interruption of essential therapy, such as mechanical ventilation or central venous catheters. Pharmacologic treatment strategies are outlined in Table 4.

RELATIONSHIP BETWEEN DELIRIUM AND DEMENTIA

Delirium and dementia are highly interrelated, yet the nature of their interrelationship remains poorly examined. Although a cause and effect relation has not been established between delirium and dementia, investigation of their intersection may yield important insights that will advance our understanding of both conditions (see Table 3). Dementia is the leading risk factor for delirium, and fully two-thirds of cases of delirium occur in patients with dementia.[1,39] Thus, the underlying vulnerability of the brain in patients with dementia may predispose them to the development of delirium as a result of insults related to acute medical illnesses, medications, or environmental perturbations. Recent studies suggest that delirium persists much longer than previously believed,[4,40-44] with symptoms in many patients lasting months or years. The existence of the well described entities of persistent delirium[4,40-44] and reversible

Table 4: Pharmacologic treatment of delirium[31]

Class and drug	*Dose*	*Adverse effect*	*Comments*
Typical			
Antipsychotic Haloperidol	0.5–1.0 mg twice daily orally, with additional doses every 4 hours as needed (peak effect, 4–6 hours) 0.5–1.0 mg intramuscularly; observe after 30–60 min and repeat if needed (peak effect, 20-40 min)	Extrapyramidal symptoms, especially if dose is >3 mg per day Prolonged QT interval on electrocardiogram Avoid in patients with withdrawal syndrome, hepatic insufficiency, neuroleptic malignant syndrome	Usually agent of choice Effectiveness demonstrated in randomized, controlled trials[20,37] Avoid intravenous use because of short duration of action
Atypical antipsychotic Risperidone Olanzapine Quetiapine	0.5 mg twice daily 2.5–5.0 mg once daily 2.5–5.0 mg once daily	Extrapyramidal effects equivalent to or slightly less than those with haloperidol Prolonged corrected QT interal on electrocardiogram	Tested only in small uncontrolled studies Associated with increased mortality rate among older patients with dementia
Benzodiazepine Lorazepam	0.5–1.0 mg orally, with additional doses every 4 hours as needed	Paradoxical excitation, respiratory depression, oversedation	Second-line agent Associated with prolongation and worsening of delirium symptoms demonstrated in clinical trial[37] Reserve for use in patients undergoing sedative and alcohol withdrawal, those with Parkinson's disease, and those with neuroleptic malignant syndrome
Antidepressant Trazodone	25–150 mg orally at bedtime	Over sedation	Tested only in uncontrolled studies

dementia[45] blurs the boundaries between these conditions. Moreover, studies have shown that delirium and dementia are both associated with decreased cerebral metabolism, cholinergic deficiency, and inflammation,[46] reflecting their overlapping clinical, metabolic, and cellular mechanisms. In fact, delirium and dementia may represent points along a continuum of cognitive disorders, rather than two entirely separate conditions.[39-48]

Does delirium contribute to dementia? Although it is not likely that the delirium itself causes the pathologic changes of dementia, there is no question that delirium contributes to worsening functional status, loss of independence, and poorer outcomes among patients with dementia.[52-56]

Delirium can alter the course of an underlying dementia, with dramatic worsening of the trajectory of cognitive decline, resulting in more rapid progression of functional losses and worse long-term outcomes. This phenomenon has been well recognized clinically in elderly patients with dementia: clinicians and family members have noted that the patients "never returned to base line" after an episode of delirium. In follow-up studies, patients in whom delirium develops have worse outcomes than those with dementia along,[49] including worsened cognitive function and increased rates of hospitalization, institutionalization, and death.[49]

Delirium may serve as an important model for research by offering a unique approach to advance our general understanding of cognitive disorders and dementias (see Table 3).[50-56] The development of delirium in certain persons may help to identify those who are vulnerable to cognitive decline through genetic predisposition or through the presence of early dementia or mild cognitive impairment that may otherwise remain unidentified. Moreover, a better understanding of the pathogenesis of delirium may help elucidate factors that led directly to neuronal injury and, thus, to permanent cognitive sequelae.[57,58] Studies investigating the pathogenesis of delirium with the use of neuropsychological testing, neuroimaging methods, electrophysiological methods, laboratory markers, genetic studies, and neuropathological approaches are greatly needed. Investigation of delirium provides an important opportunity to clarify the link between brain pathophysiology and behavioral manifestation, which might hold broader implications for other cognitive and psychiatric disorders. New prospects for therapy include strategies to increase acetylcholine activity in the brain (e.g., through the use of procholinergic agents and avoidance of highly anticholinergic drugs), the use of selective dopamine antagonist that affect D1, D2, D3 and D4 receptors differently, and the use of drugs to enhance cerebrovascular flow (e.g.

anti-inflammatory or antiplatelet agents). Finally, targeting delirium with new therapeutic approaches may offer opportunities for early intervention, preservation of cognitive reserve capacity, and prevention of permanent cognitive damage, which may potentially delay or abate the ultimate development of dementia.

REFERENCES

1. Cole MG. Delirium in elderly patients. Am J Geriatr Psychiatry. 2004;12:7-21.
2. Inouye SK, Rushing JT, Foreman MD, Palmer RM, Pompel P. Does delirium contribute to poor hospital outcomes? A three site epidemiologic study. J Gen Intern Med. 1998;12:234-42.
3. Francis J, Kapoor WN. Prognosis after hospital discharge of older medical patients with delirium. J Am Geriatr Soc. 1992;40:601-6.
4. Levkoff SE, Evans Da, Litpzin B, et al. Delirium: the occurrence and persistence of symptoms among elderly hospitalized patients. Arch Intern Med. 1992;131:334-40
5. Murray AM, Levkoff SE, Wetle TT, et al. Acute delirium and functional decline in the hospitalized elderly patient. J Gerontol. 1993;48:M181-M186.
6. O'Keeffe S, Lavan J. The prognostic significance of delirium in older hospital patients. J Am Geriatr Soc. 1997;45:174-8.
7. Administration on Aging. A profile of older Americans. Washington, DC: Centers for Medicare and Medicaid Services, 2003. (CMS publication no.03445.)
8. Inouye SK, Bogardus St Jr, Charpentier PA, et al. A multicomponent intervention to prevent delirium in hospitalized older patients. N Engl J Med. 1999;106:565-73.
9. Department of Health and Human Services. 2003 CMS statistics. Washington, DC: Centers for Medicare and Medicaid Services, 2003. (CMS publication no.03445.)
10. Agostini JV, Inouye SK. Delirium. In: Hazzard Wr, Blass JP, Halter JB, Ouslander JG, Tinetti ME (Eds). Principles of geriatric medicine and gerontology, 5th edition. New York:McGraw-Hill, 2003:1503-15.
11. Inouye SK. Delirium in hospitalized older patients. Clin Geriatr Med. 1998;14:745-64.
12. Inouye SK. Delirium in hospitalized older patients. Clin Geriatr Med. 1999;24:45-56.
13. Pisani MA, McNicoll L, Inouye SK. Cognitive impairment in the intensive care unit. Clin Chest Med. 2003;24:727-37.
14. Kiely DK, Bergmann MA, Jones RN, Murphy KM, Orav EJ, Marcantonio ER. Characteristics associated with delirium persistence among newly admitted post acute facility patients. J Gerontol A Biol Sci Med Sci. 2004;59:344-9.
15. Roche V. Etiology and management of delirium. Am J Med Sci. 2003;325:20-30
16. Bereitbart W, Stout D. Delirium in the terminally ill. Clin Geriatr Med. 2000;16:357-72.
17. Casarett D, Inouye SK. Diagnosis and management of delirium near the end of life. Ann Intern Med. 2001;135:32-40.
18. Folstein MF, Bassett SS, Romanosski AJ, Nestadt G. The epidemiology of delirium in the community: the Estern Baltimore Mental Health Survey. Int Psychogeriatr. 1991;3: 169-76.
19. Rahkonen T, Eloniemi-Sulkava U, Paanila S, Halonen P, Sivenius J, Sulkava R. Systematic intervention of supporting community care of elderly people after a delirium episode. Int Psychogeriatr. 2001;13:37-49.
20. American Psychiatric Association. Practice guideline for the treatment of patients with delirium. Am J Psychiatry. 1999;156(Suppl):1-20.
21. Moran JA, Dorevitch MI. Dellrium in the hospitalized elderly. Aust J Hosp Pharm. 2001;31:35-40.
22. Cole MG, Dendukuri N, McCusker J, Han L. An empirical study of different diagnostic criteria for delirium among elderly medical inpatients. J Neuropsychiatry Clin Neurosei. 2003;15:200-7.
23. Laurila JV, Pitkala KH, Strandberg TE, Tilvis RS. Delirium among patients with and without dementia: does the diagnosis according to the DSM-IV differ from the previous classifications? Int J Geriatr Psychiatry. 2004;19:271-7.
24. Nouye SK, Foreman MD, Mion LC, Katz KH, Cooney LM Jr. Nurses' recognition of delirium and its symptoms: comparison of nurse and researcher ratings. Arch Intern Med. 2001;161:2467-73.
25. Inouye SK, Charpentier PA. Precipitating factors for delirium in hospitalized elderly persons: predictive model and interrelationship with baseline vulnerability. JAMA 1996;275(8)31-7.
26. Gleason OC. Delirium. Am Fam Physician 2003;67:1027-34.
27. Rolfson D. The causes of delirium. In: Lindesay J, Rockwood K, Macdonald A (Eds). Delirium in old age. Oxford, England: Oxford University Press; 2002.pp.101-22.
28. Romano J, Engel GL. Delirium I: electroencephalographic data. Arch Neurol Psychiatry. 1944;51:356-77.
29. Trzepacz P, van derl Mast R. The neuropathophysiology of delirium. In: Lindesay J, Rockwood K, Macdonald A (Eds). Delirium in old age. Oxford, England: Oxford University Press; 2002.pp.51-90.
30. Burns A, Gallagley A, Byrne J. Delirium. J Neurol Neurosurg Psychiatry. 2004;75:362-7.
31. Han L, McCusker J, Cole M, Abrahamozicz M, Primeau F, Elie M, Primeau F, Elie M. Use of medications with anticholinergic effect predicts clinical severity of delirium symptoms in older medical impatients. Arch Intern Med. 2001;161:-1099-105.
32. Shigeta H, Yashui A, Numra Y, et al. Postoperative delirium and melatonin levels in elderly patients. Am J Surg. 2001;182:449-54.
33. Broadhurst C, Wilson K. Immunology of delirium: new opportunities for treatment and research. Br J Psychiatry. 2001;179:288-9.

34. Robertsson B, Blennow K, Brane G, et al. Hyperactivity in the hypothalamic pituitary adrenal axis in demented patients with delirium. In Clin Psychopharmacol. 2001;16:39-47.
35. Uno H, Ross T, Else JG, Suleman MA, Sapolsky RM. Hippocampal damage associated with prolonged and fatal stress in primates. J Neurosci. 1989;9:1705-11.
36. Meijer OC, de Kolet ER. Corticosterone and serotonergic neurotransmission in the hippocampus: functional implications of central corticosteroid receptor diversity. Crit Rev Neurobiol. 1998;12:1-20.
37. Breitbart W, Marotta R, Platt MM, et al. A double blind trial of haloperidol, chlorpromazine, and lorazepam in the treatment of delrium in hospitalized AIDs patients. Am J Psychiatry. 1996;153:231-7.
38. Marcantonio ER, Flacker JM, Wright J, Resnick NM. Reducing delirium after hip fracture: a randomized trial. J Am Geriatr Soc. 2001;49:516-22.
39. Inouye SK. Delirium and cognitive decline: does delirium lead to dementia? In: Fillit HM, Butler RN (Eds). Cognitive decline: strategies for prevention: proceedings of a White House Conference on Aging 64. London: Greenwich Medical Media; 1997.pp.85-107.
40. Rockwood K. The occurrence and duration of symptoms in elderly patients with delirium. J Gerontol Med Sci. 1993;48:M162-M166.
41. Levkoff SE, Liptzin B, Evans EA, et al. Progression and resolution of delirium in elderly patients hospitalized for acute care. Am J Geriatr Psychiatry. 1994;2:230-8.
42. Marcantonio Er, Flacker JM, Michaels M, Resnick NM, Delirium is independently associated with poor functional recovery after hip fracture. J Am Geriatr Soc. 2000;48:618-24.
43. Cole M, McCusker J, Dendukuri N, Han L. The prognostic significance of subsyndromal delirium in elderly medical inpatients. J Am Geriatr Soc. 2003;51:754-60.
44. McCusker J, Cole M, Dendukuri N, Han L, Belzili E. The course of delirium in older medical inpatients: a prospective study. J Gen Intern Med. 2003;18:696-704.
45. Clarifield AM. The reversible dementias: do they reverse? Ann Intern Med. 1988;109:476-86.
46. Eikelenboom P, Hoogendijk WJ. Do delirium and Alzheimer's dementia share specific pathogenetic mechanisms? Dement Geriatr Cogn Disord. 1999;10:319-24.
47. Jackson JC, Gordon SM, Hart RP, Hopkins RO, Ely EW. The association between delirium and cognitive decline: a review of the empirical literature. Neuropsychol Rev. 2004;14: 87-98.
48. Yokota H, Ogawa S, Jurokawa A, Yamamoto Y. Regional cerebral blood flow in delirium patients. Psychiatry Clin Neurosci. 2003;57:337-9.
49. Fick D, Foreman M. Consequences of not recognizing delirium super imposed on dementia in hospitalized elderly individuals. J Gerontol Nurs. 2000;26:30-40.
50. Rockwood K, Cosway S, Carver D, Jarrett P, Stadnkyk K, Fisk J. The risk of dementia and death after delirium. Age ageing 1999;28:551-6.
51. McCusker J, Cole M, Dendukuri N, Belzile E, Primeau F. Delirium in older medical inpatients and subsequent cognitive and functional status: a prospective study. CMAJ. 2001;165:575-83.
52. Baker FM, Wiley C, Kokmen E, Chandra V, Schoenberg BS. Delirium episodes during the course of clinically diagnosed Alzheimer's disease. J Natl Med Assoc. 1999;91: 625-30.
53. Rothschild JM, Bates DW, Le ape LL. Preventable medical injuries in older patients. Arch Intern Med. 2000;160:2717-28.
54. Gillck MR, Serrell NA, Gillick LS. Adverse consequences of hospitalization in the elderly. Sco Sci Med. 1982;16: 1033-8.
55. Williamson JW. Formulating priorities for quality assurance activity. JAMA. 1978;239:631-7.
56. Sloss EM, Solomon DH, Shekelle PG, et al. Selecting target conditions for quality of care improvement in vulnerable older adults. J Am Geriatr Soc. 2000;48:363-9.
57. Institute of Medicine (IOM) Committee on Quality of Health Care in America. Building a safer health system. Washington, DC: National Academy Press; 2000.pp.26-48.
58. Thomas EJ, Studdert DM, New-house JP, et al. Costs of medical injuries in Utah and Colorado. Inquiry. 1999;36:255-68.

CHAPTER

74 Spectrum of Tardive Syndromes: Clinical Recognition and Management

BK Singh

The discovery of tardive dyskinesia (TD) occurred more than five decades ago, about 5 years after the introduction of neuroleptic drugs into psychiatry. The original description of persistent abnormal involuntary movements induced by neuroleptic agents was published in a paper by Schonecker in 1957.[1] Since then, the phenomenon of TD altered physicians and the public to its iatrogenicity and to its medicolegal impact, further enhancing clinical awareness of a potential negative and delayed impact to these useful drugs on the nervous system. While tardive syndromes (TS) encompass all aspects of abnormal movements, tardive dyskinesia (TD) specifically refers to classical orobuccal-lingual dyskinesia associated with 'piano playing' finger movements. The involuntary movements of various phenomenology associated with neuroleptic agents are classified as TS, including classic orobuccal-lingual dyskinesia, stereotypy, dystonia, akathisia, tics, myoclonus, tremor, and parkinsonism. TS is now accepted as a separate and unique entity as a result of the principle adverse effect of long-term treatment with conventional antipsychotic agents. In this review, we discuss the clinical issues related to TS, including clinical recognition of various phenomenologies of TS, not limited to TD, and the practical management of this condition. Basic common principles of management of TS are also provided. When possible, preventive measures should be considered such as avoiding the use of neuroleptics when alternative treatments are available, limiting the course of neuroleptic treatment, and carefully watching of the earliest signs of TS. Once TS has developed, therapeutic choices often include the discontinuation of neuroleptics in patients with TS (if possible), and a determination of which medications may be considered for suppressing TS. In medically intractable cases, severe disability many force the need for chemodenervation of surgical intervention.

CLASSIFICATION OF TARDIVE SYNDROMES

Tardive syndromes (TD) refers to a group of disorders characterized by predominantly late onset and sometimes persistent involuntary movements (or a sensation of restlessness), which are caused by exposure to dopamine receptor blocking agents (DRBAs). The first international congress of movement disorders defined TD as a hyperkinetic movement that develops during treatment with neuroleptics or within 6 months of stopping the offending agent, and it must persist for at least 1 month after discontinuing all neuroleptics. A somewhat different definition by the American Psychiatric Task Force required 3 months of exposure to a DRBA for diagnosis of TD.[2,3] The Diagnostic and Statistical Manual of Mental Disorder, 4th edition (DSM-IV) criteria specifics the shortest duration of exposure to DRBAs of at least 1 month in individuals ≥60 years. The French term 'tardive' is used to denoted its late onset during the course of neuroleptic therapy, and 'dyskinesia' refers to unnatural movements which may or may not be involuntary. Generally, TD does not appear until after 1–2 years of continued neuroleptic treatment, and almost never before 3 months. Because virtually all types of movement disorders have been associated with neuroleptic therapy and this identical clinical syndrome can be induced by other agents in addition to neuroleptics (Box 1), the term 'tradive dyskinesia' is confusing and problematic. Traditionally and historically, term 'tardive dyskinesia' was used to describe a specific type of movement, characterized by oro-buccal-lingual dyskinesias.[4] There are several phenomenological distinct types of abnormal movements and they are classified into classical tardive dyskinesia, tardive stereotypy, tardive dystonia, tardive akathisia, tardive tremor, tardive myoclonus, and tardive tourettism (Box 2).[5] It remains unclear if tardive parkinsonism truly exists. The term 'classical tardive dyskinesia' will be used in this review to denoted a characteristic oro-buccal-lingual dyskinesia. Although detailed and somewhat impractical, this differentiation into specific abnormal movements gives physicians additional clues to identify a specific etiology, pathophysiologic mechanism, and specific treatment protocols in certain subgroups of populations. The combination of more than one type of hyperkinetic movements (e.g. stereotypy and dystonia) strongly suggests the diagnosis of TD.

Box 1: Drugs that are commonly associated with tardive syndromes

Phenothiazines
- Chlorpromazine
- Triflupromazine
- Thioridazine
- Mesoridazine
- Trifluoperazine
- Prochlorperazine
- Perphenazine
- Fluphenazine
- Perazine

Thioxanthenes
- Chloprothixene
- Thiothixene

Butyrophenones
- Haloperidol
- Droperidol

Diphenylbutylpiperidine
- Pimozide

Dibenzazepine
- Loxapine

Dibenzodiazepine
- Clozapine
- Quetiapine

Thienobenzodiazepine
- Olanzapine

Substituted Benzamides
- Metoclopramide
- Tiapride
- Sulpiride
- Clebopride
- Remoxipride
- Veralipride

Indolones
- Molindone

Pyrimidinone
- Risperidone

Tricyclic antidepressants
- Amoxapine

Calcium channel blockers
- Flunarizine
- Cinnarizine

Box 2: Classification of tardive syndromes

- Tardive dyskinesia
- Tardive stereotypy
- Tardive dystonia
- Tardive akathisia
- Tardive tourettism
- Tardive myoclonus
- Tardive tremor
- Tardive parkinsonism

Epidemiology and Risk Factors of TS

The most compelling evidence supporting the association between neuroleptics and TD comes from epidemiologic studies. In general, TD is the most frequently observed disorder in TS. These studies have also determined risk factors, including age, duration of treatment, and gender. While the prevalence of TD varies widely in the literature, reflecting the heterogeneity of the groups being observed as well as the various assessment method used, an average prevalence among neuroleptic treated patients, corrected for the prevalence of spontaneous dyskinesia is estimated to be between 20 and 40%.[6-9] In addition to TD, there are few studies about prevalence of other movement disorders as part of TS. Tardive dystonia has a prevalence of between 2 and 16% of neuroleptic treated patients.[10,11] The prevalence of tardive akathisia, tics, myoclonus, and tremor have been reported as 22%, 4%, 1% and 30% respectively.[10]

Aging appears to be a critical risk factor for developing TD, as the incidence increases from 5% in the younger age group (4 years old) to 12% of higher in the older age group (≥40 years old).[12] In general, at least 20% of patients treated with typical neuroleptics are affected with TD and approximately 5% are expected to develop TD during each year of neuroleptic treatment. Female gender may be a risk factor although this is not supported by incidence studies. Patients with existing movement disorders are at greater risk of developing TD with continued use of antipsychotics. Total neuroleptics load, the dose a duration of use, is considered to be a risk factor. Neuroleptics, both typical and atypical agents, induced the upregulation of D2 receptor binding, which is associated with the development of TD. However, typical neuroleptics carry a greater risk than atypical agents.[13-15] Indeed, all atypical neuroleptics have a high serotonin-to-dopamine receptor blockade ratio in the brain, and this high serotonergic blockade is thought to play a role in reducing acute extrapyramidal symptoms. Other reported risk factors are race, a diagnosis of a mood disorder, cognitive impairment, the presence of negative symptoms, alcohol and substance abuse, the use of antiparkinsonian agents and lithium, early extrapyramidal symptoms illness awareness, diabetes, and lastly, HIV seropositive status[16] (Box 3).

Classical TD

Classical TD comprises a phenomenologically distinct syndrome of TS, is the most common persistent adverse reaction to prolonged neuroleptic medication, and was the first to be identified. General characteristics are frequently observed to resemble normal movement patterns, such as chewing (rumination), bridling (retraction of the corners of the mouth) grasping or 'piano-playing movements; however,

Box 3: Risk factors of tardive syndromes

- Older age (young age in case of tardive dystonia)
- Female gender
- African American population
- Typical neuroleptics
- Higher dose and longer duration of neuroleptic use
- Pre-existing mood disorders
- Cognitive impairments
- Presence of negative symptoms
- Alcohol and substance abuse
- Use of antiparkinsonian agents and lithium
- Early extrapyramidal symptoms
- Diabetes
- HIV seropositive status

patients perform these movements involuntarily. Orofacial movements especially may be temporarily suppressed by patients themselves or when engaged to voluntary activities, such as talking or chewing. Interestingly, many patients with classical TD do not even notice their involuntary movements unless their attention is drawn to them by others.

The facial muscles, particularly the perioral and oral muscles, are commonly affected in affected in classical TD.[4-17] Dyskinesia of the tongue is characterized by a slow and repetitive retraction, or a sweeping tongue movement within the oral cavity, producing a bulge in the cheek, referred to as the 'bonbon sign'.[18] When the patient is asked to extend the tongue, irregular, worm-like contractions of the tongue muscles are frequently observed. Grimacing, with a lifting or arching of eyebrows or frowning, can also be a symptom of classical TD. Most patients exhibit uncoordinated flexion-extension movements of individual fingers, somewhat resembling guitar or piano playing movements. Dyskinesias of the legs—'stamping movements'—give the impression of slowly walking in place or shifting body weight form one foot to the other.[18] Dyskinesia of the diaphragm may lead to an irregular, uneven rhythm of speech or uncontrollable grunting and groaning. Other movements that have been describe in classical TD include hip-rocking movements, to-and-fro movements of the upper torso, head nodding, and flexion-extension movements of the toes, wrists, and ankles.

Tardive Stereotypy

Stereotypy, which is defined as a seemingly purposeful, coordinated but involuntary, repetitive, ritualistic gesture, mannerism or utterance, was reported, by Stacy et al.[19,20] and Miller et al.[21] to be the most common form of TD. Some experts suggested that tardive stereotypy is probably a more appropriate term than classical TD to describe the repetitive, rather than random, movements. However, the stereotypic movements in classical TD are very characteristic and similar in almost all patients with than disorder, differentiating it from other types of stereotypes seen in patients with autism and psychosis.[22]

Tardive Dystonia

Since the earliest reports of TD, a variety of involuntary movements in addition to the well-known orobuccal lingual masticatory movements, have been described, including dystonia. The term 'tardive dystonia' was defined by Burke et al. to represent and involuntary movement predominated by dystonia and associated with the use of DRBAs.[23] For reasons not fully understood, young adults seem to be particularly susceptible to this disorder.[19] According to Burke et al. dystonia must be present for more than a month and occur either during ongoing treatment with a DRBA or within 3 months of its discontinuation.[23] Although choreiform movements may occur, the principal movement must be dystonia. Dystonic movements in tardive dystonia are strikingly different from the classical TD. Firstly, dystonic movements, defined as a syndrome of sustained muscle contraction frequently causing twisting and abnormal postures, tend to be action specific. They occur consistently with certain actions and do not exhibit clear-cut periodicity as classical TD. Secondly, many patients with dystonia note that their movements can be partially controlled by simple tactile maneuvres, termed sensory tricks or 'geste antagoniste'. Such as touching the chin to alleviate torticollis.[24] Third, tardive dystonia occur more often among men than women, the gender at greater risk of classic TD.[25] Finally, the shorter duration for neuroleptic exposure develops tardive dystonia and it tends to occur in populations with a lower age of onset when compared with other TS.[10,26]

Without a reliable history, tardive dystonia may be indistinguishable from idiopathic torsion dystonia, including sensory tricks and distribution of dystonia. However, there are some different features of identification of these disorders (Table 1). Tardive dystonia has a special predilection for cranial and cervical muscles. When it affects the neck, it usually results in retrocollis, in contrast to laterocollis or torticollis in idiopathic cervical dystonia. When involving the trunk, it usually produces severe scoliosis or opisthotonic posturing. When involving the upper limbs, internal rotation of the arms, extension of the elbows, and flexion of the wrists are common postures in tardive dystonia.[26] The legs are only infrequently involved. Tardive dystonia often occurs with other TS, while idiopathic torsion dystonia rarely does.

Tardive Akathisia

Akathisia refers to a feeling of inner restlessness and jitteriness that is often manifested by semi-purposeful movements. Subjectively, the most common complaint is the inability

Table 1: A comparison of tardive dystonia and idiopathic torsion dystonia

Clinical features	*Tardive dystonia*	*Idiopathic torsion dystonia*
Cervical dystonic posture	Retrocollis	Torticollis, Laterocollis
Axial dystonic posture	Opisthotonic posturing	Lateral twisting of trunk
Unique characteristics: internal rotation of the arms, extension of elbows, and flexion of the wrists	Frequent in young men	None
Leg involvement	Less frequent	Frequent in primary generalized dystonia
Dystonia after voluntary action	Reduced	Exacerbate
Coexist with other tardive syndromes	Frequent	None

to keep the legs still which are associated with vague inner tension, unease, or anxiety. Objectively, patients are seen rocking from foot to foot, walking in place, grunting, moaning, or trunk rocking. In addition to its common occurrence as an acute adverse effect of neuroleptics, akathisia can become chronic (tardive akathisia).[27] Not surprisingly, tardive akathisia usually coexists with classic TD. The mean age of onset is 58 years, as the age of onset of patients to whom neuroleptics are administered typically is younger than those taking other agents.[10]

Although earlier evidence indicated a potential increased risk of suicide among patients with tardive akathisia, evidence on this association is still conflicting and requires a long-term prospective study to address this issue.[28]

Tardive Tics

Tics are brief, repetitive, temporarily suppressible movements or sounds. There are usually premonitory sensations preceding motor or vocal tics. Tics have been reported to occur in patients after exposure to DBBAs. Besides older age of onset and history of neuroleptic exposure, they are clinically indistinguishable from Tourette's syndrome.

Tardive Myoclonus

Postural myoclonus was also observed in approximately 25% of psychiatric patients who had been taking neuroleptics for at least 3 months (tardive myoclonus). It usually is prominent myoclonus in the upper extremities and is accompanied by other TS.[29]

Tardive Tremor

Tardive tremor was first described by Jankovic.[4,30] The existence of tardive tremor has been the subject of case reports.[30] High amplitude, moderate frequency, postural and resting tremor have been observed in some patients who were exposed to neuroleptics, but without signs of parkinsonism.

Tardive Parkinsonism

As noted above, the category of tardive parkinsonism is questionable, but it has been used to describe the movements of some patients who had persistent parkinsonian features several months after neuroleptic discontinuation.[31]

DIFFERENTIAL DIAGNOSIS OF TARDIVE SYNDROMES

The development of dyskinesias in a psychiatric patient is often attributed to neuroleptic therapy. Although neuroleptic exposure may be the cause of involuntary movements in the majority of psychiatric patients, other possibilities should always be considered since dyskinesias are symptoms or signs of neurological dysfunction and may stem from a variety of disparate neurological or medical disorders (Box 4).[32] Furthermore, many neurological disorder, such a Huntington's disease or Wilson's disease, may initially

Box 4: Differential diagnosis of tardive syndromes

Classical tardive dyskinesia
- Huntington's disease
- Hepatolenticular degeneration
- Drug induced dyskinesias
  - Levodopa
  - Tricyclic antidepressants
  - Selective serotonin reuptake inhibitors
  - Serotonin and norepinephrine reuptake inhibitors
  - Lithium
  - Phenytoin
- Edentulous orodyskinesia
- Spontaneous orofacial dyskinesias
- Stroke
- Immune chorea

Tardive dystonia
- Primary dystonia
- Hereodegenerative dystonia—for example, Wilson's disease
- Secondary dystonia

Tremor
- Parkinsonian tremor
- Essential tremor
- Cerebellar tremor
- Enhanced physiologic tremor
- Idiopathic tremor

manifest themselves by isolated neuropsychiatric syndromes, preceding the onset of motor abnormalities by many years.[33]

Dyskinesias are symptoms or may represent a syndrome, but they are not a diagnosis. There are no definitive clinical, laboratory, or electrophysiological criteria for a diagnosis of neuroleptic induced TD. However, some clues, if present, may provide an alternative diagnose other than TD: (1) a rapidly deteriorating course; (2) constant unilateral manifestation; (3) the presence of additional neurological signs such as dementia, sensory abnormalities, or urinary incontinence; and (4) the appearance of other physical symptoms or signs, such as jaundice, fever, skin rash, etc.

Huntington's disease (HD) is the major challenge for a differential diagnosis of TD because abnormal movements in both disorders can be phenomenologically identical and both can initially present with neuropsychiatric symptoms without motor abnormalities, However, careful observations of motor abnormalities in HD reveal different patterns, which may help distinguish it from TD. In HD, choreic movements are random, flowing from one part of the body to the other, and frequently superimposed by semi-purposeful movements in an attempt to mask involuntary movements. In contrast, choreic movements in TD are more likely to be slow, stereotypic and repetitive, often in the oral region. Furthermore, gait abnormalities, described as a stuttering choreic gait, more frequently occur with HD. Importantly, eye movement abnormalities in HD such as slow saccades have been frequently observed. Before the discovery of the HD gene, a definite diagnosis of HD would be made in the presence of: (1) a positive family history consistent with autosomal dominant inheritance; (2) progressive motor disability; and (3) mental disturbances including cognitive decline, affective disturbances, and/or changes in personality. Furthermore, in HD, progressive atrophy of the caudate nucleus if frequently observed. Which is not seen in TD.[34,35] Despite these clinical criteria, misdiagnosis occurs fairly frequently. The availability of the HD gene, especially its pathogenic mutation, has made it easier to distinguish TD from HD.

Among various dystonic syndromes, Wilson's disease figures prominently in the differential diagnosis of tardive dystonia. Although dystonia in both conditions frequently affects craniocervical regions, the presence of retrocollis or axial dystonia is highly suggestive of tardive dystonia, while oromandibular dystonia is more common in Wilson's disease. Wilson's disease is an autosomal recessive disorder and can present with a myriad of manifestations, ranging from psychiatric illness to various types of movement disorders. Wilson's disease should be considered in adolescents and adults younger than 40 years with the following: (1) elevated liver enzymes found incidentally or in the context of an acute hepatitis episode; (2) dysphagia or dysarthria not explained by other neurological disorders; (3) patients with any types of movement disorders; (4) patients with psychiatric symptoms movement disorders; (4) patients with psychiatric symptoms and liver disease; (5) adolescents with mood disorders and minor elevations of liver transaminase; (5) patients with Coomb's negative hemolytic anemia; and (7) patients with unexplained liver cirrhosis and hepatic failure.[36] Until recently, the genetic basis of Wilson's disease confirmed the link to one of the transport proteins with a defect in a p-type ATP (ATPase) involving the transport of copper across the trans-Golgi and into transport vesicles.[37,38]

Withdrawal emergent syndrome, typically seen in children, is identical to classical TD manifested in adults with exception of the more generalized movements.[39] This syndrome is referred to as withdrawal dyskinesia, occurring after an acute withdrawal of long-term use of antipsychotics. In contrast to classical TD, the random hyperkinesias seen in this syndrome primarily involved the limbs, neck, and trunk, and seldom the lower facial region, developing within a few days after discontinuation of antipsychotics. The course of illness in withdrawal emergent syndrome is shorter and more benign than classical TD and typically disappears after 3 months.

Hyperkinetic movements, identified as spontaneous dyskinesia, may occur in some elderly individuals without any known causes.[40] Interestingly these spontaneous movements are found much more frequently among neuroleptic naive schizophrenic patients than among older nonpsychiatric patients and patients with other psychiatric diagnoses. Whether the presence of spontaneous dyskinesia is intrinsic to the pathophysiology of schizophrenia or a manifestation of brain damage remains to be elucidated. In addition to neuroleptics, late onset dyskinesias can be induced by tricyclic antidepressants (TCAs), selective serotonin reuptake inhibitors (SSRIs), and serotonin and norepinephrine reuptake inhibitors (SNRIs).[41] In patients with Parkinson's disease, levodopa, and to a lesser extent the dopamine agonists, can induce dyskinesia with a fluctuating course and peripheral distribution.[42-45] Occasionally, poorly fitted dentures of loss of teeth can produce bucco-oral movements mimicking orofacial dyskinesias.[46-49]

Natural History of Tardive Syndrome

Tardive dyskinesia typically begins several years after the initiation of neuroleptic treatment. However, a period of 3 months is generally regarded as the minimum period to include the vast majority of patients in whom neuroleptics play an essential role as a causative agent. Older patients appear to develop symptoms more quickly than younger patients, perhaps as a result of neurobiological changes associated with aging.[49] In general, TD has an insidious onset, later reaching its maximal severity rapidly, and then stabilizes. Although different reports have shown the natural history of TD to persist, improve, or to have an unpredictable course, the most common course of TD by far is waxing and waning of mild-to-moderate symptoms over many years. Significant worsening after a period of stabilization is unusual. Clinical manifestations may be precipitated by a dose reduction of withdrawal of neuroleptics, especially the first several weeks,[5,50] or by concomitant administration of anticholinergics of antidepressants.[51] Five percent to 10% of patients on long-term neuroleptics develop symptoms that are severe enough to notably impair functioning. Orofacial dyskinesias can cause difficulty in eating, resulting in weight loss. Similarly, only 11% of patients improve, and remissions, if they occur, usually appear within 1–2 years after discontinuation. About 50% of patients have had relatively persistent symptoms over the course, of 5 years.[52] These data may suggest that continued treatment with neuroleptics after the development of TD is probably a reasonable option for many patients.

Pathophysiology of TS

Despite extensive research on the mechanisms of action of neuroleptics, the specific pathophysiological processes underlying movement disorders remain incompletely understood. While patients with genetic predisposition for movement disorders, neurodegenerative disorders, or pre-existing brain injury may be more susceptible in developing TS, the most accepted theories suggest the chronic exposure of neuroleptics resulted in a combination of postsynaptic dopamine receptor hypersensitivity, abnormalities of striatal GABA (g-aminobutyric acid)-containing neurons, and degeneration of striatal cholinergic interneurons.[53] Chronic blockade with neuroleptics may result in D2 receptor upregulation and increased sensitivity of the dopamine receptors.[54] In addition, the findings of degeneration of neurons in the striato-pallidal and striato-nigral GABA-aminergic pathways combined with cholinergic interneurons were also observed in animal models of TD.[53,55,56]

Management of TS

Since, by definition, TD is an iatrogenic disorder, the best management is prevention. Patients should be advised of the inherent risk of developing TD before commencing drug therapy with neuroleptics. Once a TD is encountered, removal of the etiologic agent should be seriously considered. Importantly, early detection and discontinuation of DRBAs provide a higher chance for remission, although younger are is associated with a better chance.[57] Most experts recommend neuroleptic withdrawal only in those who can tolerate it.[3] Unfortunately, the best treatment for many psychiatric disorders is the long-term administration of neuroleptics. Therefore, dose reductions and the use of the smallest effective dose is generally recommended as the next step.[3]

Atypical versus Typical Neuroleptics

As a result, patients with TD should have a greater likelihood of TD remission on atypical neuroleptics.[58-62] Other than risperidone, little information is available on the use of atypical neuroleptics in TD.[63] Recently, one multicenter, double blind trial found significant improvement of anti-dyskinetic scores in risperidone treated schizophrenic patient greater than either haloperidol or placebo. Risperidone treated patients at 6 mg per day showed the most beneficial effect on TD, with greater efficacy in the oro-buccal-lingual than the limb area.[64] Unlike the conventional and other atypical neuroleptics, clozapine is a relatively weak D2 receptor blocker and a number of small studies have demonstrated a reduction in involuntary movements for a short period with clozapine in both classical TD and tardive dystonia.[65-70] Several smaller studies reported improvement of TD after switching typical neuroleptics to olanzapine and quetiapine. Overall, the cumulative data conclude that risperidone has been shown to be effective in the treatment of TD, mainly buccolinguomasticatory dyskinesia, over an 8 weeks period.[64] Regarding clozapine, it does not worsen TD and may improve it. Despite limited evidence, some experts recommended switching from a typical neuroleptic to an atypical neuroleptic without distinguishing among atypical agents.[71] However, the decision should be based on a consideration of both the benefits and the risk to the patient for each treatment option. With atypical agents, the possible benefits of TD reduction must be balanced against the risk of side effects, including sedation, weight gain, diabetes, agranulocytosis, and psychiatric exacerbation.

In classical TD, involuntary movements often are not disabling or even bothersome to the patients and many of them seem unaware of the movements. However, the families often tend to be more distressed or upset than the patients. If this is the case, symptomatic therapy is rarely indicated although other management should be directed at trying to encourage the development of spontaneous remission or improvement through adjustment of neuroleptics as described above. Alternatively, some patients are severely distressed by the movements, and functional disabilities occur which interfere with speech and feeding including biting lips, and irregular respiration. Severe TD most commonly occurs in younger men (< 40 years) and older women (over 65 years), and often has component of dystonia. Treatment of severe TD requires continued neuroleptic therapy concomitantly with serial trials of suppressive agents.

Generally, suppressive therapy with neuroleptics is successful in 75% of patients, but the long-term safety has not been demonstrated. There are no validated guidelines to follow when choosing a suppressive agent since not a single agent has been successful in large scale, double blinded, randomized controlled trials.[72] Selection should be based on the underlying psychiatric diagnosis, risk/benefit analysis, potential side effects, and interaction with other medications. In general, therapeutic trials have attempt to manipulate one of the following neurotransmitters, including dopamine, GABA, acetylcholine, norepinephrine, and serotonin. Based on the dopamine hypersensitivity hypothesis, both typical and atypical neuroleptics may be effective in suppressing TD.[73] While its efficacy in short-term suppression has been clearly demonstrated, the therapeutic efficacy of long-term suppression (more than 8 weeks) remains unclear. High potency neuroleptics have been observed to have more suppressive effect than those of lower potency.[73] Although overall results have varied, significant improvement, particularly with dystonic features, has been observed with clozapine and risperidone.[64,74]

Dopamine Depleting Agents

The strategy of depleting dopamine without exposing the brain to DRBAs has been shown to reduced TD symptoms. Reserpine and tetrabenazine inhibit the vesicular monoamine transporter and thereby deplete presynaptic stores of dopamine. Studies of dopamine depleting medications suggest that they may alleviate symptoms in up to 50% of patients with TD.[73] Tetrabenzine has a quicker onset and shorter duration of action, with fewer peripheral catecholamine detecting effects than reserpine. In addition, both agents have has been implicated in causing TD. While larger well controlled studies are needed to validate the efficacy of tetrabenazine the limited available data support its use for TD suppression.[75]

Cholinergic versus Anticholinergic Agent

The observations that parkinsonian symptoms can be improved by dopamine agonists or cholinergic antagonists have implicated the imbalance between acetylcholine and dopamine to induce dyskinesias. As a result numerous studies have been conducted since 1970 to examine the efficacy of cholinomimetic agents or acetylcholinesterase inhibitors.[76-78] Unfortunately, a systematic review of cholinergic agents was unable to demonstrate its clear cut value in ameliorating dyskinesias. Currently, only donepezil has demonstrated some benefit in suppressing TD.[79-81] Like-wise, antichloinergics do not help or may actually worsen TD and discontinuation may be helpful in some patients. The only exception is tardive dystonia, which may improve with high doses of trihexyphenidyl.[74]

GABA Agonists

No clear evidence has been reported that GABA agonists, benzodiazepines, are effective in suppressing TD.[82] However, 40–50% of patients reported favorable outcome with clonazepam or diazepam, mainly with dystonic symptoms.[83,84] Baclofen, a GABAB-agonist, brought about significant improvements as a suppressive agent in TD when it was combined with neuroleptic agents.[85,86]

Botulinum Toxin

In addition to primary torsion dystonia, chemodenervation with botulinum toxin, mainly type A, was also considered as treatment for tardive dystonia.[87-89] The response to botulinum toxin in tardive patients was no different than the response in other forms of dystonia.[90]

Antioxidants

Chronic neuroleptic exposure has been shown to increase the turnover of dopamine in the brain, which subsequently leads to production of cytotoxic free radicals. Thus, vitamin E has been proposed as an effective treatment for TD by neuroleptic free radicals. While positive effects have been observed on patients with relatively recent onset (within 5 years), a recent large multicenter study found no significant improvement of TD with vitamin E at a daily dose of 1600 mg.[91-93] Therefore there still is no consistent evidence for suppressive benefits of vitamin E in TD. Additions to vitamin E, other antioxidants such as melatonin, vitamin B6, or eicosapentaenoic acid, are unproven in efficacy for suppressing TD.

Surgical Treatment

Recently, there have been many studies for surgical intervention in patients with TS, mainly dystonia. The optimal target of lesioning or deep brain stimulation is the globus pallidus internus. As a result, the efficacy of both pallidotomy and pallidal deep brain stimulation had shown improvement in several case reports among tardive dystonia patients. The motor beneficial effects were similar for oro-buccal-ligual dystonia and axial as well as limb dystonia.[94-97] However, pallidal surgical procedures are appropriate for severe disabling tardive dystonia patients unresponsive to other forms of therapy.

Treatment of TD is challenging and is often unsatisfactory since there are no specific antidyskinetic drugs. The severity of TD and the absolute necessity for neuroleptics often dictates the treatment approach for the disorder. Since withdrawal of the offending drug may bring full remission in some instances, this option should always be considered in all patients if at all possible. If not, as is usually the case, than a drug that may permit passive healing should be considered. While clozapine is a good choice, it is logistically difficult to use and risperidone or quetiapine might be considered as an alternative. In mid cases that do not warrant treatment, adding vitamin E may be worthwhile albeit still unproven. The dose of atypical neuroleptics should be kept as low as possible. With limited current evidence and the lack of formal guidelines, the use of suppressive agents is highly individualized. Each expert may have a different strategy and there may not be a generalized approach for all circumstances. Often, a trial of different drugs is needed before an effective one of found. The decision regarding which suppressive agent should be chosen requires a consideration of the benefits and risk to patient for each treatment option.

CONCLUSION

Tardive syndromes refers to a group of delayed onset movement disorders, not limited to classical TD, caused by DRBAs. While the most frequent manifestation of TS is characterized by oro-buccal-lingual dyskinesias, TS may exist in other forms, including stereotypy, akathisa, tics, myoclonus, tremor, and possibly parkinsonism. Many risk factors for TS have been identified, including older age, female gender, African American ethnicity, typical neuroleptics of higher dosages, longer duration of neuroleptics exposure, and pre-existing mood or psychiatric disorders. With the increasing use of neuroleptics by multiple medical specialists, TD will continue to pose a clinical dilemma and remain a major public health issue in psychiatry. Further understanding of the pathophysiology of TD will lead to further advances in discovering newer agents with lower propensity to cause TD and effective therapeutic agents to reduce symptoms lastly, physicians should always remind themselves of the adage primum non nocere (first, do not harm) when prescribing any medicine.

REFERENCES

1. Schonecker M. Paroxysmal dyskinesia as the effect of magaphen. Nervenarn. 1957;28:550-3.
2. Baldessarini RJ, Cole JO, Davis JM, et al. Tardive dyskinesia: summary of a test. Force Report of the American Psychiatric Association. Am J Psychiatry. 1980;137:1163-72.
3. Dyskinesia APATFoT. Tardive Dyskinesia: A Task Force Report of the American Psychiatric Association. Washington DC: American Psychiatric Press; 1992.
4. Jankovic J. Tardive syndromes and other drug induced movement disorders. Clin Neuropharmacol. 1995;18:197-214.
5. Fernandez HH, Friendman JH. Classification and treatment of tardive syndromes. Neurologists. 2003;9:16-27.
6. Woerner MG, Kane JM, Lieberman JA. et al. The prevalence of tardive dyskinesia. J Clin Psychopharmacol. 1991;11:34-42.
7. Yassa R, Nair NP. A 10-year follow-up study of tardive dyskinesia. Acta Psychiatry Scand. 1992;86:262-6.
8. Kane JM, Smith JM. Tardive dyskinesia: prevalence and risk factors, 1959 to 1979. Arch Gen Psychiatry. 1982;39;473-81.
9. Yassa R, Jeste DV. Gender differences in tardive dyskinesia: a clinical review of the literature. Schizophar Bull. 1992;18:701-15.
10. Orti-pareja M, Jimenez-Jimenz FJ, Vazquez A, et al. Drug-induced tardive syndromes. Parkinsonism Relat Disord. 1999;5:59-65.
11. Yassa R, Nair V, Dimitry R. Prevalence of tardive dystonia. Acta Psychiatr Scand. 1996;73:629-33.
12. Jeste DV, Wyatt RJ. Changing epidemiology of tardive dyskinesia: An overview. Am J Psychiatry. 1981;138:297-309.
13. Margolese HC, Chouinard G, Kolivakis TT. et al. Tardive dyskinesia in the era of typical and atypical antipsychotics. part:2 Incidence and management strategies in patients with schizophrenia. Can J Psychiatry. 2005;50:703-14.
14. Jeste DV. Tardive dyskinesia rates with atypical antipsychotics in adults: Prevalence and incidence. J Clin Psychiatry. 2004;65(Suppl 9):21-4.
15. Kane JM. Tardive dyskinesia rates with atyplical antipsychotics in adults: prevalence and incidence. J Clin Psychiatry. 2004;64(Suppl 9):16-20.
16. Shedlack KJ, Soldato-Couture C, Swanson CL Jr. Rapidly progressive tardive dyskinesia in AIDS. Biol Psychiatry. 1994;35:147-8.
17. Barnes TR. The present status of tardive dyskinesia and akathisia in the treatment of schizophrenia. Psychiatr Dev. 1987;5:301-19.
18. Simpson GM, Lee JH, Zoubok B, et al. A rating scale for tardive dyskinesia. Psychopharmacology. 1979;64:171-9.
19. Stacy M, Jankovic J. Tardive dyskinesia. Curr Opin Neurol Neurosurg. 1991;4:343-9.
20. Stacy, Cardoso F, Jankovic J. Tardive stereotypy and other movement; disorders in tardive dyskinesias. Neurology. 1993;43:937-41.
21. Miller LG, Jankovic J. Neurologic approach to drug induced movement disorders in 125 patients. South Med J. 1990;83:937-41.
22. Jankovic J. Stereotypies. In: Marsden CD FS, Ed. Movement disorder 3. London Butterworth-Heinemann; 1994.pp.503-17.
23. Burke RE, Fahn S, Janakovic J. et al. Tardive dystonia: late-onset and persistent dystonia caused by antipsychotic durgs. Neurology. 1982;32:335-46.
24. Bhidayasiri R, Bronstein JM. Improvement of cervical dystonia possible role of transcranial magnetic stimulation simulating sensory tricks effect. Med Hypotheses. 2005;64:941-5.
25. Kiriakakis V, Bhatia KP, Quinn NP, et al. The natural history of tardive dystonia A long-term follow-up study of 107 cases. Brain. 1998;212(Pt 11);2053-65.
26. Kang UJ, Burke RE, Fahn S. Natural history and treatment of tardive dystonia. Mov Disord. 1986;1:193-208.
27. Burke RE, Kang UJ, Jankovic J, et al. Tardive akethisia: an analysis of clinical features and response to open therapeutic trials. Mov Disord. 1989;4:157-75.
28. Hansen L, Jones RM, Kingdom D. No association between akathisia or Parkinsonism and suicidality in treatment-resistant Schizoohrenia. J Psychopharnacol. 2004;18:384-7.

29. Tominaga H, Fukuzako H, Izumi K, et al. Tardive myoclonus. Lancet. 1989;4:157-75.
30. Stacy M, Jankovic J. Tardive tremor. Mov Disord. 1992;7:53-57.
31. Marsalek M. Tardive drug indiced extrapyramioal syndromes. Pharmacopsychiatry. 2000;33(Suppl 1):14-33.
32. Hyde TM, Hotson JR, Kleinman JE. Differential diagnosis of choreiform tardive dyskinesia. J Neuropsychiatry Clin Neurosci. 1991;3:225-68.
33. Bhidayasiri R, Truong DD. Chorea and related disorders Postgrad Med J. 2004;80:527-34.
34. Stober T, Wussow W, Schimrigk K. Bicaudate diameter—the most specific and simple CT parameter in the diagnosis of Huntington's disease. Neuroradology. 1984;26:25-8.
35. McCreadie RG, Thara R, Padmavati R, et al. Structural brain differences between never-treated patients with schizophrenia, with and without dyskinesia, and normal control subjects: amagnetic resonance imaging study. Arch Gen Psychiatry. 2002; 59:332-6.
36. El-Youssef M, Wilson disease. Mayo Clin Proc. 2003;78:1126-36.
37. La Fontaine S, Mercer JF. Trafficking of the copper-ATpases. ATP7A and ATP7B: role in copper homeostasis Arch Biochem Biophys. 2007;463:149-67.
38. Tao TY, Lia F, Klomp L, et al. The Copper toxicosis gene product intreracts with the Wilson deisease proten. J Biol Chem. 2003;278:41593-6.
39. Winsberg BG, Hurwic MJ, Perel J. Neurochemistry of withdrawal emergent symptoms in children. Psychopharmacol Bull. 1977;13:38-40.
40. Weiner WJ, Klawans HL Jr. Lingual-facial-buccal movements in the elderly. Pathophysiology and treatment. J Am Geriatr Soc. 1973;21:314-17.
41. Lauterbach EC, Shillcutt SD. Dyskinesia with fluoxetine: tardive or late-onset persistent, acute norfluoxetine dyskinesia? J Clin Psychiatry. 1997;58:85-6.
42. Fabbrini G, Brotchine JM, Grandas F, et al. Levodopa induced dyskinesias. Mov Disord. 2007;22:1379-89. quiz 532.
43. Jankovic J. Motor fluctuations and dyskinesias in Parkinson's disease. Clinical manifestations. Mov Disord. 2005;20(Suppl 11):S11-16.
44. Vidailhet M, Bonnet AM, Marconi R, et al. The phenomenology of L-dopa induced dyskinesias in Parkinson's disease. Mov Disord. 1999;14(Suppl 1):13-8.
45. Bhidayasiri R, Trougn DD. Motor complications in Parkinson disease: clinical manifestations and management. J Neurol Sic. 2008:266:204-15.
46. Koller WC. Edentulous orodyskinesia. Ann Neuroli. 1983;13:97-9.
47. Blancher PJ, Popovici R, Guitard F, et al. Pain and denture condition in edentulous orodyskinesia comparisons with tardive dyskinesia and control subjects. Mov Disord. 2008;23:1837-42.
48. Chou KL, Friedman JH. Tardive syndromes in the elderly. Clin Geriat Med. 2006;22:915-33. Viii.
49. Saltz BL, Kane JM, Woerner MG, et al. Prospective study of tardive dyskinesia in the elderly. Psychopharmacol Bull. 1989;25:52-6.
50. Kane JM, Woerner M, Lieberman J. Tardive dyskinesia: prevalence, incidence, and risk factors. J Clin Psychopharmacol. 1988;8(4 suppl):52S-6s.
51. Gardos G, Cole JO, Rapkin RM, et al. Anticholinergic challenge and neuroleptic withdrawal changes in dyskinesia and symptom measues. Arch Gen Psychiatry. 1984;41:1030-5.
52. Eberhard J, Lindstrom E, Levander S. Tardive dyskinesia and antipsychotics: a 5-year longitudinal study of frequency, correlates and course. Int Clin Psychopharmacol. 2006;21:35-42.
53. Margolese HC, Chouinard G, Kolivakis TT, et al. Tardive dyskinesia in the era of typical and atypical antipsychotics. Par 1: pathophysiology and mechanisms of indication. Can J Psychiatry. 2005;50:541-7.
54. Silverstri S, Seeman MV, Negrete JC, et al. Increased dopamine D2 receptor binding after long-term treatment with antipsychotics in humans: a clinical PET study. Psychopharmacology (Berl). 2000;152:174-80.
55. Miller R, Chouinard G. Loss of striatal cholinergic neurons as a basis for tardive and L-dopa-induced dyskinesias, neuroleptic-induced supersensitivity psychosis and refractory schizophrenia. Biol Psychiatry. 1993;34:713-38.
56. Sachdev PS. The current status of tardive dyskinesia. Aust N Z J Psychiatry. 2000;34:355-69.
57. Glazer WM, Morgenstern H, Schooler N, et al. Predictors of improvement in tardive dyskinesia following discontinuation of neuroleptic medication. Br J Psychiatry. 1990;157:585-92.
58. Dalack GW, Becks L, Meador-Woodruff JH. Tardive dyskinesia, colzapine, and treatment response. Frog Neuropsychopharmacol Biol Psychiatry. 1998;22:567-73.
59. Modestin J, Stephan PL, Erni T, et al. Prevalence of extrapyramidal syndromes in psychiatric inpatients and the relationship of clozapine treatment to tardive dyskinesia. Schizophr Res. 2000;42;223-30.
60. Bassitt DP, Louza Neto MR. Clozapine efficacy in tardive dyskinesia in schizophrenic patients. Eur Arch Psychiatry Clin Neurosic. 1998;248:209-11.
61. Vesely C, Kufferie B, Brucke T, et al. Remission of severe tardive dyskinesia in a schizophrenic patient treated with the atypical antipsychotic substance quetiapine. Int Clin Psychopharmacol. 2000;15:57-60.
62. Soutullo CA, Keck PE Jr, McElroy SL. Olanzapine in the treatment of tardive dyskinesia; a report of two cases. J Clin Psychopharmacol. 1999;19:100-1.
63. Kane JM, Woerner MG, Pollack S, et al. Does clozapine cause tardive dyskinesia? J Clin Psychiatry. 1993;54:327-30.
64. Chouinard G. Effects of resperidone in tardive dyskinesia: an analysis of the Canadian multicenter nsperidone study. J Clin Psychopharmacol. 1995;15(1 Suppl 1):36S-44S.
65. Factor SA, Friedman JH. The emerging role of clozapine in the treatment of movement disorders. Mov Disord. 1997;12:483-96.

66. Simpson GM, Lee JH, Shrivastava RK. Colzapine in tardive dyskinesia. Br J Psychiatry. 1991;158:503-10.
67. Small JG, Milstein V, Marhenke JD, et al. Treatment outcome with colzapine in tardive dyskinesia, neuroleptic sensitivity, and treatment-resistant psychosis. J Clin Psychiatry. 1987;48:263-7.
68. Meltzer HY, Luchins DJ. Effect of clozapine in severe tardive dyskinesia: a case report. J Clin Psychopharmacol. 1984;4: 286-7.
69. Van Putten T, Wirshing WC, Marder SR. Tardive Meige syndrome responsive to clozacine. J Clin Psychopharmacol. 1990;10:381-2.
70. Trugman JM, Leadbetter R, Zalis ME, et al. Treatment of severe axial tardive dystonia with clozapine; Case report and hypothesis. Mov Disord. 1994;9:441-6.
71. Simpson GM. The treatment of tardive dyskinesia and tardive dystonia. J Clin Psychiatry. 2000;61(Suppl 4):39-44.
72. Soares KV. Mc Grath JJ. The treatment of tardive dyskinesia—a systematic review and meta-analysis. Schizophar Res. 1999;39: 11-16; discussion 7-8.
73. Egan MF, Apud J, Wyatt RJ. Treatment of tardive dyskinesia. Scrizoper Bull. 1997;23:583-609.
74. Bhidayasiri R, Tarsy D. Treatment of dystonia. Bpert Rev Neurotner. 2006;6:863-86.
75. Ondo WG, Hanna PA, Jankovic J. Tetrabenazine treatment for tarive dyskinesia: assessment by randomized videotape protocol. Am J Psychiatry. 1999;156:1279-81.
76. Lieberman J, Pollack S, Lesser M, et al. Pharmacologic characterization of tardive dyskinesia. J Clin Psychopharmacol. 1988;8:254-60.
77. Yagi G, Takamiya M, Kanba S, et al. Mortality rate of schizophrenic patients with tardive dyskinesia during 10 years: a controlled study. Kero J Med. 1989;38:70-2.
78. Lzumi K, Tominaga H, Koja T, et al. Mechofenotate therapy in tardive dyskinesia: a preliminary report. Biol Psychiatry. 1986; 21:151-60.
79. Bergman J, Dwolatzky T, Brettholz I, et al. Beneficial effect of donepezil in the treatment of elderly patients with tardive movement disorders. J Clin Psychiatry. 2005;66:107-10.
80. Caroff SN, Campbell EC, Havey JC. et al. Treatment of tardive dyskinesia with donepezil. J Clin Psychiatry. 2001;62: 128-9.
81. Schopick D. Donepezil and tardive dyskinesia. J Am Acad Child Adolescent Psychiatry. 2005;44:112.
82. Soares KV, McGrath JJ, Deeks JJ. Gamma-amnobutync acid agonsis for neuroleptic-induced tardive dyskinesia. Cochrance Database Syst Rev. 2001;(2):CD000203.
83. Thaker GK, Nguyen JA, Strauss ME, et al. Clonazepam treatment of tardive dyskinesia: a practical GABAmimetic strategy. Am J Psychiatry. 1990;147:445-51.
84. Singh MM, Becker RE, Pitman RK, et al. Sustained improvement of tardive dyskinesia with diazepam: indirect evidence for corticolimbic involvement. Bull. 1983;11:179-85.
85. Stewart RM, Rollins J, Beckham B, et al. Baclofen in tardive dyskinesia patients maintained on neuroleptics. Clin Neuropharmacol. 1982;5:365-73.
86. Gerlach J, Rye T, Kristjansen P. Effect of baclofen on tardive dyskinesia. Psychopharmacology (Berl). 1978;56:145-51.
87. Brashear A, Ambrosius WT, Eckert GJ, et al. Comparison of treatment of tardive dystonia and idiopathic cervical dystonia with botullnumtoxin type A. Mov Disord. 1998;13:158-61.
88. Tarsy D, Daufman D, Sethi KD, et al. An open-label study of botulinum toxin A for treatment of tardive dystonia. Clin Neuropharmacol. 1997;20:90-3.
89. Chatterjee A, Forrest Gordon M, Giladi N, et al. Botulinum toxin in the treatment of tardive dystonia. J Clin Psychopharmcol. 1997;17:497-8.
90. Jankovic J, Brin MF. Therapeutic uses of botulinum toxin. N Engl J Med. 1991;324:1186-94.
91. Egan MF, Hyde TM, Albers GW, et al. Treatment of tardive dyskinesia with vitamin E. Am J Psychiatry. 1992;149:773-7.
92. Adler LA, Peselow E, Rotrosen J, et al. Vitamin E treatment of tardive dyskinesia. Am J Psychiatry. 1993;150:1405-7.
93. Adler LA, Rotrosen J, Edson R, et al. Vitamin E treatment for tardive dyskinesia Veterans Affairs Cooperative Study #394 Study Group. Arch Gen Psychiatry. 1999;56:836-41.
94. Gruber D, Trottenberg T, Kivi A, et al. Long-term effects of pallidal deep brain stimulation in tardive dystonia. Neurology. 20009;73:53-8.
95. Trottenberg T, Volkmann J, Deuschl G, et al. Treatment of severe tardive dystonia with pallidal deep brain stimulation. Neurology. 2005;64:344-6.
96. Elthawy HA, Feinstein A, Khan F, et al. Bilateral globus pallidus internus deep brain stimulation in tardive dyskinesia: a case report. Mov Disord. 2004;19:969-72.
97. Damier P, Thobois S, Witjas T, et al. Bilateral deep brain stimulation of the globus pallidus to treat tardive dyskinesia. Arch Gen Psychiatry. 2007;64:170-6.

CHAPTER

75

Tourette's Syndrome and Other Tic Disorder

Ashok Singal

In 1885, Gilles de la Tourette (under the tutelage of Charcot at the Salpetriere in Paris, described the syndrome of tics, echolalia and coprolalia, initially in nine patients (not all of whom he had met). The same syndrome had in fact been previously described by Armand Trousseau 20 years earlier, but for some reason his description never caught on. Interest in this syndrome in Paris was heightened by contemporary descriptions of some culturally determined startle syndromes (Latah, myriachit and the "jumping Frenchmen of Maine"), all characterized by echolalia, coprolalia and automatic obedience in response to startling stimuli.[1] However, Tourette noted that the behaviors of his patients could occur without a clear stimulus.

During most of the last part of the 19th century and the first 60 years of the 20th century, psychoanalytical explanations for tics were in vogue; they appeared to many clinicians of the time as a 'breakthrough' of suppressed feelings, thoughts and behaviors. However, in 1961, Seignot reported the first successful treatment of Tourette's syndrome with haloperidol in a single case and this was followed by an explosion in biological research into the causes of the syndrome.[2] The familial and genetic aspects of Tourette's syndrome were documented over the next few years although a single gene association looks unlikely. Epidemiological studies have now suggested that Tourette's syndrome, as it is currently defined, is common in children, although often mildly expressed.[3] Associated problems with attention, concentration, obsessionality and mood changes are also frequently described. Of these, the obsessional and compulsive problems seem to be the most closely related to tics in terms of their phenomenology and etiology. Finally, research into autoimmune mechanisms has renewed interest in the relationship between Tourette's syndrome and Sydenham's chorea (St. Vitus' dance).[4]

CLINICAL FEATURES OF TICS

Tics are stereotyped movements which are jerky or dystonic. They are the clinical phenomena that form the core of Tourette's syndrome. Just before the tics, there is often a premonitory sensation—an itchy, tense or tight feeling around the area of the tics, or a mental feeling- internal tension, a desire to tic only relieved by performing the tic. The tics can be suppressed but at the expense of rising internal tension. The tic itself often brings relief from the tension while attempted tic suppression can lead to a 'rebound', when the tick is finally released, it may be more frequent and severe. Sometimes tic-like movements can be entirely voluntary, in order to reduced the premonitory sensations. Tics may be motor or phonic. They tend to occur in clusters or bouts. They can be simple (eye blinks) or complex (squatting, jumping or twirling). Diagnosis of tics in children is more difficult than in adults as premonitory sensations are harder to elicit (either they are not experienced or children find them difficult to describe).

Table 1 illustrates the main clinical phenomena which distinguish tics from the other forms of motor disorder:

- Tics can be confused with myoclonus, but this is a faster movement (which can be measured

Table 1: Features of tics compared with some other types of motor disorders

	Premonitory sensation	*Suppressible*	*Unidirectional*	*Sudden*	*Rhythmic*
Tics	+	+	+	+	–
Myoclonus	–	–	+	++	±
Dystonia	±	–	+	–	–
Chorea	–	–	+	+	–
Akathisia	+	+	±	–	±
Tremor	–	–	–	–	+

electrophysiologically), can be rhythmic and is experienced with no sensory phenomena.

- Patients may experience tics similarly to akathisia (i.e. as an urge that has to be satisfied).
- Stereotypies, often seen in patients with autism, are usually bidirectional (e.g. rocking or hand flapping) and prolonged, and do not have the same level of premonitory urge. It may be that stereotypies represent a comforting behavior which is chosen by the patient.

DSM-5 Diagnostic Criteria for Tourette's Disorder[23]
Both multiple motor and one or more vocal tics have been present at some time during the illness, although not necessarily concurrently.
The tics may wax and wane in frequency but have persisted for more than 1 year since first tic onset.
Onset is before age of 18 years
The disturbance is not attributable to the physiological effects of substance (e.g. Cocaine) or another medical condition (e.g. Huntington's disease, postviral encephalitis).

EPIDEMIOLOGY OF TIC DISORDERS

Epidemiological studies have been hampered by the lack of any external validators, by a phenotype which is on a spectrum with normal behavior, and by ascertainment bias in most of the early studies on clinic or hospital populations. Rutter's[5] 1970 study of psychiatric disorders on the Isle of Wight suggested a prevalence of tic disorders (including transient tics, chronic tic disorders of either motor or vocal type and Tourette's syndrome) of around 4% in school-aged children but clear diagnostic criteria were not used. A prevalence of 0.1% for Tourette's syndrome was found in Israeia army conscripts but some may have grown out of tics by 17 years of age and others may have disguised them in order to be conscripted.[6] A study in a mainstream school in Essex using observation and clinical examination showed a prevalence of Tourette's syndrome of nearly 3% (5 out of 167 pupils); all were mild and had not sought medical attention.[7] A number of recent community based epidemiological studies (in Sweden, Taiwan, China and USA) have indicated a prevalence of Tourette's syndrome of between 0.5% and 1% in school aged children.[3] Thus in a school of 400 children, between two and four might meet the diagnostic criteria for Tourette's syndrome, half of whom with symptoms which impair function.

DIAGNOSTIC CRITERIA OF TOURETTE'S SYNDROME

The Diagnostic and Statistical Manual, fourth edition (DSM-IV), criteria currently defining the syndrome are as follows:

- Multiple motor and one or more phonic tics
- Onset before 18 years of age
- Symptoms present for 1 year at least
- Not due to detectable neurological disorder or substance abuse.

The definition includes non-mandatory characteristics:

- Tics occur many times a day in bouts
- Tics tend to 'wax and wane', changing frequency, severity, type and location over time.

There has been argument about whether to include the idea of 'significant impairment of function' in the diagnosis, as there are many people who fulfill the current criteria but do not have any impairment of function. Many clinicians want to include impairment in the diagnostic criteria but researchers (especially geneticists) do not because to do so may cloud the search for the phenotype which most accurately reflects any underlying genetic markers. Including the 'significant impairment' criterion halves the recorded prevalence of Tourette's syndrome.

ASSOCIATED PHENOMENA

Coprolalia (swearing vocalizations as a tic) and copropraxia (swearing gestures as a tic) are the symptoms that the general public most commonly associate with Tourette's syndrome. Swearing outbursts and gestures are experience as irresistible urges but are socially, grammatically and affectively non-contextual. Patients may commonly swear between spoken sentences and attempt to disguise words and gestures (particularly changing the ends of words to make them more acceptable or disguising the word within a cough). Other patients have disguised copropraxia by turning it into a grooming behavior such as brushing their hair back. In fact, coprophenomena are seen in less than 30% of patients with tourette's attending specialist clinics.

Echophenomena are present in roughly the same proportion of patients as coprophenomena. Echolalia and echopraxia are the copying of others' speech or behavior. Echophenomena commonly also occur in autism and have been reported in dementia and following brain injury. Palilalia (rapid repetition of a word or phrase) and palipraxia (rapid repetition of an action) also occur in around 20% of clinic populations with Tourette's syndrome.

CLINICAL COURSE OF TOURETTE'S SYNDROME

The typical age of onset is between 6 years and 8 years with tics starting in the head and neck regions. Tics tend to become more complex with time. The average for the most severe tics is between 10 years and 12 years, with tics tending to improve in late adolescence or early adulthood. Moreover, in adulthood, the repertorie of tics tends to narrow and become more stable.[8] Recent follow-up studies comparing videotaped interviews of adults indicate that most people with Tourette's syndrome still do have tics even if they are not aware of them. There have been few prospective studies looking at the factors that might determine eventual remission, or whether the symptoms persist into adulthood. Poor prognosis for Tourette's syndrome in these studies was associated with tics below the head and shoulders,and with coprolalia. Poor social outcome is related to any associated problems, such as attention deficit hyperactivity disorder (ADHD).

DIFFERENTIAL DIAGNOSIS

The current classification distinguishes idiopathic tic disorders from neurological disorders in which tics are a symptom. The idiopathic tic disorders in DSM-IV are divided into:

- Transient tic disorders (lasting less than 1 year)
- Chronic multiple tics (motor or phonic but not both)
- Tourette's syndrome (onset before 18 years, motor and phonic tics, no other neurological explanation)
- Tic disorders not otherwise specified (e.g. a syndrome identical to Tourette's but onset over 18 years of age).

These distinctions do not have a clear basis in epidemiology or pathology, and the categories are open to a number of criticisms. For instance, 'transient tic disorder' can only be diagnosed when it has ceased, which diminishes its validity. One criticism of the Tourette's category, also leveled at other apparently idiopathic disorders, is that when a cause is found for some people with the syndrome (for instance, acanthocytosis or drug intoxication), they automatically cases to have it-by definition (Flow chart 1).

More recent factor analytical studies[9] have suggested reclassification along the following lines, for adults as well as children:

- Tourette's syndrome simplex (justics)
- Tourette's syndrome complex (tics plus echo-, pail-or coprophenomena)
- Tourette's syndrome plus comorbid conditions such as ADHD or autistic spectrum disorders.

Further advances in brain research will inevitably lead to a reclassification of tic disorders to more accurately reflect their biology.

OTHER CONDITIONS THAT MAY INCLUDE TICS AS A SYMPTOM

There are many other disorders of childhood and adulthood which have tics as a symptom.

- Acanthocytosis
- Drug intoxication or withdrawal (including cocaine and amphetamine)
- Lesch-Nyhan Syndrome
- Huntington's disease
- Wilson's disease
- Homocystinuria
- Tardive tics due to neuroleptics
- Cerebrovascular disease (stroke and vascular dementia)
- Cerebral palsy.

It is also possible that tics may exist as part of conversion or factitious disorders.

In most cases, the diagnosis of Tourette's syndrome can be made without extensive investigations. Factors in the history or examination which should trigger further investigation include:

- Intellectual impairment or developmental delay
- Onset of symptoms in adulthood or late life

Flow chart 1: Diagnosis of tic disorders NOS, not otherwise specified[13]

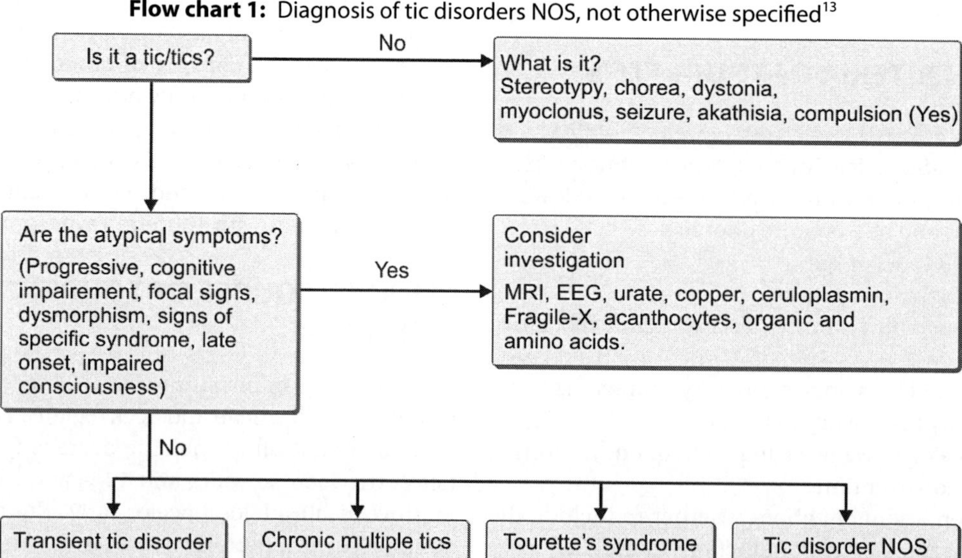

Note: Flow chart for the diagnosis and investigation of tic disorders, after which sub-classification can then be made into transient tic disorder, chronic multiple tics (motor or vocal tics but not both), Tourette's syndrome or Tourette's syndrome not otherwise specified

- Presence of myoclonus
- Progressive (rather than 'waxing and waning') course
- Impaired consciousness
- No 'sensory' symptoms
- Fixed or task specific dystonias such as writer's cramp
- Focal neurological signs
- Specific dysmorphic features (e.g. indicating fragile X or Down's syndrome)
- Short-lived period of motor disorder with long symptom free periods (could be drug intoxication).

COMORBIDITY IN TOURETTE'S SYNDROME

Studies of comorbidity are again hampered by the problem of ascertainment bias because most have been conducted in clinic settings. Clearly, both obsessive-compulsive behaviors and obsessive-compulsive disorder (OCD) are very common in Tourette's syndrome and share many clinical characteristics with tics. Both tics and compulsions are phenomena which a person feels compelled to perform, and which can be resisted at the expense of rising internal tension. Performance of both compulsions and tics lead to relief tension. May be compulsions are just more complex, more goal-directed tics. Self injurious behaviors are seen in a third clinic patients with Tourette's syndrome and they have compulsive (and sometimes symmetrical) nature:[10]

- A middle-aged man with long-standing Tourette's had a compulsion to burn his philtrum with his cigarette just after he had lit it.
- A young women with Tourette's had a compulsion to cut into her forearm (along the arm, rather than across it) and then to copy the cut exactly on the other forearm.

Interestingly, studies from the veterinary world (especially of horses) show similar patterns of tick-like and self-injurious behaviors. Attention deficit problems are also very common in Tourette's syndrome and may affect around 40% of children, at least of those attending clinics. However, some of these attentional problems may be caused by tic suppression, obsessional rumination, medications, depression or anxiety so-called 'pseudo ADH'. The recent community based epidemiological studies have, however, shown a true comorbidity with ADHD (not due to ascertainment bias or 'pseudo-ADHD').[11]

Finally, both depression and anxiety are common in people with Tourette's syndrome.

ETIOLOGY OF TOURETTE'S SYNDROME

Tics probably represent a final common pathway of a variety of developmental problems, but the etiology of Tourette's syndrome is unknown.

- Family studies show that it is to a large extent heritable alongside an early onset form of OCD; large family pedigree studies have indicated that these two disorders cluster together but the most common form of ADHD does not share genetic factors with Tourette's syndrome.[12] The largest genome-wide association study of Tourette's to date showed linkage to chromosome 2p23.2 with a lod score of 3.8 but this needs replication.[12]
- Imaging has shown changes in basal ganglia volumes and symmetries but no clear reliable abnormality.[13]
- Neuropsychological studies have shown executive function to be relatively intact but possible difficulties with implicit memory and social cognition.[14]
- Perinatal events appear to confer extra risk but are neither necessary nor sufficient for the diagnosis.
- Recent research, following the autoimmune ideas around Sydenham's chorea, has shown that people with Tourette's syndrome also have a high prevalence of antibasal ganglia antibodies, but on average every child has eight streptococcal infections and so demonstrating that this infection really is the pathological agent could be difficult. Furthermore, the technique used to measure antibasal ganglia antibodies may not be specific. Nonetheless, some centers are already using prophylactic penicillin, and trials are taking place on immune modulating therapies, with limited success so far.[15]

In conclusion, Tourette's syndrome may be the end result of a variety of abnormal brain processes but in truth the cause remains unknown.

MANAGEMENT OF TOURETTE'S SYNDROME

General Approach

Management should be holistic and factor in the quality of life of the patient and family-tics do not kill people and the syndrome is not degenerative. Most disability is social. Indeed, people with Tourette's have been quoted as saying, "If everyone had Tourette's syndrome, their would be something called "Quiet syndrome" and "I do not have Tourette's syndrome, you have intolerance syndrome". Education of the patient and family about the disorder is vital, including genetic counseling where appropriate. Close liaison with schools is important from the point of view of educating teachers about Tourette's syndrome and monitoring progress. Statements of special educational needs may be necessary. Any further treatment should be focused on the symptoms that most impair quality of life, development of learning. These may not necessarily be the tics.

Psychological Treatment

There are a number of useful psychological treatments which can be used to manage tics; currently the most common is habit reversal. This is based on the ideal that performance of the tic leads to relief and that this relief forms a reward which reinforces the behavior (which is a tic). Patients are asked to perform a competing response (for instance, if the tic is a head shake, they are asked to put their chin on their chest). The internal tension will initially rise but after a while will usually diminish. Three well designed clinical trials now support these habit reversal techniques, and there are very few adverse effects.[16]

Drug Treatments

For most people, Tourette's syndrome is a relatively self-limiting disorder and any medication should be used sparingly. Adverse effects can often impair mood, concentration and learning.

- Randomized controlled trials (RCTs) support the use of risperidone and pimozide (pimozide can affect the QT interval and there is one report of a death when it was prescribed alongside a macrolide antibiotic and led to an arrhythmia).
- One RCT supports the use of haloperidol but another demonstrates no difference between haloperidol and placebo. Most of the reports of tardive dyskinesia in Tourette's syndrome have been in relation to haloperidol, so it is definitely not for first line use.
- Sulpiride has been extensively used but there are no supporting RCTs (just one large open label study).
- Clonidine has been used in children with Tourette's syndrome and ADHD but there is no evidence for efficacy.
- Aripiprazole, a new atypical neuroleptic, has shown initial promise in the treatment of tics.
- There are some data supporting tetrabenazine in a range of hyperkinetic motor disorders but psychiatric adverse effects can be problematic.[17]

There has been controversy about whether stimulants used to treat ADHD (such as methylphenidate) make tics worse. The most recent evidence from a US Tourette's Syndrome Study group trial is that they do not. This finding needs replication.[18]

There is very little research on the treatment of OCD in the setting of Tourette's syndrome. The consensus favors treatment with selective serotonin reuptake inhibitors such as sertraline (sometimes at the upper end or the dose range) in conjunction with cognitive behavioral treatment (such as exposure and response prevention).

Botulinum Toxin

Botulinum toxin has been used to good effect in individual tics. The toxin can be injected directly into the muscle group involved in the tic. It appears to reduced premonitory sensations as well as the tics themselves. A number of cases have been reported of successful use of botulinum injections into the laryngeal muscles to minimize coprolalia.[19]

Surgery

Deep brain stimulation has now been reported in around 60 cases of severe Tourette's syndrome. The rationale is sketchy and controlled trials are infrequent.[20] The largest number of cases have had electrode implants in the ventro-oralis nucleus of the thalamus,[21] and there are approximately eight reported cases of successful implantation in the globus pallidus interna (both the 'traditional' posterior target and a more anterior 'limbic' target in some).[22] In general, results are good with few adverse effects but controlled trials are urgently needed. One emerging problem is electrode 'twiddling' as a compulsion, and this can break the leads.

REFERENCES

1. Rickards H, Woolf I, Cavanna AE. "Trousseau's disease": A description of the Gilles de la Tourette syndrome 12 years before 1885. Mov Disord. 2010 (in press).
2. Rickards EHG, Hartley NM, Robertson MM. Seignot's original paper on the treatment of Gilles de la. Tourette syndrome with haloperidol. Hist Psychiatry. 1997;vii:433-6.
3. Robertson MM. The prevalence and epidemiology of Gilles de la Tourette syndrome: Part 1: The epidemiological and prevalence studies. J Psychosom Res. 2008;65:461-72.
4. Leckman JF, Cohen, DJ, Goetz CG, et al. Tourette syndrome: pieces of the puzzle. Adv Neurol. 2001;85:369-90.
5. Rutter M, Tizard J, Yule W, et al. Isle of Wight studies 1964–1974. Psychol Med. 1976;6:313-32.
6. Apter A, Pauls DL, Bleich A, et al. An epidemiologic study of Gilles de la Tourette's syndrome in Israel. Arch Gen Psychiatry. 1993;50:734-8.
7. Mason A. Bannerjee S, Eapen V, et al. The prevalence of Tourette syndrome in a mainstream school population. J Dev Med Child Neurol. 2008;40:292-6.
8. Bloch MH, Leckman JF. Clinical course of Tourette syndrome. J Psychosom Res. 2009;67:97-501.
9. Robertson MM, Althoff RR, Hafez A, et al. Principal component analysis of a large cohort with Tourette syndrome. Br J Psychiatry. 2008;193:31-6.
10. Cavanna AE, Servo S, Monaco F, et al. The behavioural spectrum of Gilles de la Tourette syndrome. J Neuropsychiatry Clin Neurosci. 2003;21:13-23.
11. Khalifa N, VonKnorring AL. Psychopathology in a Swedist population of school children with tic disorders. J Am Acad Child Address Psychiatry. 2006;45:1346-53.
12. O'Rourke JA, Scharf JM, Yu D, et al. The genetics of Tourette syndrome: a review. J Psychosom Res. 2009;67: 533-45.
13. Peterson BS, Thomas P, Kane MJ, et al. Basal Ganglia volumes in patients with Gilles de al Tourette syndrome. Arch Gen Psychiatry. 2003;60:415-24.
14. Cavanna AE, Eday C, Rickards HE. Cognitive functioning in Tourette syndrome. Discov Med. 2009;8:191-5.

15. Martino D, Defazio G, Giovannon G. The PANDAS subgroup of tic disorders and childhood-onset obsessive-compulsive disorder. J Psychonsom Res. 2009;67: 547-57.
16. Piacentini J, Woods DW, Seahill L, et al. Behaviour therapy for children with Tourette disorder: a randomized controlled trail JAMA. 2010;303:1929-37.
17. Scahill L, Erenberg G, Berlin CM Jr, et al. Contemporary assessment and pharmacotherapy of Tourette syndrome. NeuroRx. 2006;3:192-206.
18. Kurlan R. Tourette's syndrome: are stimulants safe? Curr Neurol Neurosic Rep. 2003;3:285-8.
19. Scott BL, Jankovic J, Donovan DT. Botulinum toxin injection into vocal cord in the treatment of malignant coprolalia associated with Tourette's syndrome. Mov Disord. 1996;11: 431-3.
20. Maciunas RJ, Maddux BN, Riley DE, et al. Prospective randomized double biind trail of bilateral thalamic deep brain stimulation in adults with Tourette syndrome. J Neurosurg. 2007;107:1004-14.
21. Porta M, Sassi M, Ail F, et al. Neurosurgical treatment for Gilles de la Tourette syndrome the Italian prespective. J Psychosom Res. 2009;67:585-90.
22. Welter ML, Mallet L, Houeto JL, et al. Internal pallidal and thalamic stimulation in patients with Tourette syndrome. Arch Neurol. 2008;65:952-7.
23. American Psychiatric Association. Desk Reference to the Diagnostic Criteria from DSM-5. Washington DC. 2013.

CHAPTER 76

Gambling Disorder

JN Vyas

INTRODUCTION

Gambling in one form or another has probably pervaded every culture-archeologists have uncovered primitive dice made from the knucklebones of sheep (astralagi) in caves dating from 3500 BCE.[1] Gambling activities range from informal games of chance (e.g. sports betting) to formalized and legal options, such as destination report casinos and highly developed online gaming environments. Most recently, such legalised gambling is increasing in unprecedented amounts throughout the world. Even countries that do not offer gambling to its citizens for religious or cultural reasons sometimes allow the operation of casinos for foreign visitors (e.g. Malaysia, China, and South Korea). The desire and willingness to wager money or other items of value on randomly established outcomes seems universal. Although most individuals participate in gambling as an enjoyable social activity, a small group of people become too seriously involved in terms of time invested and money wagered and they continue to gamble despite substantial and negative personal, social, family, and financial effects.

DIAGNOSIS AND EVALUATION

Diagnostic Criteria, Classification, and Prevalence

Two categories of gambling disorders are salient in published work; pathological gambling and problem gambling. Pathological gambling is medically defined, with diagnostic criteria described in both the Diagnostic and Statistical Manual of Mental Disorders, 4th edition, text revision (DSM-IV-TR)[2] and International Classification of Diseases, 10th revision (ICD-10)[3] (Panel 1).

Both classification systems summarize pathological gambling from an atheoretical perspective (i.e. they list only objective and behavioral diagnostic criteria), and both classify pathological gambling within an impulse disorder section. The predominant diagnostic system of the two, however, is the DSM-IV concept of pathological gambling.[4] Although several popular diagnostic instruments have been based on criteria from DSM-IV or earlier versions, there is little research examining the reliability, validity, and classification accuracy of the criteria.[5] The American Psychiatric Association is in the process of evaluating how pathological gambling might be classified in the fifth edition of DSM.[6-9]

The informally defined category of problem gambling is often reported in prevalence surveys and is typically seen as a less severe form of gambling disorder. Although this category is not included in either DSM-IV or ICD-10, it has been referenced extensively among several diagnostic instruments.

Prevalence rates for pathological and problem gambling form national surveys vary worldwide. For example, past 12-month rates of problem gambling range from 0.2% in Norway to 5.3% in Hong Kong.[10] Reported rates of pathological gambling in the USA range from 0.4% to 1.1% of adults, with an additional 1.2% identified as problem gamblers.[11] Data from prevalence surveys indicate variability in rates of gambling disorders not only from difference in survey methods-such as the use of different screening techniques, timeframes (e.g. reported past year problems, lifetime problems), administration format, and response rates[12]—but also as a result of variability associated with the availability and accessibility of national prevalence rates are stable over time despite an increase in gambling opportunities,[10,14] suggesting that some type of social adaptation might take place as gambling becomes less novel in a local environment.[15]

Screening and Assessment Instruments

A range of self-report and interview assessment methods have been developed for both community and clinical populations.[5,16] The most well-known screening instrument is the South Oaks Gambling Screen (SOGS)[17] which was based on DSM-III criteria.[18] This assessment has been translated into several languages and can be administered in either self-report or interview format. The original test assessed lifetime pathological gambling, although parallel past-year

Panel 1: Criteria for diagnosis of pathological gambling, according to DSM-IV-TR and ICD-10

DSM-IV-TR criteria[2]

A Persistent and recurrent maladaptive gambling behavior is indicated if the individual has five (or more) of the following:
1. Is preoccupied with gambling?
2. Needs to gamble with increasing amount of money.
3. Has repeated unsuccessful efforts to control, cut back, or stop gambling?
4. Is restless or irritable when attempting to cut down or stop gambling?
5. Gambles as a way of escaping from problems or of relieving a dysphonic mood.
6. After losing money gambling, often returns another day to get even (i.e. "chasing one's losses").
7. Lies to conceal the extent of involvement with gambling
8 Has committed illegal acts to finance gambling?
9. Has jeopardized or lost an important relationship, job, or educational or career opportunity because of gambling?
10. Relies on others to provide money to relieve a desperate financial situation caused by gambling.

B The gambling behavior is not better accounted for by a manic episode

ICD-10 criteria[3]

A Individuals have frequent and repeated episodes of gambling despite adverse consequences.
B Individuals put their jobs at risk, acquire large debts, and line or break the law.
C Individuals have intense urges to gamble, which are difficult to control.
D Individuals have preoccupation with ideas and images of the act of gambling.
E Should be distinguished from gambling and betting (frequent gambling for excitement or in an attempt to make money), excessive gambling by manic patients, and gambling by sociopathic personalities.

DSM-5 Diagnostic criteria for gambling disorder[120] 312.31 (F63.0)

A. Persistent and recurrent problematic gambling behavior leading to clinically significant impairment of distress, as indicated by the individual exhibiting four (or more) of the following in a 12-month period:
1. Needs to gamble with increasing amounts of money in order to achieve the desired excitement.
2. Is restless or irritable when attempting to cut down or stop gambling?
3. Has made repeated unsuccessful efforts to control, cut back, or stop gambling?
4. Is often preoccupied with gambling (e.g. having persistent thoughts of relieving past gambling experiences, handicapping or planning the next venture, thinking of ways to get money with which to gamble)?
5. Often gambles when feeling distressed (e.g. helpless, guilty, anxious, depressed).
6. After losing money gambling, often returns another day to get even ("chasing" one's losses).
7. Lies to conceal the extent of involvement with gambling.
8. Has jeopardized or lost a significant relationship, job, or educational or career opportunity because of gambling?
9. Relies on others to provide money to relieve desperate financial situations caused by gambling.

B. The gambling behavior is not better explained by a manic episode.

Specify if:
Episodic: Meeting diagnostic criteria at more than one time point, with symptoms subsiding between periods of gambling disorder for at least several months.

Persistent: Experiencing continuous symptoms, to meet diagnostic criteria for multiple years

Specify if:
In early remission: After full criteria for gambling disorder were previously met, none of the criteria for gambling disorder have been met for at least 3 months but for less than 12 months.

In sustained remission: After full criteria for gambling disorder were previously met, none of the criteria for gambling disorder have been met during a period of 12 months or longer.

Specify current severity:
Mild: 4–5 criteria met
Moderate: 6–7 criteria met
Severe: 8–9 criteria met

and past-3 month versions were subsequently developed.[19,20] The past-year self-report version has indicated good overall classification accuracy (0.96), with better sensitivity (0.99) than specificity (0.75),[21] indicating that SOGS tends to more often identify false positives.

A briefer screening technique is nine-item problem gambling severity index. (A subscale of the Canadian Problem Severity Index).[22] This index assesses low-risk, moderated-risk, and problem gambling within the past year (Panel 2), has been used as a clinical screening instrument, and is increasingly used in prevalence surveys around the world (e.g. Australia, Denmark, Iceland, South Africa, and the UK). The classification accuracy of the problem gambling category has had adequate sensitivity (0.83) and excellent specificity (1.0) with use of DSM-IV classification as the criterion.[22]

A third screening instrument is the 17-item National Opinion Research Center DSM-IV Screen for Gambling Problems (NODS), which was originally developed for a US national gambling telephone survey and was based on past-year and lifetime DSM-IV diagnostic criteria for pathological gambling.[23] The total score is used to identify pathological gambling, and lower cutoffs indicated low-risk and problem gamblers. Positive psychometric information is available, although more data are needed to confirm the validity of the cutoffs in both clinical and nonclinical population.[20,23-25] A three-item short version of NODS, NODS CLiP,[11] has bad excellent sensitivity (0.94) and specificity (0.96) in US

Panel 2: Problem gambling severity index

1. Thinking about the past 12 months, have you bet more than you could really afford to lose?
2. Still thinking about the past 12 months, have you needed to gamble with larger amounts of money to get the same feeling of excitement?
3. When you gambled, did you go back another day to try to win back the money you lost?
4. Have you borrowed money or sold anything to get money to gamble?
5. Have you felt that you might have a problem with gambling?
6. Has gambling caused you any health problems, including stress or anxiety?
7. Have people criticized your betting or told you that you had a gambling problem, regardless of whether or not you through it was true?
8. Has your gambling caused any financial problems for you or your household?
9. Have you felt guilty about the way you gamble or what happens when you gamble?

Scores for the nine items are summed (never = 0; sometime = 1; most of the time = 2; almost always = 3), and the results are interpreted as follows: 0 = no problem gambling; 1–2 = low level of problems with few or no identified negative consequences: 3–7 = moderate level of problems, leading to some negative consequences; ≥ 8 = problem gambling with negative consequences and a possible loss of control.

community samples, whereas NODS CLiP provides screening for lifetime problems, a three-item Brief Biosocial Gambling Screen (BBGS;[26] figure) was recently developed with a reporting window from the past 12 months. The BBGS was derived by use of DSM-IV assessment items and data form the National Epidemiologic Survey of Alcohol and Related Conditions (NESARC).[27] With excellent sensitivity (0.96) and specificity (0.99), BBGS holds promise as a practical implement with clinical use. Neither BBGS nor NODS CLiP has been cross-validated in other national samples or validated in clinical sample.

For a more comprehensive assessment, the Gambling Treatment Outcome Monitoring System (GAMTOMS)[28] is a multidimensional self-report of interview assessment instrument. The GAMTOMS incorporates SOGS and also assesses various domains pertaining to treatment planning and outcome monitoring, including gambling frequency, mental health, financial problems, legal problems, and motivation. Additionally, this system has a ten-item DSM-IV measure that is relevant for diagnostic purposes. The GAMTOMS has been used for several psychometric evaluations in clinical samples,[28] whereby DSM-IV categorical diagnosis of pathological gambling had good sensitivity (0.96) and specificity (1.0) distinguishing SOGS-positive case from SOGS-negative cases.[5] The GAMTOMS also includes a follow-up version that measured treatment outcome via self-report.[28]

Finally, gambling behavior and expenditures can be reliably measured with a timeline follow-back interview adapted form a method sued for individuals who have problems with alcohol.[29] Typically, pharmacological treatment trials rely on the clinician-administered Yale-Brown Obsessive Compulsive Scale Modified for Pathological Gambling[30] or the self-report Gambling Symptom Assessment Scale,[31] both of which assess gambling urges and behavior and have had excellent reliability and validity.

CAUSE AND PATHOGENESIS

Demographic, Psychological, and Biological Associations

In the past two decades, researchers have identified many predictive risk factors and processes associated with the development of gambling disorders.[4,32] A substantial body of empirical work indicates that particular demographic associations-including young age, male sex, nonwhite ethnic origin, low socioeconomic status, and divorced or separated marital status-are general risk factors that are associated with gambling problems.[32,33] These findings, however, are often reported in an aggregated form, thereby failing to account for moderating variables, such as type of gambling activity. To briefly highlight this important point, the results from one study[34] indicated that, among other results, sports gamblers tended to be young men with high rates of addiction comorbidity, whereas slot machine gamblers tended to be older women with higher rates of psychiatric comorbidity and later onset of gambling.

Mental Health Comorbidity

Gambling disorders are highly comorbid with other psychiatric disorders.[32] The strongest evidence based relates to substance use disorders. In NESARC,[77] the targets psychiatric epidemiology study undertaken so far pathological gamblers had an increased risk of having a diagnosis of alcohol misuse in their lifetime by a factor of six, and an increased risk of having a substance use disorder by a factor of 4.4 compared with nongamblers. Additionally, rates of major depression and dysthymia were each about three times higher in pathological gamblers than in nongamblers, whereas rates of a manic episode were eight times higher in gamblers. Moreover, generalized anxiety disorders, panic disorder, and specific phobias were each more than three times higher in gamblers, with social phobia twice as high a risk. Modules for obsessive-compulsive and post-traumatic stress disorders were not included in the NESARC study, and evidence for the comorbidity between those disorders with pathological gambling in other published studies is mixed. In the NESARC sample, pathological gamblers also had an increased risk of having a personality disorder by a factor of about eight.

In another large-scale US national survey of mental disorders-the National Comorbidity Survey Replication (NCS-R)[35]-similar comorbidity rates of pathological gambling with psychiatric disorders were obtained. Of those with pathological gambling, the risk of having a substance use disorder was increased by 5.5 times, that for having a mood disorder was increased by 3.7 times, and that for having an anxiety disorder increased by 3.1 times. Although the bidirectional nature of the association between pathological gambling and psychiatric disorders is unclear, the NCS-R was the first study to obtain retrospective onset data, indicating that in pathological gamblers with a comorbid disorder, the onset of pathological gambling preceded the comorbid disorder 23.5% of the time, whereas pathological gambling followed the comorbid disorder 74.3% of the time. Results from the NCS-R also suggested that mood and anxiety disorders predicted the subsequent onset of pathological gambling. With regard to substance use disorders, pathological gambling more often predicted the subsequent onset of substance use disorders than vice versa.

Neurocognition

The behaviors that characterise problematic gambling (e.g. chasing losses, preoccupation with gambling, inability to stop) are impulsive in that they are often premature, poorly though out, risky, and result in deleterious long-term outcomes.[36] Deficits in aspects of inhibition. Working memory, planning, cognitive flexibility, and time management or estimation are more common individuals with pathological gambling then in healthy volunteers.[37-45] In one neuroimaging study on inhibition in pathological gambling, decreased activation in the ventrolateral prefrontal cortex was reported in problem gamblers compared with healthy controls by use of the Stroop color-word task.[46] Studies of patients, however, can often have confounds, such as treatments received and potential deleterious cognitive effects of comorbidities (e.g. depression). Furthermore, these studies do not enable characterization of the temporal association between the manifestation of cognitive deficits and clinically significant symptoms. These deficits could occur in people at risk before symptoms develop or could alternatively stem from the disorder itself, perhaps reflecting a secondary or incidental epiphenomenon.

Neurobiology

Increasing evidence implicates multiple neurotransmitter systems (e.g. dopaminerigc, serotonergic, noradrenergic, opioidergic) in the pathophysiology of gambling disorders. Dopamine is implicated in learning, motivation, and the salience of stimuli, including rewards. Alterations in dopaminergic pathways might underlie the seeking of rewards (i.e. gambling) that trigger the release of dopamine and produce feelings of pleasure.[47] Neuroimaging research suggests that the dopaminergic mesolimbic pathway from the ventral tegmental area to the nucleus accumbens might be involved in pathological gambling. Neuroimaging studies in pathological gamblers have indicated diminished ventral striatum and ventromedial prefrontal cortex and ventrolateral prefrontal cortex activity during rewarding events suggestive of a blunted neurophysiological response to rewards and losses.[48,49] Contrary to what might be expected form dopamine involvement, antagonists at dopamine D2/D3 receptors enhance gambling-related motivations and behaviors in patients with pathological gambling[50] and have no effect in the treatment of pathological gambling.[51,52] Further research is needed to clarify the precise role of dopamine in pathological gambling.

Evidence for serotonergic involvement in pathological gambling comes from preclinical research examining the effect of a serotonergic agonist in rats undertaking a gambling task.[53] A serotonergic agonist resulted in an inability to judge between expected outcomes on the basis of the relative likelihood and size of rewards and punishments.[53] Other support for dysfunction within the serotonergic system comes from human studies of pathological gamblers; decreased concentrations of platelet monoamine oxidase B (a peripheral marker of serotonergic function), low concentrations of serotonin metabolites (e.g. 5-hydroxyindoleacetic acid) in the cerebrospinal fluid, and a euphoric response to serotonergic pharmacological challenge studies.[54]

Genetic Factor

Relatively few family history or genetics studies of pathological gambling have been designed with appropriate control groups. In one small family study of probands with pathological gambling, first-degree relatives of the probands had significantly higher lifetime rates of alcohol disorders, other substance use disorders, and depression than did control individuals.[55]

Data from twin studies suggest a genetic contribution to gambling disorders.[56-62] The genetic versus environmental contributions to pathological gambling can be estimated by comparing its concordance in identical (monozygotic) and fraternal (dizygotic) twin pairs. In a study of male twins that used the Vietnam Era Twin Registry,[57] 12–20% of the genetic variation in risk for pathological gambling and 3–8% of the nonshared environmental variation in risk for pathological gambling was accounted for by risk for alcohol use disorder. Two-thirds (64%) of the co-occurrence between pathological gambling and alcohol use disorder was attributable to genes that affect both disorders, suggesting overlap in the genetically transmitted underpinnings of both conditions. A follow-up study of female twins reported that the estimate of the proportion of variation in liability for disordered gambling attributable to genetics was 49% and that there was

Flow chart 1: Brief biosocial gambling screen[26]

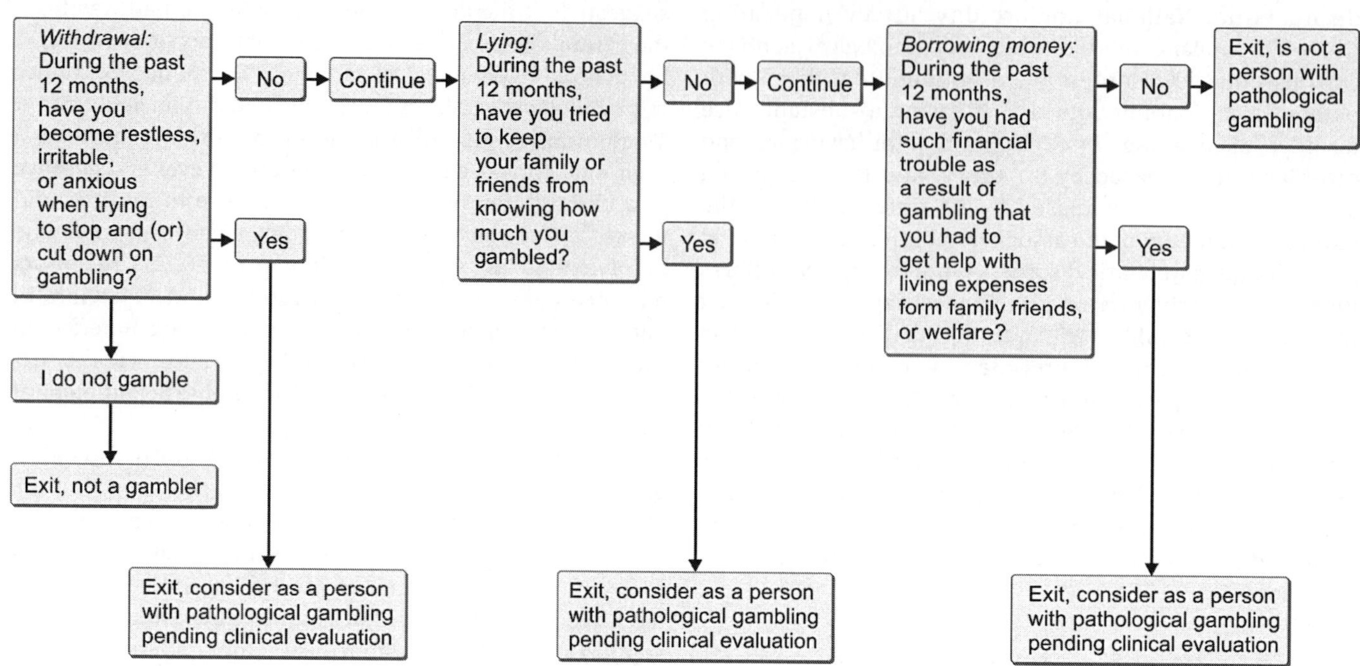

no evidence for shared environmental effects contributing to variation in disordered gambling liability.[61]

There are few molecular genetic studies of pathological gambling. The D2A1 allele of the D2 dopamine receptor gene (*DRD2*) increases in frequency from individuals with non-problematic gambling to those with pathological gambling and co-occurring pathological gambling and substance use disorders.[63] Other research has also implicated allelic variants of *DRD1* and *DRD3* as having an association with pathological gambling.[64,65]

Environmental Factors

Although many genes confer vulnerability, several environmental factors also contribute to developmental pathways of gambling disorders. The structural and situational characteristic of gambling activities (e.g. accessibility to gambling, location and type of gambling establishment, size and number of prizes, and near-miss opportunities) are important factors involved in the maintenance of gambling behavior.[13,66] Additionally, rates of early negative childhood experiences, such as abuse and trauma, seem to be higher in individuals with gambling disorders that in social gamblers, with the severity of maltreatment being associated with the severity of gambling problems and an earlier age of gambling onset.[67,68] Childhood exposure to gambling also probably affects gambling behavior later in life, as suggested by reports of association between gambling problems and parental gambling.[69,70]

Integrative Models

Two predominant integrative heuristic models have been proposed to explain the cause of gambling disorders; the biopsychosocial model[71,72] and the pathways model.[73] The biospsychosocial model is essentially predicated on a cognitive-behavioral and diathesis-stress framework, whereby predisposing factors (e.g. poor problem-solving and coping skills and genetic vulnerabilities) interact with early gambling experiences (e.g. stressful life problems, boredom) to give rise to gambling disorders (Flow chart 1). Both the biopsychosocial and pathways models describe similar factors and process involved in the development and maintenance of gambling problems. The major difference is that the biopsychocial model assumes homogeneity of gambling disorders and the pathways model postulates heterogeneity of gambling disorders manifested as three main pathways leading to three subtypes of problems gamblers: behaviorally conditioned subtype of characterised by and absence of premorbid psychopathological changes and impaired control over gambling results from the effects of conditioning, distorted cognitions, and poor decision making associated with frequent exposure to gambling. These same environmental principles are involved in the cause of the other two subtypes, although premorbid pathological changes are a complicating factor in terms of motives for gambling and course of the disorder. The emotionally vulnerable subtype has pre-existing depression, anxiety, and poor coping and problem-solving skills, and a history of trauma and gambling helps to modulate affective states. The third subtype has pre-existing impulsivity, attentional difficulties, and antisocial features, and gambling serves as a risky and exciting activity. Clinical experience suggests that there is merit to taking into account the heterogeneity of gambling disorders, and descriptive validation of the pathways model is beginning to accumulate for both adults[74] and adolescents.[75] Nevertheless, no longitudinal data are available to test the developmental aspects or treatment implications of the typology.

Natural and Treatment-assisted Recovery and Support

Pathways to Recovery

Prevalence surveys indicate that only a small proportion (<10%) of the individuals who have gambling disorders seek formal treatment.[76,77] In a recent review[78] of perceived barriers to treatment seeking, the results of studies undertaken across five countries were similar. A desire to handle the problem on their own, shame, and denial were the most frequently described reasons for individuals not accessing treatment rather than perceived or actual treatment availability. Prevalence surveys have also reported that, despite the low rate of treatment seeking, many people have recovered from gambling problems past-year. Prevalence rates of gambling disorders are consistently about two-thirds of the lifetime rates, suggesting a recovery rate of a third.[79-81] Very little longitudinal research is available about the natural course of gambling disorders. However, available data suggest that, at the individual level, gambling problems are transient and episodic.[82,83] Follow-up samples indicated that most recovered individuals have accomplished their recoveries without accessing formal treatment services,[80] which is consistent with what is report for other addictive disorders.[84] In-depth interviews with convenience samples of recovered people reveal that their recovery strategies are practical and behavior focused-including involvement in time-consuming activities that are incompatible with gambling and avoidance of conditioned cues to gamble (e.g. gambling venues and information about betting odds).[85,86] Similar recovery strategies are reported by individuals who have accessed treatment and those who recovered without the assistance of treatment.

Brief Treatment

Brief treatments are not necessarily seen as treatment by individuals who access them. In two randomized controlled trials, individuals who did not want to attend treatment, despite acknowledging a problem and meeting diagnostic criteria for pathological gambling, were specifically recruited.[87-89] A telephone-based motivational interview contact combined with a mailed self-help cognitive-behavioral therapy workbook led to good outcomes over 12-month and 24-month follow-up periods. Motivational interviewing is a therapeutic style of interacting with individuals to encourage them to focus on their personal reasons for needing to address problem behaviors, as well as to voice any factors that work against change. Resolution of people's natural ambivalence about change motivates them to take action. A similar motivational interviewing and cognitive-behavioral therapy intervention has been adapted to a web-based format in Sweden,[90] in which a therapist provides telephone support for individuals using online recovery materials. In a US randomized controlled study,[91] a 5-min session of behavioral advice and four sessions of motivational enhancement plus cognitive-behavioral therapy were equally effective for reduction of gambling in individuals not seeking treatment and were more effective than one session of motivational interviewing alone or a no treatment control. The New Zealand telephone helpline service for problem gamblers uses a randomized controlled design to evaluate the relative effectiveness of various combinations of motivational interviewing, a workbook, and booster telephone calls. Telephone gambling help lines and websites that provide treatment referral or personal support are common in many countries (e.g. the USA, Canada, Australia, and the UK) so development of evidence-based interventions with these methods of important. Another potential strategy for providing brief interventions is through gambling venue-based treatment referral and support services, which are increasingly being offered in venues such as casinos.

Psychosocial Treatment

Various treatment models have been adapted for gambling disorders. In a meta-analysis,[92] randomized trails published between 1986 and 2004 were identified. In general, psychological treatments were more effective than no treatment, both after treatment (overall effect size 2.01) and at follow-up averaging 17 months later (overall effect size 1.59). Although the author did not evaluate which specific types of treatments were more effective than others, most studies of treatment outcomes that were included in their meta-analysis were done within the behavioral, cognitive, and cognitive-behavioral formats. Another meta-analysis, which focused exclusively on the cognitive-behavioral treatment literature, included 25 studies.[93] Substantial variability in the outcomes were reported but, in general, post-treatment effects were positive for different types of therapy (e.g. behavioral, and cognitive) and method of therapy (e.g. behavioral, and cognitive) and method of therapy (e.g. individual, group, and self-directed). No randomized trials of inpatient treatment have yet been done.[94]

Behavioral models summarize gambling disorders as learned patterns of reinforcements within a functional framework (i.e. antecedents, behaviors, and consequences), and behavioral treatments focus on modifying one or more components of the functional relationship. Specifically, strategies include reducing avoidance, exposure to high-risk situations, behavioral experiments to challenge distorted thoughts, and development of skills in various areas (e.g. assertiveness, problem solving, and relaxation).

Cognitive treatment models focus specifically on modifying distorted cognitions associated with gambling.[72] including overestimating probabilities of winning, illusions of control over the outcome of a gamble, the belief that a win is due after a series of losses (i.e. the gambler's fallacy), and memory bases in favor of remembering wings.[95]

Although a few trials have evaluated the efficacy of a purely cognitive approach, the largest number and the most rigorously designed trials evaluate a combined cognitive-behavioral therapy model. Overall, although there is variability in outcomes, different research groups working in several languages in diverse areas of the world generally report positive effects.[92] Some trials have recently examined the efficacy of motivational interviewing alone or in combination with cognitive-behavioral therapy interventions. Data form a recent Swedish trial[96] showed that group cognitive-behavioral therapy and an individual motivational interview intervention had equivalent outcomes and that both were superior to a wait list control. Results from two small trails indicated that the addition of motivational interviewing to cognitive-behavioral therapy reduced treatment attrition and improved outcomes.[97,98] Dropout rates from psychosocial treatment are high so interventions that lead patients to complete treatment are potentially very valuable.

Psychopharmacological Treatment

Although no drug has received regulatory approval in any jurisdiction as a treatment for gambling disorders, there have been 18 double-blind, placebo-controlled trials of various drugs (opioid antagonists, glutamatergic agents, antidepressants, and mood stabilizers) for the treatment of pathological gambling. A meta-analysis of randomised trials included 16 outcomes studies, published between 2000 and 2006,[99] which revealed that, in general, pharmacological treatments were more effective than was placebo treatment (overall effect size 0.78). However, studies generally reported a particularly strong placebo effect, which would serve to lower the effect size of the drug, attrition rates were high in several of these trials, and several other studies have been published since 2006.

Given their ability to modulate dopaminergic transmission in the mesolimbic pathway, opioid receptor antagonists (naltrexone and nalmefene) have been investigated in the treatment of pathological gambling (Table 1). Results from two multicenter double-blind, placebo-controlled trials of nalmefene suggest efficacy of opioid antagonists in reducing the intensity of urges to gamble, gambling thoughts, and gambling behavior.[100-103] Pooled analyses of individuals who responded to opioid antagonists indicated significant reduction in gambling urges, particularly in participants with a positive family history of alcohol dependence.[104]

Because improvement in glutamatergic tone in the nucleus accumbens has been implicated in reducing the reward-seeking behavior in addictions,[105] N-acetyl cysteine, an amino acid and glutamate modulator, has been studies in the treatment of pathological gambling.[106] N-acetlycysteine had positive effects on urges and gambling behavior.[106]

Results from trials of the atypical antipsychotic olanzapine and a trial of bupropion, however, had no benefit over placebo.[51,52,107] Finally, a nontreatment trial examined the effects of an atypical stimulant, modefinil, on pathological gamblers classified according to impulsivity.[108] Highly impulsive people had decreased motivation to gamble and less risky decision making, whereas people with low impulses had increased responses. The data form this study indicate a potential direction for pharmacological research in gambling disorders-examining the relative efficacy of different drug classes in individual with related comorbid disorders (e.g. mood, bipolar, anxiety, attention deficit hyperactivity, and substance use). Thus far, there has been little research examining the effect of combining pharmacological and psychosocial treatments.[94] However, in one trial, individuals receiving cognitive-behavioral therapy for comorbid gambling and alcohol use disorders did equally well with naltrexone and placebo.[109] Finally, pharmacological studies with longer term follow-ups are needed. In an open-lable discontinuation trial of 43 men fully responding to fluvoxamine, topiramate, bupropion, or naltrexone, most responders did not relapse during a 6-month drug-free follow-up period.[110]

Gamblers Anonymous

Gamblers Anonymous self-help groups were started in 1957 in Los Angels, CA, USA and are now operating in at least 55 countries worldwide.[111] Individuals use a programme of 12 steps and 12 traditions, modified from Alcoholics Anonymous, to acknowledge powerlessness over compulsive gambling and to remain gambling free. The groups promote a sense of common purpose and understanding and reinforce each consecutive day of abstinence from gambling. As with Alcoholics Anonymous, periods of success are marked with celebrations and rewards.

There are few outcome studies evaluating the effectiveness of Gamblers Anonymous, and well controlled efficacy research has been done. Correlational data have indicated that individuals affiliated with Gamblers Anonymous have better gambling outcomes than do those who are not,[112] even when they are concurrently engaged in professions treatment.[113] However, treatment outcome studies that have

Table 1: Studies of usefulness of drugs for pathological gambling

	Dose (mg Per day)	*Number of participants*	*Response rate for drug*	*Response rate for placebo*
Naltrexone[102,103]	50–150	122	61.8%	34.2%
Nalmefene[102,103]	20–100	414	51.8%	46%
Fluvoxamine[99]	50–250	47	72%	48%
Paroxetine[99]	10–60	121	62.9%	39.7%
Sertraline[99]	50–150	60	68%	66%
Bupropion[107]	75–375	39	35.7%	47.1%
Olanzapine[54,57]	2.5–15	63	66.7%	71.4%

Data from double-blind, placebo-controlled studies. Table does not include studies using an open-label design followed by double-blind discontinuation; studies used various measures to assess response, and some studies were fixed-dose studies and others allowed for dose titration. Where two studies have been done with the same drug, the response rates reflect pooled means. In these cases, there was often one positive and one negative study, and therefore the results need to be interpreted in the context of each study's method.

used referral to Gamblers Anonymous as a comparison condition to cognitive-behavioral treatment have indicated poor attendance of Gamblers Anonymous and outcomes.[113,114]

Family Therapy

Advances in family therapy interventions for treatment of substance abuse problems have been adapted for gambling disorders. A self-help workbook, a gambling adaptation of the Community Reinforcement and Family Therapy (CRAFT) model, has been evaluated in two randomised controlled trials.[115,116] In CRAFT, concerned family members are trained to use behavioral principles to reinforce non-gambling behavior in individuals who are not addressing their gambling problem. Although positive effects for family members and their gambling relatives were reported in both trials, the most recent trial also concluded that the behavioral principles were too complex for family members to implement without the support of a therapist.[116] Moreover, in neither trial did the gambling relatives enter treatment because of the intervention, one of the main goals of CRAFT. A coping skill group therapy model developed for alcohol problems has also been evaluated for gambling. In a small randomised controlled trial, partners of individuals with gambling problems improved their ability to self-manage feelings of depression and naxieyt.[117] Finally, congruence couple therapy for gambling problems has been developed form Satir's family therapy approach. The therapeutic goal is to help individuals achieve congruence in intrapsychic, interpersonal, intergenerational, and spiritual dimensions. In an uncontrolled trial of 24 couples, positive effects on both gambling and the couple's relationships were reported.[118] In summary, the role of family therapy models in the treatment of gambling disorders remains to be studies but shows promise on the basis of this small amount of research.

Clinical Factors and Future Directions

Despite the progress that has been made into development of effective treatments for gambling disorders, several unresolved clinical issues exist. As noted in the Seminar, there is substantial comorbidity of gambling disorders and mental and substance use disorders. How concurrent disorders should be addressed in gambling treatment is not well understood and has not been empirically studied.[119]

Most of our progress in recognizing and understanding gambling disorders has been made in the past 25 years. Our knowledge continues to evolve in parallel with a burgeoning availability of gambling opportunities. Internet gambling, for example, is providing around-the-clock home access to several types of gambling activities to an increasing number of people around the world. Thus, although substantial progress has been made, this evolution warrants, and is likely to encourage, more innovative research into gambling disorders and it translation into clinical progress.

REFERENCES

1. Bernstein PL, Against the Gods: the remarkable story of risk. New York: John Willey & Sons, 1996.
2. American Psychiatric Association. Diagnostic and Statistical Manual of Mental Disorders Text Revision, 4th edn. Washington, DC: American Psychiatric Association, 2000.
3. WHO, International Classification of Disease (ICD-10): clinical descriptions and diagnostic guidelines. Geneva: World Health Organization, 1992.
4. National Research Council. Pathological gambling: a critical review. Washington, DC: National Academy Press; 1999.
5. Stinchfield R, Govoni R, Frisch GR. A review of screening and assessment instruments for problem and pathological gambling. In: Smith G, Hodgins DC, Williams RJ (Eds).

Research and Measurement Issues in Gambling Studies. Boston: Academic Press/Elsevier. 2007:180-213.

6. American Psychiatric Association. Diagnostic and Statistical Manual of Mental Disorders, 3rd edn. Washington, DC: American Psychiatric Association; 1980.
7. Lesieur HR, Rosenthal RJ. Pathological gambling: a review of the literature. J Gambl Stud. 1991;7:5-39.
8. American Psychiatric Association. DSM-5 development: pathological gambling, 2010. *http://www.dsm5.org/Proposed Revisions/Pages/ proposedrivision, aspx? rid=210#* (accessed July 25, 2012).
9. Petry NM, Pathologicla gambling and the DSM-V. Int Gambl Stud. 2010;10:113-5.
10. Wardle H, Sproston K, Orfor J, et al. British Gambling Prevalence Survey 2007. London: National Centre for Social Research; 2007.
11. Toce-Gerstein M, Gerstein DR, Volberg RA. The NODS-CLiP: a rapid screen for adult pathological and problem gambling. J Gambl Stud. 2009;25:541-55.
12. Williams RJ, Volberg RA. Impact of survey description administration format, and exclusionary criteria on population prevalence rates of problem gambling. Int Gambl Stud. 2009;9:101-7.
13. Abbott MW. Situational factors that affect gambling behavior. In: Smith G, Hodgins DC, Williams RJ (Eds). Research and measurement issues in gambling studies. San Diego, CA: Academic Press. 2007:251-78.
14. Abbott MW, Williams MM, Volberg RA. A prospective study of problem and regular nonproblems gamblers living in community. Subst Use Misuse. 2004;39:855-84.
15. Shaffer HJ, LaBrie RA, LaPlante DA. Laying the foundation for quantifying regional exposure to social phenomena: considering the cause of legalized gambling as a public health toxin. Psychol Addict Behav. 2004;18:40-8.
16. Hodgins DC, Stinchfielf R. Gambling disorders. In: Hunsley J, Mash EJ (Eds). A guide to assessments that work. New York, NY: Oxford University Press. 2008;370-88.
17. Lesieur HR, Blume SB. The South Oaks Gambling Screen (SOGS): a new instrument for the identification of pathological gamblers. Am J Psychiatry. 1987;144:1184-8.
18. Shaffer HJ, Hall MN. Updating and refining prevalence estimates of disordered gambling and behaviour in the Unites States and Canada. Can J Public Health. 2001;92:168-72.
19. Lesieur HR, Blume SB. Revising the South Oaks Gambling Screen in different settings. J Gambl Stud. 1993;9:213-23.
20. Wulfert E, Hartley J, Lee M, Wang N, Franco C, Sodano R. Gambling Screens: does shortening the time frame affect their psychometric properties? J Gambl Stud. 2005;21:521-36.
21. Stinchfield R. Reliability, validity, and classification accuracy of the South Oaks Gambling Screen (SOGS). Addict Behav. 2002;27:1-19.
22. Ferris J, Wynne H. The Canadian Problem Gambling Index: final report. Ottawa, ON: phase II final report to the Canadian Inter Provinical Task Force on Problem Gambling, 2001.
23. Gerstein D, Murphy S, Toce M, et al. Gambling impact and behaviour study: report to the National Gambling Impact Study Commission; 1999.
24. Hodgins DC. Using the NORC DSM Screen for Gambling Problems (NODS) as an outcome measure for pathological gambling: psychometric evaluation. Addict Behav. 2004;29:1685-90.
25. Wickwire EM Jr, Burke RS, Brown SA, Parker JD, Many RK, Psychometirc evaluation of the National Opinion Research Centre DSM-IV Screen for Gambling Problems (NODS). Am J Addict. 2008;17:392-5.
26. Gebauer L, LaBrie R, Shaffer HJ. Optimizing DSM-IV-TR classification accuracy: a brief biosocial screen for detecting current gambling disorders aming gamblers in the general household population. Can J Psychiatry. 2010;55:82-90.
27. Petry NM, Stinson FS, Grant BF. Comorbidity of DSM-IV pathological gambling and other psychiatric disorders: results from the National Epidemiologic Survey on Alcohol and Related Conditions. J Clin Psychiatry. 2005;66:564-74.
28. Stinchfield R, Winters KC, Botzet A, Jerstad S, Breyer J. Development and psychometric evaluation of the Gambling Treatment Outcome Monitoring System (GAMTOMS). Psychol Addict Behav. 2007;21:174-84.
29. Weinstock J, Whelan JP, Meyers AW. Behavioural assessment of gambling an application of the timeline followback method. Psychol Assess. 2004;16:72-80.
30. Hollander E, DeCaria CM, Mari E, et al. Short-term single-blind fluvoxamine treatment of pathological gambling. Am J Psychiatry. 1998;155:1781-3.
31. Kim SW, Gran JE. Potenza MN, Blanco C, Hollander E. The Gambling Symptom Assessment Scale (G-SAS): a reliability and validity study. Psychiatry Res. 2009;166:76-84.
32. Petry NM. Pathological gambling: etiology, comorbidity, and treatment, Washington, DC: American Psychological Association, 2005.
33. Toneatto T, Nguyen L. Individual characterstic and problem gambling behaviour. In: Smith G, Hodgins DC, Williams RJ, (Eds). Research and Measurement Issues in Gambling Studies. San Diego, CA: Academic Press; 2007.pp.279-303.
34. Petry NM. A comparison of treatment seeking pathological gamblers based on preferred gambling activity. Addiction. 2003;98:645-55.
35. Kessler RC, Hwang I, LaBric R, et al. DSM-IV Pathological gambling in the National Comorbidity Survey Replication. Psychol Med. 2008;38:1351-60.
36. Chamberlain SR, Sahakian BJ. The neuropsychiatry of impulsivity. Curr Opin Psychiatry. 2007;20:255-61.
37. Petry NM. Pathological gamblers with and without substance use disorders, discount delayed rewards at high rates. J Abnorm Psychol. 2001;110:482-7.
38. Regard M, Knoch D, Gutling E, Landis T. Brain damange and addictive behaviour: a neuropsychological and electroencephalogram investigation with pathologic gamblers. Cogn Behav Neurol. 2003;16:47-53.

39. Brand M, Kalbe E, Labudda K, Fujiwara E, Kessler J, Markowitsch JHJ. Decision-making impairments in patients with pathological gambling. Psychiatry Res. 2005;133:91-9.
40. Fuentes D, Tavares H, Artes R, Gorenstein C. Self-reported and neuropsychological measures of impulsivity in pathological gambling. J Int Neuropsychol Soc. 2006;12:907-12.
41. Goudriaan AE, Oosterlaan J, de Beurs E, van den Brink W. Neurocognitive functions in pathological gambling: a comparison wth alcohol dependence, Tourette syndrome and normal controls. Addiction. 2006;101:534-47.
42. Kalechstein AD, Fong T, Rosenthal RJ, Davis A, Vanyo H, Newton TF. Pathological gamblers demonstrate frontal lobe impairment consistent with that of methamphetamine-dependent individuals. J Neuropsychiatry Clin Neurosic. 2007;19:298-303.
43. Lawrence AJ, Luty J, Bogdan NA, Sahakian BJ, Clark L, Impulsivity and response inhibition in alcohol dependence and problem gambling. Psychopharmacology. 2009; 207:163-72.
44. Lawrence AJ, Luty J, Bogdan NA. Sahakian BJ, Clark L. Problem gamblers share deficits in impulsive decision-making with alcohol-dependent individuals. Addiction. 2009;104:1006-15.
45. Roca M, Torralva T, Lopez P, Cetkovich M, Clark L, Manes F. Executive functions in pathologic gamblers selected in an ecologic setting. Cogn Behav Neurol. 2008;21:1-4.
46. Potenza MN, Leung HC, Blumberg HP, et al. An FMRI Stroop task study of ventromedial prefrontal cortical function in pathological gamblers. Am J Psychiatry. 2003;160:1990-4.
47. Zack M, Poulos CX. Parallel roles for dopamine in pathological gambling and psychostimulant addiction. Curr Drug Abuse REV. 2009;2:11-25.
48. Reuter J, Raedler T, Rose M, Hand I, Glascher J, Buchel C. Pathological gambling is linked to reduced activation of the mesolimbic reward system. Nat Neurosci. 2005;8:147-8.
49. De Ruiter MB, Veltman DJ, Goudriaan AE, Oosterlaan J, Sjoerds Z, Ven den Brink W. Response perseveration and ventral perforontal sensitivity to reward and punsihment in male problem gamblers and smokers. Neuropsychopharmacology. 2007;32:1678-86.
51. Fong T, Kaleschstein A, Bernhard B, Rosental R, Rugle L. A double-blind, placebo-controlled trial of olanzapine for the treatment of video poker pathological gamblers. Pharmaco Bicohem Behav. 2008;89:298-303.
52. McElroy SL, Nelson EB, Welge JA, Kaehler L, Keck PE Jr. Olanzapine in the treatment of pathological gambling: a negative randomized placebo-controlled trial. J Clin Psychiatry. 2008;69:433-40.
53. Zeeb FD, Robbins TW. Winstanley CA. Serotonergic and dopaminergic modulation of gambling behavior as assessed using a novel rat gambling task. Neuropsychopharmacology. 2009;34:2329-43.
54. Potenza MN. The neurobiology of pathological gambling. Semin Clin Neuropsychiatry. 2001;6:217-26.
55. Black DW, Monahan PO, Temkit M, Shaw M. A family study of pathological gambling. Psychiatry Res. 2006;141:295-303.
56. Eisen SA, Lin N, Lyons MJ, et al. Familial influences on gambling behavior: an analysis of 3359 twin pairs. Addiction 1998:93:1375-84.
57. Slutske WS, Eisen S, True WR, Lyons MJ, Goldberg J, Tsuang M. Common genetic vulnerability for pathological gambling and alcohol dependence in men. Arch Gen Psychiatry. 2000;57:666-73.
58. Xian H, Scherrer JF, Slutske WS, Shah KR, Volberg R, Eisen SA. Genetic and environmental contributions to pathological gambling symptoms in a 10-year follow-up. Twin Res Hum Genet. 2007;10:174-9.
59. Potenza MN, Xian H, Shah K, Scherrer JF, Eisen SA. Shared genetic contributions to pathological gambling and major depression in men. Arch Gen Psychiatry. 2005;62:1015-21.
60. Winters KC. Rich T. A twin study of adult gambling behavior. J Gambl Stud. 1998;14:213-25.
61. Slutske WS, Zhu G, Meier MH. Mertin NG, Genetic and environmental influences on disordered gambling in men and women. Arch Gen Psychiatry. 2010;67:624-30.
62. Slutske WS. Meier MH, Zhu G, Statham DJ, Blaszczynski A, Martin NG. The Australian Twin Study of Gambling (OZ-GAM): rationale, sample description, predictors of participation, and a first look at sources of individual differences in gambling involvement. Twin Res Hum Genet. 2009;12:63-78.
63. Comings DE, Gade-Andavolu R, Gonzales N, et al. The addictive effect of neurotransmitter genes in pathological gambling. Clin Genet. 2001;60:107-16.
64. Lobo DS, Souza RP, Tong RP, et al. Association of functional variants in the dopamine D2-like receptors with risk for gambling behaviour in healthy Caucasian subjects. Biol Psychol. 2010;85:33-7.
65. Lobo DS, Kennedy JL. Genetic aspects of pathological gambling: a complex disorder with shared genetic vulnerabilities. Addiction 2009;104:1454-65.
66. Parke J, Griffiths M. The role of structural characteristics in gambling. In: Smith G, Hodogins DC, Williams RJ (Eds). Research and Measurement Issues in Gambling Studies. New York, NY: Academic Press. 2007:217-49.
67. Petry NM, Steinberg KL. Childhood maltreatment in male and female treatment-seeking pathological gambliers. Psychol Addict Behav. 2005;19:226-9.
68. Hodgins DC, Schopflocher DP, el-Guebaly N, et al. The association between childhood maltreatment and gambling problems in a community sample of adult men and women. Psychol Addict Behav. 2010;24:548-54.
69. Oei TP, Raylu N. Familial influence on offspring gambling: a cognitive mechanism for transmission of gambling behavior in families. Psychol Med. 2004;34:1279-88.
70. Schreiber L, Odlaug BL, Kim SW, Grant JE. Characteristics of pathological gamblers with a problem gambling parent. Am J Addict. 2009:18:462-9.
71. Sharpe L. A reformulate cognitive-behavioral model of problem gambling: a biopsychosocial perspective. Clin Psychol Rev. 2002;22:1-25.

72. Sharpe L, Tarrier N. Towards a cognitive-behavioural theory of problem gambling. Br J Psychiatry. 1993;162:407-12.
73. Blaszczynski A, Nower L. A pathways model of problem and pathological gambling. Addiction. 2002;97:487-99.
74. Vachon DD. Bagby RM. Pathological gambling subtypes. Psychol Ass. 2009;21:608-15.
75. Gupta R, Nower L, Derevensky JL, Blaszczynski A. Problem gambling in adolescents: an examination of the pathways model. Guelph: Ontario Problem Gambling Research Centre, 2009.
76. Slutske WS, Blaszczynski A, Martin NG. Sex differences in the rates of recovery, treatment-seeking and natural recovery in pathological gambling: results from an Australian Community-based twin survey. Twin Res Hum Genet. 2009;12:425-32.
77. Cunningham JA. Little use of treatment among problem gamblers. Psychiatr Serv. 2005;56:1024-5.
78. Suurvali H, Hodgins DC, Cunningham JA. Motivators for resolving or seeking help for gambling problems: a review of the empirical literature. J Gambl Study. 2010;26:1-33.
79. Cunningham JA, Hodgins DC. Interest in different self-help services for problem gamblers. Psychiatr Serv. 2008;59:659-96.
80. Hodgins DC, Wynne H, makarchuk K. Pathways to recovery from gambling problems: Follow-up from a general population survey. J Gambl Stud. 199;15:93-104.
81. Slutske WS. Natural recovery and treatment-seeking in pathological gambling: results of two U.S. national surveys. Am J Psychiatry. 2006;163:297-302.
82. Slutske WS, Jackson KM, Sher KJ. The natural history of problem gambling from age 8 to 29. J Abnorm Psychol. 2003;112:263-74.
83. LaPlante DA, Nelson SE, LaBrie RA, Shaffer JH. Stability and progression of disordered gambling: lessons from longitudinal studies. Can J Psychitry. 2008;53:52-60.
84. Sobell LC, Cunningham JA, Sobeel MB. Recovery from alcohol problems with and without treatment: prevalence in two population surveys. Am J Public Health. 1996;86:966-72.
85. Hodgins DC, el-Guebaly N. Natural and treatment-assisted recovery from gambling problems: a comparison of resolved and active gamblers. Addication. 2000;95:777-89.
86. Cunningham JA, Hodgins DC, Toneatto T. Natural and treatment-assisted recovery frorm gambling problems. Result form a general population survey. Sucht. 2009;55:99-103.
87. Hodgins DC, Currie SR, el-Gueblay N. Motivational enhancement and self-help treatments for problem gambling. J Consult Clin Psychol. 2001;69:50-7.
89. Hodgins DC, Currie SR, Currie G, Fick GH. A randomized clinical trial of brief motivational treatments for pathological gamblers: more is not necessarily better. J Consult Clin Psychol. 2009;77:950-60.
90. Carlbring P, Smit F. Randomized trial of internet-delivered self-help with telephone support for pathological gamblers. J Consult Clin Psychol. 2008;76:1090-94.
91. Petry NM, Weinstock J, Ledgerwood DM, Morasco B. A randomized trial of brief interventions for problem and pathological gamblers. J Consult Clin Psychol. 2008;76: 1090-4.
92. Pallesen S, Mitsem M, Kvale G, Johnsen B-H. Outocme of psychological treatments of pathological gambling: a review and meta-analysis. Addiction. 2005;100:1412-22.
93. Gooding P, Tarrier N. A systematic review and meta-analysis of cognitive-behavioural interventions to reduce problem gambling: hedging out best? Behav Res Ther. 2009;47:592-607.
94. Hoding DC, Holub A. Treatment of problem gambling. In: Smith G, Hoding DC, Williams R (Eds). Research and Measurement Issues in Gambling Studies. New York, NY: Elsevier. 2007:372-98.
95. Toneatto T. Cognitive psychopathology of problem gambling. Subst Use Misuse. 1999;34:1593-604.
96. Carlbring P, Jonsson J, Josephson H, Forsberg L. Motivational interviewing versus cognitive behavioral group therapy in the treatment of problem and pathological gambling: a randomized controlled trial. Cogn Behav Ther. 2010;39:92-103.
97. Diskin KM, Hodgins DC. A randomized controlled trial of a single session motivational intervention for concerned gamblers. Behav Res Ther. 2009;47:382-8.
98. Wulfert E, Blanchard EB, Freidenberg B, Martell R. Retaining pathological gamblers in cognitive-behavioral therapy through motivational enhancement. Behav Modif. 2006;30:315-40.
99. Pallesen S, Molde H, Arnestad HM, et al. Outcome of pharmacological treatments of pathological gambling a review and meta-analysis. J Clin Psychopharmacol. 2007;27:357-64.
100. Kim SW, Grant JE, Adson DE, Shin YC. Double-blind naltrexone and placebo comparison study in the treatment of pathological gambling. Biol Psychiatry. 2001;49:914-21.
101. Grant JE, Kim SW, Hartman BK. A double-blind, placebo-controlled study of the opiate antagonist naltrexone in the treatment of pathological gambling urges. J Clin Psychiatry. 2008;69:783-9.
102. Grant JE. Potenza MN, Hollander E, et al. Multicenter investigation of the opioid antagonist nalmefene in the treatment of pathological gambling. Am J Psychiatry. 2006;163:303-12.
103. Grant JE, Odlaug BL, Potenza MN, Hollander E, Kim SW. Nalmefene in the treatment of pathological gambling: multicentre, double-blind, placebo-controlled study. Br J Psychiatry. 2010;197:330-1.
104. Grant JE, Kim SW, Hollander E, Potenza MN. Predicting response to opiate antagonists and placebo in the treatment of pathological gambling. Psychopharmacology. 2008;200:521-7.
105. Kalivas PW, Peters J, Kanckstedt L. Animal Models and brain circuits in drug addiction. Psychopharmacology. 2008;200:521-44.

106. Grant JE, Kim SW, Odlaug BL, N-acetyl Cysteine, a glutamate-modulating agent, in the treatment of pathological gambling: a pilot study. Biol Psychiatry. 2007;62:652-7.
107. Black DW, Arndt S, Coryell WH, et al. Bupropion in the treatment of pathological gambling: a randomized, double-blind, placebo-controlled, flexible-dose study. J Clin Psychopharmacol. 2007;27:143-50.
108. Zack M, Poulos CX. Effects of the atypical stimulant modafinil on a brief gambling episode in pathological gamblers with high vs. Low impulsivity. J Psychopharmacol. 2009;23:660-71.
109. Toneatto T, Brands B, Selby P. A randomized, double-blind placebo-controlled trial of naltrexone in the treatment of concurrent alcohol use disorder and pathological gambling. Am J Addict. 2009;18:219-25.
110. Dannon PN, Lowengrub K, Musin E, Gonopolsky Y, Kotler M. 12-month follow-up study of drug treatment in pathological gamblers: a primary outcome study. J Clin Psychopharmacol. 2007;27:620-4.
111. Gamblers Anonymous. Gamblers Anonymous international directory. 6-9-2010. *http://www.gamblersanonymous.org/mtgdirTOP. html* (accessed July 25,2012).
112. Hodgins DC, Penden N, Cassidy E. The association between comorbidity and outcome in pathological gambling: a prospective follow-up of recent quitters. J Gambl Stud. 2005;21:225-71.
113. Perty NM, Ammerman Y, Bohl J, et al. Cognitive behavioral therapy for pathological gamblers. J Consult Clin Psychol. 2006;74:555-67.
114. Grant JE. Donahue CB, Odlaug BL, Kim SW, Miller MJ, Perty NM. Imaginal desensitization plus motivational interviewing for pathological gambling: randomized controlled trial. Br J Psychiatry. 2009;195:266-7.
115. Makarchuk K, Hodgins DC, Peden N. Development of a brief intervention for concerned significant others of problem gambliers. Addict Disord Their Treat. 2002;1:126-34.
116. Hodgins DC, Toneatto T, Makarchuk K, Skinner W, Vincent S. Minimal treatment approaches for concerned significant others of problem gamblers: a randomized controlled trial. J Gambl Stud. 2007;23:215-30.
117. Rychatarik RG, McGillicuddy NB. Preliminary evaluation of a coping skills training program for those with a pathological-gambling Partner. J Gambl Stud. 2006;22:165-78.
118. Lee Bk, Rovers M. Bringing torn lives together again: effects of the first congruence couple training application to clients in pathological gambling. Int Gambl Stud. 2008; 8:113-29.
119. Ladouceur R, Lachance S, Fournier PM. Is control a viable goal in the treatment of pathological gambling? Behav Res Ther. 2009; 47:189-97.
120. American Psychiatric Association. Desk Reference to the Diagnostic Criteria from DSM-5. Washington DC; 2013

CHAPTER

77 Functional Symptoms in Neurology: Mimics and Chameleons

JN Vyas, VS Chadda

INTRODUCTION

When the request came to write this review article on mimics and chameleons of functional neurological symptoms, we had to do a double take. You want us to help neurologists to avoid accidentally diagnosing functional symptoms as a disease? Are you sure you do not just mean the other way round?

Functional/psychogenic/nonorganic symptoms are customarily diagnoses that figure on the differential diagnosis of other conditions. There are plenty of cautionary tales in the literature about patients with a neurological disease misdiagnosed as 'hysterical' and 'nonorganic'. However, we are not aware of any previous review article that has tackled the issue of differential diagnosis from the perspective of functional symptoms.

It is gratifying, therefore, that the field has come sufficiently far to warrant a discussion of diagnostic pitfalls in the same terms as that for epilepsy and Alzheimer's disease, the ultimate aim being that neurologists might all one day say to themselves, 'It would be really embarrassing (or maybe I will get used) if I miss the diagnosis of functional symptoms in this patient'.

Functional symptoms are, as any general neurologist knows, very common, and are the second most common reason for a neurological outpatient consultation (in Scotland, anyway).[1] Nonepileptic attacks account for around one in seven patients in a 'first fit' clinic, and functional limb weakness is as common as multiple sclerosis.[2] They also account for a group of patients who, by self-report at least, are as physically impaired and more distressed than equivalent patients seen in neurology outpatients with disease.[3]

Most neurological symptoms can have a functional explanation. In this article, we will discuss general pitfalls in assessing and approaching patients with functional symptoms, and then discuss separately individual pitfalls of dissociative (nonepileptic) attacks, functional motor symptoms and speech/visual/cognitive symptoms.

The guiding principle of diagnosis of most functional symptoms is that there should be inconsistency during the physical examination (so-called internal inconsistency) or incongruity with recognized neurological disease. Sticking to this principle will avoid many of the pitfalls listed below. This article does not recapitulate all the positive clinical signs of inconsistency and incongruity (such as Hoover's sign for functional weakness, motor distraction tasks for functional tremor and features such as eyes closed during a generalized shaking attack), but they are available elsewhere.[4]

As in much of neurology, there are patients where there is diagnostic uncertainty; as a clinician you should always be prepared to say 'not sure'.

EIGHT SHADES OF DIAGNOSTIC CHANGE

Even when the diagnosis does appear to change over time, it is rarely as simple as, '*I thought it was functional, but actually it's multiple sclerosis*'. There are different kinds of diagnostic change with different degrees of error. As well as the most well-known type of misdiagnosis—when you look back and think, '*got that wrong*'—there are other types of change that could be construed as error when in fact they are not (Table 1).

For instance, someone presenting with functional hemiparesis who later develops motor neurone disease, may genuinely have had a functional hemiparesis, it is just that you did not detect (and were not able to detect) the comorbid neurological disease predisposing to it at the time. Alternatively, a patient presenting with a functional movement disorder may, 1 year later, have a stroke, but it still does not account for their functional movement disorder. Diagnostic disagreements, patients where the diagnosis of functional symptoms is initially in the differential but then drops out, also form part of the list of ways in which diagnoses may change over time, without there necessarily having been a 'howler'.

Table 1: A change in diagnosis does not necessarily mean you got it wrong first time around (adapted from[1] with permission)

Type of diagnostic revision	*Example*	*Degree of clinician error*
1. Diagnostic error	Patient presented with symptoms that were plausibly all due to multiple sclerosis but was diagnosed with functional symptoms. The diagnosis of multiple sclerosis had not been considered and was unexpected at follow-up	Major
2. Differential diagnostic change	Patient presented with multiple symptoms. Doctor suggested chronic fatigue syndrome as most likely but considered multiple sclerosis as a possible diagnosis. Appropriate investigations and follow-up confirmed multiple sclerosis	None to minor
3. Diagnostic refinement	Doctor diagnosed epilepsy but at follow-up the diagnosis was refined to juvenile myoclonic epilepsy	None
4. Comorbid diagnostic change	Doctor correctly identified both epilepsy and nonepileptic seizures in the same patient. At follow-up, one of the disorders had remitted	None
5. Prodromal diagnostic change	Patient presented with an anxiety state. At 1 year follow-up, she had developed Alzheimer's disease. With hindsight, anxiety was a prodromal symptom of dementia but the diagnosis could not have been made at the initial assessment as the dementia symptoms (or findings on examination or investigation) had not developed sufficiently	None
6. *De novo* development of organic disease	Patient was correctly diagnosed with chronic fatigue syndrome. During the period of follow-up, the patient developed subarachnoid hemorrhage as a completely new and unrelated condition	None
7. Disagreement between doctors–without	Patient was diagnosed at baseline with chronic fatigue syndrome and at follow-up new information at follow-up with chronic Lyme disease by a different doctor, even though there is no new information. However, if the two doctors had both met the patient at follow-up, they would still have arrived at the different diagnoses. This would be reflected in similar divided opinion among their peers	None
8. Disagreement between doctors–with	Patient was diagnosed at baseline with chronic fatigue syndrome, and at follow-up new information at follow-up with fatigue due to a Chiari malformation by a different doctor because of new information at follow-up, (in this case an MRI scan ordered at the time of the first appointment). However, the first doctor seeing the patient again at follow-up continued to diagnose chronic fatigue syndrome, believing the Chiari malformation to be an incidental finding. This would be reflected in divided opinion among their peers	None

GENERAL CLINICAL FEATURES OF MIMICS AND CHAMELEONS

Table 2 lists some factors that we often come across in patients who have been erroneously labeled as having a disease when they actually have functional symptoms, and vice versa.

'This patient is Anxious/Recently Stressed/has a Personality Disorder', So, Must have Functional Symptoms (Table 3)

Probably the most common source of diagnostic error is when the clinician pays too much attention to the patient's psychosocial history and not enough to the presenting symptom. A generation and more of doctors have been taught via psychiatric diagnostic criteria that functional neurological symptoms are a form of 'conversion disorder' and, as such, represent the conversion of recent stress into a physical symptom.

In fact, the evidence on life events is not conclusive. Some studies have found an excess of recent and more distant life events[5] compared with disease controls, but some have not.[6,7] It is clear that there are many patients with no recent life events, and many others in whom life events or stress cannot be easily related to their symptom.

Likewise, the data on comorbid psychiatric disorder (such as anxiety, panic and depression) and personality disorder (such as avoidant or borderline personality) suggest that these things are more common than in disease controls. However, many patients with functional symptoms are psychiatrically 'normal', and around a third of patients with defined neurological disease have comorbid psychiatric symptoms. The upshot of this is that it is dangerous to base your diagnosis on the psychosocial history, however tempting the narrative may appear. Just as you would not make a diagnosis of stroke because someone smokes and has high blood pressure, these features should be regarded as supporting risk factors but not diagnostic in their own right. Be particularly careful of the patient who thinks their symptoms *are* stress related, as patients with disease are more likely to present with psychosocial attributions than patients with functional symptoms.[2]

Table 2: Functional symptoms; general factors relevant to spotting mimics and chameleons

Mimics: features of neurological disease that can lead erroneously to a diagnosis of functional symptoms	*Diagnostic clues/how not to mess up*
The presence of psychiatric disorder, especially personality disorder	Detecting psychiatric comorbidity may be useful in treating the patient but should be ignored in making the diagnosis. Focus on the nature of the attack/the physical examination. Are the physical features typical of functional symptoms?
Presence of schizophrenia or other psychotic illness	Such patients seldom have functional symptoms
The patient's presenting complaint is of new onset mood or behavioral disturbance.	Patients with functional symptoms rarely complain of significant psychiatric or behavioral symptoms, for example, panic, as their primary, subjective complaint, even if it is clearly present
The presence of an obvious life event or stressor	Ignore the presence of recent stress in making the diagnosis, even if this may be relevant for treatment
Failure to consider that the patient may have functional symptoms and a neurological disease	Remember that neurological disease is one of the most powerful risk factors for developing functional symptoms. (e.g. epilepsy/nonepileptic attacks, multiple sclerosis/functional weakness, idiopathic intracranial hypertension/functional visual symptoms)
Failure to consider that the patient may have functional symptoms and a progressive neurological disease, which may be too early for you to diagnose (yet)	As above, but in some cases, especially where neuroimaging does not help, the disease may only become apparent on follow up (e.g. motor neurone disease, Wilson's disease, Alzheimer's disease, myopathy)
'Labelle indifférence'—apparent indifference to disability	This 'sexy' French concept is wedded to conversion disorder and is of no diagnostic value, probably occurring more frequently in neurological disease, especially with frontal lobe involvement[11]
Normal neuroimaging	Many neurological diseases, for instance, epilepsy, motor neurone disease, myopathy, spinocerebellar ataxia have normal brain and spine imaging. Do not rely on it alone to exclude disease

Table 3: Chameleons: features of patients with functional symptoms that can wrongly put you off the diagnosis

The patient is 'normal'/'nice'/'stoical'/'like me'	Nice people get functional symptoms too
The patient has no 'form' that is, previous functional symptoms	Patients can present with dramatic neurological functional symptoms with no prior history
The patient has not been stressed	Between 1 in 3 and 1 in 4 patients have no evidence of recent stress
The patient is not tired/ only has one symptom	Lack of fatigue or other symptoms should make you think twice about a diagnosis of functional symptoms but monosymptomatic presentations do occur
The symptoms came on after injury, minor pathological disease	Commonplace in functional symptoms[12]
The patient suggests a psychological causation	Around 1 in 4 patients with functional symptoms do think that psychological factors are relevant
The patient has an established diagnosis of 'known epilepsy', 'known MS'	Always question other people's diagnoses (and your own!)
The patient is too old	Older patients with functional symptoms often have health anxiety and comorbid disease and are probably under-recognized[8]
Incidental abnormalities on MRI (e.g. enlarged perivascular space, Chiari malformation), EEG, serology or other tests	Do not assume that all structural abnormalities are relevant

'The Patient is Too Normal/Nice/Stoical/Male/Old/'Like Me'', So, Must have a Neurological Disease

The converse and quite common pitfall is the patient with functional symptoms who has the misfortune to share the same social and demographic features of the doctor attempting to make the diagnosis. In line with the discussion above, middle-aged males, people who are 'normal', 'nice' or 'seem genuine enough' can all develop functional symptoms, even dramatic ones. Studies on older patients with nonepileptic attacks show that they have an equal sex ratio, and often suffer from potentially life-threatening disease (such as ischemic heart disease or severe asthma), triggering health anxiety that links to the attacks themselves.[8]

'I have Made a Diagnosis, There is no Need for Another One'; The Problem of Comorbidity

The children's card game 'Top Trumps' involves comparing features of cars or superheroes, like 'top speed' or 'agility' to see which one is best. In the neurological 'Top Trumps' of the outpatient clinic, functional symptoms are usually a card that neither doctor nor patient wishes to hold, since it would always be beaten on criteria of public understanding and popularity by a disease diagnosis.

Neurological diseases tend to trump functional symptoms for both neurologists and patients, but try not to play this game when making a diagnosis in clinic. Instead, be willing to make two diagnoses if necessary.

The presence of any disease, however small, therefore, tends to 'trump' the presence of functional symptoms; but the reality is that the experience of bodily dysfunction caused by neurological disease is one of the most powerful risk factors for developing functional symptoms. Many patients have two diagnoses, for instance, epilepsy and dissociative (nonepileptic) attacks; multiple sclerosis and functional limb weakness; idiopathic intracranial hypertension and functional visual symptoms. It is easy for the presence of disease to obscure the presence of functional symptoms. Conversely, recognizing the functional symptom, diagnosis can assist the patient's treatment as it will often have more potential for reversibility than the underlying disease. In our own Scottish Study of 2467 outpatients with neurological disease, around 12% also had a diagnosis of a functional symptom. In these 12% of patients, no single disease category was more common than another. In other words, patients with, for example, multiple sclerosis or Parkinson's disease, do not appear to be more prone to functional symptoms than people with epilepsy or muscle disease.[9]

Comorbidity can present concurrently, for example, a patient who presents acutely with a mild episode of demyelination in whom the clinical features of the weakness are predominantly functional. Or functional symptoms can develop as a later complication of neurological disease; with health anxiety often having a key etiological role.

More problematically, some patients, especially those with degenerative and slowly progressive conditions, may present with functional symptoms years before the clear onset of their neurological disease. In some cases, a definite functional diagnosis, such as functional paralysis can present as part of the commonly encountered 'psychiatric prodrome' in dementias. In others, the experience of having a very mild ataxia, for instance, in the very early stages of spinocerebellar ataxia, seems enough to trigger the functional symptom.

The answer is, do not play neurological top trumps! Always look for comorbid disease, even if the diagnosis of functional symptoms is clear-cut, and make two diagnoses if necessary. If there is no disease, consider whether there are features that deserve longer-term follow-up that might indicate the patient is in the early stage of a slowly progressive disease. Finally, accept that you will sometimes get it wrong, or fail to anticipate the development of a disease, however careful you are. Studies of functional symptoms from the 1970s onwards coalesce around frequencies of misdiagnosis of about 5% after 5 years.[10] This is the same rate of misdiagnosis for most neurological and psychiatric disorders, and probably at least as common as misdiagnosis of functional symptoms as disease.

DISSOCIATIVE (NONEPILEPTIC) ATTACKS

A previous article in this series discussed mimics and chameleons of epilepsy, including dissociative (non-epileptic) attacks (Table 4).[13] Looking at the problem from the other end of the telescope, several features come into view which can lead to confusion both in terms of mistakenly calling attacks nonepileptic when they are not, and missing the diagnosis of nonepileptic attacks when it is right in front of you.

The diagnosis of nonepileptic attacks should be made on the basis of objective signs, such as eyes closed, resistance to eye opening, ictal or postictal weeping and prolonged attacks.[14] The problem is that the evidence for many of these signs comes from videotelemetry studies: in the real world, witnesses, including medical ones, can be very unreliable. For example, reports of eye closure from witnesses may be close to useless when compared with video electroencephalogram (EEG) evidence.[15] Therefore, the patient's subjective seizure experience is also important in giving additional clues. Simple questions, such as whether they 'remember the shaking' can be helpful,[14] but there is also evidence that there are conversational features of seizure description typical of nonepileptic attacks, including reluctance to describe seizure symptoms, or giving a poorly detailed description.[16] Instead, patients with dissociative attacks prefer to focus on the situations in which their attacks occur and the consequences of attacks.

The main theme of the nonepileptic attack mimics is that there are types of epilepsy that look a bit weird. For example, frontal lobe seizures can be associated with retained awareness or pelvic movements that can lead to assumptions that the patient may be 'acting out' abuse.[17] It is particularly important to remember that in temporal lobe epilepsy there can be quite a long prodrome lasting minutes in which the patient may have fear and dissociative symptoms similar to a patient having a dissociative (nonepileptic) attack.[18] Although ictal fear is usually distinguishable from a panic attack by the shorter duration, associated temporal lobe features and impaired awareness,[19] this is not such an easy distinction to make with nonepileptic attacks which may have all these features.

Table 4: Dissociative (nonepileptic) attacks: mimics and chameleons

Mimics: conditions that can look like dissociative (nonepileptic) attacks	*Diagnostic clues/how not to mess up*
Generalized tonic–clonic seizure	Include: ictal guttural 'cry' (not weeping) typically at onset, stertorous breathing, eyes open
Frontal lobe seizures	Short duration (less than 30 sec) Retained awareness during seizures Shouting, truncal or cycling leg movements Onset often/mostly from sleep
Temporal lobe seizures with ictal fear	Progression to generalized convulsion. Structural cause. Many temporal lobe features (e.g. olfactory hallucinations, macropsia) can appear in a dissociative nonepileptic attack
Self-induced seizures	Some patients with epilepsy can induce their own seizures, or may manipulate their medication to do so
Autoimmune limbic encephalitis [e.g. anti-N-methyl D-aspartate (Anti-NMDA), anti-voltage gated potassium channel (Anti-VGKC)]	Patients may present with psychiatric symptoms, unusual behavior and focal seizures
Stress induced seizures or syncope	Some epileptic seizures and cardiac syncope (e.g. long QT-related) can be triggered by emotional stress

Table 5: Chameleons: features of genuine dissociative (non-epileptic) attacks that can wrongly put you off the diagnosis

Olfactory hallucinations	Reports of 'burning rubber'/ 'feces'/'chemical smell' appear quite commonly in dissociative attacks
Dissociative experiences	Depersonalization, visual and perceptual changes in dissociative attacks can sound like temporal lobe epilepsy
Eyes open	Although 'eyes closed' is a good clue, some patients with dissociative attacks do open their eyes (with rolling) during attacks
Cyanosis/breath holding	Including low oxygen saturations
Injury	Including bitten tongue (sometimes visibly), broken teeth, (recurrent) shoulder dislocation and falls on stairs all occur in dissociative attacks. Reports of injury may be more common than actual injury
Incontinence	Urinary incontinence is common and fecal incontinence does happen in dissociative attacks
Seizures arising from sleep/when alone	Occurs in dissociative attacks
Response to 'trial of antiepileptics'/relapse of attacks when antiepileptics withdrawn	Patients with dissociative attacks may experience both strong placebo effect when antiepileptics are started and nocebo effect when they are stopped
The patient in intensive care who several non-neurologist physicians and anesthetists are convinced is in status epilepticus	Prolonged events/seizure 'status' is more common in patients with dissociative attacks than in patients with epilepsy. Up to 50% of patients attending hospital in apparent refractory status have this diagnosis

The chameleons are mostly those things that people think are quite specific to epilepsy, but in reality are not, such as injury[20] (and especially report of injury), olfactory hallucinations and going blue (Table 5).

In clinical practice, it is not always possible to be sure what a patient's attack disorder is due to, even with all this information. For this reason, the careful neurologist strikes a balance between making confident diagnoses where possible, but saying 'not sure' where appropriate. In any patient, it is important not to close the book completely on the diagnosis, checking seizure descriptions at each visit, and watching out for the combination of both epilepsy and nonepileptic attacks. Trials of antiepileptic drugs should be avoided because they rarely deliver convincing answers, often increase diagnostic confusion, and may have iatrogenic effects.

FUNCTIONAL MOTOR SYMPTOMS

The diagnosis of functional motor symptoms should always be based on positive evidence on the examination of internal inconsistency (e.g. Hoover's sign for paralysis or a tremor that stops or entrains during contralateral cued rhythmical movement).[4] However, there can be difficulties in overinterpretation of these 'positive signs', and it would be unreasonable to expect them always to perform, especially in isolation. The presence of pain in a limb, inattention or neglect, or simple failure to understand the examiner's instructions, are all reasons why these signs may be falsely positive.

As with epilepsy, things that look weird, like stiff person syndrome or generalized dystonia, particularly

Table 6: Functional motor symptoms: mimics and chameleons

Mimics: conditions that can look like functional motor symptoms	*Diagnostic clues/how not to mess up*
Higher cortical gait disturbance	Do not rely on an 'odd gait' to make the diagnosis
Acute parietal stroke/pathology	May have Hoover's sign/MRI brain
Stiff person syndrome	Electrophysiology findings and antiglutamic acid decarboxylase (anti-GAD) antibodies
Dystonia (geste antagoniste), better walking backwards or running)	Familiarity with clinical presentation of organic movement disorders
Myasthenia (variability, give-way weakness)	Avoid putting diagnostic weight on edrophonium (Tensilon) test, which can be false positive (even when blinded) in patients with chronic fatigue syndrome. Strong placebo response to corticosteroids may also occur in patients with functional symptoms
Pain with weakness in limbs	Place less reliability on positive signs of functional weakness in presence of pain. Ask patient if they think pain is the reason their limb is weak
Paroxysmal dyskinesia especially with aura and urge to move	Familiarity with clinical presentation of organic movement disorders
Tics/Tourette's syndrome	Ability to suppress with rebound movements, (may be distractible)

Table 7: Chameleons: Features of functional motor symptoms that can wrongly put you off the diagnosis

Variable ankle clonus	Happens
Facial symptoms	Common
Slightly asymmetrical reflexes /mute plantar	Happens
Contractures in fixed dystonia	Happens
Migraine at onset	Migraine can trigger functional symptoms
Tremor unaffected by distraction	In chronic functional tremor motor distraction tasks sometimes no longer visibly affect the tremor. Thermography or video recording may be helpful
Urinary retention	Appears quite common in patients with acute back pain and leg weakness in the absence of structural changes.[26] Also occurs with opiate overuse
Axial 'propriospinal' myoclonus	Usually functional[27]
Convergent spasm leading to apparent sixth nerve palsy	Look for variability over the assessment or resolution with a more distant target
Lack of pain or sensory disturbance	This should make you think twice about a diagnosis of functional motor symptoms but can occur

if they are inherently somewhat variable, can fool the unwary into a diagnosis of functional symptoms. The list in Table 6 is obviously not comprehensive. Orthostatic tremor (a movement disorder only present on standing), alien limb phenomena in corticobasal degeneration, and the aura of paroxysmal kinesigenic dyskinesia, are just some of the reasons why the diagnosis of functional neurological symptoms should usually be made by a neurologist who is familiar with the breadth of unusual presentation that neurological disease has to offer.

Conversely, in patients who do have functional symptoms, there can be surprising findings (Table 7). Just as reflexes can be brisk in people who are anxious, we have seen patients with unilaterally increased reflexes as a transient phenomenon. Such reflex asymmetry was well reported in the older literature.[21] Occasionally, patients with unilateral motor symptoms also develop something that looks very similar to ankle clonus, but is variable between assessments. It is not unusual for plantars to be mute on the same side as functional hemisensory loss.

Functional facial symptoms, typically with contraction of orbicularis oculis, orbicularis oris and platysma and sometimes with jaw deviation are clinically quite common. They were well described in the older literature, and have recently been described again in more detail.[22] Since these facial symptoms lead to an appearance of weakness (even though they are due to muscle overactivity), this can lead to erroneous diagnoses of stroke if the presentation is acute.

Asymmetrical platysma contraction can arise as a functional symptom, causing facial asymmetry and diagnostic confusion. Reproduced from Fasano et al.[22] with permission.

Slightly better known, although still commonly missed, is convergence spasm, which is relatively common in patients with functional motor symptoms.[23] You can usually bring this out by asking the patient to converge on a near target for 10 sec. In convergence spasm, the convergence persists long enough to produce the appearance of impaired abduction, which can be mistaken for a sixth nerve palsy. One way around this is to go back and test eye movements without convergence, and using a more distant target at a different point in the assessment, or just to observe eye movement during the consultation, to show the inconsistency.

Contractures can cause concern about a diagnosis of functional or fixed dystonia, but these do occur in patients who have been immobile for a long time, albeit they are rare and should at least prompt some reconsideration of the diagnosis. They can be demonstrated under anesthesia.

There is insufficient space here to rehearse all the debates about the overlap between functional symptoms and complex regional pain syndrome. It is indisputably the case, however, that the functional motor symptoms seen in complex regional pain syndrome are clinically identical to those functional motor symptoms seen in patients without pain.[24,25] The debate would be a lot more interesting if advocates of the 'biological model' were not so ready to dismiss patients with 'psychogenic' symptoms as having symptoms of doubtful authenticity.

OTHER MIMICS AND CHAMELEONS

- *Laryngeal dystonia* (as seen in multiple system atrophy) can be confused with functional dysphonia when the otolaryngological assessment suggests that there is nothing wrong with the vocal cords.[27]
- *Cortical blindness* (e.g. from a stroke). Beware the patient who reports being blind but has normal pupillary reflexes and preserved optokinetic nystagmus. These patients should always earn an MRI brain scan as, occasionally, this is due to bilateral occipital pathology—cortical blindness. A subset of patients with cortical blindness think they can see even though they cannot (Anton's syndrome).[28]
- *Brain injury* (diagnosed on the basis of a poor cognitive score) can be a functional chameleon. Poor concentration and memory symptoms are common as part of the 'postconcussion syndrome' after minor head injury. Although this is sometimes partly attributable to minor injury (at least for a period of weeks), there is evidence that the 'postconcussion syndrome' arises just as commonly after trauma to other parts of the body.[28] Postconcussion syndrome is predicted by psychological factors more than by the severity of the head injury,[29] and in many cases is best seen as a generic functional response to trauma, rather than a consequence of brain injury. Some patients who present late after physical injury find their way into neuropsychological assessment. If the assessor is unwary (which may include a neuropsychologist) they may interpret poor cognitive scores as unequivocal evidence of brain injury. This is especially the case if the patient scores normally on simple screening tests of anxiety and depression. Contrary to popular belief, a low score on these does not 'filter out' patients with functional symptoms. For the neurologist, it is particularly important not to be put off a diagnosis of functional cognitive symptoms by a low score on cognitive tests such as the Addenbrooke's Cognitive Examination (ACE). Tests like this are largely validated against healthy controls, and not against patients with functional disorders. Low scores on tests of attention, memory and fluency are typical. The patient with a low ACE score who attends on their own is another clue that the symptoms may be functional. Even detailed psychometric examination has a very poor predictive validity in such patients, particularly in the absence of effort testing. The key message is that brain injury should always be diagnosed with regard to standard peri-injury clinical features, such as presence of loss of consciousness or amnesia, which often gets lost as time passes.

Psychiatric Disorders

Our bias in this article was to disentangle functional symptoms from neurological disease, but there are occasions when other psychiatric disorders need to be considered.

- *Panic attacks*. Patients with panic disorder not infrequently find their way to a neurology clinic with paresthesia or intermittent dizziness. Panic symptoms can present as unilateral paresthesia. Some patients have predominantly cardiorespiratory symptoms (chest tightness, palpitations and shortness of breath), whereas, others may have a more autonomic presentation (nausea, sweating, chills). Dissociation is often described as 'dizziness.'[30] Typically, the patient in the neurology clinic regards the intense fear as a reaction to the physical symptoms rather than a cause of the symptoms, but a subset of patients do not experience severe fear, so-called 'panic without fear.'[31]
- *Anxiety*. As with panic disorder, it is possible to have all the somatic symptoms of anxiety, fatigue, restlessness, irritability, poor concentration and insomnia, but not necessarily feel that anxious. Hyperventilation may also be unassociated with feelings of panic (and may cause unilateral paresthesia and tetany).
- *Depression* is a frequent complication of neurological disease, and often is associated with poorer than expected physical function, diffuse aches and pains and marked fatigue.
- *Body dysmorphic disorder* presents with an excessive preoccupation with a bodily part that usually works normally. It is not a common presentation in neurological settings. The conviction of the concern about the affected body part is usually very noticeable.
- *Psychosis* is rarely confused with functional symptoms. Where somatic hallucinations are present, they are

usually accompanied by bizarre and complex delusional explanations.

- *Mania* presents with increased motor activity accompanied by grandiosity and loosening of associations in language function. It is rarely confused with functional symptoms, but can be mistaken for encephalitis.
- *Alcohol misuse* (frequently covert) can present as a recurrent 'attack' disorder, with individual episodes of intoxication, and with a range of neurological complications.[32]

FACTITIOUS DISORDER AND MALINGERING

Finally, there is one last area of diagnostic overlap with functional symptoms: the patient who is deliberately assuming symptoms in order to gain medical care (factitious disorder) or some material/financial benefit (malingering).

This is something that neurologists often worry about[33] (probably more than misdiagnosis of disease). The truth is that the only way to know if someone's symptoms are consciously produced, as opposed to genuinely experienced, is to obtain either:

- A confession, or
- Evidence of a major discrepancy between reported function (what the patient tells you) and observed function (what you see the patient doing when unobserved).

In reality, such evidence rarely appears. This leaves open the possibility of exaggeration, as for any subjectively reported symptom, such as pain and depression. Evidence of lying in the past, evidence of inconsistent reporting of the history between different doctors, multiple name changes and attending multiple hospitals are clues to factitious disorder and malingering.

Some things argue against the idea that malingering is endemic—for instance, the way that patients consistently describe their subjective symptoms, have attacks when suggested during EEG, develop wear marks on their shoes, and retain disability and distress at follow-up. An important study of actigraphy in functional tremor showed that even patients who know they are being monitored are hopeless at guessing how bad their symptoms are. In this study, the 10 patients with functional tremor thought, on average, that their symptoms were present 83% of the time, when in fact they were only present 4% of the time (compared with 58% reported vs 24% observed in organic tremor).[34] In other words, the patients with functional tremor in this study probably only had the symptom when they thought about it, but this gives the illusion of the symptom being there all the time. This is a bit like assuming that the light is always on in the fridge because it appears to be so whenever you open the door!

Clinicians are sometimes asked to comment explicitly on these issues in a court setting. In personal injury settings, functional symptoms/possible functional overlay is commonplace. It is appropriate to make such diagnoses to the court, but remember that in any given individual, functional symptoms cannot be distinguished from deliberate exaggeration by clinical examination alone. Strong support of an individual's claim and testimony of their honesty in the absence of clear objective supporting evidence is a quick route to later professional embarrassment. In the context of criminal cases, diagnoses of functional symptoms are likely to only apply to fugue states and psychogenic nonepileptic attacks. Many perpetrators of violent crime report no memory of the events, but in the overwhelming majority of cases, medical explanations are not relevant. Functional diagnoses should probably not be made in this situation, and then, if they are, only where there is clear objective supporting evidence, and the diagnosis is not incompatible with the nature of the crime.

CONCLUSION

The mimics and chameleons of functional symptoms could be a whole textbook of neurology, but when things go wrong, there are some recurring themes, notably: diagnostic bias introduced by the presence or absence of psychiatric comorbidity or by life events; neurological diseases that look 'weird'; and a lack of appreciation of the more unusual features of functional symptoms themselves.

REFERENCES

1. Stone J, Carson A, Duncan R, et al. Symptoms 'unexplained by organic disease' in 1144 new neurology out-patients: how often does the diagnosis change at follow-up? Brain. 2009;132(Pt 10):2878-88.
2. Stone J, Warlow C, Sharpe M. The symptom of functional weakness: a controlled study of 107 patients. Brain. 2010; 133: 1537-51.
3. Carson A, Stone J, Hibberd C, et al. Disability, distress and unemployment in neurology outpatients with symptoms 'unexplained by organic disease'. J Neurol Neurosurg Psychiatry. 2011;82:810-13.
4. Stone J. The bare essentials: functional symptoms in neurology. Pract Neurol. 2009; 9: 179-89.
5. Sharpe D, Faye C. Non-epileptic seizures and child sexual abuse: a critical review of the literature. Clin Psychol Rev. 2006; 26: 1020-40.
6. Testa SM, Krauss GL, Lesser RP, et al. Stressful life event appraisal and coping in patients with psychogenic seizures and those with epilepsy. Seizure. 2012; 21:282-7.
7. Kranick S, Ekanayake V, Martinez V, et al. Psychopathology and psychogenic movement disorders. Mov Disord. 2011;26:1844-50.
8. Duncan R, Oto M, Martin E, et al. Late onset psychogenic nonepileptic attacks.Neurology. 2006;66:1644-7.

9. Stone J, Carson A, Duncan R, et al. Which neurological diseases are most likely to be associated with "symptoms unexplained by organic disease". J Neurol. 2012;259:33-8.
10. Stone J, Smyth R, Carson A, et al. Systematic review of misdiagnosis of conversion symptoms and "hysteria". BMJ. 2005;331:989.
11. Stone J, Smyth R, Carson A, et al. La belle indifference in conversion symptoms and hysteria: systematic review. Br J Psychiatry. 2006;188:204-9.
12. Stone J, Warlow C, Sharpe M. Functional weakness: clues to mechanism from the nature of onset. J Neurol Neurosurg Psychiatry. 2012;83:67-9.
13. Smith PE. Epilepsy: mimics, borderland and chameleons. Pract Neurol. 2012;12:299-307.
14. Avbersek A, Sisodiya S. Does the primary literature provide support for clinical signs used to distinguish psychogenic nonepileptic seizures from epileptic seizures? J Neurol Neurosurg Psychiatry. 2010; 81:719-25.
15. Syed TU, Arozullah AM, Suciu GP, et al. Do observer and self-reports of ictal eye closure predict psychogenic nonepileptic seizures? Epilepsia. 2008; 49:898-904.
16. Plug L, Reuber M. Making the diagnosis in patients with blackouts—it's all in the history.Pract Neurol. 2008.
17. Geyer JD, Payne TA, Drury I. The value of pelvic thrusting in the diagnosis of seizures and pseudoseizures. Neurology. 2000; 54: 227-9.
18. Goldstein LH, Mellers JD. Ictal symptoms of anxiety, avoidance behaviour, and dissociation in patients with dissociative seizures. J Neurol Neurosurg Psychiatry. 2006; 77:616-21.
19. Beyenburg S, Mitchell AJ, Schmidt D, et al. Anxiety in patients with epilepsy: systematic review and suggestions for clinical management. Epilepsy Behav. 2005;7:161-71.
20. Peguero E, bou-Khalil B, Fakhoury T, et al. Self-injury and incontinence in psychogenic seizures. Epilepsia. 1995;36:586-91.
21. Allen IM. Observations on the motor phenomena of hysteria. J Neurol Psychopathol. 1935;16:1-25.
22. Fasano A, Valadas A, Bhatia KP, et al. Psychogenic facial movement disorders: clinical features and associated conditions. Mov Disord. 2012;27:1544-51.
23. Fekete R, Baizabal-Carvallo JF, Ha AD, et al. Convergence spasm in conversion disorders: prevalence in psychogenic and other movement disorders compared with controls. J Neurol Neurosurg Psychiatry. 2012;83:202-4.
24. Deuschl G, Blumberg H, Lucking CH. Tremor in reflex sympathetic dystrophy. Arch Neurol. 1991;48:1247-52.
25. Schrag A, Trimble M, Quinn N, et al. The syndrome of fixed dystonia: an evaluation of 103 patients. Brain. 2004;127(Pt 10):2360-72.
26. Rooney A, Statham PF, Stone J. Cauda equina syndrome with normal MR imaging. J Neurol. 2009;256:721-5.
27. van der Salm SM, Koelman JH, Henneke S, et al. Axial jerks: a clinical spectrum ranging from propriospinal to psychogenic myoclonus. J Neurol. 2010;257:1349-55.
28. Meares S, Shores EA, Taylor AJ, et al. Mild traumatic brain injury does not predict acute postconcussion syndrome. J Neurol Neurosurg Psychiatry. 2008;79:300-6.
29. Hou R, Moss-Morris R, Peveler R, et al. When a minor head injury results in enduring symptoms: a prospective investigation of risk factors for postconcussional syndrome after mild traumatic brain injury. J Neurol Neurosurg Psychiatry. 2012;83:217-23.
30. Stone J. Dissociation: what is it and why is it important? Pract Neurol. 2006;6:308-13.
31. Kushner MG, Beitman BD. Panic attacks without fear: an overview. Behav Res Ther. 1990;28:469-79.
32. Welch KA. Neurological complications of alcohol and misuse of drugs. Pract Neurol. 2011;11:206-19.
33. Kanaan R, Armstrong D, Barnes P, et al. In the psychiatrist's chair: how neurologists understand conversion disorder. Brain. 2009;132(Pt 10):2889-96.
34. Parees I, Saifee TA, Kassavetis P, et al. Believing is perceiving: mismatch between self-report and actigraphy in psychogenic tremor. Brain. 2012;135(Pt 1):117-23.

CHAPTER 78

Nonconventional Approaches of Treatment in Psychiatry

Jayati Simlai, Sourav Khanra, Umesh S, CRJ Khess

INTRODUCTION

Throughout history there have been two separate traditional systems in the practice of medicine. One is the 'art of healing' and usually involves its own specialized brand of training and relies mainly on a prescriber's intuition and patient perceptions of successful outcomes. This system aims to use the art as a form of therapy to soothe patients' minds and bodies and help them on their path to recovery.[1] The second tradition, the 'science of healing', is based on technological and scientific ideas and leaves much less opportunity for practitioners to express an innovative and intuitive approach to medicine. Complementary and alternative medicine (CAM) is a group of nonorthodox and traditional therapies that may be used alone, or to complement orthodox or other non-orthodox therapies in the treatment and/or prevention of disease. Medications are known for their side effects, sometime fail to respond and they carry high costs. Hence, researchers are beginning to realize that CAM approaches can influence many of the regulatory systems involved in the pathogenesis of psychiatric disorders and provide new avenues for treatment. Many therapies are well known, whereas others may be exotic, mysterious or even hazardous. Relaxation techniques, massage, diet and so on could be considered to be lifestyle choices rather than true therapeutic interventions. However, it could be argued that an enhanced feeling of well-being is sufficient to warrant the inclusion of a procedure as a therapeutic intervention. Till date, more than 700 complementary and alternative therapies are practiced in developed as well as in developing regions of the world.[2] However, majority of these traditional healing practices have not been thoroughly investigated using standard research methods. Despite the paucity of robust scientific evidence complementary and alternative medicine remains popular with clients who appreciate the holistic approach and have a belief in its effectiveness.

DEFINITIONS OF CAM

The term 'complementary and alternative medicine' has been the main term used by both CAM practitioners and health providers since the early 1990s. Although not all practitioners accept that the distinction between 'complementary' and 'alternative' is valid or meaningful, much of the literature makes a firm distinction between 'complementary' medicine on the one hand and 'alternative' medicine on the other. The British Medical Association (BMA)[3] distinguishes between complementary and alternative therapies. 'Complementary' therapies are those which can work alongside and in conjunction with orthodox medical treatment. Within this category there is clearly a wide diversity of types of practice, which would include self-help therapies such as yoga; relatively noninvasive therapies such as healing and massage; and therapies such as acupuncture and chiropractic. In contrast, 'alternative' therapies could be seen as those which are given in place of orthodox medical treatment. While, clearly any nonconventional therapy could in some circumstances be used as an alternative form of treatment; for example, if a practitioner of any discipline suggested that the patient should not receive concurrent orthodox medical treatment; there are some therapies which, by their very nature, aim to replace orthodox medicine. Examples of such therapies might include herbal medicines, which are often given in place of orthodox medication, as an alternative to allopathic drugs.

In the United States, National Center of Complementary and Alternative Medicine (NCCAM)[4] makes a similar distinction to the BMA, differentiating between complementary and alternative medicine using the following definitions. Complementary medicine is used together with conventional medicine. An example of a complementary therapy is using aromatherapy to help lessen a patient's discomfort following surgery. Alternative medicine is used in place of conventional medicine. An example of an alternative therapy is using a special diet to treat cancer instead of undergoing surgery, radiation, or chemotherapy that has been recommended by a conventional doctor.

MAJOR TYPES OF CAM[4]

Alternative Medical Systems

Alternative medical systems are built upon complete systems of theory and practice. Often, these systems have evolved apart from and earlier than the conventional medical approaches of the West. Examples of alternative medical systems that have developed in Western cultures include homeopathic medicine and naturopathic medicine. Examples of systems that have developed in non-Western cultures include traditional Chinese medicine and Ayurveda.

Mind-body Interventions

Mind-body medicine uses a variety of techniques designed to enhance the mind's capacity to affect bodily function and symptoms. Some techniques that were considered CAM in the past have become mainstream (for example, patient support groups and cognitive-behavioral therapy). Other mind-body techniques are still considered CAM, including meditation, prayer, mental healing, Yoga and therapies that use creative outlets such as art, music, or dance.

Biologically-based Therapies

Biologically-based therapies in CAM use substances found in nature, such as herbs, foods and vitamins. Some examples include dietary supplements, herbal products, and the use of other so-called 'natural,' but as yet scientifically unproven therapies.

Manipulative and Body-based Methods

Manipulative and body-based methods in CAM are based on manipulation and/or movement of one or more parts of the body. Some examples include chiropractic manipulation and massage therapy.

Energy Therapies

Energy therapies involve the use of energy fields.
They are two types of energy therapies:

1. *Biofield therapies:* These are intended to affect energy fields that purportedly surround and penetrate the human body. The existence of such fields has not yet been scientifically proven. Some forms of energy therapy manipulate biofields by applying pressure and/or manipulating the body by placing the hands in, or through, these fields. Examples include Qi gong, Reiki, and Therapeutic Touch.
2. *Bioelectromagnetic-based therapies:* These involve the unconventional use of electromagnetic fields, such as pulsed fields, magnetic fields, or alternating current or direct current fields.

CLASSIFYING CAM THERAPIES ACCORDING TO ETHICAL ISSUES

Stone[5] categorized CAM disciplines by grouping therapies based on the ethical issues they raise. Researchers believe that a categorization explicitly based on ethical issues should take account of the underlying concerns, such as inherent risk and capacity to cause harm. An appreciation of this classification requires an understanding of the scope of ethics. Here, ethical considerations include the following principles:

Any form of treatment should have the capacity to benefit and not to harm. Treatment should usually be given on the basis of a voluntary, informed consent. Appropriate mechanisms should be in place in case anything goes wrong.

Stone's[5] classification therapies divides into the following six groups:

1. Hands-on therapy, includes chiropractic, massage, reflexology, aromatherapy and therapeutic touch.
2. Invasive therapies, include acupuncture or any therapy using an invasive technique.
3. Product-based therapies, include homeopathy, herbalism (Western and traditional Chinese herbal medicine), Ayurveda, Unani, aromatherapy, nutritional therapy.
4. Energy-based medicine, includes spiritual healing, reiki, therapeutic touch, acupuncture and qi gong.
5. Psychological interventions include hypnotherapy, counseling and psychotherapy.
6. Self-help techniques include yoga, biofeedback, meditation, visualization, self-hypnosis, relaxation techniques, Qi gong and autogenic training.

Each group is based on a predominant ethical concern. For example, hands-on therapies are linked by respect for bodily sovereignty and the extent to which ethicists regard the slightest 'unwanted touching' as infringement of a patient's autonomy. In hands-on therapies, autonomy and boundary issues are thus paramount as touching the patient inappropriately could lead to professional disciplinary issues. Product-based therapies are linked by their capacity to cause harm as well as good. Thus, there is a need for quality control and practitioners should give the patient adequate information about the product so they can make an informed choice about its use. The linking of product-based therapies also highlights regulatory issues, including the evidence base which is required before specific medicinal claims can be made about CAM products. Self-help techniques are linked from an ethical perspective by the extent to which patients are expected to take responsibility for themselves and the consequent sharing of responsibility for outcomes.

VARIOUS NONCONVENTIONAL APPROACHES OF TREATMENT IN PSYCHIATRY

This section would be dealing with various modalities of treatment which have been found to be efficacious in researches through the last few decades. As described earlier these modalities of treatment intend to enhance or supplement other treatments including traditional Western medicine. The list of complementary methods or modalities changes continually, as those therapies that are proven to be safe and effective become adopted into conventional health care and as new approaches to health care emerge. Including all the modalities and products would be beyond the scope of this chapter. For the sake of discussion various biological modalities, herbal products including St. John's wort, phytomedicines and adaptogens would be focused on.

BIOLOGICAL TREATMENTS

A plethora of nutrients have been tried and found to be effective in treatment of psychiatric disorders. These may include dietary modification, vitamins, minerals, etc.

Vitamins—folate, B_{12}

Extensive researches in last few decades have demonstrated that folate (vitamin B_9) and cobalamin (vitamin B_{12}) play important roles in the development and function of the central nervous system. The relationship between these two can be appreciated by similarities in clinical presentation produced by deficits and/or impaired metabolism of these two vitamins. The metabolic connection between these two is the conversion of homocysteine (Hcy) to methionine. Methionine is an essential amino acid which is the substrate of s-adenosylmethionine. Both folate and vitamin B_{12} help in the conversion of homocysteine to methionine. On the other hand s-adenosylmethionine (SAMe), produced from methionine, is an exclusive methyl donor in several methylation reaction of human body. This methylation reaction is important as it is required for normal cell function of our body. In methylation reaction, sAMe donates the methyl group to a donor molecule. The various donor molecules include DNA bases, proteins, phospholipids, neurotransmitters, free amino acids, and other compounds.[5] Active uptake of folate across the blood-brain-barrier occurs at specific folate-receptor a (FR- a) sites, localized in the choroid plexus. FR-a has a high affinity for 5-MTHF and a lower affinity for other reduced folates. Once 5-MTHF enters the cerebrospinal fluid (CSF) compartment it is transported into neuronal cells, and participates in methylation of Hcy and synthesis of methionine and SAMe.

Folate and Depression

In the late twentieth century, all surveys of folate deficiency, including those of depression, mania, schizophrenia and dementia reported low levels of serum folate. Despite various reports on association of folate and depression, very few controlled clinical trials have been designed to examine the effect of folate treatment alone on mood disorders. On the contrary, a combination of folate, vitamin B_6 and vitamin B_{12} have been investigated for their efficacy on mood disorders. One double-blind randomized, placebo-controlled trial[6] evaluated the effect of a daily supplement of 200 mg folic acid or a matched placebo in a group of 75 patients. All of them were on lithium according to research design. This study of one year duration showed that patients with the highest concentrations of plasma folate had a significant reduction in their affective morbidity. This finding persuaded the investigators to suggest that a daily supplement of 300 to 400 m g/day folic acid could be useful in long-term lithium treatment. Another large double blind randomized placebo controlled trial compared the effect of folic acid versus placebo given as an adjuvant to fluoxetine treatment in 127 depressed patients.[7] Significant reduction in Hamilton Depression Rating Scale (HAM-D) scores was observed in the folic acid plus fluoxetine group. But this was observed only in female patients. Female patients had the highest plasma folate and significantly lower plasma total homocysteine (tHcy) values after treatment compared with baseline values. Moreover, efficacy of 5-MTHF as an adjunctive therapy for SSRI resistant depression was studied in 2 randomized, double-blind, parallel sequential trials.[8] One of them showed significant decrease in HAM-D score in adjunctive therapy group. Besides this, in both trials there were no significant difference in side effects in treatment groups. But unlike SSRIs, folic acid is yet to be examined as an adjunctive treatment with other classes of antidepressants. To add to this, one double blind placebo controlled trial examined its effect in depression and schizophrenia and found improvement of clinical and social recovery in those who were folate deficient.[9]

Folate and Dementia

Several studies have shown associations between the status of these vitamins and elevated levels of plasma tHcy regarding cognitive function. One trial examined the effect of folic acid on community dwelling men and women aged between 50 and 70 years and found that 800 mg folic acid only, given daily for 3 years, improved measures of cognitive functions compared with placebo.[10] A more recent study on similar patient population showed significant improvement in cognitive function after 2 years of treatment with folic acid, vitamin B_{12}, and vitamin B_6.[11] But as a combination was used the extent of a synergistic effect could not be made out and effect due to individual components was unclear. In case of Alzheimer's disease there is inconsistent evidence for efficacy of folic acid in improving cognition. One double-blind randomized placebo-controlled trial of folate and B vitamins in subjects with Alzheimer dementia failed to show any significant effect on cognitive function.[12] However, in one study improvement was observed after 15 months in subjects having higher mini-mental state examination (MMSE) scores at baseline.[13] In summary, folate and B-vitamin treatment may slow the rate of cognitive decline in subjects less severely affected at baseline. In line with this, supplementation trials with folic acid, vitamin B_{12}, and B_6 in subjects with mild cognitive impairment (MCI) showed significant benefit in global cognition, episodic memory and semantic memory.[14] In a 24-month study, folic acid and B vitamins significantly slowed the rate of brain atrophy in subjects with MCI, an effect that was also related to baseline plasma tHcy concentrations.[15]

Vitamin B_{12} and Depression

Vitamin B_{12} deficiency has been reported in numerous studies to be associated with psychiatric disorders including depression, bipolar disorder, panic disorder, psychosis, and phobias. In one study in the Netherlands, 278 individuals older than 55 years with depressive symptoms had lower levels of plasma vitamin B_{12}.[16] In Chinese elderly subjects (n 5 669) a low level of vitamin B_{12} (<180 pmol/L) was significantly associated with depressive symptoms (odds ratio 2.68), independent of folate or tHcy levels.[17] These findings are consistent with an earlier study of 700 community-dwelling older women that found a 2-fold risk of severe depression in subjects with elevated Methylmalonic Acid levels (MMA, a marker of B_{12} deficiency).[18] However, one randomized placebo-controlled trial[19] in elderly men did not find that vitamin B_{12} supplementation for two years had any significant effect in reducing severity or incidence of depressive symptoms. On the other hand, a prospective study of 115 outpatients with major depressive disorder showed that higher vitamin B_{12} levels correlate with a better response to treatment.[20] Also, several case reports describe a lack of antidepressant response in individuals with vitamin B_{12} deficiency who showed considerable clinical improvement following supplementation with vitamin B_{12}. There is no current recommended guideline for the prophylactic use of vitamin B_{12} in the treatment of depression. Side effects of vitamin B_{12} are rare. One report found that a combination of folate, B_6, and B_{12} supplementation increased the risk of re-stenosis by 8% in men only with cardiac stents and a baseline Hcy of less than 15 mmol/L.[21] But this was not replicated in an another study.[22] Considering the low level of adverse effects, clinicians may choose to prescribe vitamin B_{12} in depressed patients or in those with low serum levels of vitamin B_{12} or elevated MMA.

Vitamin B_{12} and Dementia

The best example of association between vitamin B_{12} deficiency and dementia can be found in patients with pernicious anemia who develop a dementia syndrome that responds well to vitamin B_{12} treatment, when given before irreversible damage occurs. The relationship between low levels of serum vitamin B_{12} and cognitive function in healthy elderly subjects has been extensively studied, and the symptoms described can often overlap with those observed in dementia of the Alzheimer type. Furthermore, low serum vitamin B_{12} has been associated with greater cognitive impairment in patients with Alzheimer disease. This association is stronger when elevated plasma tHcy is present, which has been shown to be a risk factor for dementia.[5] Likewise in case of folate, vitamin B_{12} is an essential cofactor for 2 enzymes, namely methionine synthase and MMCoA mutase. High doses can help to maintain low blood levels of Hcy and MMA. Vitamin B_{12}-dependent metabolism of Hcy to methionine enhances sAMe synthesis and methylation in the same manner as folate.

S-Adenosyl Methionine

S-Adenosyl Methionine and Depression

In a meta-analysis, Bressa reviewed 25 controlled trials including a total of 791 patients. He concluded that s-adenosyl methionine (sAMe) had a significantly greater response rate than placebo and was comparable with tricyclic antidepressants.[23] In another literature review, Brown and colleagues[24] reported that sAMe had been studied in 16 open, uncontrolled trials (660 patients); 13 double blind randomized placebo-controlled trials (537 patients); and 19 controlled trials comparing sAMe with other antidepressants (1134 patients). All 16 open trials reported significant antidepressant effects. In 18 controlled trials, sAMe was as effective as tricyclics like chlorimipramine, imipramine, and nomifensine. Also side effects were less reported than other standard antidepressants. A double blind randomized placebo-controlled trial of sAMe tablets, similar to the over-the-counter dietary supplement, was administered to 73 serotonin reuptake inhibitor (SRI) nonresponders with major depressive disorders. The adjunctive oral dose of sAMe (800 mg twice daily) was shown to augment the response rates for depression at the end of the 6-week trial. In this study, the dose of sAMe was both effective and well tolerated. In an 8-week double blind randomized placebo-controlled study of 18 schizophrenic patients, oral sAMe (800 mg/day) significantly improved ameliorated aggressive symptoms.[25] Most trials of oral sAMe have been performed in patients with major depressive disorder. One limitation is that relatively small numbers of subjects (fewer than 50 patients in each therapeutic arm) were recruited into those trials. Current evidence suggests that in clinical trials the lowest dose of sAMe shown to be effective is 800 mg/day for mild to moderate depression and 1600 mg/day for severe major depressive disorder.[5]

S-Adenosyl Methionine and Dementia

Despite the lack of large well-controlled clinical trials, there is significant evidence to support the role of sAMe and methylation in dementia. Concentrations of sAMe in CSF have been reported to be significantly reduced in Alzheimer dementia. Current evidence demonstrates that administration of oral sAMe for 3 to 5 months (400 mg 3 times daily), can increase plasma and CSF concentrations and improve measures of cognitive function as well as mood and speed of mental processing. In a more recent double-blind randomized placebo-controlled trial on the use of adjunctive sAMe in 47 patients with major depressive disorder, a secondary analysis demonstrated that oral SAMe (1600 mg daily) improved memory-related cognitive symptoms such as the ability to recall information and word finding.[5]

The stimulatory effect of sAMe on central monoaminergic neurotransmitters is a likely viable mechanism underlying its antidepressant effect. There is a modest body of literature linking hypomethylation as a major biological mechanism involved in the etiology of dementia. These findings include decreased sAMe concentrations in CSF in patients with Alzheimer's disease, hypomethylation of proteins that regulate levels of brain tissue phosphorylated-Tau, and hypomethylation of genes that affect the expression of β-amyloid protein. The effect of sAMe on site-specific methylation of DNA-promoter regions that regulate gene function, and carboxymethylation of proteins that can regulate β-amyloid and phosphorylation of Tau proteins is important, because these are well-established neuropathological hallmarks of Alzheimer's disease.[5]

Essential Fatty Acids

Omega-3 Fatty Acid

Increasingly stressful twenty-first century life along with Western diet, have been postulated to contribute to psychiatric illnesses by creating a proinflammatory state. Administration of n-3FA supplements may potentially reverse this proinflammatory state by correcting the n-6FA: n-3FA ratio. The two n-3 fatty acids most relevant to psychiatry are eicosapentaenoic acid (EPA; 20:5) and docosahexaenoic acid (DHA; 22:6), both of which are found primarily in fish oil and other marine sources. Proposed mechanisms of n-3FAs for the amelioration of mood disorders include an effect on membrane-bound receptors and enzymes involved in the regulation of neurotransmitter signaling, including increased serotonergic neurotransmission and alterations in dopaminergic function, as well as regulation of calcium-ion influx through calcium channels. This process may contribute to stabilization and fluidity of neuronal membranes. Omega-3 administration may counter the impact of n-6FA–derived eicosanoids and inhibit secretion of inflammatory cytokines, resulting in decreased corticosteroid release from the adrenal gland and dampening of the mood-altering effects associated with cortisol.[5]

N-3FAs have been studied most often in mood disorders and, to a lesser degree, in schizophrenia. More than 30 controlled trials and a few open trials in the United States with EPA and/or DHA suggest that supplementation with n-3FAs at doses about 5 or more times the standard dietary intake may yield antidepressant and/or mood-stabilizing effects. Most studies have used EPA monotherapy or a combination of EPA and DHA; few studies have examined DHA alone. Various reviews and meta-analyses have been done for efficacy of n-3 fatty acids in depression.[26–28] Efficacy for perinatal depression has also been examined though findings have been inconsistent. In the first clinical trial of omega-3 for bipolar illness, Stoll and colleagues[29] administered high doses of an n-3FA mix (6.2 g/day EPA plus 3.4 g/day DHA) to 30 patients with bipolar disorder I or II in a comparison with placebo over a 4-month period. However, Keck and colleagues were unable to replicate these results in a larger-scale study.[30] Apart from mood disorders, n-3FA has been studied in psychotic illness, personality disorders and in developmental disorder as well.[5]

The omega-3s have been shown to be very safe and well tolerated. Most complaints of side effects, such as gastrointestinal upset and fishy aftertaste, tend to occur with higher doses (greater than 5 g/day). Side effects mostly happens with less pure preparations. At the more typical doses of 1 g/day with highly purified omega-3 preparations, these adverse effects are less common. There has been some concern about the possibility of bleeding with doses greater than 3 g/day, although this risk seems to be minimal, except in patients who are taking other agents that also affect platelet function.[5]

Minerals: Zinc, Iron, Copper

Zinc

Zinc is important for immune regulation, energy metabolism, sexual function, insulin storage, and macromolecule stabilization; and modulation of protein synthesis, DNA transcription, neuronal precursor cell activity, neurotrophins, neurotransmitters, and antioxidants.[5] A systematic review identified 4 eligible randomized controlled trials (RCTs) of moderate quality. In 2 studies antidepressant augmentation with zinc (7–25 mg/day) for 10 to 12 weeks significantly improved depressive symptoms in comparison with placebo add-on. However, evidence for efficacy of zinc monotherapy was insufficient. The third RCT of 674 Guatemalan elementary school children (no DSM-IV diagnosis) at risk for zinc deficiency found no effect of zinc supplementation on mental health. However, increases in serum zinc concentrations were associated with decreases in internalizing symptoms (depression and anxiety). The fourth study found weak evidence of beneficial effects of zinc on mood in nondepressed subjects.[31]

In healthy states zinc, copper, and amyloid-β (Aβ) metabolism are in a fine balance. If the balance is disturbed oxidative and cytotoxic damage happens inside brain. Zinc may protect against Aβ-mediated oxidative cytotoxicity. Paradoxically, accumulation of either zinc or Aβ could lead to zinc-induced and/or Aβ-mediated oxidative and cytotoxic damage. Parallel with this evidences zinc has been studied in Alzheimer's dementia (AD). Histopathological and case-control studies show increased levels of brain zinc, mostly in parietal lobes and reduced levels of serum zinc in patients with AD.[1] In a systematic review of 55 studies, no conclusive evidence for any effect of zinc on AD was found. In summary, zinc supplementation of antidepressants might be beneficial in the treatment of depression. Zinc alone or in combination with stimulants might improve hyperactivity and impulsivity symptoms of ADHD. Zinc is not beneficial for the treatment of dementia. Zinc may have minimal impact on intelligence quotient or mental health in children in those with zinc deficiency.[32]

Iron

Iron is essential for energy production, DNA and neurotransmitter synthesis, myelination, and phospholipid metabolism. Iron deficiency has been linked to movement disorders, including restless leg syndrome (RLS), possibly attributable to effects on dopamine synthesis. The diagnosis of iron-deficiency RLS is easily missed, particularly in children with ADHD in whom leg movements may be misinterpreted as a sign of hyperactivity. Iron deficiency is more common in children with ADHD. One study documented low levels of serum ferritin in 84% of children with ADHD compared with 18% of 27 children who did not have ADHD. Lower ferritin levels correlated with more severe cognitive deficits and ADHD ratings.[5]

Studies of iron supplementation for the treatment of RLS have shown mixed results, which may be due to lack of measurement of serum ferritin levels, differences in populations studied, poor gastrointestinal absorption or brain uptake of supplements, genetic polymorphisms, or other dietary factors. A study of intravenous ferric carboxymaltose showed significant benefits in adults with RLS and low levels of ferritin. In adolescents with iron deficiency, iron supplements improved learning and memory. In a controlled study of 23 children (age 5–8 years) with low levels of serum ferritin, iron supplementation (80 mg/day) reduced ADHD symptoms. Iron therapy was well tolerated.[33] Larger studies are needed to explore the role of iron supplements in the treatment of ADHD.

Amino Acids and its Precursors

N-Acetylcysteine

N-Acetylcysteine (NAC) is a precursor to the essential amino acid, cysteine. Unlike cysteine, NAC can penetrate the blood-brain barrier, thereby, increasing blood and brain levels of cysteine. NAC plays important roles in metabolic pathways believed to contribute to psychiatric disorders. Its effects can be summarized through following mechanisms. Firstly, it can modulate glutamatergic and dopaminergic neurotransmission through cysteine. *In vitro* studies have shown to reduce synaptic release of glutamate and an increase in dopamine release. Secondly, NAC helps in body's antioxidant mechanism by producing Glutathione (GSH) which is an essential endogenous antioxidant. Thus, in turn, NAC can reduce oxidative stress induced damage which is being thought as a culprit of many psychiatric disorders.[34]

NAC has been tried for the treatment various psychiatric disorders like in addictions, bipolar depression, schizophrenia, autism, obsessive-compulsive disorder (OCD), trichotillomania, nail biting, skin picking. Side effects of NAC are infrequent and generally mild. Overdose of NAC was associated with seizures.[11, 35–39]

Tryptophan: 5-Hydroxy-L-Tryptophan

5-Hydroxy-L-tryptophan (5-HTP) is the immediate precursor of serotonin (5-hydroxy-tryptamine; 5-HT). A review of 27 studies of 5-HTP for depression found that of the 11 double-blind randomized placebo-controlled trials, 7 reported superiority over placebo, but only 5 of these showed statistical significance. Studies have shown that 5-HTP augments the response to prescription antidepressants such as nialamide, clomipramine, and nomifensine. The average dosage of 5-HTP in adults is 200 to 300 mg/day in divided doses taken twice or 3 times per day. Limited evidence supports the use of 5-HTP as augmentation to antidepressant medications. Common side effects of 5-HTP include nausea, vomiting, and diarrhea; less frequent are headache and insomnia. There are no case reports of serotonin syndrome in humans taking 5-HTP alone or in combination with selective serotonin reuptake inhibitors. Studies report no adverse effects from a combination of 5-HTP and monoamine oxidase inhibitors.[5]

Choline and its Precursors

Choline produces acetylcholine in the body. As neurons are incapable of synthesizing choline, human body must collect it through blood stream from dietary sources. Dysfunction in cholinergic neurotransmission in the hippocampus and cortex is associated with dementia, particularly AD.[5] Supplements tested for the treatment of dementia by potentially increasing acetylcholine content and release include lecithin, cytidine diphosphocholine (CDP-choline), choline alphoscerate, and phosphatidylserine. In a systematic review of 12 randomized studies, no study showed significant objective benefit of lecithin for AD or dementia of Parkinson's disease. Only 1 trial reported significant improvement following lecithin administration for subjective memory problems.[5] A widely studied choline precursor CDP-choline (citicoline), has been comprehensively reviewed. In a cochrane systematic review of 14 studies (with up to 12 months duration) it was found that CDP-choline had an effect in improving memory and behavior, but did not have beneficial effect for attention. Several studies have demonstrated that citicoline can lead to resolution of brain edema, restoration of consciousness which in turn lead to improvement in survival. Also, several trials have consistently demonstrated a beneficial role of citicoline (usual doses of 500–2000 mg/day) in prevention of head-injury sequelae, including faster recovery of consciousness and memory function, accelerated resolution of neuropsychological disorders, shorter hospital stays, and improved EEG, quality of life, and motor recovery.[40]

Herbal Compounds

Phytomedicines

Phytomedicinal (herbal) compounds have a myriad of biological actions relevant to psychiatry. They can influence neurotransmitter systems by synthesizing neurotransmitters and their metabolizing enzymes, binding to neurotransmitters and receptors, by altering membrane transport. They can also modulate neuroendocrine systems, neuroprotection, enhance mitochondrial energy production, cellular repair, regulate gene expression, and neurogenesis.[41] Two systematic reviews found evidence for herbal supplements containing chamomile (*Matricaria Recutita*) or kava (*Piper Methysticum)* in the treatment of anxiety.[42] Anxiolytic phytomedicines usually work via gamma-aminobutyric acid (GABA) like in case conventional anxiolytic psychotropics. Increasing GABAergic action reduces CNS stimulation and amygdala overactivity (as occurs in anxiety disorders). Others which have been examined for efficacy in various psychiatric disorders are Centrophenoxine (Meclofenoxate, Lucidril), Huperzine A (*Huperzia Serrata*), Galantamine–snowdrop (*Galanthus Nivalis*), Vinpocetine (*Vinca Minor),* Arctic Root (*R. Rosea),* Maca (*Lepidium myenii*), and Theanine (*Camellia Sinensis*).[5] Evidence for the beneficial effects of herbal extracts on oxidative stress, mitochondrial energy production, cellular repair, neurotransmission, CNS activation or inhibition, neuroendocrine systems, and gene expression is expanding. Understanding the psychopharmacology and the potential clinical effects on anxiety, insomnia, cognitive function, and sexual function would enable clinicians to evaluate the supplements being taken by patients and to advise them on safety and efficacy. Future research should be carried out to improve testing constituents of herbal extracts to enhance assessment of supplement quality.

Adaptogens

Research on adaptogens are not very old in medical literature. The term adaptogen was introduced into scientific literature recently in 1958. It referred to substances that increase the "state of nonspecific resistance" during stress, based on Hans Selye's theory of stress and the general adaptation syndrome.[43] For any herb to be an adaptogenic, it should have a high level of safety and ability to normalize body functions regardless of the nature of stressors.[44] As researches progressed, Adaptogens were redefined as "metabolic regulators which increase the ability of an organism to adapt to environmental stressors and prevent damage to the organism by such stressors".[45] Though over last two decades, better quality studies have been published and reviewed the systematic comparison of clinical trials of botanicals has an important limitation. Those can be summarized as follows—herbal preparations are not absolutely identical, their compositions vary in proportions from one to another, unlike synthetic psychotropics that are bioequivalent across studies. Chemical composition of herbal preparations are dependent on many factors. They are genetic factors, environmental factors, climate, soil characteristics (pH, fertilization, heavy metals), infections (insects, pests, microbes), parts of the plant used, processing (pulverization, extraction, solvent polarity, temperature, duration, distillation, expression, fermentation, purification), storage (light, oxygen, humidity, temperature). To mention the names of various adaptogens examined in several open labeled, uncontrolled and randomized placebo-controlled double-blind clinical trials are *E senticosus*, *R Rosea* and *S chinensis.* The study population in these studies were bipolar disorder, chronic fatigue syndrome, depression, neurosis, anxiety and schizophrenia. Proposed mechanisms for effects on cognitive functions, memory, learning, and attention are associated with down regulation of cAMP followed by closure of hyperpolarization-activated channels, activation of PI3K required for long-term potentiation (learning and memory), normalization of cortisol homeostasis, genomic effects in neuroglial cells, mainly affecting energy metabolism (anabolic effect) and CNS functions, which can be associated with beneficial effects on behavioral, mental and aging related disorders.[5]

Ginkgo Biloba

Ginkgo biloba is one of the most frequently prescribed herbal preparations in various countries. Commonly it is used in any of the following three situations—cerebrovascular, peripheral vascular, or tissue damage.[46] Most randomized control trials (RCTs) use the EGb 761 which is a special extract of Ginkgo biloba to examine its efficacy in various medical and psychiatric conditions. Ginkgo's putative neuroprotective and cognitive enhancing properties in problems with memory, information processing, attention and concentration, psychomotor function, mood, fatigue, and activities of daily living, have provided support for its use in treating neurological, psychiatric, functional, and physiologic symptoms.[5] There are specific domains of cognitive functions which have been found to be yield significant effects versus placebo. These are fluid intelligence (37.8%), selective attention (43.7%), short-term and long-term verbal and visual memory (ranging from 28% to 33%) executive functions (e.g. planning 33.2%, working memory 20.7%, flexibility 24.4%, and processing speed 33.0%).[47] Common psychiatric indications include Alzheimer and age-associated dementia, normal aging, traumatic brain injury, stroke, multi-infarct dementia. Moreover, it is indicated in glutamate toxicity which is hypothesized and proven to be the mediating factor in various psychiatric illnesses.[1] In addition to dementia, Ginkgo has been examined as an add-on therapy for symptoms of schizophrenia and has shown some promise.[48] In a meta-analysis of 6 studies, 466 cases on ginkgo and 362 cases on placebo were evaluated. Scales used for assessment for various domains in symptoms of schizophrenia were Scale for the Assessment of Negative Symptoms (SANS), and the Scale for the Assessment of Positive Symptoms (SAPS) or the Brief Psychiatric Rating Scale (BPRS). Ginkgo as an add-on to antipsychotic medication produced statistically significant moderate improvement in total and negative symptoms of chronic schizophrenia, suggesting a role for Ginkgo in improving the symptoms of chronic schizophrenia.

A dosage range from 80 mg to 240 mg of dry extract divided into 2 or 3 daily doses, with an average daily dose of 120 mg has been recommended as a dietary supplement. Ginkgo seems to exert its effects through its antioxidant and anti-platelet-activating factor (anti-PAF) activity via flavones and terpene lactones, respectively. It induces modulatory effects on cerebrovasculature tone and glucose metabolism. It alters receptor/transmitter activity and electroencephalographic activity in brain. Although Gingko is generally safe, patients should be cautioned regarding possible increased risks of bleeding, particularly when Ginkgo is used with medications exerting synergistic effects.[49]

St. John's Wort

The flowering tops of *Hypericum perforatum* (St. John's wort; SJW) have been used throughout millennia for a range of nervous system conditions, including depressed mood.[50] Numerous clinical trials have consistently demonstrated the herbal medicine's efficacy in major depressive disorder (MDD).[51] Clinicians' enthusiasm for SJW started to be diminished after two randomized controlled trials (RCTs) revealed no greater efficacy than placebo. However, the findings of those studies were not purely due to a lack of antidepressant efficacy, but, instead, an increasing placebo response was appreciated.[52] A meta-analysis of RCTs involving SJW for depression conducted by Linde and colleagues[53] revealed a relative risk (RR) of 1.48 (1.23, 1.77) from 18 combined studies for response to SJW versus placebo and an equivocal effect to selective serotonin reuptake inhibitors (SSRIs) of 1.00 (0.90, 1.15). But not all studies are supportive of SJW for the treatment of MDD. In 2002, the National Institute of Mental Health (NIMH)-funded "Hypericum Depression Trial Study Group" (a 3-arm RCT; n = 340) revealed that, at the week 8 endpoint, neither SJW nor sertraline were significantly different from placebo in reducing HAMD scores.[51] SJW was examined in other depressive disorders also, such as dysthymia and seasonal affective disorder (SAD), but clear evidence of efficacy is lacking. SJW has also been studied in social phobia, obsessive-compulsive disorder (OCD), somatoform disorders, and attention-deficit hyperactivity disorder (ADHD). But the evidence does not support their efficacy.[5] Though some preclinical studies have suggested a range of neurochemical activities for antidepressant efficacy of SJW in major depressive disorder, poor bioavailability and lack of penetration across blood brain barrier make those activities futile in human studies. Most adverse effects are found to be reversible dermatologic and gastrointestinal symptoms. Possible SJW-induced mania, psychosis, and serotonin syndrome have been reported in some case reports.[48] Clinicians should be careful about potential drug interactions if using products with higher (greater than 1 mg) hyperforin, and in coadministration with other psychotropic medications. SJW should not be prescribed at higher than recommended doses and caution is advised for SJW use in persons with bipolar disorder who are not receiving a mood stabilizer.[1] Future research should explore the use of SJW in generalized anxiety and, potentially, in bipolar depression (adjunctively in patients taking mood stabilizers).

Ayurveda

Ayurveda is the most ancient and Traditional System of Medicine in India. It deals with the whole life of human being starting from birth to end of the life because Ayurveda describe the art of living and it is a science of life that reveals what is appropriate as well as auspicious for a happy and long life. The term Ayurveda is formed by the combination of two words '*Ayu*' meaning life, and '*Veda*' meaning knowledge. Ayurveda is regarded as "The Science of Life" and the practice involve the care of physical, mental and spiritual health of human being. Life according to Ayurveda is a combination of senses, mind, body and soul. Ayurveda is not only limited to body or physical symptoms but also give comprehensive knowledge about spiritual, mental and social health. Ayurveda describes three *Guna* of Mind and named as *Satwa* (Balance), *Raja* (Arrogance) and *Tama* (Indolence). Mind is called 'Manas'. Ayurveda describes that a possibility for disease is due to imbalance of the '*tamas*' or '*rajas*' in the mind which are the reactive tendencies which vitiate the mind and leading to emotional imbalance, also results in psychological disturbances, hence *Rajas* and *Tamas* are termed as '*Doshas* of mind'. Tridosha are *Vata, Pitta* and *Kapha* and these leads to unhealthy condition by the accumulation of toxins. If they are not driven out of the body in a stipulated period of time, they give rise to or may lead into various chronic mental disorders like anxiety, neurosis, depression, insomnia, etc. and if it is further ignored can turn into permanent disorder like psychosis (Unmad). According to *Charaksamhita*,[54] systematic line of mental disorders includes *Nidana Parivarjana*, (elimination of basic cause), *Daivavyapasraya chikitsa, and Yukti vyapasraya chikitsa*. '*Vyapasraya*' refers to depending on, or trusting to. *Daivavyapasraya* is literally translated to mean any therapy that depend on the '*Daivya*' (Devine) or linked to it and it is concerned to unknown circumstances, which are beyond the purview of reasoning or cannot establish on scientific basis, and hence it is just remain as spiritual therapy. As it is Magicoreligious Practice it include *Mantrah* (Incantations), *Manidharan* (Precious Stones), *Oushadam* (Amulets), *Mangalam* (Propitiatory Rites), *Balih* (Oblations), *Homah* (Sacrifice), *Upavasah* (Fasting), *Japah* (Prayer), *Vratam* (Vows). *Yuktivyapasraya (Yukti* refers to reasoning and Yuktivyapasraya is based on a rational and scientific outlook). The treatment of mental disorders is given by specific procedures known as Panchakarma and provides suitable palliative measures as drugs (*Aushadha*), psychotherapy (Sattvavajaya) and diet regimen.

Homeopathy

Homeopathy (from Greek omeos, meaning similar, and pathos, meaning suffering) is a system of medicine whose first tenet is the principle of similar. This principle was developed into a system of medicine in the nineteenth century by the renowned German physician Hahnemann. Homeopathy originally was based on the vitalistic theory. Similar to Ayurveda and traditional Chinese medicine, homeopathy emphasizes the self-healing potential of the human body and a close mind/body connection. It is based on a premise that illness is a result of an imbalance of one's vital force, or essential energetic makeup. A correctly prescribed remedy leads to a restoration of the balance and ultimately to cure. The system of homeopathy rests on 2 fundamental principles (1) similarity, whereby the indicated remedy for particular symptoms is that which elicits similar symptoms when given to a healthy person, and (2) the power of the minimum dose, whereby a substance that is repeatedly diluted and agitated is believed to preserve its effect even into "ultramolecular" solutions.[55] Randomized placebocontrolled studies suggest that homeopathy may be useful for functional somatic syndromes (fibromyalgia, chronic fatigue syndrome), conditions like anxiety, ADHD, premenstrual and sleep-related problems, its benefit is undetermined. For other common psychiatric conditions such as depression, post-traumatic stress disorder, and dementia, there are no informative data.[56] Although homeopathic medicines are well tolerated and believed to carry few side effects, there has to date been no adequate demonstration of their safety. However, rare cases of toxicity have been reported when low dilutions of arsenic, cadmium, or other heavy metals are used. It is still unknown whether a single individually chosen homeopathic medicine is more effective than a fixed-dose combination formula.

Massage Therapy

Massage therapy (therapeutic massage) is the manual manipulation of soft body tissues to enhance health and well-being. Animal behavior indicates that the application of pressure, rubbing, vibration and joint movement are used instinctively to relieve pain or respond to injury.[57] Massage therapy is one of the oldest forms of medicine known to mankind, having been practiced worldwide since ancient times. Earlier, massage was used for pain relief based on a theory of counter-irritation. Subsequently, researchers started investigating the physiological aspects of massage therapy and found that massage causes psychological changes in musculoskeletal, circulatory-lymphatic and nervous systems. Specific physiological changes includes improved connective tissue pliability and mobility, increased joint mobility, improved circulation, enhanced immune system function and reduction.[57] Massage improves elevated blood pressure and reduces heart rate and provides anxiolytic effects. Massage increases serotonin, dopamine levels and enhanced endorphin production. Field and colleagues[58,59] have documented both psychological and physiological changes with massage therapy, including improved mood, decreased anxiety and reduced levels of stress hormones (cortisol, epinephrine, norepinephrine) in childrens suffering from post-traumatic stress disorder, depression, eating disorders, chronic fatigue and fibromyalgia.

MIND-BODY MEDICINE

Mind-body medicine (MBM) has been an interesting area of researches in recent decades and is flooded with enormous literature. MBM combines characteristics of ancient traditional healing systems with the modern biomedical model to create an integrated approach to health care. MBM, as a field of medicine tries to understand various processes of the mind that influence the body. This field mostly conceptualizes the mind-body as a single entity, with the health of one part necessarily influencing the health of the other. MBM therapies include meditation, hypnosis, guided imagery, relaxation therapies, biofeedback, spiritual healing, yoga, tai chi, qigong, art therapy, light therapy and others. MBM techniques offer patients greater control over their treatment, cheaper alternatives, effective options for managing chronic conditions, and methods for maintaining wellness.[60] Various MBM therapies are as follows:

Music Therapy

Music therapy is the prescribed use of music by a qualified person to effect positive changes in the psychological, physical, cognitive or social functioning of individuals with health or educational problems. Studies with electroencephalography suggest that music creates a level of coherence between the electrical activities of different areas of the brain. The groups said to benefit from music therapy include children with developmental and learning disabilities, elderly people with mental health needs, Alzheimer's disease and other age-related conditions, people with substance abuse problems, people with physical disabilities and/or acute and chronic pain and women in labor.[61]

Meditation

Meditation is the intentional self-regulation of attention, a systematic focus on particular aspects of inner or outer experience. It has been developed in association with religious and spiritual contexts (e.g. Buddhist and Hindu rituals), the aim being to seek a full state of mind embodied in the concept of 'enlightenment'. It originated in ancient India 3000 years ago and has existed in some form in all the major religions. There are two general types, of meditation: 1. Concentration meditation and 2. Mindfulness meditation. Concentration meditation is best represented in modern medicine by transcendental meditation (TM) and the relaxation response. Mindfulness meditation is represented best by mindfulness-based stress reduction (MBSR). Common to both forms of meditation is the principle of focusing one's full mental attention on a designated object of meditation. When the mind wanders from this object, effort is made to return attention to the object. In concentration meditation, this exercise is repeated with the same object, which may be an image, a mantra (a sound repeated mentally to oneself; this is the case for the technique of TM and the relaxation response), or the physical sensation of the breath. In mindfulness meditation, the objects of meditation, after initial training with the breath, include other aspects of human experience, such as physical sensations (e.g. pain) or mental and emotional states (e.g. maladaptive thought patterns, anxiety).[61] Meditation has been extensively examined as a treatment of anxiety. Beneficial physiological effects of meditation include decreased oxygen consumption, respiratory rate and blood pressure, as well as EEG changes associated with decreased autonomic arousal. TM has been used in the reduction of stress and various anxiety states. It has also been used to reduce symptoms of anxiety and panic and help maintain these reductions in patients with generalized anxiety disorder, panic disorder or panic disorder with agoraphobia.[61] Meditation has also been proved to be effective in reducing hypercholesterolemia, hypertension, asthma, coronary artery diseases and so on.

Yoga

The Sanskrit word yoga is translated as 'union' of mind, body and spirit. Yoga is intimately connected to the religious beliefs and practices of the Indian religions and is also visible in Buddhism. Yoga involves postures, breathing exercises and meditation aimed at improving mental and physical functioning. Some practitioners understand yoga in terms of traditional Indian medicine, with the postures improving the flow of *prana* energy around the body. Others see yoga in more conventional terms of muscle stretching and mental relaxation, with an ability to improve vitality.[62] Commonly practized yoga methods are pranayama (controlled deep breathing), *asanas* (physical postures) and *dhyana* (meditation), which are mixed in varying proportions with differing philosophical ideas. Yoga is one such therapy that has low barriers to access and has strong influence on the mental states. The scientific rationale for yoga effects on the mind is also quite strong. In healthy individuals, biomarker studies suggest that yoga influences neurotransmitters, inflammation, oxidative stress, lipids, growth factors and second messengers in a manner largely similar to what has been shown for antidepressants and psychotherapy. It is hypothesized that yoga combines the effects of physical postures, which have been independently associated with mood changes and meditation which increases the levels of Brain-derived neurotrophic factor (BDNF). Sudharshana Kriya Yoga has been found to improve depressive symptoms by reducing serum cortisol levels. Other effects that have been noted include increased vagal tone, increased gamma-aminobutyric acid (GABA) levels, increase in serum prolactin and promotion of frontal electroencephalogram (EEG) alpha wave activity which improves relaxation. Lastly, prior clinical studies have noted several psychiatric conditions for which yoga has proved beneficial in conditions like schizophrenia, mood disorders, substance use disorder, anxiety disorders, obsessive compulsive disorder, attention deficit hyperactivity disorders and post-traumatic stress disorder.[62]

Hypnotherapy

Hypnotherapy is an intervention based on the use of hypnosis, a form of cognitive information processing in which a suspension of peripheral awareness and critical analysis of cognition can lead to, apparently involuntary, changes in perception, memory, mood and physiology.[63] In simpler terms hypnosis may be considered as the induction of a deeply relaxed state, with increased suggestibility and suspension of critical faculties. Hypnotherapy is often associated with the induction of a trance-like state during which behavioral modification may be suggested (e.g. stop smoking during pregnancy or reduce eating). In fact it is now more widely used as an adjunct to psychological treatments. Hypnosis may be indicated if the patient has a high ability and suggestibility to become hypnotized and has a positive attitude towards hypnosis for the treatment of a condition in which alteration of perception, memory and mood can reduce the intensity of a symptom. Thus, it may be used in suitable patients for the reduction of chronic pain, reduction in the memory of past pain, mood enhancement, anxiety as well as irritable bowel syndrome.[61]

Biofeedback

Biofeedback is a therapeutic method that gives the patient conscious control over a physiological function not normally under conscious control. It is based on operant-reinforcement principles applied to automatic musculoskeletal responses. A feedback signal alerts the participant if the physiological parameter under investigation is within expected range. Over a series of successive trails, individuals gradually gain control over the selected physiological responses and can eventually elicit the desired physiological response upon demand. This control is achieved by using technology that depends on the levels of activity of a physiological parameter, such as muscle tension, skin temperature, skin resistance or electroencephalographic activity which is presents to the patient in visual or auditory form.[61] An individual is connected to sensors that pick up signals of involuntary bodily activities. At the time of stress, these signals are recorded by the machine to inform the person how the body is handling that stress. The goal of biofeedback is to help recognize these reactions and learn to alter them through relaxation techniques. Biofeedback is useful in reducing stress as a trigger for various disorders or disease. Patients of biofeedback are usually taught various breathing techniques as a way to overcome anxiety and other stress responses.

Neurofeedback

Electroencephalography (EEG) is a technique that records the dynamic electrical activity of the cortical structure. Sustained 'shifts' in the dynamic equilibrium of electrical brain activity have been proposed as a general mechanism underlying therapeutic effects of EEG biofeedback (neuro-feedback). EEG biofeedback trains patients to notice and influence their state of alertness based on EEG measures. Numerous studies have evaluated the efficacy of EEG biofeedback as a treatment of anxiety disorders, depressed mood, attention-deficit disorder, epilepsy and migraine. Several protocols have been developed that includes sensori–motor rhythm (SMR, 12–15 Hz) for epilepsy and ADHD, alpha–theta protocol to reduce the risks of re-traumatization in post-traumatic stress disorders and in depressed alcohol dependent patients. Low Frequency Neurotherapy System (LENS), is another method that has been seen to be beneficial in ADHD, PTSD, mood disorders, pain syndromes, chronic fatigue, and fibromyalgia.[64]

Aromatherapy

The practice of using oils to treat illnesses is reputed to be at least 6000 years old that has beginning in the oriental cultures of China, India, Persia and Egypt. The earliest Hindu scriptures mention several hundred perfumes and aromatic products, classifying their use for both rituals and therapeutic applications. Aromatherapy is a branch of herbal medicine, using very concentrated plant extracts called essential oils (EOs) are inhaled or applied topically. Strictly speaking the substances used in aromatherapy are not fragrances or aromatic mixtures (as used in the perfume industry) but are volatile substances extracted from plant source which have curative property. The controlled use of EOs is done to promote balance and harmony in the body and mind. It is believed that the use of fragrant essential oils has effect on or alters a person's mood or behavior. The source of extracted essential oils includes cinnamon, orange, garlic, clove, jasmine, lavender, rose, lemon, mandarin, lemongrass, eucalyptus, geranium, peppermint, ginger, fennel, sandalwood and so on.[63] The possible neurochemical effects include; inhibition of binding of glutamate, augmentation of α-aminobutyric acid and acetylcholine receptor binding. Aromatherapy has been found to be effective in treatment of anxiety, pain, insomnia, agitation in dementia, menopausal symptoms and so on. Infrequent adverse effects of essential oils include skin allergies, phototoxic reactions, and potentiation of sedative–hypnotics when used with lavender or other oils known to have sedating effects. Pregnant women should avoid topical use of essential oil therapies because of possible toxic effects on the fetus caused by systemic absorption.[65]

Energy Medicine

Energy medicine includes a broad variety of complementary and alternative medicine therapies. The term energy medicine derives from the perceptions and beliefs of therapists and patients that there are subtle biological energies that surround and permeate the body that are alleged to sustain life. It is suggested that these energies may be accessed in various ways for diagnostic and therapeutic interventions. Some energy medicine therapies like acupuncture and homeopathy are provided by a therapist whereas others encourage patients to participate in their own healing (Reiki, Qigong).[65]

Spiritual Awareness

The important therapeutic component of energy medicine includes the spiritual awareness that is "inner sense of being a part of something vastly larger and wiser than the self." This component is especially common for various spiritual healing and self-healing approaches. Patients experiencing energy medicine treatments may report that they feel an inner peace, a spiritual guidance and a reconnection with their spiritual or religious roots. This feeling may occur with no prompting on the part of the therapist or arise out of deliberate efforts for a spiritual connection through practices of meditation and imagery. Spiritual awareness may be helpful in terminally ill patients and their families in dealing with dying.

Spiritual Healing

Energy medicine is illustrated most clearly with various forms of spiritual healing, such as Reiki, therapeutic touch and Qigong. Healers report sensations in their hands such as heat, tingling, vibration, electrical sensations or cold and patients may feel similar sensations in the part of their body being treated. Spiritual healers and many other therapists who are sensitive to bioenergies report they can palpate with their hands an energy field surrounding the body. The energy fields are believed to be templates for what occurs within the body, being shaped by genetic, psychic, emotional, and environmental factors. In addition to sensing people's conditions, healers can enhance people's states of health by interacting with various bioenergy fields. Spiritual healing is a therapy that can be given as a complement to any other therapy, with no side effects or dangerous interactions with other treatments.[63]

Chiropractic

Chiropractic is derived from Greek words *chieri,* meaning hand, and *praktikos,* meaning to perform; thus chiropractic means performed or done by hand. It is believed that when vertebrae are subluxated, dislocated or misaligned, the person experiences number of ailments, including back pain, sciatica, vision and hearing problems, muscle spasms, asthma, allergy and so on. The therapists, using the light touch with hands and manipulation of vertebra, try to regulate flows of energies that may result in indirect healing of subluxation. When the subluxation is relieved, it is thought that the body has the opportunity to heal itself. Clinical reports indicate that this method can be helpful in patients with fibromyalgia; frozen shoulder, postillness symptoms of head injury, meningitis, encephalitis, behavioral, developmental, and learning disorders in children (sometimes attributed to cranial birth injury).[63] As with spiritual healing, there are no known deleterious effects of chiropractic. Because the touch used in these therapies is light, without physical manipulation, they are considered to be safe.

Acupuncture

Acupuncture is a component of traditional Chinese medicine (TCM) in which extremely fine long needles were inserted into the skin over points corresponding to parts and functions of the body mapped out in a system of meridians. It is one of the widely practiced alternative therapies in eastern as well as Western world. These meridians are basically 'lines of energy' that runs from the head to the extremities. Along the meridians, there are acupuncture points that relate to anatomic parts and physiologic functions in various parts of the body. By stimulating these points, it is said to release unhealthy blocks in energy flows along the meridians, which in turn improves the functions of the related organs. Acupuncture points can be stimulated with needles, physical pressure, electrical stimulation or laser light. Diagnoses in acupuncture relate to whether bioenergies are flowing smoothly, blocked, or congested. It is believed that the abnormal activity in one meridian influences energy flow in other meridians. Acupuncture has been successfully used in the treatment of depression, anxiety, stress related problems and substance induced withdrawal states.[41]

Qigong

Qigong is a physical and spiritual Chinese discipline geared toward helping energy (qi) move through—out the body for optimal functioning. Often referred to as a branch of energy medicine, the qigong philosophy is that clogged, impure, or polluted qi causes disease or dysfunction and that it can be removed or cleansed so the body may be restored to health. The practice of qigong may involve breathing exercises, meditation, and hands-on manipulation of energy (or laying on of hands) along the body's meridians.[64] "Medical" Qigong may be used as a self-healing technique and as an aid to help others heal. Qigong masters, as they are known, make a conscious effort through focused mental intent, meditation, or prayer to send healing *qi* to ailing individuals, or in a technique called "external *qi* healing."

Internal qigong is a self-healing technique which involves exercises that are easily adapted to an individual's condition, strength and circumstances. Qigong has been useful in depression, anxiety, insomnia and migraine. However, unskillful or excessive practice of qigong can result in serious psychological or psychosomatic symptoms.[65] Psychotic symptoms have also been reported following erroneous Qigong and are described as a culture-bound syndrome, "qigong psychotic reaction."[64]

Reiki

Reiki is a branch of energy medicine involving intense mental focus and the laying on of hands, named from the Japanese words *rei* and *ki,* meaning 'universal life energy' or in simple terms 'healing.' Reiki's main premise is to direct or infuse healing energy to the body in order to rebalance blocked energies, release toxins, and activate innate healing capabilities. Reiki is practiced by placing hands on to the patient's body at a number of strategic points which is held for up to 3 minutes and no pressure is exerted. Energy is said to flow into the body and move to the source of the imbalance and not just to the manifesting symptoms. This practice has found to be beneficial with some circumstantial evidence from case studies especially in stress, menstrual problems, migraines, pain syndromes, anxiety, depression and insomnia.[66]

Legal and Ethical Issues

The use of nonconventional therapies in mental health care raises important legal and ethical issues for psychiatrists and other mental health professionals. The legal concerns that may arise in the practice of nonconventional therapies includes licensure, malpractice liability, professional discipline and quackery. Clinicians who recommend or prescribe nonconventional treatments often do so in the absence of professional guidance. This situation has becomes more intricate by the absence of treatment guidelines, policies, and procedures to help clinicians to deal with liability issues. From a legal perspective, the choice of treatment defines the purpose of a contract between a patient and a psychiatrist or other health care provider. There is also no clearly established legal-ethical framework that defines the scope of practice for physicians or alternative medical practitioners who treat patients using nonconventional modalities. Furthermore, substantial differences often exist between state jurisdictions for the kinds of practices that are legally sanctioned for a given alternative medical practitioner. The patient assumes responsibility for complying with prescribed treatment and notifying his or her psychiatrist or other health care provider of the adverse effects or other problems that emerge during the course of treatment. Medical practitioners who use interventions that are not recognized as falling within the scope of their professional competence may invite disciplinary action that may result in probation, suspension or withdrawal of a professional license to practice. It is, hence, advisable for psychiatrists who use nonconventional treatments to learn about all applicable restrictions imposed by their medical board on the scope of medical practices in their particular state or country.[67]

Safety

It is generally perceived by the public that CAM is entirely safe. In fact many interventions have the potential to do harm if used inappropriately, e.g. herbalism has medicines with a potential risk of intrinsic toxicity as well as possible dangerous interactions with allopathic medications being taken concurrently. Certain manipulative therapies can also cause damage if not performed correctly. The general dangers of using CAM may be categorized under two headings: direct and indirect risks.

Direct Risks

- Allergic reactions or other adverse reactions to medicines used during the practice of CAM
- Use of adulterated or poor quality preparations
- Interaction between CAM medicines and existing medication
- Manipulative or other damage caused by inexperienced practitioners.

Indirect Risks

- Patient's condition deteriorates due to inaccurate diagnosis and/or inappropriate treatment
- Serious illness not detected through lack of knowledge or experience of practitioner
- Discontinuation of prescribed orthodox medication without permission (or knowledge) of patient's doctor
- Application of alternative approach to CAM preventing consideration of other orthodox procedures
- Patient attempts to self-treat in response to media or internet when professional advice should be sought.[67]

The US Food and Drug Administration (FDA) has provided guidelines for good manufacturing practices (GMPs) pertaining to the safety, quality, consistency, and purity of natural products, including vitamins, herbals, and all nonherbal natural products. However, herbals medicines, supplements and other nonconventional biological therapies may cause adverse effects and potentially interact with other natural products or synthetic drugs with synergistic or harmful consequences. Safety information on medicinal herbs is especially incomplete with regard to young children, pregnant and nursing women and patients with significant liver or kidney disease. The paucity of reliable safety data is complicated by the absence of established standards of professional training for practitioners of many nonconventional systems of medicine. Furthermore, as noted earlier, individuals who use prescription medications frequently self-treat using herbs or other natural products without disclosing this information to their psychiatrist or family physician, resulting in unknown kinds and rates of toxic interactions and under-reporting of serious adverse effects and interactions between specific medications and natural products.[67]

Certain herbal products widely used to treat psychiatric disorders are known to have potentially serious adverse effects. For example, St. John's wort may induce mania in bipolar patients, spontaneous abortion in pregnant women or photosensitive rashes. There are few cases of mild serotonin syndrome reported with the amino acids sAMe and L-tryptophan. Patients who use SAMe or 5-HTP to augment conventional antidepressants especially selective serotonin reuptake inhibitors (SSRIs) should be closely monitored for signs of possible serotonin syndrome. Essential oils applied topically or used as aromatherapy to self-treat anxiety disorders can potentially exacerbate asthma and hypertension. The essential oils of parsley and nutmeg are known to have monoamine oxidase-inhibiting (MAOI) activity and should not be used concurrently with MAOIs as it may lead to hypertensive crises.[65]

In contrast to herbals and nonherbal natural supplements, few safety risks are associated with somatic therapies, mind-body practices, and 'energy' healing techniques. Rare cases of injury or adverse effects have been reported with nonconventional therapies that are not based on a specific biological mechanism of action, including therapeutic massage, acupuncture, yoga, qigong, and Reiki. When adverse effects occur they are generally minor and resolve when the duration or frequency of treatments is decreased. Acupuncture is sometimes associated with transient pain, tiredness, bruising, fainting, and vomiting, HIV and hepatitis-B infections and there are extremely rare case reports of pneumothorax and nerve damage. Following a Reiki treatment, some patients report residual headaches and dizziness. Mild somatic complaints associated with Reiki and other energy therapies can generally be managed by reducing the frequency or duration of sessions.[65]

Although most alternative practitioners are thoroughly trained in their respective healing traditions and dedicated to patient care, some lack the skills needed to manage serious psychiatric disorders. Nonconventionally trained practitioners sometimes give patients specific advice about medications, resulting in potentially serious safety issues when medication doses are inappropriately changed or abruptly discontinued leading to increased risk of relapse and unnecessary treatment delays. In view of these liability issues, it is always prudent to refer patients to alternative medical practitioners only after verifying their credentials, training, and reputation as competent clinicians.[66]

Advances in CAM

The following advances in CAM have been noted by Vickers:[68]

- The quantity of applied research in complementary medicine is growing rapidly and the quality is improving.
- Complementary medicine is increasingly practiced in conventional medical settings, particularly acupuncture for pain, and massage, music therapy and relaxation techniques for mild anxiety and depression.
- There is a more open attitude to complementary medicine among conventional health professionals; this is partly explained by the rise of evidence-based medicine (EBM).

COMPLEMENTARY AND ALTERNATIVE MEDICINE: INDIAN SCENARIO

Nonconventional approaches of treatment in various illnesses including psychiatric one, have been integrated in irrespective of its status in the national health care policy. The various approaches which have been practiced in this country include Ayurveda, Unani, yoga, naturopathy, homeopathy and siddha. Many of them have been mentioned above. This section would focus on rest of the approaches along with their current status in health care planning.

Naturopathy

Naturopathy is a system of man, building in harmony with the constructive principles of nature on physical, mental, moral and spiritual planes of living. It has health promotive, disease preventive, curative and restorative potential. According to the British Naturopathic Association, "Naturopathy is a system of treatment which recognizes the existence of the vital curative force within the body." It therefore, advocates aiding human system to remove the cause of disease, i.e. toxins by expelling the unwanted and unused matters from human body for curing diseases. Naturopathy considers that, except for traumatic and environmental conditions, the cause of all the disease is one, i.e. accumulation of morbid matter in the body. The treatment of all diseases is by elimination of morbid matter from the body. The practitioners consider that acute diseases are self-healing efforts of the body and chronic diseases are chronic diseases are outcome of wrong treatment and suppression of the acute diseases. They consider that nature is the greatest healer and the human body itself has the healing power to prevent itself from disease and regain health if unhealthy. Naturopathy treats the body as a whole that includes physical, mental, social and spiritual, all at the same time. Various techniques are used in naturopathy that includes diet therapy, fasting therapy, mud therapy, hydrotherapy, acupuncture, chromo therapy, magnet therapy and so on.[70]

Siddha

Siddha system is one of the oldest systems of medicine in India. The term Siddha means achievements and Siddhars were saintly persons who achieved results in medicine. Eighteen Siddhars were said to have contributed towards the development of this medical system. Siddha literature is in Tamil and it is practiced largely in Tamil speaking part of India and abroad. The Siddha system is largely therapeutic in nature. According to this system the human body is the replica of the universe and so are the food and drugs irrespective of their origin. Like Ayurveda, this system believes that all objects in the universe including human body are composed of five basic elements namely, earth, water, fire, air and sky. The food, which the human body takes and the drugs it uses are all, made of these five elements. The proportion of the elements present in the drugs vary and their preponderance or otherwise is responsible for certain actions and therapeutic results. As in Ayurveda, this system also considers that the equilibrium of humors is considered as health and its disturbance or imbalance leads to disease or sickness. This system also deals with the concept of salvation in life and claims that it is possible by medicines and meditation. This system uses metals and minerals; some are used in soluble, insoluble and vapour form. They use gold, silver, copper, tine, lead, iron, red sulphide of mercury, mercuric chloride and red oxide of mercury, etc. In addition there are drugs obtained from animal sources. The system has published a hand-book on Siddha treatment for common diseases. Siddha recognizes various types of mental disorder and has flourished in southern India.[70]

Unani

The Unani System of Medicine has a long and impressive record in India. It was introduced in India by the Arabs and Persians sometime around the eleventh century. Today, India is one of the leading countries in so for as the practice of Unani medicine is concerned. As the name indicates, Unani system originated in Greece. The foundation of Unani system was laid by Hippocrates. The system owes its present form to the Arabs who not only saved much of the Greek literature by rendering it into Arabic but also enriched the medicine of their day with their own contributions. Avicenna, one of the greatest scholars of Unani Tibb (medicine), has defined it as "Tibb is the science of which we learn the various states of body, in health and when not in health, and the means by which health is likely to be lost and, when lost, is likely to be restored." The basic theory of Unani system is based upon the well-known four humor theory of Hippocrates. According to Unani system, body is considered to be made up of the following seven components are Arkan (Elements), Mizaj (Temperament), Akhlat (Humors), Aaza (Organs), Arwah (Spirits), Quwa (Faculties) and Afaal (Functions). Prevention of disease is as much a concern of the system as curing of sickness. There is emphasis on the need for keeping water, food and air free from pollution. Exercises, rest and adequate sleep are considered necessary for maintaining good health. Various therapeutic procedures have been documented and practiced that includes regimental therapy (Ilaj-bil-Tadbir), diet therapy (Ilaj-bil-Ghiza), pharmacotherapy (Ilaj-bil-Dawa) and surgery (Ilaj-bil-Yad).[70] The system also documents extensively, the impact on health of psychological factors like happiness, sorrow, anger and provide pharmacological and psychological treatments for various mental problems.

AYURVEDA, YOGA AND NATUROPATHY, UNANI, SIDDHA AND HOMEOPATHY

With the advances in scientific treatment, there is resurgence of interest in holistic systems of health care in India especially, in the prevention and management of chronic lifestyle related noncommunicable diseases and systemic diseases.[69]

The Department of Indian Systems of Medicine and Homoeopathy (ISM&H) was established in March, 1995 and re-named as Department of Ayurveda, Yoga & Naturopathy, Unani, Siddha and Homoeopathy (AYUSH) in November, 2003 with a view to providing focused attention to development of Education & Research in Ayurveda, Yoga & Naturopathy, Unani, Siddha and Homeopathy systems. The Department has continued to lay emphasis on upgradation of AYUSH educational standards, quality control and standardization of drugs, improving the availability of medicinal plant material, research and development and awareness generation about the efficacy of the systems domestically and internationally.

Objectives of AYUSH

- To upgrade the educational standards in the Indian Systems of Medicines and Homeopathy colleges in the country.
- To strengthen existing research institutions and ensure a time-bound research program on identified diseases for which these systems have an effective treatment.
- To draw up schemes for promotion, cultivation and regeneration of medicinal plants used in these systems.
- To evolve Pharmacopoeial standards for Indian Systems of Medicine and Homeopathy drugs.

The AYUSH sector across the country supported a network of 3203 hospitals and 21351 dispensaries. The health services provided by this network largely focused on primary health care. The sector, however, has a marginal presence in secondary and tertiary health care. In the private and not-for-profit sector, there are several thousand AYUSH clinics and around 250 hospitals and nursing homes for in patient care and specialized therapies like *Panchkarma*.[69] There were preliminary efforts to integrate AYUSH in National rural health mission (NRHM) were initiated during the Tenth Plan. However, the coverage so far is not significant. Only 24.6% of the public health facilities could avail central assistance for AYUSH medicines and 8.7% PHCs, 5.8% CHCs and 13.9% District Hospitals availed the relevant centrally sponsored scheme for setting up the infrastructure required for co-location of AYUSH facilities.[70]

STANDARDIZATION AND QUALITY CONTROL OF AYURVEDA, SIDDHA, UNANI, AND HOMEOPATHY (ASU&H) DRUGS

Four different Pharmacopoeia Committees are working for preparing official formularies/pharmacopoeias to evolve uniform standards in preparation of drugs of ASU&H and to prescribe working standards for single drugs as well as compound formulations. Standards for around 40% of the raw materials and around 15% of formulations have been published by these committees. Drug Control Cell (AYUSH) is working in the Department of AYUSH to deal with the matters pertaining to licensing and regulation of Ayurvedic, Unani, and Siddha Drugs. Setting up of the Central Drug Authority for centralized licensing and enforcement of the provisions of Drugs and Cosmetics Act and Rules would go a long way in ensuring quality and safety of ASU&H drugs. Department of AYUSH intends to convert Pharmacopoeial Committees of various systems into a modern pharmacopoeial commission with adequate representation of stakeholders and to develop standards that are in line with internationally acceptable pharmacopoeial standards and quality parameters of Ayurveda, Siddha and Unani drugs.[71] In order to expand the quality control base of highest standards as per the requirement of Drugs & Cosmetics Act, 1940 and for the testing of exported/imported ASU&H drugs and for R&D purpose, it is proposed to set up hi-tech quality control laboratories under AYUSH Research Councils.[71]

Important initiatives during the 11th five year plan:

- Development of common drug testing and other infrastructure facilities for AYUSH industry clusters
- Financial assistance to ASU&H Units for capacity building to improve quality control and research and development (R&D)
- Support to centers of excellence in AYUSH education/drug development/clinical research/tertiary care
- Support for validation and revitalization of local health traditions
- Development of backward and forward linkages for *in situ* conservation and *ex situ* cultivation of medicinal plants for a sustainable ASU&H Industry
- Provision of marketing and value-added services to medicinal plant farmers
- Expansion of international cooperation and exchange program with focus on global positioning of AYUSH systems and facilitation of cooperation with other countries in the areas of AYUSH education, research, and exports.[70]

The major achievements during the 11th five-year plan are:

- Publication of pharmacopeia standards and Standard Operating Procedures (SOPs) of 152 Ayurvedic formulations
- Publication of pharmacopeial monographs of 101 single plant drugs and 21 minerals
- Publication of macro & microscopic atlases of 172 drugs
- Development of eight community herbal monographs in the format given by European Medicines Evaluation Agency (EMEA) for submission to European Union.[71]

CONCLUSION

In parallel with the advancement in molecular understanding of psychiatric illnesses, researchers have been trying to examine other nonconventional approaches in treatment for last few decades. Some of them has already been found to be having strong evidence base for their efficacy while others are struggling. Although many of the approaches mentioned and discussed, have not been generally used by clinicians in India, they can offer significant benefits for many individuals. It is expected despite continuing researches in this area, clinicians would experience dilemma of varying degree to incorporate them in day to day patient care. Yet, a knowledge and theoretical understanding of these approaches would place them in better position in mental health care. A well-informed clinician is best qualified to help patients and their families to understand and develop their alternative treatment regimens.

REFERENCES

1. Eisenberg DM, Davis RB, Ettner SL, et al. Trends in alternative medicine use in the US, 1990-1997. Results of a follow-up national survey. JAMA. 1998;280:1569-75.
2. Kayne SB (Ed). Complementary and alternative medicine, 2nd edition. 2009; London: Pharmaceutical Press.
3. British Medical Association (BMA). Complementary Medicine: New Approaches to Good Practice, 1993; London, BMA.
4. National Center of Complementary and Alternative Medicine. *www.nccam.nih.gov/health.*
5. Philip R. Muskin, Patricia L. Gerbarg, Richard P Brown (Eds). Complementary and Integrative Therapies for Psychiatric Disorders. Psychiatric Clinics of north America. 2013;36(1).
6. Coppen A, Chaudhry S, Swade C. Folic acid enhances lithium prophylaxis. [Clinical Trial Controlled Clinical Trial]. Journal of Affective Disorders. 1986;10(1):9-13.
7. Alpert JE, Mischoulon D, Rubenstein GE, Bottonari K, Nierenberg AA, Fava M. Folinic acid (Leucovorin) as an adjunctive treatment for SSRI-refractory depression. [Clinical Trial Research Support, Non-U.S. Gov't]. Annals of Clinical Psychiatry. 2002;14(1):33-8.
8. Papakostas GI, Shelton RC, Zajecka JM, Etemad B, Rickels K, Clain A, Fava M. L-methylfolate as adjunctive therapy for SSRI-resistant major depression: results of two randomized, double-blind, parallel-sequential trials. [Multicenter Study Randomized Controlled Trial Research Support, NIH,

Extramural Research Support, Non-U.S. Gov't]. Am J Psychiatry. 2012;169(12):1267-74. doi: 10.1176/appi.ajp.2012.11071114.

9. Godfrey PSA, Toone BK, Bottiglien T, Laundy M, Reynolds EH, Carney MWP, et al. Enhancement of recovery from psychiatric illness by methylfolate. The Lancet. 1990;336(8712):392-5.
10. Durga J, van Boxtel MP, Schouten EG, Kok FJ, Jolles J, Katan MB, Verhoef P. Effect of 3-year folic acid supplementation on cognitive function in older adults in the FACIT trial: a randomised, double blind, controlled trial. [Randomized Controlled Trial Research Support, Non-U.S. Gov't]. Lancet. 2007;369(9557):208-16. doi: 10.1016/S0140-6736(07)60109-3.
11. Walker JG, Batterham PJ, Mackinnon AJ, Jorm AF, Hickie I, Fenech M, Christensen H. Oral folic acid and vitamin B_{12} supplementation to prevent cognitive decline in community-dwelling older adults with depressive symptoms--the Beyond Ageing Project: a randomized controlled trial. [Randomized Controlled Trial Research Support, Non-U.S. Gov't]. Am J Clin Nutr. 2012;95(1):194-203. doi: 10.3945/ajcn.110.007799.
12. Kwok T, Lee J, Law CB, Pan PC, Yung CY, Choi KC, Lam LC. A randomized placebo controlled trial of homocysteine lowering to reduce cognitive decline in older demented people. [Randomized Controlled Trial Research Support, Non-U.S. Gov't]. Clin Nutr. 2011;30(3):297-302. doi: 10.1016/j.clnu.2010.12.004.
13. Aisen PS, Schneider LS, Sano M, et al. Alzheimer Disease Cooperative Study. High-dose B vitamin supplementation and cognitive decline in Alzheimer disease: a randomized controlled trial. JAMA. 2008;300(15):1774-83.
14. Cognitive and clinical outcomes of homocysteine-lowering B-vitamin treatment in mild cognitive impairment: a randomized controlled trial. Intern Jour of Ger Psych. 2012;27(6):592-600.
15. Smith AD, Smith SM, de Jager CA, et al. Homocysteine-lowering by B vitamins slows the rate of accelerated brain atrophy in mild cognitive impairment: a randomized controlled trial. PLoS One. 2010;5(9):e12244.
16. Tiemeier H, van Tuijl HR, Hofman A, et al. Vitamin B_{12}, folate, and homocysteine in depression: The Rotterdam Study. Am J Psychiatry. 2002;159:2099-101.
17. Ng TP, Feng L, Niti M, et al. Folate, vitamin B_{12}, homocysteine, and depressive symptoms in a population sample of older Chinese adults. J Am Geriatric Soc. 2009;57:871-6.
18. Penninx BW, Guralnik JM, Ferrucci L, et al. Vitamin B_{12} deficiency and depression in physically disabled older women: epidemiologic evidence from The Women's Health and Aging Study. Am J Psychiatry. 2000;157:715-21.
19. Hvas AN, et al. No effect of Vitamin B_{12} treatment on cognitive function and depression: a randomized placebo controlled study. Journal of Affective Disorder. 2004;81:269-73.
20. Hintikka J, Tolmunen T, Tanskanen A, et al. High vitamin B_{12} level and good treatment outcome may be associated in major depressive disorder. BMC Psychiatry. 2003;3:17.
21. Lange H, et al. Folate therapy and in-stent restenosis after coronary intervention. The New England Journal of Medicine. 2004;350:2673-81.
22. Schnyder, et al. Effects of Homocysteine Lowering Therapy with Folic Acid, Vitamin B_{12} and vitamin B_6 on clinical outcome after percutaneous coronary intervention. The Swiss heart study: A Randomized Controlled trial, Journal of American Medical Association. 2002;288:973-9.
23. Bressa GM. S-Adenosyl-l-methionine as antidepressant: meta-analysis of clinical studies; Acta Neurologica Scandinavica. Supplementum; 1994.pp.7-14
24. Brown R, Gerbarg P, Bottiglieri T. S-Adenosylmethionine in the clinical practice of psychiatry, neurology and internal medicine. Clin Pract Intern Med. 2000;1:230-41.
25. Strous RD, et al. Improvement in aggressive behaviour and quality of life impairment following S-Adenosyl methionine (sAMe) augmentation in schizophrenia; European Neuropsychopharmacology. 2009;19(1):14-22.
26. Freeman MP, Hibbeln JR, Wisner KL, et al. Omega-3 fatty acids: evidence basis for treatment and future research in psychiatry. J Clin Psychiatr. 2006;67:1954-67.
27. Lin PY, Su KP. A meta-analytic review of double-blind, placebo-controlled trials of antidepressant efficacy of omega-3 fatty acids. J Clin Psychiatry. 2007;68(7):1056-61.
28. Sublette ME, Ellis SP, Geant AL, et al. Meta-analysis of the effects of eicosapentaenoic acid (EPA) in clinical trials in depression. J Clin Psychiatry. 2011;72(12):1577-84.
29. Stoll, et al. Omega 3 fatty acids in bipolar disorder: a preliminary double blind placebo controlled trial; Archives of General Psychiatry. 1999;56(5):4-12.
30. Keck Jr PE, Mintz J, McElroy SL, Freeman MP, Suppes T, Frye MA, et al. Double-blind, randomized, placebo-controlled trials of ethyl-eicosapentanoate in the treatment of bipolar depression and rapid cycling bipolar disorder. Biological psychiatry. 2006;60(9):1020-2.
31. Lai J, Moxey A, Nowak G, et al. The efficacy of zinc supplementation in depression: systematic review of randomised controlled trials. J Affect Disord. 2012;136(1-2):e31-9.
32. Schrag M, Mueller C, Oyoyo U, et al. Iron, zinc and copper in the Alzheimer's disease brain: a quantitative meta-analysis. Some insight on the influence of citation bias on scientific opinion. Prog Neurobiol. 2011;94(3):296-306.
33. Konofal E, Lecendreux M, Deron J, et al. Effects of iron supplementation on attention deficit hyperactivity disorder in children. Pediatr Neurol. 2008;38(1):20-6.
34. Dean O, Giorlando F, Berk M. N-acetylcysteine in psychiatry: current therapeutic evidence and potential mechanisms of action. J Psychiatry Neurosci. 2011;36(2):78-86.
35. Gray KM, Carpenter MJ, Baker NL, et al. A double-blind randomized controlled trial of N-acetylcysteine in cannabis-dependent adolescents. Am J Psychiatry. 2012;169(8):805-12.
36. Schmaal L, Berk L, Hulstijn KP, et al. Efficacy of N-acetylcysteine in the treatment of nicotine dependence: a

double-blind placebo-controlled pilot study. Eur Addict Res. 2011;17(4):211-6.

37. Grant JE, Odlaug BL, Kim SW. N-acetylcysteine, a glutamate modulator, in the treatment of trichotillomania: a double-blind, placebo-controlled study. Arch Gen Psychiatry. 2009;66(7):756-63.
38. Berk M, Copolov DL, Dean O, et al. N-acetyl cysteine for depressive symptoms in bipolar disorder—a double-blind randomized placebo-controlled trial. Biol Psychiatry. 2008;64(6):468-75.
39. Berk M, Copolov D, Dean O, et al. N-acetyl cysteine as a glutathione precursor for schizophrenia—a double-blind, randomized, placebo-controlled trial. Biol Psychiatry. 2008;64(5):361-8.
40. Secades JJ. Citicoline: pharmacological and clinical review, 2010 update. Rev Neurol. 2011;52(Suppl 2):S1-62.
41. Brown RP, Gerbarg PL, Muskin PR. Alternative treatments in psychiatry. In: Tasman A, Kay J, Lieberman J (Eds). Psychiatry. 3rd edition. London: John Wiley & Sons, Ltd; 2008.pp.2318-53.
42. Sarris J, Panossian A, Schweitzer I, et al. Herbal medicine for depression, anxiety and insomnia: a review of psychopharmacology and clinical evidence. Eur Neuropsychopharmacology. 2011;21(12):841-60.
43. Panossian A, Wagner H. A review of their history, biological activity, and clinical benefits. Herbal Gram. 2011;90:52-63.
44. EMEA/HMPC/102655/2007. Reflection paper on the adaptogenic concept. London: European Medicines Agency, 2008.
45. Panossian A, Wikman G, Wagner H. Plant adaptogens III: earlier and more recent aspects and concepts on their modes of action. Phytomedicine. 1999;6:287-300.
46. Ponto LL, Schultz SK. Gingko biloba extract: review of CNS effects. Ann Clin Psychiatry. 2003;15:109-19.
47. Kaschel R. Ginkgo biloba: specificity of neuropsychological improvement? A selective review in search of differential effects. Hum Psychopharmacol. 2009;24:345-70.
48. Singh V, Singh SP, Chan K. Review and meta-analysis of usage of ginkgo as an adjunct therapy in chronic schizophrenia. Int J Neuropsychopharmacol. 2010;13:257-71.
49. Bressler R. Interactions between ginkgo biloba and prescription medications. Geriatrics. 2005;60:30-3.
50. Sarris J, Kavanagh DJ. Kava and St John's wort: current evidence for use in mood and anxiety disorders. J Altern Complement Med. 2009;15(8):827-36.
51. Hypericum Depression Trial Study Group. Effect of Hypericum perforatum (St John's wort) in major depressive disorder: a randomized controlled trial. JAMA. 2002;287(14):1807-14.
52. Fournier J, DeRubeis R, Hollon S, et al. Antidepressant drug effects and depression severity: a patient-level meta-analysis. JAMA 2010;303(1):47-53.
53. Linde K, Berner M, Kriston L. St John's wort for major depression. Cochrane Data base Syst Rev. 2008;(4):CD000448.
54. Charak Samhita. In: Yadav S (Ed). Mumbai: SBP Nirnay Sagar.
55. Jonas WB, Kaptchuk TJ, Linde K. A Critical overview of homeopathy. Ann Intern Med. 2003;138(5):393-9.
56. Davidson JR, Crawford C, Ives JA, Jonas WB. Homeopathic treatments in psychiatry: a systematic review of randomized placebo-controlled studies. J Clin Psychiatry. 2011;72(6):795-805.
57. Fritz S. Mosby's Fundamentals of Therapeutic Massage. St Louis, MO: Mosby-Year Book; 1995.
58. Field T, Seligman S, Scafaldi F, et al. Alleviating post-traumatic stress in children following Hurricane Andrew. J Appl Dev Psychol. 1996;22:607-1741.
59. Field T, Morrow C, Valdeon C, et al. Massage reduces anxiety in child and adolescent psychiatric patients. J Am Acad Child Adolesc Psychiatr. 1992;31:125-31.
60. Marwick C. Music therapists chime in with data on medical results. JAMA. 2000;283:731-3.
61. Barrows KA, Jacobs BP: Mind-body medicine. An introduction and review of the literature. Med Clin North Am. 2002; 86(1):11-31.
62. Telle S, Nilkamal S. Sciences of the mind: Ancient yoga texts and modern studies. Psychiatr Clin N Am. 2013;36:93-108.
63. Kayne SB (Ed). Complementary and alternative medicine. 2nd edition. London: Pharmaceutical Press; 2008.
64. Lake JH. Nonconventional Approaches in Mental Health Care. In: Kaplan HI, Sadock BJ (Eds). Comprehensive Textbook of Psychiatry. 9th edition. Philadelphia: Lippincott Wiliams & Wilkins; 2009.pp.2593-15.
65. Maciocia G. The Foundations of Chinese Medicine: A comprehensive text, 2nd edition. London: Churchill-Livingstone Elsevier; 2005.
66. Heller T, Treween GL, Katz J, Stone J, Spurr S (Eds). Perspectives on Complementary and Alternative Medicine. Routledge, London; 2005.pp.173-204.
67. Werneke U, Turner T, Priebe S. Complementary medicines in psychiatry: Review of effectiveness and safety. Br J Psychiatry. 2006;188:109.
68. Vickers A. Recent advances -Complementary medicine. BMJ. 2000;321:683-6.
69. Department of Ayurveda, Yoga & Naturopathy, Unani, Siddha and Homoeopathy (AYUSH), Official website. [*http://indianmedicine.nic.in/index2.asp?slid=19&sublinkid=15&lang=1*].
70. Health and Family Welfare and AYUSH. Official website of Planning Commission. Government of India. [*http://planningcommission.nic.in/plans/planrel/fiveyr/11th/11.../11v2_ch3.pdf*].
71. Steering Committee on AYUSH for 12th Five year plan. Health Division Planning Commission Government-of-India-2011. Official-website [*planningcommission.gov.in/aboutus/committee/st_ayush0903.pdf*].

CHAPTER 79

Forensic Psychiatry

GC Munjal, Niraj Ahuja

Forensic psychiatry is a subspecialty of psychiatry which usually deals with the application of psychiatric knowledge to legal issues (i.e. *psychiatry in law*) and sometimes with the application of legal knowledge to psychiatric issues (i.e. *law in psychiatry*). In short, it represents an interface between law and psychiatry.

The law can be broadly divided into two branches:

1. *Criminal law:* It defines certain acts as offences against the state and in doing so makes them punishable. The criminal law is enforced by, or on behalf of, the State.
2. *Civil law:* It defines the rights and duties of individuals in relation to each other. In this branch of law, actions are brought by individuals to establish their rights against another person, and not by the State.

Thus, forensic psychiatry can be discussed broadly under the headings of criminal responsibility, competence to stand trial (psychiatry in law; criminal law); civil responsibility (psychiatry in law; civil law); Indian Lunacy Act, Mental Health Act, Narcotic Drugs and Psychotropic Substances Act (law in psychiatry); and psychiatrist as an expert witness.

CRIMINAL RESPONSIBILITY

History of the Concept

It has been considered unjust to call a person criminal in law unless his act was voluntary and done with a guilty intent. The imbeciles, infants and deaf-mutes were not considered blameworthy for their 'crimes', in the early Jewish laws, as they lacked the necessary guilty intent.

Plato, in his 'Laws', said that "a man might conceivably commit an act of one of these kinds from insanity, or when so disordered by disease, so extremely aged, or of such tender years, as to be virtually insane". Such an offender could be exculpated, although he often had to make restitution for the damage caused by his act.

The 'Corpus Iuris Civilis', a collection of excerpts of legal knowledge complied under the Emperor Justinian in the 5th Century AD, mentions that the insane person is 'compos mentis non est' (i.e. does not have control on his mind; later known as *'non compos mentis'*) and can not understand the consequences of his acts, like an infant or a four-footed animal. Such a person was believed to have no *'culpa'* and was, therefore, not accountable in justice. Measures were suggested to ensure the care of such person and the security of those related to him.[1]

Henry de Bracton, Chief Justice of England, commented in his 'On the Laws and Customs of England' that a crime is not committed unless 'the will to harm' is present, and such an intent is lacking in young children and 'mad men'. In 1265, he devised a test to identify an insane person. Later known as the *'wild beast test'*, it provided that an insane person is one who behaves like a wild beast.

In 1349, Giovanni was exculpated for double murder on grounds of insanity, using the Justininan Corpus (Table 1). He was sent back to his family.[2] However, the family had to pay the costs of his custody. This established a precedent for the criminal responsibility of an insane person at that time. The responsibility of the family members too was clarified. They provided for the upkeep if he was imprisoned, and were responsible for his care if he was released.[3]

The 'Constitutio Criminalis Carolina', published in Germany in 1532, recognized that there were several types of homicide which were not punishable under certain conditions, one of which was an offender who was 'deprived of his understanding'.

In 1553, Fitz-Herbert formulated a rather simplified test that allowed for exculpation of one who could not "account or number 29 pence, nor tell who was his father or mother, nor how old he (was)".

In the 17th Century, Sir Matthew Hale, in the 'History of The Pleas of The Crown' opined that the defendant 'laboring under melancholy distempers' should ordinarily have an understanding equal to that possessed by a 14-year-old child to be held criminally liable. The relevant understanding pertained to the understanding of what is right and wrong (the right and wrong test). Thus, according to him, the mere presence of insanity was not sufficient to remove criminal

Table 1: Criminal responsibility: Some famous cases

No.	*Name year Place*	*Convicted for evidence in relation to crime*	*Mental disorder*	*Judicial proceedings*	*Medical witness opinion*	*Defendant's fate*	*Other remarks*
1.	Giovanni 1349 Venice	Murder of 2 men	"Clearly insane" at the time of crime, according to witnesses	Used Justinian Corpus as standard	—	Exculpated; Sent back to family in Germany	Family had to pay for the cost of custody
2.	Edward Arnold 1723 England	Firing at and wounding Lord Onslow	Had a delusion that Lord Onslow was sending devils every night to torment him	Wild beast test (Justice Tracy)	—	Guilty; sentenced to death; Death sentence commuted by personal inter-vention of Lord Onslow	—
3.	Earl Fenners 1760 England	Shooting at and killing his steward	A "fit of rage" at the time of crime	Cross-examination before House of Lords	(Dr John Munro)	Guilty; sentenced to death; Publicly hanged	—
4.	Margaret (Peg) Nicholson 1786 England	Attempting to kill King George III with a desert knife	"Clearly insane" at the time of crime and subsequently; No motive	Privy Council	Insane (Dr Munro)	King George III ordered for "humane" treatment; Committed to Bethlem hospital for life	—
5.	James Hadfield 1800 England	Firing at King George III	Insanity due to severe brain damage; fits of terrifying madness; bizarre delusions; shot at the King to guarantee his own death	Wild beast test (Council for defense-Thomas Erskine)	Insane (Dr Crichton)	Not guilty, being under the influence of insanity; Sent to Bethlem hospital	A retrospective legislation issued for commitment of insane "criminals"
6.	John Bellingham 1812 England	Shooting at and killing Chancellor of Exchequer, Spencer Percival	His insistence that Government refused to redress "unparalleled wrong" caused to him	Cross-examination	—	Guilty; sentenced to death; Hanged 7 days after the killing'	The lack of a medical witness and the final verdict were widely criticized
7.	Edward Oxford 1840 England	Firing at Queen Victoria	Had a delusion that he was acting as an instrument of a secret imaginary society	Cross-examination (Justice Denman)	Insane due to "lesion of will" (Dr Hodgkin); Physiognomy of skull debated by Dr John Connolly	Guilty but insane; Sent to Bethlem and then to Broadmoor hospital; showed no evidence of insanity in hospital	The verdict was incorporated in the Act of 1800 passed in the Hadfield case
8.	Daniel McNaughten 1843 England	Shooting at and killing PM's private secretary, Edward Drummond	Had a delusion for many years that Torries were against him and wanted to kill him; hence decided to kill the PM, Sir Robert Peel	Cross-examination (Council for defense-Alexander Cockburn)	(9 for defense and 1 for prosecution)	No guilty on grounds of insanity; Sent to Bethlem and then to Broadmoor hospital for life	Wide public outcry. Following Queen Victoria's intervention, McNaughten Rules formed

Contd...

Contd...

No.	*Name year Place*	*Convicted for evidence in relation to crime*	*Mental disorder*	*Judicial proceedings*	*Medical witness opinion*	*Defendant's fate*	*Other remarks*
9.	Burton 1863 England	Gruesome, savage killing of a boy	Had an impulse to kill someone as he wished to be hanged; hence killed the 1st person he met	Right and wrong test (Justice Wightman)	—	Guilty; sentenced to death	Criticized by Henry Maudsley in his book, 'Responsibility in Mental Disease'
10.	Federick Baker 1867 England	Murder of a little girl. Fanny Adams, and dismembering her body	"Homicidal insanity": Made an entry in his diary after the murder, "Killed a young girl; it was fine and hot"; Positive family history	Cross-examination	Insane	Guilty; sentenced to death	—
11.	James Atkinson 1858 England	Murder of his girlfriend	Killed because of "jealousy"	Cross-examination	Imbecile (Dr Forbes Winslow and others)	Not guilty due to insanity. Sent to Bethlem hospital	Verdict widely criticized both within and outside medical community
12.	George Victor Townley 1864 England	Savage stabbing of his fiancee to death	Killed because of "jealousy"	McNaughten Rules	Morally insane (Dr Forbes Winslow)	Guilty; sentenced to death; Re-examined by Lunacy Commissioner; found insane but responsible; execution stayed by Home Secretary; sent to Bethlem hospital	Because of protests, was re-examined; found to be of sound mind; served life sentence; committed suicide sometime after the final verdict
13.	Alexander Dingwall 1867 Scotland	Murder of his wife	Long history of alcoholism; otherwise sane	Cross-examination	—	Killing considered as "murder with extenuating circumstances'	1st recorded case of diminished responsibility
14.	Simon Fraser 1878 Scotland	Killing his son by banging his head against wall	"Temporary insanity" during sleep; was asleep when killed his son	Refuted the opinion	Temporary insanity	Not guilty; Acquitted on giving a pledge that he would sleep alone!	Example of somnambulism as a type of "automatism"
15.	Jack Ruby 1964 USA	Murder of Lee Harvey Oswald who assassinated President Kennedy	Psychomotor epilepsy	Cross-examination; McNaughten Rules	—	Guilty; Life sentence; Died in prison	—
16.	Peter Sutcliffe ("Yorkshire Ripper") 1981 England	Murder of 13 women and attempted murder of 7 women over years	Schizophrenia	Justice Boreham refused to accept "diminished responsibility"; cross-examination	Mentally ill; paranoid schizophrenia	Guilty; life imprisonment. Mental illness worsened in prison; transferred to Broadmoor hospital	The judge and the jury completely disregarded medical evidence

Contd...

Contd...

No.	*Name year Place*	*Convicted for evidence in relation to crime*	*Mental disorder*	*Judicial proceedings*	*Medical witness opinion*	*Defendant's fate*	*Other remarks*
17.	Hinckley Jr. 1982 USA	Attempted to murder President Ronald Reagen	—	ALI Test	Mentally ill; Personality disorder (prosecution witness); Schizophrenia (defense witnesses)	Not guilty by reason of insanity	—
18.	John Steed ("the M4 Rapist") 1986 England	Raping 4 women and murdering 1 prostitute	The manner of committing crimes	Cross-examination (Sir James Miskin)	Psychopathy	4 life sentences plus 20 years' imprisonment	Medical opinion again disregarded

responsibility. He recognized that insanity could be partial or limited. He allowed for two kinds of verdicts.[4]

1. Not guilty, and
2. Committed the act but was non-compos (mentis).

Paulus Zacchias,[5] the personal physician of the Pope in 17th Century, is considered the Father of Legal Medicine as well as the Father of Forensic Psychiatry. In 'Questiones Medico-legales,'[5] he declared that physicians should have exclusive competence in the field of pathological mental states, amentias. He provided a classification of mental disorders keeping in mind the legal issues of that time.

In this classification, the mental disorders *(amentias)* were of three types: the *fatuitas* (equivalent to mental retardation), the *insania* (disorders often presenting with lucid intervals), and the *phrenitis* (delirium without fever and without lucid intervals). The *fatuitas* were of 3 types: the *ignorantes* were incapable of inheriting land or acting as guardians, but were capable of marriage and were criminally responsible; the *fatui* were incapable of marriage or of making wills, usually; and the *stolidi* were incapable of civil obligations and were criminally not accountable. Further, criminal and civil acts committed under violent passions (a type of *insania*) could be declared void on a judge's discretion.[5]

At the end of the 18th century, the eminent philosopher Immanuel Kant[6] suggested that courts should take the opinion of a psychologist from the 'faculty of philosophy', instead of a physician in deciding the level of understanding, the capacity of judgment and the question of insanity in cases involving criminal responsibility.

Although several interesting cases can be recounted (Table 1), the first important case with regard to criminal responsibility of an insane person came to a court in 1800.[7]

Hadfield Case

James Hadfield had fought in a battle in 1794 as one of the Duke of York's bodyguards and had suffered severe brain damage as a result of sword wounds to his head. Thereafter he was subject to episodic, terrifying rage. In one such outburst, he threatened to kill his child as he heard God command him to do so.

He also developed a bizarre delusion that God was going to destroy the world and the only way to prevent it was to sacrifice his own life. Not wanting to commit the 'moral' crime of suicide, he guaranteed his death by shooting at, though missing by nearly 12 inches, King George III in the year 1800. He was caught easily and was charged with high treason.[7]

Thomas Erskine, the counsel for defense, countered *the wild beast* test with the statement that "no such madness ever existed in the world". Hadfield was able to distinguish right from wrong *(right and wrong test)* and knew the nature of his crime. Erskine argued that the act was committed under the influence of a delusion which existed at the time of the offence, and therefore he could not be considered guilty. The Lord Chief Justice Kenyon directed the jury to find him 'not guilty'.

McNaughten Case and McNaughten Rules

The Hadfield case was followed by the cases of John Bellingham who was found guilty, and of Edward Oxford who was not (Table 2). However, the case that lead to widespread public attention was that of McNaughten.[8]

Daniel McNaughten, a 29-year-old Scotsman, was probably suffering from paranoid schizophrenia.[9] For many years, he had a delusion that spies sent by Catholic priests, with the help of Tories (the party then in power in England), were constantly following him, harassing him and hatching a conspiracy against him. He also probably had auditory hallucinations of Tories accusing him of crimes of which he said he was not guilty.

Therefore, he decided to kill the Tories Prime Minister, Sir Robert Peel, making elaborate plans for the criminal act.

Table 2: The McNaughten Rules (Questions and Answers)

Q.1.	"What is the law respecting alleged crimes committed by persons afflicted with insane delusions in respect of one or more particular subjects or persons, as, for instance, where, at the time of the commission of the alleged crime, the accused knew he was acting contrary to law, but did the act complained of, with a view, under the influence of insane delusion, of redressing or avenging some supposed grievance or injury, or of producing some supposed benefit"?
A.1.	"Assuming that your Lordships' inquiries are confined to those persons who labor under such partial delusions only, are not in other respects insane, we are of opinion that (notwithstanding the accused did the act complained of with a view, under the influence of insane delusion, of redressing or avenging some supposed grievance or injury, or of producing some public benefit) he is nevertheless punishable, according to the nature of the crime committed, if he knew at the time of committing such crime that he was acting contrary to law, by which expression we understand your Lordships to mean the law of the land".
Q.2.	"What are the proper questions to be submitted to the jury when a person alleged to be afflicted with insane delusions respecting one or more particular subjects or persons, is charged with the commission of a crime (murder, for example) and insanity is set up as a defense"?
Q.3.	"In what term ought the question to be left to the jury as to the prisoner's state of mind at the time when the act was committed"?
A.2 and 3.	"As these two questions appear to us to be more conveniently answered together, we submit our opinion to be that the jury ought to be told in all cases that every man is presumed to be sane, and to possess a sufficient degree of reason to be responsible for his crimes, until the contrary is proved to their satisfaction; that to establish a defense on the ground of insanity, it must be clearly proved that, at the time of committing the act, the accused was laboring under such a defect of reason, from disease of the mind, as not to know the nature and quality of the act he was doing, or, if he did know it, that he did not know that he was doing what was wrong. The mode of putting the latter part of the question to the jury on these occasions has generally been, whether the accused at the time of doing the act knew the difference between right and wrong; which mode, though rarely if ever, leading to any mistake with the jury, is not, we conceive, so accurate when put generally and in the abstract as when put with reference to the party's knowledge of right and wrong in respect to the very act with which he is charged. If the question where to be put as to the knowledge of the land, it might tend to confound the jury by inducing them to believe that an actual knowledge of the law of the land was essential in order to lead to a conviction; whereas the law is administered on the principle that everyone must be taken conclusively to know it without proof that he does know it. If the accused was conscious that the act was one which he ought not to do, and if that act was at the same time contrary to law of the land, he is punishable. The usual course, therefore, has been to leave the question to the jury, whether the accused had a sufficient degree of reason to know that he was doing an act that was wrong; and this course we think is correct, accompanied with such observation and corrections as the circumstances of each particular may require".
Q.4.	"If a person under an insane delusion as to existing facts commits an offence in consequence thereof, is he thereby excused"?
A.4.	"The answer must of course depend upon the nature of the delusion but making the same assumption as we did before, namely, that he labors under such partial delusions only, and is not in other respects insane, we think he must be considered in the same situation as to responsibility as if the facts with respect to which the delusion exist were real. For example, if under the influence of his delusion, he supposes another man to be in the act of attempting to take away his life and he kills that man, as he supposes, in self-defense, he would be exempt from punishment. If his delusion was that the deceased has inflicted a serious injury to his character and fortune, and he killed him in revenge for such supposed injury, he would be liable to punishment".
Q.5.	"Can a medical man, conversant with the disease of insanity who never saw the prisoner previously to the trial, but who present during the whole trial and the examination of all the witnesses, be asked his opinion as to the state of prisoner's mind at the time of the commission of the alleged crime, or his opinion whether the prisoner was conscious at the time of doing the act that he was acting contrary to law, or whether he was laboring under any, and what, delusions at the time"?
A.5.	"We think that the medical man, in the circumstances supposed, can not in strictness be asked his opinion in the terms above stated, because each of these questions involves the determination of the truth of the facts deposed to, which it is for the jury to decide, and the questions are not more questions upon a matter of science, in which case such evidence is admissible. But where the facts are admitted, or not disputed, and the question becomes substantially one of science only, it may be convenient to allow the question to be put in the general form, although the same cannot be insisted on as a matter of right".

On 20th January 1843, he shot Sir Peel's Private Secretary, Edward Drummond, in the back, mistaking him for the Prime Minister.[10]

During the trial, he admitted that he 'was driven to desperation by persecution.' Ten physicians (9 for defence and 1 for prosecution) found him insane. He was found 'not guilty on grounds of insanity' and was sent to Bethlem Hospital for life.

The verdict lead to unprecedented public (and Royal) outcry.[11] The Lord Chancellor, Lord Lyndhurst put to a panel of 14 judges, 5 hypothetical questions designed to clarify the legal position. The answers, given on 19th June 1843, came to be known as the 'McNaughten Rules' (Table 2).

These rules, also known as the *legal test*, can be summarized as follows: To establish a defense on the ground of insanity, it must be clearly proved that at the time of committing the act, the party accused was laboring under such a defect to reason, from disease of the mind, as not to know the nature and quality of the act he was doing or, if he did know it, that he did not know he was doing what was wrong or contrary to the law of the land.

The irony is that if these rules were applied to the McNaughten case, he would not have been found 'not guilty.' Despite the fact that these rules came into existence in 1843 and were clearly stated, the 'insanity defense' continued to have a chequered course.

Disease of the Mind

When an insanity defense is used, it must be clearly established that a defect of reason resulted from the 'disease of the mind'. The 'disease of the mind' is a legal, and not a psychiatric, concept. The English Law recognizes as disease of the mind, any disease which is capable of producing mental dysfunction. The law is not concerned with the brain but with the mind, as the term is used in law terminology meaning reason, memory and understanding.[12]

However, when mental dysfunction is attributable to external factors (e.g. alcohol and drugs consumed voluntarily), this is not called as the disease of the mind.

The Intent

A crime is an act declared by the law of the land to be an offence at a particular time. It is a behavior which is in violation of the law and is punishable. A crime can be seen to consist of 2 main elements.[13]

1. The *actus reus* (i.e. the guilty act which is against the criminal law).
2. The *mens rea* (i.e. the intent).

Both these elements must be present before the accused can be said to have committed certain crimes (intent is not important in some crimes, like manslaughter), of which murder is the most important.

Murder is the unlawful killing of another with 'malice aforethought'. Malice aforethought occurs when there is either an intention to kill or to inflict grievous bodily harm.

All unlawful killings, which are not murder, are called manslaughter (In India, culpable homicide). Manslaughter[14] can be either,

- Involuntary, where the accused has no malice aforethought, or
- Voluntary, where the accused may have had malice aforethought but there are mitigating circumstances which reduce the offence. These circumstances are:
  - Diminished responsibility,
  - Provocation, and
  - Suicide pact.

The punishment for manslaughter is less than that for murder and does not include capital punishment.

Diminished Responsibility

The concept of diminished responsibility arose as a means of avoiding the death penalty. The first recorded case, in which the verdict was diminished or partial responsibility ('murder with extenuating circumstances'), was that of Alexander Dingwall of Scotland in 1867 (Table 1). It was subsequently used widely in the Scotland courts though it was incorporated in the English law only in the 1957 Homicide Act. It has not been incorporated in the Indian law as yet.

According to the Homicide Act 1957 of England, "when a person kills or is a party to the killing of another, he shall not be convicted of murder, if he was suffering from such abnormality of mind (whether arising from a condition of arrested or retarded development of mind or any inherent causes or induced by disease or injury) as substantially impaired his mental responsibility for his acts and omissions in doing or being a party to the killing". Here, the burden of proof is on the defense on a 'balance of probabilities' and not on 'beyond reasonable doubt' as is in other criminal cases.

The defense of diminished responsibility is usually employed in cases of 'mental unsoundness' or 'partial insanity', though not in cases of 'complete insanity' where the McNaughten rules are applicable. On the other end, this defence is also not used for simulated insanity, mild character defects, bad temper, jealousy, hatred, drug use, racial characteristics, low intelligence, poor judgment, political fanaticism and similar unfavorable personal feelings.[15]

Only 40% of those convicted of manslaughter in the years 1968 to 1977 were psychotic.[16] A majority of the remaining 60% were those with personality disorders and depression.

Irresistible Impulse Test

This is another example of diminished responsibility. As mentioned earlier, the McNaughten rule takes into account only the defects in reason. To deal with cases characterized by an incapacity to control behavior in absence of a defect of reason, a new test was devised by Issac Ray (Father of American Forensic Psychiatry) and Judge Charles Doe in 1869 (State vs Pike) in New Hampshire, USA. The test came to be known as the *irresistible impulse test* or the *New Hampshire doctrine*.

The irresistible impulse has been criticized for several reasons. It has often been asked in such cases whether the impulse was strong (and irresistible) or the offender weak (not resisting the impulse voluntarily). This is a metaphysical question for which psychiatry, as well as law, have no answer.

A popular query to resolve this issue in the past was: "would the person have yielded to that impulse had there been a policeman at his elbow" *(the policeman at the elbow test)*. Such a test has no meaning when it is recalled that Jack Ruby, Guiteau and Czolgosz (for example) killed Lee Harvey Oswald, President Garfield and President McKinley, respectively, in the presence of a myriad of police officers and security guards. In fact some have called the notion of irresistible impulse 'an incoherent piece of nonsense'.

Automatism

Automatic behavior (defined as an apparently purposeful and complex behavior which occurs without conscious control, and for which there is amnesia later) occurs in a variety of conditions which include epilepsy, somnambulism, concussion, intoxication and hypoglycemia.[17]

The English law distinguishes automatisms occurring in such conditions (known as 'non-insane automatisms') from insanity. 'Noninsane automatism' falls short of the 'disease of the mind'.

A verdict of noninsane automatism in the English law leads to acquittal and not to involuntary hospitalization as in the case of a successful insanity defense.[17]

However, the concept of automatism is very vague and unsatisfactory. The American and the Indian law have no special provision for automatism.

Infanticide

According to the English Infanticide Act 1938, "where a woman by any willful act or omission causes the death of her child under the age of 12 months, but at the time of the act or omission the balance of her mind was disturbed by reason of her not having fully recovered from the effect of giving birth to the child or by reason of the effect of lactation consequent upon the birth of the child, then she shall be guilty of infanticide".

The verdict of infanticide amounts to manslaughter, and not to murder, and calls for diminished responsibility.

Durham Rule

In 1954, Judge David Bazelon formulated the *product rule or test* in the Monte Durham case (Durham vs US) in the District of Columbia, USA. The rule said that "an accused is not criminally responsible if his unlawful act was the product of mental disease or mental defect". The term mental disease referred to mental disorder, while the term mental defect referred to mental retardation.

A lot of confusion was caused by the terms 'product', 'mental disease' and 'mental defect'. The rule was discarded 18 years later in the Brawner case (US vs Brawner, 1972) by 9 members of the Court, including Judge Bazelon.

The American Law Institute's Test of Criminal Responsibility

The American Law Institute's (ALI) test of criminal responsibility, in its Model Penal Code[18] (1960), was adopted in 1972 in the same Brawner case which discarded the Durham rule.

It states that:

- A person is not responsible for criminal conduct if at the time of such conduct, as a result of mental disease or defect, he lacks substantial capacity either to appreciate the wrongfulness of his act or to conform his behavior to the requirement of the law.
- As used here, the terms 'mental disease or defect' do not include any abnormality manifested only by repeated criminal or otherwise antisocial conduct.

Butler Report

Meanwhile in England, the Committee on Mentally Abnormal Offenders, chaired by Lord Butler, submitted its report (Butler report)[19] in 1975. The recommendations of the committee with regard to the insanity defense can be summarized as follows:

- The term 'insanity' should be replaced with 'mental disorder'.
- The insanity defense should be renamed 'not guilty with evidence of mental illness/disorder'.
- The McNaughten rules should be eliminated and replaced by a two-pronged test for *mens rea*.
  - "Did he know what he was doing was wrong".
  - Presence of severe mental illness or severe mental subnormality; with no requirement to demonstrate a causal connection between the mental abnormality and the offence, as in a severe mental disorder, a causal connection could be safely presumed.
- The burden of proof for the requisite mental state for 3 (i) should rest with the prosecution (and not the defense) just as it does with any other issue of intention.
- The concept of diminished responsibility, and of infanticide, should be abolished.
- There should be no mandatory institutionalization but court discretion to take appropriate action.

The Butler committee[19] also recommended criteria of evidence of severe mental disorder. One or more of the following characteristics should be present:

- Lasting impairment of intellectual functions shown by failure of:
  - Memory,
  - Orientation,
  - Comprehension, and
  - Learning capacity.
- Lasting alteration of mood of such degree as to give rise to delusional appraisal of the patient's situation, his past or his future, or that of others, or to lack of any appraisal.
- Delusional beliefs: persecutory, jealous or grandiose.
- Abnormal perception associated with delusional misinterpretation of events.
- Thinking so disordered as to prevent reasonable appraisal of patient's situation or reasonable communication with others.

These recommendations have not been adopted by the English law yet.

Criminal Law Revision Committee

An alternative revision, the Criminal Law Revision Committee's 14th report ('Offences Against The Person')[20] of 1980, found its way into the Law Commission's 'Codification of the Criminal Law', 1985.[21] It provides that:

- This section applies where the person who kills another is suffering from a form of mental abnormality which is a substantial enough reason to reduce his offence to manslaughter.

- 'Mental abnormality' here means mental illness, arrested or incomplete development of mind, psychopathic disorder, and any other disorder or disability of mind, except intoxication.

Hinckley Trial

In USA, the ALI test of criminal responsibility,[18] adopted in 1972, worked well enough till the famous trial of John W Hinckley Jr., who attempted to murder President Ronald Reagan. A verdict of 'not guilty by reason of insanity' was returned by the jury. The public was outraged and demanded modifications in the insanity defense.

This led to the abolition of the special verdict (insanity defense) in some US states (like Montana), and the institution of a new test of 'guilty but mentally ill' in a number of other states.[22]

The 'guilty but mentally ill' has been severely criticized as it treated the accused like any other prisoner. Also, though it recognized the accused as a mentally ill person, it still called him guilty. Thus, it is at best a poor compromise and is clearly unsatisfactory.

Comprehensive Crime Control Act

The Comprehensive Crime Control Act 1984 (USA) attempted to solve the problem by reverting to the McNaughten rule, with one change. The word 'know' was replaced by the word 'appreciate', to broaden the purely cognitive ('reason') approach of the McNaughten rule by including the emotional aspects.

Thus, the accused would be found not to have criminal responsibility if, at the time of the crime, he was suffering from mental illness such that he could not appreciate the nature and quality of his act or that what he was doing was wrong.

The Act also prohibits the psychiatrists from testifying to the ultimate question of insanity in the federal cases. This belonged only in the province of the judge or the jury.

APA and AMA Guidelines

The American Psychiatric Association (APA)[23] has recommended the following guidelines to deal with the disposition of violent insanity acquittees:

- Special legislation should be designed.
- A board, that includes psychiatrists along with other professionals, should make the confinement and release decisions, including suggestions regarding preventive detention and reconfinement.

In 1984, an APA task force[24] also suggested that the behavioral part of the ALI Standard should be eliminated and only the mental state should be addressed by psychiatrists in such cases.

The American Medical Association (AMA)[25] proposed that the insanity defense should be limited to cases in which the accused is so ill (mentally) as to lack the necessary *mens rea* (criminal intent).

Recently, the AMA and the APA attempted to collaborate on a proposal on criminal responsibility without any final resolution.

Indian Law

The Indian law regarding criminal responsibility is a direct descendent of the famous McNaughten Rule. Section 84 of the Indian Penal Code (Act 45 of 1860; IPC) states that "nothing is an offence which is done by a person who, at the time of doing it, by reason of unsoundness of mind, is incapable of knowing the nature of the act, or that he is doing what is either wrong or contrary to law".

The insanity defense is usually used in charges of murder in order to escape capital punishment. When successful, the defendant is found 'not guilty'. However, since the society must be protected against a 'lunatic', he is often kept in a safe custody which is usually an 'asylum' (mental hospital).

The law presumes every major person to be sane unless the contrary is proved to the satisfaction of the court. The burden of proof is on the defense. To benefit from this section, it must be proved that unsoundness of mind existed at the time of committing the offence. Subsequent unsoundness of mind is not a defense, though it may affect the trial.

No reference is made in this Act to lack of control, irresistible impulse, infanticide, or diminished responsibility.

The medical officer (or the psychiatrist), when called as an expert witness, usually takes the following points into consideration before deciding regarding unsoundness of mind. These include personal history, family history, past history, absence of motive, want of secrecy, lack of concealment, want of preparedness, use of needless force, multiple murders, want of accomplices, and indifference to the crime committed.[26] However, these points are only suggestive and never conclusive.

The expert evidence does not relieve the court from forming an independent opinion. In fact, the question of insanity is primarily to be decided by the court, keeping in reference the submatter evidence.

Idiots, imbeciles and persons who are deprived of all understanding and memory (like children below 7 years, or children between 7 years and 12 years of immature understanding) are clearly not criminally responsible. The vexing question of absolving the criminal responsibility is in "partial insanity" (i.e. insanity where understanding and memory are intact, and dysfunction is primarily in the delusional area, e.g. paranoid disorders). In such cases, it has been suggested that the accused should be placed as regards criminal responsibility in the same situation as if the facts of his delusions were true and real.

Therefore, if the defendant murdered somebody acting on his delusions of persecution, he would be guilty, because even if his persecutory delusions were true he could not have lawfully resorted to murder.

The following cases are examples of 'partial insanity', where Section 84 IPC can be applied:

- The accused kills another person who he thought was coming immediately to shoot him and the accused acted in self-defense, thus not knowing what he was doing was wrong or contrary to law.
- The accused killed another person under a delusion that he was (say) an earthern pot, thus not knowing what he was doing.

The insanity defense is invoked in only a small percentage of cases and is upheld in only a fraction of these. Judges (and juries) are usually skeptical. It is usually a desperation defense in criminal law when all else fails.

If the defendant is acquired on grounds of unsoundness of mind, it is required by Section 334 of the Code of Criminal Procedure 1973, that the finding state specifically whether he committed the act or not. If the act has been committed, then the Magistrate can either order for detention in safe custody or an asylum in accordance with the Indian Lunacy Act 1912, or order him to be delivered to any relative or friend on receiving application of such relative or friend (Section 335 CPC). The relative or friend has to provide sufficient security that he will be properly cared for, will be prevented from injuring himself or others, and will be produced before the court or any officer when required.

Intoxication

Section 85 and 86 of IPC provide that an accused is not criminally responsible, if the intoxicant was administered to him without his knowledge or against his will.

Thus, intoxication caused by voluntary use of alcohol or some other intoxicating drug is no excuse for the commission of a crime. However, insanity produced by drunkenness, voluntary or otherwise, (e.g. delirium tremens) absolves one from criminal responsibility, if Section 84 IPC is applicable.

COMPETENCY TO STAND TRIAL (AND SUBSEQUENT PROCEDURE)

The law provides an accused the right to consult his lawyer to ensure that fair treatment is provided under possibly hostile conditions. A defendant, who lacks the capacity to understand the nature and the object of proceedings against him, to consult his lawyer, and to assist in preparing the defense, may not be subjected to a criminal trial.

This prohibition is an understandable by-product of the ban on trials *in-absentia*. A mentally ill, and therefore incompetent, defendant, although physically present in the court, is not really offered any opportunity to defend himself. At issue is the defendant's ability to take part in the trial; his mental condition at the time of the offence has no bearing on the matter.

A test of competence, which emerged during the Dusky trial (Dusky vs US, 1960), recognizes a criminal defendent as competent to stand trial if he "has rational as well as factual understanding of the proceedings against him?"

When initiated by the prosecution, the process is often called as 'preventive detention', while when raised by the defense it is known as 'medical immunity' from trial.

The most widely used test in America is the *McGarry Instrument*,[27] developed in 1973. It is a useful, though a bit lengthy, clinical guide for the mental health professional to ascertain a defendant's competence to stand trial. It identifies 13 areas of functioning to assess the issue of competency.

The Procedure

Sections 328 to 339 of the Code of Criminal Procedure 1973 (Act 2 of 1974; CPC) relate to provisions as to accused persons of unsound mind, including fitness to stand trial and the subsequent procedure(s).

When an accused is a 'lunatic' and is consequently incapable of making his defense, the Magistrate enquires into the fact of unsoundness of mind at the first instance, including examination of the accused by a medical officer. If the Magistrate is satisfied that he is of unsound mind and thus incapable of making his defense, he postpones further proceedings in the case (Section 328, CPC).

The accused can then be either detained in safe custody (under Indian Lunacy Act 1912) or be released pending investigation or trial if bail can be taken and sufficient security is provided by a relative or friend that he will be properly cared for, will be prevented from injuring himself or others, and will be produced before the court whenever necessary.

The trial can resume if the accused ceases to be of unsound mind.

OTHER CRIMINAL LAWS RELEVANT TO PSYCHIATRY

Suicide

If a person attempts to commit suicide and does any act towards the commission of such offence, he can be punished under Section 309 IPC with simple imprisonment for a term which may extend to 1 year or with fine or with both. The offence is cognizable but bailable.

A mentally ill person is not responsible, if Section 84 IPC is applicable. Therefore, suicide is not an offence if the person at the time of committing it, by reason of mental illness, did not know what he was doing or what he was doing was either wrong or contrary to law.[28]

In April 1994, a two judge bench of Supreme Court (Justice RM Sahai and Justice BL Hansaria) had declared the offence void. They observed that "the right to live (under Article 21 of the Constitution of India) can be said to bring in its trial the right not to live a forced life". They declared Section 309 of IPC as irrational and cruel.[29]

However, in March 1996, a five judge Constitution Bench of the Supreme court, setting aside the earlier judgment, held that attempted suicide is an offence under the IPC.[29] So, the section 309 IPC continues to be valid.

Consent

Under Section 90 IPC, "a consent is not a consent....if.... given by a person who, from unsoundness of mind, or intoxication, is unable to understand the nature and consequence of that to which he gives his consent.....", or "given by a person who is under 12 years of age". The question of invalidity of consent may arise in rape, murder, grievous hurt, and abetment to suicide.

Consent to sexual intercourse given by a woman who is imbecile or lunatic, is of no avail and the act amounts to rape.

Section 89 IPC provides that an act done in good faith for the benefit of an insane person by the guardian or with consent of the guardian, is not an offence.

Right of Private Defense Against an Insane Person

Section 98 IPC states that "when an act, which would otherwise be a certain offence, is not that offence by reason of.....the unsoundness of mind or the intoxication of the person doing that act.....every person, has the same right of private defense against that act" as if it were an offence.

Miscellaneous

In addition, a mentally ill person may be involved in any crime. Some of the more commonly seen criminal acts include: unnatural offences (e.g. in sexual perversions; Section 377 IPC); affrays (e.g. in mania; Section 159 IPC); misconduct in public while drunk (e.g. in alcohol dependence; Section 510 IPC).

Civil Responsibility

Contract

A contract is an agreement enforceable by law, according to the Indian Contract Act (Act 9 of 1872). An agreement is simply an accepted proposal. Although an oral agreement is perfectly valid, writing and registration are necessary where so required.

Section 6 of the Act provides that "a proposal is revoked by the death or insanity of the proposer, if the fact.....comes to the knowledge of the acceptor before acceptance."

Section 11 of the Act states that "every person is competent to contract, who is of the age of majority......and who is of sound mind....."

Section 12 of the Act declares a person to be of sound mind for the purposes of contract "if, at the time when he makes it, he is capable of understanding it and of forming rational judgment as to its effect upon his interests."

"A person who is usually of unsound mind, but occasionally of sound mind (lucid interval), may make a contract when he is of sound mind". Similarly "a person who is usually of sound mind, but occasionally of unsound mind, may not make a contract when he is of unsound mind".

A mentally ill person is responsible for payment of necessaries purchased by him in accordance with his status and social position, whether the vendor knew his condition or not. However, he is not responsible, if:

- The order was grossly extravagant and beyond his means (e.g. in mania), or if
- The vendor took advantage of the fact of his insanity in selling those necessaries to him.

A court may, on petition of one of the partners, dissolve a firm on the ground that a partner is found to be a mentally ill person under the Mental Health Act 1987.

Marriage

The Hindu Marriage Act (Act 25 of 1955) provides for conditions for a Hindu marriage under Section 5. One of the conditions, Section 5(ii) introduced by Act 68 of 1976, states that at the time of the marriage, neither party,

- is incapable of giving a valid consent.....(due to) unsoundness of mind; or
- though capable of giving consent, has been suffering from mental disorder of such a kind or to such an extent as to be unfit for marriage and the procreation of children; or
- has been subject to recurrent attacks of insanity or epilepsy.....

Any marriage solemnized in contravention to this condition shall be voidable and may be *annulled* by a decree of nullity under Section 12 of the Act. Another ground for nullity under the same section is the fact that the consent for marriage was obtained by 'fraud', "as to any material fact or circumstance concerning the respondent", for example, the fact of mental illness or treatment for the same.

Divorce can be granted under Section 13 of the Act on a petition presented by either spouse on the ground that the other party "has been incurably of unsound mind, or has been suffering continuously or intermittently from mental disorder of such kind and to such an extent that the petitioner cannot reasonably be expected to live with the respondent" [Section 13 (iii) inserted by Act 68 of 1976].

Here, the term mental disorder means "mental illness, arrested or incomplete development of mind, psychopathic disorder or any other disorder or disability of mind and includes schizophrenia". The term psychopathic disorder here means "a persistent disorder or disability of mind (whether or not including subnormality of intelligence) which results in abnormally aggressive or seriously irresponsible conduct on the part of the other party, and whether or not it requires or is susceptible to medical treatment".

The Special Marriage Act (Act 43 of 1954) also provides that marriage can be solemnized between any two persons if at the time of marriage neither party was an idiot or a lunatic.

Under the dissolution of Muslim Marriage Act 1939, a woman married under Muslim law is entitled to obtain a decree for the dissolution of marriage on the ground of her husband being insane for a period of 2 years. The husband under the Muslim law has the power to pronounce divorce (talak) at any time, anywhere, and without assigning any reason.

Any married person may be granted divorce, under the Parsi Marriage and Divorce Act 1936, on the ground that the other party had been of unsound mind at the time of marriage (and the petitioner was ignorant of the fact) and has been habitually so till the date of petition, which should be within 3 years of the date of marriage.

Adoption

Under the Hindu Adoptions and Maintenance Act (Act 78 of 1956), any Hindu male "who is of sound mind and is not a minor" can adopt a child, with the consent of his wife unless ".....(she) has been declared by a court.....to be of unsound mind" (Section 7).

Similarly, any Hindu female "who is of sound mind", is not a minor, and is not married, can adopt a child. If she is married, then her husband"......has been declared by a court......to be of unsound mind" (Section 8).

Also, the person capable of giving in adoption of a child should be of sound mind.

Witness

Under the Indian Evidence Act 1872, a lunatic is not competent to give evidence if he is prevented by virtue of his lunacy from understanding the questions put to him and giving rational answers to them (Section 118).

However, such a person can give evidence during a lucid interval on the discretion of the judge (and the jury).

Testamentary Capacity

Testamentary disposition is regulated by the Indian Succession Act (Act 39 of 1925). Some of the salient points regarding testamentary disposition are as follows:

- A will must be in writing, though it need not be registered.
- It must be signed by *testator* in the presence of at least two witnesses.
- A legatee cannot attest a will.
- An executor(s) is appointed under the will by the testator to carry out its terms after his death.
- A will can be revoked or modified any time before the death of the testator.
- A will comes into effect after the death of the testator. It is said to speak from grave and to be 'ambulatory'.
- The testator must be of a 'sound and disposing mind'. Section 59 of the Act states that "every person of sound mind, not being a minor, may dispose of his property by will".

Explanation 4 of this section states that "no person can make a will while he is in such a state of mind, whether arising from intoxication or from illnesses or from any other cause, that he does not know what he is doing.

If a medical practitioner is called to examine a testator as to his fitness to make a valid will, the following points must be kept in mind:

- Testamentary capacity consists of:
  - An understanding of the nature of the will,
  - A knowledge of the property to be disposed of, and
  - An ability to recognize those who may have justifiable claims on his property.
- The testator should be tested on the above-mentioned points by thorough questioning.
- If the testator is seriously ill, he must be made to read out aloud the will in the presence of the doctor.
- A will is invalid if it is executed under undue influence of any other person. If there is reason to suspect that such is the case, the testator should be questioned when he is alone.
- A will is invalid under the following conditions (for example):
  - Imbecility arising from advanced age or by excessive drinking.
  - Insane delusions making the testator incapable of rational views and judgment.
- A will is valid under the following conditions (for example):
  - Deaf, dumb, or blind persons who are not thereby incapacitated for making a will and are able to know what they do by it.
  - Lucid intervals.

- If testator commits suicide immediately after making the will, in the absence of evidence of mental disorder.
- Presence of delusions not affecting in any way the disposal of the property or the persons affected by the will.

• A will may be declared invalid if the testator disposes his property in a way which he would not have done under normal conditions.

Torts

The law of torts or the law of allocation and distribution of losses is a system of laws that enables a person, who has suffered harm or injury by the acts of another, may claim damages in a civil proceeding. The law of torts is not codified like statute laws; instead common legal principles are applied.

A tort is a species of civil wrong or injury, other than a mere breach of trust or contract.

Insanity is a good defense against torts if the defendant was not competent by reason of insanity of such degree that he did not know the nature and quality of the act, or what he was doing was wrong. The mere presence of insanity is not a defense in a tort, nor is a medical certificate declaring the defendant insane.

Rights to Vote and to Stand for Election

Under Act 326 of the Constitution of India, no person declared to be of unsound mind can vote.

Under Act 102 of the Constitution of India, a person is disqualified from being chosen as or for being a Member of either House of Parliament, if he is of unsound mind and stands so declared by a competent court.

Civil Proceedings

A civil suit *by* a lunatic must be filed through a 'next friend' who is approved by the court. A suit *against* a lunatic must be filed against him represented by a *guardian ad litem*. The plaintiff must apply to the court and get a *guardian ad litem* appointed for the purposes of the suit.

If the suit is filed against a lunatic without a 'next friend' or a *guardian ad litem*, it will be struck off and the lawyer filing such a suit may be directed to pay the costs.

If the court has in inquisition proceedings earlier appointed a manager or guardian, he alone must be appointed *guardian ad litem* and the preferential "next friend".

MENTAL HEALTH ACT

Indian Lunacy Act (ILA), Act 4 of 1912, replaced the Indian Lunatic Asylums Act, Act 36 of 1858. It was enacted to govern reception, detention and care of lunatics and their property, and to consolidate and amend the laws relating to lunacy.

The Act was divided into 4 parts and 8 chapters consisting of 100 sections, in addition to 2 schedules (appendices); Schedule I has 8 forms, while Schedule II was repealed in 1914 (Act 17).

The Act provided for punishment, if two or more lunatic are illegally detained for gain in any place, not being an asylum.

The enactment of Indian Lunacy Act of 1912 was followed by opening of many new asylums, an improvement in the general conditions of asylums, and an increase in awareness regarding the prevailing situation of lunatics in such asylums. However, this Act provided for establishment of separate hospitals for Europeans and Indian patients, and separate provisions were made for them in the Act. The name lunatic asylum was changed to mental hospital in 1920.

In 1946, the Bhore Committee, the Health Survey and Development Committee, submitted its recommendations. The committee had requested Colonel M Taylor, Medical Superintendent of Ranchi European Mental Hospital (Now Central Institute of Psychiatry), to visit all the major hospitals in the country and to prepare a report. The report,[29] apart from suggesting that majority of mental hospitals in India were quite out of date and were designed for detention and safe custody without regard to curative treatment, also commented that "the cardinal points in the Indian Lunacy Act 1912, have outlived their usefulness".

The Indian Psychiatric Society, established in January 1947, was quick to react to the recommendations of Colonel Taylor and Bhore Committee. In January 1949, an adhoc drafting committee was appointed which consisted of 3 distinguished psychiatrists, namely Dr J Roy (Nagpur), Major (Dr) RB Davis (Ranchi European Mental Hospital), and Dr Hasib (Indian Mental Hospital, Ranchi). They prepared a draft bill called as the 'Indian Mental Health Act', which was redrafted and finalized in January 1950 and forwarded to Government of India.

The initial efforts of the Indian Psychiatric Society, in persuading the Government of India to amend the existing Indian Lunacy Act, failed. Nearly 10 years later, in 1959, the Director General of Health Services requested Dr David Satyanand (Medical Superintendent of Hospital of Mental Diseases, later renamed Central Institute of Psychiatry) to prepare a new modified draft. The modified draft was submitted to Government of India and the contents were discussed in a conference of Medical Superintendents, held in November 1960 at Agra.

The Ministry of Health, Government of India, appointed at 'Mental Health Advisory Committee' in September 1962. The years 1963-1966 saw formation of 4 more subcommittees on the matter but no concrete action resulted. Finally, after persistent efforts of the Indian Psychiatric Society, the Bill was introduced in the Lok Sabha in April 1978 but the Bill lapsed in 1979 when the Parliament was dissolved.

The same Bill was reintroduced in the Parliament in December 1981. After some discussion, the Bill was referred to a Joint Committee of Members of Parliament for Mental Health Bill. The committee held multiple meetings, visited mental hospitals, heard oral evidence from psychiatrists and received memoranda from several individuals. However, it took formation of one more Joint Committee in April 1985, before the two Houses in May 1986.[29]

The Mental Health Act (MHA) 1987 was finally passed by the Rajya Sabha on 26th November 1986, and by the Lok Sabha on 19th March 1987. The amendments made by the Lok Sabha were agreed to by the Rajya Sabha on 22nd April 1987. It was finally assented to by the President on 22nd May 1987 when it became the Act 14 of 1987. Later, the Government of India issued orders that the Act came in force with effect from April 1, 1993 in all the States and Union territories of India.[29]

The Act

It is an "act to consolidate and amend the law relating to the treatment and care of mentally ill persons, to make better provision with respect to their property and affairs and for matters connected therewith or incidental thereto".

The Act is divided into 10 chapters consisting of 98 sections. Chapter I (Preliminary) deals with the various definitions like cost of maintenance, inspecting officer, license, medical officer, psychiatrist, psychiatric hospital/nursing home, among others. The term 'mentally ill person' in MHA replaces the term 'lunatic' in ILA, and means "a person who is in need of treatment by reason of any mental disorder other than mental retardation". The term 'mentally ill prisoner' replaces the term 'criminal lunatic' and means "a mentally ill person for whose detention in, or removal to, a psychiatric hospital, psychiatric nursing home, jail or other place of safe custody". The terms 'psychiatric hospital' and 'psychiatric nursing home' replace the term 'asylum'.

Chapter II is a new chapter, concerned with mental health authorities. A central authority for mental health services is envisaged, under the Central Government, with the following main functions:

- In-charge of regulation, development, direction and co-ordination with respect to mental health services under the Central Government.
- Supervision of psychiatric hospitals, nursing homes and other mental health service agencies under the Central Government, and
- Advisor to the Central Government on all matters 'relating to mental health'.

A similar State authority for mental health services with similar functions is also envisaged for the various States.

Chapter III deals with psychiatric hospitals and psychiatric nursing homes. The Central and the State Government is empowered to establish or maintain psychiatric hospitals and nursing homes. There is a provision for separate hospitals for:

- Those under the age of 16 years,
- Those addicted to alcohol or other drugs which lead to behavioral changes,
- Mentally ill prisoners, and
- Any other prescribed class or category.

The establishment or maintenance of psychiatric hospitals or psychiatric nursing homes is based on the following prerequisites:

- A valid license, which is granted under the Act by the Licensing Authority on the following conditions:
  - Receipt of an application for license.
  - On enquiry, it is satisfied that such establishment or maintenance is necessary.
  - The applicant can provide the minimum facilities prescribed for admission, treatment and care of mentally ill persons.
  - The In-charge is a medical officer who is a psychiatrist.
  - The license is not transferable or heritable.
  - The license is valid for a maximum period of 5 years, after which it has to be renewed.
- The license can be revoked if the licensing authority is satisfied that:
  - The psychiatric hospital/nursing home is not being maintained by the licensee in accordance with the provisions of the Act, or
  - The maintenance is carried out in a manner detrimental to the moral, mental, or physical well-being of the inpatients.

In such a case, if the license is revoked, the inpatients can be transferred to any other specified psychiatric hospital/nursing home. There is a provision for any aggrieved person to appeal against any order to the State Government.

There is a provision for an Inspecting Officer to inspect any psychiatric hospital/nursing home, records thereof, and to visit and interview patients in private receiving treatment and care therein. Any personal records of a patient so inspected are to be kept confidential. The inspecting officer may report the matter to the licensing authority.

In case, a mentally-ill person's condition does not warrant admission, he can receive treatment as an outpatient.

Chapter IV (Admission and detention in psychiatric hospital or psychiatric nursing home) consists of 3 parts, with part III divided into 4 further subdivisions. A mentally ill person, under this Act, can be admitted in a psychiatric hospital or psychiatric nursing home in one of the following ways:

- Admission as a voluntary patient.
- Admission under special circumstances (for not more than 90 days).
- Reception order on application.
- Reception order on production of mentally ill person before Magistrate.
- Admission as inpatient after inquisition.
- Admission as a mentally ill prisoner.

A *reception order* for admission can be obtained from a Magistrate on production of the following documents.

- A petition (or application in writing).
  - Containing the particulars of the case (showing how the order is necessary),
  - Presented by husband or wife of the alleged mentally ill person (if not available, then by any other relative),
  - The petitioner being a major (not a minor), and having seen the alleged mentally ill person within 14 days before the presentation of petition.
- Supported by two medical certificates, one of which shall be from a medical practitioner in the service of Government.
  - The certificates should be on the specified forms only.
  - The certificates should be on separate sheets of paper.
  - The medical officers or practitioners filling the certificates should examine the alleged mentally ill person personally, separately and independently.
  - The medical examination should be performed within 10 days of the petition (or the order, in cases of reception order without petition).
  - The certificate must state the facts upon which the opinions have been formed, distinguishing facts observed (implying mental status examination) and facts communicated (implying history provided). No certificate should be based on only the communicated facts.
  - The certificate is equivalent to a sworn statement.

In addition, the Magistrate can order detention of an alleged mentally ill person for short periods pending report by medical officer (for a period not exceeding 10 days in aggregate) or pending his removal to psychiatric hospital or psychiatric nursing home (for a period not exceeding 30 days).

A *reception order without petition* can be issued by a Magistrate, if an officer in-charge of a police-station arrests a,

- Wandering mentally ill person, who is believed to be incapable of taking care of himself, or
- Dangerous mentally ill person, or
- Ill treated or neglected mentally ill person, or
- Mentally ill person, not under proper care and control,
- And produces him before the Magistrate. The magistrate, after examining the said mentally ill person, can have him examined by a medical officer, in addition to making any other suitable enquiries. After the medical officer issues a medical certificate, the Magistrate may then:

- Issue a reception order for admission in an asylum, or
- Send him to a licensed psychiatric hospital, if any friend or relative agree in writing to pay for his maintenance, or
- Summon a relative (who has or ought to have charge of him) and order him to properly care for the mentally ill person (subject to punishment, if he willfully disobeys the order), or
- Order a temporary detention (not exceeding 10 days at one time, and not exceeding a total period of 30 days) pending further enquiry.

A reception order is sufficient authority for conveyance, reception and detention of a mentally ill person in a psychiatric hospital. The medical officer-incharge of the psychiatric hospital is bound to comply with such an order.

The reception order ceases to have an effect:

- After 30 days of issue (unless the person is admitted), and
- After discharge from a psychiatric hospital, under the Act.

Temporary treatment order (for periods not exceeding 6 months), and Emergency admission (for periods not exceeding 72 hours) did find a mention in the Mental Health Bill, but these were removed from the finally enacted Mental Health Act, though temporary treatment order receives a brief mention in Section 20.

Voluntary admission can be effected by the medical officer in-charge of a psychiatric hospital/nursing home, if:

- A major mentally ill person (not a minor) requests for admission as a voluntary patient.
- The guardian of a minor mentally ill person requests for admission of the minor as a voluntary patient.

A comparison of the various admission and discharge procedures under the Indian Lunacy Act (ILA) and the Mental Health Act (MHA) is provided in Table 3.

Chapter V (Inspection, discharge, leave of absence and removal of mentally ill persons) is divided into 4 parts: Part I, Inspection; Part II, Discharge; Part III, Leave of absence; and Part IV, Removal.

The State/Central Government shall appoint for every psychiatric hospital and every psychiatric nursing home not less than 5 visitors, of whom at least 1 is a medical officer, preferably a psychiatrist, and 2 social workers. The Head of the Medical Services of the State (or his nominee, preferably a psychiatrist) shall be an ex-officio visitor of all psychiatric hospitals and psychiatric nursing homes in the State.

The visitors are bound to inspect the psychiatric hospital/nursing home on the following lines:

- Inspection at least once in every month.
- At least 3 visitors should be present at the joint inspection.
- Shall write their remarks in the Visitor's book regarding management and conditions of such hospital or nursing home and of the inpatients thereof.
- Shall not inspect any personal records of an inpatient which, in the opinion of the medical officer incharge, are confidential in nature.

The IG Prisons, along with at least 3 visitors, of which 1 should be a social worker, shall make a visit every 3 months to inspect the mentally ill prisoners. The medical officer incharge of a psychiatric hospital/nursing home, where a mentally ill prisoner is admitted, shall submit a special report

Table 3: Admission and Discharge Procedures in ILA and MHA: A Comparison

Type of admission	*Act*	*Admission application by*	*Court intervention*	*Medical certificate(s)*	*Admitting authority*	*Discharge application by*	*Discharge authority*	*Duration of admission*	*Type of patient**
1. Voluntary	ILA	Any lunatic			Asylum Incharge + Atleast 2 visitors Medical Officer Incharge	Voluntary Boarder	Asylum Incharge	Discharge within 24 hours of application	Voluntary
	MHA	Any (major) mentally ill person or guardian of minor mentally ill person				Patient (major) or Guardian (for minor)	Medical Officer Incharge	Discharge within 24 hours of application	
2. Under special circumstances	ILA								
	MHA	A relative or friend of mentally ill person		Two	Medical Officer Incharge	Mentally ill person, or his friend/relative	Magistrate	Not more than 90 days	Non-volitional and Involitional
3. Reception order on petition/ application	ILA	Husband, wife or nearest relative	Reception order	Two	Magistrate	1. No application 2. Petitioner 3. Inquisition	3 or more visitors Asylum Incharge Magistrate	Unspecified	Non-volitional and Involitional
	MHA	Husband, wife, or any other relative; or Medical Officer Incharge	Reception order	Two	Magistrate	1. No application 2. Petitioner 3. Mentally ill person (+ a certificate from Medical Officer Incharge) 4. Inquisition 5. A friend or relative (furnishing a bond)	Medical Officer Incharge + 2 Medical Practitioners (1 preferably a psychiatrist) Medical Officer Incharge Magistrate Magistrate Medical Officer Incharge	Unspecified	
4. Reception order without petition/On production of mentally ill person before magistrate	ILA	Report by a police officer	Reception order	One	Magistrate	1. No application 2. A friend or relative 3. Inquisition	3 or more visitors Asylum Incharge Magistrate	Unspecified	Wandering, dangerous, neglected, or cruelly treated mentally ill persons
	MHA	Report by a police officer	Reception order		Magistrate	1. No application 2. Mentally ill person (+ a certificate from Medical Officer Incharge) 3. Inquisition 4. A friend or relative	Medical Officer Incharge + 2 Medical Practitioners (1 preferably a psychiatrist) Magistrate Magistrate Medical Officer Incharge	Unspecified	

Contd...

Contd...

Type of admission	*Act*	*Admission application by*	*Court intervention*	*Medical certificate(s)*	*Admitting authority*	*Discharge application by*	*Discharge authority*	*Duration of admission*	*Type of patient**
5. Inquisition	ILA	Any relative or Advocate General or Public Curator or District Collector	Notification and Enquiry		Magistrate	Inquisition	Magistrate	Unspecified	Any lunatic/ Mentally ill person
	MHA	Any relative or Advocate General or Public Curator or District Collector	Notification and Enquiry		Magistrate	Inquisition	Magistrate	Unspecified	
6. Criminal lunatic/ Mentally Ill prisoner	ILA	Any order under S. 466 or 471 of CPC (1898); S. 30 of Prisoners Act (1900); S. 103A of Indian Army Act (1911)			The order	Visitor can recommend discharge	Under the relevant section	Unspecified	Criminal lunatic/ Mentally ill prisoner
	MHA	Any order under S. 30 of Prisoners Act (1900); S. 144 of Air Force Act (1950); S. 145 of Army Act (1950); S. 143 or 144 of Navy Act (1957); S. 330 or 335 of CPC (1973)			The order		Under the relevant section	Unspecified	

Abbreviations: ILA, Indian Lunacy Act, MHA, Mental Health Act.
*There are 3 types of patients:
1. Volitional/Voluntary (Have insight into their illness and demand admission).
2. Involitional (Lack insight into their illness and refuse admission), e.g. paranoid schizophrenia.
3. Non-Volitional (Can not give consent or refuse consent for admission), e.g. catatonic stupor, severe mental retardation.

regarding the mental and physical condition of such person once in every 6 months.

A leave of absence can be granted to any inpatient (except a mentally ill prisoner) on application by the petitioner/applicant (for admission) or by a near relative, on entering a bond (with or without sureties) with the medical officer incharge. The bond may specify that the applicant shall:

- Take proper care of the mentally ill person,
- Prevent such person from causing injury to himself or to others, and
- Bring back such person on the expiry of the leave period (or else the Magistrate shall be notified).

The maximum period of such leave is 60 days. In case the medical officer incharge refuses to grant the leave of absence, the applicant may apply to the Magistrate who is empowered to grant or refuse such leave.

If a mentally ill person (except a mentally ill prisoner) escapes from a psychiatric hospital/nursing home, he can be recaptured by authorized persons, only within 1 month of the date of escape.

Chapter IV deals with judicial inquisition regarding alleged mentally ill person possessing property, custody of his person, and management of his property. The application for holding an inquisition into the mental condition of such persons may be made by any of his relatives, or a public curator, or the Advocate General of the State, or the District Collector (when property involves land). For the purpose of holding the inquisition, the District Court may appoint 2 or more persons to act as assessors.

On the completion of the inquisition, the District court shall record its findings on 2 issues:

1. Whether the alleged mentally ill person is in fact mentally ill?
2. If mentally ill, whether he is incapable to care for himself and manage his property, or incapable of managing his property only?

The District Court can order for appointment of a Guardian (if incapable of looking after both himself and his property) or a Manager (if incapable of looking after only his property but can look after himself).

Where the District Court has reason to believe that such person has ceased to be mentally ill, it may, after an enquiry, set aside the action taken earlier.

Chapter VII deals with the liability to meet cost of maintenance of mentally ill persons detained in psychiatric hospital or psychiatric nursing home.

Chapter VIII deals with the protection of human rights of mentally ill persons. This is a new chapter in the Act. It specifies that:

- Mentally ill person shall not be subjected during treatment to any physical or mental indignity, or cruelty.
- Mentally ill person under treatment shall not be used for research purposes, unless:
  - such research is of direct benefit to him for diagnosis or treatment; or
  - written consent has been obtained from the patient (if a major, voluntary patient) or the guardian (if minor or incompetent) for such research.
- Unless otherwise specified (Section 94), no letters or other communications sent by or to a mentally ill person under treatment shall be intercepted, detained or destroyed.

The Mental Health Bill had one more sub-section restricting the use of harsh measures, mechanical restraint and solitary confinement. This sub-section has not found its way through the enactment of the Act.

Chapter IX deals with the penalties and procedure, while Chapter X deals with miscellaneous issues.

In addition, the State Mental Health Rules, 1990 (which also contains the nine important forms required by the Mental Health Act, 1987) and the Central Mental Health Authority Rules, 1990, have also been passed by the Government of India on December 29, 1990.

NARCOTIC DRUGS AND PSYCHOTROPIC SUBSTANCES ACT

Before 1985, the drug related matters were dealt with under 3 main legislations, namely:

1. The Opium Act 1857,
2. The Opium Act 1878, and
3. The Dangerous Drugs Act, 1930.

The Opium Acts dealt exclusively with matters related to opium. Therefore, it was the Dangerous Drugs Act which dealt with other drugs like cannabis and cocaine. It did not, however, deal with psychotropic substances which were covered partially under the Drugs and Cosmetics Act 1940; also, no mention was made of cannabis cultivation in the Act.

The maximum punishment, under the Dangerous Drugs Act, for the various offences related to drugs, was a simple imprisonment of 3 years (with or without fine) for the 1st offence.

However, when the drug situation in India worsened rapidly in the early 1980s due to an influx of heroin, a new legislation was necessary to cope up with the situation. This was effected by the enactment of the Narcotic Drugs and Psychotropic Substances Act in 1985.

The Act

The Narcotic Drugs and Psychotropic Substances Act (NDPSA), Act 61 of 1985 as amended up to Act 2 of 1989, along with Narcotic Drugs and Psychotropic Substances Rules (NDPSR) 1985 and Narcotic Drugs and Psychotropic Substances (Execution of Bond by Convicts or Addicts) Rules [NDPS (EBCA) R] 1985 was enacted on 16th September, 1985. It is an act to consolidate and amend the law relating to narcotic drugs, to make stringent provision for the control and regulation of operations relating to narcotic drugs and psychotropic substances, to provide for the forfeiture of property derived from, or used in illicit traffic in narcotic drugs and psychotropic substances, to implement the provisions of the International Conventions on Narcotic Drugs and Psychotropic Substances, and for matters connected therewith. The Act came in force on 14th November, 1985.

The Act consists of 6 chapters with 83 sections. Chapter I (Preliminary) deals with definitions of the various terms, some of which are:

- *Addict:* A person addicted to any narcotic drug or psychotropic substance.
- *Narcotic drug:* Coca leaf, cannabis, opium, poppy straw, and includes all manufactured drugs.
- *Manufactured drug:* All coca derivatives, medicinal cannabis, opium derivatives, poppy straw concentrate, and any other notified narcotic substance or preparation (88 have been notified).
- *Psychotropic substance:* Any substance, natural or synthetic, or any natural material, or any salt or preparation of such substance or material included in the list of psychotropic substances specified in the schedule (76 substances and their salts and preparations have been specified in the accompanying schedule).

Minimum concentrations have been specified in respect of opium preparations (not less than 0.2% of morphine, or any amount of diacetylmorphine) and coca derivatives (not less than 0.1% of cocaine) for the preparations to be considered as narcotic drugs.

Chapter II deals with authorities and officers. Among other authorities and officers, there is provision for appointment of a Narcotics Commissioner, and a Narcotic Drugs and Psychotropic Substance Consultative Committee (with a Chairman and other members, not exceeding 20) by the Central Government. There is provision under Chapter IIA for constitution of a National Fund for Control of Drug Abuse (with a Governing Body consisting of a Chairman and other members, not exceeding 6). The Central Government has constituted an authority known as the Narcotics Control Bureau (headed by a Director General), with headquarters at New Delhi and 5 zonal offices at Bombay, Calcutta, Delhi, Madras and Varanasi, on 17th March 1986 to exercise the powers and functions of the Central Government under this Act.

Chapter III deals with prohibition, control and regulation. According to Section 8, No person shall:

- Cultivate any coca, opium poppy or cannabis plant, or
- Produce, possess,.....or consume any narcotic drug or psychotropic substance, except for medicinal or scientific purposes and in the manner and to the extent provided by the Act.

Such prohibition for '*ganja*' shall take effect only from the date notified by the Central Government. There are clauses in this chapter regarding the power of Central and State Government to permit, control and regulate the narcotic drugs and psychotropic substances, including the matter of licenses.

Chapter IV deals with offences and penalties. The important offences and penalties under this chapter include:

- Punishment for contravention in relation to poppy straw; coca plant and leaves; prepared opium, opium poppy, and opium; cannabis plant (except 'ganja'); manufactured drugs: psychotropic substances:
  - *For 1st offence:* Rigorous Imprisonment (RI) for not less than 10 years (may extend to 20 years), And Fine not less than 1 Lakh rupees (may extend to 2 Lakh rupees or even more).
  - *For 2nd and subsequent conviction:* RI for not less than 15 years (may extend to 30 years), And Fine not less than 1.5 Lakh rupees (may extend to 3 Lakh rupees or even more).
- Punishment for contravention in relation to *'ganja' or cultivation of cannabis plant:*
  - *For 1st offence:* RI which may extend to 5 years, and Fine which may extend to 50,000 rupees.
  - *For 2nd and subsequent conviction:* RI which may extend to 10 years, and Fine which may extend to 1 Lakh rupees (or even more).
- Punishment for contravention in relation to *any controlled substance* (which means any substance which the Central Government may declare to be a controlled substance): RI which may extend to 10 years, and Fine which may extend to 1 Lakh rupees (or even more).
- Punishment for illegal possession in *small quantity* for personal consumption of any narcotic drug or psychotropic substance (Section 27):
  - If the narcotic drug or psychotropic substance possessed or consumed in small quantities is cocaine, morphine, heroine or any other specified substance, the punishment is imprisonment for a term which may extend to 1 year, Or Fine, Or Both.
  - If the narcotic drug or psychotropic substance possessed or consumed in small quantities is other than those specified above, the punishment is imprisonment for a term which may extend to 6 months, Or Fine, Or Both.

  The small quantities specified are:
  Heroin (250 mg); Hashish/Charas (5 g); Opium (5 g); Cocaine (125 mg); and Ganja (500 g).
  Here, the burden of proving that the substance was intended for personal use shall lie on such person.
- *Death penalty* may be given, if any person who has been convicted earlier (under Section 15 to 25, or Section 27A)

and has been subsequently convicted in relation to narcotic drugs and psychotropic substances specified below and involving quantities equal to or more that those indicated against each:

- Opium (10 kg).
- Morphine (1 kg).
- Heroin (1 kg).
- Codeine (1 kg).
- Thebaine (1 kg).
- Cocaine (500 g).
- Hashish (20 kg).
- A mixture of any of the above drugs (1.5 kg).
- LSD (0.5 kg).
- THC (0.5 kg).
- Methamphetamine (1.5 kg).
- Methaqualone (1.5 kg).
- Amphetamine (1.5 kg).
- Salts and preparations of substances mentioned in (ix) to (xiii) above (1.5 kg).

Under this Act, existence of a culpable mental state is presumed (Here 'culpable mental state' includes intention, motive, knowledge of a fact and belief in, or reason to believe a fact). It is a defense for the accused to prove the fact that he had no such mental state with respect to the act charged as an offence in that prosecution.

Every offence punishable under this Act is cognizable, and any punishment more than 5 years imprisonment is nonbailable.

Any addict convicted under Section 27 (Section on small quantities) can be, instead of being sentenced, with his consent, released for undergoing medical treatment for detoxification or deaddiction from a Government maintained or recognized hospital or institution. This can be done with regard to the addict's age, character, antecedents, or physical or mental condition, and on his entering into a bond (with or without sureties) to appear and furnish before the court within a period not exceeding 1 year, a report of his medical treatment and to abstain from commission of any offence, under this Act in the meantime. If satisfied, the court may direct the release of such an offender after due admonition and entering into another bond covering a maximum period of 3 years.

The court is empowered to publish names, places of business or residence, and nature of contravention of offenders under this chapter (except those convicted for small quantities under Section 27).

Chapter V details the procedure related to this Act, while Chapter V-A deals with forfeiture of property derived from, or used in illicit traffic. Chapter VI deals with miscellaneous issues like Central and State Government to have regard to international conventions while making rules, and power of Government to establish centers for identification, treatment, etc. of addicts.

This Act is in addition to the Customs Act 1962 and the Drugs and Cosmetics Act 1940. By enactment of this Act, the following Acts have been repealed:

- The Opium Act 1857 (Act 13 of 1857).
- The Opium Act 1978 (Act 13 of 1878).
- The Dangerous Drugs Act 1930 (Act 2 of 1930).

Narcotic Drugs and Psychotropic Substances Rules

The narcotic drugs and psychotropic substances rules (NDPSR) 1985 consists of rules of Central Government in exercise of powers conferred by NDPSA 1985. It consists of 8 chapters (with 68 sections), 3 schedules, and 7 forms. The rules refer to power of officers; and cultivation, production, manufacture, sale, export/import or transport of any narcotic drug or psychotropic substance. Schedules I-III detail the various narcotic drugs and psychotropic substances.

The various bonds to be executed under the NDPSA 1985 have been put together in the Narcotic Drugs and Psychotropic Substances (Execution of Bond by Convicts or Addicts) Rules 1985.

In addition, the Prevention of Illicit Traffic in Narcotic Drugs and Psychotropic Substances Act (PIT NDPSA) 1988, Act 46 of 1988, was enacted to "provide for detention in certain cases for the purpose of preventing illicit traffic in narcotic drugs and psychotropic substances and for matters connected therewith".

PSYCHIATRIST AS AN EXPERT WITNESS

There are 2 kinds of witnesses:

1. *Common witness,* who testifies of the facts observed by himself, and
2. *Expert witness,* who on account of his professional training is capable of deducing opinions and inferences from the facts observed by himself or noticed by others.

Any psychiatrist may become involved in legal proceedings as an expert, a medical specialist on mental disorders. The expert witness must possess some special knowledge, skill, training, or possibly experience, that helps in providing information and opinion regarding issues that lie beyond the experience and general knowledge of the judge and the jury.[30]

Many psychiatrists dislike the process of appearing as expert witnesses in courts. Some of the reasons of this state of affairs are:

- Legal process is an adversarial process, strangely opposed to the cooperative process of therapeutics (with emphasis on patient-therapist relationship) a psychiatrist is used to in his professional life.
- Psychiatry is a very inexact science; most of the opinions expressed by psychiatrists are based on subjective experience and are not readily testable by any objective criteria.

- Honest differences of opinion are inevitable in any effort to formulate complex judgments.
- Psychiatrists are not often fully conversant with the language, practices and objectives of the legal procedure in which they are participating.
- There is a common misapprehension that they must use legal language while offering testimony.
- There is a dilemma, whether to favor the patient's interests (as demanded by the patient-therapist relationship) or to give evidence against him (as legal process is an adversarial one).

The cross-examination of a witness, common or expert, is one of the most efficacious tests the law has devised for discovery of truth.[31] While testifying, common witness may be admonished by the judge to speak to the facts and to leave the opinion to the jury or the judge. However, expert witness may be permitted to express opinions related to their areas of professional expertise. While cross-examining a psychiatrist, the cross-examiner often tries to challenge the psychiatric method of gathering data and forming diagnoses.

There are certain general rules as to the evidence in relation to mental illness, which include:

- There is a presumption in favor of sanity, and the contrary must be proved to the satisfaction of the court, both in civil and criminal cases.
  However, in testamentary disposition, the onus of proving soundness of mind is on the testator.
- There is a presumption of continuity of sanity as well as insanity. The return of soundness of mind, as well as lucid interval, must be proved to the satisfaction of the court.
- An 'idiot' is presumed to be permanently of unsound mind, though there is no such presumption in case of a 'lunatic'.
- There is a presumption that a person who is congenitally deaf or dumb or blind is of unsound mind; however, this is rebuttable.

Although there are no general rules governing the role of psychiatrist as an expert witness, the following points will aid a novice in providing testimony in a court.[32]

- Speak the truth.
- Give evidence, irrespective as to whether it is likely to lead to conviction or acquittal of the accused.
- Listen closely to the questions asked. Pause a moment before answering, not only to give a clear answer but also allow the 'other party' to object to the question (if they have to).
- While answering, keep in mind the limits of the field.
- Don't use 'always' or 'never'.
- Speak slowly, distinctly and audibly.
- If there is no clear answer to the question asked, do not hesitate to say "I don't know?"
- Use plain and simple language. However, if necessary, use technical terms which may be explained at the appropriate opportunity.
- Whenever in doubt regarding the identity of a previously seen patient, do not hesitate to check the identity *vis-a-vis* the marks of identification recorded in the case notes.
- Check the case records to clarify any doubts rather than hazarding a guess.
- Do not loose temper even when roughly cross-examined.
- Avoid long discussions particularly with regard to theoretical or hypothetical arguments.
- If a passage is quoted from a textbook (or any other recognized source), take the book and check the title, the year of publication, the context of the quoted passage or any other relevant detail before answering.
  Even after reading the passage it is felt that the opinion expressed in the passage does not tally with the expert opinion given in the court, the expert can stand by his own opinion.
- Finally, it must be remembered that medical (or psychiatric) evidence, though admissible, is not conclusive. The final judgment is delivered by the judge or the jury.[33]

Mental Health Care Bill[34]

The proposed Mental Health Care Bill (MHCB), 2013 is available at the Ministry of Health and Family Welfare Website. This is elaborately stated in the chapter 'Mental Health Legislation in India'. The proposed MHCB (2013) includes 16 chapters and has 136 sections. It is a Bill that is to be provided to provide for mental health care and services for persons with mental illness. This aim in protect, promote and fulfill the rights of such persons during delivery of mental health care and services and for matters connected therewith or incidental thereto.

The details of MHCB is described in next chapter.

REFERENCES

1. Lebigrs A. Quelques Aspects de la Responsability Penale endroit Romain Classique. Paris: Presses Universitaires de France, 1967.
2. Ruggiero G. Excusable murder: Insanity and reason in early renaissance Venice. J Soc Hist. 1982;16:109-19.
3. Chaput B. Aspects de la marquinalite au Mouen Age. Paris: L' Aurore, 1983.
4. Walker N. Crime and Insanity in England. I. The Historical Perspective. Edinburgh: Edinburgh University Press, 1968.
5. Zacchias P. Quaestiones Medico-legales. Roma: Lib II, 1625.
6. Kant I. Anthropologie in Progmatischer Ansicht Abqefasst. 2nd edition. Koenigsberg: Nicolovius, 1800.
7. Smith R. Trial by Medicine: Insanity and Responsibility in Victorian Trials. New York: Columbia University Press, 1981.
8. Allderidge P. Why was McNaughten sent to Bethlem. In: West DJ, Walk A (Eds). Daniel McNaughten: His Trial and Aftermath. London: Gaskel, 1977.

9. Rollin HR. McNaughten's madness. In: West DJ, Walk A (Eds). Daniel McNaughten: His Trial and Aftermath. London: Gaskel, 1977.
10. West DJ, Walk A (Eds). Daniel McNaughten: His Trial and Aftermath. London: Gaskel, 1977.
11. Benson AC. The Letters of Queen Victoria, London, 1907.
12. Smith JC, Hogan B. Criminal Law. 4th edition. London: Butterworths, 1978.
13. Leng R. *Mens rea* and the defences to a criminal charge. In: Bluglass R, Bowden P (Eds). Principles and Practice of Forensic Psychiatry. Edinburgh: Churchill Livingstone, 1990.
14. Hamilton J. Manslaughter: assessment for the court. In: Bluglass R, Bowden P (Eds). Principles and Practice of Forensic Psychiatry. Edinburgh: Churchill Livingstone, 1990.
15. Samuels A. Mental illness and criminal liability. Med Sci Law. 1975;15:198-204.
16. Dell S. Murder Into Manslaughter. Maudsley Monograph No. 27. Oxford: Oxford University Press, 1984.
17. Fenwick P. Automatism. In: Bluglass R, Bowden P (Eds). Principles and Practice of Forensic Psychiatry: Edinburgh: Churchill Livingstone, 1990.
18. American Law Institute. Model Penal Code. Philadelphia: American Law Institute, 1960.
19. Report of the Committee on Mentally Abnormal Offenders. Cmnd 6244, HNSO, 1975.
20. Criminal Law Revision Committee. Offences Against the Person. Report No. 14 Cmnd 7844, HMSO, 1980.
21. Law Commission. Codification of the Criminal Law. Report No. 143, HMSO, 1985.
22. Weiner BA. Mental disability and the criminal law. In: Brakel SJ, Parry J, Weiner BA (Eds). The Mentally Disabled and the Law. 3rd edition. Chicago: American Bar Foundation, 1985.
23. American Psychiatric Association Work Group. Statement of the insanity defense. Am J Psychiatry. 1983;140:681.
24. American Psychiatric Association. Seclusion and Restraint: The Psychiatric Uses. Report of the APA Task Force on the Psychiatric Uses of Restraint and Seclusion. Washington DC: APA, 1984.
25. American Medical Association. Report of the Board of Trustees: Insanity defence in criminal trials and limitation of psychiatry testimony. J Am Med Assoc. 1984;251:2967.
26. Vama LP, Jha BK. Characteristics of murder in mental disorder. Am J Psychiatry. 1966;122:1296-98.
27. McGarry AL. Competency To Stand Trial and Mental Illness. Rockville: NIMH, 1973.
28. Taylor M. Report of the Health Survey and Development Committee. Vol. III. Simla: Government of India Press, 1946.
29. Shama SD, Chadda RK. Mental Hospital in India. New Delhi: IHBAS, 1996.
30. Freckleton IR. The Trial of the Expert: A Study of Expert Evidence and Forensic Experts. Melbourne: Oxford University Press, 1987.
31. Dutta AB. The Long March of Mental Health Legislation in Independent India; Dr. L. P. Shah Oration delivered at IPS-WZ Conference at Goa, 2001, published by Goa Psychiatry Society, 2001.
32. Narayan, et al. Process of amendments in MHA-87 and PWD Act-95. Indian Journal of Psychiatry 53(4), Oct-Dec 2011.
33. Trivedi JK. The mental health legislation: An ongoing debate. Indian J Psychiatry. 2002; 44:95-6.
34. The Mental Health Care Bill (2013), Available from; *http://www.mohfw.nic.in/*

FURTHER READING

1. American Psychiatric Association. Issues in Forensic Psychiatry. Washington DC: APA, 1984.
2. Anscombe GEM. Intent. Oxford: Blackwell, 1972.
3. Applebaum PS, Lidz CW, Meisel A. Informed consent: Legal Theory and Clinical practice. New York: Oxford University, Press, 1987.
4. Bluglass R, Bowden P (Eds). Principles and Practice of Forensic Psychiatry. Edinburgh: Churchill Livingstone, 1990.
5. Bowden P. Madness or badness? Br J Hosp Med. 1983;30:388-94.
6. Chiswick D. Use and abuse of psychiatric testimony. Br Med J. 1985;290:975-77.
7. Dunn J, Fahy TA. Police admissions to a psychiatric hospital. Br J Psychiatry. 1990;156:373-78.
8. Faulk M. Basic Forensic Psychiatry. Oxford: Blackwell, 1988.
9. Group for the Advancement of Psychiatry: The Mental Health Professional and Legal System. New York: Brunner/Mazel, 1991.
10. Mednick SA, Moffitt TE, Stack S. The Causes of Crime: New Biological Approaches. Cambridge: Cambridge University Press, 1987.
11. Schouten R, Gutheil TG. Aftermath of the *Rogers* decision: Assessing the costs. Am J Psychiatry. 1990;147:1348-52.
12. Simon R. Clinical Psychiatry and The Law. Washington DC: American Psychiatric Press, 1987.
13. Simon RI (Ed). American Psychiatric Press Review of Clinical Psychiatry and the Law. Washington DC: APPI, 1991.
14. Szasz TS. Psychiatric Justice. 2nd edition. Syracuse: Syracuse University Press, 1988.
15. Wilson C, Pitman P. Encyclopedia of Murder. London: Barker, 1961.

CHAPTER

80

Mental Health Legislation in India: A Critical Appraisal

Indira Sharma, Abhishek Pathak

INTRODUCTION

Mental health legislation is important for protecting the rights and dignity of persons with mental disorders and for developing accessible and effective mental health services. Mental health legislation protects mentally ill patients from harsh treatments, unnecessary institutionalization and inhumane handling as inpatients.

The Indian Lunatic Asylum Act, 1858, and Indian Lunacy Act (ILA), 1912 were the earliest mental health legislations in India. However, they primarily covered custodial aspects and gave little attention to the human rights of mentally ill patients. The ILA, 1912 has no relevance today because medical science has rapidly advanced. Mental illness is now treatable with proper and timely diagnosis. Also, the society's mood has changed and it is being realized that stigma should not be attached to mental illnesses.

After independence and formation of the Indian Psychiatric Society (IPS), ILA, 1912 was considered an inappropriate Act for mentally ill patients.[1,2] As a result the IPS submitted a draft Mental Health Bill in 1950. The Mental Health Act (MHA) received the assent of the President on 22nd May 1987, but it came into effect in all the states and union territories of India in April 1993.[3] It took around 37 years from its first draft to make it as an Act.

MENTAL HEALTH ACT, 1987

Definition of the Act:[4] "An act to consolidate and amend the law relating to the treatment and care of mentally ill persons, to make better provision with respect to their property and affairs and for matters connected there with or incidental thereto."

The MHA, 1987 is divided into 10 chapters consisting of 98 sections.

Chapter I: Deals with preliminaries of the act, definitions and provides for change of offensive terminologies used in ILA, 1912. It applies to all over India, including Jammu and Kashmir. It gives definition of various terms used like mentally ill person, psychiatric hospital (PH), psychiatric nursing homes (PNHs), psychiatrist, etc.

Change of older terminologies to newer ones is good. Mentally ill person is defined, but mental disorder as such is not defined. No difference between acute/chronic or patients with psychosis or anxiety disorders has been given. Mental retardation (MR) has been excluded from the definition of mentally ill person. This is not in keeping with international classifications, International Classification of Disorders and Diagnostic and Statistical Manual of Disorders.[4,5]

As a result, persons with severe and profound mental retardation, who need comprehensive care from mental health experts, may be deprived of the same.

Chapter II: Deals with the procedures for establishment of mental health authorities at central and state levels. Mental health authorities: (1) are in charge of regulation, development, and coordination of Mental Health (MH) Services, (2) supervise PHs, PNHs and other MH Services, (3) advice government regarding matters relating to MH and (4) and discharge other necessary functions.

Even though psychiatrists are in a better position to assess the facilities and services of psychiatric centers, there is low representation of psychiatrists in licensing authorities. This seems to be a major obstacle in the formulation and implementation of mental health policies. No provision of budget for mental services has been mentioned in the Act.

Chapter III: It lays down the guidelines for establishment and maintenance of psychiatric hospitals and nursing homes. Establishment or maintenance of psychiatric hospitals can be only with license. There is a provision for licensing authorities to process applications for license which have to be renewed every five years. Government psychiatric hospitals/nursing homes are exempted from licensing.

General nursing homes and tertiary hospitals have not been included in this Act. The minimum standards for PHs/PNHs appear to be quite unrealistic. The Act adopts different guidelines for government and private hospitals. The licensing process is tedious. It should be made hassle free. The irony is that there is no licensing for faith healers. This means that faith healers can practice without license, but for qualified psychiatrists license is mandatory.

Chapter IV: It deals with the procedures of admission and detention of mentally ill in psychiatric hospitals. A mentally ill person (a major) may make a request for admission as a voluntary patient; in case of a minor his guardian may make such a request. On such request, the medical officer in-charge (MOI), after enquiry within 24 hours, if thinks necessary, he may admit such a person. The medical officer shall discharge such patients on request by him or guardian as the case may be, within 24 hours, unless he finds such discharge against patient's interests. Such cases will be referred to medical board of two medical officers for opinion, which if decides the same, the patient can be further admitted for a period not exceeding 90 days for treatment.

There is provision of admitting mentally ill persons under special circumstances. A mentally ill may be admitted as inpatient on a request by friends or relatives. Such request should be supported by two medical certificates to the effect. In such cases medical officer in-charge may admit the patient if he thinks necessary. Admission shall be for maximum of 90 days. A mentally ill patient admitted by relative or friend can also apply to the magistrate for discharge.

A mentally ill person can also be admitted through reception order. An application for reception order may be made by the MOI of a mental hospital, or by the spouse or by any other relative of the mentally ill patient, for admission to the Magistrate. The Magistrate can pass the Reception Order (RO) or Rejection to the application. An RO is valid up to 30 days only or till discharged.

Request for admission may also be made by a police officer if such mentally ill person is dangerous to himself or others. Such persons will be discharged by magistrate on request by friends/relatives or after they are certified to be sane by the board of experts.

Also, there are guidelines for admission of mentally ill prisoners and those after inquisition. Power and duties of police officers have also been mentioned.

There are no specific criteria in the MHA, 1987 for involuntary admissions and treatment. Criteria for admission should be treatment and welfare, not dangerousness. Decision for involuntary admission and treatment should be based on advice of a qualified psychiatrist. Involvement of magistrate for further detention has made mental health services overly legal, cumbersome and less therapeutic. Section 23 of the act empowers the police officer to take in his custody a wandering patient and detain him for up to 24 hours. Detaining a mentally ill person in a police station violates human rights. There should be provision for taking such persons to a PH or a PNH where after assessment the person could be treated. Much stress is laid on hospital admission and treatment. This increases the cost of health care. No provisions are made for home and community based treatment.

Chapter V: It deals with the inspection, discharge, leaves of absence and removal of mentally ill persons. There is mention of appointment of visitors, monthly inspection by visitors and inspection of mentally ill prisoners. The MOI can order of discharge of a patient on his own, on an application by the person on whose request the admission order was made, on an undertaking of relatives or friends for the care mentally ill person, or on request of the person, if the person is subsequently found on inquisition to be of sound mind.

The MHA, 1987 is silent about the fate of patients for whom no relative turns up to take them back on discharge. Whether the patient would be detained indefinitely in the hospital and who would bear the expenses of such a case is not mentioned. No provisions are made for after discharge care and rehabilitation of patients.

Chapter VI: It deals with the judicial inquisition regarding alleged mentally ill persons possessing property, custody of the person and management of his property.

There is provision for appointment of guardian of mentally ill person and for manager for management of property.

On the MHA, 1987 it is presumed that mental illness is more or less permanent. Only in exceptional cases the person may cease to be free from mental illness (section 75). Excessive powers have been given to the manager. The manager can mortgage, create any charge on, or transfer by sale, gift, exchange or otherwise, any immovable property of the mentally person or lease out any such property for 5 years, without permission from the District Court. As of today most persons with mental illness have a good prognosis. There should be periodic review of the mental state of the person with mental illness, say every 3 months, and when the mentally person is fit to take care of himself and/property, his rights regarding the same may be restored to him.

Chapter VII: It deals with liability to meet the cost mentally ill persons detained in PH or PNH.

Cost of maintenance is to be borne by Government in certain cases when the person is detained in a PH or PNH. There is a provision by which persons legally bound to maintain mentally ill persons are not absolved from such a liability.

In the MH, 1987 there is no provision for meeting of expenses of treatment of patients with no estate or no relative. The state should be made responsible for such patients. Besides the word "detained" is derogatory as it is linked with criminality. Better term would be admitted.

Chapter VIII: It deals with the protection of human rights of mentally ill persons. There is prohibition of any research unless it is of direct benefit to the person for purposes of diagnosis and treatment. No mentally ill person shall be subjected to any indignity or cruelty. In addition, no letters or other communications, sent by or to mentally ill person under treatment, shall be intercepted, detained or destroyed.

In the MH, 1987, there is no mention of restriction on the violation of human rights outside hospitals and medical institutions by quacks and faith healers. The rights and entitlements of mentally ill persons should be specified in detail.

Chapter IX: It deals with the penalties and procedures. There are penalties for establishment of PHs and PNHs in contravention of Chapter III, for improper reception of mentally ill person and for mismanagement of property of person with mental illness and general provision for punishment of other offenses.

In the MHA, 1987 there are no provisions for punishing the relatives and officers requesting for unnecessary detention of a person to such psychiatric hospitals. There is no penalty for those who detain psychiatric patients in *dargahs*, temples other places of faith healing under inhuman conditions they are tortured and maltreated in the garb of treatment. The horrific tragedy of Erwadi is a recent glaring example of the same.

Chapter X: It deals with miscellaneous matters not covered in other chapters of the Act like provision as to bonds, report by MO, pension of mentally person payable by government; legal aid to mentally ill person at state expense in certain cases, and protection of action taken in good faith.

The positive aspects of the MHA, 1987 are:

1. Uniform Act for whole of India.
2. Replacement of offensive terminologies of ILA, 1912 by new soft and soothing terms. This has helped in upholding dignity of mentally ill patients.
3. Establishment of licensing authorities to provide a check on licensing and working of mental health hospitals.
4. Provision for establishment of new hospitals for admission, treatment and care of mentally ill persons.
5. Provision for establishing separate PHs for different categories of patients: those under the age of 16 years, those who are addicted to alcohol and other drugs which lead to behavioral changes in a person, those who have been convicted of any offence; and those belonging to such other class or category of persons as may be prescribed.
6. Provision for outpatient care thus avoiding unnecessary detention.
7. Simple procedures for admission and discharge of mentally ill persons to PHs and PNHs which does not involve magistrate and is useful in cases of emergency for admitting involuntary patients for a period of 90 days.
8. Mentally ill person to be treated without violation of human rights.
9. Patients; records considered to be confidential by MOI may not be accessible to the members of the board.
10. Appointment of guardians for maintaining property and person of a person with mental illness.
11. Provision for bearing the expenses of treatment by government in certain cases.
12. Persons legally bound to maintain mentally ill person not absolved from such liability.

MHA, 1987 is silent about certain other important issues like:

1. Suicide prevention.
2. General hospital psychiatry.
3. Integrating psychiatric care into primary care.
4. Community psychiatric treatment.
5. Consultation liaison psychiatry.
6. Abuse of psychiatry (psychiatric malpractice).
7. Confidentiality and informed consent.
8. Ethical issues related to hard to discharge patients.
9. New scientific development in the field of psychiatry.
10. Incorporating United Nations principles on the protection of human rights of persons with mental illness.

The process of amendment of the MHA, 1987 was initiated by the Government of India in 2010 which would repeal MHA, 1987. The proposed Mental Health Care Bill (MHCB), 2013 is available at the Ministry of Health and Family Welfare Website.[6] The IPS has submitted its position statement on MHCB several times to the Government.

The proposed MHCB, 2013 includes 16 chapters and has 136 sections. It is a Bill "to provide for mental health care and services for persons with mental illness and to protect, promote and fulfill the rights of such persons during delivery of mental health care and services and for matters connected therewith or incidental thereto."

The salient features of the proposed MHCB (2013)[6] are as follows with some critical comments:

1. *Definition of mental illness (Chapter I):* Mental illness means "a substantial disorder of thinking, mood, perception, orientation or memory, that grossly impairs judgement, behavior and capacity to recognize reality or ability to meet the ordinary demands of life, mental conditions associated with the abuse of alcohol and drugs, but does not include mental retardation which is a condition of arrested or incomplete development of mind of a person, specially characterized by subnormality of intelligence".

   The definition of mental illness in the MHCB is over-inclusive, and can be misinterpreted by the legal system based on personal convenience. It should be in accordance with current internationally accepted definitions. Mental retardation has been excluded even though it finds a place in International classificatory systems.
2. Determination of mental illness and capacity to make health care and treatment decisions (Chapter II).
3. *Advance directive (AD) (Chapter III):* Every person, who is not a minor, shall have a right to write an AD specifying the way the person wishes to be cared for and treated for a mental illness, and the individual(s), in order of precedence, he wants to appoint as nominated representative (NR). AD should be made in writing on a plane paper with the person's signature or thumb impression on it. AD may be made irrespective of the person's past mental illness or treatment for the same. A typical AD may be that the individual will like to be treated with only psychotherapy, not medication, nor electroconvulsive therapy (ECT) or he would like to be treated as an outpatient and not be admitted to a hospital.

Some riders apply. For example, ADs would have to be signed by a general practitioner to ensure decision making capacity at the time of writing, ADs would not be applicable during 72 hours of "emergency treatment" and all ADs of "no treatment at all" would have to be submitted to the Mental Health Review Board (MHRB) for validation. Where the mental health professional/a caregiver/a relative desires not to follow the AD an application can be made to the MHRB for its modification or cancellation.

4. *Nominated representative (NR) (Chapter IV):* Any person with mental illness who has attained the age of 18 years has the right to appoint a NR whose duty would be to support the person with mental illness in making treatment decisions. The NR would have a right to information on diagnosis and treatment, right to be involved in discharge planning, right to apply to the MH facility for admission, right to apply to the district panel of the MHRB on behalf of the person with mental illness for discharge, right to apply to the district panel of the MHRC against violation of the rights of the person with mental illness in MH facilities and right to give consent for research under certain circumstances. The NR shall have access to family or home based rehabilitation services provided to the person with mental illness.
5. *Rights of persons with mental illness (Chapter V):* 11 rights of persons with mental illness have been covered including right to: access to mental health care; community living; protection from cruel, inhuman and degrading treatment; equality and nondiscrimination; information; confidentiality; restriction on release of information in respect of mental illness, access medical records, personal contact and communication, legal aid and make complaints about deficiencies in provision of services.

   Every person shall have a right to access mental healthcare and treatment from mental health services run or funded by the appropriate government. If a particular district has no public mental health services, the individual has a right to access private services and get refunded. The governments are mandated by the bill to provide essential psychotropic medications free of cost. The insurance companies will have to consider mental illness at par with physical illnesses, and will not be allowed to include mental illness as one of the exclusion criteria.
6. *Duties of the government (Chapter VI):* The government has the duties including organization of programs for promotion mental health, creating awareness about mental health and illness, prevention of mental illness, reducing stigma associated with mental illness and to take measures for human resource development and training in mental health care
7. *Central mental health authority (Chapter VII)*
8. *State mental health authority (Chapter VIII)*
9. *Financial, accounts and audit (Chapter IX):* Deals with grants, annual and accounts of the MH authorities.
10. *Mental health establishments (MHE) (Chapter X):* MHEs have to be registered with the authority. The procedure for registration, inspection and inquiry of MHEs has been outlined. Every MHE must fulfill the minimum requirements in terms of facilities and services, qualifications for the personnel, and provision for maintenance of records and reporting. MHEs may be classified into different categories. The authority may cancel the registration of a MHE if so directed by the MHRC or a MHRB to do so. The authority can take *suo motu* cognizance of a complaint made by any person regarding with respect to nonadherence of minimum standards and order an inspection or inquiry of any MHE. An appeal to the High Court in the State can be made against an order of Authority by the MHE. Every MHE shall display within the establishment at a conspicuous place (including on its website) the contact details including address and telephone numbers of the concerned board. Also, every MHE shall provide the person with the necessary forms to apply to the concerned Board and also give free access to make telephone calls to the Board to apply for a review of the admission.
11. *Mental health review commission (MHRC) (Chapter XI):* The MHRC will be constituted by the Central Government. The latter will have its headquarters at Mumbai. The commission shall have a president (Chief Justice of a High Court or a Judge of the High Court with 5 years experience) and 4 members appointed by the President of India. Out of the 4 members, one each shall be from amongst: (1) psychiatrists (with >15 years experience), (2) persons with mental illness or representatives of persons with mental illness, (3) representatives of families and caregivers or of nongovernmental organizations (NGOs) working in mental health and (4) persons with a background of public health administration. The MHRC shall with prior concurrence of State Governments, constitute Mental Health Review Boards (MHRBs) in the districts of that state. Each Board shall consist of: (1) a Chairperson (District Judge or a person qualified to be a District Judge), (2) a representative of district administration, (3) two mental health professionals (one to be a psychiatrist) and (4) two members who are persons with mental illness, caregivers or person representing organizations of persons with mental illness or caregivers or NGOs working in the field of mental health. The commission shall function through the MHRBs.

    Any person with mental illness or his NR or a registered NGO being aggrieved with the decision of a MHE or whose rights under the Act have been violated can make an application to the MHRB for redressal or appropriate relief. An appeal against the decision of the MHRB or MHRC shall lie to the High Court of the State in which the Board is situated.
12. *Admission, treatment and discharge (Chapter XII):* Independent admissions refer to the admissions of

persons with mental illness to a MHE where the person has the capacity to make mental health care and treatment decisions and requires minimum support. If a person so admitted requests for discharge, he shall be discharged within 24 hours or else assessed and admitted as a supported patient for a maximum period of 30 days. Minors can be admitted in a mental health facility 'only' in accordance with the procedure laid down in Section 96. A minor must be accommodated separately from adults and a NR or an attendant nominated by the NR must stay with the minor in the MHE during the entire period of hospitalisation. All admissions of minors continuing till 30 days would have to be reported to the MHRB. The Board will regulate all admissions of minors beyond 30 days.

There is provision for supported admissions of persons with mental illness who do not have the capacity for independent admission, and pose a danger to themselves or others, or risk of harm to self. Treatment is to be provided after taking into account an AD, if any; or informed consent of the patient with the support of the NR. The doctor shall review the capacity of the patient to give consent every 7 days. The admission shall be limited to 30 days. All supported admissions have to be reported to the MHRB within 3 (woman or minor) to 7 days. A supported admission of a person with mental illness can continue beyond 30 days to a maximum of 180 day with approval by the Board in accordance with procedure laid down in section 99.

Emergency treatment (includes transportation to the nearest MHE for assessment), other than electroconvulsive therapy (ECT), can be provided by any registered medical practitioner, for a maximum period of 72 hours.

Prohibited treatments for persons with mental illness include ECT without the use of muscle relaxants and anesthesia, sterilization as a treatment of for mental illness and chaining in any manner. ECT for minors and psychosurgery may only be performed on prior permission of the Board. Guidelines for physical restraint and seclusion are mentioned in section 106.

Guidelines for conducting research on persons with mental illness are outlined. In case of research involving any psychological, physical, chemical or medicinal interventions to be conducted on persons who are unable to give free and informed consent, but do not resist participation in such research, permission to conduct such research must be obtained from concerned State Mental Health Authority. The State Mental Health Authority may allow the research to be conducted based on informed consent being obtained from the NRs of persons with mental illness, if the State Mental Health Authority is satisfied. There is no restriction on research based study of a person who is unable to give informed consent, so long as anonymity of the person is secured.

13. *Responsibilities of other agencies (Chapter XIII):* There is provision for treatment (including inpatient treatment) and care of persons with mental illness, who are wandering or homeless; living at home, but being neglected or ill-treated, prisoners, and those in custodial institutions. The duties of police officers, magistrate and others and procedure in this regard are outlined.
14. Restriction to discharge functions by professionals not covered by profession (Chapter XIV)
15. *Offences and penalties (Chapter XV)*
16. *Miscellaneous provisions (Chapter XVI):* Any person who attempts to commit suicide shall be shall be presumed, unless proved otherwise, to be suffering from mental illness, at the time of attempting suicide and shall not be liable to punishment under section 309. The government has a duty to provide care, treatment and rehabilitation to the person to reduce the risk of recurrence.

    ECT without the use of muscle relaxants and anesthesia, ECT to minors and sterilization of persons with mental illness intended for treatment of mental illness are prohibited in the proposed draft. Psychosurgery may only be performed on approval of the State Mental Health Authority. The bill also stipulates that ECT to minors will be given only after permission from the MHRC on a case-to-case basis.

Some important observations on the MHCB are mentioned below:

General Comments

1. The MHCB is modern in terminology.
2. Mental conditions associated with the abuse of alcohol and drugs have been clearly included in the definition of mental illness.
3. The commitment of the government to provide mental health facilities to every citizen of the country, work on promotion of mental health and preventive programs is laudable.
4. The MHCB endeavors to address the rights of persons with mental illness. AD, NR, MHRC and MHRBs are new concepts that have been introduced into the bill to meet this objective. The Bill recommends treating persons with mental illness in the least restrictive environment and also talks about reducing stigma associated with mental illness.
5. The importance given to the rights of persons with mental illness seems to be at the cost of the human right, the "right to access mental health care". AD and NR are modern concepts, which are most unsuited for India. AD seems to be a hypothetical concept as it is virtually impossible to predict well in advance the circumstances at the time of a major psychiatric illness. In most of the countries where AD has been used have had mixed results. These provisions are likely to deny many patients

appropriate and timely treatment. Since these patients lack insight during most part of illness, they can be easily cheated by so called NRs and parents would be helpless mute spectators. For most persons with mental illness in India there would be deemed NR(s), usually the legal guardian of the patient. In India, where mental health services are scarce and community mental health services almost nonexistent, families bear most of burden of mental illness and its treatment. Introducing a brand new concept which positions the family and the patient as adversaries is fraught with consequences which may do more harm to patients' interests than good.

6. Decentralization of clinical decisions relating to admission, treatment and discharge of persons with mental illness to MHRCs and MHRBs, would lead to loss of time and denial of mental health services, especially emergency treatments, to the most serious patients. This would seriously compromise their health and safety.
7. Decentralization of clinical decisions as mentioned above will compromise the autonomy of MHEs and make them inefficient. Besides, mandatory information that has to be provided by MHEs to MHRBs about admissions under sections 96, 98 (including admissions of women and minors), would not only increase the burden of work, but also add to the stigma of mental illness, which is against the spirit of the MHCB. Some checks on MHEs are welcome, but too many would result in stigma and compromise the quality of care.
8. In the MHCB restrictions are imposed on the clinical expert (psychiatrist) to make clinical decisions related to admission, treatment and discharge of persons with mental illness. The final authorities are MHRBs and MHRCs having membership that is largely non-professional. Only one expert (psychiatrist) is included. 1 paraprofessional (psychiatric social worker or psychiatric nurse or clinical psychologist) is also included, but the latter has very limited knowledge of mental illness.
9. All decisions relating to admission, treatment and discharge of persons with mental illness should be made by an expert or a body of experts in the hospital itself. Where the number of experts in a hospital is less, one or more may be co-opted from another hospital.
10. The MHCB seeks to segregate, to a large extent, mental illness and mental health care, from physical illness and physical health care, whereas the spirit of MHCB to integrate mental health services with general health care. Many patients with physical illness have comorbid mental illness and vice versa. Patients with mental illness may be admitted to medical wards (as psychiatry is a subspeciality of medicine). It would have been more appropriate to have bill applicable to medical patients.
11. Provision of emergency treatment in the first 72 hours without any hassles is a progressive step. The emergency treatment can include transportation of a patient to a mental health facility. This fills a lacuna overlooked by the architects of the previous law, which led to transporting a disturbed patient, except on a court order, illegal.
12. Major advances in mental health care have not been given due consideration. For example:
    - Present day psychiatry is concerned not only with treating unmanageable or chronically mentally ill patients, but also caters to a large number of patients ranging from mood, anxiety and somatoform disorders, to adjustment and substance use disorders, sex related issues, sleep disturbances, and learning and behavioral problems among children and adolescents.
    - There has been a major shift from "custodial care" of the treatment of chronic mental illness in mental hospitals to treatment in general hospital psychiatric units (GHPUs) resulting in destigmatizing and deinstitutionalizing of mental health care. GHPUs have also succeeded in providing comprehensive care as patient gets treatment for comorbid medical and surgical problems as well. This has led to establishment of open wards in multispecialty hospitals and has brought psychiatry into the main stream of medical care. Besides, GHPUs are supposed to maintain minimum standard of care as per laid down guidelines by different regulatory bodies. They are open to various visitors for the purpose of inspection on the behalf of MCI, RCI, Nursing Council of India and the affiliating university. Thus GHPUs should be out of the purview of MHCB.
    - Over the last two decades, there is enormous growth of mental health care facilities in the private sector. There is also recent phenomenon of setting up of Half Way Homes, Long Stay Homes, Deaddiction Centers, Rehabilitation Centers, Centers for the care of the elderly and children with behavioral problems in the private sector. Their functioning was not envisaged in the MHA, 1987. There is a need to encourage these treatment care facilities as well as regulate their functioning so that human rights abuses do not occur.
    - A major role is played by the family and relatives in the care and protection of person with mental illness. In addition to care at home, family members stay with the patients during admission in psychiatry wards in GHPUs. It is well established that treatment in the community with family's support results in better prognosis, recovery and rehabilitation, as well as reduces stigma that surrounds mental illnesses. There is a pressing need to strengthen the family institution.
    - The MHCB should distinguish between various inpatient settings. In open wards patients seeking voluntary treatment are admitted. Invariably the

patient is accompanied by relative(s) or a legal guardian who stay round the clock with the patients and are consulted and consent is obtained for all treatment related issues. There is no chance of any human rights violation. Thus there is no need of regulation of GHPUs under a separate act. On the other hand, closed wards provide involuntary admission to patients, without the requirement of family staying with the patient in the ward. Since the family members are not required to stay with the patient and he is looked after by the hospital staff, there are chances of neglect and human rights violation. Long stay facilities must be regulated by the legislation as in these cases human rights violations most commonly occur. There should be different regulations for each type of treatment setting.

- With advancements in the field of mental health including newer understanding of the causes of mental disorders and discovery of newer medications which are safe and effective, it is now possible to treat large numbers of patients with mental illness in the community utilizing the large resource of family members as caregivers.
- Many persons with severe mental illness, who are noncompliant to medication and cannot be admitted, are treated successfully as outpatients by giving antipsychotic medication in food by their family members. It is suggested that there should guidelines for involuntary (supported) for outpatient treatment as well.

13. Definition of a mental health professional for the purposes of this Act should be limited to only a qualified psychiatrist, who alone should be authorized to issue certificates with respect to mental illness. Paraprofessionals (clinical psychologists, psychiatry social workers and psychiatry nurses) or person from the judiciary or police do not have the expertise to decide on whether a person has a mental illness or not.

Specific Comments

1. In clinical practice, an acute psychotic episode often takes up to six weeks to improve, so the period in Section 98 should be at least 40 days.
2. There should a redressal system within the hospital at the place where the problems arise. A 4-step redressal system, from the **Psychiatric Team** (Consultant, junior residents, psychiatric social worker and others) to **Unit** to **Department** to **Hospital Administration**, is suggested. MHRC or MHRBs are not needed. The person with mental illness or family can always approach the Courts. If not satisfied with the decision of the redressal system.
3. A large number of patients suffering from major mental illness are not willing for treatment as they lack insight and MHCB proposes that they cannot/or it difficult to treat them against their will. This will increase violence in the community due to untreated mental disorders.
4. Mandatory documentation of all admissions, case histories, treatments and discharge should be the protocol for all PHs and PNHs, which could be checked periodically by the inspecting officer. This would offset the need for sending regular information to MHRC or MHRBs.
5. Prohibition of ECT for patients below 18 years is based on sentiments rather than on scientific evidence. ECT has been revived after intensive research by the most developed countries of the world and in these countries it used in adults as well as in minors. There is no evidence whatsoever that ECT is unsafe or has more side effects below age 18 years. It is also important to mention that in young people with catatonic schizophrenia, ECT is the treatment of choice and often life saving. These cases present as emergencies and there is no time to run around for obtaining permission. In surgical oncology mutilating surgeries are carried even when the results are not very predictable. There could be a statutory obligation to obtain confirmation from an independent psychiatrist before resorting to ECT in a minor.
6. Similarly, the prohibition of UMECT seems to be based on issues more related to popular perception rather than on scientific evidence. A specially prepared 36 paged position statement on UMECT was presented, discussed and approved at a special symposium held on January 20, 2012, at the 64th Annual National Conference of the IPS. UMECT is as efficacious as MECT (MECT). Besides, in some cases UECT is safer than MECT. Thus the ban on MECT is thus not justified. Consideration of the practical side is also necessary. In rural and remote locations anesthetists are not available even for routine surgery. Besides, many district hospitals do not have an anaesthetist. It is suggested that MECT is preferable, but UMECT can be given instead if the situation demands. Each case should be considered on its own merit.
7. Considering the shortage of anesthetists, Under Duties of Appropriate Government (Chapter VI) Government should have a duty to include, in MD (Psychiatry) course, training to give anaesthesia for modified ECT.
8. Presumption of mental illness, unless proved otherwise, in case of attempt to commit suicide by a person, who shall not be liable to punishment under 309 IPC, is most welcome research.
9. For approval of research protocols teaching institutes will face enormous burden as permission of State Mental Health Authority would have to be obtained when patients unable to give informed consent and research in future

would become a cumbersome task. Postgraduate Medical courses are under different regulatory bodies of the university (e.g. Department Research Committee, Ethical and Scientific Committee, Postgraduate Medical Board, Academic Council, etc.) and Indian Council of Medical Research. It is suggested that in the presence of internal regulatory bodies such riders should not be needed.

Recently the Standing Parliamentary Committee made minor amendments in the MHCB, 2013. The same are as follows:

1. *Section 2:* Clinical psychologists not registered with Rehabilitation Council of India, but with 2 years supervised clinical training from University Grants Commission recognized University *replaced.*
2. *Section 4:* The section 'capacity to make mental health treatment decisions'—the word "unless it is proved" *added* for assuming the lack of the capacity.
3. Making it obligatory to make an application to the Board before over-riding of an AD.
4. Making provisions for 'definition' of half way home, sheltered accommodation and supported accommodation.
5. State to ensure the coverage of mental illness by insurance policies.
6. Making changes in Section 23(2)—regarding right to confidentiality—any exception to be carefully framed.
7. Scope of misuse of medical records to be relooked and suitably addressed.
8. Section 27(2)—regarding free legal aid—to ensure that no person with mental illness is deprived of the benefit of free legal aid from legal services authority due to ignorance.
9. State MHA power to prescribe minimum standards in MHEs—*increased.*
10. Suggested inclusion of Registered Medical Practitioner in the Boards of MHRC.
11. Section 99 regarding following of AD—provision added of 'informed consent'.
12. Section 100 leave of person with mental illness from a MHE—clause 2 to 9 *deleted*—these are the provisions of being taken back by a police officer.
13. Expressed 'reservations' on ECT to minors.
14. *Deletion* of word 'Seclusion'—Now only the word Physical Restraint remains in relevant section.
15. Section 108—regarding permission of research—the words 'promoting health' *replaced* by promoting mental health'.
16. Section 113—State run custodial home—*amendment* recommended ensuring their monitoring under this Act.
17. Section—114—Clause (1)—provisions regarding divorce - *deleted.*
18. Changes suggested in case of North Eastern States
19. Clause—"Presumption of Mental Illness" in case of suicide *replaced* by Presumption of severe stress.
20. Suggestions regarding the *transition provisions* from the MHA 1987.
21. Suggestions in respect of ensuring help to State Governments, who are facing financial crunch by the Central Government to meet obligation of the Act.

CONCLUSION AND FUTURE DIRECTION

The MHCB, 2013 is major change from the MHA, 1987. The provision of the Act, except for sections 33, 45 and 73, shall come into force within a period of 9 months from the date on which it receives the assent of the President. Professionals, paraprofessionals, persons with mental illness, caregivers and other stake hold holders have mixed feelings towards it. Only time will tell to what extent the golden objectives of the Act are fulfilled in letter and spirit.

REFERENCES

1. Dutta AB. The Long March of Mental Health Legislation in Independent India; Dr. L. P. Shah Oration delivered at IPS-WZ Conference at Goa, 2001, published by Goa Psychiatry Society, 2001.
2. Narayan, et al. Process of amendments in MHA-87 and PWD Act-95. Indian Journal of Psychiatry 53(4), Oct-Dec 2011.
3. Trivedi JK. The mental health legislation: An ongoing debate. Indian J Psychiatry. 2002;44:95-6.
4. World Health Organisation. The ICD 10 Classification of Mental and Behavioural Disorders-Clinical Descriptions and Behavioural Guidelines. Geneva; WHO, 1993.
5. American Psychiatric Association. Diagnostic and Statistical Manual of Mental Disorders, 4th edition, text revision. Washington, DC: American Psychiatric Association; 2000.
6. The Mental Health Care Bill (2013) Available from *http://www.mohfw.nic.in/*

FURTHER READING

1. Chandrashekar H. Mental Health Care Act, Bulletin. 2011;1: 13-15.
2. Kala A. Time to face new realities; mental health care bill-2013. Indian J Psychiatry. 2013;55:216-9.
3. Knight B, et al. Cox, Medical Jurisprudence and Toxicology. 6th ed., Allahabad: The Law Book Company Pvt. Ltd; 1990.pp.507-8, 810.
4. Pillay VV. Textbook of Forensic Medicine and Toxicology. 14th edition, Hyderabad. Paras Medical Publishers; 2004. pp.311-2.
5. Prateek Rastogi. Mental Health Act 1987-An Analysis. JIAFM; 2005;27(3).
6. Sinha V. Mental Health Care Act: A Critical Appraisal. Indian J of Social Psychiatry. 2011;27(3-4):72-74.
7. World Health Organization Scaling up care for mental, neurological and substance use disorders (MhGAP) WHO, Geneva; 2008.

CHAPTER 81 Ethics in Psychiatry

AK Agarwal, SC Gupta

The work *ethics* has been derived from the Greek term *ethikos*, which stands for rules of conduct that govern natural disposition in human beings. Encyclopedia Britannica defines ethics as a systematic study of the ultimate problems of human conduct. These ultimate problems are concerned with the concepts of right and wrong, morality and similar other issues. *Medical ethics* is as old as the art of healing itself and the earliest code of medical ethics was formed by Hippocrates in 5th century BC. The need for medical ethics is becoming more and more acute with the rapid advancement of medical knowledge. Today organ transplant, euthanasia, and artificial prolongation of life are issues on which clear ethical guidelines are required.

Psychiatric ethics is rather of a recent origin. It was in the year 1970 that the American Psychiatric Association, for the first time, appointed a committee to develop a code of ethics. Subsequently, in 1977, the World Psychiatric Association developed a code of ethics which is known as the "Declaration of Hawaii". Indian Psychiatric Society adopted its ethical code in 1985 (Appendix 1).

There is of course no doubt that ethics is much more relevant to psychiatry, as the line of demarcation between normal and abnormal is often hazy and the appropriateness of psychiatric diagnosis and treatment can be easily questioned. Moreover, as the treatment aims at modifying behavior, it may sometimes be perceived as an implied threat because the psychiatric treatment occasionally may be utilized for controlling behavior for certain vested interests. Besides, as the psychiatric treatment involves close relationship between the patient and the therapist, it could lead to intense transference which may be maliciously utilized. Another important related issue is that as many psychiatric patients are not likely to be fully in contact with reality, they might consent to or become party to decisions which are not ultimately to their benefit. A manic patient may give a blank cheque to the therapist or he may ask the therapist to communicate certain things to others which are not in his best interest.

The main objectives of professional ethics are as under:

- To provide guidelines of conduct among the professionals themselves. It includes areas like referral from one therapist to another, giving comments on the opinion of another professional, and charging consultation fee from co-professionals and their families.
- To formulate guidelines in dealing with the patients, their relatives and third parties. The areas to which these guidelines relate are mainly the following:
  - Psychiatric diagnosis.
  - Informed consent.
  - Voluntary and involuntary treatment and hospitalization.
  - Confidentiality.
  - Respect for the patient and his human rights.
  - Third party responsibility.
  - Psychiatric research.

A brief description about each of these areas would be useful in helping the professionals to decide on the appropriateness of their behavior.

PSYCHIATRIC DIAGNOSIS

It is of interest to note that there are certain schools of thought that doubt the very existence of the discipline of Psychiatry. A Supreme Court judge in the United States recently opined that psychiatry was akin to charlatanism and that psychiatric diagnosis was no more accurate than palm reading.[1] Thomas Szasz[2] argues that there is nothing like a psychiatric illness and the so-called illnesses are actually different ways of leading life. Humanists have also raised objections, pointing out that dissenters in the various political systems are labeled as mentally sick and are sometimes incarcerated in the mental hospitals. All these instances raise the basic question regarding the boundaries of mental illness.

According to Kendell,[3] "it is worth reflecting whether the many attempts we have recently witnessed to discredit the concept of mental illness might not be a reaction to the equally absurd claim we have made that all unhappiness and all undesirable behavior are manifestations of mental illness". Recently, WHO has published the 10th revision of International Classification of Diseases, which makes the diagnosis precise and more acceptable. American Psychiatric Association has also similarly published the 5th revision of its diagnostic system, the Diagnostic and Statistical Manual (DSM-IV). Both these diagnostic systems are compatible with each other. To a large extent, this puts to end the controversy of psychiatric diagnosis. However, one should not equate a psychiatric diagnosis with legal insanity or it should not be used as a defense for reduced responsibility, because large number of psychiatric diagnoses do not fulfill the legal conditions required for insanity. Psychiatric diagnosis should only be used for clinical purposes, as it provides a reasonable guideline regarding etiology, management and prognosis.

INFORMED CONSENT

Till recently, seeking consultation itself was considered to include consent for treatment and medical men generally decided treatment which they felt to be best in the interest of patient. This method of medical practice is also known as *medical paternalism*.[4] However, during the last few decades, a greater emphasis has been laid upon the patient's human rights. The human rights of the patient should be more reasonably protected and as such the patient should be informed about the nature of illness and treatments available, so that he/she could partake in the decision-making process.[5] Consumer protection movement further compels the medical profession to provide a detailed information about these matters and obtain informed consent before undertaking any treatment for their own safeguard.

Informed consent has the following constituents:

- Information to be provided by the treating physician.
- Competence of the patient to comprehend the information provided.
- Freedom to choose.

Information to be Provided for Informed Consent

The information to be provided should include the following:

- Nature of the disorder.
- Prognosis of the disorder without treatment and with each of the alternative treatment methods.
- Treatment options available.
- Reasons for specific treatment being offered and drawbacks of the same.
- A specific statement that the consent could be withdrawn whenever the patient wishes so.

Information provided under the above headings may appear ideal but it has several practical problems. For instance, informing a patient of schizophrenia the exact prognosis of the illness at the initial stage may give rise to severe depression and may sometimes lead to adverse consequences. Information of treatment options, like drugs and ECTs, may not be fully understood by the patient and he is also likely to make decisions on the basis of certain prevailing biases and prejudices against each of these treatment methods.

Competence of Patient

Regardless of the fact that every adult individual is considered to be responsible for his behavior, competence to give informed consent is a controversial issue. The term competence in this context refers to the patient's ability to understand the nature and severity of his presenting problems, and need of suggested therapeutic help and its limitations. Whether a psychiatrically ill person is likely to possess such as ability has been debated for a long time by several researchers.

Some authors have gone to the extent to state that there is no difference between the level of comprehension of the information provided to psychiatric patients and non-psychiatric patients. However, most psychiatric patients are unable to accept that they are sick and hence, not able to give consent for their treatment. Even if they give consent it may be for wrong reasons, e.g. a manic patient may challenge the doctor to give all the drugs that he has. Such consent has no meaning. Before giving consent, patient should fully comprehend the information provided and should be able to decide on the course of treatment in an understanding manner. Before deciding whether the patient is really competent or not, a clinician should make an effort to assess the following:

- Whether the patient has comprehended the information provided? This can be done by asking a few questions on the information made available to him.
- Whether the patient is able to objectively understand that he is ill and requires treatment?
- Can he understand the nature of each treatment option and their consequences?

When all the above questions are reasonably answered to the satisfaction of the therapist, only then the consent given by the patient can be considered to be valid. Nevertheless, any patient can be treated in an emergency even without the availability of consent. For instance, the treatment of a stuporous or acutely excited patient should not be deferred on account of nonavailability of the consent.

While minors (below the age of 18 years) are not considered to be legally competent to give consent, the issue of consent in cases of minors is being seriously debated in the

West, since the children of more than 12 years may be able to understand the nature of their illness/problems and may be able to give consent.

Mental Health Act (1987) allows specified relatives to give consent for admission in mental hospitals. Using the same logic, one could also assume that specified relatives could give consent for treatment of patients on an outdoor basis. However, one should take such consent in writing and as soon as the patient is competent, his consent should be obtained.

Freedom to Choose

Informed consent *a priori* implies that the person has freedom to choose from certain available options. In a country like ours with meagre psychiatric facilities and poor economic conditions, real options are however not truly available. The patients either do not have easy access to psychiatric facilities, or if somehow they reach a facility, they have to accept whatsoever is available. It is the duty of every mental health professional to educate and inform the affected person about the treatment modalities available to him and his right to choose them.

Another issue involved with informed consent is whether the consent should be written or verbal. The written consent has a standard format. However, information about individual disease variables and treatment methods cannot be provided in it and, therefore, it is better to have a standard written information sheet, with an addition of a clause that the patient is at liberty to ask any further clarification or information.

INVOLUNTARY VERSUS VOLUNTARY TREATMENT

The humanists react with abhorrence if an individual's freedom is restricted without a justified legal process. As a large number of psychiatric patients do not consider themselves to be ill, they have to be hospitalized or treated against their will. Most of these patients are admitted as 'voluntary' or 'informal' patients, by obtaining their signatures on consent form without obtaining their real consent. Opposing the prevailing practice, Szasz[6] calls voluntary admissions an unacknowledged example of medical fraud. It is undeniable that most of the so-called voluntary patients are coerced to some extent for accepting hospitalization. This coercion may be from employer, family or medical personnel. Quite often, the voluntary patients demand discharge after a few days of hospitalization and they need to be persuaded to continue treatment. Thus, what Szasz says has an element of truth but it has to be evaluated on the principle of beneficence. Temporary hospitalization to regain sanity is a much preferable alternative to staying chronically sick but free. In this context, Peele, Chodoff and Taub[7] state that "it is a perversion and travesty to deprive these needy and suffering people of treatment in order to preserve a liberty which is in actuality so destructive as to constitute another form of imprisonment." To obviate some of these difficulties, there are certain alternatives, each of which requires a serious consideration.

Each psychiatric patient can be taken to a court of law where the evidence of his being mentally sick can be produced, and if the judge accepts that he or she is ill then he may order such a person to be admitted to a mental hospital. By a rough estimate, around 1% of the population suffers from serious psychiatric illnesses and needs hospitalization. This will mean that around 8 million persons in India need to be screened by the overburdened judiciary. Thus, recourse to nonjudicial methods for involuntary hospitalization would have to be accepted. Mental Health Act (1987) provides for involuntary hospitalization with the consent of relatives, which to a large extent obviates the need of judicial order for every patient. There could be occasional cases, where relatives seek hospitalization of the individual on account of malicious intentions. A mental health professional should be alert to such an eventuality. Even if the judiciary is able to do the needful, there is an acute shortage of hospital beds and, therefore, it would be rather impossible to provide admissions. It stands to reason then that legal recourse for involuntary treatment of mental patients is out of question and is impractical.

According to the prevailing practice of treating psychiatric patients in our country, a large number of such patients are treated as outpatients and the only available consent is that of the concerned relatives.

The Hawaii declaration of the World Psychiatric Association provides the following guidelines for such a situation: "No procedure must be performed or treatment given against or independent of a patient's own will, unless the patient lacks capacity to express his or her own wishes, or owing to psychiatric illness cannot see what is in his best interest or, for the same reason, is a severe threat to others. In these cases, compulsory treatment may or should be given, provided that it is done in the patient's best interest and over a reasonable period of time, a retroactive informed consent can be presumed and, whenever possible, consent has been obtained from someone close to the patient. As soon as the above conditions for compulsory treatment or detention no longer apply the patient must be released, unless he or she voluntary consents to further treatment. Whenever there is compulsory treatment, there must be an independent and neutral body of appeal for regular inquiry into these cases. Every patient must be informed of its existence and be permitted to appeal to it, personally or through a representative without interference by hospital staff or by anyone else". The guiding principle is that the least restrictive alternative should be used. The patient should be kept in the hospital against his will for as short a period as possible and that too according to the prevailing legal requirements.

CONFIDENTIALITY

Medical ethics, from the time of Hippocrates, have emphasized on the confidentiality in doctor-patient interaction. Anything learned during the professional relationship should not be revealed to others without the consent of the patient. Records of the patient should therefore be strictly safeguarded, so that no unauthorized person can have access to them. Unauthorized person would include any person other than the treating team and the family member on whose consent patient has been admitted. However, after having achieved recovery, if the patient advises the therapeutic team that even the admitting family member/relative should not have access to the patient's record, his wishes should be respected. The employers, insurance companies and other interested parties should be provided information after obtaining consent from the patient.

The major problems in this area may be of the following nature:

For example, when the information provided by the patient can be dangerous to others or himself. This leads to the dilemma of protective privilege versus public peril.[8] For instance, if a patient informs his therapist that he is planning to kill Mr X, should the psychiatrist inform Mr X or the police, so that protective measures could be taken? Similarly, a bus or train driver suffering from psychosis poses threat to the public safety. Again, should the psychiatrist inform or remain silent?

There cannot be a simple rule of thumb in these situations. The psychiatrist has to consider the nature and the severity of the risk involved, and then decide on an appropriate measure which may cause least breach of confidentiality. The situation may be thoroughly discussed with the close family members to arrive at an effective solution. If the situation is still intangible, one could always discuss it with a colleague to decide on an appropriate action.

Sometimes, courts summon the psychiatrist to testify. In such a situation, one should obtain the consent from the patient, and if that is not forthcoming, then one has to depose after lodging protest with the judge.

The confidentiality clause will require more careful monitoring as the new Mental Health Act has come into operation. The records of the patient may be inspected by the "inspectors" at any time. Some of these "inspectors" may not be professionally trained. Therefore, one must only record all the observations which seem to be relevant to diagnosis and treatment. Hypothetical questions and unscientific speculations may not be put on record because these may be misconstrued by the lay "inspectors".

RESPECT FOR THE PATIENT AND HIS HUMAN RIGHTS

Each patient has to be respected as an individual and the aim of the treatment should be towards an early restoration of the functioning of the individual. In achieving this objective, nothing should be done which could be perceived as violation of human rights of the individual. For instance, unnecessary restraints, keeping a person in solitary cell, and afflicting physical punishment would be considered as highly unethical practices. ECT is given sometimes as a punishment for unacceptable behavior. Such practices should be condemned.

Each patient should have facilities for basic human rights like privacy, uncensored opportunities to communicate with others, and basic requirement of food, hygiene, etc. Every treatment method should be in conformity with the basic human rights; for instance, aversive treatment methods which may inflict pain or torture have to be avoided.

THIRD PARTY RESPONSIBILITY

In the modern era, medical treatment has no longer remained within the confines of doctor-patient relationship. Many external agencies influence both the content as well as the form of treatment. In the Western countries, where insurance companies often provide funds for the treatment, they are likely to influence the policy of hospitalization and its duration. Quite often, these insurance companies provide guidelines about treatment procedures which tend to influence the therapeutic options of the treating team. In a country like ours, where most treatment facilities are government-funded, the availability of drugs and number of trained personnel could be the main factors affecting the decision-making of treatment. Lastly, but not the least, pharmaceutical companies are also nowadays indirectly influencing the treatment decisions. For instance, the extensive use of II and III generation antidepressants, which are much costlier than the tricyclic antidepressants, is a result of the third party influence. This is largely a byproduct of a spate of research and media articles glamorizing these drugs.

PSYCHIATRIC RESEARCH

Research is essential for the advancement of knowledge. However, when research is involved with human beings, certain safeguards are a must. Helsinki declaration provides detailed guidelines regarding the use of human subjects in research. Following are the main considerations:

- Any research which is not likely to directly benefit the patient should not be undertaken.

- No human subject should undergo research without adequate safeguards. The researcher has to be a protector of the interest of the patient.
- Any patient, who is not able to give informed consent, should not normally be included for purposes or research, unless such a permission has been sought from the concerned family member or relative.
- While publishing research material, one should take care that the research publication does not violate the confidentiality.

Much higher and rigorous ethical standards are required in India, because there are few legislations for the professional service and the public gives *carte blanche* (unlimited authority) to the therapist. A mechanism of inner controls has to be evolved to maintain a high standard of practice and to develop public confidence. Ethics also involves regulating the charging of fees and acceptance of gifts. India is a vast country and there cannot be any uniform rate of professional charges, but the fee should be appropriate to the local conditions and should not be increased without appropriate reason. Of course, gifts of any kind during the therapy are not permitted. Any kind of sexual advance towards the patient is strictly prohibited.

Ethics also encompasses the relationship among psychiatrists themselves. Quite often, patients hope from one psychiatrist to another and psychiatrists do accept them for further treatment. Ethically, one should entertain a patient only after a due referral from the treating psychiatrist. It is hoped that this referral practice would gradually become a norm. Another important issue may be that the psychiatrists often condone or do not react to the malpractices of their colleagues. This is often done under the misguided notion that by doing so they would be doing a disservice to the profession. On the contrary, such black sheeps in reality bring the profession to disrepute and their exposure in public would cleanse the profession. It is an ethical duty of each professional to do so.

Unfortunately, ethical issues are not given any attention in the undergraduate and postgraduate medical education. Ethical issues should be discussed formally, so that young doctors are sensitized to the kind of problems they are likely to face. There is, however, no denying the fact that the ethical practices are largely learned by the process of imitation and, as such, it is mandatory that the teachers of these young medicos should themselves put up exemplary models.

APPENDIX 1

A CODE OF ETHICS FOR PSYCHIATRISTS

A committee comprising of Prof JS Neki, Prof DN Nandi, Prof AK Agarwal, Dr VN Vahia and Dr JK Trivedi was requested to prepare the recommendations for a code of ethics for psychiatrists in India. The committee prepared the following draft recommendations, which have been approved by the Indian Psychiatric Society at its Annual Conference, 1989, held at Cuttack, Odisha (India).

Preamble

Ethics has been an essential part of the healing art. Ethical guidelines have been prepared by international and national organizations for different groups of practitioners. Each country has its own social, economical and psychological compulsions which might make it difficult to translate and practice ethical codes of other countries. Hence, this body proposes the following ethical guidelines for the members of psychiatric profession in this country.

These principles are intended to aid the psychiatrists individually and collectively, in maintaining a high level of ethical conduct. These are not laws but standards by which a psychiatrist may determine the propriety of his conduct or his relationship with patients, with members of allied professions and with the public.

Principles

Responsibility

As a practitioner, the psychiatrist must know that he bears a heavy social responsibility because he not only deals with disturbed human behavior but also to contend with intimacies of life.

As a scientist, he would serve the society through observation, investigation and experimentation, and well-planned and ethically carried out research.

Competence

The maintenance of high standards of professional competence is (the) responsibility of all psychiatrists in the interest of both the public and the profession. Psychiatrists are responsible for their own continuing education and should realize that theirs must be a lifetime learning.

As members of the profession, they will not violate ethical standards and, when such violation comes to their notice, will take steps to correct it.

Benevolence

The interest of the patient and his health will stand paramount with them in their professional practices. Personal interest would find but a secondary place. Financial arrangements will never contravene professional standards. Psychiatrists will always safeguard the interests of the patient and the profession.

Moral Standards

They will at all times be responsive to the moral codes and expectations of the community they serve, and will not let their behavior in any way malign their profession.

Patient Welfare

They will not treat a case that does not clearly fall within their competence. The ones they accept, they will treat with the best of their ability and with the highest regards for the patient's integrity and welfare, as also that of the communities in which they work.

They will terminate the clinical or consulting relationship with the patient when it is reasonably clear to them that the patient is no longer benefiting from it.

In case of referral, they will continue to feel responsible for the patient's welfare until the responsibility has been formally transferred.

Confidentiality

They will safeguard information about a patient that they have obtained in the course of their clinical work, teaching or research in order to safeguard the patient's interest and protect him from social stigma, discrimination and harm. They will treat this as a primary obligation and not reveal unto others any such information unless certain ethical conditions are met, or when there is clear and imminent danger to an individual or society and then only to the appropriate authorities or concerned co-professionals. Confidentiality of the clinical records will be meticulously guarded and identity of the patients will not be revealed even in scientific communication.

No data about a patient shall be ordinarily revealed to any agency without the consent of the patient or his family.

Recommendations

- Every person, who has attained the age of majority and who does not appear to have lost the ability of reason, shall be assumed to be capable of giving consent.
  A patient should be taken up for medical evaluation and treatment with his consent. In case a patient, because of his mental illness, is unable to express valid consent, the psychiatrist may undertake to treat him with the consent of a person close to him, who appears to be clearly interested in the welfare of the patient. The only exception to treating without consent would be an emergency situation involving an immediate threat to the life or health of patient or others. For purposes of research, the consent shall be obtained on the lines indicated above after satisfying the following:
  - The consent is entirely voluntary.
  - The patient can withdraw the consent at any stage.
  - Withdrawal of the consent shall not affect the interests of the patient.
- The decision to hospitalize a patient will essentially rest on the consideration of his welfare and will also take into consideration legal and administrative constraints as well as its social appropriateness.
- Psychiatric treatment shall be initiated only on clinical considerations and shall be in accordance with scientific knowledge and professional ethics. The patient's welfare should be the primary factor determining the choice of the treatment modality. Should the specific modality not fall within the competence of a psychiatrist, he should refer the patient to a competent colleague. The termination of therapy also shall be determined on clinical consideration. Treatment should not be permitted to continue unjustifiably or for material consideration.
  All treatment should be humane and never punitive. No psychiatrist shall refuse to treat in an emergency.
- Gift and gratifications from patients under treatment should not be accepted.
- Any kind of sexual advance towards any patient is unethical.
- In case of doubt or in situations where unconventional treatment procedures are contemplated, a second opinion must be obtained.
- It is unethical to force a contract upon a patient during treatment.
- Even when a patient has been referred by legal or administrative authority or by the employer, welfare of the patient will remain of paramount consideration. The patient should be informed of the purpose for which he is to be examined.
- Basic human rights of the mentally retarded should not be subjected to unethical abridgement. Due ethical discretion should be exercised when advising such procedures as sterilization.
- In the interest of patient and the society, drug abusers who refuse to give consent may be treated with the consent of their relatives. Efforts have to be made to motivate them for accepting treatment voluntarily.

These ethical codes have to be implemented with sincerity. It is proposed that ethical committees may be formed at central and zonal levels. These committees should consider complaints either from public or from fellow professionals and then, carefully investigate them.[9]

REFERENCES

1. Applebaum PS. The Supreme Court looks at psychiatry. Am J Psychiatry. 1984;141:827-35.
2. Szasz TS. The myth of mental illness. Am Psychol. 1960;15:113-8.
3. Kendell RE. The concept of disease and its implication for psychiatry. Br J Psychiatry. 1975;125:305-15.

4. American Psychiatric Association. Psychiatric ethics primer. Washington DC. American Psychiatric Publishing Inc. 2001.
5. Montgomery J. Health Care Law. Oxford University Press. Oxford; 2002.
6. Szasz TS. Law, Liberty and Psychiatry: An Enquiry into the Social Usage of Mental Health Practices. New York: MacMillan, 1963.
7. Peele R, Chodoff P, Taub N. Involuntary hospitalization and treatability: Observations from the District of Columbia Experience. Catholic University Law Review. 1974;23:744-53.
8. Wilkinson G, Russell FG, Marks I, et al. Case reports and confidentiality: Opinion is sought medical and legal. Br J Psychiatry. 1995;166:555-8.
9. Hope T, Savelescu J, Hendrick J. Medical ethics and law: the core curriculum. Churchil Livingstone, London; 2003.

FURTHER READING

1. American Psychiatric Association. Principles of Medical Ethics with Annotations Applicable to Psychiatry. Washington DC: American Psychiatric Press, 1986.
2. Appelbaum PS, Roth LH. Clinical issues in the assessment of competency. Am J Psychiatry. 1981;138:1462-7.
3. Carrick P. Medical Ethics in Antiquity. Boston: D. Reidel, 1985.
4. Committee on Confidentiality. Guidelines on confidentiality. Am J Psychiatry. 1987;144:1522-6.
5. Dyer AR. Ethics and Psychiatry: Toward Professional Definition. Washington DC: American Psychiatric Press, 1988.
6. Fromm E. Man for Himself: An Inquiry into the Psychology of Ethics. New York: Hart, Rinehart and Winston, 1974.
7. Group for the Advancement of Psychiatry: A Casebook in Psychiatric Ethics. GAP Report No. 129. Brunner/Mazel, 1990.
8. Lakin M. Ethical Issues in the Psychotherapies. New York: Oxford, 1988.
9. Levine M. Psychiatry and Ethics. New York: George Brazillar, 1972.
10. Redlich F, Mollica RF. Overview: Ethical issues in contemporary psychiatry. Am J Psychiatry. 1976;133:125-36.
11. Stanley BH, Stanley M. Psychiatric patients in research: Protecting their autonomy. Compr Psychiatry. 1981;22:420-7.
12. Stone AA. Ethics in biological psychiatry. In: Arieti S, Berger PA, Brodie KB (Eds). American Handbook of Psychiatry, 2nd edn, Vol. 8. Biological Psychiatry. New York: Basic Books, 1986.

CHAPTER

82

History of Psychiatry

Niraj Ahuja

Writing a history of psychiatry is a daunting task, and according to many students, so is reading it. To make this exercise simpler and more interesting, the history of psychiatry has been recounted here in a temporally sequenced and numbered manner, placing emphasis on individual names (of persons, places, books, societies and even laws) rather than on the historical trends or the *zeitgeist*. A telegraphic style has been adopted for ease in locating the various names or contributions. The history enumerated here is necessarily sketchy in detail and cannot hope to satisfy everybody. Contemporary names have been deliberately omitted as they have been discussed under the heading of current research in the various chapters of this book. Another significant omission is the current systems of classification, which have been dealt with in the various Chapters.

Ayurveda (Compiled Around 4000 BC)

- Indian system of scientific medicine and positive health.
- Psychiatry was labeled as *Bhut-Vidya*, i.e. demonology. However, it never meant that demons alone can cause mental illness. As Atreya, a sage physician, said in *Charak Samhita*, "Neither gods,... nor demons, ...(can) torment the man who is not tormented of himself."
- Heredity was believed to have an important etiological role in causation of mental disorders, as well as in determining the physique and temperament of a person.
- Five types of constitutions (*Prakriti*) were described depending on the predominance of the 3 bodily humors (*Kapha*, *Pitta* and *Vayu*). These included 3 main constitutional types (a forerunner of Kretschmer's 3 body types) and 2 types formed by a mixture of these 3 main constitutions.
- Three main types of personality were defined, namely:
  1. *Satvik*: Characterized by high intellectual and moral level. 7 subtypes were described (namely *Brahma*, *Rishi*, *Indra*, *Yama*, *Varuna*, *Kubera*, and *Gandharva*) based on the quality of gods after whom they were named.
  2. *Rajasik*: Characterized by high emotionality, passionate nature, and impulsiveness. There are 5 subtypes (namely *Asura*, *Rakshaka*, *Pisacha*, *Sarpa* and *Preta*).
  3. *Tamasik*: Equivalent to mental subnormality. 4 subtypes were described comparing the persons to birds (*Sakuna*), animals (*Pasva*), fishes (*Matsya*) and vegetables (*Vanas-patya*) depending on the severity of mental sub-normality.
- Mental disorders were believed to be caused by, either
  - *Endogenous causes:* The disorders were believed to be provoked by humors, e.g. by *Vayu* (Vatonmad, probably schizophrenia), by *Pitta* (Pittonmad, probably mania), by *Kaph* (Kaphonmad, probably depression), and by all three humors (Trishonmad, probably severe depression).
  - *Exogenous causes:* These disorders were believed to be caused by sudden fear, stress, or by influence of gods or demons (8 types were described).
- Modernistic descriptions of mental disorders (e.g. toxic disorders, paranoid states, epilepsy, alcoholism, and hysteria) were provided. For example, in *Pittonmad* (mania), the typical patient is described as a neat and clean person with a smiling and cheerful face, reciting Sanskrit *shalokas* (verses), reminding one of *daivas* (gods). Amorous tendencies of manic patients are described (as *yaksha*), as are their dancing tendencies (as *gandharvas*).
- Psychiatric patients were usually treated with sympathy and kindness. Mental disorders caused by an excess of a certain emotion were treated by an antagonistic emotion. The other methods of treatment included talismans, amulets, charms, rituals, prayers, and medications like *dhatura* and roots of 'serpentina' plant mixed with oil.
- Intractable diseases were sometimes treated by brutal treatment with scalding (by hot water, iron or oil), whipping, tying with soft bandages and confinement. Occasionally, patients were subjected to 'shock treatment' by exposure to snakes (whose poisonous fangs were removed), trained lions or elephants.

- *Sushruta* believed that passions and strong emotions could not only cause mental disorders but also physical disorders that may require surgical intervention. This was a psychosomatic viewpoint much ahead of its time.

Sage Agastya (7th Century BC)

- Indian sage; a practitioner of *Siddha* system of medicine.
- Described 18 types of mental disorders, with treatment consisting of giving *bhasam* (a kind of ash with medicinal properties).
- Wrote a treatise of mental disorders called as '*Agastiyar Kirigai Nool*'.

Alcmaeon (6th Century BC)

- A Greek physician-priest; a student of Pythagoras.
- Related sensation to brain processes, and concluded that defects in reasoning must result from brain pathology and not from abstract spiritual phenomena (as was generally believed at that time).

Jivak (5th Century BC)

- Indian physician.
- Practiced neurosurgery and performed several operations on brain.

Bhagavad Gita (4th Century BC)

- Probably the first recorded evidence of psychotherapy and counseling.
- This is also an example of crisis intervention psychotherapy (on the battlefield).
- In the process of psychotherapy, the importance of therapist-client or doctor-patient relationship (the *Guru-Chela relationship*) was emphasized.
- Although Lord Krishna egged *Arjuna* on to action (Directive psychotherapy), he did not force his ideas on Arjuna. The final decision was left to *Arjuna*, ('Do what you want to do'), which he finally took and the rest is history.

Hippocrates (460–377 BC)

- Greek physician.
- Probably he did not develop all the ideas he is credited for. Other unknown authors (along with Hippocrates) who are collectively known as '*Hippocratic authors*' possibly wrote the '*Corpus Hippocraticum*'.
- Temperaments were believed to be caused by a mixture of 4 bodily humors (blood, phlegm, yellow bile and black bile) and were called as sanguine, phlegmatic, choleric and melancholic.
- Diseases were believed to be caused by an imbalance in these bodily humors (e.g. melancholia caused by an excess of black bile).
- Attempted to classify mental disorders into categories recognizable as melancholia, postpartum psychosis, phobias, toxic delirium, senile dementia, and hysteria.
- Hysteria was believed to be caused by wandering uterus, occurring only in women. Recommended treatments included marriage and sexual intercourse.
- Refuted that epilepsy was a sacred disease and believed natural causes to be responsible for the malady.
- Stressed the importance of doctor-patient relationship.

Socrates (469–399 BC)

- Greek philosopher.
- Developed a unique method of teaching (the *Socratic Method*) in which, through questions, he drew out the truths and the understandings in the mind of a rational pupil. He talked about the 'faint, positive steps towards psychological growth, once the negative, handicapping misunderstandings had been cleared away' as a result of his sequence of questions. He called this method of counseling as '*Maieutics*'.

Plato (427–347 BC)

- Greek philosopher and rationalist.
- Believed that the mental world consists of self-existent ideas, which are wholly independent of one's life experiences. These ideas are the unchanging, basic realities. Matter depends upon ideas to lift it out of inertia and meaninglessness.
- Divided the soul or psyche into 3 parts (appetite, impulses, and reason; located respectively in abdomen, chest and head; corresponding to the three classes of citizens in his book, '*the Republic*', namely workers, soldiers, and philosophers). These have been compared to Freud's later tripartite subdivision of psyche (id, ego and superego).
- Earlier, he described 2 kinds of madness:
  1. The appetitive soul loses the domination of the rational soul.
  2. The gods inspire the madness (divine madness).
- Later, in '*Phaedrus*', he described 4 kinds of madness:
  1. Prophetic madness.
  2. Telestic or Ritual madness.
  3. Poetic madness.
  4. Erotic madness.
- In the '*Laws*', definite norms for handling a 'mental' patient are given, e.g. confinement at home, exile, and even punishment by death (in extreme cases).

Aristotle (384–322 BC)

- Greek physician; Plato's most influential student.
- Insisted that theories should be derived from observable data; thus believed in empiricism as opposed to Plato's rationalism.
- Described 'heart' as the seat of all mental functions and therefore, the major agent of causation of mental disorders.
- Described the various emotions or 'affections' (e.g. desire, joy, courage, anger, fear, hatred, and pity) in '*De Anima*' (a collection of 8 books, containing his views and theories on psychology).
- Discussed '*catharsis*' as a natural outlet for disturbing passions. Advocated that passions must be purged consistently to avoid violence.

Herophilus (335–280 BC)

- Greek physician.
- Known as the 'Father of Anatomy.'
- Refuted the theory of body humors and believed anatomic defects within the brain to be responsible for mental disorders.

King Ashoka (274–235 BC)

- Indian King; a great warrior who later embraced Buddhism.
- His regime saw establishment of many hospitals. Mentally ill were humanely cared for, along with the physically ill, in these hospitals.

Asclepiades (c150 BC)

- Roman (originally from Asia Minor) philosopher-physician.
- Rejected the doctrine of bodily humors.
- Differentiated illusions from delusions.
- Subdivided the diseases into acute and chronic.
- Advocated psychological modes of treatment and stressed the importance of environmental influences.
- His teachings led to the cult of Asclepias (or *Asclepiades*), the god of healing. The Asclepian priests used dream interpretation to suggest healing measures.

Cicero (106–43 BC)

- Roman physician.
- Provided the 1st detailed description of passions, the strongest of which was '*libido*' (violent passion).
- 1st to use the term '*libido*' in a psychological sense.

Aurelius Cornelius Celsus (25 BC–50 AD)

- Nonmedical, Roman encyclopedist.
- Described 6 types of insanity in his classic medical textbook, '*De Re Medica*';
  1. Phrenitis
  2. Melancholia
  3. Delirium
  4. Lethargus (stupor)
  5. Epilepsy
  6. 'Schizophrenia-like illness.'
- Advocated '*shocking harshly*' as a method of treatment for the mentally ill.
- This '*shock treatment*' provided a rationale for the brutal treatment of the insane for centuries to come.

Aretaeus (50–130 AD)

- Physician in Cappadocia, in Eastern Asia Minor (a part of the Roman Empire).
- Believed mental disorders to be exaggerated normal processes.
- 1st to describe mania and depression as two phases of the same disorder, occurring in the same person.
- Also described paranoid syndromes.
- Studied premorbid personalities of the mentally ill and conducted detailed follow-up studies.
- Proposed an 'eclectic' approach in treatment.

Soranus (93–138)

- Roman physician.
- Provided many accurate descriptions of mental disorders (especially delusions of grandiosity, states of stupor).
- Erroneously localized hysteria (to uterus), '*phrenitis*' (a feverish disease of 'that part of mind' localized in diaphragm or '*phren*') and hypochondriasis (to hypochondrium).
- Demonstrated that mentally ill had defective reasoning and, therefore, showed the uselessness of Celsus's harsh '*shock treatment*.'

Galen (130–200)

- Physician in Asia Minor (Now Turkey) of the Roman Empire.
- Instrumental in the 'rebirth' and propagation of the humoral theory.
- Defined hysteria as a complex, incurable disease with an unknown physical cause. He located the seat of the disorder in cerebellum, calling it the site of 'carnal love.'
- His views had widespread acceptance and hindered the development of knowledge regarding mental disorders for many centuries.

St. Augustine (354–430)

- Aurelius Augustinus, later known as St. Augustine, was born in Tagaste (Numidia, North Africa).
- Wrote the 1st book, '*Confessions*', on psychological introspection based on self-analysis, though tinged with religious overtones.
- 1st to describe vividly, and in detail, his subjective emotional experiences without any reservations. Believed to be the forerunner of existentialism, phenomenology and psychoanalysis.
- His views had tremendous influence on the Western intellectual world for at least the next 10 centuries.

Baghdad Mental Asylum (c705)

- 1st asylum for the mentally ill (exclusively), at Baghdad.
- Provided humane treatment for the insane.

Rhazes or Al Razi (865–925)

- Persian physician in the city of Baghdad.
- Known as the 'Persian Galen'.
- Believed mental disorders to have 'organic' causes.
- Proponent of psychological modes of treatment.
- Was the Physician-in-Chief of the Baghdad hospital?
- Wrote more than 200 volumes on subjects ranging from medicine and religion, to philosophy and astronomy.

Avicenna or Abu Ali Ibn Sina (980–1037)

- Persian physician.
- Recognized that emotional upsets can cause certain physical and mental disorders.
- Used psychological methods of treatment.

Constantius Africanus (1020–1087)

- A resident of Carthage (North Africa).
- Provided a detailed description of melancholia in his book, "*De Melancholia*', especially describing delusional thinking in melancholia for the 1st time.
- Like Hippocrates, believed melancholia to be caused by an excess of black bile.
- Opined that prognosis was better in acute, reactive conditions.
- Was instrumental in spreading Galenic views on depression.

Moses Maimonides (1135–1204)

- Arab scholar at Cordoba.
- Provided a detailed clinical description of depression.
- Believed in and advocated a mental hygiene program for a good mental health (a preventive approach in psychiatry).

Najabuddin Unhammad (c1222)

- Indian physician.
- Described 7 types of mental disorders:
    1. *Sauda-a-Tabee* (schizophrenia), which can become chronic, known as *Janoon* (chronic schizophrenia)
    2. *Muree Sauda* (depression)
    3. *Malikholia-a-Maraki* (delirium)
    4. *Haziyan* (paranoid state)
    5. *Ishk* (delusion of love)
    6. *Nisyan* (organic mental disorder)
    7. *Janoon* (as described above).
- Methods of treatment included bleeding and purging (at an early stage), nutritious food, massage, change of climate, avoidance of fear and irritation, soft music, pleasant surroundings, rest, fresh air, sympathy and kindness, medications, and encouragement to choose an occupation of one's own choice.

Bartholomaeus Anglicus (13th Century)

- French Monk.
- One of the 1st attempts to localize brain function (and mental disorders), e.g. imagination (and madness) to the forebrain; reason (and melancholy) to the area around the body of ventricles; and memory (and forgetfulness) to the posterior part of brain.

Valencia Mental Asylum (c1409)

- 1st European hospital devoted entirely to the mentally ill at Valencia, Spain.
- Founded by Father Gilabert Jofré (1350–1417).
- Advocated relatively humane treatment of the mentally ill.
- A separate unit for the mentally ill children was added in 1545.
- Though it was the 1st European mental asylum, Arabs built earlier asylums in Baghdad (c705), Cairo (c800), and Damascus and Aleppo (c1270).

Maulana Fazulur-lah Hakim (c1450)

- Indian physician (Hakim).
- In-charge of the 1st Indian mental asylum opened by the ruler, Mahmood Khilji (1436–1469) at Dhar (near Mandu, Madhya Pradesh), India.

Malleus Maleficarum (1487)

- A book, title of which means '*Witches' Hammer*'.
- Authored by two inquisitional Dominicans, Heinrich Kraemer and Johann Sprenger, based in Germany.
- Was encouraged by the 1484 '*Summis Desidenantes Affectibus*', in which Pope Innocent VIII exhorted the

clergy to use all means for detecting and eliminating witchcraft.

- The '*Malleus*' prescribed death by torture for the witches', as the mentally ill women were known then.
- With such a sanction from the Church, witch-hunters persecuted thousands of mentally ill, till the last recorded case in 1782.

Philippus Aureolus Paracelsus (1493–1542)

- Austrian physician, born as Theophrastus Bombastus von Hohenheim in Switzerland; later latinized his name to Paracelsus (meaning greater than Celsus).
- Provided a new classification of diseases in his book, '*On Diseases Which Deprive Man of Reason*':
  - *Vesania*: Disorders caused by poisons.
  - *Lunacy*: A periodic condition influenced by the phases of moon.
  - *Insanity*: Diseases caused by heredity.
- Believed mental disorders to be 'natural' diseases and not caused by demons. He, however, believed in bodily 'magnetism' and that lunar phenomena determined the course of an illness.
- Advocated treatment with chemicals; there was complete absence of 'psychotherapy' in his treatment.

Juan Louis Vives (1492–1540)

- Spanish philosopher.
- Wrote the 1st 'modern' Textbook of Psychology.
- Was a forerunner of Freud in emphasizing the importance of psychological associations in forming emotions?
- Believed that painful, long-forgotten memories can be recalled through *reflective association.*
- Popular for his humanitarian stance towards the mental patients.

Johann Weyer (1515–1588)

- Dutch physician.
- 1st physician whose major interest was mental disorders and can truly be called a psychiatrist.
- Regarded by some as the Father of Modern Psychiatry.
- His book, '*De Praestigiis Daemonum*'(1563), vigorously attacked the 'Malleus', refuting that the demons were the cause of mental disorders.
- Accurately described the general behavior of the mentally ill.
- Practiced psychotherapy and emphasized the importance of a good therapist-patient relationship.

Francis Bacon (1521–1626)

- Introduced the inductive method (reasoning from a particular data to a general conclusion) into science.

Bethlehem Hospital (1547)

- Founded as a priory of St Mary of Bethlehem, London, in 1247.
- Henry VIII gave it a charter as a 'hospital for the cure of lunatics' in 1547.
- Due to the disorderly condition of the hospital, its name was later corrupted to *Bedlam*, which came to mean 'madhouse' and disorderly confusion, for centuries. On several occasions, tickets were sold to the public to visit the hospital for entertainment by poking fun at the inmates.

Timothy Bright (1551–1615)

- English physician.
- Wrote the 1st treatise on mental illness by an English physician.
- Classified melancholia into 2 types:
  1. One caused by humoral imbalance, which can be treated by diet and physical means.
  2. One caused by psychological factors (by '*mind's apprehension*'), which can be treated by psychological treatment.

Felix Plater (1536–1614)

- Swiss physician.
- Classified mental disorders on the basis of observable symptoms, as:
  - *Consernatio mentis* (disturbances of consciousness).
  - *Mentis alienato* (disorders of violence, sadness, delirium, or confusion).
  - *Mentis defatigatio* (mental exhaustion).
  - *Imbecillitas mentis* (mental deficiency and dementia).
- Emphasized the importance of clinical observation over speculation in the understanding of mental disorders.
- Believed brain damage to be the chief cause of the mental disorders.
- 1st physician to separate medicine from philosophy and make it a natural science.

Reginald Scot (1538–1599)

- English physician.
- Vehement opponent of demonology.
- His book, '*Discovery of Witchcraft*', was ordered burned by King James I.

Gockel (1547–1628)

- German philosopher.
- Coined the word *psychology* in 1590.
- Emphasized the importance of mind-body relation-ship.

Robert Burton (1577–1640)

- Oxford Dean of Divinity.
- Provided a comprehensive description of melancholia in his '*The Anatomy of Melancholy*' (1621), published at first under the pseudonym *Democritus Junior*. This still remains a classic account of depressive states.

Rene Descartes (1596–1650)

- A deductive rationalist.
- Introduced the concept of *reflex arc* to explain all animal, and much human, behavior. "A sense organ is stimulated; there is a tug on the 'strings' leading to brain; animal spirits are released into hollow tubes running to the muscles; and the organism behaves. In the case of man, however, a 'dam' may be raised through the faculty of will".
- Believed that man had a '*thinking substance*', the *soul*, which did not interact with the body, thus creating a misleading mind-body dichotomy which still haunts the study of man.

Paolo Zacchia (1584–1659)

- Italian physician and lawyer.
- Probably the 1st forensic psychiatrist.
- Suggested that a physician, rather than a priest or lawyer, should evaluate a patient's responsibility for abnormal behavior.

Thomas Sydenham (1624–1689)

- English physician.
- Provided a comprehensive account of the symptomatology of hysteria, recognizing (for the 1st time) that it can occur in males too in the form of 'hypochondriacal complaints'.
- Believed hysteria to be caused by disturbed animal spirits.
- Noted that apparent organic impairment may be a symptom of hysteria.
- 1st to draw attention to the symptoms of neuroses (hysteria) while others focused exclusively on psychotic phenomena.

Baruch Spinoza (1632–1677)

- Portuguese/Dutch philosopher.
- Has been called as perhaps the greatest of pre-Freudian psychologists.
- Challenged Descartes' mind-body dualism and replaced it with a concept of *psychophysiological parallelism*, supplying the epistemological foundation of psychosomatic medicine.

Thomas Willis (1622–1675)

- English physician.
- Classified mental disorders into two types:
  1. Caused by gross brain disease (madness accompanied by delusions and hallucinations, due to vice or fault of the brain).
  2. Caused by 'disturbed animal spirits' (e.g. melancholia due to 'passions of the heart').
- Described clinical features of the known major mental disorders (1672).
- 1st to describe the circle of Willis in brain and also probably the 1st to use the term reflex action (in addition to Rene Descartes).

George Ernst Stahl (1660–1734)

- German physician.
- 1st to make a distinction between '*functional*' and '*organic*' illnesses.
- Propounded his theory of animism. According to this theory, the *soul* (*anima*) maintains body functions in health and disease.
- Mental disorders were believed to be caused by either inhibitions of '*anima*' or bodily illnesses.

George Cheyne (1671–1743)

- English physician.
- Described depression as '*the English Malady*' and said that 'there is nothing shameful about neurotic behavior'.

Francois Biossier de Sauvages (1706–1767)

- French botanist and physician.
- Arranged mental disorders' overt symptoms in a manner similar to natural scientists who systematize plants and animals. Thus, there were 2400 'different diseases' grouped into classes, orders and genera.
- This nosological work became very popular in his time.

Bombay Asylum (1745)

- 1st lunatic asylum to be built in 'modern' India, at Bombay.
- Built at the cost of Rs. 125/-; no trace of it exists today.

Pennsylvania Hospital (1751)

- 1st hospital in USA to accept the mentally ill.
- Founded at Philadelphia.

Simon Andre Tissot (1728–1797)

- Swiss physician.
- 1st medical description of masturbation, as *Onanism*.
- Emphasized the pathological effects of excessive masturbation.

William Cullen (1710–1790)

- Scottish physician.
- 1st to use the term '*neurosis*' (and the term '*neurotic*'), for diseases without fever or localized pathology.
- Authored a comprehensive text on nosology.
- Believed mental disorders to be, due to a breakdown in the nervous system; thus emphasizing the 'endogenous' nature of mental disorders.

Robert Whytt (1714–1766)

- 1st Scottish neurologist.
- Classified the neuroses into 3 types:
  1. Hysteria.
  2. Hypochondriasis.
  3. Nervous exhaustion (neurasthenia).

William Battie (1703–1776)

- English physician; Medical Superintendent of St Luke's Hospital, London.
- 1st physician to make mental disorders his full time occupation.
- Probably 1st to initiate the teaching of clinical psychiatry in England.
- 1st used '*madness*' in the title of a book, which was the 1st extensive treatise on mental disorders published in England.
- Made 'treatment of madness' a respected specialty.
- Distinguished mental disorders that arise from 'internal' causes.

John Aiken (1747–1822)

- English physician.
- Wrote the 1st book on hospitals, in which '*lunatic hospitals*' were discussed.

Williamsburg Asylum (1773)

1st asylum in USA exclusively for the care of the mentally ill, founded at Williamsburg, also known as the Eastern Asylum.

Franz Anton Mesmer (1734–1815)

- Austrian physician; later shifted to Paris.
- Borrowing from Paracelsus' notion of planetary magnetism, he believed that illness resulted from an imbalance of universal magnetic fluids. Developed the concept of *animal magnetism* (1779), which later came to be known as hypnosis.
- Used this animal magnetism in the treatment of mental disorders, either by manipulating magnetic devices or by drawing upon the magnetic forces emanating from one person to another.

Abbe de Faria (1756–1819)

- Resident of Goa, India.
- Probably learnt '*hypnosis*' from temple priests in India.
- Believed suggestion to be responsible for the phenomenon and denied the existence of any magnetic fluid.
- Arrived in Paris 4 years after the departure of Mesmer.
- There is a statue of Abbé de Faria, depicting hypnotizing a woman, in Goa.

Johann Gottfried Langermann (1768–1832)

- Superintendent of an asylum near Bayreuth, Bavaria.
- Wrote the 1st doctoral dissertation in psychiatry, 'on the method of diagnosing and treating chronic mental diseases'.
- Believed that organic 'malfunction' can occur from psychological disturbances, a psychosomatic concept.
- Was instrumental in the establishment of humanitarian hospitals at Seidburg and Leubus, in Prussia.

Calcutta Asylum (1787)

- 1st asylum in India for insane Europeans.
- Established on April 3, 1787 by Surgeon Dr George M Kenderline.
- A new asylum made in its place by Surgeon William Dick, later.
- Later in 1817, Surgeon Breadmore established the 1st private psychiatric hospital (for European patients only) in India, at the outskirts of Calcutta. This psychiatric hospital was famous for its cleanliness, good ventilation and benevolent patient care.

Vincenzo Chiarugi (1759–1820)

- Italian physician.
- Director of the Bonifacio hospital (asylum), built by the Grand Duke Peter Leopald in 1788. The Grand Duke had

earlier (1774) passed the '*Law of the Insane*' establishing the specific rules, including a mental examination, that were to be followed in cases of commitment.

- One of the 1st (5 years before Pinel) to institute humane reforms in the treatment of the mentally ill in asylums (1788).
- Classified mental illnesses into 3 types:
  1. Melancholia.
  2. Mania.
  3. Amentia.

Philippe Pinel (1745–1826)

- French physician; a student of Sauvages.
- Taking advantage of the French revolutionary emphasis on individual freedom, he dramatically removed the chains of the mentally ill at the Bicetre asylum (1793) and later at the Salpetriere asylum (c1800).
- Insisted on humane and '*moral treatment*' of the mentally ill.
- Was instrumental in making La Salpetriere a premier institution for more than a century.
- Classified mental disorders into 4 main types:
  1. Melancholia.
  2. Mania.
  3. Dementia.
  4. Idiocy.

Madras Asylum (1793)

- Private lunatic asylum opened at Kilpauk, Madras, India (sanctioned on November 15, 1793 and opened, with the bed strength of 20, on October 1, 1794).
- 1st Superintendent and owner was Surgeon Valentine Conolly, Secretary to the Medical Board, Madras.
- Replaced by Surgeon Morris Fitzgerald in 1799 (till 1802) and later by Surgeon John Goldie.
- In 1807, Surgeon James Dalton took over the asylum and expanded the bed strength to 54. There were separate buildings for European and Indian patients.
- Although in 1815, Dr John Underwood took over as the Superintendent of the 'lunatic hospital', it continued to be known as '*Dalton's madhouse*'.

Monghyr Asylum (1795)

1st lunatic asylum for insane Indian sepoys (soldiers), at Monghyr, Bihar (India). It was closed on November 1, 1821.

Johann Christian Reil (1759–1813)

- German physician.
- 1st to use the word *'Psychiatry'* (1803).
- Founded the 1st psychiatric journal, '*Magazin Fuir Die Psychische Heilkunde*' (1805).
- Performed anatomical studies of brain (1807–08).
- Founder of rational psychotherapy.
- Proposed a wide range of therapeutic measures for the mentally ill, which included music therapy, occupational therapy and drama therapy.

William Tuke (1732–1822)

- English Quaker (a religious moralist group), tea merchant and member of '*The Society of Friends*'.
- Founded the famous '*York Retreat*' (1792) for the '*moral treatment*' of mentally ill, just 4 years after King George III suffered from a depressive psychosis.
- His son (Henry Tuke) and his great grandson (Samuel Tuke) carried on his work on humanitarian attitude towards the mentally ill at the 'York Retreat' after his demise.

Joseph Guislain (1797–1860)

- Belgian physician.
- Instituted humane treatment at Ghent (Belgium).
- Known as the '*Belgian Pinel*'.

Benjamin Rush (1745–1813)

- American physician; a student of Cullen and Sydenham.
- One of the signatories of the Declaration of Independence (1776) of USA.
- Wrote the 1st systematic general Textbook of Psychiatry in USA.
- Known as the Father of American Psychiatry.
- His portrait is on the seal of the American Psychiatric Association (APA).

Thomas Sutton (1767–1835)

- English physician.
- 1st description of delirium tremens during alcohol withdrawal.

Joseph Adams (1756–1818)

- English physician.
- Emphasized the hereditary 'properties' of diseases, particularly 'madness'. Wrote the 1st textbook on this subject.
- Proposed that it was not the disease but a susceptibility to disease that was inherited; thus, prevention as well as cure was possible.

Franz Joseph Gall (1758–1828)

- Austrian physician, who later shifted to Germany.
- Founder of phrenology (i.e. mapping parts of brain, defining their psychological functions, and corresponding brain areas with protuberances of the external cranial surface), along with his disciple Johann Caspar Spurzheim (1776–1832).
- Described 27 specific organs in the human brain (1815).
- Although phrenology eventually fell into disrepute, Gall's concepts of cerebral localization gave a tremendous impetus to the development of neurology, especially in Germany.

Johann Christian Heinroth (1773–1843)

- German physician.
- 1st to use the term psychosomatic.
- 1st to hold a chair in Psychological Medicine, in the University of Leipzig.
- Authored the 1st systematic textbook of psychiatry in Germany.
- Propounded ideas that are believed by some to be forerunners of psychoanalysis.
- Said that personality is the outcome of an inner struggle between the instincts (similar to id), the self (similar to ego), and the conscience (similar to superego).

Robert Gooch (1784–1830)

- English physician.
- 1st clear account of *postpartum psychosis.*

Amariah Brigham (1798–1849)

- American psychiatrist.
- Superintendent of the 1st public institution for the mentally ill in New York State (USA), the Lunatic asylum at Utica.
- Pioneer in social psychiatry.
- Founder-Editor of the American Journal of Insanity (July 1844), which later became the American Journal of Psychiatry.
- Believed in '*moral treatment*' of a kind that later came to be known as occupational and recreational therapy.

James Prichard (1786–1848)

- English physician.
- Authored a standard Textbook of Psychiatry, reviewing almost all the existing literature.
- Described *moral insanity,* which later came to be called as psychopathy or antisocial personality.

James Esdaile (1808–1859)

- Indian surgeon.
- Performed nearly 300 major operations, using 'hypnosis', at Asansol (India), before surgical anesthesia had been discovered.

Jean Etienne Dominique Esquirol (1772–1840)

- French psychiatrist; a student of Pinel and teacher of many influential psychiatrists of the nineteenth century.
- Coined the terms *hallucination* (differentiating it from *illusion*) and *monomania* (calling it '*partial insanity*').
- Described *idiocy* in detail.
- Classified mental disorders into 2 types:
  1. *Monomania* ('partial insanity').
  2. *General 'delirium'* ('complete insanity').
- Recognized that both emotional and organic causes can lead to mental disorders.
- Proposed that '*criminally insane*' should be treated rather than punished, a truly revolutionary and humanitarian approach at that time.
- Authored a famous treatise on mental disorders, '*Des Maladies Mentalies*'.

Issac Ray (1807–1881)

- American psychiatrist.
- One of the founders of the American Psychiatric Association (the Association of Medical Superintendents of American Institutions for the Insane, as it was then known), in 1844.
- Founder of American forensic psychiatry.
- Authored the 1st treatise on forensic psychiatry in USA (1838).

Daniel Hack Tuke (1827–1895)

- English physician.
- Great-grandson of William Tuke, the founder of York Retreat.
- Authored a truly comprehensive Textbook of Psychiatry, '*Manual of Psychological Medicine*', along with John Charles Bucknill (1858).
- Also authored many dictionaries, manuals, histories, and treatises on psychiatry.

James Braid (1795–1860)

- English physician; first practiced in Calcutta (India) and then shifted to England.
- Coined the term *hypnosis*, separating it from 'animal magnetism'.

Ernst Freihern von Feuchtersleben (1806–1849)

- German psychiatrist practicing in Vienna. Later Dean of the University of Vienna Medical School.
- Coined the word *psychosis* (1845).
- Regarded by some as the Father of Psychosomatic Medicine.
- Criticizing the mind-body dichotomy, he stressed on the indivisibility of the mind-body phenomena.
- Emphasized the role of '*mind*' in producing physical illnesses and the effectiveness of psychological modes of treatment in some physical illnesses.

Wilhelm Griesinger (1817–1868)

- Professor of Neurology and Psychiatry at University of Berlin, Germany.
- Founded the specialty of Neuropsychiatry.
- Believed that all mental disorders are brain diseases (1845).
- Shifted the focus of psychiatric work from the asylum to the University, facilitating treatment, research and teaching.
- 1st full time academic psychiatrist who worked to make psychiatry a medical specialty.
- Put forward the *unitary psychosis* (*einheitspsychose*) concept.

Jacques Moreau de Tours (1804–1884)

- French psychiatrist; a student of Esquirol.
- Recognized the importance of dreams in understanding mental disorders.
- Probably the 1st to differentiate between primary and secondary thought processes.
- Has the dubious distinction of being the 1st psychiatrist to experience a drug-induced psychosis.
- Described personal experiences of taking hashish (cannabis).

Paul Briquet (1796–1881)

- French psychiatrist.
- Described hysteria in 1859, which is now known as *Briquet's syndrome* or somatization disorder.

Walter Cooper Dendy (1794–1871)

- English psychiatrist.
- Coined the term *psychotherapies* (now, psychotherapy) and defined it as prevention and remedy of disease by psychical influence.
- Believed that psychotherapy will become a valuable mode of treatment in future.

Jules Baillarger (1809–1890)

- French psychiatrist.
- Described mania and depression occurring as two phases in the same patient, as *folie a double forme* (1854) just 2 weeks before Falret described it.

Jean-Pierre Falret (1794–1870)

- French psychiatrist; Director of La Salpetriere.
- A student of Esquirol.
- Described mania and depression in the same patient, as *folie circulaire* (1854).
- Coined the word *mental alienation*, to describe mental illness; this was done to rid the patients of the social stigma attached to terms like insanity and dementia.
- Psychiatrists, thus, came to be known as *alienists*.
- Developed psychiatric interviewing techniques.
- Conducted pioneering studies on suicide.

Dorothea Lynde Dix (1802–1887)

- Massachusetts (USA) school teacher.
- Over a span of nearly 40 years, beginning in 1841, she worked towards the establishment of over 30 state supported hospitals and reforming of the asylums of Scotland and Canada.
- Was instrumental in establishing firmly the modern principle of public responsibility for the mentally ill.

Thomas Story Kirkbride (1809–1883)

- American psychiatrist.
- Superintendent of the Pennsylvania Hospital and one of the founders of the American Psychiatric Association.
- Conducted pioneering work in the care of 'chronic insanes'.

George Robinson (1821–1875)

- English physician.
- Authored the 1st book, '*On the Prevention and Treatment of Mental Disorders*' (1859) that searched past the boundaries of 'lunatic asylums', for the prevention and treatment of mental disorders.

Indian Lunatic Asylum Act (1858)

- 1st Lunacy Act in India, known as Act 36.
- Provided guidelines for the establishment of mental asylums and set procedure for admission of the mentally ill.

- Modified in 1888 by a committee appointed in the state of Bengal. The revised Act provided elaborate instructions and guidelines for admission and treatment of criminal lunatics.
- Repealed in 1912, when the new Indian Lunacy Act came into force.

Gustav Theodor Fechner (1801–1887)

- German physicist, psychologist and philosopher.
- Founder of experimental and physiological psychology.
- One of the proponents of the *Weber-Fechner psychophysical law*, along with Ernst Heinrich Weber (1795–1878).
- Authored a highly influential book, the '*Elements of Psychophysics*' (1860).

Benedict-Augustin Morel (1809–1873)

- French psychiatrist and physiologist.
- Director of La Salpetriere.
- Described for the 1st time *demence precoce*, as a mental illness that has an onset in adolescence.
- Focused on the contribution of hereditary factors in causation of mental illnesses.
- Described '*larval epilepsy*'.
- Proposed a '*theory of degeneration*' that said that insanity is caused by inherited mental degeneration that becomes worse from one generation to another, finally leading to dementia.

Forbes B Winslow (1810–1874)

- Resident of England.
- 1st to describe diagnostic psychological tests in 1860.
- Also described in detail the psychiatric interviewing.

Karl Kahlbaum (1828–1899)

- German psychiatrist.
- Classified mental disorders according to their course and outcome.
- Coined the terms, *catatonia* (1874), *symptom complex*, *verbigeration* and *cyclothymia*.
- According to him, catatonia passed through the following stages:
  - Melancholia,
  - Mania,
  - Stupor,
  - Confusion, and finally
  - Dementia.

  Any of these stages could be absent in a given case and cure can set in at any stage except the last.

Henry Maudsley (1835–1918)

- English psychiatrist.
- Believed that classification should be based on etiology.
- Attempted to integrate psychology, reflex neurophysiology and psychiatry into a single synthetic whole.
- Believed mental illnesses to be primarily organic in nature.
- His book '*Responsibility in Mental Disease*' (1874) marked a turning point in English psychiatry, as it was influential in fostering scientific conceptual systems in place of romantic, philosophical systems.
- His influence led to the founding of the famous Maudsley Hospital in London, in 1923, five years after his death.

Ewald Hecker (1843–1909)

- German psychiatrist.
- Student of Kahlbaum.
- Coined the term and described the condition, *hebephrenia* at Kahlbaum's suggestion.

Valentin Magnan (1835–1916)

- French psychiatrist.
- Used the '*theory of degeneration*' (of Morel) to explain alcoholism, obsessive compulsive disorder and delusional disorder.
- 1st to study alcoholism and narcotic addiction in a scientific manner.
- One of the 1st to provide clinical teaching demonstrations of the mentally ill in his courses.

Jean-Martin Charcot (1925–1893)

- French neurologist.
- Physician in charge of La Salpetriere from 1862 onwards.
- Conducted pioneering studies on hysteria; believed it to be an organic disease of the nervous system in which 'stigmata' and 'seizures' are triggered off by hysterongenous zones.
- Demonstrated the use of hypnosis in psychiatric treatment, especially of hysteria.
- Believed hypnotizability and suggestibility to be signs of underlying weakness of the nervous system.
- Teacher of Freud and Janet.

Hippolyte-Marie Bernheim (1840–1919)

- French psychotherapist.
- Along with Ambrose-August Liebault (1823-1904), opposed Charcot's concept of underlying weakness

of the nervous system in the phenomenon of hypnotizability.

- Conducted extensive studies on 'posthypnotic suggestion'.

Karl Wernicke (1848–1905)

- Viennese neurologist.
- Published his classic work on '*aphasia*' in 1874.
- Found the occurrence of specific memory losses with brain damage as one way to differentiate organic from functional psychoses.

Wilhelm Max Wundt (1832–1920)

- German psychologist.
- Father of scientific (and experimental) psychology.
- Opened a '*psychophysiology laboratory*' at the University of Leipzig, in 1879, to measure the '*mind*'.
- Evolved a procedure of *controlled introspection.*
- In his science of '*conscious experience*', he systematically recorded reactions to complex and impure stimuli, recognizing that consciousness was more than a product of simple sensation.

George Miller Beard (1839–1883)

- American psychiatrist.
- Introduced the concept of '*nervous exhaustion*' or *Neurasthenia*, replacing hypochondriasis.

Paul Broca (1824–1880)

1st to locate the center of motor speech, called as *Broca's area*, by examining the brain of a patient of aphasia at postmortem.

Francis Galton (1822–1911)

- Founder of *Differential psychology.*
- Established an Anthropometric Laboratory (London) in 1882.
- Constructed and used simple psychological tests for exploration of psychological traits and temperament.
- Used statistical measures in measurement of human attributes for the 1st time, following a suggestion by Quatelet, a Belgian statistician.
- Laid emphasis on individual differences rather than on group characteristics.

Baron Richard von Krafft-Ebing (1840–1902)

- Professor of Psychiatry at University of Strasbourg, Germany.
- Published a classic description of sexual aberrations and perversions (in the book, '*Psychopathia sexualis*'), which signaled a wave of research in sexual problems.
- Coined the terms, '*sadism*' and '*masochism*'.
- Conducted original research on syphilis, particularly GPI and tabes dorsalis (1897).
- Wrongly believed that masturbation causes psychosis, neurosis and homosexuality.

Hermann Emminghaus (1845–1904)

- German psychiatrist.
- Authored the 1st textbook of child psychiatry in 1887, which was unfortunately ignored at that time.

James McKeen Cattell (1860–1944)

- American psychologist.
- Student of Wilhelm Wundt at Leipzig.
- Coined the term '*Mental test*' in 1890 to reflect the quantitative or psychometric method.

Sergei Korsakov (1854–1900)

- Russian neuropsychiatrist.
- 1st described *polyneuritis psychosis* or *Korsakov's psychosis* in alcoholism.

Emil Kraepelin (1856–1926)

- German psychiatrist.
- Worked on psychiatric nosology and systematization.
- Classified major psychoses into 2 groups on the basis of prognosis and outcome.
    1. Dementia precox (later renamed schizophrenia by EugenBleuler).
    2. Manic depressive insanity (or psychoses).
- Wrote a small compendium in 1883 that went through 9 editions until 1927, when it came out in two volumes and 2500 pages. This was considered as a 'Psychiatrist's Bible' for several decades.
- Proponent of the '*empirical method*' in psychiatry.

Alfred Binet (1857–1911)

- French psychologist.
- Brought psychological tests out of the laboratory, into systematic clinical use.
- In 1905, combined several of his instruments into the 1st formal scale of general intelligence.

WR Rice (c1895)

- Surgeon General of India.
- Issued his survey of lunatic asylums in 1895; he suggested that the smaller asylums should be disbanded.
- For the 1st time suggested the importance of occupational therapy in the treatment of mentally ill.

John Hughlings Jackson (1834–1911)

- English neurologist.
- Described how neurological and psychological functions developed through evolution. The more recently developed brain parts not only were more complex but also inhibited the older parts. Diseases and external toxins (e.g. alcohol) usually involved the evolutionarily newer parts first, leading to regression to (release of) older, inferior levels of neurological and psychological function.
- Elaborated and described the concept of positive and negative symptoms, originally proposed by John Russell Reynolds (1828–1896).

Josef Breuer (1841–1925)

- Viennese neurologist.
- In 1895, published with Freud '*The Studies on Hysteria*'.

William James (1842–1910)

- Professor of psychology at Harvard.
- Wrote '*Principles of Psychology*' (1890), an influential textbook of its time.

Sigmund Freud (1856–1939)

- Austrian neurologist.
- Founder of psychoanalysis.
- His work influenced psychiatric thought for many decades.
- Moved the emphasis in psychiatry from an 'organic' to a psychological approach.
- Some of the main contributions are:
  - Interpretation of dreams.
  - Free association.
  - Psychodynamics.
  - Psychoanalysis.
  - Theory of infantile sexuality; Oedipus complex; penis envy; primal scene; stages of psychosexual development.
  - Libido theory.
  - Concepts of repression, resistance; transference; counter-transference; ego defense mechanisms.
  - Concept of psychological determinism.
  - Topographical model of mind (conscious; preconscious; unconscious).
  - Theory of instincts.
  - Structural model of mind (id; ego; superego).
  - Pleasure and reality principles.
  - Therapeutic use of couch.
  - Psychopathology of everyday life; slips of tongue.

Morton Prince (1854–1929)

- American psychiatrist and neurologist.
- Gave an early account of *multiple personality*, placing emphasis on manifestations of the unconscious and on hypnosis.

Havelock Ellis (1859–1939)

- English physician.
- Authored '*Studies in the Psychology of Sex*' in 1897.
- Proposed that homosexuality is neither a disease nor a crime but simply a congenitally acquired sexual orientation.

Pierre Janet (1859–1947)

- Professor of Psychiatry at College de France; also neurologist, philosopher and Professor of experimental psychology.
- Student of Charcot.
- Pioneer of psychodynamic psychiatry.
- Stressed the concept of *personality integration.*
- Made extensive use of the *Cathartic treatment.*
- Provided detailed clinical description of obsessive compulsive neurosis and hysteria.
- Coined the term '*psychasthenia*' for an illness in which there is dissociation of ideas due to 'weak personality integration'.
- Initiated the movement to unite clinical and academic psychiatry.

Franz Nissl (1860–1919)

- Professor of Psychiatry at University of Heidelberg (1904–1918).
- Described a method of staining neurons, called as '*Nissl's stain*'. However, he never published his work of staining methods for neurons.

Ivan Petrovich Pavlov (1849–1936)

- Russian physiologist; Professor of Physiology (1895).
- Conducted classical animal studies on *conditioned reflexes* that paved the way for the origin of learning theories.
- Received Nobel Prize in 1904 for his work on the physiology of digestion.
- Proposed that the symptoms of schizophrenia are the result of a state of inhibition of the cerebral cortex.

Walter Bradford Cannon (1871–1947)

Gave 'emergency theory' of emotions.

Lord John Morley (c1905)

- Secretary of State for India (1905).
- Psychiatry was recognized as a medical specialty for the 1st time in India (1905).
- Psychiatrists were renamed '*alienists*' and were called upon for the 1st time in India to care for the insanes in lunatic asylums.
- More 'central' asylums were proposed and established.
- A new '*lunacy act*' was contemplated which finally came out in 1912.

Alois Alzheimer (1864–1915)

- German neuropathologist.
- Reported the 1st case of progressive dementia, later to be known after him as '*Alzheimer's disease*'.

Clifford Whittingham Beers (1876–1943)

- American citizen.
- Authored '*A Mind That Found Itself*' in 1908, an autobiographical account of his treatment in '*insane asylums*'.
- Founded the '*society for mental hygiene*' with the support of such eminent men as William James and Adolf Meyer.

Eugen Bleuler (1857–1939)

- Swiss psychiatrist; Director of Burghölzli Hospital at Zurich (1898–1927).
- Coined the term 'schizophrenia' to replace 'dementia precox'; called the condition as a 'group of schizophrenias'.
- Believed that schizophrenia results from a splitting of the personality (i.e. splitting of the thought processes from emotional responses).
- Described the cardinal symptoms of schizophrenia (fundamental/accessory; primary/secondary).

Indian Lunacy Act (1912)

- Came into force in 1912, though it was first drafted in 1906. It happened in the same year (1912) when the capital of India was shifted from Calcutta to Delhi and the unification of Bengal occurred.
- Replaced the existing Indian Lunatic Asylum Act of 1858.

Kari Jaspers (1883–1969)

- German philosopher and psychiatrist.
- Belonged to the Heidelberg school, known for its studies of mental phenomena, other students were Gruhle, Schneider and Mayer-Gross.
- Has come to be seen as one of the founders of *existential psychology*.
- Worked on *Morbid Jealousy* (1910).
- In 1913, published the 1st edition of his, now classic, '*General Psychopathology*'.

Hideyo Noguchi (1876–1928)

- American bacteriologist.
- Working along with JW Moore (1913), provided a definitive demonstration that the spirochete *Treponema pallidum* (discovered by Schaudinn in 1905) causes general paresis of insane (GPI); this was the 1st time that the etiology of a major psychosis was elucidated.

Alfred Adler (1870–1937)

- Viennese student of Freud.
- 1st defector from Freudian psychoanalysis.
- Founder of the school of '*individual psychology*' (1911).
- Coined the terms *life style*, *inferiority complex*, *will to power*, *overcompensation*, *organ inferiority*, and *creative self*.

Carl Gustav Jung (1875–1961)

- Swiss psychiatrist; student of Freud.
- Founder of the school of '*analytical psychology*', a modified version of psychoanalysis.
- Originated the *word-association tests*.
- Coined the terms, *collective and personal unconscious*, *complex*, *introvert* and *extrovert*, *archetypes*, *anima* and *animus*, and *persona*.

Hermann Rorschach (1884–1922)

- Swiss psychiatrist.
- Based on an earlier observation made by Binet regarding the use of inkblots for 'personality diagnosis', he developed an '*Inkblot Test*' for psychiatric diagnosis.
- His work stimulated the development of other projective diagnostic tests.

Otto Rank (1884–1939)

- Viennese psychoanalyst; student of Freud.
- Developed the concept of *birth trauma* as the prototype of all anxiety occurring in later life.
- Advocated his approach of *will therapy*.

American Psychiatric Association (1902)

- Established in 1844 (October 16) as the Association of Medical Superintendents of American Institutions for the Insane.

- Reorganized in 1892 as the American Medico-Psychological Association.
- Renamed American Psychiatric Association in 1921.

Karl Abraham (1877–1925)

- 1st German psychoanalyst; student of Freud.
- Provided psychoanalytic description of character formation and early psychosexual development.
- Described *character types, manic-depressive psychosis, symbolism*, and *pregenital stages.*

Ernst Kretschmer (1888–1964)

- Professor of Psychiatry at University of Tubingen, Germany.
- Described the 4 constitutions (leptosomatic or asthenic, athletic, pyknic, and dysplastics) in relation to character, personality and mental illness (1924).

Grindra Shekhar Bose (1886–1959)

- Indian psychiatrist.
- Developed his own technique of psychoanalysis (1911), oblivious of Freud's work; later corresponded with Freud. He did not agree with Freud regarding the presence of 'Oedipus complex' and 'desire to be female' in Hindu male patients.
- Utilized these analytic techniques in treatment of patients.
- Developed theory of '*opposite wishes*'.
- Published the 1st psychoanalytic journal in India, '*Samiksha*', in 1921.
- Opened the 1st psychiatry unit in a general hospital in India at RG Kar Medical College, Calcutta. (1st general hospital psychiatric unit was opened by John Carswell at the Barnhill Parochial Hospital, Glasgow, England).

Jacoh Klaesi (B 1883)

Developed the '*continuous sleep treatment*', using any sedative (most often barbiturates), with an aim of producing about 20 hours of sleep per day for periods of up to 3 weeks. This treatment was believed to be useful in certain mental disorders (1922).

American Orthopsychiatric Association (1924)

Founded in 1924; dedicated to an interdisciplinary approach in the study, prevention and treatment of mental illness.

Julius Wagner von Jauregg (1857–1940)

- Austrian psychiatrist and neurologist.
- Developed '*malarial (fever) treatment*' for GPI, the 1st most successful treatment of a psychosis.
- Received Nobel Prize in 1927 for this contribution; 1st psychiatrist to receive such an honor.

Melanie Klein (1882–1960)

- English psychoanalyst.
- 1st to use psychoanalytic techniques extensively in the treatment of mentally ill children.

Karen Horney (1885–1952)

- American psychoanalyst.
- The Horney school, a Neo-Freudian school, emphasizes the importance of environmental and cultural factors in the genesis of neurosis.
- Developed a '*theory of neurosis*'.
- Opposed the Freudian theory of castration complex in women and blamed Freud for his 'sexist bias' in his theory of sexuality.

Adolf Meyer (1866–150)

- American psychiatrist.
- Was considered the Dean of American Psychiatry for several decades.
- Was famous for his '*common sense psychiatry*' approach.
- Founder of '*Psychobiology*'.

Franz Alexander (1891–1964)

- Hungarian psychoanalyst settled in USA; Professor of psychoanalysis at University of Chicago.
- Conducted the 1st systematic research on *psychosomatic illness.*
- Also worked on *brief analytic therapy.*

Gordon Willard Allport (1897–1967)

- American psychologist and educator.
- Developed a holistic psychology of human behavior and personality.
- Proposed a '*trait theory*' regarding relatively enduring personality dispositions which underlie overt behavior.

John Broadus Watson (1878–1958)

- American psychologist.
- Founder of *behaviorism* (1913); developed as an antidote for the preoccupation with 'conscious' and 'introspection' at that time; used the Pavlovian concepts.

Karl Spencer Lashley (1890–1958)

- American psychologist, bacteriologist and geneticist.
- Director of Yerkes Laboratory of Primate Biology.
- Authored numerous monographs on psychology, neurology and the biology of behavior.
- Developed a 'psychology of learning'.
- Wrote '*Brain Mechanisms and Intelligence*' (1929).

Kurt Goldstein (1876–1965)

- German Professor of Neurology (Professor of Psychiatry and Chief of Neurophysiological Laboratory later); and one of the proponents of the gestalt school.
- Believed that personality cannot be understood by studying isolated functions or behaviors because the organism operates as a unit that cannot be analyzed in terms of its parts.
- Demonstrated in several brain-damaged patients that brain damage led, not to a loss of function of the affected part but, to a reorganization of his total functioning, enabling the individual to keep his drives and goals intact though at a more primitive level.
- Described '*catastrophic reaction*' in brain-injured patients, and divided the human acts in to '*concrete*' and '*abstract*'.

Reserpine use (c1931)

- Two Indian Scientists, S Siddiqui and Rafat Siddiqui, isolated 5 alkaloids from the snakeroot plant ('*Sarpaga-ndha*'; Rauwolfia serpentina) in 1931.
- Ganesh Sen and Kartik Bose described the use of the snakeroot plant in cases of high blood pressure and also in psychoses (1931, India).

Manfred Sakel (1900–1957)

- Polish psychiatrist trained in Vienna; later settled in USA.
- Developed Insulin shock and *Insulin coma therapy* for psychoses in 1933.

Ladislas Lazio Joseph von Meduna (1896–1964)

- Hungarian born, American psychiatrist.
- Used *cardiazol* (*Metrazol*), a camphor compound, to induce convulsions in psychotic patients (1934) based on an erroneous observation that epilepsy and psychosis rarely coexist, and that psychotic symptoms often disappear following spontaneous convulsions.
- Also developed *carbon dioxide therapy*.

Antonio Caetano de Abreau Freire Egas Moniz (1874–1955)

- Portuguese neurologist.
- Performed *psychosurgery* (*prefrontal leucotomy*) along with a neurosurgeon, Almenda Lima, in psychotic patients (1936).
- Developed *cerebral angiography* as an investigative tool in neurology (1927).
- Received Nobel Prize in 1949, along with WR Hess.

Ugo Cerletti (1877–1963)

- Italian neuropsychiatrist.
- Used electrically induced convulsions, a technique developed in animals by Leduc and Robinovitch in 1900, for the treatment of psychoses (1st in schizophrenia, and later in manic depressive psychosis) in 1938 (April 15), along with Lucio Bini.
- Called this technique *Electro-shock treatment* (EST), which later came to be known as *electroconvulsive therapy* (ECT).
- Believed that the convulsions brought the patient close to a state of death, arousing extraordinary biological defenses that led in turn to therapeutic recovery.
- Propounded the '*acroagonine theory*' to explain the mechanism of action of ECT.

Lucio Bini (1908–1964)

- Italian psychiatrist.
- Used ECT, along with Ugo Cerletti, in the treatment of psychoses.
- Developed the 1st ECT machine, and the technique of bitemporal placement of electrodes.

Franz Kallman (1897–1965)

- German psychoanalyst and geneticist settled in USA.
- Established the 1st department of medical genetics in a psychiatric hospital in USA.
- Emphasized the role of genetic factors in schizophrenia.

Colonel O Berkeley Hill (c1939)

- British psychiatrist practicing in India.
- Was the Medical Superintendent of Mental Asylum at Ranchi (the Central European Hospital).
- Changed the name of mental asylums in India to '*mental hospitals*' in 1920.
- Founded the Indian Association for Mental Hygiene in 1929, which was affiliated to the National Council of

Mental Hygiene, Great Britain. This was disbanded after the retirement and, then, demise of Col. Hill.

- Opened the 1st private nursing home in India for the care of mentally ill in 1937.
- Emphasized humane treatment of mentally ill.
- Discarded seclusion of mentally ill; opened the closed doors of the wards in 1939 (this happened nearly 2–3 decades later in USA), and patients were allowed to move freely on the hospital grounds.

Lt Col CJ Lodge-Patch (c1939)

- British psychiatrist practicing in India.
- Was the Medical Superintendent of Punjab Mental Hospital, Lahore (now in Pakistan)?
- Authored an important book entitled *"A critical review of the Mental Hospitals in Punjab from 1844–1930"*, which is summarized in his excellent Article 20.
- Established the *Indian Division of the Royal Medico-Psychological Association* in 1935 along with Banarasi Das, Medical Superintendent, Mental Hospital, Agra (India).
- Was the 1st President of this 1st exclusive association of Indian psychiatrists, which began its work in 1939 (January 24). This association was disbanded in 1941 after its 2nd meeting at Agra, due to World War II.

Leo Kanner (1894–1981)

- Austrian born American psychiatrist.
- Published the 1st American Textbook on Child Psychiatry (1935).
- Described in detail for the 1st time the '*early infantile autism*' (1943) as the '*autistic disturbances of affective contact*' (*Kanner's syndrome*).

Lauretta Bender (B1897)

- American neuropsychiatrist.
- Developed the *Visual Motor Gestalt Test* (*Bender Gestalt Test*; the BG Test).
- Main area of work was child psychiatry, especially schizophrenia and brain damage.

Margaret Schoenberger Mahler (1897–1985)

- Hungarian born American psychoanalyst.
- Worked on childhood schizophrenia and described in detail the concept of *symbiotic psychosis*.
- Proposed *object relation theory* of pregenital psychosexual development.

Helen Deutsch (1884–1982)

- American psychoanalyst.
- Provided a psychoanalytical account of the psychology and life cycle of women in her book, '*The Psychology of Women*'.
- Described the '*as-if personality*'.

Anna Freud (1895–1982)

- Viennese lay analyst, who later shifted to London (1939).
- Famous daughter of Sigmund Freud.
- Worked on psychoanalysis of children and adolescents.
- Among her major contribution is '*play therapy*' for children and '*mechanisms of ego defense*'.

Indian Psychiatric Society (1947)

- Inaugurated on January 7, 1947 at Delhi, at the initiative of Major RB Davis and Lt Col RJ Rosie.
- 1st meeting held on January 2, 1948 at Patna under the chairmanship of 1st President Nagendra Nath De.

Indian Journal of Psychiatry (1949)

- Founded in 1949 as *Indian Journal of Neurology and Psychiatry* (Editor: Nagendra Nath De).
- Ceased publication in 1954 after 6 issues.
- Was renamed as *Indian Journal of Psychiatry* in 1958 and was placed under the editorship of Lt Col Bardhan, a pathologist.

John F Cade (1912–1981)

- Australian psychiatrist.
- Used lithium for the 1st time as a successful treatment in manic excitement, believing that an excess of normal metabolites such as urea or uric acid probably causes mania. Before using it in humans, he 1st injected lithium in guinea pigs and observed drowsiness (1949).
- Although discovered by Cade, the use of lithium was popularized by Mogen Schou (1954, Denmark) who also showed its effectiveness in both mania and depression. The use of lithium was approved by FDA (USA) only in 1970.

Kurt Schneider (1887–1967)

- Professor of Neurology and Psychiatry at University of Heidelberg, Germany.

- Developed a comprehensive descriptive-phenomenological psychopathology.
- Famous for his description of (*Schneiderian*) *first rank symptoms* (SFRS or FRS) in schizophrenia.

Erik H Erikson (1902–1997)

- American psychoanalyst.
- Described the stages of *life cycle*.
- Used '*psychohistory*' in the psychoanalytic study of Mahatama Gandhi and Martin Luther King, Jr.
- Described '*identity*' vs '*role confusion*'.

Jean PL Delay (B 1907)

- French psychiatrist.
- Used *chlorpromazine*, the 1st phenothiazine derivative and a drug originally synthesized for hypertensive and surgical patients, in the treatment of psychoses, along with Pierre Deniker (b 1917), also a French psychiatrist.
- Called this treatment as *hibernotherapie*.
- Coined the word '*neuroleptic*' and described the condition '*neuroleptic malignant syndrome*' (NMS), along with Deniker.

Maxwell Jones (B 1907)

- English psychiatrist at Dingleton Hospital, Melrose (Scotland).
- Originated the concept of '*therapeutic community*'.
- His views led to an era of '*social psychiatry*'.

Harry Stack Sullivan (1892–1949)

- American psychoanalyst.
- Chief proponent of the so-called '*dynamic-cultural school*' of psychoanalysis (along with Karen Horney) which emphasizes social rather than biological events, present day contacts rather than past experiences, and current interpersonal relationships rather than infantile sexuality.
- Founder of '*interpersonal school of psychiatry*'.
- Described 6 stages in personality development, each of which represents a new interpersonal constellation. These are:
  1. Infancy
  2. Childhood
  3. Juvenile period
  4. Pre-adolescence
  5. Early adolescence, and
  6. Late adolescence.

Jean Piaget (1897–1980)

- Swiss biologist and Professor of Philosophy at University of Neuchatel. Later became the Head of the departments of child psychology, history of scientific thought and experimental psychology. Then he became Professor of general psychology.
- Worked on the nature of children's intellectual development.
- Divided a child's thought development into 4 stages:
  1. Sensory-motor stage (1–2 years).
  2. Preoperational stage (2–7 years).
  3. Concrete operations stage (7–12 years).
  4. Formal operations stage (12 years-adulthood).

William H Masters (B 1915) and Virginia E Johnson (B 1925)

- American husband and wife team of therapists.
- Originated *dual sex therapy*.
- Authored very popular books on normal and inadequate human sexuality.

Konrad Lorenz (B 1903)

- Head of psychology department at University of Konigsberg. Later, Director of Max Planck Institute for the Physiology of Behavior.
- Provided a comprehensive theory of instinctive behavior based on observation of bird behavior.
- His theory was instrumental in providing a framework for the systematic growth of Ethology as a discipline.
- Shared Nobel Prize in 1973 with von Frisch and Tinbergen.

Burrhus Frederic Skinner (1904–1990)

- Experimental Psychologist at Harvard University (USA).
- Originator of the '*operant conditioning*' *model* of learning theory, the idea that seemingly spontaneous action is regulated through rewards and punishment.

Vidya Sagar

- Professor of psychiatry at Amritsar and later at Rohtak, India.
- Originator of the Camp approach in psychiatry. He put up tents in the hospital campus to cater for more patients, entrusted the nursing care to the family members who stayed with the patients. This was started at Amritsar in 1958 and then carried on to Rohtak in 1970.
- Was influential towards removing the stigma of mental illness by this new approach. Was revered by his patients.

Mental Health Act (1987)

- Drafted in 1949 at Allahabad by 3 distinguished psychiatrists: J Roy (Nagpur), RB Davis (Ranchi) and. Dr Hasib (Ranchi), appointed by the Indian Psychiatric Society.

- After a long wait of 38 years, it was finally made Act No. 14 in 1987. The Government of India passed orders that the Act would come in force from April 1, 1993 in all the States and Union Territories of India.
- The new act replaces the Indian Lunacy Act of 1912.
- Mental Health Act envisages a change in nomenclature, provision for supervision of mental hospitals, separate hospitals for special category of patients (like children, elderly), new procedures for admission and discharge, and care for the human rights of the patient.

ICD-10 Publication in 1992

Work on ICD-10 began in 1983, and the new revision was endorsed by the Forty-third World Health Assembly in May 1990. The latest version came into use in WHO Member States starting in 1994. The classification system allows more than 155,000 different codes and permits tracking of many new diagnoses and procedures, a significant expansion on the 17,000 codes available in ICD-9. Adoption was relatively swift in most of the world. Several materials are made available online by WHO to facilitate its use, including a manual, training guidelines, a browser, and files for download. Some countries have adapted the international standard, such as the "ICD-10-AM" published in Australia in 1998 (also used in New Zealand), and the "ICD-10-CA" introduced in Canada in 2000.

DSM-IV Publication in 1994

DSM-IV built upon the research generated by the empirical orientation of DSM-III. By the early 1990s, most psychiatric diagnoses had an accumulated body of published studies or data sets. Publications up through 1992 were reviewed for DSM-IV, which was published in 1994. Conflicting reports or lack of evidence were handled by data re-analyses and field trials. The National Institute of Mental Health sponsored 12 DSM-IV field trials together with the National Institute on Drug Abuse (NIDA) and the National Institute on Alcohol Abuse and Alcoholism (NIAAA). The field trials compared the diagnostic criteria sets of DSM-III, DSM-III-R, ICD-10 (which had been published in 1992), and the proposed criteria sets for DSM-IV. The field trials recruited subjects from a variety of ethnic and cultural backgrounds, in keeping with a new concern for cross-cultural applicability of diagnostic standards. In addition to its inclusion of culture-specific syndromes and disorders, DSM-IV represented much closer cooperation and coordination with the experts from WHO who had worked on ICD-10. A modification of ICD-10 for clinical practitioners, the ICD-10-CM, is scheduled to be introduced in the United States in 2004.

DSM-5 Publication in 2013

The Diagnostic and Statistical Manual of Mental Disorders, Fifth edition (DSM-5) is the 2013 update to the American Psychiatric Association's (APA) classification and diagnostic tool. The DSM-5 was published on May 18, 2013, superseding the DSM-IV-TR, which was published in 2000. The development of the new edition began with a conference in 1999, and proceeded with the formation of a Task Force in 2007, which developed and field-tested a variety of new classifications. In most respects DSM-5 is not greatly changed from DSM-IV-TR. Notable changes include dropping Asperger syndrome as a distinct classification; loss of subtype classifications for variant forms of schizophrenia; dropping the "bereavement exclusion" for depressive disorders; a revised treatment and naming of gender identity disorder to gender dysphoria, and removing the A2 criterion for post-traumatic stress disorder (PTSD) because its requirement for specific emotional reactions to trauma did not apply to combat veterans and first responders with PTSD.

BIBLIOGRAPHY

1. Ackerknecht EH. A short history of psychiatry. Trans. Wolff S. New York: Hafner, 1959.
2. Alexander FG, Selesnick ST. The History of Psychiatry. New York: Mentor, 1966.
3. Altschule M. Roots of modern psychiatry. New York: Grune and Stratton, 1957.
4. American Psychiatric Association. Desk Reference to the Diagnostic Criteria from DSM-5. Washington DC. 2013.
5. American Psychiatric Association. Diagnostic and statistical manual of mental disorders, 4th edition. American Psychiatric Association, Washington, DC. 1994.
6. Anderson RD. The history of witchcraft: A review with some psychiatric comments. Am J Psychiatry. 1970;126:1727-35.
7. Berrios GE. Historical aspects of psychoses: 19th century issues. Br Med Bull. 1987;43:484-98.
8. Berrios GE. The uses of psychiatric historiography: the 19th and 20th centuries. In: Davison K, Kerr A (Eds). Contemporary Themes in Psychiatry: A Tribute to Sir Martin Roth. London: Gaskell; 1989.pp.31-8.
9. Bromberg W. The Mind of Man: The history of psychotherapy and psychoanalysis. New York: Harper, 1959.
10. Foucault M. Madness and civilization: A history of insanity in the age of reason. New York: Pantheon Books, 1965.
11. Freeman L, Small M. The story of psychoanalysis. New York: Pocket Books, 1960.
12. Hafner H. Ernst Kreschmer 1888-1964. Psychol Med. 1990;20:487-92.
13. Hube G. Kurt Schneider: Images in Psychiatry. Am J Psychiatry. 1994;151:1492.

14. Hunter R, Macapline I. Three Hundred Years of Psychiatry, 1525-1860; A History Presented in Selected English Texts. London: Oxford University Press, 1963.
15. Kraepelin E. One Hundred Years of Psychiatry. New York: Citadel Press, 1962.
16. Leigh D. The Historical Development of British Psychiatry. New York: Pergamon, 1961.
17. Lewis A. The State of Psychiatry: Essays And Addresses. London: Routledge and Kegan Paul, 1967.
18. Lewis N. Short history of psychiatric achievement. New York: WW Norton, 1941.
19. Lodge-Patch CJ. A century of psychiatry in Punjab. J Ment Sci. 1939;05:391.
20. Mora G, Brand J (Eds). Psychiatry and Its History. Springfield: Charles C Thomas, 1970.
21. Mora G. The history of psychiatry: Its relevance for the psychiatrist. Am J Psychiatry. 1970;126:957-67.
22. Murphy C. Historical introduction to modern psychology. New York: Harcourt, 1949.
23. Peters RS (Ed). Brett's History of Psychology. New York: McMillan, 1953.
24. Sabshin M. Turning points in twentieth-century American psychiatry. Am J Psychiatry. 1990;147:1267-74.
25. Schneck S. History of psychiatry. Springfield: Charles C Thomas, 1960.
26. Selesnick ST. Historical perspectives in the development of child psychiatry. In: Masserman T (Ed). Current Theories. New York: Grune and Stratton, 1965.
27. Sharma SD. Mental hospitals in India. New Delhi: Directorate General of Health Services. 1990.
28. Siegler M, Osmond H. Models of Madness, Models of Medicine. New York: Harper Colophon Books, 1976.
29. Simon B. Mind and Madness in Ancient Greece: The Classical Roots of Modem Psychiatry. Ithaca: Cornell University Press, 1978.
30. Varma LP. History of psychiatry in India. In: Continuing Medical Education Program Booklet. Ahmedabad: Indian Psychiatric Society. 1982;1:1-14.
31. Varma LP. History of psychiatry in India and Pakistan. Indian J Neurology Psychiatry. 1953;4:26-53;4:138-64.
32. Varma LP. Psychiatry in Ayurveda. Indian J Psychiatry. 1965;VII(4):297-312.
33. Varma LP. Psychiatry in our scriptures. Patna J Med. 1969; Dec. Issue: 496-502.
34. Venkoba Rao A. History of psychiatry in India. In: Howell JG. (Ed). World history of psychiatry. New York: Brunner/Mazel, 1975.
35. Venkoba Rao A. Psychiatric thought in ancient India. Indian J Psychiatry. 1978;20:107-19.
36. Whitwell R. Historical notes on psychiatry. London: HK Lewis, 1936.
37. World Health Organization. International statistical classification of diseases and related health problems, 10th revision. WHO, Geneva; 1992
38. Zilboorg G. Henry GW. A history of medical psychology. New York: WW Norton, 1941.

Index

Page numbers followed by *f* refer to figure and *t* refer to table

A

B

C

F

G

H

I

J

K

L

M

Q

R

S

T

U

V

W

Y

Z